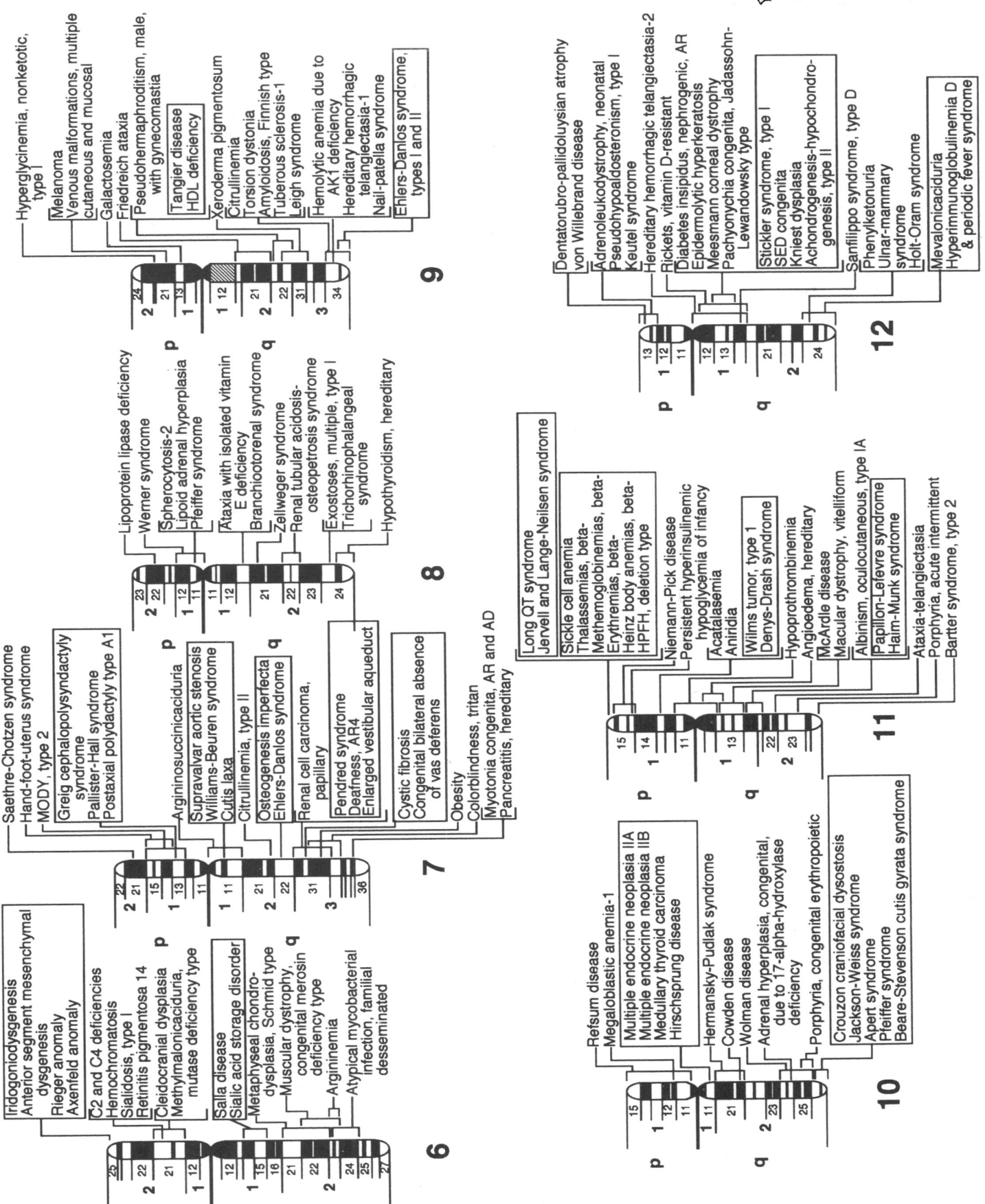

# The Metabolic &
# Molecular Bases of
# Inherited Disease

eighth edition

EDITORS

Charles R. Scriver, M.D.C.M.
Alva Professor of Human Genetics, Professor of Pediatrics, Faculty of Medicine, Professor of Biology,
Faculty of Science, McGill University; Director (retired), deBelle Laboratory of Biochemical Genetics
and Biochemical Genetics Clinical Unit, McGill University–Montreal Children's Hospital Research
Institute, McGill University Health Centre, Montreal, Quebec, Canada

Arthur L. Beaudet, M.D.
Henry and Emma Meyer Professor and Chair, Department of Molecular and Human Genetics, Professor,
Departments of Pediatrics and Molecular and Cellular Biology, Baylor College of Medicine, Houston,
Texas

William S. Sly, M.D.
Alice A. Doisy Professor of Biochemistry and Molecular Biology, Chair, Edward A. Doisy
Department of Biochemistry and Molecular Biology, Professor of Pediatrics, St. Louis University School of Medicine,
St. Louis, Missouri

David Valle, M.D.
Professor of Pediatrics and Molecular Biology, Howard Hughes Medical Institute, McKusick-Nathans Institute of Genetic
Medicine. The Johns Hopkins University School of Medicine, Baltimore, Maryland


ASSOCIATE EDITORS

Barton Childs, M.D.
Emeritus Professor of Pediatrics, The Johns Hopkins University School of Medicine, Baltimore, Maryland

Kenneth W. Kinzler, Ph.D.
Professor of Oncology, The Johns Hopkins University School of Medicine, Baltimore, Maryland

Bert Vogelstein, M.D.
Investigator, Howard Hughes Medical Institute, Clayton Professor of Oncology and Pathology, The Johns
Hopkins University School of Medicine, Baltimore, Maryland

# The Metabolic & Molecular Bases of Inherited Disease

eighth edition

## VOLUME IV

EDITORS

Charles R. Scriver, M.D.C.M.
Arthur L. Beaudet, M.D.
William S. Sly, M.D.
David Valle, M.D.

ASSOCIATE EDITORS

Barton Childs, M.D.
Kenneth W. Kinzler, Ph.D.
Bert Vogelstein, M.D.

McGraw-Hill
Medical Publishing Division

New York  St. Louis  San Francisco  Auckland  Bogotá  Caracas  Lisbon  London  Madrid  Mexico City
Milan  Montreal  New Delhi  San Juan  Singapore  Sydney  Tokyo  Toronto

# McGraw-Hill

*A Division of The* **McGraw·Hill** *Companies*

**The Metabolic and Molecular Bases of Inherited Disease, 8th Edition**

1234567890 KGPKGP 09876543210

ISBNs
0-07-913035-6
0-07-136319-X    (vol. 1)
0-07-136320-3    (vol. 2)
0-07-136321-1    (vol. 3)
0-07-136322-X    (vol. 4)
This book was set in Times Roman by Progressive Information Technologies, Inc.
The editors were Martin J. Wonsiewicz, Susan R. Noujaim, and Peter J. Boyle;
the production supervisor was Richard Ruzycka; the text designer was José R. Fonfrias;
the cover designer was Elizabeth Schmitz; Barbara Littlewood prepared the index.
Quebecor Printing/Kingsport was printer and binder.
This book is printed on acid-free paper.


**Library of Congress Cataloging-in-Publication Data**

The metabolic and molecular bases of inherited disease / editors,
   Charles R. Scriver . . . [et al.].–8th ed.
      p.;  cm.
   Includes bibliographical references and index.
   ISBN 0-07-913035-6 (set)
   1. Metabolism, Inborn errors of  2. Medical genetics.  3. Pathology, Molecular. I.
Scriver, Charles R.
   [DNLM: 1. Hereditary Diseases. 2. Metabolic Diseases. 3. Metabolism, Inborn Errors.
WD 200 M5865 2001]
RC627.8 . M47 2001
616′.042–dc21
                                     00-060957
INTERNATIONAL EDITION
ISBNs 0-07-116336-0
0-07-118833-9    (vol. 1)
0-07-118834-7    (vol. 2)
0-07-118835-5    (vol. 3)
0-07-118836-3    (vol. 4)

## Notice

Medicine is an ever-changing science. As new research and clinical experience broaden our knowledge, changes in treatment and drug therapy are required. The editors and the publisher of this work have checked with sources believed to be reliable in their efforts to provide information that is complete and generally in accord with the standards accepted at the time of publication. However, in view of the possibility of human error or changes in medical sciences, neither the editors nor the publisher nor any other party who has been involved in the preparation or publication of this work warrants that the information contained herein is in every respect accurate or complete, and they disclaim all responsibility for any errors or omissions or for the results obtained from use of the information contained in this work. Readers are encouraged to confirm the information contained herein with other sources. For example and in particular, readers are advised to check the product information sheet included in the package of each drug they plan to administer to be certain that the information contained in this work is accurate and that changes have not been made in the recommended dose or in the contraindications for administration. This recommendation is of particular importance in connection with new or infrequently used drugs.

# CONTENTS

## VOLUME I

## PART 1
## INTRODUCTION

## PART 2
## PERSPECTIVES

# PART 5
# CHROMOSOMES

# PART 6
# DIAGNOSTIC APPROACHES

# PART 7
# CARBOHYDRATES

# VOLUME II

## PART 8
## AMINO ACIDS

# PART 9
# ORGANIC ACIDS

# PART 10
# DISORDERS OF MITOCHONDRIAL FUNCTION

# VOLUME III

## PART 16
# LYSOSOMAL DISORDERS

# PART 17
# VITAMINS

# PART 20
# IMMUNE AND DEFENSE SYSTEMS

## PART 21
# MEMBRANE TRANSPORT DISORDERS

# V O L U M E   I V

## PART 22
# CONNECTIVE TISSUE

## PART 23
# CARDIOVASCULAR SYSTEM

## PART 24
# KIDNEY

## PART 25
# MUSCLE

## PART 29
## EYE

## PART 30
## MULTISYSTEM INBORN ERRORS OF DEVELOPMENT

Color plates appear between pages 1296 and 1297.

# CONTRIBUTORS

Lauri A. Aaltonen, M.D.   [34]*
Senior Fellow, Academy of Finland, Dept. of Medical Genetics,
Haartman Institute, Finland
Lauri.aaltonen@helsinki.fi

Frank Accurso, M.D.   [201]
Dept. of Pediatrics, University of Colorado School of Medicine;
Director, The Mike McMorris Cystic Fibrosis Center,
The Children's Hospital, Denver, Colorado
accurso.frank@tchden.org

Milton B. Adesnik, Ph.D.   [16]
Professor of Cell Biology, Dept. of Cell Biology, New York
University School of Medicine, New York, New York
Adesnm01@popmail.med.nyu.edu

Björn A. Afzelius, M.D.   [187]
Professor Emeritus, Wenner-Gren Institute, Stockholm University,
Arrhenius Laboratories, Stockholm, Sweden
Bjorn.Afzelius@zub.su.se

Naji Al-Dosari, M.D.   [57]
Duke University, Durham, North Carolina
naji@acpub.duke

Rando L. Allikmets, Ph.D.   [243]
Dept. of Ophthalmology, Columbia University, New York,
New York
rla22@columbia.edu

Robert J. Alpern, M.D.   [195]
Dean, Southwestern Medical School, Ruth W. and Milton P. Levy,
Sr., Chair in Molecular Nephrology, Atticus James Gill Chair in
Medical Science, Div. of Nephrology, UT Southwestern Medical
Center at Dallas, Dallas, Texas
Robert.alpern@email.swmed.edu

Wallace L.M. Alward, M.D.   [242]
Dept. of Opthalmology and Visual Sciences, University of Iowa
College of Medicine, Iowa City, Iowa
wallace-alward@uiowa.edu

Joanna S. Amberger, M.D.   [1]
McKusick-Nathans Institute of Genetic Medicine, Johns Hopkins
University School of Medicine, Baltimore, Maryland
joanna@peas.welch.jhu.edu

Donald C. Anderson, M.D.   [188]
Professor, Dept. of Pediatrics, Baylor College of Medicine, Vice
President and Chief Scientific Officer, Pharmacia & Upjohn,
Kalamazoo, Michigan
donald.c.anderson@pnu.com

Karl E. Anderson, M.D.   [124]
Professor of Preventive Medicine and Community Health, Internal
Medicine, and Pharmacology and Toxicology, Dept. of Preventive
Medicine and Community Health, University of Texas Medical
Branch, Galveston, Texas
karl.anderson@utmb.edu

Mary E. Anderson, Ph.D.   [96]
Assistant Professor, Dept. of Microbiology and Molecular Cell
Sciences, University of Memphis, Memphis, Tennessee
Mary@mmcs.memphis.edu

Generoso Andria, M.D.   [152]
Professor of Pediatrics, Department of Pediatrics, Federico II
University, Naples, Italy

Stylianos E. Antonarakis, M.D., D.Sc.   [13, 172]
Professor and Director of Medical Genetics, Div. of Medical
Genetics, University of Geneva Medical School, Geneva,
Switzerland
stylianos.antonarakis@medicine.unige.ch

Irwin M. Arias, M.D.   [125]
Professor and Chairman, Dept. of Physiology, Tufts University,
Boston, Massachusetts
irwin.arias@tufts.edu

Gerd Assmann, M.D., F.R.C.P   [118, 122, 142]
Professor of Medicine, Director, Institute for Clinical Chemistry
and Lab Medicine, Director, Institute for Arteriosclerosis
Research, Westfälische Wilhelms-University, Münster, Germany
assmann@uni-muenster.de

Arleen D. Auerbach, Ph.D.   [31]
Associate Professor, Laboratory of Human Genetics and
Hematology, The Rockefeller University, New York, New York
auerbac@rockvax.rockefeller.edu

Perti Aula, M.D.   [141, 200]
Professor of Medical Genetics, Medical Genetics Dept., University
of Helsinko, Haartman Institute, Haartmaninkatu, Finland
Perti.aula@helsinki.fi

Salvatore Auricchio, M.D.   [75]
Professor, Dept. di Pediatria, Università Federico II Napoli, Italy

Andrea Ballabio, M.D.   [149, 166, 225]
Professor of Medical Genetics, Second University of Naples,
Director, Telethon Institute of Genetics and Medicine (TIGEM),
Naples, Italy
ballabio@tigem.it

Peter G. Barth   [130]
Professor of Pediatric Neurology, University of Amsterdam
Academic Medical Centre, Emma Children's Hospital and Clinical
Chemistry, Amsterdam, The Netherlands
p.g.barth@amc.uva.nl

Stephen B. Baylin, M.D.   [58]
Professor of Oncology and Medicine, Associate Director for
Research, The Johns Hopkins Oncology Center, Baltimore,
Maryland
sbaylin@jhmi.edu

Philip A. Beachy, M.D.   [205]
Professor of Molecular Biology and Genetics, Howard Hughes
Medical Institute, The Johns Hopkins University School of
Medicine, Baltimore, Maryland
pbeachy@jhmi.edu

Arthur L. Beaudet, M.D.   [1, 229]
Henry and Emma Meyer Professor and Chair, Dept. of Molecular
and Human Genetics, Professor, Depts. of Pediatrics and
Molecular and Cellular Biology, Baylor College of Medicine,
Houston, Texas
abeaudet@bcm.tmc.edu

Michael A. Becker, M.D.   [106]
Professor of Medicine
Dept. of Medicine University of Chicago School of Medicine,
Chicago, Illinois
mbecker@medicine.bsd.uchicago.edu

*The numbers in brackets following each contributor's name refer to chapters written
or co-written by that contributor.

David M.O. Becroft, M.D. [113]
Dept. of Obstetrics and Gynecology, University of Auckland
School of Medicine, Auckland, New Zealand
David.Genevieve.Becroft@extra.co.nz

Lenore K. Beitel, Ph.D. [161]
Research Scientist, Lady Davis Institute for Medical Research,
Sir M.B. Davis–Jewish General Hospital, Montreal, Quebec,
Canada
mdtm001@musica.mcgill.ca

John W. Belmont, M.D., Ph.D. [185]
Dept. of Molecular and Human Genetics, Baylor College of
Medicine, Houston, Texas
jbelmont@bcm.tmc.edu

Merrill D. Benson, M.D. [209]
Professor of Medicine, Pathology and Medical Genetics, Dept. of
Medical and Molecular Genetics, Indiana University
School of Medicine, Indianapolis, Indiana
mdbenson@iupui.edu

Wolfgang Berger, M.D. [239]
Max-Planck-Institute for Molecular Genetics, Berlin, Germany
berger@molgen@mpg.de

Michel Bergeron, M.D. [196]
Professor of Physiology, Dept. of Physiology, Université de
Montréal, Montreal, Quebec, Canada
Bergermi@ere.umontreal.ca

Sten Erik Bergstrom, M.D. [187]
Dept. of Pediatrics, Huddinge University Hospital, Stockholm,
Sweden

Ernest Beutler, M.D. [127, 146, 182]
Chairman, Dept. of Molecular and Experimental Medicine,
Scripps Clinic and Research Foundation, La Jolla, California
beutler@scripps.edu

Daniel G. Bichet, M.D. [163]
Professor of Medicine, University of Montreal,
Director, Clinical Research Unit, Hopital du Sacre-Coeur de
Montreal, Montreal, Quebec, Canada
D-Binette@crhsc.umontreal.ca

Sandra H. Bigner, M.D. [57]
Professor of Pathology, Dept. of Pathology, Duke University
Medical Center, Durham, North Carolina
Bigne002@mc.duke.edu

David F. Bishop, Ph.D. [124]
Professor of Human Genetics, Dept. of Human Genetics, Mount
Sinai School of Medicine, New York, New York
David.bishop@mssm.edu

Ingemar Björkhem, M.D., Ph.D. [123]
Professor and Head Physician, Dept. of Medical Laboratory
Sciences and Technology, Division of Clinical Chemistry,
Karolinska Institutet, Huddinge University Hospital, Huddinge,
Sweden
Ingemar.Bjorkhem@chemlab.hs.sll.se

E. Joan Blanchette-Mackie, M.D. [145]
Chief, Sect. of Lipid Cell Biology, Laboratory of Cell
Biochemistry and Biology, National Institute of Diabetes and
Digestive and Kidney Diseases, Bethesda, Maryland
eb78u@nih.gov

Nenad Blau, M.D., Ph.D. [78]
Associate Professor, Div. of Clinical Chemistry and Biochemistry,
Dept. of Pediatrics, University Children's Hospital, Zurich,
Switzerland
blau@access.unizh.ch

Kirsten Muri Boberg, M.D., Ph.D. [123]
Dept. of Clinical Chemistry, Rikshospitalet, Oslo, Norway
kirsten.boberg@online.no

Sir Walter F. Bodmer, M.D., Ph.D., F.R.C.Path., F.R.S. [11]
Imperial Cancer Research Fund Laboratories, University of
Oxford, Institute of Molecular Medicine, John Radcliffe Hospital,
Oxford, United Kingdom
walter.bodmer@hertford.ox.ac.uk

C. Richard Boland, M.D. [32]
Professor of Medicine; Chief, Gastroenterology, University of
California, San Diego, La Jolla, California
CRBOLAND@UCSD.EDU

Dirk Bootsma, M.D. [28]
Dept. of Cell Biology and Genetics, Erasmus University,
Rotterdam, The Netherlands
Bootsma@gen.fgg.eur.nl

Thomas H. Bothwell, M.D., D.Sc. [127]
Emeritus Professor of Medicine, Honorary Professorial Research
Fellow, Faculty of Medicine, University of Witwatersrand,
Medical School, Johannesburg, South Africa
014jozo@chiron.wits.ac.za

G. Steven Bova, M.D. [56]
Assistant Professor, Depts. of Pathology, Urology and Oncology,
Johns Hopkins Hospital, Pelican Laboratory, Baltimore, Maryland
gbov@jhmi.edu

Bernard Brais, M.D., MPhil, Ph.D. [216]
Direction de L'IREP, Centre de recherche du CHUM, Hopital
Notre-Dame, Montreal, Quebec, Canada

David S. Bredt, M.D., Ph.D. [168]
Associate Professor of Physiology, Dept. of Physiology, University
of California, San Francisco
bredt@phy.ucsf.edu

Jan L. Breslow, M.D. [121]
Frederick Henry Leonhardt Professor, Director, Laboratory of
Biochemical Genetics and Metabolism, The Rockefeller
University, New York, New York
breslow@rockvax.rockefeller.edu

Martijn H. Breuning, M.D. [248]
Dept. of Clinical Genetics, Centre for Human and Clinical
Genetics, Leiden University Medical Centre, Leiden, The
Netherlands M.H.Breuning@kgc.azl.nl

H. Bryan Brewer, Jr., M.D. [118, 122]
Chief, Molecular Disease Branch, National Heart, Lung, and
Blood Institute, Bethesda, Maryland
bryan@mdb.nhlbi.nih.gov

Garrett M. Brodeur, M.D. [21, 60]
Div. of Oncology, Children's Hospital of Philadelphia,
Philadelphia, Pennsylvania
brodeur@email.chop.edu

Dieter Brömme, Ph.D. [137]
Associate Professor of Human Genetics, Mount Sinai School of
Medicine, New York, New York
brommd01@doc.mssm.edu

Michael D. Brown [105]
Assistant Professor, The Center for Molecular Medicine, Emory
University School of Medicine, Atlanta, Georgia
mdbrown@gen.emory.edu

Michael S. Brown, M.D. [120]
Regental Professor, Johnson Center for Molecular Genetics,
University of Texas Southwestern Medical Center, Dallas, Texas
mike.brown@utsouthwestern.edu

George J. Broze, Jr., M.D.   [175]
Professor of Medicine, Cell Biology and Physiology,
Washington University School of Medicine,
Barnes-Jewish Hospital at Washington University, St. Louis,
Missouri
gbroze@im.wustl.edu

John D. Brunzell, M.D.   [117]
Professor of Medicine, Program Director, General Clinical
Research Center, Dept. of Medicine, University of Washington
School of Medicine, Seattle, Washington
brunzell@u.washington.edu

Saul W. Brusilow, M.D.   [85]
Professor of Pediatrics Emeritus, The Johns Hopkins Hospital,
Baltimore, Maryland
sbru@jhmi.edu

Manuel Buchwald, O.C., Ph.D., F.R.S.C.   [31]
Professor, Molecular and Medical Genetics, University of Toronto,
Chief of Research and Director, Research Institute, Hospital for
Sick Children, Toronto, Ontario, Canada
Manuel.Buchwald@sickkids.on.ca

Peter H. Byers, M.D.   [205]
Professor, Dept. of Pathology and Medicine, Dept. of Pathology,
University of Washington, Seattle, Washington
pbyers@u.washington.edu

Daniel P Cahill, M.D., Ph.D.   [22]
Dept. of Oncology, The Johns Hopkins University School of
Medicine, Baltimore, Maryland

Paul Cairns, M.D.   [54]
Fox Chase Cancer Center, Philadelphia, Pennsylvania 19111

Giovanna Camerino, Ph.D.   [62]
Professor Biologia Generale E Genetica Medica, Universitá Di
Pavia, Pavia, Italy
camerino@unipv.it

Hubert Carchon, Ph.D.   [74]
Assistant Professor, University of Leuven, Centre for Metabolic
Disease, Leuven, Belgium
hubert.carchon@med.kuleuven.ac.be

Eugene D. Carstea, M.D.   [145]
Director, Saccomanno Research Institute,
St. Mary's Hospital and Medical Center,
Grand Junction, Colorado
gcarstea@stmarygj.com

Webster K. Cavenee, M.D.   [36]
Director, Ludwig Institute for Cancer Research, University of
California, San Diego, La Jolla, California

Aravinda Chakravarti, Ph.D.   [251]
Henry J. Knott Professor and Director, McKusick-Nathans
Institute of Genetic Medicine, Johns Hopkins University School of
Medicine, Baltimore, Maryland
aravinda@jhmi.edu

Arlene B. Chapman, M.D.   [215]
Associate Professor of Medicine, Director,
Hypertension and Renal Disease Research Center,
Emory University School of Medicine, Atlanta, Georgia
arlene_chapman@emory.org

Robert W. Charlton, M.D.   [127]
Emeritus Professor, University of Witwatersrand Medical School,
Johannesburg, South Africa
014jozo@chiron.wits.ac.za

Christiane Charpentier, Ph.D.   [66]
Biologist, INSERM-Paris France, Metabolic/Diabetes
Unit-Dept. of Pediatrics, Hopital Necker Enfants Malades, Paris,
France
Elisabeth.saudubray@nck.ap_hop_paris.fr

Yuan-Tsong Chen, M.D., Ph.D.   [71]
Professor of Pediatrics and Genetics, Chief, Div. of Medical
Genetics, Duke University Medical Center, Durham, North
Carolina
chen0010@mc.duke.edu

Russell W. Chesney, M.D.   [194]
Le Bonheur Professor and Chair, Dept. of Pediatrics, Le Bonheur
Children's Medical Center, University of Tennessee, Memphis,
Tennessee
rchesney@utmem.edu

Barton Childs, M.D.   [2, 3, 4]
Emeritus Professor of Pediatrics, The Johns Hopkins University
School of Medicine, Baltimore, Maryland

Kathleen R. Cho, M.D.   [53]
Associate Professor, Depts. of Pathology and Internal Medicine,
University of Michigan Medical School, Ann Arbor,
Michigan
kathcho@umich.edu

Streamson C. Chua, Jr.   [157]
Dept. of Medicine, Columbia University College of Physicians and
Surgeons, New York, New York

David T. Chuang, Ph.D.   [87]
Associate Professor, Dept. of Biochemistry, University of Texas
Southwestern Medical Center, Dallas, Texas
david.chuang@utsouthwestern.edu

Dominic W. Chung, Ph.D.   [171]
Dept. of Biochemistry School of Medicine, University of
Washington, Seattle, Washington
chung@u.washington.edu

Carmen Cifuentes-Diaz, Ph.D.   [231]
Laboratoire de Neurogénétique Molécularie, INSERM,
GENOPOLE, Evry, France
c.diaz@genopole.inserm.fr

James E. Cleaver, M.D.   [28]
Dept. of Dermatology, University of California at San Francisco
Cancer Center, San Francisco, California
jcleaver@cc.ucsf.edu

J.B. Clegg   [181]
Institute of Molecular Medicine, John Radcliffe Hospital, Oxford,
United Kingdom

Bruce E. Clurman, M.D.   [23]
Assistant Professor, Fred Hutchinson Cancer Research Center,
Seattle, Washington
bclurman@fhcrc.org

Anne-Marie Codori, Ph.D.   [49]
Dept. of Psychiatry and Behavioral Sciences, The Johns Hopkins
University School of Medicine, Baltimore, Maryland

Joy D. Cogan, M.D.   [162]
Research Assistant Professor of Pediatric Genetics, Div. of
Genetics, Vanderbilt University School of Medicine, Nashville,
Tennessee
joy.cogan@mcmail.vanderbilt.edu

Francis S. Collins, M.D., Ph.D.   [39]
National Human Genome Research Institute, Bethesda, Maryland
Fc23@nih.gov

Mary Ellen Conley, M.D.   [184]
St. Jude Children's Research Hospital, University of Tennessee
School of Medicine, Memphis, Tennessee
maryellen.conley@stjude.org

David N. Cooper, Ph.D.   [13]
Professor of Human Molecular Genetics, Institute of Medical
Genetics, University of Wales College of Medicine, Cardiff,
Wales, United Kingdom
cooperdn@cardiff.ac.uk

Valerie Cormier-Daire, M.D., Ph.D.   [99]
Dept. of Medical Genetics, Hopital Necker Enfants Malades,
Paris, France
cormier@necker.fr

Richard G.H. Cotton, Ph.D., D.Sc.   [1, 78]
Professor, Mutation Research Centre, Director, Mutation Research
Centre, St. Vincent's Hospital, Fitzroy, Victoria, Australia
cotton@ariel.ucs.unimelb.edu.au

Fergus J. Couch, M.D.   [47]
Assistant Professor, Dept. of Laboratory Medicine and Pathology,
Mayo Foundation and Clinic, Rochester, Minnesota
Couch.Fergus@mayo.edu

Diane Wilson Cox, M.D., Ph.D.   [219]
Professor and Chair, Dept. of Medical Genetics, Genetics Sect.
Head, Child Health, Capital Health Authority, Dept. of Medical
Genetics, University of Alberta, Edmonton, Alberta, Canada
diane.cox@ualberta.ca

Rody P. Cox, M.D., Ph.D.   [86]
Professor of Internal Medicine, Dept. of Internal Medicine,
University of Texas, Southwestern Medical Center, Attending
Physician, Parkland Memorial Hospital and St. Paul University
Hospital, Dallas, Texas
rcox@mednet.swmed.edu

William J. Craigen, M.D., Ph.D.   [14]
Dept. of Molecular and Human Genetics, Baylor College of
Medicine, Houston, Texas
wcraigen@bcm.tmc.edu

Donnell J. Creel, Ph.D.   [220]
Research Professor, Moran Eye Center, University of Utah School
of Medicine, Salt Lake City, Utah
Donnell.creel@hsc.utah.edu

Frans P.M. Cremers, Ph.D.   [236]
Associate Professor, Dept. of Human Genetics University Medical
Center Nymegen, Nymegen, The Netherlands
F.Cremers@Antrg.azn.nl

Valeria Cizewski Culotta, Ph.D.   [126]
Associate Professor, Dept. of Environmental Health Sciences,
Johns Hopkins University, School of Hygiene and Public Health,
Baltimore, Maryland
vculotta@JHSPH.edu

Garry R. Cutting, M.D.   [201]
Professor of Pediatrics and Medicine, McKusick-Nathan Institute
of Genetic Medicine, The Johns Hopkins University, Baltimore,
Maryland
gcutting@jhmi.edu

Christopher J. Danpure, Ph.D.   [133]
Professor of Molecular Cell Biology, MRC Laboratory for
Molecular Cell Biology, University College London, London,
United Kingdom
c.danpure@ucl.ac.uk

Earl W. Davie, Ph.D.   [169]
Dept. of Biochemistry School of Medicine,
University of Washington, Seattle, Washington

Alessandra d'Azzo, Ph.D.   [152]
Professor, Member, Dept. of Genetics, St. Jude Children's
Research Hospital, Memphis, Tennessee
sandra.dazzo@stjude.org

Samir S. Deeb, Ph.D.   [117, 238]
Research Professor of Medicine and Genetics, Dept. of Genetics,
University of Washington School of Medicine, Seattle, Washington
deeb@genetics.washington.edu

Robert J. Desnick, Ph.D., M.D.   [124, 137, 139, 144, 150]
Professor and Chairman, Human Genetics, Professor of Pediatrics;
Attending Physician, Dept. of Human Genetics, Mount Sinai
School of Medicine, New York, New York
rjdesnick@mcvax.mssm.edu

Harry C. Dietz, M.D.   [206]
Associate Investigator, Howard Hughes Medical Institute,
Professor, Dept. of Pediatrics, Medicine and Molecular Biology
and Genetics, McKusick-Nathan Institute of Genetic Medicine,
Johns Hopkins University School of Medicine, Baltimore,
Maryland
hdietz@jhmi.edu

Mary C. Dinauer, M.D., Ph.D.   [189]
Novz Letzter Professor of Pediatrics and Medical and Molecular
Genetics, Riley Hospital for Children, Indiana University School
of Medicine, Director, Herman B. Wells Center for Pediatric
Research, Indianapolis, Indiana
mdinauer@iupui.edu

Jiahuan Ding, M.D., Ph.D.   [101]
Director, Molecular Diagnostics, Senior Scientist, Associate
Professor, Baylor University, Waco, Texas, Institute of Metabolic
Disease, Baylor University Medical Center, Dallas, Texas
j.ding@baylordallas.edu

Michael J. Dixon, M.D.   [246]
Professor of Dental Genetics, School of Biological Sciences,
Dept. of Dental Medicine and Surgery, University of Manchester,
Manchester, United Kingdom
mdixon@fs1.scg.man.ac.uk

Patricia A. Donohoue, M.D.   [159]
Associate Professor, Dept. of Pediatrics, Div. of Endocrinology,
University of Iowa Hospitals, Dept. of Pediatrics, The Children's
Hospital of Iowa, Iowa City, Iowa
patricia-donohoue@uiowa.edu

Thaddeus P. Dryja, M.D.   [235]
Professor of Ophthalmology, Harvard Medical School, Dept. of
Ophthalmology, Massachusetts Eye and Ear Infirmary,
Boston, Massachusetts
dryja@helix.mgh.harvard.edu

Louis Dubeau, M.D., Ph.D.   [51]
Professor, Dept. of Pathology, USC/Norris Comprehensive Cancer
Center, Keck School of Medicine of USC, Los Angeles,
California
ldubeau@hsc.usc.edu

Thomas D. DuBose, Jr., M.D.   [195]
Peter T. Bohan Professor and Chair, Dept. of Internal Medicine,
Professor of Molecular and Integrative Physiology,
University of Kansas School of Medicine, Kansas City, Kansas
tdubose@kumc.edu

Jacques E. Dumont, M.D., Ph.D.   [158]
Professor of Biochemistry, Head, Institut de Recherche
interdisciplinaire, Faculté de Medecine, Université Libre de
Bruxelles, Brussels, Belgium
jedumont@ulb.ac.be

Marinus Duran, M.D. [128]
Academic Medical Center, Laboratory Genetic Metabolic
Diseases, University of Amsterdam, Amsterdam, The Netherlands
m.duram@amc.uva.nl

Michael J. Econs, M.D. [197]
Associate Professor of Medicine and Medical and Molecular
Genetics, Indiana University School of Medicine, Indianapolis,
Indiana
mecons@iupui.edu

Lora Hedrick Ellenson, M.D. [52]
Associate Professor and Director, Div. of Gynecologic Pathology,
Weill Medical College of Cornell University,
New York, New York
lhellens@med.cornell.edu

Nathan A. Ellis, M.D. [59]
Associate Member, Dept. of Human Genetics, Memorial Sloan-
Kettering Cancer Center, New York, New York
n-ellis@ski.mskcc.org

Lynne W. Elmore, Ph.D. [59]
Research Associate, Dept. of Pathology, School of Medicine,
Virginia Commonwealth University, Richmond, Virginia
LWElmore@hsc.vcu.edu

Charis Eng, M.D., Ph.D. [45]
Assoc. Professor of Medicine and Human Cancer Genetics, The
Ohio State University; Hon. Fellow, CRC, Human Cancer
Genetics Research Group, Univ. of Cambridge, United Kingdom;
Director, Clinical Cancer Genetics Program,
Ohio State University, Columbus, Ohio
Eng-1@medctr.osu.edu

Christine M. Eng, M.D. [150]
Associate Professor, Dept. of Molecular and Human Genetics,
Baylor College of Medicine, Houston, Texas
ceng@bcm.tmc.edu

Charles J. Epstein, M.D. [63]
Professor of Pediatrics, Co-Director, Program of Human Genetics,
Chief, Div. of Medical Genetics, Dept. of Pediatrics, University of
California at San Francisco, California
cepst@itsa.ucsf.edu

Charles T. Esmon, Ph.D. [170]
Head, Cardiovascular Biology Research Program, Oklahoma
Medical Research Foundation, Investigator, Howard Hughes
Medical Institute, Oklahoma Medical Research Foundation,
Oklahoma City, Oklahoma
charles-esmon@omrf.ouhsc.edu

Lindsay A. Farrer, Ph.D. [234]
Genetics Program, Boston University School of Medicine, Boston,
Massachusetts
farrer@neugen.bu.edu

Eric R. Fearon, M.D. [26]
Div. of Molecular Medicine and Genetics, University of Michigan
Medical Center, Ann Arbor, Michigan
fearon@umich.edu

Andrew P. Feinberg, M.D., M.P.H. [18]
King Fahd Professor of Medicine, Oncology and Molecular
Biology and Genetics, Johns Hopkins Medical School,
Baltimore, Maryland
afeinberg@jhu.edu

Anthony H. Fensom, Ph.D. [143]
Prince Philip Laboratory, Guy's Hospital, London, United
Kingdom

Wayne A. Fenton, Ph.D. [94, 155]
Dept. of Genetics, Yale University School of Medicine,
New Haven, Connecticut
wayne.fenton@yale.edu

Malcolm A. Ferguson-Smith, F.R.S. [62]
Professor, Dept. of Clinical Veterinary Medicine, University of
Cambridge, Centre for Veterinary Science, Cambridge,
United Kingdom

Clair A. Francomano, M.D. [210]
National Center for Human Genome Research, National Institutes
of Health, Bethesda, Maryland
clairf@nhgri.nih.giv

Deborah L. French, Ph.D. [177]
Assistant Professor of Medicine and Immunobiology,
Div. of Hematology, Mount Sinai School of Medicine, New York,
New York
dfrench@mssm.edu

Frank E. Frerman, Ph.D. [95, 103]
Professor of Pediatrics, Dept. of Pediatrics, University of Colorado
Health Science Center, Denver, Colorado
Frank.frerman@uchsc.edu

Carol Freund, Ph.D. [240]
Dept. of Clinical Bioethics, National Institutes of Health,
Bethesda, Maryland
cfreund@nih.gov

Theodore Friedmann, M.D. [107]
Dept. of Pediatric/Molecular Genetics, University of California,
San Diego, Center for Molecular Genetics, La Jolla, California
tfriedmann@ucsd.edu

Tony Frugier, MSc [231]
Laboratoire de Neurogénétique Moléculaire, INSERM,
GENOPOLE, Evry, France
t.frugier@genopole.inserm.fr

Elaine Fuchs, Ph.D. [221]
Amgen Professor of Basic Sciences, HHMI, Dept. of Molecular
Genetics and Cell Biology, University of Chicago, Chicago,
Illinois
lain@midway.uchicago.edu

Lars Fugger, M.D., Ph.D. [12]
Professor, Dept. of Clinical Immunology, Aarhus University
Hospital, Aarhus, Denmark
fugger@inet.uni2.dk

T. Mary Fujiwara, MSc [163]
Assistant Professor, Depts. of Human Genetics and Medicine,
McGill University, Div. of Medical Genetics, Montreal General
Hospital, Montreal, Quebec, Canada
fujiwara@bagel.epi.mcgill.ca

Toshiyuki Fukao, M.D., Ph.D. [102]
Department of Pediatrics, Gifu University School of Medecine,
Gifu, Japan
toshi-gif@umin.ac.jp

William A. Gahl, M.D., Ph.D. [199, 200]
Head, Sect. on Human Biochemical Genetics, Heritable Disorders
Branch, National Institute of Child Health and Human
Development, Bethesda, Maryland
bgahl@helix.nih.gov

David Gailani, M.D. [175]
Assistant Professor of Pathology and Medicine, Director, Clinical
Coagulation Laboratory, Vanderbilt Hospital, Hematology/
Oncology Div., Vanderbilt University, Nashville, Tennessee
dave.gailani@mcmail.vanderbilt.edu

Hans Galjaard, M.D., Ph.D. [152]
Professor of Clinical Genetics, Dept. of Clinical Genetics,
Erasmus University Medical Faculty, Rotterdam, The Netherlands
galjaard@algm.azr.nl

Carlos A. Garcia, M.D. [227]
Professor, Dept. of Psychiatry and Neurology, Tulane University
Health Sciences Center, New Orleans, Louisiana
cgarcia2@tulane.edu

Paolo Gasparini, M.D. [191]
Medical Genetics Service, IRCCS-Ospedale CSS, San Giovanni
Rotondo, Foggia, Italy
genetcss@fg.nettuno.it

Richard A. Gatti, M.D. [29]
Professor, Dept. of Pathology, School of Medicine, University of
California, Los Angeles, Los Angeles, California
rgatti@mednet.ucla.edu

Bruce D. Gelb, M.D. [137]
Associate Professor of Pediatrics and Human Genetics, Mount
Sinai School of Medicine, New York, New York
gelbb01@doc.mssm.edu

James L. German, III, M.D. [30]
Professor, Dept. of Pediatrics, Weill Medical College of Cornell
University, New York, New York
jlg2003@mail.med.cornell.edu

Gregory G. Germino, M.D. [215]
Associate Professor of Medicine, Div. of Nephrology, Johns
Hopkins University School of Medicine, Baltimore, Maryland
ggermino@welch.jhu.edu

Ali Gharavi, M.D. [211]
Assistant Professor of Medicine, Mount Sinai School of Medicine,
New York, New York; Visiting Assistant Professor, Dept. of
Genetics, Yale University School of Medicine, New Haven,
Connecticut
ali.gharavi@yale.edu

K. Michael Gibson, Ph.D. [91]
Director, Biochemical Genetics Laboratory, Associate Professor,
Dept. of Molecular and Medical Genetics, Biochemical Genetics
Lab, Oregon University Health Sciences, Portland, Oregon
gibsonm@ohsu.edu

Volkmar Gieselmann, M.D. [148]
Professor and Director, Biochemisches Institut, Christian-
Albrechts-Universitat Zu Kiel, Kiel, Germany
office@biochem.uni-kiel.de

Rachel H. Giles, Ph.D. [248]
Dept. of Immunology, University Medical Center Utrecht, Utrecht,
The Netherlands
R.Giles@lab.azu.nl

David Ginsburg, M.D. [178]
Warner-Lambert/Parke-Davis Professor of Medicine and Human
Genetics, Investigator, Howard Hughes Medical Institute, The
University of Michigan Medical Center, Ann Arbor, Michigan
ginsburg@umich.edu

Jonathan David Gitlin, M.D. [126]
Helene B. Roberson Professor of Pediatrics, Professor of
Pathology and Immunology, Director, Division of Pediatric
Immunology and Rheumatology, Washington University School of
Medicine, St. Louis Children's Hospital, St. Louis, Missouri
gitlin@kidsal.wustl.edu

Richard Gitzelmann, M.D. [70]
Professor Emeritus, Div. of Metabolic and Molecular Pediatrics,
University Children's Hospital, University of Zurich, Zurich,
Switzerland

M. Goedert, M.D., Ph.D. [234]
MRC Laboratory of Molecular Biology, Cambridge, England,
United Kingdom
mg@mrc-lmb.cam.ac.uk

Joseph L. Goldstein, M.D. [120]
Paul J. Thomas, Professor of Genetics and Chair, Dept. of
Molecular Genetics, University of Texas Southwestern Medical
Center, Dallas, Texas
joseph.goldstein@utsouthwestern.edu

Peter N. Goodfellow, B.Sc., D.Phil. [62]
Senior Vice President, Discovery Biopharmaceutical Research and
Development, SmithKline Beecham, Harlow, Essex,
United Kingdom
peter_n_goodfellow@sbphrd.com

Stephen I. Goodman, M.D. [95, 103]
Chief, Sect. of Genetics, Metabolism, and Birth Defects,
Professor of Pediatrics, Dept. of Pediatrics, School of Medicine,
University of Colorado Health Science Center, Denver,
Colorado
stephen.goodman@uchsc.edu

Paul Goodyer, M.D. [191]
Professor of Pediatrics, McGill University, Montreal Children's
Hospital, Nephrology Dept., Montreal, Quebec, Canada
paul.goodyer@muhc.mcgill.ca

Jerome L. Gorski, M.D. [247]
Professor of Pediatrics and Human Genetics, Director, Div. of
Pediatric Genetics, Div. of Clinical Genetics, Dept. of Pediatrics,
University of Michigan, Ann Arbor, Michigan
jlgorski@umich.edu

André Gougoux, M.D. [196]
Professor of Medicine, CHUM (Pavillon Notre Dame), Université
de Montréal, Montreal, Quebec, Canada

Stephen J. Gould, Ph.D. [129]
Associate Professor, Dept. of Biological Chemistry, The Johns
Hopkins University School of Medicine, Baltimore, Maryland
sgould@jhmi.edu

Gregory A. Grabowski, M.D. [146]
Director, Div. and Program in Human Genetics, Children's
Hospital Research Foundation, Cincinnati, Ohio
grabg0@chmcc.org

Denis M. Grant, Ph.D. [9]
Genetics and Genomic Biology Programme, Research Institute,
Hospital for Sick Children, Toronto, Ontario, Canada
grant@sickkids.on.ca

Roy A. Gravel, Ph.D. [94, 153]
Professor, Cell Biology and Anatomy, University of Calgary,
Calgary, Alberta, Canada
rgravel@ucalgary.ca

Eric D. Green, M.D., Ph.D [10]
Chief, Genome Technology Branch, Director, NIH, Intramural
Sequencing Center, National Human Genome Research Institute,
Bethesda, Maryland
egreen@nhgri.nih.gov

Daniel L. Greenberg, M.D. [169]
Dept. of Medicine, University of Washington Medical Center,
Division of Hematology, Seattle, Washington
robin@u.washington.edu

James E. Griffin, M.D. [160]
Professor of Internal Medicine, Diana and Richard C. Strauss
Professor in Biomedical Research, University of Texas
Southwestern Medical Center, Dallas, Texas
jgrif2@mednet.swmed.edu

Markus Grompe, M.D. [79]
Dept. of Molecular/Medical Genetics and Dept. of Pediatrics,
Oregon Health Sciences University, Portland, Oregon
grompem@ohsu.edu

James Gusella, M.D. [40]
Molecular Neurogenetics Unit, Massachusetts General Hospital,
Charlestown, Massachusetts

David H. Gutmann, M.D., Ph.D. [39]
Associate Professor, Director, Neurofibromatosis Program,
St. Louis Children's Hospital, Dept. of Neurology, Washington
University, St. Louis, Missouri
gutmannd@neuro.wustl.edu

Daniel A. Haber, M.D., Ph.D. [38]
Associate Professor of Medicine, Harvard Medical School,
Director, Center for Cancer Risk Analysis, Massachusetts General
Hospital Cancer Center, Lab of Molecular Genetics, Charlestown,
Massachusetts
haber@helix.mgh.harvard.edu

Theodora Hadjistilianou, M.D. [36]
Associate Professor, Dept. of Ophthalmology, University of Siena
School of Medicine, Siena, Tuscany, Italy

Judith G. Hall, M.D. [15]
Dept. of Pediatrics, British Columbia Children's Hospital,
Vancouver, British Columbia, Canada
judyhall@interchange.ubc.ca

Ada Hamosh, M.D., M.P.H. [1, 90]
Associate Professor of Pediatric, McKusick-Nathans Institute of
Genetic Medicine, The Johns Hopkins University School of
Medicine, Johns Hopkins Hospital, Baltimore, Maryland
ahamosh@jhmi.edu

Folker Hanefeld, M.D. [84]
Professor of Pediatrics and Child Neurology, Georg-August-
Universitat, Zentrum Kinderheilkunde, Abt. Padiatrie,
Schwerpunkt Neuropadiatrie, Germany

Isabel Hanson, M.D. [240]
Molecular Medicine Center, Western General Hospital,
Edinburgh, United Kingdom
isabel.hanson@ed.ac.uk

Jean-Pierre Hardelin [254]
Unite de Genetique des Deficits Sensoriels, Institut Pasteur, Paris,
France

Peter S. Harper, M.D. [217]
Professor and Consultant in Medical Genetics, University of Wales
College of Medicine, Heath Park Institute of Medical Genetics,
Cardiff, United Kingdom
harperps@cardiff.ac.uk

Curtis C. Harris, M.D. [59]
Chief, Laboratory of Human Carcinogenesis, National Cancer
Institute, Bethesda, Maryland
Curtis_Harris@NIH.GOV

Klaus Harzer, M.D. [134]
Professor, Neurochemical Laboratory, University of Tübingen,
Institut für Hirnforschung, Tübingen, Germany
hirnforschung@uni-tuebingen.de

Richard J. Havel, M.D. [114, 115]
Professor Emeritus, Cardiovascular Research Institute,
University of California School of Medicine, San Francisco,
California
dargank@curi.ucsf.edu

J. Ross Hawkins, Ph.D. [62]
Principal Scientist of Development Incyte Genomics, Ltd.
Cambridge, United Kingdom
Ross.Hawkins@incyte.com

Michael R. Hayden, M.D., ChB, Ph.D., FRCP(C), FRSC [223]
Professor of Medical Genetics, Centre for Molecular Medicine and
Therapeutics, University of British Columbia, Vancouver, British
Columbia, Canada
mrh@cmmt.ubc.ca

Vincent J. Hearing, M.D. [220]
Laboratory of Cell Biology, National Institutes of Health,
Bethesda, Maryland

Jacqueline T. Hecht, Ph.D. [210]
Dept. of Pediatrics, University of Texas Medical School,
Houston, Texas
jhecht@ped1.med.uth.tmc.edu

Peter Hechtman, Ph.D. [82]
Associate Professor of Biology, Human Genetics, and Pediatrics,
McGill University, Dept. of Biochemical Genetics, Montreal
Children's Hospital, Montreal, Quebec, Canada
Peter@uww.debelle.mcgill.ca

James F. Hejtmancik, M.D., Ph.D. [241]
National Eye Institute, National Institutes of Health, Bethesda,
Maryland
f3h@helix.nih.gov

Raoul C. M. Hennekam, Ph.D., M.D. [248, 249]
Pediatrician and Clinical Geneticist, Dept. of Pediatrics and
Institute for Human Genetics, Academic Medical Center,
University of Amsterdam, Amsterdam, The Netherlands
r.c.hennekam@amc.uva.nl

Meenhard Herlyn, Ph.D. [44]
Professor, The Wistar Institute, Philadelphia, Pennsylvania
herlynm@wistar.upenn.edu

Michael S. Hershfield, M.D. [109]
Dept. of Medicine and Biochemistry, Duke University Medical
Center, Durham, North Carolina
msh@biochem.duke.edu

Hugo S.A. Heymans [130]
Professor of Pediatrics, Director and Chairman. Emma Children's
Hospital and Clinical Chemistry, University of Amsterdam
Academic Medical Centre, Amsterdam, The Netherlands
h.s.heymans@amc.uva.nl

Howard H. Hiatt, M.D. [73]
Professor of Medicine, Harvard Medical School, Senior Physician,
Div. of General Medicine, Dept. of Medicine, Brigham and
Women's Hospital, Boston, Massachusetts
hhiatt@partners.org

D.R. Higgs [181]
Institute of Molecular Medicine, John Radcliffe Hospital, Oxford,
United Kingdom
drhiggs@molbiol.ox.ac.uk

Katherine A. High, M.D. [173]
William H. Bennett Professor of Pediatrics, UPENN School of
Medicine, Director of Research, Hematology Div., Director,
Hematology and Coagulation Laboratories, Children's Hospital of
Philadelphia, Philadelphia, Pennsylvania
high@email.chop.edu

Adrian V. S. Hill, D.Phil., D.M. [7]
Professor of Human Genetics, Wellcome Trust Centre for Human
Genetics, Headington, Oxford, United Kingdom
adrian.hill@imm.ox.ac.uk

Akira Hirono, M.D., Ph.D. [182]
Research Associate, Okinaka Memorial Institute for Medical
Research, Tokyo, Japan
Ncc01353@nifty.nc.jp

Rochelle Hirschhorn, M.D. [135]
Professor of Medicine and Cell Biology, Chief, Div. of Medical
Genetics, Dept. of Medicine, New York University School of
Medicine, New York, New York
hirscr0l@mcrcr0.med.nyu.edu

Helen H. Hobbs, M.D. [120]
Professor, Depts. of Internal Medicine and Molecular Genetics,
The University of Texas Southwestern Medical Center at Dallas,
Dallas, Texas
helen.hobbs@utsouthwestern.edu

Jan H.J. Hoeijmakers, M.D. [28]
Dept. of Cell Biology and Genetics, Erasmus University,
Rotterdam, The Netherlands
hoeijmakers@gen.fgg.eur.nl

Sandra L. Hofmann, M.D., Ph.D. [154]
Associate Professor of Internal Medicine, Hamon Center for
Therapeutic Oncology Research, University of Texas
Southwestern Medical Center, Dallas, Texas
hofmann@simmons.swmed.edu

Jeffrey M. Hoeg, M.D. [118]
Chief, Section on Molecular Biology, Molecular Disease Branch,
National Institutes of Health, Bethesda,
Maryland
Deceased 7/21/98.

Michael D. Hogarty, M.D. [21]
Div. of Oncology, The Children's Hospital of Philadelphia,
Philadelphia, Pennsylvania
hogartym@email.chop.edu

Edward J. Hollox, Ph.D. [76]
Institute of Genetics, University of Nottingham, Queens Medical
Centre Nottingham, United Kingdom
Ed.Hollox@Nottingham.ac.uk

Edward W. Holmes, M.D. [110]
Vice Chancellor and Dean, School of Medicine, University of
California, San Diego, California

John B. Holton, Ph.D. [72]
Emeritus Consultant Clinical Scientist, Clinical Biochemistry,
Southmean Hospital, Bristol, United Kingdom

John J. Hopwood, Ph.D. [149]
Professor & Head, Lysosomal Diseases Research Unit,
Dept. of Chemical Pathology, Women's and Children's Hospital,
North Adelaide, South Australia
john.hopwood@adelaide.edu.au

Ourania Horaitis, B.Sc. [1]
Co-ordinator, HUGO Mutation Database Initiative, Mutation
Research Centre, St. Vincent's Hospital, Fitzroy,
Melbourne, Victoria, Australia
horaitis@ariel.ucs.unimelb.edu.au

D. Jonathan Horsford, B.Sc. [240]
Program in Developmental Biology, Hospital for Sick Children,
Toronto, Ontario, Canada
djhors@sickkids.on.ca

Arthur L. Horwich, M.D. [85]
Professor of Genetics and Pediatrics, Investigator, HHMI, Yale
School of Medicine/HHMI, New Haven, Connecticut
horwich@csb.yale.edu

James R. Howe, M.D. [35]
Assistant Professor, Dept. of Surgery, University of Iowa College
of Medicine, Iowa City, Iowa
James_howe@uiowa.edu

Ralph H. Hruban, M.D. [50]
Professor of Pathology and Oncology, The Johns Hopkins
University, School of Medicine, Dept. of Oncology and Pathology,
Baltimore, Maryland
rhruban@jhmi.edu

Chien-an A. Hu, Ph.D. [81]
Research Associate, McKusick-Nathans Institute of Genetic
Medicine, Johns Hopkins University School of Medicine,
Baltimore, Maryland
cahu@welch.jhu.edu

Lynn D. Hudson, Ph.D. [228]
Acting Chief, Lab of Developmental Neurogenetics, National
Institute of Neurologic Disorders and Stroke, National Institutes of
Health, Bethesda, Maryland
hudsonl@ninds.nih.gov

Donald E. Hultquist [180]
Associate Chair, Dept. of Biological Chemistry, University of
Michigan Medical School, Ann Arbor, Michigan
hultquis@umich.edu

Keith Hyland, Ph.D. [78]
Associate Professor, Baylor University, Associate Professor,
University of Texas Southwestern Medical Center, Senior
Research Scientist, Baylor University Medical Center, Institute of
Metabolic Diseases, Dallas, Texas
k.hyland@baylordallas.edu

Akitada Ichinose, M.D., Ph.D. [171]
Professor and Chairman, Dept. of Molecular Pathological
Biochemistry, Yamagata University School of Medicine,
Yamagata, Japan
aichinos@med.id.yamagata-u.ac.jp

Yiannis A. Ioannou, Ph.D. [150]
Associate Professor, Dept. of Human Genetics, Mount Sinai
School of Medicine, New York, New York
yiannis.ioannou@mssm.edu

William B. Isaacs, Ph.D. [56]
Professor of Urology and of Oncology, Dept. of Urology, The
Johns Hopkins University School of Medicine, Baltimore,
Maryland
wisaacs@mail.jhmi.edu

Dirk Isbrandt, M.D. [84]
Research Scientist, Universitat Hamburg, Zentrum fur Molekulare
Neurobiologie Hamburg, Institut fur Neurale Signalverarbeitung,
Hamburg, Germany
isbrandt@uni-hamburg.de

Jaak Jaeken, M.D., Ph.D. [74, 112, 148]
Professor of Pediatrics, University of Leuven; Director, Center for
Metabolic Disease, University Hospital Gasthuisberg, Leuven,
Belgium
Jaak.jacken@uz.kuleuven.ac.be

Ernst R. Jaffe, M.D. [180]
Distinguished University Professor of Medicine Emeritus, Albert
Einstein College of Medicine, Bronx, New York
(Deceased)

Cornelis Jakobs, Ph.D. [91, 132]
Associate Professor, Head Metabolic Unit, Dept. of Clinical
Chemistry, Vrije Universiteit Medical Centre, Amsterdam,
The Netherlands
C.Jakobs@AZVU.nl

Anu Jalanko, Ph.D. [141]
Senior Scientist, Dept. of Human Molecular Genetics, National
Public Health Institute, Helsinki, Finland
Anu.jalanko@ktl.fi

Joanna C. Jen, M.D. [204]
Assistant Professor, Dept. of Neurology, UCLA School of
Medicine, Los Angeles, California
jjen@ucla.edu

Gerardo Jimenez-Sanchez, M.D., Ph.D. [3,4]
McKusick-Nathans Institute of Genetic Medicine, Johns Hopkins
University School of Medicine, Baltimore, Maryland
gjimenez@jhmi.edu

H.A. Jinnah, M.D., Ph.D. [107]
Assistant Professor, Dept. of Neurology, Johns Hopkins Hospital,
Baltimore, Maryland
hjinnah@welch.jhu.edu

Hans Joenje, Ph.D. [31]
Senior Scientist, Dept. Clinical and Human Genetics, Free
University Medical Center, Amsterdam, The Netherlands
H.Joenje.HumGen@med.vu.nl

Jean L. Johnson, M.D. [128]
Assistant Research Professor, Dept. of Biochemistry, Duke
University Medical Center, Durham, North Carolina
jean_johnson@biochem.duke.edu

Keith J. Johnson, Ph.D. [217]
Professor of Genetics, Head, Div. of Molecular Genetics, Institute
of Biomedical and Life Sciences, University of Glasgow, Glasgow,
United Kingdom
K.Johnson@bio.gla.ac.uk

Michael V. Johnston, M.D. [90]
Professor of Neurology and Pediatrics, The Johns Hopkins
University School of Medicine, Kennedy Krieger Institute,
Baltimore, Maryland
johnston@kennedykrieger.org

Michael M. Kaback, M.D. [153]
Professor, Depts. of Pediatrics and Reproductive Medicine,
University of California, San Diego, Children's Hospital and
Health Center, San Diego, California
mkaback@ucsd.edu

Steven E. Kahn, M.B., Ch.B. [67]
Associate Professor of Medicine, University of Washington, Staff
Physician, VA Puget Sound Health Care System, Seattle,
Washington
skahn@u.washington.edu

Muriel I. Kaiser-Kupfer, M.D. [241]
Chief, Ophthalmic Genetics, National Eye Institute, Bethesda,
Maryland
kaiserm@box-k.nih.gov

Anne Kallioniemi, M.D. [20]
Cancer Genetics Branch, National Human Genome Research
Institute, Bethesda, Maryland

Werner Kalow, M.D. [9]
Professor Emeritus, Dept. of Pharmacology, University of Toronto,
Toronto, Ontario, Canada
w.kalow@utoronto.ca

Naoyuki Kamatani, M.D. [108]
Professor and Director, Institute of Rheumatology, Tokyo
Women's Medical University, Tokyo, Japan
kamatani@ior.twmu.ac.jp

Alexander Kamb, Ph.D. [44]
Chief Scientific Officer, Arcaris, Inc., Salt Lake City, Utah
kamb@arcaris.com

John P. Kane, M.D., Ph.D. [114, 115]
University of California, San Francisco, California
Kane@itsa.ucsf.edu

Hitoshi Kanno, M.D., Ph.D. [182]
Assistant Professor, Dept. of Biochemistry, Nihon University
School of Medicine, Tokyo, Japan
hikanno@med.nihon-u.ac.jp

Josseline Kaplan [237]
Unite de Recherches sur les Handicaps, Genetiques de L'Enfant,
INSERM, Hôpital des Enfants Malades, Paris, Cedex, France

George Karpati, M.D., FRCP(C), FRS(C) [216]
Director, Neuromuscular Research, Dept. Neurology/
Neurosurgery, Montreal Neurological Institute, McGill University,
Montreal, Quebec, Canada
mcgk@musica.mcgill.ca

Seymour Kaufman, Ph.D. [77]
Emeritus Chief, Laboratory of Neurochemistry, National Institute
of Mental Health, National Institutes of Health, Bethesda,
Maryland
kaufman@codon.nih.gov

Haig H. Kazazian, Jr., M.D. [172]
Chairman, Dept. of Genetics, University of Pennsylvania School
of Medicine, Philadelphia, Pennsylvania
kazazian@mail.med.upenn.edu

Mark T. Keating, M.D. [203]
Professor of Medicine and Human Genetics, Eccles Institute
of Human Genetics, University of Utah/Howard Hughes Medical
Institute, Eccles Institute of Human Genetics, Salt Lake City, Utah
mark@howard.genetics.utah.edu

Richard I. Kelley, M.D., Ph.D. [249]
Associate Professor of Pediatrics, Johns Hopkins University,
Director of Metabolism, Kennedy Krieger Institute, Baltimore,
Maryland
kelle_ri@jhuvms.hcf.jhu.edu

Scott E. Kern, M.D. [50]
Associate Professor of Oncology, Johns Hopkins University
School of Medicine, Baltimore, Maryland
sk@jhmi.edu

Keith Kerstann, M.A. [105]
The Center for Molecular Medicine, Emory University School of
Medicine, Atlanta, Georgia
kkersta@gen.emory.edu

Richard A. King, M.D. [220]
Professor, University of Minnesota, Minneapolis, Minnesota
kingx002@tc.umn.edu

Kenneth W. Kinzler, Ph.D. [17, 27, 48]
Professor of Oncology, The Johns Hopkins University School of
Medicine, Baltimore, Maryland
kinzlke@jhmi.edu

D. Richard Klausner, M.D. [41]
Director, National Cancer Institute, Bethesda, Maryland
Klausner@helix.nih.gov

Michael Koenig, M.D. [232]
Professor of Medical Genetics, University of Louis Pasteur,
Strasbourg; Adjunct Director of the Genetics Diagnosis
Laboratory, Institute de Genetique et de Biologie Moleculaire et
Cellulaire, CNRS-INSERM-ULP, Illkirch, Strasbourg, France
mkoenig@igbmc.u-strasbg.fr

Thomas Kolter, Ph.D. [134]
Kekule-Institut für Organische Chemie und Biochemie, der
Reinnischen Friedrich-Wilhelms Universität Bonn, Bonn,
Germany
kolter@snchemie1.chemie.uni-bonn.de

Stuart Kornfeld, M.D. [138]
Professor of Medicine, Div. of Hematology-Oncology, Dept. of
Medicine, Washington University School of Medicine,
St. Louis, Missouri
skornfel@im.wustl.edu

Kenneth H. Kraemer, M.D. [28]
Research Scientist, Basic Research Laboratory, National Cancer
Institute, Bethesda, Maryland
kraemerk@nih.gov

Jan P. Kraus, Ph.D. [88]
Professor of Pediatrics and Cellular/Structural Biology, Dept. of Pediatrics, University of Colorado School of Medicine, Denver, Colorado
jan.kraus@uchsc.edu

Michael Krawczak, M.D. [13]
Professor, Institute of Medical Genetics, University of Wales College of Medicine, Cardiff, Wales, United Kingdom
krawczak@cardiff.ac.uk

Berry Kremer, M.D., Ph.D. [223]
Professor, Dept. of Neurology, University Medical Center Nijmegen, The Netherlands
h.kremer@czzoneu.azn.nl

Anjli Kukreja, Ph.D. [69]
Research Associate, Weill College of Medicine, Cornell University, New York
anjlik@hotmail.com

Bert N. La Du, Jr., M.D., Ph.D. [92]
Emeritus Professor of Pharmacology, Dept. of Pharmacology, University of Michigan Medical School, Ann Arbor, Michigan
bladu@umich.edu

Marie Lambert, M.D. [79]
Service de genetique medicale, Centre de recherche, Ste-Justine Hospital, Montreal, Quebec, Canada
lamberma@medclin.umontreal.ca

Risto Lappatto, M.D., Ph.D. [111]
Consultant Pediatrician, University of Helsinki, Helsinki, Finland
Risto.Lapatto@helsinki.fi

Agne Larsson, M.D., Ph.D. [96]
Professor of Pediatrics, Chairman, Dept. of Pediatrics, Children's Hospital, Karolinska Institutet, Huddinge University Hospital, Stockholm Sweden
agne.larsson@klinvet.ki.se

David H. Ledbetter, Ph.D. [65]
Professor and Chair, Dept. of Human Genetics, The University of Chicago, Chicago, Illinois
dhl@genetics.uchicago.edu

Rudolph L. Leibel, M.D. [157]
Chief, Division of Molecular Genetics, Co-Director, Naomi Berrie Diabetes Center, Professor of Pediatrics and Medicine, Columbia University College of Physicians & Surgeons, New York, New York
RL232@columbia.edu

Eran Leitersdorf, M.D. [123]
Professor of Medicine, Dorothy and Maurice Bucksbaum Chair in Molecular Genetics, Head, Center for Research, Prevention, and Treatment of Atherosclerosis, Dept. of Medicine, Hadassah University Hospital, Jerusalem, Israel
eran1@hadassah.org.il

Christoph Lengauer, M.D. [22]
The Johns Hopkins Oncology Center, Baltimore, Maryland
lengauer@jhmi.edu

Thierry Levade, Ph.D. [143]
Laboratoire de Biochemie, Maladies Metaboliques, CJF INSERM, Institut Louis Bugnard, Toulouse, France

Jacqueline Levilliers [254]
Unite de Genetique des Deficits Sensoriels, Institut Pasteur, Paris, France

Harvey L. Levy, M.D. [80, 88, 193]
Associate Professor of Pediatrics, Harvard Medical School, Senior Associate in Medicine and Genetics, Children's Hospital, Boston, Massachusetts
levy_h@al.tch.harvard.edu

Richard Alan Lewis, M.D. [243]
Professor, Dept. of Ophthalmology, Medicine, Pediatrics and Molecular Human Genetics, Baylor College of Medicine, Houston, Texas
rlewis@bcm.tmc.edu

Roland Libau, M.D. [12]
Postdoctoral Fellow, Dept. of Microbiology and Immunology, Stanford University School of Medicine, Stanford, California

Uri A. Liberman, M.D., Ph.D. [165]
Professor of Physiology and Medicine, Head, Dept. of Endocrinology and Metabolism, Rabin Medical Center, Beilinson Campus, Sackler School of Medicine, Tel-Aviv University, Petach-Tikvah, Israel
uliberman@clalit.org.il

Richard P. Lifton, M.D. [211]
Associate Investigator, Howard Hughes Medical Institute, Chair, Dept. of Genetics, Professor of Genetics, Internal Medicine & Molecular Biophysics, Yale University School of Medicine, New Haven, Connecticut
richard.lifton@yale.edu

W. Marston Linehan, M.D. [41]
Chief, Urologic Oncology Branch, National Cancer Institute, Bethesda, Maryland
Wml@nih.gov

Thomas Linke, M.D. [143]
Institute fur Organisch Chemie, Bonn, Germany

A. Thomas Look, M.D. [19]
Dept. of Experimental Oncology, St. Jude Children's Research Hospital, Memphis, Tennessee
Thomas.look@stjude.org

Marie T. Lott, M.A. [105]
Research Specialist, Supervisor, Center for Molecular Medicine, Emory University School of Medicine, Atlanta, Georgia
mtlott@gen.emory.edu

James R. Lupski, M.D., Ph.D. [65, 227, 243]
Cullen Professor of Molecular and Human Genetics and Professor of Medicine, Dept. of Molecular and Human Genetics, Baylor College of Medicine, Houston, Texas
jlupski@bcm.tmc.edu

Andreas Lux, Ph.D. [212]
Research Associate, Dept. of Genetics, Duke University Medical Center, Durham, North Carolina

Samuel E. Lux, IV, M.D. [183]
Robert A. Stranahan Professor of Pediatrics, Harvard Medical School Chief, Div. of Hematology/Oncology, Children's Hospital, Boston, Massachusetts
lux@genetics.med.harvard.edu

Lucio Luzatto, M.D., Ph.D. [179]
Scientific Director, Instituo Nazionale per la Ricerca sul Cancro, Genova, Italy
luzzatto@hp380.ist.unige.it

Stanislas Lyonnet, M.D., Ph.D. [251]
Professor of Genetics, University of Paris, Dept. de Genetique et Unite, INSERM, Hospital Necker-Enfants Malades, Paris, France
lyonnet@necker.fr

Mack Mabry, M.D. [58]
Div. of Radiology, The Johns Hopkins Hospital, Baltimore, Maryland

Mia MacCollin, M.D. [40]
Assistant Professor of Neurology, Massachusetts General Hospital, Charlestown, Massachusetts
maccollin@helix.mgh.harvard.edu

Noel Keith Maclaren, M.D. [69]
Professor of Pediatrics, Director, Juvenile Diabetes, Weill College
of Medicine, Cornell University, New York
NKMaclaren@aol.com

Edward R. B. McCabe, M.D., Ph.D [97, 167]
Professor and Executive Chair, Dept. of Pediatrics UCLA School
of Medicine; Physician-in-Chief, Mattel Children's Hospital at
UCLA, Los Angeles, California
emccabe@pediatrics.medsch.ucla.edu

Hugh O. McDevitt, M.D. [12]
Professor of Microbiology and Immunology, Stanford University
School of Medicine, Stanford, California
hughmcd@stanford.edu

Roderick R. McInnes, M.D., Ph.D. [80, 240]
University of Toronto Tanenbaum Chair in Molecular Medicine,
Professor of Pediatrics and Molecular Genetics, University of
Toronto, Head, Program in Developmental Biology, Research
Institute, Hospital for Sick Children, Toronto, Ontario, Canada
mcinnes@sickkids.on.ca

Victor A. McKusick, M.D. [1]
Professor , McKusick-Nathans Institute of Genetic Medicine,
Johns Hopkins University School of Medicine, Baltimore,
Maryland
McKusick@peas.welch.jhu.edu

Roger E. McLendon, M.D. [57]
Associate Professor; Director of Anatomic Pathology Services;
Chief, Sect. of Neuropathology, Duke University Medical Center,
Durham, North Carolina
roger.mclendon@duke.edu

Michael J. McPhaul, M.D. [160]
Professor, Dept. of Internal Medicine, Div. of Endocrinology and
Metabolism, University of Texas Southwestern Medical Center,
Dallas, Texas
mcphaul@pop3.utsw.swmed.edu

Robert W. Mahley, M.D., Ph.D. [119]
Director, Gladstone Institute of Cardiovascular Disease, Professor
of Pathology and Medicine, University of California, San
Francisco
rmahley@gladstone.ucsf.edu

David Malkin, M.D. [37]
Associate Professor of Pediatrics, University of Toronto, Program
in Cancer and Blood Research, Research Institute, Hospital for
Sick Children, Toronto, Ontario, Canada
David.malkin@sickkids.on.ca

Ned Mantei, Ph.D. [75]
Professor, Swiss Federal Institute of Technology, Institute for Cell
Biology, Zurich, Switzerland
mantei@cell.biol.ethz.ch

Douglas A. Marchuk, Ph.D. [212]
Assistant Professor, Dept. of Genetics, Duke University Medical
Center, Durham, North Carolina
march004@mc.duke.edu

Sandrine Marlin [254]
Unite de Genetique des Deficits Sensoriels, Institut Pasteur,
Paris, France

Karen L. Marsh, Ph.D. [246]
University of Manchester, School of Biological Sciences,
Manchester, United Kingdom

George M. Martin, M.D. [8]
Professor of Pathology, Adjunct Professor of Genetics, Director,
Alzheimer's Disease Research Center, Attending Pathologist,
Medical Center, University of Washington School of Medicine,
Seattle, Washington
gmmartin@u.washington.edu

Martín G. Martín, M.D. [190]
Dept. of Pediatrics, Gastroenterology, UCLA School of Medicine,
Los Angeles, California
mmartin@mednet.ucla.edu

Paula Martin, Ph.D. [214]
Dept. of Biochemistry, University of Oulu, Finland
paula.martin@oula.fi

Stephen J. Marx, M.D. [43, 165]
Chief, Genetics and Endocrinology Sect., National Institutes of
Health, Bethesda, Maryland
stephenm@intra.niddk.nih.gov

Gert Matthijs, Ph.D. [74]
Assistant Professor, Center for Human Genetics, University
Hospital of Leuven, Centre for Human Genetics, Leuven, Belgium
gert.matthijs@med.kuleuven.ac.be

Atul Mehta, M.D. [179]
Consultant Hematologist, Dept. of Hematology, Royal Free
Hospital, London, United Kingdom
atul.mehta@rfh.nthames.nhs.uk

Judith Melki, M.D., Ph.D. [231]
Neurogénétique Moléculaire, INSERM, GENOPOLE, Evry,
France
j.melki@genopole.inserm.fr

Paul S. Meltzer, M.D., Ph.D. [20]
Sect. of Molecular Cytogenetics, Lab of Cancer Genetics, National
Institutes of Health, Bethesda, Maryland

Claude J. Migeon, M.D. [159]
Professor of Pediatrics, Div. of Pediatric Endocrinology, The Johns
Hopkins University School of Medicine, Baltimore, Maryland
cmigeon@welchlink.welch.jhu.edu

Tetsuro Miki, Ph.D. [33]
Geriatric Research Education and Clinical Center, University of
Washington, Seattle, Washington

Beverly S. Mitchell [109]
Wellcome Professor of Cancer Research, University of North
Carolina, Lineberger Comprehensive Cancer Center, Chapel Hill,
North Carolina

Grant A. Mitchell, M.D. [79, 102]
Div. of Medical Genetics, Hopital Ste-Justine, Montreal, Quebec,
Canada
mitchell@justine.umontreal.ca

Shiro Miwa, M.D. [182]
Director, Okinaka Memorial Institute for Medical Research,
Tokyo, Japan

Maria Judit Molnar, M.D., Ph.D. [216]
Dept. of Neurology, Medical University of Debrecen, National
Institute of Psychiatry and Neurology, Budapest, Hungary
molnarm@jaguar.dote.hu

Jill A. Morris, Ph.D. [145]
Senior Research Biologist, Dept. of Pharmacology, Merck
Research Laboratories, West Point, Pennsylvania
jill_morris@merck.com

Ann B. Moser, BA [131]
Kennedy Krieger Institute, Baltimore, Maryland
mosera@kennedykrieger.org

Hugo W. Moser, M.D. [131, 143]
Professor of Neurology and Pediatrics, Johns Hopkins University,
Director of Neurogenetics, Kennedy Krieger Institute, Baltimore,
Maryland
moser@kennedykrieger.org

Björn Mossberg, M.D., Ph.D. [187]
Chief Physician, Dept. of Respiratory Medicine and Allerology,
Huddinge University Hospital Stockholm, Sweden
bjorn.mossberg@lungall.hs.sll.se

Arno G. Motulsky, M.D., D.Sc. [127, 238]
Professor Emeritus Active of Medicine and Genetics, Attending
Physician, University of Washington Hospital, Div. of Medical
Genetics, Dept. of Medicine, University of Washington, Seattle,
Washington
agmot@u.washington.edu

S. Harvey Mudd, M.D. [88]
Guest Scientist, Laboratory of Molecular Biology, National
Institute of Mental Health, National Institutes of Health, Bethesda,
Maryland
sbm@codon.nih.gov

Maximilian Muenke, M.D. [245, 250]
Chief, Medical Genetics Branch, National Human Genome
Research Institute, National Institutes of Health, Bethesda,
Maryland
muenke@nih.gov

Joseph Muenzer, M.D., Ph.D. [136]
Associate Professor of Pediatrics, Dept. of Pediatrics, University
of North Carolina at Chapel Hill, North Carolina
muenzer@css.unc.edu

Arnold Munnich, M.D., Ph.D. [99, 237]
Professor, Dept. of Pediatrics, INSERM, Hopital des Enfants
Malades, Hopital Necker, Paris, France
munnich@necker.fr

Jun Nakura, M.D., Ph.D. [33]
Department of Geriatric Medicine, School of Medicine, Ehime
University, Ehime, Japan
nakura@ m.ehime-u.ac.jp

Eiji Nanba, M.D. [151]
Associate Professor, Gene Research Center, Tottori University,
Yonago, Japan
enanba@grape.med.tottori-u.ac.jp

William M. Nauseef, M.D. [189]
Professor, Inflammation Program and Dept. of Medicine,
University of Iowa, Iowa City, Iowa
william-nauseef@uiowa.ed

Barry D. Nelkin, Ph.D. [58]
Associate Professor of Oncology, Johns Hopkins University
School of Medicine, Baltimore, Maryland
bnelkin@jhmi.edu

Edward B. Neufeld, Ph.D. [145]
National Heart, Lung, and Blood Institute, Bethesda, Maryland
neufelde@mail.nih.gov

Elizabeth F. Neufeld, Ph.D. [136]
Professor and Chair Biological Chemistry, Dept. of Biological
Chemistry, UCLA School of Medicine, Los Angeles, California
eneufeld@mednet.ucla.edu

Peter E. Newburger, M.D. [189]
Professor of Pediatrics and Molecular, Genetics/Microbiology;
Director, Pediatric Hematology/Oncology, University of
Massachusetts Medical School, Worcester, Massachusetts
peter.newburger@ummed.edu

Peter J. Newman, Ph.D. [177]
Senior Investigator, Vice President and Assoc. Director for
Research, The Blood Center, Milwaukee, Wisconsin
pjnewman@bcsew.edu

Irene F. Newsham, Ph.D. [36]
Dept. of Anatomy and Pathology, Medical College of Virginia,
Richmond, Virginia
inewsham@hsc.vcu.edu

Jeffrey L. Noebels, M.D., Ph.D. [230]
Professor of Neurology, Neuroscience, and Molecular and Human
Genetics, Dept. of Neurology, Baylor College of Medicine,
Houston, Texas
jnoebels@bcm.tmc.edu

Josette Noël, M.D. [196]
Assistant Professor, Dept. of Physiology, Université de Montréal,
Montreal, Quebec, Canada
josette.noel@umontreal.ca

Lawrence M. Nogee, M.D. [218]
Associate Professor, Dept. of Pediatrics, Div. of Neonatology,
Johns Hopkins University School of Medicine, Baltimore,
Maryland
lnogee@welch.jhu.edu

Virginia Nunes, Ph.D. [191]
Medical and Molecular Genetics Center, L'Hospitalet de
Llobregat, Barcelona, Catalunya, Spain
vnunes@iro.es

Robert L. Nussbaum, M.D. [252]
Chief, Genetic Diseases Research Branch, National Human
Genome Research Institute, Bethesda, Maryland
rlnuss@nhgri.nih.gov

William S. Oetting, M.D. [220]
Assistant Professor, University of Minnesota, Minneapolis,
Minnesota
bill@lenti.med.umn.edu

Harry T. Orr, M.D. [226]
University of Minnesota, Institute of Human Genetics,
Minneapolis, Minnesota
harry@lenti.med.umn.edu

Akihiro Oshima, M.D. [151]
Visiting Investigator, Dept. of Veterinary Science, National
Institute of Infectious Diseases, Tokyo, Japan
oshima@nih.go.jp

Manuel Palacín, M.D. [191]
Professor, Biochemistry and Molecular Biology, Faculty of
Biology, Dept. of Biochemistry and Physiology, University of
Barcelona, Barcelona, Spain
mnpalacin@porthos.bio.ub.es

Cristina Panozzo, Ph.D. [231]
Laboratoire de Neurogénétique Moléculaire, INSERM,
GENOPOLE, Evry, France
c.panozzo@genopole.inserm.fr

Lucie Parent, M.D. [196]
Associate Professor, Dept. of Physiology, Université de Montréal,
Montreal, Quebec, Canada
lucie.parent@umontreal.ca

Peter Parham, Ph.D. [12]
Professor of Structural Biology and of Microbiology and
Immunology, Stanford University, Stanford, California
Peropa@leland.stanford.edu

Morag Park, M.D. [25]
Molecular Oncology Group, Royal Victoria Hospital, Montreal,
Quebec, Canada
morag@lan1.molonc.mcgill.ca

Keith L. Parker, M.D., Ph.D. [159]
Professor of Internal Medicine and Pharmacology, Dept. of
Internal Medicine, UT Southwestern Medical Center, Dallas,
Texas
kparke@mednet.swmed.edu

Ramon Parsons, M.D., Ph.D. [45]
Assistant Professor, Columbia Institute of Cancer Genetics,
Columbia University, New York, New York
rep15@columbia.edu

Marc C. Patterson, M.D. [145]
Consultant, Div. of Child and Adolescent Neurology, Mayo Clinic,
Rochester, Minnesota
mpatterson@mayo.edu

Leena Peltonen, M.D., Ph.D. [141, 154]
Professor and Chair of Human Genetics, Dept. of Human
Genetics, UCLA School of Medicine, Los Angeles, California
lpeltonen@mednet.ucla.edu

Peter G. Pentchev, Ph.D. [145]
Chief, Sect. of Cellular and Molecular Pathophysiology,
Developmental and Metabolic Neurology Branch, National
Institutes of Neurological Disorders and Stroke, Bethesda,
Maryland
peter.pentchev@xtra.co.nz

Isabelle Perrault, M.D. [237]
Unite de Recherches sur les Handicaps, Genetiques de L'Enfant,
INSERM, Hôpital des Enfants Malades, Paris, France

Gloria M. Petersen, Ph.D. [49]
Professor of Clinical Epidemiology, Consultant, Mayo
Foundation, Mayo Clinic, Rochester, New York
peterg@mayo.edu

Christine Petit [254]
Unite de Genetique des Deficits Sensoriels, Institut Pasteur, Paris,
France
cpetit@pasteur.fr

Fred Petrij, M.D. [248]
Clinical Genetics Registrar, Dept. of Clinical Genetics, Erasmus
University, Rotterdam, The Netherlands
petrij@kgen.azr.nl

James M. Phang, M.D. [81]
Chief, Metabolism and Cancer Susceptibility Sect., Basic
Research Laboratory, Div. of Basic Sciences, National Cancer
Institute, Frederick, Maryland
phang@mail.ncifcrf.gov

John A. Phillips, III, M.D. [162]
Professor of Pediatrics and Biochemistry, Div. of Medical
Genetics, Vanderbilt University School of Medicine, Nashville,
Tennessee
john.phillips@mcmail.vanderbilt.edu

Joram Piatigorsky, Ph.D. [241]
Chief, Laboratory of Molecular and Developmental Biology,
National Eye Institute, Bethesda, Maryland
joramp@intra.nei.nih.gov

Leonard Pinsky, M.D. [161]
Professor, Depts. of Medicine, Human Genetics, Biology and
Pediatrics, McGill University, Lady Davis Institute for Medical
Research, Sir M.B. Davis–Jewish General Hospital, Montreal,
Quebec, Canada
rrosenzw@ldi.jgh.mcgill.ca

Eleanor S. Pollak, M.D. [173]
Assistant Professor of Pathology and Laboratory Medicine,
Hospital of the University of Pennsylvania, Associate Director,
Clinical Coagulation Laboratory, The Children's Hospital of
Philadelphia, Philadelphia, Pennsylvania
pollak@mail.med.upenn.edu

Bruce A.J. Ponder, Ph.D., F.R.C.P. [42]
CRC Professor of Oncology, University of Cambridge, Cambridge
Institute for Medical Research, Cambridge, United Kingdom
bajp@mole.bio.cam.ac.uk

Mortimer Poncz, M.D. [177]
Professor of Pediatrics, University of Pennsylvania Medical
Center, Philadelphia, Pennsylvania

Daniel Porte, Jr., M.D. [67]
Professor of Medicine, University of California San Diego;
Staff Physician, VA San Diego Health Care System, San Diego,
California
dporte@ucsd.edu
poncz@email.chop.edu

Steven M. Powell, M.D. [55]
Assistant Professor of Medicine, Div. of Gastroenterology,
University of Virginia Health Systems, Charlottesville, Virginia
SMP8N@virginia.edu

James M. Powers, M.D. [131]
Dept. of Pathology, University of Rochester Medical Center,
Rochester, New York

Richard L. Proia, Ph.D. [153]
Chief, Genetics of Development and Disease Branch, National
Institute of Diabetes and Digestive and Kidney Diseases, National
Institutes of Health, Bethesda, Maryland
proia@nih.gov

Kathleen P. Pratt, Ph.D. [171]
Instructor, Department of Biochemistry, University of Washington,
Seattle
kpratt@u.washington.edu

Stanley B. Prusiner, M.D. [224]
Director, Institute for Neurodegenerative Diseases, Professor of
Neurology and Biochemistry, Dept. of Neurology, University of
California, San Francisco, California

Louis J. Ptáček, M.D. [204]
Associate Professor, Associate Investigator, Dept. of Neurology
Human Genetics, Howard Hughes Medical Institute, University of
Utah, Salt Lake City, Utah
ptacek@genetics.utah.edu

Jennifer M. Puck, M.D. [185]
Head Chief, Immunologic Genetics Sect., National Human
Genome Research Institute, Genetics and Molecular Biology
Branch, Bethesda, Maryland
jpuck@nhgri.nih.gov

Leena Pulkkinen, Ph.D. [222]
Jefferson Institute of Molecular Medicine, Dept. of Dermatology
and Cutaneous Biology, Jefferson Medical College, Thomas
Jefferson University, Philadelphia, Pennsylvania
leena.pulkkinen@mail.tju.edu

Reed E. Pyeritz, M.D., Ph.D. [206]
Professor of Human Genetics, MCP Hahnemann School of
Medicine, Philadelphia, Pennsylvania
pyeritz@yahoo.com

Kari O. Raivio, M.D. [111]
Professor of Perinatal Medicine, School of Medicine, University of
Helsinki, Helsinki, Finland
kari.raivio@helsinki.fi

Stanley C. Rall, Jr., Ph.D. [119]
Investigator, Gladstone Institute of Cardiovascular Disease, San
Francisco, California

Bonnie W. Ramsey, M.D. [201]
Dept. of Pediatrics, University of Washington School of Medicine,
Children's Hospital Regional Medical Center, Seattle,
Washington
bramsey@u.washington.edu

Ahmed Rasheed [57]
Research Assistant Professor, Duke University Medical Center, Durham, North Carolina
a.rasheed@duke.edu

Gerald V. Raymond, M.D. [129]
Assistant Professor, Neurology, Kennedy Krieger Institute, Johns Hopkins University School of Medicine, Baltimore, Maryland
raymond@kennedykrieger.org

Andrew P. Read, MA, Ph.D., FRC Path, FmedSci [244]
Professor of Human Genetics, Dept. of Medical Genetics, St. Mary's Hospital, University of Manchester, Manchester, United Kingdom
andrew.read@man.ac.uk

Jonathan J. Rees, MBBS, FRCP [46]
Professor and Chairman, Dept. of Dermatology, The University of Edinburgh, Edinburgh, Scotland, United Kingdom
Jonathan.rees@ed.ac.uk

Samuel Refetoff, M.D. [158]
Professor of Medicine and Pediatrics, Director, Endocrinology Laboratory, Depts. of Medicine and Pediatrics and the J.P. Kennedy Jr. Mental Retardation Research Center, The University of Chicago, Chicago, Illinois
refetoff@medicine.bsd.uchicago.edu

Arnold J.J. Reuser, Ph.D. [135]
Associate Professor of Cell Biology, Erasmus University Rotterdam, Dept. of Clinical Genetics, Rotterdam, The Netherlands
reuser@ikg.fgg.eur.nl

William B. Rizzo, M.D. [98]
Professor of Pediatrics, Human Genetics, Biochemistry, and Molecular Biophysics, Dept. of Pediatrics, Medical College of Virginia, Virginia Commonwealth University, Richmond, Virginia
wrizzo@hsc.vcu.edu

James M. Roberts, M.D. [23]
Div. of Basic Sciences, Fred Hutchinson Cancer Research Center, Seattle, Washington 98104

Brian H. Robinson, Ph.D. [100]
Professor, Depts. of Biochemistry and Pediatrics, Program Head, Metabolism, Senior Scientist, Genetics and Genomic Biology, Hospital for Sick Children, Toronto, Ontario, Canada
bhr@sickkids.on.ca

Charles R. Roe, M.D. [101]
Institute of Metabolic Disease, Baylor University Medical Center, Dallas, Texas
cr.roe@baylordallas.edu

Hans-Hilger Ropers, M.D., Ph.D. [236, 239]
Professor, Dept. of Human Genetics, Max-Planck-Institute fuer Molekulare Genetik, Berlin, Germany
Ropers@molgen.mpg.de

Michael Rosenbaum, M.D. [157]
Associate Professor of Clinical Pediatrics and Clinical Medicine, Div. of Molecular Genetics, Russ Berrie Research Center, Columbia University College of Physicians and Surgeons, New York, New York
mr475@columbia.edu

David S. Rosenblatt, M.D. [94, 155]
Professor of Human Genetics, Medicine, Pediatrics, and Biology, Director, Div. of Medical Genetics, McGill University Health Centre, Royal Victoria Hospital, Montreal, Quebec, Canada
mc74@musica.mcgill.ca

Agnes Rötig, Ph.D. [99]
Dept. of Genetics, INSERM, Hopital Necker, Paris, France
roetig@necker.fr

Jayanta Roy Chowdhury, M.D., M.R.C.P. [125]
Professor of Medicine and Molecular Genetics, Dept. of Medicine and Molecular Genetics, Albert Einstein College of Medicine at Yeshiva University, Bronx, New York
chowdhur@aecom.yu.edu

Namita Roy Chowdhury, Ph.D. [125]
Professor of Medicine and Molecular Genetics, Albert Einstein College of Medicine, Bronx, New York

Jean-Michel Rozet, M.D. [237]
Unite de Recherches sur les Handicaps, Genetiques de L'Enfant, INSERM, Hôpital des Enfants Malades, Paris, France

Edward M. Rubin, M.D., Ph.D. [121]
Head, Genome Sciences Dept., Lawrence, Berkeley Laboratory, University of California at Berkeley, Berkeley, California
emrubin@lbl.gov

Charles M. Rudin, M.D. [24]
Assistant Professor of Medicine, University of Chicago Medical Center, Chicago, Illinois
crudin@medicine.bsd.uchicago.edu

Elena I. Rugarli, M.D. [225]
Researcher, Telethon Institute of Genetics and Medicine (TIGEM), Milan, Italy
rugarli@tigem.it

David W. Russell, Ph.D. [160]
Eugene McDermott Distinguished Professor of Molecular Genetics, University of Texas Southwestern Medical Center Dallas, Texas
russell@utsw.swmed.edu

Pierre Rustin, Ph.D. [99]
Dept. of Genetics, INSERM, Hopital Des Enfants-Malades, Paris, France
rustin@necker.fr

David D. Sabatini, M.D., Ph.D. [16]
Frederick L. Ehrman Professor and Chairman, Dept. of Cell Biology, New York University School of Medicine, New York, New York
Sabatd01@popmail.med.nyu.edu

Richard L. Sabina, Ph.D. [110]
Associate Professor of Biochemistry, Dept. of Biochemistry, Medical College of Wisconsin, Milwaukee, Wisconsin
sabinar@mcw.edu

J. Evan Sadler, M.D., Ph.D. [174]
Professor, Depts. Of Medicine, Biochemistry and Molecular Biophysics; Investigator, Howard Hughes Medical Institute, Washington University School of Medicine, St. Louis, Missouri
esadler@im.wustl.edu

Amrik S. Sahota, Ph.D., F.A.C.M.G. [108]
Dept. of Genetics, Nelson Biological Laboratories, Rutgers University, Piscataway, New Jersey
sahota@nel-exchange.vutgers.edu

Mika Saksela, M.D. [111]
Research Associate, Children's Hospital, University of Helsinki, Helsinki, Finland
Mika.Saksela@Helsinki.fi

Julian R. Sampson, M.D. [233]
Professor of Medical Genetics Institute of Medical Genetics, University of Wales, College of Medicine, Cardiff, United Kingdom
wmgjrs@cardiff.ac.uk

Konrad Sandhoff, Ph.D.   [134, 143, 153]
Director and Professor of Biochemistry, Kekule-Institut fur
Organische Chemie und Biochemie, Universitat Bonn, Bonn,
Germany
sandhoff@uni-bonn.de

Michael C. Sanguinetti, Ph.D.   [203]
University of Utah, Eccles Institute of Human Genetics, Salt Lake
City, Utah
mike.sanguinetti@hci.utah.edu

Silvia Santamarina-Fojo, M.D, Ph.D.   [118]
Chief, Section on Cell Biology, Molecular Disease Branch,
National Institutes of Health, Bethesda, Maryland
silvia@mdb.nhlbi.nih.gov

Carmen Sapienza, Ph.D.   [15]
Professor of Pathology and Laboratory Medicine, Associate
Director, Fels Institute for Cancer Research, Temple University
School of Medicine, Philadelphia, Pennsylvania
sapienza@unix.temple.edu

Shigeru Sassa, M.D., Ph.D. [124]
Emeritus Head, Laboratory of Biochemical Hematology,
The Rockefeller University, New York, New York
sassa@rockvax.rockefeller.edu

Jean-Marie Saudubray, M.D.   [66]
Director of the Metabolic/Diabetes Unit, Professor, Dept. of
Pediatrics, Hopital Necker Enfants Malades, Paris, France
Elisabeth.saudubray@nck.ap_hop_paris.fr

Alan J. Schafer, Ph.D.   [253]
Vice President Genetics, Incyte Genomics, Cambridge, United
Kingdom
alan.schafer@incyte.com

Gerard Schellenberg, Ph.D.   [33]
Veterans Affairs Medical Center, Seattle, Washington
zachdad@u.washington.edu

Detlev Schindler, M.D.   [139]
Director, Cell Culture, Biochemistry and Flowcytometry Div.;
Associate Professor of Human Genetics, Dept. of Human
Genetics, University of Wuerzburg, Wuerzburg, Germany
schindler@biozentrum.uni-wuerzburg.de

Jerry A. Schneider, M.D.   [199]
Professor of Pediatrics; Benard L. Maas Chair in Inherited
Metabolic Disease, Dean for Academic Affairs, Office of the
Dean, School of Medicine, University of California, San Diego
School of Medicine, La Jolla, California
jschneider@ucsd.edu

Edward H. Schuchman, Ph.D.   [144]
Professor of Human Genetics, Dept. of Human Genetics, Mount
Sinai School of Medicine, Member, Institute for Gene Therapy
and Molecular Medicine, New York, New York
schuchman@msvax.mssm.edu

C. Ronald Scott, M.D.   [89]
Professor, Dept. of Pediatrics, University of Washington School of
Medicine, Seattle, Washington
crscott@u.washington.edu

Charles R. Scriver, M.D.C.M.   [1, 5, 77]
Alva Professor of Human Genetics, Professor of Pediatrics,
Faculty of Medicine, Professor of Biology, Faculty of Science,
McGill University; McGill University-Montreal Children's
Hospital Research Institute, McGill University Health Centre,
Montreal, Quebec, Canada
mc77@musica.mcgill.ca

Udo Seedorf, M.D.   [142]
Institut fur Klinische Chemie and Laboratoriumsmedizin,
Zentrallaboratorium Westfalische Wilhelms-Universitat, Munster,
Germany
seedorfu@uni-muenster.de

Christine E. Seidman, M.D.   [213]
Investigator, Howard Hughes Medical Institute
Professor Medicine and Genetics, Director, Cardiovascular
Genetics Center, Dept. of Medicine, Brigham and Women's
Hospital, Harvard Medical School, Boston, Massachusetts
cseidman@rascal.med.harvard.edu

Jonathan G. Seidman, Ph.D.   [213]
Henrietta B. and Frederick H. Bugher Professor of Cardiovascular
Genetics, Investigator, Howard Hughes Medical Institute, Harvard
Medical School, Boston, Massachusetts

Giorgio Semenza, M.D.   [75]
Professor, Dept. of Biochemistry, Swiss Institute of Technology,
Laboratorium fur Biochemie, Zurich, Switzerland; Professor,
Dept. of Chemistry and Medical Biochemistry, University of
Milan, Milan, Italy
giorgio.semenza@unimi.it
semenza@bc.biol.ethz.ch

Gul N. Shah, Ph.D. [208]
Assistant Research Professor, Edward A. Doisy Dept. of
Biochemistry and Molecular Biology, Saint Louis University
School of Medicine, St. Louis, Missouri
shahgn@slu.edu

Lisa G. Shaffer, Ph.D.   [65]
Associate Professor, Dept. of Molecular and Human Genetics,
Baylor College of Medicine, Houston, Texas
lshaffer@bcm.tmc.edu

Larry J. Shapiro, M.D.   [166]
W.H. and Marie Wattis Distinguished Professor, Chairman, Dept.
of Pediatrics, University of California Medical Center, San
Francisco, California
Lshapiro@peds.ucsf.edu

Val C. Sheffield, M.D., Ph.D.   [242]
Professor of Pediatrics, Associate Investigator, Howard Hughes
Medical Institute, Dept. of Pediatrics, Div. of Medical Genetics,
University of Iowa Hospital and Clinic, Iowa City, Iowa
Val-sheffield@uiowa.edu

Stephanie L. Sherman, Ph.D.   [64]
Dept. of Genetics Emory University School of Medicine, Atlanta,
Georgia
ssherman@genetics.emory.edu

Vivian E. Shih, M.D.   [87]
Professor of Neurology, Harvard Medical School, Director, Amino
Acid Disorder Laboratory/Metabolic Disorders Unit,
Massachusetts General Hospital, Charlestown, Massachusetts
vshih@partners.org

John M. Shoffner, M.D.   [104]
Director, Molecular Medicine, Molecular Medicine Laboratory,
Children's Healthcare of Atlanta, Atlanta, Georgia
john.shoffner@choa.org

David Sidransky, M.D.   [54]
Dept. of Otolaryngology-HNS, The Johns Hopkins University
School of Medicine, Baltimore, Maryland
dsidrans@jhmi.edu

Olli Simell, M.D.   [83, 192]
Professor of Pediatrics, Dept. of Pediatrics, University of Turku,
Turku, Finland
Olli.simell@utu.fi

H. Anne Simmonds, Ph.D.   [108]
Purine Research Unit, Guy's Hospital, London Bridge, London,
United Kingdom
anne.simmonds@kcl.ac.uk

Ola H. Skjeldal, M.D., Ph.D.   [132]
Div. of Pediatrics, Ulleval University Hospital, Oslo, Norway
ola.skjeldal@klinmed.uio.no

William S. Sly, M.D.   [1, 138, 208]
Alice A. Doisy Professor of Biochemistry and Molecular Biology,
Chair, Edward A. Doisy Dept. of Biochemistry and Molecular
Biology, Professor of Pediatrics, St. Louis University School of
Medicine, St. Louis, Missouri
slyws@slu.edu

C. Wayne Smith, M.D.   [188]
Head, Sect. of Leukocyte Biology; Professor, Depts. of Pediatrics,
Microbiology and Immunology, Sect. of Leukocyte Biology,
Children's Nutrition Research Center, Baylor College of Medicine
Houston, Texas
cwsmith@bcm.tmc.edu

Kirby D. Smith, Ph.D. [131]
Professor of Pediatrics, Kennedy Krieger Institute,
McKusick-Nathans Institute of Genetic Medicine, The Johns
Hopkins University School of Medicine, Baltimore, Maryland
smithk@mail.jhmi.edu

Oded Sperling, Ph.D.   [198]
Professor and Chairman of Clinical Biochemistry, Dept. of
Clinical Biochemistry, Rabin Medical Center, Petah-Tikva, Israel
odeds@post.tau.ac.il

Allen M. Spiegel, M.D.   [164]
Director, National Institute of Diabetes and Digestive and Kidney
Diseases, Bethesda, Maryland
allens@amb.niddk.nih.gov

Peter H. St. George-Hyslop, M.D.   [234]
Professor, Dept. of Medicine, Center for Research in
Neurodegenerative Diseases, University of Toronto, Toronto,
Ontario, Canada
p.hyslop@utoronto.ca

Beat Steinmann, M.D.   [70]
Professor, Div. of Metabolism and Molecular Pediatrics,
University Children's Hospital, Zurich, Switzerland
beat.steinmann@kispi.unizh.ch

Sylvia Stöckler-Ipsiroglu, M.D.   [84]
Dept. of Pediatrics, University Hospital Vienna, Laboratory for
Inherited Metabolic Diseases, Wahringergurtel, Vienna,
Austria

Edwin M. Stone, M.D., Ph.D.   [242]
Dept. of Ophthalmology and Visual Sciences, University of Iowa
College of Medicine, Iowa City, Iowa
edwin-stone@viowa.edu

Pietro Strisciuglio, M.D.   [152]
Associate Professor of Pediatrics, Dept. of Pediatrics, "Magna
Graecia", Catanzaro, Italy
strisciuglio_unicz@libero.it

Sharon F. Suchy, Ph.D. [252]
Staff Scientist, Genetic Disease Research Branch, National Human
Genome Research Instit, Bethesda, Maryland
suchy@nhgri.nih.gov

Kathleen E. Sullivan, M.D., Ph.D. [186]
Assistant Professor of Pediatrics, Children's Hospital of
Philadelphia, Philadelphia, Pennsylvania

Andrea Superti-Furga, M.D.   [202]
Div. of Metabolism and Molecular Pediatrics, University of
Zurich, Universitaets-Kinderklinik, Zurich, Switzerland
asuperti@access.unizh.ch

Kinuko Suzuki, M.D.   [145, 147, 153]
Professor of Pathology and Lab Medicine, Dept. of Pathology and
Lab Medicine, School of Medicine, University of North Carolina
at Chapel Hill
kis@med.unc.edu

Kunihiko Suzuki, M.D.   [147, 153]
Director Emeritus, Neuroscience Center, Professor of Neurology
and Psychiatry, School of Medicine,
University of North Carolina at Chapel Hill, North Corolina
Kuni.Suzuki@attglobal.net

Yoshiyuki Suzuki, M.D.   [147, 151]
Professor and Director, Nasu Institute for Developmental
Disabilities, Clinical Research Center, International University of
Health and Welfare, Otawara, Japan
suzukiy@iuhw.ac.jp

Dallas M. Swallow, Ph.D.   [76]
Professor of Human Genetics, The Galton Laboratory, Dept. of
Biology, University College London, London, United Kingdom
dswallow@hgmp.mrc.ac.uk

Lawrence Sweetman, Ph.D.   [93]
Professor, Institute of Biomedical Studies, Baylor University;
Director, Mass Spectrometry Lab, Institute of Metabolic Disease,
Baylor University Medical Center, Dallas, Texas
l.sweetman@baylordallas.edu

Alan Richard Tall, M.D.   [121]
Tilden Weger Bieler Professor of Medicine, Dept. of Medicine,
Div. of Molecular Medicine, Columbia University College of
Physicians and Surgeons, New York, New York
art1@columbia.edu

Robert M. Tanguay, Ph.D.   [79]
Laboratoire de genetique cellulaire et developpementale, Pavillon
Charles-Eugene Marchand, Université Laval, Ste-Foy, Quebec,
Canada
robert.tanguay@rsvs.ulaval.ca

Robin G. Taylor, Ph.D.   [80]
Dept. of Genetics, The Hospital for Sick Children Research
Institute, Toronto, Canada
rgtaylor@alumni.haas.org

Simeon I. Taylor, M.D., Ph.D.   [68]
Lilly Research Fellow, Lilly Research Laboratories, Indianapolis,
Indiana

Harriet S. Tenenhouse, Ph.D.   [197]
Professor of Pediatrics and Human Genetics, Auxiliary Professor
of Biology, Div. of Medical Genetics,
McGill University, Montreal Children's Hospital Research
Institute, Montreal, Quebec, Canada
mdht@www.debelle.mcgill.ca

Jess G. Thoene, M.D.   [199]
Karen Gore Professor; Director, Hayward Genetics Center, Human
Genetics Program, Tulane University School of Medicine, New
Orleans, Louisiana
jthoene@mailhost.tcs.tulane.edu

George H. Thomas, Ph.D.   [140]
Professor of Pediatrics, Pathology and Medicine, The Johns
Hopkins University School of Medicine, Director of Kennedy
Krieger Institute Genetics Laboratory Baltimore, Maryland
thomasg@kennedykrieger.org

Craig B. Thompson, M.D.   [24]
Abramson Family Cancer Research Institute, University of
Pennsylvania, Philadelphia, Pennsylvania
drt@mail.med.upenn.edu

Beat Thöny, Ph.D.   [78]
Associate Professor, Division of Clinical Chemistry &
Biochemistry, Div. of Chemistry and Biochemistry, University of
Zurich, Zurich, Switzerland
bthony@kispi.unizh.ch

Roland Tisch, Ph.D.  [12]
Postdoctoral Fellow, Dept. of Microbiology and Immunology,
Stanford University School of Medicine,
Stanford, California

Jay A. Tischfield, Ph.D.  [108]
MacMillan Professor and Chair, Dept. of Genetics, Rutgers
University, Professor of Pediatrics and Psychiatry, Robert Wood
Johnson Medical School, Piscataway, New Jersey

John A. Todd, M.D.  [6]
Professor, Dept. of Medical Genetics, Cambridge University;
Institute for Medical Research, Addenbrooke's Hospital,
Cambridge, United Kingdom
john.todd@cimr.cam.ac.uk

Douglas M. Tollefsen, M.D., Ph.D.  [176]
Professor of Medicine, Hematology Div., Washington University
Medical School, St. Louis, Missouri
tollefsen@im.wustl.edu

Eileen P. Treacy, M.D.  [5]
Associate Professor of Human Genetics and Pediatrics; Director,
Biochemical Genetics Unit, Div. of Medical Genetics, Dept. of
Biochemical Genetics, Montreal Children's Hospital, Montreal,
Quebec, Canada
mcet@musica.mcgill.ca

Jeffrey M. Trent, M.D., Ph.D.  [20]
Chief, Lab of Cancer Genetics, National Human Genome
Research Institute, Bethesda, Maryland
jtrent@nih.gov

Mark A. Trifiro, Ph.D.  [161]
Associate Professor, Dept. of Medicine, McGill University;
Associate Physician, Dept. of Medicine, Lady Davis Institute for
Medical Research, Sir Mortimer B. Davis Jewish General
Hospital, Montreal, Canada, Quebec
mdtm@musica.mcgill.ca

Karl Tryggvason, M.D.  [214]
Div. Matrix Biology, Dept. of Medical Biochemistry and
Biophysics, Karolinska Institut, Stockholm, Sweden
karl.tryggvason@mbb.ki.se

William T. Tse, M.D., Ph.D.  [183]
Children's Hospital/Dana-Farber Cancer Institute, Div. of
Hematology/Oncology, Boston, Massachusetts
William_tse@dfci.harvard.edu

Edward G.D. Tuddenham, M.D.  [172]
Professor, MRC/CSC, Hammersmith Hospital, London,
United Kingdom
etuddenh@rpms.ac.uk

Eric Turk, Ph.D.  [190]
Dept. of Physiology, UCLA School of Medicine, Los Angeles,
California
eturk@mednet.ucla.edu

Linda A. Tyfield, M.D.  [72]
Consultant Clinical Scientist, Hon. Sr. Research Fellow,
Dept. of Child Health, University of Bristol, Molecular Genetics
Unit, The Lewis Laboratories, Southmead Hospital, Bristol,
United Kingdom
linda.tyfield@bristol.ac.uk

Jouni Uitto, M.D., Ph.D.  [222]
Jefferson Institute of Molecular Medicine, Dept. of Dermatology
and Cutaneous Biology, Jefferson Medical College, Philadelphia,
Pennsylvania
jouni.uitto@mail.tju.edu

Gerd M. Utermann, M.D.  [116]
Professor and Chair, Institute for Medical Biology and Human
Genetics, Leopold-Franzens University of Innsbruck, Innsbruck,
Austria
Gerd.Utermann@uibk.ac.at

David Valle, M.D.  [1, 3, 4, 5, 81, 83, 129]
Professor of Pediatrics Genetics and Molecular Biology,
Investigator Howard Hughes Medical Institute, McKusick-
Nathans Institute of Genetic Medicine, The Johns Hopkins
University, Baltimore, Maryland
dvalle@jhmi.edu

Georges Van den Berghe, M.D.  [70, 112]
Professor, Dept. of Biochemistry and Cellular Biology, University
of Louvain Medical School, Director of Research, Laboratory of
Physiological Chemistry, Christian de Duve Institute of Cellular
Pathology, Brussels, Belgium
vandenberghe@bchm.ucl.ac.be

Peter van Endert, M.D.  [12]
Postdoctoral Fellow, Dept. of Microbiology and Immunology,
Stanford University School of Medicine, Stanford,
California

Albert H. van Gennip, M.D.  [113]
Laboratory Genetic Metabole Diseases, Academic Medical
Center, University of Amsterdam, Amsterdam, The Netherlands

Veronica van Heyningen, D.Phil., F.R.S.E.  [240]
Head of Cell and Molecular Genetics Sect., MRC Human Genetics
Unit, Western General Hospital, Edinburgh, Scotland, United
Kingdom
v.vanheyningen@hgu.mrc.ac.uk

Marie T. Vanier, M.D., Ph.D.  [145]
Directeur de Recherche INSERM, Lyon-Sud Medical School,
Oullins, France
vanier@univ-lyonl.fr

André B.P. Van Kuilenburg, M.D.  [113]
Laboratory Genetic Metabole Diseases, Academic Medical
Center, University of Amsterdam, Amsterdam,
The Netherlands

Emile Van Schaftingen, M.D., Ph.D.  [74]
Professor of Biochemistry, Laboratory of Physiological Chemistry,
ICP, Universite Catholique de Louvain, Brussels, Belgium
vanschaftingen@bchm.ucl.ac.be

Gilbert Vassart, M.D., Ph.D.  [158]
Head, Dept. of Medical Genetics, Institut de Recherche
Interdisciplinaire, Universite Libre de Bruxelles, Brussels,
Belgium
gvassart@ulb.ac.be

Bert Vogelstein, M.D.  [17, 27, 48]
Investigator, Howard Hughes Medical Institute, Clayton Professor
of Oncology and Pathology, The Johns Hopkins University School
of Medicine, Baltimore, Maryland
vogelbe@welch.jhu.edu

Arnold von Eckardstein, M.D.  [122]
Institut für Klinische Chemie und Laboratoriumsmedizin,
Zentrallaboratorium, Westfälische Wilhelms-Universität Münster,
Münster, Germany
vonecka@uni-muenster.de

Kurt von Figura, Ph.D.  [84, 148]
Director and Professor, Institute of Biochemistry II Zentrum
Biochemie und Molekulare Zellbiologie Georg-August-
Universitat Gottingen, Gottingen, Germany
kfigura@gwdg.de

Tom Vulliamy, Ph.D.  [179]
Clinical Scientist, Honorary Lecturer, Dept. of Hematology,
Imperial College of School of Medicine, Hammersmith Hospital,
London, United Kingdom
t.vulliamy@ic.ac.uk

Douglas C. Wallace, Ph.D. [105]
Robert W. Woodruff, Professor of Molecular Genetics, Professor and Director, Center for Molecular Medicine, Emory University School of Medicine, Atlanta, Georgia
dwallace@gen.emory.edu

John H. Walter, M.D. [72]
Consultant Pediatrician, Willink Biochemical Genetics Unit, Royal Manchester Children's Hospital, Pendlebury, Manchester, United Kingdom
john@jhwalter.demon.co.uk

Ronald J.A. Wanders, Ph.D. [130, 132]
Professor of Clinical Enzymology and Inherited Diseases, University of Amsterdam Academic Medical Centre, Emma Children's Hospital and Clinical Chemistry, Amsterdam, The Netherlands
wanders@amc.uva.nl

Stephen T. Warren, Ph.D. [64]
Rollins Research Center, Emory University School of Medicine, Atlanta, Georgia
swarren@bimcore.emory.edu

Paul A. Watkins, M.D., Ph.D. [131]
Associate Professor, Neurology, Dept. of Neurogenetics, Kennedy Krieger Institute, Johns Hopkins University, Baltimore, Maryland
watkins@kennedykrieger.org

Sir David J. Weatherall, M.D., FRS [181]
Regius Professor of Medicine, Institute of Molecular Medicine, John Radcliffe Hospital, Headington, Oxford, United Kingdom
janet.watt@imm.ox.ac.uk

Barbara L. Weber, M.D. [47]
Professor of Medicine and Genetics; Director, Breast Cancer Program; Assoc. Director, Cancer, Control and Population Science, University of Pennsylvania Cancer Center, Philadelphia, Pennsylvania
weberb@mail.med.upenn.edu

Dianne R. Webster, Ph.D [113]
National Testing Center, Lab Plus Auckland Hospital, Auckland, New Zealand

Lee S. Weinstein, M.D. [164]
Investigator, Metabolic Disease Branch, National Institute of Diabetes and Digestive Kidney Diseases, Bethesda, Maryland

Michael J. Welsh, M.D. [201]
Investigator, Howard Hughes Medical Institute, Dept. of Internal Medicine, University of Iowa College of Medicine, Iowa City, Iowa
mjwelsh@blue.weeg.uiowa.edu

David A. Wenger, Ph.D. [147]
Professor of Neurology and Biochemistry and Molecular Pharmacology, Jefferson Medical College, Philadelphia, Pennsylvania
David.wenger@mail.tju.edu

Jeffrey A. Whitsett, M.D. [218]
Div. of Pulmonary Biology, Children's Hospital Medical Center, Cincinnati, Ohio
jeff.whitsett@chmcc.org

Michael P. Whyte, M.D. [207]
Professor of Medicine, Pediatrics, and Genetics, Div. of Bone and Mineral Diseases, Washington University School of Medicine, Barnes-Jewish Hospital, Medical Scientific Director, Center for Metabolic Bone Disease and Molecular Research, Shriners Hospital for Children, St. Louis, Missouri
mwhyte@shrinenet.org

Andrew O.M. Wilkie, M.D., F.R.C.P. [245]
Senior Research Fellow in Clinical Science, Wellcome Trust, Institute of Molecular Medicine, John Radcliffe Hospital, Headington, Oxford, United Kingdom
awilkie@worf.molbiol.ox.ac.uk

Douglas Wilkin, Ph.D. [210]
Medical Genetics Branch, National Human Genome Research Institute, Bethesda, Maryland

Huntington F. Willard, Ph.D. [61]
Henry Wilson Payne Professor and Chairman of Genetics, Director, Center for Human Genetics, Case Western Reserve University School of Medicine, Cleveland, Ohio
hfw@po.cwru.edu

Julian C. Williams, M.D., Ph.D. [93]
Associate Professor of Pediatrics, USC School of Medicine, Head, Div. Of Med. Genetics, Children's Hospital LA, Med. Dir., Dept. of Pathology and Laboratory Medicine Genetics Laboratories, Los Angeles, California
jwilliams@chlais.usc.edu

Jean D. Wilson, M.D. [160]
Charles Cameron Sprague Distinguished Chair in Biomedical Science, Clinical Professor of Internal Medicine, Dept. of Internal Medicine, University of Texas Southwestern Medical Center, Dallas, Texas
jwils1@mednet.swmed.edu

Jerry A. Winkelstein, M.D. [186]
Dept. of Pediatrics, Johns Hopkins University School of Medicine, Baltimore, Maryland
jwinkels@welchlink.welch.jhu.edu

Barry Wolf, M.D., Ph.D. [156]
Associate Chair for Research, Head, Div. of Pediatric Research, Professor, Div. of Human Genetics, University of Connecticut School of Medicine, Director of Pediatric Research, Connecticut Children's Medical Center, Hartford, Connecticut
bwolf@hsc.vcu.edu

Allan W. Wolkoff, M.D. [125]
Professor, Albert Einstein College of Medicine, Liver Research Center Bronx, New York
wolkoff@aecom.yu.edu

W.G. Wood [181]
Institute of Molecular Medicine, John Radcliffe Hospital, Oxford, United Kingdom

Ronald G. Worton, C.M., Ph.D., F.R.S.C. [216]
CEO and Scientific Director, Ottawa General Hospital Research Institute, University of Ottawa, Ottawa, Ontario, Canada
rworton@ogh.on.ca

Ernest M. Wright, D.Sc. [190]
Professor and Chair, Dept. of Physiology, UCLA School of Medicine, Los Angeles, California
ewright@mednet.ucla.edu

Charles John Yeo, M.D. [50]
Professor and Attending Surgeon, Dept. of Surgery and Oncology, The Johns Hopkins Hospital, Baltimore, Maryland
cyeo@jhmi.edu

Chang-En Yu, M.D., Ph.D. [33]
Veterans Affairs Puget Sound Health Care System, Seattle Div. and the Dept. of Medicine, University of Washington, Seattle, Washington
changeyu@u.washington.edu

Berton Zbar, M.D. [41]
Chief, Laboratory of Immunology, National Cancer Institute-Frederick Cancer, Research Facility, Frederick, Maryland
zbar@mail.ncifcrf.gov

Huda Y. Zoghbi, M.D. [226, 255]
Professor, Dept. of Pediatrics and Molecular and Human Genetics; Investigator Howard Hughes Medical Institute, Baylor College of Medicine, Houston, Texas
hzoghbi@bcm.tmc.edu

# PREFACE TO THE EIGHTH EDITION

Following "the new synthesis" of Mendelism and Darwinism, Theodosins Dobzhansky stated that biology makes sense only in the light of evolution.[1] A corollary to that opinion would say that medicine without biology does not make sense. This book, now in its eighth edition, presents evidence that biology, as we come to know it in the era of genomics, is helping to make better sense of medicine.

In its first edition,[2] this book, then known as *The Metabolic Basis of Inherited Disease* (MBID), focused almost exclusively on the Mendelian diseases falling into the category known as "inborn errors of metabolism." For the next five editions, MBID served as a medical companion to human biochemical genetics which had its own seminal text.[3] Then, to acknowledge the increasing relevance of molecular biology and molecular genetics, for the seventh edition we changed its title to: *The Metabolic and Molecular Bases of Inherited Disease* (MMBID). There were further changes in the seventh edition: complex genetic traits were increasingly recognized, cancer being a notable new section of the book, and even more so in the CD-ROM update of the print edition. Chromosomal disorders had appeared in the sixth edition and they increased their presence in the seventh, along with a chapter dedicated to imprinting.

The eighth edition of MMBID, now appearing in the first year of the twenty-first century, contains new chapters on the history of the inborn errors of metabolism (Chapter 3), their impact on health (Chapter 4) and their response to treatment (Chapter 5). This edition further reveals how genetics is contributing to the understanding of complex traits and birth defects as well as the Mendelian diseases with nominal pathways of metabolism or development. It is not surprising then that MMBID-8 should have chapters on aging and hypertension or on Hirschsprung disease, for example. In brief, this book is becoming a "textbook of medicine," as predicted by one reviewer of an earlier edition.[4]

Five questions formulated as such by Victor McKusick among others have been of abiding interest in medicine since at least the time of Osler: (1) What is the problem? (2) How did it happen? (3) What is the cause? (4) What can be done? (5) Will it happen again? The questions address the corresponding issues of diagnosis, pathogenesis, ultimate and proximal cause, treatment and prevention, and inherited risks of recurrence. As for cause, the theme of special interest shared by every entity discussed in this book is *mutation*: mutation that modifies phenotype, contributes to pathogenesis of the disease and, in various ways, identifies a key component in a "pathway" or "network" responsible for homeostasis and functional integrity.

MMBID-8 is being published as genome projects, both human and nonhuman, yield information and knowledge about the organization and nucleotide sequences of genomes. The allied field of research, now called genomics, has been called "a journey to the center of biology."[5] Comparative genomics reveals that homeostasis of energy metabolism and many aspects of intermediary metabolism are encoded in genes with a very long evolutionary history (see Chapter 4). Moreover, a number of the human disorders can be analyzed functionally in yeast in a manner some will call "biochemical genomics"[6] and there is a corresponding database cross-referencing human and yeast phenotypes.[7] Accordingly, Dobzhansky's angle of vision is increasingly validated.

At the same time, the genomes of *C. elegans* and *Drosophila* are telling us that development of multicellular organisms is controlled by the major portion of the corresponding genomes and each organism has particular programs for particular body plans.

New sections and chapters in MMBID-8 are devoted to various disorders of development in *H. sapiens*.

It follows that biology is indeed a shared language for medicine.[8] However, shared language does not preclude particular language to deal with variant phenotypes (the diseases), their clinical consequences, and the specialization in clinical expertise required to address them. In recognition of this, the book contains material in the particular languages of counseling, testing and screening, and treatment; indeed, in a language increasingly accessed on Web sites by patients who want to know. The particular language extends beyond phenotype, counseling, and so on; it reaches the patient. Every patient who has one of the so-called "single-gene" diseases described in this book has an "orphan" disease; furthermore, because of biological individuality, each patient has his or her own private (orphan) form of unhealth. In other words, this book is an ultimate guidebook for *individualized medicine*.

MMBID-8 will contribute to an instauration of the clinician-investigator, a colleague who has been much marginalized by successes in the basic science and molecular and cellular biology and the corresponding contributions to medical science. The original editions of MBID were written largely by clinician-investigators; or by basic scientists who still retained a familiarity with patients or did research that was patient-oriented and disease-oriented.[9] However, in the more recent editions of MMBID, the chapters themselves and the majority of the references cited in them were more often than not authored by persons doing basic research, sometimes rather remote from the patient's primary problem. But, as the "genome project" moves from its structural to a functional phase and into biochemical- and pharmacogenomics, the editors of MMBID recognize a need for the return of the clinician-investigator. The latter must share equal status with the basic scientist so that science can be translated quickly into benefits for patients. That is why some chapters in MMBID-8 (e.g., 66 and 99) are devoted to clinical algorithms.

The prefaces to MBID-6 and MMBID-7 described how the editors chose material for Chapters and Parts of these editions. In the seventh edition, we said: "If there is an identifiable molecular explanation for the disease — and it affects a dynamic phenotype, metabolic or otherwise — then it is a candidate for inclusion .... The expansion of topics here is selective and obviously not inclusive of all possibilities." Although MMBID-8 has not changed its title, it has changed in many other ways. It has three new associate editors (Barton Childs, Kenneth Kinzler, and Bert Vogelstein), new chapters have appeared (the total is now 255) and the number of authors now exceeds 500. That the printed and bound book exceeds 7000 pages is not really a surprise, but it is an abiding reason to have portable and online versions of the book.

A survey undertaken by some of the editors, by some of our readers and owners of the seventh edition showed that 70% used the book at least once per week. Half those persons believed the book should grow beyond its original domain; that content of MMBID-7 was appropriate; and over 90% of the readers welcomed the prospect of a Web version.

The editors intend to keep MMBID-8 "user friendly;" and also to keep it up to date. We hope a portable version of MMBID-8 will be available for those who wish to have something they can carry home; there will be a Web version. In this latter format, MMBID will become a "continuous book," able to update all material and to incorporate new topics as they become pertinent to our stated mission. Accordingly, as more and more scientific print literature goes "on line" in one format or another, MMBID will do likewise;

the web version will allow MMBID to reincarnate itself through a long and healthy life.

So much seems to change between editions of MMBID; for example, a new team — Susan Noujaim, Peter Boyle, Marty Wonsiewicz, and others at McGraw-Hill — have translated formidable stacks of typescript into a book agreeable to the publisher. On the other hand, stability can still be found in the life of this book; the editors are still working with the same colleagues: Lynne Prevost and Huguette Rizziero (CRS), Grace Watson (AB), Elizabeth Torno (WS), Sandy Muscelli (DV); while Kathy Helwig helped the new editors (BC, KK, and BV). The process of reading manuscripts and proofs was yet again lightened by the tolerant support of our families and by colleagues at the places of business.

## REFERENCES

1. Dobzhansky TH: "Nothing in biology makes sense except in the light of evolution." *Am Biol Teach* **35**:125, 1973.
2. Stanbury JB, Wyngaarden JB, Fredrickson DS (eds.): *The Metabolic Basis of Inherited Disease.* McGraw-Hill Book Co., New York. 1960.
3. Harris H: The principles of human biochemical genetics. *Frontiers of Biology* (Neuberger A, Tatum EL (eds.), Vol. 19. North Holland Pub. Co., London, 1970. North-Holland Research Monographs.
4. Childs B: Book Review. *The Metabolic Basis of Inherited Disease.* 6th ed. 2 volumes. Scriver CR, Beaudet AL, Sly WS, Valle D (eds.). *Am J Hum Genet* **46**:848, 1990.
5. Lander ES, Weinberg RA: Genomics: Journey to the center of biology. *Science* **287**:1777, 2000.
6. Carlson M: The awesome power of yeast biochemical genomics. *Trends Genet* **16**:49, 2000.
7. Bassett DE Jr., Boguski MS, Spencer F, Reeves R, Kim SH, Weaver T, Hieter P: Genome cross-referencing and XREFdb: Implications for the identification and analysis of genes mutated in human disease. *Nat Genet* **15**:339, 1997.
8. Scriver CR: American Pediatric Society Presidential Address 1995. Disease, war and biology: Language for medicine — and pediatrics. *Pediatric Res* **38**:819, 1995.
9. Goldstein JL, Brown MS: The clinical investigator: Bewitched, bothered, and bewildered — but still beloved. Editorial. *J Clin Invest* **99**:2803, 1997.

# PREFACE TO THE SEVENTH EDITION

The sixth edition of *The Metabolic Basis of Inherited Disease* experienced "transition, transformation, and challenge." Transition continues in the seventh edition with the arrival of many new authors. Challenge remains, like the mountain whose peak is never in view while the climb proceeds. And there is transformation again, not least with the title: *The Metabolic and* Molecular *Bases of Inherited Disease*. The new word is significant.

A reviewer of the sixth edition reminds us of the original plan for the book: to present "the pertinent clinical, biochemical, and genetic information concerning those metabolic anomalies grouped under Garrod's engaging term 'inborn errors of metabolism.' "[1] The term *molecular* is a belated but natural homecoming for Garrod. During his lifetime, Garrod's views grew to encompass inherited susceptibility to any disease originating in our chemical individuality. These ideas emerged fully developed, for their time, in Garrod's second book. *The Inborn Factors in Disease*. That we have been slow to perceive the reach of his thinking is a theme of his recent biographer.[2] To accept it and put it to use requires the means to test its validity. Molecular analysis of the genetic variation causing or predisposing to disease provides the opportunity. The inborn errors of metabolism are simply our most obvious illustrations of the genetic variation that affects health and the molecular underpinnings of that variation. A corresponding analysis of multifactorial diseases is the obvious next step in the understanding of disease.[3] Need we say that MMBID-7 is nothing less than a textbook of molecular medicine, encompassing the diseases about which we know most? We predict that the "classic" textbooks of medicine in the future will look more and more like MMBID.

Change in the title of MBID did something else: it solved a problem the editors created for themselves in MBID-6, again commented on by the above-mentioned reviewer.[1] When we included topics not overtly "metabolic" in the sixth edition, for example, Down and fragile X syndromes, primary ciliary dyskinesia, collagen disorders and the muscular dystrophies, we moved well beyond the canonical theme of inborn errors of *metabolism*. The nonmetabolic topics are further expanded in this edition because they conform to a *logic of disease*, as it is called by Barton Childs in Chapter 2. The manifestations of any "genetic" disease are explained by a process (pathogenesis) that originates in part or in full form an intrinsic cause (mutation); and, since genotype is one of the determinants of the phenotype (disease), it follows that diagnosis, treatment, and counseling should be motivated form the genetic point of view because the disease involves both the patient and his or her family.

If there is an identifiable molecular explanation for the disease — and it affects a dynamic phenotype, metabolic or otherwise — then it is a candidate for inclusion in the seventh edition. The expansion of topics here is selective and obviously not inclusive of all possibilities. If this were the case, the table of contents would resemble the McKusick catalog, *Mendelian Inheritance in Man*! Nevertheless, yet a further 32 chapters are new to this edition of MBID while 31 others were introduced in the sixth edition; new ideas appear again and again in virtually all "old" chapters. Will it be three volumes — or more — for the eighth edition? (A CD-ROM format is under serious consideration for the next edition.) The Summary Table, immediately preceding Chapter 1, surveys the information in MMBID-7.

In the first section of the book, the following major new themes appear:

- A logic of disease based on genetic and evolutionary concepts that challenges conventional medical thinking (Chapter 2).

- Mutational mechanisms, including dynamic mutations (elastic or unstable DNA) (Chapter 3) and the methods to detect them (Chapter 1).

- Pharmacogenetics (Chapter 4) as a classical illustration of multifactorial disease (with ultimate and proximate causes) and of the "idiosyncratic reaction to drugs" — to recall Garrod's felicitous phrase.

- Diagnostic algorithms for the patient with an inborn error of metabolism (Chapter 5).

- Mapping of genes (genomics) (Chapter 6), along with an increased awareness that mutant gene expression may involve more than conventional Mendelian inheritance: for example, imprinting and mosaicism (Chapter 7).

- How cellular organelles, protein targeting and posttranslational modification, and the HLA complex affect expression of "genetic" disease (the subjects of Chapters 8 and 9, respectively).

- Cancer appears as a major theme for the first time in this edition (Chapters 10 to 15). Cancers are products of genetic damage. Modified events in pathways release cells from the normal controls of replication and growth. The cascades of events controlled by proto-oncogenes are counterparts of Garrod's pathways of metabolism. Because cancers can involve constitutional mutations, somatic mutations, or both, they further expand the conceptual boundaries of the book.

- Processes of inactivation harbored on the X chromosome (Chapter 16) and knowledge about the testis-determining factor and primary sex reversal (Chapter 17) are topics new to the section on chromosomes, itself an innovation of the sixth edition.

An awesome expansion of information continues in old and new chapters. The new chapters include, for example, insulin gene defects (Chapter 22); a completely new look at nonketotic hyperglycinemia (Chapter 37); diseases of the mitochondrial genome (Chapter 46); the apolipoprotein (a) molecule and its association with heart disease (Chapter 58); oxalosis as a peroxisomal disorder (Chapter 75); lysosomal enzyme activator proteins (Chapter 76); Pompe disease as a disease of lysosome function (Chapter 77) rather than a disease of carbohydrate metabolism; Lowe syndrome, separated from the Fanconi syndrome, following positional cloning of the gene (Chapter 123); Marfan syndrome, a disease of fibrillin dysfunction (Chapter 135); the muscular dystrophies (Chapters 140 and 141), and hypertrophic cardiomyopathy (Chapter 142). All is not new; in recognition of tradition, the spelling of *alcaptonuria* has reverted to *alkaptonuria* (Chapter 39).

A new section on disease of the eye (Chapters 143 to 146) includes retinitis pigmentosis, choroideremia, and disorders of color vision and crystallins. Discussions of epidermolysis bullosa (Chapter 149). Huntington disease (Chapter 152), and prion-related diseases (Chapter 153) reflect emerging molecular information on diseases of skin and brain. Chapter 154, the last in the book, catches recent developments involving half a dozen diseases.

The authors of chapters about particular diseases were asked to remember the needs of physicians and families, and they provide up-to-date information on diagnosis, treatment, and counseling. (These aspects are dealt with an even greater depth in a book that functions as our companion — the excellent *Inborn Metabolic*

*Diseases: Diagnosis and Treatment*, edited by J. Fernandes, J-M. Saudubray, and K. Tada.)

Some 200 authors wrote for MBID-6; 302 have written for MMBID-7; they have achieved the continuing transformation of this text. While so much seems to change overnight in molecular biology and genetics, stability can be found in the life of this book. Gail Gavert, Mariapaz Ramos-Englis, J. Dereck Jeffers, Peter McCurdy, and their colleagues have translated formidable stacks of typescript into a book agreeable to the publisher. The editors are still working with the same colleagues: Lynne Prevost and Huguette Rizziero (CRS), Grace Watson (AB), Elizabeth Torno (WS), and Sandy Muscelli (DV), Loy Denis was again our editorial coordinator until the last stages of this edition; her successor is Catherine Watson. The process of reading manuscripts and proofs was lightened by the tolerant support of our families and by colleagues at the place of business.

As this edition went to press, Harry Harris died. A giant in our field, his imprint is apparent everywhere in the book.

## REFERENCES

1. Childs B: Book Review: *The Metabolic Basis of Inherited Disease*, 6th ed. *Am J Hum Genet* **66**:848, 1990.
2. Bearn AG: *Archibald Garrod and the Individuality of Man*. New York, Oxford University Press, 1993, 227 pp.
3. King RA, Rutter JI, Motulsky AG: *The Genetic Basis of Common Diseases*. New York, Oxford University Press, 1993, 978 pp.

# PREFACE TO THE SIXTH EDITION

This edition of *The Metabolic Basis of Inherited Disease* marks a transition, a changing of the guard, as it were, among the editors. The sixth edition also reflects a transformation in the field of endeavor it encompasses; and there is a challenge too — for future editions. Transitions can be difficult and transformations sometimes produce unhappy results; neither need be the case here. Challenges can invigorate.

## THE TRANSITION

Stanbury-Wyngaarden-'n-Fredrickson, collectively, were one famous "author" known to everyone in the field. This extraordinary editorial organism piloted the novel and timely book they had introduced and then edited through four successful editions. By a remarkable fision — or was it fusion? — the fifth edition was placed under the care of Stanbury-Wyngaarden-'n-Fredrickson, Goldstein 'n Brown. Now that giant has stepped aside, handing the challenge to a new team. The new editors have discovered how great the former ones were — if they hadn't known it before. Very large shoes had to be filled!

## THE TRANSFORMATION

The sixth edition has many new features, notably the evidence of molecular genetics in one chapter after another. If *The Metabolic Basis of Inherited Disease* has had an abiding rationale, it was that the cause of all diseases listed in it was Mendelian and the diseases (so-called inborn errors of metabolism) were exceptions to be treasured for their illumination of human biology and for the insight they gave into pathogenesis of disease. But always there was a feeling that one did not understand cause as well as one should because not much was known about the genes. That situation is changing. There are new data about loci and structures of numerous normal genes and about the mutations affecting the phenotype encoded by them.

With 31 new chapters, the book is approximately one-third larger than it was. Accordingly, this edition appears for the first time in a two-volume format. It is a change undertaken with reluctance, but size of type, weight of paper, and the like had been adapted to the limit in the previous edition to accommodate the mass of information presented there. We elected to revise and print all chapters instead of using a précis of some, as in the last edition. Authors were encouraged to focus on up-to-date material and to use previous editions as archives of older material. But the wealth of new information neutralized contraction of the old. Hence the option taken here; to divide the book into two volumes, between separate covers.

New topics in the sixth edition include the following: There is a formal discussion of gene mapping and the medical use of genome markers (Chapter 6). Down syndrome (Chapter 7) and fragile X syndrome (Chapter 8) illustrate how any genetic disorder can eventually accommodate to our views of molecular genetics. They are the thin edge of the wedge toward understanding a great deal about human genetic disease and the editors introduce these chapters with some trepidation, realizing they could well be the very thin edge of a very big wedge — one of our challenges for future editions. One new chapter (122) covers the lactose deficiency polymorphism. This disorder does not fit the paradigm of a rare inborn error because it is so common; on the other hand, it does represent a Mendelian disadaptive phenotype for some individuals. There is a whole new section on peroxisomal diseases (Chapters 57–60) and Chapter 3 covers organelle biogenesis. Contiguous gene syndromes appear in this edition for the first time. The retinoblastoma story (Chapter 9) began as a contiguous gene syndrome; the new chapter encompasses this and analogous phenomena. Chapter 5 on oncogenes is new. The genes for retinoblastoma, chronic granulomatosus disease, and Duchenne muscular dystrophy are now known through techniques of "reverse" or "indirect" genetics. They are harbingers of what is to come in other diseases and they are topics developed at some length in this edition. Two appendices to Chapter 1, experiments in this edition, list: (1) the Mendelian disorders that can be diagnosed at the DNA level through oligonucleotide probes or by tightly linked markers that associate with alleles encoding mutant gene products; useful probes and their sources are catalogued in this appendix; (2) the mapped loci and their chromosomal assignments in the most current version of Victor McKusick's famous catalog available as we went to press. Perhaps a future edition will also catalog what we know about the mutant alleles at the loci encoding disease. Meanwhile the summary table grows in Chapter 1. It was introduced for the first time in the fifth edition and it is continued here for two reasons: first to show, in a simple manner, the growth of subject material between the last and present editions; second, to show how the white spaces in the fifth edition table are being filled in.

## THE CHALLENGE

The future holds the potential for a separate chapter delineating the biochemical basis of each variant listed in McKusick's *Mendelian Inheritance in Man*. If this is the case, there will be many hundred chapters in subsequent editions of MBID. In addition, most monogenic disorders are not monogenic but modified through other loci by definable biochemical mechanisms; and most diseases are caused by polygenic and multifactorial mechanisms which also have a biochemical basis. Cytogenetic disorders have a biochemical basis as well, and in some instances the phenotypes may be determined by one or a few loci. These all represent effects of the constitutional genotypes on the phenotype, but there is also the role of somatic mutation in the pathogenesis of malignancies whether inherited or sporadic. With the explosion of information virtually assured, the challenge of how to focus and mold future editions is a daunting one.

This book has not grown unattended. In addition to the herculean efforts of some 200 authors and their assistants, others assured a safe passage during the development of the book, notably Dereck Jeffers and Gail Gavert at McGraw-Hill; Loy Denis, who served as coordinator for the editors and authors; and our own assistants: Lynne Prevost and Huguette Rizziéro (CRS), Grace Watson (AB), Elizabeth Torno (WS), and Sandy Muscelli (DV). But especially we thank our extraordinary predecessors for their nurture and care of a book many of us have come to admire and need. If this edition meets with the approval of its former editors, we will have partially done the job we acquired; the readers will ultimately decide whether it was done satisfactorily.

Last, an acknowledgment to our families; they know more about this book than they bargained for . . .!

*Charles R. Scriver*
*Arthur L. Beaudet*
*William S. Sly*
*David Valle*

# The Metabolic &
# Molecular Bases of
# Inherited Disease

eighth edition

# CONNECTIVE TISSUE

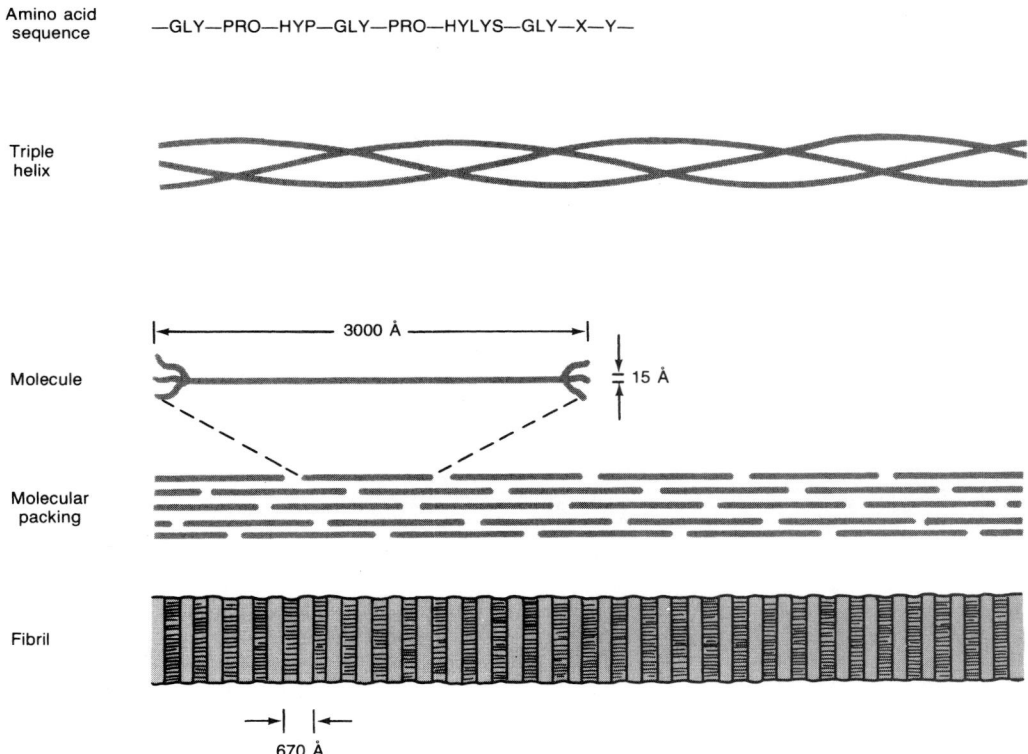

Amino acid
sequence —GLY—PRO—HYP—GLY—PRO—HYLYS—GLY—X—Y—

Triple
helix

Molecule

Molecular
packing

Fibril

3000 Å

15 Å

670 Å

Fibrillar collagen

# Disorders of Collagen Biosynthesis and Structure

*Peter H. Byers*

1. Collagen is the most abundant protein family in the mammalian body. More than 30 dispersed genes encode the protein products that form more than 19 different types of collagens that are distributed in a characteristic fashion among tissues.

2. Collagens are proteins that contain three chains wound in a triple helix. The biosynthesis is complex. Individual precursor chains are synthesized on membrane-bound polyribosomes. During transfer of the growing chain into the lumen of the rough endoplasmic reticulum, certain prolyl and lysyl residues in the triple-helical domain are hydroxylated and some hydroxylysyl residues are glycosylated. Assembly of the three chains in the rough endoplasmic reticulum is mediated by structures in the C-terminal propeptide domains of each chain and folding of the triple helix occurs from the C-terminal end of the molecule. Transport through the Golgi apparatus is accompanied by modification of oligosaccharide groups. Following secretion limited proteolysis leads to removal of the amino- and C-terminal propeptide extensions. Collagen molecules are stabilized in fibrillar structures or other meshworks through lysine-derived covalent intermolecular cross-links.

3. Disorders presently known to result from alterations in the structure and function of collagens affect the genes of collagens type I, II, III, IV, V, VI, VII, IX, X, XI, and XVII, and the enzymes lysyl hydroxylase and type I procollagen N-proteinase involved in the posttranslational modification of collagens.

4. The clinical heterogeneity apparent in the osteogenesis imperfecta (OI) phenotypes is a reflection of the underlying molecular heterogeneity. Mutations that affect the synthesis of the proα1(I) chains of type I collagen generally result in the relatively mild OI type I phenotype. Multiexon deletions or insertions in the *COL1A1* and *COL1A2* genes that encode the chains of type I collagen generally result in the lethal OI type II phenotype. The phenotypic effects of point mutations that result in substitutions for glycine residues in the triple-helical domains of proα1(I) of proα2(I) chains depend on the chain in which the mutation occurs, the location of the substitution within the chain, and the nature of the substituting amino acid.

5. The molecular basis of the Ehlers-Danlos syndrome (EDS) is heterogeneous. EDS type I and II result from mutations in the type V collagen genes and, possibly, in tenascin X. EDS type IV results from mutations that affect the synthesis, structure, or secretion of type III collagen. EDS type VI is a recessively inherited disorder that results from lack of lysyl hydroxylation. EDS type VII usually results from loss of the substrate sequence for the N-terminal procollagen protease in one of the chains of type I procollagen or from mutations in the enzyme itself.

6. Chondrodysplasias, including spondyloepiphyseal dysplasia, achondrogenesis, and some forms of Stickler syndrome result from mutations in type II collagen genes. Other forms of chondrodysplasia, Stickler syndrome type II and II, otospondyomegaepiphyseal dysplasia, and Marshall syndrome results from mutations in the closely related type XI collagen genes, while mutations in type IX collagen produce a form of multiple epiphyseal dysplasia. The nature of the phenotypic effect of these mutations depends on the character and location of the mutation in the fibrillar collagen genes in a manner similar to that seen in OI.

7. The X-linked form of Alport syndrome arises from mutations in the *COL4A5* gene with an unusual form that involves renal disease and esophageal leiomyomatosis arising from deletions involving the contiguous *COL4A5* and *COL4A6* genes. Recessive forms result from mutations in the contiguous *COL4A3* and *COL4A4* genes.

8. Bethlem myopathy results from mutations in any of the three chains of type VI collagen.

9. Mutations in type VII collagen result in the dystrophic forms of epidermolysis bullosa and other forms result from mutations in type XVII collagen genes.

10. The clinical consequences of mutations in collagen genes reflect the effects of the mutations on biosynthesis, assembly, posttranslational modification, secretion, fibrillogenesis, and interaction with other components of a complex extracellular matrix in which there is considerable molecular interaction.

A list of standard abbreviations is located immediately preceding the index in each volume. Additional abbreviations used in this chapter include: DI = dentinogenesis imperfecta; EB = epidermolysis bullosa; EDS = Ehlers-Danlos syndrome; OI = osteogenesis imperfecta; and SED = spondyloepiphyseal dysplasia. See legend to Table 205-1 for collagen nomenclature. Missense mutations are designated by the single letter codes (e.g., glycine to cysteine at codon 244 is indicated as G244C). By convention, missense mutations within the triple-helical domain of collagen chains are referred to with the reference point being the first glycine of the triple helix. Thus in the above example, G244C refers to the glycine at position 244 of the triple helix.

The collagens form a multigene family with more than 30 members, the genes for which are known to be dispersed to at least 14 chromosomes (see Table 205-1 and Fig. 205-1).[1–4] The products of these genes share important structural properties: they

**Table 205-1** Collagen Types: Their Constituent Chains, Chromosomal Locations of Their Genes, and Disorders Due to Mutations in the Genes*

| Collagen Type | Gene | Chromosomal Location | Protein | Disorders |
|---|---|---|---|---|
| I | COL1A1 | 17q21.31-q22.05 | proα1(I) | Osteogenesis imperfecta |
| | | | | Ehlers-Danlos syndrome type VIIA |
| | COL1A2 | 7q22.1 | proα2(I) | Osteogenesis imperfecta |
| | | | | Ehlers-Danlos syndrome type VIIB |
| | | | | Ehlers-Danlos syndrome type II |
| II | COL2A1 | 12q13.11-q13.2 | proα1(II) | Stickler syndrome, type I |
| | | | | Wagner syndrome type II |
| | | | | Spondylepiphyseal dysplasia congenita |
| | | | | Kniest dysplasia |
| | | | | Hypochondrogenesis |
| | | | | Achondrogenesis type II |
| | | | | Spondylo-metaphyseal-epiphyseal dysplasia (SMED), Strudwick type |
| III | COL3A1 | 2q31 | proα1(III) | Ehlers-Danlos syndrome type IV |
| | | | | Ehlers-Danlos syndrome type III (?) |
| IV | COL4A1 | 13q34 | proα1(IV) | |
| | COL4A2 | 13q34 | proα2(IV) | |
| | COL4A3 | 2q36-q37 | proα3(IV) | Alport syndrome, recessive |
| | COL4A4 | 2q36-q37 | proα4(IV) | Alport syndrome, recessive |
| | COL4A5 | Xq22 | proα5(IV) | Alport syndrome, X-linked |
| | COL4A6 | Xq22 | proα6(IV) | Alport syndrome, X-linked, leimyomatosis |
| V | COL5A1 | 9q34.2-q34.3 | proα1(V) | Ehlers-Danlos syndrome type I |
| | | | | Ehlers-Danlos syndrome type II |
| | COL5A2 | 2q31 | proα2(V) | Ehlers-Danlos syndrome type I |
| | COL5A3 | Not mapped | proα3(V) | |
| VI | COL6A1 | 21q22.3 | proα1(VI) | Bethlem myopathy |
| | COL6A2 | 21q22.3 | proα2(VI) | Bethlem myopathy |
| | COL6A3 | 2q37 | proα3(VI) | Bethlem myopathy |
| VII | COL7A1 | 3p21.3 | proα1(VII) | Epidermolysis bullosa, recessive dystrophic |
| | | | | Epidermolysis bullosa, dominant dystrophic |
| | | | | Epidermolysis bullosa, pretibial |
| VIII | COL8A1 | 3q12-q13.1 | proα1(VIII) | |
| | COL8A2 | 1p34.4-p32.3 | proα2(VIII) | |
| IX | COL9A1 | 6q13 | proα1(IX) | Multiple epiphyseal dysplasia |
| | COL9A2 | 1q33-p32.2 | proα2(IX) | Multiple epiphyseal dysplasia, type II |
| | COL9A3 | 20q13.3 | proα3(IX) | Multiple epiphyseal dysplasia, type III |
| X | COL10A1 | 6q21-q22.3 | proα1(X) | Metaphyseal chondrodysplasia, Schmid type |
| | | | | Spondylometaphysealdysplasia, Japanese type |
| XI | COL11A1 | 1p21 | proα1(XI) | Stickler syndrome, type III |
| | | | | Marshall syndrome |
| | COL11A2 | 6p21.3 | proα2(XI) | Stickler syndrome, type II |
| | | | | Otospondylomegaepiphyseal dysplasia (OSMED) |
| | | | | Weissenbacher-Zweymuller syndrome |
| | | | | Non-syndromic deafness (DFNA13) |
| XII | COL12A1 | 6 | proα1(XII) | |
| XIII | COL13A1 | 10q22 | proα1(XIII) | |
| XIV | COL14A1 | 8q23 | proα1(XIV) | |
| XV | COL15A1 | 9q21-q22 | proα1(XV) | |
| XVI | COL16A1 | 1p34 | proα1(XVI) | |
| XVII | COL17A1 | 10q24.3 | proα1(XVII) | Epidermolysis bullosa, generalized atrophic benign |
| XVIII | COL18A1 | 21q22.3 | proα1(XVIII) | |
| XIX | COL19A1 | 6q12-q14 | proα1(XIX) | |

*The nomenclature for collagens is as follows. The individual chain of each molecule is referred to as an α chain. The type of collagen is designated by a Roman numeral in parentheses, for example, (I) and the chains of a collagen type are numbered in Arabic numerals from 1 upward. The chains of type I collagen were originally numbered by their chromatographic elution during CM-cellulose column chromatography, α(I) and α2(I), respectively. This convention no longer applies and the numbering is dependent on priority of identification. The precursor chains are designated as preproα chains (with the signal sequence intact) and proα chains once the signal sequence has been removed. Proα chains from which the C-terminal, non-triple-helical precursor specific domain has been removed are called pNα chains and those from which the N-terminal precursor specific extension has been removed are called pCα chains. β-components (sometimes referred to as chains in the older literature) contain two α chains, generally cross-linked by lysine-derived covalent cross-links; γ-components are three α chains similarly linked. These terms do not refer to individual, genetically distinct chains as they often do in other protein families. The genes encoding collagen chains are referred to in the following manner: COL1A2 indicates the gene that encodes the preproα2 (A2) chain of type I collagen (COL1).

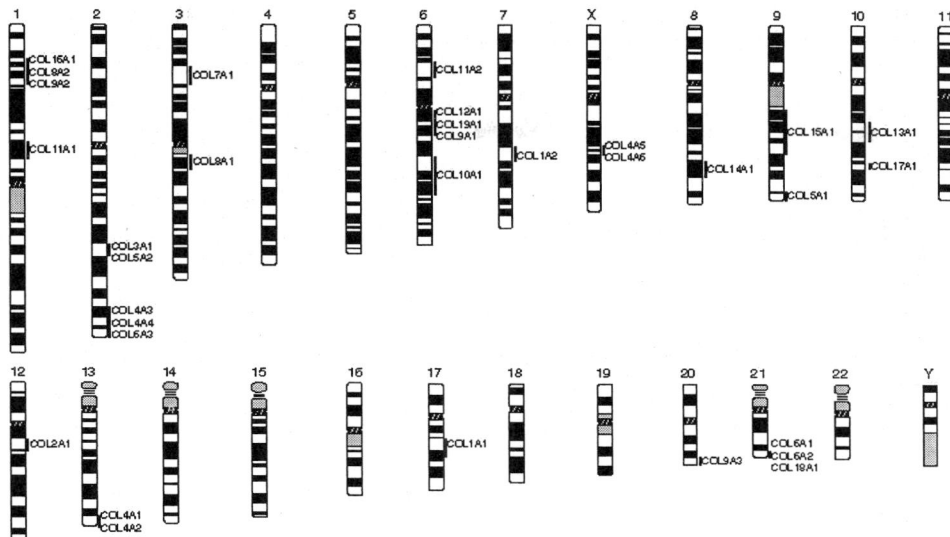

**Fig. 205-1 Chromosomal distribution of collagen genes.**

all form molecules that contain three chains (either hetero- or homotrimers, depending on collagen type) that have a triple-helical domain characterized by the repeating amino acid sequence $(Gly-X-Y)_n$; they have an abundance of the special amino acids hydroxyproline and hydroxylysine; and they play a structural role in tissues. Some other proteins; including acetylcholinesterase,[5] the C1q component of the complement cascade;[6] pulmonary surfactant proteins,[7] which are part of a set of proteins known as collectins; lectins involved in host-bacterial interactions;[8] a mannose-binding protein in serum;[9] and a gene that bears mutations that give rise to the X-linked ectodermal dysplasia syndrome;[10,11] have all appropriated stretches of the triple-helical structure, perhaps as a structural domain. Since the last edition of this chapter was written, the genes that encode all the human collagen chains that are identified at the protein level have been isolated and either completely or partially characterized. Several new collagen genes have been identified by screening of cDNA libraries and expressed sequence tagged elements from data bases, necessitating a search for function and distribution of the encoded protein. There continues to be an emphasis on understanding how mutations generate phenotype; and transgenic animals containing altered collagen genes have been used to define the role of those collagens and to identify candidate disorders for those genes. Mutations in more than half of the known collagen genes have been identified and shown to result in human genetic disease (osteogenesis imperfecta, forms of Ehlers-Danlos syndrome, several chondrodysplasias, Alport syndrome, and dystrophic forms of epidermolysis bullosa) (see Table 205-1). The models for how mutation influence the behavior of proteins and how the abnormal proteins are recognized and handled in the cell or in the matrix continue to come largely from the study of the ubiquitously expressed and readily available type I collagen producing cells. Although these studies serve as models for mutations in fibrillar collagen genes, they probably fall short in helping to understand how mutations in some of the more complex collagen genes alter molecular behavior and produce disease phenotypes.

As a family of proteins, the collagens are the most abundant in the body. The vast majority of collagen in the body is type I collagen, which is ubiquitously distributed and is the major protein in bone, skin, tendon, ligament, sclera, cornea, blood vessels, and hollow organs (Table 205-2).[12] Mutations that affect the structure or processing of the chains of type I collagen are often expressed as generalized connective tissue disorders, although the specific tissue in which the major effect is seen may vary and determine the clinical phenotype (e.g. osteogenesis imperfecta and some forms of the Ehlers-Danlos syndrome all result from mutations in type I

collagen genes).[13] With the exception of types III, V, and VI collagen, which are also distributed in virtually all tissues (little type III collagen is found in bone and cartilage), most other collagens have a tissue-specific or structure-specific distribution (see Table 205-2). Types II, IX, X, and XI collagens are found in hyaline cartilage, fibrocartilage of the intervertebral disk, and the vitreous of the eye,[12,14–16] type IV collagens are found in basement membranes,[17] and type VII collagen is found at some epithelial-mesenchymal junctions in anchoring fibril structures.[18] The recent demonstration that domains of types XV and XVIII collagens contain the endostatin sequences that are involved in the regulation of blood vessel formation demonstrates the extended array of functions of portions of these collagens.[19,20]

With the exception of collagen types I, III, V, and VI, most collagens are expressed by a limited array of fully differentiated cell types, but it is not unusual for one cell to synthesize a group of collagen types. For example, chondrocytes may express types II, IX, X, and XI but not types I and III to any appreciable extent. Although the mechanisms of such control are of great interest, there remains too little understanding of how cell and tissue specific control of expression of collagens are achieved.

As a consequence of differences in structure, expression, and tissue distribution, the collagens perform different functions; in different tissues the same collagen may perform different functions. For example, type I collagen provides tensile strength in bone, skin, and tendon but is mineralized only in bone under normal circumstances. It provides or facilitates transparency of the cornea (in part as a consequence of its fibril structure), though the sclera is opaque; and it forms hollow tubes as part of blood vessels but solid structures as part of tendons. Type IV collagen provides the major structural protein of basement membrane, does not form fibril structures, and acts as a filtration barrier in the kidney and at the dermal-epidermal junction. The functions of types II, IX, X, and XI collagens in cartilage are less clear, although in the absence of type II collagen bone does not grow normally and development is impeded because of failure of notochord formation.[21,22] Similarly, the functions of the fibrillar collagens types III and V are not clear, although analysis of the phenotypic effects of mutations in these collagens indicate that both are essential in the formation of intact tissues.[23,24] Thus collagens function in a number of ways: to provide tensile strength, to facilitate transparency, to provide form during embryonic and fetal development, to interact with other proteins to build tissues and organs, to separate cell layers during and after development, and to provide filtration barriers between spaces. It is likely that some of the functions are achieved as a direct result of collagen structure,

**Table 205-2 Collagen Types; Chain Composition, and Tissue Distribution**

| Collagen Type | Chains | Molecules | Tissue Distribution |
|---|---|---|---|
| Fibrillar Collagens | | | |
| I | $\alpha(I)$, $\alpha 2(I)$ | $\alpha 1(I)_2 \alpha 2(I)$ | Ubiquitous in hard and soft tissues, major protein of bone, skin |
| | | $\alpha 1(I)_3$ | Uncommon, found in some tumors, amniotic fluid cells |
| II | $\alpha 1(II)$ | $\alpha 1(II)_3$ | Cartilage, vitreous, intervertebral disk |
| | | See also type XI | |
| III | $\alpha 1(III)$ | $\alpha 1(III)_3$ | Soft tissues and hollow organs |
| V | $\alpha 1(V)$, $\alpha 2(V)$, $\alpha 3(V)$ | $\alpha 1(V)_2 \alpha 2(V)$ | Soft tissues, placental, vessels, chorion |
| | | $\alpha 1(V) \alpha 2(V) \alpha 3(V)$ | $\alpha 2(V)$ can substitute for the $\alpha 2(XI)$ chain in vitreous |
| | | See also type XI | |
| XI | $\alpha 1(XI)$, $\alpha 2(XI)$ | $\alpha 1(XI) \alpha 2(XI) \alpha 1(II)$ | Cartilage |
| | | $\alpha 1(XI) \alpha 2(V) \alpha 1(II)$ | Vitreous |
| Basement membrane collagens | | | |
| IV | $\alpha 1(IV)$, $\alpha 2(IV)$ $\alpha 3(IV)$, $\alpha 4(IV)$ $\alpha 5(IV)$, $\alpha 6(IV)$ | $\alpha 1(IV)_2 \alpha 2(IV)$ Others uncertain | Basement membranes |
| Fibril-associated collagens with interrupted triple helices (FACIT) | | | |
| IX | $\alpha 1(IX)$, $\alpha 2(IX)$, $\alpha 3(IX)$ | $\alpha 1(IX)$, $\alpha 2(IX) \alpha 3(IX)$ | Cartilage, vitreous |
| XII | $\alpha 1(XII)$ | $\alpha 1(XII)_3$ | Soft tissues |
| XIV | $\alpha 1(XIV)$ | $\alpha 1(XIV)_3$ | Soft tissues |
| Meshwork-forming collagaens | | | |
| VIII | $\alpha 1(VIII)$, $\alpha 2(VIII)$ | $\alpha 1(VIII)_2 \alpha 2(VIII)$ | Cornea, endothelium |
| X | $\alpha 1(X)$ | $\alpha 1(X)_3$ | Hypertrophic zone of the growth plate |
| Anchoring-fibril collagen | | | |
| VII | $\alpha 1(VII)$ | $\alpha 1(VII)_3$ | Anchoring fibrils, dermal epidermal junction |
| Microfibril-forming collagens | | | |
| VI | $\alpha 1(VI)$, $\alpha 2(VI)$, $\alpha 3(VI)$ | $\alpha 1(VI)$, $\alpha 2(VI) \alpha 3(VI)$ | Microfibrils in soft tissues and cartilage |
| Transmembrane collagens | | | |
| XIII | $\alpha 1(XIII)$ | $\alpha 1(XIII)_3$ | Cell surfaces, epithelial cells |
| XVII | $\alpha 1(XVII)$ | $\alpha 1(XVII)_3$ | Epidermal cell surfaces |
| Endostatin forming collagens | | | |
| XV | $\alpha 1(XV)$ | $\alpha 1(XV)_3$ | Endothelial cells |
| XVIII | $\alpha 1(XVIII)$ | $\alpha 1(XVIII)_3$ | Endothelial cells |
| Others | | | |
| XVI | $\alpha 1(XVI)$ | $\alpha 1(XVI)_3$ | Ubiquitous |
| XIX | $\alpha 1(XIX)$ | $\alpha 1(XIX)_3$ | Ubiquitous |

while others depend on interactions with additional matrix macromolecules.

This chapter details the molecular basis of varieties of osteogenesis imperfecta (type I collagen genes); the Ehlers-Danlos syndrome (type I and III collagen genes and posttranslational enzymes); several chondrodysplasias including achondrogenesis, hypochondrogenesis, spondyloepiphyseal dysplasia, Stickler syndrome, and multiple epiphyseal dysplasias (type II, type IX, type X, and type XI collagen genes). The effects of mutations in type IV collagen genes (Alport syndrome with different types of inheritance and accompanying phenotypes (type IV collagen genes); and dystrophic and other forms of epidermolysis bullosa (types VII and XVII collagen genes) (see Table 205-1) are discussed in other chapters (Chaps. 214 and 222). To put these disorders in perspective, the chapter begins with a review of the nature of the collagen gene family and of the biosynthesis of collagens, using type I collagen as the example. Following, there is detailed information about each disorder, including clinical presentation, natural history and genetics, the molecular basis of the clinical phenotype, treatments provided, and animal models of the conditions.

## COLLAGEN GENES

### Collagen Gene and Protein Structure

On the basis of structure there appear to be several classes of collagen genes:[3,4] (1) the fibrillar collagens, type I [*COL1A1*, *COL1A2*] type II [*COL2A1*], type III [*COL3A1*], type V [*COL5A1*, *COL5A2*, and *COL5A3*], and type XI [*COL11A1* and *COL11A2*]; (2) basement membrane collagens or type IV [*COL4A1*, *COL4A2*, *COL4A3*, *COL4A4*, *COL4A5*, and *COL4A6*]; (3) the fibril associated collagens with interrupted triple helices (FACIT) collagens, type IX [*COL9A1*, *COL9A2*, *COL9A3*], type XII

[*COL12A1*], and type XIV [*COL14A1*]; (4) network forming collagens, type VIII [*COL8A1, COL8A2*] and type X [*COL10A1*]; (5) collagens of microfibrils, type VI [*COL6A1, COL6A2,* and *COL6A3*]; and (6) the long chain collagen of anchoring fibrils with an interrupted triple helix, type VII [*COL7A1*]). The nature of the protein products are illustrated in Fig. 205-2.

## Genes that Encode the Fibrillar Collagens

The genes that encode the chains of collagen types I, II, III, V, and XI, a total of 10 distinct genes, constitute the family of fibrillar collagen genes (see Table 205-1). This family has two subsets of which the *COL5A1*,[25] and *COL11A2*[26] genes form one branch and the remainder form the second branch. Each protein is characterized by an unbroken triple-helical domain (Gly-X-Y) containing slightly more than 1000 amino acids, and the genes in the larger branch encode this structure with a set of 42 exons that contain 45, 54, 99, 108, or 162 base pairs with some variations in the genes of

the second branch. There are transition exons at both ends of the triple-helical domains. These exons contain the regions that encode the sites of proteolytic cleavage at the amino-terminal and carboxyl-terminal ends of the triple helix. There is a minor triple helix encoded by a single exon in the 5′ end of the gene, just upstream from the exon that encodes the proteolytic site at the N-terminal end of the major triple helix. The exons in the triple-helical domain begin with a glycine codon and thus end with the codon for the Y-position amino acid; exons in non-triple-helical domains may contain interrupted codons.

The organization of the genes for the two branches of the fibrillar collagen gene family is similar although the minor branch is characterized by more variation in exon size and some differences in the location of intron/exon boundaries. For much of the length of all the genes the intron-exon structure is similar; differences in the sizes of the genes are accounted for by variation in intron size. The gene that encodes the proα1(I) chain (*COL1A1*)

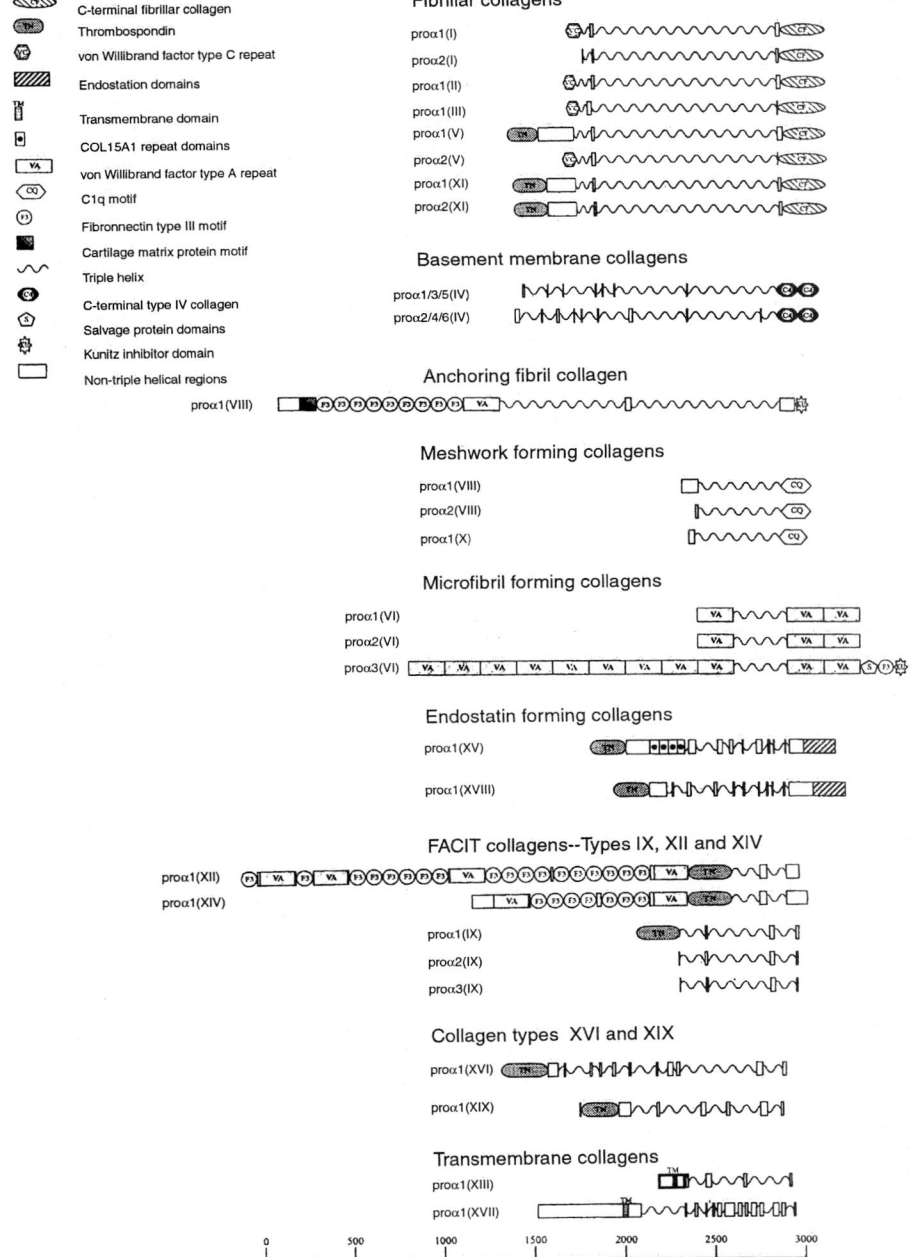

Fig. 205-2 The modular structure of collagens. Collagens share many modular motifs with other matrix proteins, as illustrated here. (*Redrawn from Brown JC, Timpl.[3] Used by permission.*)

on chromosome 17[27] is about 18 kb in length;[28] those that encode the proα2(I) chain (COL1A2)[28] on chromosome 7,[29] the proα1(II) (COL2A1) chains[30] on chromosome 12,[31] the proα1(III) chain (COL3A1) the proα2(V) chain (COL5A2) on chromosome 2,[32] and the proα1(XI) (COL11A1) on chromsome[33] chain are each about 40 kb in size. The COL5A1 gene has a huge first intron (600 to 800 kb) so the gene size is commensurately large.[25] The similar gene structure and homologies in amino acid sequence provide strong evidence for the divergence of collagen types following the evolutionary setting of gene structure. (See Table 205-1 for a compilation of collagen types, their constituent chains, collagen gene size, and their chromosomal locations.) The fibrillar collagen gene structure is present in birds and mammals, dating the emergence of the structure of the fibrillar collagen genes prior to the radiation of those two groups, more than 50 million years ago. The genes that encode the chains of the fibrillar collagens are widely dispersed among the chromosomes (Table 205-1 and Fig. 205-1).

## Basement Membrane Collagen Genes — Type IV Collagen

The genes that encode the six basement membrane nonfibrillar collagens are similar in size to those that encode most fibrillar collagens but differ somewhat in organization.[34] The exons that encode the largely triple-helical domains vary more widely in size, do not always begin with a glycine codon nor end with a codon for a Y-position amino acid, frequently split codons, and encode interruptions of the triple helix. The interruptions of triple-helical sequence when compared to the fibrillar collagen genes could be explained by small deletions, single nucleotide substitutions, and mutations at former splice junctions. Six genes that encode basement membrane collagens have been isolated and encode similar mRNAs, have similar gene structures, and have a remarkable organization. The six type IV collagen genes are organized in three tandem arrays: COL4A1 and COL4A2, are located in a head-to-head array on the distal long arm of chromosome 13,[35–37] COL4A3 and COL4A4 in a similar distribution on chromosome 2,[38,39] and the COL4A5 and COL4A6 genes have the same relationship on the long arm of the X-chromosome.[40–42] The three pairs each share a promotor element, and are transcribed from opposite strands.[34] It is likely that a single ancestral gene duplicated with an inversion and the binary structure was then propagated to other chromosomes in either a single or two separate events.

## Fibril Associated Collagens with Interrupted Triple Helices (FACIT) — Types IX, XII, and XIV

Distinct from both the fibrillar and basement membrane genes are those that encode collagenous proteins that become associated with large collagen fibrils in tissues. The first of these recognized was type IX collagen, now known to comprise three genes, each of which encodes chains that contain three triple-helical domains with interruptions. The three type IX collagen genes are dispersed to separate chromosomes.[43–45] Each chain consists of about 900 amino acids divided into seven distinct domains: three that contain triple-helical Gly-X-Y repeat motifs (the COL1, COL2, and COL3 domains that contain 134, 339, and 137 amino acids, respectively) and four noncollagenous domains (NC1, NC2, NC3, and NC4 that contain about 20, 30, 12, and 243 amino acids, respectively).[14] The NC1 domain is the most C-terminal region of each chain, the NC2 domain separates COL1 and COL2, and the NC3 domain separates COL2 and COL3. The COL3 domain contains one imperfection and the COL1 domain contains two. Type IX collagen genes are expressed in concert with those of type II collagen and the proteins are found together in cartilaginous tissues and the vitreous humor of the eye. The α2(IX) chain contains an attachment site for a glycosaminoglycan side chain that may facilitate interactions between collagens and proteoglycans in cartilage matrices.[46]

There are two additional members of the FACIT gene family, COL12A1 and COL14A1. The gene that encodes the chains of type XII collagen, COL12A1, is located on chromosome 6 in the same region as the COL9A1 gene;[47] the COL14A1 gene is at 8q23. The type XII collagen gene draws attention to the complexity of some of the collagen-related genes in that the collagenous domains are quite small in relation to the content of other domains shared by matrix proteins.[48,49] This gene also introduces the complexity of relationships that exist between collagens and other matrix proteins.[3,4] Type XII collagen is a homotrimer of α1(XII) chains and is ubiquitously distributed, paralleling the distribution of the types I, III, and V collagens, which has suggested that it may act with respect to those proteins as type IX collagens does with type II collagen. In cartilage, covalent cross-links contain sequences from types II and IX collagens, which confirms their proximity. The difference in the mass of the N-terminal end of type XII collagen compared to type IX does, however, raise questions about the precise correspondence of the two classes of molecules.

## Filament-Producing Collagen — Type VI

Two of the genes for type VI, COL6A1 and COL6A2, reside on the long arm of chromosome 21,[50–52] and the COL6A3 gene is located on chromosome 6.[53] These genes encode three chains that have a 335 or 336 amino acid triple helix, with two imperfections embedded within noncollagenous sequences.[54] The COL6A1 and COL6A2 genes encode NC2 (amino-terminal) peptides of about 235 residues and NC1 (C-terminal) peptides of about 430 residues. The COL6A3 gene encodes a protein with a homologous collagenous domain but a large (1800 amino acids) NC2 (N-terminal) domain and a NC1 domain that is twice the size of the peptides in the other two type VI collagens. The NC1 domain of the α3(VI) chain contains more than six repeats of a von Willebrand factor domain, and the C-terminal noncollagenous domain contains repeats of other types. Type VI collagen is a heterotrimer of all three chains. The monomers interact with other monomers to form partially overlapping head-to-tail dimers that interact with other dimers to produce tetramers, the base unit for forming beaded microfilaments in the matrix. These, in turn, form microfibrillar arrays in extracellular matrices of virtually all tissues and in cultured cells in vitro. The microfibrillar network formed by type VI collagen is distinct from that which contains fibrillin, the microfibrils associated with the elastic fiber network. The function of these microfibrillar structures is unknown.

## Network-Forming Collagens — Type VIII and Type X

Type VIII and type X collagens have similar coding sequences and gene structures[55–57] and encode proteins that form meshworks, similar, perhaps, to the meshwork produced by type IV collagens in basement membranes. The structure of these genes is, however, different than those of type IV collagen family. These three genes have a remarkably compact structure and encode chains that are very similar. The two COL8 genes encode chains that have a core triple-helical domain of 454 (COL8A1) and 457 residues (COL8A2) bounded by an NC1 domain (carboxyl-terminal) of 173 and 167 residues, respectively, and a slightly smaller NC2 domain (amino-terminal). The genes contain three exons with the triple helix and NC1 domains encoded by a single exon, and the NC2 domain divided between the remaining two exons. Type VIII collagen is a heterotrimer with two proα1(VIII) chains and a single proα2(VIII) chain. The chains are probably not processed in the extracellular space but, instead, the NC1 and NC2 domains participate in formation of the meshwork. The NC1 domain at the carboxyl-terminus is important for trimer formation as illustrated by the effects of mutations in that domain of the type COL10A1 gene. The structure of the COL10A1 gene is similar, differing only in the size of the respective domains.

Type VIII collagen was originally isolated from endothelial cells but is an abundant component of Descemet's membrane that separates corneal epithelium and corneal stroma. Two genes of type VIII collagen have been localized to chromosome 3 for COL8A1[55] and to chromosome 1 for COL8A2.[56]

Type X collagen is a component of hypertrophic cartilage, and although a role for endochondral bone formation has been postulated, its function remains uncertain. Only a single gene has yet been isolated that encodes type X collagen chains.

## Anchoring Fibril Collagen — Type VII

Type VII collagen is confined to anchoring fibrils at the dermal-epidermal junction and at some other basement membranes that separate epithelial and mesenchymal structures.[18,58] The protein is a large homotrimer with constituent chains of approximately 170 kDa. This protein is, like many collagens, a mosaic of collagenous and non-collagenous motifs. The gene is located on the long arm of chromosome 3 and encodes this large polypeptide with an astonishingly compact and interrupted structure: 118 exons distributed in the small domain of 30 kb — probably the most complex gene yet described.[59,60]

## Endostatin Forming Collagens

Type XV and type XVIII collagens have domains at their carboxyl-terminal ends that contain the sequences of the two major inhibitors of angiogenesis, the endostatins.[19,20,61] Both genes are strongly expressed in endothelial cells in most tissues.[62]

## Transmembrane Collagens

Two collagens are retained at the cell surface and act as transmembrane proteins, type XIII and type XVIII collagen. Both are found in epithelial cells and may act as cell-matrix ligands. Mutations in the *COL17A1* gene result in a blistering disorder but the consequences of mutations in the *COL13A1* gene have not been identified.

# COLLAGEN PROTEIN STRUCTURE

## Domain Structure of Type I Procollagen

Type I procollagen, a heterotrimer that contains two proα1(I) chains encoded by *COL1A1* and one proα2(I) chain (encoded by *COL1A2*), contains seven distinct domains, each of which has one or more functions (Figs. 205-3, 205-4). Each preproα chain is synthesized with a signal sequence of approximately 20 residues that facilitates passage across the rough endoplasmic reticulum (RER) membrane and is cleaved during transit into the RER. The proα1(I) chain contains a cysteine-rich globular extension of 86 residues, the function of which is not known; a similar sequence is missing in the proα2(I) chain. Both chains contain a 36-residue domain of 12 Gly-X-Y triplets that forms a triple helix in the intact procollagen molecule. This short triple helix has a relatively high denaturation temperature and may stabilize the N-terminal end of the molecule. There is a short, non-triple-helical telopeptide

domain that contains the site of proteolytic cleavage of the N-terminal propeptide extension and lysyl residues that become involved in intermolecular cross-links. The major triple-helical domain of both chains is 1014 residues in length and is characterized by glycine in every third position $(Gly-X-Y)_{338}$.

Hydroxyproline occupies the Y-position in about a third of the triplets and is often preceded by proline. Some lysyl residues in the Y-position are also hydroxylated but the extent of this modification is highly dependent on the collagen type. The amino acids 4-hydroxyproline and hydroxylysine are found only in the Y-position of the triple helix (a consequence of the specificity of the hydroxylating enzymes). All phenylalanine residues and virtually all leucine residues (with one exception) are found in the X-position, apparently because of severe steric hindrance to the formation of triple helix when these residues occur in the Y-position.[63] The basic residue, arginine, occurs preferentially in the Y-position; the acidic residue, glutamic acid, is found usually in the X-position, a distribution that may facilitate charge-charge interactions and increase triple helix thermal stability. A 28-residue telopeptide at the C-terminal end of the triple helix contains a lysyl residue in proα1(I), which is absent from proα2(I). This residue is involved in interchain crosslink formation; the telopeptide also contains the site at which the C-terminal procollagen peptidase cleaves. The final 220 residues of the proα chains form globular structures that contain intra- and interchain disulfide bonds. This domain facilitates chain assembly, determines the chain specificity for assembly of the type I procollagen molecule, and provides intracellular solubility.

# STRUCTURE OF THE COLLAGEN TRIPLE-HELIX

By virtue of the triple-helical structure, collagen has several unique features. The primary sequence of the α chains can be written $(Gly-X-Y)_{338}$ where X and Y can be most amino acids except tryptophan and cysteine, which are excluded from the triple helix in both chains of type I collagen; tyrosine is excluded from the triple helix of α1(I) but there is one residue in α2(I) and, as pointed out, the distribution of a small number of other unmodified residues is not symmetrical. Hydroxyproline and hydroxylysine are found only in the Y-position as a consequence of enzymatic posttranslational modification (see below). The individual α chains assume a left-handed extended polyproline-like helical structure (minor helix) that has a distance of approximately 9.5 Å between residues in equivalent position (pitch), that is the distance from one residue to the next one that sits at the same position on the side of the chain. Three chains associate to form a right-handed triple-helical structure (major helix) that has a pitch of approximately

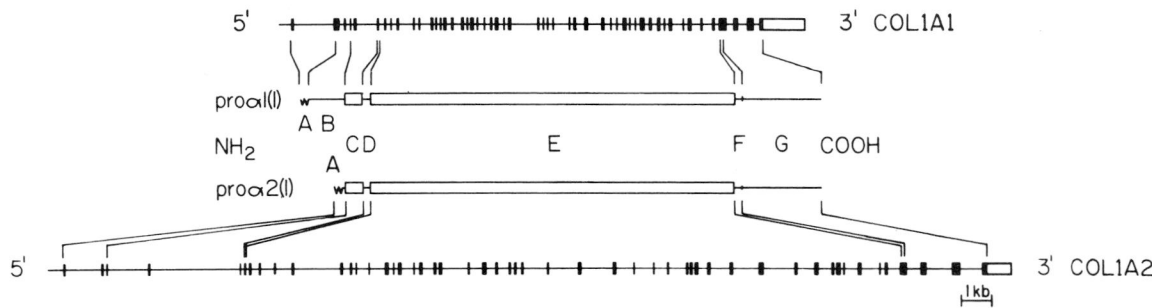

**Fig. 205-3 Fibrillar collagen gene structure.** The intron-exon structure of the prototype fibrillar collagen genes (*COL1A1* and *COL1A2*, which encode the preproα1(I) and preproα2(I) chains of type I procollagen, respectively) are represented. The exons are designated by the solid boxes or vertical lines. All the exons that encode sequences only in the triple-helical domain (exons 7 to 48) contain 45, 54, 99, 108, or 162 nucleotides; start with a glycine codon; and end with the codon for the Y-position amino acid. The organization of the other fibrillar collagen genes is similar and intron-exon boundaries and exon sizes are maintained throughout. The structure of the genes that encode the nonfibrillar collagens differs considerably. The domains in the polypeptide chains are: A = signal sequence; B = N-terminal propeptide globular domain; C = N-terminal propeptide triple-helical domain; D = N-terminal telopeptide; E = triple helix; F = C-terminal telopeptide; and G = C-terminal propeptide. (*Adapted and redrawn from Ramirez et al. Ann N Y Acad Sci 460:117, 1985. Used with permission.*)

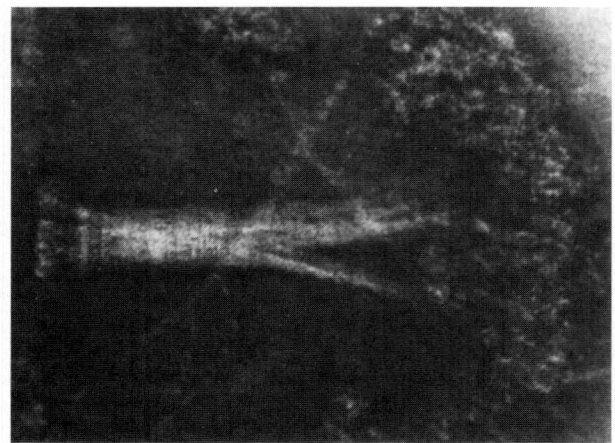

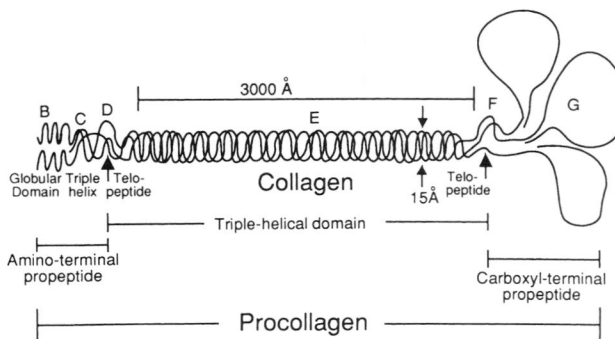

**Fig. 205-4 Electron micrograph of segment-long-spacing (SLS) aggregates of type I procollagen (top) and a model of a type I procollagen molecule (bottom). SLS aggregates were made by lateral aggregation of procollagen molecules that had been synthesized and secreted into culture medium by normal fibroblasts. Arrayed in a side-to-side orientation, the molecules are precipitated, stained, and then examined in the electron microscope. The model of type I procollagen represents the major domains of the molecule. Designations for domains B through G are as for Fig. 205-1. The signal sequence is not shown for either chain. (*Micrograph courtesy of Dr. Lynne T. Smith, University of Washington.*)**

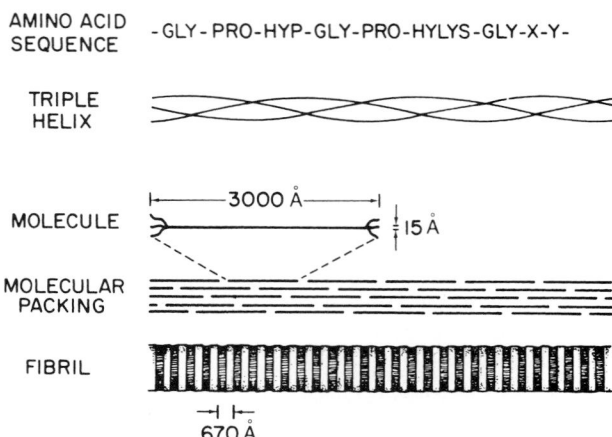

**Fig. 205-5 The hierarchical structure and organization of fibrillar collagens. The $\alpha$ chains of fibrillar collagens contain a core triple-helical domain of slightly more than 1000 residues that is characterized by the repeating triplet, Gly-X-Y (top), and in which each chain forms a left-handed helix with a pitch of 3.6 nM. Three chains form a triple-helical molecule in which they are wound in a right-handed spiral. Molecules in the matrix aggregate in an ordered fashion staggered by about a quarter of the length of the triple-helical domain. The staggered order contributes an ordered pattern of electron dense and electron lucent regions in fibrils as seen in the electron microscope and reflected in the 670 Ångstrom repeating band pattern (bottom).**

100 Å (Fig. 205-5) and resembles a relatively stiff rope with regions of flexibility. Glycine, as the smallest amino acid with no side chains, is required in every third position of each chain because space does not exist in the structure for side chains. The side chains on any substituting residue would point toward the center of the helix and not permit a triple helix to form (see "Osteogenesis Imperfecta" below). The side chains of residues in the X and Y positions are arrayed toward the external surface of the molecule. The chains are associated in such a way that the glycine residues are staggered one residue with respect to the adjacent chain. That is, a glycine of the second chain would be adjacent to the X-position residue in the first chain and the glycine of the third chain would be adjacent to the Y-position residue of the first chain.

The stability of the triple helix is provided by interchain hydrogen bonds between the amide group of glycine and the oxygen of the carbonyl group of an X-position residue on an adjacent chain.[64,65] Additional hydrogen bonds that involve the hydroxyl group of hydroxyproline and the carbonyl backbone of the chain further stabilize the molecule. In the absence of hydroxylation, the triple helix of type I collagen denatures at about 27°C;[66,67] with complete hydroxylation the denaturation temperature is about 42°C (the precise denaturation temperature depends on the manner in which it is measured). Triple-helical structure is one of the requirements for transport of type I collagen

beyond the rough endoplasmic reticulum;[68,69] thus, in its absence little or no normal collagen is secreted at normal body temperatures. It is likely that other factors, especially charge-charge interactions, contribute to the stability of the triple helix and, although recognized for some time, their importance is often overlooked.

The triple-helical structure of collagen provides resistance to degradation by most proteases, the exceptions being the specific collagenases synthesized by mesenchymal (and some epithelial) cells, and collagenases synthesized by a number of microorganisms. The resistance of the triple helix to proteases allows collagens to provide an extremely stable structure in the extracellular environment. Once denatured, the chains are exquisitely sensitive to most proteases, which ensures normal turnover.

## BIOSYNTHESIS OF COLLAGEN

The biosynthesis, processing, and secretion of collagens is a remarkably complex process that begins with highly regulated and coordinated transcription of genes for multiple chains, includes chain-specific posttranslational modifications, and ends with regulated secretion and degradation (Table 205-3).

### Control of Collagen Biosynthesis

Collagen biosynthesis is controlled at many levels and the mechanisms by which control is exerted are not completely understood. The genes of type I collagen (*COL1A1* and *COL1A2*) are located on different chromosomes and their physical relationship during the cell cycle is not known. They are present in equal numbers (one copy per haploid genome) but are transcribed with different efficiencies; *COL1A1* produces twice the steady state mRNA levels as *COL1A2*.[70] The difference results from transcriptional efficiency, not mRNA stability, and is probably not accounted for by the size of the genes. The expression of the genes is almost always coordinated and ultimately results in the synthesis of two pro$\alpha$1(I) chains for each pro$\alpha$2(I) chain. Upstream domains provide regions that control organ- or tissue-specific expression. Nucleotide sequences in the upstream sequences and in the first intron of the *COL1A1* and *COL1A2* genes of type I collagen provide positive and negative enhancers and direct tissue-specific expression of the genes.[71–79]

**Table 205-3 Nature and Location of Events during Collagen Biosynthesis**

| Event | Enzyme | Location |
|---|---|---|
| Transcription | Many | Nucleus |
| Splicing | "Splicesome-complex" | Nucleus |
| Transport | Unknown | Nucleus-cytoplasm |
| Translation | Many | Cytoplasm/RER |
| Signal cleavage | Signal peptidase | RER membrane |
| Prolyl hydroxylation | Proline 4-hydroxylase | RER lumen |
|  | Proline 3-hydroxylase | RER lumen |
| Lysyl hydroxylation | Lysyl hydroxylase | RER lumen |
| Hydroxylysyl glycosylation | Collagen glycosyltransferase | RER lumen |
| Heterosaccharide addition and modification | Collagen galactosyltransferase | RER lumen |
| Intrachain disulfide bond formation | Disulfide isomerase | RER lumen |
| Chain assembly | Not known | RER lumen |
| Interchain disulfide bond formation | Disulfide isomerase | RER lumen |
| Triple-helix propagation | Prolyl *cis-trans* isomerase | RER lumen |
| Transport to Golgi | Many (unknown) | RER/Golgi |
| Modification of heterosaccharide | Many | Golgi |
| Sulfation | Sulfotransferase | Golgi |
| Exocytosis | Many | Cell surface |
| N-terminal processing | Procollagen aminoprotease | ECM* |
| C-terminal processing | Lysyl oxidase | ECM |

*ECM = extracellular matrix.

The expression of collagen genes can be altered by a variety of growth factors[80,81] and by the presence or absence of ascorbic acid.[82] Sequences between the transcription start sites and the first translated domain of the mRNA can form stem-loop structures, which appear to influence the efficiency of translation.[83] Under some circumstances, for example in chondrocytes placed in culture, the COL1A2 gene is transcribed but the proα2(I) mRNA is inefficiently translated, apparently as a result of translational arrest.[84] There is evidence that control of translation of some collagen mRNAs can be influenced by peptides derived from the N-terminal extension of type I procollagen chains[85,86] and by sequences derived from the C-terminal propeptide extension.[87] An additional level of control is provided once the proα chains are synthesized. For heterotrimeric molecules, like type I procollagen, the relative ratios of the two chains determines the amount of the correct molecule available and because molecular stability is determined, at least in part, by prolyl hydroxylation, the activity of the enzyme can be linked to the rate of synthesis of collagen. Finally, there is a constant level of intracellular degradation of collagenous proteins through a mechanism that probably scans abnormal sequences or unfolded molecules.[88] Thus the control of collagen production occurs at many levels, some of which function in a qualitative fashion, while others provide more quantitative variation.

## Nuclear Events

Like virtually all eukaryotic mRNAs that encode secreted proteins, those encoding collagen chains are synthesized as precursors that are then spliced to remove intervening sequences, capped, polyadenylated, and transported to the cytoplasm. Splicing of the precursor mRNA is clearly a complex process as most of the genes for collagens have more than 50 exons. Some, like those that encode the chains of type VIII and type X collagens have only three, though the type VII collagen precursor RNA has 118. In the fibrillar collagen genes, splicing is orderly but is not processive, and this allocation to relative fast and relatively slowly removed introns probably contributes to some of the surprising outcomes of splice site mutations in these genes (see "Splice Site Mutations," below).[89]

## Translation

Little is known about the control of translation of collagen mRNA species. As indicated above, the formation of stem-loop structures

in mRNAs for some collagens appears to influence the efficiency of translation. The observation that cells from patients and animals with defects in cleavage of the N-terminal propeptide of type I procollagen[90,91] synthesized less type I procollagen than control cells led to attempts to determine if the decrease in synthesis resulted from feedback regulation. Isolated N-terminal propeptide extensions from proα1(I) decreased the translational efficiency of proα1(I), proα2(I), and proα1(II) mRNA in vitro. A short peptide from the pN domain of proα1(I) can virtually abolish translation at relatively high concentrations but blocks translation of all messages. Evidence has also been presented that suggests that peptides derived from the C-terminal propeptide can affect the efficiency of translation.

## Posttranslational Modification and Events in the RER Signal Sequence

The mRNA is translated on ribosomes that become membrane bound. The signal sequences of preproα1(I) and preproα2(I) are cleaved during elongation of the chains as they are transported through the membrane into the lumen of the rough endoplasmic reticulum.

**Hydroxylation of Prolyl and Lysyl Residues.** During translation, lagging about 300 residues behind assembly, Y-position prolyl and lysyl residues, N-terminal to glycyl residues in the major and minor triple-helical sequences, are hydroxylated by the enzymes prolyl 4-hydroxylase and lysyl hydroxylase, respectively.[92,93] In addition some prolyl residues in the sequence Gly-Pro-4Hypro-Gly are hydroxylated in the 3-position by the enzyme prolyl 3-hydroxylase, a distinct protein.[93] The usual substrates for these reactions are the nascent chain and the free proα chains; for prolyl 4-hydroxylase, the minimum sequence requirement is an X-Pro-Gly triplet. The extent of hydroxylation is regulated, in part, by substrate availability because the fully hydroxylated triple helix has a melting temperature of 42°C and chains in triple-helical conformation are not substrates for the hydroxylases.[93]

Prolyl 4-hydroxylase is on the inner membrane of the rough endoplasmic reticulum. It is a tetramer that contains two α-subunits and two β-subunits. The subunits have molecular weights of 64,000 (α) and 60,000 (β) and are the products of different genes. The β-subunit is protein disulfide isomerase, an enzyme that facilitates disulfide exchange in folding proteins.[93]

Like some other molecules that reside in the lumen of the rough endoplasmic reticulum (RER), the $\beta$-subunit has the C-terminal amino acid sequence Lys-Asp-Glu-Leu (KDEL, using the single letter amino acid code). This sequence interacts with KDEL receptors, integral proteins of the RER membrane to retain this class of chaperone and modifying proteins in the RER. The hydroxylating activity of the tetramer resides in the $\alpha$-subunit, which is inactive if not in the heterotetrameric form. The gene for prolyl 4-hydroxylase I is located at 10q21.3-23.1 and is within 500 kb of the *COL13A1* gene, in a telomeric direction. A second gene has been identified that has a very similar structure to the $\alpha$-subunit but a different distribution.[94] It appears to be the major enzyme in chondrocytes, cartilage, and endothelial cells.[95] Because the two gene products, type I and type II $\alpha$-subunits do not form functional heterodimers when coexpressed in insect cells, their differential tissue distribution probably reflects differential gene expression.[95] Because neither the product of the type I or type II gene contains the KDEL sequence, RER localization must be a product of interaction with the $\beta$-subunit. The binding of the substrate collagens to the active enzyme is a function of the $\alpha$-subunit through a region in the middle of the chain that has a high affinity for polyproline or Pro-Pro-Gly polymers.[96]

Lysyl hydroxylase is a homodimer, the monomer of which has a molecular weight of 85,000.[93] Three genes (*PLOD1*, *PLOD2*, and *PLOD3*)[97–101] that encode chains of lysyl hydroxylase have been isolated. It is not clear if heterodimers form. Despite similar enzymatic mechanisms, there is little sequence similarity between prolyl 4-hydroxylase and lysyl hydroxylase.[93] Like the $\alpha$-subunit of prolyl 4-hydroxylase, lysyl hydroxylase does not contain a KDEL sequence at the carboxyl-terminal end of the chain. There is an internal CDEL sequence but it is not known if it is sufficient for binding to KDEL receptors. The mechanism for RER retention is still unclear. The genes that encode the three forms of lysyl hydroxylase have been isolated and localized to nonsyntenic regions: *PLOD1* at 1q36.3-p36.2, *PLOD2* to 3q23-q24, and *PLOD3* to 7q36. It was pointed out that highly purified lysyl hydroxylase, isolated for its activity against triple-helical lysyl residues, did not hydroxylate the amino-terminal telopeptide residues that are important in intermolecular cross-link formation.[102] None of the isolated enzymes recognize this region as a substrate. Furthermore, Bruck syndrome, in which there appears to be a deficiency of telopeptide lysyl hydroxylation in bone maps to a region other than those which contain the three known enzymes.[103] Although *PLOD2* is not well expressed in marrow stromal cells (precursors to bone forming cells) or skin fibroblasts, it becomes a significant factor in the course of bone development and the synthesis of hydroxylated N-terminal cross-links.[104] The resolution of this paradox may depend on more definitive mapping of the syndrome and careful analysis of the tissue-specific substrates. Thus it remains unclear whether the explanation for very marked differences in lysyl hydroxylation of different collagens (e.g. 15 percent in types I and III, more than 90 percent in type IV) reflects rates of folding and helix formation or type-specific hydroxylases.

Prolyl 3-hydroxylase has a molecular weight of about 160,000, but the subunit composition has not been determined and the gene has not been isolated and characterized.[93] The amount of 3-hydroxyproline differs markedly among collagen types and the mechanisms that control the extent of modification have not been determined.

The three collagen hydroxylases require $Fe^{2+}$, 2-oxoglutarate, molecular oxygen ($O_2$), and ascorbate.[93] The 2-oxoglutarate is decarboxylated and oxidized to succinate; the other member of the oxygen molecule is incorporated into the prolyl residue at the 3- or 4-position or into the lysyl residue at the 5-position. The function of the ascorbate is not clear; it can be replaced by other reducing agents and it is thought that ascorbate may keep the $Fe^{2+}$ atom reduced. Ascorbate is not used stoichiometrically during reactions and there is evidence that it is important during noncoupled oxidation of 2-oxoglutarate. The role of ascorbate in providing a reducing agent for the disulfide exchange portion of prolyl 4-hydroxylase is not known.

The hydroxylation of proline in the 4-position is essential to provide thermal stability to the triple helix. The modification of the chains occurs during elongation and terminates with the formation of a stable triple helix. Hydroxylation of lysyl residues provides substrates for glycosylation and, in addition, the hydroxylysyl residues form more stable covalent cross-links than lysyl residues and are important determinants of tissue tensile strength.[105] The function of 3-hydroxyproline is unknown.

**Hydroxylysyl Glycosylation.** The glycosylation of hydroxylysyl residues in collagen requires two enzymes, hydroxylysyl galactosyltransferase and galactosylhydroxylysyl glucosyltransferase. The former transfers UDP-galactose to the oxygen on the 5-carbon of hydroxylysine in peptide linkage; $Mn^{2+}$ is probably a cofactor for the enzyme. The latter enzyme transfers UDP-glucose, also in the presence of the metal cofactor. The distribution of mono- and disaccharide is influenced by collagen type, probably by the amino acid sequence in the region of the hydroxylysyl residue. The reaction is carried out only on a non-triple-helical substrate. The functions of the carbohydrate on collagens are unknown. Carbohydrate modification may influence fibril formation, may affect collagen-cell interaction and collagen interactions with other macromolecules, and may protect modified hydroxylysyl residues from oxidation to cross-link precursors.

**Glycosylation of Asparagine Residues in the Propeptide Extensions.** Type I procollagen contains a single asparagine-linked carbohydrate group on the C-terminal propeptide of each chain.[106,107] Other procollagens may contain more units and they may be located in both non-triple-helical extension regions.[108] The carbohydrate units are synthesized on a dolichol lipid intermediate in the membrane of the RER and transferred intact to the pro$\alpha$ chains. There is initial cleavage of the terminal units while the chains are in the RER, and additional trimming and resynthesis of the structure in the Golgi apparatus, which results in a high-mannose unit.

## Assembly of the Procollagen Molecule

The assembly of the trimeric procollagen molecule faces several obstacles within the RER—failure to fold, association with incorrect partners, and rapid degradation, among others. The control of chain association and folding is made more complex because although biosynthesis and hydroxylation occur in an amino-terminal to carboxyl-terminal direction, chain association and helix propagation have the opposite polarity. The hydroxylation reactions begin while the chains are being synthesized and are completed when the molecule is assembled and the triple helix is stable. The protein HSP47, an ER-resident protein anchored by a KDEL receptor and also known as colligin, binds non-hydroxylated chains.[109] This binding is markedly reduced following prolyl hydroxylation.[110] However, as both proteins are membrane bound, and because lysyl hydroxylase is anchored to the membrane, the association of the nascent chains with these proteins may protect them from degradation and from proteolysis. Following completion of synthesis, the globular domains of the pro$\alpha$ chains are substrates for protein disulfide isomerase, the $\beta$-subunit of prolyl 4-hydroxylase, but the interaction is independent of association with the $\alpha$-subunits of the protein.[111] This protein acts as a chaperone and facilitates the formation of the correct intrachain disulfide bonds in the carboxyl-terminal propeptide.

Correct chain association is essential in cells that synthesize and secrete several types of similar collagens. For example, skin fibroblasts produce type I, type III, and type V collagen, which, among them, contain six different chains. There is flexibility in chain association, no doubt to provide different functional facets. For example, pro$\alpha$1(I) chains can form homotrimers or heterotrimers in which one pro$\alpha$1(I) is replaced by pro$\alpha$2(I). These molecules do not contain any of the other chain types. With procollagens made in cartilage and the vitreous there is more flexibility allowed. For example, the proα1(II) chain of type II collagen also interacts with the proα1(XI) and proα2(XI) to form type XI collagen.[16] In the vitreous, the proα2(V) chain substitutes for the proα2(XI) chain.[112] The specificity of interaction among chains resides in a short discontinuous set of 17 amino acids in the middle of the proα chains.[113] Swapping experiments indicate that these sequences do specify chain association. Two intrachain disulfide bonds in the fibrillar collagens stabilize the folded carboxyl-terminal propeptide structure of each chain. Once intrachain disulfide bonding is completed, the two proα1(I) chains and single proα2(I) chain associate through domains created by the correct folding of the C-terminal propeptide sequences; the order of initial association appears to be random but determines the identity of the third chain brought into the molecule. Triple helix is nucleated at the carboxyl-terminal end of that domain, probably through the interaction of sequences very rich in hydroxyproline, and is propagated toward the N-terminal end of the molecule. Within the final triple helix all the peptide bonds that involve proline are in the *trans* form but in the chains prior to that time *trans* and *cis* bonds appear in about equal proportion.[114] The propagation of the triple-helical structure requires isomerization to the *trans* form, which is accomplished, in part, by the action of the enzyme peptidyl-prolyl *cis-trans*-isomerase.[115] The triple helix has regions of high density of hydroxyproline and others of low density. The high-density regions may represent areas of secondary nucleation that are required to permit the ordered propagation of the triple helix.

## Modifications Beyond the RER and Secretion

Procollagen molecules are translocated to the Golgi where they are organized in a side-to-side packing array.[116,117] The Golgi functions in a dynamic fashion moving whole segments through and recycling membrane from the *trans* to the *cis* compartments; the contents move through in this manner rather than by sequential budding and fusion. The packaged procollagen molecules are released from the *trans*-Golgi in secretory vesicles that fuse with the cell membrane and release their contents into the extracellular environment. Exit of procollagen molecules from the RER to the Golgi is regulated by structural determinants, the most important of which is an intact triple helix. The importance of triple-helical conformation has been known for many years, but the mechanism by which a cell senses this structure is not known.

In the Golgi, heterosaccharide is trimmed, and synthesis of a high mannose structure occurs on each chain of type I procollagen. In addition, some collagens, notably type V, probably type III, and possibly type I, undergo sulfation of some tyrosine residues in the N-terminal propeptide extension;[118,119] phosphorylation of certain serine residues of the extension of proα1(I) occurs in bone.[120] The functions of the glycosylation, sulfation, and phosphorylation are not known. Inhibition of glycosylation with tunicamycin does not alter the efficiency of secretion of type I procollagen, as it does with some other matrix macromolecules.

## Extracellular Events

Once outside the cell, the fibrillar procollagens undergo proteolytic conversion to collagen, form fibrils, interact with noncollagen and collagenous proteins, and are stabilized by intermolecular cross-links. During development and at other times of rapid growth or repair, collagens are degraded in an orderly fashion; under some other circumstances degradation may be unregulated.

**Cleavage of the N-Terminal and C-Terminal Propeptides.** The conversion of procollagen to collagen occurs in the extracellular space. The peptides of type I procollagen are removed by two enzymes, procollagen N-proteinase[121–123] and procollagen C-proteinase.[124] The N-proteinase that cleaves type I procollagen also recognizes and cleaves type II procollagen, but not type III procollagen. In type I collagen the enzyme cleaves a Pro-Gln bond in the proα1(I) chains and a Ala-Gln bond in the proα2(I) chain,

both encoded in exon 6 of each gene. In both cases cyclization of the glutamine forms the N-terminal residue, pyroglutamic acid. The enzyme is an endopeptidase that requires all three chains of type I procollagen to be in register to form the substrate.[124] The propeptide is removed en-bloc without further degradation. Some is detectable in plasma but the site of further degradation and the half-life of the molecule in plasma are not known. In the procollagen molecule the propeptide probably acts to prevent or delay fibril formation and the minor triple helix may stabilize the N-terminal end of the major triple helix. The enzyme functions in the extracellular environment, probably close to the cell surface. The activity is maximal at neutral pH, and the enzyme requires a divalent cation for function. Cleavage is sequential in chains without apparent specificity as to the first reaction. The gene for the type I procollagen N-proteinase has been localized to 5q34.[123] It encodes a protein of approximately 1400 amino acids and its mutations cause dermatosparaxis in animals and Ehlers-Danlos syndrome type VIIC in humans (see "Ehlers-Danlos Syndrome" below).

Cleavage at the C-terminal site occurs at an Ala-Asp bond in both proα1(I) and proα2(I) chains. Both residues are encoded in exon 49 of the chain and reside about two dozen residues beyond the carboxyl-terminal end of the triple-helical domain. In contrast to cleavage at the N-terminal site, this reaction does not require an intact trimer. The enzyme requires a divalent cation, such as $Ca^{2+}$. There does not appear to be a preferred order for cleavage of the termini and intermediates that contain either end intact can be found in tissues and in cultured cells. Some collagens are probably not processed in tissues and some may be cleaved only at one end.

It was a surprise to find that the C-proteinase for type I procollagen was the previously identified bone morphogenetic protein, BMP-1, a member of the tolloid family of proteins involved in specification of form in many animals.[124]

## Fibril Formation

Once cleaved, fibrillar collagen molecules rapidly aggregate into ordered structures. Aggregation occurs in concert with proteolytic processing of the propeptide extensions very close to the cell membrane in invaginations of the cell surface.[125] Under these conditions the high concentration of collagen molecules drives the formation of fibrils. On the basis of electron micrographs of chick tendons it was proposed that procollagen molecules aggregate in an ordered fashion in secretory vesicles and are then reordered following secretion and cleavage of the propeptides. Although this concept was not widely accepted, recent studies of cultured cells confirm that procollagen molecules are organized in the Golgi into small aggregates.[116] Fibril formation results from aggregation of molecules in both a side-to-side format and in a longitudinal array.[126–129] The interaction of molecules is determined largely by the distribution of charged and hydrophobic groups at the surface. Collagen molecules aggregate in an ordered parallel overlapping lateral array such that adjacent molecules are staggered by slightly less than a quarter of a molecule in length (see Fig. 205-5). Fibril formation is a nonenzymatic process, and the nature of the interactions that govern fibril diameter is incompletely understood. Interactions with collagens other than type I collagen (eg., types III and V) or with proteoglycans or other glycoproteins are thought to control the rate of fibrillogenesis and ultimate fibril diameter.[130] Nonfibrillar collagens, such as type IV, type VIII, and type X collagens form meshworks, and type VI collagen forms linear microfibrils.

## Formation, Structure, and Function of Cross-Links

Collagen molecules in fibrillar array become substrates for the enzyme lysyl oxidase that oxidatively deaminates certain lysyl and hydroxylysyl residues in collagen and elastin (see Fig. 205-6).[131] There are four principal cross-linking loci in molecules of type I, II, and III collagens: a lysyl residue located nine residues from the N-terminal end of the triple helix of the chain in the telopeptide, a hydroxylysyl residue (usually glycosylated at triple-helical residue

*A*

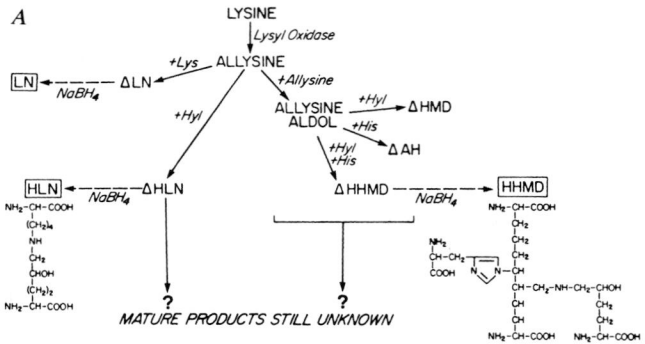

*B*

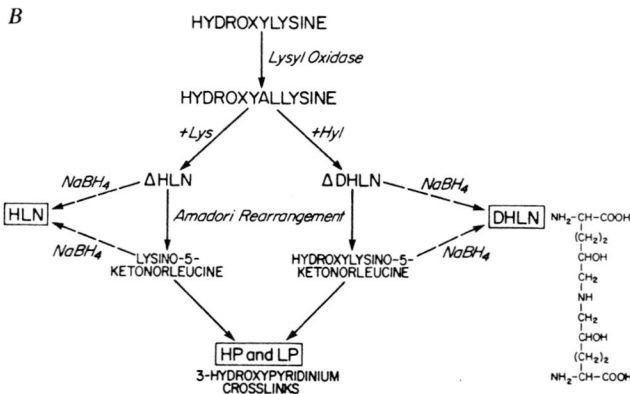

*C*

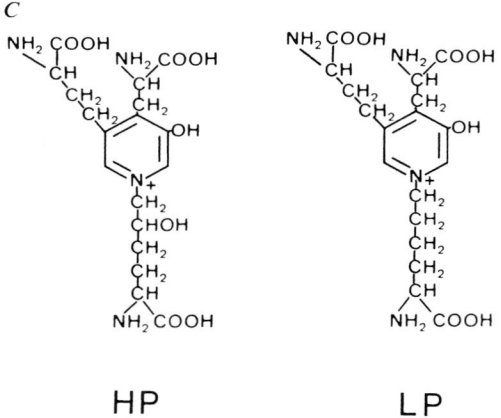

HP                    LP

**Fig. 205-6 Collagen crosslinks. *A.* Cross-links derived from oxidation of lysyl residues by lysyl oxidase. The oxidation of lysyl residues in collagen peptide linkage begins the minor cross-link pathway. The first product is allysine, which may condense with a lysyl group, an additional allysine, or hydroxylysyl to form bivalent compounds that go on to form other more complex products by addition of histidine or other residues. The structures of some compounds are known; others have not yet been identified. The intermediates can be trapped by reduction with borohydride to produce the stable products indicated. *B.* The major pathway of cross-link formation begins with the oxidation of hydroxylysyl residues in peptide linkage by lysyl oxidase to form hydroxyallysine, which may condense with lysyl or hydroxylysyl residues on other chains, rearrange, and then as shown in *C.*, add a third group to form the fluorescent 3-hydroxypyridinium (HP) and lysyl pyridinium (LP) cross-links: LN, lysinonorleucine; HLN, hyroxylysinonorleucine; HMD, hydroxymerodesmosine; HHMD, histidinylhydroxy-merodesmosine; and DHLN, dehydrolysinonorleucine. (*Courtesy of Dr. David Eyre, University of Washington.*)**

87), a glycosylated hydroxylysyl residue at triple-helical position 930, and a hydroxylysyl residue 16 amino acids from the C-terminal end of the triple helix in C-terminal telopeptide. The two non-triple-helical sites are the substrate positions of the enzymes. Because the sequences around the triple-helical residues are highly conserved among species and are virtually identical at the two sites, it is thought that this region represents the attachment site for the enzyme and explains the need for the fibrillar substrate. The lateral aggregation and staggered positions of the triple-helical residues and those in the telopeptide extensions in the collagen fibril place the relevant lysyl or hydroxylysyl residues in appropriate proximity. Lysyl oxidase activity results in formation of a reactive aldehyde (allysine or hydroxyallysine if the substrate residues are lysine or hydroxylysine, respectively) that condenses with lysyl or hydroxylysyl residues in adjacent molecules to form divalent cross-links. The enzyme does not recognize the glycosylated hydroxylysyl residues as substrate, explaining one possible function of that modification. Although divalent cross-links are first formed, there is rapid formation of more complex cross-links that stabilize collagen structures in tissues. The complex products may involve histidine or additional lysyl and hydroxylysyl residues to form three-membered cross-links among amino acids that stabilize interactions among three chains.

Lysyl oxidase functions as a monomeric enzyme glycoprotein with a molecular weight of approximately 32,000.[132,133] It requires pyridoxal and copper as cofactors, the latter probably for stability.[131] The human gene encoding lysyl oxidase has been isolated and assigned to chromosome 5q23.3-q31.2.[133] Multiple transcripts are generated from the same gene and, surprisingly, there is extensive homology of the human lysyl oxidase sequence with that of the murine ras recision gene, a gene that can reverse the ras phenotype in mouse NIH 3T3-transformed cells.[132] The consequences of these homologies are unclear at present.

Cross-linking is vitally important to provide tensile strength to tissues. Several defects that affect cross-link formation demonstrate the importance of this aspect of collagen metabolism. Indeed, virtually any mutation that alters the ability of collagens to form fibrils probably affects cross-link formation collagens and thus interferes with normal tissue function.

## INHERITED DISORDERS OF COLLAGEN BIOSYNTHESIS AND STRUCTURE

### Inheritance

Because of the complexity of collagen processing and the stringent requirements for maintenance of many structural motifs in collagen molecules, a variety of mutations that affect collagen structure or modifications result in recognizable phenotypic alterations. Most mutations in the processing enzymes result in clinically apparent phenotypes only when the defect is present in the homozygous state, as is true of most other enzymatic disorders. In contrast, most mutations that affect the structural collagen genes are phenotypically apparent in the heterozygous state. Because collagens are polymeric proteins, the effect of mutations in one allele are amplified beyond the initial expectations. For example, a mutation in a single *COL1A2* allele is represented in 50 percent of type I collagen molecules assembled (assuming that the defective chains are incorporated into molecules with normal efficiency). A mutation in a single *COL1A1* allele is represented in 75 percent of all type I collagen molecules synthesized (with the same assumption); but a mutation in *COL2A1* or *COL3A1* allele is represented in 87.5 percent of all molecules produced because they are homotrimeric molecules. Fibrillar collagens are the building blocks of extensive fibrils that depend on the uniformity of the components for their integrity. Thus, if even some abnormal molecules are incorporated into fibrils, the effects on structure can be dismayingly dramatic, further emphasizing the "dominant negative" mode of action of these mutations. In contrast, the effect of having a nonfunctional (or nonexpressed) allele is far less deleterious and would be expected to have fewer clinical consequences (see "Osteogenesis Imperfecta Type I" below, for example).

## Screening and Methods of Analysis

The first disorders of collagen processing were identified almost 30 years ago and were recognized because of the differences in the size of collagen chains in skin, in dermatosparaxis in cattle,[134] or because of altered posttranslational modification of collagen in skin in Ehlers-Danlos syndrome type VI.[135] Measurements of the relative amounts of collagens in skin were instrumental in suggesting that decreased production of type I collagen could result in the OI phenotypes.[136] Ultrastructural examination of tissues from individuals with EDS type IV suggested that structural mutations that affect secretion of collagens could produce disease following observation of markedly dilated RER in dermal fibroblasts.[137]

Characterization of macromolecules synthesized by cultured dermal fibroblastic cells rapidly became the method of choice to determine if abnormal amounts or structurally abnormal collagens were synthesized. This has demonstrated utility in some of the EDS phenotypes (some instances of EDS type I and II, EDS type IV, VI, and VII, and most of the OI phenotypes) because skin fibroblasts synthesize types I, III, and V collagens. The ease with which mutations can be identified in the coding genes depends on the effect that they have on molecular structure and processing. For example, large rearrangements resulting in longer than normal or shorter than normal chains are readily apparent when radiolabeled-proteins are examined. Certain single amino acid substitutions can also be identified in this manner, either by specific labeling (eg., with cysteine in some of the fibrillar collagens because ordinarily this amino is absent from the triple-helical domain). Dermal fibroblasts cannot be used to identify mutations in genes that are not expressed in them, unless genomic screening methods are employed.

Linkage studies were important to demonstrate that mutations in many different collagen genes resulted in their respective phenotypes. As these genes were sequenced in their entirety, direct examination of sequences, first with screening strategies and then with direct sequence analysis, has become one of the common modes of analysis.[28,138] Not all the candidate genes have been sequenced completely so intron/exon boundaries have been difficult to locate and genomic screening is not yet available—

although a wait of only another year or two should provide all these sequences.

## OSTEOGENESIS IMPERFECTA

Osteogenesis imperfecta (OI) is a heterogeneous group of inherited disorders characterized by bone fragility that is accompanied by abnormalities in teeth (dentinogenesis imperfecta), hearing loss, alterations in scleral hue, and evidence of soft tissue dysplasia (Table 205-4).[139,140] The vast majority of individuals with OI have mutations that affect the structure of genes encoding the chains of type I collagen (Fig. 205-7). The clinical heterogeneity is extensive, ranging from death in the perinatal period through marked short stature and severe bone deformity, to normal life span with only mild decrease in bone mass.[139] This heterogeneity led to many efforts to devise a classification of osteogenesis imperfecta that would predict natural history (with the attendant needs for medical intervention), determine the mode of genetic transmission, and facilitate a biochemical approach to this group of disorders. An initial attempt to classify osteogenesis imperfecta divided affected individuals into those with fractures and/or deformity at birth (OI congenita) and those who did not develop fractures or deformity until later (OI tarda).[141] This scheme was later amended to add a second tarda group to distinguish between the severe and often lethal group and those that survived. Although often helpful in predicting long-term morbidity, this division frequently provided a false sense of security because it could be difficult, several years later, to distinguish some individuals initially classified in the tarda group from those in the congenita group. Ibsen[142] in Denmark expanded the classification based on the additional criterion of the mode of inheritance of the condition. Beginning in the late 1970's Sillence and his colleagues, using radiographic, genetic, and clinical criteria, developed the classification currently in use.[139] Although the geneticists rapidly adopted this classification of OI into four major types (I-IV), it has not achieved similar popularity with orthopedic surgeons because of the difficulty in classifying many patients. The Sillence classification has been used to categorize most of the patients who have been investigated at the biochemical and genetic levels.

Classification of an essentially continuous phenotype into a small number of arbitrary groupings is fraught with difficulty and disagreement about the boundaries of types to be expected.

**Table 205-4** Osteogenesis Imperfecta: Clinical Features, Mode of Inheritance and Nature of the Mutations

| Type | Clinical Manifestations | Inheritance | Mutations |
|---|---|---|---|
| I (Mild) | Blue sclerae, bone fragility | AD | COL1A1 Null |
| II (Perinatal lethal) | Dark sclerae, severe bone fragility, absent calvarial mineralization, bony compression | AD (New mutations) | COL1A1 and COL1A2 substitutions for glycine exon-skipping paratial gene deletions |
| | | | C-terminal propeptide mutations that interfere with chain association |
| III (Deforming) | Light sclerae, bone fragility and progressive deformity, dentinogenesis imperfecta, marked short stature | AD | COL1A1 and COL1A2 substitutions for glycine exon-skipping |
| | | AR(Rare) | COL1A2 mutations that prohibit chain association |
| IV (Mild deforming) | Light sclerae, dentinogenesis imperfecta, mild short stature | AD | COL1A1 and COL1A2 substitutions for glycine exon-skipping partial gene deletions |

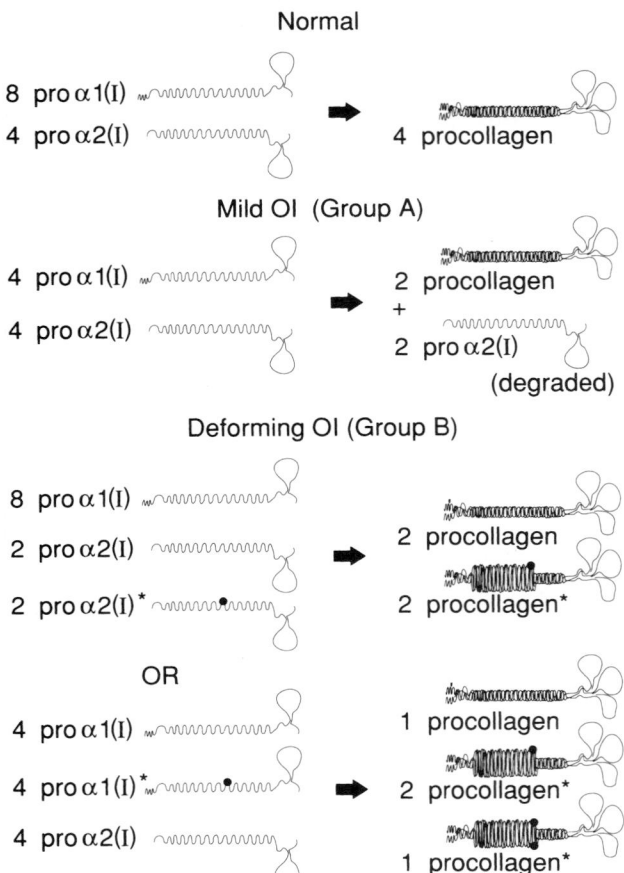

Fig. 205-7 Molecular basis of OI. In the mild dominantly inherited form of OI, OI type I, several defects in the structure of the *COL1A1* gene can lead to a decrease in the synthesis of proα1(I) chains and thus to production of less than normal amounts of type I procollagen (top). In contrast, in the other forms of OI in which bone deformity and short stature are common features, mutations within the *COL1A1* or *COL1A2* lead to the synthesis of abnormal molecules which may be poorly secreted but often interfere with the formation of a normal fibrillar structure. The mutations in the triple-helical domain are represented by the dark dots and the consequent overmodification is shown to the change in helix diameter.

Substitution for almost any glycine in the triple helix and skipping of any exon generally produces the OI phenotype. Eight substitutions of glycine (cysteine, tryptophan, arginine, serine, aspartic acid, glutamic acid, alanine, and valine) can be expected from single nucleotide substitutions in glycine codons. Codon usage in collagen genes suggests that over 2000 possible amino acid substitutions in the triple-helical domain of each type I collagen gene are likely to result in OI. Thus it is likely that even a molecular genetic classification will not be entirely adequate for prediction of natural history in part because of the enormous range of mutations. No doubt variation in other matrix components could also regulate the phenotypic expression of the primary mutation.

## Genetics and Natural History of Osteogenesis Imperfecta

**Osteogenesis Imperfecta Type I (Dominant Inheritance with Blue Sclerae).** OI type I is inherited in an autosomal dominant fashion and affected individuals typically have blue sclerae, normal teeth, and normal or near normal stature; they may experience a few or more than fifty fractures (usually of long bones) prior to puberty. It has been suggested that this group of patients could be subdivided on the basis of the absence (type IA) or presence (type IB) of dentinogenesis imperfecta (DI). Because

the presence of dentinogenesis imperfecta usually indicates the synthesis of abnormal collagen molecules, the OI type IB group would better fit in the OI type IV group if distinction between groups is made on biochemical findings rather than clinical findings alone (see "Osteogenesis Imperfecta Type IV" below).

Individuals with this type of OI occasionally have fractures in the perinatal period. Intrauterine femoral bowing and fractures at birth uncommonly can be the initial presentation. Fractures may occur first within the weeks following birth; these are sometimes associated with diaper changing but more commonly occur as children begin to walk. The most frequent bones broken are the long bones of the arms and legs, the ribs, and the small bones of the hands and feet. The fracture frequency remains steady through childhood and then decreases following the onset of puberty, suggesting that hormonal and other changes alter bone strength. Fractures heal rapidly with evidence of good callus formation, and without deformity.

The prevalence of this form of OI has been estimated at between 1 in 10,000 and 1 in 25,000, but because of the relatively mild presentation, it may be more frequent.[139,143,144] There appears to be no decrease in fertility or longevity in affected individuals. At birth, blue sclerae are readily apparent and may be darkly colored, lightening gradually to blue-grey in affected adults. Radiographic bone morphology is generally normal, although mild osteopenia may be present on radiographs and can be documented by densitometry. Height is usually within the normal range, although affected individuals may be shorter than their unaffected family members. Vertebral body morphology in the adult is normal initially but often develops the classic "cod-fish" appearance that is accompanied by loss of height in the later decades. Fracture frequency often increases following menopause in women and in the sixth to eighth decades for men. In about half the families with OI type I, affected individuals have early onset hearing loss, beginning in the late teens and leading, gradually, to profound loss by the end of the fourth to fifth decades.[145–149] The early phases of hearing loss may be primarily conductive and recent advances in design and replacement of the fractured and fused bones of the middle ear have provided significant restoration of hearing for many affected individuals.[150–152] Early hearing loss is typically high-frequency in type, and tympanometry results in a characteristic bifid compliance curve.[149] Later the hearing loss is mixed in type and surgical intervention may be less successful.[153,154] Additional clinical findings often include mild joint hypermobility and increased bruising. A variety of nonskeletal problems have been identified in individuals with OI type I, including mitral valve and aortic valvular problems, but it is likely that these are not significantly more frequent than in the general population. A small group of patients has been identified with slightly larger than normal aortic root diameters, without the risk of dissection.[155,156] Life expectancy is normal.[157]

**Diagnosis, Management, Treatment, and Prenatal Diagnosis.** The diagnosis of OI type I is first suspected clinically, usually because of the presence of a dominant family history, the observation of blue sclerae in the patient, and bone fractures, and is confirmed by measuring the production of type I procollagen by dermal fibroblasts in culture. The proportion of affected individuals who have new dominant mutations is not known. Ordinarily, about 85 percent of the collagen synthesized by cultured fibroblasts is type I procollagen and most of the remainder is type III procollagen; cells from patients with OI type I synthesize about half the normal amount of type I procollagen but a normal amount of other proteins.[158,159] In rare families, other types of mutations may be found. Diagnosis is particularly important in the newly affected infant for whom there is no family history because it can facilitate genetic counseling and help to reassure the family about prognosis. It can also remove the concern of child abuse in some families, and it may be important for families to have a letter from the child's physician stating the diagnosis.

Management of fractures is generally conservative and intramedullary rods are used only if recurrent fractures limit mobility. Several different types of medical intervention have been tried, none with notable success. In the last few years there has been increasing interest in the use of bisphosphonates, agents that interfere with bone resorption by inhibiting osteoclast activity.[160] Presentations at international meetings suggest that these agents may decrease bone turnover and increase bone mineral content in individuals with OI type I. The next few years will bring accounts of these studies and hope that intervention will decrease fractures and minimize bone loss later in life.

Prenatal identification of affected fetuses can be provided by any of several methods that identify the mutant allele including segregation studies with an appropriate family structure, identification of the nonexpressed allele in mRNA from the fetus, direct identification of the mutation, or by recognition of fracture or bowing of long bones by ultrasound.[161] Allele segregation studies or direct mutation analysis provide diagnosis at 11 to 12 weeks gestation if chorionic villus samples are used. Analysis of the amount of type I procollagen synthesized by cells cultured from chorionic villus samples taken at 9 to 10 weeks gestation could provide a means to detect affected fetuses early in gestation. However, our experience has been that the amount of type I procollagen synthesized by cultured CVS cells varies with time in culture so that the ability to identify alterations in the proportions of different molecules made by the cells may be compromised. Because of this experience, we have been reluctant to use cultured CVS cells, even with age-in-culture and gestational age-matched controls, for diagnostic studies based on protein analysis alone. Amniotic fluid cells are not useful in establishing the diagnosis at the protein level because the major population of cells that grows out does not synthesize normal type I procollagen.[162]

**Osteogenesis Imperfecta Type II (Perinatal Lethal).** OI type II, the perinatal lethal form of OI, affects between 1 in 20,000 and 1 in 60,000 infants.[139,143,144] Prematurity and low birth weight are common. Affected infants have a characteristic facial appearance with dark sclerae, beaked nose, and extremely soft calvarium. The extremities are short, the legs are bowed, and the hips are usually in a flexed and abducted (frog-leg) position; the thoracic cavity is generally very small. The radiological picture is characteristic but exhibits some heterogeneity[163] (Fig. 205-8). All infants have markedly telescoped femurs, bowed tibias, and virtual absence of calvarial mineralization. The ribs are generally beaded, although they may be broad throughout; frank fractures are rare in the newborn period and the vertebral bodies may be flattened. Death usually results from respiratory failure and frequently occurs during the first few hours following birth. More than 60 percent of infants with OI type II die during the first day, 80 percent die within the first month, and survival beyond a year must be rare. With the increasing use of routine early gestational ultrasound, first affected infants in families are being detected during the second trimester of pregnancy. It is worth noting that the subdivision of OI type II into groups A, B, and C and the identification of 4 groups with OI type II each demands too much of the supporting data.[163,164]

There was uncertainty about the mode of inheritance of OI type II. Seedorf identified instances of sibling recurrence of OI type II in which parents were not related and thought they were examples of recessive inheritance.[141] Sillence et al.[139] identified one family with multiple affected children born to normal but consanguineous parents. They were, in addition, able to cite a number of other instances of sibling recurrences, with consanguineous matings in some, to support the hypothesis of autosomal recessive inheritance of OI type II.

These assessments of the mode of inheritance of OI type II were either incorrect or incomplete. Analysis of more than 100 families into which a proband with OI type II was born,[163,165] indicated that new dominant mutation was the explanation for the phenotype in almost all instances. Although there were no

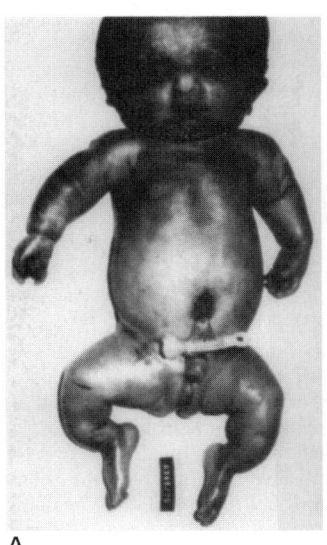 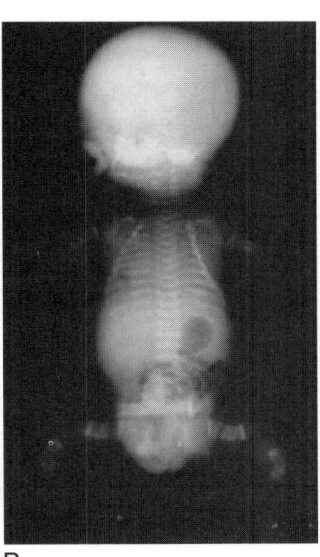

A.                                            B.

**Fig. 205-8** Clinical *A.*, and radiographic *B.*, appearance of an infant with the perinatal lethal form of osteogenesis imperfecta (OI type II). Infants with OI type II have large soft calvaria, a small thoracic cavity, short extremities with marked angulation of the lower legs, and generally have their legs in a flexed and abducted position. The x-rays demonstrate virtual absence of calvarial mineralization, shortened and markedly undermineralized bones, block shaped femurs, bowed tibias, and markedly flattened vertebral bodies.

instances of recurrence of OI type II in two studies, there were five in the third.[163,165] Biochemical analysis was consistent with heterozygosity for a mutation in a type I collagen gene and suggested that parental germline mosaicism for a mutation was the best explanation for recurrence of OI type II in most families.

The largest studies found recurrence risks of 2 to 3 percent and 6 to 7 percent among siblings. Recurrence results from parental mosaicism for the mutation that is lethal in the heterozygous. In the families in which the mutation was identified, one parent was mosaic in both germline and somatic cells, indicating that the mutation had occurred early in embryogenesis, prior to the allocation of cells to different lineages. On the basis of results to date, it appears that the mutation occurs equally in male and female embryos. In some instances, the extent of mosaicism is sufficient to result in mild features of OI (often compatible with OI type IV, see "Osteogenesis Imperfecta Type IV" below) in the mosaic parent.[166–171] Several options for prenatal diagnosis in subsequent pregnancies can now be offered to all families who have had a child with OI type II (see "Management and Prenatal Diagnosis" below).

OI type II needs to be differentiated from other lethal skeletal dysplasias (especially thanatophoric dysplasia (MIM 187600) and achondrogenesis types I and II (MIM 200600, 200610) and the autosomal recessive form of hypophosphatasia (MIM241500). While the radiographic picture of OI type II is characteristic, the ultrasound features early in pregnancy may be difficult to distinguish from other lethal forms of skeletal dysplasia. The characteristic rib abnormalities and markedly decreased calvarial mineralization are the most helpful features. Experienced pediatric radiologists generally have little trouble with the diagnosis in newborns although evaluation of x-rays of early fetuses may present problems. Nonetheless, many referral centers can provide diagnostic assistance. If there is any doubt, the diagnosis of OI type II can be confirmed by examination of the collagens synthesized by cultured fibroblastic cells from any of several tissues.

**Management and Prenatal Diagnosis.** OI type II is a lethal condition with a life expectancy ranging from minutes to months.

Death may result from pulmonary insufficiency, congestive heart failure, or infection. The most difficult management decisions occur at the birth of an affected infant when the diagnosis may not be clear and the infant has marked pulmonary insufficiency. Ordinarily, when the diagnosis is known, infants are offered supportive care and parental bonding is encouraged. Some affected infants leave the hospital and supportive care in the home is essential. Bedding that contains soft foam can decrease the fracture frequency. Because of the respiratory insufficiency many of these infants have feeding problems, and it is often difficult to maintain adequate caloric intake.

Prenatal diagnosis of OI type II has been accomplished by ultrasound screening of pregnancies between 14 to 18 weeks gestation (see above). By that age femurs are short, the thoracic cage is small, and calvarial mineralization is minimal. Analysis of chorionic villi for the presence of abnormal collagens and of collagens synthesized by cells grown from chorionic villi, or for direct mutation analysis can be used to identify an affected fetus or exclude the diagnosis. With advances in routine ultrasound scanning an increasing proportion of affected infants are being identified early in pregnancy proteins synthesized by those cells.

**Osteogenesis Imperfecta Type III (Progressive Deforming Variety).** OI type III is usually recognized at birth because of short stature and deformities resulting from in utero fractures (Fig. 205-9). There are well-documented autosomal recessive and autosomal dominant forms of OI type III, although the recessive form is rare in most populations.[172] Radiologically, at birth the calvarium is undermineralized, the ribs are thin, long bones are

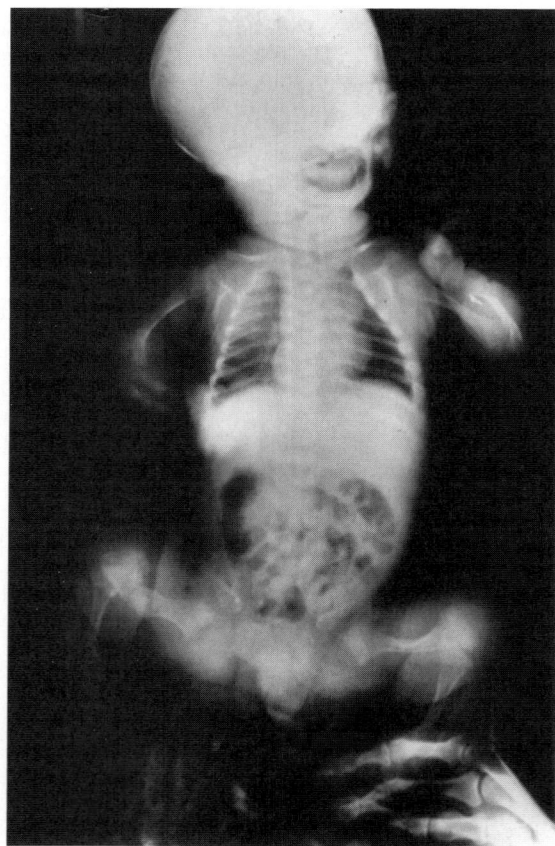

**Fig. 205-9** Radiographic features of the progressive deforming OI type III phenotype in the newborn period. Calvarial mineralization is adequate; there is deformity of the long bones and rare fractures of the thin ribs. The infant pictured in this radiograph was heterozygous for mutation that resulted in substitution of cysteine for glycine at position 526 in the COL1A1 gene. (*X-ray courtesy of Dr. Lester Weiss, Henry Ford Hospital, Detroit.*)

thin with evidence of fracture, and the skeleton is osteopenic. If no fractures are present at birth, they usually occur during the first year of life, and deformity becomes apparent during that period. Beginning between two and five years of age, unusual "cystic" structures form in the epiphyses of some long bones, especially the distal femurs.[173] These are areas in which the growth plate is markedly disrupted, probably by recurrent microfractures. As a result, bone growth is poor and marked stature results. The thin cortex results in frequent long bone fracture. Angulation deformities of the tibias and the femurs reduce the efficiency of weight bearing and increase the likelihood of fracture. Treatment is directed toward providing a more functional anatomy, and placement of intramedullary rods in long bones improves prognosis and may facilitate walking in some.[174,175] For some children, bone fragility makes independent ambulation difficult in all but the most restricted circumstances, and motorized wheelchairs provide the most mobility. Growth in these children is limited, and adult height between three feet and four feet is common. Because of the bone fragility and deformity, many children develop significant kyphoscoliosis and may progress to pulmonary insufficiency. Sclerae are often pale blue at birth and become nearly normal by puberty. Dentinogenesis imperfecta is common; the frequency of hearing loss is not known. Longevity is decreased although there appears to be a biphasic survival curve with early deaths in childhood and other deaths beginning in the fourth decade.

Initially described as an autosomal recessive condition, the OI type III phenotype is genetically heterogeneous. The autosomal recessive phenotype is the unusual form in most populations, but among South African blacks it may be the most common form of OI.[172] In families of most children with the severe deforming varieties of OI, recurrence is rare, which suggests that while there may be some recessive families, in others the condition usually results from new dominant mutations.[176] This has been confirmed in some families by birth of affected children to affected individuals and by biochemical studies (see below).

**Management, Treatment, and Prenatal Diagnosis of OI Type III.** The clinical management of children and adults with OI type III represents the most difficult challenge to physicians and others caring for individuals with OI. The primary objectives of therapy are to provide an affected individual with a satisfying and productive life. The major complications are marked short stature, severe bone fragility and deformity, and severe progressive scoliosis that can result in life-threatening cardiopulmonary decompensation.[157] The bone fractures and deformity can be managed by a combination of splinting, usual orthopedic treatment of fractures, and intramedullary rodding to provide anatomic positioning of extremities. Because of fragility, independent ambulation may be beyond the capabilities of some affected individuals. If that is the case, then efforts to provide mobility within the home and independence outside the home should be the thrust of therapy.[177] Scoliosis may be difficult to treat because of the compliant nature of bones of the ribs and their deformation with external bracing. In some instances surgical intervention can ameliorate scoliosis while in others it is of little long-term benefit.

***Treatments with Bisphosphonates.*** In the last several years there has been increased enthusiasm for treatment with bisphosphonates.[160,178–180] Reduction of bone pain, elimination of the characteristic sweating, and increased bone density are all claimed as outcomes of treatment although there are no carefully controlled studies of the effects of these drugs. Nonetheless, if they improve bone structure to the point that surgical intervention for scoliosis and respiratory insufficiency are tenable, then, even without improvement in fracture frequency or growth, these drugs hold promise. The most recent studies suggest that these drugs inhibit the mevalonate synthesis pathway and, as a consequence, interfere with protein prenylation. The major effect in bone is the reduction of the activity of osteoclasts, thus assuring less bone resorption.[181–183]

***Bone Marrow Transplantation.*** Bone marrow transplantation from matched sib donors, a far more controversial mode of therapy, has been performed in several children with severe forms of OI.[184] Although the objectives of the initial studies were to test feasibility, there have been questions raised as to whether the assessment of the children allowed that goal to be achieved.[185] A reasonable course at this point would be to determine if such studies in animal models permit engraftment of the marrow stromal cells (the source of osteoblastic precursors) prior to additional human studies.

***Prenatal Diagnosis.*** Prenatal diagnosis of OI type III by ultrasound examination of fetuses during the second trimester has been documented.[186,187] If the specific biochemical defect is known in an individual hoping to have children (in the case of the dominantly inherited forms) or in a child in a family seeking to have additional children (with recessively inherited forms or with dominantly inherited forms), the mutations can be detected in collagens synthesized by chorionic villus cells or in the DNA isolated from the tissue directly.[161] If families so choose, prenatal diagnosis by direct mutation analysis can be provided within a week of tissue availability while analysis of collagen synthesized by cultured cells takes 2 to 3 weeks after biopsy of chorionic villus.[28] Ultrasound diagnosis may not be feasible until considerably later (20 to 22 weeks).

**Osteogenesis Imperfecta Type IV.** OI type IV is a dominantly inherited disorder characterized by normal or greyish sclerae, mild to moderate deformity, and variable stature. (Fig. 205-10). Dentinogenesis imperfecta is common, but hearing loss may affect fewer than half of the affected individuals; when present both features are familial although they, like the stature of affected individuals, may vary considerably in expression. Some infants with OI type IV have fractures and deformity at birth while others have only mild to moderate femoral bowing. Birth length usually is normal, but by the age of two years height may be at or below the 25th percentile (frequently below the 10th percentile), and growth is generally along the lower percentile tracks thereafter. As in the other forms of OI, fracture frequency decreases at the time of puberty only to increase in the older age group, especially postmenopausal women. Progressive scoliosis is seen in about a third of individuals with OI type IV and may compromise pulmonary function if severe.

Although thought to be rare initially, OI type IV may be one of the more common varieties of OI.[188] Both sporadically affected individuals and large families are seen and there is significant intrafamilial and interfamilial variation. The intrafamilial variability can be striking (such that it may be difficult to decide whether the family is most appropriately classified on clinical grounds as OI type III, OI type IV, or OI type I). Several families have been identified in which a parent with OI type IV has had children with a lethal OI phenotype as a consequence of parental mosaicism for the lethal mutation.[169,170,189] Such extreme variability is rare but must be considered in counseling.

Life expectancy in this group is near normal and generally compromised only if pulmonary or cardiac function is affected by severe untreated scoliosis. The objectives of treatment and management of OI type IV are to provide maximum independence and mobility. The complications of dentinogenesis imperfecta, fracture and excessive wear of very fragile teeth can be treated by capping teeth with more solid materials. Hard polymers can be used to coat and shape teeth and improve both function and cosmetic appearance. Hearing loss, if principally conduction, can be treated surgically but if mixed or primarily sensorineural is managed with hearing aids

Prenatal diagnosis by linkage in the dominant families, direct mutation analysis, or analysis of proteins produced by cells grown from CVS biopsies are all useful strategies.[161] Ultrasound analysis is of little value because of the late appearance of bone deformity or shortness.

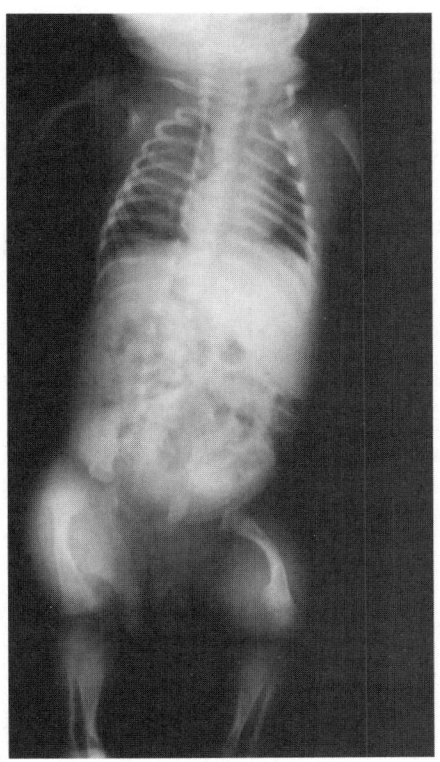

A.

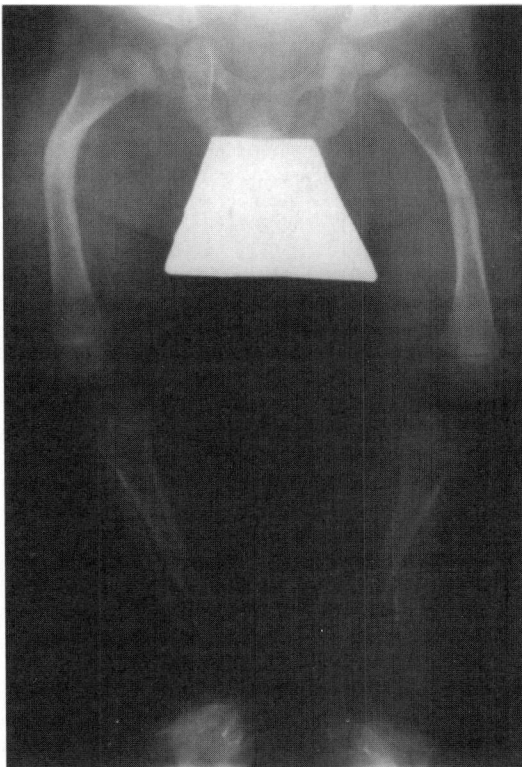

B.

**Fig. 205-10 Radiographic features of OI type IV in the newborn period *A.*, and at 8 months *B*. The most notable feature is the bowing of femurs, which gradually lessens during the first year. (*This patient is described in detail by Wenstrup et al. Hum Genet 74:47, 1986. X-rays courtesy of Dr. Alasdair Hunter, Ottawa.*)**

**Other Forms of OI.** The Sillence classification does not adequately describe all individuals with OI, a point that has become clear with more detailed clinical and molecular studies. As a consequence, additional types are being proposed although the criteria are not yet well established and the molecular bases remain unclear.[190] Other clinical phenotypes that share similarities to OI include the osteoporosis-pseudoglioma syndrome,[191-193] a recessively inherited syndrome recently mapped to 11q12-q13, juvenile osteoporosis, and maturity onset osteoporosis. In each instance, these disorders are characterized by marked osteopenia of unknown cause. There are no biochemical studies that provide clues about the nature of the mutations that result in these conditions. Bruck syndrome, characterized by an OI-like phenotype and contractures of large and small joints, may result from a defect in the hydroxylation of telopeptide lysyl residues involved in cross-link formation.[103]

Isolated dentinogenesis imperfecta (DI) is genetically distinct from the DI that accompanies some forms of OI. Linkage studies have confirmed that the mutant gene is in close proximity to the Gc locus on chromosome 4,[194-198] a region devoid of known fibrillar collagen genes. Teeth from individuals with isolated DI have been shown to lack a glycoprotein in dentin. Although the molecular mechanism by which dentinogenesis imperfecta is produced is not known, identification of a candidate protein distinct from a collagen suggests that mutations that affect the interaction of the two proteins could result in the phenotype. Thus mutations that alter collagen structure may produce OI and DI while mutations which affect the glycoprotein could produce DI but not interfere with other functions of the collagen molecule.

## MOLECULAR DEFECTS IN OSTEOGENESIS IMPERFECTA

### Biochemical and Molecular Bases of Osteogenesis Imperfecta

Now that more than 200 mutations in the type I collagen genes have been identified from people with different forms of OI, several characteristics of the genes and consequences of mutations have become clear. Although it is not yet possible to predict the phenotype knowing the mutation alone, it is clear that different classes of mutations exist and their effects on protein structure are important determinants of phenotype. Several different types of mutation give rise to OI (Fig. 205-7). Mutations that result in lack of function of single *COL1A1* alleles produce OI type I. Substitutions for glycine residues within the triple helix can result in almost any OI phenotype. The clinical effects of splice site mutations depend on their outcome, the position in the chain, and the chain in which it occurs. Finally, mutations in the C-terminal domain have different phenotypes depending on how they alter protein processing.

The type I collagen genes have more than 50 exons which in *COL1A1* occupy approximately 20 kb of genomic DNA and in *COL1A2* gene are distributed over approximately 40 kb. The triple-helical domain is encoded within 46 exons. Each one starts with a glycine codon (GGN) and ends with a codon for a Y-position amino acid of the triplet repeat structure of the chain $(Gly-X-Y)_{334}$. The exons in that domain are "cassettes" and when deletions of an entire exon occur the triplet structure is retained, although the precise sequence and placement of charged and hydrophobic residues are disrupted.[13]

Within the coding sequence of the triple-helical domains, mutation in two-ninths of all coding nucleotides ($GGN_7$, being the coding sequence for a triplet, in which G is the base guanidine) will result in substitutions for glycine and are likely to be phenotypically significant. With more than 50 exons each, mutations in any of roughly 500 bp of intron sequence in each gene would be expected to alter splicing and could give rise to identifiable phenotypes.

Although most mutations that lead to OI fall within the triple-helical domain (probably a reflection both of the density of phenotypically active sites and the length of the sequence) the carboxyl-terminal extensions of both chains are functionally important. The folding of the molecule depends on precise folding

of the primary structure of C-terminal propeptide, the formation of intrachain disulfide bonds, the interactions of the three chains of the molecule in a precise stoichiometry, and the propagation of the triple helix from the C-terminal end of the molecules. Thus an interesting array of mutations is found in this region which reflects very different effects — those on chain-chain interaction and on folding of a more globular structure.

### Substitutions for Glycine Residues in the Triple Helix

Single nucleotide substitutions within glycine codons are the most common type of mutation (Fig. 205-11). Three characteristics determine the phenotypic effects of mutations that result in substitutions for glycine residues within the triple-helical coding region of type I collagen genes: the position of the substitution, the nature of the substituting amino acid, and the chain in which the substitution occurs.[13,199,200] All the known published mutations in the type I collagen genes that give rise to OI can be found at the Database of Human Collagen Mutations (www.le.ac.uk/genetics/collagen).

First position substitutions lead to substitution of glycine by arginine, serine, cysteine, and tryptophan in approximately that order of frequency due to the number of synonymous codons, and the relative frequency of nucleotides in the third position. Second position substitutions give rise to alanine, valine, glutamic acid, and aspartic acid codons. In the proα1(I) chain, the product of the *COL1A1* gene, substitutions of valine, glutamic acid, aspartic acid, and arginine produce severe, usually lethal, phenotypes from the carboxyl-terminal end to the region of about residue 200 of the triple helix.[199,201] The severity of similar substitutions within the proα2(I) chain seems somewhat milder, perhaps because there is a single proα2(I) chain in a molecule and there are two proα1(I) chains.[199,201] Alternatively, the helix may be more tolerant of irregularity in the triple helix in the proα2(I) chain. Tryptophan substitutions are extremely rare, probably because of the rarity of GGG glycine codons. The relative frequency of substitutions by alanine, valine, glutamic acid, and aspartic acid do not correspond to codon frequencies and the reasons for the disparities are not clear.

In contrast to the gradient of effect of the large residue substitutions, substitutions by the residues with smaller hydrophilic side chains, specifically serine and cysteine, for glycine have a startlingly nonlinear effect on phenotype. These two substitutions have quite different effects within the molecule. There are no cysteine residues within the triple-helical domain of either proα1(I) or proα2(I) chains. Substitution of cysteine for glycine within proα1(I) leads to interchain, intramolecular disulfide bonds. The appearance of the new interactions between chains introduces a "kink" in the triple helix but may also serve to partially stabilize an otherwise unstable molecule and provide a new site of nucleation of triple helix formation. In contrast, serine appears to disturb triple helix shape or the rate at which helix forms, or both. Within the proα1(I) chain both substitutions result in alternating regions of lethal and nonlethal phenotypes. The density of mutations is not yet sufficient to determine if these domains of the two types of substitutions are congruent and there are few examples of different substitutions at the same residue within the triple helix. Substitutions by these two residues in the triple-helical domain of the proα2(I) chain also have a discontinuous effect on phenotype.

Substitutions for glycine residues alter the triple-helical structure[202] and delay triple helix formation. A helix appears to propagate normally from the region of nucleation at the carboxyl-terminal end to the domain of the mutation where it either ceases or slows at 37°C.[203] The effect on helical structure has been suggested by both modeling studies and by analysis of peptides with substitutions.[202,204,205] In both instances, there is a change in the pitch of the helix in the region of the substitution that propagates an altered relationship among the chains to their amino-terminal ends.

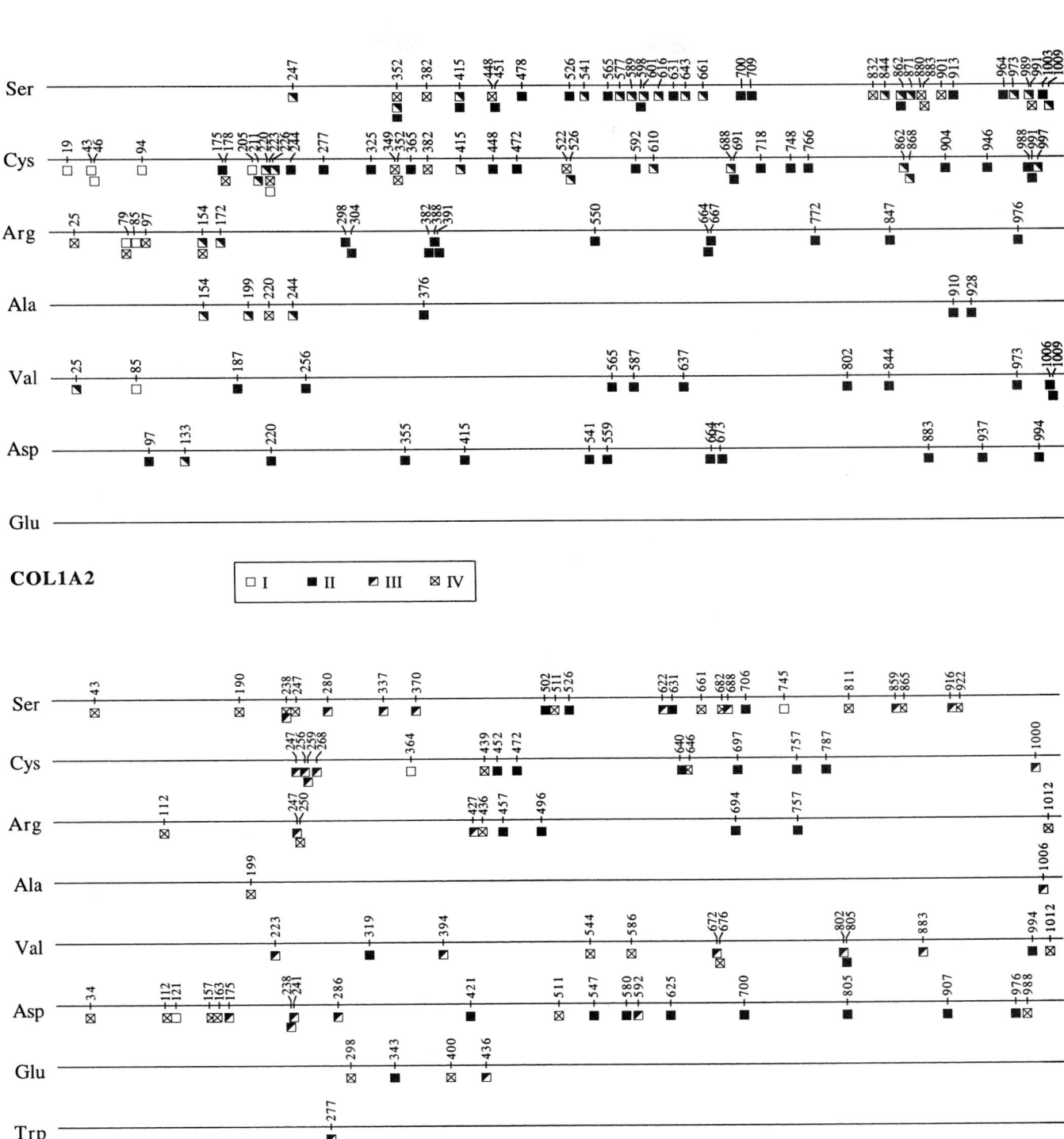

**Fig. 205-11** Summary of the effects of known point mutations that produce substitutions for glycine residues (Gly-Xaa-Yaa) within the triple-helical domains of the type I collagen genes and result in OI. The positions of the point mutations are shown along horizontal lines representing the triple-helical domain of the proα1(I) *A.*, and proα2(I) *B.*, chains. The amino acid at the left indicates the substituting residue and the number indicates the position of the glycine within the triple helix that is substituted. The first glycine of the triple helix in the proα1(I) chain (counting from the initiating methionine) is residue 179 and in the proα2(I) chain is residue 91. This nomenclature is used as shorthand to place mutations in the same relative position in the triple helix of the molecule. The phenotype is indicated below the line (see the inset box for the key). The mutations are derived from the Collagen Mutation Database, and the original references are shown there (www.le.ac.uk/genetics/collagen), or come from our unpublished collection of mutations.

Both the delay in helix formation and the change in the relationship among residues in the three chains help to explain why overmodification of lysyl residues occurs largely amino-terminal to the site of mutations. In the normal molecule, posttranslational modification continues until the triple helix is formed and stable. In the presence of mutations in the triple helix, the disruption of the helical motif does not allow the chains to come into proximity. A new site of nucleation must be found amino-terminal to the disruption and while this occurs post-translational modification continues. The association of the molecules that contain abnormal chains with the modifying enzymes is one factor that accounts for the delay in secretion.

Studies of cells that synthesize abnormal collagens and of bone from affected individuals suggest that some abnormal molecules are incorporated into the matrix, although not into the most highly cross-linked, stable portion.[206] In vitro studies of purified molecules demonstrate that inclusion of even a small proportion of molecules that harbor abnormal chains readily leads to failure of fibril formation or formation of abnormal fibrils.[207] These two types of studies have not been readily reconciled as there are abundant fibrils formed both in tissues and in cultured cells even in the presence of known mutations. Thus the precise manner in which these mutations produce a phenotype remains to be examined.

### Splice Site Mutations

Splice site mutations are the second most abundant type of mutation in type I collagen genes that result in the OI phenotypes.[201] There are two types of outcomes of splice site mutations: skipping exons or using alternate or cryptic sites. The former results in retention of the canonical triple-helical triplet structure, whereas the latter may or, more usually, do not. The effects of the use of cryptic splice sites depend on whether the spliced product can be resolved by the spliceosome and if it is in translational reading frame. Those that change reading frame and lead to a premature termination codon in the mRNA are generally unstable.

Within the *COL1A1* gene, exon-skipping mutations are generally very severe or lethal if they are located 3′ to exon 14.[199] For example, mutations in splice sites that result in skipping of exons 14, 20, 22 (Byers et al., unpublished), 27,[161] 30 (unpublished), 44,[208] and 47 (unpublished) are all associated with the OI type II phenotype. In the *COL1A2*, the chain seems more tolerant of deletions that affect sequences closer to the carboxyl terminal end of the protein as there are no lethal exon-skipping mutations 5′ of exon 27 and that mutation appears to be accompanied by a null mutation in the other allele. In both genes when exon-skipping is found in more 3′ locations, it is often associated with the simultaneous use of cryptic sites in the same allele, some of which lead to unstable mRNAs and thus, presumably, mitigate the severity of the expected phenotype.

One of the surprising features of splice site mutations in the *COL1A1* and *COL1A2* genes is that identical nucleotide substitutions in different donor or acceptor sites have different effects on the splicing process and, as a consequence, on the phenotype. A dramatic example of this disparity is the different outcomes of the IVS47+1G → A and IVS48+1G → A mutations. The former results in exon-skipping and the lethal OI type II phenotype (unpublished), and the latter results in use of cryptic donor sites, mostly within exon 48, creation of out of frame mRNAs that are subject to nonsense mediated decay, and the OI type I phenotype.[209]

The reason for the different splice outcomes was illuminated by study of cells in which an IVS8+1G → A mutation resulted in several different splice products.[89,210] These products included one in which exon 7 was redefined and exon 8 skipped, one in which exon 8 was skipped, one in which intron 8 was included, one in which intron 7 and intron 8 were included, and one in which an out-of-frame cryptic donor site in exon 8 was used. Examination of

splice order in this region revealed that normally there were two pathways, one in which intron 8 was removed prior to removal of intron 7 and the other, less frequent, in which intron 7 was removed first. In the "intron 8 first" pathway, the presence of the mutation led to splice paralysis and accumulation in the nucleus of both the single and the double intron inclusion product, and to the use of the cryptic donor site within exon 8, the product of which also accumulated in the nucleus. In the "intron 7 first" pathway, the exon 8-skip product resulted. The redefinition product may have occurred through both pathways. These studies, along with more recent ones[211] suggest that exon-skipping is the usual effect of mutations in rapidly processed introns, while more complex outcomes that reflect the use of cryptic sites derive from mutations in slowly removed introns. The appearance of multiple products from the same allele generally suggests that the introns that bear mutations vary in order of removal. The determinants of the order of intron removal remain to be identified and, once known, should provide the ability to predict outcome of splice site mutations in known genes.

Mutations that result in frame shifts in the mRNA generally result in degradation of the molecule through a process known as nonsense mediated mRNA decay and, with mutations in the *COL1A1* gene result in the OI type I phenotype. Similar mutations in the *COL1A2* gene do not have as clearly defined phenotypes in the heterozygous state. To date they are said to produce little phenotypic effect.

### Mutations in the Carboxyl-Terminal Propeptide

The carboxyl-terminal propeptides assure correct chain-chain interactions in RER in which chains of several different collagen types may coexist. The failure to find interspecies chain association, absent deliberate mutations, is a testament to the specificity of these binding domains, which appear to reside within a short, discontinuous region of the carboxyl-terminus of each chain.[113] Although no mutations in these regions have been defined that alter association specificity, mutations in other regions have been identified that either abrogate chain assembly completely or alter the efficiency of chain association. Different classes of mutations have dramatically different effects on the phenotype.

Mutations in the *COL1A1* gene that completely abolish chain recognition result in the OI type I phenotype.[212] Chain association permits molecules in which there are two or more proα1(I) chains, with the trimer that contains 2 proα1(I) chains and a single proα2(I) chain being overwhelmingly preferred. In the absence of sufficient proα1(I) chains, excess proα2(I) chains are not incorporated and are rapidly degraded. The end result is similar to failure to synthesize proα1(I) chains and the phenotype of OI type I results. The abnormal proα1(I) chains are may be degraded through the cytoplasmic proteosome system;[213] the fate of the excess proα2(I) chains is less clear.

In contrast mutations that do permit chain association usually have a highly deleterious outcome, perhaps because they entrap molecules and lead to dramatic overmodification of the unfolded portions of the triple helix. These mutations lead to activation of a separate recognition system, that of the unfolded protein response pathway. In cells that carry many of the these mutations the stress-response proteins BiP (GRP78) and GRP94 are synthesized at high levels and appear to interact with the abnormal proteins, perhaps directing them to sites of degradation as they are often short-lived.[214,215] These abnormal molecules may also be subject to degradation through the proteosome.[213]

### Null Mutations

Null mutations in the type I collagen genes have different effects. Those in the *COL1A1* gene result in OI type I in the heterozygous state. They would probably be lethal in the homozygous state, judging from the outcome in the *Mov13* mouse in which an insertional mutagen results in complete lack of expression of

*COL1A1* in bone.[216] In the *COL1A2* gene null mutations appear to have different phenotypic presentations. Homozygosity for a null at the level of chain association results in the *oim* model of OI in the mouse[217] and a similar phenotype in humans.[218] In both those examples the mRNA is stable but the proteins do not associate into molecules and are very unstable. However, if the mRNA is unstable, in humans the homozygote appears to have an EDS type II phenotype.[219] The reasons for these differences are unclear and the mechanisms of most *COL1A2* nulls at the gene level have not been identified.

The common element, regardless of how premature termination codons occur, is that the mRNA species is unstable. Although often referred to as "truncation" mutations, truncated proteins appear to be rare and, instead, haploinsufficiency appears to be the mechanism of disease pathogenesis. The site of nonsense-mediated decay remains controversial and may involve both nuclear and cytoplasmic elements.[220]

One of the common mechanisms to create new stop codons is substitution of single nucleotides within the coding regions. In some genes recurrent mutation at CpG sites (especially arginine codon, CGA) occur while in others they are more generally distributed and may affect other codons, and involve the noncoding strand. Several sites in the *COL1A1* gene have been noted to lead to these new stop codons.[28,221] Another mechanism is by the insertion or deletion of a small number of nucleotides, not divisible by 3, in the coding regions. As long as they are sufficiently distant from the constitutive translation termination codon, they almost inevitably lead to the introduction of new stop codons. Preferred sites for such mutations are in runs of single nucleotides, and mechanisms of slippage at the time of replication at or prior to meiosis likely lead to such changes. These regions are often the sites of recurrent mutations.[28,221]

### Effects of Mutations on Molecular Transport

The key to transport of type I procollagen molecules from the endoplasmic reticulum is folded status.[13] The effects of mutations vary from complete inhibition of transport to virtually undetectable delay in secretion. Substitutions for glycine are most likely to result in intracellular retention if they occur near the carboxyl-terminal end of the triple helix and if the substituting residue is bulky, for example, valine, aspartic acid, glutamic acid, and arginine. Substitutions of glycine by serine often result in relatively efficient secretion, despite overmodification and relatively carboxyl-terminal locations.[222] The reasons for the disparities in effects are not clear. Possibly the large residues exert a greater effect on folding and impair chain alignment more than small ones, as might be expected. Alternatively, there may be a greater effect on changes in helical pitch with larger residues. In any event, it is likely that these abnormal molecules are retained by association with modifying enzymes in the rough endoplasmic reticulum, prolyl and lysyl hydroxylases and protein disulfide isomerase being the best candidates.[111,223]

Mutations that result in exon-skipping or insertion or deletion of small multiples of triplets also delay secretion, largely as a result of retention in the rough endoplasmic reticulum. This has always been a result that is difficult to explain because triplet integrity is maintained. Studies of one cell strain with a 7 exon deletion from the *COL1A2* gene showed clearly that virtually all the molecules that contained the abnormal chain were retained in the rough ER.[224] Those molecules propagated helix at 37°C, but only to the region of the change in sequence—although at 4°C the helix could wind to its ends. More recent studies suggest that the pitch of the helix is different along the normal molecule.[202] The logical interpretation of these two kinds of data suggests that there is too little flexibility in these different helical motifs to allow propagation to occur efficiently. Thus, regardless of the size of discontinuity (single triplet, single exon, or multiple exon), the failure to propagate helix reflects variations in pitch. This appears

to provide a unifying model for these different extents of deletion or insertion.

### Effects of Mutations on Extracellular Fibril Formation and Mineralization

Once abnormal molecules are secreted their effects on phenotype are probably modulated through several factors: the influence of the mutation on ability to process the molecule, the effect of the processed or unprocessed procollagen on fibril formation, and the effects of altered fibril structure on mineralization.

Many mutations, even at considerable distance from the amino-terminal end of the triple helix, alter the efficiency of the N-protease, which cleaves the amino-terminal propeptide.[225,226] The propeptide is normally folded back on the helical portion. It is clear that deletion of the sequences of exon 6 of either the proα1(I) or proα2(I) chain, which contain the N-protease cleavage site, alter the structure of that fold. There are no equivalent experiments with molecules known to harbor point mutations, but some of these molecules have slowed cleavage rates. Bulky substitutions and deletions of sequence within the triple helix are more apt to alter rates than small residue substitutions. No doubt this influences fibrillogenesis.

Studies done with purified molecules indicate that not only is the rate of fibrillogenesis slowed, but also the structure of the fibrils formed is altered.[227–229] It is not clear how these findings can be readily reconciled with studies of tissues of infants and adults with OI that demonstrate normal fibrillar arrangements. Presumably the complexity of the biological system provides a buffer that facilitates fibril formation, perhaps even in the presence of abnormal fibrils.

Even when fibrils appear normal, mineralization is almost certainly disturbed. Mineral crystal size is often smaller than in normal and it is possible to capture unmineralized fibrils from these tissues.[230,231] The fragility of bone in the presence of abnormal fibrils probably reflects the altered crystal structure as well as the change in the fibrillar matrix.

### Translation of Genotype to Phenotype

Perhaps the most complex task in the study of OI is the understanding of the relationship between genotype (the specific mutation in a single host) and the phenotype in that person. The context of this difficulty is best perceived if we remember that the OI phenotype is, in fact, the physiologic response to a mutation in a single collagen allele (most of the time). This means that the entire genetic background, the product of millions of years of evolution in the context of normal collagen alleles, influences the expression of the single change. It is not surprising that it is not straightforward to find molecular correlates of clinical severity.

At the molecular level, OI falls into two different groups that have fundamentally different mechanisms of action: production of structurally normal but diminished amounts of type I procollagen, on the one hand, and production of abnormal molecules, on the other. At the clinical level, this distinction marks the divide between OI type I and all other types of OI. Yet even among those with OI type I there can be considerable difference in the clinical picture. For practical purposes OI type I results from mutations in the *COL1A1* gene that lead to premature termination codons within the mRNA from one allele. The several mechanisms by which these alleles are produced may explain some of the clinical variability. The most striking examples of molecular differences occur with splice mutations. Although those that result in use of cryptic sites that change reading frame are common, they often occur on the background of additional splice outcomes. In the event that these result in even very small amounts of in-frame deletions they could dramatically modify the phenotype.

The effects of substitutions for glycine residues within the triple-helical domain depend on the nature of the substitution, the site of substitution within the chain, and the chain in which the substitution has occurred. As indicated previously, bulky substitutions tend to have a severe or lethal outcome along the majority of the proα1(I) chain but perhaps slightly less predictably along the proα2(I) chain. In contrast, substitutions of glycine by serine or cysteine appear to have domain-specific effects, although the definition of the domains is not yet clear. Further, the regions that influence severity may vary between the two chains, as the same mutation in different chains does not always result in the identical clinical outcome.

Several points about these attempts are clear. First, there is not a saturation set of mutations. Consequently, domains are unspecified in part because the data are incomplete. Second, it may require much more complete analysis of the efficiency of secretion and the effects on fibrillogenesis and mineralization before these mutations are understood at the phenotypic level. Finally, the role of alterations in several other genes needs to be understood. Many of these issues apply for mutations in other collagen genes.

Thus while there is considerable hope that phenotype/genotype relationships will ultimately be understood, hope for any near term comprehension needs to be tempered by the reality of the number of factors that will need to be understood.

### Animal Models of OI

Three naturally occurring animal models of OI have been identified. Two herds of cattle, one first isolated in Australia[232] and a second identified in New Zealand (K. Thompson, personal communication), produced calves with a severe form of OI that was lethal in the first few weeks of life. In each herd a single (separate) bull sired the affected animals. In the Australian herd about 45 percent of calves born as a result of insemination of cows with sperm from the progenitor bull had OI, although the bull was phenotypically normal. Analysis of bone collagen from one of the calves[233] was compatible with the mutation being in a collagen gene because of the presence of normal collagen molecules and overmodified collagen molecules. These studies are consistent with a high level of parental mosaicism for the mutation that could have been limited to the germ cells. In the second herd there were also multiple recurrences of the moderately severe phenotype among calves sired by a single phenotypically normal bull. No biochemical studies have yet been completed.

A recessively inherited form of OI (*oim/oim*) results from the insertion of a single T near the end of the coding region of the *COL1A2* gene that creates a frameshift and alteration of the sequence of the chain near the C-terminal end.[217] The mRNA is stable and although the abnormal chain is synthesized, it cannot be incorporated into molecules. As a result the only type I procollagen molecules secreted are trimers of proα1(I) chains. This mouse does provide a model for the very similar human variant of OI[234,235] and provides animals in which to test a variety of therapies.

A strain of mice has been created in which a retrovirus fortuitously inserted into the first intron of one *COL1A1* allele.[236] Mice heterozygous for the insertion, known as the *Mov13* mutation, are asymptomatic except for hearing loss,[237,238] although tissues contain about half the normal amount of *COL1A1* mRNA and bones are more fragile when tested. Embryos homozygous for the insertion die at about 12 days gestation from rupture of the heart and arterial vessels.[236] Tissues contain no demonstrable type I collagen, and it has been surmised that death results from mechanical failure of the organs. Transfection of the normal *COL1A1* gene into cells grown from the embryos homozygous for the *Mov13* mutation rescues proα2(I) chains, which are otherwise rapidly degraded following synthesis.[216]

An additional transgenic mouse model of OI has been created by insertion of a *COL1A1* "minigene" in which a substantial portion of the triple-helical domain was excised.[239–241] Because some molecules are synthesized that contain the abnormal chain, this mouse may serve to test reagents that alter the production of the abnormal chain or modify the effect of incorporation of the abnormal molecules into fibrils.

Currently there are too few adequate animals models in which to do testing of therapeutic agents, such as bisphosphonates. Although there is recent progress in this regard, the need for additional models is apparent because they may provide the only way to determine the efficacy of medical therapies and to test multiple drug programs.

## EHLERS-DANLOS SYNDROME

The Ehlers-Danlos syndrome (EDS) is a heterogeneous group of generalized connective tissue disorders, the major manifestations of which are skin fragility, skin hyperextensibility, and joint hypermobility[242,243] (Table 205-5). During the last 25 years, genetic and biochemical studies have defined the molecular basis of many of these disorders. Mutations in eight separate genes have been shown to contribute to these phenotypes (see below). Correct diagnosis is important because the natural history and mode of inheritance differ among the types. For example, EDS type IV is often complicated by bowel and arterial rupture leading to a shortened life-expectancy while most other types are generally more benign.

This group of disorders has been recognized for many years, but the first formal medical descriptions appeared near the turn of the last century.[244–246] The early reports concentrated on the unusual features of the skin and on ocular abnormalities. The heterogeneity began to be appreciated about 35 years ago, and the modern classification was developed by Barabas,[247] extended by Beighton in the late 1960s[248,249] on the basis of analysis of patients with these phenotypes, and then later amplified with the insights provided by biochemical and molecular genetic studies. On clinical and genetic grounds, Beighton identified five separate types of EDS.[249] Subsequent biochemical studies identified a sixth[135] and seventh type,[250] and further clinical and biochemical studies identified additional families with diverse findings prompting the expansion of the syndrome. The issues of classification were revisited recently and a revised classification has been proposed that includes clinical and biochemical or molecular criteria for the diagnosis.[251] The discussion below is couched in terms of the former numerical classification of EDS although the revised nomenclature is presented in the table (Table 205-5) and in the descriptions of each disorder.

### Ehlers-Danlos Syndrome Type I (Gravis Variety) and Ehlers-Danlos Syndrome Type II (Mitis Variety), the Classical Forms, and Ehlers-Danlos Syndrome Type III, the Hypermobile Form

**Clinical Presentations, Natural History, and Genetics.** EDS type I is inherited in an autosomal dominant fashion and affected individuals have soft, velvety, hyperextensible skin; impressive joint hypermobility; easy bruising; and formation of thin, atrophic, "cigarette-paper" scars following trauma (Fig. 205-12) are additional cardinal features. Trauma often results in gaping wounds that bleed less than expected. Areas of repeated trauma (elbows, knees, and shins) generally have pigment deposition in addition to scarring. Molluscoid pseudotumors, small accumulations of connective tissue, form in the skin, and some individuals have palpable subcutaneous calcified nodules. Varicose veins are common. As many as half the infants with EDS type I are born 4 to 8 weeks prematurely,[252] usually because of premature rupture of the membranes. The diagnosis of EDS type I can be made in newborns but more often is not considered until children begin to crawl and stand. At that time joint hypermobility may become apparent and lead to concern because of a delay in walking. Early trauma from falling characteristically leads to scars on the forehead, shins, knees, elbows, and the under the chin. Because of repeated trauma, easy bruising, and skin fragility, the families of children with EDS type I (and several other forms of EDS and OI) may be evaluated by social service agencies for evidence of child abuse. Many individuals with EDS type I have mitral prolapse and a few may be symptomatic.[253] Structural cardiac defects are

**Table 205-5** Ehlers-Danlos Syndrome: Clinical Features, Mode of Inheritance and Biochemical Disorder

| Type | Revised Classification | Clinical Features | Inheritance | Molecular Defect |
|------|------------------------|-------------------|-------------|------------------|
| I: Gravis | Classical type | Soft, velvety, hyperextensible skin; easy bruising; "cigarette paper" scars prematurity | AD | COL5A1 and COL5A2 mutations |
| II: Mitis | Classical type | Similar to EDS type I but less severe | AD (AR, rare) | COL5A1 mutations<br><br>COL1A2 null alleles |
| III: Familial hypermobility | Hypermobile type | Soft skin, no scarring, marked large and small joint hypermobility | AD | Not known (Rare: COL3A1 G631S) |
| IV: Arterial | Arterial type | Thin, translucent skin with visible veins; marked bruising; skin and joints have normal extensibility; arterial, bowel and uterine rupture. | AD | Mutations in the COL3A1 gene that alter type III collagen synthesis, secretion and structure |
| V: X-linked | X-linked; Removed to "Other" category | Similar to EDS type II | XLR | Not known |
| VI: Ocular | Ocular, scoliotic type | Soft, velvety, hyperextensible skin; hypermobile joints, scoliosis; ocular fragility and keratoconus | AR | Lysyl hydroxylase deficiency due to mutations in the PLOD1 gene |
| VII: A and B Arthrochalasis multiplex congenita | Arthrochalasis type | Congenital hip dislocation, joint hypermobility; soft skin with normal scarring | AD | A: COL1A1 exon 6 skipping mutations that delete N-proteinase cleavage site<br>B: COL1A2 exon 6 skipping mutations that delete N-proteinase cleavage site |
| C: Dermatosparaxis | Dermatosparaxis | Very soft, fragile, bruisably skin, marked joint hypermobility, blue sclerae, small jaw, hypertrichosis | AR | C: Procollagen N-proteinase deficiency |
| VIII: Periodontal | Removed to "Other" category | Generalized periodontitis; skin similar to EDS type II | AD | Not known |
| IX: X-linked cutis laxa; occipital horn syndrome | Removed from EDS phenotypes | Soft, extensible, lax skin; bladder diverticulae and rupture; short arms, limited pronation and supination, broad clavicles, occipital horns | XLR | Abnormal intracellular copper utilization due to mutations in the ATP7A gene; allelic to Menkes syndrome |
| X: Fibronectin defect | Removed to "Other" category | Similar to EDS type II | AR | Defect in fibronectin |

probably not more common than in the general population. Scoliosis is uncommon and usually limited to the lumbar spine. The increased joint mobility is often associated with early degenerative joint disease, apparently because of the alteration in the joint mechanics, the most effective therapy for which is nonweight bearing exercises and mild anti-inflammatory agents.

Surgery in individuals with EDS type I may be complicated by increase in tissue friability and bleeding. Sutures should be left in about twice as long as usual to facilitate healing and decrease the likelihood of abnormal scar formation. The precise incidence of EDS type I is not known; estimates are on the order of 1 per 20,000. The life expectancy for individuals with EDS type I is normal.

EDS type II, also a dominantly inherited disorder, is characterized by joint laxity and by soft, hyperextensible, fragile skin. The phenotypic presentation is generally less severe than in EDS type I; prematurity is rare, varicose veins are less frequent, and skin fragility is less. Mitral valve prolapse is common, and some individuals with EDS type II develop premature degenerative arthritis. The similarity to EDS type I led to the grouping of the two as "classical" forms of EDS. Both may result from mutation in type V collagen genes although, in general, the phenotype is consistent within a family. At least one family with sufficient variability to include both phenotypes argues for the broader classification proposed recently that combines EDS type I and II into the "classical" type.[251,254]

EDS type III is a dominantly inherited disorder characterized by marked joint hypermobility, recurrent joint dislocation, and soft but not hyperextensible or fragile skin. Affected infants may be slow to walk because of joint laxity. The major complications of EDS type III are recurrent joint dislocation, which may require surgery for stabilization, and early onset degenerative joint disease. Mitral valve prolapse is frequently seen. EDS type III is probably the most common type of EDS, but precise figures are lacking and discrimination from variants of normal is often difficult.

The major differential diagnosis for EDS type I and II includes EDS types V, VI, VIII, and X (see below). EDS type III is most commonly confused with variation among normal individuals.

**Treatment and Management.** There is no specific therapy for the joint hypermobility or skin fragility in these three types of EDS. Dietary supplementation with ascorbic acid has been recommended with anecdotal reports of decreased bruising and a trend toward normalization of joint hypermobility. However, because joint mobility usually decreases with age, these reports are difficult to evaluate. Surgery is usually accomplished without major complications although sutures should remain in place for 2 to 3 times the usual time to minimize abnormal scar formation. The complications of mitral valve prolapse should be treated in the usual fashion.

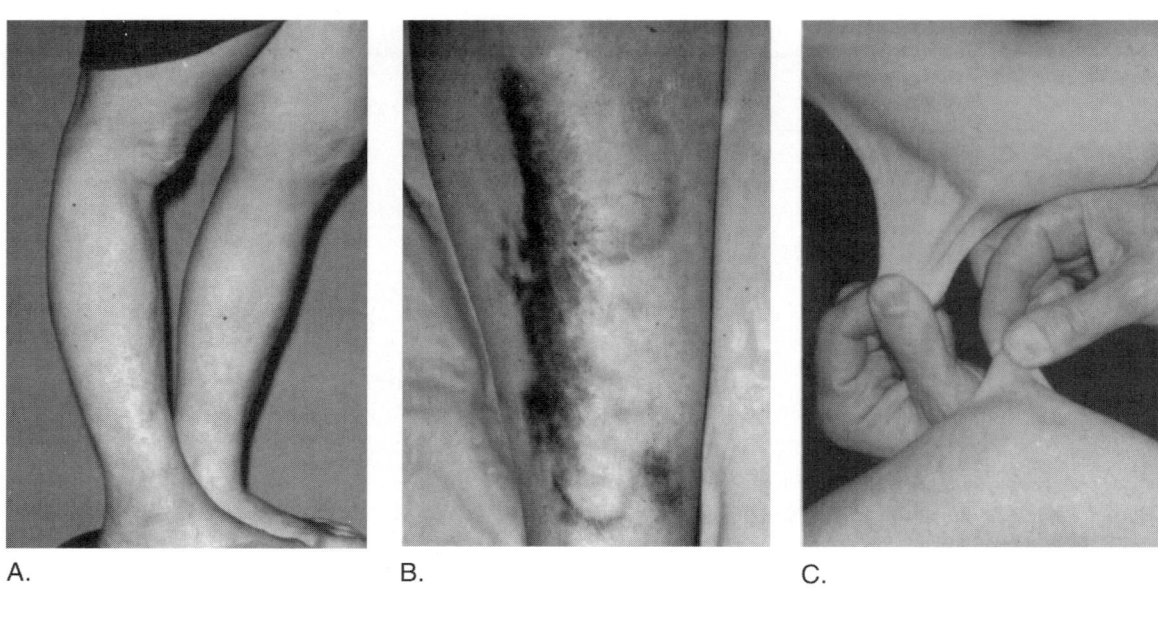

A.   B.   C.

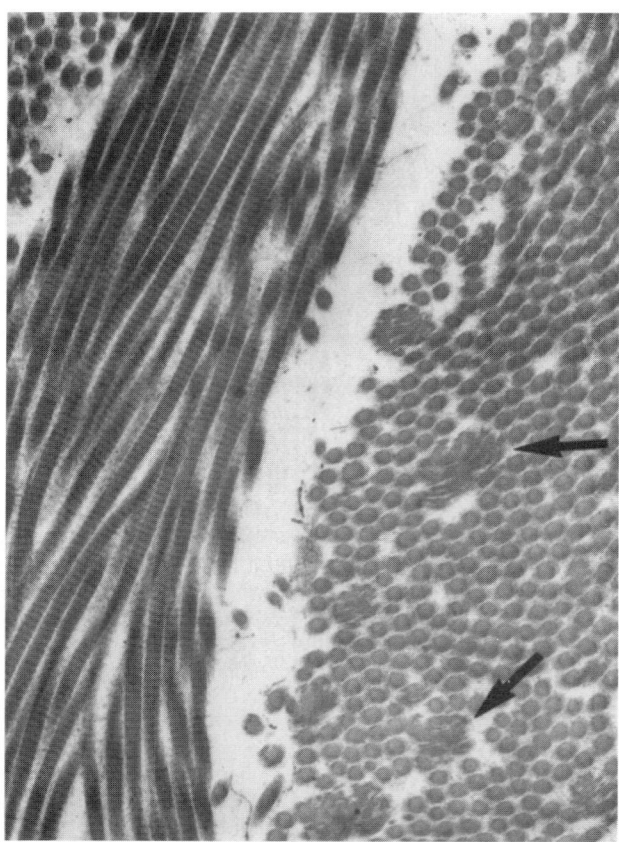

**Fig. 205-12 Clinical and electron microscopic characteristics of Ehlers-Danlos syndrome type I.** *A.* Large joint hypermobility. *B.* Cigarette paper scars and pigment accumulation in areas of repeated trauma. *C.* Skin hyperextensibility (top) with control (bottom). *(From P Bornstein, Byers PH: Collagen Metabolism. Kalamazoo, Upjohn, 1980. Used with permission.)* D. Morphological appearance of collagen fibrils in skin of an individual with Ehlers-Danlos syndrome type I. Fibrils are larger than control, and there are frequent "composite" structures (arrows). The morphological appearance of collagen in skin from individuals with EDS types II, III, VI, and X is similar to that shown here. The abnormal fibrils may be seen in other conditions. *(Courtesy of Dr. Karen A. Holbrook, University of Washington.)*

D.

### Biochemical, Genetic, and Structural Studies

*EDS Types I and II.* Studies with polymorphic markers in the *COL5A1* gene provided evidence that EDS type II[255] and mixed EDS type I/II in the same family[254,256] were linked to that locus. In some families linkage to *COL5A1*[257] or *COL5A1* and *COL5A2*[258] could be excluded. Biochemical analysis of type V collagen molecules synthesized by cultured fibroblasts supported the concept that abnormalities of these proteins contributed to the phenotype of EDS type I or II.[259] Analysis of cells from a child with EDS type II and an X/9 chromosomal translocation identified the breakpoint at 9q34 within intron 25 of the *COL5A1* gene.[260] No protein product of the truncated transcript was identified. Deletions that result from exon-skipping mutations in the region of the *COL5A1* gene that encodes the carboxyl-terminal propeptide,[258] or the triple-helical domain, and a point mutation that changed a cysteine to serine in the carboxyl-terminal propeptide[261] each result in the EDS type I or II phenotype. More recently, point mutations in the *COL5A2* gene that produced single amino acid substitutions (G934R) in the triple-helical domain[262] or exon-skipping[263] were identified in individuals with EDS type I or II.

Although the coding sequences of both *COL5A1* and *COL5A2* have been searched extensively, the yield has been surprisingly small. One recent search of 28 affected individuals identified only four mutations in the two genes (two in each).[263] The possibility that other genes might be involved was raised by linkage studies that appeared to exclude both genes[258] and the identification of a deletion of one allele of tenascin X[264] in an adolescent with Ehlers-Danlos syndrome and 21-hydroxylase deficiency. In the search for mutations in the type V collagen genes, *COL5A1* and *COL5A2*, the analyses have been done using cDNA amplified from mRNA obtained from cultured fibroblasts.

Although missense and splice site mutations in both type V collagen genes can cause the classic EDS type I and II phenotypes, it is plausible that other mutations in the genes could also play a role. The mutation that results in deletion of the sequence encoded by exon 65 of the *COL5A1* gene removed a domain that is predicted to function in chain-chain interaction during molecular assembly.[263] The chromosomal translocation resulted in failure to synthesize a peptide from one *COL5A1* allele, which, if expressed, would lack the chain assembly region of the carboxyl-terminal propeptide.[260] Together these examples suggested that other mutations that diminish the amount of proα1(V) might also result in the classical EDS phenotypes. Indeed, more recent studies now suggest that 25 to 40 percent of individuals with these phenotypes have null mutations in the *COL5A1* gene that result in loss of mRNA from one allele.[265,266] The mechanisms are similar to those found in the *COL1A1* gene in individuals with OI type I.

Biomechanical studies of skin fragments are consistent with abnormal collagen in dermis.[267] Electron microscopic studies of dermis demonstrated larger than normal collagen fibrils, frequent composite fibrils, and smaller than normal bundles[268–270] (Fig. 205-12). Type V collagen is an integral component of collagen fibrils in soft tissues. These molecules are found both at the surface of fibrils and embedded within them where they are accessible to antibodies only after partial unfolding of fibrils.[271] A portion of the large amino-terminal propeptide of the proα1(V) chain is thought to sit perpendicular to the axis of the large fibrils. In the absence of sufficient type V collagen, fibril size is increased and, on the basis of studies in affected individuals, the usual precise definition of fibril diameter is lost. While these studies indicate an abnormality in the formation of the usual dermal collagen structures they do not clarify the reason for the biomechanical abnormalities of tissues.

Two patients have been described who have joint hypermobility, hyperextensible skin, and mild aortic root dilatation and whose cultured dermal fibroblasts failed to synthesize proα2(I) chains. As a result, the cells secreted proα1(I) trimers.[219,272] These are particularly intriguing patients because of the previous description of a child with OI type III and a similar molecular phenotype.[218,234,273] The cells from the individuals with EDS did not synthesize any proα2(I) chains whereas those from the boy with OI type III synthesized chains that were not incorporated into molecules. Failure to synthesize proα2(I) chains is rare among individuals with EDS types I and II; the presence of aortic dilatation suggests that this clinical entity may have a different prognosis. It is likely due to compound heterozygosity for mutations in the *COL1A2* gene or homozygosity for mutations that lead to a null allele.

In a single family described as having EDS type III, a point mutation in a *COL3A1* allele (G637S) is thought to result in the phenotype, rather than the expected picture of EDS type IV.[274] It is not clear if this domain of the *COL3A1* gene is more amenable to substitution with more benign effects than the remainder. Perhaps, like the type I collagen chains, some regions are more likely to have benign phenotypes.

**Animal Models of EDS Types I and II.** Mink, cats, and dogs with clinical features of the EDS type I phenotype have been identified and studied in several laboratories.[275] These animals have lax joints and hyperextensible skin. Fibril structure in dermal collagen is similar to that in people with EDS type I in that mean fibril diameter is large, most fibrils are irregular, and there is an abundance of composite fibrils. The disorder is inherited in an autosomal dominant fashion in all species; the molecular basis of the disorder is not known in any.

## Ehlers-Danlos Syndrome Type IV, Vascular or Ecchymotic Type

**Clinical Presentation, Natural History, and Genetics.** EDS type IV was recognized as a distinct entity by Barabas in 1967,[247] although Sack[276] and Gottron[277] probably described the same entity a quarter century earlier. The biochemical basis of the disorder was first recognized in 1975.[278] This is a rare form of EDS, and estimates of its prevalence range from 1/100,000 to less than 1/1,000,000.[279] The disorder is the result of heterozygosity for mutations in the *COL3A1* gene, and while generally inherited in an autosomal dominant fashion,[279] it is common to encounter the first affected individuals in families. Although it has been proposed that autosomal recessive forms also exist,[280,281] these are rare, if they exist at all.

Affected individuals have thin, translucent skin through which the venous pattern over the trunk, abdomen, and extremities is visible; minimal joint hypermobility that may be limited to the small joints of the hands and feet; and easy bruising (Fig. 205-13). The skin over the face often has a parchment-like appearance, and in some individuals there is an aged or "acrogeric" character to the hands and feet; in the older European literature some individuals with "acrogeria" probably have EDS type IV.[277] There is an "EDS type IV facies" that is characterized by a "stare," a very thin nose, and the tight-skinned appearance.[282] Venous varicosities are frequent, may be severe, and appear at a young age. Even in families in which children are known to be at 50 percent risk, it is often difficult to make the diagnosis on clinical grounds in childhood unless bruising is severe or the venous pattern is particularly noticeable. Many individuals with EDS type IV are first thought to have disorders of coagulation because of the bruising.

The major clinical complications of EDS type IV are arterial rupture, spontaneous rupture of the colon, and rupture of the gravid uterus[283] and some individuals may experience all three. There does not appear to be a familial predilection for gastrointestinal complications, arterial rupture, or uterine tears, and the age of first involvement may vary from late childhood to the seventh decade, although deaths from complications in the third and fourth decade are most common.[279]

The location of arterial hemorrhage determines the presenting symptoms: stroke, intra-abdominal or intra-thoracic bleed, or limb compartmental syndrome.[279] The most common locations of arterial bleeding are in the abdominal cavity and involve the smaller arteries rather than the aorta itself. In some individuals there is evidence of aneurysm formation while in others the vessels appear normal by angiography. Arterial rupture accounts for most deaths in EDS type IV because of its frequency, the involvement of vessels from which hemorrhage is rapid, and because of the difficulty in repairing the markedly friable tissues. Surgical repair is possible but depends on early recognition of the cause of hypotension, the ability to distinguish arterial bleeding from GI tract rupture, and rapid and appropriate intervention.

Several individuals with EDS type IV have been described with carotid-cavernous sinus fistula formation and resultant unilateral exophthalmos.[284–287] Surgical repair or embolization has been attempted with success in some.

Rupture of the distal colon, usually in the sigmoid, is the most common of the bowel problems.[279] In some individuals it has been possible to identify diverticula on the antimesenteric border, but in most the bowel surface appears normal. The clinical presentation

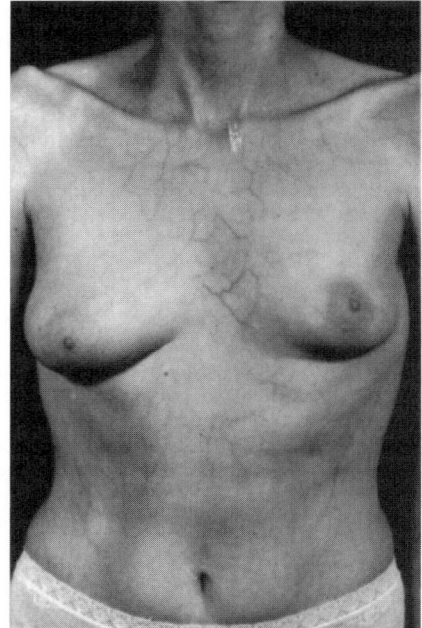

A.

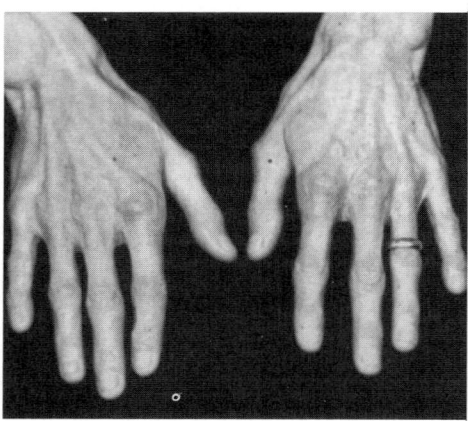

B.

**Fig. 205-13** Clinical features of Ehlers-Danlos syndrome type IV. *A.* The venous vasculature of the chest and abdomen is remarkably apparent in this 26-year-old woman with EDS type IV. *B.* Her hands have the aged appearance of acrogeria. She has a single nucleotide substitution with one *COL3A1* allele that leads to substitution of the glycine at position 1018 of the triple helix by valine (G1018V). (*From Byers et al. Hum Genet 47:141, 1979. Used with permission.*)

of bowel rupture is similar to that in individuals without EDS type IV and the surgical approach should be the same. Tissue friability and soiling of the peritoneal space are the major impediments to repair and rapid recovery. The degree of tissue friability differs among individuals and even in the same individual with aging. Descriptions of tissues with the physical characteristics of wet blotting paper are common in surgical reports. Assiduous attention to surgical technique and lavage of the peritoneal cavity with instillation of antibiotics and parenteral antibiotic therapy frequently permit rapid recovery. Following repair, recurrence of bowel rupture has been seen in some individuals, and the likelihood of repeated episodes can be minimized by removal of the distal two-thirds of the colon.

Rupture of the small bowel is rare but recurrent abdominal pain during childhood, adolescence, and adult life may result from mural hemorrhage. Bowel function is generally not compromised by these episodes, although occasionally regions of mural fibrosis

are observed at surgery or at autopsy in individuals with EDS type IV.

Uterine rupture is an uncommon complication of EDS type IV and generally occurs in the last two months of pregnancy or during labor. Uterine rupture in labor is accompanied by marked increase in abdominal pain, rapid loss of vascular volume, cessation of labor, and loss of fetal heart tones. Prompt surgical intervention is the only life-saving technique and rapid recognition of the condition is necessary. More commonly, uterine rupture is not recognized and leads to maternal and infant death. Although infrequent, the possibility of this occurrence warrants close attention to all pregnancies in women with EDS type IV and delivery in tertiary medical centers with careful monitoring during labor. The complications of pregnancy, in addition to vascular rupture and uterine rupture, include tearing of vaginal tissues during delivery. In one series, almost 20 percent of the women with EDS type IV who became pregnant died as a result of pregnancy complications. In a recent extension of that series, in which more than 180 pregnancies were identified, the mortality was more than 1/20 pregnancies.[279] The absence of such complications in another series suggested that pregnancy complications may vary in different populations,[288] which makes it difficult to estimate the overall frequency of pregnancy-related deaths.

Other complications of EDS type IV include keratoconus,[289] periodontal disease, and some birth defects.[279]

The life expectancy of individuals with EDS type IV is in the mid-40s for both men and women. Deaths in the third through the fifth decades are the rule with survival beyond sixty years of age being rare.[279]

Although initially proposed to be an autosomal recessive disorder, Ehlers-Danlos syndrome type IV is inherited in an autosomal dominant fashion. Almost half of affected individuals represent *de novo* mutations. Parental mosaicism for the mutation accounts for recurrence of the disorder among siblings whose parents are asymptomatic.

**Clinical Management.** When suspected, the diagnosis of EDS type IV should be confirmed by examining the biosynthesis of type III procollagen by cultured dermal fibroblasts or sequences of the *COL3A1* gene. The differentiation of this type of EDS from others is important because of the nature of the complications and the importance of prompt surgical intervention. No medical treatment is available currently to increase the production of normal type III collagen. The important elements of clinical management are prompt recognition of the major complications of the disorder, patient education, and clear communication between the patient and physician. A letter that summarizes the important complications of the disorder can be an important resource when affected individuals travel out of their local area.

**Biochemical and Ultrastructural Findings.** EDS type IV results from abnormalities in the structure, synthesis, or secretion of type III procollagen. At the ultrastructural level, tissues (especially dermis and vessels) from most individuals with EDS type IV have abnormal collagen fibrils and fiber bundles.[137,270,290] The dermis is often thin, collagen fiber bundles are small, and fibril diameters are either uniformly small or characterized by marked variation. Elastic fibers are abundant because of the decreased amount of collagen in the dermis. In many patients, dermal fibroblasts have dilated rough endoplasmic reticulum that contains the abnormal, poorly secreted type III procollagen species (Fig. 205-14). The biochemical abnormalities are heterogeneous. Cells from individuals in some families synthesize a normal amount of type III procollagen but secrete only 10 to 15 percent of it. The overmodified nonsecreted type III procollagen is sequestered within the rough endoplasmic reticulum and very slowly degraded. There is virtual exclusion of the abnormal molecules from the extracellular space. Studies of cell strains from other individuals demonstrate a marked reduction in the extracellular accumulation

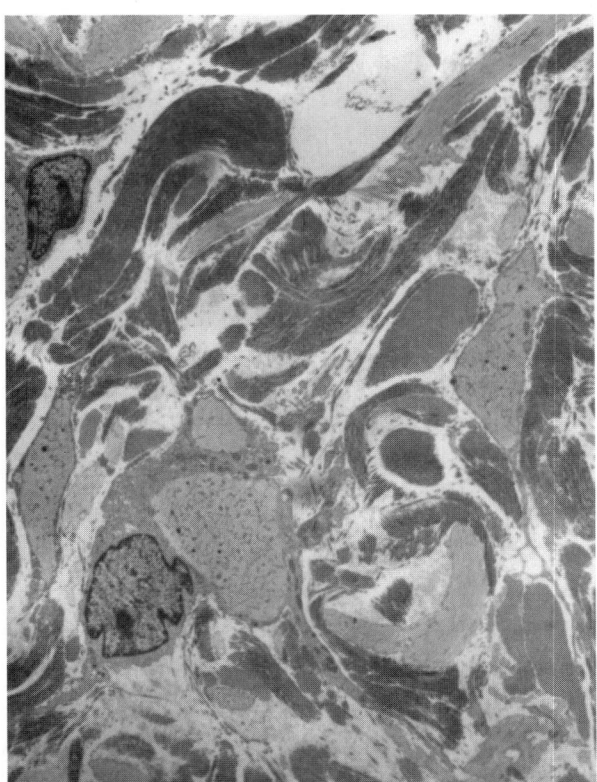

**Fig. 205-14 Morphological appearance of fibroblasts in skin of the woman with EDS type IV shown in Fig. 205-13. There is marked dilatation of the rough endoplasmic reticulum with a form of type III procollagen that cannot be secreted.** (*Courtesy of Dr. Karen A. Holbrook, University of Washington.*)

of type III collagen and procollagen but little accumulation of abnormal procollagen within the cells, probably because the abnormal molecules are more rapidly degraded within the cell. With heterozygous mutations in the *COL3A1* gene, only 12.5 percent of all molecules would contain only normal chains, if the mutation does not affect chain selection.

**Molecular Genetics of EDS type IV.** EDS type IV results from mutations within the *COL3A1* gene. Like those in the type I collagen genes that result in OI, mutations that produce substitution for glycine residues within the triple-helical domain, exon-skipping mutations within the triple-helical domain, and multiexon deletions have been identified (see Fig. 205-15). These mutations are summarized in the Collagen Mutation Data Base (www.le.ac.uk/genetics/collagen) and by Kuivaniemi et al.[201]

Substitutions for glycine residues along the length of the triple helix give rise to the EDS type IV phenotype. Between those published (summarized in the Collagen Mutation Database) and those identified in this laboratory more than 130 such mutations have been identified (Fig. 205-15). Of those identified there are 7 substitutions of cysteine for glycine, 26 substitutions by arginine, 19 by serine, 23 by aspartic acid, 27 by glutamic acid, 1 by alanine, and 27 by valine. The most common substitution is G016S, a CpG site in exon 7, of which 9 have been identified. A single substitution of tryptophan for glycine has been identified, probably a reflection of the rarity of the GGG glycine codon. The rarity of substitutions of alanine for glycine substitutions is unexplained, as is the relative paucity of substitutions of cysteine for glycine. Substitutions of glycine by alanine are uncommon in the type I collagen genes in OI, as well. A peptide that contains sequences from the proα1(I) chain with a substitution of glycine by alanine at one site does form triple helix; and x-ray crystallographic studies

of crystals demonstrate that there is a subtle alteration in the conformation with slight untwisting of the triple helix. A water bond substitutes direct hydrogen bonding within the triple helix. It is possible that collagen sequence militates against second position substitutions of C for G (GGN → GCN; gly → ala) or, alternatively, alanine may have less consequence for molecular structure so that substitutions induce a milder phenotype. At present it is not possible to identify specific relationships between the type of substitution for glycine, the position in which substitutions occur, and the nature or timing of complications.[279] Mutations that result in substitutions near the carboxyl-terminal end of the triple helix seem more likely to result in the acrogeric picture.[282] Another exception may be the case of the G637S mutation that appears to give rise to an EDS type III-like picture.[274] Substitutions for glycine are the most common of the identified mutations in the *COL3A1* gene.

Splice site mutations are the next most abundant changes that result in the EDS type IV phenotype.[201] One site, the first nucleotide of the donor splice site in intron 24 occurs as frequently as the G016S mutation. Other mutations that result in exon skipping are spread throughout the gene. In the majority of instances the mutations are in donor sites.[291] Mutations in some introns result in unusual outcomes.[292] For example donor site +1G → A mutations in most exons result in skipping of the preceding exon. However, in intron 20 a very complex mixture of outcomes (skipping, intron inclusion, use of a cryptic site within the intron, and use of a cryptic donor site in the exon) have been identified.[291,292] In intron 42 the mutation results in use of a cryptic site within the intron, addition of 30nt to the mRNA, and insertion of 10 amino acids that are not the canonical triplets.[291,292] The different outcomes of identical splice mutations may well reflect the effect of splice order, just as it appears to do in the *COL1A1* gene. Splice mutations that result in null alleles have not been encountered, although some of the mRNA species encountered with the intron 20 mutation have premature termination codons. It may well be that these have more subtle presentations at the protein level and will require increased diligence to identify.

In contrast to multiexon deletions in the *COL1A1* and *COL1A2* genes, the phenotypic consequences of these mutations in the *COL3A1* gene are not demonstrably more severe than other types of mutations in the gene.

**Prenatal Diagnosis and Recurrence.** Parental mosaicism for new dominant mutations in the *COL3A1* gene has been recognized and accounts for recurrence of the phenotype among siblings with normal parents.[293–295] Biochemical or molecular genetic prenatal diagnosis can be achieved in the same manner as outlined for OI.

**Genotype to Phenotype.** The mechanisms by which mutations in the *COL3A1* result in the EDS type IV phenotype remain unclear. In many soft tissues, type III collagen is expressed early in development and may create a scaffold for elaboration of additional structures. Type III collagen forms heteropolymeric fibrils with type I and type V collagen (probably among others) and has a role in regulation of fibril diameter. The major effect, however, still appears to be on formation of matrices that have adequate tensile strength, through mechanisms that deserve further investigation.

**Animal Models.** There are no naturally occurring animal models of EDS type IV. Homozygosity for a null *Col3a1* allele in mice leads to diminished survival and early death from arterial rupture. The heterozygotes appear to have a normal life span.[23]

## Ehlers-Danlos Syndrome Type V, the X-Linked Type

**Clinical Features, Natural History, and Genetics.** EDS type V has been used to describe two families in which the inheritance of a phenotype clinically similar to EDS type II is manifested. Intramuscular hemorrhage is a common finding and X-linked

COL3A1

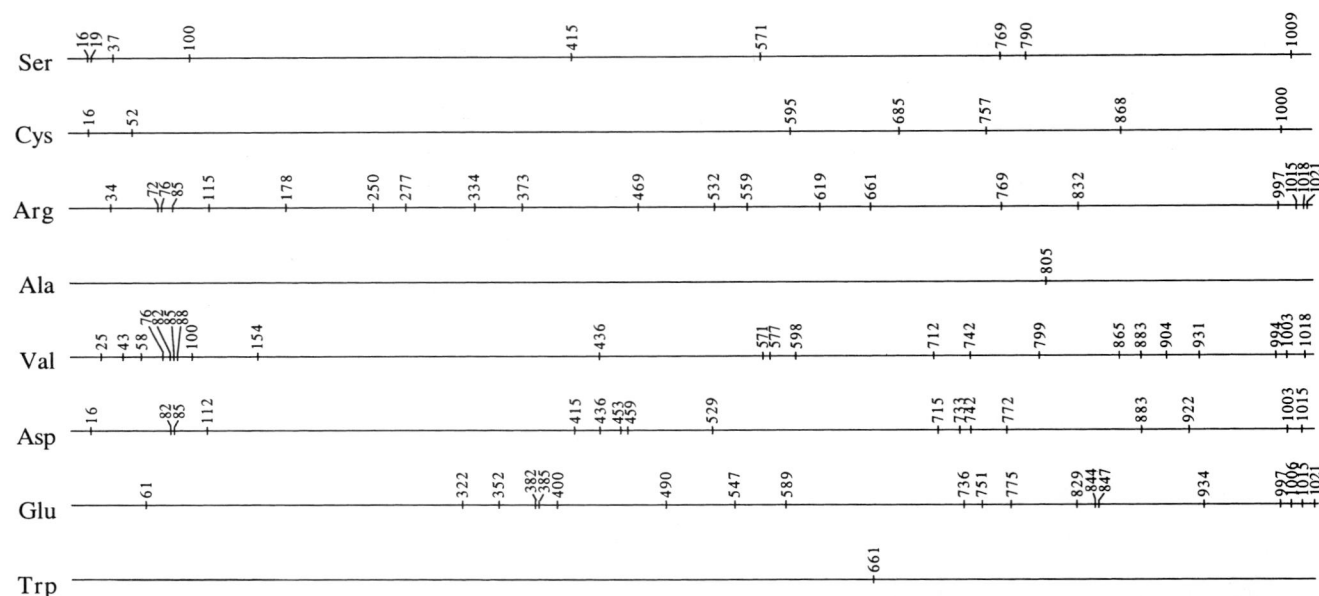

Fig. 205-15 Mutations in the *COL3A1* gene that result in substitutions for glycine in the triple-helical domain of the proα1(III) chains. The mutations are annotated in the same fashion as in Fig. 205-11. The first glycine of the triple helix is at position 168 of the proα1(III) chain. The original publications that contain the published mutations are described in the Collagen Mutation Database (www.le.ac.uk/genetics/collagen). The remaining mutations are derived from our own studies and summarized in Pepin et al.[279]

recessive inheritance, rather than variable expression of an autosomal dominant phenotype has been assumed.[242,296] The original authors suggested that the disorder is rare; Steinmann et al.[243] suggested that this entity does not currently warrant a distinct designation.

**Biochemical Studies.** In studies of cells from members of the two original families with EDS type V, the activity of lysyl oxidase in the medium was normal.[297,298] At the time the studies were done it was thought that the lysyl oxidase gene was on the X-chromosome (it is on 16). Close linkage to the Xg blood group (short arm of the X-chromosome) and to the loci for color blindness (long arm of the X-chromosome) have both been excluded.

### Ehlers-Danlos Syndrome Type VI, the Ocular-Scoliotic Type

**Clinical Features, Natural History, and Genetics.** Individuals with EDS type VI, an autosomal recessive condition,[135] often have soft, hyperextensible skin, joint hypermobility, scoliosis, ocular fragility, and a marfanoid habitus (Fig. 205-16). Microcornea and recurrent intraocular bleeding, with resultant blindness, are features in some patients. Some children have been identified because of delay in reaching major motor milestones, the result of marked joint laxity.[299] Others have been identified by screening sporadically affected individuals with EDS for decreased amounts of hydroxylysine in skin. The disorder is uncommon and about four dozen individuals have now been identified.[300–309]

Because of the relatively small number of affected individuals identified so far, the natural history of the disorder is not well understood. Three major complications have been identified: severe kyphoscoliosis, which may be resistant to external bracing or surgical intervention; blindness from globe rupture or repeated retinal hemorrhage; and morbidity or death from vascular rupture. Kyphoscoliosis is common among children ascertained due to delay in motor development, but it does not represent a universal accompaniment of the biochemical disorder. When severe, the kyphoscoliosis can lead to cardiopulmonary failure, and death has been reported in the third decade. One of the index patients with EDS type VI suffered ocular globe rupture from minimal trauma.[135] Retinal hemorrhage and GI hemorrhage have been known to affect others with EDS type VI. The proband in the second family identified with EDS type VI died in her sixth decade, probably as a result of intra-abdominal arterial rupture.[310]

The phenotype may be genetically heterogeneous because at least one family has been identified in which two affected male sibs, with normal parents, have skin and joint manifestation of EDS and are blind from retinal hemorrhage. Both have normal levels of lysyl hydroxylation in skin collagen and have normal levels of lysyl hydroxylase enzyme in cultured cells.[311]

**Clinical Management and Prenatal Diagnosis.** Because of the apparent frequency of severe kyphoscoliosis and accompanying cardiorespiratory complications, the complications of ocular globe fragility and retinal hemorrhage, and the autosomal recessive mode of inheritance of EDS type VI, it is important that this diagnosis be considered in all sporadic individuals with a compatible phenotype (e.g., EDS type II, V, X). The most expeditious method of diagnosis is the analysis of pyridinoline cross-links in urine.[312,313]

The orthopedic management of scoliosis should follow accepted orthopedic practice. The efficacy of bracing and of surgical intervention is not yet established. Routine eye exam should be recommended because of the relatively high incidence of intraocular bleeding, globe fragility, and keratoconus. While no specific therapy has been demonstrated to be effective, the use of pharmacological doses of ascorbic acid, a cofactor for lysyl hydroxylase, has been advocated, and an increase in urinary excretion of hydroxylysine has been found following long-term treatment with the vitamin.

Prenatal diagnosis by measurement of lysyl hydroxylase enzyme activity in amniotic fluid cells has been attempted in one family at risk, and the birth of an unaffected but heterozygous

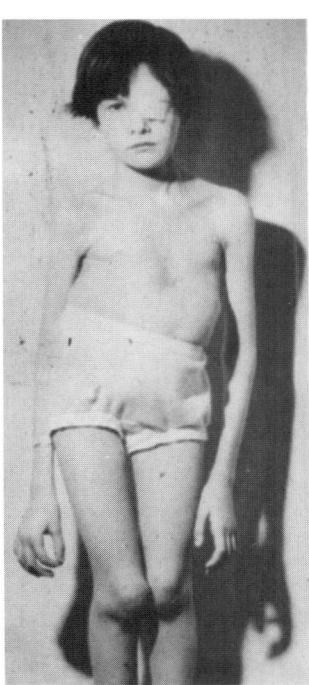

**Fig. 205-16 Clinical appearance of the index patient with Ehlers-Danlos syndrome type VI. (*Courtesy of Dr. Sheldon Pinnell, Duke University.*)**

infant was correctly predicted.[314] Amniotic fluid cells synthesize amounts of lysyl hydroxylase that are roughly equivalent to those synthesized by dermal fibroblasts. A more reliable diagnostic procedure is the identification of the causative mutation(s) in the at-risk fetus.[315]

**Biochemical and Molecular Genetic Studies.** The EDS type VI phenotype results from mutations in the *PLOD1* gene (lysyl hydroxylase 1) that lead to markedly decreased activity of the enzyme. About 20 percent of the mutations identified represent duplication of exons 10 to 16 of the gene because of Alu-Alu recombination. The majority of these alleles appear to have similar flanking polymorphisms suggesting a single or small number of originating events.[303,308,316] The other mutations identified either result in premature termination codons and unstable alleles[301,309,317] or sequence changes that might be expected to change folding or activity of the enzyme.[306,309,318,319]

The posttranslational hydroxylation of lysyl residues in types I and III collagens in skin is markedly reduced, but that of type II collagen in cartilage is normal or near normal in tissues from affected individuals in which it has been measured. It is not clear if the hydroxylation of other collagens is the consequence of enzymes encoded by the additional PLOD genes.

Decreased hydroxylation of lysyl residues in type I collagen interferes with the formation of normal cross-links among collagen molecules.[105] Although cross-links form in the absence of lysyl hydroxylation, the lysine-derived cross-links are not as stable as those derived from hydroxylysine and do not mature as readily to the multicomponent intermolecular links that stabilize molecular interactions at a larger scale. Presumably, the clinical phenotype results from the absence of the more complex cross-links.

## Ehlers-Danlos Syndrome Type VII, the Arthrochalasis Types and Dermatosparaxis

**Natural History and Genetics.** EDS type VII designates three disorders in which there are defects in the conversion of type I procollagen to collagen. In two the defects are in the substrate (EDS types VIIA and VIIB, the arthrochalasis types), and in the

third they are in the converting enzyme, procollagen N-protease (EDS type VIIC or dermatosparaxis).

EDS types VIIA and VIIB are characterized by marked joint hypermobility, multiple joint dislocations, and bilateral congenital hip dislocation (Fig. 205-17).[320,321] The hip dislocation is often difficult to reduce, even with surgery. Mild to moderate short stature is seen in some individuals and midface hypoplasia may be present. The precise prevalence of the condition is not known but it is probably uncommon. Congenital hip dislocation is one of the more frequent birth defects in the general population (with an incidence of approximately 1/500 live births), but only a small proportion of those infants has EDS type VII. Although all but two of the described individuals are sporadic in their families, all the biochemical studies are compatible with the result of dominant mutations (see below).

The major complications of EDS type VIIA and VIIB are premature degenerative joint disease. Bone fractures occur in some individuals with EDS type VIIA or VIIB.

**Biochemical Abnormalities and Molecular Genetics.** Initially, EDS type VII was thought to result from abnormalities in the enzyme that cleaves the N-terminal propeptide extension from type I procollagen,[250] analogous to a recessively inherited disorder in cattle, sheep, cats, and dogs.[134,322] Restudy of some of the original patients and detailed study of collagens synthesized by cells from several new patients demonstrated that, instead, the mutations involve the cleavage sites of the substrate proα1(I) and proα2(I) chains.[323–329] In all patients with EDS type VIIA or VIIB in which the mutation has been characterized, the mRNA from the mutant allele lacks all or most of the sequence of exon 6, the domain that encodes the cleavage site for the N-proteinase. At the genomic level, the mutations at the acceptor site result in exon-skipping, use of a cryptic site within the exon that deletes 15nt from the mRNA, or both.[320] Donor site mutations result only in skipping, and substitutions at the last nucleotide of the exon result in skipping or normal splicing with about equal frequency. In cultured cells it is possible to recognize a defect in the rate of conversion of procollagen to collagen and a retention of N-terminal propeptide extensions on the abnormal chains. The deleted sequences contain the cleavage site for the enzyme. Because the enzyme works in a concerted fashion and requires all three chains to be accessible, the *COL1A2* mutations result in abnormalities in half the molecules, and mutations in the *COL1A1* chain result in abnormalities in three-quarters of the molecules synthesized. It is likely that the phenotypic effect of the mutations derives from alterations in cross-link formation and fibrillogenesis that result in decreased tensile strength of most tissues made up principally of type I collagen.[330]

**EDS Type VIIC, Dermatosparaxis.** Search for the recessively inherited EDS type VIIC in humans came to fruition more than 20 years after the disorder was first identified in animals.[91,331] In the space of 2 years, three affected children were identified and since then three more have been found.[123,332,333] All six have skin fragility with easy bruising, extremely soft, doughy skin, marked joint laxity with delayed motor milestones, blue sclerae, micrognathia, large umbilical hernia, and mild hirsutism. One child has had a central nervous system hemorrhage in the newborn period. Otherwise, intellectual development is normal. The oldest affected individual is now in her early 20s. She has marked skin alterations but is intellectually normal. None of the affected children have had major vessel abnormalities.

Precursors to type I procollagen that contain the N-terminal propeptides accumulate in skin from affected children. Although some apparently "normal" chains are present, they probably are produced by cleavage with a separate matrix protease, as cultured cells do not convert at all.

The N-proteinase gene has been cloned and mutations in all children have been identified.[123] One is homozygous for a premature termination codon near the 3′ end of the gene but the

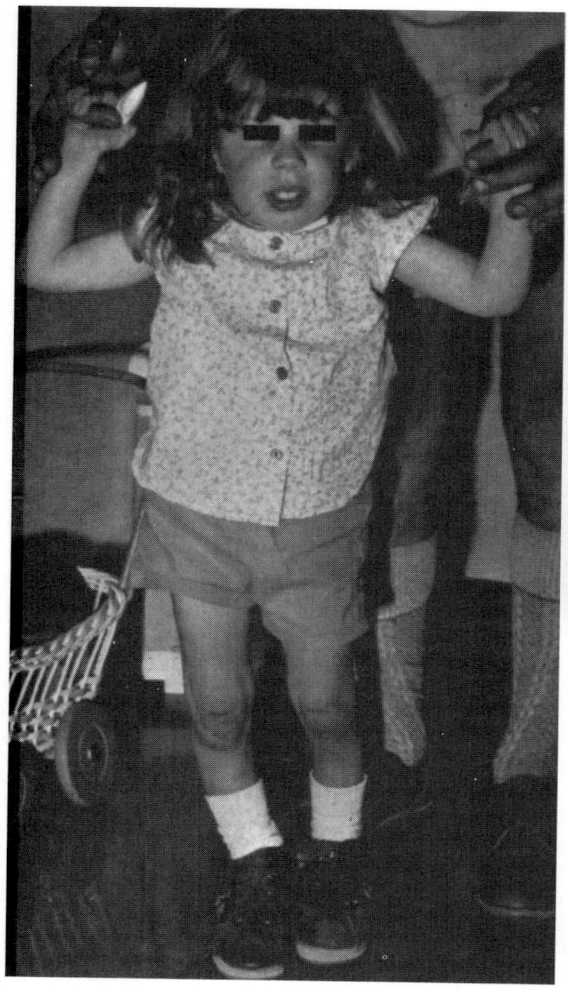

A.

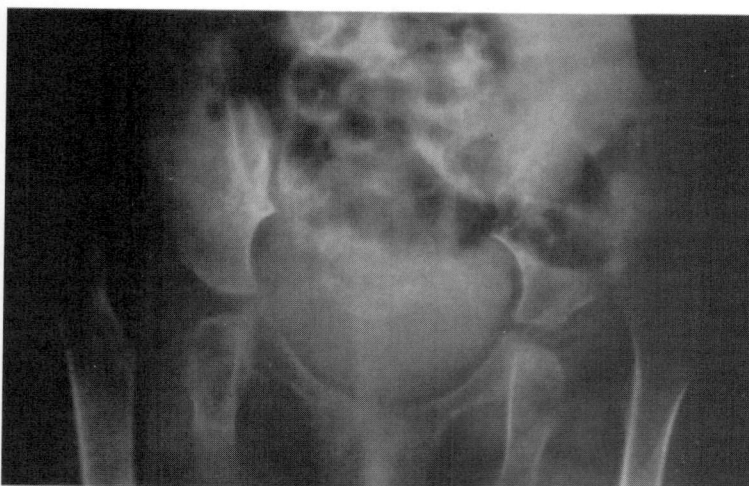

B.

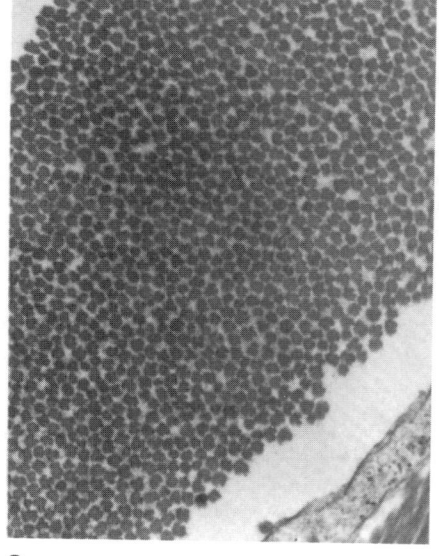

C.

Fig. 205-17 Ehlers-Danlos syndrome type VII. *A.* Clinical features of young girl with EDS type VIIA that results from heterozygous deletion of the amino acid sequences encoded by exon 6 of the *COL1A1* gene; the deletion removes the N-terminal procollagen protease cleavage site. She has mild midface hypoplasia and markedly lax ligaments. *B.* Radiograph of bilateral hip dislocation. *C.* Morphologic appearance of collagen fibrils in the child's skin in which the fibrils have an irregular shape. (*Courtesy of Dr. William Cole, Royal Children's Hospital, Melbourne.*)

others are each homozygous for a more 5' premature termination codon (Q225X). Eight or 9 of the 10 alleles are also homozygous for downstream polymorphisms in the coding region suggesting that there was a common origin of the mutation. Three of the children are of Ashkenazi Jewish origin, one is Hispanic, and the fifth is Caucasian of unknown background. In humans there are two transcripts from the gene. The Q225X mutation would affect both while the downstream mutation affects only a long transcript that appears to encode the active protease. There is no residual protease derived from the shorter product and its function remains uncertain, as there does not appear to be a clinical difference between children with the different mutations. The lack of the protease leads to retention of the N-terminal propeptide on type I procollagen and interferes with fibrillogenesis (Fig. 205-18).

**Prenatal Diagnosis of EDS Type VII.** Prenatal diagnosis for any form of EDS type VII has not been reported but, because the mutations are known, direct analysis of DNA is feasible using any of the usual substrates.

**Animal Models.** Among animals, dermatosparaxis was first recognized in cattle as a genetic disorder that affected the structure or processing of collagen.[134] Subsequently the disorder has been found in sheep, cats, and dogs. In all there is generalized skin fragility and joint laxity. Although the enzyme also cleaves type II procollagen, there have not been any bony or cartilaginous defects recognized. The picture in the affected animals is one of marked skin friability, infection, and early death from sepsis, in some settings. The historical importance of this disorder in

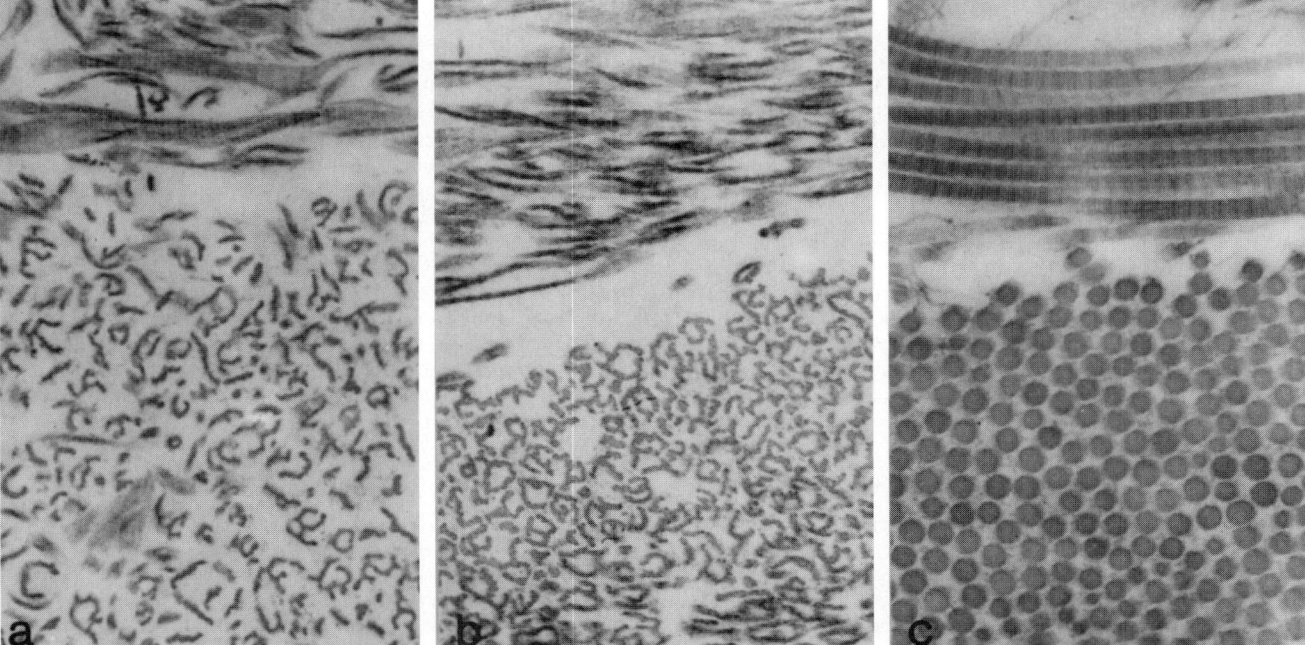

**Fig. 205-18 Electron micrograph of skin from two children (a and b) with Ehlers-Danlos syndrome type VIIC. The collagen fibrils form ribbon like structures that have a hieroglyphic character when seen in cross section, in contrast to those from the normal (c). (*Reprinted from Smith et al.*[331] *Used with permission.*)**

understanding the dynamics of collagen production is hard to overstate. The disorder was identified at a time before collagen precursors were known and thus permitted collagen precursor identification and isolation. Analysis of cells from these animals suggested that the N-terminal propeptide might have a role in feedback regulation of synthesis, although confirmation of that concept has not proved easy (see "Biosynthesis of Collagen," above). The discovery of the affected cattle truly opened the door to analysis of many different disorders of collagen production and processing.

### Ehlers-Danlos Syndrome Type VIII

EDS type VIII is characterized by bruising, soft, and hyperextensible skin, hypermobile joints, and periodontal disease.[334,335] The disorder is inherited in an autosomal dominant fashion, and loss of teeth, as a result of marked periodontal involvement, is common by the third decade. EDS type VIII is probably uncommon; no prevalence figures are available and only a few families have been described. No biochemical defects have been identified. Because gingival disease may occur in EDS type IV, it is important to exclude that diagnosis. Recent biochemical and genetic studies suggest that EDS type VIII does not result from mutations in *COL3A1*.[336]

### Ehlers-Danlos Syndrome Type IX
### (Occipital Horn Syndrome)

This disorder is now considered a variant of Menkes disease.

### Ehlers-Danlos Syndrome Type X

EDS type X is inherited in an autosomal recessive fashion and characterized by mild joint hypermobility and easy bruising. The disorder appears to result from an alteration in fibronectin that interferes with normal platelet aggregation.[337] Only one family has been identified to date. There is some uncertainty about the existence of this as a separate disorder.

### Approach to Patients with EDS

Many patients with EDS-like clinical findings do not fit the general classification scheme and, as more biochemical studies are completed, it is likely that the classification will change. From the clinical point of view, the important considerations are whether the patient has a condition inherited in an autosomal dominant, autosomal recessive, or X-linked fashion, and whether the natural history can be predicted from family studies or biochemical and molecular genetic studies. It is vital to distinguish the known, well-characterized recessively inherited disorder EDS type VI, because prenatal diagnosis is available and because orthopedic and ophthalmologic management differ from those in other varieties. It is important to identify patients with EDS type IV so that clear discussion of pregnancy risks and of problems in surgery can proceed outside the setting of emergency care.

## CHONDRODYSPLASIAS, DISORDERS OF TYPES II, IX, X AND XI COLLAGEN GENES

Cartilage derives its mechanical properties from the presence of water and of large numbers of complex macromolecules and proteoglycans. Cartilage is, however, more than a simple mechanical buffer at the ends of long bones and in intervertebral spaces. Cartilage plays an important developmental role in modeling long bone structures and in determining growth. Early in their development every long bone is laid down as an anlage that consists of cartilage. The enormous clinical range of the more than 150 chondrodysplasias attests to the large number of molecules within cartilage and to the varying effects of different mutations within them. These disorders of bone growth and structure, have been identified using radiological, clinical, genetic, and pathological features.[338] Within this array of disorders, several classes result from mutations in collagen genes, particularly those that encode type II, type IX, type X, and type XI collagens. The role of these proteins in fibril formation and their domains of expression suggest that the phenotypes should differ. Indeed, Spranger pointed out that some forms of achondrogenesis, hypochondrogenesis, spondyloepiphyseal dysplasia, Kniest syndrome, and variants of the Stickler syndrome form a continuous clinical spectrum from a radiological and clinical perspective. Other variants of Stickler syndrome and additional disorders share many other features.[339] These disorders result from abnormalities of the articular cartilage and of the vitreous humor of the eye, both tissues rich in type II and type XI collagen, and result from mutations in the *COL2A1*, *COL11A1*, and *COL11A2* genes.

In cartilage, type II, type IX, and type XI collagens form a complex network. Type II collagen is the major protein but fibrils also contain type XI molecules. The proα1(XI) chain, like the proα1(V) chain, has a long amino terminal propeptide extension. Type XI collagen is a heterotrimer of three chains—α1(XI), α2(XI), and α1(II). In the vitreous, the α2(XI) chain is substituted by the α2(V) chain. Type IX collagen, a heterotrimer of the three different chains, is thought to be linked to the outer surfaces of the type II/XI fibrils and provides an interaction with proteoglycans through a glycosaminoglycan side chain. Type X collagen is found only in the hypertrophic zone of cartilage in which the cells are at the very base of the proliferating columns at growth plates. The different distributions of these gene products account for many of the phenotypic variations that distinguish the clinical pictures of people with mutations in the genes.

## Achondrogenesis and Hypochondrogenesis

The most severe end of the spectrum of chondrodysplasias in which there is evidence of involvement of the *COL2A1* gene is the achondrogenesis type II/hypochondrogenesis group that has an incidence of approximately 1/40,000 to 60,000 births.[144] Infants with achondrogenesis type II have severe short-limbed dwarfism and die in the immediate perinatal period or *in utero*. These infants have very short limbs and trunk. The tubular bones are very short and have metaphyseal cupping. There is often absent or diminished ossification of the vertebral bodies and sacrum, and

small iliac wings with diminished ossification. The ribs are extremely short; the mineralization of the calvarium is usually normal and the calvarium is usually of normal size or large (Fig. 205-19). It may be difficult to distinguish mild hypochondrogenesis from severe spondyloepiphyseal dysplasia (SED congenita). The infants that survive to term die shortly after birth from pulmonary insufficiency. In those rare instances in which external ventilatory support has been provided survival may be extended by only a few weeks. The bony abnormalities in the hypochondrogenesis are similar but not as severe. In particular, the tubular bones are longer although the thoracic cavity remains small and death from pulmonary compromise is the rule.

At the morphologic level, chondrocytes generally have dilated rough endoplasmic reticulum and there is a paucity of identifiable collagen fibrils in the extracellular matrix.[340] The growth plate is generally very disorganized, providing an explanation for the very poor growth. Type II collagen is markedly diminished in the cartilage.

This group of disorders results from heterozygosity for mutations in the *COL2A1* gene. Several mutations have been identified, all of which disrupt the triple-helical domain, either by substitution for single glycine residues or inducing exon skipping.[201] Similar mutations can give rise to forms of SED. There are still too few mutations identified in this gene to allow clear genotype/phenotype correlations to be discerned.

## Spondyloepiphyseal Dysplasia (SED)

Spondyloepiphyseal dysplasias are a group of chondrodysplasias in which the radiological features include abnormal epiphyses,

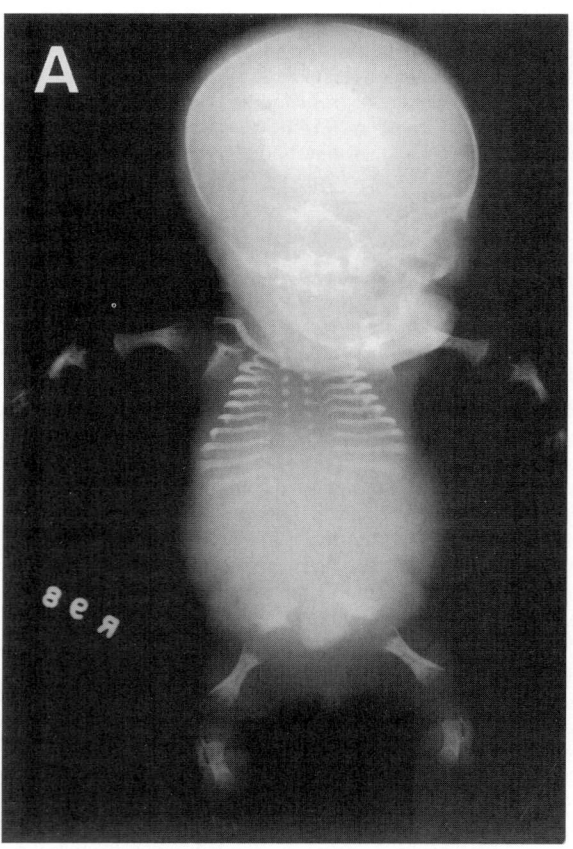
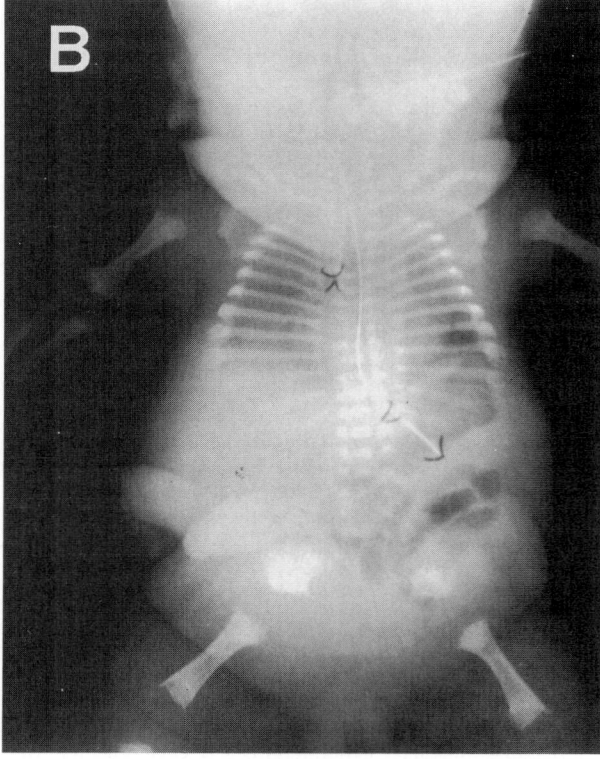

Fig. 205-19 Radiographs of achondrogenesis type II (top) and hypochondrogenesis (bottom). *A.* In achondrogenesis type II the veterbral bodies are not mineralized, the thorax is short, there is marked micromelia, small iliac wings, and concave metaphyses, seen especially here in the ulna. *B.* Hypochondroplasia. The vertebral bodies are poorly ossified and ovoid or flat, the femurs are very short with some metaphyseal irregularity, the ilia **are** hypoplastic, the pubic bones are not ossified, the ribs are short **and** the anterior metaphyses are flared. Both x-rays are from newborns. (*Radiographs courtesy of Dr. Deborah Krakow, Cedars-Sinai Medical Center, Los Angeles.*)

flattened vertebral bodies, and frequently, ocular involvement that ranges from myopia to vitreo-retinal degeneration (Fig. 205-20). There is a very marked range of clinical expression from mild short stature (SED Tarda) to very severe short stature, pulmonary compromise, and death in infancy (SED congenital).[338] Short stature is apparent at birth, the midface is flat, and cleft palate is frequent. The most striking complications include C1-C2 vertebral body subluxation and cord compression, early degenerative changes in the joints of the long bones, and myopia, vitreal degeneration, and retinal detachment. Because of the vertebral changes, the neck is very short, the chest is barrel shaped and the tubular bones of the limbs are very short although the hands and feet may be near normal in size. A waddling gait is common and varus or valgum deformities at the knee are common. Early degenerative joint disease commonly leads to joint replacement, particularly of the hip and knee. The survival is not well studied but in those with severe forms of SED it is probably decreased both from neurological and respiratory compromise.

Confirmation of the diagnosis of SED is generally dependent on radiological examination, although molecular diagnostic evaluation of the *COL2A1* gene can be done readily.[341]

Analysis of type II collagen in articular cartilage from individuals with different forms of SED demonstrated alterations in the amount and electrophoretic mobilities of the $\alpha 1(II)$ chains in those tissues, compatible with mutations in the *COL2A1* gene. Analysis of the *COL2A1* gene from several individuals with different forms of SED have identified mutations that include partial duplication of exon 48 with the resultant addition of 15 amino acids (duplication of residues 970 to 984 of the triple helix),[342] deletion of exon 48 from one allele,[343] substitutions of the glycine at positions 247,[344] 895,[345] or 997[346] in the triple helix by serine, a splice junction mutation that results in skipping the sequences of exon 20,[347] and, surprisingly, substitutions of cysteine for arginine at position 75 or 789 in the triple-helical domain.[348] The substitutions for glycine residues and alterations of sequence length clearly interfere with propagation and folding of

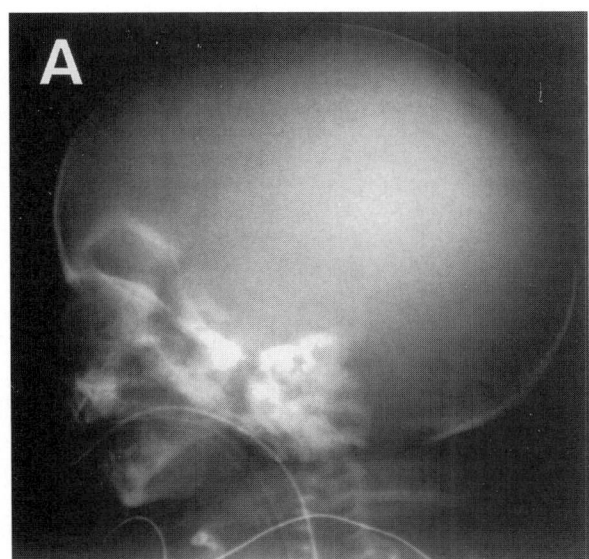

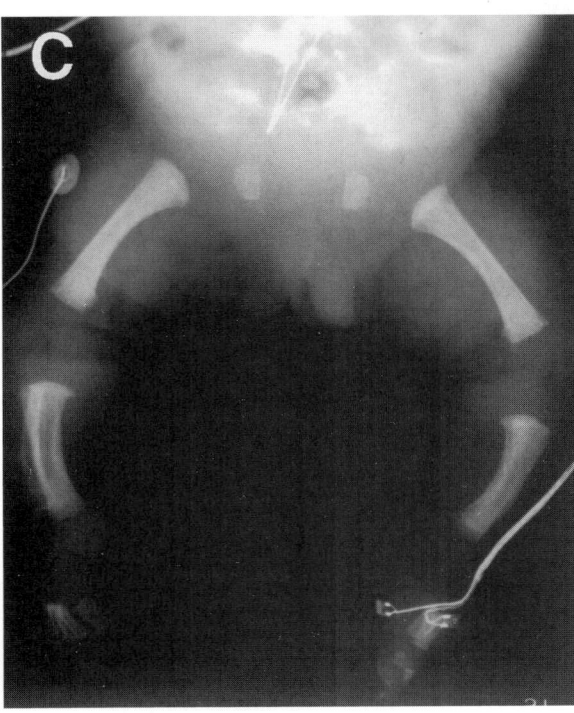

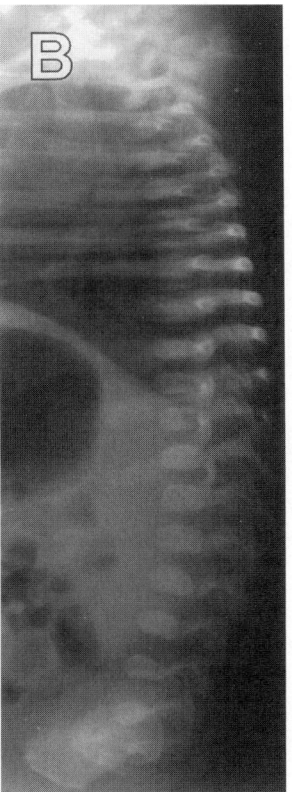

Fig. 205-20 **Spondyloepiphyseal dysplasia congenita.** *A.* There is a defect in the ossification of the cranial base. *B.* Ovoid vertebral bodies. *C.* Absent ossification of the pubis, hypoplastic ischia, delayed formation of the epiphyses, and no mineralization of the calcaneus and talus. (*Radiographs courtesy of Dr. Deborah Krakow, Cedars-Sinai Medical Center, Los Angeles.*)

the triple helix because they result in alteration of the electrophoretic mobility of the α1(II) chains in cartilage and intracellular storage visible by electron microscopy.

Substitutions for nonglycine residues within the triple-helical domain are unusual causes of identifiable phenotypes. Introduction of a cysteine residue in the triple-helical domain could have several effects. First, a subset of type II collagen molecules would have a free sulfhydryl and thus be capable of forming covalent interactions with other matrix molecules. Second, the position in the triple helix is close to a cross-link lysine and could interfere with the enzymatic stabilization of fibrils. Finally, *in* vitro experiments suggest that such substitutions can interfere with fibrillogenesis, although examination of tissues from affected individuals suggests that the proportion of mutant and normal chains is close to the expected[349].

## Kniest Dysplasia

Kniest dysplasia is a dominantly inherited disorder that can be differentiated from the other conditions that result from mutation in the *COL2A1* gene by its clinical and radiographic features. At birth infants are slightly short, have a flat midface and enlarged joints with metaphyseal flaring, prominent eyes, and may have cleft palate. High myopia is present at an early age and vitreal degeneration and retinal detachment are common so that visual loss may occur. At birth the lateral radiographs demonstrate a characteristic coronal cleft in vertebral bodies, and the long bones have a dumbbell appearance. With time the vertebral bodies become flattened and scoliosis is common. The joints at the ends of all the long bones become enlarged and there is marked widening of the epiphyseal plate prior to fusion and of the metaphyseal portion following fusion (Fig. 205-21). Degenerative changes occur early and may lead to multiple joint replacement.

Molecular defects in the *COL2A1* gene have been identified in several individuals with Kniest dysplasia. In the majority these are characterized by loss of amino acids in the region of the triple

helix encoded by exons 12 through 24 either as a consequence of mutations that predict exon-skipping,[350–353] use of a cryptic site to delete 21 coding residues, or loss of 7 amino acids from the triple helix.[354–356] Two substitutions for glycine have been identified: G103D[357] and G127D.[350] Finally, deletion of 18nt from mRNA encoded by exon 49 results in loss of residues 1007 to 1012 of the triple helix.[358] It is not clear how these disparate mutations translate into the Kniest dysplasia and what the common pathway represents. It seems possible that the effects of splice site mutations could vary, as they do in some forms of OI, such that the amount of the abnormal protein produced was far less than expected. This effect could be mediated through alternate splicing pathways in which the same mutation leads both to an unstable mRNA and an exon-skipped mRNA. Unfortunately, most studies are done at the genomic level so that little information about the effects of these mutations is available.

One important finding that links Kniest with the other disorders of type II collagen is the identification of individuals mosaic for the causative Kniest mutation who have a Stickler phenotype.[359,360]

## Stickler Syndrome

Stickler syndrome, hereditary arthro-ophthalmo-dystrophy, is an autosomal dominant disorder characterized by early degenerative joint disease in the presence of a mild epiphyseal dysplasia, vitreal degeneration, and moderate to severe myopia with retinal detachment.[361] In some individuals cleft palate and/or Pierre-Robin anomaly make diagnosis in the newborn period more apparent, but often, in the absence of family history, the diagnosis is delayed. There has been an ongoing concern about etiologic relationships among the Stickler syndrome, the Wagner syndrome, the Marshall syndrome, OSMED (oto-spondylo-megaepiphyseal dysplasia), and other disorders in which both ocular and joint manifestations are present. Molecular genetic studies completed within the last few years have done much to clarify the

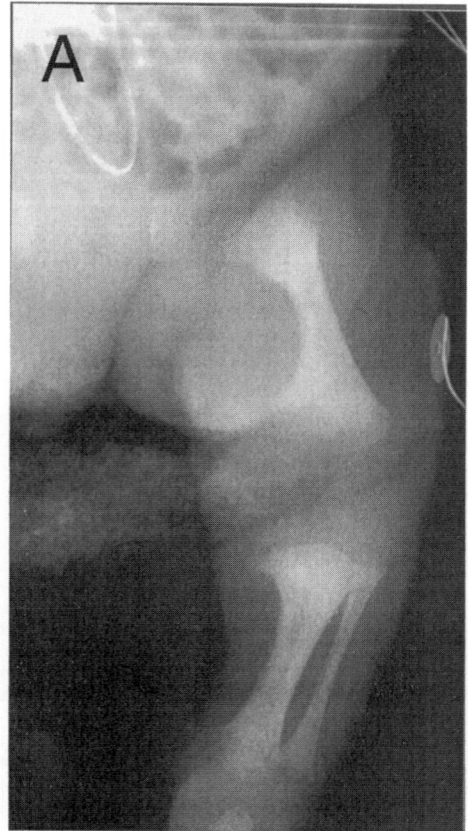
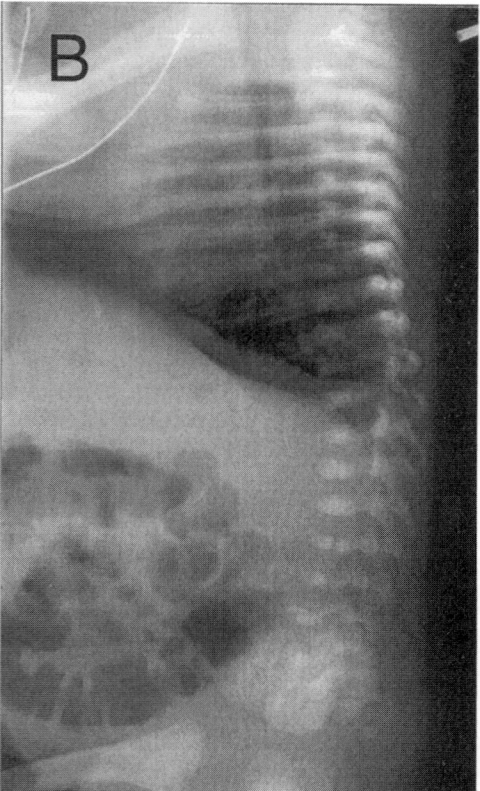

Fig. 205-21 Kniest dysplasia. *A.* The short, dumbbell appearance, a consequence of metaphyseal splaying and delayed formation of the femoral capital epiphyses in this 2-week-old are characteristic of Kniest dysplasia. *B.* The vertebral bodies in lower spine of this newborn have coronal clefts. (*Radiographs courtesy of Dr. Deborah Krakow, Cedars-Sinai Medical Center, Los Angeles.*)

relationships among these disorders and to explain the basis for both the similarities and the differences among them.

Linkage studies in families with the Stickler syndrome indicate genetic heterogeneity. In most families the phenotype is linked to the *COL2A1* locus and in these families the ocular findings are prominent. A small group of families is linked to the *COL11A1* locus and others to the *COL11A2* locus. In a small remaining group linkage appears to be excluded from all three loci.[362]

Mutations in the *COL2A1* gene have now been identified in almost two dozen families. Almost all the mutations predict a premature termination codon, either by single base substitution or by insertion or deletion of small number of nucleotides. There are several splice site mutations identified; but the outcome of most of these mutations is not known, and, given the usual types of mutations, it seems likely that the use of cryptic sites results in premature termination codons and unstable mRNAs. Point mutations that result in substitution for glycine residues are rare; when they occur they are most likely to be found near the amino-terminal end of the triple-helical domain.[201]

These findings indicate that a diminished amount of type II collagen in cartilage is sufficient to produce the Stickler syndrome and that this group of affected individuals has the complete Stickler phenotype. Similar types of mutations in the *COL11A1* and *COL11A2* genes give rise to the skeletal manifestations of Stickler syndrome, but those with mutations in the *COL11A2* gene appear to lack the ocular findings. It is likely that the substitution of the product of the *COL5A2* product for proα2(XI) in type XI collagen in the vitreous could account for this difference. This suggests that *COL5A2* mutations could be associated with ocular findings, but in the few individuals with Ehlers-Danlos syndrome type I/II in which they have been found no ocular changes have been described. *COL5A2* coding sequence abnormalities were excluded in one family in which the nonocular Stickler phenotype was shown to be excluded from the *COL2A1*, *COL11A1*, and *COL11A2* genes.[363]

Very recently the *COL11A2* gene has been found to harbor mutations that give rise to nonsyndromic deafness, *DFNA13*.[364] Although hearing loss is a component of many of the disorders of collagen genes, the finding of isolated deafness without a skeletal component is surprising. The mutations involve a substitution of cysteine for arginine within the triple-helical domain (R549C) in one family and of glutamic acid for glycine (G323E) in a second. The first is similar to the mild chondrodysplasia and early onset degenerative joint disease seen with a similar substitution in the *COL2A1* coding sequence (see below) but the latter is surprising in lacking other clinical features, considering the mutations in that gene that lead to other phenotypes.

### Chondrodysplasia with Early Arthropathy

With rare exceptions, substitutions for residues other than glycine within the triple-helical domains of fibrillar collagens are without phenotypic consequence. In several families substitutions for nonglycine residues within triple-helical domain of the proα1(II) chain produce a phenotype with normal stature but aggressive, early onset degenerative joint disease, and mild spondylodysplasia.[365–367] Substitutions of the arginine at position 519 (R519C) have been found in several independent families and results from recurrent mutation at the CpG site.[365] The age of onset of joint symptoms is often in the mid-20s and joint replacement may occur far earlier than with the usual forms of degenerative joint disease.

### Schmid Metaphyseal Chondrodysplasia, a Disorder of Type X Collagen

This disorder (MIM 156600) is thought to have been misidentified as a form of achondroplasia because of the femoral bowing and waddling gait that affected members of a multigenerational family[368] in which the first mutation in the *COL10A1* gene was identified.[369] The disorder derives its name, however, from a later description of a 6-year-old child and a probably affected mother.[370] Children with this disorder are generally of normal length at birth and begin to fall below the 5th percentile by about 2 years. They present with coxa vara, and femoral bowing is apparent by radiological examination (Fig. 205-22). The proximal and distal femoral metaphysis are widened and flared with irregularity or the surface. Tibial metaphyses are abnormal and broad. The capital femoral epiphyses are often enlarged but the pelvis and vertebral bodies are normal. Facial appearance is normal. The ribs often have anterior cupping. Final height is less than 145 cm for males and less than 140 cm for females.[371] The natural history of pelvic and knee arthropathy has not received a great deal of attention, but early replacement may be common. The lack of involvement of other bony structures reinforces the distribution of this gene product in the hypertrophic zone of the growth plates.

Mutations in the *COL10A1* gene are distributed in a highly asymmetric fashion in people with Schmid metaphyseal chondrodysplasia (Fig. 205-23). All but 2 mutations are found in the region that encodes the NC1 domain, the 161 amino acid carboxyl-terminal peptide that mediates chain association, summarized by Chan and Jacenko.[372] The other two mutations occur in the NC2 domain, the amino-terminal non-triple-helical extension at the signal peptide cleavage site.[373] The mutations in the NC1 domain include several missense mutations, frame-shift mutations that lead to altered sequence and early truncation, and nonsense mutations, all of which affect sequences in the last 100 amino acids of the chain.

The mechanism of disease production remains an area of some dispute at this point, perhaps because several mechanisms may lead to the same outcome. Type X collagen forms a meshwork in which both the amino-terminal (NC2) and carboxyl-terminal (NC1) non-helical domains participate. The missense mutations in the NC1 domain appear to alter residues that facilitate chain association.[374] Although these mutations permit trimerization, the complexes formed are less stable. The abnormal chains can associate in trimers, but those with altered sequences appear to remain associated with chaperones, specifically protein disulfide isomerase and HSP47, for longer than usual.[375] At least one of

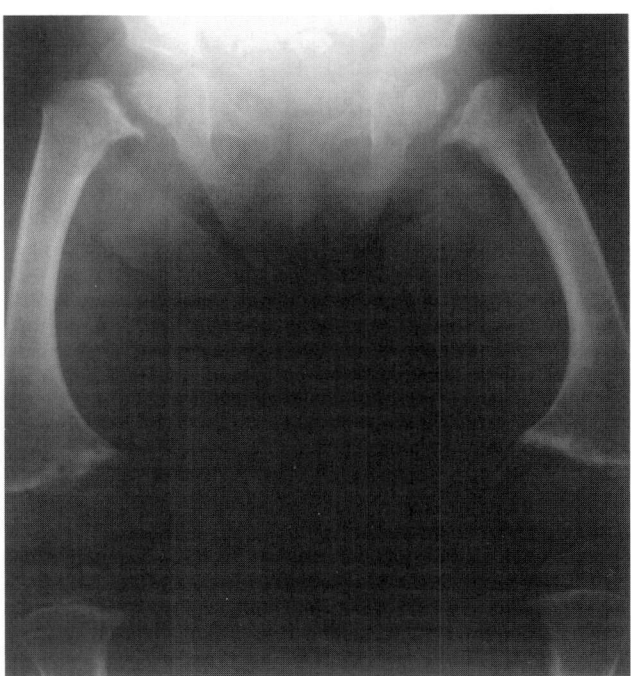

**Fig. 205-22 Metaphyseal chondrodysplasia, Schmid type. In this 2-year-old there is flaring of the proximal and distal femoral metaphyses, enlarged capital femoral epiphyses, and bowed femurs. (*Radiographs courtesy of Dr. Deborah Krakow, Cedars-Sinai Medical Center, Los Angeles.*)**

# COL10A1

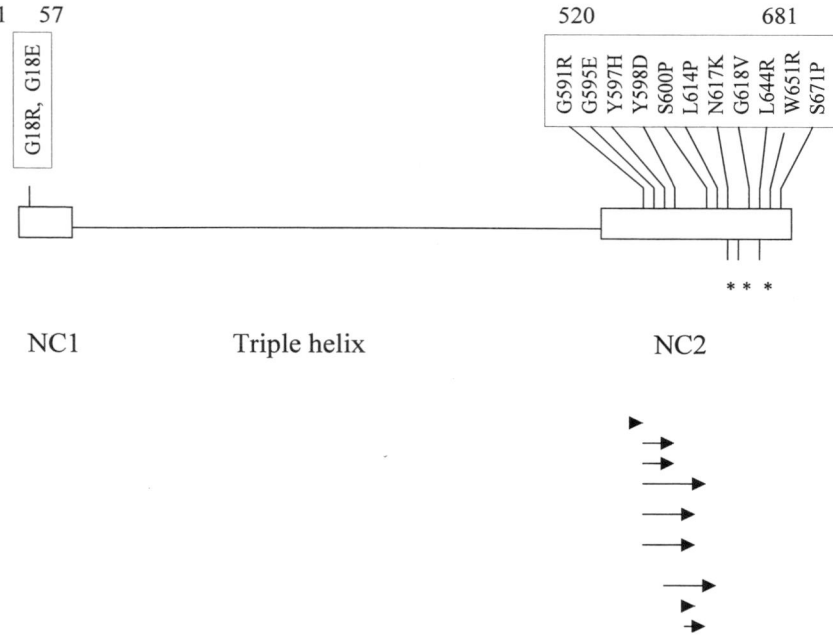

Fig. 205-23 Mutations in the *COL10A1* gene in individuals with Schmid metaphyseal chondrodysplasia.

these mutations interferes with multimer formation,[376] the initial phase of meshwork creation. Finally, a premature termination codon, Y632X, results in a markedly diminished amount of the mRNA from that allele in tissue and no evidence of the abnormal protein in the extracellular matrix.[377] The mechanism of allele loss is unclear as nonsense-mediated decay ordinarily requires at least one intron between the premature termination codon and the constitutive one, a situation not found in this instance.

The clustering of mutations in the one region is unusual for collagens. To date no mutations have been identified in the triple-helical domain, suggesting that the phenotypic consequences of such mutations are different.

**Animal Models.** There is no known naturally occurring animal model with type X collagen mutations. Mice with two separate deletions within the triple-helical domain (21 or 293 amino acids) were created, using a chicken *COL10A1* gene. These animals had marked phenotypic variability, even in the same litter, ranging from perinatal lethal to variable dwarfism with the extent of short stature correlated with growth plate involvement and, surprisingly, involvement of marrow elements and hematopoiesis.[378] The latter involvement is not part of the Schmid metaphyseal chondrodysplasia phenotype or of mice heterozygous or homozygous for *COL10A1* null alleles created by targeted mutagenesis.[379,380] Perhaps these differences provide a clue to the effects of mutations in the triple-helical domain of the molecule.

### Multiple Epiphyseal Dysplasia (MED) Due to Mutations in Two Genes of Type IX Collagen

The multiple epiphyseal dysplasias are a clinical heterogeneous group of disorders characterized clinically by early onset joint discomfort followed by degenerative changes. In some families stature is short but in other it is normal. The most commonly involved joints are the ankles, knees, and hips, although in some forms hip involvement is minimal. Linkage studies identified one locus on chromosome 1 that proved to contain the cartilage oligomeric matrix protein (COMP) in which mutations were identified.[381,382] However additional studies indicated that at least two additional loci were involved, and more recently mutations

have been identified in the *COL9A2* and *COL9A3* genes.[383–385] The mutations identified in the three families all alter the splicing of exon 3 of either the *COL9A2* or *COL9A3* gene and result in skipping of the 36nt of that exon and an in-frame deletion of 12 amino acids from the COL4 domain of the protein. Although the *COL9A1* gene has been examined in the same region, no mutations have been identified.

**Animal Model.** Homozygotes for the *Col9a1* null allele created in mice[386] fail to assemble any type IX collagen molecules, attesting to the primacy of the proα1(IX) chain in molecular assembly. The heterozygotes produce a reduced amount of normal type IX collagen and are asymptomatic but the homozygotes have early onset degenerative changes in early adulthood. They have no other phenotypic abnormalities.

## SUMMARY COMMENTS

Like many other fields, the investigation of the genetic disorders of collagen metabolism was revolutionized by the introduction of molecular genetic techniques. These techniques have facilitated the analysis of mutations in collagen genes and in the genes that encode processing enzymes, and permitted the creation of mice bearing mutations in some collagen genes (particularly *COL1A1*, *COL2A1*, *COL3A1*, *COL9A1*, and *COL10A1*) in attempts to identify candidate phenotypes for mutations in those genes. These approaches have facilitated prenatal diagnosis of a variety of disorders and enabled investigators to further explore the effects of these mutations on the abnormal proteins, both within and outside the cell. Thus the molecular pathogenesis of some collagen gene disorders, particularly some forms of osteogenesis imperfecta and Ehlers-Danlos syndrome type IV, is becoming increasingly well understood. Furthermore, the molecular studies have shown that the enormous range in severity of identifiable disorders such as OI, EDS type IV, and some chondrodysplasias, suggest that some forms of far more common disorders such as osteoporosis, arterial aneurysms, and degenerative arthropathies could be due to mutations in the same genes. Hailed as a road to therapy for some of the severe collagen gene disorders, the molecular understanding of these disorders has, to date, provided few, if any, insights into productive therapies. The prospect of specific gene-based therapy, either by targeted replacement or inhibition of expression of mutant alleles, seems remote and limited by the often generalized nature of the disorders and the necessity to affect only the mutant allele. With much of the work accomplished to identify mutations in many collagen gene disorders and the recognition of the nature of these disorders, it seems likely that attention could be profitably shifted to an analysis of productive therapies that can use the information currently being generated about the mechanisms of disease.

## ACKNOWLEDGMENTS

Original investigations were supported in part by grants from the National Institutes of Health (AR 21557 and AR 41223). I am indebted to discussion with individuals in my laboratory and to Dr. Deborah Krakow, Cedars-Sinai Medical Center, for providing the radiographs of infants and children with skeletal dysplasias.

## REFERENCES

1. Kadler K: Extracellular Matrix 1:Fibril-forming collagens. *Protein Profile* **2**:491, 1995.
2. Engel J, Prockop DJ: The zipper-like folding of collagen triple helices and the effects of mutations that disrupt the zipper. *Annu Rev Biophys Biophys Chem* **20**:137, 1991.
3. Brown JC, Timpl R: The collagen superfamily. *Int Arch Allergy Immunol* **107**:484, 1995.
4. van der Rest M, Garrone R: Collagen family of proteins. *Faseb J* **5**:2814, 1991.
5. Mays C, Rosenberry TL: Characterization of pepsin-resistant collagen-like tail subunit fragments of 18S and 14S acetylcholinesterase from Electrophorus electricus. *Biochemistry* **20**:2810, 1981.
6. Reid KB: Complete amino acid sequences of the three collagen-like regions present in subcomponent C1q of the first component of human complement. *Biochem J* **179**:367, 1979.
7. Bhattacharyya SN, Passero MA, DiAugustine RP, Lynn WS: Isolation and characterization of two hydroxyproline-containing glycoproteins from normal animal lung lavage and lamellar bodies. *J Clin Invest* **55**:914, 1975.
8. Crouch EC: Collectins and pulmonary host defense. *Am J Respir Cell Mol Biol* **19**:177, 1998.
9. Taylor ME, Brickell PM, Craig RK, Summerfield JA: Structure and evolutionary origin of the gene encoding a human serum mannose-binding protein. *Biochem J* **262**:763, 1989.
10. Kere J, Srivastava AK, Montonen O, Zonana J, Thomas N, Ferguson B, Munoz F, et al: X-linked anhidrotic (hypohidrotic) ectodermal dysplasia is caused by mutation in a novel transmembrane protein [see comments]. *Nat Genet* **13**:409, 1996.
11. Monreal AW, Zonana J, Ferguson B: Identification of a new splice form of the EDA1 gene permits detection of nearly all X-linked hypohidrotic ectodermal dysplasia mutations. *Am J Hum Genet* **63**:380, 1998.
12. Kuhn K: The classical collagens: Types I, II, and III, in Mayne R, Burgeson RE (eds): *Structure and Function of Collagen Types.* Orlando, FL, Academic Press, 1987, p 1.
13. Prockop DJ, Kivirikko KI: Collagens: Molecular biology, diseases, and potentials for therapy. *Annu Rev Biochem* **64**:403, 1995.
14. van der Rest M, Mayne R: Type IX collagen, in Mayne R, Burgeson RE (eds): *Structure and Function of Collagen Types.* Orlando, FL, Academic Press, 1987, p 195.
15. Schmid TM, Linsenmayer TF: Type X collagen, in Mayne R, Burgeson RE (eds): *Structure and Function of Collagen Types.* Orlando, FL, Academic Press, 1987, p 223.
16. Eyre D, Wu J-J: Type XI or 1a2a3a collagen, in Mayne R, Burgeson RE (eds): *Structure and Function of Collagen Types.* Orlando, FL, Academic Press, 1987, p 261.
17. Glanville RW: Type IV collagen, in Mayne R, Burgeson RE (eds): *Structure and Function of Collagen Types.* Orlando, FL, Academic Press, 1987, p 43.
18. Burgeson RE: Type VII collagen, in Mayne R, Burgeson RE (eds): *Structure and Function of Collagen Types.* Orlando, FL, Academic Press, 1987, p 145.
19. O'Reilly MS, Boehm T, Shing Y, Fukai N, Vasios G, Lane WS, Flynn E, et al: Endostatin: An endogenous inhibitor of angiogenesis and tumor growth. *Cell* **88**:277, 1997.
20. Saarela J, Ylikarppa R, Rehn M, Purmonen S, Pihlajaniemi T: Complete primary structure of two variant forms of human type XVIII collagen and tissue-specific differences in the expression of the corresponding transcripts. *Matrix Biol* **16**:319, 1998.
21. Aszodi A, Chan D, Hunziker E, Bateman JF, Fassler R: Collagen II is essential for the removal of the notochord and the formation of intervertebral discs. *J Cell Biol* **143**:1399, 1998.
22. Savontaus M, Metsaranta M, Vuorio E: Mutation in type II collagen gene disturbs spinal development and gene expression patterns in transgenic Del1 mice. *Lab Invest* **77**:591, 1997.
23. Liu X, Wu H, Byrne M, Krane S, Jaenisch R: Type III collagen is crucial for collagen I fibrillogenesis and for normal cardiovascular development. *Proc Natl Acad Sci U S A* **94**:1852, 1997.
24. Andrikopoulos K, Liu X, Keene DR, Jaenisch R, Ramirez F: Targeted mutation in the *Col5a2* gene reveals a regulatory role for type V collagen during matrix assembly. *Nat Genet* **9**:31, 1995.
25. Takahara K, Hoffman GG, Greenspan DS: Complete structural organization of the human α1(V) collagen gene (COL5A1): Divergence from the conserved organization of other characterized fibrillar collagen genes. *Genomics* **29**:588, 1995.
26. Vuoristo MM, Pihlajamaa T, Vandenberg P, Korkko J, Prockop DJ, Ala-Kokko L: Complete structure of the human COL11A2 gene: The exon sizes and other features indicate the gene has not evolved with genes for other fibriller collagens. *Ann N Y Acad Sci* **785**:343, 1996.
27. Sundar Raj CV, Church RL, Klobutcher LA, Ruddle FH: Genetics of the connective tissue proteins: assignment of the gene for human type I procollagen to chromosome 17 by analysis of cell hybrids and microcell hybrids. *Proc Natl Acad Sci U S A* **74**:4444, 1977.
28. Korkko J, Ala-Kokko L, De Paepe A, Nuytinck L, Earley J, Prockop DJ: Analysis of the COL1A1 and COL1A2 genes by PCR amplification and scanning by conformation-sensitive gel electrophoresis identifies only COL1A1 mutations in 15 patients with osteogenesis imperfecta type I: Identification of common sequences of null-allele mutations. *Am J Hum Genet* **62**:98, 1998.
29. Huerre C, Junien C, Weil D, Chu ML, Morabito M, Van Cong N, Myers JC, et al: Human type I procollagen genes are located on different chromosomes. *Proc Natl Acad Sci U S A* **79**:6627, 1982.
30. Ala-Kokko L, Kvist AP, Metsaranta M, Kivirikko KI, de Crombrugghe B, Prockop DJ, Vuorio E: Conservation of the sizes of 53 introns and over 100 intronic sequences for the binding of common transcription factors in the human and mouse genes for type II procollagen (COL2A1). *Biochem J* **308**:923, 1995.
31. Strom CM, Eddy RL, Shows TB: Localization of human type II procollagen gene (COL2A1) to chromosome 12. *Somat Cell Mol Genet* **10**:651, 1984.
32. Emanuel BS, Cannizzaro LA, Seyer JM, Myers JC: Human α1(III) and α2(V) procollagen genes are located on the long arm of chromosome 2. *Proc Natl Acad Sci U S A* **82**:3385, 1985.
33. Henry I, Bernheim A, Bernard M, van der Rest M, Kimura T, Jeanpierre C, Barichard F, et al: Mapping of a human fibrillar collagen gene, proα1(XI) (COL11A1), to the p21 region of chromosome 1. *Genomics* **3**:87, 1988.
34. Sado Y, Kagawa M, Naito I, Ueki Y, Seki T, Momota R, Oohashi T, et al: Organization and expression of basement membrane collagen IV genes and their roles in human disorders. *J Biochem (Tokyo)* **123**:767, 1998.
35. Solomon E, Hiorns LR, Spurr N, Kurkinen M, Barlow D, Hogan BL, Dalgleish R: Chromosomal assignments of the genes coding for human types II, III, and IV collagen: A dispersed gene family. *Proc Natl Acad Sci U S A* **82**:3330, 1985.
36. Emanuel BS, Sellinger BT, Gudas LJ, Myers JC: Localization of the human procollagen α1(IV) gene to chromosome 13q34 by in situ hybridization. *Am J Hum Genet* **38**:38, 1986.
37. Griffin CA, Emanuel BS, Hansen JR, Cavenee WK, Myers JC: Human collagen genes encoding basement membrane α1(IV) and α2(IV) chains map to the distal long arm of chromosome 13. *Proc Natl Acad Sci U S A* **84**:512, 1987.
38. Mariyama M, Zheng K, Yang-Feng TL, Reeders ST: Colocalization of the genes for the α3(IV) and α4(IV) chains of type IV collagen to chromosome 2 bands q35-q37. *Genomics* **13**:809, 1992.
39. Cutting GR, Kazazian HH Jr, Antonarakis SE, Killen PD, Yamada Y, Francomano CA: Macrorestriction mapping of COL4A1 and COL4A2 collagen genes on human chromosome 13q34. *Genomics* **3**:256, 1988.

40. Hostikka SL, Eddy RL, Byers MG, Hoyhtya M, Shows TB, Tryggvason K: Identification of a distinct type IV collagen α chain with restricted kidney distribution and assignment of its gene to the locus of X chromosome-linked Alport syndrome. *Proc Natl Acad Sci U S A* **87**:1606, 1990.

41. Sugimoto M, Oohashi T, Ninomiya Y: The genes COL4A5 and COL4A6, coding for basement membrane collagen chains α5(IV) and α6(IV), are located head-to-head in close proximity on human chromosome Xq22 and COL4A6 is transcribed from two alternative promoters. *Proc Natl Acad Sci U S A* **91**:11679, 1994.

42. Srivastava AK, Featherstone T, Wein K, Schlessinger D: YAC contigs mapping the human COL4A5 and COL4A6 genes and DXS118 within Xq21.3-q22. *Genomics* **26**:502, 1995.

43. Kimura T, Mattei MG, Stevens JW, Goldring MB, Ninomiya Y, Olsen BR: Molecular cloning of rat and human type IX collagen cDNA and localization of the α1(IX) gene on the human chromosome 6. *Eur J Biochem* **179**:71, 1989.

44. Warman ML, McCarthy MT, Perala M, Vuorio E, Knoll JH, McDaniels CN, Mayne R, et al: The genes encoding α2(IX) collagen (COL9A2) map to human chromosome 1p32.3-p33 and mouse chromosome 4. *Genomics* **23**:158, 1994.

45. Brewton RG, Wood BM, Ren ZX, Gong Y, Tiller GE, Warman ML, Lee B, et al: Molecular cloning of the α3 chain of human type IX collagen: Linkage of the gene COL9A3 to chromosome 20q13.3. *Genomics* **30**:329, 1995.

46. van der Rest M, Mayne R: Type IX collagen proteoglycan from cartilage is covalently cross-linked to type II collagen. *J Biol Chem* **263**:1615, 1988.

47. Oh SP, Taylor RW, Gerecke DR, Rochelle JM, Seldin MF, Olsen BR: The mouse α1(XII) and human α1(XII)-like collagen genes are localized on mouse chromosome 9 and human chromosome 6. *Genomics* **14**:225, 1992.

48. Gordon MK, Gerecke DR, Dublet B, van der Rest M, Olsen BR: Type XII collagen. A large multidomain molecule with partial homology to type IX collagen. *J Biol Chem* **264**:19772, 1989.

49. Dublet B, Oh S, Sugrue SP, Gordon MK, Gerecke DR, Olsen BR, van der Rest M: The structure of avian type XII collagen. α1(XII) chains contain 190-kDa non-triple helical amino-terminal domains and form homotrimeric molecules. *J Biol Chem* **264**:13150, 1989.

50. Weil D, Mattei MG, Passage E, N'Guyen VC, Pribula-Conway D, Mann K, Deutzmann R, et al: Cloning and chromosomal localization of human genes encoding the three chains of type VI collagen. *Am J Hum Genet* **42**:435, 1988.

51. Francomano CA, Cutting GR, McCormick MK, Chu ML, Timpl R, Hong HK, Antonarakis SE: The COL6A1 and COL6A2 genes exist as a gene cluster and detect highly informative DNA polymorphisms in the telomeric region of human chromosome 21q. *Hum Genet* **87**:162, 1991.

52. Heiskanen M, Saitta B, Palotie A, Chu ML: Head to tail organization of the human COL6A1 and COL6A2 genes by fiber- FISH. *Genomics* **29**:801, 1995.

53. Schurr E, Skamene E, Morgan K, Chu ML, Gros P: Mapping of Col3a1 and Col6a3 to proximal murine chromosome 1 identifies conserved linkage of structural protein genes between murine chromosome 1 and human chromosome 2q. *Genomics* **8**:477, 1990.

54. Timpl R, Engel J: Type VI collagen, in Mayne R, Burgeson RE (eds): *Structure and Function of Collagen Types.* Orlando, FL, Academic Press, 1987, p 105.

55. Muragaki Y, Mattei MG, Yamaguchi N, Olsen BR, Ninomiya Y: The complete primary structure of the human α1(VIII) chain and assignment of its gene (COL8A1) to chromosome 3. *Eur J Biochem* **197**:615, 1991.

56. Muragaki Y, Jacenko O, Apte S, Mattei MG, Ninomiya Y, Olsen BR: The α2(VIII) collagen gene. A novel member of the short chain collagen family located on the human chromosome 1. *J Biol Chem* **266**:7721, 1991.

57. Thomas JT, Cresswell CJ, Rash B, Nicolai H, Jones T, Solomon E, Grant ME, et al: The human collagen X gene. Complete primary translated sequence and chromosomal localization. *Biochem J* **280**:617, 1991.

58. Bruckner-Tuderman L: Biology and pathology of the skin basement membrane zone. *Matrix Biol* **18**:3, 1999.

59. Parente MG, Chung LC, Ryynanen J, Woodley DT, Wynn KC, Bauer EA, Mattei MG, et al: Human type VII collagen: cDNA cloning and chromosomal mapping of the gene. *Proc Natl Acad Sci U S A* **88**:6931, 1991.

60. Christiano AM, Hoffman GG, Zhang X, Xu Y, Tamai Y, Greenspan DS, Uitto J: Strategy for identification of sequence variants in COL7A1 and a novel 2-bp deletion mutation in recessive dystrophic epidermolysis bullosa. *Hum Mutat* **10**:408, 1997.

61. Ramchandran R, Dhanabal M, Volk R, Waterman MJ, Segal M, Lu H, Knebelmann B, et al: Antiangiogenic activity of restin, NC10 domain of human collagen XV: Comparison to endostatin. *Biochem Biophys Res Commun* **255**:735, 1999.

62. Hagg PM, Muona A, Lietard J, Kivirikko S, Pihlajaniemi T: Complete exon-intron organization of the human gene for the α1 chain of type XV collagen (COL15A1) and comparison with the homologous COL18A1 gene. *J Biol Chem* **273**:17824, 1998.

63. Salem G, Traub W: Conformational implications of amino acid sequence regularities in collagen. *FEBS Lett* **51**:94, 1975.

64. Brodsky B, Shah NK: Protein motifs. 8. The triple-helix motif in proteins. *FASEB J* **9**:1537, 1995.

65. Brodsky B, Ramshaw JA: The collagen triple-helix structure. *Matrix Biol* **15**:545, 1997.

66. Rosenbloom J, Harsch M, Jimenez S: Hydroxyproline content determines the denaturation temperature of chick tendon collagen. *Arch Biochem Biophys* **158**:478, 1973.

67. Berg RA, Prockop DJ: The thermal transition of a non-hydroxylated form of collagen. Evidence for a role for hydroxyproline in stabilizing the triple-helix of collagen. *Biochem Biophys Res Commun* **52**:115, 1973.

68. Harwood R, Grant ME, Jackson DS: The route of secretion of procollagen. The influence of αα'- bipyridyl, colchicine and antimycin A on the secretory process in embryonic-chick tendon and cartilage cells. *Biochem J* **156**:81, 1976.

69. Walmsley AR, Batten MR, Lad U, Bulleid NJ: Intracellular retention of procollagen within the endoplasmic reticulum is mediated by prolyl 4-hydroxylase. *J Biol Chem* **274**:14884, 1999.

70. de Wet WJ, Chu ML, Prockop DJ: The mRNAs for the pro-α1(I) and pro-α 2(I) chains of type I procollagen are translated at the same rate in normal human fibroblasts and in fibroblasts from two variants of osteogenesis imperfecta with altered steady state ratios of the two mRNAs. *J Biol Chem* **258**:14385, 1983.

71. Rossi P, de Crombrugghe B: Identification of a cell-specific transcriptional enhancer in the first intron of the mouse α2 (type I) collagen gene. *Proc Natl Acad Sci U S A* **84**:5590, 1987.

72. Bornstein P, McKay J, Morishima JK, Devarayalu S, Gelinas RE: Regulatory elements in the first intron contribute to transcriptional control of the human α1(I) collagen gene. *Proc Natl Acad Sci U S A* **84**:8869, 1987.

73. Chen SS, Ruteshouser EC, Maity SN, de Crombrugghe B: Cell-specific in vivo DNA-protein interactions at the proximal promoters of the proα1(I) and the proα2(I) collagen genes. *Nucleic Acids Res* **25**:3261, 1997.

74. Hasegawa T, Takeuchi A, Miyaishi O, Isobe K, de Crombrugghe B: Cloning and characterization of a transcription factor that binds to the proximal promoters of the two mouse type I collagen genes. *J Biol Chem* **272**:4915, 1997.

75. Hasegawa T, Zhou X, Garrett LA, Ruteshouser EC, Maity SN, de Crombrugghe B: Evidence for three major transcription activation elements in the proximal mouse proα2(I) collagen promoter. *Nucleic Acids Res* **24**:3253, 1996.

76. Hormuzdi SG, Penttinen R, Jaenisch R, Bornstein P: A gene-targeting approach identifies a function for the first intron in expression of the α1(I) collagen gene. *Mol Cell Biol* **18**:3368, 1998.

77. Bornstein P: Regulation of expression of the α1(I) collagen gene: A critical appraisal of the role of the first intron. *Matrix Biol* **15**:3, 1996.

78. Liska DJ, Reed MJ, Sage EH, Bornstein P: Cell-specific expression of α1(I) collagen-hGH minigenes in transgenic mice. *J Cell Biol* **125**:695, 1994.

79. Breault DT, Lichtler AC, Rowe DW: COL1A1 transgene expression in stably transfected osteoblastic cells. Relative contributions of first intron, 3'-flanking sequences, and sequences derived from the body of the human COL1A1 minigene. *J Biol Chem* **272**:31241, 1997.

80. Roberts AB, Sporn MB, Assoian RK, Smith JM, Roche NS, Wakefield LM, Heine UI, et al: Transforming growth factor type beta: Rapid induction of fibrosis and angiogenesis in vivo and stimulation of collagen formation in vitro. *Proc Natl Acad Sci U S A* **83**:4167, 1986.

81. Raghow R, Postlethwaite AE, Keski-Oja J, Moses HL, Kang AH: Transforming growth factor-beta increases steady state levels of type I procollagen and fibronectin messenger RNAs posttranscriptionally in cultured human dermal fibroblasts. *J Clin Invest* **79**:1285, 1987.

82. Murad S, Grove D, Lindberg KA, Reynolds G, Sivarajah A, Pinnell SR: Regulation of collagen synthesis by ascorbic acid. *Proc Natl Acad Sci U S A* **78**:2879, 1981.

83. Yamada Y, Mudryj M, de Crombrugghe B: A uniquely conserved regulatory signal is found around the translation initiation site in three different collagen genes. *J Biol Chem* **258**:14914, 1983.

84. Bennett VD, Adams SL: Characterization of the translational control mechanism preventing synthesis of α2(I) collagen in chicken vertebral chondroblasts. *J Biol Chem* **262**:14806, 1987.

85. Paglia L, Wilczek J, de Leon LD, Martin GR, Horlein D, Muller P: Inhibition of procollagen cell-free synthesis by amino-terminal extension peptides. *Biochemistry* **18**:5030, 1979.

86. Fouser L, Sage EH, Clark J, Bornstein P: Feedback regulation of collagen gene expression: A Trojan horse approach. *Proc Natl Acad Sci U S A* **88**:10158, 1991.

87. Aycock RS, Raghow R, Stricklin GP, Seyer JM, Kang AH: Post-transcriptional inhibition of collagen and fibronectin synthesis by a synthetic homolog of a portion of the carboxyl-terminal propeptide of human type I collagen. *J Biol Chem* **261**:14355, 1986.

88. Bienkowski RS, Curran SF, Berg RA: Kinetics of intracellular degradation of newly synthesized collagen. *Biochemistry* **25**:2455, 1986.

89. Schwarze U, Starman BJ, Byers PH: Redefinition of exon 7 in the COL1A1 gene of type I collagen by an intron 8 splice-donor-site mutation in a form of osteogenesis imperfecta: influence of intron splice order on outcome of splice-site mutation. *Am J Hum Genet* **65**:336, 1999.

90. Wiestner M, Rohde H, Helle O, Krieg T, Timpl R, Muller PK: Low rate of procollagen conversion in dermatosparactic sheep fibroblasts is paralleled by increased synthesis of type I and type III collagens. *EMBO J* **1**:513, 1982.

91. Nusgens BV, Verellen-Dumoulin C, Hermanns-Le T, De Paepe A, Nuytinck L, Pierard GE, Lapiere CM: Evidence for a relationship between Ehlers-Danlos type VII C in humans and bovine dermatosparaxis. *Nat Genet* **1**:214, 1992.

92. Vuust J, Piez KA: A kinetic study of collagen biosynthesis. *J Biol Chem* **247**:856, 1972.

93. Kivirikko KI, Pihlajaniemi T: Collagen hydroxylases and the protein disulfide isomerase subunit of prolyl 4-hydroxylases. *Adv Enzymol Relat Areas Mol Biol* **72**:325, 1998.

94. Annunen P, Helaakoski T, Myllyharju J, Veijola J, Pihlajaniemi T, Kivirikko KI: Cloning of the human prolyl 4-hydroxylase α subunit isoform α(II) and characterization of the type II enzyme tetramer. The α(I) and α(II) subunits do not form a mixed α(I)α(II)β2 tetramer. *J Biol Chem* **272**:17342, 1997.

95. Annunen P, Autio-Harmainen H, Kivirikko KI: The novel type II prolyl 4-hydroxylase is the main enzyme form in chondrocytes and capillary endothelial cells, whereas the type I enzyme predominates in most cells. *J Biol Chem* **273**:5989, 1998.

96. Myllyharju J, Kivirikko KI: Identification of a novel proline-rich peptide-binding domain in prolyl 4-hydroxylase. *EMBO J* **18**:306, 1999.

97. Passoja K, Rautavuoma K, Ala-Kokko L, Kosonen T, Kivirikko KI: Cloning and characterization of a third human lysyl hydroxylase isoform. *Proc Natl Acad Sci U S A* **95**:10482, 1998.

98. Hautala T, Byers MG, Eddy RL, Shows TB, Kivirikko KI, Myllyla R: Cloning of human lysyl hydroxylase: Complete cDNA-derived amino acid sequence and assignment of the gene (PLOD) to chromosome 1p36.3-p36.2. *Genomics* **13**:62, 1992.

99. Szpirer C, Szpirer J, Riviere M, Vanvooren P, Valtavaara M, Myllyla R: Localization of the gene encoding a novel isoform of lysyl hydroxylase. *Mamm Genome* **8**:707, 1997.

100. Valtavaara M, Papponen H, Pirttila AM, Hiltunen K, Helander H, Myllyla R: Cloning and characterization of a novel human lysyl hydroxylase isoform highly expressed in pancreas and muscle. *J Biol Chem* **272**:6831, 1997.

101. Yeowell HN, Ha V, Clark WL, Marshall MK, Pinnell SR: Sequence analysis of a cDNA for lysyl hydroxylase isolated from human skin fibroblasts from a normal donor: Differences from human placental lysyl hydroxylase cDNA. *J Invest Dermatol* **102**:382, 1994.

102. Royce PM, Barnes MJ: Failure of highly purified lysyl hydroxylase to hydroxylate lysyl residues in the non-helical regions of collagen. *Biochem J* **230**:475, 1985.

103. Bank RA, Robins SP, Wijmenga C, Breslau-Siderius LJ, Bardoel AF, van der Sluijs HA, Pruijs HE, et al: Defective collagen cross-linking in bone, but not in ligament or cartilage, in Bruck syndrome: Indications for a bone-specific telopeptide lysyl hydroxylase on chromosome 17. *Proc Natl Acad Sci U S A* **96**:1054, 1999.

104. Uzawa K, Grzesik WJ, Nishiura T, Kuznetsov SA, Robey PG, Brenner DA, Yamauchi M: Differential expression of human lysyl hydroxylase genes, lysine hydroxylation, and cross-linking of type I collagen during osteoblastic differentiation in vitro. *J Bone Miner Res* **14**:1272, 1999.

105. Eyre DR: Collagen cross-linking amino acids. *Methods Enzymol.* **144**:115, 1987.

106. Clark CC: The distribution and initial characterization of oligosaccharide units on the COOH-terminal propeptide extensions of the pro-α1 and pro-α2 chains of type I procollagen. *J Biol Chem* **254**:10798, 1979.

107. Anttinen H, Oikarinen A, Ryhanen L, Kivirikko KI: Evidence for the transfer of mannose to the extension peptides of procollagen within the cisternae of the rough endoplasmic reticulum. *FEBS Lett* **87**:222, 1978.

108. Guzman NA, Graves PN, Prockop DJ: Addition of mannose to both the amino- and carboxy-terminal properties of type II procollagen occurs without formation of a triple helix. *Biochem Biophys Res Commun* **84**:691, 1978.

109. Koide T, Asada S, Nagata K: Substrate recognition of collagen-specific molecular chaperone HSP47. Structural requirements and binding regulation. *J Biol Chem* **274**:34523, 1999.

110. Asada S, Koide T, Yasui H, Nagata K: Effect of HSP47 on prolyl 4-hydroxylation of collagen model peptides. *Cell Struct Funct* **24**:187, 1999.

111. Wilson R, Lees JF, Bulleid NJ: Protein disulfide isomerase acts as a molecular chaperone during the assembly of procollagen. *J Biol Chem* **273**:9637, 1998.

112. Mayne R, Brewton RG, Mayne PM, Baker JR: Isolation and characterization of the chains of type V/type XI collagen present in bovine vitreous. *J Biol Chem* **268**:9381, 1993.

113. Lees JF, Tasab M, Bulleid NJ: Identification of the molecular recognition sequence which determines the type-specific assembly of procollagen. *EMBO J* **16**:908, 1997.

114. Bachinger HP, Bruckner P, Timpl R, Engel J: The role of *cis-trans* isomerization of peptide bonds in the coil leads to and comes from triple helix conversion of collagen. *Eur J Biochem* **90**:605, 1978.

115. Bachinger HP: The influence of peptidyl-prolyl *cis-trans* isomerase on the in vitro folding of type III collagen. *J Biol Chem* **262**:17144, 1987.

116. Bonfanti L, Mironov AA Jr, Martinez-Menarguez JA, Martella O, Fusella A, Baldassarre M, Buccione R, et al: Procollagen traverses the Golgi stack without leaving the lumen of cisternae: Evidence for cisternal maturation. *Cell* **95**:993, 1998.

117. Trelstad RL, Hayashi K, Gross J: Collagen fibrillogenesis: Intermediate aggregates and suprafibrillar order. *Proc Natl Acad Sci U S A* **73**:4027, 1976.

118. Fessler LI, Chapin S, Brosh S, Fessler JH: Intracellular transport and tyrosine sulfation of procollagens V. *Eur J Biochem* **158**:511, 1986.

119. Fessler LI, Brosh S, Chapin S, Fessler JH: Tyrosine sulfation in precursors of collagen V. *J Biol Chem* **261**:5034, 1986.

120. Fisher LW, Robey PG, Tuross N, Otsuka AS, Tepen DA, Esch FS, Shimasaki S, et al: The Mr 24,000 phosphoprotein from developing bone is the NH2-terminal propeptide of the α1 chain of type I collagen. *J Biol Chem* **262**:13457, 1987.

121. Lapiere CM, Lenaers A, Kohn LD: Procollagen peptidase: An enzyme excising the coordination peptides of procollagen. *Proc Natl Acad Sci U S A* **68**:3054, 1971.

122. Colige A, Li SW, Sieron AL, Nusgens BV, Prockop DJ, Lapiere CM: cDNA cloning and expression of bovine procollagen I N-proteinase: A new member of the superfamily of zinc-metalloproteinases with binding sites for cells and other matrix components. *Proc Natl Acad Sci U S A* **94**:2374, 1997.

123. Colige A, Sieron AL, Li SW, Schwarze U, Petty E, Wertelecki W, Wilcox W, et al: Human Ehlers-Danlos syndrome type VII C and bovine dermatosparaxis are caused by mutations in the procollagen I N-proteinase gene. *Am J Hum Genet* **65**:308, 1999.

124. Imamura Y, Steiglitz BM, Greenspan DS: Bone morphogenetic protein-1 processes the NH2-terminal propeptide, and a furin-like proprotein convertase processes the COOH-terminal propeptide of pro-α1(V) collagen. *J Biol Chem* **273**:27511, 1998.

125. Birk DE, Trelstad RL: Extracellular compartments in tendon morphogenesis: Collagen fibril, bundle, and macroaggregate formation. *J Cell Biol* **103**:231, 1986.

126. Holmes DF, Watson RB, Chapman JA, Kadler KE: Enzymic control of collagen fibril shape. *J Mol Biol* **261**:93, 1996.

127. Kadler KE, Hojima Y, Prockop DJ: Assembly of collagen fibrils de novo by cleavage of the type I pC-collagen with procollagen C-proteinase. Assay of critical concentration demonstrates that collagen self-assembly is a classical example of an entropy-driven process. *J Biol Chem* **262**:15696, 1987.

128. Kadler KE, Hojima Y, Prockop DJ: Assembly of type I collagen fibrils *de novo*. Between 37 and 41 degrees C the process is limited by micro-unfolding of monomers. *J Biol Chem* **263**:10517, 1988.

129. Kadler KE, Hojima Y, Prockop DJ: Collagen fibrils in vitro grow from pointed tips in the C- to N-terminal direction. *Biochem J* **268**:339, 1990.

130. Danielson KG, Baribault H, Holmes DF, Graham H, Kadler KE, Iozzo RV: Targeted disruption of decorin leads to abnormal collagen fibril morphology and skin fragility. *J Cell Biol* **136**:729, 1997.

131. Smith-Mungo LI, Kagan HM: Lysyl oxidase: Properties, regulation and multiple functions in biology. *Matrix Biol* **16**:387, 1998.

132. Mariani TJ, Trackman PC, Kagan HM, Eddy RL, Shows TB, Boyd CD, Deak SB: The complete derived amino acid sequence of human lysyl oxidase and assignment of the gene to chromosome 5 (extensive sequence homology with the murine ras recision gene). *Matrix* **12**:242, 1992.

133. Hamalainen ER, Jones TA, Sheer D, Taskinen K, Pihlajaniemi T, Kivirikko KI: Molecular cloning of human lysyl oxidase and assignment of the gene to chromosome 5q23.3-31.2. *Genomics* **11**:508, 1991.

134. Lenaers A, Ansay M, Nusgens BV, Lapiere CM: Collagen made of extended α-chains, procollagen, in genetically defective dermatosparaxic calves. *Eur J Biochem* **23**:533, 1971.

135. Pinnell SR, Krane SM, Kenzora JE, Glimcher MJ: A heritable disorder of connective tissue. Hydroxylysine-deficient collagen disease. *N Engl J Med* **286**:1013, 1972.

136. Sykes B, Francis MJ, Smith R: Altered relation of two collagen types in osteogenesis imperfecta. *N Engl J Med* **296**:1200, 1977.

137. Holbrook KA, Byers PH: Ultrastructural characteristics of the skin in a form of the Ehlers- Danlos syndrome type IV. Storage in the rough endoplasmic reticulum. *Lab Invest* **44**:342, 1981.

138. Korkko J, Ritvaniemi P, Haataja L, Kaariainen H, Kivirikko KI, Prockop DJ, Ala-Kokko L: Mutation in type II procollagen (COL2A1) that substitutes aspartate for glycine α1-67 and that causes cataracts and retinal detachment: Evidence for molecular heterogeneity in the Wagner syndrome and the Stickler syndrome (arthro-ophthalmopathy) [see comments]. *Am J Hum Genet* **53**:55, 1993.

139. Sillence DO, Senn A, Danks DM: Genetic heterogeneity in osteogenesis imperfecta. *J Med Genet* **16**:101, 1979.

140. Smith R, Francis MJO, Houghton GR: The Brittle Bone Syndrome: *Osteogenesis*. London, Butterworths, 1983.

141. Seedorf KS: Osteogenesis imperfecta: a study of clinical features and heredity based on 55 Danish families. Universitetsforlaget I, Aarhus, 1949.

142. Ibsen KH: Distinct varieties of osteogenesis imperfecta. *Clin Orthop* **50**:279, 1967.

143. Andersen PE Jr, Hauge M: Osteogenesis imperfecta: A genetic, radiological, and epidemiological study. *Clin Genet* **36**:250, 1989.

144. Orioli IM, Castilla EE, Barbosa-Neto JG: The birth prevalence rates for the skeletal dysplasias. *J Med Genet* **23**:328, 1986.

145. Cox JR, Simmons CL: Osteogenesis imperfecta and associated hearing loss in five kindreds. *South Med J* **75**:1222, 1982.

146. Garretsen AJ, Cremers CW, Huygen PL: Hearing loss (in nonoperated ears) in relation to age in osteogenesis imperfecta type I. *Ann Otol Rhinol Laryngol* **106**:575, 1997.

147. Pedersen U: Hearing loss in patients with osteogenesis imperfecta. A clinical and audiological study of 201 patients. *Scand Audiol* **13**:67, 1984.

148. Quisling RW, Moore GR, Jahrsdoerfer RA, Cantrell RW: Osteogenesis imperfecta. A study of 160 family members. *Arch Otolaryngol* **105**:207, 1979.

149. Shapiro JR, Pikus A, Weiss G, Rowe DW: Hearing and middle ear function in osteogenesis imperfecta. *JAMA* **247**:2120, 1982.

150. Pedersen U, Elbrond O: Stapedectomy in osteogenesis imperfecta. *J Otorhinolaryngol Relat Spec* **45**:330, 1983.

151. Garretsen TJ, Cremers CW: Ear surgery in osteogenesis imperfecta. Clinical findings and short- term and long-term results. *Arch Otolaryngol Head Neck Surg* **116**:317, 1990.

152. Szilvassy J, Jori J, Czigner J, Toth F, Szilvassy Z, Kiss JG: Cochlear implantation in osteogenesis imperfecta. *Acta Otorhinolaryngol Belg* **52**:253, 1998.

153. Garretsen TJ, Cremers CW: Stapes surgery in osteogenesis imperfecta: Analysis of postoperative hearing loss. *Ann Otol Rhinol Laryngol* **100**:120, 1991.

154. Pedersen U: Osteogenesis imperfecta clinical features, hearing loss and stapedectomy. Biochemical, osteodensitometric, corneometric and histological aspects in comparison with otosclerosis. *Acta Otolaryngol Suppl* **415**:1, 1985.

155. White NJ, Winearls CG, Smith R: Cardiovascular abnormalities in osteogenesis imperfecta. *Am Heart J* **106**:1416, 1983.

156. Hortop J, Tsipouras P, Hanley JA, Maron BJ, Shapiro JR: Cardiovascular involvement in osteogenesis imperfecta. *Circulation* **73**:54, 1986.

157. McAllion SJ, Paterson CR: Causes of death in osteogenesis imperfecta. *J Clin Pathol* **49**:627, 1996.

158. Barsh GS, Byers PH: Reduced secretion of structurally abnormal type I procollagen in a form of osteogenesis imperfecta. *Proc Natl Acad Sci U S A* **78**:5142, 1981.

159. Rowe DW, Shapiro JR, Poirier M, Schlesinger S: Diminished type I collagen synthesis and reduced α1(I) collagen messenger RNA in cultured fibroblasts from patients with dominantly inherited (type I) osteogenesis imperfecta. *J Clin Invest* **76**:604, 1985.

160. Glorieux FH, Bishop NJ, Plotkin H, Chabot G, Lanoue G, Travers R: Cyclic administration of pamidronate in children with severe osteogenesis imperfecta. *N Engl J Med* **339**:947, 1998.

161. Pepin M, Atkinson M, Starman BJ, Byers PH: Strategies and outcomes of prenatal diagnosis for osteogenesis imperfecta: A review of biochemical and molecular studies completed in 129 pregnancies. *Prenat Diagn* **17**:559, 1997.

162. Crouch E, Bornstein P: Collagen synthesis by human amniotic fluid cells in culture: Characterization of a procollagen with three identical proα1(I) chains. *Biochemistry* **17**:5499, 1978.

163. Byers PH, Tsipouras P, Bonadio JF, Starman BJ, Schwartz RC: Perinatal lethal osteogenesis imperfecta (OI type II): A biochemically heterogeneous disorder usually due to new mutations in the genes for type I collagen. *Am J Hum Genet* **42**:237, 1988.

164. Sillence DO, Barlow KK, Garber AP, Hall JG, Rimoin DL: Osteogenesis imperfecta type II delineation of the phenotype with reference to genetic heterogeneity. *Am J Med Genet* **17**:407, 1984.

165. Thompson EM, Young ID, Hall CM, Pembrey ME: Recurrence risks and prognosis in severe sporadic osteogenesis imperfecta. *J Med Genet* **24**:390, 1987.

166. Bonaventure J, Cohen-Solal L, Lasselin C, Maroteaux P: A dominant mutation in the COL1A1 gene that substitutes glycine for valine causes recurrent lethal osteogenesis imperfecta. *Hum Genet* **89**:640, 1992.

167. Cohen-Solal L, Bonaventure J, Maroteaux P: Dominant mutations in familial lethal and severe osteogenesis imperfecta. *Hum Genet* **87**:297, 1991.

168. Cohn DH, Starman BJ, Blumberg B, Byers PH: Recurrence of lethal osteogenesis imperfecta due to parental mosaicism for a dominant mutation in a human type I collagen gene (COL1A1). *Am J Hum Genet* **46**:591, 1990.

169. Constantinou CD, Pack M, Young SB, Prockop DJ: Phenotypic heterogeneity in osteogenesis imperfecta: the mildly affected mother of a proband with a lethal variant has the same mutation substituting cysteine for α1-glycine 904 in a type I procollagen gene (COL1A1). *Am J Hum Genet* **47**:670, 1990.

170. Edwards MJ, Wenstrup RJ, Byers PH, Cohn DH: Recurrence of lethal osteogenesis imperfecta due to parental mosaicism for a mutation in the COL1A2 gene of type I collagen. The mosaic parent exhibits phenotypic features of a mild form of the disease. *Hum Mutat* **1**:47, 1992.

171. Mottes M, Gomez Lira MM, Valli M, Scarano G, Lonardo F, Forlino A, Cetta G, et al: Paternal mosaicism for a COL1A1 dominant mutation (α1 Ser-415) causes recurrent osteogenesis imperfecta. *Hum Mutat* **2**:196, 1993.

172. Beighton P, Versfeld GA: On the paradoxically high relative prevalence of osteogenesis imperfecta type III in the black population of South Africa. *Clin Genet* **27**:398, 1985.

173. Goldman AB, Davidson D, Pavlov H, Bullough PG: "Popcorn" calcifications: A prognostic sign in osteogenesis imperfecta. *Radiology* **136**:351, 1980.

174. Cole WG: Early surgical management of severe forms of osteogenesis imperfecta. *Am J Med Genet* **45**:270, 1993.

175. Cole WG: Orthopaedic treatment of osteogenesis imperfecta. *Ann N Y Acad Sci* **543**:157, 1988.

176. Lund AM, Nicholls AC, Schwartz M, Skovby F: Parental mosaicism and autosomal dominant mutations causing structural abnormalities of collagen I are frequent in families with osteogenesis imperfecta type III/IV. *Acta Paediatr* **86**:711, 1997.

177. Binder H, Conway A, Hason S, Gerber LH, Marini J, Berry R, Weintrob J: Comprehensive rehabilitation of the child with osteogenesis imperfecta. *Am J Med Genet* **45**:265, 1993.

178. Landsmeer-Beker EA, Massa GG, Maaswinkel-Mooy PD, van de Kamp JJ, Papapoulos SE: Treatment of osteogenesis imperfecta with

the bisphosphonate olpadronate (dimethylaminohydroxypropylidene bisphosphonate). *Eur J Pediatr* **156**:792, 1997.

179. Astrom E, Soderhall S: Beneficial effect of bisphosphonate during five years of treatment of severe osteogenesis imperfecta. *Acta Paediatr* **87**:64, 1998.

180. Bembi B, Parma A, Bottega M, Ceschel S, Zanatta M, Martini C, Ciana G: Intravenous pamidronate treatment in osteogenesis imperfecta. *J Pediatr* **131**:622, 1997.

181. Bergstrom JD, Bostedor RG, Masarachia PJ, Reszka AA, Rodan G: Alendronate is a specific, nanomolar inhibitor of farnesyl diphosphate synthase. *Arch Biochem Biophys* **373**:231, 2000.

182. Fisher JE, Rogers MJ, Halasy JM, Luckman SP, Hughes DE, Masarachia PJ, Wesolowski G, et al.: Alendronate mechanism of action: Geranylgeranyl, an intermediate in the mevalonate pathway, prevents inhibition of osteoclast formation, bone resorption, and kinase activation in vitro. *Proc Natl Acad Sci U S A* **96**:133, 1999.

183. Rodan GA: Bone homeostasis. *Proc Natl Acad Sci U S A* **95**:13361, 1998.

184. Horwitz EM, Prockop DJ, Fitzpatrick LA, Koo WW, Gordon PL, Neel M, Sussman M, et al: Transplantability and therapeutic effects of bone marrow-derived mesenchymal cells in children with osteogenesis imperfecta. *Nat Med* **5**:309, 1999.

185. Marini JC: Osteogenesis imperfecta calls for caution [Letter; Comment]. *Nat Med* **5**:466, 1999.

186. Aylsworth AS, Seeds JW, Guilford WB, Burns CB, Washburn DB: Prenatal diagnosis of a severe deforming type of osteogenesis imperfecta. *Am J Med Genet* **19**:707, 1984.

187. Robinson LP, Worthen NJ, Lachman RS, Adomian GE, Rimoin DL: Prenatal diagnosis of osteogenesis imperfecta type III. *Prenat Diagn* **7**:7, 1987.

188. Paterson CR, McAllion S, Miller R: Osteogenesis imperfecta with dominant inheritance and normal sclerae. *J Bone Joint Surg [Br]* **65**:35, 1983.

189. Wallis GA, Starman BJ, Zinn AB, Byers PH: Variable expression of osteogenesis imperfecta in a nuclear family is explained by somatic mosaicism for a lethal point mutation in the α1(I) gene (COL1A1) of type I collagen in a parent. *Am J Hum Genet* **46**:1034, 1990.

190. Boyde A, Travers R, Glorieux FH, Jones SJ: The mineralization density of iliac crest bone from children with osteogenesis imperfecta. *Calcif Tissue Int* **64**:185, 1999.

191. Neuhauser G, Kaveggia EG, Opitz JM: Autosomal recessive syndrome of pseudogliomantous blindness, osteoporosis and mild mental retardation. *Clin Genet* **9**:324, 1976.

192. Capoen J, De Paepe A, Lauwers H: The osteoporosis pseudoglioma syndrome. *J Belge Radiol* **76**:224, 1993.

193. Swoboda W, Grill F: The osteoporosis pseudoglioma syndrome. Update and report on two affected siblings. *Pediatr Radiol* **18**:399, 1988.

194. MacDougall M, Jeffords LG, Gu TT, Knight CB, Frei G, Reus BE, Otterud B, et al: Genetic linkage of the dentinogenesis imperfecta type III locus to chromosome 4q. *J Dent Res* **78**:1277, 1999.

195. Aplin HM, Hirst KL, Dixon MJ: Refinement of the dentinogenesis imperfecta type II locus to an interval of less than 2 centiMorgans at chromosome 4q21 and the creation of a yeast artificial chromosome contig of the critical region. *J Dent Res* **78**:1270, 1999.

196. Dean JA, Hartsfield JK Jr, Wright JT, Hart TC: Dentin dysplasia, type II linkage to chromosome 4q. *J Craniofac Genet Dev Biol* **17**:172, 1997.

197. Crosby AH, Scherpbier-Heddema T, Wijmenga C, Altherr MR, Murray JC, Buetow KH, Dixon MJ: Genetic mapping of the dentinogenesis imperfecta type II locus. *Am J Hum Genet* **57**:832, 1995.

198. Ball SP, Cook PJ, Mars M, Buckton KE: Linkage between dentinogenesis imperfecta and Gc. *Ann Hum Genet* **46**:35, 1982.

199. Byers PH: Osteogenesis imperfecta, in Royce PM, Steinmann B (eds): *Connective Tissue and its Heritable Disorders. Molecular, Genetic and Medical Aspects.* New York, Wiley-Liss, 1993, 317.

200. Marini JC, Lewis MB, Wang Q, Chen KJ, Orrison BM: Serine for glycine substitutions in type I collagen in two cases of type IV osteogenesis imperfecta (OI). Additional evidence for a regional model of OI pathophysiology. *J Biol Chem* **268**:2667, 1993.

201. Kuivaniemi H, Tromp G, Prockop DJ: Mutations in fibrillar collagens (types I, II, III, and XI), fibril-associated collagen (type IX), and network-forming collagen (type X) cause a spectrum of diseases of bone, cartilage, and blood vessels. *Hum Mutat* **9**:300, 1997.

202. Baum J, Brodsky B: Folding of peptide models of collagen and misfolding in disease. *Curr Opin Struct Biol* **9**:122, 1999.

203. Raghunath M, Bruckner P, Steinmann B: Delayed triple helix formation of mutant collagen from patients with osteogenesis imperfecta. *J Mol Biol* **236**:940, 1994.

204. Vogel BE, Doelz R, Kadler KE, Hojima Y, Engel J, Prockop DJ: A substitution of cysteine for glycine 748 of the α1 chain produces a kink at this site in the procollagen I molecule and an altered N-proteinase cleavage site over 225 nm away. *J Biol Chem* **263**:19249, 1988.

205. Bella J, Eaton M, Brodsky B, Berman HM: Crystal and molecular structure of a collagen-like peptide at 1.9 Å resolution [see comments]. *Science* **266**:75, 1994.

206. Bateman JF, Chan D, Walker ID, Rogers JG, Cole WG: Lethal perinatal osteogenesis imperfecta due to the substitution of arginine for glycine at residue 391 of the α1(I) chain of type I collagen. *J Biol Chem* **262**:7021, 1987.

207. Torre-Blanco A, Adachi E, Romanic AM, Prockop DJ: Copolymerization of normal type I collagen with three mutated type I collagens containing substitutions of cysteine at different glycine positions in the α1(I) chain. *J Biol Chem* **267**:4968, 1992.

208. Byers PH: Brittle bones — Fragile molecules: Disorders of collagen gene structure and expression. *Trends Genet* **6**:293, 1990.

209. Willing MC, Deschenes SP, Scott DA, Byers PH, Slayton RL, Pitts SH, Arikat H, et al: Osteogenesis imperfecta type I: Molecular heterogeneity for COL1A1 null alleles of type I collagen. *Am J Hum Genet* **55**:638, 1994.

210. Bateman JF, Chan D, Moeller I, Hannagan M, Cole WG: A 5' splice site mutation affecting the pre-mRNA splicing of two upstream exons in the collagen COL1A1 gene. Exon 8 skipping and altered definition of exon 7 generates truncated pro α1(I) chains with a non-collagenous insertion destabilizing the triple helix. *Biochem J* **302**:729, 1994.

211. Kuslich CD, Schwarze U, Byers PH: The order of intron removal influences the outcome of splice site mutations. *Am J Hum Genet* **65**:A80, 1999.

212. Willing MC, Cohn DH, Byers PH: Frameshift mutation near the 3' end of the COL1A1 gene of type I collagen predicts an elongated proα1(I) chain and results in osteogenesis imperfecta type I. *J Clin Invest* **85**:282, 1990.

213. Fitzgerald J, Lamande SR, Bateman JF: Proteasomal degradation of unassembled mutant type I collagen pro-α1(I) chains. *J Biol Chem* **274**:27392, 1999.

214. Chessler SD, Byers PH: BiP binds type I procollagen proα chains with mutations in the carboxyl-terminal propeptide synthesized by cells from patients with osteogenesis imperfecta. *J Biol Chem* **268**:18226, 1993.

215. Lamande SR, Chessler SD, Golub SB, Byers PH, Chan D, Cole WG, Sillence DO, et al: Endoplasmic reticulum-mediated quality control of type I collagen production by cells from osteogenesis imperfecta patients with mutations in the proα1(I) chain carboxyl-terminal propeptide which impair subunit assembly. *J Biol Chem* **270**:8642, 1995.

216. Schnieke A, Dziadek M, Bateman J, Mascara T, Harbers K, Gelinas R, Jaenisch R: Introduction of the human proα1(I) collagen gene into proα1(I)-deficient Mov-13 mouse cells leads to formation of functional mouse-human hybrid type I collagen. *Proc Natl Acad Sci U S A* **84**:764, 1987.

217. Chipman SD, Sweet HO, McBride DJ Jr, Davisson MT, Marks SC Jr, Shuldiner AR, Wenstrup RJ, et al: Defective proα2(I) collagen synthesis in a recessive mutation in mice: A model of human osteogenesis imperfecta. *Proc Natl Acad Sci U S A* **90**:1701, 1993.

218. Pihlajaniemi T, Dickson LA, Pope FM, Korhonen VR, Nicholls A, Prockop DJ, Myers JC: Osteogenesis imperfecta: Cloning of a pro-α2(I) collagen gene with a frameshift mutation. *J Biol Chem* **259**:12941, 1984.

219. Hata R, Kurata S, Shinkai H: Existence of malfunctioning proα2(I) collagen genes in a patient with a proα2(I)-chain-defective variant of Ehlers-Danlos syndrome. *Eur J Biochem* **174**:231, 1988.

220. Maquat LE: When cells stop making sense: Effects of nonsense codons on RNA metabolism in vertebrate cells. *RNA* **1**:453, 1995.

221. Willing MC, Deschenes SP, Slayton RL, Roberts EJ: Premature chain termination is a unifying mechanism for COL1A1 null alleles in osteogenesis imperfecta type I cell strains. *Am J Hum Genet* **59**:799, 1996.

222. Lightfoot SJ, Atkinson MS, Murphy G, Byers PH, Kadler KE: Substitution of serine for glycine 883 in the triple helix of the proα1(I) chain of type I procollagen produces osteogenesis imperfecta type IV and introduces a structural change in the triple helix that does not alter cleavage of the molecule by procollagen N-proteinase. *J Biol Chem* **269**:30352, 1994.

223. Chessler SD, Byers PH: Defective folding and stable association with protein disulfide isomerase/prolyl hydroxylase of type I procollagen with a deletion in the proα2(I) chain that preserves the Gly-X-Y repeat pattern. *J Biol Chem* **267**:7751, 1992.

224. Willing MC, Cohn DH, Starman B, Holbrook KA, Greenberg CR, Byers PH: Heterozygosity for a large deletion in the α2(I) collagen gene has a dramatic effect on type I collagen secretion and produces perinatal lethal osteogenesis imperfecta. *J Biol Chem* **263**:8398, 1988.

225. Vogel BE, Minor RR, Freund M, Prockop DJ: A point mutation in a type I procollagen gene converts glycine 748 of the α1 chain to cysteine and destabilizes the triple helix in a lethal variant of osteogenesis imperfecta. *J Biol Chem* **262**:14737, 1987.

226. Lightfoot SJ, Holmes DF, Brass A, Grant ME, Byers PH, Kadler KE: Type I procollagens containing substitutions of aspartate, arginine, and cysteine for glycine in the proα1(I) chain are cleaved slowly by N-proteinase, but only the cysteine substitution introduces a kink in the molecule. *J Biol Chem* **267**:25521, 1992.

227. Parkinson J, Brass A, Canova G, Brechet Y: The mechanical properties of simulated collagen fibrils. *J Biomech* **30**:549, 1997.

228. Kadler KE, Holmes DF, Trotter JA, Chapman JA: Collagen fibril formation. *Biochem J* **316**:1, 1996.

229. Kadler KE, Torre-Blanco A, Adachi E, Vogel BE, Hojima Y, Prockop DJ: A type I collagen with substitution of a cysteine for glycine-748 in the α1(I) chain copolymerizes with normal type I collagen and can generate fractal-like structures. *Biochemistry* **30**:5081, 1991.

230. Traub W, Arad T, Vetter U, Weiner S: Ultrastructural studies of bones from patients with osteogenesis imperfecta. *Matrix Biol* **14**:337, 1994.

231. Culbert AA, Lowe MP, Atkinson M, Byers PH, Wallis GA, Kadler KE: Substitutions of aspartic acid for glycine-220 and of arginine for glycine-664 in the triple helix of the proα1(I) chain of type I procollagen produce lethal osteogenesis imperfecta and disrupt the ability of collagen fibrils to incorporate crystalline hydroxyapatite. *Biochem J* **311**:815, 1995.

232. Denholm LJ, Cole WG: Heritable bone fragility, joint laxity and dysplastic dentin in Friesian calves: A bovine syndrome of osteogenesis imperfecta. *Aust Vet J* **60**:9, 1983.

233. Fisher LW, Denholm LJ, Conn KM, Termine JD: Mineralized tissue protein profiles in the Australian form of bovine osteogenesis imperfecta. *Calcif Tissue Int* **38**:16, 1986.

234. Deak SB, Nicholls A, Pope FM, Prockop DJ: The molecular defect in a nonlethal variant of osteogenesis imperfecta. Synthesis of pro-α2(I) chains which are not incorporated into trimers of type I procollagen. *J Biol Chem* **258**:15192, 1983.

235. Dickson LA, Pihlajaniemi T, Deak S, Pope FM, Nicholls A, Prockop DJ, Myers JC: Nuclease S1 mapping of a homozygous mutation in the carboxyl-propeptide-coding region of the proα2(I) collagen gene in a patient with osteogenesis imperfecta. *Proc Natl Acad Sci U S A* **81**:4524, 1984.

236. Schnieke A, Harbers K, Jaenisch R: Embryonic lethal mutation in mice induced by retrovirus insertion into the α1(I) collagen gene. *Nature* **304**:315, 1983.

237. Bonadio J, Saunders TL, Tsai E, Goldstein SA, Morris-Wiman J, Brinkley L, Dolan DF, et al: Transgenic mouse model of the mild dominant form of osteogenesis imperfecta. *Proc Natl Acad Sci U S A* **87**:7145, 1990.

238. Bonadio J, Jepsen KJ, Mansoura MK, Jaenisch R, Kuhn JL, Goldstein SA: A murine skeletal adaptation that significantly increases cortical bone mechanical properties. Implications for human skeletal fragility. *J Clin Invest* **92**:1697, 1993.

239. Pereira R, Khillan JS, Helminen HJ, Hume EL, Prockop DJ: Transgenic mice expressing a partially deleted gene for type I procollagen (COL1A1). A breeding line with a phenotype of spontaneous fractures and decreased bone collagen and mineral. *J Clin Invest* **91**:709, 1993.

240. Pereira R, Halford K, Sokolov BP, Khillan JS, Prockop DJ: Phenotypic variability and incomplete penetrance of spontaneous fractures in an inbred strain of transgenic mice expressing a mutated collagen gene (COL1A1). *J Clin Invest* **93**:1765, 1994.

241. Pereira RF, Hume EL, Halford KW, Prockop DJ: Bone fragility in transgenic mice expressing a mutated gene for type I procollagen (COL1A1) parallels the age-dependent phenotype of human osteogenesis imperfecta. *J Bone Miner Res* **10**:1837, 1995.

242. Beighton P: The Ehlers-Danlos Syndromes, in Beighton P (ed): *McKusick's Heritable Disorders of Connective Tissue*, 5th ed. St. Louis, Mosby-Year Book, 1993.

243. Steinmann B, Royce PM, Superti-Furga A: The Ehlers-Danlos Syndrome, in Royce PM, Steinmann B (eds): *Connective Tissue and its Heritable Disorders. Molecular, Genetic and Medical Aspects*. New York, Wiley-Liss, 1993, p 351.

244. Ehlers E: Cutis laxa, niegung zu haemorrhagien in der haut, lockerung mehrerer artikulationen. *Derm Zeit* **8**:173, 1901.

245. Tschernogobow A: Ein fall von cutis laxa. *Jahresb Ges Med* **27**:562, 1892.

246. Danlos M: Un cas de cutis laxa avec tumeurs par contusion chronique des coudes et des genoux (xanthome juvenile pseudodiabetique de MM Hallopeau et Mace de Lepinay). *Bull Soc Franc Derm Syph* **19**:70, 1908.

247. Barabas AP: Heterogeneity of the Ehlers-Danlos syndrome: Description of three clinical types and a hypothesis to explain the basic defect(s). *Br Med J* **2**:612, 1967.

248. Beighton P, Price A, Lord J, Dickson E: Variants of the Ehlers-Danlos syndrome. Clinical, biochemical, haematological, and chromosomal features of 100 patients. *Ann Rheum Dis* **28**:228, 1969.

249. Beighton P: *The Ehlers-Danlos Syndrome*. London, Heinemann, 1970.

250. Lichtenstein JR, Martin GR, Kohn LD, Byers PH, McKusick VA: Defect in conversion of procollagen to collagen in a form of Ehlers-Danlos syndrome. *Science* **182**:298, 1973.

251. Beighton P, De Paepe A, Steinmann B, Tsipouras P, Wenstrup RJ: Ehlers-Danlos syndromes: Revised nosology, Villefranche, 1997. Ehlers-Danlos National Foundation (USA) and Ehlers-Danlos Support Group (UK). *Am J Med Genet* **77**:31, 1998.

252. Barabas AP: Ehlers-Danlos syndrome: Associated with prematurity and premature rupture of foetal membranes; possible increase in incidence. *Br Med J* **5515**:682, 1966.

253. Leier CV, Call TD, Fulkerson PK, Wooley CF: The spectrum of cardiac defects in the Ehlers-Danlos syndrome, types I and III. *Ann Intern Med* **92**:171, 1980.

254. Burrows NP, Nicholls AC, Yates JR, Richards AJ, Pope FM: Genetic linkage to the collagen α1(V) gene (COL5A1) in two British Ehlers-Danlos syndrome families with variable type I and II phenotypes. *Clin Exp Dermatol* **22**:174, 1997.

255. Loughlin J, Irven C, Hardwick LJ, Butcher S, Walsh S, Wordsworth P, Sykes B: Linkage of the gene that encodes the α1 chain of type V collagen (COL5A1) to type II Ehlers-Danlos syndrome (EDS II). *Hum Mol Genet* **4**:1649, 1995.

256. Burrows NP, Nicholls AC, Yates JR, Gatward G, Sarathachandra P, Richards A, Pope FM: The gene encoding collagen α1(V)(COL5A1) is linked to mixed Ehlers-Danlos syndrome type I/II. *J Invest Dermatol* **106**:1273, 1996.

257. Greenspan DS, Northrup H, Au KS, McAllister KA, Francomano CA, Wenstrup RJ, Marchuk DA, et al: COL5A1: Fine genetic mapping and exclusion as candidate gene in families with nail-patella syndrome, tuberous sclerosis 1, hereditary hemorrhagic telangiectasia, and Ehlers-Danlos Syndrome type II. *Genomics* **25**:737, 1995.

258. Wenstrup RJ, Langland GT, Willing MC, D'Souza VN, Cole WG: A splice-junction mutation in the region of COL5A1 that codes for the carboxyl propeptide of proα1(V) chains results in the gravis form of the Ehlers-Danlos syndrome (type I). *Hum Mol Genet* **5**:1733, 1996.

259. Nicholls AC, McCarron S, Narcisi P, Pope FM: Molecular abnormalities of type V collagen in Ehlers Danlos syndrome. *Am J Hum Genet* **55**:A233, 1994.

260. Toriello HV, Glover TW, Takahara K, Byers PH, Miller DE, Higgins JV, Greenspan DS: A translocation interrupts the COL5A1 gene in a patient with Ehlers- Danlos syndrome and hypomelanosis of Ito. *Nat Genet* **13**:361, 1996.

261. De Paepe A, Nuytinck L, Hausser I, Anton-Lamprecht I, Naeyaert JM: Mutations in the COL5A1 gene are causal in the Ehlers-Danlos syndromes I and II. *Am J Hum Genet* **60**:547, 1997.

262. Richards AJ, Martin S, Nicholls AC, Harrison JB, Pope FM, Burrows NP: A single base mutation in COL5A2 causes Ehlers-Danlos syndrome type II. *J Med Genet* **35**:846, 1998.

263. Michalickova K, Susic M, Willing MC, Wenstrup RJ, Cole WG: Mutations of the α2(V) chain of type V collagen impair matrix assembly and produce Ehlers-Danlos syndrome type I. *Hum Mol Genet* **7**:249, 1998.

264. Burch GH, Gong Y, Liu W, Dettman RW, Curry CJ, Miller WL, Bristow J: Tenascin-X deficiency is associated with Ehlers-Danlos syndrome. *Nat Genet* **17**:104, 1997.

265. Schwarze U, Atkinson M, Hoffman GG, Greenspan DS, Byers PH: Null alleles of the COL5A1 gene of type V collagen are a cause of the classical forms of Ehlers-Danlos syndrome (types I and II). *Am J Hum Genet* **66**:1757, 2000.

266. Wenstrup RJ, Florer JB, Willing MC, Giunta C, Steinmann B, Young F, Susic M, et al.: COL5A1 Haploinsufficiency is a common molecular

mechanism underlying the classical form of EDS. *Am J Hum Genet* **66**:1766, 2000.

267. Grahame R, Beighton P: Physical properties of the skin in the Ehlers-Danlos syndrome. *Ann Rheum Dis* **28**:246, 1969.

268. Vogel A, Holbrook KA, Steinmann B, Gitzelmann R, Byers PH: Abnormal collagen fibril structure in the gravis form (type I) of Ehlers-Danlos syndrome. *Lab Invest* **40**:201, 1979.

269. Holbrook KA, Byers PH: Skin is a window on heritable disorders of connective tissue. *Am J Med Genet* **34**:105, 1989.

270. Hausser I, Anton-Lamprecht I: Differential ultrastructural aberrations of collagen fibrils in Ehlers-Danlos syndrome types I-IV as a means of diagnostics and classification. *Hum Genet* **93**:394, 1994.

271. Linsenmayer TF, Gibney E, Igoe F, Gordon MK, Fitch JM, Fessler LI, Birk DE: Type V collagen: Molecular structure and fibrillar organization of the chicken α1(V) NH2-terminal domain, a putative regulator of corneal fibrillogenesis. *J Cell Biol* **121**:1181, 1993.

272. Sasaki T, Arai K, Ono M, Yamaguchi T, Furuta S, Nagai Y: Ehlers-Danlos syndrome. A variant characterized by the deficiency of proα2 chain of type I procollagen. *Arch Dermatol* **123**:76, 1987.

273. Nicholls AC, Osse G, Schloon HG, Lenard HG, Deak S, Myers JC, Prockop DJ, et al: The clinical features of homozygous α2(I) collagen deficient osteogenesis imperfecta. *J Med Genet* **21**:257, 1984.

274. Narcisi P, Richards AJ, Ferguson SD, Pope FM: A family with Ehlers-Danlos syndrome type III/articular hypermobility syndrome has a glycine 637 to serine substitution in type III collagen. *Hum Mol Genet* **3**:1617, 1994.

275. Hegreberg GA: Animal models of collagen disease. *Prog Clin Biol Res* **94**:229, 1982.

276. Sack G: Status dysvascularis: Ein fall von besonderer zerreisslichkeit deve blutgefasse. *Dtsch Archiv Klin Med* **178**:663, 1936.

277. Gottron F: Familiare acrogeria. *Arch Dermatol Res* **181**:571, 1940.

278. Pope FM, Martin GR, Lichtenstein JR, Penttinen R, Gerson B, Rowe DW, McKusick VA: Patients with Ehlers-Danlos syndrome type IV lack type III collagen. *Proc Natl Acad Sci U S A* **72**:1314, 1975.

279. Pepin M, Schwarze U, Superti-Furga A, Byers PH: Clinical and genetic features of Ehlers-Danlos syndrome type IV, the vascular type. *N Engl J Med* **342**:673, 2000.

280. Pope FM, Martin GR, McKusick VA: Inheritance of Ehlers-Danlos type IV syndrome. *J Med Genet* **14**:200, 1977.

281. Sulh HM, Steinmann B, Rao VH, Dudin G, Zeid JA, Slim M, Der Kaloustian VM: Ehlers-Danlos syndrome type IV D: An autosomal recessive disorder. *Clin Genet* **25**:278, 1984.

282. Pope FM, Narcisi P, Nicholls AC, Liberman M, Oorthuys JW: Clinical presentations of Ehlers Danlos syndrome type IV. *Arch Dis Child* **63**:1016, 1988.

283. Rudd NL, Nimrod C, Holbrook KA, Byers PH: Pregnancy complications in type IV Ehlers-Danlos Syndrome. *Lancet* **1**:50, 1983.

284. Lach B, Nair SG, Russell NA, Benoit BG: Spontaneous carotid-cavernous fistula and multiple arterial dissections in type IV Ehlers-Danlos syndrome. Case report. *J Neurosurg* **66**:462, 1987.

285. North KN, Whiteman DA, Pepin MG, Byers PH: Cerebrovascular complications in Ehlers-Danlos syndrome type IV. *Ann Neurol* **38**:960, 1995.

286. Schievink WI, Piepgras DG, Earnest Ft, Gordon H: Spontaneous carotid-cavernous fistulae in Ehlers-Danlos syndrome Type IV. Case report. *J Neurosurg* **74**:991, 1991.

287. Halbach VV, Higashida RT, Dowd CF, Barnwell SL, Hieshima GB: Treatment of carotid-cavernous fistulas associated with Ehlers-Danlos syndrome. *Neurosurgery* **26**:1021, 1990.

288. Pope FM, Nicholls AC: Pregnancy and Ehlers-Danlos syndrome type IV. *Lancet* **1**:249, 1983.

289. Kuming BS, Joffe L: Ehlers-Danlos syndrome associated with keratoconus. A case report. *S Afr Med J* **52**:403, 1977.

290. Smith LT, Schwarze U, Goldstein J, Byers PH: Mutations in the COL3A1 gene result in the Ehlers-Danlos syndrome type IV and alterations in the size and distribution of the major collagen fibrils of the dermis. *J Invest Dermatol* **108**:241, 1997.

291. Schwarze U, Goldstein JA, Byers PH: Splicing defects in the COL3A1 gene: Marked preference for 5′ (donor) spice-site mutations in patients with exon-skipping mutations and Ehlers-Danlos syndrome type IV. *Am J Hum Genet* **61**:1276, 1997.

292. Kuivaniemi H, Kontusaari S, Tromp G, Zhao MJ, Sabol C, Prockop DJ: Identical G+1 to A mutations in three different introns of the type III procollagen gene (COL3A1) produce different patterns of RNA splicing in three variants of Ehlers-Danlos syndrome. IV. An explanation for exon skipping with some mutations and not others. *J Biol Chem* **265**:12067, 1990.

293. Kontusaari S, Tromp G, Kuivaniemi H, Stolle C, Pope FM, Prockop DJ: Substitution of aspartate for glycine 1018 in the type III procollagen (COL3A1) gene causes type IV Ehlers-Danlos syndrome: The mutated allele is present in most blood leukocytes of the asymptomatic and mosaic mother. *Am J Hum Genet* **51**:497, 1992.

294. Milewicz DM, Witz AM, Smith AC, Manchester DK, Waldstein G, Byers PH: Parental somatic and germ-line mosaicism for a multiexon deletion with unusual endpoints in a type III collagen (COL3A1) allele produces Ehlers-Danlos syndrome type IV in the heterozygous offspring. *Am J Hum Genet* **53**:62, 1993.

295. Richards AJ, Ward PN, Narcisi P, Nicholls AC, Lloyd JC, Pope FM: A single base mutation in the gene for type III collagen (COL3A1) converts glycine 847 to glutamic acid in a family with Ehlers-Danlos syndrome type IV. An unaffected family member is mosaic for the mutation. *Hum Genet* **89**:414, 1992.

296. Beighton P: X-linked recessive inheritance in the Ehlers-Danlos syndrome. *Br Med J* **2**:9, 1968.

297. Beighton P, Curtis D: X-linked Ehlers-Danlos syndrome type V: The next generation. *Clin Genet* **27**:472, 1985.

298. Siegel RC, Black CM, Bailey AJ: Cross-linking of collagen in the X-linked Ehlers-Danlos type V. *Biochem Biophys Res Commun* **88**:281, 1979.

299. Elsas LJd, Miller RL, Pinnell SR: Inherited human collagen lysyl hydroxylase deficiency: Ascorbic acid response. *J Pediatr* **92**:378, 1978.

300. Jarisch A, Giunta C, Zielen S, Konig R, Steinmann B: Sibs affected with both Ehlers-Danlos syndrome type IV and cystic fibrosis. *Am J Med Genet* **78**:455, 1998.

301. Hyland J, Ala-Kokko L, Royce P, Steinmann B, Kivirikko KI, Myllyla R: A homozygous stop codon in the lysyl hydroxylase gene in two siblings with Ehlers-Danlos syndrome type VI. *Nat Genet* **2**:228, 1992.

302. Ihme A, Risteli L, Krieg T, Risteli J, Feldmann U, Kruse K, Muller PK: Biochemical characterization of variants of the Ehlers-Danlos syndrome type VI. *Eur J Clin Invest* **13**:357, 1983.

303. Heikkinen J, Toppinen T, Yeowell H, Krieg T, Steinmann B, Kivirikko KI, Myllyla R: Duplication of seven exons in the lysyl hydroxylase gene is associated with longer forms of a repetitive sequence within the gene and is a common cause for the type VI variant of Ehlers-Danlos syndrome. *Am J Hum Genet* **60**:48, 1997.

304. Krieg T, Feldmann U, Kessler W, Muller PK: Biochemical characteristics of Ehlers-Danlos syndrome type VI in a family with one affected infant. *Hum Genet* **46**:41, 1979.

305. Pousi B, Hautala T, Heikkinen J, Pajunen L, Kivirikko KI, Myllyla R: Alu-Alu recombination results in a duplication of seven exons in the lysyl hydroxylase gene in a patient with the type VI variant of Ehlers-Danlos syndrome. *Am J Hum Genet* **55**:899, 1994.

306. Pousi B, Hautala T, Hyland JC, Schroter J, Eckes B, Kivirikko KI, Myllyla R: A compound heterozygote patient with Ehlers-Danlos syndrome type VI has a deletion in one allele and a splicing defect in the other allele of the lysyl hydroxylase gene. *Hum Mutat* **11**:55, 1998.

307. Wenstrup RJ, Murad S, Pinnell SR: Ehlers-Danlos syndrome type VI: Clinical manifestations of collagen lysyl hydroxylase deficiency. *J Pediatr* **115**:405, 1989.

308. Yeowell HN, Walker LC, Murad S, Pinnell SR: A common duplication in the lysyl hydroxylase gene of patients with Ehlers Danlos syndrome type VI results in preferential stimulation of lysyl hydroxylase activity and mRNA by hydralazine. *Arch Biochem Biophys* **347**:126, 1997.

309. Yeowell HN, Walker LC: Ehlers-Danlos syndrome type VI results from a nonsense mutation and a splice site-mediated exon-skipping mutation in the lysyl hydroxylase gene. *Proc Assoc Am Physicians* **109**:383, 1997.

310. Sussman M, Lichtenstein JR, Nigra TP, Martin GR, McKusick VA: Hydroxylysine-deficient skin collagen in a patient with a form of the Ehlers-Danlos syndrome. *J Bone Joint Surg [Am]* **56**:1228, 1974.

311. Judisch GF, Waziri M, Krachmer JH: Ocular Ehlers-Danlos syndrome with normal lysyl hydroxylase activity. *Arch Ophthalmol* **94**:1489, 1976.

312. Pasquali M, Still MJ, Vales T, Rosen RI, Evinger JD, Dembure PP, Longo N, et al: Abnormal formation of collagen cross-links in skin fibroblasts cultured from patients with Ehlers-Danlos syndrome type VI. *Proc Assoc Am Physicians* **109**:33, 1997.

313. Steinmann B, Eyre DR, Shao P: Urinary pyridinoline cross-links in Ehlers-Danlos syndrome type VI. *Am J Hum Genet* **57**:1505, 1995.

314. Dembure PP, Priest JH, Snoddy SC, Elsas LJ: Genotyping and prenatal assessment of collagen lysyl hydroxylase deficiency in a family with Ehlers-Danlos syndrome type VI. *Am J Hum Genet* **36**:783, 1984.

315. Yeowell HN, Walker LC: Prenatal exclusion of Ehlers-Danlos syndrome type VI by mutational analysis. *Proc Assoc Am Physicians* **111**:57, 1999.

316. Hautala T, Heikkinen J, Kivirikko KI, Myllyla R: A large duplication in the gene for lysyl hydroxylase accounts for the type VI variant of Ehlers-Danlos syndrome in two siblings. *Genomics* **15**:399, 1993.

317. Brinckmann J, Acil Y, Feshchenko S, Katzer E, Brenner R, Kulozik A, Kugler S: Ehlers-Danlos syndrome type VI: lysyl hydroxylase deficiency due to a novel point mutation (W612C). *Arch Dermatol Res* **290**:181, 1998.

318. Pajunen L, Suokas M, Hautala T, Kellokumpu S, Tebbe B, Kivirikko KI, Myllyla R: A splice-site mutation that induces exon skipping and reduction in lysyl hydroxylase mRNA levels but does not create a nonsense codon in Ehlers-Danlos syndrome type VI. *DNA Cell Biol* **17**:117, 1998.

319. Ha VT, Marshall MK, Elsas LJ, Pinnell SR, Yeowell HN: A patient with Ehlers-Danlos syndrome type VI is a compound heterozygote for mutations in the lysyl hydroxylase gene. *J Clin Invest* **93**:1716, 1994.

320. Byers PH, Duvic M, Atkinson M, Robinow M, Smith LT, Krane SM, Greally MT, et al: Ehlers-Danlos syndrome type VIIA and VIIB result from splice-junction mutations or genomic deletions that involve exon 6 in the COL1A1 and COL1A2 genes of type I collagen. *Am J Med Genet* **72**:94, 1997.

321. Giunta C, Superti-Furga A, Spranger S, Cole WG, Steinmann B: Ehlers-Danlos syndrome type VII: Clinical features and molecular defects. *J Bone Joint Surg Am* **81**:225, 1999.

322. Counts DF, Byers PH, Holbrook KA, Hegreberg GA: Dermatosparaxis in a Himalayan cat: I. Biochemical studies of dermal collagen. *J Invest Dermatol* **74**:96, 1980.

323. Steinmann B, Tuderman L, Peltonen L, Martin GR, McKusick VA, Prockop DJ: Evidence for a structural mutation of procollagen type I in a patient with the Ehlers-Danlos syndrome type VII. *J Biol Chem* **255**:8887, 1980.

324. Eyre DR, Shapiro FD, Aldridge JF: A heterozygous collagen defect in a variant of the Ehlers-Danlos syndrome type VII. Evidence for a deleted amino-telopeptide domain in the pro-α2(I) chain. *J Biol Chem* **260**:11322, 1985.

325. Cole WG, Chan D, Chambers GW, Walker ID, Bateman JF: Deletion of 24 amino acids from the pro-α1(I) chain of type I procollagen in a patient with the Ehlers-Danlos syndrome type VII. *J Biol Chem* **261**:5496, 1986.

326. Wirtz MK, Glanville RW, Steinmann B, Rao VH, Hollister DW: Ehlers-Danlos syndrome type VIIB. Deletion of 18 amino acids comprising the N-telopeptide region of a pro-α2(I) chain. *J Biol Chem* **262**:16376, 1987.

327. Weil D, Bernard M, Combates N, Wirtz MK, Hollister DW, Steinmann B, Ramirez F: Identification of a mutation that causes exon skipping during collagen pre-mRNA splicing in an Ehlers-Danlos syndrome variant. *J Biol Chem* **263**:8561, 1988.

328. Weil D, D'Alessio M, Ramirez F, Eyre DR: Structural and functional characterization of a splicing mutation in the pro-α2(I) collagen gene of an Ehlers-Danlos type VII patient. *J Biol Chem* **265**:16007, 1990.

329. Vasan NS, Kuivaniemi H, Vogel BE, Minor RR, Wootton JA, Tromp G, Weksberg R, et al: A mutation in the pro α2(I) gene (COL1A2) for type I procollagen in Ehlers-Danlos syndrome type VII: Evidence suggesting that skipping of exon 6 in RNA splicing may be a common cause of the phenotype. *Am J Hum Genet* **48**:305, 1991.

330. Watson RB, Holmes DF, Graham HK, Nusgens BV, Kadler KE: Surface located procollagen N-propeptides on dermatosparactic collagen fibrils are not cleaved by procollagen N-proteinase and do not inhibit binding of decorin to the fibril surface. *J Mol Biol* **278**:195, 1998.

331. Smith LT, Wertelecki W, Milstone LM, Petty EM, Seashore MR, Braverman IM, Jenkins TG, et al: Human dermatosparaxis: A form of Ehlers-Danlos syndrome that results from failure to remove the amino-terminal propeptide of type I procollagen. *Am J Hum Genet* **51**:235, 1992.

332. Fujimoto A, Wilcox WR, Cohn DH: Clinical, morphological, and biochemical phenotype of a new case of Ehlers-Danlos syndrome type VIIC. *Am J Med Genet* **68**:25, 1997.

333. Reardon W, Winter RM, Smith LT, Lake BD, Rossiter M, Baraitser M: The natural history of human dermatosparaxis (Ehlers-Danlos syndrome type VIIC). *Clin Dysmorphol* **4**:1, 1995.

334. Stewart RE, Hollister DW, Rimoin DL: A new variant of Ehlers-Danlos syndrome: An autosomal dominant disorder of fragile skin, abnormal scarring, and generalized periodontitis. *Birth Defects Orig Artic Ser* **13**:85, 1977.

335. Linch DC, Acton CH: Ehlers-Danlos syndrome presenting with juvenile destructive periodontitis. *Br Dent J* **147**:95, 1979.

336. Hartsfield JK Jr, Kousseff BG: Phenotypic overlap of Ehlers-Danlos syndrome types IV and VIII. *Am J Med Genet* **37**:465, 1990.

337. Arneson MA, Hammerschmidt DE, Furcht LT, King RA: A new form of Ehlers-Danlos syndrome. Fibronectin corrects defective platelet function. *JAMA* **244**:144, 1980.

338. Beighton P, de Paepe A, Danks D, Finidori G, Gedde-Dahl T, Goodman R, Hall JG, et al: International Nosology of Heritable Disorders of Connective Tissue, Berlin, 1986. *Am J Med Genet* **29**:581, 1988.

339. Spranger J, Winterpacht A, Zabel B: The type II collagenopathies: A spectrum of chondrodysplasias. *Eur J Pediatr* **153**:56, 1994.

340. Godfrey M, Hollister DW: Type II achondrogenesis-hypochondrogenesis: Identification of abnormal type II collagen. *Am J Hum Genet* **43**:904, 1988.

341. Ritvaniemi P, Korkko J, Bonaventure J, Vikkula M, Hyland J, Paassilta P, Kaitila I, et al: Identification of COL2A1 gene mutations in patients with chondrodysplasias and familial osteoarthritis. *Arthritis Rheum* **38**:999, 1995.

342. Tiller GE, Rimoin DL, Murray LW, Cohn DH: Tandem duplication within a type II collagen gene (COL2A1) exon in an individual with spondyloepiphyseal dysplasia. *Proc Natl Acad Sci U S A* **87**:3889, 1990.

343. Lee B, Vissing H, Ramirez F, Rogers D, Rimoin D: Identification of the molecular defect in a family with spondyloepiphyseal dysplasia. *Science* **244**:978, 1989.

344. Ritvaniemi P, Sokolov BP, Williams CJ, Considine E, Yurgenev L, Meerson EM, Ala-Kokko L, et al: A single base mutation in the type II procollagen gene (COL2A1) that converts glycine α1-247 to serine in a family with late-onset spondyloepiphyseal dysplasia. *Hum Mutat* **3**:261, 1994.

345. Winterpacht A, Hilbert K, Schwarze U, Zabel B: Non-radioactive multiplex-SSCP analysis: Detection of a new type II procollagen gene (COL2A1) mutation. *Hum Genet* **95**:437, 1995.

346. Chan D, Cole WG: Low basal transcription of genes for tissue-specific collagens by fibroblasts and lymphoblastoid cells. Application to the characterization of a glycine 997 to serine substitution in α1(II) collagen chains of a patient with spondyloepiphyseal dysplasia. *J Biol Chem* **266**:12487, 1991.

347. Tiller GE, Weis MA, Polumbo PA, Gruber HE, Rimoin DL, Cohn DH, Eyre DR: An RNA-splicing mutation (G+5IVS20) in the type II collagen gene (COL2A1) in a family with spondyloepiphyseal dysplasia congenita. *Am J Hum Genet* **56**:388, 1995.

348. Chan D, Rogers JF, Bateman JF, Cole WG: Recurrent substitutions of arginine 789 by cysteine in pro-α1 (II) collagen chains produce spondyloepiphyseal dysplasia congenita. *J Rheumatol Suppl* **43**:37, 1995.

349. Fertala A, Ala-Kokko L, Wiaderkiewicz R, Prockop DJ: Collagen II containing a Cys substitution for Arg-α1-519. Homotrimeric monomers containing the mutation do not assemble into fibrils but alter the self-assembly of the normal protein. *J Biol Chem* **272**:6457, 1997.

350. Weis MA, Wilkin DJ, Kim HJ, Wilcox WR, Lachman RS, Rimoin DL, Cohn DH, et al: Structurally abnormal type II collagen in a severe form of Kniest dysplasia caused by an exon 24 skipping mutation. *J Biol Chem* **273**:4761, 1998.

351. Fernandes RJ, Wilkin DJ, Weis MA, Wilcox WR, Cohn DH, Rimoin DL, Eyre DR: Incorporation of structurally defective type II collagen into cartilage matrix in Kniest chondrodysplasia. *Arch Biochem Biophys* **355**:282, 1998.

352. Winterpacht A, Schwarze U, Mundlos S, Menger H, Spranger J, Zabel B: Alternative splicing as the result of a type II procollagen gene (COL2A1) mutation in a patient with Kniest dysplasia. *Hum Mol Genet* **3**:1891, 1994.

353. Spranger J, Winterpacht A, Zabel B: Kniest dysplasia: Dr. W. Kniest, his patient, the molecular defect. *Am J Med Genet* **69**:79, 1997.

354. Bogaert R, Wilkin D, Wilcox WR, Lachman R, Rimoin D, Cohn DH, Eyre DR: Expression, in cartilage, of a 7-amino-acid deletion in type II collagen from two unrelated individuals with Kniest dysplasia. *Am J Hum Genet* **55**:1128, 1994.

355. Chen L, Yang W, Cole WG: Alternative splicing of exon 12 of the COL2A1 gene interrupts the triple helix of type-II collagen in the Kniest form of spondyloepiphyseal dysplasia. *J Orthop Res* **14**:712, 1996.

356. Wilkin DJ, Artz AS, South S, Lachman RS, Rimoin DL, Wilcox WR, McKusick VA, et al: Small deletions in the type II collagen triple helix produce Kniest dysplasia. *Am J Med Genet* **85**:105, 1999.

357. Wilkin DJ, Bogaert R, Lachman RS, Rimoin DL, Eyre DR, Cohn DH: A single amino acid substitution (G103D) in the type II collagen triple helix produces Kniest dysplasia. *Hum Mol Genet* 3:1999, 1994.

358. Winterpacht A, Superti-Furga A, Schwarze U, Stoss H, Steinmann B, Spranger J, Zabel B: The deletion of six amino acids at the C-terminus of the α1(II) chain causes overmodification of type II and type XI collagen: Further evidence for the association between small deletions in COL2A1 and Kniest dysplasia. *J Med Genet* 33:649, 1996.

359. Spranger J, Menger H, Mundlos S, Winterpacht A, Zabel B: Kniest dysplasia is caused by dominant collagen II (COL2A1) mutations: Parental somatic mosaicism manifesting as Stickler phenotype and mild spondyloepiphyseal dysplasia. *Pediatr Radiol* 24:431, 1994.

360. Winterpacht A, Hilbert M, Schwarze U, Mundlos S, Spranger J, Zabel BU: Kniest and Stickler dysplasia phenotypes caused by collagen type II gene (COL2A1) defect. *Nat Genet* 3:323, 1993.

361. Herrmann J, France TD, Spranger JW, Opitz JM, Wiffler C: The Stickler syndrome (hereditary arthro-ophthalmopathy). *Birth Defects Orig Artic Ser* 11:76, 1975.

362. Wilkin DJ, Mortier GR, Johnson CL, Jones MC, de Paepe A, Shohat M, Wildin RS, et al: Correlation of linkage data with phenotype in eight families with Stickler syndrome. *Am J Med Genet* 80:121, 1998.

363. Martin S, Richards AJ, Yates JR, Scott JD, Pope M, Snead MP: Stickler syndrome: Further mutations in COL11A1 and evidence for additional locus heterogeneity. *Eur J Hum Genet* 7:807, 1999.

364. McGuirt WT, Prasad SD, Griffith AJ, Kunst HP, Green GE, Shpargel KB, Runge C, et al: Mutations in COL11A2 cause non-syndromic hearing loss (DFNA13). *Nat Genet* 23:413, 1999.

365. Bleasel JF, Holderbaum D, Brancolini V, Moskowitz RW, Considine EL, Prockop DJ, Devoto M, et al: Five families with arginine 519-cysteine mutation in COL2A1:Evidence for three distinct founders. *Hum Mutat* 12:172, 1998.

366. Pun YL, Moskowitz RW, Lie S, Sundstrom WR, Block SR, McEwen C, Williams HJ, et al: Clinical correlations of osteoarthritis associated with a single-base mutation (arginine519 to cysteine) in type II procollagen gene. A newly defined pathogenesis. *Arthritis Rheum* 37:264, 1994.

367. Ala-Kokko L, Baldwin CT, Moskowitz RW, Prockop DJ: Single base mutation in the type II procollagen gene (COL2A1) as a cause of primary osteoarthritis associated with a mild chondrodysplasia. *Proc Natl Acad Sci U S A* 87:6565, 1990.

368. Stephens FE: An achondroplasic mutation and the nature of its inheritance. *J Hered* 34:229, 1943.

369. Warman ML, Abbott M, Apte SS, Hefferon T, McIntosh I, Cohn DH, Hecht JT, et al: A type X collagen mutation causes Schmid metaphyseal chondrodysplasia. *Nat Genet* 5:79, 1993.

370. Schmid F: Beitrag zur dysostosis enchondralis metaphysaria. *Mschr Kinderheilk* 97:393, 1949.

371. Lachman RS, Rimoin DL, Spranger J: Metaphyseal chondrodysplasia, Schmid type. Clinical and radiographic delineation with a review of the literature. *Pediatric Radiology* 18:93, 1988.

372. Chan D, Jacenko O: Phenotypic and biochemical consequences of collagen X mutations in mice and humans. *Matrix Biol* 17:169, 1998.

373. Ikegawa S, Nakamura K, Nagano A, Haga N, Nakamura Y: Mutations in the N-terminal globular domain of the type X collagen gene (COL10A1) in patients with Schmid metaphyseal chondrodysplasia. *Hum Mutat* 9:131, 1997.

374. Marks DS, Gregory CA, Wallis GA, Brass A, Kadler KE, Boot-Handford RP: Metaphyseal chondrodysplasia type Schmid mutations are predicted to occur in two distinct three-dimensional clusters within type X collagen NC1 domains that retain the ability to trimerize. *J Biol Chem* 274:3632, 1999.

375. McLaughlin SH, Conn SN, Bulleid NJ: Folding and assembly of type X collagen mutants that cause metaphyseal chondrodysplasia-type Schmid. Evidence for co-assembly of the mutant and wild-type chains and binding to molecular chaperones. *J Biol Chem* 274:7570, 1999.

376. Chan D, Cole WG, Rogers JG, Bateman JF: Type X collagen multimer assembly in vitro is prevented by a Gly618 to Val mutation in the α1(X) NC1 domain resulting in Schmid metaphyseal chondrodysplasia. *J Biol Chem* 270:4558, 1995.

377. Chan D, Weng YM, Graham HK, Sillence DO, Bateman JF: A nonsense mutation in the carboxyl-terminal domain of type X collagen causes haploinsufficiency in schmid metaphyseal chondrodysplasia. *J Clin Invest* 101:1490, 1998.

378. Jacenko O, LuValle PA, Olsen BR: Spondylometaphyseal dysplasia in mice carrying a dominant negative mutation in a matrix protein specific for cartilage-to-bone transition. *Nature* 365:56, 1993.

379. Kwan KM, Pang MK, Zhou S, Cowan SK, Kong RY, Pfordte T, Olsen BR, et al: Abnormal compartmentalization of cartilage matrix components in mice lacking collagen X: Implications for function. *J Cell Biol* 136:459, 1997.

380. Rosati R, Horan GS, Pinero GJ, Garofalo S, Keene DR, Horton WA, Vuorio E, et al: Normal long bone growth and development in type X collagen-null mice. *Nat Genet* 8:129, 1994.

381. Briggs MD, Choi H, Warman ML, Loughlin JA, Wordsworth P, Sykes BC, Irven CM, et al: Genetic mapping of a locus for multiple epiphyseal dysplasia (EDM2) to a region of chromosome 1 containing a type IX collagen gene. *Am J Hum Genet* 55:678, 1994.

382. Briggs MD, Mortier GR, Cole WG, King LM, Golik SS, Bonaventure J, Nuytinck L et al: Diverse mutations in the gene for cartilage oligomeric matrix protein in the pseudoachondroplasia-multiple epiphyseal dysplasia disease spectrum. *Am J Hum Genet* 62:311, 1998.

383. Holden P, Canty EG, Mortier GR, Zabel B, Spranger J, Carr A, Grant ME, et al: Identification of novel pro-α2(IX) collagen gene mutations in two families with distinctive oligo-epiphyseal forms of multiple epiphyseal dysplasia. *Am J Hum Genet* 65:31, 1999.

384. Muragaki Y, Mariman EC, van Beersum SE, Perala M, van Mourik JB, Warman ML, Hamel BC, et al: A mutation in COL9A2 causes multiple epiphyseal dysplasia (EDM2). *Ann N Y Acad Sci* 785:303, 1996.

385. Paassilta P, Lohiniva J, Annunen S, Bonaventure J, Le Merrer M, Pai L, Ala-Kokko L: COL9A3:A third locus for multiple epiphyseal dysplasia. *Am J Hum Genet* 64:1036, 1999.

386. Fassler R, Schnegelsberg PN, Dausman J, Shinya T, Muragaki Y, McCarthy MT, Olsen BR, et al: Mice lacking α1(IX) collagen develop noninflammatory degenerative joint disease. *Proc Natl Acad Sci U S A* 91:5070, 1994.

# Marfan Syndrome and Related Disorders

*Harry C. Dietz* ■ *Reed E. Pyeritz*

1. Marfan syndrome is an autosomal dominant disorder of connective tissue with systemic effects and major manifestations in the cardiovascular, musculoskeletal, and ophthalmic systems and the integument. Diagnostic criteria, based mainly on clinical findings, are reasonably successful in differentiating Marfan syndrome (MIM 154700) from related disorders, such as congenital contractural arachnodactyly, MASS phenotype, mitral valve prolapse syndrome, familial aortic aneurysm, and familial forms of ectopia lentis.

2. The basic genetic defect in Marfan syndrome involves mutations in the extracellular matrix glycoprotein fibrillin-1, encoded by *FBN1* at 15q21.1. Mutations in a highly homologous gene, *FBN2*, at 5q23-q31, cause congenital contractural arachnodactyly (MIM 121050).

3. The cardinal clinical manifestations of Marfan syndrome include tall stature with dolichostenomelia and arachnodactyly; deformity of the spine and anterior chest; joint hypermobility or contracture; dilatation and dissection of the ascending aorta; mitral valve prolapse; myopia; ectopia lentis; pneumothorax; hernias; and dural ectasia. The prevalence of Marfan syndrome is uncertain, but is at least 2 to 3 in 10,000 individuals without regard to ethnicity. One-quarter to one-third of all cases represent new mutations; germinal mosaicism, while reported, is rare. The Marfan syndrome phenotype exhibits high penetrance but highly variable expression. If untreated, the condition leads to premature death, generally from cardiovascular complications. Aggressive management can result in nearly normal life expectancy. Management must be multidisciplinary to cover all aspects of medical care, surgical intervention, and genetic counseling.

4. Among the Marfan-related conditions is congenital contractural arachnodactyly, which exhibits dolichostenomelia, progressive scoliosis, congenital joint contractures, and deformity of the helix of the ear. Some people with CCA have mitral valve prolapse but aortic dilatation or ectopia lentis should prompt consideration of Marfan syndrome. In most inherited forms of ectopia lentis, findings are limited to the eye. Some families with autosomal dominant ectopia lentis have mild skeletal and cardiovascular features suggestive of the Marfan syndrome, but do not meet diagnostic criteria; some of these families have mutations in *FBN1*. Similarly, families lacking ectopia lentis and severe skeletal features, but having mitral valve prolapse, or aortic root dilatation, or both, have been shown, in a few cases, to link to or have mutations in *FBN1*. However, some families with autosomal dominant aortic aneurysm or dissection, and many sporadic patients with aortic aneurysm do not appear to have a mutation in *FBN1*.

5. Fibrillin is a major component of the 10-nM microfibrils of extracellular matrices. The primary structure of fibrillin exhibits a multidomain organization characterized by several cysteine-rich motifs reminiscent of the epidermal growth factor module. Extracellularly, fibrillin monomers aggregate into a supramolecular structure that has a "beads on a string" appearance on transmission electron microscopy. Characterization of a variety of fibrillin mutations has emphasized the importance of the structural integrity of individual cysteine-rich repeats, as well as the requirement that the fibrillin monomer must have a certain absolute length for normal microfibril assembly.

6. In addition to being linked to the Marfan syndrome, *FBN1* has been genetically linked to dominantly inherited ectopia lentis, MASS phenotype and familial aortic aneurysm, suggesting that mutations in functionally distinct domains of this gene product may cause seemingly distinct clinical phenotypes. On the other hand, linkage between congenital contractural arachnodactyly and *FBN2* suggests that fibrillin proteins have distinct functions in different tissues.

## HISTORICAL PERSPECTIVE

In 1896, French pediatrician Antonine Bernard-Jean Marfan[1] described to his colleagues in Paris a 5-year-old girl, Gabrielle P., who was tall for her age, had disproportionately long limbs and fingers, and joint contractures of fingers and knees. Marfan used the term "dolichostenomelia" for this clinical presentation to emphasize the unusually long and narrow frame of the young girl. Six years later, Mery and Babonneix,[2] in reexamining Gabrielle, added scoliosis to the previously described skeletal abnormalities and renamed the condition "hyperchondroplasia." In the same year, another French clinician, Achard,[3] coined the term "arachnodactyly" (long, spidery fingers) in describing the clinical phenotype of a seemingly identical patient. In subsequent reports, displacement of the ocular lens (ectopia lentis) and mitral regurgitation were added to the features of the disorder.[4,5] The involvement of several mesenchymal tissues in the clinical picture of Marfan syndrome (MFS), together with the demonstration of the genetic nature of the disorder, led Weve[6] to propose in 1931, the name "dystrophia mesodermalis congenita, typus Marfanis." Seven years later, Apert[7] condensed Weve's designation to the current term, Marfan syndrome. In 1943, one year after Marfan's death, aortic dilatation, regurgitation, and dissection were added to

---

A list of standard abbreviations is located immediately preceding the index in each volume. Additional abbreviations used in this chapter include: cbEGF = calcium binding epidermal growth factor; CCA = congenital contractural arachnodactyly; EGF = epidermal growth factor; FBN1 and FBN2 = genes for fibrillin-1 and fibrillin-2, respectively; LTBP = latency-inducing transforming growth factor β-binding proteins; MAGP = microfibril-associated glycoprotein; MASS = mitral valve prolapse in association with aortic, skeletal, and skin manifestations; MFAP = microfibril-associated protein; MFS = Marfan syndrome; MVP = mitral valve prolapse; TGFβ = transforming growth factor beta; US/LS = upper-to-lower segment ratio.

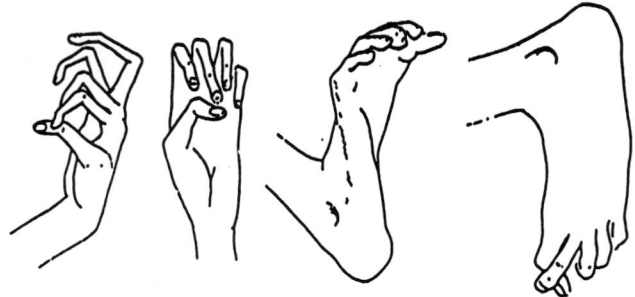

**Fig. 206-1 Depiction of the skeletal phenotype of the original case reported by Marfan showing arachnodactyly and suggesting joint contracture.**

the features of MFS.[8,9] Weve[6] also commented on the familial nature of the syndrome. In 1949, Lutman and Neel[10] examined the segregation of the skeletal and ocular features, interpreted this in terms of autosomal dominant inheritance, and concluded that the syndrome likely represented the pleiotropic effects of a single gene.

In 1955, McKusick[11] published a clinical and pathologic review of cases that was of seminal importance for three reasons. First, he showed that cardiovascular involvement was much more common in MFS than previously suspected, and that aortic complications were a leading cause of death. Second, he used MFS to introduce a nosologic idea of a "heritable disorder of connective tissue," a notion he expanded in a monograph bearing that title.[12] Finally, McKusick speculated on the fundamental defect that might cause a complex, pleiotropic phenotype similar to MFS, and suggested a defective component of the connective tissue, notably, "... the elastic fiber or a component intimately associated with elastic fiber."

During the next decade, several disorders that had been lumped with MFS were recognized as distinct based on phenotype, natural history, and genetics. Homocystinuria, a recessive condition of amino acid metabolism (see Chap. 87) and congenital contractural arachnodactyly (CCA) were most prominent.[13–16] Indeed, on reexamining the case reports on Gabrielle P., Hecht and Beals[17] emphasized the contractures of the elbows, fingers, knees, and toes (Fig. 206-1) in the absence of apparent cardiovascular or ocular difficulties, and suggested that Professor Marfan's original patient might have been affected by congenital contractural arachnodactyly (CCA), and not MFS. While plausible, the methods to detect aortic dilatation and subtle lens dislocation, even if suspected, were unavailable early in the twentieth century, and congenital contractures do occur in MFS. It is doubtful that Gabrielle, who died at 14 of presumed tuberculosis, will ever relinquish her diagnostic secret.

The 1970s and 1980s saw considerable progress in understanding the natural and clinical histories, and in expanding the range of pleiotropic involvement beyond the skeleton, heart and eye. The development of a variety of medical and surgical approaches to managing all of the clinical features resulted in improved functional capabilities and life expectancy. Recent reviews expand on these clinical issues.[18,19]

The three decades before 1990 also saw considerable activity in attempting to define the basic defect in MFS. McKusick[12] enunciated the challenge in the first edition of his monograph when he said, "What the suspensory ligament of the lens has in common with the tunica media of the aorta is obscure. If this common factor were known, the basic defect of the Marfan syndrome might be understood." Initial attention was directed to the fibrillar collagens, the most abundant structural component of the ECM, and to hyaluronic acid, the principle substance that accumulates in the media of the Marfan aorta. A wide variety of "abnormalities" of these and other components on the ECM were

reported.[20,21] All proved to be epiphenomena of the underlying defect.

In the late 1950s and early 1960s, several investigators documented the presence of extracellular microfibrils in a variety of tissues.[22–24] For example, dermatologists distinguish among elaunin, oxytalan, and elastic fibers in the skin, and each contains microfibrils. The oxytalan fibers, which extend perpendicularly across the epidermal-dermal junction, contribute to the stability of that interface. In the early 1980s, Cleary and colleagues[25] began to tease apart the components of the microfibril. In 1986, Sakai and colleagues[26] used polyclonal and monoclonal antibodies raised against microfibrils to identify a major component, a 350-kDa glycoprotein that they named fibrillin. The colocalization of fibrillin with microfibrils in both elastic and nonelastic tissues prompted a medical geneticist colleague of Lynn Sakai, David Hollister, to suggest that this macromolecule represented a candidate protein in the causation of MFS. What followed was an intense series of investigations over several years involving immunohistopathology,[27,28] biochemistry,[29,30] gene mapping of the MFS phenotype,[31–35] and gene cloning and mapping of fibrillin.[36–38] All results pointed to fibrillin as the most likely primary defect in MFS. The trail became slightly complicated by the discovery of two homologues, called fibrillin-1 and fibrillin-2, but the mapping data pointed to the loci for MFS and fibrillin-1 as being coincident.[33,37]

The first of many reports of mutations in patients with MFS in the gene for fibrillin-1 (now called *FBN1*) appeared in 1991.[39] Collectively, these studies indicate that mutations in *FBN1* are responsible for the MFS in most, if not all, cases.[40] Further studies strongly suggest that mutations in fibrillin genes may cause a variety of phenotypes, broadly belonging to the clinical spectrum of MFS-related disorders.

## GENETIC AND CLINICAL FEATURES OF MARFAN SYNDROME

The Marfan syndrome is an autosomal dominant disorder of connective tissue that occurs with an estimated frequency of 2 to 3 per 10,000 individuals. About one-quarter to one-third of newly diagnosed patients have neither parent affected with MFS, and thus their condition is most likely the result of a new germinal mutation. As with many dominant traits, advanced paternal age is found among the fathers of sporadic cases, presumably because age predisposes to *de novo* mutations in spermatocytes.[41] Most infants with a severe form of MFS are isolated cases, which is a bit tautologous because the more severe the phenotype the less the likelihood of survival to reproduction. Inheritance of mutations in *FBN1* from both parents has been suggested in a few severely affected children,[42,43] and then documented through molecular analysis.[44] Penetrance of MFS in families is high, although age-dependent; sensitive tests, such as echocardiography and slit-lamp examination of the eyes, may be required to detect subtle features at an early age. Intrafamilial variability is often impressive. As is explained subsequently, MFS is one end of a clinical spectrum resulting from mutations in *FBN1*, so the wide interfamilial variability in MFS reflects, in part, where the clinical diagnostic criteria are set along this phenotypic continuum.

The diagnosis of MFS is largely clinical and relies on the presence of a combination of manifestations in several organ systems, with some manifestations that are deemed "major" carrying particular weight (Table 206-1).[45] Major manifestations include aortic root dilatation and dissection, ectopia lentis, dural ectasia, and at least four of eight specific skeletal features. Family history of an unequivocal case of MFS as a first-degree relative of the person in whom the diagnosis is being considered is an important consideration, and results in fewer clinical findings being needed to warrant a diagnosis of MFS. However, because many of the manifestations of MFS are common in the general population (e.g., tall stature, scoliosis, pectus excavatum, mitral valve prolapse, myopia), the current criteria were designed to

**Table 206-1  Diagnostic Criteria for the Marfan Syndrome**

### Skeletal System

**Major criterion**: Presence of at least four of the following manifestations.
- Pectus carinatum
- Pectus excavatum requiring surgery
- Reduced upper to lower segment ratio or arm span to height ratio greater than 1.05
- Positive wrist and thumb signs
- Scoliosis of $\geq 20°$ or spondylolisthesis
- Reduced extension of the elbows ($< 170°$)
- Medial displacement of the medial malleolus causing pes planus
- Protrusio acetabulum of any degree (ascertained on x-ray)

**Minor criteria**
- Pectus excavatum of moderate severity
- Joint hypermobility
- Highly arched palate with dental crowding
- Facial appearance (dolichocephaly, malar hypoplasia, enophthalmos, retrognathia, down-slanting palpebral fissures)

*For the skeletal system to be involved, at least two of the components comprising the major criterion or one component comprising the major criterion plus two of the minor criteria must be present.*

### Ocular System

**Major criterion**
- Ectopia lentis

**Minor criteria**
- Abnormally flat cornea (as measured by keratometry)
- Increased axial length of globe (as measured by ultrasound)
- Hypoplastic iris or hypoplastic ciliary muscle causing a decreased miosis

*For the ocular system to be involved, at least two of the minor criteria must be present.*

### Cardiovascular System

**Major criteria**
- Dilatation of the ascending aorta with or without aortic regurgitation and involving at least the sinuses of Valsalva; or
- Dissection of the ascending aorta

**Minor criteria**
- Mitral valve prolapse with or without mitral valve regurgitation;
- Dilatation of main pulmonary artery, in absence of valvular or peripheral pulmonic stenosis or any other obvious cause, below the age of 40 years;
- Calcification of the mitral annulus below the age of 40 years; or
- Dilatation or dissection of the descending thoracic or abdominal aorta below the age of 50 years

*For the cardiovascular system to be involved a major criterion or only one of the minor criteria must be present.*

**Table 206-1  (Continued)**

### Pulmonary System

**Major criteria**
- None

**Minor criteria**
- Spontaneous pneumothorax, or
- Apical blebs (ascertained by chest radiography)

*For the pulmonary system to be involved one of the minor criteria must be present.*

### Skin and Integument

**Major criterion**
- Lumbosacral dural ectasia by CT or MRI

**Minor criteria**
- Striae atrophicae (stretch marks) not associated with marked weight changes, pregnancy or repetitive stress, or
- Recurrent or incisional herniae

*For the skin and integument to be involved the major criterion or one of the minor criteria must be present.*

### Family History

**Major criteria**
- Having a parent, child, or sib who meets these diagnostic criteria independently;
- Presence of a mutation in *FBNI* known to cause the Marfan syndrome; or
- Presence of a haplotype around *FBNI,* inherited by descent, known to be associated with unequivocally diagnosed Marfan syndrome in the family

**Minor criteria**
- None

*For the family history to be contributory, one of the major criteria must be present.*

### Requirements of the Diagnosis of the Marfan Syndrome

**For the index case**
- Major criteria in at least two different organ systems and involvement of a third organ system

---

minimize labeling people inappropriately with MFS.[46] Because of extensive intragenic heterogeneity in the cause of MFS, the large size of *FBN1*, the current inadequacy of methods to find mutations efficiently, and the fact that mutations in *FBN1* cause many of the very conditions confused with MFS, molecular diagnosis has a limited role in assigning the diagnosis in a new case. The exceptions are when a person is a direct relative of someone with MFS who has a known mutation in *FBN1*, when a person with an unclear diagnosis is found to have a mutation in *FBN1* that is known to cause MFS in an unrelated person, or when a person is part of a family suitable for linkage analysis.

## Skeletal Manifestations

People with MFS are taller at any age then their genetic background minus the mutation in *FBN1* would predict. The tall stature is due to overgrowth of the long bones, resulting in disproportionately long legs, arms and digits, which is termed *dolichostenomelia* (Fig. 206-2). Consequences are a decreased upper-to-lower segment ratio (US/LS),[47] an arm-span that exceeds body height, and arachnodactyly, which does not need to be quantified radiographically by the metacarpal index.[48,49] Another complication of overgrowth of tubular bones is deformity of the anterior chest.[50,51] The ribs can push the sternum in (pectus excavatum), out (pectus carinatum), or in on one side (typically the right costochondral junctions) and out on the other. The pathogenesis of bony overgrowth is unclear, although fibrillin-1 is present in perichondrium and periosteum.

The skull is often elongated (dolichocephaly), the face is long and narrow, the palate is narrow and highly arched, the mandible underdeveloped (retrognathism), and the teeth crowded.[52] Side-to-side curvature of the spine (scoliosis) occurs to some degree in more than half of people with MFS, tends to worsen during periods

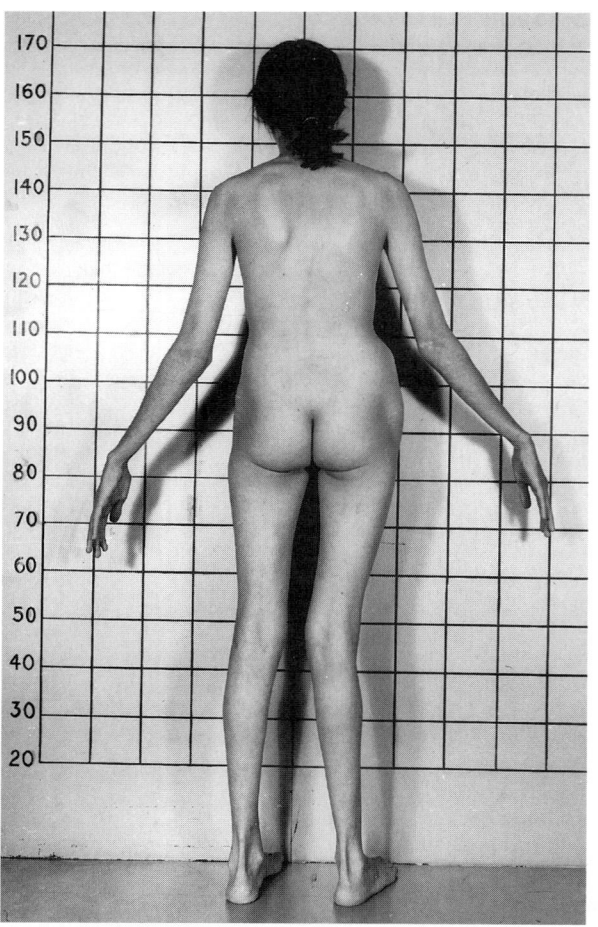

**Fig. 206-2 Skeletal features of Marfan syndrome in a 16-year-old girl. Note the long limbs that are associated with disproportionate tall stature, long fingers, scoliosis, and genu valgum.**

of rapid growth,[53–57] and occasionally develops in the young child.[58] The spine normally has cervical lordosis, upper thoracic kyphosis, and lumbar lordosis; any of these can be reversed, reduced, or accentuated in MFS. Ligamentous laxity, generalized joint hypermobility and joint pain are common in MFS,[59,60] especially of the digits, elbows, knees (genu recurvatum) and feet (pes planus) (Fig. 206-3). Joint dislocations are uncommon, although the incidences of atlantoaxial instability, spondylolisthesis, and congenital hip dislocation are increased.[57,61–64] Paradoxically, congenital joint contractures are also common in MFS, especially of the elbows and fingers, and hammer-toe deformities often develop over time. Another skeletal problem that becomes evident with age is erosion of the acetabulum (protrusio acetabuli).[65–69] In part, this tendency may reflect an underlying predisposition to osteoporosis.[70–73] With improved survival from the cardiovascular complications, people with MFS may well see an increased occurrence of degenerative skeletal problems, such as osteoarthritis, due to osteoporosis, protrusio acetabula, and joint laxity.

## Ocular Manifestations

Displacement of the lens from the center of the pupil (ectopia lentis) is the ocular hallmark of MFS, but is present in only 50 to 60 percent of affected people.[74,75] When displacement of a lens is detected in the absence of a traumatic event (the most common cause[76]), MFS should always be considered. In MFS, the ocular zonules, which attach to the limbus of the lens to the ciliary body,

become stretched and occasionally break. The lens displacement is usually upward, may be congenital, and tends to progress during periods of bodily growth (Fig. 206-4). Iridodonesis (fluttering of the iris) when the eye accommodates is a useful bedside indicator of lens dislocation, but may not be present in subtle ectopia lentis. A slit-lamp examination after maximal pupillary dilatation is an essential part of the diagnostic examination. However, because of hypoplasia of the ciliary muscle, pupillary dilatation with the usual mydriatic agents is often suboptimal.

The cornea is often flatter than normal, a finding reflected in the keratometer reading.[75] Despite the flat cornea, myopia is the most common ocular feature. Failure to detect and correct abnormal visual acuity in young children with MFS often results in persistent amblyopia. The globe is often elongated, and the greater the radius of curvature of the posterior globe, the greater the risk of spontaneous retinal detachment.[77] This serious complication also used to be associated with extirpation of the lens, but newer surgical techniques, including the implantation of artificial lenses, has mitigated this problem. Strabismus is not uncommon.[78] Glaucoma and cataract formation in middle adulthood are becoming recognized as important problems.[79]

## Cardiovascular Manifestations

Prolapse of the mitral valve (MVP), due to redundancy of the valve tissue, enlargement of the valve annulus, and elongation of the chordae tendineae, is the most common finding in childhood, and its progression to severe mitral regurgitation is the most frequent indication for cardiovascular surgery before age 10 years.[80–82] While MVP is common in the general population (3 to 5 percent of young adults) and in other connective tissue disorders (discussed later), over two-thirds of people with MFS eventually show MVP.[83] As the left ventricle enlarges, as a result of aortic regurgitation, intrinsic failure, or β-adrenergic blockade, the tension on the chordae increases and the amount of MVP may diminish.[84] Prolapse of the tricuspid valve is also common, but not nearly as much of a clinical problem. Histopathology of the atrioventricular valves shows myxomatous degeneration, with excessive accumulation of proteoglycan.[85]

The proximal portions of both the aorta (Fig. 206-5) and the main pulmonary artery progressively dilate, with onset often in utero.[86,87] These findings are highly important for both diagnosis and prognosis in MFS. Identification and monitoring of aortic root dilatation are effectively made through transthoracic echocardiography, which is also the procedure of choice for detection of MVP. As the sinus of Valsalva of the aorta enlarge, the commissures of the aortic valve stretch and eventually cause leakage of the valve (aortic regurgitation) during diastole. Before a murmur is heard, the leakage can be detected by Doppler echocardiography. Progression of the aortic regurgitation (AR) can lead to left-ventricular enlargement and failure, and before the era of effective cardiovascular surgery, AR was a common cause of death in MFS.[88] While mild pulmonic regurgitation is common, serious complications of pulmonary dilatation are rare.[89]

Dilatation of the proximal aorta occurs because of degeneration of elastic fibers in the aortic media (Fig. 206-6).[86,90] Erdheim[91] originally termed this histopathology "cystic medial necrosis," but there are neither cysts nor necrosis. Pools of hyaluronic acid are interspersed among the fragmented elastic fibers and there is a relative paucity of smooth muscle cells. Because the dilatation is gradual, and the aortic caliber does normally increase during childhood and adolescence, use of a "growth curve" for aortic diameter, in which diameter is related to body surface area, is essential for deciding whether a person's aortic caliber is greater than "normal."[92–94] The larger the diameter of the aortic root, the greater the likelihood of AR and of aortic dissection.[81,84,95,96] Today, aortic dissection, in which a separation occurs in the medial layer of the aorta, is the most common cause of death. A predisposition to dissection tracks in families, suggesting that

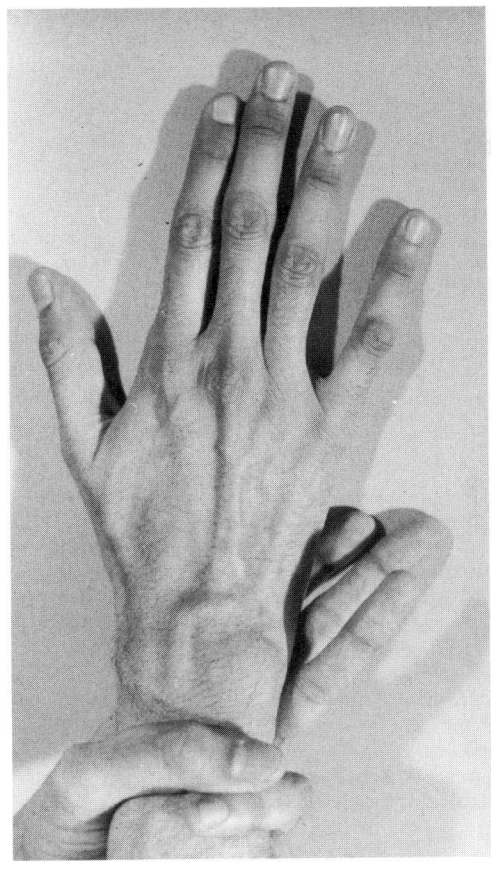

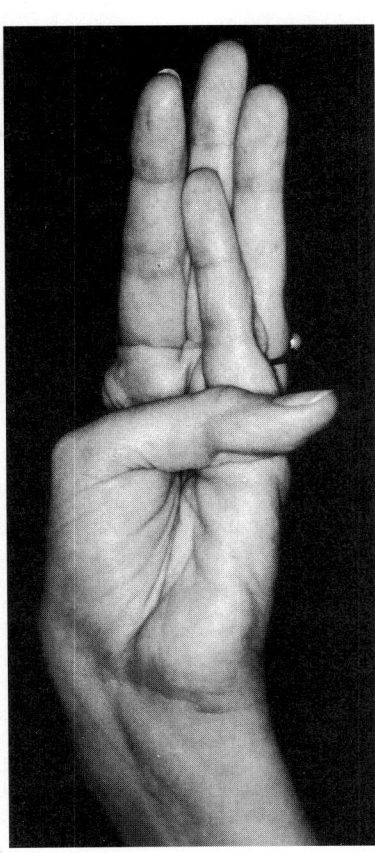

**Fig. 206-3 Adults with the Marfan syndrome demonstrating the wrist (*A*) and thumb (*B*) signs. The former is due to long digits and a paucity of skeletal muscle and fat; the latter manifests a long thumb and increased longitudinal flexibility of the hand. (*A is reproduced from Pyeritz.*[18] *Used with permission.*)**

different mutations in *FBN1* might be variably predisposing.[97–99] About 90 percent of aortic dissections begin with a tear in the intima just above the sinotubular junction (type A dissection), and then most progress distally to involve the entire aorta. Retrograde dissection with bleeding into the pericardial sac accounts for most acute mortality. About 10 percent of dissections begin in the distal

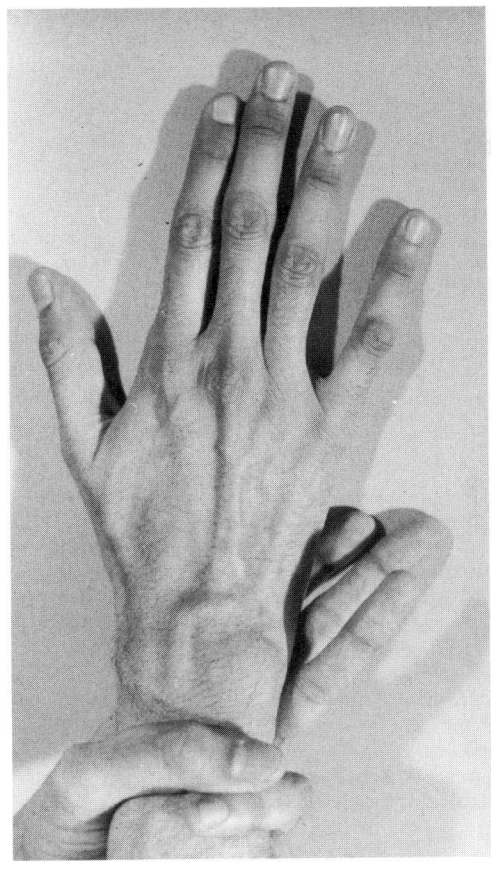

**Fig. 206-4 Superior displacement of the ocular lens in the Marfan syndrome. (*Courtesy of A.H. Child.*)**

aorta (type B dissection), usually in the proximal descending thoracic aorta. Predisposition to abdominal aortic aneurysm does not appear strong, but patients with MFS are only now routinely living into the decades in which aneurysms of the distal aorta become more common.[100,101]

Dilatation and dissection of other elastic arteries, has been reported many times in people with MFS, but nonetheless is not very likely to occur in any given patient.[102–107] Whether some mutations predispose to problems in arteries other than the aorta is unknown.

Some people with MFS are especially prone to dysrhythmia, often in association with MVP.[108] In a few patients, a primary myocardial dysfunction occurs, with a course like idiopathic dilated cardiomyopathy.[81,109]

Venous varicosities, especially of the superficial veins of the legs, are of increased frequency in MFS, but rarely cause significant problems.

## Pulmonary Manifestations

Spontaneous pneumothorax, due to rupture of an apical bleb in the lung, occurs in 4 to 5 percent of people with MFS, usually in adolescence.[110–113] Some children with severe MFS have cystic lung disease,[114] and adults may be more prone to emphysematous changes,[115–117] especially if they smoke. The combination of pectus excavatum and thoracic vertebral deformity reduce lung volumes and occasionally produce severe restrictive deficits.[117,118] Standard pulmonary function tests often misrepresent static values (forced vital capacity, total lung capacity) as abnormally low, because the standards for any patient are based on standing height; in MFS the legs are disproportionate, so the expected lung volumes are overestimated.[118] While the high proportion of elastic tissue in the lung might suggest prominent pulmonary involvement in MFS,[115,116] surprisingly little has been found to be

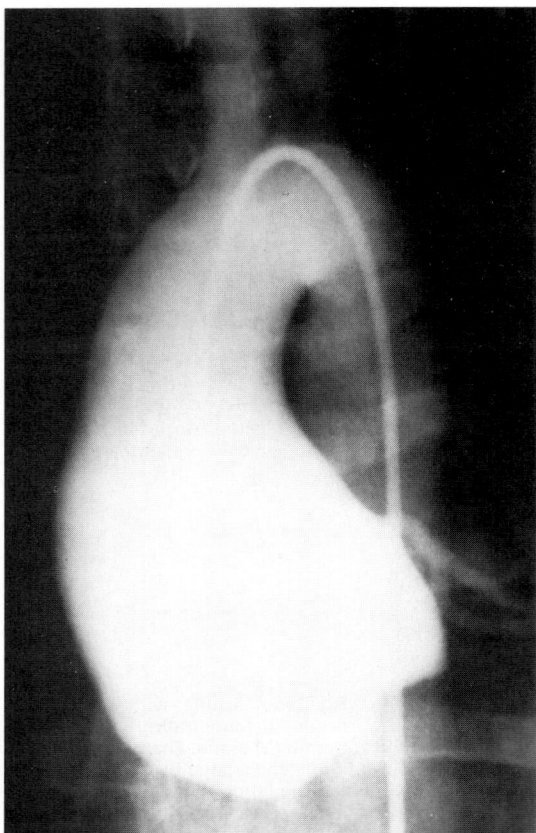

Fig. 206-5 Anteroposterior aortogram in a 21-year-old patient with Marfan syndrome. The dilatation is greatest in the sinus of Valsalva and limited to the proximal ascending aorta.

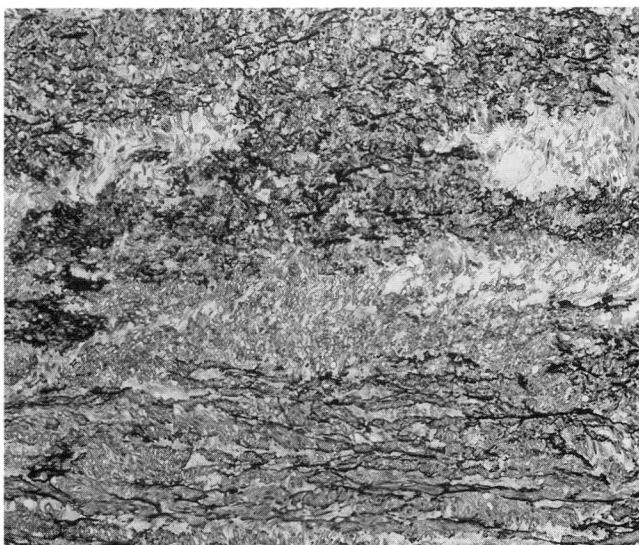

Fig. 206-6 Elastin stain of the aortic media in a patient with Marfan syndrome. Note the widespread fragmentation of elastic fibers and the accumulation of amorphous matrix components. (*Courtesy of R.H. Hruban.*)

over the thighs, shoulders, lumbar area, back and breasts; rather than fading as adolescent stretch marks often do, in MFS they mature from being violaceous to being depigmented and more extensive. Abdominal stretch marks of pregnancy (striae gravidarum) can be particularly impressive in MFS.

abnormal in dynamic lung function; however, detailed studies are lacking.

Obstructive sleep apnea may be more common in MFS due to laxity of hypopharyngeal tissue, retrognathia, or both.[52,119,120] Rapid onset of obstructive airway problems should raise concern about aortic enlargement.[121]

## Manifestations in the Integument

The dura is pure connective tissue and contains fibrillin-1. The dura stretches under the normal pressure of the cerebrospinal fluid. With upright posture, these forces are maximal in the lumbosacral region. The dura in MFS cannot prevent this pressure from eroding the bone of the vertebral bodies, which causes two manifestations (Fig. 206-7). First, the size of the neural canal increases (dural ectasia).[122–124] Second, dura containing cerebrospinal fluid erodes the neural foramina and may protrude into the pelvis as arachnoid cysts or anterior meningoceles.[123,125–129] These cysts may be misinterpreted as ovarian in origin in women with MFS. Because spinal nerve roots usually course over these cysts, pain and neurologic abnormalities in the distribution of the lower lumbar and sacral nerve roots can be difficult problems.[130]

Hernias of various types are more common in MFS. Inguinal hernias may occur in infancy or at any other time, and tend to reoccur after standard surgical repair. Hernias of the diaphragm may be congenital.[131,132] Hernias at the site of surgical incisions are also common.

The skin of some people with MFS is unusually thin, hyperelastic, or both.[59] Scars may be thin, but keloid formation does occur as well. In general, however, the skin is not unusually fragile, and no unusual attention to skin wounds is indicated. The most characteristic manifestation in the skin is the stretch mark (striae atrophicae).[133,134] These tend to begin in early adolescence

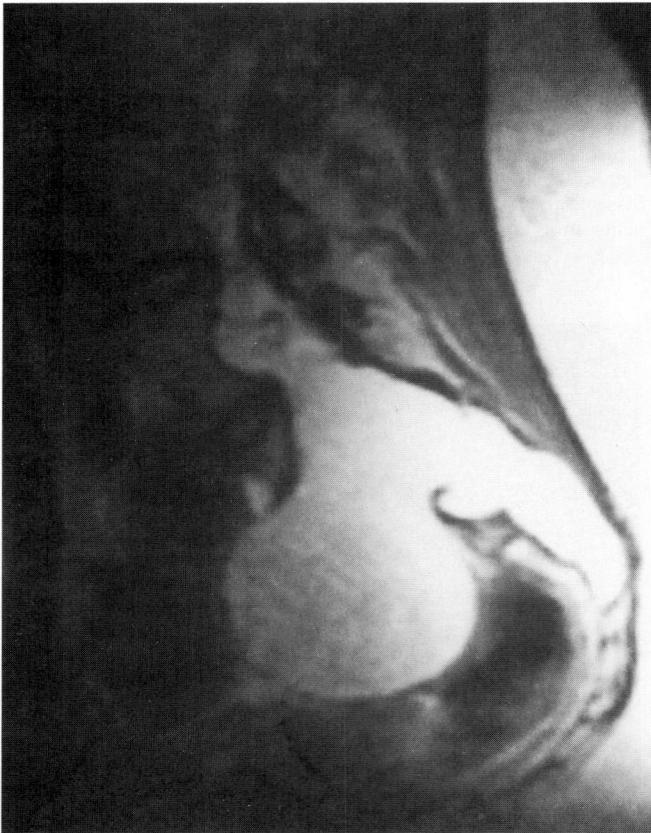

Fig. 206-7 Magnetic resonance imaging study in the parasagittal plane showing marked dural ectasia with anterior meningocele in a 25-year-old patient with Marfan syndrome. (*Reproduced from Pyeritz.*[18] *Used with permission.*)

## Other Manifestations

Skeletal muscle is underdeveloped in some people with MFS, and no amount of exertion (which is not indicated in any event because of the strain on the cardiovascular system) seems capable of causing hypertrophy. Results are a "myotonic" facial appearance and downward sloping shoulders.

Subcutaneous adipose tissue is also underdeveloped. This feature, especially when coupled with muscular hypoplasia, accounts for the asthenic appearance of some patients, especially children with severe MFS. As people with MFS age, adiposity does tend to accumulate in the truncal region.

Occasional people with MFS have cystic areas in the liver, kidneys, or both; whether these are pleiotropic manifestations remains unclear.

More children and adolescents than would be expected have difficulty with learning. This is not a problem with native intelligence;[135] rather, the prevalences of attention deficit, hyperactivity, and verbal-performance discrepancies seem to be increased.[135,136] As might be expected with any young person with an unusual appearance, chronic health problems or limitations on activity, difficulties with psychosocial coping may arise,[137] but these do not appear unique to MFS.

## Life Expectancy

In the only study of its kind, a retrospective review of age and causes of death of people with MFS, performed before medical and surgical therapy were having any positive benefit, showed an average age of death in the fourth and fifth decade, with some infants and children succumbing.[88] This represents the natural history of MFS. Most people died of complications of AR or aortic dissection.

## Management

Individuals with MFS require multidisciplinary management by a team of medical specialists, but one health professional should coordinate care.[18,81,138]

The skeletal manifestations often require no specific intervention. The spine should be evaluated at least annually in children and adolescents until growth is complete in order to detect scoliosis.[55–58] Bracing should be considered for progressive curves. Once a curve exceeds 40°, surgical stabilization is often necessary. Repair of severe pectus excavatum should be considered to improve lung volume and respiratory mechanics,[139] but in the asymptomatic person with MFS, only when growth is nearly complete to avoid recurrence.[51] Stabilization of the sternum until regeneration of the costochondral junctions occurs appears warranted; minimally invasive approaches have not been formally studied in MFS.[140] For those patients with severe pectus excavatum who also require cardiac surgery, a staged process is preferable to a combined approach.[139,141,142] Adult height can be reduced if hormonal treatment is begun before puberty.[143] No controlled trials of hormonal modulation have been reported, and girls have been treated much more frequently than boys.[47,144]

Visual acuity should be assessed as early as possible in an infant with MFS and correction instituted to avoid amblyopia.[75] Contact lenses can be tolerated despite the flat cornea.[145] The indications for surgical removal of the lens have expanded in recent years because the operation is safer and an artificial lens can be implanted.[146] People with MFS should avoid surgical correction of myopia such as radial keratometry.

The key to improving life expectancy has been prophylactic management of the cardiovascular system. The aorta gradually dilates, and the risk of complications of AR and dissection are positively associated with aortic diameter, family history of dissection and perhaps ascending aortic shape.[97–99,147] Regular assessment by transthoracic echocardiography is essential, at least annual and more frequent the larger the diameter. Chronic β-adrenergic blockade reduces the rate of dilatation and protects against dissection in many people with MFS,[148,149] although

responses among patients vary.[150,151] Routinely, people with MFS should avoid exertion at maximal capacity, isometric exertion, and contact sports.

The surest method for preventing dissection of the ascending aorta is to replace the root when it becomes moderately dilated. During the period 1975 to the present, the composite graft approach, first developed by Bentall,[152] served this purpose well.[153] Life expectancy has improved dramatically, with people having prophylactic repair now living, on average, into their seventh decade.[153,154] Surgery should be considered whenever the aortic root is greater than 55 mm in an adult, and even sooner if relatives with MFS have suffered aortic dissection.[97,99,153] People having surgery after a dissection has occurred do less well, mainly because complications from chronic dissection accrue and additional aortic surgery usually is necessary.[153,155] Indeed, if necessary, the entire aorta can be replaced in a staged series of operations.[156] Recently a valve-sparing procedure was developed that obviates replacement of the aortic valve with a prosthetic one that requires life-long anticoagulation.[157] Long-term studies are necessary to prove its efficacy,[153,158] but even now valve-sparing is a reasonable alternative for individuals who should avoid anticoagulation, such as children and women who wish to become pregnant.

The mitral valve may require surgical correction if mitral regurgitation becomes severe.[83] Valve repair is preferable to replacement because it avoids the need for anticoagulation. Despite the connective tissue defect in the mitral apparatus, valve repairs hold up well in the majority of patients including children.[82]

Pregnancy in a woman with MFS carries substantial risk,[159–161] although if the aortic diameter is 40 mm or less, the chance of ascending aortic dissection is relatively small.[162]

## ETIOLOGY AND PATHOGENESIS OF MARFAN SYNDROME

### Historical Perspective

Multiple histopathologic and clinical observations suggested a primary defect in the extracellular matrix in the Marfan syndrome. Mutations in a structural protein that contributes to higher order macroaggregates seemed likely because of autosomal dominant inheritance. Over the years, some evidence implicating most of the major classes of connective tissue has been presented. One hypothesis suggested that aortic failure results from inadequate tensile strength due to abnormal synthesis, matrix incorporation, and/or tissue homeostasis of fibrillar collagens, particularly type I.[163,164] Supporting evidence included sporadic demonstration of increased urinary excretion of hydroxyproline, increased solubility of dermal collagen, and decreased collagen cross-links.[165–167] Interest intensified after the publication of an apparent mutation in the COL1A2 gene in a Marfan patient.[168] None of the biochemical abnormalities were consistently observed in Marfan syndrome, the putative pathogenic mutation was later shown to be a neutral polymorphism, and all of the genes encoding the major fibrillar procollagens were ultimately excluded by linkage analysis.[169–174]

The observation of excessive proteoglycans and glycosaminoglycans in affected tissues fueled speculation that the basic defect in Marfan syndrome is in the ground substance.[175–179] This histopathologic observation was later associated with increased hyaluronic acid synthetase activity and decreased serum β-glucuronidase activity in patient fibroblast cultures.[180–182] Others found evidence of decreased mRNA encoding decorin, a chondroitin-dermatan sulfate proteoglycan, in a subset of patients with Marfan syndrome.[183–185] It should be noted that an accumulation of ground substance in the medial layer is a universal finding in aortic aneurysm, regardless of etiology.[186–189] Moreover, alterations of proteoglycan or glycosaminoglycan metabolism, including decreased expression of decorin, can be seen in heritable disorders of collagen metabolism and after experimental inhibition of elastin crosslinks.[190-194] Thus, it appears that these results represent nonspecific secondary pathologic or compensatory changes that can be initiated by a variety of primary disorders of connective tissue.

In 1955, McKusick suggested that the basic defect in Marfan syndrome was located in the elastic fiber.[11] Early histopathologic studies demonstrated elastic fiber fragmentation and decreased elastin content in both the skin and medial layer of the aorta.[134,179,195-198] These observations were later correlated with apparent abnormalities of elastin metabolism in Marfan patients, including decreased urinary excretion of desmosines, increased elastin solubility, decreased desmosine and isodesmosine content of extracted protein, and increased elastin susceptibility to digestion by pancreatic elastase.[197,199-202] These results suggested a decrease in the density and/or quality of elastin cross-links.

Despite early speculation to the contrary,[203] the elastin gene was a poor candidate for the site of primary mutations causing Marfan syndrome. Most significantly, the Marfan syndrome involves tissues that are devoid of elastin including the ciliary zonules and skeleton.[204] Ultrastructural, biochemical and immunologic analyses of elastic fibers demonstrated a material surrounding the amorphous component with a distinct staining pattern and susceptibility to enzymatic digestion.[24,205-207] These so-called microfibrils have a diameter of 8 to 14 nM and are constituents of all elastic tissues. Microfibrils are also widely distributed in mammalian tissues that are devoid of amorphous elastin including the oxytalan fibers intrinsic to the dermal-epidermal junction, tendons, fascia, periosteum, corneal stroma, and the adventitial layer of blood vessels; in numerous basement membranes; and in the renal glomerular mesangium. Of particular interest was the observation that the ciliary zonules that suspend the ocular lens are composed of fibrillar aggregates that demonstrate an ultrastructural appearance and biochemical profile reminiscent of elastin-associated microfibrils.[208,209] Streeten and colleagues first formally proposed an etiologic link between microfibrillar components and the Marfan phenotype after observing that an antibody prepared against sonicated bovine zonules immunolabeled both zonular and elastin-associated microfibrils with an identical periodicity.[210]

## Locus and Gene Identification

In 1986, Sakai and colleagues first identified fibrillin-1, a 350-kDa glycoprotein component of extracellular microfibrils. They demonstrated that fibrillin-1 is common to microfibrillar aggregates in all of the tissues altered in the Marfan phenotype including the vascular wall, ciliary zonules, skin, hyaline cartilage, perichondrium, and alveolar wall.[211] Subsequent immunohistochemical study of Marfan patient tissues showed that the vast majority of cases had diminished amounts of microfibrils in skin, fibroblast culture, or both (Fig. 206-8).[27,28] Examination of fibrillin-1 metabolism in cultured skin fibroblasts demonstrated diminished incorporation of fibrillin-1 into the extracellular matrix in about 85 percent of cultures derived from MFS patients.[30] In addition, some patient samples showed defects in fibrillin-1 synthesis or secretion. In 1991, linkage analysis using anonymous markers mapped the Marfan locus to the long arm of chromosome 15, allowing a tentative assignment to 15q15-q21.1.[32,33] By this time, a portion of the cDNA encoding fibrillin-1 had been isolated,[36,37] allowing the gene to be mapped to a position coincident with the Marfan locus at 15q21.1.[37-39] Mutational analysis of fibrillin-1 cDNA from patients with MFS revealed a recurrent *de novo* missense mutation in FBN1 in two unrelated individuals.[39] With a cumulative lod score in excess of 100, the linkage evidence demonstrates an absence of locus heterogeneity for the classic Marfan phenotype.[32-35,37,39,46,212-214] While published reports suggest a second locus on chromosome 3p,[215] this is based upon the analysis of a single kindred that segregates a phenotype that shows both similarities to and differences from MFS.[216] Thus, it appears that FBN1 gene mutations are the predominant, if not the sole cause of the classic disorder.

## Fibrillin-1 Gene and Protein

The 8616-bp coding sequence of the FBN1 gene is comprised of 65 exons that span approximately 200 kb of genomic DNA.[217-219] The presence of three alternatively utilized, in-frame exons upstream of the exon containing the putative initiating methionine in both the human and murine genes generated some ambiguity regarding the site of fibrillin-1 translation initiation.[217,220] The first coding exon of the porcine gene contains an in-frame termination codon upstream of the putative initiating methionine.[219] In view of the extreme amino acid conservation of fibrillin-1 among mammals, these data strongly suggest that this ATG is the only translation start site of fibrillin-1.

Fibrillin-1 is a cysteine-rich 350-kDa glycoprotein with a complex modular organization that is shared within the fibrillin family of proteins.[26,217,218,221] Differences in amino acid composition or domain content can be shown by the designation of five distinct regions of the protein (A to E; Fig. 206-9).[217,218] Exon 1 encodes a signal peptide followed by a unique, short, basic N-terminal sequence that does not show homology with other identified proteins (region A). The C-terminal sequence encoded by exons 64 and 65 (region E) is also unique, but a high concentration of basic residues and a subsequence surrounding two cysteines are conserved between fibrillin-1 and fibrillin-2.[217,218,221] Both the N- and C-termini contain propeptide cleavage sites that conform to the consensus sequence for PACE/furin-like proteases.[222-226] Exon 10 encodes region C which is extremely rich in proline residues (38 percent), as opposed to glycines in fibrillin-2.[217,218,221] Rotary shadow analysis of fibrillin monomers reveals a characteristic bend in this region.[211] This domain of fibrillin-1 may contribute to the inherent distensibility of microfibrils.[217,218] Additional analysis demonstrated that region C was sufficient to induce dimer formation of recombinant peptides, suggesting a role in nucleation during microfibrillar assembly.[227,228] This region also contains sites susceptible to cleavage by matrix metalloproteinases.[229,230] We recently appreciated that this domain contains 10 perfect tandem repeats of PXXP where P is proline and X is any residue (commonly also P):

$$\boxed{P}\,GR\,\boxed{P}\,EY\,\boxed{P}\,PP\,\boxed{P}\,LG\,\boxed{P}\,IP\,\boxed{P}\,VL\,\boxed{P}\,VP\,\boxed{P}\,GF\,\boxed{P}\,PG\,\boxed{P}\,QI\,\boxed{P}$$

This structure is common in Src homology 3 (SH3) domain ligands, but fibrillin-1 lacks the characteristic positions for interspersed and critical R and L residues.[231] Rather, this sequence appears to form a polyproline II (PPII)-helix. PPII-helices tend to be found connecting major structural parts of a molecule where their high conformational mobility confers flexibility.[232] They are frequently located on the surface of proteins where they can serve as sites of intermolecular interactions, often linking with other PPII-helices. PPII-helices are conserved in protein families and are found in all serine proteinases including neutrophil elastase, an enzyme known to cleave fibrillin-1.[232,233]

Regions B and D comprise the bulk of the protein and are encoded largely by exons 2 to 9 and 11 to 63, respectively.[218] Both regions are characterized by the repetition of cysteine-rich domains, including those that were first identified in epidermal growth factor precursor (EGF-like) and latency-inducing transforming growth factor β-binding proteins (LTBP-like). EGF-like motifs are found in many types of proteins including vitamin K-dependent clotting factors and components of the extracellular matrix. One consistent feature is the presence of six predictably spaced cysteine residues that interact via disulfide linkage (1–3, 2–4, 5–6) to form an antiparallel β-pleated sheet conformation (Fig. 206-10).[234] A subset of EGF-like domains, including 43 of 47 found in fibrillin-1, satisfy the consensus for calcium binding (cbEGF-like), an event that is required to maintain a rigid, rod-like structure for tandemly repeated motifs and to promote protein-protein interactions.[217,235-241] Briefly, calcium binding is dependent on maintenance of domain structure, as dictated by the three intradomain disulfide bonds and a number of highly conserved

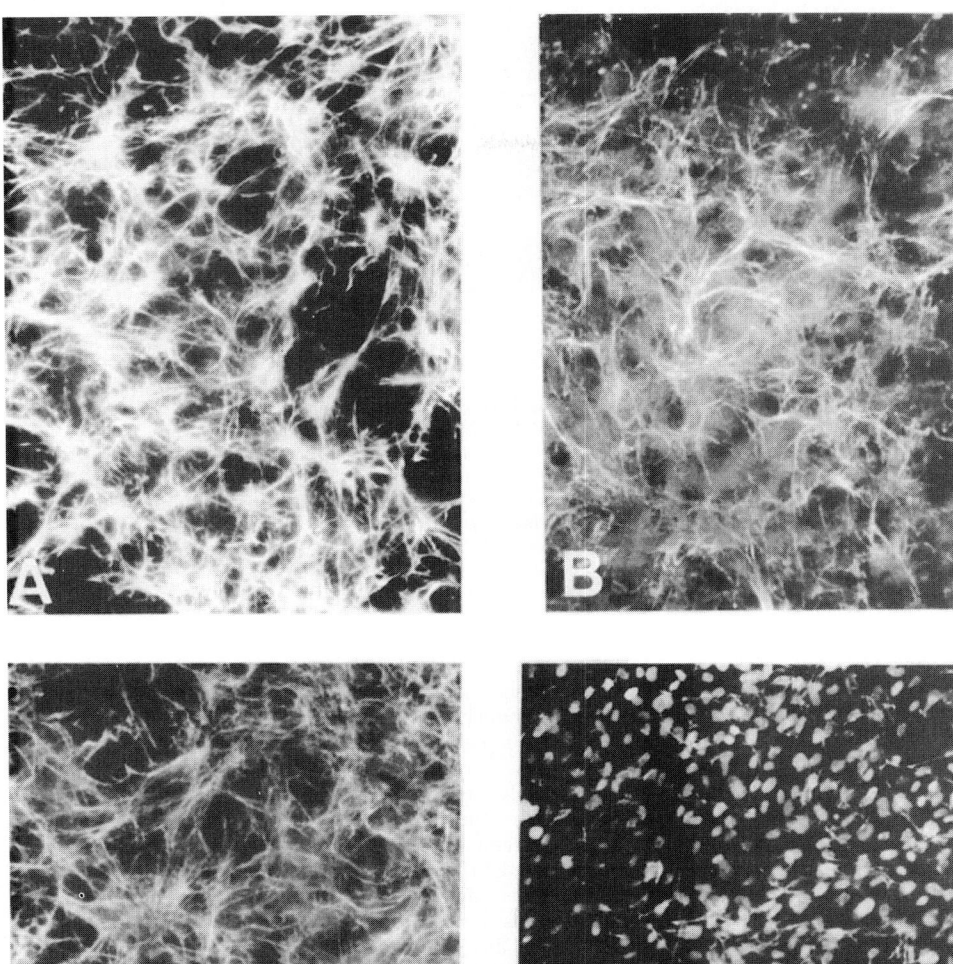

**Fig. 206-8 Immunohistochemical analysis of confluent cultured dermal fibroblasts from a normal subject (*A*), and patients with classic Marfan syndrome (*B*), nonsyndromic ascending aortic aneurysm (*C*), or neonatal presentation of severe and rapidly progressive Marfan syndrome (*D*). Panels *A* and *C* show normal abundance and architecture of immunoreactive fibrillin-1. Both samples from individuals with Marfan syndrome show abnormal fibrillin-1 content and loss of architecture of microfibrillar bundles. Note that the degree of abnormality correlates with the severity of disease in this example.**

residues that define the consensus sequence $(D/N)X(D/N)$ $(E/Q)X_n(D*/N*)X_m(Y/F)$ where $n$ and $m$ are variable and the *asterisk* indicates potential $\beta$-hydroxylation (Fig. 206-10).[242,243] Other conserved residues stabilize the calcium binding pocket at the N-terminus of an adjacent cbEGF-like domain by mediating interdomain hydrophobic packing interactions.[244,245]

LTBP-like domains contain eight conserved cysteine residues that pair via intramolecular disulfide linkage (1–3, 2–6, 4–7, 5–8).[246] While this domain contributes to the covalent association between LTBP-1 and TGF-$\beta$1 latency-associated propeptide (LAP) through disulfide bond exchange,[247,248] the ability of the seven homologous domains in fibrillin-1 to participate in intermolecular interactions has not yet been shown. The RGD sequence within the fourth LTBP-like domain of fibrillin-1 was shown to support cell adhesion through interaction with integrin alphavbeta3.[249–251] Little is known about the function of other conserved residues in LTBP-like domains. A third cysteine-rich

domain, termed the hybrid motif, occurs once in region B and once in region D, and likely manifests fusion between LTBP-like and EGF-like motifs during evolution.[218] The functional characteristics of this novel domain are entirely unexplored.

## Microfibril Assembly

Fibrillin-1 is synthesized in a precursor form which undergoes proteolytic cleavage at both the N- and C-termini.[222–226] Both processing events occur at multibasic sites that resemble the consensus sequence for PACE/furin-like proteases. Current evidence suggests that C-terminal cleavage is calcium-dependent and occurs intracellularly in a secretory pathway compartment.[225] N-terminal sequence, including the proline-rich region of fibrillin-1 and flanking cysteine-rich domains, is sufficient to induce dimer formation.[227,228] Dimers apparently form intracellularly and are stabilized by disulfide linkage.[227] Further polymerization occurs in the extracellular space, but may be dependent on the formation of

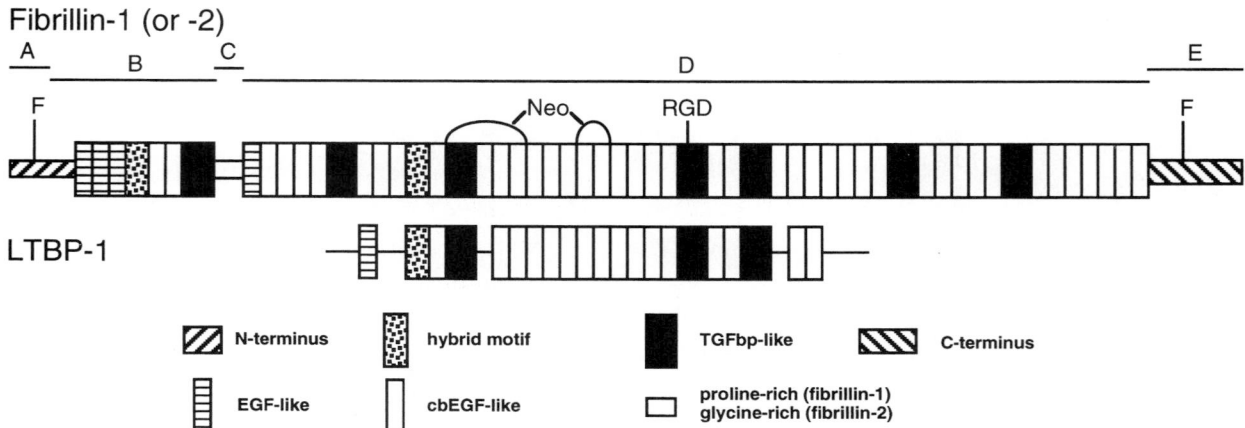

Fig. 206-9 Domain organization of fibrillin-1, fibrillin-2 and LTBP-1. Character of each domain type is shown at the bottom of the figure. Fibrillin-1 is divided into 5 regions (A-E) for purposes of discussion (see text). F, furin-like propeptide cleavage sites; Neo, regions associated with neonatal presentation of severe disease. The position of an RGD sequence in fibrillin-1 is indicated. (*Modified from a previously published version found in Nijbroek et al.[274] Used with permission.*)

intracellular intermediate structures. C-terminal sequence beyond the propeptide cleavage site appears to negatively regulate early steps in homopolymerization,[222,226] perhaps through direct intramolecular interaction with critical N-terminal domains.

Other posttranslational modification events include extensive glycosylation, beta hydroxylation of specific Asn residues within cbEGF-like domains, and calcium binding.[26,217,252] About one-third of cysteines are in the free sulfhydryl form and may participate in intermolecular interactions. Epitope mapping studies suggest that fibrillin-1 monomers self assemble into macroaggregates characterized by parallel arrays of linear extended structures with a head-to-tail orientation.[253] Adjacent monomers or microfibrillar bundles appear to connect predominantly via disulfide linkage, although transglutaminase cross-links have also been observed in tissue extracts.[254]

As previously noted, fibrillin-1 and fibrillin-2 show remarkable conservation of domain organization and sequence and both are integral components of microfibrils. Variation in the temporal and spatial pattern of expression of the two proteins, suggests that they contribute to distinct microfibrillar beds (Yin, 1995 2932).[221,255] As a general rule, fibrillin-2 expression occurs earlier in development and concentrates in elastic fiber-rich tissues at the onset of elastogenesis. Fibrillin-1 expression is seen somewhat later in morphogenesis in both elastic and non elastic tissues.

A large number of other proteins have either been extracted from or immunolocalize to extracellular microfibrils. Collectively referred to as microfibril-associated glycoproteins (MAGPs) or, more recently, microfibril-associated proteins (MFAPs), the contribution of these molecules to the structure and function of microfibrils remains largely unknown. MFAP-2 (MAGP-1) has been proposed to mediate interactions between microfibrils and other proteins including elastin and type VI collagen.[256,257] Fibulin-2 was found to directly interact with fibrillin-1, but expression of this protein is limited relative to that for fibrillin-1, dynamic in response to injury, and often concentrated at the interface between microfibrils and the amorphous elastin core.[258,259] Selected latency-inducing transforming growth factor β-binding proteins (LTBPs) may also associate with or comprise microfibrils.[260-262] It should be noted that, despite intensive investigation, only the fibrillins have been associated with MFS or related conditions. It is possible that the contribution of the other proteins to microfibrillar function is trivial or easily compensated.

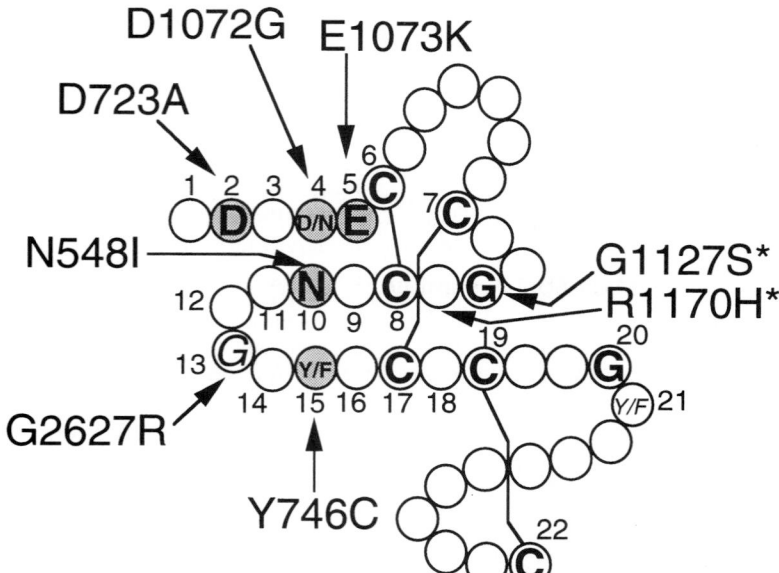

Fig. 206-10 A representative cbEGF-like domain from fibrillin-1. Residues conserved in this domain type are indicated using the single letter amino acid code. Lines indicate disulfide bonds between cysteine residues. Shading indicates the residues that comprise the calcium-binding consensus. Residues shown in italics (positions 13 and 21) are critical for interdomain hydrophobic packing. Representative mutations in FBN1 are shown. Asterisks indicate mutations associated with mild phenotypes (see text). (*Modified from a previously published version found in Dietz et al.[277] Used with permission.*)

Alternatively, in consideration of the extreme loss of microfibrillar abundance and architecture seen in MFS (see below), this phenotype may manifest a cumulative loss-of-function of many proteins. In this scenario, mutation in any given associated protein may lead to a phenotype that is not intuitively grouped with this spectrum of connective tissue disorders.

## FBN1 Mutations in Marfan Syndrome

To date, approximately 200 FBN1 mutations in patients with MFS or related phenotypes have been published or reported to an international database.[40,263–266] All mutational classes are represented. About 20 percent of mutations create premature termination codons, 10 percent perturb splicing, a handful cause small in-frame deletions or insertions, and the remainder (about 70 percent) involve missense substitutions. Greater than 90 percent of mutations are unique to single individuals or families, and the rest are only present in a handful of apparently unrelated probands. The low rate of recurrent mutations and the high degree of intrafamilial clinical variability have limited the development of clear phenotype-to-genotype correlations. The majority of missense mutations (~80 percent) occur within the 47 tandemly repeated epidermal growth factor (EGF)-like domains of fibrillin-1, of which 43 satisfy the consensus for calcium binding (cbEGF-like domains; Fig. 206-10).[242,243] Many mutations substitute one of the cysteine residues, highly conserved residues within the calcium-binding consensus sequence, or residues important for interdomain hydrophobic packing interactions.[40,238,263–266] Solving for the solution structure of a pair of cbEGF-like domains demonstrated that calcium binding is required to maintain a rigid rod-like structure for tandemly repeated motifs.[238,244] Moreover, disruption of domain folding or calcium binding has been shown to result in conformational changes and enhanced proteolytic degradation of single domains, recombinant peptides or intact monomers, as well as ultrastructural changes in microfibrils.[235,239,267–270]

It is clear that the nature of the substitution within cbEGF-like domains is not the sole determinant of phenotypic expression. For example, substitution of the highly conserved asparagine (N) residue at consensus position 10 in Fig. 206-10 can result in classic MFS (codons 548, 1893), MFS without eye involvement (codon 2144), or isolated ectopia lentis (codon 1173).[40,263] With rare exceptions,[271] substitution of one of the invariant cysteine residues in cbEGF-like domains of fibrillin-1 is associated with classic MFS of variable severity.

Few firm genotype-to-phenotype correlations have emerged. One clear exception is the clustering of mutations causing neonatal presentation of severe and rapidly progressive disease in exons 24 to 27 and 31 to 32.[272–275] Interestingly, multiple types of mutation are represented and many mutations within these intervals cause classic or even mild forms of disease.[40,263,265,271,274] As a general rule, mutations causing the in-frame loss or gain of central coding sequence, either through genomic deletions or insertions or splicing errors, are associated with more severe disease.[40,276] In contrast, many mutations that create a premature termination codon that result in rapid degradation of mutant transcripts are associated with mild conditions that may fail to meet diagnostic criteria for Marfan syndrome.[274,277–279] Individuals harboring a mutation that prevented C-terminal propeptide processing had only skeletal manifestations.[222] The mutant gene product was synthesized and secreted, but lacked the ability to interact with wild-type protein derived from the normal allele. Taken together these data suggest a dominant-negative mechanism of disease pathogenesis[40,277] that has been validated by immunohistochemical studies and biochemical characterization of cultured patient dermal fibroblasts by pulse-chase analysis. Both methods demonstrate a dramatic reduction of extracellular fibrillin-1 in the majority of patient lines, far below the 50 percent level that would be expected for an autosomal dominant disorder in which the relevant mechanism was pure haploinsufficiency.[28,30,280–282] There is some correlation between the degree of impairment of

extracellular deposition of fibrillin-1 and disease severity and clinical outcome.[282]

Although some are associated with a mild phenotype, many mutations that create premature termination codons (PTCs) and transcript instability are associated with classic Marfan syndrome. In general, the lower the residual mutant mRNA level, the less severe the phenotype, but there are clear exceptions.[283,284] One possibility is that N-terminal fragments of fibrillin-1 derived from nonsense alleles have dominant-negative activity. Alternatively, the apparent dominant-negative effect seen with heterozygous nonsense alleles may reflect a concentration-dependent decrease in the efficiency of utilization of protein derived from the normal allele.[284] In this scenario, low synthesis, secretion, or stability of mutant protein would all be expected to result in a severe decrease in the level of extracellular microfibrils below 50 percent of normal.

Beyond the few residues in each EGF-like domain that are known to have functional significance, nearly all of the intervening residues in human fibrillin-1 are identical in mouse, pig, and cow.[219,220,285] With few exceptions, missense mutations causing MFS that do not occur in cbEGF-like domains involve cysteine, proline, or glycine residues. The same is true for mutations within cbEGF-like domains that do not replace cysteine or calcium-binding consensus residues. These changes are predicted, or have been shown, to alter protein folding and stability.[238,269,286] A few mutations that occur within variable loop regions of EGF-like domains are associated with very mild forms of disease. Notably, mutation R1170H was identified in two families with minor skeletal involvement with or without mitral valve prolapse but none of the major manifestations of MFS.[284,287] Such mutations may allow the deposition of stable microfibrils with an as yet undefined but limited functional deficit.

FBN1 mutation detection in MFS is an extremely inefficient process, leading some to infer locus heterogeneity. It is difficult to reconcile this hypothesis with extensive linkage evidence for a single predominant locus at a map position coincident with FBN1.[32–35,37,39,46,212–214] In consideration of the varying patient populations and screening techniques, it is difficult to arrive at a meaningful estimate of sensitivity for mutation detection. Estimates vary between 10 percent and 80 percent.[265,274,278,288,289] In one particularly revealing study, the efficiency of screening was directly proportional to the size and degree of clinical characterization of the family,[288] ranging from 78 percent for families with four or more affected individuals to 17 percent when only one affected individual was analyzed. It is also clear that MFS was overly diagnosed prior to the establishment of stringent criteria.[45] Thus, studies that rely on historic and/or incomplete clinical data may include phenotypes other than MFS and conclude low sensitivity for mutational analysis. Mutations or rearrangements in noncoding sequence may be other contributing factors. Finally, locus heterogeneity cannot be definitively excluded.

## Higher Order Pathogenesis of MFS

It is not difficult to imagine how the incorporation of relatively few mutant monomers into microfibrils would suffice to cause global disruption of structure, stability, and function. The formation of microfibrillar aggregates and subsequent deposition of amorphous elastin are temporally and spatially linked. This association led to the hypothesis that microfibrils represent an elastin precursor or regulate elastin deposition during embryonic development.[206,207] According to this model, the deficiency in elastic fiber number and architecture observed in mature vascular lesions in MFS predominantly represents a primary failure of elastogenesis. This absence of organized elastic fibers would cause both a primary structural deficit and a diminished capacity to modulate hemodynamic stress, possibly predisposing to secondary damage. Elastic fiber formation is virtually complete after early postnatal life.[206,207,290] Fibrillin-1 and its highly homologous family member fibrillin-2 (mutated in congenital contractural arachnodactyly[291]) have distinct temporal and spatial patterns of expression, suggesting that they comprise structurally and perhaps functionally different microfibrillar beds.[220,221,255] Normally, neither protein is expressed after early childhood. Taken together, these data suggest a limited window of opportunity to intervene in the pathogenetic sequence of Marfan syndrome and bode poorly for the development of therapeutic strategies aimed at improving the integrity of elastic tissues including the aortic media.

**Animal Models.** Understanding the pathogenetic sequence leading to aneurysm in patients with MFS was impeded by the lack of ability to follow the natural history of vascular histologic changes. The analysis of mice harboring targeted Fbn1 alleles has provided new insight. An in-frame deletion through the substitution of exons 19 to 25 of Fbn1 with a neomycin resistance cassette (Neo[r]),[292] the so-called mgΔ allele, encodes a centrally truncated monomer that was expected to behave in a dominant-negative manner. However, very-low levels of mutant mRNA and protein were synthesized, due to transcriptional interference from Neo[r], with only about 5 to 10 percent expression of the mutant allele compared to its wild-type counterpart. Heterozygous mice showed only subtle skeletal abnormalities late in life.[292] Homozygous mgΔ/mgΔ animals were also born at the expected frequency, but died suddenly prior to weaning. Aortic dilatation and dissection with hemopericardium or hemothorax were seen in all homozygous mutant animals that died naturally.[292] Disruption of elastic laminae and loss of elastin content with the accumulation of amorphous matrix elements was seen in the aortic media, similar to the appearance of mature human lesions.[189] What was unexpected was the focal nature of these abnormalities (Fig. 206-11). The bulk of the aorta showed linear, uninterrupted, and parallel elastic fibers at the level of histologic resolution. These data documented that minimal microfibrillar function is sufficient to support the deposition of extended elastic structures and highlighted the prominent role of fibrillin-1 in elastic fiber homeostasis.

Early death of mgΔ/mgΔ animals prevented a complete analysis of pathologic changes leading to aneurysm formation. Important new understanding arose from the analysis of a second targeted allele (called mgR) that resulted from the insertion of Neo[r] into intron 18 without rearrangement in the coding sequence.[293] This allele is only expressed at a level approximating 15 percent of normal because of transcriptional interference. However, protein derived from the R1 allele is structurally normal. Heterozygous mgR/+ animals were phenotypically indistinguishable from wild-type littermates. Homozygous mgR/mgR mice were born without phenotypic abnormalities, but died between 3

and 6 months of age.[293] In addition to vascular disease, these animals developed bone overgrowth, most prominently in the ribs and extremities. The aortic media showed focal calcification of intact elastic laminae as early as 6 weeks of age. With increasing age, calcified segments increased in number and coalesced. Intimal hyperplasia, SMC proliferation, and excessive and disorganized deposition of matrix components were evident by 9 weeks of age. Generally, areas of adventitial inflammation coincided with calcification and intimal thickening. Finally, mixed inflammatory cells infiltration of the media with associated expression of MMPs, intense elastolysis, and structural collapse of the vessel wall were observed.[293]

A review of autopsy specimens from young patients with MFS revealed diffuse calcification and intimal hyperplasia in the aorta and other muscular arteries (our unpublished data; manuscript submitted). In addition, Takebayashi and colleagues had previously reported the accumulation of an electron-dense, granular material on the surface of and within vascular elastic fibers of MFS patients.[178,294] Although this observation, termed osmiophilic elastolysis, had been attributed to the accumulation of a peculiar elastin breakdown product, it is clear in retrospect that the authors were observing diffuse calcification of elastic structures. These observations in MFS patients do not represent normal age-dependent changes. They were seen in all medium-to-large elastic arteries that were examined and were seen in children without correlation of distribution or severity to the age of the individual (our unpublished data; manuscript submitted). It is important to note that calcification and intimal hyperplasia occur in vessels that do not dilate or dissect in MFS, suggesting that these changes do not initiate aneurysm formation.

Ultrastructural analysis has documented cellular events that precede or coincide with destructive changes in the aortic media of fibrillin-1-deficient mice. Normally, elastic laminae connect to adjacent endothelial and smooth muscle cells (SMC) through junctions composed of microfibrils,[295–297] possibly by the interaction between the RGD sequence of fibrillin-1 and integrin alphavbeta3.[249–251] These connections may contribute to the structural integrity of the vessel wall by anchoring cells and coordinating contractile and elastic tensions.[295,296] Homozygous mgR mice show a remarkably reduced number of these connections, with SMC processes directly contacting elastic lamellae (our unpublished data; manuscript submitted). Loss of physical interactions, and hence context-specifying signals, seems to induce alteration in the morphology and synthetic program of flanking cells that are typical of a dedifferentiated state. These cellular changes are concurrent with the onset of elastolysis (our unpublished data; manuscript submitted). These observations fit well with those of increased immunoreactivity for MMPs at the periphery of mature vascular lesions in patients with MFS.[298] Subsequent disruption of the internal or external elastic laminae in fibrillin-1-deficient mice permits inflammatory cell infiltration into the media, resulting in accelerated elastolysis and eventual dissection.[292,293]

Fibrillin-1-deficient mice and patients with MFS have partial but not complete loss of microfibrillar function caused by different pathogenetic mechanisms. Although FBN1 genotype clearly determines the extent of functional impairment, hemodynamic stress and/or other environmental factors may cause additional loss of residual function. Figure 206-12 reviews the various molecular mechanisms that have been shown or proposed to result in Marfan syndrome or related phenotypes. Homozygosity for a wild-type allele (+/+) is associated with a normal microfibrillar matrix and phenotype. Functional haploinsufficiency can result either when the abnormal product from the mutant allele cannot interact with normal fibrillin-1 derived from the wild-type allele, or when there is efficient degradation of mutant mRNA from heterozygous nonsense alleles. Both situations have been observed in association with mild phenotypes in which the predominant manifestations are skeletal.[222,274,277–279] Near-haploinsufficiency in mgR/+ or mgΔ/+ mice is associated with absence or limitation

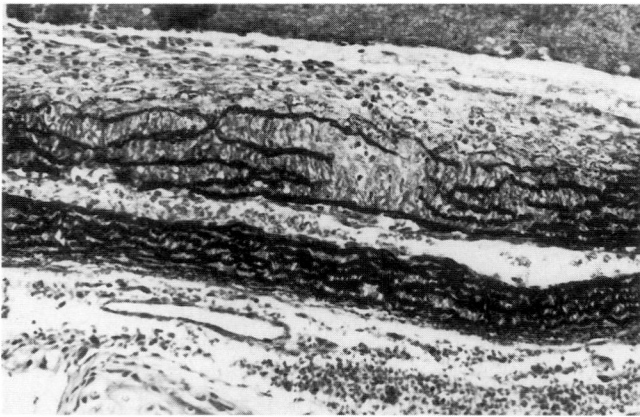

**Fig. 206-11** Elastin stain of a longitudinal section through the aortic media in a mouse homozygous for the mgΔ allele. One wall of the aorta (*top*) is thickened with focal fragmentation of elastic fibers and the accumulation of extracellular matrix. The other wall (*bottom*) shows relative preservation of architecture with long, linear, and extended elastic fibers.

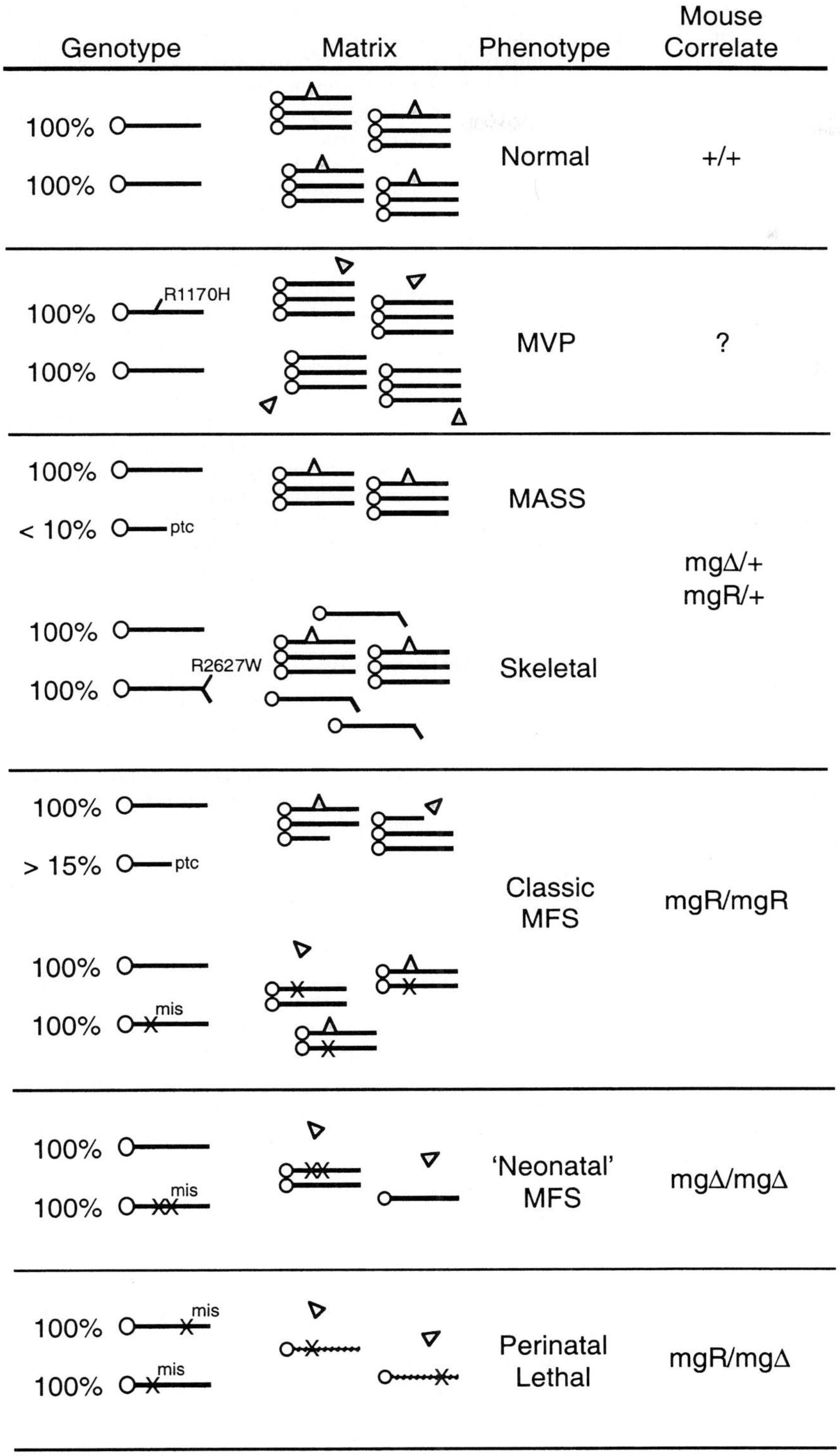

| Genotype | Matrix | Phenotype | Mouse Correlate |
|---|---|---|---|
| 100% 100% | | Normal | +/+ |
| 100% (R1170H) 100% | | MVP | ? |
| 100% < 10% (ptc) | | MASS | mgΔ/+ mgR/+ |
| 100% 100% (R2627W) | | Skeletal | |
| 100% > 15% (ptc) | | Classic MFS | mgR/mgR |
| 100% 100% (mis) | | | |
| 100% 100% (mis) | | 'Neonatal' MFS | mgΔ/mgΔ |
| 100% (mis) 100% (mis) | | Perinatal Lethal | mgR/mgΔ |

**Fig. 206-12** Genotypes and pathogenetic mechanisms in MFS and related disorders. Genotypes: + = wild-type allele; ptc = premature termination codon; X = missense mutation (mis) associated with classic MFS; XX = missense mutation associated with neonatal presentation of severe disease; each horizontal line capped by a circle represents a fibrillin-1 monomer; percent figure indicates expression level relative to a single + allele. Matrix cartoon indicates the abundance and character of microfibrils. A cluster of three aligned monomers indicates a microfibril; triangle indicates a putative interacting protein. Phenotype: MVP = mitral valve prolapse syndrome; MASS = mitral, aortic, skin, skeletal, skin phenotype (see text); Skeletal; isolated dolichostenomelia. Mouse correlate: genotypes of mice demonstrating a similar phenotype or proposed to manifest a similar pathogenetic mechanism. (*Modified from a previously published version found in Dietz et al.*[377] *Used with permission.*)

of the disease phenotype, respectively.[292,293] The extent of functional loss achieved by the dominant negative interaction in patients with missense mutations and classic MFS appears to be recapitulated in homozygous mgR mice.[293] Secondary events are required for this deficiency to become clinically manifest. The severe and rapidly progressive phenotype that manifests in the neonatal period presumably is caused by alleles with extreme dominant-negative potential.[274,276,299] This phenotype can be recapitulated by homozygosity for an allele that expresses low levels of a centrally deleted monomer in mice (mgΔ/mgΔ).[292] Additional loss of function is seen upon inheritance of two mutant human FBN1 alleles leading to either prenatal fetal loss or perinatal lethality.[44] An equally severe phenotype is seen when the mgR and mgΔ alleles occur in compound heterozygosity. These data suggest that homopolymers of mutant monomers retain more function than heteropolymers and that the proper alignment of selected domains in adjacent monomers is critical for the assembly or integrity of microfibrils.

**Regulatory Role for Microfibrils.** The extracellular matrix plays a significant role in many cellular events including differentiation, proliferation, and migration. Elastin expression may affect the phenotype of SMC in developing blood vessels and myofibroblasts in the developing lung.[300–302] To a large extent, this hypothesis is derived from an observed association between alterations in the quantity or quality of extracellular elastin and abnormalities of cellular composition and behavior. Patients with supravalvar aortic stenosis (SVAS) who are hemizygous for the elastin gene and elastin knockout mice show an abnormal proliferative and synthetic SMC phenotype, possibly related to a loss of matrix-cellular signaling.[302,303] Alternatively, phenotypic changes may simply reflect the loss of a structural constraint to cellular proliferation that is normally imposed by neighboring elastic laminae. The basis for the difference in vascular phenotypes seen in primary (SVAS) and secondary (MFS) elastin deficiency is not fully understood. Perhaps microfibrils play a structural role in the aorta independent of their association with elastin, as they do in the suspensory ligament of the ocular lens. Alternatively, the obstructive changes characteristic of SVAS may have a small developmental window. Finally, it may be that microfibrils have nonstructural functions that are critical in the development and/or homeostasis of the blood vessel wall. For example, it has been proposed that microfibrils may be active in the regulation of the local activity of TGF$\beta$.[304] This hypothesis stems from the homology between a repeated eight-cysteine domain in fibrillin-1 and a motif first observed in latency-inducing TGF$\beta$-binding proteins (LTBPs).[247] TGF$\beta$ is secreted in an inactive form resulting from its association with its processed propeptide dimer, called the latency-associated peptide (LAP).[305] This small latent complex binds to LTBPs via disulfide linkage to form the large latent complex.[305,306] The extracellular matrix regulates TGF$\beta$ activity by sequestering the large latent complex from cell surface-associated activators including plasmin and integrins alphavbeta6 and alphavbeta1.[305,307,308] There is considerable speculation, and emerging direct evidence, that complexed TGF$\beta$ interacts with microfibrils.[260,261,304,309,310] In this scenario, a genetically determined deficiency of microfibrils (Marfan syndrome) would allow excessive processing of the large latent complex resulting in an increase in TGF$\beta$ activity. The effects of TGF$\beta$ vary between tissues. In general, this multipotent cytokine inhibits cell proliferation and migration and promotes cellular differentiation and matrix deposition. Interestingly, the embryologic origin of VSMC determines the VSMC's response to TGF$\beta$.[300,311–314] VSMC derived from mesoderm that populate the descending aorta are inhibited in proliferation and migration, and have a neutral response in collagen production in response to TGF$\beta$. VSMC derived from neural crest that populate the proximal ascending aorta show opposite effects, with the induction of cellular proliferation, migration and collagen production. Thus, the histologic abnormalities that are predicted for a pathologic up-regulation of TGF$\beta$ activity would occur at the aortic segment that is uniquely predisposed for aneurysm formation in the Marfan syndrome and would closely mimic pathologic findings in fibrillin-1-deficient mice.

Analysis of the tight skin (Tsk) mouse provides further evidence for a regulatory role for microfibrils. Homozygosity for this naturally occurring mutation causes early embryonic death. Heterozygosity is associated with progressive tissue fibrosis, obstructive lung changes, and autoimmunity.[315,316] Tsk mice harbor a large genomic duplication within the Fbn1 gene resulting in the tandem repeat of exons 17 to 40 in the mRNA.[317,318] The fate of the mutant protein is the subject of ongoing investigation.[319,320] Early evidence suggested that mutant monomers interact with each other, but lack the ability to interact with normal fibrillin-1.[319] More recent results suggest that the abnormal protein is degraded near the cell surface (F. Ramirez, personal communication). It is difficult to reconcile the Tsk phenotype with an isolated deficiency of the structural role of microfibrils.

Interestingly, the duplication within the mutant protein spans the region of fibrillin-1 that shows greatest homology to the LTBPs.[317] In an in vitro binding assay, TGF$\beta$ shows increased affinity for the Tsk gene product.[320] The internally duplicated product may result in a gain-of-function, leading to excessive fibrosis and explaining the lack of significant overlap between the Tsk and MFS phenotypes. In addition, autoantibodies to fibrillin-1 have been identified in Tsk mice and in patients with scleroderma and other related connective tissue disorders.[321,322] The functional significance of this observation remains unknown.

An enhanced understanding of multiple disease processes has resulted from the study of genetic disruption of the elastin-microfibrillar array in mice. While the events and molecules that mediate the clinical expression of a deficiency in this specialized matrix have yet to be fully defined, it is important to note that selected VSMC and connective tissue abnormalities observed in MFS are also seen in common disease processes including nonsyndromic aortic aneurysm, hypertension, and atherosclerosis.[323–325] Elastic fiber calcification and degradation and intimal hyperplasia are also a component of the normal aging process. It is therefore possible that an acquired loss of elastic matrix-cell attachments, and consequent destructive changes, are integral to the pathogenesis of disorders resulting from a wide variety of genetic predispositions.

## MARFAN-RELATED CONDITIONS

The establishment of an international nosology of heritable disorders of connective tissue has recently clarified, albeit arbitrarily, the diagnostic criteria for discriminating between MFS and a collection of conditions that share certain manifestations with MFS.[45] Diagnostic distinctions have prognostic value and affect the clinical management and lifestyle of patients. The list of disorders sharing features with MFS manifestations in one or more organ system is extensive.[18,19] One can conceptualize the phenotypic relationships in several ways. A phenotypic continuum occupies but one dimension, and fails to account for the pleiotropy so characteristic of many of the conditions. Overlapping Venn diagrams extends the analysis to two dimensions but leads to rather complex interlocking structures. A display based on numeric taxonomy would be similarly limited, not that the analysis has been done. Perhaps some three-dimensional display would adequately depict the phenotypic similarities and distinctions. The following discussion describes those conditions for which at least some affected individuals and families have been associated with abnormal fibrillins.[40]

### Mitral Valve Prolapse Syndrome and MASS Phenotype

The most common clinical conundrum is determining whether a tall child or adolescent with mild skeletal features, myopia but no ectopia lentis, and mitral valve prolapse but no definite enlargement of the aortic root has MFS. Because most of the features of MFS are age-dependent, in some cases observation of the patient over time will result in a confident diagnosis of MFS. However, if major features of MFS do not emerge, and the family history reveals no close relative with MFS, what is the proper diagnosis? Faced with many such diagnostic challenges in an era before molecular understanding of MFS, Glesby and Pyeritz[93] defined a "phenotype" termed MASS (MIM 604308), for *m*itral valve prolapse, *m*yopia, minimal and nonprogressive *a*ortic root dilatation, mild *s*keletal abnormalities, and *s*triae atrophicae. MASS was not termed a "syndrome" because genetic and pathogenetic heterogeneity were assumed; however, MASS clearly is a phenotypic continuum with MFS.[81] MASS can be either a highly variable, autosomal dominant trait in a family, or it can be sporadic. Although careful prospective studies have not been performed, the perception is that important aortic and ocular problems rarely develop. MVP is usually associated with valve thickening and a tendency to progress to mitral regurgitation. The echocardiographic finding of MVP is the most common "abnormality" of the human heart.[326] The conditions and other factors that are associated with MVP are legion.[327] In the absence of contributory systemic illness or thickening of the valve (which suggests an underlying connective tissue condition), MVP is often of no or trivial concern, as is tautologically evident from the high prevalences found in some studies of 5 percent or more in young adults, especially women.[328] However, MVP has long been known to be familial (MIM 157700), and the consensus of studies has pointed to autosomal dominance with reduced penetrance.[329] Studies of probands identified through MVP have shown a higher proportion than expected with long arms, joint hypermobility, pectus excavatum, reduced thoracic kyphosis, and spontaneous pneumothorax.[330,331] This phenotype segregates in families, warranting the designation mitral valve prolapse syndrome.

**Etiology and Pathogenesis.** In a few patients with MASS phenotype, mutations in FBN1 have been identified.[274,277–279] In general, these mutations create premature termination codons that cause degradation of the mutant transcript. One PTC associated with MASS phenotype occurred in the last exon and therefore did not generate transcript instability.[274] Too few mutations have been described to determine whether the mild manifestations of the disease are determined by FBN1 genotype or by the influence of modifiers. However, the phenotype breeds true in large kindreds, supportive of the former hypothesis. Mutation R1170H is associated with dolichostenomelia with[284] or without[287] mitral valve prolapse. This and similar mutations may permit the deposition of structurally stable microfibrils that lack some functional quality such as the ability to interact with a particular protein (Fig. 206-12).[238,284] No individual in either family exhibited lens dislocation or aortic root dilatation. Finally, an individual with somatic mosaicism for a fibrillin-1 mutation had MVP with subtle skeletal manifestations.[284] When inherited through the germline, the same mutation caused classic and severe MFS.[284]

Familial MVP is a genetically heterogeneous disorder. We have excluded linkage to FBN1 in a number of large pedigrees (our unpublished data). Furthermore, a form of familial myxomatous valvular dystrophy was mapped to Xq28[332] and a locus for autosomal dominant MVP maps to 16p11.2-p12.1.[333]

## Congenital Contractural Arachnodactyly

This condition primarily affects the skeleton with contractures of the digits, elbows, and knees evident at birth, elongated long bones, and kyphoscoliosis that usually develops during childhood and progresses (Figs. 206-13 and 206-14). A peculiar abnormality of the external ear, "crumpling" of the pinna, occurs in most individuals and persists (Fig. 206-15).[15,16,334,335] Cardiovascular involvement with MVP does occur in CCA,[20,335–337] but aortic dilatation, or dissection, or ectopia lentis should suggest MFS.[338–340] Just as in MFS, CCA is inherited as an autosomal dominant trait and a large proportion of cases are sporadic, indicative of a new mutation in a parental germ cell.

In general, CCA is a milder phenotype than MFS. The joint contractures tend to improve with age, especially with physical therapy.[336] In some individuals, scoliosis has been rapidly progressive and resistant to bracing. Although its incidence has not been estimated, CCA is much less common than MFS.

**Etiology and Pathogenesis.** All families studied show linkage to the FBN2 gene on chromosome 5.[37,212] Thus far, all of the mutations identified occur in a limited region of fibrillin-2 flanked by exons 24 to 34. Mutations in the corresponding region of fibrillin-1 cause the most severe variant of MFS. The nature of mutations seen in FBN2 is very similar to that seen in FBN1, including cysteine substitutions in cbEGF-like domains and splicing mutations.[291,341–345] Multiple mutations with less-clear functional consequence precisely correspond to FBN1 mutations

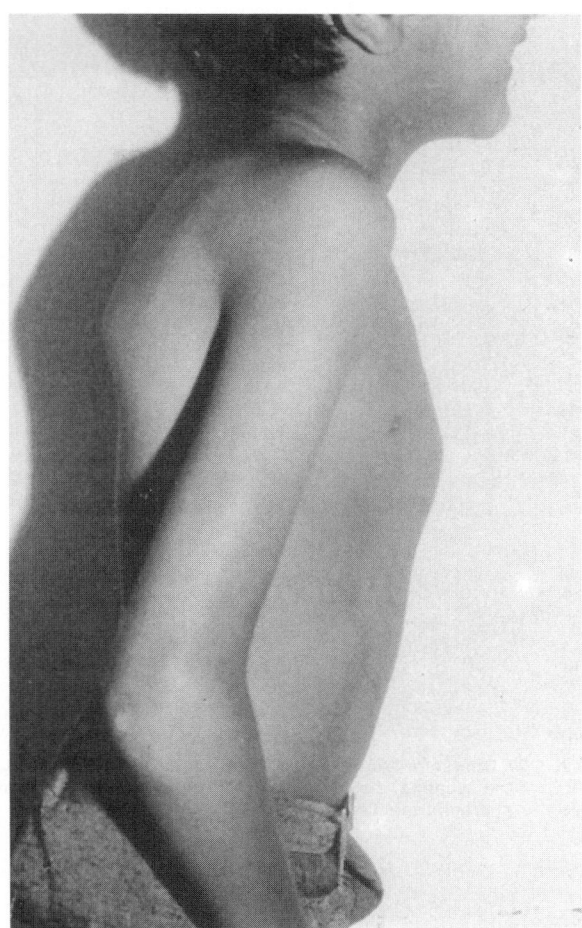

Fig. 206-13 Contracture of the elbow in an individual with congenital contractural arachnodactyly. (*From Viljoen et al.*[335] *Used with permission.*)

causing MFS.[344] Because only a small number of mutations have been identified, whether this clustering of mutations is influenced by any selection bias remains unclear. Mutations outside this region are likely either phenotypically neutral or result in a milder variant of disease. Interestingly, a fetus with an interstitial deletion of chromosome 5 encompassing the FBN2 gene showed selected

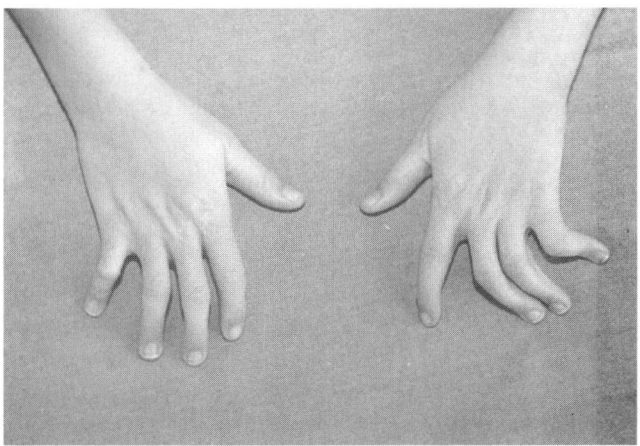

Fig. 206-14 Contracture of the fingers in an individual with congenital contractural arachnodactyly. (*Courtesy of D. Weaver.*)

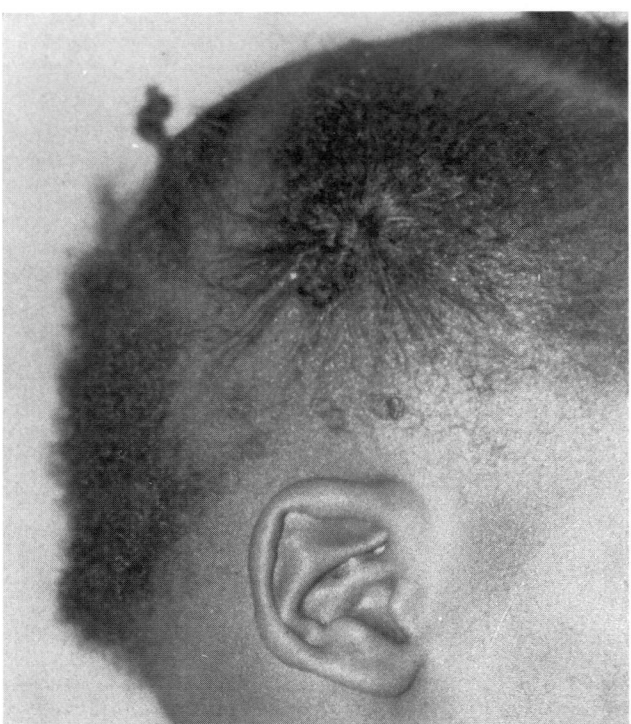

Fig. 206-15 Characteristic "crumpled" ear (incomplete development of the scapha helix) in a young girl with congenital contractural arachnodactyly.

features of CCA.[346] These observations suggest that loss-of-function may be an important pathogenetic mechanism.

## Familial Ectopia Lentis

The most common cause of ectopia lentis is trauma;[76] the next most common is MFS. Other causes of ectopia lentis include metabolic disorders that have secondary effects on ciliary zonules, such as homocystinuria (MIM 236200), hyperlysinemia (MIM 238700), sulfite oxidase deficiency (MIM 272300), and the Weill-Marchesani syndrome (MIM 277600), the cause of which remains unclear. In addition, isolated ectopia lentis can be inherited as a congenital dominant (MIM 129600), congenital recessive (MIM 225100), and adult-onset dominant trait (MIM 185450).[347] Finally, ectopia lentis et pupillae is an autosomal recessive trait (MIM 225200).[348]

In a Danish registry, the incidence of congenital ectopia lentis was 0.83 per 10,000 live births. A cause was evident in about two-thirds, with MFS accounting for two-thirds of those. Ectopia lentis et pupillae was present in 21 percent of those with a defined cause and simple dominant ectopia lentis accounted for 8 percent. Other causes were Weill-Marchesani syndrome, homocystinuria, and sulfite oxidase deficiency in about 1 percent of those patients with defined cause.[76]

**Etiology and Pathogenesis.** Linkage to FBN1 has been demonstrated for some forms of dominant ectopia lentis, including families with mild, nonspecific signs of a systemic connective tissue disorder.[212,349] To date, only a single fibrillin-1 mutation causing dominant ectopia lentis has been identified. Some members of this family had significant skeletal and skin involvement, but no individual had aortic enlargement. The mutation (E2447K) results in the substitution of lysine for a glutamic acid residue that is part of the calcium binding consensus sequence and highly conserved in cbEGF-like domains (Fig. 206-10). Interestingly, mutations at the corresponding amino acid in other fibrillin-1 cbEGF-like domains cause typical MFS.[40,263,274]

## Familial Aortic Aneurysm and Familial Aortic Dissection

The term "annuloaortic ectasia" was coined in the 1950s to describe the enlargement of the aortic root that is typical of MFS but found even more commonly in people as an isolated finding (MIM #132900). The term is something of a misnomer, because the aortic annulus rarely enlarges; any regurgitation of an otherwise normal aortic valve is due to stretching of the commissures at the sinotubular junction. Indeed, with the marked decrease in prevalence of rheumatic valvular disease, so-called idiopathic annuloaortic ectasia has become the most common cause of isolated aortic regurgitation.[350] Except in cases of inflammatory or infectious involvement of the aorta, the histopathology of the aortic wall invariably shows medial degeneration that is indistinguishable from that of MFS.[186,189] What is becoming clear only recently is the high frequency of a genetic basis for defects of the proximal aorta. The phenotypes fall into three classes, which undoubtedly overlap.

Familial aortic aneurysm shows all of the hallmarks of proximal aortic disease in the MFS.[351] Probands may show mild skeletal features of MFS, especially anterior chest and vertebral column deformity. Aortic root dilatation shows autosomal dominant inheritance with marked variability.[352] Management should follow the prescription for MFS, described above. In some,[40,353] but not all,[352,354] families, abnormalities of fibrillin are found.

Familial aortic dissection is characterized by a susceptibility to dissection of the proximal aorta with little or no preceding dilatation.[355–357] This is also an autosomal dominant disorder that is, fortunately, extremely rare. Determining who in a family may have inherited the susceptibility is quite difficult.[358] No family with aortic dissection in the absence of dilatation has been linked to FBN1 or FBN2.[40] The condition needs to be distinguished from the vascular form of Ehlers-Danlos syndrome (MIM 130050).

An association between coarctation of the aorta, bicuspid aortic valve, aneurysm of the proximal aorta, and aortic dissection has long been recognized.[359,360] The aortic dilatation was thought due to the turbulence of flow through the bicuspid valve, but some individuals with no discernible valve dysfunction develop dilatation, which suggests a fundamental defect in the aortic wall.[361] While the site of maximal dilatation of the aorta can occur at the sinuses of Valsalva, in our experience, other segments of the ascending aorta are commonly involved. No underlying cause of this conjunction of developmental defects has been discovered, although all involved segments derive from the neural crest. People with one or all parts of this triad may also show deformities of the thoracic cage reminiscent of MFS. Similarly, people ascertained through one of the cardiovascular features should be screened for the others. Furthermore, because bicuspid aortic valve is one of the defects in the "left-sided flow" spectrum of congenital heart abnormalities,[362] which shows relatively high recurrence risk,[363] echocardiographic screening of close relatives, reproductive genetic counseling, and, in selected cases, fetal echocardiography (hypoplastic left heart is at the severe end of the spectrum) are warranted.

The common finding of pleiotropic skeletal and cardiovascular manifestations in patients with ascending thoracic aortic aneurysm suggests that this is a systemic disorder of connective tissue. Valve replacement or removal of an aneurysm does not preclude subsequent involvement of other aortic segments, mandating routine follow-up. The Ross procedure should be used with caution; it might prove problematic to place a structurally predisposed segment of the pulmonary artery into the high-pressure systemic circulation. Finally, relatives of probands with bicuspid valve and aneurysm may have isolated aortic dilatation and dissection. Therefore, a negative screen for bicuspid valve does not remove the risk for the development of significant vascular disease. An indefinite period of follow-up is indicated.

**Etiology and Pathogenesis.** A few FBN1 mutations have been reported in families with ascending aortic aneurysm. The G1127S mutation was found in a large family exhibiting late onset dilatation of the aortic root.[353] Some individuals in this kindred showed fragile zonules and/or skeletal manifestations, but no individual satisfied diagnostic criteria for MFS. This glycine residue is conserved in cbEGF-like domains but has not been implicated in calcium binding or hydrophobic packing interactions. NMR analysis demonstrated defective domain folding.[286] Interestingly, an analogous mutation in a cbEGF-like domain of factor IX is associated with mild hemophilia.[364]

Mutations D1155N and P1837S were also found in individuals with ascending aortic aneurysms and skeletal involvement that failed to meet diagnostic criteria for Marfan syndrome.[365] No affected family members were available for analysis. Interestingly, many mutations at the analogous position in cbEGF-like domains as D1155N have been associated with classic MFS. Also, cells harboring mutations G1127S and D1155N showed diminished fibrillin-1 deposition in the extracellular matrix by pulse-chase analysis.[353,365] It is, therefore, difficult to postulate pathogenetic mechanisms that distinguish MFS from these cases of familial ascending aortic aneurysm.

Many families with familial ascending aortic aneurysm do not show linkage to FBN1 or the chromosome 3p locus described for a Marfan-like condition (our unpublished data).[215,366] The relevant genes have not yet been localized or identified.

## Shprintzen-Goldberg Syndrome

This condition should also be termed a phenotype, in keeping with the reasoning used for the MASS phenotype, above. The clinical features are highly variable, but the most important for diagnostic purposes include craniosynostosis and exophthalmos, arachnodactyly and camptodactyly, hernias, and muscular hypotonia. The original patients also had developmental delay,[367,368] but as more individuals are identified, it is clear that the range of intelligence includes normality.[369] A few patients with this phenotype have had severe cardiovascular involvement characteristic of MFS.[370] While most individuals have had no affected relatives, autosomal dominant and recessive inheritance have been reported.[371]

This phenotype seems heterogeneous, based on genetics and diversity of features. Greally et al. (1998)[369] suggest that in addition to craniosynostosis and other craniofacial features, the presence of dysplasia of the first and second cervical vertebrae, dilatation of the lateral ventricles and a Chiari I malformation define SGS.[369] Mergarbane and Hokayem (1998)[372] suggested that patients with SGS type I be limited to those patients with mental retardation, craniosynostosis, and skeletal changes of MFS, while SGS type II include those with normal intelligence and aortic root dilatation.[372]

**Etiology and Pathogenesis.** In one patient with SGS, a FBN1 mutation (C1223Y) was identified. This mutation involved the substitution of a cysteine residue in a cbEGF-like domain, the most common mutational class causing MFS. C1223Y was also identified in a mother and daughter diagnosed with MFS.[373] Despite suggestive evidence, the diagnosis of SGS could not be confirmed in this family. Mutation P1148A was initially identified in a patient with SGS and in individuals with ascending aortic aneurysm and their family members.[370] This mutation was subsequently identified in individuals without apparent connective tissue abnormalities, with an increased population frequency in those of Hispanic or Asian decent.[374-376] In view of the highly variable clinical presentation of individuals diagnosed with SGS, genetic heterogeneity seems certain.

## Familial Tall Stature

Completing the phenotypic spectrum of traits that mirror some of the features of MFS is this condition that involves only the

skeleton. The proband had, in addition to dolichostenomelic tall stature, minor skeletal changes of MFS, but no ocular or cardiovascular changes. A nonpolymorphic mutation in *FBN1* was found in the proband and in a number of close relatives, each of whom was tall without other features of a connective tissue disorder.[222] No systematic search for *FBN1* mutations among tall individuals has been performed.

**Etiology and Pathogenesis.** Mutation R2627W substitutes a residue that lies immediately adjacent to the consensus site for cleavage by PACE/furin-like proteases[222] and prevents C-terminal processing. The abnormal fibrillin-1 monomer is synthesized and secreted, but fails to participate in microfibrillar assembly.[222,226] These data suggest that initiation of multimerization is negatively regulated by the presence of the C-terminal propeptide. Because the proline-rich domain near the N-terminus can support dimerization,[227,228] it is appealing to suggest that this regulation involves intramolecular interactions. This may explain why mutations that truncate or substitute fibrillin-1 beyond the cleavage site can impair microfibrillar assembly and cause MFS.

## REFERENCES

1. Marfan A-B: Un cas de déformation congénitale des quatre membres plus prononcée aux extremites caractérisée par l'allongement des os avec un certain degré d'amincissement. *Bull Mem Soc Med Hop Paris* **13**:220, 1896.
2. Mery H, Babonneix L: Un cas de déformation congénitale des quatre membres: Hyperchondroplasie. *Bull Mem Soc Med Hop Paris* **19**:671, 1902.
3. Achard C: Arachnodactilie. *Bull Mem Soc Med Hop Paris* **19**:834, 1902.
4. Borger F: Uber zwei Falle von Arachnodaktylie. *Z Kinderheilkd* **12**:161, 1914.
5. Salle V: Über einen fall von angeborener abnormer grosse der extremitaen mit einem an akromegalie erinnernden symptomkomplex. *Jahrb Kinderheilkd Phys Erziehung* **75**:540, 1912.
6. Weve H: Über arachnodaktylie (dystrophia mesodermalis congenita, typus Marfan). *Arch Augenheilkd* **104**:1, 1931.
7. Apert E: Les formes frustes du syndrome dolichosténomélique de Marfan. *Nourrisson* **26**:1, 1938.
8. Etter L, Glover LP: Arachnodactyly complicated by dislocated lens and death from rupture of dissecting aneurysm of aorta. *JAPA* **123**:88, 1943.
9. Baer R, Taussig HB, Oppenheimer EH: Congenital aneurysmal dilatation of aorta associated with arachnodactyly. *Bull Johns Hopkins Hospital* **72**:309, 1943.
10. Lutman FC, Neel JV: Inheritance of arachnodactyly, ectopia lentis and other congenital anomalies (Marfan syndrome) in the E. family. *Arch Ophthalmol* **41**:276, 1949.
11. McKusick V: The cardiovascular aspects of Marfan's syndrome: A heritable disorder of connective tissue. *Circulation* **11**:321, 1955.
12. McKusick V: *Heritable Disorders of Connective Tissue*. St. Louis, CV Mosby, 1956.
13. Carson NAJ, Neill DW: Metabolic abnormalities detected in a survey of mentally backward individuals in Northern Ireland. *Arch Dis Child* **37**:505, 1962.
14. Schimke RN, McKusick VA, Huang T, Pollock AD: Homocystinuria, a study of 38 cases in 20 families. *JAMA* **193**:711, 1965.
15. Epstein C, Graham CB, Hodkin WE, Hecht F, Motulsky AG: Hereditary dysplasia of bone with kyphoscoliosis, contractures and abnormally shaped ears. *J Pediatr* **73**:379, 1968.
16. Beals R, Hecht F: Congenital contractural arachnodactyly: A heritable disorder of connective tissue. *J Bone Joint Surg* **53**:887, 1971.
17. Hecht F, Beals RK: "New" syndrome of congenital contractural arachnodactyly originally described by Marfan in 1896. *Pediatrics* **49**:574, 1972.
18. Pyeritz RE: Marfan syndrome and other disorders fibrillin, in Rimoin DL, Connor JM, Pyeritz RE (eds): *Principles and Practice of Medical Genetics*. New York, Churchill-Livingston, 1997, p 1027.
19. Pyeritz RE, Dietz HC: The Marfan syndrome and other fibrillinopathies, in Royce PM, Steinmann B (eds): *Connective Tissue and Its Heritable Disorders: Molecular, Genetics and Medical Aspects*. New York, Wiley-Liss, 1999.

20. Pyeritz RE: The Marfan syndrome, in Emery AEH, Rimoin DL (eds): *The Principles and Practice of Medical Genetics.* New York, Churchill-Livingston, 1990, p 1047.

21. Byers PH: Disorders of collagen biosynthesis and structure, in Scriver CR, Beaudet AL, Sly WS, Valle D (eds): *The Metabolic Basis of Inherited Disease.* New York, McGraw Hill, 1989, p 2805.

22. Karrer HE: The fine structure of connective tissue in the tunica propria of bronchioles. *J Ultrastruc Res* 2:29, 1958.

23. Low FN: Microfibrils: Fine filamentous components of tissue space. *Anat Rec* 142:131, 1962.

24. Ross R, Bornstein P: The elastic fiber. I. The separation and partial characterization of its macromolecular components. *J Cell Biol* 40:366, 1969.

25. Cleary E, Gibson M: Elastin-associated microfibrils and microfibrillar proteins. *Int Rev Connect Tissue Res* 10:97, 1983.

26. Sakai LY, Keene DR, Engvall E: Fibrillin, a new 350-kD glycoprotein, is a component of extracellular microfibrils. *J Cell Biol* 103:2499, 1986.

27. Hollister DW, Godfrey M, Sakai LY, Pyeritz RE: Immunohistologic abnormalities of the microfibrillar-fiber system in the Marfan syndrome. *N Engl J Med* 323:152, 1990.

28. Godfrey M, Menashe V, Weleber RG, Koler RD, Bigley RH, Lovrien E, Zonana J, Hollister DW: Cosegregation of elastin-associated microfibrillar abnormalities with the Marfan phenotype in families. *Am J Hum Genet* 46:652, 1990.

29. Maddox BK, Sakai LY, Keene DR, Glanville RW: Connective tissue microfibrils. Isolation and characterization of three large pepsin-resistant domains of fibrillin. *J Biol Chem* 264:21381, 1989.

30. Milewicz DM, Pyeritz RE, Crawford ES, Byers PH: Marfan syndrome: Defective synthesis, secretion, and extracellular matrix formation of fibrillin by cultured dermal fibroblasts. *J Clin Invest* 89:79, 1992.

31. Blanton SH, Sarfarazi M, Eiberg H, de Groote J, Farndon PA, Kilpatrick MW, Child AH, Pope FM, Peltonen L, Francomano CA, et al: An exclusion map of Marfan syndrome. *J Med Genet* 27:73, 1990.

32. Kainulainen K, Pulkkinen L, Savolainen A, Kaitila I, Peltonen L: Location on chromosome 15 of the gene defect causing Marfan syndrome [see comments]. *N Engl J Med* 323:935, 1990.

33. Dietz HC, Pyeritz RE, Hall BD, Cadle RG, Hamosh A, Schwartz J, Meyers DA, Francomano CA: The Marfan syndrome locus: confirmation of assignment to chromosome 15 and identification of tightly linked markers at 15q15-q21.3. *Genomics* 9:355, 1991.

34. Tsipouras P, Sarfarazi M, Devi A, Weiffenbach B, Boxer M: Marfan syndrome is closely linked to a marker on chromosome 15q1.5-q2.1. *Proc Natl Acad Sci U S A* 88:4486, 1991.

35. Kainulainen K, Steinmann B, Collins F, Dietz HC, Francomano CA, Child A, Kilpatrick MW, Brock DJ, Keston M, Pyeritz RE, et al: Marfan syndrome: No evidence for heterogeneity in different populations, and more precise mapping of the gene. *Am J Hum Genet* 49:662, 1991.

36. Maslen CL, Corson GM, Maddox BK, Glanville RW, Sakai LY: Partial sequence of a candidate gene for the Marfan syndrome [see comments]. *Nature* 352:334, 1991.

37. Lee B, Godfrey M, Vitale E, Hori H, Mattei MG, Sarfarazi M, Tsipouras P, Ramirez F, Hollister DW: Linkage of Marfan syndrome and a phenotypically related disorder to two different fibrillin genes. *Nature* 352:330, 1991.

38. Magenis RE, Maslen CL, Smith L, Allen L, Sakai LY: Localization of the fibrillin (FBN) gene to chromosome 15, band q21.1. *Genomics* 11:346, 1991.

39. Dietz HC, Cutting GR, Pyeritz RE, Maslen CL, Sakai LY, Corson GM, Puffenberger EG, Hamosh A, Nanthakumar EJ, Curristin SM, et al: Marfan syndrome caused by a recurrent de novo missense mutation in the fibrillin gene. *Nature* 352:337, 1991.

40. Dietz HC, Pyeritz RE: Mutations in the human gene for fibrillin-1 (FBN1) in the Marfan syndrome and related disorders. *Hum Mol Genet* 4:1799, 1995.

41. Murdoch JL, Walker BA, McKusick VA: Parental age effects on the occurrence of new mutations for the Marfan syndrome. *Ann Hum Genet* 35:331, 1972.

42. Chemke J, Nisani R, Feigl A, Garty R, Cooper M, Barash Y, Duksin D: Homozygosity for autosomal dominant Marfan syndrome. *J Med Genet* 21:173, 1984.

43. Schollin J, Bjarke B, Gustavson KH: Probable homozygotic form of the Marfan syndrome in a newborn child. *Acta Paediatr Scand* 77:452, 1988.

44. Karttunen L, Raghunath M, Lonnqvist L, Peltonen L: A compound-heterozygous Marfan patient: Two defective fibrillin alleles result in a lethal phenotype. *Am J Hum Genet* 55:1083, 1994.

45. De Paepe A, Devereux RB, Dietz HC, Hennekam RC, Pyeritz RE: Revised diagnostic criteria for the Marfan syndrome. *Am J Med Genet* 62:417, 1996.

46. Pereira L, Levran O, Ramirez F, Lynch JR, Sykes B, Pyeritz RE, Dietz HC: A molecular approach to the stratification of cardiovascular risk in families with Marfan's syndrome. *N Engl J Med* 331:148, 1994.

47. Pyeritz RE, Murphy EA, Lin SJ, Rosell EM: Growth and anthropometrics in the Marfan syndrome. *Prog Clin Biol Res* 200:355, 1985.

48. Eldridge R: The metacarpal index: A useful aid in the diagnosis of Marfan syndrome. *Arch Intern Med* 113:248, 1964.

49. Joseph KN: The metacarpal index—Obsolete in Marfan syndrome! *Skeletal Radiol* 21:371, 1992.

50. Magid D, Pyeritz RE, Fishman EK: Musculoskeletal manifestations of the Marfan syndrome: Radiologic features. *AJR Am J Roentgenol* 155:99, 1990.

51. Arn PH, Scherer LR, Haller JA Jr, Pyeritz RE: Outcome of pectus excavatum in patients with Marfan syndrome and in the general population. *J Pediatr* 115:954, 1989.

52. Westling L, Mohlin B, Bresin A: Craniofacial manifestations in the Marfan syndrome: Palatal dimensions and a comparative cephalometric analysis. *J Craniofac Genet Dev Biol* 18:211, 1998.

53. Savini R, Cervellati S, Beroaldo E: Spinal deformities in Marfan's syndrome. *Ital J Orthop Traumatol* 6:19, 1980.

54. Birch JG, Herring JA: Spinal deformity in Marfan syndrome. *J Pediatr Orthop* 7:546, 1987.

55. Robins PR, Moe JH, Winter RB: Scoliosis in Marfan's syndrome. Its characteristics and results of treatment in thirty-five patients. *J Bone Joint Surg [Am]* 57:358, 1975.

56. Sponseller PD, Hobbs W, Riley LH 3rd, Pyeritz RE: The thoraco-lumbar spine in Marfan syndrome. *J Bone Joint Surg Am* 77:867, 1995.

57. Hobbs WR, Sponseller PD, Weiss AP, Pyeritz RE: The cervical spine in Marfan syndrome. *Spine* 22:983, 1997.

58. Sponseller PD, Sethi N, Cameron DE, Pyeritz RE: Infantile scoliosis in Marfan syndrome. *Spine* 22:509, 1997.

59. Grahame R, Pyeritz RE: The Marfan syndrome: joint and skin manifestations are prevalent and correlated. *Br J Rheumatol* 34:126, 1995.

60. Pennes DR, Braunstein EM, Shirazi KK: Carpal ligamentous laxity with bilateral perilunate dislocation in Marfan syndrome. *Skeletal Radiol* 13:62, 1985.

61. Sponseller PD, Tomek IM, Pyertiz RE: Developmental dysplasia of the hip in Marfan syndrome. *J Pediatr Orthop B* 6:255, 1997.

62. Winter RB: Severe spondylolisthesis in Marfan's syndrome: Report of two cases. *J Pediatr Orthop* 2:51, 1982.

63. Levander B, Mellstrom A, Grepe A: Atlantoaxial instability in Marfan's syndrome. Diagnosis and treatment. A case report. *Neuroradiology* 21:43, 1981.

64. Taylor LJ: Severe spondylolisthesis and scoliosis in association with Marfan's syndrome. Case report and review of the literature. *Clin Orthop* 221:207, 1987.

65. Wenger DR, Ditkoff TJ, Herring JA, Mauldin DM: Protrusio acetabuli in Marfan's syndrome. *Clin Orthop* 147:134, 1980.

66. Fast A, Otremsky Y, Pollack D, Floman Y: Protrusio acetabuli in Marfan's syndrome: Report on two patients. *J Rheumatol* 11:549, 1984.

67. Kuhlman JE, Scott WW Jr, Fishman EK, Pyeritz RE, Siegelman SS: Acetabular protrusion in the Marfan syndrome. *Radiology* 164:415, 1987.

68. Steel HH: Protrusio acetabuli: its occurrence in the completely expressed Marfan syndrome and its musculoskeletal component and a procedure to arrest the course of protrusion in the growing pelvis. *J Pediatr Orthop* 16:704, 1996.

69. Kharrazi FD, Rodgers WB, Coran DL, Kasser JR, Hall JE: Protrusio acetabuli and bilateral basocervical femoral neck fractures in a patient with Marfan syndrome. *Am J Orthop* 26:689, 1997.

70. Kohlmeier L, Gasner C, Marcus R: Bone mineral status of women with Marfan syndrome. *Am J Med* 95:568, 1993.

71. Gray JR, Bridges AB, Mole PA, Pringle T, Boxer M, Paterson CR: Osteoporosis and the Marfan syndrome. *Postgrad Med J* 69:373, 1993.

72. Kohlmeier L, Gasner C, Bachrach LK, Marcus R: The bone mineral status of patients with Marfan syndrome. *J Bone Miner Res* 10:1550, 1995.

73. Tobias JH, Dalzell N, Child AH: Assessment of bone mineral density in women with Marfan syndrome. *Br J Rheumatol* 34:516, 1995.

74. Cross HE, Jensen AD: Ocular manifestations in the Marfan syndrome and homocystinuria. *Am J Ophthalmol* **75**:405, 1973.
75. Maumenee IH: The eye in the Marfan syndrome. *Trans Am Ophthalmol Soc* **79**:684, 1981.
76. Fuchs J, Rosenberg T: Congenital ectopia lentis. A Danish national survey. *Acta Ophthalmol Scand* **76**:20, 1998.
77. Dotrelova D, Karel I, Clupkova E: Retinal detachment in Marfan's syndrome. Characteristics and surgical results. *Retina* **17**:390, 1997.
78. Izquierdo NJ, Traboulsi EI, Enger C, Maumenee IH: Strabismus in the Marfan syndrome. *Am J Ophthalmol* **117**:632, 1994.
79. Izquierdo NJ, Traboulsi EI, Enger C, Maumenee IH: Glaucoma in the Marfan syndrome. *Trans Am Ophthalmol Soc* **90**:111, 1992.
80. Phornphutkul C, Rosenthal A, Nadas AS: Cardiac manifestations of Marfan syndrome in infancy and childhood. *Circulation* **47**:587, 1973.
81. Morse RP, Rockenmacher S, Pyeritz RE, Sanders SP, Bieber FR, Lin A, MacLeod P, Hall B, Graham JM Jr: Diagnosis and management of infantile Marfan syndrome. *Pediatrics* **86**:888, 1990.
82. Gillinov AM, Zehr KJ, Redmond JM, Gott VL, Deitz HC, Reitz BA, Laschinger JC, Cameron DE: Cardiac operations in children with Marfan's syndrome: Indications and results. *Ann Thorac Surg* **64**:1140, 1997.
83. Pyeritz RE, Wappel MA: Mitral valve dysfunction in the Marfan syndrome. Clinical and echocardiographic study of prevalence and natural history. *Am J Med* **74**:797, 1983.
84. Lima SD, Lima JA, Pyeritz RE, Weiss JL: Relation of mitral valve prolapse to left ventricular size in Marfan's syndrome. *Am J Cardiol* **55**:739, 1985.
85. Roberts WC, Honig HS: The spectrum of cardiovascular disease in the Marfan syndrome: A clinico-morphologic study of 18 necropsy patients and comparison to 151 previously reported necropsy patients. *Am Heart J* **104**:115, 1982.
86. Marsalese DL, Moodie DS, Vacante M, Lytle BW, Gill CC, Sterba R, Cosgrove DM, Passalacqua M, Goormastic M, Kovacs A: Marfan's syndrome: Natural history and long-term follow-up of cardiovascular involvement. *J Am Coll Cardiol* **14**:422, 1989.
87. Sisk HE, Zahka KG, Pyeritz RE: The Marfan syndrome in early childhood: Analysis of 15 patients diagnosed at less than 4 years of age. *Am J Cardiol* **52**:353, 1983.
88. Murdoch JL, Walker BA, Halpern BL, Kuzma JW, McKusick VA: Life expectancy and causes of death in the Marfan syndrome. *N Engl J Med* **286**:804, 1972.
89. Disler LJ, Manga P, Barlow JB: Pulmonary arterial aneurysms in Marfan's syndrome. *Int J Cardiol* **21**:79, 1988.
90. Schlatmann TJ, Becker AE: Pathogenesis of dissecting aneurysm of aorta. Comparative histopathologic study of significance of medial changes. *Am J Cardiol* **39**:21, 1977.
91. Erdheim J: Medionecrosis aortae idiopathica cystica. *Virchow Arch Pathol Anat* **276**:187, 1930.
92. Roman MJ, Devereux RB, Kramer-Fox R, O'Loughlin J: Two-dimensional echocardiographic aortic root dimensions in normal children and adults. *Am J Cardiol* **64**:507, 1989.
93. Glesby MJ, Pyeritz RE: Association of mitral valve prolapse and systemic abnormalities of connective tissue. A phenotypic continuum. *JAMA* **262**:523, 1989.
94. Reed CM, Richey PA, Pulliam DA, Somes GW, Alpert BS: Aortic dimensions in tall men and women. *Am J Cardiol* **71**:608, 1993.
95. Geva T, Hegesi J, Frand M: The clinical course and echocardiographic features of Marfan's syndrome in childhood. *Am J Dis Child* **141**:1179, 1987.
96. Groenink M, Rozendaal L, Naeff MS, Hennekam RC, Hart AA, van der Wall EE, Mulder BJ: Marfan syndrome in children and adolescents: Predictive and prognostic value of aortic root growth for screening for aortic complications. *Heart* **80**:163, 1998.
97. Pyeritz RE: Predictors of dissection of the ascending aorta in Marfan syndrome. *Circulation* **84**:II, 1991.
98. Roman MJ, Rosen SE, Kramer-Fox R, Devereux RB: Prognostic significance of the pattern of aortic root dilation in the Marfan syndrome. *J Am Coll Cardiol* **22**:1470, 1993.
99. Silverman DI, Gray J, Roman MJ, Bridges A, Burton K, Boxer M, Devereux RB, Tsipouras P: Family history of severe cardiovascular disease in Marfan syndrome is associated with increased aortic diameter and decreased survival. *J Am Coll Cardiol* **26**:1062, 1995.
100. Lafferty K, McLean L, Salisbury J, Cotton LT: Ruptured abdominal aortic aneurysm in Marfan's syndrome. *Postgrad Med J* **63**:685, 1987.
101. van Ooijen B: Marfan's syndrome and isolated aneurysm of the abdominal aorta. *Br Heart J* **59**:81, 1988.
102. Srinivasan R, Parvin SD, Lambert D: Spontaneously ruptured middle colic artery aneurysm in a patient with Marfan's syndrome. *Eur J Vasc Surg* **4**:317, 1990.
103. Savolainen H, Savola J, Savolainen A: Aneurysm of the iliac artery in Marfan's syndrome. *Ann Chir Gynaecol* **82**:203, 1993.
104. de Virgilio C, Cherry KJ Jr, Schaff HV: Multiple aneurysms and aortic dissection: An unusual manifestation of Marfan's syndrome. *Ann Vasc Surg* **8**:383, 1994.
105. Matsuda M, Matsuda I, Handa H, Okamoto K: Intracavernous giant aneurysm associated with Marfan's syndrome. *Surg Neurol* **12**:119, 1979.
106. van den Berg JS, Limburg M, Hennekam RC: Is Marfan syndrome associated with symptomatic intracranial aneurysms? *Stroke* **27**:10, 1996.
107. Schievink WI, Parisi JE, Piepgras DG, Michels VV: Intracranial aneurysms in Marfan's syndrome: An autopsy study. *Neurosurgery* **41**:866, 1997.
108. Chen S, Fagan LF, Nouri S, Donahoe JL: Ventricular dysrhythmias in children with Marfan's syndrome. *Am J Dis Child* **139**:273, 1985.
109. Wang SWS, Wade EG: Congestive cardiomyopathy in the Marfan syndrome: Report of two cases. *Proc Hong Kong Cardiol Soc* **7**:105, 1980.
110. Dwyer EM, Troncale F: Spontaneous pneumothorax and pulmonary disease in the Marfan syndrome. Report of two cases and review of the literature. *Ann Intern Med* **62**:1285, 1965.
111. Lipton RA, Greenwald RA, Seriff NS: Pneumothorax and bilateral honeycombed lung in Marfan syndrome. Report of a case and review of the pulmonary abnormalities in this disorder. *Am Rev Respir Dis* **104**:924, 1971.
112. Hall JR, Pyeritz RE, Dudgeon DL, Haller JA Jr: Pneumothorax in the Marfan syndrome: prevalence and therapy. *Ann Thorac Surg* **37**:500, 1984.
113. Yellin A, Shiner RJ, Lieberman Y: Familial multiple bilateral pneumothorax associated with Marfan syndrome. *Chest* **100**:577, 1991.
114. Bamforth S, Hayden MR: Pulmonary emphysema in neonate with the Marfan syndrome. *Pediatr Radiol* **18**:88, 1988.
115. Reye RD, Bale PM: Elastic tissue in pulmonary emphysema in Marfan syndrome. *Arch Pathol* **96**:427, 1973.
116. Sayers CP, Goltz RW, Mottaz J: Pulmonary elastic tissue in generalized elastolysis (cutis laxa) and Marfan's syndrome: A light and electron microscopic study. *J Invest Dermatol* **65**:451, 1975.
117. Wood JR, Bellamy D, Child AH, Citron KM: Pulmonary disease in patients with Marfan syndrome. *Thorax* **39**:780, 1984.
118. Streeten EA, Murphy EA, Pyeritz RE: Pulmonary function in the Marfan syndrome. *Chest* **91**:408, 1987.
119. Cistulli PA, Sullivan CE: Sleep-disordered breathing in Marfan's syndrome. *Am Rev Respir Dis* **147**:645, 1993.
120. Fiarcloth DN, Tenholder MF, Whitlock WL, Downs RH: Pulmonary dysfunction secondary to mandibular retrognathia in Marfan's syndrome. *Chest* **105**:1610, 1994.
121. Hargreaves MR, Gilbert TJ, Pillai R, Hart G: Large airway obstruction by a chronic dissecting aortic aneurysm in the Marfan syndrome. *Postgrad Med J* **73**:726, 1997.
122. Fishman EK, Zinreich SJ, Kumar AJ, Rosenbaum AE, Siegelman SS: Sacral abnormalities in Marfan syndrome. *J Comput Assist Tomogr* **7**:851, 1983.
123. Pyeritz RE, Fishman EK, Bernhardt BA, Siegelman SS: Dural ectasia is a common feature of the Marfan syndrome. *Am J Hum Genet* **43**:726, 1988.
124. Stern WE: Dural ectasia and the Marfan syndrome. *J Neurosurg* **69**:221, 1988.
125. Thierry A, Archimbaud JP, Fischer G, Freidel M, Mansuy L: [Anterior sacral meningocele. Review of the literature and presentation of a case.] *Neurochirurgie* **15**:389, 1969.
126. Strand RD, Eisenberg HM: Anterior sacral meningocele in association with Marfan's syndrome. *Radiology* **99**:653, 1971.
127. Smith MD: Large sacral dural defect in Marfan syndrome. A case report. *J Bone Joint Surg Am* **75**:1067, 1993.
128. Raftopoulos C, Delecluse F, Braude P, Rodesh C, Brotchi J: Anterior sacral meningocele and Marfan syndrome: A review. *Acta Chir Belg* **93**:1, 1993.
129. Davenport RJ, Chataway SJ, Warlow CP: Spontaneous intracranial hypotension from a CSF leak in a patient with Marfan's syndrome. *J Neurol Neurosurg Psychiatry* **59**:516, 1995.

130. Raftopoulos C, Pierard GE, Retif C, Braude P, Brotchi J: Endoscopic cure of a giant sacral meningocele associated with Marfan's syndrome: Case report. *Neurosurgery* **30**:765, 1992.

131. Shin MS, Mulligan SA, Baxley WA, Ho KJ: Bochdalek hernia of diaphragm in the adult. Diagnosis by computed tomography. *Chest* **92**:1098, 1987.

132. Parida SK, Kriss VM, Hall BD: Hiatus/paraesophageal hernias in neonatal Marfan syndrome. *Am J Med Genet* **72**:156, 1997.

133. Pottkotter L: Striae and systemic abnormalities of connective tissue. *JAMA* **262**:3132, 1989.

134. Pinkus H, Keech MK, Mehregan AH: Histopathology of striae distensae, with special reference to striae and wound healing in the Marfan syndrome. *J Invest Dermatol* **46**:283, 1966.

135. Hofman KJ, Bernhardt BA, Pyeritz RE: Marfan syndrome: Neuropsychological aspects. *Am J Med Genet* **31**:331, 1988.

136. Lannoo E, De Paepe A, Leroy B, Thiery E: Neuropsychological aspects of Marfan syndrome. *Clin Genet* **49**:65, 1996.

137. Van Tongerloo A, De Paepe A: Psychosocial adaptation in adolescents and young adults with Marfan syndrome: an exploratory study. *J Med Genet* **35**:405, 1998.

138. Health supervision for children with Marfan syndrome. American Academy of Pediatrics Committee on Genetics. *Pediatrics* **98**:978, 1996.

139. Scherer LR, Arn PH, Dressel DA, Pyeritz RM, Haller JA Jr: Surgical management of children and young adults with Marfan syndrome and pectus excavatum. *J Pediatr Surg* **23**:1169, 1988.

140. Nuss D, Kelly RE Jr, Croitoru DP, Katz ME: A 10-year review of a minimally invasive technique for the correction of pectus excavatum. *J Pediatr Surg* **33**:545, 1998.

141. Jones WG, Hoffman L, Devereux RB, Isom OW, Gold JP: Staged approach to combined repair of pectus excavatum and lesions of the heart. *Ann Thorac Surg* **57**:212, 1994.

142. Kalangos A, Delay D, Murith N, Pretre R, Bruschweiler I, Faidutti B: Correction of pectus excavatum combined with open heart surgery in a patient with Marfan's syndrome. *Thorac Cardiovasc Surg* **43**:220, 1995.

143. Bailey JD, Park E, Cowell C: Estrogen treatment of girls and constitutional tall stature. *Pediatr Clin North Am* **28**:501, 1981.

144. Knudtzon J, Aarskog D: Estrogen treatment of excessively tall girls with Marfan syndrome. *Acta Paediatr Scand* **77**:537, 1988.

145. Yeung KK, Weissman BA: Contact lens correction of patients with Marfan syndrome. *J Am Optom Assoc* **68**:367, 1997.

146. Omulecki W, Nawrocki J, Palenga-Pydyn D, Sempinska-Szewczyk J: Pars plana vitrectomy, lensectomy, or extraction in transscleral intraocular lens fixation for the management of dislocated lenses in a family with Marfan's syndrome. *Ophthalmic Surg Lasers* **29**:375, 1998.

147. Legget ME, Unger TA, O'Sullivan CK, Zwink TR, Bennett RL, Byers PH, Otto CM: Aortic root complications in Marfan's syndrome: Identification of a lower risk group. *Heart* **75**:389, 1996.

148. Shores J, Berger KR, Murphy EA, Pyeritz RE: Progression of aortic dilatation and the benefit of long-term beta- adrenergic blockade in Marfan's syndrome. *N Engl J Med* **330**:1335, 1994.

149. Salim MA, Alpert BS, Ward JC, Pyeritz RE: Effect of beta-adrenergic blockade on aortic root rate of dilation in the Marfan syndrome. *Am J Cardiol* **74**:629, 1994.

150. Yin FC, Brin KP, Ting CT, Pyeritz RE: Arterial hemodynamic indexes in Marfan's syndrome. *Circulation* **79**:854, 1989.

151. Haouzi A, Berglund H, Pelikan PC, Maurer G, Siegel RJ: Heterogeneous aortic response to acute beta-adrenergic blockade in Marfan syndrome. *Am Heart J* **133**:60, 1997.

152. Bentall H, De Bono A: A technique for complete replacement of the ascending aorta. *Thorax* **23**:338, 1968.

153. Gott VL, Greene PS, Alejo DE, Cameron DE, Naftel DC, Miller DC, Gillinov AM, Laschinger JC, Pyeritz RE: Replacement of the aortic root in patients with Marfan's syndrome. *N Engl J Med* **340**:1307, 1999.

154. Silverman DI, Burton KJ, Gray J, Bosner MS, Kouchoukos NT, Roman MJ, Boxer M, Devereux RB, Tsipouras P: Life expectancy in the Marfan syndrome. *Am J Cardiol* **75**:157, 1995.

155. Crawford ES: Marfan's syndrome. Broad spectral surgical treatment cardiovascular manifestations. *Ann Surg* **198**:487, 1983.

156. Crawford ES, Crawford JL, Stowe CL, Safi HJ: Total aortic replacement for chronic aortic dissection occurring in patients with and without Marfan's syndrome. *Ann Surg* **199**:358, 1984.

157. David TE: Aortic valve repair in patients with Marfan syndrome and ascending aorta aneurysms due to degenerative disease. *J Card Surg* **9**:182, 1994.

158. Gallo R, Kumar N, al Halees Z, Duran C: Early failure of aortic valve conservation in aortic root aneurysm. *J Thorac Cardiovasc Surg* **109**:1011, 1995.

159. Pyeritz RE: Maternal and fetal complications of pregnancy in the Marfan syndrome. *Am J Med* **71**:784, 1981.

160. Lipscomb KJ, Smith JC, Clarke B, Donnai P, Harris R: Outcome of pregnancy in women with Marfan's syndrome. *Br J Obstet Gynaecol* **104**:201, 1997.

161. Rasmussen LA, Lund JT, Pettersson G: [Marfan syndrome and pregnancy.] *Ugeskr Laeger* **160**:6219, 1998.

162. Rossiter JP, Repke JT, Morales AJ, Murphy EA, Pyeritz RE: A prospective longitudinal evaluation of pregnancy in the Marfan syndrome. *Am J Obstet Gynecol* **173**:1599, 1995.

163. Scheck M, Siegel RC, Parker J, Chang YH, Fu JC: Aortic aneurysm in Marfan's syndrome: Changes in the ultrastructure and composition of collagen. *J Anat* **129**:645, 1979.

164. Krieg T, Muauller PK: The Marfan's syndrome. In vitro study of collagen metabolism in tissue specimens of the aorta. *Exp Cell Biol* **45**:207, 1977.

165. Laitinen O, Uitto J, Iivanainen M, Hannuksela M, Kivirikko KI: Collagen metabolism of the skin in Marfan's syndrome. *Clin Chim Acta* **21**:321, 1968.

166. Priest RE, Moinuddin JF, Priest JH: Letter: Collagen of Marfan syndrome is abnormally soluble. *Nature* **245**:264, 1973.

167. Boucek R, Noble NL, Gunja-Smith Z, Butler WT: The Marfan syndrome: A deficiency in chemically stable collagen cross-links. *N Engl J Med* **305**:988, 1981.

168. Byers P, Siegel RC, Peterson KE, Rowe DW, Holbrook KA, Smith LT, Chang Y, Fu JCC: Marfan syndrome: An abnormal alpha 2 chain in type I collagen. *Proc Natl Acad Sci U S A* **78**:7745, 1981.

169. Phillips C, Shrago-Howe AW, Pinnell SR, Wenstrup RJ: A substitution at a non-glycine position in the triple-helical domain of pro-$\alpha$2(I) collagen chains present in an individual with a variant of the Marfan's syndrome. *J Clin Invest* **86**:1723, 1990.

170. Tsipouras P, Borresen AL, Bamforth S, Harper PS, Berg K: Marfan syndrome: Exclusion of genetic linkage to the COL1A2 gene. *Clin Genet* **30**:428, 1986.

171. Dalgleish R, Hawkins JR, Keston M: Exclusion of the $\alpha$2(I) and $\alpha$1(III) collagen genes as the mutant loci in a Marfan syndrome family. *J Med genet* **24**:148, 1987.

172. Ogilvie D, Wordsworth BP, Priestley LM, Dalgleish R, Schmidtke J, Zoll B, Sykes B: Segregation of all four major fibrillar collagen genes in the Marfan syndrome. *Am J Hum Genet* **41**:1071, 1987.

173. Francomano C, Streeten EA, Meyers DA, Pyeritz RE: Exclusion of fibrillar procollagens as causes of Marfan syndrome. *Am J Med Genet* **29**:457, 1988.

174. Kainulainen K, Savolainen A, Palotie A, Kaitila I, Rosenbloom J, Peltonen L: Marfan syndrome: Exclusion of genetic linkage to five genes coding for connective tissue components in the long arm of chromosome 2. *Hum Genet* **84**:233, 1990.

175. Hurley J: Marfan's syndrome: The nature of the aortic defect. *Aust Ann Med* **8**:45, 1959.

176. Manley G, Kent PW: Aortic mucopolysaccharides and metachromasia in dissecting aneurysm. *Br J Exp Pathol* **44**:635, 1963.

177. Bacchus H: Serum seromucoid and acid mucopolysaccharide in the Marfan syndrome. *J Lab Clin Med* **55**:221, 1960.

178. Takebayashi S, Kubota I, Takagi T: Ultrastructural and histochemical studies of vascular lesions in Marfan's syndrome, with report of 4 autopsy cases. *Acta Pathol Jpn* **23**:847, 1973.

179. Takeichi S: An autopsy case of Marfan syndrome with histochemical studies on the cardiovascular system. *Tokushima J Exp Med* **31**:33, 1984.

180. Appel A, Horwitz AL, Dorfman A: Cell-free synthesis of hyaluronic acid in Marfan syndrome. *J Biol Chem* **254**:12199, 1979.

181. Lamberg S: Stimulatory effect of exogenous hyaluronic acid distinguishes cultured fibroblasts of Marfan's disease from controls. *J Invest Dermatol* **71**:391, 1978.

182. Nakashima Y: Reduced activity of serum $\beta$-glucuronidase in Marfan syndrome. *Angiology* **37**:576, 1986.

183. Pulkkinen L, Kainulainen K, Krusius T, Makinen P, Schollin J, Gustavsson KH, Peltonen L: Deficient expression of the gene coding for decorin in a lethal form of Marfan syndrome. *J Biol Chem* **265**:17780, 1990.

184. Superti-Furga A, Raghunath M, Willems PJ: Deficiencies of fibrillin and decorin in fibroblast cultures of a patient with neonatal Marfan syndrome. *J Med Genet* **29**:875, 1992.

185. Raghunath M, Superti-Furga A, Godfrey M, Steinmann B: Decreased extracellular deposition of fibrillin and decorin in neonatal Marfan syndrome fibroblasts. *Hum Genet* **90**:511, 1993.
186. Savunen T, Aho HJ: Annulo-aortic ectasia. Light and electron microscopic changes in aortic media. *Virchows Arch A Pathol Anat Histopathol* **407**:279, 1985.
187. Nakashima Y, Shiokawa Y, Sueishi K: Alterations of elastic architecture in human aortic dissecting aneurysm. *Lab Invest* **62**:751, 1990.
188. Nakashima Y, Kurozumi T, Sueishi K, Tanaka K: Dissecting aneurysm: A clinicopathologic and histopathologic study of 111 autopsied cases. *Hum Pathol* **21**:291, 1990.
189. Trotter SE, Olsen EG: Marfan's disease and Erdheim's cystic medionecrosis. A study of their pathology. *Eur Heart J* **12**:83, 1991.
190. Turakainen H, Larjava H, Saarni H, Penttinen R: Synthesis of hyaluronic acid and collagen in skin fibroblasts cultured from patients with osteogenesis imperfecta. *Biochim Biophys Acta* **628**:388, 1980.
191. Vetter U, Fisher LW, Mintz KP, Kopp JB, Tuross N, Termine JD, Robey PG: Osteogenesis imperfecta: Changes in noncollagenous proteins in bone. *J Bone Miner Res* **6**:501, 1991.
192. Stanescu V, Stanescu R, Maroteaux P: Pathogenic mechanisms in osteochondrodysplasias. *J Bone Joint Surg [Am]* **66**:817, 1984.
193. Dyne KM, Valli M, Forlino A, Mottes M, Kresse H, Cetta G: Deficient expression of the small proteoglycan decorin in a case of severe/lethal osteogenesis imperfecta. *Am J Med Genet* **63**:161, 1996.
194. Fornieri C, Baccarani-Contri M, Quaglino D Jr, Pasquali-Ronchetti I: Lysyl oxidase activity and elastin/glycosaminoglycan interactions in growing chick and rat aortas. *J Cell Biol* **105**:1463, 1987.
195. Roark JW: The Marfan syndrome: Report of one case with autopsy, special histological study and review of the literature. *Arch Intern Med* **103**:123, 1959.
196. Kohn JL, Strauss L: Marfan's syndrome (arachnodactyly): Observation of a patient from birth until death at 18 years. *Pediatrics* **25**:872, 1960.
197. Halme T, Savunen T, Aho H, Vihersaari T, Penttinen R: Elastin and collagen in the aortic wall: changes in the Marfan syndrome and annuloaortic ectasia. *Exp Mol Pathol* **43**:1, 1985.
198. Tsuji T: Marfan syndrome: Demonstration of abnormal elastic fibers in skin. *J Cutan Pathol* **13**:144, 1986.
199. Gunja-Smith Z, Boucek RJ: Desmosines in human urine. Amounts in early development and in Marfan's syndrome. *Biochem J* **193**:915, 1981.
200. Derouette S, Hornebeck W, Loisance D, Godeau G, Cachera JP, Robert L: Studies on elastic tissue of aorta in aortic dissections and Marfan syndrome. *Pathol Biol (Paris)* **29**:539, 1981.
201. Abraham PA, Perejda AJ, Carnes WH, Uitto J: Marfan syndrome. Demonstration of abnormal elastin in aorta. *J Clin Invest* **70**:1245, 1982.
202. Perejda AJ, Abraham PA, Carnes WH, Coulson WF, Uitto J: Marfan's syndrome: Structural, biochemical, and mechanical studies of the aortic media. *J Lab Clin Med* **106**:376, 1985.
203. Rosenbloom J: Elastin: Relation of protein and gene structure to disease. *Lab Invest* **51**:605, 1984.
204. Pyeritz RE, McKusick VA: The Marfan syndrome: diagnosis and management. *N Engl J Med* **300**:772, 1979.
205. Karrer HE, Coox J: Electron microscope study of developing chick embryo aorta. *J Ultrastruct Res* **4**:420, 1961.
206. Fahrenbach WH, Sandberg LB, Cleary EG: Ultrastructural studies on early elastogenesis. *Anat Rec* **155**:563, 1966.
207. Greenlee TKJ, Ross R, Hartman JL: The fine structure of elastic fibers. *J Cell Biol* **30**:59, 1966.
208. Buddecke E, Wollensak J: [On the biochemistry of Zinn's membrane of the bovine eye.] *Z Naturforsch B* **21**:337, 1966.
209. Raviola G: The fine structure of the ciliary zonule and ciliary epithelium. With special regard to the organization and insertion of the zonular fibrils. *Invest Ophthalmol* **10**:851, 1971.
210. Streeten BW, Licari PA, Marucci AA, Dougherty RM: Immunohisto-chemical comparison of ocular zonules and the microfibrils of elastic tissue. *Invest Ophthalmol Vis Sci* **21**:130, 1981.
211. Sakai LY, Keene DR, Glanville RW, Bachinger HP: Purification and partial characterization of fibrillin, a cysteine-rich structural component of connective tissue microfibrils. *J Biol Chem* **266**:14763, 1991.
212. Tsipouras P, Del Mastro R, Sarfarazi M, Lee B, Vitale E, Child AH, Godfrey M, Devereux RB, Hewett D, Steinmann B, et al: Genetic linkage of the Marfan syndrome, ectopia lentis, and congenital contractural arachnodactyly to the fibrillin genes on chromosomes 15 and 5. The International Marfan Syndrome Collaborative Study. *N Engl J Med* **326**:905, 1992.
213. Tsipouras P, Del Mastro R, Sarfarazi M, Lee B, Vitale E, Child A, Godfrey M, Devereux R, Hewett D, Steinmann B, Viljoen D, Sykes BC, Kilkpatrick M, Ramirez F: Linkage of Marfan syndrome, dominant ectopia lentis and congenital contractural arachnodactyly to the fibrillin genes on chromosomes 15 and 5. *N Engl J Med* **326**:905, 1992.
214. Sarfarazi M, Tsipouras P, Del Mastro R, Kilpatrick M, Farndon P, Boxer M, Bridges A, Boileau C, Junien C, Hayward C, et al: A linkage map of 10 loci flanking the Marfan syndrome locus on 15q: Results of an International Consortium study. *J Med Genet* **29**:75, 1992.
215. Collod G, Babron MC, Jondeau G, Coulon M, Weissenbach J, Dubourg O, Bourdarias JP, Bonaiti-Pellie C, Junien C, Boileau C: A second locus for Marfan syndrome maps to chromosome 3p24.2-p25. *Nat Genet* **8**:264, 1994.
216. Dietz H, Francke U, Furthmayr H, Francomano C, De Paepe A, Devereux R, Ramirez F, Pyeritz R: The question of heterogeneity in Marfan syndrome. *Nat Genet* **9**:228, 1995.
217. Corson GM, Chalberg SC, Dietz HC, Charbonneau NL, Sakai LY: Fibrillin binds calcium and is coded by cDNAs that reveal a multidomain structure and alternatively spliced exons at the 5′ end. *Genomics* **17**:476, 1993.
218. Pereira L, D'Alessio M, Ramirez F, Lynch JR, Sykes B, Pangilinan T, Bonadio J: Genomic organization of the sequence coding for fibrillin, the defective gene product in Marfan syndrome. *Hum Mol Genet* **2**:961, 1993.
219. Biery NJ, Eldadah ZA, Moore CS, Stetten G, Spencer F, Dietz HC: Revised genomic organization of FBN1 and significance for regulated gene expression. *Genomics* **56**:70, 1999.
220. Yin W, Smiley E, Germiller J, Sanguineti C, Lawton T, Pereira L, Ramirez F, Bonadio J: Primary structure and developmental expression of Fbn-1, the mouse fibrillin gene. *J Biol Chem* **270**:1798, 1995.
221. Zhang H, Apfelroth SD, Hu W, Davis EC, Sanguineti C, Bonadio J, Mecham RP, Ramirez F: Structure and expression of fibrillin-2, a novel microfibrillar component preferentially located in elastic matrices. *J Cell Biol* **124**:855, 1994.
222. Milewicz DM, Grossfield J, Cao SN, Kielty C, Covitz W, Jewett T: A mutation in FBN1 disrupts profibrillin processing and results in isolated skeletal features of the Marfan syndrome. *J Clin Invest* **95**:2373, 1995.
223. Reinhardt DP, Chalberg SC, Sakai LY: The structure and function of fibrillin. *Ciba Found Symp* **192**:128, 1995.
224. Lonnqvist L, Reinhardt D, Sakai L, Peltonen L: Evidence for furin-type activity-mediated C-terminal processing of profibrillin-1 and interference in the processing by certain mutations. *Hum Mol Genet* **7**:2039, 1998.
225. Ritty TM, Broekelmann T, Tisdale C, Milewicz DM, Mecham RP: Processing of the fibrillin-1 carboxyl-terminal domain. *J Biol Chem* **274**:8933, 1999.
226. Raghunath M, Putnam EA, Ritty T, Hamstra D, Park ES, Tschodrich-Rotter M, Peters R, Rehemtulla A, Milewicz DM: Carboxy-terminal conversion of profibrillin to fibrillin at a basic site by PACE/furin-like activity required for incorporation in the matrix. *J Cell Sci* **112**:1093, 1999.
227. Trask TM, Ritty TM, Broekelmann T, Tisdale C, Mecham RP: N-terminal domains of fibrillin 1 and fibrillin 2 direct the formation of homodimers: A possible first step in microfibril assembly. *Biochem J* **340**:693, 1999.
228. Ashworth JL, Kelly V, Wilson R, Shuttleworth CA, Kielty CM: Fibrillin assembly: Dimer formation mediated by amino-terminal sequences. *J Cell Sci* **112**:3549, 1999.
229. Ashworth JL, Murphy G, Rock MJ, Sherratt MJ, Shapiro SD, Shuttleworth CA, Kielty CM: Fibrillin degradation by matrix metalloproteinases: Implications for connective tissue remodelling. *Biochem J* **340**:171, 1999.
230. Hindson VJ, Ashworth JL, Rock MJ, Cunliffe S, Shuttleworth CA, Kielty CM: Fibrillin degradation by matrix metalloproteinases: Identification of amino- and carboxy-terminal cleavage sites. *FEBS Lett* **452**:195, 1999.
231. Alexandropoulos K, Cheng G, Baltimore D: Proline-rich sequences that bind to Src homology 3 domains with individual specificities. *Proc Natl Acad Sci U S A* **92**:3110, 1995.
232. Adzhubei AA, Sternberg MJ: Conservation of polyproline II helices in homologous proteins: Implications for structure prediction by model building. *Protein Sci* **3**:2395, 1994.
233. Kielty CM, Woolley DE, Whittaker SP, Shuttleworth CA: Catabolism of intact fibrillin microfibrils by neutrophil elastase, chymotrypsin and trypsin. *FEBS Lett* **351**:85, 1994.

234. Cooke RM, Wilkinson AJ, Baron M, Pastore A, Tappin MJ, Campbell ID, Gregory H, Sheard B: The solution structure of human epidermal growth factor. *Nature* **327**:339, 1987.

235. Kielty CM, Shuttleworth CA: The role of calcium in the organization of fibrillin microfibrils. *FEBS Lett* **336**:323, 1993.

236. Rao Z, Handford P, Mayhew M, Knott V, Brownlee GG, Stuart D: The structure of a Ca(2+)-binding epidermal growth factor-like domain: its role in protein-protein interactions. *Cell* **82**:131, 1995.

237. Handford P, Downing AK, Rao Z, Hewett DR, Sykes BC, Kielty CM: The calcium binding properties and molecular organization of epidermal growth factor-like domains in human fibrillin-1. *J Biol Chem* **270**:6751, 1995.

238. Downing AK, Knott V, Werner JM, Cardy CM, Campbell ID, Handford PA: Solution structure of a pair of calcium-binding epidermal growth factor- like domains: Implications for the Marfan syndrome and other genetic disorders. *Cell* **85**:597, 1996.

239. Reinhardt DP, Mechling DE, Boswell BA, Keene DR, Sakai LY, Bachinger HP: Calcium determines the shape of fibrillin. *J Biol Chem* **272**:7368, 1997.

240. Wess TJ, Purslow PP, Sherratt MJ, Ashworth J, Shuttleworth CA, Kielty CM: Calcium determines the supramolecular organization of fibrillin-rich microfibrils. *J Cell Biol* **141**:829, 1998.

241. Cardy CM, Handford PA: Metal ion dependency of microfibrils supports a rod-like conformation for fibrillin-1 calcium-binding epidermal growth factor-like domains. *J Mol Biol* **276**:855, 1998.

242. Handford PA, Mayhew M, Baron M, Winship PR, Campbell ID, Brownlee GG: Key residues involved in calcium-binding motifs in EGF-like domains. *Nature* **351**:164, 1991.

243. Selander-Sunnerhagen M, Ullner M, Persson E, Teleman O, Stenflo J, Drakenberg T: How an epidermal growth factor (EGF)-like domain binds calcium. High resolution NMR structure of the calcium form of the NH2-terminal EGF- like domain in coagulation factor X. *J Biol Chem* **267**:19642, 1992.

244. Knott V, Downing AK, Cardy CM, Handford P: Calcium binding properties of an epidermal growth factor-like domain pair from human fibrillin-1. *J Mol Biol* **255**:22, 1996.

245. Smallridge RS, Whiteman P, Doering K, Handford PA, Downing AK: EGF-like domain calcium affinity modulated by N-terminal domain linkage in human fibrillin-1. *J Mol Biol* **286**:661, 1999.

246. Yuan X, Downing AK, Knott V, Handford PA: Solution structure of the transforming growth factor beta-binding protein-like module, a domain associated with matrix fibrils. *Embo J* **16**:6659, 1997.

247. Gleizes PE, Beavis RC, Mazzieri R, Shen B, Rifkin DB: Identification and characterization of an eight-cysteine repeat of the latent transforming growth factor-beta binding protein-1 that mediates bonding to the latent transforming growth factor-beta1. *J Biol Chem* **271**:29891, 1996.

248. Saharinen J, Taipale J, Keski-Oja J: Association of the small latent transforming growth factor-beta with an eight cysteine repeat of its binding protein LTBP-1. *Embo J* **15**:245, 1996.

249. D'Arrigo C, Burl S, Withers AP, Dobson H, Black C, Boxer M: TGF-beta1 binding protein-like modules of fibrillin-1 and -2 mediate integrin-dependent cell adhesion. *Connect Tissue Res* **37**:29, 1998.

250. Sakamoto H, Broekelmann T, Cheresh DA, Ramirez F, Rosenbloom J, Mecham RP: Cell-type specific recognition of RGD- and non-RGD-containing cell binding domains in fibrillin-1. *J Biol Chem* **271**:4916, 1996.

251. Pfaff M, Reinhardt DP, Sakai LY, Timpl R: Cell adhesion and integrin binding to recombinant human fibrillin-1. *FEBS Lett* **384**:247, 1996.

252. Glanville RW, Qian RQ, McClure DW, Maslen CL: Calcium binding, hydroxylation, and glycosylation of the precursor epidermal growth factor-like domains of fibrillin-1, the Marfan gene protein. *J Biol Chem* **269**:26630, 1994.

253. Reinhardt DP, Keene DR, Corson GM, Poschl E, Bachinger HP, Gambee JE, Sakai LY: Fibrillin-1: Organization in microfibrils and structural properties. *J Mol Biol* **258**:104, 1996.

254. Qian RQ, Glanville RW: Alignment of fibrillin molecules in elastic microfibrils is defined by transglutaminase-derived cross-links. *Biochemistry* **36**:15841, 1997.

255. Zhang H, Hu W, Ramirez F: Developmental expression of fibrillin genes suggests heterogeneity of extracellular microfibrils. *J Cell Biol* **129**:1165, 1995.

256. Brown-Augsburger P, Broekelmann T, Mecham L, Mercer R, Gibson MA, Cleary EG, Abrams WR, Rosenbloom J, Mecham RP: Microfibril-associated glycoprotein binds to the carboxyl-terminal domain of tropoelastin and is a substrate for transglutaminase. *J Biol Chem* **269**:28443, 1994.

257. Gibson MA, Kumaratilake JS, Cleary EG: Immunohistochemical and ultrastructural localization of MP78/70 (betaig-h3) in extracellular matrix of developing and mature bovine tissues. *J Histochem Cytochem* **45**:1683, 1997.

258. Reinhardt DP, Sasaki T, Dzamba BJ, Keene DR, Chu ML, Gohring W, Timpl R, Sakai LY: Fibrillin-1 and fibulin-2 interact and are colocalized in some tissues. *J Biol Chem* **271**:19489, 1996.

259. Raghunath M, Tschodrich-Rotter M, Sasaki T, Meuli M, Chu ML, Timpl R: Confocal laser scanning analysis of the association of fibulin-2 with fibrillin-1 and fibronectin define different stages of skin regeneration. *J Invest Dermatol* **112**:97, 1999.

260. Gibson MA, Hatzinikolas G, Davis EC, Baker E, Sutherland GR, Mecham RP: Bovine latent transforming growth factor beta 1-binding protein 2: Molecular cloning, identification of tissue isoforms, and immunolocalization to elastin-associated microfibrils. *Mol Cell Biol* **15**:6932, 1995.

261. Raghunath M, Unsold C, Kubitscheck U, Bruckner-Tuderman L, Peters R, Meuli M: The cutaneous microfibrillar apparatus contains latent transforming growth factor-beta binding protein-1 (LTBP-1) and is a repository for latent TGF-beta1. *J Invest Dermatol* **111**:559, 1998.

262. Nakajima Y, Miyazono K, Nakamura H: Immunolocalization of latent transforming growth factor-beta binding protein-1 (LTBP1) during mouse development: possible roles in epithelial and mesenchymal cytodifferentiation. *Cell Tissue Res* **295**:257, 1999.

263. Collod-Beroud G, Beroud C, Ades L, Black C, Boxer M, Brock DJ, Holman KJ, de Paepe A, Francke U, Grau U, Hayward C, Klein HG, Liu W, Nuytinck L, Peltonen L, Alvarez Perez AB, Rantamaki T, Junien C, Boileau C: Marfan Database (third edition): New mutations and new routines for the software. *Nucleic Acids Res* **26**:229, 1998.

264. El-Aleem AA, Karck M, Haverich A, Schmidtke J, Arslan-Kirchner M: Identification of 9 novel FBN1 mutations in German patients with Marfan syndrome. *Hum Mutat* **14**:181, 1999.

265. Liu WO, Oefner PJ, Qian C, Odom RS, Francke U: Denaturing HPLC-identified novel FBN1 mutations, polymorphisms, and sequence variants in Marfan syndrome and related connective tissue disorders. *Genet Test* **1**:237, 1999.

266. Perez AB, Pereira LV, Brunoni D, Zatz M, Passos-Bueno MR: Identification of 8 new mutations in Brazilian families with Marfan syndrome. *Hum Mutat* **13**:84, 1999.

267. Kielty CM, Shuttleworth CA: Abnormal fibrillin assembly by dermal fibroblasts from two patients with Marfan syndrome. *J Cell Biol* **124**:997, 1994.

268. Kielty CM, Phillips JE, Child AH, Pope FM, Shuttleworth CA: Fibrillin secretion and microfibril assembly by Marfan dermal fibroblasts. *Matrix Biol* **14**:191, 1994.

269. Wu YS, Bevilacqua VL, Berg JM: Fibrillin domain folding and calcium binding: Significance to Marfan syndrome. *Chem Biol* **2**:91, 1995.

270. Reinhardt DP, Ono RN, Sakai LY: Calcium stabilizes fibrillin-1 against proteolytic degradation. *J Biol Chem* **272**:1231, 1997.

271. Schrijver I, Liu W, Brenn T, Furthmayr H, Francke U: Cysteine substitutions in epidermal growth factor-like domains of fibrillin-1: Distinct effects on biochemical and clinical phenotypes. *Am J Hum Genet* **65**:1007, 1999.

272. Kainulainen K, Karttunen L, Puhakka L, Sakai L, Peltonen L: Mutations in the fibrillin gene responsible for dominant ectopia lentis and neonatal Marfan syndrome. *Nat Genet* **6**:64, 1994.

273. Wang M, Price C, Han J, Cisler J, Imaizumi K, Van Thienen MN, DePaepe A, Godfrey M: Recurrent missplicing of fibrillin exon 32 in two patients with neonatal Marfan syndrome. *Hum Mol Genet* **4**:607, 1995.

274. Nijbroek G, Sood S, McIntosh I, Francomano CA, Bull E, Pereira L, Ramirez F, Pyeritz RE, Dietz HC: Fifteen novel FBN1 mutations causing Marfan syndrome detected by heteroduplex analysis of genomic amplicons. *Am J Hum Genet* **57**:8, 1995.

275. Putnam EA, Cho M, Zinn AB, Towbin JA, Byers PH, Milewicz DM: Delineation of the Marfan phenotype associated with mutations in exons 23-32 of the FBN1 gene. *Am J Med Genet* **62**:233, 1996.

276. Liu W, Qian C, Comeau K, Brenn T, Furthmayr H, Francke U: Mutant fibrillin-1 monomers lacking EGF-like domains disrupt microfibril assembly and cause severe Marfan syndrome. *Hum Mol Genet* **5**:1581, 1996.

277. Dietz HC, McIntosh I, Sakai LY, Corson GM, Chalberg SC, Pyeritz RE, Francomano CA: Four novel FBN1 mutations: Significance for mutant transcript level and EGF-like domain calcium binding in the pathogenesis of Marfan syndrome. *Genomics* **17**:468, 1993.

278. Tynan K, Comeau K, Pearson M, Wilgenbus P, Levitt D, Gasner C, Berg MA, Miller DC, Francke U: Mutation screening of complete fibrillin-1 coding sequence: Report of five new mutations, including two in 8-cysteine domains. *Hum Mol Genet* 2:1813, 1993.

279. Hayward C, Porteous ME, Brock DJ: Identification of a novel nonsense mutation in the fibrillin gene (FBN1) using nonisotopic techniques. *Hum Mutat* 3:159, 1994.

280. Aoyama T, Tynan K, Dietz HC, Francke U, Furthmayr H: Missense mutations impair intracellular processing of fibrillin and microfibril assembly in Marfan syndrome. *Hum Mol Genet* 2:2135, 1993.

281. Aoyama T, Francke U, Dietz HC, Furthmayr H: Quantitative differences in biosynthesis and extracellular deposition of fibrillin in cultured fibroblasts distinguish five groups of Marfan syndrome patients and suggest distinct pathogenetic mechanisms. *J Clin Invest* 94:130, 1994.

282. Aoyama T, Francke U, Gasner C, Furthmayr H: Fibrillin abnormalities and prognosis in Marfan syndrome and related disorders. *Am J Med Genet* 58:169, 1995.

283. Hewett D, Lynch J, Child A, Firth H, Sykes B: Differential allelic expression of a fibrillin gene (FBN1) in patients with Marfan syndrome. *Am J Hum Genet* 55:447, 1994.

284. Montgomery RA, Geraghty MT, Bull E, Gelb BD, Johnson M, McIntosh I, Francomano CA, Dietz HC: Multiple molecular mechanisms underlying subdiagnostic variants of Marfan syndrome. *Am J Hum Genet* 63:1703, 1998.

285. Tilstra DJ, Li L, Potter KA, Womack J, Byers PH: Sequence of the coding region of the bovine fibrillin cDNA and localization to bovine chromosome 10. *Genomics* 23:480, 1994.

286. Whiteman P, Downing AK, Smallridge R, Winship PR, Handford PA: A Gly → Ser change causes defective folding in vitro of calcium-binding epidermal growth factor-like domains from factor IX and fibrillin-1. *J Biol Chem* 273:7807, 1998.

287. Hayward C, Porteous ME, Brock DJ: A novel mutation in the fibrillin gene (FBN1) in familial arachnodactyly. *Mol Cell Probes* 8:325, 1994.

288. Hayward C, Porteous ME, Brock DJ: Mutation screening of all 65 exons of the fibrillin-1 gene in 60 patients with Marfan syndrome: Report of 12 novel mutations. *Hum Mutat* 10:280, 1997.

289. Thomas JP, Pyeritz RE: Comparison of heteroduplex analysis, direct sequencing, and enzyme mismatch cleavage for detecting mutations in a large gene, FBN1. *Hum Mutat* 14:440, 1999.

290. Rosenbloom J, Abrams WR, Mecham R: Extracellular matrix 4: The elastic fiber. *FASEB J* 7:1208, 1993.

291. Putnam EA, Zhang H, Ramirez F, Milewicz DM: Fibrillin-2 (FBN2) mutations result in the Marfan-like disorder, congenital contractural arachnodactyly. *Nat Genet* 11:456, 1995.

292. Pereira L, Andrikopoulos K, Tian J, Lee SY, Keene DR, Ono R, Reinhardt DP, Sakai LY, Biery NJ, Bunton T, Dietz HC, Ramirez F: Targetting of the gene encoding fibrillin-1 recapitulates the vascular aspect of Marfan syndrome. *Nat Genet* 17:218, 1997.

293. Pereira L, Lee SY, Gayraud B, Andrikopoulos K, Shapiro SD, Bunton T, Biery NJ, Dietz HC, Sakai LY, Ramirez F: Pathogenetic sequence for aneurysm revealed in mice underexpresssing fibrillin-1. *Proc Natl Acad Sci U S A* 96:3819, 1999.

294. Takebayashi S, Taguchi T, Kawamura K, Sakata N: "Osmiophilic elastolysis" of peripheral organ arteries in patients with Marfan's syndrome. *Acta Pathol Jpn* 38:1433, 1988.

295. Davis EC: Smooth muscle cell to elastic lamina connections in developing mouse aorta. Role in aortic medial organization. *Lab Invest* 68:89, 1993.

296. Davis EC: Endothelial cell connecting filaments anchor endothelial cells to the subjacent elastic lamina in the developing aortic intima of the mouse. *Cell Tissue Res* 272:211, 1993.

297. Davis E: Immunolocalization of microfibril and microfibril-associated proteins in the subendothelial matrix of the developing mouse aorta. *J Cell Sci* 107:727, 1994.

298. Segura AM, Luna RE, Horiba K, Stetler-Stevenson W, McAllister HAJ, Willerson JT, Ferrans VJ: Immunohistochemistry of matrix metalloproteinases and their inhibitors in thoracic aortic aneurysms and aortic valves of patients with Marfan's syndrome. *Circulation* 98:II-331, 1998.

299. Milewicz DM, Duvic M: Severe neonatal Marfan syndrome resulting from a de novo 3-bp insertion into the fibrillin gene on chromosome 15. *Am J Hum Genet* 54:447, 1994.

300. Rosenquist TH, Beall AC: Elastogenic cells in the developing cardiovascular system. Smooth muscle, nonmuscle, and cardiac neural crest. *Ann N Y Acad Sci* 588:106, 1990.

301. Mariani TJ, Sandefur S, Pierce RA: Elastin in lung development. *Exp Lung Res* 23:131, 1997.

302. Li DY, Brooke B, Davis EC, Mecham RP, Sorensen LK, Boak BB, Eichwald E, Keating MT: Elastin is an essential determinant of arterial morphogenesis. *Nature* 393:276, 1998.

303. Li DY, Faury G, Taylor DG, Davis EC, Boyle WA, Mecham RP, Stenzel P, Boak B, Keating MT: Novel arterial pathology in mice and humans hemizygous for elastin. *J Clin Invest* 102:1783, 1998.

304. Dallas SL, Miyazono K, Skerry TM, Mundy GR, Bonewald LF: Dual role for the latent transforming growth factor-beta binding protein in storage of latent TGF-beta in the extracellular matrix and as a structural matrix protein. *J Cell Biol* 131:539, 1995.

305. Munger JS, Harpel JG, Gleizes PE, Mazzieri R, Nunes I, Rifkin DB: Latent transforming growth factor-beta: Structural features and mechanisms of activation. *Kidney Int* 51:1376, 1997.

306. Kanzaki T, Olofsson A, Moren A, Wernstedt C, Hellman U, Miyazono K, Claesson-Welsh L, Heldin CH: TGF-beta 1 binding protein: A component of the large latent complex of TGF-beta 1 with multiple repeat sequences. *Cell* 61:1051, 1990.

307. Munger JS, Harpel JG, Giancotti FG, Rifkin DB: Interactions between growth factors and integrins: Latent forms of transforming growth factor-beta are ligands for the integrin alphavbeta1. *Mol Biol Cell* 9:2627, 1998.

308. Munger JS, Huang X, Kawakatsu H, Griffiths MJ, Dalton SL, Wu J, Pittet JF, Kaminski N, Garat C, Matthay MA, Rifkin DB, Sheppard D: The integrin alpha v beta 6 binds and activates latent TGF beta 1:A mechanism for regulating pulmonary inflammation and fibrosis. *Cell* 96:319, 1999.

309. Hyytiainen M, Taipale J, Heldin CH, Keski-Oja J: Recombinant latent transforming growth factor beta-binding protein 2 assembles to fibroblast extracellular matrix and is susceptible to proteolytic processing and release. *J Biol Chem* 273:20669, 1998.

310. Sinha S, Nevett C, Shuttleworth CA, Kielty CM: Cellular and extracellular biology of the latent transforming growth factor-beta binding proteins. *Matrix Biol* 17:529, 1998.

311. Mii S, Ware JA, Kent KC: Transforming growth factor-beta inhibits human vascular smooth muscle cell growth and migration. *Surgery* 114:464, 1993.

312. Gadson PF Jr, Dalton ML, Patterson E, Svoboda DD, Hutchinson L, Schram D, Rosenquist TH: Differential response of mesoderm- and neural crest-derived smooth muscle to TGF-beta1:Regulation of c-myb and alpha1 (I) procollagen genes. *Exp Cell Res* 230:169, 1997.

313. Thieszen SL, Dalton M, Gadson PF, Patterson E, Rosenquist TH: Embryonic lineage of vascular smooth muscle cells determines responses to collagen matrices and integrin receptor expression. *Exp Cell Res* 227:135, 1996.

314. Topouzis S, Majesky MW: Smooth muscle lineage diversity in the chick embryo. Two types of aortic smooth muscle cell differ in growth and receptor-mediated transcriptional responses to transforming growth factor-beta. *Dev Biol* 178:430, 1996.

315. Green MC, Sweet HO, Bunker LE: Tight-skin, a new mutation of the mouse causing excessive growth of connective tissue and skeleton. *Am J Pathol* 82:493, 1976.

316. Muryoi T, Kasturi KN, Kafina MJ, Saitoh Y, Usuba O, Perlish JS, Fleischmajer R, Bona CA: Self reactive repertoire of tight skin mouse: Immunochemical and molecular characterization of anti-topoisomerase I autoantibodies. *Autoimmunity* 9:109, 1991.

317. Siracusa LD, McGrath R, Ma Q, Moskow JJ, Manne J, Christner PJ, Buchberg AM, Jimenez SA: A tandem duplication within the fibrillin 1 gene is associated with the mouse tight skin mutation. *Genome Res* 6:300, 1996.

318. Bona CA, Murai C, Casares S, Kasturi K, Nishimura H, Honjo T, Matsuda F: Structure of the mutant fibrillin-1 gene in the tight skin (Tsk) mouse. *DNA Res* 4:267, 1997.

319. Kielty CM, Raghunath M, Siracusa LD, Sherratt MJ, Peters R, Shuttleworth CA, Jimenez SA: The Tight skin mouse: Demonstration of mutant fibrillin-1 production and assembly into abnormal microfibrils. *J Cell Biol* 140:1159, 1998.

320. Saito S, Nishimura H, Brumeanu TD, Casares S, Stan AC, Honjo T, Bona CA: Characterization of mutated protein encoded by partially duplicated fibrillin-1 gene in tight skin (TSK) mice. *Mol Immunol* 36:169, 1999.

321. Murai C, Saito S, Kasturi KN, Bona CA: Spontaneous occurrence of anti-fibrillin-1 autoantibodies in tight-skin mice. *Autoimmunity* 28:151, 1998.

322. Tan FK, Arnett FC, Antohi S, Saito S, Mirarchi A, Spiera H, Sasaki T, Shoichi O, Takeuchi K, Pandy JP, Silver RM, LeRoy C, Postlethwaite

AE, Bona CA: Autoantibodies to the extracellular matrix microfibrillar protein, fibrillin-1, in patients with scleroderma and other connective tissue diseases. *J Immunol* **163**:1066, 1999.

323. Campbell JH, Tachas G, Black MJ, Cockerill G, Campbell GR: Molecular biology of vascular hypertrophy. *Basic Res Cardiol* **86**:3, 1991.
324. van Neck JW, Bloemers HP: Molecular aspects of pathological processes in the artery wall. *Mol Biol Rep* **17**:1, 1992.
325. Cowan DB, Langille BL: Cellular and molecular biology of vascular remodeling. *Curr Opin Lipidol* **7**:94, 1996.
326. Cheng TO, Barlow JB: Mitral leaflet billowing and prolapse: Its prevalence around the world. *Angiology* **40**:77, 1989.
327. Pyeritz RE: Genetics and cardiovascular disease, in Braunwald E (ed): *Heart Disease*. Philadelphia, WB Saunders, 1997, p 1650.
328. Perloff JK, Child JS, Edwards JE: New guidelines for the clinical diagnosis of mitral valve prolapse. *Am J Cardiol* **57**:1124, 1986.
329. Devereux RB, Brown WT: Genetics of mitral valve prolapse. *Prog Med Genet* **5**:139, 1983.
330. Salomon J, Shah PM, Heinle RA: Thoracic skeletal abnormalities in idiopathic mitral valve prolapse. *Am J Cardiol* **36**:32, 1975.
331. Roman MJ, Devereux RB, Kramer-Fox R, Spitzer MC: Comparison of cardiovascular and skeletal features of primary mitral valve prolapse and Marfan syndrome. *Am J Cardiol* **63**:317, 1989.
332. Kyndt F, Schott JJ, Trochu JN, Baranger F, Herbert O, Scott V, Fressinaud E, David A, Moisan JP, Bouhour JB, Le Marec H, Benichou B: Mapping of X-linked myxomatous valvular dystrophy to chromosome Xq28. *Am J Hum Genet* **62**:627, 1998.
333. Disse S, Abergel E, Berrebi A, Houot AM, Le Heuzey JY, Diebold B, Guize L, Carpentier A, Corvol P, Jeunemaitre X: Mapping of a first locus for autosomal dominant myxomatous mitral-valve prolapse to chromosome 16p11.2-p12.1. *Am J Hum Genet* **65**:1242, 1999.
334. Ramos Arroyo MA, Weaver DD, Beals RK: Congenital contractural arachnodactyly. Report of four additional families and review of literature. *Clin Genet* **27**:570, 1985.
335. Viljoen D, Ramesar R, Behari D: Beals syndrome: Clinical and molecular investigations in a kindred of Indian descent. *Clin Genet* **39**:181, 1991.
336. Anderson RA, Koch S, Camerini-Otero RD: Cardiovascular findings in congenital contractural arachnodactyly: report of an affected kindred. *Am J Med Genet* **18**:265, 1984.
337. Bell RE, Wheller JJ: Cardiac defects in a patient with congenital contractural arachnodactyly. *South Med J* **78**:742, 1985.
338. Gruber MA, Graham TP Jr, Engel E, Smith C: Marfan syndrome with contractural arachnodactyly and severe mitral regurgitation in a premature infant. *J Pediatr* **93**:80, 1978.
339. Huggon IC, Burke JP, Talbot JF: Contractural arachnodactyly with mitral regurgitation and iridodonesis. *Arch Dis Child* **65**:317, 1990.
340. Bawle E, Quigg MH: Ectopia lentis and aortic root dilatation in congenital contractural arachnodactyly. *Am J Med Genet* **42**:19, 1992.
341. Wang M, Clericuzio CL, Godfrey M: Familial occurrence of typical and severe lethal congenital contractural arachnodactyly caused by missplicing of exon 34 of fibrillin-2. *Am J Hum Genet* **59**:1027, 1996.
342. Maslen C, Babcock D, Raghunath M, Steinmann B: A rare branch-point mutation is associated with missplicing of fibrillin-2 in a large family with congenital contractural arachnodactyly. *Am J Hum Genet* **60**:1389, 1997.
343. Putnam EA, Park ES, Aalfs CM, Hennekam RC, Milewicz DM: Parental somatic and germ-line mosaicism for a FBN2 mutation and analysis of FBN2 transcript levels in dermal fibroblasts. *Am J Hum Genet* **60**:818, 1997.
344. Park ES, Putnam EA, Chitayat D, Child A, Milewicz DM: Clustering of FBN2 mutations in patients with congenital contractural arachnodactyly indicates an important role of the domains encoded by exons 24 through 34 during human development. *Am J Med Genet* **78**:350, 1998.
345. Babcock D, Gasner C, Francke U, Maslen C: A single mutation that results in an Asp to His substitution and partial exon skipping in a family with congenital contractural arachnodactyly. *Hum Genet* **103**:22, 1998.
346. Courtens W, Tjalma W, Messiaen L, Vamos E, Martin JJ, Van Bogaert E, Keersmaekers G, Meulyzer P, Wauters J: Prenatal diagnosis of a constitutional interstitial deletion of chromosome 5 (q15q13.1) presenting with features of congenital contractural arachnodactyly. *Am J Med Genet* **77**:188, 1998.
347. Jaureguy BM, Hall JG: Isolated congenital ectopia lentis with autosomal dominant inheritance. *Clin Genet* **15**:97, 1979.
348. Siemens HW: Veber die aetiologie der ectopia lentis et pupillae. *Graefes Arch Clin Exp Ophthalmol* **109**:359, 1920.
349. Edwards MJ, Challinor CJ, Colley PW, Roberts J, Partington MW, Hollway GE, Kozman HM, Mulley JC: Clinical and linkage study of a large family with simple ectopia lentis linked to FBN1. *Am J Med Genet* **53**:65, 1994.
350. Dare AJ, Veinot JP, Edwards WD, Tazelaar HD, Schaff HV: New observations on the etiology of aortic valve disease: A surgical pathologic study of 236 cases from 1990. *Hum Pathol* **24**:1330, 1993.
351. Teien D, Finley JP, Murphy DA, Lacson A, Longhi J, Gillis DA: Idiopathic dilatation of the aorta with dissection in a family without Marfan syndrome. *Acta Paediatr Scand* **80**:1246, 1991.
352. Boileau C, Jondeau G, Babron MC, Coulon M, Alexandre JA, Sakai L, Melki J, Delorme G, Dubourg O, Bonaiti-Pellie C, et al: Autosomal dominant Marfan-like connective-tissue disorder with aortic dilation and skeletal anomalies not linked to the fibrillin genes. *Am J Hum Genet* **53**:46, 1993.
353. Francke U, Berg MA, Tynan K, Brenn T, Liu W, Aoyama T, Gasner C, Miller DC, Furthmayr H: A Gly1127Ser mutation in an EGF-like domain of the fibrillin-1 gene is a risk factor for ascending aortic aneurysm and dissection. *Am J Hum Genet* **56**:1287, 1995.
354. Furthmayr H, Francke U: Ascending aortic aneurysm with or without features of Marfan syndrome and other fibrillinopathies: New insights. *Semin Thorac Cardiovasc Surg* **9**:191, 1997.
355. Hanley WB, Jones NB: Familial dissecting aortic aneurysm. A report of three cases within two generations. *Br Heart J* **29**:852, 1967.
356. Nicod P, Bloor C, Godfrey M, Hollister D, Pyeritz RE, Dittrich H, Polikar R, Peterson KL: Familial aortic dissecting aneurysm. *J Am Coll Cardiol* **13**:811, 1989.
357. Toyama M, Amano A, Kameda T: Familial aortic dissection: A report of rare family cluster. *Br Heart J* **61**:204, 1989.
358. McManus BM, Cassling RS, Soundy TJ, Wilson JE, Sears TD, Rogler WC, Buehler BA, Wolford JF, Duggan MJ, Byers PH, Fleming WH, Sanger WG: Familial aortic dissection in absence of ascending aortic aneurysms: A lethal syndrome associated with precocious systemic hypertension. *Am J Cardiovasc Pathol* **1**:55, 1986.
359. McKusick VA: Association of congenital bicuspid aortic valve and Erdheim's cystic medial necrosis. *Lancet* **1**:1026, 1972.
360. Lindsay J Jr: Coarctation of the aorta, bicuspid aortic valve and abnormal ascending aortic wall. *Am J Cardiol* **61**:182, 1988.
361. Pachulski RT, Weinberg AL, Chan KL: Aortic aneurysm in patients with functionally normal or minimally stenotic bicuspid aortic valve. *Am J Cardiol* **67**:781, 1991.
362. Clark EB, Takao A: *Developmental Cardiology: Morphogenesis and Function*. Mount Kisco, NY, Futura, 1990.
363. Gerboni S, Sabatino G, Mingarelli R, Dallapiccola B: Coarctation of the aorta, interrupted aortic arch, and hypoplastic left heart syndrome in three generations. *J Med Genet* **30**:328, 1993.
364. Denton PH, Fowlkes DM, Lord ST, Reisner HM: Hemophilia B Durham: A mutation in the first EGF-like domain of factor IX that is characterized by polymerase chain reaction. *Blood* **72**:1407, 1988.
365. Milewicz DM, Michael K, Fisher N, Coselli JS, Markello T, Biddinger A: Fibrillin-1 (FBN1) mutations in patients with thoracic aortic aneurysms. *Circulation* **94**:2708, 1996.
366. Milewicz DM, Chen H, Park ES, Petty EM, Zaghi H, Shashidhar G, Willing M, Patel V: Reduced penetrance and variable expressivity of familial thoracic aortic aneurysms/dissections. *Am J Cardiol* **82**:474, 1998.
367. Shprintzen RJ, Goldberg RB: A recurrent pattern syndrome of craniosynostosis associated with arachnodactyly and abdominal hernias. *J Craniofac Genet Dev Biol* **2**:65, 1982.
368. Furlong J, Kurczynski TW, Hennessy JR: New Marfanoid syndrome with craniosynostosis. *Am J Med Genet* **26**:599, 1987.
369. Greally MT, Carey JC, Milewicz DM, Hudgins L, Goldberg RB, Shprintzen RJ, Cousineau AJ, Smith WL Jr, Judisch GF, Hanson JW: Shprintzen-Goldberg syndrome: A clinical analysis. *Am J Med Genet* **76**:202, 1998.
370. Sood S, Eldadah ZA, Krause WL, McIntosh I, Dietz HC: Mutation in fibrillin-1 and the Marfanoid-craniosynostosis (Shprintzen-Goldberg) syndrome. *Nat Genet* **12**:209, 1996.
371. Ades LC, Morris LL, Power RG, Wilson M, Haan EA, Bateman JF, Milewicz DM, Sillence DO: Distinct skeletal abnormalities in four girls with Shprintzen-Goldberg syndrome. *Am J Med Genet* **57**:565, 1995.
372. Megarbane A, Hokayem N: Craniosynostosis and marfanoid habitus without mental retardation: Report of a third case. *Am J Med Genet* **77**:170, 1998.

373. Hewett DR, Lynch JR, Child A, Sykes BC: A new missense mutation of fibrillin in a patient with Marfan syndrome. *J Med Genet* **31**:338, 1994.

374. Wang M, Mathews KR, Imaizumi K, Beiraghi S, Blumberg B, Scheuner M, Graham JM Jr, Godfrey M: P1148A in fibrillin-1 is not a mutation anymore. *Nat Genet* **15**:12, 1997.

375. Schrijver I, Liu W, Francke U: The pathogenicity of the Pro1148Ala substitution in the FBN1 gene: Causing or predisposing to Marfan syndrome and aortic aneurysm, or clinically innocent? *Hum Genet* **99**:607, 1997.

376. Watanabe Y, Yano S, Koga Y, Yukizane S, Nishiyori A, Yoshino M, Kato H, Ogata T, Adachi M: P1148A in fibrillin-1 is not a mutation leading to Shprintzen-Goldberg syndrome. *Hum Mutat* **10**:326, 1997.

377. Dietz HC, Ramirez F, Sakai LY: Marfan's syndrome and other microfibrillar diseases. *Adv Hum Genet* **22**:153, 1994.

# Hypophosphatasia

*Michael P. Whyte*

1. Hypophosphatasia (McKusick 146300, 241500, 241510) is a metabolic bone disease that establishes a critical (but as yet undefined) role for alkaline phosphatase (ALP) in skeletal mineralization in humans. Subnormal activity of ALP in serum (hypophosphatasemia) is the biochemical hallmark and reflects a generalized deficiency of activity of the tissue-nonspecific (liver/bone/kidney) ALP isoenzyme (TNSALP). Catalysis by the tissue-specific ALP isoenzymes — intestinal, placental, and germ-cell (placental-like) ALP — is not diminished.

2. TNSALP is a zinc metalloglycoprotein that is catalytically active as a multimer of identical subunits. The bone and liver isoforms differ by post-translational modification. TNSALP is attached to the extracellular surface of plasma membranes by glycosylphosphatidylinositol linkage. The TNSALP gene is greater than 50 kb and localized on chromosome 1p36.1-34 (McKusick 171760). The tissue-specific ALP isoenzymes, perhaps including a fetal form of intestinal ALP, are encoded by a family of smaller genes on chromosome 2q34-37 (McKusick 171740, 171750, 171800, 171810).

3. Hypophosphatasia causes defective skeletal mineralization that manifests clinically as rickets in infants and children and as osteomalacia in adults. Expressivity is remarkably variable. Stillbirth can follow *in utero* disease in the perinatal ("lethal") form, which is apparent in newborns and is associated with the most severe skeletal hypomineralization and deformity. The infantile form presents as a developmental disorder by age 6 months. It can result in craniosynostosis and nephrocalcinosis from hypercalcemia and hypercalciuria and is often fatal. Premature loss of deciduous teeth, rickets, and myopathy are the cardinal clinical features of childhood hypophosphatasia. Adult hypophosphatasia typically causes recurrent metatarsal stress fractures and pseudofractures in long bones and occasionally produces arthritis from calcium pyrophosphate dihydrate (CPPD) and calcium phosphate crystal deposition. Odontohypophosphatasia refers to mildly affected individuals who have dental but no skeletal manifestations. Pseudohypophosphatasia is an extremely rare severe variant in which serum ALP activity is normal in clinical laboratory assays.

4. Three phosphocompounds (phosphoethanolamine [PEA], inorganic pyrophosphate [$PP_i$], and pyridoxal 5'-phosphate [PLP]) accumulate endogenously in hypophosphatasia and are inferred to be natural substrates for TNSALP. PLP, a cofactor form of vitamin $B_6$, collects extracellularly, but a variety of evidence shows that levels of PLP within cells are normal. This observation explains the usual absence of symptoms of deficiency or toxicity of vitamin $B_6$ in patients and indicates that TNSALP functions as an ectoenzyme. Extracellular accumulation of $PP_i$, which at low concentrations promotes calcium phosphate deposition but at high concentrations acts as an inhibitor of hydroxyapatite crystal growth, seems to account for the associated CPPD deposition, and perhaps calcific periarthritis, and the defective mineralization of bones and teeth.

5. Perinatal and infantile hypophosphatasia are transmitted as autosomal recessive traits and can be due to homozygosity or compound heterozygosity for a considerable number and variety of mutations in the TNSALP gene. Defective regulation of TNSALP gene expression or TNSALP biosynthesis may explain especially rare cases. Patients with childhood, adult, or odonto forms of hypophosphatasia can also be compound heterozygotes for TNSALP gene mutations. In some kindreds, however, mild forms of hypophosphatasia manifest with autosomal dominant inheritance. The TNSALP gene knock-out mouse is an excellent model for infantile hypophosphatasia, but prominently features lethal seizures that can be controlled with vitamin $B_6$ supplementation.

6. There is no established medical treatment. Enzyme replacement by intravenous infusion of ALP from various tissue sources has generally not been clinically helpful. Clinical and radiographic improvement occurred, despite persistent biochemical abnormalities, in the one severely affected infant treated by bone marrow and stromal cell transplantation.

7. Prenatal diagnosis of perinatal hypophosphatasia has been achieved during the second trimester with ultrasonography, radiography, and assay of ALP activity in amniocytes. During the first trimester, chorionic villus samples have been used for RFLP and TNSALP gene mutation analysis and for TNSALP activity assay. Prenatal diagnosis of the infantile form requires molecular techniques.

## BIOCHEMISTRY AND MOLECULAR BIOLOGY OF ALKALINE PHOSPHATASE

Alkaline phosphatase (ALP) (orthophosphoric-monoester phosphohydrolase, alkaline optimum, EC 3.1.3.1) is found in most plants and in all animals.[1] In humans, ALPs are encoded by at least four genes.[2–4] Three isoenzymes are expressed in a tissue-specific manner — intestinal, placental, and germ-cell (placental-like) ALP. The fourth isoenzyme is ubiquitous but abundant in liver, bone, and kidney.[2,3] Accordingly, this "liver/bone/kidney" ALP is also called tissue-nonspecific ALP (TNSALP).[3,4] There may also be a fetal intestinal ALP isoenzyme.[4] The distinctive physicochemical properties among the ALPs purified from liver, bone, and kidney are lost following digestion with glycosidases.[5]

A list of standard abbreviations is located immediately preceding the index in each volume. Additional abbreviations used in this chapter include: ALP = alkaline phosphatase; ALPL = gene mapping symbol for the TNSALP locus; CPPD = calcium pyrophosphate dihydrate; NTP-PPi-ase = nucleoside triphosphate pyrophosphatase; PEA = phosphoethanolamine; PL = pyridoxal; PLP = pyridoxal 5'-phosphate; PTH = parathyroid hormone; TmP/GFR = tubular maximum for $P_i$/glomerular filtration rate; TNSALP = tissue-nonspecific (liver/bone/kidney) ALP isoenzyme.

Thus, the various types of TNSALP constitute a family of "secondary" isoenzymes (isoforms) that differ only by posttranslational modifications involving carbohydrate residues.[6]

The TNSALP gene (McKusick 171760) is located near the end of the short arm of chromosome 1 (1p36.1-34);[7] the genes for intestinal, placental, and germ-cell ALP, and perhaps fetal intestinal ALP (McKusick 171740, 171750, 171800, 171810), are clustered near the tip of the long arm of chromosome 2 (2q34-37).[8] The human gene mapping symbol for the TNSALP locus is ALPL (ALP-liver).[4,9] Each ALP locus has been sequenced and characterized.[10-12] The TNSALP gene is more than 50 kb and contains 12 exons, 11 of which are translated to form the 507-amino-acid nascent enzyme.[3,12] The promoter region is localized within 610 nucleotides 5' to the major transcription start site.[13] TATA and Sp1 sequences appear to be important for promoter function. Basal levels of TNSALP gene expression seem to reflect inherent "housekeeping" promoter activity, whereas differential expression in various tissues may be mediated by a posttranscriptional mechanism[13] with a 5' untranslated region that differs for the bone and liver TNSALP isoforms.[14] The tissue-specific ALP genes are much smaller, primarily because of shorter introns. Amino acid profiles deduced from the human ALP cDNAs suggest 87 percent positional identity between placental and intestinal ALPs, but 50 to 60 percent identity between TNSALP and the other ALP isoenzymes.[2,3] However, the active site of TNSALP, which is encoded by six exons, reflects base sequences that have been conserved in ALPs throughout nature.[15] TNSALP seems to be the product of the ancestral gene; the tissue-specific ALP isoenzymes in man derive from a series of gene duplications.[2]

The ALPs are $Zn^{2+}$-metalloenzymes.[1,2] Catalytic activity of each isoenzyme depends on a multimeric configuration of identical subunits with molecular mass ranging from 40 to 75 kDa.[3] Each monomer has one active site and contains two $Zn^{2+}$ cations that stabilize its tertiary structure.[16] TNSALP in symmetric dimeric form has an $\alpha/\beta$ topology for each subunit with a 10-stranded $\beta$-sheet at the center.[17] Catalytic activity requires $Mg^{2+}$ as a cofactor.[1] The cDNA sequence of TNSALP predicts five potential $N$-linked glycosylation sites.[12]

N-glycosylation is necessary for enzymatic activity.[14] O-glycosylation involves the bone but not the liver form of TNSALP.[14] The ALPs are generally considered homodimeric in the circulation.[1,3] However, in tissues, ALPs may function as homotetramers attached to plasma membranes.[18]

The ALP isoenzymes have broad substrate specificity and pH optima that depend on the type and concentration of phospho-compound undergoing breakdown.[1] Hydrolytic activity cleaves phosphoesters and $PP_i$.[19] Catalysis involves phosphorylation-dephosphorylation of a serine residue; dissociation of covalently linked $P_i$ seems to be the rate limiting step. $P_i$ is a potent competitive inhibitor of ALP,[1,16] but $P_i$ may also stabilize the enzyme.[20]

Relatively little is known about the biosynthesis of ALP in higher organisms. Analysis of the human ALP gene sequences indicates that the nascent polypeptides have a short signal sequence of 17 to 21 amino acid residues[2,3] and a hydrophobic domain at their C-termini.[10-12] However, ALPs become tethered to the plasma membrane surface where they are bound to the polar head group of a phosphatidylinositol-glycan moiety and can be liberated by phosphatidylinositol-specific phospholipase.[18,21] The precise interaction with phosphatidylinositol may differ among the individual ALP isoenzymes.[21]

Although lipid-free ALP is present in plasma, the mechanism for its release from cell surfaces is poorly understood.[22] Clearance of ALP out of the circulation is presumed to occur, as for many other glycoproteins, in the liver.[23] In healthy adults, most of the ALP in serum represents approximately equal amounts of TNSALP from liver and bone tissue.[24] However, in infants and children, and particularly during the growth spurt of adolescence, blood is rich in the bone isoform of TNSALP.[1] Although some individuals (with B and O blood types and positive secretory status) increase their circulating intestinal ALP levels after a fatty meal,[1,25] the value usually represents no more than a few percent of the serum total ALP activity.[26] Placental ALP normally circulates only in women during the latter stages of pregnancy. Expression of ALP in the placenta is controlled by the fetal genome.[1] With various malignancies, however, placental ALP or germ-cell (placental-like) ALP may be detected in the blood.[2,3]

## PHYSIOLOGY OF SKELETAL FORMATION AND FUNCTION

The skeleton serves two important physiological functions. It acts throughout life as the structural framework for the body and as a metabolic reservoir for calcium, $P_i$, bicarbonate, and other ions. Skeletal development is complex and involves growth, modeling (shaping of individual bones), and remodeling (formation and resorption or "turnover" of osseous tissue).[27] Growth of bones in the extremities and elsewhere occurs by endochondral bone formation until just after puberty.[27] In healthy physes (growth plates), there is orderly proliferation, hypertrophy, and then degeneration of chondrocytes. Concurrently, deposition and then mineralization of extracellular cartilage matrix occurs (referred to as *primary spongiosa*).[27] Modeling is due to resorption of selective surfaces of individual bones as they enlarge. Remodeling is a lifelong process necessary for fracture repair and for metabolic regulation by the skeleton. Remodeling is carried out by osteoclasts and osteoblasts that are controlled by complex endocrine and paracrine systems.[27] Osteoclasts resorb the skeleton by degrading both mineral and matrix; osteoblasts synthesize bone matrix (osteoid) which subsequently mineralizes with calcium and $P_i$ deposition. Osteoclasts are abundant in acid phosphatase; chondrocytes and osteoblasts are rich in the bone isoform of TNSALP.[27]

Electron microscopy indicates that the earliest site of mineral deposition in the skeleton is within extracellular, membrane-bound structures called *matrix vesicles*.[28] Matrix vesicles were discovered as buds of chondrocyte plasmalemma, but subsequently were found in membranous and cortical bone and in fracture callus. These vesicles are rich in a variety of enzymes (including TNSALP, pyrophosphatase, and ATPase), and may contain polysaccharides, phospholipids, and glycolipids.[28] During skeletal formation, crystals of hydroxyapatite are first observed within matrix vesicles. Subsequently, these crystals grow and eventually rupture the vesicle membrane. Extravesicular crystal growth then continues and the hydroxyapatite formed is deposited into bone matrix (osteoid).[28] Accordingly, skeletal mineralization is described as *primary* (occurring in matrix vesicles until their rupture) and *secondary* (enlargement of hydroxyapatite crystals in the extracellular space).[29]

Generalized impairment of skeletal matrix mineralization in infants or children causes rickets. In adults, this disturbance manifests as osteomalacia. The principal feature that distinguishes rickets from osteomalacia is the disruption of calcification within growth plates.[27] Subnormal extracellular levels of calcium and/or $P_i$, potentially from a considerable variety of disorders (see Chaps. 165 and 197), cause nearly all forms of rickets or osteomalacia.[30] Hypophosphatasia is an interesting and instructive exception.

## PHYSIOLOGICAL ROLE OF ALKALINE PHOSPHATASE

In 1923, Robert Robison discovered that ossifying cartilage and bone from young rats and rabbits was rich in phosphatase activity. He suggested that the enzyme action conditioned skeletal mineralization by hydrolyzing some unknown phosphate ester to locally increase the concentration of free $P_i$.[31] One year later, Robison and Soames found that this catalytic reaction had a distinctly alkaline pH optimum.[32]

Soon after its discovery, however, ALP was also noted to be abundant in tissues that do not mineralize (e.g., intestine, placenta).[1] This observation challenged a role for ALP in calcification and suggested, instead, a more general purpose. Currently, the physiological roles postulated for ALP also include hydrolysis of phosphate esters to supply the nonphosphate moiety, synthesis of phosphate esters with ALP functioning as a transferase, and regulation of a variety of cellular processes in which ALP acts as a phosphoprotein phosphatase.[1] In fact, a considerable variety of hypotheses contend for how TNSALP might function in skeletal mineralization itself (Table 207-1).[33]

Robison's suggestion that ALP conditions this process by raising the concentration of $P_i$ locally was questioned in part because he did not identify the enzyme's natural substrate(s). It has been proposed that the $P_i$ donor could be nucleoside phosphate liberated by degenerating cells.[34] An important alternative hypothesis, however, suggests that ALP acts by hydrolyzing an inhibitor of mineralization.[1,33] Indeed, the discoveries that (a) $PP_i$ can impair the growth of hydroxyapatite crystals,[35] (b) ALP can function as a $PP_i$-ase,[36,37] and (c) plasma levels of $PP_i$ are increased in hypophosphatasia[38] offer a plausible candidate for this inhibitor, as well as an explanation for the major clinical feature of this enzymopathy (see below).[39] Nevertheless, it has also been suggested that ALP might act in mineralization as (a) a plasma membrane transport protein for $P_i$;[33] (b) an extracellular $Ca^{2+}$-binder that promotes calcium phosphate formation and orients hydroxyapatite crystal deposition into osteoid;[40] (c) a $Ca^{2+}/Mg^{2+}$-ATPase; or (d) a phosphoprotein phosphatase that conditions the skeletal matrix for ossification.[41] Recently, it was suggested that ALP could contribute to human aging by inducing tissue hardening and calcification.[42]

Seventy-five years after its discovery, the methods used to assay ALP activity reflect our ignorance of this enzyme's physiological function(s).[1,33,43] In both clinical and research laboratories, ALP activity is generally measured with high concentrations (mM) of artificial substrates (e.g., p-nitrophenylphosphate) in nonphysiological alkaline conditions (e.g., pH 9.2 to 10.5).[1] Such sensitive assays were developed primarily as a means to detect and follow the course of a variety of hepatobiliary and skeletal disorders by facilitating measurement of ALP activity in serum.[1] Nevertheless, the pH optimum of ALP is less alkaline for certain biochemical substrates at low concentrations, although the hydrolytic rate is reduced.[1] The potential physiological significance of this observation has been discussed.[1,33,43]

In my opinion, it is the characterization and investigation of hypophosphatasia that has provided the greatest insight into the physiological role of ALP in humans.[33,43] With identification of deactivating mutations in the TNSALP gene causing this inborn error of metabolism, there is now unequivocal evidence that TNSALP acts critically during mineralization of the skeleton and dentition in man. However, the seemingly undisturbed function of other organs/tissues in hypophosphatasia poses challenging questions about the biologic significance of TNSALP elsewhere in the body.[3,33,43]

# HYPOPHOSPHATASIA

## History

In 1948, J.C. Rathbun, a Canadian pediatrician, coined the term hypophosphatasia when he described an infant boy who developed and then died from severe rickets, weight loss, and seizures, yet whose ALP activity in serum, bone, and other tissues was paradoxically subnormal.[44] Several historical reviews mention case reports published earlier that probably depicted this condition.[45,46] In 1953, premature loss of deciduous teeth was noted to be a second major clinical feature of hypophosphatasia.[47] About 350 patients have been described in the medical literature.

Discoveries of elevated levels endogenously of three phosphocompounds (Fig. 207-1) clarified the metabolic basis for hypophosphatasia and the physiological role of TNSALP. In 1955, increased urinary concentrations of phosphoethanolamine (PEA)[48,49] pro-

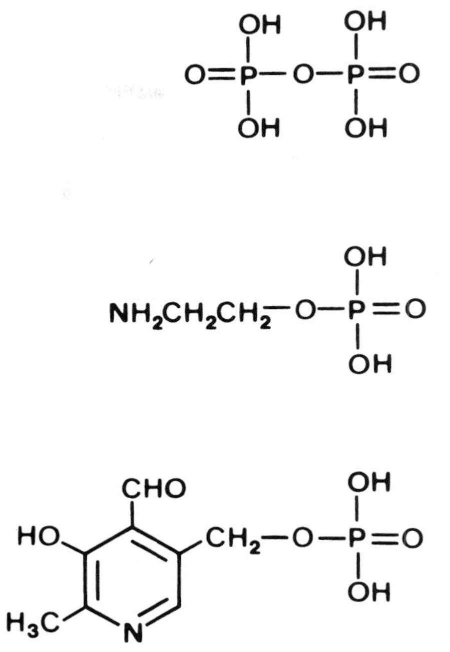

Fig. 207-1 Natural substrates for TNSALP. Three phosphocompounds appear to be natural substrates for TNSALP, because each accumulates endogenously in hypophosphatasia: inorganic pyrophosphate (PPi), phosphoethanolamine (PEA), and pyridoxal 5'-phosphate (PLP).

vided a useful biochemical marker for the disorder. In 1965 and 1971, high levels of $PP_i$ were noted in urine[50] and in blood,[38] respectively, suggesting a mechanism for the defective mineralization of hard tissues. In 1985, elevated plasma levels of pyridoxal 5'-phosphate (PLP) were found—an observation that indicated an ectoenzyme action for TNSALP[51] (see below). In 1988, the structure of the TNSALP gene was characterized[12] and the first molecular defect was discovered in hypophosphatasia.[52]

## Clinical Features

Hypophosphatasia occurs throughout the world. However, the disorder is especially prevalent in inbred Mennonite families from Manitoba, Canada, where 1 in 2500 newborns manifests severe disease and approximately 1 in 25 individuals is a carrier.[53] The incidence of severe forms in Toronto, Canada was estimated in 1957 to be 1 per 100,000 live births.[46]

Despite the presence of relatively high levels of TNSALP in bone, liver, kidney, and adrenal tissue in healthy individuals (and at least some TNSALP throughout the body), the clinical impact of hypophosphatasia predominantly disturbs the skeleton and dentition. However, the severity of expression is remarkably variable and ranges from death *in utero* to mere problems with dentition in adult life.[46,54–57] In fact, some individuals who demonstrate characteristic biochemical abnormalities may never become symptomatic.[55,56] Although hypophosphatasia generally breeds true within sibships, significantly variable clinical expression can occur in this setting as well.[55,56,58,59] Because the genetic basis for hypophosphatasia is being uncovered (see later),[15] there is promise for a molecular nosology in the future. Nevertheless, the current classification of patients for prognostication, recurrence risk estimates, and so on remains a clinical one. Several schemes have been proposed that attempt to deal with the disorder's remarkably variable expression.[46,54] Six clinical forms constitute a useful separation. The age at which lesions in bone are discovered distinguish the perinatal (lethal), infantile, childhood, and adult forms.[46,57] Patients who have only dental manifestations are regarded as having *odonto*hypophosphatasia. An especially rare variant called *pseudo*hypophosphatasia resembles infantile hypophosphatasia, except that serum ALP activity is not subnormal in the clinical laboratory (discussed below). The prognoses for these six forms of hypophosphatasia generally reflect the severity of the skeletal disease which, in turn, corresponds with the age at presentation. Usually, the younger a patient becomes symptomatic, the more severe the disorder.[33,43,46] Although this nosology is useful, there is considerable variability within each clinical form and no clear-cut separations between them.

**Perinatal (Lethal) Hypophosphatasia.** Perinatal hypophosphatasia is the most severe form. It is expressed *in utero* and can result in stillbirth. The pregnancy may be complicated by polyhydramnios. Caput membranaceum and limbs that are shortened and deformed from profound skeletal hypomineralization are noted at birth. Unusual osteochondral spurs may protrude through the skin from the midportion of the forearms and legs.[60,61] Some affected neonates live a few days, but then suffer increasing respiratory compromise from rachitic defects in the chest and from hypoplastic lungs.[62] Clinical findings also include failure to gain weight and often a high-pitched cry, irritability, periodic apnea with cyanosis and bradycardia, unexplained fever, myelophthisic anemia (perhaps from encroachment on the marrow space by excess osteoid), intracranial hemorrhage, and seizures.[54,57] Very rarely there is prolonged survival.[63]

Radiographic study of the skeleton enables perinatal hypophosphatasia to be distinguished from even the most severe types of osteogenesis imperfecta and other forms of congenital dwarfism. Indeed, the radiographic changes may be considered diagnostic.[60,61] Nevertheless, the findings can be diverse and there is marked patient-to-patient variability.[61] In some cases, the skeleton appears to be almost completely unmineralized (Fig. 207-2). In others, there is marked bony undermineralization and severe rachitic changes including irregular extensions of radiolucency into the metaphyses together with poorly ossified epiphyses. Fractures are often present. The individual membranous bones of the cranium may show calcification only at their center portions, so that the areas of unossified skull give the illusion that the cranial sutures are widely separated. However, these sutures can be functionally closed.[60] The teeth are poorly formed.[61] Other unusual features include parts of (or entire) vertebrae that appear to be missing and bony spurs that protrude laterally from the midshaft of the ulnae and fibulae.[64]

**Infantile Hypophosphatasia.** Infantile hypophosphatasia presents before 6 months of age.[46] Postnatal development often seems normal until the onset of poor feeding, inadequate weight gain, and clinical signs of rickets. The cranial sutures feel wide, but the ossification defects in the skull can cause a "functional" craniosynostosis. There may be raised intracranial pressure, with bulging of the anterior fontanel, papilledema, proptosis, mild hypertelorism, and brachycephaly. True premature fusion of the cranial sutures may occur if the patient survives infancy.[60] Blue sclerae have been reported.[65] A flail chest from rachitic deformity or rib fractures may predispose the infant to pneumonia. Hypercalcemia and hypercalciuria are common and can cause recurrent vomiting, nephrocalcinosis, and renal compromise.[46,66,67]

The radiographic features of infantile hypophosphatasia are characteristic and resemble those of the perinatal form, although they are less severe.[60] In some newly diagnosed patients, there is a seemingly abrupt transition from a normal-appearing diaphysis to a poorly calcified metaphysis. This finding is of interest because it suggests that a pathophysiological change suddenly occurred.[46] Sequential radiographic studies may disclose not only the persistent defective skeletal mineralization typical of rickets, but gradual demineralization of osseous tissue as well.[67] Skeletal scintigraphy can help demonstrate functional closure of cranial sutures, because these structures exhibit decreased tracer uptake although they appear "widened" on conventional radiography.[68]

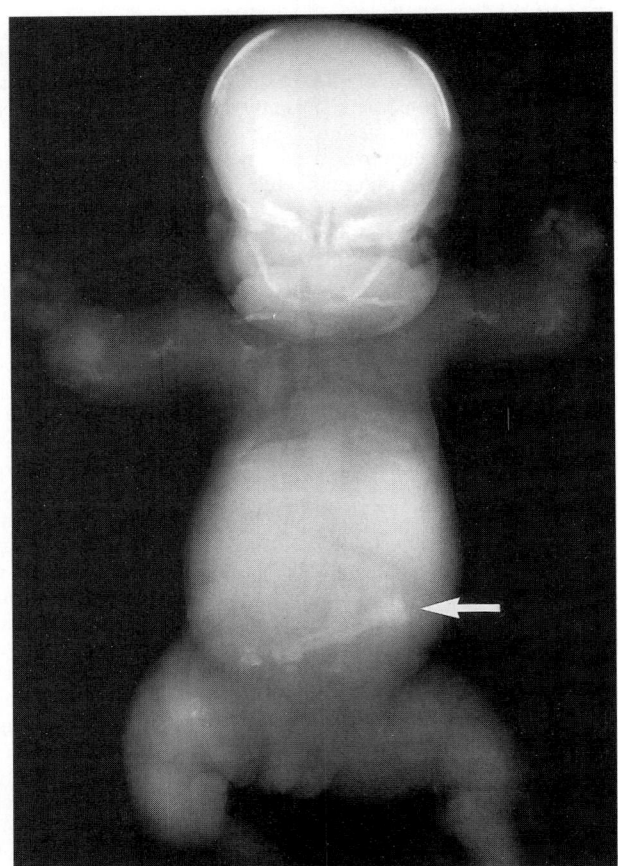

**Fig. 207-2 Perinatal hypophosphatasia. Profound hypomineralization is obvious (an umbilical clip [arrow] is more dense than the skeleton). The ends of the long bones in the upper limbs show severe rachitic change.** *Reproduced with permission from Whyte MP. Hypophosphatasia: Nature's window on alkaline phosphatase function in man, in Bilezikian J, Raisz L, Rodan G (eds.):* **Principles of Bone Biology.** *San Diego, Academic Press, p. 951, 1996.*

**Childhood Hypophosphatasia.** Childhood hypophosphatasia is also highly variable in its clinical expression.[46,62,69] Premature loss of deciduous teeth (i.e., earlier than 5 years of age) occurs with only minimal tooth root resorption because of aplasia, hypoplasia, or dysplasia of dental cementum.[70,71] Less likely, destruction of cementum has been caused by periodontal infection.[72] The lower incisors are typically lost first, and occasionally nearly the entire dentition is exfoliated. Dental radiography may show enlarged pulp chambers and root canals ("shell teeth"). Alveolar bone attrition, especially in the anterior mandible, can occur from lack of mechanical stimulation because defects in cementum prevent periodontal ligaments from properly connecting the teeth to the jaw.[73] The prognosis for the permanent dentition is generally better.[74]

In childhood hypophosphatasia, rickets often causes short stature and is associated with delayed walking and a characteristic waddling gait.[46,66] Rachitic deformities include beading of the costochondral junctions; either bowed legs or knock-knees; enlargement of the wrists, knees, and ankles from flared metaphyses; and, occasionally, a brachycephalic skull. Patients may complain of pain and stiffness, as well as isolated episodes of joint discomfort and swelling. They can have significant muscle weakness in their extremities (especially the thighs) consistent with a nonprogressive myopathy.[75]

Radiography of the metaphyses of major long bones usually reveals characteristic focal bony defects—"tongues" of radiolucency that project from growth plates into metaphyses (Fig. 207-3). This feature, if present, distinguishes hypopho-

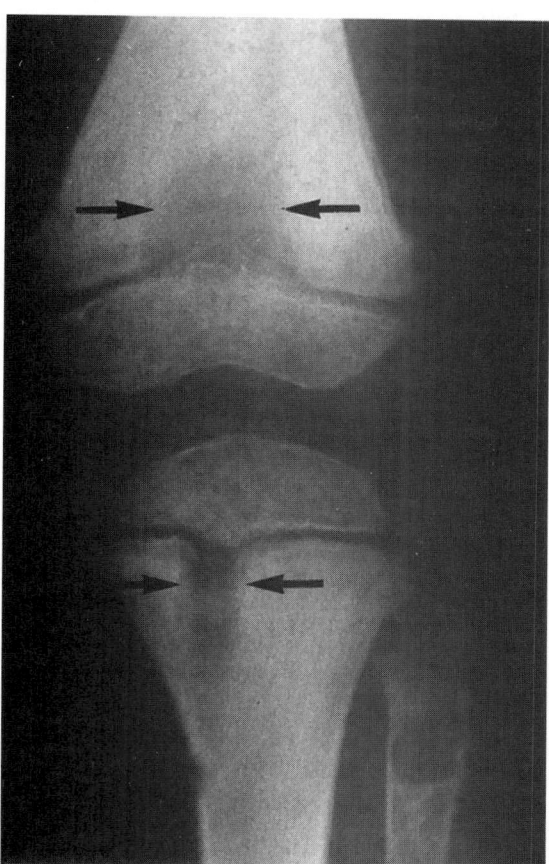

Fig. 207-3 Childhood hypophosphatasia. Posteroanterior view of the knee of a 5-year-old boy with hypophosphatasia shows growth plates that are not greatly widened, but defective endochondral bone formation is revealed by irregular radiolucencies (arrows) that project into the metaphyses. This finding is characteristic of the childhood form of hypophosphatasia.

sphatasia from other forms of rickets and metaphyseal dysplasias.[60] Epiphyseal centers of ossification may be well preserved. Functional craniosynostosis can occur in affected infants and young children despite widely "open" fontanels that are an illusion caused by hypomineralized areas of calvarium. Later, true premature bony fusion of cranial sutures may cause raised intracranial pressure, proptosis, and cerebral damage. The skull can then have a "beaten-copper" appearance.

**Adult Hypophosphatasia.** Adult hypophosphatasia usually presents during middle age.[55,56] Not infrequently, however, patients recount a history of rickets and premature loss of deciduous teeth followed by relatively good health. Subsequently, osteomalacia manifests with pain in the feet due to recurrent, poorly healing metatarsal stress fractures and discomfort in the thighs or hips due to femoral pseudofractures (Fig. 207-4). Early loss or extraction of the adult dentition is common.[55,56,76] Calcium pyrophosphate dihydrate (CPPD) deposition, occasionally with attacks of arthritis (pseudogout), troubles some patients. Others may suffer from a PP_i arthropathy. Apparently, these complications are due to increased endogenous levels of $PP_i$ (see below).[56,77] Affected individuals may also be somewhat predisposed to develop primary hyperparathyroidism (personal observation). Screening studies often reveal symptomatic or asymptomatic family members.[55,56] In some kindreds with hypophosphatasemia, there is periarticular calcium phosphate deposition that manifests clinically as "calcific periarthritis" and with ossification of ligaments (syndesmophytes) resembling spinal hyperostosis (Forestier disease).[78,79]

Radiographic study may show pseudofractures (Looser zones), a hallmark of osteomalacia. Inexplicably, these defects occur most often in the lateral cortices of the proximal femora, rather than medially as in most other types of osteomalacia.[80] There may also be osteopenia, chondrocalcinosis, features of pyrophosphate arthropathy, and perhaps calcific periarthritis.[56,78,79]

**Odontohypophosphatasia.** Odontohypophosphatasia is present when the only clinical abnormality is dental disease with radiographic and/or bone biopsy studies showing no evidence of rickets or osteomalacia. Odontohypophosphatasia may explain some cases of "early-onset periodontitis,"[81] although hereditary leukocyte abnormalities and other disorders usually account for this condition.

**Pseudohypophosphatasia.** Pseudohypophosphatasia is a particularly interesting, but especially rare, form of hypophosphatasia. The disorder was convincingly documented in two infants.[82,83] In this unusual hypophosphatasia variant, the clinical, radiographic, and biochemical findings are like those of patients who have infantile hypophosphatasia, except serum ALP activity is consistently normal or increased in assays performed in the clinical laboratory.[82,83] The enzymatic defect seems to involve a mutant TNSALP that either retains or has enhanced catalytic activity under the nonphysiological conditions of routine ALP assay procedures, but has diminished activity endogenously. As a consequence, PEA, $PP_i$, and PLP accumulate (see below).[84,85]

Some reports of pseudohypophosphatasia are not convincing[86-88] and seemingly describe individuals with hypophosphatasia for whom there had been transient normalization of serum ALP activity during fracture, illness, and so on, or, more likely,

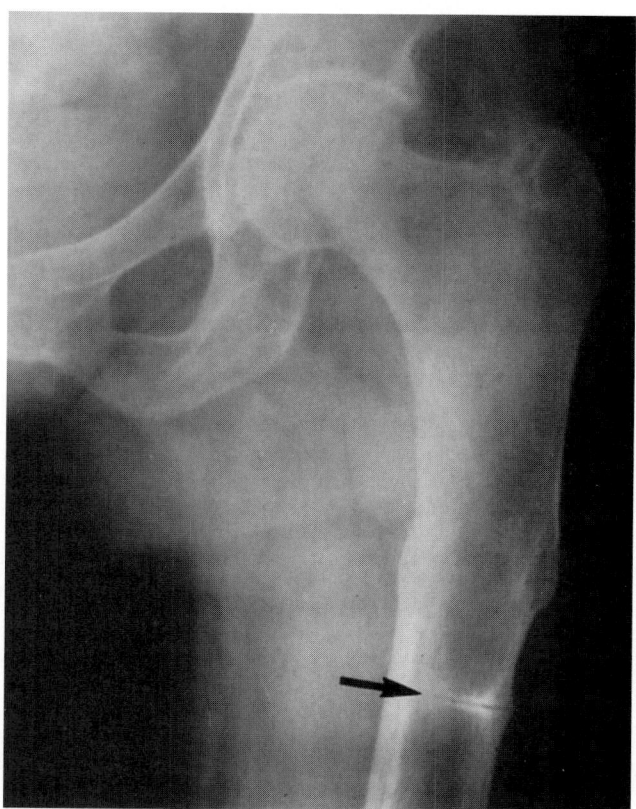

Fig. 207-4 Adult hypophosphatasia. The femur of this middle-aged woman has a pseudofracture (Looser zone) that has been unhealed for several years (arrow). These cortical bone defects characteristically form on the lateral side of the femur in adult hypophosphatasia, rather than medially as in most other forms of osteomalacia.

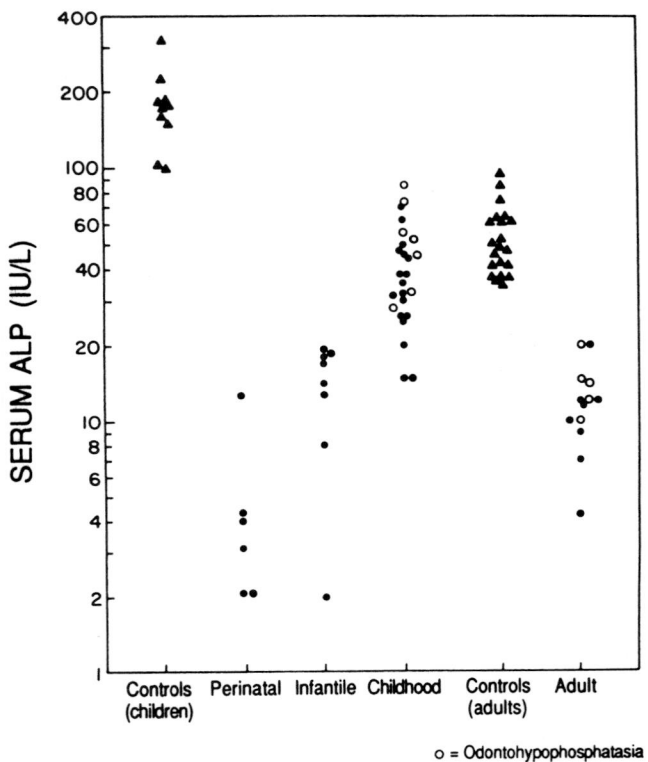

Normal Mean & Range ( ± 2 SD mean)

Children 166 (80-342)          Adults 51 (28-91)

**Fig. 207-5** Serum ALP activity in hypophosphatasia. ALP activity in serum in normal children and normal adults (▲) and in 52 patients (●, ○) from 47 families with the various clinical forms of hypophosphatasia. Note the logarithmic scale. All assays were performed at the Metabolic Research Unit, Shriners Hospital for Children, St. Louis, MO.

misinterpretation of reference ranges for serum ALP activity and/or overemphasis on the significance of a slightly elevated urinary PEA level (see below).

## Laboratory Diagnosis

**Biochemical Findings.** *ALP Activity.* Hypophosphatasia can be diagnosed with confidence when a consistent clinical history, physical findings, and radiographic changes occur with serum ALP activity that is clearly and consistently subnormal. In general, the more severe the disease the lower the serum ALP activity appropriate for age (Fig. 207-5). Even patients with odontohypophosphatasia are distinguishable from healthy individuals by their hypophosphatasemia. In the perinatal and infantile forms, hypophosphatasemia is detectable in umbilical cord blood.[66,89] In fact, in types of rickets or osteomalacia other than hypophosphatasia, serum ALP activity is typically increased.[30] Nevertheless, a variety of diagnostic pitfalls must be avoided. First, blood must be collected correctly.[90] Chelation of $Mg^{2+}$ or $Zn^{2+}$ by EDTA and other means will destroy ALP activity.[1] Second, levels of serum ALP activity must be interpreted knowing that control values vary significantly depending on age and sex; for example, infants and children have considerably higher levels (due to a relative abundance of the bone isoform of TNSALP) compared to adults. Serum ALP activity is especially high during the growth spurt of adolescence, which occurs earlier in girls than in boys.[1] Because the reference ranges cited by many clinical laboratories are, unfortunately, appropriate only for adults, some infants or

children with hypophosphatasia are mistakenly judged to have normal enzyme activity, or perhaps pseudohypophosphatasia, when the higher pediatric reference range for ALP is not provided. Third, hypophosphatasemia may occur in hypothyroidism, starvation, scurvy, severe anemia, celiac disease, Wilson disease, hypomagnesemia, or $Zn^{2+}$ deficiency and with exposure to certain drugs (glucocorticoids, chemotherapy, clofibrate, intoxication levels of vitamin D, or milk-alkali syndrome), as well as with radioactive heavy metal poisoning or massive transfusion of blood or plasma.[90,91] However, each of these clinical situations should be readily apparent. Rarely, newborns with severe osteogenesis imperfecta can have low serum ALP activity.[92] Finally, a few case reports of hypophosphatasia describe transient increases in serum ALP activity (probably the bone isoform of TNSALP) after fracture or orthopedic surgery.[55] Theoretically, conditions that increase circulating activity of any type of ALP (e.g., pregnancy, liver disease) could mask a biochemical diagnosis of hypophosphatasia.[66,93] Accordingly, in puzzling cases, documentation that serum ALP activity is low on more than one occasion during clinical stability seems advisable. Quantitation of ALP isoenzyme levels or TNSALP isoforms in serum may also be helpful. Assay of PEA, $PP_i$, and PLP levels are especially important in uncertain situations.[94]

*Minerals.* In contrast to most types of rickets or osteomalacia, neither calcium nor $P_i$ levels in serum are low in hypophosphatasia. In fact, hypercalciuria and hypercalcemia occur frequently in the infantile form of the disease.[45,54,57] In childhood hypophosphatasia, severely affected patients can have hypercalciuria but without hypercalcemia. The pathogenesis of the calcium disturbance may involve defective uptake of mineral by a poorly developing skeleton. Circulating levels of the bioactive forms of vitamin D (25-hydroxyvitamin D and 1,25-dihydroxyvitamin D) and parathyroid hormone (PTH) are usually unremarkable.[95,96] Several patients, however, reportedly had elevated serum PTH levels, but renal compromise from hypercalcemia with retention of immunoreactive PTH fragments may have been the explanation in the severe cases. Conversely, low circulating levels of PTH, possibly reflecting an abnormality in the $Ca^{2+}$-PTH feedback system, have also been described.[97]

Patients with the childhood and adult forms of hypophosphatasia have serum $P_i$ levels that are above the mean value for controls, and approximately 50 percent of patients are distinctly hyperphosphatemic. Enhanced renal reclamation of $P_i$ (increased tubular maximum for $P_i$/glomerular filtration rate; that is, TmP/GFR) accounts for this finding.[98] Conversely, especially rare hypophosphatasemic patients who are hypophosphatemic from renal $P_i$ wasting have been reported.[99,100]

*Routine Biochemical Studies.* Other standard laboratory tests, including serum parameters of liver or muscle function (e.g., bilirubin, aspartate aminotransferase, lactate dehydrogenase, creatine kinase, and aldolase), are typically unremarkable in all forms of hypophosphatasia. Increased levels of proline in blood and urine have been reported in a few patients, but the significance of this observation is not known.[101] Acid phosphatase activity in serum is generally normal,[102] but tartrate-resistant enzyme of the mononuclear/phagocyte type (band 5), possibly of osteoclast origin, has been elevated for more than a decade in the blood of one affected woman.[103]

*Phosphoethanolaminuria.* Increased urinary phosphoethanolaminuria (PEA) levels support a diagnosis of hypophosphatasia,[104] but the finding is not pathognomonic. Elevated PEA can occur in a variety of other disorders, including several metabolic bone diseases.[105] Ideally, a 24-h urine collection is assayed and PEA excretion is "normalized" to creatinine content prior to interpretation. It is important for diagnosing mild cases of hypophosphatasia to recognize that PEA levels are conditioned by age, depend on diet, follow a circadian rhythm, and have been reported

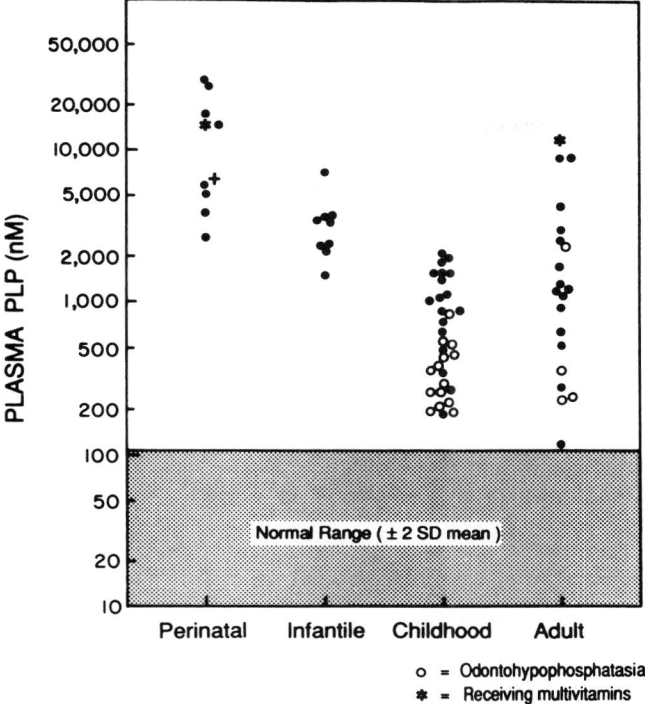

PLASMA PLP (nM)

o = Odontohypophosphatasia
✱ = Receiving multivitamins
+ = Cord blood

**Fig. 207-6 Plasma PLP levels in hypophosphatasia. PLP levels in plasma in the clinical forms of hypophosphatasia (hatched area is the normal range for children and adults). Elevated levels are present in all 71 patients (representing 60 families). In general, the plasma PLP level reflects the disease severity. Note the logarithmic scale with some overlap between the clinical forms. (Assays performed courtesy of Dr. Stephen P. Coburn, Fort Wayne State Developmental Center, Fort Wayne, IN.)**

to be normal in several mildly affected individuals.[54,106] The following reference ranges (micromoles of PEA per gram of urine creatinine) have been published: less than 15 years, 83 to 222; 15 to 30 years, 42 to 146; 31 to 41 years, 38 to 155; and over 45 years, 48 to 93.[105]

*PLP.* An increased plasma level of PLP is the most sensitive and specific TNSALP substrate marker for hypophosphatasia[51,84,107] (Fig. 207-6). Even patients with odontohypophosphatasia manifest this finding.[51] However, to exclude low-level false positive values, vitamin supplements must not be taken for 1 week before testing.[107] In general, the more severely affected the patient, the greater the elevation in the plasma PLP level. Nevertheless, overlap occurs between the clinical subtypes. Assay of plasma PLP levels after oral challenge with pyridoxine hydrochloride distinguishes patients especially well, and is helpful for identifying Canadian Mennonite carriers of severe hypophosphatasia.[108]

*PP$_i$.* Urinary PP$_i$ levels are increased in most hypophosphatasia patients,[94] but are occasionally unremarkable in mildly affected individuals.[39] Nevertheless, quantitation of urinary PP$_i$ levels has been reported to be a sensitive means for carrier detection.[109] Unfortunately, assay of PP$_i$ remains a research technique.

**Radiologic Findings.** Radiographic studies of the skeleton are diagnostic in perinatal hypophosphatasia (Fig. 207-2). In the infantile and childhood forms, characteristic abnormalities are usually demonstrated (Figs. 207-3 and 207-4) (see above). Bone scanning retains its utility for identifying fractures and may help to diagnose craniosynostosis.[68]

**Histopathologic Findings.** Abnormalities are observed primarily in the hard tissues. In severe cases, hypoplastic lungs have been found and extramedullary hematopoiesis is occasionally noted in the liver.[29,69]

*Skeleton.* In growth plates, rachitic changes are described[29,69,110] where there is disruption of the normal columnar arrangement of chondrocytes, zones of provisional calcification are widened, and areas near degenerating cartilage cells fail to calcify. However, the cellular sources of the bone isoform of TNSALP (chondrocytes and osteoblasts), as well as their matrix vesicles, are present, although with reduced levels of TNSALP activity.[29,69]

In all but the mildest cases (odontohypophosphatasia),[55] nondecalcified sections of bone reveal evidence of defective mineralization of the skeleton.[29,69,110] However, features of secondary hyperparathyroidism, which occur from hypocalcemia in most other types of rickets or osteomalacia, are generally absent. Unmineralized matrix accumulates because osteoid does not calcify properly. Cranial "sutures" that seem to be widened are not fibrous tissue, but the result of this pathologic process.[46] Impaired skeletal mineralization is confirmed when brief courses of a tetracycline are given orally prior to bone biopsy; fluorescence microscopy will fail to show characteristic fluorescent bands on bone surfaces where calcification should normally be occurring at "mineralization fronts." Some questionable cases of pseudohypophosphatasia (with normal serum ALP activity, skeletal symptoms, dental caries, elevated urinary PEA levels, and excessive amounts of osteoid in bone specimens) lack this important information from tetracycline labeling.[111] The severity of the mineralization defect in hypophosphatasia generally reflects the clinical outcome.[69] In lethal cases, even the bony structures of the middle ear can be poorly ossified.[112] Woven bone, a finding that can reflect either bone repair or defective skeletal formation, may be present.[69]

Unless histochemical studies of ALP activity are performed, the histopathologic changes of hypophosphatasia in the skeleton cannot be distinguished from most other forms of rickets or osteomalacia.[69] The numbers and morphology of osteoblasts and osteoclasts, as well as the appearance of unmineralized osteoid, vary from patient to patient. The level of ALP activity in boneÂtissue correlates inversely with the degree of osteoid accumulation.[69]

Electron microscopy of bone from cases of perinatal hypophosphatasia has shown normal distribution of proteoglycan granules, collagen fibers, and matrix vesicles in the extracellular space.[29,69] Matrix vesicles are deficient in ALP activity yet contain hydroxyapatite crystals.[110] However, in the osteoid, only isolated or tiny groups of hydroxyapatite crystals (calcospherites), frequently not associated with matrix vesicles, have been observed.[29,61,110] The significance of this observation is discussed later.

*Dentition.* Premature loss of deciduous teeth occurs in a variety of diseases (including toxicities, metabolic errors, and malignancies).[72] In hypophosphatasia, this complication is due to aplasia, hypoplasia, or dysplasia of cementum, despite the presence of cells that look like cementoblasts (Fig. 207-7).[71,74,113] The cementum may be afibrillar.[114] The magnitude of the defect varies from tooth to tooth, but generally reflects the severity of the skeletal disease. Incisors are the most vulnerable. Big pulp chambers suggest retarded dentinogenesis. Dentin tubules may be enlarged although reduced in number. The excessive width of predentin, increased amounts of interglobular dentin, and impaired calcification of cementum are analogous to the osteoidosis observed in bone. Conflicting reports concern whether the enamel is directly affected.[72,113] The histopathologic changes found in the permanent teeth seem similar, but more mild, compared to those in the deciduous teeth.[74,114] Desiccated teeth exfoliated years earlier may still be useful for microscopic examination.[115]

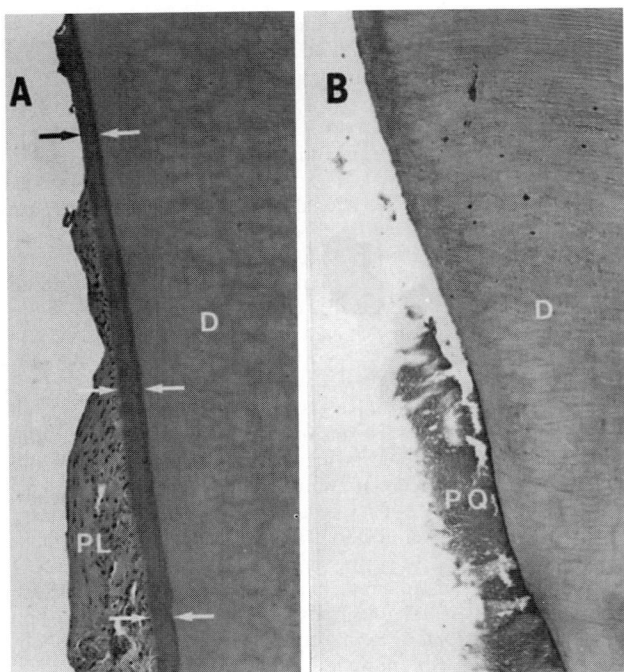

Fig. 207-7 Dental histopathology in hypophosphatasia. *A,* Decalcified section of part of the root of a maxillary incisor from a child with X-linked hypophosphatemic rickets shows primary cementum (delineated by arrows) at the tooth surface. *B,* In hypophosphatasia, cementum is absent. Magnification ×150. PL = periodontal ligament; PQ = plaque; D = dentin.

**Biochemical and Genetic Defect.** *TNSALP Deficiency.* Early on, autopsy studies of perinatal and infantile cases elucidated the enzymatic defect causing hypophosphatasia, but they also pointed to its etiology. Profound deficiency of ALP activity was documented in liver, bone, and kidney, yet ALP activity was not diminished in intestine or in placenta (fetal trophoblast).[116,117] This observation was consistent with results emerging from amino acid sequence analysis of ALPs purified from healthy human tissues,[3,33] and indicated a defect that selectively diminished the catalytic activity of all of the secondary isoforms of the TNSALP isoenzyme family.

Investigation of the cardinal biochemical feature of hypophosphatasia, hypophosphatasemia, supports the autopsy studies. There is deficient activity of both the liver and the bone isoform of TNSALP in serum.[24] However, the hypophosphatasemia does not seem to be due to enhanced clearance of TNSALP from the circulation.[55,118] The bone isoform of TNSALP (enriched in plasma from patients with Paget bone disease) and purified placental ALP have unremarkable circulating half-lives when given intravenously to severely affected infants with hypophosphatasia during attempted enzyme-replacement therapy (see below).[67] Furthermore, coincubation experiments with mixtures of serum as well as cell coculture and heterokaryon studies using fibroblasts from severely affected patients have excluded the presence of an inhibitor or the absence of an activator of TNSALP.[46,55,77,119] Instead, the hypophosphatasemia of hypophosphatasia appears to reflect failure of especially liver and bone tissue to contribute adequate amounts of TNSALP activity into the circulation. Leukocyte ALP activity, first noted to be absent in an adult with hypophosphatasia,[120] is a mixture of the TNSALP and the placental ALP isoenzymes and therefore can also be subnormal in any clinical form of the disease except perhaps pseudohypophosphatasia.[69] During pregnancy in hypophosphatasia, low levels of leukocyte ALP activity may correct due to increased placental ALP isoenzyme activity.[121]

In hypophosphatasia tissue specimens, preliminary observations using a polyclonal antibody to the liver isoform of TNSALP suggested the presence of normal amounts of enzyme protein.[122,123] However, a monoclonal antibody-based immunoassay demonstrated low levels of bone and liver TNSALP isoforms in the serum of patients with all clinical forms of hypophosphatasia except pseudohypophosphatasia.[124] This immunoassay measured dimeric TNSALP.[124] Accordingly, disruption of the immunoreactivity, and perhaps the tertiary structure of TNSALP, may occur after its release from cell surfaces in hypophosphatasia patients.[124]

In infants with hypophosphatasia, some ALP activity is detectable by sensitive methods in liver, bone, and kidney tissue and in skin fibroblasts in culture.[125,126] The ALP in the fibroblasts has different physicochemical properties when compared with the enzyme in normal cells.[125] In one case of infantile hypophosphatasia, catalytic inhibition and isoelectric focusing studies suggested that the residual ALP activity was intestinal ALP,[117] perhaps reflecting compensatory expression of an intestinal ALP gene. Indeed, studies of homogenates of small bowel mucosa from a family with a clinically mild childhood/adult form of hypophosphatasia,[127] and autopsy tissue from severely affected patients,[126] showed increased amounts of intestinal ALP. However, fibroblasts in culture from severely affected patients seem to produce low ALP activity with physicochemical properties that are TNSALP-like.[125] Nevertheless, the physicochemical and immunologic properties differ from patient to patient.[128] Accordingly, the effect of TNSALP gene mutations (see below) on circulating, as well as tissue, ALP requires further investigation.

Autopsy studies of children or adults with hypophosphatasia have not been reported. However, these nonlethal subtypes also seem to feature globally diminished TNSALP activity within tissues. TNSALP isoform activity can be deficient in serum,[24] circulating granulocytes,[69] bone,[69] and cultivated skin fibroblasts.[129] TNSALP isoform immunoreactivity in serum is also reduced in these patients.[124]

*Inheritance.* The first evidence that hypophosphatasia was a heritable disorder came when affected sibs were reported in 1950.[130] Early on, family studies of severe disease in infants or children indicated autosomal recessive inheritance. The parents of such patients often had low or low-normal levels of serum ALP activity, and PEA was detectable in their urine.[45,46] Furthermore, consanguinity was reported in some kindreds.

The inheritance pattern for the milder forms of hypophosphatasia is, however, less clear. In some reports, childhood and adult hypophosphatasia, as well as odontohypophosphatasia, are regarded as autosomal recessive conditions.[131-133] Indeed, vertical transmission of clinically apparent disease seems to be unusual.[55,56] Nevertheless, multigenerational occurrence of clinical and biochemical abnormalities of hypophosphatasia suggests that mild disease can be transmitted as an autosomal dominant trait.[55,56,74,134-136] Family studies rarely show mildly affected individuals with severe disease in their offspring.[55,136,137]

Identification of carriers for hypophosphatasia is difficult, necessitating quantitation of several biochemical markers, including urinary PP$_i$.[138] Pyridoxine loading followed by assay of plasma PLP levels is especially helpful in heterozygote detection, particularly among the Mennonite population in Canada.[108]

*Gene Defects.* Chromosomal defects have rarely been reported in hypophosphatasia. A common D/D translocation was found in 1970 in one adult patient, but it was not present in other affected family members, and was therefore presumed coincidental.[77]

Phenylketonuria was described in one infant with hypophosphatasemia, phosphoethanolaminuria, and generalized skeletal demineralization.[139] Morquio syndrome together with hypophosphatasia has occurred in a Canadian Hutterite kindred.[140] These patients, however, appear to reflect the coincidence of two autosomal recessive conditions.[140]

CHAPTER 207 / HYPOPHOSPHATASIA **5321**

In 1984, a preliminary report using skin fibroblast heterokaryons deficient in ALP activity from patients representing 10 families with perinatal or infantile hypophosphatasia described absence of complementation.[119] This observation indicated a molecular defect involving one gene locus.[119]

In 1987, genetic linkage of the Rh blood group in six inbred Mennonite kindreds from Manitoba, Canada, provided evidence that the "candidate" TNSALP gene was involved in severe hypophosphatasia in this population.[141]

In 1988, characterization of the gene encoding the TNSALP[12] isoenzyme provided the background for significant advances in our understanding of the genetic basis for hypophosphatasia.[12,142] That same year, a missense mutation of the TNSALP gene was discovered in an infant with perinatal hypophosphatasia born to second cousins in Nova Scotia.[52] The patient was homozygous and both parents carriers of a single base-transition that caused a threonine-for-alanine substitution at amino acid position 162. Site-directed mutagenesis and transfection analysis of the patient's TNSALP gene defect confirmed that the mutation diminished the enzyme's catalytic activity. Three-dimensional structure information concerning *Escherichia coli* ALP by x-ray crystallography[16] suggested that the base change compromised the spatial relationship of metal ligands to an important arginine residue at the catalytic pocket.[50] Later, this defect was shown to impair transport of the mutated enzyme leading to its intracellular aggregation.[143]

In 1992, sequence analysis of the TNSALP cDNAs of four additional unrelated patients with perinatal or infantile hypophosphatasia revealed a different missense mutation in each of the eight TNSALP alleles examined.[142] Screening of 50 unrelated patients with all clinical forms of hypophosphatasia disclosed 23 individuals with one of these defects, but in whom the nature of the other TNSALP allele was not known. Of interest, however, two sibs with typical childhood hypophosphatasia and one unrelated elderly woman with classic adult hypophosphatasia were found to be compound heterozygotes for the identical TNSALP missense mutations. This observation showed that childhood and adult hypophosphatasia can be the same disorder and can be transmitted as an autosomal recessive trait.[142] Each of these 9 TNSALP missense mutations altered an amino acid residue that is shared in mammalian TNSALPs.[15] Indeed, several of these amino acid residues are conserved even among bacteria. The three-dimensional structure of *E. coli* ALP[15,16] suggests that some of the base substitutions would disturb metal ligand-binding in the mature enzyme, but how the other mutations are deleterious was not fully understood.[15]

In 1993, homozygosity for a tenth TNSALP missense mutation was found to account for severe hypophosphatasia prevalent in Canadian Mennonites, presumably explained by a founder effect and inbreeding.[53]

In 1998, 18 TNSALP gene mutations were reported in 26 distinct chromosomes carrying a possible mutation in the TNSALP gene in 13 European families with the perinatal, infantile, or childhood form of hypophosphatasia; 15 were novel, and most were missense mutations.[144] In this study, 24 of 26 alleles had a mutation responsible for severe hypophosphatasia. In two patients, only one mutation was found, which was consistent with a possible dominant effect and a functional role for polymorphisms in the TNSALP gene.[144,145] Computer-assisted modeling of the mutated proteins did not show any obvious modification in the predicted enzyme structure except for mutation R206W that could abolish a turn between two $\beta$-sheets.[144] To date, 58 different defects have been reported in the TNSALP gene in hypophosphatasia patients,[145a] including missense, nonsense, donor splice-site, and frame-shift deletions.[52,53,63,142–151] All principal clinical forms of hypophosphatasia (perhaps also including pseudohypophosphatasia) can involve TNSALP mutations. Molecular studies from Japan suggest that even odontohypophosphatasia can be inherited as an autosomal recessive trait.[152] Genetic diagnosis of hypophosphatasia requires extensive analysis of the TNSALP gene worldwide in outbred populations.[142,144,145]

Especially rare cases of hypophosphatasia, however, may be due to a regulatory defect in the biosynthesis of TNSALP. In one boy with the infantile form, a series of IV infusions of pooled normal plasma in attempted enzyme replacement therapy was followed by a 4-month correction of hypophosphatasemia due to skeletal synthesis of the bone isoform of TNSALP.[153] Remarkable transient remineralization of osseous tissue occurred during this time. The observation could not be attributed to the infused ALP, which had a circulating half-life of just several days.[153]

Regulation of TNSALP biosynthesis may affect disease expression in other ways. Patients with the childhood form of hypophosphatasia usually have higher absolute levels of ALP activity than adult-onset cases (Fig. 207-5). Physiological decreases in individual serum (skeletal) ALP levels during the adult years possibly engender clinical reexpression of the condition. However, the degree of hypophosphatasemia (relative to the serum ALP level that is appropriate for age) is similar in affected children and adults and perhaps helps to explain the "overlap" in defining these two clinical forms of hypophosphatasia.

Recent transfection studies indicate that some TNSALP gene mutations inactivate the enzyme and lead to its intracellular accumulation.[143,144,152] Other defects may diminish expression of the mutated allele or mRNA stability.[63]

**Prognosis.** Perinatal (lethal) hypophosphatasia is almost always a fatal condition. Rarely, prolonged survival occurs.[63] Infantile hypophosphatasia has an unpredictable outcome when first diagnosed. In some patients, there is progressive skeletal deterioration;[67] in others, there is significant spontaneous improvement.[154] Sequential radiographic studies are critical for prognostication. Approximately 50 percent of these patients die from respiratory compromise and pneumonia that follow worsening skeletal disease in the chest.[46] The prognosis seems to improve after infancy. Indeed, a preliminary report from Canada suggests that in their patient population, the adult stature of survivors of infantile hypophosphatasia may be normal (although I am aware of significant exceptions in the United States). Childhood hypophosphatasia may also spontaneously improve during adolescence,[46] but recurrence of symptoms in adult life is possible, if not likely.[46,55,155] Adult hypophosphatasia causes chronic orthopedic problems after the onset of skeletal symptomatology.[46,55,80,155] Worsening osteomalacia, leading to osteopenia and fractures, can occur in affected women at menopause, and was not prevented by estrogen replacement therapy in two patients (personal observation).

**Treatment.** *Medical.* There is no established medical therapy for hypophosphatasia, although a variety of treatments have been studied.[46,55,153,156,157] Assessment of any regimen is made difficult by the uncertain clinical course of many affected individuals, some of whom improve spontaneously on radiographic study.

Traditional therapies for rickets and osteomalacia (vitamin D and mineral supplements) should be avoided, unless clear-cut deficiencies are documented, because circulating levels of calcium, $P_i$, and the vitamin D metabolites are not low. Indeed, in infantile cases, excess vitamin D could augment intestinal absorption of calcium without enhancing skeletal formation and thus cause or exacerbate hypercalcemia and hypercalciuria. However, complete restriction of vitamin D intake or exposure to sunshine should be guarded against, because superimposed vitamin D-deficiency rickets has occurred.[96] Hypercalcemia in infantile hypophosphatasia can be improved by lowering dietary calcium intake and/or with glucocorticoid therapy,[60,67] but progressive skeletal demineralization may follow.[67,155,156,158] Synthetic calcitonin treatment to control hypercalcemia and to block mineral loss may be beneficial.[159]

In theory, therapy with agents that could stimulate TNSALP biosynthesis or enhance its activity might be helpful for hypophosphatasia. Administration of cortisone to a few patients with severe disease was reportedly followed by periods of normalization of serum ALP activity and radiographic improvement,[46,156,160] but this has not been a consistent finding.[46] Brief treatments with zinc, magnesium, and an active fragment of PTH to stimulate ALP activity or synthesis have been unsuccessful.[55,153] In other metabolic bone diseases, sodium fluoride enhances osteoblast function and increases the activity of the bone form of TNSALP in serum.[161] However, an excessive amount of fluoride can itself impair skeletal mineralization and bone quality, and fluoride has not been rigorously tested in hypophosphatasia.

If extracellular accumulation of $PP_i$ is a key pathogenetic factor in hypophosphatasia (see below), reduction in endogenous $PP_i$ levels might enable skeletal mineralization to proceed normally.[33,39] In 1968, an attempt to achieve this outcome using oral $P_i$ supplementation to promote renal $PP_i$ excretion reportedly met with some radiographic success.[162] However, in subsequent studies, plasma $PP_i$ levels were found to be essentially unchanged by this treatment. In fact, increased urinary $PP_i$ levels after $P_i$ is administered orally may merely reflect enhanced renal $PP_i$ synthesis.[33,39] This therapeutic approach has been repeated, but its efficacy has not been confirmed.[50,116]

Enzyme replacement therapy for hypophosphatasia has been attempted by IV infusion of several types of ALP given to patients with the infantile form of the disease. The results generally have been disappointing. Serum from an individual with Paget bone disease given to one affected infant was associated with some radiographic improvement.[67,163] However, subsequent trials of this therapy for four patients showed no significant clinical or radiographic benefit, and their disease proved fatal.[156] Weekly intravenous infusions of fresh plasma were followed by clinical and some radiographic improvement in one patient.[164] Also, infusions of plasma from several normal individuals, which had been frozen and then pooled, were followed by transient correction of hypophosphatasemia and marked temporary clinical, radiographic, and histologic improvement in one severely affected boy (see above).[153] However, it may be that he had a unique defect in TNSALP gene regulation or TNSALP biosynthesis. Indeed, a subsequent trial of pooled plasma infusions in a different patient did not reproduce this response.[126] Recently, after a brief report that suggested that IV administration of ALP purified from liver improved the histologic appearance of bone and decreased urinary PEA levels in one patient,[165] a vigorous therapeutic attempt was conducted with IV infusion of purified placental ALP. In a study of pregnant women who were carriers for hypophosphatasia, placental ALP was shown to be catalytically active toward PEA, $PP_i$, and PLP.[166] Infusions of placental ALP caused hyperphosphatasemia, but resulted in only modest decrements of plasma PLP and urinary PEA concentrations, and no change in urinary $PP_i$ levels. Furthermore, there was no clinical or radiographic improvement for lethal disease.[167] These cumulative observations may reflect the fact that the amount of ALP in the body is much greater than levels achieved in the circulation by these treatments. Alternatively, they are consistent with a requirement for ALP to be present on cell surfaces, particularly in the skeleton, to act therapeutically.[167] In this regard, it is notable that the extreme skeletal disease characterizing perinatal hypophosphatasia occurs *in utero* in an environment that is not protective. Preliminary findings in the TNSALP gene knock-out mouse,[168] and in one patient with infantile hypophosphatasia,[169] indicate that bone marrow transplantation could be beneficial.

*Supportive.* Infants and young children with hypophosphatasia should be followed carefully for increased intracranial pressure from either "functional" or "true" premature craniosynostosis. As discussed, functional synostosis (that may require craniotomy) can occur despite the radiographic illusion of widely open fontanels.[60] Fractures in children do mend, although delayed healing after femoral osteotomy with casting has been reported.[170] In adult patients, pseudofractures may remain unchanged for years, but will not heal unless they progress to completion, or are treated orthopedically.[55] Use of intramedullary rods rather than load-sparing devices, such as plates, seems best for the prophylactic or acute surgical management of femoral fractures and pseudofractures.[80] For recurrent metatarsal stress fractures, ankle-foot orthoses are useful.

Expert dental care is especially important for affected children. Severely involved dentition can impair nutrition, and efforts to preserve teeth in position or use of complete or partial dentures may be necessary.[70,71] One study indicates that proliferation of bacteria on the tooth surface, perhaps related to deficiency of TNSALP activity in leukocytes, may contribute to loss of dentition.[114]

Symptoms from CPPD or calcium phosphate crystal deposition may respond to nonsteroidal anti-inflammatory medication.[78]

**Prenatal Diagnosis.** Assay of ALP activity in amniotic fluid is not helpful.[171] At 14 to 18 weeks of gestation, most is intestinal ALP excreted from the fetus.[172] Measurement of $\alpha$-fetoprotein in amniotic fluid, however, can help to differentiate anencephaly from severe hypophosphatasia.

The perinatal (lethal) form of hypophosphatasia has been diagnosed *in utero*.[79] During the first trimester, chorionic villus samples from 15 pregnancies were assessed utilizing a monoclonal antibody-based assay specific for TNSALP.[173,174] A precisely timed and carefully prepared specimen is required.[173,175] RFLP analysis, using a chorionic villus sample, was used successfully for a Canadian Mennonite[176] and for a Japanese family.[177] During the second trimester, perinatal hypophosphatasia has been diagnosed with ultrasonography (with attention to the limbs as well as the skull),[178] radiographic study of the fetus, and assay of ALP activity in amniotic fluid cells by an experienced laboratory.[179] An ultrasound study, however, was judged to be normal at 16 to 19 weeks of gestation in 3 cases of perinatal hypophosphatasia in which radiographic study at 38 weeks of gestation showed absence of a fetal skeleton.[180,181] Combined use of radiologic techniques, including serial ultrasonography, seems to be best. The utility of assaying cord blood ALP is untested. TNSALP gene mutation information has been used successfully to evaluate pregnancies at risk for lethal disease.[144,182,183]

Mild forms of hypophosphatasia have not been diagnosed prenatally. I am aware of two such children who reportedly had normal ultrasonography in early pregnancy. Conversely, severe bowing of the lower extremities detected by ultrasound, suggestive of a potentially lethal form of skeletal dysplasia, occurred in four pregnancies in three families in whom the deformity corrected spontaneously postnatally and the clinical phenotype otherwise was childhood hypophosphatasia.[184,185]

**Mouse Model for Hypophosphatasia.** In 1995 and 1997, two independent laboratories reported use of homologous recombination to inactivate the equivalent of the TNSALP gene in mice.[186,187]

Although there were some minor phenotypic differences, perhaps explained by the background strains,[188] the animals developed skeletal disease that resembled a form of rickets and had endogenous accumulation of PEA, $PP_i$, and PLP.[188] Homozygous knock-out mice had unremarkable skeletons at birth, suggesting *in utero* protection or redundant or back-up mechanisms for skeletal development.[186–188] A striking feature was seizures apparently due to low extracellular and tissue levels of PL leading to decreased gamma-aminobutyric acid in the brain.[186] Parenteral administration of vitamin $B_6$ was necessary to keep the animals alive. Subsequent investigation showed that the mice were an excellent model for infantile hypophosphaturia with postnatal development of defective skeletal mineralization, endogenous accumulation of PEA, $PP_i$, and PLP and, interestingly, a disturbance in epiphyseal and physeal chondrocyte development.[188]

## PHYSIOLOGICAL ROLE OF TISSUE-NONSPECIFIC ALKALINE PHOSPHATASE EXPLORED IN HYPOPHOSPHATASIA

Discovery in 1988 that mutation within the TNSALP gene can deactivate the enzyme and cause hypophosphatasia[52] proved that Robert Robison was correct.[31,32] ALP does, indeed, function critically in calcification of the skeleton (also in formation of the teeth).[33,43] The process of "secondary mineralization" of cartilage and bone seems to be the primary site of the disturbance. Hydroxyapatite crystals are found in matrix vesicles, but are deficient nearby in skeletal tissue.[29] The defects in teeth seem to be analogous to those in the skeleton.[73]

Although the liver, kidneys, and adrenals are normally rich in TNSALP activity,[1] these organs do not seem to be dysfunctional in hypophosphatasia. Notably, however, two Japanese siblings with infantile hypophosphatasia died with sudden unexplained liver failure as teenagers.[148] It has been suggested that TNSALP deficiency might diminish biosynthesis of the phospholipid surfactant and cause pulmonary atelectasis in hypophosphatasia,[66] but the respiratory problems of severely affected patients likely reflect thoracic deformity, rib fractures, and hypoplastic lungs. A variety of studies suggest that TNSALP may function in cell growth and differentiation; however, TNSALP-deficient infantile hypophosphatasia dermal fibroblasts have been shown to proliferate normally in culture.[189] Accordingly, TNSALP in humans may have little physiological importance except for formation of hard tissues.[33,43]

Two-dimensional gel electrophoresis shows that hypophosphatasia fibroblasts profoundly deficient in TNSALP activity have unremarkable profiles of plasma membrane-associated phosphoproteins.[190] This observation suggests that TNSALP does not act as a phosphoprotein phosphatase on the plasmalemma. Instead, ALPs are now being investigated for amino acid sequence domains that predict binding to other proteins (including types I, II, and X collagen), perhaps to orient TNSALP in skeletal matrix for mineral deposition.[191]

Several roles for TNSALP in calcification have been proposed that could be deranged in hypophosphatasia (see Table 207-1). As reviewed below, the discovery that PEA, PLP, and PP$_i$ accumulate endogenously, and are inferred therefore to be natural substrates for TNSALP, has been important for understanding the physiological role of TNSALP.

### Phosphoethanolamine

The discovery in 1955 that urinary PEA levels are increased in hypophosphatasia provided both a useful biochemical marker for this inborn error of metabolism and the first evidence from this disorder for a natural substrate for TNSALP.[48,49,104] Detailed studies of renal handling of PEA in healthy subjects showed that this phosphocompound is excreted when plasma levels are scarcely detectable; that is, essentially no renal threshold exists for PEA.[104] Although its metabolic origin is unclear, PEA is thought not to be a derivative of phosphatidylethanolamine — that is, not from plasma membrane phospholipid breakdown. PEA is now recognized to be a constituent of the phosphatidylinositol-glycan linkage apparatus. Accordingly, extracellular PEA could

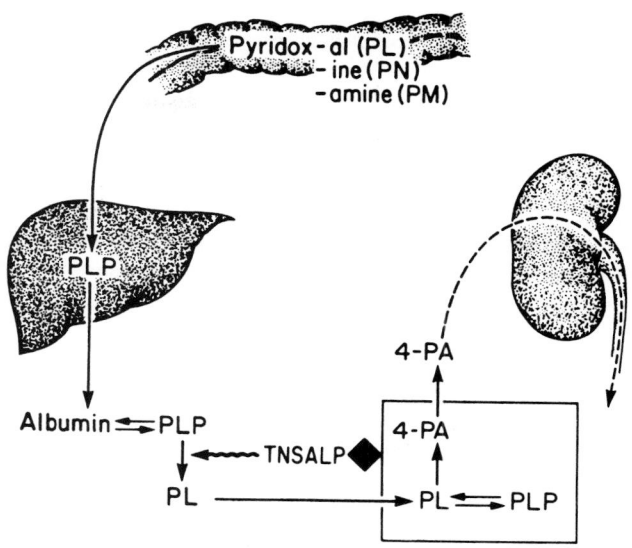

**Fig. 207-8** Role of TNSALP in vitamin $B_6$ metabolism. The various vitameric forms of vitamin $B_6$ in the diet are dephosphorylated in the gut and then absorbed into the hepatic portal circulation. In the liver, they are each converted to PLP, which is secreted bound to albumin into the plasma. Before entering tissues, plasma PLP must be dephosphorylated to PL, which can traverse membranes. 4-Pyridoxic acid (4-PA), the major degradation product of vitamin $B_6$, is excreted in the urine. High plasma levels of PLP in hypophosphatasia, yet normal plasma concentrations of pyridoxal (PL), are consistent with an ectoenzyme role for TNSALP in the extracellular dephosphorylation of PLP to PL.

derive from the degradation of these anchors of cell-surface proteins. In one family with adult hypophosphatasia,[24] urinary levels of PEA were found to correlate inversely with the activity in serum of the liver (but not the bone) isoform of TNSALP. In fact, the major source of circulating PEA reportedly is the liver,[192] which metabolizes PEA to ammonia, acetaldehyde, and P$_i$ in a reaction that is catalyzed by O-phosphorylethanolamine phosphorylase. This enzyme requires PLP as a cofactor and it has been proposed that pseudohypophosphatasia might result from its deficiency.[192]

### Pyridoxal 5'-Phosphate

Discovery in 1985 that plasma levels of PLP are increased in hypophosphatasia helped significantly to clarify the physiological role of TNSALP.[51] As reviewed in Fig. 207-8, the variety of dietary forms of vitamin $B_6$ (including pyridoxine, pyridoxal, and pyridoxamine and their phosphorylated derivatives) are converted in the liver[193] to PLP, a cofactor form of vitamin $B_6$. Organ ablation studies show that hepatic tissue is the major source of PLP in plasma. Apparently, PLP is secreted from the liver into the circulation primarily coupled to albumin.[193] A minor fraction of PLP in plasma is bound to various enzymes. Only a small amount of PLP circulates freely. Like many phosphorylated compounds, however, PLP cannot traverse plasma membranes and must first be dephosphorylated to pyridoxal (PL) before PL can enter cells. Once PL crosses plasma membranes, it is rephosphorylated to PLP or converted to pyridoxamine 5'-phosphate, which both act intracellularly as cofactors for many enzymatic reactions. Ultimately, vitamin $B_6$ is degraded to 4-pyridoxic acid, primarily in the liver, and is then excreted in the urine.[193]

Increases in plasma levels of PLP in hypophosphatasia suggest that TNSALP acts importantly in the extracellular dephosphorylation of PLP.[51,107] In fact, when serum levels of the bone or the liver TNSALP isoforms are increased by other skeletal or hepatic diseases, plasma PLP levels are decreased.[107,194] The increased

**Table 207-1** Suggested Roles for ALP in Skeletal Mineralization[202]

1. Locally increase P$_i$ levels
2. Destruction of inhibitor of hydroxyapatite crystal growth
3. Transport of P$_i$
4. Ca$^{2+}$-binding protein
5. Ca$^{2+}$/Mg$^{2+}$ATPase
6. Tyrosine-specific phosphoprotein phosphatase

plasma levels of PLP in hypophosphatasia seem to result from failure of PLP hydrolysis rather than excessive PLP production. Accordingly, plasma membrane-bound TNSALP would function as an ectoenzyme.[51,107] Consonant with this hypothesis is the clinical observation that patients with hypophosphatasia typically do not have symptoms of vitamin $B_6$ deficiency or toxicity. Dermatitis, stomatitis, peripheral neuritis, depression, or anemia—clinical hallmarks of vitamin $B_6$ deficiency[193]—are not recognized complications. Similarly, peripheral neuropathy, a manifestation of vitamin $B_6$ toxicity,[193] is not a feature of hypophosphatasia. Furthermore, biochemical studies also indicate that intracellular levels of vitamin $B_6$ are normal in hypophosphatasia. Urinary concentrations of 4-pyridoxic acid were unremarkable in four subjects examined with the childhood form of the disease.[51,126] Children with hypophosphatasia respond normally during a conventional L-tryptophan-loading test for vitamin $B_6$ deficiency (Whyte MP and Coburn SP, unpublished observation). Levels of PLP and total vitamin $B_6$ in homogenates of cultured TNSALP-deficient fibroblasts obtained from severely affected hypophosphatasia patients were normal.[194] Finally, analysis of tissues obtained at autopsy from three perinatal cases, in which plasma PLP concentrations were elevated 50 to 900 times, revealed unremarkable levels of PLP, PL, and total forms of vitamin $B_6$.[126]

Although vitamin $B_6$ deficiency has been associated with kidney stones and epilepsy is an important complication, these problems in patients with hypophosphatasia may be explained by other factors. Nephrocalcinosis in infants with hypophosphatasia is likely due to hypercalciuria. However, the possibility of altered oxalate metabolism (a consequence of vitamin $B_6$ deficiency) has not been explored.[193] The epilepsy of severely affected patients may be related to cranial deformity, hemorrhage, periodic apnea, and so on. Additionally, PEA was found to be epileptogenic when given intravenously to one such infant during a study of PEA metabolism.[195] In hypophosphatasia, normal or somewhat elevated plasma PL levels are usually observed.[51] In most patients, there seems to be sufficient extracellular dephosphorylation of PLP to PL by some mechanism to account for their normal vitamin $B_6$ status. Furthermore, in two patients with perinatal hypophosphatasia and epilepsy who had plasma PL levels below assay sensitivity, administration of vitamin $B_6$ did not correct the seizure disorder[126] (personal observation). However, lethal seizures that can be controlled by vitamin $B_6$ supplementation are a major feature of the TNSALP knock-out mouse model for infantile hypophosphatasia.[186–188] This observation increases the likelihood that some very severely affected infants with hypophosphatasia have epilepsy from altered vitamin $B_6$ metabolism.[196] Because TNSALP seems to dephosphorylate PLP to PL extracellularly, PL in the circulation could be low in such hypophosphatasia patients.

In 1985, the clinical and biochemical observations concerning vitamin $B_6$ metabolism in hypophosphatasia indicated an ectoenzyme role for TNSALP.[51] Subsequent characterization of TNSALP as a plasma membrane-bound glycoprotein, covalently linked to the polar head group of phosphatidylinositol, verified this conclusion.[197] Studies using cultivated dermal fibroblasts from patients with infantile hypophosphatasia[164] and human osteosarcoma cells show that TNSALP is attached to plasma membranes with ectotopography and dephosphorylates PLP and PEA at physiological concentrations and at physiological pH.[198,199]

### Inorganic Pyrophosphate

Discovery in 1965 that $PP_i$ levels are increased in the urine[50] in hypophosphatasia patients suggested a mechanism for the associated disorders of crystal deposition and the defective skeletal mineralization.[38,39]

At low concentrations, $PP_i$ enhances precipitation of calcium and $P_i$ to form amorphous calcium phosphate.[39] Perhaps the calcific periarthritis is explained by this action of $PP_i$.[78] CPPD deposition leading to chondrocalcinosis, pseudogout, and pyro-

phosphate arthropathy[56] likely results from failure of TNSALP to hydrolyze $PP_i$ and to destroy CPPD crystals.[19] ALP dissolves CPPD crystals in vitro.[19] This pyrophosphatase activity seems to be unrelated to its capacity to hydrolyze phosphoesters.

At high concentrations, however, $PP_i$ is known to adsorb to amorphous calcium phosphate and prevent its transformation to hydroxyapatite crystals.[38] Furthermore, adsorption of $PP_i$ to hydroxyapatite crystals impairs their growth and dissolution.[35,39] Hence, $PP_i$ accumulation surrounding matrix vesicles could be expressed clinically as rickets or osteomalacia.

Studies using TNSALP-deficient fibroblasts from perinatal and infantile hypophosphatasia patients demonstrate that these cells generate $PP_i$ at normal rates from extracellular ATP.[200] They have normal levels of nucleoside triphosphate pyrophosphatase (NTP-$PP_i$-ase) activity. Accordingly, NTP-$PP_i$-ase appears to be different from TNSALP. Furthermore, clearance studies of $^{32}PP_i$ administered to adults with hypophosphatasia indicate that the endogenous accumulation of $PP_i$ results from defective degradation rather than from increased $PP_i$ biosynthesis.[39]

### Circulating Tissue-Nonspecific Alkaline Phosphatase

A variety of evidence suggests that circulating ALP is physiologically inactive.[33] Infants with hypophosphatasia who received IV infusions of plasma from patients with Paget bone disease[155] or were given purified placental ALP[167] (so that normal or even elevated levels of ALP activity in serum were achieved, respectively) demonstrated no clinical or radiographic improvement. Furthermore, such therapy failed to substantially reduce urinary PEA or $PP_i$ levels or plasma PLP concentrations.[67,167] Accordingly, deficiency of TNSALP activity in the skeleton itself seems to account for the rickets and osteomalacia of hypophosphatasia. Interestingly, Fraser and Yendt reported in 1955 that rachitic rat cartilage would calcify in serum obtained from an infant with hypophosphatasia, yet slices of the patient's costochondral junction would not mineralize in synthetic calcifying medium or in the pooled serum of healthy children.[201] TNSALP bound to cell surfaces seems to be the physiologically active form of the enzyme.

### A MODEL FOR TISSUE-NONSPECIFIC ALKALINE PHOSPHATASE FUNCTION

Observations from hypophosphatasia can be formulated into an overview of how TNSALP might function physiologically in humans (Fig. 207-9). Increased levels of PEA, $PP_i$, and PLP endogenously in this disorder indicate that TNSALP is catalytically active toward a variety of substrates with fairly variable chemical structure (see Fig. 207-1). Clinical and biochemical investigations of vitamin $B_6$ metabolism, confirmed by subsequent cell culture studies, reveal that TNSALP is an ectoenzyme. Extracellular accumulation of PEA, $PP_i$, and PLP in hypophosphatasia is a consequence of deficient ecto-TNSALP activity. The source of the accumulated PEA is unclear, but could be the degradation of the phosphatidylinositol-glycan moiety that anchors a variety of ectoproteins to cell surfaces. Accumulation of membrane-impermeable PLP in plasma, but not in tissues, explains the absence of vitamin $B_6$ toxicity. With profound deficiency of TNSALP activity, conversion of PLP to PL may be sufficiently impaired to cause seizures. Generation of extracellular $PP_i$, perhaps from ATP, occurs normally in hypophosphatasia by the action of NTP-$PP_i$-ase. $PP_i$ accumulation reflects decreased $PP_i$ degradation extracellularly. In hypophosphatasia, calcium phosphate crystal deposition causes calcific periarthritis and CPPD precipitation results in chondrocalcinosis and/or $PP_i$ arthropathy. Calcific periarthritis reflects the effect of $PP_i$ at low concentrations to stimulate calcium phosphate precipitation. Chondrocalcinosis and $PP_i$ arthropathy occur from $PP_i$ accumulation and failure of TNSALP to hydrolyze CPPD crystals. Rickets and osteomalacia develop in hypophosphatasia from extracellular accumulation of

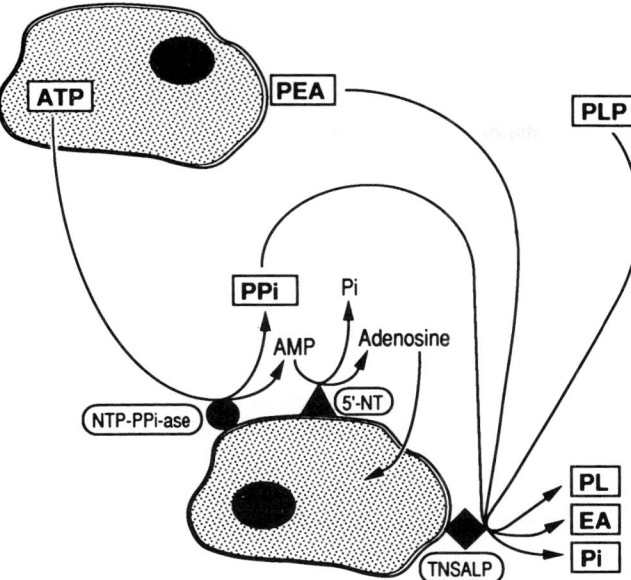

**Fig. 207-9 Metabolic basis for hypophosphatasia (hypothesis).** Extracellular generation of $PP_i$, by the action of NTP-PP$_i$-ase, is normal in hypophosphatasia, but extracellular degradation of $PP_i$, PLP, and PEA is diminished because of deficient ecto-TNSALP activity. Accumulation of $PP_i$ extracellularly accounts for the CPPD and perhaps calcium phosphate crystal deposition as well as rickets/osteomalacia.

$PP_i$ at sites of mineralization outside of matrix vesicles, because at high concentrations $PP_i$ is an inhibitor of hydroxyapatite crystal formation and growth. TNSALP appears to be physiologically active in tissues, but not in the circulation. Because three phosphocompounds (PEA, $PP_i$, PLP) are normally present in extracellular fluid at nanomolar or micromolar concentrations, TNSALP acts at substrate concentrations that are much lower than those used in routine clinical assays for ALP activity.[165] Furthermore, it is clear that TNSALP must be functional at physiological pH. Accordingly, the term "alkaline phosphatase" (never used by Robison) is a misnomer.

## REFERENCES

1. McComb RB, Bowers GN Jr, Posen S: *Alkaline Phosphatase.* New York, Plenum, 1979.
2. Harris H: The human alkaline phosphatases: What we know and what we don't know. *Clin Chim Acta* **186**:133, 1989.
3. Henthorn PS: Alkaline phosphatase, in Bilezikian J, Raisz L, Rodan G (eds): *Principles of Bone Biology.* San Diego, Academic Press, 1996, p 197.
4. McKusick VA: *Mendelian Inheritance in Man: A Catalog of Human Genes and Genetic Disorders,* 12th ed. Baltimore, Johns Hopkins University Press, 1998.
5. Moss DW, Whitaker KB: Modification of alkaline phosphatases by treatment with glycosidases. *Enzyme* **34**:212, 1985.
6. Harris H: *The Principles of Human Biochemical Genetics,* 3rd ed. Amsterdam, Elsevier/North Holland, 1980.
7. Smith M, Weiss MJ, Griffin CA, Murray JC, Buetow KH, Emanuel BS, Henthorn PS, et al.: Regional assignment of the gene for human liver/bone/kidney alkaline phosphatase to human chromosome 1p36.1-p34. *Genomics* **2**:139, 1988.
8. Griffin CA, Smith M, Henthorn PS, Harris H, Weiss MJ, Raducha M, Emanuel BS: Human placental and intestinal alkaline phosphatase genes map to 2q34-q37. *Am J Hum Genet* **41**:1025, 1987.
9. Human gene mapping. *Cytogenet Cell Genet* **40**:1, 1986.
10. Berger J, Garattini E, Hua J-C, Udenfriend S: Cloning and sequencing of human intestinal alkaline phosphatase cDNA. *Proc Natl Acad Sci U S A* **84**:695, 1987.
11. Henthorn PS, Raducha M, Edwards YH, Weiss MJ, Slaughter C, Lafferty MA, Harris H: Nucleotide and amino acid sequences of human intestinal alkaline phosphatase: Close homology to placental alkaline phosphatase. *Proc Natl Acad Sci U S A* **84**:1234, 1987.
12. Weiss MJ, Ray K, Henthorn PS, Lamb B, Kadesch T, Harris H: Structure of the human liver/bone/kidney alkaline phosphatase gene. *J Biol Chem* **263**:12002, 1988.
13. Kiledjian M, Kadesch T: Analysis of the human liver/bone/kidney alkaline phosphatase promoter in vivo and in vitro. *Nucleic Acids Res* **18**:957, 1990.
14. Nosjean O, Koyama I, Goseki M, Roux B, Komoda T: Human tissue non-specific alkaline phosphatases: Sugar-moiety-induced enzymic and antigenic modulations and genetic aspects. *Biochem J* **321**:297, 1997.
15. Henthorn PS, Whyte MP: Missense mutations of the tissue-nonspecific alkaline phosphatase gene in hypophosphatasia. *Clin Chem* **38**:2501, 1992.
16. Kim EE, Wyckoff HW: Reaction mechanism of alkaline phosphatase based on crystal structures. Two-metal ion catalysis. *J Mol Biol* **218**:449, 1991.
17. Hoylaerts MF, Millan JL: Site-directed mutagenesis and epitope-mapped monoclonal antibodies define a catalytically important conformational difference between human placental and germ cell alkaline phosphatase. *Eur J Biochem* **202**:605, 1991.
18. Hawrylak K, Stinson RA: Tetrameric alkaline phosphatase from human liver is converted to dimers by phosphatidylinositol phospholipase C. *FEBS Lett* **212**:289, 1987.
19. Xu Y, Cruz TF, Pritzker KP: Alkaline phosphatase dissolves calcium pyrophosphate dihydrate crystals. *J Rheumatol* **18**:1606, 1991.
20. Farley JR: Phosphate regulates the stability of skeletal alkaline phosphatase activity in human osteosarcoma (SaOS-2) cells without equivalent effects on the level of skeletal alkaline phosphatase immunoreactive protein. *Calcif Tissue Int* **57**:371, 1995.
21. Seetharam B, Tiruppathi C, Alpers DH: Hydrophobic interactions of brush border alkaline phosphatases: The role of phosphatidyl inositol. *Arch Biochem Biophys* **253**:189, 1987.
22. Anh DJ, Dimai HP, Hall SL, Farley JR: Skeletal alkaline phosphatase activity is primarily released from human osteoblasts in an insoluble form, and the net release is inhibited by calcium and skeletal growth factors. *Calcif Tissue Int* **62**:332, 1962.
23. Young GP, Rose IS, Cropper S, Seetharam S, Alpers DH: Hepatic clearance of rat plasma intestinal alkaline phosphatase. *Am J Physiol* **247**:G419, 1984.
24. Millan JL, Whyte MP, Avioli LV, Fishman WH: Hypophosphatasia (adult form): Quantitation of serum alkaline phosphatase isoenzyme activity in a large kindred. *Clin Chem* **26**:840, 1980.
25. Langman MJ, Leuthold E, Robson EB, Harris J, Luffman JE, Harris H: Influence of diet on the "intestinal" component of serum alkaline phosphatase in people of different ABO blood groups and secretor status. *Nature* **212**:41, 1966.
26. Mulivor RA, Boccelli D, Harris H: Quantitative analysis of alkaline phosphatases in serum and amniotic fluid: Comparison of biochemical and immunologic assays. *J Lab Clin Med* **105**:342, 1985.
27. Williams PL, Warwick R, Dyson M, Bannister LH (eds): *Gray's Anatomy,* 37th ed. Edinburgh, Churchill Livingstone, 1989.
28. Anderson HC: Molecular biology of matrix vesicles. *Clin Orthop Rel Res* **314**:266, 1995.
29. Ornoy A, Adomian GE, Rimoin DL: Histologic and ultrastructural studies on the mineralization process in hypophosphatasia. *Am J Med Genet* **22**:743, 1985.
30. Glorieux FH (ed): *Rickets.* New York, Raven, 1991.
31. Robison R: The possible significance of hexosephosphoric esters in ossification. *Biochem J* **17**:286, 1923.
32. Robison R, Soames KM: The possible significance of hexosephosphoric esters in ossification. II. The phosphoric esterase of ossifying cartilage. *Biochem J* **18**:740, 1924.
33. Whyte MP: Hypophosphatasia: Nature's window on alkaline phosphatase function in man, in Bilezikian J, Raisz L, Rodan G (eds): *Principles of Bone Biology.* San Diego, Academic Press, 1996, p 951.
34. Majeska RJ, Wuthier RE: Studies on matrix vesicles isolated from chick epiphyseal cartilage. Association of pyrophosphatase and ATPase activities with alkaline phosphatase. *Biochim Biophys Acta* **391**:51, 1975.
35. Fleisch H, Russell RGG, Straumann F: Effect of pyrophosphate on hydroxyapatite and its implications in calcium homeostasis. *Nature* **212**:901, 1966.

36. Moss DW, Eaton RH, Smith JK, Whitby LG: Association of inorganic-pyrophosphatase activity with human alkaline phosphatase preparations. *Biochem J* **102**:53, 1967.

37. Leone FA, Rezende LA, Ciancaglini P, Pizauro JM: Allosteric modulation of pyrophosphatase activity of rat osseous plate alkaline phosphatase by magnesium ions. *Int J Biochem Cell Biol* **30**:89, 1998.

38. Russell RG, Bisaz S, Donath A, Morgan DB, Fleisch H: Inorganic pyrophosphate in plasma in normal persons and in patients with hypophosphatasia, osteogenesis imperfecta, and other disorders of bone. *J Clin Invest* **50**:961, 1971.

39. Caswell AM, Whyte MP, Russell RGG: Hypophosphatasia and the extracellular metabolism of inorganic pyrophosphate: Clinical and laboratory aspects. *Crit Rev Clin Lab Sci* **28**:175, 1991.

40. de Bernard B, Bianco P, Bonucci E, Costantini M, Lunazzi GC, Martinuzzi P, Modricky C, Moro L, Panfili E, Pollesello P, Stagni N, Vittor F: Biochemical and immunohistochemical evidence that in cartilage an alkaline phosphatase is a Ca$^{2+}$-binding glycoprotein. *J Cell Biol* **103**:1615, 1986.

41. Lau KH, Farley JR, Baylink DJ: Phosphotyrosyl-specific protein phosphatase activity of a bovine skeletal acid phosphatase isoenzyme. Comparison with the phosphotyrosyl protein phosphatase activity of skeletal alkaline phosphatase. *J Biol Chem* **260**:4653, 1985.

42. Hui M, Tenenbaum HC: New face of an old enzyme: Alkaline phosphatase may contribute to human tissue aging by inducing tissue hardening and calcification. *Anat Rec* **253**:91, 1998.

43. Whyte MP: Hypophosphatasia and the role of alkaline phosphatase in skeletal mineralization. *Endocr Rev* **15**:439, 1994.

44. Rathbun JC: Hypophosphatasia, a new developmental anomaly. *Am J Dis Child* **75**:822, 1948.

45. Currarino G, Neuhauser E, Reyersback G, Sobel E: Hypophosphatasia. *AJR Am J Roentgenol* **78**:392, 1957.

46. Fraser D: Hypophosphatasia. *Am J Med* **22**:730, 1957.

47. Sobel EH, Clark LC, Fox RP, Robinow M: Rickets, deficiency of "alkaline" phosphatase activity and premature loss of teeth in childhood. *Pediatrics* **11**:309, 1953.

48. Fraser D, Yendt ER, Christie FHE: Metabolic abnormalities in hypophosphatasia. *Lancet* **1**:286, 1955.

49. McCance RA, Morrison AB, Dent CE: The excretion of phosphoethanolamine and hypophosphatasia. *Lancet* **1**:131, 1955.

50. Russell RGG: Excretion of inorganic pyrophosphate in hypophosphatasia. *Lancet* **2**:461, 1965.

51. Whyte MP, Mahuren JD, Vrabel LA, Coburn SP: Markedly increased circulating pyridoxal-5′-phosphate levels in hypophosphatasia. Alkaline phosphatase acts in vitamin B6 metabolism. *J Clin Invest* **76**:752, 1985.

52. Weiss MJ, Cole DE, Ray K, Whyte MP, Lafferty MA, Mulivor RA, Harris H: A missense mutation in the human liver/bone/kidney alkaline phosphatase gene causing a lethal form of hypophosphatasia. *Proc Natl Acad Sci U S A* **85**:7666, 1988.

53. Greenberg CR, Taylor CL, Haworth JC, Seargeant LE, Philipps S, Triggs-Raine B, Chodirker BN: A homoallelic Gly317 → Asp mutation in ALPL causes the perinatal (lethal) form of hypophosphatasia in Canadian Mennonites. *Genomics* **17**:215, 1993.

54. Taillard F, Desbois JC, Delepine N, Gretillat F, Allaneau C, Herrault A: L'hypophosphatasie affection polymorphe de frequence peut-etre sous estimee. *Med Inf (Lond)* **91**:559, 1984.

55. Whyte MP, Teitelbaum SL, Murphy WA, Bergfeld M, Avioli LV: Adult hypophosphatasia: Clinical, laboratory, and genetic investigation of a large kindred with review of the literature. *Medicine (Baltimore)* **58**:329, 1979.

56. Whyte MP, Murphy WA, Fallon MD: Adult hypophosphatasia with chondrocalcinosis and arthropathy: Variable penetrance of hypophosphatasemia in a large Oklahoma kindred. *Am J Med* **72**:631, 1982.

57. Terheggen HG, Wischermann A: Congenital hypophosphatasia. *Monatsschr Kinderheilkd* **132**:512, 1984.

58. Moore CA, Ward JC, Rivas MC, Magill HL, Whyte MP: Infantile hypophosphatasia: Autosomal recessive transmission to two related sibships. *Am J Med Genet* **36**:15, 1990.

59. Macfarlane JD, Kroon HM, van der Harten JJ: Phenotypically dissimilar hypophosphatasia in two sibships. *Am J Med Genet* **42**:117, 1992.

60. Kozlowski K, Sutcliffe J, Barylak A, Harrington G, Kemperdick H, Nolte K, Rheinwein H, Thomas PS, Uniecka W: Hypophosphatasia: Review of 24 cases. *Pediatr Radiol* **5**:103, 1976.

61. Shohat M, Rimoin DL, Gruber HE, Lachman RS: Perinatal lethal hypophosphatasia: Clinical, radiologic, and morphologic findings. *Pediatr Radiol* **21**:421, 1991.

62. Silver MM, Vilos GA, Milne KJ: Pulmonary hypoplasia in neonatal hypophosphatasia. *Pediatr Pathol* **8**:483, 1988.

63. Ozono K, Yamagata M, Michigami T, Nakajima S, Sakai N, Cai G, Satomura K, Yasui N, Okada S, Nakayama M: Identification of novel missense mutations (Phe310Leu and Gly439Arg) in a neonatal case of hypophosphatasia. *J Clin Endocrinol Metab* **81**:4458, 1996.

64. Whyte MP: Spur-limbed dwarfism in hypophosphatasia [Letter]. *Dysmorphol Clin Genet* **2**:126, 1988.

65. Brenner RL, Smith JL, Cleveland WW, Bejar RL, Lockhart WS Jr: Eye signs of hypophosphatasia. *Arch Ophthalmol* **81**:614, 1969.

66. Teree TM, Klein LR: Hypophosphatasia: Clinical and metabolic studies. *J Pediatr* **72**:41, 1968.

67. Whyte MP, Valdes R Jr, Ryan LM, McAlister WH: Infantile hypophosphatasia: Enzyme replacement therapy by intravenous infusion of alkaline phosphatase-rich plasma from patients with Paget bone disease. *J Pediatr* **101**:379, 1982.

68. Sty JR, Boedecker RA, Babbitt DP: Skull scintigraphy in infantile hypophosphatasia. *J Nucl Med* **20**:305, 1979.

69. Fallon MD, Teitelbaum SL, Weinstein RS, Goldfischer S, Brown DM, Whyte MP: Hypophosphatasia: Clinicopathologic comparison of the infantile, childhood, and adult forms. *Medicine (Baltimore)* **63**:12, 1984.

70. Kjellman M, Oldfelt V, Nordenram A, Olow-Nordenram M: Five cases of hypophosphatasia with dental findings. *Int J Oral Surg* **2**:152, 1973.

71. Lundgren T, Westphal O, Bolme P, Modeer T, Noren JG: Retrospective study of children with hypophosphatasia with reference to dental changes. *Scand J Dent Res* **99**:357, 1991.

72. Chapple IL: Hypophosphatasia: Dental aspects and mode of inheritance. *J Clin Periodontol* **20**:615, 1993.

73. Bixler D: Heritable disorders affecting cementum and the periodontal structure, in Stewart RE, Prescott GH (eds): *Oral Facial Genetics*. St. Louis, CV Mosby, 1976, p 262.

74. Lepe X, Rothwell BR, Banich S, Page RC: Absence of adult dental anomalies in familial hypophosphatasia. *J Periodontal Res* **32**:375, 1997.

75. Seshia SS, Derbyshire G, Haworth JC, Hoogstraten J: Myopathy with hypophosphatasia. *Arch Dis Child* **65**:130, 1990.

76. Wendling D, Cassou M, Guidet M: Hypophosphatasia in adults. Apropos of 2 cases. *Rev Rhum Mal Osteoartic* **52**:43, 1985.

77. O'Duffy JD: Hypophosphatasia associated with calcium pyrophosphate dihydrate deposits in cartilage. *Arthritis Rheum* **13**:381, 1970.

78. Chuck AJ, Pattrick MG, Hamilton E, Wilson R, Doherty M: Crystal deposition in hypophosphatasia: A reappraisal. *Ann Rheum Dis* **48**:571, 1989.

79. Lassere MN, Jones JG: Recurrent calcific periarthritis, erosive osteoarthritis and hypophosphatasia: A family study. *J Rheumatol* **17**:1244, 1990.

80. Coe JD, Murphy WA, Whyte MP: Management of femoral fractures and pseudofractures in adult hypophosphatasia. *J Bone Joint Surg Am* **68**:981, 1986.

81. Page RC, Baab DA: A new look at the etiology and pathogenesis of early onset periodontitis. Cementopathia revisited. *J Periodontol* **56**:748, 1985.

82. Scriver CR, Cameron D: Pseudohypophosphatasia. *N Engl J Med* **281**:604, 1969.

83. Moore CA, Wappner RS, Coburn SP, Mulivor RA, Fedde KN, Whyte MP: Pseudohypophosphatasia: Clinical, radiographic, and biochemical characterization of a second case [Abstract]. *Am J Hum Genet* **47**:A-68, 1990.

84. Cole DE, Salisbury SR, Stinson RA, Coburn SP, Ryan LM, Whyte MP: Increased serum pyridoxal-5′-phosphate in pseudohypophosphatasia [Letter]. *N Engl J Med* **314**:992, 1986.

85. Fedde KN, Cole DE, Whyte MP: Pseudohypophosphatasia: Aberrant localization and substrate specificity of alkaline phosphatase in cultured skin fibroblasts. *Am J Hum Genet* **47**:776, 1990.

86. Heaton BW, McClendon JL: Childhood pseudohypophosphatasia. Clinical and laboratory study of two cases. *Tex Dent J* **103**:4, 1986.

87. Mehes K, Klujber L, Lassu G, Kajtar P: Hypophosphatasia: Screening and family investigations in an endogamous Hungarian village. *Clin Genet* **3**:60, 1972.

88. Rubecz I, Mehes K, Klujber L, Bozzay L, Weisenbach J, Fenyvesi J: Hypophosphatasia: Screening and family investigation. *Clin Genet* **6**:155, 1974.

89. Kleinman G, Uri M, Hull S, Keene C: Perinatal ultrasound casebook. Antenatal findings in congenital hypophosphatasia. *J Perinatol* **11**:282, 1991.

90. Weinstein RS, Whyte MP: Heterogeneity of adult hypophosphatasia: Report of severe and mild cases. *Arch Intern Med* **141**:727, 1981.

91. Macfarlane JD, Souverijn JH, Breedveld FC: Clinical significance of a low serum alkaline phosphatase. *Neth J Med* **40**:9, 1992.

92. Royce PM, Blumberg A, Zurbrugg RP, Zimmermann A, Colombo J-P, Steinmann B: Lethal osteogenesis imperfecta: Abnormal collagen metabolism and biochemical characteristics of hypophosphatasia. *Eur J Pediatr* **147**:626, 1988.

93. Pillans PI, Berman P, Saunders SJ: Cholestatic jaundice with a normal serum alkaline phosphatase level: Another case of hypophosphatasia in an adult. *Gastroenterology* **84**:175, 1983.

94. Whyte MP, Chines A, Landt M, Mahuren JD, Ryan LM, Coburn SP: Hypophosphatasia: Diagnostic utility of phosphoethanolamine, inorganic pyrophosphate and pyridoxal 5′-phosphate quantitation contrasted in affected children. (In manuscript)

95. Whyte MP, Seino Y: Circulating vitamin D metabolite levels in hypophosphatasia. *J Clin Endocrinol Metab* **55**:178, 1982.

96. Opshaug O, Maurseth K, Howlid H, Aksnes L, Aarskog D: Vitamin D metabolism in hypophosphatasia. *Acta Paediatr Scand* **71**:517, 1982.

97. Taillard F, Desbois J-C, Gueris J, Delepine N, Lacour R, Gretillat F, Wyart D: Pyrophosphates inorganiques et parathormone dans l'hypophosphatasie. Etude d'une famille. *Biomed Pharmacother* **39**:236, 1985.

98. Whyte MP, Rettinger SD: Hyperphosphatemia due to enhanced renal reclamation of phosphate in hypophosphatasia [Abstract]. *J Bone Miner Res* **2(Suppl 1)**:399, 1987.

99. Nusynowitz ML: Low serum alkaline phosphatase level, hypophosphatemia, and aching extremities [Letter]. *JAMA* **242**:2800, 1979.

100. Juan D, Lambert PW: Vitamin D. Metabolism and phosphorus absorption studies in a case of coexistent vitamin D resistant rickets and hypophosphatasia, in Cohn DV, Talmage RV, Matthews JL (eds): *Hormonal Control of Calcium Metabolism.* International Congress Series 511. Amsterdam, Excerpta Medica, 1981.

101. De Vries HR, Duran M, De Bree PK, Wadman SK: A patient with hypophosphatasia and hyperprolinaemia. *Neth J Med* **21**:28, 1978.

102. Rettinger SD, Whyte MP: Normal circulating acid phosphatase activity in hypophosphatasia. *J Inherit Metab Dis* **8**:161, 1985.

103. Iqbal SJ: Persistently raised serum acid phosphatase activity in a patient with hypophosphatasia. Electrophoretic and molecular weight characterization as type 5. *Clin Chim Acta* **271**:213, 1998.

104. Rasmussen K: Phosphorylethanolamine and hypophosphatasia. Studies on urinary excretion, renal handling and elimination of endogenous and exogenous phosphorylethanolamine in healthy persons, carriers, and in patients with hypophosphatasia. *Dan Med Bull* **15(Suppl II)**:1, 1968.

105. Licata AA, Radfar N, Bartter FC, Bou E: The urinary excretion of phosphoethanolamine in diseases other than hypophosphatasia. *Am J Med* **64**:133, 1978.

106. Tecza S, Prandota J, Morawska Z, Rudzka M, Pankow-Prandota L: Hypophosphatasia with normal urinary phosphoethanolamine in a 22-month-old girl. *Pediatr Pol* **55**:791, 1980.

107. Coburn SP, Whyte MP: Role of phosphatases in the regulation of vitamin B$_6$ metabolism in hypophosphatasia and other disorders, in Leklem JE, Reynolds RD (eds): *Clinical and Physiological Applications of Vitamin B$_6$.* New York, Alan R. Liss, 1988, p 65.

108. Chodirker BN, Coburn SP, Seargeant LE, Whyte MP, Greenberg CR: Increased plasma pyridoxal-5′-phosphate levels before and after pyridoxine loading in carriers of perinatal/infantile hypophosphatasia. *J Inherit Metab Dis* **13**:891, 1990.

109. Macfarlane JD, Poorthuis BJ, Mulivor RA, Caswell AM: Raised urinary excretion of inorganic pyrophosphate in asymptomatic members of a hypophosphatasia kindred. *Clin Chim Acta* **202**:141, 1991.

110. Anderson HC, Hsu HH, Morris DC, Fedde KN, Whyte MP: Matrix vesicles in osteomalacic hypophosphatasia bone contain apatite-like mineral crystals. *Am J Pathol* **151**:1555, 1997.

111. Manicourt D, Orloff S, Taverne-Verbanck J: Osteomalacia in hyperphosphoethanolaminuria without hypophosphatasia. *Ann Endocrinol* **40**:167, 1979.

112. Nomura Y, Mori W: Hypophosphatasia: Histopathology of human temporal bones. *J Laryngol Otol* **82**:1129, 1968.

113. Beumer J III, Trowbridge HO, Silverman S Jr, Eisenberg E: Childhood hypophosphatasia and the premature loss of teeth: A clinical and laboratory study of seven cases. *Oral Surg Oral Med Oral Pathol Oral Radiol Endod* **35**:631, 1973.

114. el-Labban NG, Lee KW, Rule D: Permanent teeth in hypophosphatasia: Light and electron microscopic study. *J Oral Pathol Med* **20**:352, 1991.

115. Ramer M, Basta R, Fisher K: Childhood hypophosphatasia: A case report. *NYS Dent J* **63**:36, 1997.

116. Vanneuville FJ, Leroy JG: Enzymatic diagnosis of congenital lethal hypophosphatasia in tissues, plasma, and diploid skin fibroblasts. *J Inherit Metab Dis* **4**:129, 1981.

117. Mueller HD, Stinson RA, Mohyuddin F, Milne JK: Isoenzymes of alkaline phosphatase in infantile hypophosphatasia. *J Lab Clin Med* **102**:24, 1983.

118. Gorodischer R, Davidson RG, Mosovich LL, Yaffe SJ: Hypophosphatasia: A developmental anomaly of alkaline phosphatase? *Pediatr Res* **10**:650, 1976.

119. Whyte M, Vrabel L: Infantile hypophosphatasia: Complementation analysis with skin fibroblast heterokaryons suggests a defect(s) at a single gene locus [Abstract]. *Am J Hum Genet* **26**:209-S, 1984.

120. Beisel WR, Austern KF, Rosen H, Herndon EG: Metabolic observations in adult hypophosphatasia. *Am J Med* **29**:369, 1960.

121. Iqbal SJ: Increase in leukocyte alkaline phosphatase in a patient with hypophosphatasia during pregnancy. *J Inherit Metab Dis* **21**:83, 1998.

122. Fallon MD, Whyte MP, Weiss MJ, Harris H: Molecular biology of hypophosphatasia: A point mutation or small deletion in the bone/liver/kidney alkaline phosphatase gene results in an intact but functionally inactive enzyme [Abstract]. *J Bone Miner Res* **4**:S-304, 1989.

123. Goseki M, Oida S, Takagi Y, Okuyama T, Watanabe J, Sasaki S: Immunological study on hypophosphatasia. *Clin Chim Acta* **190**:263, 1990.

124. Whyte MP, Walkenhorst DA, Fedde KN, Henthorn PS, Hill CS: Hypophosphatasia: Levels of bone alkaline phosphatase immunoreactivity in serum reflect disease severity. *J Clin Endocrinol Metab* **81**:2142, 1996.

125. Whyte MP, Rettinger SD, Vrabel LA: Infantile hypophosphatasia: Enzymatic defect explored with alkaline phosphatase-deficient patient skin fibroblasts in culture. *Calcif Tissue Int* **40**:244, 1987.

126. Whyte MP, Mahuren JD, Fedde KN, Cole FS, McCabe ER, Coburn SP: Perinatal hypophosphatasia: Tissue levels of vitamin B$_6$ are unremarkable despite markedly increased circulating concentrations of pyridoxal-5′-phosphate (evidence for an ectoenzyme role for tissue-nonspecific alkaline phosphatase). *J Clin Invest* **81**:1234, 1988.

127. Danovitch SH, Baer PN, Laster L: Intestinal alkaline phosphatase activity in familial hypophosphatasia. *N Engl J Med* **278**:1253, 1968.

128. Fedde KN, Michell MP, Henthorn PS, Whyte MP: Aberrant properties of alkaline phosphatase in patient fibroblasts correlate with clinical expressivity in severe forms of hypophosphatasia. *J Clin Endocrinol Metab* **81**:2587, 1996.

129. Whyte MP, Vrabel LA, Schwartz TD: Alkaline phosphatase deficiency in cultured skin fibroblasts from patients with hypophosphatasia: Comparison of the infantile, childhood, and adult forms. *J Clin Endocrinol Metab* **57**:831, 1983.

130. Schneider RW, Corcoran AC: Familial nephrogenic osteopathy due to excessive tubular reabsorption of inorganic phosphate: A new syndrome and a novel mode of relief. *J Lab Clin Med* **36**:985, 1950.

131. Pimstone B, Eisenberg E, Silverman S: Hypophosphatasia: Genetic and dental studies. *Ann Intern Med* **65**:722, 1966.

132. Harris B, Robson EB: A genetical study of ethanolamine phosphate excretion in hypophosphatasia. *Hum Genet* **23**:421, 1959.

133. McCance RA, Fairweather DVI, Barrett AM, Morrison AB: Genetic, clinical, biochemical and pathological features of hypophosphatasia. *Q J Med* **25**:523, 1956.

134. Eberle F, Hartenfels S, Pralle H, Kabisch A: Adult hypophosphatasia without apparent skeletal disease: "Odontohypophosphatasia" in four heterozygote members of a family. *Klin Wochenschr* **62**:371, 1984.

135. Silverman JL: Apparent dominant inheritance of hypophosphatasia. *Arch Intern Med* **110**:191, 1962.

136. Eastman JR, Bixler D: Clinical, laboratory, and genetic investigations of hypophosphatasia: Support for autosomal dominant inheritance with homozygous lethality. *J Craniofac Genet Dev Biol* **3**:213, 1983.

137. Eastman J, Bixler D: Lethal and mild hypophosphatasia in half-sibs. *J Craniofac Genet Dev Biol* **2**:35, 1982.

138. Sorensen SA, Flodgaard H, Sorensen E: Serum alkaline phosphatase, serum pyrophosphatase, phosphorylethanolamine and inorganic pyrophosphate in plasma and urine: A genetic and clinical study of hypophosphatasia. *Monogr Hum Genet* **10**:66, 1978.

139. Blaskovics ME, Shaw KN: Hypophosphatasia with phenylketonuria. *Eur J Pediatr* **117**:265, 1974.

140. Lowry RB, Snyder FF, Wesenberg RL, Machin GA, Applegarth DA, Morgan K, Carter RJ, Toone JR, Holmes TM, Dewar RD: Morquio syndrome (MPS IVA) and hypophosphatasia in a Hutterite kindred. *Am J Med Genet* 22:463, 1985.

141. Chodirker BN, Evans JA , Lewis M, Coghlan G, Belcher E, Philipps S, Seargeant LE, Sus C, Greenberg CR: Infantile hypophosphatasia—Linkage with the RH locus. *Genomics* 1:280, 1987.

142. Henthorn PS, Raducha M, Fedde KN, Lafferty MA, Whyte MP: Different missense mutations at the tissue-nonspecific alkaline phosphatase gene locus in autosomal recessively inherited forms of mild and severe hypophosphatasia. *Proc Natl Acad Sci U S A* 89:9924, 1992.

143. Shibata H, Fukushi M, Igarashi A, Misumi Y, Ikehara Y, Ohashi Y, Oda K: Defective intracellular transport of tissue-nonspecific alkaline phosphatase with an Ala$^{162}$ → Thr mutation associated with lethal hypophosphatasia. *J Biochem* 123:968, 1998.

144. Mornet E, Taillandier A, Peyramaure S, Kaper F, Muller F, Brenner R, Bussiere P, Freisinger P, Godard J, LeMerrer M, Oury J, Plauchu H, Puddu R, Rival JM, Superti-Furga A, Touraine RL, Serre JL, Simon-Bouy B: Identification of fifteen novel mutations in the tissue-nonspecific alkaline phosphatase (TNSALP) gene in European patients with severe hypophosphatasia. *Eur J Hum Genet* 6:308, 1998.

145. Henthorn P, Ferrero A, Fedde K, Coburn S, Whyte M: Hypophosphatasia mutation D361V exhibits dominant effects both in vivo and in vitro [Abstract]. *Am J Hum Genet* 59:A-199, 1996.

145a. Whyte MP: Hypophosphatasia. In Econs MJ (ed): *The Genetics of Osteoporosis and Metabolic Bone Disease*, Totowa, New Jersey, Humana Press, p 335, 2000.

146. Fukushi M, Amizuka N, Hoshi K, Ozawa H, Kumagai H, Omura S, Misumi Y, Ikehara Y, Oda K: Intracellular retention and degradation of tissue-nonspecific alkaline phosphatase with a Gly$^{317}$ → Asp substitution associated with lethal hypophosphatasia. *Biochem Biophys Res Commun* 246:613, 1998.

147. Goseki-Sone M, Orimo H, Iimura T, Takagi Y, Watanabe H, Taketa K, Sato S, Mayanagi H, Shimada T, Oida S: Hypophosphatasia: Identification of five novel missense mutations (G507A, G705A, A748G, T1155C, G1320A) in the tissue-nonspecific alkaline phosphatase gene among Japanese patients. *Hum Mutat* (**Suppl 1**):S263, 1998.

148. Sugimoto N, Iwamoto S, Hoshino Y, Kajii E: A novel missense mutation of the tissue-nonspecific alkaline phosphatase gene detected in a patient with hypophosphatasia. *J Hum Genet* 43:160, 1998.

149. Orimo H, Hayashi Z, Watanabe A, Hirayama T, Hirayama T, Shimada T: Novel missense and frameshift mutations in the tissue-nonspecific alkaline phosphatase gene in a Japanese patient with hypophosphatasia. *Hum Mol Genet* 3:1683, 1994.

150. Orimo H, Goseki-Sone M, Sato S, Shimada T: Detection of deletion 1154-1156 hypophosphatasia mutation using TNSALP exon amplification. *Genomics* 42:364, 1997.

151. Mumm S, Jones J, Henthorn PS, Eddy MC, Whyte MP: Mutational analysis of the bone alkaline phosphatase gene in hypophosphatasia. *Bone* 5(**Suppl 1**):S281, 1998.

152. Goseki-Sone M, Orimo H, Iimura T, Miyazaki H, Oda K, Shibata H, Yanagishita M, Takagi Y, Watanabe H, Shimada T, Oida S: Expression of the mutant (1735T-DEL) tissue-nonspecific alkaline phosphatase gene from hypophosphatasia patients. *J Bone Miner Res* 13:1827, 1998.

153. Whyte MP, Magill HL, Fallon MD, Herrod HG: Infantile hypophosphatasia: Normalization of circulating bone alkaline phosphatase activity followed by skeletal remineralization. Evidence for an intact structural gene for tissue nonspecific alkaline phosphatase. *J Pediatr* 108:82, 1986.

154. Caswell AM, Russell RG, Whyte MP: Hypophosphatasia: Pediatric forms. *J Pediatr Endocrinol* 3:73, 1989.

155. Weinstein RS, Whyte MP: Fifty-year follow-up of hypophosphatasia [Letter]. *Arch Intern Med* 141:1720, 1981.

156. Whyte MP, McAlister WH, Patton LS, Magill HL, Fallon MD, Lorentz WB Jr, Herrod HG: Enzyme replacement therapy for infantile hypophosphatasia attempted by intravenous infusions of alkaline phosphatase-rich Paget plasma: Results in three additional patients. *J Pediatr* 105:926, 1984.

157. Wolfish NM, Heick H: Hyperparathyroidism and infantile hypophosphatasia: Effect of prednisone and vitamin K therapy. *J Pediatr* 95:1079, 1979.

158. Scaglione PR, Lucey JF: Further observations on hypophosphatasia. *Am J Dis Child* 92:493, 1956.

159. Barcia JP, Strife CF, Langman CB: Infantile hypophosphatasia: Treatment options to control hypercalcemia, hypercalciuria, and chronic bone demineralization. *J Pediatr* 130:825, 1997.

160. Fraser D, Laidlaw JC: Treatment of hypophosphatasia with cortisone, preliminary communication. *Lancet* 1:553, 1956.

161. Riggs BL, Seeman E, Hodgson SF, Taves DR, O'Fallon WM: Effect of the fluoride/calcium regimen on vertebral fracture occurrence in postmenopausal osteoporosis: Comparison with conventional therapy. *N Engl J Med* 306:446, 1982.

162. Bongiovanni AM, Album MM, Root AW, Hope JW, Marino J, Spencer DM: Studies in hypophosphatasia and response to high phosphate intake. *Am J Med Sci* 255:163, 1968.

163. Macpherson RI, Kroeker M, Houston CS: Hypophosphatasia. *J Can Assoc Radiol* 23:16, 1972.

164. Albeggiani A, Cataldo F: Infantile hypophosphatasia diagnosed at 4 months and surviving at 2 years. *Helv Paediatr Acta* 37:49, 1982.

165. Weninger M, Stinson RA, Plenk H Jr, Bock P, Pollack A: Biochemical and morphological effects of human hepatic alkaline phosphatase in a neonate with hypophosphatasia. *Acta Paediatr Scand Suppl* 360:154, 1989.

166. Whyte M, Landt M, Ryan L, Mulivor R, Henthorn P, Fedde K, Coburn S: Alkaline phosphatase: Placental and tissue nonspecific isoenzymes hydrolyze phosphoethanolamine, inorganic pyrophosphate, and pyridoxal 5'-phosphate (substrate accumulation in carriers of hypophosphatasia corrects during pregnancy). *J Clin Invest* 95:1440, 1995.

167. Whyte MP, Habib D, Coburn SP, Tecklenburg F, Ryan L, Fedde KN, Stinson RA: Failure of hyperphosphatasemia by intravenous infusion of purified placental alkaline phosphatase (ALP) to correct severe hypophosphatasia: Evidence against a role for circulating ALP in skeletal mineralization [Abstract]. *J Bone Miner Res* 7(**Suppl 1**):S155, 1992.

168. Fedde KN, Blair L, Terzic F, Anderson HC, Narisawa S, Millan JL, Whyte MP: Amelioration of the skeletal disease in hypophosphatasia by bone marrow transplantation using the alkaline phosphatase-knockout mouse model [Abstract]. *Am J Hum Genet* 59:A-15, 1996.

169. Whyte MP, Kurtzburg J, Gottesman GS, McAlister WH, Coburn SP, Ryan LM, Miller C, Martin PL: Marked clinical and radiographic improvement in infantile hypophosphatasia transiently after haploi-dentical bone marrow transplantation [Abstract]. *Bone* 23(**Suppl**):S191, 1998.

170. Jacobson DP, McClain EJ: Hypophosphatasia in monozygotic twins. *J Bone Joint Surg Am* 49:377, 1967.

171. Rudd NL, Miskin M, Hoar DI, Benzie R, Doran TA: Prenatal diagnosis of hypophosphatasia. *N Engl J Med* 295:146, 1976.

172. Mulivor RA, Mennuti M, Zackai EH, Harris H: Prenatal diagnosis of hypophosphatasia; genetic, biochemical, and clinical studies. *Am J Hum Genet* 30:271, 1978.

173. Warren RC, McKenzie CF, Rodeck CH, Moscoso G, Brock DJ, Barron L: First trimester diagnosis of hypophosphatasia with a monoclonal antibody to liver/bone/kidney isoenzyme of alkaline phosphatase. *Lancet* 2:856, 1985.

174. Brock DJH, Barron L: First-trimester prenatal diagnosis of hypophosphatasia: Experience with 16 cases. *Prenat Diagn* 11:387, 1991.

175. Muller F, Oury JF, Bussiere P, Lewin F, Boue J: First-trimester diagnosis of hypophosphatasia. Importance of gestational age and purity of CV samples. *Prenat Diagn* 11:725, 1991.

176. Greenberg CR, Evans JA, McKendry-Smith S, Redekopp S, Haworth JC, Mulivor R, Chodirker BN: Infantile hypophosphatasia: Localization within chromosome region 1p36.1-34 and prenatal diagnosis using linked DNA markers. *Am J Hum Genet* 46:286, 1990.

177. Kishi F, Matsuura S, Murano I, Akita A, Kajii T: Prenatal diagnosis of infantile hypophosphatasia. *Prenat Diagn* 11:305, 1991.

178. van Dongen PW, Hamel BC, Nijhuis JG, de Boer CN: Prenatal follow-up of hypophosphatasia by ultrasound: Case report. *Eur J Obstet Gynecol Reprod Biol* 34:283, 1990.

179. Kousseff BG, Mulivor RA: Prenatal diagnosis of hypophosphatasia. *Obstet Gynecol* 57(**Suppl**):9S, 1981.

180. Garber AP, Sillence DO, Lachman RS, Worthen NJ, Rimoin DL, Kaback MM, Mulivor RA: Discordance between ultrasound and radiographic/biochemical findings in the prenatal diagnosis of congenital lethal hypophosphatasia. The National Foundation March of Dimes Birth Defects Conference, 1979, p 61.

181. Hausser C, Habib R, Poitras P: Hypophosphatasia: Complete absence of the fetal skeleton. *Union Med Can* 113:978, 1984.

182. Orimo H, Nakajima E, Hayashi Z, Kijima K, Watanabe A, Tenjin H, Araki T, Shimada T: First-trimester prenatal molecular diagnosis of infantile hypophosphatasia in a Japanese family. *Prenat Diagn* **16**:559, 1996.

183. Henthorn P, Whyte M: Infantile hypophosphatasia: Successful prenatal assessment by testing for tissue-nonspecific alkaline phosphatase isoenzyme gene mutations. *Prenat Diagn* **15**:1001, 1995.

184. Pauli RM, Modaff P, Sipes SL, Whyte MP: Mild hypophosphatasia mimicking severe osteogenesis imperfecta *in utero*. Bent but not broken. *Am J Med Genet* **86**:434, 1999.

185. Moore CA, Curry CJR, Henthorn PS, Smith JA, Smith JC, O'Lague P, Coburn SP, Weaver DD, Whyte MP: Mild autosomal dominant hypophosphatasia: *In utero* presentation in two families. *Am J Med Genet* **86**:410, 1999.

186. Waymire KG, Mahuren JD, Jaje JM, Guilarte TR, Coburn SP, MacGregor GR: Mice lacking tissue non-specific alkaline phosphatase die from seizures due to defective metabolism of vitamin B6. *Nat Genet* **11**:45, 1995.

187. Narisawa S, Fröhlander N, Millán JL: Inactivation of two mouse alkaline phosphatase genes and establishment of a model of infantile hypophosphatasia. *Dev Dyn* **208**:432, 1997.

188. Fedde KN, Blair L, Silverstein J, Coburn SP, Ryan LM, Weinstein RS, Waymire K, MacGregor GR, Narisawa S, Millán JL, Whyte MP: Alkaline phosphatase-knock out mice recapitulate the metabolic and skeletal defects of infantile hypophosphatasia. *J Bone Miner Res* **14**:2015, 1999.

189. Whyte MP, Vrabel LA: Infantile hypophosphatasia fibroblasts proliferate normally in culture: Evidence against a role for alkaline phosphatase (tissue nonspecific isoenzyme) in the regulation of cell growth and differentiation. *Calcif Tissue Int* **40**:1, 1987.

190. Fedde KN, Michel M, Whyte MP: Evidence against a role for alkaline phosphatase in the dephosphorylation of plasma membrane proteins: Hypophosphatasia fibroblast study. *J Cell Biochem* **53**:43, 1993.

191. Wu LN, Genge BR, Wuthier RE: Evidence for specific interaction between matrix vesicle proteins and the connective tissue matrix. *J Bone Miner Res* **17**:247, 1992.

192. Gron IH: Mammalian O-phosphorylethanolamine phosphorylase activity and its inhibition. *Scand J Clin Lab Invest* **38**:107, 1978.

193. Dolphin D, Poulson R, Avramovic O: *Vitamin B₆ Pyridoxal Phosphate: Clinical, Biochemical, and Medical Aspects: Part B.* New York, John Wiley, 1986.

194. Whyte MP, Mahuren JD, Scott MJ, Coburn SP: Hypophosphatasia: Pyridoxal-5′-phosphate levels are markedly increased in hypophosphatasemic plasma but normal in alkaline phosphatase-deficient fibroblasts (evidence for an ectoenzyme role for alkaline phosphatase in vitamin B6 metabolism) [Abstract]. *J Bone Miner Res* **1**:92, 1986.

195. Takahashi T, Iwantanti A, Mizuno S, Morishita Y, Nishio H, Kodama S, Matsuo T: The relationship between phosphoethanolamine level in serum and intractable seizure on hypophosphatasia infantile form, in Cohn DV, Fugita T, Potts JT Jr, Talmage RV (eds): *Endocrine Control of Bone and Calcium Metabolism*, vol 8-B. Amsterdam, Excerpta Medica, p 93, 1984.

196. Posen S, Whyte M, Coburn S, Freeman R, Collins F, Fedde K, Bye A: Infantile hypophosphatasia with fatal status epilepticus [Abstract]. *J Bone Miner Res* **12(Suppl 1)**:S-528, 1997.

197. Low MG, Saltiel AR: Structural and functional roles of glycosyl-phosphatidylinositol in membranes. *Science* **239**:268, 1988.

198. Fedde KN, Lane CC, Whyte MP: Alkaline phosphatase is an ectoenzyme that acts on micromolar concentrations of natural substrates at physiologic pH in human osteosarcoma (SAOS-2) cells. *Arch Biochem Biophys* **264**:400, 1988.

199. Fedde KN, Whyte MP: Alkaline phosphatase (tissue-nonspecific isoenzyme) is a phosphoethanolamine and pyridoxal-5′-phosphate ectophosphatase: Normal and hypophosphatasia fibroblast study. *Am J Hum Genet* **47**:767, 1990.

200. Caswell AM, Whyte MP, Russell RG: Normal activity of nucleoside triphosphate pyrophosphatase in alkaline phosphatase-deficient fibroblasts from patients with infantile hypophosphatasia. *J Clin Endocrinol Metab* **63**:1237, 1986.

201. Fraser D, Yendt ER: Metabolic abnormalities in hypophosphatasia. *Am J Dis Child* **90**:552, 1955.

202. Whyte MP: Alkaline phosphatase: Physiologic role explored in hypophosphatasia, in Peck WA (ed): *Bone and Mineral Research*, vol 6. Amsterdam, Elsevier, 1989, p 175.

# The Carbonic Anhydrase II Deficiency Syndrome: Osteopetrosis with Renal Tubular Acidosis and Cerebral Calcification

*William S. Sly* ■ *Gul N. Shah*

1. The carbonic anhydrase II deficiency syndrome is an autosomal recessive disorder that produces osteopetrosis, renal tubular acidosis, and cerebral calcification. Other features include mental retardation (seen in over 90 percent of reported cases), growth failure, and dental malocclusion.

2. Complications of osteopetrosis include increased susceptibility to fractures (which do, however, heal normally) and cranial nerve compression symptoms. Anemia and other hematologic manifestations of osteopetrosis are absent.

3. The renal tubular acidosis is usually a mixed type. A distal component is evident from inability to acidify the urine, and a proximal component is evident from a lowered transport maximum for bicarbonate. Impaired respiratory compensation for the metabolic acidosis has recently been recognized.

4. Over 110 patients have been reported, all of who have a quantitative deficiency of carbonic anhydrase II activity and immunoreactivity in erythrocytes. Heterozygous carriers can be identified by simple tests. Structural gene mutations have been identified in the CA II gene of every patient analyzed genetically.

5. The carbonic anhydrase II gene is 20 kb, contains seven exons, and maps to chromosome 8q22. Sixteen distinct mutations have been identified in 110 reported patients. Nearly 65 percent of affected patients are homozygous for a splice junction mutation at the 5′ end of exon 2. Because of its prevalence among families of Arabic descent from Kuwait, Saudi Arabia, and North Africa, this mutation has been designated the "Arabic mutation." The second recurrent mutation, a frameshift in exon 7, is most prevalent in Caribbean Hispanic populations. The third recurrent mutation is His 107 → Tyr, the first reported mutation. This mutation is due to a C → T transition in exon 3 and has been found in Belgian, Italian, Japanese, and American patients. The three affected sisters in the American family were compound heterozygotes, having inherited the His 107 → Tyr mutation from their mother and a splice acceptor mutation in the 3′ end of intron 5 from their father. The remaining 13 mutations are private mutations seen in single families and all are detectable by PCR amplification and direct sequencing of various exons.

Thus, PCR-based diagnosis and prenatal diagnosis are available for the 16 known mutations.

6. Symptoms of metabolic acidosis improve with treatment, but no specific treatment is available.

## HISTORY

Albers-Schönberg first described osteopetrosis (marble bone disease) in 1904.[1] Subsequently, over 300 cases have been reported.[2] Among these, two principal types were distinguished. An autosomal dominant form was called the adult, benign form because of the relatively few symptoms and the benign course, which is compatible with normal life span. The diagnosis is often made incidentally in adults evaluated for other complaints. At the other extreme is the clinically severe, autosomal recessive form which has its onset in infancy and produces anemia, leukopenia, hepatomegaly, failure to thrive, cranial nerve symptoms, and early death. This form is often referred to as the infantile, malignant, or lethal form. Beighton and colleagues have pointed out the existence of clinically intermediate forms of osteopetrosis.[3] Although this genetic heterogeneity indicates that multiple genetic causes produce osteopetrosis, the common mechanism underlying all forms is thought to be failure of bone resorption.[4]

The association of renal tubular acidosis with osteopetrosis was reported independently from three different countries — France,[5] Belgium,[6] and the United States[7] — in 1972. These initial pedigrees suggested that the pattern of inheritance is autosomal recessive. The clinical course began with onset in infancy or early childhood. Although not entirely benign, it was much milder than the course of the recessive lethal form and was compatible with long survival. The hematologic abnormalities associated with the recessive lethal form of osteopetrosis were mild or absent. In 1980, Ohlsson et al.[8] reported the additional finding of cerebral calcification, documented by CT scans, in four children with osteopetrosis and renal tubular acidosis from Saudi Arabia. Calcification of the basal ganglia in the original American kindred was reported independently by Whyte et al. the same year.[9]

In an effort to explain the pleiotropic effects of the mutation underlying this disorder by a single enzyme defect, we postulated a defect in one of the three isozymes of carbonic anhydrase (CA I, CA II, CA III) that are known to be under separate genetic control in humans.[10–14] This hypothesis seemed attractive for two reasons:

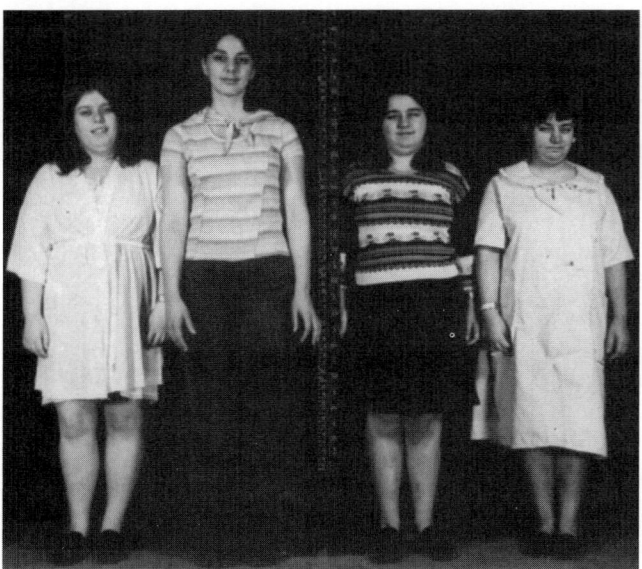

**Fig. 208-1** American family reported by Whyte et al. with the CA II deficiency syndrome.[9] From left are case 3, unaffected sister, case 2, and case 1 (propositus). This picture was taken in 1978 when the propositus was 29. Osteopetrosis had been diagnosed at age 2 years following a pathologic fracture.[9] Note short stature, unusual facial features, and squint in the three affected sisters. Cases 2 and 3 had limited vision and were considered legally blind. Vision was nearly normal in case 1. (*From Whyte et al.[9] Used by permission.*)

(a) metabolic acidosis can be produced by sulfonamide inhibitors of CA,[12] and (b) several reports had shown that CA inhibitors can block the parathyroid hormone-induced release of calcium from bone, suggesting a role for CA in bone resorption.[15–17]

The relationship of CA deficiency to cerebral calcification was less apparent, although it was known that CA II is present in brain,[18] and that CA inhibitors inhibit cerebrospinal fluid production[19] and affect electrical activity of the brain.[20] A defect in the CA II isozyme seemed most likely because this is the most widely distributed of the three known soluble isozymes of CA in human tissues[10,11] and CA II was the only soluble isozyme so far identified in renal and brain tissue.[18,21,22] In addition, a genetically determined, virtually complete absence of CA I in mature erythrocytes has no clinical consequences.[23] Because both CA I and CA II are expressed in human erythrocytes, it was possible to test this hypothesis by examining these isozymes in hemolysates of peripheral blood from the family we reported previously.[8]

In 1983, Sly et al.[24] tested this hypothesis and found that the three sisters from the original American kindred with this syndrome (Fig. 208-1) lacked carbonic anhydrase II (CA II) in their erythrocytes. Their normal appearing parents and many first-degree relatives had half-normal levels of CA II in erythrocyte lysates. These observations, coupled with CA II being the only known soluble isozyme of CA in kidney and brain, led them to propose that CA II deficiency is the primary defect in the newly recognized metabolic disorder of bone, kidney, and brain.[24]

In a subsequent report, Sly et al.[25] extended these studies to 18 additional patients in 11 unrelated families of different geographical and ethnic origins. Subsequently, Ohlsson et al.[26] reported four additional Saudi Arabian patients, including the first affected neonate, and summarized the clinical features of 21 reported patients. Cochat et al.[27] added an additional case and reviewed the clinical findings on the 30 patients reported by 1987, including a few who had not been completely described clinically. A few individual cases have been reported since, and many more have been recognized.[28–32] Whyte reviewed nearly 50 cases reported up to 1992.[32] Sixty more cases have been reported since 1992.[91–101] Deficiency of CA II was found in erythrocyte lysates of every patient so far reported with this syndrome, and structural gene

mutations have been identified in the CA II gene of every patient analyzed genetically.

## NOMENCLATURE

The syndrome of osteopetrosis with renal tubular acidosis (McKusick catalog 259730[33]) was recognized as a distinct entity in 1972.[5–7] In 1980, when Ohlsson et al.[8] pointed out that cerebral calcification was part of the syndrome, they suggested that it be referred to as marble brain disease by analogy with marble bone disease, the name given earlier to inherited forms of osteopetrosis that did not involve the brain.[2] However, because the enzymatic basis for the disorder was established,[24,25] it has been referred to as the carbonic anhydrase II deficiency syndrome.[26,33] It has also been called the Guibaud-Vainsel syndrome after the authors of the first two full reports on the disorder.[33]

## CLINICAL MANIFESTATIONS

There is considerable variability in the age of onset and the severity of clinical manifestations among the reported cases.[27] With the exception of three Hispanic patients, all had renal tubular acidosis and eventually developed osteopetrosis and cerebral calcification. Recently, Lien, Lien and Lai[102] reported that the acidosis has a respiratory component. Additional features include growth failure, mental retardation, and dental malocclusion. In some patients, bone fractures and other complications of osteopetrosis have dominated the clinical picture.[6,9] In others, symptoms of metabolic acidosis, including failure to thrive, developmental retardation, and growth retardation, have been more prominent.[5,8,27,95]

### Osteopetrosis

Osteopetrosis results from a generalized accumulation of bone mass that is secondary to a defect in bone resorption.[4] This defect prevents the normal development of marrow cavities, the normal tubulation of long bones, and the enlargement of osseous foramina. The clinical manifestations of osteopetrosis in the CA II deficiency syndrome tend to be milder than in the recessive, lethal form of osteopetrosis. They appear later,[26,27] and they also tend to improve over time.[9]

Anemia is rarely profound in patients with CA II deficiency, though three patients with anemia have been reported. Two of them were referred for bone marrow transplantation. In fact, the first reported bone marrow transplantation for osteopetrosis was done on a patient who very likely had the CA II deficiency syndrome,[34] and not the recessive lethal form of osteopetrosis, for which bone marrow transplantation has become an accepted form of therapy.[35] This patient was reported to have a favorable hematologic response, but to have been unimproved in terms of the metabolic acidosis following bone marrow transplantation.[27]

The radiologic findings in patients with CA II deficiency syndrome are not distinguishable from those in patients with other forms of osteopetrosis.[9,27,30–32] Increased bone density (Fig. 208-2), abnormal modeling, delay or failure of normal tubulation of long bones, transverse banding of metaphyses, fractures, and "bone-in-bone" appearance are all seen, as in other forms of osteopetrosis. However, the changes can vary with age. In the only neonate studied to date, the radiologic features were too subtle to justify the diagnosis at 23 days of age,[26] even though the hyperchloremic metabolic acidosis and alkaline urine were already prominent findings. This observation suggests that the osteopetrosis is a postpartum developmental abnormality that appears over the first year of life. The first patients reported by Guibaud[5,27] also had no osteopetrosis at age 4 months, but typical findings evolved and progressed over the first 3 years of life before stabilizing. In at least some patients followed into adulthood, the radiologic features of osteopetrosis, which were fully developed in childhood, improved substantially after puberty (Fig. 208-3). The radiographs may become nearly normal as the patients move into adulthood.[9]

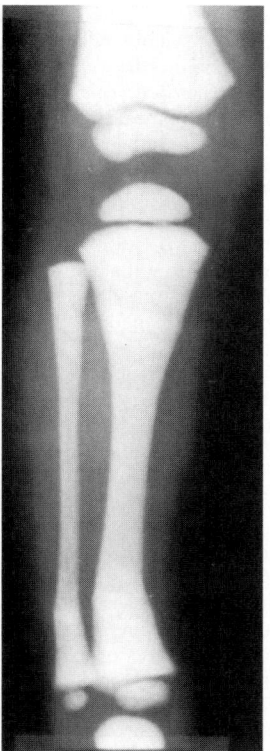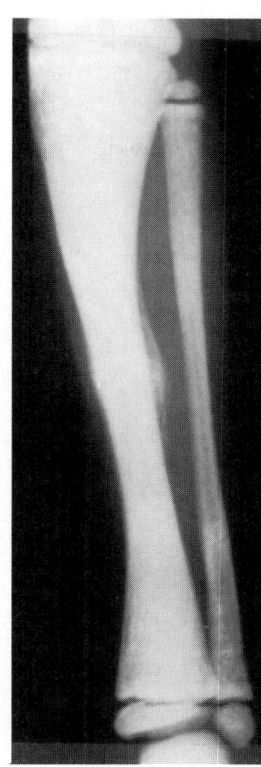

**Fig. 208-2** Anteroposterior radiographs of right tibia and fibula of case 2 at 2 years of age and left tibia and fibula of case 3 at age 6 years. Features of osteopetrosis include diffuse osteosclerosis with absence of medullary cavities and flared metaphyses containing transverse lines. Despite the increased bone density, healing fractures are evident in both radiographs.

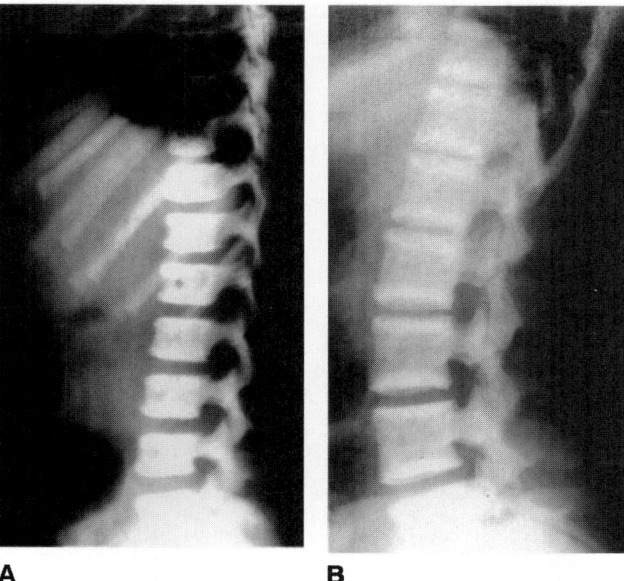

**A**  **B**

**Fig. 208-3** Patient 1, lumbar spine (lateral roentgenograms). *A*, Age 8 years. *B*, Age 25 years. Osteosclerosis diminished greatly. Persistent osteosclerosis at the vertebral end plates characterizes the "sandwich vertebrae" of osteopetrosis. (*From Whyte et al.*[9] *Used by permission.*)

Bone fractures are common in childhood in many patients, with some reporting 15 to 30 fractures by midadolescence.[6,9,36] After puberty, the frequency of bone fractures decreases. Fractures were the most prominent symptoms in the American patients[7] and the Belgian patient[6] in whom mental retardation was not present (Fig. 208-2). Fractures were not seen in Guibaud's patients who were of Arabic descent.[5]

The symptoms of cranial nerve compression secondary to osteopetrosis are milder than in the recessive, lethal form of osteopetrosis. However, the cranial nerve symptoms appear in 60 percent of reported patients.[27] Optic nerve pallor is common, but frank optic nerve atrophy is less frequent. Strabismus is also common, as is hearing impairment. Facial weakness has been noted in two reports.

## Renal Tubular Acidosis

Patients typically have metabolic acidosis, which varies considerably in type and severity in different pedigrees.[27] Metabolic acidosis was already present at 23 days of age in the first affected neonate.[26] Although one of the first patients reported had only proximal renal tubular acidosis, evidenced by low bicarbonate threshold, and had normal distal acidification,[5,27] most of the patients have a combination of proximal and distal renal tubular acidosis.[6,9,27,37,38,92] Of 26 patients in whom the renal lesion was characterized, it was believed that 5 had proximal, 5 had distal, and 12 had both proximal and distal components to their renal tubular acidosis.[26,92–94] Most patients had hyperchloremia, a normal anion gap, and inappropriately alkaline urine pH (>6.0). These findings are consistent with distal renal tubular acidosis.

Symptomatic hypokalemia has been observed in five patients.[9,27,92] Glomerular filtration rate is not reduced, and serum creatinine and blood urea nitrogen are not elevated. Recently, medullary nephrocalcinosis, which has not been described in association with CA II previously, was reported in one Kuwaiti patient. Another patient of the same ethnic background developed bilateral recurrent renal stones and hypercalciuria without nephrocalcinosis.[93] These abnormalities are isolated occurrences in children who are products of consanguineous marriages and are not considered part of the CA II deficiency syndrome. In fact, four recent reports have stressed the absence of hypercalciuria in CA II-deficient patients[6,38,103,104] and suggested that low serum calcium due to impairment in bone resorption may prevent hypercalciuria in patients with distal renal tubular acidosis secondary to CA II deficiency.

Most patients also have a reduced tubular maximum for bicarbonate. Although they usually have no bicarbonaturia when acidotic, they lose bicarbonate when plasma bicarbonate levels are raised to normal levels by loading. They do not have aminoaciduria, glycosuria, or any other manifestations of the Fanconi syndrome.

## Mental Retardation

The frequency and severity of mental retardation were not fully appreciated initially, because affected patients in two of the first four families recognized with this syndrome were not retarded.[6,7,9] However, over 90 percent of the patients reported to date have had significant mental retardation.[26,27,96,99–101] Even in the two families where intelligence was not below the normal range, some learning disabilities were observed. In most families, the mental retardation in affected patients has been severe enough to preclude education in regular schools.[27]

## Cerebral Calcification

Cerebral calcifications, evident by CT scans, were first reported by Ohlsson.[8] They were not present at birth, but appeared some time during the first decade (in one case, by 18 months).[5,25,27,105] Calcifications involved the caudate nucleus, putamen, and globus pallidus, and appeared peripherally in the periventricular and subcortical white matter (Fig. 208-4). The variability in the rate of progression of cerebral calcification in different patients has not been documented.

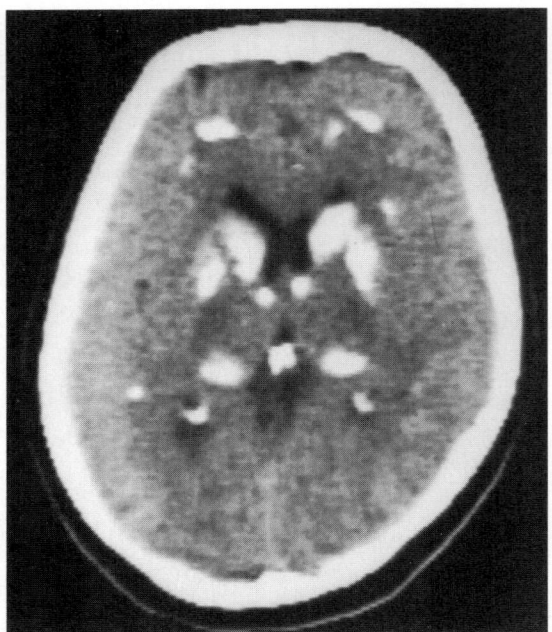

Fig. 208-4 CT scan of the head of patient 3 at 33 years of age. Scattered dense cerebral calcifications are especially prominent in the basal ganglia. (*From Sly et al.*[25] *Reprinted with permission.*)

### Growth Retardation

Growth retardation is nearly a constant finding. Almost all reported patients had short stature and many were underweight. Bone age was retarded, and corresponded to height age. Genu valgum is a common finding in older patients. At least part of the growth retardation is due to the chronic metabolic acidosis. Guibaud reported acceleration of growth following correction of the acidosis,[5] but later noted that growth retardation persisted, even after treatment.[27] Final height achieved by the patient who responded initially to correction of the acidosis was still nearly four standard deviations below normal.[5,27] Jandziszak et al. recently reported that growth hormone is low in male CA II-deficient mice, but not in females, and that long-term administration of growth hormone increases linear growth in CA II-deficient mice despite persistent acidosis.[106]

### Dental Malocclusion

Dentition was typically delayed and dental malocclusion was a prominent finding in affected patients from several families. Dental malalignment and malocclusion complicate dental hygiene, and dental caries may be severe.[9,26] Enamel hypoplasia has also been noted.[8,26]

### Other Features

Ohlsson[8,26] has reported a characteristic facies in the patients from Saudi Arabia that is present in many patients from other ethnic groups as well. These features include craniofacial disproportion with a prominent forehead and a large cranial vault relative to the size of the face. The mouth is small, and there is micrognathia. The nose is narrow, but prominent. The philtrum is short, the upper lip thin, and the lower lip thick. Squint is common and contributes to the unusual facies (Fig. 208-1).

Ohlsson et al.[26] reported findings of restrictive lung disease in two patients. Chest films showed no signs of parenchymal lung disease, but the rib cages were very dense.

Optic atrophy has been found in patients in whom the optic foramina were of normal size.[27] The mechanism of optic atrophy in these patients is unclear.

Hematologic disorders, including anemia, leukopenia, and thrombocytopenia, which are typically prominent in the recessive

malignant lethal form of osteopetrosis, are usually not seen in osteopetrotic patients with the CA II deficiency syndrome. However, anemia and hepatosplenomegaly were seen in three unrelated patients who were even considered candidates for bone marrow transplantation until the anemia and hepatosplenomegaly improved without treatment and the more benign course became apparent.

## PATHOLOGY

No autopsies have been reported on patients with the CA II deficiency syndrome. However, bone biopsies from iliac crest have been analyzed, and showed histologic features typical of osteopetrosis.[5,9,26] The cortical bone showed small Haversian systems widely separated from dense bone. The separation of cortical and cancellous was generally indistinct. Trabeculae were broad and irregular. Osteoid and normal-appearing osteoblasts were seen lining trabecular bone in several areas. On routine microscopy, osteoclast morphology was unremarkable. A minute sample of femoral cortex was obtained during open reduction of a femoral fracture. Osteoclasts were normal in appearance on light microscopy. Four osteoclasts were identified on electron microscopy, and showed a normal rim of cytoplasm adjacent to the bone surface. This "clear zone" was free of organelles. The osteoclasts appeared normal, although no "ruffled borders" were seen. In summary, the histologic findings of osteopetrosis were present, but no features appeared to distinguish the osteopetrosis of the CA II deficiency syndrome from other forms of osteopetrosis.

## PATHOGENESIS

### The Carbonic Anhydrase Gene Family

At least 11 enzymatically active CAs are recognized (referred to as CAs I, II, III, IV, VA, VB, VI, VII, IX, XII, and XIV). Several additional CA-related proteins that have complete CA domains but lack enzymatic activity because of amino acid substitutions in the active site have also been recognized. The active CAs differ considerably in tissue distribution, kinetic properties, and sensitivity to various inhibitors.

All active CAs catalyze the hydration of $CO_2$ to form bicarbonate and a proton. Considerable evidence suggests that the reaction involves two steps,[107] conversion of $CO_2$ to $HCO_3^-$, leaving $H_2O$ as a ligand on the zinc (equation 1), and transfer of proton to solvent buffer through a proton shuttle group, His64 (equation 2).

$$EZn\text{-}OH^- + CO_2 \leftrightarrow EZn\text{-}HCO_3^- \overset{+H_2O}{\leftrightarrow} EZn\text{-}H_2O + HCO_3^- \quad (1)$$

$$His64\text{-}EZn\text{-}H_2O \leftrightarrow H^+\text{-}His64\text{-}EZn\text{-}OH^- \overset{B}{\underset{BH}{\leftrightarrow}} His64\text{-}EZn\text{-}OH^- \quad (2)$$

In the first step shown in equation 1, the zinc-bound $OH^-$ adds to $CO_2$ to yield $HCO_3^-$ with a hydroxyl coordinated to the zinc. In the second step, displacement of the zinc-bound bicarbonate by a water molecule releases bicarbonate and restores zinc-bound water. The proton release reaction (equation 2), which is facilitated by His64, is the rate-limiting step for the high-activity isozymes like CA II.[108] The direction of the reaction in a given tissue or body fluid depends on the relative concentrations of $CO_2$, $HCO_3^-$, and $H^+$ ion, that is, the pH.

There is a distinctive membrane-bound CA in lung called CA IV,[40] which was shown to be identical to the membrane-bound CA in the brush border lining the lumen of the proximal tubules of the kidney.[41] The CA IV cDNA[42] and CA IV genomic organization[43] were recently reported. A distinct, secretory form of CA (CA VI) has been described in saliva of the rat,[44] human,[45] and sheep.[46] The amino acid sequence of the ovine salivary CA was recently reported and showed 33 percent sequence identity with ovine CA II, though residues involved in the active site were more highly conserved. The structure of the CA VI gene was recently published.[109] The low concentration of this isozyme in saliva is associated with prevalence of caries,[110] and it is also reported to protect gastroesophageal mucosa from acid injury.[111]

A distinct CA was reported in mitochondria in the liver and was designated CA V.[47] Since the recent report of another isozyme, CA VB, in the mitochondria of human[112] and mouse,[113] the isozyme previously designated CA V is renamed as CA VA. CA V (whether A or B is not yet established) has been shown to play a role in pyruvate decarboxylation in rat adipocytes[114] and in the regulation of glucose-stimulated insulin secretion by isolated rat islets.[115] The structure of mouse CA VA at 2.45 Å resolution[116] and its catalytic properties have been reported.[117] In addition, three membrane CAs, human CA IX[118] and CA XII,[119] as well as human[120] and mouse[121] CA XIV, were recently cloned and expressed. A role for CA IX and CA XII has been suggested in cancer because these two isozymes are up-regulated in certain forms of cancer, and CA XII has been shown to be regulated by von Hippel-Lindau tumor suppressor gene.[122]

### Chromosome Localization of CA Genes

Genetic and structural evidence suggests that the CA isozymes comprise a multilocus enzyme family derived from a common ancestral gene by gene duplications.[48] CAs I, II, and III are clustered at chromosome 8q22;[49] CA IV is assigned to 17q23;[43] and CA VI is assigned to 1p.[50] CA VA (previously CA V) is assigned to chromosome 16,[47] to which CA VII was previously mapped.[51] Newly reported mitochondrial CA VB is located on Xp22.1.[112] The chromosomal localization of CA IX is 17q21.2.[122] CA XII is mapped to chromosome 15q22.[119] CA XIV is located on chromosome 1q21.[120]

### Tissue Distribution and Properties of CA Isozymes

The kinetic parameters of the different isozymes, and their sensitivities to different inhibitors, as well as their tissue distributions, can differ markedly, indicating different physiological roles for the different isozymes.[52,53] The human CA II isozyme, whose turnover number for $CO_2$ hydration (1.3 to $1.9 \times 10^6$ sec$^{-1}$) is the highest known for any enzyme,[54,55] is widely distributed. It has been identified in erythrocytes, brain, eye, kidney, cartilage, liver, lung, skeletal muscle, pancreas, gastric mucosa, and anterior pituitary body.[39,56] The other isozymes, whose activities are lower than those of CA II, in the order CA II>CA IV>CA I>CA III>CA V, appear to have a more limited distribution.[47,57] CA I is found primarily in erythrocytes. CA III is found mainly in red skeletal muscle.[52,53] CA IV is expressed on the apical and basolateral surfaces of cells of the proximal tubule and thick ascending limb of the nephron,[41] and on the plasma face of certain endothelial surfaces including the pulmonary microvasculature,[58] the choriocapillaris,[59] and microcapillaries of brain,[60] heart, and skeletal muscle.[57,61]

CA VA is seen in liver and skeletal muscle by both western and northern blot analyses. The message for CA VA is also detectable in kidney.[113] The CA VB protein is present in heart, liver, lung, kidney, testis, and muscle, with a weaker band of the same size in other tissues. The CA VB transcripts are widely distributed with strongest signal seen in RNA from the kidney.[113] Both protein and RNA data show that CA VB is more widely distributed than CA VA. This observation suggests different physiological roles for the two mitochondrial CA isozymes. CA VI, the only secretory CA isozyme, is produced predominantly by serous acinar cells of submandibular and parotid glands.[123] Immunohistochemical studies show the presence of CA VI in the enamel pellicle.[124] In vitro studies document binding of CA VI to polished enamel. CA IX, one of the three newly discovered membrane CAs, has been found in several human carcinomas but not in corresponding normal tissues.[118,122,125] Besides stomach mucosa, basolateral surfaces of the enterocytes of duodenum and jejunum, as well as crypts of ileal mucosa, are the only normal tissues found so far to express CA IX.[118,126] The CA XII transcript has been reported in normal kidney and intestine.[119] However, in 10 percent of patients with renal cell carcinoma (RCC), the CA XII transcript was

expressed at much higher levels in RCC than in the normal surrounding kidney tissue. Ivanov et al.[122] showed high expression of CA XII in colon, kidney, and prostate; moderate expression in pancreas, testis, and ovary; and very low expression in lung and brain. Recently, CA XII was shown by immunocytochemistry to be present in normal human endometrial epithelium[127] and in normal human gut, as well as in colorectal tumors.[128] The association of CA IX and CA XII with carcinomas points to a potential role for these CA isozymes in proliferation and cancerous cell growth. CA XIV is most abundant in kidney and heart followed by skeletal muscle, brain, lung, and liver.[120,121] In situ hybridization shows that in the kidney the gene is expressed intensely in the proximal convoluted tubule, which is the major segment for bicarbonate resorption. The role of CA XIV in renal physiology remains to be established.

### The Biochemical Defect

In 1983, the three affected sisters reported initially by Sly et al.,[7] and described in detail by Whyte et al.,[9] were shown to have no detectable CA II activity in their erythrocytes.[24] CA I was present in near-normal levels. No immunoreactivity was detectable with specific antibody to CA II. The obligate heterozygote parents and several additional family members were found to have half-normal levels of CA II activity. These findings were subsequently extended to 110 similarly affected patients from mostly unrelated families of different geographic and ethnic origins. Every patient with osteopetrosis and renal tubular acidosis tested since has had undetectable levels of CA II activity.[25,27,91-101] Thus, there has been no exception to the finding of a quantitative defect in CA II in erythrocytes of patients with this syndrome.

Mutations in the structural gene for CA II (summarized below) have been found in all patients with CA II deficiency analyzed genetically.[63-65,91,95-101] Although the complete absence of CA II activity and immunoreactivity in erythrocytes are consistent findings in affected patients, it should be stressed that the residual activity in cells that continue to synthesize protein (such as osteoclasts in bone and cells in the proximal and distal tubules of the kidney) might be significantly higher than in erythrocytes. In fact, we suspect that some of the clinical heterogeneity in this syndrome may be explained by differences in residual CA II activity in bone and kidney in patients with different mutations in the structural gene for CA II.

### Pathophysiology

The finding of a quantitative defect in CA II in these patients provided an unusual opportunity to assess the function of this enzyme and to understand its importance for bone, brain, and kidney metabolism.

**Bone Metabolism.** All known forms of osteopetrosis involve the failure to resorb bone.[4] Studies showing inhibition of PTH-induced release of $Ca^{2+}$ from bone by CA inhibitors had suggested a role for CA in bone resorption.[15-17] Also, CA had been demonstrated histochemically in chick and hen osteoclasts[66] and CA II demonstrated immunohistochemically in rat[67] and human[15] osteoclasts. The osteopetrosis seen in patients with CA II deficiency provided genetic evidence for a role for CA in bone resorption, and specifically implicated the CA II isozyme.[24]

It had been suggested that CA aids the resorptive process by mediating the secretion of H$^+$.[16,67,129,130] We proposed that the role of CA II in acidifying the bone-resorbing component is an indirect one, analogous to its role in supporting the acidification of the lumen in the distal tubule of the kidney. It was recently suggested that the acidification of the bone-resorbing compartment is mediated by a proton-translocating ATPase,[68] which secretes protons into the lumen. This reaction would simultaneously generate an OH$^-$ ion in the cytoplasm for each H$^+$ translocated to the lumen. Titration of the OH$^-$ ions produced in the cytosol by CA II might be required to allow the proton-translocating ATPase to maintain the pH gradient (7.0 to 4.5) between the cytosol of the osteoclast and the bone-resorbing compartment. This could explain the pharmacologic evidence for a requirement for CA in bone resorption.[15-17] Because CA II is the only CA isozyme known to be expressed in osteoclasts,[67,68] it could also explain the osseous manifestations of CA II deficiency.

**Renal Tubular Acidosis.** Three things need explanation concerning renal metabolism in these patients. First, most CA II-deficient patients have both a proximal and a distal component to the renal tubular acidosis.[27] Second, some patients have predominantly proximal renal tubular acidosis, while in other patients, the distal renal tubular acidosis predominates.[27] Third, CA II-deficient patients have a nearly normal bicarbonaturia following ingestion or infusion of carbonic anhydrase inhibitors.[69] Some of these observations can be explained by a model in which the functions of CA II in the proximal and distal tubules are physiologically and biochemically distinct, and the major role of CA in bicarbonate reclamation is assigned not to CA II, but to CA IV, the luminal CA in the brush border of the proximal tubule.[70,71] CA IV is biochemically and immunologically distinct from CA II, and appeared to be normal in CA II-deficient patients[69] based on normal bicarbonaturia in response to infused acetazolamide. We demonstrated that the affected patients in the original American family with CA II deficiency have normal CA IV levels in their urinary membranes.[69a]

We deal first with the explanation for the proximal renal tubular acidosis. There is general agreement that renal reabsorption of bicarbonate is a major factor in acid-base homeostasis. Most of the bicarbonate reclamation takes place in the proximal tubule and is blocked by inhibitors of CA. However, two distinct CAs participate in bicarbonate reclamation by the proximal tubule, and they play separate roles in bicarbonate reclamation.

Bicarbonate reclamation depends on $H^+$ secretion, which is mediated primarily by $Na^+/H^+$ exchange in the proximal tubule but also by the $Mg^{2+}/H^+$-ATPase on the apical membrane.[72] The $H^+$ secreted into the lumen of the proximal tubule is titrated by the $HCO_3^-$ in the glomerular filtrate to produce $H_2CO_3$, which is in contact with the membrane-bound CA IV. The luminal CA IV catalyzes the dehydration of $H_2CO_3$ to $H_2O$ and $CO_2$.[73,74] The bicarbonaturia seen in response to infused acetazolamide in already acidotic CA II-deficient patients is attributed to inhibition of this luminal CA IV.[69]

The $CO_2$ produced by the CA IV-catalyzed reaction in the lumen diffuses freely into the cytosol of the proximal tubule. Here in the cytoplasm $CO_2$ encounters CA II which acts to hydrate the $CO_2$ to produce $H_2CO_3$, which dissociates spontaneously to $HCO_3^-$ and $H^+$. The $HCO_3^-$ generated from $CO_2$ in the cytosol is transported from the cytosol to the interstitial fluid or peritubular capillary by the Na-3HCO$_3$ cotransporter, completing the reclamation of the filtered bicarbonate. The $H^+$ regenerated in the cytosol by the CA II-catalyzed reaction can be secreted in exchange for $Na^+$ to initiate another round of $HCO_3^-$ reclamation.[72,74]

Thus, both the luminal CA IV and the cytosolic CA II participate in the reclamation of $HCO_3^-$ in the proximal tubule. The fact that CA II-deficient patients do not spill $HCO_3^-$ when acidotic suggests that CA II is not required for $HCO_3^-$ reclamation when patients have low bicarbonate loads, that is, when acidotic.[92] However, they have a lowered tubular maximum for bicarbonate and lose bicarbonate when the filtered load is increased by bicarbonate infusion or ingestion, indicating that CA II is required to regenerate $H^+$ for bicarbonate reclamation under normal bicarbonate loads. This requirement explains the proximal component of the renal tubular acidosis in CA II-deficient patients (Fig. 208-5A).

The prominent distal component of the renal tubular acidosis in most CA II-deficient patients, evidenced by inappropriately high urine pH values when patients are acidotic, suggests a need for CA II for distal acidification as well. This is consistent with the immunohistochemical evidence showing a much more intense

reaction for CA II in the distal tubule and the intercalated cells of the collecting ducts than in the proximal tubules.[71] Why is there normally such an abundance of CA II in the distal tubules, when most of the $HCO_3^-$ reclamation takes place in the proximal tubule? We suggest[69] that the explanation may be inferred from the analogous situation in the distal nephron and collecting system in the amphibian. In the turtle bladder, for example, the "CA-rich cells" are specialized cells that secrete $H^+$ and are capable of generating a steep pH gradient.[75,76] However, the acidification of the lumen is sensitive to inhibition by acetazolamide. It has been proposed that CA is needed in the amphibian nephron to titrate the $OH^-$ produced in the cytosol by the proton-translocating $Mg^{2+}$ ATPase. We have suggested a similar role for CA II in the distal tubule of the human kidney, that is, catalyzing the conversion of $OH^-$ and $CO_2$ to $HCO_3^-$.[69] Unless the $OH^-$ is titrated by $CO_2$, the proton-translocating ATPase cannot generate a pH gradient and acidify the lumen. The absence of CA II for this reaction in CA II-deficient patients can explain their defect in distal tubular acidification (Fig. 208-5B).

The third point, the basis for heterogeneity in the renal lesion in CA II deficiency, still requires explanation. Why is there variability in prominence of the proximal and distal lesions in different pedigrees? The explanation for this heterogeneity is still speculative. The different structural gene mutations producing CA II deficiency in different pedigrees may contribute to this heterogeneity in at least two ways. First, different mutations may affect the rate of enzyme turnover in proximal and distal tubular cells differentially, resulting in different levels of residual enzyme activity in the two different locations. Second, different structural gene mutations could affect the two different enzymatic activities in the two locations differentially. Thus, hydration of $CO_2$ to produce $H^+$ and $HCO_3^-$ in the proximal tubule and the condensation of $OH^-$ and $CO_2$ to produce $HCO_3^-$ in the distal tubule might be differentially affected by different mutations in the CA II gene. Continued delineation of the mutations in different CA II-deficient patients and studies of the enzyme produced after expression of the cloned mutant enzymes in prokaryotic and eukaryotic cells may allow one to test this hypothesis.

**Respiratory Acidosis.** Although not appreciated initially, Lien and Lai[102] pointed out that the acidosis in CA II deficiency has a respiratory component. They reported that CA II-deficient mice have a high arterial blood $PCO_2$, indicating failure of adequate compensation for metabolic acidosis. Furthermore, when the metabolic acidosis was corrected by $NaHCO_3$ infusion, the respiratory acidosis became more profound. They suggested that $CO_2$ retention in the animal was due to CA II deficiency in both erythrocytes and type II pneumocytes. Taki, Kato, and Yoshida[131] recently studied three patients with CA II deficiency and reported that all three have non-anionic gap metabolic acidosis due to renal losses of bicarbonate, but with virtually no compensatory reduction in $PCO_2$. Thus, impaired respiratory compensation for the metabolic acidosis due to $CO_2$ retention is a previously unrecognized component of the CA II deficiency syndrome, although it has not been associated with symptomatic respiratory distress.

## Brain Calcification and Cerebral Function

The mechanism of the cerebral calcification is unclear. CA II is primarily a glial enzyme that occurs predominantly in oligodendrocytes.[77] It is the only soluble carbonic anhydrase in brain homogenates. As much as 50 percent of the total CA II activity occurs in a membrane-bound or myelin-associated form.[78] The function of CA II in brain is not known. Morphologic changes in oligodendrocytes were reported in brains of CA II-deficient mice.[132] Whether the cerebral calcification in carbonic anhydrase II deficiency is a direct effect of the deficiency of CA II in the brain or an indirect effect—for example, of carbonic anhydrase deficiency in erythrocytes, or of chronic systemic acidosis—is not clear.

## Proximal Tubule

## Distal Tubule

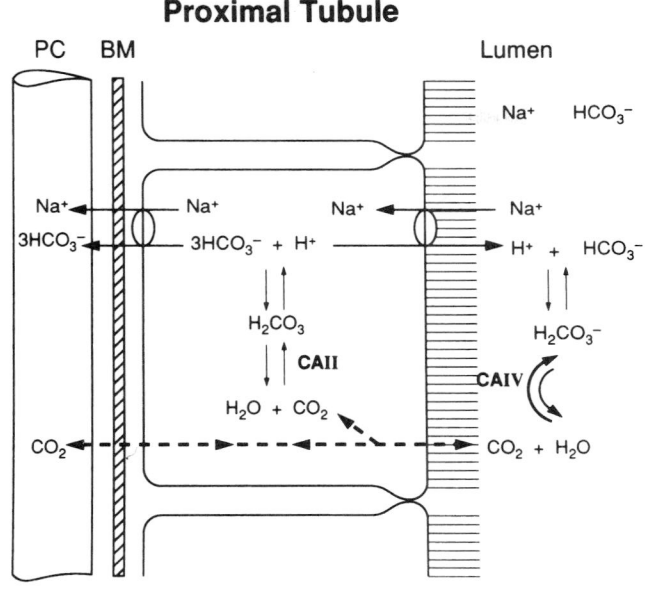

**Fig. 208-5** *A*, Proposed roles of carbonic anhydrases in bicarbonate reclamation in the proximal tubule. $Na^+$ and $HCO_3^-$ enter the lumen of the proximal tubule. $H^+$ is secreted in exchange for $Na^+$, and $H^+$ and $HCO_3^-$ are converted to $CO_2$ and $H_2O$ in a reaction catalyzed by the luminal CA (CA IV). We propose that this enzyme functions normally in CA II-deficient patients, and that its inhibition explains the positive response to acetazolamide (normal bicarbonate diuresis). $CO_2$ diffuses freely into the proximal tubular cell (and across the basement membrane [BM] and into the peritubular capillary [PC]), and is exposed to cytosolic CA II which catalyzes its rehydration to form $HCO_3^-$ and $H^+$. $3HCO_3^-$ is cotransported with $1Na^+$ by the basolateral cotransporter from the contraluminal surface of the proximal tubular cell to the peritubular capillary [PC]. The $H^+$

generated by CA II is secreted in exchange for $Na^+$ to initiate another cycle of $HCO_3^-$ reabsorption. Loss of CA II-mediated regeneration of $H^+$ is suggested as the cause of $HCO_3^-$ wasting in CA II-deficient patients. *B*, Proposed role of CA II in distal urinary acidification. The $H^+$ is secreted into the lumen by a proton-translocating $Mg^{++}$ ATPase, as in amphibians, which produces $OH^-$ in the cytosol. $CO_2$ can condense with $OH^-$ to form $HCO_3^-$ in a CA II-catalyzed reaction, and $HCO_3^-$ can be transported across the basement membrane and into the peritubular capillary. We suggest that failure to titrate the $OH^-$ limits the ability to secrete $H^+$ and acidify the urine appropriately in CA II-deficient patients. (*From Sly et al.*[69] *Used by permission.*)

While brain development and central nervous system function are not profoundly deranged in patients with this syndrome, psychomotor delay, learning disabilities, and even mental retardation are evident in most affected patients.[27] The mental retardation was not so obvious in the initial reports of patients with CA II deficiency syndrome, but it is now clear that over 90 percent of the reported patients have mental retardation severe enough to prevent school attendance. Whether this is a direct consequence of the CA II deficiency, or an indirect effect, is not yet clear.

Although CA II is the only soluble CA expressed in brain, CA IV is expressed on the plasma face of cerebral capillaries and anchored to the capillary membrane by a glycosylphosphoinositol linkage.[60]

### Growth Failure

Growth failure appears to result from the combined effects of the osteopetrosis on bone elongation, and of the chronic metabolic acidosis on general health. Correction of the acidosis has been followed by a growth spurt in one patient,[27] but the dramatic reduction in final height achieved by this patient makes it clear that the growth retardation is not due to the acidosis alone.

## GENETICS

### Inheritance

The CA II deficiency syndrome is inherited as an autosomal recessive trait. Affected patients are offspring of normal-appearing heterozygote carrier parents who have half-normal levels of CA II in their erythrocyte lysates. Heterozygotes have no symptoms and

no signs of the disorder. Males and females are affected with equal frequency and severity. Consanguinity is very common (87 percent) in parents of affected offspring.[27]

The geographic distribution of this syndrome is striking, with more than half the known cases observed in families from Kuwait, Saudi Arabia, and North Africa.[25,96,99–101] This probably results from both an increased frequency of the carbonic anhydrase II deficiency allele in these regions and an increased frequency of consanguineous marriages, particularly in the Bedouin tribes from which many of these patients originated.

### Molecular Genetics

In humans, the CA I, II, and III genes (CA1, CA2, CA3) are clustered within approximately 180 kb on chromosome 8q22.[48] The entire 20-kb CA II gene has been cloned and the intron/exon organization determined[63,64] (Fig. 208-6). The human CA II gene contains seven exons, as does the mouse gene, and intron/exon junctions 2 to 7 are conserved in all human CAs so far examined. The 5′ flanking region of the human CA II gene contains a TATA box and a possible CAAT box. It also contains nine potential Sp1 binding sites. Deletion analysis of the human 5′ promoter region showed a gradual but differential loss in promoter activity with loss of Sp1 binding sites.[79]

The full-length human cDNA has been expressed in both prokaryotic and eukaryotic cells. Although mRNA from CA II-deficient patients could not be easily obtained, knowledge of the genomic organization and of intronic sequences surrounding each exon has made mutational analysis on patient genomic DNA straightforward. Sixteen different mutations have been identified so far in CA II-deficient patients (Fig. 208-6).

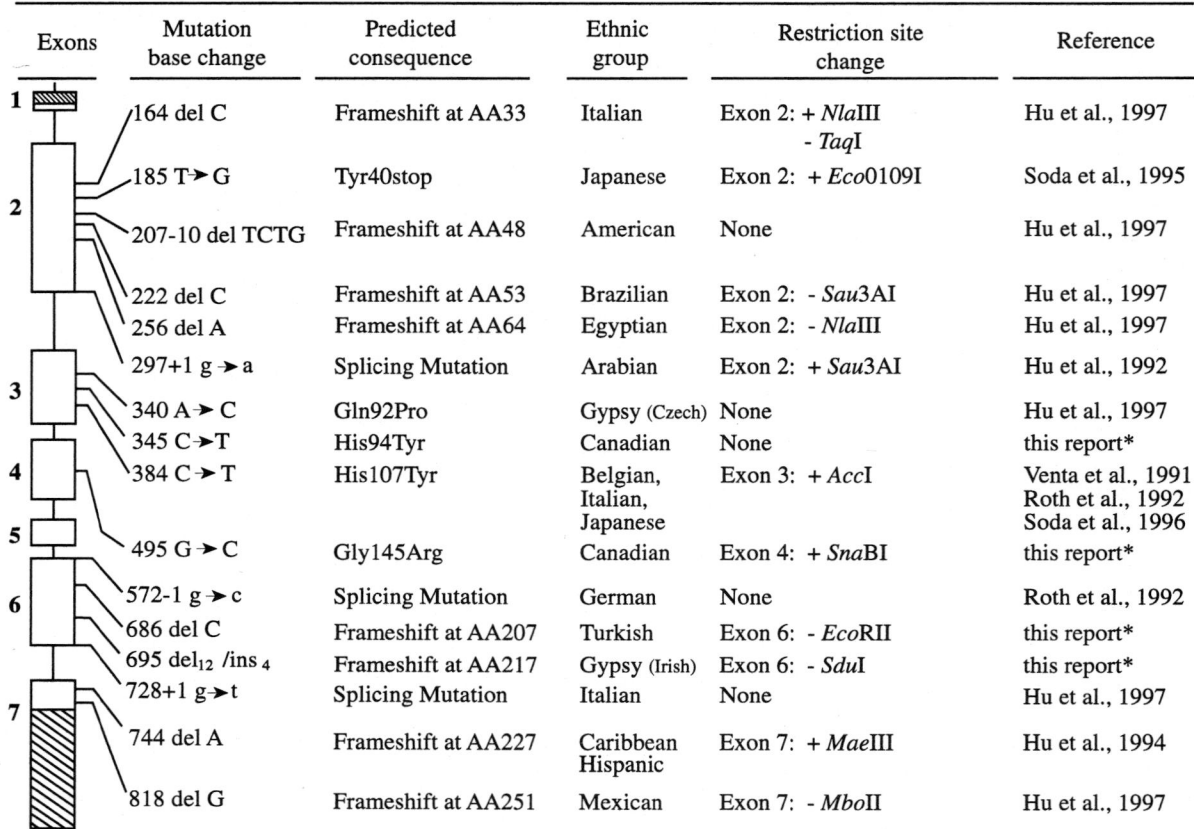

| Exons | Mutation base change | Predicted consequence | Ethnic group | Restriction site change | Reference |
|---|---|---|---|---|---|
| 1 | 164 del C | Frameshift at AA33 | Italian | Exon 2: + NlaIII − TaqI | Hu et al., 1997 |
| 2 | 185 T→G | Tyr40stop | Japanese | Exon 2: + Eco0109I | Soda et al., 1995 |
| | 207-10 del TCTG | Frameshift at AA48 | American | None | Hu et al., 1997 |
| | 222 del C | Frameshift at AA53 | Brazilian | Exon 2: − Sau3AI | Hu et al., 1997 |
| | 256 del A | Frameshift at AA64 | Egyptian | Exon 2: − NlaIII | Hu et al., 1997 |
| 3 | 297+1 g→a | Splicing Mutation | Arabian | Exon 2: + Sau3AI | Hu et al., 1992 |
| | 340 A→C | Gln92Pro | Gypsy (Czech) | None | Hu et al., 1997 |
| | 345 C→T | His94Tyr | Canadian | None | this report* |
| 4 | 384 C→T | His107Tyr | Belgian, Italian, Japanese | Exon 3: + AccI | Venta et al., 1991 Roth et al., 1992 Soda et al., 1996 |
| 5 | 495 G→C | Gly145Arg | Canadian | Exon 4: + SnaBI | this report* |
| 6 | 572-1 g→c | Splicing Mutation | German | None | Roth et al., 1992 |
| | 686 del C | Frameshift at AA207 | Turkish | Exon 6: − EcoRII | this report* |
| | 695 del₁₂ /ins₄ | Frameshift at AA217 | Gypsy (Irish) | Exon 6: − SduI | this report* |
| | 728+1 g→t | Splicing Mutation | Italian | None | Hu et al., 1997 |
| 7 | 744 del A | Frameshift at AA227 | Caribbean Hispanic | Exon 7: + MaeIII | Hu et al., 1994 |
| | 818 del G | Frameshift at AA251 | Mexican | Exon 7: − MboII | Hu et al., 1997 |

**Fig. 208-6 Sixteen structural gene mutations in CA II-deficient patients.** The human CA II gene contains seven exons and six introns. Exons 1 through 6 and coding region of exon 7 can be PCR amplified with the primers described recently.[101] Direct sequencing of each exon, in both directions, can be accomplished by using the same primers. Eleven of the 16 reported mutations either create or destroy restriction enzyme sites in various exons. Digestion of PCR-amplified exons with the appropriate restriction enzyme followed by agarose gel electrophoresis enables accurate diagnosis of these mutations.[63,65,80,100] The remaining five mutations neither introduce nor remove any restriction sites. In such cases, diagnosis can be made by PCR amplification and direct sequencing of appropriate exons.[101] In the right-hand column, "this report*" refers to reference 101.

The first mutation was identified in a Belgian patient with a C to T transition in exon 3, which results in replacement of the conserved histidine at position 107 with tyrosine (His 107 → Tyr).[63] The three affected sisters in the American family in which CA II deficiency was first reported were also found to have this mutation. However, they were compound heterozygotes, having inherited the His 107 → Tyr mutation from their mother and a splice acceptor mutation in the 3′ end of intron 5 from their father.[64] Neither the Belgian patient nor the American patients were mentally retarded. Frequent skeletal fractures were the most disabling manifestation of their disease.[28] When the CA II cDNA containing the His 107 → Tyr mutation was expressed in E. coli, the activity of the mutant protein was drastically reduced compared to that of the normal enzyme.[133] However, residual activity could be easily demonstrated in cells induced at 30°C and 20°C where a larger fraction of the expressed enzyme remained soluble (80 percent at 20°C).[63] These experiments suggested that a small amount of residual CA II activity in patients with the His 107 → Tyr mutation may allow them to escape mental retardation.[64]

The third structural gene mutation identified is a splice junction mutation at the 5′ end of intron 2, which was found in patients of Arabic descent from Kuwait, Saudi Arabia, Algeria, and Tunisia.[65,96,99–101] About 65 percent of all patients so far reported were Arabic and were severely affected. Mental retardation and metabolic acidosis were prominent in these patients, while bone fractures were less frequent.[28,65,91–93,99–101]

A novel frameshift mutation resulting from a single-base deletion in the coding region of exon 7 was found in a mildly affected Hispanic girl, who is the first patient reported with no renal tubular acidosis.[80] This single-base deletion results in a frameshift at codon 227 that changes the next 12 amino acids and introduces a UGA stop codon at codon 239. The truncated enzyme resulting from this mutation is 22 amino acids shorter than the 260 amino acids in normal CA II. When expressed in bacteria, the mutant allele produced 0.07 percent of the activity expressed by the normal allele. Unexpectedly, this mutant enzyme activity was not due to the truncated form of the mutant enzyme (27 kDa), but to a small fraction of near-normal size enzyme (29 kDa) which had about 10 percent of normal specific activity. Protein sequencing showed that the first 11 amino acids were abnormal in the 29-kDa mutant protein, as predicted by the frameshift, after which the reading frame was restored. The last 23 amino acids of the 29-kDa mutant protein were the same as in normal CA II. These results can be explained by a ribosomal -1 translational frameshift that restores the reading frame 11 codons after the original mutation and allows completion of full-length CA II.[134] Subsequently, patients referred from seven independent Hispanic families, some having severe clinical manifestations including severe renal tubular acidosis, anemia, and hepatosplenomegaly, were found by sequencing or restriction site analysis to be homozygous for the same mutation. The basis for the wide clinical variability in these patients is unclear. However, these findings raise the possibility that individual variation in efficiency of frameshift suppression may contribute to clinical heterogeneity among patients with identical frameshift mutations.

The fifth reported mutation was a nonsense mutation in exon 2 (Tyr 40 → stop) in a Japanese patient who exhibited severe mental retardation with the other features of CA II deficiency syndrome.[95]

Of the seven novel mutations reported subsequently in 1997,[100] four were deletions in exon 2. Single-bp deletions 164delC, 222delC, and 256delA were found in Italian, Belgian, and Egyptian patients, respectively. A 4-bp deletion, 207-10delTCTG, was observed in an American patient. These four deletions are predicted to cause early frameshifts at amino acids 33, 53, 64, and 48, and, in all cases, early termination of translation. Expression of two of these deletion mutations, 164delC and 222delC, in *E. coli* produced no CA activity and no detectable truncated products. Such upstream frameshifts and early terminations would predict severe clinical phenotypes for patients carrying these mutations. The phenotypes of the three patients with a single-bp deletion and the patient with the 4-bp deletion in exon 2 were indeed severe. All four patients exhibited osteopetrosis, renal tubular acidosis, and cerebral calcification in addition to mental retardation and developmental delay.

A splice junction mutation at the 5′ end of exon 6 was found in an Italian patient. This mutation also predicts a severe clinical consequence, since translation will proceed into the intron and terminate in exon 6 after translation of 24 missense amino acids. The predicted mutant protein should lack the entire 39 normal amino acid sequence at the C-terminus, which includes 13 residues conserved in all human CAs. Surprisingly, the clinical symptoms of this patient were relatively mild;[135] they included failure to thrive and hepatosplenomegaly in the first 4 months of life and a delayed psychomotor development soon afterward. At age 3 years, mild mental retardation, mild hyperchloremic (normal anion gap) acidosis with increased urine pH, generalized osteopetrosis, and scattered dense cerebral calcification (especially in basal ganglia) were reported. This milder phenotype might be attributed to residual activity of the abnormal CA II protein, but no studies have been done to test this hypothesis.

An A → C transversion at codon 92 that results in a replacement of a conserved glutamine with proline was found in a Gypsy patient from Czechoslovakia. This patient also had a severe clinical phenotype, according to the referring physician.

A single-bp deletion (818delG) at codon 251 was found in a pair of Mexican siblings. The two brothers, both homozygous for the 818delG mutation, have an unusual phenotype in that mental retardation is severe, but renal tubular acidosis is absent.[136] The elder brother was reported to have multiple fractures at the age of 8 years and the younger was diagnosed with osteopetrosis at the age of 2 years. Studies have yet to be done to characterize the residual activity and other properties of 818delG mutant protein.

Four additional novel mutations were recently identified in three families of different ethnic backgrounds.[101] The first mutation, detected in an Irish-Gypsy patient, was a del$_{12}$/ins$_4$ mutation in exon 6. Twelve bp (GCTCAAGGAACC), ranging from nucleotide 696 to nucleotide 707, are deleted and are replaced by four nucleotides (CACA). This del$_{12}$/ins$_4$ mutation causes a frameshift in codon 211 leading to a stop after 13 missense amino acids. The resulting protein lacks 37 amino acids at the C-terminus. This patient was reported to have osteopetrosis, renal tubular acidosis, and developmental delay but no mental retardation.

Another novel mutation, a single-bp deletion in exon 6, was identified in a Turkish family. A cytosine at position 686 was deleted (686delC), causing a +1 frameshift in codon 208 and incorporation of 15 missense amino acids before a stop codon. Thus, the predicted mutant protein would not only contain abnormal amino acids from position 208 to 222, but the early termination would result in a protein another 37 amino acids shorter than the normal CA II. The two affected siblings of this Turkish family, who were products of a consanguineous marriage, were severely retarded and showed other typical symptoms of CA II deficiency syndrome.

The remaining two mutations, which bring the total number of known mutations in the CA II gene to 16, were both identified in

the same Canadian family. Both are missense mutations. The paternal mutation, a C → T transition at nucleotide 345, changes an active site histidine to a tyrosine at codon 94 (His 94 → Tyr). In the mother, a nonconserved glycine at codon 145 was changed to an arginine (Gly 145 → Arg) due to a G → C transversion at nucleotide 495. Both affected sons were compound heterozygotes for His 94 → Tyr and Gly 145 → Arg mutations. When the His 94 → Tyr and Gly 145 → Arg mutations were introduced separately in human CA II cDNAs and expressed in *E. coli*, both mutant cDNAs expressed immunologically detectable products. No detectable CA II activity was observed in the Gly 145 → Arg mutant protein. Some sodium iodide-resistant and acetazolamide-inhibitable residual activity (0.24 percent of normal level) was observed in the His94Tyr mutant protein. These patients showed osteopetrosis, renal tubular acidosis, and developmental delay, but no obvious mental retardation. The residual activity provided by the His94Tyr mutant enzyme might explain the absence of mental retardation in these patients.

## DIAGNOSIS

Clinically, CA II deficiency should be suspected in any newborn infant with metabolic acidosis and failure to thrive, especially if the urine pH is alkaline. Osteopetrosis may not be present initially, but usually develops over the first year of life. If osteopetrosis and renal tubular acidosis coexist, the diagnosis is virtually certain. No patient with this combination has yet been found who does not have CA II deficiency. Cerebral calcification, evident by CT scan, is usually present by the end of the first decade.

Enzymatic confirmation can be made by quantitating the CA II level in erythrocyte lysates.[81,82] A relatively easy assay has been described which allows one to quantitate both CA I and CA II levels. This method takes advantage of the large difference in sensitivity of CA I and CA II to inhibition by sodium iodide. Normally, CA I and CA II each contribute about 50 percent of the total activity, and the CA I activity is virtually completely abolished by inclusion of 8 mM sodium iodide in the assay. One simply measures the total activity (CA I + CA II) as well as the activity seen in the presence of 8 mM sodium iodide (CA II). Patients with CA II deficiency have no iodide-resistant enzyme (i.e., no CA II). Obligate heterozygotes have about half-normal levels of iodide-resistant activity. Other assays have been described including staining of individual isozymes following electrophoresis, quantitation of CA I/CA II ratios by high-pressure liquid chromatography, and immunologic identification of the isozymes on immunodiffusion with specific antisera.[24]

Simple and accurate techniques for the identification of the structural gene mutations underlying CA II deficiency have been developed that are useful for diagnosis, genetic counseling, and prenatal diagnosis, and also for carrier detection in certain populations. As shown in Fig. 208-6, 11 of the 16 mutations in the CA II gene introduce new restriction sites or remove restriction sites present in normal CA II alleles. The Arabic mutation introduces an extra *Sau*3AI site in exon 2, the His 107 → Tyr mutation creates a new *Acc*I site in exon 3, and the Hispanic mutation creates an additional *Mae*III site in exon 7. The single-bp deletions in exon 2, 164delC and 222delC, create an *Nla*III and a *Sau*3AI restriction site in exon 2, respectively. The 256delA mutation removes an *Nla*III site.

The missense Tyr 40 → stop mutation creates an *Eco*0109I site in exon 2. The Gly 145 → Arg, the only mutation identified in exon 4, creates a *Sna*BI restriction site. Of the two frameshift mutations in exon 6, one, 686delC, removes an *Eco*RII site and the second, 695del$_{12}$/ins$_4$, creates an *Sdu*I restriction site. A single-bp deletion 818delG removes an *Mbo*II site in exon 7. Digestion of PCR-amplified genomic DNA fragments with the appropriate restriction enzymes followed by agarose gel electrophoresis allows one to make accurate diagnoses of all these mutations.[63,65,80,101] Mutations that do not create or destroy any restriction sites include the 4-bp deletion (207-10delTCTG in exon 2), two nonsense mutations (Gln 92 → Pro and His 94 → Tyr), and a splice-junction mutation at the 3' end of intron 5. In these cases, PCR amplification and direct sequencing of the appropriate exons provide a reliable two-step method of distinguishing patients, carriers, and normal individuals. This method works for prenatal diagnosis as well.[101]

## GENETIC COUNSELING

The appropriate counseling for an autosomal recessive trait is indicated. First-degree relatives can be tested for heterozygosity. Because the osteopetrosis does not appear prenatally, the diagnosis cannot be made in the fetus radiologically or by ultrasound. Carbonic anhydrase levels in erythrocytes are normally extremely low at birth, and it is unlikely that CA II deficiency could be diagnosed by measuring CA II activity in samples of fetal blood. However, prenatal diagnosis is reliable using the techniques described above under DNA diagnosis.

## TREATMENT

No specific treatment for CA II deficiency is available. Treatment for the metabolic acidosis is recommended, at least until after adolescence.[27] It appears that the renal tubular acidosis may stabilize at a milder level after puberty. Frequent fractures require conventional orthopedic management. Bone healing is usually normal. Most patients require special education because of mental retardation. There is no specific treatment for the cranial nerve abnormalities, which may lead to impaired vision, hearing deficits, and facial nerve weakness. Attention to dental hygiene is important because of the susceptibility to caries.

In the early course of the initial American family, treatment with bicarbonate was withheld for fear that the acidosis may be compensating for the osteopetrosis, and that treatment of the acidosis might aggravate the osteopetrosis with further loss of vision and hearing. However, prolonged treatment of several patients by Dr. Guibaud and colleagues appeared to have a beneficial effect on general health without any marked progression of the osteopetrosis and with no aggravation of cranial nerve symptoms.[27] It is not clear whether the development of cerebral calcification is influenced by correction of the acidosis.

Bone marrow transplantation is not usually indicated, because the hematologic manifestations for which this is usually considered appropriate in the infantile, recessive lethal form of osteopetrosis[34] are usually not present in the CA II deficiency syndrome. On the other hand, the bone manifestations should theoretically improve following bone marrow transplantation, because CA II-containing osteoclasts would be provided by stem cells from the donor marrow. However, the renal insufficiency will not improve. This was actually the observation reported in the first patient transplanted for osteopetrosis who, in retrospect, appears to have had CA II deficiency.[33] Currently, the positive improvements in the skeleton do not seem to warrant the risks and morbidity of bone marrow transplantation.

We had the opportunity to replace the CA II-deficient red cells with CA II-replete blood cells following severe uterine hemorrhage in one of the patients we followed.[83] Raising the circulating erythrocyte levels of CA II to the heterozygote range by transfusion with replete erythrocytes had no effect on plasma pH or urine pH. These observations supported the proposal that the metabolic acidosis is due to the renal CA II deficiency, and not a secondary consequence of CA II deficiency in erythrocytes.

Recently, it was shown that CA II-deficient male mice have low levels of growth hormone,[106] and long-term administration of the recombinant growth hormone to these mice caused an increase in linear growth despite persistent acidosis. In another recent report, Lai et al.[137] showed that liposome-mediated gene therapy on CA II-deficient mice with the human CA II gene substantially corrects renal tubular acidosis for up to 3 weeks. They suggest that with further refinements gene therapy can be used as a treatment for

hereditary renal tubular acidosis in humans. However, there are no reports of either growth hormone administration or gene therapy in humans for treatment of CA II deficiency syndrome.

## FUTURE PROSPECTS

Delineation of the molecular defect has made prenatal diagnosis possible in many families. The PCR-based RFLP analysis may be practical in population-based screening in certain restricted populations. Perhaps the clearest example is that of the Arabic mutation which accounts for more than 75 percent of cases reported to date. Using the PCR-based RFLP analysis, Fathallah et al. found that every affected member in 14 families in Tunisia had this mutation.[32] In families where the mutation has not been established, PCR amplification and direct sequencing of various exons can readily detect novel mutations.[101] This technique can be successfully used for prenatal diagnosis as well.

Another potentially important development is the description of a mouse with CA II deficiency.[84] The mutation was produced intentionally by exposing mice that were heterozygotes for electrophoretically distinguishable CA II gene products to a powerful mutagen and screening progeny electrophoretically for loss of one of the alleles. A null mutation was found, and a breeding colony established. The affected mouse has severe acidosis, but has not been found to have osteopetrosis or cerebral calcification. Although this animal model lacks some of the components of the human CA II deficiency syndrome, it is certain to be a profitable model for studying many facets of $CO_2$ and $HCO_3^-$ metabolism, and for studying certain experimental therapies like bone marrow replacement and gene therapy.

Finally, the remarkable utility of this human disease in shedding light on the physiological roles of the various carbonic anhydrases should stimulate clinical research aimed at identifying disorders due to deficiencies of other members of the CA gene family.[56] An inherited deficiency of CA I has already been found, and proved to have no clinical consequences.[56] This presumably reflects the fact that CA I is expressed primarily in the erythrocytes and CA II, which is expressed at normal levels in CA I-deficient patients, could more than handle the requirements for CA activity in the erythrocytes.[55] It seems possible that deficiencies for CAs III, IV, VA, VB, VI, VII, IX, XII, and XIV would produce significant clinical abnormalities. Such experiments of nature probably exist, and once they are identified, they will likely add greatly to our understanding of why we have evolved so many isozymes to catalyze a reaction as simple as the reversible hydration of $CO_2$.

## IMPLICATIONS FOR OSTEOPOROSIS

By now, there is considerable histochemical, pharmacologic, and genetic evidence that CA II plays an important role in the generation of hydrogen ion gradients, and is required for the normal function of osteoclasts in bone resorption.[85] Although osteopetrosis results from a defect in bone resorption, there are other metabolic disorders in which the reverse is true, and accelerated bone loss is the problem. Can one take advantage of the dependence on CA in the process of bone resorption to inhibit accelerated bone loss? A number of organ culture systems have been developed to study bone resorption.[55,86,87] In organ culture, $Ca^{2+}$ release from bones was shown to be hormone responsive (parathormone and dibutyryl cyclic AMP) and sensitive to inhibition by acetazolamide and other inhibitors of CA.[87-89] Animal studies have suggested that bone loss associated with disuse can be partially prevented by CA inhibitors.[90] This observation raises hope that CA inhibitors might have a role in treating common causes of bone loss like osteoporosis. One problem, however, is that chronic administration of currently available agents produces a systemic acidosis due to their actions on the kidney, and systemic acidosis itself can lead to calcium mobilization from bone. It has been suggested[87] that development of effective inhibitors that might be useful in metabolic bone disease may require development of agents that act selectively on CA II in bone, or that can be selectively targeted to bone resorbing osteoclasts to avoid inhibition of CA II in kidney and other sites.

# REFERENCES

1. Albers-Schönberg H: Rontgenbilder einer seltenen, Knochenerkrankung. *Muench Med Wochenschr* **51**:365, 1904.
2. Johnston CC Jr, Lavy N, Lord T, Vellios F, Merritt AD, Deiss WP Jr: Osteopetrosis: A clinical, genetic, metabolic, and morphologic study of the dominantly inherited, benign form. *Medicine (Baltimore)* **47**:149, 1968.
3. Beighton P, Hamersma H, Cremin BJ: Osteopetrosis in South Africa: The benign, lethal and intermediate forms. *S Afr Med J* **55**:659, 1979.
4. Marks SC Jr: Morphological evidence of reduced bone resorption in osteopetrotic (op) mice. *Am J Anat* **163**:157, 1982.
5. Guibaud P, Larbre F, Freycon M-T, Genoud J: Osteopetrose et acidose renale tubulaire: Deux cas de cette association dans une fratrie. *Arch Fr Pediatr* **29**:269, 1972.
6. Vainsel M, Fondu P, Cadranel S, Rocmans C, Gepts W: Osteopetrosis associated with proximal and distal tubular acidosis. *Acta Paediatr Scand* **61**:429, 1972.
7. Sly WS, Lang R, Aviolo L, Haddad J, Lubowitz H, McAlister W: Recessive osteopetrosis: New clinical phenotype. *Am J Hum Genet* **24(Suppl)**:34a, 1972.
8. Ohlsson A, Stark G, Sakati N: Marble brain disease: Recessive osteopetrosis, renal tubular acidosis and cerebral calcification in three Saudi Arabian families. *Dev Med Child Neurol* **22**:72, 1980.
9. Whyte MP, Murphy WA, Fallon MD, Sly WS, Teitelbaum SL, MacAlister WH, Avioli LV: Osteopetrosis, renal tubular acidosis and basal ganglia calcification in three sisters. *Am J Med* **69**:65, 1980.
10. Tashian RE: Evolution and regulation of the carbonic anhydrase isozymes, in Rattazzi MC, Scandalios JG, Whitt GS (eds): *Isozymes: Current Topics in Biological and Medical Research*, vol. 2. New York, Alan R. Liss, 1977, p 21.
11. Tashian RE, Hewett-Emmett D, Goodman M: On the evolution and genetics of carbonic anhydrases I, II, and III, in Rattazzi MC, Scandalios JG, Whitt GS (eds): *Isozymes: Current Topics in Biological and Medical Research*, vol. 7. New York, Alan R. Liss, 1983, p 79.
12. Maren TH: Carbonic anhydrase: Chemistry, physiology and inhibition. *Physiol Rev* **47**:595, 1967.
13. Lindskog S, Henderson LE, Kannan KK, Liljas A, Nyman PO, Strandberg B: Carbonic anhydrase, in Boyer PD (ed): *The Enzymes*. New York, Academic Press, 1971, p 587.
14. Pocker Y, Sarkanen SLL: Carbonic anhydrase: Structure, catalytic versatility, and inhibition. *Adv Enzymol* **47**:149, 1978.
15. Waite LC, Volkert WA, Kenny AD: Inhibition of bone resorption by acetazolamide in the rat. *Endocrinology* **87**:1129, 1970.
16. Waite LC: Carbonic anhydrase inhibitors, parathyroid hormone and calcium metabolism. *Endocrinology* **91**:1160, 1972.
17. Minkin C, Jennings J: Carbonic anhydrase and bone remodeling: Sulfonamide inhibition of bone resorption in organ culture. *Science* **176**:1031, 1972.
18. Kumpulainen T, Nystrom, SHM: Immunohistochemical localization of carbonic anhydrase isozyme C in human brain. *Brain Res* **220**:220, 1981.
19. Vogh BP: The relation of choroid plexus carbonic anhydrase activity to cerebrospinal fluid formation: Study of three inhibitors in cat with extrapolation to man. *J Pharmacol Exp Ther* **213**:321, 1980.
20. Nair V, Bau D: Studies on the functional significance of carbonic anhydrase in central nervous system. *Brain Res* **31**:185, 1971.
21. Wistrand PJ: Human renal cytoplasmic carbonic anhydrase. Tissue levels and kinetic properties under near physiological conditions. *Acta Physiol Scand* **109**:239, 1980.
22. Dobyan DC, Bulger RE: Renal carbonic anhydrase. *Am J Physiol* **243**:F311, 1982.
23. Kendall AG, Tashian RE: Erythrocyte carbonic anhydrase I: Inherited deficiency in humans. *Science* **197**:471, 1977.
24. Sly WS, Hewett-Emmett D, Whyte MP, Yu Y-SL, Tashian RE: Carbonic anhydrase II deficiency identified as the primary defect in the autosomal recessive syndrome of osteopetrosis with renal tubular acidosis and cerebral calcification. *Proc Natl Acad Sci U S A* **80**:2752, 1983.
25. Sly WS, Whyte MP, Sundaram V, Tashian RE, Hewett-Emmett D, Guibaud P, Vainsel M, Baluarte HJ, Gruskin A, Al-Mosawi M, Sakati

N, Ohlsson A: Carbonic anhydrase II deficiency in 12 families with the autosomal recessive syndrome of osteopetrosis with renal tubular acidosis and cerebral calcification. *N Engl J Med* **313**:139, 1985.
26. Ohlsson A, Cumming WA, Paul A, Sly WS: Carbonic anhydrase II deficiency syndrome: Recessive osteopetrosis with renal tubular acidosis and cerebral calcification. *Pediatrics* **77**:371, 1986.
27. Cochat P, Loras-Duclaux I, Guibaud P: Deficit en anhydrase carbonique II: Osteopetrose, acidose renale tubulaire et calcifications intracraniennes. Revue de la literature a partir de trois observations. *Pediatrie* **42**:121, 1987.
28. Strisciuglio P, Sartorio R, Pecoraro C, Lotito F, Sly WS: Variable clinical presentation of carbonic anhydrase deficiency: Evidence for heterogeneity? *Eur J Pediatr* **149**:337, 1990.
29. Bejaoui M, Kamoun A, Baraket M, Bourguiba H, Lakhoua R: Le syndrome associant: Osteopetrose, acidose tubulaire, retard mental et calcifications intracraniennes par deficit en anhydrase carbonique II. *Arch Fr Pediatr* **48**:211, 1991.
30. Schwartz GJ, Brion LP, Corey HE, Dorfman HD: Case report 668. Carbonic anhydrase II deficiency syndrome (osteopetrosis associated with renal tubular acidosis and cerebral calcification). *Skeletal Radiol* **20**:447, 1991.
31. Eddy R, Resendes M, Genant H: Case report 718. Osteopetrosis with carbonic anhydrase II deficiency. *Skeletal Radiol* **21**:135, 1992.
32. Fathallah DM, Bejaoui M, Dellagi K, Hu PY, Sly WS: A single splice junction mutation underlies the CA II deficiency syndrome in north African patients of Arab descent. *FASEB J* **7**:A813, 1993.
33. McKusick VA: Online Mendelian Inheritance in Man, OMIM 259730. http://www.hgmp.mrc.ac.uk.
34. Ballet JP, Griscelli C, Coutri SG, Milhaud G, Maroteaux P: Bone marrow transplantation in osteopetrosis. *Lancet* **2**:1137, 1977.
35. Coccia PF, Krivit W, Cervenka J, Clawson C, Kersey JH, Kim TH, Nesbit ME, Ramsay NK, Warkentin PI, Teitelbaum SL, Kahn AJ, Brown DM: Successful bone-marrow transplantation for infantile malignant osteopetrosis. *N Engl J Med* **302**:701, 1980.
36. Leone G: Osteopetrosis recessive con calcificazioni cerebrali: Studio di 3 sogetti adulti in due famiglie consanguine. *Radiol Med* **68**:373, 1982.
37. Baluarte J, Hiner L, Root A, Gruskin A: Osteopetrosis and renal tubular acidosis. *Pediatr Res* **7**:412, 1973.
38. Bregman H, Brown J, Rogers A, Bourke E: Osteopetrosis with combined proximal and distal tubular acidosis. *Am J Kidney Dis* **2**:357, 1982.
39. Tashian RE: Evolution and regulation of the carbonic anhydrase isozymes, in Rattazzi MC, Scandalios JG, Whitt GS (eds): *Isozymes: Current Topics in Biological Research*, vol. 2. New York, Alan R. Liss, 1977, p 21.
40. Zhu XL, Sly WS: Carbonic anhydrase IV from human lung: Purification, characterization, and comparison with membrane carbonic anhydrase from human kidney. *J Biol Chem* **265**:8795, 1990.
41. Brown D, Zhu XL, Sly WS: Localization of membrane-associated carbonic anhydrase type IV in kidney epithelial cells. *Proc Natl Acad Sci U S A* **87**:7457, 1990.
42. Okuyama T, Sato S, Zhu XL, Waheed A, Sly WS: Human carbonic anhydrase IV: cDNA cloning, sequence comparison, and expression in COS cell membranes. *Proc Natl Acad Sci U S A* **89**:1315, 1992.
43. Okuyama T, Batanian JR, Sly WS: Genomic organization and localization of gene for human carbonic anhydrase IV to chromosome 17q. *Genomics* **16**:678, 1993.
44. Feldstein JB, Silverman DN: Purification and characterization of carbonic anhydrase from the saliva of the rat. *J Biol Chem* **259**:5447, 1984.
45. Murakami H, Sly WS: Purification and characterization of human salivary carbonic anhydrase. *J Biol Chem* **262**:1382, 1987.
46. Fernley RT, Wright RD, Coghlan JP: Complete amino acid sequence of ovine salivary carbonic anhydrase. *Biochemistry* **27**:2815, 1988.
47. Nagao Y, Platero JS, Waheed A, Sly WS: Human mitochondrial carbonic anhydrase: cDNA cloning, expression, subcellular localization, and mapping to chromosome 16. *Proc Natl Acad Sci U S A* **90**:7623, 1993.
48. Tashian RE: Genetics of the mammalian carbonic anhydrases. *Adv Genet* **30**:321, 1993.
49. Nakai H, Byers MG, Venta PJ, Tashian RE, Shows TB: The gene for human carbonic anhydrase II (CA 2) is located at chromosome 8q22. *Cytogenet Cell Genet* **44**:234, 1987.
50. Southerland GR, Baker E, Fernandez KEW, Callen DF, Aldred P, Coghlan JP, Wright RE, Fernley RT: The genes for human carbonic anhydrase VI (CA VI) is on the tip of the short arm of chromosome 1. *Cytogenet Cell Genet* **50**:149, 1989.

51. Montgomery JC, Venta PJ, Eddy RL, Fukushima YS, Shows TB, Tashian RE: Characterization of the human gene for a newly discovered carbonic anhydrase, CA VII, and its localization to chromosome 16. *Genomics* **11**:835, 1991.

52. Caster MK, Pullan LM, Noltmann EA: The *p*-nitrophenyl phosphatase activity of muscle carbonic anhydrase. *Arch Biochem Biophys* **211**:632, 1981.

53. Sanyal G, Swenson ER, Pessah NI, Maren TH: The carbon dioxide hydration activity of skeletal muscle carbonic anhydrase: Inhibition by sulfonamides and anions. *Mol Pharmacol* **22**:211, 1982.

54. Sanyal G, Maren TH: Thermodynamics of carbonic anhydrase catalysis: A comparison between isozymes B and C. *J Biol Chem* **256**:608, 1981.

55. Wistrand PJ: The importance of carbonic anhydrase B and C for the unloading of $CO_2$ by the human erythrocyte. *Acta Physiol Scand* **113**:417, 1981.

56. Tashian RE, Hewett-Emmett D, Dodgson SJ, Forster RE, Sly WS: The value of inherited deficiencies of human carbonic anhydrase isoenzymes in understanding their cellular roles. *Ann NY Acad Sci* **429**:262, 1984.

57. Waheed A, Zhu XL, Sly WS: Membrane-associated carbonic anhydrase from rat lung. *J Biol Chem* **267**:3308, 1991.

58. Fleming RE, Crouch EC, Ruzicka CA, Sly WS: Developmentally regulated carbonic anhydrase IV gene expression in the alveolar capillary endothelium [Abstract 275]. *Pediatr Res* **332**:48A, 1993.

59. Hageman GS, Zhu XL, Waheed A, Sly WS: Localization of carbonic anhydrase IV in a specific capillary bed of the human eye. *Proc Natl Acad Sci U S A* **88**:2716, 1991.

60. Ghandour MS, Langley OK, Zhu XL, Waheed A, Sly WS: Carbonic anhydrase IV on brain capillary endothelial cells: A marker associated with the blood-brain barrier. *Proc Natl Acad Sci U S A* **89**:6823, 1992.

61. Waheed A, Zhu XL, Sly WS, Wetzel P, Gros G: Rat skeletal muscle membrane associated carbonic anhydrase is 39-kDa, glycosylated, GPI-anchored CA IV. *Arch Biochem Biophys* **294**:550, 1992.

62. Nagao Y, Srinivasan M, Platero JS, Svendrowski M, Waheed A, Sly, WS: Mitochondrial carbonic anhydrase (isozyme V) in mouse and rat: cDNA cloning, expression, subcellular localization, processing, and tissue distribution. *Proc Natl Acad Sci U S A* **91**:10330, 1994.

63. Venta PJ, Welty RJ, Johnson TM, Sly WS, Tashian RE: Carbonic anhydrase II deficiency syndrome in a Belgian family is caused by a point mutation at an invariant histidine residue (107 His → Tyr): Complete structure of the normal human CA II gene. *Am J Hum Genet* **49**:1082, 1991.

64. Roth DE, Venta PJ, Tashian RE, Sly WS: Molecular basis of human carbonic anhydrase II deficiency. *Proc Natl Acad Sci U S A* **89**:1804, 1992.

65. Hu PY, Roth DE, Skaggs LA, Venta PJ, Tashian RE, Guibaud P, Sly WS: A splice junction mutation in intron 2 of the carbonic anhydrase II gene of osteopetrosis patients from Arabic countries. *Hum Mutat* **1**:288, 1992.

66. Gay CV, Mueller WJ: Carbonic anhydrase and osteoclasts: Localization by labelled inhibitor autoradiography. *Science* **183**:432, 1974.

67. Väänänen HK, Parvinen E-K: High activity isoenzyme of carbonic anhydrase in rat calvaria osteoclasts: Immunohistochemical study. *Histochemistry* **78**:481, 1983.

68. Baron R, Neff L, Louvard D, Courtoy PJ: Cell-mediated extracellular acidification and bone resorption: Evidence for a low pH in resorbing lacunae and localization of a 100-kD lysosomal membrane protein at the osteoclast ruffled border. *J Cell Biol* **101**:2210, 1985.

69. Sly WS, Whyte MP, Krupin T, Sundaram V: Positive renal response to intravenous acetazolamide in patients with carbonic anhydrase II deficiency. *Pediatr Res* **19**:1033, 1985.

69a. Sato S, Zhu XL, Sly WS: Carbonic anhydrase isozymes IV and II in urinary membranes from carbonic anhydrase II-deficient patients. *Proc Natl Acad Sci U S A* **87**:6073, 1990.

70. Lonnerholm G: Histochemical locations of carbonic anhydrase in mammalian tissues. *Ann NY Acad Sci* **429**:369, 1984.

71. Spicer SS, Sens MA, Tashian RE: Immunocytochemical demonstration of carbonic anhydrase in human epithelial cells. *J Histochem Cytochem* **30**:864, 1982.

72. Alpern RJ, Stone DK, Rector FC Jr: Renal acidification mechanisms, in Renner BM, Rector FC Jr (eds): *The Kidney*, 4th ed. Philadelphia, WB Saunders, 1991, p 318.

73. Lucci MS, Tinker JP, Weiner IM, DuBose TD Jr: Function of proximal tubule carbonic anhydrase defined by selective inhibition. *Am J Physiol* **F245**:443, 1983.

74. DuBose TD, Pucacco LR, Carter NW: Determination of disequilibrium pH in the rat kidney in vivo: Evidence for hydrogen secretion. *Am J Physiol* **240**:F138, 1981.

75. Schwartz JH, Rosen S, Steinmetz PR: Carbonic anhydrase function and the epithelium organization of $H^+$ secretion in turtle urinary bladder. *J Clin Invest* **51**:2653, 1972.

76. Gluck S, Kelly S, Al-Awqati Q: The proton-translocating ATPase responsible for urinary acidification. *J Biol Chem* **257**:9230, 1982.

77. Kumpulainen T: Immunohistochemical localization of human carbonic anhydrase isozymes. *Ann NY Acad Sci* **429**:359, 1984.

78. Lees MB, Sapirstein VS, Reiss DS, Kolodny EH: Carbonic anhydrase and $2',3'$ cyclic nucleotide $3'$-phosphohydrolase activity in normal human brain and in demyelinating diseases. *Neurology* **30**:719, 1980.

79. Venta PJ, Montgomery JC, Hewett-Emmett D, Tashian RE: Comparison of the $5'$ regions of human and mouse carbonic anhydrase II genes and identification of possible regulatory elements. *Biochim Biophys Acta* **826**:195, 1985.

80. Hu PY, Ernst AR, Sly WS: UGA suppression of "Hispanic mutation" for CA II deficiency syndrome suggests novel mechanism for genetic heterogeneity [Abstract]. *Am J Hum Genet* **51(Suppl)**:A29, 1992.

81. Sundaram V, Rumbolo P, Grubb J, Strisciuglio P, Sly WS: Carbonic anhydrase deficiency: Diagnosis and carrier detection using differential enzyme inhibition and inactivation. *Am J Hum Genet* **38**:125, 1986.

82. Conroy CW, Maren TH: The determination of osteopetrotic phenotypes by selective inactivation of red cell carbonic anhydrase isoenzymes. *Clin Chim Acta* **152**:347, 1985.

83. Whyte MP, Hamm LL, Sly WS: Transfusion of carbonic anhydrase-replete erythrocytes fails to correct the acidification defect in the syndrome of osteopetrosis, renal tubular acidosis, and cerebral calcification (carbonic anhydrase-II deficiency). *J Bone Mineral Res* **3**:385, 1988.

84. Lewis SE, Erickson RP, Barnett LB, Venta PJ, Tashian RE: *N*-ethyl-*N*-nitrosourea-induced null mutation at the mouse Car-2 locus: An animal model for human carbonic anhydrase II deficiency syndrome. *Proc Natl Acad Sci U S A* **85**:1962, 1988.

85. Baron R: Molecular mechanisms of bone resorption by the osteoclast. *Anat Rec* **224**:317, 1989.

86. Bushinsky DA, Goldring JM, Coe FL: Cellular contribution to pH-mediated calcium flux in neonatal mouse calvariae. *Am J Physiol* **248**:F785, 1985.

87. Raisz LG, Simmons HA, Thompson WJ, Shepard KL, Anderson PS, Rodan GA: Effects of a potent carbonic anhydrase inhibitor on bone resorption in organ culture. *Endocrinology* **122**:1083, 1988.

88. Anderson RE, Jee WS, Woodbury DM: Stimulation of carbonic anhydrase in osteoclasts by parathyroid hormone. *Calcif Tissue Int* **37**:646, 1985.

89. Hall GE, Kenny AD: Bone resorption induced by parathyroid hormone and dibutyryl cyclic AMP: Role of carbonic anhydrase. *J Pharmacol Exper Ther* **238**:778, 1986.

90. Kenny AD: Role of carbonic anhydrase in bone: Partial inhibition of disuse atrophy of bone by parenteral acetazolamide. *Calcif Tissue Int* **37**:126, 1985.

91. Hu PY, Ernst AR, Sly WS, Venta PJ, Skaggs LA, Tashian RE: Carbonic anhydrase II deficiency: Single base deletion in exon 7 is the predominant mutation in Caribbean Hispanic patients. *Am J Hum Genet* **54**:602, 1994.

92. Nagai R, Kooh SW, Balfe JW, Fenton T, Halperin ML: Renal tubular acidosis and osteopetrosis with carbonic anhydrase II deficiency: Pathogenesis of impaired acidification. *Pediatr Nephrol* **11**:633, 1997.

93. Ismail EA, Abul Saad S, Sabry MA: Nephrocalcinosis and urolithiasis in carbonic anhydrase II deficiency syndrome. *Eur J Pediatr* **156**:957, 1997.

94. Ruffa G, Milanaccio C, Sbolgi P, Levato GL, Bartocci M, Galasso V, Bruschettini PL: Osteopetrosis and renal acidosis: A new case of this rare syndrome. *Minerva Pediatr* **47**:135, 1995.

95. Soda H: Carbonic anhydrase II deficiency syndrome — Clinicopathological, biochemical and molecular studies. *Kurume Med J* **41**:233, 1994.

96. Fathallah DM, Bejaoui M, Sly WS, Lakhoua R, Dellagi K: A unique mutation underlying carbonic anhydrase II deficiency syndrome in patients of Arab descent. *Hum Genet* **94**:581, 1994.

97. Soda H, Yukizane S, Yoshida I, Aramaki S, Kato H: Carbonic anhydrase II deficiency in a Japanese patient produced by a nonsense mutation (TAT→TAG) at Tyr-40 in exon 2, (Y40X). *Hum Mutat* **5**:348, 1995.

98. Soda H, Yukizane S, Yoshida I, Koga Y, Aramaki S, Kato H: A point mutation in exon 3 (His 107→Tyr) in two unrelated Japanese patients

with carbonic anhydrase II deficiency with central nervous system involvement. *Hum Genet* **97**:435, 1996.

99. Fathallah DM, Bejaoui M, Lepaslier D, Chater K, Sly WS, Dellagi K: Carbonic anhydrase II (CA II) deficiency in Maghrebian patients: Evidence for founder effect and genomic recombination at the CA II locus. *Hum Genet* **99**:634, 1997.

100. Hu PY, Lim EJ, Ciccolella J, Strisciuglio P, Sly WS: Seven novel mutations in carbonic anhydrase II deficiency syndrome identified by SSCP and direct sequencing analysis. *Hum Mutat* **9**:383, 1997.

101. Shah GN, Hu PY, Sly WS: Four novel mutations in carbonic anhydrase II deficiency syndrome identified by a new, simple two-step method. *Hum Mutat* (Submitted).

102. Lien YH, Lai LW: Respiratory acidosis in carbonic anhydrase II deficient mice. *Am J Physiol* **274**:602, 1998.

103. Donckerwolcke R, Stone P: Renal tubular acidosis and osteopetrosis. *Pediatr Nephrol* **13**:180, 1999.

104. Bourke E, Delaney VB, Mosawi M, Reavey P, Weston M: Renal tubular acidosis and osteopetrosis in siblings. *Nephron* **28**:268, 1981.

105. Jacquemin C, Mullaney P, Svedberg E: Marble brain syndrome: Osteopetrosis, renal tubular acidosis and calcification of brain. *Neuroradiology* **40**:662, 1998.

106. Jandziszak K, Suarez C, Wasserman E, Clark R, Baker B, Liu F, Hintz R, et al.: Disturbances of growth hormone-insulin-like growth factor axis and response to growth hormone in acidosis. *Am J Physiol* **275**:R120, 1998.

107. Sly WS, Hu PY: Human carbonic anhydrases and carbonic anhydrase deficiencies. *Annu Rev Biochem* **64**:375, 1995.

108. Tu CK, Silverman DN, Forsman C, Jonsson BH, Lindskog S: Role of histidine 64 in catalytic mechanism of human carbonic anhydrase II studied with a site-specific mutant. *Biochemistry* **28**:7913, 1989.

109. Jiang W, Gupta D: Structure of carbonic anhydrase VI (CA6) gene: Evidence for two distinct groups within the alpha-CA gene family. *Biochem J* **344**:385, 1999.

110. Kivela J, Parkkila S, Parkkila A-K, Rajaniemi H: A low concentration of carbonic anhydrase isozyme VI in whole saliva is associated with caries prevalence. *Caries Res* **33**:178, 1999.

111. Parkkila S, Parkkila A-K, Lehtola J, Reinila A, Sodervik HJ, Rannisto M, Rajaniemi H: Salivary carbonic anhydrase protects gastroesophageal mucosa from acid injury. *Dig Dis Sci* **42**:1013, 1997.

112. Fujikawa-Adachi K, Nishimori I, Taguchi T, Onishi S: Human mitochondrial carbonic anhydrase VB. *J Biol Chem* **274**:21228, 1999.

113. Shah GN, Hewett-Emmett D, Grubb JH, Migas MC, Fleming RE, Waheed A, Sly WS: Mitochondrial carbonic anhydrase CA VB: Differences in tissue distribution and pattern of evolution from those of CA VA suggest distinct physiological roles. *Proc Natl Acad Sci U S A* **97**:1677, 2000.

114. Hazen SA, Waheed A, Sly WS, LaNoue KF, Lynch CJ: Differentiation-dependent expression of CA V and the role of carbonic anhydrase isozymes in pyruvate carboxylation in adipocytes. *FASEB J* **10**:481, 1996.

115. Parkkila A-K, Scarim AL, Parkkila S, Waheed A, Corbett JA, Sly WS: Expression of carbonic anhydrase V in pancreatic beta cells suggests a role for mitochondrial carbonic anhydrase in insulin secretion. *J Biol Chem* **273**:24620, 1998.

116. Boriack-Sjodin PN, Heck RW, Laipis PJ, Silverman DN, Christianson DW: Structure determination of murine mitochondrial carbonic anhydrase V at 2.45-Å resolution: Implications for catalytic proton transfer and inhibitor design. *Proc Natl Acad Sci U S A* **92**:10949, 1995.

117. Heck RW, Tanhauser SM, Manda R, Tu C, Laipis PJ, Silverman DN: Catalytic properties of mouse carbonic anhydrase V. *J Biol Chem* **269**:24742, 1994.

118. Pastorek J, Pastorekova S, Callebaut I, Mornon JP, Zelnik V, Opavsky R, Zatovicova M, et al.: Cloning and characterization of MN, a human tumor-associated protein with a domain homologous to carbonic anhydrase and a putative helix-loop-helix DNA binding segment. *Oncogene* **9**:2877, 1994.

119. Tureci O, Sahin U, Vollmar E, Siemer S, Gottert E, Seitz G, Parkkila A-K, et al.: Human carbonic anhydrase XII: cDNA cloning, expression, and chromosomal localization of a carbonic anhydrase gene that is overexpressed in some renal cell carcinomas. *Proc Natl Acad Sci U S A* **95**:7608, 1998.

120. Fujikawa-Adachi K, Nishimori I, Taguchi T, Onishi S: Human carbonic anhydrase XIV (CA14): cDNA cloning, mRNA expression, and mapping to chromosome 1. *Genomics* **61**:74, 1999.

121. Mori K, Ogawa Y, Ebihara K, Tamura N, Tashiro K, Kuwahara T, Mukoyama M, et al.: Isolation and characterization of CA XIV, a novel membrane-bound carbonic anhydrase from mouse kidney. *J Biol Chem* **274**:15701, 1999.

122. Ivanov SV, Kuzmin I, Wei MH, Pack S, Geil L, Johson BE, Stanbridge EJ, et al.: Down regulation of transmembrane carbonic anhydrases in renal cell carcinoma cell lines by wild-type von Hippel-Lindau transgenes. *Proc Natl Acad Sci U S A* **95**:12569, 1998.

123. Penschow JD, Giles ME, Coghlan JP, Fernley RT: Redistribution of carbonic anhydrase VI expression from the ducts to acini during development of ovine parotid and submandibular glands. *Histochem Cell Biol* **107**:417, 1997.

124. Kivela LJ, Parkkila S, Parkkila A-K, Rajaniemi H: Salivary carbonic anhydrase isozyme VI is located in the human enamel pellicle. *Caries Res* **33**:185, 1999.

125. Parkkila S, Parkkila A-K, Haukipuro K, Pastorekova S, Pastorek J, Kairaluoma MI, Karttunen TJ: Immunohistochemical study of colorectal tumors for expression of a novel transmembrane carbonic anhydrase, MN/CA IX, with potential value as a marker of cell proliferation. *Am J Pathol* **153**:1, 1998.

126. Saarnio J, Parkkila S, Parkkila A-K, Waheed A, Casey MC, Zhou XY, Pastorekova S, et al.: Immunohistochemistry of carbonic anhydrase isozyme IX (MN/CA IX) in human gut reveals polarized expression in the epithelial cells with the highest proliferative capacity. *J Histochem Cytochem* **46**:497, 1998.

127. Karhumaa P, Parkkila, S, Tureci O, Waheed A, Grubb JH, Shah G, Parkkila A-K, et al.: Identification of carbonic anhydrase XII as the membrane isozyme expressed in the normal human endometrial epithelium. *Mol Hum Reprod* **6**:68, 2000.

128. Kivela A, Parkkila S, Saarino J, Karttunen TJ, Kivela J, Parkkila A-K, Waheed A, et al.: Expression of a novel transmembrane carbonic anhydrase isozyme XII in normal human gut and colorectal tumors. *Am J Pathol* **156**:577, 2000.

129. Schlesinger PH, Mattsson JP, Blair HC: Osteoclastic acid transport: Mechanism and implications for physiological and pharmacological regulation. *Miner Electrolyte Metab* **20**:31, 1994.

130. Felix R, Hofstetter W, Cecchini MG: Recent developments in the understanding of the pathophysiology of osteopetrosis. *Eur J Endocrinol* **134**:143, 1996.

131. Taki K, Kato H, Yoshia I: Elimination of $CO_2$ in patients with carbonic anhydrase II deficiency, with studies of respiratory function at rest. *Respir Med* **93**:536, 1999.

132. Cammer W, Zhang H, Cammer M: Glial cell abnormalities in the CNS of the carbonic anhydrase II deficient mutant mouse. *J Neurol Sci* **118**:1, 1993.

133. Tu C, Couton JM, Van Heeke G, Richards NG, Silverman DN: Kinetic analysis of a mutant (His107→Tyr) responsible for human carbonic anhydrase II deficiency syndrome. *J Biol Chem* **268**:4775, 1993.

134. Hu PY, Waheed A, Sly WS: Partial rescue of human carbonic anhydrase II frameshift mutation by ribosomal frameshift. *Proc Natl Acad Sci U S A* **92**:2136, 1995.

135. Strisciuglio P, Hu PY, Lim EJ, Ciccolella J, Sly WS: Clinical and molecular heterogeneity in carbonic anhydrase II deficiency and prenatal diagnosis in an Italian family. *J Pediatr* **132**:717, 1998.

136. Funderburk SJ: Osteopetrosis in two brothers with severe mental retardation. *Birth Defects* **11**:91, 1975.

137. Lai LW, Chan DM, Erickson RP, Hsu SJ, Lien YH: Correction of renal tubular acidosis in carbonic anhydrase II-deficient mice with gene therapy. *J Clin Invest* **101**:1320, 1998.

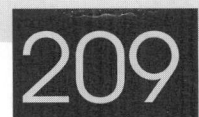

# Amyloidosis

*Merrill D. Benson*

1. Hereditary amyloidosis is characterized by the extracellular accumulation of protein fibrils having $\beta$-pleated sheet structure. Actually, hereditary amyloidosis is only one of a number of forms of amyloidosis, each characterized by the protein that is the basic subunit of the amyloid fibril. Systemic hereditary amyloidosis (involving multiple organ systems) may be associated with variant forms of transthyretin, apolipoprotein A-I, gelsolin, cystatin C, fibrinogen, or lysozyme. Other forms of systemic amyloidosis, which are not hereditary, include immunoglobulin (amyloidosis of light chain (AL), primary) amyloidosis, in which the subunit protein is the variable portion of monoclonal immunoglobulin light chain; reactive (secondary) amyloidosis, in which the subunit protein is a degradation product—amyloid A (AA)—of a serum acute-phase protein—serum amyloid A (SAA); and $\beta_2$-microglobulin (dialysis-associated) amyloidosis, in which the subunit protein is $\beta_2$-microglobulin. All forms of amyloidosis cause illness and death by physical encroachment of the deposits on normal organ structures. In autosomal dominant hereditary amyloidosis, peripheral neuropathy is the most common finding, although infiltration of vital organs, such as heart, kidney, and bowel, give various syndromes, which usually lead to death.
2. Hereditary amyloidosis is a late-onset disease with clinical symptoms beginning in most kindreds within the third to seventh decades of life. The clinical disease usually progresses over 5 to 15 years and ends with death from cardiac failure, renal failure, or malnutrition. In some kindreds, heterozygotes with late-onset disease, however, have lived past age 90. Gene prevalence is not known, because there are a number of mutations in the genes for various plasma proteins, and many of the kindreds were characterized only recently. In the United States, the prevalence of variant transthyretin genes associated with amyloidosis varies with ethnic origin. In Caucasians, the prevalence is relatively low (perhaps 1 in 100,000). In Americans of African descent, as many as 1 in 25 may have one specific transthyretin variant (Val122Ile) that causes late-onset cardiomyopathy.
3. The primary defect in autosomal dominant transthyretin amyloidosis results from one of a number of mutations in the gene for transthyretin, which is a single-copy sequence on chromosome 18. To date, 73 single amino acid substitutions in the transthyretin molecule that could be associated with hereditary amyloidosis have been found. In addition, six mutations have been described in apolipoprotein A-I,

two in gelsolin, four in fibrinogen A $\alpha$-chain, two in lysozyme, and one in cystatin C, all of which are associated with systemic amyloidosis.
4. Direct DNA tests have been developed for many of the variant genes for transthyretin, apolipoprotein A-I, gelsolin, fibrinogen, lysozyme, and cystatin C. In addition, modern molecular biology techniques can provide easy detection methods for all of the demonstrated mutations. In many cases, restriction enzyme analysis of PCR amplification products has replaced Southern blot analysis. Direct DNA sequencing based on PCR technology is used in the discovery of new mutations. DNA tests have been established for certain protein variants, and these are used for genetic counseling.
5. Prenatal diagnosis has been developed for at least two forms of transthyretin amyloidosis based on PCR technology.
6. Autosomal dominant forms of amyloidosis that are localized to one organ system include familial Alzheimer disease, hereditary cerebral hemorrhage with amyloidosis-Dutch type ($\beta$-amyloid precursor protein, $\beta$-APP), Gerstmann-Sträussler-Scheinker syndrome, Creutzfeldt-Jakob disease (prion), medullary carcinoma of the thyroid (procalcitonin), and various types of lattice corneal dystrophy (keratoepithelin).

The term amyloidosis is used to describe a number of protein deposition diseases in which homogeneous protein molecules aggregate into an ordered structure to make fibrils measuring 75 to 100 Å in cross-section and having indeterminate length.[1] These fibrils accumulate in extracellular spaces to form deposits that, because of their ordered structure, have the crystalline property of birefringence and, in addition, have selective affinities for certain histochemical dyes such as Congo red.

There are several types of amyloidosis, defined by the basic protein constituent of the fibrils. The most life threatening of these disorders are systemic with involvement of major organ systems. There are, however, localized forms of amyloidosis that, because of the specific organ involved, are also fatal. Although each type of amyloidosis is a separate disease with its own etiology and pathogenic mechanisms, all share the physicochemical properties of the amyloid fibril and cause illness in the same way. As the extracellular deposits enlarge, they displace normal tissue structures, causing disruption of cell function and ultimately cell death. The signs and symptoms of the disease depend on the strategic location and size of the fibril deposits, but the basic mechanisms and end result of their presence is the same in all types of amyloidosis. Despite this final common pathway, the etiology, pathogenesis, prognosis, and therapeutic interventions for the different forms of amyloidosis must be considered separately. To set the stage for such a discussion and prepare us for handling the rapidly accumulating data in this area, some historical perspective is important.

## HISTORY

Although amyloidosis has undoubtedly occurred for centuries, it was not until the mid-1800s that attention was brought to the

---

A list of standard abbreviations is located immediately preceding the index in each volume. Additional abbreviations used in this chapter include: AH amyloidosis = heavy chain of immunoglobulin/amyloidosis; AL amyloidosis = amyloid light chain of immunoglobulin amyloidosis; -APP = amyloid precursor protein; FAP = familial amyloid polyneuropathy; FMF = familial Mediterranean fever; HCHWA = hereditary cerebral hemorrhage with amyloid, type I and type D (Dutch); *MEFV* = familial Mediterranean fever gene; PCR-I MRA = PCR-induced mutation restriction analysis; PS-1, PS-2 = presenilin 1, presenilin 2; RBP = retinol-binding protein; SAA = serum amyloid A; TTR = transthyretin.

condition. In 1842, Rokitansky[2] wrote about the "lardaceous liver" found at autopsy in patients with chronic diseases, and Virchow (1854) subsequently showed that these tissues gave a unique color reaction with iodine and sulfuric acid.[3,4] Virchow coined the term amyloid, which means "starch-like," because of this reaction, which led him to believe that amyloid represented deposits of carbohydrates. However, in 1859, Friedreich and Kekule reported evidence that amyloid deposits were composed mainly of protein.[5] Over the next 100 years, amyloidosis associated with chronic diseases was studied histologically and epidemiologically.[6] It became obvious that some patients with amyloidosis had no predisposing illness, and that amyloidosis was occasionally seen in familial patterns. Eventually the term *primary* was applied to the apparently sporadic form of amyloidosis and secondary to amyloidosis that developed in individuals with chronic inflammatory diseases such as tuberculosis, osteomyelitis, and rheumatoid arthritis. Hereditary amyloidosis was not widely recognized as such until 1952 when Andrade published his studies of amyloidosis in families with polyneuropathy in northern Portugal.[7] Reviews of the literature show that, as early as the 1920s, familial occurrence of amyloidotic polyneuropathy had been described, but these cases were classified as primary.[8,9] Indeed, Ostertag in 1932 reported a family with hereditary amyloid nephropathy and subsequently published a very detailed study of this kindred in 1950, two years before Andrade's description of Portuguese families.[10] Ostertag was pathologist in the very clinic in Berlin that was named for Rudolph Virchow. So why do we revere Virchow for his description of amyloid, although he mistakenly thought it carbohydrate in character, and give little credit to Ostertag, who wrote one of the first descriptions of hereditary amyloidosis? The answer is as clear as the evolution of science in medicine. During the reign of Rudolph Virchow as the preeminent pathologist in the world, German medical science was at its pinnacle, and the accepted language of science was German. By the time of Ostertag's major publication 100 years later, American medical science had gained supremacy, and with it came the installation of English as the preferred scientific language. Alas, Ostertag published in German and Andrade in English.

Characterization of amyloid remained relatively static until 1959 when Cohen and Calkins[11] showed by electron microscopy that amyloid deposits were not amorphous but contained nonbranching fibrils with diameters of 75 to 100 Å and of indeterminate length. Its resistance to solubilization in practically all solvents hindered chemical characterization of this fibril material. However, by 1971, Glenner et al.[12] were able to solubilize amyloid fibrils from the tissues of patients with primary amyloidosis using strong chaotropic agents, and isolate the major subunit proteins. Amino acid sequencing revealed that these subunits were homologous to the variable segment of immunoglobulin light chains. This breakthrough in amyloid research at the chemical level was quickly followed by the demonstration that amyloid fibrils from patients with secondary amyloidosis were composed of a previously undescribed protein, which was subsequently named "amyloid A protein" (AA).[13-15] Further studies revealed that AA was derived from an acute-phase plasma protein, which was then named "serum amyloid A" (SAA).[16-22] In 1978, Costa et al. found that amyloid material from patients with hereditary amyloidosis was composed of a subunit protein which reacted with antiserum to plasma transthyretin (prealbumin).[23] The presence of transthyretin in hereditary amyloid deposits was confirmed at the structural level by 1981,[24] and since then numerous variants of this plasma protein have been found to be associated with hereditary amyloidosis.[25-30] Subsequently, various forms of other plasma proteins have been found to be associated with hereditary amyloidosis, including apolipoprotein A-I,[31] gelsolin,[32,33] the Aα-chain of fibrinogen,[34] and lysozyme.[35] In addition, advances have been made in the chemical characterization of localized forms of amyloidosis, including determination of the structure of the β-amyloid of Alzheimer plaques,[36] the prion protein of Creutzfeldt-Jakob disease and

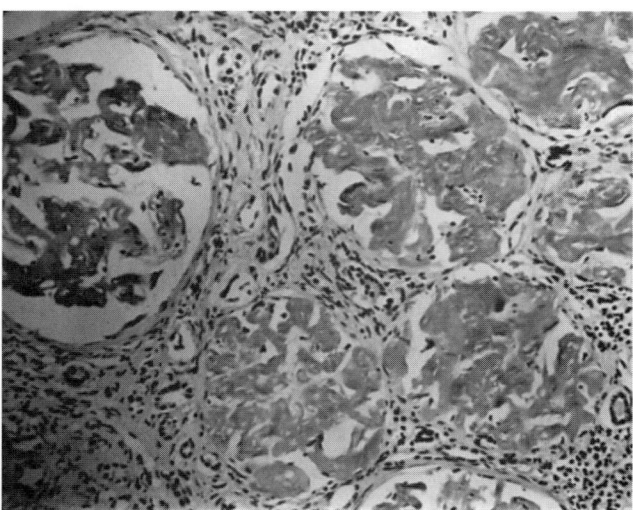

**Fig. 209-1** Amyloid deposits obliterating renal glomeruli in a patient with hereditary amyloidosis. Hematoxylin and eosin stain.

Gerstmann-Sträussler-Scheinker syndrome,[37] and the amyloid of islets of Langerhans in type 2 diabetes mellitus.[38] This brings us to the present time where we can discuss amyloidosis at the physicochemical level and consider hypotheses on the etiology and pathogenic mechanisms of the various types.

## PHYSICAL PROPERTIES OF AMYLOID FIBRILS

By light microscopy, in hematoxylin-and-eosin-stained preparations, amyloid deposits of all kinds are amorphous and eosinophilic (Fig. 209-1). The deposits are extracellular and often appear to be crowding the cells aside. This phenomenon is best appreciated in peripheral nerves, where the typical nerve bundles and Schwann cell nuclei detour around large accumulations of amyloid (Fig. 209-2). In other tissues, amyloid may accumulate along cell margins. This is seen in the liver, where columns of amyloid separate the hepatic cords, and in the heart, where cross-sectional preparations show rings of amyloid around the myocardial fibers. In some tissues, large collections of amyloid may completely lack identifiable cellular elements.

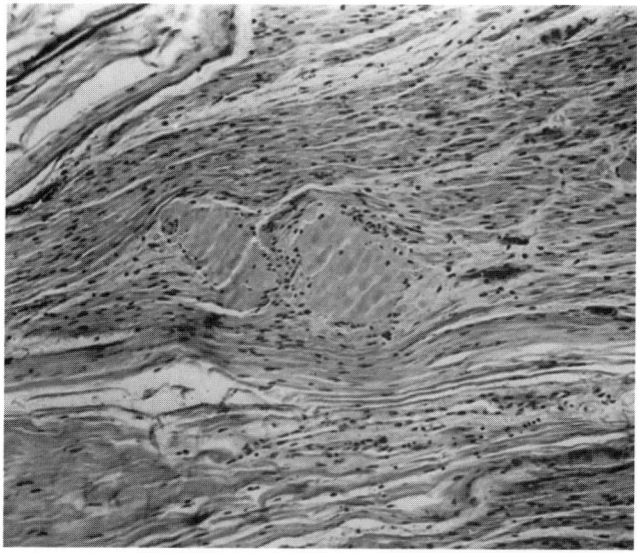

**Fig. 209-2** Amyloid deposits within peripheral nerve displacing nerve fibers and supporting cells. Congo red counterstained with hematoxylin.

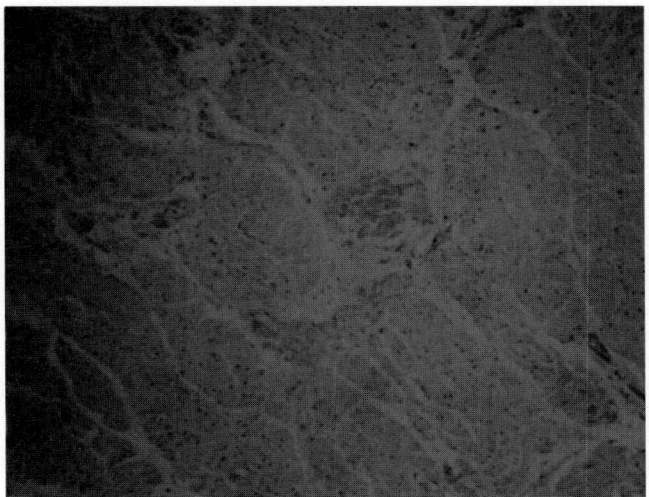

A.

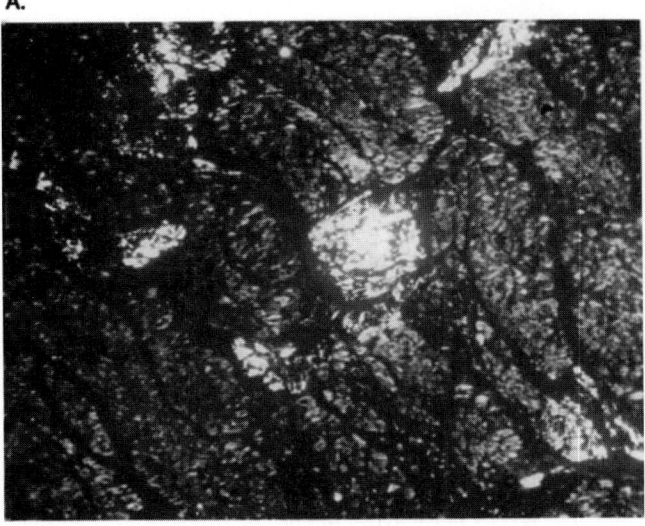

B.

**Fig. 209-3 Amyloid deposits within myocardium stained with Congo red. A, Light microscopic view. B, The same section through crossed polars. Congo red-stained amyloid deposits show green birefringence. Ring structures caused by amyloid deposits around myocardial fiber bundles also become apparent in the polarizing microscope. Congo red counterstained with hematoxylin.**

While amyloid deposits of all kinds are eosinophilic, they also have unique staining properties that are useful in diagnosis. In the past, methyl violet and crystal violet, which give metachromatic reactions with amyloid, were used to stain amyloid deposits. Now Congo red is the standard for identification of amyloid on histologic sections (Fig. 209-3).[39] In tissue sections stained with alkaline Congo red, amyloid deposits take up the dye and give a characteristic green color when viewed in the polarizing microscope. This specific marker for amyloid is due to the birefringent nature of the amyloid fibrils and to their ability to bind Congo red. Collagen is also birefringent in histologic sections, but collagen does not bind Congo red, and, therefore, the green birefringence is not seen. The fluorescent thioflavin dyes have also been used to localize amyloid but have not been universally accepted because of lack of complete specificity.

At the level of electron microscopy, amyloid deposits contain characteristic fibrillar structures, which are often in linear array, but lack of ordered structure is the rule (Fig. 209-4). Deep invaginations of the fibrils into the cytoplasmic membranes of reticuloendothelial cells are frequently seen and have been

postulated to be the sites of amyloid formation, but controversy persists on where actual fibril formation occurs. When amyloid fibrils are physically extracted from tissue deposits, negatively stained with uranyl acetate or phosphotungstic acid, and studied by high-resolution electron microscopy, the nonbranching fibrils appear to consist of at least two and perhaps several parallel subunit filaments.[40] Helical twisting of these subunits, which measure about 25 to 35 Å in width, may give a beaded appearance to the fibrils. While a fair degree of structural diversity is seen from one fibril preparation to another, no ultrastructural features that distinguish immunoglobulin, AA, or transthyretin amyloid fibrils have been reported.

The substructure of amyloid fibrils has been studied by x-ray diffraction.[41,42] While amyloid fibrils basically have a crystalline structure, which gives them their birefringence, it has not been possible to solubilize and recrystallize amyloid fibrils to study the crystal lattice by x-ray diffraction. Chemical studies suggest that other substances (e.g., proteoglycans) may be involved in fibril formation, and, therefore, fibrils are a mixture of substances other than just the basic protein subunit. X-ray powder patterns, however, are consistent with $\beta$-structure, which is the basis for developing the antiparallel $\beta$-pleated sheet model of amyloid fibrils (Fig. 209-5). This is supported by x-ray crystallographic data on two of the amyloid fibril subunit proteins — immunoglobulin light chain and transthyretin. Immunoglobulin light chain domains have an extensive antiparallel $\beta$-configuration.[43] Similarly, the transthyretin monomer has an extensive $\beta$-structure, with eight polypeptide segments running in an antiparallel fashion in two planes.[44] The tertiary structure of AA protein in reactive amyloidosis is not as well understood, and structural models suggest that $\alpha$ helices may also be involved in intrinsic fibril formation.

## OVERALL CLASSIFICATION OF THE AMYLOIDOSES

Although the term amyloid turned out to be a misnomer, we have all become accustomed to using the term amyloidosis to denote the syndromes characterized by the deposition of the $\beta$-pleated sheet fibrils. Amyloidosis is a more general term than such terms as $\beta$-fibrilloses because it can accommodate conditions such as immunoglobulin light chain deposition disease, a B-lymphocyte dyscrasia in which monoclonal light chain proteins (usually $\kappa$) accumulate in organs (often the kidneys) and result in death but evidently do not have the capability of forming fibrils.[45,46] This condition appears to be very closely related to immunoglobulin amyloidosis, because there are reports of patients who had immunoglobulin light chain deposition disease and in whom postmortem examination showed actual amyloid fibril deposits in organs other than the kidney.[47] Using the term amyloidoses to designate the entire group of protein deposition diseases, a classification has been proposed based on chemical composition of the amyloid deposits.[48] Such a classification has to be modified for clinical use, because patterns of organ involvement will continue to be important. For instance, whether an amyloidosis is systemic or localized has far-reaching significance for treatment and prognosis. Therefore, it is best to classify the systemic amyloidoses separately from the localized forms and then to use subclassifications based on chemical compositions when known.

Historically, for want of a better method, the amyloidoses were classified according to the clinical features of each syndrome. "*Primary amyloidosis*" was used to designate those syndromes in which there was no obvious predisposing disease; "*secondary amyloidosis*" referred to those cases in which there was a predisposing chronic inflammatory disease; and "*heredofamilial*" or "*hereditary amyloidosis*" was used whenever there was a definite familial pattern. A few confusing terms were used, and these need to be mentioned because they persist in the old literature. First, patients with amyloidosis associated with multiple myeloma were frequently said to have amyloidosis "secondary"

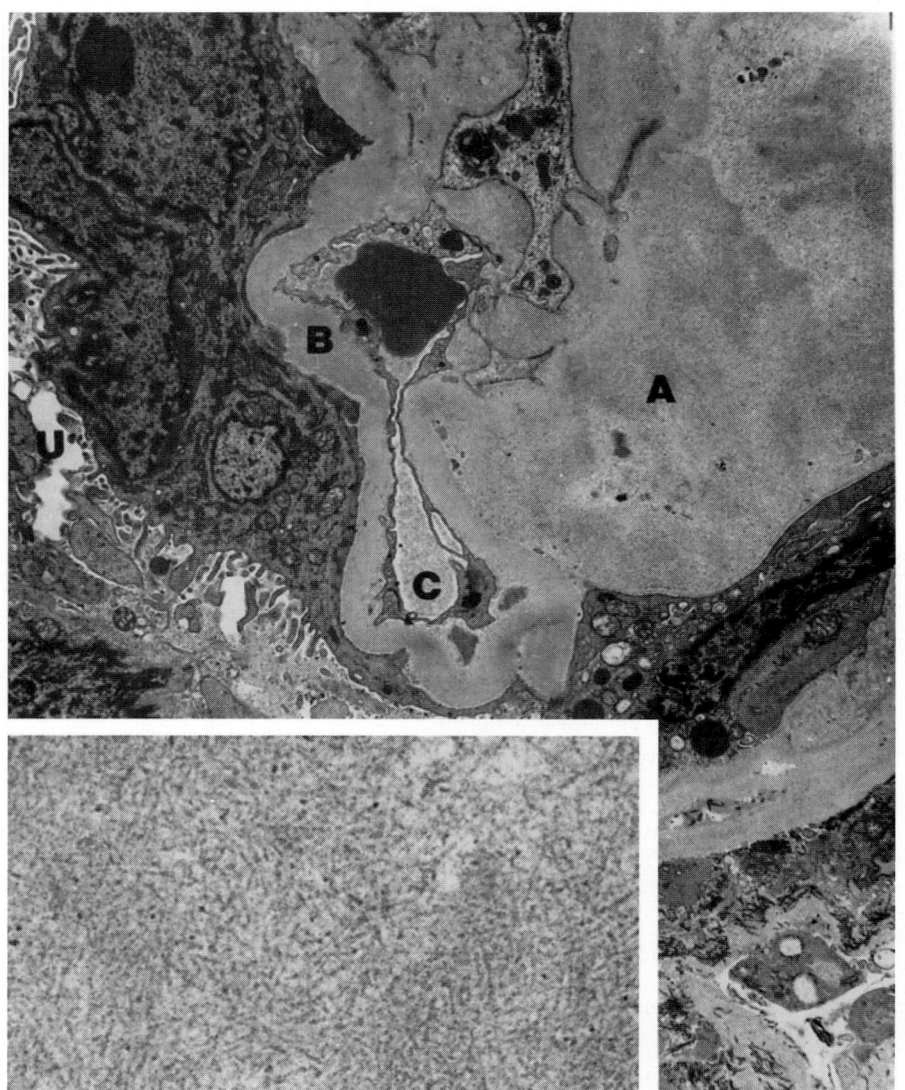

**Fig. 209-4 Electron micrograph of a renal biopsy. Amyloid deposits are present throughout the basement membrane and in adjacent structures. Inset: higher-power micrograph showing the fibrillar structures that are characteristic of all types of amyloid deposits. A = amyloid; B = basement membrane; C = capillary loop; U = urinary space.**

to multiple myeloma. The use of the term secondary in this context is unfortunate because chemical analysis now shows that myeloma-associated amyloidosis is chemically the same as primary amyloidosis. These two groups should be and are presently classified as immunoglobulin light chain amyloidosis. Further confusion was caused by the use of the term primary in some of the reports of hereditary amyloidosis.

At the present time, the best classification of the amyloidoses is based on the chemical composition of the amyloid fibrils. This is of particular value in the systemic amyloidoses, where we know the chemical composition of the deposits. A word of caution is in order, however, because there may be other forms of systemic amyloidosis, particularly in the hereditary group, for which we may find as yet undescribed amyloid subunits. In the localized forms of amyloidosis, fewer subunit proteins have been characterized biochemically, so it remains necessary to classify them by a combination of factors, including organ system involvement and chemical composition, where known. Some hereditary amyloidoses are systemic and others are localized. In the systemic group are the autosomal dominant forms, which often show peripheral neuropathy and/or cardiomyopathy, and in which many variant forms of transthyretin have been described, as well as mutations in apolipoprotein A-I, plasma gelsolin, lysozyme, cystatin C, and fibrinogen Aα-chain. In addition, there is the systemic amyloidosis associated with familial Mediterranean fever, in which the pattern

of inheritance is autosomal recessive.[49] Hereditary amyloid syndromes with localized deposits include medullary carcinoma of the thyroid,[50,51] familial cutaneous amyloidosis,[52,53] and those forms of Alzheimer disease in which there is a familial pattern.[54] Localized forms of amyloidosis without an apparent hereditary pattern include amyloid in the islets of Langerhans in diabetes mellitus, amyloid of the larynx and upper respiratory tract, the sporadic occurrence of amyloid tumors in the genitourinary tract, some cutaneous amyloidoses, nonfamilial cerebral amyloid angiopathy, and most Alzheimer disease.

## SYSTEMIC AMYLOIDOSES

Three major types of systemic amyloidosis are recognized in humans: (a) immunoglobulin (primary); (b) reactive (secondary); and (c) hereditary (Table 209-1). A fourth type, which thus far has been described only in patients with chronic renal failure, usually on hemodialysis, has deposits containing $\beta_2$-microglobulin.[55,56] While this type of amyloid deposition is predominantly restricted to bones and joints, other organ involvement has been seen.

This chapter is principally interested in the hereditary forms of amyloidosis, but it is important to understand the other types of human systemic amyloidosis for two reasons. First, at the clinical level, the different types of systemic amyloidosis may be very similar. They all may affect the same organ systems to varying

A.

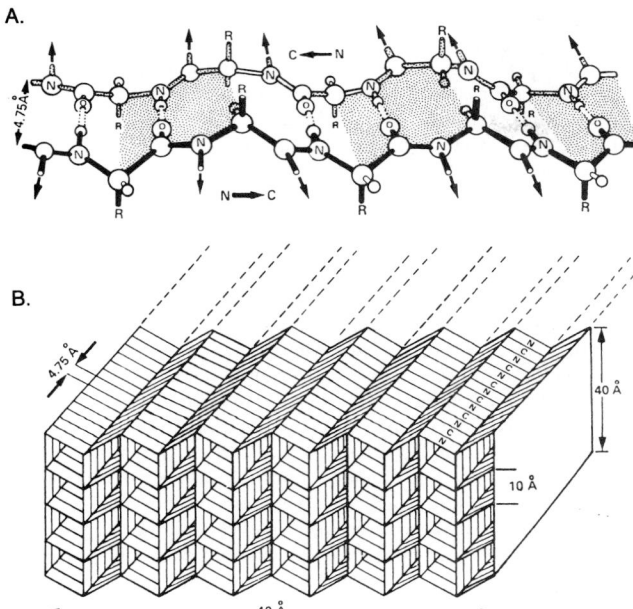

B.

**Fig. 209-5 Proposed model of antiparallel β-structure. *A,* The structural basis of the antiparallel β-sheet. The structure is formed by a single polypeptide chain that folds back on itself. The N-terminal to C-terminal directions are as shown. The strands are held together by hydrogen bonding and have an interchain distance of approximately 4.75 Å. *B,* The proposed structure of amyloid fibrils is shown with basic dimensions of 40 × 40 Å with indefinite length. Two or more of these fibrils probably associate by twisting along the long axis to form the amyloid fibril. (*Modified from Sack et al.[282] Used by permission.*)**

degrees. One form of amyloidosis can be easily mistaken for another, especially in situations where a family history is not available or informative, or when chronic inflammatory disease, which may predispose to reactive amyloidosis, is not readily apparent. Second, it is increasingly evident that there is a genetic basis for both the immunoglobulin and the reactive types of amyloidosis. The monoclonal immunoglobulin light chains that are the subunit proteins of immunoglobulin amyloidosis are the products of intricate gene rearrangement mechanisms in B-lymphocyte clones. Limited structural studies of amyloid light chain proteins suggest that only certain structures are amyloidogenic (i.e., are capable of forming amyloid fibrils). Whatever pathogenic mechanisms are involved in immunoglobulin amyloid formation, DNA rearrangements are an integral part of the process.

In reactive amyloidosis, the liver synthesizes the precursor protein SAA. Multiple genes code for this protein and, again, while structural data are limited, they suggest that certain isotypes of SAA are preferentially processed to make amyloid fibrils. While no inheritance pattern of reactive amyloidosis has been shown other than in febrile diseases such as familial Mediterranean fever and Muckle-Wells syndrome, the fact that only certain SAA gene products are associated with amyloid fibrils suggests that there is a genetic basis for reactive amyloidosis as well. Therefore, this chapter reviews the clinical, pathogenic, and biochemical aspects of the two classic forms of systemic amyloidosis before it turns attention to the hereditary amyloidoses.

## Immunoglobulin Amyloidosis

Immunoglobulin amyloidosis includes all cases in which the basic building block of the amyloid fibril is immunoglobulin light chain protein. This type is referred to as "*AL amyloidosis,*" for amyloid light chain. This group of disorders includes primary amyloidosis, as well as amyloidosis associated with multiple myeloma and other plasma cell dyscrasias, such as Waldenström macroglobulinemia and B cell lymphomas. The unifying factor in these amyloidoses is the overproduction of monoclonal immunoglobulin protein, with the light chain of the clonal product becoming the subunit of the amyloid fibril. Rarely truncated forms of immunoglobulin heavy chain proteins will form amyloid fibrils and result in systemic disease similar to AL syndromes. These have been designated AH for amyloid heavy chain,[57] and are also monoclonal plasma cell disease.

**Incidence.** Immunoglobulin amyloidosis is the most common form of systemic amyloidosis. There are no good prevalence data, but in a large medical center, there should be several patients with this disease each year.[58] Unfortunately, a fair percentage of patients with immunoglobulin amyloidosis die without the benefit of a correct diagnosis. Even when the diagnosis is made, the lack of a proven form of therapy often discourages the primary physician from referring the patient to a specialty center where that person would be entered in the published statistics. The tendency of immunoglobulin amyloidosis to affect the heart and cause heart failure or fatal arrhythmia probably adds to the number of undiagnosed cases.

**Clinical Presentation.** Immunoglobulin amyloidosis affects the mesenchyme-derived organs such as heart, skeletal muscle, and nerve. These structures are involved much more frequently than in reactive (secondary) amyloidosis. Still, the most common presentation for immunoglobulin amyloidosis is renal involvement with nephrotic syndrome.[59] Some patients present with hepatomegaly, and a small number of patients present with clotting factor X deficiency, which may be related to amyloid infiltration of the

**Table 209-1 Systemic Amyloidoses**

| Type | Previous Name(s) | Subunit Protein | Distinguishing Feature |
|---|---|---|---|
| Immunoglobulin (AL) | Primary<br>Myeloma-associated | Ig light chains (Kappa or Lambda) | Monoclonal immunoglobulin |
| Reactive (AA) | Secondary | Amyloid A | Inflammatory disease |
| Hereditary | Familial<br>Heredofamilial<br>FAP | Transthyretin<br>Apolipoprotein A-I<br>Gelsolin<br>Fibrinogen<br>Lysozyme<br>Cystatin C | Autosomal dominant |
| β2-Microglobulin (β2M) | Dialysis | β2-Microglobulin | Renal dialysis |

spleen.[60] Immunoglobulin amyloidosis is increasingly recognized in patients with cardiomyopathy, as well as in patients with life-threatening ventricular arrhythmias. Bowel involvement with chronic diarrhea and weight loss is common, and autonomic nervous system involvement with orthostatic hypotension and sexual impotence is also frequent. Vascular deposits in the skin may cause purpura. A number of patients have carpal tunnel syndrome, and some have generalized neuropathy due to amyloid infiltration of nerves.[61] These latter cases may be confused with the hereditary neuropathy syndromes (see Chap. 227).

**Laboratory Findings.** Laboratory test results will reflect which organ systems are infiltrated by amyloid. Electrocardiograms often show decreased voltage and evidence of anteroseptal myocardial infarction. Numerous studies have shown that no such infarction exists in these patients and that the septal Q waves and voltage abnormalities are most likely due to amyloid deposits in the muscle. Echocardiography may show thickened ventricular walls, but good systolic function is retained. Valve thickening is much less common in this type of amyloidosis than in the hereditary syndromes. Renal amyloid usually causes proteinuria in the nephrotic range; in later stages there is increasing azotemia. Heart failure and orthostatic hypotension can frequently cause prerenal azotemia. Protein electrophoresis and immunoelectrophoresis of serum and urine will detect monoclonal immunoglobulin components in approximately 80 percent of patients with immunoglobulin amyloidosis. The bone marrow frequently has increased numbers of plasma cells which, in classic primary amyloidosis, lack malignant features but often have increased cytoplasm, which probably indicates active immunoglobulin synthesis. The percentage of plasma cells in the bone marrow is frequently between 3 and 5 percent, but may be 20 percent or greater. In patients with overt myeloma, the plasma cells have malignant features and may constitute 50 percent or more of the bone marrow population. Recent studies using immunostaining are particularly useful in evaluating patients with immunoglobulin amyloidosis in which circulating monoclonal proteins are not detected. The demonstration that plasma cells in a bone marrow are monoclonal supports the diagnosis of AL amyloidosis. Quantitation of Bence-Jones protein in serum or urine is not always useful in distinguishing multiple myeloma from primary amyloidosis, but it is often used as one of the parameters to diagnose multiple myeloma. If multiple myeloma is present, lytic lesions in the skull or the spine may be seen on radiographs. Clinicians need to be wary, however, because amyloid deposits in such structures as the femoral head may occasionally completely replace the bone and be misinterpreted as evidence of myeloma.

**Clinical Course and Prognosis.** Immunoglobulin amyloidosis is a variable disease, with the prognosis depending on which organ system is involved. Large clinical studies have demonstrated median survival of patients with AL amyloidosis ranging from 10 to 24 months after tissue biopsy diagnosis, but for the individual patient, certain clinical parameters may offer a more definitive prognosis.[62,63] For patients with serum creatinine > 4 mg/dl or severe heart failure, a life expectancy of 6 months should be considered. Patients who present with only neuropathy or carpal tunnel syndrome may survive several years. All studies, however, show an approximate 5-year survival rate of 20 percent. Of the major types of systemic amyloidosis, the immunoglobulin type has the worst prognosis. The prognosis is especially grim for patients with multiple myeloma and amyloidosis, and many die within 6 months of diagnosis.

**Pathogenesis.** Because all immunoglobulin-type amyloid deposits are composed of monoclonal immunoglobulin light chain proteins, we know that a basic factor in the pathogenesis of this disease is the overproduction of immunoglobulin light chains by a particular B-lymphocyte clone. The factors responsible for the initiation of this process are unknown. In multiple myeloma, it

may be due to the malignant nature of the cell, but in most cases of classic primary amyloidosis, it would appear that normal metabolic processes are altered so that light chains are either overproduced or cannot be degraded completely. Clinical studies suggest that certain immunoglobulin light chains are more amyloidogenic than others. For instance, more $\lambda$ light chain proteins are associated with amyloid than $\kappa$ proteins.[1] Because the ratio of $\kappa$ to $\lambda$ in the immune system is 2:1, this suggests that $\lambda$ light chains are more amyloidogenic. This result may be partly due to the fact that free Bence-Jones proteins in plasma usually exist as dimers, and $\lambda$ light chains have a higher association constant than $\kappa$ light chains. This hypothesis is supported by studies of systemic amyloidosis due to truncated heavy chain proteins that, when analyzed, had essentially the same size and structure as an immunoglobulin light chain.[57] Because the domains of heavy and light chains are similar at the tertiary structure level, it would appear that the size of the immunoglobulin protein is a determining factor in fibril formation. Little is known about why certain monoclonal light chains deposit in any particular organ. Vascular organs such as kidney, liver, spleen, and heart are very prone to amyloid deposition, but bowel and nerve are also commonly involved. The light chain protein is usually processed when incorporated into fibrils, so that most amyloid subunit proteins include the entire variable segment of the light chain plus approximately the first tryptic peptide of the constant region. Because both the variable segment and the constant segment have extensive $\beta$-structure, they are readily incorporated into the $\beta$-pleated sheet of the amyloid fibril.[43] Practically no data are available on whether the light chains are cleaved prior to incorporation into the fibril or whether incorporation occurs and then the bulk of the constant region is clipped off during the aggregation process. Occasionally, amyloid fibrils are found in which the entire light chain is incorporated into the fibril. Thus far, no polyclonal light chains have been found incorporated in fibrils, suggesting that fibril synthesis is a very selective process.

**Treatment.** The most frequently used treatment for immunoglobulin amyloidosis is chemotherapy with alkylating agents such as melphalan coupled with prednisone.[64] This has been a standard therapy for multiple myeloma for many years and, in selected cases, appears to be effective in immunoglobulin amyloidosis. Patients with Waldenström macroglobulinemia and amyloidosis are often treated with chlorambucil. In recent years, colchicine has been added to this regimen[65] or used alone[66] because it is effective in preventing amyloid fibril formation in the murine model of amyloidosis, and also in patients with familial Mediterranean fever.[67,68] It should be noted that the murine model of amyloid is of the reactive (AA) type, as is the amyloid of familial Mediterranean fever. Use of colchicine in the other forms of systemic amyloidosis is based on the hypothesis that the drug interferes with fibril formation and not with protein synthesis. At least one clinical study has suggested that the use of colchicine may be associated with prolonged survival.[66] Trials of combination chemotherapy with drugs including vincristine, Adriamycin, bischloroethylnitrosourea (BCNU), cyclophosphamide, melphalan, and prednisone, generally failed to show advantages over treatment with the established regimen of melphalan and prednisone. Similarly, treatment with high-dose dexamethasone has not been shown to be superior to melphalan and prednisone, and gives a response in only a small percentage of cases that fail to respond to the standard treatment. Recently, several amyloid centers have established therapeutic trials of high-dose intravenous melphalan with autologous stem cell rescue for AL amyloidosis.[69] Initial results are favorable but extent of disease at the time of diagnosis and potential toxicity of this procedure often preclude undertaking this option. Treatment of AL amyloidosis with 4′-iodo-4′-deoxydoxorubicin has benefitted some patients but has not been shown to give recovery of heart, kidney, or liver function.[70] A therapeutic trial in the United States to evaluate the efficacy of this drug in AL amyloidosis was recently approved.

Numerous supportive measures have been shown to prolong the survival of patients with immunoglobulin amyloidosis. Potent diuretics can alleviate the nephrotic syndrome and congestive heart failure, and antiarrhythmia medications may prevent fatal cardiac arrhythmias. These often increase the problems of restrictive cardiomyopathy, however. Renal failure can be treated with dialysis, and some patients have received renal transplants. Cardiac transplantation has been performed in a small number of patients with varying results.[71] Transplanted organs usually develop amyloidosis if the patient lives long enough, but in selected cases survival is definitely prolonged.[72] Recent trials of organ transplantation in selected patients, coupled with high-dose melphalan therapy with autologous stem cell rescue, may offer a therapeutic option for patients who until now have had little chance for prolonging their life. In a few patients, splenectomy corrected bleeding diathesis from factor X deficiency.[73]

## Reactive Amyloidosis

Reactive (secondary) amyloidosis is usually found in individuals with chronic inflammatory disease. Many diseases will predispose to reactive amyloidosis, but the most frequent include inflammatory arthritides, such as rheumatoid or psoriatic arthritis, granulomatous bowel disease, tuberculosis, leprosy, osteomyelitis, and suppurative infections, as may be seen in patients with quadriplegia or paraplegia. Reactive amyloidosis has also been reported in patients with cystic fibrosis, systemic lupus erythematosus, and bronchiectasis. In recent years, there has been an increasing number of reports of reactive amyloidosis in intravenous drug users, presumably associated with chronic skin and other organ infection. Occasionally, reactive amyloidosis is seen in a patient with no predisposing disease. Reactive amyloidosis occurs in a familial pattern in patients with familial Mediterranean fever. This association is discussed in the sections on familial Mediterranean fever and Muckle-Wells syndrome. The acronym classification for reactive amyloidosis is AA, which stands for amyloid A to reflect the subunit protein of the fibrils.

**Incidence.** Recent studies suggest that the incidence of reactive amyloidosis is decreasing. In the early part of the twentieth century, amyloidosis was common in patients with suppurative tuberculous lesions such as empyema. A lower incidence is noted in chronic cavitary disease, and now that tuberculosis is usually treated satisfactorily, it is quite uncommon to see a patient with amyloidosis associated with tuberculosis. The incidence in patients with rheumatoid arthritis was reported to be high in the past, but more recent studies based on random intestinal biopsy report approximately 8 percent positivity. Most physicians would agree that clinically significant amyloidosis is seen in a much smaller percentage of patients with an inflammatory arthritis such as rheumatoid arthritis. The relatively high incidence in patients with quadriplegia or paraplegia persists despite the use of antibiotics. In certain equatorial parts of the world, leprosy is frequently associated with reactive amyloidosis.

**Clinical Presentation.** Reactive amyloid deposits usually involve the kidney, liver, and spleen early in the course of the disease. Many patients present with the nephrotic syndrome, and this may persist for months or years before azotemia occurs. By the time of death, major liver and spleen involvement is common. The gastrointestinal tract is commonly involved, but motility is less affected than in the immunoglobulin and hereditary amyloidoses. However, gastrointestinal bleeding, which may be life threatening, is quite frequent, and often no definite site of bleeding can be found on clinical evaluation. Cardiac and skeletal muscle are much less commonly involved, and neuropathy has not been reported. Length of survival with reactive amyloidosis depends on how early in the course the diagnosis is made. Renal disease usually progresses slowly, and a patient may be nephrotic for 3 to 5 years before becoming significantly azotemic. Hemodialysis or peritoneal dialysis may prolong life. Amyloid infiltration in blood vessel walls, however, causes increased risk of hemorrhage, and involvement of other organs such as the liver eventually leads to death.

**Pathogenesis.** The precursor protein of reactive amyloid fibrils is serum amyloid A, which is synthesized mainly in the liver.[16,20,74] There is some evidence that other tissues produce SAA, but hepatic synthesis far outweighs any other origin. SAA is both an acute-phase reactant and an apolipoprotein.[75,76] The kinetics of hepatic SAA production are very similar to those for C-reactive protein, another acute-phase reactant.[20,21] Both interleukin 1 and interleukin 6, either alone or in concert with other cytokines, stimulate hepatocytes to produce SAA by inducing the transcription of SAA genes.[77,78] In the human, there are at least four SAA genes with multiple alleles located on the short arm of chromosome 11.[79,80] Human SAA1 and SAA2 are acute-phase proteins. Each is a single polypeptide chain of 104 amino acid residues and can contribute to amyloid fibril formation.[81,82] SAA is usually proteolyzed by cleavage between residues 76 and 77 with only the 1 to 76 residue portion incorporated into amyloid fibrils, although considerable C-terminal heterogeneity for fibril subunit proteins has been described.[13,83] Human SAA4, a normal constituent of HDL, is present in serum at a higher concentration than SAA1 and SAA2, but is not induced by inflammation and does not participate in amyloid fibril formation.[84] Human SAA3 is a pseudogene.[85] The mouse has varying numbers of SAA genes (1 to 5) depending on the strain.[86] The Balb/C mouse has five recognized SAA genes including a pseudogene (SAA4) localized to chromosome 7.[87-89] Two forms of murine SAA (SAA1 and SAA2) are produced as acute-phase proteins by the liver.[86] In addition, mouse serum contains another SAA isotype (SAA5) which does not show typical acute-phase kinetics and is analogous to human SAA4.[89] The mouse SAA3 gene is expressed in extrahepatic tissues.[90] A protein analogous to murine SAA3 was found in rabbit cell culture systems and the corresponding mRNA identified.[91] The nomenclature for SAA genes and proteins in various mammalian species is a bit confusing and continues to evolve. For more information on SAA gene and protein structure the reader is referred to a review by Husby et al.[92] In the mouse, only SAA2 (which, based on gene structure, is really analogous to human SAA1) is found in amyloid fibrils.[93] This gives support to the hypothesis that the structure of the SAA subunit protein is important in amyloid fibril formation. In addition to SAA structure, there are obviously other factors that dictate AA amyloid formation. Only a minor percentage of humans with sustained high plasma levels of SAA1 and SAA2 develop amyloidosis. Some studies suggest that subjects that develop reactive amyloidosis may have a defect in normal degradation of SAA.[94] Reactive amyloidosis is the most thoroughly studied because there are several animal models of this disease that lend themselves to laboratory investigation (see "Animal Models of Amyloidosis" below).

**Treatment.** There is no specific treatment for reactive amyloidosis. Control of the chronic inflammatory processes which led to amyloidosis is a natural factor to be considered in slowing the progression of this disease. Chronic colchicine administration prevents the occurrence of reactive amyloidosis in patients with familial Mediterranean fever, but no such finding has been reported for sporadic reactive amyloidosis.[95] Suppression of chronic inflammation with antimetabolite drugs such as azathioprine and methotrexate might have a favorable effect on the overall outcome, and chlorambucil has been reported to be effective in patients with juvenile rheumatoid arthritis and reactive amyloidosis. Supportive measures are often very effective and can add significant time to survival. These include not only renal dialysis, but also the judicious use of diuretics, antibiotics, and measures to treat the primary inflammatory disease.

## β₂-Microglobulin Amyloidosis (MIM 109700)

In 1980, it was reported that carpal tunnel syndrome in patients on hemodialysis for chronic renal insufficiency was associated with amyloid deposits in the soft tissues of the wrist.[96,97] While surgical decompression of the carpal tunnel resulted in relief of symptoms, these patients frequently developed diffuse arthralgias and, particularly, pain in the shoulders with decreased range of motion. Articular erosions and radiolucent cysts within juxta-articular bone of the shoulders, hips, and wrists are frequently seen, and are due to deposition of amyloid within joint capsule, synovium, subchondral bone, and articular cartilage.[98] In addition, a number of patients have presented with destructive vertebral lesions where bone is essentially replaced by amyloid.

The incidence of amyloidosis associated with chronic hemodialysis increases with time on dialysis. As many as 70 percent of patients on dialysis for 10 years will have the carpal tunnel syndrome and radiolucent juxta-articular bone cysts that are typical of this syndrome. While most cases are associated with hemodialysis, the syndrome has now been observed in a number of patients treated with chronic ambulatory peritoneal dialysis, and it has also been reported in patients with chronic azotemia who have not been treated with dialysis.

In 1985, chemical analysis of amyloid deposits from dialysis patients resulted in the characterization of the fibril subunit protein as $\beta_2$-microglobulin.[99,100] $\beta_2$-Microglobulin is part of the HLA class I complex present on all nucleated cells. It is noncovalently associated with the heavy chain of the HLA complex. $\beta_2$-Microglobulin is present in the plasma in a monomeric form (11.8 kDa), and most of it is removed by glomerular filtration, after which proximal tubular reabsorption and degradation normally occur. Plasma levels are approximately 2 mg/liter but may be elevated up to sixtyfold in chronic uremia. While it was originally suspected that dialysis membranes were involved in generating high levels of $\beta_2$-microglobulin, it has been shown that the high plasma levels are explainable by the lack of plasma clearance and degradation.[101] The current hypothesis is that decreased renal clearance of $\beta_2$-microglobulin allows markedly elevated circulating levels of the protein and subsequent amyloid formation. It is unclear why deposits tend to occur in synovium, cartilage, and juxta-articular bone and soft tissue.

There is no specific treatment for $\beta_2$-microglobulin amyloidosis. Joint replacement has been used when destruction of the hip has occurred. Stabilizing the spine orthopedically may be necessary for destructive vertebral lesions. Some patients with this syndrome have benefited from successful renal transplantation, which presumably reestablishes normal degradation or clearance of $\beta_2$-microglobulin from the plasma. Unfortunately, many patients on chronic hemodialysis have already failed successful renal transplantation or are in an elderly group where transplantation is less indicated. Artificial means of removing $\beta_2$-microglobulin from the plasma, as by immunoabsorbent or other filtration techniques, are not yet clinically available. Recent studies with polysulfone or polyacrylonitrile dialysis membranes show improved clearance of $\beta_2$-microglobulin but the effect on amyloid deposition has not yet been determined.

## Animal Models of Amyloidosis

Systemic amyloidosis occurs in many animal species, most often as a sporadic disease, but occasionally with hereditary aspects. The amyloid fibrils from a number of species have been analyzed and shown to contain AA proteins, which revealed the reactive nature of the disease. AA proteins have been structurally characterized for the mouse, horse, cow, dog, cat, monkey, guinea pig, hamster, mink, and Pekin duck.[74,102–108] The duck, other waterfowl and the chicken are the only nonmammalian species, so far, in which AA of reactive amyloid has been characterized. In a strain of collie dogs, amyloidosis is associated with hereditary cyclic neutropenia.[109] In Abyssinian cats, amyloidosis shows a hereditary pattern.[110] Some strains of mice have spontaneous amyloid that is not of the AA type. In particular, a strain of mice showing early senescence has been shown to have amyloid fibrils composed of apolipoprotein A-II (apo A-II).[111] In this particular type of amyloidosis, an amino acid substitution (Pro5Gln) in apo A-II has

been shown to be associated with the strains that develop amyloidosis. This model may be valuable in studying senescence, but, to date, human amyloidosis related to apolipoprotein A-II has not been discovered.

Reactive amyloidosis can be induced in most mammalian species. Kuczynski first showed that amyloidosis could be caused in mice by parenteral administration of sodium caseinate.[112,113] Subsequently, the murine model of induced systemic amyloidosis was used extensively as a model of the human disease. It has many features of the human disease, with major deposition of fibrils in spleen, liver, and kidney. This form of amyloid can also be produced by administration of Freund's complete adjuvant and by chronic administration of endotoxin. Studies using this model show that interleukin 1 and interleukin 6 are generated by macrophages,[77,114,115] and these cytokines induce the liver to synthesize SAA,[22] one form of which (SAA2) is incorporated into amyloid fibrils.[93] It is interesting that of all the mammalian species studied thus far, the rat does not appear to synthesize a full-length SAA and has never been shown to develop reactive amyloidosis. The murine model of casein-induced amyloidosis has been used to show that high doses of colchicine will prevent amyloid fibril formation and that discontinuing casein administration will result in some resolution of the fibril deposits.[116]

Animal models of human immunoglobulin light chain amyloidosis have not been available for study. Despite extensive studies with myeloma proteins in mice, no strain of mice has yet been found to spontaneously develop immunoglobulin amyloid deposits. The mouse is capable of processing light chain to give amyloid deposits, however, because the administration of massive doses of human amyloid-producing Bence-Jones protein into mice results in deposition of material meeting the histologic criteria for amyloid.[117] This model has not been developed to the point where it can be used for studying human amyloid pathogenesis. Immunoglobulin amyloidosis does occur rarely in horses, dogs, and cats but it is a sporadic disease and these species have not presented a model for study of pathogenesis.[118,119]

No species other than humans has been shown to have transthyretin-type amyloidosis. Transgenic mice have been created with the methionine 30 (Met30) variant of transthyretin, and this model promises to be important in studying the pathogenesis of hereditary amyloidosis.[120,121] In transgenic mice with the Met30 transthyretin gene ligated to the metallothionein promoter, amyloid deposits were noted first in intestinal mucosa at 6 months of age.[122] These increased with age along with glomerular amyloid deposits. By 24 months of age, all glomeruli had amyloid deposits, and myocardial deposits of amyloid were also reported. Amyloid deposits were not, however, detected in peripheral nerve, which is the earliest and most common site of localization in humans.[123] Even so, this model gives a new approach to the study of pathogenesis of a hereditary disease. Recently, amyloidosis in mice carrying multiple copies of the normal human transthyretin was described. This transgenic mouse model has promise for the study of senile cardiac amyloidosis.

The development of cell culture systems for amyloid synthesis also holds promise for studying pathogenesis. While many proteins can be made to produce amyloid-like fibrils in vitro, this is usually under nonphysiological conditions and results are mainly pertinent to analysis of the role of structure in fibril formation. In vitro cell culture systems offer the opportunity to study cell uptake and enzymatic processing as well as structure of amyloid precursor proteins. Amyloid fibril synthesis from immunoglobulin light chain proteins in cultures of human kidney mesangial cells has been described.[124] Also, murine peritoneal macrophages reproducibly produce AA amyloid deposits when cultured in the presence of murine SAA2.[125,126]

## HEREDITARY AMYLOIDOSIS

Hereditary amyloidosis continues to hold a prominent position in the minds of students of amyloid. Besides presenting models for studying the role of protein structure, expression, and metabolism in the mechanism of amyloid formation, the hereditary amyloidoses allow correlation of these basic factors with clinical observations on phenotypic expression, genetic transmission, and epidemiology. This makes hereditary amyloidosis a valuable model for the study of cell processes that may be common to many forms of amyloidosis. Mutant forms of plasma transthyretin continue to be the most common cause of hereditary amyloidosis. Since the last edition of this text, the number of mutations in transthyretin that are associated with systemic amyloidosis has increased to 73. Increased numbers of mutations in other proteins associated with hereditary amyloidosis have also been discovered, including 8 mutations in apolipoprotein A-I, four in fibrinogen Aα-chain, two in lysozyme, two in gelsolin and one in cystatin C. Several mutations in the Alzheimer β-APP protein result either in cerebral amyloid plaques or cerebrovascular Congophilic angiopathy. Mutations in the prion protein are associated with familial Creutzfeldt-Jakob disease and Gerstmann-Sträussler-Scheinker syndrome, which show amyloid fibril deposits. In addition, mutations in proteins presumed to be involved in the metabolism of normal amyloid fibril precursor proteins have been discovered, including mutations in presenilin I and II which cause Alzheimer plaque formation from normal β-APP. Similar genetic factors may be involved in the amyloid formation from normal apolipoprotein A-I and transthyretin. It is obvious that the hereditary amyloidoses are truly worldwide in distribution and that they affect a much larger number of families than ever previously considered.

### The Transthyretin Amyloidoses (MIM 176300)

Most of the autosomal dominant amyloidoses characterized thus far are associated with variants of plasma transthyretin. So far, 73 mutations of transthyretin have been described, and there is likely to be more. To understand the pathogenesis of these forms of amyloidosis better, it is important to review the properties of transthyretin. Transthyretin is a normal plasma protein. It was originally called "prealbumin" or "thyroxine-binding prealbumin" because it migrates ahead of albumin on standard protein electrophoresis.[127] However, it has no structural relationship to albumin.[128] The name transthyretin (TTR) was coined because of the transport properties of the protein, which binds both thyroxine and retinol-binding protein (RBP).[129] The term transthyretin is relatively universally accepted and is in general use. However, any literature review will find many of the significant articles under the name prealbumin.

Plasma transthyretin is synthesized by the liver in a constitutive manner as a single polypeptide chain of 127 amino acid residues.[130,131] The primary structure has been known since 1974, and the secondary, tertiary, and quaternary structures were defined by x-ray diffraction.[132] The entity circulating in plasma is a tetramer ($M_r = 55,000$) composed of four identical monomers[44,132] (Fig. 209-6). Two monomers noncovalently combine to form a stable dimer, and then two dimers associate to form the tetramer with twofold symmetry. Down the center channel of the tetramer are two binding sites for thyroxine, although binding studies suggest that these sites show negative cooperativity.[133] Transthyretin also binds retinol saturated RBP ($M_r = 21,000$) to provide transport of vitamin A without loss of the small RBP molecule through the kidney.[134] RBP binds to the outside surface of transthyretin involving the isoleucine at position 84 and, while there are four potential binding sites on each tetramer, x-ray crystallography of the transthyretin and RBP complex shows that binding of one RBP molecule to the tetramer restricts binding of a second molecule to that side of the tetramer.[135-137] Therefore, only two molecules of RBP can bind to one transthyretin tetramer. The transthyretin concentration in plasma normally ranges from 20 to 40 mg/dl and has been found to be significantly depressed in individuals with malnutrition. The plasma concentration also decreases at times of acute or chronic inflammation, and, therefore, transthyretin has been called a negative acute-phase protein. Plasma levels are also significantly depressed in many

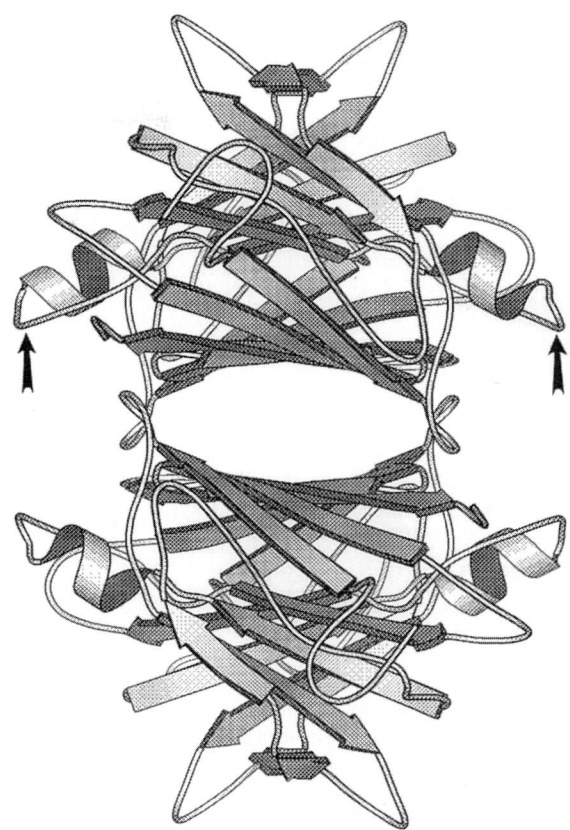

**Fig. 209-6 Computergraphic model of the transthyretin tetramer based on x-ray diffraction data.[144] Thyroxine binds to the central cavity. Rentinol-binding protein-vitamin A binds to the outside of the tetramer with amino acid Ile84 being central to the binding (arrows). Only two molecules of retinol-binding protein bind to one transthyretin tetramer because each molecule of retinol-binding protein (21,000 daltons) blocks the second potential binding site on that side of the tetramer.[137]**

patients with the transthyretin amyloidoses, but the reason for this is unclear.[138-140] The single gene for transthyretin is located on human chromosome 18.[141] Most individuals with transthyretin amyloidosis have been found to be heterozygotes having one normal transthyretin allele and one variant allele. Expression of the two alleles is probably equal, but most studies have shown more of the normal gene product in the plasma than of the variant.[142,143]

Transthyretin has extensive β-structure; the monomers have eight β-chains arranged in an antiparallel configuration in two planes (Fig. 209-7). This configuration would appear to predispose the protein toward amyloid fibril formation. Each of the amino acid substitutions that has been identified in variant transthyretins associated with hereditary amyloidosis can be hypothesized to alter the surface topography of the molecule.[144] This alteration presumably would favor aggregation and fibril formation; however, no clear unifying structural change has been noted. The identification of several transthyretin variants that do not predispose to amyloid formation has not helped clarify this problem.[145,146]

The transthyretin cDNA sequence has been reported by a number of laboratories,[141,147,148] and the complete nucleotide sequence of the transthyretin gene in humans has been reported by two laboratories (GenBank NM_000371) (Fig. 209-8).[149,150] The human gene has four exons (Fig. 209-9). Exon 1 codes for a 20-residue signal peptide and the first three amino acids of the mature protein, exon 2 codes for residues 4 to 47, exon 3, residues 48 to 92 and exon 4, residues 93 to 127. The proximal upstream 5'

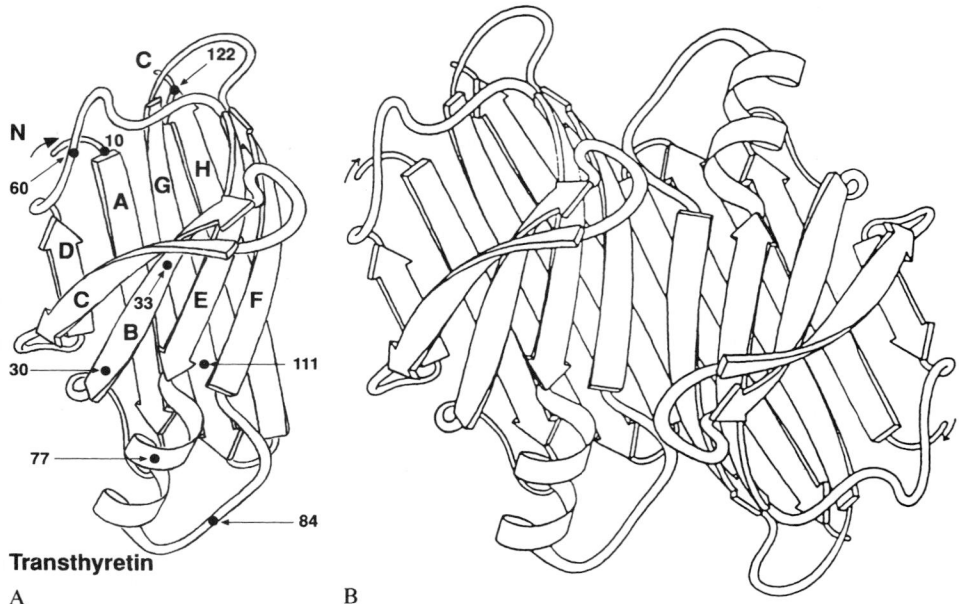

**Transthyretin**

A                    B

**Fig. 209-7** Subunit structure of transthyretin. *A,* Antiparallel β-structure of transthyretin. Eight β-strands are arranged in two parallel planes. The approximate locations of eight of the mutations associated with amyloidosis are indicated. These include the mutation (Arg10) closest to the N-terminal and the mutation (Ile122) closest to the C-terminal. These two mutations are at the ends of the ordered β-strand structure. *B,* Two prealbumin monomers associate to form a dimer. Two dimers then associate to give the tetramer depicted in Fig. 209-6. (*A modified from and B from Richardson JS: Adv Protein Chem 34:270, 1981. Used with permission.*)

region has sequences similar to those for binding the glucocorticoid receptor. However, the mouse prealbumin gene appears to have additional regulatory sequences about 2 kb upstream from the coding regions.[130,151] Transthyretin mRNA has been identified in choroid plexus of rats[152–154] and humans[155] and also in retina, so synthesis is not exclusively hepatic. It is unlikely that extrahepatic transthyretin synthesis plays a role in the systemic manifestations of amyloidosis, but leptomeningeal involvement may be related to intracranial synthesis, and vitreous amyloid may possibly be the result of local gene expression.

## Autosomal Dominant Transthyretin-Associated Amyloidosis Syndromes

**Clinical Features.** Most of the autosomal dominant amyloidoses have peripheral neuropathy as a major clinical manifestation. Thus, these disorders have also been called "familial amyloidotic polyneuropathy" (FAP). In the past, clinical classification of the syndromes was based on whether lower-extremity or upper-extremity neuropathy was the presenting symptom.[156] This criterion is less valid now, because the upper-extremity neuropathy, which is really a compression neuropathy from the carpal tunnel syndrome, has been seen in many of the recently described kindreds, sometimes before and sometimes after involvement of the lower extremities (Fig. 209-10).

The Portuguese neuropathy (FAP type I) shows the classic and most common features of hereditary amyloidosis (Fig. 209-11). The clinical disease usually starts in the third or fourth decade, although the onset of symptoms may be delayed until old age. The disease progresses over 10 to 20 years with peripheral sensorimotor neuropathy, autonomic neuropathy, and varying degrees of systemic amyloid involvement. The neuropathy starts in the lower extremities with paresthesias and often hypesthesia, which can be debilitating. Autonomic neuropathy is an early feature, and patients may present with sexual impotence or gastrointestinal dysfunction. Sensory loss in the lower extremities follows a stocking distribution, and it has been noted that temperature and pain sensations are impaired earlier than proprioception. By the time sensory loss has progressed to the level of the knees, the hands usually become involved by a sensory neuropathy with a glove distribution. Motor loss develops later and frequently results in footdrop, wristdrop, and difficulty in hand function. Trophic ulcers on the lower extremities are common and, before the advent of antibiotics, were a frequent cause of infection and death. Orthostatic hypotension is common and has profound significance

in patients with cardiac amyloid. Gastrointestinal symptoms are due mainly to nerve dysfunction with affected individuals having constipation alternating with diarrhea. Delayed gastric emptying may lead to distension of the organ and poor appetite. Cachexia is a frequent feature and may be a significant factor in mortality.

Visual involvement has been known to occur in the Portuguese syndrome but is much more frequently seen in Swedish kindreds and in the Indiana/Swiss amyloidosis (FAP II). Amyloid within the vitreous humor of the eye interferes with vision, but this can usually be corrected, at least temporarily, by surgical removal of the deposits (Fig. 209-12). The scalloped pupil deformity is another eye manifestation that has been described both in Portuguese and Swedish kindreds with FAP I, and is probably due to involvement of ciliary nerves. Autonomic neuropathy may cause urinary retention severe enough to require diversionary procedures to prevent renal damage. Hypohidrosis has also been seen.

Other clinical manifestations of hereditary amyloidosis depend on which organ systems are involved. FAP I patients (Portuguese, Swedish, Japanese) may have renal amyloid with significant protein loss and subsequent renal insufficiency. In these patients, dialysis may prolong life, but subsequent involvement of other organs is not prevented. The Indiana/Swiss kindred (FAP II), the Appalachian kindred, and several of the more recently described kindreds have severe cardiomyopathy, which is usually the cause of death. Cardiac conduction disturbances occur early and frequently require artificial pacing. The subsequent clinical picture is one of restrictive cardiomyopathy with low-output heart failure. Cardiomyopathy without peripheral neuropathy is the main feature of the amyloidosis described by Frederiksen et al., in Denmark.[157]

**Chemical Classification.** A number of transthyretin variants have been identified in the amyloid fibrils or plasma of patients with hereditary amyloidosis (Table 209-2). While the distribution of the amino acid substitutions gives no obvious clue to fibrillogenesis, all involve single amino acid substitutions that result from single nucleotide mutations in coding regions except for one which is the deletion of a codon (V122Δ).[158] The substitutions range in location from amino acid residue 10 (Cys10Arg) to residue 122 (Val122Ile) of TTR, with 27 mutations in exon 2, 32 mutations in exon 3, and 14 mutations in exon 4. No mutation in exon 1 (coding amino acids 1 through 3) has yet been discovered. These findings provide a biochemical basis for classifying the transthyretin amyloidoses and show that, although the old classification based

## TRANSTHYRETIN MUTATIONS

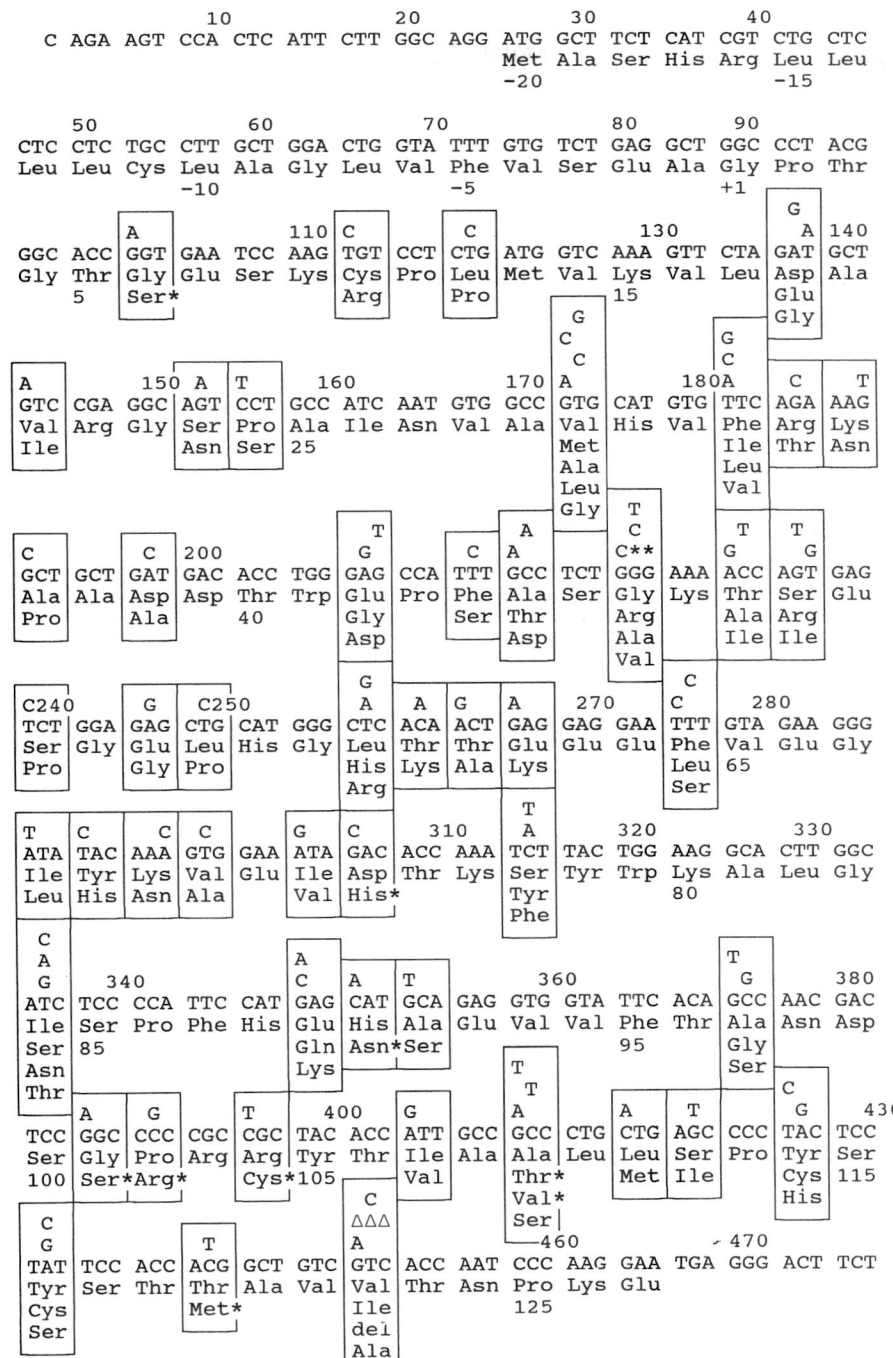

Fig. 209-8 Nucleotide sequence of transthyretin cDNA and protein amino acid sequence. Mutations shown include 66 associated with amyloidosis and 9 not associated with amyloidosis (indicated by *). Gly47Arg has been reported with both CGG and AGG codons (indicated by **). For recent mutation reports see Table 209-2.

on the clinical syndrome and ethnic origin is basically sound, there is a great deal of overlap among the syndromes. Identification of nonsymptomatic carriers of variant transthyretin genes in many of the kindreds has widened the recognized time span of clinical onset for each syndrome. The following transthyretin variants have been identified in families with hereditary amyloidosis. The clinical, geographic, and ethnic parameters that are relatively unique to each familial syndrome are emphasized to aid the clinician in recognizing and diagnosing the disease. A few additional transthyretin variants have been identified (Table 209-2), but in these, insufficient clinical data have been reported.

*Arginine 10 (C10R).* This type of systemic amyloidosis presents as a peripheral neuropathy in the sixth and seventh decades of life. The only kindred that has been described is located in Pennsylvania with ancestors of Hungarian origin.[159] No evidence for the mutation in Hungary has been found to date. In three cousins who died with this syndrome and who were studied in detail, severe cardiomyopathy and bowel dysfunction were the major factors leading to death between ages 64 and 70. This particular variant transthyretin has added importance for two reasons: (a) The mutation is the most N-terminal of all the amyloid associated mutations and is at the boundary of the less organized

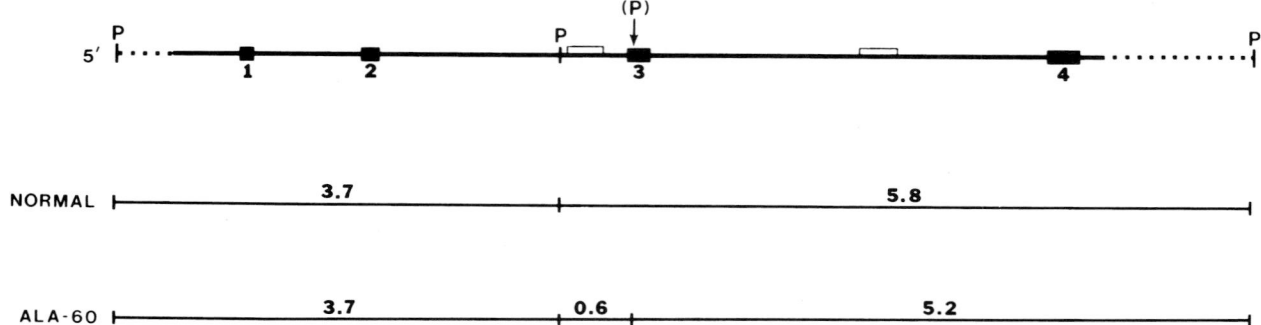

**Fig. 209-9** Drawing of human transthyretin gene showing four exons. Twenty-seven mutations associated with amyloidosis have been identified in exon 2; 32 in exon 3; and 14 in exon 4. The recognition sites for *Pvu*II are indicated (P) to show the DNA fragments generated in the Southern blot test for the Ala60 gene (see Fig. 209-16).

structure (amino acid residues 1 to 9) and highly ordered structure of the remainder of the transthyretin molecule.[132] (b) Arginine 10 replaces the only cysteine in the transthyretin molecule. This may be significant in terms of the possible involvement of disulfide linkage in amyloid fibrillogenesis.

**Proline 12 (L12P).** Subarachnoid hemorrhage at age 37 associated with leptomeningeal amyloid deposition was the presenting clinical picture in the first subject found to have this mutation. A similar clinical phenotype with subarachnoid hemorrhage has been reported with other transthyretin variants including Asp18Gly, Val30Gly, Phe64Ser, and Val122Δ.

**Glutamic Acid 18 (D18E).** This mutation was found in a 49-year-old subject from South America who had typical FAP.

**Glycine 18 (D18G).** A single Hungarian family has been described with this transthyretin variant. The clinical picture included memory loss, ataxia, hearing loss, spastic paraparesis, hallucinations, and urinary retention.[160] The mutation A to G in the second position of codon 18 abolishes an *Xba*I restriction endonuclease site.[161]

**Isoleucine 20 (V20I).** This mutation was first described in a German family, the index case was a 60-year-old man with severe cardiomyopathy and mild peripheral neuropathy.[162] It was also found in a 50-year-old man in the United States who received cardiac transplant for amyloid cardiomyopathy.[163]

**Asparagine 23 (S23N).** Severe cardiomyopathy in a man in his thirties was found to be associated with this variant transthyretin.

**Serine 24 (P24S).** Transthyretin Pro24Ser was discovered in a family with relatively late-onset amyloidosis.[164] The propositus, who was born in Kentucky, developed carpal tunnel syndrome at age 50, severe diarrhea at age 65, and died at age 70. Three brothers died of cardiac disease, and in one, cardiac amyloidosis was documented at postmortem.

The substitution of serine for proline, the result of a C → T transition in the first position of codon 24, does not give a new restriction site, so a PCR-induced mutation-restriction analysis (PCR-IMRA) (see "Detection of Gene Carriers in Hereditary Amyloidosis" below) has been used to detect the carriers of this allele.

**Methionine 30 (V30M).** The most common type of hereditary amyloidosis thus far reported is characterized by a substitution of methionine for valine at position 30 of the transthyretin molecule. This variant transthyretin has been found in many kindreds in Portugal and Japan, and also in American kindreds of Swedish, English, and Greek origin.[25,143,148,165–167] It has also been identified in Turkey, Majorca, Brazil, France, and England. While the largest numbers of patients and families have been identified in northern Portugal, the V30M allele has its highest prevalence in isolated communities in northern Sweden, where as much as 3 to 5 percent of the population may be heterozygous for the trait.[168] A number of patients homozygous for the V30M allele have been

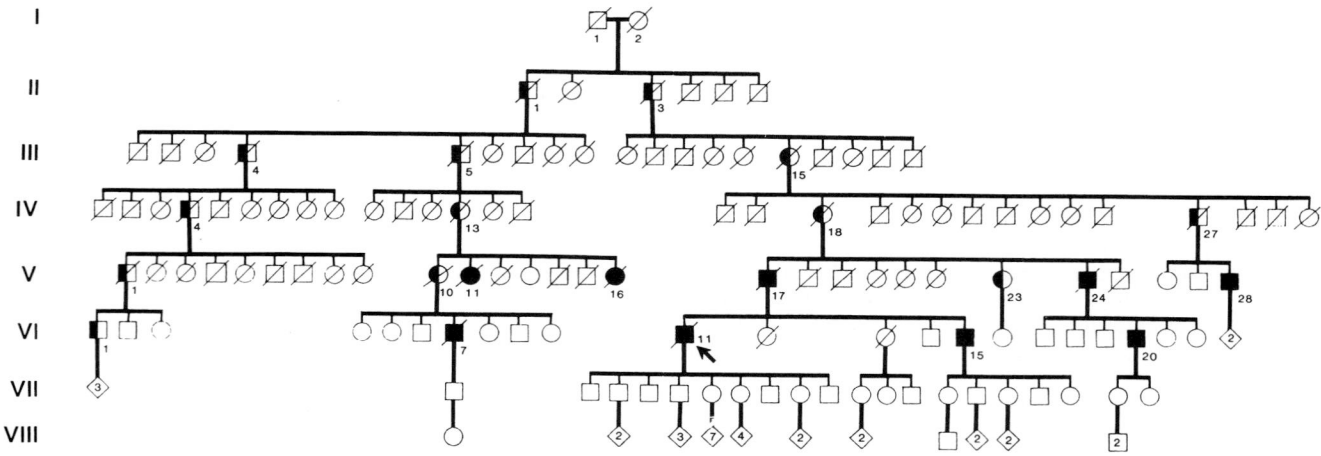

**Fig 209-10** Kindred with hereditary transthyretin amyloidosis associated with variant transthyretin showing the typical autosomal dominant pattern of inheritance. ■ = biopsy proven; □ = presumed affected; ◇ = multiple sibs, sex unspecified.

Based on the analysis

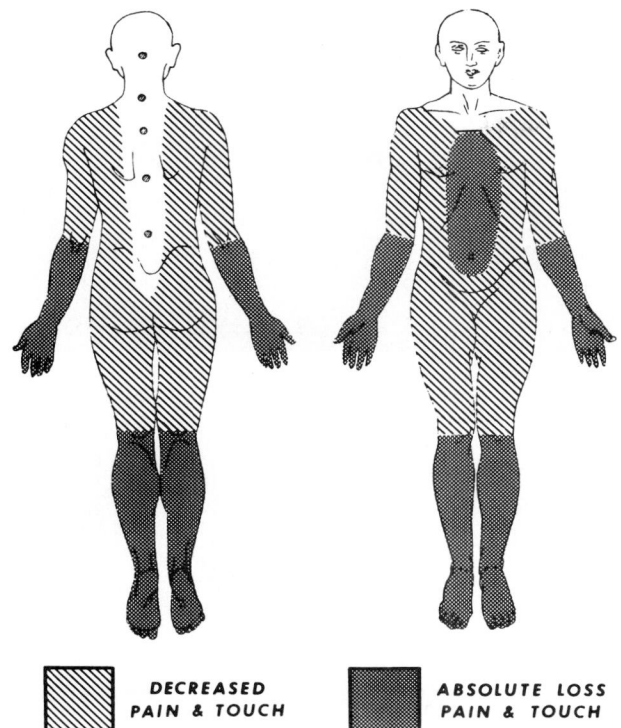

DECREASED PAIN & TOUCH    ABSOLUTE LOSS PAIN & TOUCH

**Fig. 209-11 Pattern of sensory loss in familial amyloid polyneuropathy type I.**

identified in Sweden[169] and in Turkey.[170] The onset of clinical amyloidosis and progression of the disease in these homozygous individuals does not appear to be different from that of their heterozygous kin. Clinically, most of these kindreds have been classified as FAP I with neuropathy starting in the lower extremities. Varying degrees of renal and cardiac involvement have been reported, but autonomic and gastrointestinal symptoms are present in most patients. Vitreous deposits of amyloid have been reported, as has the scalloped pupil deformity.[7] In particular, vitreous involvement appears to be much more common in the Swedish families than in the Portuguese families. Another interesting difference between Portuguese families and Swedish families with this same V30M mutation is the time of onset of disease. In Portugal, the mean age of onset is in the early thirties, with death often occurring by age 40. In Sweden, the mean age of onset of clinical disease is in the late fifties, and patients often live to the eighth decade. Mental functioning is generally not affected, but amyloid may be present in blood vessels of the central nervous system and in the leptomeninges.[171] There is evidence that the high prevalence and worldwide distribution of the V30M transthyretin mutation is in some part due to multiple mutational events. The V30M mutation was found in Japan in association with three distinct haplotypes.[172] One of these haplotypes is the same as the haplotype found in Portuguese V30M patients and Swedish V30M patients, suggesting that the gene has been spread from a common focus. The association of the V30M mutation with other haplotypes, however, suggests that separate mutation events may have occurred in Japan, and at least one V30M kindred of English origin in the United States does not share the Portugese-Swedish haplotype.[173] The idea that multiple mutational events have generated the V30M transthyretin is supported by the fact that this position is one of the mutation hot spots in the TTR coding region, where the CpG dinucleotide sequence can be altered by deamidation of a methylated cytosine.

***Alanine 30 (V30A).*** Substitution of alanine for valine at position 30 has been reported in association with systemic amyloidosis in

one family.[174] The disease had a relatively early onset in the twenties, with death in 4 to 6 years. Clinical manifestations include autonomic neuropathy with orthostasis and gastric atony, but only mild sensory neuropathy of the FAP I variety. No eye or renal involvement was clinically noted. Amyloid fibrils containing transthyretin were isolated from the heart of one individual. The T → C mutation in the second position of codon 30 gives a new *Cfo*I restriction site in exon 2.

***Leucine 30 (V30L).*** A third mutation at position 30 (Val30Leu) was discovered in a 53-year-old Japanese woman who presented with weight loss and diarrhea at age 51.[175,176] Sensory neuropathy was present in the lower extremities and sural nerve biopsy revealed deposits of amyloid which stained positively with antihuman transthyretin antibody. No vitreous opacities were reported, and there was no family history suggestive of FAP. The G → C transition in the third base of codon 30 results in a novel *Cfr*13I site, which can be used for identification of this mutation.

***Glycine 30 (V30G).*** This mutation was first identified in an American of French ancestry with vitreous opacities. It has also been found in the Ohio kindred of German origin which was reported as oculoleptomeningeal amyloidosis.[177,178] The syndrome had minor systemic amyloid and peripheral neuropathy, but was characterized by vitreous opacities and extensive leptomeningeal amyloid deposition. Dementia and ataxia are a part of the syndrome.

***Isoleucine 33 (F33I).*** This type of amyloidosis was originally called "Jewish FAP" because the only individual described with the disease was a Jewish man who was born in Poland and immigrated to Israel. The disease manifested as type I peripheral neuropathy, diarrhea, and impotence. Vitreous opacities were described between ages 25 and 30.[179] Autopsy revealed amyloid in all major organs, particularly the thyroid, kidney, spleen, and nerves. The original studies of amyloid isolated from the thyroid showed that a significant proportion of the transthyretin molecules had been cleaved between amino acid positions 48 and 49, and there was evidence for a substitution of glycine for threonine at position 49.[180] Subsequently, however, amyloid subunit protein isolated from splenic tissue showed an isoleucine substituted for phenylalanine at position 33.[181] This substitution was verified by DNA sequence studies, which failed to show any mutation in codon 49. Incidentally, the affected individual in this kindred was found to also have the TTR mutation that gives serine at position 6, which has been described by others but not in association with amyloid formation. No other kindreds with the isoleucine 33 transthyretin amyloid have been described.

***Leucine 33 (F33L).*** This mutation (Phe33Leu) was found in a middle-aged man of Polish and Lithuanian heritage who had lower limb neuropathy and cardiomyopathy.[182] There was no previous family history of amyloidosis, and no other kindreds have been identified. The T → C mutation at the first base of codon 33 gives a new *Dde*I site in exon 2.

***Valine 33 (F33V).*** This mutation was reported for a single individual in the United Kingdom with typical FAP.

***Threonine 34 (R34T).*** Three affected brothers from the Puglia area of Italy presented with polyneuropathy and restrictive cardiomyopathy after age 50.

***Asparagine 35 (K35N).*** One subject was found with this mutation producing typical amyloid polyneuropathy. This individual lived in France, but the country of origin was not determined.[183]

***Proline 36 (A36P).*** This mutation (Ala36Pro) has been described in two kindreds,[184,185] an American family of Greek origin and a Jewish family in which members died between ages 36 and 65.

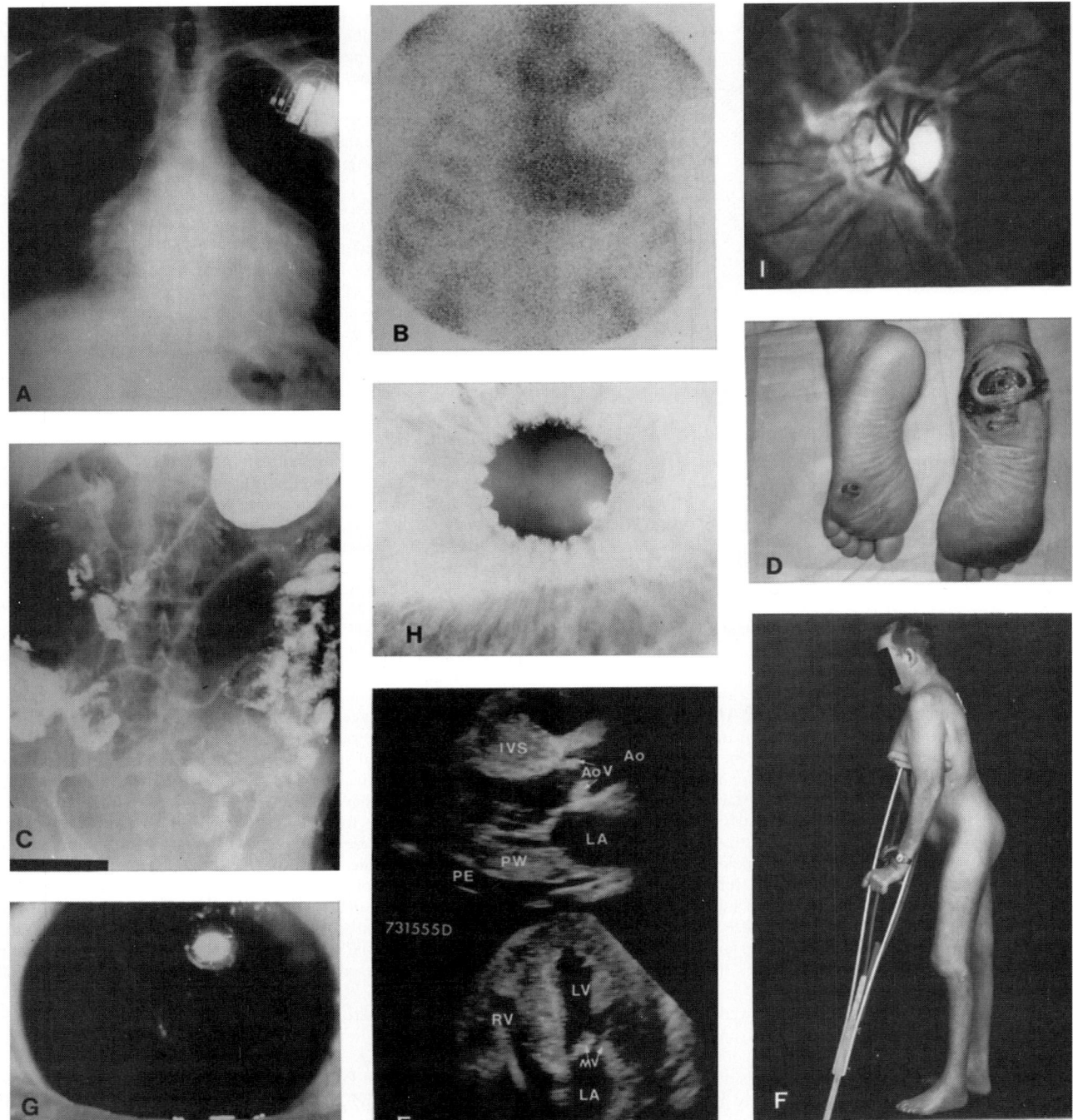

**Fig. 209-12 Clinical features of the hereditary amyloidoses.** *A,* Cardiomegaly in Ser84 amyloidosis. *B,* Technetium pyrophosphate uptake in cardiac amyloidosis. *C,* Gastric distension and dilated small bowel in Ala60 amyloidosis. *D,* Neurogenic ulcer and calcaneal osteomyelitis in Met30 amyloidosis. *E,* Two-dimensional echocardiography in Ser84 amyloidosis showing thickening intraventricular septum (IVS), left ventricular wall (PW), aortic (AOV), and mitral valves (MV), plus dilated left atrium (LA). *F,* Typical neuropathy of Met30 amyloidosis. This patient has neuropathic arthropathy (Charcot knee). *G,* Lattice corneal dystrophy of Finnish amyloidosis. *H,* Scalloped pupil in Met30 amyloidosis. *I,* Vitreous deposits in Ser84 amyloidosis.

The age of onset was 28 in one individual, and the symptoms included lower limb neuropathy, autonomic neuropathy, and vitreous opacities.

*Glycine 42 (E42G).* One kindred with glycine substituted for glutamic acid at transthyretin position 42 has been described in Japan (Toyama Prefecture).[186] At least six members of the kindred were affected with FAP, which was manifested as lower-limb neuropathy, autonomic neuropathy, cardiomyopathy, and vitreous opacities. Onset of disease was between ages 35 and 41, and major morbidity was related to restrictive cardiomyopathy. This mutation was also found in an American Caucasian family with amyloidosis that also has the nonamyloidogenic H91N mutation and in one individual from Russia. The A → G mutation at the second position of codon 42 results in a new *Cfr*13I restriction site in exon 2.

*Aspartic Acid 42 (E42D).* This mutation was discovered in one individual, age 63, with amyloid cardiomyopathy. There was no family history of amyloidosis and no neuropathy was documented.

**Table 209-2** Transthyretin Amyloidoses

| Mutation | Clinical Features* | Geographic Kindreds |
|---|---|---|
| Cys10Arg | Heart, Eye, PN | United States (PA) |
| Leu12Pro | LM | United Kingdom |
| Asp18Glu | PN | South America |
| Asp18Gly | LM | Hungary |
| Val20Ile | Heart, CTS | Germany, United States |
| Ser23Asn | Heart, PN, Eye | United States |
| Pro24Ser | Heart, CTS, PN | United States |
| Val30Met | PN, AN, Eye, LM | Portugal, Japan, Sweden, United States (FAP I) |
| Val30Ala | Heart, AN | United States |
| Val30Leu | PN, Heart | Japan |
| Val30Gly | LM, Eye | United States |
| Phe33Ile | PN, Eye | Israel |
| Phe33Leu | PN, Heart | United States |
| Phe33Val | PN | United Kingdom, Japan |
| Arg34Thr | PN, Heart | Italy |
| Lys35Asn | PN, AN, Heart | France |
| Ala36Pro | Eye, CTS | United States |
| Asp38Ala | PN, Heart | Japan |
| Glu42Gly | PN, AN, Heart | Japan, United States, Russia |
| Glu42Asp | Heart | France |
| Phe44Ser | PN, AN, Heart | United States |
| Ala45Asp | Heart, PN | United States |
| Ala45Ser | Heart | Sweden |
| Ala45Thr | Heart | United States |
| Gly47Arg | PN, AN | Japan |
| Gly47Ala | Heart, AN | Italy, Germany |
| Gly47Val | CTS, PN, AN, Heart | Sri Lanka |
| Thr49Ala | Heart, CTS | France, Italy |
| Thr49Ile | PN, Heart | Japan |
| Ser50Arg | AN, PN | Japan, French/Italian |
| Ser50Ile | Heart, PN, AN | Japan |
| Glu51Gly | Heart | United States |
| Ser52Pro | PN, AN, Heart, Kidney | England |
| Gly53Glu | LM, Heart | Basque |
| Glu54Gly | PN, AN, Eye | England |
| Leu55Arg | LM | Germany |
| Leu55Pro | Heart, AN, Eye | United States, Taiwan |
| His56Arg | Heart | United States |
| Leu58His | CTS, Heart | United States (MD) (FAP II) |
| Leu58Arg | CTS, AN, Eye | Japan |
| Thr59Lys | Heart, PN, AN | Italy |
| Thr60Ala | Heart, CTS | United States (Appalachian) |
| Glu61Lys | PN | Japan |
| Phe64Leu | PN, CTS, Heart | United States, Italy |
| Phe64Ser | LM, PN, Eye | Canada, England |
| Ile68Leu | Heart | Germany |
| Tyr69His | Eye | United States |
| Lys70Asn | Eye, CTS, PN | United States |
| Val71Ala | PN, Eye, CTS | France, Spain |
| Ile73Val | PN, AN | Bangladesh |
| Ser77Phe | | France |
| Ser77Tyr | Kidney | United States (IL, TX), France |
| Ile84Ser | Heart, CTS, Eye, LM | United States (IN), Hungary (FAP II) |
| Ile84Asn | Heart, Eye | United States |
| Ile84Thr | | Germany, United Kingdom |
| Glu89Gln | PN, Heart | Italy |
| Glu89Lys | PN, Heart | United States |
| Ala91Ser | PN, CTS, Heart | France |
| Ala97Gly | Heart, PN | Japan |
| Ala97Ser | PN, Heart | Taiwan |
| Ile107Val | Heart, CTS, PN | United States |
| Ala109Ser | | Japan |
| Leu111Met | Heart | Denmark |

**Table 209-2** (Continued)

| Mutation | Clinical Features* | Geographic Kindreds |
|---|---|---|
| Ser112Ile | PN, Heart | Italy |
| Tyr114Cys | PN, AN, Eye, LM | Japan |
| Tyr114His | CTS | Japan |
| Tyr116Cys | | France |
| Tyr116Ser | | France |
| Val122Ile | Heart | United States |
| ΔVal122 | Heart, PN | United States (Ecuador) |
| Val122Ala | Heart, Eye, PN | United States |

*AN = autonomic neuropathy; CTS = carpal tunnel syndrome; Eye = vitreous deposits; LM = leptomeningeal; PN = peripheral neuropathy

***Serine 44 (F44S).*** A single American of Irish descent has been described with peripheral neuropathy starting at age 26. When evaluated at age 32 he had severe headaches, autonomic neuropathy, hearing loss, and signs of amyloid cardiomyopathy. The serine for phenylalanine substitution is due to a thymine to cytosine mutation at the second base of codon 44 and can be detected by induced mutation restriction analysis.[187]

***Threonine 45 (A45T).*** One individual with cardiomyopathy appearing at approximately age 50 was reported to be heterozygous for a threonine substitution (Ala45Thr) at position 45 of transthyretin.[188] This individual was of Irish and Italian descent, and the family history suggested that the trait was from the Italian side of the family. Other studies of an American/Irish patient who died with restrictive cardiomyopathy showed the same mutation, but it is not known whether this single individual was a member of the previously reported kindred.

***Aspartic Acid 45 (A45D).*** This mutation associated with peripheral neuropathy and cardiomyopathy was reported from the United States. The proband was heterozygous for both A45D and the nonamyloid G6S mutation. The proband's father, who died of amyloidosis, had only the A45D mutation.

***Arginine 47 (G47R).*** The first evidence of a de novo mutation in transthyretin is represented by the arginine-for-glycine substitution at position 47.[189] The proband of the family was a 38-year-old Japanese man who showed symptoms of autonomic neuropathy at age 29. Polyneuropathy was proved by sural nerve biopsy showing amyloid deposits that stained with antitransthyretin. No vitreous opacities were noted. DNA studies of both parents and two siblings failed to show the mutation in codon 45, thus suggesting that the C-for-G transversion may be a de novo mutation.

***Alanine 47 (G47A).*** A family from Italy with cardiomyopathy and peripheral neuropathy in the fifth decade of life was found to have an alanine-for-glycine substitution at position 47.[190] Although a PCR test based on mutation-induced restriction analysis to give a novel *Msp*I site has been described, no other kindred with this mutation has yet been found.

***Valine 47 (G47V).*** This mutation was found in a Sri Lankan kindred with polyneuropathy.

***Alanine 49 (T49A).*** This mutation was found in two distinct kindreds, one in France and one in Italy, both showing cardiomyopathy.[191,192] The Italian kindred was reported to have vitreous opacities, which was not a feature in the French kindred. The French kindred, first reported in 1983, showed onset of polyneuropathy and carpal tunnel syndrome between ages 35 and 40, with subsequent development of restrictive cardiomyopathy.[193] Clinical onset of disease was at a similar age in the Italian kindred, with polyneuropathy occurring in the fifth decade of life.

***Isoleucine 49 (T49I).*** The proband in this Japanese kindred was 63 years old when she developed painful paresthesias in all extremities. A grandmother had similar neuropathy and a brother died of cardiac amyloidosis. The mutation is a C → T transition at the second base of codon 49. Original detection was by electrospray ionization mass spectrometry (ESI-MS), which revealed a 12-dalton shift in molecular mass of plasma transthyretin.[194]

***Arginine 50 (S50R).*** This mutation (Ser50Arg) was discovered in a Japanese family in which affected members presented with peripheral and autonomic neuropathy in their early forties. One man died of generalized wasting 6 years after the onset of polyneuropathy.[195] The abnormal TTR was present in serum and cardiac amyloid deposits.[196] The T → G transversion in the first position of codon 50 gives a new *Mva*I site. This mutation has also been found in a European family.[183]

***Isoleucine 50 (S50I).*** A G → T tranversion in the second position of codon 50 of TTR exon 3 giving a Ser50Ile mutation was identified in a 56-year-old Japanese woman with a 7-year history of sensorimotor and autonomic neuropathy.[197] Another report of this mutation emphasized cardiomyopathy as cause of death.[198]

***Proline 52 (S52P).*** This mutation was reported from the United Kingdom and is associated with peripheral neuropathy, autonomic neuropathy, cardiomyopathy, and renal amyloidosis.

***Proline 55 (L55P).*** Seven members of one kindred from West Virginia of Dutch and German descent showed early-onset, aggressive, systemic amyloidosis which caused peripheral neuropathy, autonomic neuropathy, and vitreous opacities.[199] Death in most individuals was from restrictive cardiomyopathy, and autopsy revealed diffuse systemic amyloid deposits. The variant is due to a T → C transition in the second position of codon 55 of transthyretin, which gives a proline substitution for leucine. In the one kindred, multiple organ system involvement was noted by age 35, and all patients had died by age 38. Over four generations anticipation was suggested, with the youngest individual affected at age 19, but there is no molecular evidence to support anticipation. This mutation was also found in a Chinese family in Taiwan with early onset amyloidosis.[200]

***Histidine 58 (L58H).*** Mahloudji et al. originally described a number of kindreds in Maryland with this form of amyloidosis.[201] It was classified as FAP II because of onset with carpal tunnel syndrome. The disease, however, has varied manifestations, with frequent painful neuropathy and relatively slow progression. Onset may be as early as the forties, but many patients live into their seventies. Death is frequently caused by cardiomyopathy, but the syndrome is distinguished from the Indiana/Swiss (I84S) form of FAP II by a lack of vitreous opacities. A T → A transversion in the second position of codon 58 results in substitution of histidine for leucine.[202] The L58H transthyretin gene has been detected in families throughout the United States.[203] Recently, the mutation was found in a family with amyloid cardiomyopathy living in the region of Germany from which the American immigrants originated in the 1740s.[204] Only one haplotype has been demonstrated in several families with this mutant transthyretin, suggesting a common origin. Recently, one individual homozygous for the L58H gene was shown to have a rapid course of generalized neuropathy with clinical presentation at age 46 and death 6 years later.[205] This is unlike the V30M and V122I TTR variants, in which homozygous individuals do not seem to have more aggressive disease.

***Arginine 58 (L58R).*** A single family was described in which a mother, age 62, and her son, age 39, had lower limb neuropathy, autonomic neuropathy, and carpal tunnel syndrome.[206] The mother had vitreous opacities noted at age 53, and the son developed

neuropathy as early as age 36. The mutation, a T → G change in the second position of codon 58, results in a new *Bha*I restriction site.

***Lysine 59 (T59K).*** Cardiac amyloidosis was the major feature in an Italian family with disease onset between 49 and 64 years.[207] The mutation is a cytosine to adenine transversion at the second base of codon 59.

***Alanine 60 (T60A).*** This type of amyloidosis (also called Appalachian amyloidosis) was originally discovered in a large kindred from West Virginia in which the disease was traced to a couple having Irish, English, and German ancestry.[208,209] Since then, the T60A transthyretin variant has been found in other U.S. families of Irish lineage, and the gene has now been reported in patients in Ireland. It is also the first mutation to be found in Australia, in a family also of Irish origin. One family of Welsh origin now in the United States has been found with this mutation. Sensorimotor neuropathy is not a prominent feature of this syndrome, although some patients have carpal tunnel syndrome. Most affected individuals have some degree of peripheral neuropathy in the lower extremities, but incapacitation is related more to bowel disease and resultant malnutrition. Sexual impotence is common. Many affected individuals die of cardiomyopathy, which usually starts after age 50 and may not begin until after age 60. The disease is progressive but may run a 10- to 20-year course. While most individuals have died in their sixties, some have been known to live past age 90. Combined heart and liver transplantation has been done in at least one individual with this disease with good outcome. Postmortem examinations have shown amyloid in nerves, heart, and thyroid (Figs. 209-13 and 209-14). Significant amyloid in liver, kidney, and spleen has not been seen. The original Appalachian kindred is very large and is dispersed throughout the United States. The gene has also been detected in a large kindred in the northeastern United States.[210] The T60A mutation is the result of an A → G transition at the first position of codon 60 and results in a new *Pvu*II restriction site in exon 3.

***Lysine 61 (E61K).*** This mutation was reported in a 62-year-old Japanese individual with diarrhea and sensorimotor neuropathy.[211]

***Leucine 64 (F64L).*** This mutation (Phe64Leu) was discovered in one individual with disease beginning at age 66 as a peripheral neuropathy involving both upper and lower extremities.[212] Cardiomyopathy was present, but no eye involvement was noted. The patient was an American of Italian descent.

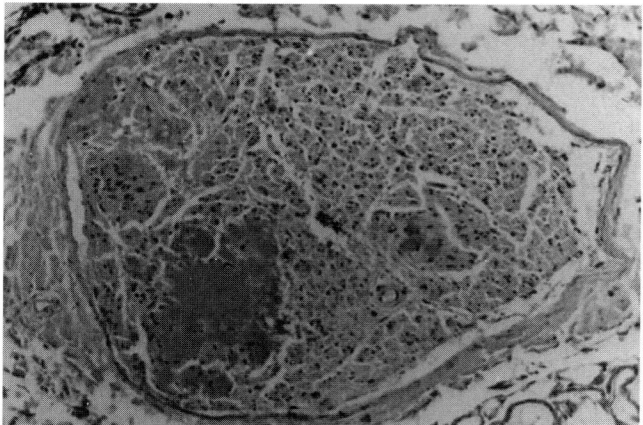

**Fig. 209-13 Section of peripheral nerve stained for transthyretin by the avidin-biotin peroxidase method. Amyloid deposits are found within the nerve structure, and the positive staining for transthyretin proves the diagnosis of hereditary amyloidosis. ×100.**

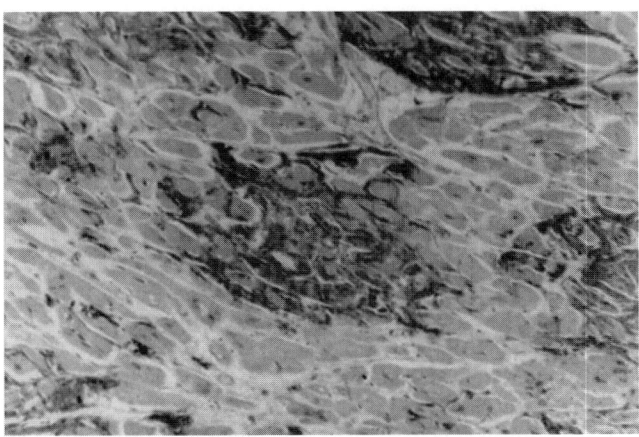

**Fig. 209-14 Section of left ventricle stained immunohistochemically using antitransthyretin. Amyloid deposits displace myocardial fibrils and also form rings around the cardiac muscle bundles. ×100.**

***Serine 64 (F64S).*** The principal feature associated with this mutation is amyloid angiopathy involving the meninges of the brain and spinal cord, retina, and peripheral nerves. Vitreous opacities were also present. Clinical features included migraine, periodic obtundation, psychosis, seizures, intracerebral hemorrhages, myelopathy, deafness, and peripheral neuropathy.[213] The syndrome was originally discovered in a Canadian family of Italian origin, but was recently found in a family in England with vitreous opacities and peripheral neuropathy. A transition of T → C at the second position of codon 64 creates a new *Hin*fI site, which can be used for PCR-based gene detection.[214]

***Leucine 68 (I68L).*** A substitution of leucine for isoleucine at position 68 of transthyretin was described in a 61-year-old German individual with cardiomyopathy.[215] The mutation, an A → T transversion in the first position of codon 68, was detected in the propositus' son, who was unaffected, but not in the propositus' mother. The propositus' father died at age 56 of an accident without symptoms of amyloidosis. While polyneuropathy was suggested by complaints of dysesthesia, neurologic examination did not reveal objective pathologic findings.

***Histidine 69 (Y69H).*** Only one family has been reported with this mutation (Tyr69His).[216] The proband noted symptoms of vitreous opacities at age 59, and amyloidosis was proved by pathologic examination of a vitrectomy specimen removed at age 62. The proband had symptoms of carpal tunnel syndrome and gastrointestinal complaints suggesting autonomic nervous system involvement. No peripheral neuropathy was noted, however. An older sibling also had vitreous opacities but died of a brain hemorrhage at age 62. The Y69H allele is the result of a T → C mutation in the first position of codon 69.

***Asparagine 70 (K70N).*** A family from New Jersey of German ancestry was found to have amyloidosis associated with a substitution of asparagine for lysine at position 70 of transthyretin.[217] This is due to an A → C transversion at the third base of codon 70. This syndrome usually presents as carpal tunnel syndrome as early as in the thirties. One individual died of renal insufficiency, but nodular glomerulosclerosis characteristic of Kimmelstiel-Wilson disease was found instead of amyloid. Amyloid vitreous opacities were a common finding in this syndrome.

***Alanine 71 (V71A).*** Val71Ala was first discovered in a family from northern France in which the proband developed carpal tunnel syndrome at age 35 and subsequently had lower limb

neuropathy at age 42.[218] The proband's father had paresthesias and diarrhea starting at age 40 and subsequently developed vitreous opacities. The V71A mutation, which is due to a C → T transition, in the second position of codon 71, has also been found in an individual in Spain.

***Valine 73 (I73V).*** This mutation was associated with FAP starting at age 50 years in multiple members of a Bangladeshi family with amyloid deposition proven in peripheral nerve. The A → G transition in the first position of codon 73 creates a new *Acc*I restriction enzyme site.[219]

***Tyrosine 77 (S77Y).*** Amyloidosis associated with the tyrosine 77 transthyretin variant was originally described in a family of German extraction from Illinois.[220] The clinical syndrome shows a lower limb neuropathy and diarrhea starting about age 50. While kidney failure has been a major cause of death, cardiomyopathy has also been noted in individuals with this mutation. This transthyretin variant has now been found with the same haplotype in several families in the United States, including a large kindred in Texas.[221] A family from northern France, however, has the S77Y transthyretin with a different haplotype, suggesting a separate mutational event.[222] The mutation, a C → T transition at the second position of codon 77, gives a new *Ssp*I restriction site.

***Serine 84 (I84S).*** Although the Indiana/Swiss kindred with amyloidosis was originally reported by Falls et al. in 1955,[223] Rukavina's description of the kindred in 1956 caused his name to be used in identifying the syndrome, which, because of presentation with carpal tunnel syndrome, was designated FAP II to distinguish it from the FAP I peripheral neuropathy syndrome.[224] Carpal tunnel syndrome occurs as early as the third decade of life, whereas infiltrative peripheral neuropathy tends to occur later in the course and can affect all extremities. Vitreous opacities are seen in essentially all affected individuals, and cardiomyopathy is the usual cause of death. Most patients die in their mid-fifties or sixties, although some individuals have reached age 80 with the help of artificial cardiac pacing. Sexual impotence is common in men, and bowel dysfunction with diarrhea and malabsorption is also common.[225]

The I84S mutation is the result of a T → G transversion in the second position of codon 84. This gives a new *Alu*I restriction site, which can be used for DNA testing.[226] Gene carriers in this kindred, both affected and presymptomatic, have significantly reduced plasma RBP concentrations. This finding agrees with structure data that show that this area of the molecule around residue 84 is involved in the interaction with RBP.[136,137,227] The depression in the serum RBP level is such that heterozygotes can usually be identified by this measurement alone. Recently a second kindred with the I84S transthyretin gene was found in Hungary; this family, which also has vitreous and cardiac amyloid, may be related to the original Swiss/German families.[228]

***Asparagine 84 (I84N).*** A second mutation in transthyretin position 84 (Ile84Asn) is due to a T → G transversion in the second position of codon 84.[229] It was reported in an individual who developed vitreous opacities at age 62. There was no family history of amyloidosis in this American family of Italian descent, although the proband's father died suddenly at age 62. Carpal tunnel syndrome developing after age 70 and mild cardiomyopathy were present in the proband. Plasma RBP concentration was found to be low as with the I84S mutation.[135]

***Threonine 84 (I84T).*** A 60-year-old German woman with cardiomyopathy and peripheral neuropathy had this mutation, a T → C transition at the second base of codon 84.

***Glutamine 89 (E89Q).*** The substitution of glutamine for glutamic acid at position 89 of transthyretin was discovered in a Sicilian family with carpal tunnel syndrome, cardiomyopathy, and neuropathy presenting in the fifth decade of life.[191] This is the result of a G → C transversion in the first position of codon 89.

***Lysine 89 (E89K).*** Peripheral neuropathy and cardiomyopathy after age 55 years characterized this disease in an American family. The mutation is a G → A transition at the first position of codon 89.[230]

***Serine 91 (A91S).*** This mutation was associated with peripheral neuropathy, carpal tunnel syndrome, and cardiomyopathy in a French family. The index case was 72 years old at presentation. The G → T transversion at the first base of codon 91 ablates a *Sph*I restriction-enzyme site.[231]

***Glycine 97 (A97G).*** This mutation in a Japanese kindred was associated with cardiomyopathy and peripheral neuropathy, but well-preserved autonomic function. Age of onset of clinical disease was 52 years with slow progression of disease.[232]

***Valine 107 (I107V).*** A 57-year-old man of English/German descent developed carpal tunnel syndrome at age 57 and, subsequently, generalized peripheral neuropathy at age 65.[233] Amyloid deposition was identified on muscle biopsy. There was no family history of amyloidosis. A TTR mutation, A → G in the first position of codon 107, predicts a valine-for-isoleucine substitution.

***Serine 109 (A109S).*** This mutation was discovered in a 75-year-old Japanese woman with peripheral neuropathy. Sural nerve biopsy confirmed amyloid deposition.[234] The G → T transversion at the first position of codon 109 abolishes a *Fnu*4H1 restriction enzyme site. It is of interest that the two other reported mutations at residue 109 are associated with euthyroid hyperthyroxinemia, but not with amyloidosis.[145]

***Methionine 111 (L111M).*** In 1962, Frederiksen et al. described a kindred in Denmark with amyloid cardiomyopathy.[157,235] No neuropathy was detected either at that time or on subsequent reexamination of the kindred. The clinical findings are those of restrictive cardiomyopathy. DNA sequencing showed a C → A transversion in the first position of codon 111, with the substitution of methionine for leucine.[236] A recent analysis of sera obtained at the time of the original report has detected the mutant transthyretin in all affected individuals.[237] No other kindreds have been discovered with this particular mutation, which is remarkable for its restriction of amyloid pathology to the heart.

***Isoleucine 112 (S112I).*** This mutation was reported from Italy. The index case was 44 years old at presentation with cardiomyopathy, peripheral neuropathy, and chronic renal failure. Several family members had disease onset at this relatively early age. The mutation is a G → T transversion at the second position of codon 112.

***Cysteine 114 (Y114C).*** Members of a kindred from Nagasaki prefecture in Japan were found to have systemic amyloidosis associated with a cysteine-for-tyrosine replacement at codon 114.[238] This is the result of an A → G change in the second position of codon 114.[239] The syndrome was manifest at age 30, with lower-limb neuropathy, autonomic neuropathy, and subsequent development of vitreous opacities. Heart failure was the most common cause of death.

***Histidine 114 (Y114H).*** This mutation was found in a Japanese kindred in Niigata prefecture with carpal tunnel syndrome, but without other features of amyloidosis.[240]

***Serine 116 (Y116S).*** A 75-year-old French man with peripheral neuropathy and carpal tunnel syndrome had amyloidosis proven by sural nerve biopsy.[231] The mutation, an A → C transversion at

the second position of codon 116 creates a new *Ear*1 restriction-enzyme site. While there was no family history of amyloidosis, a daughter and a 70-year-old sister also had the mutation.

***Isoleucine 122 (V122I).*** The Val122Ile mutation was discovered in an individual with cardiomyopathy but no family history of amyloidosis.[241] It was first believed to explain some cases of senile cardiac amyloidosis. It is particularly interesting because the first two individuals reported with this mutation were from separate families, and both were homozygous for V122I transthyretin.[242,243] Subsequently, other individuals have been discovered with cardiac amyloidosis who were heterozygous for V122I transthyretin.[244] All affected individuals so far were elderly, presenting after age 60 with cardiomyopathy, and nearly all were African-Americans. The mutation, a G → A transition in the first position of codon 122, was present in approximately 4 percent of selected African-American cohorts and may be the cause of heart failure in a significant portion of the elderly in this population.[245] Peripheral neuropathy has been reported, but is a minor clinical manifestation of this syndrome. Because transthyretin amyloidosis is an autosomal dominant trait, the high allele frequency makes this one of the most important genetic mutations in the United States. Unfortunately, the clinical disease in this population is frequently not diagnosed and, therefore, the affected individual receives less than optimal therapy. Recently, the mutation was found in populations of the west coast of Africa and in South Africa.

***delVal122 (ΔV122Δ).*** This is the first and only deletion mutation to be discovered for transthyretin. It is associated with peripheral and autonomic neuropathy and cardiomyopathy starting after age 60 years.[158] The proband immigrated to the United States from Ecuador. DNA-sequencing gels of exon 4 PCR products reveal multiple bands due to the trinucleotide deletion.

***Alanine 122 (V122A).*** This mutation was discovered in a 47-year-old American of Welsh and English descent who presented with cardiomyopathy.[246] The T → C transition at the second position of codon 122 results in the loss of a *Mae*III restriction enzyme site.

**Senile Systemic Amyloidosis.** In addition to the characterized cases of senile cardiac amyloidosis, a number of postmortem studies show a high incidence of amyloid deposits in individuals dying after age 80.[247] These deposits are often in the heart, but varying degrees of systemic involvement have also been noted.[248,249]

The term *senile systemic amyloidosis* has been used for these cases, as well as for those previously labeled senile cardiac amyloidosis.[250] Immunohistochemical studies show that a number of these cases involve transthyretin amyloid, although some studies fail to show staining with antitransthyretin antisera.[251] DNA-sequencing studies of some individuals with transthyretin cardiomyopathy without a family history of this disease failed to show mutations in the coding regions of the TTR gene.[252] This finding suggests that normal transthyretin may, in some situations, produce amyloid fibrils without the presence of a mutation.

**Transthyretin Variants Not Associated with Amyloidosis.** A number of variants of transthyretin have been reported in individuals and families without evidence of systemic amyloidosis. These have been identified either by an association with altered thyroxine binding or by an abnormal pattern on protein electrophoresis. Although routine serum electrophoresis does not identify variant forms of transthyretin, both two-dimensional polyacrylamide gel electrophoresis and a system called "hybrid isoelectric focusing" have successfully discriminated several variants from normal transthyretin.[253] In addition, advances in mass spectrometry have made detection of variant forms of transthyretin possible and may lead to discovery of more nonpathogenic variants of this plasma protein. A variant transthyretin with serine substituted for glycine at position 6 (G6S) was discovered in a family with hyperthyroxinemia.[254,255] Studies suggest that an abnormal albumin in this kindred may cause increased thyroxine binding, giving a euthyroid state; and in vitro thyroxine-binding studies on a recombinantly produced G6S variant TTR failed to show increased thyroxine binding for this variant.[256] G6S transthyretin may be a relatively common polymorphism having been reported in 12 percent of Caucasians. Amino acid substitutions at position 109 of transthyretin have also been identified in families with euthyroid hyperthyroxinemia. Ala109Thr (A109T) is the most thoroughly studied, with a fairly large kindred showing increased thyroxine binding but a euthyroid state.[257] Thyroxine-binding studies of recombinant A109T TTR demonstrate increased affinity for $T_4$,[256] and a structural basis for this increased affinity was demonstrated by solution of the x-ray structure at 1.7Å.[258] A valine substitution at position 109 has also been described in an individual with hyperthyroxinemia. Transthyretin Met119 was discovered by two-dimensional polyacrylamide gel electrophoresis in a family without any evidence of hyperthyroxinemia.[146] This TTR variant may be relatively common in the general population, but has not been associated with amyloid deposition. Transthyretin T119M, like G6S and V30M, may be the result of a mutational hot spot, where deamination of a methylated cytosine at a CpG site would lead to this mutation. A transthyretin variant with histidine substituted for aspartic acid at position 74 (D74H) was discovered in individuals without evidence of amyloidosis;[259] an asparagine for histidine at position 91 (H91N) and arginine substitution for proline at position 102 (P102R) have also been described.[260] The number of known amyloid-producing variants of transthyretin far exceeds the number of nonamyloid variants. However, no concerted effort of population screening at the DNA level has been made to discover other clinically silent variants of this protein. With such a large number of amyloid-associated variants, it would appear that the propensity for amyloid fibril formation is significantly enhanced by most perturbations in primary structure of this heavily $\beta$-structured protein.

**Pathogenesis.** The pathogenesis of transthyretin amyloidosis is not well understood; although it is obvious that certain factors such as the extensive $\beta$-conformation of the protein, its inherent structural stability, and resistance to proteolysis must play important roles in amyloid fibril formation. The discovery of single amino acid substitution variants of transthyretin led to the hypothesis that changes in the structure of the protein in some way lead to aggregation of the subunit protein molecules to form fibrils. However, determination of the tertiary structure of a number of amyloidogenic, as well as nonamyloidogenic, transthyretin variants has failed to show common factors that would predict the transition of a soluble plasma protein to insoluble amyloid fibrils. The intramolecular position and type of amino acid substitution in transthyretin are not obvious factors in pathogenesis. Mutations from neutral to charged residues, from charged to neutral residues, from hydrophobic to hydrophilic, or hydrophilic to hydrophobic, have all been discovered to be associated with amyloid formation. The mutations are distributed over most of the length of the transthyretin molecule with only the N- and C-terminal segments not having mutations associated with amyloidosis. Even so, most speculation on transthyretin amyloid fibril formation is centered on hypothesized changes in tertiary structure caused by amino acid substitutions. One hypothesis is that under acidic conditions transthyretin is converted to a conformational intermediate that then self-associates to give fibrils.[261] Another hypothesis is that amino acid substitutions cause changes in the edge strands (residues 45 to 58) of the two $\beta$-sheets that form the structural framework of the TTR molecule and this leads to molecular self-assembly giving growth of intermolecular $\beta$-sheet structures.[262] Another possible mechanism is that, rather than changes in tertiary structure that lead to aggregation, amino acid substitutions may alter metabolism of the transthyretin molecule

so the concentration or conformation of a proteolytic intermediate may be changed from the norm, and this may affect a pathway that leads to fibril formation. That normal transthyretin may generate amyloid fibrils favors this hypothesis. Some degree of intramolecular proteolysis in the process of amyloid formation is suggested by the fact that fragments of transthyretin representing amino acid residues 47 to 127, 49 to 127, and 52 to 127, are commonly found in amyloid fibrils extracted from tissues.

The liver predominantly synthesizes plasma transthyretin and this is the presumed source of substrate for amyloid deposits in the vascular tree, the heart, and the kidney. The liver and spleen, however, are rarely involved with significant amyloid deposition. The reasons for deposition in any particular organ are not readily apparent, but it is obvious that cardiac amyloid deposition is a predominant feature of many of the syndromes. The choroid plexus also synthesizes transthyretin and this may be the source for amyloid deposition in the leptomeninges. In addition, the retinal pigment epithelium synthesizes transthyretin, and this may be the source of amyloid in the vitreous of the eye. Recent reports of development of vitreous opacities in patients who have undergone orthotopic liver transplantation suggest that vitreous deposits are the result of intraocular synthesis and not hepatic synthesis. The predilection for amyloid deposition in peripheral nerves is not understood. Amyloid deposits may start as vascular deposits in vasa nervorum, but there is also evidence for significant deposition in dorsal root ganglia. This may explain the prominence of sensory neuropathy in many of the transthyretin amyloidoses.

**Treatment of Transthyretin Amyloidosis.** The only specific therapy for transthyretin amyloidosis is liver transplantation.[263,264] Replacement of the liver results in disappearance of variant transthyretin from the plasma, and presumably this would stop the synthesis of amyloid fibrils.[265] While this appears to be the case in most individuals, a few reports of progression of vitreous opacities and cardiomyopathy have tended to dampen the enthusiasm for liver transplantation.

Progression in vitreous opacities may be related to synthesis of variant transthyretin by retinal pigment epithelium. On the other hand, progression of cardiac amyloid might be related to the fact that normal transthyretin may perpetuate amyloid fibril formation which was originally initiated by a variant transthyretin protein. To date, approximately 300 individuals have received orthotopic liver transplants and the 2-year survival is approximately 78 percent. Because other liver functions in these individuals are normal, the morbidity from surgery is less than for individuals who have liver transplants for primary liver disease. Most individuals have not shown objective evidence of improved neurologic function after transplantation; however, regeneration of nerve fibers documented by sural nerve biopsy was recently reported.[266] While liver transplantation may represent a specific and essentially curative treatment for systemic amyloidosis, the cost of this procedure and present-day problems with organ procurement and tissue rejection preclude its general use and acceptance.

In addition to liver transplantation, there are nonspecific therapeutic measures that may significantly prolong the life of an individual with transthyretin amyloidosis. Renal dialysis may be used for patients who have severe nephropathy. Cardiac pacemakers have prolonged life for many individuals. Potent diuretics can significantly improve the quality of life for patients with restrictive cardiomyopathy, but frequently some degree of volume overload is necessary to maintain adequate cardiac filling and, therefore, tissue perfusion. Bowel involvement can be devastating to some individuals; the judicious use of antibiotics to reduce intestinal flora and of agents such as metoclopramide to stimulate gastric emptying has been helpful. Vitrectomy can restore vision to some patients with vitreous opacities, although all too often this is only temporary. Patients who have had a vitrectomy for amyloidosis should be observed carefully for development of secondary glaucoma, which can be painless and can cause irreversible retinal damage. Plasmapheresis has been tried in some individuals with transthyretin amyloidosis but, while anecdotal reports suggest some improvement in quality of life, no definite therapeutic advantage has been noted. Colchicine is commonly given because of the reports of its preventing amyloid in familial Mediterranean fever. There is no definite evidence that it prevents transthyretin amyloid fibril formation, but nevertheless it is frequently given in the hope that it might delay the onset or progression of amyloid formation particularly in presymptomatic carriers of mutant transthyretin genes. A very significant factor in the treatment of patients with transthyretin amyloidosis is genetic screening, which allows identification of subjects with this condition so that they can receive timely diagnosis and treatment.

## Hereditary Amyloidosis Not Associated with Transthyretin

**Apolipoprotein A-I Amyloidosis (MIM 107680).** In 1969, Van Allen et al. described a kindred from Iowa of English, Irish, and Scottish descent with autosomal dominant amyloidosis causing the nephrotic syndrome and/or renal insufficiency.[267] Individuals in their twenties have been shown to be affected, but others lived into their seventies. A striking incidence of peptic ulcer disease was seen in this syndrome. Lower-limb neuropathy is characteristic of this syndrome, which in the past was called "FAP III," although a few reports have called it "FAP IV" (Table 209-3).

Amyloid fibrils isolated from tissues of a patient with this syndrome were found to contain a degradation product of a variant form of apolipoprotein A-I (GenBank NM_000039), with arginine replacing glycine at position 26 (G26R).[31,268] While both normal and variant types of apolipoprotein A-I were demonstrated in the plasma of affected individuals, only the G26R variant arginine 26 apo A-I was found in amyloid fibril deposits. A second American kindred of Italian origin was subsequently identified with this mutation, and families in England have been described with and without neuropathy. The G26R substitution is the result of a G → C transversion in the first position of codon 26 in exon 2.[268]

A second apolipoprotein A-I mutation, Leu60Arg (L60R), was identified in an English family in which the propositus presented at age 24 with splenic and hepatic amyloidosis.[269] Subsequently, this individual developed hypertension and thrombocytopenia. Other members of the kindred presented with renal amyloidosis, but no evidence of neuropathy. Chemical analysis of amyloid fibrils revealed apo A-I degradation peptides of 88, 92, and 93 residues, whereas the original mutated apo A-I amyloid protein showed no peptides beyond residue 83 of apo A-I. No normal apolipoprotein A-I was found in the L60R amyloid fibrils.

A substitution of tryptophan by arginine at position 50 (W50R) is associated with non-neuropathic amyloidosis in a Jewish kindred. The proband presented with hepatic and renal amyloidosis. Amyloid fibrils isolated from liver contained apo A-I peptides of 1 to 86, 1 to 92, and 1 to 93 residues.[270] Two deletion mutants of apo A-I have been found in families with amyloidosis. The first has a deletion in exon 4 that results in the loss of residues 60 to 71 with insertion of two new residues Val-Thr.[271] Hepatic amyloid is the main feature of this syndrome and death, usually by the sixth decade, is from liver failure. The only family identified so far is from Spain. Another apo A-I deletion mutant with loss of amino acid residues 70 to 72 (Glu Phe Trp) was discovered in a kindred in South Africa.[272] Death is from renal failure, although liver and spleen may also be affected. A completely different clinical syndrome associated with an apo A-I variant was recently described. A substitution of proline for leucine at position 90 (L90P) results in extensive cutaneous amyloid deposition and subsequently restrictive cardiomyopathy.[273] Affected individuals in a kindred from Southern France developed skin rash by age 50 and died of heart failure by the sixth or seventh decade of life. Amyloid fibrils isolated from cardiac tissue contained a peptide of the variant apo A-I representing residues 1 to 94 with the L90P variant. Amyloid fibrils from the skin, however, contained only the normal residues 1 to 88.[274]

Apolipoprotein A-I, like transthyretin, has been associated with amyloid deposits without evidence of a variant form of the protein. Amyloid deposits that are frequently found at postmortem in the intima of the aorta contain peptides of apo A-I.[275] Unlike transthyretin, apo A-I has been found to be associated with amyloidosis in another species than humans. Pulmonary vascular deposits of amyloid in aging dogs contain N-terminal peptides of apo A-I.[276]

**Gelsolin Amyloidosis (MIM 137350).** In 1969, Meretoja described familial amyloidosis with lattice corneal dystrophy, progressive cranial neuropathy, and skin changes with various internal symptoms.[277–279] The first manifestation of the disease is a dystrophic change of the cornea due to amyloid deposition. Over several decades, thickening of the skin on the forehead and back occurs, and patients may develop facial paralysis caused by cranial neuropathies. Death related to renal and cardiac amyloid has been reported. While the largest occurrence of this type of amyloidosis is in Finland, there have been reports of patients in the United States,[280–282] Denmark, and Canada. An amyloid subunit protein of 71 amino acid residues derived from plasma gelsolin was isolated from tissues of patients with this disease and shown to

**Table 209-3** Mutant Proteins (Other Than Transthyretin) Associated with Autosomal Dominant Systemic Amyloidosis

| Protein | Mutation | Clinical Features | Geographic Kindreds |
|---|---|---|---|
| Apolipoprotein AI | Gly26Arg | PN,* nephropathy | United States |
| | Leu60Arg | Nephropathy | England |
| | Trp50Arg | Nephropathy | England |
| | del60−71 insVal/Thr | Hepatic | Spain |
| | del70−72 | Nephropathy | South Africa |
| | Leu90Pro | Cardiomyopathy, cutaneous | France |
| Gelsolin | Asp187Asn | PN,* Lattice corneal dystrophy | Finland, United States, Japan |
| | Asp187Tyr | PN* | Denmark, Czech |
| Cystatin C | Leu68Gln | Cerebral hemorrhage | Iceland |
| Fibrinogen | Arg554Leu | Nephropathy | Mexico |
| | Glu526Val | Nephropathy | United States |
| | 4904delG | Nephropathy | United States |
| | 4897delT | Nephropathy | France |
| Lysozyme | Ile56Thr | Nephropathy, petechiae | England |
| | Asp67His | Nephropathy | England |

*PN = Peripheral neuropathy

have an asparagine substituted for the aspartic acid at position 187 (D187N).[32,33,283] This substitution is caused by a G → A transition,[284,285] which has now been demonstrated in American families[286] and in a Japanese kindred.[287] So far, haplotype analysis has provided evidence for more than one mutational event leading to the various kindreds in Finland and Holland.[288] Individuals homozygous for the D187N variant have demonstrated early onset of severe renal amyloidosis.[289] Recently, a tyrosine-for-aspartate substitution at residue 187 (D187Y) was identified in kindreds from Denmark and Czechoslovakia, with syndromes similar to the amyloidosis described by Meretoja. The same mutation, a G → T transversion at the first position of codon 187, was demonstrated for both kindreds, but they had different haplotypes, suggesting separate mutational events.[288] No other families with this mutation have been identified. Recently, other types of corneal dystrophies which link to chromosome 5q31 have been found to be caused by mutations in keratoepithelin.[290,291] These diseases are not associated with systemic amyloid deposition and can be considered under localized amyloidosis.

Gelsolin is a calcium-binding protein that binds to and fragments actin filaments (GenBank NM000177).[292] There are two forms of gelsolin encoded by a single gene and derived through alternative splicing. A cytoplasmic gelsolin binds actin monomers and may have an important role in the reorganization of the cytoskeleton during receptor-mediated signaling.[293] Plasma gelsolin (93 kDa) also binds actin and presumably functions to clear actin from the plasma. The gelsolin gene is on chromosome 9 (9q32-q34) and spans approximately 70 kb.[294] The genomic structure has been partially determined and the gene shown to contain at least 14 exons. The higher molecular weight of plasma gelsolin is due to a 25-amino-acid extension at the N-terminal of the protein and is the result of alternate splicing. In the human, the plasma concentration of gelsolin is approximately 220 mg/liter. Unlike transthyretin and apolipoprotein A-I, which are synthesized mainly by the liver, plasma gelsolin is derived in large part from muscle.[295] Therefore, organ transplantation is not an option for treatment of gelsolin amyloidosis.

**Fibrinogen-Associated Amyloidosis (MIM 134820).** Mutations in the fibrinogen Aα-chain gene have been identified in individuals with familial autosomal dominant amyloidosis.[34] To date, two missense mutations and two single nucleotide deletion mutants have been found associated with amyloidosis. The disease in these families shares several features. First, it is relatively early in onset, often appearing in the patient's forties, but sometimes in the twenties or earlier. Second, the principal manifestation of the amyloidosis is nephropathy, often presenting with hypertension and proteinuria. Third, there is no peripheral neuropathy. All known amyloid associated mutations are in the protease-sensitive C-terminal region of fibrinogen Aα.

Fibrinogen is a major plasma protein that is involved in the final phase of blood coagulation. It is composed of two sets of three different polypeptide chains, α, β, and γ, which have molecular weights of 66,000, 52,000, and 46,500, respectively, and are the products of closely associated genes on chromosome 4 (see Chap. 171).[296–298] Fibrinogen is converted to insoluble fibrin by the action of thrombin and factor VIIIa. A number of mutations in the fibrinogen Aα-chain have been described in individuals with dysfibrinogenemia (Chap. 171), but none has shown an association with amyloidosis.[299] Most of these mutations are in the N-terminal end of the fibrinogen Aα-chain (GenBank NM_000508). The plasma concentration of fibrinogen is approximately 3 mg/ml, and it functions as a moderate acute-phase reactant. A substitution of leucine for arginine at residue 554 (R554L) of the fibrinogen Aα-chain was identified in amyloid fibril subunit protein isolated from kidney tissue of a Peruvian patient who died with renal amyloidosis.[34] A sister and son also had biopsy-proven amyloidosis and died with renal failure, the sister at age 28 and the son at age 24. Genomic DNA sequencing revealed a G → T transversion at nucleotide position 4993 of the fibrinogen Aα-chain gene,

corresponding to the second base of codon 554. This mutation was recently found in an African-American family and in a French family.[300,301]

Another fibrinogen Aα-chain variant with valine substituted for glutamic acid at position 526 (E526V) caused by a A → T mutation at nucleotide 1674 was discovered in two large, unrelated American kindreds with renal amyloidosis.[302] The disease in both kindreds had typical autosomal dominant inheritance, and there was no history of either neuropathy or coagulopathy. In at least one case, postmortem examination found amyloid deposition in the spleen but not the heart. Typical pathology in all individuals, however, is dense amyloid deposition in renal glomeruli. Families with the E526V fibrinogen Aα-chain amyloidosis have been found in Canada and in Germany.[303] Two single-nucleotide deletion mutations have been described in kindreds with autosomal dominant renal amyloidosis. The first is an American family with renal failure starting in middle age. This syndrome is due to a 4904delG mutation of the fibrinogen Aα-chain gene.[304] This results in a frameshift and new C-terminal sequence for the Aα-chain, 23 residues before a premature stop codon occurs (Fig. 209-15). A second deletion mutant (4897delT) was found in a French kindred.[305] This deletion leads to a similar aberrant peptide of 26 residues at the C-terminus of the Aα-chain. This last variant is of particular interest because it resulted in renal amyloidosis in one individual age 12 years and amyloid recurred in a renal graft 2 years after transplant.

**Lysozyme-Associated Amyloidosis (MIM 153450).** Two mutations in human lysozyme (GenBank M19045) have been reported to be associated with non-neuropathic systemic amyloidosis.[306] In one family, petechial skin rash from childhood and subsequent renal failure characterized the syndrome. A mutation at residue 56 of lysozyme with threonine replacing isoleucine (I56T) was found by amino acid sequencing of an amyloid fibril subunit protein isolated from renal tissue. The full-length variant lysozyme molecule was present in the amyloid deposits, and no normal lysozyme was found. The I56T change is caused by a single-base T → C transition in exon 2 of the lysozyme gene. An aspartic acid-to-histidine mutation at residue 67 (D67H) was found by DNA analysis of members of a second family with renal amyloidosis. This mutation is the result of a single-nucleotide change with a G → C transversion in the first base of codon 67. In both lysozyme mutations, the affected individuals were heterozygotes, consistent with an autosomal dominant form of amyloidosis.

Lysozyme is a bacteriolytic enzyme present in external secretions, polymorphonuclear leukocytes, and macrophages. Its biologic significance is not completely known, and polymorphic forms not associated with amyloidosis have not been described. Fibrillogenesis may be related to transition from α structure to β-conformation via unstable intermediates.[306]

**Cystatin C Amyloidosis (MIM 105150).** In 1972, Gudmundsson et al. described a syndrome of premature strokes and intracranial hemorrhage in Icelandic families.[307] The syndrome (hereditary cerebral hemorrhage with amyloid) usually occurred in the third or fourth decade of life and showed autosomal dominant inheritance. Neurologic symptoms varied, depending on the location and severity of hemorrhage and, while some individuals died abruptly, others suffered numerous nonfatal cerebral accidents over several years before death. Postmortem examinations showed amyloid primarily restricted to cerebral blood vessels; subsequent studies, however, report systemic deposits. Chemical analysis of this amyloid has shown a fibril subunit that is a degradation product of cystatin C (γ trace protein).[308] The amyloid subunit lacked the first 10 residues of cystatin C and, in addition, a glutamine was found at position 58 (residue 68 of intact cystatin C) instead of the normal leucine (L68Q).[309] DNA analysis has shown the clinical disease segregating with the L68Q substitution.[310] Individuals affected with this disease show extremely low levels of cystatin C in the cerebrospinal fluid, which provides an alternative test for detection

## AMYLOID MUTATIONS IN THE FIBRINOGEN Aα CHAIN GENE

```
                                  500                                     510                                     520
*********** CAC CCT GAT GAA GCT GCC TTC TTC GAC ACT GCC TCA ACT GGA AAA ACA TTC CCA GGT TTC TTC TCA CCT ATG TTA GGA GAG
            His Pro Asp Glu Ala Ala Phe Phe Asp Thr Ala Ser Thr Gly Lys Thr Phe Pro Gly Phe Phe Ser Pro Met Leu Gly Glu

521  Δ        Δ       T                   530                                     540                                     550
TTT GTC AGT GAG ACT GAG TCT AGG GGC TCA GAA TCT GGC ATC TTC ACA AAT ACA AAG GAA TCC AGT TCT CAT CAC CCT GGG ATA GCT GAA
Phe Val Ser Glu Thr Glu Ser Arg Gly Ser Glu Ser Gly Ile Phe Thr Asn Thr Lys Glu Ser Ser Ser His His Pro Gly Ile Ala Glu
                    Val

                Glu Leu Ser Leu Gly Ala Gln Asn Leu Ala Ser Ser Gln Ile Gln Arg Asn Pro Val Leu Ile Thr Leu Gly *

        Ala Val Arg Leu Ser Leu Gly Ala Gln Asn Leu Ala Ser Ser Gln Ile Gln Arg Asn Pro Val Leu Ile Thr Leu Gly **

551          T                            560                                     570                                     580
TTC CCT TCC CGT GGT AAA TCT TCA AGT TCA AGC AAA CAA TTT ACT AGT AGC CAG AGT TAC AAC AGA GGA GAC TCC ACA TTT GAA AGC AAG
Phe Pro Ser Arg Gly Lys Ser Ser Ser Tyr Ser Lys Gln Phe Thr Ser Ser Thr Ser Tyr Asn Arg Gly Asp Ser Thr Phe Glu Ser Lys
            Leu

581                                       590                                     600
AGC TAT AAA ATG GCA GAT GAG GCC GGA AGT GAA GCC GAT CAT GAA GGA ACA CAT AGC ACC AAG AGA GGC CAT GCT AAA TCT ***********
Ser Tyr Lys Met Ala Asp Glu Ala Gly Ser Glu Ala Asp His Glu Gly Thr His Ser Thr Lys Arg Gly His Ala Lys Ser
```

**Fig. 209-15 The C-terminal portion of the fibrinogen Aα-chain amino acid and gene sequence showing the two missense mutations associated with amyloidosis (Glu526Val and Arg554Leu) and the abnormal peptide sequences resulting from single nucleotide deletions 4904delG* and 4897delT*.**

of carriers.[311] Senile plaques containing amyloid of the type seen in Alzheimer disease are not a feature of the Icelandic amyloidosis.[312]

Cystatin C, a cysteine protease inhibitor, contains 120 amino acids in a single polypeptide chain (GenBank NM_000099). It is the product of a single-copy gene on chromosome 20. The gene, which covers approximately 7 kb, contains three exons and is expressed in many tissues, including kidney, liver, gut, pancreas, and heart.[313]

Visceral deposition of amyloid, including deposits in spleen, while not usually of clinical significance, indicates that this is a systemic form of amyloidosis. While there is no specific treatment for this form of leptomeningeal amyloidosis, it has been shown that aggregation of the variant cystatin C protein is accelerated by temperatures above 37°C and, therefore, fever may promote amyloid formation in carriers of the mutant gene.[314]

**Hereditary Cerebral Hemorrhage with Amyloid (Dutch) (MIM 104760).** Several families with congophilic angiopathy of the cerebral vessels resulting in intracerebral hemorrhage have been described in Holland. Affected members of these families have neither the cystatin C mutation described in hereditary cerebral hemorrhage with amyloid type I (HCHWA-I) nor low spinal fluid concentrations of cystatin C. Instead, amyloid isolated from leptomeninges contains the $\beta$-peptide analogous to the fibril subunit found in Alzheimer plaques and vascular deposits.[315] A glutamine substitution for glutamic acid at residue 693 (E693Q) of the 770-amino-acid form of $\beta$-amyloid precursor protein ($\beta$-APP) was found, and this mutation was corroborated at the DNA level.[316] While senile dementia is not a feature of this syndrome, there have been reports of intracerebral $\beta$-amyloid deposits demonstrated by immunohistochemistry with specific antibodies. Recently, a mutation at codon 692 (Ala692Glu; A692E) of the $\beta$-APP gene, which is also associated with cerebral hemorrhage, has been described.[317] Individuals in these families, which are also of Dutch origin, show an early-onset form of familial Alzheimer disease, as well as cerebral hemorrhage from congophilic angiopathy. Unlike cystatin C amyloidosis (HDHWA-I), the Dutch disease (HCHWA-D) appears to be a localized form of amyloidosis as are other syndromes associated with mutations in the Alzheimer $\beta$-PP protein.

**Familial Mediterranean Fever (MIM 249100).** Familial Mediterranean fever (FMF) is the only syndrome in which systemic amyloidosis appears in a definite autosomal recessive pattern. Siegal first described FMF in 1945, using the name benign paroxysmal peritonitis.[318] Other terms applied to this syndrome include familial paroxysmal polyserositis and periodic fever. Heller used the term familial Mediterranean fever and first noted the autosomal recessive inheritance.[319] A high percentage of patients with FMF develop systemic amyloidosis with prominent renal involvement.

FMF is seen most frequently in individuals of Mediterranean origin.[320,321] It is particularly prominent in Sephardic Jews and Armenians. The disease is characterized by periodic episodes of fever, which may be accompanied by signs of peritonitis, synovitis, pleuritis, or an erythematous rash. These attacks may occur within the first decade of life and usually persist throughout life. The clinical manifestations have wide variability, however, and some patients have only mild abdominal discomfort during attacks. Large joint effusions can be seen, but these usually resolve without residual effects.[322] The pathologic mechanisms underlying these attacks are unknown, and biopsies of either peritoneum or pleura show nothing more than evidence of mild inflammation. The attacks are self-limiting and usually resolve after 2 or 3 days.

FMF is transmitted as a simple autosomal recessive trait, and linkage analysis has localized the FMF gene to the short arm of chromosome 16.[323] The FMF gene frequency in Sephardic Jews has been calculated as 0.22.[324,325] FMF-type illnesses have been described in other ethnic groups, however, and in some instances autosomal dominant inheritance with incomplete penetrance cannot be excluded. While systemic amyloidosis is common in patients with FMF, the relationship between the FMF and amyloidosis is not clear.[326] The development of amyloidosis does not correlate well with numbers or degrees of febrile attacks, and indeed some members of FMF kindreds have been described with amyloidosis but without the febrile attacks.[327] The incidence of amyloidosis in FMF patients of Armenian descent is much lower than in Sephardic Jews, supporting the hypothesis that FMF and amyloidosis are two separate traits with separate genetic bases. The recent characterization of the FMF gene (*MEFV*) and identification of mutations associated with the clinical syndrome have not answered the question of variable incidence of amyloidosis in different ethnic populations. Two research groups cloned the gene for FMF and named the postulated protein pyrin and marenostrin.[328,329] Several missense mutations have been identified and segregate with the disease in large kindreds. The FMF gene (GenBank NM_000243) encodes a 3.7-kb transcript that is expressed in granulocytes. The predicted protein is a member of a family of nuclear factors homologous to the R052 autoantigen. Identified mutations in the C-terminal portion of the predicted 781-residue protein include M680I, M694V, M694I, and V726A. All were found in families with FMF and segregate with disease. While the M694V, which is most prevalent in North African Jews, has the greatest correlation with amyloidosis, it is still not clear whether the specific mutation modulates the development of amyloid. The expanding number of mutations (presently over a dozen) and the occurrence of compound heterozygotes also clouds this issue.

The amyloidosis of FMF typically has a predilection for renal involvement with nephrotic syndrome followed by azotemia. Many patients die by their early twenties. Pathologically, glomerular deposits of amyloid predominate. The spleen is commonly involved, and the thyroid may be heavily infiltrated. Vascular deposits throughout the body are common but rarely lead to organ dysfunction. Treatment with either chronic hemodialysis or peritoneal dialysis yields fair results and kidney transplantation is effective.[330] Treatment with colchicine prevents the febrile attacks in most patients and is associated with a lack of progression of amyloidosis.[331] This has led to treatment of all FMF patients with colchicine. In studies by Zemer et al., only patients who did not maintain this therapeutic regimen developed progressive renal amyloidosis.[332]

The amyloid fibrils of FMF contain protein AA, and on chemical grounds this amyloidosis is the reactive type.[13,16] The serum SAA concentration usually increases during febrile attacks and returns to normal between attacks. Because SAA levels are elevated by attacks of inflammation, it would appear that the amyloidosis of FMF is indeed a reactive type not only chemically but clinically, and that at least two determining factors act in concert. Variables that may lead to the differences in expression of the amyloidosis include: (a) penetrance of the FMF genetic trait; (b) prevalence of an amyloidogenic SAA allele (on chromosome 11) in the population at risk; and (c) environmental, dietary, and metabolic factors that may modulate the expression of the SAA genes and degradation of their protein products.

**Muckle-Wells Syndrome (MIM 191900).** In 1962, Muckle and Wells described a syndrome characterized by nerve deafness, fever, urticaria, malaise, and "augey" bouts (attacks of urticaria or angioedema-like symptoms).[333] Nephrotic syndrome developed by middle age, and affected individuals died of renal insufficiency. Postmortem studies showed glomerular amyloidosis plus involvement of the adrenals and spleen. Families with similar syndromes have been described, including one family of Norwegian descent[334] and one Irish family in which familial Hibernian fever was described.[335] While the original description supports autosomal dominant inheritance, this syndrome is similar to FMF in that the amyloid contains protein AA.[336] The gene for Muckle-Wells syndrome has been localized to chromosome 1q44;[336a] whereas the FMF gene (*MEFV*) is on chromosome 16. The gene for familial Hibernian fever has now been identified as the tumor necrosis factor alpha (TNFα) gene (chromosome 12), and several mutations are associated with the disease. It is likely that the familial fever syndromes represent an heterogeneous group of diseases with a common final pathway of clinical expression.

**Miscellaneous Hereditary Amyloidosis Syndromes.** In 1932, Ostertag described a familial syndrome of renal amyloidosis (MIM 105200).[10] More recently, Weiss and Page provided an excellent pathologic description of the nephropathy in another family.[337] The main feature is renal amyloid without neuropathy and death resulting from azotemia. At autopsy the adrenals and spleen, as well as the kidneys, may be involved with amyloid. Possible precursor proteins associated with this type of amyloidosis include mutant forms of apolipoprotein A-I,[268–274] and variants of plasma fibrinogen.[34] The family originally described by Ostertag has so far not been found, and the family of Weiss and Page, while under study, has not yet revealed the secret of their amyloidosis.

## Localized Hereditary Amyloidosis

Localized amyloidosis occurs in a number of syndromes. The first to be characterized chemically was the amyloid associated with medullary carcinoma of the thyroid (MIM 155240). This carcinoma occurs in both sporadic and autosomal dominant patterns and is frequently associated with other endocrinopathies, including pheochromocytomas.[50,51] This syndrome has been designated "multiple endocrine" neoplasia type 2 (MEN2; MIM 171400; see Chap. 42).[338] Chemically, the amyloid is composed of peptides derived from procalcitonin and is limited to the thyroid or tumor metastases.[339]

Cutaneous amyloidosis has been reported in families and may be characterized as lichenoid changes of the skin.[340–343] Cutaneous amyloidosis appeared to be autosomal dominant (MIM 105250) in a family reported by Rajagopalan and Tay,[53] but there have also been reports of X-linked disease (MIM 301220).[344] Familial bullous cutaneous amyloid (MIM 204900) infiltration has also been reported. It is possible that some of the previously described familial cutaneous forms of amyloidosis are similar to the recently discovered apolipoprotein A-I amyloidosis.[274]

Isolated atrial amyloidosis is a localized form of amyloidosis that occurs with increasing prevalence in aging hearts,[345] but is occasionally recognized in a familial pattern.[346] Small deposits of amyloid along the sarcolemma of atrial muscle cells may be observed as early as age 40, and prevalence may reach 95 percent by the ninth decade of life.[347] The hemodynamic significance of this form of amyloid is not clear, but in some families it may be associated with atrial standstill.[346]

Isolated atrial amyloid contains a 28-amino-acid residue C-terminal degradation product of atrial natriuretic peptide.[348–350] This peptide is synthesized by cardiac myocytes and may be induced as a response to congestive heart failure. This suggests that the increasing prevalence of atrial amyloidosis with age may be associated with ventricular dysfunction.[351] The familial atrial standstill syndrome, however, may show no heart failure and may be related to an unknown genetic factor.[352]

Clinically, perhaps the most important of the localized amyloidoses is Alzheimer disease, a progressive dementia characterized by accumulations of amyloid substance in the brain (see Chap. 234).[54] Amyloid deposits (plaques) in cortical tissues are associated with neurofibrillary tangles and blood vessel deposits (congophilic angiopathy), which also stain histologically as amyloid. While only 10 to 20 percent of Alzheimer disease is clearly inherited, it is a late-onset disease, and many familial cases may not be recognized.[353] The Alzheimer plaques and congophilic angiopathy deposits contain a subunit protein (amyloid β-protein or β-A4 protein) having a molecular weight of approximately 4000 and from 39 to 42 amino acid residues and representing an internal fragment of the C-terminal portion of an amyloid precursor protein (β-APP).[36] β-APP is the product of a single gene on chromosome 21q and has at least three alternatively spliced transcripts, the largest encoding a protein of 770 amino acid residues.[354–356] While most cases of Alzheimer disease are sporadic, definite autosomal dominant inheritance is seen in many kindreds, and, recently, point mutations in the β-APP gene localized to chromosome 21 that are associated with Alzheimer pathology in a small number of families were described. In particular, four different amino acid substitutions at codon 717 of β-APP were found to be associated with Alzheimer disease,[357–359] and other amino acid substitutions in the β-amyloid peptide sequence were shown to be associated with either cerebral hemorrhage as in hereditary cerebral hemorrhage with amyloid type D (HCHWA-D) or dementia.[316,317] A larger number of families with familial

Alzheimer disease have mutations in the presenilin (PS-1) gene on chromosome 14.[360] To date, over 60 PS-1 mutations have been identified in families with Alzheimer disease. Two mutations in the presenilin 2 gene on chromosome 1 have been identified, one in the Volga-German families and one in Italian families.[361,362] Several studies have reported evidence that mutations in β-APP and presenilin genes are associated with changes in β-APP protein metabolism and generation of increased amounts of the 1 to 42 amino acid residue Aβ-peptide.[363,364]

Gerstmann-Sträussler-Scheinker disease and familial forms of Creutzfeldt-Jakob disease have also been shown to be heterogeneous.[365] Each is associated with several mutations in the prion protein, which is also implicated in the transmissible forms of Creutzfeldt-Jakob disease and Kuru in humans and Scrapie in sheep (see Chap. 224).[366,367]

Type 2 (adult-onset) diabetes mellitus was shown to be associated with hyalinized pancreatic islets of Langerhans as early as 1900.[368] Subsequently, this hyalinized material was shown to meet the criteria of amyloid and, therefore, this is a form of localized amyloidosis. Little progress was made in understanding this form of amyloidosis until it was found to be associated with age-associated diabetes in cats, as well as humans and some nonhuman primates.[369] Isolation of a unique 37-amino-acid peptide, first from an insulinoma and subsequently from diabetic islets, proved that this was a new type of amyloid protein.[38,370] This peptide, which is called either islet amyloid polypeptide (IAPP) or amylin,[371] is the product of a gene on the short arm of chromosome 12.[372] It is synthesized predominantly in β-cells of the pancreas and is cosecreted with insulin, although in molar amounts 100 times less. Islet amyloid polypeptide has significant (43 to 46 percent) homology with calcitonin-gene-related peptides (CGRP) 1 and 2, which are neuropeptides encoded on chromosome 11.[373]

The functions of islet amyloid polypeptide in normal physiology are not known, although various effects on insulin secretion and function have been reported. The relation of islet amyloid polypeptide to the pathogenesis of diabetes also remains to be determined. The restriction of the islet amyloid deposits to certain species (humans, apes, and cats) and the association with glucose intolerance in these species suggests that it is of importance in diabetes. The idea that this form of amyloidosis represents a hereditary condition rests on its association with type 2 diabetes, which has obvious but unclear genetic features. So far, no polymorphisms in the coding regions of the islet amyloid polypeptide gene have been discovered to explain the development of this form of amyloid, but regulation of gene expression has been incompletely explored. Amyloid in the pancreatic islets of a South American rodent (*Octodon degus*) was shown to contain insulin instead of islet amyloid polypeptide as the fibril subunit protein.[374]

Other clinically recognized types of localized amyloidosis are associated with specific syndromes. Tumoral deposits of amyloid in the urinary tract are common and have been shown to contain immunoglobulin light chain protein.[375] Ureteral obstruction or hemorrhage from the bladder may lead to clinical recognition of these deposits.[376] Amyloid in the respiratory tract without systemic involvement has been frequently reported and has been shown to be of immunoglobulin origin.[377] Amyloid deposits in senile articular cartilage may occur with or without association of calcium pyrophosphate deposition disease.[378] It is possible that these deposits are related to the β$_2$-microglobulin articular amyloid that is seen in chronic dialysis patients, but no studies have been reported on this topic. It is also possible that these deposits may be a reactive type as is the articular AA amyloid of chickens.[379] None of these localized amyloidoses appears to be inherited, but expression may be influenced by genetic factors.

## DETECTION OF GENE CARRIERS IN HEREDITARY AMYLOIDOSIS

Identification of carriers of genes associated with amyloidosis is important for individuals who have clinical disease and those who

have not yet developed clinical evidence of amyloidosis. In the former, identification of a mutation in a gene coding for one of the amyloid-associated proteins usually allows proper diagnosis. Because the amyloidoses are heterogeneous, it is not uncommon for one syndrome to be mistaken for another. This is particularly true for distinguishing hereditary amyloidosis from the immunoglobulin type of amyloidosis. Immunoglobulin amyloidosis (AL) commonly causes cardiomyopathy with or without peripheral neuropathy, as seen in many of the transthyretin amyloidoses. Immunoglobulin amyloidosis frequently has renal involvement without neuropathy, a syndrome similar to the fibrinogen and some of the apolipoprotein A-I amyloidoses. Even the systemic manifestations of gelsolin amyloidosis may be mistaken for the AL syndrome. Because it is common to treat immunoglobulin amyloidosis with chemotherapy, it is imperative that the hereditary forms of amyloidosis be excluded from the diagnosis. Prognosis is a second major reason for distinguishing hereditary amyloid syndromes from other types of amyloidosis. The mean life span after diagnosis for individuals with AL amyloidosis is approximately 2 years. Most of the hereditary amyloidoses have a much better prognosis, with life spans of 5 to 20 years after tissue diagnosis. While the longevity with transthyretin amyloidosis may vary considerably even between families having the same mutation, disease progression is often very uniform within each kindred. Thus, attention to family histories can often lead to a more astute prognosis. For individuals in families with hereditary amyloidosis, detection of disease-associated genes is of value for genetic counseling. The autosomal dominant amyloidoses are late-onset diseases, so heterozygotes usually have their children before disease onset. Gene status may be important for family planning. While the knowledge of being a carrier of a disease-producing gene may be a heavy psychologic burden for an individual, those individuals who are found to be negative for the amyloid variant gene are often fortunate beneficiaries of DNA testing. In addition, for individuals in families with hereditary amyloidosis, genetic testing offers the opportunity to participate in the clinical research which, hopefully, will enhance recognition and subsequently therapeutic progress for these diseases.

Because many of the autosomal dominant inherited amyloidoses are associated with variant forms of plasma proteins, it is possible to detect heterozygotes by isolating and analyzing the plasma protein in question. This can be done for transthyretin, gelsolin, apolipoprotein AI, and fibrinogen with varying degrees of difficulty. A fairly small amount of plasma can be used if the test involves gel electrophoresis, as is used for variants of apolipoprotein AI or hybrid isoelectric focusing, as described for variant forms of transthyretin.[253,380] In general, these methods are not used for detecting carriers of amyloid-associated genes. One exception is the use of cyanogen bromide to cleave plasma transthyretins that have a methionine as the substituted residue.[381] This method has been used to detect the V30M transthyretin, where an efficient biochemical test uses a small amount of plasma and an antibody generated against the aberrant peptide produced by cyanogen bromide cleavage at the methionine 30 residue.[382,383] Recently, cyanogen bromide cleavage of the methionine 111 transthyretin associated with the Danish type of amyloid cardiomyopathy was used to detect the variant transthyretin in plasma samples that were stored for 30 years.[237]

DNA analysis has been used extensively for detecting variant amyloid-associated genes because it presents significant advantages: (a) only small amounts of peripheral blood are required to isolate leukocyte DNA; (b) DNA can be isolated from tissues and even histologic sections of organs from individuals who have died;[31,358] and (c) present-day DNA analysis techniques can be applied to amniocytes or chorionic villus samples obtained for prenatal diagnosis.[384,385]

Sasaki et al.[386] developed the first DNA test for the V30M transthyretin mutation using a specific restriction endonuclease and Southern blot analysis. The V30M mutation creates a recognition site for *Nsi*I, thus giving new hybridization bands on

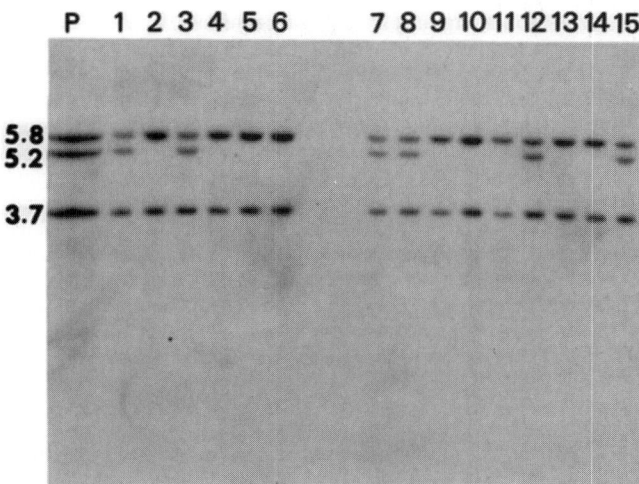

**Fig. 209-16** Southern blot analysis of members of the kindred shown in Fig. 209-10. The propositus at the left and six of his relatives have an extra 5.2-kb band which is a result of the extra *PvuII* site in the Ala60 gene. The transthyretin cDNA is the probe.

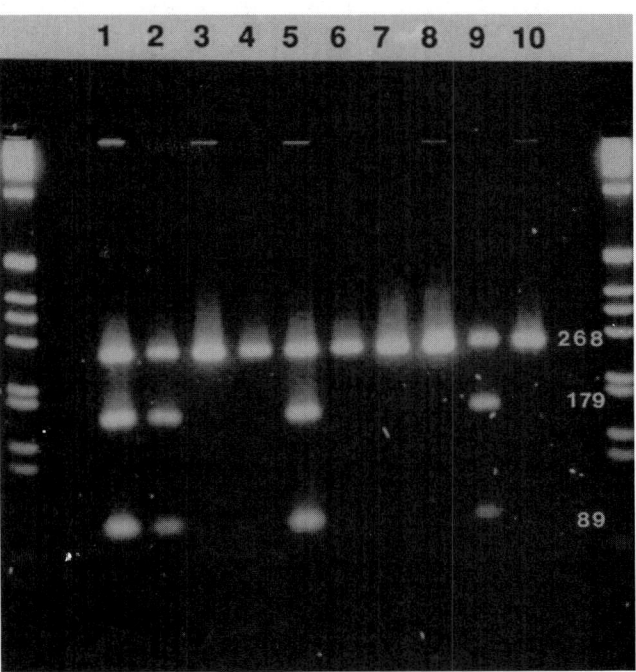

**Fig. 209-17** *PvuII* digest of the exon 3 containing amplification product for detection of the Ala60 transthyretin gene. Lanes 3, 4, 6, 7, 8, and 10: Individuals who are not carriers of the Ala60 gene; only the normal 268-bp product is observed. Lanes 1, 2, 5, and 9: Individuals who are carriers of the Ala60 gene; the normal 268-bp product, as well as 179-bp and 89-bp fragments, which result from digestion of the variant allele at the new *PvuII* site, are observed. One kilobase ladder of molecular weight markers flanks lanes 1 to 10. Fragments were separated by agarose gel electrophoresis and visualized by ethidium bromide staining. Fragment sizes are indicated in base pairs.

Southern blot analysis.[387] Similarly, the transthyretin alanine 60 variant gene can be detected using *PvuII* because the A → G change in codon 60 creates a new *PvuII* site (Fig. 209-16).[208] Southern blot analysis, however, usually requires the use of radioactive probes and relatively lengthy hybridization schedules followed by exposure of radiographic film. The use of Southern blot analysis, therefore, has given way to polymerase chain reaction (PCR) technology, in which specific coding regions of the genes are amplified in vitro and then subjected to various procedures to identify base mutations.[388]

There are four commonly used methods to detect mutations in PCR-amplified fragments of genomic DNA. The first, and most widely used, is PCR followed by restriction digestion (Table 209-4). Many of the disease-associated mutations in transthyretin result in new restriction endonuclease recognition sites. Therefore, digestion of PCR-amplified genomic fragments with the appropriate restriction endonuclease followed by size identification of the restriction fragments on ethidium bromide-stained agarose electrophoresis gels results in specific recognition of the mutation in question (Fig. 209-17). This method is applicable to the detection of both heterozygous and homozygous individuals and has been widely used for the V30M, T60A, S77Y, and I84S mutations.[388] Mutations that result in loss of a restriction enzyme recognition site can also be detected by this method, but proper controls to determine the activity of the restriction endonuclease must be included in each test. In addition, because restriction endonuclease recognition sites are usually four or six bases in length, mutations in the vicinity of the disease-causing mutation will also result in lack of digestion and, therefore, spurious results.

When a point mutation does not result in alteration of a restriction endonuclease recognition site, allele-specific oligonucleotides (ASO) have been used for hybridization to the variant gene sequence.[188,284] In this technique, the genomic coding sequence to be analyzed is amplified by PCR, and this product is then blotted onto nitrocellulose membrane and hybridized with a radiolabeled oligonucleotide specific for the mutation. Careful control of hybridization conditions differentiates between the presence of normal and variant allele products. If the proper combinations are used, homozygous and heterozygous gene products are identifiable.

Another method that is used for identifying point mutations is allele-specific PCR.[31,202] In this technique, the gene segment to be analyzed is amplified using a set of oligonucleotide primers, one of which has its 3′ nucleotide complementary to the point mutation. If, under the proper conditions, amplification occurs, the variant

**Table 209-4** Oligonucleotide Primers Used in Enzymatic Amplification of TTR Exons 2, 3, and 4 (the Pst I Recognition Site Is Underlined)

| Primer | Sequence | PCR product |
|--------|----------|-------------|
| E2LP1 | 5′-GATCCTGCAGGTTAACTTCTCACGTGTCTT-3′ | 215 basepairs containing |
| E2LP2 | 5′-AGATCTGCAGAAGTCCTGTGGGAGGGTTCT-3′ | exon 2 of TTR |
| E3LP1 | 5′-GCCACTGCAGTCCTCCATGCGTAACTTAAT-3′ | 268 basepairs containing |
| E3LP2 | 5′-ACTGCTGCAGACTGTGCATTTCCTGGAATG-3′ | exon 3 of TTR |
| E4LP1 | 5′-TCTGCTGCAGATGGATCTGTCTGTCTTCTC-3′ | 190 basepairs containing |
| E4LP2 | 5′-ATGACTGCAGATCCCTCGTCCTTCAGGTCC-3′ | exon 4 of TTR |

The 10 nucleotides at the 5′ ends (for cloning purposes) can be omitted for PCR-RFLP analysis and direct DNA sequencing.

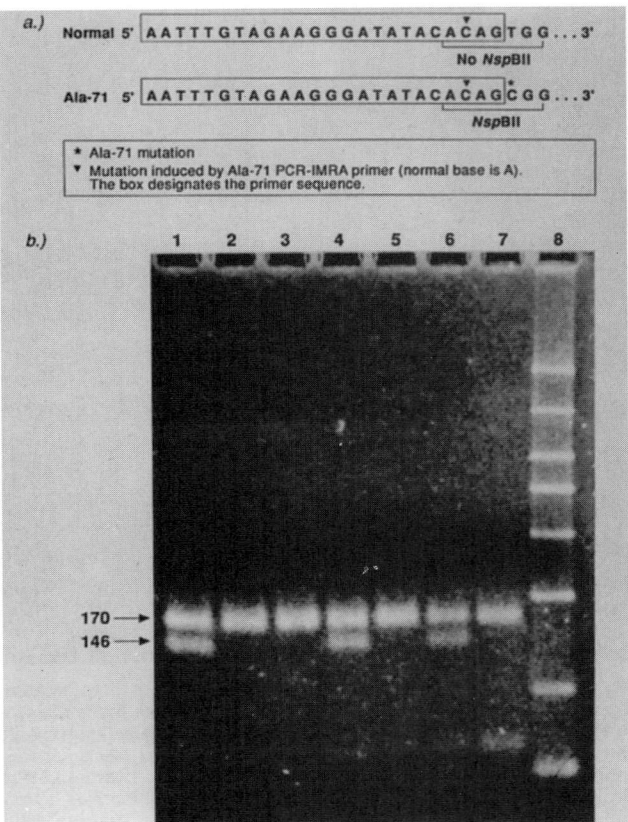

**Fig. 209-18** *A*, PCR-induced mutation restriction analysis for the transthyretin Val71Ala allele. Mutation primer is shown and used in amplification reaction with E3LP2 (see Table 209-3). *B*, Ethidium bromide-stained agarose gel of NspBII-digested PCR products. Lanes 1, 4, and 6 show both the normal 170-bp and the digested variant products, indicating heterozygosity for the Ala71 allele. Lane 8 contains size markers. PCR-IMRA = PCR-induced mutation restriction analysis.

allele is present. If no amplification occurs, the individual is assumed to lack the variant allele. This method does not identify homozygous variant individuals unless a second PCR is performed with an oligonucleotide primer that has the 3′ base complementary to the normal base at the position of the mutation.

Because there are limitations to both the ASO and the allele-specific PCR techniques, a new method has been used increasingly to identify disease-associated mutations where no novel restriction endonuclease recognition site exists. In this technique, called PCR-induced mutation restriction analysis (PCR-IMRA)[218,389] or PCR-induced restriction analysis (PIRA),[390] a restriction endonuclease recognition site is created using a mutagenesis primer that induces an enzyme site when a single base mutation is created in close proximity to the disease-associated mutation (Fig. 209-18). The mutagenesis primer is usually 20 to 25 nucleotides or more long, so that when the amplification products are digested with the specific enzyme, the resulting DNA fragments can be identified on ethidium bromide-stained agarose gels. This method is capable of differentiating normal individuals from heterozygous and homozygous carriers of the variant allele. With the large number of restriction endonucleases now commercially available, it is frequently easy to plan a mutagenesis primer to create a specific endonuclease recognition site. Occasionally, this method can be used to replace an enzyme site for an expensive enzyme with one for a much less expensive and/or more specific enzyme.[159,216]

With the expanding number of mutations in transthyretin, fibrinogen Aα-chain and other amyloid-related genes, screening of exons for mutations using single-strand conformation polymorphism (SSCP) analysis has become more popular.[300]

These DNA tests enable the application of molecular biology to the practice of clinical medicine and make the latest methods of genetic counseling and treatment available to individuals with these late-onset, genetically determined diseases. DNA tests, of course, can only identify carriers of amyloid-producing genes. While they may aid in the diagnosis and subsequent treatment, they cannot change the course of the disease in affected individuals. Even more important at this time is to find some means of modifying the disease process so that fibril synthesis is decreased or stopped. Possible answers may lie in developing methods to regulate expression of specific genes or to modify the biochemical fate of their protein products.

## REFERENCES

1. Glenner GG: Amyloid deposits and amyloidosis: The B-fibrilloses. *N Engl J Med* **302**:1283, 1333, 1980.
2. Rokitansky KF: *Handbuch der Pathologischen Anatomie*, vol 3. Vienna, Braumueller and Seidel, 1842.
3. Virchow R: Zur Cellulose-Frage. *Virchows Arch Pathol Anat* **6**:416, 1854.
4. Virchow VR: Ueber eineim Gehirn und Rueckenmark des Menschen aufgefundene Substanz mit der chemischen reaction der Cellulose. *Virchows Arch Pathol Anat* **6**:135, 1854.
5. Friedreich N, Kekule A: Zur Amyloidfrage. *Virchows Arch Pathol Anat* **16**:50, 1859.
6. Cohen AS: The constitution and genesis of amyloid. *Int Rev Exp Pathol* **4**:159, 1965.
7. Andrade C: A peculiar form of peripheral neuropathy. Familial atypical generalized amyloidosis with special involvement of the peripheral nerves. *Brain* **75**:408, 1952.
8. Debruyn RS, Stern RO: A case of the progressive hypertrophic polyneuritis of Dejerine and Sottas with pathological examination. *Brain* **52**:84, 1929.
9. Denavasquez S, Treble HA: A case of generalized amyloid disease with involvement of the nerves. *Brain* **61**:116, 1938.
10. Ostertag B: Familiere Amyloid-Erkrankung. *Z Menschl Vererbungs Konstit Lehre* **30**:105, 1950.
11. Cohen AS, Calkins E: Electron microscopic observation on a fibrous component in amyloid of diverse origins. *Nature* **183**:1202, 1959.
12. Glenner GG, Terry W, Harada M, Isersky C, Page D: Amyloid fibril proteins: Proof of homology with immunoglobulin light chains by sequence analysis. *Science* **172**:1150, 1971.
13. Levin M, Franklin EC, Frangione B, Pras M: The amino acid sequence of a major nonimmunoglobulin component of some amyloid fibrils. *J Clin Invest* **51**:2773, 1972.
14. Husby G, Sletten K, Michaelsen TE, Natvig JB: Antigenic and chemical characterization of non-immunoglobulin amyloid proteins. *Scand J Immunol* **1**:393, 1972.
15. Sletten K, Husby G: The complete amino acid sequence of non-immunoglobulin amyloid fibril protein AS in rheumatoid arthritis. *Eur J Biochem* **41**:117, 1974.
16. Levin M, Pras M, Franklin EC: Immunologic studies of the major non-immunoglobulin protein of amyloid I. Identification and partial characterization of a related serum component. *J Exp Med* **138**:373, 1973.
17. Husby G, Natvig JB: A serum component related to immunoglobulin amyloid protein AS, a possible precursor of the fibrils. *J Clin Invest* **53**:1054, 1974.
18. Rosenthal CJ, Franklin EC: Variation with age and disease of an amyloid A protein-related serum component. *J Clin Invest* **55**:746, 1975.
19. Linke RP, Sipe JD, Pollock PS, Ignaczak TF, Glenner GG: Isolation of a low molecular weight serum component antigenically related to an amyloid fibril protein of unknown origin. *Proc Natl Acad Sci U S A* **72**:1473, 1975.
20. McAdam KPWJ, Sipe JD: Murine model for human secondary amyloidosis: Genetic variability of the acute-phase serum protein SAA response to endotoxins and casein. *J Exp Med* **144**:1121, 1976.
21. Benson MD, Scheinberg MA, Shirahama T, Cathcart ES, Skinner M: Kinetics of serum amyloid protein A in casein-induced murine amyloidosis. *J Clin Invest* **59**:412, 1977.
22. Benson MD, Kleiner E: Synthesis and secretion of serum amyloid protein A (SAA) by hepatocytes in mice treated with casein. *J Immunol* **124**:495, 1980.

23. Costa PP, Figuera AS, Bravo FR: Amyloid fibril protein related to prealbumin in familial amyloidotic polyneuropathy. *Proc Natl Acad Sci U S A* **75**:4499, 1978.

24. Benson MD: Partial amino acid sequence homology between an heredofamilial amyloid protein and human plasma prealbumin. *J Clin Invest* **67**:1035, 1981.

25. Dwulet FE, Benson MD: Polymorphism of human plasma thyroxine binding prealbumin. *Biochem Biophys Res Commun* **114**:657, 1983.

26. Nakasato M, Kangawa K, Minaminoi N, Tawara S, Matsuo H, Araki S: Revised analysis of amino acid replacement in a prealbumin variant (SKO-III) associated with familial amyloidotic polyneuropathy of Jewish origin. *Biochem Biophys Res Commun* **123**:921, 1984.

27. Wallace MR, Dwulet FE, Conneally PM, Benson MD: Biochemical and molecular genetic characteristic of a new variant prealbumin associated with hereditary amyloidosis. *J Clin Invest* **78**:6, 1986.

28. Dwulet FE, Benson MD: Characterization of prealbumin variant associated with familial amyloidotic polyneuropathy type II (Indiana/Swiss). *J Clin Invest* **78**:880, 1986.

29. Nichols WC, Liepnieks JJ, McKusick VA, Benson MD: Direct sequencing of the gene for Maryland/German familial amyloidotic polyneuropathy type II and genotyping by allele-specific enzymatic amplification. *Genomics* **5**:535, 1989.

30. Benson MD, Uemichi T: Review — Transthyretin amyloidosis. *Amyloid Int J Exp Clin Invest* **3**:44, 1996.

31. Nichols WC, Dwulet FE, Liepnieks J, Benson MD: Variant apolipoprotein AI as a major constituent of a human hereditary amyloid. *Biochem Biophys Res Commun* **156**:762, 1988.

32. Maury CPJ, Alli K, Baumann M: Finnish hereditary amyloidosis. Amino acid sequence homology between the amyloid fibril protein and human plasma gelsoline. *FEBS Lett* **260**:85, 1990.

33. Haltia M, Prelli F, Ghiso J, Kiuru S, Somer H, Palo J, Frangione B: Amyloid protein in familial amyloidosis (Finnish type) is homologous to gelsolin, an actin-binding protein. *Biochem Biophys Res Commun* **167**:927, 1990.

34. Benson MD, Liepnieks J, Uemichi T, Wheeler G, Correa R: Hereditary renal amyloidosis associated with a mutant fibrinogen α-chain. *Nat Genet* **3**:252, 1993.

35. Pepys MB, Hawkins PN, Booth DR, Vigushin DM, Tennent GA, Soutar AK, Totty N, et al: Human lysozyme gene mutations cause hereditary systemic amyloidosis. *Nature* **362**:553, 1993.

36. Glenner GG, Wong CD: Alzheimer's disease: Initial report of the purification and characterization of a novel cerebrovascular amyloid protein. *Biochem Biophys Res Commun* **120**:885, 1984.

37. Tagliavini F, Prelli F, Ghiso J, Bugiani O, Serban D, Prusiner SB, Farlow MR, et al: Amyloid protein of Gerstmann-Sträussler-Scheinker disease (Indiana kindred) is an 11 kd fragment of prion protein with an N-terminal glycine at codon 58. *EMBO J* **10**:513, 1991.

38. Westermark P, Wernstedt C, Wilander E, Sletten K: A novel peptide in the calcitonin gene related family as an amyloid fibril protein in the endocrine pancreas. *Biochem Biophys Res Commun* **140**:827, 1986.

39. Puchtler H, Sweat F, Levine M: On the binding of Congo red by amyloid. *J Histochem Cytochem* **10**:355, 1962.

40. Shirahama T, Cohen AS: High-resolution electron microscopic analysis of the amyloid fibril. *J Cell Biol* **33**:679, 1967.

41. Eanes ED, Glenner GG: X-ray diffraction studies of amyloid filaments. *J Histochem Cytochem* **16**:673, 1968.

42. Bonar L, Cohen AS, Skinner MM: Characterization of the amyloid fibrils as a cross-B protein. *Proc Soc Exp Biol Med* **131**:1373, 1969.

43. Poljak RJ, Anzel LM, Ehcn BL, Phizackerley RP, Saul F: The three-dimensional structure of the Fab' fragment of a human myeloma immunoglobulin at 2.0 Å resolution. *Proc Natl Acad Sci U S A* **71**:3440, 1974.

44. Blake CCF, Geisow MJ, Swan IDA: Structure of human plasma prealbumin at 2.5 Å resolution. *J Mol Biol* **88**:1, 1974.

45. Randall RE, Williamson WC Jr, Mullinax F, Tung MX, Still WJS: Manifestations of light chain deposition. *Am J Med* **60**:293, 1976.

46. Preud'homme JL, Morel-Maroger L, Brovet JC, Cerf M, Mignon F, Guglielmi P, Seligmann M: Synthesis of abnormal immunoglobulin in lymphoplasmolytic disorders with visceral light chain deposition. *Am J Med* **69**:703, 1980.

47. Hofmann-Guilaine C, Nochy D, Jacquot C, Bariety J, Camilleri JP: Association light chain deposition disease (LCDD) and amyloidosis. *Pathol Res Pract* **180**:214, 1985.

48. WHO-IUIS Nomenclature Sub-Committee: Nomenclature of amyloid and amyloidosis. *Bull World Health Organ* **71**:105, 1993.

49. Heller H, Sohar E, Gafni J, Heller J: Amyloidosis in familial Mediterranean fever. *Arch Intern Med* **107**:539, 1961.

50. Schimke RN, Hartmann WH: Familial amyloid-producing medullary thyroid carcinoma and pheochromocytoma: Distinct genetic entity. *Ann Intern Med* **63**:1027, 1965.

51. Sipple JH: The association of pheochromocytoma with carcinoma of the thyroid gland. *Am J Med* **31**:163, 1961.

52. Sagher F, Shanon J: Amyloid cutis: Familial occurrence in three generations. *Arch Dermatol* **87**:171, 1963.

53. Rajagopalan K, Tay CH: Familial lichen amyloidosis: Report of 19 cases in 4 generations of a Chinese family in Malaysia. *Br J Dermatol* **87**:123, 1972.

54. Davies P: The genetics of Alzheimer's disease: A review and a discussion of the implications. *Neurobiol Aging* **7**:459, 1986.

55. Bardin T, Kuntz D, Zingraff J, Voisin M, Zelmar A, Lansaman J: Synovial amyloidosis in patients undergoing long-term hemodialysis. *Arthritis Rheum* **28**:1052, 1985.

56. Gejyo F, Yamada T, Odani S, Nakagawa Y, Arakawa M, Kunit-Omo T, Kataoka H, et al: A new form of amyloid protein associated with chronic hemodialysis was identified as $B_2$-microglobulin. *Biochem Biophys Res Commun* **129**:701, 1985.

57. Eulitz M, Weiss DT, Solomon A: Immunoglobulin heavy-chain-associated amyloidosis. *Proc Natl Acad Sci U S A* **87**:6542, 1990.

58. Kyle RA, Greipp PR: Amyloidosis (AL): Clinical and laboratory features in 229 cases. *Mayo Clin Proc* **58**:665, 1983.

59. Brandt KD, Cathcart ES, Cohen AS: A clinical analysis of the course and prognosis of 42 patients with amyloidosis. *Am J Med* **44**:955, 1968.

60. Greipp PR, Kyle RA, Bowie WEJ: Factor-X deficiency in amyloidosis in a critical review. *Am J Hematol* **11**:443, 1981.

61. Benson MD, Cohen AS, Brandt KD, Cathcart ES: Neuropathy, M-components and amyloid. *Lancet* **1**:10, 1975.

62. Skinner M, Anderson JJ, Simms R, Falk R, Wang M, Libbey CA, Jones LA, et al: Treatment of 100 patients with primary amyloidosis: A randomized trial of melphalan, prednisone, and colchicine versus colchicine only. *Am J Med* **100**:290, 1996.

63. Kyle RA, Gertz MA: Systemic amyloidosis. *Crit Rev Oncol Hematol* **10**:49, 1990.

64. Kyle RA, Wagoner RD, Holley KE: Primary systemic amyloidosis: Resolution of the nephrotic syndrome with melphalan and prednisone. *Arch Intern Med* **142**:1445, 1982.

65. Benson MD: Treatment of AL amyloidosis with melphalan, prednisone and colchicine. *Arthritis Rheum* **29**:683, 1986.

66. Cohen AS, Rubinow A, Anderson JJ, Skinner M, Mason JH, Libbey C, Kayne H: Survival of patients with primary (AL) amyloidosis. *Am J Med* **82**:1182, 1987.

67. Kedar (Keizman) I, Ravid M, Sohar E, Gafni J: Colchicine inhibition of casein-induced amyloidosis in mice. *Isr J Med Sci* **10**:787, 1974.

68. Shirahama T, Cohen AS: Blockage of amyloid induction by colchicine in an animal model. *J Exp Med* **140**:1102, 1974.

69. Comenzo RL, Vosburgh E, Simms RW, Bergethon P, Sarnacki D, Finn K, Duprey S, et al: Dose-intensive melphalan with blood stem cell support for the treatment of AL amyloidosis: One-year follow-up in five patients. *Blood* **38**:2801, 1996.

70. Merlini G, Ascari E, Amboldi N, Bellotti V, Arbustini E, Perfetti V, Ferrari M, et al: Interaction of the anthracycline 4'-iodo-4'-deoxydoxorubicin with amyloid fibrils: Inhibition of amyloidogenesis. *Proc Natl Acad Sci U S A* **92**:2959, 1995.

71. Pelosi Jr. F, Capehart J, Roberts WC: Effectiveness of cardiac transplantation for primary (AL) cardiac amyloidosis. *Am J Cardiol* **79**:532, 1997.

72. Dubrey S, Simms RW, Skinner M, Falk RH: Recurrence of primary (AL) amyloidosis in a transplanted heart with four-year survival. *Am J Cardiol* **76**:739, 1995.

73. Greipp PR, Kyle RA, Bowie EJW: Factor-X deficiency in primary amyloidosis: Resolution after splenectomy. *N Engl J Med* **301**:1050, 1979.

74. Benditt EP, Eriksen N, Hermodson MA, Ericsson LH: The major proteins of human and monkey amyloid substance: Common properties including unusual N-terminal amino acid sequences. *FEBS Lett* **19**:169, 1971.

75. Benditt EP, Eriksen N: Amyloid protein SAA is associated with high-density lipoproteins from human serum. *Proc Natl Acad Sci U S A* **74**:4025, 1977.

76. Benditt EP, Eriksen N, Hanson RH: Amyloid protein SAA is an apoprotein of mouse plasma high density lipoprotein. *Proc Natl Acad Sci U S A* **76**:4092, 1979.

77. Sipe JD, Vogel SN, Ryan JL, McAdams KPWJ, Rosenstreich DL: Detection of a mediator derived from endotoxin-stimulated macrophages that induces the acute phase serum amyloid A response in mice. *J Exp Med* **150**:597, 1979.

78. Morrow JF, Stearman RS, Peltzman CG, Potter DA: Induction of hepatic synthesis of serum amyloid A protein and actin. *Proc Natl Acad Sci U S A* **78**:4718, 1981.

79. Kluve-Beckerman B, Naylor SL, Marshal A, Gardner JC, Shows TB, Benson MD: Localization of human SAA gene(s) to chromosome 11 and detection of DNA polymorphisms. *Biochem Biophys Res Commun* **137**:1196, 1986.

80. Smith MW, Clark SP, Hutchinson JS, Wei YH, Churukian AC, Daniels LB, Diggle KL, et al: A sequence-tagged site map of chromosome 11. *Genomics* **17**:699, 1993.

81. Dwulet FE, Wallace DK, Benson MD: Amino acid structures of multiple forms of amyloid-related serum protein SAA from a single individual. *Biochemistry* **27**:1677, 1988.

82. Parmalee DC, Titani K, Ericsson LH, Eriksen N, Benditt EP, Walsh KA: Amino acid sequence of amyloid related apoprotein (apo SAA) from human high-density lipoproteins. *Biochemistry* **21**:3298, 1982.

83. Liepnieks JJ, Kluve-Beckerman B, Benson MD: Characterization of amyloid A protein in human secondary amyloidosis: The predominant deposition of serum amyloid A1. *Biochim Biophys Acta* **1270**:81, 1995.

84. Whitehead AS, deBeer MC, Steel DM, Rits M, Lelias JM, Lane WS, deBeer FC: Identification of novel members of the serum amyloid A protein superfamily as constitutive apolipoproteins of high density lipoprotein. *J Biol Chem* **267**:3862, 1992.

85. Kluve-Beckerman B, Drumm ML, Benson MD: Nonexpression of the human serum amyloid A three (SAA3) gene. *DNA Cell Biol* **10**:651, 1991.

86. Yamamoto K, Migita S: Complete primary structure of two major murine serum amyloids A proteins deduced from cDNA sequence. *Proc Natl Acad Sci U S A* **82**:2915, 1985.

87. Taylor BA, Rowe L: Genes for serum amyloid A proteins map to chromosome 7 in the mouse. *Mol Gen Genet* **195**:491, 1984.

88. Lowell CA, Potter DA, Stearman RS, Morrow JF: Structure of the murine serum amyloid A gene family. *J Biol Chem* **261**:8442, 1986.

89. deBeer MC, Beach CM, Shedlofsky SI, deBeer FC: Identification of a novel serum amyloid A protein (SAA) in Balb/C mice. *Biochem J* **280**:45, 1991.

90. Meek RL, Eriksen N, Benditt EP: Murine serum amyloid A₃ is a high density apolipoprotein and is secreted by macrophages. *Proc Natl Acad Sci U S A* **89**:7949, 1992.

91. Mitchell TI, Coon CI, Brinckerhoff CE: Serum amyloid A (SAA3) produced by rabbit synovial fibroblasts treated with phorbol esters or interleukin 1 induces synthesis of collagenase and is neutralized by specific antiserum. *J Clin Invest* **87**:1177, 1991.

92. Husby G, Marhaug G, Dowton B, Sletten K, Sipe JD: Serum amyloid A (SAA): biochemistry, genetics and the pathogenesis of AA amyloidosis. *Amyloid Int J Exp Clin Invest* **1**:119, 1994.

93. Hoffman JS, Ericsson LH, Eriksen N, Walsh KA, Benditt EP: Murine tissue amyloid protein AA NH2-terminal sequence identity with only one of two serum amyloid protein (Apo SAA) gene products. *J Exp Med* **159**:641, 1984.

94. Lavie G, Zucker-Franklin D, Franklin EC: Degradation of serum amyloid A protein by surface-associated enzymes of human blood monocytes. *J Exp Med* **148**:1020, 1978.

95. Zemer D, Pras M, Sohar E, Modan M, Cabili S, Gafni J: Colchicine in the prevention and treatment of the amyloidosis of familial Mediterranean fever. *N Engl J Med* **314**:1001, 1986.

96. Assenat H, Calemard E, Charra B, Laurent G, Terrat JC, Vanel T: Hemodialyse, syndrome du canal carpien et substance amyloide. *Nouv Presse Med* **9**:1715, 1980.

97. Clanet M, Mansat M, Durroux R, Testut MF, Guiraud B, Rascol A, Conte J: Syndrome du canal carpien, tenosynovite amyloide et hemodialyse periodique. *Rev Neurol (Paris)* **137**:613, 1981.

98. Bardin T, Kuntz D, Zingraff J, Voisin M-C, Zelmar A, Lansaman J: Synovial amyloidosis in patients undergoing long-term hemodialysis. *Arthritis Rheum* **28**:1052, 1985.

99. Gejyo F, Yamada T, Odani S, Nakagawa Y, Arakawa M, Kunitomo T, Kataoka H, et al: A new form of amyloid protein associated with chronic hemodialysis was identified as β₂-microglobulin. *Biochem Biophys Res Commun* **129**:701, 1985.

100. Gorevic PD, Stone TT, Stone WJ, DiRaimondo CR, Prelli FC, Frangione B: Beta-2-microglobulin is an amyloidogenic protein in man. *J Clin Invest* **76**:2425, 1985.

101. Floege J, Bartsch A, Schulze M, Shaldon S, Koch KM, Smeby C: Clearance and synthesis rates of β₂-microglobulin in patients undergoing hemodialysis and in normal subjects. *J Lab Clin Med* **118**:153, 1991.

102. Dwulet FE, Benson MD: Primary structure of amyloid fibril protein AA in azocasein-induced amyloidosis of CBA/J mice. *J Lab Clin Med* **110**:322, 1987.

103. Westermark P, Johnson KH, Westermark GT, Sletten K, Hayden DW: Bovine amyloid protein AA: Isolation and amino acid sequence analysis. *Comp Biochem Physiol* **85B**:609, 1986.

104. Benson MD, Dwulet FE, DiBartola SP: Identification and characterization of amyloid protein AA in spontaneous canine amyloidosis. *Lab Invest* **52**:448, 1985.

105. DiBartola SP, Benson MD, Dwulet FE, Cornacoff JB: Isolation and characterization of amyloid protein AA in the Abyssinian cat. *Lab Invest* **52**:485, 1985.

106. Skinner M, Cathcart ES, Cohen AS, Benson MD: Isolation and identification by sequence analysis of experimentally induced guinea pig amyloid fibrils. *J Exp Med* **140**:871, 1974.

107. Anders RF, Nordstoga K, Natvig JB, Husby G: Amyloid-related serum protein SAA in endotoxin-induced amyloidosis of the mink. *J Exp Med* **143**:678, 1976.

108. Gorevic PD, Greenwald M, Frangione B, Pras M, Franklin EC: The amino acid sequence of duck amyloid A (AA) protein. *J Immunol* **118**:1113, 1977.

109. Machado EA, Gregory RS, Jones JB, Lange RD: The cyclic hematopoietic dog: A model for spontaneous secondary amyloidosis. *Am J Pathol* **92**:23, 1978.

110. Boyce JT, DiBartola SP, Chew DJ, Gasper PW: Familial renal amyloidosis in Abyssinian cats. *Vet Pathol* **21**:33, 1984.

111. Yonezu T, Tsunasawa S, Higuchi K, Kogishi K, Naiki H, Hanada K, Sakiyama F, et al: A molecular-pathologic approach to murine senile amyloidosis. *Lab Invest* **57**:65, 1987.

112. Kuczynski MH: Neue Beitraege zur Lehre vom Amyloid. *Klin Wochenschr* **2**:727, 1923.

113. Kuczynski MH: Weitere Beitraege zur Lehre vom Amyloid 3. Mitteilung, Ueber die Rueckbildung des Amyloids. *Klin Wochenschr* **2**:2193, 1923.

114. Sipe JD, McAdams KPWJ, Uchino F: Biochemical evidence for the biphasic development of experimental amyloidosis. *Lab Invest* **38**:110, 1978.

115. Yamamoto K, Shiroo M, Migita S: Diverse gene expression for isotypes of murine serum amyloid A protein during acute phase reaction. *Science* **232**:227, 1986.

116. Shirahama T, Cohen AS: Redistribution of amyloid deposits. *Am J Pathol* **99**:539, 1980.

117. Solomon A, Weiss DT, Pepys MB: Induction in mice of human light-chain-associated amyloidosis. *Am J Pathol* **140**:629, 1992.

118. Liepnieks JJ, DiBartola SP, Benson MD: Systemic immunoglobulin (AL) amyloidosis in a cat: Complete primary structure of a feline lambda light chain. *Amyloid Int J Exp Clin Invest* **3**:177, 1996.

119. Newald TA, Murphy C, Gruys E, Weiss DT, Solomon A: Equine light-chain-associated amyloidosis. *Amyloid Int J Exp Clin Invest* **3**:183, 1996.

120. Sasaki H, Tone S, Nakazato M, Yoshioka K, Matsuo H, Kato Y, Sakaki Y: Generation of transgenic mice producing a human transthyretin variant: A possible mouse model for familial amyloidotic polyneuropathy. *Biochem Biophys Res Commun* **139**:794, 1986.

121. Araki S, Yi S, Murakami T, Watanabe S, Ikegawa S, Takahashi K, Yamamura K-I: Systemic amyloidosis in transgenic mice carrying the human mutant transthyretin (Met30) gene. *Mol Neurobiol* **8**:15, 1994.

122. Yi S, Takahashi K, Naito M, Tashiro F, Wakasugi S, Maeda S, Shimada K, et al: Systemic amyloidosis in transgenic mice carrying the human mutant transthyretin (Met30) gene. *Am J Pathol* **138**:403, 1991.

123. Kohno K, Palha JA, Miyakawa K, Saraiva MJM, Ito S, Mabuchi T, Blaner WS, et al: Analysis of amyloid deposition in a transgenic mouse model of homozygous familial amyloidotic polyneuropathy. *Am J Pathol* **150**:1497, 1997.

124. Tagouri YM, Sanders PW, Picken MM, Siegal GP, Kerby JD, Herrera GA: In vitro AL-amyloid formation by rat and human mesangial cells. *Lab Invest* **74**:290, 1996.

125. Shirahama T, Miura K, Ju S-T, Kisilevsky R, Gruys E, Cohen AS: Amyloid enhancing factor-loaded macrophages in amyloid fibril formation. *Lab Invest* **62**:61, 1990.

126. Kluve-Beckerman B, Liepnieks JJ, Wang L, Benson MD: A cell culture system for the study of amyloid pathogenesis: Characterization of amyloid formation by murine peritoneal cells maintained in the presence of recombinant serum amyloid A. *Am J Pathol* **155**:123, 1999.

127. Branch WT Jr, Robbins J, Edelhock H: Thyroxine-binding prealbumin. *J Biol Chem* **246**:6011, 1971.

128. Robbins J: Thyroxine-binding proteins. *Prog Clin Biol Res* 5:331, 1976.

129. NC-IUB and JCBN Newsletter, Nomenclature Committee of IUB. *J Biol Chem* 256:12, 1981.

130. Costa RH, Lai E, Darnell JE: Transcriptional control of the mouse prealbumin (transthyretin) gene: Both promotor sequences and a distinct enhancer are cell specific. *Mol Cell Biol* 6:4697, 1986.

131. Kanda Y, Goodman DS, Canfield RE, Morgan FJ: The amino acid sequence of human plasma prealbumin. *J Biol Chem* 249:6796, 1974.

132. Blake CCF, Geisow MJ, Oatley SJ: Structure of prealbumin: Secondary, tertiary and quaternary interactions determined by Fourier refinement at 1.8 Å. *J Mol Biol* 121:339, 1978.

133. Oatley SJ, Blaney JM, Langridge R, Kollman PA: Molecular mechanical studies of hormone-protein interactions: The interaction of T4 and T3 with prealbumin. *Biopolymers* 23:2931, 1984.

134. Goodman DS: Retinol-binding protein, prealbumin and vitamin A transport. *Prog Clin Biol Res* 5:313, 1976.

135. Waits RP, Yamada T, Uemichi T, Benson MD: Low plasma concentrations of retinol-binding protein in individuals with mutations affecting position 84 of the transthyretin molecule. *Clin Chem* 41:1288, 1995.

136. Berni R, Malpeli G, Folli C, Murrell J, Liepnieks JJ, Benson MD: The Ile84Ser amino acid substitution in transthyretin interferes with the interaction with plasma retinol-binding protein. *J Biol Chem* 269:23395, 1994.

137. Monaco HL, Rizzi M, Coda A: Structure of a complex of two plasma proteins: Transthyretin and retinol-binding protein. *Science* 268:1039, 1995.

138. Benson MD, Dwulet FE: Prealbumin and retinol binding protein serum concentrations in the Indiana type hereditary amyloidosis. *Arthritis Rheum* 26:1493, 1983.

139. Skinner M, Connors LH, Rubinow A, Libbey C, Sipe JD, Cohen AS: Lowered prealbumin levels in patients with familial amyloid polyneuropathy (FAP) and their non-affected but at risk relatives. *Am J Med Sci* 289:17, 1985.

140. Westermark P, Pitkanen P, Benson L, Vahlquist A, Olofsson BO, Cornwell GG III: Serum prealbumin and retinol-binding protein in the prealbumin-related senile and familial forms of systemic amyloidosis. *Lab Invest* 52:314, 1985.

141. Wallace MR, Naylor SL, Kluve-Beckerman B, Long GL, McDonald L, Shows TB, Benson D: Localization of the human prealbumin gene to chromosome 18. *Biochem Biophys Res Commun* 129:753, 1985.

142. Benson MD, Dwulet FE: Identification of carriers of a variant plasma prealbumin (transthyretin) associated with familial amyloidotic polyneuropathy type I. *J Clin Invest* 75:71, 1985.

143. Dwulet FE, Benson MD: Primary structure of an amyloid prealbumin and its plasma precursor in a heredofamilial polyneuropathy of Swedish origin. *Proc Natl Acad Sci U S A* 81:694, 1984.

144. Hamilton JA, Steinrauf LK, Braden BC, Liepnieks J, Benson MD, Holmgren G, Sandgren O, et al: The X-ray crystal structure refinements of normal human transthyretin and the amyloidogenic Val30 → Met variant to 1.7-Å resolution. *J Biol Chem* 268:2416, 1993.

145. Moses AC, Rosen HN, Moller DE, Tsuzaki S, Haddow JE, Lawlor J, Liepnieks JJ, et al: A point mutation in transthyretin increases affinity for thyroxine and produces euthyroid hyperthyroxinemia. *J Clin Invest* 86:2025, 1990.

146. Harrison HH, Gordon ED, Nichols WC, Benson MD: Biochemical and clinical characterization of prealbumin$^{CHICAGO}$: An apparently benign variant of serum prealbumin (transthyretin) discovered with high-resolution two-dimensional electrophoresis. *Am J Med Genet* 39:442, 1991.

147. Mita S, Maeda S, Shimada K, Araki S: Cloning and sequence analysis of cDNA for human prealbumin. *Biochem Biophys Res Commun* 124:558, 1984.

148. Sasaki H, Sakaki Y, Matsuo H, Goto I, Kuroiwa Y, Sahashi I, Takahashi A, et al: Diagnosis of familial amyloidotic polyneuropathy by recombinant DNA techniques. *Biochem Biophys Res Commun* 125:636, 1984.

149. Tsuzuki T, Mita S, Maeda S, Araki S, Shimada K: Structure of the human prealbumin gene. *J Biol Chem* 260:12224, 1985.

150. Sasaki H, Yoshioka N, Takagi Y, Sakaki Y: Structure of the chromosomal gene for human serum prealbumin. *Gene* 37:191, 1985.

151. Wakasugi S, Maeda S, Shimada K: Structure and expression of the mouse prealbumin gene. *J Biochem* 100:49, 1986.

152. Soprano DR, Herbert J, Soprano KJ, Schon EA, Goodman DS: Demonstration of transthyretin mRNA in the brain and other extrahepatic tissues in the rat. *J Biol Chem* 260:11793, 1985.

153. Dickson PW, Aldred AR, Marley PD, Guo-Fen T, Howlett GJ, Schreiber G: High prealbumin and transferrin mRNA levels in the choroid plexus of rat brain. *Biochem Biophys Res Commun* 127:890, 1985.

154. Stauder AJ, Dickson PW, Aldred AR, Schreiber G, Mendelsohn FAO, Hudson P: Synthesis of transthyretin (prealbumin) mRNA in choroid plexus epithelial cells, localized by in situ hydridization in rat brain. *J Histochem Cytochem* 34:949, 1986.

155. Dickson PW, Schreiber G: High levels of messenger RNA for transthyretin (prealbumin) in human choroid plexus. *Neurosci Lett* 66:311, 1986.

156. Andrade A, Araki S, Block WD, Cohen AS, Jackson CE, Kuroiwa Y, McKusick VA, et al: Hereditary amyloidosis. *Arthritis Rheum* 13:902, 1970.

157. Frederiksen T, Gotzsche H, Harboe N, Kiaer W, Mellemgaard K: Familial primary amyloidosis with severe amyloid heart disease. *Am J Med* 33:328, 1962.

158. Uemichi T, Liepnieks JJ, Waits RP, Benson MD: A trinucleotide deletion in the transthyretin gene (ΔV122) in a kindred with familial amyloidotic polyneuropathy. *Neurology* 48:1667, 1997.

159. Uemichi T, Murrell JR, Zeldenrust S, Benson MD: A new mutant transthyretin (Arg 10) associated with familial amyloid polyneuropathy. *J Med Genet* 29:888, 1992.

160. Garzuly F, Wisniewski T, Brittig F, Budka H: Familial meningocerebrovascular amyloidosis, Hungarian type, with mutant transthyretin (TTR Asp18Gly). *Neurol* 47:1562, 1996.

161. Vidal R, Garzuly F, Budka H, Lalowki M, Linke RP, Brittig F, Frangione B, et al: Meningocerebrovascular amyloidosis associated with a novel transthyretin missence mutation at codon 18 (TTRD18G). *Am J Pathol* 148:361, 1996.

162. Jenne DE, Denzel K, Blatzinger P, Winter P, Obermaier B, Linke RP, Altland K: A new isoleucine substitution of Val20 in transthyretin tetramers selectively impairs dimer-dimer contacts and causes systemic amyloidosis. *Proc Natl Acad Sci U S A* 93:6302, 1996.

163. Jacobson DR, Pan T, Kyle RA, Buxbaum JN: Transthyretin Ile20, a new variant associated with late-onset cardiac amyloidosis. *Hum Mutat* 9:83, 1997.

164. Uemichi T, Gertz MA, Benson MD: A new transthyretin variant (Ser24) associated with familial amyloid polyneuropathy. *J Med Genet* 32:279, 1995.

165. Saraiva MJM, Birken S, Costa PP, Goodman DS: Amyloid fibril protein in familial amyloidotic polyneuropathy, Portuguese type. *J Clin Invest* 74:104, 1984.

166. Tawara S, Nakazato M, Kangawa K, Matsuo H, Araki S: Identification of amyloid prealbumin variant in familial amyloidotic polyneuropathy (Japanese type). *Biochem Biophys Res Commun* 116:880, 1983.

167. Skinner M, Cohen AS: The prealbumin nature of the amyloid protein in familial amyloid polyneuropathy (FAP) — Swedish variety. *Biochem Biophys Res Commun* 99:1326, 1981.

168. Holmgren G, Holmberg E, Lindstrom A, Lindstrom E, Nordenson I, Sandgren O, Steen L, et al: Diagnosis of familial amyloidotic polyneuropathy in Sweden by RFLP analysis. *Clin Genet* 32:289, 1988.

169. Holmgren G, Bergstrom S, Drugge U, Lundgren E, Nording-Sikstrom C, Sandgren O, Steen L: Homozygosity for the transthyretin-Met30-gene in seven individuals with familial amyloidosis with polyneuropathy detected by restriction enzyme analysis of amplified genomic DNA sequences. *Clin Genet* 41:39, 1992.

170. Skare J, Yazier H, Erken E, Dede H, Cohen A, Milunsky A, Skinner M: Homozygosity for the Met30 transthyretin gene in a Turkish kindred with familial amyloidotic polyneuropathy. *Hum Genet* 86:89, 1990.

171. Benson MD, Cohen AS: Generalized amyloid in a family of Swedish origin. A study of 426 family members in 7 generations of a new kinship with neuropathy, nephropathy and central nervous system involvement. *Ann Intern Med* 86:419, 1977.

172. Yoshioka K, Furuya H, Sasaki H, Saraiva MJM, Costa PP, Sakaki Y: Haplotype analysis of familial amyloidotic polyneuropathy. *Hum Genet* 82:9, 1980.

173. Kincaid JC, Wallace MR, Benson MD: Late-onset familial amyloid polyneuropathy in an American family of English origin. *Neurology* 39:861, 1989.

174. Jones LA, Skare JC, Cohen AS, Harding JA, Milunsky A, Skinner M: Familial amyloidotic polyneuropathy: A new transthyretin position 30 mutation (alanine for valine) in a family of German descent. *Clin Genet* 41:70, 1992.

175. Nakazato M, Ikeda S, Shiomi K, Matsukura S, Yoshida K, Shimizu H, Atsumi T, et al: Identification of a novel transthyretin variant (Val30 → Leu) associated with familial amyloidotic polyneuropathy. *FEBS Lett* 306:206, 1992.

176. Murakami T, Atsumi T, Maeda S, Tanase S, Ishikawa K, Mita S, Kumamoto T, et al: A novel transthyretin mutation at position 30 (Leu for Val) associated with familial amyloidotic polyneuropathy. *Biochem Biophys Res Commun* **187**:397, 1992.

177. Goren H, Steinberg MC, Farboody GH: Familial oculoleptomeningeal amyloidosis. *Brain* **103**:473, 1980.

178. Petersen RB, Tresser NJ, Richardson SL, Gali M, Goren H, Gametti P: A family with oculoleptomeningeal amyloidosis and dementia has a mutation in the transthyretin gene. *J Neuropathol Exp Neurol* **54**:413, 1995.

179. Gafni J, Fischel B, Reif R, Yaron M, Pras M: Amyloidotic polyneuropathy in a Jewish family. Evidence for the genetic heterogeneity of the lower limb familial amyloidotic neuropathies. *Q J Med* **55**:33, 1985.

180. Pras M, Prelli F, Franklin EC, Frangione B: Primary structure of an amyloid prealbumin variant in familial polyneuropathy of Jewish origin. *Proc Natl Acad Sci U S A* **80**:539, 1983.

181. Nakazato M, Kangawa K, Minamino N, Tawara S, Matsuo H, Araki S: Revised analysis of amino acid replacement in a prealbumin variant (SKO-III) associated with familial amyloidotic polyneuropathy of Jewish origin. *Biochem Biophys Res Commun* **123**:921, 1984.

182. Harding J, Skare J, Skinner M: A second transthyretin mutation at position 33 (Leu/Phe) associated with familial amyloidotic polyneuropathy. *Biochim Biophys Acta* **1097**:183, 1991.

183. Reilly MM, Adams D, Booth DR, Davis MB, Said G, Laubriat-Bianchim M, Pepys MB, et al: Transthyretin gene analysis in European patients with suspected familial amyloid polyneuropathy. *Brain* **118**:849, 1995.

184. Jones LA, Skare JC, Harding JA, Cohen AS, Milunsky A, Skinner M: Proline at position 36: A new transthyretin mutation associated with familial amyloidotic polyneuropathy. *Am J Hum Genet* **48**:979, 1991.

185. Jacobson DR, Rosenthal CJ, Buxbaum JN: Transthyretin Pro 36 associated with familial amyloidotic polyneuropathy in an Ashkenazic Jewish kindred. *Hum Genet* **90**:158, 1992.

186. Uemichi T, Ueno S, Fujimura H, Umekage T, Yorifuji S, Matsuzawa Y, Tarui S: Familial amyloid polyneuropathy related to transthyretin Gly42 in a Japanese family. *Muscle Nerve* **15**:904, 1992.

187. Klein CJ, Nakamura M, Jacobson DR, Lacy MQ, Benson MD, Petersen RC: Transthyretin amyloidosis (serine 44) associated with headache, hearing loss, and peripheral neuropathy. *Neurology* **51**:1462, 1998.

188. Saraiva MJM, Almeida MR, Sherman W, Gawinowicz M, Costa P, Costa PP, Goodman DS: A new transthyretin mutation associated with amyloid cardiomyopathy. *Am J Hum Genet* **50**:1027, 1992.

189. Murakami T, Maeda S, Yi S, Ikegawa S, Kawashima E, Onodera S, Shimada K, et al: A novel transthyretin mutation associated with familial amyloidotic polyneuropathy. *Biochem Biophys Res Commun* **182**:520, 1992.

190. Ferlini A, Salvi F, Patrosso C, Fini S, Vezzoni P, Forabosco A: Gly47Ala: A new transthyretin gene mutation in hereditary amyloidosis TTR-related. *J Rheumatol* **20**:187, 1993.

191. Almeida MR, Ferlini A, Forabosco A, Gawinowicz MA, Costa PP, Salvi F, Plasmati R, et al: Two transthyretin variants (TTR Ala49 and TTR Gln89) in two Sicilian kindreds with hereditary amyloidosis. *Hum Mutat* **1**:211, 1992.

192. Benson MD II, Julien J, Liepnieks J, Zeldenrust S, Benson MD: A transthyretin variant (alanine 49) associated with familial amyloidotic polyneuropathy in a French family. *J Med Genet* **30**:117, 1993.

193. Julien J, Vital CI, Vallat JM, Lagueny A, Ferrer X: Familial amyloid neuropathy in three families of French origin. *Rev Neurol (Paris)* **139**:259, 1983.

194. Nakamura M, Yamashita T, Ando Y, Hamidi Asl K, Tashima K, Ohlsson P-I, Kususe Y, et al: Identification of a new transthyretin variant (Ile49) in familial amyloidotic polyneuropathy using electrospray ionization mass spectrometry and non-isotopic Rnase cleavage assay. *Hum Hered* **49**:186, 1998.

195. Ueno S, Uemichi T, Takahashi N, Soga F, Yorifuji S, Tarui S: Two novel variants of transthyretin identified in Japanese cases with familial amyloidotic polyneuropathy: Transthyretin (Glu42 to Gly) and transthyretin (Ser50 to Arg). *Biochem Biophys Res Commun* **169**:1117, 1990.

196. Takahashi N, Ueno S, Uemichi T, Fujimura H, Yorifuji S, Tarui S: Amyloid polyneuropathy with transthyretin Arg50 in a Japanese case from Osaka. *J Neurol Sci* **112**:58, 1992.

197. Saeki Y, Ueno S, Takahashi N, Soga F, Yanagihara T: A novel mutant (transthyretin Ile-50) related to amyloid polyneuropathy. *FEBS Lett* **308**:35, 1992.

198. Nishi H, Kimura A, Harada H, Hayashi Y, Nakamura M, Sasazuki T: Novel variant transthyretin gene (Ser50 to Ile) in familial cardiac amyloidosis. *Biochem Biophys Res Commun* **187**:460, 1992.

199. Jacobson DR, McFarlin DE, Kane I, Buxbaum JN: Transthyretin Pro55, a variant associated with early-onset, aggressive diffuse amyloidosis with cardiac and neurologic involvement. *Hum Genet* **89**:353, 1992.

200. Yamamoto K, Hsu SP, Yoshida K, Ikeda S, Nakazato M, Shiomi K, Cheng SY, et al: Familial amyloid polyneuropathy in Taiwan: Identification of transthyretin variant (Leu55 → Pro). *Muscle Nerve* **17**:637, 1994.

201. Mahloudji M, Teasdall RD, Adamkiewicz JJ, Hartmann WH, Lambird PA, McKusick VA: The genetic amyloidoses. With particular reference to hereditary neuropathic amyloidosis, type II (Indiana or Rukavina type). *Medicine* **48**:1, 1969.

202. Nichols WC, Liepnieks JJ, McKusick VA, Benson MD: Direct sequencing of the gene for Maryland/German familial amyloidotic polyneuropathy type II and genotyping by allele-specific enzymatic amplification. *Genomics* **5**:535, 1989.

203. Mendell JR, Jiang X-S, Warmolts JR, Nichols WC, Benson MD: Diagnosis of Maryland/German familial amyloidotic polyneuropathy using allele-specific, enzymatically amplified genomic DNA. *Ann Neurol* **27**:553, 1990.

204. Goebel HH, Seddigh S, Hopf HC, Uemichi T, Benson MD, McKusick VA: A European family with histidine 58 transthyretin mutation in familial amyloid polyneuropathy. *Neuromuscular Disorders* **7**:229, 1997.

205. Jacobson DR, Gorevic PD, Sack GH, Malamet RL: Homozygous transthyretin His58 associated with unusually aggressive familial amyloidotic polyneuropathy. *J Rheumatol* **20**:178, 1991.

206. Saeki Y, Ueno S, Yorifuji S, Sugiyama Y, Ide Y, Matsuzawa Y: New mutant gene (transthyretin Arg 58) in cases with hereditary polyneuropathy detected by non-isotope method of single-strand conformation polymorphism analysis. *Biochem Biophys Res Commun* **180**:380, 1991.

207. Booth DR, Tan SY, Hawkins PN, Pepys MB, Frustaci A: A novel variant of transthyretin, $59^{Thr \rightarrow Lys}$, associated with autosomal dominant cardiac amyloidosis in an Italian family. *Circulation* **91**:962, 1995.

208. Wallace MR, Dwulet FE, Conneally PM, Benson MD: Biochemical and molecular genetic characterization of a new variant prealbumin associated with hereditary amyloidosis. *J Clin Invest* **78**:6, 1986.

209. Benson MD, Wallace MR, Tejada E, Baumann H, Page B: Hereditary amyloidosis: Description of a new American kindred with late onset cardiomyopathy. *Arthritis Rheum* **30**:195, 1987.

210. Koeppen AH, Wallace MR, Benson MD, Altland K: Familial amyloid polyneuropathy: Alanine-for-threonine substitution in the transthyretin (prealbumin) molecule. *Muscle Nerve* **13**:1065, 1990.

211. Shiomi K, Nakazato M, Matsukura S, Ohnishi A, Hatanaka H, Tsuji S, Murai Y, et al: A basic transthyretin variant (GLU$^{61}$ → LYS) causes familial amyloidotic polyneuropathy: Protein and DNA sequencing and PCR-induced mutation restriction analysis. *Biochem Biophys Res Commun* **194**:1090, 1993.

212. Ii S, Minnerath S, Ii K, Dyck PJ, Sommer SS: Two-tiered DNA-based diagnosis of transthyretin amyloidosis reveals two novel point mutations. *Neurology* **41**:893, 1991.

213. Uitti RJ, Donat JR, Rozdilsky B, Schneider RJ, Koeppen AH: Familial oculoleptomeningeal amyloidosis. Report of a new family with unusual features. *Arch Neurol* **45**:1118, 1988.

214. Uemichi T, Uitti RJ, Koeppen AH, Donat JR, Benson MD: Oculoleptomeningeal amyloidosis associated with a new transthyretin variant G6S4. *Arch Neurol*, in press.

215. Almeida MR, Hesse JA, Steinmetz A, Maisch B, Altland K, Linke RP, Gawinowicz MA, et al: Transthyretin Leu 68 in a form of cardiac amyloidosis. *Basic Res Cardiol* **86**:567, 1991.

216. Zeldenrust SR, Skinner M, Harding J, Skare J, Benson MD: A new transthyretin variant (His69) associated with vitreous amyloid in an FAP family. *Amyloid Int J Exp Clin Invest* **1**:17, 1994.

217. Izumoto S, Younger D, Hays AP, Martone RL, Smith RT, Herbert J: Familial amyloidotic polyneuropathy presenting with carpal tunnel syndrome and a new transthyretin mutation, asparagine 70. *Neurology* **42**:2094, 1992.

218. Benson MD II, Turpin JC, Lucotte G, Zeldenrust S, LeChevalier, Benson MD: A transthyretin variant (alanine 71) associated with familial amyloidotic polyneuropathy in a French family. *J Med Genet* **30**:120, 1993.

219. Booth DR, Gillmore JD, Persey MR, Booth SE, Cafferty KD, Tennent GA, Madhoo S, et al: Transthyretin Ile 73Val is associated with familial amyloidotic polyneuropathy in a Bangladeshi family. *Hum Mutat* 12:135, 1998.
220. Wallace MR, Dwulet FE, Williams EC, Conneally PM, Benson MD: Identification of a new hereditary amyloid prealbumin variant, Tyr-77, associated with autosomal dominant amyloidosis. *Am J Hum Genet* 39:A22, 1986.
221. Libbey CA, Rubinow A, Shirahama T, Deal C, Cohen AS: Familial amyloid polyneuropathy. Demonstration of prealbumin in a kinship of German/English ancestry with onset in the seventh decade. *Am J Med* 76:18, 1984.
222. Satier F, Nichols WC, Benson MD: Diagnosis of familial amyloidotic polyneuropathy in France. *Clin Genet* 38:469, 1990.
223. Falls HF, Jackson JH, Carey JG, Rukavina JG, Block WD: Ocular manifestations of hereditary primary systemic amyloidosis. *Arch Ophthalmol* 54:660, 1955.
224. Rukavina JG, Block WD, Jackson CE, Falls HF, Carey JH, Curtis AC: Primary systemic amyloidosis: A review and an experimental, genetic, and clinical study of 29 cases with particular emphasis on the familial form. *Medicine* 35:239, 1956.
225. Dwulet FE, Benson MD: Characterization of a transthyretin (prealbumin) variant associated with familial amyloidotic polyneuropathy type II (Indiana/Swiss). *J Clin Invest* 78:880, 1986.
226. Wallace MR, Conneally PM, Benson MD: A DNA test for Indiana/ Swiss hereditary amyloidosis (FAP II). *Am J Hum Genet* 43:182, 1988.
227. Hamilton JA, Steinrauf LK, Braden BC, Murrell JR, Benson MD: Structural changes in transthyretin produced by the Ile84Ser mutation which result in decreased affinity for retinol-binding protein and thyroxine. *Amyloid Int J Exp Clin Invest* 3:1, 1996.
228. Zólyomi Z, Benson MD, Halász K, Uemichi T, Fekete G: Transthyretin mutation (Serine 84) associated with familial amyloid polyneuropathy in a Hungarian family. *Amyloid Int J Exp Clin Invest* 5:30, 1998.
229. Skinner M, Harding J, Skare I, Jones LA, Cohen AS, Milunsky A, Skare J: A new transthyretin mutation associated with amyloidotic vitreous opacities. Asparagine for isoleucine at position 84. *Ophthalmology* 99:503, 1992.
230. Nakamura M, Hamidi Asl K, Benson MD: A novel variant of transthyretin Glu89Lys associated with familial amyloidotic polyneuropathy. *Amyloid Int J Exp Clin Invest* 7:46, 2000.
231. Misrahi M, Plante V, Lalu T, Serre I, Adams D, Lacroix C, Said G: New transthyretin variants SER91 and SER116 associated with familial amyloidotic polyneuropathy. *Hum Mutat*, 12:71, 1998.
232. Yasuda T, Sobue G, Doyu M, Nakazato M, Shiomi K, Yanagi T, Mitsuma T: Familial amyloidotic polyneuropathy with late-onset and well-preserved autonomic function: A Japanese kindred with novel mutant transthyretin (Ala97 to Gly). *J Neurol Sci* 121:97, 1994.
233. Uemichi T, Gertz MA, Benson MD: Amyloid polyneuropathy in two German-American families: A new transthyretin variant (Val107). *J Med Genet* 31:416, 1994.
234. Date Y, Nakazato M, Kangawa K, Shirieda K, Fujimoto T, Matsukura S: Detection of three transthyretin gene mutations in familial amyloidotic polyneuropathy by analysis of DNA extracted from formalin-fixed and paraffin-embedded tissues. *J Neurol Sci* 150:143, 1997.
235. Husby G, Ranlov PJ, Sletten K, Marhaug G: The amyloid in familial amyloid cardiomyopathy of Danish origin is related to prealbumin. *Clin Exp Immunol* 60:207, 1985.
236. Nordlie M, Sletten K, Husby G, Ranløv PJ: A new preaibumin variant in familial amyloid cardiomyopathy of Danish origin. *Scand J Immunol* 27:119, 1988.
237. Ranløv I, Alves IL, Ranløv PJ, Husby G, Costa PP, Saraiva MJM: A Danish kindred with familial amyloid cardiomyopathy revisited: Identification of a mutant transthyretin-methionine111 variant in serum from patients and carriers. *Am J Med* 93:3, 1992.
238. Ueno S, Fujimura H, Yorifuji S, Nakamura Y, Takahashi M, Tarui S, Yanagihara T: Familial amyloid polyneuropathy associated with the transthyretin cys114 gene in a Japanese kindred. *Brain* 115:1275, 1992.
239. Ueno S, Uemichi T, Yorifuji S, Tarui S: A novel variant of transthyretin (Tyr114 to Cys) deduced from the nucleotide sequences of gene fragments from familial amyloidotic polyneuropathy in Japanese sibling cases. *Biochem Biophys Res Commun* 169:143, 1990.
240. Murakami T, Tachibana S, Endo Y, Kawai R, Hara M, Tanase S, Ando M: Familial carpal tunnel syndrome due to amyloidogenic transthyretin His114 variant. *Neurology* 44:315, 1994.
241. Gorevic PD, Prelli FC, Wright J, Pras M, Frangione B: Systemic senile amyloidosis. Identification of a new prealbumin (transthyretin) variant in cardiac tissue: Immunologic and biochemical similarity to one form of familial amyloidotic polyneuropathy. *J Clin Invest* 83:836, 1989.
242. Jacobson DR, Gorevic PD, Buxbaum JN: A homozygous transthyretin variant associated with senile systemic amyloidosis: Evidence for a late-onset disease of genetic etiology. *Am J Hum Genet* 47:127, 1990.
243. Nichols WC, Liepnieks JJ, Snyder EL, Benson MD: Senile cardiac amyloidosis associated with homozygosity for a transthyretin variant (Ile-122). *J Lab Clin Med* 117:175, 1991.
244. Saraiva MJM, Sherman W, Marboe C, Figueira A, Costa P, De Freitas AF, Gawinowicz MA: Cardiac amyloidosis: Report of a patient heterozygous for the transthyretin isoleucine 122 variant. *Scand J Immunol* 32:341, 1990.
245. Jacobson DR, Pastore R, Pool S, Malendowicz S, Kane I, Shivji A, Embury SH, et al: Revised transthyretin Ile122 allele frequency in African-Americans. *Hum Genet* 98:236, 1996.
246. Théberge R, Conners L, Skare J, Skinner M, Falk RH, Costello CE: A new transthyretin variant (Val122Ala) found in a compound heterozygous patient. *Amyloid Int J Exp Clin Invest* 6:54, 1999.
247. Buerger L, Braunstein H: Senile cardiac amyloidosis. *Am J Med* 28:357, 1960.
248. Pomerance A: The pathology of senile cardiac amyloidosis. *J Pathol Bacteriol* 91:357, 1966.
249. Hodkinson HM, Pomerance A: The clinical significance of senile cardiac amyloidosis: A prospective clinicopathological study. *Q J Med* 46:381, 1977.
250. Pitkanen P, Westermark P, Cornwell GG: Senile systemic amyloidosis. *Am J Pathol* 117:391, 1984.
251. Cornwell GG, Westermark P, Natvig JB, Murdoch W: Senile cardiac amyloid: Evidence that fibrils contain a protein immunologically related to prealbumin. *Immunology* 44:447, 1981.
252. Westermark P, Sletten K, Johansson B, Cornwell GG: Fibril in senile systemic amyloidosis is derived from normal transthyretin. *Proc Natl Acad Sci U S A* 87:2843, 1990.
253. Altland K, Becher P, Banzhoff A: Paraffin oil protected high resolution hybrid isoelectric focusing for the demonstration of substitutions of neutral amino acids in denatured proteins: The case of four human transthyretin (prealbumin) variants associated with familial amyloidotic polyneuropathy. *Electrophoresis* 8:293, 1987.
254. Lalloz MRA, Byfield PGH, Goel KM, Loudon MM, Thomson JA, Himsworth RL: Hyperthyroxinemia due to the coexistence of two raised affinity thyroxine-binding proteins (albumin and prealbumin) in one family. *J Clin Endocrinol Metab* 64:346, 1987.
255. Fitch NJS, Akbari MT, Ramsden DB: An inherited non-amyloidogenic transthyretin variant, [Ser6]-TTR, with increased thyroxine-binding affinity, characterized by DNA sequencing. *J Endocrinol* 129:309, 1991.
256. Murrell JR, Schoner RG, Liepnieks JJ, Rosen HN, Moses AC, Benson MD: Production and functional analysis of normal and variant recombinant human transthyretin proteins. *J Biol Chem* 267:16595, 1992.
257. Moses AC, Lawlor J, Haddow J, Jackson I: Familial euthyroid hyperthyroxinemia resulting from increased thyroxine-binding prealbumin. *N Engl J Med* 306:966, 1982.
258. Steinrauf LK, Hamilton JA, Braden BC, Murrell JR, Benson MD: X-ray crystal structure of the Ala109→Thr variant of human transthyretin which produces euthyroid hyperthyroxinemia. *J Biol Chem* 268:2425, 1990.
259. Uemichi T, Liepnieks JJ, Altland K, Benson MD: Identification of a novel non-amyloidogenic transthyretin polymorphism (His74) in the German population. *Amyloid Int J Exp Clin Invest* 1:149, 1994.
260. Almeida MR, Altland K, Rauh S, Gawinowicz M, Moreira P, Costa PP, Saraiva MJ: Characterization of a basic transthyretin variant—TTR Arg102—in the German population. *Biochem Biophys Acta* 1097:224, 1991.
261. Lai Z, Colón W, Kelly JW: The acid-mediated denaturation pathway of transthyretin yields a conformational intermediate that can self-assemble into amyloid. *Biochemistry* 35:6470, 1996.
262. Serpell LC, Goldsteins G, Dacklin I, Lundgren E, Blake CCF: The "edge strand" hypothesis: prediction and test of a mutational "hot-spot" on the transthyretin molecule associated with FAP amyloidogenesis. *Amyloid Int J Exp Clin Invest* 3:75, 1996.
263. Holmgren G, Steen L, Ekstedt J, Groth C-G, Ericzon B-G, Eriksson S, Andersen O, et al: Biochemical effect of liver transplantation in two Swedish patients with familial amyloidotic polyneuropathy (FAP-met30). *Clin Genet* 40:242, 1991.

264. Holmgren G, Ericzon B-G, Groth C-G, Steen L, Suhr O, Andersen O, Wallin BG I, et al: Clinical improvement and amyloid regression after liver transplantation in hereditary transthyretin amyloidosis. *Lancet* **341**:1113, 1993.

265. Skinner M, Lewis WD, Jones LA, Kasirsky J, Kane K, Ju S-T, Jenkins R, et al: Liver transplantation as a treatment for familial amyloidotic polyneuropathy. *Ann Intern Med* **120**:133, 1994.

266. Ikeda S-I, Takei Y-I, Yanagisawa N, Matsunami H, Hashikura Y, Ikegami T, Kawasaki S: Peripheral nerves regenerated in familial amyloid polyneuropathy after liver transplantation. *Ann Intern Med* **127**:618, 1997.

267. Van Allen MW, Frohlich JA, Davis JR: Inherited predisposition to generalized amyloidosis. *Neurology* **19**:10, 1969.

268. Nichols WC, Gregg RE, Brewer HB Jr, Benson MD: A mutation in apolipoprotein A-I in the Iowa type of familial amyloidotic polyneuropathy. *Genomics* **8**:318, 1990.

269. Soutar AK, Hawkins PN, Vigushin DM, Tennent GA, Booth SE, Hutton T, Nguyen O, et al: Apolipoprotein AI mutation Arg-60 causes autosomal dominant amyloidosis. *Proc Natl Acad Sci U S A* **89**:7389, 1992.

270. Booth DR, Tan S-Y, Booth SE, Hsuan JJ, Totty NF, Nguyen O, Hutton T, et al: A new apolipoprotein AI variant, Trp50Arg, causes hereditary amyloidosis. *Q J Med* **88**:695, 1995.

271. Booth DR, Tan S-Y, Booth SE, Tennent GA, Hutchinson WL, Hsuan JJ, Totty NF, et al: Hereditary hepatic and systemic amyloidosis caused by a new deletion/insertion mutation in the apolipoprotein AI gene. *J Clin Invest* **97**:2714, 1996.

272. Persey MR, Booth DR, Booth SE, van Zyl-Smit R, Adams BK, Fattaar AB, Tennent GA, et al: Hereditary nephropathic systemic amyloidosis caused by a novel variant apolipoprotein A-I. *Kidney Int* **53**:276, 1998.

273. Moulin G, Cognat T, Delaye J, Ferrier E, Wagschal D: Amylose disséminée primitive familiale (nouvelle forme clinique?). *Ann Dermatol Venereol* **115**:565, 1988.

274. Hamidi Asl L, Liepnieks JJ, Hamidi Asl K, Uemichi T, Moulin G, Desjoyaux E, Loire R, et al: Hereditary amyloid cardiomyopathy caused by a variant apolipoprotein A1. *Am J Pathol* **154**:221, 1999.

275. Westermark P, Mucchiano G, Marthin T, Johnson KH, Sletten K: Apolipoprotein A1-derived amyloid in human aortic atherosclerotic plaques. *Am J Pathol* **147**:1186, 1995.

276. Roertgen KE, Lund EM, O'Brien TD, Westermark P, Hayden DW, Johnson KH: Apolipoprotein A1-derived pulmonary vascular amyloid in aged dogs. *Am J Pathol* **147**:1311, 1995.

277. Meretoja J: Familial systemic paramyloidosis with lattice dystrophy of the cornea, progressive cranial neuropathy, skin changes and various internal symptoms. *Ann Clin Res* **1**:314, 1969.

278. Meretoja J: Genetic aspects of familial amyloidosis with corneal lattice dystrophy and cranial neuropathy. *Clin Genet* **4**:173, 1973.

279. Meretoja J, Teppo L: Histopathological findings of familial amyloidosis with cranial neuropathy as principal manifestation. *Acta Pathol Microbiol Immunol Scand* **79**:432, 1971.

280. Klintworth GK: Lattice corneal dystrophy. An inherited variety of amyloidosis restricted to the cornea. *Am J Pathol* **50**:371, 1967.

281. Darras BT, Adelman LS, Mora JS, Bodziner RA, Munsat TL: Familial amyloidosis with cranial neuropathy and corneal lattice dystrophy. *Neurology* **36**:432, 1986.

282. Sack GH, Dumars KW, Gummerson KS, Law A, McKusick VA: Three forms of dominant amyloid neuropathy. *Johns Hopkins Med J* **149**:239, 1981.

283. Maury CPJ: Isolation and characterization of cardiac amyloid in familial amyloid polyneuropathy type IV (Finnish): Relation of the amyloid protein to variant gelsolin. *Biochim Biophys Acta* **1096**:84, 1990.

284. Maury CPJ, Kere J, Tolvanen R, de la Chapelle A: Finnish hereditary amyloidosis is caused by a single nucleotide substitution in the gelsolin gene. *FEBS Lett* **276**:75, 1990.

285. Levy E, Haltia M, Fernandez-Madrid I, Koivunen O, Ghiso J, Prelli F, Frangione B: Mutation in gelsolin gene in Finnish hereditary amyloidosis. *J Exp Med* **172**:1865, 1990.

286. de la Chapelle A, Kere J, Sack GH Jr, Tolvanen R, Maury CPJ: Familial amyloidosis, Finnish type: G654 → A mutation of the gelsolin gene in Finnish families and an unrelated American family. *Genomics* **13**:898, 1992.

287. Sunada Y, Shimizu T, Nakase H, Ohta S, Asaoka T, Amano S, Sawa M, et al: Inherited amyloid polyneuropathy type IV (gelsolin variant) in a Japanese family. *Ann Neurol* **33**:57, 1993.

288. de la Chapelle A, Tolvanen R, Boysen G, Santavy J, Blecker-Wagemakers L, Maury CPJ, Kere J: Gelsolin-derived familial

289. Maury CPJ, Kere J, Tolvanen R, de la Chapelle A: Homozygosity for the Asn187 gelsolin mutation in Finnish-type familial amyloidosis is associated with severe renal disease. *Genomics* **13**:902, 1992.

290. Munier FL, Korvatska E, Djemaï A, Paslier DL, Zografos L, Pescia G, Schorderet DF: Kerato-epithelin mutations in four 5q31-linked corneal dystrophies. *Nat Genet* **15**:247, 1997.

291. Korvatska E, Munier FL, Djemaï A, Wang MX, Frueh B, Chiou G-Y, Uffer S, et al: Mutation hot spots in 5q31-linked corneal dystrophies. *Am J Hum Genet* **62**:320, 1998.

292. Yin HL, Kwiatkowski DJ, Mole JE, Cole FS: Structure and biosynthesis of cytoplasmic and secreted variants of gelsolin. *J Biol Chem* **259**:5271, 1984.

293. Kwiatkowski DJ, Mehl R, Yin HL: Genomic organization and biosynthesis of secreted and cytoplasmic forms of gelsolin. *J Cell Biol* **106**:375, 1988.

294. Kwiatkowski DJ, Westbrook CA, Bruns GAP, Morton CC: Localization of gelsolin proximal to ABL on chromosome 9. *Am J Hum Genet* **42**:565, 1988.

295. Kwiatkowski DJ, Mehl R, Izumo S, Nadal-Ginard B, Yin HL: Muscle is the major source of plasma gelsolin. *J Biol Chem* **263**:8239, 1988.

296. Shafer JA, Higgins DL: Human fibrinogen. *CRC Crit Rev Clin Lab Sci* **26**:1, 1988.

297. Doolittle RF, Watt KWK, Cottrell BA, Strong DD, Riley M: The amino acid sequence of the α-chain of human fibrinogen. *Nature* **280**:464, 1979.

298. Rixon MW, Chan WY, Davie EW, Chung DW: Characterization of a complementary deoxyribonucleic acid coding for the α-chain of human fibrinogen. *Biochemistry* **22**:3237, 1983.

299. Matsuda M, Yoshida N, Terukina S, Yamazumi K, Mackawa H: Molecular abnormalities of fibrinogen—the present status of structure elucidation, in Matsuda M, Iwanage S, Takada A, Henschen A (eds): *Fibrinogen 4: Current Basic and Clinical Aspects*. Amsterdam, Excerpta Medica, 1990, p 139.

300. Uemichi T, Liepnieks JJ, Gertz MA, Benson MD: Fibrinogen Aα-chain Leu554: An African-American kindred with late onset renal amyloidosis. *Amyloid Int J Exp Clin Invest* **5**:188, 1998.

301. Hamidi Asl L, Fournier V, Billerey C, Justrabo E, Chevet D, Droz D, Pecheux C, et al: Fibrinogen A α chain mutation (Arg554Leu) associated with hereditary renal amyloidosis in a French family. *Amyloid Int J Exp Clin Invest* **5**:279, 1998.

302. Uemichi T, Liepnieks JJ, Benson MD: Hereditary renal amyloidosis with a novel variant fibrinogen. *J Clin Invest* **93**:731, 1994.

303. Uemichi T, Liepnieks JJ, Alexander F, Benson MD: The molecular basis of renal amyloidosis in Irish-American and Polish-Canadian kindreds. *Q J Med* **89**:745, 1996.

304. Uemichi T, Liepnieks JJ, Yamada T, Gertz MA, Bang N, Benson MD: A frame shift mutation in the fibrinogen Aα-chain gene in a kindred with renal amyloidosis. *Blood* **87**:4197, 1996.

305. Hamidi Asl L, Liepnieks JJ, Uemichi T, Rebebou JM, Justrabo E, Droz D, Mousson C, et al: Renal amyloidosis with a frame shift mutation in fibrinogen Aα-chain producing a novel amyloid protein. *Blood* **90**:4799, 1997.

306. Booth DR, Sunde M, Bellotti V, Robinson CV, Hutchinson WL, Fraser PE, Hawkins PN, et al: Instability, unfolding and aggregation of human lysozyme variants underlying amyloid fibrillogenesis. *Nature* **385**:787, 1997.

307. Gudmundsson G, Hallgrimsson J, Jonasson TA, Bjarnason O: Hereditary cerebral hemorrhage with amyloidosis. *Brain* **95**:387, 1972.

308. Cohen DH, Feiner H, Jensson O, Frangione B: Amyloid fibril in hereditary cerebral hemorrhage with amyloidosis (HCHWA) is related to gastroentero-pancreatic neuroendocrine protein, gamma trace. *J Exp Med* **158**:623, 1983.

309. Ghiso J, Pons-Estel B, Frangione B: Hereditary cerebral amyloid angiopathy: The amyloid fibrils contain a protein which is a variant of cystatin C, an inhibitor of lysosomal cysteine proteases. *Biochem Biophys Res Commun* **136**:548, 1986.

310. Abrahamson M, Jonsdottir S, Olafsson I, Jensson O, Grubb A: Hereditary cystatin C amyloid angiopathy: Identification of the disease-causing mutation and specific diagnosis by polymerase chain reaction based analysis. *Hum Genet* **89**:377, 1992.

311. Jensson O, Luyendijk W, Petursdottir I, Arnason A, Gudmundsson G, Grubb A: Cystatin C values in the cerebrospinal fluid: Comparison between the Icelandic and the Dutch type of hereditary central nervous system amyloid angiopathy. *Acta Neurol Scand* **73**:313, 1986.

[top of right column:] amyloidosis caused by asparagine or tyrosine substitution for aspartic acid at residue 187. *Nat Genet* **2**:157, 1992.

312. Jensson O, Thorsteinsson L, Bots GTAM, Luyendijk W, Gudmunds- son G, Arnason A, Lofberg H: Immunohistochemical comparison between the Dutch and the Icelandic form of hereditary central ner- vous system amyloid angiopathy. *Acta Neurol Scand* **73**:312, 1986.
313. Abrahamson M, Olafsson I, Palsdottir A, Ulvsback M, Lundwall A, Jensson O, Grubb A: Structure and expression of the human cystatin C gene. *Biochem J* **268**:287, 1990.
314. Abrahamson M, Grugg A: Increased body temperature accelerates aggregation of the Leu68 → Gln mutant cystatin C, the amyloid- forming protein in hereditary cystatin C amyloid angiopathy. *Proc Natl Acad Sci U S A* **91**:1416, 1994.
315. van Duinen SG, Castano EM, Prelli F, Bots GTAM, Luyendijk W, Frangione B: Hereditary cerebral hemorrhage with amyloidosis in patients of Dutch origin is related to Alzheimer disease. *Proc Natl Acad Sci U S A* **84**:5991, 1987.
316. Levy E, Carman MD, Fernandez-Madrid IJ, Power MD, Lieberburg I, van Duinen SG, Bots GTAM, et al: Mutation of the Alzheimer's disease amyloid gene in hereditary cerebral hemorrhage, Dutch type. *Science* **248**:1124, 1990.
317. Hendriks L, van Duijn CM, Cras P, Druts M, van Hul W, van Harskamp F, Warren A, et al: Presenile dementia and cerebral haemorrhage linked to a mutation at codon 692 of the β-amyloid precursor protein gene. *Nat Genet* **1**:218, 1992.
318. Siegal S: Benign paroxysmal peritonitis. *Ann Intern Med* **23**:1, 1945.
319. Heller H, Sohar E, Sherf L: Familial Mediterranean fever. *Arch Intern Med* **102**:50, 1958.
320. Sohar E, Pras M, Heller J, Heller H: Genetics of familial Mediterranean fever (FMF). *Arch Intern Med* **107**:529, 1961.
321. Sohar E, Gafni J, Pras M, Heller H: Familial Mediterranean fever. *Am J Med* **43**:227, 1967.
322. Heller H, Gafni J, Michaeli D, Shahin N, Sohar E, Erlich G, Karten I, et al: The arthritis of familial Mediterranean fever (FMF). *Arthritis Rheum* **9**:1, 1966.
323. Pras E, Aksentijevich I, Gruberg L, Balow JE, Prosen L, Dean M, Steinberg AD, et al: Mapping of a gene causing familial Mediterra- nean fever to the short arm of chromosome 16. *N Engl J Med* **326**:1509, 1992.
324. Shohat M, Bu X, Shohat T, Fischel-Ghodsian N, Magal N, Nakamura Y, Schwabe AD, et al: The gene for familial Mediterranean fever in both Armenians and non-Ashkenazi Jews is linked to the α-globin complex on 16p: Evidence for locus homogeneity. *Am J Hum Genet* **51**:1349, 1992.
325. Pras M, Bronshpigel N, Zemer D, Gafni J: Variable incidence of amyloidosis in familial Mediterranean fever among different ethnic groups. *Johns Hopkins Med J* **150**:22, 1982.
326. Gafni J, Ravid M, Sohar E: The role of amyloidosis in familial Mediterranean fever: A population study. *Isr J Med Sci* **4**:995, 1968.
327. Blum A, Gafni J, Sohar E, Shibolet S, Heller H: Amyloidosis as the sole manifestation of familial Mediterranean fever (FMF). *Ann Intern Med* **57**:795, 1962.
328. The International FMF Consortium: Ancient missense mutations in a new member of the RoRet gene family are likely to cause familial Mediterranean fever. *Cell* **90**:797, 1997.
329. The French FMF Consortium: A candidate gene for familial Mediterranean fever. *Nat Genet* **17**:25, 1997.
330. Benson MD, Skinner M, Cohen AS: Amyloid deposition in a renal transplant in familial Mediterranean fever. *Ann Intern Med* **87**:31, 1977.
331. Goldstain RC, Schwabe AD: Prophylactic colchicine therapy in familial Mediterranean fever: A controlled, double-blind study. *Ann Intern Med* **81**:792, 1974.
332. Zemer D, Pras M, Sohar E, Modan M, Cabili S, Gafni J: Colchicine in the prevention and treatment of the amyloidosis of familial Mediterranean fever. *N Engl J Med* **314**:1001, 1986.
333. Muckle TJ, Wells M: Urticaria, deafness and amyloidosis: A new heredofamilial syndrome. *Q J Med* **31**:235, 1962.
334. Black JT: Amyloidosis, deafness, urticaria and limb pains: A hereditary syndrome. *Ann Intern Med* **70**:989, 1969.
335. Williamson LM, Hull D, Mehta R, Reeves WG, Robinson BHB, Toghill PJ: Familial Hibernian fever. *Q J Med* **51**:469, 1982.
336. Linke RP, Heilman KL, Nathrath WBJ, Eulitz M: Identification of amyloid A protein in a sporadic Muckle-Wells syndrome. *Lab Invest* **48**:698, 1983.
336a. Cuisset L, Drenth JP, Berthelot JM, Meyrier A, Vaudour G, Watts RA, Scott DG, Nicholia A, Pavek S, Vasseur C, Beckmann JS, Delpech M, Grateau G: Genetic linkage of the muckle-wells syndrome to chromosome 1q44. *Am J Hum Genet* **65**:1054, 1999.

337. Weiss SW, Page DL: Amyloid nephropathy of Ostertag with special reference to renal glomerular giant cells. *Am J Pathol* **72**:447, 1973.
338. Keiser HR, Beaven MA, Doppman J, Wells S, Buja LM: Sipple's syndrome: Medullary thyroid carcinoma, pheochromocytoma, and parathyroid disease. *Ann Intern Med* **78**:561, 1973.
339. Sletten K, Westermark P, Natvig JB: Characterization of amyloid fibril proteins from medullary carcinoma of the thyroid. *J Exp Med* **143**:993, 1976.
340. Eng AM, Cogan L, Gunnar RM, Blekys I: Familial generalized dyschromic amyloidosis cutis. *J Cutan Pathol* **3**:102, 1976.
341. Ozaki M: Familial Lichen Amyloidosis. *Int J Dermatol* **23**:190, 1984.
342. Newton JA, Jagjivan A, Bhogal B, McKee PH, McGibbon DH: Familial primary cutaneous amyloidosis. *Br J Dermatol* **112**:201, 1985.
343. De Pietro WP: Primary familial cutaneous amyloidosis. *Arch Dermatol* **117**:639, 1981.
344. Partington MW, Marriott PJ, Prentice RSA, Cavaglia A, Simpson NE: Familial cutaneous amyloidosis with systemic manifestations in males. *Am J Med Genet* **10**:65, 1981.
345. Cornwell GG III, Westermark P: Senile amyloidosis: A protean manifestation of the aging process. *J Clin Pathol* **33**:1146, 1980.
346. Allensworth DC, Rice GJ, Loew GW: Persistent atrial standstill in a family with myocardial disease. *Am J Med* **47**:775, 1969.
347. Steiner I: The prevalence of isolated atrial amyloid. *J Pathol* **153**:395, 1987.
348. Kaye GC, Butler MG, d'Ardenne AJ, Edmondson SJ, Camm AJ, Slavin G: Isolated atrial amyloid contains atrial natriuretic peptide: A report of six cases. *Br Heart J* **56**:317, 1960.
349. Johansson B, Wernstedt C, Westermark P: Atrial natriuretic peptide deposited as atrial amyloid fibrils. *Biochem Biphys Res Commun* **148**:1087, 1987.
350. Linke RP, Voigt C, Storkel FS, Eulitz M: N-terminal amino acid sequence analysis indicates that isolated atrial amyloid is derived from atrial natriuretic peptide. *Virchows Archiv (Berlin)* **55**:125, 1988.
351. Pucci A, Wharton J, Arbustini E, Grasso M, Diegoli M, Needleman P, Vigano M, et al: Atrial amyloid deposits in the failing human heart display both atrial and brain natriuretic peptide-like immunoreactiv- ity. *J Pathol* **165**:235, 1991.
352. Maeda S, Tanaka T, Hayashi T: Familial atrial standstill caused by amyloidosis. *Br Heart J* **59**:498, 1988.
353. Marotta CA, Majocha RE, Tate B: Molecular and cellular biology of Alzheimer amyloid. *J Mol Neurosci* **3**:111, 1992.
354. St George-Hyslop PH, Tanzi RE, Polinsky RJ, Haines JL, Nee L, Watkins PC, Myers RH, et al: The genetic defect causing familial Alzheimer's disease, maps on chromosome 21. *Science* **235**:885, 1987.
355. Tanzi RE, Gusella JF, Watkins PC, Bruns GAP, St George-Hyslop P, Van Keuren ML, Patterson D, et al: Amyloid beta protein gene: cDNA, mRNA distribution, and genetic linkage near the Alzheimer locus. *Science* **235**:880, 1987.
356. Palmert MR, Podlinsky MB, Witker DS, Oltersdorf T, Younkin LH, Selkoe DJ, Younkin SG: The β-amyloid protein precursor of Alzheimer disease has soluble derivatives found in human brain and cerebrospinal fluid. *Proc Natl Acad Sci U S A* **86**:6338, 1989.
357. Goate A, Chartier-Harlin M-C, Mullan M, Brown J, Crawford F, Fidani L, Giuffra L, et al: Segregation of a missense mutation in the amyloid precursor protein gene with familial Alzheimer's disease. *Nature* **349**:704, 1991.
358. Murrell J, Farlow M, Ghetti B, Benson MD: A mutation in the amyloid precursor protein associated with hereditary Alzheimer's disease. *Science* **254**:97, 1991.
359. Chartier-Harlin M-C, Crawford F, Houlden H, Warren A, Hughes D, Fidani L, Goate A, et al: Early-onset alzheimer's disease caused by mutations at codon 717 of the β-amyloid precursor protein gene. *Nature* **353**:844, 1991.
360. George-Hyslop P, Haines J, Rogaev E, Mortilla M, Vaula G, Pericak- Vance MA, Foncin JF, et al: Genetic evidence for a novel familial Alzheimer's disease locus on chromosome 14. *Nat Genet* **2**:330, 1992.
361. Rogaev EI, Sherrington R, Rogaeva EA, Levesque G, Ikeda M, Liang Y Chi H, et al: Familial Alzheimer's disease in kindreds with missense mutations in a novel gene on chromosome 1 related to the Alzheimer's disease type 3 gene. *Nature* **376**:775, 1995.
362. Schellenberg GD: Genetic dissection of Alzheimer disease, a heterogeneous disorder. *Proc Natl Acad Sci U S A* **92**:8552, 1995.

363. Haass C, Lemere CA, Capell A, Citron M, Seubert P, Schenk D, Lannfelt L, et al: The Swedish mutation causes early-onset alzheimer's disease by $\beta$-secretase cleavage within the secretory pathway. *Nat Med* **1**:1291, 1995.

364. Tomita T, Maruyama K, Saido TC, Kume H, Shinozaki K, Tokuhiro S, Capell A, et al: The presenilin 2 mutation (N141I) linked to familial Alzheimer disease (Volga German families) increases the secretion of amyloid $\beta$-protein ending at the 42nd (or 43rd) residue. *Proc Natl Acad Sci U S A* **94**:2025, 1997.

365. Hsiao K, Dlouhy SR, Farlow MR, Cass C, DaCosta M, Conneally PM, Hodes ME, et al: Mutant prion proteins in Gerstmann-Sträussler-Scheinker disease with neurofibrillary tangles. *Nat Genet* **1**:68, 1992.

366. Prusiner SB, DeArmond SJ: Prion protein amyloid and neurodegeneration. *Amyloid Int J Exp Clin Invest* **2**:39, 1995.

367. Prusiner SB: Novel proteinaceous infectious particles cause scrapie. *Science* **215**:136, 1982.

368. Opie EL: On relation of chronic interstitial pancreatitis to the islands of Langerhans and to diabetes mellitus. *J Exp Med* **5**:397, 1900.

369. Yano BL, Hayden DW, Johnson KH: Feline insular amyloid: Association with diabetes mellitus. *Vet Pathol* **18**:621, 1981.

370. Westermark P, Wernstedt C, Wilander E, Hayden DW, O'Brien TD, Johnson KH: Amyloid fibrils in human insulinoma and islets of Langerhans of the diabetic cat are derived from a neuropeptide-like protein also present in normal islet cells. *Proc Natl Acad Sci U S A* **84**:3881, 1987.

371. Roberts AN, Leighton B, Todd JA, Cockburn D, Schofield PN, Sutton R, Holt S, et al: Molecular and functional characterization of amylin, a peptide associated with type 2 diabetes mellitus. *Proc Natl Acad Sci U S A* **86**:9662, 1989.

372. Mosselman S, Hoppener JWM, Zandberg J, van Mansveld ADM, Geurts van Kessel AHM, Lips CJM, Jansz HS: Islet amyloid polypeptide: Identification and chromosomal localization of the human gene. *FEBS Lett* **239**:227, 1988.

373. Johnson KH, O'Brien TD, Betsholtz C, Westermark P: Biology of disease. Islet amyloid polypeptide: Mechanisms of amyloidogenesis in the pancreatic islets and potential roles in diabetes mellitus. *Lab Invest* **66**:522, 1992.

374. Nishi M, Steiner DF: Cloning of complementary DNAs encoding amyloid polypeptide, insulin, and glucagon precursors from a new world rodent, the degu, *Octodon degus*. *Mol Endocrinol* **4**:1192, 1990.

375. Hamidi Asl K, Liepnieks JJ, Bihrle R, Benson MD: Local synthesis of amyloid fibril precursor in AL amyloidosis of the urinary tract. *Amyloid Int J Exp Clin Invest* **5**:49, 1998.

376. Fujihara S, Glenner GG: Primary localized amyloidosis of the genitourinary tract: Immunohistochemical study on eleven cases. *Lab Invest* **44**:55, 1981.

377. Thompson PJ, Citron KM: Amyloid and the lower respiratory tract. *Thorax* **38**:84, 1983.

378. Athanasou NA, Sallie B: Localized deposition of amyloid in articular cartilage. *Histopathology* **20**:41, 1992.

379. Landman WJM, Peperkamp NHMT, Koch CAM, Tooten PCJ, Crauwels PAP, Gruys E: Induction of amyloid arthropathy in chickens. *Amyloid Int J Exp Clin Invest* **4**:87, 1997.

380. Altland K, Banzhoff A: Separation by hybrid isoelectric focusing of normal human plasma transthyretin (prealbumin) and a variant with a methionine for valine substitution associated with familial amyloidotic polyneuropathy. *Electrophoresis* **7**:529, 1986.

381. Benson MD, Dwulet FE: Identification of carriers of a variant plasma prealbumin (transthyretin) associated with familial amyloidotic polyneuropathy type I. *J Clin Invest* **75**:71, 1985.

382. Nakazato M, Kurihara T, Matsukura S, Kangawa K, Matsuo H: Diagnostic radioimmunoassay for amyloidotic polyneuropathy before clinical onset. *J Clin Invest* **77**:1699, 1986.

383. Saraiva MJM, Costa PP, Goodman DS: Biochemical marker in familial amyloidotic polyneuropathy, Portuguese type. *J Clin Invest* **76**:2171, 1985.

384. Nichols WC, Padilla L-M, Benson MD: Prenatal detection of a gene for hereditary amyloidosis. *Am J Med Genet* **34**:520, 1989.

385. Morris M, Nichols WC, Benson MD: Prenatal diagnosis of hereditary amyloidosis in a Portuguese family. *Am J Med Genet* **39**:123, 1991.

386. Sasaki H, Sakaki Y, Matsuo H, Goto I, Kuroiwa Y, Sahashi I, Takahashi A, et al: Diagnosis of familial amyloidotic polyneuropathy by recombinant DNA techniques. *Biochem Biophys Res Commun* **125**:636, 1984.

387. Mita S, Maeda S, Ide M, Tsuzuki T, Shimada K, Araki S: Familial amyloidotic polyneuropathy diagnosed by cloned human prealbumin cDNA. *Neurology* **36**:298, 1986.

388. Nichols WC, Benson MD: Hereditary amyloidosis: Detection of variant prealbumin genes by restriction enzyme analysis of amplified genomic DNA sequences. *Clin Genet* **37**:44, 1990.

389. Zeldenrust SR, Murrell J, Farlow M, Ghetti B, Roses AD, Benson MD: RFLP analysis for APP 717 mutations associated with Alzheimer's disease. *J Med Genet* **30**:476, 1993.

390. Jacobson DR: A specific test for transthyretin 122 (Val → Ile), based on PCR-primer-introduced restriction analysis (PCR-PIRA): Confirmation of the gene frequency in blacks. *Am J Hum Genet* **50**:195, 1992.

# Achondroplasia and Pseudoachondroplasia

*Douglas J. Wilkin* ■ *Jacqueline T. Hecht* ■ *Clair A. Francomano*

1. Achondroplasia and pseudoachondroplasia are clinically and genetically distinct phenotypes that are among the most common human disorders resulting in short stature. Both are inherited as autosomal dominant conditions. Achondroplasia, the single most common form of human dwarfism, results in most cases from one of two very specific mutations in the gene encoding fibroblast growth factor receptor 3 (*FGFR3*). Pseudoachondroplasia is caused by a variety of mutations in the gene encoding cartilage oligomeric matrix protein (*COMP*). Both disorders are characterized by short-limb dwarfism, in which the affected person's arms and legs are relatively short compared to the height of the trunk. Disorders with clinical, radiographic, and molecular features in common with achondroplasia include hypochondroplasia, thanatophoric dysplasia (TD), and severe achondroplasia with developmental delay and acanthosis nigricans (SADDAN). Similarly, pseudoachondroplasia and multiple epiphyseal dysplasia (MED) are related.

2. The clinical manifestations of achondroplasia include rhizomelic short stature, frontal bossing with midface hypoplasia, short ribs, trident hand, limited elbow extension, and hyperextensible hips and knees. Infants may have a thoracolumbar kyphosis or gibbus. Spinal stenosis is a common complication in adulthood. Less frequent complications in childhood include cervicomedullary compression secondary to a small foramen magnum, hydrocephalus, and obstructive apnea secondary to small airways. Age-specific mortality is increased in the first 4 years of life and in the fourth to fifth decades.

3. Homozygous achondroplasia is a neonatal lethal condition in which the skeletal manifestations of achondroplasia are exaggerated. Death is usually secondary to respiratory compromise or from cervical cord compression by a very small foramen magnum. In families where both parents have achondroplasia, the children are at 25 percent risk of inheriting the achondroplasia mutation from both parents, resulting in homozygous achondroplasia.

4. The phenotype of hypochondroplasia is similar to that of achondroplasia but milder in degree. The height curves overlap with those of the average population and spinal stenosis is infrequently observed. Learning disabilities may be more common among children with hypochondroplasia than among children with achondroplasia.

5. Thanatophoric dysplasia (TD), a neonatal lethal disorder, is the most severe of the *FGFR3* phenotypes. Two types, designated TDI and TDII, are distinguishable on clinical and molecular grounds. The SADDAN phenotype is a recently recognized condition in the achondroplasia family of disorders.

6. Achondroplasia, hypochondroplasia, TDI, TDII, and the SADDAN phenotype are all caused by mutations in the *FGFR3* gene. All are dominant phenotypes and most cases occur as a result of new mutation. Most, if not all, new mutations causing achondroplasia occur on the paternal allele.

7. The FGFRs are a family of four tyrosine kinase receptors. They have three immunoglobulin-like regions in the extracellular domain, a transmembrane domain, and a split intracellular tyrosine kinase domain. The different receptors bind fibroblast growth factors (FGFs) with variable affinity. Alternative splicing is a feature of FGFR RNA processing. The receptor monomers dimerize, in a step requiring heparin, before ligand may be bound. The dimerization process is promiscuous; any FGFR monomer may dimerize with any other.

8. *FGFR3* has two splice forms depending on which of two alternative exons are used for the C-terminal half of the third immunoglobulin-like domain. *FGFR3* with exon IIIb has a high ligand-specificity for acidic FGF/FGF-1 and is expressed in mouse embryo skin and epidermal keratinocytes. The splice form containing exon IIIc is expressed in developing mouse brain and in the spinal cord, as well as in cartilage rudiments of developing bone.

9. The *FGFR3* cDNA is 4.4 kb and contains an open reading frame of 2520 nucleotides, encoding an 840-amino-acid protein. The human gene is located at 4p16.3, spans 16.5 kb and has 19 exons. The two most common mutations causing achondroplasia are *FGFR3* 1138G>A and 1138 G>C, both resulting in a G380R substitution in the transmembrane domain of the receptor. Together, these two mutations account for more than 98 percent of achondroplasia cases. The tight correlation between specific mutations and their consequent phenotypes is a unique feature of the *FGFR* genes.

10. The two most common *FGFR3* mutations causing hypochondroplasia both result in N540K substitutions in the tyrosine kinase domain of the receptor. Genetic heterogeneity is an issue in hypochondroplasia, because in some families the phenotype is not linked to *FGFR3*. There is allelic heterogeneity among cases of TDI, but to date, all reported cases of TDII are caused by the K650E missense mutations in the tyrosine kinase domain of *FGFR3*. The SADDAN phenotype is caused by K650M substitutions.

---

A list of standard abbreviations is located immediately preceding the index in each volume. Additional abbreviations used in this chapter include: COMP = cartilage oligomeric matrix protein; CPAP = continuous positive airway pressure; FGF = fibroblast growth factors; FGFR3 = fibroblast growth factor receptor 3; MAP = mitogen-activated protein; MED = multiple epiphyseal dysplasia; SADDAN = severe achondroplasia with developmental delay and acanthosis nigricans; TD = thanatophoric dysplasia.

11. The *FGFR3* mutations causing achondroplasia, hypochondroplasia, thanatophoric dysplasia, and SADDAN all result in constitutive activation of the receptor. The varying degrees of severity between these phenotypes are due in part to varying degrees of ligand-independent activation of the FGF receptor by their mutations. By contrast, homozygous knockout mice entirely lacking *FGFR3* have long bone overgrowth. These observations suggest that the normal function of *FGFR3* is necessary for negative regulation of bone growth.

12. Recent molecular studies demonstrate that pseudoachondroplasia and MED are allelic disorders that result from mutations in the *COMP* gene. MED demonstrates locus heterogeneity as the phenotype results, in a few cases, from mutations in the genes encoding the alpha 2 and alpha 3 chains of type IX collagen (*COL9A2* and *COL9A3*).

13. Clinical features associated with pseudoachondroplasia include normal appearance at birth with deceleration of linear growth between the first and second years of life. The diagnosis is usually made at this time. Shortening of the extremities becomes more obvious over time. The fingers are short and there is excessive laxity of most of the joints. Multiple other skeletal features include genu valgum, genu vara, or "windswept deformities" of the legs, limitations of elbow extension, ulnar deviation of the hand, scoliosis, and odontoid hypoplasia. Osteoarthritis and painful joints are common. Developmental milestones and intelligence are normal. Radiographic features include epiphyseal and metaphyseal changes, vertebral flattening with irregular vertebral endplates, and anterior beaking of the vertebrae.

14. MED is more commonly diagnosed in mid-childhood, presenting with a waddling gate and hip pain. If short stature is present, it is usually mild. Body proportions are normal although the fingers may be short and joint laxity is often excessive. Osteoarthritis is a major complication. The radiographic features are similar to those seen in pseudoachondroplasia, but much milder in degree, with considerably less metaphyseal and vertebral involvement.

15. Both pseudoachondroplasia and MED are autosomal dominant disorders with most cases arising as a result of new mutations. In families previously thought to have a recessive form of pseudoachondroplasia, germ line mosaicism appears to explain the observation of multiple affected children in families with unaffected parents.

16. The *COMP* gene, located at 19p13.1, is composed of 19 exons and encodes a 2.4-kb mature transcript. The protein is a 540-kDa extracellular matrix glycoprotein. It is a member of the extracellular calcium-binding thrombospondin family. The mature molecule is composed of five identical subunits, each of which contains a pentamer formation domain, four EGF-like domains, seven calcium-binding domains, and a globular domain. It is found in the territorial matrix surrounding chondrocytes.

17. To date, more than 70 *COMP* mutations are known, less than 10 of which were identified in patients with MED; the remainder were identified in patients with pseudoachondroplasia. Most of the mutations occur in the calcium-binding domains. No relationship between genotype and phenotype is established; similar mutations are found in patients with pseudoachondroplasia and MED.

18. The molecular pathogenesis of pseudoachondroplasia and MED is by a dominant negative effect. Electron microscopy of growth plate cartilage in these conditions demonstrates large lamellar inclusions in the rough endoplasmic reticulum (rER), now known to contain COMP, aggrecan, and type IX collagen. The massive accumulation of these extracellular matrix proteins in the rER causes chondrocyte death in culture, suggesting that the decrease in linear growth is related to the loss of growth plate chondrocytes. Pseudoachondroplasia chondrocytes in vitro make less matrix, with diminished amounts of COMP. The osteoarthritis associated with pseudoachondroplasia and MED may result from a structurally abnormal matrix that is susceptible to early erosion.

19. Although most cases of MED result from *COMP* mutations, five cases were caused by mutations of *COL9A2*, located at 1p33-p32.2, or *COL9A3*, located at 20q13.3. For both genes, the identified mutations alter the acceptor splice site in intron 2 and lead to skipping of exon 3.

20. Genetic heterogeneity in MED and the known occurrence of germ line and somatic mosaicism in pseudoachondroplasia complicate genetic counseling for these conditions.

Achondroplasia (MIM 100800) and pseudoachondroplasia (MIM 177170) are two of the most common forms of human dwarfism. Before the late 1950s, all forms of dwarfism resulting in short-limb short-stature were called "achondroplasia." In 1959, Marateux and Lamy[1] made a distinction between pseudoachondroplasia (originally called "pseudoachondroplastic spondyloepiphyseal dysplasia") and achondroplasia because of clear-cut radiographic differences and the recognition of more subtle, but nonetheless evident, clinical differences between the two conditions. We now know that achondroplasia and pseudoachondroplasia are clinically and genetically distinct and they are discussed separately in this chapter. The chapter also discusses other phenotypes that are included in the skeletal dysplasia "families," or groups of disorders, and that are caused by mutations in the gene responsible for achondroplasia, fibroblast growth factor receptor 3 (*FGFR3*), and the gene responsible for pseudoachondroplasia, cartilage oligomeric matrix protein (*COMP*).

## ACHONDROPLASIA

### Historical Perspective

When Jurgen Spranger classified the human skeletal dysplasias in 1988,[2] he placed achondroplasia, thanatophoric dysplasia (TD; MIM 187600, 187601) and hypochondroplasia (MIM 146000) in the same family of disorders, based on the similarity among the skeletal and histologic phenotypes. While all of these disorders result in short-limb short-stature, the phenotypes range from the neonatal lethal (TD) to the relatively mild decrease in stature (hypochondroplasia), with achondroplasia representing a moderately severe phenotype in this spectrum. Progress in elucidating the molecular bases of these skeletal dysplasias has shown Spranger's clinical predictions to be correct. All three disorders in the "achondroplasia family" of skeletal dysplasias are now known to be caused by mutations in the gene encoding *FGFR3* (Table 210-1).[3–12]

### Clinical Manifestations

**Achondroplasia.** The phenotype of achondroplasia is readily recognizable in adults (Fig. 210-1) but is more subtle in the newborn (Figs. 210-2 and 210-3). The astute clinician will recognize relatively short limbs and macrocephaly with frontal bossing and midface hypoplasia in infants with achondroplasia[13] (Figs. 210-2 and 210-3). The limbs are more notably short in the proximal segment, although the entire limb is short; this is called "rhizomelic" dwarfism. Others features of the limbs include limitation of elbow extension and the so-called "trident hand" in which there is a distinct space between the distal phalanges of the third and fourth digits. Hyperextensibility of the knees and hips is common. A thoracic gibbus may be present at birth and usually resolves spontaneously coincident with the development of improved muscle tone and commencement of independent sitting.

**Table 210-1** *FGFR3* Mutations in the Achondroplasia Family of Skeletal Dysplasias

| Phenotype | Common mutation (frequency) | Less frequent mutations | References |
|---|---|---|---|
| Anchondroplasia | G380R (>97%) | G346E, G375C | 3, 4, 7, 77–85 |
| Hypochondroplasia | N540K (~50%) | I538V, N540T | 6, 7, 9 |
| TD I | R248C (~50%) | S371C, S249C, Y373C, G370C, X807G, X807R, X807C | 5, 7, 8, 10–12, 40 |
| TD II | K650E (100%) | | 5, 40 |
| SADDAN dysplasia | K650M (100%) | | 38, 39 |

Linear growth progressively falls below normal (Fig. 210-4). The growth curves for head circumference overlap with the curves for unaffected children, but true megalencephaly is often present (Fig. 210-4). There is an increased risk of intracranial bleeding during vaginal delivery.[14]

The affected newborn (Figs. 210-2 and 210-3) is often hypotonic, and muscle tone usually improves during the first and second year of life. One consequence of the low muscle tone during infancy is a delay in the development of motor milestones. Typically, intelligence is normal.[15]

Radiographic abnormalities include caudad narrowing of the vertebral interpedicular distance and a notchlike sacroiliac groove in the pelvis. The long bones are short and relatively wide, as are the tarsal and metatarsal bones and all of the phalanges[16,17] (Figs. 210-5 and 210-6).

The age-specific mortality for achondroplasia is relatively high in the first 4 years of life, approaching 7.5 percent in the first year and 2.5 percent in years 1 to 4.[18] The mortality curves approach those of unaffected children in later childhood, adolescence, and early adulthood, but climb again at the end of the fourth decade.[18] The cause of this increase in age-specific mortality in mid-adulthood is unknown.

Relatively small and tortuous eustachian tubes often result in poor drainage of the middle ear with frequent episodes of otitis media as a consequence. Many children with achondroplasia require placement of pressure-equalizing tubes. The otitis may result in compromised hearing if not recognized and treated aggressively in early childhood.

Neurologic complications may arise from a relatively small foramen magnum present in the newborn period in almost all children with achondroplasia. Compression of the cerviomedullary junction by a small foramen magnum may result in generalized hypotonia, hyperreflexia, or clonus, and/or central hypopnea or central apnea.[19] Surgical decompression of a compromised cerviomedullary junction, performed by a surgeon experienced in the procedure, has a high probability of improving neurologic function.[20] Hydrocephalus may result from stenosis of the sigmoid sinus secondary to narrowed jugular foramina.[21,22] Conventional treatment for hydrocephalus in this population is placement of a ventriculoperitoneal shunt, although venous decompression at the jugular foramen has been proposed as an alternative.[23]

In older persons, the narrow spinal canal frequently results in symptomatic thoracic and/or lumbar spinal stenosis. Initial symptoms are usually back pain and pain on walking, which is

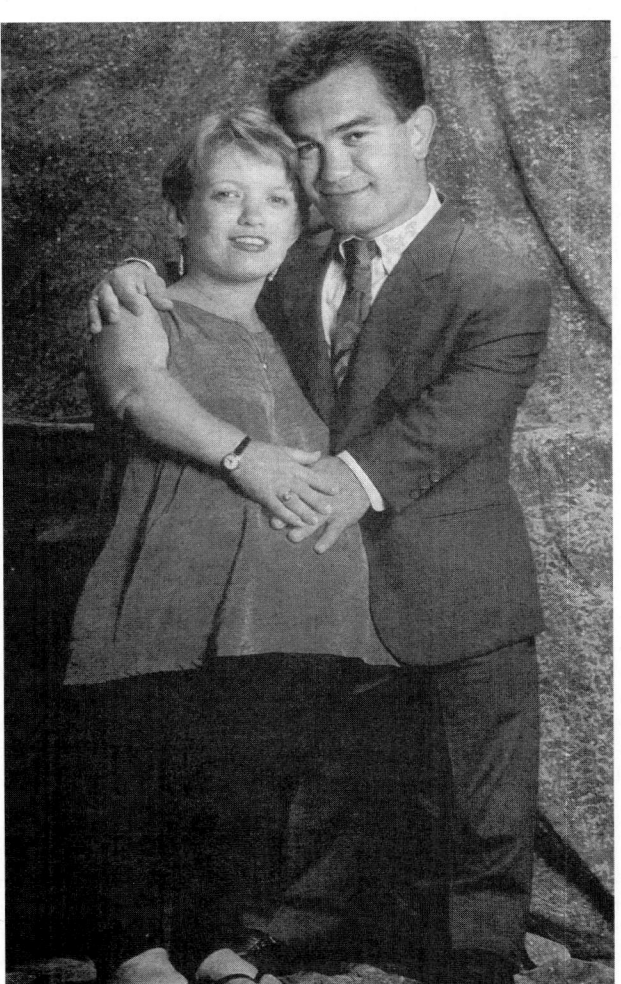

**Fig. 210-1** The typical adult achondroplasia phenotype, seen here in a husband and pregnant wife. Note the disproportionate short stature with rhizomelic (proximal) shortening of the limbs, relative macrocephaly, and midface hypoplasia.

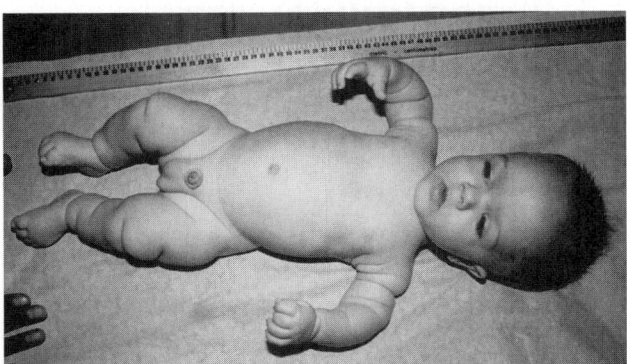

**Fig. 210-2** An infant with achondroplasia. Evident are short limbs with skin folds, small chest and protuberant abdomen, macrocephaly, and midface hypoplasia.

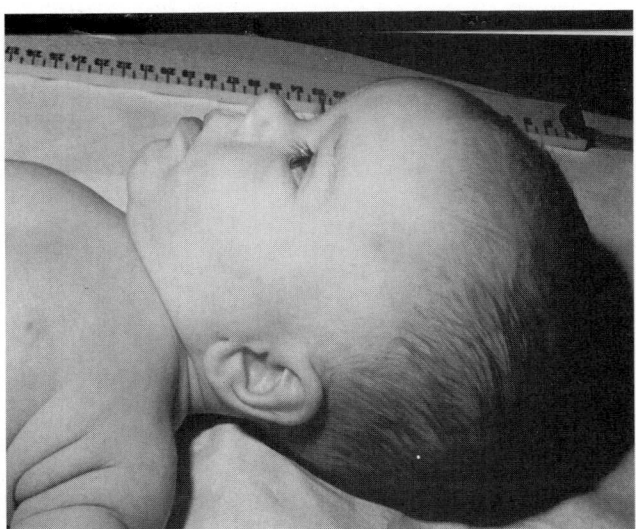

Fig. 210-3 An infant with achondroplasia illustrating macrocephaly and marked midface hypoplasia.

relieved by squatting. These may progress to unremitting pain, leg weakness, and bladder and bowel incontinence if untreated. This complication is amenable to surgical correction by spinal laminectomy.[24]

Pulmonary compromise may result from any or all of three contributing factors. A relatively small chest may lead to restrictive lung disease. Small upper airways may contribute to the development of obstructive apnea requiring treatment by continuous positive airway pressure or tracheostomy.[25–27] Finally, compression of the cervicomedullary junction may cause central hypopnea or central apnea necessitating, in the most severe instances, surgical decompression of the foramen magnum.

In older patients with achondroplasia, obesity is often a significant problem.[28,29] Up to a height of 75 cm, the mean weight:height curves are comparable for average-stature children and children with achondroplasia. Above 75 cm, the weight:height curves for achondroplasia rise significantly above those for the general population.[29] Obesity contributes to the morbidity associated with lumbar stenosis. Obesity also contributes to nonspecific joint problems and may play a role in the early mortality seen in some adults with achondroplasia.

**Homozygous Achondroplasia.** Couples in which both parents have achondroplasia are at 25 percent risk for having children who inherit two copies of the achondroplasia mutation. These children are said to have homozygous achondroplasia, or, colloquially, "double-dominant" achondroplasia.[30,31] This phenotype is almost invariably lethal within the first days to months of life. It may be difficult to distinguish clinically from thanatophoric dysplasia, but the family history is the key to this differential diagnosis. Children with homozygous achondroplasia have pronounced rhizomelic dwarfism, marked midface hypoplasia, large heads relative to the size of their bodies, and short ribs resulting in a small thorax and restrictive respiratory compromise. A small foramen magnum may also lead to lethal compression at the cervicomedullary junction.

**Hypochondroplasia.** The phenotype of hypochondroplasia is very similar to, but generally milder than, that which presents in achondroplasia (Fig. 210-7).[32,33] Affected persons have rhizomelic short-limb dwarfism, but the short stature is less extreme than in achondroplasia, and the growth curve actually overlaps the height ranges of average children. The craniofacial manifestations are not as pronounced. Head size is usually within the normal range, and there are rarely complications of cervical or lumbar spinal

stenosis. A few reports have suggested that learning disabilities may be increased among children affected by hypochondroplasia.[34,35]

**Thanatophoric Dysplasia (TD).** TD, a neonatal lethal condition, whose name means "death bearing," lies at the other end of the severity spectrum from hypochondroplasia. Almost all children with TD die in the neonatal period. There have been a few reports of survivors into the first decade.[36,37] Infants with TD have severe rhizomelic dwarfism, profound midface hypoplasia, and extremely short ribs resulting in a small thorax (Fig. 210-8). In utero hydrocephalus is common and when associated with premature fusion of the coronal and lambdoid sutures, produces a cranial deformity known as cloverleaf skull or Kleeblattschädel (Fig. 210-8). TD patients with severe bowing of the long bones usually do not have the cloverleaf skull deformity, while those with little or no bowing often have craniosynostosis and cloverleaf skull. With the advent of molecular data (see "Genetics" below), these two subgroups have been resolved into TDI and TDII, respectively. Death is thought to be respiratory, due to the small thorax and compromised upper airways, or neurologic, secondary to an extremely small foramen magnum.

**Severe Achondroplasia with Developmental Delay and Acanthosis Nigricans (SADDAN).** This phenotype, first published in 1999, is caused by a single, specific mutation in the *FGFR3* gene.[38] Affected persons have profound short stature (one affected 5-year-old child was at the 50 percent level for a 1-year-old with achondroplasia), marked craniofacial characteristics including midface hypoplasia, and severe developmental delay and eventual mental retardation (Fig. 210-9). They also develop acanthosis nigricans, a dermatologic condition resulting in thickening of the skin with hyperpigmentation in the flexion creases of the thorax and limbs. Medical complications are similar to those seen in achondroplasia, but occur earlier in life and with greater severity. Hydrocephalus and seizures occurred in all three reported children with the SADDAN phenotype.[39]

## GENETICS

All four phenotypes in the achondroplasia family of skeletal dysplasias (achondroplasia, hypochondroplasia, TD, and SADDAN) are inherited as autosomal dominant conditions caused by mutations in the *FGFR3* gene on chromosome 4p16.3. Penetrance is complete and the majority of cases result from new mutations.

The close relationship between specific mutations and specific phenotypes is unusual in the *FGFR* family of genes. Unlike most human genetic disorders, in which there is a wide range of mutations causing a similar phenotype, in this family of disorders there is a very high correlation between specific mutations and the phenotypes with which they are associated. In achondroplasia, more than 97 percent of cases are caused by one of two mutations that substitute arginine for glycine at codon 380 in the transmembrane domain of the protein (Fig. 210-10). This remarkable molecular homogeneity facilitates precise molecular diagnosis and prenatal diagnosis (Fig. 210-11). More than 80 percent of cases of hypochondroplasia are caused by mutations resulting in the substitution of asparagine for lysine at codon 540.

TD is an interesting case in point; analysis of mutation data allowed clinicians to go back to their patients and separate them into two distinct clinical subsets based on the molecular data. TDI is associated with bowed deformity of the femurs and other tubular bones, usually without cloverleaf skull, and results from mutations affecting several different domains of the FGFR3 protein (see Table 210-1). TDII, however, has straight femurs and is usually associated with craniosynostosis and cloverleaf skull. TDII is invariably caused by mutations resulting in a K650E substitution in the intracellular tyrosine kinase domain of FGFR3.[10,38,40]

To date, three cases of the SADDAN phenotype have been reported.[39,41] All three cases resulted from 1949A>T mutation at

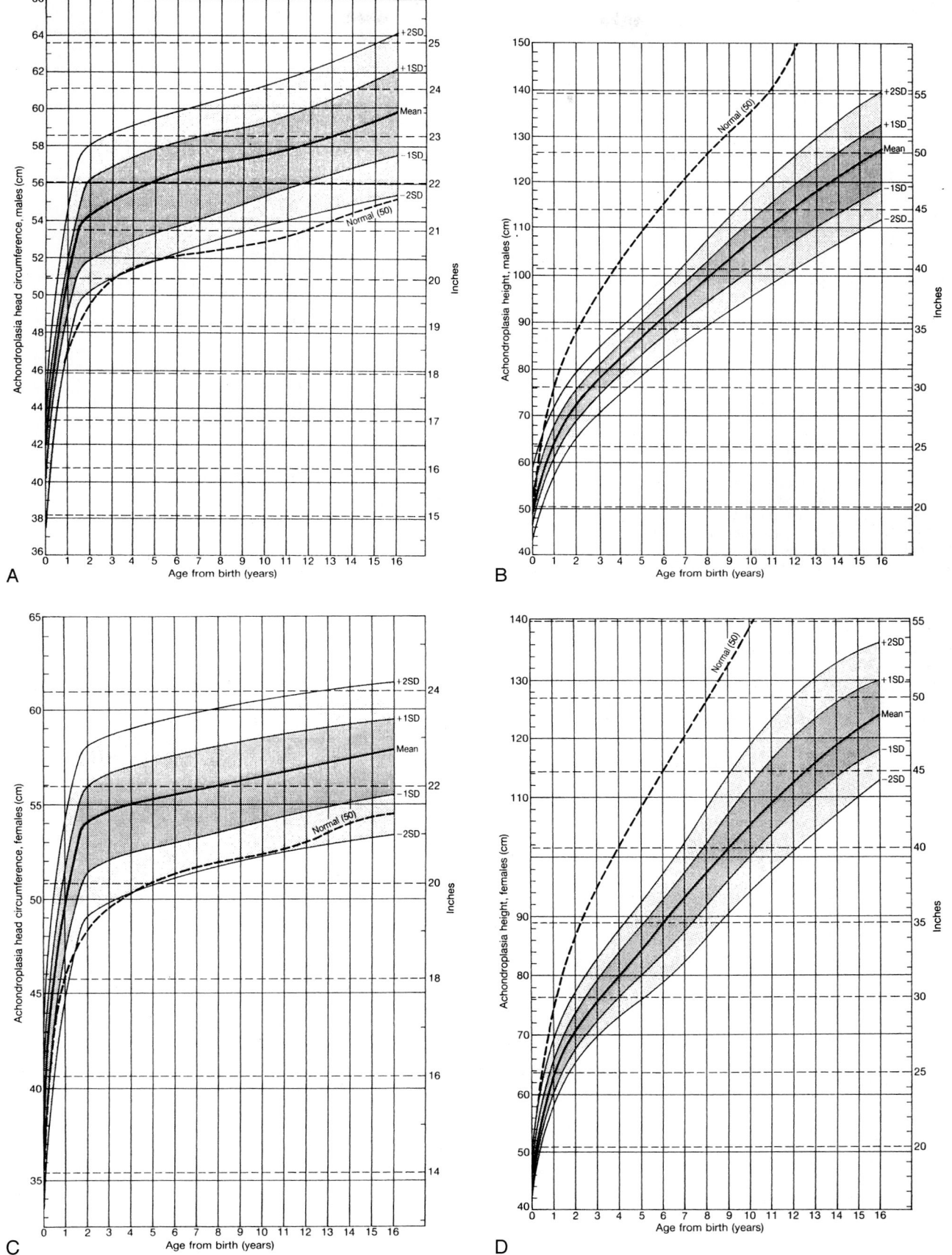

**Fig. 210-4 Growth curves for children with achondroplasia from birth to age 16 years.** *A*, Head circumference for achondroplasia males; *B*, height for achondroplasia males; *C*, head circumference for achondroplasia females; *D*, height for achondroplasia females.

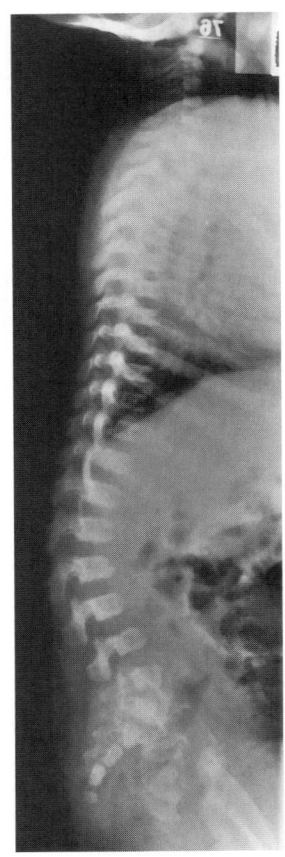

Fig. 210-5 Radiograph of the lateral spine in an infant with achondroplasia. Note the kyphotic curve in the lower lumbar region.

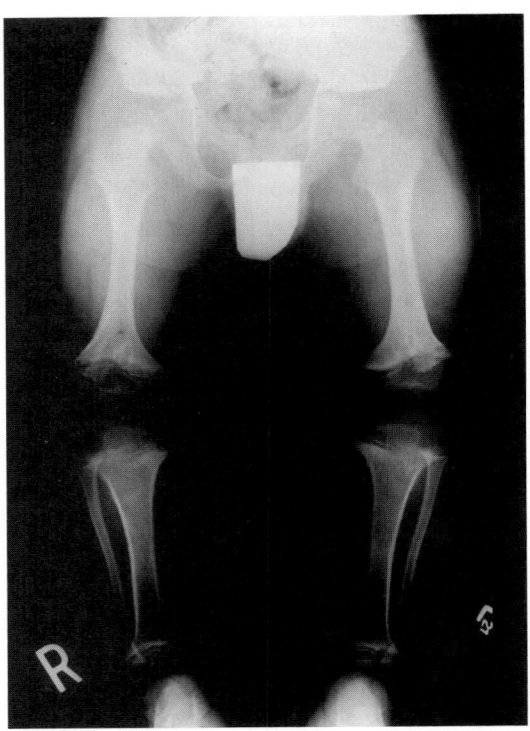

Fig. 210-6 Radiographic features of the lower limbs in a young child with achondroplasia.

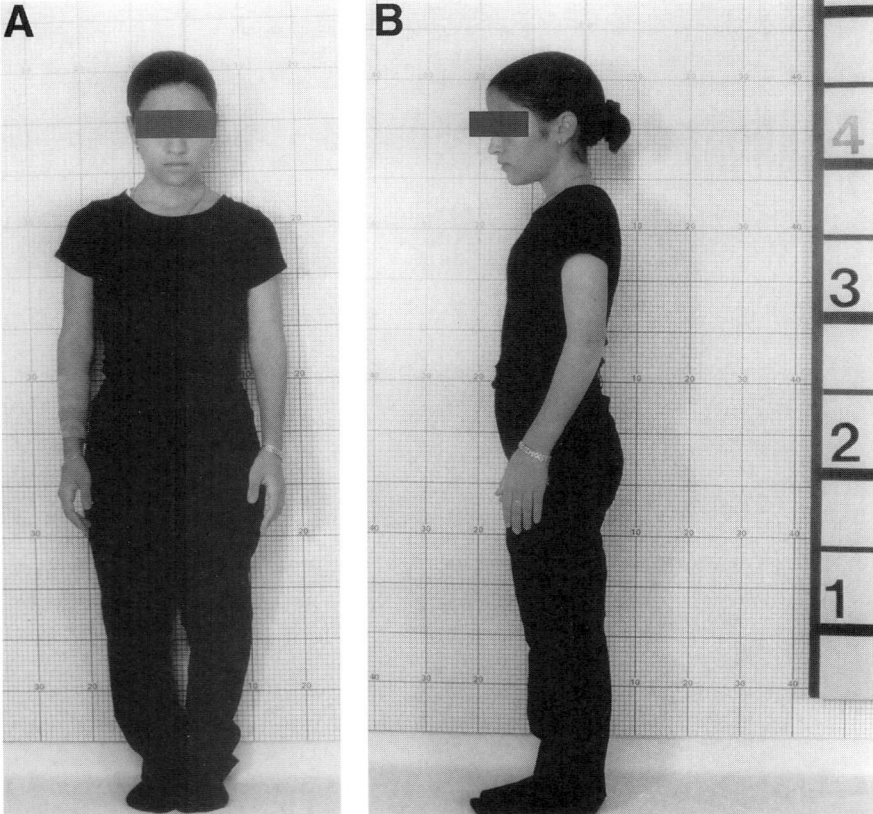

Fig. 210-7 A young girl with hypochon-droplasia. Note her less severe rhizomelia as compared to achondroplasia (*A* and *B*) and normal cranial contour (*B*).

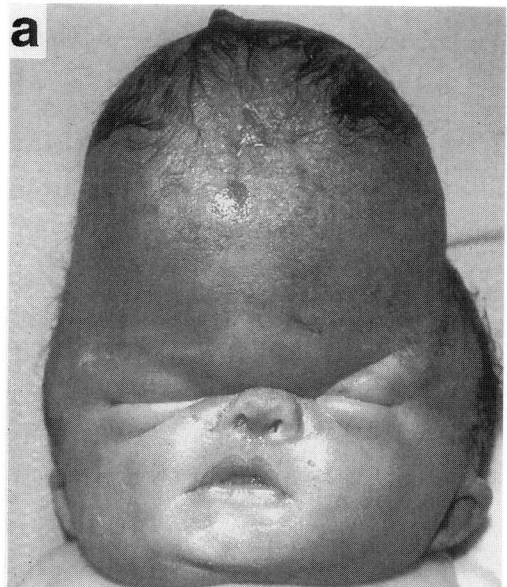

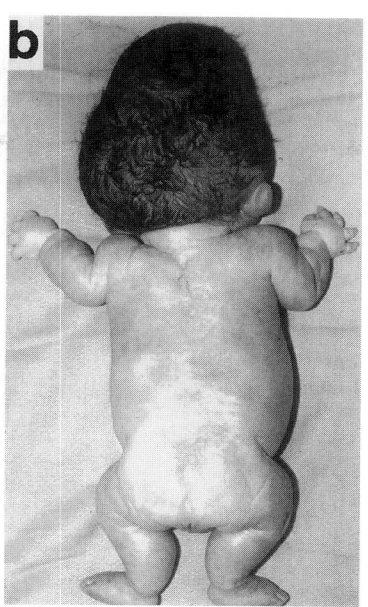

Fig. 210-8 A stillborn infant with TD. Note the severe cranial malformation (cloverleaf skull or Kleeblattschädel) (*A*) and the marked shortening of the extremities (*B*).

the same codon in which TDII mutations are found and produced a K650M substitution.

Estimates of the prevalence of achondroplasia range from 1/15,000 to 1/60,000 live births.[42-44] The estimated mutation rate is between $5.5 \times 10^{-6}$ and $2.8 \times 10^{-5}$ per gamete per generation.[31,45] Historical estimates of the prevalence of achondroplasia are likely to be inaccurate because of misdiagnoses before the delineation and widespread recognition of multiple different forms of short-limb dwarfism.

As has been the case in several different autosomal dominant conditions, studies of families with achondroplasia demonstrated that unaffected fathers of infants with achondroplasia were older, on average, than fathers of unaffected children.[45-47] A recent report demonstrated that the achondroplasia mutation was exclusively present on the paternal allele in a cohort of 40 families.[48] The advanced paternal age effect suggests that these mutations arise during spermatogenesis in the unaffected father.

The paucity of cases with familial recurrence of achondroplasia speaks against significant levels of germ line mosaicism, although there have been a few reports of multiple affected children from families with unaffected parents.[49-52] Germ line mosaicism has been demonstrated in families with recurrence of other skeletal dysplasias, including osteogenesis imperfecta[53] and pseudoachondroplasia.[54]

## FIBROBLAST GROWTH FACTOR RECEPTORS

In humans, the FGFRs are a family of four tyrosine kinase receptors (FGFR1 to 4) that bind fibroblast growth factors (FGFs) with variable affinity.[55] The FGF family of proteins consist of at least nine structurally related, heparin-binding polypeptides that play a key role in the growth and differentiation of various cells of mesenchymal and neuroectodermal origin.[56-58] FGFs are also implicated in chemotaxis, angiogenesis, apoptosis, and spatial

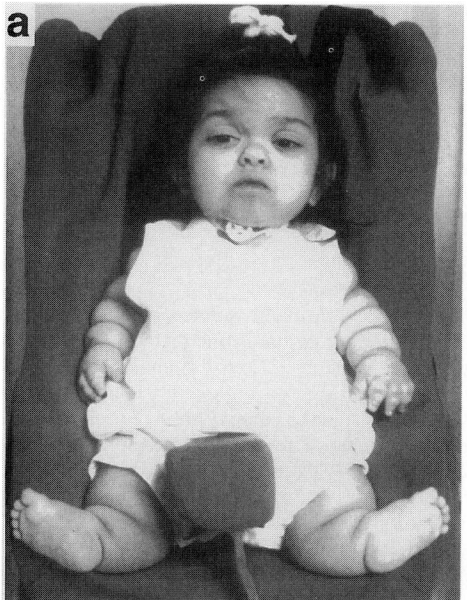

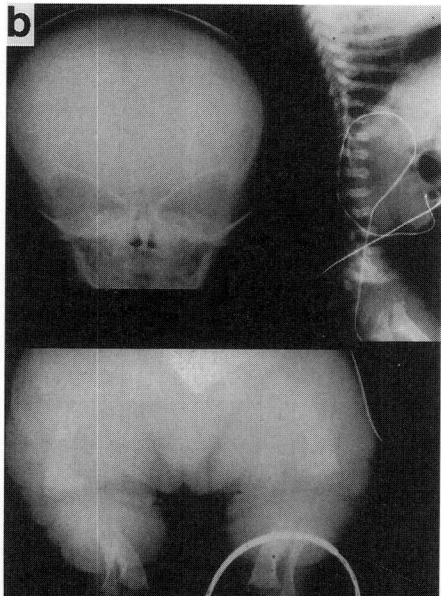

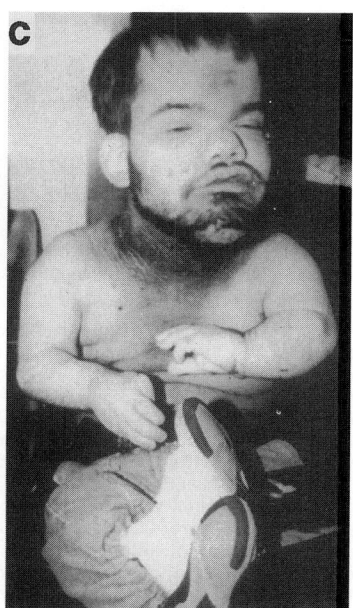

Fig. 210-9 The SADDAN phenotype in (*A*) a 5-year-old child; (*B*) her radiographs showing prominent shortening of the long bones and cranial involvement; and (*C*) in a 19-year-old male with prominent acanthosis nigricans in the cervical region.

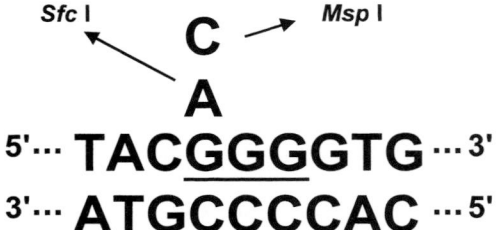

Fig. 210-10 The two common *FGFR3* mutations that cause achondroplasia both result in G380R amino acid substitutions. Shown is the sequence of the *FGFR3* gene surrounding the site of the common mutation. The underline designates the normal G380 codon. The 1138G>A mutation creates a novel *Sfc* I site; the 1138G>C mutation creates a *Msp* I site. Both mutations result in G380R.

patterning.[59,60] The prototypical FGF, FGF-2 (also called basic FGF) is a potent angiogenic protein, and stimulates smooth-muscle cell growth, wound healing, and tissue repair. FGF-2 may also stimulate hematopoiesis and may play an important role in the differentiation and/or function of the skeleton, eye, and nervous system.[55,56]

The FGFRs have a highly conserved protein structure (Fig. 210-12). The mature FGFR proteins are membrane-spanning tyrosine kinase receptors with an extracellular ligand-binding domain consisting of three immunoglobulin (Ig) domains, a transmembrane domain, and a split intracellular tyrosine kinase domain.[61] Between the first and second Ig domains is a stretch of four to eight acidic amino acids, termed the "acid box." Alternative splice sites in the *FGFR* genes result in at least 12 distinct isoforms for each gene.[62-64] Variants include those that lack one or more Ig domains, the acid box, or the transmembrane domain. Some isoforms have a truncated C-terminus, while others have regions of alternative sequence.

One specific FGFR isoform is due to the presence of an alternative splice site found in the third Ig domain (closest to the membrane) and typically contains an alternative exon for this

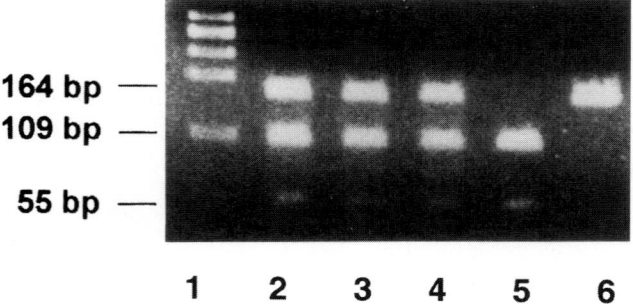

Fig. 210-11 A first trimester prenatal diagnosis in a couple in which both parents have achondroplasia due to a common 1138G>C *FGFR3* mutation. They are at risk for having an infant with homozygous achondroplasia. PCR amplification products of the region of *FGFR3* surrounding the 1138G>A mutation were digested with *Sfc* I, separated by electrophoresis on a 2 percent Nusieve/1 percent agarose gel, and visualized by ethidium bromide staining. The *FGFR3* 1138G>A mutation creates a new *Sfc* I restriction endonuclease site. When this mutation is present, *Sfc* I digestion of the 164-bp PCR product yields fragments of 109 bp and 55 bp. The mother (lane 2) and father (lane 3) show the expected pattern for *FGFR3* 1138G>C heterozygotes. The fetus (lane 4) is also a heterozygote. A sample from a homozygote for 1138>A is shown in lane 5 as a positive control while the product in lane 6 is from an average-stature individual. *Lane 1* = DNA size standards. (*Figure courtesy of G. Bellus, M.D., Ph.D.*)

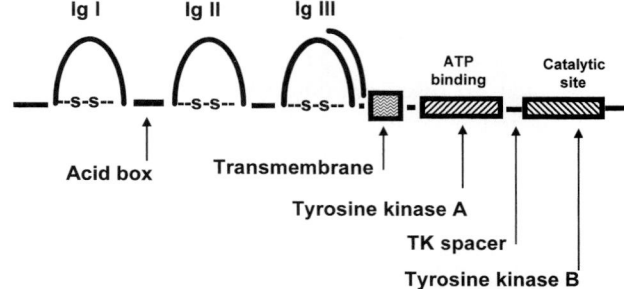

Fig. 210-12 Diagram of a prototypical FGFR protein. Three immunoglobulin-like domains (IgI to IgIII) are indicated by loops, closed with disulfide bridges. These Ig-like domains are extracellular and responsible for ligand binding. Alternative splicing in the C-terminal half of the third Ig-like loop is indicated by an extra "half" loop. The acid box is a stretch of acidic amino acids found in all FGFRs between IgI and IgII. The tyrosine kinase domains are found intracellularly. The tyrosine kinase A domain contains the ATP binding site. The tyrosine kinase B domain contains the catalytic site.

domain. The Ig domain 3 is encoded by two separate exons: exon IIIa, which encodes the N-terminal segment, and exon IIIb or IIIc, which encodes the C-terminal half.[62,63] The isoforms differ in their ligand affinity and preferential ligand binding, as well as tissue-specific expression. The FGFR3 isoform containing sequence encoded by exon IIIb has a high ligand specificity for acidic FGF-1[64] and is expressed in mouse embryo, skin, and epidermal keratinocytes.[65] The isoform containing the segment encoded by exon IIIc is present in the developing mouse brain and in the spinal cord, as well as developing bone.[65]

Developmental expression studies of *FGFR3* suggest that its protein product plays a significant role in skeletal development. Outside of the nervous system, the highest levels of *FGFR3* expression are observed in cartilage rudiments of developing bone. During endochondral ossification, *FGFR3* is expressed exclusively in resting cartilage.[65] In the mouse, *FGFR3* has a unique pattern of expression during organogenesis: early in development *FGFR3* is expressed in the germinal epithelium of the neural tube; while at 1 day postpartum and in the adult, *FGFR3* is expressed diffusely throughout the brain.[65,66] In the chick, *FGFR3* is expressed in the mesoderm of limb and feather buds.[67]

Ligand binding requires dimerization of two monomeric FGFRs and includes a heparin-binding step.[61] Promiscuous dimerization is observed; in addition to dimerizing with itself, FGFR1 may dimerize with FGFR2, 3, or 4. Similar dimerization combinations of other FGFR monomers are also possible. Differing combinations of dimers are observed in different tissues and stages of development, and this diversity of dimers probably plays an important role in skeletal differentiation.

## THE *FGFR3* GENE

A human *FGFR3* cDNA was originally isolated in the search for the Huntington disease gene on chromosome 4p16.[68] The 4.4-kb cDNA has an open reading frame of 2520 bp encoding an 840-amino-acid protein. A 3'-untranslated region of 1800 bp with a consensus polyadenylation signal sequence and a poly(A) tail follow the open reading frame. The human and mouse *FGFR3* genes have been characterized[69-71] and span 16.5 kb and 15 kb, respectively. Both are comprised of 19 exons with translation initiation and termination sites located in exons 2 and 19, respectively. The 5' flanking regions lack typical TATA and CAAT boxes. Several Sp1, AP2, Zeste, Krox 24, and IgHC.4 putative *cis*-acting elements are present in the promoter region, which is contained in a CpG island.[71,72] The promoter regions of the human and mouse *FGFR3* genes are similar, with conservation of several putative transcription factor binding sites, suggesting an important role for these elements and their corresponding transcription factors in the regulation of *FGFR3* expression.[71] The 100 bp of sequence immediately 5′ of the *FGFR3* initiation site is sufficient to confer a twenty- to fortyfold increase in transcriptional activity.[72] There is an Sp1 binding-enhancer element in intron 1, containing two purine-rich elements, between nucleotides +340 and +395. *FGFR3* sequences between −220 and +609 are sufficient to promote tissue-specific expression.[72]

At least three polymorphisms have been found within the *FGFR3* gene, in close proximity to the achondroplasia mutation site. These include a G to C transition toward the 5′ end of intron 9 that creates a PflM I site; a C to T transversion in intron 10 that creates a Pml I site; and a single G deletion in a stretch of 11 consecutive G residues in intron 9. In one analysis, 10 of 224 chromosomes (4.5 percent) had the PflM I polymorphism and 30 of 288 (10.4 percent) had the Pml I polymorphism.[48]

## MOLECULAR GENETICS OF ACHONDROPLASIA

In 1994, the gene causing achondroplasia was mapped to a region of 2.5 Mb of DNA at the telomeric end of the short arm of chromosome 4, 4p16.3.[41,73,74] The candidate region contained the *FGFR3* gene which had been cloned in the search for the Huntington disease locus in the same region.[41] Mutations in the *FGFR3* gene were found in the DNA from patients with achondroplasia within 6 months of recognition of the map location.[3,4] Soon thereafter, *FGFR3* mutations causing TD were found.[5] The identification of *FGFR3* mutations that cause hypochondroplasia[6] completed the molecular basis of the achondroplasia family of skeletal dysplasias and confirmed the allelic nature of these disorders.

The first reports of mutations in *FGFR3* causing achondroplasia[3,4] showed that 38 of 39 mutations were the same G to A transition at nucleotide 1138. The remaining mutation was a G to C transversion, also at nucleotide 1138. Both mutations result in the substitution of arginine for the glycine residue at position 380 (G380R) in the transmembrane domain of the FGFR3 protein (Fig. 210-6). Most analyses were performed on heterozygous achondroplasia patients, but the G380R mutation was also detected in several cases of homozygous achondroplasia. A larger series reported in 1995 found a G380R mutation on 153 of 154 alleles, confirming the remarkable degree of genetic homogeneity of this disorder.[75] In this later series, the 1138G > A transition accounted for 150 alleles, while the 1138G > C transversion was found in three. (The remaining proband of the 154 studied was later recognized as having SADDAN dysplasia.) Stoilov et al.[76] found the G380R mutations in 21 of 23 achondroplasia chromosomes studied.

Recent studies from Sweden, Japan, and China have demonstrated G380R mutations in almost all patients with achondroplasia.[77–82] Sixteen Swedish, 10 Chinese, and 20 Japanese achondroplasia patients were studied for the presence of *FGFR3* mutations. All of the Swedish and Chinese patients, and 18 of 20 Japanese patients were heterozygous for the 1138G>A transition.[77–82] One Japanese patient had the 1138G>C (G380R) mutation, and the final Japanese patient had a G375C mutation.[78]

Thus, almost all cases of achondroplasia are caused by the same G380R substitution. Exceptions include three cases in which the mutation was 5 codons downstream producing G375C.[78,83,84] In one such case, the radiographic features were reportedly abnormal.[79] This mutation also alters the transmembrane domain of FGFR3. One patient with a G346E mutation has also been reported.[85]

These observations, taken with the relatively high incidence of achondroplasia, suggest that nucleotide G1138 in the *FGFR3* gene is among the most mutable nucleotides in the human genome.[75] G1138 occurs in the context of a CpG dinucleotide, which might explain some of the increased incidence at this site. However, the mutation rate for G1138 is two to three orders of magnitude higher

than the rate previously reported for transversions and transitions at CpG dinucleotides.[75,86] The genotypic homogeneity of mutations in achondroplasia is unprecedented for an autosomal dominant disorder, and may explain the relative lack of phenotypic heterogeneity in affected individuals.

## Functional Consequences of *FGFR3* Mutations

All of the *FGFR3* mutations observed to date result in constitutive activation of the receptor. In vitro biochemical studies suggest that the phenotypic differences among the disorders in the achondroplasia family of skeletal dysplasias are due, at least in part, to varying degrees of ligand-independent *FGFR3* activation.

These considerations predict that loss of *FGFR3* function will result in a different phenotype. In support of this prediction, mice homozygous for a targeted total disruption of the *FGFR3* gene exhibit skeletal and inner ear defects.[87,88] The skeletal manifestations in these mice include kyphosis, scoliosis, and kinking of the tail; in addition, the long bones exhibit overgrowth, in direct contradistinction to the shortening of the long bones seen in achondroplasia and related disorders. These observations suggest that normal function of *FGFR3* is necessary for negative regulation of bone growth.[87,88] Thus, *FGFR3* mutations producing phenotypes in the achondroplasia family are thought to be gain-of-function mutations that activate, in a ligand-independent manner, the negative growth control exerted by the *FGFR3* pathway.[88,89] It will be of great interest to identify a human phenotype caused by loss of *FGFR3* function.

Based on current knowledge of the signal transduction by the FGF pathway, activation of FGFRs normally occurs only after ligand binding.[90] Functional analysis of *Xenopus FGFR1* and *FGFR2* alleles engineered to contain missense mutations analogous to those identified in human disorders including achondroplasia (G380R) and TD (K650E) demonstrated that ligand-independent FGFR activation may be a common mechanism for these disease-associated mutations.[91]

Webster et al.[92] provided additional evidence for the gain-of-function hypothesis. In an in vitro model system, profound constitutive activation of the *FGFR3* tyrosine kinase (approximately one hundredfold above the wild-type) was associated with the K650E mutation, which causes TDII.[92] Altered kinase activation was dependent on both the position of the altered amino acids, and the charge of the amino acid. The authors speculated that the TD II mutation in the *FGFR3* activation loop mimicked the conformational changes that activate the tyrosine kinase domain.[92] Ligand binding and autophosphorylation of the receptor normally initiate this activation. Using immunoprecipitation followed by an in vitro kinase assay, Webster and Donoghue[93] also found that the TD mutation resulted in increased autophosphorylation of the FGFR3 relative to wild-type receptor or that produced by the achondroplasia mutation.

Subsequently, similar constitutive *FGFR3* activation was associated with the G380R mutation causing achondroplasia.[93–96] Consistent with the relative severity of the disorders, the receptor produced by the TDII mutation (K650E) has higher autophosphorylation than that resulting from the achondroplasia mutation, suggesting that the severity of the conditions may correlate with the degree of autophosphorylation caused by the receptor mutation.[96]

The constitutive tyrosine kinase activity of *FGFR3* with the TDII mutation (K650E) specifically activates the transcription factor Stat1 (signal transducer and activator of transcription).[97] K650E-FGFR3 also induces nuclear translocation of Stat1 and expression of the cell-cycle inhibitor p21 (WAF/CIP1), resulting in cellular growth arrest. Stat1 activation and increased p21 (WAF/CIP1) expression were found in chondrocytes from a TDII fetus, but not in chondrocytes from an unaffected fetus. These observations suggested that Stat1 may mediate inhibition of bone growth retardation and that the abnormal Stat activation and p21 (WAF/CIP1) expression characteristic of TDII may be responsible for the phenotype.[97]

Additional information regarding the ligand-dependence of the mutant FGFR3 receptors comes from the studies of Thompson et al.[98] who constructed chimeric receptors containing the extracellular domain of platelet-derived growth factor fused to the transmembrane and intracellular domain of wild-type FGFR3 or FGFR3 with the rare G375C achondroplasia mutation. These chimeric receptors were expressed in PC-12 cells that respond to activation of the receptor by neurite outgrowth. Ligand-dependent autophosphorylation of the chimera receptor was observed, as was strong phosphorylation of mitogen-activated protein (MAP) kinase, phospholipase C, and Shc. Compared to cells expressing the chimeric receptor with normal FGFR3 sequences, cells expressing with the G375C-FGFR3 chimera were more responsive to ligand and had a less-sustained MAP kinase activation, which is indicative of a primed or constitutively "on" condition. This observation is consistent with the hypothesis that these mutations reduce ligand control of the FGFR3 receptor, and may provide a biochemical explanation for the observation that the TD phenotype is more severe than that of achondroplasia.[98]

Similar autonomous receptor activation has been observed as a consequence of mutations in other tyrosine kinase-kinase receptors, such as FGFR2, epidermal growth factor receptor, colony-stimulating factor 1, and the RET oncogene.[99–103]

## Implications

The identification of *FGFR3* mutation in each of the phenotypes in the "achondroplasia family" of skeletal dysplasias has had a significant impact on our understanding of these disorders. Yet these molecular findings have also raised many additional intriguing questions. Why are particular nucleotides of the *FGFR* genes so highly mutable? It seems that certain nucleotides in the *FGFR* genes are more highly susceptible to mutation than most other nucleotides in the human genome. Additionally, there is a high degree of correlation in the locations of observed mutations from one *FGFR* gene to another. This conservation of mutations at particular sites in the *FGFR* genes is an intriguing biologic phenomenon and is not yet understood at the time of this writing.

Moreover, the high degree of phenotypic specificity associated with *FGFR3* mutations is unprecedented in the study of human genetics and disease. The explanation for this remains elusive. Since the 1138G>A mutation was found in achondroplasia, similar observations of tight genotype/phenotype correlations have been made in *FGFR3* and other human *FGFR* genes causing other skeletal phenotypes, including hypochondroplasia and TD, and the Pfeiffer and Apert craniosynostosis syndromes.[5–12,104–112]

Finally, the identification of a relatively small number of mutations causing achondroplasia and related skeletal dysplasias has had an enormous impact on our ability to offer prenatal diagnosis for these disorders (Fig. 210-11). A reliable prenatal diagnosis of a *de novo* case is difficult to achieve by sonographic methods. In the face of uncertainty, physicians sometimes elect to emphasize the most severe alternative diagnoses.[113,114]

The identification of mutations responsible for the most common skeletal dysplasias has made it possible to offer mutational analysis when a short-limb disorder is detected prenatally by ultrasound. If molecular detection of the mutant allele is possible, prenatal diagnosis becomes much more reliable and informative, and parents may make informed and rational reproductive choices based on accurate diagnoses. Therefore, the high degree of specificity of the *FGFR3* 1138G>A mutation for the achondroplasia phenotype has profound implications for persons with achondroplasia, their families, and their physicians. Because the achondroplasia mutations are easily detectable by molecular means, the diagnosis is one that is performable in many molecular laboratories. One positive outcome of the ability to perform molecular diagnosis is that couples at risk for children with homozygous achondroplasia now have access to reliable prenatal diagnostic testing for this inevitably lethal condition.

# PSEUDOACHONDROPLASIA/MULTIPLE EPIPHYSEAL DYSPLASIA (MED)

## Historical Perspective

Pseudoachondroplasia and MED were previously considered to be separate disorders based on clinical and radiographic criteria. Recent molecular studies have shown that both result from mutations in *COMP*.[115,116] A few cases of MED, however, have been shown to result from mutations in *COL9A2*[117,118] and *COL9A3* genes.[119] Both pseudoachondroplasia and MED are relatively common and are easily distinguished from the more frequent skeletal dysplasia, achondroplasia.[1] Pseudoachondroplasia was first delineated at the nomenclature meetings in Paris in 1971,[120] and more recent studies have contributed to our understanding of the clinical and radiologic features and genetic mutations.

## Clinical Manifestations

**Pseudoachondroplasia.** Newborns with pseudoachondroplasia have a normal appearance, birth length, birthweight, and head circumference. The diagnosis is generally recognized between the first and second years of life when linear growth decelerates.[121] Shortening of the extremities becomes more obvious over time and a waddling gait may be another presenting feature (Fig. 210-13). Developmental milestones and intelligence are normal. The face is normal, often angular, and distinctively attractive. The fingers are short and there is excessive laxity in all the joints. Genu varum, genu valgum, or windswept deformities are common and begin in early childhood. While surgical intervention can correct these deformities, they often recur and require multiple surgical interventions to attain the correct alignment. Elbow extension is limited and ulnar deviation of the wrists is often present. Scoliosis occurs and was reported in almost half of the patients in one study.[121] Odontoid hypoplasia occurs in about 50 percent of patients with pseudoachondroplasia.[121,122] Because this abnormality of the upper cervical spine puts the affected individual at high risk for severe, even fatal, spinal cord trauma when the neck is extended (e.g., during routine exercise or during intubation for general anesthesia), all patients with pseudoachondroplasia should

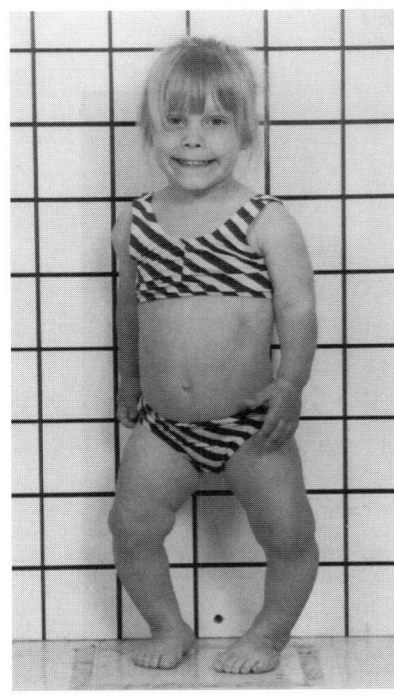

**Fig. 210-13 Typical pseudoachondroplasia in a young girl. Notice the short limbs with genu varum (bowed legs), short broad fingers, and average-size head.**

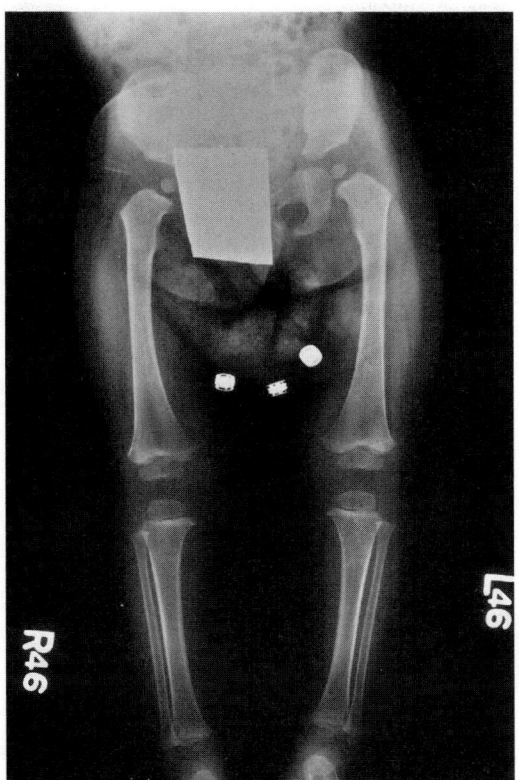

Fig. 210-14 Radiographic features of the lower extremity of a 14-month-old child with pseudoachondroplasia. Note the short femur, tibia, and fibula, and small irregular epiphyses.

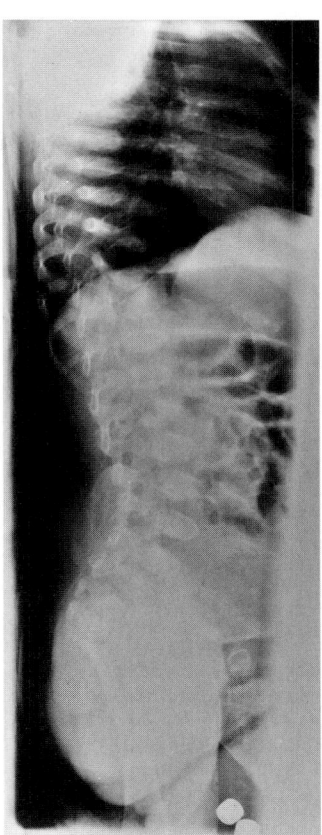

Fig. 210-15 Radiographic features of the lateral spine in a 14-month-old child with pseudoachondroplasia. Note the flattened, bullet-shaped vertebrae.

be evaluated for odontoid hypoplasia. Osteoarthritis and painful joints are common complaints in pseudoachondroplasia. The hips and knees are generally the first joints affected, but all the joints subsequently show osteoarthritic changes. One study found that 33 percent of adult individuals with pseudoachondroplasia had undergone hip replacement.[121]

Radiographic manifestations include both epiphyseal and metaphyseal abnormalities.[123] All of the tubular bones are short and the metaphyses are irregular and widened (Fig. 210-14). The epiphyses are small and fragmented and often display delayed ossification. The femoral necks are short and the capital femoral epiphyses are often small and dysplastic. The vertebrae demonstrate flattening and anterior beaking that usually resolves by adulthood (Fig. 210-15). The vertebral endplates are often irregular.

**MED.** MED usually is diagnosed in mid-childhood. The presenting symptom is usually a waddling gait and hip pain.[122] Mild short-stature may also occur. Developmental milestones and intelligence are normal. Body proportions are normal although the fingers are often short. Joint laxity may also be present. Legg-Perthes or avascular necrosis of the capital femoral epiphyses is a common complication that responds to orthopedic intervention. Osteoarthritis is a major complication beginning in the hip and knees, and, to a lesser extent, in other joints. Hip replacement is also common in MED.

The radiographic findings in MED are similar to those in pseudoachondroplasia, but much milder.[123] All of the epiphyseal centers are small and underossified, especially in the hips. There is less metaphyseal and vertebral involvement, although platyspondylia has been reported in MED.

## Genetics and Pathogenesis

Pseudoachondroplasia and MED are both well-documented autosomal dominant phenotypes with many of the cases arising as new mutations.[115,116,124,125] Molecular studies have shown that pseudoachondroplasia and MED are allelic disorders (see below). Previous studies suggested autosomal recessive forms of pseudoachondroplasia,[124] but germ line mosaicism has been shown to account for these cases (Fig. 210-16).[54,126,127]

In 1993, Briggs et al.[128] and Hecht et al.[129] mapped the pseudoachondroplasia (MED) locus to the pericentric region of chromosome 19p12-13.1. Subsequently *COMP* was mapped into the same region making it a candidate gene for pseudoachondroplasia and MED.[130] Mutation analysis confirmed this suspicion with more than 70 *COMP* mutations reported, most resulting in the pseudoachondroplasia phenotype. Less than 10 of the mutations result in the MED phenotype.[54,115,116,127,131–139] Two-thirds of the reported mutations have been identified in isolated new mutation pseudoachondroplasia patients; the remainder were identified in familial cases.

The *COMP* gene is composed of 19 exons (Fig. 210-17) that encode a 2.4-kb cDNA.[130] Most of the mutations occur in the calcium-binding domains with 30 percent being an allele with a 3-bp inframe deletion in a sequence of five GAC repeats (nucleotides 1430 to 1445) with the result that a series of 5 aspartates (codons 469 to 473) is reduced by 1.[116] Only four mutations have been found outside of these domains, and all are in exon 19, which encodes part of the globular domain. No genotype/phenotype correlation can be established as similar mutations have been described in patients with either pseudoachondroplasia or MED.[54,115,116,127,131–139]

COMP is a large, 540-kDa, extracellular matrix glycoprotein whose function is unknown[130] (Fig. 210-18). It is the fifth member of the extracellular calcium-binding thrombospondin gene family and is part of subgroup B that contains the pentameric members.[130] COMP is composed of five identical subunits,

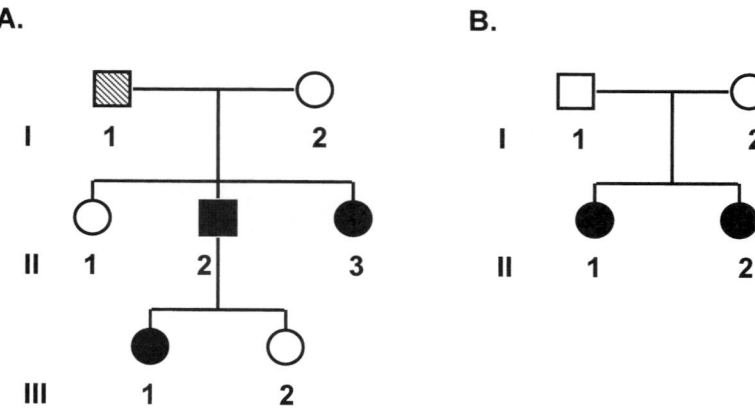

Fig. 210-16 Pseudoachondroplasia pedigrees illustrating somatic (*A*) and germ line (*B*) mosaicism. *A*, The shaded individual (I1) is of normal stature but is unable to extend his elbows completely. Mutation analysis showed a trace amount of the mutant fragment in the PCR amplified products from his lymphocyte genomic DNA. The individuals indicated by the black symbols all had typical pseudoachondroplasia and were heterozygotes for the causative mutation (see reference 54).

A. *COMP* gene exons:

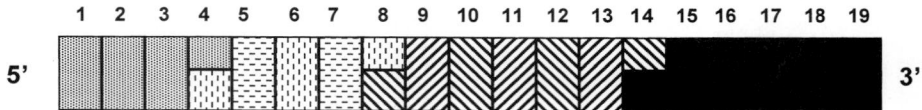

B. COMP protein domains:

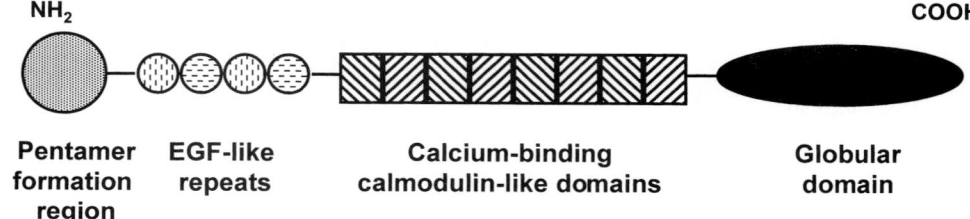

Fig. 210-17 *A*, The *COMP* gene has 19 exons. The shading indicates the functional domains of the protein encoded by each exon. Exons 1 to 4 encode the N-terminal pentamer-association domain; exons 4 to 8 encode four epidermal growth factor-like repeats; exons 8 to 14 encode eight Ca$^{++}$ binding, calmodulin-like units; and exons 14 to 19 encode a globular C-terminal domain. *B*, The COMP monomer with its functional domains.

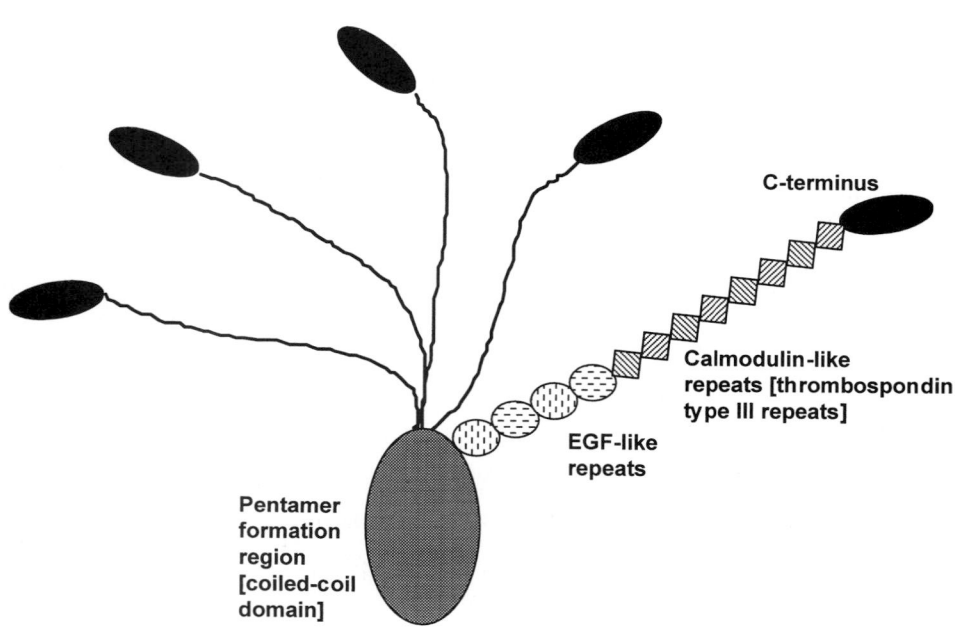

Fig. 210-18 A model of the COMP pentamer. Prominent features of the molecules include the coiled-coil domain at the N-terminus, the five flexible arms composed of a linear array of epidermal growth factor like domains and eight thrombospondin type III repeats that terminate in a globular domain at the C-terminus. Assembly of COMP requires the formation of an α-helical coiled-coil domain, which is stabilized by interchain disulfide bonds.

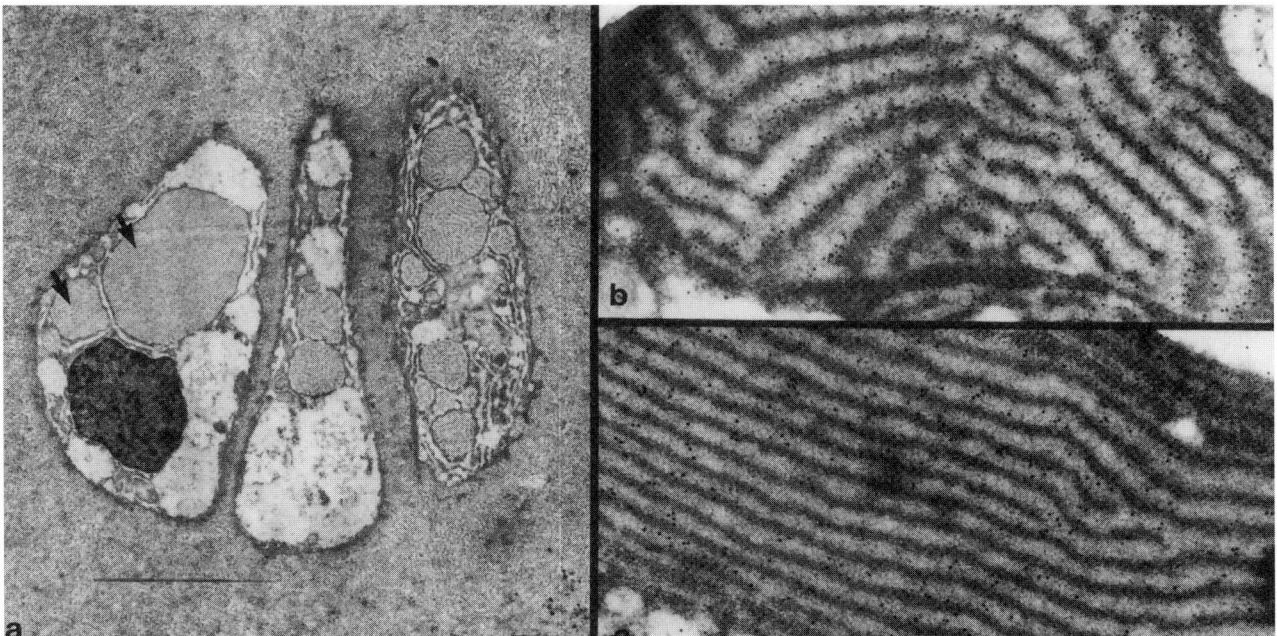

**Fig. 210-19** Ultrastructure and immunolocalization of COMP protein and type IX collagen in pseudoachondroplasia cartilage. *A*, A cluster of chondrocytes from growth plate cartilage of an individual with pseudoachondroplasia. The characteristic engorged rough endo-plasmic reticulum is apparent (*arrows*). Antibodies to COMP (*B*) and type IX collagen (*C*) localize these proteins to the dark rings of the lamellar structures within the inclusion bodies. (*From Maddox et al.[137] Reprinted with permission.*)

each containing a pentamer association domain, four EGF-like domains, seven calcium-binding domains, and a globular domain.[130] COMP is found in the territorial matrix surrounding chondrocytes[140] and has a bouquet appearance by rotary shadowing.[141]

The pathogenesis of pseudoachondroplasia and MED is a dominant negative effect as 97 percent of all COMP is predicted to have from one to five mutant subunits.[116] Studies of pseudoachondroplasia and MED growth-plate chondrocytes show large lamellar inclusions in rough endoplasmic reticulum (rER)[142-144] that contain COMP, aggrecan, and type IX collagen[134,137,145] (Figs. 210-19 and 210-20). In vitro studies of redifferentiated pseudoachondroplasia chondrocytes suggest that the massive retention of these extracellular matrix proteins compromises chondrocyte function and causes chondrocyte death.[145] These results suggest that the decrease in linear growth is related to the loss of growth-plate chondrocytes. Moreover, the pseudoachondroplasia chondrocytes appear to make smaller amounts of matrix, and the matrix contains diminished amounts of COMP. This would lead to a matrix that has less structural integrity. Thus, the short-stature phenotype results from loss of chondrocytes and the osteoarthritis results from a structurally abnormal matrix that undergoes erosion.

Germ line/somatic mosaicism in pseudoachondroplasia was first reported by Hall et al.[126] and confirmed by Ferguson[54] and Deere[127] (Fig. 210-16). Mutations in *COMP* have now been identified in four families with two affected children born to average stature parents. These results suggest that all cases of pseudoachondroplasia are secondary to mutations in *COMP* and that germ line mosaicism should be considered when counseling all isolated cases. While the exact recurrence risk is unknown, a 1 to 2 percent risk of recurrence is suggested (Hecht, unpublished results). Prenatal diagnosis is possible after the mutation is identified in the affected parent. Most of the MED cases result from mutations in *COMP* except for five cases with mutations in type 9 collagen genes.

**Type 9 Collagen Mutations.** Five MED cases with type 9 collagen mutations have been reported.[117-119] Three of these cases had mutations in *COL9A2*[117,118] and two had mutations in *COL9A3*.[119] For both genes the identified mutations alter the acceptor splice site in intron 2 with the result that exon 3 is deleted from the mature transcript. The clinical reports suggest that these alterations in type 9 collagen result in abnormalities of the hip and knee joints. Stature does not appear to be reduced. The currently available information about these families and the spectrum of the mutations is minimal. A careful phenotypic comparison of the MED patients with mutations in *COMP* to those with mutations in *COL9A2* and *COL9A3* genes is merited.

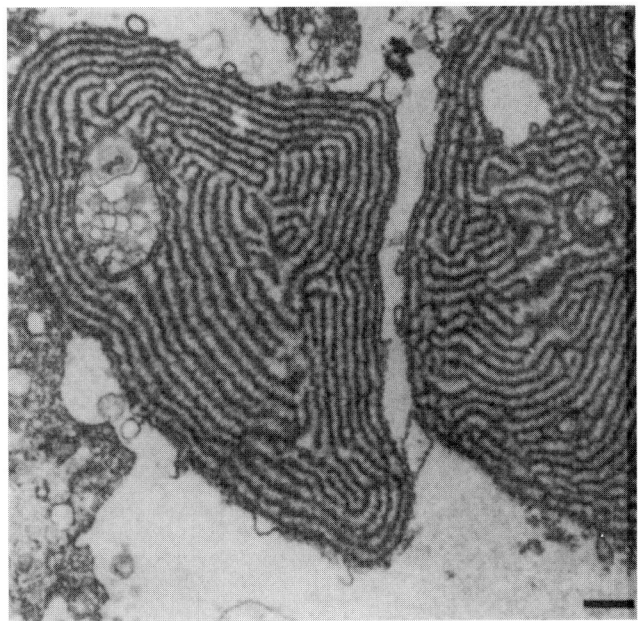

**Fig. 210-20** Isolated pseudoachondroplasia chondrocytes containing the lamellar rough endoplasmic reticulum vesicles viewed by electron microscopy. (*From Maddox et al.[137] Reprinted with permission.*)

## REFERENCES

1. Maroteaux P, Lamy M: Les formes pseudo-achondroplastiques des dysplasies spondylo-epiphysaires. *Presse Med* 67:383, 1959.
2. Spranger J: Bone dysplasia families. *Pathol Immunpathol Res* 7:76, 1988.
3. Shiang R, Thompson LM, Zhu YZ, Church DM, Fielder TJ, Bocian M, Winokur ST, Wasmuth JJ: Mutations in the transmembrane domain of FGFR3 cause the most common genetic form of dwarfism, achondroplasia. *Cell* 78:335, 1994.
4. Rousseau F, Bonaventure J, Legai-Mallet L, Pelet A, Rozet JM, Maroteaux P, Le Merrer M: Mutations in the gene encoding fibroblast receptor growth factor receptor-3 in achondroplasia. *Nature* 371:252, 1994.
5. Tavormina PL, Shiang R, Thompson LM, Zhu YZ, Wilkin DJ, Lachman RS, Wilcox WR, Rimoin DL, Cohn DH, Wasmuth JJ: Thanatophoric dysplasia (types I and II) caused by distinct mutations in fibroblast growth factor receptor 3. *Nat Genet* 9:321, 1995.
6. Bellus GA, McIntosh I, Smith EA, Aylsworth AS, Kaitila I, Horton WA, Greenhaw GA, Hecht JT, Francomano CA: A recurrent mutation in the tyrosine kinase domain of fibroblast growth factor receptor 3 causes hypochondroplasia. *Nat Genet* 10:357, 1995.
7. Bonaventur eJ, Rousseau J, Legai-Mallet L, Le Merrer M, Munnich A, Maroteaux P: Common mutations in the fibroblast growth factor receptor 3 (FGFR 3) gene account for achondroplasia, hypochondroplasia and thanatophoric dwarfism. *Am J Med Genet* 63:148, 1996.
8. Rousseau F, Saugier P, Le Merrer M, Munnich A, Delezoide AL, Maroteaux P, Bonaventure J: Stop codon FGFR3 mutations in thanatophoric dysplasia type I. *Nat Genet* 10:11, 1995.
9. Prinos P, Costa T, Sommer A, Kilpatrick MW, Tsipouras P: A common FGFR3 gene mutation in hypochondroplasia. *Hum Mol Genet* 4:2097, 1995.
10. Tavormina PL, Rimoin DL, Cohn DH, Zhu YZ, Shiang R, Wasmuth JJ: Another mutation that results in the substitution of an unpaired cystine residue in the extracellular domain of FGFR-3 in thanatophoric dysplasia type I. *Hum Mol Genet* 4:2175, 1995.
11. Rousseau F, el Ghouzzi V, Delezoide AL, Legai-Mallet L, Le Merrer M, Munnich A, Bonaventure J: Missense FGFR3 mutations create cysteine residues in thanatophoric dwarfism type I. *Hum Mol Genet* 5:509, 1996.
12. Rousseau F, Legeai-Mallet L, Le Merrer M, Munnich A, Bonaventure J: Mutations in extracellular domain of FGFR-3 produce unpaired cysteine residues in thanatophoric dysplasia type I. *Eur J Hum Gene* 4:64, 1996.
13. Rimoin DL, Lachman RS: *Genetic Disorders of the Osseous Skeleton*. St. Louis, Mosby-Yearbook, 1993.
14. Hall JG, Horton W, Kelly T, Scott CI: Head growth in achondroplasia: Use of ultrasound studies. *Am J Med Genet* 13:105, 1982.
15. Thompson NM, Hecht JT, Bohan TP, Kramer LA, Davidson K, Brandt ME, Fletcher JM: Neuroanatomic and neuropsychological outcome in school-age children with achondroplasia. *Am J Med Genet* 88:145, 1999.
16. Langer LO Jr, Baumann PA, Gorlin RJ: Achondroplasia. *Am J Roentgen* 100:12, 1967.
17. Hall JG: The natural history of achondroplasia, in Nicoletti BKS, Ascani E, et al (eds): *Human Achondroplasia: A Multidisciplinary Approach*. New York, Plenum, 1988, p 3.
18. Hecht JT, Francomano CA, Horton WA, Annegers JF: Mortality in achondroplasia. *Am J Hum Genet* 41:454, 1987.
19. Nelson FW, Hecht JT, Horton WA, Butler IJ, Goldie WD, Miner M: Neurological basis of respiratory complications in achondroplasia. *Ann Neurol* 24:89, 1988.
20. Aryanpur J, Hurko O, Francomano C, Wang H, Carson B: Craniocervical decompression for cervicomedullary compression in pediatric patients with achondroplasia. *J Neurosurg* 73:375, 1990.
21. Pierre-Kahn A, Hirsch JF, Renier D, Metzger J, Maroteaux P: Hydrocephalus and achondroplasia: A study of 25 observations. *Child's Brain* 7:205, 1980.
22. Steinbok P, Hall J, Flodmark O: Hydrocephalus in achondroplasia: The possible role of intracranial venous hypertension. *J Neurosurg* 71:42, 1989.
23. Lundar T, Bakke SJ, Nornes H: Hydrocephalus in an achondroplastic child treated by venous decompression at the jugular foramen [Case Report]. *J Neurosurg* 73:138, 1990.
24. Pyeritz RE, Sack GH Jr, Udvarhelyi GB: Thoracolumbosacral laminectomy in achondroplasia: Long-term results in 22 patients. *Am J Med Genet* 28:433, 1987.

25. Waters KA, Everett F, Sillence DO, Fagan ER, Sullivan CE: Treatment of obstructive sleep apnea in achondroplasia: Evaluation of sleep, breathing, and somatosensory-evoked potentials. *Am J Med Genet* 59:460, 1995.
26. Tasker RC, Dundas I, Laverty A, Fletcher M, Lane R, Stocks J: Distinct patterns of respiratory difficulty in young children with achondroplasia: A clinical, sleep, and lung function study. *Arch Dis Child* 79:99, 1998.
27. Mogayzel PJ Jr, Carroll JL, Loughlin GM, Hurko O, Francomano CA, Marcus CL: Sleep-disordered breathing in children with achondroplasia. *J Pediatr* 132:667, 1998.
28. Hecht JT, Hood OJ, Schwartz RJ, Hennessey JC, Bernhardt BA, Horton WA: Obesity in achondroplasia. *Am J Med Genet* 31:597, 1988.
29. Hunter AGW, Hecht JT, Scott CI Jr: Standard weight for height curves in achondroplasia. *Am J Med Genet* 62:255, 1996.
30. Hall JG, Dorst JP, Taybi H, Scott CI Jr, Langer LO Jr, McKusick VA: Two probable cases of homozygosity for the achondroplasia gene. *Birth Defects Orig Art Ser* V:24, 1969.
31. Patel MD, Filly RA: Homozygous achondroplasia: US distinction between homozygous, heterozygous, and unaffected fetuses in the second trimester. *Radiology* 196:541, 1995.
32. Hall BD, Spranger J: Hypochondroplasia: Clinical and radiological aspects in 39 cases. *Radiology* 133:95, 1979.
33. Walker BA, Murdoch JL, McKusick VA, Langer LO, Beals RK: Hypochondroplasia. *Am J Dis Child* 122:95, 1971.
34. Specht EE, Daentl DL: Hypochondroplasia. *Clin Orthop* 110:249, 1975.
35. Wynne-Davies R, Patton MA: The frequency of mental retardation in hypochondroplasia. *J Med Genet* 28:644, 1991.
36. Baker KM, Olson DS, Harding CO, Pauli RM: Long-term survival in typical thanatophoric dysplasia type 1. *Am J Med Genet* 70:427, 1997.
37. MacDonald IM, Hunter AG, MacLeod PM, MacMurray SB: Growth and development in thanatophoric dysplasia. *Am J Med Genet* 33:508, 1989.
38. Tavormina PL, Bellus GA, Webster MK, Bamshad MJ, Fraley AE, McIntosh I, Szabo J, Jiang W, Jabs EW, Wilcox WR, Wasmuth JJ, Donoghue DI, Thompson LM, Francomano CA: A novel skeletal dysplasia with developmental delay and acanthosis nigricans is caused by a Lys650Met mutation in the fibroblast growth factor receptor 3 (FGFR3) gene. *Am J Hum Genet* 64:722, 1999.
39. Bellus GA, Bamshad MJ, Przylepa KA, Dorst J, Lee RR, Hurko O, Jabs EW, Curry CJR, Wilcox WR, Lachman RS, Rimoin DL, Francomano CA: Severe achondroplasia with developmental delay and acanthosis nigricans (SADDAN): Phenotypic analysis of a new skeletal dysplasia caused by a Lys650Met mutation in fibroblast growth factor receptor 3. *Am J Med Genet* 85:53, 1999.
40. Wilcox WR, Tavormina PL, Krakow D, Kitoh H, Lachman RS, Wasmuth JJ, Thompson LM, Rimoin DL: Molecular, radiologic, and histopathologic correlations in thanatophoric dysplasia. *Am J Med Genet* 78:274, 1998.
41. Francomano CA, Ortiz de Luna RI, Hefferon TW, Bellus GA, Turner CE, Taylor E, Meyers DA, et al: Localization of the achondroplasia gene to the distal 2.5 Mb of human chromosome 4p. *Hum Mol Genet* 3:787, 1994.
42. Orioli IM, Castilla EE, Barbosa-Neto JG: The birth prevalence rates for the skeletal dysplasias. *J Med Genet* 23:328, 1986.
43. Andersen PE Jr, Hauge M: Congenital generalised bone dysplasias: A clinical, radiological, and epidemiological survey. *J Med Genet* 26:37, 1989.
44. Martinez-Frias ML, Cereijo A, Bermejo E, Lopez M, Sanchez M, Gonzalo C: Epidemiological aspects of mendelian syndromes in a Spanish population sample: I. Autosomal dominant malformation syndromes. *Am J Med Genet* 38:622, 1991.
45. Penrose LS: Parental age and mutation. *Lancet* II:312, 1955.
46. Orioli IM, Castilla EE, Scarano G, Mastroiacovo P: Effect of paternal age in achondroplasia, thanatophoric dysplasia, and osteogenesis imperfecta. *Am J Med Genet* 59:209, 1995.
47. Stoll C, Roth M-P, Bigel P: A reexamination of parental age effect on the occurrence of new mutations for achondroplasia, in Papadatos CJBC (ed): *Skeletal Dysplasias*. New York, Alan R. Liss, 1982, p 419.
48. Wilkin DJ, Szabo JK, Cameron R, Henderson S, Bellus GA, Mack ML, Kaitila I, et al: Fibroblast growth factor receptor 3 (FGFR3) mutations in sporadic cases of achondroplasia occur exclusively on the paternally derived chromosome. *Am J Hum Genet* 63:711, 1998.
49. Bowen P: Achondroplasia in two sisters with normal parents. *Birth Defects Orig Art Ser* X:31, 1974.

50. Fryns JP, Kleczkowska A, Verresen H, van den Berghe H: Germinal mosaicism in achondroplasia: A family with 3 affected siblings of normal parents. *Clin Gene* **24**:56, 1983.

51. Reiser CA, Pauli RM, Hall JG: Achondroplasia: unexpected familial recurrence. *Am J Med Genet* **19**:245, 1984.

52. Philip N, Auger M, Mattei JF, Giraud F: Achondroplasia in sibs of normal parents. *J Med Gene* **25**:857, 1988.

53. Cole WG, Dalgleish R: Perinatal lethal osteogenesis imperfecta. *J Med Genet* **32**:284, 1995.

54. Ferguson HL, Deere M, Evans R, Rotta J, Hall JG, Hecht JT: Mosaicism in pseudoachondroplasia. *Am J Med Genet* **70**:287, 1997.

55. Johnson DE, Williams LT: Structural and functional diversity in the FGF receptor multigene family. *Adv Cancer Res* **60**:1, 1993.

56. Bikfalvi A, Klein S, Pintucci G, Rifkin D: Biological roles of fibroblast growth factor-2. *Endocr Rev* **18**:26, 1997.

57. Givol D, Yayon A: Complexity of FGF receptors: Genetic basis for structural diversity. *FASEB J* **6**:3362, 1992.

58. Basilico C, Mostacelli D: The FGF family of growth factors and oncogenes. *Adv Cancer Res* **59**:115, 1992.

59. Burgess WH, Maciag T: The heparin-binding (fibroblast) growth factor family of proteins. *Ann Rev Biochem* **58**:575, 1989.

60. Laufer E, Nelson CE, Johnson RL, Morgan BA, Tabin C: Sonic hedgehog and FGF-4 act through a signaling cascade and feedback loop to integrate growth and patterning of the developing limb bud. *Cell* **79**:993, 1994.

61. Green PJ, Walsh FS, Doherty P: Promiscuity of fibroblast growth factor receptors. *Bioessays* **18**:639, 1996.

62. Chellaiah AT, McEwen DG, Werner S, Xu J, Ornitz DM: Fibroblast growth factor receptor (FGFR) 3. Alternative splicing in immunoglobulin-like domain III creates a receptor highly specific for acidic FGF/FGF-1. *J Biol Chem* **269**:11620, 1994.

63. Avivi A, Yayon A, Givo D: A novel form of FGF receptor-3 using an alternative exon in the immunoglobulin domain III. *FEBS Lett* **249**:249, 1993.

64. Wuechner C, Nordqvist AC, Winterpacht A, Zabel B, Schalling M: Developmental expression of splicing variants of fibroblast growth factor receptor 3 (FGFR3) in mouse. *Int J Dev Biol* **40**:1185, 1996.

65. Peters K, Ornitz D, Werner S, Williams L: Unique expression pattern of the FGF receptor 3 gene during mouse organogenesis. *Dev Biol* **155**:423, 1993.

66. Belluardo N, Wu G, Mudo G, Hansson AC, Pettersson R, Fuxe K: Comparative localization of fibroblast growth factor receptor-1, -2, and -3 mRNAs in the rat brain: In situ hybridization analysis. *J Comp Neurol* **379**:226, 1997.

67. Noji S, Koyama E, Myokai F, Nohno T, Ohuchi H, Nishikawa K, Taniguchi S: Differential expression of three chick FGF receptor genes, FGFR1, FGFR2 and FGFR3, in limb and feather development. *Prog Clin Biol Res* **383B**: 645, 1993.

68. Thompson LM, Plummer S, Schalling M, Altherr MR, Gusella JF, Housman DE, Wasmuth JJ: A gene encoding a fibroblast growth factor receptor isolated from the Huntington disease gene region of human chromosome 4. *Genomics* **11**:1133, 1991.

69. Wuchner C, Hilbert K, Zabel B, Winterpacht A: Human fibroblast growth factor receptor 3 gene (FGFR3): Genomic sequence and primer set information for gene analysis. *Hum Genet* **100**:215, 1997.

70. Perez-Castro AV, Wilson J, Altherr MR: Genomic organization of the mouse fibroblast growth factor receptor 3 (Fgfr3) gene. *Genomics* **30**:157, 1995.

71. Perez-Castro AV, Wilson J, Altherr MR: Genomic organization of the human fibroblast growth factor receptor 3 (FGFR3) gene and comparative sequence analysis with the mouse Fgfr3 gene. *Genomics* **41**:10, 1997.

72. McEwen DG, Ornitz DM: Regulation of the fibroblast growth factor receptor 3 promoter and intron I enhancer by Sp1 family transcription factors. *J Biol Chem* **273**:5349, 1998.

73. Le Merrer M, Rousseau F, Legeai-Mallet L, Landais JC, Pelet A, Bonaventure J, Sanak M, et al: A gene for achondroplasia-hypochondroplasia maps to chromosome 4p. *Nat Genet* **6**:318, 1994.

74. Velinov M, Slaugenhaupt SA, Stoilov I, Scott CI Jr, Gusella JF, Tsipouras P: The gene for achondroplasia maps to the telomeric region of chromosome 4p. *Nat Genet* **6**:314, 1994.

75. Bellus G, Hefferon T, Ortiz de Luna R, Hecht JT, Horton WA, Machado M, Kaitila I, et al: Achondroplasia is defined by recurrent G380R mutations in FGFR3. *Am J Hum Genet* **56**:368, 1995.

76. Stoilov I, Kilpatrick MW, Tsipouras P: A common FGFR3 gene mutation is present in achondroplasia but not hypochondroplasia. *Am J Med Genet* **55**:127, 1995.

77. Niu DM, Hsiao KJ, Wang NH, Chin LS, Chen CH: Chinese achondroplasia is also defined by recurrent G380R mutations of the fibroblast growth factor receptor-3 gene. *Hum Genet* **98**:65, 1996.

78. Ikegawa S, Fukushima Y, Isomura M, Takada F, Nakamura Y: Mutations of the fibroblast growth factor receptor-3 gene in one familial and six sporadic cases of achondroplasia in Japanese patients. *Hum Genet* **96**:309, 1995.

79. Alderborn A, Anvret M, Gustavson KH, Hagenas L, Wadelius C: Achondroplasia in Sweden caused by the G1138A mutation in FGFR3. *Acta Paediatr* **85**:1506, 1996.

80. Wang TR, Wang WP, Hwu WL, Lee ML: Fibroblast growth factor receptor 3 (FGFR3) gene G1138A mutation in Chinese patients with achondroplasia. *Hum Mutat* **8**:178, 1996.

81. Tonoki H, Nakae J, Tajima T, Shinohara N: Predominance of the mutation at 1138 of the cDNA for the fibroblast growth factor receptor 3 in Japanese patients with achondroplasia. *Jpn J Hum Genet* **40**:347, 1995.

82. Kitoh H, Nogami H, Yamada Y, Goto H, Ogasawara N: Identification of mutations in the gene encoding the fibroblast growth factor receptor 3 in Japanese patients with achondroplasia. *Congenital Anomalies* **35**:231, 1995.

83. Superti-Furga A, Eich GU, Bucher H: A glycine 375-to-cysteine substitution in the transmembrane domain of the fibroblast growth factor receptor-3 in a newborn with achondroplasia. *Eur J Pediatr* **95**:215, 1995.

84. Nishimura G, Fukushima Y, Ohashi H, Ikegawa S: Atypical radiological findings in achondroplasia with uncommon mutation of the fibroblast growth factor receptor-3 (FGFR-3) gene (Gly to Cys transition at codon 375). *Am J Med Genet* **59**:393, 1995.

85. Prinos P, Kilpatrick MW, Tsiopuras P: A novel G346E mutation in achondroplasia. *Pediatr Res* **37**:151A, 1994.

86. Green PM, Montandon AJ, Bentley DR, Ljung R, Nilsson IM, Giannelli F: The incidence and distribution of CpG⁽ᵀ⁾TpG transitions in the coagulation factor IX gene. *Nucleic Acid Res* **18**:3227, 1990.

87. Colvin JS, Bohne BA, Harding GW, McEwen DG, Ornitz DM: Skeletal overgrowth and deafness in mice lacking fibroblast growth factor receptor 3. *Nat Genet* **12**:390, 1996.

88. Deng C, Wynshaw-Boris A, Zhou F, Kuo A, Leder P: Fibroblast growth factor receptor 3 is a negative regulator of bone growth. *Cell* **84**:911, 1996.

89. Thompson LM, Raffioni S, Zhu Y-Z, Wasmuth JJ, Bradshaw RA: Biological studies of mutations in FGFR3 which cause skeletal dysplasias. *Am J Hum Genet* **59**:A161, 1996.

90. Mason IJ: The ins and outs of fibroblast growth factors. *Cell* **78**:547, 1994.

91. Neilson KM, Friesel R: Ligand-independent activation of fibroblast growth factor receptors by point mutations in the extracellular, transmembrane, and kinase domains. *J Biol Chem* **271**:25049, 1996.

92. Webster MK, Davis PY, Robertson SC, Donoghue DJ: Profound ligand-independent kinase activation of fibroblast growth factor receptor 3 by the activation loop mutation responsible for a lethal skeletal dysplasia, thanatophoric dysplasia type II. *Mol Cell Biol* **16**:4081, 1996.

93. Webster MK, Donoghue DJ: Fibroblast growth factor receptor 3 is constitutively activated by independent mechanisms in two skeletal dysplasias. *Proc Annu Meet Am Assoc Cancer Res* **37**:A264, 1996.

94. Webster MK, Donoghue DJ: Constitutive activation of fibroblast growth factor receptor 3 by the transmembrane domain point mutation found in achondroplasia. *EMBO J* **15**:520, 1996.

95. Li Y, Mangasarian K, Mansukhani A, Basilico C: Activation of FGF receptors by mutations in the transmembrane domain. *Oncogene* **14**:1397, 1997.

96. Naski MC, Wang Q, Xu J, Ornitz DM: Graded activation of fibroblast growth factor receptor 3 by mutations causing achondroplasia and thanatophoric dysplasia. *Nat Genet* **13**:233, 1996.

97. Su WC, Kitagawa M, Xue N, Xie B, Garofalo S, Cho J, Deng C, Horton WA, Fu XY: Activation of Stat1 by mutant fibroblast growth-factor receptor in thanatophoric dysplasia type II dwarfism. *Nature* **386**:288, 1997.

98. Thompson LM, Raffioni S, Wasmuth JJ, Bradshaw RA: Chimeras of the native form or achondroplasia mutant (G375C) of human fibroblast growth factor receptor 3 induce ligand-dependent differentiation of PC12 cells. *Mol Cell Biol* **17**:4169, 1997.

99. Galvin BD, Hart KC, Meyer AN, Webster MK: Constitutive receptor activation by Crouzon syndrome mutations in fibroblast growth factor receptor (FGFR)2 and FGFR2/Neu chimeras. *Proc Natl Acad Sci U S A* **93**:7894, 1996.

100. Roussel MF, Downing JR, Sherr CJ: Transforming activities of human CSF-1 receptors with different point mutations at codon 301 in their extracellular domain. *Oncogene* **5**:25, 1990.

101. Santoro M, Carlomango F, Romano A, Bottaro DP, Dothan NA, Grieco M, Frisco A, et al: Activation of RET as a dominant transforming gene by germ-line mutations of MEN2A and MEN2B. *Science* **267**:381, 1995.

102. Sorokin A, Lemmon MA, Ullrich A, Schlessinger J: Stabilization of an active dimeric form of the epidermal growth factor by introduction of an inter-receptor disulfide bond. *J Biol Chem* **269**:9752, 1994.

103. Neilson KM, Friesel RE: Constitutive activation of fibroblast growth factor receptor-2 by a point mutation associated with Crouzon syndrome. *J Biol Chem* **270**:26037, 1995.

104. Pokharel RK, Alimsardjono H, Takeshima Y, Nakamura H, Naritomi K, Hirose S, Onishi S, Matsuo M: Japanese cases of type 1 thanatophoric dysplasia exclusively carry a C to T transition at nucleotide 742 of the fibroblast growth factor receptor 3 gene. *Biochem Biophys Res Commun* **227**:236, 1996.

105. Muenke M, Gripp KW, McDonald-McGinn DM, Gaudenz K, Whitaker LA, Bartlett SP, Markowitz RI, Robin NH, Nwokoro N, Mulvihill JJ, Losken HW, Mulliken JB, Guttmacher AE, Wilroy RS, Clarke LA, Hollway G, Ades LC, Haan EA, Mulley JC, Cohen MM Jr, Bellus GA, Francomano CA, Moloney DM, Wall SA, Wilkie AO, et al: A unique point mutation in the fibroblast growth factor receptor 3 gene (FGFR3) defines a new craniosynostosis syndrome. *Am J Hum Genet* **60**:555, 1997.

106. Reardon W, Wilkes D, Rutland P, Pulleyn LJ, Malcolm S, Dean JC, Evans RD, Jones BM, Hayward R, Hall CM, Nevin NC, Baraister M, Winter RM: Craniosynostosis associated with FGFR3 pro250arg mutation results in a range of clinical presentations including unisutural sporadic craniosynostosis. *J Med Genet* **34**:632, 1997.

107. Wilkie AOM, Slaney SF, Oldridge M, Poole MD, Ashworth GJ, Hockley AD, Hayward RD: Apert syndrome results from localized mutations of FGFR2 and is allelic with Crouzon syndrome. *Nat Genet* **9**:165, 1995.

108. Rutland P, Pulleyn LJ, Reardon W, Baraitser M, Hayward R, Jones B, Malcolm S, Winter RM, Oldridge M, Slaney SF: Identical mutations in the FGFR2 gene cause both Pfeiffer and Crouzon syndrome phenotypes [Comments]. *Nat Genet* **9**:173, 1995.

109. Schell U, Hehr A, Feldman GJ, Robin NH, Zackai EH, de Die-Smulders C, Viskochil DH, Stewart JM, Wolff G, Ohashi H: Mutations in FGFR1 and FGFR2 cause familial and sporadic Pfeiffer syndrome. *Hum Mol Genet* **4**:323, 1995.

110. Jabs EW, Li X, Scott AF, Meyers G, Chen W, Eccles M, Mao JI, Charnas LR, Jackson CE, Jaye M: Jackson-Weiss and Crouzon syndromes are allelic with mutations in fibroblast growth factor receptor 2 [Erratum appears in *Nat Genet* 9(4):451, 1995]. *Nat Genet* **8**:275, 1994.

111. Reardon W, Winter RM, Rutland P, Pulleyn LJ, Jones BM, Malcolm S: Mutations in the fibroblast growth factor receptor 2 gene cause Crouzon syndrome. *Nat Genet* **8**:98, 1994.

112. Gorry MC, Preston RA, White GJ, Zhang Y, Singhal VK, Losken HW, Parker MG, Nwokoro NA, Post JC, Ehrlich GD: Crouzon syndrome: Mutations in two spliceoforms of FGFR2 and a common point mutation shared with Jackson-Weiss syndrome. *Hum Mol Genet* **4**:1387, 1995.

113. Modaff P, Horton VK, Pauli RM: Errors in the prenatal diagnosis of children with achondroplasia. *Prenat Diagn* **16**:525, 1996.

114. Mesoraca A, Pilu G, Perolo A, Novelli G: Ultrasound and molecular mid-trimester prenatal diagnosis of de novo achondroplasia. *Prenat Diagn* **16**:764, 1996.

115. Briggs MD, Hoffman SM, King LM, Olsen AS, Mohrenweiser H, Leroy JG, Mortier GR: Pseudoachondroplasia and multiple epiphyseal dysplasia due to mutations in the cartilage oligomeric matrix protein gene. *Nat Genet* **10**:330, 1995.

116. Hecht JT, Nelson LD, Crowder E, Wang Y, Elder FF, Harrison WR, Francomano CA: Mutations in exon 17B of cartilage oligomeric matrix protein (COMP) cause pseudoachondroplasia. *Nat Genet* **10**:325, 1995.

117. Muragaki Y, Mariman ECM, van Beersum SEC, Perala M, van Mourik JBA, Warman ML, Olsen BR: A mutation in the gene encoding the alpha-2 chain of the fibril-associated collagen IX, COL9A2, causes multiple epiphyseal dysplasia (EDM2). *Nat Genet* **12**:103, 1996.

118. Holden P, Canty EG, Mortier GR, Zabel B, Spranger J, Carr A, Grant ME, Loughlin JA, Briggs MA: Identification of novel pro-a2(IX) collagen gene mutations in two families with distinctive oligo-epiphyseal forms of multiple epiphyseal dysplasia. *Am J Hum Genet* **65**:31, 1999.

119. Paassilta P, Lohiniva J, Annunen S, Bonaventure J, Le Merrer M, Pai L, Ala-Kokko L: COL9A3:A third locus for multiple epiphyseal dysplasia. *Am J Hum Genet* **64**:1036, 1999.

120. McKusick VA, Scott C: A nomenclature for constitutional disorders of bone. *J Bone Joint Surg* **53A**:978, 1971.

121. McKeand J, Rotta J, Hecht JT: Natural history study of pseudoachondroplasia. *Am J Med Genet* **63**:406, 1996.

122. Wynne-Davies R, Hall CM, Young ID: Pseudoachondroplasia: Clinical diagnosis at different ages and comparison of autosomal dominant and recessive types. A review of 32 patients (26 kindred). *J Med Genet* **23**:425, 1986.

123. Langer LO Jr, Schaefer GB, Wadsworth DT: Patient with double heterozygosity for achondroplasia and pseudoachondroplasia, with comments on these conditions and the relationship between pseudoachondroplasia and multiple epiphyseal dysplasia, Fairbank type. *Am J Med Genet* **47**:772, 1993.

124. Hall JG, Dorst JP: Pseudoachondroplastic SED, recessive Maroteaux-Lamy type. *Birth Defects Orig Art Ser* **V**:254, 1969.

125. Oehlmann R, Summerville GP, Yeh G, Weaver EJ, Jimenez SA, Knowlton RG: Genetic linkage mapping of multiple epiphyseal dysplasia to the pericentromeric region of chromosome 19. *Am J Hum Gene* **54**:3, 1994.

126. Hall JG, Dorst JP, Rotta J, McKusick VA: Gonadal mosaicism in pseudoachondroplasia. *Am J Med Genet* **28**:143, 1987.

127. Deere M, Sanford T, Francomano CA, Daniels K, Hecht JT: Identification of nine novel mutations in cartilage oligomeric matrix protein in patients with pseudoachondroplasia and multiple epiphyseal dysplasia. *Am J Med Genet* **8**:486, 1999.

128. Briggs MD, Rasmussen IM, Weber JL, Yuen J, Reinker K, Garber AP, Rimoin DL, et al: Genetic linkage of mild pseudoachondroplasia (PSACH) to markers in the pericentromeric region of chromosome 19. *Genomics* **18**:656, 1993.

129. Hecht JT, Francomano CA, Briggs MD, Deere M, Conner B, Horton WA, Warman M, et al: Linkage of typical pseudoachondroplasia to chromosome 19. *Genomics* **18**:661, 1993.

130. Newton G, Weremowicz S, Morton CC, Copeland NG, Gilbert DJ, Jenkins NA, Lawler J: Characterization of human and mouse cartilage oligomeric matrix protein. *Genomics* **24**:435, 1994.

131. Deere M, Sanford T, Ferguson HL, Daniels K, Hecht JT: Identification of twelve mutations in cartilage oligomeric matrix protein (COMP) in patients with pseudoachondroplasia. *Am J Med Gene* **80**:510, 1998.

132. Ballo R, Briggs MD, Cohn DH, Knowlton RG, Beighton PH, Ramesar RS: Multiple epiphyseal dysplasia, ribbing type: A novel point mutation in the COMP gene in a South African family. *Am J Med Genet* **68**:396, 1997.

133. Briggs MD, Mortier GR, Cole WG, King LM, Golik SS, Bonaventure J, Nuytinck L, et al: Diverse mutations in the gene for cartilage oligomeric matrix protein in the Pseudoachondroplasia-multiple epiphyseal dysplasia disease spectrum. *Am J Hum Gene* **62**:311, 1998.

134. Délot E, Brodie SG, King LM, Wilcox WR, Cohn DH: Physiological and pathological secretion of cartilage oligomeric matrix protein by cells in culture. *J Biol Chem* **273**:26692, 1998.

135. Délot E, King LM, Briggs MD, Wilcox WR, Cohn DH: Trinucleotide expansion mutations in the cartilage oligomeric matrix protein (COMP) gene. *Hum Mol Genet* **8**:123, 1999.

136. Loughlin J, Irven C, Mustafa Z, Briggs MD, Carr A, Lynch A-A, Knowlton RG, Cohn DH, Sykes B: Identification of five novel mutations in cartilage oligomeric matrix protein gene in pseudoachondroplasia and multiple epiphyseal dysplasia. *Hum Mutat Suppl* **1**:S10, 1998.

137. Maddox BK, Keene DR, Sakai LY, Charbonneau NL, Morris NP, Ridgway CC, Boswell BA, Sussman MD, Horton WA, Bachinger HP, Hecht JT: The fate of cartilage oligomeric matrix protein is determined by the cell type in the case of a novel mutation in pseudoachondroplasia. *J Biol Chem* **272**:30993, 1997.

138. Susic S, McGrory J, Ahier J, Cole WG: Multiple epiphyseal dysplasia and Pseudoachondroplasia due to novel mutations in the calmodulin-like repeats of cartilage oligomeric matrix protein. *J Clin Genet* **51**:219, 1997.

139. Susic S, Ahier J, Cole WG: Pseudoachondroplasia due to the substitution of the highly conserved Asp482 by Gly in the seventh calmodulin-like repeat of cartilage oligomeric matrix protein. *Hum Mutat* **1**(**Suppl**):S125, 1998.

140. Hedbom E, Antonsson P, Hjerpe A, Aeschlimann D, Paulsson M, Rosa-Pimentel E, Sommarin Y, et al: Cartilage matrix proteins: an acidic oligomeric protein (COMP) detected only in cartilage. *J Biol Chem* **267**:6132, 1992.

141. Mîrgelin M, Heinegürd D, Engel J, Paulsson J: Electron microscopy of native cartilage oligomeric matrix protein purified from the Swarm rat chondrosarcoma reveals a five armed structure. *J Biol Chem* **267**:6137, 1992.

142. Stanescu V, Maroteaux P, Stanescu R: The biochemical defect of pseudoachondroplasia. *Eur J Pediat* **138**:221, 1982.

143. Cooper RR, Ponseti IV, Maynard JA: Pseudoachondroplastic dwarfism. A rough-surfaced endoplasmic reticulum storage disorder. *J Bone Joint Surg* **55A:** 475, 1973.

144. Maynard JA, Cooper RR, Ponseti IV: A unique rough surface endoplasmic reticulum inclusion in pseudoachondroplasia. *Lab Invest* **26**:40, 1972.

145. Hecht JT, Montufar-Solis D, Decker G, Lawler J, Daniels K, Duke PJ: Retention of cartilage oligomeric matrix protein (COMP) and cell death in redifferentiated pseudoachondroplasia chondrocytes. *Matrix Biol* **17**:625, 1998.

# CARDIOVASCULAR SYSTEM

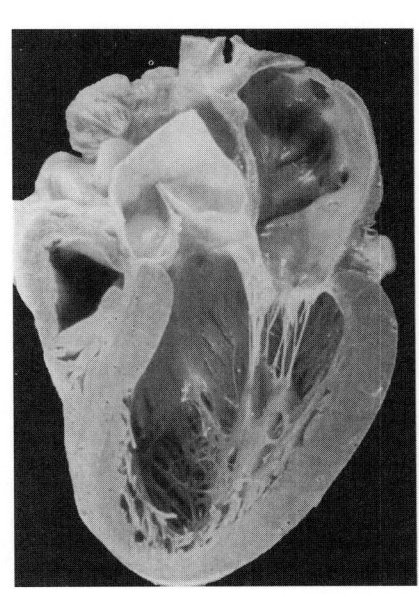
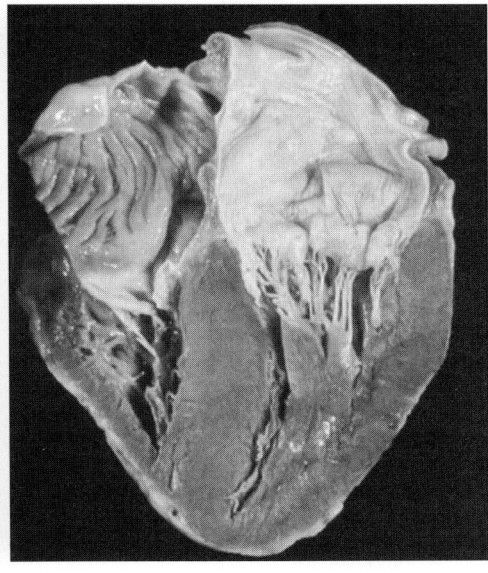

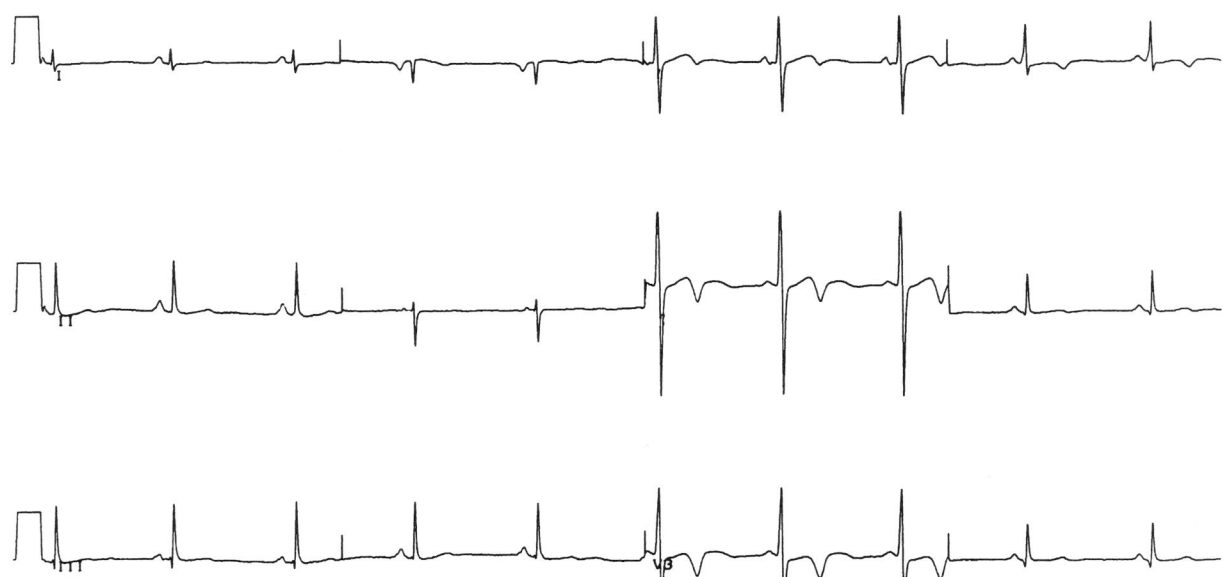

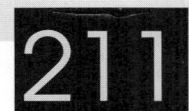

# The Inherited Basis of Blood Pressure Variation and Hypertension

*Ali Gharavi* ■ *Richard P. Lifton*

1. Blood pressure is a multifactorial quantitative trait showing a continuous distribution in the general population. The determinants of blood pressure variation include genetic and environmental factors, as well as demographic factors such as age, gender, and ethnicity. Multiple lines of evidence demonstrate the importance of heredity in blood pressure variation. Blood pressure aggregates within families, with greater concordance in biologic sibs than in adoptive sibs living in the same household. Monozygotic twins who share 100 percent of their genes show significantly greater concordance in blood pressure than do dizygotic twins who only share 50 percent of their genes. The impact of genetic factors on the development of hypertension is modified by environmental factors such as weight gain and sodium intake.

2. Blood pressure is regulated by the interplay between a large number of physiological variables. Physiological studies have not generally succeeded in identifying the initiating factors responsible for the development of high blood pressure. However, these studies indicate that the kidney plays an essential role in the long-term regulation of blood pressure. Maintenance of elevated blood pressure implicates a derangement in the renal pressure natriuresis mechanism, and disturbance in this system has been verified in humans with essential hypertension as well as in experimental models of the disease. At steady state, hypertension is characterized by a rightward resetting of the pressure natriuresis response, resulting in inappropriately elevated blood volume for the level of blood pressure. This signifies that derangements in salt handling are likely to participate in the development of hypertension. Genetic studies confirm these findings and demonstrate that mutations underlying all Mendelian forms of high and low blood pressure converge on a final common pathway: mutations that cause a net increase in salt reabsorption result in hypertension, whereas mutations that cause salt wasting produce hypotension.

3. Mendelian forms of hypertension: Glucocorticoid-remediable aldosteronism is caused by unequal crossing over, fusing regulatory sequences of the 11-beta hydroxylase onto coding sequences of the aldosterone synthase genes, resulting in ectopic production of aldosterone under the control of ACTH. Liddle syndrome is caused by activating mutations in genes encoding the beta and gamma subunits of the epithelial sodium channel in the distal nephron, leading to increased distal sodium reabsorption. Apparent mineralocorticoid excess is caused by 11-beta hydroxysteroid dehydrogenase deficiency that results in excessive stimulation of the mineralocorticoid receptor by cortisol. Activating mutations in the mineralocorticoid receptor cause hypertension with marked exacerbation during pregnancy. The hypertensive forms of congenital adrenal hyperplasia are caused by enzyme deficiencies in the steroid synthesis pathways that lead to accumulation of mineralocorticoid precursors. Finally, pseudohypoaldosteronism type II, characterized by hypertension and hyperkalemia, and the syndrome of hypertension with brachydactyly are two Mendelian disorders that have been mapped but whose molecular etiologies have not yet been defined.

4. Mendelian forms of hypotension: Pseudohypoaldosteronism type I features renal salt wasting with impaired secretion of potassium and hydrogen ions. Recessive and dominant PHA-I are caused by loss-of-function mutations in the genes encoding subunits of the epithelial sodium channel and the mineralocorticoid receptor, respectively. Congenital adrenal hyperplasia with salt wasting caused by 21-hydroxylase deficiency results in inability to produce mineralocorticoids. Gitelman syndrome, characterized by hypokalemic metabolic alkalosis, hypomagnesemia, and hypocalciuria, is a consequence of mutations in the gene encoding the thiazide-sensitive sodium chloride cotransporter, which is responsible for salt reabsorption in the distal convoluted tubule. Bartter syndrome is a genetically heterogeneous disorder characterized by impaired salt reabsorption in the thick ascending loop of Henle, hypokalemic metabolic alkalosis, and hypercalcuria. Bartter syndrome is caused by mutations in at least three genes, including those encoding the apical $Na^+$-$K^+$-$2Cl^-$ cotransporter of the renal thick ascending limb, the ATP-sensitive $K^+$ channel ROMK, and the chloride channel CLCKB.

5. Efforts to identify genetic variants that underlie blood pressure variation in the general population are currently in progress. These studies are confounded by the complexity

---

A list of standard abbreviations is located immediately preceding the index in each volume. Additional abbreviations used in this chapter include: 11BHSD = 11-beta hydroxysteroid dehydrogenase; ACE = angiotensin-converting enzyme; AME = apparent mineralocorticoid excess syndrome; AII = angiotensin II; BP = blood pressure; BMI = body mass index; CAH = congenital adrenal hyperplasia; CLCK = chloride channels; DOC = deoxycorticosterone; ENac = epithelial sodium channel; GRA = glucocorticoid remediable aldosteronism; MR = mineralocorticoid receptor; NCCT = thiazide-sensitive Na-Cl cotransporter; NKCC2 = bumetanide-sensitive $Na^+$-$K^+$-$2Cl^-$ cotransporter; PHA = pseudohypoaldosteronism; PTH-rp = parathyroid hormone-related protein; ROMK = ATP-sensitive $K^+$ channel ROMK.

of the trait, the inability to determine how many genes influence the trait in the general population, and the lack of knowledge of the magnitude of the effect imparted by any locus. Analysis of published studies reveals one promising interval on human chromosome 17 that has been identified as a blood pressure locus in rat, and shows evidence for linkage in both Mendelian and essential hypertension in humans. Additional loci have provided suggestions of linkage that remain to be confirmed. Investigation of candidate genes by studies of linkage and/or association suggests roles for a number of genes in blood pressure variation; however, the results of these studies have been inconsistent, leaving their interpretation in some doubt. The most promising of these studies suggest that common variants in the angiotensinogen and angiotensin-converting enzyme loci may impart modest effects on blood pressure in the general population.

6. Disturbances in renal salt handling mediate virtually all known forms of inherited and acquired blood pressure variation and implicate this mechanism as a final common pathway for blood pressure variation. The discovery of the genetic bases of hypertension should permit early detection of subjects at risk, offer new therapeutic approaches, and enable individualization of therapy.

With every cycle of cardiac contraction, the heart propels blood into the arterial system, resulting in delivery of oxygen and nutrients to tissues. It is intuitive that the force of cardiac contraction must be sufficient to adequately perfuse all organs, and, following Ohm's law, that the pressure generated in the arterial system is proportional to the amount of blood pumped by the heart and to the resistance to flow imparted by the arterial system. The force exerted by blood on the arterial system is referred to as blood pressure, and is typically divided into systolic and diastolic components, the former corresponding to the peak pressure generated as a bolus of blood passes through the arterial system, the latter corresponding to the trough pressure occurring after the bolus has passed.

Epidemiologic studies have documented the increased risk of a number of morbid outcomes among individuals with elevated blood pressure, including stroke, myocardial infarction, congestive heart failure, and end-stage renal disease. For example, the MRFIT study, a prospective study that screened over 350,000 males, demonstrated that cardiovascular mortality rises progressively across deciles of blood pressure level, with the relative risk of coronary heart disease death 2.9 times higher for individuals in the highest decile as compared to those in the lowest decile.[1] Hypertension is also the leading cause of stroke and the second most common cause of end-stage renal disease.[1-3] A similar graded relation was found between blood pressure level and the development of these clinical entities.[1-4] Moreover, as demonstrated by prospective randomized controlled trials, the risk of these outcomes is reduced by intervention with agents that lower blood pressure.[5-7] Thus, the diagnosis of hypertension is based on an operational definition that serves to identify individuals at increased risk of morbid outcomes and in whom intervention can reduce overall morbidity and mortality.

Based on these observational and interventional studies, individuals with blood pressures higher than 140/90 mm Hg are said to have high blood pressure, or hypertension. By this definition, hypertension affects about 25 percent of the adult population of most industrial societies and is a major cause of cardiovascular and renal disease.[8,9]

Despite remarkable progress in understanding the physiological systems that regulate blood pressure (BP), the primary determinants of BP variation in humans have proved elusive. This can partly be attributed to the fact that blood pressure as a trait can only be measured in an intact, living organism and cannot be reduced to a simple in vitro system. The many physiological systems involved in blood pressure regulation all respond to changes in their homeostasis; consequently, it is not surprising that abnormalities have been described in nearly all of these pathways in hypertensive subjects. However, determining which, if any, of these are primary underlying abnormalities, and distinguishing these from secondary adaptive or maladaptive responses has proved difficult from physiological investigation alone.

## EPIDEMIOLOGY

Epidemiologic studies have identified a large number of demographic, environmental, and genetic characteristics that contribute to blood pressure variation. These demonstrate that blood pressure is a continuously distributed quantitative trait across all age and gender groups.[8-10] BP follows a Gaussian distribution with slight skewing at the high end.[8-10] Consistent with these characteristics, cardiovascular risk associated with BP level is also continuously distributed and rises with increasing BP. Multiple large studies have convincingly demonstrated that there are no apparent threshold levels for the development of cardiovascular complications.[1-8]

### Demographic Factors

As for other traits, BP is influenced by demographic variables, including age, gender, and ethnicity. BP level rises and tracks with increasing age; longitudinal studies reveal that individuals generally remain near the same age-adjusted BP percentile throughout life.[8-11] Thus, being at the high end of the blood pressure distribution early in life is one of the most powerful predictors of hypertension in adulthood. This age-related rise in BP is a characteristic of modern societies. In contrast, in many primitive societies studied, there is little or no increase in BP with age.[12-14] Studies of migrating populations have demonstrated that this feature develops in individuals who make the transition from more primitive societies to more modern, urban settings.[10,15-17] Many possible explanations have been offered for this phenomenon, including increased salt intake, low potassium intake, higher caloric intake, more sedentary lifestyle, or increased psychosocial stress.[10] However, none of these explanations have been clearly substantiated as playing a causal role.

Gender affects blood pressure as well; BP is higher in males as compared to females until the fifth decade of life, at which time the prevalence of hypertension in women increases to nearly the same levels seen among men.[8-10] This late increase in incidence in women may reflect the loss of vascular protection afforded by estrogens.

Blood pressure also displays ethnic variability. In particular, it is higher in Blacks of African ancestry compared to Caucasians.[8-10] The higher prevalence of hypertension among Blacks appears to be confined to urban and western societies, because rural Africans have a threefold reduced incidence of hypertension as compared to urban populations.[12] In the United States, the prevalence of hypertension is 32.4 percent in non-Hispanic Blacks as compared to 23.3 percent in non-Hispanic Caucasians, a 40 percent increase.[9] In addition, hypertension occurs at an earlier age and is more severe among non-Hispanic Blacks, resulting in a much higher incidence of mortality due to cardiovascular disease.[9,10,18,19] These findings have been taken as evidence for genetic predisposition or even selection in blacks.[20] However, certain Black populations living in Africa display a very low incidence of hypertension, suggesting an interplay of demographic, environmental, and genetic factors.[11-14]

### Environmental Factors

Body mass index (BMI) and physical activity are among the strongest environmental predictors of hypertension. There is a continuous relationship between BP and BMI, even in the lowest ranges of BMI.[21-23] Consistent with this finding, there is an inverse relation between physical activity and the risk of hypertension.[24] Weight gain early in life is, therefore, one of the most potentially modifiable environmental factors for hypertension. Weight gain and obesity may contribute to the development of hypertension by promoting insulin resistance, which occurs in up to 50 percent of hypertensive subjects.[25] Population studies indicate a clustering of hyperlipidemia, diabetes, and hypertension, while family and twin studies demonstrate high concordance rates for joint occurrence of these disorders.[25–31] These findings have prompted the hypothesis that insulin resistance is a unifying mechanism underlying the clustering of these risk factors for coronary heart disease.[25] The pathogenic pathways linking insulin resistance, diabetes, hyperlipidemia, and hypertension have not yet been defined. Proposed mechanisms linking insulin resistance to hypertension include stimulation of sodium reabsorption, increased sympathetic outflow, and increased peripheral vascular resistance.[25] However, none of these pathways has been convincingly validated and the cause and effect relation between hypertension and these other diseases remains a matter of controversy. Nonetheless, these interesting associations suggest that these disorders share a common genetic underpinning that is exacerbated by the environmental exposures of industrialized societies.

Finally, the most widely studied environmental aspect of hypertension is its relationship to sodium intake. The strongest evidence for a pathogenic role of sodium in the development of hypertension stems from the INTERSALT study.[10,12] This study measured the 24-h sodium excretion in over 10,000 individuals residing in 52 differing communities worldwide and demonstrated a strong relation between Na excretion, BP level, and future risk of hypertension. This positive association was mostly derived from the data from eight communities with the lowest range of Na intake (<50 mM/day), which also demonstrated no age-related change in BP. Exclusion of these communities from the analysis abolished the relation between Na excretion and BP, suggesting a threshold effect. The relationship of salt intake to hypertension has also been documented in studies of migrating populations; immigrants switching to a diet with higher sodium content are more likely to develop hypertension.[15,16]

Experimental support for the role of $Na^+$ in hypertension emanates from studies of chimpanzees on long-term increased Na intake. Compared to control animals remaining on normal (low) Na intake, chimpanzees switching to high-Na diets develop a substantial rise in BP (systolic and diastolic blood pressures rising 33 and 10 mm Hg, respectively, after 89 weeks). These increases remitted when the diet was changed back to the normal low-salt diet.[32] Conversely, studies in humans and animal models have demonstrated that a low-Na diet results in lowering of BP in a significant number of individuals.[33,34] However, dietary Na modifies BP response only in a subset of individuals labeled as salt sensitive. Depending on the criteria used, 20 to 50 percent of hypertensive subjects can be classified as salt sensitive, although few long-term studies have been performed.[33,34]

## PHYSIOLOGY

As blood pressure must follow Ohm's law, it is apparent that its variation must ultimately be attributable to changes in cardiac output or systemic vascular resistance to blood flow. There are a number of physiological systems that impact these parameters, and their complex interactions have thwarted efforts to define the underlying primary determinants from physiological analysis alone. Some of the difficulties in identifying the initiating factor(s) from physiological studies alone are illustrated in studies of experimental models of hypertension. For example, administration of mineralocorticoids, which promote renal salt reabsorption, results in sodium retention and increased plasma volume, leading to increased cardiac output and elevation of blood pressure.[35] Over several weeks, however, the hemodynamic pattern of the hypertension evolves to one of normal cardiac output with high systemic vascular resistance. This altered hemodynamic pattern

has been attributed to autoregulation of blood flow, with tissues matching their perfusion to metabolic demand. This is accompanied by alteration in a variety of physiological alterations, and from the steady state pattern, it would be difficult to deduce the inciting cause of hypertension.

However, the seminal studies of Guyton on the renal pressure-natriuresis curve argue for the requirement of abnormalities in the kidney in the maintenance of elevated blood pressure.[36] The kidney responds to BP elevations by increasing sodium excretion, returning BP to normal. This is an extremely sensitive mechanism with nearly infinite gain as illustrated by the very steep curve relating BP to sodium excretion. Maintenance of hypertension therefore implicates a rightward resetting of the pressure-natriuresis mechanism, resulting in an inappropriate degree of sodium retention.[36–38] In addition, this concept allows for the possibility that hypertension can occur without an absolute increase in blood volume. Studies have demonstrated a negative correlation between diastolic BP and blood volume in normotensive individuals.[39] However, this inverse relationship is not present in hypertensive subjects, suggesting that plasma volume is inappropriately high for the level of BP.[39] These data are consistent with the frequent absence of suppression in plasma renin activity in hypertensive humans, again implicating a disturbance in renal salt regulation.[39–41] Abnormal pressure natriuresis has also been documented in all genetic and experimental causes of hypertension. Disturbances in the pressure-natriuresis curve are also documented in genetic models such as the Dahl salt-sensitive hypertensive rats (S). Furthermore, in these animals, transplantation of the kidney of a salt-resistant normotensive rat (R) into an S rat results in normalization of BP. Conversely, transplantation of an S kidney into an R rat results in hypertension.[42] Finally, data from human transplant recipients demonstrate lowering of BP in patients with hypertensive nephrosclerosis who received renal transplants from normotensive donors.[43] Thus, regardless of the initiating factors, the maintenance of hypertension appears to depend on the inability of the kidney to maintain an appropriate relation between sodium excretion and blood pressure. It is important to point out that there are many inputs to the determination of this aspect of renal function, including primary effectors in the kidney as well as hormonal and neural contributions to these functions.

## GENETIC EPIDEMIOLOGY

From epidemiologic data, it appears most likely that in single individuals, inheritance at multiple loci influences blood pressure. Moreover, factors other than genes, including demographic factors such as age, gender, and body mass, as well as other environmental factors, influence blood pressure. Finally, there may also be significant interactions among susceptibility factors, with both gene-gene interactions and interactions between genes and environmental factors, with particular genes imparting effects only in particular environmental conditions. A key and unanswered question remains: Is the genetic effect on blood pressure determined by a small number of genes, each accounting for a fairly large fraction of the variation in blood pressure, or by a large number of genes, each imparting a very small effect on blood pressure?

Evidence for the multifactorial determination of blood pressure in the general population first arose from the seminal studies of Hamilton and Pickering.[10] They demonstrated that BP is a continuously distributed trait within the population, with considerable familial similarity of blood pressure. Nonetheless, they recognized that there is generally no evidence for segregation of blood pressure in the offspring of hypertensive individuals, but rather that the blood pressure distribution is shifted toward higher values among all offspring. These and other studies of blood pressure resemblances within families provide estimates of heritability of blood pressure variation that typically range from 20 to 50 percent.[10,44–46] Similar conclusions can be reached through adoption and twin studies, which further validate the contribution of genetic factors to BP variation.[10] That this familial resemblance is likely attributable to the effects of shared genes rather than shared environments alone is supported by adoption studies that document greater similarity in blood pressure among biologic than among adoptive sibs living in the same household. Twin adoption studies yield similar results, with monozygotic twins, whether reared together or apart, showing greater BP concordance than do dizygotic twins.[10,47–52] Taken together, these studies provide strong evidence for an effect of genes on blood pressure in the general population; however, they do not settle the question of how many genes influence the trait, nor the magnitude of the effect imparted by any single locus. These confounding elements introduce substantial uncertainty to the best approaches to identification of underlying genes contributing to blood pressure variation.

That variation in single genes can indeed influence blood pressure has been conclusively demonstrated by the study of Mendelian disorders that dramatically alter BP homeostasis.

## MENDELIAN FORMS OF BLOOD PRESSURE VARIATION

Although rare, kindreds with these disorders can provide valuable insight into primary determinants that can alter blood pressure in humans, and that can identify pathways that when altered influence blood pressure in humans. Moreover, these studies can identify new targets for development of new antihypertensive agents. It is important to point out that these agents may be applicable to the treatment of hypertension in the general population, regardless of the role of inherited variation in the target and pathway in the general population. The studies of these Mendelian diseases follow a stereotypic path of positional cloning or identification of candidates from physiological studies. The identification of independent mutations in the same gene in different disease families that alter the function of the encoded gene product, that segregate with the disease, and that show specificity for the disease constitutes proof that a disease gene has been identified. To date, these studies have led to the identification of mutations in seven genes that cause early severe hypertension, and mutations in nine genes that push affected individuals to the opposite extreme of the blood pressure distribution, causing lower blood pressure (Table 211-1).

Intriguingly, all mutations underlying known Mendelian forms of hyper- or hypotension converge on a final common pathway, altering renal salt homeostasis. This pathway is critical for regulating intravascular volume. The kidneys normally filter up to 1.5 kg of salt per day, and maintenance of homeostasis on a 5-g salt diet consequently requires reabsorption of more than 99.5 percent of the filtered load. This homeostatic system has many components (Fig. 211-1). There are four principal pathways of renal salt reabsorption. Sixty percent of a filtered salt load is reabsorbed in the proximal tubule, mostly by Na/H exchange. Thirty percent is reabsorbed in the thick ascending limb of Henle's loop, with apical salt entry mediated by the Na-K-2Cl cotransporter, *NKCC2*. This cotransporter is the normal target for loop diuretics such as furosemide. Seven percent of a filtered load is reabsorbed by the Na-Cl cotransporter encoded by the *NCCT* gene in the distal convoluted tubule; this cotransporter is the target for thiazide diuretics. The last 2 percent of a filtered load is reabsorbed by the action of the epithelial sodium channel (ENaC) of the distal nephron. While ENaC mediates reabsorption of only a small fraction of the filtered salt load, its action is normally the major determinant of net salt balance, as this is the main regulated step.

The principal regulator of ENaC activity is the renin-angiotensin system acting through the effector hormone aldosterone. Renin secretion from cells of the juxtaglomerular apparatus of the kidney leads to increased formation of the peptide hormone angiotensin II (AII). By binding to its specific receptor in the adrenal glomerulosa, AII leads to increased secretion of the steroid

**Table 211-1** Clinical Features of Mendelian Forms of Human High and Low Blood Pressure

**HYPERTENSIVE DISORDERS**
**Glucocorticoid-remediable aldosteronism**
Autosomal dominant transmission
High or normal aldosterone levels
Suppressed plasma renin activity
Variable hypokalemic alkalosis
High levels of 18-hydroxy and 18-oxocortisol
Regulation of aldosterone secretion by ACTH

**Liddle syndrome**
Autosomal dominant transmission
Suppressed plasma renin activity
Suppressed aldosterone secretion
Variable hypokalemic alkalosis

**Syndrome of apparent mineralocorticoid excess**
Autosomal recessive transmission
Suppressed plasma renin activity
Suppressed aldosterone secretion
Hypokalemic alkalosis
Elevated cortisol:cortisone ratio

**Pseudohypoaldosteronism type II**
Autosomal dominant transmission
Hyperkalemia with normal GFR
Suppressed plasma renin activity
Renal tubular acidosis

**Steroid 11β-hydroxylase deficiency**
Autosomal recessive transmission
Hypokalemic metabolic alkalosis
Virilizing

**Steroid 17α-hydroxylase deficiency**
Autosomal recessive transmission
Hypokalemic metabolic alkalosis
Feminization (males) or lack of sexual maturation (females)

**Hypertension plus brachydactyly**
Autosomal dominant transmission
Brachydactyly
Abnormal sympathetic outflow

**HYPOTENSIVE DISORDERS**
**Pseudohypoaldosteronism type I**
Autosomal recessive or dominant transmission
Renal salt wasting
Hyperkalemia
Metabolic acidosis
Elevated plasma renin activity
Elevated aldosterone levels

**Steroid 21-hydroxylase deficiency**
Autosomal recessive transmission
Hyperkalemia and salt wasting
Androgen excess (virilizing in females, accelerated maturation in males)

**Gitelman syndrome**
Autosomal recessive transmission
Renal salt wasting
Hypokalemic alkalosis
Elevated plasma renin activity
Elevated aldosterone
Hypomagnesemia
Hypocalciuria

**Bartter syndrome**
Autosomal recessive transmission
Renal salt wasting
Hypokalemic alkalosis
Elevated plasma renin activity
Elevated aldosterone
Hypercalciuria

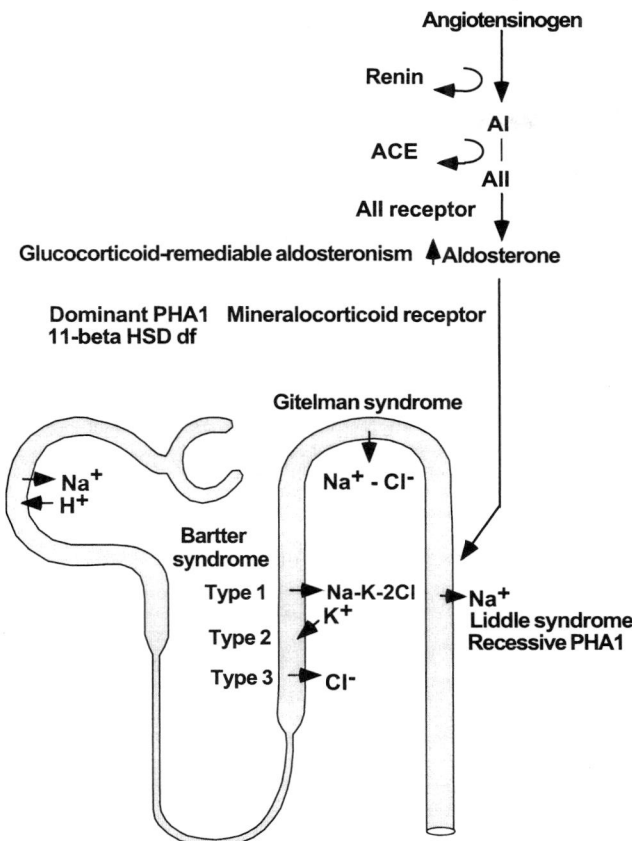

**Fig. 211-1** Mutations that alter renal salt handling. A diagram of a nephron is shown, and major mediators of renal salt reabsorption are shown. These include $Na^+/H^+$ exchange in the proximal tubule, $Na^+$-$K^+$-$2Cl^-$ cotransport in the thick ascending limb of Henle, Na-Cl cotransport in the distal convoluted tubule, and electrogenic $Na^+$ reabsorption via the epithelial sodium channel (ENaC). The role of the renin-angiotensin system in the regulation of salt homeostasis is indicated. Renin, secreted by cells of the juxtaglomerular apparatus, cleaves angiotensinogen to angiotensin I, which is further processed by angiotensin-converting enzyme (ACE) to the active hormone angiotensin II. Angiotensin II binds to specific receptors in the adrenal glomerulosa, resulting in increased secretion of the steroid hormone aldosterone. Aldosterone binds to mineralocorticoid receptors in principal cells, leading to increased activity of the epithelial sodium channel. Diseases caused by mutations in genes of these pathways are indicated.

hormone aldosterone. Aldosterone binding to the mineralocorticoid receptor in principal cells of the distal nephron results in increased ENaC activity, increasing net reabsorption of salt. The finding that mutations in many of the components of this system alter blood pressure, establishes alteration in renal salt handling as one fundamental mechanism for altering blood pressure in humans.

## Mendelian Forms of Hypertension

**Glucocorticoid-Remediable Aldosteronism (GRA).** GRA (also known as dexamethasone-suppressible aldosteronism) was one of the first investigated disorders that featured early onset of hypertension. Affected individuals have normal or elevated aldosterone levels despite suppressed plasma renin activity. Hypokalemia and metabolic alkalosis are variable findings. In addition, these patients have two features that make them unique: First, they secrete high levels of 18-hydroxycortisol and 18-oxocortisol, steroids that are secreted in negligible amounts by normal individuals.[53] Second, the secretion of aldosterone in these patients is positively regulated by adrenocorticotrophic hormone

(ACTH), rather than the usual secretagogue for aldosterone, angiotensin II. Consequently, the secretion of aldosterone can be almost completely suppressed by administration of glucocorticoids.

Recognized from its original description as a familial disorder, analysis of an extended kindred revealed that GRA is transmitted as an autosomal dominant trait with virtually complete penetrance of the high levels of 18-oxocortisol secretion. Identification of this single informative family permitted molecular genetic studies of this disease, using the abnormal steroid secretion as a Mendelian phenotype for analysis of linkage. Comparison of the inheritance of chromosome segments to the inheritance of this biochemical abnormality demonstrated precise cosegregation of GRA with a segment of chromosome 8 that normally contains two genes involved in adrenal steroid biosynthesis, aldosterone synthase and steroid 11-beta hydroxylase.[55] Aldosterone synthase mediates the two-step enzymatic conversion of corticosterone to aldosterone by oxidation of carbon 18. The gene encoding this enzyme is normally expressed in the adrenal glomerulosa under control of angiotensin II, and is not normally expressed in the adrenal fasciculata. The second gene encodes steroid 11-beta hydroxylase; this enzyme is used in the biosynthesis of cortisol in the adrenal fasciculata, and its expression is positively regulated by ACTH in adrenal fasciculata. These two genes lie in close proximity on chromosome 8, separated by only 45,000 base pairs with the same transcriptional orientation, with aldosterone synthase lying 5′ to 11-hydroxylase[56] (Fig. 211-2). These two genes recently evolved from a common ancestral gene and as a consequence show remarkable similarities in structure: the two genes share identical intron-exon organization and also share a remarkable 95 percent identity in DNA sequence across the coding region.[56] The striking similarity between these two genes is underscored by the observation that alteration of only two amino acids encoded in exon 5 are sufficient to confer 18-oxidase enzymatic activity to an otherwise normal 11-hydroxylase gene product.[58]

The finding of complete linkage of GRA to the chromosome segment containing these two genes suggested that the mutations causing this disease might lie in these genes. This has proved to be the case in this first family as well as all other GRA kindreds. The chromosome segments segregating with GRA contain three genes instead of the normal two: in addition to the two normal genes, there is a third chimeric gene that fuses the head of 11-beta hydroxylase gene onto the body of the aldosterone synthase gene (Fig. 211-2). This mutation arises from an aberrant recombination event, unequal crossing over between these highly similar genes. One of the progeny chromosomes of such an event will carry three genes instead of two.

From the structure of the duplicated gene, the pathogenesis of GRA can be deduced. Owing to the 5′ regulatory sequences from 11-beta hydroxylase, the chimeric gene is expressed in adrenal fasciculata under control of ACTH. However, by virtue of coding sequences from aldosterone synthase, including the critical residues in exon 5, the encoded protein will have aldosterone synthase enzymatic activity. The consequence is that aldosterone synthase enzymatic activity, normally confined to adrenal glomerulosa, is ectopically produced in adrenal fasciculata under control of the wrong hormone, ACTH (Fig. 211-3).

The physiological consequences of this event are predictable. This ectopic expression leads to aldosterone synthesis and secretion from adrenal fasciculata. This aldosterone secretion activates the mineralocorticoid receptor, leading to increased renal salt reabsorption by increasing the activity of the ENaC of the distal nephron; this is accompanied by increased water reabsorption to maintain normal sodium concentration in blood, resulting in expanded plasma volume. In turn, this leads to increased venous blood return to the heart, with consequent increased cardiac output, which by Ohm's law results in a rise in blood pressure.

This physiological sequence leads to counterregulatory mechanisms. The increased renal blood flow arising from the increased cardiac output leads to increased chloride delivery to the

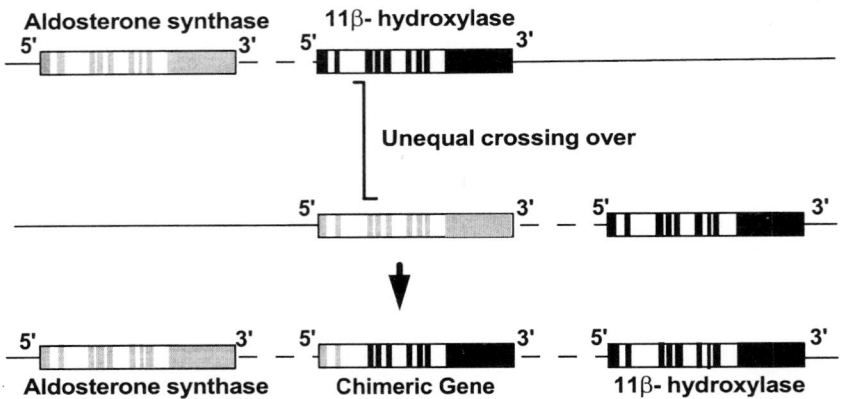

**Fig. 211-2** Glucocorticoid-remediable aldosteronism (GRA) is caused by a gene duplication affecting expression of the gene encoding aldosterone synthase. A diagram of the genomic organization of the genes encoding aldosterone synthase (*CYP11B2*) and steroid 11β-hydroxylase (*CYP11B1*) is shown. The genes have the same transcriptional orientation and identical intron-exon organization, and are separated from one another by only 45,000 base pairs on chromosome 8. Gene duplication arising from unequal crossing over between these two highly homologous genes causes GRA. In all cases, these duplicated genes fuse 5′ sequences from aldosterone synthase to distal coding sequences from aldosterone synthase, with exon 5 and beyond always derived from aldosterone synthase. The result is that the chimeric gene is expressed like the normal steroid 11β-hydroxylase gene in adrenal fasciculata but has aldosterone synthase enzymatic activity.

juxtaglomerular apparatus, with consequent suppression of secretion of active renin, and diminished formation of angiotensin II. While this turns off aldosterone secretion from adrenal glomerulosa, it does diminish secretion from adrenal fasciculata, where ACTH regulates aldosterone secretion. Consequently, at the expense of maintaining normal cortisol secretion, ACTH stimulation results in obligatory secretion of aldosterone, resulting in sustained hypertension.

The hypokalemia and metabolic alkalosis seen in affected patients can also be attributed to known physiology. ENaC is an electrogenic sodium channel, and an increase in its activity provides an increased electrical gradient for the renal secretion of $K^+$ and $H^+$, resulting in decreased concentrations of these ions in serum.

The mutations causing GRA can also explain the production of aberrant steroids by these patients. Upon its expression in adrenal fasciculata, aldosterone synthase can use cortisol as a substrate, accounting for the production of 18-hydroxycortisol and 18-oxocortisol; these steroids have both the 17-hydroxyl groups typical of glucocorticoids and oxidation at carbon 18, which is characteristic of the action of aldosterone synthase. Finally, as this mutation results in a genetic gain of function, this mutation explains the autosomal dominant transmission of GRA.

All kindreds with the GRA phenotype studied to date have chimeric gene duplications. This has led to use of a simple direct genetic test for these mutations that can easily be applied to DNA prepared from a small venous blood sample.[56] This test has extremely high sensitivity and specificity for the disease, is accurate regardless of concurrent treatment, and does not require patients to undergo further clinical evaluation.

This test has been applied to a cohort of patients referred for testing due to suspicion of an inherited form of hypertension. The

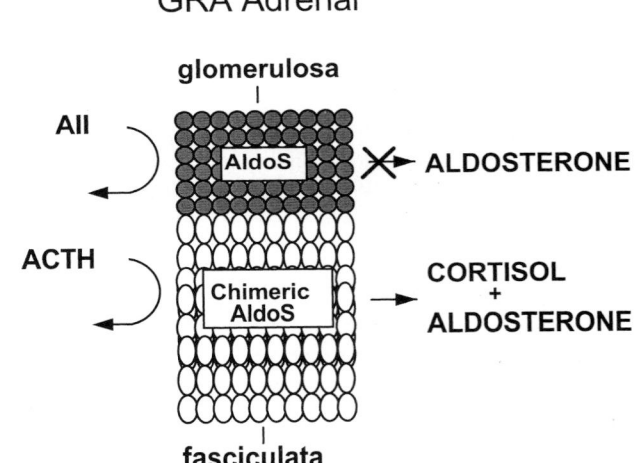

**Fig. 211-3** Ectopic secretion of aldosterone from adrenal fasciculata in glucocorticoid-remediable aldosteronism. Diagrams of the normal and GRA adrenal glands are shown. In the normal adrenal, angiotensin II (AII) stimulates secretion of aldosterone from adrenal glomerulosa through its action to increase expression of aldosterone synthase; adrenocorticotropic hormone (ACTH) increases secretion of cortisol from adrenal fasciculata via effects on the steroid 11β-hydroxylase gene. In the GRA adrenal, ACTH drives expression of the chimeric gene in adrenal fasciculata, with the consequence that aldosterone synthase enzymatic activity is ectopically produced in this part of the adrenal. The resulting volume expansion suppresses formation of AII; however, the coupling of aldosterone secretion to ACTH leads to sustained aldosterone secretion and hypertension. The abnormal steroids seen in affected patients, 18-hydroxycortisol and 18-oxocortisol, result from aldosterone synthase having access to cortisol as a substrate.

results have identified a substantial number of new kindreds with GRA, and because this is a dominant disease, many gene carriers have been identified within each kindred. Identification of gene carriers has permitted assessment of the impact of inheriting this mutation on blood pressure and clinical outcome. The results demonstrate that on average, inheritance of this gene imparts a large effect on systolic and diastolic blood pressure, averaging about 30 mm Hg. Knowledge of the underlying basis for this disease led to the ability to offer more tailored treatment of the hypertension seen in affected individuals. These patients are often labeled as having refractory hypertension; however, they generally respond well to treatment tailored to the underlying molecular defect. Treatment with salt restriction and amiloride, an ENaC antagonist, is effective, as is spironolactone. Replacement doses of exogenous glucocorticoids can turn off secretion of ACTH, thereby diminishing expression of the mutant gene and suppressing aldosterone secretion. This "pharmacologic gene therapy" can be effective, but requires careful attention to dosing of glucocorticoids.

One morbid clinical outcome predominates among GRA cases—cerebral hemorrhage before age 45. Such events have been documented in many GRA patients, a striking increase in prevalence compared with the general population.[59] Several of these hemorrhages have been documented as arising from berry aneurysms. These observations may motivate early screening for these aneurysms in affected patients.

**11-Beta Hydroxysteroid Dehydrogenase Deficiency (Apparent Mineralocorticoid Excess Syndrome).** The syndrome of apparent mineralocorticoid excess (AME), now recognized as due to 11-beta hydroxysteroid dehydrogenase (11BHSD) deficiency, results from the activation of the mineralocorticoid receptor by a nonphysiological agonist, the steroid hormone cortisol.[60,61] This is an autosomal recessive trait. Affected patients have early onset of hypertension with hypokalemia and metabolic alkalosis despite suppressed plasma renin activity and very-low aldosterone secretion. Efficacy of antagonists of the mineralocorticoid receptor in reducing blood pressure suggested a circulating mineralocorticoid as the cause of this disease; however, no abnormal steroids were identified in the serum of these patients. Nonetheless, two unique biochemical abnormalities were identified. Affected patients proved to have a strikingly elevated ratio of cortisol:cortisone in the urine.[60,61] They also had a prolonged serum half-life of cortisol. These findings of altered cortisol metabolism raised the possibility that cortisol might be acting as a mineralocorticoid in AME, consistent with a deficiency in the enzyme required for conversion of cortisol to cortisone, 11BHSD; however, the mechanism by which deficiency of this enzyme would produce increased mineralocorticoid receptor activity remained obscure.

A key to this puzzle came with the cloning of the gene encoding the mineralocorticoid receptor.[61] In vivo cortisol, circulating at concentrations up to one thousandfold higher than aldosterone, has weak mineralocorticoid activity. It consequently appeared paradoxical that in vitro cortisol proved to bind and activate the mineralocorticoid receptor with potency very similar to that of aldosterone. This paradox was resolved by the realization that in vivo activation of the mineralocorticoid receptor by cortisol is prevented by 11BHSD. 11BHSD is highly expressed in kidney, and normally oxidizes cortisol to the inactive metabolite cortisone, thereby "protecting" the receptor from activation by cortisol.

These observations predicted that patients with AME would have mutations in 11BHSD, which proved true. Cloning of the 11BHSD2 gene led to identification of a variety of loss-of-function mutations in this gene in affected patients.[59] This deficiency impairs conversion of cortisol to cortisone in the kidney, explaining the high cortisol:cortisone ratio. It also permits cortisol to act as a potent MR agonist, resulting in increased renal salt reabsorption and consequent hypertension.

The observation that under some circumstances cortisol can be a potent mineralocorticoid also explains the hypertension seen in several other disorders. For example, it was initially surprising that patients with loss-of-function mutations in the glucocorticoid receptor have marked hypertension.[64] This is explained by the extremely high cortisol levels seen in these patients; these very high levels outstrip the ability of 11BHSD to convert cortisol to cortisone, and cortisol again becomes a potent MR agonist in vivo. The hypertension seen in Cushing syndrome of cortisol excess may also be explained by this mechanism. Finally, the ability of compounds such as glycyrrhetinic acid produced from ingestion of natural licorice to inhibit 11BHSD activity accounts for the increased activation of the mineralocorticoid receptor and the hypertension resulting from their ingestion.[65]

**Hypertensive Congenital Adrenal Hyperplasia (CAH).** These autosomal recessive disorders arise from deficiencies of key adrenal enzymes in the steroid hormone biosynthetic pathway.[61] Interruption of cortisol synthesis leads to increased ACTH release, which produces adrenal hyperplasia, stimulation of the steroid biosynthetic pathway, and diversion of steroid precursors into functional pathways proximal to the block. The position of enzymatic block determines which precursors accumulate, and accounts for the presence of hyper- or hypotension and additional clinical features. Steroid 21-hydroxyl groups are normally required for activation of the mineralocorticoid receptor. Consequently, enzymatic defects proximal to this step (e.g., 21α-hydroxylase deficiency) prevent formation of active mineralocorticoids and result in salt wasting and hypotension. Conversely, mutations that impair formation of cortisol but that produce high levels of 21-hydroxylated steroids (e.g., 11β-hydroxylase or 17α-hydroxylase deficiency) lead to accumulation of precursors with mineralocorticoid activity resulting in hypertension. Additional clinical features are determined by the effects of the enzymatic defects on androgen production, with either an increase (21-hydroxylase and 11β-hydroxylase deficiency) or decrease (17α-hydroxylase) in production of these hormones.

*17α-Hydroxylase Deficiency.* This form of CAH is characterized by a[FES6] deficient conversion of pregnenolone into progesterone and androgens, resulting in absent sex hormone production.[66] Males develop feminization and pseudohermaphroditism, while females develop amenorrhea and sexual infantilism. In addition, accumulation of DOC leads to mineralocorticoid-dependent hypertension with hypokalemic metabolic alkalosis. Aldosterone levels are reduced because excess mineralocorticoid receptor stimulation leads to suppression of the renin-angiotensin axis, the main physiological regulator of aldosterone synthesis. The disease is usually diagnosed in adolescence when affected individuals fail to undergo puberty.

Many mutations in the 17α-hydroxylase (CYP17) gene on 10q24 have been described. They range from complete loss-of-function mutations to missense mutations that reduce activity.[67–69] Interestingly, CYP17 also has 17,20 lyase activity, catalyzing the conversion 17OH-pregnenolone into DHEA. A subset of patients has isolated 17,20 lyase deficiency due to mutations that selectively ablate 17,20 lyase activity required for formation of sex hormones.[70] Individuals with this subtype have intact glucocorticoid and mineralocorticoid synthesis but deficient sex hormone synthesis. Thus, blood pressure is normal but feminization occurs in males described with this subtype. The treatment for 17α-hydroxylase deficiency consists of glucocorticoid administration. In addition, women may require sex hormone administration.

*11β-Hydroxylase Deficiency.* 11β-hydroxylase deficiency results in cortisol deficiency, and accumulation of 18-deoxycortisol, deoxycorticosterone (DOC), and androgens.[70] Increased DOC leads to hypertension in a significant fraction of affected individuals with hypokalemic metabolic alkalosis due to activation of the mineralocorticoid receptor. In addition, increased androgen production results in virilizing from infancy, prompting diagnostic investigation. The diagnosis is made by finding elevated plasma

18-deoxycortisol and DOC. Occasionally, female gender is not recognized and some affected females are reared as males until puberty. This disorder has an increased prevalence in Saudi Arabia and in both Moroccan and Iranian Jews.[73]

11β-Hydroxylase deficiency is a recessive trait caused by complete or partial loss-of-function mutations in the 11β-hydroxylase gene on chromosome 8.[71–73] The usual treatment for this disorder consists of exogenous corticosteroids, which turn off secretion of ACTH, leading to reduced androgen and mineralocorticoid synthesis. Reduced mineralocorticoid production can cause some mild salt wasting, but this can be corrected by salt supplementation as needed.[71]

**Gain-of-Function Mutations in the Mineralocorticoid Receptor (MR).** The pathophysiology of GRA and 11BHSD deficiency indicate that increased activity of the mineralocorticoid receptor by any number of mechanisms is capable of leading to hypertension. These observations lead to the finding that gain-of-function mutations in the mineralocorticoid receptor itself might result in hypertension.[75] Analysis of the MR in a patient with early severe hypertension identified a mutation substituting leucine for the normal serine at codon 810 of the gene. Clinical investigation of this 15-year-old male revealed that he had suppressed renin, low aldosterone levels, and hypokalemic alkalosis, consistent with activation of the receptor. Interestingly, amino acid S810 is conserved among all members of the MR family from *Xenopus* to humans, supporting the potential functional significance of this variant.

Family studies strongly supported the significance of this mutation, revealing that all members of this family who inherited L810 had been diagnosed with hypertension before age 20, while this phenotype was absent among those who inherited two wild-type copies of MR.

Biochemical studies of the wild-type and mutant receptor in mammalian cells revealed that the mutant MR had 27 percent of maximal activity in the absence of any added steroid, consistent with either constitutive activity or activation by an endogenous ligand. Moreover, the mutant receptor was also activated by progesterone, a steroid that normally binds, but does not activate, MR. Similarly, normal antagonists of MR, such as spironolactone, also activated the mutant receptor.

Interestingly, the two women in the pedigree who have undergone pregnancy have had extremely difficult to manage hypertension throughout their pregnancies, and both had been advised not to become pregnant again. This observation is consistent with progesterone acting as an MR agonist in vivo.

These observations indicate that alteration of this single amino acid in MR results in constitutive activity and altered steroid specificity. The mechanism by which steroids that normally bind but do not activate the receptor become agonists is presently unknown.

**Liddle Syndrome.** Liddle syndrome is a rare disorder characterized by autosomal dominant transmission of early, and often severe, hypertension associated with hypokalemic metabolic alkalosis, low plasma renin activity, and suppressed aldosterone secretion.[76] The hypertension in affected patients is not ameliorated by antagonists of the mineralocorticoid receptor, but can be improved by a low-salt diet in conjunction with antagonists of ENaC. Moreover, the clinical and biochemical features of this disease can be corrected by renal transplantation, indicating that Liddle syndrome is a primary renal disease.[77]

The characterization of the extended kindred originally identified by Liddle in the 1960s provided the opportunity to perform genetic studies of this disease. In this family, the diagnosis of hypertension before the age of 20 was used as the phenotype for linkage studies, and eventually a segment of chromosome 16 was shown to completely cosegregate with early hypertension in this family, providing odds of over 1 billion to 1 in favor of this chromosome segment containing the gene for Liddle syndrome.[78] In parallel, subunits of ENaC were cloned and the channel was shown to be composed of three subunits of similar structure— each spans the plasma membrane twice with intracellular N- and C-termini. Genes encoding these subunits were localized on the human genetic map, demonstrating that the beta and gamma subunits localized to the same segment of chromosome 16 to which the gene for Liddle syndrome was linked. Ultimately, different families with Liddle syndrome were shown to harbor mutations in either the beta or the gamma ENaC subunits.[78,79] All of these initial mutations had the same consequence—they introduced premature termination codons or frameshift mutations in the cytoplasmic C-terminus of either the beta or gamma subunits, thereby eliminating the last 45 to 75 amino acids from the subunits (Fig. 211-4).

From the nature of the phenotype of patients harboring these mutations, it can be inferred that these mutations in some fashion increase renal sodium reabsorption. Expression of ENaC that contains mutant subunits demonstrated that this is the case.[81] When expressed in oocytes of the toad *Xenopus laevis*, mutant ENaC shows markedly increased amiloride-sensitive sodium current compared with oocytes expressing wild-type ENaC. To determine whether loss of specific amino acids accounts for this

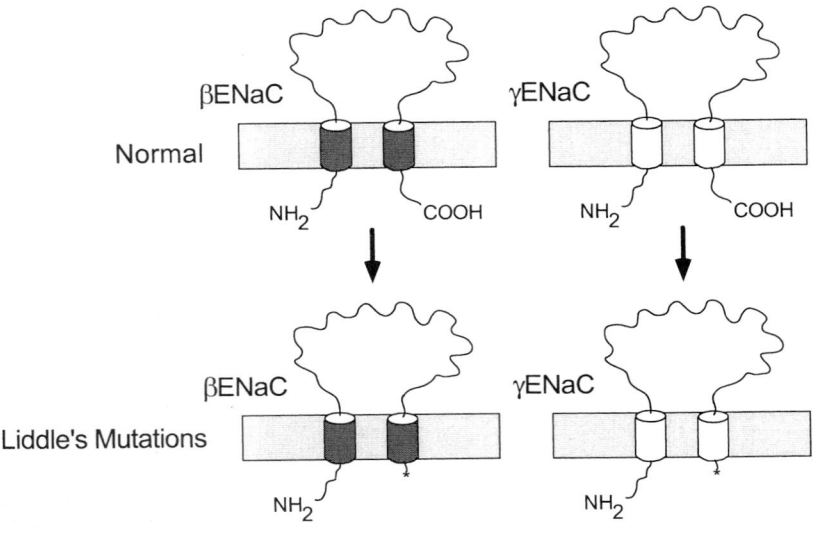

**Fig. 211-4** Mutations in the beta or gamma subunits of the epithelial sodium channel (ENaC) cause Liddle syndrome. ENaC is composed of three subunits, each of which has two membrane-spanning domains, a large extracellular loop, and short intracytoplasmic N- and C-termini. In all cases, Liddle syndrome is caused by mutations in either the beta or gamma ENaC subunit. These mutations either remove the last 45 to 75 amino acids from the C-terminus or alter single amino acids in the TPPPXY sequence conserved between these two subunits.

activation, each amino acid of the C-terminus of beta ENaC was systematically replaced with alanine and the activity of channels containing these mutant channels was tested. The results demonstrated that the only mutations that increased channel activity were those that altered amino acids of a short segment shared by the beta and gamma ENaC subunits TPPPXY.[83,84] These observations suggested that this segment is required for the normal regulation of ENaC activity, and that mutations that alter this segment acquire increased channel activity. Strong clinical corroboration of this finding came from identification of *de novo* missense mutations in ENaC in patients with Liddle syndrome; those identified to date all alter one of these same residues.[83,84]

It is noteworthy that the identified target sequence for Liddle syndrome bears similarity to the NPXY sequence initially identified in the LDL receptor as being required for the clearance of this receptor from the cell surface by endocytosis via clathrin-coated pits. This observation raised the possibility that Liddle mutations might remove this signal for clearance of ENaC from the cell surface, leading to an increased number of active channels at the cell surface. Consistent with this notion, the number of ENaC channels at the surface of oocytes expressing mutant ENaC is increased[85,86] and the cell surface half-life of mutant ENaC is markedly prolonged when compared with wild-type ENaC.[78]

If wild-type ENaC is being cleared by clathrin-mediated endocytosis, then a specific inhibitor of this process should result in prolongation of half-life and increased channel activity, producing a phenocopy of the mutant ENaC causing Liddle syndrome. It has been shown that normal activity of the protein dynamin is required for the final step in internalization of clathrin-coated pits; moreover, a well-characterized dominant negative dynamin mutation specifically arrests endocytosis via clathrin-coated pits. Expression of this dominant negative dynamin in cells expressing wild-type ENaC produces an increase in amiloride-sensitive sodium flux, an increase in the number of active channels, and a prolongation of active ENaC half-life indistinguishable from that seen with ENaC mutations found in Liddle syndrome.[78] These findings strongly suggest that the hypertension seen in patients with Liddle syndrome is attributable to an inability to normally clear ENaC from the apical surface of principal cells, resulting in increased salt balance and leading to hypertension (Fig. 211-5).

It is of further interest that a ubiquitously expressed protein, Nedd-4, contains multiple WW domains that mediate protein-protein interaction and shows highly specific binding to the PPPXY sequence of beta and gamma ENaC.[87] Nedd-4 also

contains a ubiquitin ligase domain, suggesting that Nedd-4 has a role in protein degradation. Dominant-negative Nedd-4 mutations, like dynamin mutations, lead to increased ENaC activity by prolonging half-life at the cell surface.[88] It is presently unclear whether Nedd-4 is involved in the recruitment of ENaC to clathrin-coated pits or whether it acts independently of this pathway.

In addition to these effects of Liddle mutations on the number of channels at the cell surface, there is also evidence that these mutations have independent effects on the open probability of ENaC.[89]

These findings establish that increased activity of ENaC in the absence of circulating mineralocorticoids can produce hypertension in humans.

**Pseudohypoaldosteronism Type II (PHA-II).** PHA-II is characterized by hypertension with hyperkalemia despite normal glomerular filtration. Renal tubular acidosis, hyperchloremia, and suppressed plasma renin activity are associated findings.[90] Thiazide diuretics correct these physiological abnormalities. Clinical studies show that these abnormalities are dependent on the reabsorption of sodium with chloride; if sodium is administered with sulfate as the anion, then the physiological abnormalities are corrected.

Study of eight families with this disease revealed a pattern of transmission that is consistent with autosomal dominant inheritance. Analysis of linkage in these kindreds demonstrated that the disease cannot be accounted for by mutation in the same gene in all families. Instead, the results indicate locus heterogeneity, with mutations in two different genes accounting for disease in different families, and disease in all families attributable to one of these two genes. One of these genes is located at chromosome 1q31-42, while the other lies on chromosome 17 at 17p11-q21.[91]

The identity of the underlying genes causing this disease is presently unknown. Nonetheless, it is intriguing that the chromosome 17 interval overlaps the syntenic interval of rat chromosome 10 that contains a blood pressure quantitative trait locus (QTL). Moreover, subsequent linkage studies of patients with essential hypertension suggest linkage of essential hypertension to this same chromosome interval. These observations raise the intriguing possibility that all of these loci reflect underlying mutations in orthologous genes, motivating identification of the PHA-II locus by positional cloning. Attainment of the human genome sequence will provide substrate for performing a gene-by-gene study of genes in the interval for mutations underlying PHA-II.

**Hypertension with Brachydactyly.** Hypertension with brachydactyly is a rare familial syndrome characterized by early onset of severe hypertension with shortening of phalanges and metacarpals. It was first described in a Turkish kindred residing on the northern end of the Black Sea coast. The disease is transmitted as an autosomal dominant trait with high penetrance.[92] The hypertension is not associated with any distinguishing features, such as electrolyte disturbance, salt sensitivity, or insulin resistance, and there are no other skeletal abnormalities.[92] Affected individuals exhibit a relative paucity of hypertensive end-organ damage.[92] However, MRI studies of the brain demonstrate pica loops in the posterior/inferior cerebellar arteries in affected individuals. At this time, it is unclear whether this feature is a primary pathogenic abnormality. Physiological studies of these patients suggest the hypertension is mediated via increased sympathetic activity, although they do not show preferential clinical response to antagonists of the adrenergic receptors.[92]

Genome-wide linkage analysis has mapped the disease locus to chromosome 12p12.2-11.2.[93] This interval does not contain any genes known to regulate blood pressure. It is interesting to note, however, that the gene for the parathyroid hormone related protein (PTH-rp) maps to 12p12. Gene-targeting studies demonstrate that loss of the PTH-rp gene in mice results in a skeletal phenotype similar to those observed in patients with this syndrome,[94] but no mutations in this gene have been detected in human kindreds with

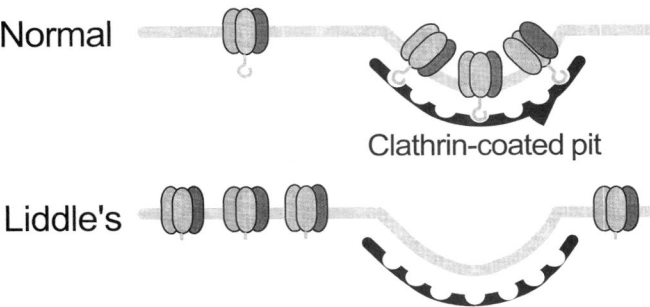

**Fig. 211-5 Increased numbers of epithelial sodium channels at the cell surface in Liddle syndrome. Mutations causing Liddle syndrome result in markedly increased numbers of channels at the cell surface, owing to a prolonged half-life of channels at the cell surface. Dominant-negative dynamin mutations result in phenocopies of Liddle syndrome, as do dominant-negative mutations of Nedd-4. Given the known role of dynamin in endocytosis via clathrin-coated pits and the known role of sequences related to the TPPPXY motif in this process, the data are consistent with the normal channel being cleared from the cell surface via this process, and Liddle syndrome resulting from failure of this normal clearance mechanism.**

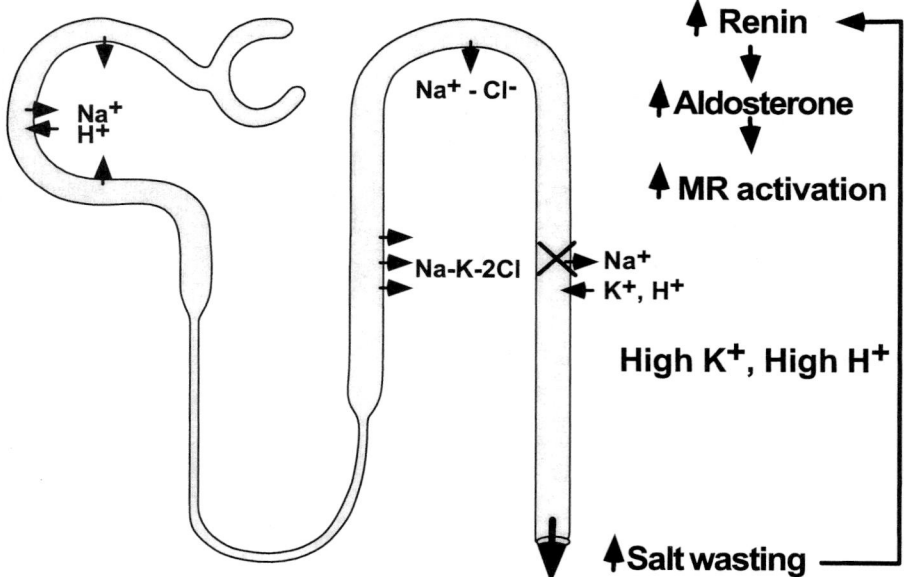

**Fig. 211-6** Pathophysiology of pseudo-hypoaldosteronism type I (PHA-I). A diagram of a nephron is shown. Recessive PHA-I is caused by mutations resulting in loss of function of the epithelial sodium channel. This leads to salt wasting and consequent activation of the renin-angiotensin system with high levels of plasma renin activity and aldosterone. This fails, however, to adequately augment renal salt reabsorption because the major target for aldosterone action, ENaC, is defective. Moreover, electrogenic $Na^+$ reabsorption via ENaC in this nephron segment provides the electrical driving force for net secretion of $K^+$ and $H^+$. The lack of normal ENaC function results in sustained renal salt wasting as well as impaired secretion of $K^+$ and $H^+$, leading to hyperkalemia and metabolic acidosis. Dominant PHA-I is caused by heterozygous loss-of-function mutations in the mineralocorticoid receptor.

this disorder. The location of the disease gene has now been narrowed to a 3-cM interval by studying additional non-Turkish kindreds with this disease, and it is likely that it will be identified soon.[95] The cloning of the gene may delineate a novel pathway for the development of hypertension in humans.

## Mendelian Forms of Hypotension

Just as there are genes that push individuals to the high end of the blood pressure distribution, there are also likely to be genes that drive blood pressures to the low end of the distribution. Identification of these genes might prove just as important in understanding mechanisms of blood pressure variation. Because of this possibility, investigators have embarked on the study of inherited forms of early severe hypotension.

**Recessive Pseudohypoaldosteronism Type I (PHA-I).** Pseudohypoaldosteronism type I is a disease of autosomal dominant, autosomal recessive, or sporadic occurrence.[96–98] This often life-threatening disease is typically characterized by severe hypotension with shock in the neonatal period in association with severe renal salt wasting despite elevated renin and aldosterone levels, hyperkalemia, and metabolic acidosis. The recessive form is typically severe and requires life-long treatment with salt supplementation and control of hyperkalemia.[98,99] In contrast, the dominant form of the disease may be severe at birth, but typically remits in the first years of life, with adult patients entirely asymptomatic, although they do have persistently elevated serum aldosterone levels.[96,100]

Investigators reasoned that because the phenotype of PHA-I looked like a mirror image of Liddle syndrome, and if Liddle syndrome is caused by gain-of-function mutations in ENaC subunits, then PHA-I might prove attributable to loss-of-function mutations in these same genes. Genetic analysis of recessive PHA-I kindreds revealed linkage to chromosome segments containing genes encoding ENaC subunits and examination of these genes identified underlying mutations in these genes. These mutations introduced premature termination codons, frameshift, and nonconservative missense mutations in ENaC residues that are conserved across long phylogenetic distances. Expression of ENaC bearing these mutations results in marked reduction in ENaC activity, indicating that these mutations result in diminished ENaC function.[101] These findings provide an explanation of the physiological and clinical features of recessive PHA-I

(Fig. 211-6). The loss of ENaC function results in salt wasting and intravascular volume depletion, which leads to increased plasma renin activity, increased formation of angiotensin II, and increased secretion of aldosterone. Although this high level of aldosterone activates the mineralocorticoid receptor, it does not appropriately augment renal sodium reabsorption because of the absence of normal ENaC, accounting for the salt wasting observed in affected patients. Importantly, sodium reabsorption via ENaC is required for establishing the electrochemical gradient permitting potassium and hydrogen ion secretion in the distal nephron. Consequently, patients deficient in ENaC activity cannot maintain normal potassium and pH homeostasis. Finally, it is noteworthy that these patients require life-long treatment for salt wasting and hyperkalemia.

In contrast to patients with recessive PHA-I, there are no mutations in ENaC subunits in patients with the dominant form of the disease.[100] As maximal activity of the epithelial sodium channel depends on aldosterone action, mutation in any gene that couples aldosterone signaling to increasing ENaC function is a logical candidate gene. The best-characterized component of this coupling mechanism is the mineralocorticoid receptor, a member of the nuclear hormone receptor family of transcription factors. Examination of this gene for mutations in kindreds with dominant PHA-I identified heterozygous premature termination, frameshift, and splice-site mutations that result in loss of function of one copy of the mineralocorticoid receptor gene. These mutations segregate with the disease and are not found among unaffected individuals, establishing that these mutations cause dominant PHA-I. In addition, some cases of sporadic PHA-I are also attributable to mutation at this locus due to *de novo* mutation.[100]

As with recessive PHA-I, the phenotype of patients with dominant PHA-I due to mutation in MR can be explained on the basis of impaired ENaC activity, in this case, secondary to an inability to adequately augment activity by stimulation with aldosterone.

The different clinical course of patients with loss-of-function mineralocorticoid receptor mutations, in contrast to that of patients with mutations that directly impair ENaC function, is illustrative. Maintenance of normal salt homeostasis in humans is highly dependent on activation of the mineralocorticoid receptor in the neonatal period, and a 50 percent decrease in receptor number cannot support normal salt homeostasis at this time. This is consistent with the very low salt content of breast milk, suggesting the need for a very efficient salt-retaining mechanism at this time. However, upon transition to the relatively high-salt diet typical of industrialized societies, dependence on aldosterone and the mineralocorticoid receptor for salt homeostasis is markedly diminished, so much so that older patients are asymptomatic and maintain normal salt homeostasis with only the biochemical trace of chronically elevated aldosterone levels.

The clinical contrast with PHA-I due to ENaC mutation is striking, as patients with ENaC mutations typically require life-long salt supplementation as well as treatment for hyperkalemia. These observations may have broad clinical relevance. Because amiloride is a poor antihypertensive diuretic agent in patients ingesting a high-salt diet, it is popularly believed that ENaC activity in this setting is normally low. If this were true, recessive PHA-I patients would be expected to be clinically normal on a typical high-salt diet. That these patients continue to have severe salt wasting that requires substantial salt supplementation and often treatment to control potassium levels, indicates that ENaC is active and required for normal salt homeostasis even on a high-salt diet. This is corroborated by biochemical studies that indicate that salt acts as a competitive antagonist with amiloride, indicating that on high-salt diets, amiloride levels are too low to inhibit ENaC. These observations indicate that new pharmacologic agents that are effective ENaC antagonists despite a high-salt diet would have potent antihypertensive diuretic activity that would be potassium sparing. Such agents might prove to be of high efficacy without the side effects that limit some other classes of antihypertensive agents.

### Hypotensive Congenital Adrenal Hyperplasia
*21-Hydroxylase Deficiency.* 21-Hydroxylase deficiency is one of the most common congenital disorders worldwide (1:15,000 live births) and comprises over 90 percent of cases of CAH.[61,71] It is caused by mutations in the steroid 21-hydroxylase (CYP21) gene, which encodes a key enzyme in cortisol synthesis. Defective activity of this enzyme leads to reduced production of the cortisol precursor, 11-deoxycortisol. This results in glucocorticoid and mineralocorticoid deficiency and virilization. The expression of the disease correlates with the activity of the enzyme and falls into distinct clinical subcategories: (a) classic salt-wasting; (b) classic virilizing; and (c) nonclassic. Patients with the classic salt-wasting form can have the most severe presentation with life-threatening hypotension and hyperkalemia at birth and prenatal virilization. The classic virilizing form presents with virilizing symptoms resulting in genital ambiguity in females and accelerated maturation in males. Finally, the nonclassic form results from partial deficiency in 21-hydroxylation. It is most commonly diagnosed in postpubertal women who present with symptoms related to hyperandrogenism such as hirsutism, oligomenorrhea, and infertility. The diagnosis is made by the detection of elevated 17-hydroxyprogesterone after ACTH stimulation.

The gene for 21-hydroxylase deficiency (CYP21) maps to 6p21, within the histocompatibility gene cluster. The gene is flanked by a nonfunctional pseudogene. The majority ( > 90 percent) of mutations in this syndrome arise from gene conversions or unequal crossing over that removes normal sequences of the bona fide gene.[102,103] Allelic variations underlying the CYP21 mutations tend to explain the clinical spectrum of disease: individuals with null mutations fall within the severe form of disease (i.e., classic salt-wasting, or classic virilizing), whereas those with missense mutations that reduce enzymatic function tend to have late-onset disease (nonclassic form).[104,105] However, considerable variation in severity of phenotype may exist within a single kindred segregating the same mutation, demonstrating that other genetic or environmental factors influence the development of disease.[106] The treatment for this condition consists of administration of corticosteroids and mineralocorticoids, which reverse the virilizing process and salt wasting.[61,71] In addition, prenatal diagnosis of disease is now available to parents with a previously diagnosed child. Prenatal treatment with dexametha-

sone can prevent the development of the virilizing and subsequent deleterious effects of hyperandrogenism.[61]

**Inherited Hypokalemic Metabolic Alkalosis without Hypertension.** Mutations that directly increase activity of ENaC all result in hypertension, and clues to the diagnosis of these patients often come from recognition of hypokalemia and metabolic alkalosis. These features arise from the increased electrical driving force for potassium and hydrogen ion secretion due to increased electrogenic sodium reabsorption via ENaC. Not all patients with inherited hypokalemic alkalosis, however, develop hypertension. In particular, patients with Gitelman and Bartter syndromes have hypokalemic alkalosis with so-called normal blood pressure. Affected patients all have renal salt wasting with high plasma renin activity and elevated aldosterone levels; this elevation in aldosterone can account for the observed hypokalemic alkalosis. However, the other clinical features seen among patients can be very diverse. For example, while some patients have low urinary calcium, others have elevated urinary calcium with or without nephrocalcinosis; some have hypomagnesemia, while others do not; some can have life-threatening disease at birth, while others are diagnosed incidentally. The uniform finding of salt wasting despite elevated aldosterone levels implied impaired renal salt handling; the finding of hypokalemic alkalosis further implied that ENaC was responding normally to aldosterone, implicating other salt-handling systems. Mutations in four different genes that underlie this trait have been identified, and the differences in the physiological functions of the underlying genes explain much of the observed variation in clinical presentation.

*Gitelman Syndrome.* Gitelman syndrome now refers to the clinical syndrome of autosomal recessive renal salt wasting with hypokalemic metabolic alkalosis, elevated plasma renin activity, and increased serum aldosterone levels in conjunction with hypomagnesemia and hypocalciuria.[106,107] Affected patients typically are diagnosed in adolescence or young adulthood with presentation including muscular pain and cramping with exercise, fatigue, and weakness. Patients rarely present in the neonatal period, and signs of intravascular volume depletion are not prominent.[108]

Genetic studies of families with this disease revealed linkage to a segment of chromosome 16 containing the gene encoding the thiazide-sensitive Na-Cl cotransporter of the distal convoluted tubule (*NCCT*).[109] Investigation of this gene in affected patients has identified a wide range of loss-of-function mutations in both copies of the gene. It appears that virtually all families with this phenotype have mutations in this gene. Studies of a large inbred kindred have demonstrated that the converse is also true, namely that virtually all patients with mutations in both copies of the gene encoding the Na-Cl cotransporter have all of the biochemical features of the disease. These findings establish that Gitelman syndrome is caused by a primary defect in renal salt reabsorption and that all of the observed clinical features must ultimately be attributable to this primary defect.

The understanding of the physiology of the Na-Cl cotransporter's role in salt homeostasis can explain many of the features of Gitelman syndrome[107,109] (Fig. 211-7). The loss-of-function mutations result in salt wasting from the distal convoluted tubule, ultimately resulting in increased aldosterone secretion, which increases $Na^+$ reabsorption via ENaC, thereby defending intravascular volume. However, because of the indirect coupling of $Na^+$ reabsorption to $K^+$ and $H^+$ secretion in the distal nephron, this augmented ENaC activity occurs at the expense of increased $K^+$ and $H^+$ secretion, accounting for the observed hypokalemia and metabolic alkalosis. These patients nonetheless have diminished net salt balance, and affected patients have reduced blood pressure compared to their unaffected relatives; this reduced blood pressure protects these individuals from development of hypertension.[110]

Other biochemical features of this disorder are surprising. These patients uniformly have hypocalciuria despite having

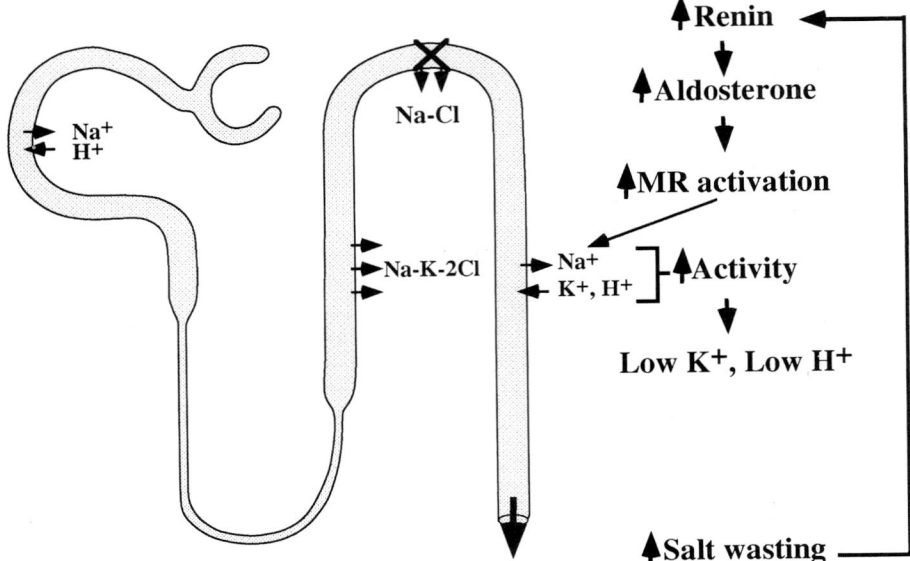

Fig. 211-7 Pathophysiology of Gitelman syndrome. A diagram of a nephron is shown. Gitelman syndrome is caused by loss-of-function mutations in the thiazide-sensitive Na-Cl cotransporter. This results in salt wasting and activation of the renin-angiotensin system. The resulting increase in electrogenic sodium reabsorption is accompanied by increased secretion of $K^+$ and $H^+$, leading to hypokalemia and metabolic alkalosis.

normal serum calcium levels.[109] Even more surprising, they also uniformly have hypomagnesemia.[109] These findings reveal unanticipated relationships between salt reabsorption in the DCT and the handling of these other electrolytes.

***Bartter Syndrome.*** Bartter syndrome now refers to a group of disorders that are unified by autosomal recessive transmission of impaired salt reabsorption in the thick ascending limb of Henle with pronounced salt wasting and hypokalemic metabolic alkalosis.[109,111] In contrast to patients with Gitelman syndrome, Bartter patients virtually always have hypercalciuria and normal magnesium levels.[108] Most affected patients present in the prenatal and neonatal period with severe intravascular volume depletion; they are often born prematurely of mothers with polyhydramnios. Prostaglandin $E_2$ levels are typically elevated. A substantial fraction of affected patients have nephrocalcinosis that can be detected at birth. Patients are often critically ill in the neonatal period, and require massive salt supplementation; treatment with cyclooxygenase inhibitors appears to have dramatic clinical benefit.

Genetic studies demonstrate that Bartter syndrome is genetically heterogeneous and have, to date, identified mutations in three different genes that cause this disease.

***Mutations in the $Na^+$-$K^+$-$2Cl^-$ Cotransporter Underlie Bartter Syndrome Type 1.*** Identification of mutations in the Na-Cl cotransporter as the basis of Gitelman syndrome, suggested the

bumetanide-sensitive $Na^+$-$K^+$-$2Cl^-$ cotransporter encoded by the gene *NKCC2* as a candidate gene for Bartter syndrome.[112,113] This cotransporter is known to be expressed on the apical surface of cells of the thick ascending limb of Henle and is the major mediator of apical salt entry in this nephron segment (Fig. 211-8). Investigators found evidence of linkage of *NKCC2* to Bartter syndrome, and then searched this gene for mutations.[114] Ultimately, a number of independent mutations that result in loss of function of the gene product that cosegregated with the disease in families were identified, demonstrating that these mutations cause the disease.[114] As for Gitelman syndrome, the salt wasting in this disorder results in activation of the renin-angiotensin system, with consequent increased distal salt reabsorption at the expense of increased renal loss of $K^+$ and $H^+$, resulting in hypokalemic alkalosis. The more severe phenotype seen in these patients compared with Gitelman syndrome can be attributed to the greater fraction of salt reabsorption mediated by this pathway. The hypercalciuria seen in these and other Bartter patients can be accounted for by the requirement of an intact salt-retaining pathway in this nephron segment for the establishment of the electrical gradient that supports paracellular $Ca^{2+}$ reabsorption.

***Mutations in the $K^+$ Channel ROMK Underlie Bartter Syndrome Type 2.*** While *NKCC2* mutations were found in some patients with Bartter syndrome, others did not have mutations in this gene, implicating other genes in this disease. Consideration of the known physiology of salt reabsorption in the TAL suggested a potential

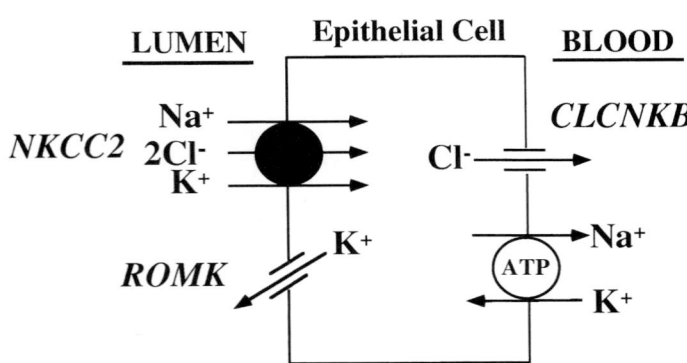

Fig. 211-8 Pathophysiology of Bartter syndrome. A diagram of a cell of the thick ascending limb of Henle is shown. Bartter syndrome is caused by mutation in any of three genes expressed in this nephron segment—the bumetanide-sensitive Na-K-2Cl cotransporter (*NKCC2*), the $K^+$ channel ROMK, or the $Cl^-$ channel (*CLCNKB*). Together these define components of the pathway by which salt is reabsorbed from the lumen and returned to the bloodstream.

candidate gene, the gene encoding the ATP-sensitive K$^+$ channel ROMK (Fig. 211-8). Fluid entering the TAL is high in sodium and chloride but low in potassium, whereas by the end of the loop, levels of sodium and chloride are much closer to that of K$^+$. Given that sodium and potassium enter cells of the TAL in nearly stoichiometric amounts, it is apparent that K$^+$ levels could be quickly depleted, long before Na$^+$ levels were reduced to the observed levels at the end of the TAL. This would place severe limits on the amount of salt that could be reabsorbed in this nephron segment. The recycling of K$^+$ back into the lumen via potassium channels permits efficient reabsorption of sodium and chloride. A candidate for this K$^+$ channel was cloned as an ATP-sensitive K$^+$ channel of the renal outer medulla, ROMK.[115,116] This gene was screened for mutations in patients with Bartter syndrome, and a subset of families who did not have mutation in *NKCC2* was found to have a loss-of-function mutation in *ROMK*.[117] This finding demonstrates the irreplaceable role of ROMK in salt reabsorption in the TAL.[117]

### Mutations in the Cl$^-$ Channel CLCKB Underlie Bartter Syndrome Type 3.

Bartter patients with mutations in NKCC2 and ROMK together account for no more than half of all Bartter patients. Linkage studies on the remaining families demonstrated that a substantial fraction was linked to a segment of chromosome 1.[118] This segment was shown to contain two genes showing high sequence similarity to the CLC family of chloride channels. These two genes, *CLCKA* and *CLCKB*, were both known to be selectively expressed in the kidney, suggesting a potential role in renal salt homeostasis.[119] The structures of these genes were determined, demonstrating that they are closely linked in genomic DNA with the same transcriptional orientation and virtually identical intron-exon organization, supporting their recent evolution from a common ancestor.[118] Examination of these genes in Bartter patients revealed loss-of-function mutations in CLCKB in a large number of kindreds.[118] In addition to premature termination, frameshift, and missense mutations, many of these mutations are deletions that remove a substantial number of exons of this gene. At least some of these deletions result from unequal crossing over between CLCKA and CLCKB, with Bartter alleles carrying only a single CLC gene that bears the 5' regulatory sequences from CLCKA.

These findings implicate mutations in this presumed Cl$^-$ channel in Bartter syndrome, and indicate that this gene product plays an irreplaceable role in renal salt reabsorption. Sodium and chloride entering cells of the TAL must exit across the basolateral surface to return to the bloodstream. Na$^+$ exits by the action of the Na$^+$-K$^+$ ATPase. The mode of exit of Cl$^-$ is speculated to occur by Cl$^-$ channels, K$^+$-Cl$^-$ cotransport, or both. The finding that patients with CLCKB mutations have Bartter syndrome implicates the gene product as a Cl$^-$ channel mediating Cl$^-$ exit in the TAL (Fig. 211-8). Loss of this channel would impair the ability to reabsorb Cl$^-$ at this site, resulting in a Bartter phenotype.

Together, mutations in NKCC2, ROMK, and CLCKB still do not account for all patients with Bartter syndrome, indicating that additional genes when mutated can produce this phenotype. One additional subset in which Bartter syndrome cosegregates with sensorineural deafness has been mapped to chromosome 1, but not yet identified at the molecular level.[120]

### Genotype-Phenotype Correlations in Gitelman and Bartter Syndromes.

The ability to sort patients with inherited salt wasting with hypokalemic alkalosis according to which mutant gene underlies the disease provides the opportunity to determine the extent to which variation in clinical features seen among patients can be attributed to underlying genetic differences. Briefly, Gitelman patients are separable from the others based on hypomagnesemia and hypocalciuria. Nephrocalcinosis can be diagnosed in a substantial fraction, but not all, of Bartter patients at birth, but is not seen in Gitelman syndrome.[110] This finding proves to be nearly universal among patients with mutations in NKCC2

and ROMK, but is present in only about 20 percent of patients with mutations in CLCKB.[118] This may be attributable to the lower levels of hypercalciuria seen in the latter patients. Interestingly, patients with ROMK mutations universally present at birth with hyperkalemia rather than hypokalemia; they evolve to hypokalemia within the first weeks to months of life. They do not, however, require K$^+$ supplementation like their counterparts with mutations in NKCC2 or CLCKB. These findings may be explained by the fact that ROMK, in addition to its use in K$^+$ recycling in the TAL, is also used for K$^+$ secretion in the distal nephron. As a result, these patients can be predisposed to hyperkalemia or hypokalemia depending on their age and specific environment.

These observations in Gitelman and Bartter syndromes illustrate the utility of genetic investigation to clarify the causation of diverse phenotypic features based on differences in the underlying disease genes.

## GENETIC STUDIES OF BLOOD PRESSURE VARIATION IN THE GENERAL POPULATION

In addition to these studies of Mendelian traits, efforts have been made to identify genes predisposing to hypertension in the general population. These have generally taken the form of candidate gene studies. Recently, however, a few genome-wide studies of essential hypertension have been completed. The success of linkage studies for investigation of complex traits depends largely on the number of loci influencing the trait, the frequencies of the susceptibility alleles, and the magnitude of the effect imparted by each in the population.[122] For traits with a $\lambda s = \approx 2$ to 3, such as essential hypertension, the standard affected relative-pair method alone may not be sufficiently robust.[122] To increase analytic power, investigators have offered a number of extensions to the standard affected relative-pair method (e.g., studying highly concordant or discordant sib pairs or twins), and these have been implemented in some of the studies performed to date.[123–127] Among these studies, several are of particular interest. The lack of consistent reproducibility of these studies highlights the difficulties in investigation of the genetics of multifactorial traits.

One of the best-studied candidate genes encodes angiotensinogen, and studies suggest a role for angiotensinogen variants in blood pressure variation.[128–130] Nonetheless, positive results have been found in some, but not all studies,[131,132] and it seems likely that common angiotensinogen variants account for at most a small fraction of the variance in blood pressure.[133] Jeunemaitre et al. first identified linkage of angiotensinogen to human hypertension in Caucasian subjects and found molecular variants associated with the disease.[128] They also showed that plasma levels of AGT are associated with a specific variant in this gene, M235T, in Caucasians, with subjects homozygous for the 235T mutation (TT genotype) having the highest angiotensinogen levels.[128] Since this initial study, linkage to this locus has been reexamined and confirmed in some, but not all, studies.[129–133] As the M235T variant is in strong disequilibrium with a variant at the −6 position upstream of the transcription initiation site, the −6 variant has been investigated for its potential functional effect, and has been shown to cause a modest increase in the rate of transcription initiation, suggesting a mechanism by which these variants lead to increased levels of angiotensinogen.[134] These studies underscore the difficulty in defining the contributions of genes with relatively small effect on the trait in the population.[122]

The angiotensin-converting enzyme (ACE) promotes the conversion of angiotensin I to angiotensin II and thus presents an attractive candidate gene for human hypertension. ACE was initially excluded as a candidate for human hypertension in a cohort of Caucasian subjects.[135] However, recent analysis of another Caucasian cohort from Rochester, MN indicated significant linkage of the ACE gene to BP variation in males.[136] This data was recently confirmed in the Framingham Heart Study, which examined BP as a quantitative trait in 1044 sib pairs and found evidence of linkage and association to the ACE locus in males.[137] An insertion/deletion (I/D) polymorphism of the ACE gene in intron 16 of the gene is associated with circulating ACE levels.[138] The polymorphism influences ACE levels in a codominant manner, with the D allele associated with increased levels. The D allele has been associated with a number of cardiovascular phenotypes, including coronary disease and left ventricular hypertrophy.[139,140] In the Framingham study, the DD and ID genotypes of the ACE polymorphism resulted in 1.2 to 1.6 increased odds of hypertension in men, respectively.[136] It is still unclear how this intronic variant influences ACE levels, but the mechanism may involve linkage disequilibrium with functional variants in the coding sequence of the ACE gene.[141] Thus, the relation of this gene to blood pressure variation merits further study.

Studies of 286 families from Australia and another study of 66 Caucasian dizygotic twins found evidence of linkage of systolic BP (multipoint LOD = 3.74; p = 0.001 and p = 0.01, respectively) to the chromosome 16 interval containing the subunits of the epithelial sodium channel mutated in Liddle syndrome.[141–144] Other studies in Caucasian, African Caribbean, and Chinese populations failed to detect linkage.[145,146] In addition, a polymorphism (threonine594 to methionine) in the $\beta$ subunit of ENaC was associated with hypertension in some small case-control studies, but the relevance of this polymorphism to BP variation has not been determined in a large population-based study.[147–149]

The chromosome 5q region harbors the gene for the $\alpha_1$- and $\beta_2$-adrenergic receptors and dopamine type 1A receptor. The most robust study to date examined 55 pedigrees with sibs discordant for BP and found modest evidence of linkage (multipoint linkage p = 0.0163) using quantitative BP levels.[154] The evidence was strongest near the $\alpha_1$-adrenergic receptor and dopamine type 1A receptor. Other studies have found evidence of linkage or association of the $\beta_2$-adrenergic receptor with a number of BP-related phenotypes, including salt sensitivity, but the results are not uniform.[155–157]

Few studies have performed genome-wide scans to search for blood pressure loci. Xu et al. performed a genome-wide screen in 564 Chinese sib pairs (concordant and discordant for BP level) but did not find any loci with significant evidence of linkage.[154] Further analysis of one suggestive region on 15q yielded a LOD score of 3.77 in subset of 53 concordant sib pairs, using an age- and weight-adjusted BP phenotype.[155] Interestingly, this 15q region was also identified (p = 0.0033) in a genome-wide scan of 53 Caucasian kindreds from Rochester, MN, selected based on having a sib pair discordant for BP level.[156] This study identified three other loci on chromosomes 5q, 6q, and 2p. However, only a locus on 6q was close to genome-wide significance levels (p = $9 \times 10^{-5}$). In addition, loci suggestive of linkage did not coincide with previously identified candidate regions.

One persistently interesting interval is a segment of chromosome 17 in humans that is syntenic to a segment of chromosome 10 in rat. This interval contains a blood pressure QTL in rat,[156,157] and the syntenic interval of chromosome 17 in human contains one of the genes for PHA-II.[91] Julier et al. examined this interval in 518 Caucasian sib pairs and found evidence suggestive of linkage 18 cM proximal to the ACE locus, although these results were not significant at the genome-wide level.[159] This locus was also tested in a smaller sample of 125 hypertensive Caucasian sib pairs and again resulted in suggestive evidence of linkage (p = $5 \times 10^{-4}$).[161] The gene(s) underlying this linkage have not been identified, but the evidence favors the existence of a BP locus in this interval. It is tempting to speculate that all of these linkages might reflect variants in the same underlying orthologous gene.

Review of these studies indicates many of the difficulties in identification of genes for multifactorial traits. In general, the studies performed have low power for linkage because of relatively small numbers of families studied, and studies of association have been plagued by lack of appropriate controls to examine population stratification and have not used within-family

tests such as transmission disequilibrium. In addition, most of these studies have also only focused on the high end of the blood pressure distribution, ignoring the fact that protective alleles that reduce BP also surely exist in the population. There is clearly a pressing need for study of large, well-phenotyped populations in whom quantitative blood pressure measures can be utilized, and in which studies of linkage, association, and transmission disequilibrium can be performed. A complementary approach combining all these study designs will maximize the chances of success.

## IMPLICATIONS

To date, investigators have identified mutations in seven genes that raise blood pressure and in nine genes that lower blood pressure in humans. The identification of these mutations provides an explanation of the clinical features and physiology of affected patients, permits use of new diagnostic tests to identify individuals with inherited susceptibility to disease, and provides the opportunity to apply therapies that are tailored to underlying physiological abnormalities in individual patients that may improve the treatment of these subjects. Moreover, these findings identify "validated targets" for development of new antihypertensive agents; that is, targets whose altered activity would have highly predictable effects.

It is noteworthy that all of these genes act in a final, common pathway, altering renal salt handling. Mutations that increase renal salt reabsorption increase blood pressure, whereas mutations that reduce reabsorption reduce blood pressure. These findings are all the more relevant as the relationship between salt and blood pressure has proved maddeningly difficult to settle from epidemiologic studies or from studies that have altered dietary salt intake. These genetic studies establish beyond doubt that primary alteration in renal salt handling alters blood pressure in humans.

This association between salt balance and blood pressure prompts one to consider the known causes of acquired forms of hypertension. These, too, can, in whole or in part, be attributed to increased net salt balance. Aldosterone-producing adenoma is one obvious example. Another is renal artery stenosis, which leads to increased plasma renin activity, ultimately increasing salt balance via increased aldosterone secretion. The excess catecholamines in pheochromocytoma increase proximal renal tubular salt reabsorption and decrease renal blood flow. At present, one can make the case that all of the known causes of hypertension act by increasing net salt balance, either by altering renal salt handling directly, or as a secondary effect of impaired renal perfusion or glomerular filtration.

These observations fit with the expectation that increased plasma volume should result in increased cardiac output and thereby raise blood pressure. Moreover, they also mesh nicely with the work of Guyton and colleagues who have argued that the active participation of the kidney is needed to sustain alteration in blood pressure.

One might logically inquire whether there has been selection bias in the diseases studied. Are there a host of additional known Mendelian forms of human hypertension that have not been studied that might identify abnormalities in other pathways? The answer is no. Of the known Mendelian forms of human hypertension, only PHA-II and the syndrome of hypertension with brachydactyly remain to be solved at the molecular level. This does, however, leave open the question of whether there may be other, as yet unrecognized, Mendelian forms of hypertension. In this regard, it is noteworthy that all of the Mendelian forms identified to date have a feature in addition to hypertension, such as hypokalemia or brachydactyly, that suggested a diagnosis other than essential hypertension. Systematic investigation of families, particularly those ascertained for early or severe hypertension, might identify additional kindreds in which hypertension segregates as a Mendelian trait.

Do abnormalities in salt handling underlie more common forms of human hypertension? Low plasma potassium is infrequently encountered in the untreated essential hypertensive population. If serum potassium is taken as a measure of distal nephron salt reabsorption, then the low prevalence of hypokalemia in essential hypertension might argue against the presence of abnormal sodium homeostasis as a contributing factor. However, the work on GRA demonstrates that increased ENaC activity need not be accompanied by hypokalemia. This suggests that other forms of aldosteronism are underdiagnosed. Indeed, recent studies using renin:aldosterone ratios are identifying an increasing number of patients whose hypertension might be attributable to previously unrecognized aldosteronism.

Studies of patients with essential hypertension have typically demonstrated hemodynamic patterns of normal cardiac output with elevated systemic vascular resistance, and this profile is *a priori* inconsistent with the pattern of increased cardiac output expected from a primary increase in renal salt reabsorption. Again, physiological work by Guyton and others on the DOCA or Goldblatt models of hypertension is illustrative: It is impossible to determine the primary underlying cause of hypertension from steady state hemodynamic profiles, as hypertension of all causes will evolve to the same pattern of hypertension dominated by high systemic vascular resistance and normal cardiac output. Consequently, it seems safe to say that the primary physiological abnormalities underlying essential hypertension are presently unknown. Nonetheless, with virtually all of the known sufficient causes of hypertension acting in the renal salt pathway, it would be surprising if this mechanism played no role in essential hypertension. In particular, from the experience with Mendelian forms of high and low blood pressure, it seems highly probable that low-renin forms of hypertension result from primary increases in renal salt reabsorption with secondary suppression of renin secretion.

Finally, the studies on Mendelian forms of BP variation have identified a number of targets for development of new or improved pharmaceutic agents. Detailed knowledge of the physiological consequences of loss of a gene product by mutation provides useful insight into what the consequences would be if that gene product's function were inhibited by a pharmacologic agent. For example, the observation that patients homozygous for mutations in the K channel ROMK results in salt wasting with relative potassium sparing provides a strong indication that a specific antagonist of this channel would have potent antihypertensive diuretic effects that would be K sparing. Moreover, the absence of phenotypic effects of these mutations in other organ systems, such as the heart and brain, indicates that a specific antagonist for this channel would not have side effects in these organs. Similarly, the phenotype of patients with recessive PHA-I resurrects ENaC as an attractive target for new antagonists that do not compete with $Na^+$; such agents are also predicted to have potent potassium-sparing antihypertensive diuretic effects. It is important to point out that just as HMGCoA reductase inhibitors are efficacious in patients who do not have mutations in the LDL receptor, the efficacy of such agents would not likely be restricted to individuals with inherited mutations in these genes.

## FUTURE DIRECTIONS

These findings in Mendelian forms of hypertension leave no doubt about the ability of genetic variation to influence blood pressure in humans. As these mutations account for only a very small fraction of variance in blood pressure, they naturally raise the question of what are the variants that account for blood pressure variation in the general population. There are several complementary approaches to this problem. The most powerful approach is to identify putative functional genetic variants and to test the possible impact of these variants on blood pressure in the general population by comparing the blood pressures of individuals with and without these variants. The impending acquisition of the human genome sequence and the ability to rapidly resequence genomic DNA will accelerate these efforts. Underlying assump-

tions in this approach are that effects at blood pressure loci are substantially determined by common variants in the population and that one can identify the correct candidate genes for testing. Performing within-family analyses can minimize confounding effects of differences in genetic background within a population. Based on the findings in Mendelian disorders, in the coming years, all of the genes whose products mediate or regulate renal salt handling will be carefully examined for molecular variants and their impact. Undoubtedly, every other gene in pathways implicated in the control of blood pressure will also be examined.

As a note of caution, one can anticipate that many claims of significant association will appear in the literature, and a major challenge will be to sort out which of these are true positive from those that are false positive. The consistent reproducibility of the findings in other studies will prove critical, and supporting data from biochemical studies and investigation of transgenic or knockout models will strengthen the argument.

In addition to such studies of association, linkage studies in either hypertensive populations or the general population have the potential to identify loci imparting significant effects on blood pressure. The major limitation of such studies will remain the unknown fraction of the variance in blood pressure accounted for by inheritance at any single locus. Consequently, the power of any study to find significant linkage is unknown *a priori*.

The other major question for such studies is which phenotypes should be employed. Exhaustive phenotyping of patients will only be better than using blood pressure alone if the phenotypes used prove to have a more homogeneous genetic basis than blood pressure itself. With the exception of the rare Mendelian disorders, few relevant phenotypes are known to meet this criterion. The results of genome-wide linkage studies are becoming available, and will prove of considerable interest. For intervals showing evidence of linkage, the availability of human genome sequence will greatly accelerate the ability to identify the underlying trait loci.

In sum, genetic approaches to hypertension are in their infancy. Nonetheless, results to date offer insight into basic disease mechanisms and physiology, provide new diagnostic tests of high specificity, and present new approaches to therapeutics. The prospects for continuing efforts in this area to have a substantial impact on the understanding, diagnosis, and treatment of this disorder are bright.

## REFERENCES

1. Neaton JD, Kuller L, Stamler J, Wentworth D: Impact of systolic and diastolic blood pressure on cardiovascular mortality, in Laragh JH, Brenner BM (eds): *Hypertension: Pathophysiology, Diagnosis and Management*, 2nd ed. New York, Raven, 1995, p 127.
2. Flack JM, Neaton J, Grimm R Jr, Shih J, Cutler J, Ensrud K, MacMahon S: Blood pressure and mortality among men with prior myocardial infarction. Multiple risk factor intervention trial research group. *Circulation* **92**:2437, 1995.
3. Kannel WB, Wolf PA, Verter J, McNamara PM: Epidemiologic assessment of the role of blood pressure in stroke: The Framingham study 1970. *JAMA* **27**:1269, 1996.
4. US Renal Data System: *1999 Annual Data Report*. The National Institute of Diabetes and Digestive and Kidney Diseases. Bethesda, MD, USRDS, July 1999.
5. MacMahon S, Rodgers A, Neal B, Chalmers J: Blood pressure lowering for the secondary prevention of myocardial infarction and stroke. *Hypertension* **29**:537, 1997.
6. Flack JM, Neaton J, Grimm R Jr, Shih J, Cutler J, Ensrud K, MacMahon S: Blood pressure and mortality among men with prior myocardial infarction. Multiple Risk Factor Intervention Trial Research Group. *Circulation* **92**:2437, 1995.
7. MacMahon S, Peto R, Cutler J, Collins R, Sorlie P, Neaton J, Abbott R, Godwin J, Dyer A, Stamler J: Blood pressure, stroke, and coronary heart disease. Part 1, Prolonged differences in blood pressure: Prospective observational studies corrected for the regression dilution bias. *Lancet* **335**:765, 1990.

8. Mosterd A, D'Agostino RB, Silbershatz H, Sytkowski PA, Kannel WB, Grobbee DE, Levy D: Trends in the prevalence of hypertension, antihypertensive therapy, and left ventricular hypertrophy from 1950 to 1989. *N Engl J Med* **340**:1221, 1999.

9. Burt VL, Whelton P, Roccella EJ, Brown C, Cutler JA, Higgins M, Horan MJ, Labarthe D: Prevalence of hypertension in the US adult population. Results from the Third National Health and Nutrition Examination Survey, 1988-1991. *Hypertension* **25**:305, 1995.

10. James GD, Baker PT: Human population biology and blood pressure: Evolutionary and ecological considerations and interpretations of population studies, in Laragh JH, Brenner BM (eds): *Hypertension: Pathophysiology, Diagnosis and Management*, 2nd ed. New York, Raven, 1995, p 115.

11. Franklin SS, Gustin W 4th, Wong ND, Larson MG, Weber MA, Kannel WB, Levy D: Hemodynamic patterns of age-related changes in blood pressure. The Framingham Heart Study. *Circulation* **96**:308, 1997.

12. Elliott P, Stamler J, Nichols R, Dyer AR, Stamler R, Kesteloot H, Marmot M: Intersalt revisited: Further analyses of 24-hour sodium excretion and blood pressure within and across populations. Intersalt Cooperative Research Group. *BMJ* **312**:1249, 1996.

13. Rodriguez BL, Labarthe DR, Huang B, Lopez-Gomez J: Rise of blood pressure with age. New evidence of population differences. *Hypertension* **24**:779, 1994.

14. Dyer AR, Elliott P, Shipley M, Stamler R, Stamler J: Body mass index and associations of sodium and potassium with blood pressure in INTERSALT. *Hypertension* **23**:729, 1994.

15. Hollenberg NK, Martinez G, McCullough M, Meinking T, Passan D, Preston M, Rivera A, Taplin D, Vicaria-Clement M: Aging, acculturation, salt intake, and hypertension in the Kuna of Panama. *Hypertension* **29**:171, 1997.

16. Klag MJ, He J, Coresh J, Whelton PK, Chen JY, Mo JP, Qian MC, Mo PS, He GQ: The contribution of urinary cations to the blood pressure differences associated with migration. *Am J Epidemiol* **142**:295, 1995.

17. Bhatnagar D, Anand IS, Durrington PN, Patel DJ, Wander GS, Mackness MI, Creed F, et al.: Coronary risk factors in people from the Indian subcontinent living in west London and their siblings in India. *Lancet* **345**:405, 1995.

18. Alderman MH, Cohen HW, Madhavan S: Related Articles Myocardial infarction in treated hypertensive patients: The paradox of lower incidence but higher mortality in young blacks compared with whites. *Circulation* **101**:1109, 2000.

19. McGee D, Cooper R, Liao Y, Durazo-Arvizu R: Patterns of comorbidity and mortality risk in blacks and whites. *Ann Epidemiol* **6**:381, 1996.

20. Grim CE, Henry JP, Myers H: High blood pressure in Blacks: Salt, slavery, survival, stress and racism, in Laragh JH, Brenner BM (eds): *Hypertension: Pathophysiology, Diagnosis and Management*, 2nd ed. New York, Raven, 1995, p 171.

21. Must A, Spadano J, Coakley EH, Field AE, Colditz G, Dietz WH: The disease burden associated with overweight and obesity. *JAMA* **282**:1523, 1999.

22. Huang Z, Willett WC, Manson JE, Rosner B, Stampfer MJ, Speizer FE, Colditz GA: Body weight, weight change, and risk for hypertension in women. *Ann Intern Med* **128**:81, 1998.

23. Curtis AB, Strogatz DS, James SA, Raghunathan TE: The contribution of baseline weight and weight gain to blood pressure change in African Americans: The Pitt County Study. *Ann Epidemiol* **8**:497, 1998.

24. Sherman SE, D'Agostino RB, Silbershatz H, Kannel WB: Comparison of past versus recent physical activity in the prevention of premature death and coronary artery disease. *Am Heart J* **138**:900, 1999.

25. Reaven GM, Lithell H, Landsberg L: Hypertension and associated metabolic abnormalities — The role of insulin resistance and the sympathoadrenal system. *N Engl J Med* **334**:374, 1996.

26. Wilson PW, Kannel WB, Silbershatz H, D'Agostino RB: Clustering of metabolic factors and coronary heart disease. *Arch Intern Med* **159**:1104, 1999.

27. Zavaroni I, Bonini L, Gasparini P, Barilli AL, Zuccarelli A, Dall'Aglio E, Delsignore R, Reaven GM: Hyperinsulinemia in a normal population as a predictor of non-insulin-dependent diabetes mellitus, hypertension, and coronary heart disease: The Barilla factory revisited. *Metabolism* **48**:989, 1999.

28. Palatini P, Vriz O, Nesbitt S, Amerena J, Majahalme S, Valentini M, Julius S: Parental hyperdynamic circulation predicts insulin resistance in offspring: The Tecumseh Offspring Study. *Hypertension* **33**:769, 1999.

29. Chen W, Srinivasan SR, Elkasabany A, Berenson GS: The association of cardiovascular risk factor clustering related to insulin resistance

30. Feinleib M, Garrison RJ, Fabsitz R, Christian JC, Hrubec Z, Borhani NO, Kannel WB, Rosenman R, Schwartz JT, Wagner JO: The NHLBI twin study of cardiovascular disease risk factors: methodology and summary of results. *Am J Epidemiol* **106**:284, 1977.

31. Vinck WJ, Vlietinck R, Fagard RH: The contribution of genes, environment and of body mass to blood pressure variance in young adult males. *J Hum Hypertens* **13**:191, 1999.

32. Denton D, Weisinger R, Mundy NI, Wickings EJ, Dixson A, Moisson P, Pingard AM, et al.: The effect of increased salt intake on blood pressure of chimpanzees. *Nat Med* **1**:1009, 1995.

33. Weinberger MH: Salt sensitivity of blood pressure in humans. *Hypertension* **27**:481, 1996.

34. Simpson FO: Blood pressure and sodium intake, in Laragh JH, Brenner BM (eds): *Hypertension: Pathophysiology, Diagnosis and Management*, 2nd ed. New York, Raven, 1995, p 273.

35. Brownie AC: The adrenal cortex in hypertension: DOCA/Salt hypertension and beyond, in Laragh JH, Brenner BM (eds): *Hypertension: Pathophysiology, Diagnosis and Management*, 2nd ed. New York, Raven, 1995, p 2127.

36. Guyton AC, Hall JE, Coleman TG, Manning RD, Norman RA: The dominant role of the kidneys in long term arterial pressure regulation in normal and hypertensive studies, in Laragh JH, Brenner BM (eds): *Hypertension: Pathophysiology, Diagnosis and Management*, 2nd ed. New York, Raven, 1995, p 1311.

37. Hall JE, Guyton AC, Brands MW: Pressure-volume regulation in hypertension. *Kidney Int* **55(Suppl)**:S35, 1996.

38. Huang M, Hester RL, Coleman TG, Smith MJ, Guyton AC: Development of hypertension in animals with reduced total peripheral resistance. *Hypertension* **20**:828, 1992.

39. Kaplan N: Primary hypertension. Pathogenesis, in Kaplan NM (ed): *Clinical Hypertension*, 7th ed. Baltimore, Williams & Wilkins, 1998, p 41.

40. Sealy JE, Lutterotti NV, Rubattu S, Campbell WG, Gahnem F, Halimi LM, Laragh JH: The greater renin system: Its prorenin-directed vasodilator limb: Relevance to diabetes mellitus, pregnancy, and hypertension, in Laragh JH, Brenner BM (eds): *Hypertension: Pathophysiology, Diagnosis and Management*, 2nd ed. New York, Raven, 1995, p 1311.

41. Blumenfeld JD, Laragh JH: Renin system analysis: A rational method for the diagnosis and treatment of the individual patient with hypertension. *Am J Hypertens* **11**:894, 1998.

42. Rettig R, Bandelow N, Patschan O, Kuttler B, Frey B, Uber A: The importance of the kidney in primary hypertension: Insights from cross-transplantation. *J Hum Hypertens* **10**:641, 1996.

43. Cowley AW Jr, Roman RJ: The role of the kidney in hypertension. *JAMA* **275**:1581, 1996.

44. An P, Rice T, Gagnon J, Borecki IB, Perusse L, Leon AS, Skinner JS, Wilmore JH, Bouchard C, Rao DC: Familial aggregation of resting blood pressure and heart rate in a sedentary population: The HERITAGE Family Study. Health, risk factors, exercise training, and genetics. *Am J Hypertens* **12**:264, 1999.

45. Wang X, Wang B, Chen C, Yang J, Fang Z, Zuckerman B, Xu X: Familial aggregation of blood pressure in a rural Chinese community. *Am J Epidemiol* **149**:412, 1999.

46. Magalhaes ME, Pozzan R, Brandao AA, Cerqueira RC, Rousoulieres AL, Szwarcwald C, Brandao AP: Early blood pressure level as a mark of familial aggregation of metabolic cardiovascular risk factors — The Rio de Janeiro Study. *J Hypertens* **16**:1885, 1998.

47. Carmelli D, Fabsitz RR, Swan GE, Reed T, Miller B, Wolf PA: Contribution of genetic and environmental influences to ankle-brachial blood pressure index in the NHLBI Twin Study. National Heart, Lung, and Blood Institute. *Am J Epidemiol* **151(5)**:452, 2000.

48. Carmelli D, Robinette D, Fabsitz R: Concordance, discordance and prevalence of hypertension in World War II male veteran twins. *J Hypertens* **12**:323, 1994.

49. Snieder H, Hayward CS, Perks U, Kelly RP, Kelly PJ, Spector TD: Heritability of central systolic pressure augmentation: A twin study. *Hypertension* **35**:574, 2000.

50. Vinck WJ, Vlietinck R, Fagard RH: The contribution of genes, environment and of body mass to blood pressure variance in young adult males. *J Hum Hypertens* **13**:191, 1999.

51. Fagard R, Brguljan J, Staessen J, Thijs L, Derom C, Thomis M, Vlietinck R: Heritability of conventional and ambulatory blood pressures. A study in twins. *Hypertension* **26**:919, 1995.

52. Hong Y, de Faire U, Heller DA, McClearn GE, Pedersen N: Genetic and environmental influences on blood pressure in elderly twins. *Hypertension* **24**:663, 1994.

53. Chu MD, Ulick S: Isolation and identification of 18-hydroxycortisol from the urine of patients with primary aldosteronism. *J Biol Chem* **257**:2218, 1982.

54. Rich GM, Ulick S, Cook S, Wang JZ, Lifton RP, Dluhy RG: Glucocorticoid-remediable aldosteronism in a large kindred: Clinical spectrum and diagnosis using a characteristic biochemical phenotype. *Ann Int Med* **116**:813, 1992.

55. Lifton RP, Dluhy RG, Powers M, Rich GM, Cook S, Ulick S, Lalouel J-M: A chimeric 11b-hydroxylase/aldosterone synthase gene causes glucocorticoid-remediable aldosteronism and human hypertension. *Nature* **355**:262, 1992.

56. Lifton RP, Dluhy RG, Powers M, et al.: Hereditary hypertension caused by chimeric gene duplications and ectopic expression of aldosterone synthase. *Nat Genet* **2**:66, 1992.

57. Mune T, Rogerson FM, Nikkila H, Agarwal AK, White PC: Human hypertension caused by mutations in the kidney isozyme of 11-hydroxysteroid dehydrogenase. *Nat Genet* **10**:394, 1995.

58. Curnow KM, Mulatero P, Emeric-Blanchouin N, Aupetit-Faisant B, Corvol P, Pascoe L: The amino acid substitutions Ser288Gly and Val320Ala convert the cortisol producing enzyme, CYP11B1, into an aldosterone producing enzyme. *Nat Struct Biol* **4**:32, 1997.

59. Litchfield WR, Anderson BF, Weiss RJ, Lifton RP, Dluhy RG: Intracranial aneurysm and hemorrhagic stroke in glucocorticoid-remediable aldosteronism. *Hypertension* **31**:445, 1998.

60. Mune T, Rogerson FM, Nikkila H, Agarwal AK, White PC: Human hypertension caused by mutations in the kidney isozyme of 11-hydroxysteroid dehydrogenase. *Nat Genet* **10**:394, 1995.

61. New MI, Wilson RC: Steroid disorders in children: Congenital adrenal hyperplasia and apparent mineralocorticoid excess. *Proc Natl Acad Sci U S A* **96**:12790, 1999.

62. Arriza JL, Weinberger C, Cerelli G, et al.: Cloning of human mineralocorticoid receptor complementary DNA: Structural and functional kinship with the glucocorticoid receptor. *Science* **230**:268, 1987.

63. Funder JW, Pearce PT, Smith R, Smith AI: Mineralocorticoid action: Target tissue specificity is enzyme, not receptor, mediated. *Science* **24**:583, 1988.

64. Karl M, Lamberts SW, Detera-Wadleigh SD, et al.: Familial glucocorticoid resistance caused by a splice site deletion in the human glucocorticoid receptor gene. *J Clin Endo Met* **76**:683, 1993.

65. Stewart PM, Wallace AM, Valentino R, Burt D, Shackleton CHL, Edwards CRW: Mineralocorticoid activity of liquorice: 11-Beta-hydroxysteroid dehydrogenase deficiency comes of age. *Lancet* **II**:821, 1987.

66. Yanase T, Simpson ER, Waterman MR: 17-Alpha-hydroxylase/17,20-lyase deficiency: From clinical investigation to molecular definition. *Endocr Rev* **12**:91, 1991.

67. Ahlgren A, Yanase T, Simpson ER, Winter JSD, Waterman MR: Compound heterozygous mutations (arg239-to-ter, pro342-to-thr) in the CYP17 (P45017-alpha) gene lead to ambiguous external genitalia in a male patient with partial combined 17-alpha-hydroxylase/17,20-lyase deficiency. *J Clin Endocr Metab* **74**:667 1992.

68. Biason A, Mantero F Scaroni C, Simpson ER, Waterman MR: Deletion within the CYP17 gene together with insertion of foreign DNA is the cause of combined complete 17-alpha-hydroxylase/17,20-lyase deficiency in an Italian patient. *Molec Endocr* **5**:2037, 1991.

69. Lin D, Harikrishna JA, Moore CCD, Jones KL, Miller WL: Missense mutation serine106-to-proline causes 17-alpha-hydroxylase deficiency. *J Biol Chem* **266**:15992, 1991.

70. Geller DH, Auchus RJ, Mendonca BB, Miller WL: The genetic and functional basis of isolated 17,20-lyase deficiency. *Nat Genet* **17**:201, 1997.

71. Wedell A: An update on the molecular genetics of congenital adrenal hyperplasia: Diagnostic and therapeutic aspects. *J Pediatr Endocrinol Metab* **11**:581, 1998.

72. Globerman H, Rosler A, Theodor R, New MI, White PC: An inherited defect in aldosterone biosynthesis caused by a mutation in or near the gene for steroid 11-hydroxylase. *New Eng J Med* **319**:1193, 1988.

73. Curnow KM, Slutsker L, Vitek J, Cole T, Speiser PW, New MI, White PC, Pascoe L: Mutations in the CYP11B1 gene causing congenital adrenal hyperplasia and hypertension cluster in exons 6, 7, and 8. *Proc Natl Acad Sci U S A* **90**:4552, 1993.

74. Geley S, Kapelari K, Johrer K, Peter M, Glatzl J, Vierhapper H, Schwarz S, Helmberg A, Sippell WG, White PC, Kofler R: CYP11B1

75. Geller DS, Farhi A, Pinkerton N, Fradley M, Moritz M, Spitzer A, Meinke G, et al.: Activating mineralocorticoid receptor mutation in hypertension exacerbated by pregnancy. *Science* **289**:119, 2000.

76. Lifton RP: Molecular genetics of human blood pressure variation. *Science* **272**:676, 1996.

77. Botero-Velez M, Curtis JJ, Warnock DG: Brief report: Liddle syndrome revisited. *New Eng J Med* **330**:178, 1994.

78. Shimkets RA, Warnock DG, Bositis C, et al.: Liddle syndrome: Heritable human hypertension caused by mutations in the beta subunit of the epithelial sodium channel. *Cell* **79**:407, 1994.

79. Hansson JH, Nelson-Williams C, Suzuki H, et al.: Hypertension caused by a truncated epithelial sodium channel gamma subunit: Genetic heterogeneity of Liddle syndrome. *Nat Genet* **11**:76, 1995.

80. Tamura H, Schild L, Enomoto N, Matsui N, Marumo F, Rossier BC: Liddle disease caused by a missense mutation of beta subunit of the epithelial sodium channel gene. *J Clin Invest* **97**:1780, 1996.

81. Schild L, Canessa CM, Shimkets RA, Gautschi I, Lifton RP, Rossier BC: A mutation in the epithelial sodium channel causing Liddle disease increases channel activity in the *Xenopus laevis* oocyte expression system. *Proc Natl Acad Sci USA* **92**: 5699, 1995.

82. Schild L, Lu Y, Gotchi I, Schneerberger G, Lifton RP, Rossier BC: Identification of a PY motif in the epithelial sodium channel subunits as a target sequence for mutations causing channel activation found in Liddle syndrome. *EMBO J* **15**:2381, 1996.

83. Tamura H, Schild L, Enomoto N, Matsui N, Marumo F, Rossier BC: Liddle disease caused by a missense mutation of beta subunit of the epithelial sodium channel gene. *J Clin Invest* **97**:1780, 1996.

84. Hansson, JH, Schild L, Lu Y, et al.: A de novo missense mutation of the B subunit of the epithelial sodium channel causes hypertension and Liddle syndrome, identifying a proline-rich segment critical for regulation of channel activity. *Proc Natl Acad Sci U S A* **92**:11495, 1995.

85. Firsov D, Schild L, Gautschi I, Merillat AM, Schneeberger E, Rossier BC: Cell surface expression of the epithelial Na channel and a mutant causing Liddle syndrome: A quantitative approach. *Proc Natl Acad Sci U S A* **93**:15370, 1996.

86. Snyder PM, Price MP, McDonald FJ, et al.: Mechanism by which Liddle syndrome mutations increase activity of a human epithelial Na(+) channel. *Cell* **83**:969, 1995.

87. Staub O, Dho S, Henry P, Correa J, Ishikawa T, McGlade J, Rotin D: WW domains of Nedd4 bind to the proline-rich PY motifs in the epithelial Na$^+$ channel deleted in Liddle syndrome. *EMBO J* **15**:2371, 1995.

88. Abriel H, Loffing J, Rebhun JF, et al.: Defective regulation of the epithelial Na$^+$ channel by Nedd4 in Liddle syndrome. *J Clin Invest* **103**:667, 1999.

89. Kellenberger S, Gautschi I, Rossier BC, Schild L: Mutations causing Liddle syndrome reduce sodium-dependent down-regulation of the epithelial sodium channel in the Xenopus oocyte expression system. *J Clin Invest* **101**:2741, 1998.

90. Gordon RD, Klemm SA, Tunny TJ, Stowasser M: Gordon's syndrome: A volume dependent form of hypertension with a genetic basis, in Laragh JH, Brenner BM (eds): *Hypertension: Pathophysiology, Diagnosis and Management*, 2nd ed. New York, Raven, 1995, p 2111.

91. Mansfield TA, Simon DB, Farfel Z, Bia M, Tucci JR, Lebel M, Gutkin M, Vialettes B, Christofilis MA, Kauppinen-Makelin R, Mayan H, Risch N, Lifton RP: Multilocus linkage of familial hyperkalaemia and hypertension, pseudohypoaldosteronism type II, to chromosomes 1q31-42 and 17p11-q21. *Nat Genet* **16**:202, 1997.

92. Schuster H, Wienker TF, Toka HR, Bahring S, Jeschke E, Toka O, Busjahn A, Hempel A, Tahlhammer C, Oelkers W, Kunze J, Bilginturan N, Haller H, Luft FC: Autosomal dominant hypertension and brachydactyly in a Turkish kindred resembles essential hypertension. *Hypertension* **28**:1085, 1996.

93. Schuster H, Wienker, TF,Bahring S, Bilginturan N, Toka, HR, Neitzel H, Jeschke E, Toka O, Gilbert D, Lowe A, Ott J, Haller H, Luft FC: Severe autosomal dominant hypertension and brachydactyly in a unique Turkish kindred maps to human chromosome 12. *Nat Genet* **13**:98, 1996.

94. Karaplis AC, Luz A, Glowacki J, Bronson RT, Tybulewicz VLJ, Kronenberg HM, Mulligan RC: Lethal skeletal dysplasia from targeted disruption of the parathyroid hormone-related peptide gene. *Genes Dev* **8**:277, 1994.

95. Bahring S, Schuster H, Wienker TF, Haller H, Toka H, Toka O, Naraghi R, Luft FC: Construction of a physical map and additional

phenotyping in autosomal-dominant hypertension and brachydactyly, which maps to chromosome 12 [Abstract]. *Am J Hum Genet* **59(Suppl)**:A55, 1996.

96. Hanukoglu A: Type I pseudohypoaldosteronism includes two clinically and genetically distinct entities with either renal or multiple target organ defects. *J Clin Endocrin Metab* **73**:936, 1991.

97. Kuhnle U, Nielsen M, Tietze HU, et al.: Pseudohypoaldosteronism in eight families: Different forms of inheritance are evidence for various genetic defects. *J Clin Endocrin Metab* **70**:638, 1990.

98. Chang SS, Grunder S, Hanukoglu A, et al.: Mutations in subunits of the epithelial sodium channel cause salt wasting with hyperkalaemic acidosis, pseudohypoaldosteronism type 1. *Nat Genet* **12**:248, 1996.

99. Kuhnle U, Nielsen M, Tietze HU, et al.: Pseudohypoaldosteronism in eight families: Different forms of inheritance are evidence for various genetic defects. *J Clin Endocrin Metab* **70**:638, 1990.

100. Geller DS, Rodriguez-Soriano J, Boado AV, Schifter S, Bayer M, Chang SS, Lifton RP: Mutations in the human mineralocorticoid receptor gene cause autosomal dominant Pseudohypoaldosteronism type I. *Nat Genet* **19**:279, 1998.

101. Chang SS, Grunder S, Hanukoglu A, et al.: Mutations in subunits of the epithelial sodium channel cause salt wasting with hyperkalaemic acidosis, pseudohypoaldosteronism type 1. *Nat Genet* **12**:248, 1996.

102. White PC, Tusie-Luna M-T, New MI, Speiser PW: Mutations in steroid 21-hydroxylase (CYP21). *Hum Mutat* **3**:373, 1994.

103. Tusie-Luna M-T, White PC: Gene conversions and unequal crossovers between CYP21 (steroid 21-hydroxylase gene) and CYP21P involve different mechanisms. *Proc Natl Acad Sci U S A* **92**:10796, 1995.

104. Speiser PW, New MI, Tannin GM, Pickering D, Yang SY, White PC: Genotype of Yupik Eskimos with congenital adrenal hyperplasia due to 21-hydroxylase deficiency. *Hum Genet* **88**:647, 1992.

105. Bachega TASS, Billerbeck AEC, Madureira G, Marcondes JAM, Longui CA, Leite MV, Arnhold IJP, Mendonca BB: Molecular genotyping in Brazilian patients with the classical and nonclassical forms of 21-hydroxylase deficiency. *J Clin Endocr Metab* **83**:4416, 1998.

106. Witchel SF, Lee PA, Suda-Hartman M, Trucco M, Hoffman EP: Evidence for a heterozygote advantage in congenital adrenal hyperplasia due to 21-hydroxylase deficiency. *J Clin Endocr Metab* **82**:2097, 1997.

107. Clive DM: Bartter syndrome: The unsolved puzzle. *Am J Kid Dis* **25**:813, 1995.

108. Simon DB, Lifton RP: The molecular basis of inherited hypokalemic alkalosis: Bartter and Gitelman syndromes. *Am J Physiol* **27**:F961, 1996.

109. Bettinelli A, Bianchetti M, Girardin E, et al.: Use of calcium excretion values to distinguish two forms of primary renal tubular hypokalemic alkalosis: Bartter and Gitelman syndromes. *J Pediatr* **120**:38, 1992.

110. Simon DB, Nelson-Williams C, Bia MJ, et al.: Gitelman variant of Bartter syndrome, inherited hypokalaemic alkalosis, is caused by mutations in the thiazide-sensitive Na-Cl cotransporter. *Nat Genet* **12**:24, 1996.

111. Cruz D, Simon DB, Gill J, Lifton RP: Reduced blood pressure in Gitelman syndrome: Study of a large extended kindred. *J Am Soc Nephrol* **9**:32A, 1998.

112. Simon DB, Lifton RP: Ion transporter mutations in Gitelman and Bartter syndromes. *Curr Opin Nephrol Hyperten* **7**:43, 1998.

113. Payne JA, Forbush B 3d: Alternatively spliced isoforms of the putative renal Na-K-Cl cotransporter are differentially distributed within the rabbit kidney. *Proc Natl Acad Sci U S A* **91**:4544, 1994.

114. Gamba G, Miyanoshita A, Lombardi M, et al.: Molecular cloning, primary structure, and characterization of two members of the mammalian electroneutral sodium-(potassium) chloride cotransporter family expressed in the kidney. *J Biol Chem* **269**:17713, 1994.

115. Simon DB, Karet FE, Hamdan JM, DiPietro A, Sanjad SA, Lifton RP: Bartter syndrome, hypokalemic alkalosis with hypercalciuria, is caused by mutations in the Na-K-2Cl cotransporter NKCC2. *Nat Genet* **13**:183, 1996.

116. Wang W, Sackin H, Giebisch G: Renal potassium channels and their regulation. *Ann Rev Physiol* **54**:81, 1992.

117. Giebisch G: Renal potassium channels: An overview. *Kidney Int* **48**:1004, 1995.

118. Simon DB, Karet FE, Rodriguez-Soriano, et al.: Genetic heterogeneity of Bartter syndrome revealed by mutations in the K$^+$ channel, ROMK. *Nat Genet* **14**:152, 1996.

119. Simon DB, Bindra RS, Mansfield TA, et al.: Mutations in the chloride channel gene, CLCNKB, cause Bartter syndrome type III. *Nat Genet* **17**:171, 1997.

120. Kieferle S, Fong P, Bens M, Vandewalle A, Jentsch TJ: Two highly homologous members of the ClC chloride channel family in both rat and human kidney. *Proc Natl Acad Sci U S A* **91**:6943, 1994.

121. Brennan TM, Landau D, Shalev H, et al.: Linkage of infantile Bartter syndrome with sensorineural deafness to chromosome 1p. *Am J Hum Genet* **62**:355, 1998.

122. Simon DB, Cruz D, Jandan J, Klein A, Yadin O, Rodriguez-Soriano J, Lifton RP: A unique phenotype of type II Bartter syndrome reveals a K$^+$ secretory defect. *J Am Soc Nephrol* **9**:111A, 1998.

123. Risch N, Merikangas K: The future of genetic studies of complex human diseases. *Science* **273**:1516, 1996.

124. Risch N, Zhang H: Extreme discordant sib pairs for mapping quantitative trait loci in humans. *Science* **268**:1584, 1995.

125. Spielman RS, McGinnis RE, Ewens WJ: Transmission test for linkage disequilibrium: The insulin gene region and insulin-dependent diabetes mellitus (IDDM). *Am J Hum Genet* **52**:506, 1993.

126. Sun F, Flanders WD, Yang Q, Khoury MJ: Transmission disequilibrium test (TDT) when only one parent is available: The 1-TDT. *Am J Epidemiol* **150**:97, 1999.

127. George V, Tiwari HK, Zhu X, Elston RC: A test of transmission/disequilibrium for quantitative traits in pedigree data, by multiple regression. *Am J Hum Genet* **1**:236, 1999.

128. Allison DB, Heo M, Kaplan N, Martin ER: Sibling-based tests of linkage and association for quantitative traits. *Am J Hum Genet* **64**:1754, 1999.

129. Jeunemaitre X, Soubrier F, Kotelevtsev YV, Lifton RP, Williams CS, Charru A, Hunt SC, Hopkins PN, Williams RR, Lalouel JM, et al.: Molecular basis of human hypertension: Role of angiotensinogen. *Cell* **71**:169, 1992.

130. Caufield M, Lavende P, Farrall M, Munroe P, et al.: Linkage of the angiotensinogen gene to essential hypertension. *N Engl J Med* **330**:1629, 1994.

131. Atwood LD, Kammerer CM, Samollow PB, Hixson JE, Shade RE, MacCluer JW: Linkage of essential hypertension to the angiotensinogen locus in Mexican Americans. *Hypertension* **30**:326, 1997.

132. Brand E, Chatelain N, Keavney B, Caulfield M, Citterio L, Connell J, Grobbee D, Schmidt S, Schunkert H, Schuster H, Sharma AM, Soubrier F: Evaluation of the angiotensinogen locus in human essential hypertension: A European study. *Hypertension* **31**:725, 1998.

133. Niu T, Xu X, Rogus J, Zhou Y, Chen C, Yang J, Fang Z, Schmitz C, Zhao J, Rao VS, Lindpaintner KV: Angiotensinogen gene and hypertension in Chinese. *J Clin Invest* **101**:188, 1998.

134. Corvol P, Persu A, Gimenez-Roqueplo AP, Jeunemaitre X: Seven lessons from two candidate genes in human essential hypertension: Angiotensinogen and epithelial sodium channel. *Hypertension* **33**:1324, 1999.

135. Inoue I, Nakajima T, Williams CS, Quackenbush J, Puryear R, Powers M, Cheng T, Ludwig EH, Sharma AM, Hata A, Jeunemaitre X, Lalouel JM: A nucleotide substitution in the promoter of human angiotensinogen is associated with essential hypertension and affects basal transcription in vitro. *J Clin Invest* **99**:1786, 1997.

136. Jeunemaitre X, Lifton RP, Hunt SC, Williams RR, Lalouel JM: Absence of linkage between the angiotensin converting enzyme locus and human essential hypertension. *Nat Genet* **1**:72, 1992.

137. Fornage M, Amos CI, Kardia S, Sing CF, Turner ST, Boerwinkle E: Variation in the region of the angiotensin-converting enzyme gene influences interindividual differences in blood pressure levels in young white males. *Circulation* **97**:1773, 1998.

138. O'Donnell CJ, Lindpaintner K, Larson MG, Rao VS, Ordovas JM, Schaefer EJ, Myers RH, Levy D: Evidence for association and genetic linkage of the angiotensin-converting enzyme locus with hypertension and blood pressure in men but not women the Framingham Heart Study. *Circulation* **97**:1766, 1998.

139. Courterousse O, Allegrini J, Lopez M, Alhenc-Gelas F: Angiotensin 1-converting enzyme in human circulating mononuclear cells: genetic polymorphism of expression in t-lymphocytes. *Biochem J* **290**:33, 1993.

140. Cambien F, Poirier O, Lecerf L, Evans A, Cambou JP, Arveiler D, Luc G, Bard JM, Bara L, Ricard S, Tiret L, Amouye P, Alhenc-Gelas F: Deletion polymorphism of the gene for angiotensin-converting enzyme is a potent risk factor for myocardial infarction. *Nature* **359**:64, 1992.

141. Shunkert H, Hense HW, Holmer SR, Stender M, Perz S, Keil U, Lorell B, Riegges GAJ: Association between angiotensin converting enzyme gene polymorphism and left ventricular hypertrophy. *N Engl J Med* **330**:1634, 1994.

142. Rieder MJ, Taylor SL, Clark AG, Nickerson DA: Sequence variation in the human angiotensin converting enzyme. *Nat Genet* **22**:59, 1999.

143. Gu L, Dene H, Deng AY, Hoebee B, Bihoreau M-T, James M, Rapp JP: Genetic mapping of two blood pressure quantitative trait loci on rat chromosome 1. *J Clin Invest* **97**:777, 1996.

144. Wong ZY, Stebbing M, Ellis JA, Lamantia A, Harrap SB: Genetic linkage of beta and gamma subunits of epithelial sodium channel to systolic blood pressure. *Lancet* **10(353)**:1222, 1999.

145. Nagy Z, Busjahn A, Bahring S, Faulhaber HD, Gohlke HR, Knoblauch H, Rosenthal M, Muller-Myhsok B, Schuster H, Luft FC: Quantitative trait loci for blood pressure exist near the IGF-1, the Liddle syndrome, the angiotensin II-receptor gene and the renin loci in man. *J Am Soc Nephrol* **10**:1709, 1999.

146. Niu T, Xu X, Cordell HJ, Rogus J, Zhou Y, Fang Z, Lindpaintner K: Linkage analysis of candidate genes and gene-gene interactions in Chinese hypertensive sib pairs. *Hypertension* **33**:1332, 1999.

147. Munroe PB, Strautnieks SS, Farrall M, Daniel HI, Lawson M, DeFreitas P, Fogarty P, Gardiner RM, Caulfield M: Absence of linkage of the epithelial sodium channel to hypertension in black Caribbeans. *Am J Hypertens* **11**:942, 1998.

148. Persu A, Barbry P, Bassilana F, Houot AM, Mengual R, Lazdunski M, Corvol P, Jeunemaitre X: Genetic analysis of the beta subunit of the epithelial Na$^+$ channel in essential hypertension. *Hypertension* **32**:129, 1998.

149. Warnock DG: T594M mutation in the ENaC beta subunit and low-renin hypertension in blacks. *Am J Kidney Dis* **34**:579, 1999.

150. Baker EH, Dong YB, Sagnella GA, Rothwell M, Onipinla AK, Markandu ND, Cappuccio FP, Cook DG, Persu A, Corvol P, Jeunemaitre X, Carter ND, MacGregor GA: Association of hypertension with T594M mutation in beta subunit of epithelial sodium channels in black people resident in London. *Lancet* **9(351)**:1388, 1998.

151. Krushkal J, Xiong M, Ferrell R, Sing CF, Turner ST, Boerwinkle E: Linkage and association of adrenergic and dopamine receptor genes in the distal portion of the long arm of chromosome 5 with systolic blood pressure variation. *Hum Mol Genet* **7**:1379, 1998.

152. Timmermann B, Mo R, Luft FC, Gerdts E, Busjahn A, Omvik P, Li GH, Schuster H, Wienker TF, Hoehe MR, Lund-Johansen P: Beta-2 adrenoceptor genetic variation is associated with genetic predisposition to essential hypertension: The Bergen Blood Pressure Study. *Kidney Int* **53**:1455, 1998.

153. Baldwin CT, Schwartz F, Baima J, Burzstyn M, DeStefano AL, Gavras I, Handy DE, Joost O, Martel T, Manolis A, Nicolaou M, Bresnahan M, Farrer L, Gavras H: Identification of a polymorphic glutamic acid stretch in the alpha2B-adrenergic receptor and lack of linkage with essential hypertension. *Am J Hypertens* **12**:853, 1999.

154. 37. Busjahn A, Li GH, Faulhaber HD, Rosenthal M, Becker A, Jeschke E, Schuster H, Timmermann B, Hoehe MR, Luft FC: Beta-2 adrenergic receptor gene variations, blood pressure, and heart size in normal twins. *Hypertension* **35**:555, 2000.

155. Xu X, Rogus JJ, Terwedow HA, Yang J, Wang Z, Chen C, Niu T, Wang B, Xu H, Weiss S, Schork NJ, Fang Z: An extreme sib-pair genome scan for genes regulating blood pressure. *Am J Hum Genet* **64**:1694, 1999.

156. Xu X, Yang J, Rogus J, Chen C, Schork N, Xu X: Mapping of a blood pressure quantitative trait locus to chromosome 15q in a Chinese population. *Hum Mol Genet* **8**:2551, 1999.

157. Krushkal J, Xiong M, Ferrell R, Sing CF, Turner ST, Boerwinkle E: Linkage and association of adrenergic and dopamine receptor genes in the distal portion of the long arm of chromosome 5 with systolic blood pressure variation. *Hum Mol Genet* **7**:1379, 1998.

158. Jacob HJ, Lindpaintner K, Lincoln SE, Kusumi K, Bunker RK, Mao Y-P, Ganten D, Dzau VJ, Lander ES: Genetic mapping of a gene causing hypertension in the stroke-prone spontaneously hypertensive rat. *Cell* **67**:213, 1991.

159. Deng Y, Rapp JP: Cosegregation of blood pressure with angiotensin converting enzyme and atrial natriuretic peptide receptor genes using Dahl salt-sensitive rats. *Nat Genet* **1**:267, 1992.

160. Julier C, Delepine M, Keavney B, Terwilliger J, Davis S, Weeks DE, Bui T, Jeunemaitre X, Velho G, Froguel P, Ratcliffe P, Corvol P, Soubrier F, Lathrop GM: Genetic susceptibility for human familial essential hypertension in a region of homology with blood pressure linkage on rat chromosome 10. *Hum Mol Genet* **6**:2077, 1997.

161. Baima J, Nicolaou M, Schwartz F, DeStefano AL, Manolis A, Gavras I, Laffer C, Elijovich F, Farrer L, Baldwin CT, Gavras H: Evidence for linkage between essential hypertension and a putative locus on human chromosome 17. *Hypertension* **34**:4, 1999.

# Hereditary Hemorrhagic Telangiectasia

*Douglas A. Marchuk* ■ *Andreas Lux*

Identified over a century ago, hereditary hemorrhagic telangiectasia (HHT), or Rendu-Osler-Weber syndrome, is an autosomal dominant condition characterized by multisystemic vascular malformations and hemorrhage from the associated vascular lesions. HHT may have first been described by Sutton[1] and in turn, Babington,[2] as a hereditary form of epistaxis. However, it was Rendu[3] who first recognized the combination of hereditary epistaxis and telangiectases as a distinct clinical entity from hemophilia. At the turn of the nineteenth century, Osler[4] and Weber[5] produced case reports of inherited epistaxis and cutaneous and/or mucocutaneous telangiectases. Shortly thereafter, Hanes[6] coined the term hereditary hemorrhagic telangiectasia using the three clinical features that at that time defined the disorder.

Although HHT occurs with a wide geographic distribution and has been described in all racial and in most ethnic groups, most of the literature describes Caucasian families. Whether this is due to an increased incidence in Caucasians or due to an ascertainment bias is uncertain. For example, careful examination of the oral and nasal mucosa, the tongue, and the conjunctiva is suggested to be important in individuals of African descent, in whom skin lesions may not be as obvious.[7] The past few decades saw increased numbers of case reports of HHT kindreds from the Far East and the Indian subcontinent, suggesting that these are due to increased awareness of the disorder.

Earlier estimates of disease prevalence were approximately 1 to 2 per 100,000. However, recent epidemiologic surveys indicate that the disorder is much more frequent than originally thought, possibly due to increased awareness of and interest in this disorder. Minimal estimates of the prevalence are 1 in 2351 individuals in the French department of Ain,[8] approximately 1 in 3500 on the Danish island of Fyn,[9] at least 1 in 16,500 in Vermont,[10] and at least 1 in 39,000 in northern England.[11] Some of these, in turn, may be low estimates as the disorder is often improperly diagnosed or missed altogether, until a life-threatening episode occurs.[10] Nonetheless, with proper physical examination and recent advances in screening for internal vascular lesions, proper diagnosis can be made in most cases. Recent studies have indicated that in HHT kindreds, penetrance is 97 percent by age 40 to 45.[8,11]

Two reports have suggested different outcomes for the homozygous state of HHT. Snyder and Doan[12] described an infant born to two HHT-affected parents, where the disease could be traced at least one generation further back for each side of the family. At birth the infant exhibited multiple cutaneous telangiectases, and died at 11 weeks of age due to hemorrhage from multiple internal "hemangiomas." The authors suggested that the child represented the homozygous state, which they felt was a lethal form of the disease. This would be partly consistent with the mouse knockout mutations for both endoglin and ALK-1, which are lethal in the homozygous state, although both mouse models exhibit embryonic lethality. Despite the severe phenotype of the infant, there is no molecular evidence that the child inherited two mutant HHT genes. In addition, the genetic heterogeneity now known to exist in HHT suggests that even if the child did inherit

mutant HHT genes from both parents, it is possible that the child was a double-heterozygote for ALK-1 and endoglin mutations. Thus, although this early case report is intriguing, it does not solve the question of the homozygous state.

On the other hand, study of a large inbred family affected with HHT led to the identification of a proposed homozygous individual who lived to adulthood.[13] Due to the high degree of consanguinity in the family, a descendant of two affected parents was identified. This male lived to adulthood and had 13 children (from multiple wives), all of whom were affected. Using Bayes theorem, the probability that he was homozygous for an HHT-causative mutation is 0.99975. This is in stark contrast to the embryonic lethal mouse homozygous endoglin and ALK-1 knockouts. Taking at face value the correct diagnoses of all 13 children of the proposed homozygous father, these data suggest crucial differences between the roles of endoglin and ALK-1 in mouse and human development.

## CLINICAL MANIFESTATIONS

HHT is characterized by vascular lesions and bleeding in a variety of organs, leading to serious morbidity and estimates of up to 10 percent mortality in affected individuals. Recently approved guidelines for diagnosis of HHT require the presence of three of the following four criteria: spontaneous recurrent epistaxis; telangiectases at characteristic sites; a visceral manifestation; and a family history of HHT.[14] However, the various organs and tissues that may contain vascular lesions give the disorder a wide range of clinical features, of which the following are characteristic. Telangiectases are red to violet lesions that appear on digits; the facial, nasal, and buccal mucosa; and the gastrointestinal tract. These lesions are dilated venules to which several arterioles make direct connections without intervening capillaries, resulting in bleeding. Epistaxis is present in up to 90 percent of the individuals and gastrointestinal tract bleeding is seen in 20 to 40 percent of patients. Hemorrhage from either site often progresses with age and can result in chronic anemia and hypoxemia. Patients requiring transfusions totaling more than 100 units of blood are well documented.[15]

Telangiectases may be the direct precursor to arteriovenous malformations (AVMs), which are commonly seen in the lung. Pulmonary AVMs consist of direct connections between a branch of a pulmonary artery and a pulmonary vein through a thin-walled aneurysm. These can result in direct right-to-left shunts and, particularly when multiple, can lead to profound dyspnea, fatigue, cyanosis, and polycythemia. Stroke is a common and serious complication because the pulmonary AVMs allow blood clots to traverse the region and be carried to the brain.[16] Brain abscesses can occur because the pulmonary AVMs also allow the passage of bacteria that can ultimately infect the brain.[16] Pregnancy is a serious risk factor for pulmonary AVMs (PAVMs) in patients with HHT, especially in the third trimester[17–20] when recurrent hemoptysis and hemothorax can occur. It is postulated that increased blood volume and/or estrogen-progesterone imbalance resulting in altered vascular tone[21] may be factors in the development of new PAVMs[22] or the growth and/or deterioration of existing lesions.[17,18]

Neurologic symptoms of HHT include migraine headache, brain abscess, transient ischemic attack, stroke, seizure, and intracerebral and subarachnoid hemorrhage. Brain abscess, transient ischemic attack, and ischemic stroke occur as neurologic sequelae of pulmonary AVMs. Subarachnoid hemorrhage, seizure, and, less commonly, paraparesis can be caused by cerebral or spinal AVMs. Cerebral vascular lesions were originally thought to involve only 5 to 10 percent of patients.[23] With the application of more sensitive screening modalities in HHT families, it appears that the frequency of cerebral vascular lesions is much greater.[24]

Gastrointestinal bleeding occurs in 10 percent to 30 percent of patients with HHT,[25-28] usually occurring much later than epistaxis, with an onset in the fourth or fifth decade.[9] In one study,[9] the median age of onset of GI bleeding was 55 years, whereas for epistaxis it was 11 years. Vascular lesions occur most frequently in the upper GI tract, predominantly in the stomach and duodenum.[9] Endoscopy reveals nodular lesions that do not differ greatly from cutaneous telangiectases, although many of the lesions were surrounded by an anemic halo. Spider nevi are not observed.

Liver involvement due to the presence of multiple AVMs or atypical cirrhosis is an important manifestation of HHT.[29,30] Retrospective estimates of liver involvement in HHT range from 8 percent[31] to 31 percent,[32] although the true prevalence remains unknown. Liver involvement in HHT can be imaged with Doppler ultrasound angiography, computed tomography (CT) with contrast enhancement, and MRI. Sonography shows increased blood flow within the dilated hepatic artery that represents a very sensitive and diagnostic parameter for hepatic involvement in HHT.[33] Angiographic and CT analysis shows that the typical features include dilated hepatic artery and hepatic veins and often multiple aneurysms of the intraparenchymal branches of the hepatic artery and both hepatoportal and hepatohepatic arteriovenous fistulae.[34] Cholestasis is often the main clinical sign that correlates with the severity of the hepatic vascular abnormalities.[33] Liver involvement may be more prevalent in a distinct genetic subtype of HHT that has yet to be genetically mapped.[35] There is some suggestion that liver involvement is not age-related and may be more prevalent in females.[33] High cardiac output caused by left-to-right shunting within the liver can lead to heart failure.[30]

## ANATOMY OF THE VASCULAR LESION

Vascular lesions seen in HHT patients range from smaller cutaneous and mucocutaneous telangiectases to larger visceral arteriovenous malformations. Early histologic descriptions of HHT-associated telangiectases showed thin-walled, dilated vessels consisting of a single layer of endothelium that lacked a connective or muscular tissue layer. The hallmark feature of the HHT-associated lesion is direct arteriovenous communication. This direct shunting of arterial blood suggests that increased blood flow through the lesion may make it prone to hemorrhage. For submucosal or subepidermal vessels, especially in the nasal passage, it appears that minor trauma or irritation can trigger hemorrhage. Various explanations have been put forward to explain the angiodysplasia seen in HHT, including endothelial cell degeneration,[36] defects in endothelial junctions,[37] lack of elastic fibers and incomplete smooth-muscle-cell coating of the vessels,[38] and weak connective tissue surrounding the vessel.[36] The recurrent hemorrhage must be related to the localized abnormality within the blood vessel because normal hemostasis and platelet function are present.[39,40]

More recent ultrastructural analysis provides a more refined view of the anatomy of the vascular lesion (Fig. 212-1). Braverman[41] studied 10 cutaneous telangiectatic lesions of HHT ranging in size from a pinpoint to 2 mm, using light and electron microscopy (EM). The lateral extent of the lesions was 6 to 10

times larger than the estimates of the size of the lesions observed clinically. The smallest and earliest detectable lesions showed a focal dilation of the postcapillary venule that retained connections to an arteriole through one or more capillaries. Under EM, the dilated postcapillary venules showed prominent stress fibers in the pericytes along their adluminal border. A perivascular infiltrate of mononuclear cells was also present. The ultrastructure of the cells suggests that the majority of these were lymphocytes with the minority being monocytes or macrophages.

Larger lesions (0.5 mm) showed a thickening of the walls of the postcapillary venules due to increased numbers of pericytes and increased luminal diameter. The arterioles were also dilated but still connected to the venules through short capillary segments. The 2-mm lesions showed marked dilation and convolution of the venules that extended through the entire dermis. The venules had 8 to 11 layers of smooth-muscle cells. Most lesions of this size had lost the intervening capillary segments that were replaced by direct arteriovenous connections. The fully developed lesion is an arteriovenous communication. The high-pressure flow into a dilated saccule without the resistance of an intervening capillary bed may cause the bleeding problems seen in HHT. Rapid flow can inhibit coagulation and lead to the profuse and prolonged bleeding characteristic of HHT. In all stages, the lesion was associated with aggregated mononuclear cells. The authors suggested that the initial lesion formation in HHT might be related to inflammation as the triggering event. Braverman did not find any evidence of abnormalities in the microvascular cells themselves; there was no endothelial necrosis, nor were there cell gaps or any other abnormalities of the pericytes or smooth-muscle cells. They suggested that the reports of HHT-associated telangiectatic vessels lacking smooth muscle and pericytes and exhibiting gaps between cells[37] were incorrectly describing lymphatic capillaries.

Braverman[42] suggests a similar outcome for microvessels injured by chronic ultraviolet light. Vessels in the dermis exhibit a widening due to the deposition of a perivascular layer of basement membrane-like material admixed with individual collagen fibers. Veil cells (flat adventitial cells) are increased in number and size. The postcapillary venules are more severely affected than terminal arterioles or capillaries. Whether or not ultraviolet light damage can trigger the cutaneous lesions seen in HHT is unknown.

## ENDOGLIN AND HHT1

In the absence of clear candidate genes for HHT, a positional cloning approach was used to identify the molecular defect. Genetic linkage for some families was established to markers on 9q33-q34.[43,44] The identification of key obligate recombinants in affected individuals from families linked to this region allowed refinement of the HHT1 locus and placed the most likely position of the HHT1 gene within a 2- to 3-cM interval between D9S60 and D9S61.[44-46] Endoglin was considered a strong candidate gene based on its location on human chromosome 9q34,[47] its precise position in the syntenic region of the mouse genome,[48] and its biologic properties. More recent physical mapping shows that the endoglin gene maps between genetic markers D9S60 and D9S61, near D9S315 and D9S112. These later markers are useful to establish or exclude linkage to this locus in new HHT families. Mutations in endoglin were subsequently identified in HHT1 kindreds.[49]

Endoglin is a homodimeric integral membrane protein expressed at high levels on human vascular endothelial cells of all blood vessels.[50] On endothelial cells, endoglin is the most abundant TGF-$\beta$-binding protein.[51] The 90-kDa endoglin protein is encoded by a gene comprising 15 exons.[52,53] In addition to the originally identified endoglin cDNA, a splice variant called S-endoglin (for short endoglin) was detected that coded for an 85-kDa protein.[54] The extracellular and transmembrane domains of S-endoglin and the longer endoglin version (L-endoglin) are identical, while the alternative splicing creates a novel, 14-amino-acid residue cytoplasmic domain for S-endoglin. These two

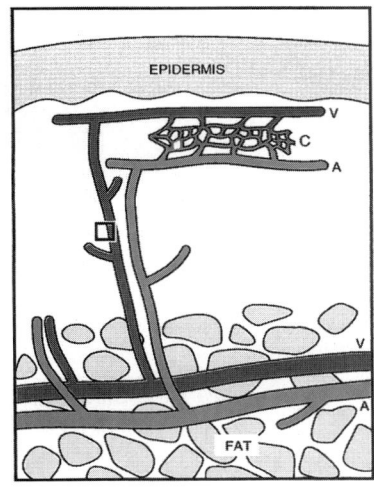
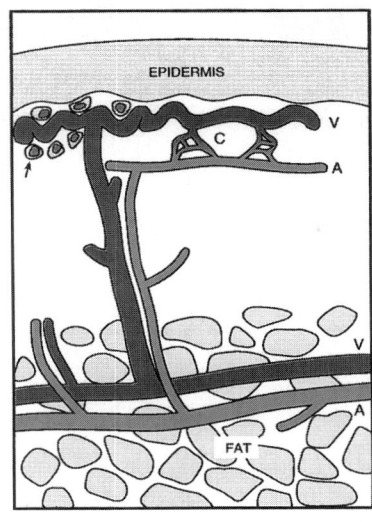
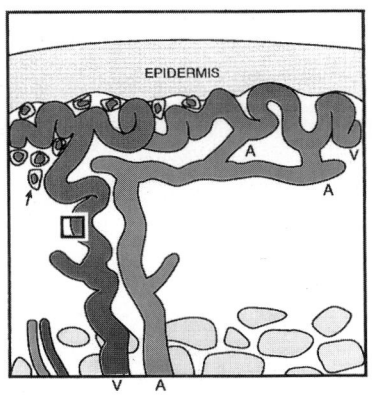
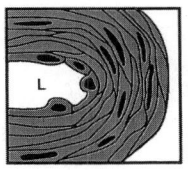
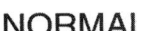

NORMAL        EARLY        LATE

**Fig. 212-1** Development of a cutaneous telangiectasis in HHT. In normal skin, arterioles (A) in the papillary dermis connect to venules (V) through multiple capillaries (C). A normal postcapillary venule (shown in cross-section in the inset) consists of the lumen (L), a single layer of endothelial cells, and two to three layers of pericytes. In the early stage of telangiectasis development, a single venule becomes dilated, but is still connected to an arteriole through one or more capillaries. A perivascular lymphocytic infiltrate is present. In the fully developed telangiectasis, the venule and its branches have become markedly dilated, elongated, and convoluted throughout the dermis. The connecting arterioles have also become dilated and these communicate directly with the venules without an intervening capillary bed. The perivascular infiltrate is still present. The dilated descending venule is markedly thickened with as many as 11 layers of smooth-muscle cells. (*Adapted from Braverman et al.*[41] *and Guttmacher et al.*[161] *Used with permission.*)

isoforms are coexpressed in different cell types, although the majority of the transcripts correspond to L-endoglin. Although the physiological distinctions between L- and S-endoglin are not yet completely known, in at least two assays of signaling, they differ in their response to ligand.[55]

Forty-one distinct mutations have thus far been identified in the endoglin gene in HHT families (Table 212-1). In all but a few cases, these mutations appear to be family specific. These include missense mutations, nonsense mutations, larger genomic deletions, splice-site changes, and small nucleotide insertions and deletions leading to frameshifts and premature stop codons. Nonsense mutations and frameshift mutations have currently been identified in exons 3 through 12, which, if translated, would produce severely truncated proteins. Expression data from a number of frameshift and nonsense mutations show that many of these create unstable messages,[53,56] and, therefore, little to no mutant proteins would be produced. Thus, these mutations are assumed to create null alleles. The identical missense mutation within the start codon of the endoglin gene has been identified in two unrelated families.[53] This mutation appears to be a null allele that eliminates the translation of the endoglin protein, similar to start codon mutations in other genetic disorders.[55,57–59] Large and small deletions of the coding region have also been described,[52] some of which are not transcribed. These are also clear examples of null alleles.

As in many genetic disorders, the missense mutations in endoglin can be instructive for understanding endoglin structure and function.[53] Two missense mutations in endoglin are within or adjacent to Cys53, suggesting that this is a critical residue involved in intra- or intermolecular disulfide bridging. In another HHT family, a conserved tryptophan at codon 149 is mutated to a cysteine. It may be significant that this mutation creates rather than destroys a cysteine, as this substitution might cause aberrant disulfide linkages. In another family, a Leu to Pro substitution disrupts a predicted alpha helix in the extracellular domain.

These missense mutations suggest that in these cases the mutant endoglin is misfolded and thus potentially nonfunctional. Expression studies show that this is the case.[60,61] In general, these missense mutations show no cell-surface expression. However, some of these mutant proteins can be expressed intracellularly and therefore might act in a dominant-negative fashion. In vitro expression in COS cells of six different missense mutations and two truncation mutations[61] revealed that the mutant proteins are misfolded and that most show no cell-surface expression when expressed alone. However, when coexpressed with wild-type endoglin, the missense mutants dimerized with the normal endoglin protein and were trafficked to the cell surface. This indicates that the normal endoglin protein can act as a chaperone for the mutant proteins by dimerizing and escorting them to the cell surface where they exist as mutant/wild-type heterodimers. With either a haploinsufficiency or dominant-negative model, each endoglin mutation would be predicted to lead to reduced levels of functional endoglin at the endothelial cell surface.

Aside from its involvement in HHT, several reports suggest that endoglin plays a key role in tumor-related angiogenesis. Elevated expression of endoglin correlates with proliferation of tumor endothelial cells[62] and higher levels of endoglin correlate with poor prognosis in breast carcinoma.[63] In vitro and in vivo studies demonstrate that antiendoglin antibodies inhibit endothelial cell growth.[64,65] In a therapeutic study, SCID mice were inoculated subcutaneously with MCF-7 human breast cancer cells and left untreated until palpable tumors of 4 to 6 mm in diameter appeared.[65] These mice were then treated three times with two different conjugated monoclonal antiendoglin antibodies.

**Table 212-1** Endoglin Mutations in HHT1 Families

**Missense mutations**

| Exon | Mutation | Effect | Reference |
|------|----------|--------|-----------|
| 1 | 2T → C | Destroys start codon | 53 |
| 2 | 155G → T | G52V | 53 |
| 2 | 157T → C | C53R | 53 |
| 4 | 447G → C | W149C | 53 |
| 4 | 479C → A | A160N | 159 |
| 5 | 662T → C | L221P | 60 |
| 7 | 917T → C | L306P | 53 |
| 9A | 1238G → T | G413V | 162 |

**Nonsense mutations**

| Exon | Mutation | Effect | Reference |
|------|----------|--------|-----------|
| 3 | 277C → T | R93X | 91 |
| 4 | 511C → T | R71X | 52 |
| 5 | 587G → A | W196X | 160 |
| 7 | 831C → G | Y277X | 49 |
| 8 | 1050T → A | C350X | 160 |
| 10 | 1414C → T | Q472X | 160 |

**Frameshift mutations: Deletions**

| Exon | Mutation | Effect | Reference |
|------|----------|--------|-----------|
| 2 | del 152 | Deletes exon 2 | 52 |
| 5 | 855del21 | Deletes RTLEWRP | 52 |
| 8 | 1089delTG | Premature stop | 91 |
| 8 | 1078delCAGA | Premature stop | 53 |
| IVS8 | del < 60kb | Deletes exons 9A-14 | 52 |
| 9A | 1186delG | Premature stop | 91 |
| 9A | 1206delG | Premature stop | 53 |
| 9A | 1267delA | Premature stop | 53 |
| 11 | 1432delAG | Premature stop | 53 |
| 11 | 1550delTG | Premature stop | 160 |
| 11 | 1553delGC | Premature stop | 49 |
| 11 | 1655delC | Premature stop | 160 |
| 12 | 1689del11 | Premature stop | 91 |

**Table 212-1** (Continued)

**Frameshift mutations: Insertions**

| Exon | Mutation | Effect | Reference |
|------|----------|--------|-----------|
| 5 | 561insCGCA | Premature stop | 91 |
| 8 | 1111insG | Premature stop | 160 |
| 11 | 1470insA | Premature stop | 91 |

**Splicing errors**

| Position | Mutation | Effect | Reference |
|----------|----------|--------|-----------|
| IVS1 + 1 | g → a | Destroys splice donor site | 162 |
| IVS3 + 1 | g → a | Deletes exon 3 | 56 |
| IVS 3 + 4 | a → g | Deletes exon 3 | 52 |
| IVS4−2 | a → g | Destroys splice acceptor site | 53 |
| IVS6−2 | a → t | ?Deletes exon 6 | 91 |
| IVS8 + 1 | g → a | 1391del24 | 52 |
| IVS9−2 | t → a | ?Deletes exon 9B | 91 |
| Exon 9B | 1311G → A | Disrupts 3′ splicing | 53 |

**Complex rearrangements**

| Exon | Mutation | Effect | Reference |
|------|----------|--------|-----------|
| 7 | 819del8, ins24 | 16-bp insertion, FS at 820 | 91 |
| 8 | del 1.5 kb | Deletes exon 8 | 52 |
| 10 | 1414delAGA, insGT | 1-bp deletion, FS at Q471 | 91 |

Long-lasting complete tumor regression (for at least 100 days) without further therapy was induced in the majority of tumor-bearing mice.

In view of the potential therapeutic applications of modulating endoglin gene expression for both HHT and possibly cancer, it is important to understand the tissue-specific expression of this gene. Two reports investigated the endoglin promoter structure.[66,67] There are several major and minor initiation transcription sites located approximately 350 to 420 nucleotides upstream of the ATG start codon. In the immediate upstream region of these initiation sites, no consensus TATA or CAAT boxes were found. The 5′-flanking region of endoglin contains several putative regulatory elements also present in other endothelial specific genes such as von Willebrand factor (VWF), P-selectin, E-selectin, VCAM-1, PECAM, VLA-4, and endothelin-1.[68–72] These consensus elements include AP-2 sites, motifs of the ets family of transcription factors, one GATA site, two NF$_\kappa$B sites, five SP1 sites, and several TGF-$\beta$ response elements including two putative SMAD sites. Various steroid-responsive elements have also been identified, and a Myc/Max site and several AP-1 and ATF/CREB sites are located further upstream.[67]

Reporter constructs using the endoglin promoter have been tested in several cell types. These constructs display endothelial-specific activity with either no expression or only basal expression in porcine and human keratinocytes, the human hepatoma cell line HepG2, the human erythroleukemia cell line K562, mouse

NIH3T3 fibroblasts, and the human cervical carcinoma cell line HeLa. The endoglin promoter is induced in the presence of TGF-$\beta$1, as suggested by the presence of the different TGF-$\beta$ response elements. In monocytes, endoglin expression can be induced either by TGF-$\beta$1 or the phorbol ester PMA. In light of the putative SMAD binding sites, it is interesting to note that SMAD3-mediated transcription can be induced by PMA. PMA addition to hematopoietic cells was found to activate a GAL4/SMAD-dependent promoter and a TGF-$\beta$-responsive promoter.[73]

Endoglin expression is also up-regulated by estradiol.[66] This is intriguing in light of the therapeutic use of estrogens to control epistaxis and gastrointestinal bleeding in HHT patients. Estrogens are thought to control hemorrhage by inducing metaplasia of normal nasal mucosa to thick layers of keratinizing squamous epithelium.[74] This presumably covers the telangiectases and protects them against local trauma. Estrogens may also modulate the expression levels of coagulation factors.[75] However, the direct modulation of endoglin levels by estrogen may play a role in its efficacy in controlling bleeding in HHT patients.

## ALK-1 AND HHT2

Locus heterogeneity for HHT was indicated by families that excluded linkage to chromosome 9q3.[44–46] A second HHT locus (HHT2) was subsequently identified in the pericentromeric region of chromosome 12.[76,77] Based on haplotype analysis and cross-overs in these 12q-linked families, a 1-cM candidate interval was established between D12S347 and D12S368. These markers are useful to establish or exclude linkage to this locus in new HHT families. A potential candidate gene, ALK-1 (activin receptor-like kinase 1), was shown to map within this interval, and mutations were identified within this gene in HHT2 families.[78]

ALK-1 is a type I cell-surface receptor for the TGF-$\beta$ superfamily of ligands. The protein is expressed primarily on

**Table 212-2  ALK-1 Mutations in HHT2 Families**

**Missense mutations**

| Exon | Mutation | Effect | Reference |
|------|----------|--------|-----------|
| 3 | 150G → T | W50C | 79 |
| 3 | 152G → A | C51Y | 80 |
| 3 | 200G → A | R67Q | 79 |
| 3 | 231C → G | C77W | 80 |
| 3 | 286A → G | N96D | 80 |
| 7 | 998G → T | S331I | 79 |
| 8 | 1120C → T | R374W | 79 |
| 8 | 1126T → G | M376R | 76 |
| 8 | 1232G → A | R411Q | 76 |
| 9 | 1207C → A | P424T | 79 |

**Nonsense mutations**

| Exon | Mutation | Effect | Reference |
|------|----------|--------|-----------|
| 4 | 423G → A | W140X | 79 |
| 4 | 475G → T | E158X | 79 |
| 7 | 924C → A | C308X | 79 |

**Frameshift mutations: Deletions**

| Exon | Mutation | Effect | Reference |
|------|----------|--------|-----------|
| 4 | 400delG | Premature stop | 80 |
| 4 | 406delGGTG | Premature stop | 80 |
| 6 | 694delTCC | Deletes Ser in frame | 76 |

**Frameshift mutations: Insertions**

| Exon | Mutation | Effect | Reference |
|------|----------|--------|-----------|
| 3 | 140insG | Premature stop | 80 |
| 7 | 865insT | Premature stop | 79 |

endothelial cells and in highly vascularized tissues.[77] The ALK-1 gene contains 10 exons, 9 of which encode the protein sequence.[79] Eighteen mutations have been identified in the ALK-1 gene in 19 different HHT families (Table 212-2), indicating that, like endoglin mutations, ALK-1 mutations are for the most part family specific. Mutations are found throughout the gene and fall into classes of nonsense, frameshift, or missense mutations, or in one case, a 3-bp in-frame deletion adjacent to the ATP binding site of the kinase domain. The nonsense and frameshift mutations are found in the extracellular domain as well as in the kinase domain. If translated, these would create truncated proteins. The strongest candidate for a null allele in the ALK-1 gene is a 1-bp insertion mutation in exon 3 (140insG).[80] This theoretic polypeptide would lack a large portion of the extracellular domain, the entire transmembrane and GS (glycine-serine) domains, and the entire serine-threonine kinase domain. RNA expression data for some of the ALK-1 nonsense and frameshift mutations show that little or no message can be detected from the mutant allele.[79] Five distinct missense mutations have been identified within the kinase domain of ALK-1. These appear at residues that are conserved in the ALK gene family and more generally in most serine-threonine kinase receptors. These data suggest that these mutations reduce or abrogate ALK-1 signaling, although these have not formally been tested in a signaling assay. Five distinct missense mutations have also been identified in the extracellular domain of ALK-1. Intriguingly, all are within or near conserved cysteine residues in the extracellular domain, suggesting that amino acid substitutions at or near these residues might interfere with critical intra- or intermolecular disulfide bridges. Three of the missense mutations in the extracellular domain were tested in a signaling assay using a chimeric ALK-1 receptor and these three abrogate signaling.[81] These data, in combination with the sum of the mutation data, suggest that most mutations create null alleles, leading to reduced signaling through the ALK-1 receptor.

## INVOLVEMENT OF OTHER GENES IN HHT

There is a single published report of an HHT family that does not map to either the endoglin or the ALK-1 loci, indicating the existence of a third gene for HHT.[35] This locus has yet to be identified or mapped to a specific chromosome. This family had an unusual presentation of liver arteriovenous malformations in many of the affected females, suggesting the possibility of a locus-specific phenotypic characteristic. However, additional families with a similar phenotype and a novel chromosome location must be identified in order to substantiate this possibility.

A number of case reports have suggested an association of generalized juvenile polyposis (JPC) and HHT, or with one feature of HHT, namely, pulmonary arteriovenous malformations.[82–86] In some of these cases, it appears that both phenotypes were passed on to a second generation. Whether this is a coincidence of two autosomal dominant disorders or a unique syndrome due to a single gene defect is uncertain. No family large enough for genetic linkage has yet been described. Some JPC families show germ line mutations in Smad4, a downstream effector of TGF-$\beta$ signaling. It is possible that the HHT/JPC kindreds harbor mutations in a different Smad or some other factor of the TGF-$\beta$-signaling pathway in common with both the colorectal epithelium and the vasculature.

Early on, a number of case reports of an association of von Willebrand disease (VWD) and HHT suggested that the two syndromes might be allelic. However, it seems that this association is rare[39] and that at least some of these reports reflect individuals with VWD who develop telangiectases, rather than individuals with both disorders.[39,87] Linkage analysis for one of these families has confirmed the latter,[88] and with the discovery of the loci for HHT1 and HHT2, it is clear now that the VWD and HHT loci are distinct. The occasional association of these two diseases might create a situation where the vascular lesions associated with HHT would show more severe bleeding due to the coagulation defect in VWD.[39] An alternative explanation is that angiodysplasia may be a feature of VWD although expressed at a lower incidence.[89] Thus, most of the case reports may have been cases of VWD with some degree of angiodysplasia such as telangiectases, which were confused with HHT.[87]

## PROSPECTS FOR MOLECULAR TESTING FOR HHT

Because the genomic structures for the endoglin and ALK-1 genes are known,[49,52,79] amplification of individual exons and DNA sequence analysis could be performed as a diagnostic test for HHT. The family-specific nature of mutations suggests that this would be labor-intensive. In addition, the possibility of large deletions would need to be investigated thoroughly before any negative result could be confirmed in new families.[52]

Measurement of endoglin expression from appropriate tissues has been exploited for diagnostic assays for HHT1. Protein expression assays have been performed on human umbilical vein endothelial cells (HUVEC) isolated from newborns of affected mothers.[90,91] This tissue is one of the few available from living patients that express high levels of endoglin protein. Using a monoclonal antibody to the endoglin protein, these studies revealed reduced endoglin protein levels in mutation carriers. This HUVEC endoglin protein expression assay has been suggested as a simple screening test for newborns in HHT kindreds.[91] Macrophages, or activated monocytes, express endoglin on the cell surface, albeit at levels greatly reduced from those of endothelial cells. Nonetheless, peripheral blood can be obtained from children or adults, and after activation of the monocytes by adherence to a plastic culture dish for approximately 24 h, these can be assayed for endoglin protein levels. This offers the possibility of diagnosis for individuals in HHT kindreds other than newborns. When these cells are isolated from known HHT1 patients, endoglin levels are approximately 50 percent that of normal.[56,90] Thus, a protein assay for HHT1 screening might also be possible for children and adults. However, endoglin levels on activated monocytes can vary widely, as hormones and other factors modulate these levels. This may limit the use of the monocyte-endoglin assay as a diagnostic tool.

To date, there has been no clear mutation-specific genotype/phenotype correlation found in HHT. A wide variability of clinical features is seen in HHT, even among members of the same family, indicating that factors other than the inherited germ line mutation determine the individual phenotype. There does appear to be a locus-specific genotype/phenotype correlation, as was first suggested by several of the original linkage reports. It now seems clear that PAVMs are significantly more common in HHT1 families than in HHT2 families.[92] However, numerous reports show that PAVMs can and do occur in HHT2 families, severely limiting the prognostic use of this correlation. It also appears that ALK-1 mutations in general can lead to a milder disease manifestation, where diagnosis may be more difficult, although, exceptions to this correlation are common. HHT2 families may also have a higher incidence of nonpenetrant mutation carriers.[76]

## PATHOPHYSIOLOGY OF HHT

### TGF-β Signaling

Endoglin and ALK-1 are receptors for members of the TGF-β superfamily of ligands. TGF-β is the prototypical member of this family of ligands that includes activins, bone morphogenetic proteins (BMP), and Mullerian inhibitory substance (MIS). These cytokines regulate many aspects of cellular function such as proliferation, differentiation, adhesion, migration, and extracellular matrix formation.[93–95] TGF-β has three distinct isoforms: β1, β2, and β3.

Signaling through TGF-β occurs via different ligand-induced heteromeric receptor complexes consisting of type I and type II transmembrane serine/threonine kinase receptors. Several authors (reviewed in references 94, 96, and 97) have proposed models for TGF-β and activin signaling. TGF-β or activin initially binds the constitutively phosphorylated type II receptor, thereby recruiting the type I receptor into the ligand/type II receptor-complex. The type I receptor is subsequently phosphorylated by the type II receptor on serine and threonine residues in its cytoplasmic juxtamembrane GS-domain.[98] The type I receptor then phosphorylates downstream signaling mediators such as members of the recently identified Smad family, which translocate to the nucleus and effect changes in gene expression (reviewed in references 99 to 101).

Smad 6 and 7, which were first identified in endothelial cells in response to fluid laminar shear stress,[102] are now known to be anti-Smads. These Smads can act as negative regulators of signaling by stable interactions with the TGF-β type I receptor (TβR-I), preventing association with the other Smads.[103,104] Whether these endothelial Smads have any role in the pathophysiology of HHT remains to be elucidated.

### Function of Endoglin

Endoglin, also called CD105, was initially identified as a surface antigen of acute lymphoblastic leukemia (ALL) cells.[105,106] It was later determined that this antigen is primarily expressed on the cell membrane of endothelial cells from all blood vessels including capillaries, arterioles, small arteries, venules, and high endothelial venules, and in umbilical cord veins.[107] Additional cell types that express endoglin include syncytiotrophoblasts, stroma cells, smooth-muscle cells, activated monocytes/macrophages, and a subpopulation of bone marrow cells.[106,108–116]

The 90-kDa endoglin protein contains 658 amino acids comprising a single transmembrane domain, a short 47-aa-long

cytoplasmic domain, and a 586-aa-long extracellular domain including the signal peptide. The extracellular domain contains 16 cysteine residues that are involved in both inter- and intramolecular disulfide bridges. Cysteine residues between residues 330 and 412 are involved in disulfide bond-aided endoglin dimerization.[61,117] There are at least four confirmed N-linked glycosylation sites (aa 58 to 60; aa 121 to 123; aa 134 to 136; aa 307 to 309)[61] and one or more O-linked glycosylation sites.[50] Mutation analyses of the N-linked glycosylation sites demonstrate that glycosylation is not a major factor in endoglin protein trafficking. One function of N-linked glycosylation of endoglin might be to stabilize the secondary and/or tertiary structure of the protein during the folding and trafficking process.

Endoglin is classified as a TGF-β type III receptor based on its sequence homology to the proteoglycan betaglycan.[118–120] Both are transmembrane receptor proteins with short cytoplasmic domains with no known active signaling function. Their transmembrane and cytoplasmic domains are 74 percent identical at the amino acid level.[119] Betaglycan is expressed on many different cell types including mesenchymal cells, epithelial cells, and neuronal cells.[119] Betaglycan binds all three TGF-β isoforms and presents the ligands to the signaling receptors TβR-II and TβR-I, increasing the signaling activity of the type I receptor.[121] Because of its sequence homology to betaglycan, a similar function was originally proposed for endoglin.

Endoglin is the most abundant TGF-β binding protein on endothelial cells,[51] and binds the β1 and β3 isoforms, but not β2. Only 1 percent of the total endoglin molecules on the endothelial cell surface are able to bind to TGF-β.[51] Despite its sequence similarities with betaglycan, endoglin appears to be an inhibitor of TGF-β signaling. In stable endoglin-transfected L6 cells, endoglin blocks both the TGF-β1-induced activation of a plasminogen activator inhibitor-1 (PAI-1) promoter reporter construct and the cell proliferation inhibitor effect of TGF-β1 on these cells.[122] Furthermore, when overexpressed in the monocyte cell line U937, endoglin inhibits the TGF-β1-induced expression of fibronectin as well as the TGF-β1-induced down-regulation of c-myc expression.[55]

Although endoglin exists primarily as a homodimer on the cell surface, it can also be found in a heteromeric complex with TβR-I, TβR-II, and ALK-1.[55,60,81,116] When coexpressed with ActR-II and ActR-IIB, endoglin can also be an activin and BMP7 receptor, respectively.[60]

Endoglin is constitutively phosphorylated on its serine residues and incubation with the protein kinase C inhibitor H-7 prevents endoglin phosphorylation.[123] After TGF-β1 treatment, endoglin becomes rapidly dephosphorylated. The regulatory role of these changes, if any, is unknown. The endoglin amino acid sequence also contains an RGD tripeptide,[50] a key recognition motif found on extracellular matrix proteins such as fibronectin, VWF, fibrinogen, type I collagen, and vitronectin. This tripeptide is recognized by integrins,[124,125] which are important factors in cell-cell adhesion. The RGD sequence of endoglin may be involved in monocyte adhesion to endothelial cells.[111] Endoglin overexpression also inhibits the migratory capacity of NCTC929 fibroblasts. This may be a consequence of reduced PAI-1 and fibronectin production impairing cell motility. Alternatively, high levels of endoglin might favor cell-cell interactions rather than migration.[126]

### Function of ALK-1

ALK-1 (also called TSR1, R3) was cloned independently by three different groups.[77,78,127] This receptor is primarily expressed in endothelial cells and, by sequence homology, is a member of the type I receptors for the TGF-β family of ligands. Depending on its glycosylation status, ALK-1 has a molecular weight of approximately 60 to 70 kDa. Initial analyses of the newly described ALK-1 receptor did not yield clear information about the corresponding ligand, the type II receptor, or the function of ALK-1 in the cell. In coexpression studies in COS cells, ALK-1 is able to bind TGF-β1 or activin when coexpressed with the type II receptors TβR-II and

ActR-II, respectively. However, neither of these complexes elicits a signal, as determined by a number of outcomes, including proliferation response, an alteration in fibronectin expression, or the ability to activate a PAI-1 promoter-based reporter gene in the mink lung cell line Mv1Lu. Nonetheless, these observations could not exclude TGF-$\beta$ and activin as ALK-1 ligands, as ALK-1 signaling initiated by these cytokines might activate other cellular responses. Using a chimeric ALK-1 receptor comprising the extracellular ligand-binding domain of ALK-1 fused to the intracellular signaling domain of T$\beta$RI, ALK-1 was shown to be a receptor for TGF-$\beta$1 and -$\beta$3 ligands, but not for TGF-$\beta$2.[81] This ligand specificity parallels that of endoglin.[51] This chimeric receptor can also signal through a third, yet unidentified, ligand, present in human serum, which is not activin A, BMP2, BMP7, or inhibin.[81] Signaling assays with coexpressed receptor pairs[81] and cross-linking studies[128] show that the corresponding type II receptor for ALK-1 for TGF-$\beta$ signaling is T$\beta$R-II, while for the signal induction by the unidentified ligand, ALK-1 probably complexes with the activin receptors ActR-II or ActR-IIB. ALK-1 appears to have a lower affinity to the TGF-$\beta$s than T$\beta$R-1 (ALK-5), as suggested by the lower signaling activity of ALK-1 compared to T$\beta$R-I.[78,81] ALK-1 signaling can inhibit the TGF-$\beta$1-induced activation of the PAI-1 promoter-reporter construct.[81]

These data suggest that one ALK-1 function is to inhibit TGF-$\beta$1-induced cellular responses in endothelial cells. With few exceptions, the endothelial cell turnover in a healthy adult organism is very low. Maintenance of this quiescent state is regulated by endogenous negative regulators. During angiogenesis, the balance between negative and positive regulators is shifted toward positive regulators. TGF-$\beta$1 can be either a negative or positive regulator and this biphasic effect on angiogenesis is dependent on TGF-$\beta$1 concentration. Therefore, endothelial response to TGF-$\beta$1 may also be concentration-dependent. This biphasic effect may be established by the use of two different receptors such as T$\beta$R-I and ALK-1, which may have different affinities for TGF-$\beta$1.

Smad2 and Smad3 usually mediate TGF-$\beta$ and activin signaling.[129–132] Smad1 and Smad5 were thought to be primarily BMP signal mediators. However, recent work suggests that these two Smads are also involved in TGF-$\beta$1 and TGF-$\beta$3 signaling.[133,134] The murine Smad5 becomes phosphorylated after TGF-$\beta$1 induction and overexpression of murine Smad5 in L6 cells results in growth arrest.[135] This is a typical effect of TGF-$\beta$ on these cells. Smad5 is also involved in the signaling pathway by which TGF-$\beta$ inhibits primitive human hematopoietic progenitor cell proliferation and Smad5 antisense oligonucleotides can interrupt this signal.[136] Although ALK-1 is a TGF-$\beta$ receptor, the ALK-1 downstream targets are Smad1 and Smad5. A constitutively active ALK-1 receptor phosphorylates Smad1.[137,138] Furthermore, TGF-$\beta$1 is able to induce Smad1 and Smad5 phosphorylation via ALK-1 (Peter ten Dijke, personal communication; also reported as unpublished data in reference 97). Studies in breast cancer cells demonstrated that TGF-$\beta$3 responses are mediated by Smad1.[133] It is possible that some of the reported Smad1 and Smad5 effects are induced by TGF-$\beta$1 via ALK-1 signaling, rather than the T$\beta$R-I receptor. Therefore, it is important to further elucidate the role of Smad1 and Smad5 in the ALK-1 signaling pathway.

## Physiological Effects of TGF-β

TGF-$\beta$ inhibits the cell division and migration of endothelial cells.[139] TGF-$\beta$-induced suppression of endothelial growth is important in branching morphogenesis of capillaries.[140] This growth inhibitory effect may also be important in the remodeling seen in vascular lesion formation in HHT.

TGF-$\beta$ also induces changes in gene expression of a number of extracellular matrix proteins. Genes that are up-regulated (in mesenchymal cells) by TGF-$\beta$ include fibronectin, a number of collagen types, biglycan, and decorin. Other known genes that are up-regulated in response to TGF-$\beta$ include inhibitors of metalloproteinases such as PAI-1 and TIMP-1. TGF-$\beta$1 is up-regulated in

repair of injury, in response to stress, and also during viral-induced pathogenesis; any of these might be a trigger for lesion formation. TGF-$\beta$1 also up-regulates synthesis and secretion of endothelin (ET-1) by vascular endothelial cells cultured in vitro.[141] ET-1 is a potent vasoconstrictor implicated in pathogenesis of hypertension and vascular remodeling, but its role in HHT has not been addressed.

Genes that are down-regulated in response to TGF-$\beta$ include plasminogen activator, collagenase, elastase, stromelysin, and c-myc. For plasminogen activator, it is intriguing that HHT-associated lesions show increased plasminogen activator levels as measured by a histochemical fibrin slide assay.[142] The fibrinolysis inhibitor, amino-caproic acid, has been, therefore, used with limited success to control hemorrhage in HHT. Because it appears that ALK-1 and endoglin inhibit TGF-$\beta$ signaling, an endoglin or ALK-1 mutation would be expected to lead to increased levels of plasminogen activator, especially at the site of a vascular lesion. This is supported by the mouse knockout of ALK-1, where mutant embryos show increased levels of plasminogen activator.[128]

The only analysis of extracellular matrix gene expression patterns in HHT was a comparative study of fibroblasts from HHT and ataxia-telangiectasia patients.[143] Although HHT fibroblasts showed a high level of fibronectin and increased levels of integrin and beta-actin mRNA expression, it is not clear whether fibroblasts would be expected to show the same effects as endothelial cells. Nonetheless, increased levels of fibronectin would be expected in HHT patient tissue if endoglin and ALK-1 play negative roles in TGF-$\beta$ signaling.

It is not yet established whether a 50 percent reduction in endoglin leads to an altered TGF-$\beta$ response. Human umbilical vein endothelial cells derived from an HHT patient with an endoglin mutation (IVS3+1, g→a; causing an exon 3 skip) did not show altered TGF-$\beta$1-induced inhibition of proliferation as compared to normal HUVECs.[56] This might suggest that this and other assays for TGF-$\beta$ signaling are not sensitive enough to unmask the defects associated with an endoglin mutation. Another possibility is that altered TGF-$\beta$ signaling may not be the underlying cause for HHT. Because ALK-1 can signal through a yet unidentified ligand, and endoglin may modulate this signal, these data might suggest that a different ligand could be involved. One scenario is that the TGF-$\beta$ signaling pathway competes with an alternative pathway for a common downstream effector. In this way, signaling through ALK-1 may inhibit TGF-$\beta$ signaling. It has been demonstrated that high levels of BMP signaling titrate Smad 4 and compete with activin signaling.[144] A similar competition for ALK-1 and endoglin may occur by the TGF-$\beta$ ligand and another ligand.

## Vascular Lesion Development

Although the mechanisms by which mutations affect endoglin and ALK-1 function are being elucidated, the factor(s) responsible for vascular lesion formation remain unknown. A reduction to 50 percent of functional endoglin or ALK-1 levels is compatible with development of a normal vascular system *in utero*, because there is no evidence of increased miscarriage in HHT families (McKinnon and Guttmacher, unpublished observations). Yet, mutation carriers are essentially at 100 percent risk to develop the vascular lesions observed in HHT. Significantly, one of the most crucial aspects of lesion development, that is, whether the lesions are congenital, has yet to be firmly determined. Although the cutaneous lesions might suggest the contrary, it is possible that the lesions are congenital and microscopic in size at birth, and increase in size with time. Whether an increase in size or *de novo* development, it appears from studies of pulmonary AVMs that a number of factors can influence the growth and/or development of vascular lesions.

Hormonal influences are one possible factor in HHT pathogenesis. Women with HHT exhibit increased epistaxis when circulating levels of endogenous estrogen are low, such as during menopause, after ovariectomy, and at the end of menstruation.[145]

Estrogen-progesterone therapy has been shown to reduce gastro-intestinal hemorrhage and epistaxis, although these observations may relate more to hemorrhage than actual lesion development. Females are also at risk for developing PAVMs during pregnancy, which suggests a more direct hormonal influence on lesion development. Hemodynamic influences are also likely to play a role in the pathogenesis of HHT. Pregnancy induces profound changes in hemodynamic flow, and these might relate to the development or exacerbation of PAVMs, especially during the third trimester.

Endothelial damage has also been postulated as a trigger for lesion formation. Menefee and colleagues[36] carried out an electron microscopic study of vascular lesions in HHT before and after therapy with synthetic estrogen/progesterone. Before treatment, the authors noted a defect in the junctions of the endothelial cells, as did Hashimoto and Pritzker,[37] but not Jahnke.[38] In addition, they found evidence for extravasation of blood in the form of erythrocytes and thrombi in the connective tissue near the vascular lesion. Because fibrin can be a matrix for endothelial budding, they proposed that repeated episodes of the sequence (endothelial break–blood leakage–fibrin framework–new endothelial out-growth from an affected vessel), might explain the development of new vascular lesions with increasing age. They identified what appeared to be degenerating or damaged endothelial cells in the vascular lesions. These sites of degeneration were proposed to result in the gaps in the lesion, where extravasation would commence. Reduced levels of surface endoglin or ALK-1 proteins might interfere with normal repair of the vessel wall, resulting in a cascade of effects ultimately changing the vascular architecture. Interestingly, after treatment with norethynodrel and mestranol, vascular integrity appeared to be restored without residual endothelial gaps or degenerative changes.[36] The mechanism whereby estrogenic hormones might influence endothelial integrity is unclear. However, it may be that up-regulation of endoglin plays some role.[66]

Another possible trigger for lesion development might be changes in hemodynamics due to obstruction of venules. This is similar to what has been proposed for vascular ectasias of the colon. Vascular ectasias of the colon are a cause of lower intestinal hemorrhage in the elderly. One theory, based on a study of cleared and injected tissues from colon specimens, suggests a model where ectasias are formed by chronic, intermittent, low-grade obstruction of submucosal veins.[146] The authors proposed that the initial effects of this obstruction were dilation and tortuosity of submucosal veins extending to venules, capillaries, and arteries of the vascular unit. The eventual loss of competency of the precapillary sphincters can result in an arteriovenous shunt. Prolonged increased flow through this shunt can lead to alterations in the arteries supplying the shunt and the veins draining it. If a similar course of events is involved in arteriovenous malformation development in HHT, it may be that the initial event is the chronic low-grade obstruction of the veins or venules.

Another model for lesion formation involves complete loss of endoglin or ALK-1 due to somatic mutation of the normal endoglin or ALK-1 allele in an endothelial cell. This two-hit hypothesis is similar to a Knudson tumor-suppressor model, but with some distinct differences. Because TGF-$\beta$ signaling in endothelial cells modulates vascular remodeling by inducing changes in the extracellular matrix,[147,148] complete loss of signaling may induce remodeling of the capillary bed to form larger vessels, rather than directly affecting the rate of endothelial cell proliferation. Additional changes in the vascular architecture such as arterialization of the venous side of the lesion may occur as a secondary response to the hemodynamic changes due to direct shunting of arterial blood into the venous return.[41] Therefore, the resulting lesion would not be a clonal expansion of the cell harboring the original somatic mutation, and thus loss of heterozygosity or lack of endoglin (or ALK-1) protein might not be evident. Neither loss of heterozygosity nor absence of endoglin immunostaining has been observed in a small number of HHT1-

associated pulmonary arteriovenous malformations (Stenzel and Marchuk, unpublished observations).

## ANIMALS MODELS OF HHT

Studies on TGF-$\beta$1 and T$\beta$R-II knockout mice demonstrate the importance of TGF-$\beta$ signaling on vascular development. Targeted disruption of the TGF-$\beta$ ligand results in defects of yolk sac vasculature, specifically disruption of cellular adhesion between the two endothelial layers of the yolk sac. Leakage of blood cells into the yolk sac is reminiscent of the HHT hemorrhage defect. This defect only occurs in 50 percent of the offspring due to strain differences that affect the stage of development where lethality occurs, indicating that the phenotype of TGF-$\beta$1 null mice is dependent on modification by other genes.[149] The type II receptor, T$\beta$R-II, is also critical for angiogenesis in the yolk sac, but not in primary vasculogenesis.[150,151] T$\beta$R-II overexpression as well as T$\beta$R-II inhibition leads to phenotypes similar to those in the T$\beta$R-II and TGF-$\beta$1 knockout (KO) mice.[152] These data suggest that TGF-$\beta$1 is necessary for the organization and maintenance of the vascular network. Furthermore, TGF-$\beta$1 is responsible for the deposition of fibronectin in the extracellular matrix to guarantee yolk sac integrity. The authors conclude that TGF-$\beta$1 signaling must be optimal and exactly balanced for normal yolk sac development. How this is achieved, through either different TGF-$\beta$ receptors, such as T$\beta$R-I and ALK-1, or by specific Smad signaling pathways, is unknown. The early death phenotype due to defects in yolk sac vascularization may mask later effects on vasculogenesis in the embryo proper. Thus, these mouse models, while providing some clues as to the role of TGF-$\beta$ signaling in angiogenesis, do not explain the nature of the defect seen in HHT.

The roles of the endoglin and ALK-1 genes in vascular development have also been probed by disruption of these genes in the mouse. For both genes, the homozygous KO mice exhibit embryonic lethality due to arrested endothelial remodeling. Three different groups have disrupted the endoglin gene.[153–155] The primary defect is maturation arrest of the primitive vascular plexus of the yolk sac into defined vessels, leading to channel dilation and rupture. Embryos show distended blood yolk sac vessels by E9.5, a lack of vascular organization by E10.5, and embryos are resorbed by E11.5. Smooth-muscle cell differentiation and recruitment to the vessels are also defective. Various heart defects have been reported, including abnormal cardiac looping, enlarged cardiac ventricles, and pericardial sac. Heart valve formation is also disrupted, with reduction in the size of the atrioventricular endocardial cushions and disorganization of the endothelial surface of the cushions. Thus, endoglin plays a crucial role in heart development.

ALK-1 homozygous null embryos also exhibit embryonic lethality due to defects in vascular development. By E9.5 they show absence of mature blood vessels in the yolk sac, and the embryos are resorbed by E10.5. Histologic analysis of the mutant embryos shows excessive fusion of capillary plexus into cavernous vessels. Hyperdilation of large vessels and deficient differentiation and recruitment of smooth muscle cells are also evident. The endocardium and myocardium are also immature, suggesting a role for ALK-1 in heart development. Transcript levels of tissue-type plasminogen activator, urokinase-type plasminogen activator, and plasminogen activator inhibitor-1 are all elevated in the embryos, in keeping with a role of the plasminogen-plasmin system in proteolysis of perivascular matrix during angiogenesis.[156,157]

The combined biochemical and mouse knockout data suggest a model for the roles of endoglin and ALK-1 in angiogenesis, and their roles in the pathogenesis of HHT (Fig. 212-2). Endothelial cells can exist either in an activation phase or a resolution phase during angiogenesis. The activation phase is characterized by endothelial cell invasion, migration into the extracellular space, subsequent proliferation, and capillary tube formation. The proteolytic degradation of the basement membrane is required to

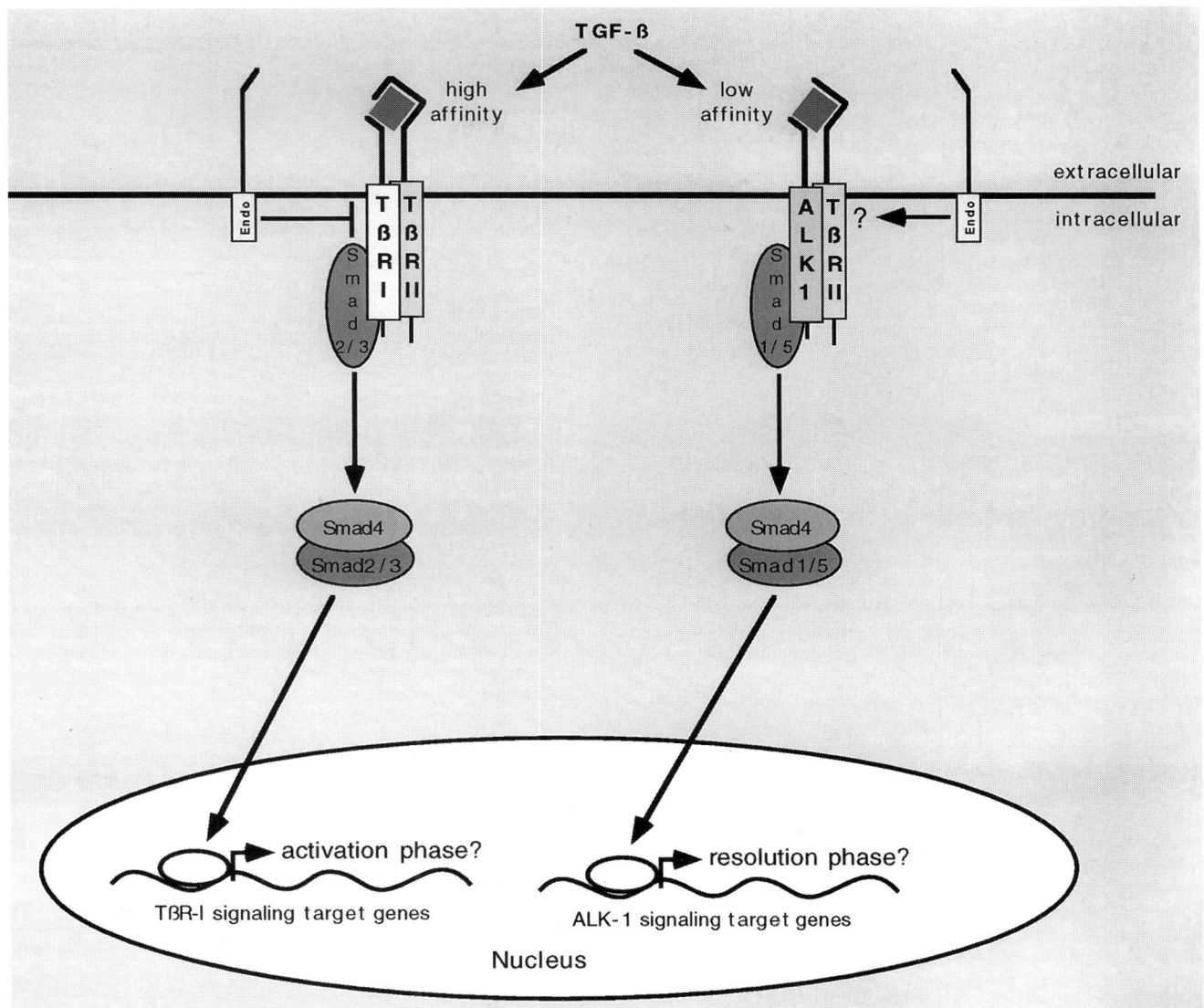

**Fig. 212-2** A model for the role of ALK-1 and endoglin in normal angiogenesis. TGF-β can signal via two distinct receptor-mediated pathways in endothelial cells. TβR-I is a high-affinity receptor that activates a pathway that includes Smad2/3 and Smad4 complexes, which may lead to transcription activation of genes involved in the activation phase of angiogenesis. ALK-1 is a lower-affinity receptor for TGF-β that signals through a pathway that includes Smad1/5 and Smad4, which may lead to transcriptional activation of genes that are involved in the resolution phase of angiogenesis. Endoglin is a negative modulator of TGF-β signaling through the TβR-I receptor, although its role in signaling via the ALK-1 receptor is less clear. Low concentrations of TGF-β ligand would favor the high-affinity TβR-I receptor, shifting the balance of signal transduction toward the activation phase of angiogenesis. High concentrations would be required to activate the ALK-1 pathway and to induce a shift to the resolution phase. Mutations in the ALK-1 gene would reduce signaling through this receptor, thus favoring signaling through the TβR-I receptor and the activation phase of angiogenesis. Mutations in endoglin would have a similar effect, removing the negative modulation of TGF-β through the TβR-I receptor, thereby shifting the balance of signal to favor the activation phase. This model assumes that endoglin enhances (or at least does not inhibit) ALK-1 receptor-mediated signaling.

initiate this process. Cessation of migration and proliferation and the reestablishment of the basement membrane characterize the resolution phase. Consistent with the biochemical data previously discussed, the ALK-1 null mice suggest that the vascular abnormalities may result from the inappropriate persistence of the activation phase of angiogenesis. Thus, ALK-1 may regulate the transition of endothelial cells from the activation to the resolution phase of angiogenesis. The biphasic effect of TGF-β on endothelial cells may also be part of this transition.[158] Low concentration of TGF-β may favor binding to the higher-affinity TβR-I receptor, which may modulate genes involved in the activation phase of angiogenesis. Higher concentrations of the TGF-β ligand may be required for binding to the lower-affinity

ALK-1 receptor, which inhibits the TβRI pathway, and thus may shift the gene expression profile to favor the resolution phase of angiogenesis.

Mutations in the ALK-1 gene would reduce signaling through this receptor, thus favoring signaling through the TβR-I receptor and the activation phase of angiogenesis. Mutations in endoglin would have a similar effect, removing the negative modulation of TGF-β through the TβR-I receptor, thereby shifting the balance of signal to favor the activation phase. This model assumes that endoglin enhances (or at least does not inhibit) ALK-1 receptor-mediated signaling.

Preliminary analyses of the heterozygotes for both ALK-1 and endoglin KO mice, the proper genetic model for the HHT phenotype, suggest that a phenotype will be less obvious and may be strain specific. No phenotype has been reported for the ALK-1 heterozygotes. A subtle phenotype of vessel dilation under the abdominal skin was noted in a few mice in one study of endoglin heterozygotes.[155] In another study, a phenotype of epistaxis and cutaneous telangiectases was apparent in a minority of endoglin heterozygotes when crossed into the inbred mouse strain background 129/Ola.[154] As previously described, strain-specific phenotypes are also seen with TGF-$\beta$1-deficient mice.[149] The existence of genetic modifiers of the mouse phenotypes is consistent with the phenotypic data in human HHT kindreds, where the phenotype can vary widely even in the same family, suggesting that other genetic and environmental factors modify the phenotype. The identification of modifier genes in the mouse should eventually lead to the examination of their human homologues in HHT kindreds.

## CONCLUSIONS

Although first described 100 years ago, little was known until recently about the molecular basis of HHT. Thus far, two genes have been identified that when mutated, give rise to this disorder. Endoglin maps to chromosome 9q33-q34 and is mutated in type 1 HHT. HHT1 families show a higher incidence of pulmonary involvement than other types of HHT families. A second gene for HHT maps to chromosome 12q13; this locus is termed type 2 HHT. The ALK-1 gene, encoding the activin receptor-like kinase 1, is mutated in HHT2. These families exhibit a lower incidence of pulmonary involvement and lower penetrance. There is evidence for a third gene with, thus far, a single family that excludes linkage to endoglin and ALK-1.

Mutations in both the endoglin and ALK-1 genes are for the most part family specific. Numerous mutations have been described in both genes that could potentially abrogate function and, in many cases, make no protein product at all. DNA sequence analysis of individual coding exons for diagnosis is possible, but labor-intensive. A diagnostic test for newborns measuring endoglin levels in umbilical vein endothelial cells, and monocytes in children or adults, may hold promise for HHT1.

Endoglin and ALK-1 are endothelial-expressed binding proteins for the family of TGF-$\beta$ ligands. It is likely that HHT pathology is caused by a defective response of endothelial cells to TGF-$\beta$1 or another ligand due to mutations in either protein. Endoglin is an accessory protein that can negatively regulate TGF-$\beta$ signaling. ALK-1 is a true receptor with a signaling function. It can signal through two TGF-$\beta$ isoforms and at least one additional unidentified ligand. ALK-1 can also down-regulate TGF-$\beta$ signaling, although the precise mechanism of this modulation is unclear. Thus, ALK-1 and endoglin may interact at the endothelial cell surface in a common signal transduction pathway involving TGF-$\beta$ or another ligand. Alternatively, ALK-1 and endoglin may act in either separate or congruent signaling pathways involving different ligands having similar effects on vascular endothelium.

The vascular lesions in HHT are localized to discrete regions within the affected tissue with no evidence of abnormal vascular structure or pathology outside the lesions themselves. This suggests that some genetic, physiologic, or mechanical event initiates the formation of each vascular lesion. The pathobiology of the disease may be related to remodeling of the vascular endothelium following an unknown initiating event. TGF-$\beta$1 mediates vascular remodeling through effects on extracellular matrix production by endothelial cells, stromal interstitial cells, smooth-muscle cells, and pericytes. Perturbations in the TGF-$\beta$ signaling pathway in HHT may lead to altered repair of vascular endothelium and remodeling of the vascular tissue via changes in expression profiles of extracellular matrix proteins.

Continued clinical research on this disorder, in combination with studies of animal models and basic biochemical characterization of the signaling pathways involved, will play an important role in elucidating the pathogenesis of HHT. In the meantime, HHT remains an intriguing puzzle whose solution promises to provide better understanding of the basic processes of vascular growth and function.

## REFERENCES

1. Sutton H: Epistaxis as an indication of impaired nutrition and degeneration of the vascular system. *Medical Mirror* **1**:769, 1864.
2. Babington B: Hereditary epistaxis [Letter]. *Lancet* **2**:362, 1865.
3. Rendu H: Epistaxis répétées chez un sujet porteur de petits angiomes cutanes et muqueux. *Gaz Hop*, 1896, p 1322.
4. Osler W: On a family form of recurring epistaxis, associated with multiple telangiectases of the skin and mucous membranes. *Bull Johns Hopkins Hosp* **12**:333, 1901.
5. Weber F: Multiple hereditary developmental angiomata (telangiectases of the skin and mucous membranes associated with recurring haemorrhages). *Lancet* **2**:160, 1907.
6. Hanes F: Multiple hereditary telangiectases causing hemorrhage (hereditary hemorrhagic telangiectasia). *Bull Johns Hopkins Hosp* **20**:63, 1909.
7. Ladipo GO: Hereditary haemorrhagic telangiectasia (Sutton-Rendu-Osler-Weber disease): first case reports in Nigerians. *Niger Med J* **8**:164, 1978.
8. Plauchu H, de Chadarevian JP, Bideau A, Robert JM: Age-related clinical profile of hereditary hemorrhagic telangiectasia in an epidemiologically recruited population. *Am J Med Genet* **32**:291, 1989.
9. Vase P, Grove O: Gastrointestinal lesions in hereditary hemorrhagic telangiectasia. *Gastroenterology* **91**:1079, 1986.
10. Guttmacher AE, McKinnon WC, Upton MD: Hereditary hemorrhagic telangiectasia: A disorder in search of the genetics community [Letter]. *Am J Med Genet* **52**:252, 1994.
11. Porteous ME, Burn J, Proctor SJ: Hereditary haemorrhagic telangiectasia: A clinical analysis. *J Med Genet* **29**:527, 1992.
12. Snyder L, Doan C: Clinical and experimental studies in human inheritance: Is the homozygous form of multiple telangiectasia lethal? *J Lab Clin Med* **29**:1211, 1944.
13. Muller JY, Michailov T, Izrael V, Bernard J: [Hereditary haemorrhagic telangiectasia in a large Saharan family: 87 cases in the same family.] *Nouv Presse Med* **7**:1723, 1978.
14. Shovlin C, Guttmacher A, Buscarini E, et al.: Diagnostic criteria for hereditary haemorrhagic telangiectasis (Rendu-Osler-Weber syndrome). *Am J Med Genet* **91**:66, 2000.
15. van Cutsem E, Rutgeerts P, Vantrappen G: Treatment of bleeding gastrointestinal vascular malformations with oestrogen-progesterone. *Lancet* **335**:953, 1990.
16. White RI Jr, Lynch-Nyhan A, Terry P, Buescher PC, Farmlett EJ, Charnas L, Shuman K, et al.: Pulmonary arteriovenous malformations: Techniques and long-term outcome of embolotherapy. *Radiology* **169**:663, 1988.
17. Gammon RB, Miksa AK, Keller FS: Osler-Weber-Rendu disease and pulmonary arteriovenous fistulas. Deterioration and embolotherapy during pregnancy. *Chest* **98**:1522, 1990.
18. Swinburne AJ, Fedullo AJ, Gangemi R, Mijangos JA: Hereditary telangiectasia and multiple pulmonary arteriovenous fistulas. Clinical deterioration during pregnancy. *Chest* **89**:459, 1986.
19. Laroche CM, Wells F, Shneerson J: Massive hemothorax due to enlarging arteriovenous fistula in pregnancy. *Chest* **101**:1452, 1992.
20. Shovlin CL, Winstock AR, Peters AM, Jackson JE, Hughes JM: Medical complications of pregnancy in hereditary haemorrhagic telangiectasia. *QJM* **88**:879, 1995.
21. Elliott JA, Rankin RN, Inwood MJ, Milne JK: An arteriovenous malformation in pregnancy: a case report and review of the literature. *Am J Obstet Gynecol* **152**:85, 1985.
22. Hoffman R, Rabens R: Evolving pulmonary nodules: multiple pulmonary arteriovenous fistulas. *Am J Roentgenol Radium Ther Nucl Med* **120**:861, 1974.
23. Roman G, Fisher M, Perl DP, Poser CM: Neurological manifestations of hereditary hemorrhagic telangiectasia (Rendu-Osler-Weber disease): Report of 2 cases and review of the literature. *Ann Neurol* **4**:130, 1978.
24. Fulbright RK, Chaloupka JC, Putman CM, Sze GK, Merriam MM, Lee GK, Fayad PB, et al.: MR of hereditary hemorrhagic telangiectasia: Prevalence and spectrum of cerebrovascular malformations. *Am J Neuroradiol* **19**:477, 1998.
25. Smith C, Bartholomew L, Cain J: hereditary hemorrhagic telangiectasia and gastrointestinal hemorrhage. *Gastroenterology* **44**:1, 1963.

26. Cachin Y, Sauvage JP, Schwaab G: [Rendu-Osler disease: Apropos of 50 cases followed at the Gustave-Roussy Institute.] *Ann Otolaryngol Chir Cervicofac* **93**:103, 1976.
27. Driscoll J, Rabe M: Hemorrhagic telangiectasis of the gastrointestinal tract, an obscure source of gastrointestinal bleeding. *Am Surg* **20**:1281, 1954.
28. Vase P, Holm M, Arendrup H: Pulmonary arteriovenous fistulas in hereditary hemorrhagic telangiectasia. *Acta Med Scand* **218**:105, 1985.
29. Martini GA: The liver in hereditary haemorrhagic teleangiectasia: An inborn error of vascular structure with multiple manifestations: A reappraisal. *Gut* **19**:531, 1978.
30. Bernard G, Mion F, Henry L, Plauchu H, Paliard P: Hepatic involvement in hereditary hemorrhagic telangiectasia: Clinical, radiological, and hemodynamic studies of 11 cases. *Gastroenterology* **105**:482, 1993.
31. Cloogman HM, DiCapo RD: Hereditary hemorrhagic telangiectasia: sonographic findings in the liver. *Radiology* **150**:521, 1984.
32. Goes E, Van Tussenbroeck F, Cottenie F, Hulstaert J, Osteaux M: Osler's disease diagnosed by ultrasound. *J Clin Ultrasound* **15**:129, 1987.
33. Buscarini E, Buscarini L, Danesino C, Piantanida M, Civardi G, Quaretti P, Rossi S, et al.: Hepatic vascular malformations in hereditary hemorrhagic telangiectasia: Doppler sonographic screening in a large family. *J Hepatol* **26**:111, 1997.
34. Rapaccini GL, Pompili M, Caturelli E, Fusilli S, Trombino C, Gomes V, Squillante MM, et al.: Ultrasound-guided fine-needle biopsy of hepatocellular carcinoma: Comparison between smear cytology and microhistology. *Am J Gastroenterol* **89**:898, 1994.
35. Piantanida M, Buscarini E, Dellavecchia C, Minelli A, Rossi A, Buscarini L, Danesino C: Hereditary haemorrhagic telangiectasia with extensive liver involvement is not caused by either HHT1 or HHT2. *J Med Genet* **33**:441, 1996.
36. Menefee MG, Flessa HC, Glueck HI, Hogg SP: Hereditary hemorrhagic telangiectasia (Osler-Weber-Rendu disease). An electron microscopic study of the vascular lesions before and after therapy with hormones. *Arch Otolaryngol* **101**:246, 1975.
37. Hashimoto K, Pritzker MS: Hereditary hemorrhagic telangiectasia. An electron microscopic study. *Oral Surg Oral Med Oral Pathol* **34**:751, 1972.
38. Jahnke V: Ultrastructure of hereditary telangiectasia. *Arch Otolaryng* **91**:262, 1970.
39. Ahr DJ, Rickles FR, Hoyer LW, O'Leary DS, Conrad ME: von Willebrand's disease and hemorrhagic telangiectasia: Association of two complex disorders of hemostasis resulting in life-threatening hemorrhage. *Am J Med* **62**:452, 1977.
40. Steel D, Bovill EG, Golden E, Tindle BH: Hereditary hemorrhagic telangiectasia. A family study. *Am J Clin Pathol* **90**:274, 1988.
41. Braverman IM, Keh A, Jacobson BS: Ultrastructure and three-dimensional organization of the telangiectases of hereditary hemorrhagic telangiectasia. *J Invest Dermatol* **95**:422, 1990.
42. Braverman IM, Sibley J, Keh-Yen A: A study of the veil cells around normal, diabetic, and aged cutaneous microvessels. *J Invest Dermatol* **86**:57, 1986.
43. McDonald MT, Papenberg KA, Ghosh S, Glatfelter AA, Biesecker BB, Helmbold EA, Markel DS, et al.: A disease locus for hereditary haemorrhagic telangiectasia maps to chromosome 9q33-34. *Nat Genet* **6**:197, 1994.
44. Shovlin CL, Hughes JM, Tuddenham EG, Temperley I, Perembelon YF, Scott J, Seidman CE, et al.: A gene for hereditary haemorrhagic telangiectasia maps to chromosome 9q3. *Nat Genet* **6**:205, 1994.
45. Heutink P, Haitjema T, Breedveld GJ, Janssen B, Sandkuijl LA, Bontekoe CJ, Westerman CJ, et al.: Linkage of hereditary haemorrhagic telangiectasia to chromosome 9q34 and evidence for locus heterogeneity. *J Med Genet* **31**:933, 1994.
46. McAllister KA, Lennon F, Bowles-Biesecker B, McKinnon WC, Helmbold EA, Markel DS, Jackson CE, et al.: Genetic heterogeneity in hereditary haemorrhagic telangiectasia: Possible correlation with clinical phenotype. *J Med Genet* **31**:927, 1994.
47. Fernandez-Ruiz E, St-Jacques S, Bellon T, Letarte M, Bernabeu C: Assignment of the human endoglin gene (END) to 9q34→qter. *Cytogenet Cell Genet* **64**:204, 1993.
48. Pilz A, Woodward K, Povey S, Abbott C: Comparative mapping of 50 human chromosome 9 loci in the laboratory mouse. *Genomics* **25**:139, 1995.
49. McAllister KA, Grogg KM, Johnson DW, Gallione CJ, Baldwin MA, Jackson CE, Helmbold EA, et al.: Endoglin, a TGF-beta binding protein of endothelial cells, is the gene for hereditary haemorrhagic telangiectasia type 1. *Nat Genet* **8**:345, 1994.
50. Gougos A, Letarte M: Primary structure of endoglin, an RGD-containing glycoprotein of human endothelial cells. *J Biol Chem* **265**:8361, 1990.
51. Cheifetz S, Bellon T, Cales C, Vera S, Bernabeu C, Massague J, Letarte M: Endoglin is a component of the transforming growth factor-beta receptor system in human endothelial cells. *J Biol Chem* **267**:19027, 1992.
52. Shovlin CL, Hughes JM, Scott J, Seidman CE, Seidman JG: Characterization of endoglin and identification of novel mutations in hereditary hemorrhagic telangiectasia. *Am J Hum Genet* **61**:68, 1997.
53. Gallione CJ, Klaus DJ, Yeh EY, Stenzel TT, Xue Y, Anthony KB, McAllister KA, et al.: Mutation and expression analysis of the endoglin gene in hereditary hemorrhagic telangiectasia reveals null alleles. *Hum Mutat* **11**:286, 1998.
54. Bellon T, Corbi A, Lastres P, Cales C, Cebrian M, Vera S, Cheifetz S, et al.: Identification and expression of two forms of the human transforming growth factor-beta-binding protein endoglin with distinct cytoplasmic regions. *Eur J Immunol* **23**:2340, 1993.
55. Lastres P, Letamendia A, Zhang H, Rius C, Almendro N, Raab U, Lopez LA, et al.: Endoglin modulates cellular responses to TGF-beta 1. *J Cell Biol* **133**:1109, 1996.
56. Pece N, Vera S, Cymerman U, White RI Jr, Wrana JL, Letarte M: Mutant endoglin in hereditary hemorrhagic telangiectasia type 1 is transiently expressed intracellularly and is not a dominant negative. *J Clin Invest* **100**:2568, 1997.
57. John SW, Scriver CR, Laframboise R, Rozen R: *In vitro* and *in vivo* correlations for I65T and M1V mutations at the phenylalanine hydroxylase locus. *Hum Mutat* **1**:147, 1992.
58. Sligh JE Jr, Hurwitz MY, Zhu CM, Anderson DC, Beaudet AL: An initiation codon mutation in CD18 in association with the moderate phenotype of leukocyte adhesion deficiency. *J Biol Chem* **267**:714, 1992.
59. Conley ME, Fitch-Hilgenberg ME, Cleveland JL, Parolini O, Rohrer J: Screening of genomic DNA to identify mutations in the gene for Bruton's tyrosine kinase. *Hum Mol Genet* **3**:1751, 1994.
60. Pece-Barbara N, Cymerman U, Vera S, Marchuk DA, Letarte M: Expression analysis of four endoglin missense mutations suggests that haploinsufficiency is the predominant mechanism for hereditary hemorrhagic telangiectasia type 1. *Hum Mol Genet* **8**:2171, 1999.
61. Lux A, Gallione CJ, Marchuk D: Expression analysis of endoglin missense and truncation mutations: insights into protein structure and disease mechanisms. *Hum Mol Genet* **9**:745, 2000.
62. Miller DW, Graulich W, Karges B, Stahl S, Ernst M, Ramaswamy A, Sedlacek HH, et al.: Elevated expression of endoglin, a component of the TGF-beta-receptor complex, correlates with proliferation of tumor endothelial cells. *Int J Cancer* **81**:568, 1999.
63. Kumar S, Ghellal A, Li C, Byrne G, Haboubi N, Wang JM, Bundred N: Breast carcinoma: vascular density determined using CD105 antibody correlates with tumor prognosis. *Cancer Res* **59**:856, 1999.
64. Maier JA, Delia D, Thorpe PE, Gasparini G: *In vitro* inhibition of endothelial cell growth by the antiangiogenic drug AGM-1470 (TNP-470) and the anti-endoglin antibody TEC-11. *Anticancer Drugs* **8**:238, 1997.
65. Matsuno F, Haruta Y, Kondo M, Tsai H, Barcos M, Seon BK: Induction of lasting complete regression of preformed distinct solid tumors by targeting the tumor vasculature using two new anti-endoglin monoclonal antibodies. *Clin Cancer Res* **5**:371, 1999.
66. Rius C, Smith JD, Almendro N, Langa C, Botella LM, Marchuk DA, Vary CPH, et al.: Cloning of the promoter region of human endoglin, the target gene for hereditary hemorrhagic telangiectasia type 1 [Citation]. *Blood* **92**:4677, 1998.
67. Graulich W, Nettelbeck DM, Fischer D, Kissel T, Muller R: Cell type specificity of the human endoglin promoter. *Gene* **227**:55, 1999.
68. Williams T, Tjian R: Analysis of the DNA-binding and activation properties of the human transcription factor AP-2. *Genes Dev* **5**:670, 1991.
69. Bassuk AG, Leiden JM: The role of Ets transcription factors in the development and function of the mammalian immune system. *Adv Immunol* **64**:65, 1997.
70. Orkin SH, Zon LI: Genetics of erythropoiesis: Induced mutations in mice and zebra fish. *Annu Rev Genet* **31**:33, 1997.
71. Baeuerle PA, T Henkel: Function and activation of NF-kappa B in the immune system. *Annu Rev Immunol* **12**:141, 1994.
72. Pugh BF, Tjian R: Mechanism of transcriptional activation by Sp1: evidence for coactivators. *Cell* **61**:1187, 1990.
73. Biggs JR, Kraft AS: The role of the Smad3 protein in phorbol ester-induced promoter expression. *J Biol Chem* **274**:36987, 1999.

74. Harrison DFN: Familial Haemorrhagic Telangiectases: 20 cases treated with systemic oestrogen. *QJM* **33**:25, 1964.

75. Geland J: Exploiting sex for therapeutic purposes. *N Eng J Med* **308**:1417, 1983.

76. Johnson DW, Berg JN, Baldwin MA, Gallione CJ, Marondel I, Yoon SJ, Stenzel TT, et al.: Mutations in the activin receptor-like kinase 1 gene in hereditary haemorrhagic telangiectasia type 2. *Nat Genet* **13**:189, 1996.

77. Attisano L, Carcamo J, Ventura F, Weis FM, Massague J, Wrana JL: Identification of human activin and TGF beta type I receptors that form heteromeric kinase complexes with type II receptors. *Cell* **75**:671, 1993.

78. ten Dijke P, Ichijo H, Franzen P, Schulz P, Saras J, Toyoshima H, Heldin CH, et al.: Activin receptor-like kinases: A novel subclass of cell-surface receptors with predicted serine/threonine kinase activity. *Oncogene* **8**:2879, 1993.

79. Berg JN, Gallione CJ, Stenzel TT, Johnson DW, Allen WP, Schwartz CE, Jackson CE, et al.: The activin receptor-like kinase 1 gene: Genomic structure and mutations in hereditary hemorrhagic telangiectasia type 2. *Am J Hum Genet* **61**:60, 1997.

80. Klaus DJ, Gallione CJ, Anthony K, Yeh EY, Yu J, Lux A, Johnson DW, et al.: Novel missense and frameshift mutations in the activin receptor-like kinase-1 in HHT. *Human Mutation: Online Mutations in Brief 164*, 1998.

81. Lux A, Attisano L, Marchuk DA: Assignment of transforming growth factor $\beta1$ and $\beta3$ and a third new ligand to the type I receptor ALK-1. *J Biol Chem* **274**:9984, 1999.

82. Cox KL, Frates RC Jr, Wong A, Gandhi G: Hereditary generalized juvenile polyposis associated with pulmonary arteriovenous malformation. *Gastroenterology* **78**:1566, 1980.

83. Conte WJ, Rotter JI, Schwartz AG, Congleton JE: Hereditary generalized juvenile polyposis, arteriovenous malformations and colonic carcinoma. *Clin Res* **30**:93A, 1982.

84. Baert AL, Casteels-Van Daele M, Broeckx J, Wijndaele L, Wilms G, Eggermont E: Generalized juvenile polyposis with pulmonary arteriovenous malformations and hypertrophic osteoarthropathy. *Am J Roentgenol* **141**:661, 1983.

85. Radin DR: Hereditary generalized juvenile polyposis: Association with arteriovenous malformations and risk of malignancy. *Abdom Imaging* **19**:140, 1994.

86. Schumacher B, Frieling T, Borchard F, Hengels KJ: Hereditary hemorrhagic telangiectasia associated with multiple pulmonary arteriovenous malformations and juvenile polyposis. *Z Gastroenterol* **32**:105, 1994.

87. Korzenik JR: Hereditary hemorrhagic telangiectasia and other intestinal vascular anomalies. *Gastroenterologist* **4**:203, 1996.

88. Iannuzzi MC, Hidaka N, Boehnke M, Bruck ME, Hanna WT, Collins FS, Ginsburg D: Analysis of the relationship of von Willebrand disease (vWD) and hereditary hemorrhagic telangiectasia and identification of a potential type IIA vWD mutation (Ile865 to Thr). *Am J Hum Genet* **48**:757, 1991.

89. Duray PH, Marcal JM Jr, LiVolsi VA, Fisher R, Scholhamer C, Brand MH: Gastrointestinal angiodysplasia: a possible component of von Willebrand's disease. *Hum Pathol* **15**:539, 1984.

90. Eiken HG, Knappskog PM, Apold J, Skjelkvale L, Boman H: A de novo phenylketonuria mutation: ATG (Met) to ATA (Ile) in the start codon of the phenylalanine hydroxylase gene. *Hum Mutat* **1**:388, 1992.

91. Cymerman U, Vera S, Pece-Barbara N, Bourdeau A, White RI Jr, Dunn J, Letarte M: Identification of hereditary hemorrhagic telangiectasia type 1 in newborns by protein expression and mutation analysis of endoglin. *Pediatr Res* **47**:24, 2000.

92. Berg JN, Guttmacher AE, Marchuk DA, Porteous ME: Clinical heterogeneity in hereditary haemorrhagic telangiectasia: Are pulmonary arteriovenous malformations more common in families linked to endoglin? *J Med Genet* **33**:256, 1996.

93. Kingsley DM: The TGF-beta superfamily: New members, new receptors, and new genetic tests of function in different organisms. *Genes Dev* **8**:133, 1994.

94. Massague J: TGF-beta signal transduction. *Annu Rev Biochem* **67**:753, 1998.

95. Sporn MB, Roberts AB: Autocrine secretion—10 years later. *Ann Intern Med* **117**:408, 1992.

96. Wrana JL, Attisano L, Wieser R, Ventura F, Massague J: Mechanism of activation of the TGF-beta receptor. *Nature* **370**:341, 1994.

97. Piek E, Westermark U, Kastemar M, Heldin CH, van Zoelen EJ, Nister M, Ten Dijke P: Expression of transforming-growth-factor (TGF)-beta receptors and Smad proteins in glioblastoma cell lines with distinct responses to TGF-beta1. *Int J Cancer* **80**:756, 1999.

98. Wieser R, Wrana JL, Massague J: GS domain mutations that constitutively activate T beta R-I, the downstream signaling component in the TGF-beta receptor complex. *EMBO J* **14**:2199, 1995.

99. Heldin CH, Miyazono K, ten Dijke P: TGF-beta signaling from cell membrane to nucleus through SMAD proteins. *Nature* **390**:465, 1997.

100. Attisano L, Wrana JL: Mads and Smads in TGF beta signaling. *Curr Opin Cell Biol* **10**:188, 1998.

101. Kretzschmar M, Massague J: SMADs: Mediators and regulators of TGF-beta signaling. *Curr Opin Genet Dev* **8**:103, 1998.

102. Topper JN, Cai J, Qiu Y, Anderson KR, Xu YY, Deeds JD, Feeley R, et al.: Vascular MADs: Two novel MAD-related genes selectively inducible by flow in human vascular endothelium. *Proc Natl Acad Sci U S A* **94**:9314, 1997.

103. Hayashi H, Abdollah S, Qiu Y, Cai J, Xu YY, Grinnell BW, Richardson MA, et al.: The MAD-related protein Smad7 associates with the TGF-beta receptor and functions as an antagonist of TGF-beta signaling. *Cell* **89**:1165, 1997.

104. Nakao A, Afrakhte M, Moren A, Nakayama T, Christian JL, Heuchel R, Itoh S, et al.: Identification of Smad7, a TGF-beta-inducible antagonist of TGF-beta signaling [Comments]. *Nature* **389**:631, 1997.

105. Quackenbush EJ, Letarte M: Identification of several cell surface proteins of non-T, non-B acute lymphoblastic leukemia by using monoclonal antibodies. *J Immunol* **134**:1276, 1985.

106. Haruta Y, Seon BK: Distinct human leukemia-associated cell surface glycoprotein GP160 defined by monoclonal antibody SN6. *Proc Natl Acad Sci U S A* **83**:7898, 1986.

107. Gougos A, Letarte M: Identification of a human endothelial cell antigen with monoclonal antibody 44G4 produced against a pre-B leukemic cell line. *J Immunol* **141**:1925, 1988.

108. Adam PJ, Clesham GJ, Weissberg PL: Expression of endoglin mRNA and protein in human vascular smooth muscle cells. *Biochem Biophys Res Commun* **247**:33, 1998.

109. Buhring HJ, Muller CA, Letarte M, Gougos A, Saalmuller A, van Agthoven AJ, Busch FW: Endoglin is expressed on a subpopulation of immature erythroid cells of normal human bone marrow. *Leukemia* **5**:841, 1991.

110. Caniggia I, Taylor CV, Ritchie JW, Lye SJ, Letarte M: Endoglin regulates trophoblast differentiation along the invasive pathway in human placental villous explants. *Endocrinology* **138**:4977, 1997.

111. Gougos A, St Jacques S, Greaves A, O'Connell PJ, d'Apice AJ, Buhring HJ, Bernabeu C, et al.: Identification of distinct epitopes of endoglin, an RGD-containing glycoprotein of endothelial cells, leukemic cells, and syncytiotrophoblasts. *Int Immunol* **4**:83, 1992.

112. Lastres P, Bellon T, Cabanas C, Sanchez-Madrid F, Acevedo A, Gougos A, Letarte M, et al.: Regulated expression on human macrophages of endoglin, an Arg-Gly-Asp–containing surface antigen. *Eur J Immunol* **22**:393, 1992.

113. Robledo MM, Hidalgo A, Lastres P, Arroyo AG, Bernabeu C, Sanchez-Madrid F, Teixido J: Characterization of TGF-beta 1-binding proteins in human bone marrow stromal cells. *Br J Haematol* **93**:507, 1996.

114. Rokhlin OW, Cohen MB, Kubagawa H, Letarte M, Cooper MD: Differential expression of endoglin on fetal and adult hematopoietic cells in human bone marrow. *J Immunol* **154**:4456, 1995.

115. St-Jacques S, Cymerman U, Pece N, Letarte M: Molecular characterization and in situ localization of murine endoglin reveal that it is a transforming growth factor-beta binding protein of endothelial and stromal cells. *Endocrinology* **134**:2645, 1994.

116. Zhang H, Shaw AR, Mak A, Letarte M: Endoglin is a component of the transforming growth factor (TGF)-beta receptor complex of human pre-B leukemic cells. *J Immunol* **156**:564, 1996.

117. Raab U, Velasco B, Lastres P, Letamendia A, Cales C, Langa C, Tapia E, et al.: Expression of normal and truncated forms of human endoglin. *Biochem J* **339**:579, 1999.

118. Lopez-Casillas F, Cheifetz S, Doody J, Andres JL, Lane WS, Massague J: Structure and expression of the membrane proteoglycan betaglycan, a component of the TGF-beta receptor system. *Cell* **67**:785, 1991.

119. Wang XF, Lin HY, Ng-Eaton E, Downward J, Lodish HF, Weinberg RA: Expression cloning and characterization of the TGF-beta type III receptor. *Cell* **67**:797, 1991.

120. Moren A, Ichijo H, Miyazono K: Molecular cloning and characterization of the human and porcine transforming growth factor-beta type III receptors. *Biochem Biophys Res Commun* **189**:356, 1992.

121. Lopez-Casillas F, Wrana JL, Massague J: Betaglycan presents ligand to the TGF beta signaling receptor. *Cell* **73**:1435, 1993.

122. Letamendia A, Lastres P, Botella LM, Raab U, Langa C, Velasco B, Attisano L, et al.: Role of endoglin in cellular responses to

transforming growth factor-beta. A comparative study with betaglycan. *J Biol Chem* **273**:33011, 1998.

123. Lastres P, Martin-Perez J, Langa C, Bernabeu C: Phosphorylation of the human-transforming-growth-factor-beta-binding protein endoglin. *Biochem J* **301**:765, 1994.

124. Ruoslahti E, Pierschbacher MD: New perspectives in cell adhesion: RGD and integrins. *Science* **238**:491, 1987.

125. Hynes RO: Integrins: A family of cell surface receptors. *Cell* **48**:549, 1987.

126. Guerrero-Esteo M, Lastres P, Letamendia A, Perez-Alvarez MJ, Langa C, Lopez LA, Fabra A, et al.: Endoglin overexpression modulates cellular morphology, migration, and adhesion of mouse fibroblasts. *Eur J Cell Biol* **78**:614, 1999.

127. He WW, Gustafson ML, Hirobe S, Donahoe PK: Developmental expression of four novel serine/threonine kinase receptors homologous to the activin/transforming growth factor-beta type II receptor family. *Dev Dyn* **196**:133, 1993.

128. Oh SP, Seki T, Goss KA, Imamura T, Yi Y, Donahoe PK, Li L, et al.: Activin receptor-like kinase 1 (ALK1) modulates TGF-beta 1 signaling in the regulation of angiogenesis. *Proc Natl Acad Sci U S A* **97**:2626, 2000.

129. Eppert K, Scherer SW, Ozcelik H, Pirone R, Hoodless P, Kim H, Tsui LC, et al.: MADR2 maps to 18q21 and encodes a TGFβ-regulated MAD-related protein that is functionally mutated in colorectal carcinoma. *Cell* **86**:543, 1996.

130. Macias-Silva M, Abdollah S, Hoodless PA, Pirone R, Attisano L, Wrana JL: MADR2 is a substrate of the TGF-beta receptor and its phosphorylation is required for nuclear accumulation and signaling. *Cell* **87**:1215, 1996.

131. Zhang Y, Feng X, We R, Derynck R: Receptor-associated Mad homologues synergize as effectors of the TGF-beta response. *Nature* **383**:168, 1996.

132. Nakao A, Roijer E, Imamura T, Souchelnytskyi S, Stenman G, Heldin CH, ten Dijke P: Identification of Smad2, a human Mad-related protein in the transforming growth factor beta signaling pathway. *J Biol Chem* **272**:2896, 1997.

133. Liu X, Yue J, Frey RS, Zhu Q, Mulder KM: Transforming growth factor beta signaling through Smad1 in human breast cancer cells. *Cancer Res* **58**:4752, 1998.

134. Yue J, Frey RS, Mulder KM: Cross-talk between the Smad1 and Ras/MEK signaling pathways for TGF-beta. *Oncogene* **18**:2033, 1999.

135. Yingling JM, Das P, Savage C, Zhang M, Padgett RW, Wang XF: Mammalian dwarfins are phosphorylated in response to transforming growth factor beta and are implicated in control of cell growth. *Proc Natl Acad Sci U S A* **93**:8940, 1996.

136. Bruno E, Horrigan SK, Van Den Berg D, Rozler E, Fitting PR, Moss ST, Westbrook C, et al.: The Smad5 gene is involved in the intracellular signaling pathways that mediate the inhibitory effects of transforming growth factor-beta on human hematopoiesis. *Blood* **91**:1917, 1998.

137. Macias-Silva M, Hoodless PA, Tang SJ, Buchwald M, Wrana JL: Specific activation of Smad1 signaling pathways by the BMP7 type I receptor, ALK2. *J Biol Chem* **273**:25628, 1998.

138. Chen YG, Massague J: Smad1 recognition and activation by the ALK1 group of transforming growth factor-β family receptors. *J Biol Chem* **274**:3672, 1999.

139. Sato Y, Rifkin DB: Inhibition of endothelial cell movement by pericytes and smooth muscle cells: activation of a latent transforming growth factor-beta 1-like molecule by plasmin during co-culture. *J Cell Biol* **109**:309, 1989.

140. Roberts AB: Molecular and cell biology of TGF-beta. *Miner Electrolyte Metab* **24**:111, 1998.

141. Kurihara H, Yoshizumi M, Sugiyama T, Takaku F, Yanagisawa M, Masaki T, Hamaoki M, et al.: Transforming growth factor-beta stimulates the expression of endothelin mRNA by vascular endothelial cells. *Biochem Biophys Res Commun* **159**:1435, 1989.

142. Kwaan HC, Silverman S: Fibrinolytic activity in lesions of hereditary hemorrhagic telangiectasia. *Arch Dermatol* **107**:571, 1973.

143. Becker Y, Tabor E, Asher Y: Ataxia-telangiectasia fibroblasts have less fibronectin mRNA than control cells but have the same levels of integrin and beta-actin mRNA. *Hum Genet* **81**:165, 1989.

144. Candia AF, Watabe T, Hawley SH, Onichtchouk D, Zhang Y, Derynck R, Niehrs C, et al.: Cellular interpretation of multiple TGF-beta signals: Intracellular antagonism between activin/BVg1 and BMP-2/4 signaling mediated by Smads. *Development* **124**:4467, 1997.

145. Koch H, Escher G, Lewis J: Hormonal management of hereditary haemorrhagic telangiectasis. *JAMA* **149**:1376, 1952.

146. Boley SJ, Sammartano R, Adams A, DiBiase A, Kleinhaus S, Sprayregen S: On the nature and etiology of vascular ectasias of the colon. Degenerative lesions of aging. *Gastroenterology* **72**:650, 1977.

147. Madri JA, Reidy MA, Kocher O, Bell L: Endothelial cell behavior after denudation injury is modulated by transforming growth factor-beta1 and fibronectin. *Lab Invest* **60**:755, 1989.

148. Merwin JR, Anderson JM, Kocher O, Van Itallie CM, Madri JA: Transforming growth factor beta 1 modulates extracellular matrix organization and cell-cell junctional complex formation during *in vitro* angiogenesis. *J Cell Physiol* **142**:117, 1990.

149. Bonyadi M, Rusholme SA, Cousins FM, Su HC, Biron CA, Farrall M, Akhurst RJ: Mapping of a major genetic modifier of embryonic lethality in TGF beta 1 knockout mice. *Nat Genet* **15**:207, 1997.

150. Dickson MC, Martin JS, Cousins FM, Kulkarni AB, Karlsson S, Akhurst RJ: Defective haematopoiesis and vasculogenesis in transforming growth factor-beta 1 knock out mice. *Development* **121**:1845, 1995.

151. Oshima M, Oshima H, Taketo MM: TGF-beta receptor type II deficiency results in defects of yolk sac hematopoiesis and vasculogenesis. *Dev Biol* **179**:297, 1996.

152. Goumans MJ, Zwijsen A, van Rooijen MA, Huylebroeck D, Roelen BA, Mummery CL: Transforming growth factor-beta signalling in extraembryonic mesoderm is required for yolk sac vasculogenesis in mice. *Development* **126**:3473, 1999.

153. Li DY, Sorensen LK, Brooke BS, Urness LD, Davis EC, Taylor DG, Boak BB, et al.: Defective angiogenesis in mice lacking endoglin. *Science* **284**:1534, 1999.

154. Bourdeau A, Dumont DJ, Letarte M: A murine model of hereditary hemorrhagic telangiectasia [Comments]. *J Clin Invest* **104**:1343, 1999.

155. Arthur HM, Ure J, Smith AJ, Renforth G, Wilson DI, Torsney E, Charlton R, et al.: Endoglin, an ancillary TGF-beta receptor, is required for extraembryonic angiogenesis and plays a key role in heart development [Citation]. *Dev Biol* **217**:42, 2000.

156. Saksela O, Rifkin DB: Cell-associated plasminogen activation: regulation and physiological functions. *Annu Rev Cell Biol* **4**:93, 1988.

157. Carmeliet P, Schoonjans L, Kieckens L, Ream B, Degen J, Bronson R, De Vos R, et al.: Physiological consequences of loss of plasminogen activator gene function in mice. *Nature* **368**:419, 1994.

158. Pepper MS, Mandriota SJ: Regulation of vascular endothelial growth factor receptor-2 (Flk-1) expression in vascular endothelial cells. *Exp Cell Res* **241**:414, 1998.

159. Yamaguchi H, Azuma H, Shigekiyo T, Inoue H, Saito S: A novel missense mutation in the endoglin gene in hereditary hemorrhagic telangiectasia. *Thromb Haemost* **77**:243, 1997.

160. McAllister KA, Baldwin MA, Thukkani AK, Gallione CJ, Berg JN, Porteous ME, Guttmacher AE, et al.: Six novel mutations in the endoglin gene in hereditary hemorrhagic telangiectasia type 1 suggest a dominant-negative effect of receptor function. *Hum Mol Genet* **4**:1983, 1995.

161. Guttmacher A, Marchuk D, White R: Current concepts: Hereditary hemorrhagic telangiectasia. *N Engl J Med* **333**:918, 1995.

162. Gallione CJ, Scheessele EA, Reinhardt D, Duits AJ, Berg JN, Westermann CJJ, Marchuk DA: Two common endoglin mutations in families with hereditary hemorrhagic telangiectasia in the Netherlands Antilles: Evidence for a founder effect. *Hum Genet* **107**:40, 2000.

# Hypertrophic Cardiomyopathy

*Christine E. Seidman* ■ *J.G. Seidman*

1. Hypertrophic cardiomyopathy is a primary disorder of ventricular muscle characterized by myocardial and myocyte hypertrophy. Disease penetrance and clinical manifestations vary considerably; some affected individuals lack symptoms, but most develop angina, dyspnea, and exercise intolerance. Sudden death, heart failure, and thromboembolic events account for the significant morbidity and mortality of hypertrophic cardiomyopathy.
2. Clinical diagnosis is based on family history, physical exam, electrocardiogram, and two-dimensional echocardiography demonstrating unexplained ventricular hypertrophy (wall thickness >13 to 15 mm in the absence of confounding factors such valvular heart disease or hypertension).
3. Hypertrophic cardiomyopathy can occur as isolated (sporadic) disease, but most often is inherited as an autosomal dominant trait (termed familial hypertrophic cardiomyopathy).
4. Cardiac pathology demonstrates increases in myocardial mass, predominantly affecting the left ventricle. Although a variety of morphologic forms of hypertrophy are recognized, asymmetric involvement of the septum is most common. Histologic findings include enlarged disorganized myocytes (disarray) interspersed with connective tissue and fibrosis.
5. The pathophysiology of hypertrophic cardiomyopathy is characterized by normal or hyperdynamic systolic function and impaired diastolic performance. Subaortic outflow tract gradients, systolic motion of the anterior mitral valve leaflet, and mitral regurgitation occur in a subset of affected individuals.
6. Familial or sporadic hypertrophic cardiomyopathy is caused by mutations in one of eight different sarcomere protein genes: cardiac actin; β-cardiac myosin heavy chain; α-tropomyosin; cardiac troponin T; cardiac troponin I; essential myosin light chain; regulatory myosin light chain; and cardiac myosin-binding protein C. At least one other disease gene (mapped to chromosome 7) remains unknown.
7. Distinct genetic etiologies of hypertrophic cardiomyopathy account for some of the variable clinical findings of disease, including age of onset of hypertrophy and survival.
8. Hypertrophic cardiomyopathy mutations rarely produce null alleles, but rather encode mutant polypeptides that are likely to be incorporated into sarcomeres. The predominant mechanism by which disease alleles perturb cardiac function therefore appears to be through dominant negative actions by mutant polypeptides.
9. Hypertrophic cardiomyopathy mutations have been genetically engineered into animals to produce relevant models for exploring the mechanisms of disease and consequences of protein mutations on sarcomere structure and function.

## OVERVIEW

Hypertrophic cardiomyopathy is a primary disorder of the myocardium characterized by an increase in heart mass (hypertrophy) that particularly affects the left ventricle (Fig. 213-1). This pathology was initially described more than 100 years ago,[1] and since then a multiplicity of descriptive names have been appended to the disease, including idiopathic subaortic stenosis, asymmetric septal hypertrophy, and hypertrophic obstructive cardiomyopathy. A modern approach to hypertrophic cardiomyopathy began when the heritable nature of the disease was recognized[2] and familial transmission defined as autosomal dominant. The development and widespread use of cardiac echocardiography over the past 25 years has, however, substantially increased clinical awareness of this disease. Current estimates indicate an incidence of hypertrophic heart disease in 1 per 500 individuals,[3] but the fraction caused by heritable gene mutations is unknown. In addition to familial disease, isolated cases of hypertrophic cardiomyopathy are also recognized.

With the application of positional cloning techniques over the past decade, considerable progress has been achieved in defining the genetic basis of hypertrophic cardiomyopathy. Although these studies have delineated large numbers of disease-causing mutations, the signals triggered by these defects and the pathways that remodel the myocardium remain unknown. Understanding how these mutations elicit a hypertrophic response is important for two reasons: First, definition of the cellular responses to these mutations could foster development of therapeutics to reduce the hypertrophic response. Second, cardiac hypertrophy is a common secondary response to a variety of other conditions, including valvular disease, hypertension, and ischemic heart disease. Delineation of the signals that trigger cardiac hypertrophy in inherited disease should lead to a better understanding of the signals that trigger cardiac hypertrophy in nongenetic conditions. Murine models of hypertrophic cardiomyopathy provide important reagents for elucidating the cellular events perturbed by gene mutations.

This chapter reviews the clinical symptoms of hypertrophic cardiomyopathy and findings on relevant diagnostic procedures, particularly electrocardiography, and echocardiography. The genetic etiologies of hypertrophic cardiomyopathy are considered, with an emphasis on the relevance that distinct mutations have in clinical phenotypes. The roles that genetically engineered mouse models have for directing future research in hypertrophic cardiomyopathy are also discussed.

## DIAGNOSIS

### Symptoms

Clinical recognition of hypertrophic cardiomyopathy is based on patient and family history, physical examination, and noninvasive cardiac assessment (electrocardiography and echocardiography). There is marked variation in the signs and symptoms of disease[4,5] and the affected individual's age, duration of disease,

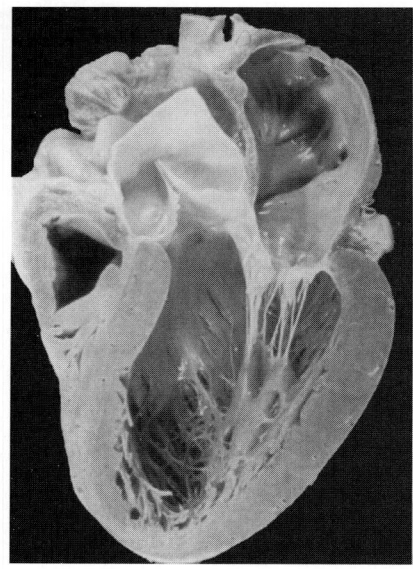
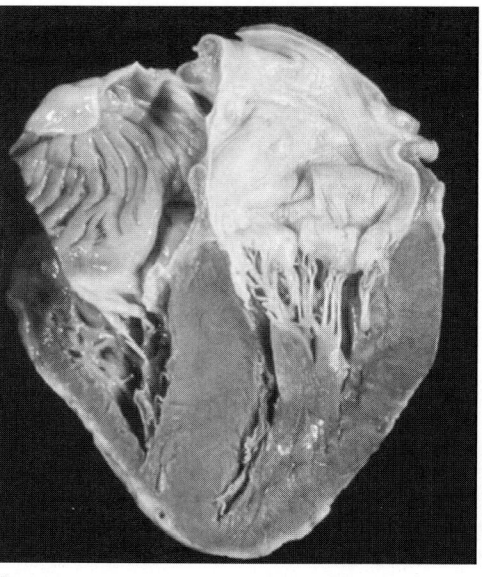

A                          B

Fig. 213-1 A comparison of normal cardiac anatomy (*A*) and the pathology of hypertrophic cardiomyopathy (*B*). Hypertrophic cardiomyopathy causes cardiomegaly (570 g; normal 270 to 360 g), biatrial (right and left) dilation, and marked increases in the interventricular and left ventricular wall thickness. Papillary muscle hypertrophy is notable.

cardiovascular hemodynamics, and genetic etiology all influence this expression. Early reports detailing the clinical manifestations of hypertrophic cardiomyopathy came from tertiary medical centers and focused on severely affected individuals. Recognition that the disorder is more common than previously suspected[3,6] now clearly indicates the marked diversity of clinical course in hypertrophic cardiomyopathy.[7] Symptoms may be absent or minimal and stable throughout life, or progress with disease duration. Early childhood years are typically asymptomatic, but by mid- to late-teenage years, and throughout adulthood, shortness of breath (dyspnea) that worsens with exertion, chest pain (angina), and palpitations become common. Palpitations can indicate benign or life-threatening arrhythmias. Atrial fibrillation is the most common arrhythmia in hypertrophic cardiomyopathy and its incidence increases with disease duration, atrial enlargement, and mitral regurgitation.[8,9] Unrecognized or untreated atrial fibrillation can cause thromboembolism and stroke, each a significant cause of comorbidity in hypertrophic cardiomyopathy. A subset of patients experience symptoms of heart failure due to the development of the dilated, burnt-out phase of disease.[10]

Hypertrophic cardiomyopathy is the most common diagnosis in sudden death of young athletes and causes premature death in approximately 2 to 4 percent of affected individuals annually.[11-13] Sudden death can be the first manifestation of disease, or can occur in established disease. Although a precise mechanism for this devastating event is often unknown, both primary arrhythmias[14,15] and hemodynamic factors[17,18] have been proposed. Recurrent syncope (loss of consciousness and hypotension), profound cardiac hypertrophy (left ventricular wall thickness > 35 mm[19]), and premature death of affected family members indicate increased risk,[20] but other clinical parameters have poor predictive values for defining the patient at risk for sudden death. An important finding from molecular studies has been recognition that genetic etiology influences survival in hypertrophic cardiomyopathy (reviewed in reference 21 and detailed below).

### Physical Exam

Physical findings in hypertrophic cardiomyopathy (detailed in reference 22) are limited to the cardiovascular exam. The cardiac exam can be normal, but often suggests hyperdynamic ventricular function. The left ventricular impulse is usually forceful, and sometimes is accompanied by a palpable S4 gallop. Outflow tract obstruction can produce a systolic murmur that radiates towards the left sternal border; notably, such murmurs increase when cardiac preload is diminished (Valsalva maneuver). Without obstruction, findings on auscultation may be limited to a systolic murmur that does not increase with provocation. Systolic murmurs that radiate into the axilla often reflect mitral regurgitation. An S4 gallop is frequently present with diastolic dysfunction. Neither the presence nor absence of cardiac findings correlates with the severity of cardiac remodeling and hypertrophy.

### Electrocardiography

The electrocardiogram is usually abnormal in hypertrophic cardiomyopathy (Fig. 213-2). Left ventricular hypertrophy is almost uniformly present and often accompanied by T wave inversion in the anterior precordial and lateral leads.[22,23] The QRS complex can be widened and exhibit a bundle branch morphology. Q waves can be prominent, and when found in the inferior (II, III, and aVF) leads, they exhibit a "pseudoinfarct" pattern. Such patterns may reflect a preponderance of electrical forces from the left ventricle.[24,25] Abnormalities of P waves (left atrial enlargement) and electrical axis (left-axis deviation), disturbances of rhythm, ectopic beats, and atrioventricular conduction delays are often present.[26] EKG abnormalities have been reported to precede echocardiographic findings in children at risk for developing hypertrophic cardiomyopathy.[27]

### Echocardiography

Echocardiography is an essential evaluation for diagnosis of hypertrophic cardiomyopathy. High-resolution, noninvasive imaging of the myocardium (Fig. 213-3) identifies and quantifies the cardinal morphologic feature of disease, ventricular hypertrophy.[22,28,29] In the absence of other etiologies (e.g., aortic valvular disease or hypertension), the demonstration of cardiac hypertrophy (ventricular wall thickness ≥13 to 15 mm) should prompt the diagnosis. The hypertrophied septum may appear inhomogeneous ("ground glass" appearance) and ventricular function is often hyperdynamic. In addition to defining the morphologic pattern of ventricular hypertrophy, echocardiographic images provide data on left atrial enlargement, systolic motion of the anterior mitral valve leaflet, mitral regurgitation, and outflow tract or midventricular gradients.[30-34] In the young, particularly prior to completion of adolescent growth, echocardiography can be normal, but most affected adults exhibit echocardiographic manifestation of disease.[19,22,26,35]

## CLINICAL GENETICS

The family history of affected individuals often indicates disease in first-degree relatives and, with appropriate diagnostic evaluation, autosomal dominant transmission of disease (Fig. 213-4) can

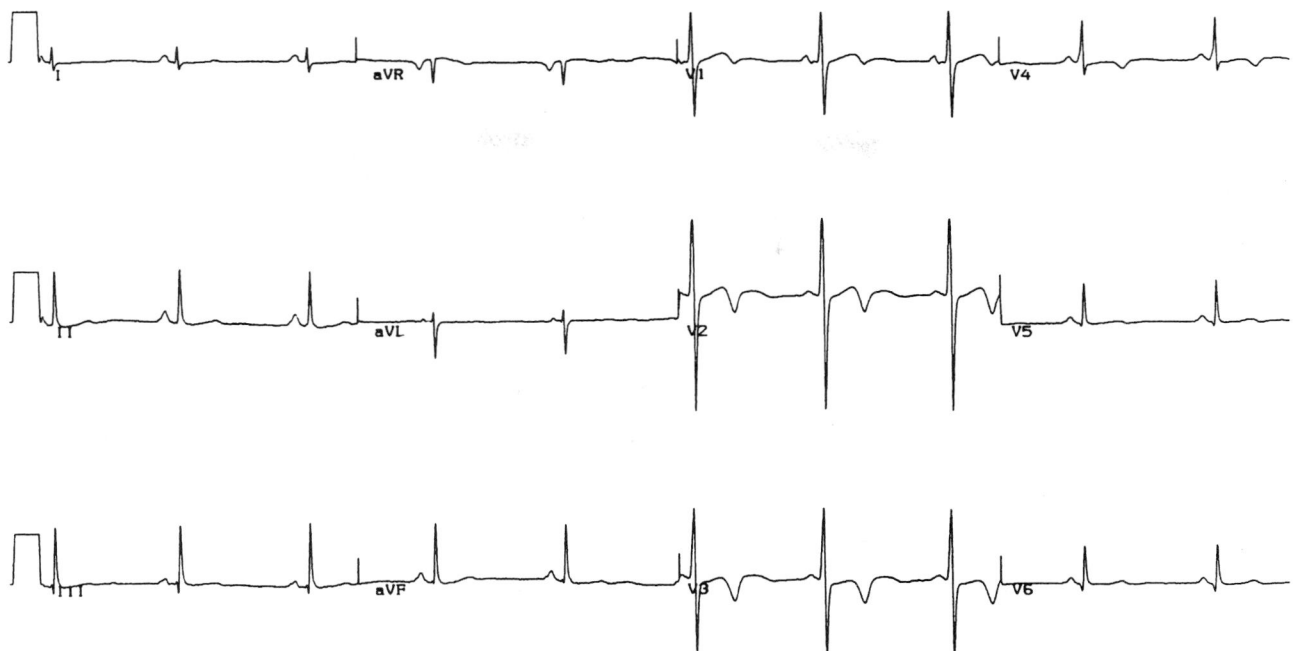

**Fig. 213-2** Twelve-lead electrocardiogram from a 29-year-old woman with familial hypertrophic cardiomyopathy caused by β-cardiac myosin heavy chain mutation Arg719Trp. Prominent voltage is evident in the precordial leads (V₁-V₃) with T wave inversion.

usually be defined.[2,35–37] Hypertrophic cardiomyopathy is also recognized as a sporadic disease (affected individuals whose parents are clinically well and do not carry a hypertrophic gene mutation); in several instances, *de novo* mutations in genes that cause familial disease have been defined.[38–40] Transmission of *de novo* mutations to offspring can establish new-onset familial disease. These data indicate a shared molecular etiology for sporadic and familial hypertrophic cardiomyopathy and underscore the need for genetic counseling of individuals with sporadic disease.

Penetrance of hypertrophic cardiomyopathy depends both on patient age and genetic etiology. Clinical disease in infants and young children at risk of inheriting the condition is unusual, but cardiac hypertrophy usually becomes evident with adolescent growth.[18] Disease penetrance is, however, dependent on genetic etiology: although most sarcomere gene mutations cause clinical disease early in adulthood, hypertrophic cardiomyopathy caused by cardiac myosin-binding protein C mutations can be delayed until after middle age.[41,42] Clinical assessment of individuals at risk for disease may, therefore, require lifelong follow-up.

## PATHOLOGY

### Anatomic Findings

Increased cardiac mass characterizes the macroscopic pathology of hypertrophic cardiomyopathy (Fig. 213-1). The pathology

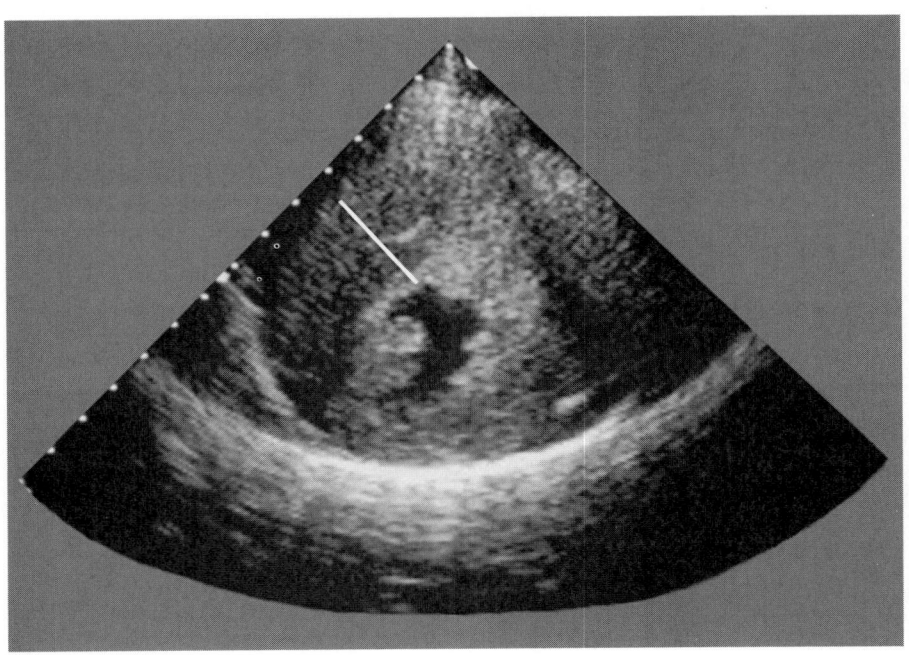

**Fig. 213-3** Short-axis two-dimensional echocardiogram view of left ventricle at the level of the papillary muscles. There is marked hypertrophy involving the interventricular septal wall (highlighted by white line) and left ventricular free wall.

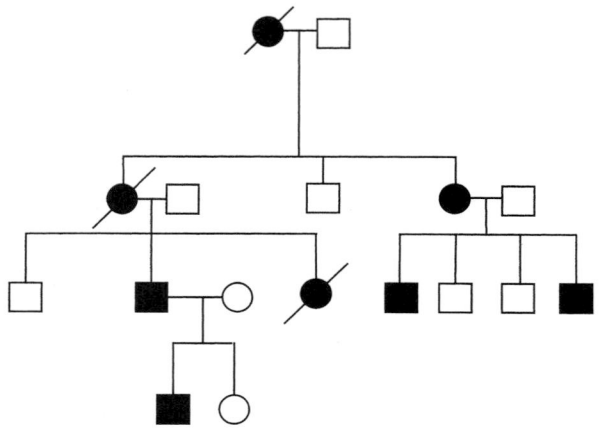

**Fig. 213-4 Autosomal dominant transmission of familial hypertrophic cardiomyopathy caused by β-cardiac myosin heavy chain mutation Arg403Gln. Three affected individuals in this kindred died suddenly, each before age 35.**

predominates in the left ventricle, but associated or isolated right ventricular hypertrophy also occurs. Most centers define cardiac hypertrophy in the adult by ventricular wall thickness ≥13 to 15 mm; in children, myocardial wall thickness must be evaluated in the context of body surface area. Abrupt transitions in wall thickness of adjacent myocardial segments are common, and substantially hypertrophied regions can be contiguous with normal myocardium. The extent and distribution of ventricular remodeling in hypertrophic cardiomyopathy varies considerably,[30,43] but usually ventricular cavity size remains normal or is small.

Of the various morphologic patterns of hypertrophic cardiomyopathy recognized,[30,31] asymmetric involvement of the interventricular septum is the most common. By convention, the asymmetric pattern is defined by a ratio of septal to posterior wall thickness that exceeds 1.5:1. Regardless of this value, however, some portion of the interventricular septum is hypertrophied in virtually all affected individuals,[44] and involved ventricular regions rarely exhibit identical or similar wall thickness.

When septal hypertrophy is marked in the subaortic valvular region (basal septum), it can be accompanied by a focal discoloration on the subaortic endocardial septal surface, a marking produced by contact between the anterior mitral valve

and septum during systole.[43] Such findings often indicate diminished area of the left ventricular outflow tract, and as such, represent morphologic manifestations associated with hemodynamic outflow obstruction.[22,45,46]

In less than one-third of affected individuals, ventricular hypertrophy is symmetric or concentric. Massive left ventricular hypertrophy ≥35 mm is more likely to be concentric or nearly so (Fig. 213-3), involving multiple ventricular segments.[47] Less-common patterns include hypertrophy restricted to the apical third of the ventricle or midventricular segment with maximal thickening at the level of the papillary muscles.[48–50]

A subset of affected individuals develops ventricular thinning and cavity enlargement late in the natural history of disease. Although this phenotype occurs in less than 10 percent of affected individuals, the development of these morphologic changes often heralds a poor prognosis and refractory cardiac failure.[51] Progressive ventricular dilation may be more common in individuals with midventricular hypertrophy.[52]

Left atrial enlargement is a prevalent finding in hypertrophic cardiomyopathy that increases with disease duration.[9,53,54] Atrial wall hypertrophy and morphologic abnormalities of the mitral wall[55,56] are frequent co-incident findings that can occur as primary manifestations of disease and secondary to hemodynamic abnormalities (especially diastolic dysfunction).

## Histopathology

The characteristic histopathology of hypertrophic cardiomyopathy is enlarged myocytes with disorganized fiber orientation (disarray) (Fig. 213-5A), interspersed intercellular connective tissue, and fibrosis.[57,58] Although myocardial fiber disarray is found in normal hearts and myocardium that hypertrophies secondary to non-genetic causes (i.e., rheumatic aortic valvular stenosis), the extent is usually far greater in hypertrophic cardiomyopathy.[59] Myocyte ultrastructure shows disarray of myofibrils and myofilaments with hyperchromatic nuclei that are sometimes bizarrely shaped. Myocardial fibrosis is typically present on light microscopy, but as in the hypertrophic response, the extent of fibrosis varies widely. Loose intercellular fibrosis is often evident in regions with myocyte hypertrophy and can contribute to the myocyte disorganization (Fig. 213-5B). When substantial, fibrosis contributes to the increased cardiac mass; when diffuse, fibrosis probably contributes to the deterioration of ventricular function. Dense focal fibrosis can sometimes appear as a macroscopic transmural scar. Another variable finding involves the intramural coronary arteries;[60] these can exhibit proliferation of collagen in the media and intima, resulting in luminal narrowing. Such

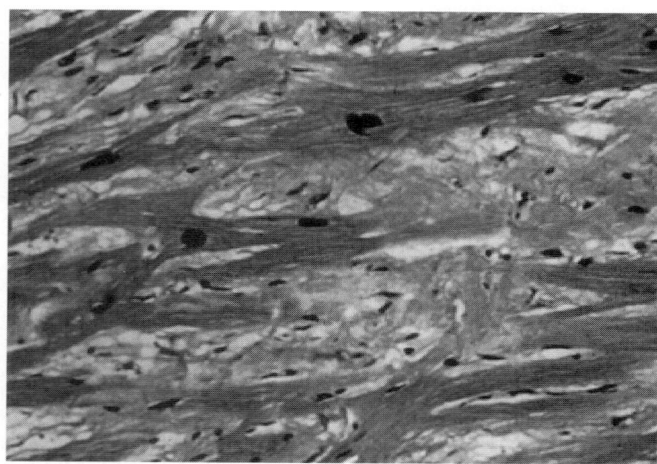

A

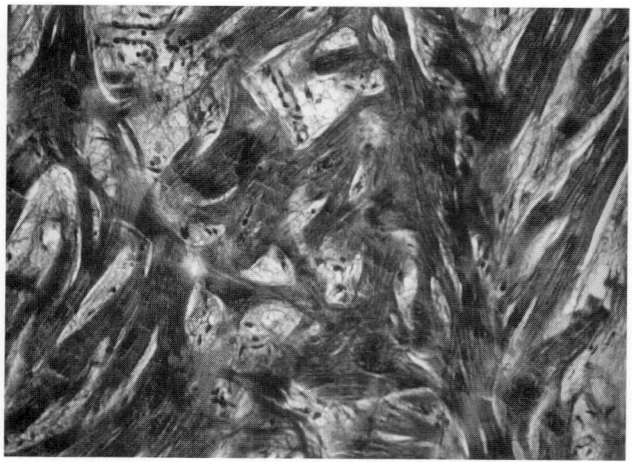

B

**Fig. 213-5 Histopathology of hypertrophic cardiomyopathy. Hematoxylin and eosin stain (A) demonstrates enlarged disorganized myocytes, with large nuclei. The prominent interspersed interstitial** fibrosis is apparent with Mason trichrome staining (B). (*Modified from Coviello et al.[98] and Geisterfer-Lowrance et al.[121] Used with permission.*)

abnormalities are most prevalent in myocardial areas with substantial hypertrophy or fibrosis and may cause regional ischemia.

## PATHOPHYSIOLOGY

### Systolic Function

Current understanding of systolic function in hypertrophic cardiomyopathy integrates data from cardiac catheterization studies and contemporary noninvasive echocardiographic investigations. Systolic function is normal but often is clinically characterized as hyperdynamic[61,62] based on physical findings and echocardiographic data of supernormal ejection fractions. Altered patterns of ventricular emptying contribute to this feature; a greater percentage of normal left ventricular stroke volume is ejected early in systole,[63] due to the distortion of ventricular morphology and/or the biophysical consequences of sarcomere protein mutations.

An intriguing feature of systolic performance in hypertrophic cardiomyopathy is the development of mid or late systolic intraventricular gradients.[22,45] These abnormalities can be of sufficient magnitude to suggest a clinical diagnosis of aortic valvular stenosis in some patients. Historic invasive hemodynamic profiling of such patients[45] clearly demonstrated that these pressure gradients originated within the outflow tract of the left ventricle, below the aortic valve. Despite considerable literature detailing the hemodynamic profile of "obstructive" hypertrophic cardiomyopathy, significant pressure gradients across the left ventricular outflow tract occur in less than 25 percent of cases.[64–66] Echocardiography and Doppler studies have helped to clarify the mechanisms for outflow tract obstruction in hypertrophic cardiomyopathy.[31,34] Subaortic gradients result from vigorous contraction of a ventricle with proximal septal hypertrophy; increased blood flow velocities establish Venturi forces that result in abnormal systolic anterior motion of the mitral valve and septal contact. While this pathophysiology is commonly labeled as "obstructive," volumetric analyses indicate that the small residual volumes that are emptied in mid to late systole in hypertrophic cardiomyopathy[63] mitigate the consequences of mitral valve-septal contact. Although elevated intraventricular pressures may be generated to eject these small volumes, the majority of stroke volume is ejected without impediment. While there is little clear evidence that "obstruction" significantly perturbs systolic performance in hypertrophic cardiomyopathy, high pressures may have detrimental effects on endocardial perfusion, cardiac energetics, and metabolism.[67]

Cardiovascular hemodynamics and pharmacologic agents can vary the magnitude of subaortic gradients in hypertrophic cardiomyopathy.[68,69] Factors that reduce ventricular preload or afterload (such as standing from a sitting or squatting position, Valsalva maneuver, exercise, administration of nitroglycerin or amyl nitrate) increase the gradient. Conversely increasing preload or afterload or reducing contractility (by squatting, passive leg elevation, handgrip, administration of phenylephrine or beta blocking drugs) diminishes outflow tract obstruction.

Prominent hypertrophy of the mid-ventricle and papillary muscles (sometimes referred to as hourglass morphology) can result in significant pressure gradients within the midventricular cavity. Molecular studies (detailed below) indicate that particular genetic etiologies of hypertrophic cardiomyopathy are more frequently associated with this finding; essential myosin light chain mutations[70] account for a small proportion of hypertrophic cardiomyopathy, but midventricular hypertrophy is particularly prevalent with these.

Mitral regurgitation is a common component of systolic dysfunction in hypertrophic cardiomyopathy. Altered myocardial geometry and pressure gradients can remodel the leaflets of the mitral valve[71,72] to become abnormally large, elongated, and redundant. With angulation of the anterior mitral valve leaflet and

systolic motion, closure can occur at the leaflet body rather than tips, thereby producing a funnel-shaped opening that directs blood toward the atria in mid and late systole. Mitral regurgitation contributes to the onset of atrial fibrillation,[54] an important comorbidity in hypertrophic cardiomyopathy.

Ten percent of individuals with hypertrophic cardiomyopathy develop significant reduction in systolic function late in the natural history of disease. Reduced ejection fractions ($<50$ percent) and ventricular wall thinning characterize this phase, thereby mimicking dilated cardiomyopathy.[51,52] The severity and duration of symptoms and degree of significant myocardial fibrosis all contribute to the development of this "burnt-out" phase of disease. Cardiac dysfunction can be so severe as to cause heart failure and necessitate transplantation.

### Diastolic Function

Impaired diastolic performance is recognized as a virtually uniform pathophysiologic finding in hypertrophic cardiomyopathy.[73–76] Importantly, myocardial diastolic dysfunction accounts for the predominant disease symptoms, dyspnea and angina.[73] Abnormal diastolic ventricular filling patterns are found in affected individuals regardless of the extent or morphologic pattern of ventricular hypertrophy. Diastolic dysfunction reflects both impaired relaxation and increased stiffness in the ventricular myocardium.[77] The time for relaxation is significantly prolonged and the profile of isovolumic relaxation assumes a linear rather than the normal exponential decay pattern. With prolonged relaxation times, early diastolic filling is impaired. Relaxation is also perturbed by the biophysical properties of the mutant sarcomere (i.e., slowed crossbridge cycling rates with prolonged activation) and altered myocyte load that can be produced by abnormal end-systolic pressure and volume, wall stress, inadequate coronary artery blood flow, and regional asynchrony of ventricular wall motion.[78,79] Increased myocardial stiffness caused by intercellular connective tissue and myocardial fiber disarray further perturbs diastolic function. A consequence of abnormal ventricular distensibility is elevation of end-diastolic ventricular pressures, despite normal or reduced ventricular volumes, which increases left atrial and pulmonary venous pressures and accounts for pulmonary congestion and dyspnea, the most common symptoms of hypertrophic cardiomyopathy.

## MOLECULAR ETIOLOGIES

Autosomal dominant transmission of hypertrophic cardiomyopathy (Fig. 213-4) implies that (a) affected individuals are heterozygous for a disease-causing mutation; (b) affected members of one family share the same mutation; (c) 50 percent of the offspring of affected individuals will inherit the disorder; and (d) males and females are equally likely to inherit the disease gene. Despite these facts, clinical studies of hypertrophic cardiomyopathy indicate considerable variation in disease penetrance and expressivity. Heterogeneity of genetic etiology is an important factor for interfamilial differences of hypertrophic cardiomyopathy. Identification of the genetic and environmental influences that affect disease expression in affected members within the same family remains an important research endeavor.[5]

Over the past decade, a large number of gene mutations that cause hypertrophic cardiomyopathy have been identified using positional cloning methods. Early investigations focused on genetic linkage (mapping) strategies to define disease loci.[80–83] Genetic mapping involves identifying DNA segments, usually identified by a sequence polymorphism that is coinherited with disease. The likelihood that a particular pattern of coinheritance would have been observed by random chance, termed LOD (logarithm of the odds), is calculated to determine the statistical significance of the observed segregation pattern. LOD scores $\geq 3$ (indicating odds $\geq 1:1000$) are considered significant. Linkage analyses of several unrelated large pedigrees with hypertrophic cardiomyopathy resulted in LOD scores $\geq 10$ (odds

**Table 213-1 Genes That Are Mutated in Hypertrophic Cardiomyopathy**

| Disease gene | Chromosome | Band | Locus | Location (cM)* | %† | Method§ |
|---|---|---|---|---|---|---|
| Cardiac troponin T | 1 | q32 | TNNT2 | 219.85 | ~15 | L |
| Essential myosin light chain | 3 | p21.2-21.3 | MYL3 | 58.748 | <1 | C |
| ? | 7 | q34 | ? | 160.300 | ? | L |
| Cardiac myosin-binding protein C | 11 | p11.2 | MYBPC3 | 57.492 | >15 | L |
| Regulatory myosin light chain | 12 | q23-24 | MYL2 | 113.441 | <1 | C |
| β-Cardiac myosin heavy chain | 14 | q11.2-13 | MYH7 | 30.027 | >35 | L |
| Cardiac actin | 15 | q14 | ACTC | 49.600 | <5 | L |
| α-Tropomyosin | 15 | q22 | TPM1 | 69.940 | <5 | L |
| Cardiac troponin I | 19 | q13.4 | TNNI3 | 62.936 | ~10 | C |

*Map location is centimorgans (cM) from p-telomere of the chromosome.
†The percentage of familial hypertrophic cardiomyopathy estimated to be caused by mutation at this locus.
§Disease genes were identified through genetic linkage analysis (L) or candidate gene (C) analysis.

≥1:10,000,000) and defined 4 distinct disease loci in the human genome. These studies provided the first evidence of genetic heterogeneity in hypertrophic cardiomyopathy and indicated that mutations in different genes could cause clinically identical disease.

Subsequent genetic linkage studies enable investigators to narrow the disease intervals for hypertrophic cardiomyopathy below 5 cM (1 cM approximates 1 million base pairs of DNA). Candidate disease genes were readily identified at four familial hypertrophic cardiomyopathy (FHC) loci: β-cardiac myosin heavy chain; cardiac troponin T; α-tropomyosin; and cardiac myosin binding protein C. The nucleotide sequences of each gene were screened and sequence variants were found in samples from affected individuals that were absent in unaffected family members and normal control samples. Sequence variants were identified in codons that are highly conserved throughout evolution and predicted to encode proteins with significantly altered structure and presumably function, thereby fulfilling standard criteria as disease-causing mutations. These genome-wide mapping strategies defined four disease genes that encode sarcomere components: β-cardiac myosin heavy chain; cardiac troponin T;

α-tropomyosin; and cardiac myosin-binding protein C (Table 213-1). Four other disease genes—cardiac actin, cardiac troponin I, regulatory myosin light chain, and essential myosin light chain—were identified by hypothesizing that mutations in other sarcomere protein genes would also cause hypertrophic cardiomyopathy. The sarcomere is the functional unit of contraction in muscle cells.

Sarcomere proteins are organized into interdigitating thick and thin filaments (Fig. 213-6) that cyclically attach and detach during contraction and relaxation, fueled by hydrolysis of ATP.[84] Most hypertrophic cardiomyopathy mutations are predicted to encode stable proteins;[85] hence, these mutations are unlikely to alter the stoichiometry of sarcomere components. Rather, these defects appear to cause disease through dominant negative mechanisms: mutant peptides are incorporated into the sarcomere and perturb function. Cardiac hypertrophy and ventricular remodeling can be viewed as compensatory responses to the biophysical consequences of a mutation and as such may provide an index to sarcomere dysfunction. A wide range of clinical responses to hypertrophic mutations is therefore not unexpected; responses might be expected to vary depending on whether the mutant peptide interferes with calcium cycling, crossbridge formation, or

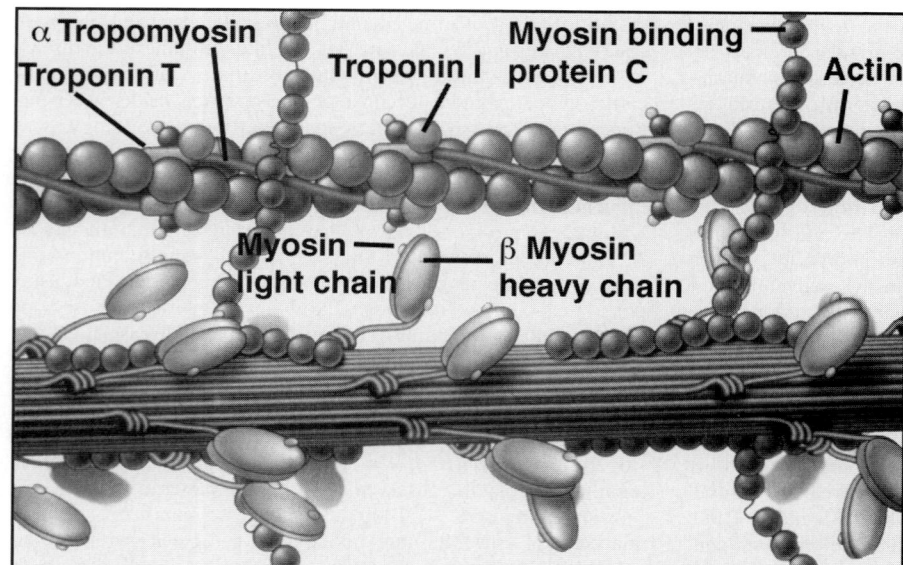

Fig. 213-6 Mutations in cardiac sarcomere proteins cause hypertrophic cardiomyopathy. Mutations in genes that encode components of the thick filament (β-cardiac myosin heavy chain, myosin essential and regulatory light chains, myosin-binding protein C) and thin filament (troponin T, troponin I, α-tropomyosin, and actin) have been identified.

A

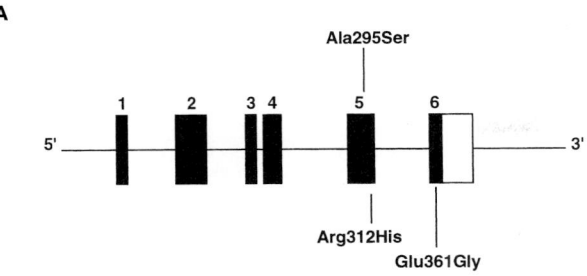

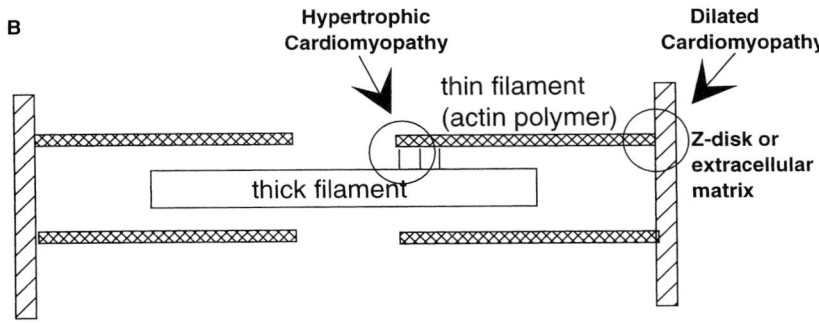

Fig. 213-7 Schematic of the cardiac actin gene and mutations that cause cardiac pathologies. *A,* Missense mutation Ala295Ser causes hypertrophic cardiomyopathy while Arg312His and Glu361Gly cause dilated cardiomyopathy. *B,* Schematic of potential interactions altered by distinct actin mutations. The hypertrophic defect may perturb force production by the sarcomere, whereas defects that cause dilated cardiomyopathy may impair force transmission to the cytoskeleton and extracellular matrix.[90]

another sarcomere function. A comprehensive understanding of hypertrophic cardiomyopathy mutations will, therefore, ultimately require integration of molecular, biophysical, and clinical data. Although this information is far from complete, more detailed insights are on the horizon, from the increasing acquisition of clinical data, in vitro structure-function analyses of sarcomere proteins, and genetic engineering of human hypertrophic cardiomyopathy mutations into murine models of disease.

## Mutations of Thin Filament Protein

Mutations in genes encoding several components of sarcomere thin filaments cause hypertrophic cardiomyopathy. Thin filament proteins including actin, tropomyosin, and the troponin complex (troponins C, I, and T) interact with the thick filament and anchor the sarcomere to the cytoskeleton (Fig. 213-6). Actin subunits polymerize to form double-helical strands: one end of actin filaments forms crossbridges with myosin, while the other end binds the sarcomere (at Z-bands) to intercalated disks via interactions with actinin (Fig. 213-7B), and to the extracellular matrix via dystrophin.[86] The helical filaments formed from tropomyosin intertwine with actin.[87] Each tropomyosin dimer spans seven actin monomers and interacts with one troponin complex. The troponin-tropomyosin complex provides a calcium-sensitive switch that regulates actomyosin crossbridge formation.[88] Troponin I is an inhibitory component; in the absence of calcium, troponin I binds actin and inhibits actomyosin ATPase activity. Calcium binding of troponin C releases actin from the troponin-tropomyosin complex and allows actin-myosin interactions. With the exception of troponin T, hypertrophic cardiomyopathy mutations have been found in each of these thin filament components.

## α-Cardiac Actin

Of the 20 actin genes in the human genome, 4 are expressed in cardiac, skeletal, or smooth muscle.[86] Human α-cardiac actin is a 375-amino-acid polypeptide protein (41 kDa) encoded in 6 exons of the cardiac actin gene (designated *ACTC*; Fig. 213-7A). α-Cardiac actin is expressed extensively throughout the myocardium and less abundantly in a variety of tissues.[89] Actin mutations are a rare cause of hypertrophic cardiomyopathy, and to date, only one mutation, Ala295Ser, has been identified.[90] The Ala295Ser mutation appears to be near a putative myosin-binding site and

produces a relatively mild form of FHC. Intriguingly, mutations in the cardiac actin gene can also cause familial dilated cardiomyopathy, a pathology characterized by chamber dilation and reduced contractile function.[91] Actin mutations that produce dilated cardiomyopathy are missense defects (Glu361Gly and Arg312Ala); these are predicted to disrupt interactions between actin filaments and the extracellular matrix (Fig. 213-7B). After comparing the clinical consequences of different actin missense mutations, Mogensen et al.[90] suggested that defects, which impair force generation and interaction with the thick filament, cause hypertrophic cardiomyopathy; mutations that impair interaction with the extracellular matrix resulted in dilated cardiomyopathy. To date, this provides the only example of distinct sarcomere mutations resulting in different clinical (dilated versus hypertrophic) phenotypes.

## α-Tropomyosin

There are four tropomyosin genes in the human genome.[87] The α-tropomyosin gene (designated *TPM1*) on chromosome 15[92] is organized into 15 exons (Fig. 213-8); alternative splicing results in transcripts encoding a 284-amino-acid polypeptide (34 kDa) found in both fast skeletal and cardiac muscle.[89] Mutations in α-tropomyosin cause only a small fraction ($<5$ percent) of hypertrophic cardiomyopathy[92] and account for both familial[94-96] and sporadic disease.[40] Studies of Finnish populations indicate a founder effect of α-tropomyosin mutation Asp175Asn; 25 percent of affected individuals shared the defect.[97] The Asp175Asn arises by a G → A transition of nucleotide residue 579, a mutation that has been observed to independently occur in affected families around the world,[98] thereby implying increased susceptibility of this residue to mutation. Notably, the severity and distribution of ventricular hypertrophy in individuals with this defect varied considerably, thus indicating that the hypertrophic response is modulated by factors other than disease-causing mutation.[5] Survival of individuals with α-tropomyosin mutations appears to be relatively good;[96,98] life expectancy is longer than that observed in individuals with mutations in cardiac troponin T or with severe β-cardiac myosin heavy chain gene mutations (Fig. 213-9).

An intriguing aspect of α-tropomyosin defects is their lack of clinical expression outside of the heart despite an abundance of α-tropomyosin in skeletal muscle. This may be related to the location of hypertrophic cardiomyopathy mutations, all of which

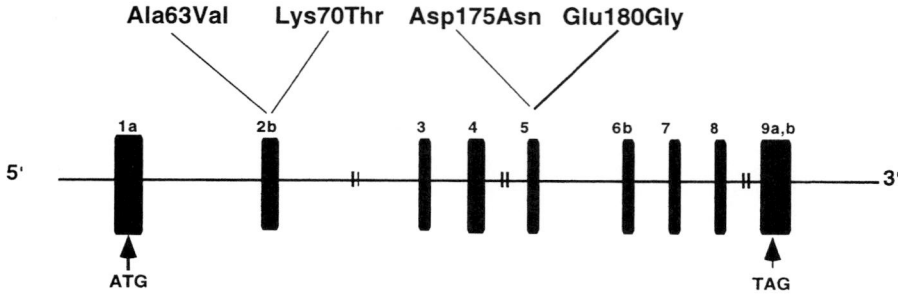

Fig. 213-8 Schematic of the α-tropomyosin gene and mutations that cause hypertrophic cardiomyopathy. Mutation of nucleotide residue 579 (Asp175Asn) has independently occurred multiple times.[98]

occur in exons that encode interactions with the cardiac-specific isoform troponin T. However, analyses of contractile parameters of skeletal muscle fibers from the vastus lateralis in individuals with the Asp175Asn mutation demonstrated differences in calcium sensitivity compared to normal muscle, although maximal force and shortening velocities were equivalent.[99] Sensitivity to calcium may be, therefore, a critical determinant in the response of cardiac versus skeletal muscle to α-tropomyosin mutation.

### Cardiac Troponin T

The cardiac troponin T gene (*TNNT2*) spans 17 kb of DNA on chromosome 1 and is one of three troponin T genes in the human genome.[100] A 288-amino-acid polypeptide (36 to 39 kDa) is encoded in 16 exons (Fig. 213-10) and several splice isoforms have been found in cardiac tissue. Approximately 15 percent of hypertrophic cardiomyopathy is caused by cardiac troponin T defects[93] and multiple disease-causing mutations have been reported.[93,94,101–103] While many are missense, splice signal mutations, insertions, and deletions have also been identified. Some defects may result in truncated polypeptides, but investigations using in vitro experimental systems suggest that both

foreshortened and missense mutant peptides are stable and perturb contractile function. Truncated mutant troponin T peptides expressed in quail myotubes were incorporated into sarcomeres and cause markedly reduced calcium-activated force generation,[104] indicating that hypertrophic cardiomyopathy mutations cause disease through a dominant negative effect on the sarcomere.

The clinical phenotype resulting from cardiac troponin T mutations is characterized by only mild to modest hypertrophy and some genetically affected adults fail to fulfill standard criteria for diagnosis. The mean maximal left ventricular wall thickness resulting from 6 different cardiac troponin T mutations was $16.7 \pm 5.5$ mm,[93] whereas the mean maximal left ventricular wall thickness observed with β-cardiac myosin heavy chain mutations was $23.7 \pm 7.7$ mm. Despite the minimal hypertrophic response produced by these mutations, shortened life expectancy and high incidences of sudden death characterize most cardiac troponin T defects[93,102] (Fig. 213-9), although "benign" mutations have been reported.[105] Troponin T mutations therefore cause significant diagnostic and management challenges for clinicians. At present neither molecular signals nor biophysical events have been defined

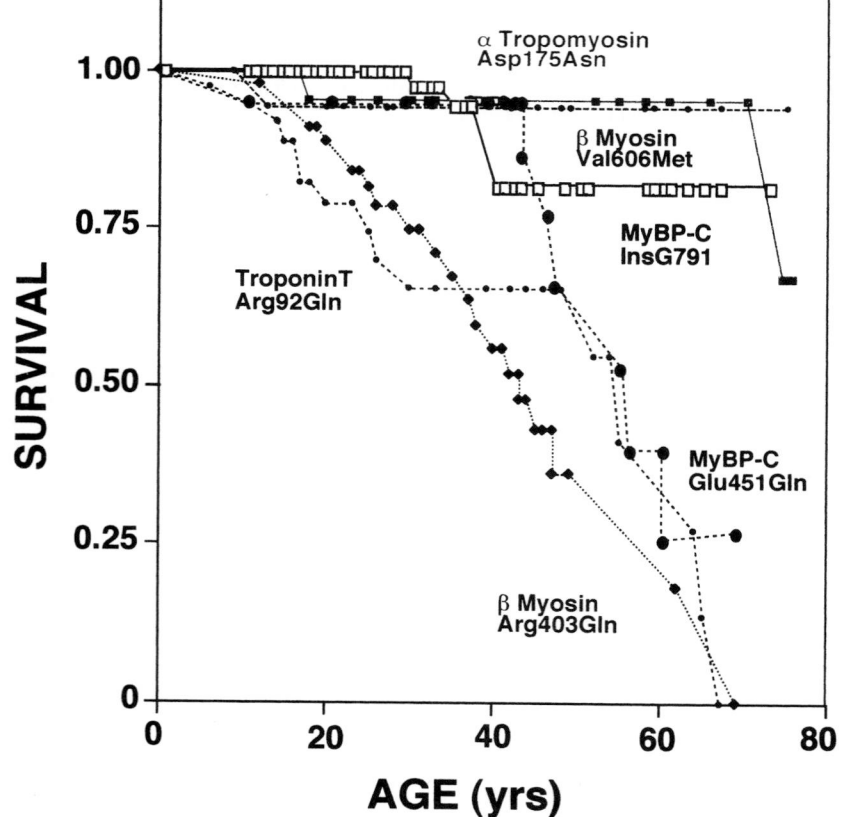

Fig. 213-9 Genetic etiology of hypertrophic cardiomyopathy influences survival. Kaplan-Meier curves demonstrate that life expectancy is similar in hypertrophic cardiomyopathy caused by α-tropomyosin mutation Asp175Asn, β-cardiac myosin heavy chain Val606Met, or myosin-binding protein C mutation InsG791, and significantly better (p < 0.001) than that observed with mutations troponin T Arg92Gln or β-cardiac myosin heavy chain Arg403Gln. (Based on data in references 41, 93, and 98.)

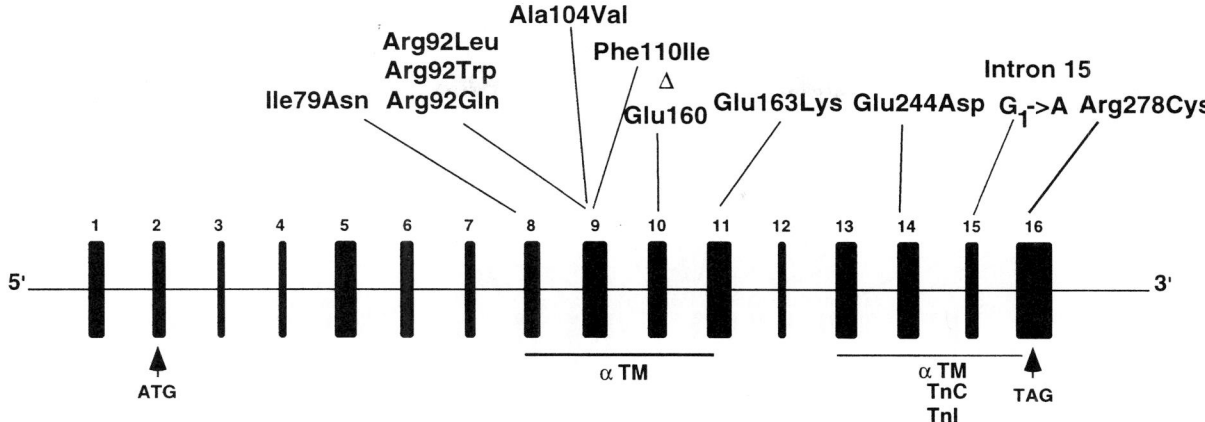

**Fig. 213-10 Schematic of the cardiac troponin T gene and mutations that cause hypertrophic cardiomyopathy. Exons that encode domains that interact with α-tropomyosin (α TM), cardiac troponin C and I (TnC and TnI, respectively) are indicated. In addition to** missense mutations, defects have been identified that are predicted to truncate the peptide (deletions [Δ] and mutations in splice signals [G₁ → A]).

that explain why these mutations produce only a modest hypertrophic response but marked electrical instability. Characterization of recently developed transgenic mice expressing mutant troponin T peptides provides important reagents for addressing these questions.

## Cardiac Troponin I

There are three troponin I genes in the human genome, but only the cardiac isoform (designated *TNTI3*) encoded on chromosome 19q13 is expressed at high levels in the myocardium. Eight exons in the cardiac troponin I gene (Fig. 213-11) encode a 210-amino-acid (27 to 31 kDa) polypeptide.[106] Direct analyses of troponin I gene sequences in hypertrophic populations indicate that less than 5 percent of disease is caused by these mutations. In most patients, disease manifestations are similar to those produced by mutations in other sarcomere protein genes, although some patients exhibit apical hypertrophy or preexcitation syndrome (Wolf-Parkinson-White syndrome).[107,108] Survival in hypertrophic cardiomyopathy due to cardiac troponin I mutations has not been assessed.

## Mutations of Thick Filament Proteins

Mutations in genes encoding components of the sarcomere thick filament are the most common cause of hypertrophic cardiomyopathy and defects have been identified in β-cardiac myosin heavy chain, regulatory myosin light chain, essential myosin light chain, and cardiac myosin binding protein C (Table 213-1). Thick filament proteins participate and modulate force generation and anchor the sarcomere to the cytoskeleton[84] (Fig. 213-6). β-Cardiac

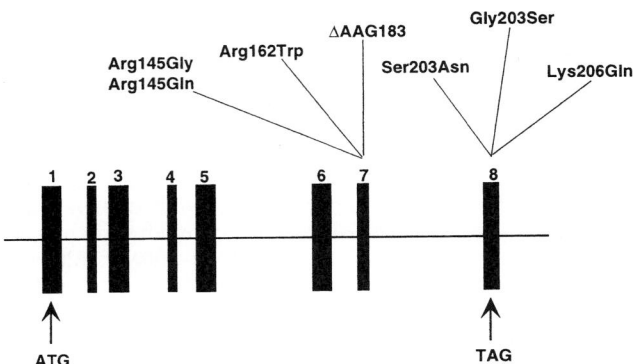

**Fig. 213-11 Schematic of the cardiac troponin I gene and mutations that cause hypertrophic cardiomyopathy. Most defects are missense, predicting a dominant negative mechanism for disease.**

myosin heavy chains are central to force production through actin-myosin interactions and ATPase activity.[109] Sequential formation and detachment of crossbridges between the myosin head and actin results in stepwise displacement of the actin filament relative to the myosin filament.[110] Hydrolysis of ATP bound to the myosin head provides energy for detachment. Myosin light chains are calcium-binding proteins that optimize both the speed and efficiency of crossbridge cycling.[111–113] Myosin-binding protein C modulates contraction by positioning the myosin head relative to the thin filament[114–116] in response to phosphorylation. This molecule is arrayed in transverse stripes of the A-bands where it tethers the sarcomere to the cytoskeleton through interactions with myosin and titin.[117]

## β-Cardiac Myosin Heavy Chain

Cardiac myosin heavy chains comprise approximately 1 percent of total myocyte protein. These large polypeptides contain 1935 amino acid residues (>200,000 kDa) that are folded into two domains (Fig. 213-12)—an N-terminal globular head region and a carboxyl rod region.[109,110] Of more than 20 myosin heavy chain genes in the genome, only two are expressed in the heart,[84] α-cardiac myosin heavy chain (*MYH6*) and β-cardiac myosin heavy chain (*MYH7*); both are encoded on chromosome 14 and separated by only 3700 bp.[118] The amino acid sequences of amino α- and β-isoforms are 92.8 percent identical, but ATPase activity and the velocity of shortening associated with these two cardiac myosin heavy chains differ considerably.[119,120] In the neonatal human cardiac ventricle, more than 60 percent of myosin heavy chains are the α-isoform. However, shortly after birth expression switches and during adult life the β-isoform predominates (greater than 90 percent) in the ventricles. By contrast, the α-cardiac myosin heavy chain remains the predominant isoform in adult human atria.[118]

Approximately 35 percent of individuals with familial hypertrophic cardiomyopathy have a β-cardiac myosin heavy chain mutation and more than 40 distinct defects have been identified.[26,27,38,39,53,123–130] *De novo* β-cardiac myosin heavy chain mutations have also been shown to account for sporadic disease.[38,39] All are missense mutations that substitute one amino acid; most are located in the globular head of the myosin heavy chain (Fig. 213-12). Like other disease alleles, myosin mutations cause hypertrophic cardiomyopathy via a dominant negative mechanism.[129–131]

The phenotype associated with myosin mutations is generally not quiescent. Clinically significant hypertrophy develops in virtually all genetically affected individuals by late adolescence, with markedly increased left ventricular wall thickness.[41,130] The

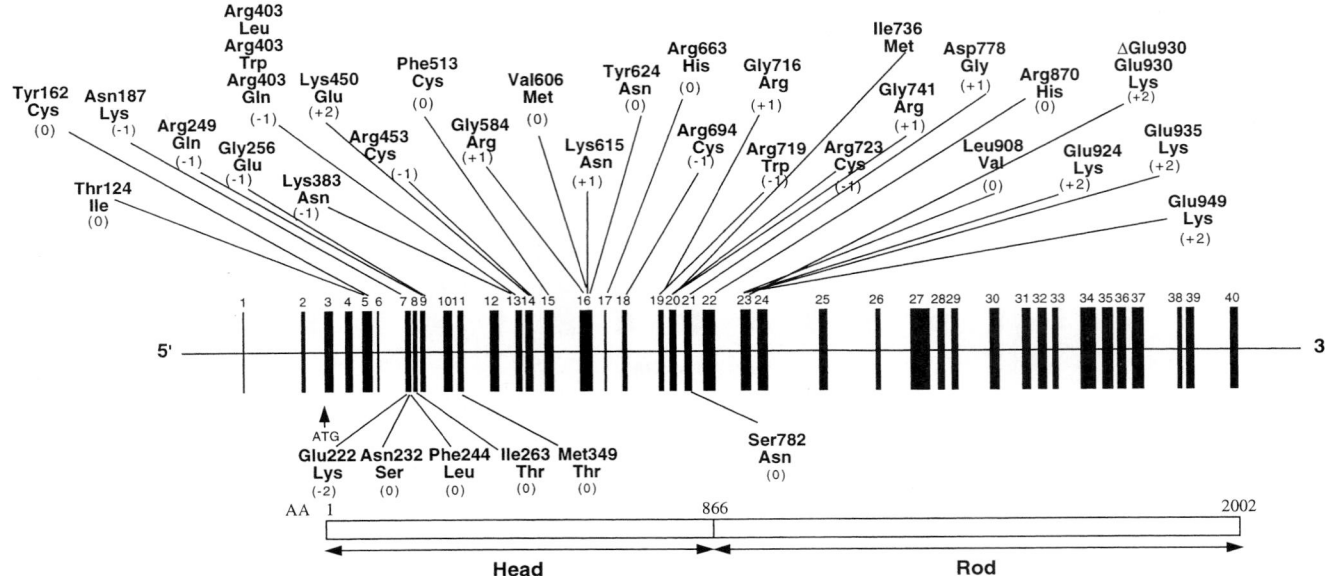

**Fig. 213-12 Missense mutations in the β-cardiac myosin heavy chain cause hypertrophic cardiomyopathy.** A schematic of the gene and encoded head and rod domains (open box) of the peptide are shown. Most defects alter sequences in the head or head-rod junction. Conservative mutations (0) may have less impact on survival than do substitutions that alter the charge of the residue (+1, +2, −1).

impact of myosin mutations on survival is variable, but several have been recognized to markedly reduce life expectancy.[53,130,132] Individuals with either the Arg403Gln or Arg719Trp mutation have an average life expectancy of 45 years, while individuals with a Val606Met missense mutation have near-normal survival (Fig. 213-9). Although many factors are likely to influence prognosis, change in charge of the substituted amino acid appears to be one important parameter. Nonconservative β-cardiac myosin heavy chain defects have a more adverse impact on survival than conservative defects, presumably because substitutions that more severely perturb myosin structure have greater impact on function.

The considerable data about the structure and biophysical and biochemical functions of myosin molecules have helped to identify potential consequences of hypertrophic mutations. The crystal structure of the S1 fragment of the globular head of chicken skeletal muscle myosin has been solved.[133] Locating hypertrophic cardiomyopathy missense mutations onto this three-dimensional structure (Fig. 213-13) reveals clustering of defects into or near four functional sites: (a) the actin binding interface; (b) the nucleotide binding site; (c) adjacent to the region connecting two reactive cysteine residues; and (d) near the interface with the essential light chain. The clinical features of disease have not been ascribed to changes in specific functional domains.

The functional effects of myosin mutations on crossbridge cycling have been assessed by in vitro translocation velocities of actin filaments on surfaces bound with mutant myosin filaments.[134,135] Initial data were difficult to interpret in that some defects (Arg403Gln and Tyr167Cys) inhibited actin translocation, whereas mutation Arg719Gln increased translocation velocities.[135] Since low levels of β-cardiac myosin heavy chains are found in skeletal muscle, analyses of soleus muscle fibers from individuals with hypertrophic cardiomyopathy also appeared promising for understanding the biophysical properties of these mutations.[136] However, isometric force generation and force-stiffness ratios in skeletal muscle fibers with different mutations also gave conflicting results: biophysical properties were reduced in muscle fibers containing the Arg403Gln mutation, but near normal in muscles bearing the Gly256Glu. Potential uncertainties associated with in vitro systems and differences that could be attributed to distinct properties of skeletal and cardiac muscle have recently been eliminated by analyses of single molecule mechanics in isolated

myocytes that contain hypertrophic cardiomyopathy mutations. Studies of the biophysical properties of myocytes derived from a genetically engineered mouse that is heterozygous or homozygous for the myosin mutation Arg403Gln demonstrated higher actin-activated ATPase activity, greater force generation, and faster actin sliding.[137]

Not only do these data provide a potential explanation for hyperdynamic function observed clinically in patients with hypertrophic cardiomyopathy, but they also further suggest that the Arg403Gln mutation causes a gain of function. Analyses of biophysical properties of other mutations that are appropriately expressed in cardiac myocytes are needed to confirm and extend these provocative data.

## Myosin Light Chains

The regulatory and essential myosin light chains decorate the head-rod junction of myosin heavy chains in cardiac sarcomeres. These light chains are members of the superfamily of "EF-hand" proteins, which contain a helix-loop-helix calcium-binding domain.[84]

The essential myosin light chain gene (*MYL3*; also known as alkali ventricular slow skeletal myosin light chain) is organized into seven exons (Fig. 213-14) encoded on chromosome 19p13.2-q13.2.[138] Essential myosin light chains contain 166 amino acids that are expressed primarily in slow skeletal muscle and ventricles. Mutations in the essential myosin light chain gene are rare causes of hypertrophic cardiomyopathy, and account for less than 1 percent of disease. An initial report suggested some defects (Arg154His and Met149Val) produced unique morphologic changes in the myocardium: prominent midventricular and papillary muscle hypertrophy variably accompanied by intraventricular gradients.[139] In addition, histologic examination of skeletal muscle biopsies from individuals with essential light chain mutations demonstrated pathologic features of primary mitochondrial disease such as ragged red fibers. Although symptoms attributed to this pathology have not been described, a subclinical skeletal myopathy appears to differentiate essential light chain mutations from other genetic etiologies of hypertrophic cardiomyopathy.

In vitro assays of the consequence of essential light chain mutations on myosin function indicate that the Met149Val defect increases actin translocation velocities.[139] Notably, the β-cardiac

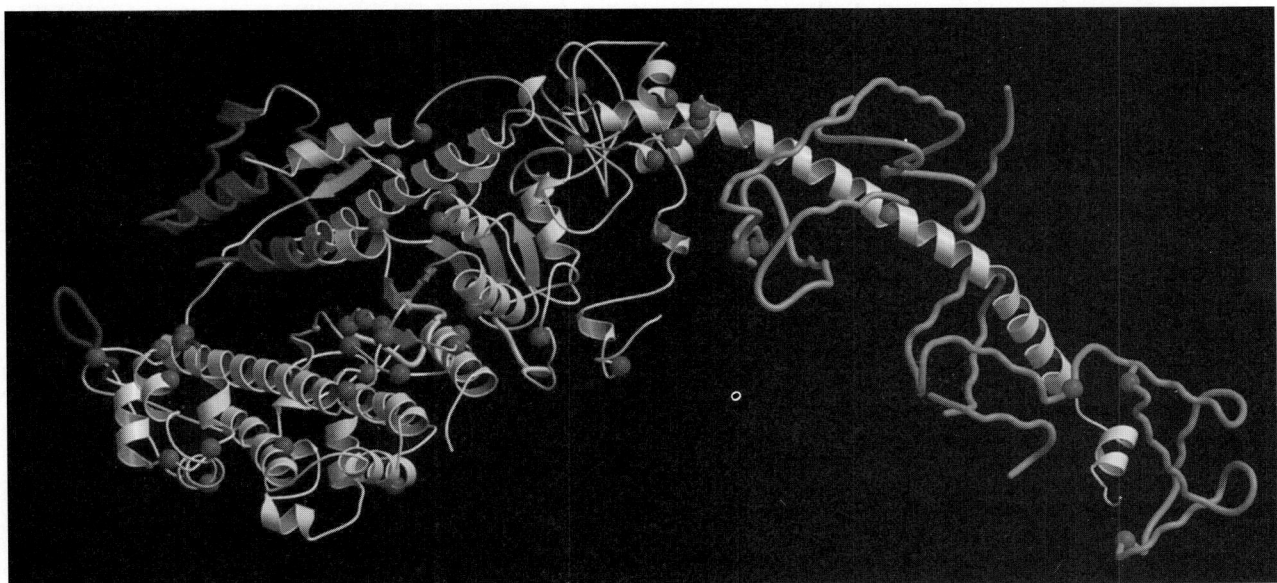

**Fig. 213-13** The location of hypertrophic cardiomyopathy mutations on a computer reconstruction of the 3-dimensional crystal structure of muscle myosin based on coordinates for chicken skeletal muscle myosin.[110] Hypertrophic cardiomyopathy mutations (red spheres) occur throughout the myosin head domain (silver). Myosin residues that interact with actin (green) or ATP (yellow) are indicated. Hypertrophic cardiomyopathy mutations that occur in the essential and regulatory light chains (turquoise and purple, respectively) are also shown. See Color Plate 11.

myosin defect (Arg719Gln) which is located in an α-helix that interfaces with the essential light chain also increases actin translocation velocities.

Atrial (MLC-2a) and ventricular slow (MLC-2s) isoforms of the regulatory myosin light chains are expressed in the myocardium; missense mutations of ventricular myosin light chains are also rare etiologies of hypertrophic cardiomyopathy.[139,140] MLC-2s is a 166-amino-acid protein encoded in seven exons of the *MYL2* gene (Fig. 213-15) on chromosome 12q2.[140,141] Of the 5 distinct mutations identified, all are missense. As with essential light chain mutations, mid-ventricular obstruction was observed in some individuals with regulatory myosin light chains defects. In contrast, mutations Phe18Leu and Arg58Gln only caused classical morphologic features of disease.[139,140]

## Cardiac Myosin-Binding Protein C

Mutations in cardiac myosin-binding protein C are prevalent causes of hypertrophic cardiomyopathy; at least 20 percent of disease is attributed to these defects.[41] The cardiac myosin-binding protein C gene (*MYBPC3*) spans 24 kb of DNA on chromosome 11p11.2 and contains 37 exons (Fig. 213-16) that encode a 1274-amino-acid (137 kDa) protein with immunoglobulin-like domains and fibronectin repeats.[117,142] Cardiac myosin-binding protein C is transversely arrayed in 7 to 9 strips separated by 43-nm intervals in the C-zone of the A-bands where it binds myosin heavy chain and titin. The molecule may provide structural integrity to the sarcomere as well as modulate myosin ATPase activity and cardiac contractility when phosphorylated by adrenergic stimulation.[114–117]

Many distinct types of mutations have been described within the cardiac myosin-binding protein C gene. In addition to missense mutations, defects in splice signals, small deletions, and insertions have been reported to cause hypertrophic cardiomyopathy.[41,142–147] Because some mutant alleles are predicted to encode truncated and possibly unstable peptides, haploinsufficiency of cardiac myosin-binding protein C has been considered one mechanism for disease. However, immunopeptide analyses of the ventricular myocardium from one affected individual showed no diminution in the levels of cardiac myosin-binding protein C in myofibrillar fractions.[145] The recent development of mice that have been engineered to express human mutations (discussed below) indicates that truncated cardiac myosin-binding protein C molecules, like other causes of hypertrophic cardiomyopathy, have a dominant negative effect on cardiac sarcomeres.

The clinical expression of either missense mutations or defects that encode truncated cardiac myosin-binding protein C peptides is similar to that observed in other genetic etiologies of hypertrophic cardiomyopathy. In contrast, the age of disease onset differs markedly (Fig. 213-17). Only half of adults under age 50 years with a cardiac myosin-binding protein C mutation had cardiac hypertrophy (wall thickness > 13 mm) and in many adults disease penetrance was incomplete through age 60.[41,83] Survival was generally better than that observed in hypertrophic cardiomyopathy caused by other sarcomere protein mutations (Fig. 213-9), but sudden death has been attributed to myosin-binding protein C defects.[41]

## Chromosome 7q3

The disease gene at one locus (chromosome 7q3) has not yet been identified.[148] This locus accounts for an unusual phenotype in which both hypertrophic cardiomyopathy and preexcitation (Wolff-Parkinson-White syndrome) segregate as an autosomal dominant trait. The natural history of disease in some affected individuals also includes progressive conduction system disease,

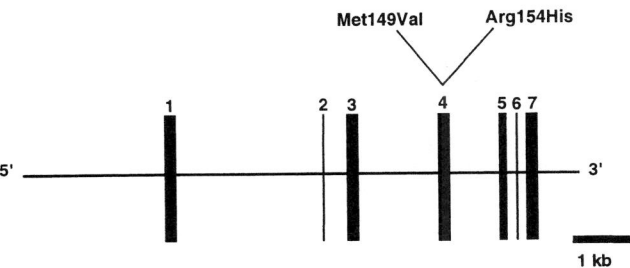

**Fig. 213-14** Schematic of the essential myosin light chain gene and two missense mutations that cause hypertrophic cardiomyopathy associated with subclinical skeletal myopathy.

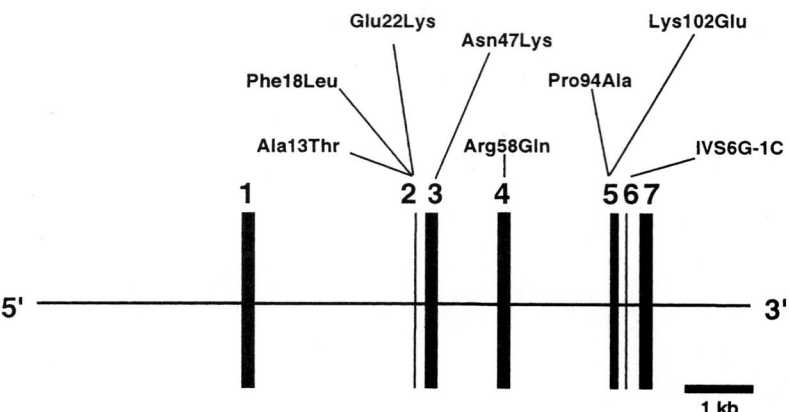

**Fig. 213-15 Schematic of the regulatory myosin light chain gene and the spectrum of mutations reported to cause hypertrophic cardiomyopathy.**

characterized by marked bradycardia and variable degrees of atrioventricular block.[148,149]

In summary, more than 100 mutations in genes encoding sarcomere proteins have been identified to cause familial and sporadic cases of hypertrophic cardiomyopathy. These defects are often family specific ("private") and, to date, compilation of the full set of gene mutations that cause hypertrophic heart disease remains a work in progress. Clinical findings associated with distinct genetic etiologies indicate that onset, severity, and morphology of hypertrophy, as well as prognosis, are all influenced by genotype. The mechanism by which hypertrophic mutations cause disease appears to be through their dominant negative impact on sarcomere function. Neither genetic studies nor the limited analyses of human cardiac tissues indicate changes in the stoichiometry of sarcomere components. Many important questions are posed by these findings: (a) Why do some sarcomere protein mutations cause more severe disease than others? (b) Why do individuals with the same mutation have a wide range of clinical features? (c) How does sarcomere dysfunction lead to myocyte hypertrophy and myocyte death? The development of mice that carry germline mutations that cause hypertrophic cardiomyopathy in humans provides the opportunity to answer these and other important questions.

## MURINE MODELS OF HYPERTROPHIC CARDIOMYOPATHY

With the identification of the genetic basis for hypertrophic cardiomyopathy, appropriate models of this pathology can be created through genetic engineering. Two different approaches have been used: transgenesis, in which a gene or cDNA encoding a mutated sarcomere component is targeted to the heart by a cardiac-specific promoter, and "knock-in" strategies in which homologous recombination is used to introduce the desired mutation into the endogenous allele of a sarcomere gene (Fig. 213-18). Transgenic approaches are technically easier and most models have been produced by this approach. A disadvantage of transgenic models is that mutant peptide expression is not regulated; levels can, therefore, be inappropriately high with the potential for producing pathology unrelated to the mutation. However, following selection of lines that exhibit equivalent expression of transgene and endogenous peptide, these models can be valuable for probing the consequences of human mutations. Knock-in mice are substantially more laborious to produce but have the advantage of maintaining endogenous regulation of mutant alleles, and may produce pathologies that more accurately reflect human disease.

Analyses of mice with mutations that cause human hypertrophic cardiomyopathy have been aided enormously by recent technologic advances in invasive and noninvasive assessment of cardiac physiology in mice. Electrocardiograms, two-dimensional echocardiograms, electrophysiologic testing, magnetic resonance imaging, and intraventricular hemodynamic profiling (Fig. 213-19) have been miniaturized to study cardiac function in mice. Application of these tools to murine models of hypertrophic cardiomyopathy has provided comprehensive approaches for assessing the consequences of sarcomere mutations on cardiac physiology.

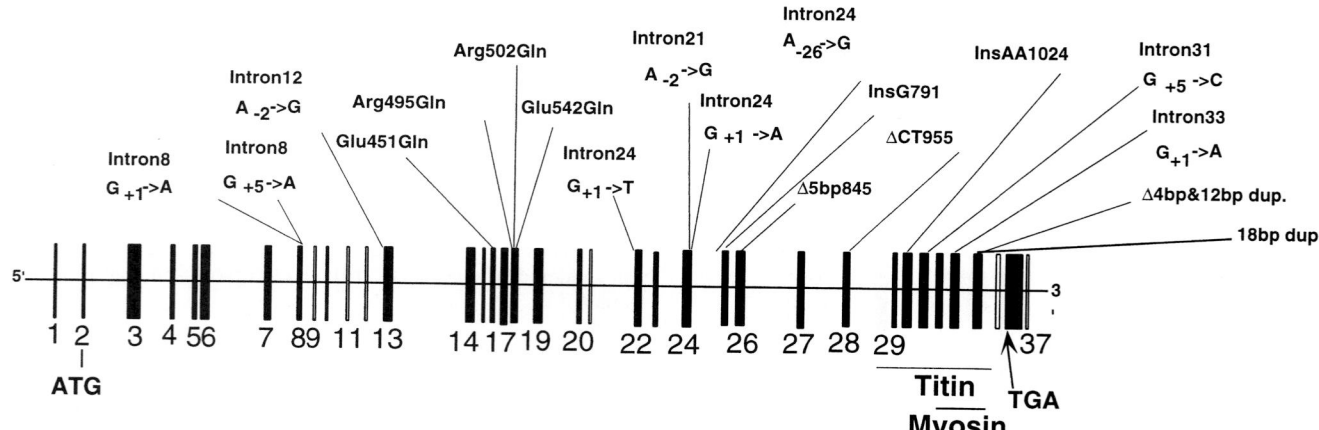

**Fig. 213-16 The genomic structure of human cardiac myosin-binding protein C gene. Missense mutations, defects in splice signals ($G_{+5} \rightarrow A$, $G_{+1} \rightarrow A$, $G_{+1} \rightarrow T$), small deletions ($\Delta$), and insertions (Ins) have been reported to cause hypertrophic cardiomyopathy. Exons that encode sequences that interact with myosin and titin are indicated.**

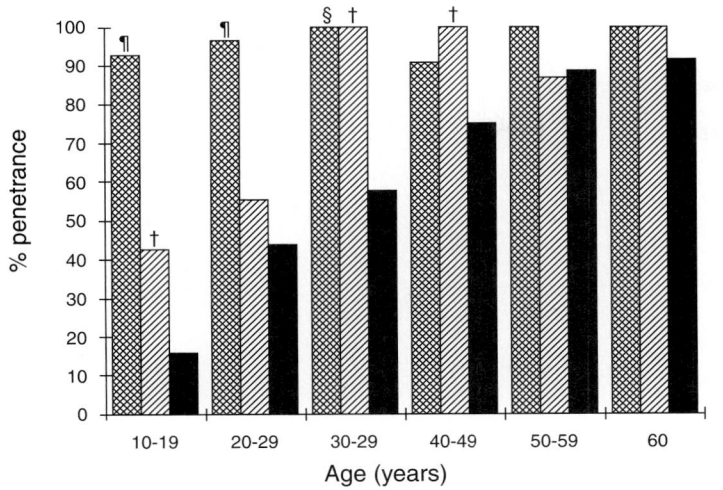

Fig. 213-17 Age-related penetrance of hypertrophic cardiomyopathy caused by mutations in different sarcomere proteins. Solid bars indicate percentages of individuals with cardiac hypertrophy at varying ages. Significant differences in the age of penetrance of cardiac myosin-binding protein C defects (right bar) versus cardiac troponin T (center bar) or β-cardiac myosin heavy chain mutations (left bar) are indicated (†, $P<0.05$; §, $P<0.005$; ¶, $P<0.0005$). (*From Niimura et al.*[41] *Used with permission.*)

Two different models of hypertrophic cardiomyopathy have been made to mimic human myosin mutations. Overexpression of a mutant rat myosin transgene,[150] targeted to the heart by the α-cardiac myosin heavy chain gene promoter, resulted in cardiac hypertrophy with disarray, injury, and replacement fibrosis. A second model, produced by homologous recombination, alters only nucleotide codon 403 of the murine α-cardiac myosin heavy chain gene[151] and is analogous to the human β-cardiac myosin heavy chain mutation Arg403Gln. (The α-cardiac myosin heavy chain gene was targeted to account for species differences in α-β-isoform expression between mice and humans.) Heterozygous mice for this mutation (α-MHC[403]) exhibit many features of the human pathology, including increased arrhythmogenicity[152] and exercise-induced sudden death.[151] Cardiac structure and function in mutant mice is normal at birth, but at adolescence, cardiac hypertrophy and histopathology progressively develop. Hemodynamic performances of α-MHC[403] mice (Fig. 213-19) show normal left ventricular contraction but perturbed (prolonged and asynchronous) relaxation proper-

ties.[153,154] Maximum rate of pressure decrease ($-dP/dT$) during relaxation is particularly attenuated from that observed in normal hearts. Biophysical studies of ventricular papillary muscle strips from α-MHC[403] mice[155,156] exhibit depression of crossbridge kinetics[75] and a reduction in developed force at high stimulation rates. These findings may account for reduced exercise capacity exhibited by α-MHC[403] mice[157] and a higher incidence of provoked arrhythmias compared to wild-type littermates.[152]

Transgenic mice expressing mutant Asp175Asn α-tropomyosin cDNAs have been used to probe the consequences of this defect on sarcomere function.[158] Abundant expression of mutant peptide led to a reciprocal diminution of endogenous levels of α-tropomyosin and worsened ventricular performance. Physiologic studies of α-tropomyosin Asp175Asn hearts showed diminished contractile function (reduced maximum rate of contraction, prolonged time to peak pressure, attenuated response to exercise, or β-adrenergic stimulation). Myofilaments containing α-tropomyosin Asp175Asn had increased calcium sensitivity and increased activation of thin

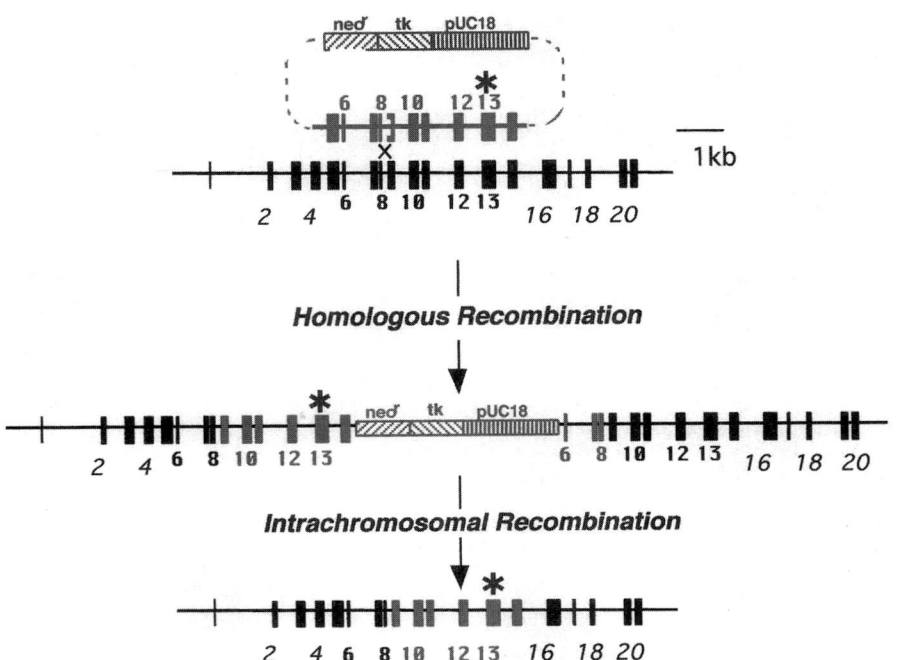

Fig. 213-18 Targeting a missense mutation to the α-cardiac myosin heavy gene of the mouse using homologous recombination. Embryonic stem cells transfected with vector pUC18 containing a fragment of the mutated gene (starred) and selectable markers (neomycin resistance = neo[r]; thymidine kinase = tk). Homologous recombination allows growth in media containing G418. Further selection with media containing FIAU allows selection of cells that undergo intrachromosomal recombination, with restitution of normal genomic structure (see Fig. 213-12) and regulated expression. (*Modified from Geisterfer-Lowrance et al.*[151] *Used with permission.*)

**A.**

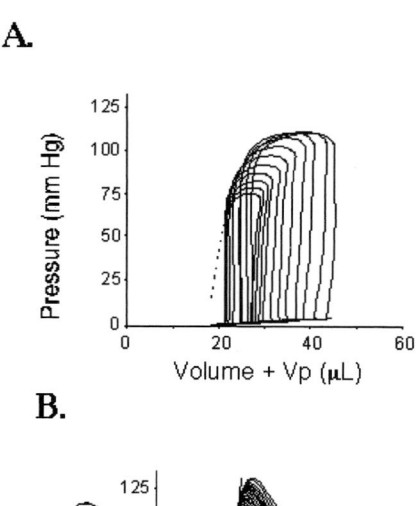

**B.**

**C.** 30

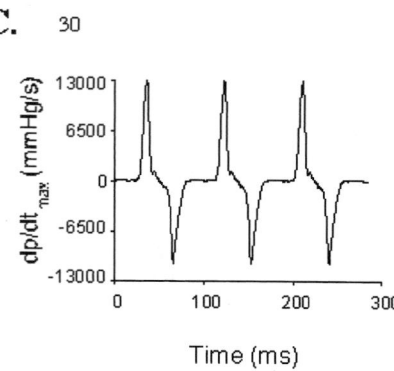

**D.**

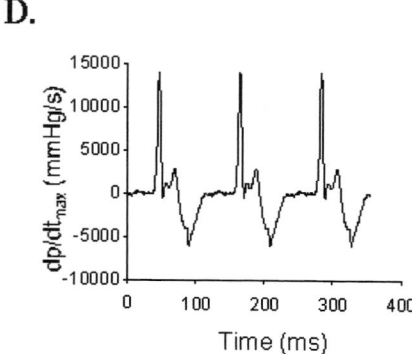

**Fig. 213-19 Cardiac function in mouse models of hypertrophic cardiomyopathy. Pressure-volume loops reveal enhanced contraction in α-MHC[403] mice (B) compared to wild-type animals (A). In contrast, relaxation (indicated by dp/dt$_{min}$ traces C, D) is markedly impaired in mutant mice. Physiologic traces from each group are comparable to data obtained in humans. (From Georgakopoulos et al.[154] Used with permission.)**

filaments, presumably due to altered interactions between mutant tropomyosin, troponin T, and actin.

Mouse models of two different human cardiac troponin T mutations have been developed. An Arg92Gln missense mutation introduced by transgenic approaches caused histopathology (myocyte disarray) and diastolic dysfunction.[159] A second transgenic model expressed a truncated cardiac troponin T; this mutation exhibited mild systolic dysfunction, markedly abnormal diastolic function, and myocellular disarray.[160] Humans with comparable troponin T mutations develop only modest hypertrophy.[93] Intriguingly, left ventricular hypertrophy was not observed in either murine model, and hearts expressing the truncated cardiac troponin T transgene were actually smaller than normal. A comparison of the molecular events triggered by troponin T versus myosin mutations may therefore uncover distinct pathways that are activated by different sarcomere defects and account for variable hypertrophic responses.

Two mouse models of cardiac myosin-binding protein C mutations have also been studied and demonstrate different mechanisms by which these gene defects cause disease. A transgenic model expressing mutant cardiac myosin-binding protein C sequences that lack domains required for binding myosin and titin[161] exhibited marked sarcomere disorganization and diminished cardiac function. Analyses of myofilaments showed inappropriate incorporation of the mutant peptide and only weak association with the contractile apparatus, causing the investigators to conclude that diminished levels of endogenous protein accounted for the pathogenic process. Studies from humans with these mutations show significant differences: symptoms are usually quite mild with disease onset late in life,[41] and myofibrillar levels of myosin-binding protein C are normal.[145] A second model was produced by mutation of the endogenous cardiac myosin-binding protein C gene that produced low-level expression of truncated peptides in sarcomere, suggesting a dominant negative mechanism for disease.[162,163] This knock-in model reproduces features of the human disease, including progressive onset of mild cardiac hypertrophy but normal cardiac

physiology.[162] The absence of a significant perturbation of ventricular function may explain the prolonged quiescence of these mutations in humans and account for late age of onset and better survival of myosin-binding protein C defects.

Further investigation of murine models for hypertrophic cardiomyopathy should more fully elucidate the mechanisms by which sarcomere protein gene mutations cause disease. In addition, these models provide sources of cardiac tissue, a reagent rarely available from human patients. Future investigations, such as transcript profiling in mutant myocardium, should foster discovery of the cellular responses to sarcomere dysfunction. Murine models will also help define factors that modulate the hypertrophic response. Human studies clearly indicate significant variation in the response to a shared sarcomere mutation, but whether this reflects the influence of background genes, environment, or lifestyles remains largely unknown. Extensive characterization of genetically identical murine models provides great opportunity to identify these and other factors that exacerbate or ameliorate disease, information that may provide new avenues for the development of therapeutics for hypertrophic cardiomyopathy.

## REFERENCES

1. Hallopeau M: Retrecissement ventriculo-aortique. *Gaz Med Paris* **24**:683, 1869.
2. Hollman A, Goodwin JF, Teare D, Renwick JW: A family with obstructive cardiomyopathy (asymmetrical hypertrophy). *Br Heart J* **22**:449, 1960.
3. Maron BJ, Gardin JM, Flack JM, Gidding SS, Kurosaki, TT, Bild DE: Prevalence of hypertrophic cardiomyopathy in a general population of young adults: Echocardiographic analysis of 4111 subjects in the CARDIA study. *Circulation* **92**:785, 1995.
4. Shapiro LM, McKenna WJ: Distribution of left ventricular hypertrophy in hypertrophic cardiomyopathy: A two-dimensional echocardiographic study. *J Am Coll Cardiol* **2**:437, 1983.
5. Marian AJ, Roberts R: Recent advances in the molecular genetics of hypertrophic cardiomyopathy. *Circulation* **92**:1336, 1995.

6. Spirito P, Chiarella F, Carratino L, Berisso, MZ, Bellotti P, Vecchio C: Clinical course and prognosis of hypertrophic cardiomyopathy in an outpatient population. *N Engl J Med* **320**:749, 1989.

7. Spirito P, Seidman CE, McKenna WJ, Maron BJ: The management of hypertrophic cardiomyopathy. *N Engl J Med* **336**:775, 1997.

8. Robinson K, Frenneaux MP, Stockins B, Karatasakis G, Poloniecki JD, McKenna WJ: Atrial fibrillation in hypertrophic cardiomyopathy: a longitudinal study. *J Am Coll Cardiol* **15**:1279, 1990.

9. Cecchi F, Montereggi A, Olivotto I, Marconi P, Dolara A, Maron BJ: Risk for atrial fibrillation in patients with hypertrophic cardiomyopathy assessed by signal averaged P wave duration. *Heart* **78**:44, 1997.

10. Hina K, Kusachi S, Iwasaki K, Nogami K, Moritani H, Kita T, Taniguchi G, et al.: Progression of left ventricular enlargement in patients with hypertrophic cardiomyopathy: incidence and prognostic value. *Clin Cardiol* **16**:403, 1993.

11. McKenna WJ, Deanfield JE: Hypertrophic cardiomyopathy: An important cause of sudden death. *Arch Dis Child* **59**:971, 1984.

12. McKenna WJ, England D, Doi YL, Deanfield JE, Oakley C, Goodwin JF: Arrhythmia in hypertrophic cardiomyopathy, I: Influence on prognosis. *Br Heart J* **46**:168, 1981.

13. Maron BJ, Cecchi F, McKenna WJ: Risk factors and stratification for sudden death in patients with hypertrophic cardiomyopathy. *Br Heart J* **72**:S13, 1994.

14. Solomon SD, Wolff S, Watkins H, Ridker PM, Come P, McKenna WJ, Seidman CE, et al.: Left ventricular hypertrophy and morphology in familial hypertrophic cardiomyopathy associated with mutations of the beta-myosin heavy chain gene. *J Am Coll Cardiol* **22**:498, 1993.

15. Counihan PJ, Fei L, Bashir Y, Farrell TG, Haywood GA, McKenna WJ: Assessment of heart rate variability in hypertrophic cardiomyopathy. Association with clinical and prognostic features. *Circulation* **88**:1682, 1993.

16. Lazzeroni E, Domenicucci S, Finardi A, Zoni A, Dodi C, Francescon P, Botti G: Severity of arrhythmias and extent of hypertrophy in hypertrophic cardiomyopathy. *Am Heart J* **118**:734, 1989.

17. Dilsizian V, Bonow RO, Epstein SE, Fananapazir L: Myocardial ischemia detected by thallium scintigraphy is frequently related to cardiac arrest and syncope in young patients with hypertrophic cardiomyopathy. *J Am Coll Cardiol* **22**:796, 1993.

18. McKenna W, Deanfield J, Faruqui A, England D, Oakley C, Goodwin J: Prognosis of hypertrophic cardiomyopathy: Role of age and clinical, electrocardiographic and hemodynamic features. *Am J Cardiol* **47**:532, 1981.

19. Spirito P, Maron BJ: Relation between extent of left ventricular hypertrophy and age in hypertrophic cardiomyopathy. *J Am Coll Cardiol* **13**:820, 1989.

20. Maron BJ, Lipson LC, Roberts WC, Savage DD, Epstein SE: "Malignant" hypertrophic cardiomyopathy: Identification of a subgroup of families with unusually frequent premature death. *Am J Cardiol* **41**:1133, 1978.

21. Louie EK, Edwards LC III: Hypertrophic cardiomyopathy. *Prog Cardiovasc Dis* **36**:275, 1994.

22. Wigle ED, Rakowski H, Kimball BP, Williams, WG: Hypertrophic cardiomyopathy: Clinical spectrum and treatment. *Circulation* **92**:1680, 1995.

23. Maron BJ, Wolfson JK, Ciro E, Spirito P: Relation of electrocardiographic abnormalities and patterns of left ventricular hypertrophy identified by 2-dimensional echocardiography in patients with hypertrophic cardiomyopathy. *Am J Cardiol* **51**:189, 1983.

24. Lemery R, Kleinebenne A, Nihoyannopoulos P, Aber V, Alfonso F, McKenna WJ: Q waves in hypertrophic cardiomyopathy in relation to the distribution and severity of right and left ventricular hypertrophy. *J Am Coll Cardiol* **16**:368, 1990.

25. Maron BJ: Q waves in hypertrophic cardiomyopathy: a reassessment. *J Am Coll Cardiol* **16**:375, 1990.

26. Charron P, Dubourg O, Desnos M, Isnard R, Hagege A, Millaire A, Carrier L, et al.: Diagnostic value of electrocardiography for familial hypertrophic cardiomyopathy in a genotyped adult population. *Circulation* **96**:214, 1997.

27. Rosenzweig A, Watkins H, Hwang D-S, Miri M, McKenna W, Traill TA, Seidman JG, et al.: Preclinical diagnosis of familial hypertrophic cardiomyopathy by genetic analysis of blood lymphocytes. *N Engl J Med* **325**:1753, 1991.

28. Lever HM, Karam RF, Currie PJ, Healy BP: Hypertrophic cardiomyopathy in the elderly: distinctions from the young based on cardiac shape. *Circulation* **79**:580, 1989.

29. Klues HG, Schiffers A, Maron BJ: Phenotypic spectrum and patterns of left ventricular hypertrophy in hypertrophic cardiomyopathy: Morphologic observations and significance as assessed by two-dimensional echocardiography in 600 patients. *J Am Coll Cardiol* **26**:1699, 1995.

30. Maron BJ, Gottdiener JS, Epstein SE: Patterns and significance of distribution of left ventricular hypertrophy in hypertrophic cardiomyopathy: A wide angle, two-dimensional echocardiographic study of 125 patients. *Am J Cardiol* **48**:418, 1981.

31. Levine RA, Lefebvre X, Guerrero JL, Vlahakes GJ, Cape EG, He S, Yoganathan AP, et al.: Unifying concepts of mitral valve function and disease: SAM, prolapse and ischemic mitral regurgitation. *J Cardiol* **24**:15, 1994.

32. McKenna WJ, Kleinebenne A, Nihoyannopoulos P, Foale R: Echocardiographic measurement of right ventricular wall thickness in hypertrophic cardiomyopathy: Relation to clinical and prognostic features. *J Am Coll Cardiol* **11**:351, 1988.

33. Maron BJ, Spirito P, Wesley Y, Arce J: Development and progression of left ventricular hypertrophy in children with hypertrophic cardiomyopathy. *N Engl J Med* **315**:610, 1986.

34. Rakowski H, Sasson Z, Wigle ED: Echocardiographic and doppler assessment of hypertrophic cardiomyopathy. *J Am Soc Echocardiogr* **1**:31, 1988.

35. Maron BJ, Moller JH, Seidman CE, Vincent GM, Dietz HC, Moss AJ, Sondheimer HM, et al.: Impact of laboratory molecular diagnosis on contemporary diagnostic criteria for genetically transmitted cardiovascular diseases: Hypertrophic cardiomyopathy, long-QT syndrome, and Marfan syndrome. *Circulation* **98**:1460, 1998.

36. Clark CE, Henry WL, Epstein SE: Familial prevalence and genetic transmission of idiopathic hypertrophic subaortic stenosis. *N Engl J Med* **289**:709, 1973.

37. Van Dorp WG, ten Cate FJ, Vletter WB, Dohmen H, Roelandt J: Familial prevalence of asymmetric septal hypertrophy. *Eur J Cardiol* **4**:349, 1976.

38. Watkins H, Thierfelder L, Hwang D-S, McKenna W, Seidman JG, Seidman CE: Sporadic hypertrophic cardiomyopathy due to de novo myosin mutations. *J Clin Invest* **90**:1666, 1992.

39. Greve G, Bachinski DL, Friedman DL, Czernuszewicz G, Anan R, Towbin JA, Seidman CE, et al.: Isolation of a de novo mutant myocardial β MHC protein in a pedigree with hypertrophic cardiomyopathy. *Hum Mol Genet* **3**:2073, 1994.

40. Watkins H, Anan R, Coviello DA, Spirito P, Seidman JG, Seidman CE: A de novo mutation in α-tropomyosin that causes hypertrophic cardiomyopathy. *Circulation* **91**:2303, 1995.

41. Niimura H, Bachinski LL, Sangwatanaroj S, Watkins H, Chudley AE, McKenna W, Kristinsson A, et al.: Mutations in the gene for cardiac myosin-binding protein C and late-onset familial hypertrophic cardiomyopathy. *N Engl J Med* **338**:1248, 1998.

42. Yu B, French JA, Carrier L, Jeremy RW, McTaggart DR, Nicholson MR, Hambly B, et al.: Molecular pathology of familial hypertrophic cardiomyopathy caused by mutations in the myosin binding protein C gene. *J Med Genet* **35**:205, 1998.

43. Wigle ED, Sasson Z, Henderson MA, Rudd TD, Fulop J, Rakowski H, Williams WG: Hypertrophic cardiomyopathy: The importance of the site and the extent of hypertrophy: A review. *Prog Cardiovasc Dis* **28**:1, 1985.

44. Semsarian C, French J, Trent RJ, Richmond DR, Jeremy RW: The natural history of left ventricular wall thickening in hypertrophic cardiomyopathy. *Aust NZ J Med* **27**:51, 1997.

45. Adelman AG, Wigle ED, Ranganathan N, Webb GD, Kidd BS, Bigelow WG, Silver MD: The clinical course in muscular subaortic stenosis: A retrospective and prospective study of 60 hemodynamically proved cases. *Ann Intern Med* **77**:515, 1972.

46. Grigg LE, Wigle ED, Williams WG, Daniel LB, Rakowski H: Transesophageal Doppler echocardiography in obstructive hypertrophic cardiomyopathy: Clarification of pathophysiology and importance in intraoperative decision making. *J Am Coll Cardiol* **20**:42, 1992.

47. Louie EK, Maron BJ: Hypertrophic cardiomyopathy characterized by extreme increase in left ventricular wall thickness: Functional and morphologic features and clinical significance. *J Am Coll Cardiol* **8**:57, 1986.

48. Falicov RE, Resnekov L, Bharati S, Lev M: Midventricular obstruction: A variant of obstructive cardiomyopathy. *Am J Cardiol* **37**:432, 1976.

49. Yamaguchi H, Ishimura T, Nishiyama S, Nagasaki FR, Nakanishi S, Takatsu F, Nishijo T, et al.: Hypertrophic nonobstructive cardiomyopathy with giant negative T-waves (apical hypertrophy): Ventriculographic and echocardiographic features in 30 patients. *Am J Cardiol* **44**:401, 1979.

50. Gaudio C, Pellicia F, Tanzilli G, Mazzarotto P, Cianfrocca C, Marino B: Magnetic resonance imaging for assessment of apical hypertrophy in hypertrophic cardiomyopathy. *Clin Cardiol* **15**:164, 1992.

51. Hecht GM, Kluse HG, Roberts WC, Maron BJ: Coexistence of sudden cardiac death and end-stage heart failure in familial hypertrophic cardiomyopathy. *J Am Coll Cardiol* **22**:489, 1993.

52. Fighali S, Krajcer Z, Edelman S, Leachman RD: Progression of hypertrophic cardiomyopathy into a hypokinetic left ventricle: Higher incidence in patients with midventricular obstruction. *J Am Coll Cardiol* **9**:288, 1987.

53. Gruver EJ, Fatkin D, Dodds GA, Kisslo J, Maron BJ, Seidman JG, Seidman CE: Familial hypertrophic cardiomyopathy and atrial fibrillation caused by Arg663His α-cardiac myosin heavy chain mutation. *Am J Cardiol* **83**:13H, 1999.

54. Cecchi F, Olivotto I, Montereggi A, Santoro G, Dolara A, Maron BJ: Hypertrophic cardiomyopathy in Tuscany: Clinical course and outcome in an unselected regional population. *J Am Coll Cardiol* **26**:1529, 1995.

55. Petrone RK, Klues HG, Panza JA, Peterson EE, Maron BJ: Significance of the occurrence of mitral valve prolapse in patients with hypertrophic cardiomyopathy. *J Am Coll Cardiol* **20**:55, 1992.

56. Klues HG, Maron BJ, Dollar A, Roberts WC: Diversity of structural mitral valve alterations in hypertrophic cardiomyopathy. *Circulation* **85**:1651, 1992.

57. St. John Sutton, MG Lee JT, Anderson KR: Histopathological specificity of hypertrophic obstructive cardiomyopathy. Myocardial fiber disarray and myocardial fibrosis. *Br Heart J* **44**:433, 1980.

58. Olsen EG: Anatomic and light microscopic characterization of hypertrophic obstructive and nonobstructive cardiomyopathy. *Eur Heart J* **4**:1, 1983.

59. Maron BJ, Roberts WC: Quantitative analysis of cardiac muscle cell disorganization in the ventricular septum of patients with hypertrophic cardiomyopathy. *Circulation* **59**:689, 1979.

60. Maron BJ, Epstein SE, and Roberts WC: Hypertrophic cardiomyopathy and transmural myocardial infarction without significant atherosclerosis of the extramural coronary arteries. *Am J Cardiol* **43**:1086, 1979.

61. Thompson DS, Naqvi N, Juul SM, Swanton RH, Coltart DJ, Jenkins BS, Webb-Peploe MM: Effects of propranolol on myocardial oxygen consumption, substrate extraction, and haemodynamics in hypertrophic obstructive cardiomyopathy. *Br Heart J* **44**:488, 1980.

62. Menges H Jr, Brandenburg RO, Brown AL Jr: The clinical, hemodynamic and pathologic diagnosis of muscular subvalvular aortic stenosis. *Circulation* **24**:1126, 1961.

63. Wilson WS, Criley JM, Ross RS: Dynamics of left ventricular emptying in hypertrophic cardiomyopathy. *Am Heart J* **73**:4, 1967.

64. Schulte HD, Bircks WH, Loesse B, Godehardt EA, Schwartzkopff B: Prognosis of patients with hypertrophic obstructive cardiomyopathy after transaortic myectomy: Late results up to twenty-five years. *J Thorac Cardiovasc Surg* **106**:709, 1993.

65. ten Berg JM, Suttorp MJ, Knaepen PJ, Ernst SM, Vermeulen FE, Jaarsma W: Hypertrophic obstructive cardiomyopathy: initial results and long-term follow-up after Morrow septal myectomy. *Circulation* **90**:1781, 1994.

66. Robbins RC, Stinson EB: Long-term results of left ventricular myotomy and myectomy for obstructive hypertrophic cardiomyopathy. *J Thorac Cardiovasc Surg* **111**:586, 1996.

67. Cannon RO III, McIntosh CL, Schenke WH, Maron BJ, Bonow RO, Epstein SE: Effect of surgical reduction of left ventricular outflow obstruction on hemodynamics, coronary flow and myocardial metabolism in hypertrophic cardiomyopathy. *Circulation* **79**:766, 1989.

68. Gilligan DM, Chan WL, Stewart R, Joshi J, Nihoyannopoulos P, Oakley CM: Cardiac responses assessed by echocardiography to changes in preload in hypertrophic cardiomyopathy. *Am J Cardiol* **73**:312, 1994.

69. Schwammenthal E, Schwatzkopff B, Block M, Johns J, Losse B, Engberding R, Borggrefe M, et al.: Doppler echocardiographic assessment of the pressure gradient during bicycle ergometry in hypertrophic cardiomyopathy. *Am J Cardiol* **69**:1623, 1992.

70. Poetter K, Jiang H, Hassanzadeh S, Master SR, Chang A, Dalakas MC, Rayment I, et al.: Mutations in either the essential or regulatory light chains of myosin are associated with a rare myopathy in human heart and skeletal muscle. *Nat Genet* **13**:63, 1996.

71. Schwammenthal E, Nakatani S, He S, Hopmeyer J, Sagie A, Weyman AE, Lever HM, et al.: Mechanism of mitral regurgitation in hypertrophic cardiomyopathy. Mismatch of posterior to anterior leaflet length and mobility. *Circulation* **98**:856, 1998.

72. Mikami T, Hashimoto, Kudo T, Sugawara T, Sakamoto S, Yasuda H: Mitral valve and its ring in hypertrophic cardiomyopathy: A mechanism creating surplus mitral leaflet involved in systolic anterior motion. *Jpn Circ J* **52**:597, 1988.

73. ten Cate FJ, Serruys PW, Mey S, Roelandt J: Effects of short-term administration of verapamil on left ventricular relaxation and filling dynamics measured by a combined hemodynamic-ultrasonic technique in patients with hypertrophic cardiomyopathy. *Circulation* **68**:1274, 1983.

74. Bonow RO, Dilsizian V, Rosing DR, Maron BJ, Bacharach SL, Green MV: Verapamil-induced improvement in left ventricular diastolic filling and increased exercise tolerance in patients with hypertrophic cardiomyopathy: short- and long-term effects. *Circulation* **72**:853, 1985.

75. Lorell BH, Paulus WJ, Grossman W, Wynne J, Cohn PF: Modification of abnormal left ventricular diastolic properties by nifedipine in patients with hypertrophic cardiomyopathy. *Circulation* **65**:499, 1982.

76. Iwase M, Sotobata I, Takagi S, Miyaguchi K, Jing HX, Yokota M: Effects of diltiazem on left ventricular diastolic behavior in patients with hypertrophic cardiomyopathy: Evaluation with exercise pulsed Doppler echocardiography. *J Am Coll Cardiol* **9**:1099, 1987.

77. Gwathmey JK, Warren SE, Briggs GM, Copelas L, Feldman MD, Phillips PJ, Callahan M Jr, et al.: Diastolic dysfunction in hypertrophic cardiomyopathy. Effect on active force generation during systole. *J Clin Invest* **87**:1023, 1991.

78. Maron BJ, Bonow RO, Cannon RO, Leon MB, Epstein SE: Hypertrophic cardiomyopathy. Interrelations of clinical manifestations, pathophysiology and therapy. *N Engl J Med* **316**:780, 844, 1987.

79. Wigle ED, Wilansky S: Diastolic dysfunction in hypertrophic cardiomyopathy. *Heart Failure* **3**:82, 1987.

80. Jarcho JA, McKenna W, Pare JAP, Solomon SD, Holcombe RF, Dickie S, Levi T, et al.: Mapping a gene for familial hypertrophic cardiomyopathy to chromosome 14q1. *N Engl J Med* **321**:1372, 1989.

81. Watkins H, MacRae C, Thierfelder L, Chou YH, Frenneaux M, McKenna W, Seidman JG, et al.: A disease locus for familial hypertrophic cardiomyopathy maps to chromosome 1q3. *Nat Genet* **3**:333, 1993.

82. Thierfelder L, MacRae C, Watkins H, Tomfohrde J, Williams M, McKenna W, Bohm K, et al.: A familial hypertrophic cardiomyopathy locus maps to chromosome 15q2. *Proc Natl Acad Sci U S A* **90**:6270, 1993.

83. Carrier L, Hengstenberg C, Beckmann JS, Guicheney P, Dufour C, Bercovici J, Dausse E, et al.: Mapping of a novel gene for familial hypertrophic cardiomyopathy to chromosome 11. *Nat Genet* **4**:311, 1993.

84. Schiaffino S, Reggiani C: Molecular diversity of myofibrillar proteins: Gene regulation and functional significance. *Physiol Rev* **76**:371, 1996.

85. Vikstrom KL, Leinwand LA: Contractile protein mutations and heart disease. *Curr Op Cell Biol* **8**:97, 1996.

86. Hamada H, Petrino MG, Kakunaga T: Molecular structure and evolutionary origin of human cardiac muscle actin gene. *Proc Natl Acad Sci U S A* **79**:5901, 1982.

87. Lees-Miller JP, Helfman DM: The molecular basis for tropomyosin isoform diversity. *Bioessays* **13**:429, 1991.

88. Zot AS, Potter JD: Structural aspects of troponin-tropomyosin regulation of skeletal muscle contraction. *Annu Rev Biophys Biophys Chem* **16**:535, 1987.

89. Schultheiss T, Lin Z, Lu MH, Murray J, Fischman DA, Weber K, Masaki T: Differential distribution of subsets of myofibrillar proteins in cardiac nonstriated and striated myofibrils. *J Cell Biol* **110**:1159, 1990.

90. Mogensen J, Klausen IC, Pedersen AK, Egebkad G, Bross P, Kruse TA, Gregersen N, et al.: α-Cardiac actin is a novel disease gene in familial hypertrophic cardiomyopathy. *J Clin Invest* **103**: R39, 1999.

91. Olson TM, Michels VV, Thibodeau SN, Tai YS, Keating MT: Actin mutations in dilated cardiomyopathy, a heritable form of heart failure. *Science* **280**:750, 1998.

92. Mogensen J, Kruse TA, Borglum AD: Refined localization of the human alpha-tropomyosin gene (TPM1) by genetic mapping. *Cytogenet Cell Genet* **84**:35, 1999.

93. Watkins H, McKenna WJ, Thierfelder L, Suk J, Anan R, O'Donoghue A, Spirito P: Mutations in the genes for cardiac troponin T and α-tropomyosin in hypertrophic cardiomyopathy. *N Engl J Med* **332**:1058, 1995.

94. Thierfelder L, Watkins H, MacRae C, Lamas R, McKenna W, Vosberg H-P, Seidman JG, et al.: α-Tropomyosin and cardiac troponin T mutations cause familial hypertrophic cardiomyopathy: A disease of the sarcomere. *Cell* **77**:1, 1994.

95. Nakajima-Taniguchi C, Matsui H, Nagata S, Kishimoto T, Yamauchi-Takihara K: Novel missense mutation in α-tropomyosin gene found in Japanese patients with hypertrophic cardiomyopathy. *J Mol Cell Cardiol* **27**:2053, 1995.

96. Yamauchi-Takihara K, Nakajima-Taniguchi C, Matsui H, Fujio Y, Kunisada K, Nagata S, Kishimoto T: Clinical implications of hypertrophic cardiomyopathy associated with mutations in the α-tropomyosin gene. *Heart* **76**:63, 1996.

97. Jaaskelainen P, Soranta M, Miettinen R, Saarinen L, Pihlajamaki J, Silvennoinen K, Tikanoja T, et al.: The cardiac beta-myosin heavy chain gene is not the predominant gene for hypertrophic cardiomyopathy in the Finnish population. *J Am Coll Cardiol* **32**:1709, 1998.

98. Coviello DA, Maron BJ, Spirito P, Watkins H, Vosberg H-P, Thierfelder L, Schoen FJ, et al.: Clinical features of hypertrophic cardiomyopathy caused by mutation of a "hot spot" in the α-tropomyosin gene. *J Am Coll Cardiol* **29**:635, 1997.

99. Bottinelli R, Coviello DA, Redwood CS, Pellegrino MA, Maron BH, Spirito P, Watkins H, et al.: A mutant tropomyosin that causes hypertrophic cardiomyopathy is expressed in vivo and associated with an increased calcium sensitivity. *Circ Res* **82**:106, 1998.

100. Farza H, Townsend PJ, Carrier L, Barton PJ, Mesnard L, Bahrend E, Forissier JF, et al.: Genomic organisation, alternative splicing and polymorphisms of the human cardiac troponin T gene. *J Mol Cell Cardiol* **30**:1247, 1998.

101. Forissier JF, Carrier L, Farza H, Bonne G, Bercovici J, Richard P, Hainque B, et al.: Codon 102 of the cardiac troponin T gene is a putative hot spot for mutations in familial hypertrophic cardiomyopathy. *Circulation* **94**:3069, 1996.

102. Moolman JC, Corfield VA, Posen B, Ngumbela K, Seidman C, Brink PA, Watkins H: Sudden death due to troponin T mutations. *J Am Coll Cardiol* **29**:549, 1997.

103. Nakajima-Taniguchi C, Matsui H, Fujio Y, Nagata S, Kishimoto T, Yamauchi-Takihara K: Novel missense mutation in cardiac troponin T gene found in Japanese patient with hypertrophic cardiomyopathy. *J Mol Cell Cardiol* **29**:839, 1997.

104. Watkins H, Seidman CE, Seidman JG, Feng HS, Sweeney HL: Expression and functional assessment of a truncated cardiac troponin T that causes hypertrophic cardiomyopathy. *J Clin Invest* **98**:2456, 1996.

105. Anan R, Shono H, Kisanuki A, Arima S, Nakao S, Tanaka H: Patients with familial hypertrophic cardiomyopathy caused by a Phe110Ile missense mutation in the cardiac troponin T gene have variable cardiac morphologies and a favorable prognosis. *Circulation* **98**:391, 1998.

106. Mogensen J, Kruse TA, Borglum AD: Assignment of the human cardiac troponin I gene (TNNI3) to chromosome 19q13.4 by radiation hybrid mapping. *Cytogenet Cell Genet* **79**:272, 1997.

107. Kimura A, Harada H, Park JE, Nishi H, Satoh M, Takahashi M, Hiroi S, et al.: Mutations in the cardiac troponin I gene associated with hypertrophic cardiomyopathy. *Nat Genet* **16**:379, 1997.

108. Klausen IC, Mogensen J, Egeblad H, Baandrup U, Borglum AD: A novel mutation in the troponin I gene is associated with sudden cardiac death in familial hypertrophic cardiomyopathy. *Am J Hum Genet* **65**:A305, 1999.

109. Sata M, Stafford WF, Mabuchi K, Ikebe M: The motor domain and the regulatory domain of myosin solely dictate enzymatic activity and phosphorylation-dependent regulation, respectively. *Proc Natl Acad Sci U S A* **94**:91, 1997.

110. Rayment I, Holden HM, Whittaker M, Yohn CB, Lorenz M, Holmes KC, Milligan RA: Structure of the actin-myosin complex and its implications for muscle contraction. *Science* **261**:58, 1993.

111. Lowey S, Waller GS, Trybus KM: Skeletal muscle myosin light chains are essential for physiological speeds of shortening. *Nature* **365**:454, 1993.

112. Trybus KM: Role of myosin light chains. *J Muscle Res Cell Motil* **15**:587, 1994.

113. Sweeney HL, Bowman BF, Stull JT: Myosin light chain phosphorylation in vertebrate striated muscle: regulation and function. *Am J Physiol* **264**:C1085, 1993.

114. Gautel M, Zuffardi O, Freiburg A, Labeit S: Phosphorylation switches specific for the cardiac isoform of myosin binding protein C: a modulator of cardiac contraction? *EMBO J* **14**:1952, 1995.

115. Weisberg A, Winegrad S: Alteration of myosin cross bridges by phosphorylation of myosin binding protein C in cardiac muscle. *Proc Natl Acad Sci U S A* **93**:8999, 1996.

116. Weisberg A, Winegrad S: Relations between crossbridge structure and actomyosin ATPase activity in rat heart. *Circ Res* **83**:60, 1998.

117. Freiburg A, Gautel M: A molecular map of the interactions between titin and myosin-binding protein C. Implications for sarcomeric assembly in familial hypertrophic cardiomyopathy. *Eur J Biochem* **235**:317, 1996.

118. Saez LJ, Gianola KM, McNally EM, Feghali R, Eddy R, Shows TB, Leinwand LA: Human cardiac myosin heavy chain genes and their linkage in the genome. *Nucleic Acids Res* **15**:5443, 1987.

119. Jaenicke T, Diederich KW, Haas W, Schleich J, Lichter P, Pfordt M, Bach A, et al.: The complete sequence of the human β-myosin heavy chain gene and a comparative analysis of its product. *Genomics* **8**:194, 1990.

120. Liew CC, Sole MJ, Yamauchi-Takihara K, Kellam B, Anderson DH, Lin LP, Liew JC: Complete sequence and organization of the human cardiac β-myosin heavy chain gene. *Nucleic Acids Res* **18**:3647, 1990.

121. Geisterfer-Lowrance AAT, Kass S, Tanigawa G, Vosberg H-P, McKenna W, Seidman CE, Seidman JG: A molecular basis for familial hypertrophic cardiomyopathy: A β-cardiac myosin heavy chain gene missense mutation. *Cell* **62**:999, 1990.

122. Dausse E, Komajda M, Dubourg O, Dufour C, Carrier L, Wisnewsky C, Bercovici J, et al.: Familial hypertrophic cardiomyopathy: Microsatellite haplotyping and identification of a hot-spot for mutations in the β-myosin heavy chain gene. *J Clin Invest* **92**:2807, 1993.

123. Anan R, Greve G, Thierfelder L, Watkins H, McKenna WJ, Solomon S, Vecchio C, et al.: Prognostic implications of novel β-myosin heavy chain mutations that cause familial hypertrophic cardiomyopathy. *J Clin Invest* **93**:280, 1994.

124. Consevage M, Salada GC, Baylen BG, Ladda RL, Rogan PK: A new missense mutation, Arg719Gln, in the β-cardiac heavy chain myosin gene of patients with familial hypertrophic cardiomyopathy. *Hum Mol Genet* **3**:1025, 1994.

125. Fananapazir L, Dalakas MC, Cyran F, Cohn G, Epstein ND: Missense mutations in the β-myosin heavy chain gene cause central core disease in hypertrophic cardiomyopathy. *Proc Natl Acad Sci U S A* **90**:3993, 1993.

126. Arai S, Matsuoka R, Hirayama K, Sakurai H, Tamura M, Ozawa T, Kimura M, et al.: Missense mutation of the β-cardiac myosin heavy chain gene in hypertrophic cardiomyopathy. *Am J Med Genet* **58**:267, 1995.

127. Nakajima-Taniguchi C, Matsui H, Eguchi N, Nagata S, Kishimoto T, Yamauchi-Takihara K: A novel deletion mutation in the β-myosin heavy chain gene found in Japanese patients with hypertrophic cardiomyopathy. *J Mol Cell Cardiol* **27**:2607, 1995.

128. Marian AJ, Yu QT, Mares A, Hill R, Roberts R, Perryman MB: Detection of a new mutation in the β-myosin heavy chain gene in an individual with hypertrophic cardiomyopathy. *J Clin Invest* **90**:2156, 1992.

129. Nishi H, Kimura A, Harada H, Koga Y, Adachi K, Matsuyama K, Koyanagi T, et al.: A myosin missense mutation, not a null allele, causes familial hypertrophic cardiomyopathy. *Circulation* **91**:2911, 1995.

130. Watkins H, Rosenzweig A, Hwang DS, Levi T, McKenna W, Seidman CE, Seidman, JG: Characteristics and prognostic implications of myosin missense mutations in familial hypertrophic cardiomyopathy. *N Engl J Med* **326**:1108, 1992.

131. Becker KD, Gottshall KR, Hickey R, Perriard JC, Chien KR: Point mutations in human β-cardiac myosin heavy chain have differential effects on sarcomeric structure and assembly: An ATP binding site change disrupts both thick and thin filaments, whereas hypertrophic cardiomyopathy mutations display normal assembly. *J Cell Biol* **137**:131, 1997.

132. Epstein ND, Cohn GM, Cyran F, Fananapazir L: Differences in clinical expression of hypertrophic cardiomyopathy associated with two distinct mutations in the beta-myosin heavy chain gene. A 908Leu-Val mutations and a 403Arg-Gln mutation. *Circulation* **86**:345, 1992.

133. Rayment I, Holden HM, Sellers JR, Fananapazir L, Epstein ND: Structural interpretation of the mutations in the β-cardiac myosin that have been implicated in familial hypertrophic cardiomyopathy. *Proc Natl Acad Sci U S A* **92**:3864, 1995.

134. Sata M, Ikebe M: Functional analysis of the mutations in the human cardiac β-myosin that are responsible for familial hypertrophic cardiomyopathy. *J Clin Invest* **98**:2866, 1996.

135. Cuda G, Fananapazir L, Epstein ND, Sellers JR: The in vitro motility activity of β-cardiac myosin depends on the nature of the β-myosin heavy chain gene mutation in hypertrophic cardiomyopathy. *J Muscle Res Cell Motil* **18**:275, 1997.

136. Lankford EB, Epstein ND, Fananapazir L, Sweeney HL: Abnormal contractile properties of muscle fibers expressing β-myosin heavy chain gene mutations in patients with hypertrophic cardiomyopathy. *J Clin Invest* **95**:1409, 1995.

137. Tyska MJ, Hayes E, Giewat M, Seidman CE, Seidman JG, Warshaw DM: Single molecule mechanics of R403Q cardiac myosin isolated from the mouse model of familial hypertrophic cardiomyopathy. *Circ Res* **86**:737, 2000.

138. Fodor WL, Darras B, Seharaseyon J, Falkenthal S, Francke U, Vanin EF: Human ventricular/slow twitch myosin alkali light chain gene: Characterization, sequence, and chromosomal location. *J Biol Chem* **264**:2143, 1989.

139. Poetter K, Jiang H, Hassanzadeh S, Master SR, Chang A, Dalakas MC, Rayment I, et al.: Mutations in either the essential or regulatory light chains of myosin are associated with a rare myopathy in human heart and skeletal muscle. *Nat Genet* **13**:63, 1996.

140. Flavigny J, Richard P, Isnard R, Carrier L, Charron P, Bonne G, Forissier JF, et al.: Identification of two novel mutations in the ventricular regulatory myosin light chain gene (MYL2) associated with familial and classical forms of hypertrophic cardiomyopathy. *J Mol Med* **76**:208, 1998.

141. Gene Map 1998. www.ncbi.nih.gov/gema98.

142. Carrier L, Bonne G, Bahrend E, Yu B, Richard P, Niel F, Hainque B, et al.: Organization and sequence of human cardiac myosin binding protein C gene (MYBPC3) and identification of mutations predicted to produce truncated proteins in familial hypertrophic cardiomyopathy. *Circ Res* **80**:427, 1997.

143. Watkins H, Conner D, Thierfelder L, Jarcho JA, MacRae C, McKenna WJ, Maron BJ, et al.: Mutations in the cardiac myosin-binding protein C gene on chromosome 11 cause familial hypertrophic cardiomyopathy. *Nat Genet* **11**:434, 1995.

144. Bonne G, Carrier L, Bercovici J, Cruaud C, Richard P, Hainque B, Gautel M, et al.: Cardiac myosin-binding protein C gene splice acceptor site mutation is associated with familial hypertrophic cardiomyopathy. *Nat Genet* **11**:438, 1995.

145. Rottbauer W, Gautel M, Zehelein J, Labeit S, Franz WM, Fischer C, Vollrath B, et al.: Novel splice donor site mutation in the cardiac myosin binding protein C gene in familial hypertrophic cardiomyopathy: Characterization of cardiac transcript and protein. *J Clin Invest* **100**:475, 1997.

146. Moolman-Smook JC, Mayosi B, Brink P, Corfield VA: Identification of a new missense mutation in MyBP-C associated with hypertrophic cardiomyopathy. *J Med Genet* **35**:253, 1998.

147. Charron P, Dubourg O, Desnos M, Bennaceur M, Carrier L, Camproux AC, Isnard R, et al.: Clinical features and prognostic implications of familial hypertrophic cardiomyopathy related to the cardiac myosin-binding protein C gene. *Circulation* **97**:2230, 1998.

148. MacRae CA, Ghaisas N, Kass S, Donnelly S, Basson CT, Watkins H, Anan R, et al.: Familial hypertrophic cardiomyopathy with Wolff-Parkinson-White syndrome maps to a locus on chromosome 7q3. *J Clin Invest* **96**:1216, 1995.

149. Mehdirad AA, Fatkin D, DiMarco JP, MacRae CA, Seidman JG, Seidman CE, Benson DW: Electrophysiologic characteristics of accessory atrioventricular connections in an inherited form of Wolff-Parkinson-White Syndrome. *J Card Electrophysiol* **10**:630, 1999.

150. Vikstrom KL, Factor SM, Leinwand LA: Mice expressing mutant myosin heavy chains are a model for familial hypertrophic cardiomyopathy. *Mol Med* **2**:556, 1996.

151. Geisterfer-Lowrance AAT, Christe M, Connor DA, Ingwall JS, Schoen RJ, Seidman CE, Seidman JG: A mouse model of familial hypertrophic cardiomyopathy. *Science* **272**:731, 1996.

152. Berul CI, Christe ME, Aronovitz, MJ, Seidman CE, Seidman JG, Mendelsohn ME: Electrophysiological abnormalities and arrhythmias in α-MHC mutant familial hypertrophic cardiomyopathy mice. *J Clin Invest* **99**:570, 1997.

153. Spindler M, Saupe KW, Christe ME, Sweeney HL, Seidman CE, Seidman JG, Ingwall JS: Diastolic dysfunction and altered energetics in the α MHC$^{403/+}$ mouse model of familial hypertrophic cardiomyopathy. *J Clin Invest* **101**:1775, 1998.

154. Georgakopoulos D, Christe ME, Giewat M, Seidman CE, Seidman JG, Kass D: The pathogenesis of familial hypertrophic cardiomyopathy: Early and evolving effects from an α cardiac myosin heavy chain missense mutation. *Nat Med* **5**:327, 1999.

155. Blanchard E, Seidman CE, Seidman JG, LeWinter M, Maughan D: Altered crossbridge kinetics in the α MHC$^{403/+}$ mouse model of familial hypertrophic cardiomyopathy. *Circ Res* **84**:475, 1999.

156. Gao WD, Perez NG, Seidman CE, Seidman CE, Marbán E: Altered cardiac excitation-contraction coupling in mutant mice with familial hypertrophic cardiomyopathy. *J Clin Invest* **103**:661, 1999.

157. Healey MJ, Fatkin D, Arroyo LH, Lee RT, Maguire CT, Bevilacqua LM, Berul CI, et al.: Exercise and beta-blocker therapy in α-myosin heavy chain mutant mice with hypertrophic cardiomyopathy. *Circulation* **98**:I-70, 1998.

158. Muthuchamy M, Pieples K, Rethinasamy P, Hoit B, Grupp IL, Boivin GP, Wolska B, et al.: Mouse model of a familial hypertrophic cardiomyopathy mutation in α-tropomyosin manifests cardiac dysfunction. *Circ Res* **85**:47, 1999.

159. Oberst L, Zhao G, Park JT, Brugada R, Michael LH, Entman ML, Roberts R, et al.: Dominant-negative effect of a mutant cardiac troponin T on cardiac structure and function in transgenic mice. *J Clin Invest* **102**:1498, 1998.

160. Tardiff JC, Factor SM, Tompkins BD, Hewett TE, Palmer BM, Moore RL, Schwartz S, et al.: A truncated cardiac troponin T molecule in transgenic mice suggests multiple cellular mechanisms for familial hypertrophic cardiomyopathy. *J Clin Invest* **101**:2800, 1998.

161. Yang Q, Sanbe A, Osinka H, Hewett TE, Klevitsky R, Robbins J: A mouse model of myosin binding protein C human familial hypertrophic cardiomyopathy. *J Clin Invest* **102**:1292, 1998.

162. McConnell BK, Jones K, Fatkin D, Arryo LH, Lee RT, Aristizabal O, Turnbull KH, et al.: Mice with a mutant myosin binding protein C gene provide a model for familial hypertrophic cardiomyopathy. *Circulation* **98**:I-625, 1998.

163. McConnell BK, Jones KA, Fatkin D, Arroyo LH, Lee RT, Aristizabal O, Turnbull DH, et al.: Dilated cardiomyopathy in homozygous myosin-binding protein-C mutant mice. *J Clin Invest* **104**:1235, 1999.

# KIDNEY

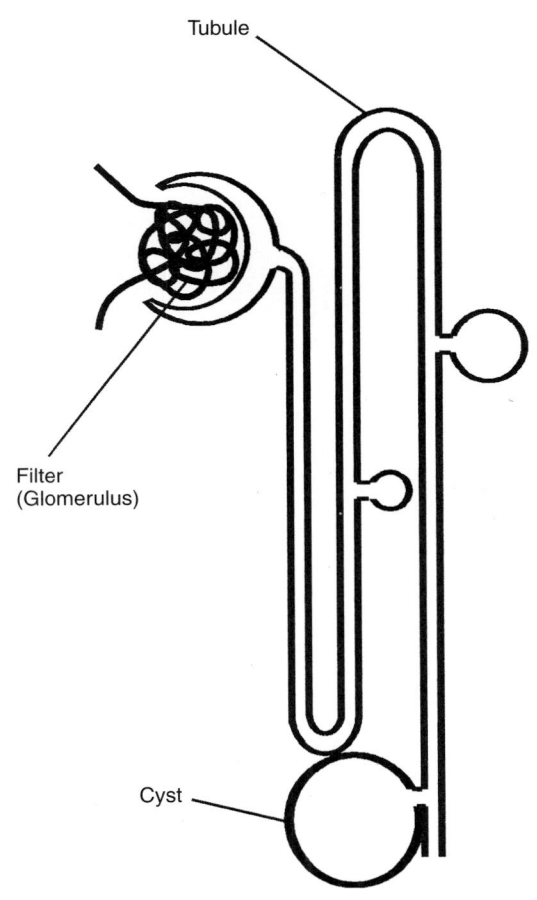

Tubule

Filter
(Glomerulus)

Cyst

# Alport Syndrome and Basement Membrane Collagen

*Karl Tryggvason* ■ *Paula Martin*

1. Alport syndrome is a progressive hereditary kidney disease characterized by hematuria, and often associated with extrarenal complications, such as sensorineural hearing loss and ocular abnormalities. By electron microscopy ultrastructural changes, including thinning, thickening, and splitting, can be seen in the glomerular basement membrane (GBM). Alport syndrome is mainly inherited as an X-linked dominant trait (MIM 301050) with mutations in the type IV collagen α5 chain gene (*COL4A5*), but both autosomal recessive (MIM 203780) and dominant forms also exist. Autosomal Alport syndrome is caused by mutations in the *COL4A3* and *COL4A4* genes encoding the type IV collagen α3 and α4 chains, respectively. Additionally, numerous deletions involving the 5′ ends of both the *COL4A6* gene and the adjacent *COL4A5* gene have been reported to cause a rare disorder, diffuse leiomyomatosis, that is associated with Alport syndrome (MIM 308940, 303631). A minority of Alport syndrome patients develop anti-GBM nephritis involving the transplanted allograft.

2. Basement membranes are thin, extracellular, sheet-like structures that separate cells of organized tissues from the interstitial connective tissue. The major complications of Alport syndrome — hematuria and proteinuria — are caused by structural alterations and consequent malfunction of the glomerular filtration barrier, especially glomerular basement membrane, a major component of the glomerular filtration barrier. The molecular structure of the GBM is much the same as that of basement membranes in other tissues. The major structural component is type IV collagen that forms a tightly cross-linked network in which a less dense laminin network is connected via entactin (nidogen) molecules.

3. Different triple-helical type IV collagen molecules are composed of six genetically distinct α-chains, namely α1(IV), α2(IV), α3(IV), α4(IV), α5(IV), or α6(IV). Each type IV collagen α-chain contains a long collagenous domain, a short noncollagenous N-terminus, and a noncollagenous domain (NC1) at the C-terminus. Type IV collagen molecules self-assemble into a complex network structure via C-terminal NC1 domains forming dimers, and at the N-termini forming tetramers. The molecular composition of different type IV collagen networks varies from tissue to tissue.

4. Type IV collagen genes are very large, the smallest one having 46 exons. An interesting feature is that the six genes are located pair-wise in three different chromosomes, sharing a common bidirectional promoter.

5. About 300 mutations have been reported in Alport syndrome patients in the *COL4A3*, *COL4A4*, and *COL4A5* genes. Different mutations cause different phenotypes, but it is difficult to predict the consequences of a certain mutation, because deletion of a whole gene does not necessarily produce a more severe phenotype than does an amino acid substitution. Immunohistologic studies of tissues from Alport syndrome patients demonstrate the existence of different α-chain networks in different tissues. Thus, differential pattern of staining in skin sections may be used to distinguish between X-linked and autosomal recessive forms of Alport syndrome.

6. Alport syndrome, which primarily affects the renal glomeruli, is an attractive disease target for gene therapy.

## CLINICAL FEATURES

### Clinical Findings

In 1927, Professor Arthur Cecil Alport first described a hereditary nephritis characterized by hematuria and sensorineural deafness as a clinical syndrome commonly referred to as Alport syndrome.[1] It is now known that Alport syndrome is clinically a very heterogeneous disease.[2,3] Patients have recurrent microscopic or gross hematuria in childhood, usually leading to end-stage renal disease (ESRD) in affected males, and, in rare cases, also in females. A large number of patients have sensorineural hearing loss affecting primarily high tones. By electron microscopy, irregular thinning and thickening of the glomerular basement membrane (GBM) with formation of longitudinal splits into thin layers with a basket-weave pattern can be observed (Fig. 214-1). These changes are most evident in male patients. Eye abnormalities, such as anterior lenticonus, premature cataracts, or perimacular retinal flecks are also frequent findings in Alport patients. Sometimes macrothrombocytopenia is also associated with the syndrome. The disease is inherited, and there is a family history in 85 percent of cases, the remaining 15 percent probably representing *de novo* mutations.[2]

### Diagnostic Criteria

Phenotypic expression of Alport syndrome is somewhat complex. The mode of transmission is heterogeneous, but most commonly it is X-linked. There is considerable heterogeneity with regard to

A list of standard abbreviations is located immediately preceding the index in each volume. Additional abbreviations used in this chapter include: 1(IV) = type IV collagen 1 chain, and other chains accordingly; AS = Alport syndrome; COL4A1 = type IV collagen 1 chain gene, and other genes accordingly; DL = diffuse leiomyomatosis; EBM = epidermal basement membrane; ESRD = end stage renal disease; GBM = glomerular basement membrane; NC1 = noncollagenous domain 1.

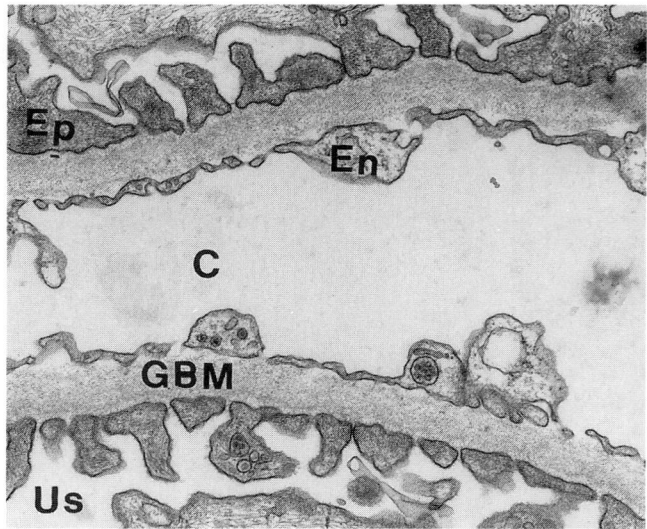

A

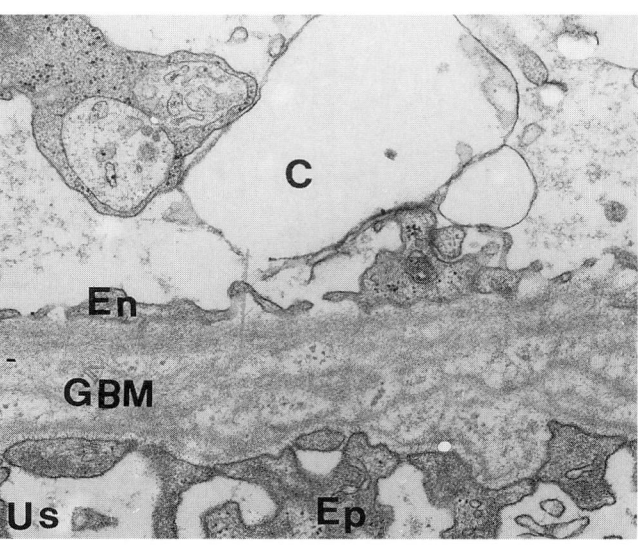

B

**Fig. 214-1** Electron microscopic picture of the glomerular basement membrane (GBM) of normal and Alport syndrome kidneys. *A,* The filtration barrier consists of the fenestrated endothelium layer (En) of the glomerular capillary (C), the ~300- to 350-nm-thick GBM, and the epithelial podocytes (Ep) partially covering the GBM on the urinary space side (Us). The podocytes are separated by an ~25-nm-wide filtration slits. Note the uniform thickness and even amorphous pattern of the GBM. *B,* Electron micrograph of a glomerular capillary loop showing characteristic glomerular basement membrane (GBM) lesions in an Alport syndrome patient. The GBM has irregular thinning and thickening, as well as lamination of the structure. C = capillary lumen; En = endothelial cell; Ep = epithelial podocyte; Us = urinary space. Magnification ×22,000. (*Courtesy of Dr. Finn P. Reinholt, Nephropathology Laboratory, Huddinge Hospital and Karolinska Institutet, Sweden.*)

onset of kidney disease, hearing loss, and other nonrenal complications. A broadly similar phenotype can be expected within a family in each affected member. Because of the heterogeneous nature, diagnosis of Alport syndrome has posed problems for physicians. In 1987, Flinter et al.[4] proposed that hematuric patients fulfilling three of four criteria — that is, positive family history, hearing loss, ocular lesions, and GBM abnormalities — could be diagnosed as having Alport syndrome. However, recent data have shown that there are numerous examples of patients with progressive renal disease and mutations in type IV collagen genes who do not fulfill these criteria. For example, inheritance cannot be demonstrated in about 15 percent of cases. Also, a proportion of patients with renal failure and mutations in type IV collagen genes do not have hearing loss or eye manifestations.[5-7] Thus, based on the new information accumulated on the disease, Gregory et al.[3] proposed a new clinical definition requiring four of the following ten criteria:

1. Family history of nephritis or unexplained hematuria in a first-degree relative or in a male relative linked through any number of females;
2. Persistent hematuria without evidence of another possibly inherited nephropathy (i.e., polycystic kidney disease, IgA nephropathy, or thin GBM disease);
3. Bilateral sensorineural hearing loss in the range of 2000 to 8000 Hz, the hearing loss develops gradually and is not present in early infancy, but commonly by age 30 years at latest;
4. A mutation in the gene encoding the α3, α4, or α5 chain of type IV collagen;
5. Immunohistochemical evidence of complete or partial lack of the Alport epitope in the GBM, epidermal basement membrane, or both;
6. Widespread GBM ultrastructural abnormalities;
7. Ocular abnormalities (anterior lenticonus, posterior subcapsular cataract, posterior polymorphous dystrophy, and retinal flecks);
8. Gradual progression to ESRD in the index case or at least two family members;
9. Macrothrombocytopenia or granulocytic inclusions; and
10. Diffuse leiomyomatosis of esophagus, female genitalia, or both.

This definition probably provides the diagnosis needed for clinical action. However, for any child who presents with visible hematuria under the age of 6 years, regardless of family history, a renal sonogram should be performed to exclude the possibility of Wilms tumor. Still, DNA analysis will always be required for the ultimate diagnosis.

### Different Forms of Alport Syndrome

**X-linked Alport Syndrome.** Alport syndrome is mainly inherited as an X-linked dominant trait, male patients being more severely affected than females. The estimated gene frequency in the intermountain west of the United States is 1:5000.[2] In Rhode Island, the incidence is about 1:10,000,[8] and in Finland, with the population of 5.1 million, about 1:53,000.[9] In 1988 and 1989, several investigators localized the defective gene for the disease to the long arm of the X chromosome.[10-12] In 1990, the *COL4A5* gene encoding the type IV collagen α5 chain was discovered and localized to the Alport gene region.[13] This was soon followed by the identification of mutations in this gene in Alport patients.[14,15] Presently, almost 300 different mutations have been identified in the type IV collagen α5 chain gene[6,7,16-20].

**Autosomal Forms of Alport Syndrome.** In about 15 percent of Alport kindreds, autosomal transmission of the disease is apparent. This includes both autosomal recessive and, in very rare cases, autosomal dominant modes of inheritance. Autosomal recessive disease is probable if there is no family history, especially if females are as severely affected as males.[21] In the much-less-common autosomal dominant form, males and females are equally severely affected, but the phenotype is milder than usually found in the X-linked form.[22] Autosomal disease is caused by mutations in the *COL4A3* and *COL4A4* genes, encoding the type IV collagen α3 and α4 chains, respectively.[23-26]

**Alport Syndrome-Associated Diffuse Leiomyomatosis.** Diffuse leiomyomatosis (DL) is a rare Alport syndrome-associated disorder characterized by benign proliferation of smooth-muscle cells in the esophageal wall.[27,28] Both sporadic and hereditary cases have been described in the literature.[28-31] In addition to the esophagus, other organs, such as the female genital tract and tracheobronchial tree, may be affected. Garcia-Torres and Guarner first described the association of Alport syndrome and diffuse leiomyomatosis (DL-AS) in 1983.[32] Numerous deletions involving the 5′ ends of both the COL4A6 gene and the adjacent COL4A5 gene are reported to cause this rare disorder. One interesting feature is that the deletion of the COL4A6 gene extends only to over the first two exons, whereas in COL4A5 the extension is variable, even up to a deletion of the whole gene.[33–35] Proposals for different molecular mechanisms have been proposed: Is there a mutation in a possible third gene around the second, large intron of COL4A6 that is behaving as a tumor-suppressor gene?[36] Might the development of DL result from the absence of an α6(IV) chain disrupting the cell-extracellular matrix interactions?[37,38] Might an abnormal, truncated COL4A6 translation product be present?[35] The clinical features and more detailed molecular genetics of DL were reviewed by Antignac and Heidet.[28]

**Alport Syndrome with Antiglomerular Basement Membrane Disease.** For an unknown reason, some Alport patients develop antibodies against renal allografts, and approximately one-third of those patients reject the transplant. This anti-GBM nephritis is a rare but dramatic feature of Alport syndrome. The onset of anti-GBM nephritis usually occurs within the first year following transplantation with eventual loss of the allograft. Unfortunately, anti-GBM nephritis recurs in most patients after retransplantation. Several researchers have studied the targets of the antibodies. The most recent study is by Brainwood et al.,[39] who showed that some of the antibodies react with the type IV collagen noncollagenous NC1 domain of the α3 chain, also known as the Goodpasture antigen;[40] some researchers identify the NC1 domain of the α5(IV) chain.[39,41,42] In spontaneous anti-GBM disease (anti-GBM or Goodpasture syndrome, MIM 233450), the major target of autoantibodies is the α3(IV) NC1 domain,[42–44] but the primary target in most Alport anti-GBM patients is the NC1 domain of the α5 chain of type IV collagen.[39]

## STRUCTURE AND MOLECULAR BIOLOGY OF THE GLOMERULAR BASEMENT MEMBRANE

Basement membranes are thin, ubiquitous, sheet-like structures located at the interphase of cells of organized tissues and the connective tissue. They are found beneath all epithelia and endothelia, as well as surrounding muscle fibers, fat cells, and peripheral nerves. Basement membranes have many important biologic roles as they provide structural support for cells; they also mediate differentiation, adhesion, and migration, as well as proliferation of cells. Additionally, they function as filters for macromolecules, as exemplified by the renal GBM, and they are important for correct tissue regeneration.[45]

The thickness of a basement membrane can vary between 50 and 350 nm, being usually 60 to 80 nm. By electron microscopy, two morphologically distinct layers, the *lamina lucida (rara)* and *lamina densa*, can be observed. Some basement membranes, such as the GBM, appear to have three layers, a subendothelial electron-translucent layer (*lamina rara interna*), an electron-dense central layer (*lamina densa*), and a subepithelial electron-translucent layer (*lamina rara externa*). This particular type of basement membrane is formed by two oppositely located cell layers, the capillary endothelium and the epithelial podocytes of the urinary space (Fig. 214-2). The three layered structure may be an artifact of the routine fixing techniques, as studies of tissue samples made with the quick-freeze method have shown the basement membranes not to contain any distinct layers.[46]

### The Glomerular Filtration Barrier

The major complications of Alport syndrome—hematuria and proteinuria—are caused by structural alterations and consequent malfunction of the glomerular filtration barrier. Primary urine is

formed by ultrafiltration of plasma in the kidney glomerulus (Fig. 214-2). There are about 1 million glomeruli per human kidney. The glomerular capillary is divided into several loops (glomerular tuft). The inner part of the capillary faces the mesangium, while the outer part forms the filter. The filtration barrier is composed of three layers: the fenestrated endothelium, the glomerular basement membrane, and the tight podocyte layer of interdigitating epithelial cells, named foot processes. The adjacent processes are separated by 20- to 30-nm-wide slit pores, or filtration slits, which contain a thin diaphragm that contains a specific protein called nephrin. The slit diaphragm forms the ultimate molecular sieve.[47,48] Under normal conditions, proteins of the size of albumin (67 kDa) or larger are not allowed to traverse the filtration barrier. Instead, an extremely high permeability to water and small solutes is obvious. Filtration across the barrier depends on the size of the molecules; that is, it is a size-dependent permeability barrier.[49] Additionally, the GBM shows selectivity according to the electrical charge of the molecules in that cationic and neutral molecules pass the membrane more easily than anionic molecules of the same size.[50]

### Molecular Composition of the Glomerular Basement Membrane

The molecular structure of the GBM is much the same as that of basement membranes in other tissues. The major structural component is type IV collagen (see "Basement Membrane Collagen" below). Type IV collagen forms a tightly cross-linked network in which less-dense laminin network is connected via entactin (nidogen) molecules (Fig. 214-3). In addition to supporting the formation of three-dimensional structure, laminin is a major adhesion molecule that also plays a role in cell differentiation and migration. Type IV collagen and laminin are both complex heterotrimeric proteins being present in numerous more or less tissue-specific isoforms. There are also other minor components, including BM40 (osteonectin, SPARC), fibulins, and agrin, that have been found in some specialized types of basement membranes.[51,52]

**Laminin.** The laminins are a group of complex extracellular glycoproteins that can be found in all basement membranes.[53–56] Laminin molecules are heterotrimers composed of α β and γ chains varying in size of 165 to 400 kDa, 140 to 220 kDa, and 130 to 220 kDa, respectively. These chains are multidomain polypeptides that share certain structural features, although they clearly form three distinct classes. To date, five α, three β, and two γ chains have been identified, these chains forming 10 or more different types of heterotrimers (isoforms).[53] The laminins have been shown to perform numerous biologic functions including cell adhesion, migration, differentiation, and proliferation.[53–55] Furthermore, as mentioned earlier, laminin is part of the structural framework[56] and, in addition to its physiological roles, it has been associated with tissue repair and in cell migration events, for example, during tumor invasion.[53,57,58]

All laminin chains have a region at the C-terminal end that assembles with the other chains to form a coiled-coil structure, the long arm. Additionally, the α chains have a large C-terminal globular domain not present in the β and γ chains. The N-termini of the chains have a varying number of cysteine-rich laminin repeats and globular domains. Knowledge of the tissue-specificity of laminin variants implies unique cell and tissue specific functions for different laminin isoforms. It is noteworthy that the β2 chain is expressed in a restricted manner during late development of the kidney, being particularly prominent in the GBM, as well as in the tubular basement membrane.[59]

**Proteoglycan.** Proteoglycans are extracellular proteins that contain large carbohydrate (glycosaminoglycan) side chains. They increase the volume of tissues by binding water through their hygroscopic properties. The basement membrane has been shown to contain proteoglycans that differ from those of other connective

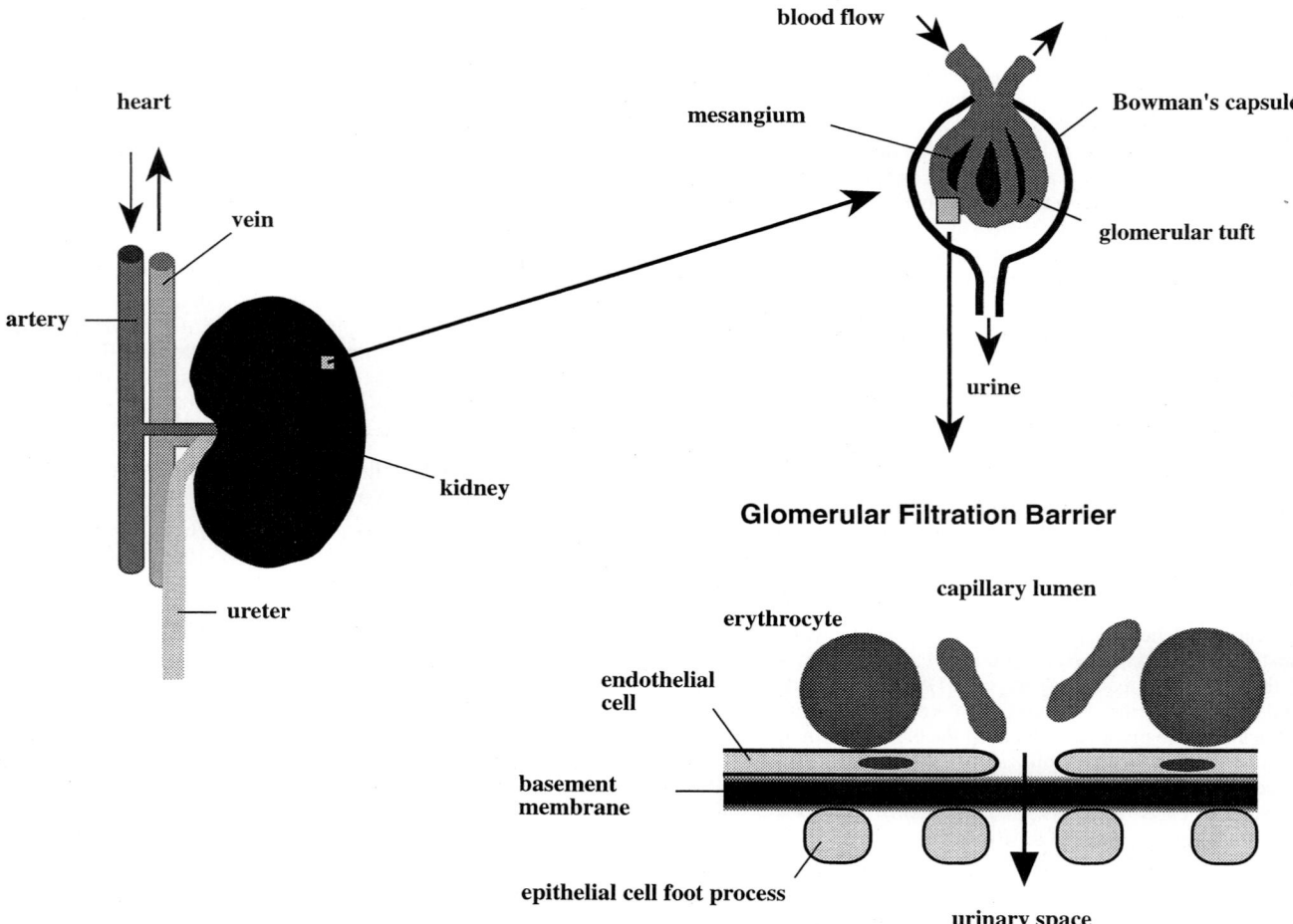

**Fig. 214-2** Illustration of the kidney, a filtration unit (glomerulus), and the glomerular filtration barrier. Each kidney contains about 1 million ball-shaped glomeruli where the filtration of blood occurs. The glomerular capillaries divide and form a set of loops (glomerular tuft) that are located inside the Bowman's capsule. The filtration of blood occurs in the capillaries so that only small proteins and waste products, together with water, can pass into the urinary space. The actual filtration barrier consists of the fenestrated capillary endothelium, the glomerular basement membrane (GBM), and the slit pores located between the foot processes of the glomerular endothelial cells. The illustrations are not drawn to scale.

tissues such as stroma and cartilage. The best studied and most abundant basement membrane proteoglycan is a large heparan sulfate proteoglycan, termed perlecan.[60] The human perlecan core protein belongs amongst the largest polypeptides in the human body with a size of 467 kDa.[61]

Perlecan is likely to serve several functions in basement membrane, but the knowledge of what they might be, is still very limited. However, Farquhar and coworkers have shown strong evidence for heparan sulfate side chains playing an important role in the selective permeability of the glomerular basement membrane due to their high anionic charge.[62–64] Loss of heparan sulfate has also been reported in the GBM in many diseases characterized by proteinuria.

**Nidogen.** Nidogen,[65] also named entactin,[66] is abundant in all basement membranes. The molecular weight of nidogen is 148 kDa, including 5 percent of carbohydrates.[67,68] Nidogen is probably essential for basement membrane function, as it appears to maintain the three-dimensional structure by linking the independent type IV collagen and laminin networks. The C-terminal end of the nidogen molecule has been shown to bind to the laminin $\gamma$1 chain,[69–71] which is present in the basement membrane of most, if not all tissues in the body. One of the three globular domains of nidogen, in turn, binds to type IV collagen.[72,73] Nidogen has been shown to also interact with the core protein of perlecan,[74] so nidogen may truly have major linking function between the various structural proteins of the basement membrane.

## BASEMENT MEMBRANE COLLAGEN

The scaffold of the basement membrane is a dense, tightly cross-linked protein network made up by type IV collagen, which is specific for the basement membrane.[75] This collagen type is a member of the collagen superfamily that contains at least 19 different types.[76] The collagens, the primary structural proteins of the body, either form extracellular fibrils or network structures that provide the main support to tissues. The collagens, other than type IV, and collagen disorders, excluding Alport syndrome, are discussed in Chap. 205.

### The α Chains of Type IV Collagen

The type IV collagen molecules that form the building blocks of the basement membrane are typical elongated triple-helical

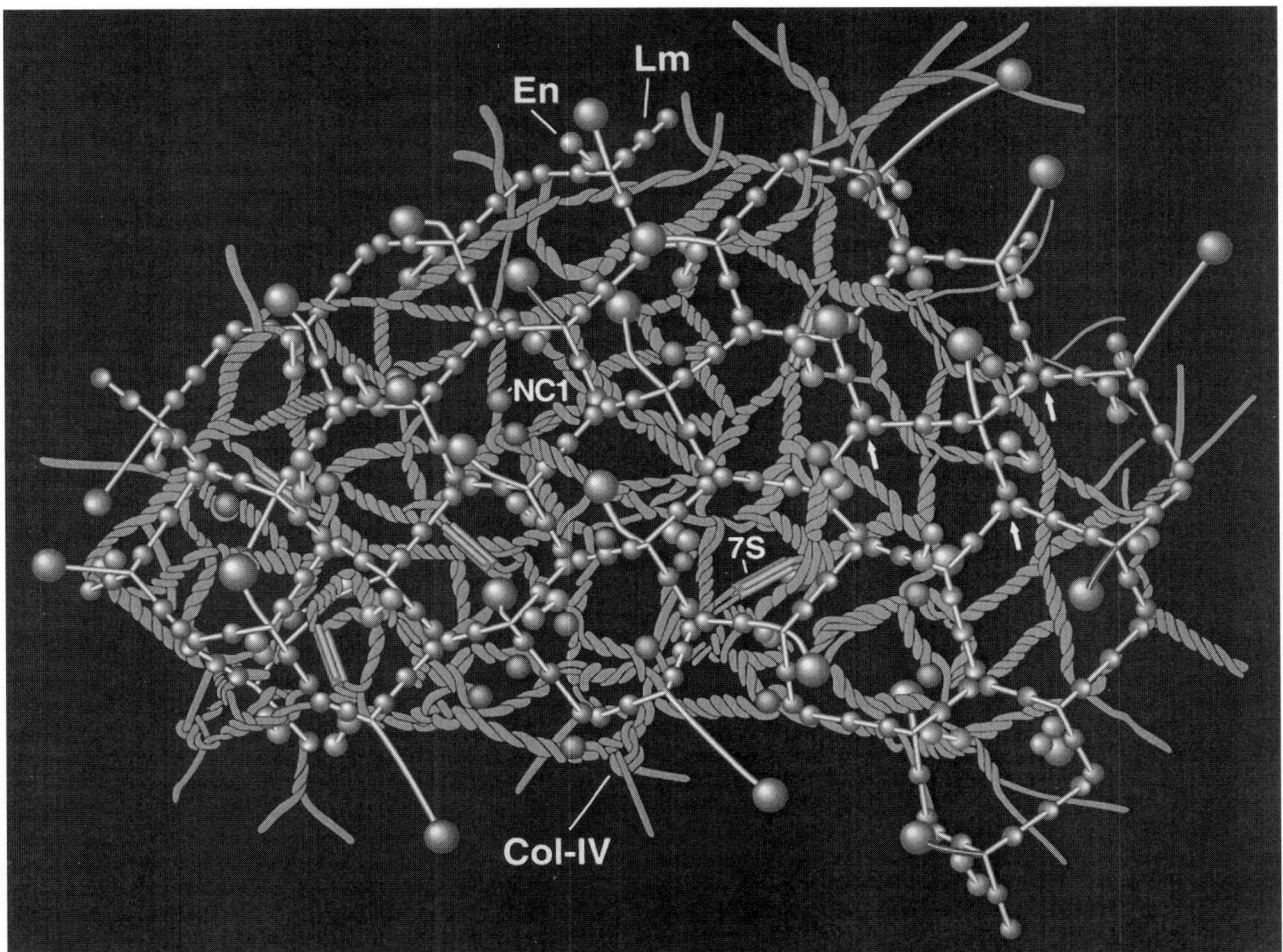

**Fig. 214-3 Hypothetical architecture of the basement membrane. Type IV collagen (Col-IV) and laminin (Lm) form double and interwoven polymer networks. The collagen scaffolding contains lateral, N-terminal tetrameric (7S), and C-terminal globular dimeric (NC1) bonds. The laminin array contains end-to-end interactions of short arms (*arrows*) and apparently long arms as well. Entactin/ nidogen (En) can bridge collagen and laminin. Heparan sulfate proteoglycan (perlecan) complexes are anchored in the network in an unknown where they interact with laminin and collagen through its polyanionic chains in an, as yet unknown. See Color Plate 12. (*Courtesy of Dr. Peter Yurchenco, Department of Pathology, Robert-Wood-Johnson Medical School, Piscataway, NJ.*)**

collagen molecules composed of three α-chains. These triple-helical molecules are composed of six genetically distinct chains — α1(IV), α2(IV), α3(IV), α4(IV), α5(IV), and α6(IV) — that can form numerous combinations. The most common isoform, present in all basement membranes, is a molecule having two α1(IV) chains and one α2(IV) chain (α1$_2$α2) for which the complete sequence have been determined in different species including man,[77,78] mouse,[79,80] and *Caenorhabditis elegans*.[81,82] Additionally, the α1(IV) sequence is known for *Drosophila*[83] and sea urchin,[84] and the α2(IV) sequence in *Ascaris suum*.[85] The primary sequences of the more tissue-specific α3(IV),[86] α4(IV),[87] α5(IV),[88,89] and α6(IV)[90,91] chains have been determined in man. The α-chains are often classified as the abundant "classical" α1(IV) and α2(IV) chains as opposed to the less abundant, tissue-specific "novel" α3(IV) to α6(IV) chains.[75]

Each type IV collagen α-chain contains a long collagenous domain of ∼1400 residues with Gly-X-Y repeats (see Chap. 205 for further structural information) that are interrupted at around 20 locations by short noncollagenous sequences, an ∼15-residue noncollagenous N-terminus, and an ∼230-residue noncollagenous domain (NC1) at the C-terminus (Fig. 214-4). The noncollagenous N-terminus and its short, neighboring, cysteine-rich collagenous sequence are referred to as the 7S domain[92]. The glycine amino acid residue in every third position of the collagenous

domain is essential, as it is the only small amino acid to fit into the center of the collagen triple helix. The interruptions in the Gly-X-Y-repeat sequence are thought to provide flexibility for the triple helical molecules. The type IV collagen α-chains are highly glycosylated, with numerous hydroxylysine-linked disaccharide units and an asparagine-linked oligosaccharide unit in the 7S domain.[93,94]

## Different Type IV Collagen Isoforms

The existence of six α-chains allows for many different kinds (isoforms) of triple-helical type IV collagen molecules that differ in type and stoichiometry of chains. As mentioned earlier, the most common form of type IV collagen, present in most basement membranes, is a heterotrimer of [α1(IV)]$_2$α2(IV).[75] Homotrimers of α1(IV) chains have also been found.[43,95] The possible combinations of the other four α-chains (α3-α6) have been intensively investigated and evidence for different networks has been presented. Heterotrimers of two α3(IV) chains and one α4(IV) chain, and homotrimers of α3(IV) chains appear to exist in the glomerular basement membrane.[43,96] Immunohistochemical stainings of kidney sections from Alport patients usually show absence of the α3(IV)-α5(IV) chains normally found in the GBM, and for a long time, the GBM was considered to contain these three chains. Recently, Gunwar et al.[97] identified a novel

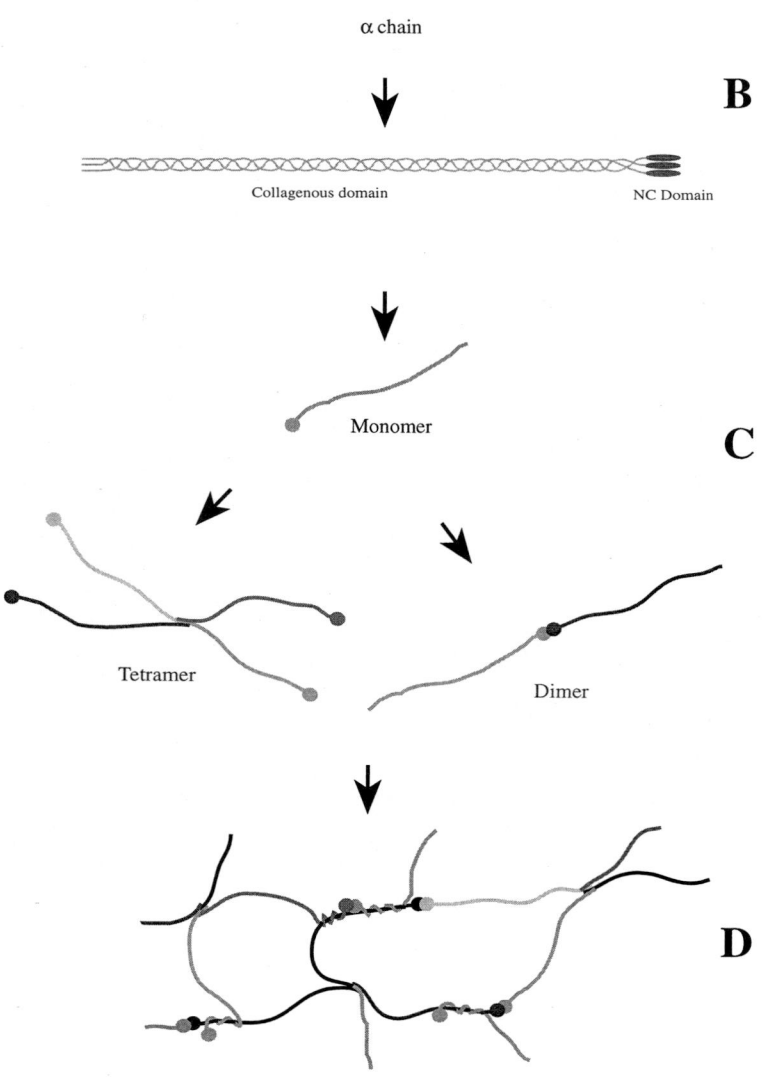

**Fig. 214-4** Illustration of the structure and supramolecular assembly of type IV collagen. *A,* Type IV collagen α chain with collagenous Gly-X-Y repeat regions interrupted by noncollagenous sequences (dark ellipsoids). *B,* The α-chains form triple-helical type IV collagen molecules (monomers) that form the building blocks of the basement membrane network. *C,* Individual monomers associate into dimers via their disulfide bonds between NC1 domains, or into tetramers through disulfide bonds between the amino termini. *D,* The supramolecular network is formed by assembly of dimers and tetramers strengthened by lateral association and partial winding of some molecules around each other.

disulfide-cross-linked α3:α4:α5 network of type IV collagen in the kidney. This finding explains several features of the GBM abnormalities in Alport syndrome.

## Network Formation

The biosynthesis of type IV collagen involves similar posttranslational modifications to those of collagenous proteins in general[98] (see Chap. 205). The secreted triple-helical type IV collagen molecules self-assemble into a complex network structure (Fig. 214-4). Several modes of interactions have been demonstrated in in vitro studies. Single triple-helical molecules associate at the C-termini (NC1- to -NC1) forming dimers and at the N-termini forming tetramers. The C-terminal associations are stabilized by interchain disulfide bonds between NC1 domains.[99] The 7S domain at the N-terminus contains four cysteine residues that participate in both intra- and intermolecular disulfide bonds.[100] In addition to end-to-end interactions, triple-helical domains wind around each other and interact with NC1 domains forming supercoiled structures.[51,100] The result is a tight three-dimensional network that serves as the major structural support for the basement membrane.

## Primary Structure of Type IV Collagen Chains

The six type IV collagen α chains all contain some distinct, highly conserved features that are presumably related, with common and unique functions of this collagen type. However, there are also distinct differences between the primary structure of some of the chains, and it is probable that some of the chain-specific features confer some biologic functions of the individual chains. Table 214-1 summarizes some major characteristics of the type IV collagen α-chains.

**C-Terminal NC1 Domain.** The noncollagenous C-terminal NC1 domains are believed to serve two major common functions among the type IV collagen α chains in all species. First, they are essential for the correct chain association that is followed by formation of the triple helix. Second, they are important for type IV collagen assembly into the network structure, during which

Table 214-1  Main Features of the Six Human Type IV Collagen α Chains and Their Genes

| α chain | Chromosome symbol | Chromosome locus | Size of the gene (kb) | Number of exons | Shortest exon (bp) | Longest exon (bp) | Residues | | | | Number of interruptions in collagenous domain | References | Gen Bank number |
|---|---|---|---|---|---|---|---|---|---|---|---|---|---|
| | | | | | | | Complete translation product | Mature α chain | Signal peptide | Collagenous domain/NC1 domain | | | |
| α1(IV) | COL4A1 | 13q34 | >100 | 52 | 27 | 213 | 1,669 | 1,642 | 27 | 1,413/229 | 21 | 77, 106–108, 111, 112, 116, 118 | Y00706 |
| α2(IV) | COL4A2 | 13q34 | >100 | 47 | 36 | 287 | 1,712 | 1,676 | 36 | 1,449/227 | 23 | 78,106–108, 112, 116 | X05610 |
| α3(IV) | COL4A3 | 2q35 | ~250 | ? | ? | ? | 1,670 | 1,652 | 28 | 1,410/232 | 23 | 86, 109, 110, 112, 119 | X80031 |
| α4(IV) | COL4A4 | 2q35 | >113 | 48 | 9 | 287 | 1,690 | 1,652 | 38 | 1,421/231 | 26 | 87, 109, 110, 112, 120 | X81053 |
| α5(IV) | COL4A5 | Xq22 | 250 | 51 | 27 | 213 | 1,685 | 1,659 | 26 | 1,430/229 | 22 | 88, 89,112, 114, 117 | U04520 |
| α6(IV) | COL4A5 | Xq22 | 425 | 46 | 36 | 222 | 1,691 | 1,670 | 21 | 1,417/228 | 25 | 90, 91, 112, 114, 117 | U04845 |

covalent disulfide bonds are formed between individual NC1 domains of two neighboring molecules (Fig. 214-4). Considering such important common functions, it is not surprising that the amino acid sequences of the NC1 domains are highly conserved between species and chain types. The NC1 domains contain ~230 residues, the sequence identity differing between 58 percent and 83 percent in man.[87] The NC1 domain sequence contains two homologous halves that rose through tandem duplication before the divergence of the $\alpha$1-like and $\alpha$2-like ancestors.[101,102] The NC1 domains contain 12 cysteines completely conserved between *Drosophila* and man, 6 cysteines being located in each symmetric half. These NC1 domain cysteines first form intradomain bonds, but during the extracellular molecular assembly there occurs a rearrangement of these bonds so that six cysteines form disulfide bonds with cysteine residues of one NC1 domain of a neighboring molecule.[103] The actual role of other individual conserved amino acids is not understood, but the maintenance of the conserved three-dimensional configuration that is required for the normal function of the NC1 domain demands a certain high degree of sequence similarity. Whether the unconserved residues confer some chain or isoform specific functions is not known.

**The Collagenous Domain.** In man, the collagenous domains of the six type IV collagen $\alpha$-chains contain between 1410 and 1449 residues (Table 214-1). The main reason for the size difference between $\alpha$-chains is the presence of 21 to 26 interruptions of varying length in the collagenous Gly-X-Y-repeat sequence. It is possible to align the Gly-X-Y-repeat sequences of all the $\alpha$-chains when one loops out the interruptions (see reference [87]). The interruptions are thought to provide the type IV collagen molecules, and thus the basement membrane, with flexibility. Several lines of evidence suggest that these interruptions are not simply randomly inserted into the chains, but that they also serve certain functions. Thus, the location and length of most of the interruptions is conserved, even between distant species. However, the strongest support for some role for the interruptions comes from the fact that numerous mutations in Alport syndrome patients simply generate interruptions into the collagenous domain by glycine substitutions.

A characteristic feature of the collagenous domain is the conservation of four cysteine residues in the 7S domain at the N-terminus. These cysteines are essential for the cross-linking of four triple-helical molecules through disulfide bonds.[99,103] The $\alpha$3(IV) and particularly the $\alpha$4(IV) chains distinguish themselves from the other $\alpha$-chains in that they contain more unconserved cysteines. Thus, the $\alpha$3(IV) contains five and the $\alpha$4(IV) chain 13 unconserved cysteines, as opposed to 2 to 3 in the other chains. This indicates that isoforms containing the $\alpha$3(IV) and $\alpha$4(IV) are more cross-linked and might be required in basement membranes that are subject to more stress than others. This hypothesis gains support from the knowledge of a developmental switch in that $\alpha$1:$\alpha$2 network is abundant in embryo and $\alpha$3:$\alpha$4:$\alpha$5 network is predominant after birth.[104,105]

# TYPE IV COLLAGEN GENES

## Evolution

The six mammalian type IV collagen genes have an exceptional arrangement in that they are located pair-wise in a head-to-head fashion on three different chromosomes.[106–110] This arrangement gives a hint of evolution of the genes from a common ancestor gene. Analysis of the sequences of the six $\alpha$ chains, together with the available data on the structure of the genes, suggest the probable evolutionary pattern of the genes. Present data predict that the first event involved a duplication and inversion of the ancestor gene at the initial locus, so that the genes came to lie head-to-head. This was followed by separation of the two genes into $\alpha$1-like and $\alpha$2-like genes. Later, the gene pair was duplicated in its entirety to another chromosome, giving rise to the *COL4A3/*

*COL4A4* gene pair (on human chromosome 2) coding for the $\alpha$3(IV) and $\alpha$4(IV) chains, respectively.[109] Still later, the original gene pair was duplicated to chromosome X to form the *COL4A5/COL4A6* gene pair coding for the $\alpha$5(IV) and $\alpha$6(IV) chains, respectively.[34] The original gene pair became the *COL4A1/COL4A2* genes on chromosome 13 that codes for the $\alpha$1(IV) and $\alpha$2(IV) chains, respectively.[111] Most probably the ancestor gene was located in an unstable region of the genome and was easily duplicated, and again these duplicates were assembled into more stable regions.[112] This is supported by the fact that a similar evolution has not taken place in lower organisms, as the two type IV collagen *COL4A1* and *COL4A2* genes in *C. elegans* are located on two different chromosomes.[113]

## Bidirectional Promoters

The 5' ends of each COL4 gene pair are adjacent to each other, separated by sequences that contain motifs involved in the gene regulation.[112] The 5' ends of the *COL4A1* and *COL4A2* genes overlap each other, and the region between the transcription start sites is only about 130 bp. These genes are transcribed from opposite DNA strands and they share a common bidirectional promoter.[106] The *COL4A5/COL4A6* gene pair is arranged similarly, but the distance between transcription start sites is longer, 442 bp. In addition, the *COL4A6* gene has two alternative promoters, indicating usage of different regulatory elements for the expression of the gene. Two distinct transcripts are established in a tissue-specific manner.[114] Studies of the murine genes have shown the bidirectional operation model for the promoter elements of the $\alpha$3(IV) and $\alpha$4(IV) genes.[115] Recently, Momota and coworkers[110] showed that the human *COL4A3* and *COL4A4* genes are also transcribed in opposite directions sharing the same promoter region. Additionally, the *COL4A4* gene has two alternative transcripts, the expression of which appears to be tissue-specific, as in *COL4A6*. One transcription start site of *COL4A4* is only 5 bp away from the transcription start site of *COL4A3* and the other starts 373 nucleotides downstream from the first. The two transcripts only differ in the 5' untranslated region, thus resulting in the same deduced amino acid sequences.

## Type IV Collagen Gene Structure

Type IV collagen genes are all very large because of the large sizes of the introns. Macrorestriction mapping studies have enabled the size of the $\alpha$1(IV) gene to be estimated as 100 to 160 kb, which is also the estimated size of the $\alpha$2(IV) gene (Table 214-1).[116] The $\alpha$5(IV) gene is about 230 to 250 kb, and the $\alpha$6(IV) gene is at least 425 kb.[117] The combined size of the *COL4A3/COL4A4* gene pair has been estimated to be about 500 kb,[109] the *COL4A4* gene being at least 113 kb.[26] The $\alpha$1(IV) gene contains 52 exons, the sizes of exons which vary from 27 to 213 base pairs.[118] The number of exons in the *COL4A2* gene is 47, the smallest being 36 bp and the largest 287 bp.[112] The exons encoding the most 3' end of the *COL4A3* and *COL4A4* genes had been characterized,[119,120] but Boye et al.[26] recently showed the *COL4A4* gene to have 48 exons, of which the smallest is 9 bp and the largest 287 bp. The type IV collagen $\alpha$5 chain gene contains 51 exons, which are almost the same size as those of the $\alpha$1(IV) gene, the smallest being 27 bp and the largest 213 bp.[89] The *COL4A6* gene contains 46 exons including exon 1' which is alternatively transcribed with exon 1 from alternative promoters. The sizes of exons vary from 36 to 222 bp (Table 214-1).[91]

# PATHOLOGY AND IMMUNOHISTOLOGY OF THE BASEMENT MEMBRANES IN ALPORT SYNDROME

## Mutations in the COL4A5 Gene

To date, numerous reports have described mutations in the *COL4A5* gene, the number already being about 300.[14–20,121] The mutations include large (14 percent) and small gene rearrangements such as deletions and insertions (3 percent in-frame, 19 percent causing frameshifts) and splicing mutations (18 percent), as well as single base changes (glycine substitutions 32 percent, other missense mutations 6 percent, and nonsense mutations 8 percent). About 85 percent of the mutations, however, are small. Furthermore, complete loss of the gene has been reported in two cases.[35,122,123] A striking finding is that the mutations identified in *COL4A5* so far are highly dispersed in this huge gene. The same mutation has been found in only a few cases in two or more unrelated kindreds. This sharply contrasts with findings in other diseases, such as cystic fibrosis where approximately 70 percent of the patients have the same mutation.[124] However, the dispersion of mutations in *COL4A5* resembles the situation reported for *osteogenesis imperfecta*, a brittle bone disease that involves a variety of mutations in type I collagen genes[125] (see Chap. 205).

**Different Effects of *COL4A5* Mutations to the Type IV Collagen.** The mutations present in the *COL4A5* gene in Alport syndrome can usually explain the structural and pathophysiological changes in the GBM. The mutations can result in changes that affect many of the steps of type IV collagen synthesis and assembly, such as: (a) the synthesis of the primary transcript; (b) posttranscriptional modification of the transcript such as splicing; (c) translation of the mRNA; (d) posttranslational modifications of nascent α-chains; (e) assembly and folding of three α-chains into a triple-helical molecule; (f) the stability of the helix structure; and (g) formation of cross-links between individual triple-helical molecules. Large gene rearrangements can result in total loss of expression of the gene and small mutations in regulatory elements can have the same effects. Large and small mutations can also affect splicing of the primary transcript. Abnormal splicing and skipping of exons can cause two types of changes. First, if the exon skipping is in-frame, the result is a shortened polypeptide so that it lacks a segment, second, if the exon skipping occurs out-of-frame, the result is a protein partially containing a nonsense amino acid sequence.

**Effects of *COL4A5* Mutations to the Type IV Collagen Network.** Mutations leading to absence of the α5(IV) chain or extensive alterations in protein size would certainly lead to abnormal structure of any type IV collagen network where the α5(IV) chain is required as a normal component. Complete loss or presence of an abnormal α5(IV) chain may explain the clinical manifestations observed in Alport syndrome. In the kidney, the α5(IV) chain is normally present only in the GBM as shown by immunostaining techniques, with a similar GBM staining pattern observed for the α3(IV) and α4(IV) chains. Although it is not known in what molecular chain combinations the α5(IV) chain is present in the GBM, it was recently shown by Gunwar et al.[97] that α3:α4:α5 network is formed in the GBM. Consequently, the absence of a normal α5 chain may weaken the structural network of the GBM in one way or another, leading to leakage of large proteins or even large blood cells into the urinary space. It is important to note, however, that heterozygous females usually exhibit only mild phenotypes and they seldom develop end stage renal disease. This suggests that the synthesis of low amounts of a normal α5(IV) chain is sufficient to maintain normal GBM function, even though the abnormal chain is present. This fact is particularly important when considering future possibilities for gene therapy through the supplementation of expression of a normal transgene in addition to that of the mutated gene.

**Single Base Mutations.** Single base mutations in exons leading to amino acid changes in the α5(IV) chain can be expected to cause the protein malfunction in most cases because such changes can affect proteins in a number of ways. The question then is how can we know whether an amino acid substitution actually causes disease instead of being silent. This is an important question, especially from a clinical point of view when making decision about the termination of pregnancy after a mutation in the fetus has been identified. Actually, this is also a very difficult question to answer. One relatively definite way of proving that a mutation is causative for the disease is to generate transgenic animals with the same mutation and observe whether it results in Alport syndrome-like phenotype. However, it is possible that a mutation causing disease in man does not cause the same disease in mice. One, therefore, has to rely on strong "circumstantial" evidence when predicting the potential pathogenic effect of mutations. Such evidence can be linkage or segregation of the mutations with the phenotype in an Alport kindred, knowledge about the role of certain amino acids for the function of the protein, or conservation of the amino acids during evolution. It is assumed that amino acid residues conserved in a protein during evolution between widely distant species have such functional importance that their substitution cannot be tolerated. If mutations occur *de novo* concurrent with the appearance of disease, they are likely to be causative.

A large number of mutations converting a glycine residue in the Gly-X-Y repeat containing collagenous domain to another amino acid have been published. These mutations can, without any doubt, affect the stability of the triple helix of the molecule because, as mentioned above, glycine is the only amino acid small enough to suit into the center of the triple helix and an uninterrupted Gly-X-Y repeat sequence is essential for the maintenance of the triple-helical conformation. The result of glycine substitution is, therefore, that the helix is destabilized, creating kinks in the molecule that are not tolerated. Although this has not been demonstrated at the protein level for type IV collagen, a number of similar glycine mutations, either inhibiting helix formation or causing kinks in the molecule have been described in type I collagen in osteogenesis imperfecta.[125]

### *COL4A5* Mutations Cause Different Phenotypes

Alport syndrome is a heterogeneous disease with onset of end-stage renal disease at varying ages and with or without manifestations such as hearing loss and deafness, ocular lesions, thrombocytopathy, and so on. Because so many mutations have been identified in the *COL4A5* gene, it is of interest from a clinical point of view to correlate them with the phenotypes they produce. However, this analysis is disappointing in the sense that it does not seem to be possible to predict the phenotype based on the type of mutation. For example, the point mutations generated by substitution of glycine residues in the collagenous domain or conserved amino acids in the NC1 domain result in a quite wide spectrum of phenotypes. Most, but not all patients have juvenile onset of end-stage renal disease, but the presence of hearing loss and ocular lesions varies between individuals.

A similar heterogeneous picture is seen for large changes in the gene. Even the entire loss of the gene does not necessarily produce more severe disease than a single glycine substitution in the collagenous domain of the α5(IV) chain. Although disappointing, this does not come as a surprise as the same phenomenon has been observed for defects in the genes for fibrillar collagens causing osteogenesis imperfecta, chondrodysplasia, Stickler syndrome, and Ehlers-Danlos syndrome.[125] A clinically important group are the ~15 percent of posttransplantation Alport patients who develop anti-GBM antibodies. Initial studies on Alport mutations and phenotypes gave hope that, based on the nature of mutation, it might be possible to predict which patients develop anti-GBM nephritis and, thus, who should obtain a transplant and who not. It seemed reasonable that a mutation deleting the highly antigenic NC1 domain of the α5(IV) chain would cause the patient to recognize the corresponding domain in the allograft as a foreign protein and should, therefore, not receive an allograft as the patient would develop anti-GBM nephritis. However, more recent data on transplanted patients with similar kinds of gene defects have shown that this explanation is not totally valid. Based on current, yet still limited knowledge, it is not possible to predict which

**Table 214-2** Distribution of the Six Type IV Collagen α Chains in Normal Tissues and in Tissues of Alport Patients

| Tissue | Normal/X-linked AS/Recessive AS | | | | | | References |
| --- | --- | --- | --- | --- | --- | --- | --- |
| | α1(IV) | α2(IV) | α3(IV) | α4(IV) | α5(IV) | α6(IV) | |
| Kidney | | | | | | | 21, 127–132, 134 |
| GBM embryonic* | + | + | − | − | − | − | |
| GBM postnatal | (+)/+/+ | (+)/+/+ | +/−/− | +/−/− | +/−/− | −/−/− | |
| Bowman's capsule | +/+/+ | +/+/+ | +/−/− | +/−/− | +/−/+ | +/−/? | |
| Distal tubules | +/+/+ | +/+/+ | +/−/− | +/−/− | +/−/+ | +/−/? | |
| Collecting ducts | + | + | − | − | + | + | |
| Mesangium | + | + | − | − | − | − | |
| Eye | | | | | | | 133 |
| Anterior lens capsule | +/+/? | +/+/? | +/−/? | +/−/? | +/−/? | ?/?/? | |
| Internal limiting membrane | + | + | + | + | + | ? | |
| Bruch's membrane | + | + | + | + | + | ? | |
| Descemet's membrane | + | + | + | + | + | ? | |
| Cochlea | + | + | + | + | + | ? | 131 |
| Skin | +/+/+ | +/+/+ | −/−/− | −/−/− | +/−/+ | +/−/? | 128, 130, 132, 134 |
| Esophagus | + | + | − | − | + | + | 131 |
| Brain | + | + | + | + | − | − | 131 |
| Lung | + | + | + | + | + | + | 131 |

*One mark indicates normal tissue distribution

patients will develop anti-GBM nephritis following kidney transplantation.

## Mutations in the COL4A3 and COL4A4 Collagen Genes in Autosomal Alport Syndrome

Although Alport syndrome is primarily considered an X-linked disorder, autosomal forms were also postulated in about 15 percent of the cases based on pedigree data.[126] Following identification of defects in the α5(IV) collagen gene in the X-linked disease, it was logical to search for mutations in autosomal disease in the COL4A3 and COL4A4 genes, encoding the α3(IV) and α4(IV) collagen chains, respectively, as these chains are also prominent in the GBM. Such mutations have now been found both in the COL4A3[23–25,126] and COL4A4[23,26] genes in several Alport kindreds. The patients have been shown to be either homozygotes or compound heterozygotes for the mutation, and the parents unaffected carriers indicating autosomal recessive pattern of inheritance. Five different mutations have been reported in the COL4A3 gene in autosomal recessive kindreds, present in either homozygous or heterozygous form. Two of these mutations are nonsense,[23,24] two are small deletions in exons,[23–25] and one is a splice-site mutation.[126] All five mutations result in premature translation stop codons, which would lead to truncated malfunctioning polypeptides. The first two mutations found in COL4A4 by Mochizuki and coworkers[23] were a nonsense mutation and a glycine substitution. Recently, Boye et al.[26] studied 31 unrelated autosomal recessive Alport syndrome patients and found 10 novel COL4A4 mutations in 8 patients. Five of these mutations create premature stop codons or a shift in the reading frame, and are, therefore, potential null mutations. One mutation probably causes a deletion of two Gly-X-Y repeats in the collagenous region, thereby shortening the protein. Two mutations affect splicing and two are missense mutations, one a glycine substitution in the collagenous region and the other a highly conserved proline to leucine substitution in the C-terminal NC1 domain. A missense mutation, substitution of evolutionarily conserved leucine to proline, was recently described in a large family with rare autosomal dominant form of Alport syndrome.[22]

## Immunohistochemistry of Alport Syndrome Affected Tissues

Immunohistochemical studies demonstrate that the six type IV collagen α chains differ quite remarkably in their tissue distribution (Table 214-2). This, in turn, suggests that the different isoforms serve different functions in vivo. The α1(IV) and α2(IV) chains that form the most common α1₂α2 isoform are present in practically all basement membranes where they are frequently the only chains present. This emphasizes a major general role of this isoform in basement membranes. The other minor chains have a highly restricted distribution.[75]

The α3, α4, and α5 chains of type IV collagen are expressed in the kidney, and their expression is highly enriched in the glomerular basement membrane, but they are also found in a subset of tubular basement membranes, such as Bowman's capsule and the distal tubules.[127,128] The α5(IV) chain is, additionally, present in the collecting ducts. Expression of the α6(IV) chain is almost identical to that of α5(IV) throughout the kidney, but it is notably absent from the GBM.[127] In many male patients with X-linked Alport syndrome the α3(IV), α4(IV), and α5(IV) chains are absent from the GBM, whereas expression of the α1(IV) and α2(IV) chains is increased.[127,129] Expression of the α6(IV) chain is normally seen in Bowman's capsules and tubules but not in such patients; this is also the case with the α3(IV), α4(IV), and α5(IV) chains.[128] Women who are heterozygous for the X-linked disease exhibit mosaic expression of the α3(IV), α4(IV), and α5(IV) chains in the GBM, while expression of the α1(IV) and α2(IV) chains is preserved.[130]

Immunohistochemical analyses of skin tissues from males with X-linked Alport syndrome have shown a complete absence of the α5(IV) and α6(IV) chains normally expressed in the skin. A discontinuous or mosaic staining for these two chains is seen in the epidermal basement membrane (EBM) of female heterozygotes.[128,131,132] Cheong et al.[133] have studied the expression of type IV collagen α chains in another Alport target tissue, the anterior lens capsule, in X-linked cases, and demonstrated the same features as in the GBM, namely, a lack of the α3(IV) to α5(IV) chains (Table 214-2).

Gubler et al. studied the distribution of different type IV collagen chains in autosomal recessive Alport syndrome.[134] Usually, no expression of the α3(IV), α4(IV), or α5(IV) chains can be seen in the GBM, but deviating from the X-linked expression pattern, the α5(IV) chain is normal in Bowman's capsule and distal tubular basement membrane. A similar expression pattern can be seen in both sexes. In addition, the α5(IV) chain shows normal staining in the EBM, while the α3(IV), α4(IV), and α5(IV) chains are absent from the GBM (Table 214-2).

This combination cannot be seen in X-linked AS, as it is well known that only the α5(IV) chain of these three is present in the epidermal basement membrane.[134] This differential pattern of staining may be a useful method for distinguishing between X-linked and autosomal recessive forms of Alport syndrome.[21]

## GENE THERAPY

To date, there is no satisfactory and curative conservative treatment available for Alport syndrome.[135,136] Patients developing end-stage renal disease are treated by hemodialysis, and by kidney transplantation whenever possible. However, about 5 percent of the transplanted patients develop anti-GBM nephritis and reject the allografted kidneys.

As a result of recent advances in molecular genetics, gene therapy may be developing into a real possibility for the future treatment of a variety of hereditary diseases. Although gene therapy has not yet come of age as a real therapeutic alternative for human diseases, extensive research efforts are being made in that direction. Alport syndrome, which primarily affects the renal glomeruli, is an attractive disease target for gene therapy for two reasons.[136] First, as it almost solely affects the kidney glomeruli; extrarenal complications not being life-threatening or occurring in all patients, the therapy can, at least initially, be targeted to the kidney alone. Second, the "isolated" kidneys, with their well-separated circulatory system, lend themselves extremely well to organ-targeted gene transfer. Extensive research still needs to be carried out before we can expect to do successful gene therapy of Alport syndrome in man, and there are numerous aspects to consider before we know whether gene therapy is even theoretically possible for this disease. The following paragraphs discuss some of the key points[136] concerning the possibility of gene therapy of Alport syndrome.

The GBM is located between layers of endothelial and epithelial cells, which are both believed to contribute to the biosynthesis of the GBM type IV collagen. Due to a lack of sensitivity, methods such as *in situ* hybridization have not confirmed whether one or both cell types produce the type IV collagen isoform α3:α4:α5, which is characteristic of the GBM. However, from the gene therapy perspective, these cells are considered the prime targets, and the gene should be efficiently transferred to these cells. Our recent work shows that it may not be an overwhelming task, as we have been able to achieve transfer of the β-galactosidase reporter gene into an estimated 85 percent of the glomeruli in pigs using an adenovirus vector (Fig. 214-5).[136] The key to this high-transfer efficacy was prolonged perfusion of the kidney, which allows for a long contact time between the cells and viruses. In contrast, intra-arterial injections of the virus have not yielded efficient gene delivery to the glomeruli, as has been noted by others.[137–139] The perfusion method is relatively easy to apply to the kidney; it can be applied *in situ*, and may also prove useful for the transfer of genes to other organs with a well-separated blood supply.

To obtain life-lasting and controlled expression of the transferred gene is a serious problem that is the main hurdle of gene therapy in general, and it poses one of the main challenges that research in this field faces today. The adenovirus used in our experiments carried out in pigs, in its current form, provides expression for only 6 to 8 weeks, as it remains extrachromosomal and is not integrated into the genome.[136] Even though the half-life of type IV collagen is estimated to be between 1 and 2 years, the treatment would need to be frequently repeated during life. This is not easy, as, at least presently, it requires an operation. Retroviruses would theoretically be better, but they cannot integrate large DNA inserts and they are only integrated into replicating DNA, which is not appropriate for the stationary glomerular cells. Therefore, successful gene therapy of Alport syndrome in man depends on future developments in research on gene transfer vectors. Reports of high-capacity adenoviral vectors may allow decreased toxicity, high transfection rates,

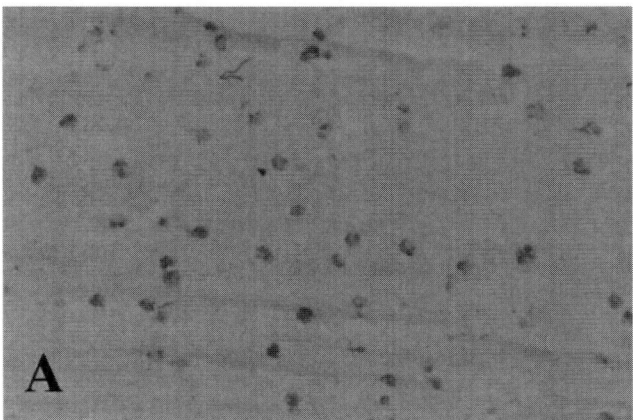

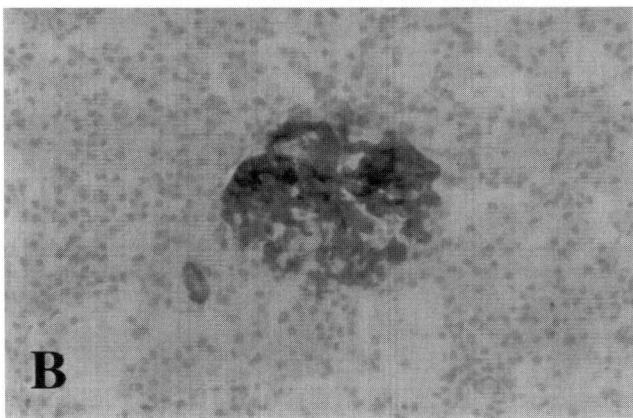

**Fig. 214-5 Expression of the β-galactosidase in pig kidneys following organ perfusion with a solution containing adenovirus with the β-galactosidase reporter gene. *A*, Intense expression can be seen in a large proportion of the glomeruli of the kidney cortex, while little, if any, expression is observed in other regions of the kidney. *B*, Expression of the reporter gene is generally achieved in all regions of the glomerulus, including the epithelial podocytes.[136]**

inclusion of natural regulatory sequences, and long duration of expression.[140]

A transferred type IV collagen cDNA or gene coupled to an appropriate promoter should be expressed in a controlled manner. Consequently, the corrected chain should be incorporated into normal α3:α4:α5 heterotrimers. The full-length α5 chain transferred by adenoviruses was already shown to be expressed in cultured cells, as well as in pig glomeruli in vivo in our experiments (unpublished data). That GBM type IV collagen is a heterotrimer is probably favorable, because it means that the limiting factor for intracellular synthesis of the trimer is likely to be the availability of the two other partner chains. Thus, if one chain is produced in excess, it will be degraded intracellularly. It has been shown that α1(IV) mRNA can exist in three- to fifteenfold excess over α2(IV) mRNA, even though the ratio of the respective chains in the protein is 2:1.[141] If production of the defective chain can be corrected to some extent, the secretion of normal molecules is likely to occur, even in the presence of some abnormal malfunctioning molecules. However, only experimental work will prove or disprove such a speculation.

Can corrected type IV collagen trimers be incorporated into the GBM to restore its structure and function? This is still an open question that has to be addressed experimentally in animal models. However, observations from heterozygous female dogs have shown that although the glomeruli are chimeric for the gene defect, it appears that normal molecules can spread within the GBM to restore its structure.[142] Thus, it can be anticipated that this may not turn out to be a major obstacle to gene therapy of Alport syndrome.

## REFERENCES

1. Alport AC: Hereditary familial congenital haemorrhagic nephritis. *BMJ* **1**:504, 1927.
2. Atkin CL, Gregory MC, Border WA: Alport syndrome, in Schrier RW, Gottschalk CW (eds): *Diseases of the Kidney*. Boston, Little, Brown, 1988, p 617.
3. Gregory MC, Terreros DA, Barker DF, Fain PN, Denison JC, Atkin CL: Alport syndrome — clinical phenotypes, incidence and pathology, in Tryggvason K (ed): *Molecular Pathology and Genetics of Alport Syndrome*. Basel, Karger, 1996, p 1.
4. Flinter FA, Bobrow M, Chantler C: Alport's syndrome or hereditary nephritis? *Pediatr Nephrol* **1**:438, 1987.
5. Tryggvason K, Zhou J, Hostikka SL, Shows TB: Molecular genetics of Alport syndrome. *Kidney Int* **43**:38, 1993.
6. Tryggvason K: Mutations in type IV collagen genes and Alport phenotypes, in Tryggvason K (ed): *Molecular Pathology and Genetics of Alport Syndrome*. Basel, Karger, 1996, p 154.
7. Heiskari N, Zhang Z, Leinonen A, et al: Identification of 17 mutations in ten exons in the COL4A5 collagen gene, but no mutations found in four exons in COL4A6. A study of 250 patients with hematuria and suspected of having Alport syndrome. *J Am Soc Nephrol* **7**:702, 1996.
8. Shaw RF, Kallen RJ: Population genetics of Alport's syndrome. Hypothesis of abnormal segregation and the necessary existence of mutation. *Nephron* **16**:427, 1976.
9. Pajari H, Kääriäinen H, Muhonen T, Koskimies O: Alport's syndrome in 78 patients: Epidemiological and clinical study. *Acta Paediatr* **85**:1300, 1996.
10. Brunner H, Schröder C, van Bennekom C, et al: Localization of the gene for X-linked Alport's syndrome. *Kidney Int* **34**:507, 1988.
11. Atkin CL, Hasstedt SJ, Menlove L, et al: Mapping of Alport syndrome to the long arm of the X chromosome. *Am J Hum Genet* **42**:249, 1988.
12. Flinter FA, Abbs S, Bobrow M: Localization of the gene for classic Alport syndrome. *Genomics* **4**:335, 1989.
13. Hostikka SL, Eddy RL, Byers MG, Höyhtyä M, Shows TB, Tryggvason K: Identification of a distinct type IV collagen alpha chain with restricted kidney distribution and assignment of its gene to the locus of X chromosome-linked Alport syndrome. *Proc Natl Acad Sci U S A* **87**:1606, 1990.
14. Barker DF, Hostikka SL, Zhou J, et al: Identification of mutations in the COL4A5 collagen gene in Alport syndrome. *Science* **248**:1224, 1990.
15. Zhou J, Barker DF, Hostikka SL, Gregory MC, Atkin CL, Tryggvason K: Single base mutation in alpha 5(IV) collagen chain gene converting a conserved cysteine to serine in Alport syndrome. *Genomics* **9**:10, 1991.
16. Renieri A, Bruttini M, Galli L, et al: X-linked Alport syndrome: An SSCP-based mutation survey over all 51 exons of the COL4A5 gene. *Am J Hum Genet* **58**:1192, 1996.
17. Kawai S, Nomura S, Harano T, Harano K, Fukushima T, Osawa G: The COL4A5 gene in Japanese Alport syndrome patients: Spectrum of mutations of all exons. The Japanese Alport Network. *Kidney Int* **49**:814, 1996.
18. Knebelmann B, Breillat C, Forestier L, et al: Spectrum of mutations in the COL4A5 collagen gene in X-linked Alport syndrome. *Am J Hum Genet* **59**:1221, 1996.
19. Lemmink HH, Schröder CH, Monnens LA, Smeets HJ: The clinical spectrum of type IV collagen mutations. *Hum Mutat* **9**:477, 1997.
20. Martin P, Heiskari N, Zhou J, et al: High mutation detection rate in the COL4A5 collagen gene in suspected Alport syndrome using PCR and direct DNA sequencing. *J Am Soc Nephrol* **9**:2291, 1998.
21. Kashtan CE, Michael AF: Alport syndrome. *Kidney Int* **50**:1445, 1996.
22. Jefferson JA, Lemmink HH, Hughes AE, Hill CM, Smeets HJM, Doherty CC, Maxwell AP: Autosomal dominant Alport syndrome linked to the type IV collagen α3 and α4 genes (COL4A3 and COL4A4). *Nephrol Dial Transplant* **12**:1595, 1997.
23. Mochizuki T, Lemmink HH, Mariyama M, et al: Identification of mutations in the α3(IV) and α4(IV) collagen genes in autosomal recessive Alport syndrome. *Nat Genet* **8**:77, 1994.
24. Lemmink HH, Mochizuki T, van den Heuvel LPWJ, et al: Mutations in the type IV collagen α3 (COL4A3) gene in autosomal recessive Alport syndrome. *Hum Mol Genet* **3**:1269, 1994.
25. Ding J, Stitzel J, Berry P, Hawkins E, Kashtan CE: Autosomal recessive Alport syndrome: Mutation in the COL4A3 gene in a womap with Alport syndrome and posttransplant antiglomerular basement membrane nephritis. *J Am Soc Nephrol* **5**:1714, 1995.
26. Boye E, Mollet G, Forestier L, et al: Determination of the genomic structure of the COL4A4 gene and of novel mutations causing autosomal recessive Alport syndrome. *Am J Hum Genet* **63**:1329, 1998.
27. Heald J, Moussalli H, Hasleton PS: Diffuse leiomyomatosis of the oesophagus. *Histopathol* **10**:755, 1986.
28. Antignac C, Heidet L: Mutations in Alport syndrome associated with diffuse esophageal leiomyomatosis, in Tryggvason K (ed): *Molecular Pathology and Genetics of Alport Syndrome*. Basel, Karger, 1996, p 172.
29. Bourque MD, Spigland N, Bensoussan AL, et al: Esophageal leiomyoma in children: Two case reports and review of the literature. *J Pediatr Surg* **24**:1103, 1989.
30. Marshall JB, Diaz-Arias AA, Bochna GS, Vogele KA: Achalasia due to diffuse esophageal leiomyomatosis and inherited as an autosomal dominant disorder. Report of a family study. *Gastroenterology* **98**:1358, 1990.
31. Rosen RM: Familial multiple upper gastrointestinal leiomyoma. *Am J Gastroenterol* **85**:303, 1990.
32. Garcia-Torres R, Guarner V: Leiomyomatosis of the esophagus, tracheo-bronchi and genitals associated with Alport type hereditary nephropathy: A new syndrome. *Rev Gastroenterol Mex* **48**:163, 1983.
33. Antignac C, Zhou J, Sanak M, et al: Alport syndrome and diffuse esophageal leiomyomatosis: deletions in the 5' end of the COL4A5 collagen gene. *Kidney Int* **42**:1178, 1992.
34. Zhou J, Mochizuki T, Smeets H, et al: Deletion of the paired α5(IV) and α6(IV) collagen genes in inherited smooth muscle tumors. *Science* **261**:1167, 1993.
35. Heidet L, Dahan K, Zhou J, et al: Deletions of both α5(IV) and α6(IV) collagen genes in Alport syndrome and in Alport syndrome associated with smooth muscle tumours. *Hum Mol Genet* **4**:99, 1995.
36. Weinberg RA: Tumor suppressor genes. *Science* **254**:1138, 1991.
37. Aumailley M, Timpl R: Attachment of cells to basement membranes. *J Biol Cell* **103**:1569, 1986.
38. Vandenberg P, Kern A, Ries A, Luchenbill-Edds L, Mann K, Kühn K: Characterization of a type IV collagen major binding site with affinity to the α1β2 and α2β1 integrins. *J Cell Biol* **113**:1475, 1991.
39. Brainwood D, Kashtan C, Gubler MC, Turner N: Targets of alloantibodies in Alport anti-glomerular basement membrane disease after renal transplantation. *Kidney Int* **53**:762, 1998.
40. Butkowski RJ, Langeveld JP, Wieslander J, Hamilton J, Hudson BG: Localization of the Goodpasture epitope to a novel chain of basement membrane collagen. *J Biol Chem* **262**:7874, 1987.
41. Kleppel MM, Fan WW, Cheong HI, Kashtan CE, Michael AF: Immunochemical studies of the Alport antigen. *Kidney Int* **41**:1629, 1992.
42. Dehan P, Weber M, Zhang X, Reeders ST, Foidart JM, Tryggvason K: Sera from patients with anti-GBM nephritis including Goodpasture syndrome show heterogenous reactivity to recombinant NC1 domain of type IV collagen α chains. *Nephrol Dial Transplant* **11**:2215, 1996.
43. Saus JJ, Wieslander J, Langeveld JPM, Quinones S, Hudson BG: Identification of the Goodpasture antigen as the α3(IV) chain of collagen IV. *J Biol Chem* **263**:13374, 1988.
44. Kalluri R, Wilson C, Weber M, Gunwar S, Chonko A, Neilson E, Hudson BG: Identification of the α3 chain of type IV collagen as the common autoantigen in antibasement membrane disease and Goodpasture syndrome. *J Am Soc Nephrol* **6**:1178, 1995.
45. Vracko R: The role of basal lamina in maintenance of orderly tissue structure, in Kühn K, Schone HH, Timpl R (eds): *New Trends in Basement Membrane Research*. New York, Raven, 1982, p 1.
46. Goldberg M, Escaig-Haye F: Is the lamina lucida of the basement membrane a fixation artefact? *Eur J Cell Biol* **42**:365, 1986.
47. Rodewald R, Karnovsky MJ: Porous substructure of the glomerular slit diaphragm in the rat and mouse. *J Cell Biol* **60**:423, 1974.
48. Ruotsalainen V, Ljunberg P, Wartiovaara J, et al: Nephrin is specifically located at the slit diaphragm of glomerular podocytes. *Proc Natl Acad Sci U S A* **96**:7962, 1999.
49. Caulfield JP, Farquhar MG: Loss of anionic sites from the glomerular basement membrane in aminonucleoside nephrosis. *Lab Invest* **39**:505, 1978.
50. Brenner BM, Hostetter TH, Humes HD: Molecular basis of proteinuria of glomerular origin. *N Engl J Med* **298**:826, 1978.

51. Yurchenco PD, O'Rear J: Supramolecular organization of basement membranes, in Rohrbach DH, Timpl R (eds): *Molecular and Cellular Aspects of Basement Membranes.* San Diego, Academic Press, 1993, p 19.

52. Timpl R, Brown J: Supramolecular assembly of basement membranes. *Bioessays* **18**:123, 1996.

53. Timpl R, Brown JC: The laminins. *Matrix Biol* **14**:275, 1994.

54. Tryggvason K: The laminin family. *Curr Opin Cell Biol* **5**:877, 1993.

55. Engel J: Laminins and other strange proteins. *Biochemistry* **31**:10643, 1992.

56. Engel J: Structure and function of laminin, in Rohrbach DH, Timpl R (eds): *Molecular and Cellular Aspects of Basement Membranes.* San Diego, Academic Press, 1993, p 147.

57. Pyke C, Romer J, Kallunki P, Lund LR, Ralfkiar E, Dano K, Tryggvason K: The gamma 2 chain of kalinin/laminin 5 is preferentially expressed in invading malignant cells in human cancers. *Am J Pathol* **145**:782, 1994.

58. Pyke C, Salo S, Ralfkiaer E, Romer J, Dano K, Tryggvason K: Laminin-5 is a marker of invading cancer cells in some human carcinomas and is coexpressed with the receptor for urokinase plasminogen activator in budding cancer cells in colon adenocarcinomas. *Cancer Res* **55**:4132, 1995.

59. Miner JH, Lewis RM, Sanes JR: Molecular cloning of a novel laminin chain, alpha 5, and widespread expression in adult mouse tissues. *J Biol Chem* **270**:28523, 1995.

60. Noonan DM, Hassell JR: Proteoglycans of basement membranes, in Rohrbach DH, Timpl R (eds): *Molecular and Cellular Aspects of Basement Membranes.* San Diego, Academic Press, 1993, p 189.

61. Kallunki P, Tryggvason K: Human basement membrane heparan sulfate proteoglycan core protein: A 467-kD protein containing multiple domains resembling elements of the low density lipoprotein receptor, laminin, neural cell adhesion molecules, and epidermal growth factor. *J Cell Biol* **116**:559, 1992.

62. Kanwar YS, Farquhar MG: Anionic sites in the glomerular basement membrane. In vivo and in vitro localization to the laminae rarae by cationic probes. *J Cell Biol* **81**:137, 1979.

63. Kanwar YS, Farquhar MG: Presence of heparan sulfate in the glomerular basement membrane. *Proc Natl Acad Sci U S A* **76**:1303, 1979.

64. Kanwar YS, Linker A, Farquhar MG: Increased permeability of the glomerular basement membrane to ferritin after removal of glycosaminoglycans (heparan sulfate) by enzyme digestion. *J Cell Biol* **86**:688, 1980.

65. Timpl R, Dziadek M, Fujiwara S, Nowack H, Wick G: Nidogen: A new, self-aggregating basement membrane protein. *Eur J Biochem* **137**:455, 1983.

66. Carlin B, Jaffe R, Bender B, Chung AE: Entactin, a novel basal lamina-associated sulfated glycoprotein. *J Biol Chem* **256**:5209, 1981.

67. Paulsson M, Dziadek M, Suchanek C, Huttner WB, Timpl R: *Nature* of sulphated macromolecules in mouse Reichert's membrane. Evidence for tyrosine O-sulphate in basement-membrane proteins. *Biochem J* **231**:571, 1985.

68. Paulsson M, Deutzmann R, Dziadek M, Nowack H, Timpl R, Weber S, Engel J: Purification and structural characterization of intact and fragmented nidogen obtained from a tumor basement membrane. *Eur J Biochem* **156**:467, 1986.

69. Mann K, Deutzmann R, Timpl R: Characterization of proteolytic fragments of the laminin-nidogen complex and their activity in ligand-binding assays. *Eur J Biochem* **178**:71, 1988.

70. Gerl M, Mann K, Aumailley M, Timpl R: Localization of a major nidogen-binding site to domain III of laminin B2 chain. *Eur J Biochem* **202**:167, 1991.

71. Mayer U, Nischt R, Poschl E, et al: A single EGF-like motif of laminin is responsible for high affinity nidogen binding. *EMBO J* **12**:1879, 1993.

72. Aumailley M, Wiedemann H, Mann K, Timpl R: Binding of nidogen and the laminin-nidogen complex to basement membrane collagen type IV. *Eur J Biochem* **184**:241, 1989.

73. Fox JW, Mayer U, Nischt R, et al: Recombinant nidogen consists of three globular domains and mediates binding of laminin to collagen type IV. *EMBO J* **10**:3137, 1991.

74. Battaglia C, Mayer U, Aumailley M, Timpl R: Basement-membrane heparan sulfate proteoglycan binds to laminin by its heparan sulfate chains and to nidogen by sites in the protein core. *Eur J Biochem* **208**:359, 1992.

75. Hudson BG, Reeders ST, Tryggvason K: Type IV collagen: structure, gene organization, and role in human diseases. Molecular basis of Goodpasture and Alport syndromes and diffuse leiomyomatosis. *J Biol Chem* **268**:26033, 1993.

76. Prockop DJ, Kivirikko KI: Collagens: Molecular biology, diseases, and potentials for therapy. *Annu Rev Biochem* **64**:403, 1995.

77. Soininen R, Haka-Risku T, Prockop DJ, Tryggvason K: Complete primary structure of the α1-chain of human basement membrane (type IV) collagen. *FEBS Lett* **225**:188, 1987.

78. Hostikka SL, Tryggvason K: The complete primary structure of the α2 chain of human type IV collagen and comparison with the α1(IV) chain. *J Biol Chem* **263**:19488, 1988.

79. Muthukumaran G, Blumberg B, Kurkinen M: The complete primary structure for the α1-chain of mouse collagen IV. Differential evolution of collagen IV domains. *J Biol Chem* **264**:6310, 1989.

80. Saus J, Quinones S, MacKrell A, Blumberg B, Muthukumaran G, Pihlajaniemi T, Kurkinen M: The complete primary structure of mouse α2(IV) collagen. Alignment with mouse α1(IV) collagen. *J Biol Chem* **264**:6318, 1989.

81. Guo X, Johnsson JJ, Kramer JM: Embryonic lethality caused by mutations in basement membrane collagen of C. elegans. *Nature* **349**:707, 1991.

82. Sibley MH, Johnson JJ, Mello CC, Kramer JM: Genetic identification, sequence, and alternative splicing of the *Caenorhabditis elegans* α2(IV) collagen gene. *J Cell Biol* **123**:255, 1993.

83. Blumberg B, MacKrell AJ, Fessler JH: Drosophila basement membrane procollagen α1(IV) collagen. II. Complete cDNA sequence, genomic structure, and general implications for supramolecular assemblies. *J Biol Chem* **263**:18328, 1988.

84. Exposito JY, D'Alessio M, DiLiberto M, Ramirez F: Complete primary structure of a sea urchin type IV collagen α chain and analyses of the 5' end of its gene. *J Biol Chem* **268**:5249, 1993.

85. Pettitt J, Kingston IP: The complete primary structure of a nematode α2(IV) collagen and the partial structural organization of its gene. *J Biol Chem* **266**:16149, 1991.

86. Mariyama M, Leinonen A, Mochizuki T, Tryggvason K, Reeders S: Complete primary structure of the human α3(IV) collagen chain: Coexpression of the α3(IV) and α4(IV) collagen chains in human tissues. *J Biol Chem* **269**:23013, 1994.

87. Leinonen A, Mariyama M, Mochizuki T, Tryggvason K, Reeders S: Complete primary structure of the human α4(IV) collagen chain: Comparison with structure and expression of the other α(IV) chains. *J Biol Chem* **269**:26172, 1994.

88. Zhou J, Hertz JM, Leinonen A, Tryggvason K: Complete amino acid sequence of the human α5(IV) collagen chain and identification of a single-base mutation in exon 23 converting glycine 521 in the collagenous domain to cysteine in an Alport syndrome patient. *J Biol Chem* **267**:12475, 1992.

89. Zhou J, Leinonen A, Tryggvason K: Structure of the human type IV collagen COL4A5 gene. *J Biol Chem* **269**:6608, 1994.

90. Zhou J, Ding M, Zhao Z, Reeders ST: Complete primary structure of the sixth chain of human basement membrane collagen, α6(IV). *J Biol Chem* **269**:13193, 1994.

91. Oohashi T, Sugimoto M, Mattei MG, Ninomiya Y: Identification of a new collagen IV chain, α6(IV), by cDNA isolation and assignment of the gene to chromosome Xq22, which is the same locus for COL4A5. *J Biol Chem* **269**:7520, 1994.

92. Timpl R: Structure and biological activity of basement membrane proteins. *Eur J Biochem* **180**:487, 1989.

93. Langeveld JPM, Noelken ME, Hard K, Todd P, Vliengenthart JFG, Rouse J, Hudson BG: Bovine glomerular basement membrane: Location and structure of the asparagine-linked oligosaccharide units and their potential role in the assembly of the 7S collagen IV tetramer. *J Biol Chem* **266**:2622, 1991.

94. Nayak BR, Spiro RG: Localization and structure of the asparagine-linked oligosaccharides of type IV collagen from glomerular basement membrane and lens capsule. *J Biol Chem* **266**:13978, 1991.

95. Haralson MA, Federspiel SJ, Martinez-Hernandez A, Rhodes RK, Miller EJ: Synthesis of [pro alpha 1(IV)]3 collagen molecules by cultured embryo-derived parietal yolk sac cells. *Biochemistry* **24**:5792, 1985.

96. Johansson C, Butkowski R, Wieslander J: The structural organization of type IV collagen. Identification of three NC1 populations in the glomerular basement membrane. *J Biol Chem* **267**:24533, 1992.

97. Gunwar S, Ballester F, Noelken ME, Sado Y, Ninomiya Y, Hudson BG: Glomerular basement membrane: Identification of a novel disulfide-cross-linked network of α3, α4 and α5 chains of type IV collagen and its implications for the pathogenesis of Alport syndrome. *J Biol Chem* **273**:8767, 1998.

98. Kivirikko KI, Myllylä R: Recent developments in posttranslational modification: intracellular processing. *Methods Enzymol* **144**:96, 1987.
99. Timpl R, Wiedemann H, van Delden V, Furthmayr H, Kühn K: A network model for the organization of type IV collagen molecules in basement membranes. *Eur J Biochem* **120**:203, 1981.
100. Siebold B, Deutzmann R, Kühn K: The arrangement of intra- and intermolecular disulfide bonds in the carboxy-terminal, non-collagenous aggregation and cross-linking domain of basement-membrane type IV collagen. *Eur J Biochem* **176**:617, 1988.
101. Pihlajaniemi T, Tryggvason K, Myers JC, et al: cDNA clones for the pro-α1(IV) chain of human type IV procollagen reveal an unusual homology of amino acid sequences in two halves of the carboxyl-terminal domain. *J Biol Chem* **260**:7681, 1985.
102. Soininen R, Chow L, Kurkinen M, Tryggvason K, Prockop DJ: The gene for the α1(IV) chain of human type IV procollagen: The exon structures do not coincide with the structural subdomains in the globular carboxy-terminus of the protein. *EMBO J* **5**:2821, 1986.
103. Siebold B, Qian R, Glanville RW et al: Construction of a model for the aggregation and cross-linking region (7S domain) of type IV collagen based upon an evaluation of the primary structure of the α1 and α2 chains in this region. *Eur J Biochem* **168**:569, 1987.
104. Miner JH, Sanes JR: Collagen IV α3, α4 and α5 chains in rodent basal laminae: Sequence, distribution, association with laminins, and developmental switches. *J Cell Biol* **127**:879, 1994.
105. Kalluri R, Shield III CF, Todd P, Hudson BG, Neilson E: Isoform switching of type IV collagen is developmentally arrested in X-linked Alport syndrome leading to increased susceptibility of renal basement membranes to endoproteolysis. *Methods Enzymol* **99**:2470, 1997.
106. Soininen R, Huotari M, Hostikka SL, Prockop DJ, Tryggvason K: The structural genes for α1 and α2 chains of human type IV collagen are divergently encoded on opposite DNA strands and have an overlapping promoter region. *J Biol Chem* **263**:17217, 1988.
107. Pöschl E, Pollner R, Kühn K: The genes for the α1(IV) and α2(IV) chains of human basement membrane collagen type IV are arranged head-to-head and separated by a bidirectional promoter of unique structure. *EMBO J* **7**:2687, 1988.
108. Burbelo PD, Martin GR, Yamada Y: α1(IV) and α2(IV) collagen genes are regulated by a bidirectional promoter and a shared enhancer. *Proc Natl Acad Sci U S A* **85**:9679, 1988.
109. Mariyama M, Zheng K, Yang-Feng TL, Reeders ST: Colocalization of the genes for the α3(IV) and α4(IV) chains of the type IV collagen to chromosome 2 bands q35-q37. *Genomics* **13**:809, 1992.
110. Momota R, Sugimoto M, Oohashi T, Kigasawa K, Yoshioka H, Ninomiya Y: Two genes, COL4A3 and COL4A4 coding for the human α3(IV) and α4(IV) collagen chains are arranged head-to-head on chromosome 2q36. *FEBS Lett* **424**:11, 1998.
111. Boyd CD, Toth-Fejel SE, Gadi IK, et al: The genes coding for human pro α1(IV) and pro α2(IV) collagen are both located at the end of the long arm of chromosome 13. *Am J Hum Genet* **42**:309, 1988.
112. Heikkilä P, Soininen R: The type IV collagen gene family, in Tryggvason K (ed): *Molecular Pathology and Genetics of Alport Syndrome*. Basel, Karger, 1996, p 105.
113. Guo X, Kramer JM: The two *Caenorhabditis elegans* basement membrane (type IV) collagen genes are located on separate chromosomes. *J Biol Chem* **264**:17574, 1989.
114. Sugimoto M, Oohashi T, Ninomiya Y: The genes COL4A5 and COL4A6, coding for basement membrane collagen chains α5(IV) and α6(IV), are located head-to-head in close proximity on human chromosome Xq22 and COL4A6 is transcribed from two alternative promoters. *Proc Natl Acad Sci U S A* **91**:11679, 1994.
115. Hlaing T, Funabiki K, Togawa M, Chapo JA, Killen PD: Molecular cloning of the murine α3(IV) and α4(IV) collagen promoter. *J Am Soc Nephrol* **5**:625, 1994.
116. Cutting GR, Kazazian HH Jr, Antonarakis SE, Killen PD, Yamada Y, Francomano CA: Macrorestriction mapping of COL4A1 and COL4A2 collagen genes on human chromosome 13q34. *Genomics* **3**:256, 1988.
117. Srivastava AK, Featherstone T, Wein K, Schlessinger D: YAC contigs mapping the human COL4A5 and COL4A6 genes and DXS118 within Xq21.3-q22. *Genomics* **26**:502, 1995.
118. Soininen R, Huotari M, Ganguly A, Prockop DJ, Tryggvason K: Structural organization of the gene for the α1(IV) chain of human type IV collagen. *J Biol Chem* **264**:13565, 1989.
119. Quinones S, Bernal D, Carcia-Sogo M, Elena SF, Saus J: Exon/intron structure of the human α3(IV) gene encompassing the Goodpasture antigen (α3(IV)NC1). Identification of a potentially antigenic region at the triple helix/NC1 domain junction. *J Biol Chem* **267**:19780, 1992.
120. Sugimoto M, Oohashi T, Yoshioka H, Matsuo N, Ninomiya Y: cDNA isolation and partial gene structure of the human α4(IV) collagen chain. *FEBS Lett* **330**:122, 1993.
121. Netzer KO, Seibold S, Gross O, Lambrecht R, Weber M: Use of psoralen-coupled nucleotide primers for screening of COL4A5 mutations in Alport syndrome. *Kidney Int* **50**:1363, 1996.
122. Antignac C, Knebelmann B, Drouot L, et al: Deletions in the COL4A5 collagen gene in X-linked Alport syndrome. Characterization of the pathological transcripts in nonrenal cells and correlation with disease expression. *Methods Enzymol* **93**:1195, 1994.
123. Netzer KO, Renders L, Zhou J, Pullig O, Tryggvason K, Weber M: Deletions of the COL4A5-gene in patients with Alport syndrome. *Kidney Int* **42**:1336, 1992.
124. Kerem B, Rommens JM, Buchanan JA, et al: Identification of the cystic fibrosis gene: Genetic analysis. *Science* **245**:1073, 1989.
125. Kuivaniemi H, Tromp G, Prockop DJ: Mutations in collagen genes: Causes of rare and some common diseases in humans. *FASEB J* **5**:2052, 1991.
126. Knebelmann B, Benessy F, Buemi M, Grünfeld JP, Gubler MC, Antignac C: Autosomal recessive (AR) inheritance in Alport syndrome (AS). *J Am Soc Nephrol* **4**:263, 1993.
127. Peissel B, Geng L, Kalluri R, et al: Comparative distribution of the α1(IV), α5(IV), and α6(IV) collagen chains in normal human adult and fetal tissues and in kidneys from X-linked Alport syndrome patients. *Methods Enzymol* **96**:1948, 1995.
128. Ninomiya Y, Kagawa M, Iyama K, et al: Differential expression of two basement membrane collagen genes, COL4A6 and COL4A5, demonstrated by immunofluorescence staining using peptide-specific monoclonal antibodies. *J Cell Biol* **130**:1219, 1995.
129. Naito I, Kawai S, Nomura S, Sado Y, Osawa G, Japanese Alport network: Relationship between COL4A5 gene mutation and distribution of type IV collagen in male X-linked Alport syndrome. *Kidney Int* **50**:304, 1996.
130. Nakanishi K, Yoshikawa N, Iijima K, et al: Immunohistochemical study of α1-5 chains of type IV collagen in hereditary nephritis. *Kidney Int* **46**:1413, 1994.
131. Zhou J, Reeders ST: The α chains of type IV collagen, in Tryggvason K (ed): *Molecular Pathology and Genetics of Alport Syndrome*. Basel, Karger, 1996, p 80.
132. Hino S, Takemura T, Sado Y, Kagawa M, Oohashi T, Ninomiya Y, Yoshioka K: Absence of α6(IV) collagen in kidney and skin of X-linked Alport syndrome patients. *Pediatr Nephrol* **10**:742, 1996.
133. Cheong HI, Kashtan CE, Kim Y, Kleppel MM, Michael AF: Immunohistologic studies of type IV collagen in anterior lens capsules of patients with Alport syndrome. *Lab Invest* **70**:553, 1994.
134. Gubler MC, Knebelmann B, Beziau A, et al: Autosomal recessive Alport syndrome: Immunohistochemical study of type IV collagen chain distribution. *Kidney Int* **47**:1142, 1995.
135. Adler SG, Cohen AH, Glassock RJ: Secondary glomerular disease, in Brenner BM (ed): *The Kidney*, 5th ed. Philadelphia, WB Saunders, 1996, p 1555.
136. Heikkilä P, Parpala T, Lukkarinen O, Weber M, Tryggvason K: Adenovirus-mediated gene transfer into kidney glomeruli using an ex vivo and in vivo kidney perfusion system — First steps towards *Gene Therapy* of Alport syndrome. *Gene Therapy* **3**:21, 1996.
137. Tomita N, Higaki J, Morishita R, Kato K, Mikami H, Kaneda Y, Ogihara T: Direct in vivo gene introduction into rat kidney. *Biochem Biophys Res Commun* **186**:129, 1992.
138. Moullier P, Friedlander G, Calise D, Ronco P, Perricaudet M, Ferry N: Adenoviral-mediated gene transfer to renal tubular cells in vivo. *Kidney Int* **45**:1220, 1994.
139. Zhu G, Nicolson AG, Cowley BD, Rosen S, Sukathme VP: In vivo adenovirus-mediated gene transfer into normal and cystic rat kidneys. *Gene Ther* **3**:298, 1996.
140. Kochanek S: High-capacity adenoviral vectors for gene transfer and somatic gene therapy. *Hum Gene Ther* **10**:241, 1999.
141. Speth C, Oberbaumer I: Expression of basement membrane proteins: Evidence for complex post-transcriptional control mechanisms. *Exp Cell Res* **204**:302, 1993.
142. Tryggvason K, Heikkilä P, Pettersson E, Tibell A, Thorner P: Can Alport syndrome be treated by gene therapy? *Kidney Int* **51**:1493, 1997.

# Autosomal Dominant Polycystic Kidney Disease

*Gregory G. Germino* ■ *Arlene B. Chapman*

1. Autosomal dominant polycystic kidney disease (ADPKD) (MIM 173900) is the most common inherited renal disease, accounting for 4.8 percent of the end-stage renal disease (ESRD) population in the United States and is a systemic disorder involving the heart, liver, cerebral vasculature, and connective tissue. Clinical manifestations of this disorder are highly variable within and between families. The average age of presentation is in the fourth decade of life with invariable penetrance by the age of 70 years.

2. Diagnosis of ADPKD relies on multiple sources of information including medical history, physical examination, laboratory evaluation, renal imaging, and genetic analysis. Gene linkage analysis provides no information concerning the clinical severity of the disorder and is used primarily for screening potentially eligible renal donors. Ultrasound in the imaging procedure of choice used to make a phenotypic diagnosis of ADPKD due to its sensitivity as well as cost and lack of invasiveness. Individuals from PKD1 families with a negative ultrasound after 30 years of age have a less than 5 percent chance of being carriers of the disease.

3. Polycystic liver disease is a common manifestation in ADPKD and is useful in differentiating ADPKD from other renal cystic disorders of the kidney. Polycystic liver disease presents approximately 10 years after renal cystic disease with women more severely affected than men. Birth control pill use, pregnancy, and postmenopausal estrogen use are associated with more progressive polycystic liver disease. Although liver cystic involvement can be massive, liver function continues to remain normal.

4. Intracranial aneurysms (ICA) occur in 8 percent of ADPKD individuals as opposed to 2 percent of the general population. ICA cluster in families with a family history of ICA and are often multiple. Smoking and hypertension are not risk factors for ICA development in ADPKD.

Individuals with a positive family history of ICA should be screened using time-of-flight three-dimensional magnetic resonance angiography. Reoccurrence of ICA is common in ADPKD individuals with a previous ICA, usually at least 3 years after the initial observation, and occurs more often in those individuals where rupture has occurred.

5. Hypertension is the most common renal complication in ADPKD occurring in 60 percent of individuals with normal renal function and is associated with a faster rate of progression to renal failure. Activation of the renin-angiotensin-aldosterone system plays an important role in the pathogenesis of hypertension in this disorder. Preliminary results from long-term studies suggest that angiotensin converting enzyme inhibition, in contrast to conventional diuretic therapy, may be beneficial in preventing progression to renal failure in this disorder.

6. Multiple therapies have been prescribed in experimental animal models of ADPKD and have shown success in slowing functional and structural progression of the disease. These therapies have not yet been successfully applied to man. Specifically, protein restriction has not demonstrated a significant impact on slowing progression to renal failure in human ADPKD. However, study design may not have been adequate to demonstrate a true benefit of this intervention.

7. Genetic linkage studies suggest there are at least three forms of ADPKD. The most common form (~85 percent), ADPKD1 (MIM 601313), results from mutation of the PKD1 gene on chromosome 16p13.3. The *PKD2* gene, on chromosome 4q22, is mutated in most of the others. A very small fraction of families have disease unlinked to markers for either locus. The three forms have nearly identical clinical phenotypes, although ADPKD2 (MIM 173910) is somewhat milder.

8. The *PKD1* gene encodes a 14-kb mRNA that is translated into a 4302-amino-acid membrane glycoprotein called polycystin-1. It is predicted to have an N-terminal extracellular domain of ~3000 residues, an odd number of transmembrane-spanning elements,[106-111] and a short cytoplasmic tail that interacts with a number of other proteins, including the *PKD2* gene product, polycystin-2. Polycystin is postulated to function as a nonkinase-type receptor for cell-cell and/or cell-matrix interactions.

9. *PKD2* encodes a 5.4-kb mRNA that is translated into a 968-amino-acid integral membrane protein predicted to have six transmembrane-spanning elements with intracellular N- and C-termini. Although polycystin-2 has modest homology to polycystin-1, it most closely resembles the family of voltage-activated calcium (and sodium) channels. Expression of a homologous gene, *PKDL*, suggests that

A list of standard abbreviations is located immediately preceding the index in each volume. Additional abbreviations used in this chapter include: ADPKD = autosomal dominant polycystic kidney disease; ADPKD1 = autosomal dominant polycystic kidney disease type 1; ADPKD2 = autosomal dominant polycystic kidney disease type 2; ESRD = end-stage renal disease; GPCR = G-protein coupled receptor; GPS = GPCR proteolytic site; GSK-3 = glycogen synthase kinase 3; JNK = c-Jun N-terminal protein kinase; LDL-A = a 40-amino-acid cysteine-rich module tandemly duplicated in the low-density lipoprotein receptor; LH2 = lipoxygenase homology 2; LOH = loss of heterozygosity; LRR = leucine-rich repeats; PKCε = protein kinase C epsilon isoform; *PKD1* = autosomal dominant polycystic kidney disease type 1 gene and gene symbol; *PKD2* = autosomal dominant polycystic kidney disease type 1 gene and gene symbol; *PKDL* = PKD2-like gene and gene symbol; REJ = receptor for egg jelly; RGS7 = regulators of G-protein signaling 7; SSCA = single-strand conformational analysis; TCF/LEF = T-cell-specific transcription factor/lymphoid enhancer-binding factor; TM = transmembrane spans; TRP = transient receptor potential; TRPC = transient receptor potential channel; *TSC2* = tuberous sclerosis type 2 gene and gene symbol; VACCα1 = voltage-activated calcium channel α1-subunit; VEO = very early onset.

polycystin-2 is likely to function as a cation channel protein.

10. The nearly identical clinical profiles that result from mutations of *PKD1* and *PKD2* suggest that their translation products are tightly linked in a common signaling pathway. A series of in vitro and in vivo studies show that the two proteins do, in fact, associate.

11. Genetic studies of cystic tissue from human ADPKD1 and ADPKD2 organs have identified clonal somatic mutations of the wild-type allele in individual cysts, suggesting a "two-hit" model of disease pathogenesis. The results of gene targeting studies of *Pkd1* and *Pkd2* in mice support this model.

12. In the murine Pkd1 and Pkd2 models, cyst formation begins at day E15. These studies suggest that loss of functional polycystin-1 or -2 below a critical threshold results in a block in the normal differentiation program of the kidney.

## CLINICAL ASPECTS OF ADPKD (MIM 173900)

Autosomal dominant polycystic kidney disease (ADPKD) is a systemic disorder occurring in 1:400 to 1:1000 individuals. It is the most common inherited renal disorder and accounts for 4.8 percent of end-stage renal disease (ESRD) in the United States.[1] Although the disease is inherited in a dominant fashion and has 90 percent penetrance in patients who live until 70 years, its phenotypic expression varies, presenting most often in the third and fourth decade of life. Diagnosis of ADPKD utilizes clinical, radiographic, and genetic information. The clinical constellation of ADPKD includes multiple manifestations in nonrenal organs such as hepatic cystic disease, intracranial aneurysms, mitral valve prolapse, and inguinal hernias.[2]

### Diagnosis of ADPKD

ADPKD is diagnosed by utilizing multiple sources of information including medical history, physical examination, laboratory evaluation, renal imaging, and genetic analysis. Whether all at-risk individuals should be screened for ADPKD can only be answered on a case-by-case basis. Importantly, many undiagnosed, yet treatable, complications are present in affected individuals who are unaware of their disease status. When 321 offspring of 46 probands greater than 15 years of age were screened for ADPKD by ultrasound, 68 (21 percent) were identified with the disorder. Of these individuals, 25 (37 percent) had one or more treatable complications at the time of diagnosis. Twenty of 68 (29 percent) had diastolic blood pressures greater than 95 mm Hg. Seven of 68 (10 percent) had documented renal insufficiency or an elevated serum creatinine concentration. Four of 68 (5 percent) had untreated urinary tract infections and 8 of 68 (12 percent) had a combination of complications.[3] Therefore, many potentially treatable medical complications due to ADPKD are not being addressed in a substantial proportion of affected individuals, perhaps because ADPKD has not been diagnosed.

Although the structure of both PKD1 and PKD2 genes has been defined,[4,5] a diagnosis of ADPKD relies more heavily on nongenetic approaches. Simple screening for *PKD1* gene mutations is difficult, as explained in subsequent sections of this chapter. *PKD2* is less complex than *PKD1* but this form of ADPKD is relatively uncommon, accounting for less than 15 percent of all individuals affected with ADPKD.[6] Therefore, a genetic diagnosis of ADPKD requires linkage analysis that relies on the presence of multiple affected members in a well-characterized family.[7]

Unfortunately, clinical application of linkage analysis in ADPKD is limited, as it is unable to predict disease severity or outcome. Even with mutational analysis, it is difficult to predict the clinical course of ADPKD. In one example, twins with some mutation had discordant phenotypes, with one having severe, in utero disease, and the other appearing clinically normal.[8] Disease severity is no more predictable within a family than between families.[9] In a phenotypically normal, at-risk fetus who is a predicted gene carrier for ADPKD based on linkage analysis or mutational analysis, the disease outcome cannot be predicted. In short, clinical characterization of the individual plays a much greater role in predicting disease outcome than the diagnosis itself. Posttest counseling, therefore, relies heavily on the clinical characteristics of the individual being tested. Patients who are potential candidates for linkage analysis include at-risk individuals considering organ donation for a family member, those who would change their family planning based on a positive diagnosis, and those who would terminate a pregnancy based on a positive diagnosis. Studies assessing attitudes toward pregnancy termination for the presence of ADPKD in a fetus have shown that the minority (< 4 percent) would change the outcome of their pregnancy while 26 percent of these individuals would terminate for other medical conditions such as Down syndrome.[10] Therefore, utilization of linkage analysis for considering pregnancy termination has limited applicability. In the majority of cases, ADPKD is diagnosed by symptoms related to advanced disease, in discovery during an evaluation as part of a family screening program, or by an incidental finding.

In asymptomatic individuals, medical history, physical examination, and laboratory evaluation may be normal, requiring renal imaging for a diagnosis of ADPKD. Although both computerized tomography (CT) and magnetic resonance imaging (MRI) can reliably identify renal cysts, ultrasound is the preferred method for diagnosing ADPKD.[11] Ultrasound is reliable, inexpensive, and does not require contrast or radiation exposure. Ultrasound findings diagnostic for ADPKD are the presence of multiple renal cysts bilaterally (Fig. 215-1), but other characteristics of ADPKD are renal enlargement and increased echogenicity depending on the stage of the disease.[12,13] The latter findings are not specific to ADPKD and can be found in conditions such as nephrotic syndrome, in other cystic diseases, such as autosomal recessive polycystic kidney disease and tuberous sclerosis, as well as in pregnancy.

The relative sensitivity of ultrasound and CT as diagnostic tools for ADPKD has been compared.[14,15] Both CT and ultrasound detect disease in 90 percent of cases; however, in 6 percent, cysts were detected by CT but not ultrasound, and in 2 percent, cysts were detected by ultrasound but not CT. CT has a small increase in sensitivity of detecting renal cysts, but given the radiation and

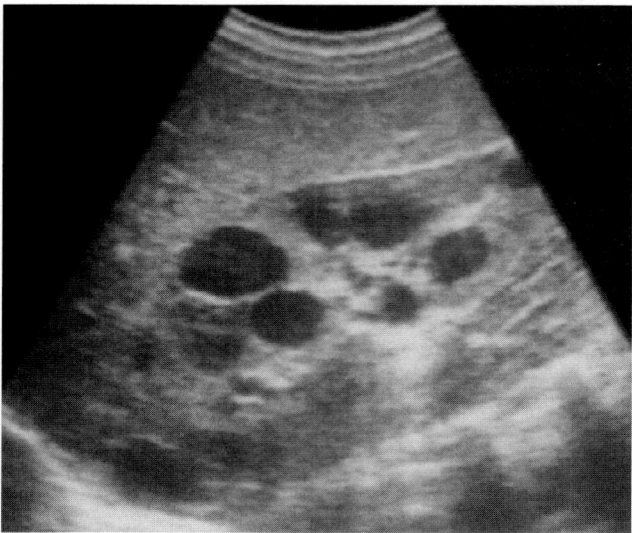

**Fig. 215-1** Longitudinal image of the right kidney in an 8-year-old girl with autosomal dominant polycystic kidney disease.

**Table 215-1** Ultrasonographic Criteria for Diagnosis of Autosomal Dominant Polycystic Kidney Disease

| Age range | Number of cysts required for a diagnosis |
|---|---|
| < 18 years | 2 cysts total |
| 18–30 years | 3 cysts total, bilateral distribution |
| 30–60 years | 4 cysts total, bilateral distribution |
| > 60 years | 8 cysts total, bilateral distribution |

radiocontrast exposure associated with CT, ultrasound is preferred for screening. The sensitivity or specificity in detecting renal cysts by MRI has not been compared to ultrasound or CT, but MRI provides similar, if not better, sensitivity than ultrasound in identifying small renal cysts and does not have as high contrast and radiation exposures as CT. Given the cost of MRI and the potential complications of scanner-related claustrophobia, ultrasound is still the first choice for diagnostic imaging in ADPKD. When a definitive diagnosis is required (e.g., for a potential renal donor for a family member with ADPKD), CT is recommended.

Two variables need to be taken into consideration when determining the reliability of ultrasound in diagnosing ADPKD. Both genetic type and age can influence the presence of renal cysts in ADPKD[16,17]. PKD2 is a less aggressive form of ADPKD with a later age of diagnosis and hypertension and the age of entry into ESRD.[16] Parfrey and associates reported that 92 percent of an expected 50 percent at-risk PKD1 patients have detectable cysts by age 30 as compared to 11 percent of PKD2 individuals.[16] Based on these data, PKD1 at-risk individuals older than 30 years of age without detectable cysts by ultrasound have < 5 percent chance of having the disease.[16,18]

In children < 16 years, simple cysts are rare, occurring in less than 0.1 percent.[19] The frequency of simple cysts increases with age occurring in 1.7 percent of individuals age 30 to 49 years, in 11.5 percent of those 50 to 70 years old, and in 22.1 percent of those older than 70 years.[20,21] Bilateral cysts are a less common occurrence, observed in only 9 percent of individuals over 70 years of age. Based on these data, the current number of cysts required for a diagnosis of ADPKD in an at-risk individual is presented in Table 215-1.

Four studies utilizing GLA and the above phenotypic criteria for a diagnosis of ADPKD in at-risk ADPKD individuals less than 30 years of age have determined the sensitivity and specificity of ultrasound in making a diagnosis early in the course of ADPKD.[13,16,17,22] Of 127 subjects studied, 16 (12.5 percent) obligatory gene carriers had a normal renal ultrasound. In one study, only 1 of 25 (4 percent) obligatory gene carriers over the age of 10 had a normal ultrasound.[13] Based on available information, ultrasound cannot reliably rule out the presence of ADPKD in individuals less than 30 years of age and follow-up screening studies are needed.

### Extra-Renal Manifestations of ADPKD

**Polycystic Liver Disease.** Despite its name, ADPKD is a systemic disorder not limited to the kidney, and polycystic liver disease is a common manifestation (Table 215-2). Hepatic cysts are a common and often differentiating feature of ADPKD compared to other cystic diseases of the kidney. Familial autosomal dominant polycystic liver disease without renal involvement and unlinked to PKD1 or PKD2 has been described.[23] Hepatic fibrosis and Caroli disease (more often associated with autosomal recessive polycystic kidney disease) have been reported in ADPKD individuals.[24,25] Hepatic cysts are rare in children but develop approximately a decade after renal cysts and are present in the majority of ADPKD individuals over 50 years of age.[26] Importantly, hepatic cystic disease tends to develop in specific sections of the liver, leaving other sections unaffected. Decreased renal function and increased renal volume are associated with the

presence and number of hepatic cysts in ADPKD.[26] Although the overall prevalence of hepatic cystic disease is the same in men and women, the number and size of liver cysts is greater in women. An increasing number of pregnancies and usage of oral contraceptive pills are both associated with increased incidence and severity of polycystic liver disease in ADPKD women.[26,27] A recent case-control study of the effects of 1 year of postmenopausal estrogen use on hepatic cyst growth revealed an increase in both cystic and noncystic hepatic parenchymal volume in ADPKD women receiving estrogen.[28]

Noncystic liver volume remains intact even in the setting of massive polycystic liver disease in ADPKD.[29] Routine laboratory values of patients with severe polycystic liver disease are not abnormal and more sophisticated measurement of hepatic blood flow and function demonstrate normal antipyrine clearances without evidence of shunting.[29]

Complications from hepatic cystic disease occur as the liver enlarges. Rarely, individuals with massive polycystic liver disease will develop hepatic venous outflow obstruction and portal hypertension.[30] Increasing abdominal pain, decreased mobility, shortness of breath and decreased appetite are all symptoms of significant polycystic liver disease. Cyst hemorrhage and cyst infection occur and present with acute upper abdominal pain and shortness of breath. In individuals with hepatic cyst infection, symptoms usually include fever and leukocytosis. Given the difficulties associated with massive hepatic cystic disease, patients may require analgesics to alleviate discomfort. In those with persistent pain, laparoscopic, percutaneous, or surgical cyst decompression, as well as hepatic resection may be beneficial.[31,32] These procedures are reserved only for those individuals whose quality of life is inadequate after a trial of rest, stretching exercises, and analgesics. Although mortality is rare with these procedures, complications, including pleural effusions, ascites, and presacral or lower extremity edema, occur 15 to 29 percent of the time. Extravascular fluid accumulation is probably due to *trans*-epithelial cyst fluid secretion from hepatic cysts that are no longer intact. Postprocedure complications occur more frequently in patients with diffuse hepatic cystic disease, than in patients with one or a few large, dominant cysts.[33]

### Other Gastrointestinal Manifestations

Multiple pancreatic cysts occur in ADPKD individuals less than 10 percent of the time; usually they are solitary.[34] Cholangiocarcinoma has been reported in individuals with ADPKD. Diverticular disease was reported to occur in 83 percent of ADPKD patients, as compared to 32 percent of non-ADPKD ESRD individuals.[35] However, prospective screening studies of asymptomatic ADPKD individuals and age and renal function-matched controls demonstrate that the frequency of diverticular disease is not increased in ADPKD individuals.[36] Complications from diverticular disease may be more common in ADPKD individuals with perforated diverticula reported to occur in approximately 25 percent of ESRD patients.[35]

### Cardiac Valvular Disease

Aortic insufficiency (12 percent) and mitral valve prolapse (26 percent) are more frequent in ADPKD individuals as compared to

**Table 215-2** Frequency of Extrarenal Manifestations in Autosomal Dominant Polycystic Kidney Disease

| Manifestation | Frequency (%) |
|---|---|
| Hepatic cysts | 75 |
| Diverticulosis coli | 70 |
| Cardiac valvular disease | 26 |
| Intracranial aneurysms | 8 |
| Inguinal hernias | 15 |

unaffected age-matched controls.[37] Mitral valve prolapse (MVP) can be associated with symptoms such as atypical chest pain and palpitations, but these symptoms rarely cause the patient harm. In an occasional individual, sustained and prolonged symptoms of shortness of breath, chest pain, or dizziness occur in association with a cardiac arrhythmia requiring medical attention and treatment. Interestingly, in two large studies, the incidence of MVP was also increased in unaffected members of ADPKD families as compared to age-matched control populations.[38,39] These findings suggest that a second modifying gene may be important in the development of MVP in this population. The incidence of bacterial endocarditis is not increased in ADPKD individuals, but antibiotic prophylaxis prior to and following dental work is recommended by the American Dental Association.

## Intracranial Aneurysms (ICA)

ICAs have been reported in ADPKD patient with mutations in either *PKD1* or *PKD2*. Although ICAs are more frequent in ADPKD patients as compared to the general population, rupture of an ICA is not the most common cause of cerebrovascular death in an ADPKD individual. Cerebrovascular hemorrhage from long-standing hypertension is more frequent, with ruptured ICA accounting for only 25 percent of all cerebrovascular deaths. Initial reports of the frequency of ruptured ICA in ADPKD patients suggested a highly variable incidence (0 to 41 percent), probably because the studies were retrospective and detection was based on symptomatic presentation.[40–45] Four prospective imaging studies using either three-dimensional time-of-flight magnetic resonance angiography (MRA), four-vessel cerebral angiography, or dynamic CT, were performed in 227 asymptomatic ADPKD individuals.[46–49] In total, 28 ICAs in 18 individuals were found, yielding a prevalence rate of 7.9 percent of ICA in asymptomatic ADPKD individuals. All of the ICAs were less than 10 mm in diameter, with a distribution predominately in the anterior portion of the circle of Willis.

These reports do not identify those who are most likely to suffer from a ruptured ICA. In the general population, ICAs rupture only 50 percent of the time. Table 215-3 compares ADPKD with asymptomatic ICA to those with ruptured ICA. Gender, age, hypertension, level of blood pressure control, and smoking were not found to be risk factors for the occurrence of ICA in ADPKD patients. However, a positive family history of ICA was more frequent in PKD individuals who had intact or ruptured ICA. In the general population, hypertension and smoking history are both associated with an increased incidence of ICA, and family history plays less of a role.[50]

Although the frequency of ICA in ADPKD is less than originally thought, rupture of an ICA is a serious and life-threatening event. The prevalence of long-term morbidity and mortality of ICA rupture in ADPKD individuals ranges from 46 to 89 percent.[51] ADPKD individuals who are acutely symptomatic with severe headaches or with neurologic findings should be screened for the presence of an ICA. However, it is not cost-effective to screen every individual with ADPKD for the presence of an ICA,[52] and an ICA has not been reported to occur in ADPKD children. Therefore, screening should not begin before the age of

21 years in an asymptomatic individual, and because a positive family history of an ICA is the only known risk factor, it is reasonable to screen only those individuals with a documented family history of an ICA. Other individuals who work at or participate in high-risk activities, such as airline piloting or deep sea diving, should also be screened for the presence of an ICA.

Time-of-flight three-dimensional MRA is the screening method of choice and can detect vascular abnormalities as small as 3 mm in diameter. Dynamic contrast CT in axial and coronal planes can be performed, but carries the risk of contrast exposure in patients who are at risk for developing contrast-induced nephrotoxicity. Data regarding comparative sensitivity in detecting ICA using cerebral angiography, MRA, or CT are limited. Both MRA and CT appear to be able to detect ICA as small as 3 mm in diameter. It is important to note that ADPKD individuals suffer from vascular complications during angiography at a greater rate than the general population (25 percent vs. 8 percent).[46] With this in mind, and given the reliability of MRA or dynamic CT imaging, angiography should not be the initial screening method in asymptomatic individuals and should be reserved for confirmation.

In individuals who have a negative initial ICA screening, there is no information about when to repeat the screen. In follow-up studies obtained less than 3 years after the initial screening, no ICAs were found. On the other hand, recurrent ICAs have been found in previously screened individuals.[53] Currently, the screening interval for an asymptomatic individual is at least 5 years.

The size and location of ICAs determine both the risk of rupture and the chances for surgical success. Risk of rupture increases dramatically when ICAs are greater than 10 mm in diameter.[54] In such patients, surgical repair is recommended. In the general population, individuals with intact an ICA < 10 mm in diameter experience no advantage with surgical intervention as compared to conservative management.[54] Whether this is applicable to the ADPKD population, especially when hypertension is present and progressive renal insufficiency can occur, is unknown. The current recommendations for screening and treatment of ICA in ADPKD individuals are provided in Fig. 215-2.

## Renal Manifestations in ADPKD

Renal manifestations of ADPKD are shown in Table 215-4. Microscopic examinations of human ADPKD nephrectomy specimens demonstrate an increased frequency of polyp formation and increased numbers of microscopic adenomas. There also is evidence for epithelial proliferation in ADPKD, but demonstration of an increased incidence of renal cell carcinoma is lacking.[55]

Cyst wall calcification is more apparent as renal insufficiency progresses and is found with increasing renal and cyst size. The majority of ADPKD subjects demonstrate a decrease in urinary citrate excretion possibly accounting for the higher frequency of renal stones found in ADPKD patients (see "Renal Complications in ADPKD" below).

Decreased urinary concentrating defect is a universal finding in ADPKD.[56] The defect is mild and is present in both children and adults with ADPKD. The cause of the urinary concentrating defect is multifactorial; vasopressin resistance at the level of the cortical collecting tubule, structural distortion of the medulla, and decreased aldolase required for the generation of a countercurrent gradient all contribute to the concentrating defect.[57]

Histopathologic examination of ADPKD nephrectomy specimens demonstrates increased number of juxtaglomerular apparatuses and renin-secreting granules.[58] There is abnormal location of renin-secreting granules along afferent arterioles and within walls of renal cysts, and active renin has been detected in the renal cyst fluid in ADPKD.[59] These abnormalities may play a role in the hypertension of ADPKD (see "Renal Complications in ADPKD" below).

Increased renal vein erythropoietin concentrations have been documented in ADPKD individuals, but frank erythropoiesis has not been described. In the Modification of Diet and Renal Disease

**Table 215-3** Characteristics of ADPKD Individuals with Intact and Ruptured Intracranial Aneurysms

| Characteristic | Intact ICA | Ruptured ICA | P value |
|---|---|---|---|
| Number of subjects | 83 | 82 | NS |
| Age, yrs | 43 | 34 | < 0.05 |
| Female (%) | 48 | 55 | NS |
| Multiple ICA (%) | 6 | 38 | < 0.05 |
| Family Hx of ICA (%) | 10 | 22 | < 0.05 |
| Recurrence rate (%) | Not applicable | 14 (10/76) | NA |

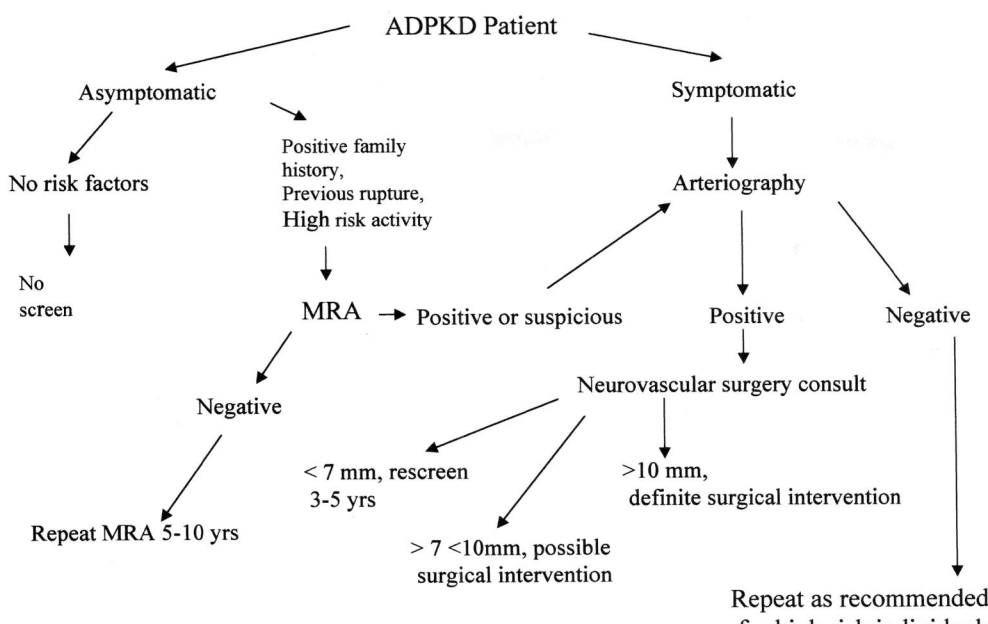

**Fig. 215-2 Algorithm for screening for intracranial aneurysms in patients with autosomal dominant polycystic kidney disease.**

(MDRD) study in which 1479 patients with multiple renal diseases and over 200 ADPKD individuals were studied, no differences in average hematocrit levels were found in ADPKD individuals as compared to those with other renal diseases.[60] One potential explanation for the lack of a difference found is the common use of angiotensin-converting enzyme inhibitors for the treatment of hypertension in ADPKD; these drugs can decrease the hematocrit levels in renin-producing ischemic kidneys (see "Renal Complications in ADPKD" below).

## Renal Complications in ADPKD

Renal complications in ADPKD are provided in Table 215-5. The most important is hypertension; it occurs in approximately 60 percent of adult ADPKD individuals with normal renal function and in 10 to 15 percent of affected children.[61,62] The average age of diagnosis of hypertension in ADPKD is early — 30 years of age.[62] ADPKD men are more often hypertensive than women and have higher blood pressures.[62] When normotensive and hypertensive ADPKD individuals with normal renal function and similar age and body mass index are compared, hypertensive ADPKD patients have larger renal volumes than their normotensive controls. In hypertensive ADPKD children, renal volume is greater than in normotensive age-matched ADPKD controls, and hypertensive ADPKD children demonstrate both larger renal volumes and a twofold greater rate of increase in renal volume over time as compared to their normotensive counterparts.[63]

In keeping with renal structural involvement playing an important role in the pathogenesis of hypertension in ADPKD, Bennett and colleagues demonstrated a significant and sustained reduction in blood pressure and the requirement for blood pressure medication in five hypertensive ADPKD individuals who underwent surgical cyst decompression for chronic abdominal and flank pain.[64] The blood pressure-lowering effects were sustained for well over 1 year, and the authors suggested that intrarenal ischemia due to cyst expansion may play a role for the development of hypertension in ADPKD. In fact, angioradiographic images of ADPKD kidneys demonstrate attenuation, narrowing, and distortion of the renal vasculature.

Both activation of the renin-angiotensin-aldosterone system and sodium retention (similar to that found in the two-kidney, two-clip or one-kidney, one-clip Goldblatt model of renal vascular hypertension) could play a role in the hypertension found in ADPKD. To test this hypothesis further, hypertensive ADPKD and essential hypertensive subjects with normal renal function, matched for blood pressure and sodium and potassium intake, were studied to determine whether activation of the renin-angiotensin-aldosterone system is present in hypertensive ADPKD individuals.[65] Subjects were evaluated during postural maneuvers and after captopril ingestion. Both plasma renin activity and plasma aldosterone concentrations were greater in the ADPKD individuals compared to the essential hypertensive controls and during acute (1-dose) and chronic (6-week) angiotensin-converting enzyme inhibition, renal

**Table 215-4** Renal Manifestations in Autosomal Dominant Polycystic Kidney Disease

|  | Manifestation | Frequency (%) |
|---|---|---|
| Anatomic | Cysts | 100 |
|  | Adenomas | 22 |
|  | Calcifications | >50 |
| Functional | Decreased concentrating ability | 100 |
|  | Decreased urinary citrate | 67 |
|  | Increased renin secretion | 70–100 |
|  | Increased erythropoietin | common |

**Table 215-5** Renal Complications in ADPKD

| Complication | Age of presentation | Frequency (%) |
|---|---|---|
| Hypertension | Adults, normal renal function | 59 |
|  | Adults, ESRD | 100 |
|  | Children | 10–15 |
| Hematuria | Adults | 50 |
| Nephrolithiasis | Adults | 25 |
| ESRD | Adults | 45% by age 60 |
| Pain syndrome | Adults | 60 |
|  | Children | 25 |

plasma flow increased and filtration fraction decreased significantly.[65,66] These data provide good circulatory and renal hemodynamic evidence for activation of the renin-angiotensin-aldosterone system in hypertension in ADPKD. Unfortunately, successful treatment of hypertension (to a level below 150/90 mm Hg) is as low as 29 percent even in ADPKD individuals with normal renal function. These data are similar to the success rate present in essential hypertensives. Moreover, a significant number of patients with ADPKD demonstrate left ventricular hypertrophy (LVH) by echocardiographic criteria.[67] Interestingly, normotensive ADPKD individuals can also demonstrate LVH, suggesting that abnormal myocardial growth responses secondary to the mutation causing ADPKD contribute to the LVH.[68] ADPKD individuals with LVH have hypertension more frequently, have higher blood pressure levels, are older, and demonstrate poorer renal function as compared to their counterparts without LVH.[67] In addition, LVH is related to an absence of the usual decline in nocturnal blood pressure and left ventricular mass index correlates with systolic blood pressure in ADPKD children.[69,70] All of these findings suggest that end-organ damage secondary to chronic blood pressure elevation contributes to the high proportion of cardiovascular deaths in this patient population.[71]

ADPKD is a disease of tubular rather than glomerular origin, so the presence of proteinuria is uncommon in this disorder: only 18 percent of 602 ADPKD individuals demonstrated detectable proteinuria (> 300 mg/day excretion).[72] However, all proteinuric ADPKD individuals were hypertensive, had larger renal volumes, and lower inulin and PAH clearances as compared to their nonproteinuric counterparts. ADPKD children with established proteinuria all have elevated blood pressure and increased renal size as compared to their nonproteinuric counterparts.[73] Proteinuria in ADPKD is associated with a more aggressive renal disease, with proteinuric individuals beginning dialysis at an earlier age.[74]

Microalbuminuria (i.e., urinary albumin excretion below the concentrations detected by the usual dipstick method) occurs in a minority of ADPKD patients.[72] Microalbuminuria is associated with higher blood pressure, increased renal volume, decreased renal function and renal plasma flow, and a more aggressive course of renal disease. Consequently, microalbuminuria is a marker for more aggressive renal disease in ADPKD. Urinary protein excretion above 2 g/day suggests a second unrelated renal disorder in the setting of ADPKD (IgA nephropathy, focal segmental glomerular sclerosis, and other glomerulopathies have been reported to occur in ADPKD patients[75]). To obtain a diagnosis in patients who present with a very high level of urinary protein excretion, an open renal biopsy should be considered.

Renal cyst infections are common in ADPKD. Patients classically present with symptoms of fever, flank, or abdominal pain on the side of the infection; occasionally, there also is nausea and vomiting. Microscopic urinalysis may be unremarkable. Positive blood cultures identify the infecting organism more often than urine cultures.[76] Most often the infection is caused by a gram-negative enteric organism from the bladder, but hematogenous spread to the kidney has also been reported.[76] Given that most cysts are not connected to a nephron, it is important to use antibiotics that provide adequate cyst penetration. Some antibiotics may not be adequate to treat cyst infections in APDKD individuals, even though the antibiotic sensitivity is appropriate, because different cysts have different transport characteristics yielding variable drug levels during a course of therapy.[77] Aminoglycosides, which are often used to treat pyelonephritis, are filtered at the glomerulus and hence will not achieve an adequate concentration in the cyst compartment. Medications that are effective in providing adequate concentrations in renal and hepatic cysts include fluoroquinolones, sulfa medications such as Bactrim, and chloramphenicol. Vancomycin will achieve adequate levels in an infected cyst in ADPKD patients.[78] Renal and hepatic cyst infections in ADPKD individuals represent closed-space infections so successful treatment depends on early recognition and an appropriately long treatment course. The minimal duration

of therapy for a cyst infection should be 14 days, and in those with poor renal function or diminished renal plasma flow, either intravenous antibiotics or a more prolonged course of oral therapy may be necessary.

Nephrolithiasis occurs in 20 to 28 percent of individuals with ADPKD.[79,80] Stone disease is most often bilateral and the frequency of nephrolithiasis increases with age; close to 40 percent of patients over 40 years of age will demonstrate stone disease.[80] Nephrolithiasis is associated with microscopic hematuria and acute flank pain in patients with ADPKD, and pain is a differentiating feature from cyst calcification, which is more common (50 percent) than renal stone (21 percent) disease.[81] Cyst wall calcification tends to occur in older individuals with bigger kidneys and worse renal function. CT and intravenous urography may be needed to locate and determine the nature of the stone or calcification; when 30 stones from 151 ADPKD patients with nephrolithiasis were analyzed, 57 percent were urate, 47 percent were calcium oxalate, 20 percent also contained calcium phosphate, and 10 percent contained struvite.[81] Distal acidification defects are thought to play a role in the stone disease in APDKD because decreased urinary pH, decreased urinary citrate excretion, and abnormal transport of ammonia are common.

## Progression to Renal Failure in ADPKD

Not all ADPKD individuals invariably progress to renal failure. The percent of subjects requiring renal replacement increases with age, with 30 to 35 percent requiring replacement at age 52, 40 to 50 percent requiring replacement at age 60, and 60 to 85 percent requiring replacement at age 70.[16,74,82] Gender is a risk factor for progression, with men entering ESRD approximately 6 years earlier than women.[83] Risk factors for progression to renal failure have been investigated and the presence of hypertension, proteinuria, large kidneys, gross hematuria in men, and more than three pregnancies in women, are all associated with a faster rate of progression to ESRD.[74,84,85] Those individuals who are diagnosed either in utero or during the first month of life have a more aggressive form of disease.[86] Importantly, hepatic cystic disease and a history of nephrectomy do not appear to place individuals at risk for progression to ESRD.[76,87]

At present, no therapy slows the progression of renal disease in ADPKD. This does not mean that all therapies are without benefit. For example, difficulty in showing a benefit of therapy on renal outcome in ADPKD individuals is related to the slowly progressive nature of the disorder (renal function is gradually lost over a number of decades). On average, a beneficial effect of dietary protein restriction or converting enzyme inhibition on renal outcome in ADPKD has not been demonstrated but both types of studies were relatively short (i.e., 2.2 years duration).[60,88] In studies of longer duration (e.g., 5 years), converting-enzyme inhibitor therapy compared to diuretic therapy was associated with a slower rate of progression of disease.[89] In another study, beta-blockade and converting-enzyme inhibitor therapy had equal efficacy in blood pressure control and the rate of renal progression in ADPKD[90] (the lack of a difference found may be because both antihypertensive agents suppress activity of the renin-angiotensin-aldosterone system). There is abundant evidence that dietary protein restriction is safe and beneficial in terms of limiting symptoms of renal insufficiency.[91] Although this may delay dialysis, there was no slowing of progressive loss of glomerular filtration rate by protein restriction in studies of PKD individuals.[60]

In animal models of ADPKD, multiple therapies have demonstrated benefit on progression of disease. In the cpk mouse model of recessive polycystic kidney disease with alterations in epidermal growth factor receptor location and function, specific tyrosine kinase inhibitors have reduced cyst growth by more than 80 percent.[92] In the Han:SPRD rat model of ADPKD, an autosomal dominant disorder with slowly progressive renal insufficiency similar to human ADPKD, dietary protein restriction, soy protein supplementation, flaxseed supplementation, blood pressure reduction, angiotensin-converting enzyme inhibition, sodium bicarbonate, lovastatin, and sodium and potassium citrate all slowed the rate of progression to renal failure as well as the rate of cyst growth.[93–99] In other inherited mouse models of polycystic kidney disease, no effect of sodium bicarbonate or citrate therapy was detectable, at least in terms of renal cystic development and progression of renal disease. This species specificity may be due to differing diets across rodent species where the mouse, unlike man, has a lower-acid-containing diet, making it more difficult to demonstrate a benefit of an alkalinizing agent. The tubular location of cysts in murine models of polycystic kidney disease differs from the Han:SPRD rat. In the mouse models, the cysts reside predominantly in the distal rather than the proximal nephron. Moreover, the acid content of the diet may have a different impact. These therapies hold hope for treatment of disease in human ADPKD, but further testing is necessary before applying them to humans.

## MOLECULAR GENETIC STUDIES

### Genetic Linkage

Linkage studies suggest that there are at least three loci responsible for ADPKD.[100–102] Mutations of *PKD1*, located at 16p13.3, account for ~85 to 95 percent of all ADPKD. Virtually all of the remaining ADPKD families have mutations of *PKD2*, which is located on chromosome 4q21-23.[6,103,104] A very small number of families have been reported in which the disease phenotype appears to be unlinked to either chromosome 16 or 4 markers.[101,105–107] This third form of ADPKD has not yet been linked to a chromosomal region, and one possible explanation is that it is a genetically heterogeneous collection. Paterson and Pei recently questioned the existence of a third form.[108] After reviewing the data for several of the families, the authors concluded that genotyping errors likely accounted for the apparent lack of linkage with chromosome 16 or 4 markers. A second family had strong evidence for bilineal disease. It is clear that the existence of a third form of ADPKD will be in question until its chromosomal position is assigned with certainty.

### PKD1 Gene Discovery

Nearly a decade had passed between the gene's initial localization in 1985 and its subsequent discovery. Two observations played key roles in ending the search. First, a major form of tuberous sclerosis (*TSC2*) was localized in the *PKD1* region by linkage analysis.[109] Second, a family was identified that had individuals with classic ADPKD as well as a child with both tuberous sclerosis and renal cystic disease.[110] Cytogenetic studies revealed that the mother and a sibling with ADPKD had balanced translocations between chromosomes 16 and 22, whereas the child with tuberous sclerosis had an unbalanced karyotype and was missing a portion of chromosome 22 as well as the telomeric portion of chromosome 16 (Fig. 215-3A). The investigators reasoned that the gene for TSC2 would be located in the portion of chromosome 16 that was lost in the child with tuberous sclerosis, while *PKD1* was likely bisected by the translocation breakpoint. Further study proved both hypotheses true, and this series of observations led to the discovery of both *TSC2* and *PKD1*.[110,111]

### PKD1 Genetic Analyses

The *PKD1* gene is relatively compact, with its 14-kb mRNA encoded by 46 exons clustered in a 53-kb genomic fragment (Fig. 215-3B).[4,110,112,113] Its genomic structure, however, has a number of features that complicate its study. Approximately 70 percent of the gene's length (exons 1 to 34, Fig. 215-3B) is replicated three to four times elsewhere on chromosome 16. The sequence identity in the replicated segments exceeds 95 percent and includes both exonic and intronic sequences. The task of developing *PKD1*-specific reagents has been further complicated by the observation that the sequences of the homologues are not identical to one another and vary from the published *PKD1* sequence in different locations.[114] Rigorous control studies are required to verify the specificity of every alleged *PKD1*-specific sequence.[115] It is not currently known whether the homologous loci have any biologic function. At least three of the loci are transcribed (mRNA of 8.5 kb, 17 kb, and 21 kb respectively on northern blot), but none have yet been shown to produce protein.[110]

A second peculiar property of the genomic organization of *PKD1* is an unusual 2.5-kb polypyrimidine tract located within intron 21.[112,113] The coding strand of this element is composed of 96 percent pyrimidines and it is the longest polypyrimidine tract yet described in the human genome. A second, much shorter element with the same sequence bias is present in an adjacent intron (intron 22). There is reason to believe that these structures may be more than interesting curiosities because similar, but much shorter, elements form triple-helical structures. Triplex DNA has been reported to regulate DNA replication and RNA transcription and processing, to induce mutations in neighboring sequences, and to enhance recombination between homologous sequences.[116–118] In the case of *PKD1*, Blaszak et al. showed that the 2.5-kb polypyrimidine-polypurine tract of intron 21 is capable of forming multiple non-B-DNA structures,[119] but it is presently unknown whether either element has any role in the transcriptional regulation of *PKD1* or in the gene's high rate of mutation (discussed below under "Mechanism of Cyst Formation"). It is interesting to note, however, that neither the polypyrimidine tracts nor the homologous loci are present within the murine *Pkd1* gene.[120]

An important practical consequence of having both the homologous loci and the polypyrimidine tracts is that mutation detection has been a very tedious and slow process.[8,110,114,115,121–133] Until recently, most of the mutations that had been described in the literature were located in the nonreplicated segment of the gene (exons 36 to 46) because it was the only region of the gene that could be easily assayed using conventional methods. Watnick et al.[115] first showed that these obstacles could be overcome using long-range PCR with widely spaced *PKD1*-specific primers, and now the entire gene can be surveyed by this approach.[119–121]

Over 60 mutations have been reported to date (www.uwcm. ac.uk/uwcm/mg/hgmd0.html), and although the data are incomplete, a few patterns are emerging. First, mutations appear to be scattered semirandomly over the gene's length. Although a major mutation hot spot or common mutation has not yet been discovered, a few areas within the gene have been found to be more prone to mutation. For example, several mutations have been reported clustered in intron 43.[124] This intron is at the lower limits of size necessary for proper splicing (75 bp) and any further deletion is capable of disrupting its correct splicing. Likewise, the replicated region of *PKD1* appears to have a somewhat disproportionately large number of mutations.[123]

Second, most mutations have been identified within a single pedigree, with very few recurrent mutations reported. The high incidence of the disease within most populations and the large number of unique mutations suggest that *PKD1* must have a high rate of mutation. The modest number of *de novo* mutations that have been described is consistent with this prediction and supports the clinical observation that a modest number of affected individuals are the first members of their family with disease.

As noted above, a few recurrent mutations have been found in apparently unrelated families. The Q4041X is the most common one yet reported, and it has been found in Spanish, British, and Italian families.[128,129] The mechanism for this mutation is likely to be slipped mispairing of an adjacent imperfect direct repeat sequence. In another example of three families sharing a 2-bp deletion in exon 15, the pedigree information is incomplete, although the data suggest that they may have different ethnic origins.[114] Interestingly, the families were recruited for study solely based on their disease phenotype (discussed below). In a final example, in two unrelated Thai families, a recurrent nonsense mutation was found that is also present in one of the homologous loci (unpublished observations, B. Phakdeekitcharoen). These data

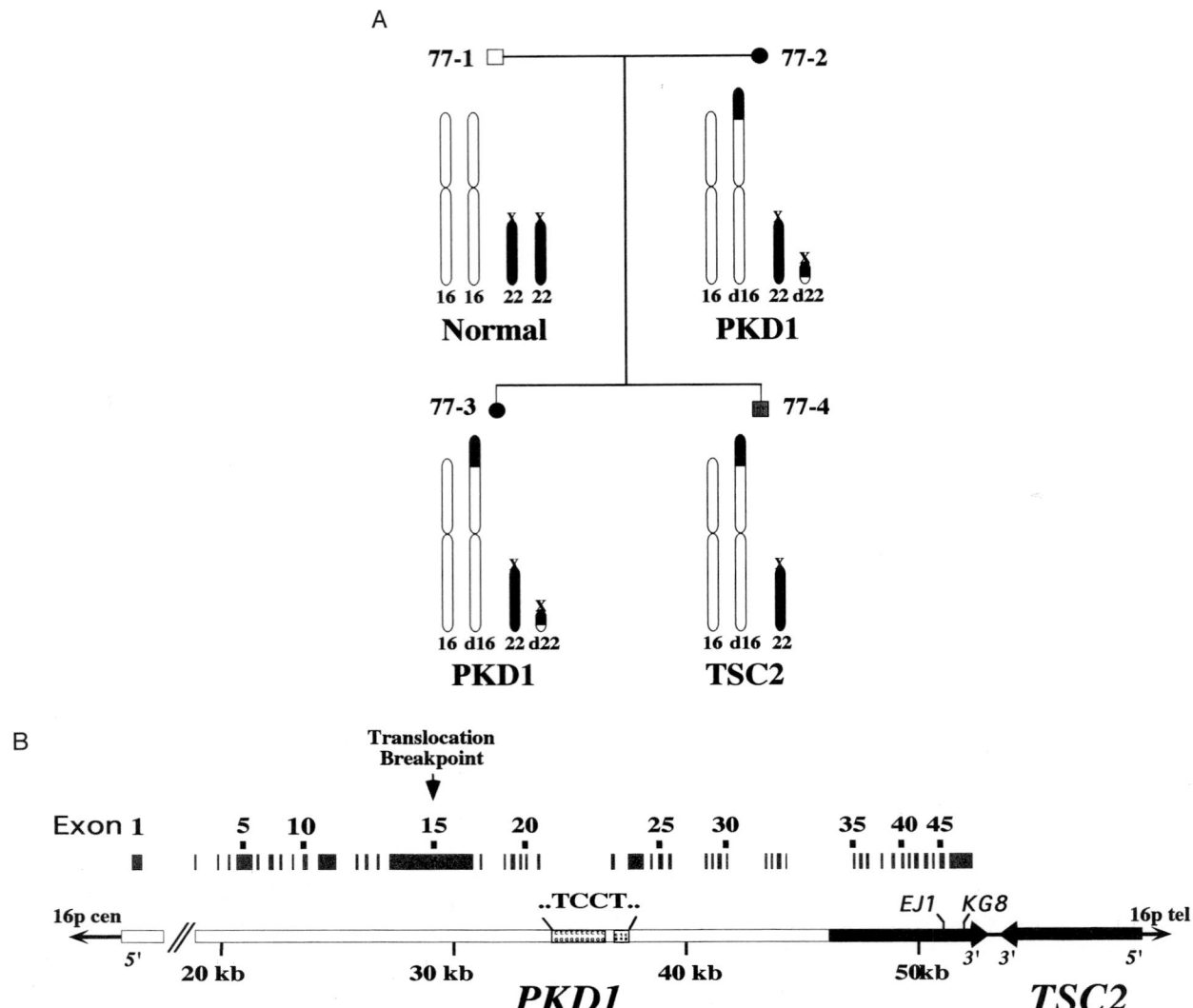

Fig. 215-3 *A*, Pedigree of the family that led to the discovery of *PKD1* and *TSC2*.[12,13] Individuals 77-2 and 77-3 have typical ADPKD and each was discovered to have a balanced chromosome 16-22 translocation disrupting the *PKD1* locus [t(16;22)(p13.3;q11.21)]. A sib of 77-3 (77-4) was found to have tuberous sclerosis and renal cystic disease and an unbalanced translocation with loss of der22 [−16−22+der(16)(16qter → 16p13.3:22q11.21 → 22qter)]. The father of 77-3 and 77-4 was unaffected with either disease. (*From Watnick and Germino.*[201] *Used with permission.*) *B*, Genomic organization of the *PKD1* gene. *PKD1* is encoded by 46 exons, represented by shaded rectangles, that extend over ~50 kb of genomic DNA on chromosome 16p13.3 (rectangular arrow). Tran-scription of the gene proceeds from its centromeric end (left) towards the telomere (right). Immediately adjacent to the 3′ end of *PKD1* is the 3′ end of the gene responsible for tuberous sclerosis 2, *TSC2*.[111] Exons 1 to 34 of *PKD1* are duplicated in multiple copies elsewhere on chromosome 16 (unfilled rectangle).[110] The gene is bisected by two polypyrimidine tracts (..TCCT..) that lie in adjacent introns (21 and 22; stippled boxes).[112,116] KG8 and *EJ1* are polymorphic markers in the 3′ end of *PKD1* that have been used for LOH studies of cystic tissue (Fig. 215-11).[187] The position of the breakpoint of the chromosome 16-22 translocation that led to the discovery of *PKD1* is as shown. (*From Watnick and Germino.*[201] *Used with permission.*)

suggest that gene conversion events may have been the mechanism responsible for their recurrent nature.

It is somewhat surprising that a subset of common mutations has not yet been identified given previous reports of linkage disequilibrium between *PKD1* and flanking genetic markers in a number of European Caucasian populations.[134–137] If linkage disequilibrium truly exists between particular genotypes and the disease in any of those groups, one would expect to find a common mutation in the same population. It is possible that the failure to find such an association is due to the incomplete status of the study. An alternative explanation is that particular haplotypes identified by the flanking markers identify a chromosome that has particular features that make it more prone to mutation. Further study is required to resolve the matter.

As noted above, the replicated region of *PKD1* appears to have a disproportionately large number of *PKD1* mutations. One mechanism that is likely responsible for at least some of this increase is gene conversion between the homologous loci and *PKD1*[138] (Fig. 215-4). Numerous polymorphisms, as well as several pathogenic mutations, are likely to have arisen by this mechanism. In one example, two families were discovered to have a nearly identical set of missense changes clustered in exon 23 that were likely the result of a gene conversion event.[138] The recurrent nonsense mutation cited above is a second example. Although the frequency with which gene conversion events between *PKD1* and its homologues actually occur is unknown, one recent study suggests that it may account for up to 25 percent of sequence variation in exons 13 to 21.[139]

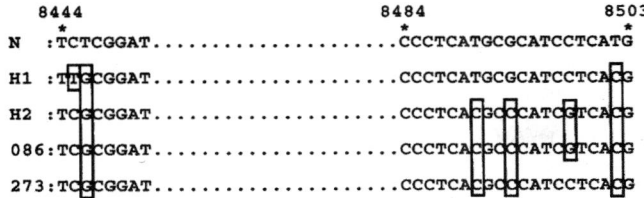

**Fig. 215-4** Examples of probable gene conversion events involving *PKD1*. Two affected individuals were discovered to have a cluster of nearly identical missense changes in exon 23 (JHU086, JHU273). Alignment of their sequences with those of two homologous loci (H1, H2) and the normal sequence (N) in the database (GenBank L33243) revealed that the sequence of JHU086 is identical to that of H2, suggesting that an H2-like locus served as template for the gene conversion event in this pedigree. Although a very similar pattern of missense changes was observed in JHU273, its sequence differs slightly from both H1 and H2, implying the existence of at least one other homologous locus. The numbers identify the position of the segment in the *PKD1* cDNA sequence. The dotted lines indicate a region of complete homology shared by the sequences while the boxes identify nucleotides that differ from the normal sequence. (*From Watnick et al.*[138] *Used with permission.*)

Most of the mutations reported to date have been small intragenic deletions, insertions, or nucleotide substitutions. Many of the mutations appear to be transcribed, but it is unknown whether any result in the synthesis of a mutant protein product in affected tissue. Preliminary in vitro studies suggest that at least some of the mutant alleles can produce stable mutant proteins (A. Bhunia, unpublished observations). The mutations are predicted to generate a wide range of mutant products, including proteins with in-frame deletions, reading frame shifts (with or without deletions or insertions), splicing abnormalities, nonsense codons, or missense changes. Most of the mutant gene products, if stable, are predicted to lack key functional domains (see below) including transmembrane-spanning regions and/or the cytoplasmic C-terminus. It is likely that even if these mutant proteins were localized correctly to the cell membrane and bound their extracellular ligands, they would be unable to transmit this information to intracellular binding partners downstream in a signaling cascade.

It is more difficult predicting the likely pathogenic effects of more subtle mutations, such as the in-frame deletions or missense substitutions. In several instances, nonconservative amino acid substitutions have been found affecting key positions within the three-dimensional structure of the PKD1 repeats.[139,140] The substitutions are predicted by computer modeling to disrupt the three-dimensional structure of polycystin-1. It is likely that some of the DNA sequence abnormalities will act indirectly by altering the gene's normal pattern of splicing or the stability of the mRNA, as has been shown for *PKD2*.[141] Functional studies are required to determine whether the remaining mutant products are less stable, processed improperly, mistargeted within the cell, or unable to bind normal ligands or interacting protein partners.

An important goal of mutation-detection studies is to determine whether particular mutations or classes of mutations correlate with the clinical presentation. In the case of ADPKD, the identification of variants associated with certain extrarenal manifestations, severe early onset disease, or the lack of renal failure would have important implications for counseling, as well as provide clues about polycystin-1 function. Unfortunately, there is little information presently available for ADPKD1. The most convincing association between presentation and genotype is that observed in a small group of children affected with severe renal cystic disease and tuberous sclerosis. Each individual was found to have large a deletion that disrupts both *PKD1* and the adjacent *TSC2* gene.[142] Watnick et al. recently reported an interesting, but less well-established, association.[114] In this study of 35 unrelated pedigrees that had individuals with either intracranial aneurysms

and/or very-early-onset disease (VEO), 3 had an identical 2-bp deletion in exon 15 (5224del2). That other studies of European populations (N = 159) failed to detect this mutation suggests that it is not a common cause of ADPKD, supporting the conclusion that the genotype may be causally associated with the phenotype.

Further evidence suggesting a possible relationship between the genotype and phenotype was recently described by Hateboer et al.[143] These investigators found interfamilial differences in a number of clinical parameters in a set of 10 large Welsh ADPKD1 families. The authors concluded that the observed interfamilial phenotypic differences were most likely due to the nature of the underlying *PKD1* mutation.

It is clear, however, that there is unlikely to be a straightforward correlation between genotype and phenotype. Mutations in diverse segments of *PKD1* have been found in severely affected individuals. Moreover, there is a range of phenotypes observed in families, including those with severely affected individuals. In the Watnick study, for example, the three pedigrees that shared the 5224del2 mutation had both classically affected individuals as well as individuals with aneurysms or early onset disease.[114] Finally, Peral et al. reported a particularly striking example of phenotypic discordance between dizygotic twins that shared an identical nonsense mutation near the 3′ end of the gene (Y3818X).[8] One child presented with VEO while the other had no evidence of cysts. In sum, it seems likely that a number of factors such as variants at other loci or environmental effects must act in concert with the primary mutation to determining clinical outcome.

Direct testing for *PKD1* mutations is currently not available as a clinical service. A number of features of the gene account for this problem. As noted above, a set of common mutations has not yet been identified. Another obstacle is the gene's very high G-C content, which makes mutation detection techniques such as single-strand conformational analysis (SSCA) less sensitive and direct DNA sequencing more prone to artifacts. The large size of *PKD1*, the presence of its homologues and its large polypyrimidine tract pose additional obstacles. Finally, it is difficult to assess the effects of many of the missense variants on protein function. Many pedigrees have been found to harbor rare missense changes that may not be seen in a population of normal controls but that also may not necessarily be pathogenic. Further study of multiple ethnic groups is required before we can establish a reliable and specific DNA-based diagnosis for ADPKD1.

## PKD2 Gene Discovery and Genetic Analysis

The genomic organization of the *PKD2* gene is far less complex than that of *PKD1*; perhaps that is why *PKD2* was discovered far more quickly. A candidate gene that had modest homology to *PKD1* was identified from a minimal genetic interval on 4q22 using positional cloning techniques.[5] A number of pathogenic, intragenic variants were found in families with chromosome 4-linked disease, confirming its identity as the gene responsible for ADPKD2. *PKD2* spans ~68 kb of genomic DNA and encodes a message of 5.4 kb composed of 15 exons.[144] Its intron-exon boundaries have been defined, but the complete genomic sequence has not yet been determined.[144]

Mutation detection of the *PKD2* gene has proceeded far more rapidly with a higher detection rate (70 to 80 percent) than for *PKD1*.[5,141,145–151] The mRNA of *PKD2* is only one-third the size of *PKD1* and the gene does not have highly homologous loci that complicate its analysis. *PKD2* also has a more balanced GC/AT content than *PKD1*, with only one exon (exon 1) that is prohibitively G-C rich. Approximately 45 *PKD2* mutations have been reported in the literature; few have been found in more than one family (www.uwcm.ac.uk/uwcm/mg/hgmd0.html). In one exception, three unrelated families were discovered to have insertions or deletions of a polyadenosine tract in exon 11, suggesting that this tract might be a relative hot spot for mutations.[146] Mutations have otherwise been generally scattered throughout most of the gene, although none have yet been reported involving exons 9, 10, or 15. The significance of this observation is unknown.

All but three of the *PKD2* mutations are predicted to result either in null alleles or in truncated proteins caused by nonsense mutations, microdeletions, microinsertions, or aberrant splicing. Given that some are predicted to be severely truncating and thus unlikely to yield a functional product, it is thought that most, if not all, will be inactivating mutations. Three missense mutations have been reported. Mutation 1532A >T results in a nonconservative substitution of an aspartic acid residue at codon 511 by valine (D511V) in the predicted third transmembrane span.[141] This aspartate is highly conserved in the family of voltage-activated cation channel subunits (to which polcystin-2 has modest homology, see below), in the *Caenorhabditis elegans PKD2* orthologue (ZK945.9), and in the *PKD2*-related PKDL protein.[152,153] Moreover, mutation of the aspartic acid residue in a K+ channel at position D258 within its S3 segment (the equivalent position of D511V in polycystin-2) results in complete loss of its activity.[154] These observations suggest that D511 also will be an inactivating mutation.

There is less information available for the other missense changes (A356P and W414G).[145,151] Both are located within the first extracellular loop of polycystin-2 but neither occurs within a known functional domain of the protein. A356 is present in mouse polycystin-2, as well as in the human *PKD2* homologue, *PKDL* but is not conserved in *C. elegans*. In contrast, W414 is highly conserved in all PKD2 family members. It is not known whether either actually results in a stable mRNA or protein. In one illustrative example, a single nucleotide substitution was found in studies of genomic DNA at position 2657A > G and was predicted to result in a single amino acid substitution (D886G).[141] RT-PCR analyses, however, failed to identify a mutant transcript with that change. Instead, a mutant product with a 37-bp deletion was discovered that resulted from activation of an upstream cryptic splice site by the 2657A > G substitution.

Unlike ADPKD1, a specific class of mutations has not yet been observed associated with a particular phenotype in ADPKD2. While one study reported finding a correlation between the location of the mutation and the severity of disease, a second failed to confirm this result.[146] It has been observed, however, that families with late onset end-stage renal disease (ESRD) may be more likely to have *PKD2* rather than *PKD1* mutations. Pei et al. selected for mutation analysis seven small ADPKD families with late onset ESRD whose pedigrees were too small to allow linkage

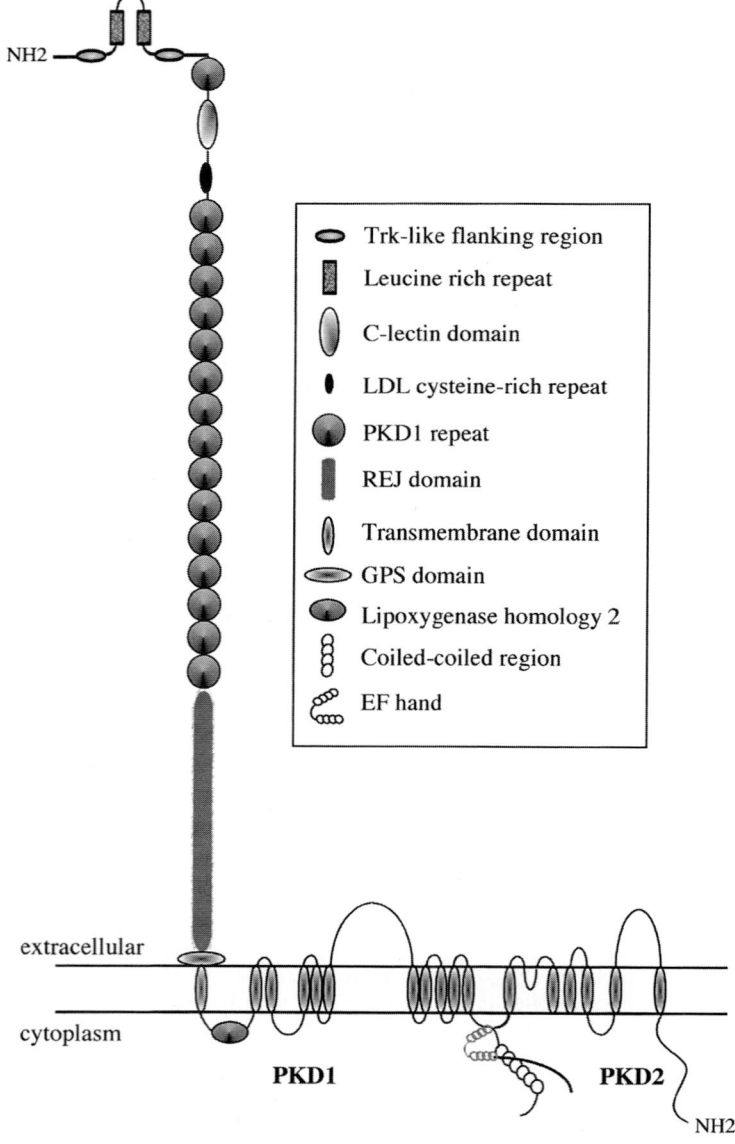

Fig. 215-5 The *PKD1* and *PKD2* gene products are integral transmembrane proteins. Polycystin-1 is predicted to have an extracellular N-terminus of ~3000 amino acids, an odd number of transmembrane-spanning elements and a short cytoplasmic C-terminus that interacts with the C-terminus of polycystin-2. It has a lengthy list of domains (shown schematically in inset box) that have been found in proteins involved in mediating cell-cell or cell matrix interactions, suggesting a similar role for polycystin-1. Polycystin-2 has homology to the voltage-activated family of calcium channels with six transmembrane spans and an EF-hand that may bind calcium and serve to regulate the channel's activity. According to the current schema, ligand binding by the extracellular N-terminus of polycystin-1 is thought to regulate the channel activity of polycystin-2. (*Modified from Watnick and Germino.[201] Used with permission.*)

testing.[146] *PKD2* mutations were identified in 5 of 7 of this group (essentially the same rate found in families with ADPKD linked to chromosome 4 markers). More extensive studies with larger datasets are required before one can use this information for counseling, but this observation may prove very helpful in guiding the selection of the appropriate test when DNA testing becomes available as a clinical service.

## PKD1 Protein Analysis

The primary peptide sequence of polycystin-1 suggests that it is likely to be a nonkinase-type membrane receptor that mediates cell-cell or cell-matrix interactions (Fig. 215-5).[4,112,113] It is predicted to have a long N-terminal extracellular domain of ~3000 amino acids followed by 7 to 11 transmembrane regions and finally a short cytoplasmic tail.[4,112,113,155,156] The cytoplasmic C-terminus is ~200 amino acids in length and has an α-helical coiled-coil structure made of five heptad repeats.[157] It has been suggested that this motif plays an essential role in mediating intracellular interactions between polycystin-1 and other signaling

molecules (see below). There are consensus sites for tyrosine and cAMP/cGMP phosphorylation nearby and these may serve to regulate the interactions.

It is presently not known what the ligands might be for the extracellular N-terminus of polcystin-1. The protein has an unusual assortment of motifs that offer tantalizing clues but no specific candidates (Fig. 215-5). The primary sequence of polycystin-1 begins with a short hydrophobic signal sequence that is followed by a pair of leucine-rich repeats (LRR). The LRRs are flanked on either side by distinctive cysteine-rich sequences that are also found in a number of other LRR-containing proteins.[158] The combination of both an amino and carboxy cysteine cluster flanking the LRRs is somewhat unusual, however, having been previously reported in only three other protein families: the trk proto-oncogenes and two developmental proteins, slit and Toll. The function of the LRRs and flanking cysteine clusters within these molecules has not been defined but they may form part of a ligand-binding region of these receptors.

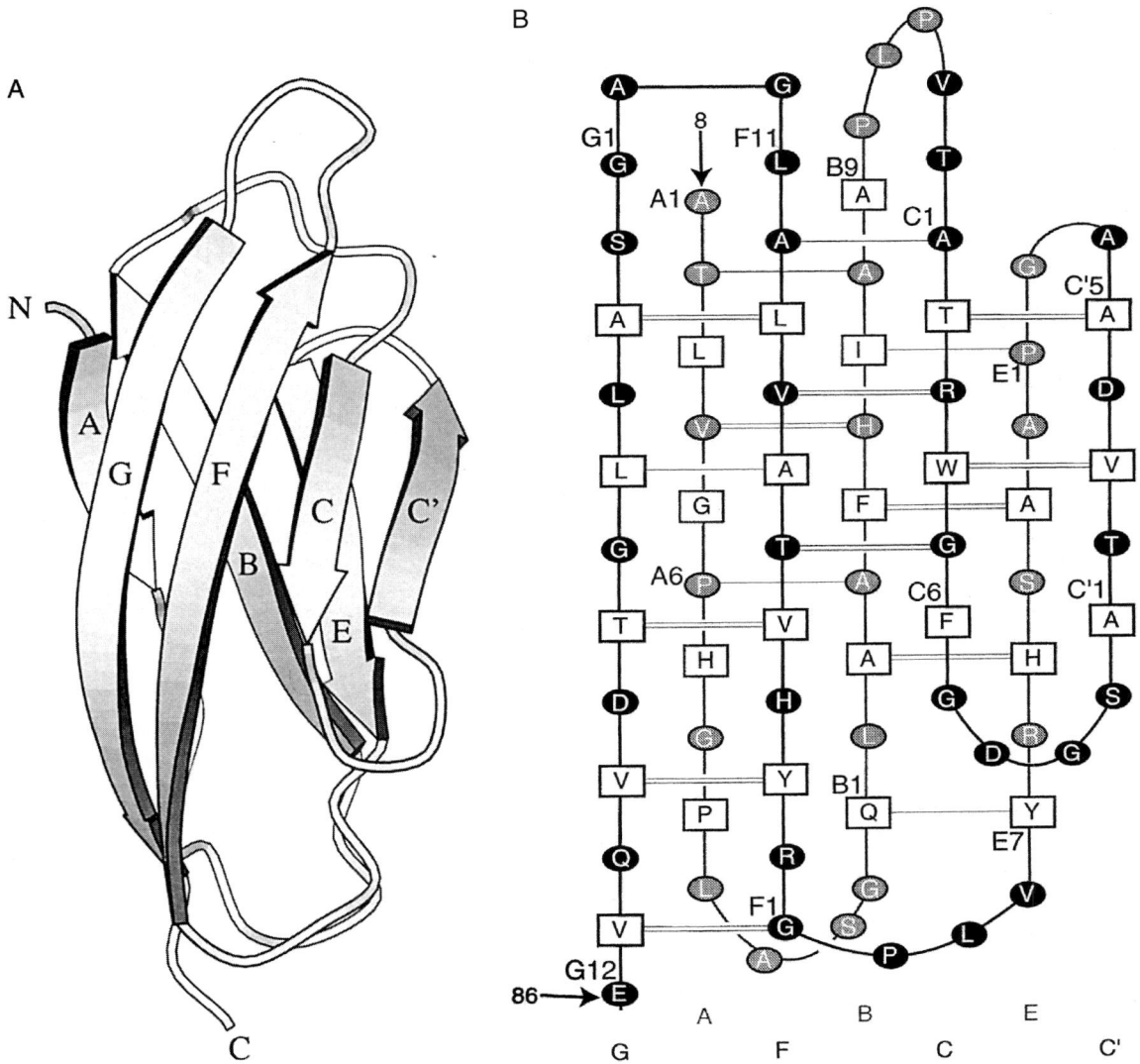

Fig. 215-6 Structural analyses of PKD domain. *A,* Secondary structure of PKD domain 1 as determined by NMR spectroscopy. The seven β-strands (labeled) form two β-sheets which are packed face to face with a well defined hydrophobic core. (*From Bycroft et al.*[140] *Used with permission.*) *B,* Diagram of the fold of PKD domain 1. The black-filled symbols identify residues that form one sheet (strands G, F, C, and C') and gray symbols identify the residues which form the other (strands A, B, and E). The one-letter code is used to identify each amino acid residue. Boxes show amino acid residues that are buried within the structure. The single and double horizontal thin lines between residues represent the main-chain hydrogen bonds that form the β-sheets. The first and last residue of each strand is identified by letter and number (e.g., G1 and G12). Loop regions of variable length connect the strands. (*From Bycroft et al.*[140] *Used with permission.*)

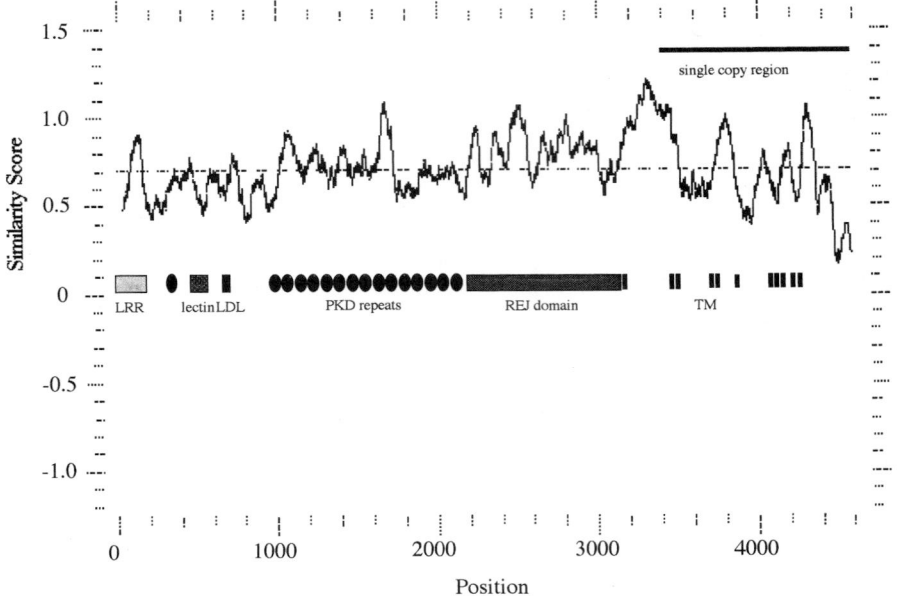

**Fig. 215-7 Similarity plot of the aligned *Fugu* and human polycystin-1 sequences.** In this figure, the amino acid position (horizontal axis) is plotted against the similarity score (y axis). A score of 1.5 represents 100 percent similarity between the two sequences, while the dashed line indicates the average degree of similarity. The approximate positions of the various domains of polycystin-1 also are shown. Regions of high similarity include the leucine rich repeats (LRRs), PKD repeat X, segments of the REJ domain, the first two intracellular loops (the first of which is the site of the LH2 domain, and the juxtamembrane portion of the cytoplasmic tail). Although the similarity score is only modest for the remainder of the C-terminus, the coiled-coil structure is highly conserved between the species. Further details of the analysis can be found in reference 156. (*From Sandford et al.*[156] *Used with permission.*)

A substantial portion of the extracellular domain of polycystin-1 is comprised of 16 copies of a repeating peptide module that is 80 to 90 amino acids in length.[4,113,140] The first unit (called a PKD domain) is positioned between the second LRR and a C-type lectin domain, and the remainder are arrayed in tandem after a single LDL-A module. This cysteine-rich domain is approximately 40 amino acids in length and is tandemly duplicated in the low-density lipoprotein receptor where it served to mediate binding to lipoproteins. It was initially thought that the PKD domain had structural properties of an immunoglobulin domain, but recent studies show that it represents a novel protein family. Bycroft et al. determined the three-dimensional structure of a representative PKD domain (domain 1) using nuclear magnetic resonance and found that it forms two β-sheets that are packed together around a well-defined hydrophobic core containing a conserved tryptophan residue[140] (Fig. 215-6*A* and *B*). Although the sequence identity between PKD1 repeat 1 and repeats 2 to 16 is low, the structure of 1 is likely to be representative because the general topography of amino acid residues for each domain is similar. The function of the

PKD repeat is unknown, although it is postulated to be a site for binding for some yet-to-be-identified factor. It has been suggested that domain 10, which is the most evolutionarily conserved from *Fugu* (puffer fish) to humans, might be the most likely to have a functional role as a ligand-binding site[140] (Fig. 215-7).

The PKD1 repeats are followed by another large segment (~1000 amino acids) that has been termed the REJ domain because it is homologous to the sea urchin sperm receptor for egg jelly (REJ).[159] The REJ receptor of sea urchin binds to matrix surrounding sea urchin eggs and the interaction results in ion-channel activation and initiation of the fertilization process.[159] It has been postulated that the REJ-matrix interaction might serve as a model for PKD1-PKD2 function because the latter has high homology to voltage-gated cation channels (see below).

Immediately preceding the first transmembrane-spanning element is a newly described GPCR proteolytic site (GPS) domain.[160] The latter was first described in G-protein-coupled receptors (GPCR). Ponting et al. reported that the GPS is highly conserved in PKD1 orthologues. The authors predict that polycystin-1 is

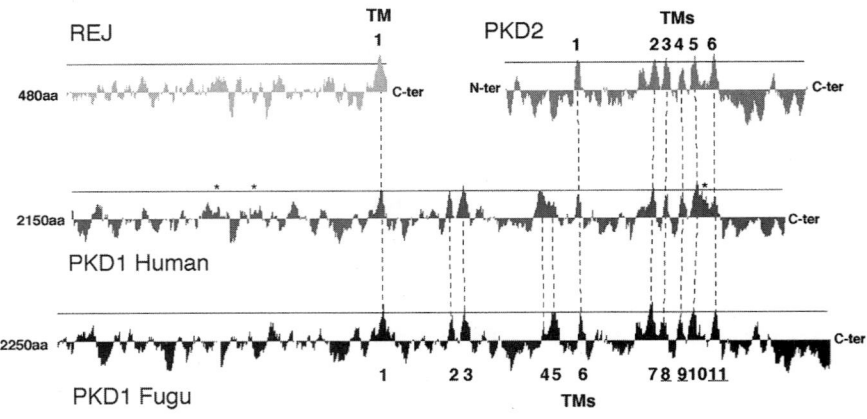

**Fig. 215-8 Comparative analysis of hydropathy plots of PKD-related proteins.** Kyte-Doolittle hydropathy plots of the C-terminal halves of human and *Fugu* polycystin-1 and REJ, as well as all of polycystin-2, are presented. The solid horizontal line in each case identifies the 2+ point of the hydrophobicity scale. Peaks that approach or exceed this value are considered possible transmembrane (TM) elements. The 11 evolutionarily conserved TM domains of human and *Fugu*

polycystin-1 predicted by this type of analysis are identified. The first TM of polycystin-1 corresponds with the single transmembrane domain of the REJ protein, while TMs 6 to 11 of polycystin-1 match TMs 1 to 6 of polycystin-2. The asterisks identify positions where earlier studies had previously placed TMs.[4] Further details of the analysis can be found in reference 156. (*From Sandford et al.*[156] *Used with permission.*)

endogenously cleaved to produce an N-terminal chain of 3048 amino acids and a C-terminal chain of 1255 residues. By analogy to other GPS proteins, it is postulated that the amino terminus is unlikely to be released postcleavage. No functional evidence in support of this model has yet been published.

The exact number of transmembrane spans (TMs) has not yet been determined, although it is universally agreed that it is very likely to be an odd number, with a consensus agreeing that it is 11. Pontig et al. suggest that TM1 of polycystin-1 may support $Ca^{2+}$ influx because a similar structure functions in this way in several other GPS-containing proteins.[160] There are no experimental data yet available to support this provocative theory. An alternative view is that the last six TMs of polycystin-1 may have channel activity. This hypothesis is based on the observation that this segment of polycystin-1 (including the corresponding intervening loops) has a modest degree of similarity with the *PKD2* gene product.[5]

Sanford et al. sought to identify important domains in polycystin-1 by assessing the degree of evolutionary conservation between the human and *Fugu* homologues[156] (Fig. 215-7). Despite being separated by nearly ~400 million years of vertebrate evolution, their overall genomic structure was very similar. The *Fugu* polycystin-1 is predicted to have 4572 amino acids with 40 percent sequence identification with and 59 percent similarity to human polycystin-1. Virtually all of the predicted functional domains were conserved between the species. Several regions had particularly high homology. The cytoplasmic region immediately adjacent to the last TM domain is 82 percent identical (88 percent similarity) over 50 amino acids in a region that includes a consensus tyrosine phosphorylation sequence, a protein kinase C phosphorylation site, and a possible binding site for G-proteins. PKD repeat 10 and several regions of the REJ domain also have very high homology and may be important sites of interaction with extracellular binding partners. A very high level of homology was unexpectedly discovered within the first cytoplasmic loop. Subsequent analyses identified a lipoxygenase homology 2 (LH2) in this region.[160] LH2 domains are noncatalytic sites present in lipoxygenases that are thought to facilitate binding of lipase and lipoxygenase substrates to the enzymes' active sites. The presence of this structure in polycystin-1 suggests a role in lipid-mediated modulation of its function. Finally, comparative analysis of the hydropathy plots of human and *Fugu* polycystin-1 identified 11 putative TM segments that are common to both, supporting the consensus model (Fig. 215-8).

There are a large number of reports describing the results of immunolocalization and immunoblot studies using either polyclonal or monoclonal α-PKD1 antibodies.[161-174] There is probably no aspect of ADPKD biology that is currently more controversial. There have been inconsistencies with respect to the nephron segments in the adult kidney and with respect to the extraepithelial cell types that express polycystin-1. There also have been disagreements over the subcellular localization of the protein, with apical, basolateral, and cytoplasmic patterns variably reported. Several studies have localized polycystin-1 to cell-cell junctions. The actual size of the protein as detected by western blot also has been disputed. Several groups have concluded that it is > 600 kDa, while most have reported a band of ~400 kDa. The inconsistent results are likely explained by either problems of antibody specificity, differences in the epitopes recognized by independently generated antibodies, different methods used to unmask epitopes, or some combination of the foregoing.

There has been general agreement on several points, however. First, it appears likely that polycystin-1 is widely expressed at low levels in many adult epithelial cell types. Second, most investigators agree that the expression of polycystin-1 is likely to be developmentally regulated with highest expression in fetal kidney and a decrease after birth. Third, most investigators agree that polycystin-1 is membrane-associated, with the majority favoring a basolateral localization. Finally, it has been uniformly observed that the amount of immunoreactivity for polycystin-1 is increased in both cystic liver and kidney.

It is noteworthy that no published study has convincingly detected either the ~3000 N-terminal or ~1200 C-terminus cleavage fragments predicted by Ponting et al. by immunoblot using antisera that recognize epitopes in the respective fragments. There are several possible explanations for this discrepancy. The cleavage may not occur, or if it does occur, it only does so under conditions not studied by these investigators. It is also possible that the cleaved fragments are unstable and rapidly degraded. If cleavage truly occurs and the products are stable, failure to detect the fragments would suggest that the antisera are not recognizing the correct protein.

## PKD2 Protein Analysis

The primary sequence of *PKD2* predicts an integral membrane protein of 968 amino acids (~110 kDa) with 6 transmembrane spanning domains nested between intracellular N- and C-termini (Figs. 215-5 and 215-8).[5] As noted above, polycystin-1 and -2 have 25 to 30 percent identity and 45 to 50 percent similarity over a 400-amino-acid segment that begins just prior to TM1 of polycystin-2 and ends just prior to TM6. Polycystin-2 has higher

**Table 215-6** Polycystin-2 Expression

| Cell type/structure | In utero expression | Postnatal expression |
|---|---|---|
| Red blood cell precursors | 3+ | 3+ |
| Mesenchymal tissues | | |
| Bone | 2+ | negative |
| Cartilage | 1+ | trace |
| Skeletal muscle | 1+ | 1+ |
| Smooth muscle | 1+ | 1+ |
| Cardiac muscle | 1+ | trace |
| Renal tissues | | |
| Mesonephros (all cells) | negative | NA |
| Metanephros | | |
| Ureteric bud | trace | negative |
| Condensing mesenchyme | negative | negative |
| Comma, S-shaped bodies | negative | negative |
| Proximal tubules | 1+ | 1+ |
| Distal tubles/MTAL | 3+ | 3+ |
| Cortical collecting ducts | NA | 2+ |
| Medullary collecting ducts | negative | 1+ |
| Glomeruli | negative | negative |
| Interstitial cells | negative | negative |
| Other epithelial tissues | | |
| Gastrointestinal epithelium | 1+ | negative |
| Endometrium | NA | negative |
| Decidualized endometrium | NA | 1+ |
| Fallopian tube epithelium | NA | negative |
| Pancreatic epithelium (exocrine) | negative | negative |
| Pulmonary parenchyma | negative | negative |
| Skin | negative | negative |
| Hepatocytes | negative | negative |
| Salivary gland | negative | negative |
| Endocrine tissues | | |
| Pancreatic islets | 1+ | 1+ |
| Pituitary | NA | 2+ |
| Adrenal cortex | 3+ (fetal adrenal cortex) | negative |
| Testes: sertoli and germ cells | NA | 1+ |
| Ovary: corpus luteum | NA | 1+ |
| Neural tissue | | |
| Neural tube | 1+ | NA |
| Forebrain | negative | negative |
| Spinal cord | negative | negative |
| Paraspinal ganglia | 1+ | trace |

sequence similarity to members of the family of voltage-gated subunits such as the $Ca^{2+}$ channel $\alpha 1E$ (VACC$\alpha$1), leading many to speculate that polycystin-2 will have ion channel activity. The region of homology begins with TM2 (S2 in the voltage-gated family members), extends into their respective cytoplasmic C-termini, and includes an EF-Hand motif. This $\alpha$-helical structure has $Ca^{2+}$ binding activity in $\sim$70 percent of the proteins in which it occurs and has been implicated in $Ca^{2+}$-sensitive inactivation of some forms of L-type VACC$\alpha$1. The EF-Hand of polycystin-2 has been shown to bind calcium in vitro, but a regulatory role has not yet been demonstrated in vivo. While polycystin-2 shares many feature with subunits of the voltage-gated channel family, its pattern of positively charged residues in TM4 (a region critical for the function of known voltage-gated channels) more closely resembles that found in some cyclic nucleotide gated channels.[156] Functional studies are required to resolve the matter.

Northern blot studies suggest that *PKD2* is ubiquitously expressed, with a high level of expression in fetal kidney and lung, and in a number of adult tissues (kidney, ovary, testis, small and large intestine, heart).[5] Immunohistochemical studies of murine tissues with polyclonal $\alpha$-polycystin-2 antisera are consistent with the mRNA studies, and suggest that the expression of polycsytin-2 is developmentally regulated[172,175] (Table 215-6). In the most complete study,[175] polycystin-2 was observed as early as the sixth embryonic day (E6) in the embryonic ectoderm and endoderm, and was present in the condensing mesenchyme of the somites and cardiac myocytes by day E9. The protein appears to be widely expressed in developing extrarenal tissues with high levels observed in red blood cell precursors, bone, and adrenal cortex. Lower levels of expression were discovered in cartilage, skeletal muscle vascular smooth muscle, the GI tract, pancreatic islets, neural tube, and paraspinal ganglia. Postnatal expression was lower in most of these tissues, with the exception of red blood cell

precursors. Moderately high levels of expression were also observed in the pituitary. Interestingly, polycystin-2 was not found using immunohistochemical techniques in the pancreas, liver, or biliary ducts although it could be detected by immunoblot.

In the developing murine kidney, only trace amounts of polycystin-2 were observed in the ureteric bud and it was absent from the condensing mesenchyme, comma and S-shaped bodies, medullary collecting ducts, the glomeruli, and interstitial cells. In contrast, moderate levels were observed in the proximal tubules, and even higher levels in the distal tubules/medullary thick-ascending limb. The pattern of staining was also different in these segments, with the protein localized to the basolateral aspect of the cell rather than the diffuse granular cytoplasmic staining observed elsewhere. In adult tissue, the intensity of Pkd2 expression in distal tubules exceeded that in any other organ or cell type (Fig. 215-9). The cortical and medullary collecting ducts also express modest amounts of the protein. In proximal tubules, the subcellular localization shifted from the diffuse cytoplasmic pattern to that observed in distal tubules, where it is localized to the basolateral membrane.

Very little information has been published on the pattern of polycystin-2 expression in human tissue. In one study of a genetically proven human ADPKD2 kidney, polycystin-2 was detected using immunohistochemical methods in a majority of cysts.[172] Interestingly, a small fraction of cysts was negative for both polycystin-1 and polycystin-2. Several other groups have reported similar findings in abstract form.

As noted above, it appears the polycystin-2 is predominantly localized to the endoplasmic reticulum (ER).[176] The protein colocalized with protein-disulfide isomerase (a resident ER protein) as determined by double-indirect immunofluorescence and codistributed with calnexin in subcellular fractionation studies of cells transfected with *PKD2* cDNA. Truncating mutations at or

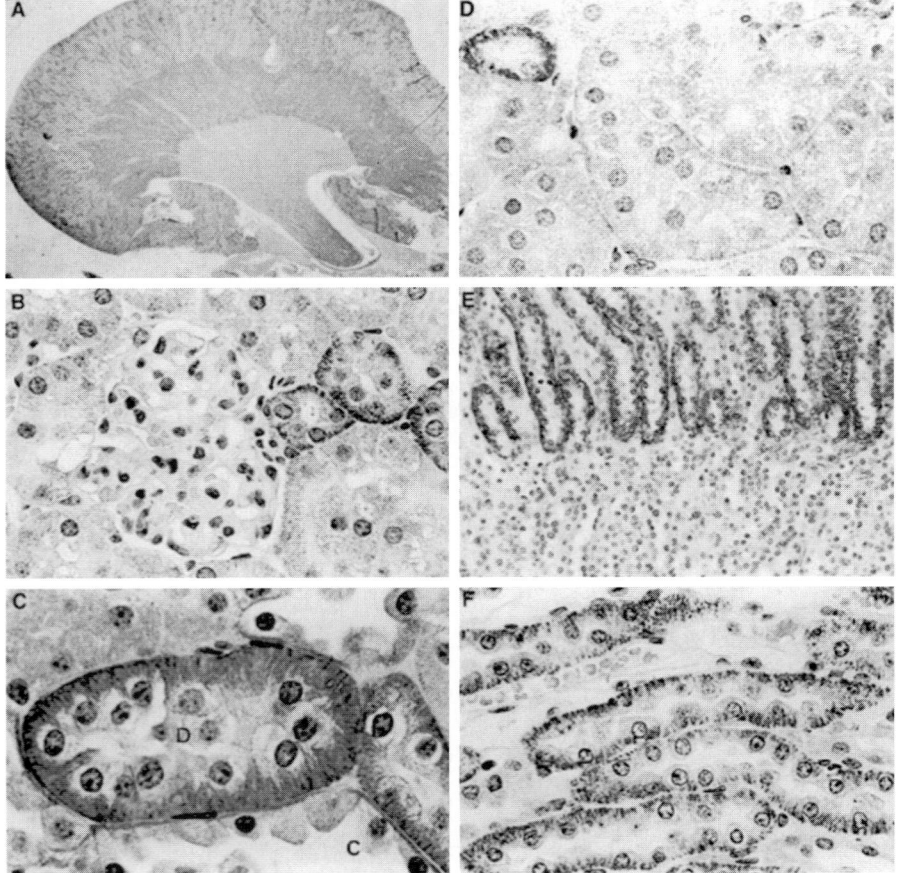

**Fig. 215-9 Polycystin-2 expression in the adult murine kidney. *A*, Whole mount of kidney from normal 4-month-old mouse stained with $\alpha$-PKD2 antisera. Pkd2 expression is limited to distal nephron segments of cortex, medullary thick-ascending limbs of inner stripe of outer medulla, and collecting tubules of papillary tip (×10). *B*, High-power view (×315) of cortex showing strong basolateral staining of distal convoluted tubules and macula densa, and faint staining in proximal tubules. *C*, Prominent basolateral staining is seen in the distal tubules ("D") while a thin line of basal positivity is seen in a cortical collecting duct ("C") (×475). *D*, Proximal tubules have slight basolateral positivity. The more intensely staining structure at top left is a distal tubule (×475). *E*, There is an abrupt transition in staining at the junction of the inner stripe of outer medulla and inner medulla that corresponds to the transition from medullary thick-ascending limbs (which stain positive) to thin-descending limbs of Henle (which stain negative) (×200). *F*, Collecting ducts of the papillary tip have strong staining for Pkd2 (×475). (*From Markowitz et al.[175] Used with permission.*)**

before Q787 result in proteins that traffic to both the ER and the plasma membrane. A 34-amino-acid region (Q787-S820) was found responsible for the exclusive localization of polycystin-2 to the ER, and it is postulated to be a binding site for some as of yet unidentified protein.

The function of polycystin-2 is unknown, but it is postulated to have ion channel activity. Overexpression of PKD2 in cells, however, has not resulted in new ion channel activity, suggesting that other factors were likely required to reconstitute this function. Polycystin-1 is a leading candidate for this role.

Recent studies suggest that PKD2 may be the prototype of a new family of channel proteins. Homologues (? orthologues) have been identified in other species, including two in *Caenorhabditis elegans*, and it is likely that the list will lengthen as the complete sequence of the various genomes becomes available. In humans, a homologue called *PKDL* has 50 percent amino acid sequence identity and 71 percent homology to *PKD2*.[152,153] It shares all of the major features of polycystin-2, including six transmembrane-spanning domains, a putative $Ca^{2+}$-binding EF hand, and a cytoplasmic coiled-coil domain. It also has been reported to be highly expressed in fetal tissues as determined by northern analysis. Mapping studies have assigned it to chromosome 10q24 and to distal chromosome 19 in the mouse. The murine homologue maps into a region that is deleted in the *kdr* (kidney and retinal defects) mutant. Human *PKDL* is an obvious candidate gene for the unlinked form of ADPKD, but studies of six unlinked ADPKD families failed to find linkage.

Oocyte expression studies using *PKDL* have provided the first experimental evidence that members of the PKD2 family are ion channels. Chen et al. showed by patch clamp experiments of frog oocytes injected with cRNA that polycystin-L is a calcium-modulated nonselective cation channel that is permeable to sodium, potassium, and calcium ions.[177] The high degree of similarity between PKD2 and PKDL suggests a similar function for polycystin-2.

## PKD Pathways

The predicted roles of polycystin-1 as a receptor and polycystin-2 as a possible $Ca^{2+}$ channel suggest that both molecules participate in signaling pathways that regulate normal renal tubule function. Given that the N-terminus of polycystin-1 has multiple potential binding sites for extracellular molecules, much attention has been focused on its cytoplasmic C-terminus as a likely transducer of extracellular signals to the intracellular milieu.

The nearly identical clinical profiles that result from mutations of *PKD1* and *PKD2* suggest that their translation products may be tightly linked in a common signaling pathway (Fig. 215-5). A series of in vitro and in vivo studies subsequently showed that the two proteins do associate.[157,178] The interaction occurs between the C-terminus of polycystin-2 and the coiled-coil domain of polycystin-1. Both naturally occurring mutations and amino acid substitutions, if introduced in such a way as to disrupt the α-helical structure of the PKD1 coiled-coil structure, are capable of abolishing the interaction. These studies suggest that one function of polycystin-1 might be to regulate the activity of polycystin-2. These data also provide the first mechanism whereby mutations of either gene could result in disease.

Four other activities have been assigned to the C-terminus of polycystin-1. First, overexpression of just this fragment of PKD1 in mammalian cells increases the kinase activity of JNK kinase, thereby triggering activation of the transcription factor AP-1.[179] This effect was nearly abrogated by dominant negative mutants of two small GTP-binding proteins, Rac-1 and Cdc42, suggesting an essential role for members of the Rho family of GTP-binding proteins in PKD-regulated pathways. Given the role of this family in the regulation of cell motility, shape, and adhesion, it is reasonable to postulate that they could be involved in the pathogenesis of cyst formation.

A second study identified within the very highly conserved segment of the C-terminus of polycystin-1, a potential 20-amino-

acid heterotrimeric G-protein activation sequence that is capable of a physical interaction in vitro with heterotrimeric G-proteins. Given that some models of polycystin-1 predict only seven TM spans, some have proposed that it may be a novel member of GPCR family.[180] It lacks, however, the additional signature features that readily identify other GPCRs, so polycystin-1 would have to be the prototype of an unusual, new class.[181]

The third putative interacting partner of the C-terminus of polycystin-1 is RGS7.[182] The latter is a member of a newly discovered family of proteins called the regulators of G-protein signaling. Members have an ~120-amino-acid domain that accelerates the intrinsic GTPase activity of Gαi and Gαq subunits, thereby causing their inactivation. Overexpression of a membrane-targeted form of the PKD1 C-terminus inhibited the degradation of overexpressed RGS7 and induced its relocalization to the membrane. The identification of a G-protein binding site near a putative site of interaction with a regulator of G-protein signaling suggests a potential key role for PKD1 in regulating G-protein signaling.

The final activity assigned to the C-terminus of polycystin-1 was also identified by its overexpression in mammalian cells. Kim et al. found by this approach that the PKD1 C-terminus is capable of stabilizing soluble endogenous β-catenin by inhibiting glycogen synthase kinase (GSK)-3b activity.[183] This resulted in the accumulation of β-catenin in both the cytoplasm and nucleus, where it interacted with members of the T-cell-specific transcription factor/lymphoid enhancer-binding factor (TCF/LEF) family of transcription factors to regulate gene transcription. They also found that microinjection of zebra fish embryos with constructs expressing the polycystin-1 C-terminus induced dorsalization. The authors suggest that one function of polycystin-1 may be to modulate Wnt signaling during renal development.

Few functional studies have been reported for polycystin-2. Tsiokas et al. identified modest homology between PKD2 and members of the mammalian transient-receptor potential-channel proteins (TRP).[184] This class of proteins is thought to be activated

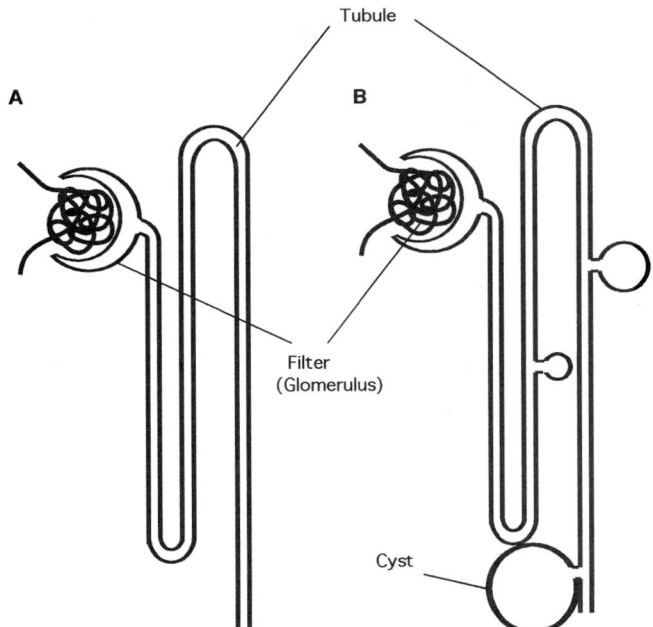

**Fig. 215-10 Illustration of the origin of tubular cysts. *A*, Cartoon of a normal nephron showing the glomerulus and its tubule. *B*, Microdissection studies of early ADPKD kidneys show that cysts begin as small focal outgrowths from any nephron segment.[186] As shown in this cartoon, more than one cyst can arise from a single nephron. (*Modified from Watnick and Germino.[201] Used with permission.*)**

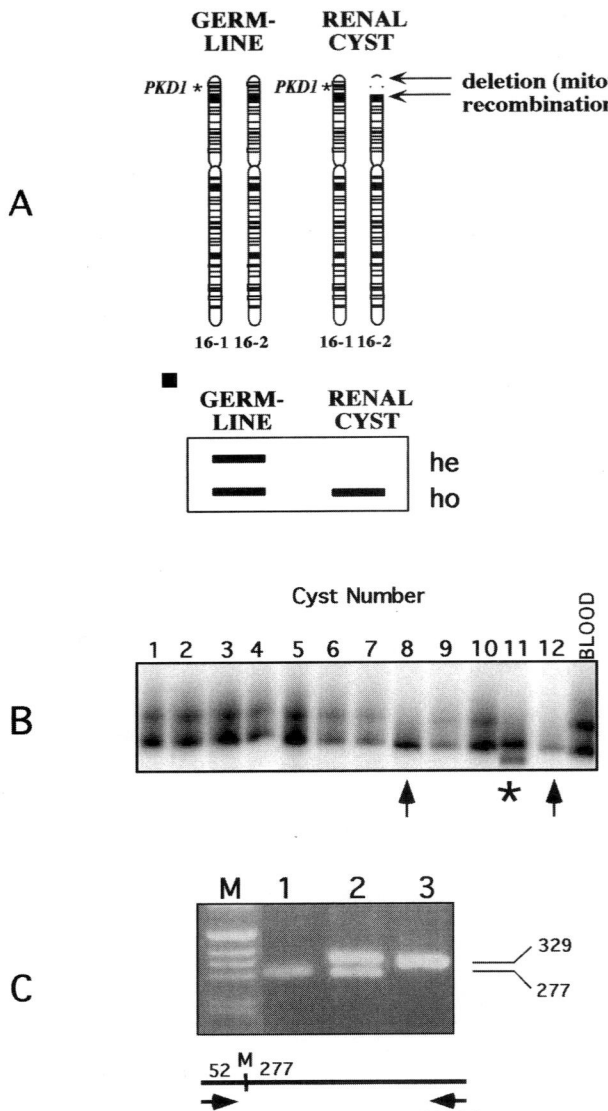

Fig. 215-11 Molecular genetic studies of cystic tissue suggest that ADPKD is a "two-hit" disease. *A*, Every cell in an individual with ADPKD1 contains two copies of chromosome 16, one of which contains a mutant copy of *PKD1* transmitted from the affected parent (*PKD1\**). Reduction to hemizygosity (via deletion) or homozygosity (via mitotic recombination[202]) for the mutant allele of *PKD1* in cystic tissue can be detected by testing for loss-of-heterozygosity (LOH) for intragenic polymorphisms. In this example, variants at the polymorphic locus *EJ1* (see Fig. 215-3 for its position) can be detected by heteroduplex analysis. Homoduplexes (Ho) appear as a single band, whereas heteroduplexes (He) have a different electrophoretic pattern on nondenaturing gels. LOH, if present in cystic tissue, results in loss of heteroduplex formation. *B*, Heteroduplex analysis of the *EJ1* locus of DNA from 12 separate liver cysts and a blood sample of an individual with ADPKD1. Although the blood sample and most of the cysts have two bands because of heteroduplex formation, cysts 8 and 12 (arrows) have only one band suggesting LOH for one of the alleles. Cyst 11 (asterisk) has a novel heteroduplex pattern suggesting an acquired mutation altering one of the alleles rather than LOH. (*Adapted from Watnick et al.[188] Used with permission.*). *C*, The germ line mutation in this individual (12589C > G) creates a premature stop codon and a new *Mael* site (M). Restriction analysis of the germ line DNA of this individual (amplified from blood) (lane 2) and cyst 12 (lane 1) shows that the germ line sample has both alleles (329 bp 277 bp), while the cyst has retained only the mutant *PKD1* (277 bp). Lane 3 shows the undigested product amplified from the blood of this individual. The 52 bp product that results from *Mael* digestion is not visible in this figure. In other studies, the novel allele detected in cyst 11 was found to result from an acquired 2 bp insertion (12,762insGC) that disrupts the reading frame of the C-terminus. (*Adapted from Watnick et al.[188] Used with permission.*).

by GPCR activation and/or depletion of $Ca^{2+}$ stores. Given that TRPs form functional homo- and heteromultimeric complexes, the investigators tested for a possible interaction between TRPs and PKD2. They found by coexpression studies that polycystin-2 can directly associate with TRPC1 but not with TRPC3, suggesting some specificity to the process. Functional studies have not yet been reported.

This same group of investigators also found that overexpression of polycystin-2 in mammalian cells resulted in AP-1 activation that was mediated by mitogen-activated kinase p38, JNK1, and protein kinase C (PKC) epsilon, a calcium-independent PKC isozyme.[185] Interestingly, treatment with a calcium chelator failed to block polycystin-2-mediated signaling in this system.

### Mechanism of Cyst Formation

An important step in determining the pathogenesis of a disease is defining the mechanism by which mutations result in an abnormal phenotype. An important clue was provided by microdissection studies of early ADPKD kidneys that showed that cysts arise as focal outgrowths from renal tubules[186] (Fig. 215-10). These observations suggested that cyst formation is likely a two-step process.

Using a novel method to isolate DNA from relatively pure populations of epithelial cells from single cysts, Qian et al.

demonstrated that renal cysts are predominantly monoclonal.[187] Furthermore, they found loss of heterozygosity (LOH) for the wild-type allele in ~15 to 20 percent of both renal and liver cysts[187,188] (Fig. 215-11). Several other groups have reported similar findings.[189,190] When techniques for *PKD1* mutation detection were applied to the genetic analysis of individual cysts, it was possible to find intragenic mutations affecting the normal allele in up to 50 percent of cysts.[188] Several studies of cystic tissue obtained from individuals with genetically proven ADPKD2 tissue have revealed similar findings.[191–193] LOH and intragenic *PKD2* mutations were consistently found disrupting the wild-type allele.

The data strongly suggest that ADPKD is another example of a "two-hit" disease as originally described by Knudson[194] (Fig. 215-12). The one "normal" allele of either *PKD1* in ADPKD1 or *PKD2* in ADPKD2 provides sufficient levels of polycystin-1 or -2 to support normal tubular maturation. Over time, however, somatic mutations of the wild-type allele are acquired, which result in a loss of functional protein below a critical level, a disruption of the signaling pathway that maintains tubular integrity, and cyst formation occurs. The time point at which somatic mutations occur (early in development vs. in adult tubules), and the rate at which they are acquired, may be critical

## A)            B)

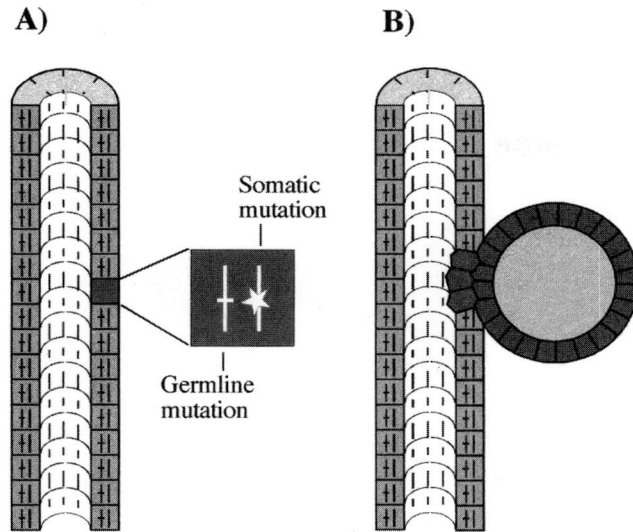

**Fig. 215-12 Knudson's "two-hit" model is the likely explanation of focal cyst formation in ADPKD. Every cell in the kidney of an individual who has inherited ADPKD has a germline mutation of *PKD1* (or *PKD2*). In most cells, the normal allele produces a sufficient amount of polycystin to allow the normal tubule differentiation program to proceed during renal development. In the fully developed organ, a single functional allele is presumably adequate to maintain normal tubular architecture. When an individual tubular cell, however, sustains a somatic mutation leading to loss of the wild-type *PKD1* (*PKD2*) allele, the level of functional protein falls below a critical threshold necessary to support differentiation (during development) or suppress proliferation (postdevelopment) leading to cystic expansion of the tubule via pathways that have not yet been identified. Simple acquired cysts, which are common in the general population and which increase in frequency with age, may be examples of random inactivation of both copies of *PKD1* or *PKD2*. (From Qian and Watnick.[203] Used with permission.)**

determinants of disease severity, and may account for the significant clinical variability that is observed. *PKD2*, which causes ADPKD with approximately one-sixth the frequency of *PKD1*, may be less mutable, and thus acquire "second hits" at a moderately lower rate, resulting in a less severe form of disease. It is also tempting to speculate that the simple cysts commonly found in the normal population may be examples of "sporadic disease" in which individual cells have acquired somatic mutations of both alleles of an ADPKD gene.

An interesting observation to consider is the high rate at which second hits must occur to account for the number of cysts that are observed in a nonproliferative tissue (adult renal epithelia has a very low proliferation index).[195] It is estimated that up to 1 percent of nephrons acquire cysts, with $10^2$ to $10^4$ cysts developing in each kidney. If each cyst is unique (as genetic studies thus far suggest), it implies a "second-hit" rate that is significantly higher than what is commonly observed with other tumor-suppressor type genes. Several possible explanations are mutually compatible. First, it is likely that, as suggested by Tishfield,[196] the somatic mutation rate is higher than is commonly recognized. Second, the kidney and liver, as the major sites of concentration and detoxification for the body, may potentially be highly exposed to mutagenizing factors. Third, the pathway regulated by *PKD1* and *PKD2* may be closely linked to the phenotype. Unlike most other tumor syndromes in which multiple genetic events are required for progression, loss of either *PKD1* or *PKD2* is sufficient to result in a disease phenotype. The pathway has a critical bottleneck with no redundancy, making it exquisitely sensitive to perturbations.

An obvious challenge to the "two-hit" model is reconciling the results of antibody studies that show an increased abundance of polycystin-1 and -2 in cystic epithelia with the molecular genetic

data that suggest show a high rate of somatic mutation.[197] In one particularly illustrative example, the authors examined tissue from individuals with known mutations of *PKD1*.[171] The samples were selected for analysis because the germ line mutation was known to cause loss of the epitope recognized by the antibodies used in the study. If either LOH or truncating mutations were an essential step in the pathogenesis of cyst formation, one would expect that most cysts should lack staining by immunohistochemical analysis. In fact, most cysts had positive staining with the antisera.

There are several possible explanations for these discrepant findings.[192] First, if the two-hit model is correct and a somatic mutation is required for each cyst to form, it is possible that most of the mutations are missense changes that inactivate the protein's function. The immunohistochemical analyses cannot distinguish between functional and nonfunctional proteins. An alternative explanation is that somatic mutations are not essential for the initiation of cyst formation but instead provide a growth advantage. Because the molecular studies were performed using material from larger cysts, it is possible that the approach introduced a bias. Finally, it is assumed that the antibodies used for the immunohistochemistry studies are specific. There is a mounting body of evidence that raises doubts about this assumption, though most of it has only been presented in abstract form. In one very provocative study, investigators performed complete mutation analysis of 28 individual PKD2 cysts. Acquired, inactivating mutations were detected in 20. The rate of detection (71 percent) is approximately equal to that of studies of germ line *PKD2* mutations. Moreover, virtually all were predicted to be truncating rather than missense changes. It is clear that further study will be required to resolve this controversy.

## ANIMAL MODELS OF ADPKD

Murine lines with targeted mutations of *Pkd1* and *Pkd2* have provided strong support for the two-hit model of cyst formation. Because there are no naturally occurring murine models of ADPKD1 or ADPKD2, investigators used homologous recombination to create the mutant alleles. In the case of ADPKD1, a mutant allele that mimicked a known truncating mutation of human exon 34[198,199] was produced. Heterozygous mice with a single mutant allele developed a few cysts, while homozygous animals developed severe cystic disease and universally died in utero or in the perinatal period. Renal development progressed normally until embryonic day 15, indicating that the earliest stages of renal development (mesonephric stages, ureteric bud outgrowth, and induction of metanephric mesenchyme) can proceed normally in the absence of polycystin-1 (Fig. 215-13). After this point, renal cysts begin appearing in the proximal tubules and rapidly progress to replace the entire renal parenchyma. Although the pattern of PKD1 antibody staining in the homozygous animals has not yet been described, a recent follow-up report suggests that most cysts present in heterozygous mutants are not immunoreactive.[199] Severe pancreatic cystic disease was also noted in the homozygous animals, although liver cysts were not observed. The cause of preterm lethality has not yet been described—renal disease in itself is an unlikely explanation.

Several different mutant murine *Pkd2* alleles have been developed.[200] In the first, a germ line null allele of *Pkd2* was generated by disruption of exon 1. Mice heterozygous for this allele ($Pkd2^{+/-}$) developed occasional renal and hepatic cysts and immunostaining studies confirmed that the cysts lacked polycystin-2. Homozygous mice ($Pkd2^{-/-}$) were not viable and died in utero. Fetal animals that survived to day E16.5 or later had severe cystic disease with multiple tubular and glomerular cysts. The cause of fetal demise was attributed to cardiac failure since cardiac defects were frequently observed.

The second murine Pkd2 line has an unstable *Pkd2* allele that contains tandem copies of the first exon of *Pkd2* ($Pkd2^{WS25}$).[200] This allele is prone to acquiring somatic mutations at a very high rate via intragenic homologous recombination. $Pkd2^{WS25/WS25}$

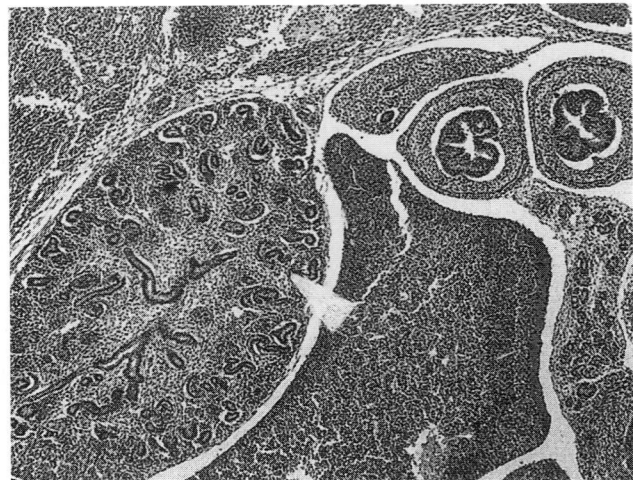

A

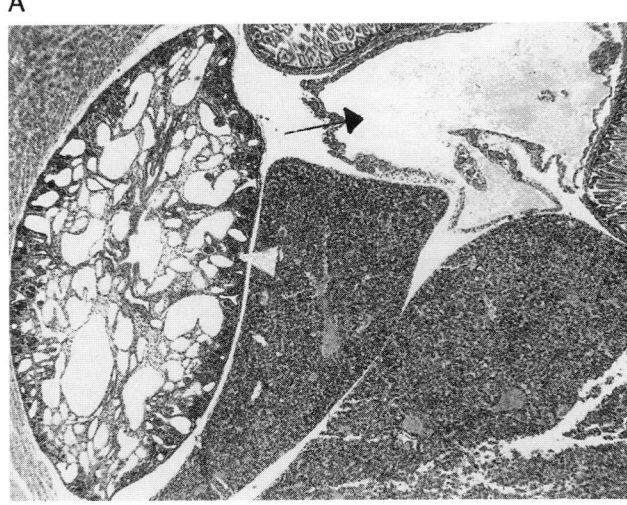

B

Fig. 215-13 Polycystins are essential for normal tubular maturation. *A*, Day E14.5 of gestation of normal murine embryo. Ureteric bud branching and induction of metanephric mesenchyme is well advanced in the kidney (arrowhead). Comma and S-shaped bodies have begun to form with more central portions of the kidney (medulla) further developed than those near the periphery (cortex). *Pkd1*$^{-/+}$ and *Pkd1*$^{-/-}$ kidneys appear to develop normally up until this stage (×50). *B*, Day E16.5 of gestation of *Pkd1*$^{-/-}$ embryo. Cysts first begin to appear at approximately day E15, primarily involving medullary segments, and become very pronounced by day 16 (white arrowhead). This stage is an important phase of tubular elongation and maturation. Also visible in this view is a massive pancreatic cyst (black arrow) which is commonly observed in *Pkd* null animals[198] (*unpublished observation*). (*Photos courtesy of K. Piontek and D. Huso, Johns Hopkins University.*)

mice developed cystic disease of variable severity (Fig. 215-14). An intercross of a *Pkd2* null allele (*Pkd2*$^{+/-}$) with mice carrying an the unstable allele (*Pkd2*$^{WS25/+}$ and *Pkd2*$^{WS25/WS25}$) produced compound *cis*-heterozygous mice (*Pkd2*$^{WS25/-}$) that consistently developed an ADPKD phenotype very similar to that observed in humans. The Pkd2$^{WS25/-}$ mice survived to birth and by 11 weeks had developed significant, bilateral renal cystic disease as well as hepatic cysts. As expected, using immunohistochemical methods, the cysts were found to lack polcycystin-2.

These animal studies suggest that loss of functional polycystin-1 or -2 below a critical threshold results in a block in the differentiation program of the kidney. Although it is highly likely that the proteins also are essential for maintenance of tubular integrity, the current models cannot adequately resolve the matter

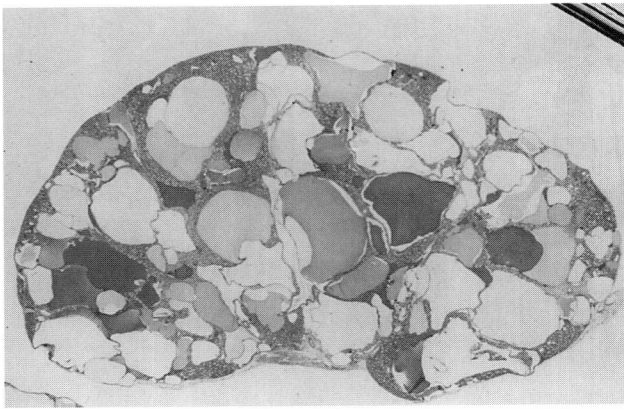

A

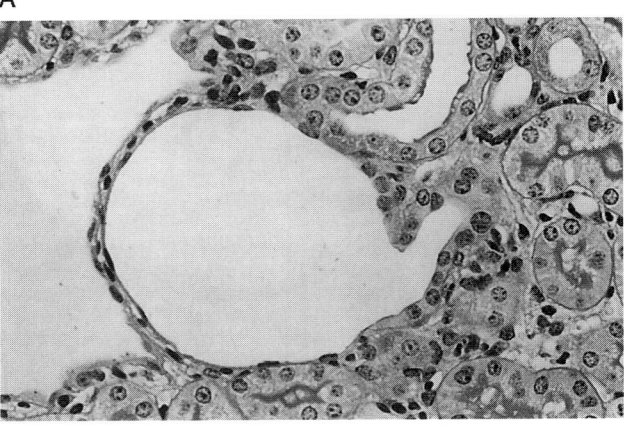

B

Fig. 215-14 Cysts arise from somatic mutation of *Pkd2* in a murine model of ADPKD2. *A*, Cross-section of an adult murine kidney removed from an animal that was homozygous for an unstable *Pkd2* allele (*Pkd2*$^{WS25/WS25}$). Severe cystic disease closely mimicking the pattern seen in human ADPKD is observed. Details of the model can be found in reference 200. *B*, Renal cysts have a focal origin as illustrated in this magnified view of a kidney section taken from a mouse with the *Pkd2*$^{WS25/WS25}$ genotype. An early cyst has begun to form as a small focal outgrowth from a segment of normal tubule. Immunohistochemical studies of similar structures using α-PKD2 antisera revealed the absence of polycystin-2 in the cyst-lining epithelia, which is consistent with homozygous inactivation of the *Pkd2* gene as the likely mechanism responsible for the focal origin. (*From Wu et al.*[200] *Used with permission.*)

because it is not known at what time point the acquired mutations actually occur in the heterozygous animals. Animals with *Pkd1* or *Pkd2* alleles that can be conditionally inactivated in a controlled fashion will resolve the issue.

## CONCLUSIONS

Discovery of the genes responsible for ADPKD has provided powerful new tools that have greatly enhanced our understanding of molecular pathogenesis and yielded some surprising new insights. ADPKD joins the lengthening list of diseases that arise through a "two-hit" mechanism. Murine lines with inactivating mutations of *Pkd1* and *Pkd2* have been created using gene-targeting techniques that have already yielded important insights into the developmental role of PKD proteins. With progressive refinements, the animal models will prove invaluable for exploring the function of the PKD proteins, identifying modifying loci, defining the pathogenesis of disease, and testing various therapeutic interventions.

There are obviously many important problems yet to be addressed. The correct localization of polycystin-1 remains uncertain and the conflicting results that have been reported must be reconciled with each other, as well as with the results of genetic studies of cystic tissue. The function of polycystin-1 and -2 must be determined and in vitro assays are required for assessing the function of either gene product. The signaling pathways regulated by either protein must be conclusively defined. Finally, better methods for accurate and rapid mutation screening of *PKD1* (and *PKD2*) are required before these tests can be implemented in the clinical arena as useful and cost-effective diagnostic tools.

From a basic science perspective, ADPKD offers a unique opportunity to investigate an aspect of renal development that is very poorly understood: the factors and signaling pathways that determine size of tubule diameter. The results of the animal studies described in the preceding section suggest that neither polycystin is essential for the earliest developmental stages of the kidney to proceed. The data suggest that loss of either in the later stages of gestation results in an apparent block in the maturation of the tubule. The genes responsible for causing ADPKD appear to regulate a critical step in the maturation pathway of tubular epithelia. Moreover, it is very likely that they play a similar role in the maintenance of mature tubular epithelia in postdevelopmental tissues. Study of ADPKD is likely to offer new insights into these fundamentally important topics.

## ACKNOWLEDGMENTS

The authors thank the numerous patients and their families who have participated in our studies as well as the various funding agencies who have supported their studies: the Polycystic Kidney Disease Research Foundation, the National Kidney Foundation, the McKutcheon Foundation, and the National Institutes of Health. GGG is the Irving Blum Scholar of the Johns Hopkins University School of Medicine.

## REFERENCES

1. Agodoa LYC, Held PJ, Port FK: *United States RDS. United States Renal Data System 1998 Annual Data Report.* Bethesda, MD, The National Institutes of Health, National Institute of Diabetes and Digestive and Kidney Diseases, 1998.
2. Gabow PA: Autosomal dominant polycystic kidney disease — More than a renal disease. *Am J Kidney Dis* **16(5)**:403, 1990.
3. Ravine D, Walker RG, Givson RN, Sheffield LJ, Kincaid-Smith P, Danks DM: Treatable complications in undiagnosed cases of autosomal dominant polycystic kidney disease. *Lancet* **337(8734)**:127, 1991.
4. Hughes J, Ward CJ, Peral B, et al: The polycystic kidney disease 1 (PKD1) gene encodes a novel protein with multiple cell recognition domains. *Nat Genet* **10**:151, 1995.
5. Mochizuki T, Wu G, Hayashi T, et al: PKD2, a gene for polycystic kidney disease that encodes an integral membrane protein. *Science* **272**:1339, 1996.
6. Kimberling WJ, Kumar S, Gabow PA, Kenyon JB, Connolly CJ, Somlo S: Autosomal dominant polycystic kidney disease: Localization of the second gene to chromosome 4q13-q23. *Genomics* **18(3)**:467, 1993.
7. Breuning MH: Improved early diagnosis of adult polycystic kidney disease with flanking DNA markers. *Lancet* **2**:1359, 1987.
8. Peral B, Ong AC, San Millan JL, Gamble V, Rees L, Harris PC: A stable, nonsense mutation associated with a case of infantile onset polycystic kidney disease 1 (PKD1). *Hum Mol Genet* **5(4)**:539, 1995.
9. Milutinovic J, Rust PF, Fialkov PJ, Adodoa LY, Phillips LA, Rudd TG, Sutherland S: Intra-familial phenotypic expression of autosomal dominant polycystic kidney disease. *Am J Kidney Dis* **19(5)**:465, 1992.
10. Sujansky E, Kreutzer SB, Johnson AM, Lezotte DC, Schrier RW, Gabow PA: Attitudes of at-risk and affected individuals regarding presymptomatic testing for autosomal dominant polycystic kidney disease. *Am J Med Genet* **35(4)**:510, 1990.
11. Begleiter Ml, Smith TH, Harris DJ: Ultrasound for genetic counseling in polycystic kidney disease. *Lancet* **2**:1073, 1977.
12. Simbaldi D, Malena S, Mangarell R, Rizzoni G: Prenatal ultrasonographic findings of dominant polycystic kidney disease and postnatal renal evolution. *Am J Med Genet* **65(4)**:337, 1996.
13. Gabow PA, Kimberling WJ, Strain JD, Manco-Johnson ML, Johnson AM: Utility of ultrasonography in the diagnosis of autosomal dominant polycystic kidney disease in children. *J Am Soc Nephrol* **8(1)**:105, 1997.
14. Levine E, Gantham JJ: The role of computed tomography in the evaluation of ADPKD. *Am J Kidney Disease* **1**:99, 1981.
15. Levine E, Grantham JJ: Diagnosis of ADPKD: Complications and radiologic recognition, in Grantham JJ, Gardner KD Jr (eds): *Problems in Diagnosis and Management of Polycystic Kidney Disease.* Kansas City, PKR Foundation, 1985.
16. Parfrey PS, Bear Jc, Morgan J, Cramer BC, McManamon PJ, Gault JH, Churchill DN, et al: The diagnosis and prognosis of autosomal dominant polycystic kidney disease. *N Engl J Med* **323(16)**:1085, 1990.
17. Elles RG, Hodgkinson KA, Mallick NP, O'Donoghue DJ, Read AP, Rimmer S, Watters EA, et al: Diagnosis of adult polycystic kidney disease by genetic markers and ultrasonographic imaging in a voluntary family register. *J Med Genet* **31**:115, 1994.
18. Gabow PA, Ikle DW, Holmes JH: Polycystic kidney disease: Prospective analysis of non-azotemic patients and family members. *Ann Intern Med* **101**:238, 1984.
19. Mir S, Rapola J, Koskimies O: Renal cysts in pediatric autopsy material. *Nephron* **33**:189, 1983.
20. Ravine D, Gibsen RN, Donlan J, Sheffield LJ: An ultrasound renal cyst prevalence survey: Specificity data for inherited renal cystic diseases. *Am J Kidney Dis* **22(6)**:803, 1993.
21. Ravine D: Evaluation of ultrasonographic diagnostic criteria for autosomal dominant polycystic kidney disease. *Lancet* **1(343)**:824, 1994.
22. Ravine D, Walker RG, Gibson RN Forrest SM, Richards RL, Friend K, Sheffield L, et al: Phenotype and genotype heterogeneity in autosomal dominant polycystic kidney disease. *Lancet* **340**:1330, 1992.
23. Lesias DM, Palmitano JA, Arrizurieta E, Kornblihtt AR, Herrera M, Bernath V, Martin RS: Isolated polycystic liver disease not linked to polycystic kidney disease 1and 2. *Dig Dis Sci* **44(2)**:385, 1999.
24. Lipschitz B, Berdon WE, Deflice AR, Levy J: Association of congenital hepatic fibrosis with ADPKD. Report of a family with review of literature. *Pediat Radiol* **23(2)**:131, 1993.
25. Jordon D, Harnaz N, Thung SN: Caroli's disease and adult polycystic kidney disease: A rarely recognized association. *Liver* **9(1)**:30, 1989.
26. Gabow PA, Johnson AM, Kaehny WD, Manco-Johnson ML, Duley IT, Everson GT: Risk factors for the development of hepatic cysts in autosomal dominant polycystic kidney disease. *Hepatology* **11**:1033, 1990.
27. Chaveau D, Pirson Y, Le Moine A, Franco D, Belghiti J, Grunfeld JP: Extrarenal manifestations in autosomal dominant polycystic kidney disease. *Adv Nephrol Necker Hosp* **26**:265, 1997.
28. Sherstha R, McKinley C, Russ P, Scherzinger A, Brunner T, Showalter R, Everson GT: Postmenopausal estrogen therapy selectively stimulates hepatic enlargement in women with autosomal dominant polycystic kidney disease. *Hepatology* **26(5)**:1282, 1998.
29. Everson GT, Scherzinger A, Berger-Leff N, Reichen J, Lezotte, Manco-Johnson M, Gabow P: Polycystic liver disease: quantification of parenchymal and cyst volumes from computed tomography images and clinical correlates of hepatic cysts. *Hepatology* **8**:1627, 1988.
30. Torres VE, Rastogi S, King BF, Stanson AW, Gross JB Jr, Nogorney DM: Hepatic venous outflow obstruction in autosomal dominant polycystic kidney disease. *J Am Soc Nephrol* **5**:1186, 1994.
31. Newman KD, Torres VE, Rakela J, Nagorney DM: Treatment of highly symptomatic polycystic liver disease: Preliminary experience with a combined hepatic resection-fenestration procedure. *Ann Surg* **212**:30, 1990.
32. Katkhouda N, Hurwitz M, Gugenheim J, Mavor E, Mason RJ, Waldrep DJ, Rivera RT, et al: Laparascopic management of benign solid and cystic lesions of the liver. *Ann Surg* **229(4)**:460, 1999.
33. Koperna T, Vogl S, Satzinger U, Schulz F: Non-parasitic cysts of the liver: Results and options of surgical treatment. *World J Surg* **21(8)**:850, 1997.
34. Torra R, Nicolau C, Badenas C, Navarro S, Perez L, Extivill X, Darnell A: Ultrasonographic study of pancreatic cysts in autosomal dominant polycystic kidney disease. *Clin Nephrol* **47(1)**:19, 1997.
35. Scheff G, Harter H, Delmez J, Knebler R: Diverticular disease in patients with chronic renal failure due to polycystic kidney disease. *Ann Intern Med* **92**:202, 1980.
36. Sharp CK, Zeligman BE, Johnson AM, Duley I, Gabow PA.: Evaluation of colonic diverticular disease in autosomal dominant polycystic kidney disease without end-stage renal disease. *Am J Kidney Dis* **34(5)**:863, 1999.

37. Leier CV, Baker PB, Kilman JW, Wooley CF: Cardiovascular abnormalities associated with autosomal dominant polycystic kidney disease. *Ann Intern Med* **100**:683, 1984.

38. Hossack KF, Leddy CL, Johnson AM, Schrier RW, Gabow PA: Echocardiographic findings in autosomal dominant polycystic kidney disease. *N Engl J Med* **319**:907, 1988.

39. Timio M, Monarca C, Pede S, Gentili S, Verdura C, Lolli S: The spectrum of cardiovascular abnormalities in autosomal dominant polycystic kidney disease: A 10-year follow-up in a five-generational kindred. *Clin Nephrol* **37(5)**:245, 1992.

40. Poutasse EF, Gardner WJ, McCormack LJ: Polycystic kidney disease and intracranial aneurysm. *JAMA* **154**:741, 1954.

41. Rengachary SS: Intracranial aneurysms and ependymal cysts, in Wilkins R, Rengachary SS (eds): *Neurosurgery.* New York, McGraw-Hill, 1985, pp 231–245.

42. Bigelow NH: The association of polycystic kidneys with intracranial aneurysms and other related disorders. *Am J Med Sci* **225**:485, 1953.

43. Wakabayashi T, Jujita S, Ohbora Y, Suyama T, Tamaki N, Matsumoto S: Polycystic kidney disease and intracranial aneurysms: Early angiographic diagnosis and early operation for the unruptured aneurysm. *J Neurosurg* **58**:488, 1983.

44. Brown RAP: Polycystic disease of the kidneys and intracranial aneurysms. The etiology and interrelationship of these conditions. Review of recent literature and report of seven cases in which both conditions coexisted. *Glasgow Med J* **32**:333, 1951.

45. Ditlefson EML, Tonjum AM: Intracranial aneurysms and polycystic kidneys. *Acta Med Scand* **168**:51, 1960.

46. Chapman AB, Rubenstein D, Hughes R, Stears JC, Earnest M, Johnson A, Gabow PA, Kaehny WD: Intracranial aneurysms in autosomal dominant polycystic kidney disease: A prospective study. *N Engl J Med* **327**:916, 1992.

47. Huston J, Torres VE, Sulivan PP, Offort KP, Weibers DO: Value of magnetic resonance angiography for the detection of intracranial aneurysms in autosomal dominant polycystic kidney disease. *J Am Soc Nephrol* **3**:1871, 1993.

48. Ruggieri PM, Poulos N, Masaryk JT, Ross SJ, Obuchowski AN, Awad AI, Braun E, et al: Occult intracranial aneurysms in polycystic kidney disease. Screening with MR Angiography. *Radiology* **191**:33, 1994.

49. Chaveau D, Pirson Y, Verellen-Dumoulin CH, Macnicol A, Gonzalo A, Grunfeld JP: Intracranial aneurysms in autosomal dominant polycystic kidney disease. *Kidney Int* **45**:1140, 1994.

50. Scheivink WI: Intracranial aneurysms. *N Engl J Med* **336**:28, 1997.

51. Chapman AB, Johnson AM, Gabow PA. Intracranial aneurysms in patients with autosomal dominant polycystic kidney disease: how to diagnose and who to screen. *Am J Kidney Dis* **22(4)**:526, 1993.

52. Butler WE, Barker FG 2d, Crowell RM: Patients with polycystic kidney disease would benefit from routine magnetic resonance angiographic screening for intracerebral aneurysms: A decision analysis. *Neurosurgery* **38**:506, 1996.

53. Chauveau D, Sirleix ME, Schillinger F, Legenre C, Gruenfeld JP: Recurrent rupture of intracranial aneurysms in autosomal dominant polycystic kidney disease. *BMJ* **301**:966, 1990.

54. The International Study of Unruptured Intracranial Aneurysms Investigators: Unruptured intracranial aneurysms, risk of rupture and risks of surgical intervention. *N Engl J Med* **339**:1725, 1998.

55. Gregoire JR, Torres V, Holley KE, Farrow GM: Renal epithelial hyperplastic and neoplastic proliferation in autosomal dominant polycystic kidney disease. *Am J Kidney Dis* **9**:27, 1987.

56. Gabow PA, Kaehny WD, Johnson AM, Duley IJ, Manco-Johnson M, Lezotte DC, Schrier RW: The clinical utility of renal concentrating capacity in polycystic kidney disease. *Kidney Int* **35(2)**:675, 1990.

57. Wilson PD, Dillingham MA, Breckon R, Anderson RJ: Defined human renal tubular epithelia in culture: growth, characterization, and hormonal response. *Am J Physiol* **248(3)**:F436.

58. Graham PC, Lindhop GBM: The anatomy of the renin secreting cell in adult polycystic kidney disease. *Kidney Int* **33**:1084, 1988.

59. Torres VE, Donovan KA, Scicli G, Holley KE, Thibodeau SN, Carretero OA, Inangami T, et al: Synthesis of renin by tubulocystic epithelium in autosomal dominant polycystic kidney disease. *Kidney Int* **42(2)**:364, 1992.

60. Klahr S, Breyer JA, Beck GJ, Dennis VS, Harman JA, Roth D, Steinman TI, et al: Dietary protein restriction, blood pressure control and the progression of polycystic kidney disease. Modification of Diet in Renal Disease Study Group. *J Am Soc Nephrol* **5(12)**:2037, 1995.

61. Fick GM, Duley IT, Johnson AM, Strain JD, Manco-Johnson ML, Gabow PA: The spectrum of autosomal dominant polycystic kidney disease in children. *J Am Soc Nephrol* **4**:1654, 1994.

62. Gabow PA, Chapman AB, Johnson AM, Tangel DJ, Duley IT, Kaehny WD, Manco Johnson et al: Renal structure and hypertension in autosomal dominant polycystic kidney disease. *Kidney Int* **38(6)**:1177, 1990.

63. Gabow PA, Johnson AM, Strain J: Children with autosomal dominant polycystic kidney disease. *J Am Soc Neph* **6(3)**:720, 1995.

64. Bennett WM, Elzinga L, Golper TA, Barry JM: Reduction of cyst volume for symptomatic management of autosomal dominant polycystic kidney disease. *J Urol* **137**:620, 1987.

65. Chapman AB, Johnson AM, Gabow PA, Schrier RW: The renin-angiotensin-aldosterone system and autosomal dominant polycystic kidney disease. *N Engl J Med* **323**:1091, 1990.

66. Watson NL, Macnicol Am, Allan PL, Wright AF: Effects of angiotensin converting enzyme inhibition in adult polycystic kidney disease. *Kidney Int* **41(1)**:206, 1992.

67. Chapman AB, Johnson AM, Rainguet S, Hossack K, Gabow P, Schrier RW: Left ventricular hypertrophy in autosomal dominant polycystic kidney disease. *J Am Soc Nephrol* **8(8)**:1292, 1997.

68. Saggar-Malik AK, Missouris CG, Gill JS, Singer DR, Markandu ND, MacGregor GA: Left ventricular mass in normotensive subjects with autosomal dominant polycystic kidney disease. *BMJ* **309(6969)**:1617, 1994.

69. Zeier M, Geberth S, Schmidt KG, Mandelbaum A, Ritz E: Elevated blood pressure profile and left ventricular mass in children and young adults with autosomal dominant polycystic kidney disease. *J Am Soc Nephrol* **3(8)**:1451, 1993.

70. Ivy DD, Shaffer EM, Johnson AM, Kimberling WJ, Dobin A, Gabow PA: Cardiovascular abnormalities in children with autosomal dominant polycystic kidney disease. *J Am Soc Nephrol* **5(12)**:2032, 1995.

71. Fick GM, Johnson AM, Hammond WS, Gabow PA: Causes of death in autosomal dominant polycystic kidney disease. *J Am Soc Nephrol* **5(12)**:2048, 1994.

72. Chapman AB, Johnson AM, Gabow PA, Schrier RW: Overt proteinuria and microalbuminuria in autosomal dominant polycystic kidney disease. *J Am Soc Nephrol* **5(6)**:1349, 1994.

73. Sharp C, Johnson A, Gabow P: Factors relating to urinary protein excretion in children with autosomal dominant polycystic kidney disease. *J Am Soc Nephrol* **10**:136, 1999.

74. Gabow PA, Johnson AM, Kaehny WD, Kimberling WJ, Lezotte DC, Duley IT, Johns RH: Factors affecting the progression of renal disease in autosomal dominant polycystic kidney disease. *Kidney Int* **41(5)**:1311, 1992.

75. Contreras G, Mercado A, Pardo V, Vaamonde CA: Nephrotic syndrome in autosomal dominant polycystic kidney disease. *J Am Soc Nephrol* **6(5)**:1354, 1995.

76. Sklar AH, Caruana RJ, Lammiers JE, Strauser GD: Renal infections in ADPKD. *Am J Kidney Dis* **10(2)**:81, 1987.

77. Muther RS, Bennett WM: Cyst fluid antibiotic concentrations in polycystic kidney disease. Differences between proximal and distal cysts. *Kidney Int* **20**:519, 1981.

78. Chapman AB, Thickman D, Gabow PA: Percutaneous cyst puncture in the treatment of cyst infection in autosomal dominant polycystic kidney disease. *Am J Kidney Dis* **16(3)**:252, 1990.

79. Torres VE, Erikson SB, Smith LH, Wilson DM, Hattery RR, Segura JW: The association of nephrolithiasis and autosomal dominant polycystic kidney disease. *Am J Kidney Dis* **11(4)**:318, 1988.

80. Torres VE, Wilson DM, Hattery RR, Segura JW: Renal stone disease in autosomal dominant polycystic kidney disease. *Am J Kidney Dis* **22(4)**:513, 1993.

81. Delakas D, Daskalopoulos HG, Gravidas A: Extracorporeal shock wave lithotripsy for urinary calculi in autosomal dominant polycystic kidney disease. *J Endourol* **11(3)**:167, 1997.

82. Churchill DN, Bear JC, Morgan J, Payne RH, McManamon PJ, Gault MH: Prognosis of adult onset polycystic kidney disease re-evaluated. *Kidney Int* **26**:190, 1984.

83. Gretz N, Zeier M, Geberth S, Strauch M, Ritz E: Is gender a determinant for evolution of renal failure? A study in autosomal dominant polycystic kidney disease. *Am J Kidney Dis* **14(3)**:178, 1989.

84. Gabow PA, Duley I, Johnson AM: Clinical profiles of gross hematuria in autosomal dominant polycystic kidney disease. *Am J Kidney Dis* **20(2)**:140, 1992.

85. Johnson AM, Gabow PA: Identification of patients with autosomal dominant polycystic kidney disease at highest risk for end-stage renal disease. *J Am Soc Nephrol* **8(10)**:1560, 1997.

86. Fick GM Johnson AM, Strain JD, Kimberling WJ, Kumar S, Manco-Johnson ML, Duley IT, Gabow PA: Characteristics of very early onset autosomal dominant polycystic kidney disease. *J Am Soc Nephrol* **3**:1863, 1993.

87. Zeier M, Geberth S, Gonzalo A, Chaveau D, Grunfeld JP, Ritz E: The effect of uninephrectomy on progression of renal failure in autosomal dominant polycystic kidney disease. *J Am Soc Nephrol* 3(5):1119, 1992.

88. Oldrizzi, Rugiu C, Maschio G: The Verona experience on the effect of diet on progression of renal failure. *Kidney Int* 36:S103, 1989.

89. Ecder T, Edelstien CL, Brsnahan GM, Johnson AM, Gabow PA, Schrier RW: Effect on renal function of diuretics versus angiotensin converting enzyme (ACE) inhibitors in hypertensive patients with autosomal dominant polycystic kidney disease (ADPKD). *J Am Soc Nephrol* 10:415, 1999.

90. Watson ML, Macnicol AM, Borg-Costanzi J: A long-term comparison of the effects on renal function of blood pressure control with either atenolol or enalapril in polycystic kidney disease. *J Am Soc Nephrol* 10:428, 1999.

91. Walser M, Mitch WE, Maroni BJ, Kopple JD: Should protein be restricted in predialysis patients? *Kidney Int* 55:771, 1999.

92. Sweeney WE, Chen Y, Nakanishi K, Frost P, Avner ED: Treatment of polycystic kidney disease with a novel tyrosine kinase inhibitor. *Kidney Int* 57(1):33, 2000.

93. Keith DS, Torres VE, Johnson CM, Holley KE: Effect of sodium chloride, enalapril and losartan on the development of polycystic kidney disease in Han:SPRD rats. *Am J Kidney Dis* 24(3):49, 1994.

94. Ogborn MR, Sareen S: Amelioration of polycystic kidney disease by modification of dietary protein intake in the rat. *J Am Soc Nephrol* 6(6):1649, 1995.

95. Ogborn MR, Bankovic-Calic N, Shoe smith C, Burst R, Peeling J: Soy protein modification of rat polycystic kidney disease. *Am J Physiol* 274:F541, 1998.

96. Tanner GA: Potassium citrate/citric acid intake improves renal function in rats with polycystic kidney disease. *J Am Soc Nephrol* 9(7):1242, 1998.

97. Gile RD, Cowley BD Jr, Gattone VH 2nd, O'Donnell MP, Swan SK, Grantham JJ: Effect of lovastatin on the development of polycystic kidney disease in the Han:SPRD rat. *Am J Kidney Dis* 26(3):501, 1995.

98. Ogborn MR, Nitschmann E, Weiler H, Leswick D, Barkovic-Calic N: Flaxseed ameliorates interstitial nephritis in rat polycystic kidney disease. *Kidney Int* 55(2):417, 1999.

99. Cowley BD Jr, Grantham JJ, Muessel MJ, Kraybill AL, Gattone VH 2d: Modification of disease progression in rats with inherited polycystic kidney disease. *Am J Kidney Dis* 27(6):865, 1996.

100. Reeders ST, Breuning MH, Davies KE, et al: A highly polymorphic DNA marker linked to adult polycystic kidney disease on chromosome 16. *Nature* 317:542, 1985.

101. Daoust MC, Reynolds DM, Bichet DG, et al: Evidence for a third genetic locus for autosomal dominant polycystic kidney disease. *Genomics* 25:733, 1995.

102. Kimberling WJ, Fain PR, Kenyon JB, et al: Linkage heterogeneity of autosomal dominant polycystic kidney disease. *N Engl J Med* 319:913, 1988.

103. Peters DJ, Sandkuijl LA: Genetic heterogeneity of polycystic kidney disease in Europe. *Contrib Nephrol* 97:128, 1992.

104. Peters DJM, Spruit L, Saris JJ, et al: Chromosome 4 localization of a second gene for autosomal-dominant polycystic kidney disease. *Nat Genet* 5:359, 1993.

105. Bogdanova N, Dworniczak B, Dragova D, et al: Genetic heterogeneity of polycystic kidney disease in Bulgaria. *Hum Genet* 95:645, 1995.

106. de Almeida S, de Almeida E, Peters D, et al: Autosomal dominant polycystic kidney disease: evidence for the existence of a third locus in a Portuguese family. *Hum Genet* 96:83, 1995.

107. Ariza M, Alvarez V, Marin R, et al: A family with a milder form of adult dominant polycystic kidney disease not linked to the PKD1 (16p) or PKD2 (4q) genes. *J Med Genet* 34:587, 1997.

108. Paterson AD, Pei Y: Is there a third gene for autosomal dominant polycystic kidney disease? *Kidney Int* 54:1759, 1998.

109. Kandt RS, Haines JL, Smith M, et al: Linkage of an important gene locus for tuberous sclerosis to a chromosome 16 marker for polycystic kidney disease. *Nat Genet* 2:37, 1992.

110. European Polycystic Kidney Disease Consortium: The polycystic kidney disease 1 gene encodes a 14 kb transcript and lies within a duplicated region on chromosome 16. *Cell* 77:881, 1994.

111. European Chromosome 16 Tuberous Sclerosis Consortium: Identification and characterization of the tuberous sclerosis gene on chromosome 16. *Cell* 75:1305, 1993.

112. Burn TJ, Connors TD, Dackowski WR, et al: The autosomal dominant polycystic kidney disease (PKD1) gene product contains a leucine-rich repeat. *Hum Mol Genet* 4:575, 1995.

113. International Polycystic Kidney Disease Consortium: Polycystic kidney disease: The complete structure of the PKD1 gene and its protein. *Cell* 81:289, 1995.

114. Watnick T, Phakdeekitcharoen B, Johnson A, et al: Mutation detection of PKD1 identifies a novel mutation common to three families with aneurysms and/or very-early-onset disease. *Am J Hum Genet* 65:1561, 1999.

115. Watnick TJ, Piontek KB, Cordal TM, et al: An unusual pattern of mutation in the duplicated portion of PKD1 is revealed by use of a novel strategy for mutation detection. *Hum Mol Genet* 6:1473, 1997.

116. Van Raay TJ, Burn TC, Connors TD, et al: A 2.5 kb polypyrimidine tract in the PKD1 gene contains at least 23 H- DNA-forming sequences. *Microb Comp Genomics* 1:317, 1996.

117. Wang G, Seidman MM, Glazer PM: Mutagenesis in mammalian cells induced by triple helix formation and transcription-coupled repair. *Science* 271:802, 1996.

118. Faruqi AF, Datta HJ, Carroll D: Triple-helix formation induces recombination in mammalian cells via a nucleotide excision repair-dependent pathway. *Mol Cell Biol* 20:990, 2000.

119. Blaszak RT, Potaman V, Sinden RR, Bissler JJ: DNA structural transitions within the PKD1 gene. *Nucleic Acids Res* 27:2610, 1999.

120. Piontek KB, Germino GG: Murine pkd1 introns 21 and 22 lack the extreme polypyrimidine bias present in human PKD1. *Mamm Genome* 10:194, 1999.

121. Peral B, Gamble V, Milan JLS, et al: Splicing mutations of the polycystic kidney disease 1 (PKD1) gene induced by intronic deletion. *Hum Mol Genet* 4:569, 1995.

122. Turco AE, Rossetti S, Bresin E, et al: A novel nonsense mutation in the PKD1 gene (C3817T) is associated with autosomal dominant polycystic kidney disease (ADPKD) in a large three-generation Italian family. *Hum Mol Genet* 4:1331, 1995.

123. Peral B, San Millan JL, Ong AC, et al: Screening the 3′ region of the polycystic kidney disease 1 (PKD1) gene reveals six novel mutations. *Am J Hum Genet* 58:86, 1996.

124. Peral B, Gamble V, San Millan JL, et al: Splicing mutations of the polycystic kidney disease 1 (PKD1) gene induced by intronic deletion. *Hum Mol Genet* 4:569, 1995.

125. Rossetti S, Bresin E, Restagno G, et al: Autosomal dominant polycystic kidney disease (ADPKD) in an Italian family carrying a novel nonsense mutation and two missense changes in exons 44 and 45 of the PKD1 Gene. *Am J Med Genet* 65:155, 1996.

126. Neophytou P, Constantinides R, Lazarou A, et al: Detection of a novel nonsense mutation and an intragenic polymorphism in the PKD1 gene of a Cypriot family with autosomal dominant polycystic kidney disease. *Hum Genet* 98:437, 1996.

127. Turco AE, Rossetti S, Bresin E, et al: Three novel mutations of the PKD1 gene in Italian families with autosomal dominant polycystic kidney disease. *Hum Mutat* 10:164, 1997.

128. Daniells C, Maheshwar M, Lazarou L, et al: Novel and recurrent mutations in the PKD1 (polycystic kidney disease) gene. *Hum Genet* 102:216, 1998.

129. Torra R, Badenas C, Peral B, et al: Recurrence of the PKD1 nonsense mutation Q4041X in Spanish, Italian, and British families. *Hum Mutat* 1(Suppl):S117, 1998.

130. Badenas C, Torra R, San Millan JL, et al: Mutational analysis within the 3′ region of the PKD1 gene. *Kidney Int* 55:1225, 1999.

131. Peral B, Gamble V, Strong C, et al: Identification of mutations in the duplicated region of the polycystic kidney disease 1 gene (PKD1) by a novel approach. *Am J Hum Genet* 60:1399, 1997.

132. Roelfsema JH, Spruit L, Saris JJ, et al: Mutation detection in the repeated part of the PKD1 gene. *Am J Hum Genet* 61:1044, 1997.

133. Thomas R, McConnell R, Whittacker J, et al: Identification of mutations in the repeated part of the autosomal dominant polycystic kidney disease type 1 gene, PKD1, by long-range PCR. *Am J Hum Genet* 65:39, 1999.

134. Pound SE, Carothers AD, Pignatelli PM, et al: Evidence for linkage disequilibrium between D16S94 and the adult onset polycystic kidney disease (PKD1) gene. *J Med Genet* 29:247, 1992.

135. Peral B, Ward CJ, San Millan JL, et al: Evidence of linkage disequilibrium in the Spanish polycystic kidney disease I population. *Am J Hum Genet* 54:899, 1994.

136. Snarey A, Thomas S, Schneider MC, et al: Linkage disequilibrium in the region of the autosomal dominant polycystic kidney disease gene (PKD1). *Am J Hum Genet* 55:365, 1994.

137. Wright GD, Hughes AE, Larkin KA, et al: Linkage disequilibrium between the CA microsatellite D16S283 and PKD1. *J Am Soc Nephrol* 5:1159, 1994.

138. Watnick TJ, Gandolph MA, Weber H, et al: Gene conversion is a likely cause of mutation in PKD1. *Hum Mol Genet* 7:1239, 1998.
139. Phakdeekitcharoen P, Watnick TJ, Ahn C, et al: 13 Novel mutations of the replicated region of PKD1 in an Asian population. Manuscript in press, *Kidney Int*, 2000.
140. Bycroft M, Bateman A, Clarke J, et al: The structure of a PKD domain from polycystin-1: implications for polycystic kidney disease. *EMBO J* 18:297, 1999.
141. Reynolds DM, Hayashi T, Cai Y, et al: Aberrant splicing in the PKD2 gene as a cause of polycystic kidney disease. *J Am Soc Nephrol* 10:2342, 1999.
142. Brook-Carter PT, Peral B, Ward CJ, et al: Deletion of the TSC2 and PKD1 genes associated with severe infantile polycystic kidney disease-a contiguous gene syndrome. *Nat Genet* 8:328, 1994.
143. Hateboer N, Lazarou LP, Williams AJ, et al: Familial phenotype differences in PKD11. *Kidney Int* 56:34, 1999.
144. Hayashi T, Mochizuki T, Reynolds DM, et al: Characterization of the exon structure of the polycystic kidney disease 2 gene (PKD2). *Genomics* 44:131, 1997.
145. Veldhuisen B, Saris JJ, de Haij S, et al: A spectrum of mutations in the second gene for autosomal dominant polycystic kidney disease (PKD2). *Am J Hum Genet* 61:547, 1997.
146. Pei Y, He N, Wang K, Kasenda M, et al: A spectrum of mutations in the polycystic kidney disease-2 (PKD2) gene from eight Canadian kindreds. *J Am Soc Nephrol* 9:1853, 1998.
147. Koptides M, Hadjimichael C, Koupepidou P, et al: Germinal and somatic mutations in the PKD2 gene of renal cysts in autosomal dominant polycystic kidney disease. *Hum Mol Genet* 8:509, 1999.
148. Pei Y, Wang K, Kasenda M, et al: A novel frameshift mutation induced by an adenosine insertion in the polycystic kidney disease 2 (PKD2) gene. *Kidney Int* 53:1127, 1998.
149. Viribay M, Hayashi T, Telleria D, et al: Novel stop and frameshifting mutations in the autosomal dominant polycystic kidney disease 2 (PKD2) gene. *Hum Genet* 101:229, 1997.
150. Xenophontos S, Constantinides R, Hayashi T, et al: A translation frameshift mutation induced by a cytosine insertion in the polycystic kidney disease 2 gene (PDK2). *Hum Mol Genet* 6:949, 1997.
151. Torra R, Viribay M, Telleria D, et al: Seven novel mutations of the PKD2 gene in families with autosomal dominant polycystic kidney disease. *Kidney Int* 56:28, 1999.
152. Nomura H, Turco AE, Pei Y, et al: Identification of PKDL, a novel polycystic kidney disease 2-like gene whose murine homologue is deleted in mice with kidney and retinal defects. *J Biol Chem* 273:25967, 1998.
153. Wu G, Hayashi T, Park JH, et al: Identification of PKD2L, a human PKD2-related gene: Tissue-specific expression and mapping to chromosome 10q25. *Genomics* 54:564, 1998.
154. Plannels-Cases R, Ferrer-Montiel AV, Patten CD, Montal M: Mutation of conserved negatively charged residues in the S2 and S3 transmembrane segments of a mammalian K+ channel selectively modulates channel gating. *Proc Natl Acad Sci U S A* 92:9422, 1995.
155. Germino GG: Autosomal dominant polycystic kidney disease: A two-hit model. *Hosp Pract* 32:81, 1997.
156. Sandford R, Sgotto B, Aparicio S, et al: Comparative analysis of the polycystic kidney disease 1 (PKD1) gene reveals an integral membrane glycoprotein with multiple evolutionary conserved domains. *Hum Mol Genet* 6:1483, 1997.
157. Qian F, Germino FJ, Cai Y, et al: PKD1 interacts with PKD2 through a probable coiled-coil domain. *Nat Genet* 16:179, 1997.
158. Kobe B, Deisenhofer J: The leucine-rich repeat: A versatile binding motif. *Trends Biochem Sci* 19:415, 1994.
159. Moy GW, Mendoza LM, Schulz JR, et al: The sea urchin sperm receptor for egg jelly is a modular protein with extensive homology to the human polycystic kidney disease protein, PKD1. *J Cell Biol* 133:809, 1996.
160. Ponting CP, Hofmann K, Bork P: A latrophilin/CL-1-like GPS domain in polycystin-1. *Curr Biol* 9:R585, 1999.
161. Ward CJ, Turley H, Ong AC, et al: Polycystin, the polycystic kidney disease 1 protein, is expressed by epithelial cells in fetal, adult, and polycystic kidney. *Proc Natl Acad Sci U S A* 93:1524, 1996.
162. Geng L, Segal Y, Peissel B, et al: Identification and localization of polycystin, the PKD1 gene product. *J Clin Invest* 98:2674, 1996.
163. Ibraghimov-Beskrovnaya O, Dackowski WR, Foggensteiner L, et al: Polycystin: In vitro synthesis, in vivo tissue expression, and subcellular localization identifies a large membrane-associated protein. *Proc Natl Acad Sci U S A* 94:6397, 1997.
164. Palsson R, Sharma CP, Kim K, et al: Characterization and cell distribution of polycystin, the product of autosomal dominant polycystic kidney disease gene 1. *Mol Med* 2:702, 1996.
165. Griffin MD, Torres VE, Grande JP, et al: Immunolocalization of polycystin in human tissues and cultured cells. *Proc Assoc Am Physicians* 108:185, 1996.
166. Geng L, Segal Y, Pavlova A, et al: Distribution and developmentally regulated expression of murine polycystin. *Am J Physiol* 272:F451, 1997.
167. Van Adelsberg J, Chamberlain S, D'Agati V: Polycystin expression is temporally and spatially regulated during renal development. *Am J Physiol* 272:F602, 1997.
168. Griffin MD, O'Sullivan DA, Torres VE, et al: Expression of polycystin in mouse metanephros and extra-metanephric tissues. *Kidney Int* 52:1196, 1997.
169. Weston BS, Jeffery S, Jeffrey I, et al: Polycystin expression during embryonic development of human kidney in adult tissues and ADPKD tissue. *Histochem J* 29:847, 1997.
170. Peters DJ, van de Wal A, Spruit L, et al: Cellular localization and tissue distribution of polycystin-1. *J Pathol* 188:439, 1999.
171. Ong AC, Harris PC, Davies DR, et al: Polycystin-1 expression in PKD1, early-onset PKD1, and TSC2/PKD1 cystic tissue. *Kidney Int* 56:1324, 1999.
172. Ong AC, Ward CJ, Butler RJ, et al: Coordinate expression of the autosomal dominant polycystic kidney disease proteins, polycystin-2 and polycystin-1, in normal and cystic tissue. *Am J Pathol* 154:1721, 1999.
173. Ong AC, Harris PC, Biddolph S, et al: Characterisation and expression of the PKD-1 protein, polycystin, in renal and extrarenal tissues. *Kidney Int* 55:2091, 1999.
174. Aguiari G, Piva R, Manzati E, et al: K562 erythroid and HL60 macrophage differentiation downregulates polycystin, a large membrane-associated protein. *Exp Cell Res* 244:259, 1998.
175. Markowitz GS, Cai Y, Li L, et al: Polycystin-2 expression is developmentally regulated. *Am J Physiol* 277(1):F17, 1999.
176. Cai Y, Maeda Y, Cedzich A, et al: Identification and characterization of polycystin-2, the PKD2 gene product. *J Biol Chem* 274:28557, 1999.
177. Chen XZ, Vassilev PM, Basora N, et al: Polycystin-L is a calcium-regulated cation channel permeable to calcium ions. *Nature* 401:383, 1999.
178. Tsiokas L, Kim E, Arnould T, et al: Homo- and heterodimeric interactions between the gene products of PKD1 and PKD2. *Proc Natl Acad Sci U S A* 94:6965, 1997.
179. Arnould T, Kim E, Tsiokas L, et al: The polycystic kidney disease 1 gene product mediates protein kinase C alpha-dependent and c-Jun N-terminal kinase-dependent activation of the transcription factor AP-1. *J Biol Chem* 273:6013, 1998.
180. Parnell SC, Magenheimer BS, Maser RL, et al: The polycystic kidney disease-1 protein, polycystin-1, binds and activates heterotrimeric G-proteins in vitro. *Biochem Biophys Res Commun* 251:625, 1998.
181. Strader CD, Fong TM, Tota MR, et al: Structure and function of G protein-coupled receptors. *Annu Rev Biochem* 63:101, 1994.
182. Kim E, Arnould T, Sellin L, et al: Interaction between RGS7 and polycystin. *Proc Natl Acad Sci U S A* 96:6371, 1999.
183. Kim E, Arnould T, Sellin LK, et al: The polycystic kidney disease 1 gene product modulates Wnt signaling. *J Biol Chem* 274:4947, 1999.
184. Tsiokas L, Arnould T, Zhu C, et al: Specific association of the gene product of PKD2 with the TRPC1 channel. *Proc Natl Acad Sci U S A* 96:3934, 1999.
185. Arnould T, Sellin L, Benzing T, et al: Cellular activation triggered by the autosomal dominant polycystic kidney disease gene product PKD2. *Mol Cell Biol* 19:3423, 1999.
186. Baert L: Hereditary polycystic kidney disease (adult form): A microdissection study of two cases at an early state of the disease. *Kidney Int* 13:519, 1978.
187. Qian F, Watnick TJ, Onuchic LF, et al: The molecular basis of focal cyst formation in human autosomal dominant polycystic kidney disease type I. *Cell* 87:979, 1996.
188. Watnick TJ, Torres VE, Gandolph MA, et al: Somatic mutation in individual liver cysts supports a two-hit model of cystogenesis in autosomal dominant polycystic kidney disease. *Mol Cells* 2:247, 1998.
189. Brasier J, Henske EP: Loss of the polycystic kidney disease (PKD1) region of chromosome 16p13 in renal cyst cells supports a loss-of-function model for cyst pathogenesis. *J Clin Invest* 99:194, 1997.
190. Koptides M, Constantinides R, Kyriakides G, et al: Loss of heterozygosity in polycystic kidney disease with a missense mutation in the repeated region of PKD1. *Hum Genet* 103:709, 1998.

191. Koptides M, Hadjimichael C, Koupepidou P, et al: Germinal and somatic mutations in the PKD2 gene of renal cysts in autosomal dominant polycystic kidney disease. *Hum Mol Genet* **8**:509, 1999.

192. Pei Y, Watnick T, He N, et al: Somatic PKD2 mutations in individual kidney and liver cysts support a "two-hit" model of cystogenesis in type 2 autosomal dominant polycystic kidney disease. *J Am Soc Nephrol* **10**:1524, 1999.

193. Torra R, Badenas C, San Millan JL, et al: A loss-of-function model for cystogenesis in human autosomal dominant polycystic kidney disease type 2. *Am J Hum Genet* **65**:345, 1999.

194. Knudson AG Jr: Mutation and cancer: statistical study of retinoblastoma. *Proc Natl Acad Sci U S A* **68**:820, 1971.

195. Qian F, Germino GG: "Mistakes happen": somatic mutation and disease. *Am J Hum Genet* **61**:1000, 1997.

196. Tischfield JA: Loss of heterozygosity or: How I learned to stop worrying and love mitotic recombination. *Am J Hum Genet* **61**:995, 1997.

197. Ong AC, Harris PC: Molecular basis of renal cyst formation-one hit or two? *Lancet* **349**:1039, 1997.

198. Lu W, Peissel B, Babakhanlou H, et al: Perinatal lethality with kidney and pancreas defects in mice with a targeted Pkd1 mutation. *Nat Genet* **17**:179, 1997.

199. Lu W, Fan X, Basora N, et al: Late onset of renal and hepatic cysts in Pkd1-targeted heterozygotes. *Nat Genet* **21**:160, 1999.

200. Wu G, D'Agati V, Cai Y, et al: Somatic inactivation of Pkd2 results in polycystic kidney disease. *Cell* **93**:177, 1998.

201. Watnick T, Germino GG: Molecular basis of autosomal dominant polycystic kidney disease. *Sem Nephrol* **19**:327, 1999.

202. Shao C, Deng L, Henegariu O, Liang L, et al: Mitotic recombination produces the majority of recessive fibroblast variants in heterozygous mice. *Proc Natl Acad Sci U S A* **96**:9230, 1999.

203. Qian F, Watnick T: Somatic mutation as mechanism for cyst formation in autosomal dominant polycystic kidney disease. *Mol Genet Metabol* **68**:237, 1999.

# MUSCLE

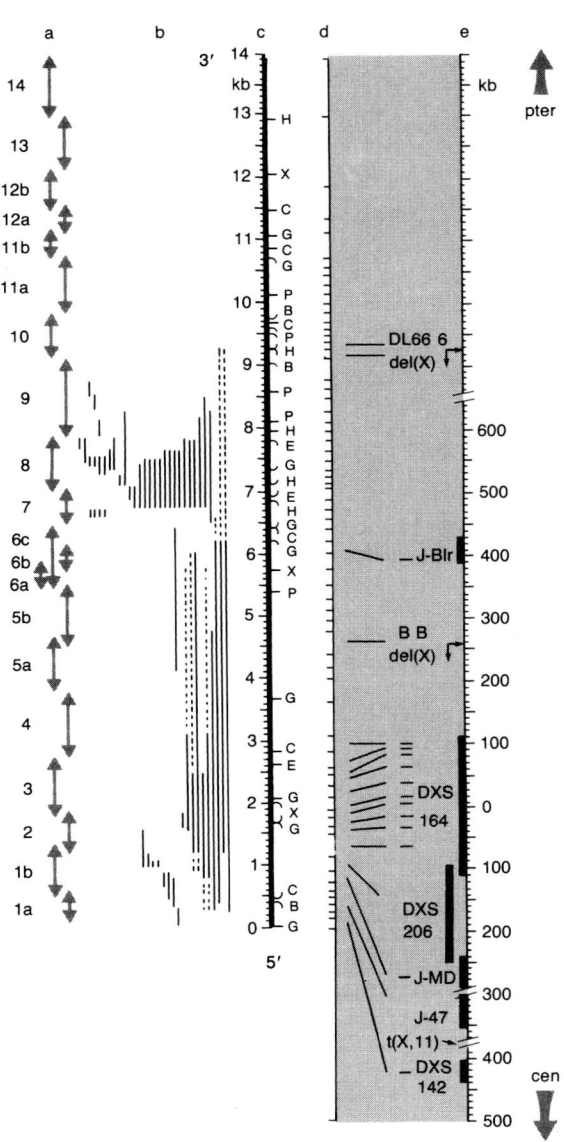

Duchenne muscular dystrophy

# The Muscular Dystrophies

*Ronald G. Worton* ■ *Maria Jutka Molnar*
*Bernard Brais* ■ *George Karpati*

1. The muscular dystrophies are a diverse group of inherited disorders characterized by progressive muscle weakness and wasting in which the primary defect becomes most symptomatic in skeletal muscle, with variable involvement of the heart. The clinical classification has been based largely on severity, distribution of affected muscles, and mode of inheritance. In the last 5 years, the molecular defect has been identified in many forms of the disease, and the clinical classification is giving way to a molecular classification.

2. Dystrophin is a high-molecular-weight cytoskeletal protein localized at the inner surface of the muscle membrane. It is part of a dystrophin-glycoprotein complex, including the dystroglycans and sarcoglycans. The complex provides a bridge across the muscle membrane, with dystrophin binding F-actin in the cytoplasm and dystroglycan binding merosin (laminin-2) in the extracellular matrix. Dystrophin deficiency results in destabilization of the complex and failure of the dystroglycans and sarcoglycans to localize in the membrane. The complex seems to be critical for the structural integrity of the muscle membrane.

3. Dystrophin is absent from the muscle of boys with Duchenne muscular dystrophy (DMD) and reduced or altered in the milder Becker muscular dystrophy (BMD) (see Tables 216-1 and 216-2 for complete lists of OMIM numbers; the corresponding GenBank numbers for cloned nucleotide sequences are given). Both are now classified as dystrophinopathies. X-linked dilated cardiomyopathy (XLDC) results from a cardiac-specific dystrophin deficiency. In each case, mutation of the large (2500-kb) dystrophin gene is responsible for the disease.

4. Several autosomal recessive forms of muscular dystrophy, including four of the eight autosomal recessive forms of limb-girdle muscular dystrophy (LGMD) have defects in the four muscle-specific sarcoglycans secondary to mutations in the corresponding genes and are now classified as sarcoglycanopathies.

5. Two other forms of autosomal recessive LGMD are due to mutations in genes unrelated to the dystrophin-glycoprotein complex. These include the gene encoding the muscle-specific, calcium-activated neutral protease calpain-3 and the gene encoding dysferlin, a protein of unknown function related to fer-1 (*Caenorhabditis elegans* spermatogenesis factor).

6. Of three known autosomal dominant forms of LGMD, the molecular defect in one is known to be in the gene encoding caveolin-3, the muscle-specific form of the principal protein component of caveolae in the plasma membrane.

7. The classic form of congenital muscular dystrophy is due to mutations in the gene encoding merosin (laminin-2) in the extracellular matrix, confirming the importance of merosin as part of the dystrophin-glycoprotein complex. Fukuyama congenital muscular dystrophy, common in Japan, is due to mutation in a gene encoding fukutin, a protein of unknown function, which results in a secondary and unexplained reduction in merosin in the extracellular matrix, the latter possibly explaining the disease phenotype.

8. Emery-Dreifuss muscular dystrophy (EDMD) is X-linked and distinct from DMD and BMD. It is caused by mutations in the ubiquitously expressed gene encoding emerin, a protein localized at the nuclear membrane of myonuclei with sequence similarity to the nuclear lamina-associated protein LAP2. Phosphorylation is critical to its putative role in anchoring the nuclear membrane to the cytoskeleton.

9. Autosomal dominant and recessive forms of oculopharyngeal muscular dystrophy (OPMD) are both caused by mutations in the gene encoding polyadenylation binding protein 2 (*PABP2*). The mutation is an expansion of a normal $(GCG)_6$ triplet repeat, resulting in an elongated polyalanine stretch at the N-terminus of the protein and presumably a conformational change that induces the formation of characteristic intranuclear filaments. Homozygosity for a $(GCG)_7$ allele is responsible for the autosomal recessive form, whereas heterozygosity for a longer expansion accounts for the autosomal dominant form.

10. Fascioscapulohumeral muscular dystrophy (FSHMD) is autosomal dominant and is due to deletion of multiple copies of a 3.2-kb tandem repeat in both sporadic and familial cases. No gene has been identified to be specifically altered in the disease, and the molecular consequences of the deletion are poorly understood.

11. With identification of the molecular defect in so many forms of muscular dystrophy, specific diagnostic tests are now available, and in familial cases, prenatal diagnosis for future pregnancies is available. A combination of DNA, RNA, and protein-based laboratory tests can be used to clearly distinguish between the many forms with overlapping phenotypes.

12. Naturally occurring animal models exist for three forms of muscular dystrophy, including the dystrophin-deficient *mdx* mouse and dog, the merosin-deficient *dy/dy* mouse, and the sarcoglycan-deficient cardiomyopathic hamster. In addition, several knock-out models have been created by homologous recombination in the mouse, and crossing with mice deficient in other molecules has resulted in

---

A list of standard abbreviations is located immediately preceding the index in each volume. Additional abbreviations used in this chapter include: DMD = Duchenne muscular dystrophy;XLDC = X-linked dilated cardiomyopathy ; BMD = Becker muscular dystrophy; LGMD = limb-girdle muscular dystrophy; CMD = congenital muscular dystrophy; FMD = Fukuyama muscular dystrophy; EDMD = Emery-Dreifuss muscular dystrophy; OPMD = oculopharyngeal muscular dystrophy; FSHMD = fascioscapulohumeral muscular dystrophy; CK = creatine kinase.

animals with severe phenotypes, useful for testing novel therapies.

13. Despite the recent progress in understanding the basic defect, the muscular dystrophies are still largely untreatable. Corticosteroids are the only pharmacologic agents that have so far shown beneficial effect for DMD, but the improvement is minimal, and side-effects preclude long-term administration. Myoblast transfer of normal myogenic cells has been tried with very limited success, but overcoming the immune rejection may lead to new clinical trials. Gene therapy is a major research activity at present, and newly developed adenoviral vectors have shown considerable promise for gene delivery with sustained activity of the transgene. There is therefore reason to be optimistic about the future for gene therapy.

The muscular dystrophies are a diverse group of inherited disorders characterized by progressive muscle weakness and wasting in which the primary defect becomes most symptomatic in skeletal muscle. Without any knowledge of the molecular or metabolic basis of the various forms of the disease, the muscular dystrophies were classified initially by clinical criteria. With the discovery of dystrophin deficiency as the cause of both Duchenne muscular dystrophy (DMD) and Becker muscular dystrophy (BMD), these forms have been classified as *dystrophinopathies*—a classification based solely on the molecular defect. In the seventh edition of this book, Chap. 140 focused on DMD and BMD because only these two forms could be characterized by their molecular defects.[1]

In the 5 years since the seventh edition was published, genetic research on muscular dystrophy has exploded to yield critical information on the molecular basis for several forms of muscular dystrophy. One of the outstanding facets of the research leading to the molecular mechanisms summarized in this chapter has been the logical and compelling way that discovery has flowed from the identification of dystrophin as the deficient or defective protein in DMD and BMD to the discovery of interacting molecules in the dystrophin-glycoprotein complex and to their demonstrated involvement in the molecular pathogenesis of several other forms of the disease. In particular, the dystroglycan complex and the sarcoglycan complex are major components of the larger molecular assembly involving dystrophin, and several autosomal recessive forms of muscular dystrophy have defects in the sarcoglycans and are now classified as *sarcoglycanopathies*.

Outside the muscle fiber, dystroglycan binds the $\alpha_2$-laminin chain of laminin-2 (merosin) in the basal lamina, and merosin defects are found in congenital muscular dystrophy. Finally, defects in molecules unrelated to the dystrophin-glycoprotein complex have been found in limb-girdle, oculopharyngeal, and Emery-Dreiffus muscular dystrophies.

One of the challenges in writing this chapter has been the need to deal with a wide variety of phenotypes and an equally large spectrum of independent but related molecular mechanisms in a logical and coherent fashion. The volume of literature on the subject is vast, and we have made no attempt to include reference to all that has been written. Our goal has been to capture the essential information and put it in a format that will allow both the novice and the veteran in the field to gain an appreciation of the current understanding of the molecular and metabolic basis of the muscular dystrophies. We begin with a brief overview of the clinical classification and then describe the dystrophin-glycoprotein complex. With this in hand, we then treat each form of muscular dystrophy in turn, providing the full clinical description, pathologic findings, and the most recent data on the molecular basis of the disease. We then end with more general sections on diagnostic workup to differentiate the various muscular dystrophies, a brief description of animal models, and an assessment of current and emerging therapeutic options.

## CLINICAL CLASSIFICATION OF THE MUSCULAR DYSTROPHIES

The muscular dystrophies are genetically determined diseases with progressive muscle weakness as the most prominent clinical manifestation. All display characteristic muscle pathology on electrical, biochemical, and histologic examination, and several also show pathologic features in organ systems other than muscle. The clinical severity varies widely and may even show variation within a single genetic type. As a group, the muscular dystrophies rank among the most frequent of inherited diseases. The inheritance pattern may be X-linked, autosomal dominant, or autosomal recessive. The major forms are listed in Table 216-1.

DMD and BMD are the classic X-linked muscular dystrophies. DMD and BMD were distinguished originally on clinical grounds, BMD having a later onset and slower rate of progression. Traditionally, those confined to a wheelchair by age 12 have been classified as DMD, and those still ambulant by age 16, as BMD. The terms *outlier* and *intermediate phenotype* have been applied to those in between. Since both diseases are due to

**Table 216-1** Clinical Classification of the Muscular Dystrophies

| Clinical Form | Abbreviation | Inheritance | Key Features |
|---|---|---|---|
| Duchenne (OMIM No. 310200) | DMD | X-linked | Severe, progressive muscle degeneration, onset ages 4–6, loss of ambulation at ages 9–12, death at ages 14–20 of respiratory failure/cardiomyopathy |
| Becker (OMIM No. 310200) | BMD | X-linked | Mild form, onset after age 16, muscle pain, dilated cardiomyopathy may require heart transplant |
| Limb-Girdle (OMIM: see Table 216-2) | LGMD | AD or AR | Severity variable, overlap DMD and BMD, involves primarily shoulder and pelvic girdle muscles |
| Congenital (classic) (OMIM 156225) | CMD | AR | Hypotonia, joint contractures, general muscle weakness, many never become ambulatory |
| Congential (Fukuyama) (OMIM 253800) | FMD | AR | Common only in Japan, similar to classic form but severe mental impairment, CNS alterations |
| Emery-Dreifuss, (OMIM 310300) | EDMD | X-linked | Contractures of elbow, neck, and spine, scapulohumeroperoneal weakness, cardiac conduction defect |
| Oculopharyngeal (OMIM: see Table 216-2) | OPMG | AD or AR | Eyelid ptosis and dysphagia, onset after age 50, |
| Fascioscapulohumeral (OMIM. 158900) | FSHMD | AD | Facial and shoulder weakness, scapular winging, variable cardiac involvement |

NOTE: AR = autosomal recessive; AD = autosomal dominant.

mutations in the dystrophin gene, they are allelic variants representing opposite ends of the clinical spectrum of the same genetic disorder.[1]

Limb-girdle muscular dystrophy (LGMD) may be inherited either as an autosomal dominant or an autosomal recessive disease. The disorder is clinically and genetically heterogeneous, the phenotype overlapping that of DMD, BMD, and spinal muscular atrophy. In some families, the term *autosomal recessive muscular dystrophy* (ARMD) has been used for essentially the same phenotype. With the identification of sarcoglycan deficiency in many LGMD and ARMD patients and defects in calpain-3, dysferlin, or caveolin-3 in others, the clinical classification is giving way to a genetic classification based on the molecular defect.

Congenital muscular dystrophy (CMD) describes a heterogeneous group of patients presenting with weakness and limb deformities in infancy. Autosomal recessive inheritance is clear in some families, and sporadic cases also may occur. A subtype found in Japan is Fukuyama muscular dystrophy (FMD). The finding of merosin deficiency in classic CMD and a defect in fukutin in FMD is the beginning of a rational classification based on the molecular defect.

Emery-Dreifuss muscular dystrophy (EDMD) is another X-linked muscular dystrophy, clinically distinct from DMD and BMD. With onset in late childhood to adulthood, cardiac arrhythmia is a distinguishing feature. The defect in the nuclear membrane protein emerin provides clues to the molecular basis of the disease.

Oculopharyngeal muscular dystrophy (OPMD) is primarily an autosomal dominant disease involving eyelid ptosis and dysphagia. Common in French Canada as a result of a founder effect, the defective gene involves an unusual triplet repeat expansion resulting in polyalanine tracts that form presumably toxic intranuclear inclusions.

Fascioscapulohumeral muscular dystrophy (FSHMD) is a dominantly inherited disorder affecting primarily facial and shoulder-girdle muscles. The genetic defect is complex and under active investigation.

## THE DYSTROPHIN-GLYCOPROTEIN COMPLEX

A schematic of the dystrophin-glycoprotein complex is shown in Fig. 216-1. The major components are dystrophin and cytoskeletal actin on the cytoplasmic face of the sarcolemma, transmembrane proteins including α-, β-, γ-, and δ-sarcoglycan plus β-dystroglycan, and α-dystroglycan and $α_2$-laminin in the extracellular matrix. The identification of this complex and its protein components has been crucial to an understanding of the molecular basis of many of the muscular dystrophies. The path of discovery began with the identification of dystrophin as the molecular defect in DMD and BMD.

## Dystrophin Isoforms and Related Protein

**The Dystrophin Gene.** Identification of the gene altered in boys with DMD was by positional cloning.[2,3] Mapping the gene relied on three lines of evidence. First, females with DMD caused by an X:autosome translocation with a chromosomal exchange point in band Xp21 suggested a DMD-related gene at this position. Nonrandom inactivation of the normal X provided an explanation for the disease in each case.[4] Second, mutations that cause the disease in males were shown to segregate with probes flanking Xp21 in families with DMD[5,6] and BMD,[7,8] providing the first indication that the genes responsible for both disorders are closely linked or identical. Finally, deletion of this region in boys with DMD as part of a contiguous gene deletion syndrome[9,10] provided the third compelling piece of evidence.

Once mapped, genomic clones were obtained from two sources: from the region of an Xp21 deletion in a contiguous gene deletion patient[11] and from the translocation junction of a t(X;21) translocation in which the *DMD* gene had recombined with a block of ribosomal RNA genes on chromosome 21.[12] Clones from these regions failed to hybridize with DNA from a subset of DMD and BMD patients, confirming that deletion of a gene in the Xp21 region is a factor in both diseases.[13,14]

The entire 2300-kb gene contains 79 exons[15] and is 100 times larger than the average human gene, half the size of the entire *Escherchia coli* genome, and larger than any chromosomes of yeast. Because of its enormous size,[16] it can be displayed by *in situ* hybridization with fluorescent DNA probes.[17] The gene is transcribed at the normal rate of about 40 nucleotides per second, requiring 16 hours to complete a transcript, and the exons are spliced together as transcription proceeds,[18] the first demonstration of cotranscriptional splicing in a mammalian cell.

The intron-exon borders have been sequenced, allowing the exons to be unambiguously numbered.[19] It is worth noting that

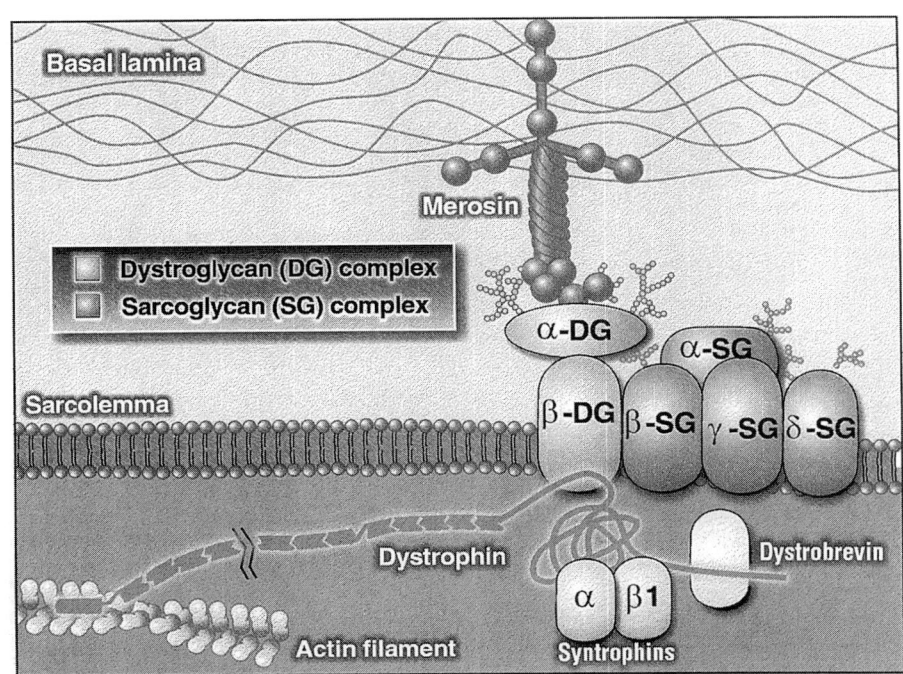

**Fig. 216-1** Schematic illustration of the dystrophin-glycoprotein complex showing the major components that are relevant to muscular dystrophy.

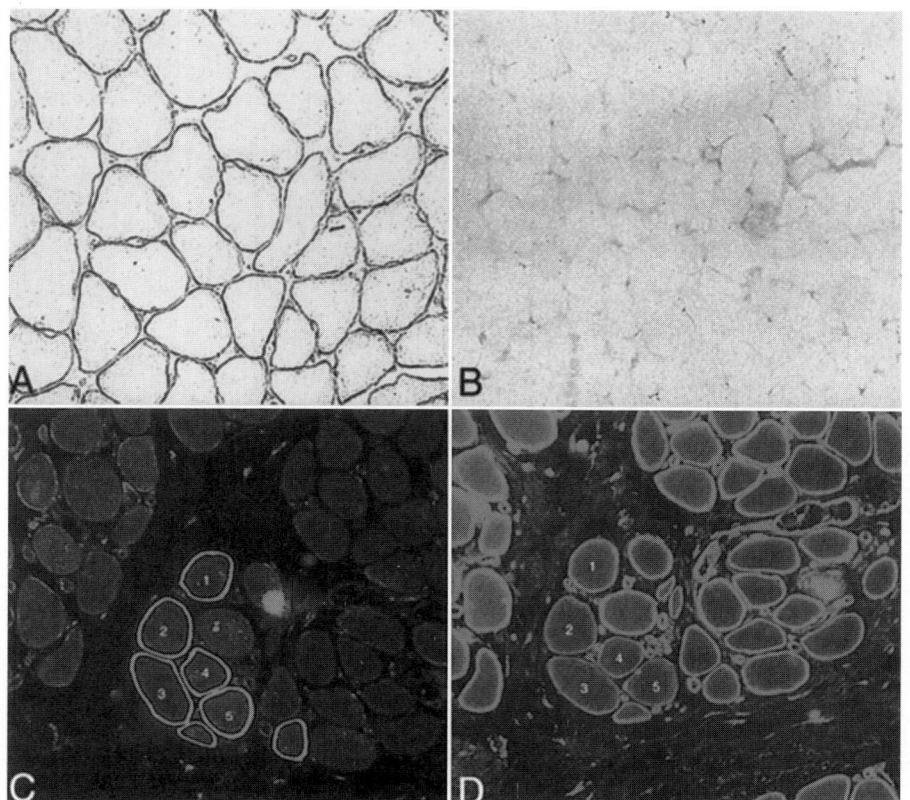

**Fig. 216-2** (*A*, *B*) Transverse cryostat sections of muscle showing immunoreactive dystrophin using a monoclonal antibody recognizing rod-domain epitopes. The bound antibodies are displayed by peroxidase reaction. (*A*) Normal muscle. (*B*) Muscle from DMD patient. (*C*, *D*) Serial sections from a DMD muscle biopsy. (*C*) Antidystrophin antibody as in *A* and *B* displayed by Cl$_3$ fluorochrome. (*D*) Antiutrophin monoclonal antibody for the N-terminus. In *C*, "revertant" fibers are shown with dystrophin immunostaining, whereas most fibers are devoid of dystrophin. In *D*, utrophin is strongly expressed in dystrophin-negative muscle fibers but weakly expressed in the revertant fibers (×160).

exons may end with the first, second, or third nucleotide of a coding triplet, and this information is valuable in determining whether or not a deletion of an exon or group of exons causes a frameshift in the mRNA. Exon-intron border types are tabulated in the seventh edition.[1]

The 13.9-kb cDNA sequence predicts a 427-kDa cytoskeletal protein of 3685 amino acids,[20] named *dystrophin* in recognition of its role in muscular dystrophy.[21] As detailed below, the protein is missing or altered in muscle from boys with DMD and BMD, *mdx* mice with a mutation in the equivalent mouse gene, and dogs with canine X-linked muscular dystrophy.

**Dystrophin Structure.** The main muscle isoform is a rod-shaped molecule about 175 nm long that contains four domains, three of which are also found in α-actinin and β-spectrin, identifying dystrophin as a member of the spectrin superfamily of cytoskeletal proteins. The N-terminal domain (amino acids 14–240) has three actin-binding sites and has been shown to bind cytoskeletal actin, as shown in Fig. 216-1.[22] The second domain (amino acids 278–3080) is rod-shaped with 24 repeats of a 109-amino-acid sequence similar to the repeats found in α-actinin and β-spectrin. It has four proline-rich "hinge regions" that may give flexibility to the rod.[23] The third domain (amino acids 3080–3360) is cysteine-rich and also bears some homology to α-actinin. The C-terminal domain is highly conserved in birds, rodents, and mammals, suggesting an important biologic role in the cell.[24] Rotary shadowed images of purified dystrophin reveal a dumbbell-shaped rodlike structure.[25]

**Dystrophin Localization.** In muscle, dystrophin constitutes about 5 percent of the membrane-associated cytoskeletal protein.[26] Western blot analysis of muscle extracts with antidystrophin antibodies reveals a greater than 400-kDa protein,[21] and immunostaining of muscle sections shows localization of dystrophin at the sarcolemmal membrane of skeletal muscle fibers[27] (Fig. 216-2*A*). As described in more detail below, dystrophin is absent from the muscle membrane of boys with DMD (see Fig. 216-2*B*) and is reduced or altered in boys with BMD. In the heart, dystrophin is strongly expressed in the Purkinje fibers.[28]

Electron microscopic localization suggests that the rod domain is 15 to 20 nm from the cytoplasmic face of the sarcolemmal membrane, with the C-terminal end closer to the membrane.[29] Colocalization of dystrophin with β-spectrin in longitudinal sections revealed a concentration of both molecules overlying the I bands in a costameric pattern, suggesting that dystrophin and spectrin, along with vinculin, may function to link the contractile apparatus to the sarcolemma.[30]

In addition to the costameric pattern at the cell surface, dystrophin is concentrated at the neuromuscular and myotendinous junctions. At the myotendinous junction, it appears to extend into the muscle away from the junction.[31] A functional role in the transmission of tension is suggested by a deficiency in attachment of actin filaments to myotendinous junctions of *mdx* mice.[32] In the neuromuscular junction, dystrophin appears concentrated at the postsynaptic membrane, specifically in the troughs of the synaptic folds,[33] where it may contribute to the stabilization of the endplate.

Dystrophin is not confined to muscle. In normal mouse brain, dystrophin is most abundant in the cerebellum, where it is found in the soma and dendrites but not axons of Purkinje cells, and in cerebral cortex, where it appears as punctate aggregates along the soma and dendrites of pyramidal neurons.[34] Since the cerebral cortex is associated with cognitive function, it is tempting to speculate that lack of dystrophin in the brain is responsible for the intellectual deficit in affected boys. In the peripheral nervous system, a short isoform of dystrophin is located along the Schwann cell membrane.[35]

The 260-kDa isoform of dystrophin (see section on isoforms below) is found in retina, at the synaptic junction in the outer plexiform layer,[36] and its deficiency in DMD patients is correlated with an abnormal electroretinogram, providing evidence for a role of dystrophin in neurotransmission.[37] The shorter, ubiquitously expressed 71-kDa isoform is also found in retina but in a different location, suggesting different functional attributes of dystrophin isoforms even within one tissue.[38]

**Dystrophin Isoforms.** Dystrophin exists in several isoforms, generated by alternative splicing and by the use of alternative promoters to initiate transcription from different places in the gene. There are at least seven tissue-specific isoforms initiated from different promoters. They include isoforms specific to muscle, brain cortex, cerebellar Purkinje cells, brain/kidney, retina, peripheral nerve, and a seventh that is expressed ubiquitously in liver and other tissues. The muscle, brain, and Purkinje cell promoters are at the 5′ end of the gene, and each has its own exon 1 that splices to exon 2 to generate a full-length isoform differing from the others only in the first few amino acids. The retina, brain/kidney, peripheral nerve, and ubiquitous promoters in introns 29, 44, 55, and 62 have first exons that splice into exons 30, 45, 56, and 63, respectively, to generate isoforms of 260, 140, 116, and 71 kDa, respectively. These short isoforms lack the actin-binding domain and all or part of the rod domain and therefore are presumed to have somewhat different function from the full-length isoforms. Greater detail on the identification and character of these isoforms is found in the seventh edition and in a recent review.[39]

Alternative splicing is most apparent at the 3′ end of the gene[40] and has been observed in skeletal, heart, and smooth muscle, in brain, and in retina. Removal of exons 71 to 74 in various combinations has been observed, but none alters the reading frame of the message and all result in near-normal dystrophin. In skeletal muscle, the "full length" mRNA is the predominant form, whereas shortened splice variants appear more often in heart.[41] Alternative splicing to remove exon 78 is more significant because it alters the reading frame of exon 79, replacing the last 14 hydrophilic amino acids with 32 hydrophobic amino acids encoded by the alternate reading frame.[41] This splicing pattern is developmentally regulated, with switching from the hydrophobic to the hydrophilic form during fetal development. An antibody directed against a synthetic peptide encoded by the alternate reading frame also detects this fetal isoform in human adult smooth muscle.[42]

**Utrophin.** The utrophin gene on chromosome 6 in human and chromosome 10 in mouse encodes a 13-kb transcript that shows extensive homology with dystrophin, suggesting derivation from a common ancestral gene.[43,44] The 395-kDa utrophin molecule is expressed in a broad range of fetal and adult tissues, including brain, heart, liver, intestine, kidney, gut, and testis. Functional similarity to dystrophin is suggested by the finding that utrophin binds to a complex of proteins and glycoproteins similar to those which bind dystrophin.[45]

In normal muscle, utrophin is localized primarily at the neuromuscular junction at the crest of the junctional folds.[46,47] However, in regenerating muscle fibers of DMD patients and in patients with inflammatory myopathies, utrophin is up-regulated and expressed throughout the extrajunctional sarcolemma.[47] It is hypothesized that in DMD this is a mitgating factor, and in a dystrophin-deficient boy who was suspected to have utrophin deficiency, the dystrophic process was particularly rapid.[48]

In otherwise normal mice, knock-out of the utrophin gene results in a relatively mild phenotype,[49,50] whereas utrophin deficiency in the *mdx* mouse aggravates the dystrophic phenotype.[51,52] Conversely, in *mdx* mice (or utrophin-deficient *mdx* mice) overexpressing utrophin from a transgene, the dystrophic phenotype is eliminated, implying that utrophin can serve as a functional surrogate of dystrophin.[53,54]

## The Dystrophin-Glycoprotein Complex

Dystrophin binds F-actin at its N-terminal end, and at the C-terminal end it is bound to a complex of proteins and glycoproteins that copurify with dystrophin from sarcolemmal membrane. In a series of elegant studies from Campbell's laboratory, several components of the dystrophin-glycoprotein complex were identified and characterized.[55,56] Antibodies are available for all the proteins in the complex, and by immunohistochemistry, all the proteins colocalize with dystrophin at the sarcolemmal membrane of muscle fibers[57] (see Fig. 216-1).

The proteins initially were referred to as *dystrophin-associated proteins* (DAPs) and *dystrophin-associated glycoproteins* (DAGs) with molecular weights of 156, 59, 40, 43, 35, and 25 kDa. Similar studies from Ozawa's laboratory identified the same proteins but assigned them different names.[58,59] The nomenclature was standardized in 1995 with recognition of the clinical importance of the molecules and the need to introduce a uniform standard.[60] By that time, the purification schemes allowed recognition of two distinct subcomplexes—the dystroglycan complex and the sarcoglycan complex.[57,61]

**F-Actin in the Dystrophin-Glycoprotein Complex.** At the N-terminal end, dystrophin binds cytoskeletal F-actin. While mutations in DMD patients that specifically remove the actin-binding sites at the N-terminal end result in a severe phenotype, the severity may be more a result of reduced levels of the protein rather than the lack of actin-binding sites. Studies in transgenic mice expressing normal levels of dystrophin, deleted for the actin-binding sites, are therefore more definitive and suggest that loss of these binding sites is compatible with a near-normal phenotype.[62,63] This raised the possibility of additional actin-binding sites elsewhere in the molecule, and indeed, such have been identified in the rod region of the protein.[64] In contrast, transgenic *mdx* mice expressing in muscle the 71-kDa isoform, which lacks both the N-terminal and rod domains, do show localization of the shortened isoform at the sarcolemma in conjunction with restoration of the glycoprotein complex, but the animals still have the dystrophic phenotype, suggesting that actin binding is critical to a normal muscle phenotype.[65]

**The Dystroglycans.** The dystroglycan complex is composed of α- and β-dystroglycan (156 and 43 kDa) derived by proteolytic processing of a single precursor protein.[66] Direct interaction between dystrophin and β-dystroglycan has been demonstrated by in vitro binding and interaction sites map within the C-terminal 15 amino acids of β-dystroglycan and within the cystine-rich domain of dystrophin.[67] β-Dystroglycan has a transmembrane domain and links to α-dystroglycan on the external side of the sarcolemma (see Fig. 216-1). Outside the muscle fiber, α-dystroglycan is highly glycosylated and binds to the α₂-laminin subunit of merosin (laminin-2) in the extracellular matrix.

Dystrophin plays a critical role in assembling or maintaining the entire complex at the sarcolemmal membrane, as evidenced by the fact that both the dystroglycans and the sarcoglycans are absent or reduced in amount at the muscle membrane of DMD patients and *mdx* mouse. Further evidence for the importance of the dystrophin-dystroglycan interaction comes from mutations that delete the binding regions. While DMD patients with C-terminal deletions that remove the dystroglycan-binding region are severely affected, this could be due to the generally reduced level of mutant protein available to the complex.[68] In transgenic *mdx* mice expressing dystrophin gene constructs that produce dystrophin molecules lacking the C-terminus or the cysteine-rich domain, the transgene fails to correct the *mdx* phenotype, demonstrating the important biologic role of these domains in preventing the characteristic muscle degeneration.[69,70]

**The Sarcoglycans.** The sarcoglycan complex of muscle is composed of four single transmembrane glycoproteins, namely, α-, β-, γ-, and δ-sarcoglycan, all of which are relatively specific for muscle.[57] The recently identified ε-sarcoglycan is expressed ubiquitously in many tissues and may have a different function.[71,72] While the members of this complex are not known to bind directly to dystrophin, dystrophin is responsible for their assembly or maintenance at the sarcolemma, since the sarcoglycan concentration at the membrane is dramatically reduced in DMD and *mdx* muscle.[57] Furthermore, they are of critical importance for biologic function of the complex, since mutations in all four muscle sarcoglycans have been shown to cause muscular dystrophy.

Most of what we know about the sarcoglycans is predicted from the nucleotide sequence of the cloned genes and their cDNAs. The predicted amino acid sequences of the α-,[73] β-,[74,75] γ-,[76] δ-,[77,78] and ε-sarcoglycans[71,72] reveal a set of proteins with no homology with other known proteins but striking similarities to one another. All have single transmembrane domains, relatively small intracellular domains, and large extracellular domains. Their molecular weights fall within a narrow range of 35 to 50 kDa, and all are glycosylated on at least one residue. All sarcoglycans contain five cysteines in the extracellular domain, and in β-, γ-, and δ-sarcoglycan, the cysteines are clustered toward the end of the extracellular domain, which in these three molecules is the C-terminal end of the protein. In contrast, the α- and ε-sarcoglycan molecules contain a signal peptide that results in the N-terminal end being extracellular. Secondary structure analysis reveals the presence of several β-pleated sheets and α-helices.[79]

**Merosin (Laminin-2) in the Basal Lamina of Muscle.** The basal lamina around muscle fibers is a specialized extracellular matrix composed of collagen, fibronectin, laminin, and proteoglycans. The matrix is a static structure that is thought to contribute to the proper migration, proliferation, and regeneration of myogenic cells during development or after injury or grafting.

Merosin, or laminin-2, is situated in the basal lamina surrounding human skeletal muscle.[80,81] Laminins are heterotrimer molecules each composed of one heavy (α) and two light (β or γ) chains[82] (see Fig. 216-1). Five different α chains, three β chains, and two γ chains are known, and different combinations of heavy and light chains gives rise to different types of laminin. Laminin-2 surrounding muscle fibers is composed of an $\alpha_2$ heavy chain combined with $\beta_1$ or $\beta_2$ and $\gamma_1$ light chains. *Merosin* is the collective name for laminins that contain an $\alpha_2$ heavy chain (i.e. laminins 2 and 4).

Merosin binds directly to specific molecules of the basal lamina, including enactin/nidogen and heparan sulfate proteoglycan/perlecan.[82] Two molecules act as muscle receptors for laminin.[83] One is α-dystroglycan, which links merosin to the dystrophin-actin complex. In addition, integrins in the muscle membrane may act as a laminin receptor based on a deficiency of $\alpha_7/\beta_1$-integrin in muscle of patients with merosin-deficient congenital muscular dystrophy.[84,85]

The gene encoding the $\alpha_2$-laminin heavy chain is very large, with 64 exons, maps to 6q2,[86] and is altered in classic congenital muscular dystrophy.

**Other Proteins in the Complex.** Also shown in Fig. 216-1 are the syntrophins (α, $\beta_1$) that directly bind to the C-terminus of dystrophin[87,88] Not shown in the figure is sarcospan, a protein with four transmembrane domains.[89] These proteins, together with dystrophin, the dystroglycans, and the sarcoglycans, constitute the core of the complex.

Dystrobrevin, the human and mouse homologue of the 87-kDa postsynaptic molecule from the Torpedo electric organ, is also closely associated with the syntrophins and dystrophin[90,91] and also may be part of a similar complex in which utrophin replaces dystrophin at the neuromuscular junction.[92,93]

Other proteins reported to be associated with the complex include the adapter protein Grb2[94] and a phosphoglucomutase-related protein,[95] but their role in the complex is not clear. The localization of neuronal nitric oxide synthase at the sarcolemma is mediated by its interaction with dystrophin and the syntrophins[96] and is missing from the sarcolemma in both DMD and BMD patients.[97,98] It therefore appears to be an integral component of the complex, and its loss in DMD and BMD is secondary to the dystrophin deficiency. Although caveolin-3 has been described as a member of the complex,[99,100] recent evidence indicates that it is not an integral component.[101]

### Function of the Glycoprotein Complex

The functions of dystrophin and its associated complex are not fully understood.[102] Dystrophin probably has multiple physiologic roles that vary according to the different isoforms in different cell types. The functional role of dystrophin in the brain and retina is undetermined, but its localization at the synaptic membrane[34] is consistent with a function in neurotransmission — perhaps stabilization of receptors, ion channels, or synaptic vesicles. The function of the short isoforms is obscure, although the 116-kDa isoform may contribute to the stabilization of sodium channels at nodes of Ranvier in peripheral nerves,[35] whereas the retinal isoform may stabilize proteins that are essential for neurotransmission in the outer plexiform layer.[36]

In skeletal muscle, the probable main role of the complex is mechanical reinforcement of the sarcolemma. The complex also may enable the sarcolemma to assume the normal folding and plication or festooning configuration in the relaxed state so that it can remain intact when muscle fibers are streched.[103] Dystrophin-deficient fibers are particularly vulnerable to lengthening contractions, and this may be at the heart of the disease pathology.[104,105]

Another suggested role for dystrophin derives from the two tryptophanes near the β-dystroglycan-binding site, consistent with a role in signal transduction.[106,107] Such signaling could lead to an abnormal control of muscle fiber caliber contributing to fiber size variation in dystrophic muscle.[108]

Another possibility is that within the complex dystrophin simply may serve as an anchor or stabilizer of the dystroglycans and sarcoglycans, reinforcing the fact that some consequences of dystrophin deficiency may reflect the loss of sarcoglycan functions. The importance of the dystroglycan-laminin interaction recently has been demonstrated by the finding that dystroglycan-laminin interactions are a prerequisite for the deposition of other basement membrane proteins.[109] This suggests that dystroglycan exerts its influence on basement membrane assembly by binding soluble laminin and organizing it on the cell surface.

Little is known about the functional role of the sarcoglycans, except that the complex is critical for normal muscle physiology, as evidenced by the mutations that result in muscular dystrophy (see below). The majority of the biologically important mutations reside in the part of the genes encoding the extracellular domains, suggesting that interactions between these domains is required for stability of the complex. We return to the role of the dystrophin-glycoprotein complex when we discuss disease pathology.

## MOLECULAR BASIS OF THE MUSCULAR DYSTROPHIES

In this section we describe for each of the muscular dystrophies the clinical, laboratory, and pathologic features of the disease and, where possible, relate these to the molecular basis of the disease.

### Duchenne and Becker Muscular Dystrophy: The Dystrophinopathies

DMD and BMD are classic X-linked recessive genetic disorders with expression essentially confined to males. The hallmark of these disorders is the genetically determined dystrophin deficiency. The incidence of DMD is approximately 28 per 100,000 male births, whereas the milder BMD has a frequency of about 5 per 100,000, for a combined incidence of 33 per /100,000, or 1 in 3000. The mutation rate calculated from the incidence figures is 1 per 10,000 for DMD, about tenfold higher than for most genetic diseases, undoubtedly a result of the large genetic target for mutations. Evidence supports equal mutation rates in male and female gametes, leading to the conclusion that about a third of DMD cases are the result of new mutation in the mother's germ line, whereas two-thirds are inherited from a carrier mother. A detailed appraisal of the literature on incidence and the mathematical derivation of the mutation rate are found in the seventh edition.[1]

Females expressing the disease are rare and are related to nonrandom inactivation of the X chromosome. In a typical DMD carrier, the X chromosome carrying the normal DMD allele is inactive in approximately 50 percent of myonuclei, providing about half the normal amount of dystrophin. This is sufficient to prevent muscle fiber necrosis as long as the normal genes are evenly distributed throughout the muscle fibers.[110] The random nature of X inactivation results in a mild clinical presentation in about 8 percent of DMD carriers,[111] whose proportion of dystrophin-positive cells is skewed below 50 percent. Nonrandom X inactivation is found in monozygotic female twins discordant for the DMD phenotype, the affected twin showing preferential inactivation of the X chromosome carrying the normal dystrophin gene.[112–114] The discordance may be related to asymmetric splitting of the inner cell mass, with the affected twin receiving the smaller cell mass and a majority of cells with the normal gene inactive. Nonrandom X inactivation also leads to DMD or BMD in females with X-autosome translocations that disrupt the dystrophin gene and at the same time trigger nonrandom inactivation of the X chromosome carrying the normal allele.[115]

### Clinical Features of DMD and BMD

*DMD.* DMD is a severe muscle-wasting disorder described by Meryon in 1852[116] and in more detail by Duchenne a few years later.[117] The phenotype is described in detail by Emery in his monograph.[111]

Boys with DMD are phenotypically unremarkable at birth, and until the ages of 3 to 5 years neither parents nor pediatrician usually recognize any abnormality. The first symptoms include slow running, difficulty in rising from a sitting position and climbing stairs, as well as a waddling gait. Initially, the calves show hypertrophy with increase of muscle fiber caliber, the cause of which is not known. In rare instances, attention is drawn to the diagnosis after general anesthesia accompanied by unexplained cardiac arrest and/or myoglobinuria—features of malignant hyperthermia.[118,119]

The progression of muscle weakness and loss of function is relentless and occurs at a predictable rate.[120,121] In these two large cohort studies, the ability to walk was lost between 9 and 12 years, and death ensued at a mean age of 17 years. Complications include contractures, particularly in the lower extremities, and thoracic scoliosis that can aggravate respiratory insufficiency. Many patients require orthopedic surgery either for release of joint contractures or for scoliosis. By the second decade, respiratory insufficiency may necessitate ventilation, particularly at night, and is the usual cause of death in the teenage years. Those who survive into the third decade with adequate lung function often develop a symptomatic cardiomyopathy.[120]

Neurologic examination reveals muscle weakness that is most prominent in the pelvic and shoulder girdles, as well as proximal lower and upper limbs and trunk erectors, particularly at the lumbar and thoracic regions.[111] This is responsible for the exaggerated lumbar lordosis and thoracolumbar scoliosis. The pelvic-girdle and proximal leg muscle weakness is responsible for the classic Gower's maneuver in rising from a sitting position on the floor. Ankle dorsiflexion is limited, and tendon reflexes are diminished. Distally, muscles are less affected, and the craniobulbar and extraocular muscles are mostly spared. A mean reduction in IQ of 20 points, with one-fifth of patients having a significant mental handicap,[122] is presumed to be due to the lack of dystrophin in the brain.[123] In a study of mental subnormality in patients with a variety of deletions, there was no clear evidence for a particular region of the dystrophin gene being specifically responsible for intelligence, and the authors speculated that the intellectual deficit may be a consequence of cerebral hypoxia due to malfunction of smooth muscle dystrophin in the brain.[124]

*BMD and Milder Phenotypes.* The clinical phenotype of BMD is distinguished from DMD by a later age of onset and slower rate of progression, with ambulation until the age of 16. Those who lose the ability to walk between the ages of 12 and 16 years are referred to as *outliers,* being neither classic DMD nor BMD. The physical examination in BMD reveals a phenotype similar to mild DMD, with a combination of axial weakness, toe walking, and muscular hypertrophy. In later life, dilated cardiomyopathy is a feature of BMD, perhaps related to the stress on the dystrophin-deficient cardiac muscle as patients remain ambulant. Muscle pain related to exercise is a prominent feature of BMD, frequently in the calf. Mental deficiency is not a factor in the disease. Rarely, onset of the disease is in the third or fourth decade of life, and ambulation is prolonged to ages 50 to 60.[125]

Cardiomyopathy is a feature of both DMD and BMD, and dystrophin deficiency has now been well documented in X-linked dilated cardiomyopathy, at least in some case the result of mutations that block dystrophin expression in the heart but not the skeletal muscle. (see below)

Dystrophin deficiency also has been described in patients with quadriceps myopathy, a slowly progressive myopathy localized to the quadriceps[126] and in otherwise normal individuals with cramps plus myoglobinuria.[127] In asymptomatic people, a moderately elevated serum creatine phosphokinase (CK) has been suggested to involve a minor defect in the dystrophin gene, but this is rarely proven.[128]

**Laboratory Investigations.** Prior to the development of molecular diagnostic tests, the diagnosis of DMD was confirmed primarily by measuring serum CK, muscle histology, and electromyography (EMG). The electromyography is characteristic, with a reduction in the duration and amplitude of motor unit action potentials and an enhanced frequency of polyphasic potentials.[129] Electrocardiography in advanced cases shows increased R/S amplitude in lead $V_1$ and deep compressed Q waves in the precordial leads.[130] Serum CK is elevated 50- to 100-fold,[131,132] the result of leakage of the muscle isoform. Measurement of CK is also of value for carrier detection, although in carrier females the range of values overlaps the normal range, making the test less than definitive. A thorough discussion of the value of CK testing is provided by Emery.[111] In most families, genetic testing, as described in a later section, provides a more reliable method of carrier identification.

In BMD patients, laboratory results are similar to those for DMD, including elevation of CK and myopathic changes on EMG.

With the discovery of the dystrophin gene and the mutations that are responsible for the disease, dystrophin analysis has become a routine part of the disease workup. This workup is described later for the muscular dystrophies as a whole.

**Classic Muscle Pathology.** In DMD, the cardinal myopathology in a proximal limb muscle biopsy is segmental necrosis of muscle fibers and subsequent regeneration of this segment.[133,134] For still unknown reason, necrotic fibers in DMD tend to occur in small groups of 3 to 10 (Fig. 216-3). Regeneration is vigorous in early stages of the disease, but as the disease progresses, regeneration becomes more and more suboptimal and produces muscle fiber segments with reduced caliber. Eventually, in individual necrotic muscle fiber segments, regeneration fails, leading to loss of muscle fibers and replacement by adipose cells and connective tissue (Fig. 216-4). The progressively impaired regenerative capacity of DMD muscle fibers may be explained by the senescence of satellite cells after having undergone many rounds of proliferation.[135,136]

The very early fine structural change that occurs prior to necrosis is a focal breach of the plasma membrane.[137,138] This begins with focal separation of the plasma membrane and basal lamina followed by dissolution of the plasma membrane[138] (Fig. 216-5). These early findings are now explained by the loss of dystrophin from the sarcolemma (see below). Such breaches can be repaired by rapid apposition of flat cistern-like membrane

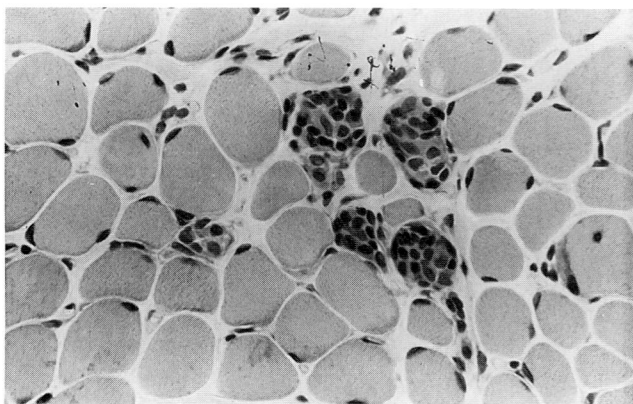

**Fig. 216-3** Cryostat section of an early-stage DMD muscle biopsy. Several necrotic fibers undergo phagocytosis. There is an abnormal variability of the muscle fiber size but relatively little endomysial connective tissue excess (modified trichrome stain; ×350).

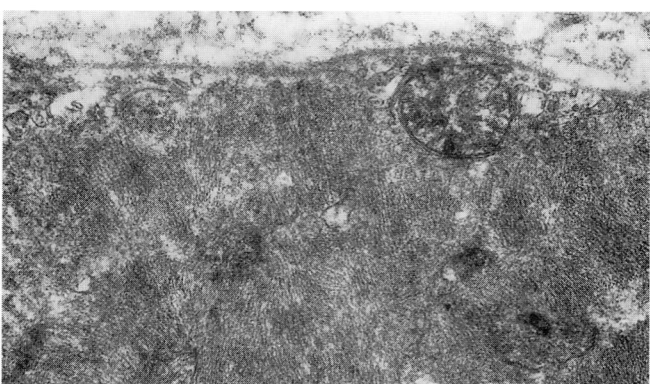

**Fig. 216-5** Electron micrograph of a DMD muscle fiber in transverse view. The fiber is in an early stage of necrosis, evidenced by the loss of plasma membrane and z discs, poor definition of myofibril, rounded mitochondria with fluffy matrix densities, but a persistent basal lamina, which is seen as a broad and diffuse line across the top of the figure. No cell membrane is seen below the basal lamina. In a neighboring necrotic segment, there was a separation of basal lamina and plasma membrane (not shown) (×28,000).

configurations to the gap. Such repaired sites are marked by focal depression of the muscle fiber surface and duplication or triplication of the basal lamina over the site of the repair.

In BMD, the muscle biopsy features variability in fiber size, muscle fibrosis, and necrosis. Internal nuclei are much more numerous, and the distinction between type I and type II fibers, often obscured in DMD, is clear in BMD. In these disorders, the muscle histology is consistent with the loss of dystrophin (DMD) or a reduction in the amount of dystrophin (BMD) at the muscle membrane, as documented below.

**Dystrophin Deficiency: The Molecular Basis of DMD and BMD.** Immunostaining of muscle sections with antidystrophin antibodies is essentially negative in DMD patients (see Fig. 216-2B),[21,139] whereas in BMD patients staining is "sporadic" or "interrupted."[140–142] A "patchy" staining, similar to that seen in BMD muscle, is also seen in other muscle disorders as well as in symptomatic carriers (Fig. 216-6). Dystrophin analysis on a muscle biopsy obtained *in utero* is also valuable for prenatal diagnosis in cases where the dystrophin gene mutation is not known.[143,144]

Presently, three useful monoclonal antibodies are commercially available for dystrophin immunostaining (Novocastra 1, 2, and 3), recognizing epitopes in the midrod, N-terminus, and C-terminus, respectively. In BMD, a given antibody may give completely

negative results if the target epitopes are missing from the truncated protein.

In both DMD and BMD muscle, small patches of positively staining fibers are seen, in which the dystrophin gene is thought to undergo a second mutation to restore the reading frame (see Fig. 216-2C). Analysis of mRNA in such "revertant" fibers has confirmed that in some cases at least a deletion of an adjacent exon restores the reading frame.[145] This has been further confirmed using exon-specific monoclonal antibodies to show that revertant fibers in a DMD patient with a deletion of exon 45 correct the frameshift by the additional deletion of exon 44.[146]

Using antibodies specific for utrophin, most DMD fibers, particularly the regenerating ones, show variable intensity of utrophin immunostaining outside the neuromuscular junction along the sarcolemma (see Fig. 216-2D).[47] This is not due to enhanced transcription but probably related to a saturation of orphaned dystrophin receptors by utrophin at the cell surface.[148] Consistent with this is the fact that revertant fibers that still have significant dystrophin in the membrane do not have such elevated levels of utrophin in the membrane (see Fig. 216-2C, D).

With the availability of antibodies against the dystroglycans and sarcoglycans, it is clear that there is a markedly attenuated immunostaining for both dystroglycans and all four sarcoglycans.[149] In contrast, merosin staining is normal. The dystroglycan and sarcoglycan depletion is clearly secondary to the dystrophin

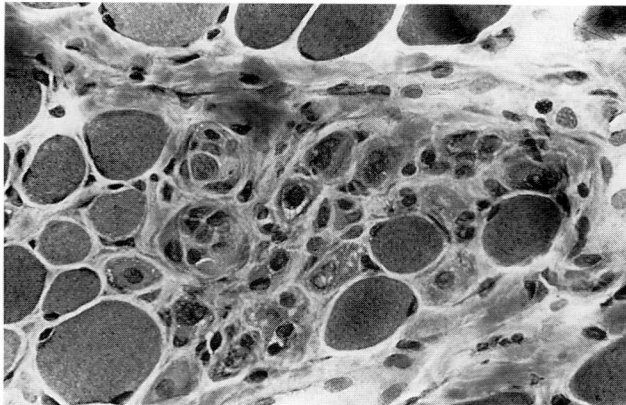

**Fig. 216-4** Cryostat section of an advanced-stage DMD muscle biopsy. A group of necrotic and regenerating muscle fibers is apparent. In addition, there is a marked variability of fiber size and conspicuous excess of endomysial connective tissue (modified trichrome stain; ×350).

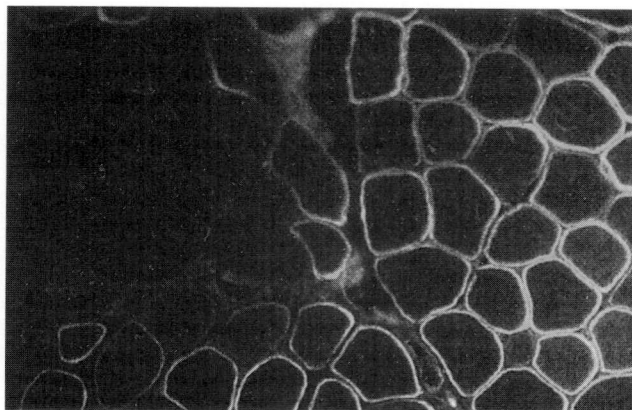

**Fig. 216-6** Dystrophin immunofluorescence from a manifesting carrier showing a cluster of dystrophin-negative muscle fibers that had normal spectrin and laminin immunostaining (×350).

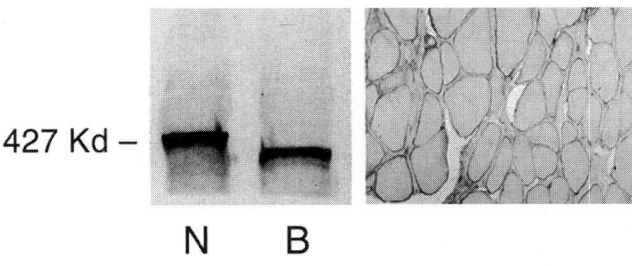

**Fig. 216-7** Immunoblot (*A*) showing normal-sized 427-kDa dystrophin from a normal muscle biopsy (N) and a lower-molecular-weight dystrophin in reduced amount from a BMD patient (*B*). Muscle biopsy from the same BMD patient shows weak and interrupted dystrophin immunoperoxidase staining (×350).

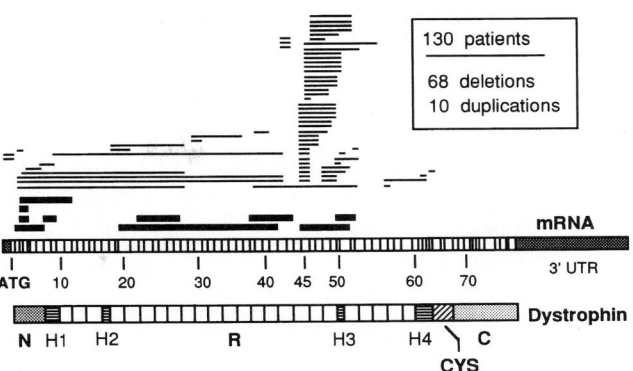

**Fig. 216-8** Schematic diagram showing the spectrum of deletions (thin bars) and duplications (thick bars) relative to the position of exons in the mRNA and to the dystrophin molecule. Each bar represents the extent of the deletion or duplication in a single patient. The hot spot for deletion around 45–52 is evident, as is the collection of larger deletions found in the 5′ half of the gene.

deficiency, since transgenic introduction of dystrophin cDNA into *mdx* mice brings about normalization of the dystrophin-associated molecules.[150] Similar results are obtained following adenovirus-mediated gene transfer of a functional utrophin gene.[151] By contrast, in primary sarcoglycan deficiency, dystrophin immunostaining is normal.[152]

By western blot, DMD patients have little or no detectable dystrophin. In contrast, most BMD patients have a reduced level of dystrophin of abnormal size due to deletion of a specific set of exons[139] (Fig. 216-7). This usually results in a patchy distribution of dystrophin in the membrane (see Fig. 216-7). With a specific monoclonal antibody and quantitative densitometry, dystrophin levels correlate with disease severity, and even severe DMD patients have detectable dystrophin of altered molecular weight.[140] Using antibodies against both ends of the protein, DMD patients have abnormal dystrophin that is detected with N-terminal but not C-terminal antibody, consistent with a truncated molecule from a frameshift mutation (see below), whereas BMD patients have dystrophin that reacts with both antibodies, consistent with a mutation that maintains the translational reading frame.[153]

**Muscle Pathology Related to Dystrophin Deficiency.** The prevailing thought is that the lack of dystrophin in muscle fibers creates a mechanically weakened sarcolemma[154,155] that becomes susceptible to focal tears on contractile activity.[105] The focal separation of the sarcolemma from the basal lamina that precedes these lesions is adequately explained by the lack of dystrophin in muscle fibers that eliminates the mechanical bridge between the actin cytoskeleton and the laminin structure of the extracellular matrix. In the absence of repair of these lesions, it is thought that calcium influx activates proteases of muscle fibers, which is an important part of the necrotic process.[156] Necrosis spreads laterally along the axis of muscle fibers until the necrotic segment is isolated from the surviving stumps by a newly formed demarcating membrane.[138,157] One might explain the fact that naturally small caliber fibers such as those in extraocular muscle or cranial muscle are spared by the fact that the relative mechanical stress per unit surface membrane area is reduced in such fibers.[158]

Underlying the dystrophin defects that are responsible for the disease pathology are the mutations in the dystrophin gene described below.

**Mutational Basis of Dystrophin Deficiency.** The loss of dystrophin at the muscle membrane is clearly related to mutations in the gene encoding dystrophin at band p21 on the X chromosome. Cloning of the dystrophin gene constituted the initial proof that deletions in the Xp21 region were associated with the disease.[14] By Southern blot analysis with a complete set of cDNA probes, the frequency of detectable deletions in DMD was estimated to be over 60 percent, and duplications were detected in 6 percent of affected boys. More recently, a number of point mutations have been described. A complete listing of dystrophin gene mutations is maintained by the

Department of Human and Clinical Genetics, Leiden University Medical Center, on the Internet (*http://www.dmd.nl*).

***Deletion.*** Deletions in the dystrophin gene are heterogeneous with respect to size and location. The largest, several thousand kilobases in size, remove neighboring genes and occur in association with a contiguous gene-deletion syndrome. Smaller deletions remove from one to a few exons, and their distribution in the gene is not random. Two deletion-rich regions are apparent in the gene, one extending over the first 20 exons and the second near the middle of the gene around exons 45 to 53[159,160] (Fig. 216-8). The clustering of the mutations allows most deletions to be detected with a set of polymerase chain reaction (PCR) reactions spanning the 18 most frequently deleted exons. These are generally carried out in two multiplex PCR reactions of 9 exons each[161–164] (Fig. 216-9).

Phenotypic severity is not simply a function of deletion size, since some deletions associated with BMD are larger than and completely encompass deletions associated with DMD. This is largely explained by the effect of the mutation on the translational reading frame of the mRNA.[165] A deletion that does not alter the reading frame generates a protein that is missing only those amino acids encoded by the deleted exons. In contrast, a frameshifting deletion creates a new reading frame after the deletion that specifies different amino acids in the protein up to an inevitable stop codon, at which point protein synthesis terminates. As summarized in the seventh edition, most frameshift deletions are found in DMD patients, whereas most nonframeshift deletions are found in BMD patients. Thus the reading frame status, which is absolutely predictable once it is known which exons are deleted, provides a valuable, though not infallible,[166] prognostic indicator for the severity of the disease.[19] Western blot analysis has confirmed that BMD patients have significant levels of dystrophin, usually of reduced size, consistent with the model[153] (see Fig. 216-7).

***Duplication.*** Duplication of one or more exons of the gene can be detected in about 6 percent of DMD patients by quantitative Southern blot.[167–169] Frame-shifting duplications occur more frequently in DMD patients, whereas duplications that do not shift the reading frame occur more often in BMD and result in an enlarged dystrophin with part of the amino acid sequence repeated in the protein.[170] However, there can be interfamilial variation in phenotype among patients with the same duplication.[171]

The mechanisms that result in duplication include both homologous and nonhomologous recombination.[172] In cases where the duplication has been traced in families, the rearrangement occurred most often in the germ line of the maternal

**Multiplex I**  **Multiplex II**

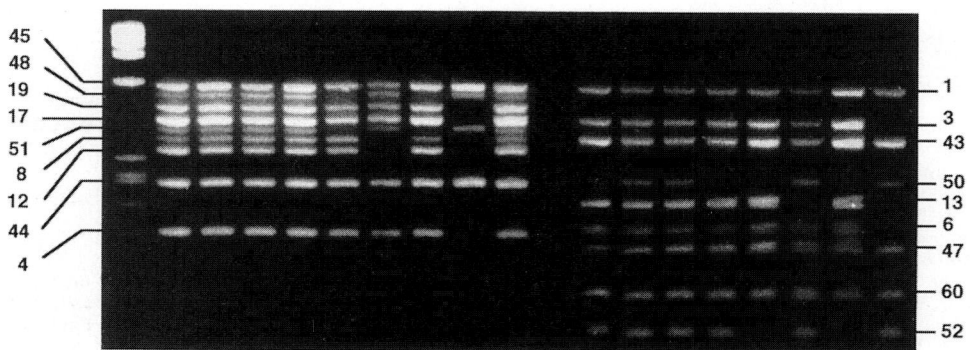

Fig. 216-9 Agarose gel electrophoresis of multiplex PCR products from blood cell DNA of four patients. Two multiplex reactions are shown. The first set of four lanes contains amplified products of exons 48, 17, 8, and 44; the second set of four lanes contains amplified products of exons 45, 19, 52, 12, and 4. In patient 1, exons 48–52 are deleted, and in patient 3, exons 45–52 are deleted. In patient 2 and in two normal controls (N), no deletions are present.

grandfather, and since males have a single X chromosome, the duplication must have occurred by unequal sister chromatid exchange.[173]

***Point Mutation.*** In the one-third of patients who do not have a large deletion or duplication spanning multiple exons, the mutations are difficult to identify due to the large size of the gene. Detection has been enhanced by the use of single-strand conformational polymorphism and heteroduplex analysis, RNA-based methods such as reverse-transcriptase PCR (RT-PCR), or the protein truncation test, as reviewed recently.[174]

These intraexon mutations, or *point mutations,* have been detected in many patients, and the first 20 to be described were tabulated in the seventh edition of this work. They included stop codons, small frameshift deletions and insertions, altered splice signals, and alterations of the muscle promoter. A 1994 review by Roberts lists 70 mutations and discusses their significance.[175] Many more have been identified since and are tabulated in the mutational data of Leiden University Medical Center (*http://www.dmd.nl*).

As of October 1998, the database listed 264 variations (154 published), of which 203 were classified as disease-causing. Ten mutations were reported twice and eight others more than twice. There were 64 small deletions and 24 insertions, plus 70 splicing alterations. The mutations are distributed throughout the gene, with no evident hot spots, and occur in almost every exon of the gene.

### X-Linked Dilated Cardiomyopathy: A Cardiac Dystrophinopathy

X-linked dilated cardiomyopathy (XLDC) segregates with the dystrophin gene[176] and is often due to mutation in the gene (for review, see references 177 and 178). The first mutations detected were in the promoter region or 5′ end of the gene.[179,180] In the case of an intron 1 splice-site alteration, the expression of the gene was eliminated in cardiac muscle, whereas the gene was expressed in skeletal muscle from the brain and Purkinje promoters, thus accounting for the cardiac-specific phenotype.[180] Examination of other patients with a disruption of exon 1 or the intron 1 enhancer[181,182] suggests that malfunction of dystrophin gene regulation may be a common feature of XLDC. Mutations that result in altered splicing that is cardiac-specific also result in XLDC.[183] Other mutations[184] listed in the Leiden University Medical Center Web site (*http://www.dmd.nl*) are not so easily explained as cardiac-specific lesions.

The role of dystrophin deficiency in cardiomyopathy was demonstrated dramatically by the finding that coxsackie virus B3-induced cardiomyopathy is a result of dystrophin cleavage by the enteroviral protease 2A, leading to disruption of the dystrophin-glycoprotein complex.[185] This is the first demonstration that dystrophin is involved in an infectious disease and that the dystrophin-glycoprotein complex is susceptible to environmentally introduced proteases.

### Sarcoglycanopathy in the Autosomal Recessive Muscular Dystrophies

LGMD may be inherited as an autosomal dominant (LGMD-1) or autosomal recessive (LGMD-2) disease. The vast majority of cases are sporadic, consistent with an autosomal recessive inheritance involving multiple loci. The disorder is clinically and genetically heterogeneous, and in some families the term *autosomal recessive muscular dystrophy* (ARMD) has been used for essentially the same phenotype. One form, with an early onset and severe phenotype, has been referred to as *severe childhood autosomal recessive muscular dystrophy* (SCARMD).

With identification of sarcoglycan deficiency in some LGMD and autosomal recessive muscular dystrophy patients, the clinical classification is giving way to a genetic classification based on the molecular defect.[186]

**Clinical Features of LGMD and the Primary Sarcoglycanopathies.** The unifying theme among LGMD patients is the initial involvement of the shoulder- and pelvic-girdle muscles with relative sparing of other muscle groups.[187–189] The phenotype, however, overlaps that of the primary dystrophinopathies, and in many patients, distinguishing this disorder from BMD is difficult.[190] The earliest symptoms are waddling gate, toe walking, exercise intolerance, and painful muscle swelling without myoglobinuria. The most common findings include increased lumbar lordosis, tight Achilles tendons, winged scapulae, and calf hypertrophy. All patients have progressive proximal muscle weakness, the hip girdle more affected than the shoulder girdle. Weakness of the neck and trunk flexors is also an early feature. The Gower maneuver is positive. The involvement of the distal muscles occurs later, and there may be cardiac involvement in the form of dilated cardiomyopathy.

Among those with demonstrated sarcoglycanopathy, the age at onset and severity of the myopathy are quite heterogeneous. Usually patients have normal early milestones, clinical signs appearing between the ages of 2 and 20 years. The most severe cases may be diagnosed as DMD-like muscular dystrophy or severe childhood autosomal recessive muscular dystrophy (SCARMD). Milder cases are most often classified as LGMD. The clinical spectrum of the sarcoglycanopathies recently has been reviewed by Angelini et al.[191]

**Laboratory Investigations.** Typical LGMD laboratory results resemble DMD or BMD. Serum CK is elevated 10- to 120-fold

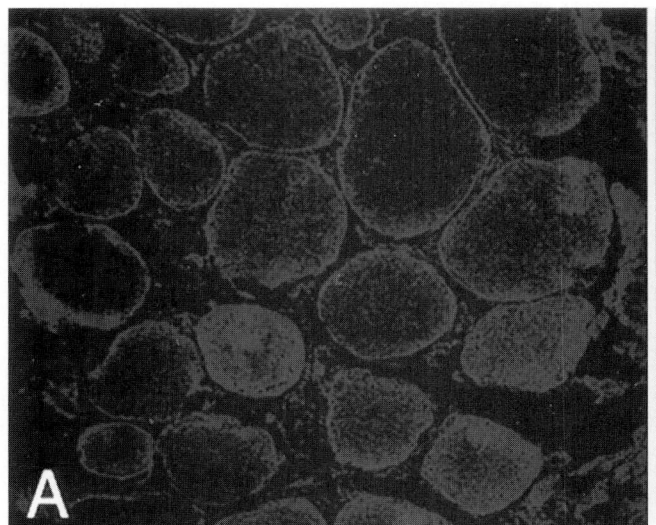
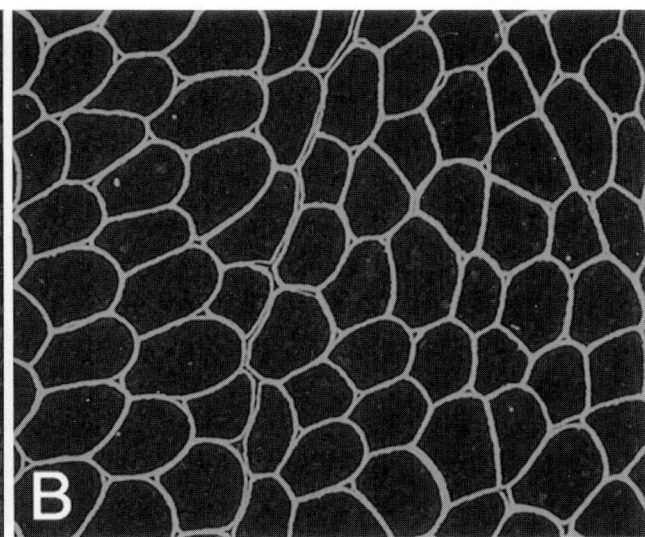

**Fig. 216-10** Immunostaining with antibody against α-sarcoglycan in muscle sections from (*A*) a 13-year-old boy who presented with a Duchenne-like muscular dystrophy and (*B*) a normal control. The patient was shown to have a missense mutation in the α-sarcoglycan gene, resulting in failure to integrate into the complex.

over normal, with no correlation between CK levels and age or functional stage. Electromyography shows typical myopathic abnormalities.

**Classic Muscle Pathology.** Muscle biopsies show dystrophic features including a wide variation in fiber size, fiber hypertrophy, and an increase in endomysial connective tissue. Necrosis and regeneration are intense, particular in young, severely affected patients. Type I fiber predominance is common.

**Sarcoglycan Deficiency in LGMD and Autosomal Recessive Muscular Dystrophy.** With the discovery of the dystrophin-glycoprotein complex, the proteins in the complex immediately became prime suspects for molecular defects leading to the autosomally inherited muscular dystrophies. A broad spectrum of patients was tested by immunostaining for dystroglycans and sarcoglycans in the muscle membrane, and as many as 30 percent were found to be deficient in all these components. In fact, a reduction in both dystroglycans and sarcoglycans at the muscle membrane of DMD patients indicates that the entire complex is unstable in the absence of dystrophin. Therefore, sarcoglycan deficiency is not by itself an indication of a primary sarcoglycanopathy. Conversely, in most cases of sarcoglycanopathies, dystrophin staining at the muscle membrane is normal, so a biopsy that is positive for dystrophin and negative for one or more sarcoglycans is indicative of a sarcoglycanopathy.[192]

The first indication for a specific deficit in the sarcoglycan complex came with the recognition of severe childhood autosomal recessive muscular dystrophy (SCARMD) patients in North Africa who had a deficiency of the 50-kDa protein that was dubbed *adhalin* from the Arabic word for muscle.[73,193] As will be seen in the section on the genetic basis of sarcoglycanopathies, the adhalin deficiency was later found to be secondary to the primary defect, since the gene for adhalin, later renamed *α-sarcoglycan,* mapped to chromosome 17, whereas the severe childhood autosomal recessive muscular dystrophy (SCARMD) locus mapped with the gene for γ-sarcoglycan on chromosome 13, and this disorder was demonstrated to be a primary γ-sarcoglycanopathy.

In patients with any primary sarcoglycanopathy, immunostaining with antibodies against α-, β-, γ-, and δ-sarcoglycans is reduced. The primary loss of any one sarcoglycan, such as α-sarcoglycan shown in Fig. 216-10, leads to the secondary reduction or absence of others.[194,195] In most cases, α-sarcoglycan is markedly deficient, which can be used as a screening procedure to detect most sarcoglycanopathies, including those resulting from a defect in the β-, γ-, and δ-sarcoglycan genes.

**The Mutational Basis of the Sarcoglycanopathies.** Deficiency in the sarcoglycans in autosomal muscular dystrophies suggested that mutations in the genes encoding these molecules might constitute the molecular basis for these disorders. We now know that patients with four different forms of LGMD, as well as autosomal recessive muscular dystrophy and the severe childhood form, all have mutations in sarcoglycan genes (Table 216-2).

In family studies, three LGMD loci have been identified in families with autosomal dominant inheritance. The LGMD-1A locus mapped to the long arm of chromosome 5,[196] and the LGMD-1B locus is mapped to the long arm of chromosome 1.[197] However, the defective genes at these loci have not been identified. The third locus, LGMD-1C, at 3p25, is the result of a defect in the caveolin-3 gene, as detailed below.

Recessive LGMD genes map to several sites revealing genetic heterogeneity, the various forms referred to as LGMD-2A, -2B, -2C, -2D, -2E, -2F, -2G, and -2H. As it became clear that several of the LGMD recessive genes comapped with the sarcoglycan genes, the latter were tested for mutations in LGMD patients, and the molecular basis of the LGMDs began to fall into place.[60,186] The genetic defects have now been determined in LGMD-2A to -2F as detailed below. The LGMD-2G and 2H genes have been mapped but not yet cloned.[198,199]

***α-Sarcoglycan Defects in Autosomal Recessive Muscular Dystrophy and LGMD-2D.*** The earliest proof that the sarcoglycans are involved in autosomal recessive muscular dystrophy came with the cloning of the gene encoding α-sarcoglycan (adhalin)[73] and its mapping to 17q.[200] Study of the gene in four affected members of a French family whose late-onset autosomal recessive muscular dystrophy mapped to chromosome 17 revealed missense mutations in both alleles.[201] Other mutations were soon described in other autosomal recessive muscular dystrophy or LGMD-2D families,[202] and in a survey of 30 patients with normal dystrophin, only one had an α-sarcoglycan gene mutation, suggesting that approximately 5 percent of non-DMD patients are defective at this locus.[152] An incidence of 5 to 10 percent primary α-sarcoglycan deficiency among dystrophin-normal muscular dystrophy patients is supported by later studies.[203,204]

By 1997, 39 distinct mutations had been identified,[205] most of which occurred in the large extracellular domain. Generally,

**Table 216-2 The Molecular Basis of the Muscular Dystrophies**

| Disease | Chromosome Location | Defective Protein | OMIM | Genbank Accession No. |
|---|---|---|---|---|
| DMD | Xp21 | Dystrophin | 310200 | NM000109 |
| BMD | Xp21 | Dystrophin | 310200 | NM000109 |
| XLDC | Xp21 | Dystrophin | 310200 | NM000109 |
| LGMD-1A | 5q22-34 | Unknown | 159000 | |
| LGMD-1B | 1q11-21 | Unknown | 159001 | |
| LGMD-1C | 3p25 | Caveolin-3 | 601253 | NM001234 |
| LGMD-2A (Amish) | 15q15-21 | Calpain-3 | 253600 | AF127765 |
| | | | 114240 | |
| LGMD-2B/Mioshi myopathy | 2p13 | Dysferlin | 253601 | NM003494 |
| | | | 603009 | |
| LGMD-2C/SCARMD | 13q12 | $\gamma$-Sarcoglycan | 253700 | NM000231 |
| LGMD-2D/ARMD | 17q12-21 | $\alpha$-Sarcoglycan | 600119 | NM000023 |
| LGMD-2E (Amish)/ARMD | 4q12 | $\beta$-Sarcoglycan | 600900 | NM000232 |
| LGMD-2F | 5q33-34 | $\delta$-Sarcoglycan | 601287 | NM000337 |
| | | | 601411 | |
| LGMD-2G | 17q11-12 | Unknown | 601954 | |
| LGMD-2H (Hutterite) | 9q31-34 | Unknown | 254110 | |
| CMD, classic | 6q2 | Merosin | 156225 | AI636560 |
| CMD, Fukuyama | 9q31-33 | Fukutin | 253800 | AB008226 |
| EDMD | Xq28 | Emerin | 310300 | NM000117 |
| OPMD | 4q11-13 | PABP2 | 164300 | NM004643 |
| | | | 257950 | |
| FSHMD | 4q | Tandem repeat | 158900 | |

surveys of patients revealed the expected correlation between the severity of the mutation, the reduction in residual level of $\alpha$-sarcoglycan in muscle, and the clinical severity.[192,206,207] However, the correlation was not absolute, since among LGMD-2D patients homozygous for the prevalent R77C mutation, both mild and severe phenotypes are found,[208,209] suggesting the existence of modifying genes. Compound heterozygotes with this allele and R34H also have shown phenotypic variability.[205] Further, in sibs homozygous for an R284C mutation, one was asymptomatic, whereas the other had mild LGMD,[210] and in a patient with a missense mutation resulting in incomplete $\alpha$-sarcoglycan deficiency (i.e., partial immunostaining), the genotype is inconsistent with a severe phenotype.[211] The updated database of mutations is found on the Leiden University Medical Center Web site (*http://www.dmd.nl*).

***β-Sarcoglycan Defects in LGMD-2E.*** Cloning of the $\beta$-sarcoglycan gene and mapping to 4q12 made it a candidate gene for LGMD-2E that had been mapped to chromosome 4 in the Amish of southern Indiana. A homozygous missense mutation in the gene of these affected individuals resulted in loss of all four sarcoglycans from the muscle membrane of affected individuals.[74] In contrast with the mild phenotype of the Amish disorder, a 3-year-old girl with moderately severe disease was found to have a stop codon and a frameshift mutation in her two alleles, indicating a possible correlation of phenotypic severity with genotype.[212] In later studies, however, the phenotype-genotype correlation failed to hold as homozygous missense mutations were found in a severely affected Brazilian family and a mildly affected Tunisian family.[75,213] Here, the hypothesis was advanced that the Arg91Pro mutation in the severe case might disrupt the $\beta$-sheet structure, whereas the more conservative Arg91Leu change in the milder case might have a smaller effect on protein structure. As with the $\alpha$-sarcoglycan gene, the $\beta$-sarcoglycan gene mutations also cluster in the extracellular domain. Some of the early cases have been reviewed,[194] and the updated database of mutations is found on the Leiden University Medical Center Web site (*http://www.dmd.nl*).

***γ-Sarcoglycan Defects in Severe Childhood Autosomal Recessive Muscular Dystrophy and LGMD-2C.*** In North Africa, Tunisian patients with severe childhood autosomal recessive muscular dystrophy initially were thought to have a defect in the $\alpha$-sarcoglycan gene, based on reduced immunostaining for $\alpha$-sarcoglycan. However, mapping of the Tunisian gene to chromosome 13[214] ruled out a genetic defect in this gene and pointed to the $\gamma$-sarcoglycan gene at 13q12. A single-base-pair deletion found in both alleles of this gene in Tunisian severe childhood autosomal recessive muscular dystrophy[76] changes the reading frame, thereby eliminating the C-terminal end of the extracellular domain. Interestingly, three of four patients have a severe phenotype, whereas one had a much milder course, raising the possibility of a modifying gene. Immunostaining with specific antibodies showed complete absence of $\gamma$-sarcoglycan and a reduction of $\alpha$- and $\beta$-sarcoglycan in the membrane, indicating destabilization of the complex. Other $\gamma$-sarcoglycan mutations in a Japanese patient[76] and in gypsies migrating out of India[215] demonstrate that alterations in this gene are not confined to Tunisia, and the lack of phenotype-genotype correlation is also seen in non-Tunisian LGMD-2C patients.[216] The updated list of mutations is found on the Leiden University Medical Center Web site (*http://www.dmd.nl*).

***δ-Sarcoglycan Defects in LGMD-2F.*** Within a year after the $\alpha$-, $\beta$-, and $\gamma$-sarcoglycanopathies were described, the $\delta$-sarcoglycan gene was cloned and mapped to 5q33[77,78] and identified as the defective gene at the LGMD-2F locus previously mapped to this location.[217–219] Again, mutations are listed on the Leiden University Medical Center Web site (*http://www.dmd.nl*).

***Sarcoglycan Defects in Cardiomyopathy.*** Cardiac manifestations are a well-known consequence of dystrophin mutations, and the finding of a sarcoglycan defect in the BIO 14.6 cardiomyopathic hamster (see below) suggested that sarcoglycan defects may be the cause of human cardiomyopathy. To date, several mutations in sarcoglycans associated with dilated cardiomyopathy have been identified in patients who first presented with LGMD,[195,220,221] but it is not much of a stretch to assume that some idiopathic cardiomyopathy may be due to sarcoglycan complex mutations.[222] The updated mutation list is on the Leiden University Medical Center Web site (*http://www.dmd.nl*).

## Calpain-3 Deficiency in LGMD-2A

The LGMD-2A locus maps to 15q15[223] and colocalized with the *CANP3* gene encoding the muscle-specific calcium-activated neutral protease calpain-3.[224] Calpain-3 is a cytosolic proteinase that may be involved in connectin/titan processing.[225-227] Fifteen different mutations in this gene were described in LGMD-2A patients, six of whom were from La Reunion Island, and a digenic inheritance model was proposed to account for several different mutations in this small inbred population.[228,229]

Additional mutations have been found in subsequent studies, and anticalpain antibodies have allowed confirmation of the protein deficiency.[230-236]

Clinically, the calpainopathy is a typical but heterogeneous limb-girdle phenotype with increased serum CK, calf hypertrophy, and weakness predominantly in the pelvic-girdle muscles. In some cases, a scapuloperoneal distribution was observed. The patients remain ambulatory into their forties.[237] The updated mutation list is on the Leiden University Medical Center Web site (*http://www.dmd.nl*).

## Dysferlin Deficiency in LGMD-2B and Myoshi Myopathy

The genes for LGMD-2B and Myoshi myopathy (MM) were both mapped to 2p12-p14,[238-241] suggesting the possibility that both arise from mutations in the same gene with the phenotype modified by additional factors. The dysferlin gene (*DYSF*) was cloned by positional cloning focusing on MM.[242,243] The large gene contains over 55 exons and produces an 8.5-kb transcript expressed strongly in skeletal muscle and heart.[243] The 2080-amino-acid protein of unknown function has significant homology with the *Caenorhabditis elegans* spermatogenesis factor fer-1.

Mutations in the dysferlin gene were found in MM and LGMD-2B patients, as well as in one patient with distal myopathy with anterior tibial onset.[243,244] Most of the mutations were predicted to cause truncation of dysferlin. One homozygous LGMD "founder" mutation was present in eight Libyan Jewish families, probably all coming from villages around Tripoli. The updated mutation list is on the Leiden University Medical Center Web site (*http://www.dmd.nl*).

## Caveolin-3 Deficiency in LGMD-1C

Two loci had been identified previously in families with autosomal dominant inheritance, the LGMD-1A gene at 5q[196] and the LGMD-1B gene at 1q11-21.[197] The genes at these loci have not been identified.

A third dominant locus, LGMD-1C, at 3p25 was identified by the finding of mutations in the *CAV3* gene encoding caveolin-3, the muscle-specific form of the principal protein component of caveolae in the plasma membrane. In two patients, heterozygous mutations at conserved amino acids in the membrane-spanning region or scaffolding domain may interfere with caveolin-3 oligomerization and disrupt caveolae.[245] Given the fact that caveolin-3 forms homo-oligomers, these variations probably exert a dominant negative effect. Other mutations in the same gene are found in homozygous form, indicating a recessive inheritance for some alleles.[100] The updated mutation list is on the Leiden University Medical Center Web site (*http://www.dmd.nl*).

Histologic and histochemical studies revealed only nonspecific changes of moderate severity. Calveolin-3 staining was reduced 90 to 95 percent, and the number and size of caveolae were abnormal. Dystrophin and sarcoglycan staining was only slightly affected.[245] This is consistent with recent evidence indicating that caveolin-3 is not an integral component of the dystrophin-glycoprotein complex.[101,246] The fact that caveolae are increased in number in DMD

patients and *mdx* mice may be related to increased expression of the *CAV3* gene.[247]

## Congenital Muscular Dystrophy Due to Merosin Deficiency

The CMDs are autosomal recessive disorders that are heterogeneous in phenotype and characterized by variable central nervous system involvement. At least four forms have been described. The classic form of CMD has no severe impairment of intellectual development and no structural abnormalities of the brain.[248] It is this form that is associated with defects in merosin.

FMD is prevalent in Japan and due to a primary deficiency in fukutin that results in a secondary merosin deficiency (see below). Muscle-eye-brain disease prevalent in Finland and Walker-Warburg disease are forms of CMD with brain and eye abnormalities.[248] The latter has been shown to have normal merosin, demonstrating that it is distinct from the classic or FMD form,[249] and linkage studies have shown that muscle-eye-brain disease is genetically distinct from FMD.[250]

**Clinical Features of Merosin-Deficient Muscular Dystrophy.** Patients with merosin deficiency are usually hypotonic at birth. Some display multiple joint contractures, and there is a generalized muscle weakness—the facial, neck, and chest musculature is variably involved. The limb muscles are more severely affected proximally than distally, and many patients never become ambulatory. The tendon reflexes are decreased or absent. Mental development is usually normal.[248]

Although merosin deficiency is normally associated with a severe phenotype, some alterations in merosin may result in a late onset (i.e., noncongenital) muscular dystrophy.[251,252]

**Laboratory Investigations.** The serum CK and aldolase levels usually are normal or mildly increased. Electromyography reveals a myopathic pattern, although peripheral nerve involvement may be present.[253] Magnetic resonance imaging (MRI) of the brain recognizes a high-density abnormality in the white matter (Fig. 216-11), perhaps related to the reduced expression of merosin in the cerebral arteries, which may become "leaky" in merosin deficiency.[254]

**Classic Muscle Pathology.** Muscle biopsy shows striking pathologic changes, consistent with a dystrophic process. An increased variation in fiber-type diameter and replacement of muscle by adipose and connective tissue are the characteristic features. Some patients showed marked inflammation in their muscle and may even present with an inflammatory myopathy.[255]

**Merosin Deficiency: The Molecular Basis of Classic CMD.** Absence of $\alpha_2$-laminin in the muscles of classic CMD was first demonstrated by Tome et al.[256] and since confirmed in many cases. Immunostaining for $\alpha_2$-laminin in muscle is completely deficient in most cases of merosin-deficient CMD (Fig. 216-12), but there are some with only partial merosin deficiency. In some patients there appears to be a compensatory increase in $\alpha_1$-laminin immunostaining. In contrast, immunostaining for dystrophin is normal, as it is for $\alpha$-, $\beta$-, $\gamma$-, and $\delta$-sarcoglycan, as well as $\beta$-dystroglycan. On Western blot analysis, merosin immunoreactivity may be negative, or in some cases a lower-molecular-weight form may be present.

Merosin is normally detectable in Schwann cell basal lamina of cutaneous nerves and in the basal lamina of the corium in the skin. In CMD patients there is no immunoreactive $\alpha_2$-laminin in these stuctures,[257-259] and skin biopsy may provide an alternative tissue to muscle for definitive diagnosis.[260]

Secondary merosin deficiency also can occur, and therefore, loss of merosin at the sarcolemma is not, of itself, diagnostic for merosin-deficient CMD. Since merosin is part of an elaborate supramolecular assembly with the dystrophin-glycoprotein complex, genetic alteration of the sarcoglycans in this complex may

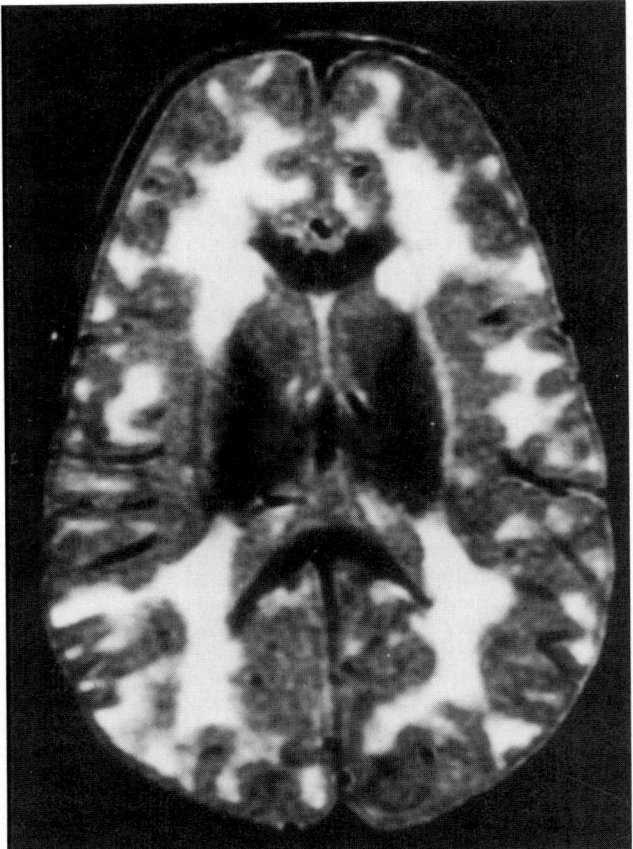

**Fig. 216-11** Computed tomographic (CT) scan (T$_2$-weighted image) of a horizontal plane of the brain shows marked hyperintense signal in the cerebral white matter in a patient with merosin-deficient CMD.

destabilize the complex and result in secondary merosin deficiency.[203] Another unexplained secondary partial merosin deficiency occurs in FMD.

**The Mutational Basis of Merosin Deficiency.** The genetic defect in merosin-negative CMD patients was shown to map to the $\alpha_2$-laminin (*LAMA2*) locus at 6q2 by homozygosity mapping.[86] Several nonsense and splice-site mutations in the *LAMA2* gene were then identified in CMD patients.[261,262] These mutations result in truncated protein removing either the short-arm domains or the

C-terminal globular domain and complete merosin deficiency. Missense mutations in the $\alpha_2$-laminin gene also have been identified in patients with partial merosin deficiency.[262,263]

Approximately 30 to 40 percent of neonatal-onset classic CMD has been shown to be due to $\alpha_2$-laminin mutations.[192,259] Merosin deficiency, however, also may be the cause of later onset forms of muscular dystrophy.[251,252] Because of the large size of the gene and the protein, the situation is similar to that in DMD, where it is difficult to screen for mutations. Most of the mutations detected to date have relied on RT-PCR to amplify the message or on single-strand conformation polymorphisms followed by sequencing. In addition, as for DMD, the protein truncation test based on *in vitro* transcription and translation of RT-PCR products is a valuable technique. The updated mutation list is on the Leiden University Medical Center Web site (*http://www.dmd.nl*).

### Fukuyama Muscular Dystrophy

FMD is one of the most common autosomal recessive disorders in Japan, with an of incidence approximately 1 per 10,000 births.[264] Affected individuals have significant mental impairment and structural changes in the central nervous system such as lissencephaly (agyria) or micropolygyria and hydrocephalus.[265–267] Initially, merosin deficiency[268] and basal lamina abnormalities[269] were described in this disease, but later this was found to be secondary to the basic defect in a gene encoding a protein termed *fukutin*. Clinical heterogeneity is recognized[270] and has been documented for patients with the fukutin deficiency.[271]

The gene was mapped to 9q31[272] and a haplotype shared by more than 80 percent of FMD chromosomes, indicating a founder effect to account for the high frequency.[264,273,274] Recently, a retrotransposal insertion of tandemly repeated sequences was identified within a candidate gene in all FMD chromosomes carrying the founder haplotype.[275] The inserted sequence is about 3 kb long and is located in the 3′ untranslated region of a gene encoding a 461-amino-acid protein. This gene is expressed in various tissues in normal individuals but not in FMD patients who carry the insertion. Two independent point mutations confirm that mutation of this gene is responsible for FMD. The predicted protein, which was termed *fukutin*, contains an N-terminal signal sequence, which together with results from transfection experiments suggests that fukutin is a secreted protein.[275]

### Emery-Dreifuss Muscular Dystrophy

Emery and Dreifuss described a mild X-linked muscular dystrophy with features similar to BMD except for early and widespread contractures and frequent cardiomyopathy.[276] Mapping of the gene to the long arm of the X chromosome firmly established it as a distinct genetic disorder, and cloning of the gene encoding the

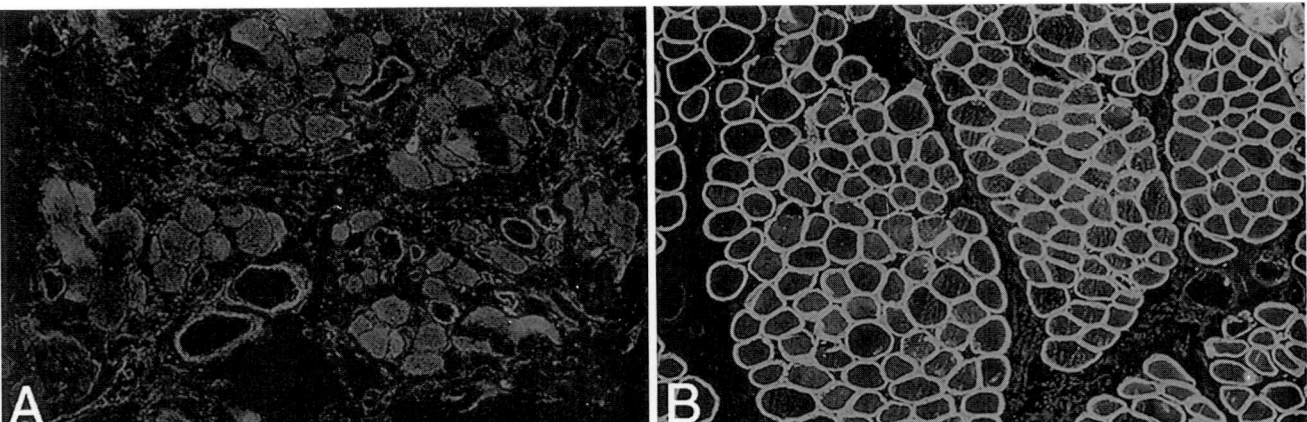

**Fig. 216-12** Immunostaining with antimerosin antibody of muscle from (*A*) merosin-deficient patient with CMD and (*B*) normal control. In the patient muscle, a few fibers retain some immunoreactive merosin (×350).

nuclear membrane protein, termed *emerin,* revealed the molecular basis of the disease.

**Clinical Features of EDMD.** The clinical features of EDMD have been reviewed in detail by Emery.[277] Onset occurs in the first decade, with toe walking, partial flexion of the elbows, and inability to fully flex the neck and spine. This distinct pattern of contractures of the heel cords, elbows, and neck extensors, associated with a scapulohumeroperoneal distribution of weakness, is an early clue to diagnosis. The neuromuscular wasting is mild and slowly progressive, with onset during adolescence, significant disability being rare before adult life. The biceps and triceps are affected first, whereas later difficulties are due mainly to weakness of the hip and knee extensors. In the lower extremities, distal muscles seem to be affected before the proximal ones, giving a humeroperoneal distribution.[276] Clinical heterogeneity is demonstrated by a report of atypical early onset disease in a boy confirmed to have a mutation in the gene encoding emerin.[278]

Another consistent feature of EDMD is a cardiac conduction defect that may, unless treated, lead to sudden death. Presymptomatic detection of heart involvement by means of regular electrocardiograms (ECGs) and the insertion of a cardiac pacemaker at an early stage may be lifesaving.[276] Cardiac risk also appears high in some but not all female carriers,[279] and in patients it may be life-threatening during anesthesia.[280]

A myopathic scapuloperoneal syndrome resembles the phenotype of EDMD, but early contractures do not occur, and cardiac conduction defects are not consistent. This and other conditions with phenotypes that overlap EDMD are tabulated by Emery.[276]

**Laboratory Investigations and Classic Muscle Pathology.** Laboratory studies in EDMD have been somewhat variable and controversial. Serum CK is usually elevated 3- to 10-fold over normal levels, considerably lower than for DMD and BMD. Disparate electromyographic results have been recorded showing both myopathic changes and evidence of denervation, even within the same individual, and muscle biopsy changes, usually consistent with a myopathy, are variable.[279] It would appear, therefore, that prime importance should be given to the clinical features of the disease, since the disparate electromyographic and histologic changes are poorly understood.[281,282]

**Emerin Deficiency: The Molecular Basis of EDMD.** In 1986, the gene for EDMD was found to be linked to the factor VIII gene at the distal end of the long arm of the X chromosome.[283-285] Subsequent studies refined the map position of the gene to Xq28, very close to the red-green color pigment (*RGCP*) gene.[286,287] The disease gene was identified by selecting candidate genes from the region and testing those expressed in skeletal and heart muscle for mutations in patients.[288]

Mutations were found in a gene encoding a novel serine-rich protein that was termed *emerin.*[289-294] The 2-kb gene has only 6 exons, making mutational analysis relatively easy, but not all patients with a diagnosis of EDMD have mutations in the emerin gene, indicating genetic heterogeneity for this disease.[289,295] The emerin gene is flanked by large inverted repeats that can recombine to delete all or part of the gene.[296,297] By 1997, 25 mutations had been described, and all abolished the synthesis of functional emerin.[298,299] The mutations are summarized in the EDMD mutation database (*http://www.path.cam.ac.uk/emd*).

Emerin is a 34-kDa protein with sequence similarity to the nuclear lamina-associated protein LAP2, and immunohistochemistry reveals that emerin localizes to the inner nuclear membrane (Fig. 216-13) via its hydrophobic C-terminal domain.[300,301] As a member of the family of type II integral membrane proteins that associate with the nuclear lamina, emerin is found not only at the nuclear rim but also at intranuclear sites, where it colocalizes with nuclear lamins B1, B2, and A/C. During mitosis, emerin is dispersed throughout the cell and then participates in the

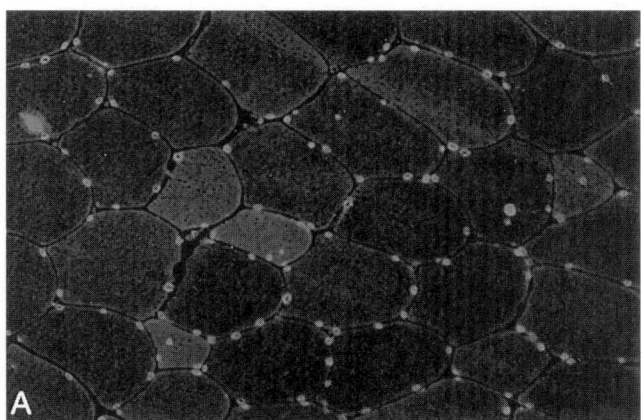

**Fig. 216-13 Immunostaining with antiemerin antibody of muscle from (*A*) normal control and (*B*) a patient with EDMD. In the control tissue, emerin is localized to the membrane of myonuclei (×350).**

reconstitution of membranes around the daughter nuclei.[302] Patient mutations that eliminate nuclear localization of the protein suggest that emerin possesses two nonoverlapping nuclear envelope targeting sequences, and altered phosphorylation patterns suggest that for emerin to function normally, it must be correctly localized, retained at the nuclear membrane, and phosphorylated by cell cycle-mediated events.[303]

The gene is expressed in many tissues of both human and mouse, and critical LAP2 phosphorylation sites are conserved.[304] In heart and cultured cardiomyocytes, emerin is associated with the intercalated disks, suggesting a role for emerin in membrane anchorage to the cytoskeleton. In heart, its specific localization to desmosomes and fasciae adherentes could account for the characteristic conduction defects.[305]

The ubiquitous expression of the gene and the localization of the protein to the nuclear membrane allow immunocytochemistry to be used as a diagnostic tool in easily accessible tissues such as skin, blood leukocytes, and cells from the oral mucosa.[306-308] In the oral mucosal cells, it appears easy to distinguish carriers with about 45 percent emerin-positive cells from normal individuals with close to 100 percent.[308] Manifesting carriers may fail to express adequate levels of emerin due to nonrandom X-inactivation.[295]

## Oculopharyngeal Muscular Dystrophy

Both autosomal dominant and recessive forms of OPMD have been documented. Originally described as a familial association of eyelid ptosis and dysphagia,[309] the autosomal dominant form of OPMD[310] has a worldwide distribution, with an estimated prevalence in France of 1 per 200,000.[311] However, it is particularly prevalent in the French-Canadian population (1 per

1000) and in Bukhara Jews living in Israel (1 per 600).[312,313] The predicted prevalence of the recessive form is 1 per 10,000.[314]

**Clinical Features of OPMD.** The hallmark of the disease is a selective progressive ptosis and dysphagia. Onset of the dominant form is usually after age 50, but the disease is fully penetrant by age 70 according to strict diagnostic criteria for dominant OPMD, including (1) a positive family history of OPMD, (2) at least one palpebral fissure at rest smaller than 9 mm (or previous corrective surgery), and (3) a swallowing time greater than 7 seconds when asked to drink 80 ml of ice-cold water.[312] Other signs in affected individuals include proximal upper extremity weakness, facial muscle weakness, limitation of upper gaze, dysphonia, proximal lower extremity weakness, and tongue atrophy and weakness.[315] The recessive OPMD clinical phenotype appears to be similar, though possibly milder.[316]

**Classic Muscle Pathology.** Pathologic findings in OPMD include rimmed vacuoles and small angulated muscle fibers.[317] Unique filamentous intranuclear inclusions identified by electron microscopy in the deltoid muscles of OPMD patients are seen in 4 to 5 percent of muscle nuclei and are considered a specific histologic marker of OPMD.[318] Pathologically, the inclusions consist of tubular filaments often arranged in palisades or tangles. The filaments are 0.25 $\mu$m in length and have an 8.5-nm external diameter and a 3-nm internal diameter. The percentage of nuclei with inclusions may correlate with the tissue expression of the mutant gene, since the more affected cricothyroid pharyngeal muscle has double the number of positive nuclei compared with the deltoid muscle of the same patient, and in homozygous OPMD patients, twice as many myonuclei show inclusions compared with heterozygous patients.[319,320] Intranuclear inclusions are also observed in recessive cases.[321]

**The Mutational Basis of OPMD.** The dominant OPMD locus was mapped to 14q11-q13 in three large French-Canadian families,[312] and linkage to the same markers was documented for families of other ethnic backgrounds,[322-325] suggesting that dominant OPMD is genetically homogeneous.

A positional cloning strategy identified the polyadenylation-binding protein 2 gene (*PABP2*) as the defective gene.[321] The characteristic mutation is an expansion of a normal (GCG)$_6$ triplet in exon 1 of the gene. In the French-Canadian families examined, OPMD is caused by a founder (GCG)$_9$ mutation. Among 81 families of different origins, the addition of 2 to 7 repeats yields mutations with 8 to 13 copies; the proportions of families with these mutations are 5 percent (GCG)$_8$, 40 percent (GCG)$_9$, 26 percent (GCG)$_{10}$, 21 percent (GCG)$_{11}$, 7 percent (GCG)$_{12}$, and 1 percent (GCG)$_{13}$. The mutations are mitotically and meiotically stable.[321]

The interfamilial phenotype variability may depend on the differences in sizes of the (GCG)$_n$ mutations, but this issue still has to be settled. The most severe cases are homozygous for a dominant OPMD mutation,[320,321] and it appears that 20 percent of the more severe cases have inherited, beside a dominant mutation, a (GCG)$_7$ polymorphism that has a 1 to 2 percent prevalence in North America, Europe, and Japan.[321]

The molecular basis of autosomal recessive OPMD in some cases is homozygosity for the (GCG)$_7$ polymorphism.[321] These cases may be underdiagnosed because of a milder phenotype and the absence of clear family history. Thus the (GCG)$_7$ allele is an example of a polymorphism that can act either as a modifier of a dominant phenotype or as a recessive mutation.

**A Model for the Molecular Basis of OPMD.** PABP2 is expressed in all tissues, but more highly in skeletal muscle. It is a nuclear protein that is involved in the second step of mRNA polyadenylation, the elongation of the poly(A) tails being dependent on PABP2 binding to the polyadenylation complex.[326-330]

The (GCG)$_6$ of the *PABP2* gene encodes a polyalanine stretch at the N-terminus of the protein, and this region is longer in the mutant-encoded protein. Brais et al.[321] have proposed a gain-of-function model in which mutant *PABP2* is a carrier of a pathogenic expanded polyalanine domain to nuclei, reminiscent of carrier models proposed in CAG repeat diseases.[331] Polyalanine oligomers are known to form $\beta$-sheet structures that are very resistant to protease digestion and chemical degradation.[332] Furthermore, polyalanine oligomers containing more than 8 alanines form fibrils spontaneously. It is proposed that beyond 10 alanines, the normal number of alanines in PABP2, the polyalanine domains polymerize to form stable $\beta$-sheets that are resistant to nuclear degradation. If these grow with time to form the OPMD intranuclear filaments that are seen on electron microscopy, it may sufficiently alter normal nuclear function to lead to cell death.[321]

## Fascioscapulohumeral Muscular Dystrophy

FSHMD is an autosomal dominant disorder with an incidence of approximately 1 per 20,000. The disease gene has not yet been identified, even though linkage of this gene to chromosome 4 has been known since 1990. Although the disease segregates as a simple Mendelian trait, the underlying molecular basis of the disease is genetically complex. The majority of patients have deletions of a 3.2-kb tandem repeat that does not appear to encode the gene, suggesting that the deletion alters chromatin structure, leading to altered expression of one or more nearby genes.

**Clinical Features of FSHMD.** Differentiation of FSHD from other types of muscular dystrophy is possible by its association with facial muscle weakness. The facial weakness is the earliest sign of disease, yet symptomatic onset is usually diagnosed with onset of shoulder weakness and scapular winging.[133] For some patients, the muscle weakness is restricted to a facioscapulohumeral distribution, but many show involvement of other skeletal muscles, preferentially the pelvic-girdle, truncal, and foot extensor muscles.[333] Cardiac involvement is variable.[334] Other clinical signs identified in patients include retinal vasculopathy, sensorineural deafness, and mental retardation.[335,336]

The onset of FSHD is highly variable but usually occurs within the second decade of life, with a penetrance of 95 percent by the age of 20.[333] A recent prospective study has established reliable measures of progression for use as outcome variables in clinical trials.[337]

At a molecular level, there is a partial correlation between the age at onset and the size of the D4Z4 deletion, larger deletions being associated with earlier onset (see below).[333,338,339] However, differential clinical expression in monozygotic twins suggests that other factors contribute to the phenotype.[340]

**The Mutational Basis of FSHMD.** Genetic linkage studies in 1990 localized the gene for FSHMD to the long arm of chromosome 4 near the telomere.[341-343] However, a detailed physical map failed to reveal the responsible gene.[344-346]

Subsequent molecular analysis detected a highly variable EcoRI polymorphism that was reduced in size in most FSHMD patients.[347,348] Further analysis attributed the DNA rearrangements to deletion of multiple copies of a 3.2-kb tandem repeat (D4Z4) in both sporadic and familial cases of FSHD.[349,350] The size of the deletion correlates with the age of onset and the severity of the phenotype[338] and is presumed to generate clinical variability between families. However, the fragment size is constant within families, implying that intrafamilial variability is due to other factors. Further studies indicated that similar repeats on 10q facilitate interchange between this region and the nearly identical region at the FSHMD locus on 4q, suggesting that translocation may be involved in the etiology of some cases.[351,352] The molecular genetics of FSHMD have been reviewed recently.[353,354]

Identification of the characteristic deletion provided the first diagnostic tool for FSHMD.[355-360] In dominant families, the genetic alteration can be used for prenatal diagnosis.[361] In sporadic cases, the mutation may be inherited from an unaffected parent with gonadal mosaicism.[362]

The related polymorphism on chromosome 10 complicates diagnosis, but sequencing the repeats identified restriction-site differences that allow the two regions to be distinguished by double digests.[363,364] Diagnosis is further complicated because subtelomeric exchanges in 20 percent of the population lead to individuals who appear "monosomic" or "trisomic" for the altered fragment.[352,365]

Each repeat contains a small open reading frame (ORF) encoding a double-homeodomain motif, but a transcript corresponding to this region has not been identified.[350] The recent discovery of a double-homeodomain gene, *DUX1*, with significant homology with this repeat ORF, expressed in skeletal and heart muscle, opens the possibility that a gene may reside within the repeats.[366]

If the repeats do not encode a gene, the disease may arise from altered expression of one or more nearby genes, a mechanism similar to telomeric silencing in yeast[367] or position-effect variegation in *Drosophila*.[368] Two genes have been identified in the 100 kb around the repeat element. One of these, *FRG1* (FSHMD region gene 1), is expressed from both alleles in patients, suggesting that it is not subjected to down-regulation,[369] and individuals who are monosomic for the region are unaffected, suggesting that haploinsufficiency is unlikely the cause of the disease.[370]

## DIAGNOSTIC WORKUP FOR THE MUSCULAR DYSTROPHIES

A practical diagnostic strategy for the muscular dystrophies is illustrated in Fig. 216-14.

### The Dystrophinopathies: DMD and BMD

**DMD Confirmation of Diagnosis.** Common practice is to follow a four-part diagnostic workup:

1. Clinical phenotype: Characteristics as above, or "outlier" with slower progression or atypical initial presentation:
   a. Slow learning/mental subnormality.
   b. Cardiac arrest during anesthesia.
   c. Malignant hyperthermia-like crisis during anesthesia.
2. Pedigree analysis: X-linked pattern of inheritance in two-thirds of cases, one-third sporadic due to new mutation.
3. Serum CK: Markedly elevated.
4. Dystrophin analysis: Confirmation of diagnosis requires one of
   a. Muscle biopsy with myopathic features and absent dystrophin. Sarcoglycan immunostaining is also reduced, secondary to the loss of dystrophin.
   b. Western blot showing absence of dystrophin.
   c. Dystrophin gene deletion or duplication detected by multiplex PCR.
   d. Point mutation detected by single-strand conformation polymorphism, heteroduplex analysis, RT-PCR, or protein truncation test, as reviewed by van Essen.[174]

**BMD Confirmation of Diagnosis.** A diagnosis of BMD is confirmed by

1. Clinical phenotype: DMD-like with later onset, loss of ambulation after age 16, slowly progressive; minor proximal muscle weakness and/or muscle cramps and/or muscle hypertrophy.
2. Pedigree analysis: X-linked pattern of inheritance in many cases.
3. Serum CK: Markedly elevated.
4. Dystrophin analysis: Confirmation of diagnosis requires one of
   a. Western blot showing reduced amount or altered size of dystrophin.
   b. Dystrophin gene deletion or duplication with unaltered reading frame, by methodologies as for DMD.

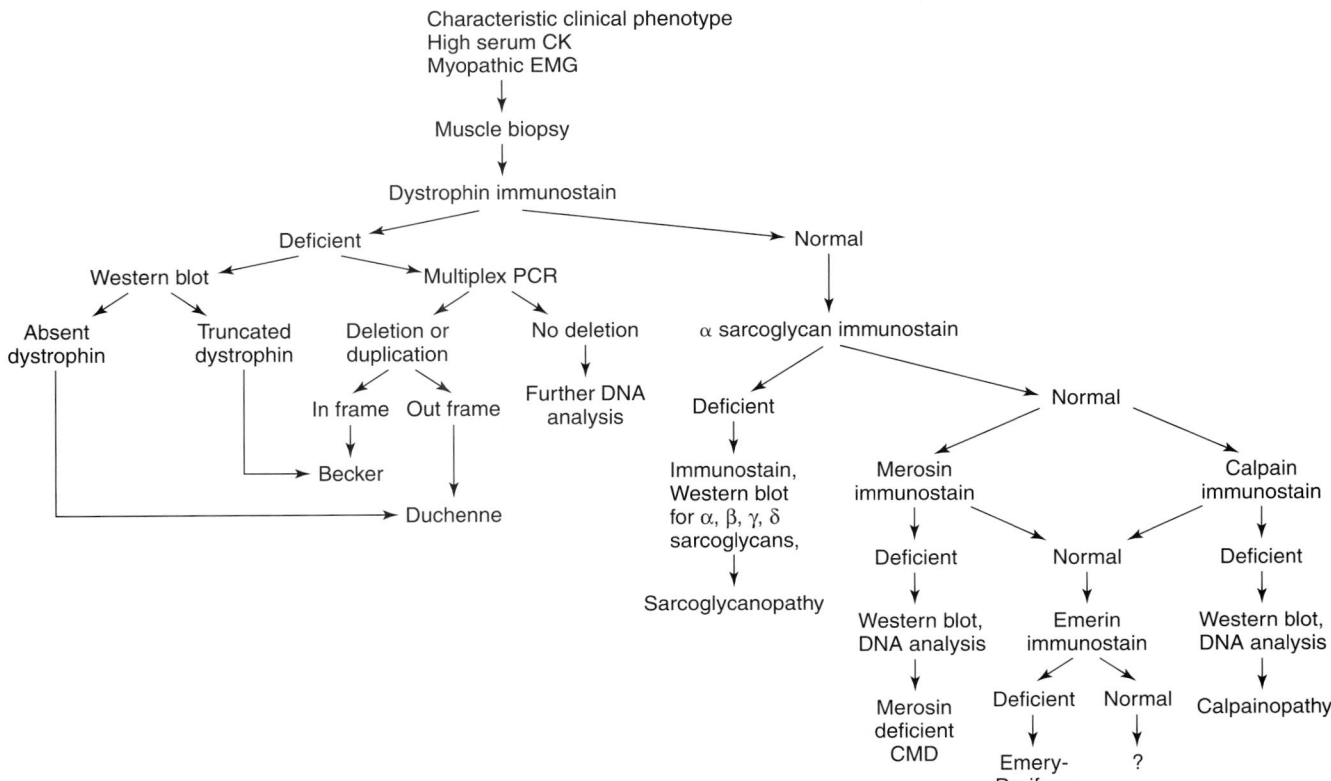

**Fig. 216-14** A flow diagram depicts a diagnostic strategy for the investigation of patients who present with a dystrophic clinical phenotype.

**DMD/BMD Carrier Identification.** Carriers are identified by

1. Pedigree analysis: May prove carrier status (e.g., affected son and brother or maternal uncle) or strongly suggest carrier status (e.g., two affected sons).
2. Serum CK: Unreliable indicator due to large overlap with normal values.
3. Muscle biopsy: Mosaic pattern of dystrophin immunostaining or quantitative western blot is inconsistent and helpful only when it reveals an altered DNA fragment.
4. If affected family member has known deletion or duplication, quantitative PCR analysis to determine copy number of the deleted/duplicated region by laser densitometry or fluorescent *in situ* hybridization is available in specialized laboratories.[371]

Note that germ-line mosaicism is a major complicating factor in carrier identification, and when present, it can result in multiple affected offspring with the same mutation from a "carrier" mother who does not display the mutation in her somatic cells. Based on estimates of frequency of gonadal mosaicism, a male fetus who carries the same X chromosome as his affected brother has an empirical risk of 10 to 30 percent of being affected.[373–376] With this risk, most genetics centers offer prenatal diagnosis to all mothers of DMD patients, regardless of proven carrier status.[377–383]

**DMD/BMD Prenatal Diagnosis.** If the gene defect is known and readily detectable:

1. Amniocentesis and mutation analysis of amniocytes, usually by multiplex PCR[379,380,382,384,385]
2. Preimplantation diagnosis by single-cell PCR of blastomer or polar body[386–389]
3. Fetal nucleated erythrocytes from maternal blood analyzed by multiplex PCR[381]

If the gene defect is not known:

1. Fetal sexing, allowing females to proceed to term
2. Fetal muscle biopsy for quantitative dystrophin analysis[143,390]

### Sarcoglycanopathies: LGMD and Other Autosomal Recessive Muscular Dystrophies

1. Clinical phenotype: DMD-like or LGMD or cardiomyopathy.
2. Pedigree analysis: Familial occurrence or inbred populations (consanguineous parents) signifies autosomal recessive inheritance.
3. Serum CK: At least 15-fold above normal.
4. Sarcoglycan analysis requires
   a. Muscle biopsy with nonspecific dystrophic features, normal immunostaining for dystrophin, but reduced immunostaining for the sarcoglycans. If both dystrophin and sarcoglycan immunostaining is normal, deficiency of calpain or caveolin is possible.
   b. Mutational analysis of the α-, β-, γ-, and δ-sarcoglycan genes is required to determine the primary defect, since a genetic defect in one sarcoglycan gene results in deficiency of all sarcoglycans at the sarcolemma.

### Merosin-Deficient Myopathies

1. Clinical phenotype: Severe CMD and peculiar white matter encephalopathy.
2. Myopathology: May show florid inflammatory myopathy, diverting attention from merosin deficiency.[390a]
3. Merosin analysis:
   a. Merosin (α₂-laminin) deficiency at the surface of muscle fibers can be demonstrated by immunocytochemistry. In FMD, due to a deficiency of fukutin, a partial and unexplained secondary merosin deficiency is present.

b. Mutational analysis to confirm primary merosin deficiency is advisable, since the disease is lethal, and prenatal diagnosis is an option considered by families. Prenatal diagnosis by mutation analysis, linkage to the *LAMA2* locus, and α₂-laminin analysis in a chronic villus biopsy have proven reliable.[262,391–394]

### Oculopharyngeal Muscular Dystrophy

1. Clinical phenotype: Varying degrees of ptosis, external ophthalmoparesis, and dysphagia. Occasionally need to differentiate OPMD from mitochondrial disease, myasthenia gravis or myasthenic syndrome, brain stem lesion, or congenital ptosis.
2. Pedigree analysis: Autosomal dominant inheritance is typical, but also recessive form.
3. Muscle biopsy: Electron microscopy of muscle biopsy reveals intranuclear inclusions. Genetic analysis now is more diagnostic.
4. Genetic analysis: GCG trinucleotide expansion in the *PAPB2* gene is a relatively easy and reliable test.[321]

### Fascioscapulohumeral Muscular Dystrophy

1. Clinical phenotype: Age at onset and extent and degree of the shoulder-girdle, truncal, and limb muscle involvement are variable; facial weakness is usually characteristic.
2. Myopathology: Not helpful, and a culprit gene and protein have not yet been identified.
3. Deletion of repeated sequences at the telomer of 4p is pathognomic for FSHMD and will differentiate it from other phenotypically similar conditions, such as scapuloperoneal muscular dystrophy, a form of familial inclusion-body myositis, and some inflammatory myopathies.

### Emery-Dreifuss Muscular Dystrophy

1. Clinical phenotype: Cardiomyopathy with atrial dilatation and early contractures at the elbows and hips is typical.
2. Pedigree analysis: If familial, it corresponds to X-linked inheritance.
3. Emerin analysis: Muscle biopsy with absence of immunoreactive emerin at the nuclear membrane or emerin deficiency by Western blot.

## ANIMAL MODELS

Animal models of muscular dystrophy share common genetic and protein alterations with the human diseases. These models can be used for the analysis of the pathogenesis of muscle fiber damage, and they serve as indispensable models for preclinical therapeutic trials.

### Dystrophin-Deficient Mouse and Dog

**The *mdx* Mouse.** There are two naturally occurring animal models of dystrophin deficiency. One is the *mdx* mouse, in which a stop codon in exon 23 results in dystrophin deficiency.[395] Dystrophin is not expressed along the surface membrane, even though the *mdx* mouse has no signs of major muscular dysfunction until late in life.[396–398] The diaphragm is an exception, and it shows early reduction of maximal force.[399]

In contrast, when utrophin-deficient "knock-out" mice, which also show a relatively normal phenotype, are crossed with *mdx* mice, the pups that are deficient in both molecules have a very severe muscle weakness.[51] The mice show joint contractures, pronounced growth retardation, and kyphosis, suggesting that in the *mdx* mouse the mild phenotype is due, at least in part, to utrophin replacement of dystrophin in the sarcolemmal membrane. A severe cardiomyopathy is also part of the phenotype.[52]

A severe dystrophic phenotype also occurs when *mdx* mice are crossed with myoD-deficient mice. In the absence of the skeletal muscle-specific transcription factor myoD, muscle regeneration is impaired, and a severe cardiomyopathy develops.[400]

**The Canine Model.** The second naturally occurring dystrophin-deficient muscular dystrophy is in the golden retriever dog, which has clinical and pathologic findings similar to DMD patients.[401-403] The disease is caused by a point mutation that induces exon skipping and creates the dystrophin deficiency in muscle fibers.[404] It is therefore an ideal model for preclinical therapeutic trials.[405,406]

### Sarcoglycan-Deficient Hamster and Mice

The BIO 14.6 cardiomyopathic hamster is a good model for the primary $\delta$-sarcoglycan-deficient muscular dystrophy. While early studies had documented a disruption of the dystrophin-glycoprotein complex in skeletal and cardiac muscle,[407,408] the $\alpha$-, $\beta$-, and $\gamma$-sarcoglycan genes were found to be normal.[409,410] The gene was mapped on hamster chromosome 9q,[411] and the candidate $\delta$-sarcoglycan gene was found to carry a mutation that results in the loss of $\delta$-sarcoglycan and disruption of the glycoprotein complex.[412] These findings make the BIO 14.6 hamster an excellent model for the study of human sarcoglycan-deficient LGMD and provides a model for the development of future strategies aimed at the treatment of human muscular dystrophy and cardiomyopathy.

Targeted gene inactivation has been used to produce a knock-out mouse with $\alpha$-sarcoglycan deficiency. Breeding to homozygosity resulted in mice that developed progressive muscular dystrophy and, in contrast to other animal models for muscular dystrophy, showed ongoing muscle necrosis with age.[413] These animals revealed loss of sarcolemmal integrity, elevated serum CK levels, and increased muscle mass. The molecular studies confirmed the absence of $\alpha$-sarcoglycan and the complete loss of the sarcoglycan complex and sarcospan from the muscle membrane.

Targeted gene inactivation also has been used to produce a knock-out mouse with $\gamma$-sarcoglycan deficiency. The mice showed pronounced dystrophic changes in early life and developed cardiomyopathy and premature death.[414] All three of these sarcoglycan-deficient animals will be important for preclinical studies on gene therapy or other therapeutic intervention.

### The Merosin-Deficient *dy/dy* Mouse

The naturally occurring *dy/dy* dystrophic mouse, known for nearly 40 years, has a much more severe phenotype than the *mdx* mouse, bearing closer resemblance to human congenital muscular dystrophy. Unlike *mdx*, it also has a dysmyelination defect that may contribute to the phenotype. The first real clue to the primary defect was the finding that the merosin gene comapped with the *dy* locus on mouse chromosome 10 and that merosin immunostaining was deficient in muscle of *dy* mice.[415,416] Follow-up with mice homozygous for the dy2J allele revealed a lower-molecular-weight merosin in the basal lamina of both skeletal muscle and peripheral nerve. The altered protein is due to a splice-site alteration that removes 57 amino acids from domain VI of the protein, presumably disrupting self-aggregation of laminin heterotrimers.[417,418]

## THERAPEUTIC APPROACHES TO THE MUSCULAR DYSTROPHIES

For genetic muscle diseases, four therapeutic approaches may be contemplated. Ideal would be a pharmacologic agent that would mitigate the deleterious consequences of a protein deficiency. Replacement of the mutant or absent protein with a normal one is another option but is not very realistic in the case of large structural proteins such as those involved in the muscular dystrophies. Up-regulation of a functional analogue of the missing protein is a particularly attractive option for DMD given the existence of the dystrophin analogue utrophin. Finally, there is gene replacement, which may be achieved by transfer of myogenic cells carrying a normal gene or by transfection of muscle with a vector containing a corrective gene capable of producing functional protein.

## Pharmacologic Approaches to the Muscular Dystrophies

Corticosteroids are the only pharmacologic agents that have so far shown beneficial effect for DMD.[419-422] Prednisone has revealed significant improvement in several parameters of muscle function in long-term studies, but side effects prevent its widespread prolonged use.[423-428] Deflazacort seems to have the beneficial effect of prednisone with somewhat fewer side effects.[429-431]

It is not clear whether glucocorticoids are helpful in the treatment of sarcoglycanopathies, although symptomatic improvement in a case of $\alpha$-sarcoglycanopathy has been reported.[210] In our experience, EDMD, FSHMD, and the merosin-deficient congenital myopathies do not respond to corticosteroid treatment. This is consistent with published reports for prednisone therapy in FSHMD patients.[432] In FSHMD, therapeutic benefit has been reported from the use of albuterol, a $\beta_2$ agonist that can produce some degree of nonspecific muscle fiber hypertrophy.[432a]

The mechanism of action of the steroid effect is still undetermined. Steroids do not work by up-regulating utrophin transcription.[148] Stabilization of the lipid bilayer of the plasma membrane has been suggested, but the amount of steroid required to produce such an effect is much higher than the therapy provides. Furthermore, immunosuppressive action of corticosteroids is unlikely to be important, since other immunosuppressive drugs are not generally useful. In myogenic cultures, steroids seem to promote myogenesis and prolong the life of myotubes.[433-435]

*In vivo*, prednisone protects rat muscle fibers against mechanically induced damage, possibly by stabilizing the muscle fiber membranes.[436] In studies with *mdx* mice, deflazacort is superior to prednisone in promoting fiber growth and muscle repair.[437,438] In DMD patients, protein degradation also may be reduced, contributing to the beneficial effect.[439]

## Gene Replacement Therapy

Gene replacement therapy may be achieved by cell-mediated gene transfer (cell therapy) or vector-mediated gene transfer (gene therapy).

**Cell-Mediated Gene Therapy.** Cell-mediated gene therapy, or cell therapy, consists of injecting normal myoblasts into a dystrophin-deficient muscle. Such myoblasts may either fuse with each other and create nascent muscle fibers with normal dystrophin content or fuse into the existing muscle fibers of the host and form mosaic muscle fibers in which there is a partial correction of dystrophin deficiency. The efficiency of such a procedure in *mdx* and *dy* mice was found to be quite promising,[397,440,441] prompting several phase 1 clinical trials.

Phase 1 clinical trials in DMD patients were disappointing, with little or no expression of dystrophin in the transplanted muscle and only borderline functional improvement in the force generation of muscle.[442-445] Only one group has continued to carry out myoblast transfer for DMD but has failed to provide convincing evidence for its effectiveness in a sizable group of patients.[446-448] Partridge recently has reviewed the state of myoblast transplantation for dystrophin replacement, and his commentary is especially useful in assessing the conflicting views.[449-452]

Assessment of the factors that caused the poor therapeutic outcome has continued in the *mdx* and *dy* mouse, and through the use of better immunosuppressive treatment, results have been improved substantially,[453,454] raising the hope that human trials will resume in the near future. For the merosin-deficient myopathies, myoblast transfer into the *dy/dy* mouse produced a partial restoration of the merosin content in the muscle fibers at the injected site.[454] Follow-up work in monkeys also has shown promise,[455,456] and use of a patient's own cells transfected with a dystrophin minigene may eliminate the immune response.[457]

**Vector-Mediated Gene Therapy.** In vector-mediated gene transfer, a dystrophin expression cassette, consisting of a truncated or full-length dystrophin cDNA driven by either a constitutive or muscle-specific promoter, is created. This cassette is incorporated into a suitable vector that is injected into the dystrophin-deficient muscle, delivering the transgene into muscle fibers. In most studies, the transgene is the truncated cDNA often referred to as a *Becker minigene*. This transgene is designed to fit into vectors with limited DNA capacity and has a portion of the dystrophin cDNA removed[458] to mimic the deleted gene identified in a patient with a mild Becker phenotype.[125] The minigene produces a reasonably functional dystrophin, as tested in transgenic *mdx* mice,[459] although it is not as good as a full-length dystrophin cDNA expressed in transgenic animals.[150]

To date, adenovirus has been the vector of choice due to its efficient delivery of its genetic payload to a broad spectrum of replicating and nonreplicating cell types. First-generation adenoviral vectors are replication defective due to removal of the E1 region and are propagated in 293 cell expressing the *E1* gene.[460] This type of vector has been used to rescue the dystrophin-glycoprotein complex by introduction of a Becker minigene into *mdx* mice,[461–464] the δ-sarcoglycan gene into the BIO 14.6 hamster,[465] and the α-sarcoglycan gene into the knock-out model of α-sarcoglycan deficiency.[413] These studies showed initial promise with virus injected directly into muscle, but the expression was short-lived, probably due to an inflammatory response and immune clearance of transduced cells related to the immunogenicity of adenovirus proteins. The loss of transgene activity was particularly apparent in mice transfected beyond the neonatal period, correlating with development of the immune system, with age-related loss of viral receptors,[466] or with loss of myoblasts that may participate in the viral transduction process.[467]

Although immunosuppression could mitigate the antiviral response, a better solution was the generation of helper-dependent adenovirus vectors. These vectors retain only those *cis*-acting elements required for virus replication and packaging, while protein-encoding genes have been removed and viral proteins are provided by a helper virus. This increased the insert capacity to 28 kb so that the full-length 14-kb dystrophin cDNA and a large muscle-specific (MCK) promoter could be accommodated.

Early attempts to develop helper-virus systems for mouse muscle were moderately successful but suffered from instability and low recovery of vector during propagation and from contaminating helper virus in the final preparation.[468–470] In the short term, the transgene was effective in correcting the dystrophic phenotype in *mdx* mice,[471] but loss of transgene activity remained a problem and was shown to be due at least in part to immunologic reaction against the product of the transgene, as evidenced by the persistent expression of a *lacZ* transgene in a *lacZ* transgenic host recipient.[472] Recently, the incorporation of *loxP* sites surrounding the helper-virus packaging signal has allowed the helper virus to be rendered unpackagable in a 293 cell expressing the Cre recombinase,[473] thereby reducing helper-virus contamination and resulting in a safer vector with enhanced transgene expression.[474]

As an alternative to vector-mediated gene delivery *in vivo*, adenovirus delivery of a dystrophin transgene to *mdx* myoblasts *in vitro* followed by myoblast transfer to muscle has shown promising results.[475] For the future, viral uptake may be enhanced by disruption of the basal lamina and by manipulating the abundance of primary adenovirus receptors at the cell surface.[476] Another major target for the future is a systemic delivery system, perhaps via the arterial route.

Other vector systems are not as well developed for gene therapy in muscular dystrophy. Herpes simplex virus-1 (HSV-1) will transfect myoblasts and differentiated myotubes in culture, but *in vivo* transfection is poor in mature muscle fibers,[477] perhaps a result of the inability of such a large viral particle to penetrate the basal lamina.[467,478–480]

Adeno-associated virus (AAV) is a promising vector for therapeutic gene transfer into mature skeletal muscle fibers, showing stable expression of a *lacZ* transgene for over a year with no indication of an inflammatory or immune response.[481] AAV is much smaller than adenovirus or HSV-1, and its uptake in mature skeletal muscle fibers is very efficient. It also has proven capacity to deliver a transgene to the heart via a coronary artery.[482] Its insert capacity is limited to 5 kb, making it a promising vector for the small sarcoglycan genes but not for larger genes.

Lipid carrier systems (liposomes) have been valuable for transfection of myogenic cells with plasmid vectors[483] but have been disappointing vehicles for delivery of genes to cultured myotubes or intact muscle fibers.[484] Success with nonviral delivery systems will require improvement of the overall efficiency of gene delivery and new approaches to target the vesicles to tissue-specific receptors.

**Up-regulation of Functional Analogues.** Up-regulation of a functional analogue is most attractive because it might be effected with small molecules. The best example of this type of therapeutic strategy involves utrophin, which is highly homologous with dystrophin in terms of molecular structure and is considered a good substitute for dystrophin.[485] Although both molecules reside in a similar molecular complex at the membrane, utrophin is normally concentrated at the neuromuscular junction and the myotendinous junction rather than throughout the sarcolemma. In DDM, there is a modest spontaneous elevation of utrophin level in the extrajunctional sarcolemma, but it is unlikely to be sufficient to rescue the muscle fibers.[486] By comparison, in *mdx* mice (or utrophin-deficient *mdx* mice) overexpressing utrophin from a transgene, the dystrophic phenotype is eliminated, implying that utrophin can serve as a functional surrogate of dystrophin.[53,54] Furthermore, adenovirus-mediated utrophin gene transfer into *mdx* mice had a similar mitigating effect on the phenotype.[151]

Together these results suggest that utrophin up-regulation by the pharmacologic enhancement of utrophin transcription and/or translation would be beneficial.

## REFERENCES

1. Worton RG, Brooke MH: The X-linked muscular dystrophies, in Scriver CR, Beaudet AL, Sly WS, Vallee D (eds): *The Metabolic and Molecular Bases of Inherited Disease*, 7th ed. New York, McGraw-Hill, 1994, p 4195.
2. Monaco AP, Kunkel LM: Cloning of the Duchenne/Becker muscular dystrophy locus. *Adv Hum Genet* 17:61, 1988.
3. Worton RG, Burghes AH: Molecular genetics of Duchenne and Becker muscular dystrophy. *Int Rev Neurobiol* 29:1, 1988.
4. Boyd Y, Buckle V, Holt S, Munro E, Hunter D, Craig I: Muscular dystrophy in girls with X;autosome translocations. *J Med Genet* 23:484, 1986.
5. Murray JM, Davies KE, Harper PS, Meredith L, Mueller CR, Williamson R: Linkage relationship of a cloned DNA sequence on the short arm of the X-chromosome to Duchenne muscular dystrophy. *Nature* 300:69, 1982.
6. Davies KE, Pearson PL, Harper PS, Murray JM, O'Brien T: Linkage analysis of two cloned DNA sequences flanking the Duchenne muscular dystrophy locus on the short arm of the human X chromosome. *Nucl Acids Res* 11:2303, 1983.
7. Kingston HM, Sarfarazi M, Thomas NS, Harper PS: Localisation of the Becker muscular dystrophy gene on the short arm of the X chromosome by linkage to cloned DNA sequences. *Hum Genet* 67:6, 1984.
8. Brown CS, Thomas NST, Sarfarazi M, Davies KE, Kunkel L, Pearson PL, Kingston HM, et al: Genetic linkage relationships of seven DNA probes with Duchenne and Becker muscular dystrophy. *Hum Genet* 71:62, 1985.
9. Francke U, Ochs HD, DeMartinville B, Giacalone J, Lindgren V: Minor Xp21 chromosome deletion in a male associated with

expression of Duchenne muscular dystrophy, chronic granulomatous disease, retinitis pigmentosa and McLeod syndrome. *Am J Hum Genet* **37**:250, 1985.

10. Wieringa B, Hustinx T, Scheres J, Renier W, ter Haar B: Complex glycerol kinase deficiency syndrome explained as X chromosomal deletion. *Clin Genet* **27**:522, 1985.

11. Kunkel LM, Monaco AP, Midlesworth W, Ochs HD, Latt SA: Specific cloning of DNA fragments absent from the DNA of a male patient with an X-chromosome deletion. *Proc Natl Acad Sci USA* **82**:4778, 1985.

12. Ray PN, Belfall B, Duff C, Logan C, Kean V, Thompson MW, Sylvester JE, et al: Cloning of the breakpoint of an X;21 translocation associated wit. *Nature* **318**:672, 1985.

13. Worton RG, Thompson MW: Genetics of Duchenne muscular dystrophy. *Annu Rev Genet* **22**:601, 1988.

14. Monaco AP, Bertelson CJ, Middlesworth W, Colletti CA, Aldridge J, Fischbeck KH, Bartlett R, et al: Detection of deletions spanning the Duchenne muscular dystrophy locus using a tightly linked DNA segment. *Nature* **316**:842, 1985.

15. Coffey AJ, Roberts RG, Green ED, Cole CG, Butler R, Anand R, Giannelli F, et al: Construction of a 2.6-Mb contig in yeast artificial chromosomes spanning the human dystrophin gene using an STS-based approach. *Genomics* **12**:474, 1992.

16. van Ommen GJ, Verkerk JM, Hofker MH, Monaco AP, Kunkel LM, Ray P, Worton R, et al: A physical map of 4 million bp around the Duchenne muscular dystroph. *Cell* **47**:499, 1986.

17. Gussoni E, Blau HM, Kunkel LM: The fate of individual myoblasts after transplantation into muscles of DMD patients. *Nature Med* **3**:970, 1997.

18. Tennyson CN, Klamut HJ, Worton RG: The human dystrophin gene requires 16 hours to be transcribed and is cotranscriptionally spliced. *Nature Genet* **9**:184, 1995.

19. Roberts RG, Coffey AJ, Bobrow M, Bentley DR: Exon structure of the human dystrophin gene. *Genomics* **16**:536, 1993.

20. Koenig M, Hoffman EP, Bertelson CJ, Monaco AP, Feener C, Kunkel LM: Complete cloning of the Duchenne muscular dystrophy (DMD) cDNA and preliminary genomic organization of the DMD gene in normal and affected individuals. *Cell* **50**:509, 1987.

21. Hoffman EP, Brown RH Jr, Kunkel LM: Dystrophin: The protein product of the Duchenne muscular dystrophy locus. *Cell* **51**:919, 1987.

22. Levine BA, Moir AJG, Patchell VB, Perry SV: Binding sites involved in the interaction of actin with the N-terminal region of dystrophin. *FEBS Lett* **298**:44, 1992.

23. Koenig M, Kunkel LM: Detailed analysis of the repeat domain of dystrophin reveals four potential hinge segments that may confer flexibility. *J Biol Chem* **265**:4560, 1990.

24. Lemaire C, Heilig R, Mandel JL: The chicken dystrophin cDNA: Striking conservation of the C-terminal coding and 3′ untranslated regions between man and chicken. *EMBO J* **7**:4157, 1988.

25. Murayama T, Sato O, Kimura S, Shimizu T, Sawada H, Maruyama K: Molecular shape of dystrophin purified from rabbit skeletal muscle myofibrils. *Proc Jpn Acad* (Series A, Series B. Physical and Biological Sciences) **66**:96, 1990.

26. Ohlendieck K, Campbell KP: Dystrophin constitutes 5 percent of membrane cytoskeleton in skeletal muscle. *FEBS Lett* **283**:230, 1991.

27. Zubrzycka-Gaarn EE, Bulman DE, Karpati G, Burghes AH, Belfall B, Klamut HJ, Talbot J, et al: The Duchenne muscular dystrophy gene product is localized in sarcolemma of human skeletal muscle. *Nature* **333**:466, 1988.

28. Bies RD, Friedman D, Roberts R, Perryman MB, Caskey CT: Expression and localization of dystrophin in human cardiac Purkinje fibers. *Circulation* **86**:147, 1992.

29. Cullen MJ, Walsh J, Nicholson LVB, Harris JB, Zubrzycka-Gaarn EE, Ray PN, Worton RG: Immunogold labelling of dystrophin in human muscle, using an antibody to the last 17 amino acids of the C-terminus. *Neuromusc Disord* **1**:113, 1991.

30. Porter GA, Dmytrenko GM, Winkelmann JC, Bloch RJ: Dystrophin colocalizes with β-spectrin in distinct subsarcolemmal domains in mammalian skeletal muscle. *J Cell Biol* **117**:997, 1992.

31. Byers TJ, Kunkel LM, Watkins SC: The subcellular distribution of dystrophin in mouse skeletal, cardiac, and smooth muscle. *J Cell Biol* **115**:411, 1991.

32. Tidball JG, Law DJ: Dystrophin is required for normal thin filament-membrane associations at myotendinous junctions. *Am J Pathol* **138**:17, 1991.

33. Huard J, Fortier L-P, Dansereau G, Labrecque C, Tremblay JP: A light and electron microscopic study of dystrophin localization at the mouse neuromuscular junction. *Synapse* **10**:83, 1992.

34. Lidov HG, Byers TJ, Watkins SC, Kunkel LM: Localization of dystrophin to postsynaptic regions of central nervous system cortical neurons. *Nature* **348**:725, 1990.

35. Byers TJ, Lidov HGW, Kunkel LM: An alternative dystrophin transcript specific to peripheral nerve. *Nature Genet* **4**:77, 1993.

36. D'Souza VN, Nguyen TM, Morris GE, Karges W, Pillers DA, Ray PN: A novel dystrophin isoform is required for normal retinal electrophysiology. *Hum Mol Genet* **4**:837, 1995.

37. Pillers DM, Bulman DE, Weleber RG, Sigesmund GA, Musarella MA, Powell PR, Murphy WH, et al: Dystrophin expression in the human retina is required for normal function as defined by electroretinography. *Nature Genet* **4**:82, 1993.

38. Howard PL, Dally GY, Wong MH, Ho A, Weleber RG, Pillers DA, Ray PN: Localization of dystrophin isoform Dp71 to the inner limiting membrane of the retina suggests a unique functional contribution of Dp71 in the retina. *Hum Mol Genet* **7**:1385, 1998.

39. Sadoulet-Puccio HM, Kunkel LM: Dystrophin and its isoforms (Review). *Brain Pathol* **6**:25, 1996.

40. Feener CA, Koenig M, Kunkel LM: Alternative splicing of human dystrophin mRNA generates isoforms at the carboxy terminus. *Nature* **338**:509, 1989.

41. Bies RD, Phelps SF, Cortez MD, Roberts R, Caskey CT, Chamberlain JS: Human and murine dystrophin mRNA transcripts are differentially expressed during skeletal muscle, heart, and brain development. *Nucl Acids Res* **20**:1725, 1992.

42. Kunkel LM, Anderson MD, Boyce FM: Dystrophin isoforms and nondeletion/duplication mutations. *Am J Hum Genet* **49**:4, 1991.

43. Tinsley JM, Blake DJ, Roche A, Fairbrother U, Riss J, Byth BC, Knight AE, et al: Primary structure of dystrophin-related protein. *Nature* **360**:591, 1992.

44. Blake DJ, Tinsley JM, Davies KE: Utrophin: A structural and functional comparison to dystrophin (Review). *Brain Pathol* **6**:37, 1996.

45. Matsumura K, Ervasti JM, Ohlendieck K, Kahl SD, Campbell KP: Association of dystrophin-related protein with dystrophin-associated proteins in mdx mouse muscle. *Nature* **360**:588, 1992.

46. Voit T, Haas K, Leger JO, Pons F, Leger JJ: Xp21 dystrophin and 6q dystrophin-related protein: Comparative immunolocalization using multiple antibodies. *Am J Pathol* **139**:969, 1991.

47. Karpati G, Carpenter S, Morris GE, Davies KE, Guerin C, Holland P: Localization and quantitation of the chromosome 6-encoded dystrophin-related protein in normal and pathological human muscle. *J Neuropathol Exp Neurol* **52**:119, 1993.

48. Chevron MP, Girard F, Claustres M, Demaille J: Expression and subcellular localization of dystrophin in skeletal, cardiac and smooth muscles during the human development. *Neuromusc Disord* **4**:419, 1994.

49. Deconinck AE, Potter AC, Tinsley JM, Wood SJ, Vater R, Young CM, Vincent A, et al: Postsynaptic abnormalities at the neuromuscular junctions of utrophin-deficient mice. *J Bacteriol* **136**:883, 1997.

50. Grady RM, Merlie JP, Sanes JR: Subtle neuromuscular defects in utrophin-deficient mice. *J Cell Biol* **136**:871, 1997.

51. Deconinck AE, Rafael JA, Skinner JA, Brown SC, Potter AC, Metzinger L, Watt DJ, et al: Utrophin-dystrophin-deficient mice as a model for Duchenne muscular dystrophy. *Cell* **90**:717, 1997.

52. Grady RM, Teng H, Nichol MC, Cunningham JC, Wilkinson RS, Sanes JR: Skeletal and cardiac myopathies in mice lacking utrophin and dystrophin: A model for Duchenne muscular dystrophy. *Cell* **90**:729, 1997.

53. Deconinck N, Tinsley J, De Backer F, Fisher R, Kahn D, Phelps S, Davies KE, et al: Expression of truncated utrophin leads to major functional improvements in dystrophin-deficient muscles of mice. *Nature Med* **3**:1216, 1997.

54. Rafael JA, Tinsley JM, Potter AC, Deconinck AE, Davies KE: Skeletal muscle-specific expression of a utrophin transgene rescues utrophin-dystrophin deficient mice. *Nature Genet* **19**:79, 1998.

55. Ervasti JM, Campbell KP: Dystrophin and the membrane skeleton. *Curr Opin Cell Biol* **5**:82, 1993.

56. Ervasti JM, Campbell KP: Membrane organization of the dystrophin-glycoprotein complex. *Cell* **66**:1121, 1991.

57. Straub V, Campbell KP: Muscular dystrophies and the dystrophin-glycoprotein complex (Review). *Curr Opin Neurol* **10**:168, 1997.

58. Arahata K, Hayashi YK, Mizuno Y, Yoshida M, Ozawa E: Dystrophin-associated glycoprotein and dystrophin co-localisation

at sarcolemma in Fukuyama congenital muscular dystrophy. *Lancet* **342**:623, 1993.

59. Yoshida M, Ozawa E: Glycoprotein complex anchoring dystrophin to sarcolemma. *J Biochem* **108**:748, 1990.
60. Worton R: Muscular dystrophies: Diseases of the dystrophin-glycoprotein complex (Comment) (Review). *Science* **270**:755, 1995.
61. Ozawa E, Noguchi S, Mizuno Y, Hagiwara Y, Yoshida M: From dystrophinopathy to sarcoglycanopathy: Evolution of a concept of muscular dystrophy (Review). *Muscle Nerve* **21**:421, 1998.
62. Corrado K, Mills PL, Chamberlain JS: Deletion analysis of the dystrophin-actin binding domain. *FEBS Lett* **344**:255, 1994.
63. Corrado K, Rafael JA, Mills PL, Cole NM, Faulkner JA, Wang KC: Transgenic *mdx* mice expressing dystrophin with a deletion in the actin-binding domain display a mild Becker phenotype. *J Cell Biol* **134**:873, 1996.
64. Rybakova IN, Amann KJ, Ervasti JM: A new model for the interaction of dystrophin with F-actin. *J Cell Biol* **135**:661, 1996.
65. Cox GA, Sunada Y, Campbell KP, Chamberlain JS: Dp71 can restore the dystrophin-associated glycoprotein complex in muscle but fails to prevent dystrophy (see comments). *Nature Genet* **8**:333, 1994.
66. Ibraghimov-Beskrovnaya O, Ervasti JM, Leveille C, Slaughter CA, Sernett SW, Campbell KP: Primary structure of dystrophin-associated glycoproteins linking dystrophin to the extracellular matrix. *Nature* **355**:696, 1992.
67. Jung D, Yang B, Meyer J, Chamberlain JS, Campbell KP: Identification and characterization of the dystrophin anchoring site on beta-dystroglycan. *J Biol Chem* **270**:27305, 1995.
68. Muntoni F, Gobbi P, Sewry C, Sherratt T, Taylor J, Sandhu SK, Abbs S, et al: Deletions in the 5' region of dystrophin and resulting phenotypes. *J Med Genet* **31**:843, 1994.
69. Phelps SF, Hauser MA, Cole NM, Rafael JA, Hinkle RT, Faulkner JA, Chamberlain JS: Expression of full-length and truncated dystrophin mini-genes in transgenic *mdx* mice. *Hum Mol Genet* **4**:1251, 1995.
70. Rafael JA, Cox GA, Corrado K, Jung D, Campbell KP, Chamberlain JS: Forced expression of dystrophin deletion constructs reveals structure-function correlations. *J Cell Biol* **134**:93, 1996.
71. Ettinger AJ, Feng G, Sanes JR: ε-Sarcoglycan, a broadly expressed homologue of the gene mutated in limb-girdle muscular dystrophy 2D [published erratum appears in *J Biol Chem* 273(31):19922, 1998]. *J Biol Chem* **272**:32534, 1997.
72. McNally EM, Ly CT, Kunkel LM: Human ε-sarcoglycan is highly related to α-sarcoglycan (adhalin), the limb girdle muscular dystrophy 2D gene. *FEBS Lett* **422**:27, 1998.
73. Roberds SL, Anderson RD, Ibraghimov-Beskrovnaya O, Campbell KP: Primary structure and muscle-specific expression of the 50-kDa dystrophin-associated glycoprotein (adhalin). *J Biol Chem* **268**:23739, 1993.
74. Lim LE, Duclos F, Broux O, Bourg N, Sunada Y, Allamand V, Meyer J, et al: Beta-sarcoglycan: Characterization and role in limb-girdle muscular dystrophy linked to 4q12. *Nature Genet* **11**:257, 1995.
75. Bonnemann CG, Passos-Bueno MR, McNally EM, Vainzof M, de Sa Moreira E, Marie SK, Pavanello RC, et al: Genomic screening for beta-sarcoglycan gene mutations: Missense mutations may cause severe limb-girdle muscular dystrophy type 2E (LGMD 2E). *Hum Mol Genet* **5**:1953, 1996.
76. Noguchi S, McNally EM, Benothmane K, Hagiwara Y, Mizuno Y, Yoshida MY, Bonnemann CG, et al: Mutations in the dystrophin-associated protein gamma-sarcoglycan in chromosome 13 muscular dystrophy. *Science* **270**:819, 1995.
77. Nigro V, Piluso G, Belsito A, Politano L, Puca AA, Papparella S, Rossi E, et al: Identification of a novel sarcoglycan gene at 5q33 encoding a sarcolemmal 35 kDa glycoprotein. *Hum Mol Genet* **5**:1179, 1996.
78. Jung D, Duclos F, Apostol B, Straub V, Lee JC, Allamand V, Venzke DP, et al: Characterization of delta-sarcoglycan, a novel component of the oligomeric sarcoglycan complex involved in limb-girdle muscular dystrophy. *J Biol Chem* **271**:32321, 1996.
79. Solovyev VV, Salamov AA: Predicting alpha-helix and beta-strand segments of globular proteins. *Comput Appl Biosci* **10**:661, 1994.
80. Engvall E: Structure and function of basement membranes (Review). *Int J Dev Biol* **39**:781, 1995.
81. Engvall E: Laminin variants: Why, where and when? *Kidney Int* **43**:2, 1993.
82. Wewer UM, Engvall E: Merosin/laminin-2 and muscular dystrophy (Review). *Neuromusc Disord* **6**:409, 1996.
83. Mercurio AM: Laminin receptors:achieving specificity through cooporation. *Trends Cell Biol* **5**:419, 1995.
84. Hodges BL, Hayashi YK, Nonaka I, Wang W, Arahata K, Kaufman SJ: Altered expression of the α7β1 integrin in human and murine muscular dystrophies. *J Cell Sci* **110**:2873, 1997.
85. Vachon PH, Xu H, Liu L, Loechel F, Hayashi Y, Arahata K, Reed JC, et al: Integrins (alpha7beta1) in muscle function and survival: Disrupted expression in merosin-deficient congenital muscular dystrophy. *J Clin Invest* **100**:1870, 1997.
86. Hillaire D, Leclerc A, Faure S, Topaloglu H, Chiannilkulchai N, Guicheney P, Grinas L, et al: Localization of merosin-negative congenital muscular dystrophy to chromosome 6q2 by homozygosity mapping. *Hum Mol Genet* **3**:1657, 1994.
87. Suzuki A, Yoshida M, Hayashi K, Mizuno Y, Hagiwara Y, Ozawa E: Molecular organization at the glycoprotein-complex-binding site of dystrophin: Three dystrophin-associated proteins bind directly to the carboxy-terminal portion of dystrophin. *Eur J Biochem* **220**:283, 1994.
88. Yang B, Jung D, Rafael JA, Chamberlain JS, Campbell KP: Identification of alpha-syntrophin binding to syntrophin triplet, dystrophin, and utrophin. *J Biol Chem* **270**:4975, 1995.
89. Crosbie RH, Heighway J, Venzke DP, Lee JC, Campbell KP: Sarcospan, the 25-kDa transmembrane component of the dystrophin-glycoprotein complex. *J Biol Chem* **272**:31221, 1997.
90. Blake DJ, Nawrotzki R, Peters MF, Froehner SC, Davies KE: Isoform diversity of dystrobrevin, the murine 87-kDa postsynaptic protein. *J Biol Chem* **271**:7802, 1996.
91. Sadoulet-Puccio HM, Khurana TS, Cohen JB, Kunkel LM: Cloning and characterization of the human homologue of a dystrophin related phosphoprotein found at the Torpedo electric organ post-synaptic membrane. *Hum Mol Genet* **5**:489, 1996.
92. Ahn AH, Freener CA, Gussoni E, Yoshida M, Ozawa E, Kunkel LM: The three human syntrophin genes are expressed in diverse tissues, have distinct chromosomal locations, and each bind to dystrophin and its relatives. *J Biol Chem* **271**:2724, 1996.
93. Yoshida M, Yamamoto H, Noguchi S, Mizuno Y, Hagiwara Y, Ozawa E: Dystrophin-associated protein A0 is a homologue of the Torpedo 87K protein. *FEBS Lett* **367**:311, 1995.
94. Yang B, Jung D, Motto D, Meyer J, Koretzky G, Campbell KP: SH3 domain-mediated interaction of dystroglycan and Grb2. *J Biol Chem* **270**:11711, 1995.
95. Moiseeva EP, Belkin AM, Spurr NK, Koteliansky VE, Critchley DR: A novel dystrophin/utrophin-associated protein is an enzymatically inactive member of the phosphoglucomutase superfamily. *Eur J Biochem* **235**:103, 1996.
96. Brenman JE, Chao DS, Gee SH, McGee AW, Craven SE, Santillano DR, Wu Z, et al: Interaction of nitric oxide synthase with the postsynaptic density protein PSD-95 and alpha1-syntrophin mediated by PDZ domains. *Cell* **84**:757, 1996.
97. Brenman JE, Chao DS, Xia H, Aldape K, Bredt DS: Nitric oxide synthase complexed with dystrophin and absent from skeletal muscle sarcolemma in Duchenne muscular dystrophy. *Cell* **82**:743, 1995.
98. Chao DS, Gorospe JR, Brenman JE, Rafael JA, Peters MF, Froehner SC, Hoffman EP, et al: Selective loss of sarcolemmal nitric oxide synthase in Becker muscular dystrophy. *J Exp Med* **184**:609, 1996.
99. Song KS, Scherer PE, Tang Z, Okamoto T, Li S, Chafel M, Chu C, et al: Expression of caveolin-3 in skeletal, cardiac, and smooth muscle cells: Caveolin-3 is a component of the sarcolemma and co-fractionates with dystrophin and dystrophin-associated glycoproteins. *J Biol Chem* **271**:15160, 1996.
100. McNally EM, de Sa M, Duggan DJ, Bonnemann CG, Lisanti MP, Lidov, HGW, et al: Caveolin-3 in muscular dystrophy. *Hum Mol Genet* **7**:871, 1998.
101. Crosbie RH, Yamada H, Venzke DP, Lisanti MP, Campbell KP: Caveolin-3 is not an integral component of the dystrophin glycoprotein complex. *FEBS Lett* **427**:279, 1998.
102. Karpati G: Recent developments in the biology of dystrophin and related molecules. *Curr Opin Neurol Neurosurg* **5**:615, 1992.
103. Hutter OF: The membrane hypothesis of Duchenne muscular dystrophy: Quest for functional evidence. *J Inher Metab Dis* **15**:565, 1992.
104. Weller B, Karpati G, Carpenter S: Dystrophin-deficient mdx muscle fibers are preferentially vulnerable to necrosis induced by experimental lengthening contractions. *J Neurol Sci* **100**:9, 1990.
105. Petrof BJ, Shrager JB, Stedman HH, Kelly AM, Sweeney HL: Dystrophin protects the sarcolemma from stresses developed during muscle contraction. *Proc Natl Acad Sci USA* **90**:3710, 1993.

106. Bork P, Sudol M: The WW domain: A signalling site in dystrophin? *Trends Biochem Sci* **19**:531, 1994.
107. Sudol M, Bork P, Einbond A, Kastury K, Druck T, Negrini M, Huebner K, et al: Characterization of the mammalian YAP (Yes-associated protein) gene and its role in defining a novel protein module, the WW domain. *J Biol Chem* **270**:14733, 1995.
108. Hardiman O: Dystrophin deficiency, altered cell signalling and fibre hypertrophy. *Neuromuscul Disord* **4**:305, 1994.
109. Henry MD, Campbell KP: A role for dystroglycan in basement membrane assembly. *Cell* **95**:859, 1998.
110. Matthews PM, Karpati G: Pattern of X-chromosome inactivation as a key determinant of the clinicopathologic phenotype of Duchenne muscular dystrophy carriers. *Neurology* **46**:1189, 1996.
111. Emery AEH: *Duchenne Muscular Dystrophy.* New York, Oxford University Press, 1993.
112. Lupski JR, Garcia CA, Zoghbi HY, Hoffman EP, Fenwick RG: Discordance of muscular dystrophy in monozygotic female twins: Evidence supporting asymmetric splitting of the inner cell mass in a manifesting carrier of Duchenne dystrophy. *Am J Med Genet* **40**:354, 1991.
113. Richards CS, Watkins SC, Hoffman EP, Schneider NR, Milsark IW, Katz KS, Cook JD, et al: Skewed X inactivation in a female MZ twin results in Duchenne muscular dystrophy. *Am J Hum Genet* **46**:672, 1990.
114. Burn J, Povey S, Boyd Y, Munro EA, West L, Harper K, Thomas D: Duchenne muscular dystrophy in one of monozygotic twin girls. *J Med Genet* **23**:494, 1986.
115. Nance WE: Do twin Lyons have larger spots? *Am J Hum Genet* **46**:646, 1990.
116. Meryon E: On granular and fatty degeneration of the voluntary muscles. *Med Chir Trans* **35**:73, 1852.
117. Duchenne GBA: Recherches sur la paralysie musculaire pseudohypertrophique ou paralysie myosclerosique. *Arch Gen Med* **11**:5, 1868.
118. Larsen UT, Juhl B, Hein Sorensen O, de Fine Olivarius B: Complications during anaesthesia in patients with Duchenne's muscular dystrophy (a retrospective study). *Can J Anaesth* **36**:418, 1989.
119. Farell PT: Anaesthesia-induced rhabdomyolysis causing cardiac arrest: Case report and review of anaesthesia and the dystrophinopathies. *Anaesth Inten Care* **22**:597, 1994.
120. Brooke MH, Fenichel GM, Griggs RC, Mendell JR, Moxley R, Florence J, King WM, et al: Duchenne muscular dystrophy: patterns of clinical progression and effects of supportive therapy. *Neurology* **39**:475, 1989.
121. Boland BJ, Silbert PL, Groover RV, Wollan PC, Silverstein MD: Skeletal, cardiac, and smooth muscle failure in Duchenne muscular dystrophy. *Pediatr Neurol* **14**:7, 1996.
122. Dubowitz V: Intellectual impairment in muscular dystrophy. *Arch Dis Child* **40**:296, 1965.
123. Lidov HG: Dystrophin in the nervous system (Review). *Brain Pathol* **6**:63, 1996.
124. Bushby KM, Appleton R, Anderson LV, Welch JL, Kelly P, Gardner-Medwin D: Deletion status and intellectual impairment in Duchenne muscular dystrophy. *Dev Med Child Neurol* **37**:260, 1995.
125. England SB, Nicholson LV, Johnson MA, Forrest SM, Love DR, Zubrzycka Gaarn EE, Bulman DE, et al: Very mild muscular dystrophy associated with the deletion of 46 percent of dystrophin. *Nature* **343**:180, 1990.
126. Sunohara N, Arahata K, Hoffman EP, Tamada H, Nishimiya J, Arikawa A, Kaido M, et al: Quadriceps myopathy: Forme fruste of Becker muscular dystrophy. *Ann Neurol* **28**:634, 1990.
127. Gospe SM Jr, Lazaro RP, Lava NS, Grootscholten PM, Scott MO, Fischbeck KH: Familial X-linked myalgia and cramps: A nonprogressive myopathy associated with a deletion in the dystrophin gene. *Neurology* **39**:1277, 1989.
128. Bushby K, Goodship J, Haggerty D, Heald A, Walls T: Duchenne muscular dystrophy and idiopathic hyperCKemia in a family causing confusion in genetic counselling (Letter; Comment). *Am J Med Genet* **66**:237, 1996.
129. Daube JR: Electrodiagnosis of muscle disorders, in Engel AG, Banker BQ (eds): *Myology.* New York, McGraw-Hill, 1986, p 1195.
130. Farrah MG, Evans EB, Vignos JP: Electrocardiographic evaluation of left ventricular function in Duchenne muscular dystrophy. *Am J Med* **69**:248, 1980.
131. Ebashi S, Toyokura Y, Momoi H, Sugita H: High creatine phosphokinase activity of sera of progressive muscular dystrophy. *J Biochem Tokyo* **46**:103, 1959.
132. Dreyfus JC, Schapira G, Demos J: Etude de la creatine kinase serique chez les myopathes et leurs families. *Rev Fr Etud Clin Biol* **5**:384, 1960.
133. Dubowitz V: *Muscle Disorders in Childhood.* Philadelphia, Saunders, 1978.
134. Dubowitz V: *Muscle Biopsy: A Practical Approach.* London, Bailliere Tindall, 1985.
135. Webster C, Blau HM: Accelerated age-related decline in replicative life-span of Duchenne muscular dystrophy myoblasts: Implications for cell and gene therapy. *Somat Cell Mol Genet* **16**:557, 1990.
136. Webster C, Filippi G, Rinaldi A, Mastropaolo C, Tondi M, Siniscalco M, Blau HM: The myoblast defect identified in Duchenne muscular dystrophy is not a primary expression of the DMD mutation: Clonal analysis of myoblasts from five double heterozygotes for two X-linked loci: DMD and G6PD. *Hum Genet* **74**:74, 1986.
137. Mokri B, Engel AG: Duchenne dystrophy: Electron microscopic findings pointing to a basic or early abnormality in the plasma membrane of the muscle fiber. *Neurology* **25**:1111, 1975.
138. Carpenter S, Karpati G: Duchenne muscular dystrophy: Plasma membrane loss initiates muscle cell necrosis unless it is repaired. *Brain* **102**:147, 1979.
139. Hoffman EP, Fischbeck KH, Brown RH, Johnson M, Medori R, Loike JD, Harris JB, et al: Characterization of dystrophin in muscle-biopsy specimens from patients with Duchenne's or Becker's muscular dystrophy. *N Engl J Med* **318**:1363, 1988.
140. Nicholson LV, Johnson MA, Gardner Medwin D, Bhattacharya S, Harris JB: Heterogeneity of dystrophin expression in patients with Duchenne and Becker muscular dystrophy. *Acta Neuropathol* **80**:239, 1990.
141. Arahata K, Hoffman EP, Kunkel LM, Ishiura S, Tsukahara T, Ishihara T, Sunohara N, et al: Dystrophin diagnosis: Comparison of dystrophin abnormalities by immunofluorescence and immunoblot analyses. *Proc Natl Acad Sci USA* **86**:7154, 1989.
142. Hoffman EP: Clinical and histopathological features of abnormalities of the dystrophin-based membrane cytoskeleton (Review). *Brain Pathol* **6**:49, 1996.
143. Evans MI, Farrell SA, Greb A, Ray P, Johnson MP, Hoffman EP: In utero fetal muscle biopsy for the diagnosis of Duchenne muscular dystrophy in a female fetus "suddenly at risk." *Am J Med Genet* **46**:309, 1993.
144. Evans MI, Hoffman EP, Cadrin C, Johnson MP, Quintero RA, Golbus MS: Fetal muscle biopsy: Collaborative experience with varied indications. *Obstet Gynecol* **84**:913, 1994.
145. Winnard AV, Mendell JR, Prior TW, Florence J, Burghes AHM: Frameshift deletions of exons 3-7 and revertant fibers in Duchenne muscular dystrophy: Mechanisms of dystrophin production. *Am J Hum Genet* **56**:158, 1995.
146. Thanh LT, Nguyen TM, Helliwell TR, Morris GE: Characterization of revertant muscle fibers in Duchenne muscular dystrophy, using exon-specific monoclonal antibodies against dystrophin. *Am J Hum Genet* **56**:725, 1995.
147. Taylor J, Muntoni F, Dubowitz V, Sewry CA: The abnormal expression of utrophin in Duchenne and Becker muscular dystrophy is age related. *Neuropathol Appl Neurobiol* **23**:399, 1997.
148. Pasquini F, Guerin C, Blake D, Davies K, Karpati G, Holland P: The effect of glucocorticoids on the accumulation of utrophin by cultured normal and dystrophic human skeletal muscle satellite cells. *Neuromusc Disord* **5**:105, 1995.
149. Ohlendieck K, Matsumura K, Ionasescu VV, Towbin JA, Bosch EP, Weinstein SL, Sernett SW, et al: Duchenne muscular dystrophy: Deficiency of dystrophin-associated proteins in the sarcolemma. *Neurology* **43**:795, 1993.
150. Cox GA, Cole NM, Matsumura K, Phelps SF, Hauschka SD, Campbell KP, Faulkner JA, et al: Overexpression of dystrophin in transgenic *mdx* mice eliminates dystrophic symptoms without toxicity. *Nature* **364**:725, 1993.
151. Gilbert R, Nalbantoglu J, Tinsley JM, Massie B, Davies KE, Karpati G: Efficient utrophin expression following adenovirus gene transfer in dystrophic muscle. *Biochem Biophys Res Commun* **242**:244, 1998.
152. Ljunggren A, Duggan D, McNally E, Boylan KB, Gama CH, Kunkel LM, Hoffman EP: Primary adhalin deficiency as a cause of muscular dystrophy in patients with normal dystrophin (see Comments). *Ann Neurol* **38**:367, 1995.
153. Arahata K, Beggs AH, Honda H, Ito S, Ishiura S, Tsukahara T, Ishiguro T, et al: Preservation of the C-terminus of dystrophin molecule in the skeletal muscle from Becker muscular dystrophy. *J Neurol Sci* **101**:148, 1991.

154. Matsumura K, Campbell KP: Dystrophin-glycoprotein complex: Its role in the molecular pathogenesis of muscular dystrophies (Review). *Muscle Nerve* **17**:2, 1994.

155. Menke A, Jockusch H: Decreased osmotic stability of dystrophin-less muscle cells from the *mdx* mouse. *Nature* **349**:69, 1991.

156. Wrogemann K, Pena SD: Mitochondrial calcium overload: A general mechanism for cell-necrosis in muscle diseases. *Lancet* **1**:672, 1976.

157. Carpenter S, Karpati G: Segmental necrosis and its demarcation in experimental micropuncture injury of skeletal muscle fibers. *J Neuropathol Exp Neurol* **48**:154, 1989.

158. Karpati G, Carpenter S: Small-caliber skeletal muscle fibers do not suffer deleteriousconsequences of dystrophic gene expression. *Am J Med Genet* **25**:653, 1986.

159. Koenig M, Beggs AH, Moyer M, Scherpf S, Heindrich K, Bettecken T, Meng G, et al: The molecular basis for Duchenne versus Becker muscular dystrophy: correlation of severity with type of deletion. *Am J Hum Genet* **45**:498, 1989.

160. Gillard EF, Chamberlain JS, Murphy EG, Duff CL, Smith B, Burghes AH, Thompson MW, et al: Molecular and phenotypic analysis of patients with deletions within the deletion-rich region of the Duchenne muscular dystrophy (DMD) gene. *Am J Hum Genet* **45**:507, 1989.

161. Chamberlain JS, Gibbs RA, Ranier JE, Nguyen PN, Caskey CT: Deletion screening of the Duchenne muscular dystrophy locus via multiplex DNA amplification. *Nucl Acids Res* **16**:11141, 1988.

162. Chamberlain JS, Farwell NJ, Chamberlain JR, Cox GA, Caskey CT: PCR analysis of dystrophin gene mutation and expression. *J Cell Biochem* **36**:255, 1991.

163. Chamberlain JS, Multicenter Study Group: Diagnosis of Duchenne and Becker muscular dystrophies by polymerase chain reaction. *JAMA* **267**:2609, 1992.

164. Beggs AH, Koenig M, Boyce FM, Kunkel LM: Detection of 98 percent of DMD/BMD gene deletions by polymerase chain reaction. *Hum Genet* **86**:45, 1990.

165. Monaco AP, Bertelson CJ, Liechti Gallati S, Moser H, Kunkel LM: An explanation for the phenotypic differences between patients bearing partial deletions of the DMD locus. *Genomics* **2**:90, 1988.

166. Malhotra SB, Hart KA, Klamut HJ, Thomas NS, Bodrug SE, Burghes AH, Bobrow M, et al: Frame-shift deletions in patients with Duchenne and Becker muscular dystrophy. *Science* **242**:755, 1988.

167. Hu XY, Burghes AH, Ray PN, Thompson MW, Murphy EG, Worton RG: Partial gene duplication in Duchenne and Becker muscular dystrophies. *J Med Genet* **25**:369, 1988.

168. Hu XY, Ray PN, Murphy EG, Thompson MW, Worton RG: Duplicational mutation at the Duchenne muscular dystrophy locus: Its frequency, distribution, origin, and phenotype-genotype correlation. *Am J Hum Genet* **46**:682, 1990.

169. Galvagni F, Saad FA, Danieli GA, Miorin M, Vitiello L, Mostacciuolo ML, Angelini C: A study on duplications of the dystrophin gene: Evidence of a geographical difference in the distribution of breakpoints by intron. *Hum Genet* **94**:83, 1994.

170. Hu X, Bulman DE, Ray PN, Worton RG: Frame-shift duplication resulting in truncated dystrophin in a patient with Duchenne muscular dystrophy. *Hum Mutat* **1**:172, 1992.

171. Toscano A, Vitiello L, Comi GP, Galvagni F, Miorin M, Prelle A, Fortunato F, et al: Duplication of dystrophin gene and dissimilar clinical phenotype in the same family. *Neuromusc Disord* **5**:475, 1995.

172. Hu XY, Ray PN, Worton RG: Mechanisms of tandem duplication in the Duchenne muscular dystrophy gene include both homologous and nonhomologous intrachromosomal recombination. *EMBO J* **10**:2471, 1991.

173. Hu XY, Burghes AH, Bulman DE, Ray PN, Worton RG: Evidence for mutation by unequal sister chromatid exchange in the Duchenne muscular dystrophy gene. *Am J Hum Genet* **44**:855, 1989.

174. van Essen AJ, Kneppers AL, van der Hout AH, Scheffer H, Ginjaar IB, ten, Kate LP, et al: The clinical and molecular genetic approach to Duchenne and Becker muscular dystrophy: An updated protocol. *J Med Genet* **34**:805, 1997.

175. Roberts RG, Gardner RJ, Bobrow M: Searching for the 1 in 2,400,000: A review of dystrophin gene point mutations (Review). *Hum Mutat* **4**:1, 1994.

176. Towbin JA, Hejtmancik JF, Brink P, Gelb B, Zhu XM, Chamberlain JS, McCabe ERB, et al: X-linked dilated cardiomyopathy: Molecular genetic evidence of linkage to the Duchenne muscular dystrophy (dystrophin) gene at the Xp21 locus. *Circulation* **87**:1854, 1993.

177. Towbin JA: The role of cytoskeletal proteins in cardiomyopathies (Review). *Curr Opin Cell Biol* **10**:131, 1998.

178. Cox GF, Kunkel LM: Dystrophies and heart disease (Review). *Curr Opin Cardiol* **12**:329, 1997.

179. Muntoni F, Cau M, Ganau A, Congiu R, Arvedi G, Mateddu A, Marrosu MG, et al: Deletion of the dystrophin muscle-promoter region associated with X-linked dilated cardiomyopathy. *N Engl J Med* **329**:921, 1993.

180. Milasin J, Muntoni F, Severini GM, Bartoloni L, Vatta M, Krajinovic M, Mateddu A, et al: A point mutation in the 5'splice site of the dystrophin gene first intron responsible for X-linked dilated cardiomyopathy. *Hum Mol Genet* **5**:73, 1996.

181. Yoshida K, Ikeda S-I, Nakamura A, Kagoshima M, Takeda S, Shoji S, Yanagisawa N: Molecular analysis of the Duchenne muscular dystrophy gene in patients with Becker muscular dystrophy presenting with dilated cardiomyopathy. *Muscle Nerve* **16**:1161, 1993.

182. Yoshida K, Nakamura A, Yazaki M, Ikeda S, Takeda S: Insertional mutation by transposable element, L1, in the DMD gene results in X-linked dilated cardiomyopathy. *Hum Mol Genet* **7**:1129, 1998.

183. Ferlini A, Galio N, Merlini L, Sewry C, Branzi A, Muntoni F: A novel Alu-like element rearranged in the dystrophin gene causes a splicing mutation in a family with X-linked dilated cardiomyopathy. *Am J Hum Genet* **63**:436, 1998.

184. Muntoni F, Di Lenarda A, Porcu M, Sinagra G, Mateddu A, Marrosu G, Ferlini A, et al: Dystrophin gene abnormalities in two patients with idiopathic dilated cardiomyopathy. *Heart* **78**:608, 1997.

185. Badorff C, Lee GH, Lamphear BJ, Martone ME, Campbell KP, Rhodes RE, Knowlton KU: Enteroviral protease 2A cleaves dystrophin: Evidence of cytoskeletal disruption in an acquired cardiomyopathy. *Nature Med* **5**:320, 1999.

186. Bushby KM, Beckmann JS: The limb-girdle muscular dystrophies: Proposal for a new nomenclature. *Neuromusc Disord* **5**:337, 1995.

187. Bushby KM: Diagnostic criteria for the limb-girdle muscular dystrophies: Report of the ENMC Consortium on Limb-Girdle Dystrophies. *Neuromusc Disord* **5**:71, 1995.

188. Bushby K: Towards the classification of the autosomal recessive limb-girdle muscular dystrophies. *Neuromusc Disord* **6**:439, 1996.

189. Bushby K: Understanding the heterogeneity of the limb-girdle muscular dystrophies (Review). *Biochem Soc Trans* **24**:489, 1996.

190. Duggan DJ, Hoffman EP: Autosomal recessive muscular dystrophy and mutations of the sarcoglycan complex. *Neuromusc Disord* **6**:475, 1996.

191. Angelini C, Fanin M, Freda MP, Duggan DJ, Siciliano G, Hoffman EP: The clinical spectrum of sarcoglycanopathies. *Neurology* **52**:176, 1999.

192. Hoffman EP, Clemens PR: HyperCKemic, proximal muscular dystrophies and the dystrophin membrane cytoskeleton, including dystrophinopathies, sarcoglycanopathies, and merosinopathies (Review). *Curr Opin Rheumatol* **8**:528, 1996.

193. Matsumura K, Tomé FMS, Collin H, Azibi K, Chaouch M, Kaplan J-C, Fardeau M, et al: Deficiency of the 50K dystrophin-associated glycoprotein in severe childhood autosomal recessive muscular dystrophy. *Nature* **359**:320, 1992.

194. Bonnemann CG, McNally EM, Kunkel LM: Beyond dystrophin: Current progress in the muscular dystrophies (Review). *Curr Opin Pediatr* **8**:569, 1996.

195. Barresi R, Confalonieri V, Lanfossi M, di Blasi C, Torchiana E, Mantegazza R, Jarre L, et al: Concomitant deficiency of beta- and gamma-sarcoglycans in 20 alpha-sarcoglycan (adhalin)-deficient patients: Immunohistochemical analysis and clinical aspects. *Acta Neuropathol* **94**:28, 1997.

196. Speer MC, Yamaoka LH, Gilchrist JH, Gaskell CP, Stajich JM, Vance JM, Kazantsev A, et al: Confirmation of genetic heterogeneity in limb-girdle muscular dystrophy: Linkage of an autosomal dominant form to chromosome 5q. *Am J Hum Genet* **50**:1211, 1992.

197. van der Kooi AJ, van Meegen M, Ledderhof TM, McNally EM, de Visser M, Bolhuis PA: Genetic localization of a newly recognized autosomal dominant limb-girdle muscular dystrophy with cardiac involvement (LGMD1B) to chromosome 1q11-21. *Am J Hum Genet* **60**:891, 1997.

198. Moreira ES, Vainzof M, Marie SK, Sertie AL, Zatz M, Passos-Bueno MR: The seventh form of autosomal recessive limb-girdle muscular dystrophy is mapped to 17q11-12. *Am J Hum Genet* **61**:151, 1997.

199. Weiler T, Greenberg CR, Zelinski T, Nylen E, Coghlan G, Crumley MJ, Fujiwara TM, et al: A gene for autosomal recessive limb-girdle muscular dystrophy in Manitoba Hutterites maps to chromosome

region 9q31-q33: Evidence for another limb-girdle muscular dystrophy locus. *Am J Hum Genet* **63**:140, 1998.

200. McNally EM, Yoshida M, Mizuno Y, Ozawa E, Kunkel LM: Human adhalin is alternatively spliced and the gene is located on chromosome 17q21. *Proc Natl Acad Sci USA* **91**:9690, 1994.

201. Roberds SL, Leturcq F, Allamand V, Piccolo F, Jeanpierre M, Anderson RD, Lim LE, et al: Missense mutations in the adhalin gene linked to autosomal recessive muscular dystrophy. *Cell* **78**:625, 1994.

202. Piccolo F, Roberds SL, Jeanpierre M, Leturcq F, Azibi K, Beldjord C, Carrie A, et al: Primary adhalinopathy: A common cause of autosomal recessive muscular dystrophy of variable severity [published erratum appears in *Nature Genet* **11**(1):104, 1995]. *Nature Genet* **10**:243, 1995.

203. Duggan DJ, Gorospe JR, Fanin M, Hoffman EP, Angelini C: Mutations in the sarcoglycan genes in patients with myopathy (see Comments). *N Engl J Med* **336**:618, 1997.

204. Hayashi YK, Arahata K: The frequency of patients with adhalin deficiency in a muscular dystrophy patient population. *Nippon Rinsho* **55**:3165, 1997 (in Japanese).

205. Carrie A, Piccolo F, Leturcq F, Detoma C, Azibi K, Beldjord CV, Merlini L, et al: Mutational diversity and hot spots in the alpha-sarcoglycan gene in autosomal recessive muscular dystrophy (*LGMD2D*). *J Med Genet* **34**:470, 1997.

206. Eymard B, Romero NB, Leturcq F, Piccolo F, Carrie A, Jeanpierre M, Collin H, et al: Primary adhalinopathy (alpha-sarcoglycanopathy): Clinical, pathologic, and genetic correlation in 20 patients with autosomal recessive muscular dystrophy. *Neurology* **48**:1227, 1997.

207. Duggan DJ, Fanin M, Pegoraro E, Angelini C, Hoffman EP: alpha-Sarcoglycan (adhalin) deficiency: Complete deficiency patients are 5 percent of childhood-onset dystrophin-normal muscular dystrophy and most partial deficiency patients do not have gene mutations. *J Neurol Sci* **140**:30, 1996.

208. Passos-Bueno MR, Bonnemann CG, Vainzof M, Moreira ED, Lidov HGWB, Denton PH, Vance JM, et al: Mild and severe muscular dystrophy caused by a single gamma-sarcoglycan mutation. *Am J Hum Genet* **59**:1040, 1996.

209. Vainzof M, Passos-Bueno MR, Canovas M, Moreira ES, Pavanello RC, Marie SK, Anderson LV, et al: The sarcoglycan complex in the six autosomal recessive limb-girdle muscular dystrophies. *Hum Mol Genet* **5**:1963, 1996.

210. Angelini C, Fanin M, Menegazzo E, Freda MP, Duggan DJ, Hoffman EP: Homozygous alpha-sarcoglycan mutation in two siblings: One asymptomatic and one steroid-responsive mild limb-girdle muscular dystrophy patient. *Muscle Nerve* **21**:769, 1998.

211. Higuchi I, Iwaki H, Kawai H, Endo T, Kunishige M, Fukunaga H, Nakagawa M, et al: New missense mutation in the alpha-sarcoglycan gene in a Japanese patient with severe childhood autosomal recessive muscular dystrophy with incomplete alpha-sarcoglycan deficiency. *J Neurol Sci* **153**:100, 1997.

212. Bonnemann CG, Modi R, Noguchi S, Mizuno Y, Yoshida M, Gussoni E, McNally EM, et al: Beta-sarcoglycan (A3b) mutations cause autosomal recessive muscular dystrophy with loss of the sarcoglycan complex [published erratum appears in *Nature Genet* **12**(1):110, 1996]. *Nature Genet* **11**:266, 1995.

213. Bonnemann CG, Wong J, Ben Hamida C, Hamida MB, Hentati F, Kunkel LM: LGMD 2E in Tunisia is caused by a homozygous missense mutation in beta-sarcoglycan exon 3. *Neuromusc Disord* **8**:193, 1998.

214. Ben Othmane K, Ben Hamida M, Pericak-Vance MA, Ben Hamida C, Blel S, Carter SC, Bowcock AM, et al: Linkage of Tunisian autosomal recessive Duchenne-like muscular dystrophy to the pericentromeric region of chromosome 13q. *Nature Genet* **2**:315, 1992.

215. Piccolo F, Jeanpierre M, Leturcq F, Dode C, Azibi K, Toutain AM, Jarre L, et al: A founder mutation in the gamma-sarcoglycan gene of gypsies possibly predated their migration out of India. *Hum Mol Genet* **5**:2019, 1996.

216. McNally EM, Duggan D, Gorospe JR, Bonnemann CG, Fanin M, Pegoraro E, Lidov HG, et al: Mutations that disrupt the carboxyl-terminus of gamma-sarcoglycan cause muscular dystrophy. *Hum Mol Genet* **5**:1841, 1996.

217. Passos-Bueno MR, Moreira ES, Vainzof M, Marie SK, Zatz M: Linkage analysis in autosomal recessive limb-girdle muscular dystrophy (AR LGMD) maps a sixth form to 5q33-34 (LGMD2F) and indicates that there is at least one more subtype of AR LGMD. *Hum Mol Genet* **5**:815, 1996.

218. Nigro Vde SβM, Piluso G, Vainzof M, Belsito A, Politano L, Puca AA, et al: Autosomal recessive limb-girdle muscular dystrophy, LGMD2F, is caused by a mutation in the delta-sarcoglycan gene. *Nature Genet* **14**:195, 1996.

219. Duggan DJ, Manchester D, Stears KP, Mathews DJ, Hart C, Hofman EP: Mutations in the delta-sarcoglycan gene are a rare cause of autosomal recessive limb-girdle muscular dystrophy (LGMD2). *Neurogenetics* **1**:49, 1997.

220. Fadic R, Sunada Y, Waclawik AJ, Buck S, Lewandoski PJ, Campbell KP, Lotz BP: Brief report: Deficiency of a dystrophin-associated glycoprotein (adhalin) in a patient with muscular dystrophy and cardiomyopathy (see Comments) [published erratum appears in *New Engl J Med* **334**(13):871, 1996]. *N Engl J Med* **334**:362, 1996.

221. van der Kooi AJ, De Voogt WG, Barth PG, Busch HF, Jennekens FG, Jongen PJ, et al: The heart in limb girdle muscular dystrophy. *Heart* **79**:73, 1998.

222. Lim LE, Campbell KP: The sarcoglycan complex in limb-girdle muscular dystrophy. *Curr Opin Neurobiol* **11**:443, 1998.

223. Allamand V, Broux O, Richard I, Fougerousse F, Chiannilkulchai N, Bourg N, Brenguier L, et al: Preferential localization of the limb-girdle muscular dystrophy type 2A gene in the proximal part of a 1-cM 15q15.1-q15.3 interval (see Comments). *Am J Hum Genet* **56**:1417, 1995.

224. Lonjou C, Collins A, Beckmann J, Allamand V, Morton N: Limb girdle muscular dystrophy type 2A (CAPN3): Mapping using allelic association. *Hum Hered* **48**:333, 1998.

225. Molinari M, Carafoli E: Calpain: A cytosolic proteinase active at the membranes (Review). *J Membr Biol* **156**:1, 1997.

226. Carafoli E, Molinari M: Calpain: A protease in search of a function? [published erratum appears in *Biochem Biophys Res Commun* **249**(2):572, 1998]. *Biochem Biophys Res Commun* **247**:193, 1998.

227. Sorimachi H, Ishiura S, Suzuki K: Structure and physiological function of calpains (Review). *Biochem J* **328**:721, 1997.

228. Richard I, Broux O, Allamand V, Fougerousse F, Chiannilkulchai N, Bourg N, Brenguier L, et al: Mutations in the proteolytic enzyme calpain 3 cause limb-girdle muscular dystrophy type 2A. *Cell* **81**:27, 1995.

229. Fardeau M, Eymard B, Mignard C, Tome FM, Richard I, Beckmann JS: Chromosome 15-linked limb-girdle muscular dystrophy: Clinical phenotypes in Reunion Island and French metropolitan communities. *Neuromusc Disord* **6**:447, 1996.

230. Anderson LV, Davison K, Moss JA, Richard I, Fardeau M, Tome FM, Hubner C, et al: Characterization of monoclonal antibodies to calpain 3 and protein expression in muscle from patients with limb-girdle muscular dystrophy type 2A. *Am J Pathol* **153**:1169, 1998.

231. Kawai H, Akaike M, Kunishige M, Inui T, Adachi K, Kimura C, Kawajiri M, et al: Clinical, pathological, and genetic features of limb-girdle muscular dystrophy type 2A with new calpain 3 gene mutations in seven patients from three Japanese families. *Muscle Nerve* **21**:1493, 1998.

232. Ono Y, Shimada H, Sorimachi H, Richard I, Saido TC, Beckmann JS, Ishiura S, et al: Functional defects of a muscle-specific calpain, p94, caused by mutations associated with limb-girdle muscular dystrophy type 2A. *J Biol Chem* **273**:17073, 1998.

233. Penisson-Besnier I, Richard I, Dubas F, Beckmann JS, Fardeau M: Pseudometabolic expression and phenotypic variability of calpain deficiency in two siblings. *Muscle Nerve* **21**:1078, 1998.

234. Spencer MJ, Tidball JG, Anderson LV, Bushby KM, Harris JB, Passos-Bueno MR, Somer H, et al: Absence of calpain 3 in a form of limb-girdle muscular dystrophy (LGMD2A). *J Neurol Sci* **146**:173, 1997.

235. Topaloglu H, Dinter P, Richard I, Aktren Z, Alehan D, Ozme S, Caglar M, et al: Calpain-3 deficiency causes a mild muscular dystrophy in childhood. *Neuropediatrics* **28**:212, 1997.

236. Dincer P, Leturcq F, Richard I, Piccolo F, Yalnizoglu D, De Toma C, Akcoren Z, et al: A biochemical, genetic, and clinical survey of autosomal recessive limb girdle muscular dystrophies in Turkey. *Ann Neurol* **42**:222, 1997.

237. Richard I, Brenguier L, Dincer P, Roudaut C, Bady B, Burgunder JM, Chemaly R, et al: Multiple independent molecular etiology for limb-girdle muscular dystrophy type 2A patients from various geographical origins. *Am J Hum Genet* **60**:1128, 1997.

238. Bashir R, Strachan T, Keers S, Stephenson A, Mahjneh I, Marconi G, Nashef L, et al: A gene for autosomal recessive limb-girdle muscular dystrophy maps to chromosome 2p. *Hum Mol Genet* **3**:455, 1994.

239. Bushby K, Bashir R, Keers S, Britton S, Zatz M, Passos-Bueno MR, Lovett M, et al: The molecular biology of *LGMD2B*: Towards the

identification of the *LGMD* gene on chromosome 2p13. *Neuromusc Disord* 6:491, 1996.

240. Passos-Bueno MR, Bashir R, Moreira ES, Vainzof M, Marie SK, Vasquez L, Iughetti P, et al: Confirmation of the 2p locus for the mild autosomal recessive limb-girdle muscular dystrophy gene (*LGMD2B*) in three families allows refinement of the candidate region. *Genomics* 27:192, 1995.

241. Bejaoui K, Hirabayashi K, Hentati F, Haines JL, Ben Hamida C, Belal S, Miller RG, et al: Linkage of Miyoshi myopathy (distal autosomal recessive muscular dystrophy) locus to chromosome 2p12-14. *Neurology* 45:768, 1995.

242. Liu J, Wu C, Bossie K, Bejaoui K, Hosler BA, Gingrich JC, Ben Hamida M, et al: Generation of a 3-Mb PAC contig spanning the Miyoshi myopathy/limb-girdle muscular dystrophy (MM/LGMD2B) locus on chromosome 2p13. *Genomics* 49:23, 1998.

243. Liu J, Aoki M, Illa I, Wu C, Fardeau M, Angelini C, Serrano C, et al: Dysferlin, a novel skeletal muscle gene, is mutated in Miyoshi myopathy and limb girdle muscular dystrophy. *Nature Genet* 20:31, 1998.

244. Bashir R, Britton S, Strachan T, Keers S, Vafiadaki E, Lako M, Richard I, et al: A gene related to *Caenorhabditis elegans* spermatogenesis factor fer-1 is mutated in limb-girdle muscular dystrophy type 2B. *Nature Genet* 20:37, 1998.

245. Minetti C, Sotgia F, Bruno C, Scartezzini P, Broda P, Bado M, Masetti E, et al: Mutations in the caveolin-3 gene cause autosomal dominant limb-girdle muscular dystrophy. *Nature Genet* 18:365, 1998.

246. Gossrau R: Caveolin-3 and nitric oxide synthase I in healthy and diseased skeletal muscle. *Acta Histochem* 100:99, 1998.

247. Vaghy PL, Fang J, Wu W, Vaghy LP: Increased caveolin-3 levels in mdx mouse muscles. *FEBS Lett* 431:125, 1998.

248. Leyten QH, Gabreels FJ, Renier WO, Ter Laak HJ: Congenital muscular dystrophy: A review of the literature (Review). *Clin Neurol Neurosurg* 98:267, 1996.

249. Voit T, Sewry CA, Meyer K, Hermann R, Straub V, Muntoni F, Kahn T, et al: Preserved merosin M-chain (or laminin-alpha 2) expression in skeletal muscle distinguishes Walker-Warburg syndrome from Fukuyama muscular dystrophy and merosin-deficient congenital muscular dystrophy (see Comments). *Neuropediatrics* 26:148, 1995.

250. Ranta S, Pihko H, Santavuori P, Tahvanainen E, de la Chapelle A: Muscle-eye-brain disease and Fukuyama type congenital muscular dystrophy are not allelic. *Neuromusc Disord* 5:221, 1995.

251. Bushby K, Anderson LV, Pollitt C, Naom I, Muntoni F, Bindoff L: Abnormal merosin in adults: A new form of late onset muscular dystrophy not linked to chromosome 6q2. *Brain* 121:581, 1998.

252. Sewry CA, Naom I, Dalessandro M, Sorokin L, Bruno S, Wilson LAD, Muntoni F: Variable clinical phenotype in merosin-deficient congenital muscular dystrophy associated with differential immuno-labelling of two fragments of the laminin alpha 2 chain. *Neuromusc Disord* 7:169, 1997.

253. Matsumura K, Yamada H, Saito F, Sunada Y, Shimizu T: Peripheral nerve involvement in merosin-deficient congenital muscular dystrophy and *dy* mouse (Review). *Neuromusc Disord* 7:7, 1997.

254. Villanova M, Malandrini A, Toti P, Salvestroni R, Six J, Martin JJ, Guazzi GC: Localization of merosin in the normal human brain: Implications for congenital muscular dystrophy with merosin deficiency. *J Submicrosc Cytol Pathol* 28:1, 1996.

255. Pegoraro E, Mancias P, Swerdlow SH, Raikow RB, Garcia C, Marks H, Crawford T, et al: Congenital muscular dystrophy with primary laminin alpha2 (merosin) deficiency presenting as inflammatory myopathy. *Ann Neurol* 40:782, 1996.

256. Tome FM, Evangelista T, Leclerc A, Sunada Y, Manole E, Estournet B, Barois A, et al: Congenital muscular dystrophy with merosin deficiency. *Comp Rendu Acad Sci* 317:351, 1994.

257. Sewry CA, D'Alessandro M, Wilson LA, Sorokin LM, Naom I, Bruno S, Ferlini A, et al: Expression of laminin chains in skin in merosin-deficient congenital muscular dystrophy. *Neuropediatrics* 28:217, 1997.

258. Marbini A, Bellanova MF, Ferrari A, Lodesani M, Gemignani F: Immunohistochemical study of merosin-negative congenital muscular dystrophy: Laminin alpha 2 deficiency in skin biopsy. *Acta Neuropathol* 94:103, 1997.

259. Sewry CA, Naom I, D'Alessandro M, Ferlini A, Philpot J, Mercuri E, Dubowitz V, et al: The protein defect in congenital muscular dystrophy. *Biochem Soc Trans* 24:281S, 1996.

260. Sewry CA, Philpot J, Sorokin LM, Wilson LA, Naom I, Goodwin FD, Dubowitz V, et al: Diagnosis of merosin (laminin-2) deficient congenital muscular dystrophy by skin biopsy. *Lancet* 347:582, 1996.

261. Helbling-Leclerc A, Zhang X, Topaloglu H, Cruaud C, Tesson F, Weissenbach J, Tome FM, et al: Mutations in the laminin alpha 2-chain gene (*LAMA2*) cause merosin-deficient congenital muscular dystrophy. *Nature Genet* 11:216, 1995.

262. Guicheney P, Vignier N, Helblingleclerc A, Nissinen M, Zhang XC, Lambert JC, Richelme C, et al: Genetics of laminin alpha 2 chain (or merosin) deficient congenital muscular dystrophy: From identification of mutations to prenatal diagnosis. *Neuromusc Disord* 7:180, 1997.

263. Nissinen M, Helbling-Leclerc A, Zhang X, Evangelista T, Topaloglu H, Cruaud C, Weissenbach J, et al: Substitution of a conserved cysteine-996 in a cysteine-rich motif of the laminin alpha$_2$-chain in congenital muscular dystrophy with partial deficiency of the protein. *Am J Hum Genet* 58:1177, 1996.

264. Kobayashi K, Nakahori Y, Mizuno K, Miyake M, Kumagai T, Honma A, Nonaka, et al: Founder-haplotype analysis in Fukuyama-type congenital muscular dystrophy (FCMD). *Hum Genet* 103:323, 1998.

265. Fukuyama Y, Osawa M, Suzuki H: Congenital progressive muscular dystrophy of the Fukuyama type: Clinical, genetic and pathological considerations. *Brain Dev* 3:1, 1981.

266. Aida N, Yagishita A, Takada K, Katsumata Y: Cerebellar MR in Fukuyama congenital muscular dystrophy: Polymicrogyria with cystic lesions. *Am J Neuroradiol* 15:1755, 1994.

267. Aida N: Fukuyama congenital muscular dystrophy: A neuroradiologic review (Review). *J Magn Reson Imag* 8:317, 1998.

268. Hayashi YK, Engvall E, Arikawa-Hirasawa E, Goto K, Koga R, Nonaka I, Sugita H, et al: Abnormal localization of laminin subunits in muscular dystrophies. *J Neurol Sci* 119:53, 1993.

269. Ishii H, Hayashi YK, Nonaka I, Arahata K: Electron microscopic examination of basal lamina in Fukuyama congenital muscular dystrophy. *Neuromusc Disord* 7:191, 1997.

270. Yoshioka M, Kuroki S: Clinical spectrum and genetic studies of Fukuyama congenital muscular dystrophy. *Am J Med Genet* 53:245, 1994.

271. Kondo-Iida E, Saito K, Tanaka H, Tsuji S, Ishihara T, Osawa M, Fukuyama Y, et al: Molecular genetic evidence of clinical heterogeneity in Fukuyama-type congenital muscular dystrophy. *Hum Genet* 99:427, 1997.

272. Toda T, Segawa M, Nomura Y, Nonaka I, Masuda K, Ishihara T, Sakai M, et al: Localization of a gene for Fukuyama type congenital muscular dystrophy to chromosome 9q31-33. *Nature Genet* 5:283, 1993.

273. Toda T, Ikegawa S, Okui K, Kondo E, Saito K, Fukuyama Y, Yoshioka M, et al: Refined mapping of a gene responsible for Fukuyama-type congenital muscular dystrophy: Evidence for strong linkage disequilibrium. *Am J Hum Genet* 55:946, 1994.

274. Miyake M, Nakahori Y, Matsushita I, Kobayashi K, Mizuno K, Hirai M, Kanazawa I, et al: YAC and cosmid contigs encompassing the Fukuyama-type congenital muscular dystrophy (FCMD) candidate region on 9q31. *Genomics* 40:284, 1997.

275. Kobayashi K, Nakahori Y, Miyake M, Matsumura K, Kondo-Iida E, Nomura Y, Segawa M, et al: An ancient retrotransposal insertion causes Fukuyama-type congenital muscular dystrophy. *Nature* 394:388, 1998.

276. Emery AE: X-linked muscular dystrophy with early contractures and cardiomyopathy (Emery-Dreifuss type). *Clin Genet* 32:360, 1987.

277. Emery AE: Emery-Dreifuss syndrome. *J Med Genet* 26:637, 1989.

278. Muntoni F, Lichtarowicz-Krynska EJ, Sewry CA, Manilal S, Recan D, Llense, Taylor J, et al: Early presentation of X-linked Emery-Dreifuss muscular dystrophy resembling limb-girdle muscular dystrophy. *Neuromusc Disord* 8:72, 1998.

279. Dickey RP, Ziter FA, Smith RA: Emery-Dreifuss muscular dystrophy. *J Pediatr* 104:555, 1984.

280. Jensen V: The anaesthetic management of a patient with Emery-Dreifuss muscular dystrophy. *Can J Anaesth* 43:968, 1996.

281. Hopkins LC, Jackson JA, Elsas LJ: Emery-Dreifuss humeroperoneal muscular dystrophy: An X-linked myopathy with unusual contractures and bradycardia. *Ann Neurol* 10:230, 1981.

282. Rowland LP, Fetell PM, Olarte M, Hays A, Singh N, Wanat FE: Emery-Dreifuss muscular dystrophy. *Ann Neurol* 5:111, 1979.

283. Thomas NS, Williams H, Elsas LJ, Hopkins LC, Sarfarazi M, Harper PS: Localisation of the gene for Emery-Dreifuss muscular dystrophy to th. *J Med Genet* 23:596, 1986.

284. Hodgson S, Boswinkel E, Cole C, Walker A, Dubowitz V, Granata C, Merlini L, et al: A linkage study of Emery-Dreifuss muscular dystrophy. *Hum Genet* **74**:409, 1986.
285. Yates JR, Affara NA, Jamieson DM, Ferguson Smith MA, Hausmanowa Petrusewicz I, Zaremba J, Borkowska J, et al: Emery-Dreifuss muscular dystrophy: Localisation to Xq27.3-qter. *J Med Genet* **23**:587, 1986.
286. Yates JRW, Warner JP, Smith JA, Deymeer F, Azulay J-P, Hausmanowa-Petrusewicz I, Zaremba J, et al: Emery-Dreifuss muscular dystrophy: Linkage to markers in distal Xq28. *J Med Genet* **30**:108, 1993.
287. Consalez GG, Thomas NS, Stayton CL, Knight SJ, Johnson M, Hopkins LC, Harper PS, et al: Assignment of Emery-Dreifuss muscular dystrophy to the distal region of Xq28: The results of a collaborative study. *Am J Hum Genet* **48**:468, 1991.
288. Bione S, Maestrini E, Rivella S, Mancini M, Regis S, Romeo G, Toniolo D: Identification of a novel X-linked gene responsible for Emery-Dreifuss muscular dystrophy. *Nature Genet* **8**:323, 1994.
289. Bione S, Small K, Aksmanovic VM, D'Urso M, Ciccodicola A, Merlini L, Morandi L, et al: Identification of new mutations in the Emery-Dreifuss muscular dystrophy gene and evidence for genetic heterogeneity of the disease. *Hum Mol Genet* **4**:1859, 1995.
290. Nigro V, Bruni P, Ciccodicola A, Politano L, Nigro G, Piluso G, Cappa V, et al: SSCP detection of novel mutations in patients with Emery-Dreifuss muscular dystrophy: Definition of a small C-terminal region required for emerin function. *Hum Mol Genet* **4**:2003, 1995.
291. Klauck SM, Wilgenbus P, Yates JR, Muller CR, Poustka A: Identification of novel mutations in three families with Emery-Dreifuss muscular dystrophy. *Hum Mol Genet* **4**:1853, 1995.
292. Yamada T, Kobayashi T: A novel emerin mutation in a Japanese patient with Emery-Dreifuss muscular dystrophy. *Hum Genet* **97**:693, 1996.
293. Wulff K, Ebener U, Wehnert CS, Ward PA, Reuner U, Hiebsch WH, Wehnert M: Direct molecular genetic diagnosis and heterozygote identification in X-linked Emery-Dreifuss muscular dystrophy by heteroduplex analysis. *Dis Mark* **13**:77, 1997.
294. Ichikawa Y, Watanabe M, Kowa H, Murayama S, Mizuno T, Komuro I, Ishiki R, et al: A Japanese family carrying a novel mutation in the Emery-Dreifuss muscular dystrophy gene. *Ann Neurol* **41**:399, 1997.
295. Manilal S, Recan D, Sewry CA, Hoeltzenbein M, Llense S, Leturcq F, Deburgrave N, et al: Mutations in Emery-Dreifuss muscular dystrophy and their effects on emerin protein expression. *Hum Mol Genet* **7**:855, 1998.
296. Small K, Iber J, Warren ST: Emerin deletion reveals a common X-chromosome inversion mediated by inverted repeats (see Comments). *Nature Genet* **16**:96, 1997.
297. Small K, Warren ST: Emerin deletions occurring on both Xq28 inversion backgrounds. *Hum Mol Genet* **7**:135, 1998.
298. Wulff K, Parrish JE, Herrmann FH, Wehnert M: Six novel mutations in the emerin gene causing X-linked Emery-Dreifuss muscular dystrophy. *Hum Mutat* **9**:526, 1997.
299. Yates JR: 43rd ENMC International Workshop on Emery-Dreifuss Muscular Dystrophy, 22 June 1996, Naarden, The Netherlands. *Neuromusc Disord* **7**:67, 1997.
300. Nagano A, Koga R, Ogawa M, Kurano Y, Kawada J, Okada R, Hayashi YK, et al: Emerin deficiency at the nuclear membrane in patients with Emery-Dreifuss muscular dystrophy. *Nature Genet* **12**:254, 1996.
301. Manilal S, Nguyen TM, Sewry CA, Morris GE: The Emery-Dreifuss muscular dystrophy protein, emerin, is a nuclear membrane protein. *Hum Mol Genet* **5**:801, 1996.
302. Manilal S, Nguyen TM, Morris GE: Colocalization of emerin and lamins in interphase nuclei and changes during mitosis. *Biochem Biophys Res Commun* **249**:643, 1998.
303. Ellis JA, Craxton M, Yates JR, Kendrick-Jones J: Aberrant intracellular targeting and cell cycle-dependent phosphorylation of emerin contribute to the Emery-Dreifuss muscular dystrophy phenotype. *J Cell Sci* **111**:781, 1998.
304. Small K, Wagener M, Warren ST: Isolation and characterization of the complete mouse emerin gene. *Mammal Genome* **8**:337, 1997.
305. Cartegni L, di Barletta MR, Barresi R, Squarzoni S, Sabatelli P, Maraldi N, Mora M, et al: Heart-specific localization of emerin: New insights into Emery-Dreifuss muscular dystrophy. *Hum Mol Genet* **6**:2257, 1997.
306. Manilal S, Sewry CA, Man N, Muntoni F, Morris GE: Diagnosis of X-linked Emery-Dreifuss muscular dystrophy by protein analysis of

leucocytes and skin with monoclonal antibodies. *Neuromusc Disord* **7**:63, 1997.
307. Mora M, Cartegni L, di Blasi C, Barresi R, Bione S, Raffaele dB, Morandi L, et al: X-linked Emery-Dreifuss muscular dystrophy can be diagnosed from skin biopsy or blood sample. *Ann Neurol* **42**:249, 1997.
308. Sabatelli P, Squarzoni S, Petrini S, Capanni C, Ognibene A, Cartegni L, Cobianchi F, et al: Oral exfoliative cytology for the non-invasive diagnosis in X-linked Emery-Dreifuss muscular dystrophy patients and carriers. *Neuromusc Disord* **8**:67, 1998.
309. Taylor EW: Progressive vagus-glossopharyngeal paralysis with ptosis: A contribution to the group of family diseases. *J Nerv Ment Dis* **42**:129, 1915.
310. Victor M, Hayes R, Adams RD: Oculopharyngeal muscular dystrophy: A familial disease of late life characterized by dysphagia and progressive ptosis of the eyelids. *New Engl J Med* **267**:1267, 1962.
311. Brunet G, Tome FMS, Samson F, Robert JM, Fardeau M: Dytrophie musculaire oculo-pharyngee: Recensement des familles francaises et etude genealogique. *Rev Neurol* **146**:425, 1990.
312. Brais B, Xie YG, Sanson M, Morgan K, Weissenbach J, Korczyn AD, Blumen SC, et al: The oculopharyngeal muscular dystrophy locus maps to the region of the cardiac α and β myosin heavy chain genes on chromosome 14q11.2-q13. *Hum Mol Genet* **4**:429, 1995.
313. Blumen SC, Nisipeanu P, Sadeh M, Asherov A, Blumen N, Wirguin Y, Khilkevich O, et al: Epidemiology and inheritance of oculopharyngeal muscular dystrophy in Israel. *Neuromusc Disord* **7**(suppl 1):S38, 1997.
314. Brais B, Bouchard JP, Gosselin F, Xie YG, Fardeau M, Tome FM, Rouleau GA, et al: Using the full power of linkage analysis in 11 French Canadian families to fine map the oculopharyngeal muscular dystrophy gene. *Neuromusc Disord* **7**(suppl 1):S70, 1997.
315. Bouchard JP, Brais B, Brunet D, Gould PV, Rouleau GA: Recent studies on oculopharyngeal muscular dystrophy in Quebec. *Neuromusc Disord* **7**(suppl 1):S22, 1997.
316. Fried K, Arlozorov A, Spira R: Autosomal recessive oculopharyngeal muscular dystrophy. *J Med Genet* **12**:416, 1975.
317. Tome FM, Chateau D, Helbling-Leclerc A, Fardeau M: Morphological changes in muscle fibers in oculopharyngeal muscular dystrophy. *Neuromusc Disord* **7**(suppl 1):S63, 1997.
318. Tome FMS, Fardeau M: Nuclear inclusions in oculopharyngeal muscular dystrophy. *Acta Neuropathol* **49**:85, 1980.
319. Coquet M, Vital C, Julien J: Presence of inclusion body myositis-like filaments in oculopharyngeal muscular dystrophy: Ultrastructural study of 10 cases. *Neuropathol Appl Neurobiol* **16**:393, 1990.
320. Blumen SC, Sadeh M, Korczyn AD, Rouche A, Nisipeanu P, Asherov A, Tome FMS: Intranuclear inclusions in oculopharyngeal muscular dystrophy among Bukhara Jews. *Neurology* **46**:1324, 1996.
321. Brais B, Bouchard JP, Xie YG, Rochefort DL, Chretien N, Tome FM, Lafreniere RG, et al: Short GCG expansions in the PABP2 gene cause oculopharyngeal muscular dystrophy [published erratum appears in *Nature Genet* **19**(4):404, 1998]. *Nature Genet* **18**:164, 1998.
322. Porschke H, Kress W, Reichmann H, Goebel HH, Grimm T: Oculopharyngeal muscular dystrophy in a northern German family linked to chromosome 14q, and presenting carnitine deficiency. *Neuromusc Disord* **7**(suppl 1):S57, 1997.
323. Stajich JM, Gilchrist JM, Lennon F, Lee A, Yamaoka L, Rosi B, Gaskell PG, et al: Confirmation of linkage of oculopharyngeal muscular dystrophy to chromosome 14q11.2-q13. *Ann Neurol* **40**:801, 1997.
324. Teh BT, Sullivan AA, Farnebo F, Zander C, Li FY, Strachan N, Schalling M, et al: Oculopharyngeal muscular dystrophy (OPMD): Report and genetic studies of an Australian kindred. *Clin Genet* **51**:52, 1997.
325. Grewal RP, Cantor R, Turner G, Grewal RK, Detera-Wadleigh SD: Genetic mapping and haplotype analysis of oculopharyngeal muscular dystrophy. *NeuroReport* **9**:961, 1998.
326. Bienroth S, Keller W, Wahle E: Assembly of a processive messenger RNA polyadenylation complex. *EMBO J* **12**:585, 1993.
327. Krause S, Fakan S, Weis K, Wahle E: Immunodetection of poly(A) binding protein II in cell nucleus. *Exp Cell Res* **214**:75, 1994.
328. Nemeth A, Krause S, Blank D, Jenny A, Jen, Lustig A, Wahle E: Isolation of genomic and cDNA clones encoding bovine poly(A) binding protein II. *Nucl Acids Res* **23**:4034, 1995.
329. Wahle E: A novel poly(A)-binding protein acts as a specificity factor in the second phase of messenger RNA polyadenylation. *Cell* **66**:759, 1991.

330. Wahle E, Lustig A, Jen, Maurer P: Mammalian poly(A)-binding protein: II. Physical properties and binding to polynucleotides. *J Biol Chem* **268**:2937, 1993.

331. Sisodia SS: Nuclear inclusions in glutamine repeat disorders: Are they pernicious, coincidental, or beneficial? *Cell* **95**:1, 1998.

332. Forood B, Perez-Paya E, Houghten RA, londelle SE: Formation of an extremely stable polyalanine B-sheet macromolecule. *Biochem Biophys Res Commun* **211**:7, 1995.

333. Lunt PW, Harper PS: Genetic counselling in facioscapulohumeral muscular dystrophy. *J Med Genet* **28**:655, 1991.

334. Laforet P, De Toma C, Eymard B, Becane HM, Jeanpierre M, Fardeau M, Duboc D: Cardiac involvement in genetically confirmed facioscapulohumeral muscular dystrophy. *Neurology* **51**:1454, 1998.

335. Funakoshi M, Goto K, Arahata K: Epilepsy and mental retardation in a subset of early onset 4q35-facioscapulohumeral muscular dystrophy. *Neurology* **50**:1791, 1998.

336. Miura K, Kumagai T, Matsumoto A, Iriyama E, Watanabe K, Goto K, Arahata K: Two cases of chromosome 4q35-linked early onset facioscapulohumeral muscular dystrophy with mental retardation and epilepsy. *Neuropediatrics* **29**:239, 1998.

337. Anonymous: A prospective, quantitative study of the natural history of facioscapulohumeral muscular dystrophy (FSHD): Implications for therapeutic trials. The FSH-DY Group. *Neurology* **48**:38, 1997.

338. Lunt PW, Jardine PE, Koch MC, Maynard J, Osborn M, Williams M, Harper PS, et al: Correlation between fragment size at D4F104S1 and age at onset or at wheelchair use, with a possible generational effect, accounts for much phenotypic variation in 4q35-facioscapulohumeral muscular dystrophy (FSHD). *Hum Mol Genet* **4**:951, 1995.

339. Brouwer OF, Padberg GW, Wijmenga C, Frants RR: Facioscapulohumeral muscular dystrophy in early childhood (Review). *Arch Neurol* **51**:387, 1994.

340. Tupler R, Barbierato L, Memmi M, Sewry CA, De Grandis D, Maraschio P, Tiepolo L, et al: Identical de novo mutation at the D4F104S1 locus in monozygotic male twins affected by facioscapulohumeral muscular dystrophy (FSHD) with different clinical expression. *J Med Genet* **35**:778, 1998.

341. Wijmenga C, Frants RR, Brouwer OF, Moerer P, Weber JL, Padberg GW: Location of facioscapulohumeral muscular dystrophy gene on chromosome 4. *Lancet* **336**:651, 1990.

342. Wijmenga C, Padberg GW, Moerer P, Wiegant J, Liem L, Brouwer OF, Milner EC, et al: Mapping of facioscapulohumeral muscular dystrophy gene to chromosome 4q35-qter by multipoint linkage analysis and *in situ* hybridization. *Genomics* **9**:570, 1991.

343. Upadhyaya M, Lunt P, Sarfarazi M, Broadhead W, Farnham J, Harper PS: The mapping of chromosome 4q markers in relation to facioscapulohumeral muscular dystrophy (FSHD). *Am J Hum Genet* **51**:404, 1992.

344. Wright TJ, Wijmenga C, Clark LN, Frants RR, Williamson R, Hewitt JE: Fine mapping of the *FSHD* gene region orientates the rearranged fragment detected by the probe p13E-11. *Hum Mol Genet* **2**:1673, 1993.

345. Wijmenga C, Wright TJ, Baan MJ, Padberg GW, Williamson R, van Ommen GJ, Hewitt JE, et al: Physical mapping and YAC-cloning connects four genetically distinct 4qter loci (D4S163, D4S139, D4F35S1 and D4F104S1) in the *FSHD* gene-region. *Hum Mol Genet* **2**:1667, 1993.

346. Weiffenbach B, Dubois J, Manning S, Ma NS, Schutte BC, Winokur ST, Altherr MR, et al: YAC contigs for 4q35 in the region of the facioscapulohumeral muscular dystrophy (*FSHD*) gene. *Genomics* **19**:532, 1994.

347. Wijmenga C, van Deutekom JC, Hewitt JE, Padberg GW, van Ommen GJ, Hofker MH, Frants RR: Pulsed-field gel electrophoresis of the D4F104S1 locus reveals the size and the parental origin of the facioscapulohumeral muscular dystrophy (*FSHD*)-associated deletions. *Genomics* **19**:21, 1994.

348. Wijmenga C, Hewitt JE, Sandkuijl LA, Clark LN, Wright TJ, Dauwerse HG, Gruter AM, et al: Chromosome 4q DNA rearrangements associated with facioscapulohumeral muscular dystrophy. *Nature Genet* **2**:26, 1992.

349. van Deutekom JC, Wijmenga C, van Tienhoven EA, Gruter AM, Hewitt JE, Padberg GW, van Ommen GJ, et al: FSHD associated DNA rearrangements are due to deletions of integral copies of a 3.2 kb tandemly repeated unit. *Hum Mol Genet* **2**:2037, 1993.

350. Hewitt JE, Lyle R, Clark LN, Valleley EM, Wright TJ, Wijmenga C, van Deutekom JC, et al: Analysis of the tandem repeat locus D4Z4

351. Cacurri S, Piazzo N, Deidda G, Vigneti E, Galluzzi G, Colantoni L, Merico B, et al: Sequence homology between 4qter and 10qter loci facilitates the instability of subtelomeric KpnI repeat units implicated in facioscapulohumeral muscular dystrophy. *Am J Hum Genet* **63**:181, 1998.

352. Lemmers RJ, van der Maarel SM, van Deutekom JC, van der Wielen MJ, Deidda, Dauwerse HG, Hewitt J, et al: Inter- and intrachromosomal sub-telomeric rearrangements on 4q35: Implications for facioscapulohumeral muscular dystrophy (FSHD) aetiology and diagnosis. *Hum Mol Genet* **7**:1207, 1998.

353. Fisher J, Upadhyaya M: Molecular genetics of facioscapulohumeral muscular dystrophy (FSHD) (Review). *Neuromusc Disord* **7**:55, 1997.

354. Tawil R, Figlewicz DA, Griggs RC, Weiffenbach B: Facioscapulohumeral dystrophy: A distinct regional myopathy with a novel molecular pathogenesis. FSH Consortium. (Review). *Ann Neurol* **43**:279, 1998.

355. Bakker E, Vanderwielen MJR, Voorhoeve E, Ippel PF, Padberg GW, Frants RR, Wijmenga C: Diagnostic, predictive and prenatal testing for faciocapulohumeral muscular dystrophy: Diagnostic approach for sporadic and familial cases. *J Med Genet* **33**:29, 1996.

356. Hsu YD, Kao MC, Shyu WC, Lin JC, Huang NE, Sun HF, Yang KD, et al: Application of chromosome 4q35-qter marker (pFR-1) for DNA rearrangement of facioscapulohumeral muscular dystrophy patients in Taiwan. *J Neurol Sci* **149**:73, 1997.

357. Nakagawa M, Matsuzaki T, Higuchi I, Fukunaga H, Inui T, Nagamitsu SY, Arimura K, et al: Facioscapulohumeral muscular dystrophy: Clinical diversity and genetic abnormalities in Japanese patients. *Intern Med* **36**:333, 1997.

358. Ohya K, Tachi N, Kozuka N, Kon S, Kikuchi K, Chiba S: Detection of the mutation in facioscapulohumeral muscular dystrophy patients. *Acta Paediatr Jpn* **39**:92, 1997.

359. Okinaga A, Matsuoka T, Umeda J, Yanagihara I, Inui K, Nagai T, Okada S: Early-onset facioscapulohumeral muscular dystrophy: Two case reports. *Brain Dev* **19**:563, 1997.

360. Zatz M, Marie SK, Cerqueira A, Vainzof M, Pavanello RC, Passos-Bueno MR: The facioscapulohumeral muscular dystrophy (*FSHD1*) gene affects males more severely and more frequently than females. *Am J Med Genet* **77**:155, 1998.

361. Rudnik-Schoneborn S, Glauner B, Rohrig D, Zerres K: Obstetric aspects in women with facioscapulohumeral muscular dystrophy, limb-girdle muscular dystrophy, and congenital myopathies. *Arch Neurol* **54**:888, 1997.

362. Roques I, Pedespan JM, Boisserie-Lacroix V, Ferrer X, Fontan D: Facioscapulohumeral myopathy and germinal mosaicism. *Arch Pediatr* **5**:880, 1998.

363. Deidda G, Cacurri S, Piazzo N, Felicetti L: Direct detection of 4q35 rearrangements implicated in facioscapulohumeral muscular dystrophy (FSHD). *J Med Genet* **33**:361, 1996.

364. Upadhyaya M, Maynard J, Rogers MT, Lunt PW, Jardine P, Ravine DH: Improved molecular diagnosis of facioscapulohumeral muscular dystrophy (FSHD): Validation of the differential double digestion for *FSHD*. *J Med Genet* **34**:476, 1997.

365. van Deutekom JC, Bakker E, Lemmers RJ, van der Wielen MJ, Bik E, Hofker MH, Padberg GW, et al: Evidence for subtelomeric exchange of 3.3 kb tandemly repeated units between chromosomes 4q35 and 10q26: Implications for genetic counselling and etiology of FSHD1. *Hum Mol Genet* **5**:1997, 1996.

366. Ding H, Beckers MC, Plaisance S, Marynen P, Collen D, Belayew A: Characterization of a double homeodomain protein (DUX1) encoded by a cDNA homologous to 3.3 kb dispersed repeated elements. *Hum Mol Genet* **7**:1681, 1998.

367. Grunstein M: Molecular model for telomeric heterochromatin in yeast. *Curr Opin Cell Biol* **9**:383, 1997.

368. Lohe AR, Hilliker AJ: Return of the H-word (heterochromatin). *Curr Opin Genet Dev* **5**:746, 1995.

369. van Deutekom JC, Lemmers RJ, Grewal PK, Van Geel M, Romberg S, Dauwerse HG, Wright TJ, et al: Identification of the first gene (FRG1) from the FSHD region on human chromosome 4q35. *Hum Mol Genet* **5**:581, 1996.

370. Tupler R, Berardinelli A, Barbierato L, Frants R, Hewitt JE, Lanzi G, Maraschio P, et al: Monosomy of distal 4q does not cause facioscapulohumeral muscular dystrophy. *J Med Genet* **33**:366, 1996.

371. Allingham-Hawkins DJ, McGlynn-Steele LK, Brown CA, Sutherland J, Ray PN: Impact of carrier status determination for Duchenne/

Becker muscular dystrophy by computer-assisted laser densitometry. *Am J Med Genet* **75**:171, 1998.

372. Calvano S, Memeo E, Piemontese MR, Melchionda S, Bisceglia L, Gasparini, Zelante L: Detection of dystrophin deletion carriers using FISH analysis. *Clin Genet* **52**:17, 1997.

373. Bakker E, Veenema H, den Dunnen JT, van Broeckhoven C, Grootscholten PM, Bonten EJ, van Ommen GJ, et al: Germinal mosaicism increases the recurrence risk for "new" Duchenne muscular dystrophy mutations. *J Med Genet* **26**:553, 1989.

374. van Essen AJ, Abbs S, Baiget M, Bakker E, Boileau C, van Broeckhoven C, Bushby K, et al: Parental origin and germline mosaicism of deletions and duplications of the dystrophin gene: A European study. *Hum Genet* **88**:249, 1992.

375. Bullock S, Felix C, Iskander-Gabra S, Davison V: Detection of germinal mosaicism in a DMD family. *Biochem Soc Trans* **24**:273S, 1996.

376. Grimm T, Meng G, Liechti-Gallati S, Bettecken T, Müller CR, Müller B: On the origin of deletions and point mutations in Duchenne muscular dystrophy: Most deletions arise in oogenesis and most point mutations result from events in spermatogenesis. *J Med Genet* **31**:183, 1994.

377. Bakker E, Bonten EJ, den Dunnen JT, Veenema H, Grootscholten PM, van Ommen GJ, Pearson PL: Carrier detection and prenatal diagnosis of Duchenne/Becker muscular dystrophy (D/BMD) by DNA-analysis. *Prog Clin Biol Res* **306**:51, 1989.

378. Bakker E, Bonten EJ, Veenema H, den Dunnen JT, Grootscholten PM, van Ommen GJ, Pearson PL: Prenatal diagnosis of Duchenne muscular dystrophy: A three-year experience in a rapidly evolving field. *J Inherit Metab Dis* **12**(suppl 1):174, 1989.

379. Prior TW: Perspectives and molecular diagnosis of Duchenne and Becker muscular dystrophies (Review). *Clin Lab Med* **15**:927, 1995.

380. Dincer P, Topaloglu H, Ayter S: DNA diagnostic tests in Xp21 dystrophy families for prenatal diagnosis. *Turk J Pediatr* **40**:347, 1998.

381. Sekizawa A, Kimura T, Sasaki M, Nakamura S, Kobayashi R, Sato T: Prenatal diagnosis of Duchenne muscular dystrophy using a single fetal nucleated erythrocyte in maternal blood. *Neurology* **46**:1350, 1996.

382. Abbs S: Prenatal diagnosis of Duchenne and Becker muscular dystrophy (Review). *Prenat Diagn* **16**:1187, 1996.

383. Gelfi C, Orsi A, Leoncini F, Righetti PG, Spiga I, Carrera P, Ferrari M: Amplification of 18 dystrophin gene exons in DMD/BMD patients: Simultaneous resolution by capillary electrophoresis in sieving liquid polymers. *Biotechnology* **19**:254, 1995.

384. Benzie RJ, Ray P, Thompson D, Hunter AG, Ivey B, Salvador L: Prenatal exclusion of Duchenne muscular dystrophy by fetal muscle biopsy. *Prenat Diagn* **14**:235, 1994.

385. Shiroshita Y, Katayama S: Prenatal diagnosis of Duchenne muscular dystrophy in the Japanese population by fluorescent CA repeat polymorphisms analysis. *J Obstet Gynaecol Res* **23**:453, 1997.

386. Grifo JA, Tang YX, Munne S, Alikani M, Cohen J, Rosenwaks Z: Healthy deliveries from biopsied human embryos. *Hum Reprod* **9**:912, 1994.

387. Liu J, Lissens W, van Broeckhoven C, Lofgren A, Camus M, Liebaers I, Van Steirteghem A: Normal pregnancy after preimplantation DNA diagnosis of a dystrophin gene deletion. *Prenat Diagn* **15**:351, 1995.

388. Liu J, Lissens W, Devroey P, Liebaers I, Van Steirteghem A: Cystic fibrosis, Duchenne muscular dystrophy and preimplantation genetic diagnosis (Review). *Hum Reprod Update* **2**:531, 1996.

389. Kristjansson K, Chong SS, Van den Veyver IB, Subramanian S, Snabes MC, Hughes MR: Preimplantation single cell analyses of dystrophin gene deletions using whole genome amplification. *Nature Genet* **6**:19, 1994.

390. Kuller JA, Hoffman EP, Fries MH, Golbus MS: Prenatal diagnosis of Duchenne muscular dystrophy by fetal muscle biopsy. *Hum Genet* **90**:34, 1992.

390a. Pegoraro E, Mancias P, Swerdlow SH, Raikow RB, Garcia C, Marks H, Crawford T, et al: Congential muscular dystrophy with primary laminin alpha2 (merosin) deficiency presenting as inflammatory myopathy. *Ann Neurol* **40**:782, 1996.

391. Voit T, Fardeau M, Tome FMS: Prenatal detection of merosin expression in human placenta. *Neuropediatrics* **25**:332, 1994.

392. Naom I, Sewry C, D'Alessandro M, Topaloglu H, Ferlini A, Wilson L, Dubowitz V, et al: Prenatal diagnosis in merosin-deficient congenital muscular dystrophy. *Neuromusc Disord* **7**:176, 1997.

393. Naom I, D'Alessandro M, Sewry C, Ferlini A, Topaloglu H, Helbling-Leclerc A, Guicheney P, et al: The role of immunocytochemistry and linkage analysis in the prenatal diagnosis of merosin-deficient congenital muscular dystrophy. *Hum Genet* **99**:535, 1997.

394. Guicheney P, Vignier N, Zhang X, He Y, Cruaud C, Frey V, Helbling-Leclerc A, et al: PCR based mutation screening of the laminin alpha2 chain gene (LAMA2): Application to prenatal diagnosis and search for founder effects in congenital muscular dystrophy. *J Med Genet* **35**:211, 1998.

395. Sicinski P, Geng Y, Ryder Cook AS, Barnard EA, Darlison MG, Barnard PJ: The molecular basis of muscular dystrophy in the *mdx* mouse: A point mutation. *Science* **244**:1578, 1989.

396. Watkins SC, Hoffman EP, Slayter HS, Kunkel LM: Dystrophin distribution in heterozygote *MDX* mice. *Muscle Nerve* **12**:861, 1989.

397. Karpati G, Pouliot Y, Zubrzycka Gaarn E, Carpenter S, Ray PN, Worton RG, Holland P: Dystrophin is expressed in mdx skeletal muscle fibers after normal myoblast implantation. *Am J Pathol* **135**:27, 1989.

398. Karpati G, Zubrzycka Gaarn EE, Carpenter S, Bulman DE, Ray PN, Worton RG: Age-related conversion of dystrophin-negative to - positive fiber segments of skeletal but not cardiac muscle fibers in heterozygote mdx mice. *J Neuropathol Exp Neurol* **49**:96, 1990.

399. Stedman HH, Sweeney HL, Shrager JB, Maguire HC, Panettieri RA, Petrof B, Narusawa M, et al: The mdx mouse diaphragm reproduces the degenerative changes of Duchenne muscular dystrophy. *Nature* **352**:536, 1991.

400. Megeney LA, Kablar B, Perry RL, Ying C, May L, Rudnicki MA: Severe cardiomyopathy in mice lacking dystrophin and MyoD. *Proc Natl Acad Sci USA* **96**:220, 1999.

401. Cooper BJ, Valentine BA: X-linked muscular dystrophy in the dog. *Trends Genet* **4**:30, 1988.

402. Kornegay JN, Tuler SM, Miller DM, Levesque DC: Muscular dystrophy in a litter of golden retriever dogs. *Muscle Nerve* **11**:1056, 1988.

403. Valentine BA, Cooper BJ, Cummings JF, de Lahunta A: Canine X-linked muscular dystrophy: Morphologic lesions. *J Neurol Sci* **97**:1, 1990.

404. Sharp NJH, Kornegay JN, Van Camp SD, Herbstreith MH, Secore SL, Kettle S, Hung W-Y, et al: An error in dystrophin mRNA processing in golden retriever muscular dystrophy, an animal homologue of Duchenne muscular dystrophy. *Genomics* **13**:115, 1992.

405. Valentine BA, Winand NJ, Pradhan D, Moise NS, de Lahunta A, Kornegay JN, Cooper BJ: Canine X-linked muscular dystrophy as an animal model of Duchenne muscular dystrophy. *Am J Med Genet* **42**:352, 1992.

406. Ervasti JM, Roberds SL, Anderson RD, Sharp NJ, Kornegay JN, Campbell KP: Alpha-dystroglycan deficiency correlates with elevated serum creatine kinase and decreased muscle contraction tension in golden retriever muscular dystrophy. *FEBS Lett* **350**:173, 1994.

407. Roberds SL, Ervasti JM, Anderson RD, Ohlendieck K, Kahl SD, Zoloto D, Campbell KP: Disruption of the dystrophin-glycoprotein complex in the cardiomyopathic hamster. *J Biol Chem* **268**:11496, 1993.

408. Mizuno Y, Noguchi S, Yamamoto H, Yoshida M, Nonaka I, Hirai S, Ozawa E: Sarcoglycan complex is selectively lost in dystrophic hamster muscle. *Am J Pathol* **146**:530, 1995.

409. Roberds SL, Campbell KP: Adhalin mRNA and cDNA sequence are normal in the cardiomyopathic hamster. *FEBS Lett* **364**:245, 1995.

410. Hanada H, Yoshida T, Pan Y, Iwata Y, Nishimura M, Shigekawa M: MRNA expression and CDNA sequences of beta- and gamma-sarcoglycans are normal in cardiomyopathic hamster heart. *Biol Pharm Bull* **20**:134, 1997.

411. Takada S, Okazaki Y, Kamiya M, Ohsumi T, Nomura O, Okuizumi H, Sasaki N, et al: Five candidate genes for hamster cardiomyopathy did not map to the cardiomyopathy locus by FISH analysis. *DNA Res* **3**:273, 1996.

412. Nigro V, Okazaki Y, Belsito A, Piluso G, Matsuda Y, Politano LN, Ventura C, et al: Identification of the Syrian hamster cardiomyopathy gene. *Hum Mol Genet* **6**:601, 1997.

413. Duclos F, Straub V, Moore SA, Venzke DP, Hrstka RF, Crosbie RH, Durbeej, et al: Progressive muscular dystrophy in alpha-sarcoglycan-deficient mice. *J Cell Biol* **142**:1461, 1998.

414. Hack AA, Ly CT, Jiang F, Clendenin CJ, Sigrist KS, Wollmann RL, McNally, et al: Gamma-sarcoglycan deficiency leads to muscle membrane defects and apoptosis independent of dystrophin. *J Cell Biol* **142**:1279, 1998.

415. Sunada Y, Bernier SM, Kozak CA, Yamada Y, Campbell KP: Deficiency of merosin in dystrophic *dy* mice and genetic linkage of laminin M chain gene to *dy* locus. *J Biol Chem* **269**:13729, 1994.

416. Xu H, Christmas P, Wu XR, Wewer UM, Engvall E: Defective muscle basement membrane and lack of M-laminin in the dystrophic *dy/dy* mouse. *Proc Natl Acad Sci USA* **91**:5572, 1994.

417. Xu H, Wu XR, Wewer UM, Engvall E: Murine muscular dystrophy caused by a mutation in the laminin alpha 2 (Lama2) gene. *Nature Genet* **8**:297, 1994.

418. Sunada Y, Bernier SM, Utani A, Yamada Y, Campbell KP: Identification of a novel mutant transcript of laminin alpha-2 chain gene responsible for muscular dystrophy and dysmyelination in *dy*(2J) mice. *Hum Mol Genet* **4**:1055, 1995.

419. Brown RH J: Prednisone therapy for Duchenne's muscular dystrophy. *N Engl J Med* **320**:1621, 1989.

420. Lord Walton: Anabolic steroids and muscular dystrophy. *Neurology* **42**:1435, 1992.

421. Khan MA: Corticosteroid therapy in Duchenne muscular dystrophy. *J Neurol Sci* **120**:8, 1993.

422. Dubrovsky AL, Angelini C, Bonifati DM, Pegoraro E, Mesa L: Steroids in muscular dystrophy: Where do we stand? *Neuromusc Disord* **8**:380, 1998.

423. Mendell JR, Moxley RT, Griggs RC, Brooke MH, Fenichel GM, Miller JP, King W, et al: Randomized, double-blind six-month trial of prednisone in Duchenne's muscular dystrophy. *N Engl J Med* **320**:1592, 1989.

424. Fenichel GM, Florence JM, Pestronk A, Mendell JR, Moxley RT, III, Griggs RC, Brooke MH, et al: Long-term benefit from prednisone therapy in Duchenne muscular dystrophy. *Neurology* **41**:1874, 1991.

425. Fenichel GM, Mendell JR, Moxley RT, III, Griggs RC, Brooke MH, Miller JP, Pestronk A, et al: A comparison of daily and alternate-day prednisone therapy in the treatment of Duchenne muscular dystrophy. *Arch Neurol* **48**:575, 1991.

426. Griggs RC, Moxley RT, III, Mendell JR, Fenichel GM, Brooke MH, Pestronk A, Miller JP: Prednisone in Duchenne dystrophy: A randomized, controlled trial defining the time course and dose response. Clinical Investigation of Duchenne Dystrophy Group. *Arch Neurol* **48**:383, 1991.

427. Griggs RC, Moxley RT, III, Mendell JR, Fenichel GM, Brooke MH, Pestronk A, Miller JP, et al: Duchenne dystrophy: Randomized, controlled trial of prednisone (18 months) and azathioprine (12 months). *Neurology* **43**:520, 1993.

428. Stern LM, Tomas FM, Burgoyne J: Monitoring the effects of prednisone in Duchenne dystrophy (Letter). *J Paediatr Child.Health* **32**:196, 1996.

429. Mesa LE, Dubrovsky AL, Corderi J, Marco P, Flores D: Steroids in Duchenne muscular dystrophy: Deflazacort trial. *Neuromusc Disord* **1**:261, 1991.

430. Angelini C, Pegoraro E, Turella E, Intino MT, Pini A, Costa C: Deflazacort in Duchenne dystrophy: Study of long-term effect [published erratum appears in *Muscle Nerve* 17(7):833, 1994]. *Muscle Nerve* **17**:386, 1994.

431. Reitter B: Deflazacort vs prednisone in Duchenne muscular dystrophy: Trends of an ongoing study. *Brain Dev* **17**(suppl):39, 1995.

432. Tawil R, McDermott MP, Pandya S, King W, Kissel J, Mendell JR, Griggs RC: A pilot trial of prednisone in facioscapulohumeral muscular dystrophy. FSH-DY Group. *Neurology* **48**:46, 1997.

432a. Kissel JT, McDermott MP, Natarajan R, Mendell JR, Pandya S, King WM, Griggs RC, Tawil R: Pilot trial of albuterol in facioscapulohumeral muscular dystrophy. FSH-DY Group. *Neurology* **50**:1402, 1998.

433. Metzinger L, Passaquin A-C, Warter J-M, Poindron P: α-Methylprednisolone promotes skeletal myogenesis in dystrophin-deficient and control mouse cultures. *Neurosci Lett* **155**:171, 1993.

434. Passaquin AC, Metzinger L, Léger JJ, Warter J-M, Poindron P: Prednisolone enhances myogenesis and dystrophin-related protein in skeletal muscle cell cultures from mdx mouse. *J Neurosci Res* **35**:363, 1993.

435. Sklar RM, Brown RH, Jr.: Methylprednisolone increases dystrophin levels by inhibiting myotube death during myogenesis of normal human muscle in vitro. *J Neurol Sci* **101**:73, 1991.

436. Jacobs SCJM, Bootsma AL, Willems PWA, Bar PR, Wokke JHJ: Prednisone can protect against exercise-induced muscle damage. *J Neurol* **243**:410, 1996.

437. Anderson JE, McIntosh LM, Poettcker R: Deflazacort but not prednisone improves both muscle repair and fiber growth in diaphragm and limb muscle in vivo in the *mdx* dystrophic mouse. *Muscle Nerve* **19**:1576, 1996.

438. McIntosh L, Granberg KE, Briere KM, Anderson JE: Nuclear magnetic resonance spectroscopy study of muscle growth, *mdx* dystrophy and glucocorticoid treatments: correlation with repair. *NMR Biomed* **11**:1, 1998.

439. Rifai Z, Welle S, Moxley RT, Lorenson M, Griggs RC: Effect of prednisone on protein metabolism in Duchenne dystrophy. *Am J Physiol* **268**:E67, 1995.

440. Partridge TA, Morgan JE, Coulton GR, Hoffman EP, Kunkel LM: Conversion of mdx myofibres from dystrophin-negative to -positive by injection of normal myoblasts. *Nature* **337**:176, 1989.

441. Law PK, Goodwin TG, Li HJ, Ajamoughli G, Chen M: Myoblast transfer improves muscle genetics/structure/function and normalizes the behavior and life-span of dystrophic mice. *Adv Exp Med Biol* **280**:75, 1990.

442. Karpati G, Ajdukovic D, Arnold D, Gledhill RB, Gittmann R, Holland P, Koch PA, et al: Myoblast transfer in Duchenne muscular dystrophy. *Ann Neurol* **34**:8, 1992.

443. Tremblay JP, Bouchard JP, Malouin F, Théau D, Cottrell F, Collin H, Rouche A, et al: Myoblast transplantation between monozygotic twin girl carriers of Duchenne muscular dystrophy. *Neuromusc Disord* **3**:583, 1993.

444. Miller RG, Sharma KR, Pavlath GK, Gussoni E, Mynhier M, Lanctot AMG, Steinman L, et al: Myoblast implantation in Duchenne muscular dystrophy: The San Francisco study. *Muscle Nerve* **20**:469, 1997.

445. Mendell JR, Kissel JT, Amato AA, King W, Signore L, Prior TW, Sahenk Z, et al: Myoblast transfer in the treatment of Duchenne's muscular dystrophy (see Comments). *N Engl J Med* **333**:832, 1995.

446. Law PK, Goodwin TG, Fang Q, Duggirala V, Larkin C, Florendo JA, Kirby DS, et al: Feasibility, safety and efficacy of myoblast transfer therapy on Duchenne muscular dystrophy boys. *Cell Transplant* **1**:235, 1992.

447. Law PK, Goodwin TG, Fang Q, Quinley T, Vastagh G, Hall T, Jackson T, et al: Human gene therapy with myoblast transfer. *Transplant Proc* **29**:2234, 1997.

448. Law PK, Goodwin TG, Fang Q, Hall TL, Quinley T, Vastagh G, Duggirala V, et al: First human myoblast transfer therapy continues to show dystrophin after 6 years. *Cell Transplant* **6**:95, 1997.

449. Partridge TA, Davies KE: Myoblast-based gene therapies (Review). *Br Med Bull* **51**:123, 1995.

450. Partridge T: The "Fantastic Voyage" of muscle progenitor cells (News). *Nature Med* **4**:554, 1998.

451. Partridge T, Beauchamp J, Morgan J, Tremblay JP, Huard J, Watt D, Wernig A, et al: Meeting of the Cell Transplantation Society in Miami (Letter, Comment). *Cell Transplant* **6**:195, 1997.

452. Partridge T, Lu QL, Morris G, Hoffman E: Is myoblast transplantation effective? (Letter). *Nature Med* **4**:1208, 1998.

453. Guerette B, Asselin I, Skuk D, Entman M, Tremblay JP: Control of inflammatory damage by anti-LFA-1: Increase success of myoblast transplantation. *Cell Transplant* **6**:101, 1997.

454. Vilquin JT, Kinoshita I, Roy B, Goulet M, Engvall E, Tome F, Fardeau M, et al: Partial laminin alpha₂ chain restoration in alpha₂ chain-deficient *dy/dy* mouse by primary muscle cell culture transplantation. *J Cell Biol* **133**:185, 1996.

455. Kinoshita I, Roy R, Dugre FJ, Gravel C, Roy B, Goulet M, Asselin I, et al: Myoblast transplantation in monkeys: control of immune response by FK506. *J Neuropathol Exp Neurol* **55**:687, 1996.

456. Skuk D, Roy B, Goulet M, Tremblay JP: Successful myoblast transplantation in primates depends on appropriate cell delivery and induction of regeneration in the host muscle. *Exp Neurol* **155**:22, 1999.

457. Moisset PA, Skuk D, Asselin I, Goulet M, Roy B, Karpati G, Tremblay JP: Successful transplantation of genetically corrected DMD myoblasts following ex vivo transduction with the dystrophin minigene. *Biochem Biophys Res Commun* **247**:94, 1998.

458. Acsadi G, Dickson G, Love DR, Jani A, Walsh FS, Gurusinghe A, Wolff JA, et al: Human dystrophin expression in mdx mice after intramuscular injection of DNA constructs. *Nature* **352**:815, 1991.

459. Wells DJ, Wells KE, Walsh FS, Davies KE, Goldspink G, Love DR, Chan-Thomas P, et al: Human dystrophin expression corrects the myopathic phenotype in mdx transgenic mice. *Hum Mol Genet* **1**:35, 1992.

460. Graham FL, Smiley J, Russel WC, Nairn R: Characteristics of a human cell line transformed by DNA from human adenovirus 5. *J Gen Virol* **36**:59, 1977.

461. Ragot T, Stratford-Perricaudet LD, Vincent N, Chafey P, Vigne E, Gilgenkrantz H, Couton D, et al: Adenovirus-mediated transfer of a

human dystrophin gene to skeletal muscle of *mdx* mouse. *Gene Ther* **1**(suppl 1):S53, 1994.

462. Clemens PR, Krause TL, Chan S, Korb KE, Graham FL, Caskey CT: Recombinant truncated dystrophin minigenes: Construction, expression, and adenoviral delivery. *Hum Gene Ther* **6**:1477, 1995.

463. Acsadi G, Lochmuller H, Jani A, Huard J, Massie B, Prescott SS, Petrof BJ, et al: Dystrophin expression in muscles of mdx mice after adenovirus-mediated in vivo gene transfer. *Hum Gene Ther* **7**:129, 1996.

464. Karpati G, Gilbert R, Petrof BJ, Nalbantoglu J: Gene therapy research for Duchenne and Becker muscular dystrophies (Review). *Curr Opin Neurol* **10**:430, 1997.

465. Holt KH, Lim LE, Straub V, Venzke DP, Duclos F, Anderson RD, Davidson BL, et al: Functional rescue of the sarcoglycan complex in the BIO 14.6 hamster using delta-sarcoglycan gene transfer. *Mol Cell* **1**:841, 1998.

466. Acsadi G, Jani A, Massie B, Simoneau M, Holland P, Blaschuk K, Karpati G: A differential efficiency of adenovirus-mediated in vivo gene transfer into skeletal muscle cells of different maturity. *Hum Mol Genet* **3**:579, 1994.

467. Feero WG, Rosenblatt JD, Huard J, Watkins SC, Epperly M, Clemens PR, Kochanek S, et al: Viral gene delivery to skeletal muscle: Insights on maturation-dependent loss of fiber infectivity for adenovirus and herpes simplex type 1 viral vectors. *Hum Gene Ther* **8**:371, 1997.

468. Kochanek S, Clemens PR, Mitani K, Chen HH, Chan S, Caskey CT: A new adenoviral vector: Replacement of all viral coding sequences with 28 kb of DNA independently expressing both full-length dystrophin and beta-galactosidase. *Proc Natl Acad Sci USA* **93**:5731, 1996.

469. Kumar-Singh R, Chamberlain JS: Encapsidated adenovirus minichromosomes allow delivery and expression of a 14 kb dystrophin cDNA to muscle cells. *Hum Mol Genet* **5**:913, 1996.

470. Haecker SE, Stedman HH, Balice-Gordon RJ, Smith DB, Greelish JP, Mitchell MA, Wells A, et al: In vivo expression of full-length human dystrophin from adenoviral vectors deleted of all viral genes. *Hum Gene Ther* **7**:1907, 1996.

471. Clemens PR, Kochanek S, Sunada Y, Chan S, Chen HH, Campbell KP, Caskey CT: In vivo muscle gene transfer of full-length dystrophin with an adenoviral vector that lacks all viral genes. *Gene Ther* **3**:965, 1996.

472. Chen HH, Mack LM, Kelly R, Ontell M, Kochanek S, Clemens PR: Persistence in muscle of an adenoviral vector that lacks all viral genes. *Proc Natl Acad Sci USA* **94**:1645, 1997.

473. Parks RJ, Chen L, Anton M, Sankar U, Rudnicki MA, Graham FL: A helper-dependent adenovirus vector system: Removal of helper virus by Cre-mediated excision of the viral packaging signal. *Proc Natl Acad Sci USA* **93**:13565, 1996.

474. Schiedner G, Morral N, Parks RJ, Wu Y, Koopmans SC, Langston C, Graham FL, et al: Genomic DNA transfer with a high-capacity adenovirus vector results in improved in vivo gene expression and decreased toxicity [published erratum appears in *Nature Genet* **18**(3):298, 1998]. *Nature Genet* **18**:180, 1998.

475. Floyd SS, Clemens PR, Ontell MR, Kochanek S, Day CS, Yang J, Hauschka SD, et al: Ex vivo gene transfer using adenovirus-mediated full-length dystrophin delivery to dystrophic muscles. *Gene Ther* **5**:19, 1998.

476. Bergelson JM, Cunningham JA, Droguett G, Kurt-Jones EA, Krithivas A, Hong JS, Horwitz MS, et al: Isolation of a common receptor for Coxsackie B viruses and adenoviruses 2 and 5. *Science* **275**:1320, 1997.

477. Huard J, Goins WF, Glorioso JC: Herpes simplex virus type 1 vector mediated gene transfer to muscle. *Gene Ther* **2**:385, 1995.

478. Huard J, Feero WG, Watkins SC, Hoffman EP, Rosenblatt DJ, Glorioso JC: The basal lamina is a physical barrier to herpes simplex virus-mediated gene delivery to mature muscle fibers. *J Virol* **70**:8117, 1996.

479. Huard J, Krisky D, Oligino T, Marconi P, Day CS, Watkins SC, Glorioso JC, et al: Gene transfer to muscle using herpes simplex virus-based vectors (Review). *Neuromusc Disord* **7**:299, 1997.

480. van Deutekom JC, Floyd SS, Booth DK, Oligino T, Krisky D, Marconi P, Glorioso JC, et al: Implications of maturation for viral gene delivery to skeletal muscle. *Neuromusc Disord* **8**:135, 1998.

481. Xiao X, Li J, Samulski RJ: Efficient long-term gene transfer into muscle tissue of immunocompetent mice by adeno-associated virus vector. *J Virol* **70**:8098, 1996.

482. Kaplitt MG, Xiao X, Samulski RJ, Li J, Ojamaa K, Klein IL, Makimura H, et al: Long-term gene transfer in porcine myocardium after coronary infusion of an adeno-associated virus vector. *Ann Thorac Surg* **62**:1669, 1996.

483. Vitiello L, Chonn A, Wasserman JD, Duff C, Worton RG: Condensation of plasmid DNA with polylysine improves liposome-mediated gene transfer into established and primary muscle cells. *Gene Ther* **3**:396, 1996.

484. Vitiello L, Bockhold K, Joshi PB, Worton RG: Transfection of cultured myoblasts in high serum concentration with DODAC:DOPE liposomes. *Gene Ther* **5**:1306, 1998.

485. Tinsley JM, Davies KE: Utrophin: A potential replacement for dystrophin? *Neuromusc Disord* **3**:537, 1993.

486. Karpati G, Acsadi G: The potential for gene therapy in Duchenne muscular dystrophy and other genetic muscle diseases. *Muscle Nerve* **16**:1141, 1993.

# Myotonic Dystrophy

*Peter S. Harper* ■ *Keith Johnson*

1. Myotonic dystrophy (MIM 160900) is the most frequent muscular dystrophy of adult life. It shows a characteristic pattern of progressive muscle weakness and wasting, together with myotonia, an electrophysiological disturbance resulting in delayed relaxation and muscle stiffness. Its progressive nature distinguishes it from other myotonic disorders. While it is the only form of muscular dystrophy showing myotonia, and even though it is a rare disorder, proximal myotonic myopathy (PROMM) (MIM 600109) was recently separated from myotonic dystrophy and is genetically, as well as clinically, distinct.

2. Myotonic dystrophy is a multisystem disorder, involving smooth and cardiac muscle, the central nervous system, and endocrine glands, and it causes cataracts. It is exceptionally variable in both severity and age at onset, the severe congenital form being frequently fatal in the neonatal period.

3. Myotonic dystrophy follows autosomal dominant inheritance, but with unusual features, notably anticipation between generations and parental origin effects; almost all congenital cases are maternally transmitted.

4. Positional cloning has isolated and characterized the myotonic dystrophy locus on chromosome 19q and has identified the responsible mutation as an expanded and unstable trinucleotide (CTG) repeat. The degree of expansion is very variable and correlates with phenotype, severe congenital cases showing several thousand repeats, while minimally affected individuals usually have less than 100 repeats. Anticipation within families also corresponds to enlargement of the molecular defect.

5. Instability of the expanded repeat sequence in germline transmission is affected by its size and by the sex of the transmitting parent, expansion being greater in male transmissions except for the largest repeats which are rarely male transmitted, agreeing with the observed parent of origin effects in the disorder. Somatic instability of the repeat is also seen in development and varies between tissues.

6. The prevalence of myotonic dystrophy varies considerably and is notably absent (with a single exception) in sub-Saharan Africa. Clinically significant mutations originate from symptomless individuals carrying expansions at the lower limit of the abnormal range; transmission through many generations with gradual increase in repeat number is likely to have preceded this and the prevalence of the disorder may be broadly related to the population frequency of alleles in the upper normal range.

7. All known cases of myotonic dystrophy show the same unstable CTG expansion, and all cases in European and Asian populations share a common haplotype, which suggests that a single original genetic event predisposing to future instability may have occurred around the time that the ancestors of present Caucasian and Asian ethnic groups migrated out of Africa. Study of the normal variation at the myotonic dystrophy locus is proving a powerful tool in understanding the process of human evolution.

8. Molecular analysis has become an essential element of clinical practice in relation to presymptomatic and prenatal detection as well as primary diagnosis. No specific pharmacologic or other therapy yet exists, but a range of important factors, notably in relation to anesthesia and the avoidance of cardiorespiratory risk factors, can help minimize morbidity and mortality. The production of transgenic animal models and other experimental approaches hold out promise for future more definitive therapy.

Myotonic dystrophy, the commonest and most variable of the adult muscular dystrophies, has long represented a major challenge to both clinicians and geneticists in attempting to explain its clinical variability and unusual inherited features. These attempts were largely unsuccessful until, in 1992, a specific mutation, within a sequence predicting function as a novel protein kinase, was isolated by positional cloning, while the nature of the mutation was recognized as an unstable trinucleotide repeat expansion. The subsequent years have seen a transformation in how we understand the disorder, especially in terms of its clinical and genetic variability, and their relationship to the underlying mutation. By contrast, our understanding of how the pathogenesis of the disease relates to the function of the myotonic dystrophy protein kinase and of other closely adjacent genes, have proved a much more difficult and complex process, providing a series of new challenges in molecular and cell biology and requiring different approaches to those used for study of the mutation.

This chapter is organized into four main sections: the clinical features of myotonic dystrophy; its genetic and mutational basis; molecular and cell biology and how this may relate to production of the disease; and approaches to molecular diagnosis and management.

## THE CLINICAL BASIS OF MYOTONIC DYSTROPHY

Myotonic dystrophy (also known as dystrophia myotonica or Steinert disease) was first delineated as a specific disorder in 1909, 30 years after the nonprogressive disorder myotonia congenita was described by Thomsen[1] on the basis of his own affected family. The initial descriptions, by Steinert in Germany[2] and by Batten and Gibb in England[3] were thorough and extensive, particularly that of Steinert; they clearly distinguished the disorders from

---

A list of standard abbreviations is located immediately preceding the index in each volume. Additional abbreviations used in this chapter include: CUGBP1 = CUG-binding protein 1; DMAHP = myotonic dystrophy associated homeodomain protein (now known as SIX5 in the databases); DMPK = myotonic dystrophy protein kinase (also known as myotonin protein kinase in some earlier papers); DMWD = new name for gene 59; ETR-3 = elav-type RNA-binding protein; GIPR = gastric inhibitory polypeptide receptor; RT-PCR = reverse transcriptase polymerase chain reaction; and SIX = gene family name derived from sine oculus of *Drosophila*. The GenBank accession numbers for the DM locus gene sequences are: X84813 = human *SIX5*; Z38015 and X84814 = mouse *SIX5*; L08835 = human *DMPK*; Z21506 = mouse *DMPK*; L19267 = *DMWD*. See reference 187 for accession numbers of trapped exons from this region.

**Table 217-1 The Inherited Myotonic Disorders**

| Disorder | Inheritance | Molecular Defect |
|---|---|---|
| Myotonic dystrophy | Autosomal dominant | Trinucleotide repeat expansion |
| Proximal myotonic myopathy (PROMM) | Autosomal dominant | Unknown (one locus mapped to chromosome 3) |
| Myotonia congenita | | |
| Thomsen disease | Autosomal dominant | Adult muscle chloride ion channel defects (both types) |
| Recessive generalized myotonia | Autosomal recessive | |
| Paramyotonia congenita | Autosomal dominant | Muscle sodium ion channel defects |
| Periodic paralysis | | |
| Normohyperkalemic (adynamia episodica) | Autosomal dominant | Muscle sodium ion channel defects |
| Hypokalemic | Autosomal dominant | Calcium ion channel defect |
| Chondrodystrophic myotonia (Schwarz-Jampel syndrome) | Autosomal recessive | Unknown |

**Table 217-2 Muscular Involvement in Myotonic Dystrophy**

Muscles most prominently affected
  Superficial facial muscles
  Levator palpebrae superioris
  Temporalis
  Sternocleidomastoids
  Distal muscles of forearm
  Dorsiflexors of foot
Other muscles commonly affected
  Quadriceps
  Diaphragm and intercostals
  Intrinsic muscles of hand and feet
  Palate and pharyngeal muscles
  Tongue
  External ocular muscles
Muscles frequently spared
  Pelvic girdle
  Hamstrings
  Soleus and gastrocnemius

Thomsen disease, and a series of subsequent studies soon provided a relatively complete clinical picture of myotonic dystrophy, to which more recent work has only added detail.

It soon became clear that myotonic dystrophy could be distinguished from other muscular dystrophies by its specific pattern of predominant muscle involvement, especially of the face, jaw, anterior neck, and distal limb muscles, as well as by the involvement of other systems and by the presence of myotonia. Cataract was found to be associated with myotonic dystrophy as early as 1912,[4] while the regular occurrence of endocrine and central nervous system changes, as well as of smooth and cardiac muscle involvement, distinguished the condition from all other myotonic disorders, as well as from the other progressive muscular dystrophies. The early clinical studies and research on myotonic dystrophy are outlined in the author's monograph on the disorder,[5] which also gives a more detailed account of the major clinical features than is possible here. The review by Harper and Rudel[6] discusses details of the neuromuscular aspects, in particular the physiological basis of myotonia. Recent molecular developments in the nonprogressive myotonias are covered fully elsewhere in this volume (see Chap. 204), and the distinguishing features from myotonic dystrophy are discussed below. Table 217-1 summarizes the principal myotonic disorders.

## Clinical Features

Myotonic dystrophy is one of the most variable disorders known, and it has presenting features that are often nonneurologic. The condition must thus be considered in a diagnostic framework much broader than that of the other muscular dystrophies. Nevertheless, the commonest symptoms are neuromuscular, principally relating to muscle weakness and myotonia, the latter being most commonly interpreted as stiffness. Table 217-2 gives the distribution of the predominant muscle involvement. It can be seen that the muscles involved contrast strikingly with those involved in the X-linked Duchenne and Becker muscular dystrophies; facioscapulohumeral dystrophy is the only autosomal dystrophy with a somewhat a similar pattern of muscle group involvement (see Chap. 216).

The mainly distal limb involvement can cause confusion with neuropathic conditions such as Charcot-Marie-Tooth disease, but the recognition of myotonia allows a specific clinical diagnosis of myotonic dystrophy to be made immediately. Involvement of facial and jaw muscles is almost invariable in myotonic dystrophy;

ptosis can be marked, while selective weakness and wasting of sternomastoid muscles is seen in the neck. Figure 217-1 illustrates some of these features.

Myotonia is most readily recognized by direct percussion of the muscles (in particular the thenar eminence) or by testing for rapid relaxation (especially of grip or, less commonly, eye closure). While most patients complain of stiffness in relation to their myotonia, this is frequently not mentioned unless directly inquired about. Some patients seem genuinely unaware that their myotonia is abnormal, while others may deliberately minimize their symptoms. The end result is that diagnosis is delayed in many patients, even when myotonia is obvious when looked for.

The extramuscular features of myotonic dystrophy are of special importance, both in the diagnosis of relatives at risk and in terms of prognosis and management of the affected individual. Some of these can be related to smooth or cardiac muscle dysfunction (Table 217-3), while others involve entirely different systems (Table 217-4).

Smooth muscle involvement may show itself in a variety of ways,[8] but esophageal dysfunction[9] may result in dysphagia and in bronchial aspiration causing pneumonia, while colonic and anal sphincter involvement[10] may give abdominal pain, severe constipation, and pseudo-obstruction,[11] and may result in unnecessary and hazardous surgery.

Cardiorespiratory problems are the main cause of death in myotonic dystrophy and require careful attention because they are often not complained of directly. A wide range of cardiac problems can occur,[12] notably arrhythmias such as atrial fibrillation and flutter, heart block, and sudden death. Anesthesia poses particular hazards[13,14] due to the combination of respiratory muscle weakness and increased sensitivity to anesthetics and muscle relaxants. Among other systemic abnormalities are cataracts, which may be the only feature of the disorder and which are characterized by highly distinctive multicolored subcortical lens opacities when viewed with the slit-lamp; a variety of endocrine changes of which testicular tubular atrophy in males is most prominent; and various degrees of central nervous system involvement ranging from increased somnolence, apathy, and mild personality abnormalities in some adults to severe mental retardation in a proportion of congenitally affected patients. Some patients presenting with these systemic features (notably cataract) may have only minimal or, occasionally, no detectable muscle abnormality even on careful investigation. Molecular diagnostics may help to confirm myotonic dystrophy in such situations, as discussed in the final section of this chapter.

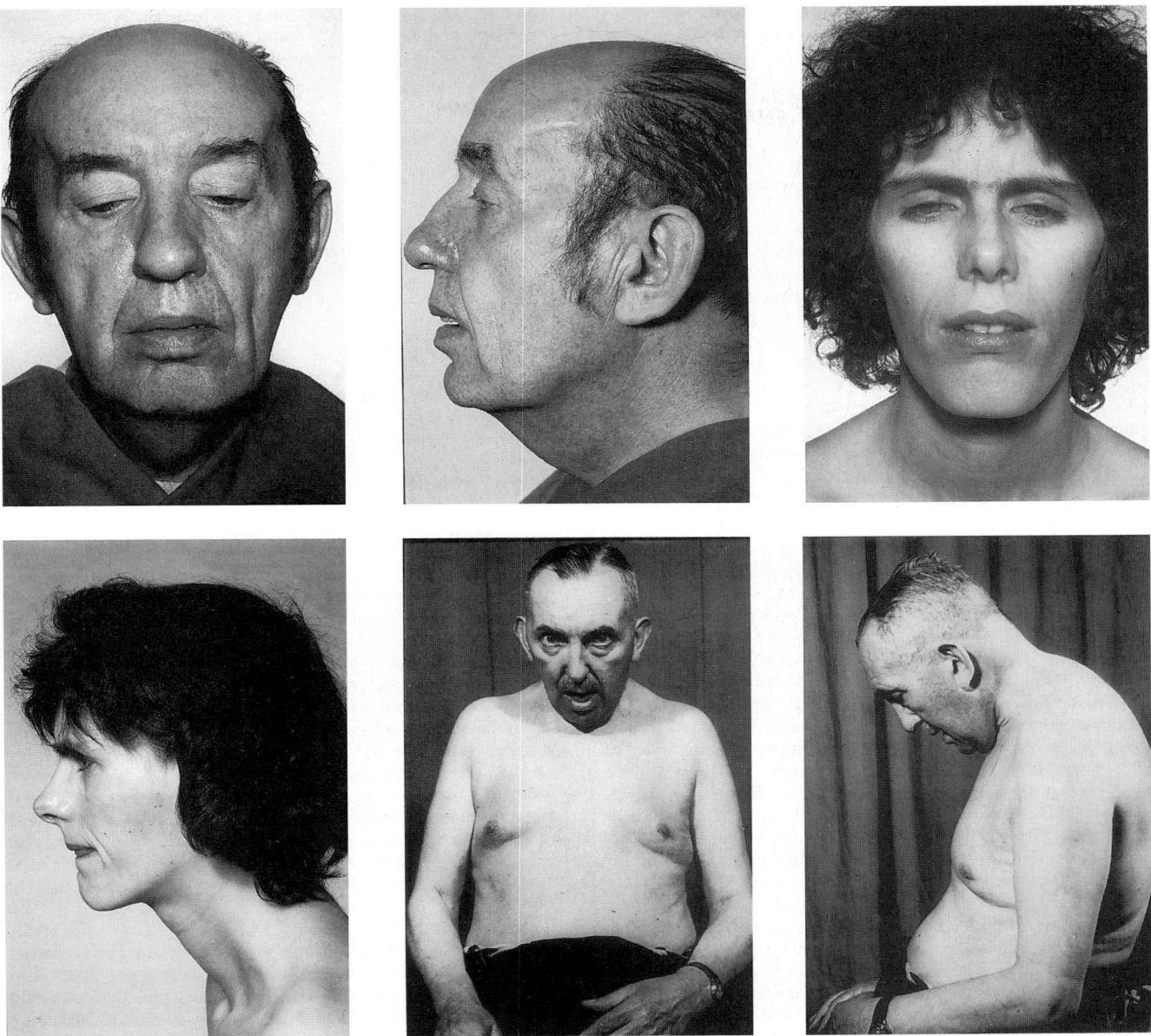

Fig. 217-1 Myotonic dystrophy in adult life. Note particularly weakness of facial and jaw muscles, ptosis, and weakness and wasting of sternomastoid muscles in the neck. (Reproduced from Harper[81] with permission.)

## Congenital Myotonic Dystrophy

**Table 217-3 Smooth and Cardiac Muscle Involvement in Myotonic Dystrophy**

| | |
|---|---|
| Gastrointestinal tract | Widespread involvement, particularly of pharynx and esophagus; colon |
| Gallbladder | Delayed emptying; high incidence of stones |
| Urinary bladder | Rarely affected |
| Ureter | Isolated instances of dilatation |
| Uterus | Uncoordinated contraction in labor and in vitro |
| Eye | Ciliary body affected; low intraocular tension |
| Heart | Conduction defects, in particular heart block; atrial arrhythmias; less commonly, cardiomyopathy |

Congenital myotonic dystrophy was first recognized by Vanier in 1960[21] and it has since become clear that it is a distinctive, frequently fatal, and far from rare form of myotonic dystrophy.[22] It is seen almost exclusively in offspring of women who are themselves affected with myotonic dystrophy.[23,24] These mothers are often only mildly affected but almost invariably show some neuromuscular abnormalities.[25]

Table 217-5 lists the main characteristics of congenital myotonic dystrophy; the features at different ages are shown in Fig. 217-2. The facial appearance is highly distinctive, largely owing to the combination of bilateral facial palsy with marked jaw weakness. The early, often intrauterine onset of muscle weakness helps to mold the craniofacial features by creating the characteristic tented upper lip and other dysmorphic features. Decreased intrauterine muscle action plays a role in many of the other features, such as the high incidence of respiratory inadequacy and pulmonary hypoplasia (caused by underdeveloped diaphragm and intercostal muscles), the occurrence of talipes and other joint

**Table 217-4 Other Systems Involved in Myotonic Dystrophy**

| System | Symptom |
|---|---|
| Eye | Cataract, retinal degeneration, ocular hypotonia, ptosis, extraocular weakness |
| Endocrine | Testicular tubular atrophy; diabetes (rarely clinically significant); sometimes abnormalities of growth hormone and other pituitary functions |
| Brain | Severe involvement in congenital form; mild mental deterioration frequent in adults; hypersomnia; sleep hypoventilation |
| Peripheral nerves | Variable and rarely clinically significant; minor sensory loss may occur |
| Skeletal | Cranial hyperostosis, air sinus enlargement; jaw and palate involvement; talipes (childhood cases); scoliosis (uncommon) |
| Skin | Premature balding; calcifying epithelioma |
| Lungs | Aspiration pneumonia from esophageal and diaphragmatic involvement; alveolar hypoventilation |

**Table 217-5 Comparative Clinical Features of Myotonic Dystrophy and Proximal Myotonic Myopathy (PROMM)**

| | Myotonic Dystrophy | PROMM |
|---|---|---|
| Neuromuscular abnormalities | | |
| Myotonia | + | + |
| Progressive muscle weakness and wasting | + | + |
| Facial weakness | + | − |
| Predominant distribution of weakness | Distal | Proximal |
| Muscle Pain | − | + |
| Other symptoms | | |
| Cardiac arrythmias | + | + |
| Cataract | + | + |
| Central nervous system involvement | + | − |
| Genetic aspects | | |
| Anticipation | + | − |
| Gene localization | 19q | Chromosome 3 (some families) |
| Specific molecular basis | Trinucleotide repeat expansion | |

contractures, the development of polyhydramnios (owing to lack of intrauterine swallowing), and the generally poor fetal movements. By contrast to the adult disorder, myotonia is inconspicuous or absent in affected infants, although it becomes more prominent as affected individuals reach later childhood.

The differential diagnosis of congenital myotonic dystrophy in the neonate relates not so much to other muscular dystrophies as to the broader group of congenital myopathies. Many patients die rapidly from respiratory inadequacy before the diagnosis can be made, but with the increasing success of neonatal intensive care, a higher proportion survives to be diagnosed. The relationship to adult myotonic dystrophy is important to recognize because the discovery of a typical adult case in the family, usually the mother or another maternal relative, confirms the diagnosis in the infant. X-linked myotubular myopathy, for which a specific gene has now been isolated,[26] is particularly likely to be confused with congenital myotonic dystrophy on the grounds of both clinical appearance and muscle pathology.[27] It is particularly important for all women with myotonic dystrophy who are considering child-bearing to understand the risk of the severe congenital form.

Molecular analysis is also proving particularly helpful in the diagnosis of congenital myotonic dystrophy, as discussed later. Many of the previously puzzling aspects of myotonic dystrophy have now been resolved by the finding that it is these patients who show the largest CTG repeat expansions (often several thousand repeats) and by the recognition that there is a limit to male transmitted expansion that is responsible for the largely maternal inheritance of this form. Nevertheless, it remains possible that other sex-related factors (such as genomic imprinting) may also be involved in producing the phenotype of congenital myotonic dystrophy. Absence of a large expansion in a suspected case would strongly suggest that another form of congenital myopathy is the cause of the problem. Detection of the molecular defect also can now be used for specific prenatal diagnosis.

## Diagnostic Tests for Myotonic Dystrophy

It is important when considering these to understand the purpose of the test. If this is genetic, such as for excluding or detecting the mutation in healthy relatives, or in prenatal diagnosis, then a genetic test is what is required; molecular analysis for the specific CTG expansion now answers these questions with a high degree of accuracy and other tests, such as slit-lamp examination of the lens, muscle biopsy, or electromyography, are normally unnecessary and sometimes misleading. On the other hand, if the question is clinical—for example, Does a known gene carrier show any

evidence of neurologic or lens abnormality?—then such clinical investigations may be very useful in determining whether or not these systems are involved. Molecular testing is now extremely helpful in primary diagnosis also, on account of its highly specific and sensitive nature. The general area of molecular diagnostics is discussed later in this chapter.

Investigations useful in the more general investigation and continuing management of myotonic dystrophy patients also include ECG, to detect cardiac arrhythmias, glucose tolerance and related endocrine studies, in view of the frequency of associated diabetes, and semen analysis if male infertility is a problem.

## Muscle Pathology

Detailed studies of muscle histology, histochemistry, and electron microscopy have given a clear picture of the changes that occur in myotonic dystrophy.[6,28] These changes are distinctive, although not totally specific. Figure 217-3 shows some of the more characteristic changes, notably increased internal nuclei, often in chains, together with ringed fibers and sarcoplasmic masses. Histochemistry shows a relative loss of type 1 fibers, while electron-microscopic changes include degeneration of microfilaments and proliferation of the sarcotubular system. More important from the viewpoint of pathogenesis are the negative ultrastructural findings, in particular absence of marked change in blood vessels and nerve endings, showing that muscle fiber itself is the principal site of the pathology.

Study of muscle from patients with congenital myotonic dystrophy shows several changes not present in adult patients.[29] The muscles are hypoplastic and the fibers have an immature appearance, with centrally placed nuclei and abundant satellite cells, suggesting arrested development rather than degeneration,[30] an important distinguishing feature from X-linked myotubular myopathy.[27] Histochemical studies show a peripheral area deficient in mitochondrial enzymes.[31]

Our understanding of the mutation and of the gene product now complements these earlier studies on the muscle pathology of myotonic dystrophy. Changes in severity of the histologic changes have been shown to be correlated with the degree of expansion of the repeat sequence,[32] but while the expansion itself is generally larger in muscle tissue than in white blood cells, there is poorer correlation with overall clinical severity, as discussed later.

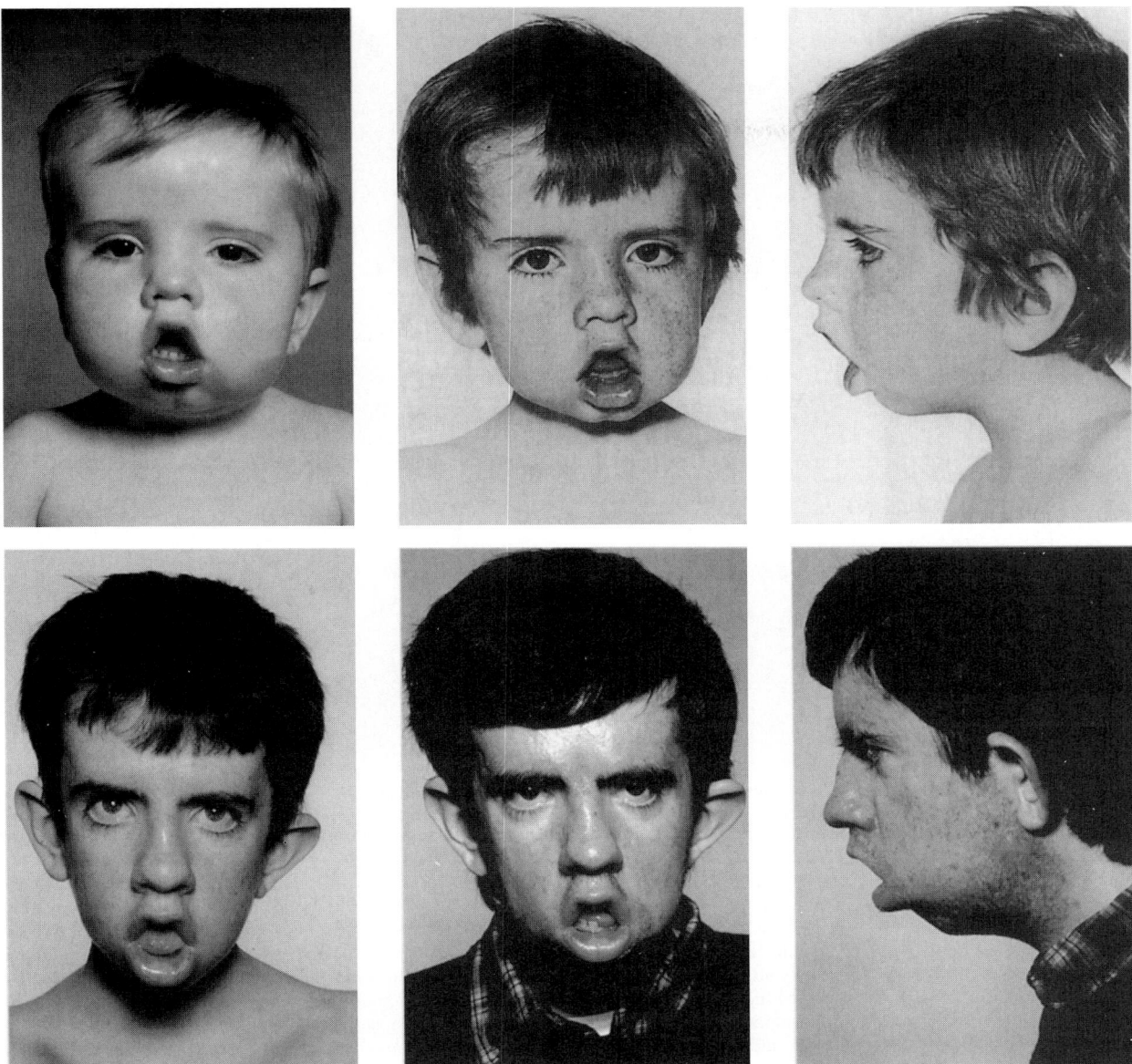

**Fig. 217-2 Congenital myotonic dystrophy.** Evolution of clinical features with age in the same patient followed over a period of 25 years. Note the facial diplegia, tented upper lip, and extreme jaw weakness. (Reproduced from Harper[81] with permission.)

Subcellular studies of the myotonic dystrophy protein kinase, although still controversial, suggest that it is a component of neuromuscular junctions[33-35] and of the sarcoplasmic reticulum.[36] In affected patients, the protein kinase is localized in the peripheral sarcoplasmic masses,[37] but whether levels are decreased or increased remains debatable.[37,38] In congenital myotonic dystrophy, the histochemical localization of myotonic dystrophy protein kinase is mainly at the sarcolemma.[39] The ways in which muscle distribution and expression of the protein are related to normal and abnormal gene function are described more fully in the section "The Molecular and Cell Biology of Myotonic Dystrophy" below. It is also important to remember that DNA analysis of stored material from a previous muscle biopsy may allow a specific diagnosis of myotonic dystrophy to be made or excluded retrospectively.

## Myotonia and Disordered Physiology in Myotonic Dystrophy

Whereas there is now considerable evidence relating nonprogressive myotonia to the dysfunction of specific muscle ion channels, notably those for sodium and chloride, the evidence for a clearly defined physiological basis for myotonia in myotonic dystrophy is much less satisfactory, with different and, in some cases, contradictory findings in different studies. So far, our new understanding of the molecular basis of myotonic dystrophy has not clearly explained the myotonia of myotonic dystrophy, but the existing evidence relating specifically to myotonic dystrophy is summarized below. Harper and Rudel[6] give a more detailed account.

The initial in vitro studies of myotonic dystrophy muscle showed a reduced resting potential across the muscle cell membrane with a raised level of intracellular sodium. A subsequent study,[40] however, found the opposite, the resting potential being high and the intracellular sodium level low. A more recent detailed study by Franke et al.[41] provides some resolution of these findings, because a reduction in resting potential was seen mainly in patients with dystrophic changes, not in those in whom myotonia was the main feature. This suggests that any change in resting membrane potential in myotonic dystrophy may be secondary to damage of muscle fibers.

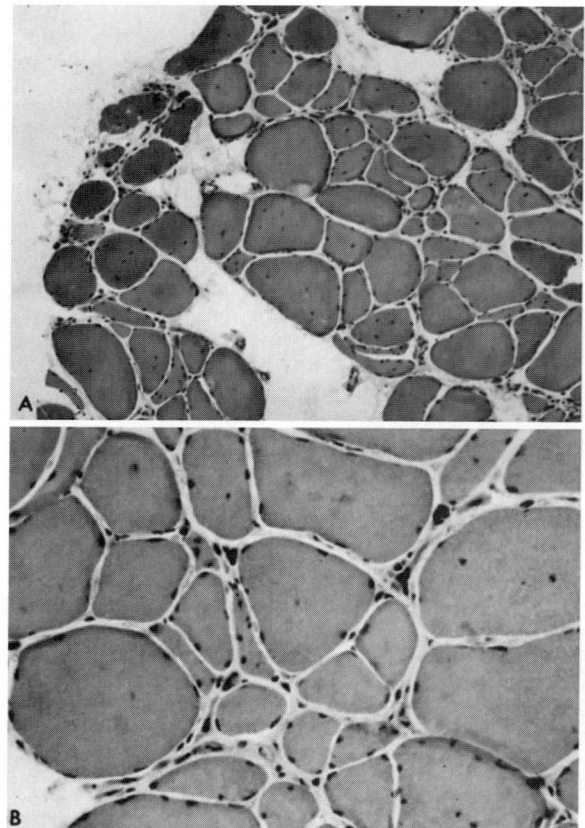

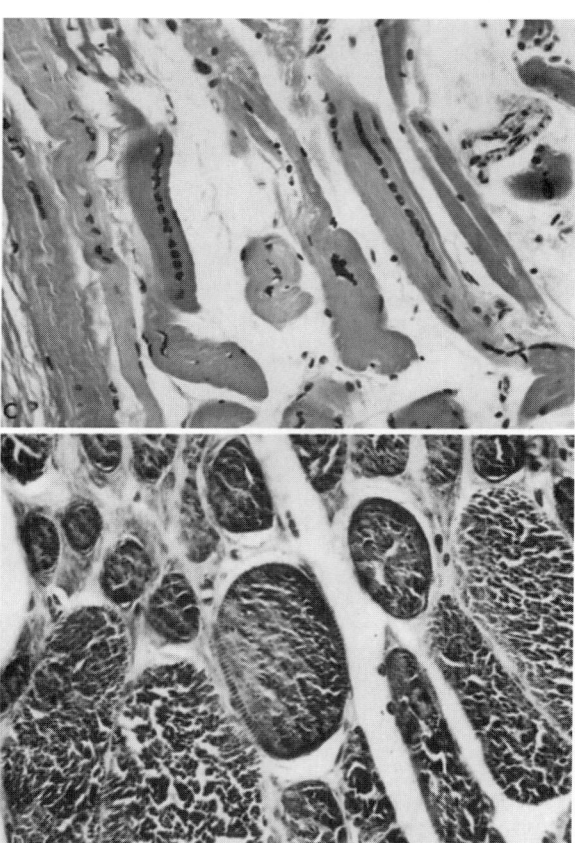

**Fig. 217-3 Changes in muscle histology in adult myotonic dystrophy.** *A.* Transverse section showing variation in fiber size and numerous internal nuclei. *B.* Higher-power transverse section showing atrophic fibers with clumped nuclei. *C.* Longitudinal section showing long chains of internal nuclei. *D.* Transverse section showing ringed fibers. (*From Harper,[5] Used by permission.*)

Reduced chloride conductance is the principal feature of the human myotonia congenita and its counterparts in the goat and the mouse, a finding that led to the hypothesis, now confirmed, that a chloride ion channel defect is responsible for this form of myotonia. In myotonic dystrophy, the results are much less clear: Lipicky found levels varying from low to normal,[40] whereas Franke et al.,[41] using resealed muscle fiber segments, found a high level in one patient with marked myotonia and normal and low levels in others. This result clearly suggests that a chloride channel defect is not the primary mechanism. Franke et al. also showed an abnormality of sodium channel function using a patch-clamp technique.

Studies of cultured muscle have also given conflicting results in myotonic dystrophy. Merickel et al.[42] found both a reduced resting potential in cultured myotonic dystrophy fibers and a decreased after-hyperpolarization, which suggests the possibility of a primary defect in potassium conductance. These findings have not been confirmed by others.[43] An interesting finding of Renaud et al.,[44] which has not yet been confirmed, was that the potassium channel receptor affected by bee venom apamin was present in myotonic dystrophy fibers, in contrast to normal adult muscle and muscle in other neuromuscular disorders. While this result could relate to the immaturity of myotonic dystrophy muscle as noted by pathology studies, it could also suggest a disturbance of potassium conductance.

The results of physiological studies on myotonic dystrophy thus remain confusing, in contrast to the clear-cut results of studies on the nonprogressive myotonias, which from the outset pointed to definite and specific ion channel defects, and which led directly to the molecular studies that confirmed the molecular basis of these myotonic disorders. However, in light of what we now know about the complexity of the molecular basis of myotonic dystrophy, these apparently confusing findings are not surprising.

## Other Myotonic Disorders

Table 217-1 summarizes the other genetic disorders in which myotonia is found; it should be emphasized that all are extremely rare in comparison with myotonic dystrophy. The nonprogressive myotonias are discussed in a separate chapter of this work (Chap. 204), but it there is rarely any difficulty in distinguishing the nonprogressive myotonias from myotonic dystrophy. Affected adults with myotonia congenita usually show no or minimal muscle weakness, and even when present it is not in the typical distribution seen in myotonic dystrophy, while systemic features are absent. Occasional myotonic dystrophy patients showing marked myotonia and little weakness can now be recognized by molecular analysis.

## Proximal Myotonic Myopathy (PROMM)

The existence of this disorder (MIM 600109) was unsuspected until after identification of the myotonic dystrophy mutation, when clinical reassessment of those few cases not showing the CTG expansion led to the realization that a group of patients actually had a clinically distinguishable albeit similar disorder.[39,40] Table 217-6 summarizes the main features in comparison with myotonic dystrophy, but the limits of the phenotype remain uncertain,[41,42] and will probably remain so until a specific molecular defect is identified.

PROMM is a progressive muscular disorder, but is usually milder than myotonic dystrophy, with slow progression, and with muscle weakness mainly proximal and sparing the face, muscle pain and stiffness may be prominent. Myotonia is often inconspicuous, but muscle biopsy somewhat resembles that seen in myotonic dystrophy. Cataract is a constant feature and in its early stages resembles the cataract of myotonic dystrophy. Inheritance is autosomal dominant, but there is no clear evidence

**Table 217-6** Congenital Myotonic Dystrophy: Major Clinical Features

Bilateral facial weakness
Hypotonia
Delayed motor development
Mental retardation
Neonatal respiratory distress
Feeding difficulties
Talipes
Hydramnios in later pregnancy
Reduced fetal movements

**Table 217-7** Inheritance of Myotonic Dystrophy — Summary of Unusual Features Requiring Explanation

Autosomal dominant inheritance — but extreme variation in expression despite lack of genetic heterogeneity.
Anticipation — progressively earlier onset and greater severity with successive generations.
Parent of origin effects — congenital form almost always maternally transmitted; first symptomatic generation usually of paternal origin.
Population variation — virtual absence in sub-Saharan Africa; isolates elsewhere with extremely high prevalence.

of anticipation. Most reported families have been small and while linkage to the myotonic dystrophy locus has been ruled out, as have the Na$^+$ and Cl$^-$ ion channel loci.[43] Some, but not all families have been localized to chromosome 3q. It will be of interest to see whether the recent chromosome 3q localization of a large kindred with the phenotype of myotonic dystrophy[44] proves also to be involved in PROMM.* It will also be important to determine whether the protein product of these genes is related to or interacts with the myotonic dystrophy protein kinase or other associated proteins. Clearly, both the phenotypic and molecular states of PROMM and other rare families that are not determined by the chromosome 19 CTG expansion will need reassessment in the light of new information.

# THE FORMAL GENETIC AND MUTATIONAL BASIS OF MYOTONIC DYSTROPHY

Our understanding of the genetics of myotonic dystrophy has been so entirely changed by the discovery that its mutational basis results from the expansion of an unstable trinucleotide repeat sequence, that it makes little sense to discuss any of the genetic aspects except in this context. However, the early studies, in particular the extensive family surveys of Fleischer,[45] Bell,[46] Thomasen,[47] and Klein,[48] were able to identify a series of unusual genetic features that demanded explanation, most of which have been resolved now that we know the mutational mechanism. These included whether autosomal dominant inheritance was an adequate explanation for the genetic basis; the extreme variability of the disorder within single families; parental origin effects in transmission of the disease, in particular the maternal transmission of congenital myotonic dystrophy; and, most notably, the phenomenon of anticipation, which required a period of 75 years from its first description in myotonic dystrophy to a satisfactory explanation for its occurrence. These aspects, summarized in Table 217-7, are considered in turn, taking the evidence from both classical formal genetic studies and from molecular analysis together. But first, the steps leading to the identification of the myotonic dystrophy gene and mutation are outlined.

## Positional Cloning of the Myotonic Dystrophy Gene

The prolonged and eventually successful gene mapping and positional cloning studies of the myotonic dystrophy region of chromosome 19 were described in detail in the previous edition of this work[49] and can now be considered as historical. Briefly, one can identify several phases of this work.

1. Early linkage studies with classical markers, allowing formation of a group of linked loci (myotonic dystrophy — Lutheran blood group — secretor locus).[50–52]
2. Assignment of the linkage group to chromosome 19.[53]
3. Detection of closely linked DNA markers[54–56] and physical mapping[57,58] of the relevant region of chromosome 19q.

4. Finding of markers showing linkage disequilibrium outside specific populations[59] and allowing detailed molecular analysis of the critical region.[60–62]
5. Discovery of the unstable DNA sequence and its trinucleotide repeat nature as the mutational basis for myotonic dystrophy.
6. Isolation of the myotonic dystrophy protein kinase gene.
7. Identification of the overlapping *DMAHP* gene (see App. I, Chap. 1) and recognition that the trinucleotide repeat mutation affects its promoter region.

In addition to allowing the discovery of the myotonic dystrophy mutation and isolation of the gene, these positional cloning studies also established several important facts that are of general importance in understanding the genetic basis of the disorder. A significant heterogeneity in terms of multiple loci was excluded by the absence of families unlinked to the chromosome 19 locus, while the existence of a common haplotype of markers in most European, Israeli, and Japanese families[59] first suggested that there might be very few original mutations. Also, the general studies of recombination along the chromosome showed that there was no extensive region of genetic instability in the neighborhood of the myotonic dystrophy gene.[63]

The disequilibrium data strongly suggested that the gene was located in a restricted region of around 200 kb.[59] This region was also suggested by individual recombinants, and the combined evidence prompted a detailed molecular analysis of this entire length of DNA. By mid-1991 this region had essentially been cloned,[61,62] and the problem was how to identify the myotonic dystrophy gene from the considerable number of genes (estimated at 10 to 20) likely to be present in this region.

Linkage disequilibrium played a further role in focusing attention on the correct region when a genomic sequence (*D19S190; 59A*) was identified[64] that showed almost complete disequilibrium with myotonic dystrophy — 74 of 75 unrelated affected patients had the same allele, in contrast to 140 of 232 normal individuals (the single apparent exception later proved to have PROMM). Because this genomic sequence was strongly conserved, it became an important candidate for the myotonic dystrophy gene.

At the end of 1991, the course of the search was radically altered by the finding that a specific abnormality was present in the DNA of individuals with myotonic dystrophy. The abnormality was seen both in a cDNA sequence[65] and in the genomic sequence 59A described above.[64] Exchange of materials by the two groups involved showed that both probes were detecting the same change, and that the abnormality, while specific to myotonic dystrophy, appeared to vary among patients, even within the same family. It was immediately recognized that this abnormality was likely to represent expansion of an unstable DNA sequence and that the sequence was probably within the myotonic dystrophy gene itself. The findings, together with those of a third group,[66] were published in *Nature* in February 1992, thus representing the successful conclusion of almost a decade of gene mapping and positional cloning studies since the original localization of the gene to chromosome 19. Table 217-8 summarizes the main properties of the unstable trinucleotide repeat sequence, which is discussed in more detail below.

*Note added in proof: Ricker et al. (*Neurology* **52**;12, 1999) have confirmed that at least some PROMM families are indeed localised to 3q.

**Table 217-8 The Myotonic Dystrophy Unstable Trinucleotide Repeat: Summary of Principal Features**

CTG repeat.

Location in 3′ untranslated region of myotonic dystrophy protein kinase gene.

Variable in normal population (less than 40 repeats).

Expansion in myotonic dystrophy extremely variable (50 to >5000 repeats).

Correlation of repeat number with severity of phenotype and early age at onset.

Intergenerational instability size and sex dependent, largely explaining observed anticipation and parent of origin effects.

Somatic instability, variable between tissues.

## An Expanded Trinucleotide Repeat Sequence in Myotonic Dystrophy

Six months prior to the recognition of the unstable sequence in myotonic dystrophy, the molecular basis of the disorder fragile X mental retardation had been found to be the presence of an expanded and unstable sequence in this gene on the X chromosome.[67] Detailed analysis of the fragile X expansion showed this sequence to be a CGG repeat.[68] Normal individuals have less than 50 copies of the repeat; clinically normal gene carriers have at least 50 copies; and clinically affected individuals have much larger expansions. The parallels with myotonic dystrophy had already been recognized at a clinical level and the identification of an unstable DNA sequence in the fragile X syndrome made it likely that a similar trinucleotide repeat sequence might be involved in myotonic dystrophy.

As indicated above, the unstable sequence was detected separately by a genomic and a cDNA clone, both of which proved to identify the same specific abnormality. Figure 217-4 illustrates the band pattern seen for the EcoRI polymorphism detected by these sequences in normal and affected individuals. The normal pattern is a two-allele insertion/deletion polymorphism with bands of 9 and 10 kb,[69,70] individuals being either heterozygous (lane 5) or homozygous for one or the other band (lane 1). In myotonic dystrophy, one normal allele is seen, but the other (invariably a 10-kb allele) is increased in size to a variable degree.

The degree of increase seen in these initial studies ranged from an extra 150 bp to as much as 6 kb additional DNA, as illustrated in Fig. 217-4. Most important, this variation was seen within single kindreds, notably between generations, as shown below in Fig. 217-6. It can immediately be appreciated that the expansion of the sequence in successive generations agrees with the clinical observation of anticipation and with the genetic stability expected from an expanded trinucleotide repeat sequence.

The confirmation of the mutational defect in myotonic dystrophy as a trinucleotide repeat expansion had to await isolation of the gene,[71-73] an event that occurred within a few months of the identification of the unstable sequence as a result of two different approaches, and the nature of which is described in more detail later. For the purposes of discussion of the mutation and its relationship to the disease, the relevant facts from these studies are that it is a CTG repeat and that it is located in the 3′ untranslated region of the gene that is now known as the myotonic dystrophy protein kinase gene (DMPK). More recently it was shown that the repeat also coincides with the regulatory sequences of a homeodomain transcription factor gene DMAHP.

## Autosomal Dominant Inheritance and Myotonic Dystrophy

It was already noted that myotonic dystrophy was proposed to follow mendelian autosomal dominant inheritance by Fleischer as long ago as 1918,[45] and that this was confirmed by the more systematic studies of Bell[46] and Thomasen,[47] both in 1948.

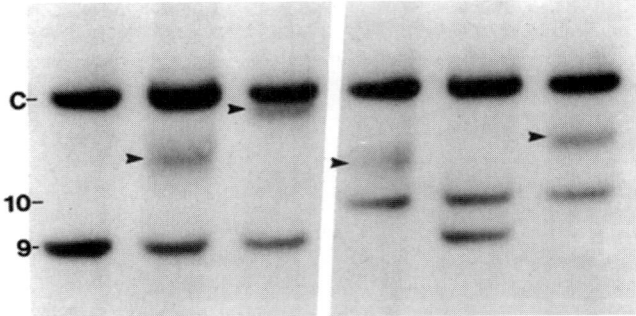

**Fig. 217-4 The unstable DNA sequence in myotonic dystrophy.** EcoRI-digested genomic DNA probed with pBB07. All individuals have a constant band of 15 kb (C). Normal individuals are either homozygous (lane 1) or heterozygous (lane 5) for bands of 9 and 10 kb. Affected individuals (lanes 2, 3, 4, 6) have one of these bands, but also show an additional larger band, whose size varies with the individual. (*Adapted from Harley et al.[64]*)

However, the emphasis since then given to the puzzling and anomalous features of inheritance in the disorder makes it necessary to reexamine whether there really is a consistent autosomal dominant foundation.

First, other patterns of mendelian inheritance can be briefly dealt with and disposed of. X-linkage is clearly ruled out by male-to-male transmission (as is mitochondrial inheritance), while autosomal recessive inheritance is made improbable by the lack of consanguinity (although the level of this varies according to the particular population) and by the transmission through successive generations.

The various studies analyzing the segregation of the disorder in families were assessed by Harper[5] who found that for both sibs and offspring of propositi, the proportion of affected offspring varied between 33.6 percent and 50.7 percent, suggesting that autosomal dominant inheritance was operating, but with a proportion of undetected gene carriers of up to 16 percent, this probably depending on the age range of the subjects and methods of the study. It should particularly be noted that no study showed a proportion of affected in significant excess of 50 percent; this was, however, strongly dependent on the propositi being removed to correct for ascertainment bias; the early study of Harper[74] for example, showed 61.3 percent affected without removing propositi, but only 42.1 percent with it done.

Following the suggestion that there might be segregation distortion and possible meiotic drive for normal polymorphic alleles at the myotonic dystrophy locus (see below), two recent studies have claimed to show anomalous segregation for the disease allele also. Both Gennarelli et al.[75] and Zatz et al.[76] found a significant excess transmission of the abnormal allele to sons. However, in neither study were propositi distinguished, a factor of especial importance in view of the sex difference, because previous studies[5] clearly showed a preferential ascertainment of affected males, again a finding that disappears when propositi are removed.

Since the identification of the CTG repeat at the myotonic dystrophy locus a series of studies has examined the segregation of normal alleles, largely as a means of explaining the generation of potentially unstable alleles to replace those lost as a result of myotonic dystrophy, a topic discussed later. Carey et al.[77] found that there was preferential transmission of large repeats (19 and above) by males; however, reanalysis of these data by Hurst et al.[78] and by Chakraborty et al.[79] both showed that there was an excess of female transmission by heterozygotes of their larger repeat number allele.

Thus, the conclusions from segregation analysis overall are that, so far as myotonic dystrophy as a disease is concerned, the pattern fits that expected for autosomal dominant inheritance, with no evidence of anomaly. For normal variation at the myotonic dystrophy locus there may be preferential transmission of larger

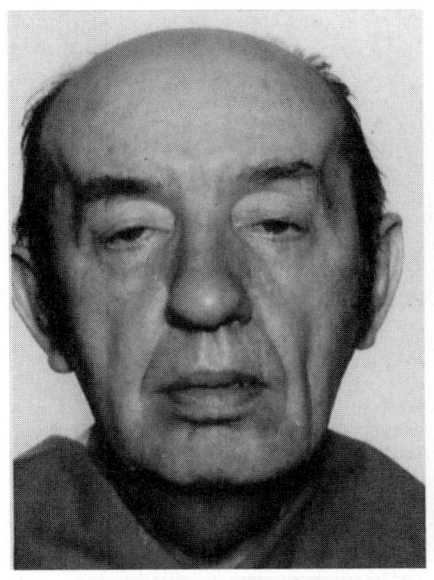
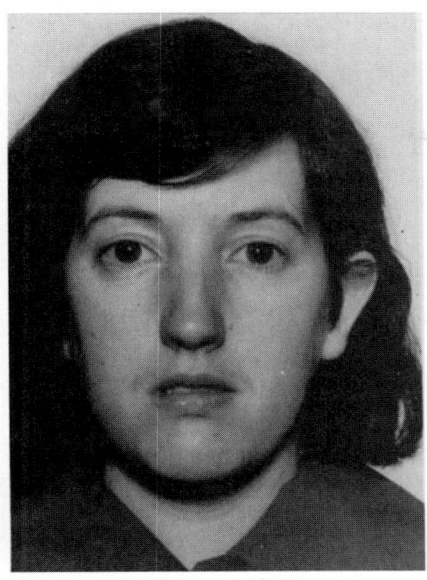
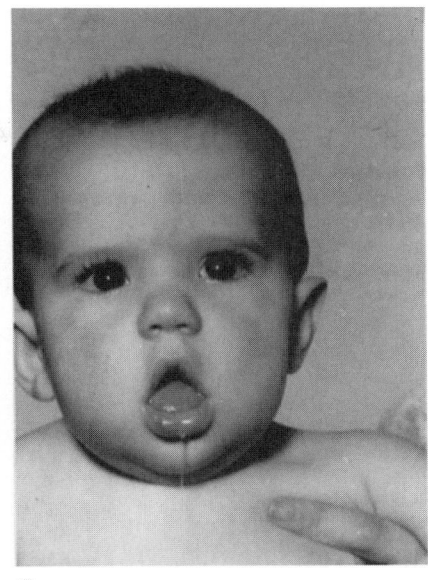

*A*                          *B*                          *C*

**Fig. 217-5** Anticipation and myotonic dystrophy. Clinical features in a three-generation family, showing the increased severity in successive generations. *A.* Grandfather (age 57). Cataracts removed at age 48. Symptoms of myotonia since age 50, but no significant disability. Ptosis, facial weakness, and myotonia on examination. Myotonic dystrophy not diagnosed until birth of affected grandson. *B.* Mother (age 24). Myotonia since late teens; weakness of face and neck present on examination, together with marked myotonia. Only diagnosed after birth of affected son (right). No cataract. *C.* Son. Congenital myotonic dystrophy. Hydramnios during pregnancy; respiratory distress at birth necessitating ventilation. Subsequent improvement, but motor and mental development remains delayed. Marked facial and jaw weakness with hypotonia.

repeat size alleles, but further data are needed to be clear about this.

## Anticipation

Anticipation has a special place in the genetics of myotonic dystrophy. Not only was it the first disorder for which it was demonstrated on the basis of valid clinical evidence, but it has always been the clearest example of the phenomenon. Full accounts of anticipation in myotonic dystrophy have been given elsewhere,[80,81] as well as of its possible role in other disorders;[82,83] anticipation is now recognized as a valuable indicator of a possible trinucleotide repeat expansion, but needs to be assessed critically.

Anticipation in myotonic dystrophy was first proposed by Fleischer in 1918,[45] on the basis of thorough genealogic and clinical studies in which he not only was able to link families through apparently unaffected individuals, but also to show that there appeared to be progression of the disease in successive generations in terms of age at onset and severity. Although the validity of this anticipation was accepted over a considerable period, the need for a biologic mechanism was questioned by Penrose in 1948,[84] who compared a series of different genetic disorders and showed varying degrees of anticipation in most, myotonic dystrophy being the most extreme example.

Penrose pointed out that a combination of ascertainment biases and variability could give the picture of apparent anticipation, and that most examples were merely the result of these biases (almost certainly a correct conclusion). For myotonic dystrophy, he suggested that an allelic modifying gene was an additional factor, together with its inherent variability. This led to the assumption that no particularly unusual biologic mechanism need be sought for anticipation in myotonic dystrophy and the subject was neglected for the next 40 years. By this time, it had become clear that the ascertainment biases were inadequate to explain the extreme anticipation seen in myotonic dystrophy;[85,86] the severe congenital form of myotonic dystrophy had been recognized and shown to be maternally transmitted and parallels had been drawn with other disorders such as fragile X mental retardation. Thus the discovery of an unstable trinucleotide repeat expansion as the basis

for both fragile X syndrome and myotonic dystrophy provided an immediate explanation for anticipation in these disorders.

The details of anticipation in relation to such factors as size of the expansion and sex of the transmitting parent are considered in the following sections, but the way in which anticipation can now be seen at the molecular as well as the clinical level is illustrated in Figs. 217-5 and 217-6, which both relate to the same family; Fig. 217-7 shows the process in a series of parent-child pairs. It can also be asked: how many generations are required for anticipation to proceed to genetic lethality in a kindred? De Die-Smulders et al.[87] examined this in a large Dutch kindred in which myotonic dystrophy had originally been described 40 years previously, and found that anticipation had resulted in almost complete extinction of the gene within five generations, although it had proceeded at a

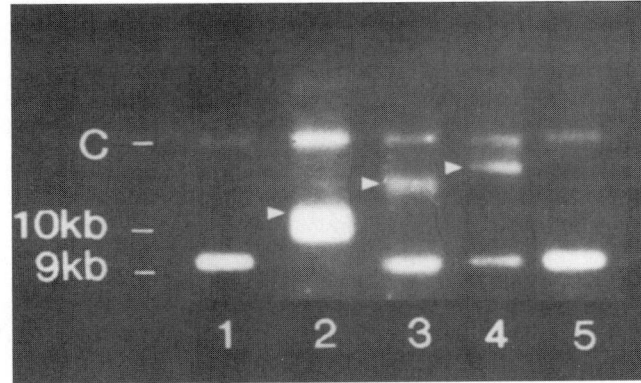

**Fig. 217-6** Anticipation and unstable DNA in myotonic dystrophy. DNA samples from the same three-generation family shown in Fig. 217-5 with myotonic dystrophy showing minimal DNA expansion in the mildly affected grandfather, lane 2 (CO.5 kb expansion), moderate expansion in the affected mother with adult onset, lane 3 (C2.5 kb), and large expansion in the congenitally affected son, lane 4 (C4 kb). Lanes 1 and 5 are from normal individuals. (*From Harley et al.*[64] *Used by permission.*)

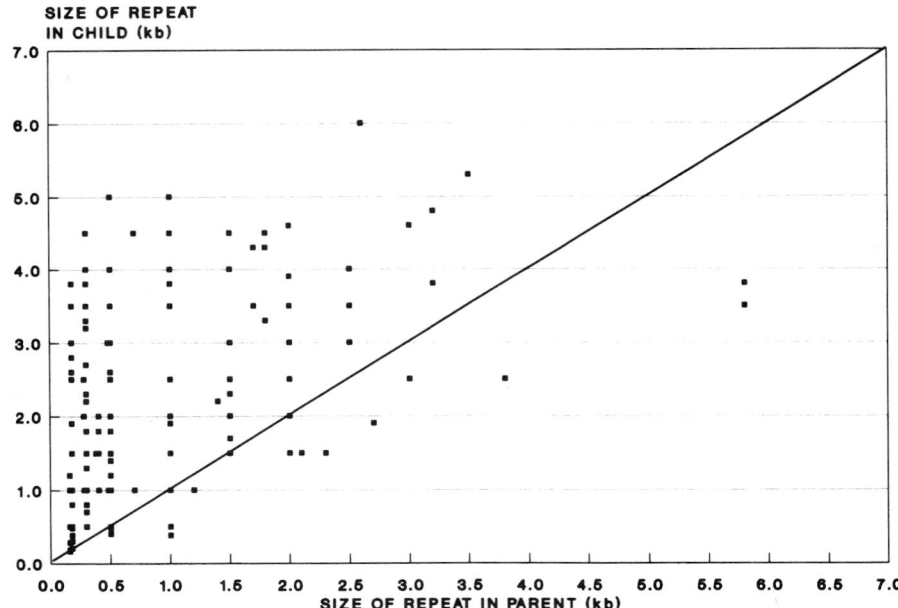

SIZE OF REPEAT
IN CHILD (kb)

SIZE OF REPEAT IN PARENT (kb)

**Fig. 217-7** Size of the CTG repeat in affected parent and offspring pairs, showing anticipation at the molecular level, with most extensions larger in the offspring than in the parent.

different rate in different branches. Infertility of male patients and mental retardation associated with congenital myotonic dystrophy were the main reasons. Interestingly, and supporting other studies, no carriers of small repeat expansions were found in the fourth and fifth generations. While this is the usual pattern seen in families, it is not invariable, as evidenced by an American kindred[88] in which relative stability was observed over three generations, with repeat numbers of 60 to 90 and no significant symptoms in most individuals.

### Genotype and Phenotype

The initial studies identifying the unstable CTG repeat in myotonic dystrophy immediately identified its variable nature within families, the relationship to anticipation, and an approximate association between degree of severity and size of the expanded sequence. Since then numerous further studies have explored the extent to which genotype and phenotype are correlated, within terms of general severity of disease and age at onset, and also in relation to specific systems clinically involved.

The main clinical categories used have been congenital myotonic dystrophy; childhood onset disease (these two frequently combined); classical adult onset of neurologic disease; and minimal disease (often cataract only) in later life. Some studies have used severity of muscle disease only. Clearly, these groupings are strongly age related, and age at onset has itself been used as an indicator, which has the advantage of being quantifiable even if approximate.

The initial study of Harley et al.[89] showed clear, though overlapping differences in expansion size for the different groups studied (Fig. 217-8). All congenital cases showed expansions of 2500 base pairs or greater, while in the minimally affected group all expansions were 250 base pairs or less, giving a complete separation of these two extreme groups. Cases with typical adult disease showed a wide variation of expansion size, overlapping with the other groups. Tsilfidis et al.[90] also showed that congenital cases were associated with the largest expansions, as did Novelli et al.,[91] Eguchi et al.[92] (in a Japanese population), and Passos-Bueno et al.[93] (in Brazilian families). For age at onset, Harley et al.[94,95] found a strong inverse correlation with expansion size (Fig. 217-9), no sex difference being found.

Gennarelli et al.[96] have attempted to express these findings in a form that expresses a probability that a given number of CTG

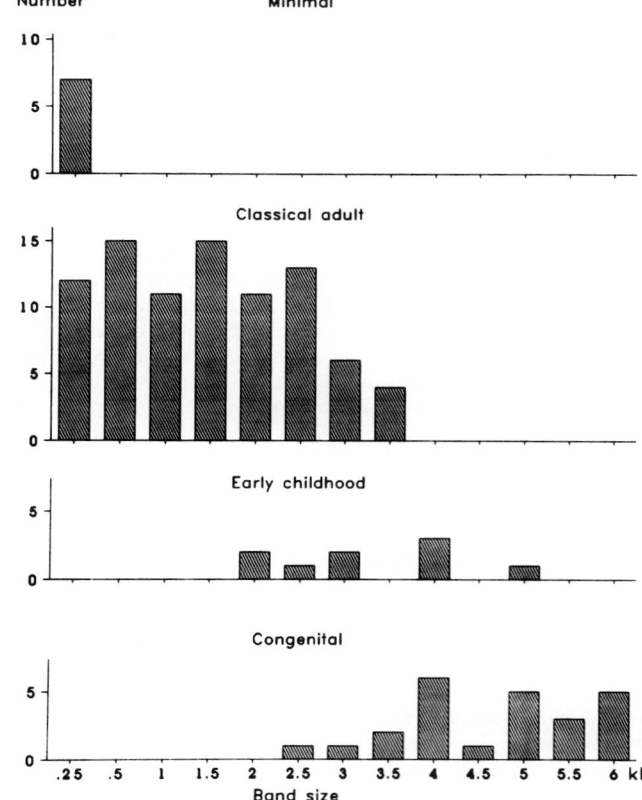

**Fig. 217-8** Size of DNA expansion in myotonic dystrophy in relation to severity of disorder. *Minimal*: Neuromuscular abnormalities absent or insignificant; cataract is the principal feature. *Classical adult*: Progressive muscle wasting with myotonia; onset in adult life. *Early childhood*: Developmental delay and other serious childhood symptoms; onset not congenital. *Congenital*: Onset of myotonic dystrophy at or before birth. DNA expansion is clearly related to these categories of severity; while individual categories show overlap, there is a distinct separation between the minimal group and those with severe childhood disease. (*From Harley et al.[89] Used by permission.*)

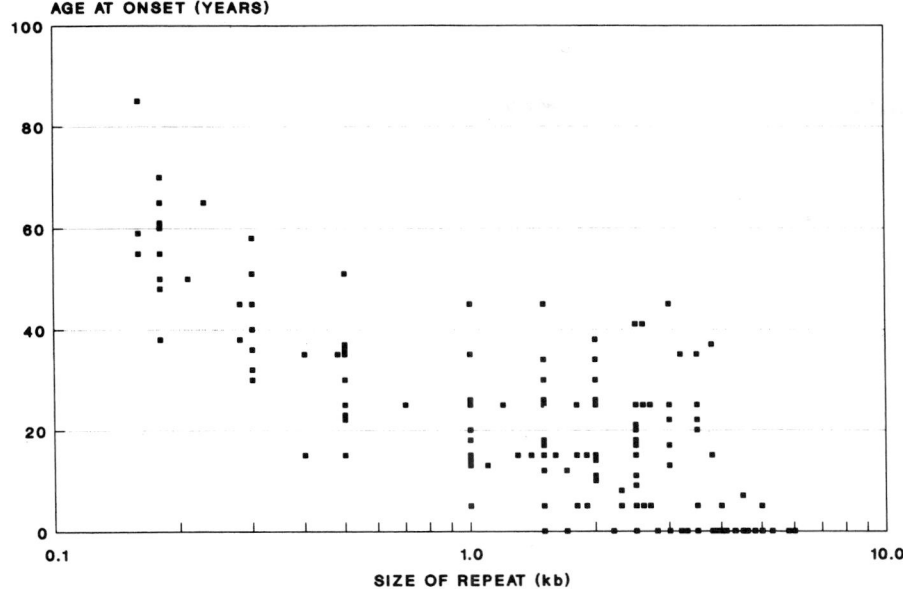

AGE AT ONSET (YEARS)

SIZE OF REPEAT (kb)

**Fig. 217-9** The relationship of the age of onset of myotonic dystrophy to the size of the CTG repeat sequence. (*From Harley et al.*[89])

repeats will result in any of three categories of severity. While their categories are mainly determined by severity of muscle disease, they approximate to the three more widely used groups of minimal, classical onset neuromuscular, and severe childhood/congenital disease, and confirm the earlier conclusions that a CTG repeat of 100 or less will almost always be associated with minimal disease, while one of 1500 or more will have a very high chance of falling into the severe category. The final section of the chapter discusses those findings useful for genetic counseling.

In addition to these phenotype-genotype studies, a number of investigators have examined the relationship to specific areas of clinical abnormality in myotonic dystrophy, particularly the nonmuscular aspects. These include central nervous system involvement, especially IQ,[97] cardiac defects,[98] and a variety of endocrine[99] and metabolic abnormalities.[100-102] Almost all have found correlations comparable to the more general studies and the main conclusion to be reached is that no single system appears to be particularly closely related to repeat number, nor to be independent of it. This finding is of relevance in terms of the possible effects of other neighboring genes in the disease pathology (see below), because it suggests that no clinical feature can be separated out that might solely result from abnormality in another gene, as is often seen in microdeletion syndromes.

While all these studies agree in showing that the myotonic dystrophy phenotype is indeed strongly correlated with genotype as defined by repeat length, they equally show that other factors must also play an important part. The practical limitations in applying the statistical correlation to prognosis in individuals have already been noted and are discussed later in relation to genetic counseling. Twin data suggest that some of the factors are developmental, while Hamshere et al.[103] suggested that the phenotype correlation with repeat number may not apply across all ranges and may relate to a threshold of repeat number influencing gene function. Clinically discordant sibs with the same repeat number have been reported,[104] while Ashizawa et al.'s[105] finding that anticipation might occur clinically even though the repeat number decreased, again indicates other important influences on phenotype. Sampling limitations and the use of different methods for determining repeat length are additional factors that need to be considered. In particular there remain doubts as to whether repeat length alone can explain the unusual clinical features and maternal transmission of congenital myotonic dystrophy.

So far these other possible factors have not been specifically identified, although an influence of the repeat number of the normal allele has been ruled out.[106] Likely future candidates might be genes interacting with *MDPK*, the immediately adjacent gene loci, and other important genes involved in muscle and central nervous system development and repair.

## Genetic Instability of the CTG Repeat: Intergenerational Aspects

The initial studies of the expanded CTG repeat in myotonic dystrophy all showed striking variation in repeat number between different individuals, even in the same family, raising immediate questions not only about the relationship with disease phenotype, but concerning the previously puzzling phenomenon of anticipation, already discussed, and the parental origin effects, especially in relation to the maternal transmission of congenital myotonic dystrophy. These aspects are examined in turn.

**Parent of Origin Effects.** Prior to discovery of the mutation, parent of origin effects in the transmission of myotonic dystrophy were well established, as already noted. In particular, the congenital form of the disorder was known almost always to be transmitted maternally, while there was a suspicion of a predominant male excess of asymptomatic or minimally affected individuals in the earliest known generation of families. A series of studies has now examined these aspects in detail and the following conclusions seem clear.

1. Congenital myotonic dystrophy, associated with the largest expansions, is indeed transmitted maternally in the overwhelming majority of cases,[23,24] but may occasionally be transmitted paternally. Ten such cases have been reported;[107-110] the clinical features of the offspring are comparable to other congenital onset patients, but the affected father does not show a tendency to particularly severe disease or early onset (in contrast to the situation for juvenile Huntington disease).

2. The majority of parent-child transmissions where the repeat size decreases are male,[105] as are the occasional instances where reversion of the expansion to the normal range has occurred.[111,112] This suggests some mechanism that limits continued expansion of the repeat in male transmission of the repeat in male transmission that is not operating in female transmission. Because studies of sperm from male patients

show a wide range of expansion sizes, there may be some selective disadvantage in fertilization by such sperm.

3. For smaller-sized repeats (less than 100 kb) expansion is greater for male transmissions than for female.[113,114]

4. Over the entire range of repeat lengths, there is no clear sex difference in expansion between the generations. Some studies have suggested a greater tendency to expansion in female transmission,[115,116] while Brunner et al.[113] found greater expansion in male transmissions overall. Harley et al.[95] found no significant sex difference when the increase was expressed as a proportion of parental repeat size. It is likely that the variable results reflect interaction of the opposite parental effects involving small and large expansions.

The predominantly male origin of the disorder in the earlier generations of families has also been confirmed in a series of studies. Harley et al. showed a significant excess of male grandparents of congenital cases, as did Lopez de Munain et al.,[117] while Brunner et al.[113] found that genealogic links between families studied predominantly involved males. Their study also showed an excess of male transmission in the initial symptomatic generation. When combined with the results of previous studies, notably those from the Quebec kindred, this male excess was significant, whereas for previous asymptomatic transmissions there was no significant sex difference.

At first sight, the parent of origin effects may appear confusing and in contrast to what is seen in other trinucleotide disorders, in particular Huntington disease, where severe juvenile cases are mainly paternally transmitted.[118] In fact, when the size-dependent nature of the parents affects is taken into consideration, any apparent conflict resolves,[119] because the size range of repeats in severe cases of the polyglutamine (CAG) repeat disorders is comparable to those of minimally affected myotonic dystrophy patients. Thus, the pattern in this expansion range for all the disorders seems to be of greater instability in male transmissions, while the unique feature of myotonic dystrophy is the occurrence and viability of individuals with exceptionally large expansions, where the mainly female transmission appears to result from some selective disadvantage of sperm carrying large expansions, probably together with increasing male infertility in this range.

**Expansion Size and Genetic Instability.** Along with the parental origin the main other factor identified as influencing instability in transmission between generations is the size of the expansion itself. A series of studies has shown that not only does the size of the expansion in the offspring correlate with that of the parent, but that it is related also to the increase between the generations, with an accelerating effect.[95,113–115,120,121] Clearly, this is an important factor underlying the clinical observation of anticipation and it is clear that this trend is already established for the range of expansion size giving clinical manifestations. The variation in rate of progression in different kindreds or branches of a kindred has already been mentioned.[110,111] What is less clear is the lower limit of significant instability—a point of practical importance in assessing risks for offspring when an individual with a borderline expansion is detected incidentally or as part of an extended family.

## Genetic Instability: Developmental and Somatic Aspects

Studies on the intergenerational variation of the myotonic dystrophy gene mutation have principally been based on comparison of the CTG expansion in blood lymphocytes of affected adults. Such studies are considerably removed from the germ line cells that are the basis for any intergenerational effects, while they give no indication as to the developmental timing of the instability that is seen. In addition, lymphocytes are not necessarily representative of other body tissues, and are certainly not the cells most closely related to the clinical abnormalities of the disorder.

Fortunately, there is now evidence available on all these aspects of genetic instability that gives us a clearer picture of the dynamics of the processes involved.

**Studies on Sperm.** While the ovum remains largely inaccessible to molecular studies, analysis of sperm allows direct analysis of the male germ line, although the azoospermia seen in many patients has been a limiting factor. Jansen et al.[122] compared sperm and blood in 24 male myotonic dystrophy patients and found that in four of nine cases, the CTG expansion was less in sperm than in blood. They also found that when the repeat length in the blood of offspring was compared to that of paternal sperm, there was an increase in six of eight cases, suggesting a significant postmeiotic contribution to the instability in the offspring. Monckton et al.[123] developed a technique for small-pool PCR analysis of sperm and other cells that enabled more detailed study and gave rather different results. In two of three males studied, there was a striking increase in the range of repeat sizes seen in sperm, including some extending down to the high normal repeat size range, even though the mean repeat size was greater in sperm than in blood. A third patient with a small expansion in blood (76 repeats) showed a greatly increased expansion in sperm (254 repeats) with none in the normal range.

While these data are still relatively few, they fit well with the clinical and overall genetic evidence on male intergenerational transmission, in particular with the greater tendency of the repeat to expand in transmission from mildly affected males with small repeats, and also with the observation that reduction in repeat size is a feature of male transmission. It is of interest whether data can be obtained from ova of affected females that will enable comparison.

**Instability and Development.** Opportunities for studying instability of the myotonic dystrophy repeat during early embryonic development are limited, but the advent of preimplantation diagnosis has shown that expansions can be detected at the blastomere stage,[124] as discussed later under "Molecular Diagnostics." However, because abnormal embryos are not implanted during IVF, this does not provide information on how the expansion might alter subsequently.

Early prenatal diagnosis using chorion villus sampling at around 10-week gestation is now an established procedure and there are several reports on the identification of fetuses with expansion of the myotonic dystrophy repeat,[125–127] including some with the very large repeats likely to have resulted in congenital myotonic dystrophy. One relevant observation on such samples is that they show little evidence of somatic variation, despite the very large number of repeats, Southern blotting showing a clear-cut band in contrast to the "smear" commonly seen in samples taken from such patients in later life.

A more detailed study of the repeat in early development was done by Worhle et al.,[126] who analyzed a range of tissues from a 13- and a 16-week-old affected fetus, both with comparable size of expansions of 4 to 6 kb. The first showed no variation between different fetal tissues, whereas in the second, there was considerable variation of repeat size. Martorell et al.[128] have taken this approach further, analyzing 7 cases of their own along with 10 previously reported cases at various stages of development from 10 weeks to the neonatal period. They confirmed that no tissue variability was seen before 13 weeks gestation, but that this was established by 16 weeks, showing no clear correlation with size of repeat.

An entirely different approach to the topic of developmental instability of the repeat sequence has come from the study of identical twins.[129–131] Five such pairs were studied by molecular techniques; clinical features were extremely similar between the twins in all cases, supporting earlier reports from before isolation of the gene. In three pairs, the expansion of the repeat sequence also appeared to be identical, but in two pairs there were considerable differences in repeat size in blood, suggesting developmental instability.

It is relevant to compare the findings on developmental instability with the situation for fragile X mental retardation, where comparably large repeat expansions are also seen. Here, no tissue differences were found during fetal development[132] and the repeat size in identical twins was the same.[133] A further difference has been in finding that affected fragile X males with a full expansion show mainly premutation ranges of repeat size in gonadal tissue.[134] This suggests that for fragile X, in contrast with myotonic dystrophy, instability is mainly prezygotic.

**Somatic Instability in Later Life.** This has been extensively studied, the main approaches being the analysis of a wide range of tissues at autopsy, the detailed comparison of muscle with blood, and the dynamics of cultured cells.

The autopsy studies on adults[122,136] have shown a wide variation in repeat numbers between tissues, this occurring to a greater degree than that already mentioned in relation to the fetal and neonatal cases. Most tissues show a greater degree of repeat expansion than seen in blood, but a consistent pattern has not emerged. One study[137] reported a smaller expansion in cerebellum than in other parts of brain and other tissues, a finding that has also been noted for Huntington disease.[138]

The repeat expansion in muscle has received particular attention, partly because of availability of biopsy material, partly because of its relevance to the disease process. It might have been thought likely that the degree of expansion in muscle would show closer correlation with severity of muscle disease than does the expansion in lymphocytes, but this has not proved to be the case. A series of studies[139–142] showed that muscle expansions are larger than in blood from the same patient, that there is considerable variation between sites, and that the correlation with severity is poorer than using blood.

The time course of genetic instability in later life was approached by studying samples (usually blood) taken at intervals. Martorell et al.[143] showed that the repeat number increased over a 5-year interval for patients with a wide range of repeat numbers, although this increase was not seen in individuals who were asymptomatic when the first sample was taken.

It is now becoming possible to study the detailed cell dynamics of genetic instability, using small-pool and single-cell PCR techniques,[123,144] and by studying cultured cells.[126,144] Monckton et al.[123] showed that a "smear" of repeat lengths seen in the blood of myotonic dystrophy patients could be resolved into a series of separate cell lines, each showing expansion from a specific starting point. There was no evidence of reduction in repeat length, agreeing with the earlier observation of a sharp lower size border of bands observed on Southern blotting and in contrast with the findings on sperm, studied by the same techniques and already mentioned. Worhle et al.[126] analyzed cultured cells from fetal tissue and showed a progressive increase in repeat length with cell proliferation following a sigmoid time course. Cell culture studies are also proving of particular importance in elucidating the mechanisms of genetic instability.

## Other Genetic Aspects

While our understanding of the genetics of myotonic dystrophy has been radically changed by the recognition of genetic instability as the underlying basis for mutation, molecular studies have also shed light on a range of other aspects that need brief noting.

**Homozygosity.** The recognition that homozygotes for Huntington disease exist and that they show no greater severity than those heterozygous for the mutation[145] has given relevance to assessing the situation for comparable homozygotes in myotonic dystrophy. Surprisingly, the first two detected by molecular studies were asymptomatic, carrying two copies of small expansions.[146] Six cases have now been reported,[147–149] only one of which appears to be more severely affected than would be expected from expansion

size.[147] Because this case resulted from an incestuous mating, other loci may have been responsible for part of the phenotype and the overall conclusion so far is that, as for Huntington disease, homozygosity does not affect the clinical phenotype. This is extremely relevant to the mechanism of gene action and would suggest that simple haploinsufficiency is not an adequate explanation for causation of the disease.

**Genetic Heterogeneity.** The involvement of more than one locus was never likely except as an extremely rare event because linkage studies over several decades showed no evidence of families clearly unlinked to the locus established on chromosome 19. This was confirmed when the unstable repeat was identified and found to be responsible for the great majority of cases. However, when the very small number of individuals not showing such a repeat expansion was studied closely, and diagnostic and technical errors discounted, it became clear that a small group of patients showed a clinical picture that was distinguishable from, although similar to, myotonic dystrophy. This disorder, now known as proximal myotonic myopathy (PROMM), was discussed earlier and may prove of considerable importance in relation to myotonic dystrophy once we know more about its molecular basis.

After PROMM families have been removed, there still remains a handful of patients whose phenotype is indistinguishable from myotonic dystrophy but who show no repeat expansion. None of these patients has so far shown any other defect in the myotonic dystrophy protein kinase or neighboring genes, but one large family[20] was recently shown to map to chromosome 3q, representing the first separate myotonic dystrophy locus. Careful clinical documentation[150] shows the classical muscle and systemic features of myotonic dystrophy, but no clear evidence of anticipation; there is no evidence so far that a trinucleotide repeat expansion is involved. What the nature of the specific gene and protein is and the extent to which this locus is involved in PROMM families are of great interest. Rare families such as this could provide the key to the specific steps in pathogenesis of myotonic dystrophy.

**Fertility.** The immense range of severity and age of onset in myotonic dystrophy makes this an extremely difficult area to study accurately. Reproduction of survivors with congenital onset is rare and many congenital cases are fatal in the neonatal period, making this form genetically lethal. At the other extreme, many patients have minimal disease with onset late in life after reproduction is complete, and such individuals often do not come to medical attention. Asymptomatic individuals now being detected who carry the mutation further complicate the situation. It can be imagined that results of studies may well depend on the different proportions of these groups that are represented in the series.

Most of the older studies, summarized by Harper,[5] showed a decreased fertility in both sexes, with an overall relative fertility two-thirds of normal. Male fertility was reduced in most series more than female, but this was largely due to a high proportion of males failing to marry. The large Quebec isolate has been the subject of particular study and offers a unique opportunity of recording fertility of earlier generations because the genealogy is completely known for the preceding 10 generations.[151] An initial study by Veillette et al.,[152] based mainly on such marriages, showed reduced fertility comparable with previous series, but when older historical periods were analyzed, no difference in fertility was found from controls in each time period.[153] It is likely that the majority of individuals included in this second study would have would have been symptomless carriers of the mutation, reinforcing the view that fertility is only likely to be impaired in those individuals with clinically significant disease.

A further factor relevant to fertility is the increased frequency of spontaneous early pregnancy loss in affected women,[154,155] something distinct from perinatal deaths due to congenital myotonic dystrophy. However, such early losses are frequently replaced and there is no evidence that they preferentially involve pregnancies carrying the myotonic dystrophy mutation.

It can be seen that analysis of fertility in myotonic dystrophy is complex and difficult to interpret; it is not only of practical relevance, however, but of theoretical importance when considering how the mutation is maintained in the face of progressive and ultimately lethal instability, a topic that forms part of the population genetic studies on the disorder, which now require discussion.

## POPULATION AND EVOLUTIONARY GENETICS

The genetics of myotonic dystrophy and of its underlying mutation have so far been considered mainly in terms of individual patients or families, but population-based studies are now providing interesting and important data that are relevant to the disease and its origins, as well as to broader questions regarding human evolution. Three related aspects of this topic are considered in turn: the diverse prevalence and its geographical variation; how the underlying repeat evolves from the normal range to clinically significant expansion; and how normal variation at the myotonic dystrophy locus throws light on human evolution.

### Prevalence of Myotonic Dystrophy

Studies have been carried out on the prevalence of myotonic dystrophy in a wide range of populations[156] and are summarized in Table 217-9. At first view, their range seems remarkably wide, but their interpretation requires considerable caution because a number of factors may influence the apparent prevalence apart from the true frequency of the disease. These include the thoroughness of the study, whether it extended to previously undiagnosed relatives, whether ascertainment was confined to neuromuscular patients, and whether the symptomless gene carriers recognized by molecular testing were included. Even when the biases are allowed for, the overall population structure may have important effects — random factors may be important in small island populations (e.g., Mallorca),[157] while rapid population expansion and founder effect is likely to have been relevant in such populations as South African Afrikaners,[158] northern Sweden,[159] and, most spectacularly, in the Saguenay-Lac St. Jean population of northern Quebec.[151] The virtual absence of the disorder in sub-Saharan African populations was originally attributed to poor ascertainment, but is now recognized to be perhaps the most significant feature of all in the worldwide variation in prevalence,[160] as noted later.

If we consider only non-African populations and discount those where the high prevalence is likely to reflect founder effect, as well as earlier studies where ascertainment was clearly incomplete, then it seems quite possible that the true prevalence does not vary greatly throughout Caucasian and Asiatic populations, apart from local concentrations due to relatively recent founder effect. Although Ashizawa et al.[160] suggested a difference between north and south Asia, apparent differences of equal magnitude are seen within Europe[161,162] and are likely to reflect the methods of study as much as the actual prevalence. This suggests a range of prevalence between 5 and 25 per 100,000, although experience with other disorders, notably Huntington disease, would indicate that the upper estimate might well be closest to the true situation because many affected individuals are overlooked in studies that are confined to primary cases.

### Origins of the Myotonic Dystrophy Mutation

This has proved a remarkably interesting and complex situation, which is not as yet fully resolved. Because the picture becomes progressively less clear the further back the process is traced, it seems sensible to work backwards in a step-by-step manner, to avoid confusion.

1. The origins of mutations causing significant disease: The discussion on anticipation and genetic instability has shown how patients with significant disease can be traced back to individuals (predominantly male) carrying small expansions (50 to 100 repeats) who have minimal disease (often cataract alone) or who may be unaffected. Clearly, such repeat expansions are already unstable, and are especially likely to expand in offspring of males.
2. Prior to this, it seems likely that small expansions can be transmitted through numerous generations by both sexes without evidence of serious instability or of clinical disease. The Saguenay kindred, where the complete genealogy has been documented, provides a striking example of this process, with a common ancestor from over 300 years ago in France and with evidence of myotonic dystrophy only appearing in numerous

**Table 217-9 Prevalence Studies in Myotonic Dystrophy**

| Country | Region | | Prevalence (per 100,000) | Cases | Total Population | Source & Data |
|---|---|---|---|---|---|---|
| European | | | | | | |
| UK | N Ireland | | 2.4 | 33 | $1.37 \times 10^6$ | Lynas[263] |
| | Wales | (South) | 7.1 | | $9.4 \times 10^3$ | MacMillan et al.[264] |
| Spain | Mallorca | | 11.0 | 60 | $5.5 \times 10^5$ | Burcet et al.[157] |
| | Guipuzcoa | Basque | 26.5 | 183 | $6.9 \times 10^5$ | Lopez de Munain et al.[162] |
| Italy | Turin | | 2.1 | 24 | $1.16 \times 10^6$ | Pinessi et al.[265] |
| | Venice | | 2.68 | | $4.1 \times 10^6$ | Mostacciulo et al.[161] |
| Germany | West | | 5.5 | | $54.6 \times 10^6$ | Grimm[266] |
| Sweden | Norbottens | | 36.5 | 95 | $2.6 \times 10^5$ | Rolander and Floderus[159] |
| Switzerland | | | 4.9 | 229 | $4.6 \times 10^6$ | Klein[48] |
| Croatia | Istria | | 18.1 | 33 | | Medica et al.[267] |
| **European Origin** | | | | | | |
| USA | Rochester | | 3.3 | 1 | $3 \times 10^4$ | Kurland[268] |
| Canada | (Saguenay) | | 189 | | $3 \times 10^5$ | Mathieu et al.[151] |
| South Africa | Transvaal Afrikaans | | 14.3 | | | Lotz and Van der Meyden[158] |
| **Non-European** | | | | | | |
| Japan | (San-In) | | 2.7 | | $1.4 \times 10^6$ | Takeshita et al.[269] |

descendant branches 10 to 12 generations later.[151] While it is possible that myotonic dystrophy might have occurred in earlier generations, there is no evidence for this, and the normal fertility of these gene carriers[153] suggests that they were clinically unaffected. That the prevalence in the population could increase to the remarkable level of almost 200 per 100,000 reflects in part the rapid expansion of this founder population, as well as that most of those transmitting the mutation in earlier generations were likely to have been healthy.

3. Once we go back beyond the era of historical records, there is strong evidence of a common origin for the myotonic dystrophy mutation extending back over the preceding millennia. This has come not so much from the mutation itself as from the conserved structure of the surrounding region of the chromosome. Even before this gene was isolated there was strong evidence of linkage disequilibrium, with a haplotype of closely linked genetic markers associated with the disease in a wide range of European, Israeli, and Japanese populations,[59,165,166] suggesting one predominant mutation. The recognition that the Alu insertion-deletion polymorphism immediately adjacent to the expanded repeat sequence showed a constant association of the 1-kb insertion (detected as a 10-kb fragment) with the disease[69,163,164] strengthened this conclusion; this finding in almost all populations worldwide provided strong evidence that a single initial event was responsible for the disorder. The alternative suggestion that this haplotype might be predisposed to recurrent mutational events has been made unlikely by the finding that the conserved haplotype extends to other markers both within the gene and outside the unstable region.[59,165]

Perhaps the strongest evidence of all for a common origin of myotonic dystrophy comes from the single and notable exception. The initial absence of the disorder in sub-Saharan Africa[166] has been noted, but a single Nigerian family, documented a considerable time ago,[167] has been restudied and found to show the typical repeat expansion, but on an entirely different haplotype background,[168] suggesting that its origin has been separate, while all other cases of myotonic dystrophy show a common origin, with the initiating event predating the divergence of Caucasian and Asian ethnic groups.

What this "event" was remains unclear. Although a gradual increase from the upper normal range into a repeat number giving instability seems likely to have happened over the succeeding millennia, it is uncertain whether the initial step was a discreet "jump" in repeat number or something entirely different that set the particular lineage along a path that would eventually lead to disease-causing instability. Evidence suggesting a "jump" comes from the study of normal variation outlined below.

## Polymorphic Variation of the Myotonic Dystrophy Repeat

All populations show marked variation in repeat length at this locus, with a basic number of 5 repeats being the commonest allele, and a trimodal distribution that includes a group of mendelian size alleles (11 to 13 repeats) and a smaller group of larger size alleles (19 to 30 repeats). Differences in the distribution between European and Japanese populations were noted at an early stage,[169] and a striking reduction in the number of larger size alleles was found in African populations.[170,171] This, along with the lack of myotonic dystrophy in sub-Saharan Africa, supports the view that the origin of the disease has been related to the presence of such normal larger alleles. Whether prevalence differences in non-African populations can be related directly to their distribution of allele sizes is less certain, though it could account for such major differences as are seen between Ashkenazi and Yemenite Jews in Israel.[172,173]

When the range of repeat numbers is examined in relation to the presence of or absence of the Alu insertion and to a wider haplotype of markers, it is found that in Caucasians and Asians, this is present in association with the 5-repeat allele and also with

the large size (19 to 30) group, but not with the immediate (11 to 13) group.[174] This supports the view that the initiating event underlying myotonic dystrophy was a "jump" involving a 5-kb allele associated with the insertion, giving rise to the group of larger alleles, from which myotonic dystrophy might eventually arise.

African populations do not show the exclusive association of haplotype with classes of repeat number and also show greater haplotype diversity,[175,176] consistent with the general evidence from mitochondrial and nuclear DNA studies that modern non-African populations are derived from a single subset of Homo sapiens in Africa that subsequently radiated throughout other parts of the world. In relation to this "out of Africa" hypothesis of human evolution, the chromosome carrying the original mutation predisposing to myotonic dystrophy in non-Africans would have occurred in this group either shortly before or after it left Africa around 100,000 years ago, and before it diverged to form present day non-African ethnic groups.[177]

## THE MOLECULAR AND CELL BIOLOGY OF MYOTONIC DYSTROPHY: GENOTYPE TO PHENOTYPE

### The Mutation and Animal Models

That point mutations in DM patients have not been detected in any of the genes at the locus indicates that the repeat expansion is the only mutation capable of giving rise to this phenotype. In the only reported *de novo* mutation causing DM in a family of sub-Saharan origin, a triplet repeat expansion was detected.[168] Although the very different haplotype on which the mutation arose obviates the predisposing haplotype hypothesis,[165] it confirms that the repeat expansion is required to generate the DM phenotype. These findings strongly implicate a more complex mechanism leading from genotype to phenotype than one might expect of a "classical" mendelian dominant trait. Indeed, it has led to considerable speculation that the mutation leads to a "field" effect at the locus, equivalent to a contiguous gene defect.[178]

Muller[180] postulated a number of mechanisms by which mutations could lead to genetic dominance, long before the realization that DNA was the genetic material. These mechanisms have been slightly modified and realized to be nonexclusive in the light of molecular data,[181] nevertheless, they remain pertinent to considering the underlying pathogenesis in DM. It seems most likely that the repeat expansion is acting at several levels within cells that are not mutually exclusive. The data support both hypomorphic (haploinsufficiency) effects on *SIX5*, and neomorphic (gain of function) effects through *DMPK* at the mRNA level. Attempts to model the disease by single-gene mutations have probably failed to recapitulate the DM phenotype in mouse because of these parallel mechanisms occurring concomitantly in patient tissues.

Hypomorphic *DMPK* mutants generated by knocking out its function in mice have produced only mild myopathic changes.[182,183] In addition, these changes are only really overt in homozygous knockout mice, indicating a recessive, rather than a dominant mode of inheritance. Moreover, none of the cardinal signs of DM were elicited in these models, which functionally were complete nulls for *DMPK* as evidenced by lack of *DMPK* mRNA and protein on northern and western blots. One hypermorphic (overexpressing) *DMPK* mutation has been reported.[183] This was generated by transgenesis to incorporate multiple copies of a human *DMPK* gene including a $(CTG)_{20}$ repeat into the mouse genome. Overexpression of *DMPK* was seen when the copy number exceeded 20 in these lines, with an associated cardiac muscle dysmorphology. The findings were of a largely disorganized myocardium, with bizarre whorling, hypertrophy, patches of degeneration with vesicular nuclei and focal fibrosis. However, cardiac function was apparently normal and no obvious parallels

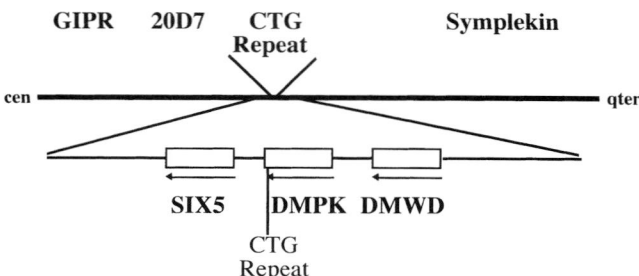

**Fig. 217-10 The location and orientation with respect to transcription of six known genes at the DM locus, based on data from reference 187 (Alwazzan et al). The position of the CTG repeat expansion in the 3'-UTR of DMPK is indicated. The database names of the genes as of April 1999 are used; prior to that time SIX5 was known as DMAHP and DMWD as N9 in mouse and 59 in human.**

with the conduction defects and fatty fibrosis seen in DM could be drawn. Neomorphic mutants, by gain of function at the transcript level have also been modeled. In these mice, ubiquitous expression of a transgene encoding a large CUG repeat in its mRNA has been generated.[184] These mice appear to model two key features of DM, the somatic heterogeneity of the repeat and the testicular atrophy. A further transgenic mouse model also recapitulates the somatic heterogeneity.[185] In this mouse, a cosmid was introduced, encompassing 40 kb of the human DM locus, inclusive of the entire 59, *DMPK*, and *SIX5* genes, and with a $(CTG)_{55}$.

All these findings from mouse models are entirely consistent with the requirement for a repeat expansion at the DM locus to generate a DM allele. To understand fully the complexity that this mutation is able to generate, we must first consider the genes present at the locus, their products, and their possible contributions to the phenotype.

### The Mutation May Affect Gene Expression at the Chromatin Level

While the repeat expansion mutation clearly explains the unusual genetic phenomena associated with the transmission of DM, the molecular mechanisms leading to specific pathophysiological changes remain obscure. The reason for this is almost certainly the nature of the location in the genome at which the mutation has arisen. The DM locus is transcriptionally very active, with a high density of transcription units, Fig. 217-10 (data from references 186 and 187). At the DM locus there is a gene approximately every 10 kb, which means the locus has a density of transcription units that is at least an order of magnitude greater than the genome average. Into this environment the repeat expansion introduces tracts of (CTG)n, which in mild cases may be only a 100 or so repeats, but in the most severe cases can be greater than 10 kb. The expanded repeat is predicted to lead to an altered chromatin structure affecting gene expression from the entire locus (reviewed in reference 179). Expanded CTG repeats are the strongest known nucleosome-positioning elements,[188] with efficiency of nucleosome formation increasing with array length. Evidence for altered chromatin structure comes from studies that detected altered DNase I hypersensitivity in muscle nuclei of three unrelated DM patients.[189] These studies showed increased resistance to DNase I and insensitivity to other nucleases of the expanded allele when compared to the wild-type allele in the same nuclei. All three patients had relatively large expansions. Stabilization of nucleosomes on the repeat array may account directly for the decrease in DNase I sensitivity or, alternatively, it may lead to the stable binding of other proteins to the region. The possibility of imprinting of the *DMPK* gene seems unlikely, given the lack of methylation differences of CpG islands comparing paternally and maternally derived alleles in congenital and adult onset cases.[190] However, methylation changes have been detected in some

congenital alleles to the 5' side of the CTG repeat with concomitant decreases in SP1 binding to the *SIX5* promoter.[191]

### Genes at the Locus and Their Possible Functions

**Myotonic Dystrophy Protein Kinase (*DMPK*).** *DMPK* is expressed in a wide range of tissues but is most predominantly found in heart, brain, muscle, and eye. The CTG repeat lies in the 3'-untranslated region (UTR) of the *DMPK* mRNA and therefore cannot directly alter the protein sequence. However, several possible mechanisms by which it affects *DMPK* gene expression have been suggested,[192] including: (a) alteration in steady state levels of *DMPK* expression; (b) interference with normal splicing patterns for *DMPK* RNA; (c) interruption of normal regulatory role of *DMPK* transcripts; and (d) change in efficiency of translation.

Conflicting data concerning the effect of the mutation on mRNA and protein levels have been published. Tissues from adult DM patients were analyzed by quantitative RT-PCR and radioimmunoassay, which showed decreased levels of mRNA and protein expression, implying that reduction in *DMPK* leads to the disease by disruption of signal transaction and amplification pathways.[193] Carango et al.[194] also reported reduction in both the synthesis and the processing of *DMPK* mRNA. However, Sabourin et al.[195] showed that *DMPK* steady state levels were markedly increased in congenital DM tissues and it was demonstrated that increases are due to elevated levels of transcripts derived from mutant *DMPK* alleles. These conflicting results may be due to differences in the tissues studied. Adult tissues were used by two groups,[193,194] whereas cells and tissues from severely affected neonates were used by the third.[195] Congenital cases are known to have different symptoms to adult onset patients; adults, for example, tend to be myotonic, whereas infants tend to be hypotonic. The control tissues also differed between the two groups, one using tissues from patients with neurologic diseases[193] and another using mRNAs from healthy adults and fetal tissues.[195] Different molecular techniques were used in the studies, adding to the difficulties in directly comparing the results.

More recently, the allele-specific expression of *DMPK* was investigated and shown not to be affected at the transcriptional level, but rather at the processing and maturation level.[196] The accumulation of transcripts from both normal and expanded alleles in patient muscle were compared with normal and myopathic controls.[197] Only a small decrease of *DMPK* RNA in the total RNA pool from muscle was found and this was not disease specific, as the myopathic controls showed a similar decrease. However, dramatic decreases of both mutant and normal *DMPK* poly (A)+ RNA were observed, and this was disease specific. The authors speculate that normal and expanded *DMPK* genes are transcribed in patient muscle, but RNA with an abnormal expansion has a dominant effect on RNA metabolism preventing the accumulation of poly(A)+ RNA. The intracellular localization of transcripts from the *DMPK* gene in fibroblasts and muscle biopsies from DM patients and normal controls was determined using a fluorochrome-conjugated probe which hybridized specifically to the CTG repeat expansion. No significant difference in the cytoplasmic location of the *DMPK* mRNA was observed.[198] The probe did, however, detect transcripts as bright foci in the nuclei of DM patient fibroblasts and muscle, but not in samples from normal controls. Using a probe that hybridized to the 5' end of the *DMPK* gene, and would therefore detect all *DMPK* sequences, as well as the expansion-specific probe, it was shown that focal accumulation of posttranscriptional RNA only occurs with transcripts from the affected allele. In the steady state, nuclear export from the affected allele does not appear to be significantly suppressed, as RNA containing the repeat is present in the cytoplasm at a level similar to that of normal RNA. However, posttranscriptional foci may inhibit other nuclear functions indirectly.

It is now believed that the earlier contradictory reports concerning the effect of the repeat expansion on *DMPK* expression were due to the use of different RNA extraction methods. Some methods remove only cytoplasmic RNA which results in a decrease in the number of *DMPK* transcripts recovered, whereas if both nuclear and cytoplasmic RNA are analyzed, an increase in the number of *DMPK* transcripts is detected, due to the their accumulation in the nuclei. More recent theories on the effect of the CTG repeat expansion at the RNA level, including the identification of CUG-binding proteins, are discussed later.

**Functional Analysis of *DMPK*.** Biochemical and histochemical studies have suggested that a 53-kDa *DMPK* product is localized at sites of cell-cell contacts in neuromuscular tissues, in particular at neuromuscular and myotendinous junctions of human and rodent skeletal muscles and intercalated disks in cardiac muscle. This indicates that *DMPK* probably plays a specialized role in intercellular communication in striated muscle. It is possible that defects in communication could lead to muscle atrophy, myotonia, and heart failure.[199] A similar-sized protein (54 kDa) that is recognized by *DMPK* antiserum has been characterized and shown to display a serine/threonine kinase activity in heart and tyrosine kinase activity in skeletal muscle.[200] Because the predicted molecular weight of *DMPK* is approximately 70 kDa, it is possible that this protein is a cross-reacting kinase species and unrelated to *DMPK*. It has been demonstrated that *DMPK* knockout mice still express this 54-kDa protein, which supports the theory that this protein is not *DMPK*.[183] A monoclonal antibody was used to identify a 64-kDa protein in type 1 skeletal muscle localized to the triadic region, and to identify a 79-kDa protein in brain.[201] Comparisons of proteolytic digests of the muscle protein and recombinant *DMPK* show similar mobilities, indicating that the 64-kDa protein is likely to be a bona fide isoform. In severely affected DM patients, redistribution of this isoform to the peripheral sarcoplasmic masses, consistent with previously reported altered localization and expression of transcripts has been seen.[195]

A panel of monoclonal antibodies has been generated in an attempt to determine the true size of the *DMPK* protein and its localization within tissues.[202] This study identified two isoforms of *DMPK* that have molecular weights of 72 and 80 kDa. The 72-kDa isoform, but not the 80-kDa isoform, was detected in all tissues tested. Previous studies have also detected doublets of approximately these molecular weights.[203,192] The presence of *DMPK* in the intercalated disks of cardiac muscle, but not in the neuromuscular junctions of skeletal muscle, was confirmed. A 55-kDa protein was detected in skeletal muscle by 2 of the 12 monoclonal antibodies, but it was not thought to be an alternatively spliced form of *DMPK* as it was not detected by antibodies raised against the coil domain. To date, no isoforms of *DMPK* lacking the coil domain have been predicted.[193,204,205]

*DMPK* is now established to be part of a distinct subfamily of protein kinases involved in cytoskeleton remodeling, with signaling via Rho. Many protein kinases interact with the GTPases Rho and cdc-42. Included in these is a subfamily of serine/threonine protein kinases that, within the catalytic cores of their kinase domains, show striking levels of similarity to *DMPK* at the amino acid sequence level. This subfamily includes myotonic dystrophy protein kinase-related Cdc-42-binding kinases (in rat MRCKs α and β[206]; in human *CDC42BPB*[207]); Genghis Khan (Gek[208]); Rho kinases[209]; and *LET502* from *C. elegans*.[210] These genes may have all evolved from a common ancestor, as they share unique three amino acid insert in their catalytic core region between subdomains VIII and IX.[207] All members of the subfamily appear to regulate morphologic changes in cells through regulating the reorganization of the actin-based cytoskeleton. This function of *DMPK* may explain independent tissue culture data obtained from transfection of myoblasts with expression constructs in which overexpression of *DMPK* inhibits terminal differentiation.[211,212] Although an independent study has reported reduced fusion only with a *DMPK* cDNA construct containing 46 repeats, a wild-type cDNA having no effect on fusion,[213] the 3'-UTR was invoked as being able to inhibit fusion in the absence

of expressed protein in one of the other studies.[211] This result may be due to effects on the neighboring gene (see below).

## Myotonic Dystrophy-Associated Homeodomain Protein (DMAHP/SIX5)

The presence of an extensive CpG island at the 3' end of *DMPK* indicated that a novel gene lay immediately downstream of the CTG repeat. This region was sequenced and murine and human sequences were found to share 86 percent identity at the putative amino acid level.[214] The CTG repeat was shown to be within a 3.5-kb CpG island. Sequence data indicated that the gene encoded a homeodomain protein and was therefore called DM locus-associated homeodomain protein (*DMAHP*). *DMAHP/SIX5* has now been identified as being one of a growing number of members of the *sine oculus*-related homeobox (SIX) subfamily of genes, so called because the founding member was the *Drosophila* eye development gene *sine oculus* (*so*). Therefore, when a murine cDNA *DMAHP* homologue was identified it was named *Six5*,[215] and this is now the official database assignment for this gene.

All members of the SIX subfamily share a region of a high-sequence homology that encodes a 60 amino acid homeodomain, and immediately upstream of the homeodomain a domain unique to the SIX subfamily, the SIX domain, which is approximately 116 amino acids. RT-PCR shows that *SIX5* is expressed in many tissues including skeletal muscle, fibroblasts, lymphocytes, heart, and brain in both normal adults and DM patients.[214] An enhancer element that controls the expression of SIX5 was identified within the DNase I hypersensitive site adjacent to the CTG repeat.[188,216] A two- to fourfold reduction in the steady state transcript levels of *SIX5* from the expanded allele compared to the normal allele of DM patient's was seen in fibroblasts and skeletal muscle cells. This implies that expansion of the CTG repeat does indeed alter local chromatin structure in such a way as to reduce expression of *SIX5*, which, in turn, is involved in the pathogenesis of DM.[216] A second group has also reported a reduction in the levels of *SIX5* mRNA synthesis from the DM allele in primary myoblast cultures and postmortem muscle, heart, and brain tissues from DM patients.[217] However, a contradictory report indicated that levels of *SIX5* expression were unchanged in cell lines from DM patients.[185] Gene expression patterns can differ between tissues and myoblast cultures and therefore gene expression data from cell lines may not be representative of what occurs in human tissue. This is partially due to the lack of innervation in cell lines. However, the dynamics of the CTG repeat are also altered in cultured lymphoblastoid cell lines from DM patients and this may affect the expression of genes that are altered by the repeat expansion.[218]

Two alternative transcripts of human *SIX5* were identified by RT-PCR.[214] One isoform contains exons A, B, and C, and the second isoform contains only exons A and C and has a different reading frame in exon C. The SIX box and homeobox are situated in exon A and are therefore encoded by both isoforms. To date, only the A-B-C isoform has been identified in mouse,[219] where it is expressed in a range of tissues during embryonic and fetal development. Provocatively, given the distribution of the main DM symptoms, the reporter gene used in this study was expressed in the developing lens, in a subset of cranial nerve nuclei (nerves V, VII, IX, and X), and in the developing forelimb, as well as in a range of other sites in parallel with pathology in patients. The expression of human *SIX5* in the eye has confirmed that it is expressed in adult lens, retina, cornea, ciliary bodies, and sclera.[220]

The A-B-C isoform is predicted to encode a protein of about 82 kDa and the A-C isoform a protein of about 36 kDa. *SIX5* lacks a consensus TATA box upstream of the open reading frame and consistent with this finding multiple transcription initiation sites have been identified in both the human and mouse genes.[216,221] The human transcriptional start sites cover a 50 to 70-bp region, are all within 400 bp of the coding region, and are in an equivalent position in the mouse gene. Transient transfection assays were used to identify regulatory regions in the mouse gene promoter region. Positive elements were identified between −434 and −344, −317 and −270, and −137 and −97, and negative elements were identified between −344 and −317 and −224 and −178. Gel retardation assays using nuclear extracts from P19 cells along with supershift assays using Sp1 and Sp3 antibodies confirmed that the three positive regulatory regions and one negative regulatory region contained Sp1/Sp3 binding elements. These Sp1/Sp3 binding sites are conserved between mouse and human, and the enhancer element in the human gene was also shown to be active in mouse.[221]

### Relationship of *SIX5* to Other Homeobox Proteins

The majority of transcription factors contain a DNA-binding domain and a transcriptional activation domain.[222] Homeobox genes encode a conserved domain of about 60 amino acids (the homeodomain) that can bind to DNA and a transcriptional activation/repression domain, thus acting as transcription factors. Recently, the *Drosophila* homeodomain protein bicoid that transcriptionally activates target genes by binding to DNA was shown to act as a repressor of translation by binding to the 3′-UTR of the cad mRNA, thus blocking the initiation of cad translation.[223] Therefore, homeodomain proteins can regulate gene expression by binding to both DNA and RNA.

*SIX1* and *SIX4* bind to the MEF3 motif in the minimal myogenin promoter.[224] This motif, TCAGGTT, is also present within the defined *SIX4* and *SIX5* binding sites in the promoter of the Na$^+$/K$^+$-ATPase subunit α-1 gene (reference 225 and K. Johnson, unpublished). It is also known that *SIX5* and *SIX4*, which are closely related to each other at the DNA and protein sequence level, bind to similar target sites.[225] In adult muscle, only a subset of fast-twitch fibers require MEF3 activation.[224,226] In DM, atrophy of slow-twitch, Type 1 fibers occurs, associated with down-regulation of genes associated with MEF3 regulatory elements in their promoters (cTnC is an example[222]). Decrease in Na$^+$/K$^+$-ATPase activity is well documented in DM muscle,[227,228] which could be due to affects mediated by *SIX5* at the promoter of the α-1 subunit gene. Haploinsufficiency of *SIX5* could also explain the expression of fetal and embryonic muscle proteins on DM adult fibers, such as the apamin receptor[229] and neural cell adhesion molecule (NCAM),[230] if its expression is required for establishment and maintenance of the adult pattern of gene expression.

### DMR-N9 (*59 gene*) and Others Within the Locus

*DMR-N9* is a murine gene that is located, with its 3′-end, 1.1-kb upstream of the DMPK gene.[204,231] This 7-kb gene contains 5 exons and codes for a 650-amino acid protein. Two regions within this gene show significant homology to WD repeats, which are highly conserved amino acid sequences found in a family of proteins involved in signal transduction of cell regulatory functions, although the actual function of *DMR-N9* is, as yet, unknown. *DMR-N9* is expressed strongly in brain and testis and could, therefore, be a candidate for involvement in mental and testicular symptoms in severe cases of DM. *59* the human homologue to *DMR-N9* has been identified and shown to be expressed in heart, brain, liver, kidney, spleen, and testis.[232] Analysis of levels of mRNA show no significant differences between DM tissues and controls, nor any differences in splicing of *59*.[186]

Other genes have been mapped within a few hundred kilobases surrounding the DM locus, including *Symplekin*, *20D7*, and *GIPR* (gastric inhibitory polypeptide receptor).[187] Symplekin is a tight-junction plaque protein that is expressed in the brain and heart as an mRNA species of about 4.5 kb. *GIPR* is involved in the stimulation and regulation of glucose-dependent insulin secretion[233] and maps 100 kb centromeric of *DMPK* (Fig. 217-10). *20D7* is transcribed in the same orientation as *Symplekin*, *59*, *DMPK*, and *SIX5*, and lies centromeric to the latter.[187] *20D7* encodes a predicted protein of 202 amino acids with no recognizable homologies or similarities within the databases, it

is expressed in testis in rat, and cDNAs were isolated form frontal cortex and substantial nigra libraries.[187]

### Effects of the Mutation at the RNA Level

Thus far, we have focused on the genes at the locus, their expression patterns, and their known or predicted functions. However, there is a growing body of evidence that part of the pathologic mechanism involves a dominant gain of function at the RNA level. This was first proposed by Eric Hoffman and colleagues[197] to explain why DMPK poly A$^+$ RNA is reduced in DM tissues yet essentially normal levels of transcripts are detected in total RNA.[196,197] This appears to be an effect on RNA processing and Timchenko and colleagues[234,235,242,244] have taken this mechanism further by proposing that the CUG repeat in the *DMPK* mRNA acts dominantly at the level of RNA processing by sequestering RNA-binding proteins. This model has now been further refined in light of the evidence that the expression of CUG-binding protein 1 (CUGBP1) is induced three- to fourfold in DM tissues.[234] Several CUG-binding proteins have been identified, including CUGBP1,[235] which is identical to a previously described human nuclear heterogeneous RNA-binding protein, hNab50. CUGBP1 appears to have specificity for RNA as it does not bind to single-stranded CTG repeats.[235,236] It contains three RNA-binding domains and is highly conserved in evolution.[237,235] In *Drosophila*, the orthologue of CUGBP1 acts in the nucleus to regulate RNA splicing,[238] but in vertebrates, CUGBP1 may act in both the nucleus and cytoplasm where it may regulate translation.[239,240] CUGBP1 has been shown to bind to pre-mRNAs that contain CUG repeats, including transcripts from the cardiac troponin T (cTnT) gene. Normal adult splicing of this pre-mRNA is altered by the binding of CUGBP1, with the inclusion of an alternative exon 5, usually not found in the adult isoform.[241] Splicing of cTnT in DM heart is abnormal when there is an increase in the amount of mRNA in which the alternative exon 5 is included. CUGBP1 RNA-binding activity is increased in DM nuclei.[235,242] Several other CUG-binding proteins have been identified, including two with molecular masses of 25 and 35 kDa, respectively from human brain[243] and an elav-type RNA-binding protein (ETR-3), which is abundant in the human heart.[244]

The complexity of the disease mechanism, potentially involving gain of function in the RNA through the CUG repeat and haploinsufficiency of *SIX5*, as well as other contributing factors, is compounded further by the heterogeneity of the repeat in somatic tissues. Adjacent cells may harbor different-sized repeats and hence provide different mechanistic contributions to their dysfunction. Even adjacent nuclei in syncytial muscle fibers could have different repeats and pathologic mechanisms. Preliminary data appear to indicate a lower repeat number threshold for nuclear retention of *DMPK* transcripts than for decrease in *DMAHP* expression using allele-specific RTPCR,[186] although this needs to be confirmed for DM tissues on more samples.

### Symptoms and Specific Gene Effects

The eye pathology is an obvious starting point for trying to assess which of the potential mechanisms give rise to particular symptoms in DM. Often, in the mildest DM cases, cataract appears to be the only obvious symptom. By analyzing the expression patterns of *DMPK* and *SIX5* in the adult human eye, it appears that the cataract is far more likely to be caused by haploinsufficiency of *SIX5* than through the RNA gain-of-function pathway. This is because *SIX5* is expressed in the adult lens, but, by a range of molecular methods, *DMPK* appears not to be so expressed,[220] although previous reports have suggested that *DMPK* is found in bovine and human lenses.[244] The reasons for this difference in observations may be due to the antibodies used or the methods of fixation of the tissues at the protein level. However, this cannot explain why there is apparently no *DMPK* mRNA in adult human lens by RT-PCR and *in situ* hybridization.[220] Two groups have independently knocked out *Six5* in the mouse with the result that hemizygous animals develop cataracts as early as 3 weeks. Thus for the first time a single gene change recapitulates one of the pathological consequences of the repeat expansion. It should be noted however that the animals do not develop any overt muscle pathology and the molecular basis of this and many other DM symptoms remains to be elucidated.[244a,244b]

## MOLECULAR DIAGNOSTICS

In addition to increasing our understanding of the genetic aspects of myotonic dystrophy, the identification of a specific mutation has had important applications in clinical practice, and provides a striking example of the power of what can be termed molecular diagnostics. Two broad areas of application are identifiable: first, that of prediction for relatives at risk, either confirming or excluding presence of the mutation; second, the use of molecular analysis as part of the primary diagnosis, usually in the absence of any clear family history of the disorder. Table 217-10 summarizes these main applications.

### Presymptomatic Detection

Prediction within families was already possible to some degree by using linked DNA markers before the mutation was identified, and extensive experience was obtained for both presymptomatic and prenatal diagnosis in this way.[246–248] However, the specificity and universal distribution of the expanded CTG repeat removed the need for studying multiple family members and rapidly replaced linkage analysis as the basis for testing.[140,249,250] For healthy relatives at risk for myotonic dystrophy, a normal molecular analysis essentially excludes the risk of developing or transmitting the disorder, although it is always wise to ensure that the mutation is indeed present in the closest affected relative, so as to exclude the possibility of misdiagnosis.

Molecular genetic services worldwide now use detection of the myotonic dystrophy mutation, an illustration not only of the power of the approach, but of the rapidity of transfer of techniques from research to service. It should be added that the research workers' willingness to allow free use of their discoveries has also helped the spread of its application.

A particularly valuable use of molecular analysis is for those relatives where equivocal or atypical clinical features have been detected on clinical assessment or by electrophysiological or ophthalmologic studies.[249] The extreme variability of the disorder makes this situation relatively frequent and some such individuals may have been told that they definitely carry a mutant allele on the basis of such information. Molecular analysis will resolve the situation, but needs to be handled carefully, especially in situations in which a person may have made important decisions over many years on the basis of believing that they carried the myotonic dystrophy gene and were likely to develop or transmit the disorder.[251]

Identification of the mutation in asymptomatic or minimally affected grandparents or other members of the older generation can be valuable in linking apparently unconnected families or in deciding which family line is at risk.[252] However, caution is again needed in such testing because these individuals will usually carry

**Table 217-10** Molecular Diagnostic Applications in Myotonic Dystrophy

---

Prediction within established family
  Presymptomatic detection in healthy relatives
  Investigation of equivocal or atypical features in relatives
  Prenatal diagnosis
  Preimplantation diagnosis
Primary molecular diagnosis
  Adult neuromuscular disorders
  Congenital myopathies
  Nonneuromuscular presentations (e.g., cataract)

---

minimally expanded repeats whose prognostic significance may be uncertain, as may the risks for having more severely affected children, while those detected may have previously had no knowledge that they were carrying a genetic mutation with potentially serious consequences to themselves and to offspring.

The issue of testing children for the myotonic dystrophy mutation is a difficult one and needs to be viewed in the more general context of childhood testing for late onset disorders.[253] There is a general consensus in the absence of clinical symptoms that such testing is best postponed to adult life, or at least until the individual can make his or her own decision. However, the variability of myotonic dystrophy, and the difficulty that may arise in deciding whether clinical symptoms are or are not related to the family disorder makes it important for each situation to be resolved on its own merits in close consultation with the family.

### Prenatal Diagnosis

The possibility of direct molecular diagnosis in early pregnancy has proved to be a major advance, although it should not be forgotten that linked markers were also useful in this[246,254] (and, indeed, that detection of the linked secretor locus gave the possibility of this approach being used as early as 1971!).[255] Prenatal diagnosis is especially requested by those couples where a previous child has died from, or is seriously affected by congenital myotonic dystrophy. In such families, the risk for a further seriously affected child is high, and prenatal diagnosis, usually by chorion villus sampling, provides an accurate method of detecting or excluding an affected pregnancy.[256,257] Such cases are almost always associated with extremely large expansions of several thousand repeats, though a precise correlation between repeat number and clinical severity is not possible. It is particularly important in prenatal diagnosis to use methods of analysis that will detect such very large expansions (see below).

### Preimplantation Diagnosis

For those couples where termination of pregnancy is unacceptable, preimplantation diagnosis offers the possibility of achieving a healthy pregnancy, while there are many others who might choose this approach in preference to prenatal diagnosis based on chorion villus sampling, if it were proven safe and effective. However, there remain major limitations in the practical use of this approach that are largely ignored by those promoting it for a wide range of genetic disorders. These limitations relate partly to the low rate of successful pregnancy as a result of in vitro fertilization and partly to the lack of evidence as to the accuracy of the molecular analysis in the preimplantation embryo.[258]

In the case of myotonic dystrophy, there are additional uncertainties relating to the timing of genetic instability in early embryonic development; clear data on preimplantation diagnosis have so far been reported by only one group,[259] which used specially adapted PCR conditions for analysis and were able to distinguish affected embryos. Problems with maternal contamination led to one diagnostic error. Several ongoing pregnancies resulting from implantation of unaffected embryos have been achieved. At present, the situation has to be regarded as still experimental, and full evaluation of all results is needed before any more general use of the approach can be decided on.

### Primary Molecular Diagnosis

The initial series of studies following isolation of the myotonic dystrophy gene showed presence of the mutation in almost all the patients studied, indicating its future usefulness as a diagnostic tool. Even the apparent exceptions proved this value because reassessment of such cases allowed the delineation of the previously unrecognized disorder, PROMM, while most of the remaining cases without a detectable mutation were shown to be misdiagnoses. Applications that have subsequently proved valuable include the differential diagnosis of puzzling adult neuromuscular disorders where myotonic dystrophy has been queried[249] and confirmation or exclusion of myotonic dystrophy as the cause of cataracts.[260] In childhood, distinction of other congenital myopathies has also proved valuable, as well as the recognition of myotonic dystrophy as a cause of such general clinical presentations as arthrogryposis or hydrops fetalis

Now that molecular testing is widely available it is worth asking whether any role remains for previously used preclinical tests such as electromyography or detection of lens opacities. Careful clinical assessment certainly remains important, and will frequently show clear abnormalities in individuals who have no symptoms; a normal clinical assessment is also important as it will allow those in whom a genetic abnormality is found, to be reassured that their current health is normal. However, a number of individuals have been erroneously labeled as affected on the basis of nonspecific lens opacities or doubtful myotonic potentials;[249] it seems unwise and unnecessary to use investigations of this type as a means of assessing genetic status when a definitive genetic test is possible.

## Diagnostic Methods

The original research studies on the molecular defect in myotonic dystrophy required adaptation to be used in a service setting. PCR-based estimation of repeat number is now the standard approach, especially for detecting small to moderate size expansions. However, the very large size of some expansions seen in myotonic dystrophy may result in failure of amplification, with only the normal allele being detected. This issue is particularly crucial in prenatal diagnosis, often done when a congenital case with a very large expansion is likely; Southern blotting has remained an essential part of the protocol here, although specially adapted PCR-based methods, capable of detecting trinucleotide expansions of all sizes, have been reported that are likely to replace this.[261,262] No failure of amplification was found in a series of 75 myotonic dystrophy patient samples with repeats of widely varying size using one of these new approaches.[261]

## Genetic Counseling

From the power and the specificity of applied molecular genetic testing described above, it might be concluded that most of the difficult genetic counseling problems previously encountered in myotonic dystrophy can now be satisfactorily resolved. This is true to a point. The options for families have certainly increased considerably as a result of genetic testing, but a number of difficulties and uncertainties remain, and testing itself can produce new problems. The difficulties encountered result from several factors, including the varying severity and phenotype of the disorder; the equally variable extent of the molecular defect; the limited correlation between phenotype and genotype; and the issues arising when individuals at risk are unaware of or do not wish to know their genetic status.

The complexity of these issues makes it unwise for molecular genetic testing to be undertaken except in the context of full discussion of the implications with those being tested. Even when molecular analysis is being used as part of primary diagnosis, the potential genetic implications of an abnormal result need clear explanation before the test is done, particularly if the patient is not aware that his or her condition might be genetic in nature. When testing individuals at risk, the possible implications for insurance and employment, the difficulty in basing any accurate clinical prognosis on the repeat number of an abnormal test result, the different implications for severity of disease in the offspring of males and females, and the possibility of systemic involvement, such as cardiac and central nervous system problems, are all important areas, quite apart from such topics as prenatal diagnosis, the testing of extended family members, and the issues related to childhood testing.

Given these and other difficulties, the process of genetic counseling in relation to myotonic dystrophy is inevitably time-consuming and demanding; there are considerable advantages for involving a specialist clinical geneticist from an early stage, but regardless of who undertakes the process it requires experience, sensitivity, and patience.

## Risk Estimates in Myotonic Dystrophy

The validity of the basic 50 percent risk estimates for first-degree relatives of patients with myotonic dystrophy was discussed earlier. This remains the starting point for all risk estimates. The following information may be useful in a variety of situations; further details can be found in the most recent edition of the monograph by Harper.[5]

1. A normal molecular analysis excludes the risk of developing or transmitting myotonic dystrophy in essentially all situations.
2. The risk of congenital myotonic dystrophy in the offspring of affected males is minimal (well under 1 percent) but not absent.
3. For women who have had a child with congenital myotonic dystrophy, almost all subsequent affected pregnancies are likely to be comparably, or at least severely affected.
4. Clinically affected women in general have around a 30 percent chance that an affected child would have congenital or severe childhood myotonic dystrophy.[264] The risk of a congenitally affected child is related to maternal repeat size; Cobo et al. found a risk of only 10 percent for those mothers with less than 300 repeats.[265] The risk of this for clinically normal women shown to have a molecular defect is considerably less, but an accurate estimate does not exist.
5. The risk for the healthy sib of a congenitally affected patient developing the disorder after childhood is low.[262] For the adult healthy sib of an adult onset case the risk of carrying the mutaiton is also low (around 10%), with about half this for developing clinically significant disease.
6. CTG repeat number provides only an approximate guide to prognosis or to pregnancy outcome.[96] Most cases with over 2000 repeats will have congenital or severe childhood onset disease; most individuals with 50 to 100 repeats will not have significant neuromuscular disease.

## Management and Therapy

Currently there is still no proven therapy that alters the natural course of myotonic dystrophy. A number of controlled trials have been carried out, but only one gives encouraging preliminary results which is of insulin-like growth factor (rhIGF-1), showing increased protein synthesis and clinical improvement in a small subset of patients.[270]

Careful general management to ensure that both patients and clinicians are fully aware of the numerous potential complication is thus all the more important; the key areas vary at different stages of life and are fully discussed in the final chapter of the author's monography.[5] Important issues include the hazards of anaesthesia and surgery and the necessary precautions to avoid these; the risk of cardiac arrhythmias; bronchial aspiration from esophageal dysfunction and colonic dilatation. Positive measures that give good results are surgery for cataracts and corrective orthopedic procedures in childhood.

Perhaps the most helpful measure of all is for patients to receive continuing medical care and supervision from a clinical team that has all-round experience and interest in myotonic dystrophy in its different aspects and for patients themselves to be fully informed about the various aspects of management and the potential problems that may arise. Awareness of the genetic risks and the range of options now available for genetic aspects of management, on which this chapter has concentrated, form an important part of helping families with this important and relatively common disorder.

## REFERENCES

1. Thomsen J: Tonische krämpfe in willkurlich beweglichen Muskeln infolge von ererbter psychischer Disposition (Ataxia muscularis). *Arch Psychiatr Nervenkr* **6**:702, 1876.

2. Steinert H: Uber das klinische und anatomische Bild des Muskelschwundes de Myotoniker. *Dtsch Z Nervenhlk* **37**:38, 1909.
3. Batten FE, Gibb HP: Myotonia atrophica. *Brain* **32**:187, 1909.
4. Curschmann H: Uber familiare atrophische Myotonie. *Dtsch Z Nerbenhlk* **45**:61, 1912.
5. Harper PS: *Myotonic Dystrophy*. 3rd ed. London, WB Saunders, 2001.
6. Harper PS, Rüdel R: Myotonic dystrophy, in Engel A (ed): *Myology*, 2d ed. New York, McGraw Hill, 1993.
7. Rüdel R, Lehman-Horn F: Non-dystrophic myotonias and periodic paralyses, in Rimoin DL, Connor JM, Pyeritz RE (eds): *Emery and Rimoin's Principles and Practice of Medical Genetics*. New York, Churchill Livingstone, 1996.
8. Ronnblom A, Forsberg H, Danielsson A: Gastrointestinal symptoms in myotonic dystrophy. *Scand J Gastroenterol* **31**(7):654, 1996.
9. Costantini M, Zaninotto G, Anselmino M, Marconi M, Iurilli V, Boccu C, Feltrin GP, Angelini C, Ancona E: Esophageal motor function in patients with myotonic dystrophy. *Dig Dis Sci* **41**(10):2032, 1996.
10. Eckardt VF, Nix W: The anal sphincter in patients with myotonic muscular dystrophy. *Gastroenterology* **100**(2):424, 1991.
11. Brunner HG, Hamel BC, Rieu P, Howeler CJ, Peters FT: Intestinal pseudo-obstruction in myotonic dystrophy. *J Med Genet* **29**(11):791, 1992.
12. Phillips MF, Harper PS: Cardiac disease in myotonic dystrophy. *Cardiovasc Res* **33**(1):13, 1997.
13. Aldridge LM: Anaesthetic problems in myotonic dystrophy — A case report and review of the Aberdeen experience comprising 48 general anaesthetics in a further 16 patients. *Br J Anaesth* **57**:1119, 1985.
14. Mathieu J, Allard P, Gobeil G, Girard M, De Braekeleer M, Begin P: Anesthetic and surgical complications in 219 cases of myotonic dystrophy. *Neurology* **49**(6):1646, 1997.
15. Harper PS. *Myotonic Dystrophy*, 2nd ed. Philadelphia, WB Saunders, 1989.
16. Lacomis D, Chad D, Smith T. Proximal weakness as the primary manifestation of myotonic dystrophy in older adults. *Muscle Nerve* **17**:687, 1994.
17. Moxley RT III, Ricker K. Proximal myotonic dystrophy. *Muscle Nerve* **18**(5):557, 1995.
18. Chad DA, Lacomis D, Skare J, Smith T. Proximal myotonic myopathy. *Muscle Nerve* **18**(5):558, 1995.
19. Fleischer B. Uber myotonische Dystrophie mit Katarakt. Albrecht von Graefes. *Arch Klin Ophalmol* **96**:91, 1918.
20. Ranum LP, Rasmussen PF, Benzow KA, Koob MD, Day JW: Genetic mapping of a second myotonic dystrophy locus. *Nat Genet* **19**(2):196, 1998.
21. Vanier TM: Dystrophia myotonica in childhood. *Br Med J* 2:1284, 1960.
22. Harper PS: Congenital myotonic dystrophy in Britain. 1. Clinical aspects *Arch Dis Child* **50**:505, 1975.
23. Harper PS, Dyken PR: Early onset dystrophia myotonica — Evidence supporting a maternal environmental factor. *Lancet* 2:53, 1972.
24. Harper PS: Congenital myotonic dystrophy in Britain II. Genetic basis. *Arch Dis Child* **50**:514, 1975.
25. Koch MC, Grimm T, Harley HG, Harper PS: Genetic risks for children of women with myotonic dystrophy. *Am J Hum Genet* **48**:1084, 1991.
26. Laporte J, Hu LJ, Kretz C, et al: A gene mutated in X-linked myotubular myopathy defines a new putative tyrosine phosphatase family conserved in yeast. *Nat Genet* **13**:175, 1996.
27. Soussi-Yanicostas N, Chevallay M, Laurent-Winter C, Tome FM, Fardeau M, Butler-Browne GS: Distinct contractile protein profile in congenital myotonic dystrophy. *Neuromuscul Disord* **1**(2):103, 1991.
28. Tohgi H, Kawamorita A, Utsugisawa K, Yamagata M, Sano M: Muscle histopathology in myotonic dystrophy in relation to age and. *Muscle Nerve* **17**(9):1037, 1994.
29. Karpati G, Carpenter S, Watters GV, Eisen AE, Andermann F: Infantile myotonic dystrophy: Histochemical and electron microscopic features in skeletal muscle. *Neurology* **23**:1066, 1973.
30. Sarnat HB, Silbert SW: Maturational arrest of fetal muscle in neonatal myotonic dystrophy. *Arch Neurol* **33**:466, 1976.
31. Farkas E, Tomé FMS, Fardeau M, Arseniio-Nunes ML, Dreyfuss P, Diebler MF: Histochemical and ultrastructural study of muscle biopsies in 3 cases of dystrophia myotonica in the newborn child. *J Neurol Sci* **21**:273, 1974.
32. Ansved T, Edstrom L, Grandell U et al: Variation of CTG-repeat number of the DMPK gene in muscle tissue. *Neuromuscul Disord* **7**:152, 1997.
33. van der Ven PF, Jansen G, van Kuppevelt TH, Perryman MB, Lupa M, Dunne PW, ter Laak HJ, Jap PH, Veerkamp JH, Epstein HF, et al: Myotonic dystrophy kinase is a component of neuromuscular junctions. *Hum Mol Genet* **2**(11):1889, 1993.
34. Maeda M, Taft CS, Bush EW, Holder E, Bailey WM, Neville H, Perryman MB, Bies RD: Identification, tissue-specific expression, and subcellular localization of the 80-kDa and 71-kDa forms of myotonic-dystrophy kinase protein. *J Biol Chem* **270**(35):20246, 1995.
35. Tachi N, Kozuka N, Ohya K, Chiba S, Kikuchi K: Expression of myotonic dystrophy protein kinase in biopsied muscles. *J Neurol Sci* **132**(1):61, 1995.
36. Shimokawa M, Ishiura S, Kameda N, Yamamoto M, Sasagawa N, Saitoh N, Sorimachi H, Ueda H, Ohno S, Suzuki K, Kobayashi T: Novel isoform of myotonin protein kinase: Gene product of myotonic dystrophy is localized in the sarcoplasmic reticulum of skeletal muscle. *Am J Pathol* **150**(4):1285, 1997.
37. Dunne PW, Ma L, Casey DL, Harati Y, Epstein HF: Localization of myotonic dystrophy protein kinase in skeletal muscle. *Cell Motil Cytoskeleton* **33**(1):52, 1996.
38. Koga R, Nakao Y, Kurano Y, Tsukahara T, Nakamura A, Ishiura S, Nonaka I, Arahata K: Decreased myotonin-protein kinase in the skeletal and cardiac muscles. *Biochem Biophys Res Commun* **202**(1):577, 1994.
39. Tachi N, Kozuka N, Ohya K, Chiba S, Kikuchi K: Immunocytochemical localization of myotonin protein kinase on muscle from patients with congenital myotonic dystrophy. *Histol Histopathol* **11**(4):869, 1996.
40. Lipicky RJ: Studies in human myotonic dystrophy, in Rowland LP (ed): *Pathogenesis of Human Muscular Dystrophy*. Amsterdam, Excerpta Medica, 1977, p 729.
41. Franke CH, Hatt H, Iaizzo PA, Lehmann-Horn F: Characteristics of $Na^+$ channels and $Cl^-$ conductance in resealed muscle fibre segments from patients with myotonic dystrophy. *J Physiol (Lond)* **425**:391, 1990.
42. Merickel M, Gray R, Chauvin P, Appel S: Cultured muscle from myotonic muscular dystrophy patients: Altered membrane electrical properties. *Proc Natl Acad Sci U S A* **78**:648, 1981.
43. Tahmoush AJ, Askansas V, Nelson PG, Engel WK: Electrophysiologic properties of a neutrally cultured muscle from patients with myotonic muscular atrophy. *Neurology* **33**:311, 1983.
44. Renaud JF, Denuelle C, Schmid-Antomarchi H, Hughes M, Serratrice G, Lazdunski M: Expression of apamin receptor in muscle of patients with myotonic muscular dystrophy. *Nature* **319**:678, 1986.
45. Fleischer B: Uber myotonischer Dystrophie mit katarakt. *Albrecht von Graefes Ztch Ophthalmol* **96**:91, 1918.
46. Bell J: Dystrophia myotonica and allied diseases, in Penrose LS (ed): *Treasury of Human Inheritance, Part V*. Cambridge, UK, Cambridge University Press, 1948.
47. Thomasen E: *Myotonia*. Aarhus, Universitetsforlaget, 1948.
48. Klein D: La dystrophie myotonique et la myotonie congenitale (Thomsen) en Suisse. *J Genet Hum* **1**(Suppl):1, 1958.
49. Harper PS: Myotonic dystrophy and other autosomal dystrophies. In: Scriver CR et al. (eds): *The Molecular and Metabolic Bases of Inherited Disease*, 7th ed. New York, McGraw Hill, 1993, p 4227.
50. Mohr J: *The Study of Linkage in Man*. Copenhagen, Munksgaard, 1954.
51. Renwick JH, Bundey SE, Ferguson-Smith MA, Izatt MM: Confirmation of the linkage of the loci for myotonic dystrophy and ABH secretion. *J Med Genet* **8**:407, 1971.
52. Harper PS, Rivas ML, Bias WBM, Hutchinson JR, Dyken PR, McKusick VA: Genetic linkage confirmed between the loci for myotonic dystrophy, ABH secretion and Lutheran blood group. *Am J Hum Genet* **24**:310, 1972.
53. Whitehead AS, Soloman E, Chambers S, Bodmer WF, Povey S, Fey G: Assignment of the structural gene for the third component of human complement to chromosome 19. *Proc Natl Acad Sci U S A* **79**:5021, 1982.
54. Shaw DJ, Meredith AL, Sarfarazi M, Huson SM, Brook JD, Myklebost O, Harper PS: The apolipoprotein CII gene: Subchromosomal localisation and linkage to the myotonic dystrophy locus. *Hum Genet* **70**:271, 1985.
55. Korneluk RG, MacKenzie AE, Nakamura Y, Dube I, Jacob P, Hunter AGW: A recording of human chromosome 19 long-arm DNA markers and identification of markers flanking the myotonic dystrophy locus. *Genomics* **5**:596, 1989.
56. Smeets B, Poddighe J, Brunner H, Ropers HH, Wieringa B: Tight linkage between myotonic dystrophy and apolipoprotein E genes. *Hum Genet* **80**(1):49, 1988.

57. Schonk D, Coerwinkel-Driessen M, van Dalen I, Oerlemans F, Smeets B, Schepens J, Hulsebos T, Cockburn D, Boyd Y, Davis M, et al: Definition of subchromosomal intervals around the myotonic dystrophy region at 19q. *Genomics* **4(3)**:384, 1989.

58. Shaw DJ, Harley HG, Brook JD, McKeithan TW: Long-range restriction map of a region of human chromosome 19. *Hum Genet* **83(1)**:71, 1989.

59. Harley HG, Brook JD, Floyd J, Rundle SA, Crow S, Walsh KV, Thibault MC, Harper PS, Shaw DJ: Detection of linkage disequilibrium between the myotonic dystrophy locus and a new polymorphic DNA marker. *Am J Hum Genet* **49(1)**:68, 1991.

60. Brook JD, Zemelman BV, Hadingham K, Siciliano MJ, Crow S, Harley HG, Rundle SA, Buxton J, Johnson K, Almond JW, et al: Radiation-reduced hybrids for the myotonic dystrophy locus. *Genomics* **13(2)**:243, 1992.

61. Jansen G, de Jong PJ, Amemiya C, Aslanidis C, Shaw DJ, Harley HG, Brook JD, Fenwick R, Korneluk RG, Tsilfidis C, et al: Physical and genetic characterization of the distal segment of the myotonic-dystrophy area on 19q. *Genomics* **13(3)**:509, 1992.

62. Shutler G, Korneluk RG, Tsilfidis C, Mahadevan M, Bailly J, Smeets H, Jansen G, Wieringa B, Lohman F, Aslanidis C, et al: Physical mapping and cloning of the proximal segment of the myotonic dystrophy gene region. *Genomics* **13(3)**:518, 1992.

63. Shutler GG, MacKenzie AE, Korneluk RG: The 1.5-Mb region spanning the myotonic dystrophy locus shows uniform recombination frequency. *Am J Hum Genet* **54(1)**:104, 1994.

64. Harley HG, Brook JD, Rundle SA, Crow S, Reardon W, Buckler AJ, Harper PS, Housman DE, Shaw DJ: Expansion of an unstable DNA region and phenotypic variation in myotonic dystrophy. *Nature* **355(6360)**:545, 1992.

65. Buxton J, Shelbourne P, Davies J, Jones C, Van Tongeren T, Aslanidis C, de Jong P, Jansen G, Anvret M, Riley B, et al: Detection of an unstable fragment of DNA specific to individuals with myotonic dystrophy. *Nature* **355(6360)**:547, 1992.

66. Aslanidis C, Jansen G, Amemiya C, et al: Cloning of the essential myotonic dystrophy region and mapping of the putative defect. *Nature* **255**:548, 1982.

67. Oberlé I, Rousseau F, Heitz D, et al: Amazing instability of a 550bp DNA segment and abnormal methylation in fragile X syndrome. *Science* **252**:1097, 1991.

68. Yu S, Pritchard M, Kremer E, et al: Fragile X genotype characterised by an unstable region of DNA. *Science* **252**:1179, 1991.

69. Crow SR, Harley HG, Brook JD, Rundle SA, Shaw DJ: Insertion/deletion polymorphism at D19S95 associated with the myotonic dystrophy CTG repeat. *Hum Mol Genet* **1(6)**:451, 1992

70. Mahadevan MS, Foitzik MA, Surh LC, Korneluk RG: Characterization and polymerase chain reaction (PCR) detection of an Alu deletion polymorphism in total linkage disequilibrium with myotonic-dystrophy. *Genomics* **15(2)**:446, 1993.

71. Brook JD, McCurrach ME, Harley HG, Buckler AJ, Church D, Aburatani H, Hunter K, Stanton VP, Thirion JP, Hudson T, et al: Molecular basis of myotonic dystrophy: Expansion of a trinucleotide (CTG) repeat at the 3′ end of a transcript encoding a protein-kinase family member. *Cell* **68(4)**:799, 1992.

72. Fu YH, Pizzuti A, Fenwick RG Jr, King J, Rajnarayan S, Dunne PW, Dubel J, Nasser GA, Ashizawa T, de Jong P, et al: An unstable triplet repeat in a gene related to myotonic muscular dystrophy. *Science* **255(5049)**:1256, 1992.

73. Mahadevan M, Tsilfidis C, Sabourin L, Shutler G, Amemiya C, Jansen G, Neville C, Narang M, Barcelo J, O'Hoy K, et al: Myotonic dystrophy mutation: An unstable CTG repeat in the 3′ untranslated region of the gene. *Science* **255(5049)**:1253, 1992.

74. Harper PS: Genetic studies in myotonic dystrophy. [DM thesis]. Oxford, UK, University of Oxford, 1972.

75. Gennarelli M, Dallapiccola B, Baiget M, Martorell L, Novelli G: Meiotic drive at the myotonic dystrophy locus [Letter]. *J Med Genet* **31(12)**:980, 1994.

76. Zatz M, Cerqueira A, Vainzof M, Passos-Bueno MR: Segregation distortion of the CTG repeats at the myotonic dystrophy locus: New data from Brazilian DM families. *J Med Genet* **34(9)**:790, 1997.

77. Carey N, Johnson K, Nokelainen P, Peltonen L, Savontaus ML, Juvonen V, Anvret M, Grandell U, Chotai K, Robertson E, et al: Meiotic drive at the myotonic dystrophy locus? [Letter; see comments]. *Nat Genet* **6(2)**:117, 1994.

78. Hurst GD, Hurst LD, Barrett JA: Meiotic drive and myotonic dystrophy [Letter; comment]. **Nat Genet 10(2)**:132, 1995.

79. Chakraborty R, Stivers DN, Deka R, Yu LM, Shriver MD, Ferrell RE: Segregation distortion of the CTG repeats at the myotonic dystrophy locus. *Am J Hum Genet* **59(1)**:109, 1996.

80. Harper PS, Harley HG, Reardon W, Shaw DJ: Anticipation in myotonic dystrophy: New light on an old problem. *Am J Hum Genet* **51**:10, 1992.

81. Harper PS: Myotonic dystrophy as a trinucleotide repeat disorder, in Wells RD, Warren ST (eds): *Genetic Instabilities and Hereditary Neurological Diseases.* New York, Academic Press, 1998, p 115.

82. McInnis MG: Anticipation: An old idea in new genes. *Am J Hum Genet* **59**:973, 1996.

83. Fraser FC: Trinucleotide repeats not the only cause of anticipation. *Lancet* **350**:459, 1997.

84. Penrose LS: The problem of anticipation in pedigrees of dystrophia myotonica. *Ann Eugen (Lond)* **14**:125, 1948.

85. Höweler CJ: *A Clinical and Genetic Study in Myotonic Dystrophy.* Thesis. Rotterdam, University of Rotterdam, 1986.

86. Howeler CJ, Busch HF, Geraedts JP, Niermeijer MF, Staal A: Anticipation in myotonic dystrophy: Fact or fiction? *Brain* **112**:779, 1989.

87. de Die-Smulders CE, Howeler CJ, Mirandolle JF, Brunner HG, Hovers V, Bruggenwirth H, Smeets HJ, Geraedts JP: Anticipation resulting in elimination of the myotonic dystrophy gene: A follow-up-study of one extended family. *J Med Genet* **31(8)**:595, 1994.

88. Simmons Z, Thornton CA, Seltzer WK, Richards CS: Relative stability of a minimal CTG repeat expansion in a large kindred with myotonic dystrophy. *Neurology* **50(5)**:1501, 1998.

89. Harley HG, Rundle SA, Reardon W, Shyring J, Crow S, Brook JD, Harper PS, Shaw DJ: Unstable DNA sequence in myotonic dystrophy. *Lancet* **339**:1125, 1992.

90. Tsilfidis C, MacKenzie AE, Mettler G, Barcelo J, Korneluk RG: Correlation between CTG trinucleotide repeat length and frequency of severe congenital myotonic dystrophy. *Nat Genet* **1(3)**:192, 1992.

91. Novelli G, Gennarelli M, Menegazzo E, Mostacciuolo ML, Pizzuti A, Fattorini C, Tessarolo D, Tomelleri G, Giacanelli M, Danieli GA, et al: (CTG)n triplet mutation and phenotype manifestations in myotonic dystrophy patients. *Biochem Med Metab Biol* **50(1)**:85, 1993.

92. Eguchi I, Koike R, Onodera O, Tanaka K, Kondo H, Tsuji S: Correlation between degrees of the CTG repeat expansion and clinical. *Rinsho Shinkeigaku* **34(2)**:118, 1994.

93. Passos-Bueno MR, Cerqueira A, Vainzof M, Marie SK, Zatz M: Myotonic dystrophy: Genetic, clinical, and molecular analysis of patients from 41 Brazilian families. *J Med Genet* **32(1)**:14, 1995.

94. Shaw DJ, Harper PS: Workshop report: Myotonic dystrophy—Advances in molecular genetics. *Neuromuscul Discord* **2**:241, 1992.

95. Imbert G, Kretz C, Johnson K, Mandel J-L: Origin of the expansion mutation in myotonic dystrophy. *Nat Genet* **4**:72, 1993.

96. Gennarelli M, Novelli G, Andreasi Bassi F, Martorell L, Cornet M, Menegazzo E, Mostacciuolo ML, Martinez JM, Angelini C, Pizzuti A, Baiget M, Dallapiccola B: Prediction of myotonic dystrophy clinical severity based on the number of intragenic [CTG](n) trinucleotide repeats. *Am J Med Genet* **65(4)**:342, 1996.

97. Turnpenny P, Clark C, Kelly K: Intelligence quotient profile in myotonic dystrophy. *J Med Genet* **31(4)**:300, 1994.

98. Melacini P, Villanova C, Menegazzo E, Novelli G, et al: Correlation between cardiac involvement and CTG trinucleotide repeat length in myotonic dystrophy. *Cardiomyopathy* **25**:239, 1995.

99. Hasegawa T, Kinoshita M, Hirose K: Multiorgan abnormalities in myotonic dystrophy—correlation among endocrine disorders, central nervous system involvements and gene analysis. *Rinsho Shinkeigaku* **35**:1, 1995.

100. Kinoshita M, Komori T, Ohtake T, Takahashi R, et al: Abnormal calcium metabolism in myotonic dystrophy as shown by the Ellsworth-Howard test and its relation to CTG triplet repeat length. *J Neurol* **244**:613, 1997.

101. Annane D, Fiorelli M, Mazoyer B, Pappata S, Eymard B, Radvanyi H, Junien C, Fardeau M, Merlet P, Gajdos P, Syrota A, Sansom Y, Duboc D: Impaired cerebral glucose metabolism in myotonic dystrophy: A triplet-size dependent phenomenon. *Neuromuscul Disord* **8(1)**:39, 1998.

102. Ito K, Takano A: Oligosaccharide abnormalities and expansion of the CTG repeat of MT-PK. *Nippon Rinsho* **55(12)**:3225, 1997.

103. Hamshere MG, Harley HG, Harper PS, Brook DJ, Brookfield JFY: Myotonic dystrophy: The correlation of (CTG) length in leucocytes with age at onset is significant only for patients with small expansions. *J Med Genet* **36**:59, 1999.

104. Novelli G, Gennarelli M, Menegazzo E, Angelini C, Dallapiccola B: Discordant clinical outcome in myotonic dystrophy relatives showing (CTG)(N) greater than 700 repeats. *Neuromuscul Disord* 5(2):157, 1995.

105. Ashizawa T, Anvret M, Baiget M, Barcelo JM, Brunner H, Cobo AM, Dallapiccola B, Fenwick RG Jr, Grandell U, Harley H, et al: Characteristics of intergenerational contractions of the CTG repeat in myotonic dystrophy. *Am J Hum Genet* 54(3):414, 1994.

106. Cipollaro M, et al: CTG repeat number in the nonaffected allele of myotonic dystrophy patients is not critical for disease expression. *Hum Biol* 69(6):887, 1997.

107. Bergoffen J, Kant J, Sladky J, McDonald-McGinn D, Zackai EH, Fischbeck KH: Paternal transmission of congenital myotonic dystrophy. *J Med Genet* 31(7):518, 1994.

108. Nakagame M, Yamada H, Higuchi I, Kaminishi Y, Miki T, Johnson K, Osame M: A case of paternally inherited congenital myotonic dystrophy. *J Med Genet* 31(5):397, 1994.

109. Ohya K, Tachi N, Chiba S, Sato T, Kon S, Kikuchi K, Imamura S, Yamagata H, Miki T: Congenital myotonic dystrophy transmitted from an asymptomatic father. *Neurology* 44(10):1958, 1994.

110. de Die-Smulders CE, et al: Paternal transmission of congenital myotonic dystrophy. *J Med Genet* 34(11):930, 1997.

111. O'Hoy KL, Tsilfidis C, Mahadevan MS, Neville CE, Barcelo J, Hunter AG, Korneluk RG: Reduction in size of the myotonic dystrophy trinucleotide repeat mutation during transmission. *Science* 259:809, 1993.

112. Brunner HG, Jansen G, Nillesen W, Nelen MR, de Die CE, Howeler CJ, van Oost BA, Wieringa B, Ropers HH, Smeets HJ: Reverse mutation in myotonic dystrophy. *N Engl J Med* 328(7):476, 1993.

113. Brunner HG, Bruggenwirth HT, Nillesen W, Jansen G, Hamel BC, Hoppe RL, de Die CE, Howeler CJ, van Oost BA, Wieringa B, et al: Influence of sex of the transmitting parent as well as of parental allele size on the CTG expansion in myotonic dystrophy. *Am J Hum Genet* 53(5):1016, 1993.

114. Ashizawa T, Dunne PW, Ward PA, Seltzer WK, Richards CS: Effects of the sex of myotonic dystrophy patients on the unstable triplet repeat in their affected offspring. *Neurology* 44(1):120, 1994.

115. Lavedan C, Hofmann-Radvanyi H, Rabes JP, Roume J, Junien C: Different sex-dependent constraints in CTG length variation as explanation for congenital myotonic dystrophy. *Lancet* 341:237, 1993.

116. Eguchi I, Tsuji S. Effect of maternal paternal transmissions in clinical manifestations of CTG repeat on myotonic dystrophy. *Nippon Rinsho* 55:3230, 1997.

117. Lopez de Munain A, Cobo AM, Poza JJ, Navarrete D, Martorell L, Palau F, Emparanza JI, Baiget M: Influence of the sex of the transmitting grandparent in congenital myotonic dystrophy. *J Med Genet* 32(9):689, 1995.

118. Harper PS (ed): *Huntington's Disease*. London, WB Saunders, 1996.

119. Harper PS. New genes for old diseases: The molecular basis of myotonic dystrophy and Huntington's disease. *J R Coll Physicians Lond* 30:221, 1996.

120. Wong LJ, Ashizawa T, Monckton DG, Caskey CT, Richards CS: Somatic heterogeneity of the CTG repeat in myotonic dystrophy is age and size dependent. *Am J Hum Genet* 56(1):114, 1995.

121. Barcelo JM, Pluscauskas M, MacKenzie AE, Tsilfidis C, Narang M, Korneluk RG: Additive influence of maternal and offspring DM-kinase gene CTG repeat lengths in the genesis of congenital myotonic dystrophy. *Am J Hum Genet* 54(6):1124, 1994.

122. Jansen G, Willems P, Coerwinkel M, Nillesen W, Smeets H, Vits L, Howeler C, Brunner H, Wieringa B: Gonosomal mosaicism in myotonic dystrophy patients: Involvement of mitotic events in (CTG)(N) repeat variation and selection against extreme expansion in sperm. *Am J Hum Genet* 54(4):575, 1994.

123. Monckton DG, Wong LJ, Ashizawa T, Caskey CT: Somatic mosaicism, germline expansions, germline reversions and intergenerational reductions in myotonic dystrophy males — Small pool PCR analyses. *Hum Mol Genet* 4(1):1, 1995.

124. Daniela R, Holding C, Kontogianni E, Monk M: Single-cell analysis of unstable genes. *J Assist Reprod Genet* 13:163, 1996.

125. Myring J, Meredith AL, Harley HG, Koch G, Norbury G, Harper PS, Shaw DJ: Specific molecular prenatal diagnosis for the CTG mutation in myotonic dystrophy. *J Med Genet* 29:785, 1992.

126. Wohrle D, Kennerknecht I, Wolf M, Enders H, Schwemmle S, Steinbach P: Heterogeneity of DM kinase repeat expansion in different fetal tissues. *Hum Mol Genet* 4(7):1147, 1995.

127. Tachi N, Ohya K, Chiba S, Sato T, Kikuchi K: Minimal somatic instability of CTG repeat in congenital myotonic dystrophy. *Pediatr Neurol* 12(1):81, 1995.

128. Martorell L, Martinez JM, Carey N, Johnson K, Baiget M: Comparison of CTG repeat length expansion and clinical progression of over a 5-year period. *J Med Genet* 32(8):593, 1995.

129. Lopez de Munain A, Cobo AM, Huguet E, Marti Masso JF, Johnson K, Baiget M: CTG trinucleotide repeat variability in identical twins with myotonic dystrophy. *Ann Neurol* 35(3):374, 1994.

130. Dubel JR, Armstrong RM, Perryman MB, Epstein HF, Ashizawa T: Phenotypic expression of the myotonic dystrophy gene in monozygotic twins. *Neurology* 42(9):1815, 1992.

131. Lopez de Munain A, Cobo AM, Huguet E, Marti Masso JF, Johnson K, Baiget M: CTG trinucleotide repeat variability in identical twins with myotonic dystrophy. *Ann Neurol* 35(3):374, 1994.

132. Imbert G, Feng Y, Nelson DL, Warren ST, Mendel JC: FM R-1 and mutations in fragile X syndrome: Molecular biology, biochemistry and genetics, in Wells RD, Warren SE (eds): *Genetic Instabilities and Hereditary Neurological Diseases*. New York, Academic Press, 1998, p 27.

133. Dubel JR, Armstrong RM, Perryman MB, et al: Phenotypic expression of the myotonic dystrophy gene in monozygotic twins. *Neurology* 42:1815, 1992.

134. Reyniers E, Vits L, De Borolle K, Van Roy B, et al: The full mutation in the FMR-1 gene of male fragile X patients is absent in their sperm. *Nat Genet* 4:143, 1993.

135. Thornton CA, Johnson K, Moxley RT 3rd: Myotonic dystrophy patients have larger CTG expansions in skeletal muscle than in leukocytes. *Ann Neurol* 35(1):104, 1994.

136. Kinoshita M, Takahashi R, Hasegawa T, et al: (CTG)n expansions in various tissues from a myotonic dystrophy patient. *Muscle Nerve* 19:240, 1996.

137. Ishii S, et al: Small increase in triplet repeat length of cerebellum from patients with myotonic dystrophy. *Hum Genet* 98(2):138, 1996.

138. Telenius H, Kremer B, Goldberg P, Theilmann J, et al, Somatic and gonadal mosaicism of the Huntington disease gene CAG repeat in brain and sperm. *Nat Genet* 6:409, 1994.

139. Ashizawa T, Dubel JR, Harati Y: Somatic instability of CTG repeat in myotonic dystrophy. *Neurology* 43(12):2674, 1993.

140. Anvret M, Ahlberg G, Grandell U, Hedberg B, Johnson K, Edstrom L: Larger expansions of the CTG repeat in muscle compared to lymphocytes. *Hum Mol Genet* 2(9):1397, 1993.

141. Thornton CA, Johnson K, Moxley RT 3rd: Myotonic dystrophy patients have larger CTG expansions in skeletal muscle than in leukocytes. *Ann Neurol* 35(1):104, 1994.

142. Ansved T, Edstrom L, Grandell U, Hedberg B, Anvret M: Variation of CTG- repeat number of the DMPK gene in muscle tissue. *Neuromuscul Disord* 7(3):152, 1997.

143. Martorell L, Martinez JM, Carey N, Johnson K, Baiget M: Comparison of CTG repeat length expansion and clinical progression of myotonic dystrophy over a 5-year period. *J Med Genet* 32(8):593, 1995.

144. Ashizawa T, Monckton DG, Vaishnav S, Patel BJ, Voskova A, Caskey CT: Instability of the expanded (CTG)n repeats in the myotonin protein. *Genomics* 36(1):47, 1996.

145. Wexler NS, Young AB, Tanzi RE, et al: Homozygotes for Huntington's disease. *Nature* 326:194, 1987.

146. Cobo A, Martinez JM, Martorell L, et al: Molecular diagnosis of homozygous myotonic dystrophy in two asymptomatic sisters. *Hum Mol Genet* 2:711, 1993.

147. Roeder E, Jain K, Timenchenko L, et al: Homozygous myotonic dystrophy. *Am J Hum Genet* 55(Suppl):A23, 1994.

148. Martorell L, Illa I, Rosell J, Benitez J, Sedano MJ, Baiget M: Homozygous myotonic dystrophy: Clinical and molecular studies of three unrelated cases. *J Med Genet* 33(9):783, 1996.

149. Murata K, Matsumura R, Murata K, Takayanagi T: [A case of dystrophia myotonica with homozygous DM kinase abnormalities]. *Rinsho Shinkeigaku* 37(6):497, 1997.

150. Day JD, Roelofs R, Leroy B, Pech I, Benzow K, Ranum LPW: Clinical and genetic characteristics of a five-generation family with a novel form of myotonic dystrophy (DM2). *Neuromuscul Disord* 9:19, 1999.

151. Mathieu J, De Braekeleer M, Prevost C: Genealogical reconstruction of myotonic dystrophy in the Saguenay-Lac-Saint-Jean area. *Neurology* 40(5):839, 1990.

152. Veillette S, Perron M, Mathieu J, La dystrophie myotonique: 2. Nuptialité, fécondité et transmission du gène. *Can J Neurol Sci* **16**:114, 1989.

153. Dao TN, Mathieu J, Bouchard JP, De Braekeleer M: Fertility in myotonic dystrophy in Saguenay-Lac-St-Jean: A historical perspective. *Clin Genet* **42(5)**:234, 1992.

154. O'Brien T, Harper PS: Reproductive problems and neonatal loss in women with myotonic dystrophy. *J Obst Gynaecol Res* **4**:170, 1984.

155. Erikson A, Forsberg H, Drugge U, Holmgren G: Outcome of pregnancy in women with myotonic dystrophy and analysis of CTG expansion. *Acta Paediatr* **84**:414, 1995.

156. Harper PS: *Myotonic Dystrophy*. London, WB Saunders, 3rd edition, in press.

157. Burcet J, Canellas F, Cavaller G, Vich M: Estudio epidemiologico de la distrofia miotonica en la isla de Mallorca. *Neurologia* **7**:61, 1992.

158. Lotz BP, Van der Meyden CH. Myotonic dystrophy. *S Afr Med J* **67**:812, 1985.

159. Rolander A, Floderus S: Dystrophia myotonica I Norbottens. *Svensk Lakartida* **58**:648, 1961.

160. Ashizawa T, Epstein HF: Ethnic distribution of myotonic dystrophy gene [Letter]. *Lancet* **338(8767)**:642, 1991.

161. Mostaccuilo ML. Barbujani G, Armani M, Danidi GA, Angelini C: Genetic epidemiology of myotonic dystrophy. *Genet Epidemiol* **4**:289, 1987.

162. Lopez de Munain A, Blanco A, Emparanza JI, Poza JJ, et al: Prevalence of myotonic dystrophy in Guipuzcoa (Basque Country, Spain). *Neurology* **43**:1573, 1993.

163. Lavedan C, Hofmann-Radvanyi H, Boileau C, Bonaiti-Pellie C, Savoy D, Shelbourne P, Duros C, Rabes JP, Dehaupas I, Luce S, et al: French myotonic dystrophy families show expansion of a CTG repeat in complete linkage disequilibrium with an intragenic 1 kb insertion. *J Med Genet* **31(1)**:33, 1994.

164. Yamagata H, Miki T, Nakagawa M, Johnson K, Deka R, Ogihara T: Association of CTG repeats and the 1-kb Alu insertion/deletion. *Hum Genet* **97(2)**:145, 1996.

165. Neville CE, Mahadevan MS, Barcelo JM, Korneluk RG: High resolution genetic analysis suggests one ancestral predisposing haplotype for the origin of the myotonic dystrophy mutation. *Hum Mol Genet* **3(1)**:45, 1994.

166. Goldman A, Krause A, Ramsay M, Jenkins T: Founder effect and prevalence of myotonic dystrophy in South Africans: Molecular studies. *Am J Hum Genet* **59(2)**:445, 1996.

167. Dada TO. Dystrophia myotonica in a Nigerian Family. *East Afr Med J* **50**:214, 1973.

168. Krahe R, Eckhart M, Ogunniyi AO, Osuntokun BO, Siciliano MJ, Ashizawa T: De novo myotonic dystrophy mutation in a Nigerian kindred. *Am J Hum Genet* **56(5)**:1067, 1995.

169. Davies J, Yamagata H, Shelbourne P, Buxton J, Ogihara T, Nokelainen P, Nakagawa M, Williamson R, Johnson K, Miki T: Comparison of the myotonic dystrophy associated CTG repeat in European and Japanese populations. *J Med Genet* **29(11)**:766, 1992.

170. Goldman A, Ramsay M, Jenkins T: Absence of myotonic dystrophy in southern African Negroids is associated with a significantly lower number of CTG trinucleotide repeats. *J Med Genet* **31(1)**:37, 1994.

171. Goldman A, Ramsay M, Jenkins T: Ethnicity and myotonic dystrophy: A possible explanation for its absence in sub-Saharan Africa. *Ann Hum Genet* **60(Pt 1)**:57, 1996.

172. Mor-Cohen R, Magal N, Gadoth N, Achiron A, Shohat T, Shohat M: The lower incidence of myotonic dystrophy in Ashkenazic Jews compared to North African Jews is associated with a significantly lower number of CTG trinucleotide repeats. *Isr J Med Sci* **33(3)**:190, 1997.

173. Korczyn AD: Neurologic genetic diseases of Jewish people. *Biomed Pharmacother* **48(8–9)**:391, 1994.

174. Imbert G, Kretz C, Johnson K, Mandel J-L: Origin of the expansion mutation in myotonic dystrophy. *Nat Genet* **4**:72, 1993.

175. Rubinsztein DC, Leggo J, Amos W, Barton DE, Ferguson-Smith MA: Myotonic dystrophy CTG repeats and the associated insertion/deletion. *Hum Mol Genet* **3(11)**:2031, 1994.

176. Zerylnick C, Torroni A, Sherman SL, Warren ST: Normal variation at the myotonic dystrophy locus in global human populations. *Am J Hum Genet* **56(1)**:123, 1995.

177. Tishkoff SA, Goldman A, Calafell F, Speed WC, Deinard AS, Bonne-Tamir B, Kidd JR, Pakstis AJ, Jenkins T, Kidd KK: A global haplotype analysis of the myotonic dystrophy locus: Implications for the evolution of modern humans and for the origin of myotonic dystrophy mutations. *Am J Hum Genet* **62(6)**:1389, 1998.

178. Winchester CL, Johnson KJ: Is myotonic dystrophy (DM) the result of a contiguous gene defect? in Wells R, Warren S (eds): *Genetic Instabilities and Hereditary Neurological Disease*, San Diego, Academic Press, 1998, p 169.

179. Deleted in proof.

180. Muller HJ: Further studies on the nature and causes of gene mutations, in Jones DF (ed): *Proceedings of the Sixth International Congress of Genetics*. Menasha, WA, Brooklyn Botanic Gardens, 1932.

181. Wilkie AO: The molecular basis of genetic dominance. *J Med Genet* **31**:89, 1998.

182. Reddy S, Smith DBJ, Rich MM, Leferovich JM, Reilly P, Davis BM, Tran K, et al: Mice lacking the myotonic dystrophy protein kinase develop a late onset progressive myopathy. *Nat Genet* **13**:325, 1996.

183. Jansen G, Groenen PJTA, Bachner D, Jap PHK, Coerwinkel M, Oerlemans F, van den Broek W, et al: Abnormal myotonic dystrophy protein kinase levels produce only mild myopathy in mice. *Nat Genet* **13**:316, 1996.

184. Monckton DG, Ashizawa T, Siciliano MJ: Murine models for myotonic dystrophy, in Wells R, Warren S (eds): *Genetic Instabilities and Hereditary Neurological Disease*, Chap. 13. San Diego, Academic Press, 1998, p 181.

185. Gourdon G, Radvanyi F, Lia AS, Duros C, Blanche M, Abitbol M, Junien C, et al: Moderate intergenerational and somatic instability of a 55-CTG repeat in transgenic mice. *Nat Genet* **15**:190, 1997.

186. Hamshere MG, Newman EE, Alwazzan M, Athwal BS, Brook, JD: Transcriptional abnormality in myotonic dystrophy affects DMPK but not neighboring genes. *Proc Natl Acad Sci U S A* **94**:7394, 1997.

187. Alwazzan M, Hamshere MG, Lennon G, Brook JD: Six transcripts map within 200 kilobases of the myotonic dystrophy expanded repeat. *Mamm Genome* **9**:485, 1998.

188. Wang YH, Griffith J: Expanded CTG triplet blocks from the myotonic dystrophy gene create the strongest known natural nucleosome positioning elements. *Genomics* **25**:570, 1995.

189. Otten AD, Tapscott SJ: Triplet repeat expansion in myotonic dystrophy alters the adjacent chromatin structure. *Proc Natl Acad Sci U S A* **92**:5465, 1995.

190. Shaw DJ, Chaudhary S, Rundle SA, Crow S, Brook JD, Harper PS, Harley HG: A study of DNA methylation in myotonic dystrophy. *J Med Genet* **30**:189, 1993.

191. Steinbach P, Glaser D, Vogel W, Wolf M, Schwemmle S: The DMPK gene of severely affected myotonic dystrophy patients is hypermethylated proximal to the largely expanded CTG repeat. *Am J Hum Genet* **62**:278, 1998.

192. Whiting EJ, Waring JD, Tamai K, Somerville MJ, Hincke M, Staines WA, Ikeda JE, et al: Characterization of myotonic dystrophy kinase (DMK) protein in human and rodent muscle and central nervous nuclei. *Hum Mol Genet* **4**:1063, 1995.

193. Fu YH, Friedman DL, Richards S, Pearlman JA, Gibbs RA, Pizzuti A, Ashizawa T, et al: Decreased expression of myotonin-protein kinase messenger RNA and protein in adult form of myotonic dystrophy. *Science* **260**:235, 1993.

194. Carango P, Noble JE, Marks HG, Funanage VL: Absence of myotonic dystrophy protein kinase (DMPK) mRNA as a result of a triplet repeat expansion in myotonic dystrophy. *Genomics* **18**:340, 1993.

195. Sabourin LA, Mahadevan MS, Narang M, Lee DSC, Surh LC, Korneluk RG: Effect of the myotonic dystrophy (DM) mutation on mRNA levels of the DM gene. *Nat Genet* **4**:233, 1993.

196. Krahe R, Ashizawa T, Abbruzzese C, Roeder E, Carango P, Giacanelli M, Funanage VL, et al: Effect of myotonic dystrophy trinucleotide repeat expansion on DMPK transcription and processing. *Genomics* **28**:1, 1995.

197. Wang J, Pegoraro E, Menegazzo E, Genarelli M, Hoop RC, Angelini C, Hoffman EP: Myotonic dystrophy: Evidence for a possible dominant-negative RNA mutation. *Hum Mol Genet* **4**:599, 1995.

198. Taneja KL, McCurrach M, Schalling M, Housman D, Singer RHF: Loci of trinucleotide repeat transcripts in nuclei of myotonic dystrophy cells and tissues. *J Cell Biol* **128**:995, 1995.

199. Van der Ven PFM, Jansen G, van Kuppevelt THMSM, Perryman MB, Lupa M, Dunne PW, ter Laak HJ, et al: Myotonic dystrophy kinase is a component of neuromuscular junctions. *Hum Mol Genet* **2**:1889, 1993.

200. Etongue Mayer P, Faure R, Bouchard J-P and Puymirat J: Characterization of a 54-kilodalton human protein kinase recognized

by an antiserum raised against the myotonin kinase. *Muscle Nerve* **21**:8, 1998.

201. Dunne PW, Ma L, Casey DL, Harati Y, Epstein HF: Localization of myotonic dystrophy protein kinase and its alteration with disease. *Cell Motil Cytoskel* **33**:52, 1996.

202. Pham YCN, thi Man N, Lam LT. and Morris GE: Localization of myotonic dystrophy protein kinase in human and rabbit tissues using a new panel of monoclonal antibodies. *Hum Mol Genet* **7**:1957, 1998.

203. Maeda M, Taft CS, Bush EW, Holder E, Bailey WM, Neville H, Perryman MB: Identification, tissue-specific expression and sub-cellular localisation of the 80-kDa and 71-kDa forms of myotonic dystrophy kinase protein. *J Biol Chem* **270**:20246, 1995.

204. Mahadevan MS, Amemiya C, Jansen G, Sabourin L, Baird S, Neville CE, Wormskamp N, et al: Structure and genomic sequence of the myotonic dystrophy (DM kinase) gene. *Hum Mol Genet* **2**:299, 1993.

205. Jansen G, Mahadevan MS, Amemiya C, Wormskamp N, Segers B, Hendriks W, O'Hoy K et al: Characterisation of the myotonic dystrophy region predicts multiple protein isoform-encoding messenger RNAs. *Nat Genet* **1**:261, 1992.

206. Leung T, Chen X, Tan I, Manser E, Lim L: Myotonic dystrophy kinase-related Cdc42-binding kinase acts as a Cdc42 effector in promoting cytoskeletal reorganisation. *Mol Cell Biol* **18**:130, 1998.

207. Moncrieff CL, Bailey MES, Morrison N, Johnson KJ: Cloning and chromosomal localisation of human Cdc42-binding protein kinase beta. *Genomics* **57**:297, 1999.

208. Luo L, Lee T, Tsai L, Tang G, Jan L, Jan YN: Genghis Khan (Gek) as a putative effector for *Drosophila* Cdc42 and regulator of actin polymerization. *Proc Natl Acad Sci U S A* **94**:12963, 1997.

209. Ishizaki T, Maekawa M, Fujisawa K, Okawa K, Iwamatsu A, Fujita A, Watanabe N: The small GTP-binding protein Rho binds to and activates a 160-kDa Ser/Thr protein kinase homologous to myotonic dystrophy kinase. *EMBO J* **15**:1885, 1996.

210. Wissmann A, Ingles I, McGhee JD, Mains PE: *Caenorhaditis elegans* LET-502 is related to Rho-binding kinases and human myotonic dystrophy kinase and interacts genetically with a homolog of the regulatory subunit of smooth muscle myosin phosphatase to affect cell shape. *Genes Dev* **11**:409, 1996.

211. Sabourin LA, Tamai K, Narang MA, Korneluk RG: Overexpression of the 3′-untranslated region of the myotonic dystrophy kinase cDNA inhibits myoblast differentiation in vitro. *J Biol Chem* **272**:29626, 1997.

212. Okoli G, Carey N, Johnson KJ, Watt DJ: Over-expression of the murine myotonic dystrophy protein kinase in the mouse myogenic C2C12 cell line leads to inhibition of terminal differentiation. *Biochem Biophys Res Commun* **246**:905, 1998.

213. Usuki F, Ishiura S, Saitoh N, Sasagawa N, Sorimachi H, Kuzume H, Maruyama K: Expanded CTG repeats in myotonin protein kinase suppresses myogenic differentiation. *Neuroreport* **8**:3749, 1997.

214. Boucher CA, King SK, Carey N, Krahe R, Winchester CL, Rahman S, Creavin T, et al: A novel homeodomain encoding gene is associated with a large CpG island interrupted by the myotonic dystrophy unstable CTG repeat. *Hum Mol Genet* **4**:1919, 1995.

215. Kawakami K, Ohto H, Takizawa T, Saito T: Identification and expression of Six family genes in mouse retina. *FEBS Lett* **393**:259, 1996.

216. Klesert TR, Otten AD, Bird TD, Tapscott SJ: Trinucleotide repeat expansion at the myotonic dystrophy locus reduces expression of DMAHP. *Nat Genet* **16**:402, 1997.

217. Thornton CA, Wymer JP, Simmons Z, McClain C, Moxley RT: III. Expansion of the myotonic dystrophy CTG reduces expression of the flanking DMAHP gene. *Nat Genet* **16**:407, 1997.

218. Ashizawa T, Monckton DG, Vaishnav S, Patel BJ, Voskova A, Caskey CT: Instability of the expanded CTG repeats in the myotonin protein kinase gene in cultured lymphoblastoid cell lines from patients with myotonic dystrophy. *Genomics* **36**:47, 1996.

219. Heath SK, Carne S, Hoyle C, Johnson KJ, Wells DJ: Characterisation of expression of mDMAHP, a homeodomain encoding gene at the murine DM locus. *Hum Mol Genet* **6**:651, 1997.

220. Winchester CL, Ferrier RK, Sermoni A, Clark BJ, Johnson KJ: Characterization of expression of DMPK and SIX5 in the human eye and implications for pathogenesis in myotonic dystrophy. *Hum Mol Genet* **8**:481, 1999.

221. Murakami Y, Ohto H, Ikeda U, Shimada K, Momoi T, Kawakami K: Promoter of mDMAHP/Six5: Differential utilization of multiple transcription initiation sites and positive/negative regulatory elements. *Hum Mol Genet* **7**:2103, 1998.

222. Engelkamp D, van Heyningen V: Transcription factors in disease. *Curr Opin Genet Dev* **6**:334, 1996, 342.

223. Dubnau J, Struhl G: RNA recognition and translational regulation by a homeodomain protein. *Nature* **379**:694, 1996, 699.

224. Spitz F, Demignon J, Porteu A, Kahn A, Concordet J-P, Daegelen D, Maire P: Expression of myogenin during embryogenesis is controlled by Six/sine oculus homeoproteins through a conserved MEF3 binding site. *Proc Natl Acad Sci U S A* **95**:14220, 1998.

224a. Kawakami K, Ohoto H, Ikeda K, Roeder RG: Structure, function and expression of a murine homeobox protein arec3, a homolog of *Drosophila* sine oculus gene product and implication in development. *Nucleic Acids Res* **24**:303, 1999.

225. Harris SE, Winchester CL, Johnson J: Functional analysis of the homeodomain protein SIX5. *Nucleic Acids Res* **28**:1871, 2000.

226. Salminen M, Lopez S, Maire P, Kahn A, Dagelen D: Fast-muscle-specific DNA-protein interactions occurring in vivo at the human aldolase A M promoter are necessary for correct promoter activity in transgenic mice. *Mol Cell Biol* **16**:76, 1996.

227. Benders AAGM, Timmermans JAH, Oosterhof A, Ter Lakk HJ, van Kuppevelt THMSM, Wevers RA and Veerkamp JH: Deficiency of Na$^+$/K$^+$-ATPase and sarcoplasmic reticulum Ca$^{2+}$-ATPase in skeletal muscle and cultured muscle cells of myotonic dystrophy patients. *Biochem J* **293**:269, 1993.

228. Damiani E, Angelini C, Pelosi M, Sacchetto R, Bortoloso E, Margreth A: Skeletal muscle sarcoplasmic reticulum phenotype in myotonic dystrophy. *Neuromuscul Disord* **6**:33, 1996.

229. Renaud JF, Desnuelle C, Schmidantomarchi H, Hughes M, Serratrice G, Lazdunski M: Expression of apamin receptor in muscles of patients with myotonic muscular dystrophy. *Nature* **319**:678, 1986.

230. Walsh FS, Moore SE, Dickson JG: Expression of membrane antigens in myotonic dystrophy. *J Neurol Neurosurg Psychiatry* **51**:136, 1988.

231. Jansen G, Bachner D, Coerwinkel M, Wormskam N, Hameister H, Wieringa B: Structural organisation and developmental expression pattern of the mouse WD-repeat gene DMR-N9 immediately upstream of the myotonic dystrophy locus. *Hum Mol Genet* **4**:843, 1995.

232. Shaw DJ, McCurrach M, Rundl, SA, Harley HG, Crow SR, Sohn R, Thirion JP, et al: Genomic organisation and transcriptional units at the myotonic dystrophy locus. *Genomics* **18**:673, 1993.

233. Brown JC, Mutt V, Penderson RA: Further purification of a polypeptide demonstrating enterogastrone activity. *J Physiol* **209**:57, 1970.

234. Timchenko LT: Human genetics '99: Trinucleotide repeats. Myotonic dystrophy: The role of RNA CUG triplet repeats. *Am J Hum Genet* **64**:360, 1999.

235. Timchenko LT, Timchenko NA, Caskey, CT, Roberts R: Novel proteins with binding specificity for DNA CTG and RNA CUG repeats: Implications for myotonic dystrophy. *Hum Mol Genet* **5**:115, 1996.

236. Timchenko LT, Miller JW, Timchenko NA, DeVore DR, Datar KV, Lin L, Roberts R et al: Identification of a (CUG)n triplet repeat RNA-binding protein and its expression in myotonic dystrophy. *Nucleic Acids Res* **24**:4407, 1996.

237. Caskey CT, Swanson MS, Timchenko LT: Myotonic dystrophy: Discussion of molecular mechanism. *Cold Spring Harbor Symp Quant Biol* **61**:607, 1996.

238. Bell LR, Horabin JI, Scedl P, Cline TW: Positive autoregulation of sex—Lethal by alternative splicing maintains the female determined state in *Drosophila*. *Cell* **65**:229, 1991.

239. Levine TD, Gao F, King PH, Andrews LG, Keene JD: Hel-N1: An autoimmune RNA-binding protein with specificity for 3′ uridylate-rich untranslated regions of growth factor mRNAs. *Mol Cell Biol* **13**:3494, 1993.

240. Myer VE, Fan XC, Steitz JA: Identification of HuR as a protein implicated in AUUUA-mediated mRNA decay. *EMBO J* **16**:2130, 1997.

241. Philips AV, Timchenko LT, Cooper TA: Disruption of splicing regulated by a CUG-binding protein in myotonic dystrophy. *Science* **280**:737, 1998.

242. Roberts R, Timchenko NA, Miller JW, Reddy S, Caskey CT, Swanson MS, Timchenko LT: Altered phosphorylation and intracellular distribution of a (CUG)n triplet repeat RNA-binding protein inpatients with myotonic dystrophy and in myotonic protein kinase knock out mice. *Proc Natl Acad Sci U S A* **94**:13221, 1997.

243. Bhagwati S, Ghatpande A, Leung B: Identification of two nuclear proteins which bind to RNA CUG repeats: Significance for myotonic dystrophy. *Biochem Biophys Res Commun* **228**:55, 1996.

244. Lu X, Timchenko NA, Timchenko LT: Cardiac elav-type RNA-binding protein (ETR-3) binds to RNA CUG triplet repeats expanded in myotonic dystrophy. *Hum Mol Genet* **8**:53, 1999.

244a. Klesert TR, Cho DH, Clark JI, Maylie J, Adelman J, Snider L, Yuen EC, Soriano P, Tapscott SJ: Mice deficient in SIX5 develop cataracts: Implications for myotonic dystrophy. *Nat Genet* **25**:105, 2000.

244b. Sarkar PS, Appukuttan B, Han J, Ito Y, Ai C, Tsai W, Cai Y, Stout JT, Reddy S: Heterozygous loss of Six5 in mice is sufficient to cause ocular cataracts. *Nat Genet* **25**:10, 2000.

245. Dunne PW, Ma L, Casey DL, Epstein HF: Myotonic protein kinase expression in human and bovine lenses. *Biochem Biophys Res Commun* **225**:281, 1996.

246. Norman AM, Floyd JL, Meredith AL, Harper PS: Presymptomatic detection and prenatal diagnosis for myotonic dystrophy. *J Med Genet* **26(12)**:750, 1989.

247. Smeets HJ, Brunner HG, Ropers HH, Wieringa B: Use of variable simple sequence motifs as genetic markers: Application to study of myotonic dystrophy. *Hum Genet* **83(3)**:245, 1989.

248. Speer MC, Pericak-Vance MA, Yamaoka L, Hung WY, Ashley A, Stajich JM, Roses AD: Presymptomatic and prenatal diagnosis in myotonic dystrophy by genetic linkage studies. *Neurology* **40(4)**:671, 1990.

249. MacMillan JC, Myring J, Harley HG, Reardon W, Harper PS, Shaw DJ: Molecular analysis for the myotonic dystrophy mutation in neuromuscular. *Neuromuscul Disord* **2(5–6)**:405, 1992.

250. Shelbourne P, Davies J, Buxton J, Anvret M, Blennow E, Bonduelle M, Schmedding E, Glass I, Lindenbaum R, Lane R, et al: Direct diagnosis of myotonic dystrophy with a disease-specific DNA marker. *N Engl J Med* **328(7)**:471, 1993.

251. Barnes PR, Hilton-Jones D, Norbury G, Roberts A, Huson SM: Incorrect diagnosis of myotonic dystrophy and its potential consequences revealed by subsequent direct genetic-analysis. *J Neurol Neurosurg Psychiatry* **57(5)**:662, 1994.

252. Reardon W, Harley HG, Brook JD, et al: Minimal expression of myotonic dystrophy: A clinical and molecular analysis. *J Med Genet* **29**:770, 1992.

253. Advisory Committee for Genetic Testing for Late Onset Disorders. London, Department of Health, 1998.

254. Reardon W, Floyd JL, Myring J, Lazarou LP, Meredith AL, Harper PS: Five years experience of predictive testing for myotonic dystrophy. *Am J Med Genet* **43(6)**:1006, 1992.

255. Harper PS, Bias WB, Hutchinson JR, McKusick VA. ABH secretor status of the fetus: A genetic marker identifiable by amniocentesis. *J Med Genet* **8**:438, 1971.

256. Myring J, Meredith AL, Harley HG, Kohn G, Norbury G, Harper PS, Shaw DJ: Specific molecular prenatal diagnosis for the CTG mutation in myotonic dystrophy. *J Med Genet* **29(11)**:785, 1992.

257. Smeets HJ, Nillesen WM, Los F, Busch HF, Korneluk RG, Wieringa B, Brunner HG: Prenatal diagnosis of myotonic dystrophy by direct mutation analysis. *Lancet* **340(8813)**:237, 1992.

258. Daniels R, Holding C, Kontogianni E, Monk M: Single-cell analysis of unstable genes. *J Assist Reprod Genet* **13(2)**:163, 1996.

259. Sermon K, Lissens W, Joris H, Seneca S, Desmyttere S, Devroey P, Van Steirteghem A, Liebaers I: Clinical application of preimplantation diagnosis for myotonic dystrophy. *Prenat Diagn* **17(10)**:925, 1997.

260. Reardon W, Macmillan JC, Myring J, Harley HG, et al: Cataract and myotonic dystrophy: The role of molecular diagnosis. *Br J Ophthalmol* **77**:579, 1993.

261. Warner JP, Barron LH, Goudie D, Kelly K, Dow D, Fitzpatrick DR, Brock DJ: A general method for the detection of large CAG repeat expansions by fluorescent PCR. *J Med Genet* **33(12)**:1022, 1996.

262. Cheng S, Barcelo JM, Korneluk RG: Characterization of large CTG repeat expansions in myotonic dystrophy alleles using PCR. *Hum Mutat* **7(4)**:304, 1996.

263. Lynas MA: Dystrophia myotonica, with special reference to Northern Ireland. *Ann Hum Genet* **21**:318, 1957.

264. MacMillan JC, Harper PS: Single-gene neurological disorders in South-Wales: An epidemiological study. *Ann Neurol* **30**:411, 1991.

265. Pinessi L, Bergamini L, Cantello R, Di Tizio C: Myotonia congenita and myotonic dystrophy: Descriptive epidemiological investigation in Turin, Italy (1955–1979). *Ital J Neurol Sci* **3**:207, 1982.

266. Grimm T: Thesis. University of Gottingen. 1975.

267. Medica I, Markovic D, Peterlin B: Genetic epidemiology of myotonic dystrophy in Istria, Croatia. *Acta Neurol Scand* **95**:164, 1997.

268. Kurland LT: Descriptive epidemiology of selected neurologic and myopathic disorders with particular reference to a survey in Rochester, Minnesota. *J Chronic Dis* **8**:378, 1958.

269. Takeshita K, Tanaka K, Makashima T, Kasagi S: Survey of patients with early onset myotonic dystrophy in the San-In district, Japan. *Jpn J Hum Genet* **26**:295, 1981.

270. Vlachopapadopoulou E, Zachwieja J, Gertner JM, Manzioe D, Bier DM, Matthews DE, Slonim AE: Metabolic and clinical response to recombinant insulin-like growth factor I in myotonic dystrophy. *J Clin Endocrin Metab* **80**:3715, 1995.

# LUNG

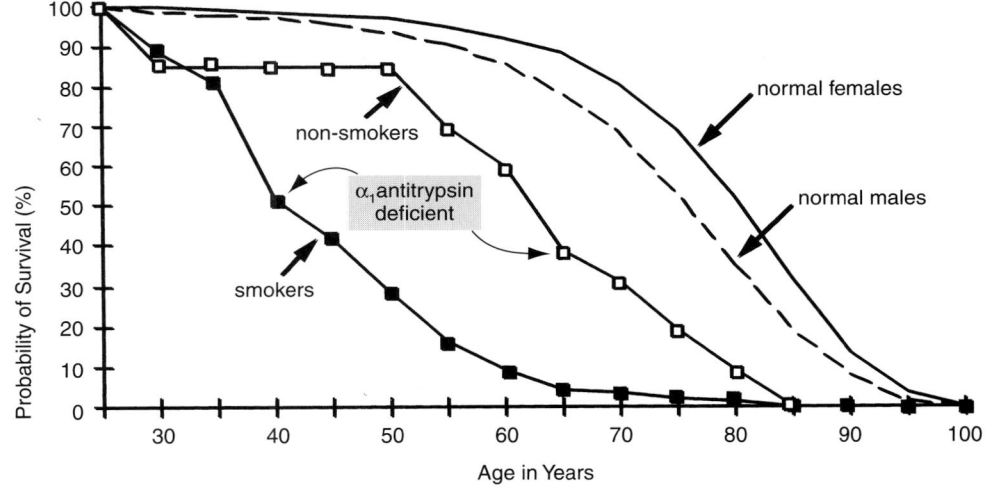

# Hereditary Surfactant Protein B Deficiency

*Jeffrey A. Whitsett ■ Lawrence M. Nogee*

Postnatal adaptation to air breathing necessitates the reduction of surface tension at the air-liquid interface in the alveoli of the lung. The rapid spreading and stability of phospholipids in pulmonary surfactant are mediated by the activity of two hydrophobic proteins, surfactant proteins B and C (SP-B and -C). Deficiency of surfactant proteins is associated with respiratory distress syndrome (RDS) in premature newborn infants, and in adults with adult respiratory distress syndrome (ARDS). While most surfactant deficiencies are secondary to prematurity or lung injury and infection, hereditary surfactant protein B deficiency, caused by mutations in the surfactant protein B gene, was recently identified as an inherited cause of respiratory failure in full-term newborn infants. This chapter describes the pathophysiology and molecular biology of hereditary SP-B deficiency.

## STRUCTURE AND FUNCTION OF SURFACTANT PROTEINS

SP-B, a 79-amino-acid amphipathic polypeptide isolated from pulmonary surfactant, is one of four distinct proteins (SP-A, SP-B, SP-C, and SP-D) that are closely associated with surfactant in the airways. SP-A and SP-D are larger, more hydrophilic proteins, and members of the collectin family of calcium-dependent, C-type mammalian lectins (see reference 1 for review). SP-A and SP-D are encoded in a gene cluster containing several ancestrally related mammalian lectins on human chromosome 10 (922 to 923).[2] Increasing evidence from gene-targeted mice demonstrates a primary role of SP-A ($M_r = 32,000-36,000$) in host defense.[3] SP-A binds and enhances both phagocytosis and killing of various viral and bacterial pathogens (see reference 4 for review). SP-D ($M_r = 43,000$) shares structural features with SP-A and binds various viruses, bacteria, and fungi.[5] Evidence from SP-D gene-targeted mice demonstrated a primary role in the regulation of surfactant lipid concentrations.[6,7] SP-D gene-targeted SP-D $-/-$ mice also develop emphysema.[6]

SP-B and SP-C are distinct and structurally unrelated proteins encoded by genes on human chromosome 2 and 8, respectively.[8,9] Both hydrophobic proteins were isolated and identified in organic solvent extracts of pulmonary surfactant, and are the major, if not sole, surface active proteins in mammalian surfactant replacement preparations presently used to treat RDS and ARDS in clinical practice. SP-C is a 33- to 34-amino-acid, extremely hydrophobic polypeptide that is produced from a preproprotein of 21,000 to 22,000 daltons.[10] The active SP-C peptide is produced only in type II epithelial cells in the lung, and is stored and secreted with surfactant phospholipids and SP-B into the alveolus. SP-C enhances the rate of spreading and stability of phospholipids

during the respiratory cycle and is the primary protein component in surfactant replacement preparations such as Survanta® and Curosurf.® While selected deficiency of SP-C has been observed in a number of term infants with respiratory failure,[11] a genetic basis of SP-C-related pulmonary disease has not yet been identified.

## BIOSYNTHESIS OF SP-B

The 79-amino-acid active SP-B peptide is produced by proteolytic processing of a 381-amino-acid precursor protein (see references 12 and 13 for review). While proSP-B is expressed in both nonciliated respiratory epithelial and type II alveolar epithelial cells, proteolytic processing of the active peptide occurs only in type II cells in the alveoli. The SP-B gene is encoded by approximately 10 kb of DNA, located on human chromosome 2p12-2p11.2, at a locus termed sftp3. The SP-B gene consists of 11 exons that are processed to a 1.9- to 2.0-kb mRNA in both bronchiolar and alveolar cells.[8] The active SP-B peptide is encoded by exons 6 and 7, and regions in both the active peptide and flanking domains of the proprotein share structural similarities to the prosaposin genes that are involved in lipid metabolism in other tissues. SP-B mRNA and proprotein are detected in human lung as early as 12 to 15 weeks of gestation, and increase dramatically in the immediate prenatal and perinatal period of development, being expressed primarily by type II epithelial cells and nonciliated bronchiolar cells in the postnatal lung. SP-B concentrations increase in amniotic fluid in association with other indices of pulmonary maturation, including the lecithin to sphingomyelin (L/S) ratio, phospholipid content, and surfactant protein A; the absence of SP-B in amniotic fluid in clinical samples is associated with increased risk for respiratory distress syndrome in preterm infants.[14] SP-B concentration in alveolar lavage fluid is relatively low in adults with adult respiratory distress syndrome (ARDS).[15]

The SP-B gene is regulated at both transcriptional and posttranscriptional levels (see reference 13 for review). SP-B mRNA content is stimulated by glucocorticoids, cAMP, and interleukin-1β (IL-1β), and inhibited by tumor necrosis factor-α (TNF-α) and transforming growth factor-β (TGF-β). At the transcriptional level, SP-B gene transcription is regulated by the interaction of both cell selective and more general transcription factors that bind to cis-acting elements in the 5′ flanking region of the SP-B gene. Lung-specific gene expression requires the activity of several transcription factors, including a homeodomain protein of the Nkx2.1 family, termed thyroid transcription factor-1 (TTF-1), and hepatocyte nuclear factor-3β (HNF-3β).[16] SP-B gene expression requires the activity of both transcription factors. TTF-1 also regulates transcriptional activity of other lung epithelial-specific genes, including surfactant proteins A and C and CCSP (Clara cell secretory protein). HNF-3β and AP-1 family members, including jun-D, as well as NF1 (nuclear factor 1) family members bind to the 5′ flanking region of the SP-B gene,

A list of standard abbreviations is located immediately preceding the index in each volume. Additional abbreviations used in this chapter include: BAL = bronchoal-veolar lavage; IL = interleukin; L/S ratio = lecithin to sphingomyelin ratio; MVB = multivesicular body; PG = phosphatidylglycerol; SP =surfactant protein; TNF = tumor necrosis factor; TGF = transforming growth factor.

and activate SP-B gene transcription. The activity of TTF-1 on SP-B transcription is further enhanced by its phosphorylation by cAMP-dependent protein kinase.[17] At the posttranscriptional level, SP-B mRNA is stabilized by glucocorticoids and destabilized by phorbol esters and TNF-α, which is likely related to changes in mRNA stability, mediated, at least in part, by actions of protein on the 3' untranslated region of the SP-B mRNA.[18]

## ROUTING, PROCESSING, AND TURNOVER OF SP-B

The SP-B mRNA encodes a 381-amino-acid proprotein, that includes an amino-terminal 22-amino-acid hydrophobic leader sequence removed during transport in the ER. ProSP-B is glycosylated and trafficked with proSP-C through the Golgi apparatus and is processed by distinct proteolytic steps, forming intermediates of 26 kDa that contain the 8.7-kDa active SP-B peptide (residues 201 to 279) and a C-terminal domain (residues 279 to 381) (see reference 19 for review). The proSP-B peptide is present in ER, Golgi, and multivesicular bodies. Proteolytic

processing to the active SP-B peptide likely occurs late in the biosynthetic pathway, during transit from the multivesicular body to the lamellar bodies. Surfactant phospholipids and surfactant proteins B and C are stored in lamellar bodies and secreted into the air space by type II epithelial cells (Fig. 218-1). The active SP-B peptide is secreted into the alveolus in association with phospholipids and associated with tubular myelin. SP-B moves to monolayers and bilayers of phospholipids at the air-liquid interface, where it enhances the rate of adsorption and stability during compression of phospholipids in surfactant. SP-B is cleared from the alveolus and recycled by type II epithelial cells and is also catabolized by the activity of alveolar macrophages. Clearance of SP-B from the airspace is similar to that of SP-A and phospholipids, being cleared from the lung with a half-life of approximately 12 h in mice.[20] A primary role of the alveolar macrophage in surfactant lipid and protein clearance was recently demonstrated in mice lacking GM-CSF (granulocyte-macrophage colony-stimulating factor) or the common β-chain of the GM-CSF receptor.[21,22] Surfactant proteins A, B, C, and D, as well as surfactant phospholipids, accumulated to large concentrations in

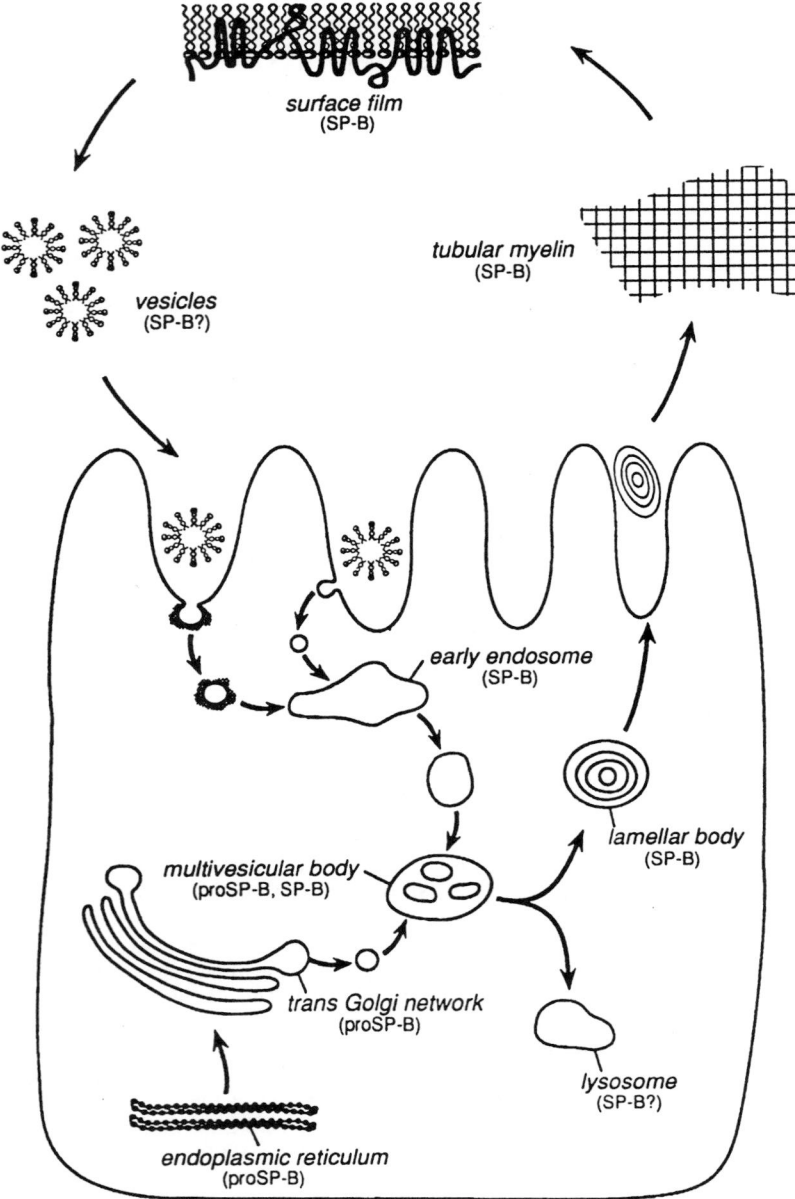

Fig. 218-1 Biosynthesis and trafficking of proSP-B and SP-B. ProSP-B is glycosylated and proteolytically processed to remove the leader sequence in the endoplasmic reticulum of type II cells. The SP-B proprotein is transported with proSP-C through the RER and Golgi to multivesicular bodies. Further proteolytic processing of proSP-B occurs during transit from multivesicular bodies to lamellar bodies, the phospholipid-rich storage organelle containing active SP-B (79 aa) and SP-C. ProSP-B is also required for correct processing of proSP-C. The active SP-B and SP-C protein are secreted into the alveolus and are associated with tubular myelin and the surfactant film that reduces surface tension at the air-liquid interface. Surfactant lipids, SP-B and SP-C, are taken up by type II cells and recycled or catabolized. Alveolar macrophages also play an important role in SP-B catabolism.

GM-CSF or GM-CSF receptor-deficient mice, causing a syndrome similar to pulmonary alveolar proteinosis in humans. Recent studies support the likelihood that defects in GM-CSF signaling are also involved in the pathogenesis of alveolar proteinosis in humans.[23]

## FUNCTIONS OF SP-B IN VIVO

Recently targeted ablation of the SP-B gene in transgenic mice provided insight into the role of SP-B in lung function and surfactant homeostasis in vivo.[24] While heterozygous SP-B +/− deficient mice survive postnatally, homozygous SP-B −/− mice died of respiratory failure in the immediate postnatal period. Abnormalities in the SP-B −/− mice were confined to the lung. While structurally normal at the light microscopic level, lungs of SP-B −/− mice failed to inflate after birth, the animals dying from a respiratory distress-like syndrome, with pathology similar to that seen in preterm infants with RDS. Lung lipid synthesis and content were unaffected in SP-B −/− mice; however, surfactant protein B and proSP-B were absent, and surfactant protein C was misprocessed to an aberrant, secreted form of approximately 12 kDa that consists of the $NH_2$-terminal domain and active SP-C peptide.[25] Thus, SP-B −/− mice are deficient in both SP-B protein intermediates and the active SP-B peptide, and are also deficient in active SP-C. At the electron microscopic level, lungs of SP-B −/− mice lack both lamellar bodies and tubular myelin. Type II epithelial cells contain abnormally large multivesicular bodies that failed to undergo fusion to form lamellar bodies (Fig. 218-2). Pressure-volume curves of newborn SP-B −/− mice demonstrated low lung volumes, lack of hysteresis, and loss of residual volume, consistent with the lack of surfactant function, typical of humans with RDS.[26] SP-B −/− mice have been corrected genetically by the expression of proSP-B in type II epithelial cells, but not by its expression in Clara cells.[27] Repletion of SP-B −/− mice with a proSP-B construct consisting of the active SP-B peptide, but lacking the C-terminal domain of the SP-B proprotein, corrected respiratory failure but caused a marked accumulation of surfactant lipids in the form of lamellar bodies in type II cells, supporting the concept that the C-terminal domain of SP-B plays an important role in the regulation of lipid synthesis and storage during lamellar body biogenesis.[28]

## HETEROZYGOTE SP-B +/− MICE ARE SUSCEPTIBLE TO LUNG INJURY

Lungs from SP-B +/− mice express 50 percent of the wild-type SP-B mRNA with resultant 50 percent reduction in SP-B content in the alveolus.[29] Mild air-trapping and decreased lung compliance were observed during pulmonary function testing of adult SP-B +/− mice. However, when SP-B +/− mice were exposed to hyperoxia, pulmonary compliance was markedly impaired. In addition, alveolar capillary leak was markedly increased and intratracheal administration of SP-B with surfactant phospholipids corrected the susceptibility of SP-B +/− mice to hyperoxia.[30] Thus, even a 50 percent reduction in SP-B concentrations in the alveolus causes susceptibility to lung injury in vivo. Because SP-B concentrations are reduced in preterm infants with RDS and in adults with ARDS, preexisting deficiency or secondary reduction in SP-B may exacerbate pulmonary dysfunction in a variety of respiratory disorders.

## HEREDITARY SP-B DEFICIENCY

The disorder was first recognized in a family in which three of six siblings succumbed to respiratory failure in the newborn period, all of whom had a selective absence of SP-B in their lung tissue as demonstrated by immunologic methods. Since its initial recognition in 1993, more than 80 term infants have been identified with respiratory failure caused by surfactant protein B deficiency. The disease was inherited in an autosomal recessive fashion, and the lack of SP-B protein in the initial kindred was caused by a

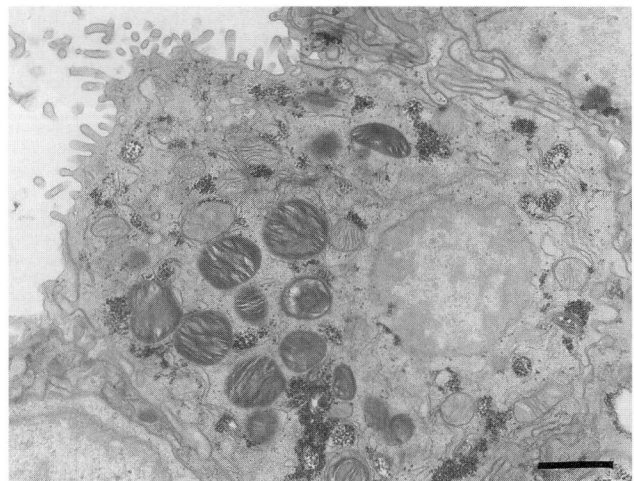
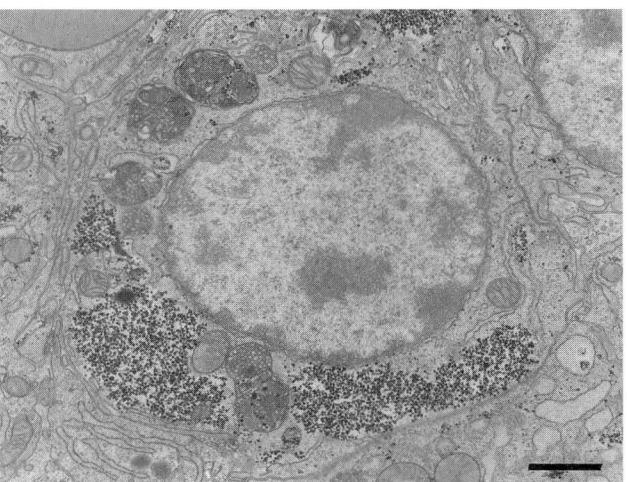

**Fig. 218-2** Ultrastructure of type II epithelial cells from normal and SP-B −/− newborn mice. Numerous lamellar bodies are located within the cytoplasm of type II cells in the normal lung (*top panel*). In contrast, lamellar bodies are absent in type II cells from SP-B-deficient mice (*bottom panel*). Large, lipid-rich, multivesicular bodies (MVB) are observed in SP-B −/− mice, demonstrating that proSP-B is required for formation of the multilamellar structures generated by fusion of lipid vesicles in the MVB. Magnification bar: 1 μM × 8000. (*Courtesy of Drs. C-L. Na and T.E. Weaver, Children's Hospital Medical Center, Cincinnati, OH.*)

substitution of three nucleotides (GAA) for a single nucleotide (C) in codon 121 of the SP-B mRNA, referred to as 121ins2. The 121ins2 mutation results in a frameshift and introduction of a premature signal for the termination of translation, and produces unstable SP-B mRNA, which is undetectable by northern blot analysis. SP-B proprotein and active peptide are undetectable in infants with the 121ins2 mutation, which is the most common mutant allele found in clinical sampling. At present, at least 22 distinct mutations, resulting in a variety of substitutions in the SP-B gene, including single-base substitutions, and in-frame deletions and insertions, are associated with clinical disease[33] (Fig. 218-3 and Table 218-1). Major deletions of the SP-B gene have not been observed to date.

## CLINICAL DIAGNOSIS

Infants affected by hereditary SP-B deficiency generally reach full term and present with respiratory distress within the first 24 h of life (Table 218-2). While the initial severity of respiratory disease

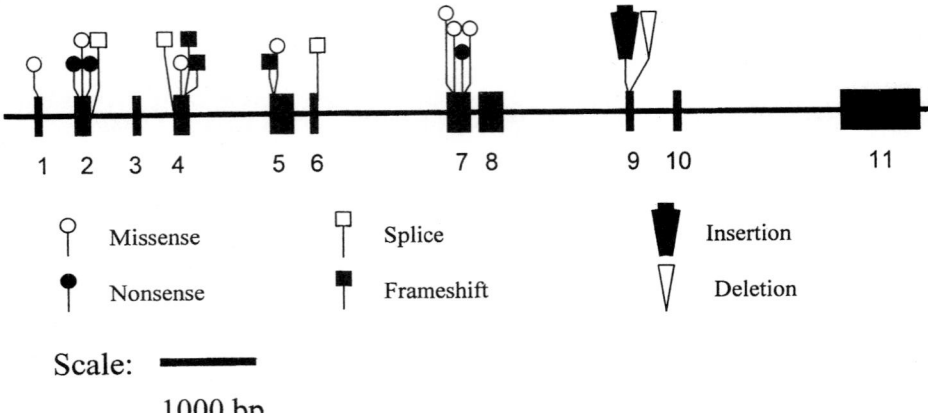

Fig. 218-3 Mutations in the human SP-B gene. The human gene consists of 11 exons, spanning approximately 10 kb on human chromosome 2. Sites of known mutations associated with respiratory disease in newborns are demarcated within exons or at splice junctions. The active SP-B peptide is encoded by exons 6 and 7.

has been variable, the degree of respiratory dysfunction usually requires ventilatory support within the first week of life. Infants typically have radiologic features consistent with RDS, lacking localized infiltrates or radiologic features of meconium aspiration. The course is often complicated by pulmonary hypertension and is often mistaken for sepsis. Replacement with exogenous surfactant preparations, including those with and without significant quantities of SP-B, usually result in only transient improvement, and have not changed the unremitting course of respiratory failure in these infants.[34] Infants with hereditary SP-B deficiency generally succumb to respiratory failure despite aggressive support with high-frequency or conventional ventilation, surfactant replacement, and extracorporeal membrane oxygenation (ECMO). The natural history includes death from respiratory disease in the first months of life, despite aggressive support. The diagnosis of hereditary SP-B deficiency may be suspected based on the typical presentation of a full-term infant with unexplained respiratory distress and a history of a previous sibling who died from neonatal respiratory disease. However, the clinical symptoms and radiographic findings are not specific, and

definitive diagnosis requires laboratory confirmation, including analysis of lung secretions (bronchoalveolar lavage [BAL] or tracheal aspirate), lung tissue, or DNA from the patient. Accurate diagnosis is essential in order to plan appropriate treatment decisions (including withdrawal of support) and to counsel parents properly regarding recurrence risk.

Lung fluid from patients with SP-B deficiency generally lacks the SP-B active peptide, as assessed by ELISA or western blot analysis, but contains abundant concentrations of surfactant protein A and aberrantly processed forms of proSP-C. These proSP-C fragments ($M_r = 9000$ to 12,000 daltons) have not been detected in normal lung tissue or observed in other clinical settings, but have been present in lungs of all patients with confirmed hereditary SP-B deficiency. Studies on phospholipid profiles of infants with hereditary SP-B deficiency are limited. Abnormalities in surfactant lipid content were observed in an infant with hereditary SP-B deficiency identified prior to birth.[34] The L/S ratio was <1.0, phosphatidylglycerol (PG) was absent, and the absence of SP-B and presence of aberrantly processed SP-C peptides were observed in amniotic fluid. In general, lung fluid from affected infants has also been deficient in PG.

If lung tissue is available, the diagnosis of SP-B deficiency may be suspected from findings of alveolar proteinosis. Distal lung spaces are often distended with granular-appearing eosinophilic proteinaceous material that stains positively with PAS reagent and contains desquamated cells and macrophages trapped within the proteinaceous debris. However, changes of alveolar proteinosis are not specific for hereditary SP-B deficiency. Similarly, findings typical of infants with severe respiratory distress treated by chronic ventilation, such as bronchopulmonary dysplasia and interstitial fibrosis, are frequently seen. Immunohistochemical

**Table 218-1 Sites and Consequences of Mutations Causing Hereditary SP-B Deficiency**

| Mutations | Effect |
|---|---|
| 121ins2 (C → GAA) | frameshift, termination |
| W39X | stop |
| W60X | stop |
| c.379delT | frameshift |
| c.415insAA | frameshift |
| c.209 + 4A → G | frameshift (skip exon 2) |
| C248X | stop |
| c.282-2delA | skip exon 4 |
| c.696G → A | splicing |
| L13P | Leu → Pro |
| C100G | Cys → Gly |
| C49R | Cys → Arg |
| C235R | Cys → Arg |
| R252C | Arg → Cys |
| c.1043ins3 (CCG) | insert Pro |
| c.1048del12 | delete Gln-Leu-Leu-Thr |
| c.147delC | frameshift |
| c.378delC | frameshift |
| c.479G → T | |

NOTE: In the left column, a lower case "c" before a number represents the codon position in the cDNA.

**Table 218-2 Clinical Characteristics and Laboratory Findings in Hereditary SP-B Deficiency**

Clinical
  Full-term infant with severe idiopathic RDS
  Refractory to conventional therapy
  Autosomal recessive inheritance
  Family history of neonatal lung disease

Laboratory Findings
  Absent or decreased alveolar (lung fluid) SP-B
  Alveolar protein accumulation—SP-A, aberrant proSP-C
  Pulmonary alveolar proteinosis appearance
  Absent or decreased proSP-B in alveolar type II cells
  Absent lamellar bodies and tubular myelin
  Mutations in the SP-B gene

staining for the surfactant protein allows for definitive diagnosis. Staining for mature SP-B is absent or markedly reduced, while staining for SP-A and proSP-C is robust. In particular, extracellular staining for proSP-C has correlated with the presence of aberrantly processed SP-C peptides, and has been a reliable indicator of hereditary SP-B deficiency. Staining for proSP-B is more variable, depending on the particular mutation(s) responsible for disease. At the ultrastructural level, tubular myelin in the air spaces and lamellar bodies within type II epithelial cells are entirely lacking in lungs from SP-B-deficient patients.[35] While the lack of lamellar bodies and the presence of enlarged multivesicular bodies appear to be characteristic of hereditary SP-B deficiency, the utility of ultrastructural analyses in the diagnosis has not been rigorously sevaluated.

DNA analysis allows for precise identification of SP-B mutant alleles, and has been useful for diagnosis, counseling, and making treatment decisions. The finding of a common mutation accounting for almost 70 percent of the mutant alleles identified to date, in conjunction with the low frequency of this allele in the population, make genetic diagnosis feasible. However, because at least 20 other mutations have been identified, the majority of which have only been found in one kindred, the sensitivity of genetic testing is limited.

## GENETICS OF HEREDITARY SP-B DEFICIENCY

The 121ins2 mutation, a frameshift mutation in exon 4, is recognized as the most common mutation causing respiratory failure in infants with hereditary SP-B deficiency. Analysis of DNA from more than 40 patients demonstrates that the 121ins2 accounts for approximately two-thirds of mutant alleles.[36] Approximately 50 percent of affected infants were homozygous for the 121ins2, 30 percent were heterozygous for the 121ins2 and another mutation, and the remainder of infants with hereditary SP-B deficiency were homozygous for distinct mutations (Nogee et al., unpublished observations). At present, 22 mutant alleles have been identified in infants with respiratory failure caused by SP-B deficiency (Fig. 218-3 and Table 218-1). In all cases identified to date, the mutant alleles were inherited in an autosomal recessive fashion. The mechanism for a common mutation is not known. The occurrence of this mutation arising *de novo* has not been reported, and most of the patients with this mutation have been of northern European descent, supporting the hypothesis of a common ancestral origin to account for the finding of a common mutation. However, at least two other frameshift mutations (c.378delC, c.379delT) (the lower case "c" before the number represents the codon position in the cDNA) have been identified within 5 bases of the location of the 121ins2 mutation, suggesting that this region of the SP-B gene may be particularly susceptible to mutation.

Most of the mutations in the SP-B gene identified to date are frameshift and nonsense mutations resulting in the lack of SP-B mRNA, SP-B proprotein, and the active SP-B peptide. However, mutations have been identified that caused single amino acid substitutions and in-frame deletions or insertions, and resulted in production of proSP-B or small amounts of mature SP-B peptides that have been identified immunohistochemically or by western blot analysis. While complete absence of SP-B causes severe pulmonary disease, several infants with mutations leading to reduced or dysfunctional SP-B have been identified who had somewhat milder clinical disease.[37,38] The amount of SP-B in lung tissue of these infants was <10 percent of that observed in control tissues, and this partial deficiency of SP-B resulted from single amino acid substitutions. The production of aberrantly processed proSP-C peptides, as detected by immunohistochemistry or by western blot of lung tissue or bronchoalveolar lavage material, is associated with all mutations causing hereditary SP-B deficiency studied to date. The amount of aberrantly processed SP-C peptides may vary inversely with the amounts of mature SP-B peptides produced.

While the typical clinical syndrome of SP-B deficiency has been inherited in an autosomal recessive fashion, at least one infant with a transient deficiency of SP-B associated with a missense mutation on his maternally inherited SP-B allele has been reported. This infant initially had undetectable levels of SP-B in BAL fluid that increased as his lung function and clinical status improved. No clear disease-causing mutations were identified on the paternally derived allele, although it remains possible that this allele contained a mutation important for proper SP-B regulation of expression. In general, carriers for one abnormal SP-B allele have not had lung disease by history, and, in a recent study, adult carriers of the 121ins2 mutation did not have pulmonary function tests that differed from a control population,[39] although the number of patients studied was small. However, given the observations that heterozygous SP-B-deficient mice have half-normal levels of SP-B mRNA and protein, and that 8 percent of mature SP-B was insufficient to prevent fatal lung disease in a human infant, it is likely that there is a critical level of SP-B expression needed for proper lung function. The susceptibility of the heterozygous SP-B-deficient mice to oxygen toxicity, and the finding of transient disease in a human infant heterozygous for an SP-B gene mutation, support the notion that carrying even one abnormal SP-B allele could predispose an individual to lung disease in situations associated with reduced SP-B expression, such as premature birth or infection.

At present, the frequency of SP-B mutations in the general population is unknown, but is likely to be relatively rare. While hereditary SP-B is presently the most common genetic cause of respiratory failure in term newborn infants, the clinical syndrome is relatively rare. DNA testing using DNA from affected individuals, parents, and siblings has been used for the diagnosis of hereditary SP-B deficiency, and the detection of the 121isn2 mutation has been useful in prenatal and postnatal diagnosis. The use of PCR and restriction analysis for a unique restriction site in the SP-B gene introduced by the 121ins2 mutation may allow for rapid, specific, and noninvasive diagnoses of affected infants, allowing for appropriate treatment decisions. However, the heterogeneity of mutant SP-B alleles limits the sensitivity of prenatal and postnatal genetic screening for the disease. Several polymorphisms, both in coding and noncoding sequences in the SP-B gene, have been described that are not clearly directly related to pulmonary disease. It is, at present, unknown whether these polymorphisms may contribute to or help identify susceptibility to pulmonary disease.[40]

## THERAPY OF HEREDITARY SP-B DEFICIENCY

Without aggressive respiratory support SP-B deficiency is rapidly fatal, and has generally resulted in death in the first months of life even with aggressive respiratory support. Infants with hereditary SP-B deficiency die from respiratory failure, bronchopulmonary dysplasia, and pulmonary hypertension. Some SP-B-deficient infants have improved with administration of glucocorticoids, which may augment SP-B production. Such treatment seems most likely to benefit those infants whose mutations allow for some SP-B production, although the long-term prognosis for infants with partial SP-B deficiency remains poor. Intratracheal administration of replacement surfactant containing exogenous SP-B generally either does not work or only transiently improves lung function in affected infants. While the outlook for infants who are completely SP-B deficient is poor, support for infants suspected of being SP-B deficient should not be withdrawn until the diagnosis is confirmed, given the possibility of transient deficiency. Because SP-B deficiency generally results in disruption of intracellular lipid and protein trafficking secretion, correction of the disorder requires the intracellular expression of proSP-B. The only currently available means for accomplishing this is lung transplantation, which has successfully prolonged and improved the quality of life of a limited number of SP-B-deficient infants.[41] However, lung transplantation is expensive, only available at a limited number of medical centers, and the availability of donor lungs is limited. Moreover, the long-term term consequences of lung transplantation for these infants remain unknown. The ability to transfer the SP-B gene to respiratory epithelial cells may offer new approaches for treatment of hereditary SP-B deficiency in the future.

## ACKNOWLEDGMENTS

This work was supported by National Institutes of Health grants HL38859 and SCOR HL56387 to JAW, and HL54703 and HL54187 to LMN.

## REFERENCES

1. Thiel S, Reid K: Structures and functions associated with the group of mammalian lectins containing collagen-like sequences. *FEBS Lett* 250:78, 1989.
2. Hoover RR, Floros J: Organization of the human SP-A and SP-D loci at 10q22-q23. *Am J Respir Cell Mol Biol* 18:353, 1998.
3. LeVine AM, Bruno MD, Huelsman KM, Ross GF, Whitsett JA, Korfhagen TR: Surfactant protein-A-deficient mice are susceptible to group B streptococcal infection. *J Immunol* 158:4336, 1997.
4. Haagsman HP: Interactions of surfactant protein A with pathogens. *Biochim Biophys Acta* **1408**:264, 1998.
5. Reid KBM: Interactions of surfactant protein D with pathogens, allergens and phagocytes. *Biochim Biophys Acta* **1480**:290, 1998.
6. Korfhagen TR, Sheftelyevich V, Burhans MS, Bruno MD, Ross GF, Wert SE, Stahlman MT, et al.: Surfactant protein-D regulates surfactant phospholipid homeostasis in vivo. *J Biol Chem* 273:28438, 1998.
7. Botas C, Poulain F, Akiyama J, Brown C, Allen L, Goerke J, Clements J, et al.: Altered surfactant homeostasis and alveolar type II cell morphology in mice lacking surfactant protein D. *Proc Natl Acad Sci U S A* 95:11869, 1998.
8. Pilot-Matias TJ, Kister SE, Fox JL, Kropp K, Glasser SW, Whitsett JA: Structure and organization of the gene encoding human pulmonary surfactant proteolipid SP-B. *DNA* 8:75, 1989.
9. Glasser SW, Korfhagen TR, Perme CM, Pilot-Matias TJ, Kister SE, Whitsett JA: Two genes encoding human pulmonary surfactant proteolipid SP-C. *J Biol Chem* 263:10326, 1988.
10. Glasser SW, Korfhagen TR, Weaver TE, Clark J, Pilot-Matias T, Meuth J, Fox JL et al.: cDNA, deduced polypeptide structure and chromosomal assignment of human pulmonary surfactant proteolipid: SPL(pVal). *J Biol Chem* 263:9, 1988.
11. Wert SE, Profitt SA, Whitsett JA, Nogee LM: Reduced surfactant protein C expression in full-term infants with respiratory distress syndrome. *Pediatr Res* 43:303A, 1998.
12. Glasser SW, Korfhagen TR, Weaver T, Pilot-Matias T, Fox JL, Whitsett JA: cDNA and deduced amino acid sequence of human pulmonary surfactant-associated proteolipid SPL(Phe). *Proc Natl Acad Sci U S A* 84:4007, 1987.
13. Whitsett JA, Nogee LM, Weaver TE, Horowitz AD: Human surfactant protein B structure, function, regulation and genetic disease. *Physiol Rev* 75:749, 1995.
14. Pryhuber GS, Hull WM, Fink I, McMahan MJ, Whitsett JA: Ontogeny of surfactant proteins A and B in human amniotic fluid as indices of fetal lung maturity. *Pediatr Res* 30:597, 1991.
15. Gregory TJ, Longmore WJ, Moxley MA, Whitsett JA, Reed CR, Fowler AA, Hudson LD, et al.: Surfactant chemical composition and biophysical activity in acute respiratory distress syndrome. *J Clin Invest* 88:1976, 1991.
16. Bohinski RJ, Huffman JA, Whitsett JA, Lattier DL: cis-Active elements controlling lung cell specific expression of human pulmonary surfactant protein B gene. *J Biol Chem* 268:11160, 1993.
17. Yan C, Whitsett JA: Protein kinase A activation of the surfactant protein B gene is mediated by phosphorylation of thyroid transcription factor 1. *J Biol Chem* 272:17327, 1997.
18. Pryhuber GS, Church SL, Kroft T, Panchal A, Whitsett JA: The 3' untranslated region of surfactant protein B mRNA mediates inhibitory effects of TPA and TNA-α on SP-B expression. *Am J Physiol* 267:L16, 1994.
19. Weaver TE: Synthesis, processing and secretion of surfactant proteins B and C. *Biochim Biophys Acta* **1408**:173, 1998.
20. Ikegami M, Jobe AH: Surfactant protein metabolism in vivo. *Biochim Biophys Acta* **1408**:218, 1998.
21. Dranoff G, Crawford AD, Sadelain M, Ream B, Rashid A, Bronson RT, Dickersin GR, et al.: Involvement of granulocyte-macrophage colony-stimulating factor in normal pulmonary homeostasis. *Science* **264**:713, 1994.
22. Cooke KR, Nishinakamura R, Martin TR, Kobzik L, Brewer J, Whitsett JA, Bungard D, et al.: Persistence of pulmonary and abnormal lung function in IL-3/GM-CSF/IL-5βc receptor-deficient mice despite correction of alveolar proteinosis after BMT. *Bone Marrow Transplant* **20**:657, 1997.
23. Dirksen U, Nishinakamura R, Groneck P, Hattenhorst U, Nogee L, Murray R, Burdach S: Human pulmonary alveolar proteinosis associated with a defect in GM-CSF/IL/IL-5 receptor common β chain expression. *J Clin Invest* **100**:2211, 1997.
24. Clark JC, Wert SE, Bachurski CJ, Stahlman MT, Stripp BR, Weaver TE, Whitsett JA: Targeted disruption of the surfactant protein B gene disrupts surfactant homeostasis, causing respiratory failure in newborn mice. *Proc Natl Acad Sci U S A* 92:7794, 1995.
25. Vorbroker DK, Profitt SA, Nogee LM, Whitsett JA: Aberrant processing of surfactant protein C (SP-C) in hereditary SP-B deficiency. *Am J Physiol* 268:L647, 1995.
26. Tokieda K, Whitsett JA, Clark JC, Weaver TE, Ikeda K, Jobe AH, Ikegami M, et al.: Pulmonary dysfunction in neonatal SP-B-deficient mice. *Am J Physiol* 273:L875, 1997.
27. Lin S, Na C-L, Akinbi HT, Apsley KS, Whitsett JA, Weaver TE: Surfactant protein B (SP-B) −/− mice are rescued by restoration of SP-B expression in alveolar type II cells but not Clara cells. *J Biol Chem* 274:19168, 1999.
28. Akinbi HT, Breslin JS, Ikegami M, Iwamoto HS, Clark JC, Whitsett JA, Jobe AH, et al.: Rescue of SP-B knockout mice with a truncated SP-B proprotein: Function of the C-terminal propeptide. *J Biol Chem* 272:9640, 1997.
29. Clark JC, Weaver TE, Iwamoto HS, Ikegami M, Jobe AH, Hull WM, Whitsett JA: Decreased lung compliance and air trapping in heterozygous SP-B-deficient mice. *Am J Respir Cell Mol Biol* 16:46, 1997.
30. Tokieda K, Whitsett JA, Bachurski C, Wert SE, Hull WM, Iwamoto HS: SP-B deficient mice are susceptible to hyperoxic lung injury. *Am J Respir Cell Mol Biol* 21:463, 1999.
31. Nogee LM, deMello DE, Dehner LP, Colten HR: Brief report: deficiency of pulmonary surfactant protein B in congenital alveolar proteinosis. *N Engl J Med* 328:406, 1993.
32. Nogee LM, Garnier G, Dietz HC, Singer L, Murphy AM, deMello DE, Colten HR: A mutation in the surfactant protein B gene responsible for fatal neonatal respiratory disease in multiple kindreds. *J Clin Invest* **93**:1860, 1994.
33. Nogee LM, Wert SE, Proffit SA, Hull WM, Whitsett JA: Allelic heterogeneity in hereditary surfactant protein B (SP-B) deficiency. *Am J Respir Crit Care Med* 161:973, 2000.
34. Hamvas A, Cole F S, deMello D, Moxley M, Whitsett JA, Colten HR, Nogee LM: Failure of surfactant replacement in an infant with surfactant protein-B deficiency. *J Pediatr* 125:356, 1994.
35. deMello DE, Heyman S, Phelps DS, Hamvas A, Nogee L, Cole S, Colten HR: Ultrastructure of lung in surfactant protein B deficiency. *Am J Respir Cell Mol Biol* 11:230, 1994.
36. Nogee LM: Genetics of the hydrophobic surfactant proteins. *Biochim Biophys Acta* **1408**:323, 1998.
37. Klein JM, Thompson MW, Snyder JM, George TN, Whitsett JA, Bell EF, McCray PB, et al.: Transient surfactant protein B deficiency in a term infant with severe respiratory failure. *J Pediatr* 132:244, 1998.
38. Ballard PL, Nogee LM, Beers MF, Ballard RA, Planer BC, Polk L, deMello DE, et al.: Partial deficiency of surfactant protein B in an infant with chronic lung disease. *Pediatrics* 96:1046, 1995.
39. Yusen RD, Cohen AH, Hamvas A: Normal lung function in subjects heterozygous for surfactant protein-B deficiency. *Am J Respir Crit Care Med* 159:411, 1999.
40. Kala P, TenHave T, Nielsen H, Dunn M, Floros J: Association of pulmonary surfactant protein A (SP-A) gene and respiratory distress syndrome: Interaction with SP-B. *Pediatr Res* 43:169, 1998.
41. Hamvas A, Nogee LM, Mallory GB, Spray TL, Huddleston CB, August LP, Dehner DE, et al.: Lung transplantation for treatment of infants with surfactant protein B deficiency. *J Pediatr* 130:231, 1997.

# $\alpha_1$-Antitrypsin Deficiency

*Diane Wilson Cox*

1. $\alpha_1$-Antitrypsin ($\alpha_1$AT), a glycoprotein of molecular mass 52 kDa, is a major plasma serine protease inhibitor (serpin). The major physiological substrate is elastase, particularly in the lower respiratory tract.

2. The locus (PI locus) for $\alpha_1$AT is on chromosome 14 at 14q32.1, in a cluster of sequence-related genes, which includes those for corticosteroid-binding globulin, $\alpha_1$-antichymotrypsin, protein C inhibitor, and kallistatin. The gene is 12.2 kb long and contains six introns. $\alpha_1$AT produced in hepatocytes has a 1.4-kb mRNA transcript, while macrophages and the cornea have a longer RNA transcript, beginning in exons 5' to the first exon for hepatocyte $\alpha_1$AT.

3. $\alpha_1$AT shows considerable genetic variability, having more than 70 genetic variants (PI types), many of which have been sequenced. The majority of variants are associated with quantitatively and qualitatively normal $\alpha_1$AT. Further variation can be revealed at the DNA level, where a number of restriction enzymes reveal polymorphisms.

4. The *PI*Z* allele is the most common deficiency variant. PI ZZ homozygotes have 15 to 20 percent of the normal plasma concentration of $\alpha_1$AT, with a corresponding reduced concentration in bronchoalveolar lavage fluid. The deficiency is due to lack of secretion of Z $\alpha_1$AT from the hepatocyte, where inclusions are formed in the rough endoplasmic reticulum. There are several rare deficiency types, including those that show lack of secretion, and those that have no product (null or Q0).

5. Liver inclusions are formed because of a tendency for Z $\alpha_1$AT to self-aggregate. This occurs because the mobile reactive center loop of one protein molecule inserts into that of another molecule, instead of its own, especially at body temperature.

6. A deficiency of $\alpha_1$AT results in a protease/protease inhibitor imbalance in the lung, allowing destruction of the alveolar wall. The resultant obstructive lung disease is the most prevalent clinical manifestation of $\alpha_1$AT deficiency. Basal lung regions are most severely affected. In nonsmokers, onset of dyspnea occurs at a mean age of 45 to 50 years, and in smokers at about 35 years of age. Smokers show a considerably increased rate of lung destruction and have a poorer survival rate than nonsmokers with the deficiency. Smoking enhances oxidation and inactivation of $\alpha_1$AT in the lung.

7. Symptoms of liver abnormalities in infancy are expressed in about 17 percent of all individuals with $\alpha_1$AT deficiency. Only a few percent of all patients with the deficiency have a poor prognosis following early liver symptoms. Other genetic and environmental factors may influence the prognosis.

8. $\alpha_1$AT appears to be involved in regulation of the immune system, perhaps through the production of proteases by T cells. The deficiency state may contribute to diseases with an immune component. Response to inflammation is also impaired.

9. Prenatal diagnosis can be carried out using the polymerase chain reaction, followed by using synthetic oligonucleotide probes, digests with restriction enzymes, or sequencing.

10. Avoidance of smoking is important preventative therapy. Replacement therapy with $\alpha_1$AT, by infusion or aerosol, is effective at increasing protease inhibition in the pulmonary alveoli. Antioxidants could potentially delay lung and liver destruction. Lung and liver transplants offer potential therapy for end-stage destruction of these organs.

$\alpha_1$-Antitrypsin ($\alpha_1$AT) (GenBank accession no. K01396) plays a central role as a protease inhibitor in controlling tissue degradation. $\alpha_1$AT, as a major protease inhibitor in human plasma, can complex with a broad spectrum of proteases including elastase, trypsin, chymotrypsin, thrombin, and bacterial proteases. The most important inhibitory action is that against leukocyte elastase, a protease that degrades elastin of the alveolar walls as well as other structural proteins of a variety of tissues. Studies of the deficiency state, which began with the astute observation of an abnormal protein pattern on electrophoresis, has led us to a better understanding of the pathogenesis of pulmonary emphysema and the role of protease inhibitors in other disease states.

$\alpha_1$AT, isolated by Schultze et al. as $\alpha_1$-3,5-glycoprotein[1] was later named $\alpha_1$-antitrypsin, as most of the serum trypsin inhibitory activity was associated with the $\alpha_1$-globulin fraction. $\alpha_1$AT became of clinical interest when Laurell, on examination of protein electrophoretic patterns, noted that a number of patients lacked an $\alpha_1$-globulin band. $\alpha_1$AT deficiency (MIM 107400) was found to occur in a number of patients with early onset emphysema[2] and was associated with a low serum trypsin inhibitory activity. (For a review of the early discovery, see Eriksson.[3]) The codominant nature of the trait was expressed as a partial deficiency of serum trypsin inhibitory activity in heterozygotes, and a marked deficiency in homozygotes. $\alpha_1$AT is associated with progressive obstructive pulmonary disease, with preferential destruction in the bases of the lungs in both males and females, beginning in the second and third decades, and particularly in smokers.

At about the same time, Fagerhol and Braend observed electrophoretic variation in the prealbumin (Pr) region, using starch gel electrophoresis, and these bands were shown to be $\alpha_1$AT.[4] Pi (now PI), for protease inhibitor, was chosen in recognition that $\alpha_1$AT was an effective inhibitor for other proteases in addition to trypsin. The extensive polymorphism of $\alpha_1$AT was detected by a starch gel electrophoresis system developed by Fagerhol,[5] now replaced by high-resolution isoelectric focusing in polyacrylamide gels.

Another observation of major importance came in 1969, with the report by H. Sharp and coworkers that $\alpha_1$AT deficiency was associated with liver disease in children.[6] We now know that the liver disease does not usually have the poor prognosis that was first suspected.

The association between $\alpha_1$AT deficiency and obstructive lung disease has led to extensive studies of the mechanisms of protease tissue destruction, and the important role of a balance between proteases and their inhibitors. Studies of $\alpha_1$AT have also examined the role of protease inhibitors in immune mechanisms, nondisjunction, and recombination. The extensive genetic variation has led to population and evolution studies. The deficiency state results from abnormal plasma protein secretion from the hepatocyte, and the study of the basic defect enhances our understanding of glycoprotein secretion mechanisms. Studies at the molecular level provide possibilities for examining recombination events within and around a cluster of genes forming a protease inhibitor complex. (For general reviews, see references 7 to 10.)

For some of the other plasma protease inhibitors, such as $\alpha_2$-macroglobulin, kallistatin, and $\alpha_1$-antichymotrypsin, a deficiency state has not yet been discovered, although a partial deficiency of the latter has been observed and may be associated with disease.[11] In future years, the other protease inhibitors will no doubt prove to be as complex and interesting.

## PHYSIOLOGY OF $\alpha_1$-ANTITRYPSIN

### Function of $\alpha_1$-Antitrypsin

$\alpha_1$AT inhibits a broad spectrum of serine proteases. Because of its efficiency of inhibition, broad substrate specificity, and ready access to tissue, $\alpha_1$AT plays an important role, particularly in the lung, in defending tissues from proteolysis. $\alpha_1$AT inhibits most serine proteases tested to date, including pancreatic and neutrophil elastase, neutrophil cathepsin G, pancreatic trypsin and chymotrypsin, collagenase from skin and synovia, acrosin, kallikrein, urokinase, and renin, and proteases within the clotting and fibrinolytic systems, such as plasmin, thrombin, factor XI, and Hageman factor cofactor (see reference 12). Some of these inhibitor activities may reflect only in vitro phenomena with no physiological importance because of the presence of other more potent inhibitors for each specific protease.

$\alpha_1$AT complex formation results in inactivation of the protease and proteolytic cleavage of the inhibitor. The rate of inactivation of $\alpha_1$AT with specific proteases varies considerably, but is greatest with neutrophil elastase, for which the association constant is $6.5 \times 10^7$/M/sec, more than $10^6$ times higher than that with thrombin.[12] Evidence for the important role of $\alpha_1$AT as a neutrophil elastase inhibitor (reviewed in reference 13), is provided by many studies showing the effectiveness of human neutrophil elastase at inducing emphysema in experimental animals. Study of these animal models has demonstrated that the destruction of elastin fibers is of primary importance for producing the lung degradation typical of emphysema. $\alpha_1$AT provides approximately 90 percent of the antielastase activity in plasma. The other plasma inhibitor of elastase, $\alpha_2$-macroglobulin, is largely inaccessible to the lower respiratory tract, because of its high molecular mass of 725 kDa.

Although a number of proteases in the clotting cascade are inhibited by $\alpha_1$AT, these reactions do not appear to be of prime physiological significance, probably because of the presence of other more effective inhibitors. Individuals with $\alpha_1$AT deficiency have not been reported to have abnormalities in coagulation or fibrinolysis. However, the change of only one amino acid at the active center (in PI$_{PITTSBURGH}$) converts $\alpha_1$AT into a potent inhibitor of thrombin and factor XI, producing a severe bleeding disorder during acute phase response.[14]

$\alpha_1$AT increases during the acute phase response, providing protection for tissues during inflammation.

### Function in the Immune Response

A number of studies have shown that proteases and their inhibitors affect the immune response. Trypsin and chymotrypsin act as mitogens on B lymphocytes. Trypsin, neutrophil elastase, and cathepsin G can substitute for helper T cells in B-cell mitogen assays. Mouse thymocytes are triggered to synthesize DNA by neutrophils or macrophages, or substances released from them. Enhanced lymphocyte responsiveness to phytohemagglutinin, observed in $\alpha_1$AT-deficient individuals, decreases with the addition of highly purified $\alpha_1$AT.[15] $\alpha_1$AT has been reported to inhibit antibody-dependent cell-mediated cytotoxicity, T-cell-mediated

cytotoxicity, and natural killer activity. $\alpha_1$AT has a direct effect on adherent cells, but not on proliferating T cells. This potential for increased T-helper activity and B-cell activation could lead to the exaggerated cell-mediated immunity and marked acceleration of delayed hypersensitivity responses, which have been demonstrated in vivo.[16] In addition to mitogenic activity, proteases also cleave IgG, liberating the Fc fragment, which can augment lymphocyte response.[15] The mechanism and extent of involvement of $\alpha_1$AT in immune regulation still needs clarification.

### Synthesis

$\alpha_1$AT is synthesized mostly in the parenchymal cells of the liver. Analysis of tissue RNA indicates that in addition to the production of $\alpha_1$AT in liver, there are low levels of production in kidney, lung, and intestine.[17] In studies of transgenic mice, $\alpha_1$AT production (both mRNA and protein) was observed in chondrocytes, thymic epithelial cells and Hassall bodies, macrophages in lymphoid tissue of the small intestine, gastric and small intestinal crypt epithelial cells, renal distal tubule brush border, and the lining of pulmonary alveoli.[17-19] The function and importance of $\alpha_1$AT in kidney and intestine are yet to be discovered. $\alpha_1$AT is expressed in the colonic epithelial tumor cell line, CaCo$_2$, a cell that differentiates into ileal-like cells, and in jejunum.[20] Expression occurs in intestinal villus enterocytes and in Paneth cells.[21]

Cultured human fetal liver cells synthesize and secrete $\alpha_1$AT. The secretion of $\alpha_1$AT is suppressed by increasing concentrations of $\alpha_1$AT in the medium, suggesting a feedback control mechanism.[22] Further support for feedback control comes from transgenic mice. With high production due to many gene copies, $\alpha_1$AT accumulates in aggregated form in the hepatocytes within a subset of distended cisternae of the rough endoplasmic reticulum, and secretion of murine $\alpha_1$AT decreases.[23]

The production of $\alpha_1$AT by monocytes and alveolar macrophages may be important in regulation of local tissue injury. Although the amount of $\alpha_1$AT produced is very small, macrophage production could be important in the defense system of the lung. Transcription and translation of the $\alpha_1$AT gene, followed by posttranslational processing, and secretion of $\alpha_1$AT in a functionally active form, has been demonstrated in human peripheral blood monocytes and in macrophages from bronchoalveoli and from breast milk.[24] Breast milk production is particularly high in the early postpartum period (0.3 to 0.6 g/liter).[25]

The catabolic rate of the normal type of $\alpha_1$AT in plasma has been estimated at 6.7 days.[26] Removal of 20 percent and 100 percent of the sialic acid residues reduced the half life to 4.0 and 0.8 days, respectively.[27]

### Plasma Concentration

The average plasma concentration of $\alpha_1$AT in healthy individuals (PI type MM) has been estimated to be 1.3 g/liter[28] However, concentration varies according to PI type. The concentration of $\alpha_1$AT in plasma can be measured either by immunochemical or functional methods (see Cox et al.[29] for details). Automated nephelometric methods are convenient for immunologic quantification; radial immunodiffusion and electroimmunoassay are also appropriate. The results of immunologic methods show considerable variability between laboratories because of differences in commercial standards, which tend to be falsely high. For this reason, laboratories may express normal values as percent of a normal pool of a large number of normal healthy individuals not pregnant or on medication. A standard from the American Pathological Association can be purchased commercially. The normal value has been calculated to be 1.3 g/liter based on a highly purified standard.[30]

Immunologic and functional assays usually correlate well; the latter, however, include a component due to $\alpha_2$-macroglobulin activity, and therefore do not specifically measure $\alpha_1$AT. Functional assays, which evaluate inhibition of trypsin or elastase, usually use synthetic substrates such as $\alpha$-N-benzoyl-DL-arginine-p-nitroanilide (BAPNA) for trypsin[31] and N-tert-butoxycarbonyl-

L-alanine-*p*-nitrophenyl-ester (NBA)[32] or *N*-succinyl-L-alanyl-L-alanyl-L-alanyl-L-alanine-*p*-nitroanilide (SLAPN)[33] for elastase.

As an acute phase protein, $\alpha_1$AT can show a fourfold increase in plasma concentration during infection. A marked increase in concentration occurs in a wide range of inflammatory conditions, in cancer, and in liver disease. Modest increases are induced by estrogen during pregnancy or when administered as therapy. In addition to the inherited deficiency, low levels of $\alpha_1$AT occur in the respiratory distress syndrome in newborns, severe protein-losing conditions, to terminal liver failure, and during the course of cystic fibrosis.

## STRUCTURE OF $\alpha_1$-ANTITRYPSIN

### Protein Structure

$\alpha_1$AT is a glycoprotein consisting of a single polypeptide chain of 394 residues, a carbohydrate content of 12 percent, and a resulting molecular mass of 52 kDa, isoelectric point 4.4 to 4.7. Methods for purification and details of characterization of the protein have been reviewed.[34] The small size of the protein enables diffusion through interstitial body fluids and into tissues such as the lung. A somewhat larger molecule, including a 24-residue hydrophobic signal peptide, is produced in the liver and in vitro.[35,36]

$\alpha_1$AT, while not crystallizable in its active form, crystallizes after proteolytic cleavage at the reactive site[37] forming a more stable relaxed (R) form.[38] Analysis of the crystal structure indicates that the single polypeptide chain is organized into well-defined secondary structural elements: three $\beta$ sheets and eight $\alpha$ helixes. The first 150 residues preferentially form the $\alpha$ helixes. $\alpha_1$AT contains one cysteine residue. No disulfide bridge is present in the protein, although the thiol group can form a disulfide bond with other proteins, such as immunoglobulin $\alpha$ heavy chain and immunoglobulin $\kappa$ light chain. Such protein binding can also produce artifacts on isoelectric focusing, which disappear when $\alpha_1$AT is exposed to a reducing agent.

### Microheterogeneity

$\alpha_1$AT is modified during transition through the endoplasmic reticulum of the hepatocyte. Some of this modification is reflected in microheterogeneity, observed in acid starch gel and agarose electrophoresis, and in polyacrylamide isoelectric focusing, as typical for glycoproteins when near their isoelectric point. Eight bands were originally noted, numbered from 1 (anodal) to 8 (cathodal); bands 4 and 6 contain 40 and 35 percent, respectively, of the total $\alpha_1$AT[4], with isoelectric points of 4.52 and 4.59[28] (Fig. 219-1). Much of the heterogeneity is due to differences in the type of carbohydrate side chains. Three carbohydrate side chains per molecule are attached at asparagine residues 46, 83, and 247.[39] The carbohydrate chains may be biantennary or triantennary, terminating in two or three *N*-acetyl-neuraminic acid residues.[40,41] The two minor cathodal components (7 and 8) have the same carbohydrate structure as the major bands (4 and 6), but the first five amino acids (Glu-Asp-Pro-Glu-Gly) have been removed, apparently by posttranslational cleavage.[41] Alterations in the usual pattern of microheterogeneity are observed in newborns and upon estrogen administration, with an increased percentage in bands 6 and 8 relative to bands 4 and 7. During inflammation or with high levels of estrogen, 80 percent of the increase in concentration of plasma $\alpha_1$AT occurs in bands 2 and 4, which is explained by the replacement of biantennary by triantennary oligosaccharides.[41]

### Reactive Site

Protease inhibition by $\alpha_1$AT occurs by formation of a tightly bound 1:1 complex between $\alpha_1$AT and the target protease, which can be one of a number of serine proteases, but is mainly elastase. Specificity is determined by crucial amino acids in the reactive site of $\alpha_1$AT. The methionine residue, at position 358 close to the C-terminus of the molecule,[42] is important for functional activity (Fig. 219-2).[43] In intact inhibitor, a strand containing the methionine residue is exposed on the surface of the molecule in a loop formation, fitting precisely the conformation of the reactive

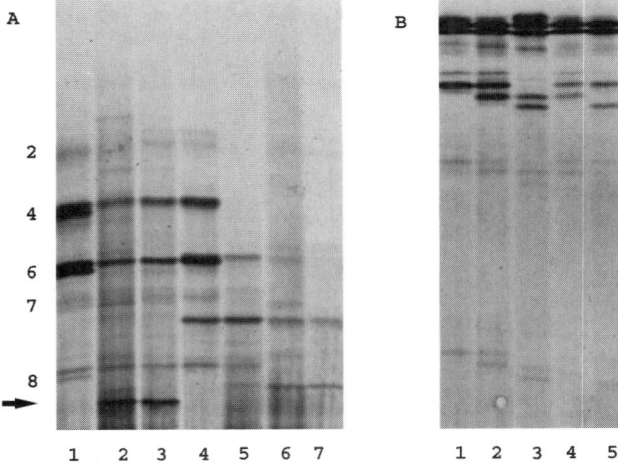

**Fig 219-1** Selected PI variants observed in human sera using isolectric focusing, polyacrylamide gel. Anode is at the top. *A*, Routine PIEF, as described,[65,69] but using Pharmalyte pH 4.5 to 5.5. Lane 1 = M1M2; 2 = M1Z; 3 = M1; 4 = M1S; 5 = SZ; 6 = ZZ with pronounced anodal components similar to position of S; 7 = ZZ. Dots indicate major Z bands (bands 4 and 6). Lanes 2 and 3 have a cathodal component (arrow) occasionally found in patients with liver disease. *B*, Increased separation of PI M variants by PIEF, with an ultranarrow immobilized pH gradient, 4.5 to 4.75. Lane 1 = M1; 2 = M1M3; 3 = M2M3; 4 = M1M4; 5 = M1M2. (*From Weidinger and Cleve.*[68] *Used by permission.*)

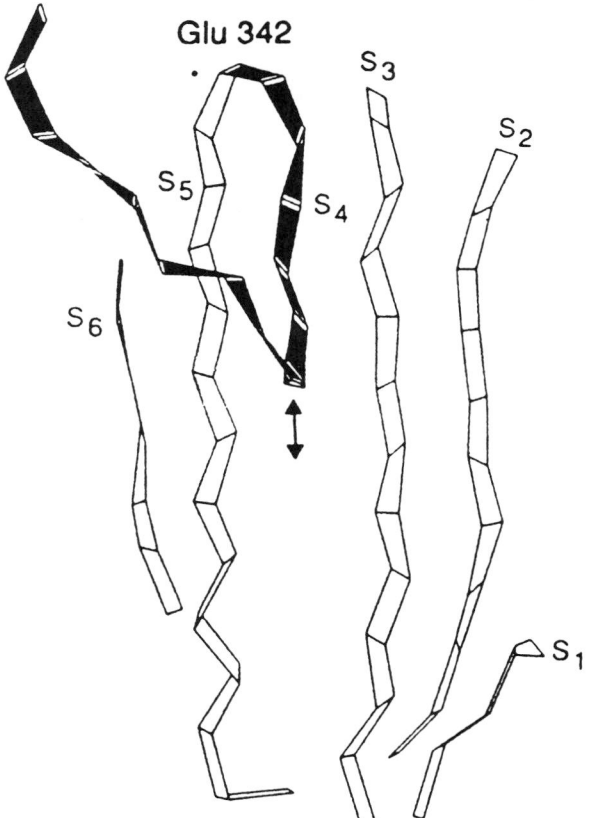

**Fig 219-2** Reactive center loop, showing gap formed in the A sheet. Loop is hinged and can fold into gap. In Z protein, another Z molecule enters the gap. (*From Lomas et al.*[121] *Used by permission. Photograph courtesy of R. W. Carrell.*)

**Table 219-1** Reactive Centers of Selected Protease Inhibitors

| Inhibitor | Substrate | Reactive center* | | | | | |
|---|---|---|---|---|---|---|---|
| | | $P_1$ | $P_{1'}$ | $P_{2'}$ | $P_{3'}$ | $P_{4'}$ | $P_{5'}$ |
| Human $\alpha_1$AT | Elastase | Met | Ser | Ile | Pro | Pro | Glu |
| Human $\alpha_1$-antichymotrypsin | Chymotrypsin | Leu | Ser | Ala | Leu | Val | Glu |
| Mouse $\alpha_1$AT | Elastase | Tyr | Ser | Met | Pro | Pro | Ile |
| Mouse contrapsin† | Trypsin | Lys | Ala | Ile | Leu | Pro | Ala |
| Human antithrombin III | Thrombin | Arg | Ser | Leu | Asn | Pro | Asn |

\* From Hill et al.[47]
† Possibly $\alpha_1$-antichymotrypsin homologue.

site of the target protease.[44] The insertion of a single residue, threonine 345, into sheet A is required for activity of $\alpha_1$AT. Proteolytic cleavage at the reactive site causes release of the strand and its subsequent incorporation into $\beta$ sheet A.[37] The exposed position of the reactive site enables ready access for oxidation. According to this model, methionine, when oxidized to methionine sulfoxide, can no longer physically complex with elastase and $\alpha_1$AT becomes inactive.[45] The association constant for oxidized $\alpha_1$AT is 1000 times lower than for native $\alpha_1$AT.[12] In some situations, the release of oxygen radicals from leukocytes and the subsequent oxidation of methionine may be advantageous, for example, by enabling local tissue breakdown in areas of inflammation.[46]

The reactive sites of several of the serine protease inhibitors are similar to each other, as well as to those of low molecular weight plant-protease inhibitors. Substrate specificity is determined by the composition of the reactive site (Table 219-1).[47] The specificity for methionine at amino acid 358 was proven in the rare natural mutant of $\alpha_1$AT, PI$_{\text{PITTSBURGH}}$, in which arginine is substituted for methionine 358.[48] This mutant lacks inhibition of porcine pancreatic elastase, and becomes a highly effective inhibitor of thrombin.

### Gene Sequence and Structure

The $\alpha_1$AT gene is 12.2 kb in length, including a 1434-bp coding region, and 6 introns[36] (Fig. 219-3A). The largest intron, 5.3 kb in

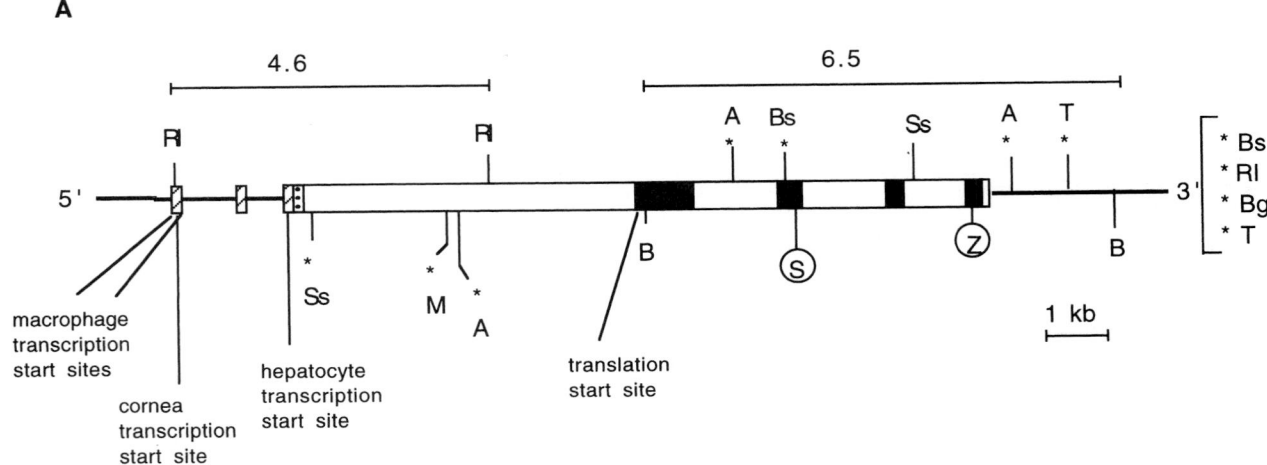

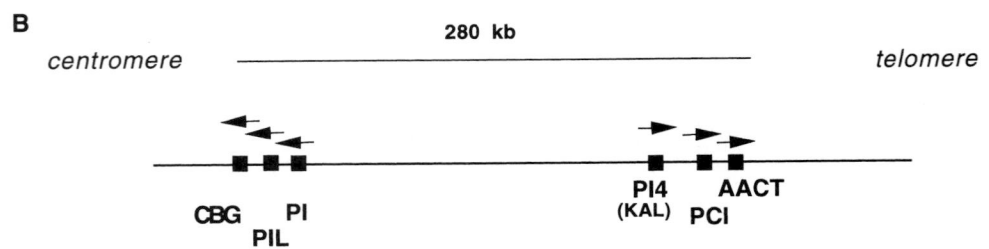

**Fig 219-3** *A*, $\alpha_1$AT gene and flanking regions. Coding regions are solid, introns open, untranslated dotted rectangles. Cross-hatched regions are exons of macrophage DNA. Asterisk indicates sites of polymorphisms for the following restriction enzymes (those in square bracket at the right indicate polymorphisms in the 3' homologous region): A = *Ava*II; Bg = *Bgl*II; Bs = *Bst*II; Ma = *Mae*III; = *Taq*I; RI = *Eco*RI; Ss = Sst site; S and Z circled-sites of mutations in PI S and PI Z, respectively. Genomic probes, 4.6 and 6.5 kb, are indicated. Position of CA repeat is 5' of first RI site. *B*, Cluster of PI and other loci in the serpin superfamily cluster on chromosome 14, as determined by pulsed field gel electrophoresis. Arrows indicate direction of transcription. PII = PI-like, CBG = corticosteroid-binding globulin; PI4 = kallistatin; PIC = protein C inhibitor; AACT = $\alpha_1$-antichymotrypsin. (*Based on data from Billingsley et al.,*[57] *Byth et al.,*[58] *and Rollini et al.*[59])

length, between exons 1C and 2, contains a 143-amino acid open reading frame, an *Alu* sequence, and a pseudo-transcription-initiation site. This open reading frame does not appear to be an actual protein-coding region. In hepatocytes, the region beginning 721 kb 5' to the transcription start site in exon 1C is necessary for efficient expression of the $\alpha_1$AT gene and for cell-specific expression.[49] There are three monocyte and one corneal transcription initiation sites 5' to the hepatocyte initiation site (Fig. 219-3A), producing longer RNA transcripts, although all have the same translation start sites.[17,50,51] Each of the transcription start sites has its own promoter, regulating tissue-specific expression. The upstream start sites are used during inflammation, and particularly in response to the acute phase mediator interleukin 6 (IL-6).[50]

DNA and protein-sequencing studies revealed homology between other protease inhibitors as well as other plasma proteins, comprising the family of serpins, or serine protease inhibitors.[38,52] Human $\alpha_1$AT shares 42 to 50 percent homology, both in nucleotide and protein sequence, with $\alpha_1$AT, protein C inhibitor, thyroxine-binding globulin, and corticosteroid-binding globulin.[53] The position and size of introns is quite different between the various members of the serpin family and evolution of the family members appears to be most related to requirements for tertiary structure.[54]

## Localization of the Structural Gene

The PI locus, encoding $\alpha_1$AT, was localized to chromosome 14 by linkage to the immunoglobulin heavy chain region using inherited markers of the Gm system,[55] and was physically mapped to chromosome band 14q32.1.[56] The PI locus lies within a cluster of homologous genes, of which the closest are corticosteroid-binding globulin (CBG) and an apparently nonfunctional gene, PI-like (PIL locus).[57,58] Another group of genes in the cluster are $\alpha_1$-antichymotrypsin (AACT), blood coagulation factor protein C inhibitor (PCI), and kallistatin (PI4)[57,59] (Fig. 219-3B).

## GENETIC VARIATION

### Genetic (PI) Variants

There are many inherited variants of $\alpha_1$AT. *PI*M* (standard allele nomenclature), which can be further classified into subtypes, is the most common allele in all populations described to date. The *PI*S* allele reaches polymorphic frequencies in many populations, as does the *PI*Z* allele, which produces a deficiency of $\alpha_1$AT.

In addition to common variants of $\alpha_1$AT, more than 60 rare variants of $\alpha_1$AT have been identified. The inheritance is described as codominant, as expression of both alleles can be observed in the heterozygote by various electrophoretic techniques. The PI variants, initially identified primarily by the method of acid starch gel electrophoresis developed by Fagerhol, were named in order of their mobility: F (fast), M (medium), S (slow), and Z (the most cathodal).[5] Additional variants were given alphabetic designations according to their mobility in starch. In 1974, isoelectric focusing in polyacrylamide was used for resolution of PI variants.[60-62] Nomenclature guidelines were established, with the position by isoelectric focusing as the criterion for designation of subsequent variants.[63] Birthplace names were used to designate the more rare alleles, abbreviated to the first three letters of the place of origin name. Alleles at the PI locus are designated *PI*M*, *PI*S*, and so forth. Phenotypes are designated as PI MZ, PI M (or MM if confirmed in family studies). Genotype is indicated as *PI*M/PI*Z*, and so forth. Alleles that produce no detectable $\alpha_1$AT in serum were originally designated as *PI** null, with genotypes –, PI M –, and so forth. According to general nomenclature guidelines, the null alleles are designated *PI*Q0*, followed by a place name as for the other variants.

Earlier methods for identification of PI variants, including starch gel electrophoresis, isoelectric focusing, and agarose electrophoresis, have been reviewed.[64] Isoelectric focusing offers increased resolution of the variants, better reproducibility, and the possibility of typing many (up to 50) samples on a single gel. A suitable method for PI typing by isoelectric focusing has been described[65] and many modifications have been developed. Narrow-range ampholytes improved the resolving power of isoelectric focusing and are available commercially, as stock or in commercially prepared gels. The use of ultrathin isoelectric focusing gels and a narrow pH gradient, for example, 4.2 to 4.9,[66] appears to produce resolution similar to that of immobilized gradients.[67] Typical results using isoelectric focusing and narrow-range ampholytes for the most clinically important PI variants are shown in Figure 219-1A.[63,67,68] The improved resolution obtainable with immobilized pH gradients and the additional, probably rare, identifiable M subtypes are shown in Figure 219-1B. Figure 219-4[63] indicates the relative position by isoelectric focusing of a number of the variants, which should serve as guidelines for those wishing to identify unusual variants. Lists of variants, with references, have been published.[69,70]

The normal ranges for PI types commonly found in the population are as follows, expressed as percent of a normal plasma pool $\pm$ 1 standard deviation:[71,72] M, $100 \pm 23.5$; MZ, $64 \pm 15.2$; MS, $86 \pm 20.5$, or according to the international standard, means of 1.3, 0.83, and 1.12, respectively. Most of the quantitative variation is accounted for by PI type.[73] Most PI variants are associated with normal concentrations of $\alpha_1$AT. The exceptions are

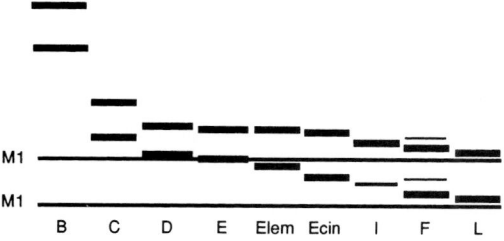

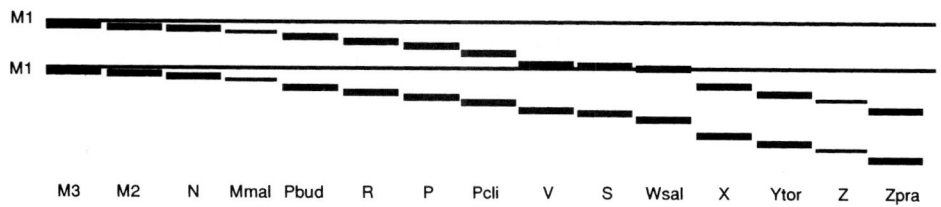

Fig 219-4 Diagram of selected anodal (top row) and cathodal (bottom row) PI variants by isoelectric focusing in acrylamide. Solid lines indicate position of two major bands of M1. Anode at top. References are found in Cox et al.[63]

**Table 219-2 Sequenced Normal "Nondeficiency" $\alpha_1$-Antitrypsin Variants**

| PI Type | Amino acid number | Exon | Ancestral allele | Normal amino acid | DNA codon | Mutant amino acid | DNA codon* |
|---|---|---|---|---|---|---|---|
| M1val (and Z) | 213 | 3 | M1val213 | Val | GTG | | |
| M1ala | 213 | 3 | M1ala213 | Ala | GCG | | |
| M3 | 376 | 5 | M1val213 | Glu | GAA | Asp | GAC |
| M2 | 101 | 2 | M3 | Arg | CGT | His | CAT |
| M4 | 101 | 2 | M1val213 | Arg | CGT | His | CAT |
| F | 223 | 3 | M1val213 | Arg | CGT | Cys | TGT |
| P$_{SAINTALBANS}$ | 256 (silent) | 3 | M1val213 | Asp | GAT | Asp | GAC |
| | 341 | 5 | | Asp | GAC | Asn | AAC |
| V$_{MUNICH}$ | 2 | 2 | M1val213 | Asp | GAT | Ala | GCT |
| X | 204 | 3 | M1val213 | Glu | GAG | Lys | (AAG) |
| X$_{CHRISTCHURCH}$ | 363 | 5 | | Glu | GAG | Lys | (AAG) |
| Pittsburg | 358 | 5 | | Met | ATG | Arg | (AGG) |
| **Reduced Plasma Concentration** | | | | | | | |
| I | 39 | 2 | M1val213 | Arg | CGC | Cys | TGC |
| S | 264 | 3 | M1val213 | Glu | GAA | Val | GTA |
| P# | 256 | 3 | M1val213 | Asp | GAT | Val | GTT |
| M$_{MINERALSPRINGS}$ | 67 | 2 | M1ala213 | Gly | GGG | Glu | GAG |
| W$_{BETHESDA}$ | 336 | 5 | M1ala213 | Ala | GCT | Thr | ACT |

*Codons in parentheses are predicted as most likely from amino acid sequence.
#Identical sequence reported for Q0$_{CARDIFF}$ and P$_{LOWELL}$.

PI I, associated on average with 68 percent of the normal concentration of $\alpha_1$AT,[74] PI S at 60 percent of normal,[71] W$_{BETHESDA}$,[75] and PI P at 30 percent of normal.[76] (A number of variants with a mobility relatively close to P have a normal concentration of $\alpha_1$AT.) PI S, P, and W$_{BETHESDA}$ show increased intracellular degradation. Most electrophoretic variants tested to date have normal functional capacity,[77] but the rare variant M$_{MINERAL SPRINGS}$ has a modest reduction of inhibitory function. These variants have been reported to be associated with emphysema only in combination with a true deficiency variant, and are classified here as normal variants. The types considered to be associated with high risk for disease all have less than 20 percent of the normal concentration of $\alpha_1$AT, and are discussed subsequently.

Not all variations observed electrophoretically are due to genetic differences. The cysteine in $\alpha_1$AT appears able to react with a variety of other plasma components to produce artifacts, which usually disappear by reduction of plasma samples prior to isoelectric focusing.[65] Anodal variants are observed in patients with liver disease and can be mistaken for the F or E variants. A variant cathodal to Z has been described in a child with cytomegalovirus and fatty liver[78] and is also noted in other patients, predominantly those with liver disease (Fig. 219-3A). Binding of $\alpha_1$AT to bile acids[79] could cause some of the abnormal gel bands. Sometimes the additional bands that appear to be $\alpha_1$AT are due to other proteins and are not observed when immunofixation is used. Repeat testing of patients frequently indicates the transitory nature of these unusual patterns. Family studies are a prerequisite to show that variants are truly genetic.

## Amino Acid/DNA Sequence of PI Variants

The amino acid sequence has been determined for a number of types of $\alpha_1$AT, either directly or by DNA sequence analysis. The mutations identified are listed in Table 219-2. An alanine-valine substitution at amino acid position 213 is common.[42,80] The alanine substitution is found in about 34 percent of PI*M1 alleles[80,81] and differentiates two subtypes of M1 — M1(Ala213) and M1(Val213). The PI*Z allele has the Ala213 substitution; however, PI types M2, M3, and S all have valine at position 213.[80,81] Variants with similar electrophoretic properties do not necessarily have the same mutation.

The modest reduction in plasma concentration associated with the S variant is due to slight changes in internal hydrogen bonds and salt bridge linkages, which result in a mild delay in secretion.[82] The Z$_{BRISTOL}$ mutation causes interference with glycosylation at amino acid residue 83. This is not a deficiency variant.[83]

## Population Studies

Distribution of the PI alleles has now been determined for many populations. In all populations, PI*M is the most common allele. Early population studies carried out by starch gel electrophoresis, which could have underestimated PI*Z frequency, showed a low frequency of variants in Finns, Lapps, and Asians, and a high frequency of PI*S in Spanish and Portuguese.[84,85] In later studies, PI typing was carried out by acid starch gel electrophoresis with crossed immunoelectrophoresis or by isoelectric focusing. A number of the population studies, up to 1985, have been summarized.[64,70,86] Data from selected population studies, including PI M subtype frequencies, are presented in Table 219-3, which shows only a few of the populations studied to illustrate the major population differences. The frequency of PI*M1 is the highest in all populations studied; PI*M2 is the next most frequent and PI*M3 is relatively uncommon. The additional subtype alleles, PI*M4 and others, are identifiable by high resolution methods.[68] The PI*S allele is rare or absent in Black and Oriental populations, highest in Spain and Portugal, next most frequent in France, and low generally in other parts of Europe. The frequency of PI*Z (discussed subsequently) is highest in Scandinavian countries, present throughout Caucasian populations, including those of the Middle East,[87] and absent from Oriental and Black populations, except in those populations known to have admixture, as in the United States.

## DNA Polymorphisms

In addition to the extensive variation found in the protein by electrophoretic methods, further variation is found in the DNA sequence within and surrounding the $\alpha_1$AT gene, recognized by various restriction enzymes, producing RFLPs (restriction-fragment-length polymorphisms), which are easily converted to single nucleotide polymorphisms (SNPs) for use with polymerase chain reaction (PCR). Polymorphic sites are shown in Figure 219-3A.

**Table 219-3** Allele Frequencies in Selected Populations*

| Population origin | No. tested | PI alleles | | | | | |
|---|---|---|---|---|---|---|---|
| | | M1 | M2 | M3 | S | Z | Other |
| Denmark | 909 | 0.728 | 0.136 | 0.082 | 0.022 | 0.023 | 0.009 |
| Netherlands | 357 | 0.679 | 0.147 | 0.129[†] | 0.029 | 0.013 | 0.003 |
| Portugal | 900 | 0.510 | 0.260 | 0.053 | 0.150 | 0.009 | 0.018 |
| U.S. (White) | 904 | 0.724 | 0.137 | 0.095 | 0.023 | 0.014 | 0.007 |
| U.S. (Black) | 549 | 0.982 | — | — | 0.015 | 0.004 | — |
| China[‡] | 1010 | 0.709 | 0.209 | 0.070 | — | — | 0.012 |
| Japan | 746 | 0.786 | 0.153 | 0.062 | — | — | — |

* References are listed in Cox.[132]
† Frequency of *PI*M3* plus *PI*M4*.
‡ Mean of five Chinese populations.

Three polymorphisms lie within the first intron, using the restriction enzymes *Sst*I, *Msp*I, and *Ava*II.[88] These show weaker linkage disequilibrium than expected, suggesting that this may be a region of increased recombination.[88,89] Polymorphisms are detected 3′ of intron 1, using the restriction enzymes *Ava*II, *Mae*III, *Bst*EII, *Taq*I, and *Eco*RI. The allele frequencies are shown in Table 219-4. *Ava*II detects polymorphisms in both the $\alpha_1$AT gene and in the homologous sequence, and was the first enzyme to show a unique DNA haplotype for PI ZZ individuals.[88]

When amino acid 213 is alanine, as found in Z and a portion of M1 $\alpha_1$AT, a restriction site for *Bst*EII[80] and *Mae*III[89] is not present as it is in those PI types with valine at amino acid 213. A *Taq*I polymorphism, proposed to lie in a region influencing gene expression, is located in the flanking region immediately 3′ to the $\alpha_1$AT gene.[90,91]

Most of the polymorphisms detected in the 6.5-kb region 3′ of intron 1 do not lie within the $\alpha_1$AT gene, but in the downstream homologous sequence. There is extensive linkage disequilibrium throughout the $\alpha_1$AT gene.[89] The most useful combination of polymorphic sites 3′ to intron 1 are those detecting variation within the $\alpha_1$AT gene (e.g., *Ava*II, *Mae*III, or *Bst*EII) in combination with a polymorphic site in the downstream region which does not show complete association,[89] such as *Taq* I or *Bgl*II.

DNA polymorphisms and haplotypes are of particular interest for evolutionary studies. A specific DNA haplotype is associated with the *PI*Z* allele and indicates a single origin for all *PI*Z* alleles.[88] The DNA haplotype is the same irrespective of ethnic group within northern Europe, and independent of the presence or type of clinical disease.[88] There appears to have been an early division between M1 subtypes because the M1A (M1A1a213) subtype, which has preceded the occurrence of the Z allele, has the same amino acid at 213[80,89] as found in the baboon.[92] M1(Val213) appears to have evolved into other PI subtypes such as M2, M3, and S.[8,89] Specific DNA haplotypes are associated with each of the protein variants and can be used to identify the evolutionary pathways.[89] They have also been useful for the identification of rare deficiency alleles.[93]

Highly polymorphic CA repeats have been identified 5′ of the PI locus and close to the genes for $\alpha_1$-antichymotrypsin and protein C inhibitor,[58] which will be useful both for linkage and for disease association studies (Table 219-4, Fig. 219-3B).

## $\alpha_1$-ANTITRYPSIN DEFICIENCY

There is no firm evidence that any of the alleles with a modest reduction in the plasma concentration of $\alpha_1$AT (Table 219-2) are associated with disease. Even in association with the *PI*Z* allele, the risk for disease does not appear to be appreciable. Risk is presented in discussions of the associated diseases. This section considers the alleles that produce a marked deficiency of $\alpha_1$AT.

### Deficiency Due to *PI*Z* Allele

The most common of the deficiency alleles is *PI*Z*, and the majority of individuals with $\alpha_1$AT deficiency are of PI type ZZ. As noted from population studies of PI variants, the *PI*Z* allele

**Table 219-4** Allele Frequencies for DNA Polymorphisms

| Probe or locus | Restriction enzyme | Alleles | | Allele frequency* | | | Heterozygosity |
|---|---|---|---|---|---|---|---|
| | | No | Size | + | − | 0 | |
| 4.6 | *Sst*I | 2 | 1.8, 1.9 kb | 0.69 | 0.31 | — | 0.43 |
| | *Msp*I | 2 | 0.95, 0.98 kb | 0.47 | 0.53 | — | 0.49 |
| | *Ava*II | 2 | 0.9, 1.1 kb | 0.65 | 0.35 | — | 0.45 |
| 6.5 | *Mae*III | 2 | 2.3, 2.5 bk | 0.71 | 0.29 | — | 0.68 |
| | *Mae*III (3′) | 2 | 0.5, 0.7 kb | 0.65 | 0.35 | — | |
| | *Ava*II (5/7) | 2 | 0.48, 0.68 kb | 0.22 | 0.78 | — | 0.61 |
| | *Ava*II (1/4)(3′) | 2 | 0.72, 2.7 kb | 0.29 | 0.71 | | |
| | *Taq*I | 2 | 1.4, 2.0 kb | 0.97 | 0.03 | — | 0.63 |
| | *Taq*I (3′) | 3 | 4.8, 6.7, 0 kb | 0.53 | 0.26 | 0.21 | |
| | *Eco*RI (3′) | 2 | 5.7, 8.6 kb | 0.23 | 0.77 | — | 0.35 |
| CBG | | 2 | 186–190 bp | | | | 0.32 |
| PI | | 18 | 155–189 bp | | | | 0.90 |
| PCI | | 15 | 128–156 bp | | | | 0.80 |
| AACT | | 17 | 141–173 bp | | | | 0.90 |

* + = Presence of restriction site; − = absence of site; 0 = no fragment.
RFLP data are from Cox et al.,[88,89] except *Eco*RI from Hodgson and Kalsheker;[91] microsatellite data from Byth et al.[58]

appears to be restricted to Caucasians, and occurs in Blacks and Orientals apparently only in populations with white admixture. The estimated frequency of the *PI*Z* allele in North American Caucasian populations is 0.0122, corresponding to a frequency of PI ZZ homozygotes of 1 in 6700.[93] The frequency of *PI*Z* is higher in Scandinavia: 0.018, as calculated from 200,000 Swedish newborns in a national screening program.[94]

## Plasma Concentration of $\alpha_1$AT

The plasma concentration of $\alpha_1$AT associated with PI type ZZ in adults is usually in the range of 12 to 24 percent of normal (0.16 to 0.31 g/liter) (mean $18 \pm 5$ percent of normal, or 0.23 g/liter).[95] However, for children or infants with liver disease, the concentrations of $\alpha_1$AT are frequently higher, and can rise to 40 percent of normal.[96] The mean plasma concentration in 75 PI ZZ children ($17 \pm 3$ percent) was similar to that of adults.[97]

## Diagnosis

$\alpha_1$AT deficiency should be considered in the differential diagnosis of patients with emphysema, jaundice in infancy, liver disease in childhood, and liver disease in adults.

Immunologic assays are the most specific assays for $\alpha_1$AT and should be used in those clinical conditions with a relatively high probability of $\alpha_1$AT deficiency. Functional assay results include a portion of inhibitory capacity due to other inhibitors such as $\alpha_2$-macroglobulin, which can prevent diagnosis of the deficiency. As a screening technique the $\alpha_1$-globulin peak in protein electrophoresis is usually, but not necessarily, absent or markedly reduced. Computer printouts of scans may be unreliable due to technical error in reading the baseline.

To confirm the diagnosis of $\alpha_1$AT deficiency, PI typing must be carried out. The plasma concentration below which PI typing is carried out must be high enough to avoid missing affected individuals. Because patients with inflammation or liver disease, particularly children, may have a concentration of $\alpha_1$AT of up to $\approx$40 percent of normal, PI typing for plasma with less than 40 percent of the normal mean concentration should detect all individuals of PI type ZZ or with rare deficiency alleles.

In place of PI typing by isoelectric focusing, DNA methods are used in some laboratories. Using PCR, the appropriate region of exon 5 can be amplified and the Z mutation tested by using labeled oligonucleotide probes.[98,99] Alternatively, a primer designed with a nucleotide substitution can create a *Taq*I site in the normal allele, but not in the Z form,[100,101] an approach also used with the enzyme *Xmn*I for the S mutation.[101] A disadvantage of this molecular approach is that a few percent of the deficiency alleles will be misclassified as M, because all of the rare deficiency alleles will appear as normal. Misclassification of the deficiency alleles results in deficient individuals being misclassified as heterozygotes. For this reason, the isoelectric focusing method of PI typing is preferable. Although rare deficiency alleles might be missed by the latter method, a deficient individual will not be misclassified. The direct assays on DNA are rapid, require very little test material, and are suitable for population screening.

## Liver Inclusions

Normal $\alpha_1$AT is secreted rapidly from the liver. Z-type $\alpha_1$AT is retained in hepatocytes, forming intracytoplasmic inclusions, which are a characteristic sign of $\alpha_1$AT deficiency.[102] Features of the inclusions have been described in detail[103] and are shown in Figure 219-5. Several histochemical stains can identify the hepatocyte inclusions. By routine hematoxylin-eosin, the inclusions appear as round to oval, slightly eosinophilic, hyalin-like globules, localized predominantly in periportal hepatocytes. With

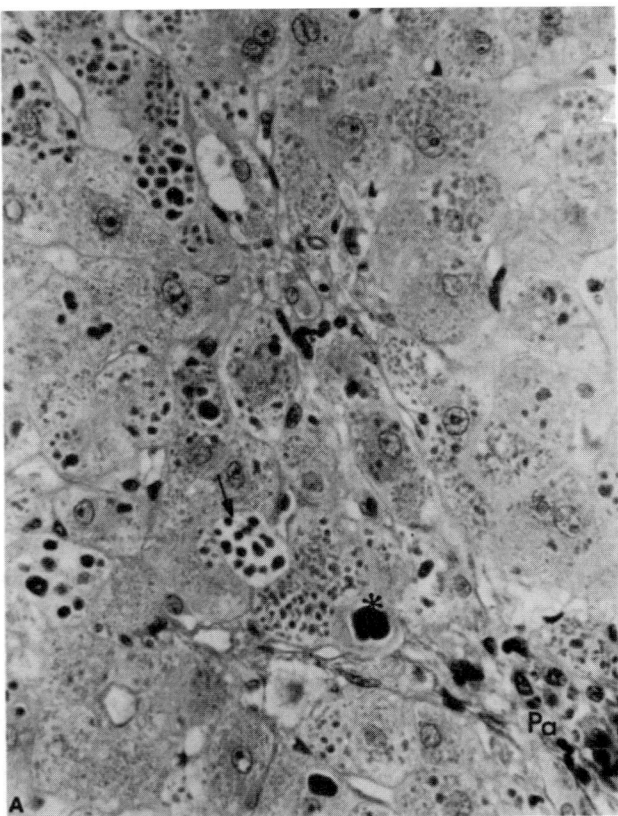
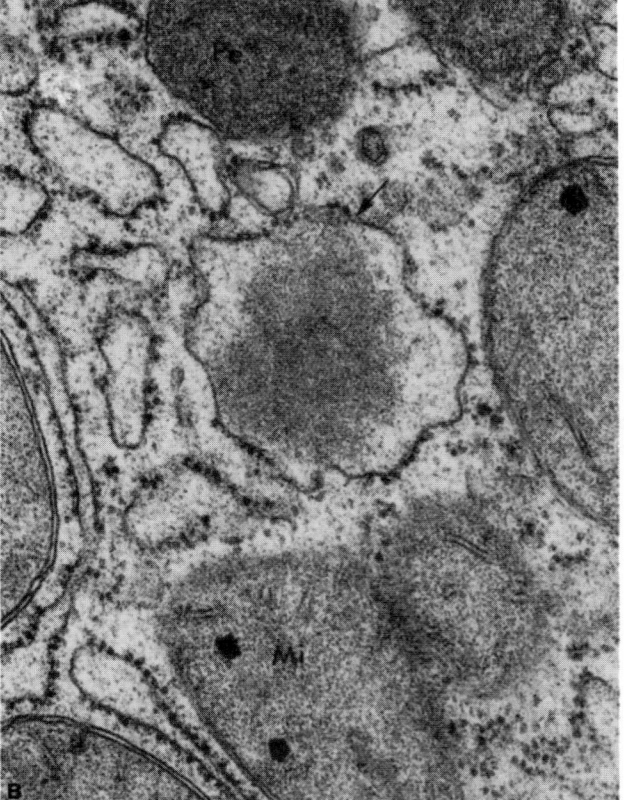

**Fig 219-5** Appearance of hepatic inclusions with PAS-D stain. Arrow indicates multiple small inclusions of $\alpha_1$AT; asterisk indicates large inclusion. Fibrosis is noted in the portal area (Pa). (PAS-D; $\times$800). *B*, Hepatic inclusion as seen with electron microscope (EM). Arrow indicates inclusion formed from dilation of rough endoplasmic reticulum, with numerous ribosomes visible on the outer membrane. Mi = mitochondria; Pe = peroxysome. $\times$70,000. (*Photographs courtesy of E. Cutz,*[103] *Used by permission.*)

PAS stain following diastase treatment (PAS-D), the inclusions are easily visualized as brilliant pink globules of various sizes. Large inclusions can be up to 15 μM in diameter. In infants with $\alpha_1$AT deficiency, the inclusions may be fine and granular. Large inclusions stain brick red with Masson trichrome stain and dark purple with phosphotungstic acid-hematoxylin (PTAH) stain.

The presence of $\alpha_1$AT in the inclusions can be demonstrated by direct immunofluorescence, with fluorescent- or peroxidase-labeled $\alpha_1$AT antibody on frozen sections.[102,103] Formalin-fixed tissue can be used after paraffin imbedding and is improved with predigestion with trypsin.[104] Immunologic identification of $\alpha_1$AT is useful for confirming the presence of $\alpha_1$AT, particularly where other liver inclusions are present. By electron microscopy, the inclusions appear as moderately electron-dense membrane-bound masses within the membranes of the endoplasmic reticulum (ER), particularly in rough endoplasmic reticulum.[103]

There is considerable variability in the extent of inclusion formation. In general, the number and size of liver inclusions increases with age.[103] The presence of inclusions indicates only the presence of at least one *PI\*Z* allele. In individuals heterozygous for $\alpha_1$AT deficiency, PI MZ, inclusions in the liver vary considerably in amount, and may be numerous and large in the presence of liver disease. Heterozygotes cannot be differentiated from homozygous-deficient individuals by an examination of liver inclusions.

In patients with chronic liver disease, liver inclusions in the periportal granules are almost always due to the presence of a deficiency allele for $\alpha_1$AT (Z or similar type of rare deficiency allele). This is not true in end-stage liver disease and in nonhepatic cancer in which $\alpha_1$AT can be stimulated by tumor necrosis factor.[105] In one study, one-third of patients with cirrhosis had PAS-D inclusions in the absence of a deficiency variant.[106] Typical inclusions can be seen with any severe systemic disease where the rate of $\alpha_1$AT exceeds the capacity of processing enzymes involved in secretion.[106,107] Occasionally, small scattered globules or deposits of lipofuscin are observed as PAS-D globules with no $\alpha_1$AT retention.[108]

## The Basic Defect

Recent advances have increased our understanding, at the molecular level, of the basic defect leading to the plasma deficiency of $\alpha_1$AT. The portion of Z $\alpha_1$AT secreted into the plasma has a nearly normal specific elastase inhibitory capacity.[77] The association constants of $\alpha_1$AT with neutrophil elastase are similar for M and monomer Z $\alpha_1$AT: $5.3 \pm 0.06 \times 10^7$ and $1.2 \pm 0.02 \times 10^7 M^{-1} s^{-1}$, respectively, for M and Z.[109] Protease inhibitor complexes are tight for both M and Z $\alpha_1$AT. Z $\alpha_1$AT has a normal rate of synthesis[110] and a half-life of 5.2 days, not significantly different from that of M$\alpha_1$AT.[26] These observations all suggest that the defect lies in secretion, consistent with accumulation of $\alpha_1$AT in liver inclusions. PI Z individuals also show the secretion defect of $\alpha_1$AT in monocytes.[111]

The inclusions in the liver do not readily dissociate, but when solubilized, Z $\alpha_1$AT binds elastase and is functionally active as an inhibitor.[112] The Z $\alpha_1$AT in the liver inclusions has an abnormal carbohydrate composition, lacking terminal *N*-acetyl-neuraminic acid and having a mannose-rich core, typical of incompletely processed glycoproteins.[112–114] Incomplete processing is, however, secondary to the basic defect, because reduced secretion in comparison with M $\alpha_1$AT also occurs when Z mRNA is injected into *Zenopus* oocytes.[115] Following up on an observation made during protein purification, Z $\alpha_1$AT was noted to have a strong tendency to aggregate, even in plasma.[116] Aggregation was particularly pronounced in the presence of pH and salt concentrations typical of the hepatic intracellular fluid and was predicted to cause the hepatic inclusions.[116] Studies of production of M and Z $\alpha_1$AT in oocytes showed that the secretion defect is independent of glycosylation.[115] In the Z protein, lysine replaces glutamic acid in normal M $\alpha_1$AT at position 342.[117,118] Glutamic acid is involved in a salt bridge important for stabilization of the molecule and occurs

at a sharp bend in the major B-sheet.[37] When lysine 290, the other component of the 290–342 salt bridge was altered to glutamic acid by site directed mutagenesis, secretion of $\alpha_1$AT was nearly normal after injection of mRNA into oocytes,[119] indicating that alteration at the critical bend by lysine is more important than the salt bridge for normal folding.

The Glu342 residue of M $\alpha_1$AT is located at a hinge region of the reactive center loop (Fig. 219-1). The reactive center loop is mobile, and capable of adopting varying configurations; under mild denaturing conditions, the loop locks into the A sheet, forming a thermostable inactive protein.[120] When the temperature is elevated to 37°C under these same conditions, the reactive center loop of one $\alpha_1$AT molecule inserts into the A sheet of a second molecule. The phenomenon has been called loop-sheet polymerization[109] but is actually a complex formation, or aggregation, as no chemical bonds are involved. Replacement of hinge residue 342 in Z $\alpha_1$AT apparently enables the A sheet to open, making the molecule a receptor for dimerization.[121] This explanation is supported by the circular dichroism spectrum of Z $\alpha_1$AT.[121] The same type of aggregation has been shown to occur spontaneously with the deficiency variant PI $M_{MALTON}$.[122] The extent of polymerization of Z $\alpha_1$AT is temperature dependent, with acceleration at 41°C, and is also concentration dependent.[121] Any increase in body temperature, for example, during inflammation and fever, could increase the aggregation of liver Z $\alpha_1$AT. Furthermore, because $\alpha_1$AT is an acute phase protein, an increase in production during inflammation or other stress could also contribute to aggregation of liver Z $\alpha_1$AT. M protein will also self-aggregate when the temperature is raised to 41°C and particularly when the concentration of $\alpha_1$AT is increased.[109]

Accumulation of Z $\alpha_1$AT appears to proceed slowly and continuously, counteracted by degradation of the abnormal protein. Our knowledge of the process by which abnormally folded proteins are degraded has increased, particularly with the studies of the abnormal protein resulting from the delta F508 mutation in cystic fibrosis, in which mutant protein also accumulates within cells. Z $\alpha_1$AT in the lumen of the endoplasmic reticulum interacts with the transmembrane molecular chaperone calnexin, and induces the polyubiquitination of calnexin in the proteasome proteolytic pathway.[123] Assembly of abnormally folded $\alpha_1$AT with calnexin was shown, in hepatoma cells, to require cotranslational trimming of glucose from asparagine-linked oligosaccharides, in studies of another abnormally folded variant.[124]

## Rare Deficiency Alleles

Deficiency alleles include the spectrum from those producing an amount of plasma $\alpha_1$AT similar to that of the *PI\*Z* allele, to those that produce no detectable $\alpha_1$AT by standard methods.

**Alleles Expressing Detectable $\alpha_1$AT.** Several deficiency alleles have been reported in which the plasma concentration is detectable by standard methods, generally in the range of about 2 to 15 percent of normal. The site of each mutation is listed in Table 219-5. All have an electrophoretic mobility different from that of the PI Z variant.[93] PI $Z_{AUGSBURG}$ (same as PI $Z_{TUNBRIDGEWELLS}$) and PI $Z_{WREXHAM}$ have the Z mutation as well as another benign amino acid difference. PI $M_{MALTON}$ is associated with PAS-positive hepatocyte inclusions identical to those found in association with PI Z;[108] like Z, the protein has a tendency to aggregate.[116] $M_{NICHINAN}$ has the $M_{MALTON}$ mutation in addition to a benign alteration at residue 148.[125] $S_{IIYAMA}$ also aggregates and forms liver inclusions,[126] and has been shown in a yeast system to be abnormally unstable.[127] Amino acid residues 52 and 53 are altered in the latter three variants. These mutations cause a displacement of the B helix that forms the base of the gap in the A sheet for the reactive center loop (Fig. 219-1). PI $M_{DUARTE}$ migrates electrophoretically similarly to PI M,[128] and the isoelectric point is similar to that of M3.[93] PAS-D globules were present in the liver,[128] indicating that this deficient variant also has, like Z and

**Table 219-5** Deficiency Alleles of $\alpha_1$-Antitrypsin

| Allele | Plasma conc'n (% normal) | Amino acid # | Exon | Normal Codon | Normal aa | Mutant Codon | Mutation | |
|---|---|---|---|---|---|---|---|---|
| Z_WREXHAM | | −19 | | TCG | Ser | TTG | Leu | S(−19)L |
| M_PROCIDA | 4 | 41 | 2 | CTG | Leu | CCG | Pro | L41P |
| M_PALERMO (213val root) | | 51/52 | 2 | TTC | Phe | | delete | F51/52del |
| M_MALTON (m2 root) | 12 | 51/52 | 2 | TTC | Phe | | delete | F51/52del |
| M_NICHINAN | <15 | 52 | 2 | TTC | Phe | | delete | F52del |
| | | 148 | 2 | GGG | Gly | AGG | Arg | G148R |
| S_IIYAMA | | 53 | 2 | TCC | Ser | TTC | Phe | S53F |
| Z_AUGSBURG | <15 | 342 | 5 | GAG | Glu | AAG | Lys | E342K |
| Z | 18 | 342 | 5 | GAG | Glu | AAG | Lys | E342K |
| M_HEERLEN | 2 | 369 | 5 | CCC | Pro | CTC | Leu | P369L |
| **Null** | | | | | | | | |
| Q0_ISOLA DI PROCIDA | 0 | | 2–5 | | | delete ex2–5 | delete 17 kb | |
| Q0_RIEDENBURG | 0 | | 2–5 | | | delete ev2–5 | delete 15 kb | |
| Q0_LISBON | | 68 | 2 | AAC | Thr | ATC | Ile | T68I |
| Q0_LUDWIGSHAFEN | 0 | 92 | 2 | ATC | Ile | AAC | Asn | I92N |
| Q0_NEWPORT | 0 | 115 | 2 | GGC | Gly | AGC | Ser | G115S |
| Q0_GRANITEFALLS | 0 | 160/161 | 2 | TACGTG | Tyr-Val | TAGTG | delete, stop | Y160X |
| Q0_TRANSFERASE | 0 | 194 | 3 | TGG | Trp | TGA | stop | W194X |
| Q0_BELLINGHAM | 0 | 217 | 3 | AAG | Lys | TAG | stop | K217X |
| Q0_CARDIFF | 0 | 256 | 3 | GAT | Asp | GTT | Val | D256V |
| Q0_HONGKONG | 0 | 317/318 | 4 | CTCTCC | Leu-Ser | CTCC | delete, stop aa 334 | L317L |
| Q0_MATTAWA | 0 | 353 | 5 | TTA | Leu | TTTA | insert, stop aa 376 | L353F |
| Q0_BOLTON | 0 | 362 | 5 | CCCG | Pro | CCG | delete, stop aa 373 | P362P |
| Q0_SAARBRÜCKEN | 0 | 362 | 5 | CCC | Pro | CCCC | insert, stop aa 376 | P362P |
| Q0_CLAYTON | 0 | 362 | 5 | CCC | Pro | CCCC | insert, stop aa 376 | P362P |

References are in text and in Brantley et al.,[8] Fraizer et al.,[136] and Faber et al.[138]

M_MALTON, a defect in secretion from the liver. M_HEERLEN[129] and M_PROCIDA[130] each have mutations involving a proline residue, which could affect stability and lead to intracellular degradation.

The non-Z deficiency alleles are found at low frequencies. PI*M_MALTON and PI*M_DUARTE occur at about 1/100th and 1/200th the frequency of the PI*Z allele, respectively.[93] The presence of these and other deficiency alleles must be considered when no Z $\alpha_1$AT is observed in plasma from a patient with an apparent deficiency. These and other alleles produce $\alpha_1$AT inclusions in the liver, particularly in heterozygotes, in the presence of an apparently normal M phenotype. Some of the mutant products may be detectable by isoelectric focusing, even in the presence of a normal M allele, and particularly by using immunofixation. Family studies should help to confirm the presence of a rare deficiency allele. Unless their presence has been definitely excluded, these rare alleles should be considered as the most likely cause of inclusions other than PI*Z. In Asian populations that lack the PI*Z allele, other rare deficiency alleles may be present; for example, the S_IIYAMA variant appears to be the most prevalent variant in Japan.[131]

**The Null (Q0) Alleles.** The null alleles result in the most severe deficiency, arbitrarily defined as those producing less than 1 percent of the normal amount of plasma $\alpha_1$AT. These alleles are designated as PI*Q0 and homozygous phenotypes designated as PI Q0Q0. While the PI*Z allele has been reported only in Caucasian populations, the null alleles are widespread. In our series of 112 patients with $\alpha_1$AT deficiency, we estimated the frequency of all null alleles to be $1.7 \times 10^{-4}$, about 1/100th the frequency of the PI*Z allele in a North American Caucasian population and similar to the frequency of PI*M_MALTON.[93] The PI Q0 variants are listed in Table 219-5.

Obstructive airways disease occurs as early as the second or third decade, even in nonsmokers.[132] Data indicate that null homozygotes have more severe obstructive airways disease than

individuals of PI type ZZ whose low concentrations of $\alpha_1$AT apparently provide some protection to lung tissue.[133] These individuals particularly may benefit from the new therapy methods that are under development. The presence of even trace amounts of $\alpha_1$AT in null homozygotes may help prevent the formation of $\alpha_1$AT antibodies during long-term augmentation therapy.

There are a variety of null mutants, each with the final result of interference with the production of $\alpha_1$AT. The most common defect is a premature stop codon, although other mechanisms are reported, such as intracellular degradation (Q0_HONGKONG;[134] Q0_MATTAWA[135]), alteration of tertiary structure (Q0_LUDWIGSHAFEN[136]), or complete deletion of the $\alpha_1$AT coding exons (Q0_ISOLA DI PROCIDA[137]) (for further details, see references 93, 136, and 138). The use of DNA haplotypes, as described for studies of normal alleles of $\alpha_1$AT, can be useful in delineating different null alleles, as each null allele usually occurs on a specific haplotype background.[93]

### Selective Mechanisms for Deficiency Alleles

Because the combined frequency of PI*Q0 alleles is about $1.7 \times 10^{-4}$, the frequency of each allele should be considerably less. If selective advantage has allowed the frequency of the PI*Z allele to increase, then it is interesting that the frequency of other deficiency alleles has not similarly increased. Possible explanations are that the PI*Z allele has some unique selective advantage in comparison with other deficiency alleles, that other deficiency alleles have arisen much more recently than PI*Z, or that chance factors have been responsible for the increase in PI*Z.

DNA haplotypes indicate a single origin for the PI*Z allele, with a subsequent spread of the mutation through northern Caucasian populations.[88] Possible mechanisms for increasing the PI*Z allele frequency are increased fertility of heterozygotes or preferential survival of heterozygotes. Preferential survival from tuberculosis has been suggested as a possible selection pressure.[139] This is entirely speculative at present, although data showing that an increased frequency of MZ individuals among older blood donors, who were adults prior to tuberculosis therapy,[140] are supportive.

# OBSTRUCTIVE LUNG DISEASE

## Clinical Features

Chronic obstructive pulmonary disease (COPD), specifically emphysema, is the most prevalent clinical disorder associated with $\alpha_1$AT deficiency. In 33 patients reported by Eriksson in 1965,[141] the first symptoms of pulmonary disease occurred below 40 years of age in 60 percent of patients and below 50 years of age in 90 percent of patients. The association with $\alpha_1$AT deficiency was confirmed in many subsequent studies. The early studies, suggesting a high proportion of emphysema in patients with $\alpha_1$AT deficiency, were biased by the ascertainment of patients because of their illness. Now it is appreciated that $\alpha_1$AT deficient patients who avoid smoking have a much delayed onset of clinical symptoms and may have an almost normal life span.

Surveys from several countries of groups of patients with COPD are in agreement with the initial report[2] that only 1 or 2 percent of all patients have $\alpha_1$AT deficiency (earlier studies are reviewed in references 86 and 142). The frequency may be considerably higher: 18 percent of patients with emphysema in one study, when the referral pattern favored young and more severely affected patients.[72] The male:female ratio is at least 2:1,[143] which may be related to smoking exposure.

Emphysema associated with $\alpha_1$AT deficiency typically involves the basal more than the apical regions of the lungs. Although most patients present with emphysema, some present with symptoms of bronchial asthma or chronic bronchitis.[143] Thoracic radiographs show a symmetric decrease in peripheral vasculature that is most prominent in the lower lungs, but only in those patients with well-established emphysema and not in asymptomatic individuals.[144] High-resolution CT scans identify changes in pulmonary structure in patients with $\alpha_1$AT deficiency.[145] Radioisotope ventilation and perfusion scans are usually abnormal and may show slight abnormalities in asymptomatic patients.[144] Changes in lung mechanics are similar to those found in other patients with emphysema, with reduction in lung volumes and expiratory flow rates. The decreased expiratory flow rate can be attributed to loss of elastic recoil. The most sensitive parameters for detecting abnormalities in asymptomatic $\alpha_1$AT-deficient patients have been reported to be closing volume, nitrogen washout volume, and lung mechanics. Clinical features of pulmonary disease were discussed extensively in an earlier edition of this text.[13]

## Age of Onset and Course of Obstructive Lung Disease

The onset and severity of disease symptoms show considerable variability. Smoking is the major factor influencing the course of disease. Of patients identified through an affected relative, female patients tend to show less-rapid deterioration of lung function with age[143] and better survival.[146] Reports of emphysema in children with $\alpha_1$AT deficiency are extremely rare; the emphysema in these patients is likely due to the coexistence of other genetic abnormalities.[147] In a follow-up of 103 16-year-olds identified through a neonatal screening program in Sweden, no significant differences in lung function were observed when compared with age-matched controls. Of 17 PI ZZ children 7 to 18 years of age, mostly ascertained through neonatal jaundice, 1 (18 years of age) had hyperinflation with mild expiratory obstruction.[148] In another study of 59 patients with liver disease, of whom 28 had $\alpha_1$AT deficiency PI type ZZ, patients with $\alpha_1$AT deficiency tended to have higher lung volumes than those of healthy controls or children with extrahepatic biliary atresia.[149] Factors that predispose to liver disease may also predispose to lung disease. Children with liver disease and $\alpha_1$AT deficiency should be followed closely as potential candidates for augmentation therapy if their liver disease does not lead to transplantation.

Unbiased survival figures for patients with $\alpha_1$AT deficiency are unknown, because many PI ZZ individuals are never identified. Survival to the sixth and seventh decade is possible. The most extensive survival data were obtained from Sweden[146] and are summarized in Figure 219-6. Mortality figures differ markedly for smokers and nonsmokers. About 98 percent of nonsmoking females and 65 percent of nonsmoking males were alive at age 55, whereas only 30 percent and 18 percent of females and males, respectively, who smoke were alive at the same age. However, the figures shown here are biased because these patients have been ascertained through hospital admissions or clinics. The prognosis, particularly in nonsmokers, is probably better than indicated by the Swedish study. A study of 54 patients with $\alpha_1$AT deficiency, in which 28 of the patients were not ascertained through the presence of COPD or other lung problems, indicates that the risk for developing COPD has been overestimated.[150] Of the $\alpha_1$AT-deficient patients between 30 and 60 years of age and not ascertained through COPD, only 1 in 3, almost all smokers, had developed COPD. Nonsmokers may have a late age of onset, and $\alpha_1$AT deficiency should be considered as a positive factor for emphysema in elderly nonsmokers.[151]

Smoking has a major effect on both the age of onset of pulmonary symptoms and on the course of pulmonary deterioration. Onset of dyspnea appears to be rare before 40 years of age in

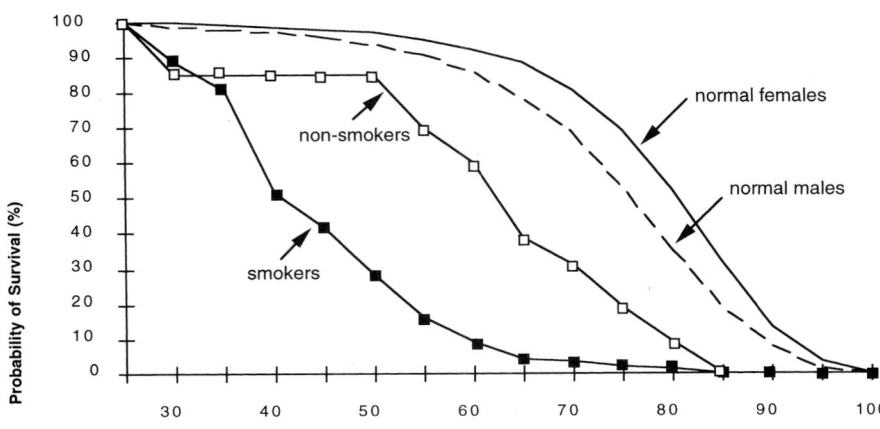

Fig 219-6 Cumulative probability of survival to specified ages for normal males, normal females, PI ZZ smokers, and PI ZZ nonsmokers as indicated in upper right. (*Based on data published by Larrson.*[146])

nonsmokers.[146] In a review of patients from the literature (30 nonsmokers and 84 smokers), the mean age of onset of dyspnea was 35 years in smokers and 44 years in nonsmokers.[152] A study of 33 patients with emphysema and $\alpha_1$AT deficiency in New Zealand indicated a mean age for onset of dyspnea of 32 years in smokers and 51 years in nonsmokers.[153] Lung function deteriorates continually with time as the alveolar walls are destroyed. The rate of deterioration of lung function, as measured by decline in $FEV_1$ (volume of air expired during the first second of forced vital capacity) shows a marked difference between $\alpha_1$AT-deficient smokers and nonsmokers. In a study of 65 PI ZZ Danish patients (60 percent of the group identified because of symptoms), the age to reach 50 percent of predicted $FEV_1$ was 17 years greater in those who had never smoked than in smokers.[154] The decline in $FEV_1$ was 86 ml/year for 18 Danish nonsmokers, 52 ml/year for 100 exsmokers, and 132 ml/year for 43 current smokers.[155] Results from the United States $\alpha_1$Antitrypsin Registry have shown a mean decline of 57.5 ml per year among 208 nonsmokers, 52.0 ml per year in 697 exsmokers, and 104.8 ml per year in 22 current smokers.[156] The rate of decline was found to be greater for males than for females. Effects of smoking could be particularly detrimental in $\alpha_1$AT deficiency, as in normal individuals, when begun during adolescence, as attainment of maximal lung function is prevented.[157]

A direct measure of the presence of a peptide produced by elastase activity could be useful in identifying individuals most likely to develop severe lung disease.[158] This assay measures the amount of a specific fragment cleaved from fibrinogen, releasing a fibrinogen A-containing fragment, $\alpha1-21$. The mean plasma levels were increased in PI MZ individuals, with considerable overlap, and the majority of PI ZZ individuals had a plasma concentration above the normal upper limit. Smokers had particularly elevated levels of the peptide. There was an inverse relationship between peptide levels in nonsmoking PI ZZ patients and percent of predicted forced expiratory volume in 1 s (FEV$_1$ percent), a measure of the extent of airway obstruction.

### The Role of Proteases in Lung Destruction

The alveolar destruction characteristic of emphysema is generally considered to be due to an imbalance between proteolytic enzymes, particularly elastase, and their inhibitors. Support for this concept is derived from numerous experimental animal studies and from the studies of patients with $\alpha_1$AT deficiency. Because of its small molecular size, $\alpha_1$AT enters lung tissue and has been recovered in bronchoalveolar lavage fluid. A plasma deficiency of $\alpha_1$AT is also reflected as a deficiency of $\alpha_1$AT in the lung.[159] The absence of adequate inhibitor allows continued destruction of lung tissue. In PI ZZ-associated emphysema, $\alpha_1$AT in the lung has been demonstrated to be in the functionally inactive polymer form.[160] Direct evidence for the complexing of $\alpha_1$AT with elastase in the lung has been provided by the finding of elastase-$\alpha_1$AT complexes in bronchial lavage fluid of normal smokers and nonsmokers, accounting for less than 1 percent of the total $\alpha_1$AT in the fluid.[161]

The role of $\alpha_1$AT as the major inhibitor of elastase at the epithelial lining was demonstrated in a homozygous null individual, in whom the antineutrophil elastase capacity of lavage fluid was less than 15 percent of normal.[162] Other potential elastase inhibitors in lung tissue, such as a low molecular weight protease inhibitor[163,164] or locally produced $\alpha_2$-macroglobulin,[165] apparently make a minor contribution.

Elastase appears to play a role in neonatal respiratory distress syndrome,[166] a condition for which $\alpha_1$AT administration may be useful.[167]

### Mechanisms of Exacerbation of Lung Destruction by Smoking

Mechanisms of lung destruction in normal smokers would be expected to have an even more detrimental effect in those with $\alpha_1$AT deficiency. An important mechanism for the increased

destruction of lung tissue in smokers appears to be oxidation, because oxidation of methionine residues interferes dramatically with complex formation of $\alpha_1$AT with elastase. Because the gas phase of tobacco smoke is rich in oxidizing agents, a direct effect of smoke on $\alpha_1$AT could be anticipated. In vitro, both a crude tar fraction of cigarette smoke and aqueous extracts of freshly generated cigarette smoke significantly inactivate $\alpha_1$AT (see review in reference 168).

Some in vivo studies assessing smoking effects show a decrease of elastase inhibitor activity in serum from smokers as compared with nonsmokers; other studies have not shown a difference. In view of the generous supply of antioxidants in plasma, a measurable effect on $\alpha_1$AT in plasma seems unlikely. A study of acute effects of smoking showed no increase in elastase-like enzyme activity in smokers, but an increase in immunologic elastase levels indicated the possible release of neutrophil elastase in the bronchoalveolar lavage fluid.[169] Slight inactivation of $\alpha_1$AT was noted in lavage fluid immediately after smoking.[170] $\alpha_1$AT with oxidized methionine and reduced inhibitory activity has been recovered from lungs of smokers.[171]

In addition to oxidation effects, smoking acts on neutrophils, which are present in increased numbers in smokers. Smoking triggers neutrophils to release elastase, as well as myeloperoxidase, which inactivates $\alpha_1$AT.[172,173] This helps account for the increased amount of proteolytically cleaved $\alpha_1$AT in smokers.[174] Smoking acts directly on elastin by impairing its cross-linking.[175]

### Other Factors Influencing the Extent of Lung Destruction

**Genetic Factors.** A number of population studies indicate that respiratory symptoms show familial aggregation (see the review in reference 176) and genetic factors no doubt influence disease severity in $\alpha_1$AT deficiency. In a study of 256 monozygotic and 158 dizygotic adult twins, a large proportion of measured variability in pulmonary function tests was accounted for by genetic influences.[176] In $\alpha_1$AT deficiency, the presence of emphysema in a parent, or the presence of asthma, appears to increase the risk for development of COPD.[150]

The absence of the restriction site for $TaqI$, 3' of the $\alpha_1$AT gene (Fig. 219-3A) has been reported as associated with an approximately threefold risk for COPD: 17 percent of patients with COPD versus 5 percent of the general population.[177,178] This mutation apparently occurs in an enhancer region for $\alpha_1$AT at a binding site for the transcription factor octamer-1 (Oct-1), and results in a loss of cooperativity with the tissue-specific factor NF-IL6. This, in turn, interferes with the IL6 response, leading to reduced acute phase response.[179] A significant difference in the frequency of the $TaqI$ ($-$) allele was noted between Black and Caucasian South Africans, 24.1 percent and 6 percent, respectively, highlighting the importance of careful ethnic matching of patient groups.[180]

A number of metabolic parameters may have a hereditary component and could alter susceptibility to lung destruction. These include the number of neutrophils, the extent of elastase released from neutrophils, and the differences in elastase quality or quantity within neutrophils. Any increase in the protease content of neutrophils, particularly elastase, might be expected to increase the rate of lung degradation. Studies to compare neutrophil proteases in COPD, and in individuals of PI type MZ and ZZ, all with appropriate controls, have not shown pronounced differences in neutrophil elastase concentration between individuals with normal lung function and those with COPD. Detrimental effects could be produced by increased production of myeloperoxidase causing local inactivation of $\alpha_1$AT, low levels of catalase (which blocks $H_2O_2$ production by myeloperoxidase), low concentrations of antioxidants, or characteristics of lung tissue that result in susceptibility to degradation. Most of these factors have not been adequately investigated.

**Antioxidant Status.** Oxidation appears to play an important role in proteolytic degradation of the lung, therefore antioxidants should play an important role in limiting this destruction. The damaging effects of chemical oxidants, such as those from cigarette smoke, and those produced by neutrophils could be modified by antioxidants present in lung tissue. Normal plasma and tissue components that may contribute to antioxidant activity include ascorbate, ceruloplasmin, transferrin, vitamin E, reduced glutathione (through the activity of glutathione peroxidase), NADPH reductase, methionine sulfoxide reductase, and superoxide dismutase. The total antioxidant activity of plasma is somewhat reduced in smokers as compared with nonsmokers,[181,182] and those with a family history of lung disease may also have reduced plasma antioxidants.[181] In vitro studies of the antioxidants ascorbate, cysteine, and dapsone demonstrate that all of these can protect $\alpha_1$AT loss of inhibitory activity due to activated neutrophils, but are not able to activate $\alpha_1$AT once inactivation has occurred.[183] The protective effects of these antioxidants are proposed to be related to their ability to scavenge superoxide and oxidants generated by the neutrophils. Vitamin E is particularly important as a tissue antioxidant, and may act predominantly on cell membranes. Animal experiments demonstrate that vitamin E neutralizes free radicals, decreases lung susceptibility to oxidant injury, and reduces damage from smoke and alveolar macrophages (see the review in reference 184). Serum levels of vitamin E and the oxidative metabolite vitamin E quinone are similar in young asymptomatic smokers and nonsmokers. Smokers, however, show markedly less vitamin E and vitamin E quinone in bronchoalveolar lavage fluid than nonsmokers, possibly due to increased oxidative metabolism of vitamin E in smokers,[184] a difference only partly corrected by vitamin E supplementation. These studies suggest that vitamin E is an important antioxidant in the lower respiratory tract, which could modify tissue destruction.

## Risk for Lung Disease in Heterozygotes

The assessment of risk for MZ heterozygotes is important because they constitute 2 to 5 percent of most populations. Surveys of patients with COPD have generally shown a two- to threefold increase of individuals of PI type MZ in comparison with those of PI type M (see the review in reference 185). These studies usually have not distinguished smokers from nonsmokers. In studies of PI MZ subjects with appropriate PI MM control subjects, slight or no differences in elastic recoil were noted in nonsmokers.[186,187] A 10-year longitudinal study of nonsmoker PI MZ individuals initially presenting with exertional dyspnea showed a significant decrease in lung function tests reflecting elastic recoil, but no decrease in $FEV_1$.[188] In contrast, PI MZ smokers showed a significant loss of elastic recoil and other abnormalities of lung function.[186,189,190] Longitudinal studies in Sweden over 6 years showed significantly increased lung destruction; mean annual reduction in $FEV_1$ in PI MZ smokers versus nonsmokers was 75 and 40 ml/year, respectively.[191] Although an increased loss of lung elasticity has been demonstrated, even PI MZ smokers usually do not develop sufficient impairment to be recognized as clinically affected. In certain families, other genetic predisposing factors may interact with $\alpha_1$AT heterozygosity to produce clinical disease.

Individuals of PI type SZ should have only a slightly greater risk than those of PI type MZ, and few have been reported in surveys of patients with COPD. Isolated reports suggest that smokers particularly may have a tendency for impaired lung function.[192]

Although the *PI*F allele is not associated with a decrease of $\alpha_1$AT concentration, PI FM heterozygotes may be more susceptible to pulmonary function impairment, particularly when exposed to industrial pollutants.[193] $\alpha_1$AT of the F type, which has an extra cysteine residue, appears to have an increased tendency to oxidation, noted by its altered electrophoretic pattern after sample aging,[69] and this increased tendency to oxidation may

make PI FM individuals susceptible to lung destruction in a polluted environment.

## LIVER DISEASE

### Childhood Onset

An association of $\alpha_1$AT deficiency and liver disease in children was first reported by Sharp and colleagues.[6] When originally reported, the prognosis for liver disease with $\alpha_1$AT deficiency was believed to be poor because all the patients identified had cirrhosis. Later studies showed the prognosis to be more favorable. The features of liver disease in $\alpha_1$AT deficiency have been discussed in several reviews.[194-197]

Liver abnormalities occur in only a portion of infants of PI type ZZ. In a screening program of 200,000 Swedish newborns, followup was carried out on 120 children of PI type ZZ and 2 children of PI type is $Z_{Q0}$. Approximately 18 percent of PI Z children developed clinically recognizable liver abnormalities: 7.3 percent had prolonged obstructive jaundice with marked evidence of liver disease, 4.1 percent had prolonged jaundice with mild liver disease, and 6.4 percent had other abnormalities suggestive of liver disease such as hepatomegaly, splenomegaly, unexplained failure to thrive, or stated history of prolonged jaundice without medical documentation.[198] A screening of infants with conjugated hyperbilirubinemia in England suggests a similar incidence, with 1 PI ZZ infant with liver abnormalities in 19,200 newborns, or 1 PI ZZ infant in 3,400 newborns.[199]

The most common sign of liver abnormality associated with $\alpha_1$AT deficiency is the "neonatal hepatitis syndrome," characterized by conjugated hyperbilirubinemia and raised serum aminotransferases, frequently with hepatosplenomegaly. Varying degrees of failure to thrive have been noted. The serum bilirubin concentration can be very high, rising to 12 to 17 mg/dl (normal less than 1).[198,200] Signs of cholestasis generally appear between 4 days and 2 months of age, and can persist for period of a few weeks to up to 8 months.[96,200] Cholestasis in $\alpha_1$AT deficiency may be severe enough to cause acholic stools, as in extrahepatic biliary atresia. $\alpha_1$AT deficiency should always be considered in a child with prolonged jaundice (conjugated hyperbilirubinemia) of unexplained origin, and PI typing should be an early diagnostic procedure. From 14 to 29 percent of infants with neonatal hepatitis have been found to have $\alpha_1$AT deficiency, PI type ZZ.[96,200] While presentation as neonatal hepatitis is the most common, hepatomegaly without jaundice in infancy or childhood, or hematemesis can be the presenting symptoms.

The pathologic features of $\alpha_1$AT deficiency associated with liver disease in children have been reviewed.[96,103] Typical PAS-D-positive inclusions, described previously, are observed in children with liver disease. They may be difficult to identify in percutaneous liver biopsy specimens from infants, and are not observed before 12 weeks of age.[199] Liver biopsies from young, asymptomatic children usually show only very small inclusions by PAS-D stain, but more extensive deposition by immunofluorescence. The amount and size of liver inclusions shows no clear correlation with severity of liver disease. Livers of older PI Z patients, particularly those in whom cirrhosis develops, contain larger amounts of $\alpha_1$AT, and inclusions usually occupy 50 to 80 percent of the parenchyma. Regenerative nodules may contain focal depositions of $\alpha_1$AT, while others may show no depositions.

In those children presenting with neonatal hepatitis, the constant histopathologic features include intrahepatic cholestasis, varying degrees of hepatocellular injury, and moderate fibrosis with inflammatory cells in portal areas. Giant cell transformation is common. Initial liver biopsy occasionally shows marked ductular proliferation with bile plugging suggestive of biliary atresia, in the presence of a normal extrahepatic biliary tree,[96] or with patent narrowed extrahepatic bile ducts.[201] Some infants have a significant decrease in the number of interlobular bile ducts. In infants who later develop cirrhosis, liver biopsies show moderate to heavy periportal inflammatory cell infiltrate and hepatocyte swelling with patchy necrosis, but no evidence of cholestasis. In infants whose liver disease apparently resolved, the main abnormality observed on later biopsy was mild to moderate portal fibrosis with a few inflammatory cells; none of these children showed hepatocellular necrosis, cholestasis, or bile ductular changes.[96]

Once the diagnosis of $\alpha_1$AT deficiency is established, liver biopsy is usually unnecessary. Biopsy is useful in establishing a long-term prognosis because portal fibrosis and ductular proliferation appear less frequently in patients with a favorable course of the disease. However, even patients with these liver abnormalities can have a favorable outcome.[202] Earlier onset and longer persistence of jaundice may occur in children who progress to an unfavorable outcome in some studies,[201] but this is not the case in all studies.[96] The level of liver enzymes, such as serum alanine aminotransferase and serum glutamyl transpeptidase, can be very high in PI ZZ infants,[198,200] and the degree of elevation does not appear to be correlated with prognosis. Gamma glutamyl transpeptidase ($\gamma$GT), in the cell membrane of a number of tissues, is useful as a measure of the extent of bile duct damage, and is typically elevated in $\alpha_1$AT deficiency.[203] Persistent elevation of liver enzymes at greater than three times the normal upper limit tends to be associated with a poor prognosis,[198,201,202,204] but elevation up to this level is not.[204] From birth through 8 years of age, many children who appear to be clinically well still have an elevation of liver-derived serum enzymes. In the Swedish study, the serum concentration of alanine aminotransferase was above the normal limit in 46 percent of children at 4 years of age, but had decreased to 12 percent by 12 years of age.[205] Measurement of urinary bile acids has been suggested to be useful for evaluating liver status in affected children.[206] Total bile acids remained consistently high in children whose early liver abnormalities progressed to cirrhosis.

## Pathogenesis of Liver Disease

Although the structural defect leading to aggregation of Z $\alpha_1$AT is known, less is known about the actual cause of liver injury. The damage could be a result of the presence of inclusions in the liver, the deficiency of the inhibitor in plasma, or both (see the reviews in references 196, 207, and 208).

A favored hypothesis is that $\alpha_1$AT, accumulated in the endoplasmic reticulum of hepatocytes, directly causes the liver injury. Intracellular accumulation of $\alpha_1$AT increases lysosomal enzyme activity,[209] which could contribute to liver damage. Prior to development of cirrhosis, cell necrosis was observed only in periportal hepatocytes with $\alpha_1$AT inclusions.[210] Transgenic mice expressing and storing mutant Z allele in the liver have been produced.[19,211] In one study, transgenic mouse lines were established with multiple copies of human $\alpha_1$AT M or Z gene per mouse genome.[19] Livers from both M and one Z (five copies of the gene/mouse genome) were similar, with a few abnormal findings. However the second Z line (12 copies) showed abundant material in the liver, and areas of liver cell necrosis. The changes in this Z line were suggested to resemble those seen in neonatal hepatitis in humans. However, as there were 12 copies of the Z allele per haploid mouse genome, this may not represent the analogous human situation. Runting was observed in this line of mice, which was later found to be strain specific.[212] No evidence of hepatitis virus was found in this colony. In another study of transgenic mice, Carlson et al.[211] studied the offspring of three lines of transgenic M mice and three lines of transgenic Z mice, the latter carrying 1, 10, and more than 10 copies of the Z gene respectively. This study was complicated because the mice carried the mouse hepatitis virus, which produced occasional necrotic and inflammatory regions in a number of mice, but the effects of the virus were shown to be no different in Z than in M transgenic mice. Inflammation and necrosis were significantly increased in mice with 10 or more copies of the Z gene. An increase in fibrosis

did not reach statistical significance in PI Z mice versus their controls ($p = 0.08$). The pathology score was increased only slightly for those mice carrying one copy of the Z gene ($p < 0.028$). If the effects of the hepatitis virus can be ignored, then the conclusion from these studies is that fibrosis, necrosis, and inflammation can be produced in the liver when a sufficiently large store of inclusion granules is present. Cholestasis was not observed. The effect of an elevation in body temperature upon Z transgenic mice is of interest. While there may be differences between the susceptibility of mouse and human livers, this exaggerated model of $\alpha_1$AT retention may provide support for the inclusions themselves as the pathologic factor in later childhood and adult liver disease, where storage of the inclusion granules is pronounced. However, other predisposing factors may be involved in infants, in whose livers $\alpha_1$AT granules are scarce. Granules are absent until 12 weeks of age,[199] after the typical presenting time for neonatal jaundice.

The liver involvement could be caused by a direct injury to the hepatocytes due to excessive uninhibited protease activity, enhanced by subsequent release of high levels of oxygen free radicals. Phagocytic cells and bacteria present in the gastrointestinal tract produce large amounts of proteases, which are transported by the portal circulation to the liver. Bacterial proteases destroy cells in several ways, including inactivation of the complement system, direct inactivation of serum protease inhibitors,[213] and, perhaps most important, the generation of superoxide radicals leading to the formation of hydrogen peroxide ($H_2O_2$),[214,215] which can produce hepatic injury. This oxidant-generating system is normally kept in check by antioxidant enzymes such as superoxide dismutase, catalase, and glutathione peroxidase. These enzymes may differ in their quantities in different individuals. An imbalance in these factors might lead to the production of liver disease in some individuals with $\alpha_1$AT deficiency. Newborn mammals have a very low level of superoxide dismutase, which increases dramatically after birth.[216] This suggests that infants would be particularly susceptible to the initiation of liver damage.[217] Environmental stresses also differ among individuals. Children with impaired biliary secretion may develop deficiencies of fat-soluble vitamins. A deficiency of vitamin E in the liver could lead to excessively high oxidant levels, promoting hepatocyte membrane damage. These speculations suggest further avenues for research and provide a rationale for the use of antioxidant therapy.

An autoimmune type of cellular damage could also be considered, with abnormal $\alpha_1$AT in hepatic inclusions stimulating an immune response. As hepatocytes containing $\alpha_1$AT are destroyed, the abnormal $\alpha_1$AT may be released and recognized as a foreign antigen. The $\alpha_1$AT in inclusions has some unique antigenic sites as compared with normal M $\alpha_1$AT, because monoclonal antibody specific for Z $\alpha_1$AT has been produced.[218] Glomerular lesions found in patients with $\alpha_1$AT deficiency and cirrhosis are suggestive of an autoimmune response.[219] Increased activation of complement components could account for the evidence of complement activation found in children with $\alpha_1$AT deficiency and liver disease.[220]

Studies of cell fibroblasts transfected with the mutation PI Z gene suggest a possible difference between PI ZZ individuals who develop liver disease and those who do not. A lag in degradation of the mutant protein in cell lines from patients with liver disease suggests an inherent problem in the degradation mechanism for abnormally folded protein.[221] However, there is probably no simple single answer for the susceptibility of certain individuals to liver disease in infancy. The liver injury could result from a combination of a slow degradation pathway, inadequate antioxidant protection from the effects of absorbed uninhibited proteases, subsequent damage and weakening of the cell membrane due to the oxidant free radicals, further destruction of the weakened cells by the presence of inclusions of $\alpha_1$AT, or an autoimmune effect from the eventual leakage of abnormal Z protein from the liver inclusions.

The presence of liver conclusions is generally held responsible for adult-onset liver disease. Viral infection was believed to be a contributing factor in a study of 54 Austrian ZZ patients with liver disease, of whom 78 percent were positive for viral markers.[222]

## Prognosis for Childhood Liver Disease

Contrary to the initial indications of a poor prognosis in children with $\alpha_1$AT deficiency and early liver symptoms, it now appears that at least two-thirds of children show recovery from their liver damage.[96] In a retrospective study from England, 20 of 82 children (24.4 percent) developed cirrhosis, 19 had a persistently raised level of liver enzymes associated with clinical normality, and 23 had no evidence of liver disease.[223] The clinical presentation, course, and outcome of the disease was reviewed in 98 patients (54 males, 55.1 percent) from 81 families in the United States seen over a period of 20 years.[224] This was a biased group, as many of the patients were referred because of deteriorating health or need for liver transplantation. In this group, an elevation of alanine aminotransferase (ALT) at the time of initial evaluation was associated with a poor outcome, as was a decrease in total inhibitory capacity of plasma (combination of $\alpha_1$AT and $\alpha_2$-macroglobulin protease inhibitory capacity). Kidney disease occurred in 9 females and 6 males (17 percent), usually membranoproliferative glomerulonephritis. Pulmonary symptoms developed in 18 percent, with the mean age of onset at 7 years, usually as asthma or obstructive lung disease detected in pulmonary function tests. Major infections occurred in 14 boys and 7 girls, with spontaneous bacterial peritonitis as the most common complication and *Pneumococcus* and *Escherichia coli* the most common organisms involved. The outcome tended to be poorer in females than in males. Dietary history was available for relatively few patients, with 14 patients breast-fed for at least 2 months, and 39 formula-fed since birth. There was no statistical difference in outcome, but the period of breast-feeding was very short. The initial indicators of poor prognosis were a serum bilirubin that remained high, low total inhibitory protease inhibitor capacity, and a high alanine aminotransferase level. At The Hospital for Sick Children in Toronto, Canada, we estimated that, at most, 37 percent of a series of PI ZZ children with liver abnormalities in the early months of life developed chronic severe liver disease, a figure that may be biased upwards because of ascertainment of more severely affected children early in the study.[96,225] Of 122 PI Z (including two PI $Z_{Q0}$) $\alpha_1$AT-deficient children identified from the Swedish screening program and followed to 8 years of age, 2 of 14 children with prolonged obstructive jaundice died of liver cirrhosis. An additional PI ZZ child with clinical symptoms of neonatal liver disease without jaundice died of aplastic anemia at 4 years of age, with incipient liver cirrhosis at autopsy. Serum glutamic-oxaloacetic transaminase (SGOT) was elevated in 40 percent of the clinically healthy PI ZZ children. Liver cirrhosis with early death therefore occurred in only 3 of 122 PI ZZ children (2.4 percent), or in 13.6 percent of those PI Z children with clinical evidence of liver abnormalities in infancy.[226]

Specific factors predisposing to the development of progressive disease in the 20 to 30 percent of children who develop neonatal hepatitis have not been identified. A poorer prognosis for males has been suggested,[198,226] but is not consistent in all series.[96,223,227] Hepatitis B virus infection, a suggested triggering factor for liver disease in PI ZZ infants,[228] has not been noted in other studies.[96,198,224] The potential effects of damage from oxygen radicals led to a study to treat heterozygotes (PI MZ) with vitamin E from infancy.[217] Such infants, who were found to be at risk for subclinical hepatic involvement manifested only by an increase in liver enzymes, showed, up to 2 months of age, an improvement in liver function when treated with vitamin E supplementation. These data suggest that supplementation of vitamin E might also be useful for infants homozygous for $\alpha_1$AT deficiency (PI ZZ). Vitamin E therapy has also been shown to improve liver function in children with cholestasis.[229]

Studies on the aggregation of Z proteins in the liver indicate that this process is enhanced by an increase in temperature. Therefore, there is a rationale for prompt treatment of inflammatory illnesses that may lead to fever. This should help to prevent the production of this acute phase reactant, which is accompanied by increased storage in the liver leading to further liver damage.

The risk for progression of the liver disease was reported to be reduced in infants who are breast fed during the first month of life as compared with those who are bottle fed.[230] Human milk has a high concentration of $\alpha_1$AT, particularly in the first week of lactation, and a breast-fed infant can have an intake of 100 to 400 mg/24h.[25] In the prospective Swedish study in which PI ZZ infants were identified through screening, 8 of 71 infants (11.3 percent) breast fed for more than 1 month, and 12 of 47 infants (25.5 percent) breast fed for less than 1 month, developed clinical signs of liver disease, and liver function tests were less abnormal than for the bottle-fed infants.[231] These differences were statistically significant. However, the two children who died of cirrhosis were both breast fed for more than 1 month (T. Sveger, personal communication). A rationale for the effectiveness of breast feeding has been proposed by which protease inhibitors in human milk help limit protease uptake and subsequent transport to the liver via the portal circulation.[232] Breast feeding does not offer absolute protection against the development of severe liver disease, but may decrease the likelihood of showing initial signs of liver abnormality and lead to a better prognosis. Further data are required to resolve this issue.

The previously suggested genetic factors may be important in determining the prognosis in children with liver abnormalities in infancy. Sibship data from ours and other series reporting a number of sibs of probands with liver disease have been reviewed.[233] In these studies, 32 families were reported in which one or more sibs were born in a family with a PI ZZ child with liver abnormalities. In 15 families in which a PI ZZ sib was born after a proband with resolved or no liver disease, 13 percent of subsequent sibs developed liver disease. In 17 families in which the PI ZZ proband developed severe liver disease, 40 percent of subsequent PI ZZ sibs developed severe liver disease. Twelve families had more that one child affected in the U.S. series, and severe liver disease occurred in 21 percent of sibs.[224] The rate of occurrence for development of severe liver disease in a subsequent sib varies considerably between studies, with the highest risk, 67 percent, reported from the U.K.[223] The risk of severe liver disease in a subsequent sib of a proband with resolved or no liver disease may not differ significantly from that of the general population, which is estimated to be about 2 percent.[226] In view of the great variability between studies, further follow-up studies with larger numbers are needed, and present risk estimates must be considered as approximate. There may be a tendency for sibs to follow the same clinical disease course, but normal healthy children with no liver involvement can be born after PI ZZ children who have severe liver disease.

## Adult Onset

Cirrhosis and fibrosis of the liver were noted in Swedish adults with $\alpha_1$AT deficiency.[234] In a series of 246 Swedish PI ZZ patients ascertained through hospital admissions, 12 percent overall and 19 percent over 50 years of age were found to have liver cirrhosis.[146] In a series of 115 adults with $\alpha_1$AT deficiency, 5.2 percent were affected with liver disease: 3.5 percent had biopsy or autopsy-proven cirrhosis and another 1.7 percent had definite biochemical evidence of liver disease.[235] When these patients were classified by sex and age, the risks for development of liver disease for males and females, respectively, were: age 20 to 40 years, 1.9 and 2.2 percent, age 41 to 50 years, 6.2 and 3.2 percent, age 51 to 60 years, 15.4 and 0 percent. These numbers are approximate because of the small numbers in each class; no corresponding figures for the normal population are available. However, these numbers indicate an appreciable risk for the development of cirrhosis, particularly in males over 50 years of age, and usually in those without a history of neonatal hepatitis. The liver disease in adults appears to show rapid progression; in most patients, death occurred within 2 years of the diagnosis of cirrhosis.[235,236] Perhaps the cirrhosis is advanced before diagnosis, with symptoms of cirrhosis having been masked by the presence of fatigue and dyspnea from pulmonary disease. Alcohol consumption does not appear to have been an important factor in the production of liver disease. In view of the appreciable risk for development of liver disease, particularly in males, avoidance of significant amounts of alcohol and environmental toxins is prudent.

### Therapy for Liver Disease

Supportive management is similar of other types of liver disease—optimal nutrition, prevention of fat-soluble vitamin deficiency, and diuretic treatment for ascites when required. As in any type of obstructive liver disease, copper accumulates in the liver and can cause damage by the production of free radicals. Therefore, antioxidant therapy is a rational addition to treatment. The majority of children with early liver symptoms spontaneously recover and liver failure may never occur.

Liver transplantation, the preferred surgical treatment for advanced liver disease, can provide a cure because the $\alpha_1AT$ produced is that of the donor. In 1988, the reported 5-year survival after transplant for 29 children and 10 adults with $\alpha_1AT$ deficiency with liver disease was 72 and 60 percent, respectively.[237] In 1994, survival rates were 90 percent at 1 year and 80 percent at 5 years.[238] Use of living related donors for liver transplant allows longer-term follow-up of slowly progressive disease, if a related liver donor is available.

Because the cause of progressive liver disease in certain PI ZZ children is unknown, there is no obvious rationale for replacement therapy with $\alpha_1AT$. If the protease load from the intestine is crucial in the early weeks of life, then this is the period in which replacement therapy might be considered. Oral therapy could be useful, if there is some purpose for the high level of $\alpha_1AT$ in human milk. The effects of therapy would be difficult to monitor, because the majority of children recover spontaneously from their liver abnormalities.

Therapeutic recombinant DNA approaches are discussed at the end of this chapter.

### Primary Liver Carcinoma

$\alpha_1AT$ deficiency appears to be associated with a small risk for developing hepatocellular carcinoma (hepatoma), with or without cirrhosis. Bile duct carcinoma has also been reported, and may be a consequence of $\alpha_1AT$ storage in bile ducts.[236] Of 246 PI Z patients over 20 years of age admitted to Swedish hospitals, hepatoma was present in 3 percent,[146] possibly an underestimate, as 46 percent of the patients were less than 50 years of age. A significant increase in primary liver cancer was observed in Sweden only in males with $\alpha_1AT$ deficiency, in comparison with population controls.[239] Among a series of 140 adult Canadian patients of PI type Z,[235] 2 had hepatoma—1 had cirrhosis without lung disease and 1 had lung disease without liver disease. These data suggest that primary liver carcinoma apparently can occur in $\alpha_1AT$-deficient individuals without preexisting cirrhosis and may be due to the accumulation of $\alpha_1AT$ in the liver. $\alpha$-Fetoprotein, usually elevated in hepatoma, is infrequently elevated in PI ZZ or MZ patients with hepatoma.[240]

In studies in which PI typing of patients with hepatoma has been carried out, homozygotes have not been found, consistent with the rarity of $\alpha_1AT$ deficiency in the population and the associated small risk for developing hepatoma.[241] $\alpha_1AT$ deficiency (homozygous or heterozygous) was not found in a series of 58 Black South Africans with hepatoma,[242] but *PI*Z is not found in Black populations. Studies of pathologic tissues have yielded conflicting and unreliable results. Such studies are difficult to interpret because PI MZ individuals do not always show PAS granules in the liver, and tumor tissues can show PAS-D granules where no such granules are present in the nontumor tissue.[243]

In summary the data suggest a small increase in risk, at least in males, for hepatocellular carcinoma or hepatoma, associated with $\alpha_1AT$ deficiency, usually in association with cirrhosis.

### Risk for Heterozygotes

**PI Type SZ Heterozygotes.** A number of isolated cases of liver disease occurring in individuals of PI type SZ have been reported and have led to the conclusion by some that these individuals are at increased risk for liver disease.[244] The reports of isolated cases in both adults and children can be explained by chance, because about 1 in 700 to 1 in 1500 of the general population is of PI type SZ. The strongest evidence for lack of risk for childhood disease comes from the Swedish screening study, which has shown a modest elevation of liver enzymes in a portion of children of PI type SZ during the early months of life, but with no clinical abnormalities or elevation of liver enzymes by 8 years of age.[226] Screening of 857 Swedish adults with liver disease revealed 7 of PI type SZ when 1 was expected, suggesting a possible increased risk for PI SZ adults.[240] Smaller studies have not confirmed this association.

**PI Type MZ Heterozygotes.** An increased risk for PI MZ individuals to develop cirrhosis has been suggested. Because 2 to 4 percent of Caucasian populations are of PI type MZ, chance associations with liver disease are expected. In surveys, appropriate PI typing must be carried out, as it is not possible to determine the phenotype based on PAS-D-positive inclusions in the liver. Individuals of both PI type MZ and ZZ can have inclusions. Furthermore, the presence of the electrophoretic band migrating cathodal to a major band of Z $\alpha_1AT$ can cause misidentification of a "Z" component (Fig. 219-3A).

In a screening study of almost 15,000 newborns in Italy, liver function tests were done on 101 PI MZ and 135 PI MS infants.[217] Aspartate aminotransferase (AST), alanine aminotransferase (ALT), and $\gamma$-glutamyltransferase (GGT) all appeared to be similarly sensitive to the assessment of liver damage. Elevation of liver enzymes, as a sign of hepatic dysfunction, was observed in PI MZ individuals: in 19 percent at 2 months, 8 percent at 5 months, and 1 percent at 12 months of age. Similarly, in 135 PI MS infants, abnormalities were observed in 15 percent at 2 months, 7 percent at 5 months, and none at 12 months of age. The concentration of plasma $\alpha_1AT$ was similar in those with normal and abnormal tests of liver function. Uninhibited proteolytic enzymes in the liver of individuals with a partial deficiency may allow cellular damage, perhaps through the production of highly reactive superoxide radicals.

In adults as well, a partial deficiency of $\alpha_1AT$ may play a small role in the development of liver disease. Among 335 patients with a variety of liver diseases, 3.3 percent were of PI type MZ as compared with 2.9 percent of normal healthy blood donors.[245] However, when examined by specific type of liver disease, none of 53 patients with autoimmune chronic active hepatitis were of PI type MZ; 2 of 18 patients (11.1 percent) with cryptogenic cirrhosis, 3 of 79 (3.8 percent) with alcoholic liver cirrhosis, 2 of 36 (5.6 percent) with primary sclerosing cholangitis, and 1 of 26 (3.9 percent) with primary biliary cirrhosis were of PI type MZ. In a study in France of 159 adults with liver cirrhosis, 132 of whom had chronic alcoholism, a small and nonsignificant increase in the number of PI MZ individuals in both alcoholic and nonalcoholic groups was found.[246] In a study in Spain of 157 alcoholic patients with cirrhosis, a significant increase in individuals of PI type MZ, but not type MS, was found (7 percent in cirrhotic patients, 1.7 percent in controls).[247] Of 857 Swedish patients with liver disease, 7.6 percent, rather than the expected 4.8 percent, were identified using a monoclonal antibody for detecting PI Z and were confirmed as of PI type MZ.[240] This difference, similar to those in previous studies, was significant with the larger patient group. In a U.S. liver transplant center, PI MZ was found at in increased frequency in cryptogenic liver disease and with hepatitis C.[248] Measurement of the concentration of serum $\alpha_1AT$ was not helpful in identifying adult patients of PI type MZ, because of the acute phase nature of $\alpha_1$AT.[249]

In summary, most studies suggest a small increase in risk for liver disease in individuals heterozygous for $\alpha_1$AT deficiency. Environmental agents, such as viruses or alcohol, can perhaps trigger liver damage in susceptible individuals. In a study of 164 patients, PI ZZ homozygotes and Z heterozygotes, mostly MZ, viral infections and alcohol appeared to play a prominent role in initiation of liver disease.[250] Most studies in which PI typing rather than liver inclusions has been the basis for diagnosis indicate that PI MZ individuals are not at increased risk for hepatoma.[241,251]

## OTHER DISEASE ASSOCIATIONS

A variety of disorders, other than liver and lung disease, have been reported to show an association with $\alpha_1$AT deficiency or other variants. These disorders are generally associated with inflammatory response, and/or hyperactivity of the immune system. The basis for hyperactivity of the immune system has been discussed previously (see "Function in the Immune Response"). Further aspects of associations with immune disorders have been reviewed.[16] The increased susceptibility may be further enhanced by a decreased ability to control local inflammation. Disease associations could also be due to potential variants in adjacent genes of the serine protease inhibitor cluster; those of corticosteroid-binding protein may be particularly relevant.

### Disorders with Immune Response and Inflammatory Components

**Kidney Disease.** Membranoproliferative glomerulonephritis (MPGN) was noted in patients with $\alpha_1$AT deficiency and liver disease[219,252,253] and may be a relatively frequent occurrence in such patients. Low levels of complement C3 were reported in two of these patients and circulating immune complex was reported in the one patient tested.[253] Nephropathy was noted in 79 percent of 19 patients of PI type ZZ with chronic liver disease.[254] Seven had mesangiocapillary glomerular nephritis and six had focal segmental mesangial proliferative glomerulonephritis, which was found at similar frequency in patients with chronic liver disease due to other causes. These authors noted that glomerular lesions might be present, even in the presence of normal urinalysis, and that the type of nephropathy is variable. In agreement with earlier studies by Moroz et al.,[219] the nephropathy was accompanied by granular $\alpha_1$AT deposit at the subendothelial region of the glomerular basement membrane. Deposits of immunoglobulins IgG, M, and A, and of C3, frequently found in cases of MPGN, were also identified[96] and may represent an immune response to the abnormal circulating PI Z protein, following hepatic destruction.[219] Multiple immune complex disorders were reported in two adults with $\alpha_1$AT deficiency, obstructive lung disease, progressive glomerulonephritis, and, in addition, mild liver disease and necrotizing angiitis,[255] or cutaneous vasculitis and colitis.[256] Abnormal $\alpha_1$AT from liver inclusions probably participates in the formation of an immune complex. All of the children in whom MPGN was identified had severe liver disease, suggesting that the kidney abnormality was a consequence of the liver disease. This is supported by the report of MPGN in one patient with liver disease being cured following liver transplantation.[257] In a study of 246 hospitalized Swedish PI Z patients, 37 (15 percent) showed signs of glomerular renal damage, indicated by constant or recurrent proteinuria or hematuria;[146] 3 patients (1 percent) developed advanced renal failure. The probability for PI Z patients to develop severe renal disease appears to be low, although its association with liver disease in this condition may be relatively high. $\alpha_1$AT deficiency is not a common cause of MPGN; among 53 patients with idiopathic MPGN, none were homozygous or heterozygous for PI Z.[253]

**Panniculitis.** Panniculitis is characterized by inflammation of the panniculus adiposis, the fat layer under the dermis. The risk for

patients with $\alpha_1$AT deficiency to develop panniculitis must be relatively small as the condition has not been identified in surveys of patients of PI type ZZ. On the other hand, a large number of cases have now been reported of severe ulcerative panniculitis associated with $\alpha_1$AT deficiency. Among five patients with panniculitis, two patients with severe panniculitis had $\alpha_1$AT deficiency.[258] Two of three sibs of PI type ZZ were reported to have panniculitis.[259] In a study of 96 patients with panniculitis, 15.6 percent were found to be $\alpha_1$AT deficient, as defined by the serum concentration.[260] Splaying of neutrophils between collagen bundles in the reticular dermis is specific to $\alpha_1$AT deficiency.[261] Administration of purified $\alpha_1$AT was successful in the treatment of two particularly severe cases of panniculitis; doxycycline, a tetracycline that inhibits collagenase activity, has also been effective.[262]

While $\alpha_1$AT is unlikely to be a primary cause of panniculitis, in the presence of triggering agents, among them histoplasmosis,[263] patients of PI type ZZ appear to be have impaired ability to control the inflammation.

**Rheumatoid Arthritis.** An increased frequency of the heterozygous deficiency PI types MZ and SZ was reported in adults with rheumatoid arthritis.[264] Subsequent studies were done in different populations with conflicting results. This disagreement could be due to geographical difference, but is more likely due to differences in patient selection. No increase in Z heterozygotes was found in studies of patients not selected for disease severity. However, in a Swedish study, in which all 200 patients had erosive rheumatoid arthritis, an increase in Z heterozygotes was found.[265] A significant increase in PI MZ patients was shown in three British studies[266–268] and in Australia.[16] These data seem to be compatible with our conclusion that an increased frequency of Z heterozygosity occurs particularly in individuals with seropositive erosive arthritis.[269] In the Swedish study of 246 hospitalized PI Z patients, 4.4 percent had rheumatoid arthritis and another 3 percent had a history of considerable joint pain with no confirmed diagnosis.[146] We conclude that tissue destruction occurs more readily in the PI Z heterozygote because of inadequate $\alpha_1$AT present in the joint fluid to prevent leukocyte elastase, cathepsin G, and collagenase from attacking the structural proteins of joint cartilage.[269] An increased frequency of PI FM, confirmed by family studies,[270] may be significant because of the increased sensitivity of the F variant to oxidation.[77]

A numerical but nonsignificant increase in Z heterozygotes was found in children with juvenile rheumatoid arthritis,[269] and a study of more severely affected British children showed a significantly increased frequency of PI type MZ.[271] Juvenile arthritis consists of a number of different subgroups, and perhaps some but not all of these subgroups show increased susceptibility.

**Other Disorders Associated with PI MZ or ZZ.** A variety of inflammatory conditions are associated with $\alpha_1$AT deficiency. Anterior uveitis, an immunologically mediated inflammatory eye disease, has been reported to be associated with an increased frequency of Z heterozygotes,[272,273] as well as with an increase in PI type MS in the latter study. The association was not confirmed in a study of 57 Caucasian American patients.[274] These discrepancies may be due to the type of patients selected. In posterior uveitis, 2 of 16 patients were of PI type MZ;[273] further studies of these types of patients are required. A PI ZZ child with corneal ulceration had markedly reduced $\alpha_1$AT in tears.[275] $\alpha_1$AT is expressed in the cornea normally.[51] Systemic vasculitis,[276] persistent cutaneous vasculitis,[277] and fatal Wegener granulomatosis[278] have been reported in PI ZZ individuals. Isolated cases of PI ZZ individuals with panarteritis in association with emphysema and glomerular nephritis,[255] Hashimoto thyroiditis,[279] and severe combined immunodeficiency,[280] have been reported.

The isolated reports of idiopathic hemochromatosis in PI MZ heterozygotes and in homozygotes[281,282] may be due to chance association, or hemochromatosis could promote cirrhosis when coexisting with $\alpha_1$AT deficiency. In a Canadian study of 15 patients, 3 were of PI type MZ.[283] The PI Z gene, as detected by a monoclonal antibody, has not been found in either the heterozygous or homozygous state in 27 male patients with idiopathic hemochromatosis, all from the same region of Sweden.[284]

## Malignancy

Studies have been done on a number of malignant conditions in addition to hepatoma. In a study of patients with bladder carcinoma, a significant increase in PI*Z and decrease in PI*M3 were found in comparison with controls.[285] PI*M3 was also decreased in a series of lymphoma and leukemia patients. A protease-protease inhibitor imbalance could affect tumor invasiveness. A mechanism for involvement of PI*M3 is not apparent. Because M3 is not always readily differentiated from PI*M1, particularly when the plasma concentration is elevated, care must be taken to avoid technical artifacts.

## Other Associations

Various disorders affecting artery integrity have been described.[286] Uninhibited elastase activity could lead to arterial weakening, accounting for the increase in PI type MZ in 47 patients with abdominal aortic aneurysm (11 percent vs. 2 to 4 percent in the general population).[287] Fibromuscular dysplasia of the carotid artery has been described in PI MZ patients.[288]

Proteolytic enzymes are involved in fertilization in cell division and could potentially be disturbed in the presence of inadequate protease inhibition.[289] This may explain the slight increase in twinning associated with MZ[290] and MS[291] heterozygotes.

## PRENATAL DIAGNOSIS

Direct DNA mutation analysis is now the preferred approach, using PCR-based methods.[292] Amniocytes or chorion villi can be the source of fetal DNA. Reliable PI typing is a crucial first step in prenatal diagnosis to determine that both parents have the Z allele and that there is no rare deficiency or null allele present in either parent.

### Risk for an Affected Fetus

For parents of PI type MZ with no affected offspring, the risk for a PI ZZ child to develop severe liver disease is the general population risk of 2 percent, with an overall risk of 0.5 percent. For PI type MZ parents who have had a child with liver abnormalities, the risk for a PI ZZ child to have severe liver disease is influenced by the course of liver disease in the previous child; from 13 percent if the liver disease has resolved, to as much as 40 percent if severe liver disease is present.[233] The basis for these recurrence risks is discussed in the section on childhood liver disease above.

### Direct Mutation Detection

Synthetic oligonucleotide probes that recognize the single Z base pair substitution can be used. This method requires that the presence of a Z allele be definitely established in both parents, as the probes will not recognize the rare deficiency mutations. Specific oligonucleotide probes have been prepared at the Z mutant site in amino acid 342 for normal M and Z deficiency DNA sequences[293] and were initially used for prenatal diagnosis on a genomic fragment cut with a specific restriction enzyme.[294] PCR offers a major improvement. The appropriate region of exon 5 can be amplified by PCR, and the Z mutation detected by the use of oligonucleotide probes labeled with $^{32}$P[98] or with biotin.[99] A similar approach, using specific oligonucleotide probes, can also be used where one of the rare variants of $\alpha_1$AT has been detected. As an alternate method for the Z mutation, a primer designed with a nucleotide substitution can create a TaqI site in the normal allele, but not in the Z form,[100,101] an approach also used with the enzyme XmnI for the S mutation.[101] A potential concern about this approach is that failure of digestion of the DNA sample for

technical reasons could lead to misinterpretation of an M sample as Z. This could be overcome by incorporation of another TaqI restriction site in the designed primer as a positive control. An advantage of the method is simplicity and lack of requirement for labeled oligonucleotide.

If previous PI typing in the family has indicated the presence of a rare deficiency allele or a PI null allele for which the mutation is unknown, DNA polymorphisms can be used for prenatal diagnosis by following segregation of markers in the family. Genomic probes used for diagnosis of $\alpha_1$AT deficiency lie within the gene and detect polymorphisms of both $\alpha_1$AT and the $\alpha_1$AT-homologous region. $\alpha_1$AT deficiency is unusual in that the DNA haplotype associated with the PI*Z allele is specific and unique. Studies of parents and sibs are theoretically unnecessary, although in practice such studies are advisable because of the possibility of rare exceptions.

## POPULATION SCREENING

The screening of 200,000 Swedish infants demonstrates that newborn screening is feasible.[94,198] In this study, a disc was punched from a dried blood sample on filter paper and eluted for semiquantitative assay of both $\alpha_1$AT and of transferrin, as an internal standard, by electroimmunoassay. Infants with less than 40 percent of normal $\alpha_1$AT had a blood sample drawn for PI typing. The majority of the infants ascertained in this way were found to be of PI type ZZ; 28 percent of those PI typed were of PI type SZ. Although electroimmunoassay was used in this population screening, automated nephelometry could be used for the quantification of $\alpha_1$AT and transferrin. The screening program could be conveniently carried out on the same dried blood spots used for tests of newborns for phenylketonuria. PI typing can be carried out on the dried blood samples by using silver stain following isoelectric focusing.[295]

At present, the main value of a population screening program is to counsel the parents to encourage their affected children to avoid smoking later in life. The message of avoidance of smoking must be reinforced directly with the children as they reach their teenage years. Even with such reinforcement, we do not know whether young adults who are then healthy will avoid smoking. Because of the known increased risk of respiratory disease in children of cigarette smokers, parents of children with $\alpha_1$AT deficiency should be advised not to smoke. Results from the Swedish study suggest children, but not their parents, can be influenced to avoid smoking.[296] The data are very clear, as discussed, in indicating that if smoking is avoided, the onset of obstructive pulmonary disease will be considerably delayed.

An extensive follow-up of psychologic consequences of the Swedish screening program indicated that most parents initially perceived $\alpha_1$AT deficiency as an imminent and serious threat to their child's health.[297] These negative feelings persisted in 58 percent of mothers and 44 percent of fathers 5 to 7 years after the initial identification of $\alpha_1$AT deficiency.[298] If population screening is undertaken in newborns, parents should be informed that the testing is to be undertaken and should be informed of the presence of the deficiency in their infant by an individual knowledgeable about the condition. Although specific treatment is not available for children with signs of liver disease, administration of antioxidants and encouragement of breast-feeding may help to alter the course of disease. Repeated long-term follow-up beyond the first year of life may be unnecessary for those children who show no signs of liver disturbance. Some provision must be made for later reinforcement of the need for avoidance of smoking, which may be difficult in families with a high degree of mobility.

While screening during the newborn period, in combination with other neonatal screening, is probably the most efficient time to screen, a screening program later in childhood may be more effective in encouraging the child to avoid smoking later in life.

# TREATMENT

## Preventative Therapy for Lung Destruction

The most effective therapy for the lung destruction of $\alpha_1$AT deficiency is prevention, mainly through avoidance of smoking. Although the Swedish follow-up study of children that had been identified as newborns indicated little impact upon the smoking habits of parents, children, aware of their deficiency at an early age, were shown to smoke less than normal controls. Of 50 children followed 18 to 20 years after initial diagnosis in a newborn screening program, 12 percent reported they had previously or currently smoked, and 5 of these 6 smoking children had one or both parents who smoked. Among 48 control children, 36 percent had smoked or were currently smoking.[296]

In the earliest studies of $\alpha_1$AT deficiency, subjects were ascertained mainly through pulmonary clinics, leading to the impression that most individuals with the deficiency would eventually develop emphysema. However, the outlook for those with $\alpha_1$AT deficiency now appears to be more positive. In order to prevent lung destruction, the most important message for patients with the deficiency is to avoid exposure to smoke at all ages. In those individuals who begin to show relatively early signs of lung destruction, the rate of destruction may be slowed by the restoration of the protease-inhibitor balance in the lung through administration of suitable protease inhibitors.

$\alpha_1$AT is known to be inactivated by oxidation. Therefore, consideration should be given to maintaining maximal antioxidant activity in lung tissue. Vitamin E status may be important in determining individual susceptibility to lung destruction. Administration of vitamin E in doses that adequately cover the daily requirements could help to protect from lung disease; vitamin E is not adequately considered as a form of preventative therapy.

## Augmentation Therapy

The adult human lung has a limited capacity for self-repair, therefore emphysema, once established, cannot be reversed. The rationale of augmentation therapy is to increase the $\alpha_1$AT plasma concentration, and subsequently that of the lower lung, to protective levels to delay the rate of lung deterioration or, if administered early, to prevent it. PI type SZ individuals, who appear to have an adequate level of projection against lung disease except in some smokers, have approximately 40 percent, or 0.52 g/liter, of plasma $\alpha_1$AT. The protective plasma level is therefore considered to be 0.52 g/liter (0.57 g/liter or 11 µM, by the NIH standard[95]) (see the reviews in references 299 and 300).

Methods to augment lung $\alpha_1$AT also have application to cystic fibrosis, to help combat excessive proteolysis enhanced by the associated chronic inflammation.[300] In low-birth weight newborns, who have a high proteolytic burden on the lungs, augmentation therapy may help prevent bronchopulmonary dysplasia.[167]

**Infusion Therapy.** The only currently approved therapy for $\alpha_1$AT deficiency is the augmentation of serum levels by the infusion of purified human $\alpha_1$AT. Administration of 60 mg/kg weekly increased levels of serum and lung $\alpha_1$AT and of antineutrophil elastase to an appropriate protective level.[301] The equivalent dose administered biweekly[302] or monthly[303] maintained an appropriate plasma level of $\alpha_1$AT most of the time, although the latter dose requires a delivery time of from 6 to 8 h to avoid cardiovascular compromise.

A randomized clinical trial, predicted to require 500 patients and controls studied for a 3-year period to show a 40 percent decrease in the decline of $FEV_1$, was not considered to be feasible.[304] Therefore, patient registries were established in the United States and Europe to monitor patients receiving augmentation therapy. Studies assessing the effects of augmentation therapy include 927 patients from the U.S. registry,[156] 97 untreated patients from the Danish registry who were compared with 198 treated patients from the German registry,[305] and an extended group of additional German patients to a total of 400,[306] reported in a separate study. Patients in all studies were of PI type ZZ or equivalent. In the Danish and German studies, patients were all exsmokers. In the U.S. study, surprisingly, 10 percent of those treated were current smokers. Survival over a period of at least 6 months was assessed in the U.S. study. There was a significant improvement only for patients with an $FEV_1$ of 35 to 49 percent, but not for those with lower or higher $FEV_1$s; however, this change in relative risk was slight in comparison with the effects of education, which presumably reflects socioeconomic status. Because all patients in the German group received therapy, there were no controls, so the Danish group, none of whom received therapy, was used as the control population. For both the U.S and European studies, there was improvement in the rate of decline of $FEV_1$ by about 25 percent in both studies, but only for those with an $FEV_1$ of about 30 to 65 percent. The decline in $FEV_1$ for untreated patients in whom the initial $FEV_1$ was less than 30 percent predicted, was 31 to 46 ml/year with no therapy, 36 to 44 ml/year with therapy. With an $FEV_1$ in the midrange (30 to 65 percent in Europe; 35 to 79 percent predicted in United States), the rate of decline was 83 to 93 ml/year with no treatment, 64 to 66 ml/year with treatment. For a comparison, the current smokers in the U.S. studies had a mean decline of 108 ml/year. For individuals with an initial $FEV_1$ of greater than or equal to 80 percent, there was no improvement in the rate of decline. All figures had large standard deviations, indicating the high degree of variability between individuals. Although these studies suggest that augmentation therapy may be useful in at least some individuals, there are many questions still to be answered and factors to be considered. Because of the high degree of variability in decline of lung function, documentation of the rate of decline of lung function in any particular patient should provide a rational basis for deciding when and if to begin therapy.

There is no evidence that the protective level must be maintained at all times. Patients with $\alpha_1$AT deficiency have been shown to have little or no free elastase activity in lung lavage, except during periods of respiratory infection.[208] This suggests that augmentation therapy might be effective when administered only during times of stress or that a lower dose might be used if supplemented during infection.[307] Unfortunately, no information has been reported on the use of antioxidants by patients in the registry. Nutritional and antioxidant status might well be an important factor in maintaining a slow decline in lung function. The replacement therapy is costly and, given this low decline of lung function in some patients, may not be required continuously for all.

**Aerosol Therapy.** Because the lungs are, in most cases, the only major organ to be significantly damaged by elastase degradation, an efficient approach to therapy is to deliver $\alpha_1$AT directly to the lungs. Effective aerosol therapy depends on delivery of appropriate size droplets to the lung alveoli. Studies in sheep demonstrated that aerosolized $\alpha_1$AT passed through the lower respiratory tract epithelium and gained access to the interstitium of the alveolar walls.[308] These investigators also showed that aerosolized M-type $\alpha_1$AT could be demonstrated in the serum of Z-type individuals. Aerosol administration of 100 mg twice daily raised the $\alpha_1$AT level in both lung and plasma to levels in the upper range of normal and well beyond the protective level, with no adverse clinical reactions.[299] The half-time in the lungs after a single dose of 200 mg was 69.2 hours, and for antineutrophil elastase activity, 53.2 hours.[309] This approach requires only about 10 percent of the purified $\alpha_1$AT used for intravenous administration and warrants further study. This may prove an economically feasible approach, in combination with antioxidant administration, for the treatment of $\alpha_1$AT deficiency.

**Recombinant $\alpha_1$AT for Augmentation Therapy.** Because of the requirements for large amounts of $\alpha_1$AT and the potential risk of infection in using human blood products, large-scale synthesis of human $\alpha_1$AT through recombinant DNA methodology is potentially useful. Normal human $\alpha_1$AT can be produced at a high level in both yeast and *Escherichia coli*; the side chains, however, are completely lacking and the stability and half-life are considerably reduced. A modified $\alpha_1$AT, with valine substituting for methionine 385 in the active center, shows effective resistance to oxidation, but has a half-life of only 8.5 h in the rabbit, in comparison with the normal human $\alpha_1$AT of 2.2 days.[310] Aerosol administration of recombinant $\alpha_1$AT, which could be administered frequently, might make this form usable for treatment.[303]

Transgenic animals may be able to provide the large amounts of $\alpha_1$AT necessary for augmentation therapy. The $\alpha_1$AT gene spliced to the gene for $\beta$ lactoglobin was injected into sheep embryos, resulting in adult sheep able to produce as much as 35 g of human $\alpha_1$AT per liter of milk.[311] This approach, if proven safe from animal pathogens, avoids the potential risk of HIV and other human viruses that could inadvertently contaminate the product made from human blood.

### Gene Therapy for $\alpha_1$AT Deficiency

$\alpha_1$AT deficiency has provided a useful model for the testing of gene therapy approaches. This approach involves alteration of the host cells by addition of a normal $\alpha_1$AT gene to the host genome (see the review in reference 300). Three vector systems — plasmid, retrovirus, and replication-deficient adenovirus — have been evaluated. The general gene therapy approach of removing cells from the patient, modifying the normal cell, and reintroducing the modified cell to the patient is difficult where the product must be targeted to the lung. Plasmids are relatively inefficient in gene transfer and are sometimes linked to a ligand to target to a particular cell type. A concern with the use of retroviral vectors is the possibility of targeting a gene involved in tumorigenesis, leading to malignancy. Adenovirus, a virus that causes upper and lower respiratory tract infections in humans, has avidity for epithelia of the respiratory tract, and most of the retrovirus DNA remains extrachromosomal. The vector does not require host cell replication for gene expression, thus bypassing the problem of slow replication of endothelial cells. Potential risks have not been fully evaluated.

Using a retroviral vector, the $\alpha_1$AT gene has been introduced into mouse fibroblasts, which, when transplanted into the peritoneum of nude mice, produced human $\alpha_1$AT in serum and in epithelial lining fluid of the lung.[312] Studies in rats have demonstrated that adenovirus vector can transfer the $\alpha_1$AT gene to respiratory epithelium where it is secreted on both the air and interstitial surfaces.[313] Data from these studies suggest that gene transfer into pulmonary arteries and capillaries could provide a source of secreted $\alpha_1$AT.

Another approach to gene therapy is the transfer of genes into the liver. General approaches have been reviewed.[314] Transfer of genes into the hepatocytes could create a source of $\alpha_1$AT to prevent the lung, and possibly liver, damage associated with $\alpha_1$AT deficiency, if circulating levels of $\alpha_1$AT were sufficiently high. The $\alpha_1$AT gene could be introduced into hepatocytes from an affected individual, which could then be returned to the peripheral circulation of the donor. Transfection with an adenovirus has achieved expression of $\alpha_1$AT in rat liver, transiently and at low levels.[315] DNA was present in episomes, which remained relatively stable and continued to produce $\alpha_1$AT for at least 4 months, after hepatocyte regeneration was induced by partial hepatectomy.[316] Targeted homologous recombination was also demonstrated in HepG2 cells, which would enable substitution of normal for an abnormal gene in the hepatocyte.[317] Gene expression in the liver has been obtained through direct injection of DNA into the liver[318] and by in vitro gene transfer into hepatocytes by small liposomes.[319] The transfection of an $\alpha_1$AT gene into human hepatocytes with a subsequent level, perhaps low, of production of $\alpha_1$AT is technically feasible. A high level of expression would not be required to protect from the development of emphysema. However, it is not known whether this approach would help avoid

liver disease, if the liver disease is due to the storage of inclusions. There may be easier ways to protect susceptible individuals, particularly through environmental manipulation. On the other hand, as this approach develops, it may become a feasible treatment for null homozygotes. Long-term therapy with injection, or gene therapy, for null homozygotes needs to be approached with caution due to the possibility of an immune reaction to replacement $\alpha_1$AT protein. However, the presence of even trace amounts of endogenous $\alpha_1$AT may help prevent the formation of antibodies against $\alpha_1$AT.

$\alpha_1$AT deficiency has provided a useful model for the testing of various types of gene therapy. However at a practical level, the much more simple approaches of $\alpha_1$AT infusion or delivery by aerosol, and/or antioxidant therapy may be more feasible and cost effective.

### Lung Transplantation

Lung transplantation has become a feasible treatment in selected patients with end-stage lung disease. While double-lung transplantation was initially believed to be necessary for patients with chronic obstructive pulmonary disease, excellent success has been obtained with single and bilateral sequential transplantation.[320,321] Among 66 lung-transplant recipients of whom 19 had $\alpha_1$AT deficiency with emphysema, the actuarial survival at 1 year was 82 percent for bilateral lung transplant recipients and 90 percent for the single-lung transplant recipients.[320] In another group of 23 patients undergoing single-lung transplantation, of whom 5 had $\alpha_1$AT deficiency, surgical procedures were slightly different and the selection criteria less stringent, resulting in an actuarial survival rate of 77 percent at 1 year and 73 percent at 2 years.[322] The 2-year survival of PI ZZ patients is almost 100 percent until $FEV_1$ falls below one-third of predicted normal, at which point mortality increases exponentially reaching 50 percent at an $FEV_1$ of 15 percent predicted. Transplantation is, therefore, an appropriate option when the $FEV_1$ falls below 30 percent.[323] This is considered a feasible approach for patients less than 60 years of age.

### ACKNOWLEDGMENTS

This chapter is dedicated to the late Andrew Sass-Kortsak, M.D., F.R.C.P. (C), my teacher, mentor, and friend, who was responsible for initiation of my studies of $\alpha_1$AT and who provided continuous support for many years. I acknowledge with thanks Colleen Dawson, Susan Kenney, Deepak Kamnasaran, John Forbes, and Anna Minarchi for assistance in manuscript preparation.

### REFERENCES

1. Schultze HE, Gollner I, Heide K, Schonenberger M, Schwick G: Zur Kenntnis der alpha globuline des menschlichen normalserums. *Z Naturforsch* **10**:463, 1955.
2. Laurell C-B, Eriksson S: The electrophoretic $\alpha_1$-globulin pattern of serum in $\alpha_1$-antitrypsin deficiency. *Scand J Clin Lab Invest* **15**:132, 1963.
3. Eriksson S: Discovery of $\alpha_1$-antitrypsin deficiency. *Lung* **168(Supp)**: 523, 1990.
4. Fagerhol MK, Laurell C-B: The polymorphism of "prealbumins" and $\alpha_1$-antitrypsin in human sera. *Clin Chim Acta* **16**:199, 1967.
5. Fagerhol MK: Serum Pi types in Norwegians. *Acta Path Microbiol Scand* **70**:421, 1967.
6. Sharp HL, Bridges RA, Krivit W: Cirrhosis associated with $\alpha_1$-antitrypsin deficiency: A previously unrecognized inherited disorder. *J Lab Clin Med* **73**:934, 1969.
7. Hutchison DC: The epidemiology of $\alpha_1$-antitrypsin deficiency. *Lung* **168(Supp)**:535, 1990.
8. Brantly M, Nukiwa T, Crystal RG: Molecular basis of $\alpha_1\alpha$-antitrypsin deficiency. *Am J Med* **84**:13, 1988.
9. Crystal RG: $\alpha_1$-antitrypsin deficiency, emphysema, and liver disease. Genetic basis and strategies for therapy. *J Clin Invest* **85**:1343, 1990.
10. Blank CA, Brantly M: Clinical features and molecular characteristics of $\alpha$1-antitrypsin deficiency [published erratum appears in *Ann Allergy*

*Asthma Immunol* 72:305, 1994]. *Ann Allergy Asthma Immunol* **72**:105, 1994.

11. Lindmark B, Svenonius E, Eriksson S: Heterozygous $\alpha_1$-antichymotrypsin and Pi Z $\alpha_1$-antitrypsin deficiency. Prevalence and clinical spectrum in asthmatic children. *Allergy* **45**:197, 1990.

12. Beatty K, Bieth J, Travis J: Kinetics of association of serine proteinases with native and oxidized $\alpha_1$-proteinase inhibitor and $\alpha_1$-antichymotrypsin. *J Biol Chem* **255**:3931, 1980.

13. Gadek JE, Crystal RG: $\alpha_1$-antitrypsin deficiency, in Stanbury JB, Wyngaarden JB, Fredrickson DS, Goldstein JL, Brown MS (eds): *Metabolic Basis of Inherited Disease.* New York, McGraw-Hill, 1983, p 1450.

14. Scott CF, Carrell RW, Glaser CB, Kueppers F, Lewis JH, Colman RW: $\alpha_1$-antitrypsin-Pittsburgh. A potent inhibitor of human plasma factor X1a, Kallikrein and factor XII. *J Clin Invest* **77**:631, 1986.

15. Folds JD, Prince II, Spitznagel JK: Limited cleavage of human immunoglobulins by elastase of human neutrophil polymorphonuclear granulocytes. Possible modulator of immune complex disease. *Lab Invest* **39**:313, 1978.

16. Breit SN, Wakefield D, Robinson JP, Luckhurst E, Clark P, Penny R: The role of $\alpha_1$-antitrypsin deficiency in the pathogenesis of immune disorders. *Clin Immunol Immunopathol* **35**:363, 1985.

17. Kelsey GD, Povey S, Bygrave AE, Lovell-Badge RH: Species- and tissue-specific expression of human $\alpha_1$-antitrypsin in transgenic mice. *Genes Develop* **1**:161, 1987.

18. Sifers RN, Carlson JA, Clift SM, Demayo FJ, Bullock DW, Woo SLC: Tissue specific expression of the human $\alpha_1$-antitrypsin gene in transgenic mice. *Nucleic Acids Res* **15**:1459, 1987.

19. Dycaico JM, Grant SGN, Felts K, et al: Neonatal hepatitis induced by $\alpha_1$-antitrypsin: A transgenic mouse model. *Science* **242**:1409, 1988.

20. Perlmutter DH, Daniels JD, Auerbach HS, De Schryver-Kecskemeti K, Winter HS, Alpers HA: The $\alpha_1$-antitrypsin gene is expressed in a human intestinal epithelial cell line. *J Biol Chem* **264**:9485, 1989.

21. Molmenti EP, Perlmutter DH, Rubin DC: Cell-specific expression of $\alpha_1$-antitrypsin in human intestinal epithelium. *J Clin Invest* **92**:2022, 1993.

22. Eriksson S, Alm R, Astedt B: Organ cultures of human fetal hepatocytes in the study of extra- and intracellular $\alpha_1$-antitrypsin. *Biochim Biophys Acta* **542**:496, 1978.

23. Sifers RN, Rogers BB, Hawkins HK, Finegold MJ, Woo SLC: Elevated synthesis of human $\alpha_1$-antitrypsin hinders the secretion of murine $\alpha_1$-antitrypsin from hepatocytes of transgenic mice. *J Biol Chem* **264**:15696, 1989.

24. Perlmutter DH, Cole FS, Kilbridge P, Rossing TH, Colten HR: Expression of the $\alpha_1$-proteinase inhibitor gene in human monocytes and macrophages. *Proc Natl Acad Sci U S A* **82**:795, 1985.

25. Davidson LA, Lonnerdal B: Fecal $\alpha_1$-antitrypsin in breast-fed infants is derived from human milk and is not indicative of enteric protein loss. *Acta Paediatr Scand* **79**:137, 1990.

26. Laurell C-B, Nosslin B, Jeppsson J-O: Catabolic rate of $\alpha_1$-antitrypsin of Pi type M and Z in man. *Clin Sci Mol Med* **52**:457, 1977.

27. Jeppsson J-O, Laurell C-B, Nosslin B, Cox DW: Catabolic rate of $\alpha_1$-antitrypsin of Pi types s and $M_{MALTON}$ and of asialylated M protein in man. *Clin Sci Mol Med* **55**:103, 1978.

28. Jeppsson J-O, Laurell C-B, Fagerhol MK: Properties of isolated $\alpha_1$-antitrypsin of Pi types M, S and Z. *Eur J Biochem* **83**:143, 1978.

29. Cox DW, Billingsley GD, Siewertsen MA: $\alpha_1$-Antitrypsin, in Hommes FA (ed): *Techniques in Diagnostic Human Biochemical Genetics: A Laboratory Manual.* New York, Alan R. Liss, 1991, p 473.

30. Whicher JT, Ritchie RF, Johnson AM, et al: New international reference preparation for proteins in human serum (RPPHS). *Clin Chem* **40**:934, 1994.

31. Erlanger BF, Kokowsky N, Cohen W: The preparation and properties of two new chromogenic substrates of trypsin. *Arch Biochem* **95**:271, 1961.

32. Visser L, Blout E: The use of p-nitrophenyl N-tert-butyloxycarbonyl-l-alaninate as substrate for elastase. *Biochim Biophys Acta* **268**:257, 1972.

33. Beatty K, Robertie P, Senior RM, Travis J: Determination of oxidized $\alpha_1$-proteinase inhibitor in serum. *J Lab Clin Med* **100**:186, 1982.

34. Travis J, Salvesen GS: Human plasma proteinase inhibitors. *Ann Rev Biochem* **52**:655, 1983.

35. Carlson J, Stenfo J: The biosynthesis of rat $\alpha_1$-antitrypsin. *J Biol Chem* **257**:12987, 1982.

36. Long GL, Chandra T, Woo SLC, Davie EW, Kurachi K: Complete sequence of the cDNA for human $\alpha_1\alpha$-antitrypsin and the gene for the S variant. *Biochem* **23**:4828, 1984.

37. Loebermann H, Tokuoka R, Deisenhofer J, Huber R: Human $\alpha_1$-proteinase inhibitor. Crystal structure analysis of two crystal modifications, molecular model and preliminary analysis of the implications for function. *J Mol Biol* **177**:531, 1984.

38. Carrell RW, Pemberton PA, Boswell DR: The serpins: Evolution and adaptation in a family of protease inhibitors. *Cold Spring Harb Symp Quant Biol* **52**:527, 1987.

39. Vaughan L, Lorier MA, Carrell RW: $\alpha_1$-Antitrypsin microheterogeneity isolation and physiological significance of isoforms. *Biochim Biophys Acta* **701**:339, 1982.

40. Chan SK, Rees DC, Li S-C, Li Y-T: Linear structure of oligosaccharide chains in $\alpha_1$-protease inhibitor isolated from human plasma. *J Biol Chem* **251**:471, 1976.

41. Jeppsson J-O, Lilja H, Johansson M: Isolation and characterization of two minor fractions of $\alpha_1$-antitrypsin by high-performance liquid chromatographic chromatofocusing. *J Chromatog* **327**:173, 1985.

42. Carrell RW, Jeppsson J-O, Laurell C-B, et al: Structure and variation of human $\alpha_1$-antitrypsin. *Nature* **298**:329, 1982.

43. Johnson D, Travis J: Structural evidence for methionine at the reactive site of human $\alpha_1$-proteinase inhibitor. *J Biol Chem* **253**:7142, 1978.

44. Laskowski J, Kato I: Protein inhibitors of proteinases. *Ann Rev Biochem* **49**:593, 1980.

45. Johnson D, Travis J: The oxidative inactivation of human $\alpha_1$-proteinase inhibitor. *J Biol Chem* **254**:4022, 1979.

46. Carrell RW, Owen MC: Plakalbumin, $\alpha_1$-antitrypsin, antithrombin and the mechanism of inflammatory thrombosis. *Nature* **317**:730, 1985.

47. Hill RE, Shaw PH, Boyd PA, Baumann H, Hastie ND: Plasma protease inhibitors in mouse and man: Divergence within the reactive centre regions. *Nature* **311**:175, 1984.

48. Owen MC, Brennan SO, Lewis JH, Carrell RW: Mutation of antitrypsin to antithrombin: $\alpha_1$-Antitrypsin-Pittsburgh (358 Met $\rightarrow$ Arg), a fatal bleeding disorder. *N Engl J Med* **309**:694, 1983.

49. Ciliberto G, Dente L, Cortese R: Cell-specific expression of a transfected human $\alpha_1$-antitrypsin gene. *Cell* **4**:531, 1985.

50. Hafeez W, Ciliberto G, Perlmutter DH: Constitutive and modulated expression of the human $\alpha_1$-antitrypsin gene. Different transcriptional initiation sites used in three different cell types. *J Clin Invest* **89**:1214, 1992.

51. Li Y, Zhou L, Twining SS, Sugar J, Yue BY: Involvement of Sp1 elements in the promoter activity of the alpha1-proteinase inhibitor gene. *J Biol Chem* **273**:9959, 1998.

52. Potempa J, Korzus E, Travis J: The serpin superfamily of proteinase inhibitors: Structure, function, and regulation. *J Biol Chem* **269**:15957, 1994.

53. Underhill DA, Hammond GL: Organization of the human corticosteroid binding globulin gene and analysis of its 5'-flanking region. *Genomics* **3**:1448, 1989.

54. Wright HT: Introns and higher-order structure in the evolution of serpins. *J Mol Evol* **36**:136, 1993.

55. Gedde-Dahl T, Fagerhol MK, Cook PJL, Noades J: Autosomal linkage between the Gm and Pi loci in man. *Ann Hum Genet* **35**:393, 1972.

56. Schroeder WT, Miller MF, Woo SLC, Saunders GF: Chromosomal localization of the human $\alpha_1\alpha$-antitrypsin gene (PI) to 14q31-32. *Am J Hum Genet* **37**:868, 1985.

57. Billingsley GD, Walter MA, Hammond GL, Cox DW: Physical mapping of four serpin genes: $\alpha_1$-Antitrypsin, $\alpha_1$-antichymotrypsin, corticosteroid-binding globulin, and protein C inhibitor, within a 280-kb region on chromosome 14q32.1. *Am J Hum Genet* **52**:343, 1993.

58. Byth BC, Billingsley GD, Cox DW: Physical and genetic mapping of the serpin gene cluster at 14q32.1: Allelic association and a unique haplotype associated with $\alpha_1$-antitrypsin deficiency. *Am J Hum Genet* **55**:126, 1994.

59. Rollini P, Fournier RE: A 370-kb cosmid contig of the serpin gene cluster on human chromosome 14q32.1: Molecular linkage of the genes encoding $\alpha_1$-antichymotrypsin, protein C inhibitor, kallistatin, $\alpha_1$-antitrypsin, and corticosteroid-binding globulin. *Genomics* **46**:409, 1997.

60. Allen RC, Harley RA, Talamo RC: A new method for determination of $\alpha_1$-antitrypsin phenotypes using isoelectric focusing on polyacrylamide gel slabs. *Am J Clin Pathol* **62**:732, 1974.

61. Arnaud P, Chapuis-Cellier C, Creyssel R: Polymorphisme de l'$\alpha_1$-antitrypsin plasmatique (système Pi). Mise en évidence par électrofocalisation sur gel de polyacrylamide. *C R Soc Biol* Paris **168**:58, 1974.

62. Lebas J, Hayem A, Martin JP: Etude des variants génétiques de l'$\alpha_1$-antitrypsin en immunofocalisation bidimensionelle. *C R Acad Sci Paris* **258**:2359, 1974.

63. Cox DW, Johnson AM, Fagerhol MK: Report of nomenclature meeting for α₁-antitrypsin. INSERM. Rouen/Bois-Guillaume-1978. *Hum Genet* 53:429, 1980.

64. Fagerhol MK, Cox DW: The Pi polymorphism: Genetic, biochemical and clinical aspects of human α₁-antitrypsin, in Advances, in Harris H, Hirschhorn K, (eds): *Human Genetics Vol 11.* New York, Plenum Press, 1981, p 1.

65. Jeppsson J-O, Franzen B: Typing of genetic variants of α₁-antitrypsin by electrofocusing. *Clin Chem* 28:219, 1982.

66. Budowle B, Murch RS: A high resolution, rapid procedure for α₁-antitrypsin phenotyping. *Electrophoresis* 6:523, 1985.

67. Weidinger S, Cleve H: Hybrid isoelectric focusing for classification of α₁-antitrypsin variants. *Prot Biol Fluids* 34:863, 1986.

68. Weidinger S, Cleve H: High resolution of α₁-antitrypsin PI M subtypes by isoelectric focusing with a modified immobilized pH gradient. *Electrophoresis* 5:223, 1984.

69. Cox DW: New variants of α₁-antitrypsin: Comparison of PI typing techniques. *Am J Hum Genet* 33:354, 1981.

70. Kamboh MI: Biochemical and genetic aspects of human serum α₁-proteinase inhibitor protein. *Dis Markers* 3:135, 1985.

71. Fagerhol MK: Quantitative studies on the inherited variants of serum α₁-antitrypsin. *Scand J Clin Lab Invest* 23:97, 1969.

72. Cox DW, Hoeppner VH, Levison H: Protease inhibitors in patients with chronic obstructive pulmonary disease: The α₁-antitrypsin heterozygote controversy. *Am Rev Respir Dis* 113:601, 1976.

73. Martin NG, Clark P, Ofulue AF, Eaves LJ, Corey LA, Nance WE: Does the PI polymorphism alone control α₁-antitrypsin expression? *Am J Hum Genet* 40:267, 1987.

74. Arnaud P, Chapuis-Cellier C, Vittoz P, Fudenberg H: Genetic polymorphism of serum α₁-protease inhibitor (α₁-antitrypsin): Pi I, a deficient allele of the Pi system. *J Lab Clin Med* 92:177, 1978.

75. Holmes MD, Brantly ML, Fells GA, Crystal RG: α₁-antitrypsin W_BETHESDA: Molecular basis of an unusual α₁-antitrypsin deficiency variant. *Biochem Biophys Res Commun* 170:1013, 1990.

76. Fagerhol MK, Hauge HE: The PI phenotype MP Discovery of a ninth allele belonging to the system of inherited variants of serum α₁-antitrypsin. *Vox Sang* 15:396, 1968.

77. Billingsley GD, Cox DW: Functional assessment of genetic variants of α₁-antitrypsin. *Hum Genet* 61:118, 1982.

78. Hug G, Chuck G, Bowles B: α₁-antitrypsin phenotype: Transient cathodal shift in serum of infant girl with urinary cytomegalovirus and fatty liver. *Pediatr Res* 16:192, 1982.

79. Janciauskiene S, Eriksson S: The interaction of hydrophobic bile acids with the α₁-proteinase inhibitor. *FEBS Lett* 343:141, 1994.

80. Nukiwa T, Brantly M, Ogushi F, et al: Characterization of the M1(ala213) type of α₁-antitrypsin, a newly recognized, common "normal" α₁-antitrypsin haplotype. *Biochem J* 26:5259, 1987.

81. Cox DW, Billingsley GD: Restriction enzyme MaeIII for prenatal diagnosis of α₁-antitrypsin deficiency. *Lancet* ii:741, 1986.

82. Teckman JH, Perlmutter DH: The endoplasmic reticulum degradation pathway for mutant secretory proteins α₁-antitrypsin Z and S is distinct from that for an unassembled membrane protein. *J Biol Chem* 271:13215, 1996.

83. Lovegrove JU, Jeremiah S, Gillett GT, Temple IK, Povey S, Whitehouse DB: A new α₁-antitrypsin mutation, Thr-Met 85 (PI Z_BRISTOL) associated with novel electrophoretic properties. *Ann Hum Genet* 61:385, 1997.

84. Fagerhol MK, Laurell C-B: The Pi system-inherited variants of serum α₁-antitrypsin in progress, in Steinberg A, Bearn A (eds): *Medical Genetics Vol. VII.* New York, Grune and Stratton, 1970, p 96.

85. Kellermann G, Walter H: Investigations on the population genetics of the α₁-antitrypsin polymorphism. *Humangenetik* 10:145, 1970.

86. Lieberman J: α₁-antitrypsin deficiency and related disorders. *Princ Prac Med Genet* 2:911, 1983.

87. Warsy AS, El-Hazmi MAF, Sedrani SH: α₁-antitrypsin phenotypes in Saudi Arabia: A study in the central province. *Ann Saudi Med* 11:159, 1993.

88. Cox DW, Woo SLC, Mansfield T: DNA restriction fragments associated with α₁-antitrypsin indicate a single origin for deficiency allele PI Z. *Nature* 316:79, 1985.

89. Cox DW, Billingsley GD, Mansfield T: DNA restriction site polymorphisms associated with the α₁-antitrypsin gene. *Am J Hum Genet* 41:891, 1987.

90. Matteson KJ, Ostrer H, Chakravarti A, et al: A study of restriction fragment length polymorphisms at the human α₁-antitrypsin locus. *Hum Genet* 69:263, 1985.

91. Hodgson I, Kalsheker N: DNA polymorphisms of the human α₁-antitrypsin gene in normal subjects and in patients with pulmonary emphysema. *J Med Genet* 24:47, 1987.

92. Kurachi K, Chandra T, Friezner Degen SJ, et al: Cloning and sequence of cDNA coding for α₁-antitrypsin. *Proc Natl Acad Sci U S A* 78:6826, 1981.

93. Cox DW, Billingsley GD: Rare deficiency types of α₁-antitrypsin: Electrophoretic variation and DNA haplotypes. *Am J Hum Genet* 44:844, 1989.

94. Laurell C-B, Sveger T: Mass screening of newborn Swedish infants for α₁-antitrypsin deficiency. *Am J Hum Genet* 27:213, 1975.

95. Brantly ML, Wittes JT, Vogelmeier CF, Hubbard RC, Fells GA, Crystal RG: Use of a highly purified α₁-antitrypsin standard to establish ranges for the common normal and deficient α₁-antitrypsin phenotypes. *Chest* 100:703, 1991.

96. Moroz SP, Cutz E, Cox DW, Sass-Kortsak A: Liver disease associated with α₁-antitrypsin deficiency in childhood. *J Pediatr* 88:19, 1976.

97. Sveger T: Plasma protease inhibitors in α₁-antitrypsin-deficient children. *Pediatr Res* 19:834, 1985.

98. Bruun Petersen K, Bruun Petersen G, Dahl R, et al: α₁-antitrypsin alleles in patients with pulmonary emphysema, detected by DNA amplification (PCR) and oligonucleotide probes. *Eur Respir J* 5:531, 1992.

99. Gregersen N, Winter V, Petersen KB, et al: Detection of point mutations in amplified single copy genes by biotin-labelled oligonucleotides: Diagnosis of variants of α₁-antitrypsin. *Clin Chim Acta* 182:151, 1989.

100. Dry PJ: Rapid detection of α₁-antitrypsin deficiency by analysis of a PCR-induced TaqI restriction site. *Hum Genet* 87:742, 1991.

101. Andresen BS, Knudsen I, Jensen PKA, Rasmussen K, Gregersen N: Two novel nonradioactive polymerase chain reaction-based assays of dried blood spots, genomic DNA, or whole cells for fast, reliable detection of Z and S mutations in the α₁-antitrypsin gene. *Clin Chem* 38:2100, 1992.

102. Sharp HL: α₁-antitrypsin deficiency. *Hosp Pract* 5:83, 1971.

103. Cutz E, Cox DW: α₁-antitrypsin deficiency: The spectrum of pathology and pathophysiology, in Rosenberg HS, Bolande RP (eds): *Perspectives in Pediatric Pathology,* New York, Masson, 1979, p 1.

104. Huang S-N, Minassian H, More JD: Application of immunofluorescent staining on paraffin sections improved by trypsin digestion. *Lab Invest* 35:383, 1976.

105. Darlington GJ, Wilson DR, Lachman LB: Monocyte conditioned medium, interleukin-1 and tumour necrosis factor stimulate the acute phase response in human hepatoma cells in vitro. *J Cell Biol* 103:787, 1986.

106. Carlson J, Eriksson S, Hagerstrand I: Intra- and extracellular α₁-antitrypsin in liver disease with special reference to Pi phenotype. *J Clin Pathol* 34:1020, 1981.

107. Iezzoni JC, Gaffey MJ, Stacy EK, Normansell DE: Hepatocytic globules in end-stage hepatic disease: Relationship to α₁-antitrypsin phenotype. *Am J Clin Pathol* 107:692, 1997.

108. Roberts EA, Cox DW, Medline A, Wanless IR: Occurrence of α₁-antitrypsin deficiency in 155 patients with alcoholic liver disease. *Amer J Clin Path* 82:424, 1984.

109. Lomas DA, Evans DL, Stone SR, Chang WW, Carrell RW: Effect of the Z mutation on the physical and inhibitory properties of α₁-antitrypsin. *Biochem* 32:500, 1993.

110. Errington DM, Bathurst IC, Janus ED, Carell RW: In vitro synthesis of M and Z forms of human α₁-antitrypsin. *FEBS Lett* 148:83, 1982.

111. Gross V, vom Berg D, Kreuzkamp J, et al: Biosynthesis and secretion of M- and Z-type α₁-proteinase inhibitor by human monocytes. Effect of inhibitors of glycosylation and of oligosaccharide processing on secretion and function. *Biol Chem Hoppe Seyler* 371:231, 1990.

112. Bathurst IC, Travis J, George PM, Carrell RW: Structural and functional characterization of the abnormal Z α₁-antitrypsin isolated from human liver. *FEBS Lett* 177:179, 1984.

113. Eriksson S, Larsson C: Purification and partial characterization of PAS-positive inclusion bodies from the liver in α₁-antitrypsin deficiency. *N Engl J Med* 292:176, 1975.

114. Hercz A, Katona E, Cutz E, Wilson JR, Barton M: α₁-antitrypsin: The presence of excess mannose in the Z variant isolated from liver. *Science* 201:1229, 1978.

115. Foreman RC, Judah JD, Colman A: Xenopus oocytes can synthesize but do not secrete the Z variant of human α₁-antitrypsin. *FEBS Lett* 168:84, 1984.

116. Cox DW, Billingsley GD, Callahan JW: Aggregation of plasma Z type α₁-antitrypsin suggests basic defect for the deficiency. *FEBS Lett* 205:255, 1986.

117. Jeppsson J-O: Amino acid substitution Gly-Lys in $\alpha_1$-antitrypsin Pi Z. *FEBS Lett* **65**:195, 1976.

118. Yoshida L, Lieberman J, Gaidulis L, Ewing C: Molecular abnormality of human $\alpha_1$-antitrypsin variant (Pi Z) associated with plasma activity deficiency. *Proc Natl Acad Sci U S A* **73**:1324, 1976.

119. Foreman RC: Disruption of the Lys 290-Glu 342 salt bridge in human $\alpha_1$-antitrypsin does not prevent its synthesis and secretion. *FEBS Lett* **216**:79, 1987.

120. Carrell RW, Evans DL, Stein PE: Mobile reactive centre of serpins and the control of thrombosis. *Nature* **353**:576, 1991.

121. Lomas DA, Evans DL, Finch JT, Carrell RW: The mechanism of Z $\alpha_1$-antitrypsin accumulation in the liver. *Nature* **357**:605, 1992.

122. Lomas DA, Elliott PR, Sidhar SK, et al: $\alpha_1$-antitrypsin $M_{MALTON}$ (Phe52-deleted) forms loop-sheet polymers in vivo. Evidence for the C sheet mechanism of polymerization. *J Biol Chem* **270**:16864, 1995.

123. Qu D, Teckman JH, Omura S, Perlmutter DH: Degradation of a mutant secretory protein, $\alpha_1$-antitrypsin Z, in the endoplasmic reticulum requires proteosome activity. *J Biol Chem* **271**:22791, 1996.

124. Liu Y, Choudhury P, Cabral CM, Sifers RN: Intracellular disposal of incompletely folded human $\alpha_1$-antitrypsin involves release from calnexin and post-translational trimming of asparagine-linked oligosaccharides. *J Biol Chem* **272**:7946, 1997.

125. Matsunaga E, Shiokawa S, Nakamura H, Maruyama T, Tsuda K, Fukumaki U: Molecular analysis of the gene of the $\alpha_1$-antitrypsin deficiency variant, $M_{NICHINAN}$. *Am J Hum Genet* **46**:602, 1990.

126. Seyama K, Nukiwa T, Takabe K, Takahashi H, Miyake K, Kira S: Siiyama[CHE10] (serine 53 (TCC) to phenylalanine 53 (TTC)). A new $\alpha_1$-antitrypsin-deficient variant with mutation on a predicted conserved residue of the serpin backbone. *J Biol Chem* **266**:12627, 1991.

127. Kang HA, Lee KN, Yu MH: Folding and stability of the Z and S(iiyama) genetic variants of human $\alpha_1$-antitrypsin. *J Biol Chem* **272**:510, 1997.

128. Lieberman J, Gaidulis L, Klotz SD: A new deficient variant of $\alpha_1$-antitrypsin ($M_{DUARTE}$). Inability to detect the heterozygous state by antitrypsin phenotyping. *Am Rev Respir Dis* **113**:31, 1976.

129. Hofker MH, Nukiwa T, Van Paassen HMB, et al: A pro → leu substitution in codon 369 in the $\alpha_1$-antitrypsin deficiency variant PI MHeerlen. *Hum Gen* **81**:264, 1989.

130. Takahashi H, Nukiwa T, Satoh K, et al: Characterization of the gene and protein of the $\alpha_1$-antitrypsin "deficiency" allele Mprocida. *J Biol Chem* **263**:15528, 1988.

131. Seyama K, Nukiwa T, Souma S, Shimizu K, Kira S: $\alpha_1$-Antitrypsin-deficient variant Siiyama (Ser53[TCC] to Phe53[TTC]) is prevalent in Japan. Status of $\alpha_1$-antitrypsin deficiency in Japan. *Am J Respir Crit Care Med* **152**:2119, 1995.

132. Cox DW: $\alpha_1$-Antitrypsin deficiency, in Scriver CR, Beaudet al, Sly WS., Valle D (eds): *The Metabolic Basis of Inherited Disease.* 6th Ed. New York, McGraw-Hill, 1989, p 2409.

133. Cox DW, Levison H: Emphysema of early onset associated with a complete deficiency of $\alpha_1$-antitrypsin (null homozygotes). *Am Rev Respir Dis* **137**:371, 1988.

134. Sifers RN, Brashears-Macatee S, Kidd VJ, Muensch H, Woo SLC: A frameshift mutation results in a truncated $\alpha_1$-antitrypsin that is retained within the rough endoplasmic reticulum. *J Biol Chem* **263**:7330, 1988.

135. Curiel D, Brantly M, Curiel E, Stier L. Crystal RG: $\alpha_1$-antitrypsin deficiency caused by the $\alpha_1$-antitrypsin Null$_{MATTAWA}$ gene. An insertion mutation rendering the $\alpha_1$-antitrypsin gene incapable of producing $\alpha_1$-antitrypsin. *J Clin Invest* **83**:1144, 1989.

136. Fraizer GC, Siewertsen MA, Hofker MH, Brubacher MG, Cox DW: A null deficiency allele of $\alpha_1$-antitrypsin, Q$_{OLUDWIGSHAFEN}$, with altered tertiary structure. *J Clin Invest* **86**:1878, 1990.

137. Takahashi H, Crystal RG: $\alpha_1$-antitrypsin Null(isola di procida): an $\alpha_1$-Antitrypsin deficiency allele caused by deletion of all $\alpha_1$-antitrypsin coding exons. *Am J Hum Genet* **47**:403, 1990.

138. Faber J-P, Poller W, Weidinger S, et al: Identification and DNA sequence analysis of 15 new $\alpha_1$-antitrypsin variants, including two PI*Q0 alleles and one deficient PI*M allele. *Am J Hum Genet* **55**:1113, 1994.

139. Carrell RW: $\alpha_1$-Antitrypsin, emphysema and smoking. *N Z Med J* **97**:327, 1984.

140. Pierce JA, Eradio B, Dew TA: Antitrypsin phenotypes in St. Louis. *JAMA* **238**:609, 1975.

141. Eriksson S: Studies in $\alpha_1$-antitrypsin deficiency. *Acta Med Scand* **177(Supp 432)**:5, 1965.

142. Morse JO: $\alpha_1$-Antitrypsin deficiency. *N Engl J Med* **299**:1045, 1978.

143. Tobin MJ, Cook PJL: Hutchison DCS: $\alpha_1$-antitrypsin deficiency: The clinical and physiological features of pulmonary emphysema in subjects homozygous for Pi type Z. *Br J Dis Chest* **77**:14, 1983.

144. Lieberman J, Winter B, Sastre A: Alpha$_1$-antitrypsin Pi types in 965 COPD Patients. *Chest* **89**:370, 1986.

145. Rienmuller RK, Behr J, Kalender WA, et al: Standardized quantitative high resolution CT in lung diseases. *J Comput Assist Tomogr* **15**:742, 1991.

146. Larsson C: Natural history and life expectancy in severe $\alpha_1$-antitrypsin deficiency, Pi Z. *Acta Med Scand* **204**:345, 1978.

147. Cox DW, Talamo RC: Genetic aspects of pediatric lung disease. *Pediatr Clin North Am* **26**:467, 1979.

148. Wiebicke W, Niggemann B, Fischer A: Pulmonary function in children with homozygous $\alpha_1$-protease inhibitor deficiency. *Eur J Pediatr* **155**:603, 1996.

149. Hird MF, Greenough A, Mieli Vergani G, Mowat AP: Hyperinflation in children with liver disease due to $\alpha_1$-antitrypsin deficiency. *Pediatr Pulmonol* **11**:212, 1991.

150. Silverman EK, Pierce JA, Province MA, Rao DC, Campbell EJ: Variability of pulmonary function in $\alpha_1$-antitrypsin deficiency: Clinical correlates. *Ann Intern Med* **111**:982, 1989.

151. Jack CI, Evans CC: Three cases of $\alpha_1$-antitrypsin deficiency in the elderly. *Postgrad Med J* **67**:840, 1991.

152. Kueppers F, Black LF: $\alpha_1\alpha$-antitrypsin and its deficiency. *Am Rev Respir Dis* **110**:176, 1974.

153. Janus ED, Phillips NT, Carrell RW: Smoking, lung function, and $\alpha_1$-antitrypsin deficiency. *Lancet* **i**:152, 1985.

154. Evald T, Dirksen A, Keittelmann S, Viskum K, Kok Jensen A: Decline in pulmonary function in patients with $\alpha_1$-antitrypsin deficiency. *Lung* **168(Supp)**:579, 1990.

155. Seersholm N, Kok-Jensen A, Dirksen A: Decline in FEV1 among patients with severe hereditary $\alpha_1$-antitrypsin deficiency type Pi Z. *Am J Respir Crit Care Med* **152**:1922, 1995.

156. $\alpha_1$-Antitrypsin Deficiency Registry Study Group: Survival and FEV$_1$ decline in individuals with severe deficiency of $\alpha_1$-antitrypsin. *Am J Respir Crit Care Med* **158**:49, 1998.

157. Tager IB, Munoz A, Rosner B, Weiss ST, Carey V, Speizer FE: Effect of cigarette smoking on the pulmonary function of children and adolescents. *Am Rev Respir Dis* **131**:752, 1985.

158. Weitz JI, Silverman EK, Thong B, Campbell EJ: Plasma levels of elastase-specific fibrinopeptides correlate with proteinase inhibitor phenotype. Evidence for increased elastase activity in subjects with homozygous and heterozygous deficiency of $\alpha_1$-proteinase inhibitor. *J Clin Invest* **89**:766, 1992.

159. Gadek JE, Hunninghake GW, Fells GA, Zimmerman RL, Keogh BA, Crystal RG: Evaluation of the protease-antiprotease theory of human destructive lung disease. *Bull Eur Physiopathol Respir* **16**:27, 1980.

160. Elliott PR, Bilton D, Lomas DA: Lung polymers in Z $\alpha_1$-antitrypsin deficiency-related emphysema. *Am J Respir Cell Mol Biol* **18**:670, 1998.

161. Jochum M, Pelletier A, Boudier C, Pauli G, Bieth JG: The concentration of leukocyte elastase $\alpha_1$-proteinase inhibitor complex in bronchoalveolar lavage fluids from healthy human subjects. *Am Rev Respir Dis* **132**:913, 1985.

162. Wewers MD, Casolaro MA, Crystal RG: Comparison of $\alpha_1$-antitrypsin levels and antineutrophil elastase capacity of blood and lung in a patient with the $\alpha_1$-antitrypsin phenotype null-null before and during $\alpha_1$-antitrypsin augmentation therapy. *Am Rev Respir Dis* **135**:539, 1987.

163. Gauthier F, Frysmark U, Ohlsson K, Bieth JG: Kinetics of the inhibition of leukocyte elastase by the bronchial inhibitor. *Biochem Biophys Acta* **700**:178, 1982.

164. Stockley RA, Morrison HM, Smith S, Tetley T: Low molecular mass bronchial proteinase inhibitor and $\alpha_1$-proteinase inhibitor in sputum and bronchoalveolar lavage. *Hoppe Seyler Z Physiol Chem* **365**:587, 1984.

165. Brissenden JE, Cox DW: $\alpha_2$-Macroglobulin production by cultured human fibroblasts. *Som Cell Genet* **8**:289, 1982.

166. Brus F, van Oeveren W, Okken A, Oetomo SB: Number and activation of circulating polymorphonuclear leukocytes and platelets are associated with neonatal respiratory distress syndrome severity. *Pediatrics* **99**:672, 1997.

167. Stiskal JA, Dunn MS, Shennan AT, et al: $\alpha_1$-Proteinase inhibitor therapy for the prevention of chronic lung disease of prematurity: A randomized, controlled trial. *Pediatrics* **101**:89, 1998.

168. Janoff A: Elastases and emphysema. Current assessment of the protease-antiprotease hypothesis. *Am Rev Respir Dis* **132**:417, 1985.

169. Fera T, Abboud RT, Richter A, Johal SS: Acute effect of smoking on elastase-like esterase activity and immunologic neutrophil elastase levels in bronchoalveolar lavage fluid. *Am Rev Respir Dis* **133**:568, 1986.

170. Abboud RT, Fera T, Richter A, Tabona MZ, Johal SS: Acute effect of smoking on the functional activity of $\alpha_1$-protease inhibitor in bronchoalveolar lavage fluid. *Am Rev Respir Dis* **131**:79, 1985.

171. Carp H, Miller F, Hoidal JR, Janoff A: Potential mechanism of emphysema: $\alpha_1$-Proteinase inhibitor recovered from lungs of cigarette smokers contains oxidized methionine and has decreased elastase inhibitory capacity. *Proc Natl Acad Sci U S A* **79**:2041, 1982.

172. Matheson NR, Wong PS, Travis J: Enzymatic inactivation of human $\alpha_1$-proteinase inhibitor by neutrophil myeloperoxidase. *Biochem Biophys Res Commun* **88**:402, 1979.

173. Clark RA, Stone PJ, Hag AE, Calore JD, Franzblau C: Myeloperoxidase-catalyzed inactivation of $\alpha_1\alpha$-protease inhibitor by human neutrophils. *J Biol Chem* **256**:3348, 1981.

174. Stockley RA, Afford SC: Qualitative studies of lung lavage $\alpha_1$-proteinase inhibitor. Hoppe-Seyler'. *Hoppe-Seyler's Z Physiol Chem* **365**:503, 1984.

175. Laurent P, Janoff A, Kagan HM: Cigarette smoke blocks cross-linking of elastin in vitro. *Am Rev Respir Dis* **127**:189, 1983.

176. Redline S, Tishler PV, Lewitter FI, Tager IB, Munoz A, Speizer FE: Assessment of genetic and nongenetic influences on pulmonary function. A twin study. *Am Rev Respir Dis* **135**:217, 1987.

177. Kalsheker NA, Watkins GL, Hill S, Morgan K, Stockley RA, Fick RB: Independent mutations in the flanking sequence of the $\alpha_1$-antitrypsin gene are associated with chronic obstructive airways disease. *Dis Markers* **8**:151, 1990.

178. Poller W, Meisen C, Olek K: DNA polymorphisms of the $\alpha_1$-antitrypsin gene region in patients with chronic obstructive pulmonary disease. *Eur J Clin Invest* **20**:1, 1990.

179. Morgan K, Scobie G, Marsters P, Kalsheker NA: Mutation in an $\alpha_1$-antitrypsin enhancer results in an interleukin-6 deficient acute-phase response due to loss of cooperativity between transcription factors. *Biochim Biophys Acta* **1362**:67, 1997.

180. Green SL, Gaillard MC, Dewar JB, Ludewick H, Song E. Feldman C: Differences in the prevalence of a *Taq*I RFLP in the 3' flanking region of the $\alpha_1$-proteinase inhibitor gene between asthmatic and non-asthmatic black and white South Africans. *Clin Genet* **52**:162, 1997.

181. Taylor JC, Madison R, Kosinska D: Is antioxidant deficiency related to chronic obstructive pulmonary disease? *Am Rev Respir Dis* **134**:285, 1986.

182. Galdston M, Feldman JG, Levytska V, Magnusson B: Antioxidant activity of serum ceruloplasmin and transferrin available iron-binding capacity in smokers and nonsmokers. *Am Rev Respir Dis* **135**:783, 1987.

183. Theron A, Anderson R: Investigation of the protective effects of the antioxidants ascorbate, cysteine, and dapsone on the phagocyte-mediated oxidative inactivation of human $\alpha_1$-protease inhibitor in vitro. *Am Rev Respir Dis* **132**:1049, 1985.

184. Pacht ER, Kaseki H, Mohammed JR, Cornwell DG, Davis WB: Deficiency of vitamin E in the alveolar fluid of cigarette smokers. Influence on alveolar macrophage cytotoxicity. *J Clin Invest* **77**:789, 1986.

185. Sandford AJ, Weir TD, Pare PD: Genetic risk factors for chronic obstructive pulmonary disease. *Eur Respir J* **10**:1380, 1997.

186. Cooper DM, Hoeppner VH, Cox DW, Zamel N, Bryan AC, Levison H: Lung function in $\alpha_1$-antitrypsin heterozygotes (Pi type MZ). *Am Rev Respir Dis* **110**:708, 1974.

187. Bruce RM, Cohen BH, Diamond EL, et al: Collaborative study to assess risk of lung disease in Pi MZ phenotype subjects. *Am Rev Respir Dis* **130**:386, 1984.

188. Tarjan E, Magyar P, Vaczi Z, Lantos A, Vaszar L: Longitudinal lung function study in heterozygous Pi MZ phenotype subjects. *Eur Respir J* **7**:2199, 1994.

189. Tattersall SF, Pereira RP, Hunter D, Blundell G, Pride NB: Lung distensibility and airway function in intermediate $\alpha_1$-antitrypsin deficiency (Pi MZ). *Thorax* **34**:637, 1979.

190. Larsson C, Eriksson S, Dirksen H: Smoking and intermediate $\alpha_1$-antitrypsin deficiency and lung function in middle-aged men. *BMJ* **2**:922, 1977.

191. Eriksson S, Lindell SE, Wiberg R: Effects of smoking and intermediate $\alpha_1$-antitrypsin deficiency (Pi MZ) on lung function. *Eur J Respir Dis* **67**:279, 1985.

192. Larsson C, Dirksen H, Sunström G, Eriksson S: Lung function studies in asymptomatic individuals with moderately (Pi SZ) and severely (Pi Z) reduced levels of $\alpha_1$-antitrypsin. *Scand J Resp Dis* **57**:267, 1976.

193. Beckman G, Stjernberg NL, Eklund A: Is the PiF allele of $\alpha_1$-antitrypsin associated with pulmonary disease? *Clin Genet* **25**:491, 1984.

194. Hussain M, Mieli Vergani G, Mowat AP: $\alpha_1$-Antitrypsin deficiency and liver disease: Clinical presentation, diagnosis and treatment. *J Inherit Metab Dis* **14**:497, 1991.

195. Povey S: Genetics of $\alpha_1$-antitrypsin deficiency in relation to neonatal liver disease. *Mol Biol Med* **7**:161, 1990.

196. Perlmutter DH: The cellular basis for liver injury in $\alpha_1$-antitrypsin deficiency. *Hepatology* **13**:172, 1991.

197. Teckman JH, Qu D, Perlmutter DH: Molecular pathogenesis of liver disease in $\alpha_1$-antitrypsin deficiency. *Hepatology* **24**:1504, 1996.

198. Sveger T: Liver disease in $\alpha_1$-antitrypsin deficiency detected by screening of 200,000 infants. *N Engl J Med* **294**:1316, 1976.

199. Malone M, Mieli Vergani G, Mowat AP, Portmann B: The fetal liver in Pi ZZ $\alpha_1$-antitrypsin deficiency: A report of five cases. *Pediatr Pathol* **9**:623, 1989.

200. Cottrall K, Cook PJL, Mowat AP: Neonatal hepatitis syndrome and $\alpha_1$-antitrypsin deficiency: An epidemiological study in south-east England. *Postgrad Med J* **50**:376, 1974.

201. Odievre M, Martin JP, Hadchouel M, Alagille D: $\alpha_1$-Antitrypsin deficiency and liver disease in children: Phenotypes, manifestations, and prognosis. *Pediatrics* **57**:226, 1976.

202. Nebbia G, Hadchouel M, Odievre M, Alagille D: Early assessment of evolution of liver disease associated with $\alpha_1$-antitrypsin deficiency in childhood. *J Pediatr* **102**:661, 1983.

203. Maggiore G, Bernard O, Hadchouel M, Lemonnier A, Alagille D: Diagnostic value of serum gamma-glutamyl transpeptidase activity in liver diseases in children. *J Pediatr Gastroenterol Nutr* **12**:21, 1991.

204. Sveger T, Thelin T: Four-year-old children with $\alpha_1$-antitrypsin deficiency: Clinical follow-up and parental attitudes towards neonatal screening. *Acta Pediatr Scand* **70**:171, 1981.

205. Sveger T: The natural history of liver disease in $\alpha_1$-antitrypsin deficient children. *Acta Paediatr Scand* **77**:847, 1988.

206. Karlaganis G, Nemeth A, Hammarskjold B, Strandvik B, Sjovall J: Urinary excretion of bile alcohols in normal children and patients with $\alpha_1$-antitrypsin deficiency during development of liver disease. *Eur J Clin Invest* **12**:399, 1982.

207. Schwarzenberg SJ, Sharp HL: Pathogenesis of $\alpha_1$-antitrypsin deficiency-associated liver disease, 1990. *J Pediatr Gastroenterol Nutr* **10**:5, 1990.

208. Mowat AP: Alpha$_1$-antitrypsin deficiency (PiZZ): Features of liver involvement in childhood. *Acta Paediatr Suppl* **393**:13, 1994.

209. Bathurst IC, Errington DM, Foreman RC, Judah JD, Carrell RW: Human Z $\alpha_1$-antitrypsin accumulates intracellularly and stimulates lysosomal activity when synthesized in the Xenopus oocyte. *FEBS Lett* **183**:304, 1985.

210. Hultcrantz R, Mengarelli S: Ultrastructure liver pathology in patients with minimal liver disease and $\alpha_1$-antitrypsin deficiency: A comparison between heterozygous and homozygous patients. *Hepatology* **4**:937, 1984.

211. Carlson JA, Rogers BB, Sifers RN, et al: Accumulation of Pi Z $\alpha_1$-antitrypsin causes liver damage in transgenic mice. *J Clin Invest* **83**:1183, 1989.

212. Dycaico MJ, Felts K, Nichols SW, Geller SA, Sorge JA: Neonatal growth delay in $\alpha_1$-antitrypsin disease. Influence of genetic background. *Mol Biol Med* **6**:137, 1989.

213. Maeda H, Molla A: Pathogenic potentials of bacterial proteases. *Clin Chim Acta* **185**:357, 1989.

214. Weiss SJ: Oxygen, ischemia and inflammation. *Acta Physiol Scand* **126**:9, 1986.

215. Comporti M: Lipid peroxidation and cellular damage in toxic liver injury. *Lab Invest* **53**:599, 1985.

216. Pittschieler K, Lebenthal E, Bujanover Y, Petell JK: Levels of Cu-Zn and Mn superoxide dismutase in rat liver during development. *Gastroenterology* **100**:1062, 1991.

217. Pittschieler K: Oxidative radicals and liver involvement of infants with $\alpha_1$-antitrypsin deficiency. *Padiatr Pathol* **26**:235, 1991.

218. Wallmark A, Alm R, Eriksson S: Monoclonal antibody specific for the mutant Pi Z $\alpha_1$-antitrypsin and its application in an ELISA procedure for identification of Pi Z gene carriers. *Proc Natl Acad Sci U S A* **81**:5690, 1984.

219. Moroz SP, Cutz E, Balfe JW, Sass-Kortsak A: Membranoproliferative glomerulonephritis in childhood cirrhosis associated with $\alpha_1$-antitrypsin deficiency. *Pediatrics* **57**:232, 1976.

220. Littleton ET, Bevis L, Hansen LJ, et al: $\alpha_1$-antitrypsin deficiency, complement activation, and chronic liver disease. *J Clin Pathol* **44**:855, 1991.

221. Wu Y, Whitman I, Molmenti E, Moore K, Hippenmeyer P, Perlmutter DH: A lag in intracellular degradation of mutant $\alpha_1$-antitrypsin correlates with the liver disease phenotype in homozygous Pi ZZ $\alpha_1$-antitrypsin deficiency. *Proc Natl Acad Sci U S A* **91**:9014, 1994.

222. Propst A, Propst T, Ofner D, Feichtinger H, Judmaier G, Vogel W: Prognosis and life expectancy on $\alpha_1$-antitrypsin deficiency and chronic liver disease. *Scand J Gastroenterol* **30**:1108, 1995.

223. Psacharopoulos HT, Mowat AP, Cook PJL, Carlille PA, Portmann B, Rodeck CH: Outcome of liver disease associated with $\alpha_1$-antitrypsin deficiency (Pi Z). *Arch Dis Child* **58**:882, 1983.

224. Ibarguen E, Gross CR, Savik SK, Sharp HL: Liver disease in $\alpha_1$-antitrypsin deficiency: Prognostic indicators. *J Pediatr* **117**:864, 1990.

225. Cox DW: $\alpha_1$-Antitrypsin deficiency, in, MM Fisher, CC Roy (eds): *Pediatric Liver Disease: Hepatology Research and Clinical Issues*, vol 5. New York, Plenum Press, 1983, pp 271–282.

226. Sveger T: Prospective study of children with $\alpha_1$-antitrypsin deficiency: Eight-year-old follow-up. *J Pediatr* **104**:91, 1984.

227. Alagille D: $\alpha_1$-Antitrypsin deficiency. *Hepatology* **4(Supp)**:11, 1984.

228. Porter CA, Mowat AP, Cook PJL, Haynes DWG, Shilkin KB, Williams R: $\alpha_1$-Antitrypsin deficiency and neonatal hepatitis. *BMJ* **3**:435, 1972.

229. Sokol RJ, Heubi JE, Mcgraw C, Balistreri WF: Correction of vitamin E deficiency in children with chronic cholestasis. II. Effect on gastrointestinal and hepatic function. *Hepatology* **6**:1263, 1986.

230. Udall JN, Dixon M, Newman AP, Wright JA: Liver disease in $\alpha_1$-antitrypsin deficiency: A retrospective analysis of the influence of early breast- vs bottle-feeding. *JAMA* **253**:2679, 1985.

231. Sveger T: Breast-feeding, $\alpha_1$-antitrypsin deficiency, and liver disease? *JAMA* **254**:3036, 1985.

232. Udall JN, Bloch KJ, Walker WA: Transport of proteases across neonatal intestine and development of liver disease in infants with $\alpha_1$-antitrypsin deficiency. *Lancet* **I**:1441, 1982.

233. Cox DW, Mansfield T: Prenatal diagnosis of $\alpha_1$-antitrypsin deficiency and estimates of fetal risk for disease. *J Med Genet* **24**:52, 1987.

234. Berg NO, Eriksson S: Liver disease in adults with $\alpha_1$-antitrypsin deficiency. *N Engl J Med* **287**:1264, 1972.

235. Cox DW, Smyth S: Risk for liver disease in adults with $\alpha_1$-antitrypsin deficiency. *Am J Med* **74**:221, 1983.

236. Eriksson S, Hagerstrand I: Cirrhosis and malignant hepatoma in $\alpha_1$-antitrypsin deficiency. *Acta Med Scand* **195**:451, 1974.

237. Esquivel CO, Marino IR, Fioravanti V, VanThiel DH: Liver transplantation for metabolic disease of the liver. *Gastroenterol Clin North Am* **17**:167, 1988.

238. Casavilla A, Gordon R, Van Thiel DH, Starzl TE: Lack of association between HLA antigen DR3 and $\alpha_1$-antitrypsin deficiency in liver transplant recipients. *Dig Dis Sci* **38**:1489, 1993.

239. Eriksson S, Carlson J, Velez R: Risk of cirrhosis and primary liver cancer in $\alpha_1$-antitrypsin deficiency. *N Engl J Med* **314**:736, 1986.

240. Carlson J, Eriksson S: Chronic 'cryptogenic' liver disease in malignant hepatoma in intermediate $\alpha_1$-antitrypsin deficiency identified by a PI Z-specific monoclonal antibody. *Scand J Gastroenterol* **20**:835, 1985.

241. Rabinovitz M, Gavaler JS, Kelly RH, Prieto M, Van Thiel DH: Lack of increase in heterozygous $\alpha_1$-antitrypsin deficiency phenotypes among patients with hepatocellular and bile duct carcinoma. *Hepatology* **15**:407, 1992.

242. Theodoropoulos A, Fertakis A, Archimandritis A, Kapordelis C, Angelopoulos B: $\alpha_1$-antitrypsin phenotypes in cirrhosis and hepatoma. *Acta Gastroenterol* **23**:114, 1976.

243. Palmer PE, Ucci AA, Wolfe HJ: Expression of protein markers in malignant hepatoma. Evidence for genetic and epigenetic mechanisms. *Cancer* **45**:1424, 1980.

244. Nukiwa T, Brantly M, Garver R, et al: Evaluation of "at risk" $\alpha_1$-antitrypsin genotype SZ with synthetic oligonucleotide gene probes. *J Clin Invest* **77**:528, 1986.

245. Bell H, Schrumpf E, Fagerhol MK: Heterozygous MZ $\alpha_1$-antitrypsin deficiency in adults with chronic liver disease. *Scand J Gastroenterol* **25**:788, 1990.

246. Morin T, Feldmann G, Martin J-P, Rueff B, Benhamou J-P, Ropartz C: Heterozygous $\alpha_1$-antitrypsin deficiency and cirrhosis in adults, a fortuitous association. *Lancet* **1**:250, 1975.

247. Lareu MV, Alvarez-Prechous A, Pardinas C, Concheiro L, Carracedo A: Genetic markers in alcoholic liver cirrhosis. *Hum Hered* **42**:235, 1992.

248. Eigenbrodt ML, McCashland TM, Dy RM, Clark J, Galati J: Heterozygous $\alpha_1$-antitrypsin phenotypes in patients with end stage liver disease. *Am J Gastroenterol* **92**:602, 1997.

249. Brind AM, Bassendine MF, Bennett MK, James OF: $\alpha_1$-Antitrypsin granules in the liver-always important? *QJM* **76**:699, 1990.

250. Propst T, Propst A, Dietze O, Judmaier G, Braunsteiner H, Vogel W: High prevalence of viral infection in adults with homozygous and heterozygous $\alpha_1$-antitrypsin deficiency and chronic liver disease. *Ann Intern Med* **117**:641, 1992.

251. Schleissner IA, Cohen AH: $\alpha_1$-Antitrypsin deficiency and hepatic carcinoma. *Am Rev Respir Dis* **111**:863, 1975.

252. Milford Ward A, Pickering JD, Shortland JR: The renal manifestations of Pi Z, in Martin J-P (ed): *L'$\alpha_1$-antitrypsine et le Système Pi*. Paris, INSERM, 1975, p 131.

253. Strife CF, Hug G, Chuck G, McAdams AJ, Davis CA. Kline JJ: Membrano-proliferative glomerulonephritis and $\alpha_1$-antitrypsin deficiency in children. *Pediatrics* **71**:88, 1983.

254. Davis ID, Burke B, Freese D, Sharp HL, Kim Y: The pathologic spectrum of the nephropathy associated with $\alpha_1$-antitrypsin deficiency. *Hum Pathol* **23**:57, 1992.

255. Miller F, Kuschner M: $\alpha_1$-Antitrypsin deficiency, emphysema, necrotizing angiitis and glomerulonephritis. *Am J Med* **46**:615, 1969.

256. Lewis M, Kallenbach J, Zaltzman M, et al: Severe deficiency of $\alpha_1$-antitrypsin associated with cutaneous vasculitis, rapidly progressive glomerulonephritis, and colitis. *Am J Med* **79**:489, 1985.

257. Elzouki AN, Lindgren S, Nilsson S, Veress B, Eriksson S: Severe $\alpha_1$-antitrypsin deficiency (Pi Z homozygosity) with membranoproliferative glomerulonephritis and nephrotic syndrome, reversible after orthotopic liver transplantation. *J Hepatol* **26**:1403, 1997.

258. Rubinstein HM, Jaffer AM, Kudrna JC, et al: $\alpha_1$-Antitrypsin deficiency with severe panniculitis. *Ann Intern Med* **86**:742, 1977.

259. Breit SN, Clark P, Robinson JP, Luckhurst E, Dawkins RL: Penny R: Familial occurrence of $\alpha_1$-antitrypsin deficiency and Weber-Christian disease. *Arch Dermatol* **119**:198, 1983.

260. Smith KC, Su WP, Pittelkow MR, Winkelmann RK: Clinical and pathologic correlations in 96 patients with panniculitis, including 15 patients with deficient levels of $\alpha_1$-antitrypsin. *J Am Acad Dermatol* **21**:1192, 1989.

261. Geller JD, Su WP: A subtle clue to the histopathologic diagnosis of early $\alpha_1$-antitrypsin deficiency panniculitis. *J Am Acad Dermatol* **31**:241, 1994.

262. Humbert P, Faivre B, Gibey R, Agache P: Use of anti-collagenase properties of doxycycline in treatment of $\alpha_1$-antitrypsin deficiency panniculitis. *Acta Derm Venereol Suppl (Stockh)* **71**:189, 1991.

263. Pottage JC Jr, Trenholme GM, Aronson IK, Harris AA: Panniculitis associated with histoplasmosis and $\alpha_1$-antitrypsin deficiency. *Am J Med* **75**:150, 1983.

264. Cox DW, Huber O: Rheumatoid arthritis and $\alpha_1$-antitrypsin. *Lancet* **I**:1216, 1976.

265. Beckman G, Beckman L, Bjelle A, Rantapaa Dahlqvist S: $\alpha_1$- Antitrypsin types and rheumatoid arthritis. *Clin Genet* **25**:496, 1984.

266. Geddes DM, Webley M, Brewerton DA, et al: $\alpha_1$-antitrypsin phenotypes in fibrosing alveolitis and rheumatoid arthritis. *Lancet* **2**:1049, 1977.

267. Buisseret PD, Pembrey ME, Lessof MH: $\alpha_1$-Antitrypsin phenotypes in rheumatoid arthritis and ankylosing spondylitis. *Lancet* **2**:1358, 1977.

268. Arnaud P, Galbraith RM, Faulk WP, Black C: Pi phenotypes of $\alpha_1$-antitrypsin in southern England: Identification of M subtypes and implications for genetic studies. *Clin Genet* **15**:406, 1979.

269. Cox DW, Huber O: Association of severe rheumatoid arthritis with heterozygosity for $\alpha_1$-Antitrypsin deficiency. *Clin Genet* **17**:153, 1980.

270. Abboud RT, Chalmers A, Gofton JP, Richter AM, Enarson DA: Relationship between severity of rheumatoid arthritis and serum $\alpha_1$-antitrypsin. *J Rheumatol* **18**:1490, 1992.

271. Arnaud P, Galbraith R, Faulk WP, Ansell BM: Increased frequency of the MZ phenotype of $\alpha_1$-protease inhibitor in juvenile chronic polyarthritis. *J Clin Invest* **60**:1442, 1977.

272. Brewerton DA, Webley M, Murphy AH, Milford Ward AM: The $\alpha_1$-antitrypsin phenotype MZ in acute anterior uveitis. *Lancet* **1**:1103, 1978.

273. Wakefield D, Breit SN, Clark P, Penny R: Immunogenetic factors in inflammatory eye disease. Influence of HLA-B27 and $\alpha_1$-antitrypsin phenotypes on disease expression. *Arthritis Rheum* **25**:1431, 1982.

274. Brown WT, Mamelok AE, Bearn AG: Anterior uveitis and $\alpha_1$-antitrypsin. *Lancet* **2**:646, 1979.

275. Manners RM, Donaldson ML, Low C, Fenton PJ: Corneal ulceration in a patient with $\alpha_1$-antitrypsin deficiency. *Br J Ophthalmol* **78**:653, 1994.

276. Mazodier P, Elzouki AN, Segelmark M, Eriksson S: Systemic necrotizing vasculitides in severe $\alpha_1$-antitrypsin deficiency. *QJM* **89**:599, 1996.

277. Brandrup F, Ostergaard PA: $\alpha_1$-antitrypsin deficiency associated with persistent cutaneous vasculitis. *Arch Dermatol* **114**:921, 1978.

278. Elzouki AN, Segalmark M, Mazodier P, Eriksson S: Wegener's granulomatosis in a patient with severe Pi ZZ $\alpha_1$-antitrypsin deficiency [letter]. *QJM* **89**:877, 1996.

279. Nicholls MG, Janus ED: Hashimoto's thyroiditis and homozygous $\alpha_1$-antitrypsin deficiency. *Aust NZ J Med* **3**:516, 1973.

280. Gelfand EW, Cox DW, Lin MT, Dosch H-M: Severe combined immune-deficiency disease in a patient with $\alpha_1$-antitrypsin deficiency. *Lancet* **2**:202, 1979.

281. Anand S, Schade R, Bendetti C, et al: Idiopathic hemochromatosis and $\alpha_1$-antitrypsin deficiency: Coexistence in a family with progressive liver disease in the proband. *Hepatology* **3**:714, 1983.

282. Eriksson S, Lindmark B: A Swedish family with $\alpha_1$-antitrypsin deficiency, hemochromatosis, haemoglobinopathy D and early death in liver cirrhosis. *J Hepatol* **2**:65, 1986.

283. Rabinovitz M, Gavaler JS, Kelly RH, Van Thiel DH: Association between heterozygous $\alpha_1$-antitrypsin deficiency and genetic hemochromatosis. *Hepatology* **16**:145, 1992.

284. Eriksson S, Lindmark B. Olsson S: Lack of association between hemochromatosis and $\alpha_1$-antitrypsin deficiency. *Acta Med Scand* **219**:291, 1986.

285. Benkmann HG, Hanssen HP, Ovenbeck R, Goedde HW: Distribution of $\alpha_1$-antitrypsin and haptoglobin phenotypes in bladder cancer patients. *Hum Hered* **37**:290, 1987.

286. Cox DW: $\alpha_1$-Antitrypsin: A guardian of vascular tissue. *Mayo Clin Proc* **69**:1123, 1994.

287. Cohen JR, Sarfati I, Ratner L, Tilson D: $\alpha_1$-antitrypsin phenotypes in patients with abdominal aortic aneurysms. *J Surg Res* **49**:319, 1990.

288. Schievink WI, Katzmann JA, Piepgras DG: $\alpha_1$-antitrypsin deficiency in spontaneous intracranial arterial dissections. *Cerebrovasc Dis* **8**:42, 1998.

289. Aarskog D, Fagerhol MK: Protease inhibitor (Pi) phenotypes in chromosome aberrations. *J Med Genet* **7**:367, 1970.

290. Lieberman J, Borhani NO, Feinleib M: $\alpha_1$-antitrypsin deficiency in twins and parents-of-twins. *Clin Genet* **15**:29, 1979.

291. Clark P, Martin NG: An excess of the Pi$^S$ allele in dizygotic twins and their mothers. *Hum Genet* **61**:171, 1982.

292. Saiki RK, Bugawan TL, Horn GT, Mullis KB, Erlich HA: Analysis of enzymatically amplified $\beta$-globin and HLA-DQa DNA with allele-specific oligonucleotide probes. *Nature* **324**:163, 1986.

293. Kidd VJ, Wallace RB, Itakura K, Woo SLC: $\alpha_1$-antitrypsin deficiency detection by direct analysis of the mutation in the gene. *Nature* **304**:230, 1983.

294. Kidd VJ, Golbus MS, Wallace RB, Itakura K, Woo SLC: Prenatal diagnosis of $\alpha_1$-antitrypsin deficiency by direct analysis of the mutation site in the gene. *N Engl J Med* **310**:639, 1984.

295. Jeppsson J-O, Sveger T: Typing of genetic variants of $\alpha_1$-antitrypsin from dried blood. *Scand J Clin Lab Invest* **44**:413, 1984.

296. Thelin T, Sveger T, McNeil TF: Primary prevention in a high-risk group: Smoking habits in adolescents with homozygous alpha1-antitrypsin deficiency (ATD). *Acta Paediatr* **85**:1207, 1996.

297. Thelin T, McNeil TF, Aspegren-Jansson E, Sveger T: Psychological consequences of neonatal screening for alpha1-antitrypsin deficiency. Parental reactions to the first news of their infants' deficiency. *Acta Paediatr Scand* **74**:787, 1985.

298. Thelin T, McNeil TF, Aspegren-Jansson E, Sveger T: Identifying children at high somatic risk: Parents' long-term emotional adjustment to their children's alpha1-antitrypsin deficiency. *Acta Psychiatr Scand* **72**:323, 1985.

299. Hubbard RC, Crystal RG: Augmentation therapy of $\alpha_1$-antitrypsin deficiency. *Eur Respir J Suppl* **9**:44s, 1990.

300. Crystal RG: Gene therapy strategies for pulmonary disease. *Am J Med* **92**:44S, 1992.

301. Wewers MD, Casolaro MA, Sellers SE, et al: Replacement therapy for alpha$_1$-antitrypsin deficiency associated with emphysema. *N Engl J Med* **316**:1055, 1987.

302. Barker AF, Iwata-Morgan I, Oveson L, Roussel R: Pharmacokinetic study of alpha$_1$-antitrypsin infusion in alpha$_1$-antitrypsin deficiency. *Chest* **112**:607, 1997.

303. Hubbard RC, McElvaney NG, Sellers SE, Healy JT, Czerski DB, Crystal RG: Recombinant DNA-produced alpha1-antitrypsin administered by aerosol augments lower respiratory tract anti-neutrophil elastase defenses in individuals with alpha1-antitrypsin deficiency. *J Clin Invest* **84**:1349, 1989.

304. Burrows B: A clinical trial of efficacy of antiproteolytic therapy: Can it be done? *Am Rev Respir Dis* **127**:S42, 1983.

305. Seersholm N, Wencker M, Banik N, et al: Does $\alpha_1$-Antitrypsin augmentation therapy slow the annual decline in FEV$_1$ in patients with severe hereditary $\alpha_1$-antitrypsin deficiency? Wissenschaftliche Arbeitsgemeinschaft zur Therapie von Lungenerkrankungen (WATL) $\alpha_1$-AT study group. *Eur Respir J* **10**:2260, 1997.

306. Wencker M, Banik N, Buhl R, Seidel R, Konietzko N: Long-term treatment of $\alpha_1$-antitrypsin deficiency-related pulmonary emphysema with human $\alpha_1$-antitrypsin. Wissenschaftliche Arbeitsgemeinschaft zur Therapie von Lungenerkrankungen (WATL)-$\alpha_1$-AT-study group. *Eur Respir J* **11**:428, 1998.

307. Pierce JA: $\alpha_1$-Antitrypsin augmentation therapy [editorial; comment]. *Chest* **112**:872, 1997.

308. Hubbard RC, Crystal RG: Strategies for aerosol therapy of $\alpha_1$-antitrypsin deficiency by the aerosol route. *Lung* **168**:565, 1990.

309. Vogelmeier C, Kirlath I, Warrington S, Banik N, Ulbrich E, du Bois RM: The intrapulmonary half-life and safety of aerosolized alpha1-protease inhibitor in normal volunteers. *Am J Respir Crit Care Med* **155**:536, 1997.

310. Travis J, Owen MC, George P, et al: Isolation and properties of recombinant DNA produced variants of human $\alpha_1$-proteinase inhibitor. *J Biol Chem* **260**:4384, 1985.

311. Cherfas J: Sheep to produce $\alpha_1$-antitrypsin. *BMJ* **304**:527, 1992.

312. Garver RI, Chytil A, Courtney M, Crystal RG: Clonal gene therapy: Transplanted mouse fibroblast clones express human $\alpha_1$-antitrypsin gene in vivo. *Science* **237**:762, 1987.

313. Rosenfeld MA, Siegfried W, Yoshimura K, et al: Adenovirus-mediated transfer of a recombinant $\alpha_1$-antitrypsin gene to the lung epithelium in vivo. *Science* **252**:431, 1991.

314. Adams RM, Soriano HE, Wang M, Darlington G, Steffen D, Ledley FD: Transduction of primary human hepatocytes with amphotropic and xenotropic retroviral vectors. *Proc Natl Acad Sci U S A* **89**:8981, 1992.

315. Jaffe HA, Danel C, Longenecker G, et al: Adenovirus-mediated in vivo gene transfer and expression in normal rat liver. *Nat Genet* **1**:372, 1992.

316. Wilson JM, Grossman M, Cabrera JA, Wu CH, Wu GY: A novel mechanism for achieving transgene persistence in vivo after somatic gene transfer into hepatocytes. *J Biol Chem* **267**:11483, 1992.

317. Savransky E, Hytiroglou P, Harpaz N, Thung SN, Johnson EM: Correcting the Pi Z defect in the $\alpha_1$-antitrypsin gene of human cells by targeted homologous recombination. *Lab Invest* **70**:676, 1994.

318. Hickman MA, Malone RW, Lehmann-Bruinsma K, et al: Gene expression following direct injection of DNA into liver. *Hum Gene Ther* **5**:1477, 1994.

319. Alino SF, Crespo J, Bobadilla M, Lejarreta M, Blaya C, Crespo A: Expression of human $\alpha_1$-antitrypsin in mouse after in vivo gene transfer to hepatocytes by small liposomes. *Biochem Biophys Res Commun* **204**:1023, 1994.

320. Trulock EP, Cooper JD, Kaiser LR, Pasque MK, Ettinger NA, Dresler CM: The Washington University-Barnes Hospital experience with lung transplantation. Washington University Lung Transplantation Group. *JAMA* **266**:1943, 1991.

321. Trulock EP: Lung transplantation for COPD. *Chest* **113**:269S, 1998.

322. Calhoon JH, Grover FL, Gibbons WJ, et al: Single lung transplantation. Alternative indications and technique. *J Thorac Cardiovasc Surg* **101**:816, 1991.

323. Seersholm N, Dirksen A, Kok-Jensen A: Airways obstruction and two-year survival in patients with severe alpha$_1$-antitrypsin deficiency. *Eur Respir J* **7**:1985, 1994.

# SKIN

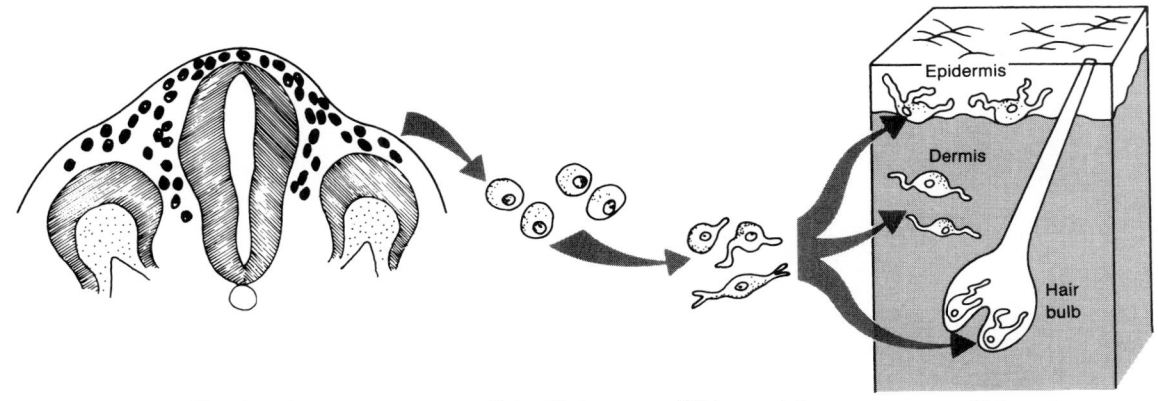

Neural crest          Melanoblasts     "Melanogonia"     Melanocytes

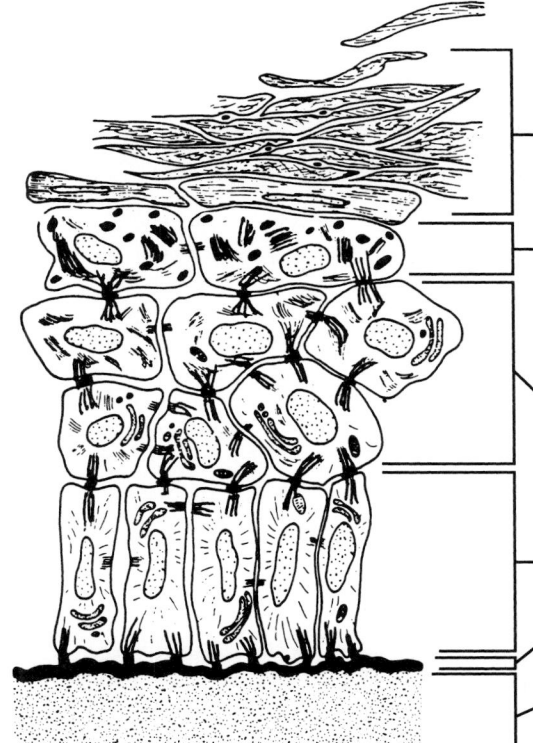

**Stratum corneum**

**Granular layers**

Filaggrin is made and macrofibrils form. Cornified envelope forms. Lipids are released to fill intercellular spaces.

**Spinous layers**

Filaments begin to aggregate. Envelope proteins and K1/K10 are synthesized

**Basal layers**

Keratin filaments are dispersed. K5/K14 are made.

**Basement membrane**

**Vascular connective tissue**

(dermis)

# Albinism

Richard A. King ■ Vincent J. Hearing
Donnell J. Creel ■ William S. Oetting

1. Melanocytes represent a relatively small subpopulation of cells, yet they are exclusively responsible for producing the melanin that accounts for virtually all visible pigmentation in the skin, hair, and eyes. Normal pigmentation requires a number of critical steps during development and a large number of genes have been shown to participate in those processes either directly or indirectly. Mutations in many of these genes produce clinical conditions of hypopigmentation, such as albinism and piebaldism.

2. Melanocytes in the skin interact with other types of cells either directly, as in the transfer of melanin granules to keratinocytes, or indirectly, as in the response to factors produced by other cells that influence the proliferation and/or pigmentation of melanocytes. Factors that regulate such melanocyte functions include environmental factors such as ultraviolet light, hormones, growth factors, cytokines, and a number of other modulators present in the milieu of the skin.

3. Tyrosinase is the critical enzyme to melanin production by virtue of its catalytic function in the hydroxylation of tyrosine, the rate-limiting reaction in the melanin biosynthetic pathway. However, there are a number of post-tyrosinase factors and enzymes that regulate the quality and quantity of melanins produced, and presumably their functional characteristics as well; included in that list are melanogenic inhibitors and other melanogenic enzymes that can modify the chemical and physical properties of melanins.

4. Two distinct types of melanins can be produced in melanocytes; these are termed eumelanins, which are black and/or brown, and pheomelanins, which are yellow and/or red. The chemical and physical characteristics, such as ultraviolet absorption, color, and solubility, of the two types of melanins are significantly different, although very little is known at present about determinants that modulate pheomelanogenesis within melanocytes.

5. The tyrosinase gene family currently contains three members: tyrosinase (TYR), tyrosinase-related protein 1 (TYRP1, also known as TRP1 and gp75), and tyrosinase-related protein 2 (DCT, also known as TRP2, TYRP2, and Tyrp2). All three genes encode proteins with similar amino acid sequences but bind different divalent metal cations, which provides them with their distinct catalytic properties. The protein products of these three loci are thought to be involved in the multicomponent melanogenic complex in the melanosome.

6. The tyrosinase locus (TYR) has been mapped to chromosome 11q14-21; the gene is more than 65 kb in length and has 5 exons. It is the human ortholog of the murine albino locus. The TYRP1 locus (orthologous to the murine brown locus) has been mapped to chromosome 9p23; TYRP1 has been shown to be important in stabilizing tyrosinase activities in human and murine melanosomes, and in mice, Tyrp1 functions as a DHICA oxidase. The DCT locus (orthologous to the murine slaty locus) has been mapped to chromosome 13q31-32, and functions as DOPAchrome tautomerase in humans and in mice.

7. The P gene, the human ortholog of the murine pink-eyed dilution gene, has been mapped to chromosome 15q11-12. The product of this gene is localized to the melanosomal membrane, where it is thought to function in ion transport to maintain an acidic pH in the melanosome. The Pmel17 gene, the human ortholog of the murine silver gene, is involved in premature graying in mice; this locus is thought to function as a melanosomal structural matrix protein important to the polymerization of melanin. The melanocyte stimulating hormone receptor (MC1R) gene, the POMC gene and the agouti gene regulate whether black/brown eumelanin or red/yellow pheomelanin is produced.

8. The human KIT gene, which codes for a mast/stem cell growth factor, has been mapped to chromosome 4q11-13; mutations in the KIT gene are responsible for piebaldism. The PAX3 gene has been mapped to chromosome 2q35; mutations of the PAX3 and MITF genes are responsible for Waardenburg syndrome.

9. Albinism represents a group of inherited abnormalities that present with congenital hypopigmentation that can involve the skin, hair, and eyes (oculocutaneous albinism or OCA) or can be limited primarily to the eyes (ocular albinism or OA). The definition of albinism includes specific changes in the optic system, including reduced retinal pigment with foveal hypoplasia, and misrouting of the optic fibers at the chiasm. These features must be present to make a diagnosis of albinism. Other common features include nystagmus, strabismus, and translucent irides.

10. OCA and OA are defined by the locus involved. OCA is autosomal recessive in inheritance; rare families with autosomal dominant OCA have been incompletely reported. OA is X-linked.

11. OCA1 is produced by mutations of the tyrosinase gene, and is separated into two subtypes related to the amount and the type of residual enzyme activity. Mutant alleles

Note to Readers: Human gene symbols are all uppercase italics (e.g., TYR); murine gene symbols are first letter uppercase, remainder lowercase italics (e.g., Tyr).

A list of standard abbreviations is located immediately preceding the index in each volume. Additional abbreviations used in this chapter include: ACTH = adrenocorticotropic hormone; ASP = agouti signal protein; BAER = brainstem auditory evoked response; CHS = Chediak-Higashi syndrome; DCT = dopachrome tautomerase, TRP2, Tyrp2; DHI = 5,6-dihydroxyindole; DHICA = 5,6-dihydroxyindole-2-carboxylic acid; DOPA = 3,4-dihydroxyphenylalanine; HPS = Hermansky-Pudlak syndrome; MC1R = melanocortin receptor 1; MSH = α-melanocyte stimulating hormone, melanotropin; OA = ocular albinism; OCA = oculocutaneous albinism; PDGFRT = platelet derived growth factor receptor, TYR = tyrosinase; TYRP1 = tyrosinase related protein 1, TRP1, gp75; and WS = Waardenburg syndrome.

associated with no tyrosinase activity produce OCA1A (the classic *tyrosinase-negative* OCA). Mutant alleles associated with some residual activity produce OCA1B with a broad phenotypic range. Many mutations of the tyrosinase gene have been identified in OCA1, and most affected individuals are compound heterozygotes.

12. OCA2 is produced by mutations of the human *P* gene. The phenotypic variability in pigmentation is broad. A distinct *tyrosinase-positive* OCA phenotype is seen in African and African-American individuals. "Brown OCA" also results from mutations of the *P* gene. The hypopigmentation in Prader-Willi syndrome and Angelman syndrome is also related to the *P* gene, but the mechanism is unknown.

13. OCA3 (Rufous OCA) is produced by mutation of the *TYRP1* gene. This type of albinism has been reported in African and African-American individuals, but clinical descriptions in other populations are not available.

14. Hermansky-Pudlak syndrome (HPS) (MIM 203300) is an infrequent autosomal recessive syndrome that presents with OCA, a mild bleeding diathesis, and a ceroid storage disease. Platelets lack dense bodies. Pulmonary fibrosis and granulomatous colitis occurs and can be severe. The *HPS1* gene responsible for most HPS in Puerto Rico maps to 10q24. Chediak-Higashi syndrome (CHS) presents with hypopigmentation associated with an increased susceptibility to bacterial infections. Several types of cells, including melanocytes, contain giant granules, indicating a basic abnormality in membrane formation. The *CHS1* gene maps to 1q43.

15. Ocular albinism (OA1) is produced by the *OA1* gene on Xp22. Cutaneous pigment appears normal in OA1, but cutaneous and ocular melanocytes contain giant melanosomes. Heterozygous females often have retinal and iris pigment changes from mosaicism from X-inactivation.

16. Proper evaluation and management of individuals with albinism includes correct diagnosis, counseling, skin care, and ophthalmologic care.

Melanin pigment in the skin, hair, and eyes represents one of the most visible markers of human variation, and disorders with hypopigmentation have long fascinated scientists and those interested in human biology. Albinism represents the extreme of these disorders, having reduced amounts of melanin synthesis in all parts of the involved tissues, in comparison to disorders such as piebaldism and Waardenburg syndrome in which the reduction in melanin is patchy and discrete. Albinism itself is heterogeneous, however, and can be separated clinically into those types that primarily involve the eyes (ocular albinism or OA) (MIM 300650) and those types that involve the skin and the hair as well as the eyes (oculocutaneous albinism or OCA) (MIM 203100).

Albinism is usually recognized because of visible reduction in melanin in the hair and skin associated with poor vision or reduced acuity. The historically earliest written records include descriptions of individuals with albinism, primarily with a total lack of visible melanin pigment.[1] Reports multiplied with the advent of world exploration and travel, and the subsequent description of different world ethnic groups. As new continents and peoples were visited, the beliefs about and toward individuals with albinism were found to vary and, in some places, to assume a mythologic aura. The familial nature of albinism was recognized almost as early as albinism itself, making this one of the first genetic conditions to be recognized.

Sir Archibald Garrod who included albinism (actually oculocutaneous albinism) as one of the four originally described inborn errors of metabolism provided the first scientific approach to human albinism. His clear insight into the nature of this condition as an enzyme defect preceded the actual biochemical demonstration of the lack of enzyme (tyrosinase) activity by many decades. Confusion about the true nature of albinism existed in the years before and after Garrod's work, however, because of variation in the phenotype. An individual with no cutaneous and ocular pigment was easily recognized as having albinism, and this was called "complete," "total," "universal," or "perfect" albinism, or oculocutaneous albinism. Individuals who had the ocular features of albinism but who had some cutaneous pigment (i.e., not a total absence of pigment) presented a problem and confusing terms such as "incomplete," "partial," or "imperfect" albinism were used. Statistical analyses of the frequency of consanguinity in families with albinism suggested genetic heterogeneity, and the identification of normally pigmented children arising from the mating of two individuals with albinism provided proof of genetic heterogeneity through genetic complementation.[1]

The problems of classification and heterogeneity persisted, however, until Witkop and colleagues developed the hairbulb test.[2] This test, in which freshly plucked hairbulbs were incubated in tyrosine or DOPA, separated oculocutaneous albinism into "tyrosinase-negative" and "tyrosinase-positive" types based on the absence or presence of melanin developing in the hairbulb after incubation. The families that demonstrated complementation were shown to be matings between an individual who had "ty-neg" and one who had "ty-pos" albinism, indicating that different genes were responsible for these two "types" of albinism. An additional albinism gene was responsible for X-linked ocular albinism, as this type of albinism could be separated by phenotype and inheritance pattern. The next phase of albinism research was based on the idea that a specific type of OCA, if carefully delineated, would result from a genetic alteration at a separate and distinct genetic locus. More than 85 different genetic loci were known to influence coat color in the mouse, and it seemed reasonable to assume that mutations at many of these loci would produce a distinct type of OCA. Clinical and biochemical changes were used to define more than 10 separate phenotypes (e.g., tyrosinase-negative, minimal pigment, platinum, yellow, autosomal recessive ocular albinism, and so on) and the classification of OCA became confusing, overlapping, and was generally useless in the clinical setting. Most importantly, this approach was wrong. Most genes that influence coat color in the mouse affect the development and distribution of the melanocyte and the type of melanin rather than the amount of melanin synthesized in the melanocyte, and mutations of these loci do not produce albinism.

Molecular studies have defined five loci that are associated with the development of OCA, and one with OA, and correlations between the genotype and the phenotype show that the phenotypic range for OCA at several of these loci is broad and includes many of the "distinct" types of OCA previously described in the literature. This chapter describes the progress that has occurred in pigment biology in the past decade, and particularly since the last edition. The basic biology of the pigment system is described, followed by a description of the known biochemistry and molecular biology of melanin synthesis. The second half of the chapter reviews the present basic and clinical knowledge of the various types of albinism. Many of the original references before 1990 are available in Chap. 119 of the 6th edition and Chap. 147 of the 7th edition of this book.[1,3]

## THE MELANOCYTE AND MELANOGENIC APPARATUS

### Overview

Melanocytes represent a relatively small subpopulation of cells present in the skin of mammals, yet they produce the melanin which accounts for virtually all visible pigmentation in that tissue (reviewed in references 4 to 7). Melanocytes are dendritic cells that derive from two different embryonic tissues: the neural crest or the optic cup. Melanocytes originating in the neural crest migrate to three principal locations: the skin (at the epidermal/dermal

**Table 220-1  Summary of Known Genes that Affect Mammalian Pigmentation**

| Murine Locus | Human Locus | Human Chromosome | Associated Disease | Protein Encoded | Function in Pigmentation |
|---|---|---|---|---|---|
| **Tissue Level** | | | | | |
| dom white-spotting (W) | KIT | 4q12 | piebaldism | tyrosine kinase receptor | melanoblast migration signal |
| steel (Sl) | MGF | 12q22 | piebaldism (putative) | KIT ligand | melanoblast migration signal |
| patch (Ph) | PDGFRA | 4q12 | piebaldism (putative) | PDGF receptor α | melanoblast development |
| splotch (Sp) | PAX3 | 2q35 | Waardenburg syndrome types 1 & 3 | PAX3 transcription factor | neural tube development/ microphthalmia |
| (mi) | MITF | 3p12-14 | Waardenburg syndrome type 2 | bHLH transcription factor | melanocyte survival |
| dom (dom) | SOX10 | 22q13 | Hirschsprung disease type 2 | HMG box transcription factor | neural crest development |
| piebald lethal (s¹) | EDNRB | 13q22 | Hirschsprung disease type 2 | endothelin receptor B | melanoblast differentiation |
| lethal spotting (ls) | EDN3 | 20q13.2 | Hirschsprung disease type 1 (putative) | endothelin 3 (EDNRB ligand) | melanocyte differentiation |
| **Cellular Level** | | | | | |
| beige (bg) | CHS1 | 1q42.1-q42.2 | Chediak-Higashi syndrome | LYST membrane protein | lysosome/melanosome structure/function |
| pale ear (eᵖ) | HPS1 | 10q24 | Hermansky-Pudlak syndrome | HPS membrane protein | lysosome/melanosome structure/function |
| pallid (pa) | EPB42 | 15q15-q21 | platelet storage pool disease | protein 4.2 pallidin | lysosome/melanosome structure/function |
| mottled (Mo) | ATP7A | Xq12-q13 | Menkes disease | ATP7A copper transport protein | tyrosinase metal ligand |
| dilute (d) | MYH12 | 15q21 | Griscelli disease | myosin type VA | melanosome movement |
| extension (e) | MC1R | 16q24.3 | hair color/skin type | MSH receptor (MC1R) | eumelanogenic stimulation |
| agouti (A) | ASIP | 20q11.2 | hair color/skin type | agouti signal protein (ASP) | pheomelanogenic stimulation |
| POMC | POMC | 2p23.3 | hair color/skin type | proopiomelanocortin (MSH) | eumelanogenic stimulation |
| pearl (pe) | HPS2 | 5q | Hermansky-Pudlak syndrome | b3A subunit-Adapter Complex 3 | vesicular transport |
| **Melanosomal Level** | | | | | |
| albino (c) | TYR | 11q14-21 | oculocutaneous albinism type 1 (OCA1) | tyrosinase | melanogenic enzyme |
| pinkeyed-dilution (p) | P | 15q11-13 | oculocutaneous albinism type 2 (OCA2) | P protein | melanosomal membrane protein |
| brown (b) | TYRP1 | 9q23 | oculocutaneous albinism type 3 (OCA3) | tyrosinase related protein 1 (TRP1) | melanosomal enzyme/ stabilizing factor |
| OA1 (moa) | OA1 | Xp22.3-22.2 | ocular albinism type 1 (OA1) | membrane protein | melanosomal membrane protein |
| silver (si) | Pmel17 | 12q13-14 | hair silvering (putative) | gp 100/silver protein | melanosomal matrix protein |
| slaty (slt) | DCT | 13q23 | unknown | tyrosinase related protein 2 (TRP2) | DOPAchrome tautomerase |
| MART1 | MART1 | unknown | Vogt-Koyanagi-Harada syndrome | membrane protein | melanosomal protein |

border), the eyes (in the choroid and iris stroma), and the hair follicles. Melanocytes in the retinal pigment epithelium are derived from neuroectoderm as cells originating from the outer layer of the developing optic vesicle. Melanin is produced by melanocytes in specific subcellular membrane-bound organelles called melanosomes. Melanin has several functions: (a) as a barrier against ionizing radiation; (b) as a participant in developmental processes; (c) as a cosmetic entity; and (d) as a potential scavenger of cytotoxic radicals and intermediates.

Normal pigmentation requires a number of critical and precise steps, including melanoblast development in the neural crest and migration of those cells to disparate parts of the body, arrest of melanoblast migration at appropriate sites, and, finally, survival, proliferation, differentiation, and function of melanocytes in those tissues. It is little wonder that mammalian pigmentation is regulated at many different levels and is influenced, either directly

or indirectly, by many genes. In the mouse, for example, hundreds of different mutations have been identified that alter pigmentation at more than 85 distinct genetic loci; about 25 percent of these genes have been cloned to date. In each instance noted thus far, an analogous and highly homologous gene is also expressed by human melanocytes, which suggests that these gene products are important to human melanocyte function. Table 220-1 presents a list of mouse pigment genes and their human orthologs; the terminology found in that Table is used throughout this chapter.

## Melanoblast/Melanocyte Development and Tissue Distribution

A number of loci regulate early stages in melanoblast development, migration, and differentiation; mutations in those loci typically lead to aberrant distribution and/or function of melanocytes in specific tissues. Genes that affect pigmentation at this level generally encode growth factor receptors (or their ligands) or transcription factors important for gene expression.

**The KIT, MCF and PDGFRT Genes.** Mutations in the *dominant white spotting* locus (*W*) in mice produce white patches in which the melanocytes are absent, and have effects on hematopoiesis and gametogenesis during embryonic development and in adult life. The *W* locus has been shown to be allelic with the *c-kit* proto-oncogene, which encodes a tyrosine kinase cell surface receptor.[1] The human *KIT* gene maps to 4q11-q13, the gene product is a mast/stem cell growth factor receptor, and mutations of this gene affect the development and/or migration of melanocytes and produce piebaldism.[8,9] The human *KIT* cDNA and gene has been isolated and sequenced;[8] it has 21 exons and is 34 kb in length. The gene organization is almost identical to the FMS proto-oncogene on chromosome 4, and there is evidence of alternative splicing of its mRNA.[10] There is also a similarity between promoters of the *KIT* gene and the tyrosinase and brown (*Tyrp1*) genes, and this may be evidence of a common melanocyte promoter. Mutations of the murine *c-kit* locus affect erythropoiesis, germ cell development, and melanogenesis, while mutations of the *KIT* locus in humans produce piebaldism only with no effects on erythropoiesis or gametogenesis.[11] Expression of the c-kit receptor is not only important during embryologic development, but it also plays a role in melanocyte survival and function in adults.[12–14] Activation of the c-kit receptor in melanocytes has been linked to the MAP kinase intracellular signaling pathway.[15,16] The patch gene in mice (analogous to the human *PDGFRT* locus) has also been associated with development of melanoblasts and the piebald phenotype.[17]

The ligand for the c-kit tyrosine kinase receptor is the mast cell growth factor (MCF, alternatively called SCF, stem cell factor, or SL, steel factor) which is encoded by the steel locus (*Sl*) in mice.[1] Mutations at the *Sl* locus prevent binding of the c-kit ligand to its receptor, which results in an aberrant pigmented phenotype similar to that seen in *W* locus mutant loci. The steel phenotype also affects erythropoiesis and germ cell development, as observed in *W* locus mutants.[18–22] This gene has not yet been cloned in humans, but mutations in the human steel homologue are expected to have a piebald phenotype.

**The PAX3 and MITF Genes.** The Splotch (*Sp*) phenotype in mice, which produces areas of hypopigmentation and has chromosomal homology between mouse chromosome 1 (which contains the *Sp* locus) and human chromosome 2 (to which WS type I maps) was used to identify a gene involved in melanocyte development.[23–25] Mutations of the *Sp* gene in mice produce areas of hypopigmentation on the abdomen and neural tube defects, such as spina bifida and exencephaly, but do not appear to affect the mouse inner ear.[26] The *pax-3* locus was shown to be located at the same area as the *Sp* locus on mouse chromosome 1 and mutations of the *pax-3* gene were shown to produce the *Sp* phenotype.[27] The human ortholog of *pax-3* has been isolated (*PAX3*); it contains 3 exons and belongs to a paired domain family of DNA binding proteins that contain sequences homologous to a homeobox gene (*prd*) from *Drosophila melanogaster*.[28,29] PAX3 contains three functional domains, a paired box, a conserved octapeptide, and a homeobox domain, as is observed in pax-3. The *pax-3* gene plays a role in the pattern formation in the developing neural crest of the mouse embryo. The high degree of similarity between the *pax-3* gene and the human ortholog *PAX3* makes it likely that the *PAX3* gene product has a similar function in the development of the human neural crest. The dominant nature of mutations associated with this gene is most likely due to insufficient dosage of the functional protein.

Another transcription factor involved in melanoblast development and melanocyte function, known as microphthalmia-associated transcription factor (MITF), has been identified, and mutations at this locus produce WS type 2. The CANNTG motif, found on many pigment-cell-specific genes (such as tyrosinase, as

discussed below), binds a family of transcription factors, characterized by the presence of a conserved helix-loop-helix structure required for DNA binding and activation.[30] MITF and the murine homologue, microphthalmia (Mitf), containing a basic helix-loop-helix-leucine zipper motif, are expressed by melanocytes, and binds to both the M-box and E-box regions (see genes involved in albinism below).[31–35] Activation of *Mitf* is associated with the regulation of cAMP levels from MC1R activation (see below), and is important in the expression of the tyrosinase gene, as well as other melanogenic genes.[35–38] Up-regulation of *Mitf* expression has been linked to the MAP kinase pathway, and thus to c-kit activation;[15,16] it has also been linked to activation of the MC1R receptor.[39] Three forms of MITF have been described.[40] One form, MITF-M, is exclusively expressed in melanocytes, and a second isoform, MITF-A, which differs in the amino-terminus, is found in the retinal pigment epithelium, providing a model for the differential expression of tyrosinase in those two tissues. A third form, MITF-H, does not appear to be involved in promoter activities for *TYR* or *TYRP1*. Mutations in *Mitf/MITF* are associated with melanoblast dysfunction in mice[41–43] and with WS type 2 in humans.[44–46]

**The Sox 10, EDNRB, and EDN3 Genes.** The Sox10 protein (encoded at the Dominant megacolon or *Dom* locus in mice) is a Sry-related HMG box transcription factor expressed in melanocytes and other neural crest derivatives during embryologic development.[47] Glial cells in the peripheral and central nervous systems during late development and in adults also express it. The mutation of *Sox10* found in *Dom* mice is a frameshift mutation that renders the mutant protein inactive.[48] *Dom* mutants of mice have served as models for Hirschsprung disease (MIM 142623) and other studies confirm that the human ortholog of *Dom*, termed *SOX10*, is indeed the locus associated with this disease. Mutations in *SOX10* have been identified in Hirschsprung disease type 2 (MIM 600155) patients, resulting in abrogation of transcriptional activation potential.[49]

Another form of Hirschsprung disease type 1 results from mutations of the gene for the endothelin-B receptor (*EDNRB*) or its ligand, endothelin 3 (*ET3*).[50,51] Recent studies show that the locus encoding EDNRB is the piebald-lethal locus in mice (*EDNRB* in humans), and the ligand, ET3, is encoded by the lethal spotting locus in mice (*EDN3* in humans).[52,53] Endothelins are important intracellular signaling factors between keratinocytes and melanocytes, particularly in response to UV light, but their role during embryologic development is not yet known.

## Melanocyte Function at the Cellular Level

A number of genes interact, at least in part, in the regulation of melanocyte function at the cellular level. In general, these act specifically in melanocytes or are also functional in other cell types in addition to melanocytes. Those that are specific for melanocytes typically are localized in melanosomes, the pigmented organelles found only in melanocytes, and genes that function at that level are discussed in this section.

**The CHS1, HPS1, ATP7A, MYH12, and Pallid Genes.** Melanosomes are now known to be specialized lysosomes, sharing many of the lysosomal proteins, as well as proteins associated with melanin formation that are present only in melanosomes.[54,55] Therefore, mutations in the genes encoding normal lysosomal proteins affect lysosomal function, pigmentation, and the functions of other organelles (such as dense bodies in platelets) that may share the lysosomal biogenetic pathway. Mutations in several "lysosomal" genes give rise to various forms of albinism, such as CHS and HPS (see CHS and HPS discussion below). Mutations in several other "lysosomal" genes have effects on pigmentation and give rise to diseases such as Menkes disease (MIM 309400) and Griscelli disease (MIM 214450) (discussed below), which are not considered to be forms of albinism. In addition to such lysosomal/melanosomal genes, there are a large number of other genes that encode melanocyte receptors important to melanocyte function and response to the environment (such as the MC1R, the endothelin receptors, βFGF receptor, c-kit receptor, and so on). Ligands that originate from external sources and activate or inactivate these receptors are also important; they include such factors as MSH, agouti signal protein (ASP), endothelins, MCF, and βFGF.

The beige gene in mice has long been known to be a model for CHS. The beige gene was recently cloned, as was the orthologous *CHS1* gene in humans.[56] Immunohistochemistry analysis of the beige protein shows that it is a cytosolic protein, expressed in most tissues, with no measurable membrane association.[57,58] It was hypothesized that the beige protein is involved in vesicle fission, including lysosomes, instead of vesicle fusion. The protein product contains 1545 amino acids and has been identified as a lysosomal trafficking regulator (LYST), which would explain the abnormal trafficking of melanogenic proteins found in melanocytes. Molecular, genetic and clinical aspects of CHS1 are discussed in detail below.

HPS (MIM 203300) is an uncommon type of albinism, but studies in two populations (Puerto Rico and Switzerland)[59,60] have mapped the locus for HPS in these populations to chromosome 10q23.[61,62] The pale ear locus is the murine homologue.[63,64] Searches of protein databases have not revealed any similarities of HPS to known proteins and its function is currently unknown. Initial analysis using confocal immunofluorescence has shown both a cytoplasmic and membrane associated distribution of the protein suggesting the possible existence of a soluble and insoluble forms of the protein, as would be expected by the two identified transcripts for the *HPS* gene.[65–67] Molecular, genetic, and clinical aspects of HPS1 are discussed in detail below.

Other important loci that affect common cellular proteins and influence pigmentation include the *ATP7A* (mottled in mice) and *MYH12* (dilute in mice) loci. The mottled locus in mice and the *ATP7A* locus in humans are homologous and encode a copper transport protein.[68–71] Mutations in those loci affect copper import into cells, and since this metal is a required ligand for tyrosinase (see below), alterations in its function adversely affect pigmentation.[72] Such mutations are responsible for Menkes disease.[73]

The dilute (*d*) locus of mice has been cloned and identified as a novel type-V heavy-chain myosin.[74] This protein has a critical function in transport of melanosomes from the perinuclear area, and mutations at this locus affect melanosomal movement to the dendrites, which is necessary for transfer to keratinocytes.[75–81] The human ortholog has been cloned (termed *MYH12*) and

encodes a protein with similar structure and function.[82] Mutations in this locus have been associated with Griscelli disease.[83–85]

Mutations of the pallid (*pa*) locus of mice lead to dilution of pigment in the hair and bleeding disorders; pallid is one of 14 known genes in the mouse that are associated with such defects.[86] The protein encoded by this locus is termed protein 4.2 (pallidin), and the gene has been cloned and sequenced.[87] The pallidin protein is associated with lysosomes, platelets, and melanosomes, which is consistent with its phenotypic effects. It is a protein of 691 residues, and shares significant sequence homology with the human erythrocyte protein 4.2. Recently, however, the pallid locus being the homologue of the membrane protein 4.2 locus has been questioned, and future studies are necessary to resolve this issue.[88]

## The Melanocyte Environment

Mammalian pigmentation does not depend solely on the production of melanin by melanocytes, but requires interaction with keratinocytes and other cell types, for signaling factors that influence melanocyte activity and for uptake of melanin granules, which influences visible color. Ocular melanocytes are distributed to the choroid, iris, and retina, where they are relatively dormant in that their rates of melanogenesis are low after fetal development, and the pigment synthesized is not secreted, but remains within the melanocyte. In contrast, melanocytes that reside in the skin and in hair follicles are highly secretory. Within hair follicles, melanocytes typically transfer melanosomes to emerging hair shafts, giving the hair visible color.[1] Melanocytes in the skin reside at the dermal:epidermal junction and secreted melanosomes are passed by neighboring keratinocytes (the predominant cell type in the epidermis), as depicted in Fig. 220-1. Melanosomes ingested by keratinocytes are further processed, degraded, and redistributed, either in smaller pieces and/or in larger complexes that eventually result in visible skin color. The association of the melanocyte and its neighboring keratinocytes has been called the "epidermal melanin unit," but this is somewhat of a misnomer because melanocytes interact with many types of cells in the skin in addition to keratinocytes. Epidermal melanocytes are highly responsive cells that continually sample their environment and modulate their levels of proliferation or melanogenesis in response to changing conditions. In sum, the melanocyte is in a highly dynamic equilibrium with different cell types in its immediate environment, all of which participate in determining its melanocytic activity. Those ligands and their receptors all play roles in regulating melanocyte function and their

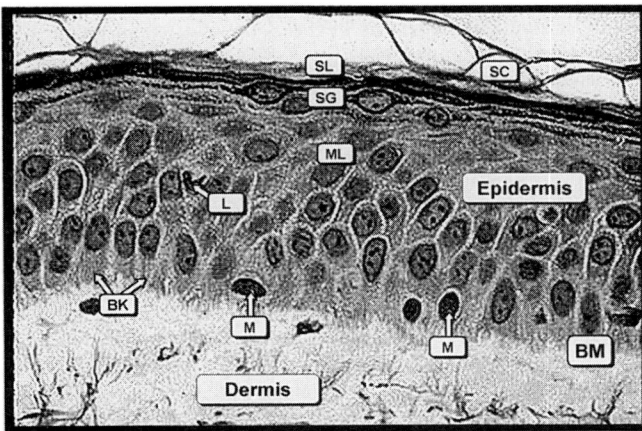

interleukins  leukotrienes  endothelins    vitamins A, D  interferons  prostaglandins    retinoids, neurotropins  growth factors {bFGF, PDGF, MSGF & SLF}

**Epidermal Cells**
**Keratinocytes**
**Melanocytes**
**Langerhans cells**

**Dermal Cells**
**Fibroblasts**
**Inflammatory cells**
**Endothelial cells**
**Mast cells**

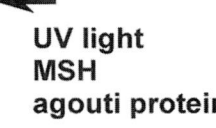

**UV light**
**MSH**
**agouti protein**

**Fig. 220-1** Melanocyte functional unit. The skin is a complex system influenced by many external environmental factors. The melanocyte functional unit consists of melanocytes (M), keratinocytes (BK), and Langerhans cells (L). The melanocytes reside in the basal layer with dendritic projections into the stratum spinosum of the epidermis.

encoding genes are obviously important to pigmentation. Three such genes have proven to be especially important in this regard.

**The *MC1R*, *POMC*, and *ASP* Genes and Their Role in Skin and Hair Color.** A number of biologic activities in mammalian pigmentation have been attributed to the action of α-melanocyte stimulating hormone (MSH, also known as melanotropin), including the promotion of melanocyte proliferation and dendricity, an increase in tyrosinase transcription, translation and catalytic activity, as well as a general increase in melanin biosynthesis. MSH is encoded by the *POMC* locus, and originally was thought to be expressed solely by the pituitary. However, it is now known that many tissues express *POMC*, including keratinocytes and melanocytes in the skin.[89-91] Once translated, POMC is cleaved by specific proteases into adrenocorticotropic hormone (ACTH) and a number of melanotropins, known as αMSH, βMSH, and γMSH. Each of these derivatives, including ACTH, work through binding to, and activation of, one or more types of melanocortin receptors (MC1R, MC2R, and so on); MC1R expression is thought to be limited to melanocytes.[92,93] Mutations in *POMC* have multiple effects in mice and humans, including effects on pigmentation, which are associated with the production of red hair.[94,95]

As noted above, MSH effects on melanocytes result when MSH binds to and activates the MC1R, a G-protein-coupled receptor, which increases intracellular cAMP concentration, and which, in turn, stimulates melanocyte differentiation. It is thought that many of the environmental factors that stimulate pigmentation, including ultraviolet light, do so by promoting expression and/or function of the MC1R or by activating the cAMP pathway downstream.[96] Recently, the mouse and the human *MC1R* genes were cloned, mapped, and sequenced,[97-99] and found to be 76 percent identical and colinear throughout the amino acid sequence. The *MC1R* locus is part of a subfamily that includes the ACTH receptor, the cannabinoid receptor, and other melanocortin receptors, all of which are G-protein-coupled receptors.

Alleles of the extension locus (which encodes MC1R in mice) range from the most dominant allele (*E*), which results in completely black mice, to the most recessive allele (*e*), which results in completely yellow mice.[100] The *recessive yellow* allele (*e*) is the result of a frameshift mutation that produces a nonfunctional protein, whereas the *sombre* (*E<sup>so</sup>*) allele, which results from a point mutation, produces a constitutively activated MC1R. The biochemical mechanisms involved with producing the various types of melanins are discussed later in this chapter. Mutations in *MC1R* and *POMC* do not produce albinism, but they are responsible for variations in hair and skin color in mammals. Although MC1R function is necessary for eumelanin synthesis in cutaneous and follicular melanocytes, retinal melanocytes will produce eumelanin even in the absence of functional *MC1R*, as seen in *e/e* mice, which suggests that there are other mechanisms that can regulate this control point. There are a number of polymorphisms of the *MC1R* gene in humans,[101] and several specific mutations that affect MC1R function, which are correlated with the red hair/fair skin phenotype.[94,95,102-106] It has also been postulated that such mutations may be associated with a predisposition to skin cancer.[107,108]

The agouti gene (*a*) has also been cloned and mapped in mice and in humans (where it is termed *ASIP*).[109-112] This product of this locus affects the switch from eumelanogenesis to pheomelanogenesis through its competitive interaction with MC1R. There are more than 18 different alleles described at the murine agouti locus and some of the alleles have severe pleiotropic effects that include obesity and lethality. The wild type (*A/A*) allele has black-and yellow-banded hair, whereas *a/a* mice contain only black hair and *A<sup>y</sup>/a* mice contain only yellow hair. The *A* locus appears to affect tyrosinase activity with *A<sup>y</sup>/a* mice having only 25 to 35 percent of the activity of *a/a*. Homozygous *A<sup>y</sup>/A<sup>y</sup>* is lethal and the great variation in alleles on pigment production has led some to hypothesize that the *A* locus is a complex locus consisting of several genes; however, the cloning of the agouti gene has shown that it encodes a single gene product (ASP).[112-114] The gene is 18 kb in length and contains 4 exons; it produces a 0.8-kb transcript and normal transcripts are expressed by cells in hair follicles and in the epidermis. The gene is not expressed in melanocytes, as shown by the presence of ASP in *W/W<sup>v</sup>* mice that lack dermal melanocytes. ASP is a polypeptide of 131 amino acids with a central region rich in basic amino acids and a cysteine-rich C-terminus. Like the steel factor, ASP acts as a ligand, which competes with MSH for binding to the MC1R.[115-120] Increased expression of the agouti gene is correlated with increased production of pheomelanin pigment, obesity, diabetes, and other pleiotropic effects.[121-124] Binding of MSH to MC1R results in dramatic stimulation of melanogenic activity, primarily through up-regulation of transcription of tyrosinase,[125-127] the end result being an increase in eumelanin production. ASP has competing effects on melanocytes, turning off the expression of all known eumelanogenic genes, including *Tyrp1*, *Dct*, *p*, and *Pmel17*, and significantly down-regulating tyrosinase.[117,128-130] Modulation of the expression of *MITF* is involved in these responses, as are other transcription factors.[43,117,131]

## Melanocyte Function at the Subcellular Level

**The *TYR*, *TYRP1*, *DCT*, *PMEL17*, *OA1* and *MART1* Genes and Their Role in Melanosome Function.** The biochemical machinery to produce melanin is confined within membrane-bound organelles called melanosomes, as shown in Fig. 220-2 (reviewed in references 132 to 134). Because many intermediates in the melanin biosynthetic pathway are potentially cytotoxic, the integrity of the melanosome and its limiting membrane may be important to minimizing these cytotoxic effects. Many mutations at the brown/*Tyrp1*, slaty/*Dct*, and silver/*Pmel17* loci in mice disrupt melanosome structure and result in premature death of mutant melanocytes. The melanosome initially evolves from the smooth endoplasmic reticulum as a cytoplasmic, membrane-bound vesicle with an amorphous interior. In this state, the organelle is referred to as a stage I premelanosome, and does not contain any of the melanogenic enzymes required for melanin synthesis.[135-138] However, the P protein and Pmel17 protein are structural components of Stage I premelanosomes.[139-142]

Tyrosinase, TYRP1, and DCT are synthesized on ribosomes, transported through the rough endoplasmic reticulum to the Golgi (GERL) apparatus where post-translational processing continues. Tyrosinase is glycosylated *en route* to the active face of the Golgi, secreted within coated vesicles into the cytoplasmic milieu, and then transported to premelanosomes where the vesicles fuse with the limiting membrane. The melanogenic enzymes (at least those that have been characterized to date) are localized within the melanosomal membrane with their catalytic centers facing inward, and active melanogenesis begins following fusion of the coated vesicles with the melanosome. At this stage, the premelanosome has an internal matrix, but contains no melanin, and is known as a stage II melanosome.

Tyrosinase is catalytically competent to produce pigment while in transit through the Golgi apparatus and coated vesicles, and it is unclear how melanogenesis is delayed until its arrival at the melanosome *in vivo*. It has been proposed that melanogenic inhibitors are responsible for preventing melanin production until incorporation within the melanosome, but this has not been satisfactorily resolved. The mechanism involved is an important issue because alterations in this process may result in various types of hypopigmentation conditions where active tyrosinase is present, yet no melanin is produced, such as in different types of oculocutaneous albinism. Following initiation of melanogenesis, melanin is deposited uniformly within the melanosome (stage III melanosome), and the opacity of the organelle gradually increases until eventually all substructure is obscured, leaving only the electron-dense mature melanin granule visible (stage IV melanosome). The different stages of melanosome development are

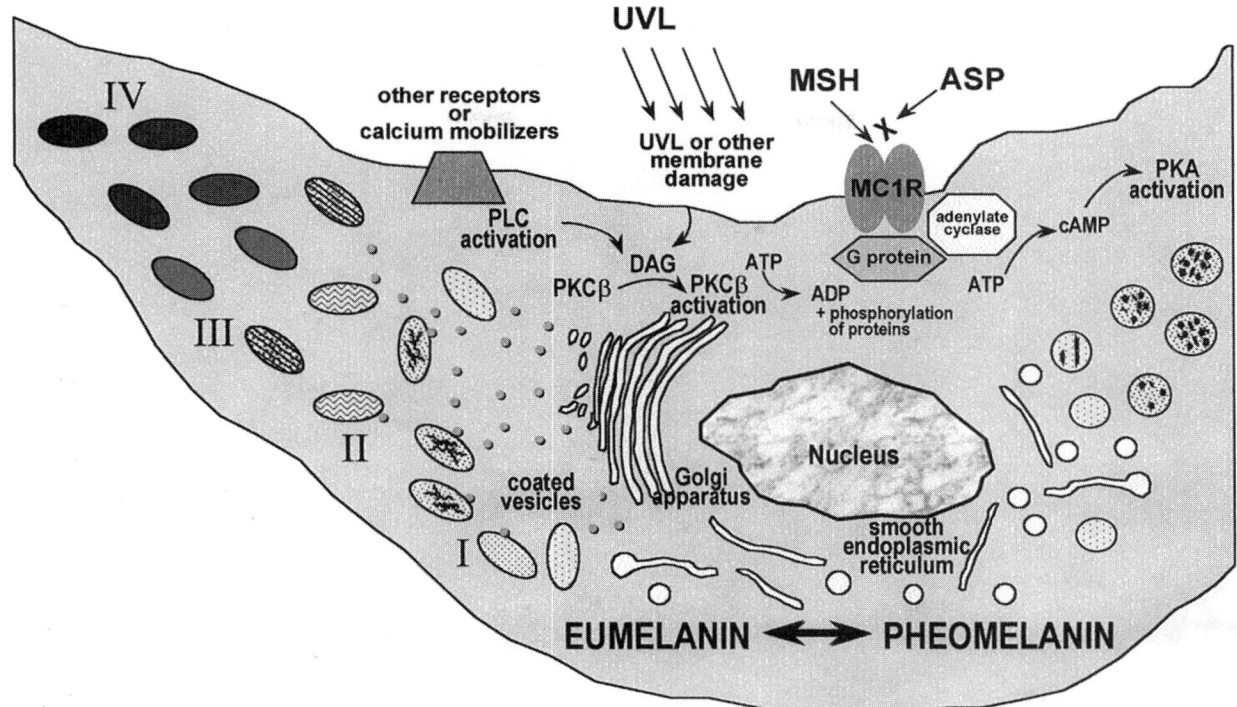

**Fig. 220-2 Melanosomal biogenesis.** The coated vesicles contain tyrosinase and other enzymatic components. The fusion of the coated vesicles with the premelanosome (I) derived from the SER allows melanogenesis to proceed. Stages I to IV of premelanosome/melanosome development are labeled. Eumelanosomal and pheomelanosomal biogenesis are shown.

shown in Fig. 220-3. During this process, the melanosome steadily moves away from the perinuclear region towards the periphery of the melanocyte, where it is passed to keratinocytes and eventually degraded.

***Tyrosinase Gene Family.*** The three genes, albino or *c* locus, brown or the *b* locus, and slaty or the *slt* locus in the mouse, and their human *TYR*, *TYRP1*, and *DCT* homologues, code for proteins with very similar nucleotide and amino acid sequences and make up the tyrosinase gene family. The product of the *TYRP1* locus has approximately 40 percent amino acid identity to *TYR*, and product of the *DCT* locus has a 50 percent amino acid identity to *TYRP1* and a 32 percent identity to *TYR*. That the cDNA for two of these loci were initially isolated using tyrosinase antibodies and cDNA expression libraries and that tyrosinase antiserum recognizes all three shows that they must have common epitopes.

The similarity of these three proteins is revealed in several shared domains. The protein products of the 3 loci contain an amino acid signal sequence, 15 conserved cysteine residues, 2 putative copper binding regions, a transmembrane region, and a cytoplasmic tail at the C-terminal of the protein. A cysteine-rich domain similar to that found in the EGF-family,[143] a motif that may be involved in protein-protein interaction, is also present in all three proteins. All three proteins are enzymes involved in the melanogenic pathway, and mutations in two loci, *TYR* and *TYRP1*, are responsible for different types of albinism (OCA1 and OCA3, respectively).

## BIOCHEMISTRY OF MELANIN SYNTHESIS

The chemical reactions involved in the production of melanin from the amino acid tyrosine are relatively straightforward, and were actually described many decades ago, but only recently was the underlying complexity of the regulatory controls involved in melanin synthesis described.[1] The melanin biosynthetic pathway is shown in Fig. 220-4. Several of the unusual properties of the

melanin biopolymer confound attempts at definitive structural analysis by conventional chemical methods and the characterization of melanin structure is still actively investigated. In addition, many of the melanogenic intermediates are highly unstable and their ability to rapidly auto-oxidize to form melanin has also hampered such analyses.

## Enzymatic Components

The copper-containing enzyme tyrosinase (EC 1.14.18.1) is critical to melanin formation due to its ability to catalyze the first reaction in the biosynthetic sequence, the hydroxylation of tyrosine. Traditionally, the product of this reaction has been thought to be L-3,4-dihydroxyphenylalanine (DOPA), but recent evidence suggests the product may be the next intermediate in the pathway, DOPAquinone.[106,144,145] This first reaction is the most critical because the spontaneous rate of tyrosine hydroxylation is negligible, and this represents the rate-limiting step in the pathway. DOPAquinone spontaneously cyclizes to form an indole ring as found in leucoDOPAchrome and DOPAchrome. Without further catalytic intervention, DOPAchrome spontaneously loses its carboxyl group to produce 5,6-dihydroxyindole (DHI), which, in turn, rapidly oxidizes to indole-5,6-quinone. Early studies suggested that melanin consisted of an homogeneous polymer of indole-5,6-quinone, but recent evidence suggests that melanins are much more heterogeneous in nature and probably consist of mixtures of several other intermediates in the pathway.[4,106,146] Melanin synthesis will occur spontaneously in the test tube once DOPAquinone is formed, but other constraints are put on these reactions *in vivo*. A number of additional factors that regulate the flow of this pathway are now characterized, including other enzymes (i.e., DCT, TYRP1, and Pmel17),[147–151] the availability of reactive sulfhydryls (e.g., cysteine),[152–156] melanogenic inhibitors,[147,151,157] and perhaps other regulatory factors. The genes for several of these melanogenic factors have been cloned, providing a glimpse of the complex mechanisms responsible for the production of different types of pigmentation. Perhaps more

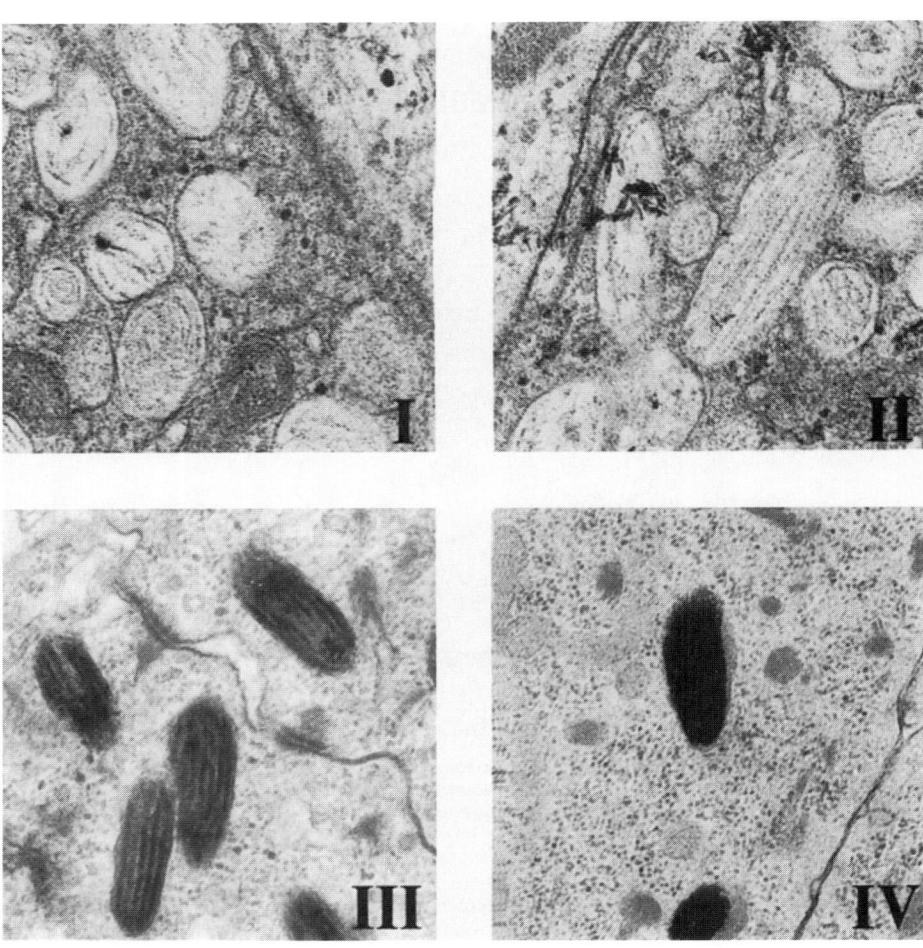

Fig. 220-3 Melanosome melanization. Ultrastructure of eumelanosome development. The maturation of melanosomes occurs in four stages: stages I, II, and III premelanosomes, and stage IV fully melanized melanosome.

importantly, it is now possible to begin understanding the molecular lesions responsible for many abnormal pigmentation conditions, such as oculocutaneous albinism.

## Eumelanin Versus Pheomelanin Synthesis

There are two distinct types of melanins that can be produced in mammalian melanocytes: eumelanin (black and/or brown in color) and pheomelanin (red and/or yellow in color).[4,158–160] The commitment to produce either type of melanin is made following the generation of DOPAquinone. If sulfhydryl groups, typically cysteine, are available, they will stoichiometrically react with the DOPAquinone and generate cysteinylDOPAs.[154,161,162] Cysteinyl-DOPAs then undergo a series of poorly understood reactions that result in the cyclization of a second ring (not of the indole type) and subsequent polymerization into a high-molecular-weight biopolymer. Pheomelanins have properties distinct from eumelanin, including a greater solubility and distinct appearance. Eumelanin and pheomelanin synthesis are obviously dependent on the expression of transporters in the melanosomal membrane and such activities have indeed been found;[138,156,163–165] it will be important in the future to characterize the role that melanosomal membrane transport of melanogenic substrates plays in regulating pigmentation. Those studies further suggest that it is cysteine, rather than glutathione, that is transported to the melanosome and is thus the physiological precursor of pheomelanins. It is not yet known whether enzymes are involved in the further metabolism of the cysteinylDOPAs and their derivatives. It seems a reasonable expectation, however, that regulatory factors similar to those of eumelanogenesis will eventually be identified for pheomelanogenesis.

In the absence of sulfhydryls, eumelanins will be produced following the generation of DOPAquinone. LeucoDOPAchrome

forms spontaneously and is quickly converted to DOPAchrome, which represents yet another key regulatory point in the pathway. DOPAchrome will spontaneously decarboxylate to form 5,6-dihydroxyindole (DHI), although in the presence of certain divalent metal cations (e.g., $Co^{++}$, $Mg^{++}$, and $Fe^{++}$) and/or the enzyme DCT, the carboxylated intermediate 5,6-dihydroxyindole-2-carboxylic acid (DHICA) is produced.[143,166–169] Because DHI and DHICA are not interconvertible, the carboxyl content of melanin is essentially determined at this step. There are at least two subsequent catalytic steps that follow the production of DHI and/or DHICA. Tyrosinase is able to oxidize DHI, which would be expected in light of the similarity between this reaction and DOPA oxidation; this has been shown for the mouse and human enzyme.[170,171] However, mouse tyrosinase is unable to oxidize DHICA, and murine TYRP1 acts in this capacity.[172–174] Interestingly, however, human TYRP1 is unable to utilize DHICA as a substrate, but human tyrosinase is able to act as a DHICA oxidase.[175] This brings into question the relative importance of TYRP1 (associated with OCA3 as discussed below) at the catalytic level. It may well be that TYRP1's ability to stabilize the melanogenic enzyme complex, and thus significantly enhance tyrosinase activity, is its most important function.[134,173,176] The final known catalytic function in the melanin biosynthetic pathway is the DHI/DHICA polymerase function that has been ascribed to Pmel17.[139,140,177,178] Pmel17 is known to be a structural matrix protein of eumelanosomes and seems to serve as a polymerization phase upon which melanin is deposited.[140,179]

Mammalian melanins contain significant levels of carboxylated and decarboxylated intermediates,[106,136,146,180–184] although it is not known how this influences their structure and/or function. DCT expression and catalytic function regulates the ratio of DHI

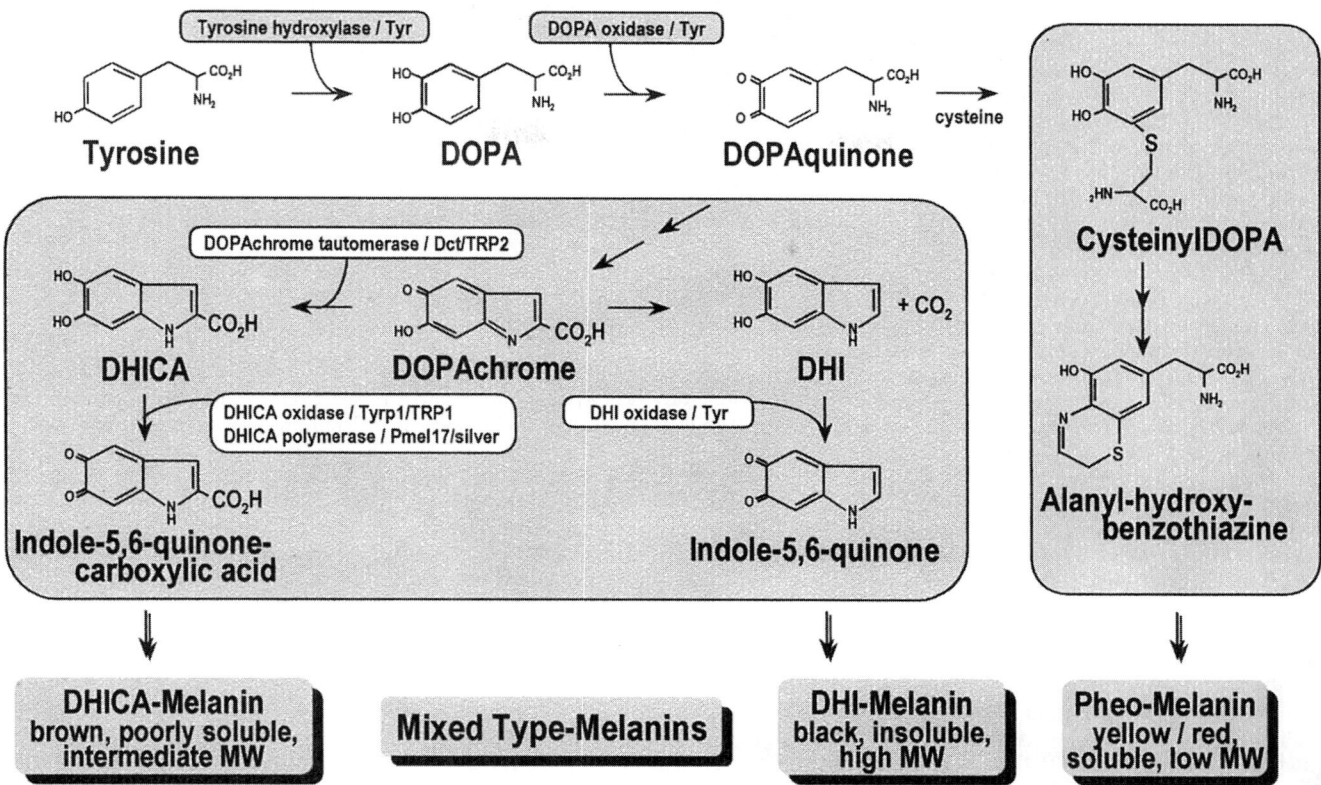

**Fig. 220-4 Melanin biosynthetic pathway.** The melanin pathway presents a summary of the known reactions and regulatory enzymes in eumelanogenesis and pheomelanogenesis.

and DHICA melanins produced. In humans, eu- and pheomelanins can be produced within the same melanocyte, and can be complexed within the same biopolymer, which is then called "mixed melanin." Studies currently underway on the contribution of the various intermediates (e.g., with or without sulfhydryl and/ or carboxyl groups) to the structure and function of melanin should provide important insights into the understanding of other regulatory controls of this pathway and the functional significance of each component.

## Melanogenic Determinants of Melanin Formation

Four direct catalytic activities (tyrosinase, DCT/DOPAchrome tautomerase, TYRP1/DHICA oxidase, and Pmel17/DHI-DHICA

polymerase) and several other regulatory factors have been identified in the melanin biosynthetic pathway within the melanosome, as shown in Fig. 220-5. Tyrosinase is absolutely essential for melanin production (as discussed above), while other melanogenic factors distal to tyrosinase modify the type of melanins produced.

**Tyrosinase.** Tyrosinase is an unusual enzyme in that it has three distinct catalytic functions. The most critical function is the hydroxylation of tyrosine because this is the rate-limiting reaction in the melanin synthetic pathway. Murine and human tyrosinase also use DOPA and DHI as substrates for oxidase activities (Fig. 220-4). It has been suggested, based on kinetic data, that the

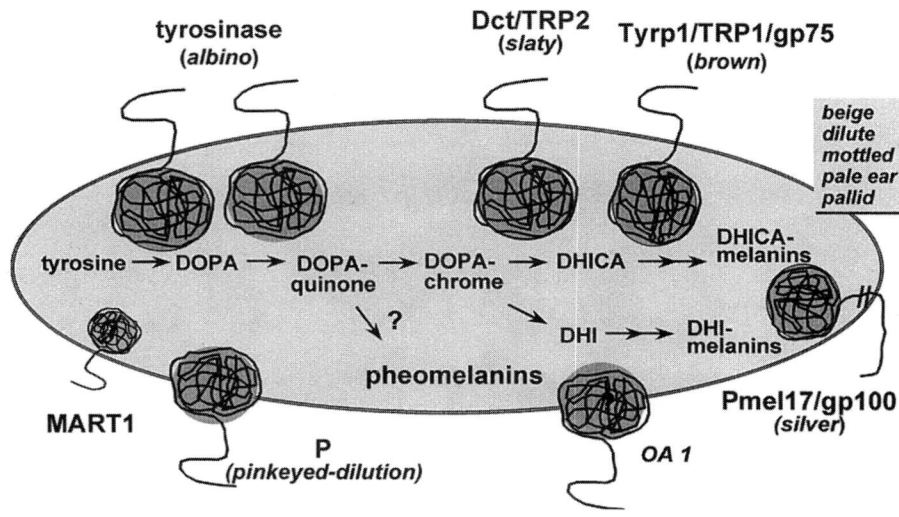

**Fig. 220-5 Melanogenic complex.** The biosynthesis of melanin is the result of several enzymes and other factors working together as a complex in the melanosome. Tyrosinase controls the rate-limiting reaction. Other enzymes and factors affect the type and amount of melanin formed.

various activities of tyrosinase reside at different sites on the enzyme, and recent biochemical evidence on the catalytic functions of various mutant human tyrosinases supports that interpretation.[171] Another distinctive characteristic of mammalian tyrosinase is its highly stereospecific requirement for DOPA as a cofactor to optimize the hydroxylation of tyrosine; rates of tyrosine hydroxylation in the absence of added cofactor are negligible. DOPA is thought to accumulate slowly from reactions further down the pathway until a catalytic concentration is achieved.[106,145,185]

Tyrosinase is synthesized as a nascent protein of approximately 60 kDa, which is glycosylated *en route* to the melanosome to a final size of approximately 75 kDa. Tyrosinase is an extremely stable protein that is highly resistant to attack by heat or by proteases, and it has an unusually long biologic half-life (~10 h in vivo). It has a relatively low isoelectric point (pH 4.3) and is bound to the melanosomal membrane with its catalytic center facing inwards. Many, if not all, of these physical characteristics of the enzyme are consistent with the structural features predicted by the coding sequence of the gene. Tyrosinase has two putative copper-binding motifs that are thought to be important to its catalytic function; recent studies show that mouse and human tyrosinases bind copper,[186] but that TYRP1 and DCT do not to a significant extent.[187] Such copper binding is important to catalytic function, and mutations that disrupt this copper binding destroy catalytic function.[186] Although tyrosinase expression is relatively specific for the melanocyte, recent studies suggest that it might also be expressed in some types of neurons, although this remains controversial.[188–190]

**DCT/DOPAchrome Tautomerase.** DCT functions in the specific conversion of DOPAchrome to the carboxylated derivative DHICA, rather than to the decarboxylated intermediate DHI, which would be formed in its absence. This specific catalytic function has been shown for the mouse and human enzyme.[148,191] Although DCT has two metal-binding motifs that are very similar to those functional in binding of copper to tyrosinase, these motifs in DCT do not bind copper, but bind zinc instead.[187,192,193] No doubt it is the bound zinc that gives this enzyme its distinct catalytic function. DCT is expressed in melanocytes where it localizes to the melanosomal membrane, but it is also synthesized in the developing forebrain of mice;[194] the reason for this is currently unknown but it has been suggested that DCT may be required in neurons to scavenge cytotoxic byproducts of the catecholamine biosynthetic pathway.[133,195] The size of the nascent form of DCT is close to that of tyrosinase (~65,000) as is its fully glycosylated size (~80,000). As noted above, however, its catalytic function is quite distinct from that of tyrosinase, and, in spite of their amino acid sequence relatedness, neither enzyme has detectable levels of the other's catalytic activity. DOPAchrome tautomerase does not seem to be as biologically stable as tyrosinase, is more labile to treatment with heat or proteases, and its activity follows a different response pattern to MSH stimulation than does that of tyrosinase.

**TYRP1/DHICA Oxidase.** A novel activity termed *DHICA oxidase* has been identified as a specific melanogenic activity. In mice, this enzyme activity is tentatively assigned to TYRP1, the product of the brown locus.[173,174,196,197] Although mouse tyrosinase can employ DHI as a substrate for its oxidase activity, it cannot use DHICA, whereas mouse TYRP1 is more efficient using DHICA than DHI. Interestingly, human tyrosinase can use DHICA as a substrate and human TYRP1 does not have this catalytic function.[175] Metal ligand studies of divalent cations bound to TYRP1 are inconclusive to date, but iron is a suggested possibility.[187] Tyrp1 in mice and in human melanocytes seems to have a common and important function in stabilizing the melanogenic complex in melanosomes, and its role in stabilizing tyrosinase may be more important than its catalytic function in determining levels of melanin produced.[134,173,198,199]

**Pmel17/DHI-DHICA Polymerase.** Pmel17 encodes a protein that is 668 amino acids long with a molecular weight of 70,944, including the putative signal peptide. The protein has several potential glycosylation sites and a hydrophobic region at the C-terminal end, indicating that it may be membrane bound. Studies show that expression of this protein is inducible by MSH and IBMX.[200] The Pmel17 protein was recently characterized as a polymerase, which can promote melanin production from DHI or DHICA.[178,201] Pmel17 is an abundant molecule localized in melanosomes, and in view of the often toxic effects of mutations in that locus, one possible biologic role for Pmel17 is in cellular protection from the cytotoxic intermediates of melanin synthesis.

## Other Determinants of Melanin Formation

**Phenylalanine Hydroxylase (MIM 261600).** Although the biochemical scheme of melanin formation traditionally begins with tyrosine, recent evidence suggests that tyrosine levels available for melanogenesis within melanocytes are controlled, at least in part, by phenylalanine hydroxylase, an enzyme that converts phenylalanine to tyrosine.[202] The importance of this enzyme has not yet been fully evaluated, but one of the pleiotropic manifestations of phenylketonuria, in which this enzyme activity is compromised, is hypopigmentation, suggesting that it is an important consideration.

**Membrane Transport.** An important level of regulation of melanogenesis might also occur at the melanosomal membrane where substrates of melanogenesis, such as cysteine and tyrosine, must be transported. Because such substrates cannot cross the membrane in the absence of a transport system, this might be actively regulated. Indeed, recent studies show that there are active and specific transporters of cysteine and tyrosine in the melanosomal membrane,[156,163,164] and that this might be actively regulated in response to physiological stimuli.[165] It was originally postulated that the P protein, which bears significant homology to small molecule membrane transporters,[203] might function in this regard. However, cysteine and tyrosine transport in pink mutant mouse melanocytes were shown to be comparable to those in melanocytes wild-type at that locus.[138,156,163] However, a recent study has put forth the interesting postulate that the P protein functions as a proton pump, which is important in maintaining the acidic nature of the melanosomes.[204] Mutations in P might, therefore, affect intramelanosomal pH and thus have dramatic consequences on catalytic functions and melanin synthesis, as well as targeting of melanosomal proteins.

**Sulfhydryl Metabolism.** Enzymes that regulate the intracellular and/or intramelanosomal concentrations of sulfhydryl compounds such as cysteine and glutathione can influence melanin synthesis by forcing the reaction toward or away from pheomelanin.[152,153,205] Among such enzymes are glutathione reductase[206,207] and γ-glutamyl transpeptidase;[208,209] however, the specific role of these enzymes in melanogenesis is not established. It is expected that additional enzymes will be identified for more distal reactions in the pheomelanin pathway.

**Peroxidase and Catalase.** The ability of peroxidase to oxidize DHI to indole-5,6-quinone has also been documented[210,211] and its potential role in melanogenesis is under investigation.[212–214] A melanosomal-specific catalase has also been suggested to participate in the melanogenic process, although its potential function in the pathway is not altogether clear.[215,216]

**Melanogenic Inhibitors.** Many types of natural and synthetic melanogenic inhibitors have been described.[147,151,157,217,218] Because the primary substrate of the melanogenic pathway, tyrosine, is a naturally occurring amino acid, many peptides and polypeptides may function as competitive inhibitors of tyrosinase if they have an exposed tyrosine or phenylalanine residue. In addition, there are other types of naturally occurring inhibitors of melanogenesis that are endogenous to melanocytes, and many laboratories are currently trying to characterize the structures and functions of those that may be biologically significant.

## GENES INVOLVED IN ALBINISM

Analysis of the coat color mutations of the mouse has provided a wealth of information on the genetics and biology of pigmentation. Over 85 loci have been described that affect melanocyte development, migration, and melanogenesis.[219,220] Recently, the transcripts, as well as the genomic sequences for several of these genes, have been isolated (Table 220-1). The products of these genes include enzymes, structural proteins, and regulatory proteins. Although humans do not have a "coat," the function of both the mouse and the human gene products has nearly always been identical. How the mouse mutations affect the coat-color phenotype has been useful in understanding how mutations in the human homologues will affect human pigmentation. At present, six loci responsible for albinism have been isolated in humans. The following is an overview of these pigment genes and their role in melanogenesis as it is currently envisioned.

### Tyrosinase Gene (*TYR*)

Tyrosinase is the key enzyme in the melanin biosynthetic pathway as discussed above. The murine tyrosinase cDNA was initially isolated using two different methodologies; a mouse melanocyte cDNA expression library probed with mouse tyrosinase antiserum, and a cDNA library probed with synthetic oligonucleotides that correspond to partial amino acid sequences of tyrosinase as determined from cyanogen bromide fragments of purified tyrosinase.[221] Subsequently, screening of a human melanocyte cDNA library with hamster tyrosinase antiserum isolated a human cDNA.[222] The authenticity of these clones was proven by comparing the predicted amino acid sequence of the tyrosinase cDNA to the amino acid sequence of isolated tyrosinase from both mouse[221] and human.[223,224] Bouchard et al. reported the full-length human cDNA sequence.[225]

The tyrosinase locus (*TYR*) in humans maps to chromosome 11q14-21.[1] The human and murine tyrosinase genes contain 5 exons spanning more than 80 kb with sizes ranging from 819 bp for exon 1 to 148 nucleotides for exon 3.[226,227] The lengths of introns 3 and 4 are approximately 15 kb, intron 1 is about 19 kb, and intron 2 approximately 30 kb.[228]

The 5′-upstream promoter region of the human tyrosinase gene contains four transcriptional start sites with the major site −79 bp from the ATG start codon and minor sites at −75 , −46, and −42 bp.[227,229] There are also several common *cis*-regulatory elements, including a putative TATA box (−106 bp) and CAATT box (−199 bp) as well as a 230-bp repeat sequence of $(GA:TC)_n$ located 713 bp upstream of the translational start site. This highly polymorphic repeat sequence can assume a hinged-DNA structure, which may play a role in regulation of expression.[229]

Twelve different alternatively spliced tyrosinase gene transcripts have been found in the mouse and 41 percent of all tyrosinase transcripts are alternatively spliced.[230] These alternate transcripts arise from exon skipping, usage of alternative 5′ and/or 3′ splice sites, or by retention of intron sequences.[230] Alternative splicing of the tyrosinase mRNA has also been demonstrated in human melanoma melanocytes.[231,232] In many cases, the alternatively spliced tyrosinase mRNAs lack important functional domains, such as the copper B region, and it is likely that these alternate mRNAs, if translated, do not act as functional tyrosinase molecules. Expression studies with alternative murine transcripts found that they do not produce proteins with tyrosinase activity.[226,233] Whether the alternatively spliced tyrosinase mRNAs encode a useful product for the melanocyte is unknown at this time.

Six polymorphisms are linked to the tyrosinase gene;[1] two produce amino acid substitutions. The Y/S192 polymorphism

affects an *Mbo*I restriction endonuclease site and the serine residue (TCT; presence of the *Mbo*I site) is found in all populations, whereas the tyrosine residue (TAT; absence of the *Mbo*I site) is found in only the non-Oriental population.[234,235] The R/Q402 polymorphism also has only one allele in the Oriental population.[236] In contrast to this, both alleles of the polymorphisms near the CCAATT box that affects a *Taq*I site have been found in all racial groups.[237] The 230-bp repeat sequence of (GA:TC)n located 713 bp upstream of the translational start site has multiple alleles.[238,239] There are also two restriction fragment length polymorphisms (RFLPs) flanking exon 1, with one detected with *Taq*I and the other with *Bgl*II.[1]

A second tyrosinase cDNA hybridization site in human genomic DNA is called the tyrosinase-related gene (*TYRL*).[1] This locus consists of a truncated tyrosinase gene containing only exons 4 and 5, as well as the entire fourth intron and part of the third. Sequence analysis shows *TYR* and *TYRL* to be very similar, with 98 percent nucleotide homology for both exons 4 and 5. Analysis of nonhuman primates shows that gorilla DNA contains the *TYRL* locus but not the chimpanzee, and, therefore, the formation of the *TYRL* locus appears to have occurred relatively recently.[240] There is no transcript product of the *TYRL* locus detectable in human melanocytes, indicating that the *TYRL* locus probably does not express a functional product.[241]

The regulatory regions of the tyrosinase gene are complex. The expression of the gene is limited to melanocytes and at specific times during development, and regulatory regions must confer both cell and temporal specific expression of pigment genes for normal pigmentation to occur. Transgenic expression studies using only 270 bp of the mouse tyrosinase 5′ promoter region have provided cell-type specificity, allowing melanocyte-specific expression in dermal melanocytes (which are neural crest-derived) and in the melanocytes of the pigmented epithelium of the retina (which are derived from the optic cup), as well as faithful temporal regulation, although the coat of these animals had uneven distribution of pigment.[242,243] Positive and negative regulatory sequences have been identified in this 270-bp region.[34] The critical *cis*-acting regulators in this region are located between −270 and −80 bp from the start codon. An element −183 bp upstream of the start codon, TATCAATTAG, was found to bind a transcription factor termed HMG-1 (high mobility group protein) and its isoform HMG-Y.[244] HMG-1(Y) is thought to be involved in nucleosome phasing, a mechanism maintaining the undifferentiated state of chromatin. This protein may alter the structure of promoter regions or facilitate the binding and activity of other *trans*-acting factors at the tyrosinase promoter. At present, the binding of HMG-1(Y) has only been demonstrated by *in vitro* studies and further confirming work is needed.

Another important regulatory element, a 6-bp CATGTG motif, is found at −104 bp from the start codon and is labeled the "M"-box (for *m*elanocyte) or the tyrosinase proximal element (TPE).[33,34,245] The M-box element has been found in the mouse and human tyrosinase promoter, as well as in the 5′ promoter region in the mouse and human tyrosinase-related proteins 1 and 2 genes (*TYRP1* and *DCT/TYRP2*).[32,245–248] Another location of this element at −12 bp to −7 of the tyrosinase gene has been termed the "E"-box.[33] The CANNTG motif is a binding site for MITF, a member of the basic-helix-loop-helix (bHLH) family of transcription factors.[30–33,35,249] Yasumoto et al. (1995) showed that an 82-bp *cis*-acting region, which contains the CATGTG motif (position −12 to −7; E-box) and the M-box (positions −107 to −97), are involved in *trans*-activation of the tyrosinase gene, suggesting that MITF is a common *trans*-acting factor regulating transcription of the pigment cell-specific genes. Murine Mitf and human MITF also increase tyrosinase, *TYRP1*, and *DCT* gene transcription preferentially in melanin-producing cells.[36,250] A second factor, termed a "ubiquitous transcription factor," was found to bind the M-box, but its role in activating melanocyte-specific transcription is unknown.[245] Although the M-box is implicated as an important regulatory sequence in the tyrosinase promoter, the deletion of the two M-box sequences in transgenic mice only reduces pigment production to 10 to 20 percent of wild-type controls, but does not eliminate pigment production, indicating the existence of other regulatory elements.[34] Evidence of other regulatory sequences, and the *trans*-acting factors that bind to these sequences, is associated with the *TYRP1* gene promoter (see *TYRP1* section) and may also exist in the tyrosinase promoter.[251]

A more distal region between −2020 to −1739 bp from the transcriptional start site contains an important enhancer.[252,253] The enhancing sequences are localized to a 39-bp core element that directs the melanoma cell-specific expression of a reporter gene under the control of this element.[252] This region is termed the tyrosinase distal element (TDE) and contains a copy of the M-box element.[31] Expression studies show that the TDE location is the strongest of the three M-box locations, with the proximal M-box elements being much weaker.[31]

An even more distal *cis*-acting regulatory region has been found 12 to 15 kb from the initiation codon.[254,255] This region was shown to contain two DNase I hypersensitive sites (HS-site) within a 200-bp region in melanoma cells, but not in other cell types.[256] These two DNase I hypersensitive sites were found to be rearranged in the hypopigmented *chinchilla*-mottled ($c^m$) mouse, indicating the importance of these sites for the proper regulation of tyrosinase.[254] The first binding site (hs1) contains the palindrome TGACTTTGTCA which resembles the binding motif to both a CREB (cAMP-responsive element binding) transcription factor and AP-1 (activator protein-1).[256] The inclusion of this region in transgenic mice enhanced tyrosinase expression.[255] Interestingly, tyrosinase expression is enhanced in neural-crest-derived melanocytes but not in neuro-ectoderm-derived melanocytes, indicating differential regulation of tyrosinase expression of these two cell lineages.[255]

The proper regulation of the tyrosinase gene requires the coordinated effort of negative and positive regulatory elements for the proper control of tyrosinase expression. As indicated above, these regulatory elements are located both proximal (i.e., the E-box; −6 bp) and distal (i.e., HS-site; 12 to 15 kb) to the transcription start site. For true wild-type expression of the tyrosinase gene, the insertion of the entire mouse tyrosinase gene into a tyrosinase-deficient albino mouse using a yeast artificial chromosome is necessary.[257,258] This transgene contained the entire coding region (80 kb) and 155 kb of the upstream sequences, and its expression was found to be position independent and copy number dependent. The resulting pigmented transgenic mice were indistinguishable from wild-type, revealing the importance of both the proximal and distal regulatory elements for proper control of tyrosinase expression.

Expression of the tyrosinase gene can be influenced by a number of different external signals. Tyrosinase activity, as well as tyrosinase mRNA transcription levels, are thought to be increased by MSH, cyclic AMP analogs or compounds that elevate cAMP levels in cells (i.e., isobutylmethylxanthine or IBMX), forskolin, and cholera toxin.[1] MSH and IBMX together increase tyrosinase transcriptional activity six- to sevenfold over either stimulant alone. Increased cAMP levels also up-regulate *TYRP1* and *DCT* expression, showing that this is a common mechanism for regulating pigment-specific genes. Increased intracellular levels of cAMP produce an increase in melanization and a decrease in cell proliferation, and fetal melanocytes will resume growth when cAMP inducers are removed. The cAMP level is influenced by means of a cAMP-dependent protein kinase (PKA) pathway. Repressing this pathway using a PKA peptide inhibitor (PKI) can reverse the melanization. Increases in cAMP levels also increase murine *Mitf* expression, as well as increasing its binding to *Tyrp1* and *Dct* M-box elements, providing the possibility that cAMP stimulation of melanogenesis occurs through Mitf.[35]

Ultraviolet B (UVB) radiation is another important regulator of melanogenesis.[1] UVB radiation is responsible for both an up-regulation of melanogenesis and an arrest of melanocyte cell division.[259,260] The increased pigmentation has two phases: immediate and delayed tanning.[261] The immediate phase results from a redistribution of preexisting melanosomes in the melanocyte, and possibly activation of preexisting tyrosinase enzyme. The delayed tanning phase is thought to involve the expression of pigment-specific genes, and analysis of UVB-induced gene transcripts shows that the expression of many genes are either up-regulated or down-regulated. There are several possible mechanisms to explain how UVB promotes melanogenesis. UVB radiation may mediate its response by increasing MSH receptor activity. UVB radiation of melanocytes results in a redistribution of MSH receptors from an internal to an external location in the cell,[262] and irradiation of keratinocytes and melanocytes causes the release of MSH and ACTH, which may, in turn, increase cAMP levels in surrounding melanocytes.[260] Another possible mechanism relates the increase in melanin biosynthesis to a response to DNA damage, associated with the release of the photoproduct, dimeric pTpT.[263–265] Thymidine dinucleotides, released after repair of DNA photodamage, will stop cell division at S phase and increase melanogenesis. Introduction of pTpT dimers to growth media mimics the effects of UVB radiation.[264] A third possible mechanism is the nitric oxide and cGMP signal transduction pathway.[266] The cGMP levels increase with UVB, along with an increase in melanogenesis, and inhibitors of guanylate cyclase inhibit this effect. Furthermore, introduction of nitric oxide in melanocyte cell cultures increases melanogenesis, and nitric oxide synthase inhibitors inhibit this. It is possible that these pathways, or others yet to be identified, are responsible for UVB signal transduction.

Tyrosinase activity and subsequent melanin biosynthesis can be increased, without an increase in tyrosinase gene expression, through post-translational activation of preexisting tyrosinase enzyme. Tyrosinase exists in several isoforms resulting mainly from post-translational glycosylation.[1] Stimulation of N-glycosylation may be involved in tyrosinase activation,[267] and studies in which glycosylation was inhibited resulted in a decrease in melanogenesis.[268] Melanoma x macrophage-fusion hybrids result in an increase in N-glycosylation and in tyrosinase activity, and the tyrosinase activity is sensitive to glycosylation inhibitors.[267] N-glycosylation may be an important regulatory pathway for MSH induced melanogenesis.[267]

Down-regulation of tyrosinase mRNA transcription occurs in the presence of compounds such as retinoic acid, the tumor promoter 12-O-tetradecanoylphorbol-13-acteate (TPA) or insulin, and this happens even in the presence of MSH.[269] Addition of retinoic acid to murine melanoma cells is associated with inhibition of melanogenesis, and a selective increase of protein kinase Ca (PKCα)PKC activity, whereas the transcription of other subspecies of PKC, d, e and z are not altered.[270] Inhibition of melanogenesis by TPA, even in the presence of increased levels of cAMP, also appears to be linked to the activity of PKC. Bertolotto showed that TPA activation of isoform PKCα leads to a decrease in the binding of MITF and subsequent reduction in tyrosinase expression and melanogenesis.[250] Since Gruber showed that overexpression of PKCα results in an increase of tyrosinase expression the exact role of PKC in regulation of melanogenesis is not clear.[271] Cells transfected with a plasmid containing the PKCα gene increased cell doubling time and melanogenesis. The role of PKCα as a promoter of tyrosinase activity was supported by Mahalingam et al. who showed that depletion of PKC activity by phorbol dibutyrate (PDBu) reduces tyrosinase expression and melanogenesis.[272] Treatment of melanocytes with TPA produces an initial short-term increase in PKC activity followed by a reduction of PKC activity and subsequent reduction of tyrosinase activity. The inhibition of tyrosinase expression by PDBu appears to be due to a decrease in the binding of MITF to the M-box.[272] Further studies are necessary to determine whether altered MITF binding is due to altered expression or protein modification, and to characterize the role of PKC in the regulation of melanogenesis.

## Tyrosinase Related Protein-1 Gene (*TYRP1*)

The brown locus of the mouse on chromosome 4 and the human ortholog on chromosome 9 encodes tyrosinase-related protein 1 (*tyrp1* in the mouse and *TYRP1* in humans).[273,274] A truncated brown pseudogene exists, but there is no evidence for a human *TYRP1* pseudogene.[247]

Mutations of the brown locus in mice reduce the amount of tyrosinase activity in the melanocyte and reduce the amount of eumelanin synthesis resulting in a brown mouse instead of a black mouse.[219] The common brown allele, resulting in a brown rather than a black coat, contains a cysteine to tyrosine amino acid substitution at codon 86 with normal levels of *TYRP1* expression.[274,275] Mice with a complete deletion of the brown locus are fully viable and have a coat that is indistinguishable in color from the classic brown mouse, showing that the brown mutation produces a null phenotype.[274] There are several interesting alleles at the brown locus that alter the pigment phenotype by a variety of genetic mechanisms. The *Cordovan-Harwell* allele results in an intermediate level of pigment formation associated with low levels of presumably normal *tryp1* mRNA. The *White-based* brown allele is dominant and appears to act by killing the melanocytes.[274] This allele has a gross rearrangement of the locus and may cause inappropriate transcription of other genes that produce a product that is toxic to the melanocyte. The *Light* allele is also dominant, but is the result of a point mutation thought to produce a neomorph, a mutation that confers a new function to the protein.[276] Electron microscopy of melanocytes from 7-day-old mice with this mutation shows a disruption of the melanosome structure, possibly by destabilization of the melanosomal matrix. It is hypothesized that this destabilization results in the release of cytotoxic pigment intermediates, which result in melanocyte death.

The structure of the *Tyrp1/TYRP1* gene varies from that of the tyrosinase gene.[246,247] The gene contains 8 exons and is 15 to 18 kb in length.[277,278] The entire sequence of the *TYRP1* gene has been determined and two dinucleotide repeats, one LINE-1 repeat element close to the transcriptional start site and one *Alu* I sequence has been identified.[278] The human cDNA shares about 93 percent identity with the mouse *Tyrp1* cDNA.[279,280] The human cDNA codes for a polypeptide of 537 amino acids with a molecular weight of 60,000 daltons and has been mapped to human chromosome 9p23.[281] The mature TYRP1 protein is a *trans*-membrane melanosomal glycoprotein with a molecular weight of 75,000 daltons. Mutations of *TYRP1* produce OCA3 or rufous oculocutaneous albinism, but there is no evidence of a role for this enzyme in the regulation of normal pigment variation.[282,283] An analysis of 100 normally pigmented Caucasians with differing hair pigment has shown no detectable polymorphisms that alter the amino acid sequence of the protein.[278] Like tyrosinase, this gene produces alternatively spliced transcripts,[247] but their significance is currently unknown.

The brown/*Tyrp1* locus contains several positive and negative regulatory elements in the promoter.[245,247,284,285] The minimum promoter in the murine *Tyrp1* gene, to confer cell-type specific expression, is between −44 bp and +107 bp from the start codon. The human *TYRP1* gene promoter includes the transcriptional initiation site 20 bp downstream of the TATAAA box and the first exon that appears to act as an enhancer, increasing transient expression sixteen- to twentyfold in both melanoma cells and HeLa cells.[277] Removal of the first intron, even when 3 kb of the upstream *TYRP1* promoter region is retained, reduced expression to background levels,[285] but the precise role of the first intron in gene expression is not clear, because other investigators have shown that it is not necessary for *TYRP1* expression in cultured cells.[246,284]

In the mouse, Mitf has been shown to bind to the *Tyrp1* M-box, *trans*-activating the expression of *Tyrp1* with a subsequent

increase in the levels of cAMP. By itself, however, this element cannot confer cell-specific expression of pigment genes in melanocytes.[251,286] First, Mitf is found in cells both expressing and not expressing pigment specific genes.[245,246] Second, the M-box can activate transcription of reporter genes in multiple cell types, revealing that *trans*-acting factors able to interact with the M-box are not melanocyte specific. Finally, removal of the M-box in the tyrosinase promoter does not completely eliminate tyrosinase gene expression. If the binding of the Mitf *trans*-acting factor to the M-box was the main driving force for melanocyte-specific expression of pigment genes, then none of these three phenomena should occur.

The melanocyte-specific factor (MSF) protein may play the role of a melanocyte-specific *trans*-acting factor. MSF is found only in the melanocyte and can act both as a positive-acting transcription factor and an antirepressor.[251] MSF appears to bind to two negative regulatory elements, one at −237 termed MSEu and the second located next to the initiation site termed MSEi.[251] Both of these sites contain a 6-bp motif GTGTGA. These sites were found to bind the Brachyury-related transcription factor (Tbx2), a repressor of *Tyrp1* expression. The binding of MSF to these two elements competes with the binding of Tbx2, allowing MSF to act both as an antirepressor and promoter of *Tyrp1* expression.[287] A complex model of *Tyrp1* expression has emerged that includes Mitf binding to the M-box, oct binding to the octamer motif (see below), and transcription factors binding to the TATA element.[251] In this model, the presence of MSF allows *Tyrp1* expression to occur by promoting the binding to MSEu and MSEi, and preventing the binding to Tbx2. In the absence of MSF, Tbx2 binds to both MSEi and MSEu, resulting in repression of *Tyrp1* expression. This repression occurs in melanoma and in melanocyte cell lines. It still needs to be determined whether MSF and Tbx2 interact with the promoters of other pigment-specific genes. If they do, modulation of the expression of both MSF and Tbx2 may be the means by which the melanocyte controls melanin pigment biosynthesis. *Tyrp1/TYRP1* expression is found only in cells containing eumelanin, whereas tyrosinase is found in cells containing either pheomelanin and/or eumelanin, showing that *TYR* and *TYRP1* can also be differentially expressed. This adds an additional layer of complexity to the regulation of the expression of pigment genes.[288]

Octamer-binding protein (OCT-1) is another potential *trans*-acting factor that regulates pigment gene expression. This factor binds to the sequence ATTTGAAT, a nonconsensus octamer motif found in the murine *Tyrp1* promoter.[245] Addition of anti-OCT-1 POU antibody inhibited factors from binding to this domain, suggesting that OCT-1 was the responsible binding factor. The region including the E-box was identified as a binding region for the OCT-1 transcription factor.[33] Other transcription factors, such as N-Oct-3 and N-Oct-5, are expressed at high levels in melanoma cells and may also be involved in mechanisms controlling the transcription of pigment specific genes.[285]

An interesting question for all proteins involved in melanogenesis is how intracellular sorting of these proteins and the targeting to the melanosome occurs. It has been proposed that the melanogenic enzymes, including tyrosinase, are transported from the Golgi to the melanosome by coated vesicles.[1] The amino acid sequence of TYRP1 contains a hexapeptide sequence, QPLLTD, located in the cytoplasmic tail at the carboxy end of the protein. This motif is important in the correct intracellular sorting of TYRP1 for movement from the endoplasmic reticulum to the Golgi, and from the Golgi to the melanosome.[289,290] Elimination of the di-leucine signal resulted in transport to the cell surface, instead of to the melanosome.[290] A small percentage (2 percent) of TYRP1 is found on the cell surface of melanocytes and is a truncated form of TYRP1 that lacks the transmembrane region including the di-leucine signal.[291] This soluble form of TYRP1 on the cell surface may explain the presence of the human melanoma autoantigenic glycoprotein 75 (gp75) antibodies found in the serum of patients with melanoma. The EXXXLL motif mediates the binding of AP-3, which may be involved in the intracellular sorting of proteins to lysosomes and melanosomes.[292] The EXXXPLL motif is present, in a similar location, in several melanosomal proteins including tyrosinase, OCA2 protein, and Pmel17, and represents a common intracellular sorting signal for melanosome-specific proteins.

### Pink-Eyed Dilution Gene (P)

The human ortholog of the pink-eyed dilution (p) locus of the mouse maps to chromosome 15q11.2-q12, a region that is associated with Prader-Willi (MIM 176270) and Angelman syndromes (MIM 105830) and that is linked to oculocutaneous albinism type 2 (OCA2).[293–295] The human cDNA is highly homologous to the mouse cDNA, exhibiting 84 percent identity for amino acids.[296]

The human P gene consists of 25 exons (exon 1 is noncoding) and spans a region between 250 and 600 kb.[203] The transcript of the P gene is 3.4 kb and encodes a protein of 838 amino acids.[296] This protein appears to be an integral membrane protein with 12 putative transmembrane regions, several N-glycosylation sites and potential protein kinase C phosphorylation sites.[203,296] The proximal promoter region contains several possible binding sites for transcription factors including several AP2 sites, one AP4 site, and three SP1 motifs.[203] No apparent TATA or CCAAT motif has been identified.

Initially, it was hypothesized that this protein may be involved in tyrosine transport to the melanosome, in part due to a reported 21 percent identity to a tyrosine-specific transport protein from *Escherichia coli*.[203,296] It has been shown that melanosomes do contain a tyrosine transport system that is temperature specific, stereospecific for L-tyrosine and other neutral amino acids, saturable with an apparent $K_m$ for tyrosine transport of 54 μM and resembles the rat thyroid FRTL-5 lysosomal system h.[163,164] Counter transport studies of p-deficient murine melanosomes show no perturbation of tyrosine transport showing that the p gene product is not part of this tyrosine transport system.[138,163] A recent report has shown that the murine p protein may act as an ionic transport protein and be responsible for the regulation of melanosomal pH.[204] The pH of the melanosome is normally acidic favoring optimal tyrosinase activity, and the P gene may be responsible for this.[297,298]

### Hermansky Pudlak Syndrome Gene (HPS1)

Hermansky-Pudlak syndrome (HPS) (MIM 203300) is a very rare type of albinism, but two isolated populations in Puerto Rico and Switzerland, provided an opportunity to map one of the HPS loci (HPS1) to chromosome 10q23.[60–62] Both mapping strategies were based on a common founder for the mutated gene in these two isolates. The syntenic murine region contains the *pale ear* (ep) and *ruby eye* (ru), two candidate mouse models for HPS, and ep is the murine homologue of HPS1.[63,64] The gene consists of 20 exons and spans 30.5 kb.[299] In the initial isolation of the HPS1 gene, a 3.6-kb transcript was identified that encodes a 700-amino acid protein with a size of 79.3 kDa.[63,299] Mutations in the 3' portion of this gene were associated with the HPS phenotype, indicating that this was the correct transcript responsible for the HPS phenotype.[63] A second 1.5-kb transcript of the HPS1 gene that encodes a 324-amino acid protein was also identified.[67] The two cDNA transcripts are from the same gene and result from alternative splicing.[67] Both transcripts are polyadenylated, and contain transmembrane domains and a putative melanosomal localization signal. The 3.6-kb transcript codes for a transmembrane protein containing two transmembrane domains, where the 1.5-kb transcript is missing the transmembrane domain in the carboxy end of the protein. There are no homologies between the putative HPS1 gene product and known proteins and its function are currently unknown. Initial analysis using confocal immunofluorescence has shown a cytoplasmic and membrane-associated distribution of the protein, suggesting a soluble and nonsoluble

protein as would be expected by the two identified transcripts for the HPS1 gene.[65]

Primer extension analysis revealed a single major transcription start site with two minor sites.[299] There are two TATA boxes, with the proximal site most likely being the active one. Several other putative transcriptional motifs were found in this area, but none are melanocyte specific.[299] Several tissues are affected by mutations in the HPS1 gene, and, not unexpectedly, the HPS1 gene is expressed in a number of different cell types, including melanocytes, megakaryocytes (progenitors of platelets), kidney, liver, and lung tissue.[63]

There are 14 murine loci that are associated with HPS-like phenotypes.[300] It is not known whether the products of all 14 loci are involved in the same metabolic pathway, but this may indicate the complexity of the process altered by mutations in the HPS locus. Analysis of HPS patients in Puerto Rico locus heterogeneity with affected individuals having no mutations in the HPS1 gene.[301] Furthermore, preliminary reports have linked the human homologue of the murine *pearl* locus on chromosome 5q to another type of HPS.[302]

### Chediak Higashi Syndrome (MIM 214500) Gene (CHS1)

The CHS gene (CHS1) has been mapped to chromosome 1q43 using the mouse beige locus on chromosome 13 as a probe,[56,303] and the gene has been isolated and sequenced.[303,304] The CHS1 gene also expresses two transcripts, a 6-kb transcript encoding a protein of 1990 amino acids and a 13-kb transcript encoding a protein of 3801 amino acids.[303] The CHS1 gene contains a stathmin-like sequence as well as several HEAT repeats and WD40 repeats.[56,303] There is also a region conserved between the HPS1 gene and the CHS1 gene called the BEACH domain.[56]

Immunohistochemistry analysis of the beige protein shows that is a cytosolic protein, expressed in most tissues, with no measurable membrane association.[57,304] It was hypothesized that the beige protein is involved in vesicle fission, including lysosomes, instead of vesicle fusion.

The mRNA is ubiquitously expressed in all mouse and human tissues tested and alternative splicing has been observed, producing transcripts from 12 to 14 kb to 3 to 4 kb. The 3 to 4 kb transcripts are thought to be the functionally important transcript products. The protein product contains 1545 amino acids and has been identified as a lysosomal trafficking regulator (LYST). This would explain the abnormal trafficking of melanogenic proteins found in the melanocytes. Several mutations in the mouse have been described.[304] The $bg^{11}$ is a 5-kb deletion at the 3' end of the gene that disrupts three exons, which would result in a truncated protein with probable splicing abnormalities as well. The $bg^{21}$ mutation has a drastically reduced level of transcription, due to a 116-bp insertion of a LINE1 sequence in the coding region producing a truncated protein.[303] The $bg^{8j}$ allele has a nucleotide substitution of a C to T at bp 2027, producing a nonsense mutation that is predicted to lack 1442 amino acids.[304]

### Ocular Albinism (OA1) (MIM 300500)

The ocular albinism type 1 gene (OA1; Nettleship-Falls X-linked OA) maps to chromosome Xp22.[305,306] Both the human (OA1) and the murine (Moa1) genes have been isolated.[307,308] In humans, the OA1 gene is divided into 9 exons within a 40-kb region.[307] The gene codes for a protein of 424 amino acids that contains several putative transmembrane regions.[307,309,310] The amino acid sequence does not share identity with any known proteins and its function is unknown. The gene is expressed almost exclusively in the retinal pigment epithelium[307] and cutaneous melanocytes,[310] and at a much lower level in the brain and adrenal tissues.[307] Although the clinical manifestations involve primarily the eye, the protein is a membrane glycoprotein localized to the melanosome in ocular and cutaneous melanocytes, indicating OA1 is really a type of OCA with changes in the eye and skin melanocytes.[310]

## ALBINISM

### Definition

Albinism represents a group of genetic abnormalities of melanin synthesis associated with a normal number and structure of melanocytes in the skin and eye.[1] A precise definition is important in understanding the difference between true albinism and other conditions that include some type of hypopigmentation in the phenotype. For this chapter, the term *albinism* is used to define disorders with a congenital reduction in melanin synthesis that is associated with specific ocular changes that are the result of reduced amounts of melanin in the developing eye. Reduced melanin synthesis in the melanocytes of the skin, hair, and eyes is termed oculocutaneous albinism (OCA), while reduced melanin synthesis primarily involving the retinal pigment epithelium of the eyes is termed ocular albinism (OA). The presence of cutaneous or ocular hypopigmentation, the color of the hair or the skin, or the presence or absence of the ability to tan, however, are not sufficient to define the type of albinism. For example, individuals with some types of OCA can appear to have relatively normal cutaneous pigment with tanning as a child or an adult, suggesting a diagnosis of OA, yet careful molecular analysis shows that they actually have a pigmenting type of OCA. A generalized reduction in skin pigment without ocular changes should be referred to as cutaneous hypopigmentation rather than albinism or cutaneous albinism, because there is no ocular involvement. Terms such as partial, incomplete, or imperfect albinism are not founded on genetic principles and should not be used.

### The Optic System

The abnormalities in the eye and the optic system in albinism (Table 220-2) are *specific* and *necessary* for the diagnosis or definition of albinism.[1,311] These abnormalities are common to all types of albinism, including OCA and OA, and appear to be related to the reduction in melanin during embryonic development and postnatal life. In general, the ocular changes are not clinically observable in heterozygotes for autosomal recessive OCA. In contrast, 80 to 90 percent of the obligate female heterozygotes for X-linked recessive OA have observable changes in ocular pigment.[312] Iris melanin is normally found in the stromal melanocytes and the posterior pigment epithelium, the latter being a continuation of the ciliary body.[1] The iris has a blue color without the formation of stromal pigment, and a normal amount of melanin in the posterior surface makes the iris opaque. The stromal melanocytes originate from the neural crest and have characteristics that are similar to melanocytes in the skin and hair follicles, while the melanocytes on the posterior iris surface are neural ectoderm in origin.[1] The reduction of melanin in the stroma and the posterior epithelial layer in albinism results in a translucent iris that transmits light through the iridial tissue on globe transillumination (Fig. 220-6).

The retinal pigmented epithelium (RPE) acquires melanin early in embryogenesis and has important functions in postnatal life, which are necessary for visual function.[313] Pigment is also present in the choroid below the retina. RPE melanin is greatly reduced or absent in albinism, making the retina transparent.[1,314,315] As a result, the choroidal blood vessels are seen below the retina on

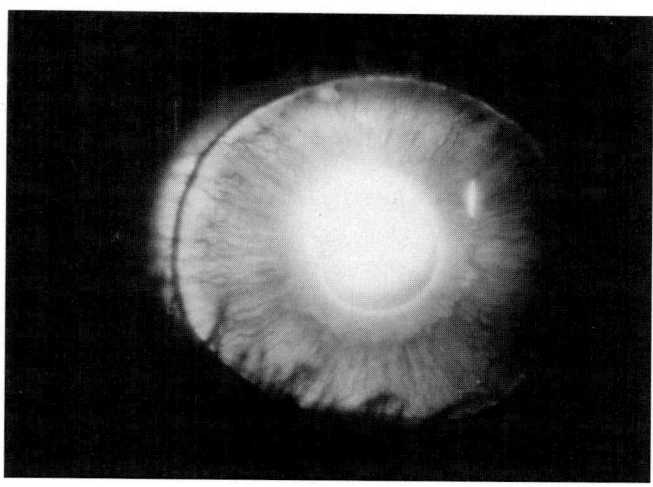

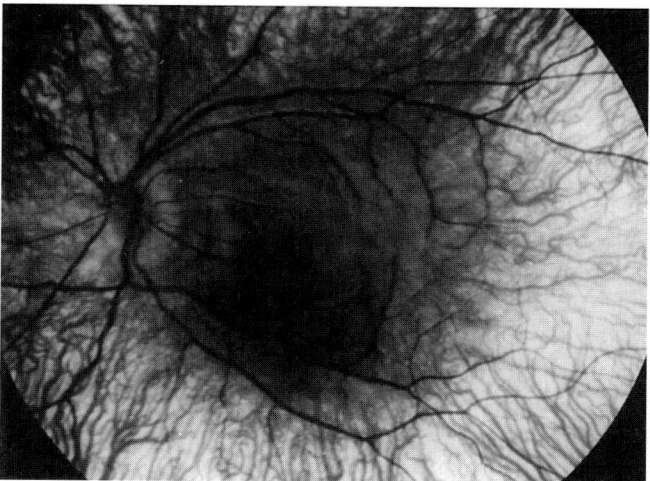

**Fig. 220-6 Ocular changes in albinism.** *Upper*: Translucent iris with globe transillumination. *Lower*: Fundus photograph showing lack of retinal melanin pigment and visualization of the choroidal blood vessels. There is no foveal reflex and no visual evidence of foveal development. The retinal vessels project through the foveal area. Both photographs are from individuals with OCA.

**Table 220-2 Characteristic Changes in the Optic System in Albinism**

Reduction in iris pigment—translucent iris
Reduction in retinal pigment—choroidal vessels visible
Foveal hypoplasia—reduced visual acuity
Misrouting of the optic nerves at the chiasm
Nystagmus
Alternating strabismus
Hyperopia or myopia and astigmatism

ophthalmoscopic examination (see Fig. 220-6). Despite the lack of melanin, most of the functions of the RPE are intact and the retina is able to receive and process light. The electroretinogram is normal.[316] Significant functional abnormalities that are associated with a moderate to marked reduction in visual acuity are present, however, in the fovea.[1,3,311] The albinotic fovea is hypoplastic with a reduced or absent foveal reflex.[1] It has been estimated that the cone density of the central retina is reduced with cones spaced three to four times farther apart than the normal pigmented retina.[317,318] The result of abnormal foveal development is reduced acuity that cannot be corrected to normal with corrective lenses. Visual acuity in albinism ranges from 20/400 to 20/40+, and is usually 20/200 to 20/100. Many individuals with albinism have myopia, hyperopia, or astigmatism, and correction of these abnormalities often improves acuity modestly. The foveal hypoplasia does not interfere with color vision, which is normal in albinism.[1]

The most striking optic system change in albinism is the abnormal decussation and misrouting of the optic fibers at the chiasm. In a mature eye that was pigmented during development, the nerve fibers of the nasal retina cross at the chiasm and terminate in the contralateral-lateral geniculate nucleus, while the fibers of the temporal retina do not cross and terminate in the ipsilateral-lateral geniculate.[1,3,311] In humans, the ratio of

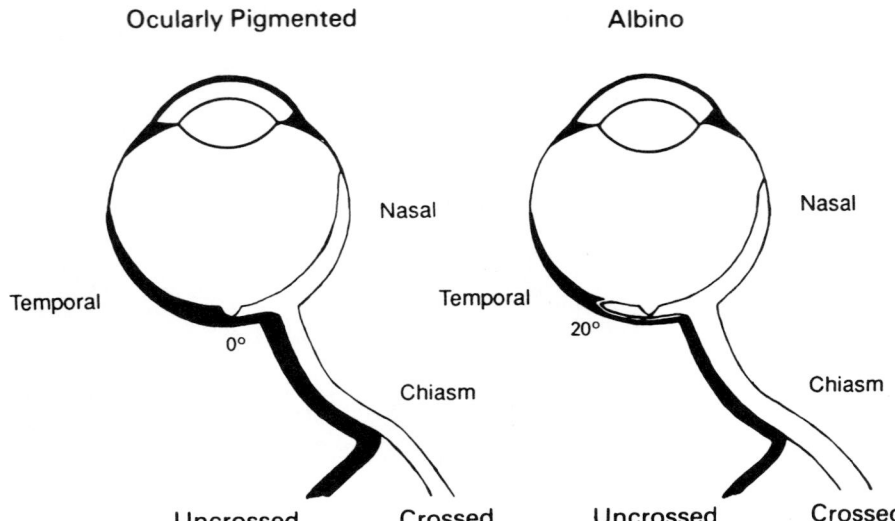

Ocularly Pigmented    Albino

Nasal · Temporal · Chiasm · 0° · Uncrossed · Crossed
Nasal · Temporal · 20° · Chiasm · Uncrossed · Crossed

**Fig. 220-7** Distribution of retinal ganglion fibers in an eye with normal pigment (left) and an eye with albinism (right). With normal ocular pigment, the nasotemporal border corresponds to the fovea, with the temporal fibers projecting to the ipsilateral geniculate nucleus and the nasal fibers projecting to the contralateral lateral geniculate nucleus. With albinism, the nasotemporal border is shifted 20° or more into the temporal retina, resulting in the majority of retinal ganglion fibers crossing at the chiasm and projecting to the contralateral geniculate nucleus. (*From Creel et al.*[319] *Used by permission of Aeolus Press.*)

contralateral (crossed) to ipsilateral (uncrossed) fibers is approximately 55:45. This correlates with overlapping visual fields, bilateral optic cortex input from each eye, and stereoscopic vision. This ratio is greatly altered in albinism in humans and in all other albino mammals tested. The proportion of crossed fibers probably exceeds 90 percent in all mammals with albinism.

The abnormal decussation is due to misrouting of the temporal nerve fibers of the retina. These fibers project to the contralateral rather than to the ipsilateral geniculate, resulting in a reduction of ipsilaterally projecting fibers, as shown in Fig. 220-7.[1,319] The temporal fibers projecting to the contralateral geniculate lead to disorganization and fragmentation of the dorsal lateral geniculate and to altered representation of the visual field in the geniculate and the optic cortex. The effects of the changes on retinal fiber projections are a loss of stereoscopic depth perception and an intermittent and alternating suppression of the vision in one eye producing an alternating strabismus.[315] The strabismus does not usually require surgical correction; amblyopia does not develop in most cases.

The misrouting of the optic fibers at the chiasm can be detected clinically by recording monocular visual evoked responses (VERs).[1] The response to flash- or pattern-onset stimuli is recorded with right and left occipital electrodes.[320] Using monocular stimulation, there will be a significant polarity reversal in VER components in the 50- to 150-ms time epoch, if the patient has abnormal decussation. This test is often used to establish a diagnosis of albinism in children (including neonates) or adults with unusual pigmentation. The diagnosis of OCA or OA cannot be made without clinical (reduced stereoacuity) or electrophysiological (asymmetric visual evoked potential) evidence of misrouting; an asymmetric visual evoked potential is the gold standard for making the diagnosis of albinism in questionable cases. Congenital nystagmus due to causes other than hypopigmentation does not produce an asymmetric visual evoked potential.[321,322]

In humans, the optic nerve projections develop early in embryogenesis and misrouting in albinism develops in the first trimester of a pregnancy, while the fovea develops late in fetal development and the foveal hypoplasia would be a late prenatal to postnatal event. The pathophysiological mechanisms of the foveal hypoplasia or the misrouting of the retinal nerve fibers are unknown. Both appear to correlate with a reduction or an absence of melanin in the eye at the appropriate time of development, rather than being a pleiotropic effect of the responsible gene mutation, because the genes responsible for the different types of OCA and OA encode proteins of widely different functions (such as an enzyme or a membrane transporter).[323] The formation of the retinal pigment epithelium in monkeys occurs primarily before birth, with little cell division in the postnatal period.[324] Studies

also show that the formation of the retinal pigment epithelium starts near the fovea and proceeds to the periphery, with a faster but shorter rate of formation centrally, suggesting that the presence or absence of melanin in these cells could affect the development of the fovea differently than it affects development of the rest of the retina.[323]

The misrouting also correlates with a reduction or an absence of melanin in the eye during early embryogenesis.[325,326] Melanin may play a direct role in the development of the optic projections;[327,328] indirect effects of melanin topography, timing, or the presence of chemical signals in the developing optic chiasm have been suggested.[319,329–331] There is also evidence that the albino gene may act by specifying the proportion of retinal ganglion cells that cross at the chiasm.[332] Current evidence suggests that the gene responsible for the albinism alters optic nerve development through its action in the developing retina rather than at other positions along the developing optic nerve.[333,334] Insertion of a functional tyrosinase transgene in transgenic mice and rabbits generated from albino strains corrected the optic misrouting normally observed in these animals.[335,336]

**Nystagmus.** Nystagmus is present in all but a few individuals with albinism.[1] The mechanism responsible for the nystagmus is not fully understood. The presence of foveal hypoplasia and reduced acuity with poor fixation may be responsible in part, but the nystagmus in albinism is often present at or shortly after birth, a time when the normally pigmented fovea is maturing, suggesting that a lack of normal foveal function may not be critical in the development of the nystagmus.[337] Abnormal development of the ocular motor system associated with the disorganization of the midbrain, and lateral geniculate nucleus and its projections to the optic cortex are thought to play a more central role in the development of nystagmus in albinism. Individuals with albinism often have a head posture that slows the nystagmus, with some improvement in vision.[338,339] Individuals with albinism are usually not aware of their nystagmus and do not see constant motion in their vision.

Foveal hypoplasia with reduced visual acuity, misrouting of the optic nerves at the chiasm, or other changes in the eye in albinism, such as refractory errors or intraocular light scatter, may all contribute to the development of nystagmus. The effects of the changes in foveal development have been studied in a small number of individuals with albinism with experiments that control for the nystagmus and increased light scattering. These studies show that foveal hypoplasia with reduced cone density is the major effector of reduced acuity, and that the changes in albinism suggest arrested ocular development.[317,318] Contrast sensitivity function has been studied in more than 30 individuals with albinism. These studies show that the nystagmus and the resulting continuous retinal image motion do have a profound effect on the visual quality in albinism, even though the abnormalities in foveal development are the limiting factor.[338,339] It is clear that the ocular changes in albinism are complex and no one change is the predominant cause of the visual abnormalities that are found.

**Visual Refractive Error.** Many individuals with albinism have high refractive errors of approximately 10 diopters or more of either myopia or hyperopia, as well as astigmatism,[1,3,340] and there is some evidence that the type of refractive error is reflective of the type of albinism present.[341] Correct refractive development of the eye and postnatal eye growth appear to be regulated by the quality of the images received by the retina.[342,343] When the retina receives a defocused image, the eye will attempt to compensate by changing the shape of the globe (elongate or shorten in focal length) to improve image quality.[344] This partly explains the refractive errors found in individuals with albinism. The genetic and experiential factors that set the growth pattern that determines the shape of the eye are unknown. It is likely that in the eye in albinism, the changes in focal length and cornea of the eye generally fail to sufficiently correct image quality, and at the end of this growth sequence the eye remains in an anomalous shape, resulting in significant refractive errors.

## The Auditory System

There are also changes in the auditory system associated with albinism.[1] Pigmented melanocytes are found in the inner ear. In the cochlea, they are found in the stria vascularis, which provides the driving current for the hair cells of the sensory receptors in the inner ear. Although there is interspecies variation in most species (including humans), the melanocytes are usually found to have an intimate relationship with the strial capillaries, and they may play a role in the microcirculation of the inner ear. The number of amelanotic melanocytes, termed "intermediate cells," appears to be normal in the cochlea in individuals with albinism. The cell volume of intermediate cells is reduced in albinotic as compared with pigmented cochleae. The diminution in melanocyte volume is accompanied by both a larger volume of an adjacent cell type, the marginal cells, and a greater resting endocochlear potential in the albino inner ear.[345–347] These findings point to differences in structure and function of the cochlea in albinism that appear to be related to the presence of amelanotic melanocytes.

Differences in the albino cochlea also exist as a decrease in the proliferative capacity of the intermediate cells.[348] The intermediate cells in the normally pigmented stria vascularis undergo continuous baseline mitosis, forming melanocytes at a rate that appears comparable to the melanocytes in the skin. The decreased proliferation of the intermediate cells in the albino cochlea suggests that the process of melanogenesis itself increases the rate by which melanocytes are formed, as observed in the normally pigmented stria vascularis.[349] The diminished proliferative potential of the albino intermediate cells may help to identify pigment-dependent mechanisms that regulate intermediate cell structure and function in the stria vascularis, as well as those that play a role in the response of the stria to various ototoxic events.

The absence of melanin pigment in the inner ear makes animals with albinism more susceptible to noise-induced hearing loss,[350] although in humans, the only definitive demonstration related to this is evidence of prolonged temporary threshold shift following exposure to noise.[1] Threshold shifts occur in all humans, but are greatest in individuals with little pigment. Animal studies indicate that the absence of melanin pigment in the inner ear may make the albino individual more susceptible to some ototoxic drugs, such as gentamicin, that may be normally detoxified due to melanin pigment's ability to inactivate polycationic drugs.[1,351]

Individuals with albinism and animal models of albinism have abnormal brainstem auditory evoked responses (BAER). The abnormal components of BAER are the potentials associated with the superior olivary complex in the brainstem. Studies of the

**Table 220-3** Estimated Prevalence of Albinism

| Population | Type | Prevalence | Reference |
|---|---|---|---|
| World Survey | All types | 1:10–20,000 | 494 |
| United States | | | |
|   Caucasian | | | |
| | All OCA | 1:18,000 | 3 |
| | OCA1 | 1:28,000 | 3 |
| | OCA2 | 1:10,000 | 3 |
|   African-American | | | |
| | All OCA | 1:10,000 | 3 |
| | OCA1 | 1:28,000 | 3 |
| | OCA2 | 1:10,000 | 3 |
|   Amerindian | | | |
|     Hopi | OCA2 | 1:227 | 495 |
|     Zuni | OCA2 | 1:240 | 496 |
|   General | | | |
| | OA1 | 1:50,000–150,000 | 497 |
| Africa | | | 948 |
|   Cameroon | OCA2 | 1:7900 | 499 |
|   South Africa | OCA1 | Rare | 500 |
| | OCA2 | 1:3900 | 500 |
| | OCA3 | 1:8500 | 411 |
|   Tanzania | OCA2 | 1:1429 | 373 |
|   Zimbabwe | OCA2 | 1:2833 | 375 |

neuronal cross-sectional area ("cell size") in the superior olive of the albino animals show significantly reduced cell size, on the order of 25 to 45 percent. Whether these differences are due to dysfunction in the albino cochlea or to pleiotropic effects of the albino mutation unrelated to effects of pigmentation remains unknown.

## OCULOCUTANEOUS ALBINISM

### Classification of Albinism

Oculocutaneous albinism is the most common inherited disorder of generalized hypopigmentation, with an estimated frequency of 1:20,000 in most populations.[1,3] The estimated prevalence for different albinism types in various populations is given in Table 220-3. OCA has been described in all ethnic groups and in all animal species, making it one of the most widely distributed genetic abnormalities in the animal kingdom. The different types of albinism, based on the genetic locus involved, are given in Table 220-4 and the clinical features of each type of OCA are given in Table 220-5. All types of OCA are autosomal recessive in inheritance. Mutations of the genes responsible for the different types of albinism are available at the HUGO Mutation Database Initiative affiliated Web site on albinism (www.cbc.umn.edu/tad).

### OCA1 (MIM 203100): Tyrosinase-Related Oculocutaneous Albinism

One of the two most common types of albinism is tyrosinase-related OCA (also known as tyrosinase-deficient OCA[352]), produced by loss of function of the melanocytic enzyme tyrosinase resulting from mutations of the tyrosinase gene. Classic OCA, with a total absence of melanin in the skin, hair, and eyes is the most obvious type of OCA1, but a wide phenotypic spectrum of OCA1 has been identified with tyrosinase gene mutations. This correlates to some degree with the well-characterized allelic series of mutations at the c-locus (tyrosinase locus) in the mouse.[219] The different phenotypes of OCA1 are dependent on the amount or type of residual enzyme produced by the mutant alleles, as well as the constitutional pigment background of the family. The range in the phenotype extends from total absence to near normal skin, hair and iris pigmentation, but the presence of the ocular changes always identify an individual as having albinism.

**Table 220-4** Genetic Classification of Oculocutaneous and Ocular Albinism

| Type | Subtype | Gene Locus | Includes | Mechanism for Albinism |
|---|---|---|---|---|
| OCA1 | OCA1A | TYR | Tyrosinase-negative OCA | Inactive/missing tyrosinase |
| | OCA1B | TYR | Minimal pigment OCA | Partially active tyrosinase |
| | | | Platinum OCA | |
| | | | Yellow OCA | |
| | | | Temperature-sensitive OCA | |
| | | | Autosomal recessive OA (some) | |
| OCA2 | ?OCA2A | P | Tyrosinase-positive OCA | ? Intramelanosomal pH |
| | ?OCA2B | P | Brown OCA | |
| | | | Autosomal recessive OA (some) | |
| OCA3 | | TYRP1 | Rufous/red OCA | Unknown |
| HPS | | HPS1 | Hermansky-Pudlak syndrome | ? Vesicular transport |
| HPS | | ADTB3A | Hermansky-Pudlak syndrome | Vesicular transport |
| CHS | | CHS1 | Chediak-Higashi syndrome | Unknown |
| OA1 | | OA1 | X-linked OA | Unknown |

An important *clinical characteristic of OCA1 that helps distinguish individuals with OCA1 from those with OCA2* is the presence of marked hypopigmentation at birth in OCA1. Most individuals affected with OCA1 have white hair, milky white skin, and blue eyes at birth. During the first and second decade of life, some individuals with OCA1 develop hair, skin, and eye pigment (OCA1B), while others do not develop any pigment (OCA1A).

The ultrastructural architecture of the skin and hairbulb melanocyte is normal in OCA1.[1,3] The structure, including the internal matrix, of the melanosome is normal. In OCA1A, there is no melanin within the melanocyte, and all melanosomes are stage I or II premelanosomes. No melanin forms after DOPA or tyrosine incubation. In OCA1B, the melanosomes contain melanin and are a mixture of partially melanized stage III premelanosomes and fully melanized stage IV melanosomes, depending on the amount of pigment that has formed.

**OCA1A.** Individuals with OCA1A or the classic *tyrosinase-negative* OCA do not synthesize melanin in their skin, hair, or eyes at any time during their life, resulting in a characteristic pheno-

type, as shown in Fig. 220-8. They are born with white hair and skin, and blue eyes, and there is no change as they mature.[1] They never develop melanin in these tissues. The phenotype is the same in all ethnic groups and at all ages. With time, the hair may develop a more intense rather than a translucent white or a slight yellow tint, but this appears to be denaturing of the hair protein related to sun exposure or to the use of different shampoos. The irides are translucent, appear pink early in life, and often turn a gray-blue color with time. No pigmented lesions develop in the skin, although amelanotic nevi can be present.

**OCA1B.** The OCA1B phenotype is produced by mutations that result in enzyme with residual activity (leaky or hypomorphic alleles) rather than a total loss of activity (null alleles). The variation in the phenotype of OCA1B is broad and extends from very little cutaneous pigment to nearly normal skin and hair pigment.[340] Fig. 220-9 shows the phenotypic range of OCA1A and OCA1B in relation to normal pigmentation. Previous editions of this book have included clinical and biochemical descriptions of yellow, minimal pigment, platinum, and temperature-sensitive OCA as

**Table 220-5** Clinical Characteristics of the Different Types of Albinism

| Characteristic | OCA1 OCA1A | OCA1 OCA1B | OCA2 | OCA3 | HPS | CHS | OA1 |
|---|---|---|---|---|---|---|---|
| **Hair Color** | | | | | | | |
| At birth | White | White | Pigmented | Pigmented | Pigmented | Pigmented | Pigmented |
| Mature | White | Light blond to brown* | Yellow to blond to brown* | Ginger to brown | Yellow to blond to brown | Blond | Normal |
| **Skin Color** | | | | | | | |
| General | Milky white Pink as baby | White | White to brown | Reddish brown | White | White | Normal |
| Tan | No | Possible | No | Possible | No | Unknown | Normal |
| Pigmented nevi and freckles | No | Yes | Yes | Yes | Yes | Yes | Normal |
| **Iris** | | | | | | | |
| Color | Blue to gray | Blue/tan | Blue/tan | Hazel/brown | Blue/tan | Blue/brown | Blue/brown |
| Translucency | ++++ | + to ++++ | + to ++++ | 0 to +++ | + to ++++ | ++ to +++ | 0 to ++ |
| Nystagmus | Yes | Yes | Yes | Not always | Yes | Not always | Yes |
| Visual acuity | Reduced | Reduced | Reduced | Normal/reduced | Reduced | Unknown | Reduced |
| Retinal pigment | Absent | 0 to ++ | 0 to ++ | +++ to ++++ | 0 to ++ | 0 to +++ | Absent |
| Foveal hypoplasia | Yes | Yes | Yes | No | Yes | Unknown | Yes |
| Optic tract misrouting | Yes | Yes | Yes | Absent or present | Yes | Unknown | Yes |
| Life span | Normal | Normal | Normal | Unknown | Can be reduced | Reduced | Normal |

*In OCA1B, the eyelash hair color is often darker than the scalp hair. In OCA2, the eyelash hair and the scalp hair have the same color.

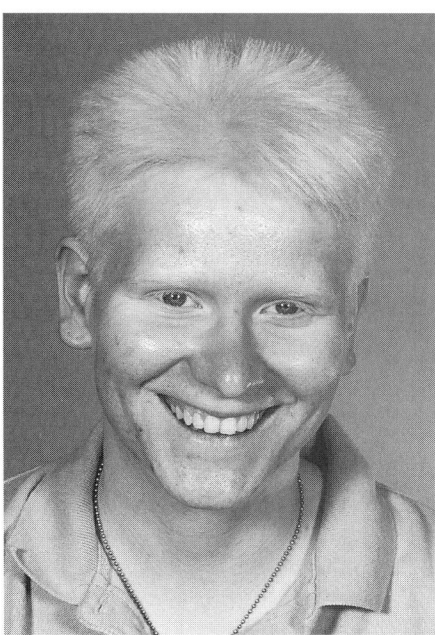

Fig. 220-8 Young female with OCA1A. No melanin pigment is present. This is the classic *tyrosinase-negative* OCA phenotype. See Color Plate 13.

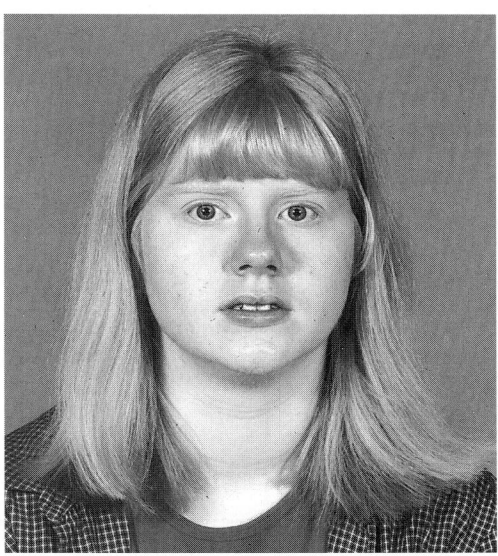

Fig. 220-10 Young female with OCA1B. The hair was white at birth. This patient now has golden blond hair, dark eyelashes, blue irides, and white skin that tans with sun exposure. See Color Plate 14.

separate and/or distinct entities, but it is now accepted that these are part of the OCA1B spectrum. OCA1B also includes some individuals who were previously classified as having autosomal recessive ocular albinism. Mutations coding for enzyme with differing amounts of residual activity are the primary cause of this variation, and a moderate amount of residual activity can lead to near normal cutaneous pigmentation and the mistaken diagnosis of ocular albinism. Ethnic and family pigment patterns can also influence the phenotype, and hair color can light red or brown in some families where this is the predominant pigment pattern.

The original OCA1B phenotype was called yellow albinism (or yellow mutant albinism) because of the color of the hair of affected individuals.[1] The hair color is the result of pheomelanin synthesis, and the predominance of this type of melanin reflects the reduced function of tyrosinase leading to reduced amounts of dopaquinone associated with the high affinity of dopaquinone for sulfhydryl compounds resulting in cysteinyldopa and pheomelanin formation. Individuals who had less hair and eye pigment were classified as minimal pigment or platinum OCA, while those who had peripheral but little central pigment were classified as temperature-sensitive OCA.[1]

The majority of individuals with OCA1B have very little or no pigment at birth and are born with white hair. They develop

varying amounts of melanin in the hair and the skin in the first or second decade, as shown in Fig. 220-10. In some cases, the melanin develops within the first year or even the first months of life. The hair color changes from white to light yellow, light blond or golden blond first, and eventually can turn dark blond or brown in the adolescent and the adult. In comparison to the pale blond or yellow hair with many individuals with OCA2, the blond hair color in OCA1B often has a distinct golden quality. The irides can develop visible light tan or brown pigment, sometimes limited to the inner third of the iris, while iris pigment may be seen with globe transillumination when the iris appear blue. Some degree of iris translucency, as demonstrated by slit-lamp examination, is usually present. Many individuals with OCA1B will tan with sun exposure. Pigmented (melanotic) and pink (amelanotic) nevi and freckles on exposed areas can develop with time.

One of the more interesting variations of OCA1B is the temperature-sensitive phenotype.[1] The pigmentation that develops after birth has an unusual distribution that is dependent on temperature. Axillary and scalp hair is white, while pigmented arm and leg hair develop. The irides remain blue. This type of OCA1B is analogous to the Siamese cat and the Himalayan mouse, and results from a mutation that makes the tyrosinase enzyme sensitive to higher temperature. Melanin synthesis occurs in the cooler but not the warmer areas of the body, such as the arms and legs, in a pattern similar to the Siamese cat.

### Molecular Pathogenesis of OCA1

Mutations of the tyrosinase gene on chromosome 11q are responsible for OCA1.[1,228,239,340,352–367] At present 88 missense, 57 missense, 13 nonsense, 15 frameshift mutations, 2 splice-site mutations, and an entire gene deletion that have been reported in the tyrosinase gene associated with OCA1 (Fig. 220-11).[362] A listing of all known mutations of the human tyrosinase gene with the appropriate references is available (www.cbc.umn.edu/tad).[362] The majority of these mutations have been found in individuals with OCA1A. The mutant alleles in OCA1A are thought to be associated with a complete lack of tyrosinase activity due to production of an inactive tyrosinase enzyme, and expression studies of some of these mutations have exhibited null enzymatic activity.[171] Many individuals with OCA1A are compound heterozygotes with different maternal and paternal mutations and affected individuals have been found with all combinations of missense, nonsense, and frameshift mutations. Approximately 20 percent of all individuals in which the entire coding region was

## Tyrosinase activity

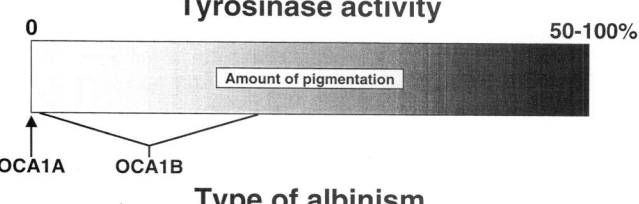

Fig. 220-9 Phenotypic range of OCA1, based on tyrosinase activity. Individuals with 50 percent (heterozygous) to 100 percent (homozygous normal) of normal activity have normal cutaneous pigmentation. Individuals with no enzyme activity (OCA1A; homozygous for one or compound heterozygous for two null alleles) are unable to synthesize melanin. Individuals with one (compound heterozygous with homologous null allele) or two (homozygous for one or compound heterozygous for two) residual-activity alleles form minimal to nearly normal amounts of cutaneous pigment.

# Missense Mutations

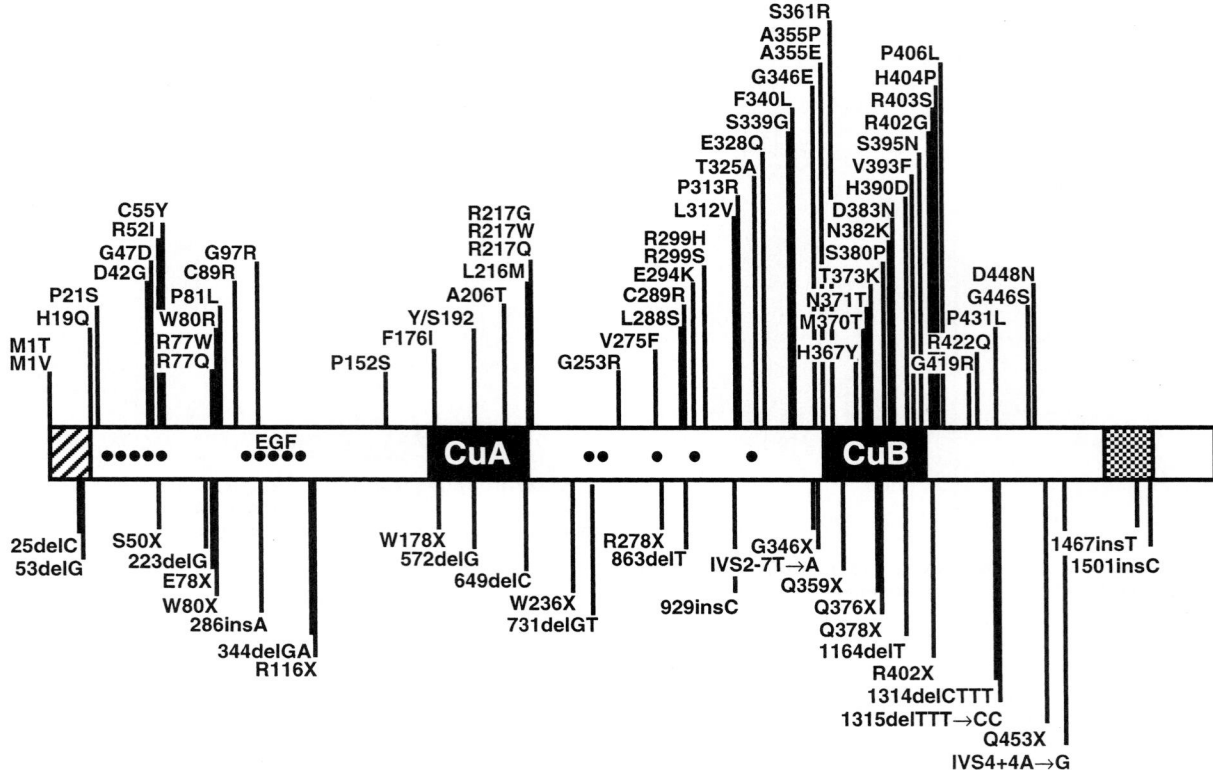

# Nonsense, Frameshift and Splice Site Mutations

**Fig. 220-11 Location of the mutations of the *TYR* gene associated with OCA1. The coding region of the *TYR* gene (529 amino acids) is shown. Striped region is the signal peptide; CuA and CuB are the copper-binding regions; the checkered box is the *trans*-membrane region. Black circles are the location of cysteine residues and the** **EGF is an epidermal growth factor-like region. Missense mutations are on indicated on the top and nonsense, frameshift, and splice site mutations are indicated on the bottom. (*From Oetting et al.[362] Used by permission of John Wiley and Sons, Inc.*)**

sequenced as well as flanking intron sequences have shown only one mutation. In all instances, the correct nucleotide is present on the homologous allele showing that these individuals are compound heterozygotes. The second mutation could be within a regulatory region not sequenced, or within the intron sequences where it produces a cryptic splice site or affects an intronic transcriptional regulator.

The majority of these mutations are found in Caucasian individuals but mutations unique to other racial groups have been identified. Two frequent mutations in the Japanese population include a missense mutation at codon 77 (R77Q) resulting in an arginine to glutamine substitution and a single base insertion of a cytosine at codon 310 (929insC) resulting in a premature termination at codon 316.[368] Mutations have also been reported in African-Americans, Afghans, Pakistanis, Moroccans, Koreans, Hmongs, and Chinese populations.[362]

Several different mutations have been found in individuals who have OCA1B.[1] This type of OCA was first described in the Amish and analysis of the original families have shown that the affected individuals in this population are homozygous for a codon 406 missense mutation resulting in a proline to leucine substitution (P406L). Because the OCA1B phenotype varies in families containing individuals homozygous for the P406L mutation as well as in individuals who are compound heterozygotes, it appears that other familial pigment genes can influence the effect these mutations have on pigmentation. Expression studies of the P406L mutation in HeLa cells showed tyrosinase enzymatic activity was

greatly reduced.[171,369] One mutation, an arginine to glutamic acid substitution at codon 422 (R422Q), results in a temperature-sensitive enzyme.[1] Expression studies using both hairbulb tyrosinase and transfected cells with the R422Q mutation showed a tyrosinase molecule that was inactivated by temperatures above 35°C.

Analysis of the distribution of the in the tyrosinase gene found that the missense mutations cluster in four areas, as shown in Fig. 220-11. Two of these clusters are found in the putative copper A and copper B binding regions. The third cluster is in the amino terminal end of the enzyme in exon I, and the fourth cluster is in exon IV next to the copper B binding region. It is thought that the clusters define functional areas of the tyrosinase enzyme.[1]

There are several mechanisms on how these mutations may cause a loss of enzymatic activity. Mutations in the putative copper A or copper B binding region could alter binding of this metal to the enzyme, leading to loss of activity. The A206T mutation in the copper A binding site affects a highly conserved motif (Pro-X-Phe-X-X-X-His), substituting a threonine for an alanine located between the proline and phenylalanine residues. The mutation F176I in the copper A binding region affects a phenylalanine in a motif (Phe-X-X-X-His) that is conserved in the copper binding centers found in tyrosinase and hemocyanin.[233,370] Computer modeling of the secondary structure of the copper B binding region has shown that mutations in this area (N371T, T373K, N382K, and D383N) affect a loop structure between the two α-helix regions responsible for correct orientation of the histidine ligands and the copper atoms.[371] Missense mutations at these locations alter the predicted secondary structure, especially within the α-helical domains.[371] Studies directly analyzing copper binding by tyrosinase show that the A206T mutation in the copper A binding site and the T373K mutation in the copper B binding site interfere with copper binding in the enzyme.[186] This is also true of any of the three histidine ligands of the copper B binding region thought to be involved in the binding of the copper atom. The juxtaposition of the two copper atoms is critical because of the need to form a peroxide with dioxygen, which is necessary for catalytic function. Any alteration of the histidine location that would affect the copper-to-copper distance is likely to render the enzyme inactive.

A second possible mechanism is that these mutations may disrupt substrate-binding domains and again reduce or eliminate enzyme function.[1] Analysis of the missense mutations H390A and P406L revealed normal to supernormal copper binding, but the mutant protein still lacked enzymatic activity, showing that amino acid residues involved in other aspects of the catalytic site, such as substrate binding, are also critical for normal enzymatic activity.[186] The binding of tyrosine or DOPA would have to occur next to the copper atoms, and if these amino acids are involved in this function, even a slight change in the chemical nature of an amino acid side chain in this region might alter substrate binding, reducing enzymatic activity. This may be the case with the cluster at the amino terminal of the enzyme (codons 42 to 89). One mutation in this cluster, R77Q, results in the removal of a positively charged amino acid (arginine) and is substituted by an uncharged amino acid (glutamine). The role of arginine in the active site as an anionic binding site has been reported in over 100 enzymes, and chemical modification of this residue results in inactivation of the enzyme. Removal of the arginine at codon 77 (and the charged group of this amino acid) may disrupt the interaction of the tyrosine substrate or dopa cofactor at the active site, resulting in an inactive enzyme. At present, there is only one mutation within the Epidermal Growth Factor (EGF)-like region, and this may suggest that this region is not critically important in the biology of tyrosinase.

Several of these missense mutations occur at CpG dinucleotides. The CpG dinucleotide is a mutational hot spot caused by methylation-mediated deamination of 5-methyl cytosine and is responsible for 35 percent of all single base pair substitutions causing human genetic disease. Most of the nucleotide substitutions occur at guanidine residues with the second highest percentage occurring at cytosine residues.[1] This distribution of nucleotide substitutions is identical to that found in other genes associated with human genetic disease.

Fifteen different frameshift mutations have been identified in OCA1, and analysis of the flanking sequences shows that many of these mutations are within repetitive sequences suggesting the mechanism of their formation. Streisinger and others have shown that frameshift mutations occur with high frequency in regions that contain repeated base sequences.[1] In areas of repetitive nucleotides where L (the length of the paired but misaligned stretch of bases) is equal to or greater than 4, deletion mutations have been found to be two to four times more likely than addition mutations.

## OCA2 (MIM 203200): P-Related Oculocutaneous Albinism

Individuals with albinism who have pigmented hair and eyes have long been identified, particularly in the African and African-American population, but not well characterized.[1] The first major insight into the separation of OCA into different types was provided by the hairbulb incubation test.[372] The presence of normally pigmented offspring from a mating between two individuals with OCA (now classified as OCA1 and OCA2) provided evidence for genetic heterogeneity and complementation at two independent pigment loci.

As a generalization that helps separate OCA2 from OCA1, individuals with OCA2 have some hair pigment at birth and iris

pigment at birth or early in life. The hair pigment may be difficult to discern in a young child who has little hair, and it may not be possible to distinguish between truly white hair and very light yellow/blond hair without taking a hair cutting and observing the hair color against a dark background (not all parents are willing to have hair removed when there is very little). As with OCA1B, localized (nevi, freckles, and lentigines) skin pigment can develop, often in sun-exposed regions of the skin, but tanning is usually absent. It has been suggested that the ethnic and constitutional pigment background of an affected individual has a greater effect on the variation in pigmentation in OCA2 than in OCA1, but this does not appear to be true now that the phenotypic range of OCA1B can be appreciated. Both OCA1B and OCA2 have a broad phenotypic range that, in part, reflects the constitutional pigment background of the affected individual. There may be some accumulation of pigment in the hair with age in OCA2, but this is much less pronounced than in OCA1B, and many individuals with OCA2 have the same hair color throughout life. OCA2 is the most common type of OCA in the world, primarily because of the high frequency in equatorial Africa.[373–377] The diagnosis of "tyrosinase-positive" OCA is often used for individuals with OCA2, but this term fits best with the common OCA2 presentation in African and African-American individuals.

**OCA2 Phenotype.** In Caucasian individuals, the hair can be very lightly pigmented at birth, having a light yellow or blond color, or more pigmented with a definite blond, golden blond, or even red color. The normal delayed maturation of the pigment system (i.e., very blond or towheaded as a child with later development of dark blond or brown hair) and lack of hair in many normally pigmented northern European children, can make it difficult to distinguish OCA1 from OCA2 in the first few months of life; the skin is white, does not appear to have generalized pigment, and does not usually tan with sun exposure. The iris color is blue-gray or lighted pigmented, and the degree of translucency on globe transillumination correlates with the amount of iris pigment present. With time, pigmented nevi and pigmented dendritic freckles may be seen in exposed areas with repeated sun exposure. The hair in Caucasian individuals may slowly turn darker through the first two or more decades of life (Fig. 220-12).

The classic *tyrosinase-positive* OCA phenotype is a distinctive OCA2 phenotype in African-American and African individuals, which may, in part, result from the existence of a single

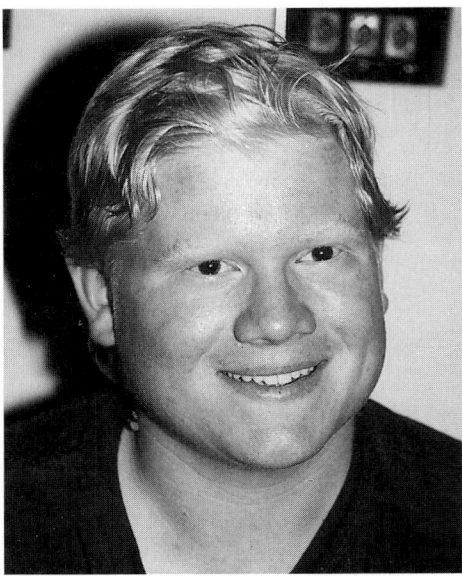

**Fig. 220-12** Young male with OCA2. Hair was light yellow at birth. This individual has yellow/blond scalp and eyelash hair, white skin, and blue irides. The skin does not tan. See Color Plate 15.

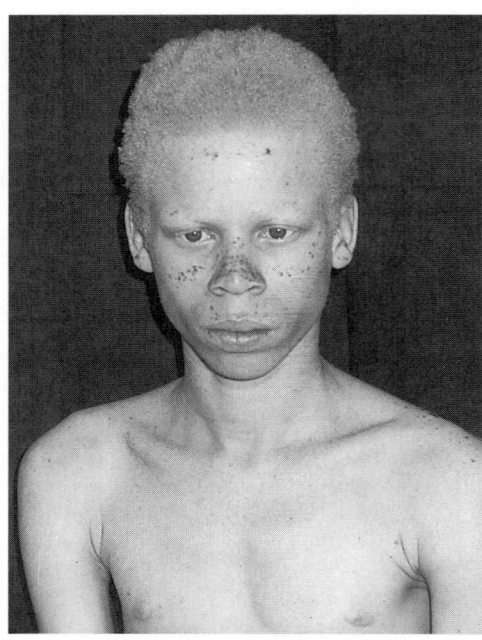

**Fig. 220-13 Young Nigerian male with classic *tyrosinase-positive* OCA phenotype. Scalp and eyelash hair are yellow. The skin is white and does not tan. See Color Plate 16.**

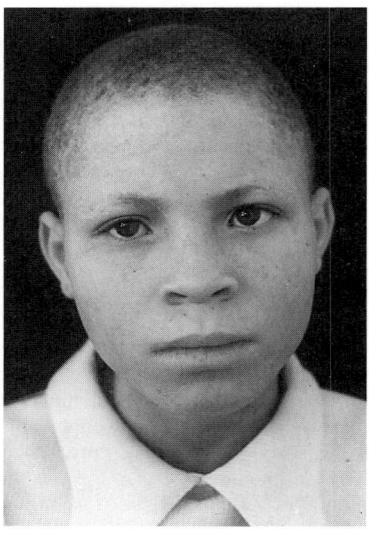

**Fig. 220-14 Young Nigerian female with Brown OCA. Hair, skin, and irides are light brown. See Color Plate 17.**

common deletion mutation throughout many parts of sub-Sahara Africa.[1,373–377] The hair is yellow at birth and remains yellow through life, although the color may turn darker (Fig. 220-13). Interestingly, the hair can turn lighter in older individuals, and this probably represents the normal graying with age. The skin is creamy white at birth and changes little with time, and generalized pigment does not appear to be present in the skin. Pigmented nevi, lentigines, and freckles develop in some individuals,[378] but the skin usually does not tan. The development of well-demarcated pigmented lesions (called dendritic freckles, lentigines, or ephelides), usually on sun-exposed areas of the skin, may reflect a separate genetic susceptibility as these lesions only appear to develop in some OCA2 families and not in others.[295,378,379] The presence of pigmented freckles is associated with a lower risk of skin cancer in South African individuals, and may reflect the presence of photoprotective melanin in the skin.[378,379] The irides in this classic type of OCA2 are blue/gray or lightly pigmented (usually a hazel or tan color, and often with the majority of the pigment forming on the inner third of the iris).

**Phenotypic Variation in OCA2.** Molecular studies are now helping to define the characteristics of the OCA2 phenotype. The pigmentation pattern in African-Americans includes more than the classic "tyrosinase-positive" phenotype in that some individuals with OCA2 (defined as having pigmented hair at birth and the ocular features of albinism) have brown, ginger, auburn, or red hair. Some of this variation may reflect genetic admixture in this population, and some may reflect allelic heterogeneity resulting from differential effects of *P* gene mutations on the function of the P protein. One African-American individual with OCA2 was reported with a mild phenotype similar to that expected for autosomal recessive ocular albinism,[380] suggesting that this is part of the phenotypic range of OCA2, as well as OCA1B. "Autosomal recessive ocular albinism" is most likely not a distinct type of albinism but rather a part of the phenotypic range of the different types of OCA.

**Brown OCA (MIM 203290).** The product of the *P* gene plays a role in ion transport into the melanosome and maintenance of the intramelanosomal acidic pH,[204,381] and studies of human albinism and coat color changes in the mouse suggest that the *P* gene

product has its primary function in the formation of eumelanin.[142,382] Mutations of the *P* gene, as seen in the classic "tyrosinase-positive" phenotype in human OCA2 are associated with the development of pheomelanin and a deficiency in eumelanin. Another type of OCA called "Brown OCA" has been described in the African and African-American populations in which the amount of eumelanin in the skin and hair is reduced but not absent.[1,383] Early studies in Nigeria suggested the "brown OCA" segregated as a single gene and did not appear to be part of the spectrum of the more common "tyrosinase-positive OCA" in that population,[384] but recent studies in South Africa show that "brown OCA" maps to the OCA2 locus and is part of the phenotypic spectrum of this type of albinism. Ramsay and coworkers carried out linkage analysis on five families containing individuals with "brown OCA" and found linkage to the *P* gene on chromosome 15q.[383] As with OCA1B, the brown phenotype may arise from a mutation of the *P* gene that reduces but does not extinguish the function of the P protein (i.e., a leaky mutation).

In African and African-American individuals with the "brown OCA" phenotype, the hair and skin color are light brown, and the irides are gray to tan at birth (Fig. 220-14).[1] With time there is little change in skin color, but the hair may turn darker and the irides may accumulate more tan pigment. The skin does not burn and will tan on sun exposure. Affected individuals are recognized as having albinism because they have all of the ocular features of albinism. The iris has punctate and radial translucency, and moderate retinal pigment is present. Visual acuity ranges from 20/60 to 20/150. The phenotype is not well defined in Caucasian individuals, but most likely includes moderate amounts of skin, hair, and eye pigmentation associated with the ocular features of albinism in an individual who was born with moderate amounts of pigment in these tissues.

**Prader-Willi Syndrome (MIM 176270).** There is an association between the hypopigmentation found with Prader-Willi and Angelman syndromes and OCA2. Prader-Willi syndrome is a developmental syndrome that includes neonatal hypotonia, hyperphagia and obesity, hypogonadism, small hands and feet, and mental retardation associated with characteristic behavior (reviewed in references 385 and 386). Approximately 70 percent of individuals with Prader-Willi syndrome have an interstitial *de novo* microdeletion of chromosome 15q11-13, and most of those without a deletion of the paternal chromosome 15 have uniparental disomy for the maternal chromosome 15 or an imprinting defect.[387,388]

## Missense Mutations

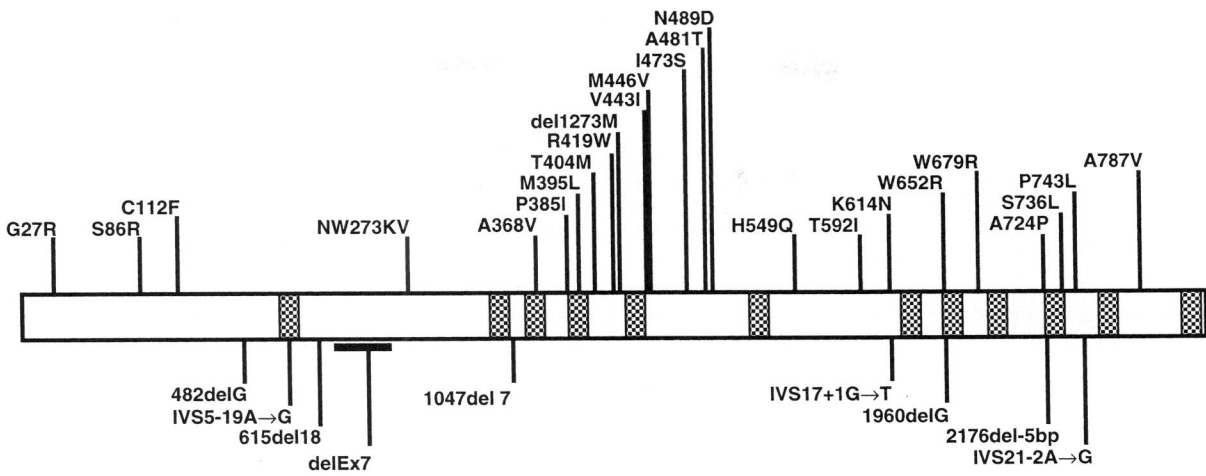

## Frameshift and Splice Site Mutations

**Fig. 220-15** Location of the mutations of the *P* gene associated with OCA2. The coding region of the *P* gene (838 amino acids) is shown. The checked boxes are the putative *trans*-membrane domains.

Missense mutations are indicated on the top and nonsense, frameshift, and splice-site mutations are indicated on the bottom. (*From Oetting et al.*[362] *Used by permission of John Wiley and Sons, Inc.*)

Approximately 50 percent or more of individuals with Prader-Willi syndrome (PWS) are hypopigmented but do not have the typical ocular features of albinism, while a smaller number have OCA and PWS.[385,389–393] For those without obvious OCA, hair and skin are lighter than unaffected family members, and childhood nystagmus and strabismus are common but often transient.[1] The irides are pigmented with some translucency on globe transillumination, and retinal pigment is reduced in amount. Although funduscopic examination does not show classic changes of foveal hypoplasia, the fovea may not appear entirely normal. Visual evoked potential studies revealed optic tract misrouting similar to that found in albinism in some individuals with Prader-Willi syndrome and hypopigmentation,[394] but this has not been universally found.[320,395] Part of the discrepancy may arise from the technique used, but part may be an effect of biologic differences in individuals with Prader-Willi syndrome.[319] The presence of hypopigmentation correlates with the presence of the 15q deletion, but the mechanism responsible for the reduction in melanin is unknown.[390,391,393,396]

Some individuals with Prader-Willi syndrome have OCA2 with cutaneous hypopigmentation associated with all of the typical ocular features of albinism.[389–391] These individuals have been found to have a deletion mutation on the paternal chromosome 15 (accounting for their Prader-Willi syndrome and for their paternal *P* gene mutation) and a maternal *P* gene mutation, making them compound heterozygotes for *P* gene mutations.

**Angelman Syndrome (MIM 105830).** Hypopigmentation is present in more than 50 percent of individuals with Angelman syndrome.[396–399] Angelman syndrome is a complex developmental disorder that includes developmental delay and severe mental retardation, microcephaly, neonatal hypotonia, ataxic movements, and inappropriate laughter. The majority of individuals with Angelman syndrome have an interstitial deletion of chromosome 15q11-13, with the remainder having a single gene abnormality, an imprinting defect, or uniparental disomy for the paternal chromosome 15.[387] In Angelman syndrome, the hypopigmentation is characterized by light skin and hair. There may be a history of nystagmus or strabismus, and iris translucency and reduced retinal pigment may be present. No analysis of the optic tract organization is available. It is expected that individuals with Angelman

syndrome having OCA2 will be described because of the location of the *P* gene in the Prader-Willi/Angelman syndrome region of chromosome 15. The presence of hypopigmentation in Angelman syndrome correlates with the presence of a 15q deletion.[396,399,400]

### Molecular Pathogenesis of OCA2

The most prevalent mutation of the *P* gene associated with OCA2 is a deletion of exon 7. This is a 2.7-kb deletion that includes the entire coding sequence of exon 7 and the flanking intronic sequences, and is thought to be of African origin.[374] This deletion is most common among the Bantu-speaking people of southern Africa with an allele frequency of 77 percent in individuals with OCA2 from Tanzania, 92 percent in Zimbabwe, 79 percent in Zambia, 33 percent in Central African Republic, and 65 percent in Cameroon.[373–375,401–404] The allele frequency among southern African Bantu-speaking people is estimated to be 1.3 percent,[404] while the frequency among African-Americans is estimated to be between 0.5 percent and 0.2 percent.[401] Haplotype analysis suggests that the 2.7-kb deletion mutation is old and arose before the Bantu-speaking people of southern Africa diverged from the middle Benue Valley between Nigeria and Cameroon approximately 3000 years age.[404]

Other reported mutations include 23 missense mutations, 4 frameshift mutations, 3 splice-site mutations, and 2 inframe deletions.[362,373,380,402,405,406] The locations of these mutations are shown in Fig. 220-15. The missense mutations of the *P* gene, unlike tyrosinase, do not cluster in defined regions. Most of the missense mutations are between or at the border of the transmembrane domains in the central region of the protein. The *P* gene has 36 reported polymorphisms, 20 of which are in the coding region and 6 result in amino acid substitutions.[203,362] This is a much greater number than that found in the tyrosinase gene, with its six reported polymorphisms. There is no functional assay of the P protein and the differentiation between pathogenic mutations and polymorphisms at present can only be accomplished by a transfection assay of *p*-deficient mouse melanocytes.[407]

### OCA3 (MIM 203290): TYRP1-Related Oculocutaneous Albinism

The characterization of the human phenotype associated with mutations of the *TYRP1* gene is new and evolving (and surprising).

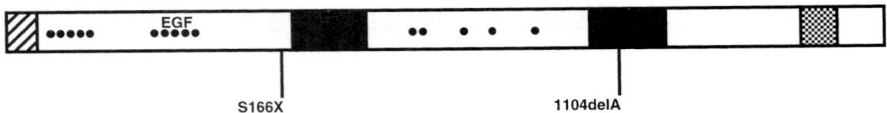

## Nonsense and Frameshift Mutations

**Fig. 220-16** Location of the mutations of the *TYRP1* gene associated with OCA3. The coding region of the *TYRP1* gene (537 amino acids) is shown. Striped region is the signal peptide; black regions are putative metal binding regions; the checkered box is the *trans*-membrane region. Black circles are the location of cysteine residues conserved in the family of tyrosinase-related proteins and the EGF is a epidermal growth factor-like region. Nonsense and frameshift mutations are indicated on the bottom. (*From Oetting et al.*[362] *Used by permission of John Wiley and Sons, Inc.*)

The *Tyrp1* gene maps to the brown locus in the mouse, and mutations at this locus change the mouse coat color from black to brown (see above). The DHICA oxidase function in the eumelanin pathway of the melanocyte is tentatively assigned to TYRP1,[174,197,408] and it has been shown that *Tyrp1* cDNA transfection to melanocytes derived from the brown mouse can induce the formation of black/dark brown melanin.[174,197,408]

**OCA3 Phenotype.** The first evidence that variations in human pigmentation are related *TYRP1* gene mutations came from studies of an African-American twin boy who had light brown skin, light brown hair, and blue-gray irides as a newborn, while his fraternal twin brother had normal pigmentation.[282] The affected twin had nystagmus and it was felt that the clinical presentation was consistent with "brown OCA" as described above. Biochemical and molecular studies showed that melanocytes from the affected twin contained no *TYRP1* mRNA, produced reduced amounts of insoluble melanin, and appeared brown rather than the black color found in control melanocytes in culture.[282] The affected twin was found to be homozygous for a single base deletion in codon 368 of the *TYRP1* gene (1104delA) on chromosome 9p[281] and the authors concluded that mutations of this gene produced a third type of OCA. This family was unfortunately lost to follow-up and the phenotype of this boy could not be followed.

The phenotype associated with mutations of the *TYRP1* gene became more obvious when another type of OCA known as "rufous" or "red OCA" was mapped to the *TYRP1* locus on chromosome 9p in the South African population, and the same deletion mutation (1104delA) of the *TYRP1* gene was found to account for 50 percent of the mutations in the study population (19 of 38 affected chromosomes).[283] Rufous or red OCA is now classified as OCA3 and this OCA type has only been partially characterized. Individuals with OCA who have red hair and reddish-brown pigmented skin have been reported in Africa and in New Guinea,[283,409,410] but clinical descriptions are incomplete, little biochemical data are available, and similar phenotypes in the U.S. population have not been identified and reported. The cases are described in the literature as "red," "rufous," or "xanthous" albinism. Individuals with OCA1 or OCA2 who have red hair are also recognized, but the reddish-brown skin pigment is usually not present, and they should not be confused with OCA3.

The phenotype of OCA3 in South African individuals includes red or reddish brown skin, ginger or reddish hair, and hazel or brown irides.[410] All of the ocular features of albinism are not always present, however, as many do not have iris translucency, nystagmus, strabismus, or foveal hypoplasia. This is similar to the hypopigmentation in Prader-Willi syndrome and Angelman syndrome associated with the *P* gene (see above). No misrouting of the optic nerves has been demonstrated by a visual evoked potential, suggesting either that this is not a true type of albinism as defined in this chapter, or that the hypopigmentation is not sufficient to consistently alter optic nerve development.[410] The ultrastructural analysis of hairbulb and skin melanocytes show eumelanosomes and pheomelanosomes in various stages of melanization, suggesting that the red color results from pheomelanin synthesis, as pheomelanosomes are absent in normally pigmented black skin and hairbulbs.[410] In New Guinea, the described phenotype includes reddish-brown skin, deep mahogany hair, reddish brown to brown irides with some translucency, and normal retinal pigment and foveal development.[409] Congenital nystagmus is present in this population but does not segregate specifically with the red phenotype. At this time, the phenotype for TYRP1-related OCA in the Caucasian and the Asian populations is unknown.

### Molecular Pathogenesis of OCA3

Two mutations in the *TYRP1* gene have been found in OCA3, S166X, and 1104delA, and both are truncating mutations (Fig. 220-16).[282,411] The 1104delA mutation accounted for 50 percent and the S116X mutation accounted for 45 percent of the OCA3 mutations in this sample of 19 individuals with rufous OCA3. Individuals homozygous for each of the mutations, as well as individuals who were compound heterozygotes for both, were identified. Because the loss of TYRP1 enzymatic activity in the mouse does not lead to a loss, but only a change in the amount or biochemical character of eumelanin, it is expected that mutations in the *TYRP1* gene will result in a less-severe phenotype than those related to null mutations of the tyrosinase or the *P* gene. Four polymorphisms in the *TYRP1* gene have also been reported. Two of the polymorphisms are within the coding region, but do not result in changes in the amino acid sequence.[411]

The study population in South Africa also included three individuals with a phenotype that was not typical for brown OCA2 or red OCA3.[411] Two sibs had skin similar to rufous OCA3 but lighter in color, and "straw-yellow" scalp hair more typical of OCA2.[411] Most interestingly, the sibs were compound heterozygotes for *TYRP1* gene mutations (S166X/1104delA) and heterozygous for the common 2.7-kb deletion mutation of the *P* gene (see above), suggesting that altered function of the P protein may modify the pigment phenotype in the presence of *TYRP1* gene mutations.

### Hermansky-Pudlak Syndrome

Hermansky-Pudlak syndrome is a complex autosomal recessive disorder that includes the triad of OCA, a mild bleeding diathesis resulting from storage-pool-deficient platelets, and a ceroid storage disease affecting primarily the lungs and the gut. The manifestation of OCA in HPS is similar to OCA1B or OCA2, as described above. Hermansky and Pudlak first described this condition in two Czechoslovakian individuals in 1959, and it has subsequently been recognized throughout the world, with the majority of affected individuals in the Puerto Rican population.[1,3] HPS is not common, except in the latter population, and does not constitute a major type of OCA in most populations. In Puerto Rico, however, the frequency is approximately 1:1800.[59] HPS is not found at an increased frequency on other Caribbean islands.

HPS is not a single entity but a phenotypic description for a collection of disorders that include the combination of OCA, storage-pool-deficient platelets, and ceroid production, the latter likely a reflection of abnormal lysosomal metabolism. There are 14 loci in the mouse that give a murine HPS phenotype of coat color reduction, storage-pool-deficient platelets, and lysosomal

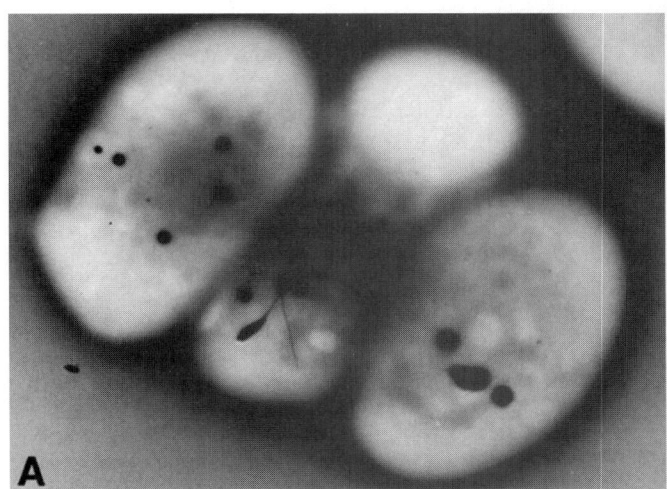

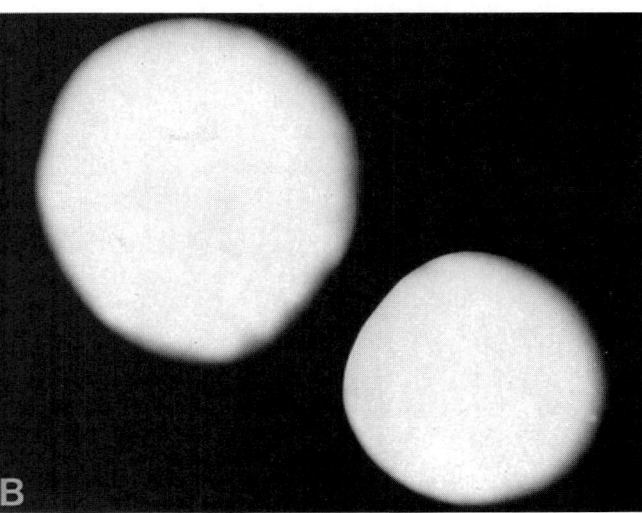

Fig. 220-17 Platelet whole mounts. *A*, Platelets from a normal individual left in contact with a form var-coated grid for 1 min and air-dried, showing 23 dense bodies. On average, four to eight dense bodies per platelet can be visualized in normal platelets with this method. *B*, Platelets from an individual with HPS using the same technique, showing no dense bodies. ×15,000. (*From Witkop et al.*[489] *Used by permission of the American Journal of Hematology.*)

dysfunction, and it is expected that mutations of many of these loci will be associated with the HPS phenotype in humans.[300] Mutations of two of these loci have already been identified (*pale ear*[64,412], *pearl*[302]) and a further locus has been associated with Chediak-Higashi syndrome (*beige*[413,414]). Individuals with HPS have also been identified who do not have mutations of any of the identified loci to date.[301,415]

The OCA in HPS is associated with the formation of cutaneous and ocular pigment, but the amount is variable. Some affected individuals have marked cutaneous hypopigmentation similar to that of OCA1A, others have white skin and yellow or blond hair similar to OCA1B or OCA2, and others have only moderate cutaneous hypopigmentation, suggesting OA rather than OCA. The variation can be seen within families as well as between families. Affected individuals in Puerto Rico have hair color that varies from white to yellow to brown.[1,415] Skin color is creamy white and definitely lighter than normally pigmented individuals in this population. Freckles are often present in the sun-exposed regions (face, neck, arms, and hands), often coalescing into large areas that look like normal dark-skin pigment, but tanning does not occur. Pigmented nevi are common. Iris translucency is present and correlates with iris color which varies from blue to brown,[416] and all of the ocular features of albinism (i.e., nystagmus, alternating strabismus, reduced acuity, foveal hypoplasia) are present. Visual acuity ranges from 20/50 to 20/400.[315,415,416] The presence of OCA may not be obvious in a Puerto Rican individual with brown hair, skin pigment in exposed areas, and brown eyes unless the cutaneous pigmentation is compared to unaffected family members (who are generally darker in pigment) and unless the ocular features of albinism are recognized. Affected individuals have been identified in other populations infrequently, and the phenotype shows the same degree of variation in pigmentation as is found in Puerto Rico.[60,417,418] Hair color varies from white to brown, and this correlates with the ethnic group. The skin is white and does not tan. Eye color varies from blue to pigmented. Excellent clinical photographs are available in several recent references.[415,419]

The bleeding diathesis in HPS is related to a deficiency of storage granules in the platelets (i.e., storage-pool-deficient platelets), as shown in Fig. 220-17. The storage granules or dense bodies are reduced in number or are absent, and this is associated with a deficiency of serotonin, adenine nucleotides, and calcium in the platelet.[1,3] As a result, HPS platelets do not show irreversible secondary aggregation when stimulated with agents that normally produce this response. This deficiency produces mild hemorrhagic

episodes in many affected individuals, including easy brusibility, epistaxis, hemoptysis, gingival bleeding with brushing or dental extraction, and postpartum bleeding.[415] Major bleeding events do occur, can be life-threatening, and may require transfusions, or treatment with desmopressin or cautery.[415]

The third part of the HPS triad is the production of autofluorescent ceroid material.[3] This is a yellow waxy material that can be found in urine of affected individuals, and is present in many tissues throughout the body when analyzed at autopsy.[420] The origin of the ceroid is unknown. Chemical analysis suggests that it arises from lipid peroxidation, and may be a manifestation of lysosomal dysfunction in humans.[3,420,421] The accumulation of ceroid in the lungs and gastrointestinal tract is associated with the clinical manifestations involving these tissues, and an obvious hypothesis is that ceroid leads to the manifestations of disease in these tissues, but this has not been proven. Ceroid is also present in the kidneys and the heart, but renal and cardiac functions are normal.[415,420]

The most severe clinical manifestations of HPS are related to the pulmonary and gastrointestinal changes. Interstitial pulmonary fibrosis has been described in many individuals with HPS, although the actual prevalence is unknown.[1,3,415,422] The fibrosis results in moderate to severe restrictive lung disease, and this is a frequent cause of death. A recent study of 49 individuals with HPS (28 Puerto Rican, 21 non-Puerto Rican) shows that homozygosity for the common 16-bp duplication mutation (described below) of the *HPS1* gene in individuals from Puerto Rico is associated with an increased frequency of clinically significant restrictive lung disease, as measured by pulmonary function tests and high-resolution computed tomography of the lungs.[415] Analysis of bronchoalveolar lavage fluid has shown the presence of PDGF (platelet derived growth factor) in affected and obligate heterozygotes, suggesting that this growth factor could be responsible for the development of the fibrosis.[422] The development of granulomatous colitis, presenting with abdominal pain and bloody diarrhea in a child or an adult, has also been described in many individuals with HPS.[1] The etiology of the colitis is unknown, and immunologic studies do not show an abnormality. The presence of ceroid material in the epithelial cells of the gut suggests that this material may be involved in the development of the colitis, but this has not been proven.

## Molecular Pathogenesis of HPS

Two loci are associated with human HPS: *HPS1* on chromosome 10q, and HPS2 on chromosome 5q. The murine homologue to

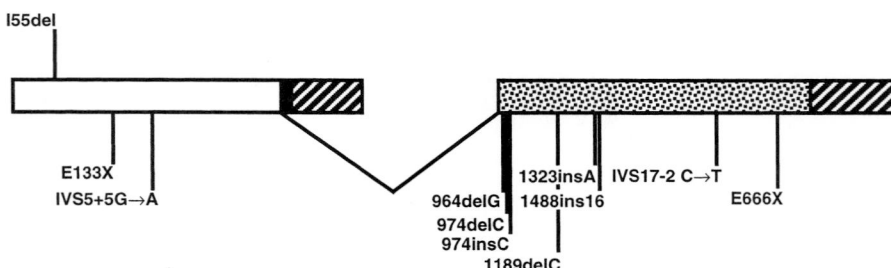

**Missense Mutations**

**Nonsense, Frameshift and Splice Site Mutations**

Fig. 220-18 Location of the mutations of the *HPS1* gene associated with Hermansky-Pudlak syndrome. Both of the *HPS1* gene transcripts that result from alternative splicing (black line) are shown. The nonfilled region represents the common coding sequences for both transcripts. The black region represents the coding region unique to the short transcript (1.5 kb). The stippled region represents the coding region unique to the large transcript (3.6 kb). Striped regions represent the 3′ untranslated region (UTR) of the transcripts. Missense mutations are indicated on the top and nonsense; frameshift, and splice-site mutations are indicated on the bottom. (*From Oetting et al.*[362] *Used by permission of John Wiley and Sons, Inc.*)

*HPS1* is *pale ear* (*ep*), and for *HPS2* it is *pearl* (*pe*).[300] Eleven mutations in the *HPS1* gene have been identified (Fig. 220-18). Nine of the mutations result in a truncated protein product. The other two mutations consist of a deletion of an isoleucine at codon 55 (I55del) and a splice-site mutation (IVS5 + 5G → A).[362] All but one (E133X) of the truncating mutations are in the unique sequence of the long transcript and none have been identified in the unique sequence of the short transcript. The most common mutation is a 16-bp duplication in exon 15 found in affected individuals in the northwestern region of Puerto Rico.[63] All individuals from Puerto Rico with mutations in the *HPS1* gene are homozygous for this mutation.[415]

Three frameshift mutations cluster in a mutational "hot spot" in exon 11 at codons 321 to 322.[423] This region consists of two sets of repeats, a sequence of six guanines, and eight cytosines divided by an CA dinucleotide. The frameshift mutations lie either within the run of guanines or cytosines. One frameshift mutation, 974insC, is the most common non-Puerto Rican mutation.[423] Haplotype analysis shows that this mutation has occurred on at least two separate occasions.[63] The individual with the I55del mutation was homozygous for this mutation and had a very mild phenotype, whereas the individual with the IVS5+5G → A mutation had a more typical HPS phenotype.[63] It has been hypothesized that the location of the truncating mutation correlates with the clinical severity of the HPS.[63] Mutations that lead to a longer protein that can be inserted into a membrane may disrupt structure or function of the tissue more than mutations that lead to a smaller protein that is lost and not inserted into a membrane.[63,419] The *HPS1* gene has 23 identified polymorphisms. Nine of these are within the coding region, four of which result in amino acid substitutions.

To date, mutations of the *HPS2* gene, the human homologue of the murine *pearl* gene, have been reported for two brothers.[302] The brothers had reduced skin and hair pigmentation, ocular features of albinism, absent platelet dense bodies, as well as persistent neutropenia associated with frequent respiratory tract infections and otitis media. The β3A subunit of the adaptor complex-3 (AP-3) is part of the mechanism facilitating vesicle budding from the *trans*-Golgi, indicating a primary role for vesicular transport dysfunction in HPS.[302,419,424] The putative location of the HPS2 gene is on chromosome 5q.[300]

### Chediak-Higashi Syndrome (CHS) (MIM 214500)

Chediak-Higashi syndrome is a rare autosomal recessive syndrome that consists of increased susceptibility to bacterial (primarily staphylococcal and streptococcal) infections, immune

defects, hypopigmentation, neurologic abnormalities, and the presence of giant peroxidase-positive lysosomal granules in peripheral blood granulocytes.[425] As with HPS, the hypopigmentation is the result of a primary defect that affects many cell types, including the melanocyte. The skin, hair, and eye pigment is reduced or diluted in CHS, but the affected individuals often do not have obvious albinism and the hypopigmentation may only be noted when compared to other family members. Hair color is light brown to blond, and the hair has a metallic silver-gray sheen. The skin is creamy white to slate gray. Iris pigment is present and nystagmus and photophobia may be present or absent.[1] Histologic studies of the eye in CHS show reduced iris pigment, a marked reduction in retinal pigment granules, and infiltration of the choroid with reticuloendothelial cells. Visual evoked potential studies show misrouting of the optic fibers. Bone marrow transplantation has been used to correct the hematologic manifestations of CHS, but this has no effect on the pigmentation.[426]

The primary defect in CHS is unknown. The susceptibility to bacterial infections appears to be the result of the abnormal granules in the neutrophils and other cells.[1,65] The hypopigmentation also arises from the formation of abnormal granules. Giant melanosomes form in the melanocyte and are unable to be transferred to the surrounding keratinocytes, leading to abnormal melanosome distribution and hypopigmentation. The pigment granules in the hair shaft are large and irregular in comparison to normally pigmented hair from an unaffected individual, and this pathologic change has been used to make a prenatal diagnosis of CHS.[427] The *beige* (*bg*) mouse is the murine model of CHS.[56,303,304,428,429] The *CHS1* gene encodes a protein with homology to a number of anonymous open reading frames and it has been suggested that the function of the beige/CHS protein is involved in vesicular transport,[56] which explains the defective vesicular transport to and from lysosomes and the aberrant compartmentalization of lysosomal and granular enzymes in this condition.[56]

### Molecular Pathogenesis of CHS

Eight mutations have been identified in the *CHS1* gene associated with Chediak-Higashi syndrome, including five frameshift and four nonsense mutations. There were also two patients that had unknown mutations that resulted in a reduction of mRNA levels.[430] Unlike the mutations of the *HPS1* gene, all but one of the *CHS1* gene mutations, 9590delA, were found in the common region of the two *CHS1* gene transcripts (Fig. 220-19). The 9590delA mutation in the long transcript is associated with a typical CHS phenotype similar to that seen with truncating

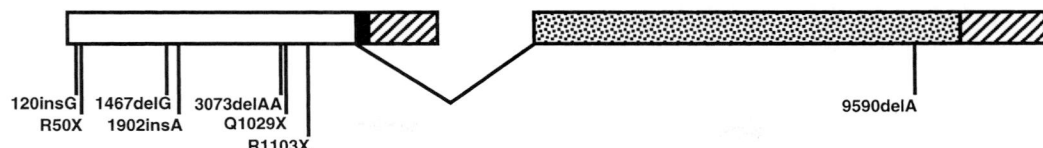

## Nonsense and Frameshift Mutations

**Fig. 220-19** Location of the mutations of the *CHS1* gene associated with Chediak-Higashi syndrome. This figure shows both of the *CHS1* gene transcripts that result from alternative splicing (black line). The nonfilled region represents the common coding sequences for both transcripts. The black region represents the coding region unique to the short transcript (6 kb; codes for 1990 amino acids). The stippled region represents the coding region unique to the large transcript (13 kb; codes for 3801 amino acids). Striped regions represent the 3′ untranslated region (UTR) of the transcripts. Missense mutations are indicated on the top and nonsense; frameshift and splice-site mutations are indicated on the bottom. (*From Oetting et al.[362] Used by permission of Wiley, Inc.*)

mutations in the common region, suggesting that mutations of the large transcript product may be all that is required for the CHS clinical phenotype.[414]

## OCULAR ALBINISM

Albinism in which the hypopigmentation is limited primarily to the eye is considerably less common than OCA 1 or OCA2, although the true prevalence is unknown (Table 220-4). Although the hypopigmentation in OA is clinically limited to the eye, changes in the cutaneous pigment system may also be present when the ultrastructure of these tissues is analyzed.

### OA1: X-Linked Recessive OA (MIM 300500)

**OA1 Phenotype.** OA1, which is known as the Nettleship-Falls type of OA, is X-linked recessive in inheritance.[1] Affected Caucasian males have irides that are blue to brown with variable translucency on globe transillumination, and all of the optic changes of albinism are present.[431–433] In African-American males, iris color is usually brown and there is little iris translucency. In Japanese affected males, iris color is brown and there is no iris translucency.[432] The skin and hair of Caucasian and Japanese males with OA1 is normally pigmented, while many African-American individuals may have scattered hypopigmented macules.

Heterozygous females can be clinically detected because of a mosaic pattern of ocular pigment that results from random X-inactivation.[1] A variegated pattern of retinal pigment and punctate areas of iris translucency are seen in approximately 80 percent of obligate heterozygotes females.[312] A small number of heterozygous females have ocular changes of albinism including nystagmus and reduced acuity that are thought to be the result of nonrandom patterns of X inactivation. Unilateral changes are occasionally observed in heterozygous females.[434]

Melanocytes are normal in OA1, but there are changes in the melanosomes.[1] Melanocytes in the skin, hair follicles, iris, and retina contain normal-sized melanosomes and large melanosomes called giant melanosomes, macromelanosomes, or melanin macroglobules. The giant melanosomes are also found in the melanocytes from the majority of obligate heterozygous females.[312] It is interesting that the OA1 gene product is a glycoprotein that is expressed at high levels in the retinal pigment epithelium and in the cutaneous melanocyte, where it localizes to the melanosomal membrane.[307,310] To date there is no explanation for why only a subset of melanosomes are abnormal in OA1. The melanosome defect in OA1 is systemic, affecting melanosomal biogenesis in the skin, as well as the eye, indicating that OA1 is actually a type of OCA in which the major manifestations are in the eye.

### Molecular Pathogenesis of OA1

The identified *OA1* gene mutations include 12 missense mutations, 1 nonsense mutation, 4 frameshift mutations, 1 3-bp deletion, 2 splice-site mutations, and 14 large deletions.[307,309,435–437] The missense mutations are located throughout the central coding region with some clustering between the first and second transmembrane regions (Fig. 220-20). The 14 deletions included 3 of exon 1, 2 of exon 2, 2 of exon 4, 6 that spanned exons 2 to 8, and 1 that deleted the entire gene.[435,436] Exon 2 is flanked by two Alu repeats in intron 1 and one Alu repeat in intron 2, providing a mechanism for the deletion of this exon.[309] The deletion of the entire gene produced a typical OA1 phenotype.[436] Additional missense mutations must be identified before structure/function analysis is available.

### Autosomal Recessive Ocular Albinism

Ocular albinism presenting in females and males in a sibship has been described as autosomal recessive ocular albinism.[1] This was

## Missense Mutations

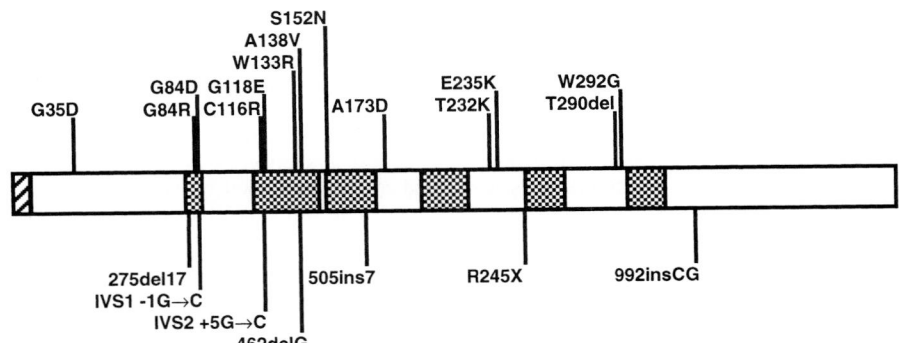

**Fig. 220-20** Location of the mutations of the OA1 gene associated with X-linked ocular albinism. The coding region of the OA1 gene (424 amino acids) is shown. The checkered boxes are putative *trans*-membrane regions. Missense mutations are indicated on the top and nonsense, frameshift, and splice-site mutations are indicated on the bottom. (*From Oetting et al.[362] Used by permission of John Wiley and Sons, Inc.*)

## Nonsense, Frameshift and Splice Site Mutations

described before the availability of molecular analysis, and recent studies suggest that true autosomal recessive ocular albinism may not exist. The phenotypic range of OCA1 and OCA2 is broad, and includes many individuals who would be included in this group.[340,356,380,438,439] For example, individuals who are diagnosed with autosomal recessive ocular albinism have been found to be compound heterozygotes with one pathologic and one functionally significant polymorphic mutation in codon 402 of the tyrosinase gene, indicating that this is actually OCA1.[356] One interesting family has been described in which affected individuals have Waardenburg syndrome type II and an apparent ocular albinism that affected males and females in four generations.[439] The Waardenburg syndrome was produced by a mutation of the *MITF* gene that segregated with this phenotype, while the hypopigmentation was again associated with heterozygosity or homozygosity for the codon 402 functional polymorphism of the *TYR* gene. Not all individuals who have apparent ocular albinism and minimal cutaneous hypopigmentation have been found to have mutations of the *TYR* or the *P* gene, however, and it is possible that the other pigment loci to be identified in the future will produce an ocular albinism phenotype.[440] Until additional loci are found, families with an autosomal recessive ocular albinism presentation should be evaluated for OCA1 or OCA2; the majority will fit in one of these two OCA types.

### Ocular Albinism and Deafness

Rare families have been described with ocular albinism and deafness.[1,439] One large Afrikaner family with X-linked OA and late-onset sensorineural deafness segregating together was reported in 1984.[441] Macromelanosomes were demonstrated in skin from affected males and obligate heterozygous females, and the clinical features of albinism were consistent with OA1. The locus for this condition maps to chromosome Xp22.3, indicating overlap with OA1.[441] It has not been established whether this syndrome of OA and deafness is part of the OA1 spectrum or related to a contiguous gene defect in this family. A family that contained three generations of males and females affected with congenital deafness and ocular albinism has been described, but little information on this family is available.[442]

### Åland Island Eye Disease/Forsius-Erickson Ocular Albinism

Forsius and Erickson described a family with X-linked tapetoretinal degeneration.[443] The locus was mapped to Xq12-21.[444,445] The clinical presentation includes nystagmus, myopia, astigmatism, foveal hypoplasia, reduced visual acuity, pigmentary changes in the retina, and changes in color vision. The optic nerves are normal and no misrouting is present.[446] This entity is described as a type of ocular albinism (MIM 300600) but it does not fit the criteria used in this chapter. This is most likely a primary photoreceptor abnormality.

## OTHER CONDITIONS WITH ALBINISM AND HYPOPIGMENTATION

### Autosomal Dominant OCA

Families demonstrating autosomal dominant expression of OCA or cutaneous hypopigmentation have been described, but characterization is incomplete and most do not fit the criteria for albinism.[447–449] In general, affected individuals have light skin that tans, light hair, and reduced iris pigment, but the ocular changes of albinism (reduced acuity, nystagmus, etc.) are often lacking. One French family had cutaneous hypopigmentation associated with skin melanocytes containing small melanosomes in three generations, suggesting a primary abnormality of melanosome structure.[448] A mother and son had ocular changes of albinism with the cutaneous albinism, while the mother's sib and father only had the hypopigmentation. Interestingly, the son also had Prader-Willi syndrome. A second family included

affected parents and children and normal grandparents.[447] Molecular analysis of OCA1 and OCA2 indicates that most families thought to have a dominant expression of OCA actually have mutations of the tyrosinase or the *P* gene with affected individuals in several sequential generations. The final characterization of dominant OCA awaits the careful evaluation of families with a clear autosomal dominant expression of OCA.

### Generalized Cutaneous Hypopigmentation (Albinoidism)

The term albinoidism refers to generalized cutaneous hypopigmentation in the absence of ocular changes of albinism.[450] This is not a very precise term, it is confusing because of its similarity to albinism, and it probably has no place in the clinical lexicon. A more correct term is generalized cutaneous hypopigmentation. The molecular investigation of generalized cutaneous hypopigmentation is just beginning. Families with generalized cutaneous hypopigmentation have been described, however, and have the potential of representing new genetically distinct syndromes. Several examples are given in the following paragraphs. Clinical syndromes that include cutaneous spotting (localized hypopigmentation) are described in the next section.

**Tietz Syndrome (MIM 103500).** In 1963, Tietz described a family with generalized cutaneous hypopigmentation and no evidence of ocular changes of albinism.[451] The original description of the hypopigmentation included "typical albino skin" with light/blond hair and blue eyes. Affected family members also had deafness and there was cosegregation of the hypopigmentation and hearing loss in multiple generations with a dominant pattern of inheritance. Recent analysis of this family identified a mutation (N207K) of the *MITF* gene that segregates with the hypopigmentation/deafness.[452] Further description of the hypopigmentation included white hair at birth that gradually became pigmented to a blond color, blue irides with an "albinoid" fundus, but no nystagmus or other ocular changes. An additional family presenting with generalized cutaneous hypopigmentation and deafness associated with a *MITF* gene mutation (DelR217) has been described.[453] The generalized cutaneous hypopigmentation in this family was not characterized, but the hair of an 18-month-old child was auburn, while that of his mother had been auburn until the development of premature graying at 16 years of age. Both families have a phenotype that is distinct from type 2A Waardenburg syndrome (see below), but are likely to be part of the spectrum of this diagnostic category.

**Oculocerebral Syndrome with Hypopigmentation (Cross Syndrome) (MIM 257800).** Cross syndrome presents with generalized cutaneous hypopigmentation and neurologic abnormalities that include developmental delay, mental retardation, spasticity, athetoid movements, muscle atrophy, and growth retardation.[1,454,455] The features of this syndrome are quite variable and all cases may not represent the same entity. The cutaneous hypopigmentation is generalized but variable in degree, and the hair has a white, silver, or silver-gray appearance.[456,457] Some of the affected individuals have had ocular changes of albinism, suggesting a diagnosis of OCA1 or OCA2 rather than hypopigmentation limited to the hair and skin.[458]

**Griscelli Syndrome (MIM 214450).** Griscelli et al. reported two girls with hypopigmentation characterized as silver-gray hair and scattered hypopigmented areas surrounded by normal or hyperpigmented skin.[459] No ocular features of albinism were present, even though the term "partial albinism" was used in the title of the paper. Both had neutropenia, thrombocytopenia, absent delayed hypersensitivity, and hypogammaglobulinemia, and repeated infections; one girl died with sepsis. Parents and sibs were normal and inheritance appeared to be autosomal recessive. Melanin was irregularly distributed in the skin with large clumps. Melanocyte number and size were normal. Melanocytes were full of normal-sized pigmented melanosomes and few were passed to keratino-cytes. Hair shafts contained large clumps of pigment, primarily in the medullar zone, interspersed with normal-sized pigment granules, and produced the silver-gray sheen. Additional cases have been reported, with further characterization of this syndrome.[460–465] The majority of reported cases are Arab. Skin pigment varies from normal to patchy or generalized hypopigmentation. Neurologic symptoms include seizures, ataxia, dysmetria, intention tremor, hemiparesis, and psychomotor deterioration. An accelerated phase develops, similar to that with CHS, associated with sepsis, fever, and death. Bone marrow transplantation eliminates the immunodeficiency, but has no effect on pigmentation.[83] This syndrome is very similar to the findings in the dilute mouse.[459] The dilute locus encodes myosin-Va, a member of the unconventional myosin family.[74] Griscelli syndrome maps to chromosome 15q21, the location of the myosin-Va (*MYO5a*) gene, and mutations of this gene have been found in four families, indicating the class V myosins are involved in membrane transport and organelle trafficking.[84]

**OCA, Black Locks, and Cell Migration Disorder.** Two families have been described with an autosomal recessive syndrome of OCA and deafness.[466] The OCA (MIM 227010) is unusual in that there are patches of pigmented hair (black locks) in the scalp. One child also had a severe defect of intestinal innervation. These changes are suggestive of a neural crest migration defect, but the gene has not been identified.

**Cutaneous Pigment Abnormalities and Deafness.** A large Moroccan Sephardic family included multiple males who had irregular skin pigmentation and deafness expressed in an X-linked recessive pattern.[467] The hair was white and the skin had well-demarcated white and hyperpigmented patches. The eyes were normal with no evidence of the changes of albinism. The gene for this syndrome was mapped to chromosome Xq24-26.[468,469] It has been proposed that this syndrome is an X-linked dominant form of type II Waardenburg syndrome.[470] This syndrome does not fit the criteria of albinism used in this chapter because of the lack of ocular changes.

### Localized Hypopigmentation

There are a variety of conditions that present with localized hypopigmentation. The general cutaneous pigment is normal, but variably sized patches of white skin are present at birth or develop with time. The ocular features of albinism, including nystagmus, reduced retinal pigment, and misrouting of the optic fibers at the chiasm, are absent in these conditions (i.e., they are not types of albinism), but the iris pigment may be reduced. Two conditions with congenital presentation are discussed below.

**Piebaldism (MIM 172800).** Piebaldism presents with a characteristic pattern of white forelock and multiple symmetrical white or depigmented macules. This condition has been reported in the literature under a variety of names, including partial albinism, familial white spotting, white forelock, or piebaldism.[1] The white forelock is usually present at birth or early in life, and can be only a few strands or a large patch of white hair. The underlying skin is white. The white macules are found on the face, trunk, and extremities, and the hair growing from them is white. Melanocytes are absent in the white patches of skin and the hair follicles of the white hair. Piebaldism is autosomal dominant in inheritance.

Mutations of the *KIT* gene are responsible for piebaldism.[9,471–476] The human *KIT* gene has 21 exons and is 70 kb in length.[8,473] The gene organization is almost identical to the FMS proto-oncogene on chromosome 4. The *KIT* transcript is 5 kb in length, codes for 976 amino acids, and produces a protein of 145 kDa. There are three major domains of the KIT protein: an extracellular domain containing the ligand binding site (the steel factor; see below); an intracellular domain containing the tyrosine kinase site; and a *trans*-membrane region between these two

domains. There are still unresolved differences between the phenotype of mutations in the murine *c-kit* gene and the *KIT* locus of humans. Murine mutations include the involvement of erythropoiesis, germ cell development, and melanogenesis, while piebaldism in humans involves only melanogenesis.[11]

The ligand in the murine *c-kit* gene is the hematopoietic growth factor (KL), or murine stem cell factor (SCF), encoded by the steel locus (*Sl*) in the mouse.[477–480] This gene has been identified as the mast cell growth factor (MGF) in humans. Mutations at the *Sl* locus prevent binding of the *c-kit* ligand to the receptor resulting in a pigmented phenotype as seen in *W* locus mutant loci.[478,479] The steel phenotype also affects erythropoiesis and germ cell development as observed with the *W* locus. The human MGF has been mapped to chromosome 12q22. At present, there are no reported mutations of this gene or associated phenotypes.

Several mutations have been found in the human *KIT* gene associated with piebaldism. As was found in the mouse, these different mutations result in a spectrum of phenotypes ranging from mild to severe forms of piebaldism.[481] The majority of the mutations affect either the tyrosine kinase activity or the transmembrane domain, and are associated with the more severe phenotypes.[473] Mutations associated with mild phenotypes are located within the extracellular ligand-binding domain. The mutations associated with the mild phenotype are mostly frame-shift mutations, resulting in the production of a truncated protein missing most of the protein. This produces haploinsufficiency for KIT-dependent signal transduction. The more severe forms are caused by frameshift or missense mutations producing a nonfunctional protein that can combine with either other nonfunctional proteins or the product from the normal allele producing a nonfunctional heterodimer. This results in a 75 percent reduction of functional receptor dimer, producing a dominant negative affect.[473] Other mutations may result in differing levels of stability for the mutated protein and may account for the variability in the phenotype for these mutant alleles.

**Waardenburg Syndrome (MIM 193500).** The combination of lateral displacement of the inner ocular canthi with a broad base of the nose, white forelock (poliosis), heterochromatic irides (different color of the two irides), hyperplasia of the medial portion of the eyebrows, and congenital sensorineural hearing loss, is known as Waardenburg syndrome (WS).[482,483] Four types of WS are described: WS type I with lateral displacement of the inner canthi (telecanthus); WS type II without telecanthus; WS type III with limb muscle hypoplasia and joint contractures; and WS type IV with Hirschsprung disease.[483] Types I to III are autosomal dominant, while type IV is autosomal recessive in inheritance. The clinical manifestations are varied and diverse, and excellent reviews are available.[483]

Mutations in two genes are responsible for Waardenburg syndrome: the *PAX3* gene for WS types I and III, and the *MITF* gene for WS type II. The *PAX3* gene contains 3 exons and codes for a protein with 836 amino acids. Analysis of individuals with WS revealed 50 different *PAX3* gene mutations, including missense, nonsense, and frameshift mutations.[483] The mutations for the most part cluster in either the paired box domain or the homeobox domain, and can be divided into three classes. The first class alters the paired domain of the protein. These mutations affect the amino acids that make contact with important DNA at the protein-DNA binding regions such as the *Pax1* gene mutation in the mouse that causes the undulated (un) phenotype.[484,485] In the *Pax1* gene, a glycine to serine missense mutation alters the protein-DNA binding properties of this protein. The second class of mutations does not affect the paired domain but eliminates the conserved octapeptide and homeobox domain, and is important for DNA binding. The third class results from frameshift, nonsense, and splice-site mutations, and produces a truncated protein product.[29,486] There are reports of heterogeneity of WS, and this may be the result of different alleles of the *PAX3* gene resulting in different phenotypes.[487] The hypothesis is that the *PAX* gene family, and probably the *PAX3* gene, encode nuclear *trans*-acting transcriptional factors that regulate several target genes. Different mutations, especially missense mutations, may vary the DNA binding or the specificity of the DNA binding, and thus produce the different phenotypes observed.

Mutations in the *MITF* gene on chromosome 3p are responsible for Waardenburg type II.[453,482,488] The gene contains 9 exons and codes for a 419-amino acid that is a basis helix-loop-helix-leucine zipper (bHLH-ZIP) transcription factor. There are 11 mutations reported, the majority located in either the basic domain, the helix-loop-helix domain, or the leucine zipper domain, with 5 being missense mutations.[483] These mutations would most likely result in loss of function, affecting the ability of the protein to bind to DNA regulatory sites, resulting in a haploinsufficiency of the protein product.[44]

## EVALUATION AND MANAGEMENT OF ALBINISM

Proper evaluation and management of individuals with albinism are critical to their normal growth and development and eventual adult life. Affected individuals have only hypopigmentation and the associated ocular (and auditory) changes; there are no changes in other functions of the brain. Specifically, mental retardation is not part of albinism; another explanation must be considered for a child or adult with developmental delay or mental retardation. Other medical problems have been reported with different types of albinism, but most of these examples appear to be cosegregation of two conditions in a family. There are several specific areas of concern for individuals with albinism: correct diagnosis, skin care, and ophthalmologic care.

### Diagnosis

The diagnosis of albinism is established when an individual with oculocutaneous or ocular hypopigmentation is found to have the ocular changes as described above. Nystagmus, reduced retinal pigment, reduced acuity, and misrouting of the optic fibers at the chiasm are present to different degrees in all patients with albinism and the diagnosis cannot be made without these characteristic findings. Iris pigment is variable in amount in OCA and OA, and the iris translucency can vary from complete transillumination to punctate translucent areas. It is occasionally necessary to perform a visual evoked potential study to demonstrate misrouting of the optic fibers when an individual presents with moderately reduced cutaneous and retinal pigment and nystagmus. The demonstration of misrouting is the most critical diagnostic criteria, and the diagnosis of albinism cannot be made without clinical or electrophysiological evidence of this. In most cases, the finding of nystagmus, alternating strabismus, foveal hypoplasia, reduced acuity, and reduced depth perception are sufficient for the diagnosis and an evoked potential study is not necessary.

An individual with OCA can be classified as OCA1 or OCA2 by clinical and molecular criteria. The medical history is important. Almost all individuals with OCA1, even when they have OCA1B and form moderate amounts of hair and iris pigment as they mature, have white or nearly white hair and white skin at birth. The hairbulb incubation test and the hairbulb tyrosinase assay were used to distinguish OCA1 from OCA2 in the past, but they are not precise and overlap exists. Hairbulb analysis is no longer part of the analysis of a child or an adult with OCA. Molecular analysis provides the most accurate method of diagnosis, and should be considered if the correct diagnosis or family counseling are in question.

The diagnosis of OA1 is made when a male presents with typical features of this condition, and the family history and maternal examination are consistent with this diagnosis. With no family history of OA and a normal maternal eye examination, it is necessary to demonstrate the presence of macromelanosomes in skin or hairbulbs of the affected male to make this diagnosis. Electron microscopic examination of skin or hairbulb melanocytes is the preferred method for this analysis.

The diagnosis of HPS should be considered with any individual who has OCA and evidence of unusual bleeding or bruising. It is not necessary to evaluate all individuals with OCA, because HPS is not common, but the diagnosis needs to be considered in all Puerto Rican individuals with OCA. Several methods have been used to make the diagnosis of HPS, and the most reliable is the demonstration of a lack of dense bodies in platelets.[489] Aspirin or aspirin-like medications must be withheld from all individuals with HPS, and should be avoided in individuals, particularly children, with OCA.

Prenatal diagnosis of OCA1 has been performed using skin biopsy and molecular analysis.[490–492]

### Skin Care

Individuals with albinism who have cutaneous hypopigmentation need to protect their skin from ultraviolet radiation. Physical methods, including long-sleeve shirts, long pants, and hats with a wide brim are excellent for this, but are often underutilized because of fashion or age. Sunscreens are very effective in protecting the skin and should be employed whenever possible. The Sun Protection Factor (SPF) rating of a sunscreen should be greater than 30 for good protection.

Some general information is helpful. The latitude is important in ultraviolet exposure, and an individual in New Jersey can tolerate more sun than one in Florida. Sand reflects ultraviolet rays and it is possible to burn when sitting in the shade on a beach. The greatest intensity of ultraviolet light occurs at the summer solstice, and between the hours of 10 AM and 2 PM standard time, and protection or avoidance of the sun in these periods can greatly reduce ultraviolet exposure.

### Ophthalmologic Care

All individuals with albinism need regular eye care. Hyperopia, myopia, and astigmatism are common and need to be corrected to obtain the best corrected visual acuity. Correction should be reevaluated on an annual basis, starting early in life. Surgery has been used successfully in albinism to reduce nystagmus, but the role of surgery in the regular care of affected individuals is unknown.[493]

Children with albinism should be placed in a regular classroom provided that the teacher and the school gives specific attention to their special needs for vision. Braille training is rarely necessary. Teachers should be instructed to use high-contrast written materials. Copies of the teacher's board notes allow the child to read the material as it is presented to the class. Large type books are available for many regular textbooks. Children with albinism should be expected to participate in all school activities, including physical education, field trips, and extracurricular activities.

### Counseling

A booklet entitled "Facts About Albinism" is available on the home page for the International Albinism Center at the University of Minnesota (www.cbc.umn.edu/iac). All families should be informed about NOAH, the national organization of albinism and hypopigmentation (www.albinism.org). A national NOAH meeting for families is held every 2 years, and provides an excellent place for parents to talk with other parents, and for affected children and teens to interact and talk about the different issues of having albinism. The HPS Network (www.medhelp.org/web/hpsn.htm) provides information and support for individuals and families with HPS.

## REFERENCES

1. King RA, Hearing VJ, Creel DJ, Oetting WS. Albinism, in Scriver CR, Beaudet AL, Sly WS, Valle D (eds): *Metabolic and Molecular Bases of Inherited Disease*, 7th ed. New York, McGraw-Hill, 1995, p 4353.
2. Witkop CJ, Van Scott EJ, Jacoby GA: Evidence for two forms of autosomal recessive albinism in man. *Proc Second Intern Cong Hum Genet* 2:1064, 1961.

3. Witkop CJ, Quevedo WC, Fitzpatrick TB, King RA: Albinism, in Scriver CR, Beaudet AL, Sly WS, Valle D (eds): *The Metabolic Basis of Inherited Diseases*, 6th ed. New York, McGraw-Hill, 1989, p 2905.

4. Prota G: *Melanins and Melanogenesis.* New York, Academic Press, 1992.

5. Nordlund JJ, Ortonne J-P: The normal color of human skin, in Nordlund JJ, Boissy RE, Hearing VJ, King RA, Ortonne J-P (eds): *The Pigmentary System. Physiology and Pathophysiology.* New York, Oxford University Press, 1998, p 475.

6. Jackson IJ: Homologous pigmentation mutations in human, mouse and other model organisms. *Hum Mol Genet* **6**:1613, 1997.

7. Boissy RE: Extracutaneous melanocytes, in Nordlund JJ, Boissy RE, Hearing VJ, King RA, Ortonne J-P (eds): *The Pigmentary System. Physiology and Pathophysiology.* New York, Oxford University Press, 1998, p 59.

8. Yarden Y, Kuang W-J, Yang-Feng T, Coussens L, Munemitsu S, Dull TJ, Chen E, Schlessinger J, Francke U, Ullrich A: Human proto-oncogene *c-kit*: A new cell surface receptor tyrosine kinase for an unidentified ligand. *EMBO J* **6**:3341, 1987.

9. Giebel LB, Spritz RA: Mutation of the *KIT* (mast/stem cell growth factor receptor) proto-oncogene in human piebaldism. *Proc Natl Acad Sci U S A* **88**:8696, 1991.

10. Hayashi SI, Kunisada T, Ogawa M, Yamaguchi K, Nishikawa SI: Exon skipping by mutation of an authentic splice site of *c-kit* gene in *W/W* mouse. *Nucleic Acid Res* **19**:1267, 1991.

11. Spritz RA: Lack of apparent hematologic abnormalities in human patients with *c-kit* (stem cell factor receptor) gene mutations. *Blood* **79**:2497, 1992.

12. Duttlinger R, Manova K, Berrozpe G, Chu TY, DeLeon V, Timokhina I, Chaganti RSK, Zelenetz AD, Bachvarova RF, Besmer P: The Wsh and Ph mutations affect the *c-kit* expression profile: *c-kit* misexpression in embryogenesis impairs melanogenesis in Wsh and Ph mutant mice. *Proc Natl Acad Sci U S A* **92**:3754, 1995.

13. Luo D, Chen H, Searles G, Jimbow K: Coordinated mRNA expression of c-kit with tyrosinase and TRP-1 in melanin pigmentation of normal and malignant human melanocytes and transient activation of tyrosinase by Kit/SCF-R. *Melanoma Res* **5**:303, 1995.

14. Norris A, Todd C, Graham A, Quinn AG, Thody AJ: The expression of the *c-kit* receptor by epidermal melanocytes may be reduced in vitiligo. *Brit J Dermatol* **134**:299, 1996.

15. Hemesath TJ, Price ER, Takemoto C, Badalian T, Fisher DE: MAP kinase links the transcription factor microphthalmia to *c-kit* signalling in melanocytes. *Nature* **391**:298-301, 1998.

16. Price ER, Ding H, Badalian T, Bhattacharya S, Takemoto C, Yao T, Hemesath TJ, Fisher DE: Lineage-specific signaling in melanocytes: *c-kit* stimulation recruits p300/CBP to microphthalmia. *J Biol Chem* **273**:17983, 1998.

17. Wehrle-Haller B, Morrison-Graham K, Weston JA: Ectopic c-kit expression affects the fate of melanocyte precursors in patch mutant embryos. *Devel Biol* **177**:463, 1996.

18. Besmer P, Manova K, Duttlinger R, Huang EJ, Packer A, Gyssler C, Bachvarova RF: The kit-ligand (steel factor) and its receptor *c-kit*/W: Pleiotropic roles in gametogenesis and melanogenesis. *Development* **1993(Suppl)**:125, 1993.

19. Morrison-Graham K, Weston JA: Transient steel factor dependence by neural crest-derived melanocyte precursors. *Devel Biol* **159**:346, 1993.

20. Reid K, Nishikawa SI, Bartlett PF, Murphy M: Steel factor directs melanocyte development in vitro through selective regulation of the number of *c-kit*+ progenitors. *Devel Biol* **169**:568, 1995.

21. Wehrle-Haller B, Weston JA: Soluble and cell-bound forms of steel factor activity play distinct roles in melanocyte precursor dispersal and survival on the lateral neural crest migration pathway. *Development* **121**:731, 1995.

22. Guo CS, Wehrle-Haller B, Rossi J, Ciment G: Autocrine regulation of neural crest cell development by steel factor. *Devel Biol* **184**:61, 1997.

23. Asher JH, Friedman TB: Mouse and hamster mutants as models for Waardenburg syndromes in humans. *J Med Genet* **27**:618, 1990.

24. Moase CE, Trasler DG: Splotch locus mouse mutants: Models for neural tube defects and Waardenburg syndrome type I in humans. *J Med Genet* **29**:145, 1992.

25. Tassabehji M, Read AP, Newton VE, Harris R, Balling R, Gruss P, Strachan T: Waardenburg's syndrome patients have mutations in the human homologue of the *Pax-3* paired box gene. *Nature* **355**:635, 1992.

26. Steel KP, Smith RJH: Normal hearing in Splotch (Sp/+), the mouse homologue of Waardenburg syndrome type 1. *Nat Genet* **2**:75, 1992.

27. Epstein DJ, Vekemans M, Gros P: Splotch (Sp2H), a mutation affecting development of the mouse neural tube, shows a deletion within the paired homeodomain of Pax-3. *Cell* **67**:767, 1991.

28. Burri M, Tromvoukis Y, Bopp D, Frigerio G, Noll M: Conservation of the paired domain in metazoans and its structure in three isolated human genes. *EMBO J* **8**:1183, 1989.

29. Morell R, Friedman TB, Moeljopawiro S, Hartono S, Asher JH Jr: A frameshift mutation in the HuP2 paired domain of the probable human homolog of murine *Pax-3* is responsible for Waardenburg syndrome type 1 in an Indonesian family. *Hum Mol Genet* **1**:243, 1992.

30. Hodgkinson CA, Moore KJ, Nakayama A, Steingrimsson E, Copeland NG, Jenkins NA, Arnheiter H: Mutations at the mouse microphthalmia locus are associated with defects in a gene encoding a novel basic-helix-loop-helix-zipper protein. *Cell* **74**:395, 1993.

31. Yasumoto K, Yokoyama K, Shibata K, Tomita Y, Shibahara S: Microphthalmia-associated transcription factor as a regulator for melanocyte-specific transcription of the human tyrosinase gene. *Mol Cell Biol* **14**:8058, 1994.

32. Hemesath TJ, Steingrimsson E, McGill G, Hansen MJ, Vaught J, Hodgkinson CA, Arnheiter H, Copeland NG, Jenkins NA, Fisher DE: *Microphthalmia*, a critical factor in melanocyte development, defines a discrete transcription factor family. *Genes Dev* **8**:2770, 1994.

33. Bentley NJ, Eisen T, Goding CR: Melanocyte-specific expression of the human tyrosinase promoter: Activation by the microphthalmia gene product and role of the initiator. *Mol Cell Biol* **14**:7996, 1994.

34. Ganss R, Schütz G, Beermann F: The mouse tyrosinase gene. Promoter modulation by positive and negative regulatory elements. *J Biol Chem* **269**:29808, 1994.

35. Bertolotto C, Bille K, Ortonne JP, Ballotti R: Regulation of tyrosinase gene expression by cAMP in B16 melanoma cells involves two CATGTG motifs surrounding the TATA box: Implication of the microphthalmia gene product. *J Cell Biol* **134**:747, 1996.

36. Yasumoto K, Mahalingam H, Suzuki H, Yoshizawa M, Yokoyama K, Shibahara S: Transcriptional activation of the melanocyte-specific genes by the human homolog of the mouse microphthalmia protein. *J Biochem* **118**:874, 1995.

37. Bertolotto C, Busca R, Abbe P, Bille K, Aberdam E, Ortonne JP, Ballotti R: Different *cis*-acting elements are involved in the regulation of TRP1 and TRP2 promoter activities by cyclic AMP: pivotal role of M boxes (GTCATGTGCT) and of microphthalmia. *Mol Cell Biol* **18**:694, 1998.

38. Bertolotto C, Abbe P, Hemesath TJ, Bille K, Fisher DE, Ortonne JP, Ballotti R: Microphthalmia gene product as a signal transducer in cAMP-induced differentiation of melanocytes. *J Cell Biol* **142**:827, 1998.

39. Price ER, Horstmann MA, Wells AG, Weilbaecher KN, Takemoto CM, Landis MW, Fisher DE: aMSH signaling regulates expression of microphthalmia, a gene deficient in Waardenburg syndrome. *J Biol Chem* **273**:33042, 1998.

40. Amae S, Fuse N, Yasumoto K, Sato S, Yajima I, Yamamoto H, Udono T, Durlu YK, Tamai M, Takahashi K, Shibahara S: Identification of a novel isoform of microphthalmia-associated transcription factor that is enriched in retinal pigment epithelium. *Biochem Biophys Res Commun* **247**:710, 1998.

41. Motohashi H, Hozawa K, Oshima T, Takeuchi T, Takasaka T: Dysgenesis of melanocytes and cochlear dysfunction in mutant microphthalmia (mi) mice. *Hear Res* **80**:10, 1994.

42. Opdecamp K, Nakayama A, Nguyen MTT, Hodgkinson CA, Pavan WJ, Arnheiter H: Melanocyte development in vivo and in neural crest cell cultures: Crucial dependence on the Mitf basic-helix-loop-helix-zipper transcription factor. *Development* **124**:2377, 1997.

43. Aberdam E, Bertolotto C, Sviderskaya EV, de Thillot V, Hemesath TJ, Fisher DE, Bennett DC, Ortonne JP, Ballotti R: Involvement of microphthalmia in the inhibition of melanocyte lineage differentiation and of melanogenesis by agouti signal protein. *J Biol Chem* **273**:19560, 1998.

44. Nobukuni Y, Watanabe A, Takeda K, Skarka H, Tachibana M: Analyses of loss-of-function mutations of the MITF gene suggest that haploinsufficiency is a cause of Waardenburg syndrome type 2A. *Am J Hum Genet* **59**:76, 1996.

45. Tachibana M, Takeda K, Nobukuni Y, Urabe K, Long JE, Meyers KA, Aaronson SA, Miki T: Ectopic expression of MITF, a gene for Waardenburg syndrome type 2, converts fibroblasts to cells with melanocyte characteristics. *Nat Genet* **14**:50–54, 1996.

46. Watanabe A, Takeda K, Ploplis B, Tachibana M: Epistatic relationship between Waardenburg syndrome genes MITF and PAX3. *Nat Genet* **18**:283, 1998.

47. Southard-Smith EM, Kos L, Pavan WJ: Sox10 mutation disrupts neural crest development in Dom Hirschsprung mouse model. *Nat Genet* **18**:60, 1998.
48. Herbarth B, Pingault V, Bondurand N, Kuhlbrodt K, Hermans-Borgmeyer I, Puliti A, Lemort N, Goossens M, Wegner M: Mutation of the Sry-related Sox10 gene in Dominant megacolon, a mouse model for human Hirschsprung disease. *Proc Natl Acad Sci U S A* **95**:5161, 1998.
49. Kuhlbrodt K, Schmidt C, Sock E, Pingault V, Bondurand N, Goossens M, Wegner M: Functional analysis of Sox10 mutations found in human Waardenburg-Hirschsprung patients. *J Biol Chem* **273**:23033, 1998.
50. Puffenberger EG, Kauffman ER, Bolk S, Matise TC, Washington SS, Angrist M, Weissenbach J, Garver KL, Mascari M, Ladda R, Slaugenhaupt SA, Chakravarti A: Identity-by-descent and association mapping of a recessive gene for Hirschsprung disease on human chromosome 13q22. *Hum Mol Genet* **3**:1217, 1994.
51. Puffenberger EG, Hosoda K, Washington SS, Nakao K, deWit D, Yanagisawa M, Chakravarti A: A missense mutation of the endothelin-B receptor gene in multigenic Hischsprung's disease. *Cell* **79**:1257, 1994.
52. Hosoda K, Hammer RE, Richardson JA, Greenstein Baynash A, Cheung JC, Giaid A, Yanagisawa M: Targeted and natural (piebald-lethal) mutations of endothelin-B receptor gene produce megacolon associated with spotted coat color in mice. *Cell* **79**:1267, 1994.
53. Pavan WJ, Tilghman SM: Piebald lethal (sl) acts early to disrupt the development of neural crest-derived melanocytes. *Proc Natl Acad Sci U S A* **91**:7159, 1994.
54. Diment S, Eidelman M, Rodriguez GM, Orlow SJ: Lysosomal hydrolases are present in melanosomes and are elevated in melanizing cells. *J Biol Chem* **270**:4213, 1995.
55. Orlow SJ: Melanosomes are specialized members of the lysosomal lineage of organelles. *J Invest Dermatol* **105**:3, 1995.
56. Nagle DL, Karim MA, Woolf EA, Holmgren L, Bork P, Misumi DJ, McGrail SH, Dussault BJ, Perou CM, Boissy RE, Duyk GM, Spritz RA, Moore KJ: Identification and mutation analysis of the complete gene for Chediak-Higashi syndrome. *Nat Genet* **14**:307, 1996.
57. Perou CM, Leslie JD, Green W, Li L, McVey Ward D, Kaplan J: The beige/Chediak-Higashi syndrome gene encodes a widely expressed cytosolic protein. *J Biol Chem* **272**:29790, 1997.
58. Napolitano A, Vincensi MR, d'Ischia M, Prota G: A new benzothiazole derivative by degradation of pheomelanins with alkaline hydrogen peroxide. *Tetrahedron Lett* **37**:6799, 1996.
59. Witkop CJ, Babcock MN, Rao GHR, Gaudier F, Summers CG, Shanahan F, Harmon KR, Townsend D, Sedano HO, King RA, Cal SX, White JG: Albinism and Hermansky-Pudlak syndrome in Puerto Rico. *Bol Asoc Med P R* **82**:333, 1990.
60. Schallreuter KU, Frenk E, Wolfe LS, Witkop CJ, Wood JM: Hermansky-Pudlak syndrome in a Swiss population. *Dermatology* **187**:248, 1993.
61. Fukai K, Oh J, Frenk E, Almodovar C, Spritz RA: Linkage disequilibrium mapping of the gene for Hermansky-Pudlak syndrome to chromosome 10q23.1-23.3. *Hum Mol Genet* **4**:1665, 1995.
62. Wildenberg SC, Oetting WS, Almadovar C, Krumwiede M, White JG, King RA: A gene causing Hermansky-Pudlak syndrome in a Puerto Rican population maps to chromosome 10q2. *Am J Hum Genet* **57**:755, 1995.
63. Oh J, Bailin T, Fukai K, Feng GH, Ho L, Mao J, Frenk E, Tamura N, Spritz RA: Positional cloning of a gene for Hermansky-Pudlak syndrome, a disorder of cytoplasmic organelles. *Nat Genet* **14**:300, 1996.
64. Feng GH, Bailin T, Oh J, Spritz RA: Mouse pale ear (ep) is homologous to human Hermansky-Pudlak syndrome and contains a rare "AT-AC" intron. *Hum Mol Genet* **6**:793, 1997.
65. Spritz RA, Oh J, Luo Z-X, Feng GH, Bordini B: Genetic and functional studies of Hermansky-Pudlak syndrome [Abstract]. *Pigment Cell Res* **11**:176, 1998.
66. Kemp EH, Gawkrodger DJ, Watson PF, Weetman AP: Immunoprecipitation of melanogenic enzyme autoantigens with vitiligo sera: evidence for cross-reactive autoantibodies to tyrosinase and tyrosinase-related protein-2 (TRP-2). *Clin Exp Immunol* **109**:495, 1997.
67. Wildenberg SC, Fryer JP, Gardner JM, Oetting WS, Brilliant MH, King RA: Identification of a novel transcript produced by the gene responsible for the Hermansky-Pudlak syndrome in Puerto Rico. *J Invest Dermatol* **110**:777, 1998.
68. Chelly J, Tumer Z, Tonnesen T, Petterson A, Ishikawa-Brush Y, Tommerup N, Horn N, Monaco AP: Isolation of a candidate gene for

Menkes disease that encodes a potential heavy metal binding protein. *Nat Genet* **3**:14, 1993.
69. Davies K: Cloning the Menkes disease gene. *Nat Genet* **3**:91, 1993.
70. Mercer JFB, Livingston J, Hall B, Paynter JA, Begy C, Chandrasekharappa S, Lockhart P, Grimes A, Bhave M, Siemieniak D, Glover TW: Isolation of a partial candidate gene for Menkes disease by positional cloning. *Nat Genet* **3**:20, 1993.
71. Vulpe C, Levinson B, Whitney S, Packman S, Gitschier J: Isolation of a candidate gene for Menkes disease and evidence that it encodes a copper-transporting ATPase. *Nat Genet* **3**:7, 1993.
72. Camakaris J, Danks DM, Ackland L, Cartwright E, Borger P, Cotton RGH: Altered copper metabolism in cultured cells from human Menkes' syndrome and mottled mouse mutants. *Biochem Genet* **18**:117, 1980.
73. Peterson J, Drolet BA, Esterly NB: Menkes' kinky hair syndrome. *Pediatr Dermatol* **15**:137, 1998.
74. Mercer JA, Seperack PK, Strobel MC, Copeland NG, Jenkins NA: Novel myosin heavy chain encoded by murine dilute coat color locus. *Nature* **349**:709, 1991.
75. Espreafico EM, Cheney RE, Matteoli M, Nascimento AAC, DeCamilli PV, Larson RE, Mooseker MS: Primary structure and cellular localization of chicken brain myosin-V (p190), an unconventional myosin with calmodulin light chains. *J Cell Biol* **119**:1541, 1993.
76. Provance DW, Wei M, Ipe V, Mercer JA: Cultured melanocytes from dilute mutant mice exhibit dendritic morphology and altered melanosome distribution. *Proc Natl Acad Sci U S A* **93**:14554, 1996.
77. Nascimento AAC, Amaral RG, Bizario JCS, Larson RE, Espreafico EM: Subcellular localization of myosin-V in the B16 melanoma cells, a wild-type cell line for the dilute gene. *Mol Biol Cell* **8**:1971, 1997.
78. Wei Q, Wu X, Hammer JA: The predominant defect in dilute melanocytes is in melanosome distribution and not cell shape, supporting a role for myosin V in melanosome transport. *J Muscle Res Cell Motil* **18**:517, 1997.
79. Wu X, Bowers B, Wei Q, Kocher R, Hammer JA: Myosin V associates with melanosomes in mouse melanocytes: Evidence that myosin V is an organelle motor. *J Cell Sci* **110**:847, 1997.
80. Lambert JM, Onderwater J, Haeghen YV, Vancoillie G, Koerten HK, Mommaas AM, Naeyaert JM: Myosin V colocalizes with melanosomes and subcortical actin bundles not associated with stress fibers in human epidermal melanocytes. *J Invest Dermatol* **111**:835, 1998.
81. Rogers SL, Gelfand VI: Myosin cooperates with microtubule motors during organelle transport in melanophores. *Curr Biol* **8**:161, 1998.
82. Engle LJ, Kennett RH: Cloning, analysis, and chromosomal localization of myoxin (MYH12), the human homologue to the mouse dilute gene. *Genomics* **19**:407, 1994.
83. Schneider LC, Berman RS, Shea CR, Perez-Atayde AR, Weinstein H, Geha RS: Bone marrow transplantation (BMT) for the syndrome of pigmentary dilution and lymphohistiocytosis (Griscelli's syndrome). *J Clin Immunol* **10**:146, 1990.
84. Pastural E, Barrat FJ, Dufourcq-Lagelouse R, Certain S, Sanal O, Jabado N, Seger R, Griscelli C, Fischer A, de Saint Basile G: Griscelli disease maps to chromosome 15q21 and is associated with mutations in the myosin-Va gene. *Nat Genet* **16**:289, 1998.
85. Mancini AJ, Chan LS, Paller AS: Partial albinism with immunodeficiency: Griscelli syndrome—Report of a case and review of the literature. *J Am Acad Dermatol* **38**:295, 1998.
86. White RA, Peters LL, Adkison LR, Korsgren C, Cohen CM, Lux SE: The murine pallid mutation is a platelet storage pool disease associated with the protein 4.2 (pallidin) gene. *Nat Genet* **2**:80, 1992.
87. Korsgren C, Cohen CM: cDNA sequence, gene sequence, and properties of murine pallidin (band 4.2), the protein implicated in the murine pallid mutation. *Genomics* **21**:478, 1994.
88. Gwynn B, Korsgren C, Cohen CM, Ciciotte SL, Peters LL: The gene encoding protein 4.2 is distinct from the mouse platelet storage pool deficiency mutation pallid. *Genomics* **42**:532, 1997.
89. Farooqui JZ, Medrano EE, Abdel-Malek ZA, Nordlund JJ: The expression of proopiomelanocortin and various POMC-derived peptides in mouse and human skin. *Ann N Y Acad Sci* **680**:508, 1993.
90. Chakraborty AK, Funasaka Y, Slominski A, Ermak G, Hwang J, Pawelek JM, Ichihashi M: Production and release of proopiomelanocortin (POMC) derived peptides by human melanocytes and keratinocytes in culture: Regulation by ultraviolet B. *Biochim Biophys Acta* **1313**:130, 1996.
91. Slominski A, Ermak G, Hwang J, Mazurkiewicz J, Corliss D, Eastman A: The expression of proopiomelanocortin (POMC) and of corticotropin releasing hormone receptor (CRH-R) genes in mouse skin. *Biochim Biophys Acta* **1289**:247, 1996.

92. Suzuki I, Cone RD, Im S, Nordlund JJ, Abdel-Malek ZA: Binding of melanotropic hormones to the melanocortin receptor MC1 on human melanocytes stimulates proliferation and melanogenesis. *Endocrinology* **137**:1627, 1996.
93. Yang YK, Dickinson C, Haskell-Luevano C, Gantz I: Molecular basis for the interaction of [Nle4,d-Phe7]melanocyte stimulating hormone with the human melanocortin-1 receptor (melanocyte a-MSH receptor). *J Biol Chem* **272**:23000, 1997.
94. Krude H, Biebermann H, Luck W, Horn R, Brabant G, Gruters A: Severe early-onset obesity, adrenal insufficiency and red hair pigmentation caused by POMC mutations in humans. *Nat Genet* **19**:155, 1998.
95. Box NF, Wyeth JR, O'Gorman LE, Martin NG, Sturm RA: Characterization of melanocyte stimulating hormone receptor variant alleles in twins with red hair. *Hum Mol Genet* **6**:1891, 1997.
96. Chakraborty A, Slominski A, Ermak G, Hwang J, Pawelek JM: Ultraviolet B and melanocyte-stimulating hormone (MSH) stimulate mRNA production for aMSH receptors and proopiomelanocortin-derived peptides in mouse melanoma cells and transformed keratinocytes. *J Invest Dermatol* **105**:655, 1995.
97. Mountjoy KG, Robbins LS, Mortrud MT, Cone RD: The cloning of a family of genes that encode the melanocortin receptors. *Science* **257**:1248, 1992.
98. Chhajlani V, Wikberg JES: Molecular cloning and expression of the human melanocyte stimulating hormone receptor cDNA. *FEBS Lett* **309**:417, 1992.
99. Gantz I, Yamada T, Tashiro T, Konda Y, Shimoto Y, Miwa H, Trent JM: Mapping of the gene encoding the melanocortin-1 (α-melanocyte stimulating hormone) receptor (MC1R) to human chromosome 16q24.3 by fluorescence in situ hybridization. *Genomics* **19**:394, 1994.
100. Chabot B, Stephenson DA, Chapman VM, Besmer P, Bernstein A: The proto-oncogene *c-kit* encoding a transmembrane tyrosine kinase receptor maps to the mouse W locus. *Nature* **335**:88, 1988.
101. Koppula SV, Robbins LS, Lu D, Baack E, White CR Jr, Swanson NA, Cone RD: Identification of common polymorphisms in the coding sequence of the human MSH receptor (MC1R) with possible biological effects. *Hum Mutat* **9**:30, 1997.
102. Valverde P, Healy E, Jackson I, Rees JL, Thody AJ: Variants of the melanocyte-stimulating hormone receptor gene are associated with red hair and fair skin in humans. *Nat Genet* **11**:328, 1995.
103. Hunt G, Todd C, Thody AJ: Unresponsiveness of human epidermal melanocytes to melanocyte stimulating hormone and its association with red hair. *Mol Cell Endocrinol* **116**:131, 1996.
104. Smith R, Healy E, Siddiqui S, Flanagan N, Steijlen PM, Rosdahl I, Jacques JP, Rogers S, Turner R, Jackson IJ, Birch-Machin MA, Rees JL: Melanocortin 1 receptor variants in an Irish population. *J Invest Dermatol* **111**:119, 1998.
105. Sturm RA, Box NF, Ramsay M: Human pigmentation genetics: The difference is only skin deep. *Bioessays* **20**:712, 1998.
106. Riley PA: Melanin. *Int J Biochem Cell Biol* **29**:1235, 1997.
107. Valverde P, Healy E, Sikkink S, Haldane F, Thody AJ, Carothers A, Jackson IJ, Rees JL: The Asp84Glu variant of the melanocortin 1 receptor (MC1R) is associated with melanoma. *Hum Mol Genet* **5**:1663, 1996.
108. Ichii-Jones F, Lear JT, Heagerty AHM, Smith AG, Hutchinson PE, Osborne J, Bowers B, Jones PW, Davies E, Ollier WER, Thomson W, Yengi L, Bath J, Fryer AA, Strange RC: Susceptibility to melanoma: Influence of skin type and polymorphism in the melanocyte stimulating hormone receptor gene. *J Invest Dermatol* **111**:218, 1998.
109. Bultman SJ, Michaud EJ, Woychik RP: Molecular characterization of the mouse agouti locus. *Cell* **71**:1195, 1992.
110. Miller MW, Duhl DMJ, Vrieling H, Cordes SP, Ollmann MM, Winkes BM, Barsh GS: Cloning of the mouse *agouti* gene predicts a secreted protein ubiquitously expressed in mice carrying the *lethal yellow* mutation. *Genes Dev* **7**:454, 1993.
111. Kwon HY, Bultman SJ, Loffler C, Chen WJ, Furdon PJ, Powell JG, Usala AL, Wilkison W, Hansmann I, Woychik RP: Molecular structure and chromosomal mapping of the human homolog of the agouti gene. *Proc Natl Acad Sci U S A* **91**:9760, 1994.
112. Wilson BD, Ollmann MM, Kang L, Stoffel M, Bell GI, Barsh GS: Structure and function of ASP, the human homolog of the mouse *agouti* gene. *Hum Mol Genet* **4**:223, 1995.
113. Shtolko VN, Koltover VK, Ilin AV, Vasileva LS, Bogdanov GN: Structural factors and the DOPA oxidase activity of membrane-bound tyrosinase. *Dokl Akad Nauk SSSR* **244**:1009, 1979.
114. Townsend SE, Allison JP: Tumor rejection after direct costimulation of CD8+ T cells by B7-transfected melanoma cells. *Science* **259**:368, 1993.
115. Lu D, Willard D, Patel IR, Kadwell S, Overton L, Kost T, Luther M, Chen W, Woychik RP, Wilkison WO, Cone RD: Agouti protein is an antagonist of the melanocyte-stimulating-hormone receptor. *Nature* **371**:799, 1994.
116. Blanchard SG, Harris CO, Ittoop ORR, Nichols JS, Parks DJ, Truesdale AT, Wilkison WO: Agouti antagonism of melanocortin binding and action in the B16 F10 murine melanoma cell line. *Biochemistry* **34**:10406, 1995.
117. Furumura M, Sakai C, Abdel-Malek Z, Barsh GS, Hearing VJ: The interaction of agouti signal protein and melanocyte stimulating hormone to regulate melanin formation in mammals. *Pigment Cell Res* **9**:191, 1996.
118. Siegrist W, Willard DH, Wilkison WO, Eberle AN: Agouti protein inhibits growth of B16 melanoma cells in vitro by acting through melanocortin receptors. *Biochem Biophys Res Commun* **218**:171, 1996.
119. Graham A, Wakamatsu K, Hunt G, Ito S, Thody AJ: Agouti protein inhibits the production of eumelanin and phaeomelanin in the presence and absence of a melanocyte stimulating hormone. *Pigment Cell Res* **10**:298, 1997.
120. Ollmann MM, Lamoreux ML, Wilson BD, Barsh GS: Interaction of agouti protein with the melanocortin 1 receptor in vitro and in vivo. *Genes Dev* **12**:316, 1998.
121. Vrieling H, Duhl DMJ, Millar SE, Miller KA, Barsh GS: Differences in dorsal and ventral pigmentation result from regional expression of the mouse agouti gene. *Proc Natl Acad Sci U S A* **91**:5667, 1994.
122. Yen TT, Gill AM, Frigeri LG, Barsh GS, Wolff GL: Obesity, diabetes, and neoplasia in yellow Avy/– mice: Ectopic expression of the agouti gene. *FASEB J* **8**:479, 1994.
123. Manne J, Argeson AC, Siracusa LD: Mechanisms for the pleiotropic effects of the agouti gene. *Proc Natl Acad Sci U S A* **92**:4721, 1995.
124. Michaud EJ, Mynatt RL, Miltenberger RJ, Klebig ML, Wilkinson JE, Zemel MB, Wilkison WO, Woychik RP: Role of the agouti gene in obesity. *J Endocrinol* **155**:207, 1997.
125. Jiménez M, Kameyama K, Maloy WL, Tomita Y, Hearing VJ: Mammalian tyrosinase: Biosynthesis, processing and modulation by melanocyte stimulating hormone. *Proc Natl Acad Sci U S A* **85**:3830, 1988.
126. Burchill SA, Marks JM, Thody AJ: Tyrosinase synthesis in different skin types and the effects of α-melanocyte stimulating hormone and cyclic AMP. *J Invest Dermatol* **95**:558, 1990.
127. Burchill SA, Ito S, Thody AJ: Effects of melanocyte-stimulating hormone on tyrosinase expression and melanin synthesis in hair follicular melanocytes of the mouse. *J Endocrinol* **137**:189, 1993.
128. Kobayashi T, Vieira WD, Potterf SB, Sakai C, Imokawa G, Hearing VJ: Modulation of melanogenic protein expression during the switch from eu- to pheomelanogenesis. *J Cell Sci* **108**:2301, 1995.
129. Sakai C, Ollmann M, Kobayashi T, Abdel-Malek ZA, Muller J, Vieira WD, Imokawa G, Barsh GS, Hearing VJ: Modulation of murine melanocyte function in vitro by agouti signal protein. *EMBO J* **16**:3544, 1997.
130. Suzuki I, Tada A, Ollmann M, Barsh GS, Im S, Lamoreux ML, Hearing VJ, Nordlund JJ, Abdel-Malek ZA: Agouti signalling protein inhibits melanogenesis and the response of human melanocytes to α-melanotropin. *J Invest Dermatol* **108**:838, 1997.
131. Furumura M, Sakai C, Potterf SB, Vieira W, Barsh GS, Hearing VJ: Characterization of genes modulated during pheomelanogenesis using differential display. *Proc Natl Acad Sci U S A* **95**:7374, 1998.
132. Hearing VJ, King RA: Determinants of skin color: Melanocytes and melanization, in Levine N (ed): *Pigmentation and Pigmentary Abnormalities*. New York, CRC Press, 1993.
133. Urabe K, Aroca P, Hearing VJ: From gene to protein: Determination of melanin synthesis. *Pigment Cell Res* **6**:186, 1993.
134. Winder AJ, Kobayashi T, Tsukamoto K, Urabe K, Aroca P, Kameyama K, Hearing VJ: The tyrosinase gene family: Interactions of melanognic proteins to regulate melanogenesis. *Cell Mol Biol Res* **40**:613, 1994.
135. Orlow SJ, Boissy RE, Moran DJ, Pifko-Hirst S: Subcellular distribution of tyrosinase and tyrosinase-related protein-1: Implications for melanosomal biogenesis. *J Invest Dermatol* **100**:55, 1993.
136. Prota G, Lamoreux ML, Muller J, Kobayashi T, Napolitano A, Vincenzi R, Sakai C, Hearing VJ: Comparative analysis of melanins and melanosomes produced by various coat color mutations. *Pigment Cell Res* **8**:153, 1995.
137. Jimbow K, Gomez PF, Toyofuku K, Chang D, Miura S, Tsujiya H, Park JS: Biological role of tyrosinase related protein and its biosynthesis

and transport from TGN to stage 1 melanosome, late endosome, through gene transfection study. *Pigment Cell Res* **10**:206, 1997.

138. Potterf SB, Furumura M, Sviderskaya EV, Sakai C, Bennett DC, Hearing VJ: Normal tyrosine transport and abnormal tyrosinase routing in pinkeyed-dilution melanocytes. *Exp Cell Res* **244**:319, 1998.
139. Zhou B-K, Kobayahi T, Donatien PD, Bennett DC, Hearing VJ, Orlow SJ: Identification of a melanosomal matrix protein encoded by the murine *si* (silver) locus using "organelle scanning." *Proc Natl Acad Sci U S A* **91**:7076, 1994.
140. Kobayashi T, Urabe K, Orlow SJ, Higashi K, Imokawa G, Kwon BS, Potterf B, Hearing VJ: The Pmel 17/*silver* locus protein: Characterization and investigation of its melanogenic function. *J Biol Chem* **269**:29198, 1994.
141. Zhou BK, Kobayashi T, Donatien PD, Bennett DC, Hearing VJ, Orlow SJ: Identification of a melanosomal matrix protein encoded by the murine (si) silver locus using "organelle scanning." *Proc Natl Acad Sci U S A* **91**:7076, 1994.
142. Lamoreux ML, Zhou B-K, Rosemblat S, Orlow SJ: The pinkeyed-dilution protein and the eumelanin/pheomelanin switch: In support of a unifying hypothesis. *Pigment Cell Res* **8**:263, 1995.
143. Tsukamoto K, Jackson IJ, Urabe K, Montague PM, Hearing VJ: A second tyrosinase-related protein, TRP2, is a melanogenic enzyme termed DOPAchrome tautomerase. *EMBO J* **11**:519, 1992.
144. Riley PA: Mechanistic aspects of the control of tyrosinase activity. *Pigment Cell Res* **6**:182, 1993.
145. Cooksey CJ, Garratt PJ, Land EJ, Pavel S, Ramsden CA, Riley PA, Smit NPM: Evidence of the indirect formation of the catecholic intermediate substrate responsible for the autoactivation kinetics of tyrosinase. *J Biol Chem* **272**:26226, 1997.
146. Ito S: Biochemistry and physiology of melanin, in Levine N (ed): *Pigmentation and Pigmentary Disorders.* Boca Raton, CRC Press, 1993, p 33.
147. Kameyama K, Takemura T, Hamada Y, Sakai C, Kondoh S, Nishiyama S, Urabe K, Hearing VJ: Pigment production in murine melanoma cells is regulated by tyrosinase, tyrosinase-related protein 1 (TRP1), DOPAchrome tautomerase (TRP2) and a melanogenic inhibitor. *J Invest Dermatol* **100**:126, 1993.
148. Kroumpouzos G, Urabe K, Kobayashi T, Sakai C, Hearing VJ: Functional analysis of the *slaty* gene product (TRP2) as DOPAchrome tautomerase, and the effect of a point mutation on its catalytic function. *Biochem Biophys Res Commun* **202**:1060, 1994.
149. Albino AP, Lloyd KO, Ikeda H, Old LJ: Biochemical analysis of a 130,000 MW glycoprotein on human melanoma cells. *J Immunol* **131**:1595, 1983.
150. Hoon DSB, Banez M, Okun E, Morton DL, Irie RF: Modulation of human melanoma cells by interleukin-4 and in combination with γ-interferon or α-tumor necrosis factor. *Cancer Res* **51**:2002, 1991.
151. Kameyama K, Sakai C, Kuge S, Nishiyama S, Tomita Y, Ito S, Wakamatsu K, Hearing VJ: Expression of tyrosinase, tyrosinase-related proteins 1 and 2 (TRP1 and TRP2), silver protein and α melanogenic inhibitor regulates melanogenesis in human melanoma cells. *Pigment Cell Res* **8**:97, 1995.
152. Benathan M, Labidi F: Cysteine-dependent 5-S-cysteinyldopa formation and its regulation by glutathione in normal epidermal melanocytes. *Arch Dermatol Res* **288**:697, 1996.
153. del Marmol V, Ito S, Bouchard B, Libert A, Wakamatsu K, Ghanem G, Solano F: Cysteine deprivation promotes eumelanogenesis in human melanoma cells. *J Invest Dermatol* **107**:698, 1996.
154. Ozeki H, Ito S, Wakamatsu K, Ishiguro I: Chemical characterization of pheomelanogenesis starting from dihydroxyphenylalanine or tyrosine and cysteine. Effects of tyrosinase and cysteine concentrations and reaction time. *Biochim Biophys Acta* **1336**:539, 1997.
155. Potterf SB, Benathan M, Sahai C, Furumura M, Hearing VJ: Regulation of melanin precursor ratios: Melanosomal transport of cysteine and glutathione [Abstract]. *Pigment Cell Res* **10**:113, 1997.
156. Potterf SB, Virador V, Wakamatsu K, Furumura M, Santis C, Ito S, Hearing VJ: Cysteine transport in melanosomes from murine melanocytes. *Pigment Cell Res* **12**:4, 1999.
157. Ohyama Y, Mishima Y: Isolation and characterization of high molecular weight melanogenic inhibitors naturally occurring in melanoma cells. *Pigment Cell Res* **6**:7, 1993.
158. Thody AJ, Higgins EM, Wakamatsu K, Ito S, Burchill SA, Marks JM: Pheomelanin as well as eumelanin is present in human epidermis. *J Invest Dermatol* **97**:340, 1991.
159. Hunt G, Kyne S, Ito S, Wakamatsu K, Todd C, Thody AJ: Eumelanin and pheomelanin contents of human epidermis and cultured melanocytes. *Pigment Cell Res* **8**:202, 1995.

160. Ozeki H, Ito S, Wakamatsu K, Thody AJ: Spectrophotometric characterization of eumelanin and pheomelanin in hair. *Pigment Cell Res* **9**:265, 1996.
161. Ito S, Imai Y, Jimbow K, Fujita K: Incorporation of sulfhydryl compounds into melanins in vitro. *Biochim Biophys Acta* **964**:1, 1988.
162. Jara JR, Aroca P, Solano F, Martínez-Liarte JH, Lozano JA: The role of sulfhydryl compounds in mammalian melanogenesis: the effect of cysteine and glutathione upon tyrosinase and the intermediates of the pathway. *Biochim Biophys Acta* **967**:296, 1988.
163. Gahl WA, Potterf B, Durham-Pierre D, Brilliant MH, Hearing VJ: Melanosomal tyrosine transport in normal and pink-eyed dilution murine melanocytes. *Pigment Cell Res* **8**:229, 1995.
164. Potterf SB, Muller J, Bernardini I, Tietze F, Kobayashi T, Hearing VJ, Gahl WA: Characterization of a melanosomal transport system in murine melanocytes mediating entry of the melanogenic substrate tyrosine. *J Biol Chem* **271**:4002, 1996.
165. Potterf SB, Hearing VJ: Tyrosine transport into melanosomes is increased following stimulation of melanocyte differentiation. *Biochem Biophys Res Commun* **248**:795, 1998.
166. Palumbo A, d'Ischia M, Misuraca G, Prota G: Effect of metal ions on the rearrangement of DOPAchrome. *Biochim Biophys Acta* **925**:203, 1987.
167. Leonard LJ, Townsend D, King RA: Function of DOPAchrome oxidoreductase and metal ions in DOPAchrome conversion in the eumelanin pathway. *Biochemistry* **27**:6156, 1988.
168. Pawelek JM: DOPAchrome conversion factor functions as an isomerase. *Biochem Biophys Res Commun* **166**:1328, 1990.
169. Palumbo A, Solano F, Misuraca G, Aroca P, García-Borrón JC, Lozano JA, Prota G: Comparative action of DOPAchrome tautomerase and metal ions on the rearrangement of DOPAchrome. *Biochim Biophys Acta* **1115**:1, 1991.
170. Korner AM, Pawelek JM: Mammalian tyrosinase catalyzes three reactions in the biosynthesis of melanin. *Science* **217**:1163, 1982.
171. Tripathi RK, Hearing VJ, Urabe K, Aroca P, Spritz RA: Mutational mapping of the catalytic activities of human tyrosinase. *J Biol Chem* **267**:23707, 1992.
172. Tutic M, Schirmer RH, Werner D: Cloning and sequencing of mammalian glutathione reductase cDNA. *Eur J Biochem* **188**:523, 1990.
173. Kobayashi T, Urabe K, Winder AJ, Tsukamoto K, Brewington T, Imokawa G, Potterf SB, Hearing VJ: The DHICA oxidase activity of TRP1 and interactions with other melanogenic enzymes. *Pigment Cell Res* **7**:227, 1994.
174. Kobayashi T, Urabe K, Winder AJ, Jiménez-Cervantes C, Imokawa G, Brewington T, Solano F, García-Barron JC, Hearing VJ: Tyrosinase-related protein 1 (TRP1) functions as a DHICA oxidase in melanin biosynthesis. *EMBO J* **13**:15818, 1994.
175. Boissy RE, Sakai C, Zhao H, Kobayashi T, Hearing VJ: Human tyrosinase related protein-1 (TRP-1) does not function as a DHICA oxidase in contrast to murine TRP-1. *Exp Dermatol* **7**:198, 1998.
176. Kobayashi T, Bennett DC, Imokawa G, Hearing VJ: Tyrosinase stabilization by the brown locus protein (TRP1). *J Biol Chem* **273**:31801, 1998.
177. Donatien PD, Orlow SJ: Interaction of melanosomal proteins with melanin. *Eur J Biochem* **232**:159, 1995.
178. Chakraborty AK, Platt JT, Kim KK, Kwon BS, Bennett DC, Pawelek JM: Polymerization of 5,6-dihydroxyindole-2-carboxylic acid to melanin by the pMel17/silver locus protein. *Eur J Biochem* **232**:257, 1996.
179. Lee ZH, Hou L, Moellmann G, Kuklinska E, Antol K, Fraser M, Halaban R, Kwon BS: Characterization and subcellular localization of human Pmel17/silver, a 100-kDa (pre)melanosomal membrane protein associated with 5,6-dihydroxyindole-2-carboxylic acid (DHICA) converting activity. *J Invest Dermatol* **106**:605, 1996.
180. Prota G: Melanins, melanogenesis and skin photoprotection. *Eur J Cancer* **30A**:553, 1994.
181. Ozeki H, Ito S, Wakamatsu K, Hirobe T: Chemical characterization of hair melanins in various coat-color mutants of mice. *J Invest Dermatol* **105**:361, 1995.
182. Ozeki H, Ito S, Wakamatsu K: Chemical characterization of melanins in sheep wool and human hair. *Pigment Cell Res* **9**:51, 1996.
183. Hearing VJ: The regulation of melanin formation, in Nordlund JJ, Boissy RE, Hearing VJ, King RA, Ortonne J-P (eds): *The Pigmentary System. Physiology and Pathophysiology,* New York, Oxford University Press, 1998, p 423.
184. Ito S: Advances in chemical analysis of melanins, in Nordlund JJ, Boissy RE, Hearing VJ, King RA, Ortonne J-P (eds): *The Pigmentary*

*System. Physiology and Pathophysiology.* New York, Oxford University Press, 1998, p 439.

185. Riley PA: The evolution of melanogenesis, in Zeise L, Chedekel MR, Fitzpatrick TB (eds): *Melanin: Its Role in Human Photoprotection*, Overland Park, KS, Valdenmar, 1995, p 1.

186. Spritz RA, Ho L, Furumura M, Hearing VJ: Mutational analysis of copper binding by human tyrosinase. *J Invest Dermatol* **109**:207, 1997.

187. Furumura M, Solano F, Matsunaga N, Sakai C, Spritz RA, Hearing VJ: Metal ligand binding specificities of the tyrosinase related proteins. *Biochem Biophys Res. Commun* **242**:579, 1998.

188. Tief K, Hahne M, Schmidt A, Beermann F: Tyrosinase, the key enzyme in melanin synthesis, is expressed in murine brain. *Eur J Biochem* **241**:12, 1996.

189. Tief K, Schmidt A, Beermann F: New evidence for presence of tyrosinase in substantia nigra, forebrain and midbrain. *Mol Brain Res* **53**:307, 1998.

190. Ikemoto K, Nagatsu I, Ito S, King RA, Nishimura A, Nagatsu T: Does tyrosinase exist in neuromelanin-pigmented neurons in the human substantia nigra? *Neurosci Lett* **253**:198, 1998.

191. Cassady JL, Sturm GE: Sequence of the human dopachrome tautomerase-encoding *TRP-2* cDNA. *Gene* **143**:295, 1994.

192. Solano F, Martinez-Liarte JH, Jimenez-Cervantes C, Garcia-Borron JC, Lozano JA: Dopachrome tautomerase is a zinc-containing enzyme. *Biochem Biophys Res Commun* **204**:1243, 1994.

193. Solano F, Martinez-Liarte JH, Jiménez-Cervantes C, García-Borrón JC, Jara JR, Lozano JA: Molecular mechanism for catalysis by a new zinc-enzyme: DOPAchrome tautomerase. *Biochem J* **313**:447, 1996.

194. Steel KP, Davidson DR, Jackson IJ: TRP2/DT, a new early melanoblast marker, shows that steel growth factor (*c-kit* ligand) is a survival factor. *Development* **115**:1111, 1992.

195. Urabe K, Aroca P, Tsukamoto K, Mascagna D, Palumbo A, Prota G, Hearing VJ: The inherent cytotoxicity of melanin precursors: A revision. *Biochim Biophys Acta* **1221**:272, 1994.

196. Jiménez-Cervantes C, Solano F, Lozano JA, García-Borrón JC: The DHICA oxidase activity of the melanosomal tyrosinases LEMT and HEMT. *Pigment Cell Res* **7**:298, 1994.

197. Kobayashi T, Urabe K, Winder A, Tsukamoto K, Brewington T, Imokawa G, Potterf B, Hearing VJ: DHICA oxidase activity of TRP1 and interactions with other melanogenic enzymes. *Pigment Cell Res* **7**:227, 1994.

198. Tsukamoto K, Urabe K, Kameyama K, Hearing VJ: Interactions of melanogenic proteins in the tyrosinase family to regulate melanogenesis. *Pigment Cell Res* **5**:97, 1992.

199. Winder A, Kobayashi T, Tsukamoto K, Urabe K, Aroca P, Kameyama K, Hearing VJ: The tyrosinase gene family—Interactions of melanogenic proteins to regulate melanogenesis. *Cell Mol Biol* **40**:613, 1994.

200. Kwon BS, Halaban R, Kim GS, Usack L, Pomerantz SH, Haq AK: A melanocyte-specific complementary DNA clone whose expression is inducible by melanotropin and isobutylmethyl xanthine. *Mol Biol Med* **4**:339, 1987.

201. Chakraborty AK, Park KC, Kwon BS, Hearing VJ, Pawelek JM: Stable activity is associated with Pmel-17 gene expression. *Pigment Cell Res* **5**:84, 1992.

202. Schallreuter KU, Wood JM, Pittelkow MR, Gutlich M, Lemke KR, Rodl W, Swanson NN, Hitzemann K, Ziegler I: Regulation of melanin biosynthesis in the human epidermis by tetrahydrobiopterin. *Science* **263**:1444, 1994.

203. Lee T-S, Nicholls RD, Jong MTC, Spritz RA: Organization and sequence of the human P gene and identification of a new family of tranport proteins. *Genomics* **26**:354, 1995.

204. Puri N, Brilliant MH: The function of the pink-eyed dilution protein [Abstract]. *Pigment Cell Res* **11**:174, 1998.

205. Granholm DE, Reese RN, Granholm NH: Agouti alleles alter cysteine and glutathione concentrations in hair follicles and serum of mice (Ay/a, AwJ/AwJ, and a/a). *J Invest Dermatol* **106**:559, 1996.

206. Prota G: Cysteine and glutathione in mammalian pigmentation, in Cavallini D, Gaull G, Zappia V (eds): *Natural Sulfur Compounds*. New York, Plenum Press, 1980, p 391.

207. Benedetto JP, Ortonne JP, Voulot C, Khatchadourian C, Prota G, Thivolet J: Role of thiol compounds in mammalian melanin pigmentation. II. Glutathione and related enzymatic activities. *J Invest Dermatol* **79**:422, 1982.

208. Mojamdar MV, Ichihashi M, Mishima Y: γ-Glutamyl transpeptidase, tyrosinase, and 5-S-cysteinylDOPA production in melanoma cells. *J Invest Dermatol* **81**:119, 1983.

209. Chakraborty C, Hatta S, Ichihashi M, Hayashibe K, Mishima Y: Effects of L-glutamine on tyrosinase and γ-glutamyl transpeptidase of B-16 melanoma cells in culture. *J Dermatol* **15**:1, 1988.

210. Mondal M, Banerjee PK: Role of peroxidase in melanogenesis: Search for a control mechanism. *Ind J Biochem Biophys* **18**:380, 1981.

211. d'Ischia M, Napolitano A, Prota G: Peroxidase as an alternative to tyrosinase in the oxidative polymerization of 5,6-dihydroxyindoles to melanin(s). *Biochim Biophys Acta* **1073**:423, 1990.

212. Palumbo A, Jackson IJ: Peroxidase activity in the ink gland of Sepia officinalis and partial nucleotide sequence of a candidate cDNA encoding the enzyme. *Biochim Biophys Acta* **1247**:173, 1995.

213. Okun MR: The role of peroxidase in mammalian melanogenesis: A review. *Physiol Chem Phys Med NMR* **28**:91, 1996.

214. Gesualdo I, Aniello F, Branno M, Palumbo A: Molecular cloning of a peroxidase mRNA specifically expressed in the ink gland of Sepia officinalis. *Biochim Biophys Acta* **1353**:111, 1997.

215. Lindbladh C, Rorsman H, Rosengren E: The effect of catalase on the inactivation of tyrosinase by ascorbic acid and by cysteine or glutathione. *Acta Derm Venereol Suppl (Stockh)* **63**:209, 1983.

216. Halaban R, Moellmann GE: Murine and human b locus pigmentation genes encode a glycoprotein (gp75) with catalase activity. *Proc Natl Acad Sci U S A* **87**:4809, 1990.

217. Daquinag AC, Nakamura S, Takao T, Shimonishi Y, Tsukamoto T: Primary structure of a potent endogenous dopa-containing inhibitor of phenol oxidase from Musca domestica. *Proc Natl Acad Sci U S A* **92**:2964, 1995.

218. Farooqui JZ, Robb E, Boyce ST, Warden GD, Nordlund JJ: Isolation of a unique melanogenic inhibitor from human skin xenografts: Initial in vitro and in vivo characterization. *J Invest Dermatol* **104**:739, 1995.

219. Silvers WK: *The Coat Colors of Mice. A Model for Mammalian Gene Action and Interaction.* New York, Springer-Verlag, 1979.

220. Mouse Genome Informatics: *Mouse Genome Database (MGD).* Bar Harbor, ME, The Jackson Laboratory, 1998.

221. Yamamoto H, Takeuchi S, Kudo T, Makino K, Nakata A, Shinoda T, Takeuchi T: Cloning and sequencing of mouse tyrosinase cDNA. *Jpn J Genet* **62**:271, 1987.

222. Kwon BS, Haq AK, Pomerantz SH, Halaban R: Isolation and sequence of a cDNA locus for human tyrosinase that maps at the mouse c-albino locus. *Proc Natl Acad Sci U S A* **84**:7473, 1987.

223. Wittbjer A, Dahlback B, Odh G, Rosengren AM, Rosengren E, Rorsman H: Isolation of human tyrosinase from cultured melanoma cells. *Acta Derm Venereol Suppl (Stockh)* **69**:125, 1989.

224. Wittbjer A, Odh G, Rosengren AM, Rosengren E, Rorsman H: Isolation of soluble tyrosinase from human melanoma cells. *Acta Derm Venereol Suppl (Stockh)* **70**:291, 1990.

225. Bouchard B, Fuller BB, Vijayasaradhi S, Houghton AN: Induction of pigmentation in mouse fibroblasts by expression of human tyrosinase cDNA. *J Exp Med* **169**:2029, 1989.

226. Ruppert S, Müller G, Kwon BS, Schütz G: Multiple transcripts of the mouse tyrosinase gene are generated by alternative splicing. *EMBO J* **7**:2715, 1988.

227. Giebel LB, Strunk KM, Spritz RA: Organization and nucleotide sequences of the human tyrosinase gene and a truncated tyrosinase-related segment. *Genomics* **9**:435, 1991.

228. Schnur RE, Selling BT, Holmes SA, Wick PA, Tatsumura YO, Spritz RA: Type I oculocutaneous albinism associated with a full-length deletion of the tyrosinase gene. *J Invest Dermatol* **106**:1137, 1996.

229. Kikuchi H, Miura H, Yamamoto H, Takeuchi T, Dei T, Watanabe M: Characteristic sequences in the upstream region of the human tyrosinase gene. *Biochim Biophys Acta* **1009**:283, 1989.

230. Porter S, Mintz B: Multiple alternatively spliced transcripts of the mouse tyrosinase-encoding gene. *Gene* **97**:277, 1991.

231. Shibahara S, Tomita Y, Tagami H, Muller RM, Cohen T: Molecular basis for the heterogeneity of human tyrosinase. *Tohoku J Exp Med* **156**:403, 1988.

232. Fryer JP, King RA, Oetting WS: Analysis of splice site mutations in individuals with OCA1 using illegitimate transcription as a source of tyrosinase RNA in lymphocytes. *Pigment Cell Res* **5(Suppl)**:34, 1996.

233. Müller G, Ruppert S, Schmid E, Schütz G: Functional analysis of alternatively spliced tyrosinase gene transcripts. *EMBO J* **7**:2723, 1988.

234. Giebel LB, Spritz RA: RFLP for *Mbo*I in the human tyrosinase (TYR) gene detected by PCR. *Nucleic Acid Res* **18**:3103, 1990.

235. Johnston JD, Winder AJ, Breimer LH: An *Mbo*I polymorphism at codon 192 of the human tyrosinase gene is present in Asians and Afrocaribbeans. *Nucleic Acid Res* **20**:1433, 1992.

236. Tripathi RK, Giebel LB, Strunk KM, Spritz RA: A polymorphism of the human tyrosinase gene is associated with temperature-sensitive enzymatic activity. *Gene Expr* **1**:103, 1991.

237. Oetting WS, Roed CM, Mentink MM, King RA: PCR detection of a Taq1 polymorphism at the CCAATT box of the human tyrosinase (TYR) gene. *Nucleic Acid Res* **19**:5800, 1991.

238. Morris SW, Muir W, St Clair D: Dinucleotide repeat polymorphism at the human tyrosinase gene. *Nucleic Acid Res* **19**:6968, 1991.

239. Oetting WS, Witkop CJ, Brown SA, Colomer R, Fryer JP, Bloom KE, King RA: A frequent mutation in the tyrosinase gene associated with type I-A (tyrosinase-negative) oculocutaneous albinism in Puerto Rico. *Am J Hum Genet* **52**:17, 1993.

240. Oetting WS, Stine OC, Townsend D, King RA: Evolution of the tyrosinase related gene (TYRL) in primates. *Pigment Cell Res* **6**:171, 1993.

241. Takeda A, Matsunaga J, Tomita Y, Tagami H, Shibahara S: Nucleotide sequence of the putative human tyrosinase pseudogene. *Tohoku J Exp Med* **163**:295, 1991.

242. Kluppel M, Beermann F, Ruppert S, Schmid E, Hummler E, Schütz G: The mouse tyrosinase promoter is sufficient for expression in melanocytes and in the pigmented epithelium of the retina. *Proc Natl Acad Sci U S A* **88**:3777, 1991.

243. Beermann F, Schmid E, Ganss R, Schütz G, Ruppert S: Molecular characterization of the mouse tyrosinase gene: pigment cell specific expression in transgenic mice. *Pigment Cell Res* **5**:295, 1992.

244. Sato S, Miura H, Yamamoto H, Takeuchi T: Identification of nuclear factors that bind to the mouse tyrosinase gene regulatory region. *Pigment Cell Res* **7**:279, 1994.

245. Lowings P, Yavuzer U, Goding CR: Positive and negative elements regulate a melanocyte-specific promoter. *Mol Cell Biol* **12**:3653, 1992.

246. Jackson IJ, Chambers DM, Budd PS, Johnson R: The tyrosinase-related protein-1 gene has a structure and promoter sequence very different from tyrosinase. *Nucleic Acid Res* **19**:3799, 1991.

247. Shibahara S, Taguchi H, Muller RM, Shibata K, Cohen T, Tomita Y, Tagami H: Structural organization of the pigment cell-specific gene located at the brown locus in mouse. Its promoter activity and alternatively spliced transcript. *J Biol Chem* **266**:15895, 1991.

248. Sturm RA, O'Sullivan BJ, Box NF, Smith AG, Smit SE, Puttick ERJ, Parsons PG, Dunn IS: Chromosomal structure of the human TYRP1 and TYRP2 loci and comparison of the tyrosinase-related protein gene family. *Genomics* **29**:24, 1995.

249. Ganss R, Schmidt A, Schütz G, Beermann F: Analysis of the mouse tyrosinase promoter in vitro and in vivo. *Pigment Cell Res* **7**:275, 1994.

250. Bertolotto C, Bille K, Ortonne J-P, Ballotti R: In B16 melanoma cells, the inhibition of melanogenesis by TPA results from PKC activation and diminution of microphthalmia binding to the M-box of the tyrosinase promoter. *Oncogene* **16**:1665, 1998.

251. Yavuzer U, Goding CR: Melanocyte-specific gene expression: Role of repression and identification of a melanocyte-specific factor, MSF. *Mol Cell Biol* **14**:3494, 1994.

252. Shibata K, Muraosa Y, Tomita Y, Tagami H, Shibahara S: Identification of a cis-acting element that enhances the pigment cell-specific expression of the human tyrosinase gene. *J Biol Chem* **267**:20584, 1992.

253. Ponnazhagan S, Hou L, Kwon BS: Structural organization of the human tyrosinase gene and sequence analysis and characterization of its promoter region. *J Invest Dermatol* **102**:744, 1994.

254. Porter S, Larue L, Mintz B: Mosaicism of tyrosinase-locus transcription and chromatin structure in dark vs light melanocyte clones of homozygous chinchilla-mottled mice. *Dev Genet* **12**:393, 1991.

255. Porter SD, Meyer CJ: A distal tyrosinase upstream element stimulates gene expression in neural-crest-derived melanocytes of transgenic mice: Position-independent and mosaic expression. *Development* **120**:2103–2111, 1994.

256. Ganss R, Montoliu L, Managhan AP, Schütz G: A cell-specific enhancer far upstream of the mouse tyrosinase gene confers high level and copy number-related expression in transgenic mice. *EMBO J* **13**:3083, 1994.

257. Schedl A, Beermann F, Thies E, Montoliu L, Kelsey G, Schütz G: Transgenic mice generated by pronuclear injection of a yeast artificial chromosome. *Nucleic Acid Res* **20**:3073, 1992.

258. Schedl A, Montollu L, Kelsey G, Schütz G: A yeast artificial chromosome covering the tyrosinase gene confers copy number-dependent expression in transgenic mice. *Nature* **362**:258, 1993.

259. Abdel-Malek ZA, Swope V, Smalara D, Babcock G, Dawes S, Nordlund JJ: Analysis of the UV-induced melanogenesis and growth arrest of human melanocytes. *Pigment Cell Res* **7**:326, 1994.

260. Im S, Moro M, Peng F, Medrano EE, Cornelius J, Babcock G, Nordlund JJ, Abdel-Malek ZA: Activation of the cyclic AMP pathway by α-melanotropin mediates the response of human melanocytes to ultraviolet B radiation. *Cancer Res* **58**:47, 1998.

261. Gilchrest BA, Park HY, Eller MS, Yaar M: Mechanisms of ultraviolet light-induced pigmentation. *Photochem Photobiol* **63**:1, 1996.

262. Chakraborty AK, Orlow SJ, Bolognia J, Pawelek JM: Structural/functional relationships between internal and external MSH receptors: Modulation of expression in Cloudman melanoma cells by UVB radiation. *J Cell Physiol* **147**:1, 1991.

263. Eller MS, Ostrom K, Gilchrest BA: DNA damage enhances melanogenesis. *Proc Natl Acad Sci U S A* **93**:1087, 1996.

264. Pedeux R, Al-Irani N, Marteau C, Pellicier F, Branche R, Ozturk M, Franchi J, Dore JF: Thymidine dinucleotides induce S phase cell cycle arrest in addition to increased melanogenesis in human melanocytes. *J Invest Dermatol* **111**:472, 1998.

265. Goukassian DA, Eller MS, Yaar M, Gilchrest BA: Thymidine dinucleotide mimics the effect of solar simulated irradiation on p53 and p53-regulated proteins. *J Invest Dermatol* **112**:25, 1999.

266. Romero-Graillet C, Aberdam E, Biagoli N, Massabni W, Ortonne JP, Ballotti R: Ultraviolet B radiation acts through the nitric oxide and cGMP signal transduction pathway to stimulate melanogenesis in human melanocytes. *J Biol Chem* **271**:28052, 1996.

267. Sodi SA, Chakraborty AK, Platt JT, Kolesnikova N, Rosemblat S, Keh-Yen A, Bolognia JL, Rachkovsky ML, Orlow SJ, Pawelek JM: Melanoma x macrophage fusion hybrids acquire increased melanogenesis and metastatic potential: Altered *N*-glycosylation as an underlying mechanism. *Pigment Cell Res* **11**:299, 1998.

268. Takahashi H, Parsons PG: Rapid and reversible inhibition of tyrosinase activity by glucosidase inhibitors in human melanoma cells. *J Invest Dermatol* **98**:481, 1992.

269. Fuller BB, Niekrasz I, Hoganson GE: Down-regulation of tyrosinase mRNA levels in melanoma cells by tumor promoters and by insulin. *Mol Cell Endocrinol* **72**:81, 1990.

270. Oka M, Ogita K, Saito N, Mishima Y: Selective increase of the α subspecies of protein kinase C and inhibition of melanogenesis induced by retinoic acid in melanoma cells. *J Invest Dermatol* **100(Suppl)**:204s, 1998.

271. Gruber JR, Ohno S, Niles RM: Increased expression of protein kinase Ca plays a key role in retinoic acid-induced melanoma differentiation. *J Biol Chem* **267**:13356, 1992.

272. Mahalingam H, Watanabe A, Tachibana M, Niles RM: Characterization of density-dependent regulation of the tyrosinase gene promoter: Role of protein kinase C. *Exp Cell Res* **237**:83, 1997.

273. Jackson IJ: A cDNA encoding tyrosinase-related protein maps to the brown locus in mice. *Proc Natl Acad Sci U S A* **85**:4392, 1988.

274. Jackson IJ, Chambers DM, Rinchik EM, Bennett DC: Characterization of TRP-1 mRNA levels in dominant and recessive mutations at the mouse brown (b) locus. *Genetics* **126**:451, 1990.

275. Zdarsky E, Favor J, Jackson IJ: The molecular basis of brown, an old mouse mutation, and of an induced revertant to wild-type. *Genetics* **126**:443, 1990.

276. Johnson R, Jackson IJ: Light is a dominant mouse mutation resulting in premature cell death. *Nat Genet* **1**:226, 1992.

277. Shibata K, Takeda K, Tomita Y, Tagami H, Shibahara S: Downstream region of the human tyrosinase-related protein gene enhances its promoter activity. *Biochem Biophys Res Commun* **184**:568, 1992.

278. Box NF, Wyeth JR, Mayne CJ, O'Gorman LE, Martin NG, Sturm RA: Complete sequence and polymorphism study of the human TYRP1 gene encoding tyrosinase-related protein 1. *Mam Genome* **9**:50, 1998.

279. Cohen T, Muller RM, Tomita Y, Shibahara S: Nucleotide sequence of the cDNA encoding human tyrosinase-related protein. *Nucleic Acid Res* **18**:2807, 1990.

280. Urquhart A: Human tyrosinase-like protein (TYRL) carboxy terminus: Closer homology with the mouse protein than previously reported. *Nucleic Acid Res* **19**:5803, 1991.

281. Murty VVVS, Bouchard B, Mathew S, Vijayasaradhi S, Houghton AN: Assignment of the Human *TYRP* (brown) locus to chromosome region 9p23 by nonradioactive *in situ* hybridization. *Genomics* **13**:227, 1992.

282. Boissy RE, Zhao H, Oetting WS, Austin LM, Wildenberg SC, Boissy YL, Zhao Y, Strum RA, Hearing VJ, King RA, Nordlund JJ: Mutation in and lack of expression of tyrosinase-related protein-1 (TRP-1) in melanocytes from an individual with brown oculocutaneous albinism: A new subtype of albinism classified as "OCA3." *Am J Hum Genet* **48**:1145, 1996.

283. Manga P, Kromberg J, Box N, Strum R, Jenkins T, Ramsay M: Rufous oculocutaneous albinism is caused by mutations of the TRP1 gene on chromosome 9p [Abstract]. *Brazil J Genet* **19**:180, 1996.

284. Yamamoto H, Kudo T, Masuko N, Miura H, Sato S, Tanaka M, Tanaka S, Takeuchi S, Shibahara S, Takeuchi T: Phylogeny of regulatory regions of vertebrate tyrosinase genes. *Pigment Cell Res* **5**:284, 1992.

285. Sturm RA, O'Sullivan BJ, Thomson JAF, Jamshidi N, Pedley J, Parsons P: Expression studies of pigmentation and POU-domain genes in human melanoma cells. *Pigment Cell Res* **7**:235, 1994.

286. Fisher F, Crouch DH, Jayaraman P-S, Clark W, Gillespie DAF, Goding CR: Transcription activation by Myc and Max: Flanking sequences target activation to a subset of CACGTG motifs in vivo. *EMBO J* **12**:5075, 1993.

287. Carreira S, Dexter TJ, Yavuzer U, Easty DJ, Goding CR: Brachyury-related transcription factor Tbx2 and repression of the melanocyte-specific TRP-1 promoter. *Mol Cell Biol* **18**:5099, 1998.

288. del Marmol V, Ito S, Jackson I, Vachtenheim J, Berr P, Ghanem G, Morandini R, Wakamatsu K, Huez G: TRP-1 expression correlates with eumelanogenesis in human pigment cells in culture. *FEBS Lett* **327**:307, 1993.

289. Vijayasaradhi S, Xu Y, Bouchard B, Houghton AN: Intracellular sorting and targeting of melanosomal membrane proteins: Identification of signals for sorting of the human brown locus protein, gp75. *J Cell Biol* **130**:807, 1995.

290. Xu Y, Vijayasaradhi S, Houghton AN: The cytoplasmic tail of the mouse brown locus product determines intracellular stability and export from the endoplasmic reticulum. *J Invest Dermatol* **110**:324, 1998.

291. Xu Y, Vijayasaradhi S, Takechi Y, Houghton AN: Sorting and secretion of a melanosome membrane protein, gp75/TRP1. *J Invest Dermatol* **109**:788, 1997.

292. Honing S, Sandoval IV, von Figura K: A di-leucine-based motif in the cytoplasmic tail of LIMP-II and tyrosinase mediates selective binding of AP-3. *EMBO J* **17**:1304, 1998.

293. Gardner JM, Nakatsu Y, Gondo Y, Lee S, Lyon MF, King RA, Brilliant MH: The mouse pink-eyed dilution gene: Association with human Prader-Willi and Angelman syndromes. *Science* **257**:1121, 1992.

294. Brilliant MH: The mouse pink-eyed dilution locus: A model for aspects of Prader-Willi syndrome, Angelman syndrome and a form of hypomelanosis of Ito. *Mam Genome* **3**:187, 1992.

295. Ramsay M, Colman MA, Stevens G, Zwane E, Kromberg J, Farrah M, Jenkins T: The tyrosinase-positive oculocutaneous albinism locus maps to chromosome 15q11.2-q12. *Am J Hum Genet* **51**:879, 1992.

296. Rinchik EM, Bultman SJ, Horsthemke B, Lee S, Stunk KM, Spritz RA, Avidano KM, Jong MTC, Nicholls RD: A gene for the mouse pink-eyed dilution locus and for human type II oculocutaneous albinism. *Nature* **361**:72, 1993.

297. Devi CC, Tripathi C, Ramaiah A: pH-dependent interconvertible allosteric forms of murine melanoma tyrosinase: Physiological implications. *Eur J Biochem* **166**:705, 1987.

298. Seiji M, Iwashita S: Intracellular localization of tyrosinase and site of melanin formation in melanocytes. *J Invest Dermatol* **45**:305, 1965.

299. Bailin T, Oh J, Feng GH, Fukai K, Spritz RA: Organization and nucleotide sequence of the human Hermansky-Pudlak syndrome (HPS) gene. *J Invest Dermatol* **108**:923, 1997.

300. Swank RT, Novak E, McGarry MP, Rusiniak ME, Feng L: Mouse models of Hermansky Pudlak syndrome: A review. *Pigment Cell Res* **11**:60, 1998.

301. Hazelwood S, Shotelersuk V, Wildenberg SC, Chen D, Iwata F, Kaiser-Kupfer MI, White JG, King RA, Gahl WA: Evidence for locus heterogeneity in Puerto Ricans with Hermansky-Pudlak syndrome. *Am J Hum Genet* **61**:1088, 1997.

302. Gahl WA, Dell'Angelica E, Shotelersuk V, Bonifacino JS: A human disorder due to mutant b3A subunit of adaptor complex-3: Failed vesicle formation in brothers with Hermansky-Pudlak syndrome (HPS) [Abstract]. *Am J Hum Genet* **63**:A2, 1998.

303. Barbosa MDFS, Nguyen QA, Tchernev VT, Ashley JA, Detter JC, Blaydes SM, Brandt SJ, Chotai D, Hodgman C, Solari RCE, Lovett M, Kingsmore SF: Identification of the homologous beige and Chediak-Higashi syndrome genes. *Nature* **382**:262, 1996.

304. Perou CM, Moore KJ, Nagle DL, Misumi DJ, Woolf EA, McGrail SH, Holmgren L, Brody TH, Dussault BJ, Monroe CA, Duyk GM, Pryor RJ, Li L, Justice MJ, Kaplan J: Identification of the murine *beige* gene by YAC complementation and positional cloning. *Nat Genet* **13**:303, 1996.

305. Bergen AAB, Samanns C, Schuurman EJM, van Osch L, van Dorp DB, Pinckers AJLG, Bakker E, Gal A, van Ommen GJB, Bleeker-Wagemakers EM: Multipoint linkage analysis in X-linked ocular albinism of the Nettleship-Falls type. *Hum Genet* **88**:162, 1991.

306. Schnur RE, Nussbaum RL, Anson-Cartwright L, McDowell C, Worton RG, Musarella MA: Linkage analysis in X-linked ocular albinism. *Genomics* **9**:605, 1991.

307. Bassi MT, Schiaffino MV, Renieri A, De Nigris F, Galli L, Bruttini M, Gebbia M, Bergen AAB, Lewis RA, Ballabio A: Cloning of the gene for ocular albinism type 1 from the distal short arm of the X chromosome. *Nat Genet* **10**:13, 1995.

308. Newton J, Orlow SJ, Barsh GS: Isolation and characterization of a mouse homolog of the X-linked ocular albinism (OA1) gene. *Genomics* **37**:219, 1996.

309. Schiaffino MV, Bassi MT, Galli L, Renieri A, Bruttini M, De Nigris F, Bergen AAB, Charles SJ, Yates JRW, Meindl A, Lewis RA, King RA, Ballabio A: Analysis of the OA1 gene reveals mutations in only one-third of patients with X-linked ocular albinism. *Hum Mol Genet* **4**:2319, 1995.

310. Schiaffino MV, Baschirotto C, Pellegrini G, Montalti S, Tacchetti C, De Luca M, Ballabio A: The ocular albinism type 1 gene product is a membrane glycoprotein localized to melanosomes. *Proc Natl Acad Sci U S A* **93**:9055, 1996.

311. King RA, Oetting WS, Creel DJ, Hearing V: Abnormalities of pigmentation, in Rimoin DL, Connor JM, Pyeritz RE (eds): *Emery and Rimoin's Principles and Practice of Medical Genetics*, 3rd ed. New York, Churchill Livingstone, 1997, p 1171.

312. Charles SJ, Moore AT, Grant JW, Yates JRW: Genetic counseling in X-linked ocular albinism. Clinical features of the carrier state. *Eye* **6**:75, 1992.

313. Zinn KM, Benjamin-Henkind J: Retinal pigment epithelium, in Duane TD, Jaeger EA (eds): *Biomedical Foundations of Ophthalmology*. Hagerstown, MD, Harper & Row, 1986, p 1.

314. Abadi R, Pascal E: The recognition and management of albinism. *Ophthalmic Physiol Opt* **9**:3, 1989.

315. Summers CG, Knobloch WH, Witkop CJ, King RA: Hermansky-Pudlak syndrome: Ophthalmic findings. *Ophthalmology* **95**:545, 1988.

316. Wack MA, Peachey NS, Fishman GA: Electroretinographic findings in human oculocutaneous albinism. *Ophthalmology* **96**:1778, 1989.

317. Wilson HR, Mets MB, Nagy SE, Kressel AB: Albino spatial vision as an instance of arrested visual development. *Vision Res* **28**:979, 1988.

318. Wilson HR, Mets MB, Nagy SE, Ferrera VP: Spatial frequency and orientation tuning of spatial visual mechanisms in human albinos. *Vision Res* **28**:991, 1988.

319. Creel DJ, Summers CG, King RA: Visual anomalies associated with albinism. *Ophthalmic Pediatr Genet* **11**:193, 1990.

320. Fitzgerald K, Cibis GW: The value of flash visual evoked potentials in albinism. *J Pediatr Ophthalmol Strabismus* **31**:18, 1994.

321. Shallo-Hoffmann J, Apkarian P: Visual evoked response asymmetry only in the albino member of a family with congenital nystagmus. *Invest Ophthalmol Vis Sci* **34**:682, 1993.

322. Bouzas EA, Caruso RC, Drews-Bankiewicz MA, Kaiser-Kupfer MI: Evoked potential analysis of visual pathways in human albinism. *Ophthalmology* **101**:309, 1994.

323. Ilia M, Jeffery G: Delayed neurogenesis in the albino retina: Evidence of a role for melanin in regulating the pace of cell generation. *Brain Res Dev Brain Res* **95**:176, 1996.

324. Rapaport DH, Rakic P, Yasamura D, LaVail MM: Genesis of the retinal pigment epithelium in the macaque monkey. *J Comp Neurol* **363**:359, 1995.

325. Rachel RA, Mason CA: Relationship between tyrosinase/melanin levels at birth and retinal pathways in dark-eyed albino mice [Abstract]. *Pigment Cell Res* **10**:119, 1997.

326. Guillery RW, Mason CA, Taylor JS: Developmental determinants at the mammalian optic chiasm [Review]. *J Neurosci* **15**:4727, 1995.

327. Silver J, Sapiro J: Axonal guidance during development of the optic nerve: The role of pigmented epithelia and other extrinsic factors. *J Comp Neurol* **202**:521, 1981.

328. Strongin AC, Guillery RW: The distribution of melanin in the developing optic cup and stalk and its relation to cellular degeneration. *J Neurosci* **1**:1193, 1981.

329. Colello RJ, Jeffery G: Evaluation of the influence of optic stalk melanin on the chiasmatic pathways in the developing rodent visual system. *J Comp Neurol* **305**:304, 1991.

330. Webster MJ, Shatz CJ, Silver J: Abnormal pigmentation and unusual morphogenesis of the optic stalk may be correlated with retinal axon misguidance in embryonic Siamese cats. *J Comp Neurol* **269**:592, 1988.

331. Wizenmann A, Thanos S, Boxberg YV, Bonhoeffer F: Differential reaction of crossing and non-crossing rat retinal axons on cell

membrane preparations from the chiasm midline; an in vitro study. *Development* **117**:725, 1993.

332. Marcus RC, Wang L-C, Mason CA: Retinal axon divergence in the optic chiasm: Midline cells are unaffected by the albino mutation. *Development* **122**:859, 1996.

333. Chan SO, Baker GE, Guillery RW: Differential action of the albino mutation on two components of the rat's uncrossed retinofugal pathway. *J Comp Neurol* **336**:362, 1993.

334. Mason CA, Sretavan DW: Glia, neurons, and axon pathfinding during optic chiasm development [Review]. *Curr Opin Neurobiol* **7**:647, 1998.

335. Jeffery G, Schütz G, Montoliu L: Correction of abnormal retinal pathways found with albinism by introduction of a functional tyrosinase gene in transgenic mice. *Devel Biol* **166**:460, 1994.

336. Jeffery G, Brem G, Montoliu L: Correction of retinal abnormalities found in albinism by introduction of a functional tyrosinase gene in transgenic mice and rabbits. *Devel Brain Res* **99**:95, 1997.

337. Collewijn H, Apkarian P, Spekreijse H: The oculomotor behaviour of human albinos. *Brain* **108**:1, 1985.

338. Abadi RV, Pascal E: Visual resolution limits in human albinism. *Vision Res* **31**:1445, 1991.

339. Abadi RV, Dickinson CM, Pascal E, Papas E: Retinal image quality in albinos. A review. *Ophthalmic Pediatr Genet* **11**:171, 1990.

340. Summers CG, Oetting WS, King RA: Diagnosis of oculocutaneous albinism with molecular analysis. *Am J Ophthalmol* **121**:724, 1996.

341. Käsman B, Ruprecht KW: Might the refractive state in oculocutaneous albino patients be a clue for distinguishing between tyrosinase-positive and tyrosinase-negative forms of oculocutaneous albinism? *German J Ophthalmol* **5**:422, 1997.

342. Laties AM, Stone RA: Some visual and neurochemical correlates of refractive development. *Vis Neurosci* **7**:125, 1991.

343. Troilo D: Neonatal eye growth and emmetropisation — A literature review. *Eye* **6**:154, 1992.

344. Diether S, Schaeffel F: Local changes in eye growth induced by imposed local refractive error dispute active accommodation. *Vision Res* **37**:659, 1997.

345. Conlee JW, Jensen RP, Parks TN, Creel DJ: Turn-specific and pigment-dependent differences in the stria vascularis of normal and gentamicin-treated albino and pigmented guinea pigs. *Hear Res* **55**:57, 1991.

346. Conlee JW, Bennett ML: Turn-specific differences in the endocochlear potential between albino and pigmented guinea pigs. *Hear Res* **65**:141, 1993.

347. Gill SS, Salt AN: Quantitative differences in endolymphatic calcium and endocochlear potential between pigmented and albino guinea pigs. *Hear Res* **113**:191, 1997.

348. Conlee JW, Gerity LC, Bennett ML: Ongoing proliferation of melanocytes in the stria vascularis of the adult guinea pig. *Hear Res* **79**:115, 1994.

349. Pawelek JM, Bolognia J, McLane J, Murray M, Osber MP, Sominski A: A possible role for melanin precursors in regulating both pigmentation and proliferation of melanocytes. *Prog Clin Biol Res* **256**:143, 1988.

350. Barrenas M-L: Hair cell loss from acoustic trauma in chloroquine-treated red, black, and albino guinea pigs. *Audiology* **36**:187, 1997.

351. Szymanski MD, Henry KR, Buchting FO: Albino and pigmented gerbil auditory function: Influence of genotype and gentamycin. *Audiology* **33**:63, 1994.

352. Park S-K, Lee K-H, Park K-C, Lee J-S, Spritz RA, Lee S-T: Prevalent and novel mutations of the tyrosinase gene in Korean patients with tyrosinase-deficient oculocutaneous albinism. *Mol Cells* **7**:187, 1997.

353. Park KC, Chintamaneni CD, Halaban R, Witkop CJ, Kwon BS: Molecular analyses of a tyrosinase-negative albino family. *Am J Hum Genet* **52**:406, 1993.

354. Oetting WS, King RA: Molecular basis of type 1 (tyrosinase-related) oculocutaneous albinism: Mutations and polymorphisms of the human tyrosinase gene. *Hum Mutat* **2**:1, 1993.

355. Oetting WS, Fryer JP, King RA: A dinucleotide deletion (−DGA115) in the tyrosinase gene responsible for type I-A (tyrosinase negative) oculocutaneous albinism in a Pakistani individual. *Hum Mol Genet* **2**:1047, 1993.

356. Fukai K, Holmes SA, Lucchese NJ, Siu VM, Weleber RG, Schnur RE, Spritz RA: Autosomal recessive ocular albinism associated with a functionally significant tyrosinase gene polymorphism. *Nat Genet* **9**:92, 1995.

357. Oetting WS, Fryer JP, Oofuji Y, Middendorf LR, Brumbaugh JA, Summers CG, King RA: Analysis of tyrosinase gene mutations using direct automated infrared fluorescence DNA sequencing of amplified exons. *Electrophoresis* **15**:159, 1994.

358. Park KC, Kim KH, Lee YS, Kwon BS: Single-strand conformation polymorphism analysis of point mutation in a tyrosinase-negative oculocutaneous albino. *J Inherit Metab Dis* **17**:123, 1994.

359. Breimer LH, Winder AF, Jay B, Jay M: Initiation codon mutation of the tyrosinase gene as a cause of human albinism. *Clin Chim Acta* **227**:17, 1994.

360. Spritz RA: Molecular genetics of oculocutaneous albinism. *Semin Dermatol* **12**:167, 1993.

361. Tripathi RK, Bundey S, Musarella MA, Droetto S, Strunk KM, Holmes SA, Spritz RA: Mutations of the tyrosinase gene in Indo-Pakistani patients with type I (tyrosinase-deficient) oculocutaneous albinism (OCA). *Am J Hum Genet* **53**:1173, 1993.

362. Oetting WS, King RA: Molecular basis of albinism: Mutations and polymorphisms of pigmentation genes associated with albinism. *Hum Mutat* **13**:99, 1999.

363. Spritz RA, Oh J, Fukai K, Holmes SA, Ho L, Chitayat D, Frabce TD, Musarella MA, Orlow SJ, Schnur RE, Weleber RG, Levin AV: Novel mutations of the tyrosinase (*TYR*) gene in type I oculocutaneous albinism. *Hum Mutat* **10**:171, 1997.

364. Gershoni-Bursch R, Rosenmann A, Droetto S, Holmes S, Tripathi RK, Spritz RA: Mutations of the tyrosinase gene in patients with oculocutaneous albinism from various ethnic groups in Israel. *Am J Hum Genet* **54**:586, 1994.

365. Breimer LH, Winder AF, Panayiotidis P, Jay M, Moore A, Jay B: A trinucleotide deletion together with a base duplication event at codon 439 in the human tyrosinase gene identifies a mutational hotspot. *Clin Chim Acta* **243**:35, 1995.

366. Oetting WS, Fryer JP, King RA: Mutations in brief: Mutations of the human tyrosinase gene associated with tyrosinase related oculocutaneous albinism (OCA1). *Hum Mutat* **12**:433, 1998.

367. Matsunaga J, Dakeishi-Hara M, Miyamura Y, Nakamura E, Tanita M, Satomura K, Tomita Y: Sequence-based diagnosis of tyrosinase-related oculocutaneous albinism: Successful sequence analysis of the tyrosinase gene from blood spots dried on filter paper. *Dermatology* **196**:189, 1998.

368. Matsunaga J, Dakeishi M, Shimizu H, Tomita Y: R278TER and P431L mutations of the tyrosinase gene exist in Japanese patients with tyrosinase-negative oculocutaneous albinism. *J Dermatol Sci* **13**:134, 1996.

369. Giebel LB, Tripathi RK, Strunk KM, Hanifin JM, Jackson CE, King RA, Spritz RA: Tyrosinase gene mutations associated with type IB ("yellow") oculocutaneous albinism. *Am J Hum Genet* **48**:1159, 1991.

370. Volbeda A, Hol WG: Crystal structure of hexameric haemocyanin from Panulirus interruptus refined at 3.2 A resolution. *J Mol Biol* **209**:249, 1989.

371. Oetting WS, King RA: Analysis of mutations in the copper B binding region associated with type I (tyrosinase-related) oculocutaneous albinism, in Takeuchi T (ed): *Molecular Biology of Pigmentation.* Copenhagen, Munksgaard, 1992, p 274.

372. Witkop JC: Albinism, in Harris H, Hirschhorn K (eds): *Advances in Human Genetics*, Vol. 2, New York, Plenum Press, 1971, p 61.

373. Spritz RA, Fukai K, Holmes SA, Luande J: Frequent intragenic deletion of the P gene in Tanzanian patients with type II oculocutanoeus albinism (OCA2). *Am J Hum Genet* **56**:1320, 1995.

374. Durham-Pierre D, Gardner JM, Nakatsu Y, King RA, Francke U, Ching A, Aquaron R, del Marmol V, Brilliant MH: African origin of an intragenic deletion of the human P gene in tyrosinase-positive oculocutaneous albinism. *Nat Genet* **7**:176, 1994.

375. Puri N, Durham-Pierre D, Aquaron R, Lund PM, King RA, Brilliant MH: Type 2 oculocutaneous albinism (OCA2) in Zimbabwe and Cameroon: Distribution of the 2.7-kb deletion allele of the P gene. *Hum Genet* **100**:651, 1997.

376. Kedda MA, Stevens G, Manga P, Vilijoen C, Jenkins T, Ramsay M: The tyrosinase-positive oculocutaneous albinism gene shows locus homogeneity on chromosome 15q11-q13 and evidence of multiple mutations in southern African Negroids. *Am J Hum Genet* **54**:1078, 1994.

377. Stevens G, van Beukering J, Jenkins T, Ramsay M: An intragenic deletion of the P gene is the common mutation causing tyrosinase-positive oculocutaneous albinism in southern African Negroids. *Am J Hum Genet* **56**:586, 1995.

378. Bothwell JE: Pigmented skin lesions in tyrosinase-positive oculocutaneous albinos: A study in black South Africans. *Int J Dermatol* **36**:831, 1994.

379. Kromberg JGR, Castle D, Zwane EM, Jenkins T: Albinism and skin cancer in southern Africa. *Clin Genet* **36**:43, 1989.

380. Lee S-T, Nicholls RD, Schnur RE, Guida LC, Lu-Kuo J, Spinner NB, Zackai EH, Spritz RA: Diverse mutations of the *P* gene among African-Americans with type II (tyrosinase-positive) oculocutaneous albinism (OCA2). *Hum Mol Genet* **3**:2047, 1994.

381. Bhatnagar V, Anjaiah S, Puri N, Arudhra Darshanam BN, Ramaiah A: pH of melanosomes of B16 murine melanoma is acidic: Its physiological importance in the regulation of melanin biosynthesis. *Arch Biochem Biophys* **307**:183, 1993.

382. Barsh GS: The genetics of pigmentation: From fancy genes to complex traits. *TIG* **12**:299, 1996.

383. Manga P, Ramsay M, Kromberg J, Jenkins T: Brown oculocutaneous albinism is allelic to tyrosinase-positive oculocutaneous albinism in southern African Negroids [Abstract]. *Am J Hum Genet* **55**:A194, 1995.

384. King RA, Rich SS: Segregation analysis of brown oculocutaneous albinism. *Clin Genet* **29**:496, 1986.

385. Cassidy SB: Prader-Willi syndrome. *J Med Genet* **34**:917, 1997.

386. Cassidy SB, Schwartz S: Prader-Willi and Angelman syndromes: Disorders of genomic imprinting. *Medicine* **77**:140, 1998.

387. Horsthemke B, Dittrich B, Buiting K: Imprinting mutations on chromosome 15 [Review]. *Hum Mutat* **10**:329, 1997.

388. Nicholls RD, Saitoh S, Horsthemke B: Imprinting in Prader-Willi and Angelman syndromes. *TIG* **14**:194, 1998.

389. Lee S-T, Nicholls RD, Bundey S, Laxova R, Musarella M, Spritz RA: Mutations of the P gene in oculocutaneous albinism, ocular albinism, and Prader-Willi syndrome plus albinism. *N Engl J Med* **330**:529, 1994.

390. Nicholls RD, Bailin T, Mascari MJ, Butler MG, Spritz RA: Hypopigmentation in the Prader-Willi syndrome correlates with P gene deletion but not with haplotype of the hemizygous P allele. *Am J Hum Genet* **59**:A39, 1996.

391. Spritz RA, Bailin T, Nicholls RD, Lee S-T, Park SK, Mascari MJ, Butler MG: Hypopigmentation in the Prader-Willi syndrome correlates with P gene deletion but not with haplotype of the hemizygous P allele. *Am J Med Genet* **71**:57, 1997.

392. Gillessen-Kaesbach G, Robinson W, Lohmann D, Kaya-Westerloh S, Passarge E, Horsthemke B: Genotype-phenotype correlation in a series of 167 deletion and non-deletion patients with Prader-Willi syndrome. *Hum Genet* **96**:638, 1995.

393. Cassidy SB, Forsythe M, Heeger S, Nicholls RD, Schork N, Benn P, Schwartz S: Comparison of phenotype between patients with Prader-Willi syndrome due to deletion 15q and uniparental disomy 15. *Am J Med Genet* **68**:433, 1997.

394. Creel DJ, Bendel CM, Wiesner GL, Wirtschafter JD, Arthur DC, King RA: Abnormalities of the central visual pathways in Prader-Willi syndrome associate with hypopigmentation. *N Engl J Med* **314**:1606, 1986.

395. Apkarian P, Spekreijse H, van Swaay E, van Schooneveld M: Visual evoked potentials in Prader-Willi syndrome. *Doc Ophthalmol* **71**:355, 1989.

396. Saitoh S, Buiting K, Cassidy SB, Conroy JM, Driscoll DJ, Gabriel JM, Gillessen-Kaesbach G, Glenn CC, Greenswag LR, Horsthemke B, Kondo I, Kuwajima K, Niikawa N, Rogan PK, Schwartz S, Seip J, Williams CA, Nicholls RD: Clinical spectrum and molecular diagnosis of Angelman and Prader-Willi syndrome patients with an imprinting mutation. *Am J Med Genet* **68**:195, 1997.

397. Buntinx IM, Hennekam RC, Brouwer OF, Stroink H, Beuten J, Mangelschots K, Fryns JP: Clinical profile of Angelman syndrome at different ages. *Am J Med Genet* **56**:176, 1995.

398. Saitoh S, Harada N, Jinno Y, Hashimoto K, Imaizumi K, Kuroki Y, Fukushima Y, Sugimoto T, Renedo M, Wagstaff J: Molecular and clinical study of 61 Angelmen syndrome patients. *Am J Med Genet* **52**:158, 1994.

399. Bürger J, Kunze J, Sperling K, Reis A: Phenotypic differences in Angelman syndrome patients: Imprinting mutations show less frequent microcephaly and hypopigmentation than deletions. *Am J Med Genet* **66**:221, 1996.

400. Smith A, Wiles C, Haan E, McGill J, Wallace G, Dixon J, Selby R, Colley A, Marks R, Trent RJ: Clinical features of 27 patients with Angelman syndrome resulting from DNA deletion. *J Med Genet* **33**:107, 1996.

401. Durham-Pierre D, King RA, Naber JM, Laken S, Brilliant MH: Estimation of carrier frequency of a 2.7-kb deletion allele of the P gene associated with OCA2 in African-Americans. *Hum Mutat* **7**:370, 1996.

402. Spritz RA, Lee S-T, Fukai K, Brondum-Nielsen K, Chitayat D, Lipson MH, Musarella MA, Rosenmann A, Weleber RG: Novel mutations of

the P gene in type II oculocutaneous albinism (OCA2). *Hum Mutat* **10**:175, 1997.

403. Lund PM, Puri N, Durham-Pierre D, King RA, Brilliant MH: Oculocutaneous albinism in an isolated Tonga community in Zimbabwe. *J Med Genet* **34**:733, 1997.

404. Stevens G, Ramsay M, Jenkins T: Oculocutaneous albinism (OCA2) in sub-Saharan Africa: Distribution of the common 2.7-kb P gene deletion mutation. *Hum Genet* **99**:523, 1997.

405. Lee S-T, Nicholls RD, Bundey S, Laxova R, Musarella M, Spritz RA: Mutations of the P gene in oculocutaneous albinism, ocular albinism, and Prader-Willi Syndrome. *N Engl J Med* **330**:529, 1994.

406. Oetting WS, Gardner JM, Fryer JP, Ching A, Durham-Pierre D, King RA, Brilliant MH: Mutations in brief: Mutations of the human P gene associated with type II oculocutaneous albinism (OCA2). *Hum Mutat* **12**:4333, 1998.

407. Sviderskaya EV, Bennett DC, Ho L, Bailin T, Lee S-T, Spritz RA: Complementation of hypipgmentatin in *p*-mutant (*pink-eyed Dilution*) mouse melanocytes by normal human *P* cDNA, and defective complementation by OCA2 mutant sequences. *J Invest Dermatol* **108**:30, 1997.

408. Jiménez-Cervantes C, Solano F, Kobayashi T, Urabe K, Hearing VJ, Lozano JA, García-Borrón JC: A new enzymatic function in the melanogenic pathway: The 5.6-dihydroxyindole-2-carboxylic acid oxidase activity of tyrosinase-related protein-1 (TRP-1). *J Biol Chem* **269**:17993, 1994.

409. Hornabrook RW, McDonald WI, Carroll RL: Congenital nystagmus among the red-skins of the highlands of Papua New Guinea. *Br J Ophthalmol* **64**:375, 1980.

410. Kromberg JGR, Castle DJ, Zwane EM, Bothwell J, Kidson S, Bartel P, Phillips JI, Jenkins T: Red or rufous albinism in southern Africa. *Ophthalmic Pediatr Genet* **11**:229, 1990.

411. Manga P, Kromberg JG, Box NF, Sturm RA, Jenkins T, Ramsay M: Rufous oculocutaneous albinism in southern African blacks is caused by mutations in the TYRP1 gene. *Am J Hum Genet* **61**:1095, 1997.

412. Gardner JM, Wildenberg SC, Keiper NM, Novak EK, Rusiniak ME, Swank RT, Puri N, Finger JN, Hagiwara N, Lehman AL, Gales T, Bayer ME, King RA, Brilliant MH: The mouse pale ear (*ep*) mutation is the homologue of Hermansky-Pudlak syndrome (HPS). *Proc Natl Acad Sci U S A* **94**:9238, 1997.

413. Spritz RA: Molecular genetics of Hermansky-Pudlak and Chediak-Higashi syndromes. *Platelets* **9**:21, 1998.

414. Karim MA, Nagle DL, Kandil HH, Bürger J, Moore KJ, Spritz RA: Mutations in the Chediak-Higashi syndrome gene (CHS1) indicate requirement for the complete 3801 amino acid CHS protein. *Hum Mol Genet* **6**:1087, 1997.

415. Gahl WA, Brantly M, Kaiser-Kupfer MI, Iwata F, Hazelwood S, Shotelersuk V, Duffy LF, Kuehl EM, Troendle J, Bernardini I: Genetic defects and clinical characteristics of patients with a form of oculocutaneous albinism (Hermansky-Pudlak syndrome). *N Engl J Med* **338**:1258, 1998.

416. Izquierdo NJ, Townsend W, Maumenee Hussels IE: Ocular findings in the Hermansky-Pudlak syndrome. *Trans Am Ophth Soc* **93**:191, 1995.

417. Hermansky F, Pudlak P: Albinism associated with hemorrhagic diathesis and unusual pigmented reticular cells in the bone marrow: Report of two cases with histochemical studies. *Blood* **14**:162, 1959.

418. Frenk E, Lattion F: The melanin pigmentary disorder in a family with Hermansky-Pudlak syndrome. *J Invest Dermatol* **78**:141, 1982.

419. Shotelersuk V, Hazelwood S, Larson D, Iwata F, Kaiser-Kupfer MI, Kuehl E, Bernardini I, Gahl WA: Three new mutations in the gene causing Hermansky-Pudlak syndrome: Clinical correlations. *Mol Genet Metab* **64**:99, 1998.

420. Ohbayashi C, Kanomata N, Imai Y, Ito H, Shimasaki H: Hermansky-Pudlak syndrome: A case report with analysis of auto-fluorescent ceroid-like pigments. *Gerontol* **41(Suppl 2)**:297, 1995.

421. Sakuma T, Monma N, Satodate R, Satoh T, Takeda R, Kuriya S-I: Ceroid pigment deposition in circulating blood monocytes and T lymphocytes in Hermansky-Pudlak syndrome: An ultrastructural study. *Pathol Int* **45**:866, 1995.

422. Harmon KR, Witkop CJ, White JG, King RA, Peterson M, Moore D, Tashjian J, Marinelli WA, Bitterman PB: Pathogenesis of pulmonary fibrosis—PDGF precedes structural alterations in the Hermansky-Pudlak syndrome. *J Lab Clin Med* **123**:617, 1994.

423. Oh J, Ho L, Ala-Mello S, Amato D, Armstrong L, Bellucci S, Carakushansky G, Ellis JP, Fong C-T, Green JS, Heon E, Legius E, Levin AV, Nieuwenhuis HK, Pinckers A, Tamura N, Whiteford ML, Yamasaki H, Spritz RA: Mutation analysis of patients with

Hermansky-Pudlak syndrome: A frameshift hot spot in the HPS gene and apparent locus heterogeneity. *Am J Hum Genet* **62**:593, 1998.

424. Kantheti P, Qiao X, Diaz ME, Peden AA, Meyer GE, Carskadon SL, Kapfhamer D, Sufalko D, Robinson MS, Noebels JL, Burmeister M: Mutations in AP-3 d in the *mocha* mouse links endosomal transport to storage deficiency in platelets, melanosomes, and synaptic vesicles. *Neuron* **21**:111, 1998.

425. Spritz RA: Genetic defects in Chediak-Higashi syndrome and the *beige* mouse. *J Clin Immunol* **18**:97, 1998.

426. Haddad E, Le Deist F, Blanche S, Benkerrou M, Rohrlich P, Vilmer E, Griscelli C, Fischer A: Treatment of Chediak-Higashi syndrome by allogenic bone marrow transplantation: Report of 10 cases. *Blood* **85**:3328, 1995.

427. Durandy A, Breton-Goriust J, Guy-Grand D, Dumez C, Griscelli C: Prenatal diagnosis of syndromes associating albinism and immune deficiencies (Chediak-Higashi syndrome and variant). *Prenat Diagn* **13**:13, 1993.

428. Novak EK, Hui SW, Swank RT: Platelet storage pool deficiency in mouse pigment mutations associated with seven distinct genetic loci. *Blood* **63**:536, 1984.

429. Fukai K, Oh J, Karim MA, Moore KJ, Kandil HH, Ito H, Burger J, Spritz RA: Homozygous mapping of the gene for Chediak-Higashi syndrome to chromosome 1q42-q44 in a segment of conserved synteny that includes the mouse *beige* locus (*bg*). *Am J Hum Genet* **59**:620, 1996.

430. Barbosa MDFS, Barrat FJ, Tchernev VT, Nguyen QA, Mishra VS, Colman SD, Pastural E, Dufourcq-Lagelouse R, Fischer A, Holcombe RF, Wallace MR, Brandt SJ, Saint Basile G, Kingsmore SF: Identification of mutations in two major mRNA isoforms of the Chediak-Higashi syndrome gene in human and mouse. *Hum Mol Genet* **6**:1091, 1997.

431. Charles SJ, Green JS, Grant JW, Yates JRW, Moore AT: Clinical features of affected males with X-linked ocular albinism. *Br J Ophthalmol* **77**:222, 1993.

432. Shiono T, Tsunoda M, Chida Y, Nakazawa M, Tamai M: X-linked ocular albinism in Japanese patients. *Br J Ophthalmol* **79**:139, 1995.

433. Schnur RE, Wick PA, Bailey C, Rebbeck T, Weleber RG, Wagstaff J, Grix AW, Pagon RA, Hockey A, Edwards MJ: Phenotypic variability in X-linked ocular albinism: Relationship to linkage genotypes. *Am J Hum Genet* **55**:484, 1994.

434. Shiono T, Mutoh T, Chida Y, Tamai M: Ocular albinism with unilateral sectorial pigmentation in the fundus. *Br J Ophthalmol* **78**:412, 1994.

435. Schnur RE, Gao M, Wick PA, Keller M, Benke PJ, Edwards MJ, Grix AW, Hockey A, Jung JH, Kidd KK, Kistenmacher M, Levin AV, Lewis RA, Musarella MA, Nowakowski RW, Orlow SJ, Pagon RS, Pillers D-AM, Punnett HH, Quinn GE, Tezcan K, Wagstaff J, Weleber RG: *OA1* mutations and deletions in X-linked ocular albinism. *Am J Hum Genet* **62**:800, 1998.

436. Tijmes NT, Bergen AAB, de Jong PTVM: Paucity of signs in X-linked ocular albinism with a 700-kb deletion spanning the OA1 gene. *Br J Ophthalmol* **82**:457, 1998.

437. Muroya K, Ogata T, Matsuo N, Nagai T, Franco B, Ballabio A, Rappold G, Sakura N, Fukushima Y: Mental retardation in a boy with an interstitial deletion of Xp22.3 involving STS, KAL1, and OA1: Implications for the MRX locus. *Am J Med Genet* **64**:583, 1996.

438. Spritz RA: Molecular genetics of oculocutaneous albinism. *Hum Mol Genet* **3**:1469, 1994.

439. Morell R, Spritz RA, Ho L, Pierpoint J, Guo W, Friedman TB, Asher JH: Apparent digenic inheritance of Waardenburg syndrome type 2 (WS2) and autosomal recessive ocular albinism (AROA). *Hum Mol Genet* **6**:659, 1997.

440. Rose NC, Menacker SJ, Schnur RE, Jackson L, McDonald-McGinn DM, Stump T, Emanuel BS, Zackai EH: Ocular albinism in a male with del (6)(q13-q15): Candidate region for autosomal recessive ocular albinism? *Am J Med Genet* **42**:700, 1992.

441. Winship IM, Babaya M, Ramesar RS: X-linked ocular albinism and sensorineural deafness: Linkage to Xp22.3. *Genomics* **18**:444, 1993.

442. Lewis RA: Ocular albinism and deafness. *Am J Hum Genet* **30**:57A, 1978.

443. Forsius H, Eriksson AW: Tapeto-retinal degenerations with varying clinical features in Åland islanders. *J Med Genet* **7**:200, 1970.

444. Alitalo T, Kruse TA, Forsius H, Eriksson AW, de la Chapelle A: Localization of the Åland Island eye disease locus to the pericentromeric region of the X chromosome by linkage analysis. *Am J Hum Genet* **48**:31, 1991.

445. Schwartz M, Rosenberg T: Åland Island disease linkage data. *Genomics* **10**:327, 1991.

446. van Dorp DB, Eriksson AW, Delleman JW, van Vliet AGM, Collewijn H, van Balen ATM, Forsius HR: Åland Island disease: No albino misrouting. *Clin Genet* **28**:526, 1985.

447. Bergsma DR, Kaiser-Kupfer M: A new form of albinism. *Am J Ophthalmol* **77**:837, 1974.

448. Frenk E, Calame A: Familial oculocutaneous hypopigmentation of dominant transmission due to a disorder in melanocyte formation. Association of Prader-Willi syndrome with a chromosome abnormality in one of the subjects involved. *Schweiz Med Wochenschr* **107**:1964, 1977.

449. Fitzpatrick TB, Jimbow K, Donaldson DD: Dominant oculocutaneous albinism. *Br J Dermatol* **91(Suppl 10)**:23, 1974.

450. Cockayne EA: *Inherited Abnormalities of the Skin and Its Appendages.* Oxford, Oxford University Press, 1933.

451. Tietz W: A syndrome of deaf-mutism associated with albinism showing autosomal dominant inheritance. *Am J Hum Genet* **15**:259, 1963.

452. Smith SD, Kenyon JB, Kelley PM, Hoover D, Comer B: Tietz syndrome (hypopigmentation/deafness) caused by mutations of MITF [Abstract]. *Am J Hum Genet* **61(Suppl)**:A347, 1997.

453. Amiel J, Watkin PM, Tassabehji M, Read AP, Winter RM: Mutation of the MITF gene in albinism-deafness syndrome (Tietz syndrome). *Clin Dysmorphol* **7**:17, 1998.

454. Fryns JP, Dereymaeker AM, Heremans G, Marien J, van Hauwaert J, Turner G, Hockey A, van den Berghe H: Oculocerebral syndrome with hypopigmentation (Cross syndrome). Report of two siblings born to consanguineous parents. *Clin Genet* **34**:81, 1988.

455. Tezcan I, Demir E, Asan E, Kale G, Muftuoglu SF, Kotiloglu E: A new case of oculocerebral hypopigmentation syndrome (Cross syndrome) with additional findings (a review). *Clin Genet* **51**:118, 1997.

456. Preus M, Fraser FC, Wiglesworth FW: An oculocutaneous hypopigmentation syndrome. *J Genet Hum* **31**:323, 1983.

457. Courtens W, Broeckx W, Ledoux M, Vamos E: Case report: Oculocutaneous hypopigmentation syndrome (Cross syndrome) in a Gypsy child. *Acta Paediatr Scand* **78**:806, 1989.

458. White CP, Waldron M, Jan JE, Carter JE: Oculocerebral hypopigmentation syndrome associated with Bartter syndrome. *Am J Med Genet* **46**:592, 1993.

459. Griscelli C, Durandy A, Guy-Grand D, Daguillard F, Herzog C, Prunieras M: A syndrome associating partial albinism and immunodeficiency. *Am J Med* **65**:691, 1978.

460. Harfi HA, Brismar J, Hainau B, Sabbah R: Partial albinism, immunodeficiency, and progressive white matter disease: A new primary immunodeficiency. *Allergy Proc* **13**:321, 1992.

461. Haraldson A, Weemaes CMR, Bakkeren JAJM, Happle R: Griscelli disease with cerebral involvement. *Eur J Pediatr* **150**:419, 1991.

462. Klein C, Philippe N, Le Deist F, Fraitag S, Prost C, Durandy A, Fischer A, Griscelli C: Partial albinism with immunodeficiency (Griscelli syndrome). *J Pediatr* **125**:886, 1994.

463. Hurvitz H, Gillis R, Klaus S, Klar A, Gross-Kieselstein F, Okun E: A kindred with Griscelli disease: Spectrum of neurological involvement. *Eur J Pediatr* **152**:402, 1993.

464. Brismar J, Harfi HA: Partial albinism with immunodeficiency: A rare syndrome with prominent posterior fossa white matter changes. *AJNR Am J Neuroradiol* **13**:387, 1992.

465. Gögüs S, Topçu M, Küçükali T, Akçören Z, Berkel I, Ersoy F, Günay M, Saatçi I: Griscelli syndrome: Report of three cases. *Pediatr Pathol Lab Med* **15**:309, 1995.

466. Gross A, Kunze J, Maier RF, Stoltenburg-Didinger G, Grimmer I, Obladen M: Autosomal recessive neural crest syndrome with *a*lbinism, *b*lack locks, *c*ell migration disorder of the neurocytes of the gut, and *d*eafness: ABCD syndrome. *Am J Med Genet* **56**:322, 1995.

467. Ziprkowski L, Krarowski A, Adam A, Costeff H, Sade J: Partial albinism and deaf mutism. *Arch Dermatol* **86**:530, 1962.

468. Litvak G, Sandkuyl L, Buchris V, Hildesheimer M, Shiloh Y: Localization of X-linked albinism-deafness syndrome (ADFN) to Xq by linkage with DNA markers [Abstract]. *Cytogenet Cell Genet* **46**:652, 1987.

469. Shiloh Y, Litvak G, Ziv Y, Lehner T, Sandkuyl L, Hildesheimer M, Buchris V, Cremers FPM, Szabo P, White BN, Holden JJA, Ott J: Genetic mapping of X-linked albinism-deafness syndrome (ADFN) to Xq26.3-q27.1. *Am J Hum Genet* **47**:20, 1990.

470. Zlotogora J: X-linked albinism-deafness syndrome and Waardenburg syndrome type II: A hypothesis [Letter]. *Am J Med Genet* **59**:386, 1995.

471. Spritz RA, Giebel LB, Holmes SA: Dominant negative and loss of function mutations of the *c-kit* (mast/stem cell growth factor receptor)

proto-oncogene in human piebaldism. *Am J Hum Genet* **50**:261, 1992.

472. Spritz RA, Holmes SA, Ramesar R, Greenberg J, Curtis D, Beighton P: Mutations of the *KIT* (mast/stem cell growth factor receptor) proto-oncogene account for a continuous range of phenotypes in human piebaldism. *Am J Hum Genet* **51**:1058, 1992.

473. Spritz RA: Molecular basis of human piebaldism. *J Invest Dermatol* **103(Suppl)**:137S, 1994.

474. Spritz RA, Holmes SA, Itin P, Kuster W: Novel mutations of the KIT (mast/stem cell growth factor receptor) proto-oncogene in human piebaldism. *J Invest Dermatol* **101**:22, 1993.

475. Spritz RA, Droetto S, Fukushima Y: Deletion of the KIT and PDGFRA genes in a patient with piebaldism. *Am J Med Genet* **44**:492, 1992.

476. Ezoe K, Holmes SA, Ho L, Bennett CP, Bolognia JL, Brueton L, Burn J, Falabella R, Gatto EM, Ishii N, Moss C, Pittelkow MR, Thompson E, Ward KA, Spritz RA: Novel mutations and deletions of the KIT (steel factor receptor) gene in human piebaldism. *Am J Hum Genet* **56**:58, 1995.

477. Williams DE, Eisenman J, Baird A, Rauch C, Van Ness K, March CJ, Park LS, Martin U, Mochizuki DY, Boswell HS, Burgess GS, Cosman D, Lyman SD: Identification of a ligand for the *c-kit* proto-oncogene. *Cell* **63**:167, 1990.

478. Flanagan JG, Leder P: The kit ligand: A cell surface molecule altered in steel mutant fibroblasts. *Cell* **63**:185, 1990.

479. Zsebo KM, Williams DA, Gelssler EN, Broudy VC, Martin FH, Atkins HL, Hsu RY, Birkett NC, Okino KH, Murdock DC, Jacobsen FW, Langley KE, Smith KA, Takeishi T, Cattanach BM, Galli SJ, Suggs SV: Stem cell factor is encoded at the Sl locus of the mouse and is the ligand for the *c-kit* tyrosine kinase receptor. *Cell* **63**:213, 1990.

480. Huang E, Nocka K, Beler DR, Chu TY, Buck J, Lahm HW, Wellner D, Leder P, Besmer P: The hematopoietic growth factor KL is encoded by the Sl locus and is the ligand of the *c-kit* receptor, the gene product of the *W* locus. *Cell* **63**:225, 1990.

481. Reith AD, Rottapel R, Giddens E, Brady C, Forrester L, Bernstein A: W mutant mice with mild or severe developmental defects contain distinct point mutations in the kinase domain of the *c-kit* receptor. *Genes Dev* **4**:390, 1990.

482. Tassabehji M, Newton VE, Liu X-Z, Brady A, Donnai D, Krajewska-Walasek M, Murday V, Norman A, Obersztyn E, Reardon W, Rice JC, Trembath R, Wieacker P, Whiteford M, Winter R, Read AP: The mutational spectrum in Waardenburg syndrome. *Hum Mol Genet* **4**:2131, 1995.

483. Read AP, Newton VE: Waardenburg syndrome. *J Med Genet* **34**:656, 1997.

484. Chalepakis G, Fritsch R, Fickenscher H, Deutsch U, Goulding M, Gruss P: The moleculaar basis of the *undulated/Pax-1* mutation. *Cell* **66**:873, 1991.

485. Hill R, van Heyningen V: Mouse mutations and human disorders are paired. *TIG* **8**:119, 1992.

486. Tassabehji M, Read AP, Newton VE, Patton M, Gruss P, Harris R, Strachan T: Mutations in the PAX3 gene causing Waardenburg syndrome type 1 and type 2. *Nat Genet* **3**:26, 1993.

487. Bard LA: Heterogeneity in Waardenburg's syndrome: Report of a family with ocular albinism. *Arch Ophthalmol* **96**:1193, 1978.

488. Tassabehji M, Newton VE, Read AP: Waardenburg syndrome type 2 caused by mutations in the human microphthalmia (*MITF*) gene. *Nat Genet* **8**:251, 1994.

489. Witkop CJ, Krumwiede M, Sedano H, White JG: The reliability of absent platelet dense bodies as a diagnostic criterion for Hermansky-Pudlak syndrome. *Am J Hematol* **26**:305, 1987.

490. Shimizu H, Niizeki H, Suzumori K, Aozaki R, Kawaguchi R, Hikiji K, Nishikawa T: Prenatal diagnosis of oculocutaneous albinism by analysis of the fetal tyrosinase gene. *J Invest Dermatol* **103**:104, 1994.

491. Shimizu H: Technical advances in prenatal diagnosis of tyrosinase-negative oculocutaneous albinism. *Acta Derm Venereol* **77**:10, 1997.

492. Kikuchi A, Shimizu H, Nishikawa T: Epidermal melanocytes in normal and tyrosinase-negative oculocutaneous albinism fetuses. *Arch Dermatol Res* **287**:529, 1995.

493. Davis PL, Baker RS, Piccione RJ: Large resection nystagmus surgery in albinos: Effect on acuity. *J Pediatr Ophthalmol Strabismus* **34**:279, 1997.

494. Pearson K, Nettleship E, Usher CH: *A monograph on albinism in man: Drapers' company research memoirs, biometric series VI.* London, Department of Applied Mathematics, Dulau and Co., Limited, 1911.

495. Woolf CM: Albinism among Indians in Arizona and New Mexico. *Am J Hum Genet* **17**:23, 1965.

496. Witkop CJ, Niswander JD, Bergsma DR, Workman PL, White JG: Tyrosinase positive oculocutaneous albinism among the Zuni and the Brandywine triracial isolate: Biochemical and clinical characteristics and fertility. *Am J Phys Anthropol* **36**:397, 1972.

497. van Dorp DB: Albinism, or the NOACH syndrome (The book of Encoh c.v. 1-20). *Clin Genet* **31**:228, 1987.

498. O'Donnell FE, Green WR: The eye in albinism, in Duane TD (ed): *Clinical Ophthalmology*, Vol. 4. Philadelphia, JB Lippincott, 1989, p 1.

499. Aquaron R: Oculocutaneous albinism in Cameroon: A 15-year follow-up study. *Ophthalmic Pediatr Genet* **11**:255, 1990.

500. Kromberg JGR, Jenkins T: Prevalence of albinism in the South African Negro. *S Afr Med J* **13**:383, 1982.

# Disorders of Intermediate Filaments and Their Associated Proteins

*Elaine Fuchs*

1. Eukaryotic cytoskeletons are composed of three filament networks. Actin microfilaments (6 nm) and microtubules (30 nm) are composed of proteins that are highly conserved in evolution from yeast to humans. Intermediate filaments (IFs, 10 nm), on the other hand, first appeared in evolution among the brachiopods and seem to have evolved to serve the specialized architectural requirements of higher eukaryotic cells. They constitute a superfamily of more than 40 proteins, which are differentially expressed in most, if not all, cells of higher organisms.

2. Despite their diversity in amino acid sequence, all IF proteins have a common secondary structure, consisting of a central, α-helical rod domain and flanking nonhelical head (N-terminal) and tail (C-terminal) segments. IF proteins form parallel, coiled-coil dimers, and more than 10,000 of these are needed to make each 10-nm filament. Dimers associate in a head-to-tail fashion to make linear arrays, which then pack laterally as two antiparallel chains arranged to form apolar protofilaments (2–3 nm). Two protofilaments intertwine to form protofibrils (4.5 nm), and approximately four of these then constitute the overall 10-nm diameter of the IF.

3. IF proteins have been subdivided into five distinct subtypes. Type I and II IF proteins are the keratins, which form obligatory heteropolymers in vitro in the absence of other auxiliary proteins or factors. Approximately 30 keratins of two distinct types are coexpressed as pairs in epithelial cells at various stages of differentiation and development. In the epidermis, keratins K5 and K14 are the major structural proteins of basal cells. As keratinocytes commit to terminal differentiation, they switch off expression of this pair and switch on expression of keratins K1 and K10, which constitute approximately 85 percent of total protein in the fully differentiated squame.

4. The first disorder of keratin to be genetically defined was epidermolysis bullosa simplex of the Dowling-Meara type (D-M EBS) (OMIM Nos. 148066 and 131760), a blistering skin disease where the innermost basal cells of the epidermis rupture and degenerate upon mechanical stress. This form of EBS is typified by clumps or aggregates of keratin material in basal epidermal cells. The elucidation of the genetic basis of EBS as a disorder of keratins K5 (OMIM No. 148040) and K14 (OMIM No. 148066) represents a novel example of the use of reverse genetics, beginning with the cloning of the basal cell keratin cDNAs and genes, defining key residues important for K5 and K14 filament assembly, engineering dominant negative-acting K14 mutants, discovering that these mutant genes cause EBS in transgenic mice, and finally focusing on human EBS and demonstrating that patients with this disorder have mutations in key residues critical for filament formation. Classic genetics substantiate the reverse genetic findings: Human families with any of four different subtypes of EBS-Dowling-Meara, Koebner (OMIM No. 131900), Weber-Cockayne (OMIM No. 131800), and mottled pigmentation (OMIM No. 131960) have genetic defects that map to either chromosome 12 or chromosome 17, at locations where the respective genes for K5 and K14 reside.

5. Many point mutations in the genes encoding K5 and K14 genes have now been found in patients with EBS, and the location of the mutation in the keratin polypeptides correlates well with earlier predictions based on random mutagenesis studies. In humans and in mice, severity in phenotype correlates with the degree to which a particular mutation affects 10-nm filament assembly, with the most severely disrupting mutations giving rise to defects in filament elongation and the milder mutations affecting lateral interactions within the filament. EBS with mottled pigmentation differs in that the location of the mutation resides in a region of K5 that is involved in connecting keratin IFs to desmosomes and possibly to other proteins/ organelles within the basal epidermal cell.

6. The advantage in a reverse genetic approach is that once the paradigm for a keratin disorder had been determined, a list could be made of additional disorders likely to involve defects in one or more of the 30 different keratin genes within the human genome. From a study of EBS, it was predicted that keratin disorders should have the following in common: cytolysis of a subset of epithelial cells sharing a common pattern of keratin expression, cytolysis as a consequence of mild physical stress, clumps or aggregates of keratin protein in the cells undergoing degeneration, and little or no involvement of epithelial cells that do not express the keratin(s) of interest. Since all epithelial cells express a

---

A list of standard abbreviations is located immediately preceding the index in each volume. Nonstandard abbreviations used in this chapter include: IF = intermediate filament; EBS = epidermolysis bullosa simplex; EBS-MP = epidermolysis bullosa simplex with mottled pigmentation; EBS-K = epidermolysis bullosa simplex Koebner; EBS-WC = epidermolysis bullosa simplex Weber-Cockayne; EBS-DM = epidermolysis bullosa simplex Dowling-Meara; EH = epidermolytic hyperkeratosis; PPK = palmoplantar keratoderma; PC = pachyonychia congenita; ALS = amyotrophic lateral sclerosis.

type I keratin that maintains a structurally important arginine that is also a genetic hotspot, even a residue likely to be mutated could be predicted.

7. The first keratin disorder shown to fit the paradigm set by EBS is epidermolytic hyperkeratosis (EH), a skin disorder showing normal basal cells but degenerating suprabasal cells leading to crusting of the skin over mechanically stressed regions such as elbows and knees. Since epidermal cells make a switch in keratin expression as they commit to terminal differentiation and move outward toward the skin surface, it was correctly predicted and subsequently demonstrated that EH is a genetic disorder involving mutation in the genes for K1 and K10. The most frequent mutation found in these patients is the highly conserved arginine residue near the N-terminal end of the rod domain of K10. A milder form of EH affecting only the uppermost suprabasal layers has been shown to involve both mild mutations in the genes for K1 or K10 and severe mutations in the gene for K2e, a keratin expressed later during differentiation. A rare form of the clinically mosaic disorder, referred to as *epidermal nevus with EH involvement,* was demonstrated to be a genetically mosaic disorder involving K10 and/or K1 mutations. Other diseases that fit the paradigm for a genetic disorder of keratin and that have been shown to involve mutations in keratins include white sponge nevus (WSN), an esophageal and oral epithelial disorder involving K4 and K13 mutations; pachyonychia congenita (PC), a hair and nail disorder involving K6 and K16 mutations; monilethrix, a brittle hair disorder involving defects in the Ha and Hb hair-specific keratins; and Meesman's corneal dystrophy, a degenerative disorder of the cornea involving mutations in the genes for K12 and K3. Some correlations have been found between cirrhosis of the liver and genetic differences in K8 and K18, but as yet, functional and genetic evidence is lacking to ascertain whether these differences are causative.

8. Since keratin mutations in humans give rise to epithelial cells displaying perturbations in IF architecture and mechanical fragility, it seems likely that defects in other IF gene family members will generate similar problems in other cell types. In this regard, it was shown recently that mice that are null for the gene encoding desmin, the IF protein of muscle cells, exhibit generalized muscle weakness and degeneration. Furthermore, desmin mutations recently were discovered in several patients suffering from generalized myopathies and who have disorganization within their muscle Z-bands, the residence of desmin IFs.

9. While studies involving genetic disorders of keratin are relatively new, the field has opened up exciting new prospects for elucidating the genetic bases of other human diseases that are typified by alterations in IF networks and cell degeneration. It seems likely that many of these diseases will either involve IF gene defects or defects in proteins or organelles that associate with 10-nm filaments. In this regard, it has been discovered that functional loss of the *bullous pemphigoid antigen 1 (BPAG1)* gene is responsible for EBS and rapid degeneration of the sensory neurons in mice, a condition referred to as *dystonia musculorum (dt/dt).* A similar disorder in humans, *EBS with muscular dystrophy,* has been shown to arise from functional loss of the *plectin* gene, sharing a high degree of sequence identity with the *BPAG1* gene. The proteins encoded by these genes are part of a growing group of IF linker proteins that function to connect the IF network to different cellular junctions and/or organelles. Taken together, the study of IF disorders and disorders of their associated proteins overtly illustrates the power of combining classic genetic approaches with reverse approaches (involving cell biology and transgenic mouse technology) in understanding the genetic bases of human diseases.

## THE EPIDERMIS AND ITS APPENDAGES: PROGRAMS OF TERMINAL DIFFERENTIATION AND DIFFERENTIAL KERATIN EXPRESSION

The epidermis and its appendages provide the protective interface between various traumas of the environment and the body.[1] The epidermis manifests its protective role by building a three-dimensional network of interconnected keratinocytes, each containing an extensive cytoskeleton of specialized 10-nm keratin filaments encased by a membranous envelope of highly cross-linked proteins. How the epidermis produces its armor is considerably simpler than the program of differentiation carried out by its appendages (Fig. 221-1). In the epidermis, the innermost basal layer maintains stem cells that periodically give rise to transiently proliferating cells that populate the basal layer. As cells commit to differentiate terminally, they exit the basal layer and begin their journey to the skin surface. In transit, they undergo a series of morphologic and biochemical changes culminating in the production of dead, flattened, enucleated squames, which are sloughed from the skin surface and continually replaced by inner cells differentiating outward.

Basal epidermal cells adhere to a basement membrane composed of extracellular matrix (ECM).[2] Their adhesion is weakly achieved through $\alpha_3\beta_1$, an integrin that plays a role in organizing ECM[3] and in maintaining the population of epidermal stem cells[4,5] (for review, see ref. 6). The lion's share of cell-substratum adhesion in the epidermis is provided by specialized, calcium-activated adhesion plaques called *hemidesmosomes.*[7-11] Hemidesmosomes contain unique anchoring proteins, including the $\alpha_6\beta_4$ integrin heterodimer, and two proteins, BPAG2 and BPAG1e, identified as autoimmune antigens from sera of patients with bullous pemphigoid (BP). BPAG2 is a transmembrane protein with an extracellular domain belonging to the collagen family.[12,13] BPAG1e is intracellular and attaches keratin filaments to the hemidesmosome.[14,15] Recently, the antigen for the HD1 hemidesmosomal antibody was identified as plectin, another intermediate filament (IF) linker protein.[16,17] Both integrin heterodimers are linked to the growth factor-signaling pathways that operate in epidermal basal cells.[18-21]

Basal cells interact laterally and suprabasally with their neighbors through calcium-activated membranous plaques called *desmosomes.*[8,22] Despite their ultrastructural similarity to hemidesmosomes, desmosomes are composed of distinct proteins, including desmogleins and desmocollins, which are members of the cadherin family, and plakophilin and plakoglobin, which are members of the armadillo family of proteins.[8,22] In contrast to classic adherens junctions that link to the actin cytoskeleton, desmosomes attach to the keratin filament cytoskeleton through plakophilin and desmoplakin, a protein related to BPAG1e.[23-26] Thus keratin filaments form a cytoskeletal network through their attachments to hemidesmosomes and desmosomes.

Basal cells of surface stratified squamous epithelia display a keratin network composed of the type II keratin K5 (58 kDa) and the type I keratin K14 (50 kDa)[27-30] (see the following section and Table 221-1 for a taxonomy of keratins discussed in this chapter). In the epidermis, these keratins constitute approximately 15 to 25 percent of basal cell protein. As basal epidermal cells differentiate, they down-regulate expression of K5/K14 and induce expression of a new set of differentiation-specific keratins.[27-29] For most body regions, the type II keratins K1 (67 kDa) and K2e (65 kDa) and the type I keratin K10 (56.5 kDa) are expressed.[27-29] K1 and K10 are expressed as epidermal cells committed to differentiate; K2e is a later marker of epidermal

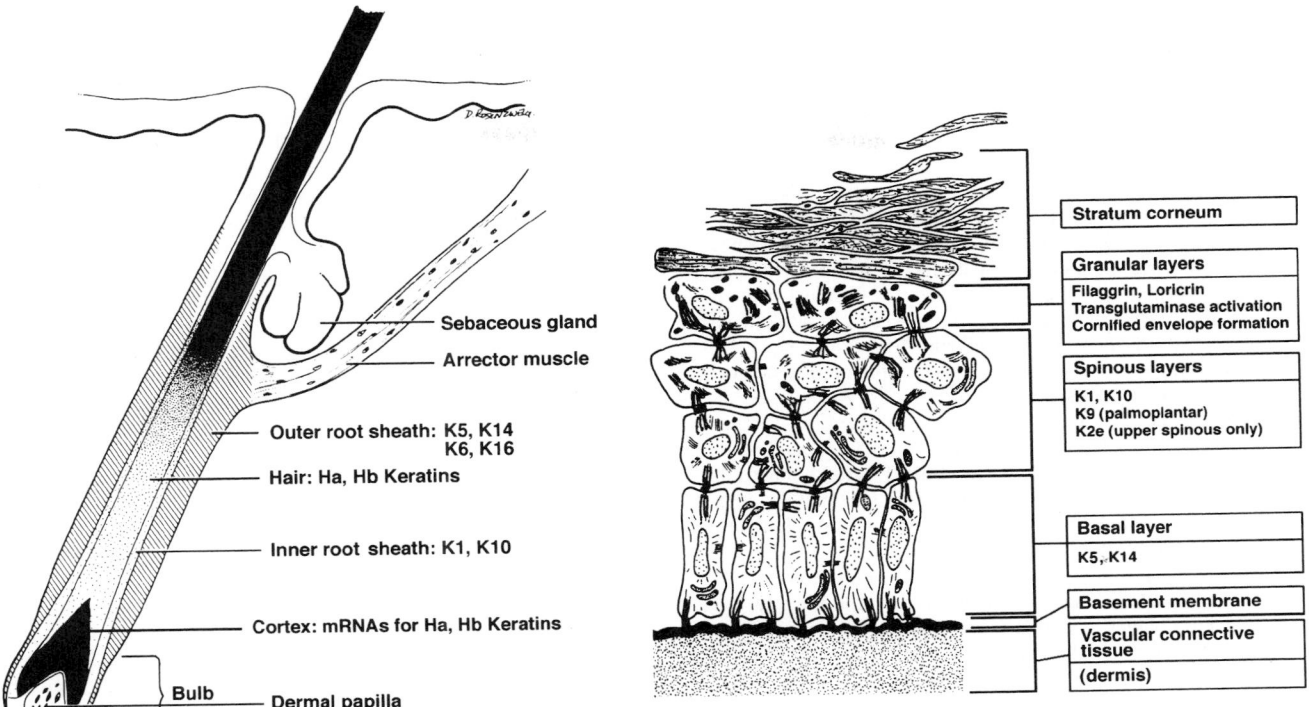

**Fig. 221-1** Keratin expression in epidermis and its appendages. (*Left*) The hair follicle and its program of keratin gene expression. Permanent segments are the sebaceous glands (K5/K14 positive), upper outer root sheath (including the bulge, K5/K14 positive), and mesenchymally derived dermal papilla (vimentin-positive); all are established during embryonic follicle morphogenesis. The lower portion cycles throughout postnatal life by a process involving transient stimulation of bulge stem cells by dermal papilla. Matrix cells express little keratin; they are transit amplifying cells that differentiate upward in concentric rings of cells, giving rise to precortex cortex and medulla (hair shaft), Ha and Hb keratin positive, differentiation. and surrounded by inner root sheath cells (K1/K10 expressing) and outer root sheath cells (K5/K14 positive). (*Right*) Schematic outlining the basic features of terminal differentiation in epidermis and the program of keratin gene expression. Outermost layer of cells is skin surface. As epidermal cells leave the basal layer and commit to terminally differentiate, they switch from expressing K5 and K14 to K1 and K10. Later in differentiation, they express K2e additionally. Palmoplantar skin is distinct in that it expresses K9 suprabasally in addition to the other differentiation-specific keratins. During wounding and in hyperproliferative disorders, K6 and K16 are expressed transiently in the suprabasal layers.

differentiation.[31] In palmar and plantar skin, an additional type I keratin, K9 (63 kDa), is expressed suprabasally.[27,28,32]

Even though terminally differentiating cells are postmitotic, they are nevertheless metabolically active, and the differentiation-associated changes in keratin expression are regulated transcriptionally.[33] In the inner spinous layers, keratins are a mixture of residual K5/K14 and newly synthesized differentiation-specific keratins. As spinous cells continue their path to the skin surface, they devote most of their protein-synthesizing machinery to manufacturing keratins. Keratins are highly stable in filament form, and K1 and K10 eventually constitute more than 85 percent of the total protein of a fully differentiated squame. Although the functional significance of the keratin switch has not yet been resolved unequivocally, K1/K10 filaments aggregate to form tonofibrillar (keratin) bundles, which are thicker than tonofilament (keratin) bundles in basal cells (for review, see ref. 34). Bundling of K1/K10 filaments also takes place in vitro and appears to depend on the pair(s) of keratins.[35] The increase in filament bundling may enhance the ability of keratins to be among the few survivors of the terminal differentiation process.

As spinous cells reach the granular layer, they undergo a final tailoring in protein synthesis, producing filaggrin, a histidine-rich basic protein that may be involved in bundling tonofibrils into large macrofibrillar cables.[36] This process may impart to keratin filaments their final protection against the destructive phase that soon ensues. Several other changes occur in the later stages of

**Table 221-1  Properties and Distribution of Intermediate Filament (IF) Proteins**

| IF Protein | Subtype | Mass (kDa) | Approx. No. | Tissue Distribution |
|---|---|---|---|---|
| Keratin | I | 40–63 | 15 (K9–K20; Ha1–Ha4) | Epithelia |
| Keratin | II | 53–67 | 15 (K1–K8; Hb1–Hb4) | Epithelia |
| Vimentin | III | 57 | 1 | Mesenchymal cells |
| Desmin | III | 53–54 | 1 | Myogenic cells |
| Glial fibrillary acidic protein | III | 50 | 1 | Glial cells and astrocytes |
| Peripherin, $\alpha$-internexin | III | 57 | 1 | Peripheral neurons |
| Neurofilament | IV | 62–210 | 3 | Neurons of central and peripheral nerves |
| Lamin proteins | V | 60–70 | 3 | All cell types |
| Nestin | VI | 240 | 1 | Neuronal stem cells |

differentiation. Membrane-coating granules, made earlier, fuse with the plasma membrane and release lipids into intercellular spaces of granular and stratum corneum cells (for review, see ref. 37). In addition, a complex array of proteins is deposited on the inner surface of the plasma membrane.[38] Some of these proteins, such as involucrin, are rich in glutamine and lysine residues and are made early during differentiation (see refs. 38 and 39 and the references therein). Others, such as loricrin, and a group of small proline-rich proteins are synthesized later.[40–42] As each differentiating cell becomes permeable during the destructive phase, a calcium influx activates epidermal transglutaminase, which then catalyzes formation of $\gamma$-glutamyl $\varepsilon$-lysine isopeptide bonds.[38,43–46] The envelope proteins thus are crosslinked into a cage to contain the keratin macrofibrils (for review, see ref. 47). The keratin filaments are also crosslinked to the cornified envelope through specific residues that protrude along the surface of the keratin filaments.[48] As lytic enzymes are released, all vestiges of metabolic activity terminate, and the resulting flattened squames are merely cellular skeletons, chock full of keratin macrofibrils. The stratum corneum, composed of squames sealed together by lipids, is an impermeable fortress, keeping microorganisms out and essential bodily fluids in.[49]

Terminal differentiation continues in the epidermis throughout life. It takes approximately 2 to 4 weeks for an epidermal cell to leave the basal layer and reach and be sloughed from the skin surface. Thus the adult epidermis is rejuvenated every few weeks.

Hair follicles and epidermis both originate from a single-layered embryonic ectoderm (for review, see ref. 50). In the adult, the lower portion of each hair follicle undergoes cycles of growth and regression, a process triggered by periodic contact with specialized mesenchyme or dermal papilla at the base of the follicle (see Fig. 221-1). Each time the follicle regresses, the developmentally fixed population of dermal papilla cells contracts upward, coming into contact with the base of the epithelial follicle's permanent segment, referred to as the *bulge*. By an as yet unidentified mechanism, dermal papilla cells stimulate the stem cells residing within the bulge to proliferate and initiate a new hair cycle.[51–53]

At the base of the follicle is a bulb of relatively undifferentiated matrix keratinocytes that remain cloaked about the dermal papilla (see Fig. 221-1). These cells originate from the bulge stem cell population; they are highly proliferative and express little keratin. Surrounding the bulb is a single layer of outer root sheath (ORS) cells, which stratifies above the bulb; these cells are less differentiated than basal epidermal cells, but they are proliferative and express K5 and K14. In addition, the inner layers of the ORS synthesize K6 and K16, keratins that in the epidermis are only induced on wound healing or in disease proliferation states.[54,55]

Depending on their spatial position within the hair bulb, matrix cells will differentiate to give rise to the inner root sheath (IRS), and the hair shaft. IRS cells express K1 and K10 and to some extent resemble differentiating epidermal cells.[56] The innermost matrix cells produce cortex cells that express the mRNAs for the hair-specific keratins.[57,58] These cells eventually move upward through the center of the follicle to form the medulla or hair shaft, which breaks the skin surface (see Fig. 221-1). For the duration of transient matrix cell proliferation, terminally differentiated hair cell ghosts continue to exit the skin in the form of the hair.

## KERATIN EXPRESSION IN OTHER EPITHELIA

Keratins constitute a large family of more than 30 different proteins (40–67 kDa) that are differentially expressed in most, if not all, epithelial tissues of the body. Like the keratins of epidermis, keratins are typically expressed as pairs (for review, see ref. 28). K5 and K14 are broadly expressed and can be found in stem and dividing cells of nearly all surface stratified squamous epithelia, including the cornea.[30] As corneal cells terminally differentiate, they express the genes encoding K3 and K12, and in this way they differ from the epidermis and its appendages.[54]

Internal tissues, including tongue and anal and vaginal epithelia, are also rich in K14 and K5.[30] As these cells differentiate, they express K6 and K16, again setting them apart from many other stratified tissues.[28,59] The esophagus expresses K5 and K14, but K15 is actually the predominant type I keratin here.[60,61] K15 is also found in dividing cells of external stratified tissues, but it is a minor component of surface epithelia.[61]

Finally, K5 and K14 are expressed in a number of nonstratified squamous epithelia, including the myoepithelial cells of the mammary glands, salivary glands, and sweat glands, the reticular cells and Hassel's corpuscles of the thymus.[28]

In contrast to stratified squamous epithelia, nearly all simple epithelial tissues, including liver, mesothelium, and intestinal epithelia, express K8 and K18, and in some situations, they also express K7 and K19.[28,62] K7 is a marker of mesothelium, whereas K19 has been tauted as a keratin expressed often in transitional epithelia.[63,64]

## THE KERATINS

### Protein and 10-nm Filament Structure

Keratins belong to the IF superfamily of proteins, which all have the capacity to assemble into 10-nm filaments (for reviews, see refs. 65–67). Based on amino acid sequence, IF proteins (40–240 kDa) have been subdivided into distinct types, of which keratins constitute type I and type II (Table 221-1). Members within a type share 50 to 99 percent sequence identity, whereas members of different types share 25 to 35 percent identity. The typifying feature of IF polypeptides is a central $\alpha$-helical rod domain, which can be subdivided into four smaller regions, referred to as 1A, 1B, 2A, and 2B. Within these helixes, sequences have heptad repeats of hydrophobic residues. Separating the helixes are short linker regions that interrupt the heptad repeat and helix continuity. In cytoskeletal IF proteins, the central domain encompasses 310 amino acids, whereas for the nuclear lamins, this length is increased by an insertion of 42 amino acids (6 heptads). Homology between different IF proteins is particularly high at the start of helix 1A and at the end of helix 2B. Flanking the rod domain are nonhelical amino (head) and carboxy (tail) domains that are variable in size and in sequence among all IF proteins, even within a single type. This variability in end domains accounts for much of the wide variability in size of IF proteins, despite their otherwise similar secondary structure. An outline of the secondary structure of IF proteins is shown in Fig. 221-2A.

The sequences of IF proteins are compatible with the subunit structures that these proteins form. While the roles of the linker sequences that segment the rod remain to be elucidated, the unique $\alpha$-helical heptad repeat structure of the rod generates a surface stripe of hydrophobicity, enabling two IF proteins to intertwine in a coiled-coil fashion, aligned in parallel and in register (reviewed in refs. 68–71). These dimers are likely to be further stabilized by periodic ionic interactions. While most IF proteins can form homodimers, keratins form obligatory heterodimers composed of type I and type II proteins.[72–74]

Tetramers form readily in vivo and in vitro, and all IF dimers appear to align in an antiparallel fashion, forming an apolar structure (for review, see ref. 70). The most stable tetramer configuration seems to be a partially staggered arrangement of dimers, overlapping at their amino ends of the rod (see refs. 72, 75, and 76 and the references therein). However, dimers aligned in exact register also have been observed, and there is some evidence that both configurations may play a role in filament assembly at least in vitro (see refs. 72, 76, and 77 and the references therein).

Figure 221-2B illustrates a model of the assembly of an IF. The mechanisms leading to higher-ordered packing of IF subunits are complex. Scanning transmission electron microscopy has revealed that approximately 32 polypeptides contribute to the overall width of most 10-nm filaments, although some polymorphism in mass-per-unit width has been described.[69,78] Each filament is subdivided

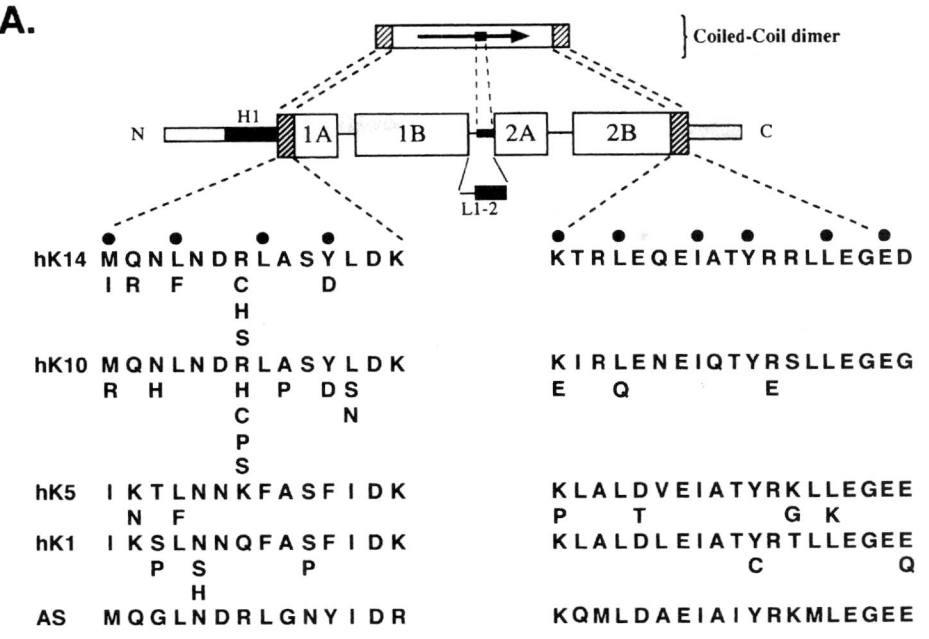

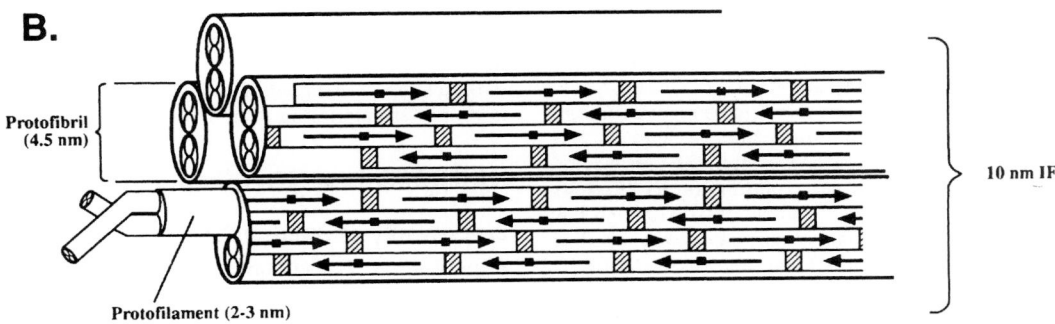

**Fig. 221-2 Model of 10-nm filament assembly. (*A*) Structure of the coiled-coil dimer subunit of an IF, with chains aligned in parallel (arrow points to C-terminus). Hatched bars denote highly conserved ends of the rod domain, whose sequences for the four major human epidermal keratin proteins and for a distantly related snail IF protein (AS) are indicated. The mutations within these regions were identified as individual point substitutions in the respective keratin proteins, as described in the text. Mutations in all keratin disorders tend to concentrate in these rod-end segments. Overhead dots denote the heptad repeats, where most first and fourth residues** throughout the coiled-coil segments are hydrophobic. The rod domain is subdivided into four α-helical segments, 1A, 1B, 2A, and 2B, separated by short helix-disrupting linker segments, of which L12 is the most important. The rod is flanked by nonhelical head (N) and tail (C) domains. H1 sequences are more highly conserved than the rest of the head segment. (*B*) Model of 10-nm filament assembly depicting the inner structure of a 10-nm filament. (*Model is adapted from that previously described by Fuchs,[312] with permission from the Journal of Cell Biology.*)

into approximately four intertwined protofibrils (4.5 nm), which in turn are composed of approximately two protofilaments (2–3 nm). Protofilaments thus can accommodate two linear chains of dimers aligned in a head-to-tail fashion. The precise arrangement of subunits in IF has been difficult to assess because many of the lateral and end-to-end interactions occur under similar conditions. However, it has been proposed that the linear arrays of dimers are arranged antiparallely and in a staggered array within the protofilament and that the unstaggered alignment occurs at a higher level of lateral alignment.[77] In vitro, in the absence of auxiliary proteins or factors, assembly of approximately 20,000 IF proteins can take place to form a single IF of 10 to 20 mm in length.

## Mutagenesis Studies I: Importance of the Rod Domain in 10-nm Filament Structure

In the mid-1980s, investigators began to assess the sequences required for IF formation. Initially, mutant IF cDNAs were expressed in transfected cultured cells, and perturbations in IF networks were visualized using indirect double immunofluores-

cence. Later, wild-type and mutant IF proteins were expressed in bacteria, purified by anion-exchange chromatography, and assayed by in vitro IF assembly. Relevant to the epidermis, many of these experiments were conducted using the human keratins K5 and K14.[72,79–82] Additional studies were conducted on simple epithelial keratins[83–86] and other IF proteins (see refs. 87–91 and the references therein).

Given the appreciable degree of sequence conservation among all IF rod domains, the universal importance of this segment in 10-nm filament structure is not surprising. From secondary structure analyses alone, it is clear that the rod domain is involved in formation of the coiled-coil dimer.[71,92] The ability of different IF proteins to recognize their respective partners in dimer and tetramer formation is also imparted by sequences in the rod. Removing a portion of the rod from an IF protein does not necessarily prevent it from forming dimers and tetramers,[81] but such deletions do interfere with filament formation in vivo and in vitro.[79–90] In many cases, these mutants interfere with filament elongation.[81]

The individual roles of amino acids within the rod have been explored through point mutagenesis studies. Amino acid substitutions in the highly conserved ends of the rod domain are often severely deleterious to filament formation both in vivo[82,85,87] and in vitro.[82,84] In contrast, even helix-disrupting residues such as proline sometimes can be tolerated within the central portion of the rod without gross perturbations to 10-nm filament structure.[82]

## Mutagenesis Studies II: Importance of Head and Tail Domains in 10-nm Filament Assembly

The highly divergent nonhelical head and tail domains of IF seem specifically tailored to suit particular 10-nm filament networks in different tissues. Given the obligatory heteropolymeric nature of keratin IF, this adds even more to the diversity of head and tail sequences and contributes to differences between the functions of these domains in keratin filaments versus other IFs. In this regard, experiments focusing on IF end domains are often applicable only to a single IF subgroup or in some instances to a single IF protein.

For keratins, the major findings obtained with tailless, headless, and tailless/headless epidermal proteins are consistent with results from similar filament assembly studies conducted with simple epithelial proteins. One general role that seems to be shared among the tail domains of keratins is to stabilize protein-protein interactions between IF subunits.[52,83,86] Thus, while tailless keratins can assemble into 10-nm structures, they often do so only under conditions that provide additional stabilization, such as elevated ionic strength. Moreover, the absence of a tail domain is less deleterious to stabilization when only one of the two keratin types in the filament is tailless.[52,83] Similar results have been obtained for type III and type IV IF proteins missing at least a part of their tail domain (see refs. 89, 90, and 93).

The role of the keratin head domain seems to be more complex. A headless K14 can assemble into filaments, at least in the presence of wild-type K5.[80,81] In contrast, even in the presence of wild-type K14, K5 requires at least a portion of its head to assemble into 10-nm filaments[52] (see also ref. 94). Although the precise function of the K5 head domain remains to be elucidated, it may play some role in the spatial alignment of subunits during IF assembly.[52] Whether the head domains of other type II keratins play a similar role is unresolved.[83,85]

The head and tail domains of nonkeratin IF proteins seem to impart a greater dynamic instability to 10-nm filament networks than is typical of keratins.[88–91,93] Specific sites have been identified in type III IF nonhelical domains that may interact with the rod, perhaps regulating the assembly process.[95,96] In addition, head and tail domains of type III and type V IF proteins contain specific phosphorylation sites that appear to play a role either in cdc2 kinase-mediated reorganization of IFs during mitosis or in other models of filament dynamics (for review, see ref. 97). It is interesting that keratins do not have the sequences that target the types III and V proteins for cell cycle-mediated phosphorylation and disassembly. Moreover, in epidermal cells, a keratin network persists throughout the cell cycle. This said, it is nevertheless possible that the stability of keratin filament networks in vivo may be influenced by phosphorylation.

The functions of head and tail domains are likely to extend beyond mere 10-nm filament structure. It is known that at least a portion of these ends protrudes along the surface of IFs,[98] thereby coating the IFs with different sequences. Thus it seems likely that end domains are involved in intracellular interactions between IFs and other organelles or structures, including the nucleus and plasma membrane.[99] A compelling study regarding tail function comes from a report by Bader et al.,[85] revealing that tailless K8/K19 filaments concentrate in the nucleus of transfected fibroblast cultures. These authors have suggested that some protein(s) or other factor(s) interacts with tail domains to maintain cytoplasmic localization of the keratin filament network. For the epidermal keratins, the head domain of the type II keratins seemed to be important in interacting with desmoplakin,[25,100] and in differentiating cells, this domain is crosslinked specifically to the cornified envelope.[44,48,101] The extent to which this and other segments of the keratins may be involved in making other cytoskeletal connections within the keratinocyte remains to be determined.

## Keratin Gene Structure and Chromosomal Organization

Many keratin genes have now been sequenced, and they have similar structures.[68] Most human type I keratin genes reside on chromosome 17,[102–106] and most human type II keratin genes are on chromosome 12.[104–109] Most important, the functional genes for the epidermal keratins K14 and K10 reside at 17q12 to q21,[102,104] and many other skin type I genes are clustered in this same region.[102,104,107] Similarly, the genes for the type II epidermal keratins K5 and K1 are clustered at the q11 to q14 band region of chromosome 12.[104,107,108]

Studies have localized epidermal type I keratin genes to murine chromosome 11, at a homologous syntenic region of human chromosome 17, and the epidermal type II keratin genes to murine chromosome 15, at a homologous syntenic region of human chromosome 12.[110] The murine homologues of the type I and type II human keratin genes map in close proximity to four dominant mutations, *Ve, Re, Bsk,* and *Reden,* known to cause abnormal hair and epidermal development (see refs. 110 and 111 and the references therein). Moreover, additional mutations affecting the development of epidermis and its appendages map to the equivalent segment of mouse chromosome 15. It is not yet known whether keratin gene mutations are the cause of these skin diseases, nor is it known whether there are human counterparts to the diseases. However, given the findings with epidermolysis bullosa simplex and epidermolytic hyperkeratosis (see below), this is clearly an interesting avenue for future research.

## INHERITED DISORDERS OF KERATIN

### Epidermolysis Bullosa Simplex

**Classification.** Epidermolysis bullosa simplex (EBS) (OMIM No. 148066) is a group of rare genetic skin diseases affecting 1 in 40,000 persons. It is typified by intraepidermal blistering due to cell degeneration within the basal layer.[112] In most cases, the diseases are autosomal dominant, although recessive cases have been reported.[113–116] Clinical manifestations are often present at birth, with blistering occurring on mild physical trauma. Blisters heal, often without scarring. Hyperpigmentation also has been reported at sites of previous blisters (see ref. 117 and the references therein). In the clinical subtype referred to as *epidermolysis bullosa simplex with mottled pigmentation* (EBS-MP) (OMIM No. 131960), patients display numerous hyperpigmented spots over their body surface, giving the skin a mottled appearance.[1] Additional curious features of EBS are that clinical manifestations improve with age and that the severity of blistering decreases during periods of fever (severe forms) but increases during warmer weather (milder forms).

EBS has been subdivided into three major and several minor subtypes[118,119] (Table 221-2). The Weber-Cockayne type (OMIM No. 131800) is the mildest form of the disease. Blisters are usually confined to palmar and plantar regions of the body, and not surprisingly, the onset of the disease is often most apparent when a child begins to walk[120] (Fig. 221-3A). As judged by ultrastructural analysis, basal cell cytolysis is evident, albeit sparse, over whole-body trunk regions. Cell rupturing occurs in a defined zone, beneath the nucleus and above the hemidesmosomes, i.e., within a domain where cytoskeleton must span the greatest distance between nucleus and plasma membrane[121] (Fig. 221-4A,B). Keratin filaments often appear nearly normal, and as in all EBS subtypes, suprabasal layers are unperturbed, indicating a normal differentiation process.[121]

In epidermolysis bullosa simplex Koebner (EBS-K) (OMIM No. 131900), blistering is more generalized than in epidermolysis

**Table 221-2** Clinical Features of the Major Subtypes of EBS

| | EBS Subtype | | | | |
| | Weber-Cockayne | Koebner | Dowling-Meara | Mottled Pigmentation | Muscular Dystrophy |
|---|---|---|---|---|---|
| OMIM number | 131800 | 131900 | 131760 | 131960 | 226670 |
| Mode of inheritance | Dominant | Dominant | Dominant | Dominant | Recessive |
| Onset | 1–5 yr | 0–6 mo. | Birth | 1–5 yr | Birth |
| Distribution | Palmoplantar | Generalized | Generalized | Generalized | Generalized |
| Cutaneous anomalies | | | | | |
|   Blisters | + | ++ | ++++ | + | ++ |
|   Hyperpigmentation | − | Rare | Rare | +++ | Rare |
|   Nail dystrophy | +/− | +/− | +++ | +/− | +/− |
|   Mechanical fragility | + | ++ | +++ | + | ++ |
| Oral cavity anomalies | | | | | |
|   Erosions | + | + | +++ | + | + |
|   Dental hypodontia | − | − | + | − | − |
|   Corneal dystrophy | − | − | ++ | − | − |
| Muscular dystrophy | − | − | − | − | Mild |

NOTE: OMIM entries (http://www.ncbi.nlm.nih.gov.min) for the clinical phenotypes are as follows (see text as well):

| | |
|---|---|
| 113800 | Bullous erythroderma ichthyosiformis congenita of Brocq |
| 131760 | EBS herpetiformis (Dowling-Meara type) |
| 131800 | EBS of hands and feet (Weber-Cockayne type) |
| 131900 | EBS (Koebner type) |

| | |
|---|---|
| 131950 | EBS (Ogna type) |
| 131960 | EBS with mottled pigmentation |
| 226670 | EBS and limb-girdle muscular dystrophy |

The corresponding affected proteins are also listed, for example: 148040, keratin 5; 148066, keratin 14; 113810, Bullous pemphigoid antigen 1 (BPAG 1).

bullosa simplex Weber-Cockayne (EBS-WC).[122] However, as in all forms of EBS, cytolysis typically is most extensive in areas susceptible to mechanical trauma, and this includes palmar and plantar epidermis. Noncutaneous involvement is rare in EBS-K, and when it occurs, it is usually the nails that become loosened when subjected to physical stress. Oral blistering has been reported.

Epidermolysis bullosa simplex Dowling-Meara (EBS-DM) (OMIM Nos. 131760 and 148066) is the most severe form of EBS[118,122–124] (see Fig. 221-3B). This disease is apparent at birth, and the incidence of neonatal death can be appreciable. Blistering is extensive and can occur over the entire body trunk and proximal extremities, often in herpetiform clusters.[122] In severe cases, denuding of skin also can occur. Plaquelike hyperkeratoses with extensive lamellar exfoliation also occur, particularly on the hands and feet.[125] Nail dystrophy, loss, and regrowth, oral mucosal blistering, and tooth destruction are relatively frequent. In addition, other superficial stratified squamous epithelia, such as the cornea, also can be affected, albeit to a lesser extent.[114,122,125–129]

The major ultrastructural feature of EBS-DM that distinguishes it from other EBS subtypes is the appearance of clumps or aggregates of keratin filaments within the basal cell cytoplasm[118,125,130] (see Fig. 221-4C). In some cases, these aggregates are so amorphous that it is not clear whether keratins are in filamentous form. In other cases, the filamentous nature of the keratins is evident. EBS keratin filament clumps are recognized by antibodies against K14 or K5, indicating that the aggregates are composed of these keratins[131,132] (see Fig. 221-4D,E). As in other EBS subtypes, the organization of hemidesmosomes and desmosomes and the program of terminal differentiation appear normal.

A few forms of EBS do not fit into the three classic subtypes. Like other EBS subtypes, EBS Ogna (OMIM No. 131950) exhibits blistering due to cytolysis in the basal layer. However, in this subtype, small traumatic blood blebs have been observed on the distal extremities, elicited by short-acting trauma and serous seasonal blistering of the hands and feet and occasionally elsewhere.[126] The relation of EBS Ogna to other subtypes is unknown, although genetic linkage to the glutamic pyruvic transaminase locus on chromosome 8q has been reported.[133,134] In addition to EBS Ogna, there are some reported cases of autosomal recessive EBS associated with appreciable extracutaneous disease, including anemia, neuromuscular disease or

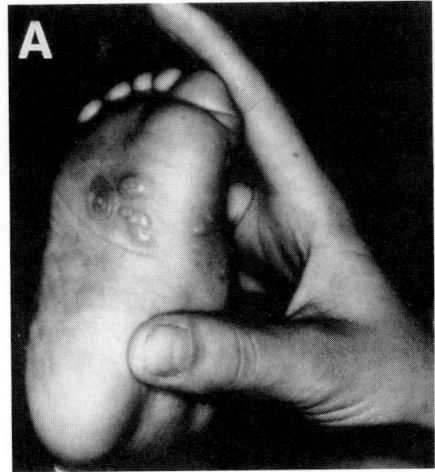
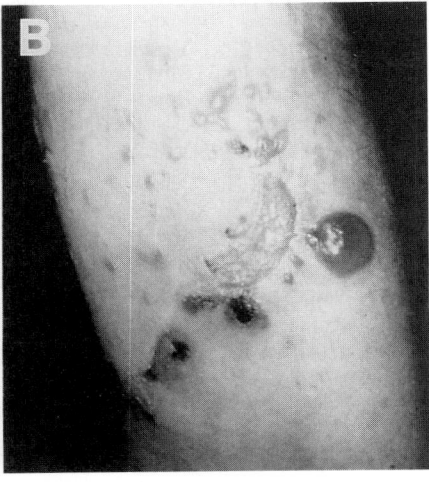

**Fig. 221-3** Clinical features of epidermolysis bullosa simplex. (*A*) Weber-Cockayne EBS. Note plantar blisters. (*B*) Dowling-Meara EBS. Note dermatitis herpetiformis-like clustering of blisters on leg. (*Courtesy of Dr. Amy S. Paller, Northwestern University.*)

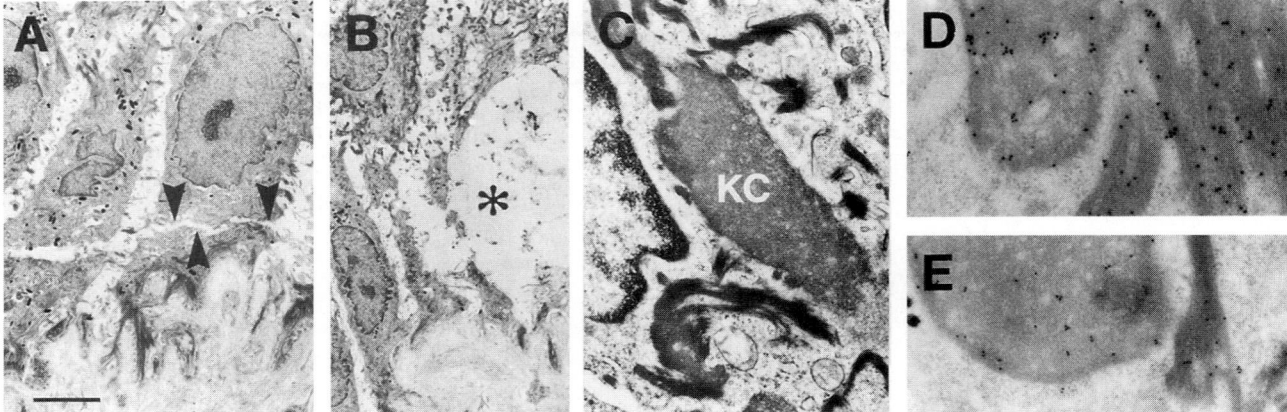

Fig. 221-4 Ultrastructural appearance of keratin in basal epidermal cells of EBS patients. (*A*) Basal layer of skin from EBS-WC patient depicting split in basal cells beneath nucleus and above hemidesmosomes (arrowheads). (*B*) Basal cell from same patient as in *A*, this time exhibiting signs of cytolysis (asterisk). (*C*). Keratin filament clumping (KC) in basal cell of skin from EBS-DM patient. (*D, E*)

Immunogold labeling of keratin filament clumps with specific antibodies against the basal epidermal keratins K14 (*D*) or K5 (*E*). N, nucleus. Bar represents 4 mm for *A*, 5 mm for *B*, 0.8 mm for *C*, and 0.4 mm for *D* and *E*. (*Courtesy of Drs. Q.-C. Yu and P.A. Coulombe, University of Chicago; see also refs. 125, 131, and 132.*)

muscular dystrophy, growth retardation, and infant mortality.[116] Recently, investigators have begun to explore the genetic bases of some of these more complex forms of EBS.

**EBS: Studies Leading to the Genetic Basis of the Disease.** The pioneering electron microscopy studies of Anton-Lamprecht provided the first insights that EBS might be a keratin disorder.[121,125,130,135] In careful ultrastructural studies of skin biopsies of EBS-DM patients, keratin filament clumping seemed to occur at the beginning of the pathogenetic process. Since clumping of keratin filaments preceded blister formation and cytolysis, it was argued that EBS was likely to arise from structural defects in keratin.[130]

In the 1980s, the implications of these elegant electron microscopic studies received little attention in the literature, since most studies focused on an interesting earlier theory by Pearson[136] that cytolytic enzymes may be responsible for the blistering in EBS. Indeed, many of the biochemical reports published during that decade seemed consistent with this hypothesis. In one study, deficient levels of galactosylhydroxylysyl glucosyltransferase, an enzyme of collagen synthesis, were found in affected members of one EBS family.[137] In another set of studies, there was controversy about whether skin fibroblast cultures from patients with EBS-K did[138] or did not[139] exhibit decreased levels of gelatinase. In one report, blister fluid from a patient with EBS was able to induce intraepidermal blistering in the basal layer of a normal skin explant culture, and follow-up studies suggested that the active factor in the blister fluid was a neutral protease (see ref. 140 and the references therein). Finally, in another study, it was discovered that clinically uninvolved skin from patients with EBS had an abnormal staining pattern with peanut agglutinin, indicating that one or more glycosylated cell membrane components may be present in reduced amounts in EBS skin.[141] In contrast, immunofluorescence staining patterns obtained with antibodies against various epidermal keratins appeared normal,[141,142] providing seemingly additional support against the notion that EBS was a structural defect in keratin.

In the 1990s, attention again turned to the possibility that EBS may have as its genetic basis defects in keratin. Kitajima et al.[143] demonstrated that keratinocytes cultured from patients with EBS-DM have a perturbed keratin network, similar to that of keratinocytes transfected with mutant K14 genes.[79,80] Then, using a reverse genetic approach, Vassar et al.[131] introduced a mutant human keratin K14 gene into the germ line of transgenic mice. The encoded truncated K14 protein had been shown previously to perturb keratin filament network formation severely in keratino-

cytes both in culture[79] and in in vitro assembly.[81] In mice, the human keratin gene was appropriately expressed in the basal layer of the epidermis and other stratified squamous epithelia (see ref. 131 and the references therein). Mice expressing the truncated human K14 gene but not the wild-type human K14 gene exhibited nearly all the phenotypic, morphologic, and biochemical traits characteristic of EBS-DM, including total-body trunk blistering (Fig. 221-5*A*), basal cell cytolysis, and keratin filament clumping in the basal cell cytoplasm, with an otherwise normal program of terminal differentiation.[131] These mice also had oral blistering and a high rate of neonatal death.

When transgenic mice were engineered that either expressed low levels of keratin mutants that severely disrupted keratin filament assembly or high levels of mutants that mildly disrupted keratin filament assembly, they had a phenotype more similar to EBS-WC, with blistering predominantly over their front paws.[144] As in EBS-WC and EBS-K, the epidermis of these mice still showed basal cell cytolysis, but in this case keratin filament clumping was not observed.[144] Thus multiple mutations in a single gene, namely, the gene encoding K14, could give rise to phenotypes characteristic of most, if not all, of the major EBS subtypes, thereby suggesting a possible genetic relation among EBS subtypes. Collectively, the transgenic mouse studies provided compelling evidence that (1) structural defects in the genes encoding K14 and K5 could generate an EBS phenotype and (2) the degree to which a specific K14 or K5 mutant perturbed 10-nm filament assembly correlated with the corresponding severity of the EBS phenotype.

**Most Forms of Human Epidermolysis Bullosa Simplex Map to Chromosomes 17 and 12 and Arise from Mutations in the Genes Encoding K14 and K5.** While transgenic mouse studies suggested that EBS may be a disease of K14 (OMIM No. 148066) or K5 (OMIM No. 148040) gene mutations, initial chromosomal mapping did not support this notion.[133,134,145,146] However, two of these studies applied to EBS Ogna, a form of EBS that may be genetically distinct from the other forms,[133,134] and the logarithm of odds (lod) scores from the other early studies left chromosomal assignments questionable. Later studies using improved markers showed that the genetic defect of several EBS-K and EBS-WC families mapped to human chromosomes 17 or 12[147–153] at locations corresponding to the loci for epidermal types I and II keratin gene clusters, respectively.[102,104,107,108]

Unequivocal evidence that human EBS can arise from genetic defects in K14 and K5 came from sequencing the corresponding genes from normal and EBS patients and from conducting a

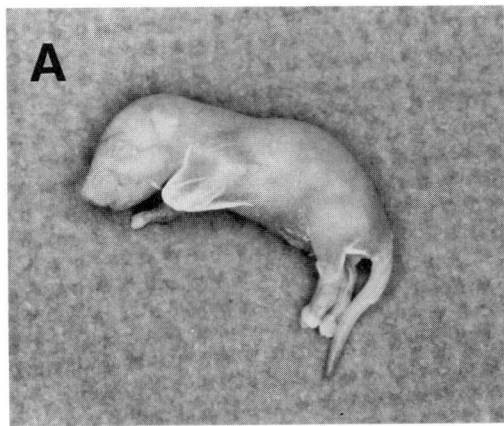

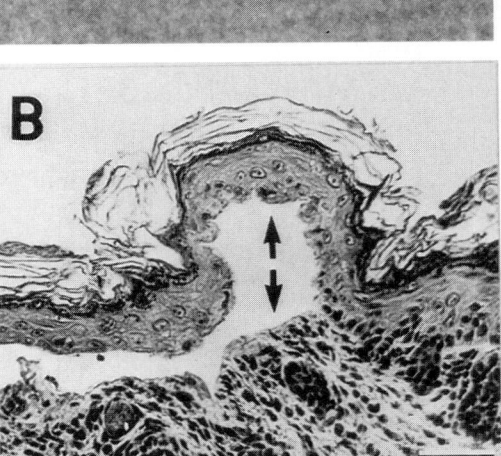

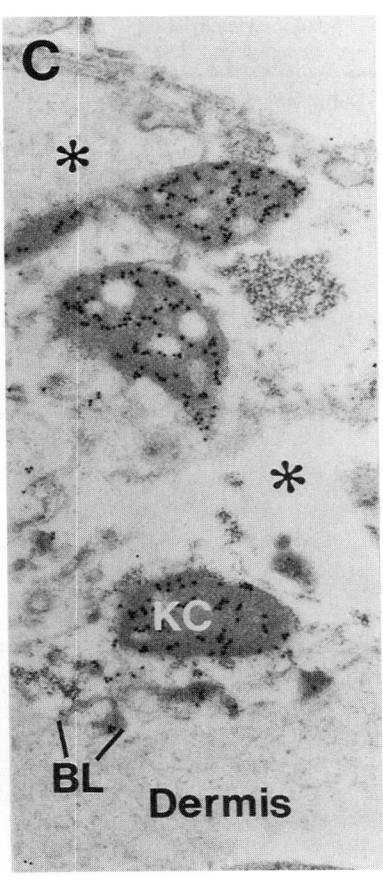

**Fig. 221-5** Transgenic mice expressing a severely disrupting mutant human K14 gene displays characteristics of EBS-DM. (*A*) Newborn transgenic mouse expressing comparable to wild-type levels of the mutant.[131] Mice display gross skin blistering over their entire body trunk in response to mild physical trauma, in this case due to the birth process. (*B*) Histopathology of the skin depicts cell cytolysis in the basal layer, giving rise to the blister. (*C*) Immunoelectron microscopy of the skin from the mouse labeled with antibodies against K5 (shown) and K14 (not shown). Note clumping of keratin filaments (KC) and cytolysis (asterisks) in the basal cells, the hallmark of human EBS-DM. BL, basal lamina. Bar represents 100 mm in *B* and 0.5 mm in *C*. (*From Fuchs,[313] by permission from Annual Reviews, Inc.*)

functional analysis of the defects. In the first studies, two patients with spontaneous cases of EBS-DM were found to have single point mutations in amino acid 125 of K14, giving rise to *R125C* and *R125H* mutations,[154] and affected members of a family with EBS-K had an *L384P* mutation in K14.[147] In the following year, affected members of a family with EBS-DM were shown to have an *E475G* mutation in K5.[155] Soon after, the mildest form, EBS-WC, was shown to be a disorder of K5 or K14.[149,150,156] Additional mutations have now been reported for all three subtypes of EBS,[151,157–175] and several rare cases of recessive EBS also have been shown to have point mutations in the gene encoding K14.[150a,153,177–179] The locations of some of these mutations are indicated in Fig. 221-2, and a comprehensive list of mutations and their corresponding positions within the keratin polypeptides is provided in Table 221-3. Intriguingly, the majority of EBS-DM patients have a mutation in arginine 125 of K14.[154,162,165,170] This residue is encoded by CGC and typically is mutated either to a cysteine (TGC) or a histidine (CAC) residue. These genetic substitutions therefore are candidates for mutation by methylation and deamination of a CpG dinucleotide in either the coding or noncoding strands, respectively. This natural method of hotspot mutagenesis can play a major role in human genetic diseases,[212] as it appears to be doing in EBS.

Functional evidence demonstrates that the keratin point mutations found in the three major subtypes of EBS are responsible for generating the phenotype.[144,150,168,213] In these studies, mutations were genetically engineered into an epitope-tagged but otherwise wild-type human K14 or K5 cDNA. When expressed in transfected human epidermal cells, the EBS mutant keratins caused perturbations in the filament networks similar to those detected in cells cultured from the patients (Fig. 221-6). In addition, bacteria expressing K14 and K4 EBS mutants had perturbed filament assembly with their wild-type counterparts in vitro, in a fashion similar to the altered filaments formed with

keratins isolated from the EBS patients (Fig. 221-7). Overall, there was a good correlation between the severity of the EBS disease, the location of the EBS point mutation with respect to keratin structure, and the degree to which a particular mutation perturbed filament assembly.[213] The *R125C* and *R125H* mutations are among the most deleterious to 10-nm filament structure of all EBS mutations thus far described. Thus this arginine is both a hotspot for genetic mutagenesis and in a critical position for IF assembly.

An unusual and rare form of EBS is EBS-MP, typified by generalized blistering and hyperpigmented spots over the body surface.[117] EBS-MP was shown recently to be a disorder of keratins K5 and K14.[152] Intriguingly, affected members of two different, seemingly unrelated families with EBS-MP have a defect that maps to chromosome 12q11-q13 and carry a P24 L mutation in one of their two K5 alleles. A patient with a sporadic case of EBS-MP also was reported with this same mutation.[176] This mutation is not present in unaffected family members, nor in the normal population, providing strong evidence that this K5 mutation is responsible for the EBS-MP phenotype. Only conserved between K5 and K6, and not among any of the other type II keratins, P24 is in the nonhelical head domain of K5 and only mildly perturbs the length of 10-nm keratin filaments assembled in vitro.[152] However, this part of the K5 head domain protrudes on the filament surface and is known to participate in interactions between desmosomes and keratin filaments.[25,100] Perturbations in such interactions could lead to aberrations in cytoskeletal architecture within the basal epidermal cells, and this, in turn, may cause microblistering and generate spots of hyperpigmentation. Alternatively, this domain of K5 could associate with other proteins/organelles within the basal cell cytoplasm. It is possible, for instance, that this mutation perturbs either longevity of melanin granules in basal epidermal cells or, alternatively, the efficiency of melanin granule transfer from melanocytes to basal keratinocytes. Either of these alterations

**Table 221-3** Mutations Found in Patients with Disorders of Keratin

| Gene | Disease | Mutation | Domain | Reference |
|------|---------|----------|--------|-----------|
| K14 | EBS-DM | K116N | 1A | 175d |
| K14 | EBS-WC | M119I | 1A | 164 |
| K14 | EBS-K-hom | M119I | 1A | 175 |
| K14 | EBS-DM | M119T | 1A | 175c |
| K14 | EBS-DM | Q120R | 1A | 164 |
| K14 | EBS-K | L122F | 1A | 163 |
| K14 | EBS-DM | N123S | 1A | 175d |
| K14 | EBS-DM | R125H (9) | 1A | 154, 158, 159 |
| K14 | EBS-DM | R125C (7) | 1A | 154, 158, 164, 165 |
| K14 | EBS-DM | R125S | 1A | 164 |
| K14 | EBS-DM | Y129D | 1A | 168 |
| K14 | EBS-DM | L143P | 1A | 175d |
| K14 | EBS-rec | E144A | 1A | 177 |
| K14 | EBS-rec | 3'splice | 1B | 179 |
| K14 | EBS-WC | V270M | L12 | 156 |
| K14 | EBS-K | M272R | L12 | 160 |
| K14 | EBS-K | A274D (1) | L12 | 164 |
| K14 | EBS-DM | A274D (2) | L12 | E Hutton & E Fuchs unpublished, 164 |
| K14 | EBS-hom | W305X | 2B | 153 |
| K14 | EBS-K | ΔE375 | 2B | 180 |
| K14 | EBS-K | I377N | 2B | 164 |
| K14 | EBS-K | L384P (2) | 2B | 147, 165 |
| K14 | EBS-WC | R388C | 2B | 164 |
| K5 | EBS-MP | P24L(3) | N-term | 152, 176 |
| K5 | EBS-DM | Δ30 aa | H1/1A | 177 |
| K5 | EBS-WC | I161S (8) | H1 | 149, 167 |
| K5 | EBS-K-hom | K173N | 1A | 171 |
| K5 | EBS-DM | L174F | 1A | 173 |
| K5 | EBS-DM | N176S | 1A | 175d |
| K5 | EBS-WC | N193K | 1A | 169 |
| K5 | EBS-K | V325A | L12 | 175b |
| K5 | EBS-WC | M327T | L12 | 150, 169 |
| K5 | EBS-WC | N329K | L12 | 150 |
| K5 | EBS-WC | D328V | L12 | 166 |
| K5 | EBS-WC | R331C | L12 | 156 |
| K5 | EBS-K | L463P (2) | 2B | 157 |
| K5 | EBS-WC | L463P | 2B | 174 |
| K5 | EBS-DM | I466T | 2B | 176a |
| K5 | EBS-DM | E475G | 2B | 155 |
| K5 | EBS-DM | E477K | 2B | 172 |
| K10 | EH | M150R | 1A | 181 |
| K10 | EN | M150R | 1A | 182 |
| K10 | EH | N154H | 1A | 183 |
| K10 | EH | R156H (5) | 1A | 174, 183–188, 193c |
| K10 | EN | R156H | 1A | 182 |
| K10 | EH | R156C (2) | 1A | 181, 183 |
| K10 | EN | R156C | 1A | 182 |
| K10 | EH | R156P | 1A | 189 |
| K10 | EH | R156S | 1A | 189 |
| K10 | EH | A158P | 1A | 190 |
| K10 | EH | Y160D | 1A | 183 |
| K10 | EH | Y160N | 1A | 186 |
| K10 | EH | L161S | 1A | 185, 187 |
| K10 | EH-mild | K439E | 2B | 181 |
| K10 | EH | L442Q | 2B | 183 |
| K10 | EH | I446T | 2B | 193a |
| K10 | AEI | R449E | 2B | 191 |
| K1 | PPK-mild | K73I | V1 | 192 |
| K1 | EH-mild | R178P | H1 | 194 |
| K1 | EH-mild | V154G | H1 | 194 |

**Table 221-3** (Continued)

| Gene | Disease | Mutation | Domain | Reference |
|------|---------|----------|--------|-----------|
| K1 | EH-mild | L160P | H1 | 194 |
| K1 | EH | S185P | 1A | 189, 193 |
| K1 | EH | N187S (2) | 1A | 189, 193 |
| K1 | EH | N187H | 1A | 184 |
| K1 | EH | S192P | 1A | 181 |
| K1 | EH | D340V | L12 | 193b |
| K1 | EH | E477D | 2B | 193d |
| K1 | EH | I479F | 2B | 193e |
| K1 | EH | I479T | 2B | 193e |
| K1 | EH | Y481C | 2B | 181 |
| K1 | EH | E489Q | 2B | 185 |
| K9 | EPPK | M156V (2) | 1A | 195, 199a |
| K9 | EPPK | M156T | 1A | 199a |
| K9 | EPPK | L159V | 1A | 196 |
| K9 | EPPK | N160Y | 1A | 127 |
| K9 | EPPK | N160K | 1A | 197 |
| K9 | EPPK | N160S | 1A | 198 |
| K9 | EPPK | R162Q (3) | 1A | 197, 199a, 199b |
| K9 | EPPK | R162W (6) | 1A | 197–200, 199b |
| K9 | EPPK | L167S | 1A | 199 |
| K9 | EPPK | Q171P | 1A | 195 |
| K2e | IBS (EH) | Q187P | 1A | 201 |
| K2e | IBS | I188N | 1A | 193g |
| K2e | IBS | N192Y | 1A | 193h |
| K2e | IBS | E482K | 2B | 193h |
| K2e | IBS | T485P | 2B | 190 |
| K2e | IBS | L490P | 2B | 193f |
| K2e | IBS | E493D | 2B | 193f |
| K2e | IBS | E493K (8) | 2B | 77, 186, 189, 201, 193f |
| K2e | IBS | E494K | 2B | 77, 193f |
| K6a | PC | ΔN170 | 1A | 202 |
| K16 | PC | L130P | 1A | 203 |
| K17 | PC-JL | N92S (5) | 1A | 204, 205a |
| K17 | PC-JL | N92D | 1A | 203 |
| K17 | PC-JL | N92H | 1A | 204 |
| K17 | PC-JL | R94H (2) | 1A | 204, 205 |
| K17 | PC-JL | R94C (2) | 1A | 205a |
| K17 | PC-JL | Y98D | 1A | 204 |
| Hb6 | Monilethrix | E410K (3) | 2B | 207 |
| Hb6 | Monilethrix | E410D (2) | 2B | 207, 207a |
| Hb6 | Monilethrix | E413K (5) | 2B | 207b |
| Hb1 | Monilethrix | E403K | 2B | 206 |
| Hb1 | Monilethrix | E402K | 2B | 207c |
| K13 | WSN | L:P | 1A | 208 |
| K4 | WSN | ΔN | 1A | 209 |
| K12 | MCD | R135G | 1A | 210 |
| K12 | MCD | R135I | 1A | 210 |
| K12 | MCD | R135T | 1A | 176 |
| K12 | MCD | L140R | 1A | 210 |
| K12 | MCD | V143L | 1A | 176 |
| K12 | MCD | Y428D | 2B | 210 |
| K3 | MCD | E509K | 2B | 176 |
| K18 | CC | H127L | 1A | 211 |

NOTE: EBS, epidermolysis bullosa simplex; WC, Weber-Cockayne; DM, Dowling-Meara; K, Koebner; MP, mottled pigmentation; EH, epidermolytic hyperkeratosis; AEI, annular epidermolytic ichthyosis; EN, epidermal nevi of the epidermolytic hyperkeratosis type; IBS, ichthyosis bullosa of Siemens; WSN, white sponge nevus; MCD, Meesmann's corneal dystrophy; PC-JL, pachyonychia congenita of the Jackson-Lawler type; CC, cryptogenic cirrhosis of the liver.

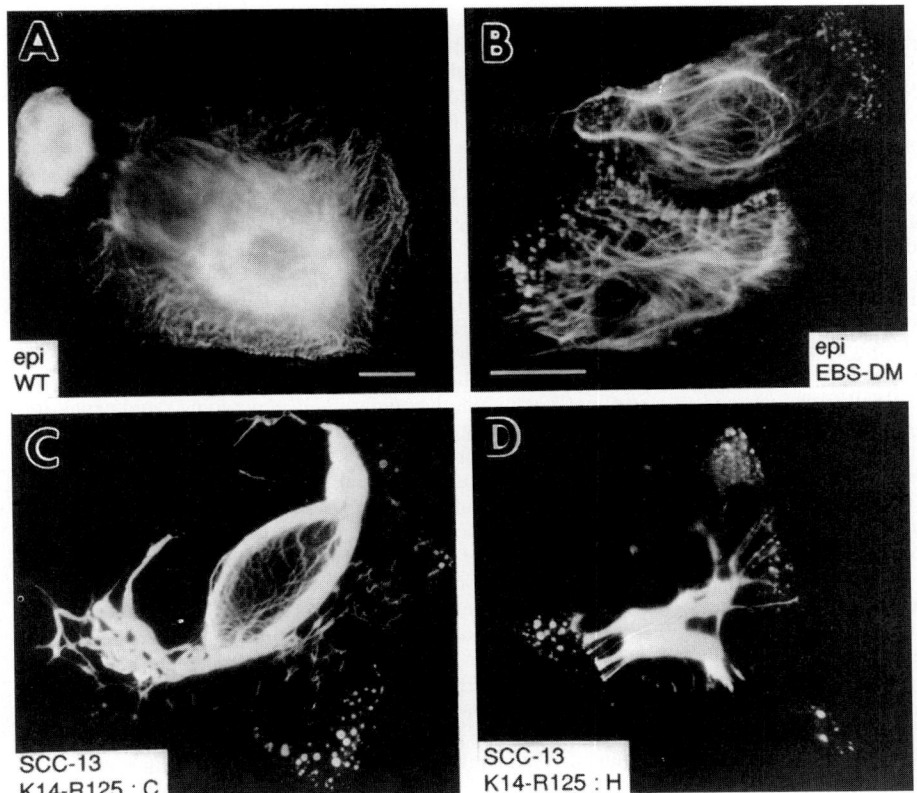

Fig. 221-6 The keratin filament network is perturbed in basal keratinocytes from EBS patients and from transient transfection of a dominant negative-acting keratin mutant transgene. Cultured human epidermal keratinocytes from primary skin cultures of wild-type (epi WT, frame *A*) and an EBS-DM patient (epi EBS-DM, frame *B*) were stained with an antibody specific for the basal keratin network. Cultured human epidermal keratinocytes (SCC-13) were transiently transfected with transgenes encoding the K14 *R125C* (frame *C*) and the K14 *R125H* (frame *D*) mutant keratins, with a small epitope tag to detect the transgene product. Forty-eight hours after transfection, cells were stained with an antibody specific for the epitope tag (shown) and with an anti-basal keratin antibody (not shown). (Note the aberrant keratin networks in frames *B-D*). Note also that the keratin mutants acted in a dominant-negative fashion, integrating into the endogenous keratin network and disrupting it. (*From Letai et al.[82] Used by permission from the Journal of Cell Biology.*)

could lead to variability in the number or distribution of melanin granules in the epidermal cells of these patients. Whether these findings on EBS-MP are relevant to a role for IFs in organelle distribution and organization within cells awaits future study.

**Combining Cell Biology and EBS Biology.** The myriad of molecular studies already conducted on K14 and K5 provides us with additional insights into clinical and genetic aspects of EBS. As alluded to earlier, we can now predict where additional EBS mutations are likely to be found. The locations of K14 and K5 point mutations in EBS-DM correlate with amino acids known to be critical for IF assembly in vitro,[82,84,91] and the arginine so frequently mutated in keratin K14 of EBS-DM patients is highly conserved, being arginine even in a snail IF protein,[144] and is

located near the N-terminus of helix 1A, in a region known to be essential for 10-nm filament structure (see Table 221-3).

In fact, the great majority of EBS-DM patients thus far analyzed have mutations either in the N-terminal end of helix 1A or the C-terminal end of helix 2B[154,155,158,159,162–164,170,172,173] (see Table 221-3). Chemical crosslinking studies indicate that these sequences interact with one another, suggesting that they mediate the head-to-tail interactions necessary to form linear arrays of dimer chains within each protofilament[75–77] (see also ref. 66). In addition, these regions are also predicted to come into close contact with each other at higher-order levels.[76,77] Dual participation in elongation and lateral packing of subunits could explain why the ends of the coiled-coil rod segment of IF proteins are so highly evolutionary conserved and so essential for IF structure.

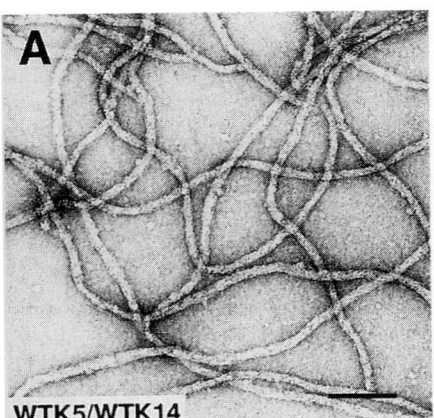
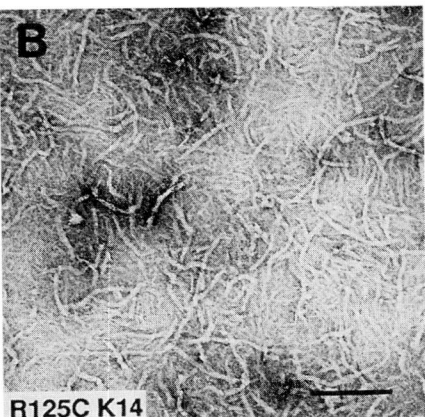
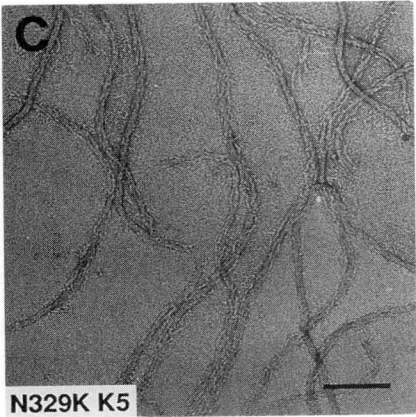

Fig. 221-7 Severity of skin blistering in EBS patients correlates with location of mutation and degree to which the mutation perturbs 10-nm keratin filament assembly. Genetically engineered human EBS-DM mutant K14 *R125C*, EBS-WC mutant K5 *N329K*, and wild-type K14 and K5 were expressed in bacteria, purified, and used in filament reconstitution assays as described.[72] Filaments were reconstituted from (*A*) wild-type K14 and K5; (*B*) K14 *R125C* and wild-type K5; (*C*) K5 *N329K* and wild-type K14. Bar represents 100 nm. (*Similar to those previously described in Chan et al.[150] Used by permission from the Journal of Cell Science.*)

In contrast to the EBS-DM mutations, the EBS-K mutations reside in less conserved α-helical segments of the rod domain[151,160,161,165,171,198] (see Table 221-3). Interestingly, a number of these EBS-K mutations are prolines. A priori, while a proline in the coiled-coil segment of a rod may be expected to perturb IF structure dramatically, in fact, proline residues can be accommodated at a number of central positions within the K14 (and presumably K5) rod domain with only a rather subtle effect on filament assembly.[82] Finally, it is intriguing that in most EBS-WC patients studied thus far, mutations reside outside the α-helical segments.[149,150,156,166,167,169,174] Affected members of two families have the same mutation, *I161:S*, in the nonhelical head domain of K5.[149] Not only is this region critical for filament assembly,[52] but it is also a region regulated by phosphorylation in the lamins and type III IF proteins.[91,97] It remains to be determined whether this site is phosphorylated in these EBS-WC patients and, if so, whether the phosphorylation contributes to filament destabilization. A major finding to come out of combined molecular and clinical studies is that even subtle perturbations to IF structure in vitro can cause EBS in vivo. Continued mapping of mutations in these mild EBS cases should afford additional insights into amino acids that are critical for more subtle features of IF structure.

Given that the pattern of mutations found in EBS patients correlates well with in vitro mutagenesis studies, it seems likely that as additional EBS mutations are mapped, the pattern will continue. Thus we may expect to find more EBS-DM mutations in conserved residues within the rod ends, with less severe EBS cases mapping to regions of K5 and K14 that do not have as severe an effect on filament assembly.

In addition to enabling predictions about the possible locations of future EBS mutations, the cell biology has provided an understanding of many previously unexplained aspects of human EBS. The autosomal dominance arises because mutant keratins are able to recognize their obligatory heterotypic partners and act in a dominant-negative fashion to perturb keratin network formation. The disease is manifested predominantly in the basal layer of the epidermis because K14 and K5 are expressed only in basal cells.[27,30] If cells can escape lysis, then they recover when they commit to differentiate terminally because they down-regulate K5/K14 expression and induce K1/K10 expression.[27] In severe cases of EBS, clinical manifestations can occur in other stratified squamous epithelia, including nail, oral mucosa, and cornea, because these cells also express K5 and K14, albeit to a lesser extent in other tissues than in epidermis.[30] Esophageal involvement has not been described in severe EBS-DM patients in part because K14 is mutated most frequently in these patients, and K15 is the predominant type I keratin expressed in the esophagus.[61]

A major question concerns why EBS cells are prone to cytolysis. A number of findings point to the hypothesis that without a proper keratin network, cells become fragile and prone to breakage on mechanical stress. Functional demonstration of this has come through the identification and analysis of mice and humans that are null for K14 expression and that lack a typical basal cell keratin network.[61,150,153,178,179] Since K5 and K14 form obligatory heterodimers, in the absence of K14, K5 cannot assemble into keratin filaments.[72] While K15 is present, it is in very low abundance, forming wispy filaments within the basal epidermal cells.[61,150,179] In the absence of a proper keratin network, epidermal cells rupture on mild mechanical stress. Interestingly, the patients and the mice lacking K14 expression have less severe blistering than those harboring severely disrupting dominant-negative mutations, suggesting that aggregates of insoluble keratin exacerbate the cell degeneration in autosomal dominant EBS cases.

Another feature of EBS is that blisters generally heal without scarring. In mice, it was shown that during the wound-healing process, basal cells flatten, reduce their level of K5 and K14 synthesis, and do not lyse.[144] In addition, when EBS keratinocytes are allowed to flatten out on the surface of a cell culture dish, they are no longer as susceptible to lysis as they are when in tissue.[144,154] Collectively, these results support the notion that lysis is a mechanical trauma-dependent phenomenon, one likely to occur from a direct compromise to mechanical integrity, and that mechanical stress may be greater when cells are cuboidal or columnar than when cells are flattened. If enzymatic aberrancies occur secondarily in EBS as a consequence of keratin filament disorganization and subsequent blister formation,[137,138,140–142] these changes are not likely to be essential to the initial rupture process.

Another interesting feature of EBS is that the phenotypic aspects of EBS-DM and EBS-K improve with age. What accounts for this difference? It is likely that mechanical stress on basal cells is greatest during development. In neonatal skin, the papillary tips and rete pegs anchoring the epidermis to the dermis are much smaller. In addition, the epidermis is undergoing rapid expansion, and the underlying support structures for the epidermis are not fully formed. Maturation is thus likely to improve the mechanical strength of the skin in general, and this may lessen basal cell fragility. Additionally, it may be that the internal mechanical strength of a basal cell may increase during development, perhaps as a consequence of as yet unidentified biochemical changes in the cytoskeleton and/or the plasma membrane.

Paradoxical questions are: Why does EBS-DM improve with fever? And why does EBS-K get worse during summer months? At the moment, we can only speculate. In this regard, however, it seems plausible that heat could cause temperature-sensitive changes in the mechanical integrity of a cell, particularly if membrane fluidity plays a role in this process. Furthermore, it is known that induction of heat-shock proteins can induce alterations in keratin filament networks, at least in simple epithelial cells.[214] Finally, the stability of the keratin network or its interaction(s) with other cellular components could change in a temperature-dependent fashion. In this regard, it was found in two phenotypically diverse cases of EBS that the keratin mutations resulted in a thermoinstability of the IF cytoskeleton in vivo and in vitro.[215]

**Diagnosis and Therapy of EBS.** Methods for diagnosis of EBS are quite good, and a preliminary diagnosis often can be made through a routine patient examination. Blistering at birth or in early childhood, lesions on mild physical trauma, and healing without scarring are signs that a patient may have EBS. However, ultrastructural analysis of a skin biopsy from a lesion is essential for accurate diagnosis, since the hallmarks of EBS, namely, intraepidermal cytolysis of the basal cell layer without perturbations in the suprabasal layers, often can be missed by clinical or light microscopic examinations.

Certain broad distinctions between the mildest and most severe EBS subtypes sometimes can be made by visual analysis. The mildest form of EBS, EBS-WC, is largely restricted to palmar and plantar areas, although some minor blistering can occur elsewhere. In contrast, the EBS-K and EBS-DM subtypes exhibit more generalized blistering over body trunk areas, including palmar and plantar blistering. EBS-DM is often more severe than EBS-K and frequently is typified by dermatitis herpetiformis-like (clustered) lesions and cutaneous and oral cavity anomalies (see Table 221-2). However, according to a recently agreed on classification,[119] the most distinctive feature of EBS-DM is the unique tonofilament clumping in the cytoplasm of basal cells, readily assessed only by ultrastructural analysis. Since cases with severe blistering and no tonofilament clumping can occur (AS Paller, E Fuchs, unpublished results, 1994; see also ref. 130), distinction between EBS-DM and EBS-K is reliant on ultrastructural analysis.

The accumulation of genetic data has made it possible to develop DNA screening methods for the diagnosis of EBS and for genetic testing within an affected family. Given that most EBS-DM mutations are clustered at the ends of the K5 and K14 rods, it is possible to rapidly identify the key mutation within most EBS-DM families, through the use of either polymerize chain reaction

(PCR) analysis and sequencing of genomic DNA or, alternatively, through immunologic tools to distinguish the wild-type from the mutant sequences at the ends of the α-helical rod domains (see ref. 155). These methods can be applied to formalin-fixed and paraffin-embedded sections, making genetic analysis feasible without additional blood and/or tissue biopsies.[165] Once the location of an EBS mutation has been identified in an affected parent, DNA probes can be used to diagnose the disease from genomic DNA isolated from chorionic villus samples. This is an improvement over previously employed methods of electron microscopy of fetal skin biopsies (for reviews, see refs. 216–218). Finally, as in vitro methods are developed to distinguish normal and mutant embryos, it may be possible in the future to eliminate the disease in future offspring of an EBS family.

The clinical treatment of children with EBS-DM represents the most difficult challenge to physicians and others caring for individuals with this disease. The primary objectives are to provide affected babies with the greatest protection against physical trauma and bacterial infections during their first few years of life. In the most severe cases, this generally means application of topical antibiotics to guard against infection, protecting affected areas with bandages, and continual care. Since blistering is exacerbated by heat, a cool environment is also important, particularly for EBS-K patients. In most cases, blistering improves with age, even in the most severe cases. Therapeutic methods have been largely ineffective.[219]

Now that the relation between keratin mutations and EBS has been established, what are the prospects for future improved therapeutic methods? It is too early to say. However, one finding from transgenic mouse studies suggests that EBS may be a disease amenable to gene therapy. In mosaic transgenic mice, in which the mutant human keratin gene is integrated into the mouse's chromosomal DNA after the first cell division of the embryo, only a fraction of the transgenic animal's epidermal cells contained the mutant gene, whereas the remainder were wild type.[131] Interestingly, within a relatively short period, these animals recovered and appeared healthy. Subsequent analysis of the skin revealed no evidence of mutant keratin transgene expression (R Vassar, E Fuchs, unpublished data, 1991).

Given these findings, it appears that there is a strong selection pressure against autolysing EBS cells. When healthy wild-type cells are seeded in the presence of mutant EBS cells, the healthy cells seem to rapidly replace basal layer vacancies left by cytolysed EBS cells. This could explain why no clinically mosaic disorders of EBS have been described. It also suggests that gene therapy may be a feasible approach for future treatment of EBS-DM patients. By developing methods to engineer out or replace the mutant keratin gene in cells cultured from an EBS patient, cultured now-healthy epidermal skin grafts could then replenish badly affected areas. The technology to culture human epidermal cells from patients is already well established and has been adapted for severely burned individuals, in which sheets of keratinocytes cultured from a patient's skin are grafted back onto the same patient.[220] Thus the rate-limiting step for gene therapy in EBS will be to develop the technology for rapidly engineering out a defective keratin gene from the cultured keratinocytes. This could be helpful in extremely severe incidences of EBS, in which the disease can be life-threatening. Whether this will be possible or feasible should be answered within the next decade.

## Genetic Disorders of Suprabasal Keratins

A number of autosomal dominant skin diseases involve disorganization of keratin filaments in the suprabasal layers of the epidermis. Some of these, such as Hailey-Hailey disease and Darier disease, exhibit anomalies in desmosomes or other structures, in addition to the aberrations in keratin filament organization (see refs. 208 and 221–224 and the references therein). These disorders do not involve mutations in keratin. Other diseases, however, exhibit suprabasal alterations in keratin filament organization that are extraordinarily similar to the basal

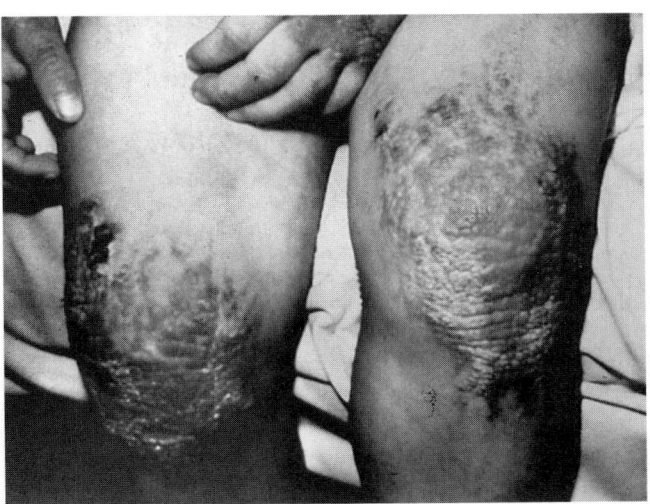

**Fig. 221-8 Clinical features of EH (bullous congenital ichthyosiform erythroderma). Note verrucous thickening of knee skin around flexural area and defects in the epidermal barrier.** *(Courtesy of Dr. Amy S. Paller, Northwestern University.)*

cell layer aberrancies that occur in EBS. Given the switches in keratin expression that take place as epidermal cells commit to differentiate terminally, diseases involving suprabasal keratin abnormalities were prime candidates for having defects in the genes encoding the terminal differentiation-specific keratins.

**Complexity and Characteristics of Epidermolytic Hyperkeratosis and Its Related Disorders.** Epidermolytic hyperkeratosis (EH) (OMIM No. 113800), previously called *bullous congenital ichthyosiform erythroderma,* is a rare form of ichthyosis.[225,226] Like EBS, it is an autosomal dominant disease, with clinical manifestations usually present at birth (Fig. 221-8). The histopathology of EH is typified by (1) a normal but hyperproliferative basal epidermal layer, (2) keratin filament clumping and perinuclear shells of tonofilament aggregates in suprabasal cells, (3) vacuolization and cytolysis in suprabasal layers, beginning in the lower spinous layers and increasing during terminal differentiation, (4) a markedly thickened granular layer and stratum corneum, and (5) keratohyalin granules of irregular shape and size[130,226,227] (Fig. 221-9). These features are also typical of several other autosomal dominant diseases, including ichthyosis hystrix Curth-Macklin[228–230] epidermolytic palmoplantar keratoderma,[231–233] epidermolytic leukoplakia,[234] and ichthyosis bullosa of Siemens.[235,236] The distinctions between bullous congenital ichthyosiform erythroderma (EH) and epidermolytic palmoplantar keratoderma of the Voerner type are somewhat similar to the distinctions between generalized EBS and EBS-WC. EH is typified by verrucous thickening with a predisposition to suprabasal blistering. This occurs over entire body trunk regions, with the flexural regions being the most affected. In contrast, epidermolytic palmoplantar keratoderma is typified by hyperkeratotic palms and soles, also accompanied by painful fissuring. While EH is not associated with all cases of keratoderma, there are a number of cases referred to as *epidermolytic palmoplantar keratoderma* in which features of EH are seen.

The distinctions between bullous congenital ichthyosiform erythroderma and some EH-related diseases are even more subtle. Ichthyosis hystrix Curth-Macklin may have morphologic features resembling EH, but with a distinctly different appearance of keratin filament organization yielding concentric perinuclear shells and no keratin filament clumping.[135,228,237] However, perinuclear shells of keratin filaments also have been seen in the suprabasal layers of skin from patients with EH.[130,135,227,229] Similarly, ichthyosis bullosa of Siemens has been distinguished by the presence of cytolysis only in the very superficial layers of the

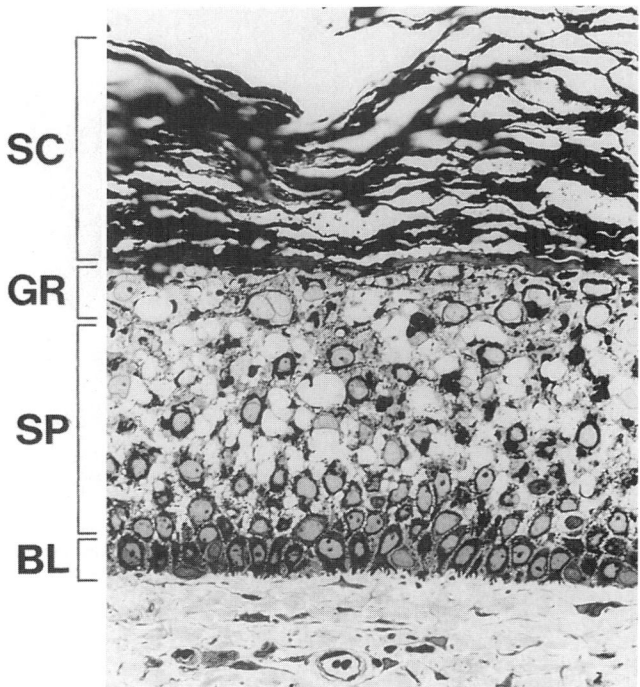

**Fig. 221-9 Morphologic appearance of EH skin. Shown is a semithin section (0.75 mm) of skin from a patient with severe EH. Basal layer (BL) is normal. Spinous layers (SP), granular layers (GR), and stratum corneum (SC) display cytolysis and hyperthickening.** (*Courtesy of Dr. Q-C Yu and Dr. E. Fuchs.*)

showed that a truncated human K10 transgene expressed in mice resulted in all the pathobiologic and biochemical characteristics of EH, including keratin filament clumping and perinuclear filament shells restricted to suprabasal layers, hyperproliferation within the basal epidermal layer, seemingly binucleate cells in the suprabasal layers, suprabasal degeneration, and gross thickening of the stratum corneum.[130,227,238,239] The alterations in keratin filament network were anticipated based on the knowledge of 10-nm filament assembly. The nuclear aberrations could be explained by distortion of suprabasal nuclei caused by disorganization of the keratin filament network or by the notion that the keratin filament network may provide a supportive scaffold to the nucleus and perhaps to other cytoplasmic organelles and that when this scaffold is perturbed, the shape and/or structural integrity of the organelles is compromised.[159] The hyperproliferation could arise from an attempt to restore the barrier function of the epidermis, compromised by suprabasal cell degeneration. This also would explain the increased thickening within the stratum corneum. Thus all the classic features of EH could be both understood and generated as a consequence of a suprabasal keratin mutation.

Indeed, in 1992, chromosomal linkage analysis confirmed that EH is a keratin disorder,[240–242] and point mutations were found in the genes encoding K10 and K1 in six patients with EH[184,185,194] (see Fig. 221-2 and Table 221-3). Interestingly, in two unrelated families[184] and in one spontaneous case,[185] affected EH members had the same *R156H* mutation in the equivalent arginine so frequently mutated in K14 in EBS patients. Thus a genetic hotspot exists in an essential and conserved residue of the type I keratin family; by virtue of the differential expression of type I keratin genes, this residue, when mutated, becomes the culprit underlying the genetic basis for a number of different genetic disorders in humans.

Of the other three EH mutations reported in 1992, two are in residues located in the highly conserved ends of the keratin rod domain.[185] Only one mutation occurred outside the rod ends, and interestingly, this mutation was *L160P* in the nonhelical head domain of K1 in a mild EH case.[194] This region of type II keratins may be important in 10-nm filament assembly.[52,149,243]

A number of additional EH cases have been analyzed, and most, if not all, involve K1 or K10 mutations.[181,183,187,189–191,193–193a–e] Like EBS, there is a correlation between the severity of the disease and the location of point mutations within the keratin polypeptides.[181,183,193,194] This said, genetic modifiers may exist, since not all mutations manifest themselves in an identical fashion, and clinical variation does occur among both EH and EBS cases with identical mutations.

epidermis and by lichenification and superficially denuded areas (*mauserung*).[236] However, initiation of cytolysis in EH can vary, ranging from the first suprabasal layer to nearly the granular layer.[135] Given the significant parallels in the histopathologies of these diseases, it seemed likely that at least some of these disorders would be genetically similar.

**Genetic Basis of EH.** A clue to the genetic basis for EH stems from the striking similarity between keratin filament clumping in suprabasal cells of EH skin and in basal cells of EBS skin[130] (Fig. 221-10). These clumps labeled with antibodies against the suprabasal keratins[184] (see Fig. 221-10). Functional studies

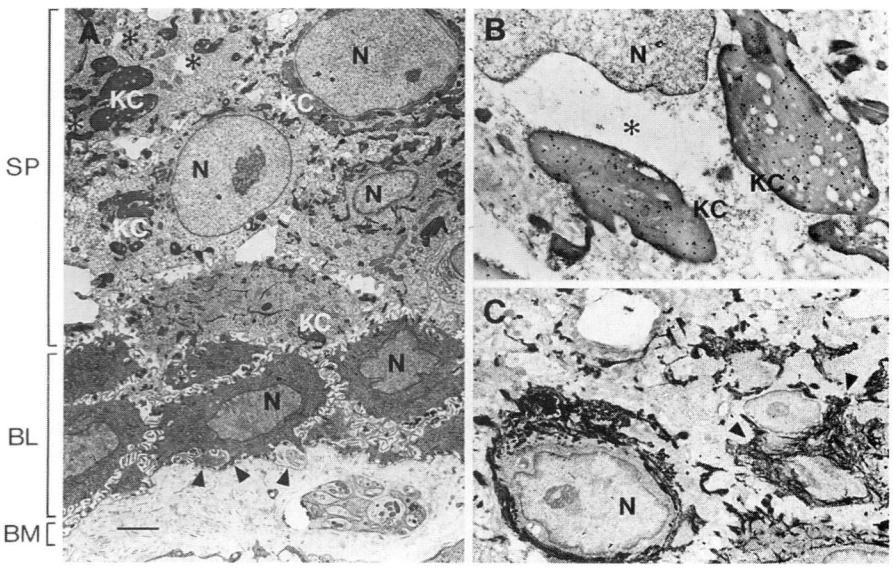

**Fig. 221-10 Ultrastructural appearance of epidermal cells of a patient with EH. (*A*) Epidermis of EH patient, with normal basal cells but keratin filament clumping (KC) and cytolysis (asterisks) in spinous cells. (*B*) Immunogold labeling with antibodies against K1 showing that the clumps are composed of suprabasal keratins. (*C*) Perinuclear shell of keratin aggregates in suprabasal cell of epidermis from EH patient. N, nucleus. Bar represents 2.3 mm for *A*, 0.8 mm for *B*, and 1.8 mm for *C*. (*From Syder et al.,*[181] *with permission from the Journal of Clinical Investigation.*)

In the last 5 years, the classification of ichthyosis bullosa of Siemens as a mild form of EH has been justified genetically. As in EH, some of these patients have mutations within the genes encoding K1 or K10.[181] In such cases, the mutations seem to reside in residues outside the highly conserved ends of the coiled-coil rod domain. A mild EH case formerly classified as annular epidermolytic ichthyosis also was found to have a K10 mutation in the nonhelical N-terminal end of K10.[191] This said, many of the analyzed cases of ichthyosis bullosa of Siemens involve K2e, the keratin expressed late during terminal differentiation.[31] In these cases, mutations are in residues that can cause greater perturbations in IF assembly.[82,186,190,193f–h,201]

**Epidermolytic Palmoplantar Keratoderma: A Specialized Form of EH.** A new consideration for EH not relevant for EBS is that in palmar/plantar skin there is a unique keratin, K9, expressed suprabasally only in these body sites.[27,32] Indeed, most cases of epidermolytic palmoplantar keratoderma (PPK) have been found to arise from K9 mutations,[161,196–200,244] and not surprisingly, many involve the equivalent genetic hotspot for the *R125* residue in K14[197,199,200] (see Table 221-3). Consistent with the mutational analysis, chromosomal mapping has shown that the disorder is predominantly one involving a defect on chromosome 17, the locus for the *KRT9* gene.[161,198,245]

There are noncytolytic forms of PPK, and while some do not appear to involve keratin mutations,[195,244] affected members of one family with this form of PPK have a point mutation in a lysine residue located near the N-terminal end of the head domain of K1.[192] In the 10-nm filament, this portion of the head domain is thought to protrude along the filament surface,[98] and the equivalent lysine residue in K5 is in a domain that participates in the direct association between desmoplakin and keratin.[25] In K1, this residue is a target for the transglutaminase enzymes that crosslink the keratin filaments to the cornified envelope.[48]

**Epidermal Nevi of the EH Type: A Mosaic Form of EH.** A form of epidermal nevi displays clinically mosaic cutaneous patterns that resemble that of EH.[246–249] Offspring of epidermal nevus patients may exhibit generalized EH. In a study of three families, parents with extensive epidermal nevi and their offspring with EH were analyzed clinically, histologically, and genetically.[182] Genomic DNAs of EH offspring were found to have specific K10 mutations that cause perturbations in IF assembly. The EH patients in each of the families had an *M150T, R156C,* or *R156H* mutation, respectively. The corresponding affected parent with epidermal nevi had the same mutation as the offspring, but the mutation was underrepresented in blood and fibroblast DNA and was absent in keratinocyte DNA from the clinically unaffected regions of the body. The mutation was only present in a 1:1 ratio in the keratinocyte DNA from clinically affected areas. Taken together, these findings demonstrated that epidermal nevus of the EH type arises from a postzygotic mutation in K1/K10. This was the first demonstration of genetic mosaicism underlying a clinically mosaic disorder (see ref. 250).

It is intriguing that no mosaic disorder of EBS has been described. The explanation for this is likely to reside in the fact that EBS is a keratin disorder of basal epidermal cells, which divide laterally. In mosaic EBS skin, the wild-type basal cells can divide and replace the cytolysing EBS cells. In contrast, EH is a keratin disorder of suprabasal cells. In mosaic EH skin, the mutant cells express the phenotype only after they have triggered to terminally differentiate and are locked in an upward mode of movement. Thus columns of clinically mutant and clinically normal epidermis are generated.

## Additional Disorders of Keratin

There are more than 30 keratin genes in the human genome, and once EBS had been established as a phenotype generated by mutant basal epidermal cell keratins, it was immediately predicted that there would be other human disorders involving some of the other differentially expressed keratins.[131] A genetic disorder of keratin is predicted to display the following key features: (1) cell degeneration within a group of epithelia sharing a common pattern of keratin gene expression, (2) clumping or abnormalities in the keratin IF network of the affected cells, and (3) an increase in cell cytolysis on mechanical trauma. Based on this paradigm, EH had been correctly predicted to be a disorder of keratins K1 and K10, and epidermolytic PPK had been correctly predicted to be predominantly a disorder of K9.

Pachyonychia congenita (PC) is an autosomal dominant disorder characterized by a thickening of the skin that surrounds the hair follicles and accompanied by defects in nails and oral tissues.[1] It is also associated with ultrastructural abnormalities in keratin filaments, leading it to be classified clinically as a keratinization disorder. Given the keratin filament abnormalities and the location of the keratinocytes that exhibit signs of degeneration in PC, PC fits the paradigm to be a disorder of K6, K16, and K17. It is now known that PC genetically maps to the type I and type II keratin gene clusters on chromosomes 17 and 12, respectively,[251,252] and also harbors mutations in each of these three genes in different PC families[202–205,205a–c,252,253] (see Table 221-3). Interestingly, missense K17 mutations have been described in PC patients with the Jackson-Lawler form of the disease, and the mutations are accompanied by multiple pilosebaceous cysts and natal teeth and hair abnormalities.[204]

Transgenic mouse studies on K6 and K16 confirm that the phenotypic abnormalities observed in PC patients are rooted in the keratin mutations found in their genomic DNA.[254] The additional complexities seen in the Jackson-Lawler form of this disease can be explained by the pattern of expression of K17, which differs from that of K16 and K6.[255,256] This said, it was discovered recently that a mutation in human K6b produces a phenocopy of the K17 Jackson-Lawler form of PC.[205]

Monilethrix is a rare autosomal dominant hair disease typified by beaded or moniliform hair as a consequence of periodic thinning of the hair shaft.[1] These structural defects in the hair result in fragility, and the hairs are brittle and break easily. Given these characteristics, the disorder fits the paradigm for a hair keratin mutation.

Several cases of monilethrix have been linked to the keratin gene cluster on chromosome 12q13,[257] and in the past few years, causative heterozygous mutations have been identified in the type II hair-specific keratins Hb6 and Hb1.[206,207,207a–c] While very few cases thus far have been analyzed genetically, affected members of two families and an unrelated individual had an Hb6 *E410K* mutation, another family had an *E410D* mutation in the same hair keratin, and a second family had a lysine substitution in the corresponding glutamic acid residue of a similar hair keratin, Hb1. Located near the end of the α-helical coiled-coil rod domain, this glutamic acid residue is highly conserved, and mutations in it have been identified in other keratin disorders. Whether it is a particular genetic hotspot for the hair keratins must await analyses of additional monilethrix families. Whether this residue may have a special importance in forming the specialized macrofibils within the differentiated hair cells will require further exploration of hair keratin filament assembly and of the various hair keratin-associated proteins. In this regard, it is interesting that hair keratin filament structure may differ somewhat from that of conventional IFs.[66,78]

White sponge nevus (WSN) is a rare autosomal dominant disorder typified by thick white plaques in the oral (primarily buccal) mucosa, occasionally accompanied by esophageal, genital, and/or rectal involvement. Thickening of the epithelium, degeneration of the suprabasal cells, and clumps or aggregates of keratin filaments signify this disorder as a candidate for a keratin defect.[258,259] Based on the distribution of clinical abnormalities and the particular cells involved, defects in K4 and K13 were expected.[28] Indeed, K4 and K13 mutations in WSN patients have been identified by several laboratories,[208,209] and ablation of the gene encoding K4 in mice gives rise to internal epithelial defects.[209]

Meesmann's corneal dystrophy is an autosomal dominant disorder characterized by intraepithelial cytolysis and keratin filament clumping within the differentiating cells of the cornea.[260] Given the corneal-specific expression of K3 and K12, it was not surprising to find that this disorder involves mutations within these proteins.[210a,210b] Thus far, mutations have been found either in K3 (*E509K*) or in K12 (*R135G, R135I, R135T, L140R, V143L,* and *Y429D*). As expected, all these mutations reside at either the N- or C-terminal ends of the coiled-coil rod domains of these keratins. Functional analysis has been conducted, and mice that are null for K12 display fragile corneas.[261]

In summary, genetic evidence has now implicated most of the keratins in various human cytoskeletal disorders, all of which share striking similarities at the histologic level. A few keratins still remain without well-established links to human disease. One pair of major interest is K8 and K18, the major keratins of simple epithelia. Recently, a K18 *H127L* mutation was described in a patient with cryptogeneic cirrhosis of the liver,[211] and transgenic mice expressing a mutant K18 develop chronic hepatitis and have an increased susceptibility to drug-induced hepatotoxicity.[262,263]

Moreover, K8/18 hyperphosphorylation seems to play a role in protecting the liver cells from a variety of cellular stresses, as judged by the facts that (1) this process occurs naturally in animals exposed to hepatotoxins and (2) transgenic mice expressing a phosphorylation-defective mutant K18 are more sensitive to hepatotoxin-mediated degeneration.[263] While promising, it has not yet been demonstrated unequivocally that K8/18 mutations underlie the cause of some types of liver degenerative disorders. In the one case identified with a putative mutant K18, the substitution was not in the region that might obviously affect phosphorylation. This may be predicted on the basis of studies in the past year, and this should be an interesting field to follow in future years.

## DISORDERS OF OTHER INTERMEDIATE FILAMENT PROTEINS

A summary of the currently known genetic disorders of IF proteins and their mutated genes is given in Table 221-4. It is reasonable to predict that other naturally occurring IF gene defects exist in the human population, given that nearly all cells of the body express these cytoskeletal genes. In particular, muscle and nervous system cells have developed elaborate IF networks, and disrupting or ablating these networks may be expected to be deleterious in a fashion similar to that seen in the skin. Such is the case for the muscle-specific IF protein desmin, which, when targeted in mice, gives rise to null embryos that die from complications in heart development and from generalized muscle weakness.[264–266] In addition, there is an autosomal dominant human disorder, congenital distal myopathy, for which heart muscle cell degeneration associated with aberrations in the desmin IF network have been described.[267–269] In one study, neither linkage nor mutations were found between the desmin locus on chromosome 2 and several families affected by a type of cardiomyopathy associated with aberrations in muscle Z-bands, where desmin is located.[270] Recently, however, two independent studies identified amino acid substitutions and/or deletions in the desmin α-helical rod domains of patients who suffered from more generalized myopathies with cardiovascular complications.[271,272] Interestingly, in two of the three families, clinical defects were observed only when both desmin alleles were affected. Functional studies conducted on the family with a 7-amino-acid residue deletion in the coiled-coil segment of helix 1B indicated that this change was grossly deleterious to the ability of desmin to assemble into an IF network in vivo and in vitro, providing compelling evidence that this change is functionally responsible for the abnormalities observed in the Z-bands of the patient and the resulting muscle weakness.[272] Moreover, when wild-type desmin and mutant desmin were combined in a 1:1 ratio, the aberrations in IF assembly were lessened, providing an explanation for why no major clinical features were detected in the heterozygous carriers within the family (Fig. 221-11). Taken together, these findings provide the first direct evidence that a mutation in desmin can cause human myopathies, and this paves the way for future studies in this area.

Neurofilament IFs are the major structural components of the large myelinated axons of motor neurons, and several neurologic disorders fit the paradigm for a genetic disorder of IFs. Amyotrophic lateral sclerosis (ALS), also known as Lou Gehrig's disease; infantile spinal muscular atrophy; and hereditary sensory motor neuropathy are all characterized clinically by progressive muscle denervation and atrophy arising from motor neuron degeneration. Most important, aggregates of neurofilament proteins and aberrant accumulation of neurofilaments in motor neuron cell bodies are associated with these disorders. Mice engineered to express a mutant neurofilament transgene exhibit pathologic features of ALS, including axonal and perikaryal swellings, slowed axonal transport, and selective degeneration of spinal motor neurons, resulting in neurogenic atrophy of the skeletal muscle.[273–275] Despite this remarkable parallel, a recent analysis of 100 familial and 75 sporadic ALS cases revealed no evidence for mutations in neurofilament genes that may account for the aberrations observed in neurofilament networks in ALS patients.[276] Thus, while a few ALS cases may arise from neurofilament defects,[276a,276b] they are likely to be a minority of cases.

The relation between defects in other IF genes and pathology is still in its infancy. However, wherever tested, gross perturbations

**Table 221-4** Genetic Disorders of IFs and Their Cytoskeletal Networks

| Disorder | Cells Involved | Species | Genes Mutated | References |
|---|---|---|---|---|
| EBS | Basal epidermal | human, mouse | K5, K14 | 148, 155, 156 |
| EBS with muscular dystrophy | Basal epidermal | human | Plectin | 290–292, 296 |
| EBS with sensory neuron degeneration | Basal epidermal, dorsal root ganglia | mouse | BPAG1 | 286, 287 |
| EH, PPK | Suprabasal, epidermal | human, mouse | K1, K10, K2e, K9 | 162, 185, 186, 195, 314 |
| Pachyonychia congenita | Nails, hair | human | K6, K16, K17 | 203, 204 |
| White sponge nevus | Esophagus, oral epithelia | human | K4, K13 | 209, 210 |
| Meesmann's corneal dystrophy | Corneal epithelia | human | K3, K12 | 315 |
| Monilethrix | Hair | human | Keratin Hb6 | 208 |
| Chronic hepatitis, cryptogenic cirrhosis | Liver | mouse human | K18 | 212, 262 |
| Colorectal hyperplasia | Colon | mouse | K8 (null) | 315 |
| Motor neuron disease | Motor neurons | mouse | NFL | 273–275 |
| Generalized myopathy | Muscle | human, mouse | desmin | 271, 272, 265, 266 |

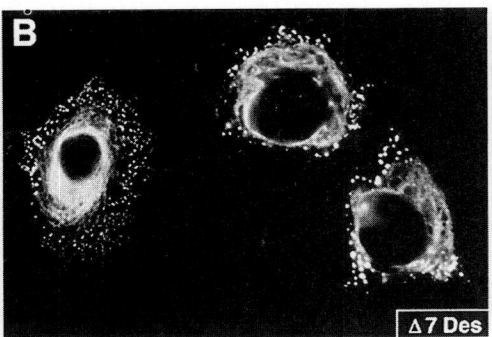
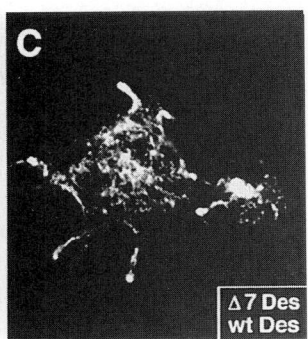

**Fig. 221-11** Perturbations in desmin filament network formation in cells expressing a recombinant desmin protein harboring a 7-amino-acid deletion found in a patient with severe generalized myopathy. MCF-7 breast epithelial cells possess an IF network of keratin filaments. Since keratin and desmin do not copolymerize, they can be used to examine *de novo* assembly of desmin IFs. Recently, a patient with severe generalized myopathy and Z-band abnormalities was found to lack the wild-type desmin gene altogether and instead express only a mutant desmin gene encoding a 7-amino-acid residue deletion within helix 1B.[272] Heterozygous carriers within the family showed no overt phenotype. To determine whether this mutation was causative for the myopathy in the patient, MCF-7 cells were transfected with mammalian expression vectors capable of expressing either (*A*) wild-type desmin, (*B*) the 7-amino-acid deletion mutant of desmin, or (*C*) a mixture of wild-type and mutant desmin. Forty-eight hours after transfection, cells were fixed and stained with antidesmin antibody, and labeling was visualized with a fluorescently tagged secondary antibody. Transfected cells are shown. Note that D7Des alone cannot form a proper IF network and instead produces punctate labeling at the cell periphery. In contrast, wt Des and a mixture of wt Des and D7Des assemble into a filamentous network. Bar represents 20mm. (*From Munoz-Marmol et al.*[272] *Used with permission from the Proceedings of the National Academy of Sciences.*)

in IF networks seem to be incompatible with cell survival. In some cases such as the lens epithelium, it does not really seem to matter what disrupting IF is expressed there. Thus overexpression of dominant-negative and/or wild-type vimentin, desmin, and neurofilament genes in the lens of mouse eyes has resulted in cataract formation.[277–279] Given that ablation of vimentin, the natural IF protein for the lens, produces mice with no tendency to develop cataracts,[280] it would appear that it is the production of insoluble aggregates, rather than loss of the IF network per se, that is the pathologic demon in this process. Notably, mice lacking either vimentin[280] or glial fibrillary acidic protein[281,282] developed normally and without any obvious phenotype. This said, by 18 months of age, glial fibrillary acidic protein (GFAP) null mice began to exhibit major defects in myelination, leading to structural and functional defects in the white matter of the brain and in the blood-brain barrier.[283]

A similar situation recently has been uncovered in axons, where ablating the neurofilament cytoskeleton in mice also can cause some, albeit relatively mild, axonal degeneration (for review, see ref. 67). The late onset of overt neuronal defects in the neurofilament null mice is in contrast to the ALS phenotype generated within 3 months of age by a dominant-negative disrupting neurofilament mutant. Thus, despite the documented function for some IFs in resisting stress,[61,264,266,284] this function may be more important in some cells than in others.

Gene knockout and transgenic technology has given us additional surprises regarding the functions, or lack thereof, of IF networks. Even though overexpression of wild-type, foreign IF networks in some cells, e.g., the lens, is problematic for their function, overexpression of up to 10 times the physiologic levels of wild-type vimentin leads to no detectable morphologic abnormalities during the early stages of *Xenopus* embryogenesis,[285] and the creation of a dense neurofilament network in transgenic mouse kidney is without apparent consequence.[279] In addition, the targeted removal of vimentin and glial filament protein resulted in mild alterations at best, considering the abundance of these proteins within specialized cells of the body. Do these studies mean that IFs are dispensable in some cases? Clearly, redundancy is always a formal possibility. However, at least in the case of neurofilaments, more than 90 percent of the IF network can be missing in mice without gross phenotypic defects, indicating that if there is compensation in the younger animals, it must be by other cytoskeletal components in these cells.

Several factors argue that even in cases where the IF network appears to be largely dispensable, they are likely to have crucial roles when the lifetime of a human is considered. Analysis of function in a laboratory mouse is likely not a fair comparison to the role of some IFs in nature. Indeed, in humans, neurons are significantly longer and undergo significantly more bending and mechanical stress than neurons in a mouse, particularly when it is considered that the mouse is confined to a relatively small space. In addition, the recent studies of the Peterson group indicate that even where neurofilaments appeared to be dispensable early in life, there were clear complications as these animals aged. Additional specialized roles, perhaps in axonal regrowth on injury, may surface when such functions are tested. Similarly, for the GFAP and vimentin knockouts, marked abnormalities have now been found in cells where none were noticed in the first round of characterizations.[283] Thus, while all IF networks may not be as essential to the daily rigors of life as is the epidermal or the desmin IF network, most, if not all, IF cytoskeletons of higher eukaryotic cells have evolved to serve specialized and important functions.

## PROTEINS THAT MAKE CONNECTIONS TO IF NETWORKS: NEW INSIGHTS INTO DEGENERATIVE DISORDERS OF THE CYTOSKELETON

Given the consequences of a disorganized IF cytoskeleton, it is not surprising that eukaryotic cells have evolved mechanisms for keeping IFs anchored. As outlined previously, IFs attach to desmosomes and hemidesmosomes in stratified epithelia. Several proteins have been described that can function as cytoskeletal linker proteins to mediate the association between IFs and these membranous plaques. They include three related large coiled-coil proteins—BPAG1e, desmoplakin, and plectin—and one protein—plakophilin—that is a member of the armadillo family of cell-cell adhesion and signal-transduction proteins.

The first hint that this group of IF linker proteins may be physiologically important came from Guo et al.,[286] who used gene targeting to ablate the *BPAG1* gene in mice. In the absence of BPAG1e, IFs were severed from the hemidesmosomes, generating an intracellular zone of mechanical fragility and an EBS phenotype. Since BPAG1e was known to be restricted to stratified epithelia, it came as a major surprise that a relatively modest genetic manipulation at the *BPAG1* locus resulted in neurofilament disorganization and gross degeneration of the sensory neurons in these mice.[286] Serendipitously, the *BPAG1* null mutation led to the discovery of the genetic basis for a well-known mouse neurologic mutant, *dystonia musculorum* (*dt/dt*), independently shown by positional cloning to arise from *BPAG1* gene defects.[287] This also led to the discovery of novel neural isoforms encoded by the *BPAG1* gene, which contained the IF linking domain of BPAG1e but in addition had an actin-binding domain not found in BPAG1e.[15,287] The function(s) of BPAG1n seems to go beyond simply anchoring IFs to the cortical actin cytoskeleton of the axons, however, because double knockout mice, missing both the core subunit of neurofilaments and the *BPAG1* gene, still show a marked dystonic phenotype, even though mice lacking the core subunit of neurofilaments appear quite healthy.[287]

Humans with EBS and sensory neuron degeneration have not yet been described. However, a few patients have been described with EBS and muscular dystrophy.[115] Relevant to this fact is that the neural isoform of BPAG1 shares a high degree of similarity to plectin, but unlike BPAG1, which is expressed in epidermis and in sensory neurons, plectin is expressed in epidermis and muscle.[288,289] On the realization that the *dt/dt* mouse is a recessive mutant of BPAG1, plectin immediately became a candidate for the underlying genetic basis of EBS with muscular dystrophy. Indeed, it is now well established that this human disorder involves recessive or compound heterozygous null mutations in plectin.[290–295,295a,295b] The plectin null mouse also has been generated, and it provides functional evidence that basal epidermal cell and muscle cell degeneration is a direct consequence of an absence of plectin.[296] Biochemical and cell biology studies on plectin have raised the possibility that BPAG1n and plectin may be general cytoskeletal linker proteins connecting not only actin and IFs but also microtubules (see refs. 287b, 289 and 297 and the references therein). This finding enhances the possible importance to medicine of future studies aimed at exploring the size of this as yet small family of IF linker proteins.

What about possible disorders of desmosome-IF linkages? A priori, providing anchorage at three sides of the cell rather than one, severing these connections in epidermis would be expected to be more severe than breaking hemidesmosome-IF connections. A second consideration is that desmoplakin is broadly expressed in all cell types that have desmosomes, making it unlikely that humans can survive without desmoplakin. Plakophilin 1 is somewhat more restricted in its expression and is predominantly expressed in suprabasal epidermal cells.[298] Interestingly, a compound heterozygous null mutation in plakophilin 1 was described recently in a patient with congenital ectodermal dysplasia (CED),[299] a genetic skin disorder typified by cell degeneration in the suprabasal epidermal layers. CED differs from EH in that desmosomes are dramatically reduced in numbers and keratin clumping is not seen at the ultrastructural level. Given that plakophilin 1 is a keratin filament-desmosome-associated protein,[26,300] it seems likely that these mutations underlie the cause of CED, although functional studies have not yet been conducted.

## CONCLUSION

This chapter has focused on cytoskeletal disorders of IFs and their associated proteins. Many of these disorders involve skin abnormalities; the reader is referred elsewhere for recent studies on noncytoskeletal genetic skin diseases, in particular, other forms of epidermolysis bullosa, that are due to defects in other structural proteins such as collagen VII (see Chap. 222), laminins, and integrins.[301–305] For other cytoskeletal disorders, it is suggested that the reader examine the chapters dealing with muscular dystrophy[306,307] (see Chap. 216), and cardiomyopathies[308–310] (see Chap. 213).

The past decade has brought answers to questions about the elusive functions of IFs. It is quite remarkable that as first suggested by Lazarides[311] many years ago, IFs truly seem to be surfacing as the mechanical integrators of the cytoplasm. Key

genetic evidence now supports this notion and strengthens the view that IFs are central to cytoarchitecture and structural integrity. In some cells, such as the fibroblast, glial cell, and neuron, IFs do not seem to be as critical to cellular function as in others, such as the epidermal keratinocyte. However, in virtually every cell thus far examined, perturbations in the IF network, either through genetic mutation in the IF genes themselves or through mutation in IF-associated proteins, appear to cause tissue degeneration and human disease. This field is still in its infancy, with much of the research stemming from work conducted in the 1990s. Indeed, it was only in 1991 that EBS, the first genetic disorder of an IF protein, was established. Thus, while IFs and their associated proteins are now squarely on the map of interesting cytoskeletal proteins with essential and important functions in cells and clear relevance to human genetic disease, our knowledge is still at the surface of the IF, with a deeper understanding awaiting to unravel in the years to come.

## ACKNOWLEDGMENTS

I thank Dr. Pierre A. Coulombe (Johns Hopkins University Medical School) and Dr. Q.-C. Yu (Howard Hughes Medical Institute, University of Chicago) for providing electron micrographs and Dr. Amy S. Paller (Northwestern Medical School) for providing clinical photographs. I also thank Dr. Ingrun Anton-Lamprecht (Institut fur Ultrastruktur-forschung der Haut, Hautklinik der Ruprecht-Karls-Universitaet, Heidelberg, Germany), Dr. Amy S. Paller, and Dr. Pierre Coulombe for their helpful comments. Finally, I would like to express my sincere gratitude to the members of my laboratory, past and present, who have so enthusiastically devoted their time and scientific expertise to enhancing our understanding of keratin filament structure and function and its relation to human skin diseases.

## REFERENCES

1. Fitzpatrick TB, Eisen AZ, Wolff K, Freedberg IM, Austen KF (eds): *Dermatology in General Medicine*, 4th ed, vol 1. New York, McGraw-Hill, 1993.
2. Burgeson RE, Christiano AM: The dermal-epidermal junction. *Curr Opin Cell Biol* **9**:651, 1997.
3. DiPersio CM, Hodivala-Dilke KM, Jaenisch R, Kreidberg JA, Hynes RO: Alpha 3 beta 1 integrin is required for normal development of the epidermal basement membrane. *J Cell Biol* **137**:729, 1997.
4. Jones PH, Watt FM: Separation of human epidermal stem cells from transit amplifying cells on the basis of differences in integrin function and expression. *Cell* **73**:713, 1993.
5. Jones PH, Harper S, Watt FM: Stem cell patterning and fate in human epidermis. *Cell* **80**:83, 1995.
6. Fuchs E, Dowling J, Segre J, Lo SH, Yu QC: Integrators of epidermal growth and differentiation: distinct functions for beta 1 and beta 4 integrins. *Curr Opin Genet Dev* **7**:672, 1997.
7. Borradori L, Sonnenberg A: Hemidesmosomes: Roles in adhesion, signaling and human diseases (review). *Curr Opin Cell Biol* **8**:647, 1996.
8. Green KJ, Jones JC: Desmosomes and hemidesmosomes: Structure and function of molecular components. *FASEB J* **10**:871, 1996.
9. Dowling J, Yu QC, Fuchs E: Beta 4 integrin is required for hemidesmosome formation, cell adhesion and cell survival. *J Cell Biol* **134**:559, 1996.
10. Georges-Labouesse E, Messaddeq N, Cadalbert L, Dierich A, Le Meur M: Absence of integrin alpha 6 leads to epidermolysis bullosa and neonatal death in mice. *Nature Genet* **13**:370, 1996.
11. van der Neut R, Krimpenfort P, Calafat J, Niessen CM, Sonnenberg A: Epithelial detachment due to absence of hemidesmosomes in integrin beta 4 null mice. *Nature Genet* **13**:366, 1996.
12. Giudice GJ, Emery DJ, Diaz LA: Cloning and primary structural analysis of the bullous pemphigoid autoantigen BP180. *J Invest Dermatol* **99**:243, 1992.
13. Li K, Tamai K, Tan E, Uitto J: Cloning of type XVII collagen: Complementary and genomic DNA sequences of mouse 180-kilodalton bullous pemphigoid antigen (BPAG2) predict an interrupted collagenous domain, a transmembrane segment, and unusual

features in the 5′-end of the gene and the 3′-untranslated region of the mRNA. *J Biol Chem* **268**:8825, 1993.

14. Amagai M, Klaus-Kovtun V, Stanley JR: Autoantibodies against a novel epithelial cadherin in pemphigus vulgaris, a disease of cell adhesion. *Cell* **67**:869, 1991.
15. Yang Y, Dowling J, Yu QC, Kouklis P, Cleveland DW, Fuchs E: An essential cytoskeletal linker protein connecting actin microfilaments to intermediate filaments. *Cell* **86**:655, 1996.
16. Wiche G, Gromov D, Donovan A, Castanon MJ, Fuchs E: Expression of plectin mutant cDNA in cultured cells indicates a role of COOH-terminal domain in intermediate filament association. *J Cell Biol* **121**:607, 1993.
17. Reznickez GA, de Pereda JM, Reipert S, Wiche G: Linking integrin α₆β₄-based cell adhesion to the intermediate filament cytoskeleton: Direct interaction between the β₄ subunit and plectin at multiple molecular sites. *J Cell Biol* **141**:209, 1998.
18. Wary KK, Mainiero F, Isakoff SJ, Marcantonio EE, Giancotti FG: The adaptor protein Shc couples a class of integrins to the control of cell cycle progression. *Cell* **87**:733, 1996.
19. Shaw LM, Rabinovitz I, Wang H, Toker A, Mercurio AM: Activation of phosphoinositide 3-OH kinase by the α₆β₄ integrin promotes carcinoma invasion. *Cell* **91**:949, 1997.
20. Cardone MH, Salvesen GS, Widmann C, Johnson G, Frisch SM: The regulation of anoikis: MEKK-1 activation requires cleavage by caspases. *Cell* **90**:315, 1997.
21. Hughes PE, Renshaw MW, Pfaff M, Forsyth J, Keivens VM, Schwartz MA, Ginsberg MH: Suppression of integrin activation: a novel function of a Ras/Raf-initiated MAP kinase pathway. *Cell* **88**:521, 1997.
22. Garrod D, Chidgey M, North A: Desmosomes: Differentiation, development, dynamics and disease. *Curr Opin Cell Biol* **8**:670, 1996.
23. Stappenbeck TS, Bornslaeger EA, Corcoran CM, Luu HH, Virata ML, Green KJ: Functional analysis of desmoplakin domains: Specification of the interaction with keratin versus vimentin intermediate filament networks. *J Cell Biol* **123**:691, 1993.
24. Stappenbeck TS, Lamb JA, Corcoran CM,Green KJ: Phosphorylation of the desmoplakin COOH terminus negatively regulates its interaction with keratin intermediate filament networks. *J Biol Chem* **269**:29351, 1994.
25. Kouklis P, Hutton E, Fuchs E: Making the connection: Keratin intermediate filaments and desmosomes proteins. *J Cell Biol* **127**:1049, 1994.
26. Smith E, Fuchs E: Defining desmoplakin's interactions with desmosomes. *J Cell Biol* **141**:1229, 1998.
27. Fuchs E, Green H: Changes in keratin gene expression during terminal differentiation of the keratinocyte. *Cell* **19**:1033, 1980.
28. Moll R, Franke W, Schiller D, Geiger B, Krepler R: The catalog of human cytokeratins: Patterns of expression in normal epithelia, tumors and cultured cells. *Cell* **31**:11, 1982.
29. Roop DR, Huitfeldt H, Kilkenny A, Yuspa SH: Regulated expression of differentiation-associated keratins in cultured epidermal cells detected by monospecific antibodies to unique peptides of mouse epidermal keratins. *Differentiation* **35**:143, 1987.
30. Nelson W, Sun TT: The 50- and 58-kilodalton keratin classes as molecular markers for stratified squamous epithelia: Cell culture studies. *J Cell Biol* **97**:244, 1983.
31. Collin C, Moll E, Kubicka S, Ouhayoun JP, Franke WW: Characterization of human cytokeratin 2, an epidermal cytoskeletal protein synthesized late during differentiation. *Exp Cell Res* **202**:132, 1992.
32. Knapp AC, Franke WW, Heid H, Hatzfeld M, Jorcano JL, Moll R: Cytokeratin no. 9, an epidermal type I keratin characteristic of a special program of keratinocyte differentiation displaying body site specificity. *J Cell Biol* **103**:657, 1986.
33. Stellmach V, Leask A, Fuchs E: Retinoid-mediated transcriptional regulation of keratin genes in human epidermal and squamous cell carcinoma cells. *Proc Natl Acad Sci USA* **88**:4582, 1991.
34. Montagna W, Lobitz WC (eds): *The Epidermis.* New York, Academic Press, 1964.
35. Eichner R, Sun TT, Aebi U: The role of keratin subfamilies and keratin pairs in the formation of human epidermal intermediate filaments. *J Cell Biol* **102**:1767, 1986.
36. Dale BA, Holbrook KA, Steinert PM: Assembly of stratum corneum basic protein and keratin filaments in macrofibrils. *Nature* **276**:729, 1978.
37. Schurer NY, Plewig G, Elias PM: Stratum corneum lipid function. *Dermatologica* **183**:77, 1991.

38. Rice RH, Green H: Presence in human epidermal cells of a soluble protein precursor of the cross-linked envelope: Activation of the cross-linking by calcium ions. *Cell* **18**:681, 1979.
39. Simon M, Green H: Enzymatic cross-linking of involucrin and other proteins by keratinocyte particulates in vitro. *Cell* **40**:677, 1985.
40. Mehrel T, Hohl D, Rothnagel JA, Longley MA, Bundman D, Cheng C, Lichti U, Bisher ME, Steven AC, Steinert PM: Identification of a major keratinocyte cell envelope protein, loricrin. *Cell* **61**:1103, 1990.
41. Jarnik M, Kartasova T, Steinert PM, Lichti U, Steven AC: Differential expression and cell envelope incorporation of small proline-rich protein 1 in different cornified epithelia. *J Cell Sci* **109**:1381, 1996.
42. Steinert PM, Kartasova T, Marekov LN: Biochemical evidence that small proline-rich proteins and trichohyalin function in epithelia by modulation of the biomechanical properties of their cornified cell envelopes. *J Biol Chem* **8**:11758, 1998.
43. Steinert PM, Marekov KB: The proteins elafin, filaggrin, keratin intermediate filaments, loricrin, and small proline-rich proteins 1 and 2 are isodipeptide cross-linked components of the human epidermal cornified cell envelope. *J Biol Chem* **270**:17702, 1995.
44. Steinert PM, Marekov LN: Direct evidence that involucrin is a major early isopeptide cross-linked component of the keratinocyte cornified cell envelope. *J Biol Chem* **272**:2021, 1997.
45. Candi E, Melino G, Mei G, Tarcsa E, Chung SI, Marekov LN, Steinert PM: Biochemical, structural, and transglutaminase substrate properties of human loricrin, the major epidermal cornified cell envelope protein. *J Biol Chem* **270**:26382, 1995.
46. Robinson NA, Eckert RL: Identification of transglutaminase-reactive residues in S100A11. *J Biol Chem* **273**:2721, 1998.
47. Greenberg CS, Birckbichler PJ, Rice RH: Transglutaminases: Multifunctional cross-linking enzymes that stabilize tissues. *FASEB J* **5**:3071, 1991.
48. Candi E, Tarcsa E, Digiovanna JJ, Compton JG, Elias PM, Marekov LN, Steinert PM: A highly conserved lysine residue on the head domain of type II keratins is essential for the attachment of keratin intermediate filaments to the cornified cell envelope through isopeptide crosslinking by transglutaminases. *Proc Natl Acad Sci USA* **95**:2067, 1998.
49. Hardman MJ, Sisi P, Banbury DN, Byrne C: Patterned acquisition of skin barrier function during development. *Development* **125**:1541, 1998.
50. Hardy MH: The secret life of the hair follicle. *Trends Genet* **8**:159, 1992.
51. Cotsarelis G, Sun TT, Lavker RM: Label-retaining cells residue in the bulge area of pilosebaceous unit: Implications for follicular stem cells, hair cycle, and skin carcinogenesis. *Cell* **61**:1329, 1990.
52. Wilson AK, Coulombe PA, Fuchs E: The roles of K5 and K14 head, tail and R/KLLEGE domains in keratin filament assembly in vitro. *J Cell Biol* **119**:401, 1992.
53. Kobayashi K, Rochat A, Barrandon Y: Segregation of keratinocyte colony-forming cells in the bulge of the rat vibrissa. *Proc Natl Acad Sci USA* **90**:7391, 1993.
54. Schermer A, Galvin S, Sun TT: Differentiation-related expression of a major 64K corneal keratin in vivo and in culture suggests limbal location of corneal epithelial stem cells. *J Cell Biol* **103**:49, 1986.
55. Mansbridge JN, Knapp AM: Changes in keratinocyte maturation during wound healing. *J Invest Dermatol* **89**:253, 1987.
56. Stark HJ, Breitkreutz D, Limat A, Bowden P, Fusenig NE: Keratins of the human hair follicle: "Hyperproliferative" keratins consistently expressed in outer root sheath cells in vivo and in vitro. *Differentiation* **35**:236, 1987.
57. Lynch MH, O'Guin WM, Hardy C, Mak L, Sun TT: Acidic and basic hair/nail ("hard") keratins: Their colocalization in upper cortical and cuticle cells of the human hair follicle and their relationship to "soft" keratins. *J Cell Biol* **103**:2593, 1986.
58. Kopan R, Fuchs E: A new look into an old problem: keratins as tools to investigate determination, morphogenesis, and differentiation in skin. *Genes Dev* **3**:1, 1989.
59. Sun TT, Eichner R, Schermer A, Cooper D, Nelson WG and Weiss: The transformed phenotype. *Cancer Cell* **1**:169, 1984.
60. Leube RE, Bader BL, Bosch FX, Zimbelmann R, Achtstaetter T, Franke WW: Molecular characterization and expression of the stratification-related cytokeratin 4 and 15. *J Cell Biol* **106**:1249, 1988.
61. Lloyd C, Yu QC, Cheng J, Turksen K, Degenstein L, Hutton E, Fuchs E: The basal keratin network of stratified squamous epithelia: defining K15 function in the absence of K14. *J Cell Biol* **129**:1329, 1995.

62. Wu YJ, Parker LM, Binder NE, Becktt MA, Sinard JH, Griffiths CT, Rheinwald JG: The mesothelial keratins: A new family of cytoskeletal proteins identified in cultured mesothelial cells. *Cell* **31**:693, 1982.

63. Lindberg K, Rheinwald JG: Suprabasal 40 kd keratin (K19) expression as an imunohistologic marker of premalignancy in oral epithelium. *Am J Pathol* **134**:89, 1989.

64. Bader BL, Franke WW: Cell-type specific and efficient synthesis of human keratin 19 in transgenic mice. *Differentiation* **45**:109, 1990.

65. Fuchs E: Keratins and the skin (review). *Annu Rev Cell Dev Biol* **11**:123, 1995.

66. Parry DA: Protein chains in hair and epidermal keratin IF: Structural features and spatial arrangements. *EXS* **78**:177, 1997.

67. Fuchs E, Cleveland D: A structural scaffolding of intermediate filaments in health and disease. *Science* **279**:514, 1998.

68. Albers K, Fuchs E: The molecular biology of intermediate filament proteins. *Int Rev Cytol* **134**:243, 1992.

69. Aebi U, Haner M, Troncoso J, Eichner R, Engel A: Unifying prinicples in intermediate filament (IF) structure and assembly. *Protoplasma* **145**:73, 1988.

70. Fuchs E, Weber K: Intermediate filaments: Structure, dynamics, function, and disease. *Annu Rev Biochem* **63**:345, 1994.

71. Conway JF, Parry DAD: Intermediate filament structure: 3. Analysis of sequence homologies. *Int J Biol Macromol* **10**:79, 1988.

72. Coulombe P, Fuchs E: Elucidating the early stages of keratin filament assembly. *J Cell Biol* **111**:153, 1990.

73. Hatzfeld M, Weber K: The coiled coil of in vitro assembled keratin filaments is a heterodimer of type I and II keratins: Use of site-specific mutagenesis and recombinant protein expression. *J Cell Biol* **110**:1199, 1990.

74. Steinert PM: The two-chain coiled-coil molecular of native epidermal keratin intermediate filaments is a type I-type II heterodimer. *J Biol Chem* **265**:8766, 1990.

75. Geisler N, Schunemann J, Weber K: Chemical cross-linking indicates a staggered and antiparallel protofilament of desmin intermediate filaments and characterizes one higher-level complex between protofilaments. *Eur J Biochem* **206**:841, 1992.

76. Steinert PM, Marekov LN, Fraser RDB, Parry DAD: Keratin intermediate filament structure: Crosslinking studies yield quantitative information on molecular dimensions and mechanisms of assembly. *J Mol Biol* **230**:436, 1993.

77. Heins S, Wong PC, Muller S, Goldie K, Cleveland DW, Aebi U: The rod domain of NF-L determines neurofilament architecture, whereas the end domains specify filament assembly and network formation. *J Cell Biol* **123**:1517, 1993.

78. Jones LN, Simon M, Watts NR,. Booy FP, Steven AC, Parry DA: Intermediate filament structure: hard alpha-keratin. *Biophys Chem* **68**:83, 1997.

79. Albers K, Fuchs E: The expression of mutant epidermal keratin cDNAs transfected in simple epithelial and squamous cell carcinoma lines. *J Cell Biol* **105**:791, 1987.

80. Albers K, Fuchs E: Expression of mutant keratin cDNAs in epithelial cells reveals possible mechanisms for initiation and assembly of intermediate filaments. *J Cell Biol* **108**:1477, 1989.

81. Coulombe P, Chan YM, Albers K, Fuchs E: Deletions in epidermal keratins leading to alterations in filament organization in vivo and in intermediate filament assembly in vitro. *J Cell Biol* **111**:3049, 1990.

82. Letai A, Coulombe P, Fuchs E: Do the ends justify the mean? Proline mutations at the ends of the keratin coiled-coil rod segment are more disruptive than internal mutations. *J Cell Biol* **116**:1181, 1992.

83. Lu X, Lane EB: Retrovirus-mediated transgenic keratin expression in cultured fibroblasts: Specific domain functions in keratin stabilization and filament formation. *Cell* **62**:681, 1990.

84. Hatzfeld M, Weber K: Modulation of keratin intermediate filament assembly by single amino acid exchanges in the consensus sequence at the C-terminal end of the rod domain. *J Cell Sci* **99**:351, 1991.

85. Bader BL, Magin TM, Freudemann M, Stumpp S, Franke WW: Intermediate filaments formed *de novo* from tail-less cytokeratins in the cytoplasm and in the nucleus. *J Cell Biol* **115**:1293, 1991.

86. Hatzfeld M, Weber L: Tailless keratins assemble into regular intermediate filaments in vitro. *J Cell Sci* **97**:317, 1990.

87. Loewinger L, McKeon F: Mutations in the nuclear lamin proteins resulting in their aberrant assembly in the cytoplasm. *Eur Mol Biol Organ J* **7**:2301, 1988.

88. Raats JMH, Pieper FR, Vree Egberts WTM, Verrijp KN, Ramaekers FCS, Bloemendal H: Assembly of amino terminally deleted desmin in vimentin-free cells. *J Cell Biol* **111**:1971, 1990.

89. Gill SR, Wong PC, Monteiro MJ, Cleveland DW: Assembly properties of dominant and recessive mutations in the small mouse neurofilament (NF-L) subunit. *J Cell Biol* **111**:2005, 1990.

90. Wong, PC, Cleveland DW: Characterization of dominant and recessive assembly defective mutations in mouse neurofilament NF-M. *J Cell Biol* **111**:1987, 1990.

91. Heald R, McKeon F: Mutations of phosphorylation sites in lamin A that prevent nuclear lamina disassembly in mitosis. *Cell* **61**:579, 1990.

92. Hanukoglu I, Fuchs E: The cDNA sequence of a type II cytoskeletal keratin reveals constant and variable structural domains among keratins. *Cell* **33**:915, 1983.

93. Kaufmann E, Weber K, Geisler N: Intermediate filament forming ability of desmin derivatives lacking either the amino-terminal 67 or the carboxy-terminal 27 residues. *J Mol Biol* **185**:733, 1985.

94. Hatzfeld M, Burba M: Function of type I and type II keratin head domains: Their role in dimer, tetramer and filament formation. *J Cell Sci* **107**:1959, 1994.

95. Birkenberger L, Ip W: Properties of the desmin tail domain: Studies using synthetic peptides and antipeptides antibodies. *J Cell Biol* **111**:2063, 1990.

96. Kouklis PD, Papamarcaki T, Merdes A, Georgatos SD: A potential role for the COOH-terminal domain in the lateral packing of type III intermediate filaments. *J Cell Biol* **114**:773, 1991.

97. Eriksson JE, Opal P, Goldman RD: Intermediate filament dynamics. *Curr Opin Cell Biol* **4**:99, 1992.

98. Steinert PM, Rice DRR, Trus ACS: Complete amino acid sequence of a mouse epidermal keratin subunit and implications for the structure of intermediate filaments. *Nature* **302**:794, 1983

99. Georgatos SD, Blobel G: Two distinct attachment sites for vimentin along the plasma membrane and the nuclear envelope in avian erythrocytes: A basis for a vectorial assembly of intermediate filaments. *J Cell Biol* **105**:105, 1987.

100. Kowalczyk AP, Bornslaeger EA, Borgwardt JE, Palka HL, Dhaliwal AS, Corcoran CM, Denning MF, Green KJ: The amino-terminal domain of desmoplakin binds to plakoglobin and clusters desmosomal cadherin-plakoglobin complexes. *J Cell Biol* **139**:773, 1997.

101. Steinert PM, Marekov LN: The proteins elafin, filaggrin, keratin intermediate filaments, loricrin, and small proline-rich proteins 1 and 2 are isodipeptide cross-linked components of the human epidermal cornified cell envelope. *J Biol Chem* **270**:17702, 1995.

102. Rosenberg M, RayChaudhury A, Shows TB, LeBeau MM, Fuchs E: A group of type I keratin genes on human chromosome 17: Characterization and expression. *Mol Cell Biol* **8**:722, 1988.

103. Bader BJ, Jahn L, Franke WW: Low level expression of cytokeratins 8, 18, and 19 in vascular smooth muscle cells of human umbilical cord and in cultured cells derived therefrom, with an analysis of the chromosomal locus containing the cytokeratin 19 gene. *Eur J Cell Biol* **47**:300, 1988.

104. Lessin SR, Huebner K, Isobe M, Croce CM, Steinert PM: Chromosomal mapping of human keratin genes: Evidence of non-linkage. *J Invest Dermatol* **91**:572, 1988.

105. Romano V, Bosco P, Rocchi M, Costa G, Leube RE, Franke WW, Romeo G: Chromosomal assignments of human type I and type II cytokeratin genes to different chromosomes. *Cytogenet Cell Genet* **48**:148, 1988.

106. Rogers MA, Nischt R, Korge B, Krieg T, Fink TM, Lichter P, Wnter H, Schweizer J: Sequence data and chromosomal localization of human type I and type II hair keratin genes. *Exp Cell Res* **220**:357, 1995.

107. Popescu NC, Bowden PE, DiPaolo JA: Two type II keratin genes are localized on human chromosome 12. *Hum Genet* **82**:109, 1989.

108. Rosenberg M, Fuchs E, Le Beau MM, Eddy R, Shows TB: Three epidermal and one epithelial keratin gene map to human chromosome 12. *Cell Cytogenet* **57**:33, 1991.

109. Yoon SJ, LeBlanc-Straceski J, Ward D, Krauter K, Kucherlapati R: Organization of the human keratin type II gene cluster of 12q13. *Genomics* **24**:502, 1994.

110. Nadeau JH, Berger FG, Cox DR, Crosby JL, Davisson MT, Ferrara D, Fuchs E, Hart C, Hunihan L, Lalley PA, Langley SH, Martin GR, Nichols L, Phillips SJ, Roderick TH, Roop DR, Ruddle FH, Skow LC, Compton JG: A family of type I keratin genes and the homeobox-2 gene complex are closely linked to the rex locus on mouse chromosome 11. *Genomics* **5**:454, 1989.

111. Hart CP, Compton JG, Langley SH, Hunihan L, LeClair KP,. Zelent A, Roderick TH, Ruddle FH: Genetic linkage analysis of the murine developmental mutant velvet coat (*Ve*) and the distal chromosome 15

developmental genes *Hox-3.1, Rar-g, Wnt-1,* and *Krt-2. J Exp Zool* **263**:83, 1992.

112. Pearson RW, Spargo B: Electron microscope studies of dermal-epidermal separation in human skin. *J Invest Dermatol* **36**:213, 1961.
113. Salih MAM, Lake BD, Hag MAEL, Atherton DJ: Lethal epidermolytic epidermolysis bullosa: A new autosomal recessive type of epidermolysis bullosa. *Br J Dermatol* **113**:135, 1985.
114. Neilsen PB, Sjolund E: Epidermolysis bullosa simplex localisata associated with anodontia, hair and nail disorders: A new syndrome. *Acta Derm Venereol (Stockh)* **65**:526, 1985.
115. Niemi KM, Sommer H, Kero M, Kanerva L, Haltia M: Epidermolysis bullosa simplex associated with muscular dystrophy with recessive inheritance. *Arch Dermatol* **124**:551, 1988.
116. Fine JD, Stenn J, Johnson L, Wright R, Bock HGO, Horiguchi Y: Autosomal recessive epidermolysis bullosa simplex. *Arch Dermatol* **125**:931, 1989.
117. Fischer T, Gedde-Dahl T: Epidermolysis bullosa simplex and mottled pigmentation: A new dominant syndrome. *Clin Genet* **15**:228, 1979.
118. Gedde-Dahl T, Anton-Lamprecht I: *Principles and Practice in Medical Genetics: Epidermolysis Bullosa.* New York, Churchill-Livingstone 1981.
119. Fine JD, Bauer EA, Briggaman RA, Carter DM, Eady RAJ, Esterly NB, Holbrook KA, Hurwitz S, Johnson L, Lin A, Pearson R, Sybert VP: Revised clinical and laboratory criteria for subtypes of inherited epidermolysis bullosa. *J Am Acad Dermatol* **24**:119, 1991.
120. Cockayne EA: Recurrent bullous eruption of the feet. *Br J Dermatol* **55**:358, 1938.
121. Haneke E, Anton-Lamprecht I: Ultrastructure of blister formation in epidermolysis bullosa hereditaria: V. Epidermolysis bullosa simplex localista type Weber-Cockayne. *J Invest Dermatol* **78**:219, 1982.
122. Gedde-Dahl T: *Paediatrische Dermatologie: Classification of Epidermolysis Bullosa.* New York, Schattauer Verlag, 1978.
123. Dowling GB, Meara RH: Epidermolysis bullosa resembling juvenile dermatitis herpetiformis. *Br J Dermatol* **66**:139, 1954.
124. Gedde-Dahl T: Sixteen types of epidermolysis bullosa: On the clinical discrimination, therapy and prenatal diagnosis. *Acta Derm Venereol (Stockh)* **95**:74, 1981.
125. Anton-Lamprecht I, Schnyder UW: Epidermolysis bullosa herpetiformis Dowling-Meara: Report of a case and pathogenesis. *Dermatologica* **164**:221, 1982.
126. Gedde-Dahl T: Phenotype-genotype correlations in epidermolysis bullosa. *Birth Defects* **7**:107, 1971.
127. Granek H, Baden HP: Corneal involvement in epidermolysis bullosa simplex. *Arch Ophthalmol* **98**:469, 1980.
128. Buchbinder LH, Lucky AW, Ballard E, Stanley JR, Stolar E, Tabas M, Bauer EA, Paller AS: Severe infantile epidermolysis bullosa simplex: Dowling-Meara type. *Arch Dermatol* **122**:190, 1986.
129. Hacham-Zadeh S, Rappersberger K, Livshin R, Konrad K: Epidermolysis bullosa herpetiformis Dowling-Meara in a large family. *J Am Acad Dermatol* **18**:702, 1988.
130. Anton-Lamprecht I: Genetically induced abnormalities of epidermal differentiation and ultrastructure in ichthyoses and epidermolysis: Pathogenesis, heterogeneity, fetal manifestation, and prenatal diagnosis. *J Invest Dermatol* **81**:149s, 1983.
131. Vassar R, Coulombe PA, Degenstein L, Albers K, Fuchs E: Mutant keratin expression in transgenic mice causes marked abnormalities resembling a human genetic skin disease. *Cell* **64**:365, 1991.
132. Ishida-Yamamoto A, McGrath JA, Chapman SJ, Leigh IM, Lane EB, Eady RAJ: Epidermolysis bullosa simplex (Dowling-Meara type) is a genetic disease characterized by an abnormal keratin-filament network involving keratins K5 and K14. *J Invest Dermatol* **97**:959, 1991.
133. Olaisen B, Gedde-Dahl T: GPT-epidermolysis bullosa simplex (EBS Ogna) linkage in man. *Hum Hered* **23**:189, 1973.
134. Gedde-Dahl T, Olaisen B, Aarum G, Brevik K, Bye R: Linkage relations of chromosome 16 marker PGP to GPT: EBS1 and unassigned markers. *Cytogenet Cell Genet* **37**:474, 1984.
135. Anton-Lamprecht I: In Papadimitriou JF, Henderson DW, Spagnolo DV (eds): *Diagnostic Ultrastructure of Non-neoplastic Diseases.* Edinburgh, Churchill-Livingstone, 1992, pp 459–550.
136. Pearson RW: *Dermatology in General Medicine: The Mechanobullous Disease (Epidermolysis Bullosa),* 1st ed. New York, McGraw-Hill, 1971.
137. Savolainen ER, Kero M, Pihlajaniemi T, Kivirikko KI: Deficiency of galactosylhydroxylysyl glucosyltransferase, an enzyme of collagen synthesis, in a family with dominant epidermolysis bullosa simplex. *N Engl J Med* **304**:197, 1981.

138. Sanchez G, Seltzer JL, Eisen AZ, Stapler P, Bauer EA: Generalized dominant epidermolysis bullosa simplex: Decreased activity of a gelatinolytic protease in cultured fibroblasts as a phenotypic marker. *J Invest Dermatol* **83**:576, 1983.
139. Winberg JO, Real D, Gedde-Dahl T: Gelatinase expression in generalized epidermolysis bullosa simplex fibroblasts. *J Invest Dermatol* **87**:326, 1986.
140. Takamori K, Ikeda S, Naito K, Ogawa H: Proteases are responsible for blister formation in recessive dystrophic epidermolysis bullosa and epidermolysis bullosa simplex. *Br J Dermatol* **112**:533, 1985.
141. Fine JD, Griffith RD: A specific defect in glycosylation of epidermal cell membranes: Definition in skin from patients with epidermolysis bullosa simplex. *Arch Dermatol* **121**:1292, 1985.
142. Tidman MJ, Eady RA, Leigh IM, MacDonald DM: Keratin expression in epidermolysis bullosa simplex (Dowling-Meara). *Acta Derm Venereol (Stockh)* **68**:15, 1988.
143. Kitajima Y, Inoue S, Yaoita H: Abnormal organization of keratin intermediate filaments in cultured keratinocytes of epidermolysis bullosa simplex. *Arch Dermatol Res* **281**:5, 1989.
144. Coulombe PA, Hutton ME, Vassar R, Fuchs E: A function for keratins and a common thread among different types of epidermolysis bullosa simplex diseases. *J Cell Biol* **115**:1661, 1991.
145. Mulley JC, Nicholls CM, Propert DN, Turner T, Sutherland GR: Genetic linkage analysis of epidermolysis bullosa simplex, Koebner type. *Am J Med Genet* **19**:573, 1984.
146. Humphries MM, Sheils D, Lawler M, Farrar GJ, McWilliam P, Kenna P, Bradley DG, Sharp EM, Gaffney EF, Young M, Uitto J, Humphries P: Epidermolysis bullosa: Evidence for linkage to genetic markers on chromosome 1 in a family with the autosomal dominant simplex form. *Genomics* **7**:377, 1990.
147. Bonifas JM, Rothman AL, Epstein EH: Epidermolysis bullosa simplex: Evidence in two families for keratin gene abnormalities. *Science* **254**:1202, 1991.
148. Ryynanen M, Knowlton RG, Uitto J: Mapping of epidermolysis bullosa simplex mutation to chromosome 12. *Am J Hum Genet* **49**:978, 1991.
149. Chan YM, Yu QC, Fine JD, Fuchs E: The genetic basis of Weber-Cockayne epidermolysis bullosa simplex. *Proc Natl Acad Sci USA* **90**:7414, 1993.
150. Chan YM, Yu QC, Christiano A, Uitto J, Fuchs E: Mutations in the non-helical linker segment L1-2 of keratin 5 in patients with Weber-Cockayne epidermolysis bullosa simplex. *J Cell Sci* **107**:765, 1994.
150a. Chan Y, Anton-Lamprecht I, Yu QC, Jackel A, Zabel B, Ernst JP, Fuchs E: A human keratin 14 "knockout": The absence of K14 leads to severe epidermolysis bullosa simplex and a function for an intermediate filament protein. *Genes Dev* **8**:2574, 1994.
151. McKenna KE, Hughes AE, Bingham EA, Nevin NC: Linkage of epidermolysis bullosa simplex to keratin gene loci. *J Med Genet* **29**:568, 1992.
152. Uttam J, Hutton E, Coulombe P, Anton-Lamprecht I, Yu QC, Gedde-Dahl T, Fine JD, Fuchs E: The genetic basis of epidermolysis bullosa simplex with mottled pigmentation. *Proc Natl Acad Sci USA* **93**:9079, 1996.
153. Corden LD, Mellerio JE, Gratian MJ, Eady RA, Harper JI, Lacour M, Magee G, Lane EB, McGrath JA, McLean WH: Homozygous nonsense mutation in helix 2 of K14 causes severe recessive epidermolysis bullosa simplex. *Hum Mutat* **11**:279, 1998.
154. Coulombe PA, Hutton ME, Letai A, Hebert A, Paller AS, Fuchs E: Point mutations in human keratin 14 genes of epidermolysis bullosa simplex patients: Genetic and functional analyses. *Cell* **66**:1301, 1991.
155. Lane EB, Rugg EL, Navsaria H, Leigh IM, Heagerty AHM, Ishida-Yamamoto A, Eady RAJ: A mutation in the conserved helix termination peptide of keratin 5 in hereditary skin blistering. *Nature* **356**:244, 1992.
156. Rugg EL, Morley SM, Smith FJD, Boxer M, Tidman MJ, Navsaria H, Leigh IM, Lane EB: Missing links: Weber-Cockayne keratin mutations implicate the L12 linker domain in effective cytoskeleton function. *Nature Genet* **5**:294, 1993.
157. Dong W, Ryynanen M, Uitto J: Identification of a leucine-to-proline mutation in the keratin 5 gene in a family with the generalized Koebner type of epidermolysis bullosa simplex (EBS). *Hum Mutat* **2**:94, 1993.
158. Stephens K, Sybert VP, Wijsman EM, Ehrlich P, Spencer A: A keratin 14 mutational hot spot for epidermolysis bullosa simplex, Dowling-Meara: Implications for diagnosis. *J Invest Dermatol* **101**:240, 1993.

159. Fuchs E, Coulombe PA: Of mice and men: Genetic skin diseases of keratin. *Cell* **69**:899, 1992.

160. Humphries MM, Sheils DM, Farrar GJ, Kumar-Singh R, Kenna PF, Mansergh FC, Jordan SA, Young M, Humphries P: A mutation (Met→Arg) in the type I keratin (K14) gene responsible for autosomal dominant epidermolysis bullosa simplex. *Hum Mutat* **2**:37, 1993.

161. Torchard D, Blanchet-Bardon C, Serova O, Langbein L, Narod S, Janin N, Goguel AF, Bernheim A, Franke WW, Lenoir GM, and Feunteun J: Epidermolytic palmoplantar keratoderma cosegregates with a keratin 9 mutation in a pedigree with breast and ovarian cancer. *Nature Genet* **6**:106, 1994.

162. Sybert VP, Stephens K: A keratin 14 mutational hot spot for epidermolysis bullosa simplex, Dowling-Meara: Implications for diagnosis (letter, comment). *J Invest Dermatol* **102**:822, 1994.

163. Yamanishi K, Matsuki M, Konishi K, Yasuno H: A novel mutation of leu122 to Phe at a highly conserved hydrophobic residue in the helix initiation motif of keratin 14 in epidermolysis bullosa simplex. *Hum Mol Genet* **3**:1171, 1994.

164. Chen H, Bonifas JM, Matsumura K, Ikeda S, Leyden WA: Keratin 14 gene mutations in patients with epidermolysis bullosa simplex. *J Invest Dermatol* **105**:629, 1995.

165. Hachisuka H, Morita M, Karashima T, Sasai Y: Keratin 14 gene point mutation in the Kobner and Dowling-Meara types of epidermolysis bullosa simplex as detected by the PASA method. *Arch Dermatol Res* **287**:142, 1995.

166. Matsuki M, Hashimoto K, Yoshikawa K, Yasuno H, Yamanishi K: Epidermolysis bullosa simplex (Weber-Cockayne) associated with a novel missense mutation of Asp328 to Val in Linker 12 domain of keratin 5. *Hum Mol Genent* **4**:1999, 1995.

167. Ehrlich P, Sybert VP, Spencer A, Stephens K: A common keratin 5 gene mutation in epidermolysis bullosa simplex-Weber-Cockayne. *J Invest Dermatol* **104**:877, 1995.

168. Chan YM, Cheng J, Gedde-Dahl T, Niemi KM, Fuchs E: Genetic analysis of a severe case of Dowling-Meara epidermolysis bullosa simplex. *J Invest Dermatol* **106**:327, 1996.

169. Humphries MM, Mansergh FC, Kiang AS, Jordan SA, Sheils DM, Martin MJ, Farrar GJ, Kenna PF, Young MM, Humphries P: Three keratin gene mutations account for the majority of dominant simplex epidermolysis bullosa cases within the population of Ireland. *Hum Mutat* **8**:57, 1996.

170. Umeki K, Nomura K, Harada K, Hashimoto I: A keratin K14 gene mutation in a Japanese patient with the Dowling-Meara type of epidermolysis bullosa simplex. *J Dermatol Sci* **11**:64, 1996.

171. Stephens K, Zlotogorski A, Smith L, Ehrlich P, Wijsman E, Livingston RJ, Sybert VP: Epidermolysis bullosa simplex: A keratin 5 mutation is a fully dominant allele in epidermal cytoskeleton function. *Am J Hum Genet* **56**:577, 1995.

172. Stephens K, Ehrlich P, Weaver M, Le R, Spencer A, Sybert VP: Primers for exon-specific amplification of the KRT5 gene: Identification of novel and recurrent mutations in epidermolysis bullosa simplex patients. *J Invest Dermatol* **108**:349, 1997.

173. Nomura K, Shimizu H, Meng X, Umeki K, Tamai K, Sawamura D, Nagao K, Kawakami T, Nishikawa T, Hashimoto I: A novel keratin K5 gene mutation in Dowling-Meara epidermolysis bullosa simplex. *J Invest Dermatol* **107**:253, 1996.

174. Nomura K, Umeki K, Meng X, Tamai K, Sawamura D, Hosokawa M, Miyazawa T, Funayama M, Hashimoto I: A keratin K5 mutation (Leu463→Pro) in a family with the Weber-Cockayne type of epidermolysis bullosa simplex. *Arch Dermatol Res* **289**:493, 1997.

175. Hu Z, Smith L, Martins S, Bonifas JM, ChenH, Epstein EH: Partial dominance of a keratin 14 mutation in epidermolysis bullosa simplex: Increased severity of disease in a homozygote. *J Invest Dermatol* **109**:360, 1997.

175a. Irvine AD, McKenna KE, Bingham A, Nebiv NC, Hughes AE: A novel mutation in the helix termination peptide of keratin 5 causing epidermolysis bullosa simples Dowling-Meara. *J Invest Dermatol* **109**:815, 1997.

175b. Galligan P, Listwan P, Siller GM, Rothangel JA: A novel mutation in the L12 domain of keratin 5 in the Kobner variant of epidermolysis bullosa simplex. *J Invest Dermatol* **111**:524, 1998.

175c. Shemanko CS, Mellerio JE, Tidman MJ, Lane EB, Eady RA: Severe palmo-plantar hyperkeratosis in Dowling-Meara epidermolysis bullosa simplex caused by a mutation in the keratin 14 gene (*KRT14*). *J Invest Dermatol* **111**:893, 1998.

175d. Sorensen CB, Ladekjaer-Mikkelsen AS, Andersen BS, Brandrup F, Veien NK, Buus SK, Anton-Lamprecht I, Kruse TA, Jensen PK,

Eiberg H, Bolund L, Gergersen N: Identification of novel and known mutations in the genes for keratin 5 and 14 in Danish patients with epidermolysis bullosa simplex: Correlation between genotype and phenotype. *J Invest Dermatol* **112**:184, 1999.

176. Irvine AD, McKenna KE, Jenkinson H, Hughes AE: A mutation in the V1 domain of keratin 5 causes epidermolysis bullosa simplex with mottled pigmentation. *J Invest Dermatol* **108**:809, 1997.

177. Hovnanian A, Pollack E, Hilal L, Rochat A, Prost C, Barrandon Y, Goossens M: A missense mutation in the rod domain of keratin 14 associated with epidermolysis bullosa simplex. *Nature Genet* **3**:327, 1993.

178. Rugg EL, McLean WHI, Lane EB, Pitera R, McMillan JR, Dopping-Hepenstal PJC, Navsaria HA, Leigh IM, Eady RAJ: A functional "knockout" of human keratin 14. *Genes Dev* **8**:2563, 1994.

179. Jonkman MF, Heeres K, Pas HH, van Luyn MJA, Elema ED, Corden LD, Smith FJD, McLean WHI, Ramaekers FCS, Burton M, Scheffer H: Effects of keratin 14 ablation on the clinical and cellular phenotype in a kindred with recessive epidermolysis bullosa simplex. *J Invest Dermatol* **107**:764, 1996.

180. Chen MA, Bonifas JM, Matsumara K, Blumenfeld A, Epstein EH: A novel three-nucleotide deletion in the helix 2B region of keratin 14 in epidermolysis bullosa simplex: Delta E375. *Hum Mol Genet* **2**:1971, 1993.

181. Syder AJ, Yu QC, Paller AS, Giudice G, Pearson R, Fuchs E: Genetic mutations in the K1 and K10 genes of patients with epidermolytic hyperkeratosis: Correlation between location and disease severity. *J Clin Invest* **93**:1533, 1994.

182. Paller AS, Syder AJ, Chan YM, Yu QC, Hutton E, Tadini G, Fuchs E: A direct link between clinical and genetic mosaicism: The genetic basis of a form of epidermal nevus. *N Engl J Med* **331**:1408, 1994.

183. Chipev CC, Yang J-M, Di Giovanna JJ, Steinert PM, Marekov L, Compton JG, Bale SJ: Preferential sites in keratin 10 that are mutated in epidermolytic hyperkeratosis. *Am J Hum Genet* **54**:179, 1994.

184. Cheng J, Syder AJ, Yu QC, Letai A, Paller AS, Fuchs E: The genetic basis of epidermolytic hyperkeratosis: A disorder of differentiation-specific epidermal keratin genes. *Cell* **70**:811, 1992.

185. Rothnagel JA, Dominey AM, Dempsey LD, Longley MA, Greenhalgh DA, Gagne TA, Huber M, Frenk E, Hohl D, Roop DR: Mutations in the rod domains of keratins 1 and 10 in epidermolytic hyperkeratosis. *Science* **257**:1128, 1992.

186. Rothnagel JA, Traupe H, Wojcik S, Huber M, Hohl D, Pittelkow MR, Saeki H, Ishibashi Y, Roop DR: Mutations in the rod domain of keratin 2e in patients with ichthyosis bullosa of Siemens. *Nature Genet* **7**:485, 1994.

187. Huber M, Scaletta C, Benethan M, Frenk E, Greenhalgh DA, Rothnagel JA, Roop DR, Hohl D: Abnormal keratin 1 and 10 cytoskeleton in cultured keratinocytes from epidermolytic hyperkeratosis caused by keratin 10 mutations. *J Invest Dermatol* **102**:691, 1994.

188. Chipev CC, Steinert PM, Woodworth CD: Characterization of an immortalized cell line from a patient with epidermolytic hyperkeratosis. *J Invest Dermatol* **106**:385, 1996.

189. McLean WHI, Eady RAJ, Dopping-Hepenstal PJC, McMillan JR, Leigh IM, Navsaria HA, Higgins C, Harper JI, Paige DG, Morley SM, Lane EB: Mutations in the rod 1A domain of keratins 1 and 10 in bullous congenital ichthyosiform erythroderma (BCIE). *J Invest Dermatol* **102**:24, 1994.

190. Yang JM, Yoneda K, Morita E, Imamura S, Nam K, Lee ES, Steinert PM: An alanine to proline mutation in the 1A rod domain of the keratin 10 chain in epiermolytic hyperkeratosis. *J Invest Dermatol* **109**:692, 1997.

191. Joh GY, Traupe H, Metze D, Nashan D, Huber M, Hohl D, Longley MA, Rothnagel JA, Roop DR: A novel dinucleotide mutation in keratin 10 in the annular epidermolytic ichthyosis variant of bullous congenital ichthyosiform erythroderma. *J Invest Dermatol* **108**:357, 1997.

192. Kimonis V, GiGiovanna JJ, Yang JM, Doyle SZ, Bale SJ, and Compton JG: A mutation in the V1 end domain of keratin 1 in non-epidermolytic palmar-plantar keratoderma. *J Invest Dermatol* **103**:764, 1994.

193. Yang JM, Chipev CC, DiGiovanna JJ, Bale SJ, Marekov LN, Steinert PM, Compton JG: Mutations in the H1 and 1A domains in the keratin 1 gene in epidermolytic hyperkeratosis. *J Invest Dermatol* **102**:17, 1994.

193a. Suga Y, Duncan KO, Heald PW, Roop DR: A novel helix termination mutation in keratin 10 in annular epidermolytic ichthyosis, a variant of bullous congenital ichthyosiform erythroderma. *J Invest Dermatol* **111**:1220, 1998.

193b. Kremer H, Lavrijsen AP, McLean WH, Lane EB, Melchers D, Ruiter DJ, Mariman EC, Steijlen PM: An atypical form of bullous congenital ichthyosiform erythroderma is caused by a mutation in the L12 linker region of keratin 1. *J Invest Dermatol* **111**:1224, 1998.

193c. Yang JM, Nam K, Kim SW, Jung SY, Min HG, Yeo UC, Park KB, Lee JH, Suhr KB, Park JK, Lee ES: Arginine in the beginning of the 1A rod domain of the keratin 10 gene is the hot spot for the mutation in epidermolytic hyperkeratosis. *J Invest Dermatol Sci* **119**:126, 1999.

193d. Yang JM, Nam K, Kim HC, Lee JH, Park JK, Wu K, Lee ES, Syeinert PM: A novel glutamic acid to aspartic acid mutation near the end of the 2B rod domain in the keratin 1 chain in epidermolytic hyperkeratosis. *J Invest Dermatol* **112**:376, 1999.

193e. Sybert VP, Francis JS, Corden LD, Smith LT, Weaver M, Stephens K, McLean WH: Cyclic ichthyosis with epidermolytic hyperkeratosis: A phenotype conferred by mutations in the 2B domain of keratin K1. *Am J Hum Genet* **64**:732, 1999.

193f. Yang JM, Lee ES, Kang HJ, Choi GS, Yoneda K, Jung SY, Park KB, Steinert PM, Lee ES: A glutamate to lysine mutation at the end of 2B rod domain of keratin 2e gene in ichthyosis bullosa of Siemens. *Acta Derm Verereol (Stockh)* **78**:417, 1998.

193g. Arin MJ, Longley MA, Epstein EH Jr, Scott G, Goldsmith LA, Rothangel JA, Roop DR: A novel mutation in the 1A domain of keratin 2e in ichthyosis bullosa of Siemens. *J Invest Dermatol* **112**:380, 1999.

193h. Smith FJ, Maingi C, Covello SP, Higgins C, Schmidt M, Lane EB, Uitto J, Leigh IM, McLean WH: Genomic organization and fine mapping of the keratin 2e gene (*KRT2E*): K2e V1 domain polymorphism and novel mutations in ichthyosis bullosa of Siemens. *J Invest Dermatol* **111**:817, 1998.

194. Chipev CC, Korge BP, Markova N, Bale SJ, DiGiovanna JJ, Compton JG, Steinert PM: A leucine → proline mutation in the H1 subdomain of keratin 1 causes epidermolytic hyperkeratosis. *Cell* **70**:821, 1992.

195. Hennies HC, Kuster W, Mischke D, Reis A: Localization of a locus for the striated form of palmoplantar keratoderma to chromosome 18q near the desmosomal cadherin gene cluster. *Hum Mol Genet* **4**:1015, 1995.

196. Endo H, Hatamochi A, Shinkkai H: A novel mutation of a leucine residue in coil 1A of keratin 9 in epidermolytic palmoplantar keratoderma. *J Invest Dermatol* **109**:113, 1997.

197. Reis A, Hennies HC, Langbein L, Digweed M, Mischke D, Drechsler M, Schrock E, Royer-Pokora B, Franke W, Sperling K, Kuster W: Keratin 9 gene mutations in epidermolytic palmoplantar keratoderma (EPPK). *Nature Genet* **6**:174, 1994.

198. Bonifas JM, Matsumura K, Chen MA, Berth-Jones J, Hutchison PE, Zloczower M, Fritsch PO, Epstein EHJ: Mutations of keratin 9 in two families with palmoplantar epidermolytic hyperkeratosis. *J Invest Dermatol* **103**:474, 1994.

199. Rothnagel JA, Wojcik S, Liefer KM, Dominey AM, Huber M, Hohl D, Roop DR: Mutations in the 1A domain of keratin 9 in patients with epidermolytic palmoplantar keratoderma. *J Invest Dermatol* **104**:430, 1995.

199a. Covello SP, Irvine AD, McKenna KE, Munro CS, Nevin NC, Smith FJ, Uitto J, McLean WH: Mutations in keratin K9 in kindreds with epidermolytic palmoplantar keratoderma and epidemiology in Northern Ireland. *J Invest Dermatol* **111**:1207, 1998.

199b. Yang JM, Lee S, Kang HJ, Lee JH, Yeo UC, Son IY, Park KB, Steinert PM, Lee ES: Mutations in the 1A rod domain segment of the keratin 9 gene in epidermolytic palmoplantar kerstoderma. *Acta Derm Verereol (Stockh)* **78**:412, 1998.

200. Navsaria HA, Swensson O, Ratnavel RC, Shamsher M, McLean WH, Lane EB, Griffiths D, Eady RA, Leigh IM: Ultrastructural changes resulting from keratin-9 gene mutations in two families with epidermolytic palmoplantar keratoderma. *J Invest Dermatol* **104**:425, 1995.

201. Kremer H, Zeeuwen P, McLean WH, Mariman EC, Lane EB, van de Kerkhof CM, Ropers HH, Steijlen PM: Ichthyosis bullosa of Siemens is caused by mutations in the keratin 2e gene. *J Invest Dermatol* **103**:286, 1994.

202. Bowden PE, Haley JL, Kansky A, Rothnagel JA, Jones DO, Turner RJ: Mutation of a type II keratin gene (K6a) in pachyonychia congenita. *Nature Genet* **10**:363, 1995.

203. McLean WH, Rugg EL, Lunny DP, Morley SM, Lane EB, Swensson O, Dopping-Hepenstal PJ, Griffiths WA, Eady RA, Higgins C: Keratin 16 and keratin 17 mutations cause pachyonychia congenita. *Nature Genet* **9**:273, 1995.

204. Smith, FJ, Corden LD, Rugg EL, Ratnavel R, Leigh IM, Moss C, Tidman MJ, Hohl D, Huber M, Kunkeler L, Munro CS, Lane EB,

McLean WB: Missense mutations in keratin 17 cause either pachyonychia congenita type 2 or a phenotype resembling steatocystoma multiplex. *J Invest Dermatol* **108**:220, 1997.

205. Hohl D: Steatocystoma multiplex and oligosymptomatic pachyonychia congenita of the Jackson-Sertoli type. *Dermatology* **195**:86, 1997.

205a. Covello SP, Smith FJ, Sillevis Smitt JH, Paller AS, Munro CS, Jonkman MF, Uitto J, McLean WH: Keratin 17 mutations cause either steatocystoma multiplex orpachyonychia congenita type 2. *Br J Dermatol* **139**:475, 1998.

205b. Fujimoto W, Nakanishi G, Hirakawa S, Nakanishi T, Shima T, Takigawa M, Arata J: Pachyonychia congenita type 2: Keratin 17 mutation in a Japanese case. *J Am Acad Dermatol* **38**:1007, 1998.

205c. Smith FJ, Jonkman MF, van Goor H, Coleman CM, Covello SP, Uitto J, McLean WH: A mutation in human keratin K6b produces a phenocopy of the K17 disorder pachyonychia congenita type 2. *Hum Mol Genet* **7**:1143, 1998.

206. Winter H, Rogers MA, Gebhardt M, Wollina U, Boxall L, Chitayat D, Babul-Hirji R, Stevens HP, Zlotogorski A, Schweizer J: A new mutation in the type II hair cortex keratin hHb1 involved in the inherited hair disorder monilethrix. *Hum Genet* **101**:165, 1997.

207. Winter H, Rogers MA, Langbein L, Stevens HP, Leigh IM, Labreze C, Roul S, Taieb A, Krieg T, Schweizer J: Mutations in the hair cortex keratin hHb6 cause the inherited hair disease monilethrix. *Nature Genet* **16**:372, 1997.

207a. Zlotogorski A, Horev L, Glaser B: Monilethrix: A keratin hHb6 mutation is co-dominant with variable expression. *Exp Dermatol* **7**:268, 1998.

207b. Korge BP, Healy E, Munro CS, Punter C, Birch-Machin M, Holmes SC, Darlington S, Hamm H, Messenger AG, Rees JL, Traupe H: A mutational hotspot in the 2B domain of human hair basic keratin 6 (hHb6) in monilethrix patients. *J Invest Dermatol* **111**:896, 1998.

207c. Winter H, Labreze C, Chapalain V, Surleve-Bazeille JE, Mercier M, Rogers MA, Taieb A, Schweizer J: A variable monilethrix phenotype associated with a novel mutation, Glu402Lys, in the helix termination motif of the typeII hair keratin hHb1. *J Invest Dermatol* **111**:169, 1998.

208. Richard G, DeLaurenzi V, Didona B, Bale SJ, Compton JG: Keratin 13 point mutation underlies the hereditary mucosal epithelia disorder white sponge nevus. *Nature Genet* **11**:453, 1995.

209. Rugg EL, McLean WHI, Allison WE, Lunny DP, Macleod RI, Felix DH, Lane EB, Munro CS: A mutation in the mucosal keratin K4 is associated with oral white sponge nevus. *Nature Genet* **11**:450, 1995.

209a. Ness SL, Edelmann W, Jenkins TD, Liedtke W, Rustgi AK, Kucherlapati R: Mouse keratin 4 is necessary for internak spithelial integrity. *J Biol Chem* **273**:23904, 1998.

210a. Nishida K, Honma Y, Dota A, Kawasaki S, Adachi W, Nakamura T, Quantock AJ, Hosotani H, Yamamoto S, Okada M, Shimomura Y, Kinoshita S: Isolation and chromosomal localization of a cornea-specific human keratin 12 gene and detection of four mutations in Meesmann's corneal epithelial dystrophy. *Am J Hum Genet* **61**:1268, 1997.

210b. Irvine AD, Corden LD, Swensson O, Swensson B, Moore JE, Frazer DG, Smith FJ, Knowlton RG, Christophers E, Rochels R, Uitto J, McLean WH: Mutations in cornea-specific keratin K3 or K12 genes cause Meesmann's corneal dystrophy. *Nature Genet* **16**:184, 1997.

211. Ku NO, Wright TL, Terrault NA, Gish R, Omary MB: Mutation of human keratin 18 in association with cryptogenic cirrhosis. *J Clin Invest* **99**:19, 1997.

212. Cooper DN, Youssoufian H: The CpG dinucleotide and human genetic disease. *Hum Genet* **78**:151, 1988.

213. Letai A, Coulombe PA, McCormick MB, Yu QC, Hutton E, Fuchs E: Disease severity correlates with position of keratin point mutations in patients with epidermolysis bullosa simplex. *Proc Natl Acad Sci USA* **90**:3197, 1993.

214. Shyy TT, Asch BB, Asch HL: Concurrent collapse of keratin filaments, aggregation of organelles, and inhibition of protein synthesis during the heat shock response in mammary epithelial cells. *J Cell Biol* **108**:997, 1989.

215. Morley SM, Dundas SR, James JL, Gupta T, Brown RA, Sexton CJ, Navsaria HA, Leigh IM, Lane EB: Temperature sensitivity of the keratin cytoskeleton and delayed spreading of keratinocyte lines derived from EBS patients. *J Cell Sci* **108**:3463, 1995.

216. Anton-Lamprecht I: Prenatal diagnosis of genetic disorders of the skin by means of electron microscopy. *Hum Genet* **59**:392, 1981.

217. Eady RA: Fetoscopy and fetal skin biopsy for prenatal diagnosis of genetic skin disorders. *Semin Dermatol* **7**:2, 1988.

218. Sybert VP, Holbrook KA, Levy M: Prenatal diagnosis of severe dermatologic diseases. *Adv Dermatol* **7**:179, 1992.

219. Fine JD, Johnson LB, Wright JT: Inherited blistering diseases of the skin. *Pediatrician* **18**:175, 1991.

220. Green H: Cultured cells for the treatment of disease. *Sci Am* **265**:96, 1991.

221. Burge SM, Garrod DR: An immunohistological study of desmosomes in Darier's disease and Hailey-Hailey disease. *Br J Dermatol* **124**:242, 1991.

222. Ishibashi Y, Kajiwara Y, Andoh I, Inoue Y, Kukita A: The nature and pathogenesis of dyskeratosis in Hailey-Hailey's disease and Darier's disease. *J Dermatol* **11**:335, 1984.

223. Monk S, Sakuntabhai A, Carter SA, Bryce SD, Cox R, Harrington L, Levy E, Ruiz-Perez VL, Katsantoni E, Kodvawala A, Munro CS, Burge S, Larregue M, Nagy G, Rees JL, Lathrop M, Monaco AP, Strachan T, Hovnanian A: Refined genetic mapping of the Darier locus to a < 1-cM region of chromosome 12q24.1, and construction of a complete, high-resolution P1 artificial chromosome/bacterial artificial chromosome contig of the critical region. *Am J Hum Genet* **62**:890, 1998.

224. Ikeda S, Shigihara T, Ogawa H, Haake A, Polakowska R, Roublevskaia I, Wakem P, Goldsmith LA, Epstein E: Narrowing of the Darier disease gene interval on chromosome 12q. *J Invest Dermatol* **110**:847, 1998.

225. Frost P, Van Scott EJ: Ichthyosiform dermatoses: Classification based on anatomic and biometric observations. *Arch Dermatol* **94**:113, 1966.

226. Ackerman AB: Histopathologic concept of epidermolytic hyperkeratosis. *Arch Dermatol* **102**:253, 1970

227. Wilgram GF, Caulfield JB: An electron microscopic study of epidermolytic hyperkeratosis. *Arch Dermatol* **94**:127, 1966.

228. Anton-Lamprecht I, Curth HO, Schnyder UW: Ultrastructure of inborn errors of keratinization: II. Ichthyosis hystrix type Curth-Macklin. *Arch Dermatol Res* **246**:77, 1973.

229. Anton-Lamprecht I, Schnyder UW: Ultrastructure of inborn errors of keratinization. *Arch Derm Forsch* **250**:207, 1974.

230. Curth HO, Macklin MT: The genetic basis of various types of ichthyosis in a family group. *Am J Hum Genet* **6**:371, 1954.

231. Voerner H: Zur Kenntris des Keratoma hereditarium palmare et plantare. *Arch Dermatol Syphilol* **56**:3, 1901.

232. Fritsch P, Hoenigsmann H, Jaschke E: Epidermolytic hereditary palmoplantar keratoderma. *Br J Dermatol* **99**:561, 1978.

233. Klaus S, Weinstein GD, Frost P: Localized epidermolytic hyperkeratosis. *Arch Dermatol* **101**:272, 1970.

234. Kolde G, Vakilzadeh F: An ultrastructural study of epidermolytic leukoplakia. *Arch Dermatol Res* **275**:86, 1983.

235. Siemens HW: The as yet undescribed regular dominant form of bullous congenital ichthyosiform erythroderma. *Hautarzt* **21**:252, 1970.

236. Traupe H, Kolde G, Hamm H, Happle R: Ichthyosis bullosa of Siemens: A unique type of epidermolytic hyperkeratosis. *J Am Acad Dermatol* **14**:1000, 1986.

237. Ollendorff-Curth H, Allen FH, Schnyder UW, Anton-Lamprecht I: Follow-up of a family group suffering from ichthyosis hystrix type Curth-Macklin. *Hum Genet* **17**:37, 1972.

238. Fuchs E, Esteves RA, Coulombe PA: Transgenic mice expressing a mutant keratin 10 gene reveal the likely genetic basis for Epidermolytic Hyperkeratosis. *Proc Natl Acad Sci USA* **89**:6906, 1992.

239. Bickenbach JR, Longley MA, Bundman DS, Dominey AM, Bowden PE, Rothnagel JA, Roop DR: A transgenic mouse model that recapitulates the clinical features of both neonatal and adult forms of the skin disease epidermolytic hyperkeratosis. *Differentiation* **61**:129, 1996.

240. Compton JG, DeGiovanna JJ, Santucci SK, Kearns KS, Amos CI, Abangan DL, Korge BP, McBride OW, Steinert PM, Bale SJ: Linkage of epidermolytic hyperkeratosis to the type II keratin gene cluster on chromosome 12q. *Nature Genet* **1**:301, 1992.

241. Bonifas JM, Bare JW, Chen MA, Lee MK, Slater CA, Goldsmith LA, Epstein EH Jr: Linkage of the epidermolytic hyperkeratosis phenotype and the region of the type II keratin gene cluster on chromosome 12. *J Invest Dermatol* **99**:524, 1992.

242. Pulkkinen L, Christiano AM, Knowlton RG, Uitto J: Epidermolytic hyperkeratosis (bullous congenital ichthyosiform erythroderma): Genetic linkage to chromosome 12q in the region of the type II keratin gene cluster. *J Clin Invest* **91**:357, 1993.

243. Steinert PM, Parry DAD: The conserved H1 domain of the type II keratin 1 chain plans an essential role in the alignment of nearest neighbor molecules in mouse and human keratin 1/keratin 10 intermediate filaments at the two- to four-molecular level of structure. *J Biol Chem* **268**:2878, 1993.

244. Magro CM, Baden LA, Crowson AN, Bowden PE, Baden HP: A novel nonepidermolytic palmoplantar keratoderma: A clinical and histopathologic study of six cases. *J Am Acad Dermatol* **37**:27, 1997.

245. Reis A, Kuster W, Eckardt R, Sperling K: Mapping of a gene for epidermolytic palmoplantar keratoderma to the region of the acidic keratin gene cluster at 17q12-q21. *Hum Genet* **90**:113, 1992.

246. Lorette G, Fetissoff F, Grangeponte MC, et al. Érythrodermie ichtyosiforme congénitale bulleuse chez une fille naevus verruquex épidermolytique chez son pére. *Ann Dermatol Venereol* **111**:858, 1984.

247. Bonafe JL, Blanchet-Bardon C, Christol B, Rolland M: Naevus verruqueux systématise épidermolytique et érythrodermie ichtyosiforme cong énitale bulleuse. *Ann Dermatol Venereol* **114**:916, 1987.

248. Happle R: Akanthokeratolytischer epidermaler navus: Vererbbar ist die akanthokeratolyse, nicht der navus. *Hautartz* **40**:117, 1990.

249. Nazzaro V, Ermacora E, Santucci E, Caputo R: Epidermolytic hyperkeratosis: Generalized form in children from parents with systematized linear form. *Br J Dermatol* **122**:417, 1990.

250. Moss C, Jones DO, Blight A, Bowden PE: Birthmark due to cutaneous mosaicism for keratin 10 mutation. *Lancet* **345**:596, 1995.

251. Munro CS, Carter S, Bryce S, Hall M, Rees JL, Kunkeler L, Stephenson A, Strachan T: A gene for pachyonychia congenita is closely linked to the keratin gene cluster on 17q12-q21. *J Med Genet* **31**:675, 1994.

252. Smith FJD, Jonkman MF, van Goor H, Coleman CM, Covello, SP, Uitto J, McLean WHI: A mutation in human keratin K6b produces a phenocopy of the K17 disorder pachyonychia congenita type 2. *Hum Mol Genet* **7**:1143, 1998.

253. Fujimoto W, Nakanishi G, Hirakawa S, Nakanishi T, Shimo T, Takigawa M, Arata J: Pachyonychia congenita type 2: Keratin 17 mutation in a Japanese case. *J Am Acad Dermatol* **38**:1007, 1998.

254. Takahashi K, Coulombe PA: A transgenic mouse model with an inducible skin blistering disease phenotype. *Proc Natl Acad Sci USA* **93**:14776, 1996.

255. Panteleyev AA, Paus R, Wanner R, Nurnberg W, Eichmuller S, Thiel R, Zhang J, Henz BM, Rosenbach T: Keratin 17 gene expression during the murine hair cycle. *J Invest Dermatol* **108**:324, 1997.

256. Tomkova H, Fujimoto W, Arata J: Expression of keratins (K10 and K17) in steatocystoma multiplex, eruptive vellus hair cysts, and epidermoid and trichilemmal cysts. *Am J Dermatopathol* **19**:250, 1997.

257. Stevens HP, Kelsell DP, Bryant SP, Bishop DT, Dawber RP, Spurr NK, Leigh IM: Linkage of monilethrix to the trichocyte and epithelial keratin gene cluster on 12q11-q13. *J Invest Dermatol* **106**:795, 1996.

258. Whitten JB: The electron microscopic examination of congenital keratoses of the oral mucous membranes: I. White sponge nevus. *Oral Surg Oral Med Oral Pathol* **29**:69, 1970.

259. McGininis JP, Turner JE: Ultrastructure of the white spong nevus. *Oral Surg Oral Med Oral Pathol* **40**:644, 1975.

260. Alkemade PP, Balen AT van: Hereditary epithelial dysrophy of the cornea; meemsman type. *Br J Ophthalmol* **50**:603, 1966.

261. Kao WW, Liu CY, Converse RL, Shiraishi A, Kao CW, Ishizaki M, Doetschman T, Duffy J: Keratin 12-deficient mice have fragile corneal epithelia. *Invest Ophthalmol Vis Sci* **37**:2572, 1996.

262. Ku NO, Michie S, Oshima RG, Omary MB: Chronic Hepatitis, hepatocyte fragility, and increased soluble phosphoglycokeratins in transgenic mice expressing a keratin 18 conserved arginine mutant. *J Cell Biol* **131**:1303, 1995.

263. Ku N, Michie SA, Soetikno RM, Resurreccion EZ, Broome RL, Oshima RG, Omary MB: Susceptibility to hepatotoxicity in transgenic mice that express a dominant-negative human keratin 18 mutant. *J Clin Invest* **98**:1034, 1996.

263a. Ku NO, Michie SA, Soetikno RM, Resurreccion EZ, Broome RL, Omary MB: Mutation of a major keratin phosphorylation site predisposes to hepatotoxic injury in transgenic mice. *J Cell Biol* **143**:2023, 1998.

264. Li Z, Colucci-Guyon E, Pincon-Raymond M, Mericskay M, Pournin S, Paulin D, Babinet C: Cardiovascular lesions and skeletal myopathy in mice lacking desmin. *Dev Biol* **175**:362, 1996.

265. Li Z, Mericskay M, Agbulut O, Butler-Browne G, Carlsson L, Thornell LE, Babinet C, Paulin D: Desmin is essential for the tensile strength and integrity of myofibrils but not for myogenic commit-

ment, differentiation, and fusion of skeletal muscle. *J Cell Biol* **139**:129, 1997.

266. Milner DJ, Weitzer G, Tran D, Bradley A, Capetanaki Y: Disruption of muscle architecture and myocardial degeneration in mice lacking desmin. *J Cell Biol* **134**:1255, 1996.

267. Horowitz SH, Schmalbruch H: Autosomal dominant distal myopathy with desmin storage: A clinicopathologic and electrophysiologic study of a large kinship. *Muscle Nerve* **17**:151, 1994.

268. Muntoni F, Catani G, Mateddu A, Rimoldi M, Congiu T, Faa G, Marrosu MG, Cianchetti C, Porcu M: Familial cardiomyopathy, mental retardation and myopathy associated with desmin-type intermediate-filaments. *Neuromusc Dis* **4**:233, 1994.

269. Cameron CH, Mirakhur M, Allen IV: Desmin myopathy with cardiomyopathy. *Acta Neuropathol* **89**:560, 1995.

270. Vicart P, Dupret JM, Hazan J, Li Z, Gyapay G, Krishnamoorthy R, Weissenbach J, Fardeau M, Paulin D: Human desmin gene:cDNA sequence, regional localization and exclusion of the locus in a familial desmin-related myopathy. *Hum Genet* **98**:422, 1996.

271. Goldfarb LG, Park KY, Cervenakova L, Gorokhova S, Lee HS, Vasconcelos O, Nagle JW, Semino-Mora C, Sivakumar K, Dalakas MC: Missense mutations in desmin associated with familial cardiac adn skeletal myopathy. *Nature Genet* **19**:402, 1998.

272. Munoz-Marmol AM, Strasser G, Isamat M, Coulombe P, Yang Y, Roca X, Vela E, Mate JL, Coll J, Fernandez-Figueras MT, Navas-Palacios JJ, Ariza A, Fuchs E: A dysfunctional desmin mutation in a patient with severe generalized myopathy. *Proc Natl Acad Sci USA* **95**:11312, 1998.

273. Xu Z, Cork LC, Griffin JW, Cleveland DW: Increased expression of neurofilament subunit NF-L produces morphological alterations that resemble the pathology of human motor neuron disease. *Cell* **73**:23, 1993.

274. Cote F, Collard JF, Julien JP: Progressive neuronopathy in transgenic mice expressing the human neurofilament heavy gene: A mouse model of amyotrophic lateral sclerosis. *Cell* **73**:35, 1993.

275. Lee MK, Marszalek JR, Cleveland DW: A mutant neurofilament subunit causes massive, selective motor neuron death: Implications for the pathogenesis of human moter neuron disease. *Neuron* **13**:975, 1994.

276. Vechio JD, Bruijn LI, Xu Z, Brown RH, Cleveland DW: Sequence variants in human neurofilament proteins: Absence of linkage to familial amyotrophic lateral sclerosis. *Ann Neurol* **40**:603, 1996.

276a. Tomkins J, Usher P, Slade JY, Ince PG, Curtis A, Bushby K, Shaw PJ: Novel insertion in the KSP region of the neurofilament heavy gene in amyotrophic lateral sclerosis (ALS). *Neuroreport* **9**:3967, 1998.

276b. Julien JP, Mushynski WE: Neurofilaments in health and disease. *Prog Nucl Acid Res Mol Biol* **61**:1, 1998.

277. Capetanaki Y, Smith S, Heath JP: Overexpression of the vimentin gene in transgenic mice inhibits normal lens cell differentiation. *J Cell Biol* **109**:1653, 1989.

278. Dunia I, Pieper F, Manenti S, Vandekamp A, Devilliers G, Benedetti EL, Bloemendal H: Plasma membrane-cytoskeleton damage in eye lenses of transgenic mice expressing desmin. *Eur J Cell Biol* **53**:59, 1990.

279. Monteiro JM, Hoffman PN, Gearhart JD, Cleveland DW: Expression of NF-L in both neuronal and nonneuronal cells of transgenic mice: Increased neurofilament density in axons without affecting caliber. *J Cell Biol* **111**:1543, 1990.

280. Colucci-Guyon E, Portier MM, Dunia I, Paulin D, Pournin S, Babinet C: Mice lacking vimentin develop and reproduce without an obvious phenotype. *Cell* **79**:679, 1994.

281. Pekny M, Leveen P, Pekna M, Eliasson C, Berthold CH, Westermark B, Betsholtz X: Mice lacking glial fibrillary acidic protein display astrocytes devoid of intermediate filaments but develop and reproduce normally. *Eur Mol Biol Org J* **14**:1590, 1995.

282. McCall MA, Gregg RG, Behringer RR, Brenner M, Delaney CL, Galbreath EJ, Zhang CL, Pearce RA, Chiu Sy, Messing A: Targeted deletion in astrocyte intermediate filament (Gfap) alters neuronal physiology. *Proc Natl Acad Sci USA* **93**:6361, 1996.

283. Liedtke W, Edelmann W, Bieri PL, Chiu FC, Cowan NJ, Kucherlapati R, Raine CS: GFAP is necessary for the integrity of CNS white matter architecture and long-term maintenance of myelination. *Neuron* **17**:607, 1996.

284. Janmey PA, Euteneuer U, Traub P, Schliwa M: Viscoelastic properties of vimentin compared with other filamentous biopolymer networks. *J Cell Biol* **113**:155, 1991.

285. Christian JL, Edelstein NG, Moon RT: Overexpression of wild-type and dominant negative mutant vimentin subunits in developing xenopus embryos. *New Biol* **2**:700, 1990.

286. Guo L, Degenstein L, Dowling J, Yu QC, Wollmann R, Perman B, Fuchs E: Gene targeting of *BPAG1*: Abnormalities in mechanical strength and cell migration in stratified squamous epithelia and severe neurologic degeneration. *Cell* **81**:233, 1995.

287. Brown A, Bernier G, Mathieu M, Rossant J, Kothary R: The mouse dystonia musculorum gene is a neural isoform of bullous pemphigoid antigen 1. *Nature Genet* **10**:301, 1995.

287a. Eyer J, Cleveland DW, Wong PC, Peterson AC: Pathogenesis of two axonopathies does not require axonal neurofilaments. *Nature* **391**:584, 1998.

287b. Fuchs E, Yang Y: Crossroads on cytoskeletal highways. *Cell* **98**:547, 1999.

288. Foisner R, Feldman B, Sander L, Seifert G, Artleib U, Wiche G: A panel of monoclonal antibodies to rat plectin: Distinction by epitope mapping and immunoreactivity with different tissues and cell lines. *Acta Histochem* **96**:421, 1994.

289. Foisner R, Bohn W, Mannweiler K, Wiche G: Distribution and ultrastructure of plectin arrays in subclones of rat glioma C6 cells differing in intermediate filament protein (vimentin) expression. *J Struct Biol* **115**:304, 1995.

290. McLean WH, Pulkkinen L, Smith FJ, Rugg EL, Lane EB, Bullrich F, Burgeson RE, Amano S, Hudson DL, Owaribe K, McGrath JA, McMillan JR, Eady RA, Leigh IM, Christiano AM, Uitto U: Loss of plectin causes epidermolysis bullosa with muscular dystrophy: cDNA cloning and genomic organization. *Genes Dev* **10**:1724, 1996.

291. Smith FJ, Eady RA, Leigh IM, McMillan JR, Rugg EL, Kelsell DP, Bryant SP, Spurr NK, Geddes JF, Kirtschig G, Milana G, de Bono AG, Owaribe K, Wiche G, Pulkkinen L, Uitto J, McLean WH, Lane EB: Plectin deficiency results in muscular dystrophy with epidermolysis bullosa. *Nature Genet* **13**:450, 1996.

292. Gache Y, Chavanas S, Lacour JP, Wiche G, Owaribe K, Meneguzzi G, Ortonne JP: Defective expression of plectin/HD1 in epidermolysis bullosa simplex with muscular dystophy. *J Clin Invest* **97**:2289, 1996.

293. Chavanas S, Pulkkinen L, Gache Y, Smith FJ, McLean WH, Uitto J, Ortonne JP, Meneguzzi G: A homozygous nonsense mutation in the *PLEC1* gene in patients with epidermolysis bullosa simplex with muscular dystrophy. *J Clin Invest* **98**:2196, 1996.

294. Pulkkinen L, Smith FJ, Shimizu H, Murata S, Yaoita H, Hachisuka H, Nishikawa T, McLean WH, Uitto J: Homozygous deletion mutations in the plectin gene (*PLEC1*) in patients with epidermolysis bullosa simplex associated with late-onset muscular dystrophy. *Hum Mol Genet* **5**:1539, 1996.

295. Mellerio JE, Smith FJ, McMillan JR, McLean WH, McGrath JA, Morrison GA, Tierney P, Albert DM, Wiche G, Leigh IM, Geddes JF, Lane EB, Uitto J, Eady RA: Recessive epidermolysis bullosa simplex associated with plectin mutations: Infantile respiratory complications in two unrelated cases. *Br J Dermatol* **137**:898, 1997.

295a. Takizawa Y, Shimizu H, Rouan F, Kawai M, Udono M, Pulkkinen L, Mishikawa T, Uitto J: Four novel plectin gene mutations in Japanese patients with epidermolysis bullosa with muscular dystrophy disclosed by heteroduplex scanning and protein truncation tests. *J Invest Dermatol* **112**:109, 1999.

295b. Dang M, Pulkkinen L, Smith FJ, McLean WH, Uitto J: Novel compound heterozygous mutations in the plectin gene in epidermolysis bullosa with muscular dystrophy and the use of protein truncation test for detection of premature termination codon mutations. *Lab Invest* **78**:195, 1998.

296. Andra K, Lassmann H, Bittner R, Shorny S, Fassler R, Propst F, Wiche G: Targeted inactivation of plectin reveals essential function in maintaining the integrity of skin, muscle, and heart cytoarchitecture. *Genes Dev* **11**:3143, 1997.

297. Svitkina T, Verkhovsky A, Borisy G: Plectin sidearms mediate interaction of intermediate filaments with microtubules and other components of the cytoskeleton. *J Cell Biol* **135**:991, 1996.

298. Moll I, Kurzen H, Langbein L, Franke WW: The distribution of the desmosomal protein, plakophilin 1, in human skin and skin tumors. *J Invest Dermatol* **108**:139, 1997.

299. McGrath JA, McMillan JR, Shemanko CS, Runswick SK, Leigh IM, Lane EB, Garrod DR, Eady RAJ: Mutations in the plakophilin 1 gene result in ectodermal dysplasia/skin fragility syndrome. *Nature Genet* **17**:240, 1997.

300. Hatzfeld M, Kristjansson GI, Plessman U, Weber K: Band 6 protein, a major constituent of desmosomes from stratified epithelia, is a novel member of the armadillo multigene family. *J Cell Sci* **107**:2259, 1994.

301. Burgeson RE: Type VII collagen, anchoring fibrils, and epidermolysis bullosa. *J Invest Dermatol* **101**:252, 1993.

302. Epstein EH:Molecular genetics of epidermolysis bullosa. *Science* **256**:799, 1992.

303. Christiano AM, Greenspan DS, Hoffman GG, Zhang X, Tamai Y, Lin AN, Dietz HC, Hovnanian A, Uitto J: A missense mutation in type VII collagen in two affected siblings with recessive dystrophic epidermolysis bullosa. *Nature Genet* **1**:62, 1993.

304. Ryynanen M, Ryynanen J, Sollberg S, Iozzo RV, Knowlton RG, Uitto J: Genetic linkage of type VII collagen (COL7A1) to dominant dystrophic epidermolysis bullosa in families with abnormal anchoring fibrils. *J Clin Invest* **89**:974, 1992.

305. Marinkovich MP, Verrando P, Keene DR, Meneguzzi G, Lunstrum GP, Ortonne JP, Burgeson RE: Basement membrane proteins kalinin and nicein are structurally and immunologically identical. *Lab Invest* **69**:295, 1993.

306. Campbell KP: Three muscular dystrophies: Loss of cytoskeleton-extracellular matrix linkage. *Cell* **80**:675, 1995.

307. Worton R: Muscular dystrophies: diseases of the dystrophin-glycoprotein complex. *Science* **270**:755, 1995.

308. Seidman CE, Seidman JG: Mutations in cardiac myosin heavy chain genes cause familial hypertrophic cardiomyopathy. *Mol Biol Med* **8**:159, 1991.

309. Keating MT, Sanguinetti MC: Molecular genetic insights into cardiovascular disease. *Science* **272**:681, 1996.

310. Spirito P, Seidman CE, McKenna WJ, Maron BJ: The management of hypertrophic cardiomyopathy. *N Engl J Med* **336**:775, 1997.

311. Lazarides E: Intermediate filaments as mechanical integrators of cellular space. *Nature* **283**:249, 1980

312. Fuchs E: Intermediate filaments and disease: Mutations that cripple cell strength. *J Cell Biol* **125**:511, 1994.

313. Fuchs E: The cytoskeleton and disease: Genetic disorders of the intermediate filaments. *Annu Rev Genet* **30**:197, 1996.

314. Reis A, Hennies HC, Langbein L, Digweed M, Mischke D, Drechsler M, Schrock E, Royer-Pokora B, Franke W, Sperling K, Kuster W: Keratin 9 gene mutations in epidermolytic palmoplantar keratoderma (EPPK). *Nature Genet* **6**:174, 1994.

315. Baribault H, Penner J, Iozzo RV, Wilson-Heiner M: Colorectal hyperplasia and inflammation in keratin 8-deficient FVB/N mice. *Genes Dev* **8**:2964, 1994.

# Epidermolysis Bullosa: The Disease of the Cutaneous Basement Membrane Zone*

*Jouni Uitto* ■ *Leena Pulkkinen*

1. Epidermolysis bullosa (EB) is a group of genodermatoses that manifest with skin fragility as the unifying diagnostic feature, in association with a number of extracutaneous manifestations. The inheritance can be either autosomal dominant or autosomal recessive. The clinical severity of different variants of EB is highly variable, and in some severe cases, the disease can lead to early demise during the postnatal period. EB has been classified, on the basis of the level of tissue separation within the dermal-epidermal basement membrane zone (BMZ), to four broad categories: the simplex, hemidesmosomal, junctional, and dystrophic variants.

2. Tissue separation in various forms of EB occurs within the cutaneous BMZ, which consists of several attachment complexes forming an intricate network necessary for stable association of the epidermis to the underlying dermis. A defect in this network structure can result in fragility of skin and manifest clinically as a form of EB.

3. Hemidesmosome-anchoring filament complexes are attachment structures at the dermal-epidermal junction extending from the intracellular milieu of basal keratinocytes to the extracellular matrix of the dermal-epidermal basement membrane. Hemidesmosomes (HD) contribute to the stable association of the lower part of epidermis to the underlying basement membrane. At least four distinct proteins, plectin, BP230, BP180, and the $\alpha6\beta4$ integrin, which represent five different gene products, are critical components of the HDs.

4. Laminins 5, 6, and 7 of the laminin family of proteins are critical components of the cutaneous BMZ. The major component, laminin 5, consists of three polypeptide subunits ($\alpha3$, $\beta3$, and $\gamma2$), which are all necessary for the stable assembly of this trimeric molecule traversing the lamina lucida-lamina densa interface.

5. Type VII collagen is the major, if not the exclusive, component of the anchoring fibrils, attachment structures extending from the lower part of the lamina densa to the underlying dermis. Type VII collagen polypeptides, the $\alpha1(VII)$ chains, are encoded by a complex gene, COL7A1, which consists of 118 distinct exons, the largest number in any gene characterized thus far. The individual $\alpha1(VII)$ collagen polypeptides consist of a central collagenous domain flanked by a large ($\sim145$-kDa) amino-terminal noncollagenous (NC-1) domain and a smaller ($\sim18$-kDa) carboxy-terminal non-collagenous (NC-2) domain. In the extracellular space, the individual type VII collagen molecules align into anti-parallel dimers with overlapping C-terminal ends, and these dimer molecules laterally assemble into functional anchoring fibrils.

6. Cloning of the genes expressed in the cutaneous BMZ has led to development of strategies to screen genome for mutations in different variants of EB. In addition to direct sequencing of PCR-amplified cDNA and genomic sequences, novel screening technologies have been adopted, including heteroduplex scanning of PCR products for sequence variants by conformation-sensitive gel electrophoresis and the protein truncation test, which has been applied to find mutations causing premature termination codon (PTC) for translation.

7. The dystrophic forms of EB (DEB), characterized by sublamina densa tissue separation and abnormalities in the anchoring fibrils, result from mutations in the type VII collagen gene (COL7A1). In the severely scarring Hallopeau-Siemens variant of recessively inherited DEB (HS-RDEB; MIM 226600), a characteristic genetic lesion is premature termination codon mutations in both COL7A1 alleles. In the milder scarring, mitis-type of RDEB (M-RDEB), a frequent mutation is a missense mutation or in-frame deletion in either one or both alleles. A characteristic lesion in dominantly inherited DEB (DDEB; MIM 131750 and 131850) is a glycine substitution

---

*GenBank accession numbers for genes of the cutaneous basement membrane zone (BMZ): *LAMA3* (X85108, X85107); *LAMC2* (U43327, U311787–U31201); *LAMB3* (L25541, U17744–U17760); *ITGB4* (X51841, U66529–U66541); *ITGA6* (X59512; AF166335–AF166343); *COL7A1*(L02870, L23982); *PLEC1* (Z54367, U53204, U53834, U63609–U63610); *BPAG1* (L11690, M69225); *BPAG2* (U76564–U76604); *KRT5* (U05838–U05849); KRT5(NM000526).

A list of standard abbreviations is located immediately preceding the index in each volume. Additional abbreviations used in this chapter include: AF = anchoring fibrils; BMZ = basement membrane zone; BP180 = the 180-kDa bullous pemphigoid antigen; BP230 = the 230-kDa bullous pemphigoid antigen; CSGE = conformation-sensitive gel electrophoresis; DDEB = dominant dystrophic epidermolysis bullosa; DEB = dystrophic epidermolysis bullosa; EB = epidermolysis bullosa; EB-MD = epidermolysis bullosa with late-onset muscular dystrophy; EB-PA = epidermolysis bullosa with pyloric atresia; EBS = epidermolysis bullosa simplex; EBS-DM = epidermolysis bullosa simplex-Dowling-Meara; EBS-K = epidermolysis bullosa simplex-Köbner; EBS-MP = epidermolysis bullosa simplex with mottled pigmentation; EBS-WC = epidermolysis bullosa simplex-Weber-Cockayne; GABEB = generalized atrophic benign epidermolysis bullosa; H-JEB = Herlitz type of junctional epidermolysis bullosa; HD = hemidesmosomes; HD-EB = hemidesmosomal variants of epidermolysis bullosa; HS-RDEB = Hallopeau-Siemens variant of recessive dystrophic epidermolysis bullosa; JEB = junctional epidermolysis bullosa; LD = lamina densa; LL = lamina lucida; M-RDEB = mitis variant of recessive dystrophic epidermolysis bullosa; NC-1 = noncollagenous domain-1; NC-2 = noncollagenous domain-2; PGD = preimplantation genetic diagnosis; PTC = premature termination codon; PTT = protein truncation test; SBDP = sub-basal dense plate; SLS = segment-long-spacing; TF = tonofilaments.

mutation in the collagenous domain of type VII collagen, which causes EB phenotype through dominant negative interference. However, not all glycine substitution mutations are dominant, and some of them can be recessive resulting in a clinical phenotype only when homozygous or compound heterozygote with a PTC. Collectively, the combination of mutations and their positions along the type VII collagen polypeptide result in abnormalities in anchoring fibrils with variable degrees of severity within the spectrum of DEB.

8. Mutations in the laminin 5 genes, *LAMA3*, *LAMB3,* and *LAMC2*, encoding the subunit polypeptides of α3, β3, and γ2, respectively, have been demonstrated in the Herlitz variant of junctional EB (H-JEB; MIM 226700). These genetic lesions are invariably PTC mutations. Although PTCs in any of the three genes can lead to similar phenotype, most (~80 percent) of these mutations reside in *LAMB3*, which is explained in part by the presence of two recurrent "hotspot" mutations, R635X and R42X. Missense mutations in the laminin 5 genes have been disclosed in cases with milder, nonlethal JEB.

9. A novel category, the hemidesmosomal variants of EB (HD-EB), was recently established. In these patients, tissue separation occurs at the basal cell/lamina lucida interface at the level of hemidesmosomes. Three clinical variants are recognized, and distinct mutations in the respective hemidesmosomal genes have been encountered. Specifically, generalized atrophic benign EB (GABEB; MIM 226650) is due to mutations in the gene encoding the 180-kDa bullous pemphigoid antigen (BP180), a transmembrane collagen designated as type XVII collagen *(BPAG2/ COL17A1).* Epidermolysis bullosa with congenital pyloric atresia (EB-PA; MIM 226730) is due to mutations in the α6β4 integrin genes, *ITGA6* and *ITGB4*, respectively. EB associated with late-onset muscular dystrophy (EB-MD, MIM 226670) results from mutations in the plectin gene *(PLEC1),* a multifunctional adhesion protein expressed both in the epidermis and the sarcolemma of the muscle.

10. Examination of the repertoire of mutations disclosed in ten distinct genes in different variants of EB adds to our understanding of the complexity of the cutaneous BMZ. The information of the nature of the genetic lesions also explains the phenotypic variability of different subtypes of EB.

11. The impact of molecular genetics of EB on patient care is already evident in terms of improved genetic counseling and refined classification with prognostic implications. The knowledge of candidate protein/gene systems and identification of specific mutations in such genes has paved the way to establish DNA-based prenatal testing for severe forms of EB. This information is also critical for development of emerging technologies, such as pre-implantation genetic diagnosis (PGD) and gene therapy, for EB.

## DIAGNOSTIC FEATURES OF EB

### Clinical Findings

Epidermolysis bullosa (EB) is a group of heritable mechanobullous disorders, with highly variable clinical severity. In its most severe forms, EB can cause demise during the early postnatal period, while the milder variants are characterized by protracted skin involvement that does not affect the overall life span of the affected individuals. The inheritance can be either autosomal dominant or autosomal recessive.[1-3] The unifying diagnostic feature of various forms of EB is fragility of skin, which manifests

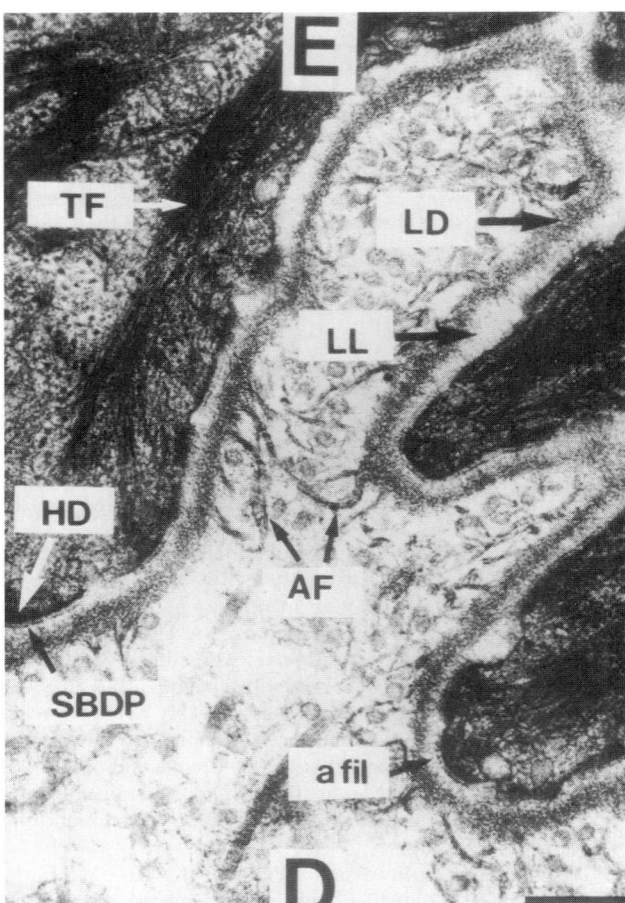

Fig. 222-1. Transmission electron microscopy of the cutaneous basement membrane zone separating the epidermis (E) from the dermis (D). Note that the dermal-epidermal basement membrane consists of two layers, the lamina densa (LD) and the lamina lucida (LL). Within the epidermal keratinocytes, tonofilaments (TF) associate with hemidesmosomes (HD), which consist of intracellular inner and outer plaques (white arrow) and a sub-basal dense plate (SBDP). Anchoring filaments (a fil) are fine, thread-like structures traversing the lamina lucida under the hemidesmosomes. Anchoring fibrils (AF) extend from the lamina densa to the underlying dermis. (*Figure courtesy of Dr. John A. McGrath, St. Johns Institute of Dermatology, London.*)

in the affected individuals as blistering and erosions as a result of mechanical trauma. In addition to skin involvement, a variety of extracutaneous manifestations can be encountered in different forms of EB; these include corneal erosions, enamel hypoplasia, nail dystrophy, scarring alopecia, erosions in the tracheal epithelium, development of esophageal strictures, congenital pyloric atresia, and late-onset muscular dystrophy.[1]

### Classification

EB has traditionally been divided into three broad categories, based on the level of tissue separation within the dermal-epidermal basement membrane zone (BMZ) (see Fig. 222-1 and 222-2). Specifically, in the simplex forms of EB, tissue separation occurs in the basal keratinocytes on the epidermal side of the basement membrane; in the junctional forms of EB, blister formation occurs in the lamina lucida of the dermal-epidermal basement membrane itself; and in the dystrophic, severely scarring forms of EB, tissue cleavage occurs at the dermal side of the cutaneous BMZ (Table 222-1). In addition, a fourth broad category, the hemidesmosomal variants of EB (HD-EB), was recently introduced.[4] In the latter patients, tissue separation occurs at the basal cell/lamina lucida

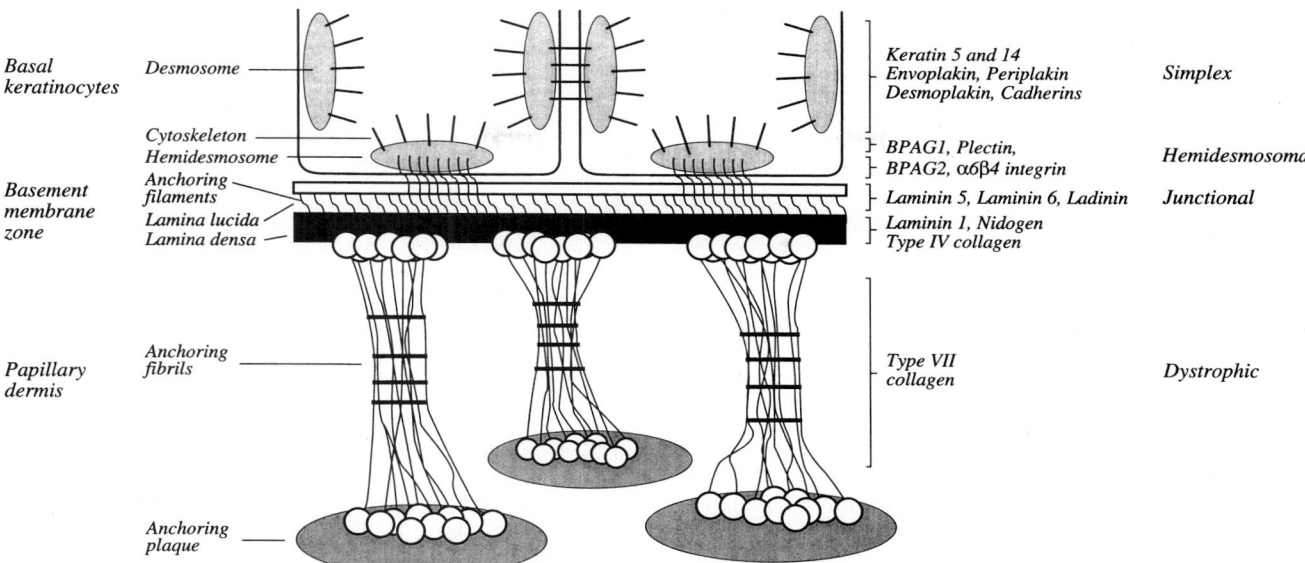

**Fig. 222-2.** Dermal-epidermal basement membrane zone depicting basal keratinocytes, which are separated from the papillary dermis by a dermal-epidermal basement membrane (compare with Fig. 222-1). Ultrastructurally detectable attachment complexes, which form an intricate network extending from the intracellular milieu of basal keratinocytes across the dermal-epidermal basement membrane to the upper papillary dermis, are indicated on the left. The protein components residing at the distinct levels of the basement membrane zone are indicated on the right. The levels of tissue separation in the simplex, hemidesmosomal, junctional and dystrophic forms of epidermolysis bullosa are also indicated on the right. (*Modified from Uitto and Christiano.*[46] *Used with permission.*)

interface at the level of hemidesmosomes. Molecular genetic studies on different variants of EB have thus far demonstrated mutations in ten distinct genes encoding the structural components of the cutaneous BMZ (see Table 222-1). Thus, the molecular heterogeneity of the cutaneous BMZ, the cutaneous and extracutaneous expression patterns of the affected genes, combined with the type, location, and distribution of the mutations, and superimposed on the individuals' genetic background, result in pathologic manifestations that explain the variability within the clinical spectrum of EB.[5]

## MOLECULAR COMPLEXITY OF THE CUTANEOUS BMZ

Significant progress was recently made in understanding the structural components of the epithelial basement membranes, primarily through cloning of the corresponding genes. Furthermore, sublocalization of the macromolecular components to specific attachment complexes was aided by immunohistochemistry and immunoelectron microscopy. Finally, the functionality of many of these BMZ components was deciphered through

**Table 222-1**  Molecular Heterogeneity of Epidermolysis Bullosa

| Variant of EB* | Cleavage plane | Mutated genes |
|---|---|---|
| EBS | Basal keratinocytes | |
| Dominant EBS-WC | | *K5, K14* |
| Dominant EBS-MP | | *K5* |
| Dominant EBS-K | | *K5, K14* |
| Recessive EBS-K | | *K14* |
| Recessive EBS-WC like | | *K14* |
| HD-EB | Hemidesmosome-lamina lucida interface | |
| EB-MD | | *PLEC1* |
| EB-PA | | *ITGA6, ITGB4* |
| GABEB | | *BPAG2/COL17A1* |
| JEB | Lamina lucida | |
| Herlitz-JEB | | *LAMA3, LAMB3, LAMC2* |
| Nonlethal JEB | | *LAMA3, LAMB3, LAMC2* |
| DEB | Papillary dermis | |
| DDEB | | *COL7A1* |
| HS-RDEB | | *COL7A1* |
| M-RDEB | | *COL7A1* |

* EB, epidermolysis bullosa; EBS, EB simplex; EBS-DM, EBS-Dowling-Meara; EBS-K, EBS-Köbner; EBS-WC, EBS-Weber-Cockayne; EBS-MP, EBS with mottled pigmentation; HD-EB, hemidesmosomal variants of EB; EB-MD, EB with muscular dystrophy; EB-PA, EB with pyloric atresia; GABEB, generalized atrophic benign EB; JEB, junctional EB; DEB, dystrophic EB; DDEB, dominant DEB; HS-RDEB, Hallopeau-Siemens recessive DEB.

development of cell biological model systems, breeding of transgenic animals, utilization of yeast two-hybrid systems, and examination of the mutation database in diseases such as EB.

Early evidence for the complexity of the cutaneous BMZ was gained by transmission electron microscopy of the cutaneous BMZ, which revealed a complex adhesion zone with several morphologically recognizable attachment structures.[6] These attachment structures include (a) hemidesmosomes that extend from the intracellular milieu of basal keratinocytes to the extracellular matrix of the lamina lucida; (b) anchoring filaments, thread-like structures that traverse the lamina lucida and extend to the underlying lamina densa; and (c) anchoring fibrils, attachment complexes that extend from the lower portion of the lamina densa to the underlying mesenchyme (Fig. 222-1). Based on detailed ultrastructural and biochemical analyses of the molecular components of these attachment structures, a concept of an intricate network traversing from the intracellular milieu of epidermal keratinocytes to the upper papillary dermis has been proposed (Fig. 222-2; and reference 4). Perturbations in this network structure, such as absence of a critical protein component due to a genetic lesion, or compromised protein-protein interactions due to mutations causing conformational changes, could result in fragility of the cutaneous BMZ and manifest clinically as a form of EB.

## MOLECULAR COMPONENTS OF THE HEMIDESMOSOMES

It is currently known that hemidesmosomes are composed of at least four distinct proteins that display defined interactions with each other, as well as with other components of the BMZ.[7] The hemidesmosomal inner plaque consists of two proteins, the 230-kDa bullous pemphigoid antigen (BP230, BPAG1) and plectin, a multifunctional adhesion molecule. Both of these proteins belong to the plakin family, which are widely expressed, cytoskeleton-associated proteins that are versatile in their binding functions.[8-10] The plakin proteins have been identified within the basal keratinocytes in association with desmosomes and/or hemidesmosomes where their function appears to relate to the binding of intermediate filaments. (For details of the intermediate filament-associated proteins, see Chap. 221.)

The outer plaque of hemidesmosomes contains at least two components, the 180-kDa bullous pemphigoid antigen (BP180, BPAG2) and the $\alpha6\beta4$ integrin. These transmembrane proteins play a major role as attachment molecules anchoring the basal keratinocytes to the underlying basement membrane.

### The 230-kDa Bullous Pemphigoid Antigen

One of the hemidesmosomal inner plaque proteins, the 230-kDa bullous pemphigoid antigen (BP230), was initially identified as an autoantigen in an acquired blistering skin disease, bullous pemphigoid, but particular insight into the function of this protein was gained by development of transgenic mice with the ablated gene *Bpag1*. Specifically, *Bpag1* $-/-$ mice demonstrated that this protein plays a critical role in binding of intermediate keratin filaments to hemidesmosomes.[11] No heritable disease has been shown to result from mutations in the *BPAG1* gene as yet.

### Plectin

Another hemidesmosomal protein is plectin, which consists of a family of widely expressed, cytoskeleton-associated proteins that are versatile in their binding activities.[8] Plectin was initially isolated as a high-molecular-weight protein that copurified with the type III intermediate-filament protein vimentin and was subsequently found to bind a number of intermediate-filament proteins, including keratins. Immunohistochemical analyses have shown that plectin is widely expressed in a variety of epithelial and mesenchymal tissues, including the skin and muscle.[12] Within the cells, plectin is found in association with cell membranes and

junctional complexes, and it colocalizes with intermediate filaments, as well as stress fibers and focal contacts.

Cloning of human plectin cDNA and genomic sequences[13,14] revealed that the primary polypeptide is approximately 500 kDa in size and molecular analyses of plectin also revealed considerable heterogeneity due to alternative splicing and alternatively transcribed 5′ exon of the gene.[10] Attesting to the importance of plectin as an adhesion molecule are the observations that mutations in the plectin gene *(PLEC1)* underlie a form of EB associated with muscular dystrophy (see below).

### The 180-kDa Bullous Pemphigoid Antigen

BPAG2 was initially characterized as an autoantigen in bullous pemphigoid, a blistering skin disease, and subsequent cloning of the corresponding gene *BPAG2* revealed that the protein is a collagen. It was shown that BP180 has an amino-terminal globular domain while the C-terminal segment has 15 characteristic collagenous Gly-X-Y repeat sequences separated by short noncollagenous segments. Furthermore, cloning analyses and cell biological studies demonstrated that BP180 has a transmembrane domain, and that the amino-terminal globular domain resides in the cytoplasm of the basal keratinocytes.[15-17] Thus, BP180 is a transmembrane collagen, designated as type XVII collagen, in type II transmembrane topography.[16] Attesting to the functional importance of BP180/type XVII collagen as a structural component of the cutaneous BMZ is the observation that mutations in the corresponding gene, *BPAG2/COL17A1*, result in a heritable blistering skin disorder, generalized atrophic benign EB (GABEB) (see below).

### The $\alpha6\beta4$ Integrin

The $\alpha6\beta4$ integrin, a dimeric transmembrane protein, is characteristically expressed in a variety of epithelial tissues, including human skin and the gastrointestinal tract. Its function is to provide integrity for BMZ by interacting with other hemidesmosomal components, such as plectin and BP180, in the intracellular milieu, and to serve as a receptor for laminin 5, an extracellular BMZ protein.[7,18-21] The recent findings that mutations in either the $\alpha6$ or the $\beta4$ subunit gene *(ITGA6* or *ITGB4)* result in a variant of EB associated with congenital pyloric atresia (EB-PA) (see below) emphasize the importance of the $\alpha6\beta4$ integrin in cutaneous BMZ biology.

## LAMININS OF THE CUTANEOUS BMZ

In addition to the hemidesmosomal components, a number of lamina lucida/lamina densa proteins have been identified in the cutaneous BMZ. One of the best-characterized BMZ proteins is laminin 5, a member of the laminin family of proteins, which consists of the $\alpha3$, $\beta3$, and $\gamma2$ chains encoded by the distinct genes *LAMA3, LAMB3,* and *LAMC2,* respectively.[22] Recent immunoelectron microscopic studies suggest that laminin 5 is located in the lower lamina lucida extending down to lamina densa,[23] where it has been shown to bind type VII collagen.[24] In addition, two other members of the laminin family, laminins 6 and 7 with chain compositions $\alpha3\beta1\gamma1$ and $\alpha3\beta2\gamma1$, respectively, have been identified in the cutaneous BMZ covalently adducted to laminin 5.[25] The importance of laminin 5 is emphasized by the fact that mutations in genes encoding any of its three polypeptides, $\alpha3$, $\beta3$ and $\gamma2$, can result in the fragility of skin and other specialized epithelia in the junctional variants of EB (see below).

## TYPE VII COLLAGEN — THE ANCHORING FIBRIL PROTEIN

### Primary Sequence and the Domain Organization

Type VII collagen, a homotrimer of three $\alpha1$(VII) chains, was initially characterized as "long-chain collagen," because of its relatively long structure in comparison to classic fibrillar

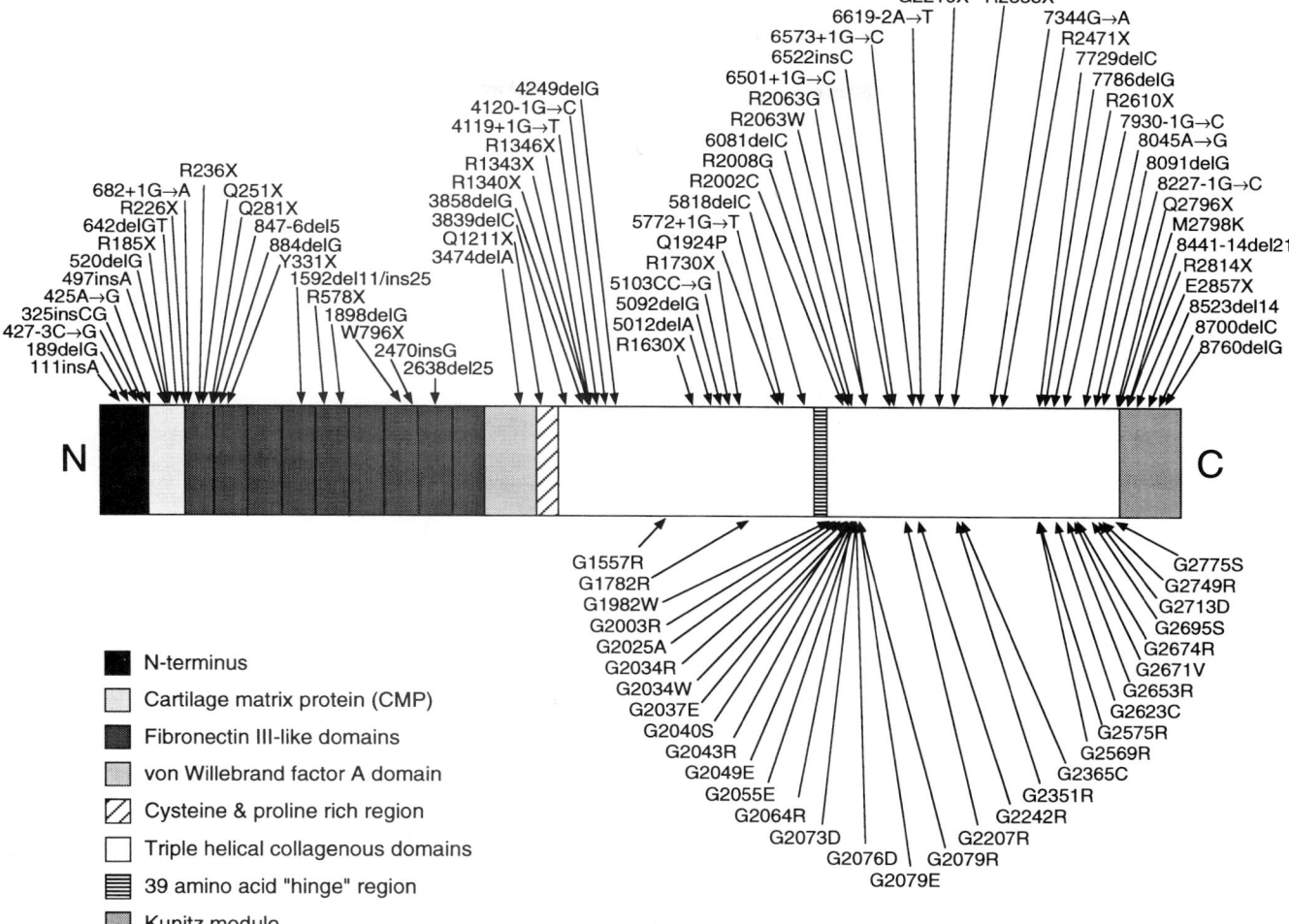

**Fig. 222-3.** Structural organization of the α1(VII) polypeptide of type VII collagen, as deduced by molecular cDNA cloning, and the distribution of *COL7A1* mutations identified in dystrophic variants of EB along the polypeptide. The pro α1(VII) chain consist of a triple-helical collagenous domain, which contains imperfections or interruptions in the Gly-X-Y repeat sequence, including a 39-amino acid "hinge" region. Noncollagenous amino-terminal NC1 and C-terminal NC2 segments flank the collagenous domain. The NC1 domain consists of submodules with homology to known adhesive proteins, as indicated at the lower-left corner. The NC2 domain has a segment with homology with the Kunitz protease-inhibitor molecule. The arrows indicate the positions of distinct genetic mutations that have been disclosed in the *COL7A1* gene. The mutations depicted above the type VII collagen molecule are primarily nonsense mutations or small insertions or deletions that result in frameshift and premature termination codon of translation. These mutations are characteristically associated with recessively inherited variants of dystrophic EB. The mutations shown below the type VII collagen molecule are glycine substitution mutations affecting the collagenous domain of the molecule. The majority of these mutations cause a dominantly inherited dystrophic EB, as a result of dominant negative interference. However, as indicated in the text, some of the glycine substitution mutations are recessive. (*Modified from Uitto.*[111] *Used with permission.*)

collagens.[26] Subsequent cloning of the type VII collagen cDNA and gene *(COL7A1)* indicated that each α1(VII) chain consists of 2944 amino acids, with a calculated molecular mass of ~300 kDa.[27,28] Examination of the segment-long-spacing (SLS) aggregates of type VII collagen suggested morphologic similarities with anchoring fibrils, and it was subsequently demonstrated that type VII collagen is the major, if not the exclusive, component of these attachment complexes.[29]

Examination of the cloned type VII collagen cDNA sequences revealed that this collagen consists of a 1530-amino acid collagenous segment characterized by Gly-X-Y repeat sequences, which, however, contain several imperfections or interruptions, including a 39-amino acid noncollagenous segment in the middle of the collagenous domain (Fig. 222-3). The central collagenous segment is flanked by noncollagenous domains, the larger (NC-1), ~145 kDa, residing at the amino-terminal end, while the smaller noncollagenous domain (NC-2), ~18 kDa, is C-terminal (Fig. 222-3).[30] Initial cDNA cloning of type VII collagen revealed

that the NC-1 domain consists of submodules with homology to known adhesive proteins, including cartilage matrix protein, nine consecutive fibronectin type III-like domains, and a segment with homology to the von Willebrand factor A domain (Fig. 222-3).[30–32] The NC-2 domain has a segment with homology to the Kunitz protease inhibitor, but its functionality has not been established.[33]

### Assembly of Anchoring Fibrils

During the extracellular assembly of anchoring fibrils, individual type VII collagen molecules align into antiparallel dimers that overlap at their C-terminal ends, and this alignment is stabilized by intermolecular disulfide bonds (Fig. 222-4). During the subsequent supramolecular assembly, a large number of type VII collagen dimers laterally associate to form structures morphologically recognized as anchoring fibrils (Fig. 222-4). Intertwining of the anchoring fibrils between interstitial collagen fibers, which consist primarily of type I, III, and V collagens, provides stable

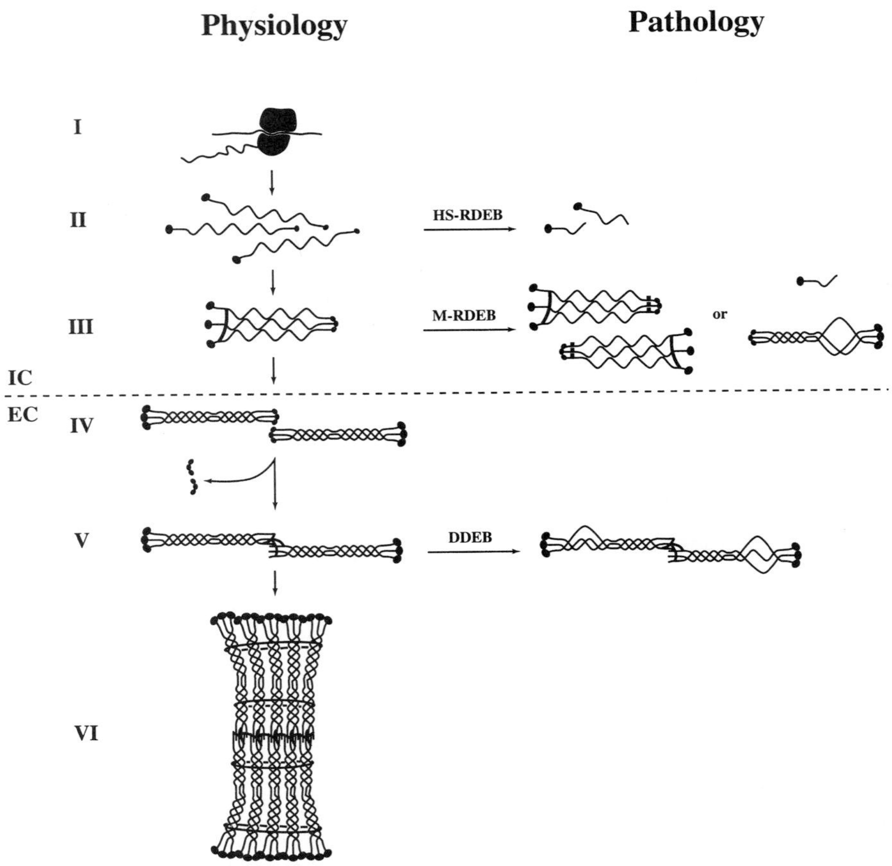

**Physiology**                    **Pathology**

Fig. 222-4. Physiology and pathology of type VII collagen. Synthesis of pro α1(VII) collagen polypeptides and their assembly into anchoring fibrils is depicted at the left side of the figure. The mRNA, ~9 kb in size, is translated on the ribosomes of cells, such as basal keratinocytes, synthesizing type VII collagen (I). Within the intracellular space (IC) three of these polypeptide chains associate and assemble into a triple-helical type VII collagen molecule, which is then secreted (II and III). In the extracellular space (EC) two triple-helical type VII collagen molecules align into an antiparallel dimer in tail-to-tail orientation with overlapping C-terminal ends (IV). The molecules are processed by proteolytic removal of the NC-2 domains (•), and the association of the dimer is stabilized by disulfide bonding (V). A large number of the dimer molecules laterally assemble in register into anchoring fibrils which contain, at both ends, intact amino-terminal NC1 domains with adhesive properties (VI). In the presence of a mutation in the *COL7A1* gene, type VII collagen pathology can manifest as different variants of dystrophic EB. For example, PTCs result in the synthesis of truncated polypeptides unable to form anchoring fibrils, and cause severe Hallopeau-Siemens type of recessive dystrophic EB (HS-RDEB). In the milder, recessively inherited forms of dystrophic EB, known as the Mitis variant (M-RDEB), missense mutations either in a homozygous state or compound heterozygous with a premature termination codon mutation *in trans* can prevent the assembly of type VII collagen dimers. In case of dominantly inherited dystrophic EB (DDEB), a characteristic mutation is a glycine substitution within the collagenous domain of type VII collagen, which interferes with the packing of the anchoring fibrils and/or compromises the stability of the triple-helical conformation of the type VII collagen molecule. (*From Järvikallio et al.*[36] *Used with permission.*)

association of the lower portion of the dermal-epidermal basement membrane to the underlying dermis. The functional importance of the anchoring fibrils has been confirmed by demonstration of a large number of mutations in the VII collagen gene *(COL7A1)* in patients with dystrophic forms of EB (see below and Fig. 222-3).

## MUTATION DETECTION STRATEGIES FOR EB

Mutations in ten distinct genes of the cutaneous BMZ have now been identified in different variants of EB (Table 222-1). In most cases, these genes were identified as candidate gene/protein systems based on ultrastructural and/or immunohistochemical observations.[4]

### Heteroduplex Scanning

Initial studies identifying mutations in different forms of EB utilized RT-PCR and direct sequencing of the cDNAs. It became quickly evident, however, that many of the mRNA transcripts are relatively large, and the corresponding gene structures were found to be complex, thus rendering mutation search by direct sequencing of the genes time-consuming and expensive. These

difficulties are exemplified by type VII collagen, which is encoded by an mRNA transcript with an open reading frame of ~8.9 kb.[27] At the same time, the corresponding gene, *COL7A1*, which is ~32 kb in size, consists of 118 separate exons, the largest number of exons in any gene published thus far.[28] Consequently, several streamlined strategies were adopted for identification of mutations in EB. For example, to identify type VII collagen mutations, a heteroduplex scanning strategy was developed which is based on amplification of *COL7A1* exons directly from genomic DNA utilizing a total of 72 primer pairs which are placed on flanking intronic sequences.[34] These primers reliably amplify all coding sequences from the *COL7A1* gene in PCR products varying from 196 to 589 bp in size. These PCR products are then subjected to heteroduplex scanning by conformation-sensitive gel electrophoresis (CSGE),[35] which, in case of heterozygous sequence variants, displays clearly detectable heteroduplex bands. This is followed by direct automated sequencing of the PCR products displaying heteroduplexes. If the sequence variants are potentially pathogenic mutations, their inheritance in the family can be examined by restriction enzyme digestions or by allele-specific oligonucleotide hybridizations. This methodology is able to detect approximately

80 percent of all single base-pair substitutions or small insertions or deletions in the *COL7A1* gene,[36] and this overall strategy has been successful in identification of well over 150 distinct mutations in *COL7A1* in the dystrophic forms of EB (see Fig. 222-3). Furthermore, similar scanning strategies were recently developed for identification of mutations in other candidate genes in different variants of EB, including the laminin 5 genes, *LAMA3*, *LAMB3*, and *LAMC2*; *COL17A1* encoding the type XVII collagen; *ITGA6* and *ITGB4*, which encode the α6 and β4 integrin subunits; and *PLEC1* encoding plectin.[4,37]

## Protein Truncation Test

An alternate mutation detection strategy is based on protein truncation test (PTT) particularly applied to find mutations in the plectin gene *(PLEC1)* in a variant of EB with late-onset muscular dystrophy (EB-MD).[38] *PLEC1* consists of 33 exons, but the two most 3′ exons (nos. 32 and 33), which are 3.3 and 6.2 kb in size, account for ~75 percent of the coding sequence of the gene.[13,14] Initial attempts to reliably amplify exon 32 and 33 sequences for heteroduplex analysis revealed difficulties, primarily due to the highly repetitive and GC-rich nature of this part of the gene, and their amplification in overlapping PCR products, < 500 bp in size, requires 37 separate PCR reactions. Therefore, PTT[39,40] has been adopted to search for mutations within these two large exons.[41,42] For this purpose, exon sequences are PCR amplified using genomic DNA as a template with forward primers containing T7 promoter and the codon for the first methionine in addition to the sequence homologous to *PLEC1*, and the reverse primers containing an in-frame stop codon. The PCR products, up to 6 kb in size, are then subjected to coupled transcription/translation with radiolabeled methionine. Examination of the radiolabeled translation products by polyacrylamide gel electrophoresis enables detection of truncated polypeptides due to translation stop codon mutations in the corresponding PCR product, which can be defined by subsequent nucleotide sequencing. PTT has been a useful complementary technology, clearly successful in disclosing mutations in the plectin gene in patients with EB-MD, especially because most of the *PLEC1* mutations, identified so far, are stop codon mutations and they reside within exon 32.[38]

## MOLECULAR PATHOLOGY OF TYPE VII COLLAGEN IN DYSTROPHIC FORMS OF EB

### Morphology of Anchoring Fibrils

The progress made in defining the molecular basis of various forms of EB is perhaps best illustrated by the dystrophic variants of EB (DEB), a subgroup of diseases with either an autosomal dominant or autosomal recessive inheritance pattern.[43] A decade ago, little was known of the molecular mechanisms of DEB, but transmission electron microscopy had revealed abnormalities in anchoring fibrils that are morphologically altered, reduced in number, or entirely absent in patients affected with DEB.[44,45] Furthermore, immunohistochemistry of the skin in patients with the most severe forms of DEB, the recessively inherited Hallopeau-Siemens variant (HS-RDEB), revealed entirely negative staining for type VII collagen epitopes.[2] Based on these observations, we proposed that type VII collagen is the gene/protein system at fault in DEB.[46]

### Genetic Linkage Analyses

Mapping of the *COL7A1* gene to human chromosome 3p21[47,48] and identification of both intragenic and flanking polymorphic markers[27] provided us with tools to establish a strong genetic linkage between the type VII collagen gene locus and DEB, in both dominantly and recessively inherited forms of the disease[49–51] (for a summary, see reference 52). Initial linkage studies utilizing intragenic polymorphisms or flanking microsatellite markers suggested that both genetic forms of DEB were linked to *COL7A1* locus at 3p21.1.[49–51,53–55] Specifically, the combined

LOD score in recessively inherited families reported thus far (n=54) is 10.6 at $\theta = 0$; and the corresponding value for dominantly inherited families (n=14) is 41.4 at $\theta = 0$.[52] Thus far, there is no report of a family that has been excluded from the *COL7A1* locus.

## PTC Mutations in the Type VII Collagen Gene (*COL7A1*) in Recessive DEB

With the advent of streamlined mutation detection strategies, as outlined above, a number of mutations in the type VII collagen gene have been disclosed in different variants of DEB. Careful examination of the *COL7A1* mutations (see Fig. 222-3) reveals that most of the mutations in recessively inherited forms of EB are nonsense mutations or small insertions or deletions that lead to frameshift and premature termination codon (PTC) for translation (see Fig. 222-3).[36,56–60] In general, PTCs are associated with reduced levels of the corresponding mRNA transcripts due to nonsense-mediated mRNA decay.[61,62] These PTC mutations are silent in the heterozygous state, but when homozygous or combined with another PTC mutation *in trans*, the consequences are severe in terms of skin fragility, as illustrated by HS-RDEB (Fig. 222-5). In spite of the extreme fragility of skin and development of joint contractures and esophageal strictures, the patients with HS-RDEB usually survive to the adolescent life. A major concern is, however, development of squamous cell carcinomas, which grow and metastasize unusually fast, and can lead to the demise of the affected individuals even during the second or third decade of life.

The PTC mutations disclosed thus far in *COL7A1* are distributed along the entire type VII collagen molecule and most of them are family specific (Fig. 222-3). However, certain recurrent mutations have been disclosed in unrelated families. For example, in a cohort of 23 British patients, two mutations, R578X and 7786delG, were found with an allelic frequency of 6/46 and 7/46, respectively.[63] Haplotype analysis of these families indicated that the mutations arose on similar allelic backgrounds in different patients, consistent with propagation of the mutated allele in the British gene pool. These, and other recurrent mutations within certain ethnic groups, will have implications for streamlined mutation detection. Specifically, because such mutations frequently alter a restriction enzyme site, the patients should be first screened for the presence or absence of these mutations by respective endonuclease digestions, before embarking on comprehensive mutation detection by heteroduplex analysis.

### Glycine Substitution Mutations in *COL7A1*

A number of missense mutations have also been identified in *COL7A1* in patients with DEB (see Fig. 222-3). A frequent missense mutation results in substitution of a glycine residue within the collagenous domain of type VII collagen by another amino acid, and these glycine substitution mutations cause, in most cases, a dominantly inherited disease through dominant negative interference[64–68] (Fig. 222-6). However, not all glycine substitution mutations are dominant, and in several cases, they lead to clinical manifestations only when in homozygous state or when combined with a PTC in the other *COL7A1* allele.[65] Although other collagen genes were previously shown to harbor either dominant or recessive mutations,[69] *COL7A1* is unique among the collagen genes in that a single class of mutations — in this case, a glycine substitution in the triple-helical region of the type VII collagen gene — can cause either dominantly or recessively inherited forms of DEB. Careful examination of the glycine substitution mutations along the entire triple-helical domain of type VII collagen does not reveal obvious position dependence with regard to the mode of inheritance in patients with these mutations (see Fig. 222-3). The apparent lack of positional effects of the glycine substitutions along the entire collagenous domain of type VII collagen could be explained by considering the collagenous region as an ensemble of cooperative triple-helical blocks, some of them more critical than others for the overall

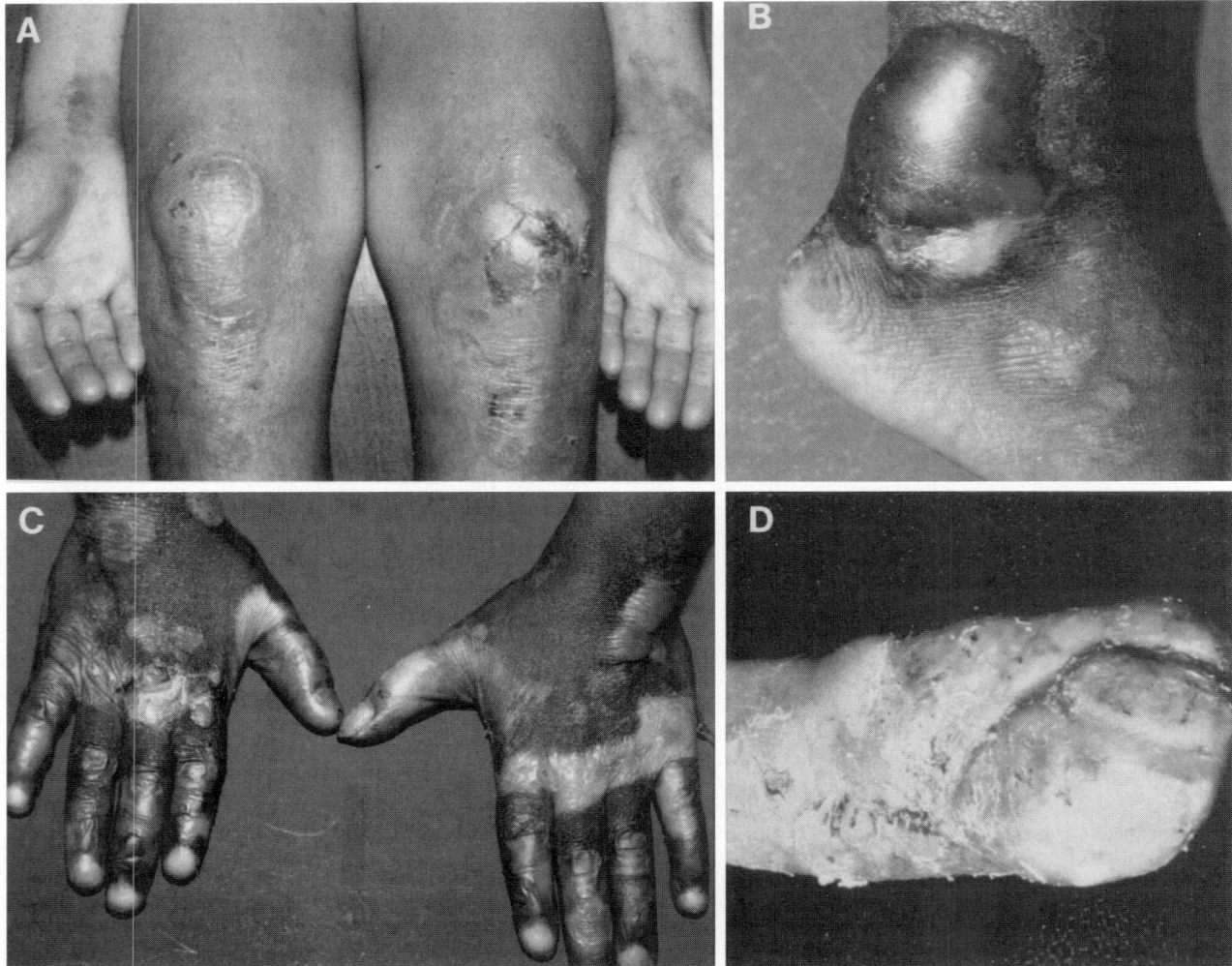

**Fig. 222-5. The spectrum of clinical severity in the dystrophic forms of EB.** In milder cases, as exemplified by a patient with dominant dystrophic EB (A), the blisters and erosions are primarily on the pressure points as shown on hands and knees. In milder recessively inherited variants of DEB, such as the Mitis RDEB, blistering can occur as a result of minor trauma (B) and often results in extensive scarring, which, however, does not lead to fusion of the digits (C). In the most severe cases with recessively inherited DEB (the Hallopeau-Siemens variants), profound scarring can lead to mutilating fusion of the digits (D). The latter patients are also prone to development to rapidly growing and aggressively metastasizing squamous cell carcinomas.

function of this protein. Thus, the specific location of the glycine substitution within a particular triple-helical submodule, rather than its position along the entire collagenous domain, might be more critical in determining its impact on the overall stability of the molecule.

Another class of mutations impacts splicing of the transcripts of the type VII collagen gene, which consists of a total of 118 exons. Many of these mutations reside within the consensus splice junctions causing aberrant splicing events that result either in skipping of exons or activation of cryptic splice sites. In many cases, the aberrantly spliced transcripts are out-of-frame and result in PTCs, thus giving rise to truncated translation products similar to nonsense mutations and causing a recessively inherited, often severe, phenotype. In some cases, the exon skipping is in-frame and results in the synthesis of internally truncated type VII collagen polypeptides. If the deletion occurs within the central collagenous domain, the noncollagenous extensions are intact and serve their adhesive functions. Thus, the anchoring fibrils may be morphologically altered, yet partially functional, causing a milder disease.

Quite recently, interesting cases of DEB with intraexonic deletions affecting exon 87 have been elucidated.[70] In these cases, the deletions are distant from the consensus splice sites, yet they cause in-frame skipping of the corresponding exon, resulting in synthesis of shortened type VII collagen polypeptides, which alter, in a dominant manner, anchoring fibril formation and cause dominant DEB.

## Genotype/Phenotype Correlations in Dystrophic EB

Examination of the *COL7A1* mutation database has enabled us to begin to develop genotype/phenotype correlations, and certain general rules are emerging. For example, it is clear that in the majority of the cases with severe, mutilating HS-RDEB, the genetic lesions consist of PTC mutations in both alleles.[43,59] These mutations predict synthesis of truncated type VII collagen polypeptides that are unable to assemble into functional anchoring fibrils (Fig. 222-6). In addition, as a consequence of PTCs, decay of mRNA is accelerated resulting in reduced levels of the corresponding transcripts.[61] Consequently, little if any of the truncated polypeptides are synthesized, thus explaining the entirely negative immunohistochemical staining for type VII collagen epitopes in HS-RDEB. As a result, anchoring fibrils are absent leading to severe fragility of the skin.

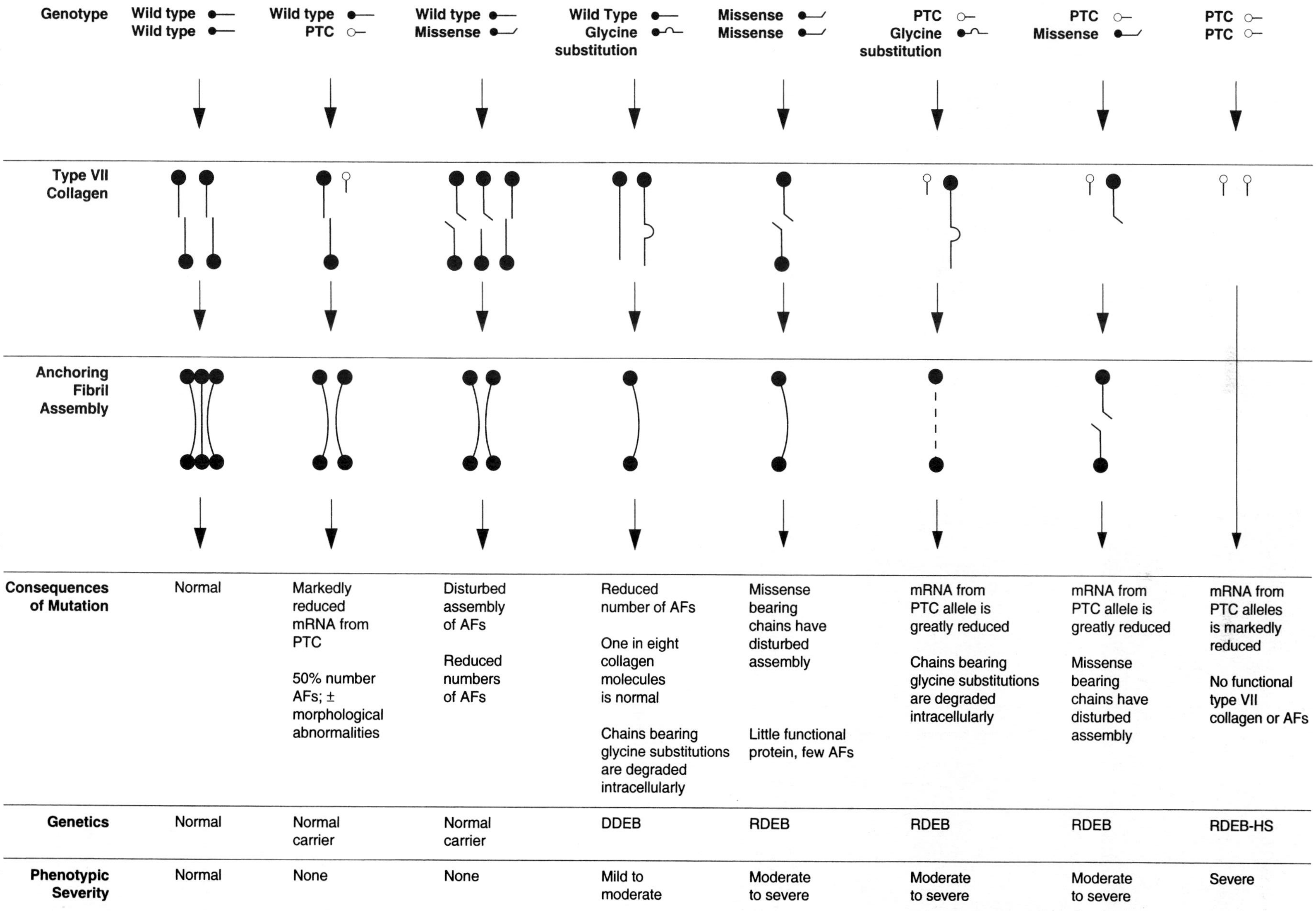

Fig. 222-6. Potential genotype/phenotype correlations in the dystrophic variants of epidermolysis bullosa, based on analysis of the *COL7A1* mutation database. (*From Christiano and Uitto.*[106] *Used with permission.*)

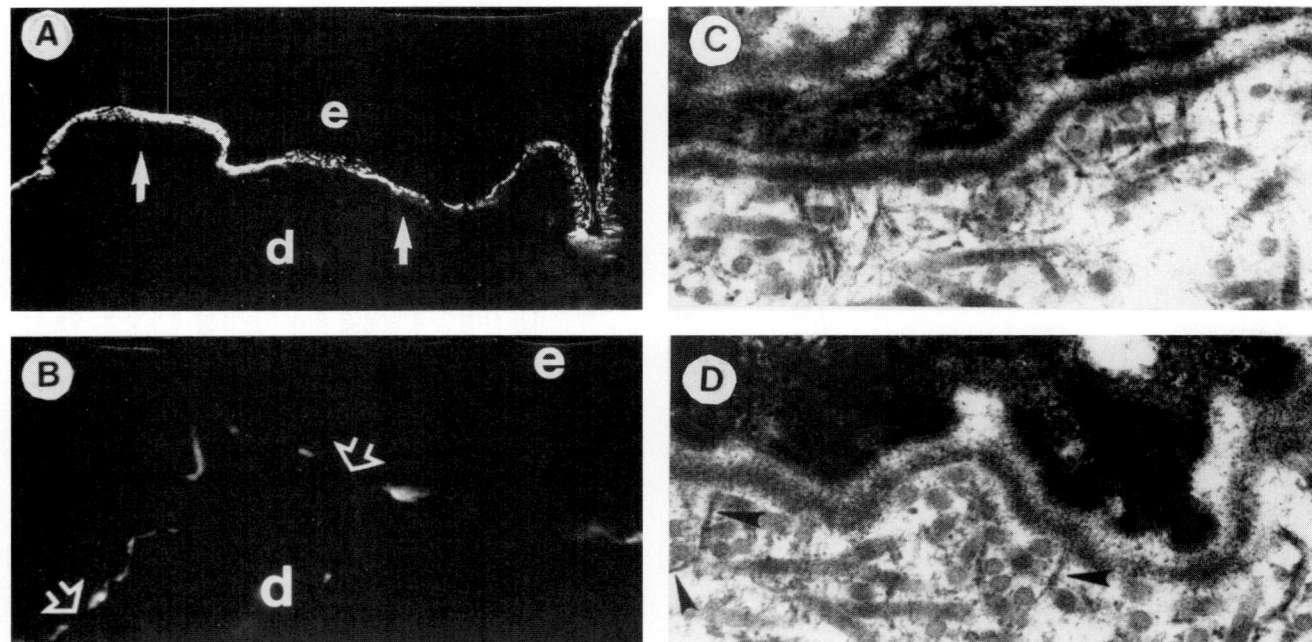

**Fig. 222-7.** Immunohistochemical staining of the skin for type VII collagen and transmission electron microscopy of the dermal-epidermal junction in a patient with the relatively mild Mitis variant of recessive dystrophic EB. Immunohistochemistry of normal skin (A) shows linear staining at the cutaneous basement membrane zone separating from epidermis (e) from the underlying dermis (d) (arrows). The staining in the patient (B) is positive, yet markedly attenuated and patchy (open arrows). Transmission electron microscopy of normal skin (C) reveals a large number of anchoring fibrils extending from the lamina densa to the underlying dermis, while in the patient's skin (D), only a few relatively thin anchoring fibrils can be seen.

[α1(VII)]₃

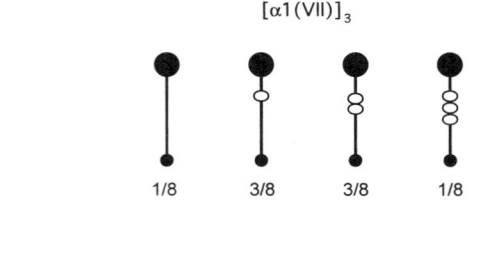

[α1(VII)]₃-dimers

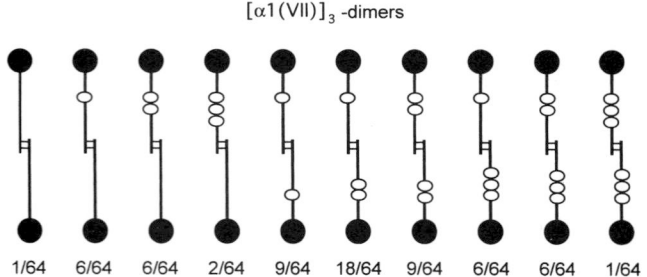

**Fig. 222-8.** Stoichiometry of normal and mutated type VII collagen molecules, [α1(VII)]₃, (upper panel), and the [α1(VII)]₃ dimer molecules (lower panel) assembled in dominantly inherited dystrophic EB with a glycine substitution mutation, assuming equal expression of both the wild-type and the mutated allele. Type VII collagen molecules consist of a central triple-helical collagenous domain ( | ) flanked by noncollagenous amino terminal NC1 (●) and carboxy-terminal NC2 (•) domains. Two of the [α1(VII)]₃ molecules form an antiparallel dimer stabilized by intermolecular disulfide bonding. In DEB, molecules containing 1, 2, or 3 mutated polypeptides with a glycine substitution (o) combine with normal molecules. One of 8 (12.5 percent) [α1(VII)]₃ collagen molecules have three normal polypeptides, whereas only 1 of 64 (1.6 percent) dimer molecules are entirely normal. (*From Kon et al.*[66] *Used with permission.*)

In the milder M-RDEB, the genetic lesion is frequently a missense mutation or in-frame deletion either in one or both alleles, as exemplified by a homozygous methionine-to-lysine substitution in one of the first cases in which the mutations in *COL7A1* were delineated.[71] In such cases, full-length type VII collagen polypeptides are synthesized, but the missense mutation, frequently affecting a critical amino acid, can alter the conformation of the protein and interferes with the assembly and packing of type VII collagen molecules into anchoring fibrils (Fig. 222-6). In the latter case, however, some ultrastructurally recognizable anchoring fibrils, although often morphologically altered, can be detected (Fig. 222-7). This notion is consistent with positive, yet frequently attenuated, immunohistochemical staining of the skin for type VII collagen epitopes (Fig. 222-7). Also, the clinical severity is less pronounced and manifests with a relatively mild blistering phenotype.

Finally, the characteristic genetic lesion in DDEB is a glycine substitution mutation within the collagenous domain of the pro α1(VII) chain. The mutated polypeptides are full-length and thus capable of assembling into triple-helical collagen molecules, but the presence of the glycine substitution destabilizes the triple helix (Fig. 222-6). Thus, the mutated polypeptides cause a dominantly inherited disease through dominant negative interference. In the context of DDEB, it should be noted that type VII collagen is a homotrimer consisting of three identical proα1(VII) chains.[22] Assuming equal level of expression from both the mutant and wild-type allele, one of eight trimeric collagen molecules (12.5 percent) is expected to consist exclusively of normal polypeptides (Fig. 222-8).[72] When these individual type VII collagen molecules align to the antiparallel dimers, only 1 of 64 (1.6 percent) dimer molecules is entirely normal (Fig. 222-8). Nevertheless, these normal type VII collagen molecules are apparently capable of forming anchoring fibrils, which are, however, thin and markedly reduced in number due to faulty assembly of mutated molecules. The presence of these structures explains positive, yet frequently attenuated, immunohistochemical staining reaction, as well as relatively mild clinical presentation in dominantly inherited forms of the disease.

## LAMININ 5 MUTATIONS IN JUNCTIONAL EB

The progress in understanding the molecular basis of the other major forms of EB has been equally striking. An example is the Herlitz type of junctional EB (H-JEB), a severe, recessively inherited condition that frequently results in premature demise of the affected individuals within a few months of birth (Fig. 222-9). Tissue separation occurs in the middle of the cutaneous BMZ at

the level of lamina lucida (Fig. 222-9). Initial clues assisting in identification of the candidate genes for mutations in this condition also came from ultrastructural and immunohistochemical studies. These studies demonstrated abnormalities in the hemidesmosome-anchoring filament complexes, and immunostaining of the skin of patients affected with H-JEB revealed absence of laminin 5.[6,73] Subsequently, more than 60 distinct mutations encoding the polypeptide subunits of laminin 5 have been identified in the three genes *LAMA3*, *LAMB3*, and *LAMC2*.[37] Characteristically, PTCs in both alleles of any of these three laminin 5 genes signifies poor prognosis due to absence of laminin 5 in the skin of the affected individuals. Again, missense mutations in one or both alleles are

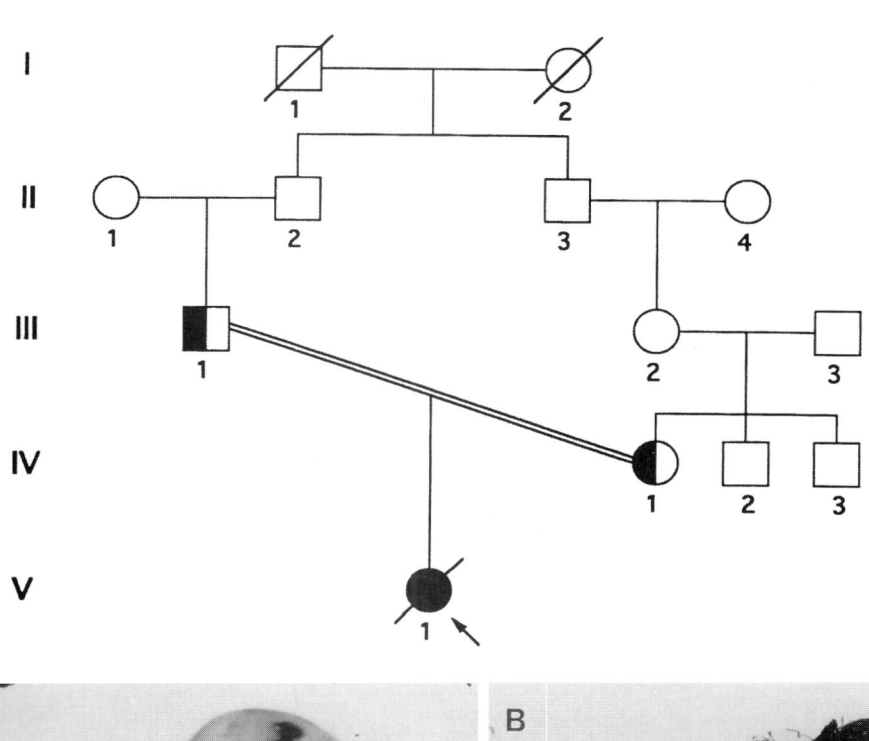

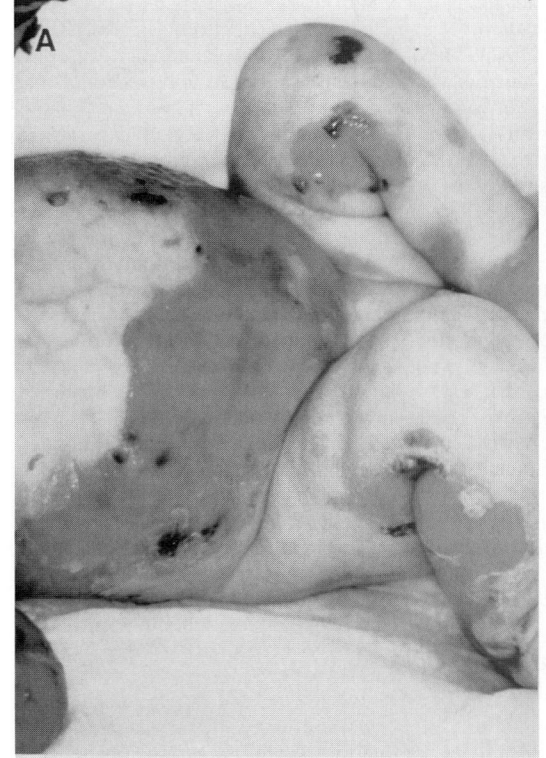

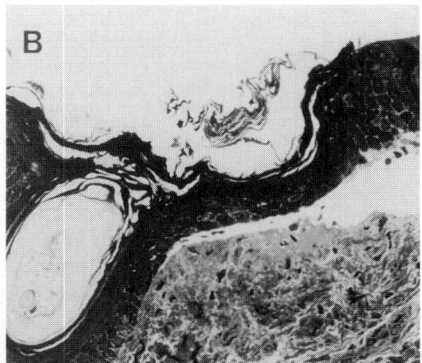

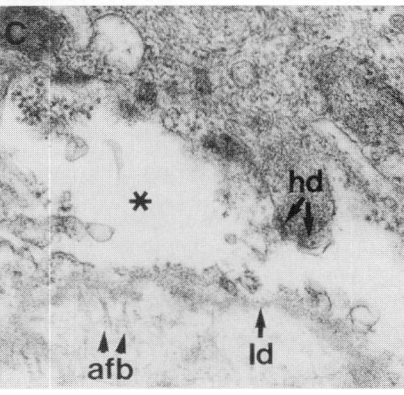

Fig. 222-9. Features of Herlitz junctional epidermolysis bullosa. The proband (arrow) is the first child of clinically normal parents who are related (upper panel). This newborn was noted to have extensive blistering and erosions of the skin (A); she died during the early postnatal period. Histopathology revealed noninflammatory blistering at the dermal-epidermal junction (B). Transmission electron microscopy revealed that blister formation (*) occurs within the lamina lucida, while the lamina densa (ld) and the anchoring fibrils (afb) are normal. Hemidesmosomes (hd) are hypoplastic (C).

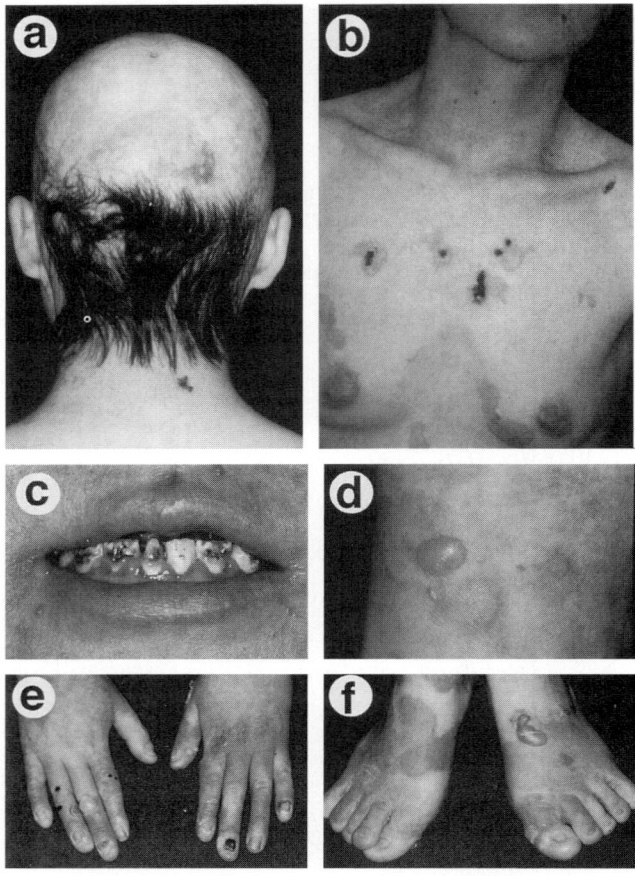

**Fig. 222-10. Clinical features of generalized atrophic benign EB (GABEB), a hemidesmosomal variant of EB. Note scarring alopecia (a), enamel hypoplasia (c), and nail dystrophy (e), in addition to extensive blistering and erosions of the skin (b, d, and f). (*Figure courtesy of Dr. Hiroshi Shimizu, Hokkaido University School of Medicine, Sapporo*).**

associated with a relatively mild phenotype characterized by life-long blistering, loss of hair and nails, and presence of dental abnormalities (see Fig. 222-10).[74–76]

Although laminin 5 mutations have been demonstrated in all three genes encoding the subunit polypeptides, the overwhelming majority (~80 percent) of these mutations reside in *LAMB3*.[37] The preponderance of *LAMB3* mutations can be explained, at least in part, by two recurrent "hotspot" mutations, R635X and R42X,[77,78] which have been demonstrated in a number of individuals; in fact, these two mutations account for approximately half of all *LAMB3* mutations disclosed thus far. Both the R635X and R42X mutations result from a C → T transition, which illustrates the hypermutability of 5-methylcytosine to thymine.[79] Identification of these two predominant mutations has led to a streamlined mutation detection strategy in families with H-JEB that first analyzes the *LAMB3* gene for these two "hotspot" mutations by restriction enzyme digestions (see Fig. 222-11), followed by heteroduplex scanning of the *LAMB3* exons.[80] If the results on *LAMB3* are negative, similar mutation detection strategies have been developed for *LAMC2* and *LAMA3*.[81,82]

The search for mutations in patients with H-JEB has also disclosed novel mechanisms for the disease. Specifically, two recent cases were associated with a rare non-Mendelian inheritance pattern, uniparental disomy.[83,84] In both families, the mother was a heterozygous carrier, while the patient was homozygous for a nonsense mutation in the *LAMB3* gene at chromosomal locus 1q32. The father in both families had wild-type *LAMB3* alleles, and nonpaternity was excluded by haplotype analysis. Microsatellite analysis revealed that both patients had inherited two

chromosome 1 homologues from the mother, while the paternal chromosome 1 was absent (Fig. 222-12). Thus, H-JEB phenotype in these cases was caused by reduction to homozygosity of the maternal mutation, most likely as a result of nondisjunction during the first meiotic cell division preceded by recombinational events.

## MOLECULAR PATHOLOGY OF HEMIDESMOSOMAL VARIANTS OF EB

### *COL17A1* Mutations in Generalized Atrophic Benign EB

The hemidesmosomal variants of EB (HD-EB) manifest clinically in three forms: generalized atrophic benign epidermolysis bullosa (GABEB), EB with pyloric atresia (EB-PA), and EB with late-onset muscular dystrophy (EB-MD). Clues as to the candidate gene/protein systems at fault in these conditions came from immunofluorescence observations on the skin of the affected individuals. This is exemplified by patients with generalized atrophic benign EB (GABEB) characterized by life-long blistering of the skin associated with nail dystrophy, enamel hypoplasia, and localized alopecia of the eyelids.[85,86] Electron microscopic examination of the skin revealed abnormalities in the hemidesmosomes which were rudimentary, and immunohistochemical staining of the patients' skin with an antibody recognizing the 180-kDa bullous pemphigoid antigen (BP180) was entirely negative at the dermal-epidermal junction, while staining of a parallel section with an antibody recognizing laminin 5 was normal.[87,88] These observations clearly suggested that the gene encoding the 180-kDa bullous pemphigoid antigen *BPAG2*, also known as type XVII collagen, is a candidate gene for mutations in GABEB. Following cloning of this gene and elucidation of its intron/exon organization, mutation detection strategies were developed that were able to pinpoint specific genetic lesions in this gene in GABEB patients.[89–91] The majority of these mutations result in PTCs due to nonsense mutations or small insertions or deletions in the *BPAG2* gene.[4]

An extremely interesting case with mutations in *BPAG2/COL17A1* was recently reported by Jonkman et al.[91] The proband, a 28-year-old female, demonstrated characteristic features of GABEB, including generalized blistering, universal alopecia, pigmentary changes, dental abnormalities, and nail dystrophy. Careful examination of her skin revealed patches of clinically unaffected areas in a symmetrical, leaf-like pattern on the hands and upper arms. Collectively, these patches covered about 10 percent of the total body surface area. Immunofluorescence staining using anti-BP180/type XVII collagen antibody was negative in clinically affected skin, while in clinically unaffected patches the expression was present in approximately 50 percent of the basal cells in groups of about 10 to 50 adjacent cells. Staining for other hemidesmosomal components showed normal continuous pattern of the dermal-epidermal junction. The proband's skin in the affected area depicted compound heterozygous mutations (1706delA/R1226X) in the *BPAG2/COL17A1* gene, while the clinically normal areas showed the presence of the maternal mutation (R1226X) only, accompanied by loss of heterozygosity along a track of at least 381 bp in revertant keratinocytes derived from the clinically unaffected skin. Thus, this case represents a revertant mosaicism of a compound heterozygous proband with the autosomal recessive genodermatosis GABEB.[91] It should be noted that the survival of genotypically heterozygous cells in the skin of this patient with compound heterozygous mutations in the *BPAG2/COL17A1* gene attest to the feasibility of ex vivo gene therapy for potential treatment of the affected individuals.

### The α6β4 Integrin Gene Mutations in EB with Pyloric Atresia

Another hemidesmosomal variant of EB is associated with congenital intestinal abnormalities, such as pyloric or duodenal

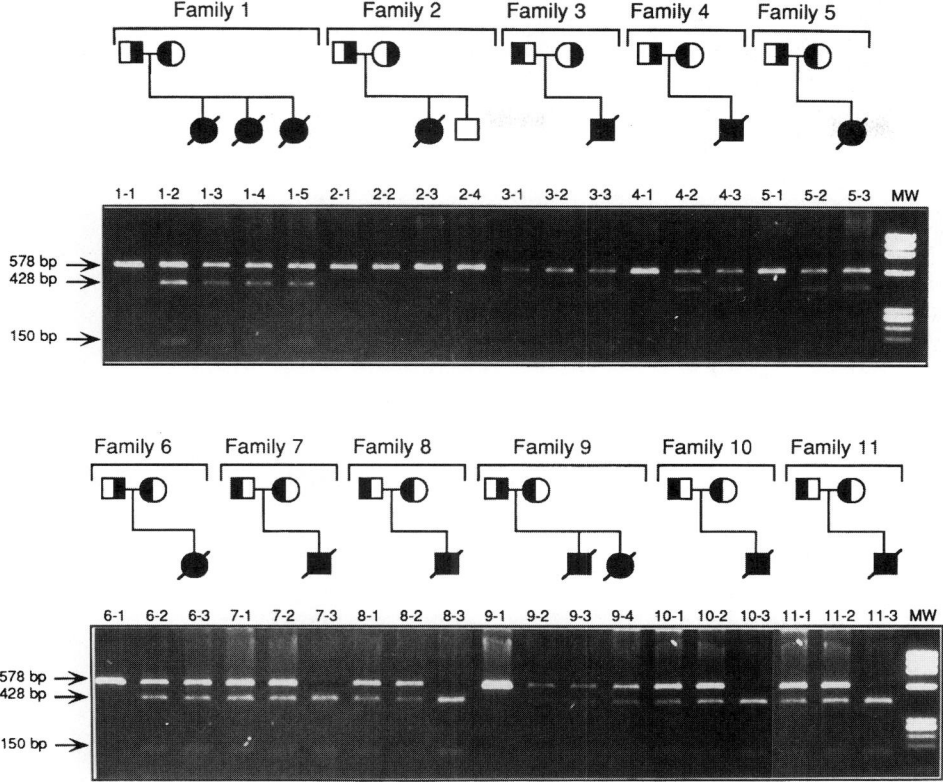

**Fig. 222-11. Restriction-enzyme digestion screening for the recurrent mutation R635X in the *LAMB3* gene of laminin 5 in 11 European families with Herlitz junctional epidermolysis bullosa. PCR products spanning exon 14 of the *LAMB3* gene were digested with the restriction enzyme *Bgl*II, followed by analysis on 2 percent agarose gel. The 578-bp band corresponds to the normal allele, which is digested to 428-bp and 150-bp bands in the mutant allele. (*From Pulkkinen et al.*[78] *Used with permission.*)**

atresia. In most cases, this condition is lethal during the early postnatal period and the affected children die from complications, in spite of surgical intervention to correct the intestinal abnormalities. However, nonlethal cases of EB-PA have also been recognized, and in some cases, the skin involvement is relatively mild, occasionally not noted until the second year of life.[92,93] Histopathology of the lesional skin reveals noninflammatory tissue separation at the level of the cutaneous BMZ, and transmission electron microscopy of the nonblistered skin shows poorly formed hemidesmosomes (Fig. 222-13). Early immunohistochemical findings also indicated that the expression of $\alpha6\beta4$ integrin is markedly reduced or entirely absent in the skin of the affected individuals with EB-PA.[94] Subsequently, a number of mutations in the genes encoding either one of the two subunits of the $\alpha6\beta4$ integrin (*ITGA6* and *ITGB4*) were demonstrated.[4] In most lethal cases, the mutations consist of PTC codons resulting in the absence of the corresponding polypeptide due to accelerated mRNA decay mechanism, or the truncated polypeptides are nonfunctional and sensitive to protein degradation. Our recent findings have also disclosed several missense mutations within the $\beta4$ integrin gene in patients presenting with different degrees of clinical severity varying from lethal phenotypes to very mild EB-PA.[92,93,95] It is of interest that three of six missense mutations characterized thus far are cysteine substitutions in the extracellular domain of the $\beta4$ integrin subunit, suggesting that these mutations may alter the formation of intra- or intermolecular disulfide bonds, possibly disrupting ligand binding or affecting noncovalent association between the $\alpha6$ and $\beta4$ subunits. Collectively, these results support the overall notion that *ITGB4* mutations underlie most cases of EB-PA, and that missense mutations are primarily associated with the nonlethal phenotypes. It should be noted, however, that mutations in the $\alpha6$ integrin subunit gene, *ITGA6*, have also been reported in two cases with EB-PA, the clinical

phenotype being indistinguishable from the lethal cases caused by mutations in *ITGB4*.[96,97]

## Plectin Mutations in EB with Muscular Dystrophy

EB-MD, a distinct hemidesmosomal variant, manifests with relatively mild blistering noted at birth and is associated with late-onset muscular dystrophy (Fig. 222-14). This phenotypic constellation was initially puzzling, and it was suggested that the occurrence of these two relatively rare clinical conditions (EB and MD) might be coincidental, because no clear molecular explanation could be presented.[98] It was recently demonstrated, however, that mutations in the gene for plectin *(PLEC1)*, which is normally expressed both in the skin and muscle, underlie this variant of EB.[38]

Clues to the molecular basis of EB-MD were first derived from immunofluorescence findings in the skin of these patients. Specifically, immunostaining with a monoclonal antibody HD-121, which recognizes the plectin variant HD1 expressed in association with hemidesmosomes,[99] revealed negative staining pattern at the dermal-epidermal BMZ; muscle staining of these patients was also negative.[100,101] Subsequent cloning of the human plectin gene[13,14] enabled development of mutation detection strategies that have proven successful in identifying mutations in patients with EB-MD. Specifically, use of direct RT-PCR, heteroduplex scanning, or protein truncation test, followed by direct nucleotide sequencing, has enabled identification of mutations in both alleles in ten probands in EB-MD.[38,41,42,101,102] Seven of these cases have been homozygous for the mutation, often associated with consanguinity in the family, while three cases were compound heterozygotes. In all cases, the mutations consisted of small insertions, deletions, or nonsense mutations, and all but one cause PTCs. The only exception to this rule is a family with two affected sisters who demonstrated a homozygous

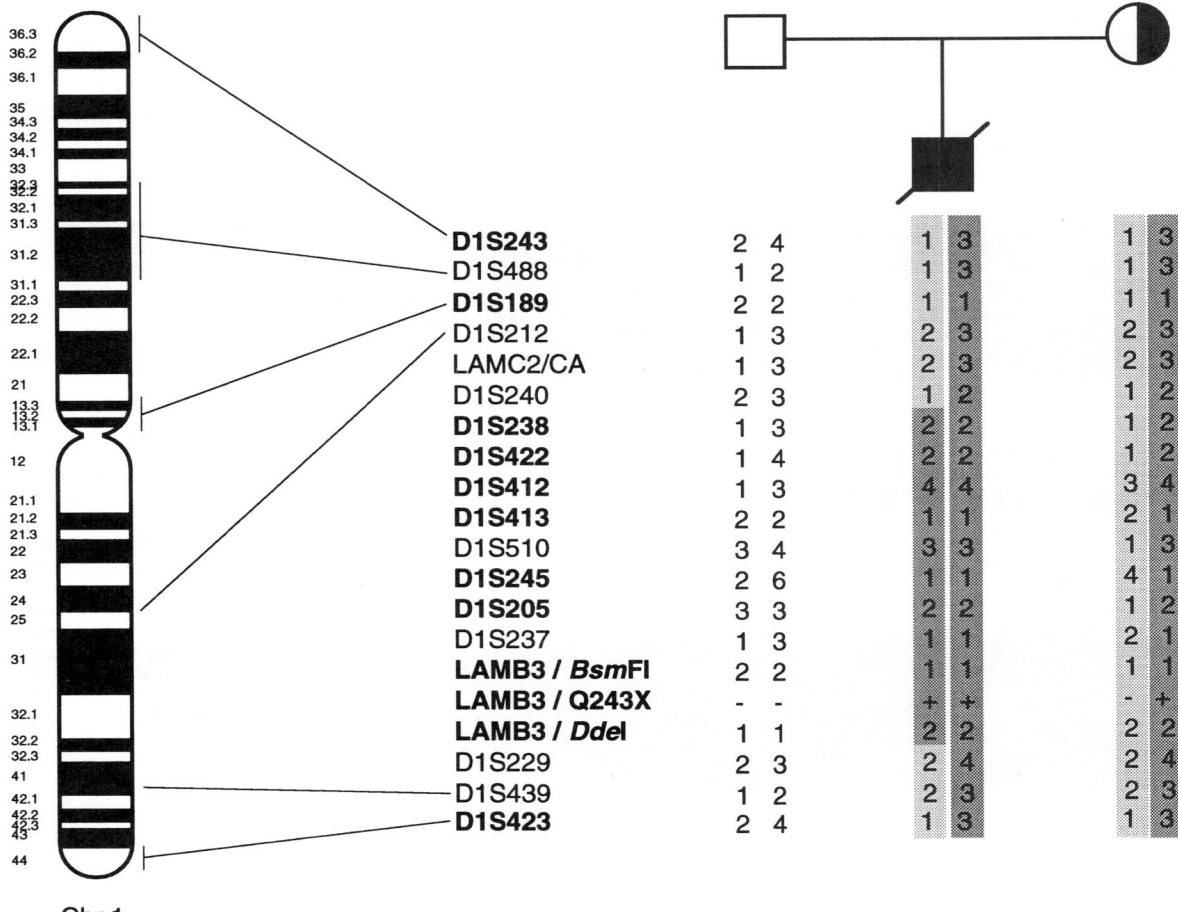

**Fig. 222-12. Uniparental disomy in a patient with Herlitz junctional EB.** The proband, a newborn male, was the first child of clinically unaffected parents. The proband died during the early postnatal period. Mutation analysis revealed that the proband was homozygous for a *LAMB3* mutation Q243X, and the mother was heterozygous carrier of the same mutation, while the father was shown not to carry this mutation; haplotype analysis excluded nonpaternity. Genotype analysis of chromosome 1, using polymorphic markers shown on the left, demonstrates that the proband inherited two maternal chromosome 1 homologues (indicated by different shaded backgrounds). In addition, the proband was homozygous for a region of maternal chromosome 1 spanning ~35 cM, including the mutant *LAMB3* locus. Thus, the proband has primary uniparental heterodisomy and partial isodisomy (also known as meroisodisomy) of chromosome 1. (*From Pulkkinen et al.[83] Used with permission.*)

in-frame deletion of 9 bp within exon 22, resulting in deletion of three amino acids.[102] Comparison of the sequence in the human and mouse plectin gene revealed 96 percent similarity and 92 percent identity in this particular exon containing the 9-bp deletion, and the deleted amino acids, QEA, reside within a stretch of 23 identical amino acids.[102] These observations suggested that the QEA sequence plays a critical role in the function of plectin. It should be noted that the 9-bp deletion occurred within a sequence where the corresponding segment was tandemly repeated, thus suggesting a slipped mispairing of DNA as the basis of this mutation.

EB-MD is a clinical constellation of skin blistering present at birth and late-onset muscle weakness that is progressive and leads eventually to the patients being wheelchair bound.[38] The involvement of muscle in this disease can be explained by the observations that plectin is also expressed in the sarcolemma and the Z-lines, and staining with plectin antibodies, which yields clearly positive reaction in control muscle, is negative in patients with EB-MD.[101] An unexplained feature of this disease is the age of the onset of muscle involvement which has been reported to take place as early as at 2 years of age, while in some cases, muscle weakness has not been noted until the third or fourth decade of life.[38] Examination of the mutation database has not provided clues to genotype/phenotype correlations, and therefore

the role of modifying genes, hormonal regulation, and/or life-style variables in affecting the severity of the disease, cannot be excluded.

## CONCLUSIONS ABOUT THE MOLECULAR HETEROGENEITY OF EB

Mutations in ten different genes expressed within the dermal-epidermal junction have been conclusively demonstrated in various variants of EB (Table 222-1). Examination of the existing patient database is enabling us to develop an understanding of the genotype/phenotype correlations, but additional information is clearly required to draw definitive conclusions about the consequences of the mutations at the level of mRNA stability, protein folding, and supramolecular assembly of the basement membranes. Nevertheless, demonstration of these mutations in EB adds to our understanding of the complexity of the cutaneous BMZ and yields novel information on the role of individual components in providing functional stability to the dermal-epidermal junction.

Collectively, the type and combination of mutations in the ten different genes predict, in general terms, the clinical severity, the phenotypic constellation, and the natural history of the disease. The clinical severity of EB represents, however, a continuum in the spectrum of clinical manifestations. It is the precise nature of the

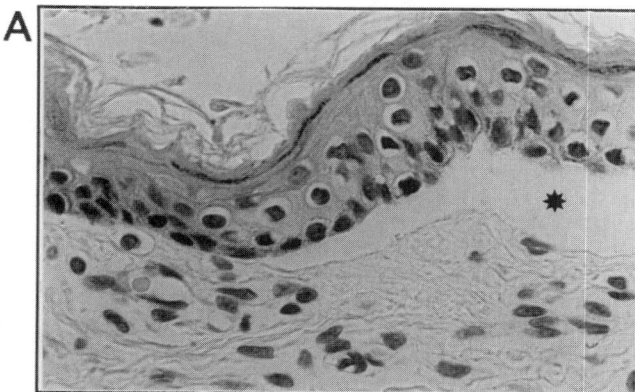

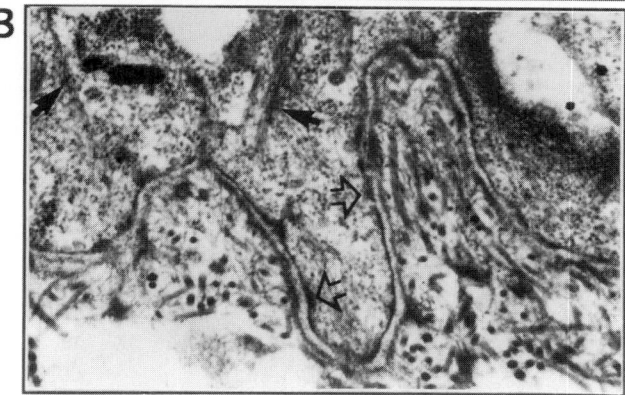

Fig. 222-13. Histopathology and transmission electron microscopy of the skin of an infant affected with epidermolysis bullosa with pyloric atresia (EB-PA). (*A*) Histopathology demonstrates dermal-epidermal tissue separation at the basement membrane zone (*). (*B*) Transmission electron microscopy demonstrates poorly formed rudimentary hemidesmosomes (open arrows) within the cutaneous basement membrane zone. Mutation analysis showed that the patient was a compound heterozygote for a 2-bp deletion mutation (120delTG) and a missense mutation (C245G) in the *β*4 integrin gene (ITGB4). (*Modified from Pulkkinen et al.*[95] *Used with permission.*)

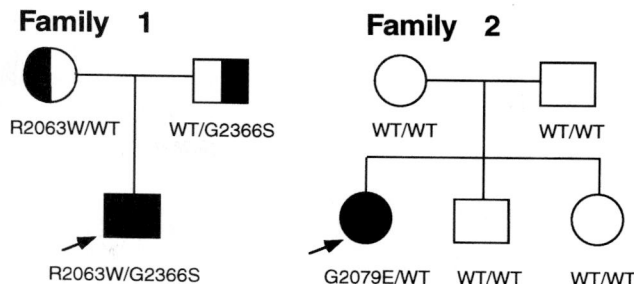

Fig. 222-15. Demonstration that glycine substitution mutations can be either recessive (Family 1) or dominant (Family 2). The proband in Family 1 is a compound heterozygote for two missense mutations, while the father carrying the glycine substitution mutation (G2366S) is clinically unaffected. The proband in Family 2 is heterozygous for the glycine substitution mutation (G2079E), while the parents are both phenotypically and genotypically normal. The proband represents a de novo case of dominant dystrophic EB (*From Hashimoto et al.*[104] *Used with permission.*)

genetic lesions, their positions along the affected gene, and the dynamic interplay of the mutant alleles on the individuals' genetic background that will determine the precise phenotype of the patient.

## TRANSLATION OF THE BASIC RESEARCH TO CLINICAL CARE

More than 300 pathogenic mutations have been disclosed thus far in various forms of EB.[37,60] Although this progress has clearly enhanced our understanding of the complexity of the cutaneous BMZ, it also raises these critical questions: What are the benefits of this progress in basic research on EB to the patients and their families? How can we translate this basic information into improved patient care? Immediate benefits have already been materialized through improved, molecularly based diagnosis with a refined classification, which allows better prognostication

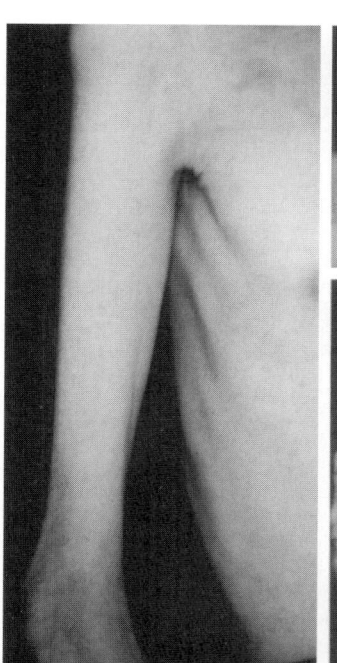

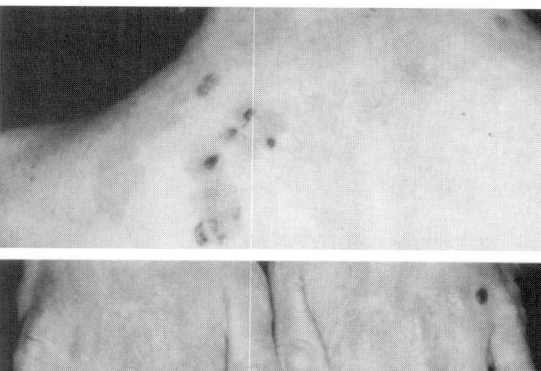

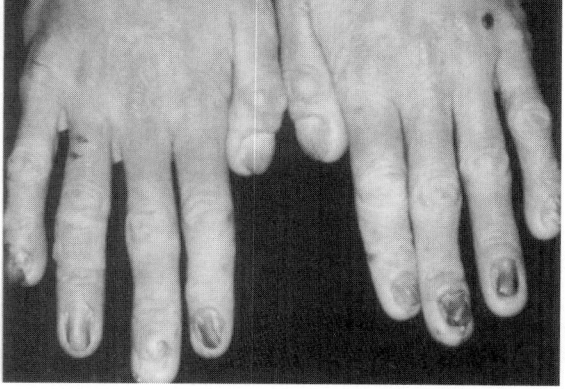

Fig. 222-14. Clinical features of a patient with epidermolysis bullosa with muscular dystrophy. Note the blisters and erosions and the dystrophy of the nails. The patient has a marked wasting of the muscles in the upper arm and in the intercostal areas reflecting severe muscle weakness. (*From Pulkkinen et al.*[102] *Used with permission.*)

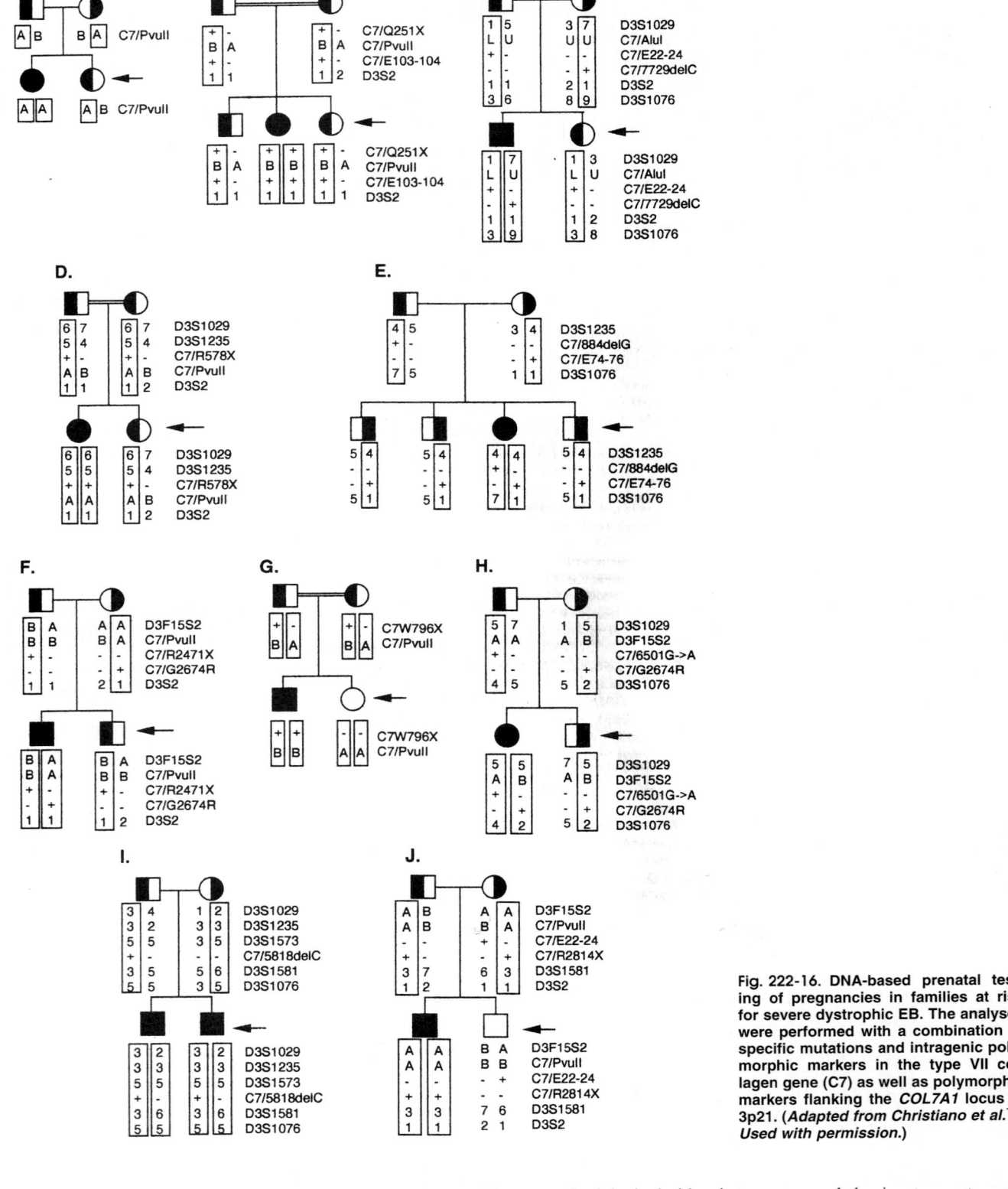

Fig. 222-16. DNA-based prenatal testing of pregnancies in families at risk for severe dystrophic EB. The analyses were performed with a combination of specific mutations and intragenic polymorphic markers in the type VII collagen gene (C7) as well as polymorphic markers flanking the *COL7A1* locus at 3p21. (*Adapted from Christiano et al.*[107] *Used with permission.*)

regarding the severity and the progress of the disease, with profound implications for genetic counseling.[103]

## Clinical Implications for Genetic Counseling

The dystrophic forms of EB are an example of the utilization of the results of molecular analyses to improve genetic counseling. DEB can be inherited either in an autosomal dominant or autosomal recessive fashion, but sporadic "de novo" cases with subsequent dominant inheritance have also been reported. The diagnosis of classic HS-RDEB in a patient with severe, mutilating scarring, with clinically unaffected parents, is usually made without difficulty. Similarly, inheritance of a blistering tendency and a relatively mild scarring phenotype in a vertical pattern, with multiple affected family members in several generations, enables unequivocal diagnosis of dominantly inherited DEB.

The difficulties arise during the diagnosis and ascertainment of the inheritance pattern in patients with a relatively mild phenotype and clinically normal parents. By ultrastructural analyses, these patients often demonstrate the presence, but in a reduced number, of anchoring fibrils (Fig. 222-15). Consequently, these cases are often diagnosed as dominant DEB, presumed to be due to a new dominant mutation or reflecting parental germline mosaicism.[104] This diagnosis obviously has serious implications in terms of genetic counseling of the affected individuals. If their disease is truly a new dominant mutation, the risk of their offspring being affected is one in two (50 percent). In contrast, in case of a recessively inherited disease, the risk of their offspring being affected is approximately as low as in the general population (< 0.1 percent), with the exception of consanguineous matings.

Careful determination of the genotype and mutation analysis of several patients with relatively mild disease and ultrastructurally detectable anchoring fibrils with positive immunofluorescence staining for type VII collagen, has demonstrated that many of them are compound heterozygotes or have homozygous missense mutations inherited in a recessive manner (see Fig. 222-15). In our survey of a cohort of more than 150 families, in which we have thus far identified 108 distinct *COL7A1* mutations, only 4 patients appear to be de novo dominant mutations.[66,68]

Based on these considerations, it appears appropriate to consider each "new" case as a recessively inherited condition for genetic counseling purposes, unless the case is proven to be a dominant mutation by molecular genetic analysis, although the mode of inheritance can be inferred for certain only by careful examinations of the proband's and the parents' *COL7A1*.

### DNA-Based Prenatal Testing and Preimplantation Genetic Diagnosis

Another consequence of the identification of specific mutations in BMZ genes in EB is the development of DNA-based prenatal testing in families at risk for recurrence of severe forms of this disease. Such testing can be performed from chorionic villus samples as early as the 10th week of gestation or from amniocentesis performed at the 12th week. In fact, prenatal testing strategies are already established for application to families at risk for the severe Hallopeau-Siemens type of recessive dystrophic EB or for Herlitz type of junctional EB.[105-108] Furthermore, prenatal predictions in cases with EB-PA have also been performed.[93,95] In case of the dystrophic forms of EB, prenatal diagnosis can be based, in addition to direct demonstration of the mutation, on haplotype analyses using intragenic or flanking polymorphic markers based on the assumption that all cases of DEB are due to mutations in the *COL7A1* gene (see Fig. 222-16). In contrast, prenatal testing for Herlitz junctional EB or for EB-PA has to be based on identification of specific mutations in the family, because three (*LAMA3*, *LAMB3*, and *LAMC2*) or two (*ITGA6* and *ITGB4*) genes, respectively, which are in different chromosomal regions, can harbor the mutations.

An extension of prenatal testing is the development of preimplantation genetic diagnosis (PGD), a technique that has been successfully applied to a variety of other genetic diseases in the past.[109] PGD is performed in conjunction with in vitro fertilization and the fertilized embryos are allowed to grow to the eight-cell stage level, at which time one cell is removed for mutation analysis. Embryos lacking the mutation can then be implanted in the uterus to establish pregnancy, which is routinely performed as part of the in vitro fertilization procedure. Couples with a child previously affected with EB can now initiate the next pregnancy by knowing that there are ways to learn the EB genotype of the fetus in the early stages of pregnancy, or even before the pregnancy is initiated.

### Prospects of Gene Therapy for EB

The current treatment of EB is rather ineffective and nonspecific, aimed primarily at reduction of trauma to the skin and prevention of bacterial infections. In the case of severe, recessive, dystrophic EB, vigilant survey for epithelial metaplasia and squamous cell carcinoma is implicated. The future prospects of the treatment of EB relate to the development of successful gene therapy approaches. This could involve ex vivo manipulation of cultured cells in a manner that a mutation is corrected, followed by grafting of the cells on the eroded areas of skin. Alternatively, direct application of DNA into the skin could be used in attempts to elicit genetic reversal of the underlying mutation.[110] Despite the skin being an attractive target organ for gene therapy due to its accessibility, concerns about the efficiency of gene therapy approaches have been raised as regards the methods of delivery, targeting of the epidermal stem cell population, sustained expression of the transgene, and long-term safety. Although successful application of gene therapy for treatment of EB may still be several years away, rapid development of new technologies, such as the use of ribozymes or application of chimeric RNA/DNA nucleotides for correction of the mutation by homologous recombination, hold promise for breakthroughs that will lead to durable gene therapy for these devastating skin diseases in the near future.

## ACKNOWLEDGMENTS

The authors thank Carol Kelly for excellent assistance. The original studies by the authors were supported by the United States Public Service, National Institutes of Health grant PO1-AR38923, the Dermatology Foundation, and the Dystrophic Epidermolysis Bullosa Research Association of America.

## REFERENCES

1. Fine J-D, Bauer EA, McGuire J, Moshell A: *Epidermolysis Bullosa. Clinical, epidemiologic, and laboratory advances and the findings of the National Epidermolysis Bullosa Registry.* Baltimore, MD, The Johns Hopkins University Press, 1999.
2. Bruckner-Tuderman L: Epidermolysis bullosa, in: Royce PM, Steinmann B (eds): *Connective Tissue and Its Heritable Disorders: Molecular, Genetic and Medical Aspects.* New York, Wiley-Liss, 1993, p 507.
3. Christiano AM, Uitto J: Molecular complexity of the cutaneous basement membrane zone. Revelations from the paradigms of epidermolysis bullosa. *Exp Dermatol* 5:1, 1996a.
4. Pulkkinen L, Uitto J: Hemidesmosomal variants of epidermolysis bullosa. Mutations in the α6β4 integrin and the 180-kDa bullous pemphigoid antigen/type XVII collagen genes. *Exp Dermatol* 7:46, 1998.
5. Uitto J, Pulkkinen L, McLean WHI: Epidermolysis bullosa: A spectrum of clinical phenotypes explained by molecular heterogeneity. *Mol Med Today* 3:457, 1997.
6. Eady RA, McGrath JA, McMillan JR: Ultrastructural clues to genetic disorders of skin: The dermal-epidermal junction. *J Invest Dermatol* 103:13S, 1994.
7. Borradori L, Sonnenberg A: Hemidesmosomes: Roles in adhesion, signaling and human diseases. *Curr Opin Cell Biol* 8:647, 1996.
8. Wiche G, Plectin: general overview and appraisal of its potential role as a subunit of the cytomatrix. *CRC Crit Rev Biochem* 24:41, 1989.
9. Green KJ, Virata MLA, Elgart GW, Stanley JR, Parry DAD: Comparative structural analysis of desmoplakin, bullous pemphigoid antigen and plectin — Members of a new gene family involved in organization of intermediate filaments. *Int J Macromol* 14:145, 1992.
10. Elliott CE, Becker B, Oehler S, Castanon MJ, Hauptmann R, Wiche G: Plectin transcript diversity: Identification and tissue distribution of variants with distinct first coding exons and rodless isoforms. *Genomics* 42:115, 1997.
11. Guo L, Degenstein L, Dowling J, Yu Q, Wollman R, Perman B, Fuchs E: Gene targeting of BPAG1: Abnormalities in mechanical strength and cell migration in stratified epithelia and neurologic degeneration. *Cell* 81:233, 1995.

12. Wiche G, Krepler R, Artlieb U, Pytela R, Denk H: Occurrence and immunolocalization of plectin in tissues. *J Cell Biol* **97**:887, 1983.

13. Liu CG, Maercker C, Castanon MJ, Hauptmann R, Wiche G: Human plectin—Organization of the gene, sequence-analysis, and chromosome localization (8q24). *Proc Natl Acad Sci U S A* **93**:4278, 1996.

14. McLean WHI, Pulkkinen L, Smith FJD, Rugg EL, Lane EB, Bullrich F, Burgeson RE, et al: Loss of plectin causes epidermolysis bullosa with muscular dystrophy: cDNA cloning and genomic organization. *Genes Dev* **10**:1724, 1996.

15. Giudice G, Emery DJ, Diaz LA: Cloning and primary structural analysis of the bullous pemphigoid autoantigen BP180. *J Invest Dermatol* **99**:243, 1992.

16. Li K, Tamai K, Tan EML, Uitto J: Cloning of type XVII collagen. Complementary and genomic DNA sequences of mouse 180-kDA bullous pemphigoid antigen (BPAG2) predict an interrupted collagenous domain, a transmembrane segment, and unusual features in the 5′-end of the gene and the 3′-untranslated region of the mRNA. *J Biol Chem* **268**:8825, 1993.

17. Hopkinson SB, Baker SE, Jones JCR: Molecular genetic studies of a human epidermal autoantigen (the 180-kDa bullous pemphigoid antigen/BP180): Identification of functionally important sequences within the BP180 and α6 integrin. *J Cell Biol* **130**:117, 1995.

18. Aho S, Uitto J: Direct interaction between the intracellular domains of bullous pemphigoid antigen 2 (BP180) and β4 integrin, hemidesmosomal components of basal keratinocytes. *Biochem Biophys Res Commun* **243**:694, 1998.

19. Niessen CM, Hulsman EHM, Oomen LCJM, Sonnenberg K, Sonnenberg A: A minimal region on the integrin β4 subunit that is critical to its localization in hemidesmosomes regulates the distribution of HD1/plectin in COS-7 cells. *J Cell Sci* **110**:1705, 1997.

20. Carter WG, Ryan MC, Gahr PJ: Epiligrin, a new cell adhesion ligand for integrin α3β1 in epithelial basement membranes. *Cell* **65**:599, 1991.

21. Xia Y, Gill SG, Carter WG: Anchorage mediated by integrin α6β4 to laminin 5 (epiligrin) regulates tyrosine phosphorylation of a membrane-associated 80-kDa protein. *J Cell Biol* **132**:727, 1996.

22. Burgeson RE, Chiquet N, Deutzmann R, Ekblom P, Engel J, Kleinman H, Martin GR, et al: A new nomenclature for laminins. *Matrix Biol* **14**:209, 1994.

23. Masunaga T, Shimizu H, Ishiko A, Tomita Y, Aberdam D, Ortonne J-P, Nishikawa T: Localization of laminin-5 in the epidermal basement membrane. *J Histochem Cytochem* **44**:1223, 1996.

24. Rousselle P, Keene DR, Ruggiero F, Champliaud M-F, van der Rest M, Burgeson RE: Laminin 5 binds to NC-1 domain of type VII collagen. *J Cell Biol* **138**:719, 1997.

25. Champliaud MF, Lunstrum GP, Rousselle P, Nishiyama T, Keene DR, Burgeson RE: Human amnion contains a novel laminin variant, laminin 7, which, like laminin 6, covalently associates with laminin 5 to promote stable epithelial-stromal attachment. *J Cell Biol* **132**:1189, 1996.

26. Burgeson RE: Type VII collagen, anchoring fibrils, and epidermolysis bullosa. *J Invest Dermatol* **101**:252, 1993.

27. Christiano AM, Greenspan DS, Lee S, Uitto J: Cloning of human type VII collagen. Complete primary sequence of the α1(VII) chain and identification of intragenic polymorphisms. *J Biol Chem* **269**:20256, 1994.

28. Christiano AM, Hoffman GG, Chung-Honet LC, Lee S, Cheng W, Uitto J, Greenspan DS: Structural organization of the human type VII collagen gene *(COL7A1)*, comprised of more exons than any previously characterized gene. *Genomics* **21**:169, 1994.

29. Keene DR, Sakai LY, Lunstrum GP, Morris NP, Burgeson RE: Type VII collagen forms an extended network of anchoring fibrils. *J Cell Biol* **104**:611, 1987.

30. Christiano AM, Rosenbaum LM, Chung-Honet LC, Parente MG, Woodley DT, Pan T-C, Zhang X, et al: The large non-collagenous domain (NC-1) of type VII collagen is amino-terminal and chimeric. Homology to cartilage matrix protein, the type III domains of fibronectin and the A domains of von Willebrand factor. *Hum Molec Genet* **1**:475, 1992.

31. Gammon WR, Abernethy ML, Padilla KM, Prisayanh PS, Cook ME, Wright J, Briggaman RA, et al: Noncollagenous (NC1) domain of collagen VII resembles multidomain adhesion proteins involved in tissue-specific organization of extracellular matrix. *J Invest Dermatol* **99**:691, 1992.

32. Tanaka T, Takahashi K, Furukawa F, Imamura S: Molecular cloning and characterization of type VII collagen cDNA. *Biochem Biophys Res Commun* **183**:958, 1992.

33. Greenspan DS: The carboxyl-terminal half of type VII collagen, including the non-collagenous NC-2 domain and intron/exon organization of the corresponding region of the *COL7A1* gene. *Hum Mol Genet* **2**:273, 1993.

34. Christiano AM, Hoffman GG, Zhang X, Xu Y, Tamai Y, Greenspan DS, Uitto J: A strategy for identification of sequence variants in *COL7A1* and a novel 2-bp deletion mutation in recessive dystrophic epidermolysis bullosa. *Human Mutat* **10**:408, 1997.

35. Ganguly A, Rock MJ, Prockop DJ: Conformation-sensitive gel electrophoresis for rapid detection of single-base differences in double-stranded PCR products and DNA fragments. *Proc Natl Acad Sci U S A* **90**:10325, 1993.

36. Järvikallio A, Pulkkinen L, Uitto J: Molecular basis of dystrophic epidermolysis bullosa: Mutations in the type VII collagen gene *(COL7A1)*. *Hum Mutat* **10**:338, 1997.

37. Pulkkinen L, Uitto J, Christiano AM: The molecular basis of the junctional forms of epidermolysis bullosa, in Fine J-D, Bauer EA, McGuire J, Moshell A (eds): *Epidermolysis Bullosa: Clinical, Epidemiologic and Laboratory Advances, and the Findings of the National Epidermolysis Bullosa Registry.* Baltimore, MD, The Johns Hopkins University Press, 1999, 300–325.

38. Uitto J, Pulkkinen L, Smith FJD, McLean WHI: Plectin and human genetic disorders of the skin and muscle. The paradigm of epidermolysis bullosa with muscular dystrophy. *Exp Dermatol* **5**:237, 1996.

39. Hogervorst FB, Cornelis RS, Bout M, van Vliet M, Oosterwijk JC, Olmer R, Bakker B, et al: Rapid detection of BRCA1 mutations by the protein truncation test. *Nat Genet* **10**:208, 1995.

40. Plummer SJ, Anton-Culver H, Webster L, Noble B, Liao S, Kennedy A, Belinson J, et al: Detection of BRCA1 mutations by the protein truncation test. *Hum Mol Genet* **4**:1989, 1995.

41. Dang M, Pulkkinen L, Smith FJD, McLean WHI, Uitto J: Novel compound heterozygous mutations in the plectin gene in epidermolysis bullosa with muscular dystrophy (EB-MD), and use of protein truncation test for detection of premature termination codon mutations. *Lab Invest* **78**:195, 1998.

42. Takizawa Y, Shimizu H, Rouan F, Kawai M, Udono M, Pulkkinen L, Nishikawa T, et al: Four novel plectin gene mutations in Japanese patients with epidermolysis bullosa with muscular dystrophy disclosed by heteroduplex scanning and protein truncation test. *J Invest Dermatol* **112**:109, 1999.

43. Uitto J, Pulkkinen L, Christiano AM: Molecular basis of the dystrophic and junctional forms of epidermolysis bullosa: Mutations in the type VII collagen and kalinin (laminin-5) genes. *J Invest Dermatol* **103**:39S, 1994.

44. Tidman MJ, Eady RAJ: Evaluation of anchoring fibrils and other components of the dermal-epidermal junction in dystrophic epidermolysis bullosa by quantitative ultrastructural technique. *J Invest Dermatol* **84**:374, 1985.

45. McGrath JA, Ishida-Yamamoto A, O'Grady A, Leigh IM, Eady RAJ: Structural variations in anchoring fibrils in dystrophic epidermolysis bullosa: Correlation with type VII collagen expression. *J Invest Dermatol* **100**:366, 1993.

46. Uitto J, Christiano AM: Molecular genetics of the cutaneous basement membrane zone. Perspectives on epidermolysis bullosa and other blistering skin diseases. *J Clin Invest* **90**:687, 1992.

47. Parente MG, Chung LC, Ryynänen J, Woodley DT, Wynn KC, Bauer EA, Mattei M-G, et al: Human type VII collagen: cDNA cloning and chromosomal mapping of the gene. *Proc Natl Acad Sci U S A* **88**:6931, 1991.

48. Greenspan DS, Byers MG, Eddy RL, Hoffman GG, Shows TB: Localization of the human collagen gene *COL7A1* to 3p21.3 by fluorescence *in situ* hybridization. *Cytogenet Cell Genet* **62**:35, 1993.

49. Ryynänen M, Knowlton RG, Parente MG, Chung LC, Chu M-L, Uitto J: Human type VII collagen: Genetic linkage of the gene *(COL7A1)* on chromosome 3 to dominant dystrophic epidermolysis bullosa. *Am J Hum Genet* **49**:797, 1991.

50. Ryynänen M, Ryynänen J, Sollberg S, Iozzo RV, Knowlton RG, Uitto J: Genetic linkage of type VII collagen *(COL7A1)* to dominant dystrophic epidermolysis bullosa in families with abnormal anchoring fibrils. *J Clin Invest* **89**:974, 1992.

51. Hovnanian A, Duquesnoy P, Blanchet-Bardon C, Knowlton RG, Amselem S, Lathrop M, Dubertret L, et al: Genetic linkage of recessive dystrophic epidermolysis bullosa to the type VII collagen gene. *J Clin Invest* **90**:1032, 1992.

52. Uitto J, Christiano AM: Molecular basis for the dystrophic forms of epidermolysis bullosa: Mutations in the type VII collagen gene. *Arch Dermatol Res* **287**:16, 1994.

53. Gruis NA, Bavinck JN, Steijlen PM, van der Schroeff JG, van Haeringen A, Happle R, Mariman E, et al: Genetic linkage between the collagen VII (*COL7A1*) gene and the autosomal dominant form of dystrophic epidermolysis bullosa in two Dutch kindreds. *J Invest Dermatol* **99**:528, 1992.

54. Al-Imara L, Richards AJ, Eady RA, Leigh IM, Farrall M, Pope FM: Linkage of autosomal dominant dystrophic epidermolysis bullosa in three British families to the marker D3S2 close to the *COL7A1* locus. *J Med Genet* **29**:381, 1992.

55. Dunnill MGS, Richards AJ, Milana G, Mollica F, Atherton D, Winship I, Farral IM, et al: Genetic linkage to the type VII collagen gene (*COL7A1*) in 26 families with generalized recessive dystrophic epidermolysis bullosa and anchoring fibril abnormalities. *J Med Genet* **31**:745, 1994.

56. Christiano AM, Anhalt G, Gibbons S, Bauer EA, Uitto J: Premature termination codons in the type VII collagen gene (*COL7A1*) underlie severe, mutilating recessive dystrophic epidermolysis bullosa. *Genomics* **21**:160, 1994.

57. Hovnanian A, Hilal L, Blanchet-Bardon C, de Prost Y, Christiano AM, Uitto J, Goossens M: Recurrent nonsense mutations within the type VII collagen gene in patients with severe recessive dystrophic epidermolysis bullosa. *Am J Hum Genet* **55**:289, 1994.

58. Hovnanian A, Rochat A, Bodemer C, Petit E, Rivers CA, Prost C, Fraitag S, et al: Characterization of 18 new mutations in *COL7A1* in recessive dystrophic epidermolysis bullosa provides evidence for distinct molecular mechanisms underlying defective anchoring fibril formation. *Am J Hum Genet* **61**:599, 1997.

59. Uitto J, Hovnanian A, Christiano AM: Premature termination codon mutations in the type VII collagen gene (*COL7A1*) underlie severe recessive dystrophic epidermolysis bullosa. *Proc Assoc Am Phys* **107**:245, 1995.

60. Uitto J, Pulkkinen L, Christiano AM: The molecular basis of the dystrophic forms of epidermolysis bullosa, in: Fine J-D, Bauer EA, McGuire J, Moshell A (eds): *Epidermolysis Bullosa: Clinical, Epidemiologic and Laboratory Advances, and the Findings of the National Epidermolysis Bullosa Registry.* Baltimore, MD, The Johns Hopkins University Press, 1999, 326–350.

61. Cui Y, Hagan KW, Zhang S, Peltz SW: Identification and characterization of genes that are required for the accelerated degradation of mRNAs containing a premature translational termination codon. *Genes Dev* **9**:423, 1995.

62. Christiano AM, Amano S, Eichenfield LF, Burgeson RE, Uitto J: Premature termination codon mutations in the type VII collagen gene (*COL7A1*) result in nonsense-mediated mRNA decay and absence of functional protein. *J Invest Dermatol* **109**:390, 1997.

63. Mellerio JE, Dunnill MGS, Allison W, Ashton GHS, Christiano AM, Uitto J, Eady RAJ, McGrath JA: Two recurrent mutations in the type VII collagen gene (*COL7A1*) in British patients with recessive dystrophic epidermolysis bullosa. *J Invest Dermatol* **109**:246, 1997.

64. Christiano AM, Ryynänen M, Uitto J: Dominant dystrophic epidermolysis bullosa: Identification of a glycine-to-serine substitution in the triple-helical domain of type VII collagen. *Proc Natl Acad Sci U S A* **91**:3549, 1994.

65. Christiano AM, McGrath JA, Tan KC, Uitto J: Glycine substitutions in the triple-helical region of type VII collagen result in a spectrum of dystrophic epidermolysis bullosa phenotypes and patterns of inheritance. *Am J Hum Genet* **58**:671, 1996.

66. Kon A, Nomura K, Pulkkinen L, Sawamura D, Hashimoto I, Uitto J: Novel glycine substitution mutations in *COL7A1* reveal that the Pasini and Cockayne-Touraine variants of dominant dystrophic epidermolysis bullosa are allelic. *J Invest Dermatol* **109**:684, 1997.

67. Kon A, Pulkkinen L, Ishida-Yamamoto, Hashimoto I, Uitto J: Novel *COL7A1* mutations in dystrophic forms of epidermolysis bullosa. *J Invest Dermatol* **111**:534, 1998.

68. Rouan F, Pulkkinen L, Jonkman MF, Bauer JW, Cserhalmi-Friedman PB, Christiano AM, Uitto J: Novel and de novo glycine substitution mutations in the type VII collagen gene (*COL7A1*) in dystrophic epidermolysis bullosa: Implications for genetic counseling. *J Invest Dermatol* **111**:1210, 1998.

69. Kuivaniemi H, Tromp G, Prockop DJ: Mutations in collagen genes: Causes of rare and some common diseases in humans. *FASEB J* **5**:2052, 1991.

70. Sakuntabhai A, Hammami-Hauasli N, Bodemer C, Rochat A, Prost C, Barrandon Y, de Prost Y, et al: Deletions within *COL7A1* exons distant from consensus splice sites alter splicing and produce shortened polypeptides in dominant dystrophic epidermolysis bullosa. *Am J Hum Genet* **63**:737, 1998.

71. Christiano AM, Greenspan DS, Hoffman GG, Zhang X, Tamai Y, Lin AN, Dietz HC, et al: A missense mutation in type VII collagen in two affected siblings with recessive dystrophic epidermolysis bullosa. *Nat Genet* **4**:62, 1993.

72. Stolle CA, Pyeritz RE, Myers JC, Prockop DJ: Synthesis of an altered type III procollagen in a patient with type IV Ehlers-Danlos dyndrome. *J Biol Chem* **260**:1937, 1985.

73. Verrando P, Blanchet-Bardon C, Pisani A, Thomas L, Cambazard F, Eady RAJ, Schofield O, et al: Monoclonal antibody GB3 defines a widespread defect of several basement membranes and a keratinocyte dysfunction in patients with lethal junctional epidermolysis bullosa. *Lab Invest* **64**:85, 1991.

74. McGrath JA, Pulkkinen L, Christiano AM, Leigh IM, Eady RAJ, Uitto J: Altered laminin 5 expression due to mutations in the gene encoding the β3 chain (*LAMB3*) in generalized atrophic benign epidermolysis bullosa. *J Invest Dermatol* **104**:467, 1995.

75. McGrath J, Christiano AM, Pulkkinen L, Eady RAJ, Uitto J: Compound heterozygosity for nonsense and missense mutations in the *LAMB3* gene in nonlethal junctional epidermolysis bullosa. *J Invest Dermatol* **106**:775, 1996.

76. Pulkkinen L, Jonkman MF, McGrath JA, Kuijpers A, Paller AS, Uitto J: *LAMB3* mutations in generalized atrophic benign epidermolysis bullosa: Consequences at the mRNA and protein levels. *Lab Invest* **78**:859, 1998.

77. Kivirikko S, McGrath JA, Pulkkinen L, Uitto J, Christiano AM: Mutational hotspots in the *LAMB3* gene in the lethal (Herlitz) type of junctional epidermolysis bullosa. *Hum Mol Genet* **5**:231, 1996.

78. Pulkkinen L, Meneguzzi G, McGrath JA, Xu Y, Blanchet-Bardon C, Ortonne J-P, Christiano AM, et al: Predominance of the recurrent mutation R635X in the *LAMB3* gene in European patients with Herlitz junctional epidermolysis bullosa has implications for mutation detection strategy. *J Invest Dermatol* **109**:232, 1997.

79. Cooper DN, Youssoufian H: The CpG dinucleotide and human genetic disease. *Hum Genet* **78**:151, 1988.

80. Pulkkinen L, McGrath JA, Christiano AM, Uitto J: Detection of sequence variants in the gene encoding the β3 chain of laminin 5 (*LAMB3*). *Hum Mutat* **6**:77, 1995.

81. Pulkkinen L, McGrath J, Airenne T, Haakana H, Tryggvason K, Kivirikko S, Meneguzzi G, et al: Detection of novel *LAMC2* mutations in Herlitz junctional epidermolysis bullosa. *Mol Med* **3**:124, 1997.

82. Pulkkinen L, Cserhalmi-Friedman PB, Tang M, Ryan MC, Uitto J, Christiano AM: Molecular analysis of the human laminin α3a chain gene (*LAMA3*a): A strategy for mutation identification and DNA-based prenatal diagnosis in Herlitz junctional epidermolysis bullosa. *Lab Invest* **78**:1067, 1998.

83. Pulkkinen L, Bullrich F, Czarnecki P, Weiss L, Uitto J: Maternal uniparental disomy of chromosome 1 with reduction to homozygosity of the *LAMB3* locus in a patient with Herlitz junctional epidermolysis bullosa. *Am J Hum Genet* **61**:611, 1997d.

84. Takizawa Y, Pulkkinen L, Shimizu H, Nishikawa T, Uitto J: Maternal uniparental meroisodisomy in the *LAMB3* region of chromosome 1 results in lethal junctional epidermolysis bullosa. *J Invest Dermatol* **110**:828, 1998b.

85. Hashimoto I, Schnyder UW, Anton-Lamprecht I: Epidermolysis bullosa hereditaria with junctional blistering in an adult. *Dermatologica* **152**:72, 1976.

86. Hintner H, Wolff K: Generalized atrophic benign epidermolysis bullosa. *Arch Dermatol* **118**:375, 1982.

87. Jonkman MF, de Jong MC, Heeres K, Pas HH, van der Meer JB, Owaribe K, Martinez de Velasco AM, et al: 180-kDa bullous pemphigoid antigen (BP180) is deficient in generalized atrophic benign epidermolysis bullosa. *J Clin Invest* **95**:1345, 1995.

88. Pohla-Gubo G, Lazarova Z, Giudice GJ, Liebert M, Grassegger A, Hintner H, Yancey KB: Diminished expression of the extracellular domain of bullous pemphigoid antigen 2 (BPAG2) in the epidermal basement membrane of patients with generalized atrophic benign epidermolysis bullosa. *Exp Dermatol* **4**:199, 1995.

89. McGrath JA, Gatalica B, Christiano AM, Li K, Owaribe K, McMillan JR, Eady RAJ, et al: Mutations in the gene encoding the 180-kDa bullous pemphigoid antigen (BPAG2), a hemidesmosomal transmembrane collagen (type XVII), in generalized atrophic benign epidermolysis bullosa. *Nat Genet* **11**:83, 1995.

90. Gatalica B, Pulkkinen L, Li K, Kuokkanen K, Ryynänen M, McGrath JA, Uitto J: Cloning of the human type XVII collagen gene

(COL17A1) and detection of novel mutations in generalized atrophic benign epidermolysis bullosa. *Am J Hum Genet* **60**:352, 1997.

91. Jonkman MF, Scheffer H, Stulp R, Pas HH, Nijenhuis M, Heeres K, Owaribe K, et al: Revertant mosaicism in epidermolysis bullosa caused by mitotic gene conversion. *Cell* **88**:543, 1997.

92. Pulkkinen L, Bruckner-Tuderman L, August C, Uitto J: Compound heterozygosity for missense (l156P) and nonsense (R554X) mutations in the β4 integrin gene (*ITGB4*) underlies mild, non-lethal phenotype of epidermolysis bullosa with pyloric atresia. *Am J Pathol* **152**:935, 1998.

93. Pulkkinen L, Rouan F, Bruckner-Tuderman L, Wallerstein R, Garzon M, Brown T, Smith L, et al: Novel *ITGB4* mutations in lethal and non-lethal variants of epidermolysis bullosa with pyloric atresia: Missense vs. nonsense. *Am J Hum Genet* **63**:1376, 1998.

94. Brown TA, Gil SG, Sybert VP, Lestringant GG, Tadini G, Caputo R, Carter WG: Defective integrin α6β4 expression in the skin of patients with junctional epidermolysis bullosa and pyloric atresia. *J Invest Dermatol* **107**:384, 1996.

95. Pulkkinen L, Kim D-U, Uitto J: Epidermolysis bullosa with pyloric atresia: Novel mutations in the β4 integrin gene (*ITGB4*). *Am J Pathol* **152**:157, 1998.

96. Pulkkinen L, Kimonis VE, Xu Y, Spanou EN, McLean WHI, Uitto J: Homozygous α6 integrin mutation in junctional epidermolysis bullosa with congenital duodenal atresia. *Hum Molec Genet* **6**:669, 1997.

97. Ruzzi L, Gagnoux-Palacious L, Pinola M, Belli S, Meneguzzi G, D'Alessio M, Zambruno G: A homozygous mutation in the integrin α6 gene in junctional epidermolysis bullosa with pyloric atresia. *J Clin Invest* **99**:2826, 1997.

98. Niemi K-M, Somer H, Kero M, Kanerva L, Haltia M: Epidermolysis bullosa simplex associated with muscular dystrophy with recessive inheritance. *Arch Dermatol* **124**:551, 1988.

99. Hieda Y, Nishizawa Y, Uematsu J, Owaribe K: Identification of a new hemidesmosomal protein, HD1: A major high molecular mass component of isolated hemidesmosomes. *J Cell Biol* **116**:1497, 1992.

100. Gache Y, Chavanas S, Lacour JP, Wiche G, Owaribe K, Meneguzzi G, Ortonne JP: Defective expression of plectin in epidermolysis bullosa simplex with muscular dystrophy. *J Clin Invest* **97**:2289, 1996.

101. Smith FJD, Eady RAJ, Leigh IM, McMillan FRY, Rugg EL, Kelsell DP, Bryant SP, et al: Plectin deficiency results in muscular dystrophy with epidermolysis bullosa. *Nat Genet* **13**:450, 1996.

102. Pulkkinen L, Smith FJD, Shimizu H, Murata S, Yaoita H, Hachisuka H, Nishikawa T, et al: Homozygous deletion mutations in the plectin gene (PLEC-1) in patients with epidermolysis bullosa simplex associated with late-onset muscular dystrophy. *Hum Mol Genet* **5**:1539, 1996.

103. Christiano AM, Uitto J: Impact of molecular genetic diagnosis on dystrophic epidermolysis bullosa. *Curr Opin Derm* **3**:225, 1996.

104. Hashimoto I, Kon A, Tamai K, Uitto J: Diagnostic dilemma of "sporadic" cases of dystrophic epidermolysis bullosa: A new dominant or Mitis recessive mutation? *Exp Dermatol* **8**:140, 1999.

105. Hovnanian A, Hilal L, Blanchet-Bardon C, Bodemer C, de Prost Y, Stark CA, Christiano AM, et al: Prenatal diagnosis of the Hallopeau-Siemens form of recessive dystrophic epidermolysis bullosa by type VII collagen gene analysis in six pregnancies at risk of recurrence. *J Invest Dermatol* **104**:456, 1995.

106. Christiano AM, Uitto J: Molecular diagnosis of inherited skin diseases: The paradigm of dystrophic epidermolysis bullosa. *Adv Dermatol* **11**:199, 1996.

107. Christiano AM, LaForgia S, Paller AS, McGuire J, Shimizu H, Uitto J: Prenatal diagnosis for recessive dystrophic epidermolysis bullosa in ten families by mutation and haplotype analysis in the type VII collagen gene (*COL7A1*). *Mol Med* **2**:59, 1996.

108. Christiano AM, Pulkkinen L, McGrath JA, Uitto J: Mutation-based prenatal diagnosis of Herlitz junctional epidermolysis bullosa. *Prenat Diag* **17**:343, 1997c.

109. McGrath JA, Handyside AH: Preimplantation genetic diagnosis of severe inherited skin diseases. *Exp Dermatol* **7**:65, 1998.

110. Khavari PA, Krueger GG: Cutaneous gene therapy. *Dermatol Clin* **15**:27, 1997.

111. Uitto J: Clinical implications of basic research on heritable skin diseases. *J Dermatol* **21**:690, 1997.

# NEUROGENETICS

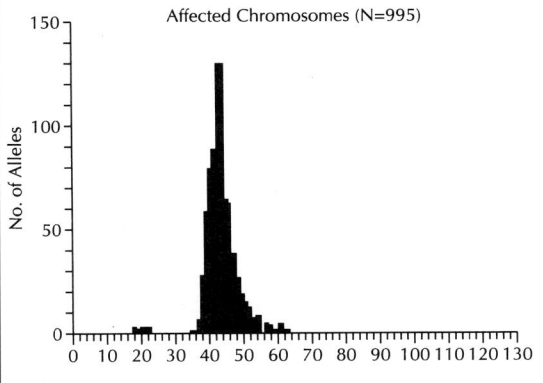

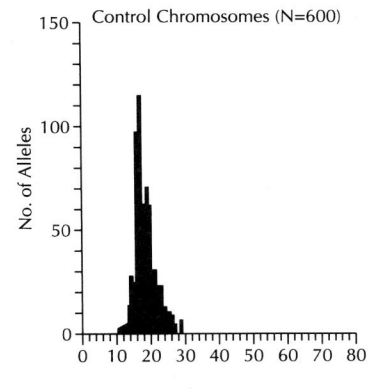

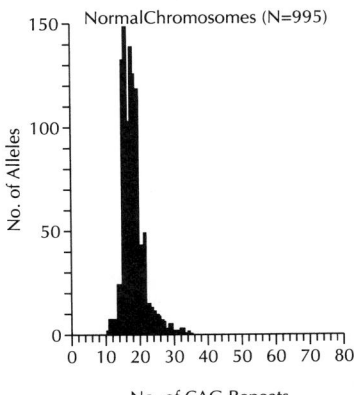

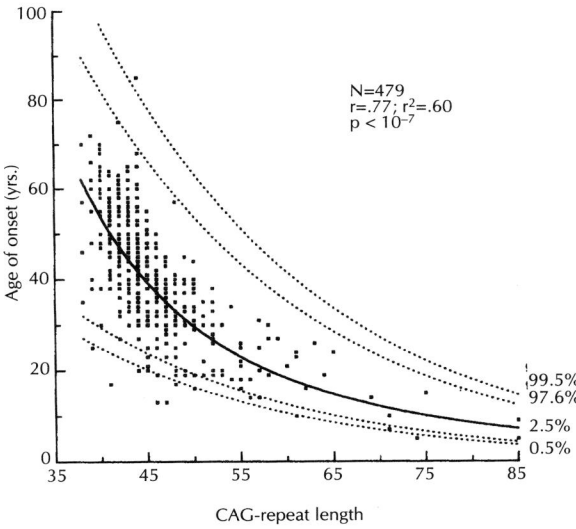

Huntington disease and CAG repeats

# Huntington Disease

*Michael R. Hayden* ■ *Berry Kremer*

1. Huntington disease (OMIM 143100) is a slowly progressive autosomal dominant neurodegenerative disease. Onset is usually in adult life, with a mean of around 40 years. However, onset before age 20 or after age 60 is well described. The disease progresses inexorably, with death occurring approximately 18 years from the time of onset. Prevalence is between 3 and 7 per 100,000 in populations of western European descent, but Huntington disease (HD) has been described in populations of many different ancestries.

2. The neuropathologic hallmark of the disease is neuronal loss and gliosis in the caudate nucleus and the putamen (the striatum), with resulting atrophy. Medium-sized striatal neurons that contain gamma-aminobutyric acid and enkephalin or gamma-aminobutyric acid and substance P as their neurotransmitters are selectively depleted. Other, neurochemically distinct striatal neuronal populations are spared, such as large aspiny acetylcholinesterase-containing neurons or NADPH-diaphorase neurons with somatostatin and neuropeptide Y. Apart from the striatum, the whole brain undergoes generalized atrophy. No specific pathologic changes have been found outside the central nervous system.

3. Clinical manifestations consist of gradually evolving involuntary movements, progressive dementia, and psychiatric disturbances, especially mood disorder and personality changes. Chorea is the most prominent abnormality, but parkinsonism, dystonia, and involuntary motor impairment all may be present. Minor motor abnormalities, including clumsiness, hyperreflexia, and eye movement disturbances, often appear as early manifestations of HD. Patients with onset before age 20 frequently have prominent bradykinesia, rigidity, epilepsy, severe dementia, and a shorter duration of illness. In contrast, cognitive decline is often less severe in patients with onset aftetr age 60.

4. In 1993, a novel gene containing a CAG trinucleotide repeat that is expanded on HD chromosomes was identified. This highly polymorphic CAG repeat located in the 5′ end of the gene has been shown to range between 10 and 29 copies on normal chromosomes, whereas it is expanded to a range of 36 to 121 on HD chromosomes. The vast majority of patients with the clinical diagnosis of HD have expansion of the CAG repeat. Age of onset shows a highly significant association with the length of the CAG repeat.

5. The biochemical defect underlying HD is unknown. Recent data suggest that cells die via apoptotic pathways. Cleavage of huntingtin, the polypeptide product of the HD gene, into a smaller fragment containing the expanded polyglutamine tract appears to be an important step in pathogenesis of the illness. There is no known treatment to retard disease progression. Neuroleptic medication is able to alleviate choreic movements to some extent, but side effects may be severe. Antidepressant therapy may be helpful in the early stages to alleviate the mood disorder.

## HISTORICAL BACKGROUND

How did this disease get its name? At the age of 21, only a year after graduating from Columbia University as a doctor, George Huntington presented his paper on chorea to the Meigs and Mason Academy of Medicine in Middleport, Ohio (Fig. 223-1). The text of the lecture appeared in the *Medical and Surgical Reporter* of Philadelphia on April 13, 1872.[1] After a general discussion on the subject of childhood chorea, Huntington provided in approximately 1200 words the most comprehensive description of hereditary chorea. Sir William Osler, professor of medicine at John Hopkins University in Baltimore, remarked (1894) that "there are few instances in the history of medicine in which a disease has been more graphically or more briefly described."[2] This account of the disorder was immediately abstracted into German,[3] with the result that Huntington's name very quickly became attached to the disease in different parts of the world, including Germany,[4] France,[5] Italy,[6] and England.[7]

Both his father and grandfather were medical doctors, and Huntington reported in 1910[8] that his grandfather had observed patients with inherited chorea when he had moved to East Hampton, New York, in 1797. George Huntington was only 8 years old when he first saw patients with this disorder while riding with his father on his professional rounds in East Hampton. He wrote out the original draft on chorea, and it was revised by his father, whose penciled remarks are still visible in the margins of the original manuscript.[9] The eventual delineation of the disorder therefore was the outcome of the cooperation between three generations of doctors in the Huntington family. An extract from Huntington's original and only contribution to medical literature, which encompassed the major features of this disease, is cited here:

> The hereditary chorea as I shall call it is confined to certain and fortunately few families and has been transmitted to them as an heirloom from generations way back in the dim past. It is spoken of by those in whose veins the seeds of the disease are known to exist with a kind of horror and not at all alluded to except through dire necessity, with it being mentioned as "that disorder." It is attended generally by all the symptoms of common chorea only in an aggravated degree, hardly ever manifesting itself until adult or middle life and then coming on gradually but surely, increasing by degrees and often occupying years in its development until the hapless sufferer is but a quivering wreck of his former self. There are three marked peculiarities in this disease: (1) its hereditary nature, (2) a tendency to insanity and suicide, and (3) its manifesting itself as a grave disease only in adult life.
>
> 1. Of its hereditary nature. When either or both the parents have shown manifestations of the disease and more especially when these manifestations have been of a serious nature, one

A list of standard abbreviations is located immediately preceding the index in each volume. Nonstandard abbreviations used in this chapter include: HD = Huntington's disease; DRPLA = dentorubropallidoluysian atrophy; GABA = gamma-aminobutyric acid; GPe = external part of the globus pallidus; GPi = internal part of the globus pallidas; EAAs = excitatory amino acids; NMDA = N-methyl-D-aspartate; AMPA = α-amino-3-hydroxy-5-methylisoxale-4-propionic acid. Gen Bank accession number L12392.

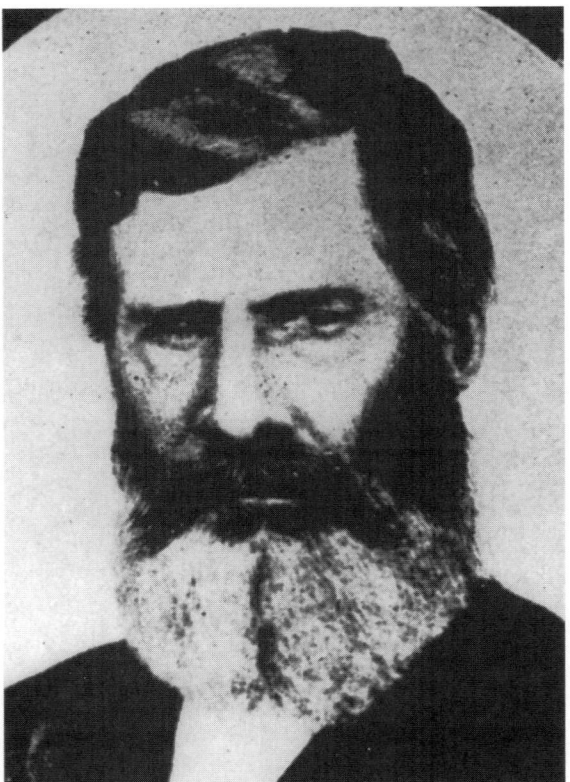

Fig. 223-1 Photograph of George Huntington.

or more of the offspring almost invariably suffer from the disease if they live to adult age. But if by any chance these children go through life without it, the thread is broken and the grandchildren and great grandchildren of the original sufferers may rest assured that they are free of the disease.

2. The tendency to insanity and sometimes that form of insanity which leads to suicide is marked. I know of several instances of suicide in people suffering from this form of chorea, or who belonged to families in which the disease existed.

3. Its third peculiarity is its coming on at least as a grave disease only in adult life. I do not know of a single case that has shown any marked signs of chorea before the age of thirty or forty years while those who pass the fortieth year without symptoms of the disease are seldom attacked. I've never known a recovery even an amelioration of symptoms in this form of chorea; when once it begins, it clings to the bitter end.

No treatment seems to be of any avail, and indeed nowadays, its end is so well known to the sufferer and his friends that medical advice is seldom sought. It seems at least to be one of the incurables.[1]

## THE HUNTINGTON DISEASE GENE

The Huntington disease (HD) gene is located on chromosome 4p16.3,[10] encompasses 67 exons, and spans over 200 kb.[11] It is ubiquitously expressed as two transcripts 10.3 and 13.6 kb in length that differ in the size of the 3′ UTR.[12] Structural analysis of the promoter region is consistent with it being a housekeeping gene.[13]

The HD gene lacks homology to any previously characterized gene and encodes a protein of 3144 amino acids with a predicted molecular mass of 348 kDa. The polyglutamine tract starts at residue 18 and is followed by a stretch of 29 consecutive prolines. The region downstream of the polyglutamine tract contains a HEAT repeat,[14] which consists of 40 loosely conserved amino acids repeated multiple times in tandem, and is proposed to be involved in protein-protein interactions. Huntingtin contains a basic peptide region PIRRKGKEK (amino acids 1182–1190), which when fused to bacterial β-galactosidase is sufficient to localize the protein to the nucleus in human 293 cells[15] (Fig. 223-2). This peptide contains an N-terminal proline residue followed by a hexapeptide motif that contains 4 basic amino acids and fulfills the sequence criteria proposed for a nuclear localization signal. The physiologic significance of these findings for huntingtin is not clear.

The rodent and the pufferfish homologues of the HD gene have been cloned.[16–19] The human and the mouse genes are 90 percent homologous with a high degree of sequence identity in the 5′ and 3′ UTRs. The pufferfish homologue is also highly conserved with 69 percent identity to the HD gene at the nucleotide level. The first 17 amino acids show 100 percent conservation between Fugu, human, and mouse peptide sequences. The murine CAG tract encodes only 7 glutamines and is interrupted by a CAA. The glutamine repeat in the pufferfish is 4 amino acids long and is encoded by two CAG and two CAA. The high degree of conservation across species suggests that the normal function of huntingtin is essential. This also has been demonstrated unequivocally by embryonic lethality in mice deficient in huntingtin at about embryonic day 8.[20–22]

### The Mutation Underlying HD

The mutation underlying HD is an expansion of a CAG/ polyglutamine tract in the first exon.[10] The CAG repeat length is highly polymorphic in the population, and the repeat size in the normal and affected ranges from 10 to 35 (median 18) and 36 to 121 (median 40), respectively.[23,24] Adult-onset patients usually have an expansion from 40 to 55, whereas juvenile-onset patients have expansions above 60. There is a well-established inverse correlation between CAG repeat length and age of onset[25]

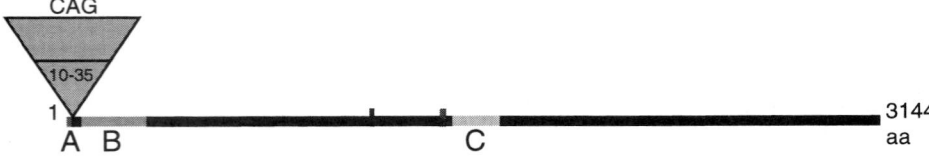

## Percentage Identity and Homology to Human Huntingtin

| | Overall | | A:1-17 aa | | B: 56-301 aa | | C: 1462-1642 aa | |
|---|---|---|---|---|---|---|---|---|
| | Identity | Homo | Identity | Homo | Identity | Homo | Identity | Homo |
| Mouse | 91 | 95 | 100 | 100 | 97 | 99 | 99 | 100 |
| Rat | 86 | 91 | 100 | 100 | 93 | 95 | 99 | 100 |
| Fugu | 80 | 90 | 100 | 100 | 82 | 92 | 95 | 98 |

Homo: Homology

Fig. 223-2 Comparison of amino acids from different portions of human, mouse, rat, and pufferfish huntingtin showing highly conserved regions of the protein.

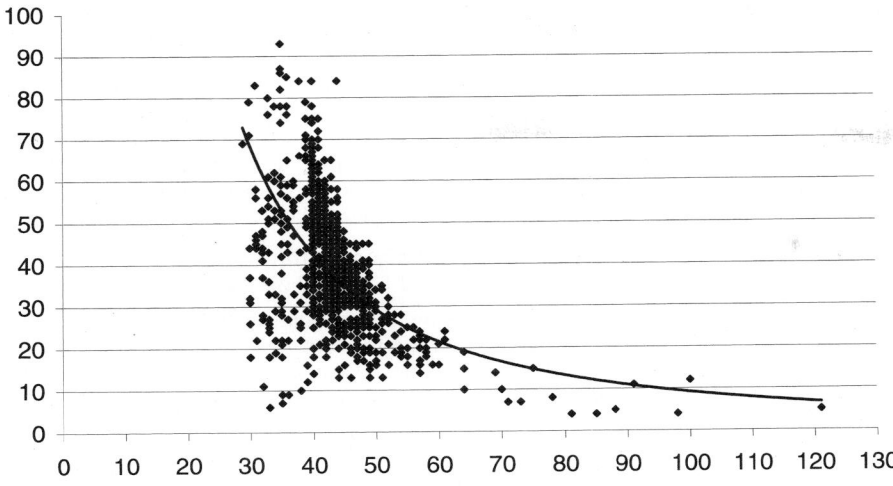

**Fig. 223-3** There is a strong inverse correlation between CAG repeat length and age at onset.

(Fig. 223-3). Translation of the protein is a requirement for the disease phenotype.[26]

## EPIDEMIOLOGY

### Prevalence and Incidence Studies: How Frequent Is This Illness?

Many different surveys presented from different parts of the world, including northwest Europe, the United Kingdom, Scandinavia, North America, Australia, Japan, and South Africa, have led to a general agreement that the frequency of HD in populations of western European descent is between 3 and 7 affected individuals per 100,000 population. The most recent epidemiologic survey that was performed in Europe, a study from Northern Ireland, yielded a 1991 prevalence rate of 6.4 per 100,000.[27] In this study, all prevalent cases were genotyped to obtain a certain diagnosis. One retrospective review of health care records in Olmsted County, Minnesota, yielded an average annual incidence rate for the period 1950 to 1989 of 0.3 [95 percent Confidence Interval (CI), 0.1–0.5] per 100,000 person-years for definite cases, and 0.6 (95 percent CI, 0.3–0.9) if probable cases were included.[28] This study did not use genotypic case ascertainment.

A few geographic areas show particularly high or low prevalence of HD. HD appears to be particularly uncommon in Japan[29] and among African blacks.[30] The prevalence of HD in Japan has been estimated at between 0.1 and 0.38 per 100,000, which is just below the prevalence in Finland of 0.5 per 100,000.[31] This prevalence is between 10 and 20 times less common than that seen in most Western countries (Table 223-1). Extensive studies in South Africa revealed that the disease is approximately 40 times less frequent in African blacks than in South African whites. Earlier studies from the United States[32,33] also showed that this disorder was approximately 3 times less frequent in American blacks than whites. However, a more detailed study by Folstein et al.[34] revealed that a prevalence in blacks was quite similar to

that seen in whites in the state of Maryland. In this study, multiple sources for ascertainment were used. However, the low prevalence of HD in Japan and Finland and in South African blacks clearly is not the result of underestimates but represents real differences in genetic background.[35,36]

Most genealogic studies have indicated that migration from northwest Europe was a primary factor responsible for the spread of the gene for HD around the world. A low prevalence of the disorder would be expected in those populations which have their origins outside Europe. For example, in Hong Kong, a 1991 prevalence of 2.5 affected individuals per 100,000 has been observed, and it has been suggested that the gene was introduced into the coastal population from Europe.[35–38]

The prevalence of HD exceeds 15 per 100,000 in five areas listed in Table 223-2. An important factor to be considered when assessing prevalence in a particular region is the total size of the surveyed population. In a small population, the presence of a few affected individuals will raise the disease prevalence.

This is obvious in the study of the Moray Firth area of Scotland, where a total of 5 affected individuals resulted in a calculated prevalence of 560 per 100,000 because the total of inhabitants in this region was under 1000. Similarly, an artificially high prevalence was found in Mauritius.[39]

The highest frequency of HD in the world in a larger population occurs in Venezuela at the edge of Lake Maracaibo.[40,41] The gene was introduced into this isolated community sometime in the early nineteenth century. The gene frequency has increased rapidly as a

**Table 223-1** Areas of Low Prevalence of Huntington's Disease

| Location | Author(s) | Rate (per 100,000) | No. of Patients | Population Size* |
|---|---|---|---|---|
| Japan | Kishimoto | 0.38 | 13 | 3,916,922 |
| Finland | Palo | 0.5 | 26 | ±4,900,000 |
| African blacks | Hayden | 0.06 | 11 | 16,640,314 |

*Calculated from data provided.

**Table 223-2** Areas of High Prevalence of Huntington's Disease

| Location | Author(s) | Rate (per 100,000) | No. of Patients | Population Size |
|---|---|---|---|---|
| North Sweden | Sjörgren | 144 | 18 | ±12,500 |
| Tasmania, Australia | Brothers | 174 | 105 | 60,344 |
| | Pridmore | 12.1 | 54 | ±447,000 |
| Moray Firth, Scotland | Lyon | 560 | 5 | 896 |
| Lake Maracaibo, Zulia, Venezuela | Avila-Giron | ±700 | 28 | ±4,000 |
| Mauritius (Caucasian) | Hayden | 46 | 16 | ±132,000 |

SOURCE: Used with permission from Hayden.[50]

result of the aggregation of affected persons in this relatively isolated area.

This population has offered a unique research opportunity for investigation of the natural history of this disorder as well as the understanding of the clinical features of the homozygous form of HD.[42] Identification of this large family with HD served to confirm the suspected linkage to G8, which was the initial discovery of linkage for the gene for HD to a polymorphic genetic marker on 4p. It was this family as well that allowed identification in 1993 of the unstable CAG repeat in the IT15 gene that causes the disease.[10]

While there have been numerous studies on the epidemiology of HD in most Western countries, there are regions for which information is extremely scanty. These include the Middle East and most of Asia. By now, patients with HD, diagnosed by an expanded CAG repeat, have been described in the former Soviet Union, Saudi Arabia, Egypt, Japan, Hong Kong, Taiwan, and mainland China, but the prevalence in these countries, as well as the ancestral origin of the gene, remains unknown.[35,43–46]

Since direct assessment of the CAG repeat in the huntingtin gene has become established for diagnostic purposes, numerous new families with HD have been identified. Individuals with late-onset HD, those with predominantly psychiatric manifestations, and individuals with new mutations for whom clinical diagnosis was difficult can now be diagnosed accurately. Therefore, the prevalence of the disease ultimately may turn out to be higher than previously estimated.

## Mortality Data

Mortality data are a poor indication of the frequency of the illness primarily due to underreporting. This has been particularly exacerbated since January 1, 1979, when HD was classified under the International Statistical Classification of Diseases (ISC) as the rubric 333.4, of which the 333 root is often the only one completed. Under the latter code are included many other diseases that occur with greater frequency than HD. Therefore, ISC data are of less value when trying to assess the number of deaths due to HD.

Detailed comparison of death rates due to HD for different countries has revealed that the similar results for northwest Europe and for U.S. whites range between 1 and 2.27 deaths per million of the population per year.[47] Careful analysis of mortality data for HD between 1968 and 1974 in the United States[48] revealed major variations in rates, with the highest being reported from South Dakota, Wyoming, and New Hampshire. North Dakota, Alaska, and Hawaii had no deaths coded for HD. These differences again may reflect biases of ascertainment with a small number of deaths in very small populations. Highly mortality rates in the states of California, Oregon, and Washington may reflect a true increase in prevalence in that part of the country.

## CLINICAL FEATURES: NATURAL HISTORY

### Age at Onset

HD is a slowly progressive disorder of insidious onset. A broad definition of age at onset is the first time any neurologic or psychiatric symptoms appear that represent a permanent change from the normal state. However, with this interpretation, estimation of the age of onset may be most difficult. Doctors seldom witness the earlier signs and symptoms of HD, and assessment of these early and insidious changes often depends on the patient themselves or their family. In some families, denial of early HD is commonplace, with acknowledgment of the presence of the disorder only in a more advanced form, whereas in others, any restlessness or clumsiness is ascribed to onset of the illness. In either situation, age at onset is commonly miscalculated. Moreover, in the various studies, either the onset of involuntary movements, the occurrence of minor motor abnormalities that precede these movements, the onset of depression, or the onset of mental alterations has been used to determine retrospectively the initial manifestations.

HD may start at any age. The youngest patient ever described was 2 years old when the disease started,[49] whereas some patients were noted to first develop signs of the disease in their mideighties.[49–51] Even within families, remarkable differences between individuals in disease onset were observed. Although in a majority of families the onset of affected individuals tended to be similar, many individual families were observed in which the disease tended to occur earlier in successive generations, a phenomenon called *anticipation*.[52]

## The Relationship between Trinucleotide (CAG) Repeat Length and Clinical Features of HD

A significant correlation between the number of CAG repeats and the age at onset of HD was demonstrated.[24,53–55] This association is present irrespective of the mode of clinical presentation at the time of onset. The number of trinucleotide repeats in the upper allele account for up to 70 percent of the variation in the age at onset.[24] Repeat length, however, is not indicative of any particular clinical phenotype because there is no independent association between any particular clinical feature of the illness and the number of repeats.

Is it possible to predict the age at which, in an individual, the signs and symptoms of HD will start? As was already pointed out in the initial studies that examined genotype-phenotype correlations, the scatter around the regression curve was too large to make meaningful predictions for individuals.[24,53–55] Another consideration is that in all series up to now, these curves have been constructed from a population of affected individuals, whereas asymptomatics gene carriers are not represented. Thus such a curve cannot be used in a situation in which an asymptomatic carrier requests information about when the disease is expected to start.

A useful approach to this problem has been to construct Kaplan-Meier curves (or life tables) that provide the likelihood of being affected at a particular age for any CAG size.[25] This is a refinement of an approach that was already provided by Harper et al.,[56] who prior to the discovery of CAG repeat expansion constructed a table that provided age-specific risk estimates (see Tables 223-3 and 223-4).

Many of these studies may be confounded by not including carefully ascertained at-risk persons with CAG expansion who are

**Table 223-3** Risk for a Healthy Subject at 50 percent Prior Risk of HD Carrying the HD Gene at Different Ages

| Age (years) | Risk (%) |
|---|---|
| 20.0 | 49.6 |
| 22.5 | 49.3 |
| 25.0 | 49.0 |
| 27.5 | 48.4 |
| 30.0 | 47.6 |
| 32.5 | 46.6 |
| 35.0 | 45.5 |
| 37.5 | 44.2 |
| 40.0 | 42.5 |
| 42.5 | 40.3 |
| 45.0 | 37.8 |
| 47.5 | 34.8 |
| 50.0 | 31.5 |
| 52.5 | 27.8 |
| 55.0 | 24.8 |
| 57.5 | 22.1 |
| 60.0 | 18.7 |
| 62.5 | 15.2 |
| 65.0 | 12.8 |
| 67.5 | 10.8 |
| 70.0 | 6.2 |
| 72.5 | 4.6 |

SOURCE: Adapted with permission from Harper and Newcombe.[56]

**Table 223-4  Observed Age at Onset by CAG Repeat Size**

| CAG Repeat Size | Median Age at Onset (years) | Range of Age at Onset (95% Confidence Intervals) (years) |
|---|---|---|
| 39 | 66 | 59–72 |
| 40 | 59 | 56–61 |
| 41 | 54 | 52–56 |
| 42 | 49 | 48–50 |
| 43 | 44 | 42–45 |
| 44 | 42 | 40–43 |
| 45 | 37 | 36–39 |
| 46 | 36 | 35–37 |
| 47 | 33 | 31–35 |
| 48 | 32 | 30–34 |
| 49 | 28 | 25–32 |
| 50 | 27 | 24–30 |

SOURCE: Reprinted with permission from Brinkaman et al.[25]

asymptomatic. Recently, one study including such persons showed that it is possible to use CAG size to predict with narrow confidence limits expected age at onset.[25] This study, if validated, also may provide useful information for design of clinical trials by facilitating selection of asymptomatic patients specifically according to their age and CAG size such that reduced sample size and duration of the trial is necessary to assess potential efficacy of a medication.

These recent data suggest that it may be possible to provide some information to persons at risk with regard to ranges or expected ages at onset for persons with particular CAG repeat lengths. However, these ranges are only an estimate for the population as a whole, and therefore, appropriate counseling to explain the details of such information is necessary.[25]

What else may explain the variance in onset? Genetic factors are likely to operate, as can be demonstrated by varying onset ages in family members with similar CAG sizes. However, the genes responsible are not known. One early publication suggested the length of the CAG repeat on the non-HD chromosome as a codeterminant, particularly in individuals who inherited this chromosome from their fathers.[54] This finding has never been replicated afterwards. Rubinsztein et al.,[57] in a comprehensive search for additional genetic factors, identified genotype variation in the kainate GluR6 receptor as a factor, which, in their material, would explain 13 percent of additional onset age variation. If this finding would be confirmed by others, it would support the role of excitotoxicity as a pathogenic mechanism in HD (see below).

In studies conducted prior to discovery of the HD gene and its mutation, the distribution of onset of signs or symptoms has been noted to be more or less normal, with a mean of around 40 and a standard deviation of approximately 10 years.[49,50] A major problem when considering population surveys of mean onset age is the truncated interval of observation that may artificially lower the age at onset because this may contain no information from asymptomatic heterozygotes who have not yet manifested signs of the disorder at the time of the study.[58]

To correct the problem of truncated intervals of observation, Wendt et al.[59] restricted their analysis to cohorts born 60 years prior to the time of data analysis and reported a mean age at onset of 43.97, which is higher than other studies. When the study of Newcombe et al.[58] was limited to persons born before 1909, the mean age at onset was 48.4 years. A successive decrease in the mean age at onset occurred as one got closer to the current time of analysis. Similarly, in the study of Adams et al.,[60] the mean age at onset in the total sample of 611 patients was 38.6 years. However, restriction of the analysis to persons born in 1920 resulted in a mean age at onset of 43.7 years. In a series of 800 deceased Dutch patients, a much higher mean age, of 55.8 years (SD 13.5 years) was observed.[61] Therefore, the mean age at onset in most of the studies may have

been underestimated as a result of the effect of the truncated intervals of observation. The proportion of people developing HD at an advanced age may be higher than previously estimated.

## Age at Death

While the age at death is a specific point in time, a survey of the mean ages at death in a population would be subject to the same biases of ascertainment as seen with age at onset; e.g., the assessment of a recent cohort would not include those who are longer survivors.

The mean age at death in different studies varies from a low of 51.4[62] to a high of 62.9 years.[63] In all instances, those studies with lower ages at death have had lower ages at onset, suggesting that this does not reflect variation in duration of the disease. The mean age at death in Tasmania is the oldest reported for any geographic region and is consistent with the finding of mean age at onset of 48.3 years in that region. The largest study of HD mortality and causes of death recently reported was based on the national data made available through the U.S. National Center of Health Statistics for all causes of death reported on death certificates.[47] In this study of 3058 persons, the mean age at death was 56.5 years. The leading causes of death in persons with HD were pneumonia (33 percent) and heart disease (24 percent).[64,65] Suicide only represented between 1 to 3 percent of deaths but is likely to be underreported. If one assumes death due to suicide in all cases in which accidental poisonings and violence were reported, this would account for approximately 8 percent of deaths. Pneumonia occurs five times more commonly in HD patients than in controls and is likely to be secondary to the significant dysphagia that results in choking and aspiration pneumonia.

## Duration of HD and Rate of Progression

The duration of HD is estimated by subtracting the age at onset from age at death. In contrast to the considerable differences in the age at onset and age at death in different studies, there are no significant variations in duration of disease, which is around 15 years, with no differences between the sexes.[49,50] For example, in a retrospective study of a cohort of 1106 patients, a median disease duration of 16.2 years (range 2–45 years) was found. Almost 20 percent of the patients survived the onset of choreatic movements for more than 23 years.[61] One lesson from these studies would be that even though the mean duration in many different studies has been quite consistent, there are marked individual variations, extending up to as much as 40 years from time of onset on rare occasions. It would appear that in some families, HD follows a milder course with longer survival. A second lesson would be that survival with HD has not significantly changed over the past 50 years, which reflects the failure of medical therapy to delay disease progression.

The factors that are associated with longer survival and disease progression in families are not yet clear, but again, CAG size may play a role. In a 2-year longitudinal study, patients with repeat sizes of 37 to 46 were found to deteriorate less rapidly on a quantified neurologic examination score, an activities of daily living assessment, and a cognitive measurement than those with CAG repeat sizes of 47 and over.[66] Other authors using different measurements of decline were unable to observe such a correlation.[67,68] For example, in a cohort of 50 patients who were followed prospectively for at least a few years, the major index of disease progression, namely, a total functional capacity scale, did not reveal a relationship between functional deterioration and CAG repeat size.[69]

## CLINICAL MANIFESTATIONS: SIGNS AND SYMPTOMS

HD is characterized clinically by a progressive illness that consists of motor abnormalities (predominantly associated with the extrapyramidal motor system), cognitive alterations, and psychiatric dysfunction (Fig. 223-4).

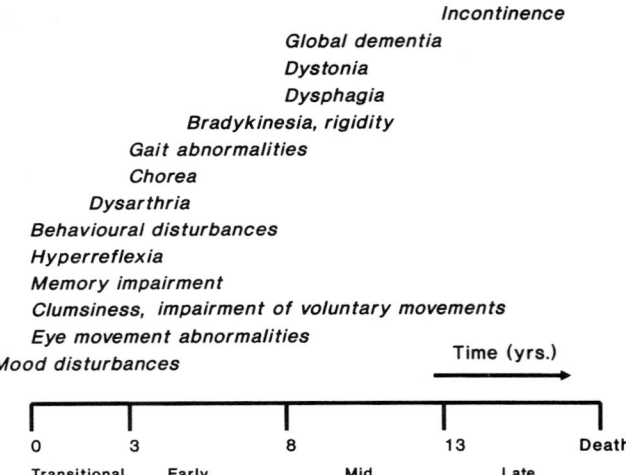

Incontinence
Global dementia
Dystonia
Dysphagia
Bradykinesia, rigidity
Gait abnormalities
Chorea
Dysarthria
Behavioural disturbances
Hyperreflexia
Memory impairment
Clumsiness, impairment of voluntary movements
Eye movement abnormalities
Mood disturbances

Time (yrs.)

0    3         8         13        Death
Transitional  Early     Mid       Late

**Fig. 223-4 Clinical phases and associated signs and symptoms in the natural history of Huntington's disease.**

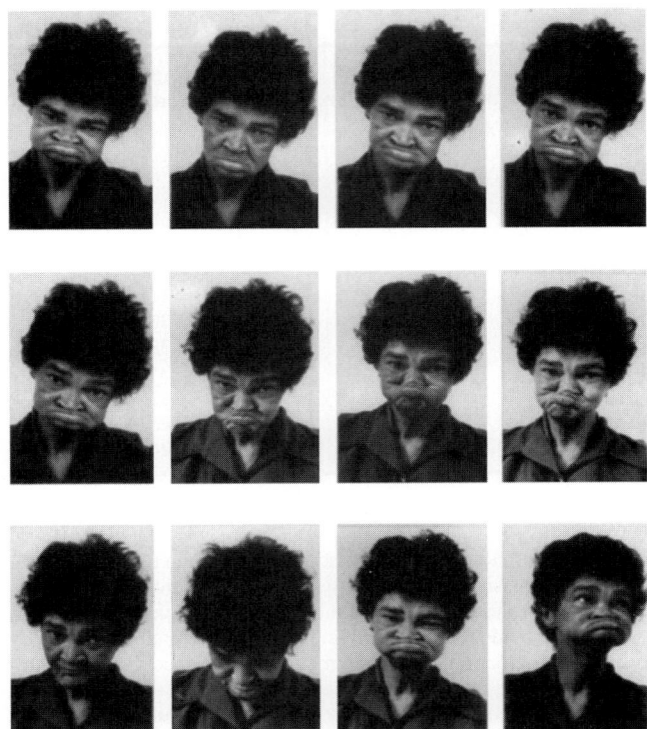

**Fig. 223-5 Orofacial dyskinesia in a patient with Huntington's disease. (*From Hayden*[50] *with permission.*)**

## Presenting Signs and Symptoms

HD does not have a specific single presenting sign or symptom. In the earliest phases, there is an insidious and slow deterioration of intellectual function as well as mild personality change. A most comprehensive way of assessing the signs and symptoms of HD is to follow a cohort for an extended period of time. The longitudinal study of the kindred in Venezuela[70] has clearly demonstrated that patients pass through a zone of onset that represents a transitional state from the normal presymptomatic phase to the time at which the diagnosis can be made clearly on neurologic examination. This zone of onset during which the diagnosis of HD cannot be made unequivocally is frequently witnessed by changes in caudate metabolic rates of glucose, as seen on positron-emission tomography (PET).[71,72]

The clear appearance of such extrapyramidal signs as chorea, hypokinesia, rigidity, or dystonia marks a phase in the disease progression, not the beginning of disease. In recent years, the longitudinal study of a large cohort of at-risk people in Venezuela,[70] follow-up of individuals in predictive testing programs, and application of PET scanning to individuals without overt chorea have provided valuable information on the earliest clinical manifestations of the disease. Most individuals will display minor motor abnormalities initially. These include general restlessness, abnormal eye movements or impaired optokinetic nystagmus, hyperreflexia, impaired finger tapping or rapid alternating hand movements, and excessive and inappropriate movements of the fingers, hands, or toes during emotional stress,[70,73] as well as mild dysarthria. Minor motor abnormalities usually precede the obvious signs of extrapyramidal dysfunction by at least 3 years.[70] Persons with a completely normal neurologic examination have a 3 percent chance of being diagnosed within the next 3 years.[70]

## Extrapyramidal Motor Signs

**Chorea.** Chorea is the major motor sign of the disease, hence the old name *Huntington's chorea*. These involuntary movements are continuously present during waking hours, cannot be suppressed voluntarily by the patient, and worsen during stress. Although the pattern of the movements may differ between affected patients, they occur in individual patients in a stereotypic manner. Choreic movements of the face are common and present as pouting of the lips, irregular grimacing, twitching of the cheeks, and alternate lifting of the eyebrows and frowning (Fig. 223-5). The neck is often involved, causing forward or backward bending of the head or rotation. Choreic movements of the trunk move the body in different directions. Breathing may become irregular. In the limbs,

there is frequent flexion and extension of the fingers. The legs may be alternately crossed and uncrossed and the toes flexed and extended. Chorea is a feature of HD in over 90 percent of patients, increasing during the first phase (~10 years) of the patients' illness. With advancing duration, features of bradykinesia, rigidity, and dystonia become more evident.[41,50,74] Chorea is seen less frequently in patients with juvenile-onset[50,75] disease and rarely may be absent in adult-onset patients.[76]

**Bradykinesia and Rigidity.** Bradykinesia and rigidity, best known as the core features of Parkinson's disease, are infrequent in the early phases of adult-onset HD. However, they appear gradually until they often dominate the final stages of the illness, in which the patient will become severely rigid and grossly akinetic.[41,70,73] Early in the illness, bradykinesia alone may contribute to an impairment in voluntary motor performance.[77] Some patients display a significant decrease in overall daytime motor activity suggestive of hypokinesia.[78] A minority of adult patients start with rigidity and severe hypokinesia that has been described as the *Westphal variant* of the disease.[79,80] In both juvenile and adult rigid cases, a coarse resting tremor, distinct from a parkinsonian tremor, may complement the clinical picture.[76,81] The use of neuroleptic drugs, intended to suppress choreic movements, may aggravate the existing bradykinesia and rigidity.

**Dystonia.** Dystonia, characterized by slow abnormal movements and abnormal posturing, is infrequent in the early symptomatic period but worsens and becomes a prominent feature toward the later stages of the illness.[41,81] These extrapyramidal motor abnormalities are the most specific signs of the disease and, in most clinical situations, reliable indicators of the fact that the disease is present in an individual.

## Other Motor Abnormalities

*Oculomotor disturbances* are among the earliest signs and are present in the vast majority of affected patients.[82,83] Saccades display the earliest abnormalities, with inability to suppress reflexive glances to suddenly appearing novel stimuli and delayed initiation of voluntary saccades.[84] Later in the disease, slowing of saccades may be seen in up to 75 percent of symptomatic individuals,[82,83] especially in early-onset cases[85] more particularly affecting the vertical rather than horizontal movements. Impaired pursuit with saccadic intrusions, impairment of gaze fixation due to distractability, slowing of optokinetic nystagmus, and inability to suppress blinking during saccades also may occur.[70,82,83,85,86] Conjugate gaze disturbances may be prominent in rigid cases.[82]

A nonspecific but early sign is impairment of *voluntary motor function*.[77,86,87] Patients and their families describe clumsiness in common daily activities. Clear abnormalities of rapid alternating movements already may be observed in the transitional phase. Disturbances in motor speed, fine motor control, and gait correlate with disease progression and appear to be better measures of duration of illness than chorea.[88] Clumsiness may increase with deterioration of functional capacity.[41]

*Hyperactive reflexes* occur early in up to 90 percent of patients, whereas clonus and extensor plantar responses occur late and are less frequent.[41,50] Again, these latter phenomena are predominant in juvenile and advanced adult cases.[41] Frontal release reflexes such as snouting, sucking, or grasping typically accompany significant cognitive decline.

*Gait disturbances* ultimately result in severe disability.[50,79] Subtle changes in gait may be observed early in the illness, including difficulty with tandem walking, sudden stopping on command, and turning.[89] With more advanced disease, walking difficulties are more pronounced. As a consequence, patients experience frequent falls with significant associated morbidity and often ultimate confinement to a wheelchair. Gait disturbances exist at least partially independent from chorea, since neuroleptic treatment that suppresses choreic movements does not improve the gait disturbance.[89]

Most patients display *speech abnormalities*,[50] that are present early in the illness.[41,90,91] Initially, mild disturbance of clarity appears, but this is aggravated by changes in rate and rhythm of speech as the disease progresses.

*Dysphagia*, or swallowing impairment, generally occurs later in progression of the illness. Initially this primarily may affect intake of fluids but later also will affect intake of solids. Choking with aspiration secondary to dysphagia is a common cause of morbidity.

## Cognitive Disturbances

A global decline in cognitive capabilities ultimately is present in all HD patients.[79] While global measurements of cognitive function initially may be preserved,[92-95] a typical pattern of decline becomes apparent very early in the disease, including slowness of thought, altered personality, affective changes, and impaired ability to integrate new knowledge. The designation *subcortical dementia* evokes anatomic correlations, but its main value is to stress the difference from the pattern of dementia occurring in Alzheimer's, Pick's, or Creutzfeldt-Jakob disease. In these, aphasia, alexia, agnosia, and apraxia are prominent, whereas they are rare in HD.[96,97]

*Memory impairment* is common early in the disease and often is one of the patient's presenting symptoms.[92] Visuospatial memory is particularly affected, involving visual retention,[95] whereas verbal memory remains fairly preserved until late.[95,98,99] For example, patients have difficulty reproducing geometric designs but may remember facts, words, or stories. This deficit may be part of the more encompassing defect in visuospatial processing described below.[100] Retrieval of information is impaired,[101,102] but verbal cues, priming, and sufficient time may lead to partial or correct recall.[93,98,103,104] Recall of recent and remote events is equally impaired.[93,105]

The learning and acquiring of new motor skills (procedural memory) is also affected in HD.[106-108] In contrast to other amnestic syndromes, orientation in both time and place remains intact until late in the illness.[109]

*Attention and concentration* are affected early,[95] resulting in easy distractibility by interfering stimuli. Difficulty in performing sustained simple motor tasks such as gazing laterally, sticking out the tongue, or tightly closing the eyelids may be a manifestation of this distractibility rather than motor disturbance. Problems with organizing, sequencing, and planning; inability to coordinate and initiate complex actions; and inability to maintain a mental set or organize cognitive strategies constitute other early impairments.[92-94,110] Particularly difficult for HD patients to perform are tasks that require the shifting of attention.[100,111] For example, patients will explain that they are unable to watch TV and talk at the same time, a task that requires a constant shift of attention from TV to the conversation and back. These functions traditionally have been ascribed to circuitry in which the frontal lobe plays an important role.

*Language and related functions* remain intact. Although speech production and fluency may be severely reduced, the dementia of HD is nonphasic.[92] Dysarthria, slowness, and lack of initiative interfere significantly with fluency and spontaneous speech,[112] but semantic and syntactic structure, word finding, and speech comprehension remain intact until the final stages of the disease.[76,90] Difficulties in writing and recognition of objects have been ascribed to defective nonlinguistic modalities, such as visuoperceptual analysis, attention and concentration, and overall cognition.[90,92,112,113] In contrast, simple naming of daily objects, as tested in the Mini Mental State Examination, may remain intact until the latest stages of the disease.[109]

Expression and perception of the musical, tonal, rhythmic, nonlinguistic aspects of language (*prosody*), which are functions of nondominant hemisphere structures (analogous to those mediating language in the dominant hemisphere), are impaired in affected HD patients.[114]

Specialized neuropsychological tests reveal impaired *visuospatial abilities*, particularly in later stages of the disease.[92,100] However, patients are oriented to time and place, able to dress themselves, and have no obvious spatial neglect until late in the illness. Clearly, in comparison with Alzheimer's disease, visuospatial disturbances are relatively preserved in HD.[76] Similarly, a patient's insight into his or her deteriorating cognitive abilities, which is absent in Alzheimer's disease, remains intact.

Various groups have addressed the issue of whether asymptomatic gene carriers do display subtle cognitive defects. The issue is that cognitive defects may precede the recognizable motor abnormalities by years. Individuals with an expanded CAG repeat may be identified who perform poorly on tests of executive functions and memory tasks, and their performance may be related to the size of their CAG expansion.[115] These individuals have a total lack of motor or psychiatric signs. But alternatively, many individuals with expanded repeats may perform perfectly equal or superior to matched controls. Only close to the estimated age at onset as predicted by CAG repeat length[25] will minor deficits in selected cognitive domains become apparent.[116] These findings illustrate two issues: Individual gene carriers pass through a truly asymptomatic phase, and HD may start with nonspecific cognitive abnormalities rather than the motor abnormalities that allow a definite diagnosis.

## Psychiatric Disturbances

Although psychiatric disturbances are as characteristic for the disease as motor and cognitive abnormalities, these appear less consistently[92] and are not necessarily related to the severity of motor abnormalities, cognitive changes, or CAG repeat size.[117-119] In rare families, psychosis and a schizophrenia-like disorder may be a consistent first manifestation of the disease.[120] However, due to the nonspecific nature, the occurrence of a psychiatric episode should never be considered as the onset of the disease.

Changes in *mood and affect* are common, ranging from anxiety and ill-defined irritability to prolonged periods of depression.[76,121] Suicide is more common in HD patients than in the affected population and may be a significant cause of death of patients in their earlier stages.[122] Manic or hypomanic episodes also occur with increased frequency. Approximately 10 percent of patients have transient episodes of increased activity, pressured speech, uncharacteristic cheerfulness, and transient return of sexual interest after a long period of libido loss and impotence.[76] Affective syndromes may precede the first signs of motor impairment by many years[76] and usually do not manifest for the first time late in the illness.[123]

*Behavioral disturbances,* as evidenced by apathy, aggressive behavior, sexual disinhibition, and alcohol abuse, are other symptoms seen in HD patients.[121] They may be either a manifestation of the progressive cognitive decline or, alternatively, manifestations of the mood disturbances, especially if they are reversible and related to the premorbid personality.[124]

*Delusions* are common, occurring in up to 50 percent of the patients with advanced disease.[121] They may be seen in depressive or manic episodes, or they may be isolated and frequently are paranoid in nature. In contrast, *hallucinations* are less common.[50]

## Other Abnormalities

*Weight loss* and striking emaciation are features of late HD.[79] Clinical follow-up[125] and anthropometric studies[126] with dietary assessment[127] all show that the vast majority of HD patients lose weight in the course of the disease. This weight loss may occur in conjunction with adequate dietary intake[125,127] or even increased carbohydrate intake.[126]

*Sleep* may be disturbed in advanced disease, with frequent nocturnal sleeplessness and reversal of the day-night pattern of sleep.[128] In early disease, sleep is essentially normal.[128–130] Choreic movements disappear during sleep.

Approximately 20 percent of all patients are *incontinent* of urine and feces in the terminal phases of the illness, whereas in early symptomatic persons, incontinence rarely occurs.[50] In incontinent patients with frequency, urgency, and nocturia, detrusor hyperreflexia without sphincter dyssynergia is apparent. Choreatic contractions have been recorded electromyographically from the perineal musculature in affected patients.[131]

It has been suggested that patients are abnormally sensitive to barbiturate *anesthesia* and may exhibit prolonged apnea,[132–134] but these reports have been disputed.[135–137] The weight loss and poor general condition of these patients may make them susceptible to the adverse effects of anesthesia.

**Assessment of Functional Decline.** Questionnaires have been developed that rate disability in terms of how the patient functions in his or her daily life.[138,139] An example is shown in Table 223-5. Simple to score, the results of these disability rating scales correlate strongly with various clinical parameters of disease progression.[41,70,73]

Chorea, unless very severe, does not appear to constitute a major impairment to normal function. Neuroleptic drugs that suppress choreic movements do not improve the functional ratings.[140] Furthermore, during the late stages, a diminished severity of choreatic movements without improvement in function is apparent. These findings caution against the use of neuroleptic medication in the later stages of illness.

## Early- and Late-Onset Disease

*Juvenile cases* with onset before age 20 constitute approximately 10 percent of all patients with HD. The youngest patient described had onset at age 3.[49,51] In line with the general (inverse) relation between onset age and length of the CAG repeat, juvenile cases have the longest repeats, with sizes typically exceeding 50 triplets.

In contrast to adult cases, bradykinesia and rigidity are conspicuous from early in the illness, dominating the neurologic findings in about 50 percent of patients.[49–51,79,141,142] Chorea is present in almost all patients but is often of short duration and is superseded by rigidity.[50] Frequent falls, dysarthria, clumsiness, hyperreflexia, and oculomotor disturbances are frequent in children with HD and occur early. Although it has been suggested that cerebellar dysfunction as elicited from the neurologic examination may be observed in juvenile patients,[41,50] we have never seen ataxia in HD. Mental deterioration is first manifested by declining school performance. Over the years, a severe progressive dementia develops.

Epileptic seizures, occurring with a similar frequency in adult HD patients as in the general adult population (1 percent),[50] are more common in early-onset patients, with an estimated 30 to 50 percent of juvenile patients affected.[50,51,143] Partial or generalized, tonic-clonic, or absence seizures all may appear. Seizures should be differentiated from myoclonic jerks, which also occur rarely in adult patients.[144] The epilepsy of juvenile HD patients is often difficult to control.

Thus the overall clinical picture of juvenile HD suggests more severe disease than in adult patients, and this clinical impression is supported by the presence of longer triplet repeat sizes in the huntingtin gene.

In contrast, the manifestations in *late-onset disease* are less severe. Approximately 25 percent of all patients will display first signs and symptoms after age 50, and in these patients, the disease will follow slower progression than usual, although the number of years they survive after disease onset may not be much different from that of patients with earlier-onset disease.[139,145] Chorea is the presenting motor disorder, and gait disturbances and dysphagia are common, though not severe. Cognitive impairment, although invariably present, may be less debilitating than in younger patients, and psychiatric manifestations may occur less often.[139,145] Families have been described in which cognitive deterioration and mental changes seemed to be totally absent, chorea in old age being the exclusive manifestation of the

**Table 223-5** Functional Designation of Patients with Huntington's Chorea

| Stage | Engagement in Occupation Score | Capacity to Handle Financial Affairs Score | Capacity to Manage Domestic Responsibility Score | Capacity to Perform Activities of Daily Living Score | Care Can Be Provided at Score |
|---|---|---|---|---|---|
| Stage 1 Usual level | 3 Full | 3 Full | 2 Full | 3 Full | 2 Home |
| Stage 2 Lower level | 2 Requires slight help | 2 Full | 2 Full | 3 Full | 2 Home |
| Stage 3 Marginal | 1 Requires major help | 1 Impaired | 1 Mildly impaired | 2 Mildly impaired | 2 Home |
| Stage 4 Unable | 0 Unable | 0 Unable | 0 Moderately impaired | 1 Moderately impaired | 1 Home extended care facility |
| Stage 5 Unable | 0 Unable | 0 Unable | 0 Severely impaired | 0 Unable | 0 Total care facility only |

SOURCES: From Shoulson and Fahn[138]; adapted from Hayden.[50]

disease.[146] An older onset is associated with a slower disease progression, as measured by functional disability.[139] This generally milder form of the disease is associated with shorter repeat lengths.[145,147]

## CLINICAL FEATURES: DIAGNOSIS

### Diagnosis of HD

Prior to discovery of the HD gene, a definite diagnosis of HD would be made in the presence of (1) a positive family history, consistent with autosomal dominant inheritance, (2) progressive motor disability involving both involuntary and voluntary movement, and (3) mental disturbances including cognitive decline, affective disturbances, and/or changes in personality. Despite these criteria, misdiagnosis occurred fairly frequently. In a community-based survey in the state of Maryland, 11 percent of 212 patients had previously received another (false) diagnosis, whereas 15 percent could not be confirmed to have HD on closer examination.[75] In an older unselected autopsy series, 7 percent of the patients diagnosed as having HD had some other neurologic condition.[148]

At present, a diagnosis can be made with virtually 100 percent certainty when the clinical demonstration of signs that are consistent with HD can be matched by the demonstration of an expanded CAG repeat in the huntingtin gene. Even in the absence of a positive family history, this approach will lead to the correct diagnosis. Molecular DNA diagnosis, based on polymerase chain reaction (PCR) amplification of the expanded repeat has a sensitivity and specificity of almost 100 percent.[23] Therefore, HD currently should only be diagnosed in the presence of an expanded repeat.

Only when patients demonstrate minor motor abnormalities, subtle cognitive changes, or psychiatric episodes while lacking the specific extrapyramidal motor abnormalities does the question arise as to whether the disease has begun. Demonstration of the presence of an expanded CAG repeat in an as yet completely asymptomatic person should never be confounded with making a diagnosis of HD. Such persons do not suffer from a disease.

### Differential Diagnosis

Due to the enormous advance in accuracy of making a diagnosis of HD that nowadays can be obtained with molecular testing, the consideration of an extensive differential diagnosis is no longer particularly relevant. Only in case of hereditary or sporadic chorea without CAG expansion should an extensive list of diseases be considered.[149] Only a few disorders that may closely mimic HD will be considered here.

Among the patients with noninherited chorea, those with *tardive dyskinesia* may resemble HD patients closely, particularly if the underlying psychiatric disorder and associated cognitive changes are taken into consideration. The absence of an expanded CAG repeat will exclude HD.

*Benign hereditary chorea* (OMIM 118700 for the common autosomal dominant form, 215450 for a rare, possibly recessive form) is usually nonprogressive without dementia. However, in rare instances, the phenotype may be more severe. In most families, autosomal dominant heredity can be demonstrated. This disease is, in all likelihood, different from HD at the molecular level, since patients and families have failed to demonstrate the mutation seen in HD.[23,150,151]

*Neuroacanthocytosis* (OMIM 100500) is inherited as an autosomal dominant trait. However, the occurrence of muscle wasting, absent lower limb tendon reflexes, clinical and electrophysiologic signs of motor neuropathy, epilepsy, orolingual dystonia, self-mutilation, and only mild dementia aid in the differentiation from HD. Laboratory findings are typical acanthocytes in a thick wet blood smear and an elevated serum creatine kinase level.[152]

*Dentatorubropallidoluysian atrophy* (DRPLA); (OMIM 125370) may closely resemble HD, and sometimes neuropathology may provide the only distinction.[153] The similarities extend to the molecular level; the disorder is caused by an expanded CAG repeat in the DRPLA gene on chromosome 12, which can be simply demonstrated.[154,155] Although the disease is extremely rare in patients of non-Japanese descent, European Caucasian families have been described, as well as a black American family.

*Senile chorea* was a diagnosis reserved for patients with late-onset (typically after age 60) chorea. Often these patients show mild cognitive defects as well, but only about half of them turn out to have HD.[156,157]

### Laboratory Investigations

For clinical purposes, the single most important investigation of a patient with a clinical suspicion of HD is the assessment of CAG repeat length in the huntingtin gene. Using PCR primers that closely flank the CAG repeat and exclude the adjacent CCG repeat, the length of the repeat can be assessed accurately. With these primers, one is able to determine the limits in a very large series of almost 1000 patients.[23] All affected individuals had CAG repeat sizes on the affected allele of 36 or higher, whereas controls had sizes ranging from 10 to 29 (median, 18). A group of individuals from HD families had intermediate repeat sizes that ranged from 30 to 35. Despite the fact that the individual was not affected by HD, these alleles showed instability in meiotic transmission. Therefore, for diagnostic purposes, a repeat length of 36 or longer, in the presence of a typical clinical syndrome, should be confirmatory of the diagnosis of HD.

No additional investigations need to be performed for strict diagnostic purposes. Competent neuropsychological testing, a comprehensive psychiatric assessment, or a complete neurologic examination may clarify doubts about the exact clinical symptomatology, but having resolved these issues, the diagnosis should be clear. There is currently no strict diagnostic indication for computed tomography (CT), magnetic resonance imaging (MRI), or neurophysiologic investigations. [18F] Deoxyglucose PET may be considered if a suspicion of very early disease is present (Fig. 223-6). The demonstration of caudate hypometabolism may be considered a sign of impending disease.[71,72]

## GENETICS

HD is inherited as an autosomal dominant trait. This implies that the gene is transmitted by parents of either sex to children of either sex. Each child of an affected parent has an even chance of inheriting the gene.

### Reduced Penetrance

In the past it has been stated repeatedly that HD is completely penetrant. However, it is now evident that only a proportion of patients with CAG between 36 and 41 may manifest within their expected lifespan.[25,158,159] The exact frequency of nonpenetrance is uncertain, but as the CAG is closer to 36, a greater proportion of persons would not be expected to manifest signs of the disease in their lifetimes.

### Homozygosity for HD

Offspring of two parents affected with HD are rare, and only a few occurrences of this nature have been well documented. In one Venezuelan family, 4 of the 14 siblings were shown by DNA segregation analysis to be homozygous for the DNA haplotype with which the HD gene was segregating.[42] Interestingly, there were no clinical features that would distinguish these persons from heterozygotes for this illness.

Therefore, the homozygous form for HD may be different from other autosomal dominant inherited disorders such as familial hypercholesterolemia or hereditary hemorrhagic telangiectasia, where homozygotes have a much more severe manifestation of the illness or even other trinucleotide expansion disease such as

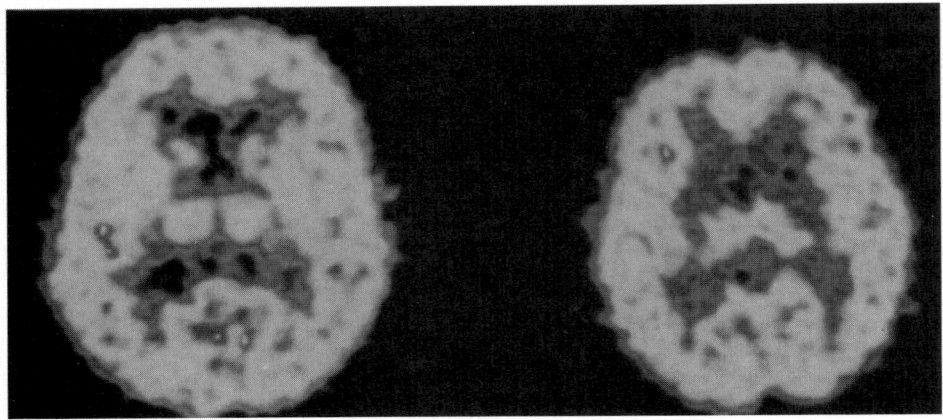

Fig. 223-6 Positron-emission tomographic scan using [$^{18}$F] deoxyglucose showing marked hypometabolism in the caudate nucleus and the putamen in a patient (right) as compared with a control subject (left). The basal ganglia were of normal size on a CT scan.

SCA3, where the homozygote is more seriously affected than the heterozygote.[160]

## Molecular Analysis of New Mutations

New mutations causing HD were proposed to be exceedingly rare, with the mutation rate estimated as the lowest for any human genetic disease.[49,161] Recent data contradict this view, with clear demonstration of the sequence of molecular events underlying new mutations for HD. In these instances, new mutations arise from intermediate alleles with CAG lengths of 29 to 35 that expand as transmission through the male germ line.[159,162]

These findings have significant genetic implications for family members of sporadic cases, in particular for siblings of such affected persons. In the past, there was no appreciation that the unaffected siblings of a sporadic HD patient might indeed have an increased risk of manifesting with HD in the future because they also may inherit an expanded HD allele. Similarly, children of unaffected siblings are also at slightly increased risk of having children with HD. This latter risk would depend on whether the intermediate allele undergoes expansion during transmission through the male germ line. Female siblings who carry the intermediate allele, however, have not been shown to pass on an expanded allele resulting in HD in their offspring.[163]

## Molecular Analysis of Juvenile HD

Juvenile HD shows remarkable features with respect to the sex of the transmitting parent. While the sex incidence for juvenile HD is equal, approximately 80 percent of juvenile patients inherit the defective gene from their father.[49] For children who have onset at up to 10 years of age (childhood onset), approximately 90 percent inherit the gene from their father, whereas approximately 75 percent of persons with adolescent onset (11–20 years) have paternal descent.[50]

Different factors have been proposed to account for this finding. Maternal protective factors mediated through mitochondria or other cytoplasmic influences are compatible with the results of some studies that have shown a greater correlation for age at onset between mother-child than for father-child pairs.[164] Imprinting[165] and, more recently, selective amplification of repeat sequences within the genome were suggested as mechanisms to explain the paternal transmission effect.[166]

The predominance of paternal descent in juvenile HD is not in accordance with classic Mendelian genetics and until the discovery of the gene remained a statistical fact with no adequate biologic explanation. It has however been shown that the size of the CAG repeat may expand and that the CAG repeat is most unstable, leading to amplification when transmitted through the male germ line, with earlier onset in such children.[166,167]

A strong biologic correlate for juvenile HD is the size of the CAG repeat, which is influenced primarily by the sex of the affected parent.[166]

## THE GENE PRODUCT

### Regional and Cellular Distribution of HD mRNA and Protein

Northern blot and in situ hybridization analysis indicates that the 10.3- and 13.6-kb transcripts are expressed in many tissues, with higher expression of the longer transcript in brain.[10,12,168,169] HD mRNA is expressed in both neural and nonneural tissues, with high levels of expression in neurons, testes, ovaries, and lung.[168–170] HD mRNA levels are low in pancreas, smooth muscle, and liver.[168] These studies suggest that selective neuronal loss in HD cannot be explained by differential expression of the HD gene in different tissues.

Similar to RNA studies, protein studies also indicate ubiquitous expression of huntingtin.[171,172] An approximately 350-kDa protein is detected in rodent neural and nonneural tissues, in various human cell lines, and in adult human peripheral tissues and brain.[171–173] Huntingtin expression is high in brain, moderate in testes, and low in other peripheral tissues. In brain, huntingtin is detected mainly in neurons.[171,172]

Two recent studies show that huntingtin expression in the nervous system may be more heterogeneous than suggested by earlier studies.[174,175] Both studies show that striatal interneurons that are spared in HD have low levels of expression of huntingtin. However, huntingtin immunoreactivity is confined primarily to neurons and neuropils in the matrix area in humans[174] and predominantly in the striosomes (patch), with much less immunoreactivity in matrix, in rat brain.[175] Neuropathologic studies have suggested that striatal matrix is affected in HD to a greater extent than striosomes,[176] but striosomes may be the earliest affected region.[177] These studies suggest that huntingtin is expressed at higher levels in neurons that die selectively in HD.

### Mutant versus Wild-Type Huntingtin Expression

Mutant huntingtin can be distinguished from the wild-type protein on Western blot by virtue of its anomalous migration.[171,173,178–181] However, similar regional distribution of both mutant and wild-type protein is evident. There is no evidence for reduced production or increased turnover of the mutant protein.[178,180] The accessibility of different epitopes targeted by antibodies used in the experiments may be affected differently by the polyglutamine expansion.

### Subcellular Distribution

Both nuclear and cytosolic localizations have been reported.[15,171,172,182–185] Using immunocytochemical and biochemical studies, huntingtin has been detected in both cytoplasm and nucleus in cultured human and mouse cells.[15,182,183]

However, immunohistochemical studies in human, monkey, and rat show that huntingtin is present exclusively in the neuronal cytoplasm, enriched in nerve endings, and associated with synaptic vesicles.[171,172,184,185] Biochemical data also suggest that wild-type and mutant huntingtin are present in cytosolic soluble fractions and microsomal membranes and associated with the cytoskeleton.[172,184,186] In affected human brains, mutant huntingtin is translocated into the nucleus.

## Interacting Proteins

Several proteins that interact directly with huntingtin have now been described.[187-193] Four of these proteins have been identified either using N-terminal portions of huntingtin containing the polyglutamine tract in yeast two-hybrid screens or by searching for proteins that interact directly with the polyglutamine tract itself using biochemical methods. However, it should be remembered that huntingtin is a large protein of 348 kDa and is likely to have an expansive repertoire of interacting proteins. Indeed, in gel filtration and Western blot studies under nondenaturing conditions, huntingtin migrates in a large (> 1000-kDa) complex, indicating the possibility of many direct or indirect interacting proteins.[192]

## NEUROPATHOLOGIC AND NEUROCHEMICAL ALTERATIONS

The most characteristic neuropathologic abnormalities are neuronal loss and concomitant gliosis in the caudate nucleus and, to a somewhat lesser extent, the putamen (together called the *neostriatum*). However, the pathology is not restricted to the neostriatum. The globus pallidus, various cortical areas, and several subcortical structures are affected. The evolution of the neuropathologic striatal abnormalities also follows a characteristic course; the sequence of extrastriatal neurodegeneration has not yet been established. The relation that has been established for CAG length and clinical course is reflected (and in all likelihood has its origin) in the relationship between CAG length and neuropathologic alterations.

## Striatal Changes

Since the descriptions of Anglade,[194] Jelgersma,[195] and Alzheimer,[196] atrophy of the caudate nucleus and the putamen (the neostriatum) has been considered the most characteristic pathologic feature of the disease.[79] Yet the severity of neostriatal abnormalities is highly variable. In a series of 163 clinically diagnosed patients, 13 lacked macroscopically visible atrophy, whereas in 18 patients the caudate was extremely shrunken and the putamen markedly atrophic[176] (Fig. 223-7). This variability is reported in all large series.[197-200]

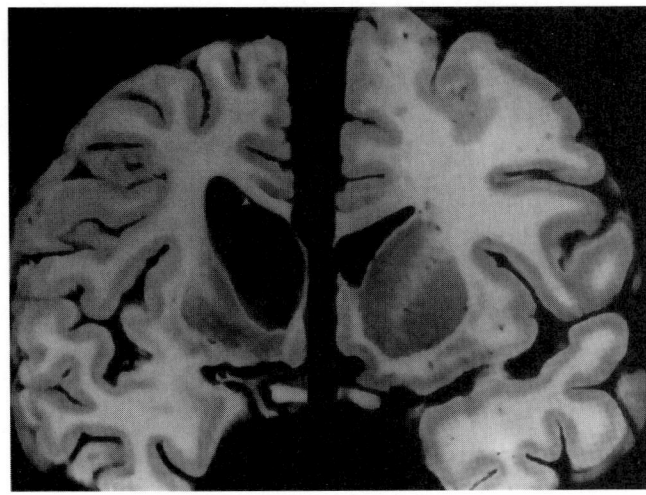

**Fig. 223-7 Coronal brain sections. Severe striatal atrophy in the brain of a patient with HD (left) compared with a control (right).**

Microscopically, the neostriatal atrophy is characterized by neuronal loss and gliosis,[79,176] which again may be highly variable (Fig. 223-8). Full appreciation of neuronal loss, however, can only be obtained by cell counting. In these instances, even in the absence of caudate abnormalities macroscopically, regional loss of up to 40 percent of the normal neurons may be found.[201] Medium- and small-sized neurons, which are the most abundant class in human striatum,[202] disappear, whereas larger neurons appear relatively preserved.[79,198,203,204] The remaining neurons often show irregular loss and pallor of the cytoplasm, some shrinkage, and pyknosis of the nucleus.[198]

Employing in situ labeling techniques of internucleosomal DNA fragmentation, numerous neurons that contain labeled DNA fragments can be found.[205,206] This finding has been interpreted as implying apoptosis as the mode of neuronal death in HD. However, these techniques do label randomly fragmented DNA, as well as internucleosomally cleaved DNA. The number of labeled neurons in these studies was so high that not all of them could possibly represent apoptotic neurons.

Ultrastructural (electron microscopic) studies of the caudate may reveal abnormalities in the nucleus and nucleolus, the endoplasmic reticulum, ribosomes, the Golgi apparatus, mitochondria, and lysosomes.[207] In affected neurons, both degenerative and

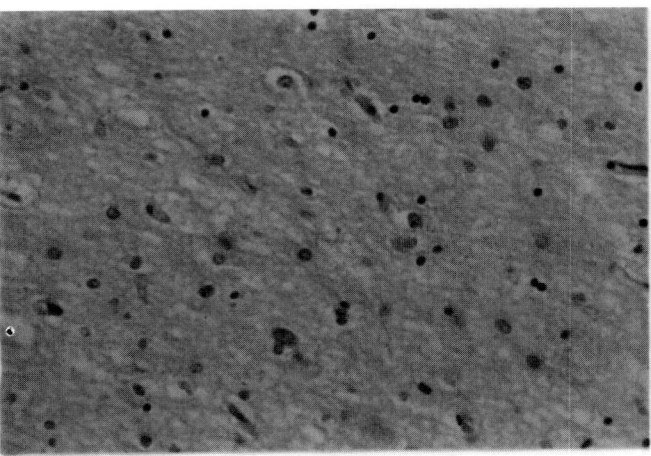
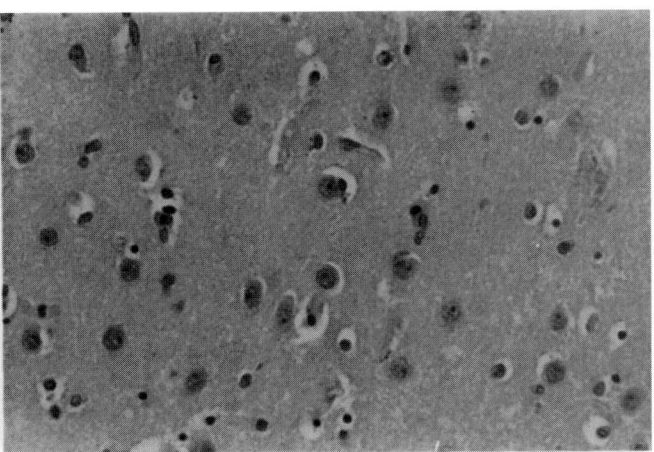

*A*

*B*

**Fig. 223-8 Microscopic view showing severe neuronal loss, increased density of glial cells, and rarefaction of the neuropil in the striatum of a patient with HD (*A*) as compared with a control (*B*).**

regenerative changes can be observed. In Golgi, stains of medium-sized spiny neurons, abnormal dendritic branching, elongation and abnormal recurvations of distal dendrites, and alterations in spine densities were visualized.[208,209] Intense immunohistochemical labeling of abnormally shaped neurites by both nonphosphorylated and phosphorylated antineurofilament antibodies,[210] displacement of calbindin (D28k) immunostaining toward the distal dendrites,[209] and increased expression of neural cell adhesion molecule immunoreactivity in the HD neostriatum[210] all may be additional manifestations of these changes. Since proliferation of dendrites occurs more frequently in moderately affected patients, with loss of dendrites in the severely affected, it has been suggested that neuritic growth actually may precede neuronal loss.[209]

Recently, aggregates of truncated peptide fragments that contain the expanded polyglutamine tract have been identified in various cellular localizations in both degenerating striatal neurons and in neurons outside susceptible areas.[184,211] They may be found in the nucleus, in the cytoplasm, or in dystrophic neurites, and they immunostain with antibodies against 5′ huntingtin peptide fragments and ubiquitin.[212] Aggregates were demonstrated initially in a transgenic mouse model of the disease,[212] but now they have been detected in the human condition as well.

Gliosis particularly manifest by astrocytosis may be prominent. In the HD neostriatum, an increased density of fibrillary astrocytes is found.[176,200] These astrocytes express glial fibrillary acidic protein (GFAP), have nuclei that appear larger and more vesicular than normal,[198,213] and possess an increased number of bundles of glial filaments in astrocytic processes on electron microscopic examination[214] (Fig. 223-9). Fibrillary astrocytosis is often easier to appreciate than mild neuronal loss.[176] It is currently unknown whether the increased density in astrocytes, as well as oligodendrocytes, represents a truly increased total number[201] or in reality obscures a normal or even decreased number of cells,[204,215] compacted in a smaller volume of shrunken tissue.

No specific cellular markers characteristic of HD have been found. Accumulation of lipofuscin in remaining neurons and astrocytes[79,198,207,213] is evident, as well as an increased neostriatal iron content,[199,213,216] probably stored in siderophages in the perivascular spaces,[198] corpora amylacea,[213] and synaptic terminals.[217] Neurons displaying nuclear membrane indentations[218,219] have all been noted to accompany the neostriatal neuronal loss and gliosis in affected human brains and in transgenic mice expressing exon 1 of the HD gene. None of these phenomena, however, is specific to HD.

Although the neostriatum is the most severely and obviously affected structure in the brains of HD patients, it is not uniformly atrophied. The caudate seems more affected than the putamen.[176,200] The nucleus accumbens is least affected.[176,198,219] Within the caudate, a gradient of atrophic changes can be discerned. The tail is more affected than the body, and the head displays the least changes. The mediodorsal parts of the caudate initially are more affected than the ventrolateral parts, but ultimately, the caudate becomes diffusely atrophic.[176] Within the putamen, a similar gradient exists, with the posterior putamen being most affected and the anterior ventral putamen least involved.[220]

The earliest and most extensively affected neurons are the medium-sized spiny neurons that express gamma-aminobutyric acid (GABA) and enkephalin (Enk) or GABA and substance P as their neurotransmitter.[221] Their cell bodies are located in the striatal matrix, and they project to the external part of the globus pallidus (GPe) or to the internal part of the globus pallidus (GPi) and the substantia nigra, pars reticulata (SNr) (GABA/Subst P)[222,223] (see Fig. 223-9). The GABA/Enk projection to the GPe may be more severely affected than the GABA/Subst P projection to the GPi.[224] The substance P projection to the SN pars compacta, originating from striosomes,[222] appears to be involved in the disease process only in the later stages.[224] A decreased number of fibers immunoreactive for enkephalin and substance P in the GPe and SNr, respectively, was already observable in the brain of an asymptomatic individual at high risk for having inherited the HD gene.[225,226] Transcription of enkephalin and substance P mRNA may precede actual cell loss, which suggests that these neurons may go through a phase of "illness" before dying.[227]

Medium-sized and large neurons containing the enzyme NADPH-diaphorase (recently identified as a nitric oxide synthase)[228] remain intact.[229] These neurons contain somatostatin and neuropeptide Y as their neurotransmitter and are localized in the striatal matrix,[230,231] probably serving as interneurons. Similar to neurons that die, decreased expression of nitric oxide synthase and somatostatin is seen in these neurons. It is unknown whether this is associated with impending degeneration or merely down-regulation of activity in an altered environment.[232] Another relatively spared group consists of large aspiny acetylcholine esterase (AChE)–containing and locally arborizing interneurons[233] that are not localized in any particular compartment. Again, it should be appreciated that the absence of studies applying formal morphometric methods precludes the assessment of whether these "resistant" neurons do not die at all or only less rapidly than their vulnerable counterparts.

The globus pallidus (GP) may show a general volume reduction as large as the neostriatum.[203,234] Part of this reduction is due to loss of striatopallidal fibers.[200,224] Demyelinization of remaining fibers, with astrocytosis and crowding of oligodendrocytes, is common. The large neurons in the GPe appear shrunken and laden with lipofuscin, whereas GPi neurons seem affected only in severe cases.[79]

## Changes in Extrastriatal Structures

The selective nature of neuronal loss may be demonstrated by the patterns of cell loss within the neostriatum. However, other regions of the brain are also affected. Macroscopically, the whole brain often appears atrophic, with narrowed gyri, widened sulci, and a reduction in brain weight, sometimes by as much as 400 g.[79,200,234]

Cortical atrophy with changes in neocortical architecture has been reported frequently.[79,194–197,235] Morphometric analysis of 30 HD brains revealed up to 30 percent reduction in mean cortical area and a reduction to 16 percent of cortical ribbon thickness associated with increasing severity of the neostriatal changes.[234] The normal layered architecture is preserved, but alterations occur in layers III, V, and VI,[79,198,200,236] with layer IV possibly also involved.[79,198,237] Ganglion cells in these layers appear shrunken, basophilic, and abnormally shaped,[197,198,235] with ultrastructural changes similar to the striatum.[207,238] The major class of neurons affected is the large pyramidal projection neurons[236] that express nonphosphorylated neurofilament epitopes.[239] Loss of their extensive cortical dendritic arborizations may explain part of the general decrease in cortical thickness and volume. Neuropeptide Y–containing cortical interneurons, in contrast, are spared,[239] as are the large Betz cells in the precentral gyrus that give rise to descending corticobulbar and corticospinal connections.[200,235]

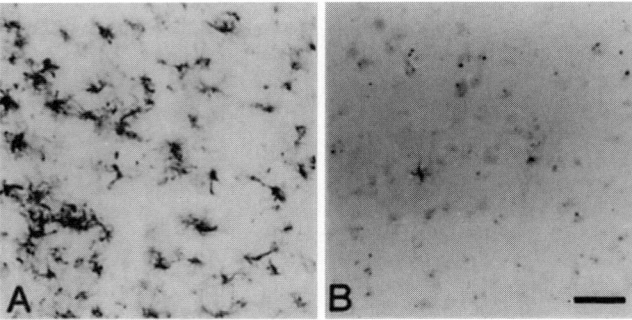

**Fig. 223-9** Immunohistochemistry for glial fibrillary acidic protein (GFAP) showing densely staining fibrillary astrocytes in the caudate of an HD patient (*A*) but not in a control (*B*).

Gliosis in the cortex is less conspicuous.[200] However, on counting, both astrocyte and oligodendrocyte densities were found to be significantly increased in all cortical layers.[240] Astrocytic changes were visible on electron microscopy, with lipofuscin accumulation and prominent bundles of glial filaments in astrocytic processes as the most characteristic changes.[238]

In mildly affected patients, the cortical changes are patchy, whereas in severely affected patients, they are spread throughout the whole cortex.[197] The changes may be most marked in the neocortical frontal areas,[235] with the parietal and temporal lobes equally affected.[198] Changes in the occipital lobe vary from mild to severe.[198,235] Hippocampal changes usually are less pronounced than in the neocortex.[198] A recent finding is the severe cell loss in the entorhinal cortex.[241]

Cortical changes in HD do not differ qualitatively from those seen in senile and other atrophies.[198,221] In some instances, senile plaques and neurofibrillary tangles may be found in neocortical and limbic areas of the brains of elderly HD patients.[200,242–244] The patchy nature of the cortical changes in less severely affected patients may lead to underrepresentation due to sampling errors. What is certain, however, is that at least one neuronal population, the large projection neurons, is predictably affected. Since this population makes up a much smaller part of the cortex than the medium-sized spiny neurons in the neostriatum, the apparent atrophy in the cortex is less impressive.

The diminution in size of the subcortical white matter and the reduced size of the corpus callosum support the described loss of cortical projection neurons.[198,234] The amygdala, although reduced in cross-sectional area,[234] is microscopically well preserved, with only a few instances of slight astrocytosis and some neuronal atrophy.[198] The thalamus, similar to most structures, may be reduced in proportion to the rest of the brain.[204,234] The density of small neurons in the ventrobasal complex is considerably reduced (50 percent), whereas the large neurons persist normally. Astrocytosis in defined thalamic nuclei may be present.[79,198,200] The subthalamic nucleus, which receives significant projections from the cerebral cortex and from the GPe, projects to the GPe, GPi, neostriatum, and substantia nigra[245] and may be significantly reduced (−23 percent) in volume but not in absolute number of nerve cells.[204] In contrast to variable changes in other extrastriatal structures, the hypothalamic lateral nucleus is severely atrophied.[246,247] Morphometric analysis has revealed a consistent reduction (−90 percent) of the normal neuronal content of about 60,000, with less than 2000 neurons remaining.[248,249] Accompanied by gliosis, the atrophic process seems similar to that in the neostriatum.[248]

Some brain regions typically remain unaffected. Brain stem nuclei including the substantia nigra, pars compacta, and neurons of the ventral tegmental mesencephalic area (with dopamine as a neurotransmitter), the locus coeruleus (norepinephrine), the raphe nuclei (serotonin), the tuberomammillary nucleus (histamine), and the large cholinergic basal forebrain neurons of the substantia innominata, including the basal nucleus of Meynert, are generally intact.[200,217,248–251] However, in severely demented patients, there may be neuronal loss in the locus coeruleus,[252] whereas cell loss in the substantia nigra is absent or only mild.[79,198,200]

Gross cerebellar atrophy is rare,[253] but some cerebellar changes are well established[79,198] and are especially prominent in early-onset patients.[143,254] However, even in adult patients, the density of cortical Purkinje cells often may be decreased to, on average, half the value of age-matched controls.[255] This decrease bears no obvious relation to the general brain atrophy.[255] The dentate nucleus is often depleted,[29,32] but the fastigial nucleus is usually normal.[200]

## Diagnostic Accuracy

In general, the combination of clinical signs and neuropathologic examination is sensitive and a very specific approach to the diagnosis of HD. In a large series of 157 patients in whom a clinical diagnosis was confirmed by a postmortem detection of CAG expansion, a neuropathologic diagnosis was made in 153.[256]

## Relation between CAG Repeat Length and Neuropathologic Changes

The relation between CAG and clinical characteristics of the disease was established immediately after the discovery of the gene. Since the clinical features of HD ultimately are determined by the changes in brain function, a relation between CAG size and neuropathologic changes may be postulated. Strong correlations were indeed detected when CAG repeat size was related to striatal neuronal counts or to neuropathologic grade[176] when corrections for age at death or for duration of disease were introduced.[257,258] CAG length typically explained about 80 percent of the variance in neuropathologic alterations, which should be considered a remarkably strong biologic effect.

## PATHOPHYSIOLOGY OF HD

Several recent reports have highlighted a morphologic feature in many of the polyglutamine expansion disorders. Intracellular aggregates have been found in neurons of affected patients,[184] murine[218] and in vitro models of HD,[259–262] SCA1,[263] SCA3,[264] SBMA,[265,266] and DRPLA.[211,267] The specific composition of these aggregates is unknown, but recent evidence showed that truncated polyglutamine fragments are associated with an increased frequency of aggregate formation. This raised the possibility that aggregates are in some way associated with cell death.

However, recent findings in human studies showed that aggregates are present in numerous cells where cell death does not occur or occurs less frequently. This includes regions outside the cerebral cortex and basal ganglia in patients with HD, such as the cerebellum, and also regions outside the CNS such as peripheral tissues, including muscle and the pancreas.

Certain factors are key to the formation of aggregates. First, expansion of the polyglutamine tract is required for aggregate formation. Aggregates are never observed in vitro, in cells transfected with polyglutamine-containing proteins with polyglutamine tracts below the disease threshold,[259,261,264] and aggregates are also never observed in brains of unaffected individuals.[184,211]

Aggregates may occur both within the nucleus and in extranuclear locations (Fig. 223-10). For example, in HD, neurons of adult patients frequently have dystrophic neurites containing aggregates.[184] While the precise composition of these aggregates is unknown, what is known is that all these intracellular aggregates in each of these diseases stain with ubiquitin antibodies, suggesting that these aggregates are at least likely to be ubiquitinated.[184,211,218,264] It has been shown previously that huntingtin is ubiquitinated in vivo,[189] and as is well known for ubiquitin-containing proteins, their ongoing metabolism is likely to occur through the proteasome.

Recently it has been shown for ataxin-1 that components of the proteosome do localize within the aggregates.[268]

Preliminary information suggests that decreasing aggregate formation by preventing cleavage by caspase-3 is associated with decreasing aggregate formation and reduced toxicity in vitro.[265] These data are consistent with the concept that proteolytic cleavage by caspases or other proteases may be important in the generation of smaller polyglutamine-containing proteins that have a greater propensity for aggregate formation in the presence of an expanded polyglutamine tract. The data are particularly pertinent because it has been shown previously that huntingtin, the androgen receptor, antrophin-1, and ataxin-3 are cleaved by one or more caspases, liberating a protein fragment containing the polyglutamine tract. Cleavage of each of these proteins occurs in apoptotic extracts using purified recombinant caspases.[269] The finding that all these polyglutamine-containing proteins are caspase substrates suggests that cleavage of the parent protein could be a common mechanism for generating truncated fragments of these proteins,

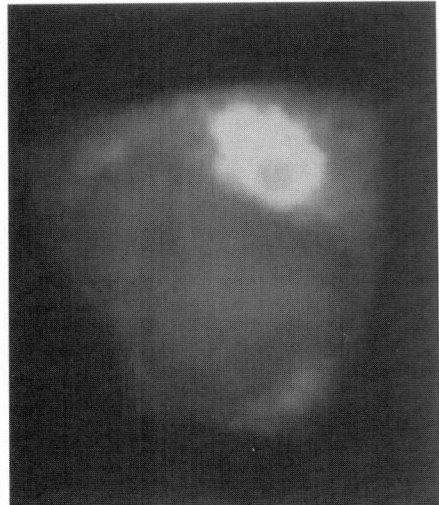 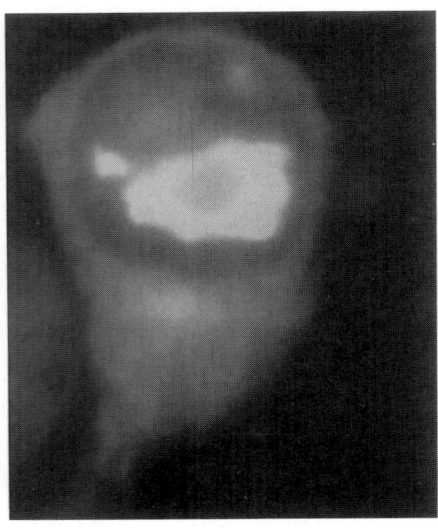

**Fig. 223-10** Perinuclear and intranuclear aggregates in 293T cells transfected with full-length and truncated HD cDNAs with 128 glutamine repeats.

with each protein having different substrate specificity and susceptibility to specific proteolytic cleavage.

Data suggesting that the expanded CAG repeat can cause pathology in the context of any protein come from recent innovative studies that have resulted from the creation of mice expressing a long polyglutamine tract within the mouse hypoxanthine phosphoribosyl transferase gene.[270] These mice normally have no particular phenotype. However, in the presence of an expanded polyglutamine tract in this exogenous site within the *HPRT* gene, these mice develop neuronal intranuclear aggregates and have significant neurologic and neuropathologic changes associated with neuronal intracellular aggregate formation. These in vivo results show that the expanded polyglutamine tract can make innocent proteins neurotoxic.

Recent data however also suggest that the aggregates are markers for toxicity but are not directly causative of neurotoxicity. Aggregates occur in neurons that do not undergo cell death. Furthermore, mice expressing full-length huntingtin[270a] and mice expressing ataxin 1 lacking the self-association region[270b] of the protein develop specific neuronal loss characteristic of the disease in the absence of aggregates. Clearly, aggregates are not required for neuronal loss.

### Animal Models

An interesting animal model of HD was constructed using exon 1 of huntingtin with a very long expanded repeat.[212] These animals developed behavioral syndromes similar to HD, including incoordination, abnormal involuntary movements, seizures, and weight loss. However, unlike HD patients, they have not shown specific neuronal cell loss in the striatum. These data are consistent with the idea that neuronal dysfunction, rather than neuronal death, may be responsible for many of the symptoms of the polyglutamine diseases.

Other approaches to creating an animal model for HD have now been undertaken using a full-length construct encoding the full-length protein with an expanded polyglutamine tract. Mice expressing the full-length protein under control of the endogenous promoter (YAC transgene a knock-in mice[270c,270d]) as well as the CHV promoter have been generated.[270e] Mice with features most reminiscent of the neuropathology of HD are seen in the YAC transgenic mice which carry the full genomic sequence of the human HD gene in the context of a normal and expanded polyglutamine tract.

In the latter, hyperactivity and selective neuronal loss involving predominantly the medium spiny neurons of the caudate nucleus together with cleavage of huntingtin are evident. This model clearly highlights the importance of protein context in mediating selectivity of neuronal loss and indicates that cleavage

of huntingtin with translocation of N-Terminal fragment into the nucleus represents an important step in the pathogenesis of HD.

### Clinicopathologic Correlations

Striatal atrophy has long been postulated to be responsible for the occurrence of choreic movements in HD. However, only recently have the distinct features of the disease been more definitely related to the particular pattern of pathologic changes.

Significant correlations have been found between the severity of caudate atrophy as seen on CT and impairment of daily activities, various neuropsychological test scores, total neurologic impairment, and eye-movement abnormalities.[110,271] Both the absence[110] and the presence[272] of a relationship between voluntary motor impairment and chorea score, on the one hand, and caudate atrophy, on the other, have been reported. PET scanning also has provided new insights. Chorea, voluntary motor abnormalities, and slowing of saccades have been shown to correlate more closely with putamen hypometabolism of glucose than with caudate metabolism. In contrast, memory abnormalities (as measured by the Wechsler Memory Scale) were found significantly associated with caudate but not with putaminal hypometabolism.[273]

These findings are consistent with the current notion, derived from both neuroanatomic[274] and neurophysiologic data,[275] that the caudate nucleus is predominantly involved in cognitive and complex associative processing, whereas the putamen is involved in sensorimotor processing.[275,276]

Lesions of the striatum generally fail to produce chorea in experimental animals.[275] However, lesions of the subthalamic nucleus (STN), accidental in humans or experimental in monkeys, produce severe choreatic movements (called *hemiballismus*) in the contralateral side of the body. It is therefore possible that dysfunction (not atrophy) of the STN is the primary pathophysiologic condition contributing to chorea in HD. This dysfunction then would be caused by a tonically exaggerated inhibition of the nucleus by GABA-ergic projections originating from the external part of the globus pallidus. The inhibitory activity of these pallidal neurons themselves is normally inhibited by the GABA-enkephalin-containing medium-sized spiny projection neurons of the striatum[277,278] (Fig. 223-11).

Striatal GABA-enkephalin projections to the GPe degenerate earlier than striatal GABA-substance P projections to the GPi[279] (see Fig. 223-9). While the initial degeneration of the former may cause chorea, the later disappearance of the projections to the GPi may be responsible for the gradually increasing bradykinesia.[280] Thus the feature that discriminates rigid from choreic patients seems to be the extent of involvement of the striatal GABA–substance P projections to the GPi. In rigid patients they

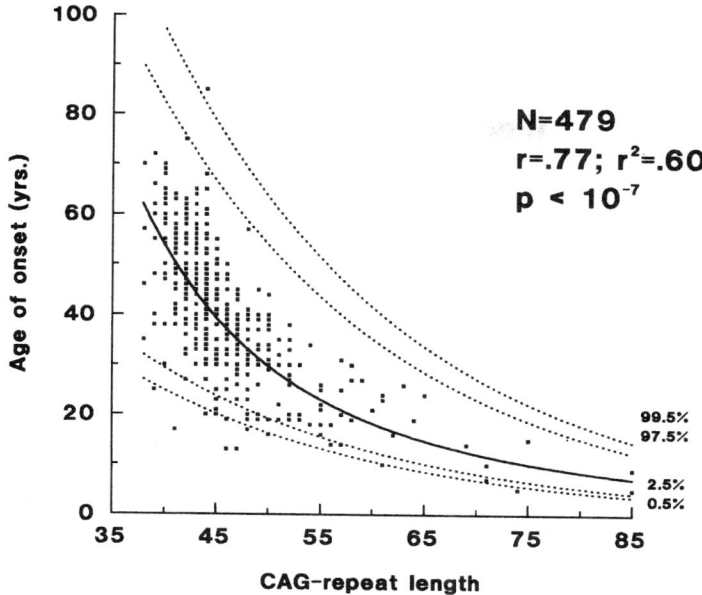

N=479
r=.77; r²=.60
p < 10⁻⁷

**Fig. 223-11** Schematic representation of neuronal connections in the basal ganglia in a normal person (left) and a person with HD (right). Inhibitory neurons and their connections are in black; excitatory neurons are in white. Dopamine probably exerts both excitatory and inhibitory effects. The GABA/Enk neurons projecting from the striatum are first affected in HD. As a result, inhibitory GABA neurons in the external part of the globus pallidus become hyperactive, depressing the activity of glutamatergic neurons in the subthalamic nucleus. *Glu*, glutamate; *GABA*, gamma-aminobutyric acid; *DA*, dopamine; *Enk*, enkephalin; *SP*, substance P.

degenerate together with GABA-enkephalin projections, whereas in choreic patients they are relatively spared.[280]

Delayed initiation and other abnormalities of saccades may result from overinhibition of neurons in the tectum mesencephali. This overinhibition is caused by the action of GABA-ergic afferent neurons from the substantia nigra, pars reticulata, that are normally inhibited by striatal GABA–substance P–containing projections.[277] This class of neurons seems to degenerate earlier than the GABA–substance P neurons to the GPi and may be affected as early as the GABA-enkephalin projections to the GPe,[224,225,281] explaining the occurrence of saccadic abnormalities already in the transitional period.

Alterations in dopaminergic neurotransmission in the degenerating neostriatum have been implicated in the appearance of choreic movements. Arguments in support of this are the contrast between the hyperkinesia in HD and the hypokinesia in Parkinson's disease (the classic dopamine-deficient basal ganglia disorder), the normal or increased dopamine concentrations in the neostriatum of HD patients,[282] the provocation of choreic movements by dopamine-enhancing drugs in patients with advanced Parkinson's disease or tardive dyskinesia, the exacerbation of choreic movements in HD patients receiving dopamine agonists,[283] and the observed suppression of involuntary movements of HD patients by neuroleptic drugs, i.e., dopamine receptor blocking agents.

Dopamine is thought to inhibit striatal GABA-enkephalin neurons and may stimulate GABA–substance P neurons.[284] This may explain the partial success of neuroleptic treatment of chorea, since the dopamine-induced suppression of remaining GABA-enkephalin neurons will be diminished.

Although a PET study of patients with juvenile-onset HD suggested deficient nigrostriatal dopaminergic neurotransmission,[285] striatal dopamine concentrations and cerebro spinal fluid (CSF) homovanillic acid (a dopamine metabolite) levels in rigid patients were similar to those in choreic patients.[282,286] Tyrosine hydroxylase immunoreactive neurons in the substantia nigra are preserved.[280] Thus, unlike Parkinson's disease, parkinsonism in HD is not clearly caused by a deficient nigrostriatal system.

## Why Do Neurons Die in HD? The Excitotoxic Hypothesis

The excitotoxic hypothesis of neuronal loss in HD proposes that endogenously produced excitatory amino acids (EAAs), or closely related substances, physiologically involved in neurotransmission damage and kill neurons that are chronically exposed to their effects.[287] Neurons affected are those which possess receptors for EAA neurotransmitters, including the N-methyl-D-aspartate (NMDA), the α-amino-3-hydroxy-5-methylisoxazole-4-propionic acid (AMPA), and the kainate receptor.

The potential pathogenic role of excitotoxic mechanisms in the HD neostriatum is supported by different observations. Injections of kainic acid, a glutamate analogue, in the rat striatum destroyed almost all neurons, whereas glial cells and afferents remained intact.[288,289] The NMDA agonists quinolinic acid and L-homocystic acid, as well as NMDA itself, produce striatal damage that closely mimics the structural and neurochemical changes of HD.[290] EAA receptors are abundant in the striatum, and NMDA, AMPA, and kainate binding are significantly decreased in HD patients.[291] In a presymptomatic individual carrying the HD gene, NMDA-receptor binding was already found to be decreased.[225] In primates with striatal excitotoxin lesions, levodopa may result in dyskinesias.[292,293] The hypothalamic lateral tuberal nucleus, prominently involved in HD, has NMDA and AMPA receptors as well.[294] All these findings support the hypothesis of EAA-mediated, and particularly NMDA-mediated, cell death in HD.

Yet several problems currently hamper the excitotoxic hypothesis in HD. Excitotoxic mechanisms clearly play a role in acute exposure to excitotoxins.[295] It is more difficult, however, to assess experimentally their role in chronic disease. Some of the early experiments with quinolinic acid injections could not be reproduced.[296] The excitotoxin itself has not been identified. Most important, the presence of EAA receptors alone provides insufficient explanation for neuronal death in HD. Many apparently unaffected neuronal populations elsewhere in the brain do contain EAA receptors, e.g., in the hippocampus, the amygdala, the cerebellum, or the frontal cortex.[297,298] Even if careful morphometrics would show some neuronal loss in these areas, the extent of the damage does not resemble that in the striatum. Apparently, other factors must be operative that either protect EAA receptor-bearing neurons against the effects of the HD gene or render striatal and some other neuronal populations, like the lateral tuberal nucleus, especially vulnerable. These factors could be the nature of their afferents, abnormal metabolism of regional EAA-like substances, different EAA receptor subtypes, abnormal mitochondrial energy metabolism in postsynaptic cells, or deficiencies in intracellular calcium-clearing mechanisms[279] (Fig. 223-12). The theory of EAA-mediated neuronal loss in HD

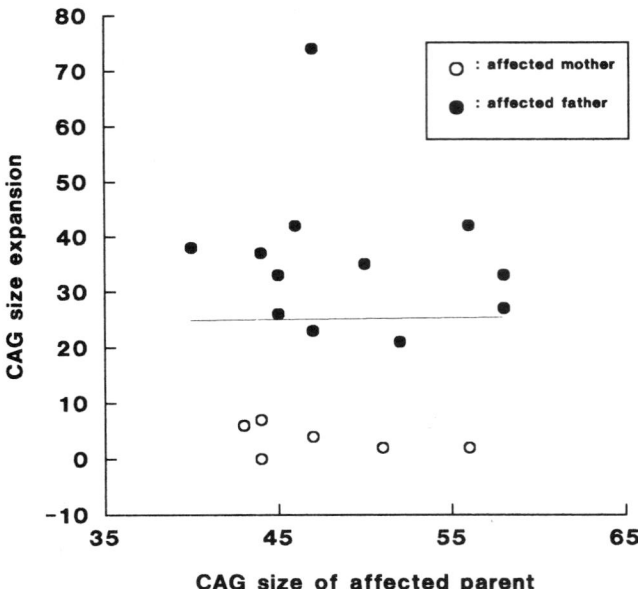

**Fig. 223-12 Some suggested mechanisms of excitatory amino acid neurotoxicity.**

supports drug trials aimed at protecting the remaining neurons from the deleterious effects of excitatory amino acids.

### Genetic Counseling

The geneticist and genetic counselor commonly encounter a healthy person at risk for HD who wants to know his or her risk for having inherited the illness. In this particular instance, it is most important to recognize that the risk varies taking into account the subject's age. For a person in early adult life with an affected parent, the risk is very close to 50 percent. However, by the time the person has reached beyond the age of 60, the risk will have decreased considerably. The risk for a healthy subject at 50 percent prior risk of carrying the HD gene at different ages is shown in Table 223-3 and is based on the life-table analysis of data from South Wales.[56]

Familial aggregation of age at onset also can be taken into account in assessing the risk at an asymptomatic individual who has a parent affected with HD. This has been investigated thoroughly for siblings of persons with juvenile HD.[299] Therefore, both familial aggregation age at onset and age of the person at risk for HD should be taken into account when deriving risks for asymptomatic individuals for having inherited the HD gene. More recently, the use of CAG-repeat size to predict age of onset in an asymptomatic individual has been assessed providing estimates with relatively narrow confidence limits[25] (Table 223-4). These data, with appropriate counseling, are likely to be useful for patients requesting predictive testing for HD.

### Predictive Testing

Predictive testing for HD has been offered in different parts of the world for several years. Prior to the introduction of these programs, research protocols were developed to evaluate the psychological impact of receiving either an increased or decreased risk result.[300–303] There was major concern that an increased risk result would precipitate catastrophic reactions such as emotional breakdown or suicide.

The psychological impact on those undergoing testing has been studied. Prior to and in the first days after receiving a result, the emotional stress is formidable, particularly in those who are told they have the HD mutation.[304] In this vulnerable situation, severe adverse reactions have occurred, most likely in those with some evidence of clinical depression.[305] Those with a decreased risk

result adjust and may benefit from the reduction of uncertainty, whereas even in some, distress may remain.[304,306] Overall, those undergoing testing seem to do remarkably well over a period of a few years.[303,307] However, individuals may develop problems years after an increased risk result.[308] Such reactions may be indistinguishable from the psychiatric problems that are part of the HD clinical spectrum or even from the common risk of psychiatric problems in the general population. From a clinical point of view, these results emphasize the need for professional counseling and support in those undergoing testing, particularly in the first weeks or months following the disclosure of a result. Moreover, they underscore the necessity of comprehensive testing protocols in centers that offer such predictive testing.[309]

The demand for predictive testing has been lower than expected in studies conducted prior to the advent of predictive testing.[301,310,311] In those countries in which protocols are widely available in general, less than 20 percent of persons at risk have requested testing. In addition, prenatal testing for HD is not a frequently chosen option.[312] Only 7 of 38 persons who became pregnant while part of a predictive testing program chose to participate in prenatal testing. The most frequently cited reason for declining prenatal testing was the hope for the development of a cure in time for their children.[313]

The demand for predictive testing is likely to increase as new approaches to therapy are developed. However, the possibility of effective therapy that may arise as a result of the cloning of the gene for HD is likely to reduce further the demand for prenatal testing, since termination of a pregnancy for a curable or potentially treatable adult-onset illness is likely to be even less acceptable. This would be similar to the very low demand for prenatal testing for other late-onset autosomal dominant disorders such as polycystic kidney disease, for which there are some effective therapies that may retard progression of the illness. The long-term effects of predictive testing for HD are not known, and there is a continued need for longitudinal investment to examine the psychological and social effects of testing and to collect data that best predict responses to change in risk status.

## MANAGEMENT

Drug therapy for the management of HD is limited to symptomatic treatment. Choreic movements can be suppressed partially by neuroleptics, whereas hypokinesia and rigidity may be ameliorated by antiparkinsonian agents. Psychiatric disturbances may react well to psychotropic drugs. Cognitive impairment is not amenable to drug treatment. Successful symptomatic treatment, however, does not lead to a significant improvement in functional capacity. Therefore, an important part of management is to help the patient and the family cope with the disease. Effective therapy to retard disease progression has not yet been achieved, although recent pathophysiologic insights suggest novel approaches. These include transplantation of fetal cells into the basal ganglia.

### Nonpharmacologic Management

It should be stressed that the contribution of nonpharmacologic approaches to the general well-being of HD patients is more important than medication. For those patients still living in the community, the close attention of family and friends, the family doctor, the social worker, or a public health nurse will be increasingly required. While there are obvious declines in functional capacity, patients with HD in many instances can remain in partial employment and fulfill domestic responsibilities until far into the illness. Premature withdrawal from these activities may further exacerbate the feelings of inadequacy and loss of power associated with the illness.

Physical therapy generally is useful for patients. Initially, it should be directed at maintaining activity, but in the final stages, the prevention of painful contractures will be most important. Speech therapy can help the patient in communication and may improve swallowing. An occupational therapist can provide valuable advice regarding domestic adaptations such as toilet and bathing facilities. If gait problems are prominent, a wheel chair will be required. Walking canes are often of limited value. Because of the frequent weight loss, nutrition requires close attention, and a high-calorie, high-protein diet may be required. Extensive nursing care plans have been described.[50,314]

Attention also should be paid to the well-being of family members. Apart from possibly being at risk for HD, they also suffer from their daily burden of providing adequate care for the patient. Intermittent, temporary relief from this burden through respite care may encourage them to continue. A crisis at home is the most common reason for forced institutionalization of HD patients. Activities for affected persons such as day care, or holiday camps have provided important relief for caregivers and great enjoyment for affected persons.

Many of these options will depend on the society in which the patients live. The advice, help, and expertise of the national lay societies, therefore, are indispensable in accumulating knowledge about the specific problems and opportunities for people with HD in their country.

## Symptomatic Treatment of Involuntary Movements

The most widely used drugs to suppress choreatic movements are dopamine receptor blocking neuroleptics such as phenothiazines or butyrophenones. The phenothiazine compound perphenazine was recommended in the United States as the first choice for this purpose in the past.[315] Haloperidol in low doses,[316] pimozide, or substituted benzamides such as sulpiride[317] or tiapride[298,318] are suitable alternatives. Tetrabenazine, a synthetic benzoquinolizine, with the reserpine-like property of depleting presynaptic mono-amines, may be even more effective.[319–322] This drug, however, is not registered in many countries. The ultimate choice of the neuroleptic will depend to a large extent on the individual clinician's experience with these drugs. Depot neuroleptics to suppress chorea should be avoided (Table 223-6).

Drugs are only partially successful in suppressing chorea. Moreover, although they suppress involuntary movements, they do not improve the patient's functional capacity[140,317,323] or fine motor performance.[88] Side effects may be prominent and confer additional disability on the patient. Drowsiness, dry mouth, blurred vision, constipation, or difficulties on micturition are well-known parasympatholytic effects of these drugs. Tetrabenazine, although in general remarkably well tolerated,[324] may cause depression. All neuroleptics may aggravate parkinsonian signs. Acute dystonia[325] or rigidity[326] and akathisia may occur early during treatment. Obviously, these side effects are difficult to discriminate from the extrapyramidal movement disorder of HD, causing in some instances considerable diagnostic uncertainty.

### Table 223-6 Drugs that May Be Useful in the Treatment of HD

| Compound | Recommended Daily Dose for | | |
| --- | --- | --- | --- |
| | Chorea | Psychosis | Depression |
| **Neuroleptics** | | | |
| Perphenazine | 2–8 mg | 2–16 mg | |
| Sulpiride | 300–1200 mg | 300–2000 mg | |
| Tiapride | 300–1200 mg | — | |
| Haloperidol | 2–10 mg | 2–16 mg | |
| Pimozide | 2–8 mg | 2–16 mg | |
| Tetrabenazine | 25–100 mg | — | * |
| **Antidepressants** | | | |
| Amitryptiline | | | 25–100 mg |
| Imipramine | | | 25–200 mg |
| Fluoxetine | | | 20–80 mg |
| Amoxepine | | | 30–90 mg |

*Stop when depression occurs.

Neuroleptic drug treatment does not improve swallowing, speaking, or walking difficulties and may in fact aggravate these through its parasympatholytic and parkinsonian effects.[89,327] In juvenile patients, neuroleptics may complicate the treatment of epilepsy. The neuroleptic malignant syndrome has been described in an HD patient receiving dopamine-depleting agents.[328]

Therefore, drug treatment of chorea should only be undertaken in those with severe movements. A crucial question prior to implementation of drug therapy is whether the movements are causing significant concern to the patient. A low initial dose, gradual increments, and frequent reassessments are required. Determining when the maximal effect is obtained is difficult but can be monitored clinically. When a certain dose is exceeded, no further suppression of chorea will occur.[316] Side effects may even further limit reaching maximal effect. The use of standardized assessments such as the quantified neurologic examination,[98] the chorea score,[329] the functional capacity scale,[138] or video may be helpful in objectively monitoring drug efficacy. A proposed list of drugs useful in HD is given in Table 223-6.

Apart from neuroleptics, many other drugs have been proposed to ameliorate dyskinesia, but their effects have been observed in a few patients only and have not been substantiated by formal trials. These drugs include low-dose bromocriptine,[330,331] apomorphine,[332,333] transdihydrolisuride,[334] benzodiazepines,[335] isoniazid,[336,337] baclofen,[338,339] lithium,[340] and corticosteroids.[341]

## Symptomatic Treatment: Pharmacotherapy of Hypokinesia and Rigidity

Levodopa and anticholinergics may ameliorate rigidity and bradykinesia.[50,327] They will, however, exacerbate chorea. Their effect on overall functional capacity has not been evaluated. Their greatest use is for predominantly rigid cases of early onset. In the individual patient, the contribution of neuroleptic medication to hypokinesia and rigidity should be assessed before starting antiparkinsonian agents.

## Pharmacotherapy of Psychiatric Disturbances

Depression may contribute to early disability,[140] and suicide occurs with increased frequency.[122] Antidepressant therapy is warranted whenever symptoms of depression become recognizable. This class of drugs is still frequently underused in the management of HD. Antidepressants fail to delay the progressive deterioration of functional capacity[140] but may provide valuable and important temporary symptomatic relief. Conventional tricyclic antidepressants, such as amitryptiline or imipramine, have proven to be useful.[342] In general, insufficient experience with the modern noradrenergic (mianserin) or serotoninergic (fluvoxamin, fluoxetin, and paroxetin) antidepressants exists, but there are no reasons to exclude them from use. In nondepressed patients, fluoxetine did not improve the functional capacity or cognitive and behavioral ratings.[343] It should be borne in mind that the effects of antidepressant treatment may only become apparent after 3 weeks. The experience with mono amine oxidase (MAO) inhibitors in HD patients is limited, but they may be effective where classic antidepressants have failed.[344] Electroconvulsive therapy may have a role as the final treatment of intractable depression.[342]

Benzodiazepines will be the first choice in anxious or irritable patients. Neuroleptics may helpful for the aggressive patient. Propranolol has been used to treat aggressive behavior in patients with organic brain disease, including HD,[345,346] but paradoxical reactions, i.e., increased aggressive behavior, to these agents have been reported.[346,347] The usefulness of lithium for mood disorders or aggression in HD patients has not yet been formally established. The need for monitoring, careful dosing, and repeated blood sampling may make it less suitable for HD patients.[342] A new drug to treat mania is carbamazepine, but its effects in HD are unknown.[123] Sexual disinhibition also may respond well to low doses of neuroleptics.

In patients with hallucinations or delusions, the classic neuroleptic drugs (see above) are probably as efficacious as in non-HD patients. The dosages required will be higher than used to treat chorea. Tetrabenazine is not indicated in this condition. Depot neuroleptics should be avoided because the ability to respond immediately to the advent of side effects is limited. Clozapine, in line with its current status, may be effective in otherwise intractable psychoses but requires extra precautions.[348]

### Symptomatic Treatment: Antiepileptic Drugs

Epilepsy in juvenile HD patients requires similar drugs as in other forms of convulsive disorders, such as carbamazepine, Dilantin, or valproic acid. Seizures are often difficult to control. Blood levels have to be monitored regularly because it may be difficult to discern toxic side effects. Moreover, long-term weight loss will tend to increase blood concentrations. Standard values for optimal therapeutic concentrations can be applied.

### Retarding Disease Progression

The excitotoxic hypothesis is currently an accepted model for neurodegeneration in HD (see section on pathophysiology). This concept has stimulated attempts to block the neurotoxic effects of glutamate or other excitotoxic amino acids. Thus far, the only reported trial used baclofen to retard disease progression because this drug inhibits corticostriatal glutamate release and displayed some protective effects against kainic acid in animal models of HD. Follow-up of 60 patients for at least 30 months in a double-blind, placebo-controlled study failed to show any effect of the drug.[339] Attempts to influence excitatory amino acid transmission, however, remain attractive.

In a double-blind, placebo-controlled trial we studied the effects of the novel antiepileptic drug lamotrigine, which possesses glutamate release-blocking properties, in 55 patients with early disease, but we failed to detect any retardation of disease progression[349] although symptomatic relief was reported. An alternative approach has been to enhance striatal metabolism and to antagonize free-radical formation. A randomized trial of idebenone, an antioxidant and enhancer of oxidative metabolism, failed to retard disease progression in a group of 91 patients.[350] A problem in all these studies has been the limited sample size, which raised issues of statistical power. Therefore, a multicenter trial is being undertaken (CARE-HD) that, based on preliminary short-term tolerability and efficacy studies, investigates the effect of coenzyme Q and remacemide combined on disease progression.[351,352]

### Restorative Treatment: Transplantation

Since the prognosis for HD patients is serious and medical therapy to retard disease progression is currently lacking, transplantation of neuronal precursor cells into the striatum of HD patients is undergoing consideration as a treatment modality. Grafting immature neuronal precursor cells into the HD striatum, in order to restore functional circuitry, is currently a goal of a number of research programs. Basic issues to be addressed include, among others, the type of neurons to be transplanted (human fetal striatal cells versus xenografts), the timing of the dissection, the necessity of immunosuppression, normal versus abnormal differentiation of transplanted cells, and the histologic and functional reestablishment of normal striatal structures.[353] In animals with excitotoxic lesions, species-specific allografts as well as xenografts (e.g., human fetal striatal cells) appear to be able to differentiate into recognizable striatal tissues, with restoration of aspects of motor function in the animals.[353–355] However, these results are not unequivocal, and doubts remain whether the behavior of the grafts has been completely characterized.[356]

Apart from these issues, recommendations need to be agreed on regarding the selection, pretransplantation testing, and post-transplantation follow-up of feasible patients. Such recommendations have indeed been proposed.[353,357] Several centers have started such trials, and more than 290 patients have received fetal striatal grafts. Early reports suggest that the procedure was well tolerated by patients.[358]

## REFERENCES

1. Huntington G: On chorea. *Med Surg Rep* **26**:317, 1872.
2. Osler W: *On Chorea and Choreiform Affections.* Philadelphia, Blakistan, 1894.
3. Kussmaul A, Nothnagel CWH: *Virchow-Hirsch's Yahrbuch für 1872.* New York, 1872, p 175.
4. Huber A: Chorea hereditaria der Erwachsenen (Huntington's chorea). *Virchows Arch Pathol Anat* **108**:267, 1887.
5. Klippel M, Ducellier F: Un cas de chorée hereditaire de l'adulte (maladie de Huntington). *EMBO* **8**:716, 1888.
6. Seppili G: Corea ereditaria (Corea d'Huntington—corea cronica progressiva). *Riv Sper Freniat* **13**:453, 1888.
7. Suckling CW: Hereditary chorea (Huntington's disease). *Br Med J* **2**:1039, 1889.
8. Huntington G: Recollections of Huntington's chorea as I saw it as East Hampton, Long Island, during my boyhood. NY Neurological Society, Dec 1909. *J Nerv Ment Dis* **37**:255, 1910.
9. De Jong RN: The history of Huntington's chorea in the United States of America, in Barbeau A, Chase TN, Paulson GW (eds): *Advances in Neurology,* Vol 1. New York, Raven Press, 1973, p 19.
10. Huntington's Disease Collaborative Research Group: A novel gene containing a trinucleotide repeat that is expanded and unstable on Huntington's disease chromosomes. *Cell* **72**:971, 1993.
11. Ambrose CM, Duyao MP, Barnes G, et al: Structure and expression of the Huntington's disease gene: Evidence against simple inactivation due to an expanded CAG repeat. *Somat Cell Mol Genet* **20**:27, 1994.
12. Lin B-Y, Rommens JM, Graham RK, et al: Differential 3′ polyadenylation of the Huntington disease gene results in two mRNA species with variable tissue expression. *Hum Mol Genet* **2**:1541, 1993.
13. Lin B, Nasir J, Kalchman MA, et al: Structural analysis of the 5′ region of mouse and human Huntington disease genes reveals conservation of putative promoter region and di- and trinucleotide polymorphisms. *Genomics* **25**:707, 1995.
14. Andrade MA, Bork P: HEAT repeats in the Huntington's disease protein (letter). *Nature Genet* **11**:115, 1995.
15. Bessert DA, Gutridge KL, Dunbar JC, Carlock LR: The identification of a functional nuclear localization signal in the Huntington disease protein. *Mol Brain Res* **33**:165, 1995.
16. Lin B, Nasir J, MacDonald H, et al: Sequence of the murine Huntington disease gene: Evidence for conservation, alternate splicing and polymorphism in a triplet (CCG) repeat. *Hum Mol Genet* **3**(1):85, 1994.
17. Barnes GT, Duyao MP, Ambrose CM, et al: Mouse Huntington's disease gene homolog (*Hdh*). *Somat Cell Mol Genet* **20**:87, 1994.
18. Schmitt I, Bachner D, Megow D, et al: Expression of the Huntington disease gene in rodents: Cloning the rat homologue and evidence for downregulation in non-neuronal tissues during development. *Hum Mol Genet* **4**:1173, 1995.
19. Baxendale S, Abdulla S, Elgar G, et al: Comparative sequence analysis of the human and pufferfish Huntington's disease genes. *Nature Genet* **10**:67, 1995.
20. Nasir S, Floresco SB, O'Kusky JR, et al: Targeted disruption of the murine Huntington disese gene results in early postimplantation embryonic lethality and behavioral and morphological abnormalities in heterozygotes. *Cell* **81**:811, 1995.
21. Duyao MP, Auerbach AB, Ryan A, et al: Inactivation of the mouse Huntington's disease gene homolog Hdh. *Science* **269**:407, 1995.
22. Zeitlin S, Liu J-P, Chapman DL, Papaioannou VE, Efstratiadis A: Increased apoptosis and early embryonic lethality in mice nullizygous for the Huntington's disease gene homologue. *Nature Genet* **11**:155, 1995.
23. Kremer B, Goldberg YP, Andrew SE, et al: A worldwide study of the Huntington's disease mutation: The sensitivity and specificity of measuring CAG repeats. *New Engl J Med* **330**:1401, 1994.
24. Andrew SE, Goldberg YP, Kremer B, et al: The relationship between trinucleotide (CAG) repeat length and clinical features of Huntington disease. *Nature Genet* **4**:398, 1993.
25. Brinkman RR, Mezei MM, Thielmann J, Almqvist E, Hayden MR: The likelihood of being affected with Huntington disease by a

particular age for a specific CAG size. *Am J Hum Genet* **60**:1202, 1997.

26. Goldberg YP, Kalchman MA, Metzler M, et al: Absence of disease phenotype and intergenerational stability of the CAG repeat in transgenic mice expressing the human Huntington disease transcript. *Hum Mol Genet* **5**:177, 1996.
27. Morrison PJ, Johnston WP, Nevin NC: The epidemiology of Huntington's disease in Northern Ireland. *J Med Genet* **32**:524, 1995.
28. Kokmen E, Ozekmekci FS, Beard CM, O'Brien PC, Kurland LT: Incidence and prevalence of Huntington's disease in Olmsted County, Minnesota (1950 through 1989). *Arch Neurol* **51**:696, 1994.
29. Kishimoto K, Nakamura M, Sotokawa Y: Population genetics study: Huntington's chorea in Japan. *Ann Rep Res Inst Environ Med* **9**:195, 1957.
30. Hayden MR, MacGregor JM, Beighton PH: The prevalence of Huntington's chorea in South Africa. *S Afr Med J* **58**:193, 1980.
31. Palo J, Somer H, Ikonen E, Karila L, Peltonen L: Low prevalence of Huntington's disease in Finland. *Lancet* **2**:805, 1987.
32. Reed TE, Chandler JH, Hughes EM, Davidson RT: Huntington's chorea in Michigan: I. Demography and genetics. *Am J Hum Genet* **10**:201, 1958.
33. Kurtzke JF, Anderson VE, Beebe GW, et al: Report of workgroup on epidemiology, biostatistics and population genetics, in *Commission for the Control of Huntington's Disease and its Consequences*, Vol III/I. DHEW Publication (NIH) 718–1503. Washington, US Government Printing Office, 1977, p 133.
34. Folstein SE, Chase GA, Wahl WE, McDonnell AM, Folstein MF: Huntington disease in Maryland: Clinical aspects of racial variation. *Am J Hum Genet* **41**:168, 1987.
35. Squitieri F, Andrew SE, Goldberg YP, et al: DNA haplotype analysis of Huntington disease reveals clues to the origins and mechanisms of CAG expansion and reasons for geographic variations of prevalence. *Hum Mol Genet* **3**(12):2103, 1994.
36. Almqvist E, Spence N, Nichol K, et al: Ancestral differences in the distribution of the XDX 2642 glutamic acid polymorphism is associated with varying CAG repeat length on normal chromosomes: Insights into the genetic evolution of Huntington disease. *Hum Mol Genet* **4**(2):207, 1995.
37. Chang CM, Yu YL, Fong KY, et al: Huntington's disease in Hong Kong Chinese: Epidemiology and clinical picture. *Clin Exp Neurol* **31**:43, 1994.
38. Leung CM, Chan YW, Chang CM, Yu YL, Chen CN: Huntington's disease in Chinese: A hypothesis of its origin. *J Neurol Neurosurg Psychiatry* **55**:681, 1992.
39. Hayden MR: *Huntington's chorea in South Africa*. Ph.D. thesis, University of Cape Town, Cape Town, South Africa, 1979.
40. Avila-Giron R: Medical and social aspects of Huntington's chorea in the State of Zulia, Venezuela, in Barbeau A, Chase TN, Paulson GW (eds): *Advances in Neurology*, Vol 1. New York, Raven Press, 1973, p 261.
41. Young AB, Shoulson I, Penney JB, et al: Huntington's disease in Venezuela: Neurologic features and functional decline. *Neurology* **36**:244, 1986.
42. Wexler NS, Young AB, Tanzi RE, et al: Homozygotes for Huntington's disease. *Nature* **326**:194, 1987.
43. Illarioshkin SN, Igarashi S, Onodera O, et al: Trinucleotide repeat length and rate of progression of Huntington's disease. *Ann Neurol* **36**:630, 1994.
44. Kandil MR, Tohamy SA, Fattah MA, Ahmed HN, Farwiez HM: Prevalence of chorea, dystonia and athetosis in Assiut, Egypt: A clinical and epidemiological study. *Neuroepidemiology* **13**:202, 1994.
45. Bohlega S, McLean D, Omer S, et al: Huntington's disease in Saudi Arabia (letter, comment). *J Med Genet* **32**:325, 1995.
46. Nakashima K, Watanabe Y, Kusumi M, et al: Epidemiological and genetic studies of Huntington's disease in the San-in area of Japan. *Neuroepidemiology* **15**:126, 1996.
47. Lanska DJ, Lavine L, Lanska MJ, Schoenberg BS: Huntington's disease mortality in the United States. *Neurology* **38**:769, 1988.
48. Hogg JE, Massey EW, Schoenberg BS: Mortality from Huntington's disease in the United States. *Adv Neurol* **23**:27, 1979.
49. Harper PS: *Huntington's Disease*. Philadelphia, Saunders, 1991.
50. Hayden MR: *Huntington's Chorea*. Berlin, Springer-Verlag, 1981.
51. Osborne JP, Munson P, Burman D: Huntington's chorea: Report of 3 cases and review of the literature. *Arch Dis Child* **57**:99, 1982.
52. Howeler CJ, Busch HF, Geraedts JP, Niermeijer MF, Staal A: Anticipation in mytonic dystrophy: Fact or fiction? *Brain* **112**:779, 1989.

53. Norremolle A, Riess O, Epplen JT, Fenger K, Hasholt L, Sorenson SA: Trinucleotide repeat elongation in the Huntington gene in Huntington disease patients from 71 Danish families. *Hum Mol Genet* **2**:1475, 1993.
54. Snell RG, MacMillan JC, Cheadle JP, et al: Relationship between trinucleotide repeat expansion and phenotypic variation in Huntington's disease. *Nature Genet* **4**:393, 1993.
55. Duyao M, Ambrose C, Myers R, et al: Trinucleotide repeat length instability in Huntington disease. *Nature Genet* **4**:387, 1993.
56. Harper PS, Newcombe RG: Age at onset and life table risks in genetic counselling for Huntington's disease. *J Med Genet* **29**:239, 1992.
57. Rubinsztein DC, Leggo J, Chiano M, et al: Genotypes at the GluR6 kainate receptor locus are associated with variation in the age of onset of Huntington disease. *Proc Natl Acad Sci USA* **94**:3872, 1997.
58. Newcombe RG: A life table for onset of Huntington's chorea. *Ann Hum Genet* **45**:375, 1981.
59. Wendt GG, Landzettel I, Unterreiner I: Erkrankungsalter bei der Huntingtonschen chorea. *Acta Genet (Basel)* **9**:18, 1959.
60. Adams P, Falek A, Arnold J: Huntington disease in Georgia: Age at onset. *Am J Hum Genet* **43**:695, 1988.
61. Roos RA, Hermans J, Vegter-van der Vlis M, van Ommen GJ, Bruyn GW: Duration of illness in Huntington's disease is not related to age at onset. *J Neurol Neurosurg Psychiatry* **56**:98, 1993.
62. Brothers CRD: Huntington's chorea in Victoria and Tasmania. *J Neurol Sci* **1**:405, 1964.
63. Pridmore SA: The prevalence of Huntington's disease in Tasmania. *Med J Aust* **153**:133, 1990.
64. Lanska DJ, Lanska MJ, Lavine L, Schoenberg BS: Conditions associated with Huntington's disease at death: A case-control study. *Arch Neurol* **45**:878, 1988.
65. Haines JL, Conneally PM: Causes of death in Huntington disease as reported on death certificates. *Genet Epidemiol* **3**:417, 1986.
66. Brandt J, Bylsma FW, Gross R, Stine OC, Ranen NG, Ross CA: Trinucleotide repeat length and clinical progression in Huntington's disease. *Neurology* **46**:527, 1996.
67. Ashizawa T, Wong LJ, Richards CS, Caskey CT, Jankovic J: CAG repeat size and clinical presentation in Huntington's disease. *Neurology* **44**:1137, 1994.
68. Claes S, Van Zand K, Legius E, et al: Correlations between triplet repeat expansion and clinical features in Huntington's disease. *Arch Neurol* **52**:749, 1995.
69. Kieburtz K, MacDonald M, Shih C, et al: Trinucleotide repeat length and progression of illness in Huntington's disease. *J Med Genet* **872**, 1994.
70. Penney JB Jr., Young AB, Shoulson I, et al: Huntington's disease in Venezuela: 7 years of follow-up on symptomatic and asymptomatic individuals. *Mov Disord* **5**:93, 1990.
71. Hayden MR, Hewitt J, Stoessel AJ, Clark C, Moennich D, Martin WR: The combined use of positron emission tomography and DNA polymorphisms for preclinical detection of Huntington's disease. *Neurology* **37**:1441, 1987.
72. Grafton ST, Mazziotta JC, Pahl JJ, et al: A comparison of neurological, metabolic, structural, and genetic evaluations in persons at risk for Huntington's disease. *Ann Neurol* **28**:614, 1990.
73. Young AB, Penney JB: Striatal inhomogeneities and basal ganglia function. *Mov Disord* **1**:3, 1986.
74. Wallace DC, Hall AC: Evidence of genetic heterogeneity in Huntington's chorea. *J Neurol Neurosurg Psychiatry* **35**:789, 1972.
75. Folstein SE, Leigh RJ, Parhad IM, Folstein MF: The diagnosis of Huntington's disease. *Neurology* **36**:1279, 1986.
76. Folstein SE: *Huntington's Disease: A Disorder of Families*. Baltimore, Johns Hopkins University Press, 1989.
77. Thompson PD, Berardelli A, Rothwell JC, et al: The coexistence of bradykinesia and chorea in Huntington's disease and its implications for theories of basal ganglia control of movement. *Brain* **111**:223, 1988.
78. van Vugt JP, van Hilten BJ, Roos RA: Hypokinesia in Huntington's disease. *Mov Disord* **11**:384, 1996.
79. Bruyn GW: Huntington's chorea: Historical, clinical and laboratory synopsis, in Vinken PJ, Bruyn GW (eds): *Diseases of the Basal Ganglia: Handbook of Clinical Neurology* Vol 6. Amsterdam, North Holland, 1968, p 298.
80. Westphal CFO: Über eine dem Bilde der cerebrospinalen grauen Degeneration ähnliche Erkrankung des centralen Nervensystems ohne anatomischen Befund, nebst einigen Bemerkungen über paradoxe Contraction. *Arch Psychiatrie Nervenkr* **14**:87–95 and 767–773, 1883.

81. Bittenbender JB, Quadfasel FA: Rigid and akinetic forms of Huntington's chorea. *Arch Neurol* **7**:275, 1962.

82. Beenen N, Buttner U, Lange HW: The diagnostic value of eye movement recordings in patients with Huntington's disease and their offspring. *Electroencephalogr Clin Neurophysiol* **63**:119, 1986.

83. Oepen G, Clarenbach P, Thoden U: Disturbance of eye movements in Huntington's chorea. *Arch Psychiatrie Nervenkr* **229**:205, 1981.

84. Lasker AG, Zee DS: Ocular motor abnormalities in Huntington's disease. *Vision Res* **37**:3639, 1997.

85. Lasker AG, Zee DS, Hain TC, Folstein SE, Singer HS: Saccades in Huntington's disease: Slowing and dysmetria. *Neurology* **38**:427, 1988.

86. Tian JR, Zee DS, Lasker AG, Folstein SE: Saccades in Huntington's disease: Predictive tracking and interaction between release of fixation and initiation of saccades. *Neurology* **41**:875, 1991.

87. Hefter H, Hömberg V, Lange HW, Freund HJ: Impairment of rapid movement in Huntington's disease. *Brain* **110**:585, 1987.

88. Folstein SE, Jensen B, Leigh RJ, Folstein MF: The measurement of abnormal movement: Methods developed for Huntington's disease. *Neurobehav Toxicol Teratol* **5**:605, 1983.

89. Koller WC, Trimble J: The gait abnormality of Huntington's disease. *Neurology* **35**:1450, 1985.

90. Podoll K, Caspary P, Lange HW, Noth J: Language functions in Huntington's disease. *Brain* **111**:1475, 1988.

91. Coleman R, Anderson D, Lovrien E: Oral motor dysfunction in individuals at risk of Huntington disease. *Am J Med Genet* **37**:36, 1990.

92. Caine ED, Fisher JM: Dementia in Huntington's disease, in Vinken PJ, Bruyn GW, Klawans HL, Frederiks JAM (eds): *Handbook of Clinical Neurology*, Vol 46, revised Series 2: Neurobehavioural Disorders. Amsterdam, Elsevier, 1985, p 305.

93. Brandt J, Butters N: The neuropsychology of Huntington's disease. *Trends Neurosci* **9**:118, 1986.

94. Jason GW, Pajurkova EM, Suchowersky O, et al: Presymptomatic neuropsychological impairment in Huntington's disease. *Arch Neurol* **45**:769, 1988.

95. Pillon B, Dubois B, Ploska A, Agid Y: Severity and specificity of cognitive impairment in Alzheimer's, Huntington's, and Parkinson's diseases and progressive supranuclear palsy. *Neurology* **41**:634, 1991.

96. Albert ML, Feldman RG, Willis AL: The subcortical dementia of progressive supranuclear palsy. *J Neurol Neurosurg Psychiatry* **37**:121, 1974.

97. Cummings JL, Benson DF: Subcortical dementia: Review of an emerging concept. *Arch Neurol* **41**:874, 1984.

98. Folstein SE: Appendix 1: The documentation of clinical features of Huntington's disease: Clinical assessment instruments, in *Huntington's Disease: A Disorder of Families*. Baltimore, Johns Hopkins University Press, 1989, p 189.

99. Fisher JM, Kennedy JL, Caine ED, Shoulson I: Dementia in Huntington disease: A cross-sectional analysis of intellectual decline. *Adv Neurol* **38**:229, 1983.

100. Lawrence AD, Sahakian BJ, Hodges JR, Rosser AE, Lange KW, Robbins TW: Executive and mnemonic functions in early Huntington's disease. *Brain* **119**:1633, 1996.

101. Wilson RS, Como PG, Garron DC, Klawans HL, Barr A, Klawans D: Memory failure in Huntington's disease. *J Clin Exp Neuropsychol* **9**:147, 1987.

102. Massman PJ, Delis DC, Butters N, Levin BE, Salmon DP: Are all subcortical dementias alike? Verbal learning and memory in Parkinson's and Huntington's disease patients. *J Clin Exp Neuropsychol* **12**:729, 1990.

103. Scholz OB, Berlemann C: Memory performance in Huntington's disease. *Int J Neurosci* **35**:155, 1987.

104. Randolph C: Implicit, explicit, and semantic memory functions in Alzheimer's disease and Huntington's disease. *J Clin Exp Neuropsychol* **13**:479, 1991.

105. Beatty WW, Salmon DP, Butters N, Heindel WC, Granholm EL: Retrograde amnesia in patients with Alzheimer's disease or Huntington's disease. *Neurobiol Aging* **9**:181, 1988.

106. Heindel WC, Butters N, Salmon DP: Impaired learning of a motor skill in patients with Huntington's disease. *Behav Neurosci* **102**:141, 1988.

107. Heindel WC, Salmon DP, Butters N: The biasing of weight judgments in Alzheimer's and Huntington's disease: A priming or programming phenomenon. *J Clin Exp Neuropsychol* **13**:189, 1991.

108. Knopman D, Nissen MJ: Procedural learning is impaired in Huntington's disease: Evidence from the serial reaction time task. *Neuropsychologia* **29**:245, 1991.

109. Brandt J, Folstein SE, Folstein MF: Differential cognitive impairment in Alzheimer's disease and Huntington's disease. *Ann Neurol* **23**:555, 1988.

110. Starkstein SE, Brandt J, Folstein S, et al: Neuropsychological and neuroradiological correlates in Huntington's disease. *J Neurol Neurosurg Psychiatry* **51**:1259, 1988.

111. Georgiou N, Bradshaw JL, Phillips JG, Chiu E: The effect of Huntington's disease and Gilles de la Tourette's syndrome on the ability to hold and shift attention. *Neuropsychologia* **34**:843, 1996.

112. Wallesch CW, Fehrenbach RA: On the neurolinguistic nature of language abnormalities in Huntington's disease. *J Neurol Neurosurg Psychiatry* **51**:367, 1988.

113. Hodges JR, Salmon DP, Butters N: The nature of the naming deficit in Alzheimer's and Huntington's disease. *Brain* **114**:1547, 1991.

114. Speedie LJ, Brake N, Folstein SE, Bowers D, Heilman KM: Comprehension of prosody in Huntington's disease. *J Neurol Neurosurg Psychiatry* **53**:607, 1990.

115. Hahn-Barma V, Deweer B, Durr A, et al: Are cognitive changes the first symptoms of Huntington's disease? A study of gene carriers. *J Neurol Neurosurg Psychiatry* **64**:172, 1998.

116. Campodonico JR, Codori AM, Brandt J: Neuropsychological stability over two years in asymptomatic carriers of the Huntington's disease mutation. *J Neurol Neurosurg Psychiatry* **61**:621, 1996.

117. Caine ED, Shoulson I: Psychiatric syndromes in Huntington's disease. *Am J Psychiatry* **140**:728, 1983.

118. Zappacosta B, Monza D, Meoni C, et al: Psychiatric symptoms do not correlate with cognitive decline, motor symptoms, or CAG repeat length in Huntington's disease. *Arch Neurol* **53**:493, 1996.

119. Weigell-Weber M, Schmid W, Spiegel R: Psychiatric symptoms and CAG expansion in Huntington's disease. *Am J Med Genet* **67**:53, 1996.

120. Lovestone S, Hodgson S, Sham P, Differ AM, Levy R: Familial psychiatric presentation of Huntington's disease. *J Med Genet* **33**:128, 1996.

121. Morris M, Tyler A: Psychiatric aspects of Huntington's disease, in Harper PS (ed): *Huntington's Disease*. London, Saunders, 1991, p 205.

122. Farrer LA: Suicide and attempted suicide in Huntington disease: implications for preclinical testing of persons at risk. *Am J Med Genet* **24**:305, 1986.

123. Folstein SE: The psychopathology of Huntington's disease. *Res Publ Assoc Res Nerv Ment Dis* **69**:181, 1991.

124. Burns A, Folstein S, Brandt J, Folstein M: Clinical assessment of irritability, aggression, and apathy in Huntington and Alzheimer disease. *J Nerv Ment Dis* **178**:20, 1990.

125. Sanberg PR, Fibiger HC, Mark RF: Body weight and dietary factors in Huntington's disease patients compared with matched controls. *Med J Aust* **1**:407, 1981.

126. Farrer LA, Yu PL: Anthropometric discrimination among affected, at-risk, and not-at-risk individuals in families with Huntington disease. *Am J Med Genet* **21**:307, 1985.

127. Morales LM, Estévez J, Suarez H, Villalobos R, Chacin de Bonilla L, Bonilla E: Nutritional evaluation of Huntington disease patients. *Am J Clin Nutr* **50**:145, 1989.

128. Hansotia P, Wall R, Berendes J: Sleep disturbances and severity of Huntington's disease. *Neurology* **35**:1672, 1985.

129. Bollen EL, Den Heijer JC, Ponsioen C, et al: Respiration during sleep in Huntington's chorea. *J Neurol Sci* **84**:63, 1988.

130. Emser W, Brenner M, Stober T, Schimrigk K: Changes in nocturnal sleep in Huntington's and Parkinson's disease. *J Neurol* **235**:177, 1988.

131. Wheeler JS, Sax DS, Krane RJ, Siroky MB: Vesico-urethral function in Huntington's chorea. *Br J Urol* **57**:63, 1985.

132. Davies DD: Abnormal response to anaesthesia in a case of Huntington's chorea. *Br J Anaesth* **38**:490, 1966.

133. Gualandi W, Bonfanti G: A case of prolonged apnea in Huntington's chorea. *Acta Anaesthesiol* **19**(suppl 6):235, 1968.

134. Blanloeil Y, Bigot A, Dixneuf B: Anaesthesia in Huntington's chorea. *Anaesthesia* **37**:695, 1982.

135. Farina J, Rauscher LA: Anaesthesia and Huntington's chorea: A report of two cases. *Br J Anaesth* **49**:1167, 1977.

136. Browne MG, Cross R: Huntington's chorea. *Br J Anaesth* **53**:1367, 1981.

137. Browne MG: Anaesthesia in Huntington's chorea. *Anaesthesia* **38**:65, 1982.

138. Shoulson I, Fahn S: Huntington disease: Clinical care and evaluation. *Neurology* **29**:1, 1979.

139. Myers RH, Sax DS, Schoenfeld M, et al: Late onset of Huntington's disease. *J Neurol Neurosurg Psychiatry* **48**:530, 1985.

140. Shoulson I: Huntington disease: Functional capacities in patients treated with neuroleptic and antidepressant drugs. *Neurology* **31**:1333, 1981.

141. Markham CH, Knox JW: Observations on Huntington's chorea in childhood. *J Pediatr* **67**:46, 1965.

142. Oliver J, Dewhurst K: Childhood and adolescent forms of Huntington's disease. *J Neurol Neurosurg Psychiatry* **32**:455, 1969.

143. Jervis GA: Huntington's chorea in childhood. *Arch Neurol* **9**:244, 1963.

144. Vogel CM, Drury I, Terry LC, Young AB: Myoclonus in adult Huntington's disease. *Ann Neurol* **29**:213, 1991.

145. James CM, Houlihan GD, Snell RG, Cheadle JP, Harper PS: Late-onset Huntington's disease: A clinical and molecular study. *Age Ageing* **23**:445, 1994.

146. Britton JW, Uitti RJ, Ahlskog JE, Robinson RG, Kremer B, Hayden MR: Hereditary late-onset chorea without significant dementia: Genetic evidence for substantial phenotypic variation in Huntington's disease. *Neurology* **45**:443, 1995.

147. Kremer B, Squitieri FS, Telenius H, et al: Molecular analysis of late onset Huntington disease. *J Med Genet* **30**:991, 1993.

148. Bird ED: The brain in Huntington's chorea. *Psychol Med* **8**:357, 1978.

149. Padberg G, Bruyn GW: Chorea—Differential diagnosis, in Vinken PJ, Bruyn GW, Klawans HL (eds): *Handbook of Clinical Neurology*, Vol 5, No 49: Extrapyramidal Disorders. Amsterdam, Elsevier, 1986, p 549.

150. Meszaros K, Brucke T, Fuchs K, et al: Normal CAG repeats in the Huntington gene in a family with benign familial chorea (letter). *Psychiatri Genet* **6**:91, 1996.

151. Hageman G, Ippel PF, van Hout MS, Rozeboom AR: A Dutch family with benign hereditary chorea of early onset: Differentiation from Huntington's disease. *Clin Neurol Neurosurg* **98**:165, 1996.

152. Hardie RJ, Pullon HWH, Harding AE, et al: Neuroacanthocytosis: A clinical, haematologic and pathological study of 19 cases. *Brain* **114**:12, 1991.

153. Iiuzuka R, Hirayama K, Maehara K: Dentato-rubro-pallido-luysian atrophy: A clinicopathological study. *J Neurol Neurosurg Psychiatry* **47**:1288, 1984.

154. Koide R, Ikeuchi T, Onodera O, et al: Unstable expansion of CAG repeat in hereditary dentatorubral-pallidoluysian atrophy (DRPLA). *Nature Genet* **6**:9, 1994.

155. Nagafuchi S, Yanagisawa H, Ohsaki E, et al: Structure and expression of the gene responsible for the triplet repeat disorder, dentatorubral and pallidoluysian atrophy (DRPLA). *Nature Genet* **8**:177, 1994.

156. Shinotoh H, Calne DB, Snow B, et al: Normal CAG repeat length in the Huntington's disease gene in senile chorea. *Neurology* **44**:2183, 1994.

157. Garcia-Ruiz PJ, Gomez-Tortosa E, del Barrio A, et al: Senile chorea: A multicenter prospective study. *Acta Neurol Scand* **95**:180, 1997.

158. McNeil SM, Novelletto A, Srinidhi J, et al: Reduced penetrance of the Huntington's disease mutation. *Hum Mol Genet* **6**:775, 1997.

159. Myers RH, MacDonald ME, Koroshetz WJ, et al: *De novo* expansion of a (CAG)$_n$ repeat in sporadic Huntington's disease. *Nature Genet* **5**:168, 1993.

160. Zlotogora J: Dominance and homozygosity. *Am J Med Genet* **68**:412, 1997.

161. Vogel F, Motuksky AG: *Human Genetics*. New York, Springer-Verlag, 1986.

162. Goldberg YP, Kremer B, Andrew SE, et al: Molecular analysis of new mutations causing Huntington disease: Intermediate alleles and sex of origin effects. *Nature Genet* **5**:174, 1993.

163. Goldberg YP, McMurray CT, Zeisler J, et al: Increased instability of intermediate alleles in families with sporadic Huntington disease compared to similar sized intermediate alleles in the general population. *Hum Mol Genet* **4**(10):1911, 1995.

164. Ridley RM, Frith CD, Crow TJ, Conneally PM: Anticipation in Huntington's disease is inherited through the male line but may originate in the female. *J Med Genet* **25**:589, 1988.

165. Reik W: Genomic imprinting: A possible mechanism for the parental origin effect in Huntington's chorea. *J Med Gen* **25**:805, 1988.

166. Telenius H, Kremer HPH, Theilmann J, et al: Molecular analysis of juvenile Huntington disease: The major influence on (CAG)$_n$ repeat length is the sex of the affected parent. *Hum Mol Genet* **2**:1535, 1993.

167. Kremer B, Almqvist E, Theilmann J, et al: Sex dependent mechanisms for expansions and contractions of the CAG repeat on affected Huntington disease chromosomes. *Am J Hum Genet* **57**:343, 1995.

168. Strong TV, Tagle DA, Valdes JM, et al: Widespread expression of the human and rat Huntington's disease gene in brain and nonneural tissues. *Nature Genet* **5**:259, 1993.

169. Li SH, Schilling G, Young III WS, et al: Huntington's disease gene (IT15) is widely expressed in human and rat tissues. *Neuron* **11**:985, 1993.

170. Landwehrmeyer GB, McNeil SM, Dure LS 4, et al: Huntington's disease gene: Regional and cellular expression in brain of normal and affected individuals. *Ann Neurol* **37**:218, 1995.

171. Trottier Y, Devys D, Imbert G, et al: Cellular localization of the Huntington's disease protein and discrimination of the normal and mutated form. *Nature Genet* **10**:104, 1995.

172. Gutekunst CA, Levey AI, Heilman CJ, et al: Identification and localization of huntingtin in brain and human lymphoblastoid cell lines with anti-fusion protein antibodies. *Proc Natl Acad Sci USA* **92**:8710, 1995.

173. Huq A, Hackam AS, Graham RK, Wellington CL, Hayden MR: Molecular pathogenesis of Huntington's disease: Biochemical studies of huntingtin, in Wells RD, Warren ST, Sarmiento M (eds): *Genetic Instabilities and Hereditary Neurological Diseases*. London, Academic Press, 1998, p 325.

174. Ferrante RJ, Gutekunst CA, Persichetti F, et al: Heterogeneous topographic and cellular distribution of huntingtin expression in the normal human neostriatum. *J Neurosci* **17**:3052, 1997.

175. Kosinski CM, Cha J-H, Young AB, et al: Huntingtin immunoreactivity in the rat neostriatum: Differential accumulation in projection and interneurons. *Exp Neurol* **144**:239, 1987.

176. Vonsattel JP, Myers RH, Stevens TJ, Ferrante RJ, Bird ED, Richardson EP Jr: Neuropathological classification of Huntington's disease. *J Neuropathol Exp Neurol* **44**:559, 1985.

177. Hedreen JC, Folstein SE: Early loss of neostriatal striosome neurons in Huntington's disease. *J Neuropathol Exp Neurol* **54**:105, 1995.

178. Aronin N, Chase K, Young C, et al: CAG expansion affects the expression of mutant huntingtin in the Huntington's disease brain. *Neuron* **15**:1193, 1995.

179. Persichetti F, Ambrose CM, Ge P, et al: Normal and expanded Huntington's disease gene alleles produce distinguishable proteins due to translation across the CAG repeat. *Mol Med* **1**:374, 1995.

180. Persichetti F, Carlee L, Faber PW, et al: Differential expression of normal and mutant huntington's disease gene alleles. *Neurobiol Dis* **3**:183, 1996.

181. Ide K, Nukina N, Masuda N, Goto J, Kanazawa I: Abnormal gene product identified in Huntington's disease lymphocytes and brain. *Biochem Biophys Res Commun* **209**:1119, 1995.

182. Hoogeveen AT, Willemsen R, Meyer N, et al: Characterization and localization of the Huntington disease gene product. *Hum Mol Genet* **2**:2069, 1993.

183. De Rooij KE, Dorsman JC, Smoor MA, Den Dunnen JT, van Ommen GJ: Subcellular localization of the Huntington's disease gene product in cell lines by immunofluorescence and biochemical subcellular fractionation. *Hum Mol Genet* **5**:1093, 1996.

184. DiFiglia M, Sapp E, Chase KO, et al: Aggregation of huntingtin in neuronal intranuclear inclusions and dystrophic neurites in brain. *Science* **277**:1990, 1997.

185. Sharp AH, Loev SJ, Schilling G, et al: Widespread expression of Huntington's disease gene (IT15) protein product. *Neuron* **14**:1065, 1995.

186. Wood JD, MacMillan JC, Harper PS, Lowenstein PR, Jones AL: Partial characterisation of murine huntingtin and apparent variations in the subcellular localisation of huntingtin in human, mouse and rat brain. *Hum Mol Genet* **5**:418, 1996.

187. Kalchman MA, Koide HB, McCutcheon K, et al: *HIP1*, a human homolog of *S. cerevisiae Sla2p*, interacts with membrane-associated huntingtin in the brain. *Nature Genet* **16**:44, 1997.

188. Li XJ, Li SH, Sharp AH, et al: A huntingtin-associated protein enriched in brain with implications for pathology. *Nature* **378**:398, 1995.

189. Kalchman MA, Graham RK, Xia G, et al: Huntingtin is ubiquitinated and interacts with a specific ubiquitin conjugating enzyme. *J Biol Chem* **271**:19385, 1996.

190. Burke JR, Enghild JJ, Martin ME, et al: Huntingtin and DRPLA proteins selectively interact with the enzyme GAPDH. *Nature Med* **2**:347, 1996.

191. Wanker EE, Rovira C, Scherzinger E, et al: HIP1: A huntingtin interacting protein isolated by the yeast two-hybrid system. *Hum Mol Genet* **6**:487, 1997.

192. Bao J, Sharp AH, Wagster MV, et al: Expansion of polyglutamine repeat in huntingtin leads to abnormal protein interactions involving calmodulin. *Proc Natl Acad Sci USA* **93**:5037, 1996.

193. Liu YF, Deth RC, Devys D: SH3 domain-dependent association of huntingtin with epidermal growth factor receptor signaling complexes. *J Biol Chem* **272**:8121, 1997.

194. Anglade M: Une autopsie de chorée de Huntington. *Gaz Hebd Sci Med Bordeaux* **27**:89, 1906.

195. Jelgersma G: Die anatomische Veränderungen bei Paralysis agitans und chronbnischer Chorea. *Verh Ges Dtsch Naturf Crtz* **2**:383, 1908.

196. Alzheimer A: Über die anatomische Gründlage der Huntington'schen Chorea und der choreatischen Bewegungen überhaupt. *Neurol Zentralbl* **30**:891, 1911.

197. Dunlap CB: Pathologic changes in Huntington's chorea with special reference to the corpus striatum. *Arch Neurol Psychiatry (Chicago)* **18**:867, 1927.

198. McCaughey WTE: The pathologic spectrum of Huntington's chorea. *J Nerv Ment Dis* **133**:91, 1961.

199. Earle KM: Pathology and experimental models of Huntington's chorea, in Barbeau A, Chase TM, Paulson GW (eds): *Huntington's Chorea 1872–1972: Advances in Neurology*. New York, Raven Press, 1973, p 341.

200. Forno LS, Jose C: Huntington's chorea: A pathological study, in Barbeau A, Chase TN, Paulson GW (eds): *Huntington's Chorea 1872–1972: Advances in Neurology*. New York, Raven Press, 1973, p 453.

201. Myers RH, Vonsattel JP, Paskevich PA, et al: Decreased neuronal and increased oligodendroglial densities in Huntington's disease caudate nucleus. *J Neuropathol Exp Neurol* **50**:729, 1991.

202. Graveland GA, Williams RS, DiFiglia M: A Golgi study of the human neostriatum: Neurons and afferent fibers. *J Comp Neurol* **234**:317, 1985.

203. Dom R, Baro F, Brucher JM: A cytometric study of the putamen in different types of Huntington's chorea, in Barbeau A, Chase TN, Paulson GW (eds): *Huntington's Chorea 1982–1972: Advances in Neurology*. New York, Raven Press, 1973, p 369.

204. Lange H, Thorner G, Hopf A, Schroder KF: Morphometric studies of the neuropathological changes in choreatic diseases. *J Neurol Sci* **28**:401, 1976.

205. Dragunow M, Faull RL, Lawlor P, et al: In situ evidence for DNA fragmentation in Huntington's disease striatum and Alzheimer's disease temporal lobes. *Neuro report* **6**:1053, 1995.

206. Portera-Cailliau C, Hedreen JC, Price DL, Koliatsos VE: Evidence for apoptotic cell death in Huntington disease and excitotoxic animal models. *J Neurosci* **15**:3775, 1995.

207. Roizin L, Stellar S, Liu JC: Neuronal nuclear-cytoplasmic changes in Huntington's chorea: Electron microscope investigations, in Chase TN, Wexler NS, Barbeau A (eds): *Huntington's Disease: Advances in Neurology*. New York, Raven Press, 1979, p 95.

208. Graveland GA, Williams RS, DiFiglia M: Evidence for degenerative and regenerative changes in neostriatal spiny neurons in Huntington's disease. *Science* **227**:770, 1985.

209. Ferrante RJ, Kowall NW, Richardson EP Jr: Proliferative and degenerative changes in striatal spiny neurons in Huntington's disease: A combined study using the section-Golgi method and calbindin D28k immunocytochemistry. *J Neurosci* **11**:3877, 1991.

210. Nihei K, Kowall NW: Neurofilament and neural cell adhesion molecule immunocytochemistry of Huntington's disease striatum. *Ann Neurol* **31**:59, 1992.

211. Becher MW, Kotzuk JA, Sharp AH et al: Intranuclear neuronal inclusions in Huntington's disease and dentatorubral and palidoluysian atrophy: Correlation between the density of inclusions and *IT15* CAG triplet repeat length. *Neurobiol Dis* **4**:387, 1998.

212. Mangiarini L, Sathasivam K, Seller M, et al: Exon 1 of the HD gene with an expanded CAG repeat is sufficient to cause a progressive neurological phenotype in transgenic mice. *Cell* **87**:493, 1996.

213. Klintworth GK: Huntington's chorea: Morphologic contributions of a century, in Barbeau A, Chase TN, Paulson GW (eds): *Huntington's Chorea 1872–1972: Advances in Neurology*. New York, Raven Press, 1973, p 353.

214. Forno LS, Norville RL: Ultrastructure of the neostriatum in Huntington's disease, in Chase TN, Wexler NS, Barbeau A (eds): *Huntington's Disease: Advances in Neurology*. New York, Raven Press, 1979, p 123.

215. Lange HW: Quantitative changes of telencephalon, diencephalon, and mesencephalon in Huntington's chorea, postencephalitic, and idiopathic parkinsonism. *Verh Anat Ges* **75**:923, 1981.

216. Dexter DT, Carayon A, Javoy-Agid F, et al: Alterations in the levels of iron, ferritin and other trace metals in Parkinson's disease and other neurodegenerative diseases affecting the basal ganglia. *Brain* **114**:1953, 1991.

217. Averback P: Lesions of the nucleus ansae peduncularis in neuropsychiatric disease. *Arch Neurol* **38**:230, 1981.

218. Davies SW, Turmaine M, Cozens BA, et al: Formation of neuronal intranuclear inclusions (NII) underlies the neurological dysfunction in mice transgenic for the HD mutation. *Cell* **90**:537, 1997.

219. Roos RA, Bots GT, Hermans J: Quantitative analysis of morphological features in Huntington's disease. *Acta Neurol Scand* **73**:131, 1986.

220. Roos RA, Pruyt JF, de Vries J, Bots GT: Neuronal distribution in the putamen in Huntington's disease. *J Neurol Neurosurg Psychiatry* **48**:422, 1985.

221. Kowall NW, Ferrante RJ, Martin JB: Patterns of cell loss in Huntington's disease. *Trends Neurosci* **10**:24, 1987.

222. Graybiel AM: Neurotransmitters and neuromodulators in the basal ganglia. *Trends Neurosci* **13**:244, 1990.

223. Smith AD, Bolam JP: The neural network of the basal ganglia as revealed by the study of synaptic connections of identified neurons. *Trends Neurosci* **13**:259, 1990.

224. Reiner A, Albin RL, Anderson KD, D'Amato CJ, Penney JB, Young AB: Differential loss of striatal projection neurons in Huntington disease. *Proc Natl Acad Scie USA* **85**:5733, 1988.

225. Albin RL, Young AB, Penney JB, et al: Abnormalities of striatal projection neurons and *N*-methyl-D-aspartate receptors in presymptomatic Huntington's disease. *New Engl J Med* **322**:1293, 1990.

226. Albin RL, Qin Y, Young AB, Penney JB, Chesselet MF: Preproenkephalin messenger RNA-containing neurons in striatum of patients with symptomatic and presymptomatic Huntington's disease: An in situ hybridization study. *Ann Neurol* **30**:542, 1991.

227. Augood SJ, Faull RL, Love DR, Emson PC: Reduction in enkephalin and substance P messenger RNA in the striatum of early grade Huntington's disease: A detailed cellular in situ hybridization study. *Neuroscience* **72**:1023, 1996.

228. Hope BT, Michael GJ, Knigge KM, Vincent SR: Neuronal NADPH-diaphorase is a nitric oxide synthase. *Proc Natl Acad Sci USA* **88**:2811, 1991.

229. Ferrante RJ, Kowall NW, Beal MF, Richardson EP Jr, Bird ED, Martin JB: Selective sparing of a class of striatal neurons in Huntington's disease. *Science* **230**:561, 1985.

230. Dawbarn D, De Quidt ME, Emson PC: Survival of basal ganglia neuropeptide Y–somatostatin neurones in Huntington's disease. *Brain Res* **340**:251, 1985.

231. Ferrante RJ, Kowall NW, Beal MF, Martin JB, Bird ED, Richardson EP Jr: Morphologic and histochemical characteristics of a spared subset of striatal neurons in Huntington's disease. *J Neuropathol Exp Neurol* **46**:12, 1987.

232. Norris PJ, Waldvogel HJ, Faull RL, Love DR, Emson PC: Decreased neuronal nitric oxide synthase messenger RNA and somatostatin messenger RNA in the striatum of Huntington's disease. *Neuroscience* **72**:1037, 1996.

233. Ferrante RJ, Beal MF, Kowall NW, Richardson EP Jr, Martin JB: Sparing of acetylcholinesterase-containing striatal neurons in Huntington's disease. *Brain Res* **411**:162, 1987.

234. de la Monte SM, Vonsattel JP, Richardson EP Jr: Morphometric demonstration of atrophic changes in the cerebral cortex, white matter, and neostriatum in Huntington's disease. *J Neuropathol Exp Neurol* **47**:516, 1988.

235. Stone TT, Falstein EI: Pathology of Huntington's chorea. *J Nerv Ment Dis* **88**:602–626, 1938.

236. Sotrel A, Paskevich PA, Kiely DK, Bird ED, Williams RS, Myers RH: Morphometric analysis of the prefrontal cortex in Huntington's disease. *Neurology* **41**:1117, 1991.

237. Savvopoulos S, Golaz J, Bouras C, Constantinidis J, Tissot R: Huntington chorea. Anatomoclinical and genetic study of 17 cases. *Encephale* **16**:251, 1990.

238. Tellez-Nagel I, Johnson AB, Terry RD: Studies on brain biopsies of patients with Huntington's chorea. *J Neuropathol Exp Neurol* **33**:308, 1974.

239. Cudkowicz M, Kowall NW: Degeneration of pyramidal projection neurons in Huntington's disease cortex. *Ann Neurol* **27**:200, 1990.

240. Zalneraitis EL, Landis DMD, Richardson EP, Selkoe DJ: A comparison of astrocytic structure in cerebral cortex and striatum in Huntington disease. *Neurology* **31**(suppl 1):151–150, 1981.

241. Braak H, Braak E: Allocortical involvement in Huntington's disease. *Neuropathol Appl Neurobiol* **18**:539, 1992.

242. McIntosh GC, Jameson HD, Markesbery WR: Huntington disease associated with Alzheimer disease. *Ann Neurol* 3:545, 1978.
243. Reyes MG, Gibbons S: Dementia of the Alzheimer's type and Huntington's disease. *Neurology* 35:273, 1985.
244. Bruyn GW, Roos RA: Senile plaques in Huntington's disease: A preliminary report. *Clin Neurol Neurosurg* 92:329, 1990.
245. Parent A: Extrinsic connections of the basal ganglia. *Trends Neurosci* 13:254, 1990.
246. Wahren W: Anatomy of the hypothalamus, in Schaltenbrand G, Bailey P (eds): *Introduction to Sterotaxis with an Atlas of the Human Brain*. Stuttgart, Georg Thieme, 1959, p 119.
247. Wahren M, Trzepacz PT: Zur pathoklise des Nucleus Tuberis lateralis. *Progr Brain Res* 5:161, 1964.
248. Kremer HP, Roos RA, Dingjan G, Marani E, Bots GT: Atrophy of the hypothalamic lateral tuberal nucleus in Huntington's disease. *J Neuropathol Exp Neurol* 49:371, 1990.
249. Kremer HP, Roos RA, Dingjan GM, Bots GT, Bruyn GW, Hofman MA: The hypothalamic lateral tuberal nucleus and the characteristics of neuronal loss in Huntington's disease. *Neurosci Lett* 132:101, 1991.
250. Tagliavini F, Pilleri G: Basal nucleus of Meynert: A neuropathological study in Alzheimer's disease, simple senile dementia, Pick's disease and Huntington's chorea. *J Neurol Sci* 62:243, 1983.
251. Clark AW, Parhad IM, Folstein SE, et al: The nucleus basalis in Huntington's disease. *Neurology* 33:1262, 1983.
252. Zweig RM, Ross CA, Hedreen JC, et al: Locus coeruleus involvement in Huntington's disease. *Arch Neurol* 49:152, 1992.
253. Rodda RA: Cerebellar atrophy in Huntington's disease. *J Neurol Sci* 50:147, 1981.
254. Byers RK, Gilles FH, Fung C: Huntington's disease in children: Neuropathologic study of four cases. *Neurology* 23:561, 1973.
255. Jeste DV, Barban L, Parisi J: Reduced Purkinje cell density in Huntington's disease. *Exp Neurol* 85:78, 1984.
256. Xuereb JH, MacMillan JC, Snell R, Davies P, Harper PS: Neuropathological diagnosis and CAG repeat expansion in Huntington's disease. *J Neurol Neurosurg Psychiatry* 60:78, 1996.
257. Furtado S, Suchowersky O, Rewcastle B, Graham L, Klimek ML, Garber A: Relationship between trinucleotide repeats and neuropathological changes in Huntington's disease. *Ann Neurol* 39:132, 1996.
258. Penney JB Jr., Vonsattel JP, MacDonald ME, Gusella JF, Myers RH: CAG repeat number governs the development rate of pathology in Huntington's disease. *Ann Neurol* 41:689, 1997.
259. Martindale D, Hackam AS, Wieczorek A, et al: Length of the protein and polyglutamine tract influence localization and frequency of intracellular aggregates of huntingtin. *Nature Genet* 18:150, 1998.
260. Li S.-H., Li X-J: Aggregation of N-terminal huntingtin is dependent on the length of its glutamine repeats. *Hum Mol Genet* 7:777, 1998.
261. Hackam AS, Singaraja R, Wellington CL, et al: The influence of huntingtin protein size on nuclear localization and cellular toxicity. *J Cell Biol* 141:1097, 1998.
262. Cooper JK, Schilling G, Peters MF, et al: Truncated N-terminal fragments of huntingtin with expanded glutamine repeats form nuclear and cytoplasmic aggregates in cell culture. *Hum Mol Genet* 7:783, 1998.
263. Skinner PJ, Koshy BT, Cummings CJ, et al: Ataxin-1 with an expanded glutamine tract alters nuclear matrix-associated structures. *Nature* 389:971, 1997.
264. Paulson HL, Perez MK, Trottier Y, et al: Intranuclear inclusions of expanded polyglutamine protein in spinocerebellar ataxia type 3. *Neuron* 19:333, 1997.
265. Ellerby LM, Hackam AS, Propp SS, Ellerby HM, Rabizadeh S, Trifiro MA, Pinsky L, Wellington CL, Salvesen GS, Hayden MR, Bredesen DE: Kennedy's disease: Caspase cleavage of the androgen receptor is a crucial event in cytotoxicity. *J Neurochem* 1999.
266. Merry DE, Kobayashi Y, Bailey CK, Taye AA, Fischbeck KH: Cleavage, aggregation and toxicity of the expanded androgen receptor in spinal and bulbar muscular atrophy. *Hum Mol Genet* 7:693, 1998.
267. Igarashi S, Koide R, Shimohata T, et al: Suppression of aggregate formation and apoptosis by translutaminase inhibitors in cells expressing truncated DRPLA protein with an expanded polyglutamine stretch. *Nature Genet* 18:111, 1998.
268. Cummings CJ, Mancini MA, Antalffy B, DeFranco DB, Orr HT, Zoghbi HY: Chaperone suppression of aggregation and altered subcellular proteasome localization imply protein misfolding in SCA1. *Nature Genet* 19:148, 1998.

269. Wellington CL, Ellerby LM, Hackam AS, et al: Caspase cleavage of gene products associated with triplet expansion disorders generates truncated fragments containing the polyglutamine tract. *J Biol Chem* 273:9159, 1998.
270. Ordway JM, Tallaksen-Greene S, Gutekunst C-A, et al: Ectopically expressed CAG repeats cause intranuclear inclusions and a progressive late onset neurological phenotype in the mouse. *Cell* 91:753, 1997.
270a. Hodgson JG, Agopyan N, Gutekunst JA, Leavitt PR, et al: A YAC mouse model for Huntington's disease with full-length mutant huntingtin, cytoplasmic toxicity, and selective striatal neurodegeneration. *Neuron* 23:181, 1999.
270b. Klement IA, Skinner RJ, Kayto HD, et al: Ataxin-1 nuclear localization and aggregation: Role in polyglutamine-induced disease in SCA1 transgenic mice. *Cell* 95:41, 1998.
270c. Shelbourne PF, Killeen N, Herner RF, et al: A Huntington's disease CAG expansion at the murine *Hdh* locus is unstable and associated with behavioral abnormalities in mice. *Hum Mol Genet* 8:763, 1999.
270d. Wheeler V, Auoba W, White J, Srinidhi J, et al: Length-dependent gametic CAG repeat instability in the Huntington's disease knock-in mouse. *Hum Mol Genet* 8:115, 1999.
270e. Reddy LH, Williams M, Chasles V, et al: Behavioral abnormalities and selective neuonal loss in HD transgenic mice expressing full-length *HD* cDNA. *Nat Genet* 17:404, 1997.
271. Bamford KA, Caine ED, Kido DK, Plassche WM, Shoulson I: Clinical-pathologic correlation in Huntington's disease: A neuropsychological and computed tomography study. *Neurology* 39:796, 1989.
272. Young AB, Penney JB, Starosta-Rubinstein S, et al: PET scan investigations of Huntington's disease: Cerebral metabolic correlates of neurological features and functional decline. *Ann Neurol* 20:296, 1986.
273. Berent S, Giordani B, Lehtinen S, et al: Positron emission tomographic scan investigations of Huntington's disease: Cerebral metabolic correlates of cognitive function. *Ann Neurol* 23:541, 1988.
274. Parent A: *Comparative Neurobiology of the Basal Ganglia*. New York, J Wiley, 1986.
275. DeLong MR, Georgopoulos AP: Motor functions of the basal ganglia, in Brooks VB (ed): *Handbook of Physiology: The Nervous System II*. Washington, American Physiology Society, 1981, p 1017.
276. Alexander GE, Crutcher MD: Functional architecture of basal ganglia circuits: Neural substrates of parallel processing. *Trends Neurosci* 13:266, 1990.
277. Albin RL, Young AB, Penney JB: The functional anatomy of basal ganglia disorders. *Trends Neurosci* 12:366, 1989.
278. DeLong MR: Primate models of movement disorders of the basal ganglia. *Trends Neurosci* 13:281, 1990.
279. Albin RL, Greenamyre JT: Alternative excitotoxic hypothesis. *Neurology* 42:733, 1992.
280. Albin RL, Reiner A, Anderson KD, Penney JB, Young AB: Striatal and nigral neuron subpopulations in rigid Huntington's disease: Implications for the functional anatomy of chorea and rigidity-akinesia. *Ann Neurol* 27:357, 1990.
281. Albin RL, Reiner A, Anderson KD, et al: Preferential loss of striato-external pallidal projection neurons in presymptomatic Huntington's disease. *Ann Neurol* 31:425, 1992.
282. Spokes EG: Neurochemical alterations in Huntington's chorea: A study of post-mortem brain tissue. *Brain* 103:179, 1980.
283. Klawans HL, Paulson GW, Ringel SP, Barbeau A: Use of L-dopa in the detection of presymptomatic Huntington's chorea. *New Engl J Med* 286:1332, 1972.
284. Gerfen CR: The neostriatal mosaic: multiple levels of compartmental organization. *Trends Neurosci* 15:133, 1992.
285. Stoessl AJ, Martin WR, Hayden MR, et al: Dopamine in Huntington disease: Studies using positron emission tomography. *Neurology* 36:310, 1986.
286. Kurlan R, Goldblatt D, Zaczek R, et al: Cerebrospinal fluid homovanillic acid and parkinsonism in Huntington's disease. *Ann Neurol* 24:282, 1988.
287. DiFiglia M: Excitotoxic injury of the neostriatum: a model for Huntington's disease. *Trends Neurosci* 13:286, 1990.
288. Coyle JT, Schwartz R: Lesion of striatal neurones with kainic acid provides a model for Huntington's chorea. *Nature* 263:244, 1976.
289. McGeer EG, McGeer PL: Duplication of biochemical changes of Huntington's chorea by intrastriatal injections of glutamic and kainic acids. *Nature* 263:517, 1976.

290. Beal MF, Ferrante RJ, Swartz KJ, Kowall NW: Chronic quinolinic acid lesions in rats closely resemble Huntington's disease. *J Neurosci* 11:1649, 1991.
291. Dure LS, Young AB, Penney JB: Excitatory amino acid binding sites in the caudate nucleus and frontal cortex of Huntington's disease. *Ann Neurol* 30:785, 1991.
292. Kanazawa I, Tanaka Y, Cho F: Choreic movements induced by unilateral kainate lesions of the striatum and L-dopa administration in monkey. *Neurosci Lett* 71:241, 1985.
293. Hantraye P, Riche D, Maziere M, Isacson O: A primate model of Huntington's disease: Behavioral and anatomical studies of unilateral excitotoxic lesions of the caudate-putamen in the baboon. *Exp Neurol* 108:91, 1990.
294. Kremer B, Tallaksen-Greene SJ, Albin RL: AMPA and NMDA binding sites in the hypothalamic lateral tuberal nucleus: implications for Huntington's disease. *Neurology* 43:1593, 1993.
295. Choi DW, Rothman SM: The role of glutamate neurotoxicity in hypoxic-ischemic neuronal death. *Annu Rev Neurosci* 13:171, 1990.
296. Beal MF: Does impairment of energy metabolism result in excitotoxic neuronal death in neurodegenerative illnesses? *Ann Neurol* 31:119, 1992.
297. Cotman CW, Monaghan DT, Ottersen OP, Storm-Mathisen J: Anatomical organization of excitatory amino acid receptors and their pathways. *Trends Neurosci* 7:273, 1987.
298. Deroover J, Baro F, Bourguignon RP, Smets P: Tiapride versus placebo: A double-blind comparative study in the management of Huntington's chorea. *Curr Med Res Opin* 9:329, 1984.
299. Hayden MR, Soles JA, Ward RH: Age of onset in sibling of persons with juvenile Huntington disease. *Clin Genet* 27:117, 1985.
300. Skraastad MI, Verwest A, Bakker E, et al: Presymptomatic, prenatal, and exclusion testing for Huntington disease using seven closely linked DNA markers. *Am J Med Genet* 39:217, 1991.
301. Craufurd D, Dodge A, Kerzin-Storrar L, Harris R: Uptake of presymptomatic predictive testing for Huntington's disease. *Lancet* 2:603, 1989.
302. Brandt J, Quaid KA, Folstein SE, et al: Presymptomatic diagnosis of delayed-onset disease with linked DNA markers: The experience in Huntington's disease. *JAMA* 261:3108, 1989.
303. Wiggins S, Whyte P, Huggins M, et al: The psychological consequences of predictive testing for Huntington disease. *New Engl J Med* 327:1401, 1992.
304. Tibben A, Timman R, Bannink EC, Duivenvoorden HJ: Three-year follow-up after presymptomatic testing for Huntington's disease in tested individuals and partners. *Health Psychol* 16:20, 1997.
305. Lawson K, Wiggins S, Green T, Adam S, Bloch M, Hayden MR: Adverse psychological events occurring in the first year after predictive testing for Huntington's disease: The Canadian Collaborative Study Predictive Testing. *J Med Genet* 33:856, 1996.
306. Huggins M, Bloch M, Wiggins S, et al: Predictive testing for Huntington disease in Canada: Adverse effects and unexpected results in those receiving a decreased risk. *Am J Med Genet* 42:508, 1992.
307. Decruyenaere M, Evers-Kiebooms G, Boogaerts A, et al: Prediction of psychological functioning one year after the predictive test for Huntington's disease and impact of the test result on reproductive decision making. *J Med Genet* 33:737, 1996.
308. Taylor CA, Myers RH: Long-term impact of Huntington disease linkage testing. *Am J Med Genet* 70:365, 1997.
309. World Federation of Neurology: Research Committee Research Group on Huntington's Chorea: Ethical issues policy statement on Huntington's disease molecular genetics predictive test. *J Neurol Sci* 94:327, 1989.
310. Meissen GJ, Berchek RL: Intended use of predictive testing by those at risk for Huntington disease. *Am J Med Genet* 26:283, 1987.
311. Mastromauro C, Myers RH, Berkman B: Attitudes toward pre-symptomatic testing in Huntington disease. *Am J Med Genet* 26:271, 1987.
312. Tyler A, Quarrell OW, Lazarou LP, Meredith AL, Harper PS: Exclusion testing in pregnancy for Huntington's disease. *J Med Genet* 27:488, 1990.
313. Adam S, Wiggins S, Whyte P, et al: Five year study of prenatal testing for Huntington disease: Demand, attitudes and psychological assessment. *J Med Genet* 30:549, 1993.
314. Drapo PJ: Huntington's disease: The nursing process. *J Adv Nurs* 6:377, 1981.
315. Shoulson I, Caine E, Fahn S, et al: Clinical care of the patient and family with Huntington's disease, in *Commission for the Control of Huntington's Disease and Its Consequences*. Washington, Department of Health, Education and Welfare, National Institute of Health, 1977, p 421.
316. Barr AN, Fischer JH, Koller WC, Spunt AL, Singhal A: Serum haloperidol concentration and choreiform movements in Huntington's disease. *Neurology* 38:84, 1988.
317. Quinn N, Marsden CD: A double blind trial of sulpiride in Huntington's disease and tardive dyskinesia. *J Neurol Neurosurg Psychiatry* 47:844, 1984.
318. Roos RA, Buruma OJ, Bruyn GW, Kemp B, van der Velde EA: Tiapride in the treatment of Huntington's chorea. *Acta Neurol Scand* 65:45, 1982.
319. Swash M, Roberts AH, Zakko H, Heathfield KW: Treatment of involuntary movement disorders with tetrabenazine. *J Neurol Neurosurg Psychiatry* 35:186, 1972.
320. McLellan DL, Chalmers RJ, Johnson RH: A double-blind trial of tetrabenazine, thiopropazate, and placebo in patients with chorea. *Lancet* 1:104, 1974.
321. Asher SW, Aminoff MJ: Tetrabenazine and movement disorders. *Neurology* 31:1051, 1981.
322. Jankovic J, Orman J: Tetrabenazine therapy of dystonia, chorea, tics, and other dyskinesias. *Neurology* 38:391, 1988.
323. Girotti F, Carella F, Scigliano G, et al: Effect of neuroleptic treatment on involuntary movements and motor performances in Huntington's disease. *J Neurol Neurosurg Psychiatry* 47:848, 1984.
324. Mikkelsen BO: Tolerance of tetrabenazine during long-term treatment. *Acta Neurol Scand* 68:57, 1983.
325. Schott K, Ried S, Stevens I, Dichgans J: Neuroleptically induced dystonia in Huntington's disease: A case report. *Eur Neurol* 29:39, 1989.
326. Moss JH, Stewart DE: Iatrogenic parkinsonism in Huntington's chorea. *Can J Psychiatry* 31:865, 1986.
327. Shoulson I: Care of patients and families with Huntington's disease, in Marsden CD, Fahn S (eds): *Movement Disorders*. London, Butterworths, 1982, p 277.
328. Burke RE, Fahn S, Mayeux R, Weinberg H, Louis K, Willner JH: Neuroleptic malignant syndrome caused by dopamine-depleting drugs in a patient with Huntington disease. *Neurology* 31:1022, 1981.
329. Marsden CD, Quinn N: Appendix 6, in Lader MH, Richens A (eds): *Methods in Cliical Pharmacology: Central Nervous System*. London, Macmillan, 1981.
330. Frattola L, Albiazzati MG, Spano PF, Trabucchi M: Treatment of Huntington's chorea with bromocriptine. *Acta Neurol Scand* 56:37, 1977.
331. Kartzinel R, Perlow MD, Carter AC, Chase TN, Calne DB, Shoulson I: Metabolic studies with bromocriptine in patients with idiopathic parkinsonism and Huntington's chorea. *Trans Am Neurol Assoc* 101:53, 1976.
332. Tolosa ES, Sparber SB: Apomorphine in Huntington's chorea: Clinical observations and theoretical considerations. *Life Sci* 15:1371, 1974.
333. Corsini GU, Onali P, Masala C, Cianchetti C, Mangoni A, Gessa G: Apomorphine hydrochloride-induced improvement in Huntington's chorea: Stimulation of dopamine receptor. *Arch Neurol* 35:27, 1978.
334. Bassi S, Albizzati MG, Corsini GU, et al: Therapeutic experience with transdihydrolisuride in Huntington's disease. *Neurology* 36:984, 1986.
335. Peiris JB, Boralessa H, Lionel ND: Clonazepam in the treatment of choreiform activity. *Med J Aust* 1:225, 1976.
336. Perry TL, Wright JM, Hansen S, MacLeod PM: Isoniazid therapy for Huntington's disease, in Chase TN, Wexler NS, Barbeau A (eds): *Huntington's Disease: Advances in Neurology*, Vol 2. New York, Raven Press, 1979, p 785.
337. McLean DR: Failure of isoniazid therapy in Huntington disease. *Neurology* 32:1189, 1982.
338. Paulson GW: Lioresal in Huntington's disease. *Disord Nerv Sys* 37:465, 1976.
339. Shoulson I, Odoroff C, Oakes D, et al: A controlled clinical trial of baclofen as protective therapy in early Huntington's disease. *Ann Neurol* 25:252, 1989.
340. Schou M: Lithium in the treatment of other psychiatric and nonpsychiatric disorders. *Arch Gen Psychiatry* 36:856, 1979.
341. Brown WT, Sanberg PR, McGeer PL: Corticosteroids and chorea. *Arch Neurol* 36:452, 1979.

342. Folstein S, Folstein M: Diagnosis and treatment of Huntington's disease. *Compr Ther* **7**:60, 1981.

343. Como PG, Rubin AJ, O'Brien CF, et al: A controlled trial of fluoxetine in nondepressed patients with Huntington's disease. *Mov Disord* **12**:397, 1997.

344. Ford MF: Treatment of depression in Huntington's disease with monoamine oxidase inhibitors. *Br J Psychiatry* **149**:654, 1986.

345. Greendyke RM, Schuster DB, Wooton JA: Propranolol in the treatment of assaultive patients with organic brain disease. *J Clin Psychopharmacol* **4**:282, 1984.

346. Stewart JT: Paradoxical aggressive effect of propranolol in a patient with Huntington's disease. *J Clin Psychiatry* **48**:385, 1987.

347. von Hafften AH, Jensen CF: Paradoxical response to pindolol treatment for aggression in a patient with Huntington's disease. *J Clin Psychiatry* **50**:230, 1989.

348. Sajatovic M, Verbanac P, Ramirez LF, Meltzer HY: Clozapine treatment of psychiatric symptoms resistant to neuroleptic treatment in patients with Huntington's chorea. *Neurology* **41**:156, 1991.

349. Kremer B, Clark CM, Almqvist EW, et al: The Lamotrigine-HD Trial: Influence on progression of early Huntington disease. *Neurology* **53**:1000, 1999.

350. Ranen NG, Peyser CE, Coyle JT, et al: A controlled trial of idebenone in Huntington's disease. *Mov Disord* **11**:549, 1996.

351. Kieburtz K, Feigin A, McDermott M, et al: A controlled trial of remacemide hydrochloride in Huntington's disease. *Mov Disord* **11**:273, 1996.

352. Feigin A, Kieburtz K, Como P, et al: Assessment of coenzyme Q10 tolerability in Huntington's disease. *Mov Disord* **11**:321, 1996.

353. Shannon KM, Kordower JH: Neural transplantation for Huntington's disease: Experimental rationale and recommendations for clinical trials. *Cell Transplant* **5**:339, 1996.

354. Pundt LL, Kondoh T, Conrad JA, Low WC: Transplantation of human striatal tissue into a rodent model of Huntington's disease: Phenotypic expression of transplanted neurons and host-to-graft innervation. *Brain Res Bull* **39**:23, 1996.

355. Grasbon-Frodl EM, Nakao N, Lindvall O, Brundin P: Developmental features of human striatal tissue transplanted in a rat model of Huntington's disease. *Neurobiol Dis* **3**:299, 1997.

356. Brundin P, Fricker RA, Nakao N: Paucity of P-zones in striatal grafts prohibit commencement of clinical trials in Huntington's disease. *Neuroscience* **71**:895, 1996.

357. Quinn N, Brown R, Craufurd D, et al: Core assessment program for intracerebral transplantation in Huntington's disease (CAPIT-HD). *Mov Disord* **11**:143, 1996.

358. Kopyov OV, Jacques S, Lieberman A, Duma CM, Eagle KS: Safety of intrastriatal neurotransplantationfor Huntington's disease patients. *Exp Neurol* **149**:97, 1998.

# Prion Diseases

*Stanley B. Prusiner*

1. Prions are novel transmissible pathogens causing a group of invariably fatal neurodegenerative diseases that present as genetic, infectious, or sporadic disorders, all of which involve modification of the prion protein (PrP).
2. Prion diseases of humans are referred to as Creutzfeldt-Jakob disease (CJD), Gerstmann-Sträussler-Scheinker disease (GSS), fatal familial insomnia (FFI), fatal sporadic insomnia (FSI), and kuru. In animals, the prion diseases are called scrapie of sheep and goats, bovine spongiform encephalopathy (BSE), chronic wasting disease (CWD) of mule deer and elk, feline spongiform encephalopathy (FSE), and transmissible mink encephalopathy (TME).
3. Prions are devoid of nucleic acid and seem to be composed exclusively of a modified protein (PrP$^{Sc}$) that is derived from the normal, cellular isoform (PrP$^C$). Through a posttranslational process, PrP$^C$ is refolded into PrP$^{Sc}$ during which the protein acquires a high $\beta$-sheet content.
4. PrP$^C$ might function as a Cu(II) metalloprotein and may have a vital role in copper homeostasis.
5. Prion diseases are caused by the accumulation of PrP$^{Sc}$. In accord with the autosomal dominant inheritance of familial prion diseases caused by mutations of the PrP gene, PrP$^{Sc}$ represents a gain of dysfunction.
6. The species of a particular prion is encoded by the sequence of the chromosomal PrP gene of the mammal in which it last replicated.
7. The length of the incubation time for infectious prion diseases is inversely proportional to the level of expression of PrP$^C$ and directly related to the level of protease-sensitive PrP$^{Sc}$. For a particular strain of prions, protease-resistant PrP$^{Sc}$ accumulates to a given level in the central nervous system followed by the onset of neurologic dysfunction.
8. In contrast to pathogens carrying a nucleic acid genome, prions appear to encipher strain-specified properties in the tertiary structure of PrP$^{Sc}$. Transgenetic studies argue that PrP$^{Sc}$ acts as a template upon which PrP$^C$ is refolded into a nascent PrP$^{Sc}$ molecule through a process facilitated by another protein.
9. The prion-like behavior of two yeast proteins whose phenotypes are transmitted nonchromosomally to their progeny has extended the generality of the prion concept.
10. Knowledge about prions has important implications for understanding the structural plasticity of proteins as well as a wide variety of degenerative diseases.

A list of standard abbreviations is located immediately preceding the index in each volume. Additional abbreviations used in this chapter include: AD = Alzheimer's disease; BSE = bovine spongiform encephalopathy; CJD = Creutzfeldt-Jakob disease; sCJD = sporadic CJD; fCJD = familial CJD; iCJD = iatrogenic CJD; vCJD = (new) variant CJD; CWD = chronic wasting disease; FFI = fatal familial insomnia; FSE = feline spongiform encephalopathy; GSS = Gerstmann-Sträussler-Scheinker disease; HGH = human growth hormone; PrP = prion protein; PrP$^C$ = cellular PrP isoform; PrP$^{Sc}$ = disease-causing PrP isoform; Prnp = PrP gene in mice; PRNP = PrP gene in humans; Prnp$^{0/0}$ = ablation of both PrP alleles; sFI = sporadic fatal insomnia; TME = transmissible mink encephalopathy; Tg = transgenic.

## INTRODUCTION

Prions cause neurodegeneration. The diseases caused by prions are unusual in that they can manifest as genetic, sporadic, and infectious disorders of the central nervous system (CNS). Investigations of prion diseases in humans have been greatly facilitated by studies of prion diseases in animals.

The prion diseases of humans are frequently referred to as Creutzfeldt-Jakob disease (CJD), Gerstmann-Sträussler-Scheinker disease (GSS), fatal familial insomnia (FFI), and kuru (Table 224-1). The prion diseases of animals include scrapie of sheep and goats, bovine spongiform encephalopathy (BSE), chronic wasting disease (CWD), and transmissible mink encephalopathy (TME).

Because prions and the mechanism of disease pathogenesis are unprecedented, classification of the prion diseases has been quite varied. For many years, the human prion diseases were classified as neurodegenerative disorders of unknown etiology based on pathologic changes being confined to the CNS. With the transmission of kuru and CJD to apes, investigators began to view these diseases as CNS infectious illnesses caused by slow viruses.[1] Although the familial nature of a subset of CJD cases was well described, the significance of this observation became more obscure with the transmission of CJD to animals.[2,3] Eventually, the meaning of heritable CJD became clear with the discovery of mutations in the PrP gene of these patients.[4,5]

The history of prions is a fascinating saga in the annals of biomedical science. For nearly five decades, with no clue as to the cause, physicians watched patients with a CNS degeneration called Creutzfeldt-Jakob disease die, often within a few months of its onset.[6-8] CJD destroys the brain while the body remains unaware of this process. No febrile response, leucocytosis or pleocytosis, or humoral immune response is mounted in response to this devastating disease. Despite its recognition as a distinct clinical entity, CJD remained a rare disease; first, it was the province of neuropsychiatrists, and later it was the province of neurologists and neuropathologists. Although multiple cases of CJD were recognized in families quite early on,[2,9-17] this observation did little to advance understanding of the disorder.

The unraveling of the etiology of CJD is a wonderful story that has many threads, each representing a distinct piece of the puzzle. An important observation was made by Igor Klatzo in 1959, when he recognized that the neuropathology of kuru resembled that of CJD;[18] the same year, William Hadlow suggested that kuru, a disease of New Guinea highlanders, was similar to scrapie, a hypothesis also based on light microscopic similarities.[19] But Hadlow's insight was much more profound because he suggested that kuru is a transmissible disease like scrapie, and that demonstration of the infectivity of kuru could be accomplished using chimpanzees because they are so closely related to humans. He also noted that many months or years might be required before clinically recognizable disease would be seen in these inoculated non-human primates. Moreover, he argued that brain tissue from patients dying of kuru should be homogenized and injected intracerebrally into chimpanzees, as was often done in studies of sheep scrapie.

At the time Hadlow's hypothesis was set forth, it was thought that scrapie was caused by a "slow virus." Bjorn Sigurdsson coined the term "slow virus" in 1954, based on his studies in

**Table 224-1** The Prion Diseases

| Disease | Host | Mechanism of Pathogenesis |
|---|---|---|
| **A.** Kuru | Fore people | Infection through ritualistic cannibalism |
| iCJD* | Humans | Infection from prion-contaminated HGH, dura mater grafts, etc. |
| vCJD | Humans | Infection from bovine prions? |
| fCJD | Humans | Germ line mutations in PrP gene |
| GSS | Humans | Germ line mutations in PrP gene |
| FFI | Humans | Germ line mutation in PrP gene (D178N, M129) |
| sCJD | Humans | Somatic mutation or spontaneous conversion of $PrP^C$ into $PrP^{Sc}$? |
| sFI | Humans | Somatic mutation or spontaneous conversion of $PrP^C$ into $PrP^{Sc}$? |
| **B.** Scrapie | Sheep | Infection in genetically susceptible sheep |
| BSE | Cattle | Infection with prion-contaminated MBM |
| TME | Mink | Infection with prions from sheep or cattle |
| CWD | Mule deer, elk | Unknown |
| FSE | Cats | Infection with prion-contaminated beef |
| Exotic ungulate encephalopathy | Greater kudu, nyala, oryx | Infection with prion-contaminated MBM |

* Abbreviations: BSE, bovine spongiform encephalopathy; CJD, Creutzfeldt-Jakob disease; sCJD, sporadic CJD; fCJD, familial CJD; iCJD, iatrogenic CJD; vCJD, (new) variant CJD; CWD, chronic wasting disease; FFI, fatal familial insomnia; FSE, feline spongiform encephalopathy; sFI, sporadic fatal insomnia; GSS, Gerstmann-Sträussler-Scheinker disease; HGH, human growth hormone; MBM, meat and bone meal; TME, transmissible mink encephalopathy.

Iceland on scrapie and visna of sheep.[20] Although Hadlow suggested that kuru, like scrapie, was caused by a slow virus, he did not perform the experiments required to demonstrate this phenomenon.[19,21] In fact, 7 years were to pass before the transmissibility of kuru was established by passaging the disease to chimpanzees,[22] and it wasn't until 1968 that the transmission of CJD to chimpanzees after intracerebral inoculation was reported.[1]

An early clue to unusual properties of the scrapie agent emerged from studies of 18,000 sheep that were inadvertently inoculated with the scrapie agent or slow virus as it was referred to at that time. These animals had been vaccinated against louping ill virus with a formalin-treated suspension of ovine brain and spleen that, as was subsequently shown, had been contaminated with the scrapie agent.[23] Three different batches of vaccines were administered, and 2 years later, 1500 sheep developed scrapie. These findings demonstrated that the scrapie agent is resistant to inactivation by formalin, unlike most viruses, which are readily inactivated by such treatment.

The unusual biological properties of the scrapie agent were no less puzzling than the disease process itself, for the infectious agent caused a devastating degeneration of the CNS in the absence of an inflammatory response.[24,25] Although the immune system remained intact, its surveillance system was unaware of a raging infection. The infectious agent that causes scrapie, now generally referred to as a "prion," achieved status as a scientific curiosity when its extreme resistance to ionizing and ultraviolet irradiation was discovered.[26-28] Later, similar resistance to inactivation by UV and ionizing radiation was reported for the CJD agent.[29] Tikvah Alper's radiation-resistance data on the scrapie agent evoked a torrent of hypotheses concerning its composition. Suggestions as to the nature of the scrapie agent ranged from small DNA viruses to membrane fragments to polysaccharides to proteins, the last of which eventually proved to be correct.[30-36]

Because the scrapie agent had been passaged from sheep into mice,[37] scrapie was the most amenable of these diseases to study experimentally. While the agents causing scrapie, CJD, and kuru were for many years thought to be different slow viruses, we now know that prions cause all these disorders and that this distinction was artificial.

Studies of prions have wide implications ranging from basic principles of protein conformation to the development of effective therapies for prion diseases.[38] In this chapter, the structural biology of prion proteins as well as the genetics and molecular neurology of prion diseases are introduced. How information is enciphered within the infectious prion particle is described.

## Neurodegenerative Diseases

Over the past two decades, advances in our understanding of the prion diseases have helped refine our definition of neurodegenerative diseases. Maladies such as Alzheimer disease, Parkinson disease, and amyotrophic lateral sclerosis are often referred to as the common neurodegenerative diseases. Examples of less prevalent neurodegenerative diseases are fronto-temporal dementia, Huntington disease, and the prion diseases (Table 224-2). With the exception of Huntington disease, a minority of all the above neurodegenerative disorders exhibit an autosomal dominant pattern of inheritance and the majority are sporadic. In all of these illnesses, including Huntington disease, the onset of CNS dysfunction is usually seen in adults and the neurologic deterioration is progressive.

Abnormal protein deposits are found in all these diseases and the pathogenic process seems to evade immune surveillance. In Alzheimer disease and the prion diseases, amyloid plaques are found but the proteins in these plaques are different. In Parkinson disease, Lewy bodies are often found, while in Huntington disease protein aggregates in the nuclei of some neurons can be observed.

**Table 224-2** Neurodegenerative Diseases

| Neurodegenerative Disease | CNS Protein Deposits | Mutant Genes in Familial Disorders |
|---|---|---|
| Prion diseases | $PrP^{Sc}$, PrP amyloid plaques | PrP |
| Alzheimer disease (AD) | $A\beta$, $A\beta$ amyloid plaques, Tau, neurofibrillary tangles | APP, PS1, PS2, ApoE* |
| Parkinson disease | α-synuclein, Lewy bodies | α-Synuclein, Parkin |
| Amyotrophic lateral sclerosis (ALS) | | SOD |
| Frontotemporal dementia (FTD) | Tau fibrils | Tau |
| Huntington disease (HD) | HD, nuclear HD aggregates | HD |

* ApoE genotype modulates the age of onset of both familial and sporadic AD.

In all of these diseases, astrocytic gliosis is seen. In some of these diseases, vacuolation in the neuropil is seen, but the most prominent vacuolation can be seen in the prion diseases where vacuoles may coalesce to create spongiform change. The degree of spongiform change is quite variable while the extent of reactive gliosis correlates with the degree of neuron loss in CJD.[39] This feature of the prion diseases has prompted some investigators to refer to the prion diseases as the spongiform encephalopathies or the transmissible spongiform encephalopathies (TSEs). The term TSE probably creates confusion because it emphasizes the transmissible aspect of prion diseases even though infectious prion diseases in humans are quite rare.

Within the context of the diseases described above (Table 224-2), neurodegeneration is defined as a pathogenic process producing neuronal dysfunction and often neuronal loss accompanied by astrocytic gliosis but no inflammatory response.

## THE PRION CONCEPT

Prions are unprecedented infectious pathogens that are devoid of nucleic acid and seem to be composed exclusively of a modified isoform of PrP designated $PrP^{Sc}$. The normal, cellular PrP, denoted $PrP^{C}$, is converted into $PrP^{Sc}$ through a process whereby a portion of its α-helical and coil structure is refolded into the β sheet.[40] This structural transition is accompanied by profound changes in the physicochemical properties of the PrP. The amino acid sequence of $PrP^{Sc}$ corresponds to that encoded by the PrP gene of the mammalian host in which it last replicated. In contrast to pathogens with a nucleic acid genome that encode strain-specific properties in genes, prions encipher these properties in the tertiary structure of $PrP^{Sc}$.[41–44] Transgenetic studies argue that $PrP^{Sc}$ acts as a template upon which $PrP^{C}$ is refolded into a nascent $PrP^{Sc}$ molecule through a process facilitated by another protein.

Perhaps, the best current working definition of a prion is a proteinaceous infectious particle that lacks nucleic acid.[43] Because prions appear to be composed entirely of a protein that adopts an abnormal conformation, it is not unreasonable to think of prions as infectious proteins.[40,42] However, the possibility of a small ligand bound to $PrP^{Sc}$ as an essential component of the infectious prion particle cannot be eliminated.

In a broader view, prions are elements that impart and propagate variability through multiple conformers of a normal cellular protein. The species of a particular prion is encoded by the sequence of the chromosomal PrP gene of the mammal in which it last replicated. In contrast to pathogens with a nucleic acid genome that encode strain-specific properties in genes, prions seem to encipher these properties in the tertiary structure of $PrP^{Sc}$.[41–44]

The discovery that mutations of the PrP gene cause dominantly inherited prion diseases in humans linked the genetic and infectious forms of prion diseases and presented another hurdle for investigators, who continued to argue that prion diseases are caused by viruses. More than 20 mutations of the PrP gene are now known to cause the inherited human prion diseases and significant genetic linkage has been established for five of these mutations.[4,45–48] The prion concept readily explains how a disease can manifest as both a heritable and an infectious illness. Moreover, the hallmark common to all of the prion diseases, whether sporadic, dominantly inherited, or acquired by infection, is that they involve the aberrant metabolism of the prion protein.[49]

Although $PrP^{Sc}$ is the only *known* component of the infectious prion particles, these unique pathogens share several phenotypic traits with other infectious entities such as viruses. Because some features of the diseases caused by prions and viruses are similar, some scientists have difficulty accepting the existence of prions despite a wealth of scientific data supporting this concept.[50–53]

### Prions Are Distinct from Viruses

Like viruses, prions are infectious because they stimulate a process whereby more of the pathogen is produced. As prions or viruses accumulate in an infected host, they eventually cause disease. Both prions and viruses exist in different varieties or subtypes that are called strains. But many features of prion structure and replication distinguish them from viruses and all other known infectious pathogens.

Prions differ from viruses and viroids because they lack a nucleic acid genome that directs the synthesis of their progeny. Prions are composed of an abnormal isoform of a cellular protein, whereas most viral proteins are encoded by the viral genome and viroids are devoid of protein.

Prions can exist in multiple molecular forms, whereas viruses exist in a single form with a distinct ultrastructural morphology. Prions have no constant structure, in marked contrast to viruses. Prion infectivity has been detected in fractions containing particles with an extremely wide range of sizes.[54–56] Initially, the small size of prions as determined by ionizing radiation inactivation studies[26] was confusing because scrapie infectivity was clearly associated with larger particles.[57] Eventually, aggregation due to hydrophobic interactions between $PrP^{Sc}$ molecules was found to be responsible for such anomalous behavior.[55]

Prions are nonimmunogenic, in contrast to viruses, which almost always provoke an immune response. Prions do not elicit an immune response because $PrP^{C}$[58,59] renders the host tolerant to $PrP^{Sc}$. In contrast, the foreign proteins of viruses that are encoded by the viral genome often elicit a profound immune response. Thus, it seems unlikely that vaccination, which has been so effective in preventing many viral illnesses, will be a useful strategy for preventing or treating prior diseases.

The phenomenon of prion strains has posed a profound conundrum with respect to how prions might be composed of only host-encoded $PrP^{Sc}$ molecules and yet exhibit diversity. An enlarging body of data argues that strains of prions are enciphered in the conformation of $PrP^{Sc}$; in contrast, strains of viruses and viroids have distinct nucleic acid sequences that produce pathogens with different properties. Many investigators argued for a nucleic acid genome within the infectious prion particle while others contended for a small noncoding polynucleotide of either foreign or cellular origin,[60–65] but no nucleic acid was found despite intensive searches using a wide variety of techniques and approaches.[66,67] Based on a wealth of evidence, it is reasonable to assert that such a nucleic acid has not been found because it does not exist.

That many of the prion diseases were discovered prior to our current understanding of prion biology has created confusion in an environment where decisions of great economic and political consequence, and possibly of public health import, are being made. For example, scrapie of sheep and BSE have different names; yet they are the same disease in two different species. Both scrapie and BSE are prion diseases that differ from each other in only two respects: First, the sheep PrP sequence differs from that of cattle at 7 or 8 positions out of 270 amino acids,[68,69] giving rise to different $PrP^{Sc}$ molecules in each. Second, some aspects of each disease are determined by the particular prion strain that infects a given host.

Understanding prion strains and the "species barrier" is of paramount importance with respect to the BSE epidemic in Britain in which more than 170,000 cattle have died over the past decade.[70] Brain extracts from eight cattle with BSE all gave the same patterns of incubation times and vacuolation of the neuropil when inoculated in a variety of inbred mice.[71,72] Incubation times and profiles of neuronal vacuolation have been used for three decades to study prion strains. Brain extracts prepared from three domestic cats, one nyala, and one kudu, all of which died with a neurologic illness, produced incubation times and lesion profiles indistinguishable from those found in the BSE cattle. Cats and exotic ungulates such as the kudu presumably developed prion disease from eating food containing bovine prions.[73–75]

### Discovery of the Prion Protein

The discovery of the prion protein transformed research on scrapie and related diseases.[76,77] It provided a molecular marker that was subsequently shown to be specific for these illnesses and identified

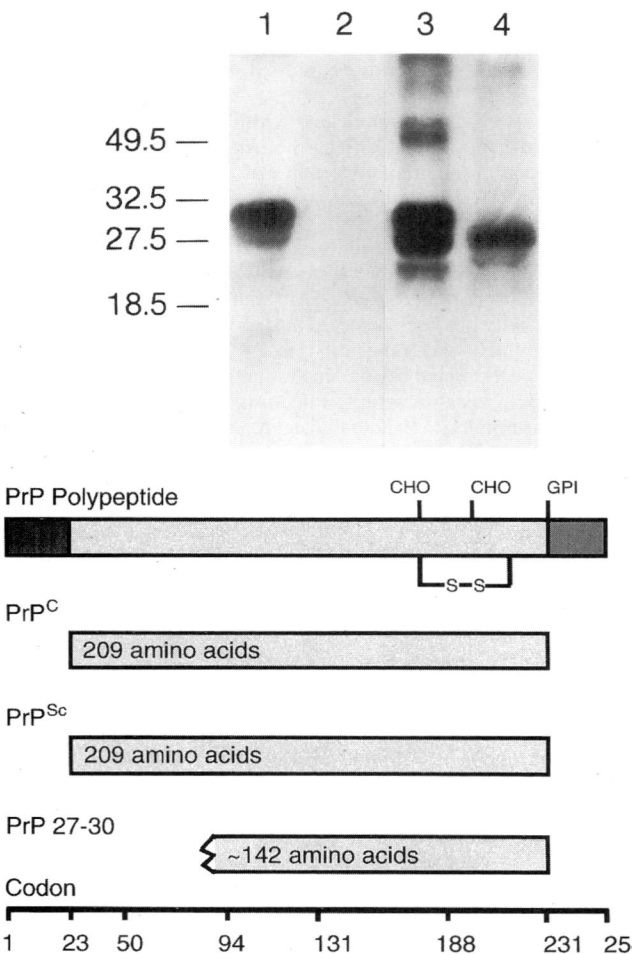

Fig. 224-1 Prion protein isoforms. *A,* Western immunoblot of brain homogenates from uninfected (lanes 1 and 2) and prion-infected (lanes 3 and 4) Syrian hamsters. Samples in lanes 2 and 4 were digested with 50 μg/ml of proteinase K for 30 min at 37°C. PrP$^C$ in lanes 2 and 4 was completely hydrolyzed under these conditions, whereas approximately 67 amino acids were digested from the NH$_2$-terminus of PrP$^{Sc}$ to generate PrP 27-30. After polyacrylamide gel electrophoresis (PAGE) and electrotransfer, the blot was developed with anti-PrP R073 polyclonal rabbit antiserum. Molecular size markers are in kilodaltons (kDa). *B,* Bar diagram of SHaPrP, which consists of 254 amino acids. After processing of the NH$_2$- and C-termini, both PrP$^C$ and PrP$^{Sc}$ consist of 209 residues. After limited proteolysis, the NH$_2$-terminus of PrP$^{Sc}$ is truncated to form PrP 27-30, which is composed of approximately 142 amino acids. *(Reprinted with permission from Les Prix Nobel 268, Prusiner SB: Prions. Copyright 1998 The Nobel Foundation.)*

the major, and possibly the only, component of the prion particle. The protease-resistant fragment of the scrapie isoform of the prion protein, designated PrP 27-30, was discovered by enriching fractions from Syrian hamster (SHa) brain for scrapie infectivity.[76,77] PrP 27-30 has an apparent molecular weight ($M_r$) of 27 to 30 kDa (Fig. 224-1).

From 1960 to 1980 there were many unsuccessful attempts to purify the scrapie agent or to identify a biochemical marker that copurified.[54,78–90] Studies on the sedimentation properties of scrapie infectivity in mouse spleens and brains suggested that hydrophobic interactions were responsible for the nonideal physical behavior of the scrapie particle.[91,92] Indeed, the scrapie agent presented a biochemical nightmare: infectivity was spread from one end to the other of a sucrose gradient and from the void volume to fractions eluting at 5 to 10 times the included volume of

chromatographic columns. Such results demanded new approaches and better assays. Only the development of improved bioassays allowed purification of the infectious pathogen that causes scrapie and CJD.[93,94]

Enriching fractions from the brains of scrapie-infected Syrian hamsters for infectivity yielded the single protein PrP 27-30. PrP 27-30 was later found to be the protease-resistant core of PrP$^{Sc}$.[95,96] Copurification of PrP 27-30 and scrapie infectivity demands that the physicochemical properties, as well as antigenicity, of these two entities be similar.[97] The results of a wide array of inactivation experiments demonstrated the similarities in the properties of PrP 27-30 and scrapie infectivity.[98,99] To explain these findings in terms of the virus hypothesis, it is necessary to postulate either a virus that has a coat protein that is highly homologous with PrP or a virus that binds tightly to PrP$^{Sc}$. In either case, the PrP-like coat proteins or the PrP$^{Sc}$/virus complexes must display properties indistinguishable from PrP$^{Sc}$ alone. The inability to inactivate preparations highly enriched for scrapie infectivity by procedures that modify nucleic acids was interpreted as evidence against the existence of a scrapie-specific nucleic acid.[27,100] To explain the findings in terms of a virus, one must argue that PrP$^{Sc}$ or an as yet undetected PrP-like protein of viral origin protects the viral genome from inactivation.

**Determination of the N-Terminal Sequence of PrP 27-30.** The molecular biology and genetics of prions began with the purification of PrP 27-30, significantly to allow determination of its NH$_2$-terminal amino acid sequence.[95] Multiple signals in each cycle of the Edman degradation suggested that either multiple proteins were present in these "purified fractions" or a single protein with a ragged NH$_2$-terminus was present. When the signals in each cycle were grouped according to their intensities of strong, intermediate, and weak, it became clear that a single protein with a ragged NH$_2$-terminus was being sequenced (Fig. 224-2). Determination of a single, unique sequence for the NH$_2$-terminus of PrP 27-30 permitted the synthesis of isocoding mixtures of oligonucleotides that were subsequently used to identify incomplete PrP cDNA clones from hamster[101] and mouse.[102] cDNA clones encoding the entire open reading frames (ORF) of SHa and Mo PrP were eventually recovered.[96,103]

## Prion Protein Isoforms

PrP mRNA levels are similar in normal, uninfected, and scrapie-infected tissues.[102] This finding produced skepticism about whether PrP 27-30 was related to the infectious prion particle. Nevertheless, the search for a protein encoded by the PrP mRNA revealed a protease-sensitive protein, designated PrP$^C$, that is soluble in nondenaturing detergents.[101,104]

PrP$^C$ and PrP$^{Sc}$ have the same covalent structure and each consists of 209 amino acids in Syrian hamsters (Fig. 224-1). The

| Relative Amount | Amino Acid Sequence [a] |
|---|---|
| 1 | G-Q-GG-G-T-H-N-Q-W-N-K-P-S-K |
| 0.4 | X-X-X-T-H-N-X-W-X-K-P |
| 0.2 | X-X-P-W-X-Q-X-X-X-T-H-X-Q-W |

[a] Single-letter amino acid code. X = amino acid not determined at that cycle.

Fig. 224-2 Interpreted amino acid sequence of the N-terminus of PrP 27-30. The "ragged ends" of PrP 27-30 are shown. Single letter amino acid code. X = amino acid not detected at that cycle.[95] (Reprinted with permission from Prusiner SB, Groth DF, Bolton DC, Kent SB, Hood LE: Purification and structural studies of a major scrapie prion protein. *Cell* 38:127, 1984. Copyright 1984 Cell Press.)

N-terminal sequencing, the deduced amino acid sequences from PrP cDNA, and immunoblotting studies argue that PrP 27-30 is a truncated protein of about 142 residues that is derived from PrP$^{Sc}$ by limited proteolysis of the N-terminus.[95,96,101,103,104]

In general, ~$10^5$ PrP$^{Sc}$ molecules correspond to one ID$_{50}$ unit of prions using the most sensitive bioassay.[77,99] PrP$^{Sc}$ is probably best defined as the abnormal isoform of the prion protein that stimulates conversion of PrP$^C$ into nascent PrP$^{Sc}$, accumulates, and causes disease. Although resistance to limited proteolysis has proved to be a convenient tool for detecting PrP$^{Sc}$, not all PrP$^{Sc}$ molecules possess protease resistance.[44,105,106] Some investigators equate protease resistance with PrP$^{Sc}$; this erroneous view has been compounded by the use of the term "PrP-res."[107]

Although both insolubility and protease resistance were used in initial studies to differentiate PrP$^{Sc}$ from PrP$^C$,[104] subsequent investigations showed that these properties are only surrogate markers, as are high $\beta$-sheet content and polymerization into amyloid.[99,108–113] When these surrogate markers are present, they are useful, but their absence does not establish the lack of prion infectivity. PrP$^{Sc}$ is usually not detected by western immunoblotting if less than $10^5$ ID$_{50}$ units/ml of prions are present in a sample.[114] Furthermore, PrP$^{Sc}$ from different species may exhibit different degrees of protease resistance.

In our experience, the method of sample preparation from scrapie-infected brain also influences the sensitivity of PrP$^{Sc}$ immunodetection, partly because PrP$^{Sc}$ is not uniformly distributed in the brain.[115,116] Some experiments in which PrP$^{Sc}$ detection proved problematic in partially purified preparations[117,118] were repeated with crude homogenates where PrP$^{Sc}$ was readily measured.[119,120]

**PrP$^C$ Is a Cu(II) Metalloprotein.** The discovery of PrP$^C$ under the circumstances where a disease process was being investigated gave no clue as to the function of this highly conserved protein.[121] Although the discovery that PrP$^C$ carries a glycosylphosphatidyl[121] inositol (GPI) moiety provided insight into the subcellular trafficking of this protein, it did not reveal the function of PrP.[122,123] The high histidine content of PrP raised the possibility that immobilized metal ion affinity chromatography (IMAC) might be employed in its purification.[124] IMAC with Cu$^{2+}$ proved efficacious in the purification of PrP$^C$ under nondenaturing conditions, leading to a comparison of the secondary structures of PrP$^C$ and PrP$^{Sc}$.[40,125] Synthetic peptides corresponding to His, Gly, and Pro rich octarepeats at the N-terminus of PrP was shown to bind Cu$^{2+}$,[126] but the significance of this finding was unclear because these octarepeats are hydrolyzed by proteinase K when PrP$^{Sc}$ is converted to PrP 27-30 under conditions where scrapie prion infectivity is preserved

In studies on the binding of Cu$^{2+}$ to recombinant Syrian hamster (SHa) PrP [SHaPrP(29-231)] and synthetic peptides corresponding to the N-terminal octarepeats, we found an extreme degree of specificity for this divalent cation.[127] In contrast to Cu$^{2+}$, the metal ions Ca$^{2+}$, Co$^{2+}$, Mg$^{2+}$, Mn$^{2+}$, Ni$^{2+}$, and Zn$^{2+}$ all failed to bind SHaPrP(29-231) at a concentration of 20 μM. Half maximal binding of Cu$^{2+}$ to SHaPrP(29-231) was observed at 14 μM. These studies suggested that Cu$^{2+}$ is coordinated by two His residues and the carbonyl oxygens of two glycines in the octarepeats and raised the possibility that the seemingly unstructured N-terminus of SHaPrP(29-231)[128] was likely to be more ordered in the presence of Cu$^{2+}$.[129,130]

## NOMENCLATURE

A listing of the different prion diseases is given in Table 224-1. Although the prions that cause TME and BSE are referred to as TME prions and BSE prions, this may be unjustified because both are thought to originate from the oral consumption of scrapie prions in sheep-derived foodstuffs and because many lines of evidence argue that the only difference among the various prions is the sequence of PrP, which is dictated by the host and not the prion itself.

**Table 224-3** Glossary of Prion Terminology

| Term | Description |
| --- | --- |
| Prion | A *proteinaceous infectious* particle that lacks nucleic acid. Prions are composed largely, if not entirely, of PrP$^{Sc}$ molecules. |
| PrP$^{Sc}$ | Abnormal, pathogenic isoform of the prion protein that causes sickness. This protein is the only identifiable macromolecule in purified preparations of prions. |
| PrP$^C$ | Cellular isoform of the prion protein. |
| PrP 27-30 | Digestion of PrP$^{Sc}$ with proteinase K generates PrP 27-30 by hydrolysis of the N-terminus. |
| PRNP | Human PrP gene located on chromosome 20. |
| *Prnp* | Mouse PrP gene located on syntenic chromosome 2. *Prnp* controls the length of the prion incubation time and is congruent with the incubation time genes *Sinc* and *Prn-i*. PrP-deficient (*Prnp$^{0/0}$*) mice are resistant to prions. |
| PrP amyloid | Fibril of PrP fragments derived from PrP$^{Sc}$ by proteolysis. Plaques containing PrP amyloid are found in the brains of some mammals with prion disease. |
| Prion rod | An amyloid polymer composed of PrP 27-30 molecules. Created by detergent extraction and limited proteolysis of PrP$^{Sc}$. |
| protein X | A hypothetical macromolecule that is thought to act like a molecular chaperone in facilitating the conversion of PrP$^C$ into PrP$^{Sc}$. |

The human prions present a similar semantic conundrum. Transmission of human prions to laboratory animals produces prions carrying PrP molecules with sequences dictated by the PrP gene of the host, not that of the inoculum.

To simplify the terminology, the generic term PrP$^{Sc}$ is suggested in place of such terms as PrP$^{CJD}$, PrP$^{BSE}$, and PrP$^{res}$.[131] To distinguish PrP$^{Sc}$ found in humans or cattle from that found in other animals, HuPrP$^{Sc}$ or BoPrP$^{Sc}$ is suggested instead of PrP$^{CJD}$ or PrP$^{BSE}$, respectively (Table 224-3). Once human prions, and thus HuPrP$^{Sc}$ molecules, are passaged into animals, the prions and PrP$^{Sc}$ are no longer of the human species unless they were formed in an animal expressing a HuPrP transgene.

The "Sc" superscript of PrP$^{Sc}$ was initially derived from the term *sc*rapie because scrapie was the prototypic prion disease. Because all of the known prion diseases (Table 224-1) of mammals involve aberrant metabolism of PrP similar to that observed in scrapie, the "Sc" superscript is suggested for all abnormal, pathogenic PrP isoforms.[131] In this context, the "Sc" superscript is used to designate the scrapie-like isoform of PrP; for those who desire a more general derivation, "Sc" can equally well be derived from the term "prion *s*i*c*kness" or "di*s*ease *c*ausing" (Table 224-3).

In the case of mutant PrPs, the mutation and any important polymorphism can be denoted in parentheses following the particular PrP isoform. For example in FFI, the pathogenic PrP isoform is referred to as PrP$^{Sc}$ or HuPrP$^{Sc}$; alternatively, if it were important to identify the mutation, then it is written as HuPrP$^{Sc}$(D178N, M129) (Table 224-4). The term PrP$^{res}$ or PrP-res is derived from the protease *res*istance of PrP$^{Sc}$, but protease resistance, insolubility, and high $\beta$-sheet content should be only considered as surrogate markers of PrP$^{Sc}$ because one or more of these may not always be present. Whether PrP$^{res}$ is useful in denoting PrP molecules that have been subjected to procedures that modify their resistance to proteolysis but which have not been demonstrated to convey infectivity or cause disease, remains debatable.

**Table 224-4 Examples of Human PrP Gene Mutations Found in the Inherited Prion Diseases**

| Inherited Prion Disease | PrP Gene Mutation |
|---|---|
| Gerstmann-Sträussler-Scheinker disease | PrP P102L* |
| Gerstmann-Sträussler-Scheinker disease | PrP A117V |
| Familial Creutzfeldt-Jakob disease | PrP D178N, V129 |
| Fatal familial insomnia | PrP D178N, M129* |
| Gerstmann-Sträussler-Scheinker disease | PrP F198S* |
| Familial Creutzfeldt-Jakob disease | PrP E200K* |
| Gerstmann-Sträussler-Scheinker disease | PrP Q217R |
| Familial Creutzfeldt-Jakob disease | PrP octarepeat insert* |

*Signifies genetic linkage between the mutation and the inherited prion disease.[4,45–47,159]

The term PrP* is used in two different ways. First, it is used to identify a fraction of PrP^Sc molecules that are infectious.[132] Such a designation is thought to be useful because there are $\sim 10^5$ PrP^Sc molecules per infectious unit.[77,99] Second, PrP* is used to designate a metastable intermediate of PrP^C that is bound to protein X.[133] It is noteworthy that neither a subset of biologically active PrP^Sc molecules nor a metastable intermediate of PrP^C has been identified to date.

In mice, the PrP gene denoted *Prnp* is now known to be identical with two genes denoted *Sinc* and *Prn-i* that are known to control the length of the incubation time in mice inoculated with prions.[134,135] These findings permit a welcome simplification. A gene designated *Pid-1* on mouse chromosome 17 also appears to influence experimental CJD and scrapie incubation times, but information on this locus is limited.

Distinguishing among CJD, GSS, and FFI is increasingly difficult with the recognition that fCJD, GSS, and FFI are autosomal dominant diseases caused by mutations in the PRNP gene (Table 224-4). Initially, it was thought that a specific PrP mutation was associated with a particular cliniconeuropathologic phenotype, but an increasing number of exceptions are being recognized. Multiple examples of variations in the cliniconeuropathologic phenotype within a single family, in which all affected members carry the same PrP mutation, have been recorded. Most patients with a PrP mutation at codon 102 present with ataxia and have PrP amyloid plaques; such patients are generally given the diagnosis of GSS, but some individuals within these families present with dementia, a clinical characteristic that is usually associated with CJD. One suggestion is to label these inherited disorders as "prion disease" followed by the mutation in parentheses, while another suggestion is to use the terms fCJD and GSS followed by the mutation. In the case of FFI, describing the D178N mutation and M129 polymorphism seems unnecessary because this is the only known mutation-polymorphism combination that gives the FFI phenotype.

The terminology for prions is still evolving (Table 224-3). While some terms are borrowed from infectious diseases caused by viruses, others are borrowed from genetics, and still others are borrowed from the biology of protein structure as well as neuropathology. This new area of biological investigation, which has such diverse roots, creates some unique problems with terminology.

# HUMAN PRION DISEASES

The human prion diseases present as infectious, genetic, and sporadic disorders.[136] This unprecedented spectrum of disease presentations demanded a new mechanism; prions provide a conceptual framework, within which this remarkably diverse spectrum can be accommodated.

Most humans afflicted with prion disease present with rapidly progressive dementia, but some manifest cerebellar ataxia. Although the brains of patients appear grossly normal on post-

mortem examination, they usually show spongiform degeneration and astrocytic gliosis under the light microscope (Fig. 224-3). In all cases of GSS and variant (v) CJD, PrP amyloid plaques are found.[137] Before PrP immunostaining was available, histochemical staining was used to examine brains from kuru patients where $\sim 70$ percent of cases were thought to have amyloid plaques.[18] The presence or absence of PrP amyloid plaques in sporadic and inherited CJD is quite variable.[138]

Human prion disease should be considered in any patient, who develops a progressive subacute or chronic decline in cognitive or motor function. Typically, adults between 40 and 80 years of age are affected.[3] The young age of people who have died of vCJD in Britain and France raises the possibility that these individuals were infected with bovine prions that contaminated beef products.[137,139,140] Over 100 young adults have also been diagnosed with iatrogenic CJD, 4 to 30 years after receiving human growth hormone (HGH) or gonadotropin derived from cadaveric pituitaries.[141–143] The longest incubation periods (20 to 30 years) are similar to those associated with more recent cases of kuru.[144,145]

## Sporadic CJD

Sporadic forms of prion disease comprise most cases of CJD and possibly a few cases of Gerstmann-Sträussler-Scheinker disease (GSS) (Table 224-1A).[4,146,147] In these patients, mutations of the PrP gene are not found. How prions causing disease arise in patients with sporadic forms is unknown; hypotheses include horizontal transmission of prions from humans or animals,[148] somatic mutation of the PrP gene, and spontaneous conversion of PrP^C into PrP^Sc.[136,149] Because numerous attempts to establish an infectious link between sporadic CJD and a preexisting prion disease in animals or humans have been unrewarding, it seems unlikely that transmission features in the pathogenesis of sporadic prion disease.[150–154]

## Inherited Prion Diseases

To date, 20 different mutations in the human PrP gene resulting in nonconservative substitutions have been found that segregate with the inherited prion diseases (Fig. 224-4B). Familial CJD cases suggested that genetic factors might influence pathogenesis,[2,10,14] but this was difficult to reconcile with the transmissibility of fCJD and GSS.[16] The discovery of genetic linkage between the PrP gene and scrapie incubation times in mice[155] raised the possibility that mutation might feature in the hereditary human prion diseases. The P102L mutation was the first PrP mutation to be genetically linked to CNS dysfunction in GSS (Fig. 224-4B)[4] and has since been found in many GSS families throughout the world.[156–158] Indeed, a mutation in the protein-coding region of the PrP gene has been found in all reported kindreds with familial human prion disease; besides the P102L mutation, genetic linkage has been established for four other mutations (Table 224-4).[45–47,159]

Tg mouse studies confirmed that mutations of the PrP gene can cause neurodegeneration. The P102L mutation of GSS was introduced into the MoPrP transgene and five lines of Tg(MoPrP-P101L) mice expressing high levels of mutant PrP developed spontaneous CNS degeneration consisting of widespread vacuolation of the neuropil, astrocytic gliosis, and numerous PrP amyloid plaques similar to those seen in the brains of humans who die from GSS(P102L).[105,106,160] Brain extracts prepared from spontaneously ill Tg(MoPrP-P101L) mice transmitted CNS degeneration to Tg196 mice, but contained no protease-resistant PrP.[105,106] The Tg196 mice do not develop spontaneous disease but express low levels of the mutant transgene MoPrP-P101L and are deficient for mouse PrP (Prnp^{0/0}).[129] These studies, combined with the transmission of prions from patients who died of GSS to apes and monkeys[16] or to Tg(MHu2M-P101L) mice,[161] demonstrate that prions are generated *de novo* by mutations in PrP. Additionally, brain extracts from patients with some other inherited prion diseases, such as fCJD(E200K) or FFI, transmit disease to Tg(MHu2M) mice.[42] An artificial set of mutations in a PrP transgene consisting of A113V, A115V, and

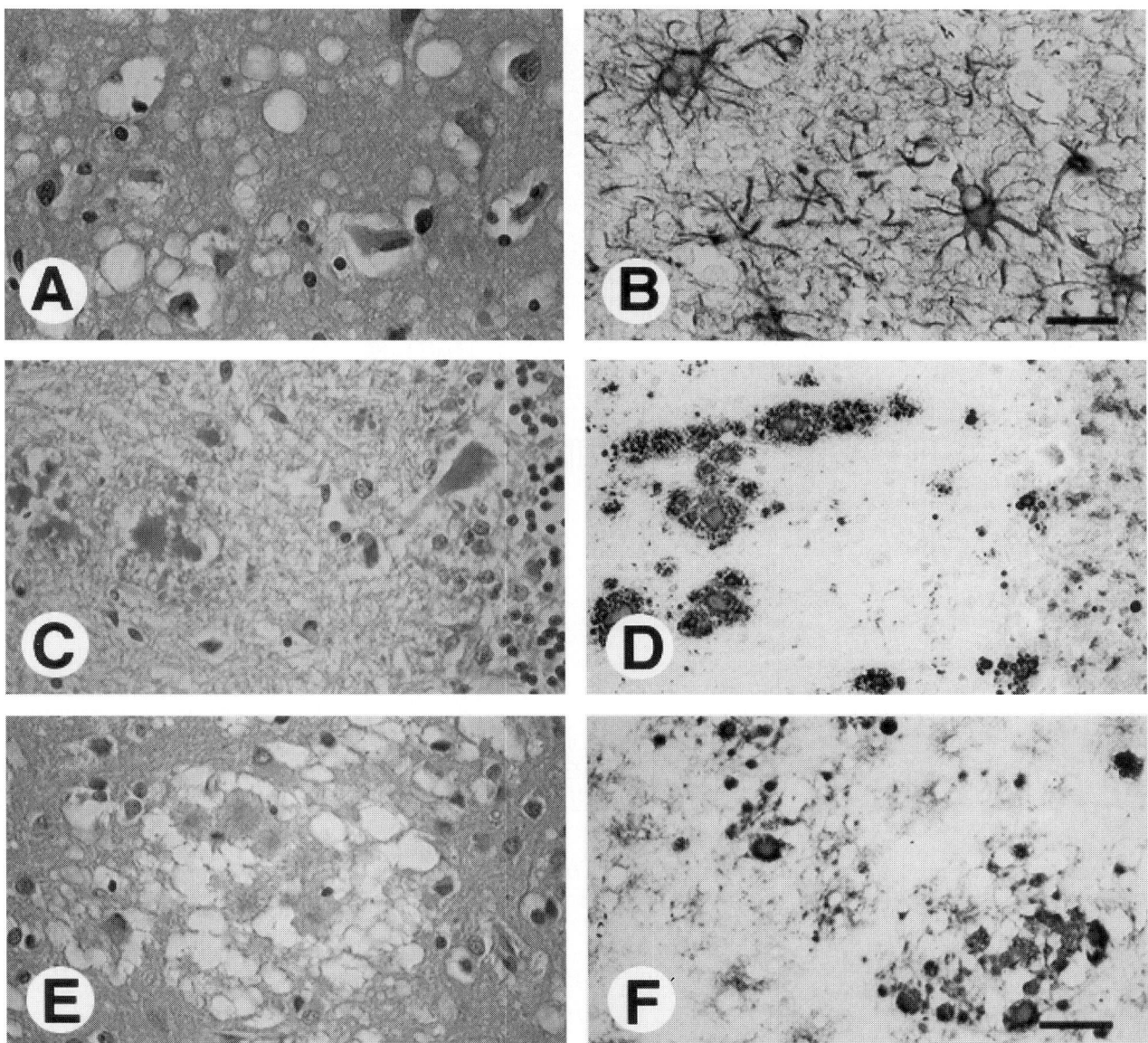

Fig. 224-3 Neuropathology of human prion diseases. *A,* Sporadic CJD, cerebral cortex stained with hematoxylin and eosin showing widespread spongiform degeneration *B,* Sporadic CJD, cerebral cortex immunostained with anit-GFAP antibodies demonstrating the widespread reactive gliosis. *C,* GSS, cerebellum with most of the GSS-plaques in the molecular layer (left 80 percent of micrograph) and many but not all are periodic acid Schiff (PAS) reaction positive. Granule cells and a single Purkinje cell are seen in the right 20 percent of the panel. *D,* GSS, cerebellum at the same location as panel C with PrP immunohistochemistry after the hydrolytic autoclaving reveals more PrP plaques than seen with the PAS reaction. *E,*

Variant CJD, cerebral cortex stained with hematoxylin and eosin shows that the plaque deposits are uniquely located within vacuoles. With this histology, these amyloid deposits have been referred to as "florid plaques." *F,* Variant CJD, cerebral cortex stained with PrP immunohistochemistry after hydrolytic autoclaving reveals numerous PrP plaques often occurring in clusters as well as minute PrP deposits surrounding many cortical neurons and their proximal processes. Bar in E=50 μm and applies also to panels A, B, and C. Bar in F is 100 μm and applies also to panel D. Stephen J. DeArmond produced these photomicrographs. (*Reprinted with permission from Alzheimer Disease. Copyright 1999 Lippincott-Raven Publishers.*)

A118V produced neurodegeneration in neonatal mice; these Val substitutions were selected for their propensity to form a β sheet.[162,163] In preliminary studies, brain extracts from these mice transmitted disease to hamsters and to Tg mice expressing a chimeric SHa/Mo PrP.

**Genetic Disease that Is Transmissible.** Had the PrP gene been identified in families with prion disease by positional cloning or through the purification and sequencing of PrP in amyloid plaques before brain extracts were shown to be transmissible, the prion concept might have been more readily accepted. Within that scenario, it seems likely that we would have explored the possibility that the mutant protein, upon inoculation in a

susceptible host, stimulated production of more of a similar protein. Postulating an infectious pathogen with a foreign genome would have been the least likely candidate to explain how a genetic disease could be experimentally transmissible.

**GSS and Genetic Linkage.** The discovery that GSS, which was known to be a familial disease, could be transmitted to apes and monkeys was first reported when many still thought that scrapie, CJD, and related disorders were caused by viruses.[16] Only the discovery that a proline (P) → leucine (L) mutation at codon 102 of the human PrP gene was genetically linked to GSS permitted the unprecedented conclusion that prion disease can have both genetic and infectious etiologies.[4,136] In that study, the codon 102

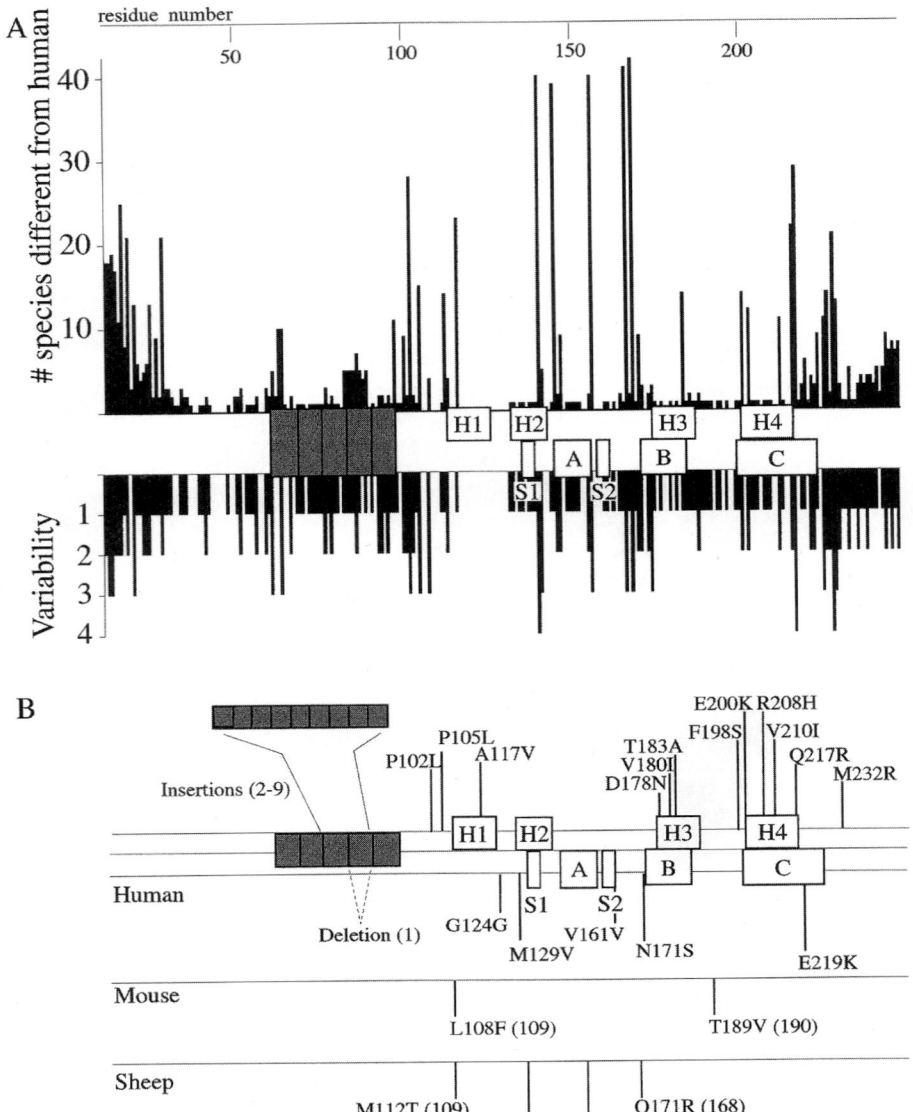

**Fig. 224-4 Species variations and mutations of the prion protein gene.** *A,* Species variations. The x-axis represents the human PrP sequence, with the five octarepeats and H1–H4 regions of putative secondary structure shown, as well as the three α helices, A, B, and C, and the two β strands, S1 and S2. Vertical bars above the axis indicate the number of species that differ from the human sequence at each position. Below the axis, the length of the bars indicates the number of alternative amino acids at each position in the alignment. *B,* Mutations causing inherited human prion disease and polymorphisms in human, mouse, and sheep. Above the line of the human sequence are mutations that cause prion disease. Below the lines are polymorphisms, some of which are known to influence the onset as well as the phenotype of disease. Paul Bamborough and Fred E. Cohen compiled the data. (*Reprinted with permission from Prusiner SB: Prion disease and the BSE crisis. Science 278:245, Prion disease and the BSE crisis stanley B. Prusiner 1997. Copyright 1997 American Association for the Advancement of Science.*)

mutation was linked to development of GSS with a logarithm of the odds (Lod) score exceeding 3, demonstrating a tight association between the altered genotype and the disease phenotype (Table 224-4). This mutation may be caused by the deamination of a methylated CpG in a germ line PrP gene, which results in the substitution of a thymine (T) for cytosine (C). This mutation has been found in many families in numerous countries, including in the original GSS family.[156–158]

**fCJD Caused by Octarepeat Inserts.** An insert of 144 bp containing 6 octarepeats at codon 53, in addition to the 5 octarepeats that are normally present, was described in patients with CJD from 4 families residing in southern England.[5,47] Genealogic investigations show that all four families are related, arguing for a single founder born more than two centuries ago. The Lod score for this extended pedigree exceeds 11. Studies from several laboratories demonstrate that inserts of two, four, five, six, seven, eight, or nine octarepeats in addition to the normal five are found in individuals with inherited CJD (Fig. 224-4*B*).[5,164]

**fCJD in Libyan Jews.** The unusually high incidence of CJD among Israeli Jews of Libyan origin was thought to be due to the

consumption of lightly cooked sheep brain or eyeballs.[165] Molecular genetic investigations revealed that Libyan and Tunisian Jews with fCJD have a PrP gene point mutation at codon 200 resulting in a Glu → Lys substitution (Fig. 224-4*B*).[149,166] The E200K mutation has been genetically linked to the mutation with a Lod score exceeding 3[159] and the same mutation has also been found in patients from Orava in north central Slovakia,[166] in a cluster of familial cases in Chile,[167] and in a large German family living in the United States.[224]

Most patients are heterozygous for the mutation and thus, express both mutant and wild-type (wt) PrP^C. In the brains of patients who die of fCJD(E200K), the mutant PrP^Sc is both insoluble and protease-resistant while much of wt PrP differs from both PrP^C and PrP^Sc in that it is insoluble but readily digested by proteases. Whether this form of PrP is an intermediate in the conversion of PrP^C to PrP^Sc remains to be established.[169]

**Penetrance of fCJD.** Life table analyses of carriers harboring the codon 200 mutation exhibit complete penetrance.[170,171] In other words, if the carriers live long enough, they all eventually develop prion disease. Some investigators have argued that the inherited prion diseases are not fully penetrant and thus, an environmental factor such as the ubiquitous "scrapie virus" is required for illness to be manifest; but as reviewed above, no viral pathogen has been found in prion disease.[167,172]

**Fatal Familial Insomnia.** Studies of inherited human prion diseases demonstrate that changing a single polymorphic residue at position 129 in addition to the D178N pathogenic mutation alters the clinical and neuropathologic phenotype. The D178N mutation combined with a Met encoded at position 129 results in a prion disease called fatal familial insomnia (FFI).[173,174] In this disease, adults generally over age 50 present with a progressive sleep disorder and usually die within about a year.[175] In their brains, deposition of PrPSc is confined largely within the anteroventral and the dorsal medial nuclei of the thalamus. The D178N mutation has been linked to the development of FFI with a Lod score exceeding 5.[46] More than 30 families worldwide with FFI have been recorded.[176] In contrast, the same D178N mutation with a Val encoded at position 129 produces fCJD in which the patients present with dementia, and widespread deposition of PrPSc is found postmortem.[177] The first family to be recognized with CJD has been found to carry the D178N mutation.[2,178]

### Human PrP Gene Polymorphisms

At PrP codon 129, an amino acid polymorphism for the Met → Val has been identified (Fig. 224-4*B*).[179] This polymorphism appears capable of influencing prion disease expression in inherited forms, as well as in iatrogenic and sporadic forms, of prion disease.[173,180,181] A second polymorphism resulting in an amino acid substitution at codon 219 (Glu → Lys) has been reported to occur with a frequency of ~12 percent in the Japanese population but not in Caucasians.[182,183] Lys at 219 appears to protect against CJD by acting as a dominant negative and thus, preventing PrPC with a Glu at 219 from being converted to PrPSc.[183a] A third polymorphism results in an amino acid substitution at codon 171 (Asn → Ser),[184] which lies adjacent to the protein X binding site. This polymorphism has been found in Caucasians, but has not been studied extensively and is not known to influence the binding of PrPC to protein X.[185] A fourth polymorphism is the deletion of a single octarepeat (24 bp), which has been found in 2.5 percent of Caucasians.[186–188] In another study of over 700 individuals, this single octarepeat was found in 1 percent of the population.[189]

Studies of Caucasian patients with sCJD have shown that most are homozygous for Met or Val at codon 129.[180] This contrasts with the general population, in which frequencies for the codon 129 polymorphism in Caucasians are 12 percent V/V, 37 percent M/M, and 51 percent M/V.[190] In contrast, the frequency of the Val allele in the Japanese population is much lower,[191,192] and heterozygosity at codon 129 (M/V) is more frequent (18 percent) in CJD patients than in the general population where the polymorphism frequencies are 0 percent V/V, 92 percent M/M, and 8 percent M/V.[193]

Although no specific mutations have been identified in the PrP gene of patients with sporadic CJD,[194] homozygosity at codon 129 in sCJD[180] is consistent with the results of Tg mouse studies. The finding that homozygosity at codon 129 predisposes to sCJD supports a model of prion production that favors PrP interactions between homologous proteins, as appears to occur in Tg mice expressing SHaPrP inoculated with either hamster prions or mouse prions,[49,195,196] as well as Tg mice expressing a chimeric SHa/Mo PrP transgene inoculated with "artificial" prions.[197]

### Infectious Prion Diseases

The infectious prion diseases include kuru of the Fore people in New Guinea where prions were transmitted by ritualistic cannibalism.[148,198,199] With the cessation of cannibalism at the urging of the colonial government and missionaries, kuru began to decline long before it was known to be transmissible. Sources of prions causing infectious CJD on several different continents include improperly sterilized depth electrodes, transplanted corneas, HGH and gonadotrophin derived from cadaveric

pituitaries, and dura mater grafts.[200] As noted above, many young adults have developed CJD after treatment with cadaveric HGH.[141–143] Dura mater grafts implanted during neurosurgical procedures seem to have caused more than 60 cases of CJD; these incubation periods range from 1 year to more than 14 years.[201–203]

### Variant Creutzfeldt-Jakob Disease (vCJD)

Studies of the prion diseases have taken on new significance with the recent reports of ~30 cases of an atypical variant Creutzfeldt-Jakob disease (vCJD) in teenagers and young adults.[137,139,204,205] To date, all of these cases have been reported from Britain, with the exception of one case from France. It now seems likely that bovine prions passed to humans through the consumption of tainted beef products.[206,207] How many cases of vCJD caused by bovine prions will occur in the years ahead and the magnitude of the problem is unknown.[140] These tragic cases have generated a continuing discourse concerning mad cows, prions, and the safety of the human and animal food supplies throughout the world. Untangling politics and economics from the science of prions seems to have been difficult in disputes between Great Britain and other European countries over the safety of beef and lamb products.

## MOLECULAR GENETICS OF EXPERIMENTAL PRION DISEASE

Once a PrP cDNA probe became available, molecular genetic studies were undertaken to determine whether the PrP gene controls scrapie incubation times in mice. Independent of the enriching of brain fractions for scrapie infectivity that led to the discovery of PrPSc, the PrP gene was shown to be genetically linked to a locus controlling the incubation time.[155] Subsequently, mutation of the PrP gene was shown to be genetically linked to the development of familial prion disease.[4] At the same time, expression of a Syrian hamster (SHa) PrP transgene in mice was shown to render the animals highly susceptible to SHa prions, which demonstrated that expression of a foreign PrP gene could abrogate the species barrier.[195] Later, PrP-deficient (Prnp0/0) mice were found to be resistant to prion infection and, as expected, failed to replicate prions.[58,208] The results of these studies indicated PrP must play a central role in the transmission and pathogenesis of prion disease. Equally important, the results helped establish that the abnormal isoform is an essential component of the prion particle.[49]

### PrP Gene Dosage Controls Length of Incubation Time

Scrapie incubation times in mice were used to distinguish prion strains and to identify a gene controlling its length.[60,209] This gene was initially called *Sinc* based on genetic crosses between C57Bl and VM mice that exhibited short and long incubation times, respectively.[60] Because the distribution of VM mice was restricted, we searched for another mouse with long incubation times. I/Ln mice proved to be a suitable substitute for VM mice; eventually, it was found that I/Ln and VM mice derived from a common ancestor. Subsequently, the PrP gene was shown to control the length of the scrapie incubation time in mice.[134,135]

### Overexpression of wt PrP Transgenes

Mice were constructed expressing different levels of the wt SHaPrP transgene.[195] Inoculation of these Tg(SHaPrP) mice with SHa prions demonstrated abrogation of the species barrier resulting in abbreviated incubation times due to a nonstochastic process.[196] The length of the incubation time after inoculation with SHa prions was inversely proportional to the level of SHaPrPC in the brains of Tg(SHaPrP) mice.[196] Bioassays of brain extracts from clinically ill Tg(SHaPrP) mice inoculated with mouse (Mo) prions revealed that only Mo prions but no SHa prions were produced. Conversely, inoculation of Tg(SHaPrP) mice with SHa prions led only to the synthesis of SHa prions. Thus, the rate of PrPSc synthesis appears to be a function of the level of PrPC expression in Tg mice; however, the level to which PrP^Sc accumulates appears to be independent of PrP^C concentration.[196]

### PrP-Deficient Mice

The development and life span of two lines of Prnp^0/0 mice were indistinguishable from controls,[129,210] while another line exhibited ataxia and Purkinje cell degeneration at ~70 weeks of age.[211] The Purkinje cell degeneration exhibited by the third line of Prnp^0/0 mice is not due to a deficiency of PrP^C, but results from altered regulation of a PrP paralogue, doppel.[210a]

In two Prnp^0/0 lines with normal development, altered sleep-wake cycles[212] and synaptic behavior in brain slices have been reported,[213,214] but the synaptic changes could not be confirmed by others.[215,216]

Prnp^0/0 mice are resistant to prions.[58,208] Prnp^0/0 mice were sacrificed 5, 60, 120, and 315 days after inoculation with RML prions and brain extracts bioassayed in CD-1 Swiss mice. Except for residual infectivity from the inoculum detected at 5 days after inoculation, no infectivity was detected in the brains of Prnp^0/0 mice.[58] One group of investigators found that Prnp^0/0 mice inoculated with RML prions and sacrificed 20 weeks later had $10^{3.6}$ ID$_{50}$ units/ml of homogenate by bioassay.[208] Others have used this report to argue that prion infectivity replicates in the absence of PrP.[50,52] Neither we nor the authors of the initial report could confirm the finding of prion replication in Prnp^0/0 mice.[58,217]

To control the expression of PrP^C in Tg mice, a tetracycline transactivator (tTA) driven by the PrP gene control elements and a tTA-responsive operator linked to a PrP gene were used.[218] Adult Tg mice showed no deleterious effects upon repression of PrP^C expression by >90 percent by oral doxycycline, but the mice developed progressive ataxia at ~50 days after inoculation with prions unless maintained on doxycycline.[219] Although Tg mice on doxycycline accumulated low levels of PrP^Sc, they showed no neurologic dysfunction indicating that low levels of PrP^Sc can be tolerated. Use of the tTA system to control PrP expression allowed production of Tg mice with high levels of PrP that otherwise cause many embryonic and neonatal deaths. Measurement of PrP^Sc clearance in Tg mice should be possible in facilitating the development of pharmacotherapeutics.

## PRION PROTEIN STRUCTURE

Once cDNA probes for PrP became available, the PrP gene was found to be constitutively expressed in adult, uninfected brain.[101,102] This finding eliminated the possibility that PrP^Sc stimulated production of more of itself by initiating transcription of the PrP gene as proposed nearly two decades earlier.[32] Determination of the structure of the PrP gene eliminated a second possible mechanism that might explain the appearance of PrP^Sc in brains already synthesizing PrP^C. Because the entire protein-coding region was contained within a single exon, there was no possibility that the two PrP isoforms were the products of alternatively spliced mRNAs.[96] Next, a posttranslational chemical modification that distinguishes PrP^Sc from PrP^C was considered, but none was found in an exhaustive study,[220] and we considered it likely that PrP^C and PrP^Sc differed only in their conformations, a hypothesis that was proposed earlier.[32]

When the secondary structures of the PrP isoforms were compared by optical spectroscopy, they were found to be markedly different.[40] Fourier transform infrared (FTIR) and circular dichroism (CD) spectroscopy studies showed that PrP^C contains about 40 percent α helix and little β sheet, while PrP^Sc is composed of about 30 percent α helix and 45 percent β sheet.[40] That the two PrP isoforms have the same amino acid sequence runs counter to the widely accepted view that the amino acid sequence specifies only one biologically active conformation of a protein.[221]

Prior to comparative studies on the structures of PrP^C and PrP^Sc, metabolic labeling studies showed that the acquisition of PrP^Sc protease resistance is a posttranslational process.[222] In a search for chemical differences that would distinguish PrP^Sc from PrP^C, we

identified ethanolamine in hydrolysates of PrP 27-30, which signaled the possibility that PrP might contain a glycosylphosphatidyl inositol (GPI) anchor.[122] Both PrP isoforms were found to carry GPI anchors and PrP^C was found on the surface of cells where it could be released by cleavage of the anchor. Subsequent studies showed that PrP^Sc formation occurs after PrP^C reaches the cell surface[223] and is localized to caveolae-like domains.[123,224]

## Computational Models and Optical Spectroscopy

Modeling studies and subsequent nuclear magnetic resonance (NMR) investigations of a synthetic PrP peptide containing residues 90 to 145 suggested that PrP^C might contain an α helix within this region (Fig. 224-4A).[225] This peptide contains the residues 113 to 128 that are most highly conserved among all species studied (Fig. 224-4A) and correspond to a transmembrane region of PrP, which was delineated in cell-free translation studies. A transmembrane form of PrP was found in brains of patients with Gerstmann-Sträussler-Scheinker disease (GSS) caused by the A117V mutation and in Tg mice overexpressing either mutant or wt PrP.[163] That no evidence for an α helix in this region has been found in NMR studies of recombinant PrP in an aqueous environment[128,226,227] suggests that these recombinant PrPs correspond to the secreted form of PrP that was also identified in the cell-free translation studies. This contention is supported by studies with recombinant antibody fragments (Fabs) showing that GPI-anchored PrP^C on the surface of cells exhibits an immunoreactivity profile similar to that of recombinant PrP prepared with an α-helical conformation.[59,228]

Models of PrP^Sc suggest that formation of the disease-causing isoform involves refolding of a region corresponding roughly to residues 108 to 144 into β sheets;[229] the single disulfide bond joining the C-terminus helices would remain intact because the disulfide is required for PrP^Sc formation (Fig. 224-5D).[112] Deletion of each of several regions of putative secondary structure in PrP, except for the NH$_2$-terminal 66 amino acids (residues 23 to 88) and a 36–amino acid stretch (Mo residues 141 to 176), prevented formation of PrP^Sc as measured in scrapie-infected cultured neuroblastoma cells.[112] With α-PrP Fabs selected from phage-display libraries and two monoclonal antibodies (MAB) derived from hybridomas, a major conformational change that occurs during conversion of PrP^C into PrP^Sc has been localized to residues 90 to 112.[228] Studies with an α-PrP IgM MAB, which was reported to immunoprecipitate PrP^Sc selectively,[230] support this conclusion. While these results indicate that PrP^Sc formation involves a conformational change at the NH$_2$-terminus, mutations causing inherited prion diseases have been found throughout the protein (Fig. 224-4B). Interestingly, all of the known point mutations in PrP with biological significance occur either within or adjacent to regions of putative secondary structure in PrP, and as such appear to destabilize the structure of PrP^C.[225,226]

## NMR Structure of Recombinant PrP

The NMR structure of recombinant SHaPrP(90-231) was determined after the protein was purified and refolded (Fig. 224-5A). Residues 90 to 112 are not shown because marked conformational heterogeneity was found in this region while residues 113 to 126 constitute the conserved hydrophobic region that also displays some structural plasticity.[227] Although some features of the structure of rPrP(90-231) are similar to those reported earlier for the smaller recombinant MoPrP(121-231) fragment,[226] substantial differences were found. For example, the loop at the NH$_2$-terminus of helix B is defined in rPrP(90-231) but is disordered in MoPrP(121-231); in addition, helix C is composed of residues 200 to 227 in rPrP(90-231) but extends only from 200 to 217 in MoPrP(121-231). The loop and the C-terminal portion of helix C are particularly important as described below (Fig. 224-5B). Whether the differences between the two recombinant PrP fragments are due to (a) their different lengths, (b) species-specific differences in sequences, or (c) the conditions used for solving the structures remains to be determined.

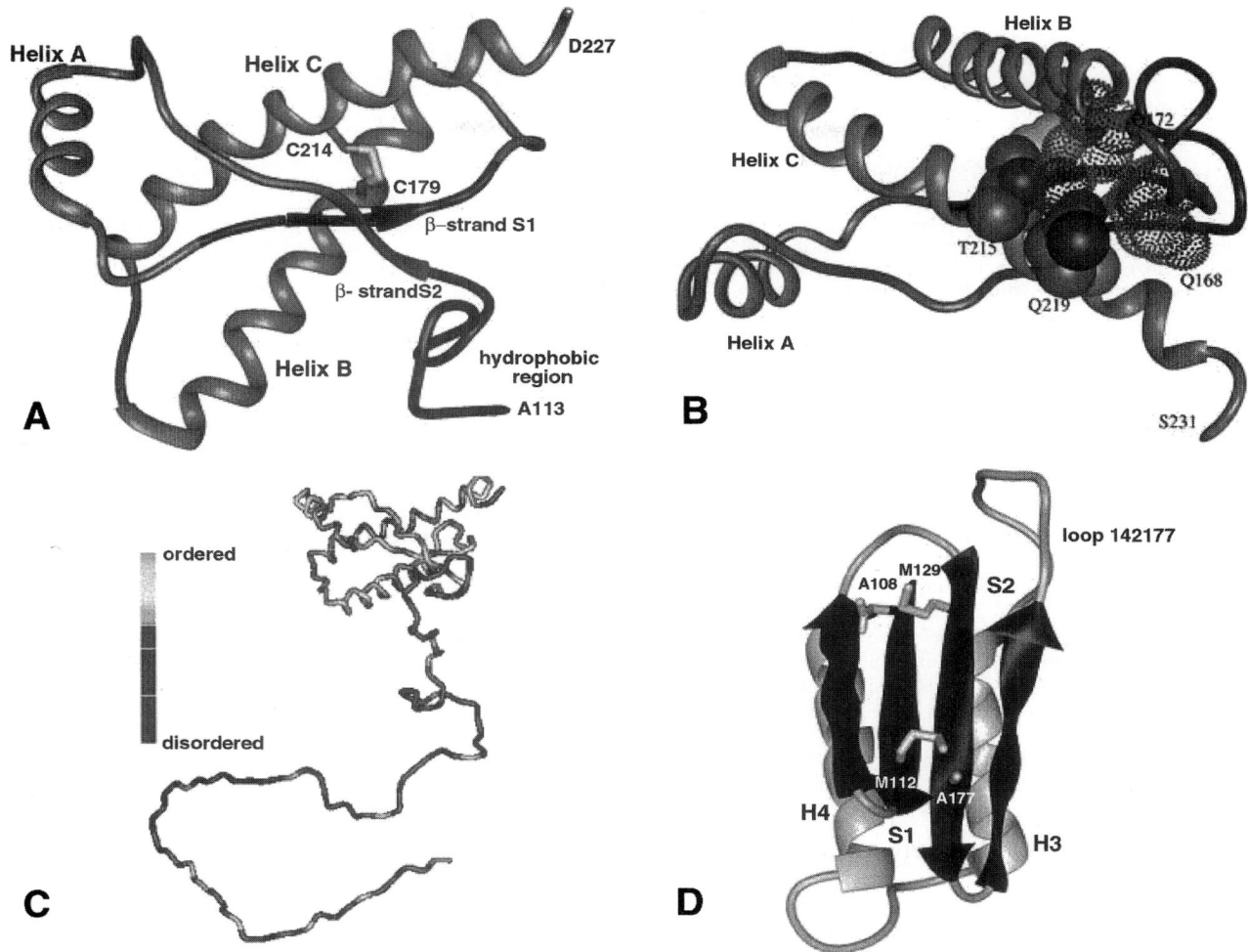

Fig. 224-5 Structures of prion proteins. *A*, NMR structure of Syrian hamster (SHa) recombinant (r) PrP(90-231). Presumably, the structure of the α-helical form of rPrP(90-231) resembles that of PrP^C. rPrP(90-231) is viewed from the interface where PrP^Sc is thought to bind to PrP^C. α Helices A are formed by residues 144-157, B by 172-193, and C by 200-227; the residues Cys179 and Cys214 form a disulfide bond; the conserved hydrophobic region is composed of residues 113-126; β strand S1 encompasses residues 129-134 and β-strand S2 residues 159-165; the arrows span residues 129-131 and 161-163, as these show a closer resemblance to β sheet.[227] *B*, NMR structure of rPrP(90-231) is viewed from the interface where protein X is thought to bind to PrP^C. Protein X appears to bind to the side chains of residues that form a discontinuous epitope. Some amino acids are in the loop composed of residues 165-171 and at the end of helix B (Gln168 and Gln172 with a low-density van der Waals rendering), whereas others are on the surface of helix C (Thr215 and Gln219 with a high-density van der Waals rendering).[185] (Reprinted with permission from *Science* 278:245, 1997. Copyright 1997 American Association for the Advancement of Science) *C*, Diagram shows the flexibility of the polypeptide chain for PrP(29-231).[29] The structure of the portion of the protein representing residues 90-231 was taken from the coordinates of PrP(90-231).[227] The remainder of the sequence was hand-built for illustration purposes only. The color scale corresponds to the heteronuclear {1H}-15H NOE data: dark gray for the lowest (most negative) values, where the polypeptide is most flexible, to light gray for the highest (most positive) values in the most structured and rigid regions of the protein. (Reprinted with permission from *Proc. Natl Acad Sci U S A* 94:13452, 1997. Copyright 1997 National Academy of Sciences.) *D*, Plausible model for the tertiary structure of human PrP^Sc.[229] S1 β strands are 108 to 113 and 116 to 122; S2 β-strands are 128 to 135 abd 138 to 144; α-helices H3 (residues 178-191) and H4 (residues 202-218) in light gray. Four residues—Asn 108, Met 122, Met 129, and Ala 133—implicated in the species barrier are shown. (Reprinted with permission from *Science* 278:245, 1997. Copyright 1997 American Association for the Advancement of Science).

Recent NMR studies of full-length MoPrP(23-231) and SHaPrP(29-231) have shown that the NH$_2$-termini are highly flexible and lack identifiable secondary structure under the experimental conditions employed (Fig. 224-5C).[128] Studies of SHaPrP(29-231) indicate transient interactions between the C-terminal end of helix B and the highly flexible, NH$_2$-terminal random-coil containing the octarepeats (residues 29 to 125).[128]

## PRION REPLICATION

In an uninfected cell, PrP^C with the wt sequence has been proposed to exist in equilibrium in its monomeric α-helical, protease-sensitive state or bound to protein X (Fig. 224-6). We denote the conformation of PrP^C that is bound to protein X as PrP*;[133] this conformation is likely to be different from that determined under aqueous conditions for monomeric recombinant PrP. The PrP*/protein X complex binds PrP^Sc, creating a replication-competent assembly. Order of addition experiments demonstrate that for PrP^C, protein X binding precedes productive PrP^Sc interactions.[185] A conformational change takes place wherein PrP, in a shape competent for binding to protein X and PrP^Sc, represents the initial phase in the formation of infectious PrP^Sc.

Several lines of evidence argue that the smallest infectious prion particle is an oligomer of PrP^Sc that may be as small as a dimer.[231] On purification, PrP^Sc tends to aggregate into insoluble multimers that can be dispersed into liposomes.[97] Whether

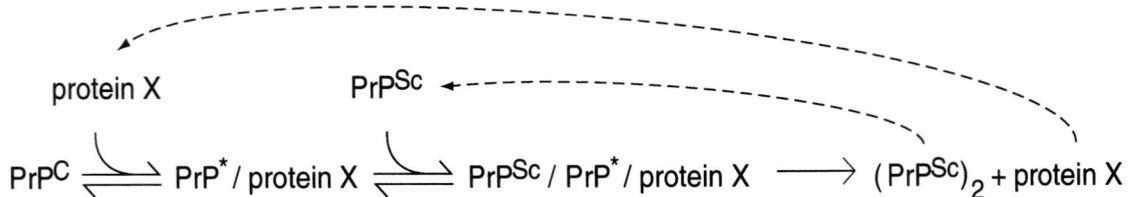

**Fig. 224-6** Diagram shows the template-assisted PrP^Sc formation. In the initial step, PrP^C binds to protein X to form the PrP*/protein X complex. Next, PrP^Sc binds to PrP* that has already formed a complex with protein X. When PrP* is transformed into a nascent molecule of PrP^Sc, protein X is released and a dimer of PrP^Sc remains. The inactivation target size of an infectious prion suggests that it is composed of a dimer of PrP^Sc.[231] In the model depicted here, a fraction of infectious PrP^Sc dimers dissociate into uninfectious monomers as the replication cycle proceeds while most of the dimers accumulate in accord with the increase in prion titer that occurs during the incubation period. Another fraction of PrP^Sc is cleared, presumably by cellular proteases. The precise stoichiometry of the replication process remains uncertain. (*Reprinted with permission from Prusiner SB, Scott MR, DeArmond SJ, Cohen FE: Prion protein biology. Cell 93:337, 1998. Copyright 1998 Cell Press.*)

insolubility is a prerequisite for PrP^Sc formation or prion infectivity, as suggested by some investigators,[232,233] who favor a nucleation-polymerization mechanism, remains to be established.

In attempts to form PrP^Sc *in vitro*, PrP^C has been exposed to 3M GdnHCl and then diluted tenfold prior to binding to PrP^Sc.[234,235] Based on these results, we presume that exposure of PrP^C to GdnHCl converts it into a PrP*-like molecule. Whether this PrP*-like protein is converted into PrP^Sc is unclear. Although the PrP*-like protein bound to PrP^Sc is protease resistant and insoluble, this protease-resistant PrP has not been reisolated in order to assess whether it was converted into PrP^Sc. It is noteworthy that recombinant PrP can be refolded into either α-helical or β-sheet forms, but none has been found to possess prion infectivity as judged by bioassay.

### Cell Biology of PrP^Sc Formation

In scrapie-infected cells, PrP^C molecules destined to become PrP^Sc exit to the cell surface prior to conversion into PrP^Sc.[122,222,223] Like other GPI-anchored proteins, PrP^C appears to reenter the cell through a subcellular compartment bounded by cholesterol-rich, detergent-insoluble membranes which might be caveolae or early endosomes.[123,224,236–238] Within this cholesterol-rich, nonacidic compartment, GPI-anchored PrP^C can be either converted into PrP^Sc or partially degraded.[123] Subsequently, PrP^Sc is trimmed at the N-terminus in an acidic compartment in scrapie-infected cultured cells to form PrP 27-30.[239] In contrast, N-terminal trimming of PrP^Sc is minimal in the brain, where little PrP 27-30 is found.[109]

### Inherited and Sporadic Prion Diseases

For inherited and sporadic prion diseases, the major question is how the first PrP^Sc molecules are formed. Once these molecules are formed, replication presumably follows the mechanism outlined for infectious disease. Several lines of evidence suggest that PrP^Sc is more stable than PrP^C and a kinetic barrier precludes the formation of PrP^Sc under normal conditions. In the case of the initiation of inherited prion diseases, the barrier to PrP^Sc formation must be lower for the mutant (ΔPrP^C) than the wt and thus ΔPrP* can spontaneously rearrange to form ΔPrP^Sc. While some of the known mutations appear to be destabilizing to the structure of PrP^C, we lack useful information about the structure of the transition state for either the mutant or wt sequences. Studies of PrP in the brains of patients, who were heterozygous for the E200K mutation revealed ΔPrP^Sc(E200K) molecules that were both detergent insoluble and resistant to limited proteolysis while most wt PrP were detergent insoluble but protease-sensitive.[169] These results suggest that in familial (f) CJD(E200K), insoluble wt PrP might represent a form of PrP*.[169] In studies with CHO cells, expression of ΔPrP(E200K) was found to be accompanied by the posttranslational acquisition of resistance to limited proteolysis,[240] but whether such cell lines expressing ΔPrP(E200K) produce infectious prions is unknown. It is noteworthy that levels of proteinase K used in the studies where ΔPrP(E200K) was expressed in CHO cells were lower by a factor of 10 to 100 as compared to digestions of PrP^Sc derived from brain or ScN2a cells. Whether these alterations in the properties of ΔPrP(E200K) in CHO cells provide evidence for ΔPrP* or such changes lie outside the pathway of ΔPrP^Sc(E200K) formation remains to be determined.

Initiation of sporadic disease may follow from a somatic mutation and thus, follow a path similar to that for germ-line mutations in inherited disease. In this situation, the mutant PrP^Sc must be capable of co-opting wt PrP^C, a process known to be possible for some mutations (e.g., E200K, D178N) but less likely for others (e.g., P102L).[42,161] Alternatively, the activation barrier separating wt PrP^C from PrP^Sc could be crossed on rare occasions when viewed in the context of a population. Most individuals would be spared while presentations in the elderly with an incidence of ~1 per million would be seen.

### Mechanism of Prion Propagation

From the foregoing formalism, we can ask, "What is the rate-limiting step in prion formation?" First, we must consider the impact of the concentration of PrP^Sc in the inoculum, which is inversely proportional to the length of the incubation time. Second, we must consider the sequence of PrP^Sc that forms an interface with PrP^C. When the sequences of the two isoforms are identical, the shortest incubation times are observed. Third, we must consider the strain-specific conformation of PrP^Sc. Some prion strains exhibit longer incubation times than others; the mechanism underlying this phenomenon is not understood. From these considerations, there exists a set of conditions, under which initial PrP^Sc concentrations can be rate limiting. These effects presumably relate to the stability of the PrP^Sc, its targeting to the correct cells and subcellular compartments, and its capability to be cleared. After infection in a cell is initiated, PrP^Sc production is operative and the following discussion of PrP^Sc formation seems most applicable. If the assembly of PrP^Sc into a specific dimeric or multimeric arrangement were difficult, then nucleation-polymerization (NP) formalism would be relevant. In NP processes, nucleation is the rate-limiting step and elongation or polymerization is facile. These conditions are frequently observed in peptide models of aggregation phenomena;[233] however, studies with Tg mice expressing foreign PrP genes suggest that a different process is occurring. From investigations with mice expressing both the SHaPrP transgene and the endogenous MoPrP gene, it is clear that PrP^Sc provides a template for directing prion replication, where a template is defined as a catalyst that leaves its imprint on the product of the reaction.[196] Inoculation of these mice with SHaPrP^Sc leads to the production of nascent SHaPrP^Sc and not MoPrP^Sc. Conversely, inoculation of the Tg(SHaPrP) mice with MoPrP^Sc results in MoPrP^Sc formation and not SHaPrP^Sc. Even stronger evidence for templating has emerged from studies of prion strains passaged in Tg(MHu2M)Prnp$^{0/0}$ mice expressing a chimeric Hu/MoPrP gene as described in more detail below.[42,43] Even though the conformational templates were initially generated with PrP$^{Sc}$ molecules having different sequences in patients with inherited prion diseases, these templates are sufficient to direct replication of distinct PrP$^{Sc}$ molecules when the amino acid sequences of the substrate PrPs are identical. If the formation of this template were rate limiting, then an NP model could apply. However, studies of PrP$^{Sc}$ formation in ScN2a cells point to a distinct rate-limiting step.

Cell biologic and transgenetic investigations argue for the existence of a chaperone-like molecule referred to as protein X that is required for PrP$^{Sc}$ formation.[161] As described below, mutagenesis experiments have created dominant negative forms of ΔPrP$^C$ that inhibit the formation of wt PrP$^{Sc}$ by binding protein X.[185,233A] This implies that the rate-limiting step *in vivo* in prion replication, under conditions where PrP$^{Sc}$ is sufficient, must be the conversion of PrP$^C$ to PrP* because a dominant negative derived from a single-point mutation could gate only a kinetically critical step in a cellular process. In the template-directed model, the conversion of PrP$^C$ to PrP* is a first order process. By contrast, NP processes follow higher order kinetics ([monomer]$^m$ where m is the number of monomers in the nucleus). The experimental implications of these rate relationships are apparent in transgenic studies; if first order kinetics operate, halving the gene dose (hemizygotes) should double the incubation time, whereas doubling the dose of a transgene array should halve the time to disease. This quantitative behavior has been observed in several studies in mice with altered levels of PrP expression.[58,134,196,241] The existence of prion strains that are conformational isoforms of PrP$^{Sc}$ with distinct structures, incubation times, and neurohistopathology must also be considered in an analysis of the kinetics of PrP$^{Sc}$ accumulation. Because the rate-limiting step in PrP$^{Sc}$ formation cannot involve the unique template provided by a strain, differential rates of intercellular spread, cellular uptake, and clearance seem most likely to account for the variation in incubation times. This is consistent with the different patterns of protease sensitivity and glycosylation for distinct prion strains.[41,42,242–244]

We hasten to add, however, that NP models can provide a useful description of other biologic phenomena. Under conditions when the monomer is relatively rare and/or the conformational change is facile (e.g., short peptides), the NP model dominates. However, when the monomer is sufficiently abundant and/or the conformational conversion is difficult to accomplish, the template-assistance formalism provides a more likely description of the process.

### Evidence for Protein X

Protein X was postulated to explain the results on the transmission of human (Hu) prions to Tg mice (Table 224-5).[161,245] Mice expressing both Mo and HuPrP were resistant to Hu prions while those expressing only HuPrP were susceptible. These results argue that MoPrP$^C$ inhibited transmission of Hu prions; that is, the formation of nascent HuPrP$^{Sc}$. In contrast to the foregoing studies, mice expressing both MoPrP and chimeric MHu2MPrP were

susceptible to Hu prions, and mice expressing MHu2MPrP alone were only slightly more susceptible. These findings contend that MoPrP$^C$ has only a minimal effect on the formation of chimeric MHu2MPrP$^{Sc}$.

When the data on Hu prion transmission to Tg mice were considered together, the data suggested that MoPrP$^C$ prevented the conversion of HuPrP$^C$ to PrP$^{Sc}$ by binding to another Mo protein but had little effect on the conversion of MHu2M to PrP$^{Sc}$. We interpreted these results in terms of MoPrP$^C$ binding to this Mo protein with a higher affinity than does HuPrP$^C$. We postulated that MoPrP$^C$ had little effect on the formation of PrP$^{Sc}$ from MHu2M (Table 224-5) because MoPrP and MHu2M share the same amino acid sequence at the C-terminus. This also suggested that MoPrP$^C$ only weakly inhibited transmission of SHa prions to Tg(SHaPrP) mice because SHaPrP is more closely related to MoPrP than is HuPrP.

Using scrapie-infected mouse neuroblastoma cells transfected with chimeric Hu/Mo PrP genes, we extended our studies of protein X. Substitution of a Hu residue at position 214 or 218 prevented PrP$^{Sc}$ formation (Fig. 224-5B).[185] The side chains of these residues protrude from the same surface of the C-terminus α helix, forming a discontinuous epitope with residues 167 and 171 in an adjacent loop. Substitution of a basic residue at positions 167, 171, or 218 prevented PrP$^{Sc}$ formation; these mutant PrPs appear to act as "dominant negatives" by binding protein X and rendering it unavailable for prion propagation.[185,233a] Our findings seem to explain the protective effects of basic polymorphic residues in PrP of humans and sheep.[246–248]

**Is Protein X a Molecular Chaperone?** Because PrP undergoes a profound structural transition during prion propagation, it seems likely that other proteins, such as chaperones, participate in this process. Whether protein X functions as a classical molecular chaperone or participates in PrP binding as part of its normal function but can also facilitate pathogenic aspects of PrP biology is unknown. Interestingly, scrapie-infected cells in culture display marked differences in the induction of heat-shock proteins,[249] and Hsp70 mRNA has been reported to increase in scrapie of mice.[250] While attempts to isolate specific proteins that bind to PrP have been disappointing,[251] PrP has been shown to interact with Bcl-2, Hsp60, and the laminin receptor protein by two-hybrid analysis in yeast.[252,253] Although these studies are suggestive, no molecular chaperone involved in prion formation in mammalian cells has been identified.

## STRAINS OF PRIONS

The existence of prion strains raises the question of how heritable biological information can be enciphered in any molecule other than nucleic acid.[60] Incubation times and the distribution of neuronal vacuolation have defined strains or varieties of prions.[60,254] Subsequently, the patterns of PrP$^{Sc}$ deposition were found to correlate with vacuolation profiles and these patterns were also used to characterize strains of prions.[115,243,255]

The typing of prion strains in C57Bl, VM, and F1(C57Bl × VM) inbred mice began with isolates from sheep with scrapie. The

**Table 224-5** Evidence for Protein X from Transmission Studies of Human Prions*

| Inoculum | Host | MoPrP gene | Incubation Time [days±SEM] | (n/n$_0$) |
|---|---|---|---|---|
| sCJD | Tg(HuPrP) | Prnp$^{+/+}$ | 721 | (1/10) |
| sCJD | Tg(HuPrP)Prnp$^{0/0}$ | Prnp$^{0/0}$ | 263±2 | (6/6) |
| sCJD | Tg(MHu2M) | Prnp$^{+/+}$ | 238±3 | (8/8) |
| sCJD | Tg(MHu2M)Prnp$^{0/0}$ | Prnp$^{0/0}$ | 191±3 | (10/10) |

* Data with inoculum RG from reference 161.

**Table 224-6** Distinct Prion Strains Generated in Humans with Inherited Prion Diseases and Transmitted to Transgenic Mice[*]

| Inoculum | Host Species | Host PrP Genotype | Incubation Time | | PrP$^{Sc}$ (kDa) |
| | | | [days±SEM] | (n/n$_0$) | |
|---|---|---|---|---|---|
| None | Human | FFI(D178N, M129) | | | 19 |
| FFI | Mouse | Tg(MHu2M) | 206±7 | (7/7) | 19 |
| FFI → Tg(MHu2M) | Mouse | Tg(MHu2M) | 136±1 | (6/6) | 19 |
| None | Human | fCJD (E200K) | | | 21 |
| fDJD | Mouse | Tg(MHu2M) | 170±2 | (10/10) | 21 |
| fCJD → Tg(MHu2M) | Mouse | Tg(MHu2M) | 167±3 | (15/15) | 21 |

[*] Data from reference 42.

prototypic strains called Me7 and 22A gave incubation times of ∼150 and ∼400 days in C57Bl mice, respectively.[60] The PrPs of C57Bl and I/Ln (and later VM) mice differ at two residues and control incubation times.[134,135]

Until recently, support for the hypothesis that the tertiary structure of PrP$^{Sc}$ enciphers strain-specific information[49] was minimal except for the DY strain isolated from mink with transmissible encephalopathy.[41] PrP$^{Sc}$ in DY prions showed diminished resistance to proteinase K digestion as well as an anomalous site of cleavage. The DY strain presented a puzzling anomaly because other prion strains exhibiting similar incubation times did not show this altered susceptibility to proteinase K digestion of PrP$^{Sc}$.[209] Also notable was the generation of new strains during passage of prions through animals with different PrP genes.[209]

### PrP$^{Sc}$ Conformation Enciphers Variation in Prions

Persuasive evidence that strain-specific information is enciphered in the tertiary structure of PrP$^{Sc}$ comes from transmission of two different inherited human prion diseases to mice expressing a chimeric MHu2M PrP transgene.[42] In FFI, the protease-resistant fragment of PrP$^{Sc}$ after deglycosylation has an $M_r$ of 19 kDa, whereas in fCJD(E200K) and most sporadic prion diseases, it is 21 kDa.[256] This difference in molecular size was shown to be due to different sites of proteolytic cleavage at the NH$_2$-termini of the two human PrP$^{Sc}$ molecules reflecting different tertiary structures.[256] These distinct conformations were not unexpected because the amino acid sequences of the PrPs differ.

Extracts from the brains of FFI patients transmitted disease into mice expressing a chimeric MHu2M PrP gene about 200 days after inoculation and induced formation of the 19-kDa PrP$^{Sc}$; whereas fCJD(E200K) and sCJD produced the 21-kDa PrP$^{Sc}$ in mice expressing the same transgene.[42] On second passage, Tg(MHu2M) mice inoculated with FFI prions showed an incubation time of ∼130 days and a 19-kDa PrP$^{Sc}$, while those inoculated with fCJD(E200K) prions exhibited an incubation time of ∼170 days and a 21-kDa PrP$^{Sc}$ (Table 224-6).[43] The experimental data demonstrate that MHu2MPrP$^{Sc}$ can exist in two different conformations based on the sizes of the protease-resistant fragments; yet, the amino acid sequence of MHu2MPrP$^{Sc}$ is invariant.

The results of our studies argue that PrP$^{Sc}$ acts as a template for the conversion of PrP$^C$ to nascent PrP$^{Sc}$. Imparting the size of the

protease-resistant fragment of PrP$^{Sc}$ through conformational templating provides a mechanism for both the generation and propagation of prion strains.

Interestingly, the protease-resistant fragment of PrP$^{Sc}$ after deglycosylation with an $M_r$ of 19 kDa has been found in a patient who died after developing a clinical disease similar to FFI. Because both PrP alleles encoded the wt sequence and a Met at position 129, we labeled this case sporadic fatal insomnia (sFI). At autopsy, the spongiform degeneration, reactive astrogliosis, and PrP$^{Sc}$ deposition were confined to the thalamus.[257] These findings argue that the clinicopathologic phenotype is determined by the conformation of PrP$^{Sc}$ in accord with the results of the transmission of human prions from patients with FFI to Tg mice.[42]

### Interplay Between the Species and Strains of Prions

Studies on the role of the primary and tertiary structures of PrP in the transmission of disease give new insights into the pathogenesis of the prion diseases. The amino acid sequence of PrP encodes the species of the prion (Table 224-7),[161,195] and the prion derives its PrP$^{Sc}$ sequence from the last mammal, in which it was passaged.[209] While the primary structure of PrP is likely to be the most important or even sole determinant of the tertiary structure of PrP$^C$, existing PrP$^{Sc}$ seems to function as a template in determining the tertiary structure of nascent PrP$^{Sc}$ molecules as they are formed from PrP$^C$.[49,133] In turn, prion diversity appears to be enciphered in the conformation of PrP$^{Sc}$ and prion strains may represent different conformers of PrP$^{Sc}$.[41,42,209]

### Evidence for Different Conformations of PrP$^{Sc}$ in Eight Prion Strains

Using a highly sensitive conformation-dependent immunoassay for measurement of PrP$^{Sc}$ in tissue homogenates, eight different prion strains passaged in Syrian hamsters were examined.[44] Brains from Syrian hamsters were collected when the animals displayed signs of neurologic dysfunction; the incubation times for the prion strains varied from 70 to 320 days. Most of the PrP in the brains of Syrian hamsters with signs of neurologic disease was PrP$^{Sc}$ as defined by the β-sheet conformation. The level of PrP$^{Sc}$ in the brains of these clinically ill animals exceeded that of PrP$^C$ by three- to tenfold (Fig. 224-7A). The highest levels of PrP$^{Sc}$ were found in the brains of Syrian hamsters infected with the

**Table 224-7** Influence of Prion Species and Strain on Transmission from Syrian Hamsters to Hamsters and Mice[*]

| Inoculum | Recipient | Sc237 Strain Incubation Time [days ± S.E.M.] (n/n$_o$) | 139 H Strain |
|---|---|---|---|
| SHa → SHa | SHa | 77±1(48/48) | 167±1 (94/94) |
| SHa → SHa | non-Tg mice | >700 (0/9) | 499±15 (11/11) |
| SHa → SHa | Tg(SHaPrP)81 mice | 75±2(22/22) | 110±2 (19/19) |

[*] The *species* of prion is *encoded* by the primary structure of PrP$^{Sc}$ and the *strain* of prion is *enciphered* by the tertiary structure of PrP$^{Sc}$. We recognize that the primary structure, as well as posttranslational chemical modifications, determine the tertiary structure of PrP$^C$, but we contend that the conformation of PrP$^C$ is modified by PrP$^{Sc}$ as it is refolded into a nascent molecule of PrP$^{Sc}$.[42]

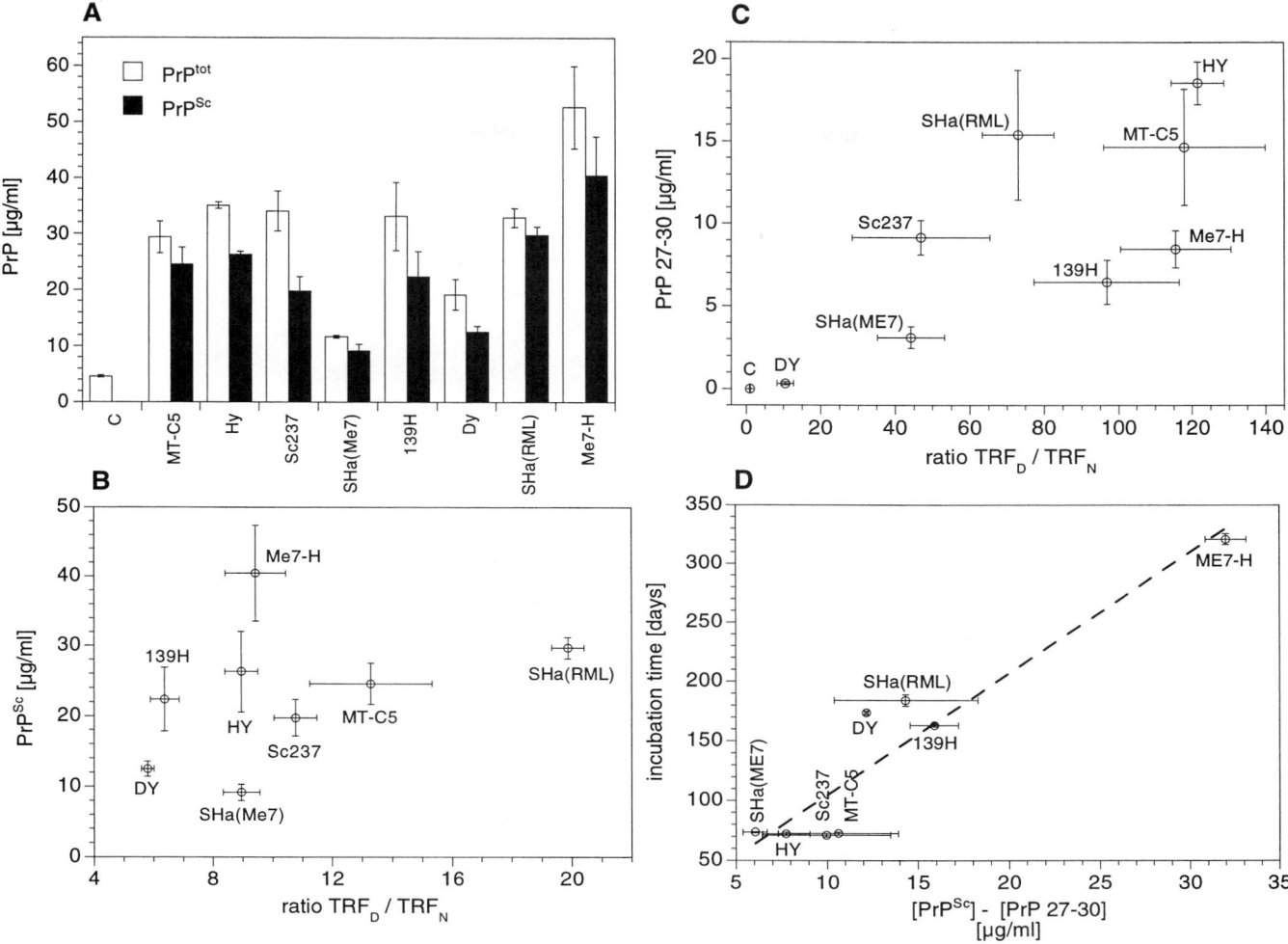

**Fig. 224-7 Eight prion strains distinguished by the conformation-dependent immunoassay.** *A*, Concentration of total PrP and PrP$^{Sc}$. The columns and bars represent the average ± SEM obtained from three different brains of LVG/LAK Syrian hamsters infected with different prion strains and measured in three independent experiments. *B*, Ratio of antibody binding to denatured/native PrP and a function of concentration of PrP$^{Sc}$ in the brains of Syrian hamsters infected with different prion strains. Concentration of PrP$^{Sc}$ (formula 1) and the ratio of antibody binding to denatured/native PrP were measured by the conformation-dependent immunoassay. *C*, Brain

homogenates of Syrian hamsters inoculated with different scrapie strains and uninoculated controls, denoted C, were digested with 50 μg/ml of proteinase K for 2 h at 37°C prior to the conformation-dependent immunoassay. *D*, Incubation time plotted as a function of the concentration of the proteinase K-sensitive fraction of PrP$^{Sc}$ ([PrP$^{Sc}$]-[PrP 27-30]). (Reprinted with permission from Safer J, Wille H, Itri V, Groth D, Serban H, Torchia M, Cohen FE, Prusiner SB. Eight prion strains have PrP$^{Sc}$ molecules with different conformation. *Nat Med* 4:1157, 1998. Copyright 1998 Nature Medicine.)

Me7-H strain; in contrast, the lowest levels were found in the brains of Syrian hamsters inoculated with the SHa(Me7) strain (Fig. 224-7A). Interestingly, the Me7-H and SHa(Me7) strains, which were both derived from Me7 passaged in mice,[209,258] possessed similar denatured/native PrP ratios, but they accumulated PrP$^{Sc}$ to quite different levels (Fig. 224-7A and B). The highest denatured/native PrP ratio of all tested strains was SHa(RML).

The apparent independence of the ratio of denatured/native PrP from the concentration of PrP$^{Sc}$ became apparent after plotting both parameters in a single graph (Fig. 224-7B). Each strain occupied a unique position, indicating differences in the conformation of accumulated PrP$^{Sc}$. Because the PrP$^C$ concentration in each strain was ≤5 μg/ml and the PrP ratio for PrP$^C$ was ≤1.8, the expected impact of the presence of PrP$^C$ on the final PrP ratio was ≤15 percent.

Because only the most tightly folded conformers of PrP$^{Sc}$ are likely to be protease resistant, we digested each of the brain homogenates with proteinase K prior to measuring the ratio of denatured/native PrP (Fig. 224-7C). As shown, the positions of

many strains changed when the protease-sensitive conformers of PrP$^{Sc}$ were enzymatically hydrolyzed (Fig. 224-7C). Most notable was the DY strain, which was readily detectable before limited proteolysis by immunoassay (Fig. 224-7B) but became almost undetectable after digestion (Fig. 224-7C), in accord with earlier Western blot studies.[41,259] Equally important, strains such as Sc237 and HY were marginally separated prior to proteinase K digestion (Fig. 224-7B) but became quite distinct afterwards (Fig. 224-7C). These findings argue that Sc237 and HY are distinct strains even though they exhibit similar incubation times of ~70 days when passaged in Syrian hamsters.[209] It is noteworthy that limited proteolysis of PrP$^{Sc}$ from Sc237- and HY-infected brains produced PrP 27-30 proteins that were indistinguishable by migration in SDS-PAGE as detected by western immunoblotting.[209]

When the incubation times of these eight strains were plotted as a function of either the concentration of PrP$^{Sc}$ or PrP 27-30, no relationship could be discerned. Incubation times were also plotted as a function of the ratio of denatured/native PrP and again, no correlation could be found.

To assess the fraction of PrP$^{Sc}$ that is sensitive to proteolysis during limited digestion with proteinase K, we subtracted the protease-resistant PrP 27-30 fraction (Fig. 224-7*C*) from the total PrP$^{Sc}$ (Fig. 224-7*B*) for each of the eight prion strains. It was asked whether the proteinase K-sensitive fraction of PrP$^{Sc}$ ([PrP$^{Sc}$]-[PrP 27-30]) might reflect those PrP$^{Sc}$ molecules that are most readily cleared by cellular proteases. The clearance of PrP$^{Sc}$ is of considerable interest with respect to control of the length of the incubation time and other phenotypic features of prion strains.[260] When the [PrP$^{Sc}$]-[PrP 27-30] fraction was plotted as a function of the incubation time, a linear relationship was found with an excellent correlation coefficient (r = 0.94) (Fig. 224-7*D*).

The above results demonstrate that eight different strains possess at least eight different conformations (Fig. 224-7*B* and *C*). Additional data argue that each strain is composed of a spectrum of conformations as revealed by limited protease digestion and GdnHCl denaturation studies.[44] These findings contrast with the recently held notion that the primary structure of a protein determines a single tertiary structure.[221]

How many formations can PrP$^{Sc}$ adopt? The conformation-dependent immunoassay described here provides a rapid tool capable of discriminating between the secondary and tertiary structures of a substantial number of PrP$^{Sc}$ molecules.

As noted above for studies of strains passaged from humans with fCJD(E200K) and FFI, PrP$^{Sc}$ must act as a template in the replication of nascent PrP$^{Sc}$ molecules. Also as discussed above, it seems likely that the binding of PrP$^C$ or a metastable intermediate PrP* to protein X is the initial step in PrP$^{Sc}$ formation and that this is the rate-limiting step in prion replication.[185,260,261] PrP$^{Sc}$ interacts with PrP$^C$ but not protein X in the PrP$^C$/protein X complex. When PrP$^C$ or PrP* is converted into a nascent PrP$^{Sc}$ molecule, protein X is released.

It also follows from these observations that the different incubation times of various prion strains should arise predominantly from distinct rates of PrP$^{Sc}$ clearance rather than from the different rates of PrP$^{Sc}$ formation.[260] Thus, prion strains that are readily cleared should have prolonged incubation times, while those that are poorly cleared should display abbreviated incubation periods. This hypothesis was investigated by relying upon the difference in brain PrP$^{Sc}$ concentrations before and after proteinase K treatment as a surrogate for *in vivo* clearance of each prion strain. When clearance as approximated by [PrP$^{Sc}$]-[PrP 27-30] was plotted as a function of the incubation time for eight strains, a linear relationship was found (Fig. 224-7*D*). It is important to recognize that proteinase K sensitivity is an imperfect model for *in vivo* clearance and that only one strain with a long incubation time (exceeding 300 days) has been studied.

It has been suggested that Asn-linked CHOs specify prion strains,[242] but this proposal is difficult to reconcile with the addition of high mannose oligosaccharides to Asn-linked consensus sites on PrP in the ER and subsequent remodeling of the sugar chains in the Golgi.[262] Modification of the complex CHOs attached to PrP$^C$ is clearly completed prior to the PrP$^C$ trafficking to the cell surface,[222,223] which indicates that the Asn-linked CHOs of PrP$^{Sc}$ do not instruct the addition of such complex-type sugars to PrP$^C$.[262a]

Mutagenesis of the complex-type sugar attachment sites seemed to increase PrP$^{Sc}$ formation in cultured cells,[263] but resulted in prolonged incubation times in Tg mice and differences in the patterns of PrP$^C$ distribution and PrP$^{Sc}$ deposition in mice expressing mutant PrPs.[243] These studies suggest that Asn-linked glycosylation might alter the stability of PrP, particularly that of PrP$^{Sc}$, which results in various patterns of PrP$^{Sc}$ deposition. Thus, different clearance rates of PrP$^{Sc}$ may be important in determining both the strain-specific neuropathology and the length of the incubation time.[260]

## Mechanism of Selective Neuronal Targeting

In addition to incubation times, neuropathologic profiles of spongiform change have been used to characterize prion strains.[254]

However, recent studies argue that such profiles may not be an intrinsic feature of strains.[243,264] The mechanism, by which prion strains modify the pattern of spongiform degeneration, was perplexing because earlier investigations had shown that PrP$^{Sc}$ deposition precedes neuronal vacuolation and reactive gliosis.[115] When FFI prions were inoculated in Tg(MHu2M) mice, PrP$^{Sc}$ was confined largely to the thalamus (Fig. 224-8*A*), as is the case for FFI in humans.[42] In contrast, fCJD(E200K) prions inoculated in Tg(MHu2M) mice produced widespread deposition of PrP$^{Sc}$ throughout the cortical mantle and many of the deep structures

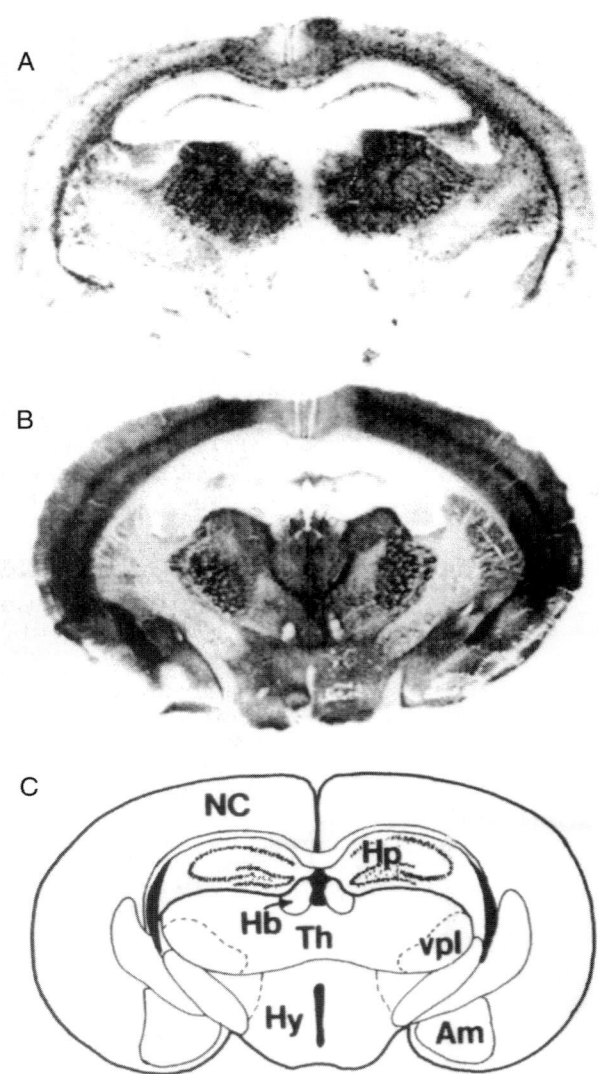

**Fig. 224-8** Regional distribution of PrP$^{Sc}$ deposition in Tg(MHu2M)Prnp$^{0/0}$ mice inoculated with prions from humans who died of inherited prion diseases. Histoblot of PrP$^{Sc}$ deposition in a coronal section of a Tg(MHu2M)Prnp$^{0/0}$ mouse through the hippocampus and thalamus.[42] *A*, The Tg mouse was inoculated with brain extract prepared from a patient who died of FFI. *B*, The Tg mouse was inoculated with extract from a patient with fCJD(E200K). Cryostat sections were mounted on nitrocellulose and treated with proteinase K to eliminate PrP$^C$.[116] To enhance the antigenicity of PrP$^{Sc}$, the histoblots were exposed to 3-guanidinium isothiocyanate before immunostaining using α-PrP 3F4 MAB.[319] *C*, Labeled diagram of a coronal section of the hippocampus/thalamus region. NC, neocortex; Hp, hippocampus; Hb, habenula; Th, thalamus; vpl, ventral posterior lateral thalamic nucleus; Hy, hypothalamus; Am, amygdala. (Reprinted with permission from Prusiner SB, Scott MR, DeArmond SJ, Cohen FE: Prion protein biology. *Cell* 93:337, 1998. Copyright 1998 Cell Press.)

of the central nervous system (Fig. 224-8*B*), as is seen in fCJD(E200K) of humans. To examine whether the diverse patterns of PrP$^{Sc}$ deposition are influenced by Asn-linked glycosylation of PrP$^{C}$, we constructed Tg mice expressing PrPs mutated at one or both of the Asn-linked glycosylation consensus sites.[243] These mutations resulted in aberrant neuroanatomic topologies of PrP$^{C}$ within the central nervous system, whereas pathologic point mutations adjacent to the consensus sites did not alter the distribution of PrP$^{C}$. Tg mice with a mutation of the second PrP glycosylation site exhibited prion incubation times of > 500 days and unusual patterns of PrP$^{Sc}$ deposition. Glycosylation can modify the conformation of PrP and affect either the turnover of PrP$^{C}$ or the clearance of PrP$^{Sc}$. Regional differences in the rate of deposition or clearance would result in specific patterns of PrP$^{Sc}$ accumulation.

## PRION DISEASES OF ANIMALS

The prion diseases of animals include scrapie of sheep and goats, bovine spongiform encephalopathy, transmissible mink encephalopathy, chronic wasting disease of mule deer and elk, feline spongiform encephalopathy, and exotic ungulate encephalopathy (Table 224-1*B*).

### Sheep and Cattle PrP Gene Polymorphisms

Parry argued that host genes were responsible for the development of scrapie in sheep. He was convinced that natural scrapie is a genetic disease that could be eradicated by proper breeding protocols.[265,266] He considered its transmission by inoculation of importance primarily for laboratory studies and communicable infection of little consequence in nature. Other investigators viewed natural scrapie as an infectious disease and argued that host genetics only modulates susceptibility to an endemic infectious agent.[267]

In sheep, polymorphisms at codons 136, 154, and 171 of the PrP gene that produces amino acid substitutions have been studied with respect to the occurrence of scrapie (Fig. 224-4*B*).[68,268–270] Studies of natural scrapie in the United States have shown that ~85 percent of the afflicted sheep are of the Suffolk breed. Only those Suffolk sheep homozygous for Gln (Q) at codon 171 developed scrapie, although healthy controls with QQ, QR, and RR genotypes were also found.[246,247,270–276] These results argue that susceptibility in Suffolk sheep is governed by the PrP codon 171 polymorphism. In Cheviot sheep, the PrP codon 171 polymorphism has a profound influence on susceptibility to scrapie, as in the Suffolk breed, and codon 136 seems to play a less pronounced role.[277,278]

In contrast to sheep, different breeds of cattle have no specific PrP polymorphisms. The only polymorphism recorded in cattle is a variation in the number of octarepeats: most cattle, like humans, have five octarepeats but some have six;[69,279] however, the presence of six octarepeats does not seem to be overrepresented in BSE.[69,279,280]

### Bovine Spongiform Encephalopathy

Prion strains and the species barrier are of paramount importance in understanding the BSE epidemic in Britain, in which it is estimated that almost one million cattle were infected with prions.[281,282] The mean incubation time for BSE is about 5 years. Therefore, most cattle did not manifest disease because they were slaughtered between 2 and 3 years of age.[283] Nevertheless, more than 175,000 cattle, primarily dairy cows, died of BSE over the past decade.[281] BSE is a massive common-source epidemic caused by meat and bone meal fed primarily to dairy cows.[282,284] The meat and bone meal was prepared from the offal of sheep, cattle, pigs, and chickens as a high-protein nutritional supplement. In the late 1970s, the hydrocarbon-solvent extraction method used in the rendering of offal began to be abandoned resulting in meat and bone meal with a much higher fat content.[284] It is now thought that this change in the rendering

process allowed scrapie prions from sheep to survive rendering and to be passed into cattle. Alternatively, bovine prions were present at low levels prior to modification of the rendering process and with the processing change, survived in sufficient numbers to initiate the BSE epidemic when inoculated back in cattle orally through meat and bone meal. Against the latter hypothesis is the widespread geographical distribution throughout England of the initial 17 cases of BSE, which occurred almost simultaneously.[282,285,286] Furthermore, there is no evidence of a preexisting prion disease of cattle, either in Great Britain or elsewhere.

**Origin of BSE Prions.** The origin of the bovine prions causing BSE cannot be determined by examining the amino acid sequence of PrP$^{Sc}$ in cattle with BSE because the PrP$^{Sc}$ in these animals has the bovine sequence whether the initial prions in meat and bone meal came from cattle or sheep. The bovine PrP sequence differs from that of sheep at seven or eight positions.[68,69,279] In contrast to the many PrP polymorphisms found in sheep, only one PrP polymorphism has been found in cattle. Although most bovine PrP alleles encode five octarepeats, some encode six. PrP alleles encoding six octarepeats do not seem to be overrepresented in BSE (Fig. 224-4*B*).[280]

Brain extracts from BSE cattle cause disease in cattle, sheep, mice, pigs, and mink after intracerebral inoculation,[206,287–290] but prions in brain extracts from sheep with scrapie fed to cattle produced illness substantially different from BSE.[291] However, no exhaustive effort has been made to test different strains of sheep prions or to examine the disease following bovine to bovine passage. The annual incidence of sheep with scrapie in Britain over the past two decades has remained relatively low (J. Wilesmith, unpublished data). In July 1988, the practice of feeding meat and bone meal to sheep and cattle was banned. Recent statistical analysis argues that the epidemic is now disappearing as a result of this ruminant feed ban,[281] which is reminiscent of the disappearance of kuru in the Fore people of New Guinea.[148,199]

**Monitoring Cattle for BSE Prions.** Although many plans have been offered for the culling of older cattle in order to minimize the spread of BSE,[281] it seems more important to monitor the frequency of prion disease in cattle as they are slaughtered for human consumption. No reliable, specific test for prion disease in live animals is available, but immunoassays for PrP$^{Sc}$ in the brainstems of cattle might provide a reasonable approach to establishing the incidence of subclinical BSE in cattle entering the human food chain.[116,230,279,292–294] Determining how early in the incubation period PrP$^{Sc}$ can be detected by immunologic methods is now possible because a reliable bioassay was created by expressing the BoPrP gene in Tg mice.[295,295a] Prior to development of Tg(BoPrP)Prnp$^{0/0}$ mice, non-Tg mice inoculated intracerebrally with BSE brain extracts required more than 300 days to develop disease.[52,206,296,297] Depending on the titer of the inoculum, the structures of PrP$^{C}$ and PrP$^{Sc}$, and the structure of protein X, the number of inoculated animals developing disease can vary greatly. Some investigators have stated that transmission of BSE to mice is quite variable with incubation periods exceeding 1 year,[52] while others report low prion titers in BSE brain homogenates[296,297] compared to rodent brain scrapie.[78,94,298,299]

**Have Bovine Prions Been Transmitted to Humans?** In 1994, the first cases of CJD in teenagers and young adults that were eventually labeled new variant (v) CJD occurred in Great Britain.[137] In addition to the young age of these cases,[204,205] the brains of these patients showed numerous PrP amyloid plaques surrounded by a halo of intense spongiform degeneration.[300] These unusual neuropathologic changes have not been seen in CJD cases in the United States, Australia, or Japan.[300,301] Both macaque monkeys and marmosets developed neurologic disease several years after inoculation with bovine prions,[302] but only the macaques exhibited numerous PrP plaques similar to those found in vCJD[303] (R. Ridley and H. Baker, unpublished data).

The restricted geographical occurrence and chronology of vCJD have raised the possibility that BSE prions have been transmitted to humans. That only ~70 vCJD cases have been recorded and the incidence has remained relatively constant make establishing the origin of vCJD difficult. No set of dietary habits distinguishes vCJD patients from apparently healthy people. Moreover, there is no explanation for the predilection of vCJD for teenagers and young adults. Why have older individuals not developed vCJD-based neuropathologic criteria? It is noteworthy that epidemiological studies over the past three decades failed to find evidence for transmission of sheep prions to humans.[151–154] Attempts to predict the future number of cases of vCJD, assuming exposure to bovine prions prior to the offal ban, have been uninformative because so few cases of vCJD have occurred.[140,304,305] Are we at the beginning of a human prion disease epidemic in Britain similar to those seen for BSE and kuru or will the number of vCJD cases remain small as seen with iatrogenic CJD (iCJD) caused by cadaveric HGH?[142,143]

**Strain of BSE Prions.** Was a particular conformation of bovine PrP$^{Sc}$ selected for heat-resistance during the rendering process and then reselected multiple times as cattle infected by ingesting prion-contaminated meat and bone meal were slaughtered and their offal rendered into more meat and bone meal? Recent studies of PrP$^{Sc}$ from brains of patients who died of vCJD show a pattern of PrP glycoforms different from those found for sporadic CJD (sCJD) or iCJD.[207,242] But the utility of measuring PrP glycoforms is questionable in trying to relate BSE to vCJD[244,306] because PrP$^{Sc}$ is formed after the protein is glycosylated[222,223] and enzymatic deglycosylation of PrP$^{Sc}$ requires denaturation.[262,307] Recently, it has been possible to establish a relationship between the conformations of PrP$^{Sc}$ from cattle with BSE and those from humans with vCJD by using Tg mice expressing bovine PrP.[295a] A relationship between vCJD and BSE has been suggested earlier based on the finding of similar incubation times in non-Tg RIII mice of ~310 days after inoculation with Hu or Bo prions.[206]

## FUNGAL PRIONS

Although prions were originally defined in the context of an infectious mammalian pathogen,[100] it is now becoming widely accepted that prions are elements that impart and propagate variability through multiple conformers of a normal cellular protein. Such a mechanism must surely not be restricted to a single class of transmissible pathogens. Indeed, it is likely that the original definition will need to be extended to encompass other situations where a similar mechanism of information transfer occurs.

Two prion-like determinants, [URE3] and [PSI], have been described in yeast; in another fungus, a third denoted [Het-s*] was reported.[308–310] Studies of candidate prion proteins in yeast may prove particularly helpful in the dissection of some of the events that feature in PrP$^{Sc}$ formation. Interestingly, different strains of yeast prions have been identified.[311] Conversion to the prion-like [PSI] state in yeast requires the molecular chaperone Hsp104; however, no homologue of Hsp104 has been found in mammals.[309] The NH$_2$-terminal prion domains of Ure2p and Sup35 that are responsible for the [URE3] and [PSI] phenotypes in yeast have been identified. In contrast to PrP, which is a GPI-anchored membrane protein, both Ure2p and Sup35 are cytosolic proteins.[312] When the prion domains of these yeast proteins were expressed in *E. coli*, the proteins were found to polymerize into fibrils with properties similar to those of proteolytically trimmed PrP and other amyloids.[313]

Whether prions explain some other examples of acquired inheritance in lower organisms is unclear.[314] For example, studies on the inheritance of positional order and cellular handedness

on the surface of small organisms demonstrate the epigenetic nature of these phenomena, but the mechanism remains unclear.[315]

## PRION DISEASES ARE DISORDERS OF PROTEIN CONFORMATION

The study of prions has taken several unexpected directions over the past three decades. The discovery that prion diseases in humans are uniquely both genetic and infectious has greatly strengthened and extended the prion concept. To date, 20 different mutations in the human PrP gene, all resulting in nonconservative substitutions, have been found to either be linked genetically to or segregate with the inherited prion diseases (Fig. 224-4B, Table 224-4). Yet, the transmissible prion particle is composed largely, if not entirely, of an abnormal isoform of the prion protein designated PrP$^{Sc}$.[49]

Understanding how PrP$^C$ unfolds and refolds into PrP$^{Sc}$ is of paramount importance in transferring advances in the prion diseases to studies of other degenerative illnesses. The mechanism by which PrP$^{Sc}$ is formed must involve a templating process where existing PrP$^{Sc}$ directs the refolding of PrP$^C$ into a nascent PrP$^{Sc}$ with the same conformation. Undoubtedly, molecular chaperones of some type participate in a process that appears to be associated with caveolae-like domains of the cell. Studies of prion-like proteins in yeast may prove particularly helpful in dissecting some of the events that feature in PrP$^{Sc}$ formation.[308]

### Therapeutic Approaches to Prion Diseases

It seems likely that it will be possible to design effective therapeutics for prion diseases as our understanding of prion propagation increases. Because people at risk for inherited prion diseases can now be identified decades before neurologic dysfunction is evident, the development of an effective therapy for these fully penetrant disorders is imperative. Although we have no way of predicting the number of individuals who may develop neurologic dysfunction from bovine prions in the future, seeking an effective therapy now seems most prudent.[43,140] Interfering with the conversion of PrP$^C$ into PrP$^{Sc}$ seems to be the most attractive therapeutic target. Either stabilizing the structure of PrP$^C$ via the formation of a PrP$^C$-drug complex or modifying the action of protein X, which might function as a molecular chaperone (Figs. 224-5B and 224-6), are reasonable strategies. Recent studies demonstrate it is reasonable to design a drug that mimics the structure of PrP$^C$ with basic polymorphic residues that prevents scrapie and CJD.[316] Because PrP$^{Sc}$ formation seems limited to caveolae-like domains,[123,224] drugs designed to inhibit this process need not penetrate the cytosol of cells but they do need to be able to enter the central nervous system. Alternatively, drugs that destabilize the structure of PrP$^{Sc}$ might also prove useful.[317]

The production of domestic animals that do not replicate prions may also be important with respect to preventing prion disease. Sheep encoding the R/R polymorphism at position 171 seem to be resistant to scrapie;[246,247] presumably, this was the genetic basis of James Parry's scrapie eradication program in Great Britain 30 years ago.[265] An effective approach using dominant negatives for producing prion-resistant domestic animals, including sheep and cattle, might be the expression of PrP transgenes encoding R171 as well as additional basic residues at the protein X binding site (Fig. 224-5B).[185,233a,316] Such an approach can be readily evaluated in Tg mice. If it is shown to be effective, it could be instituted by artificial insemination of sperm from males homozygous for the transgene. Less practical is the production of PrP-deficient cattle and sheep. Although such animals would not be susceptible to prion disease,[58,208] they might suffer some deleterious effects from ablation of the PrP gene.[211–213,216]

Whether gene therapy for the human prion diseases will prove feasible using the dominant-negative approach described above for prion-resistant animals depends on the availability of efficient vectors for delivery of the transgene to the central nervous system.

# CONCLUSION

Although the study of prions has taken several unexpected directions over the past three decades, a novel and fascinating story of prion biology is emerging. Investigations of prions have elucidated a previously unknown mechanism of disease in humans and animals. While learning the details of the structures of PrPs and deciphering the mechanism of $PrP^C$ transformation into $PrP^{Sc}$ is important, the fundamental principles of prion biology have become reasonably clear. Although some investigators prefer to view the composition of the infectious prion particle as unresolved,[51-53] such a perspective denies an enlarging body of data, none of which refutes the prion concept. Moreover, the discovery of prion-like phenomena mediated by proteins unrelated to PrP in yeast and other fungi serves not only to support the prion concept but also to widen it.

The discovery that prion diseases in humans are uniquely both genetic and infectious greatly strengthened and extended the prion concept. To date, 20 different mutations in the human PrP gene, all resulting in nonconservative substitutions, have been found either to be linked genetically to or to segregate with the inherited prion diseases (Fig. 224-4*B*, Table 224-4). Yet, the transmissible prion particle is composed largely, if not exclusively, of an abnormal isoform of the prion protein designated $PrP^{Sc}$.[49]

## Aberrant PrP Metabolism

The hallmark of all prion diseases—whether sporadic, dominantly inherited, or acquired by infection—is that they involve the aberrant metabolism and resulting accumulation of the prion protein (Table 224-1).[49] The conversion of $PrP^C$ into $PrP^{Sc}$ involves a conformation change whereby the $\alpha$-helical content diminishes and the amount of $\beta$-sheet increases.[40] These findings provide a reasonable mechanism to explain the conundrum presented by the three different manifestations of prion disease.

Understanding how $PrP^C$ unfolds and refolds into $PrP^{Sc}$ is of paramount importance in transferring advances in the prion diseases to studies of other degenerative illnesses. The mechanism, by which $PrP^{Sc}$ is formed, must involve a templating process whereby existing $PrP^{Sc}$ directs the refolding of $PrP^C$ into a nascent $PrP^{Sc}$ with the same conformation. Not only will a knowledge of $PrP^{Sc}$ formation help in the rational design of drugs that interrupt the pathogenesis of prion diseases, but it may also open new approaches to deciphering the causes of and to developing effective therapies for the more common neurodegenerative diseases including Alzheimer disease, Parkinson disease, and amyotrophic lateral sclerosis (ALS). Indeed, the expanding list of prion diseases and their novel modes of transmission and pathogenesis (Table 224-1), as well as the unprecedented mechanisms of prion propagation and information transfer, indicate that much more attention to these fatal disorders of protein conformation is urgently needed.

But prions may have even wider implications than those noted for the common neurodegenerative diseases. If we think of prion diseases as disorders of protein conformation and do not require the diseases to be transmissible, then what we have learned from the study of prions may reach far beyond these illnesses.

## Conformational Diversity

The discovery that proteins may have multiple biologically active conformations may prove no less important than the implications of prions for diseases. How many different tertiary structures can $PrP^{Sc}$ adopt? This query addresses the issue of the limits of prion diversity and also applies to proteins as they normally function within the cell or act to affect homeostasis in multicellular organisms. The expanding list of chaperones that assist in the folding and unfolding of proteins promises much new knowledge about this process. For example, it is now clear that proproteases can carry their own chaperone activity where the *pro* portion of the protein functions as a chaperone in *cis* to guide the folding of the proteolytically active portion before it is cleaved.[318] Such a

mechanism might well feature in the maturation of polypeptide hormones. Interestingly, mutation of the chaperone portion of prosubtilisin resulted in the folding of a subtilisin protease with different properties than the one folded by the wt chaperone. Such chaperones have also been shown to work in *trans*.[318] Besides transient metabolic regulation within the cell and hormonal regulation of multicellular organisms, it is not unreasonable to suggest that assembly of proteins into multimeric structures such as intermediate filaments might be controlled at least in part by alternative conformations of proteins. Such regulation of multimeric protein assemblies might occur either in the proteins that form the multimers or the proteins that function to facilitate the assembly process. Additionally, apoptosis during development and throughout adult life might also be regulated at least in part by alternative tertiary structures of proteins.

## Shifting the Debate

The wealth of data establishing the essential role of PrP in the transmission of prions and the pathogenesis of prion diseases has provoked consideration of how many biological processes are controlled by changes in protein conformation. The extreme radiation resistance of the scrapie infectivity suggested that the pathogen causing this disease and related illnesses would be different from viruses, viroids, and bacteria.[27] Indeed, an unprecedented mechanism of disease has been revealed, in which an aberrant conformational change in a protein is propagated. The future of this emerging area of biology should prove even more interesting and productive as many new discoveries are reported.

## ACKNOWLEDGMENTS

I thank Drs. Fred Cohen, Stephen DeArmond, Jiri Safar, and Michael Scott for helpful discussions. This research was supported by grants from the National Institute of Aging and the National Institute of Neurologic Diseases and Stroke of the National Institutes of Health, International Human Frontiers of Science Program, and American Health Assistance Foundation, as well as by gifts from the Sherman Fairchild Foundation, Keck Foundation, G. Harold and Leila Y. Mathers Foundation, Bernard Osher Foundation, John D. French Foundation, and Centeon.

## REFERENCES

1. Gibbs CJ Jr, Gajdusek DC, Asher DM, Alpers MP, Beck E, Daniel PM, Matthews WB: Creutzfeldt-Jakob disease (spongiform encephalopathy): Transmission to the chimpanzee. *Science* **161**:388, 1968.
2. Meggendorfer F: Klinische und genealogische Beobachtungen bei einem Fall von spastischer Pseudosklerose Jakobs. *Z. Gesamte Neurol. Psychiatr* **128**:337, 1930.
3. Roos R, Gajdusek DC, Gibbs CJ Jr: The clinical characteristics of transmissible Creutzfeldt-Jakob disease. *Brain* **96**:1, 1973.
4. Hsiao K, Baker HF, Crow TJ, Poulter M, Owen F, Terwilliger JD, Westaway D, Ott J, Prusiner SB: Linkage of a prion protein missense variant to Gerstmann-Sträussler syndrome. *Nature* **338**:342, 1989.
5. Owen F, Poulter M, Lofthouse R, Collinge J, Crow TJ, Risby D, Baker HF, Ridley RM, Hsiao K, Prusiner SB: Insertion in prion protein gene in familial Creutzfeldt-Jakob disease. *Lancet* **1**:51, 1989.
6. Creutzfeldt HG: Über eine eigenartige herdförmige Erkrankung des Zentralnervensystems. *Z Gesamte Neurol Psychiatrie* **57**:1, 1920.
7. Jakob A: Über eigenartige Erkrankungen des Zentralnervensystems mit bemerkenswertem anatomischen Befunde (spastische Pseudosklerose-Encephalomyelopathie mit disseminierten Degenerationsherden). *Z Gesamte Neurol Psychiatrie* **64**:147, 1921.
8. Kirschbaum WR: *Jakob-Creutzfeldt Disease.* Amsterdam, Elsevier, 1968.
9. Kirschbaum WR: Zwei eigenartige Erkrankungen des Zentralnervensystems nach Art der spastischen Pseudosklerose (Jakob). *Z Ges Neurol Psychiatr* **92**:175, 1924.
10. Stender A: Weitere Beiträge zum Kapitel "Spastische Pseudosklerose Jakobs." *Z Gesamte Neurol Psychiatr* **128**:528, 1930.

11. Davison C. Rabiner AM: Spastic pseudosclerosis (disseminated encephalomyelopathy; corticopal-lidospinal degeneration). Familial and nonfamilial incidence (a clinico-pathologic study). *Arch Neurol Psychiatry* **44**:578, 1940.

12. Jacob H, Pyrkosch W, Strube H: Die erbliche Form der Creutzfeldt-Jakobschen Krankheit. *Arch Psychiatr Zeitsch Neurol* **184**:653, 1950.

13. Friede RL, DeJong RN: Neuronal enzymatic failure in Creutzfeldt-Jakob disease. A familial study. *Arch Neurol* **10**:181, 1964.

14. Rosenthal NP, Keesey J, Crandall B, Brown WJ: Familial neurological disease associated with spongiform encephalopathy. *Arch Neurol* **33**:252, 1976.

15. Masters CL, Gajdusek DC, Gibbs CJ Jr, Bernouilli C, Asher DM: Familial Creutzfeldt-Jakob disease and other familial dementias: An inquiry into possible models of virus-induced familial diseases, in Prusiner SB, Hadlow WJ (eds): *Slow Transmissible Diseases of the Nervous System*, Vol 1. New York, Academic Press, 1979, p 143.

16. Masters CL, Gajdusek DC, Gibbs CJ Jr: Creutzfeldt-Jakob disease virus isolations from the Gerstmann-Sträussler syndrome. *Brain* **104**:559, 1981.

17. Masters CL, Gajdusek DC, Gibbs CJ Jr: The familial occurrence of Creutzfeldt-Jakob disease and Alzheimer's disease. *Brain* **104**:535, 1981.

18. Klatzo I Gajdusek DC, Zigas V: Pathology of kuru. *Lab Invest* **8**:799, 1959.

19. Hadlow WJ: Scrapie and kuru. *Lancet* **2**:289, 1959.

20. Sigurdsson B: Rida, a chronic encephalitis of sheep with general remarks on infections which develop slowly and some of their special characteristics. *Br Vet J* **110**:341, 1954.

21. Hadlow WJ: Neuropathology and the scrapie-kuru connection. *Brain Pathol* **5**:27, 1995.

22. Gajdusek DC, Gibbs CJ Jr, Alpers M: Experimental transmission of a kuru-like syndrome to chimpanzees. *Nature* **209**:794, 1966.

23. Gordon WS: Advances in veterinary research. *Vet.. Res..* **58**:516, 1946.

24. Zlotnik I: The pathology of scrapie: a comparative study of lesions in the brain of sheep and goats. *Acta Neuropathol (Berl) [Supp]* **1**:61, 1962.

25. Beck E, Daniel PM, Parry HB: Degeneration of the cerebellar and hypothalamo-neurohypophysial systems in sheep with scrapie, and its relationship to human system degenerations. *Brain* **87**:153, 1964.

26. Alper T, Haig DA, Clarke MC: The exceptionally small size of the scrapie agent. *Biochem Biophys Res Commun* **22**:278, 1966.

27. Alper T, Cramp WA, Haig DA, Clarke MC: Does the agent of scrapie replicate without nucleic acid? *Nature* **214**:764, 1967.

28. Latarjet R, Muel B, Haig DA, Clarke MC, Alper T: Inactivation of the scrapie agent by near monochromatic ultraviolet light. *Nature* **227**:1341, 1970.

29. Gibbs CJ Jr, Gajdusek DC, Latarjet R: Unusual resistance to ionizing radiation of the viruses of kuru, Creutzfeldt-Jakob disease. *Proc Natl Acad Sci U S A* **75**:6268, 1978.

30. Pattison IH: Experiments with scrapie with special reference to the nature of the agent and the pathology of the disease, in Gajdusek DC, Gibbs CJ Jr, Alpers MP: *Slow, Latent and Temperate Virus Infections, NINDB Monograph 2*. Washington, DC, US Government Printing, 1965, p 249.

31. Gibbons RA, Hunter GD: Nature of the scrapie agent. *Nature* **215**:1041, 1967.

32. Griffith JS: Self-replication and scrapie. *Nature* **215**:1043, 1967.

33. Pattison IH, Jones KM: The possible nature of the transmissible agent of scrapie. *Vet Rec* **80**:1, 1967.

34. Hunter GD, Kimberlin RH, Gibbons RA: Scrapie: A modified membrane hypothesis. *J Theor Biol* **20**:355, 1968.

35. Field EJ, Farmer F, Caspary EA, Joyce G: Susceptibility of scrapie agent to ionizing radiation. *Nature* **222**:90, 1969.

36. Hunter GD: Scrapie: A prototype slow infection. *J Infect Dis* **125**:427, 1972.

37. Chandler RL: Encephalopathy in mice produced by inoculation with scrapie brain material. *Lancet* **1**:1378, 1961.

38. Prusiner SB: Prions, in Frängsmyr T: *Les Prix Nobel*. Stockholm, Sweden, Almqvist & Wiksell International, 1998, p 268.

39. Masters CL, Richardson EP Jr: Subacute spongiform encephalopathy Creutzfeldt-Jakob disease — The nature and progression of spongiform change. *Brain* **101**:333, 1978.

40. Pan KM, Baldwin M, Nguyen J, Gasset M, Serban A, Groth D, Mehlhorn I, Huang Z, Fletterick RJ, Cohen FE, Prusiner SB: Conversion of $\alpha$-helices into $\beta$ sheets features in the formation of the scrapie prion proteins. *Proc Natl Acad Sci U S A* **90**:10962, 1993.

41. Bessen RA, Marsh RF: Distinct PrP properties suggest the molecular basis of strain variation in transmissible mink encephalopathy. *J Virol* **68**:7859, 1994.

42. Telling GC, Parchi P, DeArmond SJ, Cortelli P, Montagna P, Gabizon R, Mastrianni J, Lugaresi E, Gambetti P, Prusiner SB: Evidence for the conformation of the pathologic isoform of the prion protein enciphering and propagating prion diversity. *Science* **274**:2079, 1996.

43. Prusiner SB: Prion diseases and the BSE crisis. *Science* **278**:245, 1997.

44. Safar J, Wille H, Itri V, Groth D, Serban H, Torchia M, Cohen FE, Prusiner SB: Eight prion strains have PrP$^{Sc}$ molecules with different conformations. *Nat Med* **4**:1157, 1998.

45. Dlouhy SR, Hsiao K, Farlow MR, Foroud T, Conneally PM, Johnson P, Prusiner SB, Hodes ME, Ghetti B: Linkage of the Indiana kindred of Gerstmann-Sträussler-Scheinker disease to the prion protein gene. *Nat Genet* **1**:64, 1992.

46. Petersen RB, Tabaton M, Berg L, Schrank B, Torack RM, Leal S, Julien J, Vital C, Deleplanque B, Pendlebury WW, Drachman D, Smith TW, Martin JJ, Oda M, Montagna P, Ott J, Autilio-Gambetti L, Lugaresi E, Gambetti P: Analysis of the prion protein gene in thalamic dementia. *Neurology* **42**:1859, 1992.

47. Poulter M, Baker HF, Frith CD, Leach M, Lofthouse R, Ridley RM, Shah T, Owen F, Collinge J, Brown G, Hardy J, Mullan MJ, Harding AE, Bennett C, Doshi R, Crow TJ: Inherited prion disease with 144 base pair gene insertion. 1. Genealogical and molecular studies. *Brain* **115**:675, 1992.

48. Gabizon R, Rosenman H, Meiner Z, Kahana I, Kahana E, Shugart Y, Ott J, Prusiner SB: Mutation in codon 200 and polymorphism in codon 129 of the prion protein gene in Libyan Jews with Creutzfeldt-Jakob disease. *Philos Trans R Soc Lond B Biol Sci* **343**:385, 1994.

49. Prusiner SB: Molecular biology of prion diseases. *Science* **252**:1515, 1991.

50. Chesebro B, Caughey B: Scrapie agent replication without the prion protein? *Curr Biol* **3**:696, 1993.

51. Manuelidis L, Fritch W: Infectivity and host responses in Creutzfeldt-Jakob disease. *Virology* **216**:46–59, 1996.

52. Lasmézas CI, Deslys J-P, Robain O, Jaegly A, Beringue V, Peyrin J-M, Fournier J-G, Hauw J-J, Rossier J, Dormont D: Transmission of the BSE agent to mice in the absence of detectable abnormal prion protein. *Science* **275**:402, 1997.

53. Chesebro B: Prion diseases: BSE and prions: Uncertainties about the agent. *Science* **279**:42, 1998.

54. Kimberlin RH, Millson GC, Hunter GD: An experimental examination of the scrapie agent in cell membrane mixtures. III. Studies of the operational size. *J Comp Pathol* **81**:383, 1971.

55. Prusiner SB, Hadlow WJ, Garfin DE, Cochran SP, Baringer JR, Race RE, Eklund CM: Partial purification and evidence for multiple molecular forms of the scrapie agent. *Biochemistry* **17**:4993, 1978.

56. Diringer H, Kimberlin RH: Infectious scrapie agent is apparently not as small as recent claims suggest. *Biosci Rep* **3**:563, 1983.

57. Rohwer RG: Scrapie infectious agent is virus-like in size and susceptibility to inactivation. *Nature* **308**:658, 1984.

58. Prusiner SB, Groth D, Serban A, Koehler R, Foster D, Torchia M, Burton D, Yang S-L, DeArmond SJ: Ablation of the prion protein (PrP) gene in mice prevents scrapie and facilitates production of anti-PrP antibodies. *Proc Natl Acad Sci U S A* **90**:10608, 1993.

59. Williamson RA, Peretz D, Smorodinsky N, Bastidas R, Serban H, Mehlhorn I, DeArmond SJ, Prusiner SB, Burton DR: Circumventing tolerance to generate autologous monoclonal antibodies to the prion protein. *Proc Natl Acad Sci U S A* **93**:7279, 1996.

60. Dickinson AG, Meikle VMH, Fraser H: Identification of a gene which controls the incubation period of some strains of scrapie agent in mice. *J Comp Pathol* **78**:293, 1968.

61. Dickinson AG, Outram GW: Genetic aspects of unconventional virus infections: The basis of the virino hypothesis, in Bock G, Marsh J: *Novel Infectious Agents and the Central Nervous System. Ciba Foundation Symposium 135*. Chichester, UK, John Wiley and Sons, 1988, p 63.

62. Kimberlin RH: Reflections on the nature of the scrapie agent. *Trends Biochem Sci* **7**:392, 1982.

63. Kimberlin RH: Scrapie and possible relationships with viroids. *Semin Virol* **1**:153, 1990.

64. Bruce ME, McConnell I, Fraser H, Dickinson AG: The disease characteristics of different strains of scrapie in *Sinc* congenic mouse lines: implications for the nature of the agent and host control of pathogenesis. *J Gen Virol* **72**:595, 1991.

65. Weissmann C: A "unified theory" of prion propagation. *Nature* **352**:679, 1991.
66. Kellings K, Meyer N, Mirenda C, Prusiner SB, Riesner D: Further analysis of nucleic acids in purified scrapie prion preparations by improved return refocussing gel electrophoresis (RRGE). *J Gen Virol* **73**:1025, 1992.
67. Kellings K, Prusiner SB, Riesner D: Nucleic acids in prion preparations: Unspecific background or essential component? *Philos Trans R Soc Lond B Biol Sci* **343**:425, 1994.
68. Goldmann W, Hunter N, Manson J, Hope J: The PrP gene of the sheep, a natural host of scrapie. *Proceedings of the VIIIth International Congress of Virology, Berlin, Aug. 26-31*:284, 1990.
69. Goldmann W, Hunter N, Martin T, Dawson M, Hope J: Different forms of the bovine PrP gene have five or six copies of a short, G-C-rich element within the protein-coding exon. *J Gen Virol* **72**:201, 1991.
70. Wells GAH, Wilesmith JW: The neuropathology and epidemiology of bovine spongiform encephalopathy. *Brain Pathol* **5**:91, 1995.
71. Bruce M, Chree A, McConnell I, Foster J, Pearson G, Fraser H: Transmission of bovine spongiform encephalopathy and scrapie to mice: strain variation and the species barrier. *Philos Trans R Soc Lond B Biol Sci* **343**:405, 1994.
72. Bruce ME: Strain typing studies of scrapie and BSE, in Baker HF, Ridley RM (eds): *Methods in Molecular Medicine: Prion Diseases.* Totowa, NJ, Humana Press, 1996, p 223.
73. Jeffrey M, Wells GAH: Spongiform encephalopathy in a nyala (*Tragelaphus angasi*). *Vet Pathol* **25**:398, 1988.
74. Wyatt JM, Pearson GR, Smerdon TN, Gruffydd-Jones TJ, Wells GAH, Wilesmith JW: Naturally occurring scrapie-like spongiform encephalopathy in five domestic cats. *Vet Rec* **129**:233, 1991.
75. Kirkwood JK, Cunningham AA, Wells GAH, Wilesmith JW, Barnett JEF: Spongiform encephalopathy in a herd of greater kudu (*Tragelaphus strepsiceros*): Epidemiological observations. *Vet Rec* **133**:360, 1993.
76. Bolton DC, McKinley MP, Prusiner SB: Identification of a protein that purifies with the scrapie prion. *Science* **218**:1309, 1982.
77. Prusiner SB, Bolton DC, Groth DF, Bowman KA, Cochran SP, McKinley MP: Further purification and characterization of scrapie prions. *Biochemistry* **21**:6942, 1982.
78. Hunter GD, Millson GC, Chandler RL: Observations on the comparative infectivity of cellular fractions derived from homogenates of mouse-scrapie brain. *Res Vet Sci* **4**:543, 1963.
79. Hunter GD, Millson GC: Studies on the heat stability and chromatographic behavior of the scrapie agent. *J Gen Microbiol* **37**:251, 1964.
80. Hunter GD, Millson GC: Attempts to release the scrapie agent from tissue debris. *J Comp Pathol* **77**:301, 1967.
81. Hunter GD, Gibbons RA, Kimberlin RH, Millson GC: Further studies of the infectivity and stability of extracts and homogenates derived from scrapie affected mouse brains. *J Comp Pathol* **79**:101, 1969.
82. Hunter GD, Kimberlin RH, Millson GC, Gibbons RA: An experimental examination of the scrapie agent in cell membrane mixtures. I. Stability and physicochemical properties of the scrapie agent. *J Comp Pathol* **81**:23, 1971.
83. Millson G, Hunter GD, Kimberlin RH: An experimental examination of the scrapie agent in cell membrane mixtures. II. The association of scrapie infectivity with membrane fractions. *J Comp Pathol* **81**:255, 1971.
84. Marsh RF, Semancik JS, Medappa KC, Hanson RP, Rueckert RR: Scrapie and transmissible mink encephalopathy: Search for infectious nucleic acid. *J Virol* **13**:993, 1974.
85. Millson GC, Hunter GD, Kimberlin RH: The physico-chemical nature of the scrapie agent, in Kimberlin RH (ed): *Slow Virus Diseases of Animals and Man.* New York, Elsevier, 1976, p 243.
86. Siakotos AN, Gajdusek DC, Gibbs CJ Jr, Traub RD, Bucana C: Partial purification of the scrapie agent from mouse brain by pressure disruption and zonal centrifugation in sucrose-sodium chloride gradients. *Virology* **70**:230, 1976.
87. Marsh RF, Malone TG, Semancik JS, Lancaster WD, Hanson RP: Evidence for an essential DNA component in the scrapie agent. *Nature* **275**:146, 1978.
88. Gibbs CJ Jr, Gajdusek DC: Atypical viruses as the cause of sporadic, epidemic, and familial chronic diseases in man: slow viruses and human diseases, in Pollard M (ed): *Perspectives in Virology*, Vol. 10. New York, Raven Press, 1978, p 161.
89. Millson GC, Manning EJ: The effect of selected detergents on scrapie infectivity, in Prusiner SB, Hadlow WJ (eds): *Slow Transmissible Diseases of the Nervous System*, Vol. 2. New York, Academic Press, 1979, p 409.
90. Marsh RF, Malone TG, Semancik JS, Hanson RP: Studies on the physicochemical nature of the scrapie agent, in Boese A (ed): *Search for the Cause of Multiple Sclerosis and Other Chronic Diseases of the Central Nervous System.* Weinheim, Germany, Verlag Chemie, 1980, 314.
91. Prusiner SB: An approach to the isolation of biological particles using sedimentation analysis. *J Biol Chem* **253**:916, 1978.
92. Prusiner SB, Garfin DE, Baringer JR, Cochran SP, Hadlow WJ, Race RE, Eklund CM: Evidence for multiple molecular forms of the scrapie agent, in Stevens J, Todaro G, Fox CF (ed): *Persistent Viruses.* New York, Academic Press, 1978, p 591.
93. Prusiner SB, Groth DF, Cochran SP, Masiarz FR, McKinley MP, Martinez HM: Molecular properties, partial purification, and assay by incubation period measurements of the hamster scrapie agent. *Biochemistry* **19**:4883, 1980.
94. Prusiner SB, Cochran SP, Groth DF, Downey DE, Bowman KA, Martinez HM: Measurement of the scrapie agent using an incubation time interval assay. *Ann Neurol* **11**:353, 1982.
95. Prusiner SB, Groth DF, Bolton DC, Kent SB, Hood LE: Purification and structural studies of a major scrapie prion protein. *Cell* **38**:127, 1984.
96. Basler K, Oesch B, Scott M, Westaway D, Wälchli M, Groth DF, McKinley MP, Prusiner SB, Weissmann C: Scrapie and cellular PrP isoforms are encoded by the same chromosomal gene. *Cell* **46**:417, 1986.
97. Gabizon R, McKinley MP, Groth D, Prusiner SB: Immunoaffinity purification and neutralization of scrapie prion infectivity. *Proc Natl Acad Sci U S A* **85**:6617, 1988.
98. McKinley MP, Bolton DC, Prusiner SB: A protease-resistant protein is a structural component of the scrapie prion. *Cell* **35**:57, 1983.
99. Prusiner SB, McKinley MP, Bowman KA, Bolton DC, Bendheim PE, Groth DF, Glenner GG: Scrapie prions aggregate to form amyloid-like birefringent rods. *Cell* **35**:349, 1983.
100. Prusiner SB: Novel proteinaceous infectious particles cause scrapie. *Science* **216**:136, 1982.
101. Oesch B, Westaway D, Wälchli M, McKinley MP, Kent SBH, Aebersold R, Barry RA, Tempst P, Teplow DB, Hood LE, Prusiner SB, Weissmann C: A cellular gene encodes scrapie PrP 27-30 protein. *Cell* **40**:735, 1985.
102. Chesebro B, Race R, Wehrly K, Nishio J, Bloom M, Lechner D, Bergstrom S, Robbins K, Mayer L, Keith JM, Garon C, Haase A: Identification of scrapie prion protein-specific mRNA in scrapie-infected and uninfected brain. *Nature* **315**:331, 1985.
103. Locht C, Chesebro B, Race R, Keith JM: Molecular cloning and complete sequence of prion protein cDNA from mouse brain infected with the scrapie agent. *Proc Natl Acad Sci U S A* **83**:6372, 1986.
104. Meyer RK, McKinley MP, Bowman KA, Braunfeld MB, Barry RA, Prusiner SB: Separation and properties of cellular and scrapie prion proteins. *Proc Natl Acad Sci U S A* **83**:2310, 1986.
105. Hsiao KK, Groth D, Scott M, Yang S-L, Serban H, Rapp D, Foster D, Torchia M, DeArmond SJ, Prusiner SB: Serial transmission in rodents of neurodegeneration from transgenic mice expressing mutant prion protein. *Proc Natl Acad Sci U S A* **91**:9126, 1994.
106. Telling GC, Haga T, Torchia M, Tremblay P, DeArmond SJ, Prusiner SB: Interactions between wild-type and mutant prion proteins modulate neurodegeneration in transgenic mice. *Genes Dev* **10**:1736, 1996.
107. Caughey B, Neary K, Butler R, Ernst D, Perry L, Chesebro B, Race RE: Normal and scrapie-associated forms of prion protein differ in their sensitivities to phospholipase and proteases in intact neuroblastoma cells. *J Virol* **64**:1093, 1990.
108. Caughey BW, Dong A, Bhat KS, Ernst D, Hayes SF, Caughey WS: Secondary structure analysis of the scrapie-associated protein PrP 27-30 in water by infrared spectroscopy. *Biochemistry* **30**:7672, 1991.
109. McKinley MP, Meyer RK, Kenaga L, Rahbar F, Cotter R, Serban A, Prusiner SB: Scrapie prion rod formation in vitro requires both detergent extraction and limited proteolysis. *J Virol* **65**:1340, 1991.
110. Gasset M, Baldwin MA, Fletterick RJ, Prusiner SB: Perturbation of the secondary structure of the scrapie prion protein under conditions that alter infectivity. *Proc Natl Acad Sci U S A* **90**:1, 1993.
111. Safar J, Roller PP, Gajdusek DC, Gibbs CJJ: Thermal-stability and conformational transitions of scrapie amyloid (prion) protein correlate with infectivity. *Protein Sci* **2**:2206, 1993.
112. Muramoto T, Scott M, Cohen F, Prusiner SB: Recombinant scrapie-like prion protein of 106 amino acids is soluble. *Proc Natl Acad Sci U S A* **93**:15457, 1996.

113. Riesner D, Kellings K, Post K, Wille H, Serban H, Groth D, Baldwin MA, Prusiner SB: Disruption of prion rods generates 10-nm spherical particles having high α helical content and lacking scrapie infectivity. *J Virol* **70**:1714, 1996.

114. Lasmézas CI, Deslys JP, Demaimay R, Adjou KT, Hauw J-J, Dormont D: Strain specific and common pathogenic events in murine models of scrapie and bovine spongiform encephalopathy. *J Gen Virol* **77**:1601, 1996.

115. DeArmond SJ, Mobley WC, DeMott DL, Barry RA, Beckstead JH, Prusiner SB: Changes in the localization of brain prion proteins during scrapie infection. *Neurology* **37**:1271, 1987.

116. Taraboulos A, Jendroska K, Serban D, Yang S-L, DeArmond SJ, Prusiner SB: Regional mapping of prion proteins in brains. *Proc Natl Acad Sci U S A* **89**:7620, 1992.

117. Czub M, Braig HR, Diringer H: Pathogenesis of scrapie: Study of the temporal development of clinical symptoms of infectivity titers and scrapie-associated fibrils in brains of hamsters infected intraperitoneally. *J Gen Virol* **67**:2005, 1986.

118. Xi YG, Ingrosso L, Ladogana A, Masullo C, Pocchiari M: Amphotericin B treatment dissociates in vivo replication of the scrapie agent from PrP accumulation. *Nature* **356**:598, 1992.

119. Jendroska K, Heinzel FP, Torchia M, Stowring L, Kretzschmar HA, Kon A, Stern A, Prusiner SB, DeArmond SJ: Proteinase-resistant prion protein accumulation in Syrian hamster brain correlates with regional pathology and scrapie infectivity. *Neurology* **41**:1482, 1991.

120. McKenzie D, Kaczkowski J, Marsh R, Aiken J: Amphotericin B delays both scrapie agent replication and PrP-res accumulation early in infection. *J Virol* **68**:7534, 1994.

121. Büeler H, Fischer M, Lang Y, Bluethmann H, Lipp H-P, DeArmond SJ, Prusiner SB, Aguet M, Weissmann C: Normal development and behaviour of mice lacking the neuronal cell-surface PrP protein. *Nature* **356**:577, 1992.

122. Stahl N, Borchelt DR, Hsiao K, Prusiner SB: Scrapie prion protein contains a phosphatidylinositol glycolipid. *Cell* **51**:229, 1987.

123. Taraboulos A, Scott M, Semenov A, Avrahami D, Laszlo L, Prusiner SB: Cholesterol depletion and modification of COOH-terminal targeting sequence of the prion protein inhibits formation of the scrapie isoform. *J Cell Biol* **129**:121, 1995.

124. Sulkowski E: The saga of IMAC and MIT. *Bioessays* **10**:170, 1989.

125. Pan K-M, Stahl N, Prusiner SB: Purification and properties of the cellular prion protein from Syrian hamster brain. *Protein Sci* **1**:1343, 1992.

126. Hornshaw MP, McDermott JR, Candy JM, Lakey JH: Copper binding to the N-terminal tandem repeat region of mammalian and avian prion protein: Structural studies using synthetic peptides. *Biochem Biophys Res Commun* **214**:993, 1995.

127. Stöckel J, Safar J, Wallace AC, Cohen FE, Prusiner SB: Prion protein selectively binds copper-II-ions. *Biochemistry* **37**:7185, 1998.

128. Donne DG, Viles JH, Groth D, Mehlhorn I, James TL, Cohen FE, Prusiner SB, Wright PE, Dyson HJ: Structure of the recombinant full-length hamster prion protein PrP(29-231): The N terminus is highly flexible. *Proc Natl Acad Sci U S A* **94**:13452, 1997.

129. Waggoner DJ, Drisaldi B, Bartnikas TB, Casareno RL, Prohaska JR, Gitlin JD, Harris DA: Brain copper content and cuproenzyme activity do not vary with prion protein expression level. *J Biol Chem* **275**:7455, 2000.

130. Viles JH, Cohen FE, Prusiner SB, Goodin DB, Wright PE, Dyson HJ: Copper binding to the prion protein: Structural implications of four identical cooperative binding sites. *Proc Natl Acad Sci U S A* **96**:2042, 1999.

131. Prusiner SB, Baron H, Carlson G, Cohen FE, DeArmond SJ, Gabizon R, Gambetti P, Hope J, Kitamoto T, Kretzschmar HA, Laplanche J-L, Tateishi J, Telling G, Will R: Prions, in *Virus Taxonomy. 7th Report of the International Committee on Taxonomy of Viruses.* San Diego, Academic Press, 1999.

132. Weissmann C: Spongiform encephalopathies—The prion's progress. *Nature* **349**:569, 1991.

133. Cohen FE, Pan K-M, Huang Z, Baldwin M, Fletterick RJ, Prusiner SB: Structural clues to prion replication. *Science* **264**:530, 1994.

134. Carlson GA, Ebeling C, Yang S-L, Telling G, Torchia M, Groth D, Westaway D, DeArmond SJ, Prusiner SB: Prion isolate specified allotypic interactions between the cellular and scrapie prion proteins in congenic and transgenic mice. *Proc Natl Acad Sci U S A* **91**:5690, 1994.

135. Moore RC, Hope J, McBride PA, McConnell I, Selfridge J, Melton DW, Manson JC: Mice with gene targeted prion protein alterations show that *Prn-p, Sinc* and *Prni* are congruent. *Nat Genet* **18**:118, 1998.

136. Prusiner SB: Scrapie prions. *Annu Rev Microbiol* **43**:345, 1989.

137. Will RG, Ironside JW, Zeidler M, Cousens SN, Estibeiro K, Alperovitch A, Poser S, Pocchiari M, Hofman A, Smith PG: A new variant of Creutzfeldt-Jakob disease in the UK. *Lancet* **347**:921, 1996.

138. DeArmond SJ, Prusiner SB: Prion diseases, in Lantos P, Graham D: *Greenfield's Neuropathology*, 6th ed. London, Edward Arnold, 1997, p 235.

139. Chazot G, Broussolle E, Lapras CI, Blättler T, Aguzzi A, Kopp N: New variant of Creutzfeldt-Jakob disease in a 26-year-old French man. *Lancet* **347**:1181, 1996.

140. Cousens SN, Vynnycky E, Zeidler M, Will RG, Smith PG: Predicting the CJD epidemic in humans. *Nature* **385**:197, 1997.

141. Koch TK, Berg BO, DeArmond SJ, Gravina RF: Creutzfeldt-Jakob disease in a young adult with idiopathic hypopituitarism. Possible relation to the administration of cadaveric human growth hormone. *N Engl J Med* **313**:731, 1985.

142. Billette de Villemeur T, Deslys J-P, Pradel A, Soubrié C, Alpérovitch A, Tardieu M, Chaussain J-L, Hauw J-J, Dormont D, Ruberg M, Agid Y: Creutzfeldt-Jakob disease from contaminated growth hormone extracts in France. *Neurology* **47**:690, 1996.

143. PHS: *Report on Human Growth Hormone and Creutzfeldt-Jakob Disease.* Bethesda, MD, Public Health Service Interagency Coordinating Committee, 1997.

144. Gajdusek DC, Gibbs CJ Jr, Asher DM, Brown P, Diwan A, Hoffman P, Nemo G, Rohwer R, White L: Precautions in medical care of and in handling materials from patients with transmissible virus dementia (CJD). *N Engl J Med* **297**:1253, 1977.

145. Klitzman RL, Alpers MP, Gajdusek DC: The natural incubation period of kuru and the episodes of transmission in three clusters of patients. *Neuroepidemiology* **3**:3, 1984.

146. Gerstmann J, Sträussler E, Scheinker I: Über eine eigenartige hereditär-familiäre Erkrankung des Zentralnervensystems zugleich ein Beitrag zur frage des vorzeitigen lokalen Alterns. *Z Neurol* **154**:736, 1936.

147. Masters CL, Harris JO, Gajdusek DC, Gibbs CJ Jr, Bernouilli C, Asher DM: Creutzfeldt-Jakob disease: Patterns of worldwide occurrence and the significance of familial and sporadic clustering. *Ann Neurol* **5**:177, 1978.

148. Gajdusek DC: Unconventional viruses and the origin and disappearance of kuru. *Science* **197**:943, 1977.

149. Hsiao K, Meiner Z, Kahana E, Cass C, Kahana I, Avrahami D, Scarlato G, Abramsky O, Prusiner SB, Gabizon R: Mutation of the prion protein in Libyan Jews with Creutzfeldt-Jakob disease. *N Engl J Med* **324**:1091, 1991.

150. Bobowick AR, Brody JA, Matthews MR, Roos R, Gajdusek DC: Creutzfeldt-Jakob disease: A case-control study. *Am J Epidemiol* **98**:381, 1973.

151. Malmgren R, Kurland L, Mokri B, Kurtzke J: The epidemiology of Creutzfeldt-Jakob disease, in Prusiner SB, Hadlow WJ: *Slow Transmissible Diseases of the Nervous System*, Vol 1. New York, Academic Press, 1979, p 93.

152. Brown P, Cathala F, Raubertas RF, Gajdusek DC, Castaigne P: The epidemiology of Creutzfeldt-Jakob disease: Conclusion of 15-year investigation in France and review of the world literature. *Neurology* **37**:895, 1987.

153. Harries-Jones R, Knight R, Will RG, Cousens S, Smith PG, Matthews WB: Creutzfeldt-Jakob disease in England and Wales, 1980-1984: A case-control study of potential risk factors. *J Neurol Neurosurg Psychiatry* **51**:1113, 1988.

154. Cousens SN, Harries-Jones R, Knight R, Will RG, Smith PG, Matthews WB: Geographical distribution of cases of Creutzfeldt-Jakob disease in England and Wales 1970–84. *J Neurol Neurosurg Psychiatry* **53**:459, 1990.

155. Carlson GA, Kingsbury DT, Goodman PA, Coleman S, Marshall ST, DeArmond S, Westaway D, Prusiner SB: Linkage of prion protein and scrapie incubation time genes. *Cell* **46**:503, 1986.

156. Doh-ura K, Tateishi J, Sasaki H, Kitamoto T, Sakaki Y: Pro → Leu change at position 102 of prion protein is the most common but not the sole mutation related to Gerstmann-Sträussler syndrome. *Biochem Biophys Res Commun* **163**:974, 1989.

157. Goldgaber D, Goldfarb LG, Brown P, Asher DM, Brown WT, Lin S, Teener JW, Feinstone SM, Rubenstein R, Kascsak RJ, Boellaard JW, Gajdusek DC: Mutations in familial Creutzfeldt-Jakob disease and Gerstmann-Sträussler-Scheinker's syndrome. *Exp Neurol* **106**:204, 1989.

158. Kretzschmar HA, Honold G, Seitelberger F, Feucht M, Wessely P, Mehraein P, Budka H: Prion protein mutation in family first

reported by Gerstmann, Sträussler, and Scheinker. *Lancet* **337**:1160, 1991.

159. Gabizon R, Rosenmann H, Meiner Z, Kahana I, Kahana E, Shugart Y, Ott J, Prusiner SB: Mutation and polymorphism of the prion protein gene in Libyan Jews with Creutzfeldt-Jakob disease (CJD). *Am J Hum Genet* **53**:828, 1993.

160. Hsiao KK, Scott M, Foster D, Groth DF, DeArmond SJ, Prusiner SB: Spontaneous neurodegeneration in transgenic mice with mutant prion protein. *Science* **250**:1587, 1990.

161. Telling GC, Scott M, Mastrianni J, Gabizon R, Torchia M, Cohen FE, DeArmond SJ, Prusiner SB: Prion propagation in mice expressing human and chimeric PrP transgenes implicates the interaction of cellular PrP with another protein. *Cell* **83**:79, 1995.

162. Scott MR, Nguyen O, Stöckel J, Tatzelt J, DeArmond SJ, Cohen FE, Prusiner SB: Designer mutations in the prion protein promote β-sheet formation in vitro and cause neurodegeneration in transgenic mice [Abstract]. *Protein Sci* **6**(Supp 1):84, 1997.

163. Hegde RS, Mastrianni JA, Scott MR, DeFea KA, Tremblay P, Torchia M, DeArmond SJ, Prusiner SB, Lingappa VR: A transmembrane form of the prion protein in neurodegenerative disease. *Science* **279**:827, 1998.

164. Goldfarb LG, Brown P, McCombie WR, Goldgaber D, Swergold GD, Wills PR, Cervenakova L, Baron H, Gibbs CJJ, Gajdusek DC: Transmissible familial Creutzfeldt-Jakob disease associated with five, seven, and eight extra octapeptide coding repeats in the *PRNP* gene. *Proc Natl Acad Sci U S A* **88**:10926, 1991.

165. Kahana E, Milton A, Braham J, Sofer D: Creutzfeldt-Jakob disease: Focus among Libyan Jews in Israel. *Science* **183**:90, 1974.

166. Goldfarb LG, Mitrova E, Brown P, Toh BH, Gajdusek DC: Mutation in codon 200 of scrapie amyloid protein gene in two clusters of Creutzfeldt-Jakob disease in Slovakia. *Lancet* **336**:514, 1990.

167. Goldfarb LG, Brown P, Mitrova E, Cervenakova L, Goldin L, Korczyn AD, Chapman J, Galvez S, Cartier L, Rubenstein R, Gajdusek DC: Creutzfeldt-Jacob disease associated with the PRNP codon 200^(Lys) mutation: An analysis of 45 families. *Eur J Epidemiol* **7**:477, 1991.

168. Bertoni JM, Brown P, Goldfarb L, Gajdusek D, Omaha NE: Familial CreutzfeldtJakob disease with the PRNP codon 200^(Lys) mutation and supranuclear palsy but without myoclonus or periodic EEG complexes [Abstract]. *Neurology* **42**(No. 4, Supp 3):350, 1992.

169. Gabizon R, Telling G, Meiner Z, Halimi M, Kahana I, Prusiner SB: Insoluble wild-type and protease-resistant mutant prion protein in brains of patients with inherited prion disease. *Nat Med* **2**:59, 1996.

170. Chapman J, Ben-Israel J, Goldhammer Y, Korczyn AD: The risk of developing Creutzfeldt-Jakob disease in subjects with the *PRNP* gene codon 200 point mutation. *Neurology* **44**:2243, 1994.

171. Spudich S, Mastrianni JA, Wrensch M, Gabizon R, Meiner Z, Kahana I, Rosenmann H, Kahana E, Prusiner SB: Complete penetrance of Creutzfeldt-Jakob disease in Libyan Jews carrying the E200K mutation in the prion protein gene. *Mol Med* **1**:607, 1995.

172. Goldfarb L, Korczyn A, Brown P, Chapman J, Gajdusek DC: Mutation in codon 200 of scrapie amyloid precursor gene linked to Creutzfeldt-Jakob disease in Sephardic Jews of Libyan and non-Libyan origin. *Lancet* **336**:637, 1990.

173. Goldfarb LG, Petersen RB, Tabaton M, Brown P, LeBlanc AC, Montagna P, Cortelli P, Julien J, Vital C, Pendelbury WW, Haltia M, Wills PR, Hauw JJ, McKeever PE, Monari L, Schrank B, Swergold GD, Autilio-Gambetti L, Gajdusek DC, Lugaresi E, Gambetti P: Fatal familial insomnia and familial Creutzfeldt-Jakob disease: Disease phenotype determined by a DNA polymorphism. *Science* **258**:806, 1992.

174. Medori R, Montagna P, Tritschler HJ, LeBlanc A, Cortelli P, Tinuper P, Lugaresi E, Gambetti P: Fatal familial insomnia: A second kindred with mutation of prion protein gene at codon 178. *Neurology* **42**:669, 1992.

175. Lugaresi E, Medori R, Montagna P, Baruzzi A, Cortelli P, Lugaresi A, Tinuper P, Zucconi M, Gambetti P: Fatal familial insomnia and dysautonomia with selective degeneration of thalamic nuclei. *N Engl J Med* **315**:997, 1986.

176. Gambetti P, Parchi P, Petersen RB, Chen SG, Lugaresi E: Fatal familial insomnia and familial Creutzfeldt-Jakob disease: Clinical, pathological and molecular features. *Brain Pathol* **5**:43, 1995.

177. Goldfarb LG, Haltia M, Brown P, Nieto A, Kovanen J, McCombie WR, Trapp S, Gajdusek DC: New mutation in scrapie amyloid precursor gene (at codon 178) in Finnish Creutzfeldt-Jakob kindred. *Lancet* **337**:425, 1991.

178. Kretzschmar HA, Neumann M, Stavrou D: Codon 178 mutation of the human prion protein gene in a German family (Backer family): sequencing data from 72-year-old celloidin-embedded brain tissue. *Acta Neuropathol (Berl)* **89**:96, 1995.

179. Owen F, Poulter M, Collinge J, Crow TJ: Codon 129 changes in the prion protein gene in Caucasians. *Am J Hum Genet* **46**:1215, 1990.

180. Palmer MS, Dryden AJ, Hughes JT, Collinge J: Homozygous prion protein genotype predisposes to sporadic Creutzfeldt-Jakob disease. *Nature* **352**:340, 1991.

181. Collinge J, Palmer MS: Human prion diseases, in Collinge J, Palmer MS (eds): *Prion Diseases.* Oxford, UK, Oxford University Press, 1997, p 18.

182. Kitamoto T, Tateishi J: Human prion diseases with variant prion protein. *Philos Trans R Soc Lond B Biol Sci* **343**:391, 1994.

183. Furukawa H, Kitamoto T, Tanaka Y, Tateishi J: New variant prion protein in a Japanese family with Gerstmann-Sträussler syndrome. *Mol Brain Res* **30**:385, 1995.

183a. Kaneko K, Ball HL, Wille H, Zhang H, Groth D, Torchia M, Tremblay P, Safar J, Prusiner SB, DeArmond SJ, Baldwin MA, Cohen FE: A synthetic peptide initiates Gerstmann-Straussler-Scheinker (GSS) disease in transgenic mice. *J Mol Biol* **295**:997, 2000.

184. Fink JK, Peacock ML, Warren JT, Roses AD, Prusiner SB: Detecting prion protein gene mutations by denaturing gradient gel electrophoresis. *Hum Mutat* **4**:42, 1994.

185. Kaneko K, Zulianello L, Scott M, Cooper CM, Wallace AC, James TL, Cohen FE, Prusiner SB: Evidence for protein X binding to a discontinuous epitope on the cellular prion protein during scrapie prion propagation. *Proc Natl Acad Sci U S A* **94**:10069, 1997.

186. Laplanche J-L, Chatelain J, Launay J-M, Gazengel C, Vidaud M: Deletion in prion protein gene in a Moroccan family. *Nucleic Acids Res* **18**:6745, 1990.

187. Vnencak-Jones CL, Phillips JA: Identification of heterogeneous PrP gene deletions in controls by detection of allele-specific heteroduplexes (DASH). *Am J Hum Genet* **50**:871, 1992.

188. Cervenáková L, Brown P, Piccardo P, Cummings JL, Nagle J, Vinters HV, Kaur P, Ghetti B, Chapman J, Gajdusek DC, Goldfarb LG: 24-nucleotide deletion in the *PRNP* gene: Analysis of associated phenotypes, in Court L, Dodet B (eds): *Transmissible Subacute Spongiform Encephalopathies: Prion Diseases.* Paris, Elsevier, 1996, p 433.

189. Palmer MS, Mahal SP, Campbell TA, Hill AF, Sidle KCL, Laplanche J-L, Collinge J: Deletions in the prion protein gene are not associated with CJD. *Hum Mol Genet* **2**:541, 1993.

190. Collinge J, Palmer MS, Dryden AJ: Genetic predisposition to iatrogenic Creutzfeldt-Jakob disease. *Lancet* **337**:1441, 1991.

191. Doh-ura K, Kitamoto T, Sakaki Y, Tateishi J: CJD discrepancy. *Nature* **353**:801, 1991.

192. Miyazono M, Kitamoto T, Doh-ura K, Iwaki T, Tateishi J: Creutzfeldt-Jakob disease with codon 129 polymorphism (Valine): A comparative study of patients with codon 102 point mutation or without mutations. *Acta Neuropathol (Berl)* **84**:349, 1992.

193. Tateishi J. Kitamoto T: Developments in diagnosis for prion diseases. *Br Med Bull* **49**:971, 1993.

194. Goldfarb LG, Brown P, Goldgaber D, Asher DM, Rubenstein R, Brown WT, Piccardo P, Kascsak RJ, Boellaard JW, Gajdusek DC: Creutzfeldt-Jakob disease and kuru patients lack a mutation consistently found in the Gerstmann-Sträussler-Scheinker syndrome. *Exp Neurol* **108**:247, 1990.

195. Scott M, Foster D, Mirenda C, Serban D, Coufal F, Wälchli M, Torchia M, Groth D, Carlson G, DeArmond SJ, Westaway D, Prusiner SB: Transgenic mice expressing hamster prion protein produce species-specific scrapie infectivity and amyloid plaques. *Cell* **59**:847, 1989.

196. Prusiner SB, Scott M, Foster D, Pan K-M, Groth D, Mirenda C, Torchia M, Yang S-L, Serban D, Carlson GA, Hoppe PC, Westaway D, DeArmond SJ: Transgenetic studies implicate interactions between homologous PrP isoforms in scrapie prion replication. *Cell* **63**:673, 1990.

197. Scott M, Groth D, Foster D, Torchia M, Yang S-L, DeArmond SJ, Prusiner SB: Propagation of prions with artificial properties in transgenic mice expressing chimeric PrP genes. *Cell* **73**:979, 1993.

198. Alpers MP: Kuru: implications of its transmissibility for interpretation of its changing epidemiological pattern, in Bailey OT, Smith DE (eds): *The Central Nervous System, Some Experimental Models of Neurological Diseases.* Baltimore, Williams and Wilkins, 1968, p 234.

199. Alpers M: Epidemiology and clinical aspects of kuru, in Prusiner SB, McKinley MP (eds): *Prions — Novel Infectious Pathogens Causing Scrapie and Creutzfeldt-Jakob Disease*. Orlando, Academic Press, 1987, p 451.

200. Brown P, Preece MA, Will RG: "Friendly fire" in medicine: Hormones, homografts, and Creutzfeldt-Jakob disease. *Lancet* **340**:24, 1992.

201. Esmonde T, Lueck CJ, Symon L, Duchen LW, Will RG: Creutzfeldt-Jakob disease and lyophilised dura mater grafts: Report of two cases. *J Neurol Neurosurg Psychiatry* **56**:999, 1993.

202. Lane KL, Brown P, Howell DN, Crain BJ, Hulette CM, Burger PC, DeArmond SJ: Creutzfeldt-Jakob disease in a pregnant woman with an implanted dura mater graft. *Neurosurgery* **34**:737, 1994.

203. Centers for Disease Control: Creutzfeldt-Jakob disease associated with cadaveric dura mater grafts — Japan, January 1979-May 1996. *MMWR Morb Mortal Wkly Rep* **46**:1066, 1997.

204. Bateman D, Hilton D, Love S, Zeidler M, Beck J, Collinge J: Sporadic Creutzfeldt-Jakob disease in a 18-year-old in the UK [Letter]. *Lancet* **346**:1155, 1995.

205. Britton TC, Al-Sarraj S, Shaw C, Campbell T, Collinge J: Sporadic Creutzfeldt-Jakob disease in a 16-year-old in the UK [Letter]. *Lancet* **346**:1155, 1995.

206. Bruce ME, Will RG, Ironside JW, McConnell I, Drummond D, Suttie A, McCardle L, Chree A, Hope J, Birkett C, Cousens S, Fraser H, Bostock CJ: Transmissions to mice indicate that "new variant" CJD is caused by the BSE agent. *Nature* **389**:498, 1997.

207. Hill AF, Desbruslais M, Joiner S, Sidle KCL, Gowland I, Collinge J, Doey LJ, Lantos P: The same prion strain causes vCJD and BSE. *Nature* **389**:448, 1997.

208. Büeler H, Aguzzi A, Sailer A, Greiner R-A, Autenried P, Aguet M, Weissmann C: Mice devoid of PrP are resistant to scrapie. *Cell* **73**:1339, 1993.

209. Scott MR, Groth D, Tatzelt J, Torchia M, Tremblay P, DeArmond SJ, Prusiner SB: Propagation of prion strains through specific conformers of the prion protein. *J Virol* **71**:9032, 1997.

210. Manson JC, Clarke AR, Hooper ML, Aitchison L, McConnell I, Hope J: 129/Ola mice carrying a null mutation in PrP that abolishes mRNA production are developmentally normal. *Mol Neurobiol* **8**:121, 1994.

210a. Moore RC, Lee IY, Silverman GL, Harrison PM, Strome R, Heinrich C, Karunaratne A, Pasternak SH, Chisthti MA, Liang Y, Mastrangelo P, Wang K, Smit AF, Katamine S, Carlson GA, Cohen FE, Prusiner SB, Melton DW, Tremblay P, Hood LE, Westaway D: Ataxia in prion protein (PrP)-deficient mice is associated with upregulation of the novel PrP-like protein doppel. *J Mol Biol* **292**:797, 1999.

211. Sakaguchi S, Katamine S, Nishida N, Moriuchi R, Shigematsu K, Sugimoto T, Nakatani A, Kataoka Y, Houtani T, Shirabe S, Okada H, Hasegawa S, Miyamoto T, Noda T: Loss of cerebellar Purkinje cells in aged mice homozygous for a disrupted PrP gene. *Nature* **380**:528, 1996.

212. Tobler I, Gaus SE, Deboer T, Achermann P, Fischer M, Rülicke T, Moser M, Oesch B, McBride PA, Manson JC: Altered circadian activity rhythms and sleep in mice devoid of prion protein. *Nature* **380**:639, 1996.

213. Collinge J, Whittington MA, Sidle KC, Smith CJ, Palmer MS, Clarke AR, Jefferys JGR: Prion protein is necessary for normal synaptic function. *Nature* **370**:295, 1994.

214. Whittington MA, Sidle KCL, Gowland I, Meads J, Hill AF, Palmer MS, Jefferys JGR, Collinge J: Rescue of neurophysiological phenotype seen in PrP null mice by transgene encoding human prion protein. *Nat Genet* **9**:197, 1995.

215. Herms JW, Kretzschmar HA, Titz S, Keller BU: Patch-clamp analysis of synaptic transmission to cerebellar Purkinje cells of prion protein knockout mice. *Eur J Neurosci* **7**:2508, 1995.

216. Lledo P-M, Tremblay P, DeArmond SJ, Prusiner SB, Nicoll RA: Mice deficient for prion protein exhibit normal neuronal excitability and synaptic transmission in the hippocampus. *Proc Natl Acad Sci U S A* **93**:2403, 1996.

217. Sailer A, Büeler H, Fischer M, Aguzzi A, Weissmann C: No propagation of prions in mice devoid of PrP. *Cell* **77**:967, 1994.

218. Gossen M, Bujard H: Tight control of gene expression in mammalian cells by tetracycline-responsive promoters. *Proc Natl Acad Sci U S A* **89**:5547, 1992.

219. Tremblay P, Meiner Z, Galou M, Heinrich C, Petromilli C, Lisse T, Cayetano J, Torchia M, Mobley W, Bujard H, DeArmond SJ, Prusiner SB: Doxycycline control of prion protein (PrP) transgene expression modulates prion disease in mice. *Proc Natl Acad Sci U S A* **95**:12580, 1998.

220. Stahl N, Baldwin MA, Teplow DB, Hood L, Gibson BW, Burlingame AL, Prusiner SB: Structural analysis of the scrapie prion protein using mass spectrometry and amino acid sequencing. *Biochemistry* **32**:1991, 1993.

221. Anfinsen CB: Principles that govern the folding of protein chains. *Science* **181**:223, 1973.

222. Borchelt DR, Scott M, Taraboulos A, Stahl N, Prusiner SB: Scrapie and cellular prion proteins differ in their kinetics of synthesis and topology in cultured cells. *J Cell Biol* **110**:743, 1990.

223. Caughey B, Raymond GJ: The scrapie-associated form of PrP is made from a cell surface precursor that is both protease- and phospholipase-sensitive. *J Biol Chem* **266**:18217, 1991.

224. Gorodinsky A, Harris DA: Glycolipid-anchored proteins in neuroblastoma cells form detergent-resistant complexes without caveolin. *J Cell Biol* **129**:619, 1995.

225. Huang Z, Gabriel J-M, Baldwin MA, Fletterick RJ, Prusiner SB, Cohen FE: Proposed three-dimensional structure for the cellular prion protein. *Proc Natl Acad Sci U S A* **91**:7139, 1994.

226. Riek R, Hornemann S, Wider G, Billeter M, Glockshuber R, Wüthrich K: NMR structure of the mouse prion protein domain PrP(121-231). *Nature* **382**:180, 1996.

227. James TL, Liu H, Ulyanov NB, Farr-Jones S, Zhang H, Donne DG, Kaneko K, Groth D, Mehlhorn I, Prusiner SB, Cohen FE: Solution structure of a 142-residue recombinant prion protein corresponding to the infectious fragment of the scrapie isoform. *Proc Natl Acad Sci U S A* **94**:10086, 1997.

228. Peretz D, Williamson RA, Matsunaga Y, Serban H, Pinilla C, Bastidas RB, Rozenshteyn R, James TL, Houghten RA, Cohen FE, Prusiner SB, Burton DR: A conformational transition at the N terminus of the prion protein features in formation of the scrapie isoform. *J Mol Biol* **273**:614, 1997.

229. Huang Z, Prusiner SB, Cohen FE: Scrapie prions: A three-dimensional model of an infectious fragment. *Fold Design* **1**:13, 1995.

230. Korth C, Stierli B, Streit P, Moser M, Schaller O, Fischer R, Schulz-Schaeffer W, Kretzschmar H, Raeber A, Braun U, Ehrensperger F, Hornemann S, Glockshuber R, Riek R, Billeter M, Wuthrick K, Oesch B: Prion (PrP<sup>Sc</sup>)-specific epitope defined by a monoclonal antibody. *Nature* **389**:74, 1997.

231. Bellinger-Kawahara CG, Kempner E, Groth DF, Gabizon R, Prusiner SB: Scrapie prion liposomes and rods exhibit target sizes of 55,000 Da. *Virology* **164**:537, 1988.

232. Gajdusek DC: Transmissible and non-transmissible amyloidoses: Autocatalytic post-translational conversion of host precursor proteins to β-pleated sheet configurations. *J Neuroimmunol* **20**:95, 1988.

233. Caughey B, Kocisko DA, Raymond GJ, Lansbury PT Jr: Aggregates of scrapie-associated prion protein induce the cell-free conversion of protease-sensitive prion protein to the protease-resistant state. *Chem Biol* **2**:807, 1995.

233a. Zulianello L, Kaneko K, Scott M, Erpel S, Han D, Cohen FE, Prusiner SB: Dominant-negative inhibition of prion formation diminished by deletion mutagenesis of the prion protein. *J Virol* **74**:4351, 2000.

234. Kocisko DA, Come JH, Priola SA, Chesebro B, Raymond GJ, Lansbury PT Jr, Caughey B: Cell-free formation of protease-resistant prion protein. *Nature* **370**:471, 1994.

235. Kaneko K, Wille H, Mehlhorn I, Zhang H, Ball H, Cohen FE, Baldwin MA, Prusiner SB: Molecular properties of complexes formed between the prion protein and synthetic peptides. *J Mol Biol* **270**:574, 1997.

236. Vey M, Pilkuhn S, Wille H, Nixon R, DeArmond SJ, Smart EJ, Anderson RG, Taraboulos A, Prusiner SB: Subcellular colocalization of the cellular and scrapie prion proteins in caveolae-like membranous domains. *Proc Natl Acad Sci U S A* **93**:14945, 1996.

237. Kaneko K, Vey M, Scott M, Pilkuhn S, Cohen FE, Prusiner SB: COOH-terminal sequence of the cellular prion protein directs subcellular trafficking and controls conversion into the scrapie isoform. *Proc Natl Acad Sci U S A* **94**:2333, 1997.

238. Naslavsky N, Stein R, Yanai A, Friedlander G, Taraboulos A: Characterization of detergent-insoluble complexes containing the cellular prion protein and its scrapie isoform. *J Biol Chem* **272**:6324, 1997.

239. Caughey B, Raymond GJ, Ernst D, Race RE: N-terminal truncation of the scrapie-associated form of PrP by lysosomal protease(s): Implications regarding the site of conversion of PrP to the protease-resistant state. *J Virol* **65**:6597, 1991.

240. Lehmann S, Harris DA: Two mutant prion proteins expressed in cultured cells acquire biochemical properties reminiscent of the scrapie isoform. *Proc Natl Acad Sci U S A* **93**:5610, 1996.

241. Büeler H, Raeber A, Sailer A, Fischer M, Aguzzi A, Weissmann C: High prion and PrP^Sc levels but delayed onset of disease in scrapie-inoculated mice heterozygous for a disrupted PrP gene. *Mol Med* **1**:19, 1994.

242. Collinge J, Sidle KCL, Meads J, Ironside J, Hill AF: Molecular analysis of prion strain variation and the aetiology of "new variant" CJD. *Nature* **383**:685, 1996.

243. DeArmond SJ, Sánchez H, Yehiely F, Qiu Y, Ninchak-Casey A, Daggett V, Camerino AP, Cayetano J, Rogers M, Groth D, Torchia M, Tremblay P, Scott MR, Cohen FE, Prusiner SB: Selective neuronal targeting in prion disease. *Neuron* **19**:1337, 1997.

244. Somerville RA, Chong A, Mulqueen OU, Birkett CR, Wood SCER, Hope J: Biochemical typing of scrapie strains. *Nature* **386**:564, 1997.

245. Telling GC, Scott M, Hsiao KK, Foster D, Yang S-L, Torchia M, Sidle KCL, Collinge J, DeArmond SJ, Prusiner SB: Transmission of Creutzfeldt-Jakob disease from humans to transgenic mice expressing chimeric human-mouse prion protein. *Proc Natl Acad Sci U S A* **91**:9936, 1994.

246. Hunter N, Goldmann W, Benson G, Foster JD, Hope J: Swaledale sheep affected by natural scrapie differ significantly in PrP genotype frequencies from healthy sheep and those selected for reduced incidence of scrapie. *J Gen Virol* **74**:1025, 1993.

247. Westaway D, Zuliani V, Cooper CM, Da Costa M, Neuman S, Jenny AL, Detwiler L, Prusiner SB: Homozygosity for prion protein alleles encoding glutamine-171 renders sheep susceptible to natural scrapie. *Genes Dev* **8**:959, 1994.

248. Shibuya S, Higuchi J, Shin R-W, Tateishi J, Kitamoto T: Protective prion protein polymorphisms against sporadic Creutzfeldt-Jakob disease. *Lancet* **351**:419, 1998.

249. Tatzelt J, Zuo J, Voellmy R, Scott M, Hartl U, Prusiner SB, Welch WJ: Scrapie prions selectively modify the stress response in neuroblastoma cells. *Proc Natl Acad Sci U S A* **92**:2944–2948, 1995.

250. Kenward N, Hope J, Landon M, Mayer RJ: Expression of polyubiquitin and heat-shock protein 70 genes increases in the later stages of disease progression in scrapie-infected mouse brain. *J Neurochem* **62**:1870, 1994.

251. Oesch B, Teplow DB, Stahl N, Serban D, Hood LE, Prusiner SB: Identification of cellular proteins binding to the scrapie prion protein. *Biochemistry* **29**:5848, 1990.

252. Kurschner C, Morgan JI: Analysis of interaction sites in homo- and heteromeric complexes containing Bcl-2 family members and the cellular prion protein. *Mol Brain Res* **37**:249, 1996.

253. Rieger R, Edenhofer F, Lasmézas CI, Weiss S: The human 37-kDa laminin receptor precursor interacts with the prion protein in eukaryotic cells. *Nat Med* **3**:1383, 1997.

254. Fraser H, Dickinson AG: The sequential development of the brain lesions of scrapie in three strains of mice. *J Comp Pathol* **78**:301, 1968.

255. Bruce ME, McBride PA, Farquhar CF: Precise targeting of the pathology of the sialoglycoprotein, PrP, and vacuolar degeneration in mouse scrapie. *Neurosci Lett* **102**:1, 1989.

256. Monari L, Chen SG, Brown P, Parchi P, Petersen RB, Mikol J, Gray F, Cortelli P, Montagna P, Ghetti B, Goldfarb LG, Gajdusek DC, Lugaresi E, Gambetti P, Autilio-Gambetti L: Fatal familial insomnia and familial Creutzfeldt-Jakob disease: Different prion proteins determined by a DNA polymorphism. *Proc Natl Acad Sci U S A* **91**:2839, 1994.

257. Mastrianni JA, Nixon R, Layzer R, Telling GC, Han D, DeArmond SJ, Prusiner SB: Prion protein conformation in a patient with sporadic fatal insomnia. *N Engl J Med* **34**:1630, 1999.

258. Kimberlin RH, Walker CA, Fraser H: The genomic identity of different strains of mouse scrapie is expressed in hamsters and preserved on reisolation in mice. *J Gen Virol* **70**:2017, 1989.

259. Bessen RA, Marsh RF: Biochemical and physical properties of the prion protein from two strains of the transmissible mink encephalopathy agent. *J Virol* **66**:2096, 1992.

260. Prusiner SB, Scott MR, DeArmond SJ, Cohen FE: Prion protein biology. *Cell* **93**:337, 1998.

261. Cohen FE, Prusiner SB: Pathologic conformations of prion proteins. *Annu Rev Biochem* **67**:793, 1998.

262. Endo T, Groth D, Prusiner SB, Kobata A: Diversity of oligosaccharide structures linked to asparagines of the scrapie prion protein. *Biochemistry* **28**:8380, 1989.

262a. Rudd PM, Endo T, Colominas C, Groth D, Wheeler SF, Harvey DJ, Wormald MR, Serban ZH, Prusiner SB, Kobata A, Dwek RA: Glycosylation differences between the normal and pathogenic prion protein isoforms. *Proc Natl Acad Sci U S A* **96**:13044, 1999.

263. Taraboulos A, Rogers M, Borchelt DR, McKinley MP, Scott M, Serban D, Prusiner SB: Acquisition of protease resistance by prion proteins in scrapie-infected cells does not require asparagine-linked glycosylation. *Proc Natl Acad Sci U S A* **87**:8262, 1990.

264. Carp RI, Meeker H, Sersen E: Scrapie strains retain their distinctive characteristics following passages of homogenates from different brain regions and spleen. *J Gen Virol* **78**:283, 1997.

265. Parry HB: Scrapie: A transmissible and hereditary disease of sheep. *Heredity* **17**:75, 1962.

266. Parry HB: *Scrapie Disease in Sheep.* New York, Academic Press, 1983.

267. Dickinson AG, Young GB, Stamp JT, Renwick CC: An analysis of natural scrapie in Suffolk sheep. *Heredity* **20**:485, 1965.

268. Goldmann W, Hunter N, Foster JD, Salbaum JM, Beyreuther K, Hope J: Two alleles of a neural protein gene linked to scrapie in sheep. *Proc Natl Acad Sci U S A* **87**:2476, 1990.

269. Laplanche J-L, Chatelain J, Beaudry P, Dussaucy M, Bounneau C, Launay J-M: French autochthonous scrapied sheep without the 136Val PrP polymorphism. *Mammalian Genome* **4**:463, 1993.

270. Clousard C, Beaudry P, Elsen JM, Milan D, Dussaucy M, Bounneau C, Schelcher F, Chatelain J, Launay JM, Laplanche JL: Different allelic effects of the codons 136 and 171 of the prion protein gene in sheep with natural scrapie. *J Gen Virol* **76**:2097, 1995.

271. Goldmann W, Hunter N, Smith G, Foster J, Hope J: PrP genotype and agent effects in scrapie: Change in allelic interaction with different isolates of agent in sheep, a natural host of scrapie. *J Gen Virol* **75**:989, 1994.

272. Belt PBGM, Muileman IH, Schreuder BEC, Ruijter JB, Gielkens ALJ, Smits MA: Identification of five allelic variants of the sheep PrP gene and their association with natural scrapie. *J Gen Virol* **76**:509, 1995.

273. Ikeda T, Horiuchi M, Ishiguro N, Muramatsu Y, Kai-Uwe GD, Shinagawa M: Amino acid polymorphisms of PrP with reference to onset of scrapie in Suffolk and Corriedale sheep in Japan. *J Gen Virol* **76**:2577, 1995.

274. Hunter N, Moore L, Hosie BD, Dingwall WS, Greig A: Association between natural scrapie and PrP genotype in a flock of Suffolk sheep in Scotland. *Vet Rec* **140**:59, 1997.

275. Hunter N, Cairns D, Foster JD, Smith G, Goldmann W, Donnelly K: Is scrapie solely a genetic disease? *Nature* **386**:137, 1997.

276. O'Rourke KI, Holyoak GR, Clark WW, Mickelson JR, Wang S, Melco RP, Besser TE, Foote WC: PrP genotypes and experimental scrapie in orally inoculated Suffolk sheep in the United States. *J Gen Virol* **78**:975, 1997.

277. Goldmann W, Hunter N, Benson G, Foster JD, Hope J: Different scrapie-associated fibril proteins (PrP) are encoded by lines of sheep selected for different alleles of the *Sip* gene. *J Gen Virol* **72**:2411, 1991.

278. Hunter N, Foster JD, Benson G, Hope J: Restriction fragment length polymorphisms of the scrapie-associated fibril protein (PrP) gene and their association with susceptiblity to natural scrapie in British sheep. *J Gen Virol* **72**:1287, 1991.

279. Prusiner SB, Fuzi M, Scott M, Serban D, Serban H, Taraboulos A, Gabriel J-M, Wells G, Wilesmith J, Bradley R, DeArmond SJ, Kristensson K: Immunologic and molecular biological studies of prion proteins in bovine spongiform encephalopathy. *J Infect Dis* **167**:602, 1993.

280. Hunter N, Goldmann W, Smith G, Hope J: Frequencies of PrP gene variants in healthy cattle and cattle with BSE in Scotland. *Vet Rec* **135**:400, 1994.

281. Anderson RM, Donnelly CA, Ferguson NM, Woolhouse MEJ, Watt CJ, Udy HJ, MaWhinney S, Dunstan SP, Southwood TRE, Wilesmith JW, Ryan JBM, Hoinville LJ, Hillerton JE, Austin AR, Wells GAH: Transmission dynamics and epidemiology of BSE in British cattle. *Nature* **382**:779, 1996.

282. Nathanson N, Wilesmith J, Griot C: Bovine spongiform encephalopathy (BSE): Cause and consequences of a common source epidemic. *Am J Epidemiol* **145**:959, 1997.

283. Stekel DJ, Nowak MA, Southwood TRE: Prediction of future BSE spread. *Nature* **381**:119, 1996.

284. Wilesmith JW, Ryan JBM, Atkinson MJ: Bovine spongiform encephalopathy—Epidemiologic studies on the origin. *Vet Rec* **128**:199, 1991.

285. Wilesmith JW: The epidemiology of bovine spongiform encephalopathy. *Semin Virol* **2**:239, 1991.

286. Kimberlin RH: Speculations on the origin of BSE and the epidemiology of CJD, in Gibbs CJ Jr (ed): *Bovine Spongiform*

*Encephalopathy: The BSE Dilemma.* New York, Springer, 1996, p 155.

287. Fraser H, McConnell I, Wells GAH, Dawson M: Transmission of bovine spongiform encephalopathy to mice. *Vet Rec* 123:472, 1988.

288. Dawson M, Wells GAH, Parker BNJ: Preliminary evidence of the experimental transmissibility of bovine spongiform encephalopathy to cattle. *Vet Rec* 126:112, 1990.

289. Dawson M, Wells GAH, Parker BNJ, Scott AC: Primary parenteral transmission of bovine spongiform encephalopathy to the pig. *Vet Rec* 127:338, 1990.

290. Bruce M, Chree A, McConnell I, Foster J, Fraser H: Transmissions of BSE, scrapie and related diseases to mice [Abstract]. *Proceedings of the IXth International Congress of Virology, Glasgow, Scotland, Aug. 9–12*:93, 1993.

291. Robinson MM, Hadlow WJ, Knowles DP, Huff TP, Lacy PA, Marsh RF, Gorham JR: Experimental infection of cattle with the agents of transmissible mink encephalopathy and scrapie. *J Comp Pathol* 113:241, 1995.

292. Hope J, Reekie LJD, Hunter N, Multhaup G, Beyreuther K, White H, Scott AC, Stack MJ, Dawson M, Wells GAH: Fibrils from brains of cows with new cattle disease contain scrapie-associated protein. *Nature* 336:390, 1988.

293. Serban D, Taraboulos A, DeArmond SJ, Prusiner SB: Rapid detection of Creutzfeldt-Jakob disease and scrapie prion proteins. *Neurology* 40:110, 1990.

294. Grathwohl K-UD, Horiuchi M, Ishiguro N, Shinagawa M: Sensitive enzyme-linked immunosorbent assay for detection of PrP$^{Sc}$ in crude tissue extracts from scrapie-affected mice. *J Virol Methods* 64:205, 1997.

295. Scott MR, Safar J, Telling G, Nguyen O, Groth D, Torchia M, Koehler R, Tremblay P, Walther D, Cohen FE, DeArmond SJ, Prusiner SB: Identification of a prion protein epitope modulating transmission of bovine spongiform encephalopathy prions to transgenic mice. *Proc Natl Acad Sci U S A* 94:14279, 1997.

295a. Scott MR, Will R, Ironside J, Nguyen HO, Tremblay P, DeArmond SJ, Prusiner SB: Compelling transgenetic evidence for transmission of bovine spongiform encephalopathy to humans. *Proc Natl Acad Sci U S A* 96:15137, 1999.

296. Taylor KC: The control of bovine spongiform encephalopathy in Great Britain. *Vet Rec* 129:522, 1991.

297. Fraser H, Bruce ME, Chree A, McConnell I, Wells GAH: Transmission of bovine spongiform encephalopathy and scrapie to mice. *J Gen Virol* 73:1891, 1992.

298. Eklund CM, Kennedy RC, Hadlow WJ: Pathogenesis of scrapie virus infection in the mouse. *J Infect Dis* 117:15, 1967.

299. Kimberlin R, Walker C: Characteristics of a short incubation model of scrapie in the golden hamster. *J Gen Virol* 34:295, 1977.

300. Ironside JW: The new variant form of Creutzfeldt-Jakob disease: A novel prion protein amyloid disorder [Editorial]. *Amyloid: Int J Exp Clin Invest* 4:66, 1997.

301. Centers for Disease Control: Surveillance for Creutzfeldt-Jakob Disease—United States. *MMWR Morb Mortal Wkly Rep* 45:665, 1996.

302. Baker HF, Ridley RM, Wells GAH: Experimental transmission of BSE and scrapie to the common marmoset. *Vet Rec* 132:403, 1993.

303. Lasmézas CI, Deslys J-P, Demaimay R, Adjou KT, Lamoury F, Dormont D, Robain O, Ironside J, Hauw J-J: BSE transmission to macaques. *Nature* 381:743, 1996.

304. Collinge J, Palmer MS, Sidle KC, Hill AF, Gowland I, Meads J, Asante E, Bradley R, Doey LJ, Lantos PL: Unaltered susceptibility to BSE in transgenic mice expressing human prion protein. *Nature* 378:779, 1995.

305. Raymond GJ, Hope J, Kocisko DA, Priola SA, Raymond LD, Bossers A, Ironside J, Will RG, Chen SG, Petersen RB, Gambetti P, Rubenstein R, Smits MA, Lansbury PT Jr, Caughey B: Molecular assessment of the potential transmissibilities of BSE and scrapie to humans. *Nature* 388:285, 1997.

306. Parchi P, Capellari S, Chen SG, Petersen RB, Gambetti P, Kopp P, Brown P, Kitamoto T, Tateishi J, Giese A, Kretzschmar H: Typing prion isoforms [Letter]. *Nature* 386:232, 1997.

307. Haraguchi T, Fisher S, Olofsson S, Endo T, Groth D, Tarantino A, Borchelt DR, Teplow D, Hood L, Burlingame A, Lycke E, Kobata A, Prusiner SB: Asparagine-linked glycosylation of the scrapie and cellular prion proteins. *Arch Biochem Biophys* 274:1, 1989.

308. Wickner RB: [URE3] as an altered URE2 protein: Evidence for a prion analog in *Saccharomyces cerevisiae*. *Science* 264:566, 1994.

309. Chernoff YO, Lindquist SL, Ono B, Inge-Vechtomov SG, Liebman SW: Role of the chaperone protein Hsp104 in propagation of the yeast prion-like factor [*psi*$^{+}$]. *Science* 268:880, 1995.

310. Coustou V, Deleu C, Saupe S, Begueret J: The protein product of the *het-s* heterokaryon incompatibility gene of the fungus *Podospora anserina* behaves as a prion analog. *Proc Natl Acad Sci U S A* 94:9773, 1997.

311. Derkatch IL, Chernoff YO, Kushnirov VV, Inge-Vechtomov SG, Liebman SW: Genesis and variability of [*PSI*] prion factors in *Saccharomyces cerevisiae*. *Genetics* 144:1375, 1996.

312. Wickner RB: A new prion controls fungal cell fusion incompatibility [Commentary]. *Proc Natl Acad Sci U S A* 94:10012, 1997.

313. Paushkin SV Kushnirov VV, Smirnov VN, Ter-Avanesyan MD: In vitro propagation of the prion-like state of yeast Sup35 protein. *Science* 277:381, 1997.

314. Landman OE: The inheritance of acquired characteristics. *Annu Rev Genet* 25:1, 1991.

315. Frankel J: Positional order and cellular handedness. *J Cell Sci* 97:205, 1990.

316. Perrier V, Wallace AC, Kaneko K, Safar J, Prusiner SB, Cohen FE: Mimicking dominant negative inhibition of prion replication through structure-based drug design. *Proc Natl Acad Sci U S A* 97:6073, 2000.

317. Supattapone S, Nguyen HO, Cohen FE, Prusiner SB, Scott MR: Elimination of prions by branched polyamines and implications for therapeutics. *Proc Natl Acad Sci U S A* 96:14529, 1999.

318. Shinde UP, Liu JJ, Inouye M: Protein memory through altered folding mediated by intramolecular chaperones. *Nature* 389:520, 1997.

319. Kascsak RJ, Rubenstein R, Merz PA, Tonna-DeMasi M, Fersko R, Carp RI, Wisniewski HM, Diringer H: Mouse polyclonal and monoclonal antibody to scrapie-associated fibril proteins. *J Virol* 61:3688, 1987.

# Kallmann Syndrome

*Andrea Ballabio* ▪ *Elena I. Rugarli*

1. **Kallmann syndrome is an inherited disorder characterized by the association of hypogonadotropic hypogonadism, due to gonadotropin-releasing hormone (GnRH) deficiency, with inability to smell (anosmia). These symptoms are the result of a defect in migration and targeting of two specific neuronal subpopulations, the GnRH producing neurons and the olfactory neurons.**
2. **Autosomal dominant (MIM 147950), autosomal recessive (MIM 244200), and X-linked recessive inheritance patterns have been described in Kallmann syndrome, indicating the presence of genetic heterogeneity. Deletion mapping and positional cloning efforts in the distal short arm of the X chromosome (Xp22.3) led to the isolation of the gene involved in the X-linked type of Kallmann syndrome (KAL) (MIM 308700). Patients with Kallmann syndrome who carry deletions in the Xp22.3 region may have contiguous gene syndromes and may, therefore, display the phenotype of several X-linked disorders associated with Kallmann syndrome.**
3. **In addition to deletions, several point mutations in the KAL gene have been identified in patients with isolated Kallmann syndrome.**
4. **The KAL gene encodes a secreted protein of 680 amino acids that shares significant similarities with protease inhibitors and neural-cell adhesion molecules (cDNA GenBank M97252).**
5. **The characterization of KAL spatiotemporal expression pattern in human and chick embryos has provided important clues to the understanding of Kallmann syndrome pathogenesis. Within the olfactory system, the gene is expressed by the olfactory bulb, which represents the target of the olfactory axons.**
6. **It appears likely that the primary defect in Kallmann syndrome is an abnormality of olfactory system development affecting axonal targeting and/or synaptogenesis.**

## CLINICAL FEATURES, DIAGNOSIS, AND THERAPY

In 1856, Maestre de San Juan observed the association of hypogonadism with olfactory system abnormalities.[1] Later de Morsier described, under the term *olfactogenital dysplasia*, a series of patients with hypogonadism and anosmia who had various abnormalities of the olfactory system associated with multiple malformations.[2,3] Kallmann first identified the inherited nature of this condition in 1944.[4] Subsequently, the term Kallmann syndrome (KS) came to designate an inherited disorder characterized by the association of hypogonadotropic hypogonadism and anosmia.

A list of standard abbreviations is located immediately preceding the index in each volume. Additional abbreviations used in this chapter include: FN = fibronectin; FSH = follicle-stimulating hormone; GnRH = gonadotropin-releasing hormone; KAL or *KAL* = Kallmann syndrome protein or gene symbol, respectively; KAL-X = Kallmann gene on the X chromosome; KAL-Y = Kallmann pseudogene on the Y chromosome; KALc = chicken Kallmann gene or protein; KS = Kallmann syndrome; LH = luteinizing hormone; NCAM = neural-cell adhesion molecule.

The hypogonadism in KS is due to a reduced secretion of gonadotropin-releasing hormone (GnRH) by the hypothalamus.[5] The degree of GnRH deficiency in KS patients is variable, ranging from complete deficiency, in which both follicle-stimulating hormone (FSH) and luteinizing hormone (LH) levels are low and there is no evidence of sexual maturation, to partial deficiency, in which FSH secretion predominates, allowing a certain degree of germinal-cell maturation in the testis but resulting in incomplete sexual development.[6] Typical patients with KS have an eunuchoid habitus. Gynecomastia, micropenis, and cryptorchidism have been reported in some cases.[7]

The other cardinal feature of patients with KS is the presence of nonselective anosmia or hyposmia. Therefore, a precise determination of the olfactory threshold in patients with hypogonadotropic hypogonadism is of fundamental importance in confirming the diagnosis of KS.

Table 225-1 shows the complete spectrum of clinical features associated with KS. Additional features found in several patients with KS include synkinesia (mirror movements), pes cavus, high arched palate, and unilateral renal agenesis.[8–11] Hardelin et al. demonstrated that these features represent pleiotropic effects of point mutations in the X-linked KS gene.[12,13] Mirror movements occur in 85 percent of males with X-linked KS. When asked to perform unilateral intentional movements, patients with synkinesia move muscles of the contralateral side together with the primary movement. Synkinesia was suggested to arise from the lack of the fibers that typically cross within the corpus callosum and inhibit the contralateral uncrossed pyramidal tract.[14] Danek et al. measured movement-related cortical potentials in families with X-linked KS and demonstrated a complete correlation between the presence of the KS phenotype and bilaterality of evoked motor responses.[15] A recent neurophysiologic study concluded that patients with X-linked KS have a novel ipsilateral corticospinal tract, most likely resulting from a lack of decussation of the corticospinal tract at the level of the pyramids.[16] However, both PET[17] and functional MR imaging studies[18] suggest that bilateral activation of the primary motor cortices could contribute to the presence of mirror movements.

Additional neurologic symptoms described in some patients with KS include eye-movement abnormalities, cerebellar ataxia, gaze-evoked horizontal nystagmus,[10,11] sensorineural deafness,[9] spatial-attention abnormalities,[19] spastic paraplegia,[20] and mental retardation.[8] Moreover, somatic defects, such as cleft lip and palate, and congenital heart defects have been described.[9,11,21]

Occasional patients with KS also manifest features of other distinct X-linked diseases such as ichthyosis, chondrodysplasia punctata, mental retardation, short stature, and ocular albinism. This combination of disorders results from deletions of the distal short arm of the human X chromosome, leading to a contiguous gene syndrome (see Chap. 65).[22]

Patients with KS usually present at puberty with a delay in the appearance of secondary sex characteristics. Laboratory tests reveal low serum concentrations of FSH and LH[6] and very low levels of testosterone in males or of estradiol in females. Differentiation between KS and delayed puberty requires a complete family history and a thorough assessment of olfactory function, which can be tested by the method proposed by Henkin

**Table 225-1 Clinical Features Associated with Kallmann Syndrome**

Cardinal features found in most patients with Kallmann syndrome
   Hypogonadotropic hypogonadism
   Anosmia
Pleiotropic effects of mutations in the KAL gene
   Synkinesia (mirror movements)
   Unilateral renal agenesis
   High arched palate
   Pes cavus
Rare features observed in a few cases
   Eye-movement abnormalities
   Cerebellar ataxia
   Gaze-evoked horizontal nystagmus
   Sensorineural deafness
   Spatial-attention abnormalities
   Spastic paraplegia
   Mental retardation
   Cleft lip and palate
Features found in patients with Xp22.3 deletions
    (contiguous gene syndrome)
   Ichthyosis
   Mental retardation
   Chondrodysplasia punctata
   Short stature
   Ocular albinism

and Bartter[23] or by the Smell Identification Test.[24] Sporadic cases of KS may be difficult to differentiate from idiopathic hypogonadotropic hypogonadism because of the variability in expression of anosmia in KS.[25] Hypogonadotropic hypogonadism can also be due to central nervous system tumors, histiocytosis, radiation therapy, idiopathic hypopituitary dwarfism, Prader-Willi syndrome, Laurence-Moon-Biedl syndrome, chronic diseases, malnutrition, anorexia nervosa, or hypothyroidism. All of these disorders are easily distinguishable from KS.[6]

Treatment for KS is directed toward restoration of normal gonadal steroid levels to allow sexual maturation and induce fertility. The exogenous administration of testosterone is usually effective in inducing virilization. Achieving fertility, however, requires administration of gonadotropins or GnRH. Controversy exists regarding the effectiveness of gonadotropin versus GnRH replacement therapy in hypogonadotropic males, as reviewed elsewhere.[26] Combined gonadotropin replacement by administration of human chorionic gonadotropin (hCG) and human menopausal gonadotropin (hMG) appears to be the most common treatment for hypogonadotropic hypogonadism. Comparable results have been obtained with either subcutaneous or intramuscular administration. Subcutaneous applications, however, seem to be preferred because they are less painful and can be done by the patient.[27] Response to gonadotropin therapy varies considerably among individuals.[27] Although pulsatile subcutaneous administration of GnRH is the most physiological treatment,[28] the need for a programmable infusion pump makes this therapy difficult to carry out and often decreases compliance. Hormonal replacement therapy, either by gonadotropins or GnRH, is required over many months, because shorter treatments usually fail to induce normal sexual development and spermatogenesis. The patient's compliance and his desire for fertility play a fundamental role in achieving successful treatment.

## HISTOPATHOLOGY

Maestre de San Juan was the first to describe the presence of anatomic defects of the olfactory system in patients with hypogonadism and anosmia.[1] More recent anatomic studies of patients with KS revealed the absence or hypoplasia of olfactory bulbs and tracts.[29-31] In addition, biopsies of nasal mucosa from patients with KS revealed a mixture of immature olfactory neurons and degenerating axons with functionally mature cells in the olfactory epithelium.[32,33]

The first clue to the pathogenesis of KS came from the observation of a developmental relationship between GnRH-secreting neurons and the olfactory system. Two independent studies performed in mice demonstrated that GnRH-secreting neurons share a common origin and migration pathway with olfactory axons during development (Fig. 225-1).[34,35]

Immunohistochemistry and mRNA in situ hybridization studies were performed in mouse embryos using anti-GnRH antibodies and a GnRH probe, respectively. These studies demonstrated that GnRH neurons originate in the olfactory placode, which is a discrete thickening of the head ectoderm that goes on to form the olfactory epithelium. During development, GnRH neurons migrate along the olfactory, terminalis, and vomeronasal nerves, traverse both the cribriform plate and the meninges, enter the forebrain, and eventually reach their final destination in the hypothalamus.[34,35] It was evident from these data that interactions between the olfactory axons and the olfactory bulb were of essential importance for GnRH neuronal migration. Therefore, the hypothesis was formulated that KS was due to a defect in a molecule involved in the migration of olfactory axons.[34]

The concept that migration of GnRH neurons depends on contact between olfactory axons and the olfactory bulb was substantiated by data obtained from the study of a 19-week-old human fetus with X-linked KS.[30] In this fetus, olfactory axons developed normally and started their migration toward the forebrain but arrested prematurely in the meninges, between the cribriform plate and the forebrain, ending in a tangle of nerve fibers and connective tissue. Immunohistochemical analysis, using human anti-GnRH antibodies, revealed that the majority of GnRH neurons were located at the dorsal surface of the cribriform plate, in the region where olfactory, terminalis, and vomeronasal nerves ended their migration. A similar analysis, performed in three age-

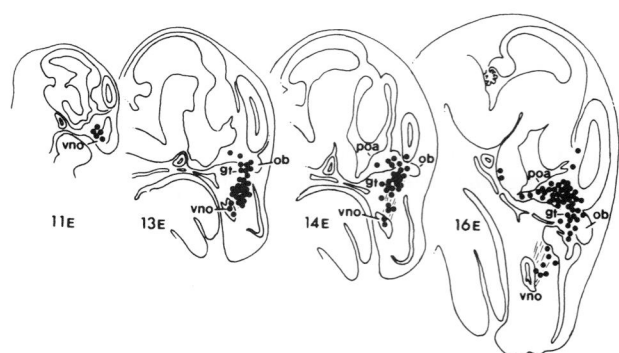

**Fig. 225-1** Migratory route of GnRH-immunoreactive neurons from derivatives of the medial olfactory placode to the forebrain is shown in microprojection drawings in the sagittal plane of 6-μm sections through the whole heads of fetal mice on embryonic (E) days 11, 13, 14, and 16. The black dots represent GnRH-immunoreactive neurons. On day 11, GnRH-immunoreactive cells are seen in the anlage of the vomeronasal organ and medial wall of the olfactory placode. On day 13, most of the GnRH cells are seen on the nasal septum, with the nervus terminalis and the vomeronasal nerves, and on day 14, most of these cells are in the ganglion terminale and in the central roots of the nervus terminalis. The 16-day-old fetal brain had most GnRH neurons arching through the forebrain into the hypothalamus and preoptic areas. gt = ganglion terminale; ob = olfactory bulb; poa = preoptic area; vno = vomeronasal organ. (*From Schwanzel-Fukuda M, Pfaff D.[34] Used by permission of Nature.*)

matched normal fetuses, showed that all GnRH neurons had reached their final destination in the hypothalamus. This study supported the hypothesis (as did previous investigations) that the contact between olfactory axons and the olfactory bulb was an essential factor in GnRH neuronal migration.[30]

MRI studies have been performed in patients with KS.[36–39] This method provides accurate in vivo imaging of the neuroanatomic defect and appears, therefore, to be a very useful diagnostic tool.[39] Using MRI, aplasia or hypoplasia of olfactory sulci and of olfactory bulbs and tracts can be detected in all KS patients examined. Interestingly, one of these studies[37] demonstrated by MRI the presence of an abnormal mass of heterotopic soft tissue located between the upper nasal vault and the forebrain. This mass might represent the radiologic correlate of the dysplastic tangle of nerve fibers that Schwanzel-Fukuda et al. observed in a KS fetus.[30]

## GENETICS

The incidence of KS has been estimated to be 1:10,000 in males and 1:50,000 in females.[40] Therefore, KS is the most common type of isolated gonadotropin deficiency. Autosomal dominant, autosomal recessive, and X-linked recessive inheritance patterns have been described, indicating the presence of genetic heterogeneity.[9,41] The five- to sixfold excess of male over female patients suggests that the X-linked form is the most frequent. Penetrance is not always complete in KS, and identical twins discordant for KS have been described.[42] Expressivity is also variable in KS, with both interfamilial and intrafamilial variability of the phenotype described by several groups.[9,41,43,44]

To date, there are no genetic mapping data on the autosomally inherited forms of KS, although four patients with KS who were carrying chromosomal rearrangements have been identified. The identified chromosomal rearrangements are a balanced translocation involving chromosome breaks at 7q22 and 12q24;[45] an extra metacentric chromosome of unknown origin;[46] a balanced complex rearrangement involving chromosome breaks at 3q13, 9q13q21, and 12q15;[47] and a balanced translocation involving chromosomes 1 and 10.[48] These translocations may be causally associated with KS and, therefore, may pinpoint map locations of autosomal genes involved in KS. Early reports can be found in which features of KS are described as part of complex X-linked syndromes.[10,49–54] A constant clinical feature in these cases was the presence of X-linked ichthyosis, a dermatologic condition characterized by dark scaly skin due to steroid sulfatase deficiency (see Chap. 166). Although most of these patients had both hypogonadotropic hypogonadism and anosmia, a diagnosis of KS was not made, perhaps due to the complexity of the observed phenotype. In some of these patients, a translocation involving the

distal short arm of the X chromosome (Xp22.3) and the long arm of the Y chromosome (Yq11) was detected.[52,53]

In 1986, the study of a family in which several affected males had hypogonadotropic hypogonadism, anosmia, and ichthyosis, led to the hypothesis that these males were affected by a contiguous gene syndrome, in which a codeletion of adjacent KS and steroid sulfatase genes on the X chromosome resulted in simultaneous expression of KS and ichthyosis (see Fig. 166-9 in Chap. 166).[55] This led to the first tentative chromosomal assignment of the X-linked KS gene to the region of the steroid sulfatase gene in Xp22.3.[55] In keeping with this hypothesis, Southern blot analysis using a steroid sulfatase cDNA probe[56] (Fig. 225-2) subsequently demonstrated a deletion of the steroid sulfatase gene in the DNA of these patients.[57] Linkage analysis in families with isolated KS confirmed the map assignment of the X-linked KS gene (KAL) to the Xp22.3 region.[58]

## THE X-LINKED KALLMANN SYNDROME GENE (KAL)

Molecular characterization of patients with contiguous gene syndromes carrying deletions and translocations involving the Xp22.3 region permitted the construction of a deletion map of this region and the assignment of KAL to a specific interval within this map.[59] A candidate KAL gene was isolated from this interval by two independent groups using a positional cloning strategy.[60,61] Evidence that this gene was the KAL gene came from the molecular analysis of two brothers with KS carrying a small (3-kb) intragenic deletion, removing the C-terminal region of the predicted protein product (Fig. 225-3).[62]

The KAL gene is expressed by both the active and the inactive X chromosomes;[60] it has a closely related nonfunctional homologue on the long arm of the Y chromosome (Yq11.2),[63,64] and it is highly conserved in many distantly related species except mice and hamsters.[65] All these features are not unique to KAL because they are shared by most of the genes localized in Xp22.3 and may be the result of recent evolutionary changes undergone by the X chromosome.[63]

The KAL cDNA sequence analysis has provided insights into the pathogenesis of KS. The gene encodes a 680-amino acid protein that shares homologies with several molecules involved in neural development. These homologies are summarized in Table 225-2. The N-terminal part of the protein contains a cysteine-rich domain, referred to as a *four-disulfide core* domain, which is found in a number of proteins, such as protease inhibitors and neurophysins.[66] This finding is intriguing because proteases (e.g., plasminogen activator-like proteases) regulate adhesion of axons to specific components of the extracellular matrix, thus facilitating their elongation. Protease inhibitors may, therefore, modulate this interaction, as it has been demonstrated for molecules belonging to the serpin family.[67–72]

The C-terminal two-thirds of KAL protein contains regions of significant similarity with the fibronectin (FN) type III repeat, first detected in fibronectin, and also found in several neural-cell adhesion molecules,[73] and in receptor-linked protein kinases and phosphatases.[74] Many of these molecules containing FN type III repeats are implicated in neuronal migration and axonal growth and guidance.[75–78] The specific function of FN type III repeats in these molecules is not known. The association of a four-disulfide core domain with FN type III repeats seems to be unique to KAL.

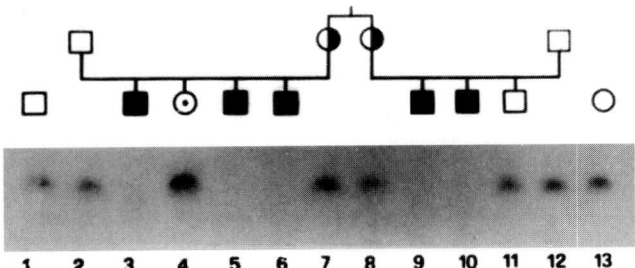

**Fig. 225-2** Autoradiograph of a Southern blot and pedigree of a family with X-linked ichthyosis associated with Kallmann syndrome. The pedigree is mounted so that each lane is below the symbol identifying the individual whose DNA was run in that lane. The first and last lanes contain male and female controls, respectively. The probe used was a steroid sulfatase cDNA clone.[56] A deletion of the steroid sulfatase gene is evident in the lanes corresponding to all affected individuals from this family. (*From Ballabio et al.[57] Used by permission of Human Genetics.*)

## MOLECULAR BASIS OF X-LINKED KALLMANN SYNDROME

A study of over 70 unrelated cases of isolated KS showed evidence of a deletion in KAL in only 1 family. While in some of the sporadic cases this likely reflects the fact that KS is genetically heterogeneous, deletions appear to be infrequent in X-linked KS.[62]

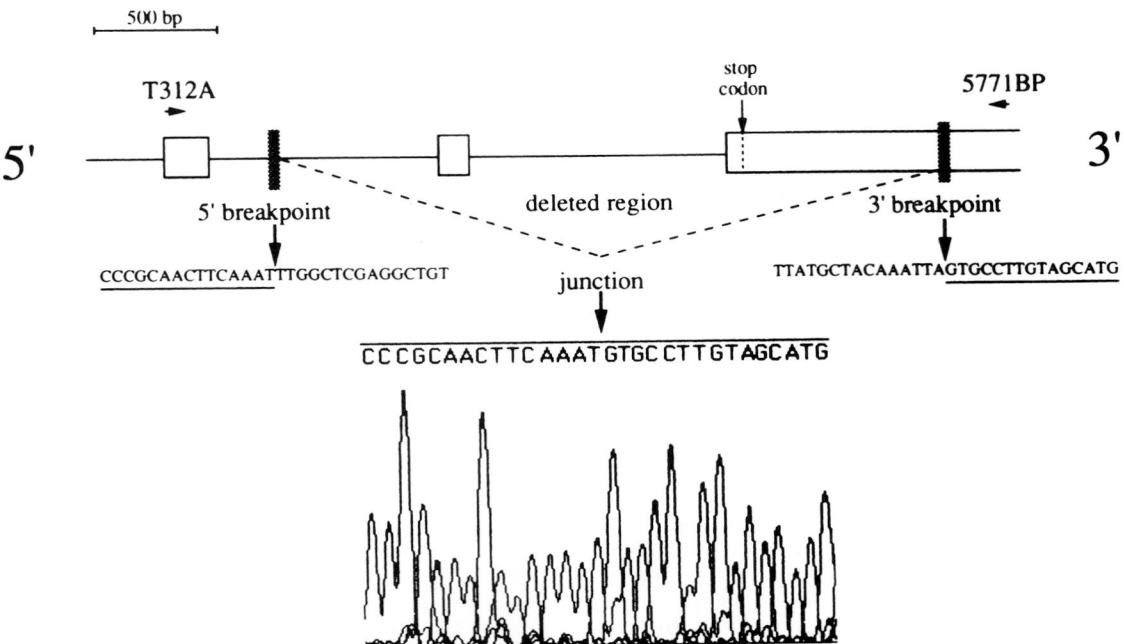

500 bp

T312A

stop codon

5771BP

5'

T312A

5' breakpoint

CCCGCAACTTCAAATTTGGCTCGAGGCTGT

deleted region

junction

3' breakpoint

3'

TTATGCTACAAATTAGTGCCTTGTAGCATG

CCCGCAACTTCAAATGTGCCTTGTAGCATG

**Fig. 225-3** Representation of the 3' end of the KAL gene and of the genomic region involved in a deletion detected in a family with X-linked Kallmann syndrome.[62] The sizes of the exons (open rectangles) and of the introns (solid lines) were derived by both sequencing and restriction mapping. The position of the stop codon at the end of KAL open reading frame is indicated. The 5' and 3' boundaries of the deleted region are indicated by hatched bars. The positions of two oligonucleotide primers (T312A and 5771BP) used for PCR amplification of the patient's DNA are indicated at the top. The sequences of 5' and the 3' deletion breakpoints in normal DNA are shown under each position. The nucleotides retained in the DNA of patients 1 and 2 are underlined. The sequence chromatogram of the junction fragment is shown at the bottom. The arrows indicate the breakpoints. (*From Bick et al.*[62] *Used by permission of The New England Journal of Medicine.*)

Mutation detection strategies have relied on a detailed characterization of the KAL gene structure. The KAL gene contains 14 exons spanning approximately 210 kb on Xp22.3.[63,64] The KAL homologue on the Y chromosome (KAL-Y) shares a very high degree of similarity with KAL but lacks exons 3, 8, and 9 and contains several stop and frameshift mutations (Fig. 225-4). This high degree of X-Y sequence similarity is present also in intronic regions and is not limited to KAL, but is shared by a large genomic region in which both the steroid sulfatase and KAL genes are located. In one patient with KS, it was demonstrated that

**Table 225-2** Molecules Sharing Homology with KAL

| 4-Disulfide Core Domain | Fibronectin Type III Repeat |
|---|---|
| Protease inhibitors | Neural-cell adhesion molecules |
|   Elafin |   Axonal glycoprotein TAG-1 |
|   Antileukoproteinase I |   Neural-cell adhesion molecule L1 |
|   ATPase inhibitor |   Neural-cell surface F3 |
|   Chelonianin |   contactin |
| Others |   Integrin $\beta$4 subunit |
|   Whey acidic protein | Protein kinases |
|   Neurophysin |   Twitchin |
|   WDNM (cDNA from |   Myosin-light-chain kinase |
|     nonmetastatic |   ROS proto-oncogene tyrosine kinase |
|     mammary adenocarcinoma) |   Insulin receptor-related receptor eck |
| | Tyrosine phosphatases |
| |   Leukocyte antigen-related protein |
| |   Protein-tyrosine-phosphatase delta |
| |   Protein-tyrosine-phosphatase DLAR |
| |   (Drosophila leukocyte common antigen related) |
| |   Protein-tyrosine-phosphatase DPTP |
| |   (Drosophila protein tyrosine phosphatase) |
| | Others |
| |   Fibronectin |
| |   Adenylate cyclase |
| |   C protein |

Bibliography is available in references 60 and 61.

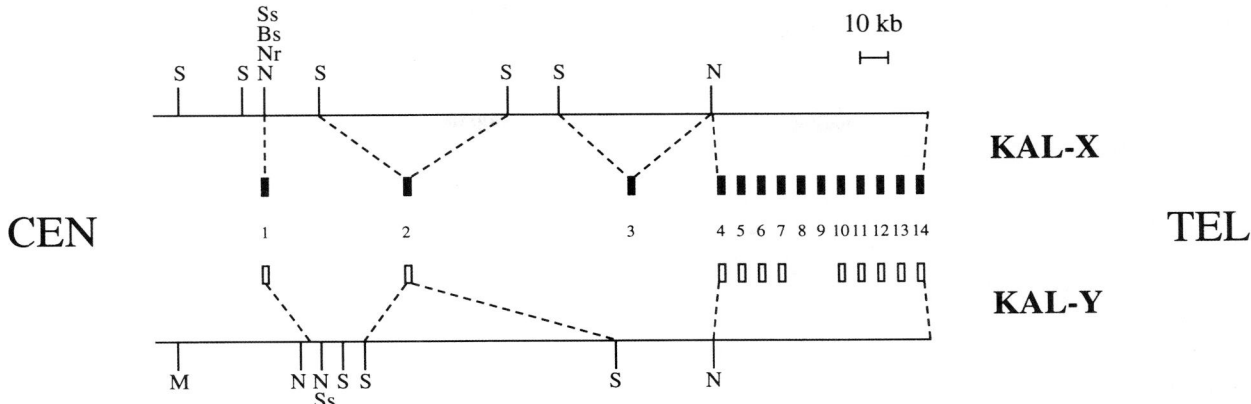

**Fig. 225-4** Genomic structure of KAL-X and KAL-Y.[63] The long-range restriction maps of the regions spanning KAL-X and KAL-Y were determined by PFGE on the YAC contigs. The restriction sites are: Bs = BssHII; M = MluI; N = NotI; Nr = NruI; S = SalI; Ss = SstI. Each exon of KAL-X and KAL-Y was localized within these maps by Southern blot analysis. Exons from KAL-X and KAL-Y are indicated as solid and open boxes, respectively. Dashed lines indicate the restriction fragment to which each exon has been localized. Exons 3, 8, and 9 are missing from KAL-Y. (*From Incerti et al.[63] Used by permission of Nature Genetics.*)

abnormal pairing and exchange between the X and Y copies of KAL resulted in an X/Y translocation, which created a nonfunctional KAL X/Y fusion gene.[79]

The presence of a nonfunctional KAL homologue on the Y chromosome hampered mutation-scanning strategies because most mutation-scanning strategies rely on the amplification of patients' genomic DNA. Therefore, primers and PCR conditions were carefully designed to minimize cross-amplification of Y-derived sequences[64] (and Meitinger T, et al., personal communication).

**Table 225-3** Mutations in the *KAL* Gene

| Patient | Nucleotide substitution | Amino acid change | Exon |
|---------|------------------------|-------------------|------|
| 1[*] | 711G > A | W237X | 5 |
| 2[*,†] | 769C > T | R257X | 6 |
| 3[*,†] | 774G > A | W258X | 6 |
| 4[*] | 1261C > T | Q421X | 9 |
| 5[*] | 1267C > T | R423X | 9 |
| 6[†] | 784C > T | R262X | 6 |
| 7[‡] | 984C > G | Y328X | 7 |
| 8[*] | 801T > A | N267K | 6 |
| 9[‡] | 1551C > G | F517L | 11 |
| 10[§] | 1540G > A | E514K | 11 |
| 11[*] | 831delC | fs | 6 |
| 12[*] | 1016–1017insA | fs | 7 |
| 13[†] | 1297–1298insAG | fs | 9 |
| 14[‡] | 1392–1405del | fs | 10 |
| 15[¶] | 1698delC | fs | 12 |
| 16[*] | IVS12-1G > A | sa | |
| 17[**] | IVS5-1G > T | sa | |
| 18[‡] | 1201–1207, IVS8+1+2del | sd | 8 |
| 19[††] | 102–103ins | fs | 1 |
| 20[¶] | deletion of exon 1 | | |
| 21[¶] | deletion exon 11 | | |
| 22[§] | deletion of exons 3–5 | | |

[*] mutations reported by Hardelin et al;[12], [†] T. Meitinger et al., personal communication; [‡] mutations reported by Georgopoulos et al;[81] [§] mutations reported by Maya-Nunez et al;[83] [¶] mutations reported by Quinton et al;[80] [**] mutations reported by O'Neill et al;[82] [††] mutation reported by Gu et al.[84] Abbreviations: fs = frameshift; sa = splice acceptor; sd = splice donor.

The results of mutation detection studies are summarized in Table 225-3[12,13,80–84] (and Meitinger T, et al., personal communication). A high degree of heterogeneity of mutations was found, although the same missense mutation, consisting of a G to A substitution at codon 514 turning glutamic acid into lysine, was recently identified in six unrelated patients of the same ethnic origin.[83] Several stop codon mutations were identified, probably representing null alleles and resulting in a complete loss of function of KAL protein. In some patients, missense and splice-site mutations were identified in regions of putative functional importance (based on sequence homology data). Some of the patients in whom point mutations were identified displayed, in addition to KS, mirror movements, pes cavus, high arched palate, and unilateral renal aplasia. This finding indicates that these additional features probably represent pleiotropic effects of KAL gene defects (see Table 225-1) and suggests that KAL plays a role in various developmental systems.[12,13]

Based on these data, molecular diagnosis can now be offered to families with X-linked KS in which a specific mutation is identified. In families in which the mutation has not yet been identified, male individuals can be tested for deletions by Southern blotting, using KAL cDNA as a probe before proceeding to sequence-based mutation detection. Patients with KS displaying complex phenotypes should undergo chromosome analysis, and their DNA should be tested with KAL and other Xp22.3 markers in order to detect a contiguous gene syndrome (see Chap. 65). There has been one report of prenatal diagnosis of KS in a fetus with a Xp22.3 contiguous-gene syndrome.[31]

## KAL FUNCTIONAL STUDIES AND A PATHOGENETIC MODEL OF KALLMANN SYNDROME

The characterization of the KAL spatiotemporal expression pattern has provided important clues to the understanding of the molecular pathogenesis of Kallmann syndrome. The chicken homologue of KAL (KALc) was isolated in order to study the developmental expression pattern of this gene.[65,85] The entire coding region of KALc was sequenced and compared to its human homologue.[65] The predicted protein product of KALc shows 77 percent amino acid identity with the human protein (84 percent when conservative substitutions are included); this value increases to over 90 percent in regions spanning the putative functional domains.[65]

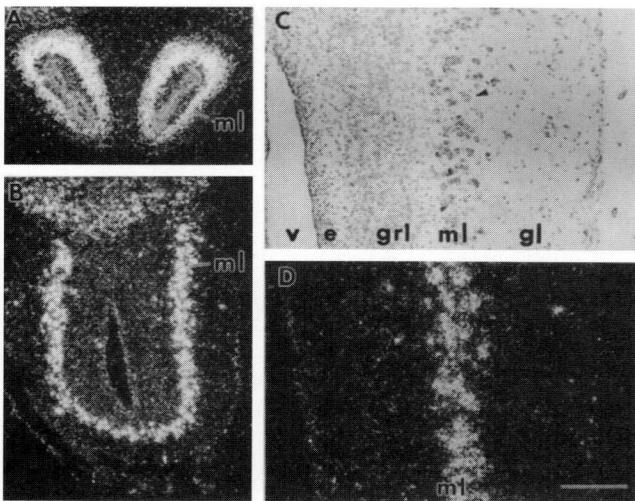

**Fig. 225-5 Expression of the chicken Kallmann syndrome gene (KALc) during the development of the olfactory system.**[65] *A,* Transverse section through both olfactory bulbs of a 7.5-day-old chick embryo. In situ hybridization reveals high levels of KALc expression in the mitral cell layer. *B,* Transverse section through the olfactory bulb of a newly hatched chicken (21 days). *C,* Neighboring section of panel D stained with thionin. *D,* Enlarged view of panel B. The KALc-positive area in the olfactory bulb corresponds to the mitral-cell layer. e = ependymal layer; gl = glomerular layer; grl = granule-cell layer; ml = mitral-cell layer; v = lateral ventricle. Scale bar is equal to 100 μm for panels C and D and to 250 μm for panels A and B. (*From Rugarli et al.*[65] *Used by permission of Nature Genetics.*)

RNA in situ hybridization studies were performed in chick embryos using KALc as a probe (Fig. 225-5).[65,85] Neither the olfactory epithelium nor the meningeal tissue through which the olfactory axons migrate expresses the gene at any developmental stage. Within the olfactory system, KALc expression was first detected in the presumptive bulb region at day 7 of chick embryonal development. As the olfactory bulb acquires its characteristic structure, KALc expression increases and persists in adult chickens. In the bulb, the gene is expressed by the mitral cells, which are the secondary sensory neurons forming synapses with the olfactory axons. Up-regulation of transcription is seen when the first synaptic contacts between the olfactory axons and mitral cells are established. KAL expression in the olfactory bulb was found to be independent of innervation from the olfactory nerve, as shown by experiments in which the chick olfactory placode was removed early during development[86] (Fig. 225-6).

Prominent expression was also found in the Purkinje cells of the cerebellum.[65,85] This pattern of expression could be related to the occurrence of cerebellar symptoms in KS patients. Multiple additional sites of KALc expression were detected, both within and outside the nervous system. During early chick development KAL expression was shown in various endodermal and mesodermal derivatives.[87] In the brain, KALc mRNA was detected in the oculomotor nucleus primordium, ectostriatum, trigeminal motor nucleus, and choroid plexus. Other tissues expressing KALc include the developing limb buds, mesonephros and metanephros, facial mesenchyme, and retina.[65,85,88]

KAL expression in human was detected as early as day 45 of embryonic development by RT-PCR in the spinal cord, mesonephros, and metanephros.[89] In situ hybridization of older fetuses (11- and 19-weeks old) revealed expression in both the olfactory bulb and the cerebellum.[86,89] Table 225-4 shows a tentative correlation between some of the sites of KAL expression and KS symptoms.

Additional insights into the putative function of KAL were obtained by biochemical characterization of the protein. Features of the predicted KAL protein, such as the presence of a leader peptide and the absence of transmembrane domains, or of sequences indicative of a phosphoinositol linkage to the membrane, suggested that it was secreted in the extracellular matrix. This was then demonstrated by overexpressing the KAL protein in eukaryotic cells and by analyzing the endogenous protein with specific antibodies. KAL is a glycosylated protein with an apparent electrophoresis motility of approximately 100 kDa[90,91] (Fig. 225-7). The protein is secreted in the extracellular matrix, where it behaves as a peripheral membrane protein. Heparan-sulfate glycosaminoglycans were shown to be

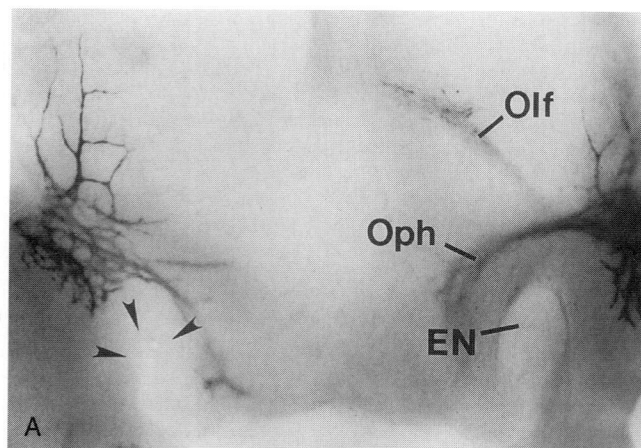

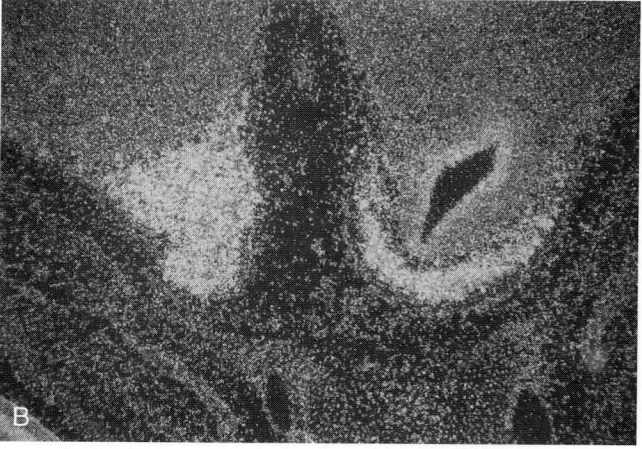

**Fig. 225-6 Effect of olfactory placode removal on the development of the chicken olfactory system and on the expression of KALc in the olfactory bulb.** *A,* Manipulated chick embryo analyzed at stage 25 by whole-mount immunostaining of the head using the antibody 3A10, which recognizes a neurofilament-associated protein. The olfactory nerve (Olf) is completely missing from the experimental side (left) and the external nares (EN) is smaller than on the control side. *B,* Manipulated embryo subjected to in situ hybridization at stage 36. The normal KALc expression pattern in the mitral cell layer of the olfactory bulb is seen on the control side (right). KALc is highly expressed on the manipulated side (left) in a stunted protrusion (*From Lutz et al.*[85] *Used by permission of Human Molecular Genetics.*)

**Table 225-4 Tentative Correlation Between *KAL* Expression Pattern and Kallmann Syndrome Phenotype**

| Expression Pattern | | Clinical Features |
|---|---|---|
| Olfactory bulb (mitral cells) | ↔ | Anosmia |
| Cerebellum (Purkinje cells) | ↔ | Cerebellar dysfunction |
| Oculomotor nucleus | ↔ | Eye-movement defects |
| Mesonephros/metanephros | ↔ | Unilateral renal aplasia |
| Facial mesenchyme | ↔ | Cleft palate |

ligands of the protein in a cell expression system.[91] Function of the KAL protein might therefore be regulated through binding to proteoglycans, as has been shown for other extracellular matrix (ECM) molecules. In cell expression systems, KAL protein undergoes proteolytic cleavage to yield a diffusible component[90,91] (Fig. 225-7). Although this processing has been observed so far only in cell culture conditions, it is closely reminiscent of that previously demonstrated in cell adhesion molecules with FNIII repeats, such as the chick Bravo/NrCAM,[92] neurofascin,[93] and Ng-CAM[94] molecules, and the mouse L1.[95] Distribution of the KAL protein in chick was analyzed by immunohistochemistry in the cerebellum, olfactory bulb, striatum, and optic tectum. Strong labeling was found to be restricted to definitive neuronal cell populations, such as Purkinje cells in the cerebellum and mitral cells in the olfactory bulb, both on cell bodies and axonal processes, thus confirming previous finding by RNA in situ hybridization[91] (Fig. 225-8). A recent study showed that KAL is an adhesion molecule for a variety of neuronal and non-neuronal cell types in vitro.[96] The adhesion properties of KAL appear to be dependent on the presence of heparan sulfate and chondroitin

sulfate glycosaminoglucans at the cell surface and to be mainly attributed to a 32 amino acid sequence located within the first fibronectin-like type III repeat of the protein. The same study reports that purified KAL protein, when absorbed to a culture dish, can promote attachment of mouse cerebellar neurons and stimulate axon outgrowth. However, when neurons were plated on stable cell lines producing KAL, an overall decrease in axon extension was noted. One possible explanation for these findings is that KAL may act to stimulate axon growth when added to cultures in a uniform concentration, but when provided as a discontinuous substrate in high local concentrations may induce cessation of axon growth.

KS was the first neuronal migration defect in vertebrates for which the gene has been identified. Since then, the genes for X-linked hydrocephalus,[97,98] lissencephaly/Miller-Dieker,[99] X-linked lissencephaly, and double-cortex syndrome[100,101] have been isolated. Although the molecules involved in these diseases are all very different, it is intriguing that X-linked hydrocephalus is due to mutations in L1, which is a cell-adhesion molecule with FNIII repeats. Despite an enormous amount of knowledge that has accumulated in the last few years on diffusible guidance cues playing a role in axon guidance,[102] the mechanism by which lack of KAL causes defective targeting of olfactory axons and migration of GnRH neurons remains elusive.

Fig. 225-9 depicts a tentative pathogenic model for KS. According to this model, the primary defect in KS is an abnormality of olfactory system development that affects axonal targeting and/or synaptogenesis, rather than neuronal migration directly. KAL protein may be a substrate adhesion molecule of the extracellular matrix mediating interactions between dendrites of mitral cells in the olfactory bulb and incoming olfactory axons. Because these interactions are essential for olfactory bulb morphogenesis, the absence of KAL prevents the bulb from acquiring its normal structure. The migration defect of GnRH

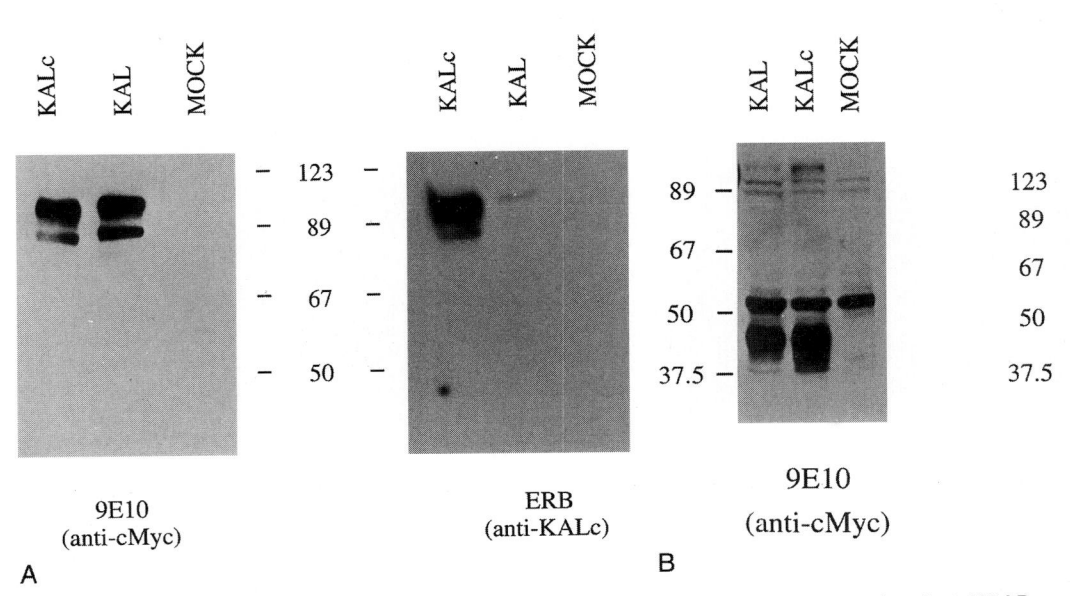

**Fig. 225-7 Biochemical analysis of recombinant KAL *A,* Western blot analysis of peripheral membrane proteins isolated from COS 7 cells transfected with the pMT21-KAL^myc and pMT21-KALc^myc constructs and from Mock-transfected cells. Analysis was carried out with Mab 9E10 directed against the myc tag, and with anti-KAL-specific antisera (ERB). KAL and KALc are detected as two distinct bands with an apparent molecular weight of 100 and 85 kDa with each antibody. The ERB antisera cross reacts at low affinity with the human KAL protein: by overexposing the blot, it is possible to distinguish the most abundant 100 kDa component. *B,* Western blot analysis of glycoproteins secreted in the conditioned medium from COS 7 cells transfected with the pMT21-KAL^myc and pMT21-KALc^myc constructs and from Mock-transfected cells. Analysis was carried out with Mab 9E10 and ERB antisera. Both Mab 9E10 and ERB antisera detect an abundant secreted 45-kDa glycoprotein in transfected cells. A very low amount of the 100 kDa KAL and KALc component is detected with the 9E10 Mab. (*From Rugarli et al.*[89] *Used by permission of Human Molecular Genetics.)*

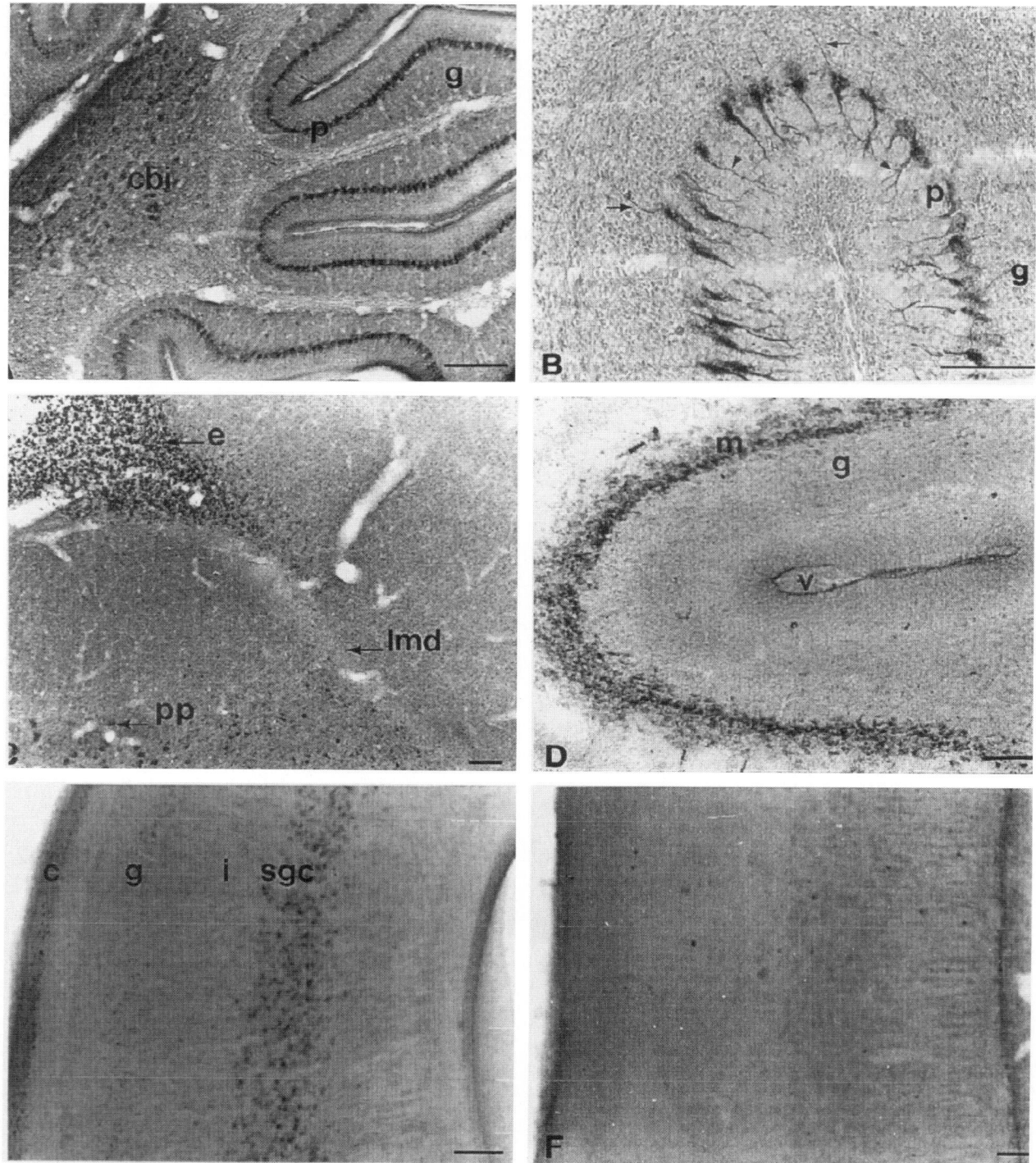

**Fig. 225-8** Distribution of KALc protein in several structures of the central nervous system of the chick embryo at ED 18. *A* and *B*, In the cerebellar cortex, the immunostaining is restricted to the Purkinje cells (p); the soma, the axon (arrows) and the dendrites (arrowheads) of these neurons are labeled. Several cell bodies in the nucleus cerebellaris internus (cbi) are stained. g = granular layer. *C*, In the striatum, the labeling concerns ectostriatum (e) and paleostriatum primitivum (pp). lmd = lamina medullaris dorsalis. *D*, In the olfactory bulb, only the mitral cell body layer (m) is labeled. g = granular layer; v = ventricule. *E* and *F*, In the tectum, the labeling is restricted to the stratum griseum centrale (sgc) and to laminae c, g, and i of the stratum griseum et fibrosum superficiale. Bars = 100 μm. (*From Soussi-Yanicostas et al.*[90] *Used by permission of Journal of Cell Science.*)

neurons in KS would, therefore, be a secondary effect caused by lack of a "migration route" for GnRH neuronal migration that is normally provided by the contact between olfactory nerves and forebrain.[88,103] It is likely that several different molecules are involved in the establishment of proper interactions between olfactory axons and the olfactory bulb and in the migration process of GnRH neurons. For example, immunohistochemical data suggest that the neural-cell adhesion molecule NCAM plays a role in the formation of a scaffold of cells and axons that link the olfactory epithelium with the forebrain.[104] The genes involved in

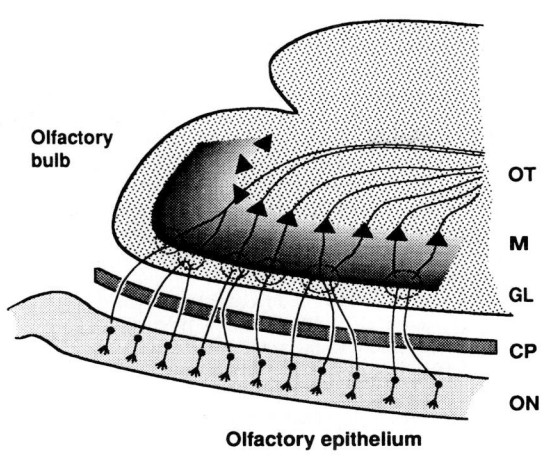
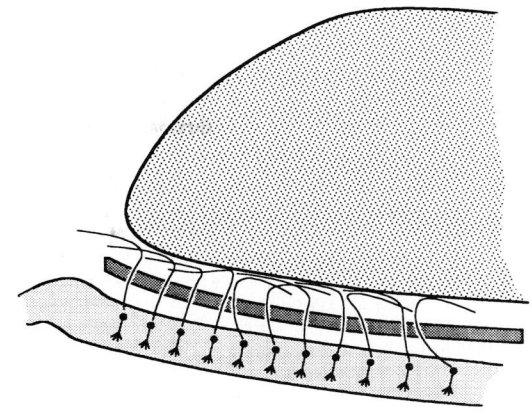

## NORMAL

Fig. 225-9 Model for KAL function and KS pathogenesis. In normal individual axons of olfactory neurons (ON) traverse the cribriform plate (CP) to reach the olfactory bulb. Within the glomerular layer of the bulb (GL), they make synapses with dendrites of mitral cells (M), whose axons will form the olfactory tracts (OT). A tentative model is proposed in which the KAL protein (shaded area) is secreted by the mitral cells and is required in the glomerular layer for the establishment/maintenance of proper interactions with olfactory axons. In

## KALLMANN SYNDROME

KS, KAL protein is absent; therefore, olfactory axons cannot interact properly with their target, ending their migration between the cribriform plate and the forebrain. The migration defect of GnRH neurons in KS would be a secondary effect caused by lack of contact between olfactory nerves and forebrain, resulting in the absence of a "migration route." (*From Rugarli and Ballabio.[101] Used by permission of the Journal of the American Medical Association.*)

the autosomal types of Kallmann syndrome may encode additional factors participating in this fascinating developmental system.

## ACKNOWLEDGMENTS

We thank Drs. B. Lutz, and G. Eichele for helpful comments and for providing Fig. 225-5, and Dr. C. Petit for providing Fig. 225-8.

## REFERENCES

1. Maestre de San Juan A: Teratologia: Falta total de los nervios olfactorios con anosmian en un individuo en quien existia un atrofia congentia de los testiculos y miembro viril. *El Siglo Med* **3**:211, 1856.
2. de Morsier G: Etudes sur les dysraphies cranio-encephaliques. 1. Agenesie des lobes olfactifs (telencephaloschizis lateral) et des commissures calleuse et anterieure (telencephaloschizis median). La dysplasie olfacto-genitale. *Schweiz Arch Neurol Neurochir Psychiat* **74**:309, 1954.
3. de Morsier G: Median cranioencephalic dysraphias and olfactogenital dysplasia. *World Neurol* **3**:485, 1962.
4. Kallmann F, Schoenfeld WA, Barrera SE: The genetic aspects of primary eunuchoidism. *Am J Ment Defic* **48**:203, 1944.
5. Naftolin F, Harris GW, Bobrow M: Effect of purified luteinizing hormone releasing factor on normal and hypogonadotropic anosmic men. *Nature* **232**:496, 1971.
6. Griffin JE, Wilson JD: Disorders of the testes and the male reproductive tract, in Wilson JD, Foster DW (eds): *Williams Textbook of Endocrinology,* 8th ed. Philadelphia, WB Saunders, 1992, p 822.
7. Turner RC, Bobrow LG, MacKinnon PCB, Bonnar J, Hockaday TDR, Ellis JD: Cryptorchidism in a family with Kallmann's syndrome. *Proc R Soc Med* **67**:33, 1974.
8. Wegenke JD, Uehling DT, Wear JB Jr, Gordon ES, Bargman JG, Deacon JSR, Herrmann JPR, Opitz JM: Familial Kallmann syndrome with unilateral renal aplasia. *Clin Genet* **7**:368, 1975.
9. White BJ, Rogol AD, Brown SK, Lieblich JM, Rosen SW: The syndrome of anosmia with hypogonadotropic hypogonadism: A genetic study of 18 new families and a review. *Am J Med Genet* **15**:417, 1983.
10. Sunohara N, Sakuragawa N, Satoyoshi E, Tanae A, Shapiro LJ: A new syndrome of anosmia, ichthyosis, hypogonadism, and various neurological manifestations with deficiency of steroid sulfatase and arylsulfatase C. *Ann Neurol* **19**:174, 1986.
11. Schwankhaus JD, Currie J, Jaffe MJ, Rose SR, Sherins RJ: Neurologic findings in men with isolated hypogonadotropic hypogonadism. *Neurology* **39**:223, 1989.
12. Hardelin J-P, Levilliers J, Blanchard S, Carel J-C, Leutenegger M, Pinard-Bertelletto J-P, Bouloux P, Petit C: Heterogeneity in the mutations responsible for X chromosome-linked Kallmann syndrome. *Hum Mol Genet* **2**:373, 1993.
13. Hardelin J-P, Levilliers J, del Castillo I, Cohen-Salmon M, Legouis R, Blanchard S, Compain S, Bouloux P, Kirk J, Moraine C, Chaussain J-L, Weissenbach J, Petit C: X chromosome-linked Kallmann syndrome: Stop mutations validate the candidate gene. *Proc Natl Acad Sci U S A* **89**:8190, 1992.
14. Nass R: Mirror movement asymmetries in congenital hemiparesis: The inhibition hypothesis revisited. *Neurology* **35**:1059, 1985.
15. Danek A, Heye B, Schroedter R: Cortically evoked motor responses in patients with Xp22.3-linked Kallmann's syndrome and in female gene carriers. *Ann Neurol* **31**:299, 1992.
16. Mayston MJ, Harrison LM, Quinton R, Stephens JA, Krams M, Bouloux P-MG: Mirror movements in X-linked Kallmann's syndrome: I. A neurophysiological study. *Brain* **120**:1199, 1997.
17. Krams M, Quinton R, Mayston MJ, Harrison LM, Dolan RJ, Bouloux P-MG, Stephens JA, Frackowiak RSJ, Passingham RE: Mirror movements in X-linked Kallmann's syndrome: II. A PET study. *Brain* **120**:1217, 1997.
18. Leinsinger GL, Heiss DT, Jassoy AG, Pfluger T, Hahn K, Danek A: Persistent mirror movements: Functional MR imaging of the hand motor cortex. *Radiology* **203**:545, 1997.
19. Kertzman C, Robinson DL, Sherins RJ, Schwankhaus JD, McClurkin JW: Abnormalities in visual spacial attention in men with mirror movements associated with isolated hypogonadotropic hypogonadism. *Neurology* **40**:1057, 1990.
20. Tuck RR, O'Neill BP, Gharib H, Mulder DW: Familial spastic paraplegia with Kallmann's syndrome. *J Neurol Neurosurg Psychiatry* **46**:671, 1983.
21. Cortez AB, Galindo A, Arensman FW, Van Dop C: Congenital heart disease associated with sporadic Kallmann syndrome. *Am J Med Genet* **46**:551, 1993.
22. Ballabio A, Andria G: Deletions and translocations involving the distal short arm of the human X chromosome: review and hypotheses. *Hum Mol Genet* **1**:221, 1992.
23. Henkin RI, Bartter FC: Studies on olfactory thresholds in normal man and in patients with adrenal cortical insufficiency: The role of adrenal cortical steroids and of serum sodium concentration. *J Clin Invest* **45**:1631, 1966.

24. *The Smell Identification Test Administration Manual.* Haddonfield, NJ, Sensonics, 1983.

25. Spratt DI, Carr DB, Merriam GR, Scully RE, Rao PN, Crowley WF Jr: The spectrum of abnormal patterns of gonadotropin-releasing hormone secretion in men and idiopathic hypogonadotropic hypogonadism: Clinical and laboratory correlations. *J Clin Endocrinol Metab* **64**:283, 1987.

26. Giusti M, Cavagnaro P: Update on pulsatile luteinizing hormone-releasing hormone therapy in males with idiopathic hypogonadotropic hypogonadism and delayed puberty. *J Endocrinol Invest* **14**:419, 1991.

27. Saal W, Happ J, Cordes U, Baum RP, Schmidt M: Subcutaneous gonadotropin therapy in male patients with hypogonadotropic hypogonadism. *Fertil Steril* **56**:319, 1991.

28. Hurley DM, Clarke IJ, Shelton R, Burger HG: Subcutaneous administration of gonadotropin-releasing hormone: Absorption kinetics and gonadotropin responses. *J Clin Endocrinol Metab* **65**:46, 1987.

29. Males JL, Townsend JL, Schneider RA: Hypogonadotropic hypogonadism with anosmia- Kallmann's syndrome. *Arch Intern Med* **131**: 501, 1973.

30. Schwanzel-Fukuda M, Bick D, Pfaff DW: Luteinizing hormone-releasing hormone (LHRH)-expressing cells do not migrate normally in an inherited hypogonadal (Kallmann) syndrome. *Molec Brain Res* **6**:311, 1989.

31. Bick DP, Schorderet DF, Price PA, Campbell L, Huff RW, Shapiro LJ, Moore CM: Prenatal diagnosis and investigation of a fetus with chondrodysplasia punctata, ichthyosis, and Kallmann syndrome due to an Xp deletion. *Prenat Diagn* **12**:19, 1992.

32. Schwob JE, Leopold DA, Mieleszko-Szumowski KE, Emko P: Histopathology of olfactory mucosa in Kallmann's syndrome. *Ann Otol Rhinol Laryngol* **102**:117, 1993.

33. Rawson NE, Brand JG, Cowart BJ, Lowry LD, Pribitkin EA, Rao VM, Restrepo D: Functionally mature olfactory neurons from two anosmic patients with Kallmann syndrome. *Brain Res* **681**:58, 1995.

34. Schwanzel-Fukuda M, Pfaff DW: Origin of luteinizing hormone-releasing hormone neurons. *Nature* **338**:161, 1989.

35. Wray S, Grant P, Gainer H: Evidence that cells expressing luteinizing hormone-releasing hormone mRNA in the mouse are derived from progenitor cells in the olfactory placode. *Proc Natn Acad Sci U S A* **86**:8132, 1989.

36. Klingmüller D, Dewes W, Krahe T, Brecht G, Schweikert H-U: Magnetic resonance imaging of the brain in patients with anosmia and hypothalamic hypogonadism (Kallmann's syndrome). *J Clin Endocrinol Metab* **65**:581, 1987.

37. Truwit CL, Barkovich AJ, Grumbach MM, Martini JJ: MR imaging of Kallmann syndrome, a genetic disorder of neuronal migration affecting the olfactory and genital systems. *Am J Neuroradiol* **14**:827, 1993.

38. Knorr JR, Ragland RL, Brown RS, Gelber N: Kallmann's syndrome: MR findings. *Am J Neuroradiol* **14**:845, 1993.

39. Bick DP, Ballabio A: Bringing Kallmann syndrome into focus. *Am J Neuroradiol* **14**:852, 1993.

40. Jones J, Kemman E: Olfacto-genital dysplasia in the female. *Obstet Gynecol Annu* **5**:443, 1976.

41. Hermanussen M, Sippell WG: Heterogeneity of Kallmann's syndrome. *Clin Genet* **28**:106, 1985.

42. Hipkin LJ, Casson IF, Davis JC: Identical twins discordant for Kallmann's syndrome. *J Med Genet* **27**:198, 1990.

43. Parenti G, Carrozzo R, Ghezzi M, Di Maio S, Ballabio A, Andria G: Molecular studies on the clinical heterogeneity in a family with X-linked ichthyosis and Kallmann syndrome. *Am J Hum Genet* **49(Supp)**:155, 1991.

44. Parenti G, Rizzolo MG, Ghezzi M, Di Maio S, Sperandeo MP, Incerti B, Franco B, Ballabio A, Andria G: Variable penetrance of hypogonadism in a sibship with Kallmann syndrome due to a deletion of the KAL gene. *Am J Med Genet* **57**:476, 1995.

45. Best LG, Wasdahl WA, Larson LM, Sturlaugson J: Chromosome abnormality in Kallmann syndrome. *Am J Med Genet* **35**:306, 1990.

46. Ventruto V, Cali A, Farina L, Festa B, Ricciardi I, Sebastio L: A case of hypogonadotrophic hypogonadism with anosmia (Kallmann's syndrome) in a male, with familial incidence of a small metacentric chromosome (47, XY, mat?+). *J Med Genet* **13**:71, 1976.

47. Casamassima AC, Wilmot PL, Vibert BK, Shapiro LR: Kallmann syndrome associated with complex chromosome rearrangement. *Am J Med Genet* **45**:539, 1993.

48. Schinzel A, Lorda-Sanchez I, Binkert F, Carter NP, Bebb CE, Ferguson-Smith MA, Eiholzer U, Zachmann M, Robinson WP:

Kallmann syndrome in a boy with a t(1;10) translocation detected by reverse chromosome painting. *J Med Genet* **32**:957, 1995.

49. Lynch HT, Ozer F, McNutt CW, Johnson JE, Jampolsky NA: Secondary male hypogonadism and congenital ichthyosis: Association of two rare genetic diseases. *Am J Hum Genet* **12**:440, 1960.

50. Perrin JCS, Idemoto JY, Sotos JF, Maurer WF, Steinberg AG: X-linked syndrome of congenital ichthyosis, hypogonadism, mental retardation and anosmia. *Birth Defects* **XII**:267, 1976.

51. Abe K, Matsuda I, Matsuura N, Murayama T, Uzuki K, Endo M, Miyakoshi M, Okuno A: X-linked ichthyosis, bilateral cryptorchidism, hypogenitalism and mental retardation in two siblings. *Clin Genet* **9**:341, 1976.

52. Tiepolo L, Zuffardi O, Fraccaro M, di Natale D, Gargantini L, Müller CR, Ropers H-H: Assignment by deletion mapping of the steroid sulfatase X-linked ichthyosis locus to Xp22.3. *Hum Genet* **54**:205, 1980.

53. Metaxotou C, Ikkos D, Panagiotopoulou P, Alevizaki M, Mavrou A, Tsenghi C, Matsaniotis N: A familial X/Y translocation in a boy with ichthyosis, hypogonadism and mental retardation. *Clin Genet* **24**:380, 1983.

54. Andria G, Ballabio A, Parenti G, Di Maio S, Piccirillo A: Steroid sulphatase deficiency is present in patients with the syndrome "Ichthyosis and male hypogonadism" and with "Rud syndrome." *J Inherit Metab Dis* **7**:159, 1984.

55. Ballabio A, Parenti G, Tippett P, Mondello C, Di Maio S, Tenore A, Andria G: X-linked ichthyosis due to steroid sulphatase deficiency associated with Kallmann syndrome (hypogonadotropic hypogonadism and anosmia): Linkage relationships with Xg and cloned DNA sequences from the distal short arm of the X chromosome. *Hum Genet* **72**:237, 1986.

56. Ballabio A, Parenti G, Carrozzo R, Sebastio G, Andria G, Buckle V, Fraser N, Craig I, Rocchi M, Romeo G, Jobsis AC, Persico MG: Isolation and characterization of a steroid sulphatase cDNA clone: Genomic deletions in patients with X-chromosome-linked ichthyosis. *Proc Nat Acad Sci U S A* **84**:4519, 1987.

57. Ballabio A, Sebastio G, Carrozzo R, Parenti G, Piccirillo A, Persico MG, Andria G: Deletions of the steroid sulphatase gene in "classical" X-linked ichthyosis and in X-linked ichthyosis associated with Kallmann syndrome. *Hum Genet* **77**:338, 1987.

58. Meitinger T, Heye B, Petit C, Levilliers J, Golla A, Moraine C, Dallapiccola B, Sippell WG, Murken J, Ballabio A: Definitive localization of X-linked Kallman syndrome (hypogonadotropic hypogonadism and anosmia) to Xp22.3: Close linkage to the hypervariable repeat sequence CRI-S232. *Am J Hum Genet* **47**:664, 1990.

59. Ballabio A, Bardoni B, Carrozzo R, Andria G, Bick D, Campbell L, Hamel B, Ferguson-Smith MA, Gimelli G, Fraccaro M, Maraschio P, Zuffardi O, Guioli S, Camerino G: Contiguous gene syndromes due to deletions in the distal short arm of the human X chromosome. *Proc Natl Acad Sci U S A* **86**:10001, 1989.

60. Franco B, Guioli S, Pragliola A, Incerti B, Bardoni B, Tonlorenzi R, Carrozzo R, Maestrini E, Pieretti M, Taillon-Miller P, Brown CJ, Willard HF, Lawrence C, Persico MG, Camerino G, Ballabio A: A gene deleted in Kallmann's syndrome shares homology with neural cell adhesion and axonal path-finding molecules. *Nature* **353**:529, 1991.

61. Legouis R, Hardelin J-P, Levilliers J, Claverie J-M, Compain S, Wunderle V, Millasseau P, Le Paslier D, Cohen D, Caterina D, Bougueleret L, Delemarre-Van de Waal H, Lutfalla G, Weissenbach J, Petit C: The candidate gene for the X-linked Kallmann syndrome encodes a protein related to adhesion molecules. *Cell* **67**:423, 1991.

62. Bick D, Franco B, Sherins RJ, Heye B, Pike L, Crawford J, Maddalena A, Incerti B, Pragliola A, Meitinger T, Ballabio A: Intragenic deletion of the *KALIG-1* gene in Kallmann's syndrome. *N Engl J Med* **326**:1752, 1992.

63. Incerti B, Guioli S, Pragliola A, Zanaria E, Borsani G, Tonlorenzi R, Bardoni B, Franco B, Wheeler D, Ballabio A, Camerino G: Kallmann syndrome gene on the X and Y chromosomes: Implications for evolutionary divergence of human sex chromosomes. *Nat Genet* **2**:311, 1992.

64. del Castillo I, Cohen-Salmon M, Blanchard S, Lutfalla G, Petit C: Structure of the X-linked Kallmann syndrome gene and its homologous pseudogene on the Y chromosome. *Nat Genet* **2**:305, 1992.

65. Rugarli EI, Lutz B, Kuratani SC, Wawersik S, Borsani G, Ballabio A, Eichele G: Expression pattern of the Kallmann syndrome gene in the olfactory system suggests a role in neuronal targeting. *Nat Genet* **4**:19, 1993.

66. Drenth J, Low BM, Richardson JS, Wright CS: The toxin-agglutinin fold. *J Biol Chem* **255**:2652, 1980.

67. McGuire PG, Seeds NW: Degradation of underlying extracellular matrix by sensory neurons during neurite outgrowth. *Neuron* 4:633, 1990.
68. Monard D: Cell-derived proteases and protease inhibitors as regulators of neurite outgrowth. *Trends Neurosci* 11:541, 1988.
69. Letourneau PC, Condic ML, Snow DM: Extracellular matrix and neurite outgrowth. *Curr Opin Genet Dev* 2:625, 1992.
70. Osterwalder T, Contartese J, Stoeckli ET, Kuhn TB, Sonderegger P: Neuroserpin, an axonally secreted serine protease inhibitor. *EMBO J* 15:2944, 1996.
71. Krueger SR, Ghisu G-P, Cinelli P, Gschwend TP, Osterwalder T, Wolfer DP, Sonderegger P: Expression of neuroserpin, an inhibitor of tissue plasminogen activator, in the developing and adult nervous system of the mouse. *J Neurosci* 17:8984, 1997.
72. Lüthi A, van der Putten H, Botteri FM, Mansuy IM, Meins M, Frey U, Sansig G, Portet C, Schmutz M, Schröder M, Nitsch C, Laurent J-P, Monard D: Endogenous serine protease inhibitor modulates epileptic activity and hippocampal long-term potentiation. *J Neurosci* 17:4688, 1997.
73. Lander AD: Understanding the molecules of neural cell contacts: Emerging patterns of structure and function. *Trends Neurosci* 12:189, 1989.
74. Fischer EH, Charbonneau H, Tonks NK: Protein tyrosine phosphatases: a diverse family of intracellular and transmembrane enzymes. *Science* 253:401, 1991.
75. Dodd J, Jessell TM: Axon guidance and the patterning of neuronal projections in vertebrates. *Science* 242:692, 1988.
76. Reichardt LF, Tomaselli KJ: Extracellular matrix molecules and their receptors: Functions in neural development. *Ann Rev Neurosci* 14:531, 1991.
77. Chiquet M, Wehrle-Haller B, Koch M: Tenascin (cytotactin): An extracellular matrix protein involved in morphogenesis of the nervous system. *Semin Neurosci* 3:341, 1991.
78. Hynes RO, Lander AD: Contact and adhesive specificities in the associations, migrations, and targeting of cells and axons. *Cell* 68:303, 1992.
79. Guioli S, Incerti B, Zanaria E, Bardoni B, Franco B, Taylor K, Ballabio A, Camerino G: Kallmann syndrome due to a translocation resulting in an X/Y fusion gene. *Nat Genet* 1:337, 1992.
80. Quinton R, Duke VM, de Zoysa PA, Platts AD, Valentine A, Kendall B, Pickman S, Kirk JM, Besser GM, Jacobs HS, Bouloux PM: The neuroradiology of Kallmann's syndrome: A genotypic and phenotypic analysis [published erratum appears in *J Clin Endocrinol Metab* 81(10):3614, 1996]. *J Clin Endocrinol Metab* 81:3010, 1996.
81. Georgopoulos NA, Pralong FP, Seidman CE, Seidman JG, Crowley WF Jr, Vallejo M: Genetic heterogeneity evidenced by low incidence of KAL-1 gene mutations in sporadic cases of gonadotropin-releasing hormone deficiency. *J Clin Endocrinol Metab* 82:213, 1997.
82. O'Neill MJ, Tridjaja B, Smith MJ, Bell KM, Warne GL, Sinclair AH: Familial Kallmann syndrome: A novel splice acceptor mutation in the KAL gene. *Hum Mutat* 11:340, 1998.
83. Maya-Nunez G, Zenteno JC, Ulloa-Aguirre A, Kofman-Alfaro S, Mendez JP: A recurrent missense mutation in the KAL gene in patients with X-linked Kallmann's syndrome. *J Clin Endocrinol Metab* 83:1650, 1998.
84. Gu W-X, Colquhoun-Kerr JS, Knopp P, Bode HH, Jameson JL: A novel aminoterminal mutation in the KAL-1 gene in a large pedigree with X-linked Kallmann syndrome. *Mol Genet Metab* 65:59, 1998.
85. Legouis R, Ayer-Le Lievre C, Leibovici M, Lapointe F, Petit C: Expression of the KAL gene in multiple neuronal sites during chicken development. *Proc Nat Acad Sci U S A* 90:2461, 1993.
86. Lutz B, Kurantani S, Rugarli EI, Wawersik S, Wong C, Bieber FR, Ballabio A, Eichele G: Expression of the Kallmann syndrome gene in human fetal brain and in the manipulated chick embryo. *Hum Mol Genet* 3:1717, 1994.

87. Legouis R, Hardelin JP, Petit C, Ayer Le Lievre C: Early expression of the KAL gene during embryonic development of the chick. *Anat Embryol (Berl)* 190:549, 1994.
88. Lutz B, Rugarli EI, Eichele G, Ballabio A: X-linked Kallmann syndrome: A neuronal targeting defect in the olfactory system? *FEBS Lett* 325:128, 1993.
89. Duke VM, Winyard PJD, Thorogood P, Soothill P, Bouloux PMG, Woolf AS: *KAL*, a gene mutated in Kallmann's syndrome, is expressed in the first trimester of human development. *Mol Cell Endocrinol* 110:73, 1995.
90. Rugarli EI, Ghezzi C, Valsecchi V, Ballabio A: The Kallmann syndrome gene product expressed in COS cells is cleaved on the cell surface to yield a diffusible component. *Hum Mol Genet* 5:1109, 1996.
91. Soussi-Yanicostas N, Hardelin J-P, del Mar Arroyo-Jimenez M, Ardouin O, Legouis R, Levilliers J, Traincard F, Betton J-M, Cabanie L, Petit C: Initial characterization of anosmin-1, a putative extracellular matrix protein synthesized by definite neuronal cell population in the central nervous system. *J Cell Sci* 109:1749, 1996.
92. Kayyem JF, Roman JM, de la Rosa EJ, Schwarz U, Dreyer WJ: Bravo/Nr-CAM is closely related to the cell adhesion molecules L1 and Ng-CAM and has a similar heterodimer structure. *J Cell Biol* 118:1259, 1992.
93. Volkmer H, Hassel B, Wolff JM, Frank R, Rathjen FG: Structure of the axonal surface recognition molecule neurofascin and its relationship to a neural subgroup of the immunoglobulin superfamily. *J Cell Biol* 118:149, 1992.
94. Burgoon MP, Grumet M, Mauro V, Edelman GM, Cunningham BA: Structure of the chicken neuron-glia cell adhesion molecule, Ng-CAM: Origin of the polypeptides and relation to the Ig superfamily. *J Cell Biol* 112:1017, 1991.
95. Faissner A, Teplow DB, Kübler D, Keilhauer G, Kinzel V, Schachner M: Biosynthesis and membrane topography of the neural cell adhesion molecule L1. *EMBO J* 4:3105, 1985.
96. Soussi-Yanicostas N, Faivre-Sarrailh C, Hardelin J-P, Levilliers J, Rougon G, Petit C: Anosmin-1 underlying the X chromosome-linked Kallmann syndrome is an adhesion molecule that can modulate neurite growth in a cell-type specific manner. *J Cell Sci* 111:2953, 1998.
97. Rosenthal A, Jouet M, Kenwrick S: Aberrant splicing of neural cell adhesion molecule L1 mRNA in a family with X-linked hydrocephalus. *Nat Genet* 2:107, 1992.
98. Van Camp G, Vits L, Coucke P, Lyonnet S, Schrander-Stumpel C, Darby J, Holden J, Munnich A, Willems PJ: A duplication in the *L1CAM* gene associated with X-linked hydrocephalus. *Nat Genet* 4:421, 1993.
99. Reiner O, Carrozzo R, Shen Y, Wehnert M, Faustinella F, Dobyns WB, Caskey CT, Ledbetter DH: Isolation of a Miller-Dieker lissencephaly gene containing G protein β-subunit-like repeats. *Nature* 364:717, 1993.
100. des Portes V, Pinard JM, Billuart P, Vinet MC, Koulakoff A, Carrié A, Gelot A, Dupuis E, Motte J, Berwald-Netter Y, Catala M, Kahn A, Beldjord C, Chelly J: A novel CNS gene required for neuronal migration and involved in X-linked subcortical laminar heterotopia and lissencephaly syndrome. *Cell* 92:51, 1998.
101. Gleeson JG, Allen KM, Fox JW, Lamperti ED, Berkovic S, Scheffer I, Cooper EC, Dobyns WB, Minnerath SR, Ross ME, Walsh CA: *Doublecortin*, a brain-specific gene mutated in human X-linked lissencephaly and double cortex syndrome, encodes a putative signaling protein. *Cell* 92:63, 1998.
102. Tessier-Lavigne M, Goodman CS: The molecular biology of axon guidance. *Science* 274:1123, 1996.
103. Rugarli EI, Ballabio A: Kallmann syndrome: from genetics to neurobiology. *JAMA* 270:2713, 1993.
104. Schwanzel-Fukuda M, Abraham S, Crossin KL, Edelman GM, Pfaff DW: Immunocytochemical demonstration of neural cell adhesion molecule (NCAM) along the migration route of luteinizing hormone-releasing hormone (LHRH) neurons in mice. *J Comp Neurol* 321:1, 1992.

# Spinocerebellar Ataxias

*Huda Y. Zoghbi* ■ *Harry T. Orr*

1. The dominantly inherited spinocerebellar ataxias (SCAs) are a heterogeneous group of neurologic disorders characterized by variable degrees of degeneration of the cerebellum, spinocerebellar tracts, and brain stem neurons. The inter- and intrafamilial variability of clinicopathologic findings hampered the classification of this group of diseases until the 1990s, during which the discovery of the genetic bases of many of the SCAs provided a means of distinguishing among them.

2. The mutational locus has been mapped for 10 SCAs: SCA1, SCA2, Machado-Joseph disease (MJD)/SCA3 (sometimes referred to here simply as SCA3), SCA4, SCA5, SCA6, SCA7, SCA8, SCA10, and dentatorubropallidoluysian atrophy (DRPLA). The clinical features shared among these SCAs are ataxia, dysarthria, and eventual bulbar dysfunction. Variable features include ophthalmoparesis (common in SCA1, 2, 3, and 7); hyporeflexia (common in SCA2 and 4); dementia (more frequent in SCA2 and common in DRPLA); dystonia and rigidity (occasional in SCA1 and common in MJD/SCA3); choreoathetosis and myoclonus (common in DRPLA); spasticity (SCA1, 3, and DRPLA); bulging eyes and fasciculations (MJD/SCA3); neuropathy (most common in SCA4 but can be seen in SCA1, 2, and 3); seizures (common in SCA10 and DRPLA); and macular degeneration and extraneuronal involvement (unique to SCA7). Neuroimaging studies demonstrate cerebellar atrophy in SCA1, 2, 3, 6, 7, and DRPLA; cortical atrophy in SCA2, 7, and DRPLA; and brain stem atrophy in SCA1, 2, 3, 7, and DRPLA. Calcification of the basal ganglia and leukodystrophic changes occur in DRPLA. Nerve conduction abnormalities occur in SCA1, 2, and 3, and are most common in SCA4. Visual evoked potentials are abnormal in SCA7, and the EEG is abnormal in DRPLA. Purkinje cell and dentate neuron degeneration is severe in SCA1, 2, 6, 7, and DRPLA, but modest in MJD/SCA3. Degeneration of the inferior olive is common in SCA1, 2, 6, and 7. Loss of brain stem neurons is common in SCA1, 2, 3, 6, and DRPLA. Basal ganglia degeneration is pronounced in DRPLA and variable in MJD/SCA3. Macular degeneration and hypomyelination of the optic tract are unique to SCA7.

3. The mutational basis of SCA1, SCA2, MJD/SCA3, SCA6, SCA7, and DRPLA is the expansion of a translated trinucleotide (CAG) repeat that encodes for a polyglutamine tract in the relevant protein. SCA8 is caused by expansion of a CTA/CTG repeat that does not appear to be translated. Expanded disease alleles typically contain 34 to 84 CAG repeats in SCA1, 2, 3, and DRPLA. In SCA6, the pathogenic range is 21 to 33, and in SCA7 it is 35 to 306. For SCA8 the expanded range varies from 110 to 130 in kindreds with established linkage to the SCA8 locus, but has been found to exceed 575 repeats in some affected patients.

4. The gene products mutated in most of the SCAs — ataxin-1, ataxin-2, ataxin-3, ataxin-7, and atrophin-1 — are novel proteins of unknown function. The gene product mutated in SCA6 is the $\alpha_{1A}$ voltage-gated calcium channel (CACN1A1). The distribution of the proteins varies: ataxin-1 is predominantly nuclear in neurons, but cytoplasmic in peripheral cells. Ataxin-7 is a nuclear protein; ataxin-2, ataxin-3, atrophin-1, and CACN1A1 are cytoplasmic. In affected neurons, ataxin-1, ataxin-3, ataxin-7, and atrophin-1 aggregate in single large nuclear inclusions that stain positively for ubiquitin. Ataxin-2 does not form nuclear aggregates but appears to accumulate in the cytoplasm of affected neurons. The translation of the mutant proteins and their altered subcellular distribution support the hypothesis that the pathogenesis is mediated at the protein level.

5. The dynamic nature of the mutations in the SCAs (the expansion of unstable trinucleotide repeats) explains a clinical feature common to this group of diseases: genetic anticipation. The intergenerational repeat instability frequently leads to further expansion, particularly when paternally inherited, leading to earlier onset and more severe clinical course. In each of these diseases, there is an inverse correlation between the number of the repeats and the age of onset. However, the age of onset for a certain expanded range varies, depending on the protein context. Small expansions in CACN1A1 cause neuronal degeneration, whereas larger expansions are required to promote the other SCAs. Similarly sized expanded alleles appear to produce an earlier age of onset in SCA2 than in SCA1, DRPLA, or MJD/SCA3. Very large expansions in excess of 200 repeats have been seen in SCA7, and these typically lead to a severe infantile phenotype that involves nonneuronal tissues (e.g., the heart) as well.

6. The mutations identified to date account for approximately 65 to 70 percent of all dominantly inherited ataxias. The prevalence of the various SCAs varies considerably among different populations. MJD/SCA3 appears to be the most prevalent disease in all ethnic groups, accounting for 25 to 35 percent of all dominant ataxias. In Caucasians, SCA1 and SCA2 are the second most common diseases, whereas in Japan DRPLA and SCA6 are more prevalent. SCA7 is reasonably common, accounting for at least 10 percent of all dominant ataxias. There is a close association between the

---

A list of standard abbreviations is located immediately preceding the index in each volume. Additional abbreviations used in this chapter include: CACN1A1, *CACN1A* = α$_{1A}$ voltage-gated calcium channel protein and gene, respectively; DRPLA, *DRPLA* = dentatorubropallidoluysian atrophy disease and gene, respectively; EA2 = episodic ataxia type 2; GAPDH = glyceraldehyde 3-phosphate dehydrogenase; HDJ-2/HSDJ = human DnaJ-2/Homosapien DnaJ; HRS = Haw-River syndrome; Hsp 40, Hsp 70 = 40-kDa and 70-kDa heat-shock proteins, respectively; LANP, *LANP, Lanp* = leucine-rich acidic nuclear protein, human gene, mouse gene, respectively; MJD = Machado-Joseph disease; MN-SCA1 = Minnesota SCA1 kindred; NLS = nuclear localizing signal; Pcp2/L7 = Purkinje cell protein 2; PHAPI = putative HLA DR associated protein I; RAPID = repeat analysis, pooled isolation and detection; SCA1, SCA2, etc. = spinocerebellar ataxia 1, 2, etc. (disease in Roman font and gene in italics); TX-SCA1 = Texas SCA1 kindred.

**prevalence of the different SCAs and the frequencies of large normal alleles in various ethnic populations.**

7. **Pathogeneses of the SCAs share two features: the expansion of the polyglutamine tract and accumulation of the mutant protein. The data point to a gain-of-function mechanism whereby the mutant protein becomes toxic to neurons. Studies of transgenic animal models support such a mechanism and demonstrate that neuronal dysfunction rather than neuronal death precedes the clinical phenotype. The SCA1 mouse model also demonstrates that nuclear localization of ataxin-1 is necessary for the pathogenesis to occur, and visible aggregation of ataxin-1 is not essential to initiate SCA1 pathogenesis. Studies in cell culture demonstrate that the Hsp40 chaperone HDJ-2/HSDJ decreases the size and frequency of ataxin-1 and ataxin-3 aggregates, supporting the hypothesis that protein misfolding is involved in the aggregation of mutant protein with expanded polyglutamine tracts.**

8. **The selective degeneration of only a subset of neurons in each of the SCAs, despite widespread expression of the disease-causing gene, remains to be explained. Possible factors include different levels of expression and/or processing of the mutant polyglutamine proteins in various cell types and protein-protein interactions with cell-specific proteins. In the case of SCA1, for example, the temporal and cellular expression patterns and subcellular distribution of the leucine-rich acidic nuclear protein (LANP) parallel that of ataxin-1; that LANP interacts more strongly with mutant than normal ataxin-1 suggests that it may play a role in SCA1 pathogenesis.**

9. **Now that the gene products for several SCAs are in hand and knowledge about the fate of the mutant proteins is rapidly accumulating, the possibility of identifying proteins and/or compounds that could modulate the course of the diseases and slow their progression is not far-fetched.**

The inherited spinocerebellar ataxias (SCAs) are a heterogeneous group of neurologic disorders characterized by variable degrees of degeneration of the cerebellum, spinal tracts, and brain stem.[1,2] Friedreich was the first to report an inherited ataxia;[3] thirty years later, in 1893, Marie[4] reported a hereditary ataxia distinct from that described by Friedreich. This clinical entity, then referred to as "Marie's ataxia," was characterized by late onset of symptoms, increased deep tendon reflexes, and an autosomal dominant pattern of inheritance. By the turn of the twentieth century, Holmes realized that the cases described by Marie were clinically and pathologically heterogeneous.[5] Several studies attempting to classify the dominantly inherited SCAs were published (see reviews[6,7]), but, given the inter- and intrafamilial variability of clinicopathologic findings, a consistent classification system proved elusive. Indeed, there were instances in which patients from the same kindred were classified under two or more distinct types of SCA.[8] It was not until the genetic bases of these diseases were discovered that it became possible to differentiate among the inherited ataxias with accuracy.

The first subtype of SCA to be identified based on genetic mapping data was SCA type 1 (SCA1), which maps to the short arm of human chromosome 6.[9,10] Over the course of the past decade, the loci for nine additional SCAs were mapped (Table 226-1). Mapping and/or cloning the genes responsible for 10 SCAs permitted analysis and clearer differentiation of the clinical features seen in each subtype. Some clinical features are common to all the SCAs, such as ataxia and dysarthria, but there are variable features seen either in some subtypes or in some families with a specific subtype. The variable features include ocular dysfunction, extrapyramidal signs, pyramidal signs, peripheral neuropathy, intellectual impairment, and seizures (Table 226-2). To provide a reliable account of the clinical features for each

**Table 226-1** Gene Loci for Various SCAs

| Locus | MIM | Chromosome | Year Cloned | GenBank |
|---|---|---|---|---|
| SCA1 | 164400 | 6p23 | 1993 | X79204 |
| SCA2 | 183090 | 12q24 | 1996 | U70323 |
| SCA3/MJD | 109150 | 14q24.3-q31 | 1994 | U64821 |
| SCA4 | 600223 | 16q22 | | |
| SCA5 | 600224 | 11p11-q11 | | |
| SCA6 | 183086 | 19p13 | 1997 | U79666 |
| SCA7 | 164500 | 3p12-p21.1 | 1998 | AJ000517 |
| SCA8 | 271245 | 13q21 | 1999 | |
| SCA9 | Unassigned | (not yet published) | | |
| SCA10 | 603516 | 22q13-ter | | |
| DRPLA | 125370 | 12q | 1994 | D38529 |

subtype, the following clinical data have been extracted only from studies in which the genetic mapping information confirmed the subtype.

## CLINICAL FEATURES AND GENETIC MAPPING STUDIES

### Spinocerebellar Ataxia Type 1 (MIM 164400)

The first clinical description of a kindred that was later proven to have SCA1 was published by Gray and Oliver in 1941.[11] The authors documented an autosomal dominant mode of inheritance and provided a thorough clinical description. When J. W. Schut reported the results of detailed clinical studies on the same kindred[12] in 1950, he distinguished between four clinical forms of the disease based on the degree of incoordination and the activity of deep tendon reflexes. Schut later reported further findings after a 25-year follow-up of 25 affected members from the same family, which is now referred to as the Minnesota (MN-SCA1) kindred.[13] Over the past 25 years detailed clinical descriptions of several other SCA1 kindreds have been published.[14–29] Certain salient features can be culled from these reports: there is extensive interfamilial and intrafamilial variability, and all affected individuals from the reported families suffered from ataxia, dysarthria, and eventual bulbar dysfunction.

In the early stages of the disease, patients with SCA1 report slight gait and limb incoordination, slurred speech, and deteriorating handwriting. In the family described by Schut,[13] a cough, which seems to represent a throat-clearing attempt, often preceded the onset of the disease. Hypermetric saccades and nystagmus may also be noted in the early stages. As the disease progresses, hyperreflexia may be detected, the ataxia worsens, and other cerebellar signs such as dysmetria, dysdiadochokinesia, hypotonia, and the rebound phenomenon become apparent. Optic nerve atrophy and variable degrees of ophthalmoparesis may be seen in some patients. Mild sphincter disturbances such as urinary urgency occur frequently. Amyotrophy, decreased or absent deep tendon reflexes, and loss of proprioception or vibration sense may occur in the middle or late stages of the disease. Mild cognitive dysfunction, manifested as emotional lability, decreased attention and abstractional abilities, and reduction in recent and remote memory,

**Table 226-2** Common and Variable Features Among the Ataxias

| Common | Cerebellar signs (ataxia, dysarthria) |
|---|---|
| Variable | Extracerebellar signs: ocular dysfunction, extrapyramidal and pyramidal signs, peripheral neuropathy, intellectual impairment, seizures |

has been documented in some SCA1 patients.[30,31] The degree of cognitive impairment correlates with the severity of disease but does not seem to interfere with quotidian life. Extrapyramidal signs, including dystonic posturing and choreiform movements, have been observed in the later stages of the disease in some individuals. In the final stage of the disease, brain stem involvement causes facial weakness and bulbar signs, including tongue atrophy and fasciculations, severe dysarthria, and dysphagia. Frequent choking spells occur as the patient loses the ability to cough effectively; the most common causes of death are aspiration and pneumonia.

The typical age of onset for SCA1 is the third or fourth decade, but early onset in the first decade has been documented in several families.[12,16,22,28] Anticipation—the earlier onset of symptoms with a concomitant increase in the severity of the phenotype in later generations—has also been observed.[12,16,20,22,26,28] The disease typically progresses over a 10 to 15-year period, but anticipation causes more rapid degeneration, as has been described in juvenile-onset cases.[16]

## Spinocerebellar Ataxia Type 2 (MIM 183090)

In 1989, Orozco and colleagues described a form of dominantly inherited SCA that occurs in an estimated frequency of 41 per 100,000 in the province of Holguine in Cuba.[32] Genetic mapping studies using DNAs from the Cuban kindreds localized the *SCA2* gene to chromosome 12q23-q24.[33] Additional mapping studies confirmed that SCA2 occurs in families of diverse ethnic backgrounds.[27,29,34–39] The clinical features of this disorder include ataxia and dysarthria, with the majority of the patients exhibiting extremely slow saccades. Typically, nystagmus precedes the slow eye movements. Hyporeflexia and ophthalmoparesis occur in over half of the patients. There are no documented cases of retinopathy or optic atrophy, and pyramidal signs and Parkinsonian features are rare.[34–39] Chorea and supranuclear ophthalmoparesis have been observed in a few members of some SCA2 families.[39,40] Dementia has also occurred in members of some families, but was an early manifestation in all symptomatic members of one kindred.[37,40] Dysphagia and bulbar failure occur in the late stages of the disease.

## Machado-Joseph Disease / Spinocerebellar Ataxia Type 3 (MIM 109150)

Machado-Joseph disease (MJD) derives its name from two families afflicted with multisystem degenerative disease of the nervous system. This dominantly inherited disorder was initially observed in families of Portuguese-Azorean origin (approximately 1:4000 Azoreans are affected[41–43]), but subsequently it was described in families that have no Portuguese ancestry.[44–47] Takiyama and colleagues mapped the *MJD* gene in Japanese families to human chromosome 14q24.3-q32.[48] Additional mapping studies in Portuguese-Azorean kindreds confirmed the mapping of *MJD* to 14q.[49,50]

Attempts were made to divide MJD into clinical subtypes based on different combination of clinical findings and age of onset.[42,51–53] But because of the considerable phenotypic variability, different "subtypes" were seen within the same family; indeed, affected individuals often evolved from one "subtype" to another, thereby rendering such clinical subclassifications problematic, if not entirely useless.

Stevanin and collaborators mapped the gene in a family with a dominantly inherited ataxia to chromosome 14q24.3-qter.[54] They designated the new locus as SCA3 because they found that the clinical features in that family bore less resemblance to MJD than SCA1. The documented clinical features of MJD were progressive ataxia; amyotrophy; external ophthalmoplegia; bulging eyes; muscle weakness; facial and lingual fasciculations; neuropathy; Parkinsonism; and spasticity. Some of the of the motor abnormalities, such as dystonia, bradykinesia, and rigidity, respond to levodopa. Stevanin noted patients with SCA3 to have progressive ataxia and dysarthria, amyotrophy, and supranuclear ophthalmo-

plegia, but with increased reflexes, nystagmus, and decreased vibration sense. Dementia, dystonia, and extrapyramidal rigidity are found in less than 20 percent of the patients and optic atrophy is rare. As the disease progresses, sphincter abnormalities and swallowing difficulties develop.[55–59] Several studies have since demonstrated that MJD and SCA3 are caused by the same mutation within the *MJD1* gene (see MJD/SCA3 under "Molecular Bases of Spinocerebellar Ataxias" below), which only emphasizes the clinical heterogeneity associated with this mutation.

## Spinocerebellar Ataxia Types 4 (MIM 600223) and 5 (MIM 600224)

SCA4 is characterized by progressive cerebellar ataxia, dysarthria, loss of vibration and position sense, areflexia, and extensor plantar reflexes. Some patients suffer from distal weakness; oculomotor signs are rare. The disease onset is typically in the fourth or fifth decade but earlier onset has been seen in successive generations, suggesting anticipation.[60] A genome-wide linkage analysis localized the *SCA4* gene to a 10-cM region on human chromosome 16q22.1 very close to *D16S397* and between *D16S514* and *D16S512*.[60]

SCA5 presents the mildest form of dominantly inherited ataxia. Patients suffer from mild disturbances of gait and limb coordination that worsen with age. The absence of bulbar findings in adult-onset SCA5 patients explains why these patients typically have normal life spans. Two juvenile-onset cases have been reported, which suggests that anticipation occurs in SCA5 as well.[21] The *SCA5* gene maps to the centromeric region of human chromosome 11.[21]

## Spinocerebellar Ataxia Type 6 (MIM 183086)

Patients with SCA6 typically develop gait and limb ataxia and dysarthria. Horizontal gaze-evoked nystagmus is quite common, and many patients have limitations of eye movements on upward and lateral gaze. Dysphagia is a frequent problem in patients who have had the disease more than 5 years. Very mild neuropathy-minimal distal wasting and decreased ankle jerks-is seen in some patients. One notable difference between SCA6 and most other ataxias is the complete absence of extrapyramidal signs, spasticity, intellectual impairment, and visual deficits.[61–71] The mapping of the SCA6 gene to human chromosome 19p13 came as a result of identifying the mutation, a CAG-repeat expansion within the $\alpha_{1A}$-voltage dependent calcium channel (*CACNA1A*).[61] Missense, splice, and protein truncating mutations in *CACNA1A* have been reported in episodic ataxia type 2 (EA2) and familial hemiplegic migraine (see Chap. 204).[72–75] It is interesting that some patients with SCA6 experience episodic ataxia in the early stages of their disease, as this raises the possibility that SCA6 and EA2 may be different points along a phenotypic continuum of the same disease.[61,66,73]

## Spinocerebellar Ataxia Type 7 (MIM 164500)

SCA7 patients may first present with cerebellar ataxia or visual deficits.[76–78] Approximately half develop both symptoms simultaneously; among the remaining half, the majority present with cerebellar ataxia and may maintain normal vision for decades. The minority who first present with visual deficits usually develop ataxia within a few years.[77] The decreased visual acuity is secondary to progressive pigmentary macular degeneration; the earliest finding is dyschromatopsia in the blue-yellow axis. When the patients become symptomatic they complain of progressive loss of central vision but note that peripheral and night visions are intact. Funduscopic exam reveals loss of foveal reflex and increased macular pigmentation. Secondary optic atrophy occurs in the later stages of the disease. The visual loss usually progresses to bilateral blindness. Additional features of SCA7 include increased reflexes and spasticity, slow saccades, ophthalmoplegia, and hearing deficits. Extrapyramidal signs such as orofacial dyskinesias, choreoathetosis, dystonia, limb rigidity, and tremors occur in some patients.[77,78] Behavioral disturbances such as auditory hallucinations, progressive psychosis, and delusions have been reported in some patients.[78] There are three infants known to have SCA7 (two molecularly proven and one very likely given the family history of ataxia and maculopathy) who, in addition to the visual and neuronal deficits, had somatic features: severe hypotonia, patent ductus arteriosus, congestive heart failure, and death in the first year of life. These infants represent a distinct phenotype resulting from the severe anticipation seen in SCA7 (see "Genotype/Phenotype Correlations" below).[76,78,79] The *SCA7* gene was mapped to human chromosome 3p12-p21.1 using multiple independent kindreds of different ethnic backgrounds.[80–82]

### Spinocerebellar Ataxia Type 8 (MIM 271245)

The usual age of onset for SCA8 is adulthood, with symptoms appearing any time between 18 and 65 years of age. Ataxia, dysarthria, nystagmus, and limb spasticity are the primary features of the disease. Some patients develop occasional choking spells, and many have diminished vibration sense. Although the disease usually progresses slowly, some severely affected patients become nonambulatory by the fourth to sixth decade.[83] The *SCA8* gene, discovered after the identification of an expanded trinucleotide repeat in symptomatic patients, maps to human chromosome 13q21 (see SCA8 under "Molecular Bases of Spinocerebellar Ataxias" below).

### Spinocerebellar Ataxia Type 9 (No MIM entry)

There is no clinical disorder or genetic locus assigned yet.

### Spinocerebellar Ataxia Type 10 (No MIM entry)

SCA10 distinguishes itself clinically from the other SCAs by causing complex partial seizures in addition to ataxia. Some patients develop unsteady gait as the first symptom, while others present with seizures. The age of onset is usually the third or fourth decade, and earlier onset in successive generations has been documented.[84,85] Dysarthria and dysphagia develop, as with the other SCAs. Seizures become generalized in some patients. Two research teams recently mapped the *SCA10* locus to chromosome 22q13-qter in families of Hispanic origin. It would be interesting to determine whether the families represent two branches deriving from a single ancestry.[84,85]

### Dentatorubropallidoluysian Atrophy (DRPLA) (MIM 125370)

In 1975, Smith described a number of patients who suffered from combined degeneration of the cerebellum and basal ganglia. He labeled this clinical entity dentatorubropallidoluysian atrophy because similar pathologic changes affected the cerebellifugal and pallidofugal pathways.[86] The hereditary nature of DRPLA was confirmed by Naito et al. through detailed clinical, genetic, and neuropathologic studies of five Japanese families that suffered from familial myoclonus and choreoathetosis.[87] Most patients present with dysarthria, gait ataxia, and tremors. They subsequently develop pyramidal signs, choreiform movements, opsoclonus, dystonia, ballismus, and myoclonus. The majority of patients develop epilepsy, and dementia occurs in the later stages of the disease.[87,88]

Age of onset and clinical features are quite variable in DRPLA. Symptoms may begin in childhood or as late as the seventh decade. Patients with juvenile onset present with myoclonus, epilepsy, and variable degrees of mental retardation or dementia. The seizures may be induced by photic, tactile, or auditory stimuli. Anticipation has been documented in DRPLA, and the disease is more rapidly progressive in juvenile cases, who typically die 10 to 20 years after onset from bulbar dysfunction and respiratory failure.[87–90] DRPLA is most prevalent in Japan, with an estimated frequency of one per million,[91] but has been observed in kindreds of Maltese, African-American, and Caucasian backgrounds.[89,90,92] The family described by Burke et al. had been diagnosed as having Haw-River syndrome (HRS) until the DRPLA mutation was found to be the basis of the neurodegeneration in this family.

HRS was described in a single African-American kindred that lived near the Haw River in central North Carolina. Patients from this family share many clinical features with DRPLA patients except that they do not develop myoclonic epilepsy. They do show evidence of demyelination of the subcortical white matter, basal ganglia calcifications, and neuroaxonal dystrophy.[92] The DRPLA gene, identified using a candidate gene approach, maps to human chromosome 12q.[93]

## NEUROIMAGING, NEUROPHYSIOLOGICAL, AND NEUROPATHOLOGIC STUDIES

### Neuroimaging

Neuroimaging studies have been done in patients with molecularly proven SCA diagnosis. In general, both CT and MRI scans demonstrate cerebellar atrophy in all SCA and DRPLA patients. The degree of cerebellar atrophy might vary within the same family and between different subtypes. Cerebellar atrophy may be more pronounced and appear earlier in SCA2 than in SCA1, SCA3, SCA6, and SCA7.[27,29,39,68,71,77,94] Cerebellar MRI findings in SCA3 are quite variable, ranging from normal to moderate atrophy. Enlargement of the fourth ventricle is apparent in most SCAs, while enlargement of the lateral and third ventricles is more typical of SCA2 and DRPLA. Marked brain stem atrophy is detected in SCA1, SCA2, and SCA7 but is variable in SCA3 and absent in SCA6, even in patients with swallowing difficulties.[29,39,64–66,68,71,77,94] Cerebral atrophy is minimal in most SCAs but has been noted in SCA2 and infantile SCA7.[37,78] In DRPLA, there are variable degrees of cerebral, cerebellar, basal ganglia, and brain stem atrophy in all patients. In addition, DRPLA patients with late-onset disease often have symmetrical high-signal lesions on MRI in the cerebral white matter and brain stem suggestive of leukodystrophic changes, and some have calcifications of the basal ganglia.[89,90,95]

### Neurophysiology

Peripheral neuropathy is present in a substantial number of patients with SCA1, 2, 3, and 6, and is common in patients with SCA4. Hence, many of the SCA patients have some nerve conduction abnormalities including slower nerve conduction velocities and decreased evoked muscle and sensory nerve action potentials.[21,29,44] These abnormalities are most pronounced in SCA2, SCA3, and SCA1, and are less frequent in SCA6.[27,96] Unlike the other SCAs, SCA4 invariably causes prominent axonal sensory neuropathy, and the sural sensory nerve action potentials are absent in more than 90 percent of the patients.[60] In SCA7 patients, visual evoked potentials are abnormal in all patients, and the electroretinogram shows abnormal scotopic responses with preservation of the photic responses late in the disease.[77] The interictal electroencephalogram (EEG) is normal in SCA10; there are no data yet about the EEG during seizures in these patients. In DRPLA, the EEG typically shows a slow and disorganized background rhythm with generalized bursts of spike and wave activity.[87–89] The paroxysmal discharges in DRPLA are easily induced by photic stimulation.[88,89]

### Neuropathology

The predominant neuropathologic findings in SCA1 are cerebellar atrophy with severe loss of Purkinje cells, dentate nucleus neurons, and neurons in the inferior olive and cranial nerve nuclei III, IV, IX, X, and XII. Eosinophilic spheres, also known as torpedoes, are present in the internal granule cell layer and some are related to Purkinje cell bodies (Fig. 226-1). The dorsal and ventral spinocerebellar tracts and dorsal columns are demyelinated; gliosis of the molecular layer of the cerebellum is marked, while gliosis of the anterior horn of the spinal cord is more mild.[14,15,18,94,97] In SCA2, the cerebellum and brain stem are quite atrophied, showing severe degeneration of Purkinje and granule cells along with conspicuous neuronal loss and gliosis in the inferior olive and

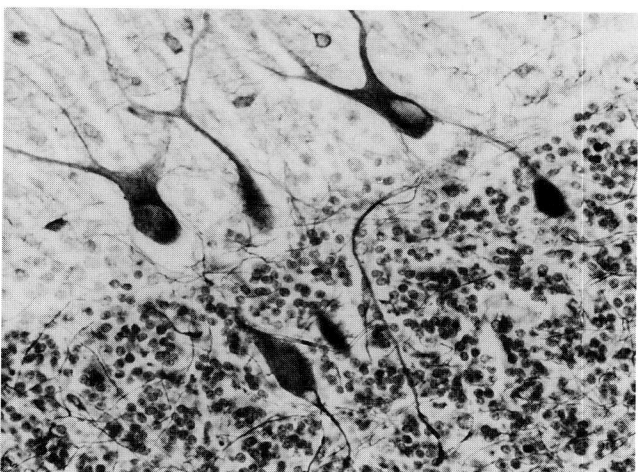

**Fig. 226-1** A section of the cerebellum stained with Sevier-Munger preparation from the brain of a 10-year-old SCA1 patient with 82 CAG repeats who died after 6 years of symptoms. Three Purkinje cells are in a state of degeneration with their axons showing torpedoes in the internal granule cell layer. (Courtesy of Dr. Dawna Armstrong.)

pons. Atrophy of the frontotemporal lobes, as well as degeneration of the substantia nigra, has been reported.[32,37] In MJD/SCA3, the degeneration is most prominent in the basal ganglia, brain stem, and spinal cord. Neuronal loss is mild in the cerebellum and not typical in the inferior olives.[59,98–101] Neuropathologic findings in SCA6 include marked cerebellar atrophy and mild atrophy of the brain stem. There is severe loss of cerebellar Purkinje cells with moderate loss of cerebellar granule cells, dentate nucleus neurons, and neurons of the inferior olive.[61,67] The predominant neuronal loss in SCA7 occurs in the cerebellum, inferior olive, and some cranial nerve nuclei. There is hypomyelination of the optic tract and some gliosis of the lateral geniculate body and visual cortex.[77,102] The neuropathology of DRPLA is quite extensive: pronounced neuronal loss in the cerebral cortex, globus pallidus, striatum, cerebellar cortex, and the subthalamic (Luys body), red, and dentate nuclei. There is intense fibrillary gliosis at the sites of neuronal degeneration; severe demyelination and axonal degeneration in the superior cerebellar peduncle is common and in some families it is also observed in the subcortical white matter along with calcification of the basal ganglia.[86–88,92]

## MOLECULAR BASES OF SPINOCEREBELLAR ATAXIAS

The mutational basis of those SCAs for which the genes have been isolated is the expansion of an unstable trinucleotide repeat. The genes involved in each of the diseases are quite different and share no homology with each other outside of the repeat sequence. The

following section summarizes data on the mutations and gene products for each SCA whose gene has been cloned (Table 226-3).

### Spinocerebellar Ataxia Type 1

In 1991, the *SCA1* gene was closely linked to the marker D6S89 in 6p22-p23.[103,104] Subsequent genetic and physical mapping data localized the candidate *SCA1* region to 1.2 Mb of DNA.[105] Because of the anticipation observed in the MN-SCA1 and TX-SCA1 kindreds,[12,16] it was proposed that SCA1 is caused by expansion of trinucleotide repeats. A focused search for such repeats led to the identification of a highly polymorphic CAG repeat (heterozygosity rate of 84 percent) that was unstable and expanded on SCA1 chromosomes.[106] The CAG repeat lies in the coding region of the gene and encodes a glutamine tract.[106] Normal alleles contain 6 to 44 repeats, whereas disease alleles contain 39 to 82 repeats.[21,22,26,107] Normal alleles with 21 or more CAG repeats are interrupted with 1 to 4 CAT repeat units encoding histidine; in contrast, SCA1 alleles contain only uninterrupted CAG repeat tracts.[22,107,108] The CAT interruption most likely contributes to maintaining CAG repeat tract stability.[109] Somatic mosaicism is observed in SCA1 particularly in sperm cells. It is interesting that in the cerebellum (the tissue with the highest number of neurons which are postmitotic) the repeat sizes are consistently smaller, suggesting that expansions are more likely to occur in tissues that have higher proportions of dividing cells.[109] Analysis of intergenerational instability of normal SCA1 alleles did not reveal any variation in repeat numbers in over 1000 meioses. In contrast, 65 percent of the expanded SCA1 alleles are unstable, with the majority of paternal transmissions showing an expansion (average +3.3 repeats), and maternal transmissions showing contractions (average − 0.4 repeat).[22,108]

The *SCA1* gene is widely expressed. The 11-kb transcript is organized into nine exons: seven 5′ untranslated exons and a very long 3′ untranslated region containing 7277 bp.[110] These exons span approximately 450 kb on 6p22-p23.[110] The coding region, which spans 2448 bp, is in exons 8 and 9. The *SCA1* gene product, ataxin-1, is a novel protein that shares no homology with other proteins and contains no motifs that yield clues as to its function. Wild-type ataxin-1 is predicted to encode 792 to 830 amino acids, depending on the size of the repeat tract.[110] The murine homolog of the *SCA1* gene shares a similar genomic structure, and the protein is highly homologous to the human protein (89 percent identity); a notable difference in the mouse is the presence of two glutamines and three prolines in place of the long glutamine repeat.[111] Wild-type ataxin-1 is predicted to be approximately 87 kDa but has an altered electrophoretic mobility, probably because of the glutamine tract. The mutant protein is translated, and its electrophoretic mobility varies according to the number of CAG repeats[97] (Fig. 226-2). Immunoblot and immunohisto-chemical analyses using antibodies raised to different regions of ataxin-1 revealed that the level of the protein in the central nervous system is two to four times that found in peripheral tissues. In lymphoblasts, heart, skeletal muscle, and liver, the protein is localized to the cytoplasm; in neurons it is predominantly nuclear,

**Table 226-3** Molecular Bases of the SCAs

| Disease | Gene Product | Normal (CAG)n | Expanded (CAG)n | Protein localization | Special features |
|---|---|---|---|---|---|
| SCA1 | ataxin-1 | 6–44 | 39–82 | nuclear in neurons | normal alleles > 21 repeats interrupted with 1–4 CAT units |
| SCA2 | ataxin-2 | 17–31 | 36–63 | cytoplasmic | normal alleles interrupted with 1–2 CAA units |
| MJD/SCA3 | ataxin-3 | 12–41 | 62–84 | cytoplasmic | |
| SCA6 | CACNA1A | 4–18 | 21–33 | cell membrane | |
| SCA7 | ataxin-7 | 4–35 | 37–306 | nuclear | intermediate alleles 28–35 |
| SCA8 | repeat not translated | 16–91 | 110–130 | | repeat configuration (CTA)nCTGCTA(CTG)n |
| DRPLA | atrophin-1 | 6–36 | 49–84 | cytoplasmic | |

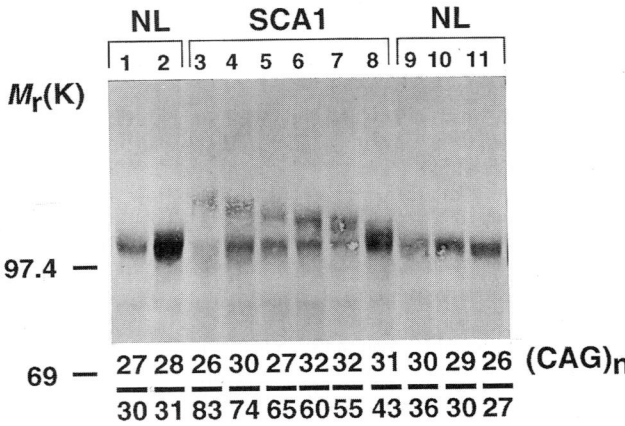

**Fig. 226-2** Expression analysis of ataxin-1 in lymphoblasts from normal (NL, lanes 1 to 2 and 9 to 11) and SCA1 patients (lanes 3 to 8). The size of the upper band, corresponding to the mutant protein, varies with the size of the CAG repeat in the *SCA1* allele. The number of CAG repeats in both alleles is shown below each lane. (*From Servadio et al.[97] Used with permission of Nature Genetics.*)

with some cytoplasmic staining in Purkinje cells and brain stem nuclei.[97,112–114] The immunolocalization patterns of ataxin-1 are similar in SCA1 patients with the exception of large nuclear ataxin-1 aggregates in the basis pontis[112,114] (Fig. 226-3).

To gain insight into the normal function of ataxin-1, Matilla et al. generated mice lacking ataxin-1. *Sca1* null mice are viable and fertile. Mice either heterozygous or homozygous for the null mutation displayed no ataxia, indicating that SCA1 is not caused by the loss of normal ataxin-1 function. They did, however, demonstrate impaired spatial and motor learning and decreased paired-pulse facilitation in CA1 area of the hippocampus. Ataxin-1 may thus play a role in synaptic plasticity and some learning tasks.[115]

### Spinocerebellar Ataxia Type 2

The *SCA2* gene was first mapped in 1993[33] and subsequently confirmed in many kindreds of diverse ethnic backgrounds.[27,34–39] Anticipation in SCA2 was first reported in a multigenerational Italian kindred in which 14 offspring of 15 parent-child pairs showed earlier disease onset.[34] The candidate SCA2 region

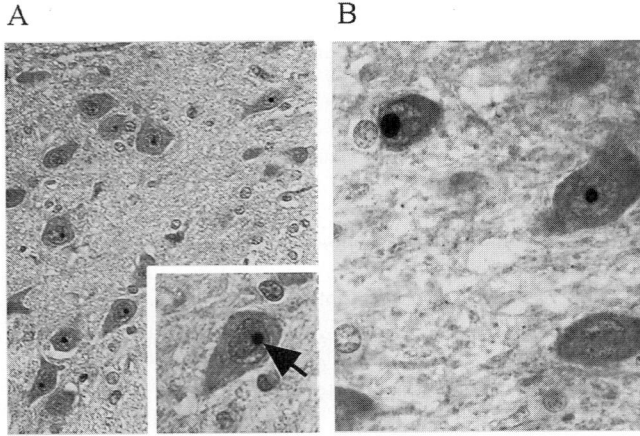

**Fig. 226-3** Immunohistochemical staining of pontine neurons using anti-ataxin-1 (*A*) and anti-ubiquitin (*B*) antibodies from the same 10-year-old SCA1 patient as in Fig. 226-1. Intense immunostaining for both antibodies is noted in a single large nuclear inclusion in each neuron. Inset shows a magnified neuron; white arrow points to the inclusion. (*Courtesy of Christopher Cummings.*)

was narrowed to a 1-cM interval through careful analysis of recombination events in the large Cuban kindred.[116]

The *SCA2* gene was identified using three independent strategies. The first approach used a monoclonal antibody that detects expanded polyglutamine tracts. This monoclonal antibody, 1C2, was raised against the polyglutamine-containing TATA binding protein and has been shown to selectively detect expanded repeats containing more than 35 glutamines in Huntington disease, SCA1, and SCA3 patients.[117] Using this antibody, Trottier and colleagues demonstrated that patients with SCA2 have protein with an expanded polyglutamine tract approximately 150 kDa in size. Imbert and colleagues used this antibody to screen a cDNA library prepared from lymphoblastoid cell lines of SCA2 patients and identified clones containing the *SCA2* cDNA.[118] Surprisingly, the *SCA2* cDNA they identified contained only a normal-sized CAG repeat. Amplification of this CAG repeat in SCA2 patients confirmed the expansion within the identified gene.

Pulst and collaborators identified the *SCA2* gene using a combination of positional cloning and candidate gene approaches.[119] Sanpei and colleagues used a novel strategy which they named DIRECT (direct identification of repeat expansion and cloning technique). This strategy involves the use of a probe with an expanded CAG tract, which is then labeled to a highly specific activity and used in Southern blot analysis of DNAs from patients and unaffected individuals. This approach identifies expanded CAG repeats based on the hybridization of the probe to larger fragments upon analysis with a variety of restriction enzymes. Subsequently, the restriction fragments are cloned by preparing a genomic library from the patients using the appropriate restriction enzymes.[120]

The *SCA2* cDNA identified from these three studies encodes a novel protein named ataxin-2, with a predicted molecular weight of 140 kDa. The protein does not share any homology with proteins of known function, but it does share sequence homology with another novel protein designated ataxin-2-related protein as well as the mouse *Sca2* gene product.[119] The *SCA2* gene is widely expressed in brain, heart, placenta, liver, skeletal muscle, and pancreas, and the transcript is estimated to be 4.5 kb.[118–120] The *SCA2* CAG repeat is not as polymorphic as those that undergo expansion in other neurodegenerative diseases. Two alleles of 22 and 23 repeats account for the majority of alleles (greater than 95 percent),[63,118–121] although normal alleles containing as few as 15 or as many as 32 repeats have been documented. The repeat configuration is interrupted by two CAA sequences on normal alleles, but on expanded alleles, it is a perfect CAG repeat tract. The size range for expanded alleles is 36 to 63 repeats; the majority of the disease alleles are between 36 and 43 repeats. Allele sizes in the 32 to 34 range have been identified in patients from SCA2 families who carry the disease haplotype but whose clinical status is normal at the time of evaluation. It is not yet clear whether these alleles are in the pathogenic range. The incidence of the SCA2 mutation in sporadic ataxia patients is quite low; in a series of 842 sporadic ataxia patients, only two patients were found to have expansions of 41 and 49 repeats.[63] In a second series reported by Cancel and colleagues, 2 of 90 patients with sporadic progressive ataxia had alleles with 37 and 39 repeats.[121]

### Machado-Joseph Disease/Spinocerebellar Ataxia Type 3

The MJD/SCA3 gene was identified using a candidate gene approach. Kawaguchi et al.[122] proposed that the most likely mutational mechanism is the expansion of a CAG repeat, as in Huntington disease and SCA1. Using an oligonucleotide probe with 13 CAG repeats, the investigators screened a human brain cDNA library and identified cDNA clones that contained CAG repeats. In one of the clones, the CAG repeat was found to be in the C-terminal portion of the open reading frame and was predicted to code for glutamine. This cDNA was labeled *MJD1* and mapped to human chromosome 14q32.1 by fluorescence *in situ* hybridization. The mapping of the *MJD* locus to chromosome

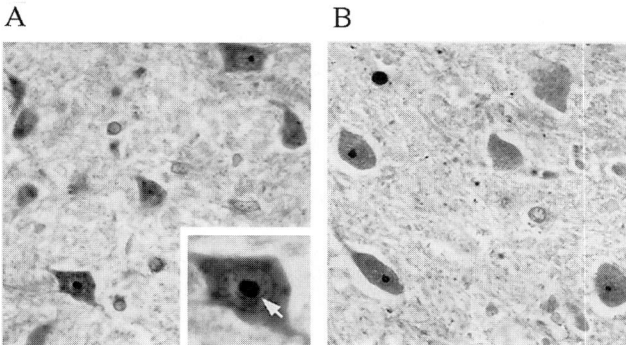

**Fig. 226-4 Immunohistochemical staining in ventral pons from an SCA3 patient using anti-ataxin-3 (*A*) and anti-ubiquitin (*B*) antibodies. The patient had 80 CAG repeats and died at 37 years of age. Immunoreactive nuclear inclusions are apparent in the neurons. Inset shows a magnified neuron, with a white arrow pointing to the inclusion. (*Courtesy of Dr. Henry Paulson.*)**

14q24.3-q32.1 by linkage analysis[48] rendered the *MJD1* gene an excellent candidate for this disorder. Amplification of this CAG repeat in normal individuals revealed that it was polymorphic, and in Japanese families with a clinical and pathologic diagnosis of MJD, repeat expansions were detected in all affected individuals.[122] Mapping of the *SCA3* locus to human 14q24.3-32.1 raised the possibility that the *MJD1* CAG repeat is likely to be expanded in SCA3 families. Analysis of this repeat in SCA3 families confirmed that SCA3 and MJD are caused by the same mutation within *MJD1*, and emphasized the marked clinical heterogeneity associated with this mutation.[55–59,123,124]

The size of the CAG tract ranges from 12 to 41 repeats on normal chromosomes and from 62 to 84 repeats on disease chromosomes,[55,57–59] making MJD/SCA3 one of the few trinucleotide repeat diseases in which there is a distinct gap between normal and affected repeat sizes. Extensive haplotype analysis on MJD/SCA3 families from various ethnic backgrounds did not support the presence of a common founder chromosome, so it is accepted that the MJD/SCA3 mutations have occurred independently in various parts of the world. Intergenerational instability of the MJD CAG repeats is quite common, with CAG length varying from −8 to about +5 repeats between parent and offspring. This intergenerational instability is more pronounced when paternally transmitted. Repeat sizes in various brain regions of affected individuals tend to be similar, although in the cerebellum the repeat number is typically smaller, suggesting limited somatic mosaicism in this disorder.[125] The *MJD1* gene encodes an intracellular protein of unknown function with a predicted size of 42 kDa.[122] The *MJD1* gene product ataxin-3 is predominantly a cytoplasmic protein, although occasionally it has been found within the nucleus in patient tissues[126] (Fig. 226-4). Ataxin-3 does not share homology with any other protein outside of the glutamine tract and is predicted to contain a nuclear localization signal.[127] Both the transcript and the protein are widely expressed without any evidence supporting higher levels in tissues that are affected in MJD/SCA3.

## Spinocerebellar Ataxia Type 6

The gene for spinocerebellar ataxia type 6 was identified using a candidate gene approach and a strategy of screening human brain cDNA libraries with a (CTG)$_7$ repeat oligonucleotide probe. A cDNA containing a polymorphic CAG repeat was identified by sequencing analysis to be the human $\alpha_{1A}$-voltage-dependent calcium channel (*CACNA1A*). Genotypic analysis of a large number of DNA samples from patients with late-onset neurodegenerative diseases and from normal ethnically-matched control individuals revealed that the CAG repeat sequence was expanded in eight families diagnosed with autosomal dominant cerebellar ataxia.[61] In this study, affected individuals had larger repeats,

ranging in size from 21 to 27, compared to the 475 nonataxia individuals with repeats in the 4 to 16 range. Careful analysis of the cDNA variants encoding for the $\alpha_{1A}$-voltage-dependent calcium channel revealed that there are several isoforms and that the CAG repeat lies within the coding region in three of the isoforms and is predicted to encode a glutamine tract. Although the size of the expansion was relatively small compared to other CAG expansions in previously cloned genes of other neurodegenerative diseases, Zhuchenko and colleagues concluded that the modest expansion in the *CACNA1A* CAG repeat is a primary cause of one form of cerebellar ataxia, which was then designated spinocerebellar ataxia type 6.

Subsequent to this initial report, several studies confirmed the finding that SCA6 is indeed caused by modest polyglutamine expansions in the human $\alpha_{1A}$-voltage-dependent calcium channel. At this time the pathogenic range for the repeat is 21 to 33, while normal alleles range in size from 14 to 18 repeats.[62–66,68,69,71,128–130]

The SCA6 CAG repeat differs from other disease-causing CAG repeats in that the expansion is small and the repeat is relatively stable. However, this repeat must undergo some expansion, given the finding of alleles with 20 or more repeats in ataxic patients. Intergenerational instability is rarely observed in the SCA6 repeat; in an evaluation of over 50 parent-child transmissions, only one expansion event was found (a 24 repeat expanded to 26 in a father-son pair).[62]

Voltage-sensitive calcium channels are multimeric complexes made of an $\alpha_{1A}$ subunit, which is sufficient to form the channel structure, and $\alpha_2$, $\delta$, and $\beta$ subunits, which are regulatory.[131] The $\alpha_{1A}$ subunit encodes P and Q type calcium channels that were identified in cerebellar Purkinje cells and granule neurons, respectively.[132,133] The $\alpha_{1A}$ subunit gene is expressed abundantly in the central nervous system, with the highest levels found in the cerebellum.[134]

Mutations in the $\alpha_{1A}$-voltage-dependent calcium channel have been identified in other neurologic disorders, such as hereditary paroxysmal cerebellar ataxia (also known as episodic ataxia type 2) and familial hemiplegic migraine. Murine mutations in this subunit are found in the tottering and tottering-leaner mice, which suffer from ataxia and seizures[72,134] (see Chap. 204). The mutations in familial hemiplegic migraine and episodic ataxia type 2 include missense mutations and a splicing mutation that leads to a truncated protein product. The mechanisms by which the various mutations in this channel cause disease have not been determined. For familial hemiplegic migraine and episodic ataxia, it is possible that the mutations cause haplo-insufficiency of the gene product or cause the mutant product to act in a dominant-negative manner. It is possible that the expansion alters the normal physiology of the channel, disrupting calcium homeostasis. Alternatively, the CAG repeat expansion may confer a novel toxic function onto the protein, as it does in other polyglutamine neurodegenerative disorders.

## Spinocerebellar Ataxia Type 7

The *SCA7* gene was mapped to human chromosome 3 by three independent groups, and subsequently localized to a 12-cM region in 3p12-p13.[80–82,135] Using a combination of positional cloning and candidate gene sequencing, the *SCA7* gene was isolated by David et al. in 1997.[135] The authors searched for CAG repeat sequences in overlapping YAC clones from the candidate SCA7 region and identified sequences containing 10 uninterrupted CAG repeats in a 579-bp open reading frame. This directed search for CAG repeats was initiated because of earlier studies using the 1C2 monoclonal antibody demonstrating the presence of a protein ranging in size from 130 to 180 kDa in SCA7 patients.[117,136] Amplification of the CAG repeat from unaffected individuals and SCA7 patients confirmed the presence of an expansion in all affected individuals.[135]

The *SCA7* gene was also identified using an approach directed at isolating expanded trinucleotide repeats and the corresponding flanking sequences.[137] The approach was dubbed RAPID, for *repeat analysis, pooled isolation and detection* (of individual clones containing expanded trinucleotide repeats). In a third strategy by Del Favero and colleagues, the *SCA7* gene was identified using a combination of genomic sequencing and exon trapping from YACs spanning the SCA7 candidate region. The authors identified expressed sequences corresponding to the *SCA7* cDNA and assembled cDNA contigs that span the *SCA7* gene. Overlapping cDNA clones spanning approximately 3969 bp of sequence revealed an open reading frame predicted to encode a protein of 892 amino acids that was designated ataxin-7. The polyglutamine tract is in the N-terminal region (codons 30 to 39). Ataxin-7 contains a nuclear localization signal consensus sequence, but shares no significant homology with known proteins. The transcript, which measures about 7.5 kb, is expressed ubiquitously, with the highest expression levels in heart, placenta, skeletal muscle, and pancreas. The relative levels in brain, liver, and kidney are lower than in heart and skeletal muscle. Within the central nervous system, the *SCA7* transcript is expressed at higher levels in the cerebellum than in other tissues. The SCA7 CAG repeat is polymorphic, ranging in size from 4 to 35 repeats on normal alleles; approximately 75 percent contain 10 repeats. All normal alleles contain pure CAG tracts without any evidence of interruption.[76–78,130,135,138–140]

SCA7 patients carry expansions ranging in size from 37 to 306 repeats. Alleles ranging in size from 34 to 36 repeats have been observed in individuals who are at risk but asymptomatic at the time of evaluation.[78,138] Intermediate alleles have been shown to expand into pathogenic range upon intergenerational transmission. For example, two alleles containing 35 and 38 CAG repeats expanded to 57 and 47 repeats, respectively, during paternal transmissions. These expansions resulted in the SCA7 phenotype in successive generations.[141]

Typically, larger expansions are paternally inherited and result from significant intergenerational repeat instability. Indeed, the SCA7 repeat is perhaps one of the most unstable CAG repeats described to date. Somatic mosaicism of this repeat has also been demonstrated in leukocyte DNA. The largest known intergenerational repeat expansion enlarged the CAG tract by 263 repeats in a father-to-son transmission.[78] Although paternal transmission causes much greater expansions, the disease is more often observed upon maternal transmission. This suggests that paternally transmitted alleles may be embryonic-lethal or are at a disadvantage for fertilization.[78,138]

### Spinocerebellar Ataxia Type 8

The molecular basis of SCA8 was determined using a direct approach aimed at identifying expanded trinucleotide repeats in families with dominantly inherited ataxias. Using RAPID analysis, expanded CAG repeats were identified in a large family with dominantly inherited progressive ataxia. A 1.15-kb *Eco*RI fragment containing the expansion was cloned, and trinucleotide repeats consisting of 80 uninterrupted CAG repeats followed by a stretch of 11 TAG repeats were identified.[83]

There was no open reading frame in either orientation, suggesting that this repeat was not translated. Further analysis of the transcriptional orientation of the sequence containing the repeat revealed that the repeat lies within a transcript that does not contain any coding sequence, and the actual configuration of the repeat is CTA/CTG. Over 1200 alleles from the general population were analyzed, and the range of the repeats from these normal alleles was 16 to 91 for the combined CTA/CTG nucleotides, with more than 99 percent of these alleles containing 16 to 34 combined repeats. Among ataxia patients from the large SCA8 kindred, the allele sizes range from 110 to 130 combined repeats (107 to 129 CTG repeats alone). All individuals with a CTG repeat tract longer than 107 were clinically affected, with the exception of one individual who had 140 CTG repeats but remained asymptomatic at 42 years of age. Large changes in repeat size were noted upon intergenerational inheritance of this

repeat, and these changed ranged from −86 to +7 repeats on paternal transmissions and −7 to +575 on maternal transmissions. The three largest expansions, estimated at +250, +350, +575, were seen on maternal transmission of the repeat. These very large expansions were seen in individuals from small ataxia kindreds for which linkage to human chromosome 13 could not be confirmed because of the small size of the kindreds, but these patients do have progressive ataxia. There were no changes in the SCA8 repeat size according to DNA isolated from peripheral blood and buccal tissue. No other tissue was tested to ascertain whether somatic instability occurs in this disorder.

The SCA8 transcript could not be detected on Northern blot analysis, but a weak signal was detected in multiple tissues by RNA dot blot analysis. Careful analysis of the transcript as well as the genomic sequences flanking the repeat provided no evidence of open reading frames. It is interesting that an adjacent transcript was identified immediately upstream of the SCA8 transcript and that this transcript encodes a protein that contains 575 amino acids and is highly homologous to the *Drosophila* kelch protein. The 5′ end of the sense transcript encoding the kelch protein overlaps with the 5′ end of the antisense SCA8 transcript. About 508 base pairs overlap between the *SCA8* antisense transcript and the .5-kbp sense mRNA. The SCA8 CTG repeat is present in the antisense transcript but is not contained within the sense transcript. These findings are quite interesting and at this time the relationship between the trinucleotide repeat and the functional regulation of either the antisense or sense transcript is not understood. SCA8 at this point remains unique in that it is caused by large expansion of CTG repeats that have not been shown to be translated.[83]

### Dentatorubropallidoluysian Atrophy

The finding of anticipation in DRPLA raised the possibility that this disorder is caused by unstable expansion of CAG repeats. To test this directly, Koide et al. used two approaches. First, they isolated cDNA clones carrying CAG repeats. They then analyzed polymorphic repeats within novel genes that were isolated by other investigators. Analysis of the CAG repeat within one such gene in DRPLA patients, known as CTG-B37 and isolated by Li et al.,[142] revealed expanded alleles in the 54 to 75 range on all DRPLA chromosomes.[93] Additional studies by several other investigators confirmed that this repeat is indeed expanded in patients with DRPLA and in those with variable clinical presentations such as Haw-River syndrome.[92,143] These studies confirmed that the normal range for the DRPLA repeat is 6 to 36 and the expanded range is 49 to 84. Intergenerational instability was greater in paternal transmissions than in maternal transmissions. These large expansions are obviously the basis of the clinical anticipation in this disease.[93,143]

It is interesting that the segregation rate of transmission of a mutant DRPLA allele is not equal to that of a wild-type DRPLA allele in paternal transmission. Analysis of Japanese families revealed that the mutant alleles were transmitted significantly more often than normal alleles in paternal transmissions.[143] The authors concluded that this gender-specific segregation distortion is most likely due to meiotic drive in DRPLA. Somatic mosaicism occurs in various tissues, but it is interesting that the repeat sizes were consistently smaller in the cerebellar and cerebral cortices than in cerebellar and cerebral white matter. These data suggest that somatic mosaicism may correlate inversely with the number of neurons in the tissue analyzed. Cortical tissue contains a higher density of postmitotic neurons, which may explain the lower degree of somatic mosaicism in these tissues.[144]

The *DRPLA* cDNA is predicted to code for 1185 amino acids; the CAG repeat is located 1462 base pairs downstream from the methionine initiation codon and is predicted to encode a polyglutamine tract. There are both a polyserine and a polyproline tract near the polyglutamine tract, but neither is polymorphic. The *DRPLA* gene product, atrophin-1, is widely expressed and shares no homology with other known proteins. Both the *DRPLA* transcript and protein are transcribed and translated in tissues from DRPLA patients.[145] Atrophin-1 is distributed throughout the cytoplasm in neurons and peripheral tissues of both unaffected and affected individuals.[145,146]

## GENOTYPE/PHENOTYPE CORRELATIONS

Molecular analysis in a large number of families with dominantly inherited ataxias confirms the significant degree of inter- and intrafamilial clinical variability among the ataxias. Nevertheless, analysis of repeat size and symptomatology in patients with a dominantly inherited ataxia has clearly demonstrated an inverse relationship between the size of the repeat and the age of onset (and, in SCA1 and 7, age of death). This inverse relationship has been demonstrated for all of the dominant inherited ataxias, but the contribution of the repeat size to age of onset varies according to subtype. For example, in SCA1 and SCA7 over 70 percent of the age of onset variability is accounted for by the number of CAG repeats, while in MJD/SCA3 the contribution of the repeat size is estimated to be about 45 to 48 percent. Furthermore, it is clear from careful study of the various kindreds that other factors, probably both environmental and genetic, contribute to the onset of disease.

Despite this strong inverse correlation between the size of repeat and age of onset, similar repeat sizes exert different toxic effects depending on the protein context. For example, a repeat size in the 50 to 60 range causes juvenile onset disease in SCA2, adult onset disease in SCA1, and no disease at all in SCA3 (Fig. 226-5A). Similarly, 70 to 80 repeats causes juvenile-onset SCA1 but adult onset disease in SCA3. Although the size of the repeat does correlate with the age of onset, other features of the protein must play an important role in mediating the toxicity of the expanded polyglutamine tract. This phenomenon is pronounced in SCA6, in which, although the expanded repeats are relatively small (ranging from 21 to 33), a change in the size of a repeat by one or two trinucleotides may alter the onset by almost one decade (Fig. 226-5B). Again, the data from SCA6 suggest that any repeat expansion is quite toxic within the context of the $\alpha_{1A}$-voltage-dependent calcium channel.

The additional important clinical correlate of CAG repeat size expansion is the fact that the anticipation can now clearly be explained by instability of these repeats. In all of these diseases, the earlier age of onset and the more severe clinical phenotype in later generations have been demonstrated to result from larger repeat expansions. For SCA1, the juvenile-onset disease is characterized by severe brain stem dysfunction in addition to the cerebellar symptoms. This brain stem dysfunction occurs quite early in the course of the juvenile disease, leading to death within 4 to 5 years after the onset of symptoms. For MJD/SCA3, larger repeat sizes are associated with early onset by the second decade and with predominantly pyramidal and extrapyramidal abnormalities. Moderate expansions typically cause disease in the third or fourth decade and are associated with cerebellar and pyramidal signs; extrapyramidal signs are quite infrequent. Smaller expansions typically cause late-onset disease in the fifth to seventh decade and manifest themselves predominantly in cerebellar signs and peripheral neuropathy.

The variability in the clinical phenotype of SCA7 is particularly well correlated with the size of the CAG repeat. Three different manifestations of SCA7 have been characterized, each clearly related to a specific range of repeats. Thirty to 40 SCA7 repeats cause disease after 20 years of age; 50 to 80 repeats cause disease between 5 and 20 years of age, and typically with visual deficits in addition to the cerebellar symptoms. Patients with more than 100 repeats have an infantile onset occurring shortly after birth or in the first few months of life. Some of these patients manifest features that involve nonneuronal tissue, for example, patent ductus arteriosus and congestive heart failure. Two infantile cases with more than 200 repeats died by 7 months of age.

A correlation between the size of the repeat and the clinical phenotype has also been observed in DRPLA. Larger expansions lead to juvenile onset disease characterized by epilepsy, myoclo-

nus, and developmental delay. These patients will have some ataxia and choreoathetosis, but it is the mental deficiency and the myoclonus and epilepsy that are most prominent. In adult onset cases, epilepsy may be seen in patients who had onset in their twenties, but typically those that have later onset usually suffer from ataxia and choreoathetosis and some may have mild dementia.

Gene dosage effects for the CAG expansions vary among trinucleotide repeat disorders. For SCA1, two cases have been confirmed to carry an expanded CAG repeat on both chromosomes. In both of these patients, the age of onset, rate of progression of disease, and clinical manifestation corresponded to what would be expected from the larger repeat size.[26] However, for SCA2, MJD/SCA3, SCA6, and DRPLA, homozygosity for the expansion causes earlier onset disease. In the case of DRPLA, homozygosity yields a clinical phenotype more typical of the juvenile onset disease: epilepsy, mental retardation, ataxia, and severe spastic paraparesis.[62,120,147–149] This gene dosage effect is not common to all triplet repeat disorders; it has not, for example, been observed in Huntington disease.[150]

The incidence of sporadic cases in the dominantly inherited spinocerebellar ataxias is rare. However, molecularly proven expansions in patients born to asymptomatic parents have been observed in SCA2, SCA6, and DRPLA. In a study by Riess and colleagues, 2 of 842 sporadic ataxia patients had an expansion of 41 and 49 repeats, respectively, for the SCA2 locus.[63] Genotyping for the SCA 6 mutation identified sporadic cases in two independent studies. These patients had quite late onset of disease and a very mild course of progression, raising the possibility that their parents did have the small expansion but developed no symptoms prior to their death from unrelated causes.[63,66] One DRPLA patient developed generalized epilepsy, ataxia, and choreoathetosis, and was found to carry an expanded allele with 62 repeats in the DRPLA gene. This patient's father showed no symptoms of DRPLA even at 66 years of age, so the patient was initially considered a sporadic case because of (apparently) negative family history. Molecular analysis, however, documented that the father had an expanded allele of 57 repeats. Most such "sporadic" cases are likely the offspring of parents that carry expanded alleles in a range that may not be penetrant at the time of the evaluation of the parent (or prior to their death).[143]

Although in each of these spinocerebellar ataxias there is involvement of cerebellar Purkinje cells or dentate neurons or both, it is clear that there is a component of cell specificity that confers distinctive features on some of these diseases. Dementia in SCA2 suggests cortical involvement; dystonia, rigidity, and Parkinsonism in SCA3 hint at basal ganglia abnormalities; severe macular degeneration is unique to SCA7. In DRPLA the presence of myoclonic epilepsy and mental retardation as well as choreoathetosis suggests that basal ganglionic and cortical dysfunction occur in this disease. Interestingly, when the expansions are very large, leading to severe juvenile-onset disease, there is significant overlap in the phenotypes of these disorders. Juvenile cases of SCA1 manifest not only the characteristic ataxia and brain stem dysfunction, but also some cognitive impairment and dystonic features. Juvenile-onset Huntington patients develop dystonia and seizures in addition to the classical phenotype of chorea and dementia seen in adult patients (see Chap. 223). This loss of cell specificity with large expansions is ntriguing, and hints that toxicity is probably much more widespread through neuronal subtypes that are normally spared when the repeat sizes are in the moderate range. Even more interesting, the very massive expansions observed in SCA7 cause not only loss of neuronal specificity but also involvement of nonneuronal tissue (e.g., the heart).

## PREVALENCE OF THE ATAXIAS AND DIAGNOSTIC CONSIDERATIONS

The prevalence of the dominantly inherited spinocerebellar ataxias varies considerably among different populations. MJD/SCA3 appears to be the most prevalent ataxia in all ethnic groups,

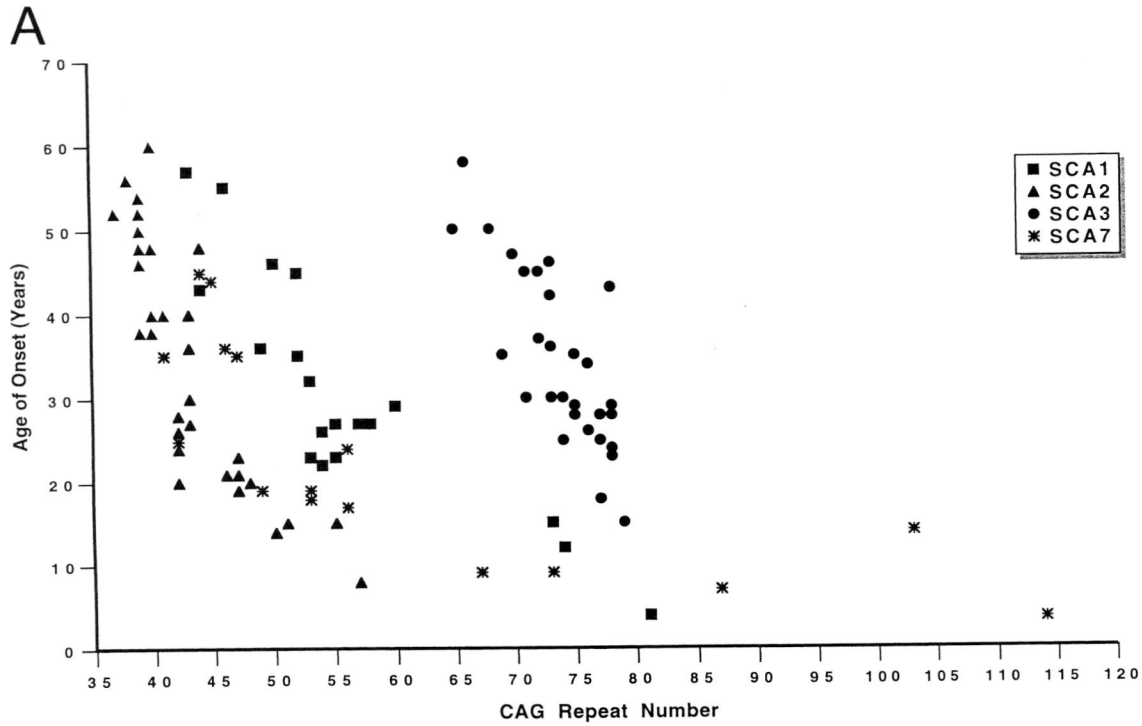

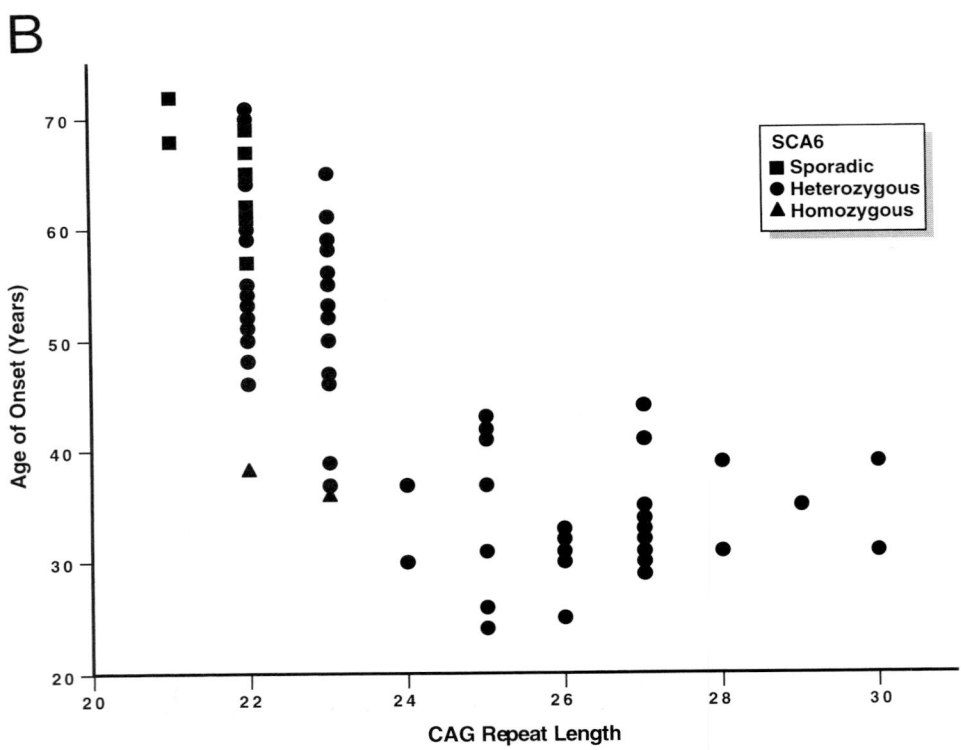

**Fig. 226-5** Relationship between age of onset and size of CAG repeat in SCA1, 2, 3, and 7 (*A*), and SCA6 (*B*). An inverse correlation is apparent between the size of the repeat and the age of onset for each SCA. However, the degree of impact of the repeat expansion on age of onset varies for each disease. Data for SCA1 are from the TX-SCA kindred; data for SCA2 are from Sanpei et al;[120] data for the SCA3 are from seven kindreds studied in the Zoghbi laboratory; data for SCA7 are from Benton et al;[78] data for SCA6 are from Zuchenko et al.,[61] Matsumura et al.,[64] Stevanin et al.,[65] Geschwind et al.,[66] Matsuyama et al.,[62] and Riess et al.[63]

accounting for 25 to 35 percent of all dominant ataxias. In Caucasian populations, SCA1 and SCA2 appear to be the second most common ataxias, whereas in Japanese populations DRPLA and SCA6 are the more prevalent ataxias. Although the DRPLA mutation has been observed in some Caucasian and African-American kindreds, the majority of DRPLA families are of Japanese descent. There are no extensive data on prevalence for SCA7 and SCA8 to date, but SCA7 appears to be a reasonably

**Table 226-4** Prevalence of SCAs

|           | Europe | Japan | US   |
|-----------|--------|-------|------|
| SCA1      | 21%    | 3%    | 6%   |
| SCA2      | 11%    | 6%    | 16%  |
| MJD/SCA3  | 31%    | 39%   | 17%  |
| SCA6      | 6%     | 10%   | 14%  |
| SCA7      | *      | *     | 10%  |
| SCA8      | *      | *     | 3%   |
| DRPLA     | <1%    | 18%   | *    |
| Undetermined | 31% | 24%   | 34%  |
| Number of families | 415 | 377 | 339 |

* No data

Data are from Reiss et al.[63], Watanabe et al.[68], Schöls et al.[71], Benton et al.[78], and Moseley et al.[130], additional data kindly provided by Drs. Stefan Pulst, Gen Sobue, and Thomas Klockgether.

**Table 226-5** Differentiating Features that Help Narrow the Choice of Molecular Test

| Symptoms | Likeliest Cause |
|----------|-----------------|
| Ataxia and dysarthria | any SCA |
| Myoclonus, slow saccades, areflexia | SCA2 |
| Bulging eyes, faciolingual fasciculations, extrapyramidal signs | SCA3/MJD |
| Late onset, slowly progressive or apparently sporadic onset ataxia | SCA6 |
| Macular degeneration | SCA7 |
| Choreoathetosis, myoclonic epilepsy, dementia | DRPLA |
| Generalized of complex partial seizures | SCA10* |

* Molecular test not yet available

common cause of dominantly inherited ataxia, possibly accounting for at least 10 percent of all ataxias (see Table 226-4). It is quite encouraging that more than 65 to 70 percent of all dominantly inherited ataxias can now be diagnosed molecularly. The remaining 30 to 35 percent will likely prove to be trinucleotide repeat expansions as well.

Takano et al.[151] proposed that the frequencies of normal alleles with relatively large numbers of CAG repeats are related to the prevalence rates of various spinocerebellar ataxias in different ethnic populations. To test this hypothesis, they investigated the relative prevalence of SCA1, SCA2, SCA3, SCA6, and DRPLA in 202 Japanese and 177 Caucasian families, and evaluated the distribution of the number of CAG repeats at these loci in normal individuals. The frequency of normal SCA1 and SCA2 alleles containing more than 30 or 22 repeats, respectively, is higher in Caucasians than in Japanese, which is consistent with the finding that relative prevalence of SCA1 and SCA2 was much higher in Caucasian pedigrees (10 percent and 14 percent, respectively) than in Japanese pedigrees (3 percent and 5 percent, respectively). Conversely, the prevalence of MJD/SCA3, SCA6, and DRPLA was much higher in the Japanese kindreds (43 percent, 11 percent, and 20 percent, respectively) than in Caucasian pedigrees (30 percent, 5 percent, and 0 percent, respectively). Confirming Takano's hypothesis, the frequencies of large normal alleles containing more than 27 repeats for the *MJD1* gene, more than 13 repeats for the *SCA6* gene, and more than 17 repeats for *DRPLA* gene were significantly higher in Japanese than in Caucasians. These data suggest a close association between the prevalence of the dominantly inherited ataxias and the frequencies of large normal alleles in various ethnic populations.

When the clinician is faced with a patient with progressive spinocerebellar ataxia, the clinician has several molecular tests from which to choose. There are some criteria that may help narrow the choice of the molecular test, based on the available phenotype-genotype correlations (Table 226-5). Nevertheless, it must be remembered that these criteria may not apply to an individual patient. An astute clinician can usually probe into family history, however, and excavate some useful information about ethnic background or clinical manifestations of disease in other family members.

## PATHOGENESIS OF THE SPINOCEREBELLAR ATAXIAS

SCA1 to 3, 6, and 7 are caused by the expansion of an unstable trinucleotide CAG repeat that encodes a tract of polyglutamines in the mutant protein. Even though there are no sequence similarities among the proteins encoded by these SCA genes, the diseases are thought to share a common pathogenesis at the protein level. Thus, models to explain the pathogenic mechanism behind each disease focus on the protein encoded by the disease-causing allele and, in particular, on the expanded polyglutamine tract within the protein. The models all posit that the mutation confers a toxic "gain-of-function"; that is, disease develops because of the expression of a mutant form of the protein, not because the protein loses its normal function.

### Studies on SCA Patient Material

One of the most important pieces of information regarding the mechanism of pathogenesis for the SCAs is that each of these disorders is inherited as a dominant disease. Several pathogenic mechanisms may result in a dominant disorder; one common mechanism is the expression of a mutant protein (rather than loss of function of the normal protein, as occurs in haploinsufficiency). In the case of SCA1, this point is illustrated by the fact that disease develops only as a consequence of the expansion of a polyglutamine tract within the *SCA1* gene on chromosome 6p23.[106] A heterozygous deletion of the *SCA1* gene does not result in SCA1, but may contribute to mental retardation and seizures in 6p deletion syndromes.[152,153]

A second important observation from patient studies is that for each of the polyglutamine-based SCAs examined, the mutant protein is detected in patient material and varies in size according to the length of the CAG repeat.[97,117,126,154,155] This clearly demonstrates that expansion of the CAG tract causes an increased number of glutamine residues. Importantly, it is also consistent with a model of pathogenesis based on a toxic gain-of-function by the protein with an expanded number of glutamines.

Immunohistochemical studies using patient material have been performed to determine the subcellular localization of both wild-type and mutant proteins encoded by the SCA mutant alleles. For SCA1, both the normal and mutant ataxin-1 are localized to neuronal nuclei throughout the brain in normal as well as affected individuals.[97] In Purkinje cells, a primary cellular site of SCA1 pathology, cytoplasmic protein was detected to a lesser extent. Peripheral tissues expressing ataxin-1 have a cytoplasmic localization. The protein encoded by the *SCA7* gene is found predominantly within the nucleus in all cell types examined.[117] In contrast, ataxin-2, ataxin-3, and atrophin-1 appear to normally be predominantly cytoplasmic.[126,146,154,155] *SCA6* encodes the $\alpha_{1A}$-voltage-dependent calcium channel, which has four transmembrane domains, and thus localizes to the plasma membrane.[61]

One aspect of the subcellular distribution for four of the SCA polyglutamine proteins is the localization of mutant proteins to ubiquitinated microscopic nuclear inclusions or aggregates within neuronal nuclei (Figs. 226-3 and 226-4). Nuclear inclusions containing the polyglutamine protein have been detected in brains of SCA1,[112] MJD/SCA3,[156] SCA7,[139] and DRPLA[157] patients. In some diseases, nuclear inclusions are found only in neurons in regions of the brain affected by the disease, for example, SCA1, MJD/SCA3, and DRPLA. Interestingly, in SCA7 patient material, ataxin-7-containing nuclear inclusions were not restricted to sites of severe neuronal loss associated with disease. Nuclear inclusions are not seen in SCA2 brain samples, but there is a clear increase in ataxin-2 immunostaining in Purkinje cells and dentate neurons, suggesting that there might be cytoplasmic accumulation of the mutant protein.[155] The dramatic presence of nuclear inclusions in brain material from SCA patients has led to the suggestion that protein aggregation is a critical molecular component of disease.[152,158] Furthermore, the presence of ubiquitin, a molecule that normally modifies and tags proteins targeted for proteolysis,[159] in the nuclear inclusions suggests that the formation of these aggregates is due to protein misfolding, and this misfolding may alter cellular degradation of the polyglutamine protein and possibly other cellular proteins.

To ascertain directly whether nuclear aggregates of a polyglutamine protein altered the cellular distribution of proteasomes, brain tissue from an SCA1 patient was examined immunohistochemically.[114] In brain regions affected by SCA1, ataxin-1 nuclear aggregates were intensely stained by antisera to the 20S subunit of the proteasome. Because alterations in proteasome function are usually associated with increased expression of the stress-response or heat-shock chaperone proteins, the subcellular distribution of the Hsp40 and Hsp70 families of chaperones were also assessed in an SCA1 brain. Ataxin-1 nuclear aggregates in neurons in the nucleus points centralis, a region affected in SCA1, were found to be positive for Hsp40, HDJ-2/HSDJ. In control human brain, Hsp40 immunohistochemical staining was cytoplasmic. Only minimal immunostaining for the constitutive form of Hsp70 was detectable. The localization of Hsp40 to the nuclear ataxin-1 aggregates supports the hypothesis that protein misfolding is responsible for the presence of the ataxin-1 aggregates in SCA1 patient brains. Furthermore, the ubiquitination of the aggregates and the association of the 20S proteasomes with the nuclear aggregates imply that nuclear proteasome-dependent protein degradation may be altered in SCA1.[114] These observations regarding SCA1 aggregates have recently been corroborated by SCA3 studies in which a fraction of the SCA3 inclusions stained positively with antibodies corresponding to Hsp40, Hsp70, and the 20S proteasome.[160] One important conclusion to be drawn from analyses of the subcellular distribution of the polyglutamine proteins in SCA patient material is that the nucleus is the primary site of pathogenesis in most of these diseases. Only in SCA2 and SCA6 does the pathogenesis seem to occur primarily in the cytoplasm.

## Cellular Models of SCA Pathogenesis

Examining polyglutamine proteins in cultured cell lines is proving to be an important strategy for assessing the behavior and properties of SCA mutant proteins. Analysis of the subcellular pattern of ataxin-1 expression upon transfection of the SCA1 gene into COS cells also revealed a predominately nuclear localization.[112] Ataxin-1 with an expanded number of glutamines formed nuclear aggregates that were larger than those aggregates seen in COS cells transfected with a wild-type allele of SCA1. In transfected kidney epithelial 293T cells, normal ataxin-3 with 27 repeats, as well as expanded ataxin-3 with 78 repeats, distributed diffusely throughout the cytoplasm.[156] Interestingly, transfected 293T cells expressing a C-terminal fragment of ataxin-3 containing the glutamine repeat localized to large cytoplasmic and occasionally nuclear aggregates. Furthermore, the expression of a truncated form of ataxin-3 with an expanded number of glutamines induced cell death in 293T cells. COS-7 cells expressing truncated forms of atrophin-1 with expanded polyglutamine stretches had filamentous peri- and intranuclear aggregates and eventually underwent apoptosis.[157] It is interesting that the cell death was partially suppressed by the addition of transglutaminase inhibitors, suggesting that the transglutaminase reaction may be involved in atrophin-1 aggregation and cell death.

Tait et al. found that full-length ataxin-3 localized primarily to the nucleus in transfected COS-7 and neuroblastoma cells.[127] These investigators also suggested that ataxin-3 associated with the nuclear matrix of COS-7 cells. Ataxin-1 has also been found associated with the nuclear matrix in transfected COS-1 cells.[112] In the case of ataxin-1, colocalization studies showed that mutant ataxin-1 causes a specific redistribution of the nuclear matrix-associated domain, promyelocytic oncogenic domain, containing the promyelocytic leukemia protein in transfected COS-1 cells. These data for ataxin-1 and ataxin-3 further support the concept that expression of a mutant SCA protein perturbs the ability of the nucleus to function properly.

Using transfected HeLa cells, Cummings et al. demonstrated that overexpression of the HDJ-2/HSDJ chaperone decreased the size and frequency of mutant ataxin-1 nuclear aggregates.[114] This result strongly indicated that misfolding of mutant ataxin-1 is involved in aggregation and that the cellular levels of a chaperone may directly regulate the propensity of an expanded polyglutamine protein to aggregate. Similarly, overexpression of HDJ-2/HSDJ in cells transfected with mutant ataxin-3 reduced the frequency of aggregate formation.[160] Thus, the studies performed to date on cultured cells expressing mutant forms of ataxin-1 and ataxin-3 demonstrate that SCA pathogenesis involves misfolding of the mutant protein in the nucleus that could then alter proteolytic processing of the mutant protein, thereby disrupting nuclear function. Central to this model are the ubiquitinated nuclear aggregates of the mutant SCA proteins. However, the precise role of these nuclear aggregates in pathogenesis is unclear from either the patient or cultured cell studies.

A key aspect of SCA pathogenesis that must be addressed by any model is the selective pathology seen in only a subset of neurons despite the broad expression pattern of each gene. One explanation for this might be that cell-specific proteins mediate pathogenesis through an interaction with each disease protein. For SCA1, the yeast two-hybrid approach has identified proteins that interact with ataxin-1.[161–163] Yeast expressing either a wild-type or mutant allele of ataxin-1 were transformed with human and mouse brain cDNA libraries. From the yeast two-hybrid screen using an adult human brain cDNA library, over 100 clones that encoded a protein capable of interacting equally well with wild-type and mutant ataxin-1 were identified.[161] Of these, a substantial number were found to encode ataxin-1. Thus, this approach led to the conclusion that the ataxin-1 protein is able to form multimers with itself. Further analysis of deletion mutants of ataxin-1 in the yeast two-hybrid system mapped this self-association region to a stretch between amino acids 495 and 605, beyond the polyglutamine stretch.

In a second yeast two-hybrid screen using a mouse brain cDNA library, the leucine-rich acidic nuclear protein (LANP) was identified as an ataxin-1 interacting protein.[162] Previously, in situ hybridization studies demonstrated expression of murine Lanp mRNA in cerebellar Purkinje cells and granule neurons, and that the highest level of Lanp expression occurs in Purkinje cells around postnatal day 14,[164] the same time of the transient burst of Sca1 expression in the mouse.[111] LANP has been previously isolated from peripheral tissues using a variety of independent strategies. Vaesen et al. purified it as a putative HLA DR-associated protein I (PHAPI) from lymphoblastoid cells based on its association with a peptide fragment from HLA-DR2.[165] The same protein was also isolated as phosphoprotein 32 (pp32) and found to inhibit the formation of transformed foci in rat embryo fibroblasts when cotransfected with a variety of oncogenes.[166] Li et al. suggested that LANP is a phosphatase 2A inhibitor.[167] More recently, mapmodulin, a protein proposed to modulate the binding of microtubule-associated proteins to microtubules, was shown to have the identical peptide sequence as PHAPI and LANP.[168]

Immunohistochemical staining for LANP in mouse cerebellar cortex confirmed its predominant expression by Purkinje cells and localized it to the nuclei of these cells.[162] Given the very high level of LANP expression within the nuclei of cerebellar Purkinje cells, this protein must have some role in Purkinje cell function that is probably distinct from some of the cytoplasmic functions proposed in peripheral dividing cells.

Immunofluorescence studies revealed that in transfected COS cells, LANP colocalized to the nuclear aggregates containing either wild-type or mutant ataxin-1.[162]

The yeast two-hybrid approach was used to define the regions of ataxin-1 that interact with LANP and to determine whether the strength of this interaction is influenced by the number of glutamines within ataxin-1.[162] From these studies, it appears that ataxin-1 interacts with LANP through the polyglutamine tract and via sequences located between residues 570 to 816. Furthermore, the strength of interaction between LANP and ataxin-1 containing 82 glutamines (82Q) was significantly higher than with ataxin-1 containing 30 glutamines (30Q), suggesting that LANP may also be involved in SCA1 pathogenesis. The temporal and subcellular pattern of LANP and ataxin-1 expression, combined with the cellular distribution of LANP expression, argue strongly that this interaction is an important component of the selective neuronal degeneration in SCA1.

An interaction between the glycolytic enzyme glyceraldehyde-3-phosphate dehydrogenase (GAPDH) was also demonstrated using the yeast two-hybrid approach.[163] Burke et. al. demonstrated that GAPDH interacts with huntingtin and atrophin-1.[169] Because GAPDH is a regulatory enzyme in glycolysis, it is tempting to propose that the binding of mutant ataxin-1 or atrophin-1 to GAPDH may have deleterious effects on its function, decreasing ATP production, and subsequently leading to neuronal degeneration.[169] However, several important considerations render this hypothesis less likely. First, the cellular levels of GAPDH are much higher than the cellular levels of any of the polyglutamine proteins. Thus, it is unlikely that a stoichiometric interaction between SCA proteins and GAPDH would impair the function of GAPDH to a physiologically relevant degree. In addition, GAPDH, a regulatory enzyme in the glycolytic conversion of glucose to pyruvic acid, is widely expressed throughout the brain. Yet, each SCA is characterized by a unique cellular pathologic pattern. It is not clear how the interaction of a polyglutamine protein with the ubiquitously expressed GAPDH would affect only a specific subset of neurons. Therefore, it seems that if the interaction of ataxin-1 with GAPDH is involved in SCA1 pathogenesis, it is most likely one component of a complex pathway that occurs well after pathogenesis is initiated.

## Animal Models of the SCAs

**SCA1.** The first transgenic mouse model of a SCA utilized the strong Purkinje cell-specific regulatory elements from the Pcp2/L7 gene to direct expression of the human *SCA1* cDNA transgenes encoding the entire ataxin-1 protein.[170] Transgenic lines were established expressing high levels of either a wild-type allele of SCA1 with 30 repeats or an expanded allele with 82 repeats. Only animals from transgenic lines expressing the expanded 82 CAG repeat *SCA1* transgene developed severe ataxia and pathologic changes within their cerebellar Purkinje cells. These studies demonstrated that pathologic changes are induced specifically by the expression of an intact, expanded *SCA1* allele. In contrast, although they manifested hippocampal and cerebellar learning difficulties, mice homozygous for a null mutation within their *Sca1* gene failed to develop the ataxia and Purkinje cell pathology seen in transgenic mice expressing a mutant *SCA1* allele.[115] This clearly demonstrated that SCA1 pathogenesis requires the expression a mutant allele of SCA1 and does not ensue with the loss of ataxin-1 function.

In SCA1 transgenic mice, normal ataxin-1 localized to several ~0.5 μM nuclear aggregates. Expanded ataxin-1, on the other hand, localized to a single ~2 μM ubiquitinated nuclear aggregate, as it does in patient material.[112] These aggregates also stained positive for the 20S proteasome and the HDJ-2/HSDJ (Hsp40) chaperone protein.[114] The appearance of single nuclear aggregates in SCA1 transgenic mice carrying the expanded ataxin-1 allele preceded the onset of ataxia by approximately 6 weeks. Thus, the SCA1 transgenic mice manifest the cellular pathologic features found in patients.

To gain insight into disease progression in the SCA1 transgenic mice, animals were examined at various ages for neurologic alterations and morphologic changes at the cellular level.[171] SCA1 transgenic animals expressing an expanded allele with 82 repeats progressively lost cerebellar function. Cerebellar impairment in 5-week-old mice was limited to decreased ability to improve motor performance over 4 days of successive trials on a rotating rod; the mice showed no gait abnormalities, and were normal in motor activity, balance, and coordination. But by 12 weeks, this slight motor skill impairment became full-blown ataxia.

No histologic alterations were detectable during the first 3 weeks of postnatal life in the SCA1 mice. At the time of impaired motor learning on the rotating rod apparatus (5 to 6 weeks of age), the Purkinje cells showed cytoplasmic vacuoles, a loss of proximal dendritic branches, and a decrease in the number of dendritic spines, indicating that mutant ataxin-1 may impair the maintenance of dendritic arborization. By the time ataxia was severe (12 to 15 weeks), there were numerous morphologic abnormalities in the Purkinje cells, but little evidence of cell loss. Expression of full-length mutant ataxin-1 in cells vulnerable to the human disease evidently can disrupt cellular function enough to cause ataxia without killing the affected neuronal population. This is an important finding, as the neurologic phenotype in SCA patients had long been assumed to result from apoptosis. The Purkinje cell loss that does occur in late-stage disease most likely results from the dysfunction already begun in earlier stages.

One striking neuropathologic feature of SCA1 transgenic mice is the movement of the Purkinje cell bodies away from their typical location at the interface of the molecular and granule cell layer into the intermediate level of the molecular layer. This heterotopia is not due to a developmental abnormality: histologic examination of young animals revealed no heterotopia in the early stages of the disease, but it is frequent by the time of overt ataxia.

A more likely explanation for the occurrence of heterotopic Purkinje cells is based on the appearance of the dendritic changes earlier in the course of the disease. Postmortem studies of the cerebellum in patients with SCA1 have shown structural abnormalities of Purkinje cells as well as cell loss. Using Golgi techniques and immunohistochemical methods, Ferrer et al.[172] and Koeppen et al.[173] described dendritic simplification with loss of spines similar to that found in the SCA1 transgenic mice. A hallmark of SCA1 pathology is the occurrence of frequent proximal axonal dilatations (torpedoes), a feature not found in the SCA1 mice. It is clear from autopsy studies of SCA1 patients that morphologic alterations antedate cell death in at least some of the Purkinje cells of these patients.

Having demonstrated the characteristics of disease in transgenic mouse models of SCA1,[170,171] subsequent studies examined the molecular and cellular aspects of ataxin-1 that are critical for pathogenesis. The first series of experiments addressed the importance of the subcellular localization of ataxin-1. Histologic analyses revealed that ataxin-1 is predominantly a nuclear protein.[97] Typically, the cellular transport machinery recognizes a target protein by its nuclear localization signal (NLS), and then moves the protein from the cytoplasm to the nucleus through pores in the nuclear envelope.[174] Although NLSs can be quite variable in appearance, many of these peptide motifs conform to the consensus cluster of arginines and lysines found in SV40 T antigen.[175] Two possible NLSs of this type were found in the ataxin-1 amino acid sequence: one near the N-terminus at lysine 15, and one near the C-terminus at lysine 772.[176] Analysis of the role of these putative NLSs in ataxin-1 nuclear transport was carried out in transfected COS cells. The C-terminal motif at lysine 772, but not the N-terminal element, is, indeed, a functional NLS.

Klement et al. studied transgenic mice expressing ataxin-1(82Q) with a mutated nuclear localization sequence, ataxin-1K772T. These mice failed to develop Purkinje cell pathology and associated motor dysfunction, and no ataxin-1 aggregates formed in the cytoplasm. Thus, nuclear localization is critical for pathogenesis and ataxin-1 aggregation. Furthermore, these data demonstrate that the mutation exerts its toxic effects at the protein, not the RNA, level.[176] In a second series of transgenic mice, ataxin-1 (77Q) containing a deletion of amino acids within the self-association region was expressed within the nuclei of Purkinje cells.[176] These mice developed ataxia and Purkinje cell pathology similar to the original SCA1 mice — with no evidence of nuclear ataxin-1 aggregation. Thus, although nuclear localization of ataxin-1 is necessary, nuclear aggregation of ataxin-1 is not required to initiate pathogenesis in transgenic mice.

The best available model of SCA1 pathogenesis proposes that sequences within the ataxin-1 protein, in addition to the polyglutamine tract, are critical in specifying the site and course of disease. The deleterious effects leading to SCA1 symptoms are initiated by the localization of ataxin-1 to the nucleus. Once there, the mutant form of ataxin-1 misfolds and is altered in its distribution. The nuclear distribution of ataxin-1 may depend on residues within the self-association region as well as the length of the polyglutamine tract, because deletion of ataxin-1's self-association domain compromises its ability to form nuclear aggregates in COS cells despite its nuclear localization. In the nucleus, ataxin-1 interacts with LANP and probably other proteins. It is likely that changes in nuclear architecture and the interaction of mutant ataxin-1 with other nuclear proteins alter gene expression, all of which may well lead to neuronal dysfunction, symptomatology, and, eventually, neuronal loss. Thus, while the expanded polyglutamine tract is clearly critical for pathogenesis, additional segments of ataxin-1 are just as significant. The extent to which this model of SCA1 pathogenesis may be applicable to other SCAs and polyglutamine disorders remains to be seen.

**SCA3.** Ikeda and colleagues established transgenic mice expressing full-length and truncated versions of the MJD/SCA3 protein also using the Pcp-2/L7 promoter region.[177] In independent transgenic lines, they obtained expression of *MJD1* cDNA transgenes encoding full-length and truncated proteins with 79 glutamine residues (designated MJD79 and Q79C, respectively, by the authors) as well as a truncated protein with 35 glutamine residues (Q35C). The Q35C and Q79C proteins contained a fragment comprising the polyglutamine tract and 42 residues C-terminal to glutamine repeat (hence the C designation). In addition, transgenic animals expressing only a 79-glutamine residue tract (Q79) were produced using the Pcp-2/L7 promoter region. Animals from both the Q79C and Q79 lines developed ataxia rapidly, by 4 weeks of age. None of the animals containing the full-length MJD79 or the truncated Q35C constructs was ataxic by 23 or 32 weeks of age, respectively.

Histologic examination of an 8-week-old Q79C transgenic animal revealed that although the cerebellum maintained its fundamental structure, it occupied only about 15 percent of its normal volume. All three layers of the cerebellum were affected. The molecular layer showed substantial thinning; the Purkinje cells were shrunken, had attenuated dendrites, and showed reduced calbindin immunoreactivity; the granule cell layer showed a significant reduction in cell number, with many of the existing cells displaying an altered, shrunken morphology.

The expanded polyglutamine tract can thus, on its own, induce Purkinje cell death and ataxia. However, in contrast to the SCA1 transgenic animals, the SCA3 transgenic mice developed ataxia as a direct result of Purkinje cell *loss*. Ikeda and colleagues proposed that a truncated form of *MJD1* — and perhaps other polyglutamine repeat-containing proteins — is more potent at inducing cell death than its full-length counterpart. Furthermore, they hypothesized that a cell-specific proteolytic cleavage of the mutant protein exposes a subset of cells to the detrimental effects of an elongated polyglutamine tract. The finding that ataxin-3 can be cleaved by a caspase,[178] a member of a family of cysteine proteases involved in apoptosis, is consistent with the possibility that ataxin-3 exerts its toxicity after cleavage and release of a polyglutamine tract. Further support for this model was provided by the report that a C-terminal fragment of ataxin-3 containing an expanded polyglutamine tract formed cytoplasmic and nuclear aggregates and was cytotoxic in transfected 293T cells.[156] However, to date there is no direct evidence that cleavage of ataxin-3 is critical for MJD/SCA3 pathogenesis.

## CONCLUDING REMARKS, MANAGEMENT, AND COUNSELING

The dominantly inherited spinocerebellar ataxias share many properties in addition to their overlapping clinical and neuropathologic features. (a) A new class of mutation that involves the expansion of a trinucleotide repeat causes them all, and the dynamic nature of this mutation explains the genetic anticipation seen in this group of diseases. (b) The mutant genes are translated, except for *SCA8*, and appear to be responsible for the neuronal dysfunction. The glutamine expansion most likely alters the conformation of the protein, which in turn might lead to aberrant protein-protein interactions and/or protein misfolding. (c) The presence of protein aggregates in the nuclei of neurons affected by SCA1, 3, 7, and DRPLA suggests that the misfolded protein might be resistant to degradation. The recent finding that members of the chaperone family of proteins and the proteasome colocalize with the mutant protein aggregates raises interesting possibilities about the roles of protein misfolding and proteolysis in SCA pathogenesis. (d) The selective neuronal degeneration in each disease is probably due to varying levels of the mutant protein in each cell group, and specific protein-protein interactions unique to the vulnerable neurons.

At this date, management is confined to supportive care. Tremor-controlling drugs do not work very well for cerebellar tremors; no dietary factor has been shown to curtail symptoms, nor has exercise or physical therapy been shown to stem the progression of incoordination or muscle weakness. Nonetheless, patients should, as much as possible, maintain activity and a desirable weight, if only because after they are wheelchair-bound, they become susceptible to so many secondary problems.

In the meantime, diagnosis of the SCAs has been greatly facilitated by the cloning of the respective genes. Patients no longer need undergo extensive and costly work-ups; a simple, inexpensive molecular test provides certain diagnosis for those who manifest symptoms. More importantly, patients and their relatives have the option of seeking genetic counseling. For presymptomatic family members, genetic testing needs to be proffered with great caution and sensitivity. The test may simply replace fear of the unknown with fear of the known. Career, family, and financial decisions are all affected. Until there is a viable treatment, it is likely that only a minority of patients will want to know or be able to handle knowing. Our best hope lies in future studies using the tools of cell biology, biochemistry, and genetics, which should provide insight into the pathogenesis of these diseases and uncover therapeutic options that could slow the progression of the disease.

## ACKNOWLEDGMENTS

The authors gratefully acknowledge Blanca E. Lopez for her patience and expertise with references; Vicky Brandt for her editorial commitment to clarity; and to the NIH/NINDS and Howard Hughes Medical Institute for making our work possible.

## REFERENCES

1. Greenfield JG: *The Spino-Cerebellar Degenerations.* Springfield, IL, Charles C. Thomas, 1954.
2. Koeppen AH, Barron KD: The neuropathology of olivopontocerebellar atrophy, in Duvoisin RC, Plaitakis A (eds): *The Olivopontocerebellar Atrophies.* New York, Raven, 1984, p 13.
3. Friedreich N: Über degenerative Atrophie der spinalen Hinterstrange. *Virchows Arch Pathol Anat* **26**:433, 1863.

4. Marie P: Sur l'heredoataxie cerebelleuse. *Semin Med (Paris)* **13**:444, 1893.

5. Holmes G: An attempt to classify cerebellar disease with a note on Marie's hereditary cerebellar ataxia. *Brain* **30**:545, 1907.

6. Harding AE: The clinical features and classification of the late onset autosomal dominant cerebellar ataxias: A study of eleven families, including descendants of the "Drew family of Walworth." *Brain* **105**:1, 1982.

7. Zoghbi HY: The spinocerebellar degenerations, in Appel SH (ed): *Current Neurology*. St. Louis, Mosby-Year Book, 1991, p 121.

8. Konigsmark BW, Weiner LP: The olivopontocerebellar atrophies: A review. *Medicine (Baltimore)* **49**:227, 1970.

9. Yakura H, Wakisaka A, Fujimoto S, Itakura K: Hereditary ataxia and HLA genotypes. *N Engl J Med* **291**:154, 1974.

10. Jackson JF, Currier RD, Terasaki PI, Morton NE: Spinocerebellar ataxia and HLA linkage: Risk prediction by HLA typing. *N Engl J Med* **296**:1138, 1977.

11. Gray RC, Oliver CP: Marie's hereditary cerebellar ataxia (olivoponto-cerebellar atrophy). *Minn Med* **24**:327, 1941.

12. Schut JW: Hereditary ataxia: Clinical study through six generations. *Arch Neurol Psychiatr* **63**:535, 1950.

13. Schut LJ: Schut family ataxia, in de Jong J (ed): *Handbook of Clinical Neurology; Volume 16: Hereditary Neuropathies and Spinocerebellar Atrophies*. Amsterdam, Elsevier, 1991, p 481.

14. Currier RD, Glover G, Jackson JF, Tipton AC: Spinocerebellar ataxia: Study of a large kindred. *Neurology* **22**:1040, 1972.

15. Nino HE, Noreen HJ, Dubey DP: A family with hereditary ataxia: HLA typing. *Neurology* **30**:12, 1980.

16. Zoghbi HY, Pollack MS, Lyons LA, Ferell RE, Daiger SP, Beaudet AL: Spinocerebellar ataxia: Variable age of onset and linkage to human leukocyte antigen in a large kindred. *Ann Neurol* **23**:580, 1988.

17. Keats BJB, Pollack MS, McCall A, Wilensky MA, Ward LJ, Lu M, Zoghbi HY: Localization of the gene for spinocerebellar ataxia to the short arm of chromosome 6 in a kindred for which close linkage to HLA is excluded. *Am J Hum Genet* **49**:972, 1991.

18. Spadaro M, Giunti P, Lulli P, Frontali M, Jodice C, Cappellacci S, Morellini M, et al: HLA-linked spinocerebellar ataxia: A clinical and genetic study of large Italian kindreds. *Acta Neurol Scand* **85**:257, 1992.

19. Bryer A, Martell RW, du Toif ED, Beighton P: Adult onset spinocerebellar ataxia linked to HLA in a South African kindred of mixed ancestry. *Tissue Antigens* **40**:111, 1992.

20. Matilla T, Volpini V, Genis D, Rosell J, Corral J, Davalos A, Molins A, et al: Presymptomatic analysis of spinocerebellar ataxia type 1 (SCA1) via the expansion of the *SCA1* CAG-repeat in a large pedigree displaying anticipation and parental male bias. *Hum Mol Genet* **2**:2123, 1993.

21. Ranum LPW, Chung M-y, Banfi S, Bryer A, Schut LJ, Ramesar R, Duvick LA, et al: Molecular and clinical correlations in spinocerebellar ataxia type 1 (SCA1): Evidence for familial effects on the age of onset. *Am J Hum Genet* **55**:244, 1994.

22. Jodice C, Malaspina P, Persichetti F, Novelletto A, Spadaro M, Giunti P, Morocutti C, et al: Effect of trinucleotide repeat length and parental sex on phenotypic variation in spinocerebellar ataxia 1. *Am J Hum Genet* **54**:959, 1994.

23. Giunti P, Sweeney MG, Spadaro M, Jodice C, Novelletto A, Malaspina P, Frontali M, et al: The trinucleotide repeat expansion on chromosome 6p (SCA1) in autosomal dominant cerebellar ataxias. *Brain* **17**:645, 1994.

24. Dubourg O, Dürr A, Cancel G, Stevanin G, Chneiweiss H, Penet C, Agid Y, et al: Analysis of the SCA1 CAG repeat in a large number of families with dominant ataxia: Clinical and molecular correlations. *Ann Neurol* **37**:176, 1995.

25. Kameya T, Abe K, Aoki M, Sahara M, Tobita M, Konno H, Itoyama Y: Analysis of spinocerebellar ataxia type 1 (SCA1)-related CAG trinucleotide expansion in Japan. *Neurology* **45**:1587, 1995.

26. Goldfarb LG, Vasconcelos O, Platonov FA, Lunkes A, Kipnis V, Kononova S, Chabrashvili T, et al: Unstable triplet repeat and phenotypic variability of spinocerebellar ataxia type 1. *Ann Neurol* **39**:500, 1996.

27. Bürk K, Abele M, Fetter M, Dichgans J, Skalej M, Laccone F, Didierjean O, et al: Autosomal dominant cerebellar ataxia type I clinical features and MRI in families with SCA1, SCA2 and SCA3. *Brain* **119**:1497, 1996.

28. Filla A, De Michele G, Campanella G, Perretti A, Santoro L, Serlenga L, Ragno M, et al: Autosomal dominant cerebellar ataxia type I. Clinical and molecular study in 36 Italian families including a comparison between SCA1 and SCA2 phenotypes. *J Neurol Sci* **142**:140, 1996.

29. Schöls L, Amoiridis G, Buttner T, Przuntek H, Epplen JT, Riess O: Autosomal dominant cerebellar ataxia: Phenotypic differences in genetically defined subtypes? *Ann Neurol* **42**:924, 1997.

30. Kish GJ, El-Awar M, Schut L, Leach L, Oscar-Berman M, Freedman M: Cognitive deficits in olivopontocerebellar atrophy: Implications for the cholinergic hypothesis of Alzheimer's dementia. *Ann Neurol* **24**:200, 1988.

31. Trojano L, Chiacchio L, Grossi D, Pisacreta AI, Calabrese O, Castaldo I, De Michele G, et al: Determinants of cognitive disorders in autosomal dominant cerebellar ataxia type 1. *J Neurol Sci* **157**:162, 1998.

32. Orozco G, Estrada R, Perry TL, Arana J, Fernandez R, Gonzalez-Quevedo A, Galarraga J, et al: Dominantly inherited olivopontocerebellar atrophy from eastern Cuba. Clinical, neuropathological, and biochemical findings. *J Neurol Sci* **93**:37, 1989.

33. Gispert S, Twells R, Orozco G, Brice A, Weber J, Heredero L, Scheufler K, et al: Chromosomal assignment of the second locus for autosomal dominant cerebellar ataxia (SCA2) to chromosome 12q23-24.1. *Nat Genet* **4**:295, 1993.

34. Pulst SM, Nechiporuk A, Starkman S: Anticipation in spinocerebellar ataxia type 2. *Nat Genet* **5**:8, 1993.

35. Belal S, Cancel G, Stevanin G, Hentati F, Khati C, Ben Hamida C, Auburger G, et al: Clinical and genetic analysis of a Tunisian family with autosomal dominant cerebellar ataxia type 1 linked to the SCA2 locus. *Neurology* **44**:1423, 1994.

36. Lopes-Cendes I, Andermann E, Attig E, Cendes F, Bosch S, Wagner M, Gerstenbrand F, et al: Confirmation of the SCA-2 locus as an alternative locus for dominantly inherited spinocerebellar ataxias and refinement of the candidate region. *Am J Hum Genet* **54**:774, 1994.

37. Dürr A, Smadja D, Cancel G, Lezin A, Stevanin G, Mikol J, Bellance R, et al: Autosomal dominant cerebellar ataxia type I in Martinique (French West Indies). Clinical and neuropathological analysis of 53 patients from three unrelated SCA2 families. *Brain* **118**:1573, 1995.

38. Filla A, De Michele G, Banfi S, Santoro L, Perretti A, Cavalcanti F, Pianese L, et al: Has spinocerebellar ataxia type 2 a distinct phenotype? Genetic and clinical study of an Italian family. *Neurology* **45**:793, 1995.

39. Sasaki H, Fukazawa T, Wakisaka A, Hamada K, Hamada T, Koyama T, Tsuji S, et al: Central phenotype and related varieties of spinocerebellar ataxia 2 (SCA2): A clinical and genetic study with a pedigree in the Japanese. *J Neurol Sci* **144**:176, 1996.

40. Geschwind DH, Perlman S, Figueroa CP, Treiman LJ, Pulst SM: The prevalence and wide clinical spectrum of the spinocerebellar ataxia type 2 trinucleotide repeat in patients with autosomal dominant cerebellar ataxia. *Am J Hum Genet* **60**:842, 1997.

41. Nakano KK, Dawson DM, Spence A: Machado disease. A hereditary ataxia in Portuguese emigrants to Massachusetts. *Neurology* **22**:49, 1972.

42. Rosenberg RN, Nyhan WL, Bay C, Shore P: Autosomal dominant striatonigral degeneration: A clinical, pathologic and biochemical study of a new genetic disorder. *Neurology* **26**:703, 1976.

43. Sequeiros J: Machado-Joseph Disease: Epidemiology, genetics, and molecular epidemiology, in Lechtenberg R (ed): *Handbook of Cerebellar Diseases*. New York, Marcel Dekker, 1993, p 345.

44. Healton EB, Brust JC, Kerr DL, Resor S, Penn A: Presumably Azorean disease in a presumably non-Portuguese family. *Neurology* **30**:1084, 1980.

45. Sakai T, Ohta M, Ishino H: Joseph disease in a non-Portuguese family. *Neurology* **33**:74, 1983.

46. Livingstone IR, Sequeiros J: Machado-Joseph disease in an American-Italian family. *J Neurogenet* **1**:185, 1984.

47. Goldberg-Stern H, D'Jaldetti R, Melamed E, Gadoth N: Machado-Joseph (Azorean) disease in a Yemenite Jewish family in Israel. *Neurology* **44**:1298, 1994.

48. Takiyama Y, Nishizawa M, Tanaka H, Kawashima S, Sakamoto H, Karube Y, Shimazaki H, et al: The gene for Machado-Joseph disease maps to human chromosome 14q. *Nat Genet* **4**:300, 1993.

49. St. George-Hyslop P, Rogaeva E, Huterer J, Tsuda T, Santos J, Haines JL, Schlumpf K, et al: Machado-Joseph disease in pedigrees of Azorean descent is linked to chromosome 14. *Am J Hum Genet* **55**:120, 1994.

50. Sequeiros J, Silveira I, Maciel P, Coutinho P, Manaia A, Gaspar C, Burlet P, et al: Genetic linkage studies of Machado-Joseph disease with chromosome 14q STRPs in 16 Portuguese-Azorean kindreds. *Genomics* **21**:645, 1994.

51. Coutinho P, Andrade C: Autosomal dominant system degeneration in Portuguese families of the Azores Islands: A new genetic disorder involving cerebellar, pyramidal, extrapyramidal, and spinal cord motor functions. *Neurology* **28**:703, 1978.

52. Rosenberg RN: Dominant ataxias. *Res Publ Assoc Res Nerv Ment Dis* **60**:195, 1983.

53. Barbeau A, Roy M, Cunha L, de Vincente AN, Rosenberg RN, Nyhan WL, MacLeod PL, et al: The natural history of Machado-Joseph disease. An analysis of 138 personally examined cases. *Can J Neurol Sci* **11**:510, 1984.

54. Stevanin G, Chneiweiss H, Le Guern E, Ravise N, Dürr A, Penet C, Agid Y, et al: Genetic heterogeneity of autosomal dominant cerebellar ataxia type I: Evidence for the existence of a third locus. *Hum Mol Genet* **2**:1483, 1993.

55. Giunti P, Sweeney MG, Harding AE: Detection of the Machado-Joseph disease/spinocerebellar ataxia three trinucleotide repeat expansion in families with autosomal dominant motor disorders, including the Drew family of Walworth. *Brain* **118**:1077, 1995.

56. Matilla T, McCall A, Subramony SH, Zoghbi HY: Molecular and clinical correlations in spinocerebellar ataxia type 3 and Machado-Joseph disease. *Ann Neurol* **38**:68, 1995.

57. Maruyama H, Nakamura S, Matsuyama Z, Sakai T, Doyu M, Sobue G, Seto M, et al: Molecular features of the CAG repeats and clinical manifestation of Machado-Joseph disease. *Hum Mol Genet* **4**:807, 1995.

58. Maciel P, Gaspar C, DeStefano AL, Silveira I, Coutinho P, Radvany J, Dawson DM, et al: Correlation between CAG repeat length and clinical features in Machado-Joseph disease. *Am J Hum Genet* **57**:54, 1995.

59. Dürr A, Stevanin G, Cancel G, Duyckaerts C, Abbas N, Didierjean O, Chneiweiss H, et al: Spinocerebellar ataxia 3 and Machado-Joseph disease: Clinical, molecular and neuropathological features. *Ann Neurol* **39**:490, 1996.

60. Flanigan K, Gardner K, Alderson K, Galser B, Otterud B, Leppert MF, Kaplan C, et al: Autosomal dominant spinocerebellar ataxia with sensory axonal neuropathy (SCA4): Clinical description and genetic localization to chromosome 16q22.1. *Am J Hum Genet* **59**:392, 1996.

61. Zhuchenko O, Bailey J, Bonnen P, Ashizawa T, Stockton DW, Amos C, Dobyns WB, et al: Autosomal dominant cerebellar ataxia (SCA6) associated with small polyglutamine expansions in the $\alpha_{1A}$-voltage-dependent calcium channel. *Nat Genet* **15**:62, 1997.

62. Matsuyama Z, Kawakami H, Maruyama H, Izumi Y, Komure O, Udaka F, Kameyama M, et al: Molecular features of the CAG repeats of spinocerebellar ataxia 6 (SCA6). *Hum Mol Genet* **6**:1283, 1997.

63. Riess O, Schols L, Bottger G, Nolte D, Vieira-Saecker AMM, Schimming C, Kreuz F, et al: SCA6 is caused by moderate CAG expansion in the $\alpha_{1A}$-voltage-dependent calcium channel gene. *Hum Mol Genet* **6**:1289, 1997.

64. Matsumura R, Futamura N, Fujimoto Y, Yanagimoto S, Horikawa H, Suzumura A, Takayanagi T: Spinocerebellar ataxia type 6: Molecular and clinical features of 35 Japanese patients including one homozygous for the CAG repeat expansion. *Neurology* **49**:1238, 1997.

65. Stevanin G, Dürr A, David G, Didierjean O, Cancel G, Rivaud S, Tourbah A, et al: Clinical and molecular features of spinocerebellar ataxia type 6. *Neurology* **49**:1243, 1997.

66. Geschwind DH, Perlman S, Figueroa KP, Karrim J, Baloh RW, Pulst SM: Spinocerebellar ataxia type 6. Frequency of the mutation and genotype-phenotype correlations. *Neurology* **49**:1247, 1997.

67. Ikeuchi T, Takano H, Koide R, Horikawa Y, Honma Y, Onishi Y, Igarashi S, et al: Spinocerebellar ataxia type 6: CAG repeat expansion in $\alpha_{1A}$ voltage-dependent calcium channel gene and clinical variations in Japanese population. *Ann Neurol* **42**:879, 1997.

68. Watanabe H, Tanaka F, Matsumoto M, Doyu M, Ando T, Mitsuma T, Sobue G: Frequency analysis of autosomal dominant cerebellar ataxias in Japanese patients and clinical characterization of spinocerebellar ataxia type 6. *Clin Genet* **53**:13, 1998.

69. Yabe I, Sasaki H, Matsuura T, Takada A, Wakisaka A, Suzuki Y, Fukazawa T, et al: SCA6 mutation analysis in a large cohort of the Japanese patients with late-onset pure cerebellar ataxia. *J Neurol Sci* **156**:89, 1998.

70. Takiyama Y, Sakoe K, Namekawa M, Soutome M, Esumi E, Ogawa T, Ishikawa K: A Japanese family with spinocerebellar ataxia type 6 which includes three individuals homozygous for an expanded CAG repeat in the SCA6/CACNL1A4 gene. *J Neurol Sci* **158**:141, 1998.

71. Schöls L, Kruger R, Amoiridis G, Przuntek H, Epplen JT, Riess O: Spinocerebellar ataxia type 6: Genotype and phenotype in German kindreds. *J Neurol Neurosurg Psychiatry* **64**:67, 1998.

72. Ophoff RA, Terwindt GM, Vergouwe MN, van Eijk R, Oefner PJ, Hoffman SMG, Lamerdin JE, et al: Familial hemiplegic migraine and episodic ataxia type-2 are caused by mutations in the CA$^2$ channel gene CACNL1A4. *Cell* **87**:543, 1996.

73. Jodice C, Mantuano E, Veneziano L, Trettel F, Sabbadini G, Calandriello L, Francia A, et al: Episodic ataxia type 2 (EA2) and spinocerebellar ataxia type 6 (SCA6) due to CAG repeat expansion in the CACNA1A gene on chromosome 19p. *Hum Mol Genet* **6**:1973, 1997.

74. Yue Q, Jen JC, Nelson SF, Baloh RW: Progressive ataxia due to a missense mutation in a calcium-channel gene. *Am J Hum Genet* **61**:1078, 1997.

75. Terwindt GM, Ophoff RA, Haan J, Vergouwe MN, van Eijk R, Frants RR, Ferrari MD: Variable clinical expression of mutations in the P/Q-type calcium channel gene in familial hemiplegic migraine. *Neurology* **50**:1105, 1998.

76. Johansson J, Forsgren L, Sandgren O, Brice A, Holmgren G, Holmberg M: Expanded CAG repeats in Swedish spinocerebellar ataxia type 7 (SCA7) patients: Effect of CAG repeat length on the clinical manifestation. *Hum Mol Genet* **7**:171, 1998.

77. David G, Dürr A, Stevanin G, Cancel G, Abbas N, Benomar A, Belal S, et al: Molecular and clinical correlations in autosomal dominant cerebellar ataxia with progressive macular dystrophy (SCA7). *Hum Mol Genet* **7**:165, 1998.

78. Benton CS, de Silva R, Rutledge SL, Bohlega S, Ashizawa T, Zoghbi HY: Molecular and clinical studies in SCA-7 define a broad clinical spectrum and the infantile phenotype. *Neurology* **51**:1081, 1998.

79. Neetens A, Martin JJ, Libert J: Autosomal dominant cone dystrophy-cerebellar atrophy (ADCoCA) (modified ADCA HardingII). *Neuro-ophthalmology* **10**:261, 1990.

80. Gouw LG, Kaplan CD, Haines JH, Digre KB, Rutledge SL, Matilla A, Leppert M, et al: Retinal degeneration characterizes a spinocerebellar ataxia mapping to chromosome 3p. *Nat Genet* **10**:89, 1995.

81. Benomar A, Krols L, Stevanin G, Cancel G, Le Guern E, David G, Ouhabi H, et al: The gene for autosomal dominant cerebellar ataxia with pigmentary macular dystrophy maps to chromosome 3p12-p21.1. *Nat Genet* **10**:84, 1995.

82. Holmberg M, Johansson J, Forsgren L, Heijbel J, Sandgren O, Holmgren G: Localization of autosomal dominant cerebellar ataxia associated with retinal degeneration and anticipation to chromosome 3p12-p21.1. *Hum Mol Genet* **4**:1441, 1995.

83. Koob MD, Moseley ML, Schut LJ, Benzow KA, Bird TD, Day JW, Ranum LPW: An untranslated CTG expansion causes a novel form of spinocerebellar ataxia (SCA8). *Nat Genet* **21**:379, 1999.

84. Zu L, Figueroa KP, Grewal R, Pulst SM: Mapping of a new autosomal dominant spinocerebellar ataxia to chromosome 22. *Am J Hum Genet* **64**:594, 1999.

85. Matsuura T, Achari M, Khajavi M, Bachinski LL, Zoghbi HY, Ashizawa T: Mapping of the gene for a novel spinocerebellar ataxia with pure cerebellar signs and epilepsy. *Ann Neurol* **45**:407, 1999.

86. Smith JK: Dentatorubropallidoluysian atrophy, in Vinken PJ, Bruyn GW (eds): *Handbook of Clinical Neurology*. Amsterdam, North-Holland, 1975, p 519.

87. Naito H, Oyanagi S: Familial myoclonus epilepsy and choreoathetosis: Hereditary dentatorubral-pallidoluysian atrophy. *Neurology* **32**:798, 1982.

88. Takahashi H, Ohama E, Naito H, Takeda S, Nakashima S, Makifuchi T, Ikuta F: Hereditary dentatorubral-pallidoluysian atrophy: Clinical and pathologic variants in a family. *Neurology* **38**:1065, 1988.

89. Warner TT, Williams L, Harding AE: DRPLA in Europe. *Nat Genet* **6**:225, 1994.

90. Potter NT, M.A. M, Zimmerman AW, Eisenstadt ML, Anderson IJ: Molecular and clinical findings in a family with dentatorubral-pallidoluysian atrophy. *Ann Neurol* **37**:273, 1995.

91. Miwa S: Triplet repeats strike again. *Nat Genet* **6**:3, 1994.

92. Burke JR, Wingfield MS, Lewis KE, Roses AD, Lee JE, Hulette C, Pericak-Vance MA, et al: The Haw River Syndrome: Dentatorubro-pallidoluysian atrophy (DRPLA) in an African-American family. *Nat Genet* **7**:521, 1994.

93. Koide R, Ikeuchi T, Onodera O, Tanaka H, Igarashi S, Endo K, Takahashi H, et al: Unstable expansion of CAG repeat in hereditary dentatorubral-pallidoluysian atrophy (DRPLA). *Nat Genet* **6**:9, 1994.

94. Bebin EM, Bebin J, Currier RD, Smith EE, Perry TL: Morphometric studies in dominant olivopontocerebellar atrophy. *Arch Neurol* **47**:188, 1990.

95. Uyama E, Kondo I, Uchino M, Fukushima T, Murayama N, Kuwano A, Inokuchi N, et al: Dentatorubral-pallidoluysian atrophy (DRPLA): Clinical, genetic, and neuroradiologic studies in a family. *J Neurol Sci* **130**:146, 1995.

96. Nagai Y, Azuma T, Funauchi M, Fujita M, Umi M, Hirano M, Matsubara T, et al: Clinical and molecular genetic study in seven Japanese families with spinocerebellar ataxia type 6. *J Neurol Sci* **157**:52, 1998.

97. Servadio A, Koshy B, Armstrong D, Antalfy B, Orr HT, Zoghbi HY: Expression analysis of the ataxin-1 protein in tissues from normal and spinocerebellar ataxia type 1 individuals. *Nat Genet* **10**:94, 1995.

98. Woods BT, Schaumburg HH: Nigro-spino-dentatal degeneration with nuclear ophthalmoplegia. A unique and partially treatable clinico-pathological entity. *J Neurol Sci* **17**:149, 1972.

99. Sachdev HS, Forno LS, Kane CA: Joseph disease: A multisystem degenerative disorder of the nervous system. *Neurology* **32**:192, 1982.

100. Yuasa T, Ohama E, Harayama H, Yamada M, Kawase Y, Wakabayashi M, Atsumi T, et al: Joseph's disease: Clinical and pathological studies in a Japanese family. *Ann Neurol* **19**:152, 1986.

101. Takiyama Y, Oyanagi S, Kawashima S, Sakamoto H, Saito K, Yoshida M, Tsuji S, et al: A clinical and pathologic study of a large Japanese family with Machado-Joseph disease tightly linked to the DNA markers on chromosome 14q. *Neurology* **44**:1302, 1994.

102. Martin JJ, Van Regemorter N, Krols L, Brucher JM, de Barsy T, Szliwowski H, Evrard P, et al: On an autosomal dominant form of retinal-cerebellar degeneration: An autopsy study of five patients in one family. *Acta Neuropathol* **88**:277, 1994.

103. Zoghbi HY, Jodice C, Sandkuijl LA, Kwiatkowski Jr TJ, McCall AE, Huntoon SA, Lulli P, et al: The gene for autosomal dominant spinocerebellar ataxia (SCA1) maps telomeric to HLA complex and is closely linked to the D6S89 locus in three large kindreds. *Am J Hum Genet* **49**:23, 1991.

104. Ranum LPW, Duvick LA, Rich SS, Schut LJ, Litt M, Orr HT: Localization of the autosomal dominant, HLA-linked spinocerebellar ataxia (SCA1) locus in two kindreds within an 8cM subregion of chromosome 6p. *Am J Hum Genet* **49**:31, 1991.

105. Banfi S, Chung MY, Kwiatkowski TJ, Jr., Ranum LP, McCall AE, Chinault AC, Orr HT, et al: Mapping and cloning of the critical region for the spinocerebellar ataxia type 1 gene (SCA1) in a yeast artificial chromosome contig spanning 1.2 Mb. *Genomics* **18**:627, 1993.

106. Orr H, Chung M-y, Banfi S, Kwiatkowski Jr TJ, Servadio A, Beaudet AL, McCall AE, et al: Expansion of an unstable trinucleotide (CAG) repeat in spinocerebellar ataxia type 1. *Nat Genet* **4**:221, 1993.

107. Quan F, Janas J, Popovich BW: A novel CAG repeat configuration in the SCA1 gene: Implications for the molecular diagnostics of spinocerebellar ataxia type 1. *Hum Mol Genet* **4**:2411, 1995.

108. Chung M-y, Ranum LPW, Duvick L, Servadio A, Zoghbi HY, Orr HT: Analysis of the CAG repeat expansion in spinocerebellar ataxia type I: Evidence for a possible mechanism predisposing to instability. *Nat Genet* **5**:254, 1993.

109. Chong SS, McCall AE, Cota J, Subramony SH, Orr HT, Zoghbi HY: Gametic and somatic tissue-specific heterogeneity of the expanded *SCA1* CAG repeat in spinocerebellar ataxia type 1. *Nat Genet* **10**:344, 1995.

110. Banfi S, Servadio A, Chung M-y, Kwiatkowski Jr TJ, McCall AE, Duvick LA, Shen Y, et al: Identification and characterization of the gene causing type 1 spinocerebellar ataxia. *Nat Genet* **7**:513, 1994.

111. Banfi S, Servadio A, Chung M-y, Capozzoli F, Duvick LA, Elde R, Zoghbi HY, et al: Cloning and developmental expression analysis of the murine homolog of the spinocerebellar ataxia type 1 gene (*Sca1*). *Hum Mol Genet* **5**:33, 1996.

112. Skinner PJ, Koshy B, Cummings C, Klement IA, Helin K, Servadio A, Zoghbi HY, et al: Ataxin-1 with extra glutamines induces alterations in nuclear matrix-associated structures. *Nature* **389**:971, 1997.

113. Koshy BT, Matilla A, Zoghbi HY: Clues about the pathogenesis of SCA1 from biochemical and molecular studies of ataxin-1, in Wells RD, Warren ST (eds): *Genetic Instabilities and Hereditary Neurological Disorders*. San Diego, Academic Press, 1998, p 241.

114. Cummings CJ, Mancini MA, Antalffy B, DeFranco DB, Orr HT, Zoghbi HY: Chaperone suppression of aggregation and altered subcellular proteasome localization imply protein misfolding in SCA1. *Nat Genet* **19**:148, 1998.

115. Matilla A, Roberson ED, Banfi S, Morales J, Armstrong DL, Burright EN, Orr HT, et al: Mice lacking ataxin-1 display learning deficits and decreased hippocampal paired-pulse facilitation. *J Neurosci* **18**:5508, 1998.

116. Gispert S, Lunkes A, Santos N, Orozco G, Ha-Hao D, Ratzlaff T, Aguiar J, et al: Localization of the candidate gene D-amino oxidase outside the refined I-cM region of spinocerebellar ataxia 2. *Am J Hum Genet* **57**:972, 1995.

117. Trottier Y, Lutz Y, Stevanin G, Imbert G, Devys D, Cancel G, Saudou F, et al: Polyglutamine expansion as a pathological epitope in Huntington's disease and four dominant cerebellar ataxias. *Nature* **378**:403, 1995.

118. Imbert G, Saudou F, Yvert G, Devys D, Trottier Y, Garnier J-M, Weber C, et al: Cloning of the gene for spinocerebellar ataxia 2 reveals a locus with high sensitivity to expanded CAG/glutamine repeats and high instability. *Nat Genet* **14**:285, 1996.

119. Pulst S-M, Nechiporuk A, Nechiporuk T, Gispert S, Chen X-N, Lopes-Cendes I, Pearlman S, et al: Identification of the SCA2 gene: Moderate expansion of a normally biallelic trinucleotide repeat. *Nat Genet* **14**:269, 1996.

120. Sanpei K, Takano H, Igarashi S, Sato T, Oyake M, Sasaki H, Wakisaka A, et al: Identification of the spinocerebellar ataxia type 2 gene using a direct identification of repeat expansion and cloning technique, DIRECT. *Nat Genet* **14**:277, 1996.

121. Cancel G, Dürr A, Didierjean O, Imbert G, Burk K, Lezin A, Belal S, et al: Molecular and clinical correlations in spinocerebellar ataxia 2: A study of 32 families. *Hum Mol Genet* **6**:709, 1997.

122. Kawaguchi Y, Okamoto T, Taniwaki M, Aizawa M, Inoue M, Katayama S, Kawakami H, et al: CAG expansions in a novel gene for Machado-Joseph disease at chromosome 14q32.1. *Nat Genet* **8**:221, 1994.

123. Cancel G, Abbas N, Stevanin G, Dürr A, Chneiweiss H, Neri C, Duyckaerts C, et al: Marked phenotypic heterogeneity associated with expansion of a CAG repeat sequence at the spinocerebellar ataxia 3/Machado-Joseph disease locus. *Am J Hum Genet* **57**:809, 1995.

124. Stevanin G, Cassa E, Cancel G, Abbas N, Durr A, Jardim E, Agid Y, et al: Characterisation of the unstable expanded CAG repeat in the MJD1 gene in four Brazilian families of Portuguese descent with Machado-Joseph disease. *J Med Genet* **32**:827, 1995.

125. Lopes-Cendes I, Maciel P, Kish S, Gaspar C, Robitaille Y, Clark HB, Koeppen AH, et al: Somatic mosaicism in the central nervous system in spinocerebellar ataxia type 1 and Machado-Joseph disease. *Ann Neurol* **40**:199, 1996.

126. Paulson HL, Das SS, Crino PB, Perez M, Patel SC, Gotsdiner D, Fischbeck KH, et al: Machado-Joseph disease gene product is a cytoplasmic protein widely expressed in brain. *Amer Neur Assoc* **41**:453, 1997.

127. Tait D, Riccio M, Sittler A, Scherzinger E, Santi S, Ognibene A, Maraldi NM, et al: Ataxin-3 is transported into the nucleus and associates with the nuclear matrix. *Hum Mol Genet* **7**:991, 1998.

128. Leggo J, Dalton A, Morrison PJ, Dodge A, Connarty M, Kotze MJ, Rubinsztein DC: Analysis of spinocerebellar ataxia types 1, 2, 3, and 6, dentatorubral- pallidoluysian atrophy, and Friedreich's ataxia genes in spinocerebellar ataxia patients in the UK. *J Med Genet* **34**:982, 1997.

129. Zoghbi HY: CAG Repeats in SCA6: Anticipating new clues. *Neurology* **49**:1196, 1997.

130. Moseley ML, Benzow KA, Schut LJ, Bird TD, Gomez CM, Barkhaus PE, Blindauer KA, et al: Incidence of dominant spinocerebellar and Friedreich triplet repeats among 361 ataxia families. *Neurology* **51**:1666, 1998.

131. Catterall WA: Structure and function of voltage-gated ion channels. *Ann Rev Biochem* **64**:493, 1995.

132. Llinas RR, Sugimori M, Cherksey B: Voltage-dependent calcium conductances in mammalian neurons. The P channel. *Ann N Y Acad Sci* **560**:103, 1989.

133. Zhang JF, Randall AD, Ellinor PT, Horne WA, Sather WA, Tanabe T, Schwarz TL, et al: Distinctive pharmacology and kinetics of cloned neuronal $Ca^2$ channels and their possible counterparts in mammalian CNS neurons. *Neuropharmacology* **32**:1075, 1993.

134. Fletcher CF, Lutz CM, O'Sullivan TN, Shaughnessy JD, Hawkes R, Frankel WN, Copeland NG, et al: Absence epilepsy in Tottering mutant mice is associated with calcium channel defects. *Cell* **87**:607, 1996.

135. David G, Abbas N, Stevanin G, Durr A, Yvert G, Cancel G, Weber C, et al: Cloning of the SCA7 gene reveals a highly unstable CAG repeat expansion. *Nat Genet* **17**:65, 1997.

136. Stevanin G, Trottier Y, Cancel G, Durr A, David G, Didierjean O, Burk K, et al: Screening for proteins with polyglutamine expansions in autosomal dominant cerebellar ataxias. *Hum Mol Genet* **5**:1887, 1996.

137. Koob MD, Benzow KA, Bird TD, Day JW, Moseley ML, Ranum LP: Rapid cloning of expanded trinucleotide repeat sequences from genomic DNA. *Nat Genet* **18**:72, 1998.

138. Gouw LG, Castaneda MA, McKenna CK, Digre KB, Pulst SM, Perlman S, Lee MS, et al: Analysis of the dynamic mutation in the SCA7 gene shows marked parental effects on CAG repeat transmission. *Hum Mol Genet* 7:525, 1998.

139. Holmberg M, Duyckaerts C, Dürr A, Cancel G, Gourfinkel-An I, Damier P, Faucheux B, et al: Spinocerebellar ataxia type 7 (SCA7): A neurodegenerative disorder with neuronal intranuclear inclusions. *Hum Mol Genet* 7:913, 1998.

140. Del-Favero J, Krols L, Michalik A, Theuns J, Lofgren A, Goossens D, Wehnert A, et al: Molecular genetic analysis of autosomal dominant cerebellar ataxia with retinal degeneration (ADCA type II) caused by CAG triplet repeat expansion. *Hum Mol Genet* 7:177, 1998.

141. Stevanin G, Giunti P, Belal GDS, Dürr A, Ruberg M, Wood N, Brice A: De novo expansion of intermediate alleles in spinocerebellar ataxia 7. *Hum Mol Genet* 7:1809, 1998.

142. Li S-H, McInnis MG, Margolis RL, Antonarakis SE, Ross C: Novel triplet repeat containing genes in human brain: Cloning, expression, and length polymorphisms. *Genomics* 16:572, 1993.

143. Ikeuchi T, Koide R, Tanaka H, Onodera O, Igarashi S, Takahashi H, Kondo R, et al: Dentatorubral-pallidoluysian atrophy: Clinical features are closely related to unstable expansions of trinucleotide (CAG) repeat. *Ann Neurol* 37:769, 1995.

144. Takano H, Onodera O, Takahashi H, Igarashi S, Yamada M, Oyake M, Ikeuchi T, et al: Somatic mosaicism of expanded CAG repeats in brains of patients with dentatorubral-pallidoluysian atrophy: Cellular population-dependent dynamics of mitotic instability. *Am J Hum Genet* 58:1212, 1996.

145. Yazawa I, Nukina N, Hashida H, Goto J, Yamada M, Kanazawa I: Abnormal gene product identified in hereditary dentatorubral-pallidoluysian atrophy (DRPLA) brain. *Nat Genet* 10:99, 1995.

146. Knight SP, Richardson MM, Osmand AP, Stakkestad A, Potter NT: Expression and distribution of the dentatorubral-pallidoluysian atrophy gene product (atrophin-1/drplap) in neuronal and non-neuronal tissues. *J Neurol Sci* 146:19, 1997.

147. Kawakami H, Maruyama H, Nakamura S, Kawaguchi Y, Kakizuka A, Doyu M, Sobue G: Unique features of the CAG repeats in Machado-Joseph disease. *Nat Genet* 9:344, 1995.

148. Sobue G, Doyu M, Nakao N, Shimada N, Mitsuma T, Maruyama H, Kawakami S, et al: Homozygosity for Machado-Joseph disease gene enhances phenotypic severity [Letter]. *J Neurol Neurosurg Psychiatry* 60:354, 1996.

149. Kurohara K, Kuroda Y, Maruyama H, Kawakami H, Yukitake M, Matsui M, Nakamura S: Homozygosity for an allele carrying intermediate CAG repeats in the dentatorubral-pallidoluysian atrophy (DRPLA) gene results in spastic paraplegia. *Neurology* 48:1087, 1997.

150. Wexler NS, Young AB, Tanzi RE, Travers H, Starosta-Rubinstein S, Penney JB, Snodgrass SR, et al: Homozygotes for Huntington's disease. *Nature* 326:194, 1987.

151. Takano H, Cancel G, Ikeuchi T, Lorenzetti D, Mawad R, Stevanin G, Didierjean O, et al: Close associations between prevalences of dominantly inherited spinocerebellar ataxias with CAG-repeat expansions and frequencies of large normal CAG alleles in Japanese and Caucasian populations. *Am J Hum Genet* 63:1060, 1998.

152. Davies SW, Beardsall K, Turmaine M, DiFiglia M, Aronin N, Bates GP: Are neuronal intranuclear inclusions the common neuropathology of triplet-repeat disorders with polyglutamine-repeat expansions? *Lancet* 351:131, 1998.

153. Davies AF, Mirza G, Sekhon G, Turnpenny P, Leroy F, Speleman F, Law C, et al: Delineation of two distinct 6p deletion syndromes. *Hum Genet* 104:64, 1999.

154. Wang G, Ide K, Nukina N, Goto J, Ichikawa Y, Uchida K, Sakamoto T, et al: Machado-Joseph disease gene product identified in lymphocytes and brain. *Biochem Biophys Res Commun* 233:476, 1997.

155. Huynh DP, Del Bigio MR, Ho DH, Pulst SM: Expression of ataxin-2 in brains from normal individuals and patients with Alzheimer's disease and spinocerebellar ataxia 2. *Ann Neurol* 45:232, 1999.

156. Paulson HL, Perez MK, Trottier Y, Trojanowsk JQ, Subramony SH, Das SS, Vig P, et al: Intranuclear inclusions of expanded polyglutamine protein in spinocerebellar ataxia Type 3. *Neuron* 19:333, 1997.

157. Igarashi S, Koide R, Shimohata T, Yamada M, Hayashi Y, Takano H, Date H, et al: Suppression of aggregate formation and apoptosis by transglutaminase inhibitors in cells expressing truncated DRPLA protein with an expanded polyglutamine stretch. *Nat Genet* 18:111, 1998.

158. Ross CA: Intranuclear neuronal inclusions: A common pathogenic mechanism for glutamine-repeat neurodegenerative diseases? *Neuron* 19:1147, 1997.

159. Hochstrasser M: Ubiquitin-dependent protein degradation. *Annu Rev Genet* 30:405, 1996.

160. Paulson HL: Protein fate in neurodegenerative proteinopathies: Polyglutamine diseases join the (mis)fold. *Am J Hum Genet* 64:339, 1999.

161. Burright EN, Davidson JD, Duvick LA, Koshy B, Zoghbi HY, Orr HT: Identification of a self-association region within the *SCA1* gene product, ataxin-1. *Hum Mol Genet* 6:513, 1997.

162. Matilla T, Koshy B, Cummings CJ, Isobe T, Orr HT, Zoghbi HY: The cerebellar leucine-rich acidic nuclear protein interacts with ataxin-1. *Nature* 389:974, 1997.

163. Koshy B, Matilla T, Burright EN, Merry DE, Fischbeck KH, Orr HT, Zoghbi HY: Spinocerebellar ataxia type-1 and spinobulbar muscular atrophy gene products interact with glyceraldehyde-3-phosphate dehydrogenase. *Hum Mol Genet* 5:1311, 1996.

164. Matsuoka K, Taoka M, Satozawa N, Nakayama H, Ichimura T, Takahashi N, Yamakuni T, et al: A nuclear factor containing the leucine-rich repeats expresses in murine cerebellar neurons. *Proc Natl Acad Sci U S A* 91:9670, 1994.

165. Vaesen M, Barnikol-Watanabe S, Gotz H, Awni LA, Cole T, Zimmermann B, Kratzin HD, et al: Purification and characterization of two putative HLA class II associated proteins: PHAPI and PHAPII. *Biol Chem Hoppe Seyler* 375:113, 1994.

166. Chen TH, Brody JR, Romantsev FE, Yu JG, Kayler AE, Voneiff E, Kuhajda FP, et al: Structure of pp32, an acidic nuclear protein which inhibits oncogene-induced formation of transformed foci. *Mol Biol Cell* 7:2045, 1996.

167. Li M, Makkinje A, Damuni Z: Molecular identification of I1PP2A, a novel potent heat-stable inhibitor protein of protein phosphatase 2A. *Biochemistry* 35:6998, 1996.

168. Ulitzur N, Humbert M, Pfeffer SR: Mapmodulin: A possible modulator of the interaction of microtubule- associated proteins with microtubules. *Proc Natl Acad Sci U S A* 94:5084, 1997.

169. Burke JR, Enghild JJ, Martin ME, Jou Y-S, Myers RM, Roses AD, Vance JM, et al: Huntingtin and DRPLA proteins selectively interact with the enzyme GAPDH. *Nat Med* 2:347, 1996.

170. Burright EN, Clark HB, Servadio A, Matilla T, Feddersen RM, Yunis WS, Duvick LA, et al: SCA1 transgenic mice: A model for neurodegeneration caused by an expanded CAG trinucleotide repeat. *Cell* 82:937, 1995.

171. Clark HB, Burright EN, Yunis WS, Larson S, Wilcox C, Hartman B, Matilla A, et al: Purkinje cell expression of a mutant allele of *SCA1* in transgenic mice leads to disparate effects on motor behaviors, followed by a progressive cerebellar dysfunction and histological alterations. *J Neurosci* 17:7385, 1997.

172. Ferrer I, Genis D, Davalos A, Bernado L, Sant F, Serrano T: The Purkinje cell in olivopontocerebellar atrophy: A Golgi and immunocytochemical study. *Neuropathol Appl Neurobiol* 20:38, 1994.

173. Koeppen AH: The Purkinje cell and its afferents in human hereditary ataxia. *J Neuropathol Exp Neurol* 50:505, 1991.

174. Kalderon D, Roberts BL, Richardson WD, Smith AE: A short amino acid sequence able to specify nuclear location. *Cell* 39:499, 1984.

175. Boulikas T: Nuclear localization signals (NLS). *Crit Rev Eukaryot Gene Expr* 3:193, 1993.

176. Klement IA, Skinner PJ, Kaytor MD, Yi H, Hersch SM, Clark HB, Zoghbi HY: Ataxin-1 nuclear localization and aggregation: Role in polyglutamine-induced disease in SCA1 transgenic mice. *Cell* 95:41, 1998.

177. Ikeda H, Yamaguchi M, Sugai S, Aze Y, Narumiya S, Kakizuka A: Expanded polyglutamine in the Machado-Joseph disease protein induces cell death in vitro and in vivo. *Nat Genet* 13:196, 1996.

178. Wellington CL, Ellerby LM, Hackam AS, Margolis RL, Trifiro MA, Singaraja R, McCutcheon K, et al: Caspase cleavage of gene products associated with triplet expansion disorders generates truncated fragments containing the polyglutamine tract. *J Biol Chem* 273:9158, 1998.

# Charcot-Marie-Tooth Peripheral Neuropathies and Related Disorders

*James R. Lupski* ■ *Carlos A. Garcia*

1. Charcot-Marie-Tooth (CMT) (MIM 118220) polyneuropathy syndrome represents a clinically and genetically heterogeneous group of disorders of the peripheral nerve. Two major types are distinguished by measuring motor nerve conduction velocities (NCV). CMT1 is a demyelinating neuropathy characterized by symmetrically slowed motor NCV (usually <38 m/s). Microscopic sections of peripheral nerve in CMT1 patients reveal onion bulb formation. CMT2 is an axonal neuropathy associated with normal or near normal NCV with decreased amplitudes and axonal loss on nerve biopsy. CMT1, which is more common and usually autosomal dominant, generally presents in the second or third decade and is associated with slowly progressive symmetric distal muscle weakness and atrophy, gait disturbance, and absent stretch reflexes. CMT2 is autosomal dominant and usually manifests later in life. Different genetic subtypes of both CMT1 and CMT2 can be further delineated based on genetic linkage analysis and mapping to distinct loci.

2. Hereditary neuropathy with liability to pressure palsies (HNPP) (MIM 162500) is a demyelinating neuropathy whose neuropathologic hallmark is sausage-like thickening of myelin sheaths (tomacula). Electrophysiological findings include mildly slowed NCV and conduction blocks. The clinical manifestations are typically episodic, nonsymmetric palsies, that may be precipitated by trauma or compression. Multifocal neuropathies, especially entrapment neuropathies such as carpal tunnel syndrome, may be manifestations of HNPP.

3. Dejerine-Sottas syndrome (DSS) (MIM 145900) is a clinically distinct entity that is more severe than CMT. DSS has earlier onset of clinical symptoms that include delayed motor milestones, more significant slowing of NCV, more pronounced demyelination, and more numerous onion

bulbs than observed in CMT. Congenital hypomyelinating neuropathy (CHN) is distinguished from DSS by its congenital manifestation and, in some cases, by absence of myelin. Roussy-Levy syndrome (RLS) (MIM 180800) combines sensory ataxia and tremor with a CMT1 phenotype but may not represent a distinct clinical entity.

4. Most CMT1 patients have DNA rearrangements as the molecular cause of their disease. A 1.5-Mb tandem duplication, the CMT1A duplication, accounts for approximately 70 percent of CMT1 cases. A deletion of the same 1.5-Mb region in chromosome 17p12 is found in >85 percent of patients with HNPP. The CMT1A duplication and HNPP deletion result from unequal crossing over and reciprocal homologous recombination involving a 24-kb repeat—CMT1A-REP—that flanks the 1.5-Mb region. A meiotic recombination hotspot occurs within CMT1A-REP. The majority of the *de novo* duplication and deletion events occur in meiosis of the male germ cells.

5. The CMT1A and HNPP phenotypes result from a gene dosage effect. CMT1A is due to trisomic overexpression of the peripheral myelin protein-22 gene, *PMP22*, whereas HNPP results from monosomic underexpression of *PMP22*. In rare patients without the CMT1A duplication or HNPP deletion, *PMP22* point mutations can cause disease. Null alleles or haploinsufficiency cause HNPP, while gain-of-function or dominant-negative missense amino acid substitution results in CMT1A or DSS.

6. Mutations in myelin protein zero (*MPZ*), connexin 32 (*Cx32*) or gap junction protein β1 (*GJB1*), and early growth response 2 (*EGR2*, the human *Krox-20* homologue) genes can also cause CMT1 (*MPZ*, *Cx32*, *EGR2*), DSS (*MPZ*, *EGR2*), or CHN (*MPZ*, *EGR2*). Mutation of *Cx32* causes the X-linked form of CMT. Thus, these myelinopathies appear to represent a spectrum of related disorders resulting from myelin dysfunction. Each of these genes (*PMP22*, *Cx32*, *MPZ*, and *EGR2*) are expressed in myelinating Schwann cells so that mutations probably exert their effects on Schwann cells and may perturb axon-glia interactions.

7. Spontaneous murine mutants *Trembler* (*Tr*) and allelic *Tr^J*, as well as transgenic and knockout rodents, have been instrumental in identifying myelinopathy associated disease genes and determining the molecular, cellular, and pathophysiological consequences of mutations or altered dosage of these genes.

8. Clinical variability is the rule in inherited neuropathies. Discordance is even noted in identical twins with the CMT1A duplication. *De novo* CMT1A duplication is

A list of standard abbreviations is located immediately preceding the index in each volume. Additional abbreviations used in this chapter include: CHN = congenital hypomyelinating neuropathy; *COX10* = gene for cytochrome c oxidase, subunit *X* encoding heme A:farnesyltransferase; CMT = Charcot-Marie-Tooth; CMT1A-REPs = CMT1A region-specific low-copy repeats; *Cx32* = connexin 32; DSS = Dejerine-Sottas syndrome; *EGR2* = early growth response 2 gene/protein; GJB1 = gap junction protein, β1; HMSNI, HMSNII, etc. = hereditary motor and sensory neuropathy types I, II, etc.; HNPP = hereditary neuropathy with liability to pressure palsies; MITE = *mariner* insect transposon-like element; *MPZ*, MPZ = myelin protein zero gene/protein; m/s = meters per second; NCV = nerve conduction velocities; *PMP22, Pmp22*, PMP22 = peripheral myelin protein-22 human gene/mouse gene/protein; PNS = peripheral nervous system; RLS = Roussy-Levy syndrome; RecBCD = homologous recombination pathway in *E. coli*; *Tr, Tr^J* = two trembler alleles in mouse.

frequently found in sporadic CMT1. DSS and RLS can also be associated with CMT1A duplication. Multifocal neuropathy, autosomal dominant carpal tunnel syndrome, and CMT1 can also be associated with the HNPP deletion. These inherited demyelinating neuropathies can be difficult to distinguish from acquired demyelinating neuropathies. Because of the clinical heterogeneity, the clinical workup of a patient with peripheral neuropathy requires molecular definition. Determining an exact molecular etiology enables a precise and secure diagnosis, provides prognostic information, allows proper genetic counseling, and makes possible the design and implementation of rational therapeutic strategies.

Hereditary peripheral neuropathies are common human genetic conditions. These clinically and genetically heterogeneous disorders produce progressive deterioration of the peripheral nerves with secondary muscle wasting and weakness in a distal distribution. The core of knowledge and characterization of these neuropathies has expanded from the clinical description of the disorders, to the delineation of electrophysiological and neuropathologic findings distinguishing demyelinating and axonal forms, to the identification of specific genes responsible for these diseases, and to the elucidation of novel mutational mechanisms including duplication and gene dosage. The study of these disorders also enabled the identification of structural features of the genome that predispose the specific DNA rearrangements.[1] The application of molecular genetic techniques has resulted in a more comprehensive understanding of peripheral nerve biology that has important clinical implications. Various aspects of peripheral nerve function and dysfunction have been reviewed extensively.[2–34] This chapter focuses on the integration of clinical experience with molecular genetic data regarding the following inherited peripheral neuropathies: Charcot-Marie-Tooth disease[35,36] types 1 and 2 (CMT1 and CMT2), also known as hereditary motor and sensory neuropathy types I and II (HMSNI and HMSNII);[37–39] the Dejerine-Sottas syndrome (DSS),[40] also known as hereditary motor and sensory neuropathy type III (HMSNIII); hereditary neuropathy with liability to pressure palsies (HNPP);[41] congenital hypomyelinating neuropathy (CHN);[42,43] and clinical variants of CMT such as Roussy-Levy syndrome (RLS).[44]

## CLINICAL PHENOTYPES

### Charcot-Marie-Tooth (CMT)

Persons with CMT usually present in the first or second decade in life with slowly progressive atrophy and weakness of the distal musculature of the legs and feet followed in most cases by involvement of the hands.[45–47] There is a wide range in age-of-onset, involvement, severity, and rate of progression even within the same family. Electrophysiological and nerve biopsy findings define two distinct phenotypes. CMT1, the demyelinating form, is characterized by slowing of the motor nerve conduction velocities (usually < 38 m/s); hypertrophy of the peripheral nerves sometimes is evident by physical examination. Onion bulb formation and segmental demyelination are seen on neuropathologic examination. Repeated cycles of demyelination and reparative remyelination give the circumferentially directed Schwann cells and their processes the appearance of onion bulbs.[48] CMT2, the neuronal or axonal form, is characterized by normal or mild slowing of nerve conduction velocities with decreased amplitudes, normal size nerves, absent or few onion bulbs, and no evidence of segmental demyelination.

The clinical heterogeneity of CMT is illustrated by the presence of genotypically affected adult individuals who show no symptoms of the disease and have a normal neurologic examination, including the ability to walk on their heels and normal deep tendon reflexes. However, they usually have slowed

**Table 227-1 CMT Clinical Features**

Foot deformity (*pes cavus, pes planus, equinovarus*)
Hammer toes
Gait disturbance (steppage gait)
Loss of balance
Distal muscle weakness
Peroneal muscular atrophy
Cold intolerance
Difficulty with fine-finger movements
Toe walking
Inability to walk on heels
Absent or diminished deep tendon reflexes (DTRs)

motor NCV by 2 years of age. Infants and children manifest the disease with toe walking and tight heel cords; some are born with foot deformities including clubfeet. Older patients present because of abnormalities of gait, foot deformities, or loss of balance (Table 227-1).[46]

Muscle weakness starts in the feet and legs. Early signs of CMT include difficulty or inability to walk on the heels and tight heel cords. Weakness of the anterior lower leg muscles diminishes the ability to dorsiflex the feet and results in frequent tripping and ankle injuries. As the foot drop progresses in severity, patients compensate by flexing the hip with each step giving a "steppage" or "equine gait." Although not observed at all ages, *pes cavus* deformity develops with disease progression as a result of muscle imbalance between the extrinsic and intrinsic muscles of the foot; that is, the plantar fascia and plantar ligaments connecting the bones of the feet tighten and pull the ends of the foot together producing a high arch. However, *pes planus* (flat foot) is also seen in CMT patients. Varus deformities of the heel also develop with disease progression due to an imbalance between the strong tibialis posterior muscle that inverts the foot and the weak peroneal longus and brevis that evert the foot. Peroneal nerve involvement also causes atrophy of the peroneal muscles and is responsible for the alternative diagnostic name, *peroneal muscular atrophy*.[36] Claw or hammer toe, a condition in which the toes initially are flexed voluntarily to improve gait but then become rigid, causes irritation to the top of the toes as they rub against the shoe. Painful calluses also develop on the lateral plantar surface that rubs against the shoes. These foot deformities make it difficult for the patient to find shoes that fit properly. Leg cramps and lumbar pain are also frequent complaints after long walks. Poor tolerance to cold weather is probably due to loss of muscle mass.

In severe cases of CMT, the most significant finding is weakness and wasting of the intrinsic muscles of the hand. This usually occurs late in the course of the disease and the severity of hand weakness is not usually related to that of leg weakness or atrophy. The initial preservation of the extrinsic forearm muscles produces an overly extended joint at the base of the fingers and the wasting of the intrinsic hand muscles produce the flexion of the middle and distal joints. The thumb lies flat in the plane of the hand instead of opposing the other fingers. These features give the appearance of a "claw hand" and can explain the frequent complaints concerning difficulty opening jars, turning doorknobs, and holding writing and eating utensils. Patients also have difficulty with fine finger movements (e.g., manipulating zippers and buttons) and approximation of the thumb with the other fingers. Hand involvement may occur earlier and be more pronounced with the X-linked form of CMT.

Muscle stretch reflexes disappear early in the ankles and later in the patella and upper limbs. The plantar responses are frequently flexor or show no response, especially as the peroneal innervation is lost. Mild sensory loss to pricking pain in the legs in a stocking distribution may be seen in some patients. Decreased vibratory sense is frequent. Patients also complain of numbness and tingling in their feet and hands but paresthesias are not as common as in acquired neuropathies.

**Table 227-2 CMT-Associated Findings**

|  | Frequency |
| --- | --- |
| Enlarged nerves | 20–25% |
| Tremor | 25–40% |
| Hip dysplasia | ? |
| Pulmonary dysfunction | Rare |

Associated findings (Table 227-2) may include enlarged nerves, tremor, hip dysplasia, and pulmonary dysfunction. Enlarged nerves, which are seen in 20 to 25 percent of patients, are unrelated to the age of the patient or the severity of the disease. The greater auricular nerve may be seen in the lateral surface of the neck in slender patients. Thickened ulnar and peroneal nerves may be palpated 1 or 2 inches above the ulnar groove and behind the head of the fibula, respectively. Tremor is not a complaint but when specifically asked, 25 to 40 percent of patients respond positively.[46,49] The tremor is usually noted in the mid-thirties and is not related to the severity of disease. Hip dysplasia may be severe but is usually asymptomatic or minimally symptomatic until adolescence. Surgical intervention is sometimes indicated if significant pain and or gait disturbance is associated with the hip dysplasia.[50] Pulmonary function tests in some patients with CMT show only mild nonprogressive impairment. Restrictive lung disease is usually not a major problem in patients with CMT1.[51] Pregnancy and delivery may exacerbate weakness in 50 percent of the patients with early onset disease, but not in patients with late onset disease. This deterioration is temporary in one-third of the patients, but persists in two-thirds. However, the rate of obstetric complications is the same as in the normal population. No identified factor, such as age at delivery and interval between onset of disease and delivery, predict progression of pregnancy-related CMT1 symptoms.[52] Some medications and certain neurotoxic substances such as excess alcohol may aggravate the neuropathy in patients with CMT. CMT patients are very sensitive to small doses of vincristine.[53–57]

Restless leg syndrome, an irresistible urge to move the legs because of dysesthetic sensations when sitting or lying down, occurs with a high frequency (37 percent) in patients with CMT2.[58] The restless leg syndrome is not found in CMT1 patients. Restless leg syndrome may be idiopathic or associated with several medical conditions including various forms of peripheral neuropathy. Axonal atrophy seems to represent a significant nerve fiber change in restless leg syndrome.[59]

## Hereditary Neuropathy with Liability to Pressure Palsies (HNPP)

Also called familial recurrent polyneuropathy or tomaculous neuropathy, HNPP was originally described in a family in which individuals in three generations had recurrent peroneal neuropathy after kneeling to dig potatoes.[60] The slowly progressive neuropathy of HNPP is milder than that of CMT. It is, however, usually episodic in nature rather than continuous. Clinical manifestations consist of periodic episodes of numbness, muscular weakness, atrophy, and, in some cases, palsies after relatively minor trauma or compression of the peripheral nerves, typically at common sites of compressive neuropathies.[41,61] The median, radial, ulnar, peroneal, and axillary nerves are most commonly affected. Electrophysiological studies can show conduction blocks at the site of compression and many patients have diffuse and mild slowing of the NCV indicative of subclinical demyelinating neuropathy. Nerve biopsies reveal demyelination and remyelination with tomacula or sausage-like thickening of the myelin sheath.[41]

## Dejerine-Sottas Syndrome (DSS)

DSS or HMSNIII was originally described as an interstitial hypertrophic neuropathy of infancy.[40] It is a more severe demyelinating neuropathy than CMT1.[62] The disease usually begins in infancy, as evidenced by delayed motor milestones, and it is generally associated with severe pathologic alterations and nerve conduction velocity abnormalities ($<6$ to 12 m/s).[63] The cerebrospinal fluid proteins can be elevated.

## Congenital Hypomyelinating Neuropathy (CHN)

CHN is characterized by infantile hypotonia, distal muscle weakness, areflexia, and markedly slow NCVs ($<10$ m/s). In severe cases, joint contractures or arthrogryposis multiplex congenita have been described.[43,64] In less severe cases, it is difficult to differentiate CHN from DSS. Some authors have considered both DSS and CHN as forms of HMSNIII.[62] The nerve biopsies show hypomyelination (few thin myelin lamellae) without active myelin breakdown products and early onion bulb formations. However, there are several histologic phenotypes for DSS and CHN.[42,64]

## Roussy-Levy Syndrome (RLS)

RLS was described in patients presenting with *pes cavus*, distal limb weakness, areflexia, distal sensory loss, sensory gait ataxia, and tremor.[44] It is controversial whether RLS represents a clinical entity distinct from CMT or a clinical variant.

## GENETICS OF CHARCOT-MARIE-TOOTH PERIPHERAL NEUROPATHIES

CMT is the most common inherited peripheral neuropathy with an estimated prevalence of ~1/2500.[65] Prevalence estimates for hereditary motor and sensory neuropathies have ranged from 0.14 to $2.8 \times 10^{-4}$ and revealed it to be the most frequently occurring inherited neuromuscular disease.[66] CMT can occur sporadically or as an autosomal dominant, autosomal recessive, or X-linked trait. Autosomal dominant inheritance is the most commonly observed pattern.

In 1939, William Allan used CMT as a model disease to illustrate two striking phenomena regarding the relation of hereditary patterns to clinical severity.[67] First, as with many diseases due to a single defective gene, a survey of 50 to 100 families revealed three patterns of inheritance: autosomal dominant, autosomal recessive, and X-linked[67] with different families revealing distinct patterns of inheritance. This may represent one of the first insights into genetic heterogeneity. Second, the pattern of inheritance correlated with the age-of-onset and the clinical severity.[67] Families with autosomal recessive patterns usually had an earlier age-of-onset, a uniform clinical presentation, and a more severe phenotype. In contrast, the families with autosomal dominant disease usually had later onset, greater clinical heterogeneity, and milder disease.

Genetic linkage studies[68–91] have identified at least nine loci for CMT1 and four for CMT2 (Table 227-3). Six of the genes associated with CMT1, and recently one gene for CMT2, have been identified.[91a] Isolation of the genes from other mapped and unmapped loci will likely provide substantial insights into development, structure, function, and maintenance of the peripheral nervous system.

## DNA REARRANGEMENTS CAUSING CMT AND RELATED NEUROPATHIES

Remarkably, one of the most common autosomal dominant disorders affecting humans is usually not caused by a mutation in a single gene, but by a duplication of a 1.5-Mb genomic segment resulting in three copies of a normal gene. Although at least eight loci are associated with a CMT1 phenotype, 70 to 90 percent of patients have the CMT1A duplication as the cause of their disease. Furthermore, *de novo* duplication accounts for a substantial fraction of sporadic CMT cases. Deletion of the same genomic segment that is duplicated in CMT1 leads to a clinically distinct neuropathy—HNPP. Thus, DNA rearrangements, the

**Table 227-3 Genetic Loci Associated with the CMT Phenotype**

| Phenotype | Linked locus | inheritance | Genome location | MIM | Gene | Protein |
|-----------|--------------|-------------|-----------------|-----|------|---------|
| CMT1 | CMT1A | AD | 17p12 | 118220 | *PMP22* | PMP22 |
|  | CMT1B | AD | 1q21.1q23.3 | 118200 | *MPZ* | P₀ |
|  | CMT1C | AD | not 17 not 1 | 601098 |  |  |
|  | CMT1X | X-linked | Xq13 | 304040 | *Cx32 (GJB1)* | connexin-32 |
|  | — | AD | 10q21q22 | 129010 | *EGR2** | EGR2 |
|  | CMT4A | AR | 8q13q21.1 | 214400 |  |  |
|  | HMSNL | AR | 8q24.3 | 601455 | *NDRG1* | NDRG1 |
|  | — | AR | 5q23q33 | 601596 |  |  |
|  | CMT4B | AR | 11q23 | 601382 | *MTMR2* | Myotubularin related protein |
| CMT2 | CMT2A | AD | 1p36p35 | 118210 |  |  |
|  | CMT2B | AD | 3q13q22 | 600882 |  |  |
|  | CMT2D | AD | 7p14 | 601472 |  |  |
|  | CMT2E | AD | 8p21 | 162280 | *NEFL* | neurofilament |

*EGR2* was identified by a candidate-gene approach and not by linkage analysis and positional cloning.

CMT1A duplication and the HNPP deletion, account for the majority of patients with inherited neuropathy (Fig. 227-1).

### CMT1A Duplication

In 1990, it became evident that the majority of families segregating autosomal dominant CMT1 were linked to 17p12.[71–79] This locus was designated type 1A or CMT1A. A submicroscopic duplication was identified independently by two groups[92,93] using multiple molecular methods. The novel molecular findings suggesting duplication included: (a) The presence of three informative alleles by polymorphic dinucleotide repeat analysis and RFLP analysis in affected individuals; (b) the identification of a 500-kb patient-specific junction fragment by pulsed-field gel electrophoresis (PFGE); and (c) duplication of probes detected by interphase

fluorescence in situ hybridization (FISH). The CMT1A duplication was initially identified in Americans of French-Acadian and Ashkenazi Jewish descent[92] as well as Belgian and Dutch families.[93] It was subsequently identified in Australian,[94] British,[95] Danish,[96] French,[97] Italian,[98,99] Swedish,[100] Asian,[101] and all other world populations[102] investigated. The detection of the same size junction fragment in multiple patients of different ethnic origin by PFGE suggested (a) that a precise recombination event generated the CMT1A duplication and (b) that a structural feature of the genome at that locus might be responsible for the recurrent events resulting in duplication.

The CMT1A duplication is stable in both meiosis and mitosis.[92,103] Its presence correlates with the diagnostic gold standard of slowed motor nerve conduction velocities.[104] It is an

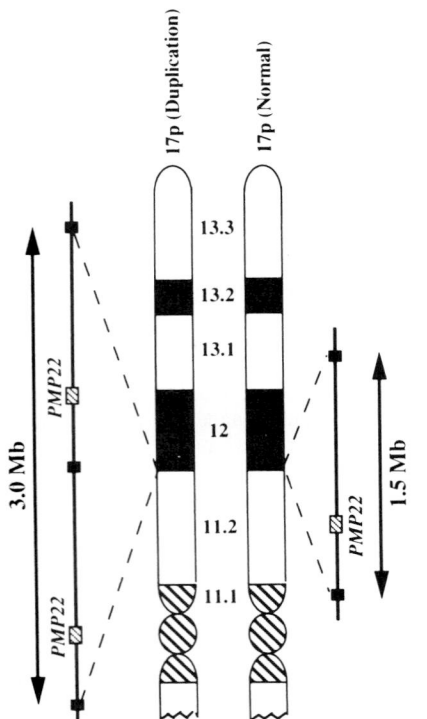

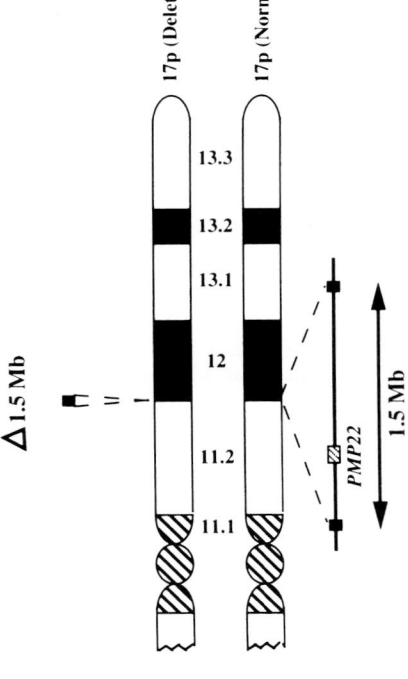

Fig. 227-1 Structure of CMT1A duplication and HNPP deletion. Ideogram of the short arm of chromosome 17 is depicted with the centromeric region denoted by a circle with cross-hatching. Both chromosome homologues are shown with the normal chromosome on the right and the rearranged chromosome on the left. The dashed lines depict an enlargement of the submicroscopic region involved in the DNA rearrangement. Bold rectangles represent the CMT1A-REP repeat while the hashed rectangle depicts the *PMP22* gene. Note the CMT1A duplication is a 3-Mb tandem duplication with three copies of CMT1A-REP and two copies of *PMP22*. The HNPP deletion is deleted for the *PMP22* gene and 1.5 Mb of surrounding genomic DNA, but retains one copy of a recombinant CMT1A-REP.

**CMT1A Duplication**

**HNPP Deletion**

**A**

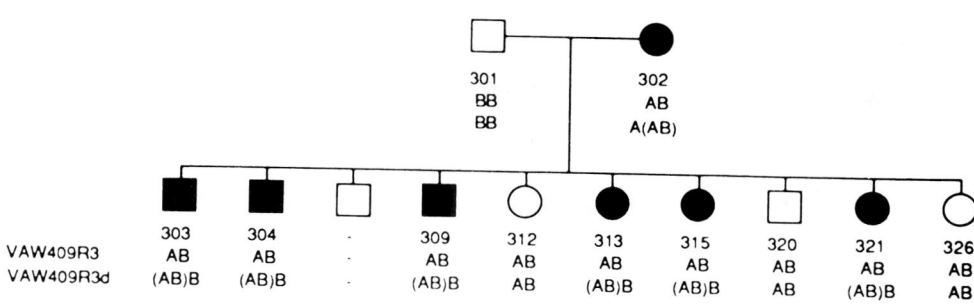

**B**

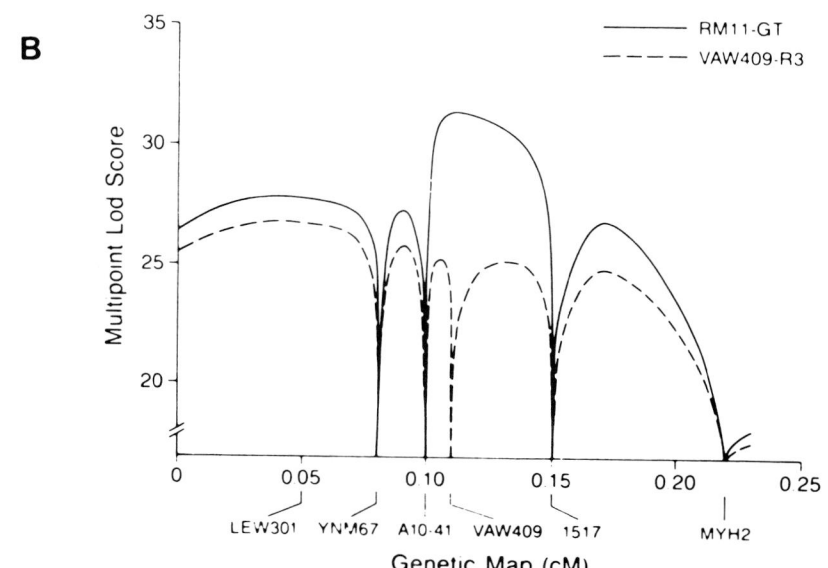

Fig. 227-2 Consequences of duplication mutation on linkage analysis. *A*, A nuclear family of pedigree HOU85 showing the misclassification of the VAW409R3 *MspI* RFLP. Shown below the pedigree symbol in descending order are the identification numbers of the individual and the VAW409R3 genotype scored without and with consideration of dosage alleles, respectively. Segregation of marker alleles demonstrates that individual 85-302 carries the A allele on the CMT1A chromosome if dosage is ignored but the AB allele on the CMT1A chromosome if dosage is considered. Individuals 85-312, 85-320, and 85-326 appear as recombinants with VAW409R3; however, VAW409R3d shows that this is due to misclassification. *B*, Multipoint linkage mapping of CMT1A on a genetic map of chromosome 17p. The locus positions of the markers are indicated on the horizontal axis. The height of the curves represents the relative likelihood of location (LOD score) at any specified point along the map. When dosage differences are ignored (dashed curve), the most likely position of the CMT1A gene is proximal to LEW301; the RM11-GT marker data (solid curve), however, clearly place CMT1A at the VAW409R3 marker locus. (*From Lupski et al.*[92] *Used with permission.*)

excellent biologic marker for the disease because it is the causative genetic event. The CMT1A duplication was responsible for 68 percent of the first 75 North American families studied[105] and 70.7 percent of 819 unrelated CMT1 European patients.[102] A new mutation was first observed in a French-Acadian kindred in which a female CMT proband with nine unaffected siblings had affected children with two different partners. The inheritance of CMT1 in this family was consistent with an autosomal dominant pattern.[76] Molecular demonstration of a *de novo* duplication was first shown by informative polymorphic alleles in a European family; the segregation of marker genotypes suggested unequal crossing over in meiosis.[93]

The CMT1A duplication is a common finding in sporadic CMT1 cases.[106] It was found in 9 of 10 sporadic cases in one study[107] and 76.5 percent of 51 sporadic cases where the parents were clinically and electrophysiologically normal.[102] In autosomal dominant CMT1A families, the new mutation individual can often times be readily identified from pedigree analysis suggesting a recent origin of the duplication in that family. The prevalence of *de novo* duplication in CMT1 pedigrees is estimated at between 5 and 9 percent of families[102,105,108] in most studies, but up to 26.5 percent in one series.[109]

**Consequences of the Duplication on Linkage Analysis.** The failure of traditional linkage analysis to account for dosage differences in two allele systems (RFLP or STR) leads to misinterpretation of parental origins of alleles.[92] These errors

appear as multiple, clustered (within sibships) recombination events that reduce the LOD score and increase the recombination value between the disease locus and the marker.[92,94] More importantly, when the errors are included, multipoint linkage analysis can seriously distort the map position of the disease locus[92,110] (Fig. 227-2).

**Structure of the Duplicated Genomic Region.** The CMT1A duplication was originally estimated to represent a large DNA rearrangement based on the physical distance between genetic markers revealing RFLP dosage differences in CMT1 patients.[92,111,112] Physical mapping with PFGE demonstrated that the duplication is a tandem repeat of a 1.5-Mb monomer unit resulting in a 3.0-Mb rearrangement.[113] There is a large discrepancy between the physical and genetic distances in this region (~1 Mb versus 4 to 14 cM) strongly suggesting increased recombination, that is, a recombination hotspot.[92,111,113] Physical analysis also revealed proximal 17p region-specific low-copy repeats (CMT1A-REPs) that flank the 1.5-Mb unit.[113] Nucleotide sequence showed both proximal (located on the centromeric side) and distal (located on the telomeric side) CMT1A-REPs to be 24,011 bp with 98.7 percent sequence identity (GenBank U71218 and U71217).[114] Both copies of CMT1A-REP contain the same coding exon (exon VI) of the human *COX10* gene, which encodes heme A:farnesyltransferase;[114] however, the *COX10* gene only traverses distal CMT1A-REP and the last coding exon of *COX10* is located within the genomic region that is duplicated in

CMT1A.[114,115] Analysis of proximal CMT1A-REP showed that it likely arose by duplication of the distal CMT1A-REP (see "Primate Origin of CMT1A-REP" below) and that the *COX10* exon within it is a "pseudoexon."[115] Remarkably, proximal CMT1A-REP also contains the 3′ end of a gene, which is transcribed from the opposite strand as the ORF in the *COX10* pseudoexon VI.[116] Thus, the CMT1A-REP genomic duplication has resulted in the evolution of a new gene of unknown function.

The 1.5-Mb region was estimated to contain some 25 to 50 genes based on the estimated 50 to 100,000 genes in the $3 \times 10^9$ bp human genome. Five of these genes have been identified by physical mapping, including part of *COX10*, to be within the 1.5-Mb region.[117,118]

**Homozygous CMT1A Duplication.** Homozygous expression of a dominant gene for CMT1 was originally proposed based on a severe phenotype in the offspring of CMT1 parents.[119] Subsequent molecular studies on several families confirmed homozygosity for the duplication in severely affected offspring and heterozygosity in more mildly affected parents;[92,104] however, the severity of the disease among homozygous patients is variable.[120,121] Patients with homozygous duplication usually present with a DSS phenotype.[119]

**Mosaicism for CMT1A Duplication.** Mosaicism for the CMT1A duplication has been reported in two cases.[122,123] In one well-documented case, in which mosaicism was proven using independent molecular methods on multiple tissues, the patient had a milder clinical phenotype than an affected parent with the duplication.[123,124] However, the clinical findings in this mosaic patient were within the broad range of variation observed with heterozygous duplication. In this case, the mechanism proposed to lead to mosaicism was a reversion of the duplication in early embryogenesis. There is no evidence for germline mosaicism of the CMT1A duplication as is expected with the proposed meiotic origin of the duplication.

### HNPP Deletion

HNPP has a clinical, pathologic, and electrophysiological phenotype that is distinct from the one observed with CMT1A duplication (Table 227-4). The HNPP locus was mapped to proximal chromosome 17p. The disease was shown to be associated with a large interstitial deletion in three unrelated pedigrees, and a de novo deletion was demonstrated for one sporadic case.[125] The deletion spanned ~1.5 Mb and included all the markers mapping within the CMT1A duplication.[125] Furthermore, the HNPP deletion breakpoints map to the same intervals as those in the CMT1A duplication. The deletion results in a lack of transmission of alleles to affected offspring such that the failure to recognize the deletion may lead to erroneous exclusion of paternity or maternity.[125]

The HNPP deletion was identified in families of different ethnic origin who segregated autosomal dominant HNPP,[126–131] and in sporadic HNPP.[125,129] A common junction fragment was defined in all patients by pulsed-field gel electrophoresis, and the uniformity in size suggested that a precise recombination event generated the recurrent deletion.[130–132]

### Molecular Mechanism for Generating the CMT1A Duplication and HNPP Deletion

**Reciprocal Homologous Recombination.** In the first molecular description of a patient with a *de novo* CMT1A duplication, studies of marker genotypes showed that the duplication arose by meiotic unequal crossing over.[93] Subsequent physical analysis of the CMT1A genomic region revealed a large low-copy repeat sequence—CMT1A-REP—that flanked the duplicated region. Misalignment of the proximal CMT1A-REP with the distal CMT1A-REP mediated the unequal crossing over via homologous recombination.[113] This unequal crossing-over model predicted a tandem CMT1A duplication structure with three copies of

**Table 227-4 Contrasting Features of CMT1A and HNPP**

| | CMT1A | HNPP |
|---|---|---|
| Clinical | Symmetric, slowly progressive | Asymmetric episodic |
| Antecedent | None | Motor nerve compression or trauma |
| Potential early signs | Mild delay in achieving motor milestones Idiopathic toe walking of childhood Absent deep tendon reflexes | None |
| Presentation | Distal muscle weakness and atrophy Dropped foot Abnormal gait Foot deformity (*pes caves* > *pes planus*) | Pressure palsies Focal neuropathy Carpal tunnel syndrome |
| Electrophysiological | Slow NCV | Conduction block |
| Neuropathology | Onion bulb | Tomacula |
| Molecular | Duplication | Deletion |

CMT1A-REP. The three copies of CMT1A-REP in the CMT1A duplication were shown by Southern blot analysis[113] and were visualized directly by FISH on stretched chromosome fibers.[133] The tandem or direct nature of the CMT1A duplication was shown by both PFGE and FISH.[113,134] Furthermore, the model predicted a reciprocal deletion of the same genomic region that is duplicated in CMT1A[113] (Fig. 227-3). The HNPP deletion was proposed to represent the reciprocal of the CMT1A duplication.[125] Identification of both the predicted junction fragment in HNPP patients by PFGE and a single copy of CMT1A-REP on the HNPP deletion chromosome supported this hypothesis.[135] Observations regarding the dosage of CMT1A-REP-specific restriction fragments suggested that the CMT1A duplication and HNPP deletion arose from recombination events within a limited region of CMT1A-REP.[135] This was the first evidence for a recombination hotspot within CMT1A-REP that was associated with the unequal crossing over.[135–137]

**Recombination Hotspot Associated with CMT1A Duplication and HNPP Deletion.** The high degree of sequence identity (> 98 percent) between the proximal and distal CMT1A-REPs[114,138] strongly indicates that the crossover occurs within a region of homology by homologous recombination. The sequence differences between proximal and distal CMT1A-REP were used to design experiments to investigate the strand exchange within the recombinant CMT1A-REP. This approach enabled the prediction of junction fragments that could be assayed by conventional Southern blot analysis. In the majority of patients with CMT1A duplication or HNPP deletion, the strand exchange occurred within a limited region of CMT1A-REP and defined a recombination hotspot.[138] This recombination hotspot was found in several different populations[138–144] (Table 227-5). Direct observation of human recombination products was attained by DNA sequence analysis of the recombinant CMT1A-REP in multiple patients.[145,146] The recombination hotspot region delineated in HNPP deletion patients[145] and CMT1A duplication patients[146]

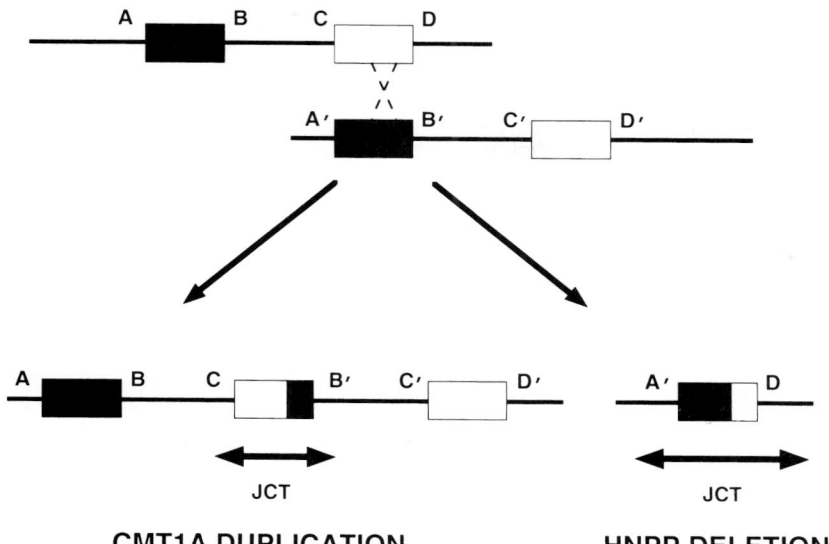

Fig. 227-3 Unequal crossing over resulting in CMT1A duplication and HNPP deletion. Misaligned chromosome 17 homologues with distal CMT1A-REP (open rectangles) paired with proximal CMT1A-REP (closed rectangles) are shown. The A, B, C, D represent unique sequence flanking the CMT1A-REP while A′, B′, C′, and D′ represent these sequences from the homologous chromosome. The dashed line represents the crossing over, or strand exchange, with the products of recombination shown at the end of the single-headed arrows. The structure of the CMT1A duplication and HNPP deletion are depicted below with the unique junction fragments (JCT) resulting from the rearranged chromosome shown with double-headed arrows.

**CMT1A DUPLICATION**

**HNPP DELETION**

overlapped and occurred in a segment of approximately 500 bp within the 24,011 bp of homology between CMT1A-REPs. Analysis of independent recombinant CMT1A-REP sequences showed patches of distal CMT1A-REP sequence interspersed with proximal sequence similar to that observed with gene conversion.[145] This finding is consistent with a double-strand break-model and resolution of a Holliday structure.[145,145a]

**A *mariner* DNA Transposon and Other Potential *cis*-Acting Recombinogenic Sequences Near the Recombination Hotspot.** Nucleotide sequences of the recombination hotspot within CMT1A-REP provided information to search for *cis*-acting DNA sequences that might stimulate localized homologous recombination similar to the Chi sequence of *E. coli*.[147] Chi sites are octameric nucleotide sequences in DNA that stimulate the RecBCD pathway of homologous recombination in *E. coli*.[147] Stimulation is maximal at the Chi site but is asymmetric and decreases by approximately a factor of 2 for each 2 to 3 kb to one side. Chi stimulates recombination through interaction with the RecBCD enzyme.[147] Chi enhances the level of hybrid DNA or heteroduplexes with one strand from each parent molecule.[148]

In the DNA sequence surrounding the recombination hotspot, there is no significant increase in sequence identity between the proximal and distal CMT1A-REP at the crossover site when compared to the surrounding sequence. This observation suggested that some other signal must be present at or near the site of strand exchange for homologous recombination to occur with an approximately 50:1 preference within the hotspot region as opposed to random sites surrounding 24 kb of homology.[138] Database searches identified a DNA transposon of the *mariner* family (MITE = *mariner* insect transposon-like element) near the

recombination hotspot.[138] The transposase-coding region of MITE contains frameshift mutations so that it does not encode an active transposase. However, 1 of the more than 100 *mariner* elements of this class within the human genome[149] hypothetically could encode a transposase that could initiate a double-strand break to stimulate homologous recombination. The present model consists of (a) a double-strand break initiated by a *trans*-acting mariner transposase, (b) patch repair by a misaligned CMT1A-REP sequence, and (c) resolution of the heteroduplex within the recombination hotspot.[8,138] However, to date there is no experimental evidence for an active *mariner* transposase in the human genome.

Other *cis*-acting sequences near the recombination hotspot that might stimulate homologous recombination have been proposed. A sequence with 7/8-bp homology to the Chi octamer[146] has been identified, but a single mismatch of Chi renders it inactive in bacteria.[147] A clustering of five minisatellite-like sequences was proposed as a unique characteristic of CMT1A-REP and minisatellites have been shown to enhance recombination at a distance.[146] A 13-nucleotide sequence highly homologous to a region of the 289-bp MT sequence involved in recombination in mice and a 15-nucleotide sequence found in the 1649-bp *Lmp2* murine hotspot were also identified.[146] None of these sequences have been implicated previously in human recombination events;[146] therefore, functional studies will be required to determine exactly what stimulates homologous recombination at the hotspot in CMT1A-REP.

The minimal efficient processing segment (MEPS) required for homologous recombination in cultured mouse cells is between 132 and 232 bp of complete shared sequence identity between recombining homologues.[150,151] A search for sequence identity of >200 bp shared by the misaligned proximal and distal 24-kb CMT1A-REPs revealed 18 sites, 7 of which have >300 bp of identity, that may be potential regions of exchange.[145] One of the three largest stretches of identity is a 456-bp region located within the 557-bp recombination hotspot. This is the closest stretch of >200 bp of sequence identity in proximity to the end of the MITE element previously implicated as a potential site of double-strand break that stimulates recombination in this region.[138] This is perhaps the first time that a correlation has been made between sites of frequent unequal crossing-over events and a potential minimal processing segment for efficient meiotic homologous recombination in humans. This preferred region of exchange may potentially help in defining the boundaries for a minimal efficient processing segment in human meiotic recombination.[145]

**Table 227-5 Recombination Hotspot in World Populations**

| Population | Patient crossover in hotspot | Total patients examined | Percent in hotspot |
|---|---|---|---|
| North American | 143 | 177 | 80% |
| European | 123 | 162 | 76% |
| French | 86 | 114 | 75% |
| Japanese | 68 | 88 | 77% |
| Chinese | 27 | 31 | 87% |
| TOTALS | 447 | 572 | 78% |

**Parent of Origin Preference for the Recombination.** The parental origin of duplication was initially studied in nine sporadic CMT patients.[152] In all cases, the mutation was the product of an unequal exchange between chromosome homologues (interchromosomal), as opposed to between chromatids of a single chromosome (intrachromosomal), during spermatogenesis.[152] Both the *de novo* CMT1A duplication[36,96,105,106,108] and the HNPP deletion[125,126,128,131,140] occur preferentially on the paternally inherited chromosome suggesting that male specific factor(s) promote the duplication or deletion during gametogenesis. However, rare *de novo* duplication[106,108] and deletions[124,153] of maternal origin indicate that these events are not solely associated with male meiosis.[8] The preponderance of paternally derived *de novo* duplication has also been hypothesized to be related to the difference between the mechanisms of sperm and egg production.[154]

Further studies of *de novo* duplications and deletions confirmed a preponderance (24 of 28) of paternal interchromosomal events.[155] In contrast, in the four informative analyses of maternally derived DNA rearrangements, two CMT1A duplications and two HNPP deletions, the rearrangements were intrachromosomal events.[155] The intrachromosomal events were proposed to result from unequal sister chromatid exchange or, in the case of deletion, potentially from excision of intrachromatidal loops.[155] These observations suggest that unequal crossing over may occur more frequently in male gametogenesis.

**Primate Origin of CMT1A-REP.** CMT1A-REP sequences are not detected in mice and hamsters, suggesting that a recent evolutionary event was responsible for the genomic duplication resulting in the two copies of CMT1A-REP.[113] Studies in primates indicate that the duplicated copy of CMT1A-REP originated between chimpanzee and gorilla speciation.[144,156] Three observations suggest that the distal CMT1A-REP was the progenitor copy: (a) the proximal CMT1A-REP has interrupted a large region-specific low copy number repeat;[113] (b) although each CMT1A-REP contains exon VI of the heme A:farnesyltransferase (*COX10*) gene, the remaining exons of *COX10* span only the distal CMT1A-REP;[114,115] and (c) the *Alu* sequence at the telomeric end of the proximal CMT1A-REP is truncated.[156]

## Abnormal Gene Dosage Causes CMT1A

Three models were initially proposed to explain how the CMT1A duplication might affect a "CMT gene" and result in disease. These models included (a) gene dosage, (b) gene interruption, and (c) position effect.[92] The gene-dosage model proposes that the presence of three copies of a "CMT gene" (instead of the usual two) is sufficient to cause disease. The gene-interruption model proposes that the junction of the CMT1A duplication would interrupt a gene and that this insertional mutation would be responsible for the phenotype. The position-effect model posited that a putative CMT gene is adjacent to different regulatory sequences as a consequence of the CMT1A duplication. The finding of a more severe phenotype in a patient homozygous for the duplication suggested that gene dosage may be important to the clinical manifestations of CMT1;[92,104] however, further support for this model was provided by the evaluation of patients with chromosomal duplications and genetically engineered mice.

**dup(17)p12 and CMT1.** To investigate further a potential role for gene dosage in the CMT1A phenotype, a patient with a cytogenetically visible duplication of the short arm of chromosome 17 [dup(17)p11.2p12] was examined for signs of CMT1 with objective electrodiagnostic techniques.[157] This patient had developmental delay and multiple congenital anomalies including complex congenital heart disease, dysmorphic features, abnormal dentition, a right floating thumb, and minor skeletal anomalies. Such a clinical picture of multisystem involvement is expected in an individual with a chromosomal abnormality. However, in addition to the above features, the motor NCV of each nerve tested

was 17 to 20 m/s (normal >38 m/s), which is diagnostic of CMT1.[157] Similarly, a patient with trisomy for the entire short arm of chromosome 17, due to an unbalanced translocation inherited from his phenotypically normal balanced carrier father, also had electrophysiologic studies and a neurologic examination consistent with demyelinating neuropathy or CMT1.[158] Other patients with cytogenetically visible duplication of proximal 17p enabled mapping of the dosage sensitive CMT1A gene to 17p12.[159] The patients whose cytogenetically visible duplication included 17p12 had electrophysiologic findings consistent with CMT1A.[159] The breakpoints of the duplication in these rare patients with cytogenetically visible alterations were distinct, and therefore would not be interrupting the same gene. Moreover, because the position of a CMT gene with respect to nearby sequence would be different for the different size alterations, a position effect cannot be involved. The diagnosis of CMT1 in persons with three copies of 17p12 and without the CMT junction strongly favors the gene dosage model over the other two models as causative in CMT1.

**PMP22: A Dosage Sensitive Myelin Gene.** The identification of the dosage-sensitive gene within chromosome 17p12 responsible for CMT1A was greatly aided by parallel studies in the mouse models for CMT1 and DSS. The animal models, *trembler* (*Tr*) and *trembler^J* (*Tr^J*), display the electrophysiological features of symmetrically slowed motor NCV and the pathologic finding of demyelinating neuropathy including onion bulbs. *Tr* and *Tr^J* both map to a region of mouse chromosome 11, which maintains conserved synteny with human 17p. *Tr* and *Tr^J* result from point mutations in the *Pmp22* (peripheral myelin protein-22) gene.[160,161] The human *PMP22* gene (GenBank L03203) mapped within the CMT1A duplication region;[134,162–164] however, the majority of CMT1A patients have three normal copies of this gene. Thus, an apparent conundrum existed because the mouse phenotype was associated with point mutation of *Pmp22*, while the human disease appeared to be due to increased dosage of a region that contained a presumably wild-type *PMP22*.[165]

Previous data had revealed that ~30 percent of CMT1 patients did not have the CMT1A duplication.[105] Analysis of *PMP22* coding sequence in a nonduplication family linked to 17p12 markers,[166] and in a sporadic CMT1 family,[167] identified a cosegregating *PMP22* alteration and a *de novo PMP22* mutation, respectively. Interestingly, in one family the PMP22 mutation (L16P) was identical to that found in the *Tr^J* mouse.[166] Subsequently, *PMP22* point mutations were identified in patients with the Dejerine-Sottas syndrome (DSS).[168] One DSS patient had a missense amino acid substitution (G150D) identical to that observed in the *Tr* mouse.[169]

The clinical phenotype of CMT1 results when one of the *PMP22* alleles is mutated or when there are three copies of *PMP22*. Likewise, deletion of one copy of *PMP22* causes the HNPP phenotype. Substantial data support that *PMP22* is the dosage-sensitive gene responsible for CMT1A and HNPP.[10,144] First, in extremely rare neuropathy cases with smaller duplications[152,170,171] or deletion,[172] the *PMP22* gene was encompassed by the alternative-sized rearrangement. Second, the *PMP22* mRNA was elevated in CMT1A duplication patients by RT-PCR of sural nerve biopsies when compared to another control myelin gene. This increase in *PMP22* mRNA was specific to CMT1A duplication patients compared to those with nonduplication neuropathies;[173] other studies, however, have not observed a direct correlation between duplication and increased *PMP22* gene expression in patients of different ages.[174–176] Third, *PMP22* mRNA was shown to be decreased in patients with the HNPP deletion[177] and the *PMP22* mRNA expression level correlated with the neuropathy disability score.[178] Fourth, quantitative immunohistochemical[179] and ultrastructural immunogold labeling[180] showed increased PMP22 protein in CMT1A duplication patients and decreased PMP22 protein in HNPP deletion patients.

Animal models, including two different transgenic mice and a rat model, that overexpress *Pmp22* recapitulate the phenotypic

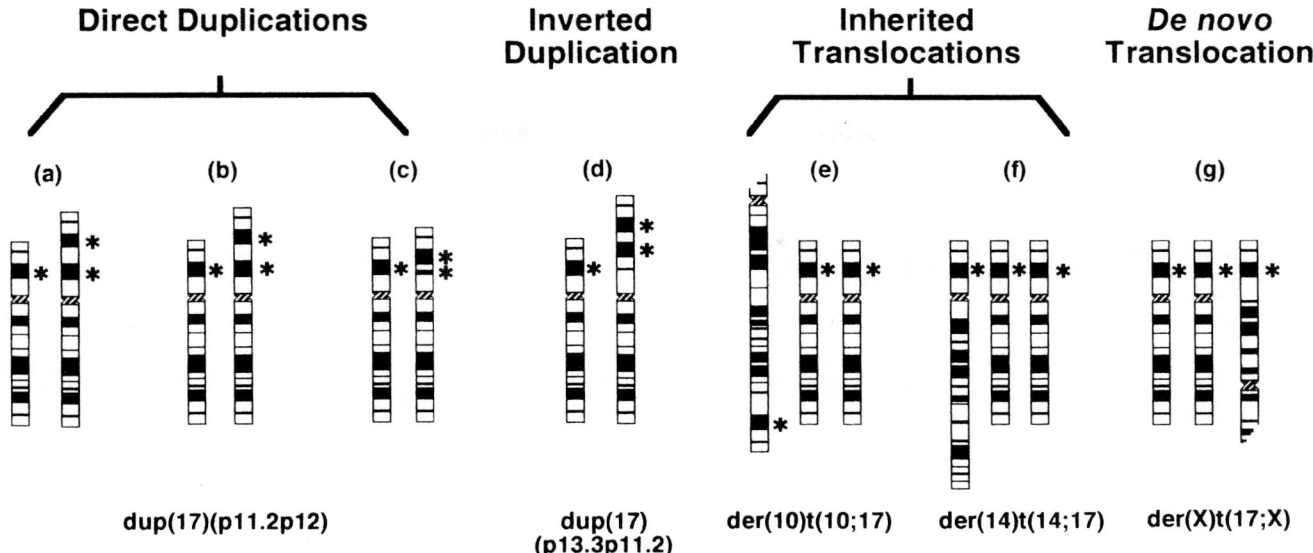

| Direct Duplications | | | Inverted Duplication | Inherited Translocations | | De novo Translocation |
|---|---|---|---|---|---|---|
| (a) | (b) | (c) | (d) | (e) | (f) | (g) |
| dup(17)(p11.2p12) | | | dup(17) (p13.3p11.2) | der(10)t(10;17) | der(14)t(14;17) | der(X)t(17;X) |

**Fig. 227-4 Chromosomal aberrations and CMT1A.** Partial karyotypes showing chromosome 17 from seven patients with chromosomal abnormalities who manifest CMT1 as part of their complex clinical phenotype. The G-banded patterns are shown for each normal chromosome 17 (left) and derivative 17 (right) with the rearrangements described below each set. The asterisk (*) represents the location of the *PMP22* gene. Derivative chromosomes are as follows: der(10) = der(10) t(10;17)(q26.3; p11.2) mat; der(14) = der(14) t(14;17)(p11;p11)pat; der(X) = der(X) t(17;X)(p22.1;p11.2). Note that all patients with chromosomal syndromes that duplicated 17p12 have three copies of the *PMP22* gene and manifest a CMT1 phenotype. *(Figure courtesy of Dr. Lisa Shaffer.)*

features of CMT1.[181-183] Within these models, the levels of *PMP22* expression correlate with the degree of demyelination and reduction in NCV.[184] Similarly, the homozygous *PMP22* knockout mouse model recapitulates the human HNPP phenotype including the pathologic finding of tomacula of peripheral nerves.[185] The heterozygous *Pmp22* knockout mice have a progressive demyelinating tomaculous neuropathy.[186] A transgenic antisense mouse model also displays the clinical, electrophysiological, and pathologic hallmarks of HNPP.[187]

Further evidence supporting *PMP22* gene dosage as a mechanism for CMT1A was the absence of mutations in the coding region of *PMP22* in the youngest CMT1A duplication patient from each of seven different families and in two sporadic CMT1A duplication patients.[188] Also, consistent with *PMP22* haploinsufficiency causing HNPP, nondeletion HNPP patients have nonsense and frameshift *PMP22* mutations that are presumably null alleles.[189,190] Interestingly, Pelizaeus-Merzbacher disease, a central nervous system dysmyelinating disorder (Chap. 228) results in many cases from duplication of the *PLP* gene encoding proteolipid protein.[191-193]

**Bridging the Gap Between Chromosomal Syndromes and Mendelian Disorders.** Traditionally, disorders that segregate as Mendelian traits result from mutations in single genes. In contrast, chromosomal syndromes have been thought to result from the effects of many genes within or flanking the region of the chromosomal abnormality.[24] Although the effects of gene-dosage imbalance in chromosomal syndromes were already appreciated,[194] the concept of "gene dosage" or gene copy number effects was crystallized by findings at the CMT1A locus in 17p12. A submicroscopic DNA duplication is transmitted as a dominant trait and is responsible for the segregation of the CMT1A neuropathy phenotype indicated by electrophysiological studies revealing slowed motor NCVs. Although the 3-Mb duplication contains several genes, only *PMP22* appears to be dosage sensitive. Patients with cytogenetically visible chromosomal duplications involving this genomic region also have slowed motor NCV as a distinct part of their more complex phenotype.[157-159,195-197] As long as the 17p12 region of the genome has three copies instead of the normal two, then part of the phenotype

will include slowed motor NCV. The extra copy of 17p12 can derive from chromosomal interstitial duplications, inverted duplication, as well as inherited or *de novo* translocations (Fig. 227-4). Thus, manifesting a simple Mendelian disorder versus a chromosomal syndrome may reflect the size of the DNA rearrangement and the number of dosage-sensitive genes contained within the duplicated or deleted genomic segment.[24]

## MYELIN GENE MUTATIONS AND MYELINOPATHIES

Mutations in four different genes — *PMP22*, *MPZ*, *Cx32*, and *EGR2* — have been associated with myelinopathies. The proteins encoded by these genes are distinct, but each is expressed by myelinating Schwann cells. *PMP22* and *MPZ* appear to encode compact myelin structural proteins (recent evidence suggests an association between these two proteins in PNS myelin[197a]); *Cx32* encodes a noncompact myelin gap junction protein that is responsible for direct transport of small molecules across the myelin sheath (Fig. 227-5);[198] and *EGR2* encodes a transcription factor required for myelin gene expression that appears to be important for myelin development and maintenance. A comprehensive mutation database for myelinopathy associated mutations is available (http://molgen-www.uia.ac.be/CMTMutations/).

### PMP22

***PMP22* Gene and Protein Structure.** The *PMP22* (GenBank L03203) cDNA was isolated as an axon-regulated Schwann cell transcript, encoding a myelin membrane protein, that is downregulated after sciatic nerve injury[199-202] and independently from a cDNA library of human fetal spinal cord.[203] It was recognized to be identical to *gas-3*, a growth arrest-specific gene.[202,204] It has also been designated CD25 and SR13. The *PMP22* gene contains four coding exons and is regulated by two alternatively used promoters.[205,206] It is expressed predominantly in the peripheral nerve,[162,205] but also in other nonneural tissues during development and in the adult.[207]

The PMP22 protein is an integral membrane glycoprotein with four proposed transmembrane domains. It has a mass of ~22 kDa (an 18-kDa core polypeptide and 4 kDa of carbohydrates linked to

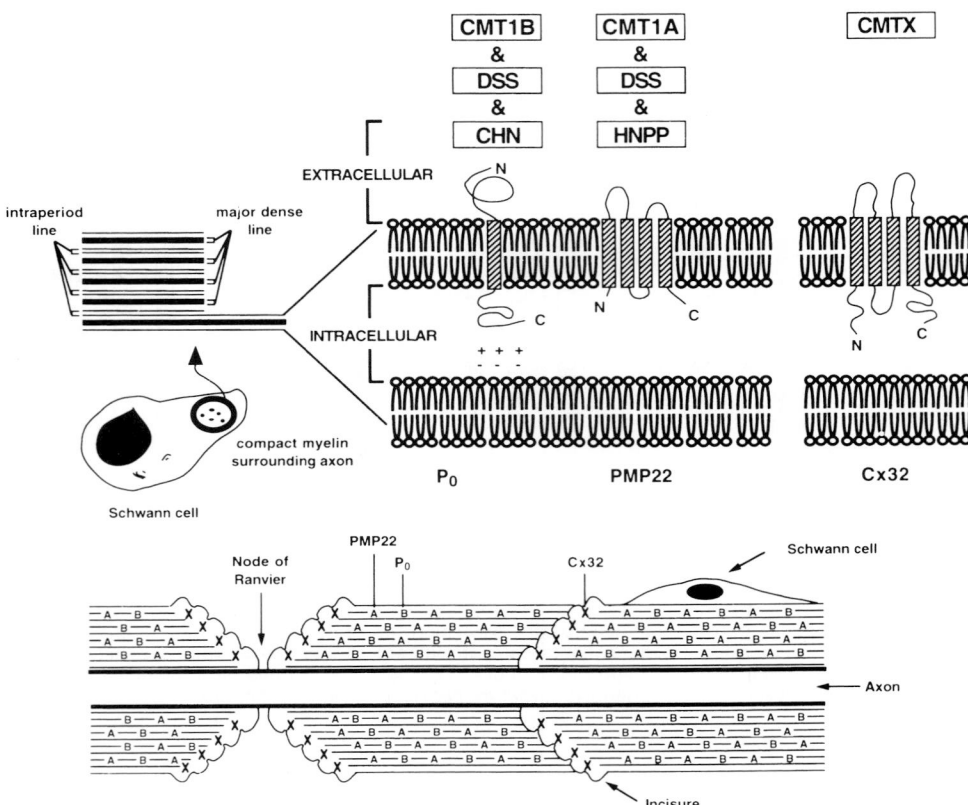

**Fig. 227-5 Myelin proteins and myelinopathies.** A Schwann cell and the structure of compact myelin with the intraperiod and major dense lines (above left). The detailed blow-up depicts the structure of the compact myelin membrane proteins $P_0$ and PMP22, as well as the noncompact myelin protein Cx32, with their major associated disease phenotypes in rectangles. A side view of the peripheral nerve with axon and myelin demonstrating the distribution of myelin protein $P_0$ (B), PMP22(A) in the compact myelin and Cx32(X) in the noncompact myelin (below). *(Adapted from Roa and Lupski.[198] Used with permission.)*

an asparagine residue). The glycosylated portion contains an L2/HNK-1 epitope.[208,209] This epitope is implicated in intercellular recognition, interaction, and adhesion processes. PMP22 comprises 2 to 5 percent of PNS myelin[210] and is found uniformly in compact, but not noncompacted, regions of myelin.[200,210,211] Although ultrastructural studies of uncompacted myelin lamellae in nerves obtained from HNPP patients suggest a structural role for PMP22, the exact function of PMP22 remains unknown.[212] An alternative proposed function is regulation of Schwann-cell growth and differentiation,[213,214] as suggested by the initial identification of *PMP22* as a growth-arrest specific gene. Some investigators suggest a dual role as a structural protein important to myelin compaction and as a regulatory protein important in myelin development and maintenance.[28] Whether PMP22 has a regulatory role in addition to its structural function remains elusive. Nevertheless, mutation studies of other myelin structural proteins (*MPZ, Cx32*) reveal dramatic effects on myelin development and maintenance.

***PMP22* Mutations and Myelinopathies.** *PMP22* point mutations have been associated with CMT1, DSS, and HNPP.[166–169,215–229] These mutations include mostly missense amino acid substitutions, but deletion of a single amino acid and a few frameshift mutations have also been reported (Fig. 227-6). Codon position 72 has been suggested to be a mutation hotspot because of four independent reports of the same mutation. This mutation occurs at a CpG dinucleotide. Most mutations occur in amino acids comprising the putative transmembrane domains. Eleven of the 24 mutations are *de novo* and associated with sporadic disease. All alterations except one are associated with disease in the heterozygous state and thus are dominant alleles. Most *PMP22* mutations result in a more severe neuropathy than that associated with the CMT1A duplication: 13 of 26 with DSS and many of the CMT1 mutations convey a more severe CMT phenotype.

Three mutations (L6fs, V30M, and G94fs) are associated with HNPP. L6fs is a null allele that causes a classic HNPP

phenotype.[189] G94fs results in a mixed HNPP and CMT1 phenotype[190,230] because 23 patients from 6 families[228] showed clinical, electrophysiological and morphologic characteristics of HNPP but neuropathologic features of CMT1. The V30M mutation, which causes a mild HNPP phenotype and HNPP in nerve xenograft studies, is a conservative substitution at the junction of the first transmembrane domain and the extracellular loop.[229]

The T118M alteration, also located at the border of an extracellular loop and transmembrane domain, has been proposed to be either a recessive pathogenic mutation[132] or a benign variant.[231] It was identified as a recessive pathogenic mutation due to a severe CMT1 phenotype in a patient who was a compound heterozygote for this allele and an HNPP deletion. This patient was clinically distinct from her HNPP-affected children who inherited only the HNPP deletion, and from her son who had normal electrophysiological studies and who was heterozygous for the T118M allele.[132] The same alteration was alternatively interpreted as a benign variant after its identification in two unaffected parents of sporadic CMT1 cases while being absent in one of the affected individuals.[231] Interestingly, overexpression of the T118M mutation in NIH3T3 cells showed a reduced ability to trigger apoptosis as compared to wild-type *PMP22*, but apoptosis occurred when coexpressed with wild-type *PMP22*.[232] In contrast, other disease-associated *PMP22* alleles have a dominant effect because their reduced ability to trigger apoptosis is not abrogated by coexpression of wild-type *PMP22*. These data support the hypothesis that the T118M variant is recessive and disease causing, because like other disease-causing *PMP22* alleles, it has an effect on the regulation of susceptibility to apoptosis. Recent in vitro experiments suggest that impaired intracellular trafficking is a common disease mechanism for *PMP22* point mutations causing peripheral neuropathies.[232a] These experiments provide independent evidence that T118M affects *PMP22* function and is not a benign alteration.[232a] Nevertheless, identification of a recessive CMT1 patient or unaffected individual who is homozygous for the

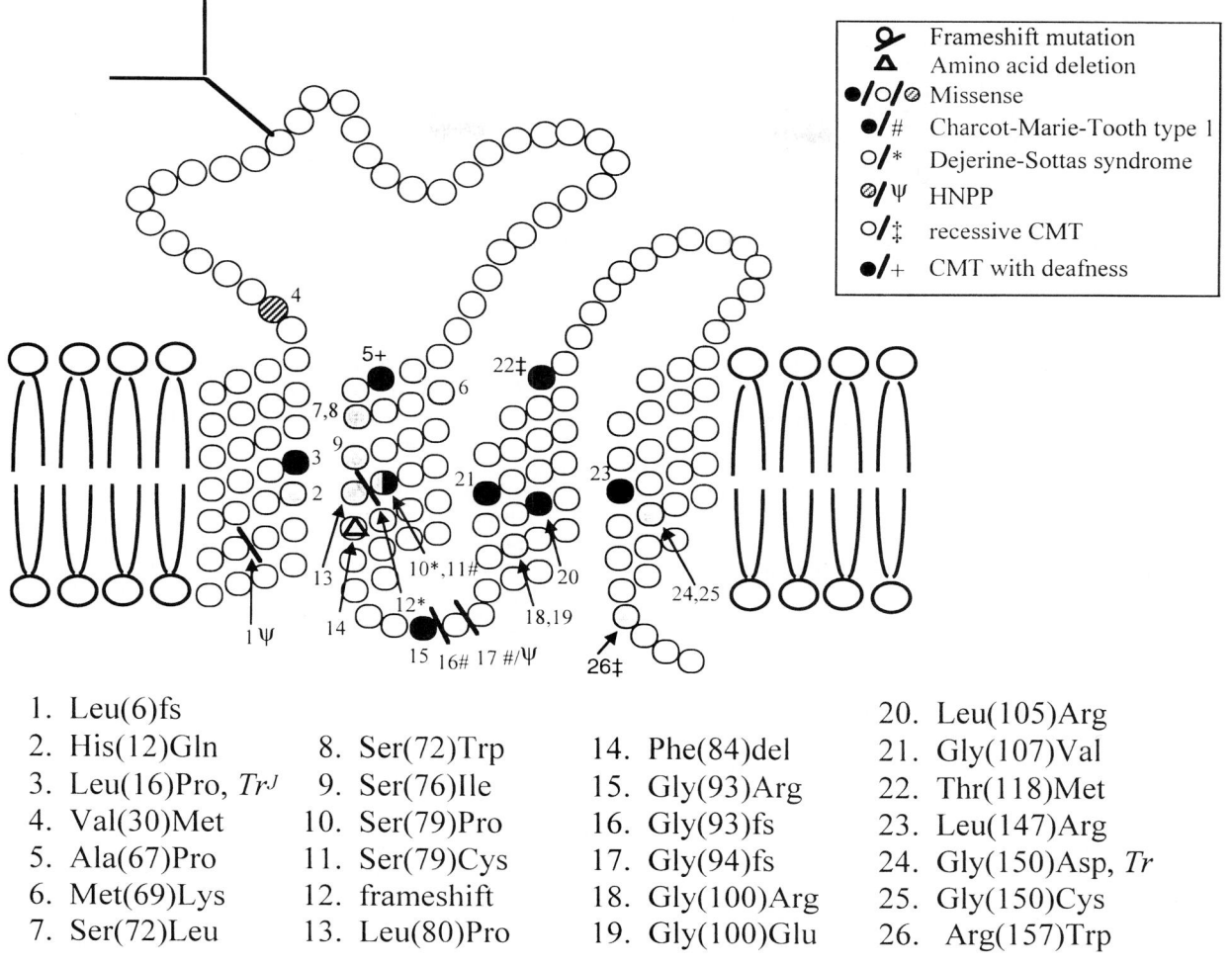

|  | Frameshift mutation |
| --- | --- |
|  | Amino acid deletion |
| ●/○/⊘ | Missense |
| ●/# | Charcot-Marie-Tooth type 1 |
| ○/* | Dejerine-Sottas syndrome |
| ⊘/ψ | HNPP |
| ○/‡ | recessive CMT |
| ●/+ | CMT with deafness |

1. Leu(6)fs
2. His(12)Gln
3. Leu(16)Pro, *Tr*<sup>J</sup>
4. Val(30)Met
5. Ala(67)Pro
6. Met(69)Lys
7. Ser(72)Leu
8. Ser(72)Trp
9. Ser(76)Ile
10. Ser(79)Pro
11. Ser(79)Cys
12. frameshift
13. Leu(80)Pro
14. Phe(84)del
15. Gly(93)Arg
16. Gly(93)fs
17. Gly(94)fs
18. Gly(100)Arg
19. Gly(100)Glu
20. Leu(105)Arg
21. Gly(107)Val
22. Thr(118)Met
23. Leu(147)Arg
24. Gly(150)Asp, *Tr*
25. Gly(150)Cys
26. Arg(157)Trp

**Fig. 227-6** Myelinopathy associated *PMP22* mutations. The four predicted transmembrane domains of PMP22 are shown with individual amino acids represented as open circles. Specific mutations are delineated below with the associated phenotype shown by symbols depicted in the upper right. Essentially all mutations are in transmembrane domains. Identical mutations to the spontaneous mouse models *Tr* (mutation 3) and *Tr*<sup>J</sup> (mutation 23) have been identified in a severe CMT1 family and DSS family respectively.

T118M variant is required to definitively answer the question of whether the T118M amino acid substitution is a recessive mutation or benign variant.

A recessive R157W mutation of *PMP22* was associated with DSS, in three affected siblings from consanguineous parents.[233] Heterozygous parents with this mutation were asymptomatic with normal NCV. A different missense amino acid substitution at the identical position, R157G, was also reported in the hemizygous state associated with CMT1.[234] The compound heterozygous CMT1 individual had the R157G allele on one chromosome and the HNPP deletion on the other homologous chromosome. Molecular modeling localizes this mutation to the intracellular domain of *PMP22*. The genotype R157G/def thus appears to convey a more severe phenotype than wt/def (CMT1 vs. HNPP) while R157W/wt and R157G/wt have normal phenotypes consistent with a recessive gain-of-function mechanism. This recessive gain-of-function mechnanism is consistent with the PMP22 protein potentially having multimeric interactions.

***PMP22* Mutations and Disease Mechanisms.** Studies of mouse models and of cell culture systems have shown that PMP22 mutations function as gain-of-function mutations, dominant-negative mutations, or both. The fact that the *Tr* mutant, *Pmp22*<sup>Tr/+</sup> mouse (GenBank M32240 for mouse *Pmp22*), displays severe hypomyelination while the heterozygous *Pmp22*<sup>+/−</sup>

knockout mice show focal hypermyelination suggests that *Tr*-PMP22 behaves as a gain-of-function or dominant-negative mutation and not as a null allele.[235] Consistent with this gain-of-function hypothesis, *Pmp22*<sup>Tr/−</sup> mice show severe hypomyelination, while *Pmp22*<sup>−/−</sup> mice have focal hypermyelination.[235] However, an overlapping dominant-negative effect is suggested by the increasing myelin deficiency with increasing numbers of *Tr* alleles; that is, *Pmp22*<sup>Tr/Tr</sup> has a more severe phenotype than *Pmp22*<sup>Tr/−</sup>.[235] The hypomyelination observed in the *Tr*<sup>Ncnp</sup> allele, an in-frame deletion of the second transmembrane domain and a part of the third transmembrane domain, also supports a gain-of-function mechanism.[236]

Two contrasting observations have been made with Pmp22 mutations. In the first situation, the Tr protein alters protein trafficking and exhibits a dominant-negative effect on wild-type Pmp22[237] in *Tr* animals and transfected cells.[232] In the second situation, the distribution of Tr and Tr<sup>J</sup> mutant proteins differ from that of wild-type Pmp22, but neither Tr nor Tr<sup>J</sup> proteins have a dominant-negative effect on the cellular distribution of wild-type Pmp22[238] suggesting that impaired trafficking of mutated Pmp22 effects Schwann cell physiology leading to myelin instability and loss.[238]

Three observations support altered trafficking and a dominant-negative effect of mutant Pmp22 protein. First, Pmp22 immuno-reactive proteins accumulate in the ER/Golgi of Schwann cells of

*Tr* mice.[237,238] Second, Tr protein is retained in the ER of transfected COS-7 and cultured Schwann cells.[237] The retention is hypothesized to be due to protein misfolding and/or impaired processing. Third, the cotransfection of wild-type Pmp22 and the Tr[J] mutant Pmp22, each with different epitope tags, demonstrated that Tr[J] protein, unlike Pmp22, does not reach the cell membrane but accumulates in the intermediate compartment,[239] and that Tr[J] protein causes some, but not all, of the wild-type Pmp22 to be diverted from its normal trafficking pathway and retained in the intermediate compartment.[239] An alternative cellular mechanism suggests that mutant Pmp22 protein is incorporated into the plasma membrane, decreasing myelin stability.[240] This hypothesis is supported by the findings that the endosomal/lysosomal pathway is up-regulated and there is an accumulation of myelin proteins (PMP22, MBP and $P_0$) in the endosomes/lysosomes.[240]

The human *PMP22* loss-of-function point mutations result in HNPP while presumably gain-of-function or dominant-negative alleles result in CMT1 or DSS. Regardless of the exact mechanism by which the latter mutations produce a severe neuropathy, it is obvious that the stoichiometry of *PMP22* is crucial for myelin function and maintenance. The major genetic mechanism for disease is not aberrant protein, but altered PMP22 dosage.[10]

## MPZ

***MPZ* Gene and Protein Structure.** The cDNA for the major structural protein of the peripheral myelin sheath, $P_0$, was isolated by differential screening and hybrid selection[241] (GenBank NM000530). The *MPZ* gene encoding human $P_0$ contains six coding exons and is regulated by a single promoter.[242] The *MPZ* promoter is often utilized as a Schwann cell-specific expression promoter in cells and transgenic mice.[243] Multiple regulatory elements control transcription of *MPZ*.[244] The gene maps to 1q22-q23 (242) where the CMT1B locus (Table 227-3) was assigned.

$P_0$ is a 28-kDa protein expressed exclusively by myelinating Schwann cells and accounts for > 50 percent of the total PNS myelin protein.[245] $P_0$ is an integral membrane protein, and is localized to compact myelin. It consists of a single membrane-spanning region, a large hydrophobic glycosylated immunoglobulin-like extracellular domain, and a smaller basic intracellular domain[241] (Fig. 227-5). The immunoglobulin-like extracellular domain is necessary for cell adhesion[246,247] and plays a significant role in the formation and compaction of the intraperiod line.[246,248] It contains an asparagine-linked glycosylation site that carries the L2/HNK-1 adhesive carbohydrate epitope.[249] Membrane juxtaposition in the extracellular space of PNS myelin is thought to be mediated by homophilic interactions of the $P_0$ extracellular domain (Fig. 227-5), while apposition of the cytoplasmic faces of the membrane is thought to be mediated by the intracellular domains.[241] The intracellular domain is extremely basic and has been shown to participate in electrostatic interactions with the opposing anionic lipid bilayer to help in the formation of the major dense line[250,251] (Fig. 227-5).

The crystal structure of the rat $P_0$ extracellular domain (97 percent identical to human $P_0$) consists of alternatively oriented cyclic tetramers, which are comprised of $P_0$ protomers arranged head-to-tail about a fourfold axis.[252] Each tetramer is related to four others of opposite orientation through protomer-protomer interfaces, which generates a network of molecules with half emanating from one membrane surface and the other half from the opposite surface.[252] The interactions between opposing membrane faces have some similarities that have been likened to a "molecular velcro."[10] Outwardly pointing tryptophan side chains extend from the apices of each tetramer and may intercalate into the opposing membrane surface.[252] Molecular modeling predicted some amino acids critical to homophilic interactions even prior to the availability of crystal structure information.[253] The dimensions of the crystal model correspond with the dimensions of PNS myelin as determined by independent methods.

***MPZ* Mutations and Myelinopathies.** *MPZ* mutations were originally identified in families that showed linkage to chromosome 1,[254,255] the first CMT locus mapped in the human genome.[70] Subsequently, *MPZ* mutations were also found in patients with DSS[256] and CHN,[257] and in some patients having a phenotype consistent with CMT2.[257,258] Interestingly, a *MPZ* mutation, N102K, has been identified in the original family studied by Roussy and Lévy suggesting this represents a clinical variant of CMT1.[258a] More than 50 different myelinopathy-associated mutations in *MPZ* have been described[259-285] (Fig. 227-7). The majority of the myelinopathy-associated mutations are missense mutations, but amino acid deletions, frameshift, and nonsense mutations also occur. Many mutations are *de novo* and all of the mutations that have been reported to date are dominant. Germ line mosaicism for one *MPZ* point mutation was reported in association with a DSS phenotype in two sisters.[258] Most mutations occur in the extracellular domain, in contrast to *PMP22* in which the majority of mutations affect the four putative transmembrane domains.

Some mutations of *MPZ* suggest an underlying genetic mechanism. The codon for Arg69 (codon 98 if one includes the signal peptide in the numbering scheme) is proposed to have a high frequency of mutation based on the identification of three different mutations in 4 of 20 unrelated French CMT1 families without the CMT1A duplication.[272] This high frequency of mutations occurs at a CpG dinucleotide. It is of interest that four different missense amino acid substitutions (R69H, R69S, R69P, R69C) and three different clinical phenotypes have been reported with mutations at this codon. The identical missense amino acid substitution R69C has been alternatively reported with DSS,[271] CHN,[283] and a severe CMT1B[276] phenotype. The R69C, R69S,[257] and R69H mutations[271] have clinically distinct phenotypes.

Some *MPZ* mutations involve more than one amino acid; usually these amino acids are adjacent, but in one case of DSS, three separate *de novo* mutations were identified on the same chromosome.[280] These three mutations did not occur in CpG dinucleotides, there is no significant secondary structure, which argues against correction of a quasipalindrome as a mechanism for multiple point mutations, and there are no known pseudogenes to participate in a gene conversion event. One potential mechanism for multiple point mutations is defective repair of a deleted region.

Selected mutations provide insights into the role of $P_0$ in myelin structure, glycosylation requirements for function, and survival of the organism. The identification of a heterozygous $P_0$ mutation associated with congenital hypomyelination suggests that a severe allele of a major myelin protein component can have dramatic effects on myelin structure and formation.[257] The identical mutation, Q186X, was also identified in another case of CHN.[281] This study used a polyclonal antibody directed against the entire $P_0$ peptide to show that almost all myelinated fibers expressed the protein normally.[281] Mutation of the single glycosylation site in $P_0$ resulted in a relatively mild CMT1B phenotype,[265] but this may not be too surprising because homophilic adhesive interactions of $P_0$ are not dependent on glycosylation as shown by studies in heterologous cell systems.[246,248,286,287] Homozygous mutation of *MPZ* has been reported twice (F35del, G74fs) and in both instances caused DSS;[257,270] the early frameshift mutation, G74fs, is likely a null allele suggesting that absence of $P_0$ is compatible with survival.

The crystal structure of the $P_0$ extracellular domain allows predictions of how mutations might affect processing, structure, and interactions, and enables attempts at correlation with disease severity. Different $P_0$ mutations at specific amino acid positions can lead to distinct phenotypes, and these provide an excellent model to examine how disease severity may correlate with mutation effect.[252,257] At positions 34 and 69, changes to cysteine are associated with a DSS phenotype while other substitutions produce CMT1. Outwardly pointing thiols hypothetically produce a dominant-negative effect through the formation of disulfide aggregates in the extracellular space, and disrupt myelin structure

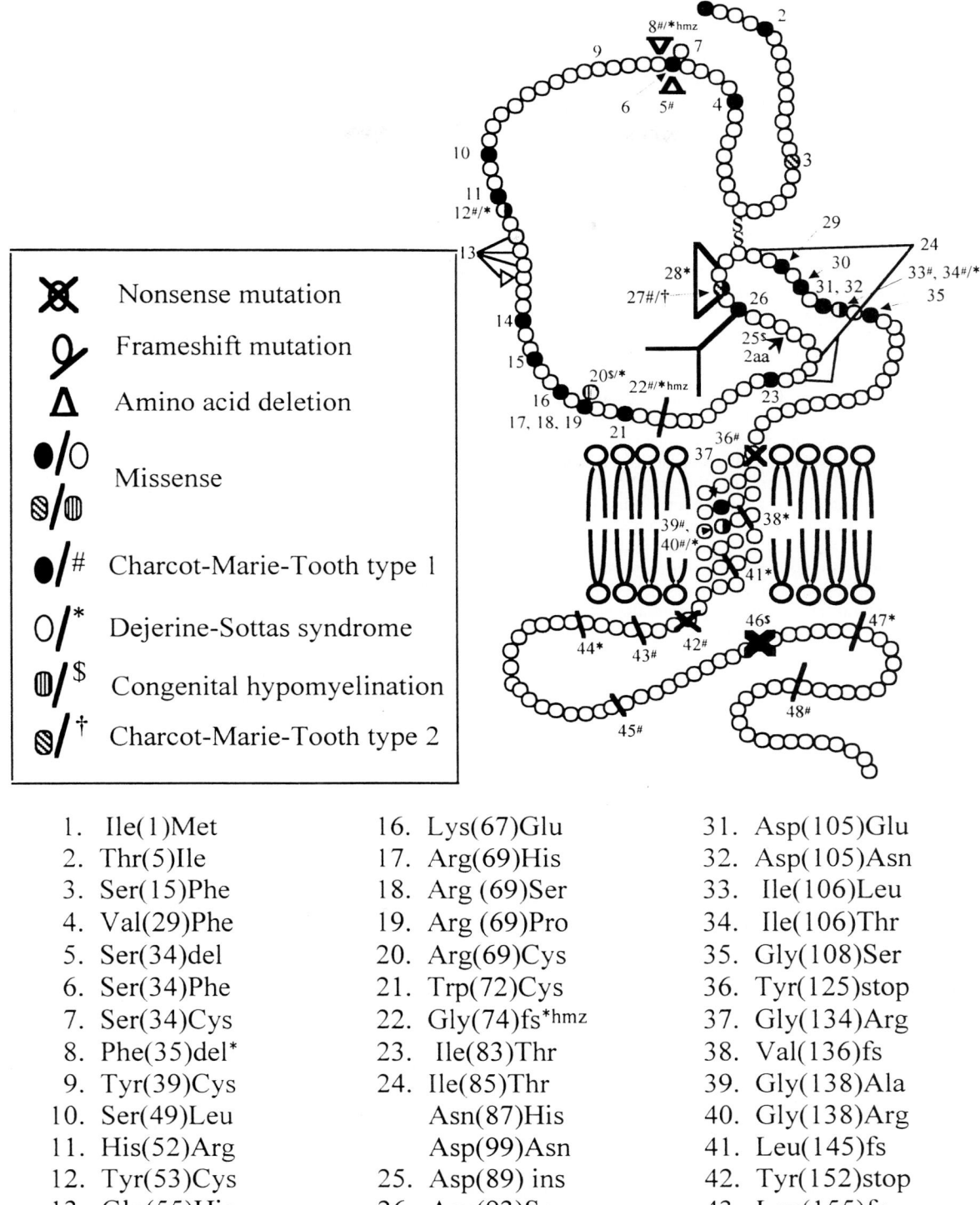

Nonsense mutation

Frameshift mutation

Amino acid deletion

●/○ Missense

⊗/⧅

●/# Charcot-Marie-Tooth type 1

○/* Dejerine-Sottas syndrome

⧅/$ Congenital hypomyelination

⊗/† Charcot-Marie-Tooth type 2

1. Ile(1)Met
2. Thr(5)Ile
3. Ser(15)Phe
4. Val(29)Phe
5. Ser(34)del
6. Ser(34)Phe
7. Ser(34)Cys
8. Phe(35)del*
9. Tyr(39)Cys
10. Ser(49)Leu
11. His(52)Arg
12. Tyr(53)Cys
13. Gln(55)His
    Pro(56)Leu
    Tyr(57)Phe
    Ile(58)del
14. Asp(61)Glu
15. Gly(64)Glu

16. Lys(67)Glu
17. Arg(69)His
18. Arg (69)Ser
19. Arg (69)Pro
20. Arg(69)Cys
21. Trp(72)Cys
22. Gly(74)fs*hmz
23. Ile(83)Thr
24. Ile(85)Thr
    Asn(87)His
    Asp(99)Asn
25. Asp(89) ins
26. Asn(93)Ser
27. Thr(95)Met
28. Thr(95)del
    Phe(96)del
29. Lys(101)Arg
30. Pro(103)Leu

31. Asp(105)Glu
32. Asp(105)Asn
33. Ile(106)Leu
34. Ile(106)Thr
35. Gly(108)Ser
36. Tyr(125)stop
37. Gly(134)Arg
38. Val(136)fs
39. Gly(138)Ala
40. Gly(138)Arg
41. Leu(145)fs
42. Tyr(152)stop
43. Leu(155)fs
44. Ala(159)fs
45. Lys(175)fs
46. Gln(186)stop
47. Ala(192)fs
48. Val(203)fs

**Fig. 227-7 Myelinopathy-associated *MPZ* mutations. The single predicted transmembrane domain, extracellular immunoglobulin-like domain and intracellular domain are shown for the protein P₀. Single amino acid positions are shown as open circles. Specific mutations are delineated below with the mutation type and manifested phenotype shown in the key in the upper left. Note that most mutations occur in the extracellular domain. However, the severity of the phenotype conveyed by the majority of mutations in the intracellular domain suggest an important function for this part of the P₀ molecule (amino acid numbering based on processed protein; * = phenotype seen when homozygous for mutation).**

by forming abnormal $P_0$ complexes.[257] Less severe CMT1-associated mutations at positions 34 and 69 may constitute loss-of-function alleles or weaker dominant-negative alleles.[257] Furthermore, the identification of nonsense mutations at positions 125 and 152 in patients with a CMT1 phenotype supports the postulate that alleles conveying a milder phenotype may represent loss-of-function alleles, because the truncated proteins may be unstable and never reach the membrane.[257] This model of disease severity associated with degree of dominant-negative effect has been supported by functional studies of *MPZ* mutations in cell surface localization and adhesion studies using *Drosophila* S2 and mammalian CHO (Chinese hamster ovary) cells.[286,287]

No crystal structure information is available for the $P_0$ intracellular domain but the severity of the phenotype associated with intracellular mutations suggests that this domain of $P_0$ plays an important functional role for myelin. Five of seven intracellular mutations cause a severe myelinopathy phenotype. In these cases, the mutant $P_0$ apparently exerts a dominant-negative effect. Supporting this contention is the observation that a $P_0$ protein truncated within the intracellular domain reaches the cell surface and inhibits extracellular domain adhesion in a cell adhesion assay.[288] The cytoplasmic domain of the myelin $P_0$ protein influences the adhesive interactions of its extracellular domain.[289]

In summary, *MPZ* mutations are a less common cause of myelinopathy than the CMT1A duplication and the HNPP deletion, but they appear to be more common than *PMP22* point mutations. Different *MPZ* point mutations may behave as loss-of-function, gain-of-function, or dominant-negative alleles. *De novo* point mutations have been identified in cases of sporadic neuropathy.

**Mouse Models for $P_0$ Deficiency.** A murine knockout of *MPZ* demonstrates that $P_0$ is essential for normal compaction and maintenance of the peripheral myelin sheath and the continued integrity of the associated axon.[290] $P_0$-deficient mice show myelin degeneration in peripheral nerves characteristic of inherited human neuropathies.[291] $P_0^{-/-}$ animals show hypomyelination by day 4 with subsequent demyelination and impaired nerve conduction. $P_0^{+/-}$ mice show normal myelination but develop progressive demyelination after 4 months of age. This demonstrates that only half the normal dose of $P_0$ is sufficient to begin myelination, but apparently is not enough to support myelin maintenance at a later age. The pathology of homozygous and heterozygous $P_0$ mutants resembles that of severely affected DSS and the CMT1B patients, respectively.[291] Motor NCV also resemble those observed in humans with *MPZ* mutations.[292] Interestingly, $P_0^{+/-}$ mice develop a peripheral neuropathy that resembles chronic inflammatory demyelinating polyneuropathy (CIDP). By 1 year of age, the mice develop severe, asymmetric slowing of motor nerves with temporal dispersion or conduction block, that are features of acquired demyelinating neuropathies including chronic inflammatory demyelinating polyneuropathy.[293]

### Cx32

***Cx32* Gene and Protein Structure.** The *Cx32* gene encoding connexin 32, also known as *GJB1* encoding gap junction protein $\beta_1$, has two exons. The entire coding sequence and 3' untranslated region are contained within the second exon[21] (GenBank NM-000166). In humans, *Cx32* maps to Xq13.1. There are two alternative *Cx32* promoters but only one is active in the peripheral nerve.[294,295]

Connexin 32 is a gap junction protein that belongs to a large family of at least 13 different mammalian genes. Six connexins form a hemichannel (connexon) in the cell membrane and two connexons between two apposed cells produce a functional channel that allows the rapid transport of ions and small molecules.[296] *Cx32* is expressed in myelinating Schwann cells and is localized to noncompact myelin in the paranode and Schmitt-Lanterman incisures.[295] *Cx32* gap junctions connect the layers of the Schwann cell cytoplasm and shorten the diffusion

pathway for nutrients and ions between the Schwann cell body and the periaxonal cytoplasm by more than one thousandfold.[297] Video microscopy of intracellularly injected dyes demonstrate that functional gap junctions are present within the myelin sheath.[298] *Cx32* expression is linked to myelin formation and is dependent on axonal signals.[299,300] Although *Cx32* is expressed in the liver, pancreas, stomach, kidney, and uterus,[297] no phenotypic abnormalities have been detected in these organs in Charcot-Marie-Tooth disease (CMTX) patients.

***Cx32* Mutations and X-Linked Neuropathy.** *Cx32* was identified as the gene responsible for X-linked dominant CMTX by a positional candidate approach.[297] Mutations of *Cx32* were identified in seven of the original eight X-linked CMT families examined.[297] To date, over 200 different *Cx32* mutations have been described.[301–323] The majority of *Cx32* mutations are missense mutations, but amino acid deletions, frameshift, and nonsense mutations also occur. The mutations occur throughout the entire Cx32 protein structure (Fig. 227-8), and unlike PMP22 and $P_0$, are not concentrated in transmembrane domains or extracellular domains. Two noncoding region mutations have also been reported in the nerve-specific *Cx32* promoter[310] and in the 5' untranslated region of exon 1b.[310,322] Each mutation results in a CMT phenotype that is usually more severe in males than in females. Nevertheless, the severity of the CMTX phenotype in males can vary markedly. The severity of the phenotype has not been correlated with the effect a *Cx32* mutation has on protein function.

**Functional Consequences of *Cx32* Mutations.** One kindred has been identified with a deletion of the *Cx32* gene.[324] How other *Cx32* mutations cause demyelination is unknown. This issue has been investigated in a variety of expression systems and four distinct effects of *Cx32* mutations have been identified: (a) altered intracellular trafficking of mutant Cx32 protein causing accumulation in a cellular compartment; (b) failure to synthesize stable protein; (c) inability to form functional channels; and (d) abnormalities of pore size or gating.

Altered trafficking and localization to the cytoplasm, as determined by indirect immunofluorescence using laser confocal microscopy, was shown for the mutants G12S, E186K, S208K, and R142W.[325] The cytoplasmic immunoreactivity colocalized with the Golgi apparatus and/or the ER. This could result in a potentially toxic cytoplasmic accumulation of Cx32 in cells. Toxic interactions with other proteins, such as chaperones or proteins of the trafficking machinery, might also occur in compartments in which mutant Cx32 accumulates. Mutant Cx32 could have dominant-negative effects on other connexins, but dominant-negative interactions between normal and mutant Cx32 are not likely to exist in myelinating Schwann cells, even in women, because Cx32 is subject to X-inactivation.[325] Cx32 accumulation and evidence of cytoplasmic accumulation of other mutated myelin proteins[237] suggested that diseases affecting myelinating cells may share a common pathophysiology.[325] The immunocytochemical localization technique defined two other classes of mutants. One which expressed mRNA but no protein, and the other in which at least some Cx32 is properly routed to the cell surface (R15Q, V63I, V139M, R220X).[325] It was proposed that the mutant Cx32 is incorporated into the plasma membrane but is not capable of forming functional gap junctions.[325]

The ability of CMTX mutant proteins to form homotypic channels (i.e., both connexons are composed of the same connexin) has been tested using the paired *Xenopus* oocyte expression system. Three mutations (R142W, E186K, and 175fs) behaved as loss-of-function alleles and did not produce functional channels.[326] In a subsequent study, 7 of the 11 mutations (R22G, R22P, L90H, V95M, P172S, E208L, and Y211X) did not induce the formation of homotypic channels and thus behaved as loss-of-function mutations.[327] Four mutations (L56F, E102G, 111del6, and R220X) assembled homotypic channels efficiently and

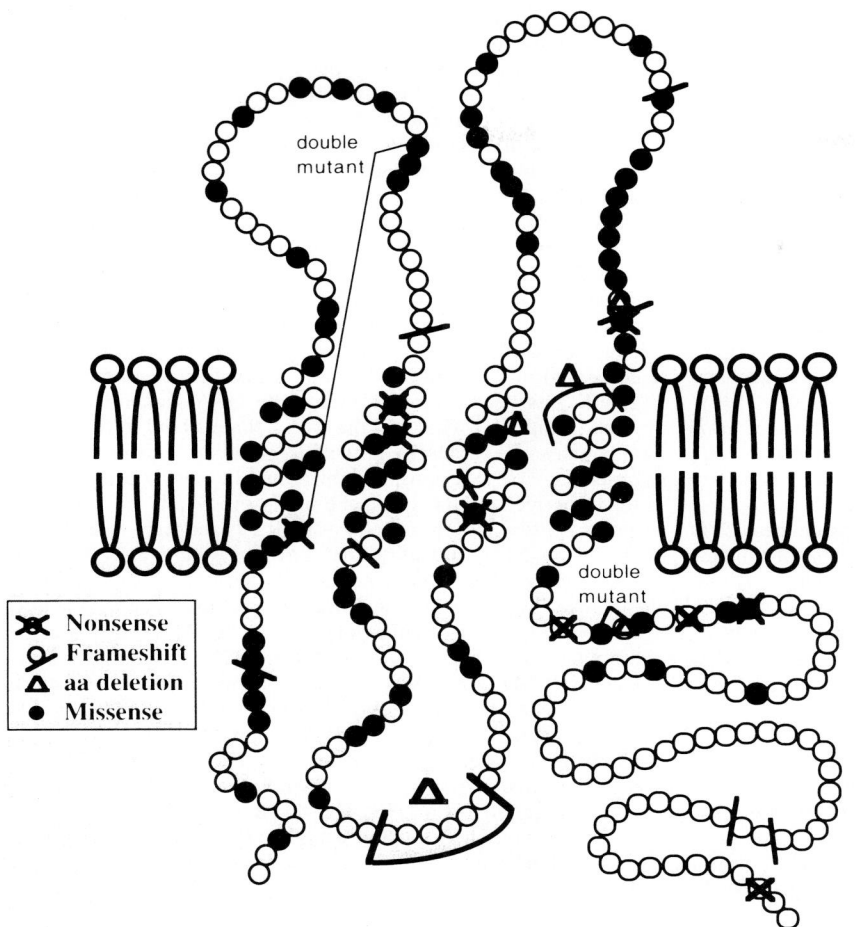

**Nonsense**
**Frameshift**
**aa deletion**
**Missense**

**Fig. 227-8 Myelinopathy-associated *Cx32* mutation. The four transmembrane domains of *Cx32* are shown with individual amino acids represented as open circles. Note that all types of mutations occur (missense > frameshift > nonsense > amino acid deletions), these mutations occur throughout the *Cx32* molecule, and each results in a CMT1 phenotype.**

induced conductance levels of the same order of magnitude as those developed by homotypic pairs expressing wild-type Cx32,[327] but exhibited altered gating properties when compared to wild-type controls.[327]

In a HeLa cell system, the function of *Cx32* mutations found in X-linked CMT were tested for their ability to form functional gap junctions among themselves and to inactivate wild-type Cx32 by a dominant-negative mechanism.[328] Four mutations (C60F, V139M, R215W, and R220X) restored gap junctional intercellular communication. When transfected with wild-type *Cx32*, each mutant Cx32 — except R220X — inhibited the gap junctional intercellular communication suggesting a dominant-negative effect.[328]

The analysis of the channel properties of mutations was analyzed in mouse Neuro-2A cell lines. Several mutations (V38M, P87A, E102G, 111del6, S26L, I30N, M34T, V35M) form functional channels when expressed either homotypically or heterotypically with Cx32 in pairs of *Xenopus* oocytes. The observation that five mutations (S26L, I30N, P87A, E102G, and 111del6) formed functional gap junctions whose voltage dependence did not differ substantially from wild-type *Cx32* suggested that alterations in junctional permeability might be responsible for the loss of Cx32 function underlying CMTX. Single-channel studies of two mutations in Neuro-2A cells demonstrated reduced junctional permeability caused by a decrease in either pore size (S26L) or open channel probability (M34T).[329] It was proposed that the permeation of second messengers such as cAMP through reflexive gap junctions between adjacent cytoplasmic loops of myelinating Schwann cells was likely to be reduced in these channels. Thus, these mutations could impair the transduction of signals arising from normal glial-neuronal interactions and thereby cause demyelination and axonal degeneration.[329]

Functional abnormalities of CMTX caused by *Cx32* mutations (C53S and P172R) were examined in transfected C6 glioma cells. Immunocytochemical and dye-transfer studies showed a lack of cell-to-cell communication because of failure to incorporate mutant Cx32 protein in the cell membrane[330] but the mutations did not interfere with cell proliferation or the expression of a myelin-specific gene (*PLP*).

The effect of the *Cx32* missense mutation E102G was tested in vivo in a nerve myelination system by a nerve xenograft from humans to nude mice. Host mouse axons regenerate through the donor human graft and are remyelinated by human Schwann cells. Ultrastructural analysis showed that Schwann cells with the E102G mutation have a profound effect on nude mice axons, while the myelination did not appear to be affected.[331] Those effects consisted of an increase in neurofilament density, a depletion of microtubules associated with fragmentation of smooth axonal reticulum, and increased vesicles and mitochondria. Thus, the Cx32 E1026 mutation appears to impair a modulatory function of Schwann cells on axons resulting in profound cytoskeletal alterations leading to distal axonal degeneration. These observations suggest a role of impaired Schwann cell-axon interactions in the pathogenesis of hereditary neuropathies.[331]

**Mouse Models for *Cx32* Deficiency.** *Cx32*-deficient mice develop a late onset and progressive neuropathy with features of demyelination and remyelination, such as onion bulbs and abnormally thin myelin.[332,333] Noncompacted aspects of myelin, such as enlarged periaxonal collars of Schwann cell cytoplasmic swelling, may represent pathological alteration caused by a compromised homeostasis of ions as a result of reduced "spatial buffering" of ions after neuronal activity.[4,332] Interestingly, demyelination was much less pronounced in sensory nerves and dorsal roots, as has been described for $P_0^{+/-}$ and $Pmp22^{+/-}$ mice.[332,333] However, the underlying cellular and molecular differences between sensory and motor fibers have not yet been determined. Similar to the findings in CMTX patients, electrophysiologic studies of Cx32-deficient mice demonstrated mild axonal loss, reflected by decreased amplitudes.[332]

A transgenic mouse was recently constructed with a frameshift mutation (175fs) that had been identified in a large CMTX family.[44] Adult transgenic animals showed no pathologic features of the peripheral nerves indicating that the 175fs mutation results in a loss-of-function without additional toxic effects.[334] In contrast, when transgenic mice expressing mutant (R142W) or wild-type human *Cx32* were compared, the nerves from transgenic lines expressing R142W had decreased levels of Cx32 on western blots, aberrant localization of Cx32 protein by immunohistochemistry, and progressive demyelination with age.[335] Thus, the R142W mutant protein had dominant effects that were distinct from overexpression. These transgenic experiments confirm in vitro studies that demonstrate that different Cx32 mutations may behave as loss-of-function or as dominant-negative alleles.

In summary, functional studies of disease-associated *Cx32* mutations suggest that most alleles behave as loss-of-function mutation because (a) the mRNA or protein is unstable, or (b) the protein is made but does not form a functional channel, or (c) a functional channel is formed but it has altered gating properties. However, some mutant alleles can have a dominant-negative effect potentially by sequestering or interacting with other connexins.

### EGR2

**EGR2 Gene and Protein Structure.** *EGR2* is a member of a multigene family encoding $Cys_2His_2$ type zinc-finger proteins that play a role in the regulation of cellular differentiation and proliferation.[336,337] The mouse orthologue, *Egr2* (also known as *Krox20*), was initially identified as an immediate-early response gene encoding a protein that binds DNA in a sequence-specific manner and acts as a transcription factor.[338–341] Stable expression of *Egr2* is specifically associated with myelination in the peripheral nervous system.[342] To date, three transcription factors have been implicated in the establishment of myelinating Schwann cells: PAX3, a paired domain-containing protein; SCIP (suppressed cAMP-inducible POU), a POU homeodomain protein; and KROX20/EGR2.[343] PAX3 is involved in differentiating embryonic Schwann cells, whereas SCIP is produced at high levels only during a short phase of glial development in the central and peripheral nervous system. After the onset of myelination, *Pax3* is expressed in nonmyelinating Schwann cells and *Krox20* expression is restricted to myelinating Schwann cells.

$Egr2^{-/-}$ ($Krox20^{-/-}$) mice display disrupted hindbrain segmentation and development[344,345] and a block of Schwann cell differentiation at an early stage.[346] Schwann cells ensheath individual axons but fail to form the spiral of membrane that becomes the myelin sheath.[346] Based on these observations, Egr2 potentially activates genes required for peripheral nerve myelination, but none of these downstream genes have been identified. SCIP-null mice have a strikingly similar phenotype to that of Krox-20 null mice, with arrested Schwann cell differentiation.[347]

**EGR2 Mutations and Myelinopathies.** The human *EGR2* gene contains two coding exons (GenBank AF139463) and maps to chromosome 10q21q22. One apparent recessive and four different dominant missense mutations have been identified in *EGR2* associated with myelinopathy phenotypes, including CHN, DSS, and CMT1[348–350] (Fig. 227-9). In contrast to the homozygous knockout mouse, no hindbrain segmentation defects were noted. The differences in clinical severity and inheritance pattern can conceivably be explained by the location of the mutations and their differing effect on protein structure and function. The I268N mutation, which behaves as a recessive allele and causes CHN, occurs within an inhibitory domain that binds two repressors, NAB1[351] and NAB2.[352] Both repressors inhibit the transcriptional

activity of multiple members of this immediate-early response gene family, including *Egr1* (also known as Krox24/NGFIA/Zif268) and *Egr2*. Mutation of this conserved Ile residue to Phe in Egr1 abolishes the inhibitory effect of NAB1 and NAB2 and increases by fifteenfold the transcriptional activity of a reporter gene.[353] Similarly, the I268N mutation disrupts repressor interactions.[354] Thus, the loss of repression could result in increased expression of a dosage-sensitive PNS gene, which, in turn, might cause CHN in the same way that increased dosage of *PMP22* expression by the CMT1A duplication results in CMT1.[10]

Mutations within the region encoding the zinc-finger domain effect the DNA-binding properties of EGR2.[348,354] These mutations cause a phenotype in the heterozygous state, thus act as dominant alleles. The $Cys_2His_2$ class of zinc-fingers usually has a conserved motif of 28 to 30 amino acids. Egr2 has two types of zinc-fingers that bind to different 3-bp DNA sequences. Type 1 fingers bind 5'-GCG-3' and the type 2 fingers bind to 5'-GGG-3', although some variability in the DNA binding sequence has been observed.[355] The residues that make up the α-helix are important for DNA recognition within the major groove.[356–359] Conserved amino acids within the α-helix of EGR2[340] and Egr1[360] have been shown by NMR modeling and x-ray crystallography to either hydrogen-bond with the donor sites on guanine or support DNA-binding interactions. The myelinopathy-associated mutations occur in these key amino acids[348–350] (Fig. 227-9). Mutation of arginine in zinc finger 3 (R409W) of EGR2[348] (Fig. 227-9), which causes a CMT1 phenotype, has been shown, in Egr1, to result in loss of DNA-binding ability.[361] Intriguingly, alteration of the corresponding arginine in zinc-finger 2 of *EGR2* also results in a CMT1 phenotype.[350] The mutation in finger 1 (R359W) was found as a *de novo* mutation independently in a Belgian[349] and an Italian[350] family with DSS. The myelinopathy-associated *EGR2* mutations alter DNA binding with the amount of residual binding directly correlating with disease severity.[354] These observations are consistent with the hypothesis that dominant mutations cause a more severe myelinopathy (CHN and DSS) owing to dominant-negative effects, while a loss-of-function mutation, as evidenced by absence of DNA binding, results in a milder CMT1 phenotype.[354]

## OTHER CMT GENES

Recently, three additional genes have been identified wherein mutations can result in CMT. *NDRG1* encodes *N-myc downstream regulated gene 1*, is ubiquitously expressed, and has been proposed to play a role in growth arrest and cell differentiation, possibly as a signaling protein shuttling between the cytoplasm and the nucleus.[364a] *MTMR2* encodes myotubularin related protein-2, a dual specificity phosphatase (DSP).[364b] Both of these genes are associated with recessive forms of CMT1. The first CMT2 gene to be identified, encodes the neurofilament light protein (NF-L; gene symbol) *NEFL* (Table 227-3).[91a,364c]

## MOUSE MODELS FOR MYELINOPATHIES

As mentioned throughout this chapter, mouse models of both spontaneously occurring mutations and engineered animals have been instrumental in delineating pathophysiologic mechanisms and the role of these genes in myelin development and maintenance (Table 227-6). Many mouse myelin gene mutations are genetically authentic models for specific human myelinopathies.[362] Animals heterozygous or homozygous for point mutations or null alleles, as well as transgenics overexpressing Pmp22, have highlighted the important effects of gene dosage.

## CLINICAL APPLICATIONS OF MOLECULAR FINDINGS

Molecular studies have uncovered the genetic basis of myelinopathies in a significant percentage of patients. The majority of CMT1 patients have the CMT1A duplication. In CMT1 patients

**A.**

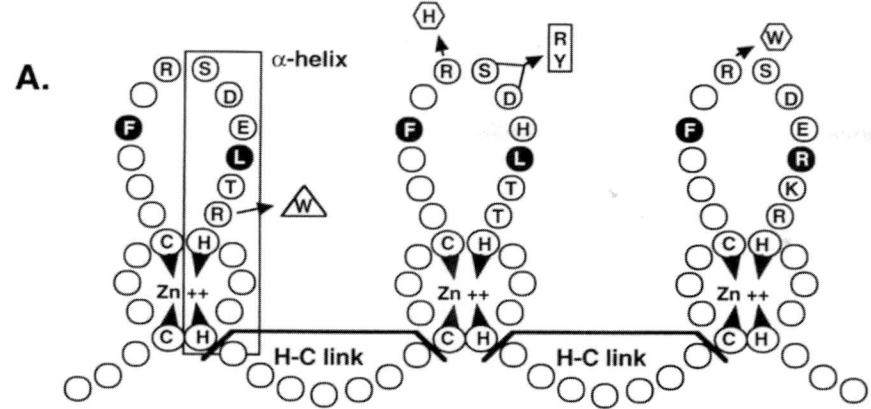

**B.**

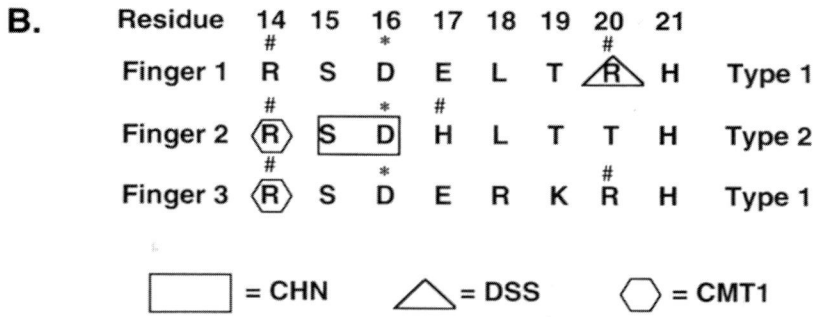

☐ = CHN    △ = DSS    ⬡ = CMT1

**C.**

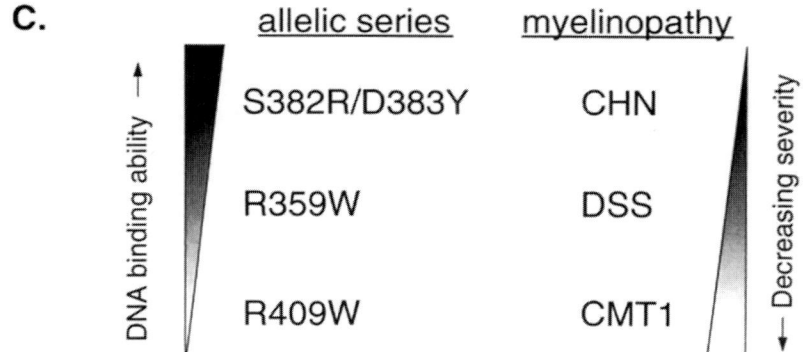

Fig. 227-9 Myelinopathy associated *EGR2* (*Krox20*) mutations. *A*, Structure of *EGR2* (*Krox20*) Zn-finger domain showing the crucial amino acids (circles) comprising the protein fingers required for DNA contact. The cysteine and histidine amino acids chelating Zn to form the three fingers are shown. *B*, Shown are the amino acids that comprise the α-helix of each finger (indicated by rectangle in *A*). The positions of four different myelinopathy associated missense amino acid substitutions and their conveyed phenotypes are shown. *C*, Results of functional studies correlate residual binding with increasing myelinopathy severity suggesting dominant-negative effects.

without the CMT1A duplication, point mutations can be found in *Cx32*, *MPZ*, *PMP22*, or *EGR2* (Table 227-7). Dejerine-Sottas syndrome has been associated with point mutations in *PMP22*, *MPZ*, and *EGR2*. In addition, most patients with homozygous duplication, and rarely patients with heterozygous duplication,[273] present with DSS. Congenital hypomyelinating neuropathy is a clinically and genetically heterogeneous condition, but some cases are caused by point mutations in *MPZ* or *EGR2*. In general, DNA rearrangements, the HNPP deletion, and the CMT1A duplication, convey milder myelinopathy phenotypes than point mutations in the genes for myelin structural proteins *MPZ*, *PMP22*, *Cx32*, or the transcription factor gene *EGR2*. Point mutations that behave as loss-of-function alleles result in milder myelinopathy phenotypes than those with dominant-negative effects.

### Clinical Variability of Expression

Variable clinical expression is a prominent feature of CMT and related disorders.[45] To date, five different clinical phenotypes have been associated with the CMT1A duplication (Table 227-7). The

majority of individuals with the CMT1A duplication present with a classical CMT1 phenotype. However, Dejerine-Sottas syndrome has been associated with heterozygous duplication,[273] as well as with homozygous duplication.[103,104,119–121] CMT1A duplication has also been reported in patients with the diagnoses of Roussy-Levy syndrome,[363,364] calf hypertrophy,[365,366] and scapuloperoneal atrophy or Davidenkow syndrome.[367,368] Pressure palsies have also been reported as the initial presentation in a case of late onset CMT1A associated with the CMT1A duplication.[369]

There can be a wide variation in clinical severity for CMT even within a specific molecular subtype. A study of 63 unrelated CMT1A duplication patients revealed interfamilial variability. The average median and ulnar motor NCVs were $20.8 \pm 6.0$ m/s and $19.9 \pm 7.2$ m/s, respectively. These values were not significantly different from those for CMT1 patients without the CMT1A duplication, for whom the average value for median motor NCV was $20.9 \pm 7.4$ m/s and the average ulnar motor NCV was $20.2 \pm 7.9$ m/s.[105] However, the range of motor NCV for both median and ulnar nerves was from 10 to 40 m/s.[105]

**Table 227-6** Mouse Models for Human Myelinopathies

**Spontaneously occurring**

| Mouse allele | Gene/mutation | Human phenotype model |
|---|---|---|
| Tr | Pmp22/(Leu16Pro) | CMT1 |
| Tr[1] | Pmp22/(Gly150Asp) | DSS |
| Tr[Nemp] | Pmp22 amino acid deletion | DSS |

**Knockout mice**

| Human gene | Mouse genotype | Human phenotype model |
|---|---|---|
| MPZ | $P_0^{+/-}$ | CMT1 |
| | $P_0^{-/-}$ | DSS/CHN |
| PMP22 | Pmp22[+/−] | HNPP* |
| | Pmp22[−/−] | DSS/CHN |
| Cx32 | Cx32[−] | CMT1X |
| EGR2 | Egr2[+/−] | |
| | Egr2[−/−] | CHN |

**Transgenic rodents**

| Pmp22 | over expressing mice | CMT1 |
|---|---|---|
| Pmp22 | over expressing rat | CMT1 |

*Pmp22 antisense mouse model produces an HNPP phenotype.

Electrophysiological studies on five large families in which molecular studies were performed demonstrated a similar wide range of motor NCV within single families.[104] Among the CMT1A duplication patients, median conduction velocities varied widely, ranging from 10.4 to 42.0 m/s. Large differences in conduction velocity were seen within families; the widest range of velocities was 26.6 m/s in one family, while the mean range for the five families was 20.3 m/s.[104] No correlation was observed between median forearm conduction velocity and age among CMT1A patients overall or within any family[104] as was found prior to molecular characterization of CMT subtypes.[370]

Clinical variability was even reported in two pairs of identical twins from two unrelated families with the CMT1A duplication.[371] In both sets, the less-affected twin had a greater degree of palpable nerve enlargement, suggesting either a protective effect of interstitial nerve hypertrophy on axon function or, alternatively, that hypertrophy may reflect a better ability to restore lost function through mechanisms such as remyelination. However, there was remarkable congruity of conduction velocities between the left and the right side of each twin and between twin brothers. The similarity and symmetry of the electrophysiological deficit contrast with the variable and asymmetric clinical presentation. Variability of clinical expression in these patients with identical duplications suggests the action of stochastic factors or, more likely, environmental modulation of disease severity.[371]

Clinical and electrophysiological investigation and nerve biopsies on 61 CMT1A duplication patients revealed 50 with a typical CMT1 phenotype, but 8 were classified as having Roussy-Levy syndrome. Three patients had associated pyramidal signs and one of these three patients had a complicated neuropathy with signs of cerebellar and bulbar involvement.[363] Median motor nerve conduction velocities were 19.9 ± 1.3 m/sec, with a range of 5 to 34 m/sec. Thus, the CMT1A duplication gives rise to a range of phenotypes and not solely to a CMT syndrome.[363]

A clinical and electrophysiological study of 119 CMT1A duplication patients demonstrated that the onset of the first functional manifestation was in the first decade in 50 percent of cases and before the age of 20 years in 70 percent of cases.[372] The predominant clinical signs were muscle weakness and wasting in

the lower limbs. Functional disability was mild, 96 percent of patients were autonomous while 25 percent were asymptomatic and diagnosed by systematic family investigation.[372] Early age at onset and greatly reduced median motor NCV were predictive of a more severe course; that is, the earlier the onset, the more reduced the median nerve NCV and the higher the functional disability after adjustment for disease duration. Cross-sectional analysis of neurologic deficit, functional deficit, and NCVs according to disease duration showed that regardless of age at onset, the disease associated with CMT1A duplication is a clinically progressive disorder.[372]

The HNPP deletion is usually associated with hereditary neuropathy with liability to pressure palsies[125–131] (Table 227-7). However, there also may be substantial clinical variability.[125–131,373] Many individuals with the deletion may remain asymptomatic even in adulthood, which can present a diagnostic problem for the clinician and family.

There can be variability in the susceptibility to minimal trauma in HNPP. Patients may have painless brachial plexus neuropathy or conduction blocks lasting more than 9 years as the unique clinical manifestation of the disease.[373] The only clinical complaint in some individuals with the HNPP deletion has been carpal tunnel syndrome.[374] In one study of multifocal neuropathy, usually not considered a genetic disorder, 50 percent of patients had the HNPP deletion and half of these individuals had no family history of neuropathy.[375] The HNPP deletion has also been identified in some patients with CMT1 referred for molecular testing.[376]

Different point mutations in the same gene have been associated with distinct demyelinating neuropathies, further emphasizing the clinical variability and phenotypic overlap in these disorders (Table 227-7). Some Cx32 mutations,[91] particularly in females, and some MPZ mutations[257,282,377–379] have been identified in patients with a clinical and electrophysiological diagnosis of CMT2. In the case of one mutation of MPZ (T124M),

**Table 227-7** Mutations Involving Myelin Genes and Associated Neuropathies

| Mutation | Clinical phenotypes |
|---|---|
| CMT1A duplication | Charcot-Marie-Tooth disease type 1 (CMT1) |
| | Roussy-Levy syndrome (RLS) |
| | Dejerine-Sottas syndrome (DSS) |
| | HMSNI with calf hypertrophy |
| | Scapuloperoneal atrophy (Davidenkow syndrome) |
| HNPP deletion | Hereditary neuropathy with liability to pressure palsies (HNPP) |
| | Multifocal neuropathy |
| | CMT1 |
| | Carpal tunnel syndrome |
| PMP22 point mutation | CMT1 |
| | DSS |
| | HNPP |
| | CHN |
| MPZ point mutation | CMT1 |
| | DSS |
| | CHN |
| | CMT2 |
| | RLS |
| Cx32 point mutation | CMT1 |
| | CMT2 (females) |
| EGR2 point mutation | CHN |
| | DSS |
| | CMT1 |

the phenotype is characterized by late onset, marked sensory abnormalities and sometimes deafness and pupillary abnormalities that are irregular and unresponsive to light (Argyll-Robertson pupils).[379] A unique point mutation (A67P) in the *PMP22* gene is associated with Charcot-Marie-Tooth disease and deafness.[380] Sensorineural deafness is also a feature associated with a connexin 32 mutation (R142Q).[381] Central nervous system findings, as indicated by pathologic changes in visually evoked potentials (VEPs), brain stem auditory evoked potentials (BAEPs), and central motor evoked potentials (CMEPs) were also recently reported in association with a N205S connexin 32 mutation.[382]

## Penetrance

Early clinical studies documented an age-dependent penetrance to the autosomal dominant CMT1 phenotype.[383] In 15 unrelated families, the average age of onset was 12.2 years. The penetrance was 28 percent in the first decade, but essentially complete by the third decade. Although the clinical manifestation of CMT1 can have marked variability of expression and marked differences in the age-of-onset of symptoms,[46] the electrophysiological abnormalities are completely penetrant at an early age.[384] NCV studies on CMT1A duplication families demonstrate complete penetrance of the electrophysiological phenotype by as early as 2 years and confirm the reliability of NCV in establishing the affection status in CMT1A.[104] Normal NCV in a single nerve can reliably exclude CMT1, but evaluation of several nerves and nerve segments to establish uniformity of conduction slowing is important in making the diagnosis.[385]

## Longitudinal Studies

Very few long-term follow-up studies are available since the description of the molecular basis of inherited peripheral neuropathies. A longitudinal study spanning 22 years in a family with the CMT1A duplication revealed that motor conduction velocities and clinical motor exam did not change significantly over 22 years.[386] The average change in median motor NCVs was −2.2 m/s (20.5 m/s in 1967 to 18.3 m/s in 1990). The average change in peroneal motor NCVs was −3.0 m/s (18.3 m/s in 1967 to 15.3 m/s in 1990). The average change in median nerve distal latencies over the same time period was also minimal (7.7 ms to 8.2 ms). Only one in eight patients showed mild objective increase in limb weakness, while subjective symptoms of gradual worsening of leg strength were noted in half the patients over the same period. The finding that conduction studies remain fairly constant in a 22-year longitudinal follow-up of patients with CMT1A further support a primary, inherited, disturbance of myelination that expresses itself in childhood and is nonprogressive after childhood by NCV measurements. However, the mild subtle progression of subjective leg weakness supports the hypothesis of a very slowly progressive distal axonal degeneration that is either secondary to chronic loss of myelin or an underlying independent axonopathy.[386] Recent experiments transplanting nerve grafts from CMT1A duplication and HNPP deletion patients to nude mice reveal axonal abnormalities in the regenerating mouse axons.[387] These alterations demonstrate that axon-Schwann cell interactions are perturbed within the CMT1A and HNPP grafts, presumably as a result of local manifestations of the genetically abnormal Schwann cell.[388]

A 20-year observation of the first family with CMT1B due to a *MPZ* mutation demonstrated the long-term phenotypic consequences on the peripheral nervous system of a specific point mutation in the $P_0$ myelin protein.[389] Affected individuals generally showed an early age-of-onset, often indicated by delayed ability to walk. Proximal muscle weakness of the lower extremities was common and often marked, but the individuals remained ambulatory and there was no decrease in life span. Motor nerve conduction velocities of the fastest fibers were severely slowed (mean, 9 to 11 m/s). Nerve histology, at autopsy from a family member who died at age 92 years from pneumonia following a hemorrhagic cerebral infarction, demonstrated a diffuse disorder

of myelinated fibers secondarily involving the posterior columns and anterior horn cells of the spinal cord but without other involvement of the central nervous system. Some nerves revealed severe endoneural fibrosis, but even those fibrotic nerves showed relatively good preservation of axons, suggesting that axonal degeneration even after long-standing demyelination was not a prominent feature. Variability of disability between family members suggested that genetic and environmental factors in addition to $P_0$ mutation played a role in the lifetime phenotype.

Longitudinal clinical and electrophysiological evaluation of CMT1A in infancy and early childhood showed that all affected children had abnormal NCV from 2 years of age.[390] In most CMT1A patients, the symptoms appear in early childhood, but the florid clinical picture did not occur until the second decade of life.[390]

## MOLECULAR DIAGNOSTICS FOR CMT AND RELATED NEUROPATHIES

The elucidation of the molecular mechanisms for these disorders has important clinical implications for the diagnosis, prognosis, genetic counseling, and rational approaches to future therapies for patients with peripheral neuropathies.[391] The CMT1A duplication and HNPP deletion are examples in humans of consistent large DNA rearrangements that can act as biologic markers for their respective diseases. These disorders are excellent models for investigating methods of detecting large DNA rearrangements responsible for human diseases. Several different methods have been applied to identify the CMT1A duplication and HNPP deletion. As is the case for any laboratory diagnostic technique, each method has inherent advantages and limitations—issues that may be particularly complex for large DNA rearrangements.[391] Nevertheless, DNA diagnosis is playing an increasingly prominent role in the evaluations of patients with peripheral neuropathy. In fact, many investigators advocate reclassification of these neuropathic disorders based on the molecular defect involved.[3,392]

Initial methods described to detect the CMT1A duplication included: (a) dosage differences of RFLP alleles in heterozygous individuals;[92,93] (b) the presence of three alleles at a highly polymorphic locus detected by PCR or Southern blot analysis;[92,93] (c) rearrangement-specific junction fragments detected by Southern blot analysis of PFGE-separated genomic DNA;[92] and (d) two-color FISH.[92] Subsequently, other methods to identify the presence of the CMT1A duplication have been based on quantitative measurement of duplicated DNA by Southern blot analysis,[393] PCR detection of three alleles by using multiple polymorphic simple sequence repeats,[394] and, more recently, the detection by conventional Southern blot analysis[138] or specific PCR amplification[395] of a junction fragment associated with a recombination hotspot. Quantitative measurements of band intensities for dosage analysis is the least robust method for determining the presence of duplication and should be replaced by alternative methods. Methods that utilize polymorphic markers rely on the informativeness of the marker, which for three alleles, depends on the heterozygosity, the number of alleles at a specific locus, and the distribution of these alleles in the population.[105] This strategy is unattractive because it may not detect the rearrangement in all cases. Likewise, methods directed at detecting crossovers within the recombination hotspot region would not detect the estimated 20 to 25 percent of duplications with strand exchanges outside the hotspot region.

For optimal detection of the CMT1A duplication and the HNPP deletion, a binary test based on the detection of the presence or absence of a band or signal is preferable to an assay based on a quantitative measurement of dosage, or to an assay that detects only a subset of rearrangements. The most informative and reliable diagnostic methods for identifying the CMT1A duplication and HNPP deletion depend on directly or indirectly determining the number of copies of the *PMP22* gene. Detection of a rearrangement-specific junction fragment utilizing PFGE is a

**Table 227-8 Selected Neuropathy Phenotypes and Molecular Diagnostic Testing to Consider**

| | | CHN | DSS | CMTX | RLS | CMT1 | CMT2 | HNPP | Multifocal neuropathy |
|---|---|---|---|---|---|---|---|---|---|
| **Rearrangements** | CMT1A duplication | | X | | X | X | | | |
| | HNPP deletion | | | | | X | | X | X |
| **Point mutations** | Cx32 | | | X | | X | X | | |
| | MPZ | X | X | | X | X | X | | |
| | PMP22 | X | X | | | X | | X | |
| | EGR2 | X | X | | | X | | | |

well-documented method[376] as is molecular cytogenetic testing with a *PMP22* probe by FISH.[396] The latter is particularly amenable to prenatal diagnostic testing.[396,397] Importantly, the PFGE and FISH test will detect both the CMT1A duplication and the HNPP deletion.

DNA sequencing is currently the method of choice for the detection of point mutations in *Cx32*, *MPZ*, *PMP22*, and *EGR2*. Denaturing high performance liquid chromatography (DHPLC) may be an alternative scanning method to detect point mutations. Future diagnostic testing might include a DNA chip able to detect point mutations in these genes, as well as others yet to be identified. Such technology will not detect the DNA rearrangements that are the most frequent molecular basis of CMT and related neuropathies.

## EVALUATION OF PATIENTS WITH CMT OR RELATED PERIPHERAL NEUROPATHY

Molecular diagnostic testing should be considered in CMT and related peripheral neuropathies[391] (Table 227-8). These disorders can present with an extremely variable clinical picture. The detection of the CMT1A duplication, HNPP deletion, or point mutations (*Cx32*, *MPZ*, *PMP22*, or *EGR2*) in a sample of peripheral blood, amniocytes, or chorionic villi, establishes the exact molecular form of the disease in a family.[391] Moreover, such a detection makes it possible to diagnose or exclude the diagnosis in other family members, enables prenatal diagnosis, and may provide prognostic information. Both prenatal[397,398] and preimplantation diagnoses[399] of CMT1A duplications have been reported. The diagnosis of CMT1A and HNPP should be considered even in the absence of a family history, given the high mutation rate and *de novo* mutations in sporadic cases. The CMT1A duplication should be ruled out in any patient who has an unexplained neuropathy or family history of neuropathy prior to the initiation of the cancer chemotherapy with vincristine because of the devastating consequences of vincristine in CMT patients.[57]

Patients who do not have the CMT1A duplication should be screened initially for *Cx32* mutations, the next most frequent cause of CMT1 that accounts for 5 to 10 percent of patients.[102] This information is also clinically relevant for genetic counseling and for estimates of recurrence risk because it establishes X-linked inheritance in the family. Of course, in the presence of definitive male-to-male transmission, there is no need to evaluate for *Cx32* mutations.

In a CMT patient without the CMT1A duplication or *Cx32* mutation, molecular analysis for *MPZ*, *PMP22*, or *EGR2* mutations may be undertaken. Alterations in these three genes can account for a significant proportion of such patients. Persons with point mutations in these genes usually manifest more clinically severe disease. Although there are no specific molecular tests available for CMT2, *Cx32* mutations (particularly in females), and *MPZ* mutations should be considered in some patients.

The HNPP deletion should be excluded in all patients with a recurrent demyelinating mononeuropathy or polyneuropathy of undetermined etiology. Early diagnosis of HNPP promotes preventive measures to avoid nerve pressure or trauma to areas such as elbows, wrist, and fibular neck. The HNPP deletion should also be considered in patients diagnosed with chronic inflammatory demyelinating polyneuropathy, primarily thought to be an acquired neuropathy, because of similar electrodiagnostic features including conduction blocks.

Patients with a severe early onset neuropathy, such as DSS or CHN, should be evaluated for point mutations in *MPZ*, *PMP22*, or *EGR2*. Sporadic cases can be associated with *de novo* point mutations in these genes (Fig. 227-10).

## THERAPY

The plan for a therapeutic regimen begins with establishing an accurate diagnosis.[400] Genetic counseling of adult patients or the parents of an affected child should be based on the inheritance pattern. Patients considering a family should be informed of the chances of having an affected child. However, the positive

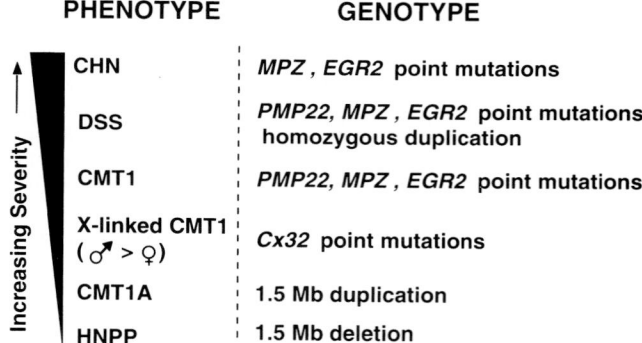

Fig. 227-10 Phenotype/genotype correlations for myelinopathies. Myelinopathy phenotypes are shown on the left, decreasing in severity from top to bottom of the figure. On the right, are the specific genotypes usually associated with the given phenotype in the same horizontal line. Note males (♂) with X-linked CMT have a more severe phenotype than females. The figure represents general trends, but inherited peripheral neuropathies can have significant clinical variability.

aspects of normal life expectancy, the lack of central nervous system involvement, and that a patient can have a family, maintain gainful employment, and lead a fulfilling life should be emphasized.

Symptomatic treatment may have a substantial impact on quality of life.[400] Medications that may be of use include nonsteroidal anti-inflammatory medication and analgesics to relieve lower back and leg pain. $\beta$-Blockers can decrease the tremor associated with CMT. Coffee and nicotine can aggravate the tremor. Medications that can worsen the neuropathy, potentially any drug with neurotoxic side effects, and excess alcohol should be avoided. Maintenance of a normal weight is recommended to reduce strain on weight-bearing muscles and joints. Physical and occupational therapy should be directed toward maintaining function and comfort, ensuring safety, and protecting joints.[401] High-top shoes or boots can stabilize weak ankles and improve gait. Ankle-foot orthosis (AFOs) can minimize the steppage gait. Surgical intervention may be needed for foot and hand abnormalities, and sometimes for hip dysplasia. Additional information for families and professionals can be obtained from the two patient support groups: CMT Association (www.charcot-marie-tooth.org/) and CMT International (www.cmtint.org).

Future therapies may include antisense and antigene technologies, including ribozymes, in patients overexpressing *PMP22* due to the CMT1A duplication. Some forms of gene-replacement therapies might be utilized in patients in whom disease is secondary to loss-of-function mutations. Other molecular therapeutic modalities may be directed at preventing toxic buildup of aberrant and wild-type proteins in the subcellular compartments. In addition, some forms of therapy could be directed at modulating disease severity by identifying and altering environmental influences on disease expression in order to mitigate the effects of mutation.

## CONCLUSIONS

Substantial progress has been made in determining the molecular genetic bases of CMT and related inherited peripheral neuropathies. The identification of large molecular rearrangements as mechanisms for human disease led to the definition of genomic architecture that predisposes such rearrangements and the role of recombination in human mutation. Unique genomic structural features have since been described in other microdeletion and microduplication syndromes.[1,402] Furthermore, the study of CMT1A and HNPP and other microdeletions and microduplications demonstrated the important role of gene dosage in causing a disease phenotype. Investigations of patients with dup(17)p12 and CMT1, as part of their complex phenotype, have demonstrated the overlap between the seemingly disparate genetic disease categories of Mendelian disorders and chromosomal syndromes.

Genetic dissection of the CMT and related neuropathy phenotypes has illustrated that both allelic variations and locus heterogeneity can be responsible for a spectrum of clinical phenotypes, which may include entities thought to be acquired. These studies confirm the long-held suspicion that inherited peripheral neuropathies are the clinical manifestations of peripheral nerve dysfunction resulting from abnormalities in Schwann cells and their myelin sheath. They also highlight the intimate interactions between axon and glia.

These new findings have provided the clinician with powerful molecular tools to diagnose and better define the inheritance and prognosis of the various peripheral neuropathy phenotypes. As such, the introduction of these molecular techniques into the daily practice of medicine irreversibly changed these clinical specialties. It has enabled, for the first time, the classification of the peripheral neuropathies based on the molecular etiology, rather than on subjective clinical features. Finally, understanding the molecular mechanisms leading to these disorders and elucidating the function of these various genes should allow the development of

novel therapeutic strategies that would result in effective treatment for these patients.

## REFERENCES

1. Lupski JR: Genomic disorders: Structural features of the genome can lead to DNA rearrangements and human disease traits. *Trends Genet* **14**:417, 1998.
2. Parry GJ (ed): *Charcot-Marie-Tooth Disorders: A Handbook for Primary Care Physicians.* Upland, PA, Charcot-Marie-Tooth Association, 1995.
3. Harding AE: From the syndrome of Charcot, Marie and Tooth to disorders of peripheral myelin proteins. *Brain* **118**:809, 1995.
4. Spray DC, Dermietzel R: X-linked dominant Charcot-Marie-Tooth disease and other potential gap-junction diseases of the nervous system. *Trends Neurosci* **18**:256, 1995.
5. Midroni G, Bilbao JM: Genetically determined neuropathies, chapter 19 in: *Biopsy Diagnosis of Peripheral Neuropathy.* Boston, MA, Butterworth-Heinemann, 1995, p 353.
6. Zorick TS, Lemke G: Schwann cell differentiation. *Curr Opin Cell Biol* **8**:870, 1996.
7. Pareyson D, Taroni F: Deletion of the *PMP22* gene and hereditary neuropathy with liability to pressure palsies. *Curr Opin Neurol* **9**:348, 1996.
8. Warner LE, Reiter LT, Murakami T, Lupski JR: Molecular mechanisms for Charcot-Marie-Tooth disease and related demyelinating peripheral neuropathies. *Cold Spring Harb Symp Quant Biol* **61**:659, 1996.
9. Murakami T, Garcia CA, Reiter LT, Lupski JR: Reviews in molecular medicine: Charcot-Marie-Tooth disease and related inherited neuropathies. *Medicine* **75**:233, 1996.
10. Lupski JR: Charcot-Marie-Tooth disease: A gene-dosage effect. *Hosp Pract* **32**:83, 1997.
11. De Jonghe P, Timmerman V, Nelis E, Martin J-J, Van Broeckhoven C: Charcot-Marie-Tooth disease and related peripheral neuropathies. *J Periph Nerv Sys* **2**:370, 1997.
12. Taylor V, Suter U: Molecular biology of axon-glia interactions in the peripheral nervous system. *Prog Nucleic Acid Res Mol Biol* **56**:225, 1997.
13. Martini R, Schachner M: Molecular bases of myelin formation as revealed by investigations on mice deficient in glial cell surface molecules. *Glia* **19**:298, 1997.
14. Quarles RH: Glycoproteins of myelin sheaths. *J Mol Neurosci* **8**:1, 1997.
15. Scherer SS: Molecular genetics of demyelination: New wrinkles on an old membrane. *Neuron* **18**:13, 1997.
16. Suter U: Myelin: Keeping nerves well wrapped up. *Curr Biol* **7**:R21, 1997.
17. Martini R: Animal models for inherited peripheral neuropathies. *J Anat* **191**:321, 1997.
18. Chance PF: Inherited demyelinating neuropathy: Charcot-Marie-Tooth disease and related disorders, in Rosenberg RN, Prusiner SB, DiMauro S, Barchi RL (eds): *The Molecular and Genetic Basis of Neurological Disease.* Boston, MA, Butterworth-Heinemann, 1997, p 807.
19. Scherer SS, Asbury AK: Inherited axonal neuropathies and the molecular biology of peripheral neuropathies, in Rosenberg RN, Prusiner SB, DiMauro S, Barchi RL (eds): *The Molecular and Genetic Basis of Neurological Disease.* Boston, MA, Butterworth-Heinemann, 1997, p 817.
20. Müller HW, Suter U, Van Broeckhoven C: Advances in Charcot-Marie-Tooth disease research: Cellular function of CMT-related proteins, transgenic animal models, and pathomechanisms. *Neurobiol Dis* **4**:215, 1997.
21. Bone LJ, Deschênes SM, Balice-Gordon RJ, Fischbeck KH, Scherer SS: Connexin 32 and X-linked Charcot-Marie disease. *Neurobiol Dis* **4**:221, 1997.
22. Mendell JR: Charcot-Marie-Tooth neuropathies and related disorders. *Semin Neurol* **18**:41, 1998.
23. Reilly MM: Genetically determined neuropathies. *J Neurol* **245**:6, 1998.
24. Lupski JR: Charcot-Marie-Tooth disease: Lessons in genetic mechanisms. *Mol Med* **4**:3, 1998.
25. Timmerman V, Nelis E, De Jonghe P, Martin J-J, Van Broeckhoven C: Hereditary neuropathies, in Emery AEH (ed): *Neuromuscular Disorders: Clinical and Molecular Genetics Chichester*, UK, John Wiley & Sons, 1998, p 487.

26. Lupski JR: Charcot-Marie-Tooth disease and related peripheral neuropathies, in Jameson JL (ed): Totowa, NJ, Humana Press, 1998, p 921.

27. Lupski JR: Molecular genetics of peripheral neuropathies, in Martin JB (ed): *Scientific American Neurology.* New York, Scientific American, 1998, p 239.

28. Naef R, Suter U: Many facets of the peripheral myelin protein *PMP22* in myelination and disease. *Microsc Res Tech* **41**:359, 1998.

29. Sommer L, Suter U: The glycoprotein P$_0$ in peripheral gliogenesis. *Cell Tissue Res* **292**:11, 1998.

30. Nelis E, Haites N, Van Broeckhoven C: Mutations in the peripheral myelin genes and associated genes in inherited peripheral neuropathies. *Hum Mutat* **13**:11, 1999.

31. Lupski JR: Charcot-Marie-Tooth polyneuropathy: Duplication, gene dosage, and genetic heterogeneity. *Pediatr Res* **45**:1, 1999.

32. Warner LE, Garcia CA, Lupski JR: Hereditary peripheral neuropathies: Clinical forms, genetics, and molecular mechanisms. *Annu Rev Med* **50**:263, 1999.

33. Shy ME, Kamholz J, Lovelace RE: Introduction to the Third International Symposium on Charcot-Marie-Tooth disorders. *Ann N Y Acad Sci* **833**:xiii, 1999.

33a. Schenone A, Mancardi GL: Molecular basis of inherited neuropathies. *Curr Opin Neurol* **12**:603, 1999.

34. Nelis E, Timmerman V, De Jonghe P, Van Broeckhoven C, Rautenstrauss B: Molecular genetics and biology of inherited peripheral neuropathies: A fast moving field. *Neurogenetics* **2**:137, 1999.

35. Charcot J-M, Marie P: Sur une forme particulière d'atrophie musculaire progressive, souvent familiale, dèbutant par les pieds, et les jambes et atteignant plus tard les mains. *Rev Med* **6**:97, 1886.

36. Tooth H: *The Peroneal Type of Progressive Muscular Atrophy.* London, HK Lewis, 1886.

37. Dyck PJ, Lambert EH: Lower motor and primary sensory neuron disease with peroneal muscular atrophy I. Neurologic, genetic and electrophysiological findings in hereditary polyneuropathies. *Arch Neurol* **18**:603, 1968.

38. Dyck PJ, Lambert EH: Lower motor and primary sensory neuron disease with peroneal muscular atrophy II. Neurologic, genetic and electrophysiological findings in various neuronal degenerations. *Arch Neurol* **18**:619, 1968.

39. Thomas PK, Calne DB, Stewart G: Hereditary motor and sensory neuropathy (peroneal muscular atrophy). *Ann Hum Genet* **38**:111, 1974.

40. Dejerine JJ, Sottas J: Sur la nevrite interstitielle hypertophique et progressive de l'enfance. *Comp Rend Seanc Soc Biol* **45**:63, 1893.

41. Windebank AJ: Inherited recurrent focal neuropathies, in Dyck PJ, Thomas PK, Griffin JW, Low PA, Poduslo JF (eds): *Peripheral Neuropathy.* Philadelphia, WB Saunders, 1993, p 1137.

42. Harati Y, Butler IJ: Congenital hypomyelinating neuropathy. *J Neurol Neurosurg Psychiatry* **48**:1269, 1985.

43. Charnas L, Trapp B, Griffin J: Congenital absence of peripheral myelin: Abnormal Schwann cell development causes lethal arthrogryposis multiplex congenita. *Neurology* **38**:966, 1988.

44. Roussy G, Lévy G: Sept cas d'une maladie particulière. *Rev Neurol* **1**:427, 1926.

45. Garcia CA: A clinical review of Charcot-Marie-Tooth. *Ann N Y Acad Sci* **883**:69, 1999.

46. Lupski JR, Garcia CA, Parry GJ, Patel PI: Charcot-Marie-Tooth polyneuropathy syndrome: Clinical, electrophysiologic, and genetic aspects, in Appel S (ed): *Current Neurology.* Chicago, Mosby-Yearbook, 1991, p 1.

47. Harding AE, Thomas PK: The clinical features of hereditary motor and sensory neuropathy types I and II. *Brain* **103**:259, 1980.

48. Chou SM: Immunohistochemical and ultrastructural classification of peripheral neuropathies with onion-bulbs. *Clin Neuropathol* **11**:109, 1992.

49. Cardoso FDC, Jankovic J: Hereditary motor-sensory neuropathy and movement disorders. *Muscle Nerve* **16**:904, 1993.

50. Kumar SJ, Marks HG, Bowen JR, MacEwen GD: Hip dysplasia associated with Charcot-Marie-Tooth disease in the older children and adolescent. *J Pediatr Orthop* **5**:511, 1985.

51. Eichaker PQ, Spiro A, Sherman M, Lazar E, Reichel J, Dodick F: Respiratory muscle dysfunction in HMSN-I. *Arch Intern Med* **148**:1739, 1988.

52. Rudnick-Shoneborn S, Rohrig D, Nicholson G, Zerres K: Pregnancy and delivery in CMT disease type 1. *Neurology* **43**:2011, 1993.

53. Weiden PL, Wright SE: Vincristine neurotoxicity. *N Engl J Med* **286**:1369, 1972.

54. Hogan-Dann CM, Fallmeth WG, McGuire SA, Kiley VA: Polyneuropathy following vincristine therapy in two patients with Charcot-Marie-Tooth syndrome. *JAMA* **252**:2862, 1984.

55. McGuire SA, Gospe SM Jr, Dahl G: Acute vincristine neurotoxicity in the presence of hereditary motor and sensory neuropathy type I. *Med Pediatr Oncol* **17**:520, 1989.

56. Igarashi M, Thompson EI, Rivera GK: Vincristine neuropathy in type I and type II Charcot-Marie-Tooth disease (hereditary motor sensory neuropathy). *Med Pediatr Oncol* **25**:113, 1995.

57. Graf WD, Chance PF, Lensch MW, Eng LJ, Lipe HP, Bird TD: Severe vincristine neuropathy in Charcot-Marie-Tooth disease type 1A. *Cancer* **77**:1356, 1996.

58. Gemignani F, Marbini A, Di Giovanni G, Salih S, Terzano MG: Charcot-Marie-Tooth disease type 2 with restless leg syndrome. *Neurology* **52**:1064, 1998.

59. Iannaccone S, Zucconi M, Marchettini P, Ferini-Strambi L, Nemi R, Quattrini A, Palazzi S, et al: Evidence of peripheral axonal neuropathy in primary restless legs syndrome. *Mov Disord* **10**:2, 1995.

60. De Jong JGY: Over families met hereditaire dipositie tot het optreden van neuritiden gecorreleered met migraine. *Psychiatr Neurol Bull* **50**:60, 1947.

61. Davies DM: Recurrent peripheral nerve palsies in a family. *Lancet* **2**:266, 1954.

62. Dyck PJ, Chance P, Lebo R, Carney JA: Hereditary motor and sensory neuropathies, in Dyck PJ, Thomas PK, Griffin JW, Low PA, Poduslo JF (eds): *Peripheral Neuropathy*, 3rd ed. Philadelphia, WB Saunders, 1993, p 1094.

63. Ouvrier RA, McLeod JG, Conchin TE: The hypertrophic forms of hereditary motor and sensory neuropathy: A study of hypertrophic Charcot-Marie-Tooth disease (HMSN type I) and Dejerine-Sottas disease (HMSN type III) in childhood. *Brain* **110**:121, 1987.

64. Boylan KB, Ferriero DM, Greco CM, Sheldon RA, Dew M: Congenital hypomyelination neuropathy with arthrogryposis multiplex congenita. *Ann Neurol* **31**:337, 1991.

65. Skre H: Genetic and clinical aspects of Charcot-Marie-Tooth's disease. *Clin Genet* **6**:98, 1974.

66. Emery AEH: Population frequencies of inherited neuromuscular diseases—A world survey. *Neuromuscul Disord* **1**:19, 1991.

67. Allan W: Relation of hereditary pattern to clinical severity as illustrated by peroneal atrophy. *Arch Intern Med* **63**:1123, 1939.

68. Gal A, Mücke J, Theile H, Wieacker PF, Ropers H-H, Wienker TF: X-linked dominant Charcot-Marie-Tooth disease: Suggestion of linkage with a cloned DNA sequence from the proximal Xq. *Hum Genet* **70**:38, 1985.

69. Beckett J, Holden JJA, Simpson NE, White BN, MacLeod PM: Localization of X-linked dominant Charcot-Marie-Tooth disease (CMT2) to Xq13. *J Neurogenet* **3**:225, 1986.

70. Bird TD, Ott J, Giblett ER: Evidence for linkage of Charcot-Marie-Tooth neuropathy to the Duffy locus on chromosome 1. *Am J Hum Genet* **34**:388, 1982.

71. Vance JM, Nicholson GA, Yamaoka LH, Stajich J, Stewart CS, Speer MC, Hung W-Y, et al: Linkage of Charcot-Marie-Tooth neuropathy type 1a to chromosome 17. *Exp Neurol* **104**:186, 1989.

72. Raeymaekers P, Timmerman V, De Jonghe P, Swerts L, Gheuens J, Martin J-J, Muylle L, et al: Localization of the mutation in an extended family with Charcot-Marie-Tooth neuropathy (HMSNI). *Am J Hum Genet* **45**:953, 1989.

73. Middleton-Price HR, Harding AE, Monteiro C, Berciano J, Malcolm S: Linkage of hereditary motor and sensory neuropathy type I to the pericentromeric region of chromosome 17. *Am J Hum Genet* **46**:92, 1990.

74. McAlpine PJ, Feasby TE, Hahn AF, Komarnicki L, James S, Guy C, Dixon M, et al: Localization of a locus for Charcot-Marie-Tooth Neuropathy type 1a (*CMT1A*) to chromosome 17. *Genomics* **7**:408, 1990.

75. Timmerman V, Raeymaekers P, De Jonghe P, De Winter G, Swerts L, Jacobs K, Gheuens J, et al: Assignment of the Charcot-Marie-Tooth neuropathy type 1 (CMT 1a) gene to 17p11.2-p12. *Am J Hum Genet* **47**:680, 1990.

76. Patel PI, Franco B, Garcia CA, Slaugenhaupt SA, Nakamura Y, Ledbetter DH, Chakravarti A, et al: Genetic mapping of autosomal dominant Charcot-Marie-Tooth disease in a large French-Acadian kindred: Identification of new linked markers on chromosome 17. *Am J Hum Genet* **46**:801, 1990.

77. Patel PI, Garcia C, Montes de Oca-Luna R, Malamut RI, Franco B, Slaughenhaupt S, Chakravarti A, et al: Isolation of a marker linked to Charcot-Marie-Tooth disease type 1A gene by differential *Alu*-PCR of human chromosome 17-retaining hybrids. *Am J Hum Genet* **47**:926, 1990.

78. Vance JM, Barker D, Yamaoka LH, Stajich JM, Loprest L, Hung W-Y, Fischbeck K, et al: Localization of Charcot-Marie-Tooth disease type 1a (CMT1A) to chromosome 17p11.2. *Genomics* **9**:623, 1991.

79. Chance PF, Matsunami N, Lensch W, Smith B, Bird TD: Analysis of the DNA duplication 17p11.2 in Charcot-Marie-Tooth neuropathy type 1 pedigrees: Additional evidence for a third autosomal CMT1 locus. *Neurology* **42**:2037, 1992.

80. Bergoffen J, Trofatter J, Pericak-Vance MA, Haines JL, Chance PF, Fischbeck KH: Linkage localization of X-linked Charcot-Marie-Tooth disease. *Am J Hum Genet* **52**:312, 1993.

81. Ben Othmane K, Middleton LT, Loprest LJ, Wilkinson KM, Lennon F, Rozear MP, Stajich JM, et al: Localization of a gene (CMT2A) for autosomal dominant Charcot-Marie-Tooth disease type 2 to chromosome 1p and evidence of genetic heterogeneity. *Genomics* **17**:370, 1993.

82. Ben Othmane K, Hentati F, Lennon F, Ben Hamida C, Blel S, Roses AD, Pericak-Vance MA, et al: Linkage of a locus (CMT4A) for autosomal recessive Charcot-Marie-Tooth disease to chromsome 8q. *Hum Mol Genet* **2**:1625, 1993.

83. Kwon JM, Elliott JL, Yee W-C, Ivanovich J, Scavarda NJ, Moolsintong PJ, Goodfellow PJ: Assignment of a second Charcot-Marie-Tooth type II locus to chromosome 3q. *Am J Hum Genet* **57**:853, 1995.

84. Takashima H, Nakagawa M, Nakahara K, Suehara M, Matsuzaki T, Higuchi I, Higa H, et al: A new type of hereditary motor and sensory neuropathy linked to chromosome 3. *Ann Neurol* **41**:771, 1997.

85. Vance JM, Speer MC, Stajich JM, West S, Wolpert C, Gaskell P, Lennon F, et al: Misclassification and linkage of hereditary sensory and autonomic neuropathy type 1 as Charcot-Marie-Tooth disease, type 2B. *Am J Hum Genet* **59**:258, 1996.

86. LeGuern E, Guilbot A, Kessali M, Ravisé N, Tassin J, Maisonobe T, Grid D, et al: Homozygosity mapping of an autosomal recessive form of demyelinating Charcot-Marie-Tooth disease to chromosome 5q23-q33. *Hum Mol Genet* **5**:1685, 1996.

87. Ionasescu V, Searby C, Sheffield VC, Roklina T, Nishimura D, Ionasescu R: Autosomal dominant Charcot-Marie-Tooth axonal neuropathy mapped on chromosome 7p (CMT2D). *Hum Mol Genet* **5**:1373, 1996.

88. Bolino A, Brancolini V, Bono F, Bruni A, Gambardella A, Romeo G, Quattrone A, et al: Localization of a gene responsible for autosomal recessive demyelinating neuropathy with focally folded myelin sheaths to chromosome11q23 by homozygosity mapping and haplotype sharing. *Hum Mol Genet* **5**:1051, 1996.

89. Kalaydjieva L, Hallmayer J, Chandler D, Savov A, Nikolova A, Angelicheva D, King RHH, et al: Gene mapping in gypsies identifies a novel demyelinating neuropathy on chromosome 8q24. *Nat Genet* **14**:214, 1996.

90. Ionasescu VV, Kimura J, Searby CC, Smith WL, Ross MA, Ionasescu R: A Dejerine-Sottas neuropathy family with a gene mapped on chromosome 8. *Muscle Nerve* **19**:319, 1996.

91. Timmerman V, De Jonghe P, Spoelders P, Simokovic S, Löfgren A, Nelis E, Vance J, et al: Linkage and mutation analysis of Charcot-Marie-Tooth neuropathy type 2 families with chromosomes 1p35-p36 and Xq13. *Neurology* **46**:1311, 1996.

91a. Lupski JR: Axonal Charcot-Marie-Tooth disease and the neurofilament light gene (*NF-L*). *Am J Hum Genet* **67**:8, 2000.

92. Lupski JR, Montes de Oca-Luna R, Slaughenhaupt S, Pentao L, Guzzetta V, Trask BJ, Saucedo-Cardenas O, et al: DNA duplication associated with Charcot-Marie-Tooth disease type 1A. *Cell* **66**:219, 1991.

93. Raeymaekers P, Timmerman V, Nelis E, De Jonghe P, Hoogendijk JE, Baas F, Barker DF, et al: Duplication in chromosome 17p11.2 in Charcot-Marie-Tooth neuropathy type 1a (CMT1a). *Neuromuscul Disord* **1**:93, 1991.

94. Nicholson GA, Kennerson ML, Keats BJB, Mesterovic N, Churcher W, Barker D, Ross DA: Charcot-Marie-Tooth neuropathy type 1A mutation: Apparent crossovers with D17S122 are due to a duplication. *Am J Med Genet* **44**:455, 1992.

95. Hallam PJ, Harding AE, Berciano J, Barker DF, Malcolm S: Duplication of part of chromosome 17 is commonly associated with hereditary motor and sensory neuropathy type I (Charcot-Marie-Tooth disease type 1). *Ann Neurol* **31**:570, 1992.

96. Hertz JM, Børglum AD, Brandt CA, Flint T, Bisgaard C: Charcot-Marie-Tooth disease type 1A: The parental origin of a *de novo* 17p11.2-p12 duplication. *Clin Genet* **46**:291, 1994.

97. Brice A, Ravisé N, Stevanin G, Gugenheim M, Bouche P, Penet C, Agid Y, et al: Duplication within chromosome 17p11.2 in 12 families of French ancestry with Charcot-Marie-Tooth disease type 1a. *J Med Genet* **29**:807, 1992.

98. Bellone E, Mandich P, Mancardi GL, Schenone A, Uccelli A, Abbruzzese M, Sghirlanzoni A, et al: Charcot-Marie-Tooth (CMT) 1a duplication at 17p11.2 in Italian families. *J Med Genet* **29**:492, 1992.

99. Guzzetta V, Santoro L, Gasparo-Rippa P, Ragno M, Vita G, Caruso G, Andria G: Charcot-Marie-Tooth disease: Molecular characterization of patients from central and southern Italy. *Clin Genet* **47**:27, 1995.

100. Holmberg BH, Holmgren G, Nelis E, Van Broeckhoven C, Westerberg B: Charcot-Marie-Tooth disease in northern Sweden: Pedigree analysis and the presence of the duplication in chromosome 17p11.2. *J Med Genet* **31**:435, 1994.

101. Ohnishi A, Li L-Y, Fukushima Y, Mori T, Mori M, Endo C, Yoshimura T, et al: Asian hereditary neuropathy patients with peripheral myelin protein-22 gene aneuploidy. *Am J Med Genet* **59**:51, 1995.

102. Nelis E, Van Broeckhoven C: Estimation of the mutation frequencies in Charcot-Marie-Tooth disease type 1 and hereditary neuropathy with liability to pressure palsies: A European collaborative study. *Eur J Hum Genet* **4**:25, 1996.

103. Lupski JR, Pentao L, Williams LL, Patel PI: Stable inheritance of the CMT1A DNA duplication in two patients with CMT1 and NF1. *Am J Med Genet* **45**:92, 1993.

104. Kaku DA, Parry GJ, Malamut R, Lupski JR, Garcia CA: Nerve conduction studies in Charcot-Marie-Tooth polyneuropathy associated with a segmental duplication of chromosome 17. *Neurology* **43**:1806, 1993.

105. Wise CA, Garcia CA, Davis SN, Heju Z, Pentao L, Patel PI, Lupski JR: Molecular analyses of unrelated Charcot-Marie-Tooth (CMT) disease patients suggest a high frequency of the CMT1A duplication. *Am J Hum Genet* **53**:853, 1993.

106. Mancardi GL, Uccelli A, Bellone E, Sghirlanzoni A, Mandich P, Pareyson D, Schenone A, et al: 17p11.2 duplication is a common finding in sporadic cases of Charcot-Marie-Tooth type 1. *Eur Neurol* **34**:135, 1994.

107. Hoogendijk JE, Hensels GW, Gabreëls-Festen AAWM, Gabreëls FJM, Janssen EAM, De Jonghe P, Martin J-J, et al: De novo mutation in hereditary motor and sensory neuropathy type 1. *Lancet* **339**:1081, 1992.

108. Blair IP, Nash J, Gordon MJ, Nicholson GA: Prevalence and origin of de novo duplications in Charcot-Marie-Tooth disease type 1A: First report of a de novo duplication with a maternal origin. *Am J Hum Genet* **58**:472, 1996.

109. Bort S, Martínez F, Palau F: Prevalence and parental origin of *de novo* 1.5-Mb duplication in Charcot-Marie-Tooth disease type 1A. *Am J Hum Genet* **60**:230, 1997.

110. Matise TC, Chakravarti A, Patel PI, Lupski JR, Nelis E, Timmerman V, Van Broeckhoven C, et al: Detection of tandem duplications and implications for linkage analysis. *Am J Hum Genet* **54**:1110, 1994.

111. Raeymaekers P, Timmerman V, Nelis E, Van Hul W, De Jonghe P, Martin J-J, Van Brockhoven C, et al: Estimation of the size of the chromosome 17p11.2 duplication in Charcot-Marie-Tooth neuropathy type 1a (CMT1A). *J Med Genet* **29**:5, 1991.

112. Hoogendijk JE, Hensels GW, Zorn I, Valentijn L, Janssen EAM, de Visser M, Barker DF, et al: The duplication in Charcot-Marie-Tooth disease type 1a spans at least 1100 kb on chromosome 17p11.2. *Hum Genet* **88**:215, 19911.

113. Pentao L, Wise CA, Chinault AC, Patel PI, Lupski JR: Charcot-Marie-Tooth type 1A duplication appears to arise from recombination at repeat sequences flanking the 1.5-Mb monomer unit. *Nat Genet* **2**:292, 1992.

114. Reiter LT, Murakami T, Koeuth T, Gibbs RA, Lupski JR: The human *COX10* gene is disrupted during homologous recombination between the 24-kb proximal and distal CMT1A-REPs. *Hum Mol Genet* **6**:1595, 1997.

115. Murakami T, Reiter LT, Lupski JR: Genomic structure and expression of the human heme A:farnesyltransferase (*COX10*) gene. *Genomics* **42**:161, 1997.

116. Kennerson ML, Nassif NT, Dawkins JL, DeKroon RM, Yang JG, Nicholson GA: The Charcot-Marie-Tooth binary repeat contains a gene transcribed from the opposite strand of a partially duplicated region of the *COX10* gene. *Genomics* **46**:61, 1997.

117. Murakami T, Lupski JR: A 1.5-Mb cosmid contig of the CMT1A duplication/HNPP deletion critical region in 17p11.2-p12. *Genomics* **34**:128, 1996.

118. Murakami T, Sun ZS, Lee CC, Lupski JR: Isolation of novel genes from the CMT1A duplication/HNPP deletion critical region in 17p11.2-p12. *Genomics* **39**:99, 1997.

119. Killian JM, Kloepfer HW: Homozygous expression of a dominant gene for Charcot-Marie-Tooth neuropathy. *Ann Neurol* **5**:515, 1979.

120. Sturtz FG, Latour P, Mocquard Y, Cruz S, Fenoll B, LeFur JM, Mabin D, et al: Clinical and electrophysiological phenotype of a homozygously duplicated Charcot-Marie-Tooth (type 1A) disease. *Eur Neurol* **38**:26, 1997.

121. LeGuern E, Gouider R, Mabin D, Tardieu S, Birouk N, Parent P, Bouche P, et al: Patients homozygous for the 17p11.2 duplication in Charcot-Marie-Tooth type 1A disease. *Ann Neurol* **41**:104, 1997.

122. Sorour E, Thompson P, MacMillan J, Upadhyaya M: Inheritance of CMT1A duplication from a mosaic father. *J Med Genet* **32**:483, 1995.

123. Liehr T, Rautenstrauss B, Grehl H, Bathke KD, Ekici A, Rauch A, Rott H-D: Mosaicism for the Charcot-Marie-Tooth disease type 1A duplication suggests somatic reversion. *Hum Genet* **98**:22, 1996.

124. Grehl H, Rautenstrauss B, Liehr T, Bickel T, Ekici A, Bathke K, Neundörfer B: Clinical and morphological phenotype of HMSN 1A mosaicism. *Neuromuscul Disord* **7**:27, 1997.

125. Chance PF, Alderson MK, Leppig KA, Lensch MW, Matsunami N, Smith B, Swanson PD, et al: DNA deletion associated with hereditary neuropathy with liability to pressure palsies. *Cell* **72**:143, 1993.

126. Verhalle D, Löfgren A, Nelis E, Dehaene I, Theys P, Lammens M, Dom R, et al: Deletion in the CMT1A locus on chromosome 17p11.2 in hereditary neuropathy with liability to pressure palsies. *Ann Neurol* **35**:704, 1994.

127. Le Guern E, Sturtz F, Gugenheim M, Gouider R, Bonnebouche C, Ravisé N, Gonnaud P-M, et al: Detection of deletion within 17p11.2 in 7 French families with hereditary neuropathy with liability to pressure palsies (HNPP). *Cytogenet Cell Genet* **65**:261, 1994.

128. Mariman ECM, Gabreëls-Festen AAWM, van Beersum SEC, Valentijn LJ, Baas F, Bolhuis PA, Jongen PJH, et al: Prevalence of the 1.5-Mb 17p deletion in families with hereditary neuropathy with liability to pressure palsies. *Ann Neurol* **36**:650, 1994.

129. Reisecker F, Leblhuber F, Lexner R, Radner G, Rosenkranz W, Wagner K: A sporadic form of hereditary neuropathy with liability to pressure palsies: Clinical, electrodiagnostic, and molecular genetic findings. *Neurology* **44**:753, 1994.

130. Lorenzetti D, Pareyson D, Sghirlanzoni A, Roa BB, Abbas NE, Pandolfo M, Di Donato S, et al: A 1.5-Mb deletion in 17p11.2-p12 is frequently observed in Italian families with hereditary neuropathy with liability to pressure palsies. *Am J Hum Genet* **56**:91, 1995.

131. Timmerman V, Löfgren A, Le Guern E, Liang P, De Jonghe P, Martin J-J, Verhalle D, et al: Molecular genetic analysis of the 17p11.2 region in patients with hereditary neuropathy with liability to pressure palsies (HNPP). *Hum Genet* **97**:26, 1996.

132. Roa BB, Garcia CA, Pentao L, Killian JM, Trask BJ, Suter U, Snipes GJ, et al: Evidence for a recessive *PMP22* point mutation in Charcot-Marie-Tooth disease type 1A. *Nat Genet* **5**:189, 1993.

133. Rautenstrauss B, Fuchs C, Liehr T, Grehl H, Murakami T, Lupski JR: Visualization of the CMT1A duplication and HNPP deletion by FISH on stretched chromosome fibers. *J Periph Nerv Sys* **2**:319, 1997.

134. Valentijn LJ, Bolhuis PA, Zorn I, Hoogendijk JE, van den Bosch N, Hensels GW, Stanton Jr VP, et al: The peripheral myelin gene *PMP22/GAS-3* is duplicated in Charcot-Marie-Tooth disease type 1A. *Nat Genet* **1**:166, 1992.

135. Chance PF, Abbas N, Lensch MW, Pentao L, Roa BB, Patel PI, Lupski JR: Two autosomal dominant neuropathies result from reciprocal DNA duplication/deletion of a region on chromosome 17. *Hum Mol Genet* **3**:223, 1994.

136. LeGuern E, Gouider R, Lopes J, Abbas N, Gugenheim M, Tardieu S, Ravisé N, et al: Constant rearrangement of the CMT1A-REP sequences in HNPP patients with a deletion in chromosome 17p11.2: A study of 30 unrelated cases. *Hum Mol Genet* **4**:1673, 1995.

137. Vandenberghe A, Latour P, Chauplannaz G, Chapon F, Pouget J, Dumas R, Laguenay A, et al: Molecular diagnosis of Charcot-Marie-Tooth 1A disease and hereditary neuropathy with liability to pressure palsies by quantifying CMT1A-REP sequences: Consequences of recombinations at variant sites on chromosome 17p11.2-12. *Clin Chem* **42**:1021, 1996.

138. Reiter LT, Murakami T, Koeuth T, Pentao L, Muzny DM, Gibbs RA, Lupski JR: A recombination hotspot responsible for two inherited peripheral neuropathies is located near a *mariner* transposon-like element. *Nat Genet* **12**:288, 1996.

139. Kiyosawa H, Lensch MW, Chance PF: Analysis of the CMT1A-REP repeat: Mapping crossover breakpoints in CMT1A and HNPP. *Hum Mol Genet* **4**:2327, 1995.

140. Timmerman V, Rautenstrauss B, Reiter LT, Koeuth T, Löfgren A, Liehr T, Nelis E, et al: Detection of the CMT1A/HNPP recombination hotspot in unrelated patients of European decent. *J Med Genet* **34**:43, 1997.

141. Lopes J, LeGuern E, Gouider R, Tardieu S, Abbas N, Birouk N, Gugenheim M, et al: Recombination hot spot in a 3.2-kb region of the Charcot-Marie-Tooth type 1A repeat sequences: New tools for molecular diagnosis of hereditary neuropathy with liability to pressure palsies and of Charcot-Marie-Tooth type 1A. *Am J Hum Genet* **58**:1223, 1996.

142. Yamamoto M, Yasuda, Hayasaka K, Ohnishi A, Yoshikawa H, Yanagihara T, Ikegami T, et al: Locations of crossover breakpoints within the CMT1A-REP repeat in Japanese patients with CMT1A and HNPP. *Hum Genet* **99**:151, 1997.

143. Chang J-G, Jong Y-J, Wang W-P, Wang J-C, Hu C-J, Lo M-C, Chang C-P: Rapid detection of a recombinant hotspot associated with Charcot-Marie-Tooth disease type 1A duplication by a PCR-based DNA test. *Clin Chem* **44**:270, 1998.

144. Boerkoel CF, Inoue K, Reiter LT, Warner LE, Lupski JR: Molecular mechanisms for CMT1A duplication and HNPP deletion. *Ann N Y Acad Sci* **883**:22, 1999.

145. Reiter LT, Hastings PJ, Nelis E, DeJohnge P, Van Broeckhoven C, Lupski JR: Human meiotic recombination products revealed by sequencing a hotspot for homologous strand exchange in multiple HNPP patients. *Am J Hum Genet* **62**:1023, 1998.

145a. Lopes J, Tardieu S, Silander K, Blair I, Vandenberghe A, Palau F, Ruberg M, et al: Homologous DNA exchanges in humans can be explained by the yeast double-strand break repair model: A study of 17p11.2 rearrangements associated with CMT1A and HNPP. *Hum Mol Genet* **8**:2285, 1999.

146. Lopes J, Ravisé N, Vandenberghe A, Palau F, Ionasescu V, Mayer M, Lévy N, et al: Fine mapping of *de novo* CMT1A and HNPP rearrangements within CMT1A-REPs evidences two distinct sex-dependent mechanisms and candidate sequences involved in recombination. *Hum Mol Genet* **7**:141, 1998.

147. Smith GR: Chi sites and their consequences, in deBruijn F, Lupski JR, Weinstock GM (eds): *Bacterial Genomes: Physical Structure and Analysis*. New York, Chapman & Hall, 1998, p 49.

148. Rosenberg SM: Chi-stimulated patches are heteroduplex, with recombinant information on the phage lambda *r* chain. *Cell* **48**:855, 1987.

149. Reiter LT, Liehr T, Rautenstrauss B, Robertson HM, Lupski JR: Human recombination-associated genetic disorders appear to coincide with locations of *mariner* transposons. *Genome Res* **9**:839, 1999.

150. Liskay RM, Letsou A, Stachelek JL: Homology requirement for efficient gene conversion between duplicated chromosomal sequences in mammalian cells. *Genetics* **115**:161, 1987.

151. Waldman AS, Liskay RM: Dependence of intrachromosomal recombination in mammalian cells on uninterrupted homology. *Mol Cell Biol* **8**:5350, 1988.

152. Palau F, Löfgren A, De Jonghe P, Bort S, Nelis E, Sevilla T, Martin J-J, et al: Origin of the *de novo* duplication in Charcot-Marie-Tooth disease type 1A: Unequal nonsister chromatid exchange during spermatogenesis. *Hum Mol Genet* **2**:2031, 1993.

153. LeGuern E, Gouider R, Ravisé N, Lopes J, Tardieu S, Gugenheim M, Abbas N, et al: A *de novo* case of hereditary neuropathy with liability to pressure palsies (HNPP) of maternal origin: A new mechanism for deletion in 17p11.2? *Hum Mol Genet* **5**:103, 1996.

154. Mandich P, Bellone E, Schenone A, Mancardi G, Abbruzzese M, Ajmar F: De novo duplication in Charcot-Marie-Tooth type 1A. *Am J Hum Genet* **59**:739, 1996.

155. Lopes J, Vandenberghe A, Tardieu S, Ionasescu V, Lévy N, Wood N, Tachi N, et al: Sex-dependent rearrangements resulting in CMT1A and HNPP. *Nat Genet* **17**:136, 1997.

156. Kiyosawa H, Chance P: Primate orgin of the CMT1A-REP repeat and analysis of a putative transposon-associated recombinational hotspot. *Hum Mol Genet* **5**:745, 1996.

157. Lupski JR, Wise CA, Kuwano A, Pentao L, Parke JT, Glaze DG, Ledbetter DH, et al: Gene dosage is a mechanism for Charcot-Marie-Tooth disease type 1A. *Nat Genet* **1**:29, 1992.

158. Chance PF, Bird TD, Matsunami N, Lensch MW, Brothman AR, Feldman GM: Trisomy 17p associated with Charcot-Marie-Tooth neuropathy type 1A phenotype: Evidence for gene dosage as a mechanism in CMT1A. *Neurology* **42**:2295, 1992.

159. Roa BB, Greenberg F, Gunaratne P, Sauer CM, Lubinsky MS, Kozma C, Meck JM, et al: Duplication of the *PMP22* gene in 17p partial trisomy patients with Charcot-Marie-Tooth type 1A neuropathy. *Hum Genet* **97**:642, 1996.

160. Suter U, Welcher AA, Özcelik T, Snipes GJ, Kosaras B, Francke U, Billings-Gagliardi S, et al: *Trembler* mouse carries a point mutation in a myelin gene. *Nature* **356**:241, 1992.

161. Suter U, Moskow JJ, Welcher AA, Snipes GJ, Kosaras B, Sidman RL, Buchberg AM, et al: A leucine-to-proline mutation in the putative first transmembrane domain of the 22-kDa peripheral myelin protein in the *trembler-J* mouse. *Proc Natl Acad Sci U S A* **89**:4382, 1992.

162. Patel PI, Roa BB, Welcher AA, Schoener-Scott R, Trask BJ, Pentao L, Snipes GJ, et al: The gene for the peripheral myelin protein PMP22 is a candidate for Charcot-Marie-Tooth disease type 1A. *Nat Genet* **1**:159, 1992.

163. Timmerman V, Nelis E, Van Hul W, Nieuwenhuijsen BW, Chen KL, Wang S, Ben Othman K, et al: The peripheral myelin protein gene *PMP22* is contained within the Charcot-Marie-Tooth disease type 1A duplication. *Nat Genet* **1**:171, 1992.

164. Matsunami N, Smith B, Ballard L, Lensch MW, Robertson M, Albertsen H, Hanemann CO, et al: Peripheral myelin protein-22 gene maps in the duplication in chromosome 17p11.2 associated with Charcot-Marie-Tooth 1A. *Nat Genet* **1**:176, 1992.

165. Lupski JR: An inherited DNA rearrangement and gene dosage effect are responsible for the most common autosomal dominant peripheral neuropathy: Charcot-Marie-Tooth disease type 1A. *Clin Res* **40**:645, 1992.

166. Valentijn LJ, Baas F, Wolterman RA, Hoogendijk JE, van den Bosch NHA, Zorn I, Gabreëls-Festen AAWM, et al: Identical point mutations of *PMP22* in Trembler-J mouse and Charcot-Marie-Tooth disease type 1A. *Nat Genet* **2**:288, 1992.

167. Roa BB, Garcia CA, Suter U, Kulpa DA, Wise CA, Mueller J, Welcher AA, et al: Charcot-Marie-Tooth disease type 1A: Association with a spontaneous point mutation in the *PMP22* gene. *N Engl J Med* **329**:96, 1993.

168. Roa BB, Dyck PJ, Marks HG, Chance PF, Lupski JR: Dejerine-Sottas syndrome associated with point mutation in the peripheral myelin protein 22 (*PMP22*) gene. *Nat Genet* **5**:269, 1993.

169. Ionasescu VV, Searby CC, Ionasescu R, Chatkupt S, Patel N, Koenigsberger R: Dejerine-Sottas neuropathy in mother and son with same point mutation of *PMP22* gene. *Muscle Nerve* **20**:97, 1997.

170. Ionasescu VV, Ionasescu R, Searby C, Barker DF: Charcot-Marie-Tooth neuropathy type 1A with both duplication and non-duplication. *Hum Mol Genet* **2**:405, 1993.

171. Valentijn LJ, Baas F, Zorn I, Hensels GW, de Visser M, Bolhuis PA: Alternatively sized duplication in Charcot-Marie-Tooth disease type 1A. *Hum Mol Genet* **2**:2143, 1993.

172. Chapon F, Diraison P, Lechevalier B, Chazot G, Viader F, Bonnebouche C, Vandenberghe A, et al: Hereditary neuropathy with liability to pressure palsies with a partial deletion of the region often duplicated in Charcot-Marie-Tooth disease, type 1A. *J Neurol Neurosurg Psychiatry* **61**:535, 1996.

173. Yoshikawa H, Nishimura T, Nakatsuji Y, Fujimura H, Himoro M, Hayasaka K, Sakoda S, et al: Elevated expression of messenger RNA for peripheral myelin protein 22 in biopsied peripheral nerves of patients with Charcot-Marie-Tooth disease type 1A. *Ann Neurol* **35**:445, 1994.

174. Hanemann CO, Stoll G, D'Urso D, Fricke W, Martin JJ, Van Broeckhoven C, Mancardi GL, et al: Peripheral myelin protein-22 expression in Charcot-Marie-Tooth disease type 1a sural nerve biopsies. *J Neurosci Res* **37**:654, 1994.

175. Hanemann CO, Stoll G, Müller HW: *PMP22* expression in CMT1a neuropathy. *Ann Neurol* **37**:136, 1995.

176. Kamholz J, Shy M, Scherer S: Elevated expression of messenger RNA for peripheral myelin protein 22 in biopsied peripheral nerves of patients with Charcot-Marie-Tooth disease type 1A. *Ann Neurol* **36**:451, 1994.

177. Schenone A, Nobbio L, Mandich P, Bellone E, Abbruzzese M, Aymar F, Mancardi GL, et al: Under expression of messenger RNA for peripheral myelin protein 22 in hereditary neuropathy with liability to pressure palsies. *Neurology* **48**:445, 1997.

178. Schenone A, Nobbio L, Caponnetto C, Abbruzzese M, Mandich P, Bellone E, Ajmar F, et al: Correlation between PMP-22 messenger RNA expression and phenotype in hereditary neuropathy with liability to pressure palsies. *Ann Neurol* **42**:866, 1997.

179. Gabriel J-M, Erne B, Pareyson D, Sghirlanzoni A, Taroni F, Steck AJ: Gene dosage effects in hereditary peripheral neuropathy. *Neurology* **49**:1635, 1997.

180. Vallat J-M, Sindou P, Preux P-M, Tabaraud F, Milor A-M, Couratier P, LeGuern E, et al: Ultrastructural *PMP22* expression in inherited demyelinating neuropathies. *Ann Neurol* **39**:813, 1996.

181. Huxley C, Passage E, Manson A, Putzu G, Figarella-Branger D, Pellissier JF, Fontés M: Construction of a mouse model of Charcot-Marie-Tooth disease type 1A by pronuclear injection of human YAC DNA. *Hum Mol Genet* **5**:563, 1996.

182. Magyar JP, Martini R, Ruelicke T, Aguzzi A, Adlkofer K, Dembic Z, Zielasek J, et al: Impaired differentiation of Schwann cells in transgenic mice with increased *PMP22* gene dosage. *J Neurosci* **16**:5351, 1996.

183. Sereda M, Griffiths I, Pühlhofer A, Stewart H, Rossner MJ, Zimmermann F, Magyar JP, et al: A transgenic rat model of Charcot-Marie-Tooth disease. *Neuron* **16**:1049, 1996.

184. Huxley C, Passage E, Robertson AM, Youl B, Huston S, Manson A, Sabéran-Djoniedi D, et al: Correlation between varying levels of PMP22 expression and the degree of demyelination and reduction in nerve conduction velocity in transgenic mice. *Hum Mol Genet* **7**:449, 1998.

185. Adlkofer K, Martini R, Aguzzi A, Zielasek J, Toyka KV, Suter U: Hypermyelination and demyelinating peripheral neuropathy in *Pmp22*-deficient mice. *Nat Genet* **11**:274, 1995.

186. Adlkofer K, Frei R, Neuberg DH-H, Zielasek J, Toyka KV, Suter U: Heterozygous peripheral myelin protein 22-deficient mice are affected by a progressive demyelinating tomaculous neuropathy. *J Neurosci* **17**:4662, 1997.

187. Maycox PR, Ortuño D, Burrola P, Kuhn R, Bieri PL, Arrezo JC, Lemke G: A transgenic mouse model for human hereditary neuropathy with liability to pressure palsies. *Mol Cell Neurosci* **6**:405, 1997.

188. Warner LE, Roa BB, Lupski JR: Absence of PMP22 coding region mutations in CMT1A duplication patients: Further evidence supporting gene dosage as a mechanism for Charcot-Marie-Tooth disease type 1A. *Hum Mutat* **8**:362, 1996.

189. Nicholson GA, Valentijn LJ, Cherryson AK, Kennerson ML, Bragg TL, DeKroon RM, Ross DA, et al: A frameshift mutation in the PMP22 gene in hereditary neuropathy with liability to pressure palsies. [Erratum *Nat Genet* **7**:113, 1994.] *Nat Genet* **6**:263, 1994.

190. Young P, Wiebusch H, Stogbauer F, Ringelstein B, Assman G, Funke H: A novel frameshift mutation in *PMP22* accounts for hereditary neuropathy with liability to pressure palsies. *Neurology* **48**:450, 1997.

191. Woodward K, Malcolm S: Proteolipid protein gene Pelizaeus-Merzbacher disease in humans and neurodegeneration in mice. *Trends Genet* **15**:125, 1999.

192. Woodward K, Kendall E, Vetrie D, Malcolm S: Pelizaeus-Merzbacher disease: Identification of Xq22 proteolipid-protein duplications and characterization of breakpoints by interphase FISH. *Am J Hum Genet* **63**:207, 1998.

193. Inoue K, Osaka H, Imaizumi K, Nezu A, Takanashi J-i, Arii J, Murayama K, et al: Proteolipid protein gene duplications causing Pelizaeus-Merzbacher disease: Molecular mechanism and phenotypic manifestations. *Ann Neurol* **45**:624, 1999.

194. Epstein CJ: *The Consequences of Chromosome Imbalance: Principles, Mechanisms, and Models.* Cambridge, UK, Cambridge University Press, 1986.

195. Upadhyaya M, Roberts SH, Farnham J, MacMillan JC, Clarke A, Heath JP, Hodges ICG, et al: Charcot-Marie-Tooth disease 1A (CMT1A) associated with a maternal duplication of chromosome 17p11.2 → 12. *Hum Genet* **91**:392, 1993.

196. Pellegrino JE, Pellegrino L, Spinner NB, Sladky J, Chance PF, Zackai EH: Developmental profile in a patient with monosomy 10q and Dup(17p) associated with a peripheral neuropathy. *Am J Med Genet* **61**:377, 1996.

197. King PH, Waldrop R, Lupski JR, Shaffer LG: Charcot-Marie-Tooth phenotype produced by a duplicated *PMP22* gene as part of a 17p trisomy-translocation to the X chromosome. *Clin Genet* **54**:413, 1998.

197a. D'Urso D, Erhardt P, Müller HW: Peripheral myelin protein 22 and protein zero: A novel association in peripheral nervous system myelin. *J Neurosci* **19**:3396, 1999.

198. Roa BB, Lupski JR: Molecular genetics of Charcot-Marie-Tooth neuropathy, in Harris H, Hirschhorn K (eds): *Advances in Human Genetics*. New York, Plenum Press, 1994, p 117.

199. Spreyer P, Kuhn G, Hanemann CO, Gillen C, Schaal H, Kuhn R, Lemke G, et al: Axon-regulated expression of a Schwann cell transcript that is homologous to a "growth arrest-specific" gene. *EMBO J* **10**:3661, 1991.

200. Welcher AA, Suter U, De Leon M, Snipes GJ, Shooter EM: A myelin protein is encoded by the homologue of a growth arrest-specific gene. *Proc Natl Acad Sci U S A* **88**:7195, 1991.

201. Martinotti A, Cariani CT, Melani C, Sozzi G, Spurr NK, Pierotti MA, Colombo MP: Isolation and mapping to 17p12-13 of the human homologous of the murine growth arrest specific Gas-3 gene. *Hum Mol Genet* **5**:331, 1992.

202. Manfioletti G, Ruaro ME, Del Sal G, Philipson L, Schneider C: A growth arrest-specific (*gas*) gene codes for a membrane protein. *Mol Cell Biol* **10**:2924, 1990.

203. Hayasaka K, Himoro M, Nanao K, Sato W, Miura M, Uyemura K, Takahaski E, et al: Isolation and sequence determination of a cDNA encoding PMP-22 (PAS-II/SR13/GAS-3) of human peripheral myelin. *Biochem Biophys Res Commun* **186**:827, 1992.

204. Schneider C, King RM, Philipson L: Genes specifically expressed at growth arrest of mammalian cells. *Cell* **54**:787, 1988.

205. Suter U, Snipes GJ, Schoener-Scott R, Welcher AA, Pareek S, Lupski JR, Murphy RA, et al: Regulation of tissue-specific expression of alternative peripheral myelin protein-22 (*PMP22*) gene transcripts by two promoters. *J Biol Chem* **269**:25795, 1994.

206. Bosse F, Zoidl G, Wilms S, Gillen CP, Kuhn HG, Muller HW: Differential expression of two mRNA species indicates a dual function of peripheral myelin protein *PMP22* in cell growth and myelination. *J Neurosci Res* **37**:529, 1994.

207. Baechner D, Liehr T, Hameister H, Altenberger H, Grehl H, Suter U, Rautenstrauss B: Widespread expression of the peripheral myelin protein-22 gene (*Pmp22*) in neural and non-neural tissues during murine development. *J Neurosci Res* **42**:733, 1995.

208. Snipes GJ, Suter U, Welcher AA, Shooter EM: Characterization of a novel peripheral nervous system myelin protein (PMP-22/SR13). *J Cell Biol* **117**:225, 1992.

209. Snipes GJ, Suter U, Shooter EM: Human peripheral myelin protein-22 carries the L2/HNK-1 carbohydrate adhesion epitope. *J Neurochem* **61**:1961, 1993.

210. Pareek S, Suter U, Snipes GJ, Welcher AA, Shooter EM, Murphy RA: Detection and processing of peripheral myelin protein PMP22 in cultured Schwann cells. *J Biol Chem* **268**:10372, 1993.

211. Haney C, Snipes GJ, Shooter EM, Suter U, Garcia CA, Griffin JW, Trapp BD: Ultrastructural distribution of *PMP22* in Charcot-Marie-Tooth disease type 1A. *J Neuropathol Exp Neurol* **55**:290, 1996.

212. Yoshikawa H, Dyck PJ: Uncompacted inner myelin lamellae in inherited tendency to pressure palsy. *J Neuropathol Exp Neurol* **50**:649, 1991.

213. Hanemann CO, Müller HW: Pathogenesis of Charcot-Marie-Tooth 1A (CMT1A) neuropathy. *Trends Neurosci* **21**:282, 1998.

214. Zoidl G, Blass-Kampmann S, D'Urso D, Schmalenbach C, Müller HW: Retroviral-mediated gene transfer of the peripheral myelin protein PMP22 in Schwann cells: modulation of cell growth. *EMBO J* **14**:1122, 1995.

215. Nelis E, Timmerman V, De Jonghe P, Van Broeckhoven C: Identification of a 5' splice site mutation in the PMP22 gene in autosomal dominant Charcot-Marie-Tooth disease type 1. *Hum Mol Genet* **3**:515, 1994.

216. Ionasescu VV, Ionasescu R, Searby C, Neahring R: Dejerine-Sottas disease with de novo dominant point mutation of the PMP22 gene. *Neurology* **45**:1766, 1995.

217. Ohnishi A: Clinical, pathologic and molecular genetic studies of patients with hereditary motor and sensory neuropathy (HMSN). *Rinsho Shinkeigaku* **35**:1438, 1995.

218. Gabreëls-Festen AAWM, Bolhuis PA, Hoogendijk JE, Valentijn LJ, Eshuis EJHM, Gabreëls FJM: Charcot-Marie-Tooth disease type 1A: Morphological phenotype of the 17p duplication versus PMP22 point mutations. *Acta Neuropathol* **90**:645, 1995.

219. Valentijn LJ, Ouvrier RA, van den Bosch NHA, Bolhuis PA, Baas F, Nicholson GA: Déjérine-Sottas neuropathy is associated with a de novo PMP22 mutation. *Hum Mutat* **5**:76, 1995.

220. Ionasescu VV, Searby C, Greenberg SA: Dejerine-Sottas disease with sensorineural hearing loss, nystagmus, and peripheral facial nerve weakness: De novo point mutation of the PMP22 gene. *J Med Genet* **33**:1048, 1996.

221. Navon R, Seifried B, Gal-On NS, Sadeh M: A new point mutation affecting the fourth transmembrane domain of PMP22 results in

222. Bort S, Sevilla T, Garcia-Planells J, Blesa D, Paricio N, Vílchez JJ, Prieto F, et al: Dejerine-Sottas neuropathy associated with *de novo* S79P mutation of the peripheral myelin protein 22 (PMP22) gene. *Hum Mutat* **1(Suppl)**:S95, 1997.

223. Ionasescu VV, Searby CC, Ionasescu R, Reisin R, Ruggieri V, Arberas C: Severe Charcot-Marie-Tooth neuropathy type 1A with 1-base pair deletion and frameshift mutation in the peripheral myelin protein 22 gene. *Muscle Nerve* **20**:1308, 1997.

224. Marrosu MG, Vaccargiu S, Marrosu G, Vannelli A, Cianchetti C, Muntoni F: A novel point mutation in the peripheral myelin protein 22 (*PMP22*) gene associated with Charcot-Marie-Tooth disease type 1A. *Neurology* **48**:489, 1997.

225. Tyson J, Ellis D, Fairbrother U, King RHM, Muntoni F, Jacobs J, Malcolm S, et al: Hereditary demyelinating neuropathy of infancy: A genetically complex syndrome. *Brain* **120**:47, 1997.

226. Ikegami T, Ikeda H, Mitsui T, Hayasaka K: Novel mutations of the myelin $P_0$ gene in a pedigree with Charcot-Marie-Tooth disease type 1B. *Am J Med Genet* **71**:246, 1997.

227. Marques W, Thomas PK, Sweeney MG, Carr L, Wood NW: Dejerine-Sottas neuropathy and PMP22 point mutations: A new base pair substitution and a possible "hot spot" on Ser72. *Ann Neurol* **43**:680, 1998.

228. Lenssen PPA, Gabreëls-Festen AAWM, Valentijn LJ, Jongen PJH, van Beersum SEC, van Engelen BGM, van Wensen PJM, et al: Hereditary neuropathy with liability to pressure palsies: Phenotypic differences between patients with the common deletion and a PMP22 frameshift mutation. *Brain* **121**:1451, 1998.

229. Sahenk Z, Chen L, Freimer M: A novel *PMP22* point mutation causing HNPP phenotype: Studies on nerve xenografts. *Neurology* **51**:702, 1998.

230. Pareyson D, Botti S, Sghirlanzoni A, Taroni F: *PMP22* frameshift mutation and hereditary neuropathy with liability to pressure palsies. *Neurology* **49**:1478, 1997.

231. Nelis E, Holmberg B, Adolfsson R, Holmgren G, Van Broeckhoven C: PMP22 Thr(118)Met: Recessive CMT1 mutation or polymorphism? *Nat Genet* **15**:13, 1997.

232. Fabbretti E, Edomi P, Brancolini C, Schneider C: Apoptotic phenotype induced by overexpression of wild-type gas3/PMP22: Its relation to the demyelinating peripheral neuropathy CMT1A. *Genes Dev* **9**:1846, 1995.

232a. Naef R, Suter U: Impaired intracellular trafficking is a common disease mechanism of *PMP22* point mutations in peripheral neuropathies. *Neurobiol Dis* **6**:1, 1999.

233. Parman Y, Planté-Bordeneuve V, Guiochon-Mantel A, Eraksoy M, Said G: Recessive inheritance of a new point mutation of the *PMP22* gene in Dejerine-Sottas disease. *Ann Neurol* **45**:1999.

234. Numakura C, Lin C, Oka N, Akiguchi I, Hayasaka K: Hemizygous mutation of the PMP22 gene associated with Charcot-Marie-Tooth disease type 1. *Ann Neurol* **47**:101, 2000.

235. Adlkofer K, Naef R, Suter U: Analysis of compound heterozygous mice reveals that the *Trembler* mutation can behave as a gain-of-function allele. *J Neurosci Res* **49**:671, 1997.

236. Suh J-G, Ichihara N, Saigoh K, Nakabayashi O, Yamanishi T, Tanaka K, Wada K, et al: An in-frame deletion in peripheral myelin protein-22 gene causes hypomyelination and cell death of the Schwann cells in the new *Trembler* mutant mice. *Neurosci* **79**:735, 1997.

237. Naef R, Adlkofer K, Lescher B, Suter U: Aberrant protein trafficking in *Trembler* suggests a disease mechanism for hereditary human peripheral neuropathies. *Mol Cell Neurosci* **9**:13, 1997.

238. D'Urso D, Prior R, Greiner-Petter R, Gabreëls-Festen AAWM, Müller HW: Overloaded endoplasmic reticulum-Golgi compartments, a possible pathomechanism of peripheral neuropathies caused by mutations of the peripheral myelin protein PMP22. *J Neurosci* **18**:731, 1998.

239. Tobler AR, Notterpek L, Naef R, Taylor V, Suter U, Shooter EM: Transport of trembler-J mutant peripheral myelin protein 22 is blocked in the intermediate compartment and affects the transport of the wild type protein by direct interaction. *J Neurosci* **19**:2027, 1999.

240. Notterpek L, Shooter EM, Snipes GJ: Upregulation of the endosomal-lysosomal pathway in the Trembler-J neuropathy. *J Neurosci* **17**:4190, 1997.

241. Lemke G, Axel R: Isolation and sequence of a cDNA encoding the major structural protein of peripheral myelin. *Cell* **40**:501, 1985.

242. Hayasaka K, Himoro M, Wang Y, Takata M, Minoshima S, Shimizu N, Miura M, et al: Structure and chromosomal localization of the gene encoding the human myelin protein zero (MPZ). *Genomics* **17**:755, 1993.

243. Messing A, Behringer RR, Hammang JP, Palmiter RD, Brinster RL, Lemke G: $P_0$ promoter directs expression of reporter and toxin genes to Schwann cells of transgenic mice. *Neuron* **8**:507, 1992.
244. Brown AM, Lemke G: Multiple regulatory elements control transcription of the peripheral myelin protein zero gene. *J Biol Chem* **272**:28939, 1997.
245. Lemke G: Unwrapping the genes of myelin. *Neuron* **1**:535, 1988.
246. Filbin MT, Walsh FS, Trapp BD, Pizzey JA, Tennekoon GI: Role of myelin $P_0$ protein as a homophilic adhesion molecule. *Nature* **344**:871, 1990.
247. Zhang K, Merazga Y, Filbin MT: Mapping the adhesive domains of the myelin $P_0$ protein. *J Neurosci Res* **45**:525, 1996.
248. D'Urso D, Brophy PJ, Staugaitis SM, Gillespie CS, Frey AB, Stempak JG, Colman DR: Protein zero of peripheral nerve myelin: Biosynthesis, membrane insertion, and evidence for homotypic interaction. *Neuron* **2**:449, 1990.
249. Bollensen E, Schachner M: The peripheral myelin glycoprotein $P_0$ expresses the L2/HNK-1 and L2 carbohydrate structures shared by neural adhesion molecules. *Neurosci Lett* **82**:77, 1987.
250. Ding Y, Brunden KR: The cytoplasmic domain of myelin glycoprotein $P_0$ interacts with negatively charged phospholipid bilayers. *J Biol Chem* **269**:10764, 1994.
251. Martini R, Mohajeri MH, Kasper S, Giese KP, Schachner M: Mice doubly deficient in the genes for $P_0$ and myelin basic protein show that both proteins contribute to the formation of the major dense line in peripheral nerve myelin. *J Neurosci* **15**:4488, 1995.
252. Shapiro L, Doyle JP, Hensley P, Colman DR, Hendrickson WA: Crystal structure of the extracellular domain from $P_0$, the major structural protein of peripheral nerve myelin. *Neuron* **17**:435, 1996.
253. Kirschner DA, Szumowski K, Gabreels-Festen AAWM, Hoogendijk JE, Bolhuis PA: Inherited demyelinating peripheral neuropathies: Relating myelin packing abnormalities to $P_0$ molecular defects. *J Neurosci Res* **46**:502, 1996.
254. Hayasaka K, Himoro M, Sato W, Takada G, Uyemura K, Shimizu N, Bird TD, et al: Charcot-Marie-Tooth neuropathy type 1B is associated with mutations of the myelin $P_0$ gene. *Nat Genet* **5**:31, 1993.
255. Kulkens T, Bolhuis PA, Wolterman RA, Kemp S, te Nijenhuis S, Valentijn LJ, Hensels GW, et al: Deletion of the serine 34 codon from the major peripheral myelin protein $P_0$ gene in Charcot-Marie-Tooth disease type 1B. *Nat Genet* **5**:35, 1993.
256. Hayasaka K, Himoro M, Sawaishi Y, Nanao K, Takahashi T, Takada G, Nicholson GA, et al: De novo mutation of the myelin $P_0$ gene in Dejerine-Sottas disease (hereditary motor and sensory neuropathy type III). *Nat Genet* **5**:266, 1993.
257. Warner LE, Hilz M, Appel SH, Killian JM, Kolodny EH, Karpati G, Carpenter S, et al: Clinical phenotype of different *MPZ* mutations may include Charcot-Marie-Tooth type 1B, Dejerine-Sottas, and congenital hypomyelination. *Neuron* **17**:451, 1996.
258. Marrosu MG, Vaccargiu S, Marrosu G, Vannelli A, Cianchetti C, Muntoni F: A novel point mutation in the myelin protein zero (MPZ) gene responsible for a form of hereditary axonal neuropathy (Charcot-Marie-Tooth type 2). *J Peripher Nerv Syst* **2**:396, 1997.
258a. Planté-Bordeneuve V, Guiochon-Mantel A, Lacroix C, Lapresle J, Said G: The Roussy-Lévy family: From original description to the gene. *Ann Neurol* **46**:770, 1999.
259. Himoro M, Yoshikawa H, Matsui T, Mitsui Y, Takahashi M, Kaido M, Nishimura T, et al: New mutation of the myelin $P_0$ gene in a pedigree of Charcot-Marie-Tooth neuropathy type 1. *Biochem Mol Biol Int* **31**:169, 1993.
260. Hayasaka K, Ohnishi A, Takada G, Fukushima Y, Murai Y: Mutation of the myelin $P_0$ gene in Charcot-Marie-Tooth neuropathy type 1. *Biochem Biophys Res Commun* **194**:1317, 1993.
261. Hayasaka K, Takada G, Ionasescu VV: Mutation of the myelin $P_0$ gene in Charcot-Marie-Tooth neuropathy type 1B. *Hum Mol Genet* **2**:1369, 1993.
262. Nelis E, Timmerman V, De Jonghe P, Muylle L, Martin J-J, Van Broeckhoven C: Linkage and mutation analysis in an extended family with Charcot-Marie-Tooth disease type 1B. *J Med Genet* **31**:811, 1994.
263. Nelis E, Timmerman V, De Jonghe P, Vandenberghe A, Pham-Dinh D, Dautigny A, Martin J-J, et al: Rapid screening of myelin genes in CMT1 patients by SSCP analysis: Identification of new mutations and polymorphisms in the $P_0$ gene. *Hum Genet* **94**:653, 1994.
264. Rautenstrauss B, Nelis E, Grehl H, Pfeiffer RA, Van Broeckhoven C: Identification of a de novo insertional mutation in $P_0$ in a patient with

a Déjérine-Sottas syndrome (DSS) phenotype. *Hum Mol Genet* **3**:1701, 1994.
265. Blanquet-Grossard F, Pham-Dinh D, Dautigny A, Latour P, Bonnebouche C, Corbillon E, Chazot G, et al: Charcot-Marie-Tooth type 1B neuropathy: Third mutation at serine 63 codon in the major peripheral myelin glycoprotein $P_0$ gene. *Clin Genet* **48**:281, 1995.
266. Latour P, Blanquet F, Nelis E, Bonnebouche C, Chapon F, Diraison P, Ollagnon E, et al: Mutations in the myelin protein zero gene associated with Charcot-Marie-Tooth disease type 1B. *Hum Mutat* **6**:50, 1995.
267. Roa BB, Warner LE, Garcia CA, Russo D, Lovelace R, Chance PF, Lupski JR: Myelin protein zero (*MPZ*) gene mutations in non-duplication type 1 Charcot-Marie-Tooth disease. *Hum Mutat* **7**:36, 1996.
268. Bellone E, Mandich P, James R, Nelis E, Lamba LD, Van Broeckhoven C, Ajmar F: Identification of a 4 bp deletion (1560del4) in $P_0$ gene in a family with severe Charcot-Marie-Tooth disease. *Hum Mutat* **7**:377, 1996.
269. Gabreëls-Festen AAWM, Hoogendijk JE, Meijerink PHS, Gabreëls FJM, Bolhuis PA, van Beersum S, Kulkens T, et al: Two divergent types of nerve pathology in patients with different $P_0$ mutations. *Neurology* **47**:761, 1996.
270. Ikegami T, Nicholson G, Ikeda H, Ishida A, Johnston H, Wise G, Ouvrier R, et al: A novel homozygous mutation of the myelin $P_0$ gene producing Dejerine-Sottas disease (hereditary motor and sensory neuropathy type III). *Biochem Biophys Res Commun* **222**:107, 1996.
271. Meijerink PHS, Hoogendijk JE, Gabreels-Festen AAWM, Zorn I, Veldman H, Baas F, de Visser M, et al: Clinically distinct codon 69 mutations in major myelin protein zero in demyelinating neuropathies. *Ann Neurol* **40**:672, 1996.
272. Rouger H, LeGuern E, Gouider R, Tardieu S, Birouk N, Gugenheim M, Bouche P, et al: High frequency of mutations in codon 98 of the peripheral myelin protein $P_0$ gene in 20 French CMT1 patients. *Am J Hum Genet* **58**:638, 1996.
273. Silander K, Meretoja P, Nelis E, Timmerman V, Van Broeckhoven C, Aula P, Savontaus M-L: A de novo duplication in 17p11.2 and a novel mutation in the $P_0$ gene in two Dejerine-Sottas syndrome patients. *Hum Mutat* **8**:304, 1996.
274. Tachi N, Kozuka N, Ohya K, Chiba S, Sasaki K, Uyemura K, Hayasaka K: A new mutation of the $P_0$ gene in patients with Charcot-Marie-Tooth disease type 1B: Screening of the $P_0$ gene by heteroduplex analysis. *Neurosci Lett* **204**:173, 1996.
275. Ikegami T, Nicholson G, Ikeda H, Ishida A, Johnston H, Wise G, Ouvrier R, et al: De novo mutation of the myelin $P_0$ gene in Dejerine-Sottas disease (hereditary motor and sensory neuropathy type III): Two amino acid insertion after Asp 118. *Hum Mutat* **1(Suppl)**:S103, 1997.
276. Komiyama A, Ohnishi A, Izawa K, Yamamori S, Ohashi H, Hasegawa O: De novo mutation ($Arg^{98} \rightarrow Cys$) of the myelin $P_0$ gene and uncompaction of the major dense line of the myelin sheath in a severe variant of Charcot-Marie-Tooth disease type 1B. *J Neurol Sci* **149**:103, 1997.
277. Schiavon F, Rampazzo A, Merlini L, Angelini C, Mostacciuolo ML: Mutations of the same sequence of the myelin $P_0$ gene causing two different phenotype. *Hum Mutat* **1**:S217, 1997.
278. Sorour E, MacMillan J, Upadhyaya M: Novel mutation of the myelin $P_0$ gene in a CMT1B family. *Hum Mutat* **9**:74, 1997.
279. Tachi N, Kozuka N, Ohya K, Chiba S, Sasaki K: Tomaculous neuropathy in Charcot-Marie-Tooth disease with myelin protein zero gene mutation. *J Neurol Sci* **153**:106, 1997.
280. Warner LE, Shohat M, Shorer Z, Lupski JR: Multiple de novo *MPZ* ($P_0$) mutations in a sporadic Dejerine-Sottas case. *Hum Mutat* **10**:21, 1997.
281. Mandich P, Mancardi GL, Varese A, Soriani S, Di Maria E, Bellone E, Bado M, Gross L, Windebank AJ, Ajmar F, Schenone A: Congenital hypomyelination due to myelin protein zero Q215X mutation. *Ann Neurol* **45**:676, 1999.
282. Pareyson D, Sghirlanzoni A, Bolti S, Ciano C, Fallica E, Mora M, Taroni F: Charcot-Marie-Tooth disease type 2 and $P_0$ gene mutations. *Neurology* **52**:1110, 1999.
283. Phillips JP, Warner LE, Lupski JR, Garg BP: Congenital hypomyelinating neuropathy: Two cases with long-term clinical follow-up, genetic analysis, and literature review. *Pediatr Neurol* **20**:226, 1999.
284. Nakagawa M, Suehara M, Saito A, Takashima H, Umehara F, Saito M, Kanzato N, et al: A novel *MPZ* gene mutation in dominantly inherited neuropathy with focally folded myelin sheaths. *Neurology* **52**:1271, 1999.

285. Takashima H, Nakagawa M, Kanzaki A, Yawata Y, Horikiri T, Matsuzaki T, Suehara M, et al: Germline mosaicism of MPZ gene in Dejerine-Sottas syndrome (HMSN III) associated with hereditary stomatocytosis. *Neuromuscul Disord* **9**:232, 1999.

286. Zhang K, Filbin MT: Myelin $P_0$ protein mutated at Cys 21 has a dominant-negative effect on adhesion of wild-type $P_0$. *J Neurosci Res* **53**:1, 1998.

287. Ekici AB, Fuchs C, Nelis E, Hillenbrand R, Schachner M, Van Broeckhoven C, Rautenstrauss B: An adhesion test system based on Schneider cells to determine genotype-phenotype correlations for mutated $P_0$ proteins. *Genet Anal* **14**:117, 1998.

288. Wong M-H, Filbin MT: Dominant-negative effect on adhesion by myelin $P_0$ protein truncated in its cytoplasmic domain. *J Cell Biol* **134**:1531, 1996.

289. Wong M-H, Filbin MT: The cytoplasmic domain of the myelin $P_0$ protein influences the adhesive interactions of its extracellular domain. *J Cell Biol* **126**:1089, 1994.

290. Giese KP, Martini R, Lemke G, Soriano P, Schachner M: Mouse $P_0$ gene disruption leads to hypomyelination, abnormal expression of recognition molecules, and degeneration of myelin and axons. *Cell* **71**:565, 1992.

291. Martini R, Zielasek J, Toyka KV, Giese KP, Schachner M: Protein zero ($P_0$)-deficient mice show myelin degeneration in peripheral nerves characteristic of inherited human neuropathies. *Nat Genet* **11**:281, 1995.

292. Zielasek J, Martini R, Toyka KV: Functional abnormalities in $P_0$-deficient mice resemble human hereditary neuropathies linked to $P_0$ gene mutations. *Muscle Nerve* **19**:946, 1996.

293. Shy ME, Arroyo E, Sladky J, Menichella D, Jiang H, Wenbo X, Kamholz J, et al: Heterozygous $P_0$ knockout mice develop a peripheral neuropathy that resembles chronic inflammatory demyelinating polyneuropathy (CIDP). *J Neuropathol Exp Neurol* **56**:811, 1997.

294. Neuhaus IM, Dahl G, Werner R: Use of alternate promoters for tissue-specific expression of the gene coding for connexin32. *Gene* **158**:257, 1995.

295. Neuhaus IM, Bone L, Wang S, Ionasescu V, Werner R: The human connexin32 gene is transcribed from two tissue-specific promoters. *Biosci Rep* **16**:239, 1996.

296. Bruzzone R, Ressot C: Connexins, gap junctions, and cell-cell signalling in the nervous system. *Eur J Neurosci* **9**:1, 1997.

297. Bergoffen J, Scherer SS, Wang S, Scott MO, Bone LJ, Paul DL, Chen K, et al: Connexin mutations in X-linked Charcot-Marie-Tooth disease. *Science* **262**:2039, 1993.

298. Balice-Gordon RJ, Bone LJ, Scherer SS: Functional gap junctions in the Schwann cell myelin sheath. *Cell Biol* **142**:1095, 1998.

299. Scherer SS, Deschenes SM, Xu Y-t, Nelles E, Grinspan JB, Fischbeck KH, Paul DL: Connexin32 is a myelin-related protein in the PNS and CNS. *J Neurosci* **15**:8281, 1995.

300. Chandross KJ, Roy C, Dermietzel R, Kessler JA, Spray DC: Functions of Schwann cell gap junctions in normal and pathologic nerve. *J Gen Physiol* **104**:29a, 1994.

301. Fairweather N, Bell C, Cochrane S, Chelly J, Wang S, Mostacciuolo ML, Monaco AP, et al: Mutations in the connexin 32 gene in X-linked dominant Charcot-Marie-Tooth disease (CMTX1). *Hum Mol Genet* **3**:29, 1994.

302. Orth U, Fairweather N, Exler M-C, Schwinger E, Gal A: X-linked dominant Charcot-Marie-Tooth neuropathy: Valine-38-methionine substitution of connexin32. *Hum Mol Genet* **3**:1699, 1994.

303. Ionasescu V, Searby C, Ionasescu R: Point mutations of the connexin32 (GJB1) gene in X-linked dominant Charcot-Marie-Tooth neuropathy. *Hum Mol Genet* **3**:355, 1994.

304. Cherryson AK, Yeung L, Kennerson ML, Nicholson GA: Mutational studies in X-linked Charcot-Marie-Tooth disease (CMTX) [Abstract]. *Am J Hum Genet* **55( Suppl)**:1261, 1994.

305. Ionasescu V, Searby C, Ionasescu R, Meschino W: New point mutations and deletions of the connexin 32 gene in X-linked Charcot-Marie-Tooth neuropathy. *Neuromuscul Disord* **5**:297, 1995.

306. Bone LJ, Dahl N, Lensch MW, Chance PF, Kelly T, Le Guern E, Magi S, et al: New connexin32 mutations associated with X-linked Charcot-Marie-Tooth disease. *Neurology* **45**:1863, 1995.

307. Niewiadomski LA, Kelly TE: X-linked Charcot-Marie-Tooth disease: Molecular analysis of interfamilial variability. *Am J Med Genet* **66**:175, 1996.

308. Gupta S, Benstead T, Neumann P, Guernsey D: A point mutation in codon 3 of connexin-32 is associated with X-linked Charcot-Marie-Tooth neuropathy. *Hum Mutat* **8**:375, 1996.

309. Ionasescu V, Ionasescu R, Searby C: Correlation between connexin 32 gene mutations and clinical phenotype in X-linked dominant Charcot-Marie-Tooth neuropathy. *Am J Med Genet* **63**:486, 1996.

310. Ionasescu VV, Searby C, Ionasescu R, Neuhaus IM, Werner R: Mutations of the noncoding region of the connexin32 gene in X-linked dominant Charcot-Marie-Tooth neuropathy. *Neurology* **47**:541, 1996.

311. Oterino A, Montón FI, Cabrera VM, Pinto F, Gonzalez A, Lavilla NR: Arginine-164-tryptophan substitution in connexin32 associated with X linked dominant Charcot-Marie-Tooth disease. *J Med Genet* **33**:413, 1996.

312. Ressot C, Latour P, Blanquet-Grossard F, Sturtz F, Duthel S, Battin J, Corbillon E, et al: X-linked dominant Charcot-Marie-Tooth neuropathy (CMTX): New mutations in the connexin32 gene. *Hum Genet* **98**:172, 1996.

313. Schiavon F, Fracasso C, Mostacciuolo ML: Novel missense mutation of the connexin32 (GJB1) gene in X-linked dominant Charcot-Marie-Tooth neuropathy. *Hum Mutat* **8**:83, 1996.

314. Tan CC, Ainsworth PJ, Hahn AF, MacLeod PM: Novel mutations in the connexin 32 gene associated with X-linked Charcot-Marie-Tooth disease. *Hum Mutat* **7**:167, 1996.

315. Yoshimura T, Ohnishi A, Yamamoto T, Fukushima Y, Kitani M, Kobayashi T: Two novel mutations (C53S, S26L) in the connexin32 of Charcot-Marie-Tooth disease type X families. *Hum Mutat* **8**:270, 1996.

316. Silander K, Meretoja P, Pihko H, Juvonen V, Issakainen J, Aula P, Savontaus M-L: Screening for connexin 32 mutations in Charcot-Marie-Tooth disease families with possible X-linked inheritance. *Hum Genet* **100**:391, 1997.

317. Janssen EAM, Kemp S, Hensels GW, Sie OG, de Die-Smulders CEM, Hoogendijk JE, de Visser M, et al: Connexin32 gene mutations in X-linked dominant Charcot-Marie-Tooth disease (CMTX1). *Hum Genet* **99**:501, 1997.

318. Latour P, Fabreguette A, Ressot C, Blanquet-Grossard F, Antoine J-C, Calvas P, Chapon F, et al: New mutations in the X-linked form of Charcot-Marie-Tooth disease. *Eur Neurol* **37**:38, 1997.

319. Nelis E, Simokovic S, Timmerman V, Löfgren A, Backhovens H, De Jonghe P, Martin JJ, et al: Mutation analysis of the connexin32 (Cx32) gene in Charcot-Marie-Tooth neuropathy type 1: Identification of five new mutations. *Hum Mutat* **9**:47, 1996.

320. Sillén A, Annerén G, Dahl N: A novel mutation (C201R) in the transmembrane domain of connexin32 in severe X-linked Charcot-Marie-Tooth disease. *Hum Mutat* **1(Suppl)**:S8, 1998.

321. Wicklein EM, Orth U, Gal A, Kunze K: Missense mutation (R15W) of the connexin32 gene in a family with X chromosomal Charcot-Marie-Tooth neuropathy with only female family members affected. *J Neurol Neurosurg Psychiatry* **63**:379, 1997.

322. Flagiello L, Cirigliano V, Strazzullo M, Cappal V, Ciccodicola A, D'Esposito M, Torrente I, et al: Mutation in the nerve-specific 5′ non-coding region of *Cx32* gene and absence of specific mRNA in a CMT1X Italian family. *Hum Mutat* **195**:1, 1998.

323. Rouger H, LeGuern E, Birouk N, Gouider R, Tardieu S, Plassart E, Gugenheim M, et al: Charcot-Marie-Tooth disease with intermediate motor nerve conduction velocities: Characterization of 14 Cx32 mutation in 35 families. *Hum Mutat* **10**:443, 1997.

324. Ainsworth PJ, Bolton CF, Murphy BC, Stuart JA, Hahn AF: Genotype/phenotype correlation in affected individuals of a family with a deletion of the entire coding sequence of the connexin 32 gene. *Hum Genet* **103**:242, 1998.

325. Deschênes SM, Walcott JL, Wexier TL, Scherer SS, Fischbeck KH: Altered trafficking of mutant connexin32. *J Neurosci* **17**:9077, 1997.

326. Bruzzone R, White TW, Scherer SS, Fischbeck KH, Paul DL: Null mutations of connexin32 in patients with X-linked Charcot-Marie-Tooth disease. *Neuron* **13**:1253, 1994.

327. Ressot C, Gomès D, Dautigny A, Pham-Dinh D, Bruzzone R: Connexin32 mutations associated with X-linked Charcot-Marie-Tooth disease show two distinct behaviors: Loss of function and altered gating properties. *J Neurosci* **18**:4063, 1998.

328. Omori Y, Mesnil M, Yamasaki H: Connexin 32 mutations from X-linked Charcot-Marie-Tooth disease patients: Functional defects and dominant negative effects. *Mol Biol Cell* **7**:907, 1996.

329. Oh S, Ri Y, Bennett MVL, Trexler EB, Verselis VK, Bargiello TA: Changes in permeability caused by connexin 32 mutations underlie X-linked Charcot-Marie-Tooth disease. *Neuron* **19**:927, 1997.

330. Yoshimura T, Satake M, Ohnishi A, Tsutsumi Y, Fujikura Y: Mutations of connexin-32 in Charcot-Marie-Tooth disease type X interfere with cell-to-cell communication but not cell proliferation and myelin-specific gene expression. *J Neurosci Res* **51**:154, 1998.

331. Sahenk Z, Chen L: Abnormalities in the axonal cytoskeleton induced by a connexin32 mutation in nerve xenografts. *J Neurosci Res* **51**:174, 1998.

332. Anzini P, Neuberg DH-H, Schachner M, Nelles E, Willecke K, Zielasek J, Toyka KV, et al: Structural abnormalities and deficient maintenance of peripheral nerve myelin in mice lacking the gap junction protein connexin 32. *J Neurosci* **17**:4545, 1997.

333. Scherer SS, Xu Y-T, Nelles E, Fischbeck EK, Willecke K, Bone LJ: Connexin32-null mice develop demyelinating peripheral neuropathy. *Glia* **24**:8, 1998.

334. Abel A, Bone LJ, Messing A, Scherer SS, Fischbeck KH: Studies in transgenic mice indicate a loss of connexin 32 function in X-linked Charcot-Marie-Tooth disease. *J Neuropath Exp Neurol* **58**:702, 1999.

335. Scherer SS, Bone LJ, Abel A, Deschênes SM, Balice-Gordon R, Fishbeck K: The role of the gap junction protein connexin32 in the pathogenesis of X-linked Charcot-Marie-Tooth disease, in Cardew G (ed): *Gap Junction-Mediated Intercellular Signalling in Health and Disease*. Novartis Foundation Symposium Vol. 219. New York, John Wiley & Sons, 1999, p. 175.

336. Joseph LJ, Le Beau MM, Jamieson GA Jr, Acharya S, Shows TB, Rowley JD, Sukhatme VP: Molecular cloning, sequencing, and mapping of *EGR2*, a human early growth response gene encoding a protein with "zinc-binding finger" structure. *Proc Natl Acad Sci U S A* **85**:7164, 1988.

337. Rangnekar VM, Aplin AC, Sukhatme VP: The serum and TPA responsive promoter and intron-exon structure of *EGR2*, a human early growth response gene encoding a zinc finger protein. *Nucleic Acids Res* **18**:2749, 1990.

338. Chavrier P, Zerial M, Lemaire P, Almendral J, Bravo R, Charnay P: A gene encoding a protein with zinc fingers is activated during G0/G1 transition in cultured cells. *EMBO J* **7**:29, 1988.

339. Chavrier P, Janssen-Timmen U, Mattéi M-G, Zerial M, Bravo R, Charnay P: Structure, chromosome location, and expression of the mouse zinc finger gene *Krox-20*: Multiple gene products and coregulation with the protoncogene c-*fos*. *Mol Cell Biol* **9**:787, 1989.

340. Vesque C, Charnay P: Mapping functional regions of the segment-specific transcription factor Krox-20. *Nucleic Acids Res* **20**:2485, 1992.

341. Nardelli J, Gibson TJ, Vesque C, Charnay P: Base sequence discrimination by zinc-finger DNA-binding domains. *Nature* **349**:175, 1991.

342. Zorick TS, Syroid DE, Arroyo E, Scherer SS, Lemke G: The transcription factors SCIP and Krox-20 mark distinct stages and cell fates in Schwann cell differentiation. *Mol Cell Neurosci* **8**:129, 1996.

343. Kioussi C, Gruss P: Making of a Schwann. *Trends Genet* **12**:84, 1996.

344. Swiatek PJ, Gridley T: Perinatal lethality and defects in hindbrain development in mice homozygous for a targeted mutation of the zinc finger gene *Krox20*. *Genes Dev* **7**:2071, 1993.

345. Schneider-Maunoury S, Topilko P, Seitanidou T, Levi G, Cohen-Tannoudji M, Pournin S, Babinet C, et al: Disruption of *Krox-20* results in alteration of rhombomeres 3 and 5 in the developing hindbrain. *Cell* **75**:1199, 1993.

346. Topilko P, Schneider-Maunoury S, Levi G, Baron-Van Evercooren A, Chennoufi ABY, Seitanidou T, Babinet C, et al: *Krox-20* controls myelination in the peripheral nervous system. *Nature* **371**:796, 1994.

347. Bermingham JR Jr, Scherer SS, O'Connell S, Arroyo E, Kalla K, Powell FL, Rosenfeld MG: Tst-1/Oct-6/SCIP regulates a unique step in peripheral myelination and is required for normal respiration. *Genes Dev* **10**:1751, 1996.

348. Warner LE, Mancias P, Butler IJ, McDonald CM, Keppen L, Koob KG, Lupski JR: Mutations in the early growth response 2 (*EGR2*) gene are associated with hereditary myelinopathies. *Nat Genet* **18**:382, 1998.

349. Timmerman V, De Jonghe P, Ceuterick C, De Vriendt E, Debrabandere S, Löfgren A, Nelis E, et al: A novel dominant mutation in the early growth response 2 (*EGR2*) gene associated with a Dejerine-Sottas syndrome (DSS) phenotype. *Neurology* **52**:1827, 1999.

350. Botti S, Pareyson D, Sghirlanzoni A, Nemni R, Riva D, Taroni F: Mutations in the transcription factor *EGR2* in patients with severe hereditary demyelinating neuropathies. *Am J Hum Genet* **63**:A352, 1998.

351. Russo MW, Sevetson BR, Milbrandt J: Identification of NAB1, a repressor of NGFI-A- and Krox20-mediated transcription. *Proc Natl Acad Sci U S A* **92**:6873, 1995.

352. Svaren J, Sevetson BR, Apel ED, Zimonjic DB, Popescu NC, Milbrandt J: NAB2, a corepressor of NGFI-A (Egr-1) and Krox20, is

induced by proliferative and differentiative stimuli. *Mol Cell Biol* **16**:3545, 1996.

353. Russo MW, Matheny C, Milbrandt J: Transcriptional activity of the zinc finger protein NGFI-A is influenced by its interaction with a cellular factor. *Mol Cell Biol* **13**:6858, 1993.

354. Warner LE, Svaren J, Milbrandt J, Lupski JR: Functional consequences of mutations in the early growth response 2 (*EGR2*) gene correlate with severity of human myelinopathies. *Hum Mol Genet* **8**:1245, 1999.

355. Swirnoff AH, Milbrandt J: DNA-binding specificity of NGFI-A and related zinc finger transcription factors. *Mol Cell Biol* **15**:2275, 1995.

356. Lee MS, Gippert GP, Soman KV, Case DA, Wright PE: Three-dimensional solution structure of a single zinc finger DNA-binding domain. *Science* **245**:635, 1989.

357. Brown RS, Argos P: Fingers and helices. *Nature* **324**:215, 1986.

358. Berg JM: Proposed structure for the zinc-binding domains from transcription factor IIIA and related proteins. *Proc Natl Acad Sci U S A* **85**:99, 1988.

359. Gibson TJ, Postma JPM, Brown RS, Argos P: A model for the tertiary structure of the 28 residue DNA-binding motif ("zinc finger") common to many eukaryotic transcriptional regulatory proteins. *Protein Eng* **2**:209, 1988.

360. Pavletich NP, Pabo CO: Zinc finger-DNA recognition: crystal structure of a Zif268-DNA complex at 2.1Å. *Science* **252**:809, 1991.

361. Wilson TE, Day ML, Pexton T, Padgett KA, Johnston M, Milbrandt J: In vivo mutational analysis of the NGFI-A zinc fingers. *J Biol Chem* **267**:3718, 1992.

361a. Kalaydjieva L, Gresham D, Gooding R, Heather L, Baas F, de Jonge R, Blechschmidt K, et al: N-myc downstream-regulated gene 1 is mutated in hereditary motor and sensory neuropathy-Lom. *Am J Hum Genet* **67**:47, 2000.

361b. Bolino A, Muglia M, Conforti FL, LeGuern E, Salih MAM, Georgiou D-M, Christodoulou K, et al: Charcot-Marie-Tooth type 4B is caused by mutations in the gene encoding the myotubularin-related protein-2. *Nat Genet* **25**:17, 2000.

361c. Mersiyanova IV, Perepelov AV, Polyakov AV, Sitnikov VF, Dadali EL, Oparin RB, Petrin AN, et al: A new variant of Charcot-Marie-Tooth disease type 2 is probably the result of a mutation in the neurofilament-light gene. *Am J Hum Genet* **67**:37, 2000.

362. Werner H, Jung M, Klugman M, Sereda M, Griffith IR, Nave K-A: Mouse models of myelin diseases. *Brain Pathol* **8**:771, 1998.

363. Thomas PK, Marques W Jr, Davis MB, Sweeney MG, King RHM, Bradley JL, Muddle JR, et al: The phenotypic manifestations of chromosome 17p11.2 duplication. *Brain* **120**:465, 1997.

364. Auer-Grumbach M, Strasser-Fuchs S, Wagner K, Körner E, Fazekas F: Roussy-Lévy syndrome is a phenotypic variant of Charcot-Marie-Tooth syndrome IA associated with a duplication on chromosome 17p11.2. *J Neurol Sci* **154**:72, 1998.

365. Uncini A, Di Muzio A, Chiavaroli F, Gambi D, Sabatelli M, Archidiacono N, Antonacci R, et al: Hereditary motor and sensory neuropathy with calf hypertrophy is associated with 17p11.2 duplication. *Ann Neurol* **35**:552, 1994.

366. Krampitz DE, Wolfe GI, Fleckenstein JL, Barohn RJ: Charcot-Marie-Tooth disease type 1A presently as calf hypertrophy and muscles cramps. *Neurology* **51**:1508, 1998.

367. Harding AE, Thomas PK: Distal and scapuloperoneal distribution of muscle involvement occurring within a family with type I hereditary motor and sensory neuropathy. *J Neurol* **224**:17, 1980.

368. Ronen GM, Lowry N, Wedge JH, Sarnat HB, Hill A: Hereditary motor sensory neuropathy type I presenting as scapuloperoneal atrophy (Davidenkow syndrome) electrophysiological and pathological studies. *Can J Neurol Sci* **13**:264, 1986.

369. Abe Y, Ikegami T, Hayasaka K, Tanno Y, Watanabe T, Sugiyama Y, Yamamoto T: Pressure palsy as the initial presentation in a case of late-onset Charcot-Marie-Tooth disease type 1A. *Intern Med* **36**:501, 1997.

370. Gutmann L, Fakadej A, Riggs JE: Evolution of nerve conduction abnormalities in children with dominant hypertrophic neuropathy of the Charcot-Marie-Tooth type. *Muscle Nerve* **6**:515, 1983.

371. Garcia CA, Malamut RE, England JD, Parry GS, Liu P, Lupski JR: Clinical variability in two pairs of identical twins with the Charcot-Marie-Tooth disease type 1A duplication. *Neurology* **45**:2090, 1995.

372. Birouk N, Gouider R, Le Guern E, Gugenheim M, Tardieu S, Maisonobe T, Le Forestier N, et al: Charcot-Marie-Tooth disease type 1A with 17p11.2 duplication: Clinical and electrophysiological phenotype study and factors influencing disease severity in 119 cases. *Brain* **120**:813, 1997.

373. Cruz-Martínez A, Bort S, Arpa J, Duarte J, Palau F: Clinical, genetic and electrophysiologic correlation in hereditary neuropathy with liability to pressure palsies with involvement of *PMP22* gene at chromosome 17p11.2. *Eur J Neurol* **4**:274, 1997.

374. Potocki L, Chen K-S, Koeuth T, Killian J, Iannaccone ST, Shapira SK, Kashork CD, et al: DNA rearrangements on both homologues of chromosome 17 in a mildly delayed individual with a family history of autosomal dominant carpal tunnel syndrome. *Am J Hum Genet* **64**:471, 1999.

375. Tyson J, Malcolm S, Thomas PK, Harding AE: Deletions of chromosome 17p11.2 in multifocal neuropathies. *Ann Neurol* **39**:180, 1996.

376. Roa BB, Ananth U, Garcia CA, Lupski JR: Molecular diagnosis of CMT1A and HNPP. *Lab Med Int* **12**:22, 1995.

377. Sghirlanzoni A, Pareyson D, Balestrini MR, Bellone E, Berta E, Ciano C, Mandich P, et al: HMSN III phenotype due to homozygous expression of a dominant HMSN II gene. *Neurology* **42**:2201, 1992.

378. Marrosu MG, Vaccargiu S, Marrosu G, Vannelli A, Cianchetti C, Muntoni F: Charcot-Marie-Tooth disease type 2 associated with mutation of the myelin protein zero gene. *Neurology* **50**:1397, 1998.

379. De Jonghe P, Timmerman V, Ceuterick C, Nelis E, De Vriendt E, Löfgren A, Vercruyssen A, et al: The Thr124Met mutation in the peripheral myelin protein zero (MPZ) is associated with a clinically distinct Charcot-Marie-Tooth phenotype. *Brain* **122**:281, 1999.

380. Kovach MJ, Lin J-P, Bodyadjiev S, Campbell K, Mazzeo L, Herman K, Rimer LA, et al: A unique point mutation in the *PMP22* gene is associated with Charcot-Marie-Tooth disease and deafness. *Am J Hum Genet* **64**:1580, 1999.

381. Stojkovic T, Latour P, Vandenberghe A, Hurtevent JF, Vermersch P: Sensorineural deafness in X-linked Charcot-Marie-Tooth disease with connexin 32 mutation (R142Q). *Neurology* **52**:1010, 1999.

382. Bahr M, Andres F, Timmerman V, Nelis ME, Van Broeckhoven C, Dichgans J: Central visual, acoustic, and motor pathway involvement in a Charcot-Marie-Tooth family with an Asn205Ser mutation in the connexin 32 gene. *J Neurol Neurosurg Psychiatry* **66**:202, 1999.

383. Bird TD, Kraft GH: Charcot-Marie-Tooth disease: Data for genetic counseling relating age to risk. *Clin Genet* **14**:43, 1978.

384. Nicholson GA: Penetrance of the hereditary motor and sensory neuropathy Ia mutation: assessment by nerve conduction studies. *Neurology* **41**:547, 1991.

385. Kaku DA, Parry GJ, Malamut R, Lupski JR, Garcia CA: Uniform slowing of conduction velocities in Charcot-Marie-Tooth polyneuropathy type 1. *Neurology* **43**:2664, 1993.

386. Killian JM, Tiwari PS, Jacobson S, Jackson RD, Lupski JR: Longitudinal studies of the duplication form of Charcot-Marie-Tooth polyneuropathy. *Muscle Nerve* **19**:74, 1996.

387. Sahenk Z, Chen L, Mendell JR: Effects of *PMP22* duplication and deletions on the axonal cytoskeleton. *Ann Neurol* **45**:16, 1999.

388. Scherer S: Axonal pathology in demyelinating diseases. *Ann Neurol* **45**:6, 1999.

389. Bird TD, Kraft GH, Lipe H, Kenney KL, Sumi SM: Clinical and pathological phenotype of the original family with Charcot-Marie-Tooth type 1B: A 20-year study. *Ann Neurol* **41**:463, 1997.

390. García A, Combarros O, Calleja J, Berciano J: Charcot-Marie-Tooth disease type 1A with 17p duplication in infancy and early childhood: A longitudinal clinical and electrophysiologic study. *Neurology* **50**:1061, 1998.

391. Lupski JR: DNA diagnostics for Charcot-Marie-Tooth disease and related inherited neuropathies. *Clin Chem* **42**:995, 1996.

392. Ouvrier R: Correlation between the histopathologic, genotypic, and phenotypic features of hereditary peripheral neuropathies in childhood. *J Child Neurol* **11**:133, 1996.

393. Hensels GW, Janssen EAM, Hoogendijk JE, Valentijn LJ, Baas F, Bolhuis PA: Quantitative measurement of duplicated DNA as a diagnostic test for Charcot-Marie-Tooth disease type 1A. *Clin Chem* **39**:1845, 1993.

394. Blair IP, Kennerson ML, Nicholson GA: Detection of Charcot-Marie-Tooth type 1A duplication by the polymerase chain reaction. *Clin Chem* **41**:1105, 1995.

395. Stronach EA, Clark C, Bell C, Löfgren A, McKay NG, Timmerman V, Van Broeckhoven C, et al: Novel PCR-based diagnostic tools for Charcot-Marie-Tooth type 1A and hereditary neuropathy with liability to pressure palsies. *J Peripher Nerv Syst* **4**:117, 1999.

396. Shaffer LG, Kennedy GM, Spikes AS, Lupski JR: Diagnosis of CMT1A duplications and HNPP deletions by interphase FISH: Implications for testing in the cytogenetics laboratory. *Am J Med Genet* **69**:325, 1997.

397. Kashork CD, Lupski JR, Shaffer LG: Prenatal diagnosis of Charcot-Marie-Tooth disease type 1A by interphase fluorescence *in situ* hybridization. *Prenat Diagn* **19**:446, 1999.

398. Navon R, Timmerman V, Löfgren A, Liang P, Nelis E, Zeitune M, Van Broeckhoven C: Prenatal diagnosis of Charcot-Marie-Tooth disease type 1A (CMT1A) using molecular genetic techniques. *Prenat Diagn* **15**:633, 1995.

399. De Vos A, Sermon K, Van de Velde H, Joris H, Vandervorst M, Lissens W, Mortier G, et al: Pregnancy after preimplantation genetic diagnosis for Charcot-Marie-Tooth disease type 1A. *Mol Hum Reprod* **4**:978, 1998.

400. Garcia CA: Familial neuropathies, in Johnson RT, Griffin JW (eds): *Current Therapy in Neurologic Disease*, 5th ed. St. Louis, Mosby-Year Book, 1997, p 386.

401. Njegovan ME, Leonard EI, Joseph FB: Rehabilitation medicine approach to Charcot-Marie-Tooth disease. *Pediatr Podiatry* **14**:99, 1997.

402. Mazzarella R, Schlessinger D: Pathological consequences of sequence duplications in the human genome. *Genome Res* **8**:1007, 1998.

# Pelizaeus-Merzbacher Disease and the Allelic Disorder X-linked Spastic Paraplegia Type 2

*Lynn D. Hudson*

1. Pelizaeus-Merzbacher disease (PMD) (MIM 312080), together with the allelic disorder spastic paraplegia type 2 (SPG2) (MIM 312920), which also maps to Xq22, are leukodystrophies of widely varying severity. PMD is characterized chiefly by impaired motor development that presents within the first year and progresses throughout life: nystagmus, ataxia, spasticity, and mental retardation are usually encountered. SPG2 patients display spasticity of the lower limbs. In patients with the complicated form of SPG2, cerebellar ataxia, sensory loss, nystagmus, and optic atrophy may also be present.

2. A loss of myelin is evident by MRI or histopathology in both PMD and SPG2, and a loss of oligodendrocytes is obvious in the severe connatal form of PMD. Abnormal central nervous system conduction velocities, as analyzed by evoked potentials, reflect the myelin defect.

3. Mutations in the X-linked PLP gene (GenBank M27110), which encodes the major central nervous system myelin protein (PLP) and its alternatively spliced isoform DM20, are responsible for the pathogenesis of PMD and SPG2. Females are affected only infrequently in PMD, but in the relatively mild SPG2 the PLP mutation can act semidominantly.

4. Animal models exist that have the identical mutation found in the human form of the disease: the *jimpy^msd* mouse for the connatal form of PMD and the *jimpy^rsh* mouse for the complicated form of SPG2.

5. PLP is a gene subject to dosage control, as overexpression of PLP is the most common type of mutation in PMD. Transgenic mice carrying multiple copies of PLP mimic the phenotype of PLP duplications found in the classical form of PMD.

6. At a cellular level, the extent of pathophysiology in PMD/SPG2 can be correlated with the type of mutation in the PLP gene. In the most severe mutations (the connatal form of PMD), nascent PLP and DM20 accumulate in the rough endoplasmic reticulum of oligodendrocytes and trigger apoptosis. Less severe mutations spare DM20, which can traffic to the sites of myelin assembly and participate in

myelin sheath formation. Abnormal PLP and DM20 proteins generate phenotypes that span the PMD/SPG2 spectrum, while either too much or too little of these lipoproteins leads to intermediate phenotypes, such as the classical form of PMD or the complicated form of SPG2.

## HISTORY AND CLASSIFICATION

Friedrich Pelizaeus published the first clinical picture of Pelizaeus-Merzbacher disease in 1885, and managed to pinpoint the mode of inheritance by including a quote from the affected family "that the disease is passed on by the mother but does not hurt her."[1] Twenty-five years later, Ludwig Merzbacher documented a widespread loss of myelin in the cortical white matter of the original family examined by Pelizaeus.[2] A high degree of similarity of what is now known as the classical form of Pelizaeus-Merzbacher disease was found among the 12 male family members, with onset in the first months of life. Initially, the disease manifested itself by aimless, wandering eye movements, followed by nystagmus. Infants failed to develop normal head control, displayed tremors or shaking movements of the head, and may have had microcephaly. The disease was slowly progressive, with additional signs including bradylalia, scanning speech, ataxia and intention tremor of the upper limbs, spastic contractions of the lower limbs, athetotic movements, mild dementia, and death in the second decade.[1,2]

Franz Seitelberger reported a much more severe disorder, detectable at birth, in which the nearly complete absence of myelin sheaths was accompanied by a profound loss of myelin-forming cells (oligodendrocytes) in the central nervous system.[3] Seitelberger correctly identified both this connatal form (type II) and the classical form (type I) of PMD as leukodystrophies; that is, conditions in which the absence of myelin is primary. Although originally described as a "demyelinating" (destruction of myelin) disorder, the pathology of the connatal form of PMD is that of a "dysmyelinating" (inability to form normal myelin) disease. A transitional intermediate (type III) between the classical and connatal forms of PMD has also been described,[4,5] but the extensive overlap of this type with the classical and connatal forms, together with intrafamilial heterogeneity in the clinical findings of all types (particularly with respect to the age of death and the extent of cerebellar dysfunction), speaks for limiting the classification to the classical and connatal forms of PMD. Additional variants have been described,[5] but the absence of X-linkage in these disorders genotypically distinguishes them from PMD.

A list of standard abbreviations is located immediately preceding the index in each volume. Additional abbreviations used in this chapter include: DM20 = an isoform of proteolipid protein with a MW of 20 kDa; PLP = proteolipid protein; PMD = Pelizaeus-Merzbacher disease; RER = rough endoplasmic reticulum; SPG2 = X-linked spastic paraplegia type 2.

A distinct clinical entity, X-linked spastic paraplegia type 2 (SPG2), was recently discovered by Odile Boespflug-Tanguy and colleagues to be an allelic disorder with PMD.[6] A combination of studies led to this unexpected finding: (a) the mapping of SPG2 to the Xq21 region, where linkage studies had previously placed PMD; (b) commonalities in the clinical presentation of PMD and the complicated form of SPG2, namely spasticity, nystagmus, cerebellar ataxia, and a pyramidal syndrome; (c) the detection of hypomyelination in a complicated form of SPG2; and (d) the observation that several PMD families included a family member diagnosed as having the rare spastic paraplegia disorder.[7] The X-linked form of spastic paraplegia type 2 exists as either a complicated form or a pure one in which the clinical phenotype is confined to lower limb spasticity. Both the pure and complicated forms of SPG2 arise from mutations in the gene encoding the myelin proteolipid protein (PLP), the same gene affected in PMD.[6–12] The detection of families in which PMD and SPG2 coexist[7,8] emphasizes the clinical continuum of these disorders, all of which share a phenotype of spasticity and hypomyelination.

## CLINICAL FEATURES

The common feature of lower limb spasticity unites the four clinically distinct categories of PMD/SPG2. Distinguishing features among the PMD/SPG2 subtypes include the presence or absence of nystagmus, cerebellar signs, optic atrophy, laryngeal stridor, dystonia, and the extent of developmental delays due to motor impairment.[7,14,15] The severity of the disease ranges from the most severely affected connatal form of PMD, the classical form of PMD, the complicated form of SPG2, and to the least affected pure form of SPG2.

### Pelizaeus-Merzbacher: Connatal (Type II) Form

The connatal form of PMD is apparent within the first few months after birth, and affected males display a nearly complete lack of psychomotor development.[4,5,16–19] Progression of the disease is rapid, with death usually occurring in the first decade. Severe feeding problems and extrapyramidal dyskinesia are early indicators of the connatal form of PMD. Prominently featured are nystagmus (roving, horizontal, or rotatory), titubation, dysarthria, optic atrophy, seizures, ataxia, and spasticity that progresses to contractures in the extremities.[4,7,14–19] The movement disorder includes head-nodding, eye-rolling, involuntary jerking of the head, eyes, or limb, and continuous random uncoordinated movement. Laryngeal stridor is often seen in these patients.[17,18]

### Pelizaeus-Merzbacher: Classical (Type I) Form

Onset of the classical form of PMD is usually noted within the first year of life, with motor handicaps as the outstanding feature.[1,2,7,14,15,17–19] Unlike the connatal form of PMD, classical types can improve in performance up to 10 to 12 years of age before a slow deterioration ensues with death occurring in mid adulthood.[7] Nystagmus is evident early, together with generalized hypotonia, slowness of motor development, head tremor, and trunk ataxia. Nystagmus may disappear on maturation, and bilateral optic atrophy may develop. Spasticity and pathologic reflexes of the lower limbs, ataxia, athetotic movements of the upper extremities, and dysarthria accompany the delayed motor development. Speech and motor deficits make it difficult to determine the extent of mental retardation.

In a mild variety of classical PMD associated with duplications of the PLP gene, the age of onset is unchanged, but the life expectancy is extended to 60 years, indicating that the progression of the disease is comparatively slow in this type of PLP mutation.[20] Nystagmus, pyramidal tract signs, and cerebellar involvement are all evident shortly after birth in these families, but features such as laryngeal stridor, optic atrophy, and dementia are not commonly encountered.[20]

## SPG2: Complicated Form

All forms of the rare SPG2 display spasticity and weakness in the lower extremities, but the complicated form has additional signs in common with PMD, which may include nystagmus, optic atrophy, ataxia, and cerebellar syndrome of the upper limbs with dysarthria.[6,7,11,13,21,22] Unlike PMD, no hypotonia, choreoathetosis, or bobbing movements of the head or trunk are evident. Patients with the complicated form of SPG2 have slowly progressive weakness and spasticity of the lower extremities, and at the onset of the disease (2 to 5 years) may appear to have the pure form of SPG2. Nystagmus occurs at a later onset than PMD, and only half of the patients have optic atrophy. Patients may be delayed in the age of walking (15 to 36 months), but can walk unaided for a long period. Mental retardation, when present, is mild, and most patients attend school.[6]

## SPG2: Pure Form

The pure form of SPG2 presents with spasticity of gait and increased deep tendon reflexes, all in the absence of other neurologic deficits.[9,11,12] The age of onset can range from toddler to teen years within a family. Like the complicated form of SPG2, the pure form is slowly progressive and the life span is nearly normal. Cognitive function is normal. More spasticity is seen in the legs than in the arms, and intention tremors may also be present.

## NEUROIMAGING, NEUROPATHOLOGY AND NEUROPHYSIOLOGY

The myelin sheath in the central nervous system is a specialized extension of the oligodendrocyte plasma membrane that successively enwraps axons, thereby permitting fast saltatory conduction of nerve impulses. Myelin formation begins prenatally, but the most rapid changes in myelination occur within the first eight postnatal months.[23,24] In general, sensory pathways tend to myelinate prior to motor pathways (unlike the peripheral nervous system). While central nervous system myelination is largely complete at the age of 2, myelination in regions of the cerebral hemispheres involved in higher-level associative functions and sensory discrimination progresses over a decade.[24] Mutations in myelin proteins that compromise the synthesis of a normal myelin sheath are, therefore, expected to present at an early developmental stage as "dysmyelinating" (inability to form normal myelin) disorders. PMD patients, for the most part, exhibit the neuroimaging and neuropathologic features of dysmyelinating disorders, in which a reduction in the amount of myelin (hypomyelination) is apparent early and signs of myelin breakdown may be prominent subsequently. "Demyelinating" (destruction of myelin) disorders are ones in which problems arise not in the synthesis but in the maintenance of myelin sheaths. Mutations that have only subtle effects on myelin structure may permit an ostensibly "normal" myelin sheath to be synthesized, but this sheath may be structurally unsound and therefore more susceptible to turnover, which can present as a demyelinating disorder.

All forms of PMD/SPG2 have hypomyelination, a feature that can be detected by magnetic resonance imaging (MRI), pathologic exam of central nervous system tissue, and/or analysis of central evoked potentials.[4,7,14,15,17,18] MRI typically shows diffuse hyperintense white matter signal in T2-weighted images, as apparent in Fig. 228-1. PMD patients generally have a homogeneous pattern of myelin loss throughout the central nervous system, with the less-affected classical PMD patients displaying small scattered areas of normal signal resembling the "tigroid pattern" described in the histopathology of the disease.[25] The MRI abnormalities can be detected in PMD patients with the severe connatal form of the disease as early as 3 months of age.[26] MRI diffusion-weighted images can be used to distinguish between dysmyelinating and demyelinating lesions—dysmyelinating lesions maintain diffusional anisotropy, whereas demyelinating

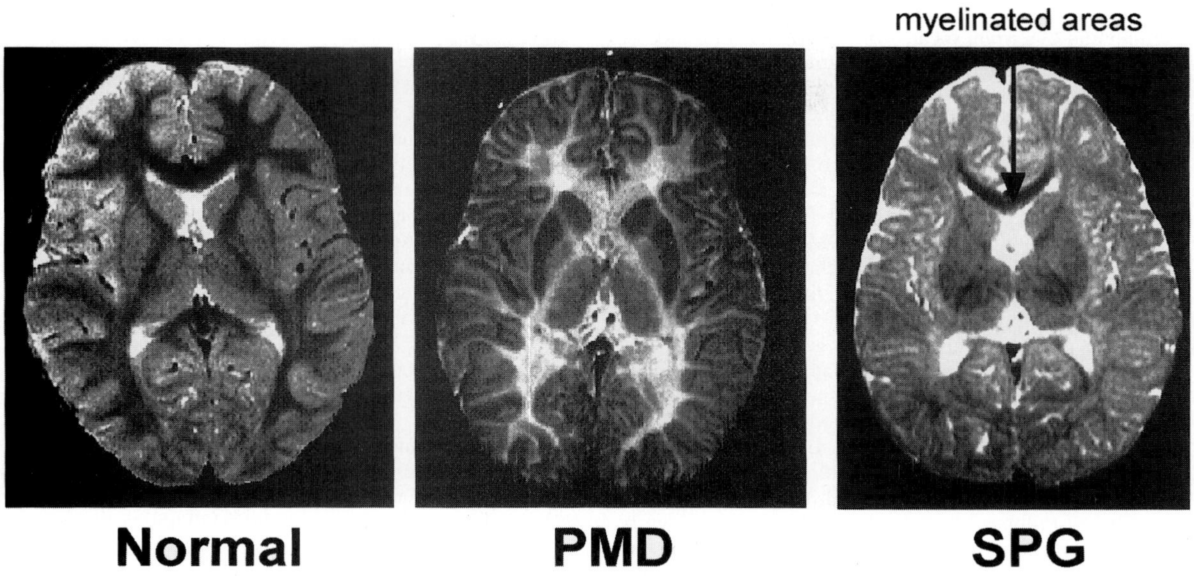

myelinated areas

**Normal**        **PMD**        **SPG**

**Fig. 228-1.** Pathology of SPG2 and PMD detected by MRI. T$_2$-weighted cerebral MRI images of a normal (3 years of age), PMD-affected (3 years of age), and SPG-affected (10 years of age) boy. In the white matter of the PMD-affected boy, a diffuse high-intensity signal is present instead of a diffuse hyposignal (seen in the normal control) that occurs when myelination has been normally achieved. Some myelinated areas (arrow) are observed in the white matter of the SPG-affected patient. (*Provided by and used with permission of Dr. O. Boespflug-Tanguy, INSERM, Cedex, France*).

lesions lose it.[27] This technique has been applied to a PMD patient who displayed the diffusional anisotropy of a dysmyelinating lesion.[27] SPG2 patients often show a heterogeneous, patchy pattern consisting of occasional extensively myelinated regions (arrow in Fig. 228-1),[7] generally with a later onset and a more variable presentation than in PMD patients. The pure and complicated forms of SPG2 are not distinguishable by MRI, as both have a diffuse hyperintense signal in white matter, and the less clinically severe pure form of SPG2 can present with a global lack of myelination, sparing of only a few transverse fibers in the pons.[12]

On histopathologic exam, the striking loss of white matter in PMD can be seen even without the benefit of dyes that stain myelin. Connatal forms of PMD may have a nearly complete absence of myelin, with few degradation products apparent.[4] Islands of myelin are preserved in the classical form of PMD, giving rise to the characteristic "tigroid" appearance. The myelin sheaths in such islands appear abnormal and remnants of myelin are found in vacuoles of surrounding cells, including astrocytes. Fibrillary gliosis occurs in affected areas, and some hypertrophic astrocytes are evident. Axonal pathology and neuronal loss can occur in affected areas.[4,17] Oligodendrocytes can be reduced in number, and often show abnormal cytoplasmic inclusions and condensed chromatin granules in the nuclei characteristic of apoptotic cells.[28] The lack of myelin extends to the grey matter, where a small number of oligodendrocytes normally reside. The peripheral nervous system is normally myelinated, although a PMD family with a mild form of the disease was recently found to have a loss of peripheral myelinated fibers, detectable degradation of myelin sheaths, and a slowing of peripheral nerve conduction.[29]

As anticipated in disorders of defective central nervous system myelination, PMD patients have extensive conduction slowing involving the brain stem to the cerebrum.[7,14,15,17,18,30-33] Conduction blocks are prominent in motor rather than sensory systems, as seen by electrophysiologic findings with brain stem auditory, somatosensory, motor, and visual evoked potentials. The visual evoked potentials can be particularly informative in young infants.[30] SPG patients also have abnormal central nervous system conduction velocities.[6,7]

## GENETICS AND MOLECULAR BIOLOGY OF PMD/SPG2

### The Proteolipid Protein (PLP) Gene Encodes a Major Myelin Protein

The most abundant protein in central nervous system myelin is proteolipid protein (PLP). An integral membrane protein, PLP is one of nature's most hydrophobic proteins due to the high content of hydrophobic amino acids (50 percent) and an unusual degree of fatty acid acylation (Fig. 228-2).[34,35] Despite the difficulties of working with a protein that is soluble only in organic solvents, Stoffel and coworkers managed to pinpoint the location of the covalently linked long chain fatty acids and to elucidate the

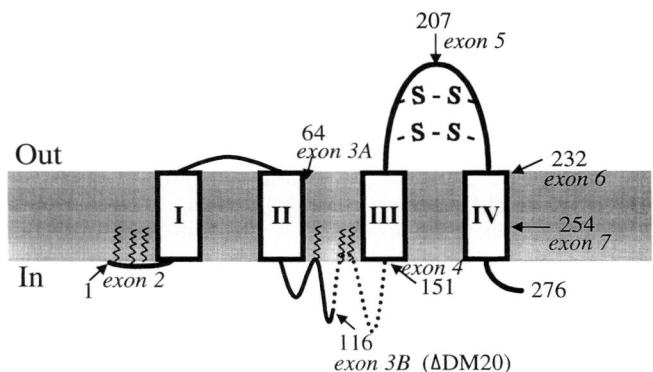

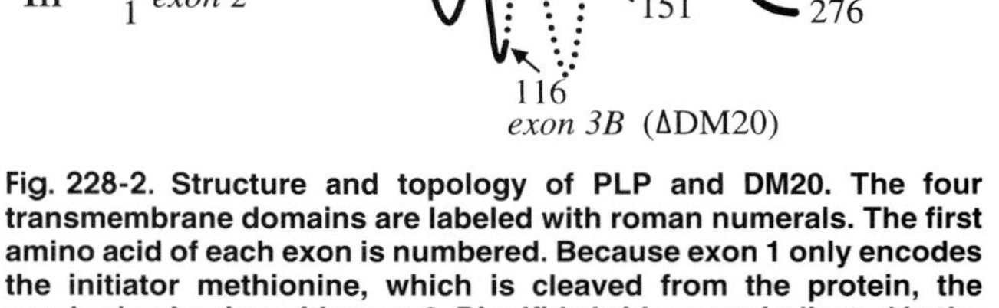

**Fig. 228-2.** Structure and topology of PLP and DM20. The four transmembrane domains are labeled with roman numerals. The first amino acid of each exon is numbered. Because exon 1 only encodes the initiator methionine, which is cleaved from the protein, the numbering begins with exon 2. Disulfide bridges are indicated in the large extracellular loop, and the fatty acids are denoted by squiggly lines. The exon 3B region that is deleted in DM20 is shown as a dotted line. During compaction of the layers of myelin membrane, the inside of the membrane becomes the major dense line and the outside becomes the intraperiod line of the myelin sheath. (*Adapted from Weimbs and Stoffel.*[36])

structure of PLP, which features four transmembrane domains with both the amino and C-termini located on the intracellular face of the membrane (Fig. 228-2).[34,36] Further structural studies have confirmed and extended the Stoffel model by demonstrating that the alternatively spliced isoform of PLP named DM20 shares the topology delineated for PLP.[37] DM20 is missing part of the intracellular loop that contains two of the six acylation sites (Fig. 228-2), which may account for the altered conformation and physical properties observed for DM20.[35,37,38] The overall structure and individual regions of PLP/DM20 resemble channel-forming regions of the nicotinic acetylcholine and glutamate receptor complexes,[39] and ionophoretic activity of PLP has been demonstrated in reconstituted systems.[35,38]

PLP is an exceptionally well-conserved gene: No amino acid differences exist between mouse, rat, and man, and no amino acid polymorphisms have been detected in any species. A single gene composed of 7 exons spread over 18 kb encodes PLP/DM20.[40–43] The first exon ends with the initiator methionine, which is cleaved off the nascent PLP/DM20 protein. The third exon contains an internal splice donor site, which is used to generate DM20 transcripts. The PLP locus is transcriptionally active in early prenatal development, at which time alternative splicing favors the DM20 transcript. Maturing oligodendrocytes orchestrate the expression of PLP/DM20 together with the other myelin proteins and lipids.[44] PLP/DM20 is synthesized in the rough endoplasmic reticulum and transported in vesicles to the sites of myelin assembly. Like PLP, DM20 is an abundantly produced myelin protein, with an estimated 1.6 ratio of PLP to DM20 protein.[45] DM20 has been proposed to facilitate, or chaperone, the movement of PLP to the cell surface.[46–49] In addition to being expressed in oligodendrocytes, the PLP gene is transcriptionally active in the myelin-forming cells of the peripheral nervous system, the Schwann cells,[50] where the predominant isoform expressed is DM20.[51] Schwann cell expression of PLP/DM20 is an order of magnitude lower than that observed in oligodendrocytes, and most of the proteins produced are not normally incorporated into the myelin sheath.[52] A low level of PLP expression also occurs outside of the nervous system, in the heart[53] and fetal thymus.[54]

## Animal Models of Pelizaeus-Merzbacher Disease/SPG2

Several of the animal models of PMD/SPG2 have the same mutation as in the human disease: *jimpy*[msd] for the connatal form of PMD[55,56] and *jimpy*[rsh] for the complicated form of SPG2.[8,10,57] The *jimpy*[msd] and *jimpy*[rsh] are alleles of *jimpy*, a strain in which hemizygous males containing the jimpy mutation display ataxia, tremor, and ultimately seizures commencing with the general onset of central nervous system myelination.[58] All of the mutant PLP animals have varying degrees of hypomyelination.[59] One of the most severely affected mutants, the *jimpy* mouse, has only 1.6 percent of control myelin in the spinal cord.[60] The biochemical profiles reflect the lack of myelin, with dramatic reductions in all myelin proteins. The residual myelin is in the patchy pattern seen as the "tigroid" pathology of PMD patients. The occasional myelin sheath may appear well-compacted but the intraperiod line, which is formed when the extracellular faces of oligodendrocyte plasma membrane are fused, can be abnormally condensed.[59] Most of the point mutations in the PLP gene feature a reduced number of mature oligodendrocytes, accompanied by a proliferation of immature oligodendrocytes and noticeable oligodendrocyte cell death.[61] A unique oligodendrocyte abnormality, grossly distended rough endoplasmic reticulum (RER), is present in several of the animal mutants (the *myelin deficient* rat and *shaking pup*).[59] This swelling of the RER may represent a general block or retardation in protein transport from the RER due to the abnormal folding and accumulation of the abundantly synthesized mutant PLP/DM20 protein. Distended RER has also been detected in oligodendrocytes from a PMD patient.[62] The other cell types in the central nervous system are secondarily affected in animals with PLP point mutations. Astrocytic hypertrophy is predominant, with

a peculiar invasion of astrocytic processes evident between the axon and the myelin sheath. Excessive numbers of microglia are found in the white matter during the period of the most cell death, a time consistent with a role for microglia in disposing of cell debris. Neuronal abnormalities, which appear subsequent to the myelin loss, include an accumulation of axonal organelles that are often segregated into giant spheroids.[59]

Moderate phenotypes predominate in the *rumpshaker* mouse (*jimpy*[rsh]),[57] the animal model for SPG2,[7,8,10] and the *paralytic tremor* rabbit.[63] Animals are long-lived and reproduce normally. In *jimpy*[rsh], oligodendrocytes are not subject to premature death and do not display cytoplasmic abnormalities. The astrocyte and microglial populations are likewise normal. Much more myelin is present in *jimpy*[rsh] mice,[57] but the myelin sheaths are structurally unstable.[64] The DM20 isoform is much less affected than PLP in *jimpy*[rsh] mice, as the myelin sheaths contain mutant DM20 but no PLP.[57]

Transgenic mice that are engineered as null for PLP/DM20 expression are only mildly affected.[65–67] Oligodendrocytes do not undergo premature cell death as in *jimpy* and *jimpy*[msd] mice. Nonetheless, the absence of PLP/DM20 noticeably alters compaction of the myelin sheath, an effect that is magnified with age.[65–67] The PLP-deficient mice suggest that neither PLP nor DM20 is essential for the normal development or differentiation of oligodendrocytes in rodents. A developmental role for PLP/DM20 had previously been indicated by the early expression of DM20 in wild-type mice and the paucity of mature oligodendrocytes in *jimpy* and *jimpy*[msd] mice with PLP point mutations. It is likely that other lipoproteins can partially substitute for PLP/DM20 in the transgenic null mice. Indeed, a proteolipid protein gene family exists, as identified by the cloning of a homologous neuronal membrane glycoprotein named M6/EMA[68,69] and related proteins expressed in sharks and rays.[39] The deletion of the PLP gene in man appears to have more serious phenotypic consequences (i.e., the classical form of PMD)[70] than those observed in transgenic mouse models, perhaps because the compensatory mechanism of alternative lipoprotein expression is not as effective in man.

The overexpression of PLP/DM20 in transgenic mice, on the other hand, has pronounced effects on myelination.[71–73] Multiple copies of the PLP gene on an autosome create severe hypomyelination, astrocytosis, and premature death. While the impact on PLP/DM20 mRNA levels was minor, little PLP protein was incorporated into myelin. Thus, increased PLP dosage leads to a translational or posttranslational arrest of PLP expression. Although the animal model differs from the duplications of the PLP gene found in a majority of patients with the classical form of PMD[7,14,20,74–77] in that three to seven copies of the PLP gene were present in the mouse, a similar phenotype occurs in both cases of PLP overexpression.

## X-linked Pattern of Inheritance

Two approaches led to the discovery of PLP mutations in PMD, and both were dependent on the assignment of PLP to the X chromosome in man[78,79] and mouse.[79,80] The first relied on the detection of a splicing defect in the PLP gene of *jimpy* mice[80–83] as the impetus for sequencing the PLP gene of PMD patients that had the same behavioral, biochemical, and morphologic profiles as *jimpy* mice.[43,84] A single base mutation substituting a charged amino acid for tryptophan in one of the transmembrane domains of PLP was found in this PMD family.[43] A large duplication of the Xq13-q22 region, which included PMD among the clinical phenotypes,[85] together with the mapping of PLP to the Xq21.2-q23 region[79] and linkage studies placing the PMD phenotype within that interval, enabled Hodes and coworkers to identify a point mutation in the PLP gene that segregated with the PMD phenotype.[86] Nearly 40 distinct point mutations in the coding regions or splice sites of the PLP gene have been subsequently identified in PMD or SPG families (Table 228-1), yet less than a quarter of the PMD/SPG patients have identifiable sequence

**Table 228-1**  **Mutations in the Proteolipid Protein Gene**

| Mutation Type | Exon | DM20 Spared | Clinical Phenotype | Affected Females | Animal Disorder | References |
|---|---|---|---|---|---|---|
| *Missense* | | | | | | |
| M0I | 1 | | PMD: Classical | + | | 89 |
| P14L | 2 | | PMD: Connatal | +¶ | | 86, 91 |
| F31V | 2 | | PMD | | | 103 |
| H36P | 2 | | | | *shaking* pup | 106 |
| H36Q | 2 | | | | *paralytic tremor* rabbit | 63 |
| A38S | 2 | | | | *jimpy*⁴ᴶ | 107 |
| T42I | 2 | | PMD | | | 108 |
| L45R | 2 | | PMD | | | 109 |
| F50S | 2 | | PMD | | | 7 |
| G73R | 3A | | PMD | | | 110 |
| T74P | 3A | | | | *myelin-deficient* rat | 111, 112 |
| T115K* | 3A | | PMD: Classical | + | | 90 |
| H139Y | 3B | + | SPG2: Complicated | + | | 6 |
| K150N* | 3B | +* | PMD | | | 101, 102 |
| T155I | 4 | | PMD: Classical | | | 113, 114 |
| W162R | 4 | | PMD: Connatal | | | 43 |
| V165E | 4 | | PMD: Classical | | | 92 |
| S169F | 4 | | SPG2: Pure | | | 12 |
| T181P | 4 | | PMD: Connatal | | | 115 |
| I186T | 4 | | SPG2: Complicated | | *jimpy*ʳˢʰ mouse | 10, 13, 57 |
| D202N | 4 | | PMD | | | 7 |
| D202H | 4 | | PMD: Classical | | | 110 |
| Y206C | 4 | | PMD | | | 99 |
| V208N | 5 | | PMD | | | 116 |
| P210L | 5 | | PMD | | | 116 |
| P215S | 5 | | PMD: Classical | | | 117 |
| G216S | 5 | | PMD: Connatal | | | 118, 119 |
| V218F | 5 | | PMD: Classical | | | 120 |
| G220C | 5 | | PMD: Connatal | | | 100 |
| L223P | 5 | | PMD: Connatal | | | 115 |
| S225P | 5 | | SPG2: Pure | | | 9 |
| F236S | 6 | | SPG2: Complicated | | | 121 |
| A241P | 6 | | PMD: Connatal | | | 122 |
| A242V | 6 | | PMD: Connatal | | *jimpy*ᵐˢᵈ mouse | 55, 56 |
| A248P | 6 | | PMD | | | 123 |
| *Nonsense* | | | | | | |
| W144X | 3B | + | SPG2/PMD | + | | 11, 93 |
| E233X | 6 | | SPG2/PMD | + | | 8 |
| *Frameshift* | | | | | | |
| del G3 | 1 | | PMD: Classical | +§ | | 29 |
| del/ins 583-9 | 4 | | PMD | | | 124 |
| insG772 | 7 | | PMD: Classical | | | 125 |
| *Deletions* | | | | | | |
| T117-V165 | 3B, 4 | | PMD: Connatal | | | 126 |
| A170-P172 | 4 | | PMD: Classical | | | 102 |
| entire gene | 1–7 | | PMD: Classical | | transgenic knockouts | 65–67, 70 |
| *Duplications* | | | | | | |
| entire gene | 1–7 | | PMD: Classical | | transgenic overexpressors | 20, 71–77 |
| *Splice sites* | | | | | | |
| A438T, exon 3B | 3 | +? | PMD | | | 127 |
| G → T, intron 3 | 4 | | PMD | | | 128 |
| A → G, intron 4 | 5 | | | | *jimpy* mouse | 81–83 |

The initiator methionine is numbered as amino acid zero, as the terminal methionine is removed from the protein following translation. The nucleotide sequencing numbering is according to Hodes et al.¹⁵ Mutations that should spare DM20 are indicated by +. Deletions are abbreviated del and insertions, ins.
* Splicing is anticipated to be affected in these mutations, as the base change alters the donor splice site at the 3′ end of either exon 3A (T115K) or exon 3B (K150N).
? This mutation would create an ideal consensus splice site AG | GT in the region of exon 3 where intra-exonic splicing normally occurs to generate the DM20 spliced isoform.
¶ Only a single female was affected in this large pedigree.
§ With a peripheral nervous system neuropathy.
An updated database of mutations in the PLP gene is available at http://www.med.wayne.edu/Neurology/plp.html

alterations in these regions.[7,13,14] The discovery by Malcolm and coworkers that PLP is a gene subject to dosage control[75] led to the current estimate that over half of PMD patients have duplications of the PLP gene.[7,14,20,74–77] There is also a significant fraction of PMD patients with no detectable PLP mutations, although a tight linkage exists between the PMD phenotype and markers of the Xq22 region in these families.[7,13,14,87] Given that the PLP gene dosage is strictly controlled, the mutations in these families probably reside in the *cis* regulatory elements that influence the levels of PLP gene expression. Linkage studies also figured prominently in the discovery that SPG2 results from mutations in the PLP gene.[6,9] Two loci on the X chromosome are associated with spastic paraplegia, SPG-1 resulting from mutations in the L1 neuronal cell adhesion molecule at Xq28 and SPG-2, which mapped to the PLP gene.[6,7,9,88]

PMD is usually inherited as an X-linked recessive.[7,13,14] No clinical phenotype or abnormal neuroimaging has been found in any mother carrying a PLP duplication. However, an occasional family with point mutations in the PLP gene will include affected female relatives.[6–8,11,29,89–93] Females heterozygous for PLP mutations are mosaics: one population of oligodendrocytes expresses normal PLP and synthesizes normal myelin sheaths, while the other population expresses a mutant form of PLP which, if these abnormal oligodendrocytes survive, would generate a defective sheath. The lack of phenotype in the vast majority of PMD female carriers can be attributed to the same phenomenon observed in female heterozygous *jimpy* mice or *myelin-deficient* rats, in which the dying mutant oligodendrocytes are gradually replaced by normal oligodendrocytes.[59,94] Most of the remaining population consequently consists of genotypically normal oligodendrocytes by early adulthood. Adult *myelin-deficient/+* females are morphologically and phenotypically normal with the possible exception of regions such as the optic nerve, where the migration of oligodendrocyte progenitors into the nerve occurs during only a brief window of time.[94] If enough normal progenitors do not enter the optic nerve in early development, there may not be enough normal cells to compensate for the apoptotic *myelin-deficient* oligodendrocytes. Another scenario that accounts for a PMD phenotype in females is unfortunate lyonization of the affected X chromosome, yielding only a very small population of normal oligodendrocyte progenitors to seed the central nervous system. Nonrandom inactivation of the affected X chromosome (the Lyon effect) occurs infrequently, and therefore is not expected to account for families with a large number of affected females. A family where the Lyon effect is a plausible explanation for an affected female is the large, multigeneration Indianapolis kindred with the connatal form of PMD in which only a single female was affected.[86,91]

Families with mild cases of PMD/SPG2 may paradoxically have more females involved, as the mutant oligodendrocytes can survive in these patients. Because the mutant oligodendrocytes are not overrun by normal oligodendrocytes in early development, they compete with the normal oligodendrocytes for axons and proceed to elaborate myelin sheaths that are structurally flawed. Over time, these sheaths are susceptible to degradation, a situation yielding a progressive loss of myelin characteristic of a "demyelinating" disease. The resultant clinical phenotype is that of an adult-onset neurodegenerative disorder with variable symptoms of spastic paraplegia[7] and/or PMD.[6–8,11,90,92,93] Over half of the SPG2 families, as well as null mutations, which give rise to a mild classical form of PMD, have affected females,[8,11,13,14,89,92,93] indicating a semidominant pattern of X-linked inheritance in these families (Table 228-1).

## Correlation of Phenotype and Genotype

Mutations at the PLP locus give rise to a clinical continuum ranging from a lack of motor development and early death in the severe connatal form of PMD to mild gait disturbances in the pure form of SPG2. While any sequence alteration in the PLP gene appears to yield a phenotype, the most dramatic disruption of

myelination occurs with certain missense mutations (Table 228-1). A model accounting for the distress inflicted on oligodendrocytes by missense mutations in PLP/DM20 has been formulated by Gow and Lazzarini, based on their observations that the intracellular trafficking of mutant PLP proteins is disrupted in transfected cells or in affected oligodendrocytes.[47,95] Mutant PLP gene products accumulate at their site of synthesis in the RER,[47,95] previously detected as grossly distended RER in PMD and in the animal models.[59] Point mutations in PLP/DM20 that eliminate the export of both DM20 and PLP from the RER are ones that create the most severe, connatal form of PMD, whereas mutations that selectively arrest PLP transport while allowing mutant DM20 to traffic to the plasma membrane result in the less severe classical form of PMD or spastic paraplegia.[47] Excessive amounts of misfolded proteins in the RER can lead to apoptosis of differentiated oligodendrocytes following axonal contact and up-regulation of myelin protein synthesis.[95] The toxic effects of mutant PLP and DM20 proteins are further illustrated by the inability of normal PLP/DM20 to correct the dysmyelinating phenotype in transgenic models[96,97] and by the enhanced survival of cultured affected oligodendrocytes treated with PLP/DM20 antisense oligodeoxynucleotides.[98]

Missense mutations are distributed equally between the transmembrane sections of PLP and the remainder of the protein. Nonetheless, mutational hot spots are evident. For the regions of the protein not embedded in the membrane, 70 percent of the missense mutations occur in the large extracellular loop derived from exons 4 and 5 (schematized in Fig. 228-2 and listed as D202N through S225P in Table 228-1). This loop, which in compact myelin would be located within the intraperiod line, may participate in protein-protein interactions crucial for myelin maintenance. Only three of the missense mutations in the PLP gene represent conservative amino acid changes, one of which (A242V) creates the most devastating impact on myelin formation in mouse and man,[55,56] and another (H139Y) that presents at the other end of the clinical spectrum with spastic paraplegia.[6] The remainder of the missense mutations impart obvious changes to the PLP structure; examples include the Y206C[99] and G220C[100] mutations, which would introduce cysteine residues into the disulfide bridge-containing large extracellular loop (Fig. 228-2). The two missense mutations that least perturb the structure of PLP/DM20, as judged by the very mild phenotype of the pure form of SPG2 in these cases, are located in the third transmembrane domain (S169F)[12] and the large extracellular loop (S225P)[9] of PLP and DM20.

Missense and nonsense mutations that affect PLP transcripts but spare the alternatively spliced DM20 isoform of PLP (H139Y[6] and W144X[11], in Table 228-1) create the much less severe disorder of SPG2. The form of SPG2 in these patients is the complicated one, probably due to the presence of abnormal PLP proteins in oligodendrocytes. An additional missense mutation which is present in the exon exclusive to PLP transcripts, but at the very end of the exon 3B (K150N[101,102] of Table 228-1), also alters the donor splice site and is anticipated to affect the synthesis of both PLP and DM20. This mutation does, in fact, produce the more severe phenotype of PMD.

The overexpression (e.g., duplications) or underexpression (e.g., null mutations or deletions of the entire gene) of PLP/DM20 generally manifests with less extreme phenotypes than the expression of abnormal proteins (e.g., the missense, frameshift, and splice-site mutations). These intermediate phenotypes range from the classical form of PMD to the complicated form of SPG2. Both the mutation of the initiator methionine[89] and a complete deletion of the PMD gene[70] give rise to a long-lived classical form of PMD. These loss-of-function mutations reveal that PLP/DM20 performs an essential role in myelination that cannot be compensated by other proteolipid proteins in humans. The transgenic models of loss-of-function mutations with normal numbers of mature oligodendrocytes, on the other hand, show that PLP/DM20 is not required for oligodendrocyte development or maturation, and reinforce the notion that many point mutations in PLP/DM20 poison oligodendrocytes through a general block in protein transport from the RER. Too much PLP can similarly undermine myelination, as seen by the duplication of the PLP gene in the majority of PMD patients.[7,14,20,74–77] While one extra copy of PLP yields the classical form of PMD, additional copies create the features of the connatal form of PMD, as characterized in a patient with a possible triplication of the PLP gene.[75–77] The correlation between copy number and severity of disease has also been documented in the transgenic mouse overexpressors.[71–73]

Myelination is a unique process that demands coordinate transcriptional and translational controls both to synthesize the vast quantities of myelin proteins and to assemble the appropriate proportions of each myelin protein into the myelin sheath.[44] It comes as no surprise that PLP, the most abundantly produced gene in central nervous system myelin, is a gene that is subject to dosage control. An analogous situation occurs in the peripheral nervous system, where duplication of one of the myelin genes expressed by Schwann cells, peripheral myelin protein 22 (PMP22), results in the myelin disorder of Charcot-Marie-Tooth disease type 1A.[105] Dosage control does not operate on all of the genes encoding myelin proteins, as no dysmyelination occurs when another major central nervous system protein (myelin basic protein) is overexpressed in transgenic mice.[104] Perhaps a single myelin gene, acting as a kind of pacemaker, is key to balancing the production levels of the other myelin constituents. Such a pacemaker role for myelination in the central nervous system would be carried out by the PLP gene, and for the PNS, PMP22 might be the regulator.

No change at the PLP locus, however subtle, goes unnoticed. The dramatic range of clinical phenotypes can be explained largely by the extent of apoptosis: mutations that highly induce the apoptotic pathway cause the most derangement. The loss of oligodendrocytes is much more debilitating than the loss of myelin sheaths or the manufacture of abnormal myelin, a phenomenon confirmed by other myelin gene mutants[104] that may point to nervous system functions of oligodendrocytes extending beyond myelin formation. Oligodendrocytes may supply the neurons that they ensheath with essential cytokines, and in the absence of these trophic molecules, neurons eventually degenerate. The cellular pathology of PMD/SPG2 illustrates how mutations that generate the mildest phenotypes in affected male patients are also the ones most likely to create problems for the "carrier" mothers. In these cases, the mutant oligodendrocytes survive in the female heterozygotes and contribute to myelin sheath formation. The abnormal myelin is unstable and breaks down over time, resulting in a late onset degenerative disorder with variable symptoms. The aversion of the PLP gene to change must be factored into therapeutic proposals for PMD/SPG2. With the exception of the loss of function mutations in the PLP gene, the PLP mutations behave dominantly within the oligodendrocyte population in which they are expressed, favoring strategies to disable the defective gene or eliminate expression of the extra copy of the PLP gene. Supplying a wild-type PLP gene can be especially problematic because of the strict dosage control displayed by PLP. The animal models of PMD/SPG2 are valuable resources for working through the special challenges posed by genes such as PLP whose expression is highly regulated. Indeed, the recent success by Duncan and coworkers in transplanting oligodendrocyte precursor cells in these animal models[129] highlights a promising approach for treating myelin deficiencies.

## REFERENCES

1. Pelizaeus F: Über eine eigentumliche Form spastischer Lühmung mit Zerebralerscheinungen auf hereditürer Grundlage (multiple Sklerose). *Arch Psychiatr Nervenkr* **16**:698, 1885.
2. Merzbacher L: Eine eigenartige familiüre Erkrankungsform (Aplasia axialis extracorticalis congenita). *Z Gesamte Neurol Psychaitr* **3**:1, 1910.
3. Seitelberger F: Die Pelizaeus-Merzbacher Krankheit, Klinisch-anatomische Untersuchungen zum Prolbem ihrer Stellung unter den diffusen Sklerosen. *Wien Z Nervenheilkd* **9**:228, 1954.
4. Seitelberger F: Pelizaeus-Merzbacher disease, in Vinken PJ, Bruyn GW (eds): *Handbook of Clinical Neurology. Leucodystrophies and Poliodystrophies*, Vol 10. Amsterdam, North Holland, 1970, p 150.
5. Roizin L, Haymaker W, D'Amelio F, Adams RD, Willson N, Kaufman MA: Disease states involving the white matter of the central nervous system, in Haymaker W, Adams RD (eds): *Histology and Histopathology of the Nervous System*, Vol 1. Springfield, IL, C.C. Thomas, 1982, p 1375.
6. Saugier-Veber P, Munnich A, Bonneau D, Rozet JM, Le Merrer M, Gil R, Boespflug-Tanguy O: X-linked spastic paraplegia and Pelizaeus-Merzbacher disease are allelic disorders at the proteolipid protein locus. *Nat Genet* **6**:257, 1994.
7. Nave KA, Boespflug-Tanguy O: X-linked developmental defects of myelination: From mouse mutants to human genetic diseases. *Neuroscientist* **2**:33, 1996.
8. Bond C, Si X, Crisp M, Wong P, Paulson G, Boesel C, Dlouhy S, et al: Family with Pelizaeus-Merzbacher disease/X-linked spastic paraplegia and a nonsense mutation in exon 6 of the proteolipid protein gene. *Am J Med Genetics* **71**:357, 1997.
9. Cambi F, Tang XM, Cordray P, Fain PR, Keppen LD, Barker, DF: Refined genetic mapping and proteolipid protein mutation analysis in X-linked pure hereditary spastic paraplegia. *Neurology* **46**:1112, 1996.
10. Kobayashi H, Hoffman EP, Marks HG: The rumpshaker mutation in spastic paraplegia. *Nat Genet* **7**:351, 1994.
11. Osaka H, Kawanishi C, Inoue K, Uesugi H, Hiroshi K, Nishiyama K, Yamada Y, et al: Novel nonsense proteolipid protein gene mutation as a cause of X-linked spastic paraplegia in twin males. *Biochem Biophys Res Commun* **215**:835, 1995.
12. Hodes ME, Hadjisavvas A, Butler IJ, Aydanian A, Dlouhy SR: X-linked spastic paraplegia due to a mutation (C506T; Ser169Phe) in exon 4 of the proteolipid protein gene (PLP). *Am J Med Genet* **75**:516, 1998.
13. Naidu S, Dlouhy SR, Geraghty M, Hodes ME: A male child with the *rumpshaker* mutation, X-linked spastic paraplegia/Pelizaeus-Merzbacher disease and lysinuria. *J Inherit Metab Dis* **20**:811, 1997.
14. Hodes ME: Pelizaeus-Merzbacher disease, in: Gilman S, Goldstein GW, Waxman SG (eds): *Neurobase*, 4th ed. San Diego, CA, Arbor Publishing, 1998.
15. Hodes, ME, Pratt VM, Dlouhy SR: The genetics of Pelizaeus-Merzbacher disease. *Dev Neurosci* **15**:383, 1993.
16. Cassidy S, Sheehan N, Farrell D, Grunnet M, Holmes G, Zimmerman A: Connatal Pelizaeus-Merzbacher disease: An autosomal recessive form. *Pediatr Neurol* **3**(5):300, 1987.
17. Zeman W, DeMyer W, Falls JS: Pelizaeus-Merzbacher disease: A study in nosology. *J Neuropathol Exp Neurol* **23**:334, 1964.
18. Boulloche J, Aicardi J: Pelizaeus-Merzbacher disease: Clinical and nosological study. *J Child Neurol* **1**:233, 1986.
19. Scheffer I E, Baraitser M, Wilson J, Harding B, Kendall B, Brett EM: Pelizaeus-Merzbacher disease: Classical or connatal? *Neuropediatrics* **22**:71, 1991.
20. Sistermans E, deCoo R, DeWijs I, Van Oost B: Duplication of the proteolipid protein gene is the major cause of Pelizaeus Merzbacher disease. *Neurology* **50**:1749, 1998.
21. Johnston AW, McKusick VA: A sex-linked recessive form of spastic paraplegia. *Am J Hum Genet* **14**:83, 1962.
22. Bonneau D, Rozet JM, Bulteau C, Berthier M, Mettey R, Gil R, Munnich A, et al: X-linked spastic paraplegia (SPG2): Clinical heterogeneity at a single gene locus. *J Med Genet* **30**:381, 1993.
23. Tanaka S, Mito T, Takashima S: Progress of myelination in the human fetal spinal nerve roots, spinal cord and brainstem with myelin basic protein immunohistochemistry. *Early Hum Dev* **41**(1):49, 1995.
24. Volpe, J: Neuonal Proliferation, migration, organization and Myelination, in *Neurology of the Newborn*, 3d ed. Philadelphia, WB Saunders, 1995, p.74.
25. Caro PA, Marks HG: Magnetic resonance imaging and computed tomography in Pelizaeus-Merzbacher disease. *Magn Reson Imaging* **8**:8128, 1990.
26. Andre M, Monin P, Moret C, Brown M, Picard L: Pelizaeus-Merzbacher disease. Contribution of magnetic resonance imaging to an early diagnosis. *J Neuroradiol* **17**:216, 1990.
27. Ono J, Harada K, Mano T, Sakurai K, Okada S: Differentiation of dys- and demyelination using diffusional anisotropy. *Pediatr Neurol* **16**(1):63, 1997.

28. Koeppen A: Pelizaeus-Merzbacher disease: X-linked proteolipid protein deficiency in the human central nervous system, in Martenson R (ed): *Myelin: Biology and Chemistry.* Boca Raton, FL, CRC Press, 1992; p 703.

29. Garbern JY, Cambi F, Tank X-M, Sima AAF, Vallat JM, Bosch EP, Lewis R, et al: Proteolipid protein is necessary in peripheral as well as central myelin. *Neuron* **19**:205, 1997.

30. Apkarian P, Koetsveld-Baart JC, Barth PG: Visual evoked potential characteristics and early diagnosis of Pelizaeus-Merzbacher disease. *Arch Neurol* **50**:981, 1993.

31. Markand ON, Garg BP, DeMyer WE, Warren C, Worth RM: Brain stem auditory, visual and somatosensory evoked potentials in leukodystrophies. *Electroencephalogr Clin Neurophysiol* **54**:39, 1982.

32. Garg, BP, Markand ON, DeMyer WE: Usefulness of BAER studies in the early diagnosis of Pelizaeus-Merzbacher disease. *Neurology* **33**:955, 1983.

33. Nezu A: Neurophysiological study in Pelizaeus-Merzbacher disease. *Brain Dev* **17**:175, 1995.

34. Stoffel W, Schroder W, Hillen H, Deutzmann R: The primary structure of bovine brain myelin lipophilin (proteolipid apoprotein). *Hoppe-Seyler's Z Physiol Chem* **364**:1455, 1983.

35. Lees, MB, Bizzozero OA: Structure and acylation of proteolipid protein, in Martenson RE (ed): *Myelin: Biology and Chemistry.* Ann Arbor, Michigan, CRC Press, 1992, p 237.

36. Weimbs T, Stoffel W: Proteolipid protein (PLP) of CNS myelin: Positions of free disulfide-bonded, and fatty acid thioester-linked cysteine residues and implications for the membrane topology of PLP. *Biochemistry* **1**:12289, 1992.

37. Gow A, Gragerov A, Gard A, Colman D, Lazzarini R: Conservation of topology, but not conformation, of the proteolipid proteins of the myelin sheath. *J Neuroscience* **17**:181, 1997.

38. Helynck G, Luu B, Nussbaum J-L, Picken D, Skalidis G, Trifilieff E, Van Dorsselaer P, et al: Brain proteolipids: isolation, purification and effect on ionic permeability of membranes. *J Biochem* **133**:689, 1983.

39. Kitagawa K, Sinoway MP, Yang C, Gould RM, Colman DR: A proteolipid protein gene family: Expression in sharks and rays and possible evolution from an ancestral gene encoding a pore-forming polypeptide. *Neuron* **11**:433, 1993.

40. Diehl H-J, Schaich M, Budzinski R-M, Stoffel W: Individual exons encode the integral membrane domains of human myelin proteolipid protein. *Proc Natl Acad Sci U S A* **83**:9807, 1986.

41. Macklin WB, Campagnoni CS, Deininger PL, Gardinier MV: Structure and expression of the mouse myelin proteolipid protein gene. *J Neurosci Res* **18**:383, 1987.

42. Ikenaka K, Furuichi T, Iwasaki Y, Moriguchi A, Okano H, Mikoshiba K: Myelin proteolipid protein gene structure and its regulation of expression in normal and *jimpy* mutant mice. *J Mol Biol* **199**:587, 1988.

43. Hudson LD, Puckett C, Berndt J, Chan J, Gencic S: Mutation of the proteolipid protein gene PLP in a human X chromosome-linked myelin disorder. *Proc Natl Acad Sci U S A* **86**:8128, 1989.

44. Hudson LD, Ko N, Kim J: Control of myelin gene expression, in Richardson WD, Jessen KR (eds): *Glial Cell Development: Basic Principles and Clinical Relevance.* London, Bios Scientific Pub, 1995, p 101.

45. Schindler P, Luu B, Sorokine O, Trifilieff E, Van Dorsselaer A: Developmental study of proteolipids in bovine brain: A novel proteolipid and DM-20 appear before proteolipid protein (PLP) during myelination. *J Neurochem* **55**:2079, 1990.

46. Sinoway MP, Kitagawa K, Timsit S, Hashim GA, Colman DR: Proteolipid protein interactions in transfectants: Implications for myelin assembly. *J Neurosci Res* **37**:441, 1994.

47. Gow A, Lazzarini RA: A cellular mechanism governing the severity of Pelizaeus- Merzbacher disease. *Nat Genet* **13**:422, 1996.

48. Tosic M, Gow A, Dolivo M, Domanska-Janik K, Lazzarini RA, Matthieu JM : Proteolipid/DM-20 proteins bearing the paralytic tremor mutation in peripheral nerves and transfected Cos-7 cells. *Neurochem Res* **21**:423, 1996.

49. Tosic M, Matthey B, Gow A, Lazzarini RA, Matthieu JM: Intracellular transport of the DM-20 bearing shaking pup (shp) mutation and its possible phenotypic consequences. *J Neurosci Res* **50**:844, 1997.

50. Puckett C, Hudson LD, Ono K, Friedrich V, Benecke J, Dubois-Dalcq M, Lazzarini RA: Myelin-specific proteolipid protein is expressed in myelinating Schwann cells but is not incorporated into myelin sheaths. *J Neurosci Res* **18**:511, 1987.

51. Pham-Dinh D, Birling, MC, Roussel G, Dautigny A, Nussbaum JL: Proteolipid DM-20 predominates over PLP in peripheral nervous system. *Molecular Neurosci* **2**:89, 1991.

52. Anderson TJ, Montague P, Nadon N, Nave KA, Griffiths IR: Modification of Schwann cell phenotype with PLP transgenes: evidence that the PLP and DM20 isoproteins are targeted to different cellular domains. *J Neurosci Res* **50**(1):13, 1997.

53. Campagnoni CW, Garbay B, Micevych P, Pribyl T, Kampf K, Handley VW, Campagnoni AT: DM20 mRNA splice product of the myelin proteolipid protein gene is expressed in the murine heart. *J Neurosci Res* **33**:148, 1992.

54. Pribyl TM, Campagnoni CW, Kampf K, Kashima T, Handley VW, McMahon J, Campagnoni AT: Expression of the myelin proteolipid protein gene in the human fetal thymus. *J Neuroimmunol* **67**:125, 1996.

55. Gencic S, Hudson LD: Conservative amino acid substitution in the myelin proteolipid protein of *jimpy*^msd mice. *J Neurosci* **10**:117, 1990.

56. Yamamoto T, Nanba E, Zhang H, Sasaki M, Komaki H: *Jimpy*^msd mouse mutation and connatal Pelizaeus-Merzbacher disease. *Am J Med Genet* **75**:439, 1998.

57. Schneider A, Montague P, Griffiths I, Fanarraga M, Kennedy P, Brophy P, Nave KA: Uncoupling of hypomyelination and glial cell death by a mutation in the proteolipid protein gene. *Nature* 758, 1992.

58. Sidman RL, Dickie MM, Appel SH: Mutant mice (quaking and jimpy) with deficient myelination in the central nervous system. *Science* **144**:309, 1964.

59. Duncan ID: Inherited disorders of myelination of the central nervous system, in Kettenman H, Ransom BR (eds): *Neuroglia.* New York, Oxford University Press, 1995, p 990.

60. Duncan ID, Hammang JP: Myelination in the jimpy mouse in the absence of PLP. *Glia* **2**:148, 1989.

61. Knapp PE, Skoff RP, Redstone DW: Oligodendroglial cell death in jimpy mice: An explanation for the myelin deficit. *J Neurosci* **6**:2813, 1986.

62. Adachi M, Schneck L, Tori J, Volk BW: Histochemical, ultrastructural, and biochemical studies of a case with leukodystrophy due to congenital deficiency of myelin. *J Neuropathol Exp Neurol* **29**:601, 1970.

63. Tosic M, Dolivo M, Domanska-Janik K, Matthieu JM: Paralytic tremor (pt): A new allele of the proteolipid protein gene in rabbits. *J Neurochem* **63**:2210, 1994.

64. Karthigasan J, Evans EL, Vouyiouklis DA, Inouye H, Borenshteyn N, Ramamurthy GV, Kirschner DA: Effects of rumpshaker mutation on CNS myelin composition and structure. *J Neurochem* **66**:338, 1996.

65. Boisson D, Stoffel W: Disruption of the compacted myelin sheath of axons of the central nervous system in proteolipid protein-deficient mice. *Proc Natl Acad Sci U S A* **91**:11709, 1994.

66. Boisson D, Bussow H, D'Urso D, Muller H-W, Stoffel W: Adhesive properties of proteolipid protein are responsible for the compaction of CNS myelin sheaths. *J Neurosci* **15**:5502, 1995.

67. Klugmann M, Schwab MH, Pühlhofer A, Schneider A, Zimmermann F, Griffiths IR, Nave KA: Assembly of CNS myelin in the absence of proteolipid protein. *Neuron* **18**:59, 1997.

68. Yan Y, Lagenaur C, Narayanan V: Molecular cloning of M6: Identification of a PLP/DM-20 gene family. *Neuron* **11**:423, 1993.

69. Baumrind N, Parkinson D, Wayne D, Heuser J, Pearlman A: EMA: A developmentally regulated cell-surface glycoprotein of CNS neurons that is concentrated at the leading edge of growth cones. *Dev Dyn* **194**:311, 1993.

70. Raskind WH, Williams CA, Hudson LD, Bird TD: Complete deletion of the proteolipid protein gene (PLP) in a family with X-linked Pelizaeus-Merzbacher disease. *Am J Hum Genet* **49**:1355, 1991.

71. Kagawa T, Ikenaka K, Inoue Y, Kuriyama S, Tsujii T, Nakao J, Nakajima K, et al: Glial cell degeneration and hypomyelination caused by overexpression of the myelin proteolipid protein gene. *Neuron* **13**:427, 1994.

72. Readhead C, Schneider A, Griffiths I, Nave KA: Premature arrest of myelin formation in transgenic mice with increased proteolipid protein gene dosage. *Neuron* **12**:583, 1994.

73. Inoue Y, Kagawa T, Matsumura Y, Ikenaka K, Mikoshiba K: Cell death of oligodendrocytes or demyelination induced by overexpression of proteolipid protein depending on expressed gene dosage. *Neurosci Res* **25**:161, 1996.

74. Inoue K, Osaka H, Sugiyama N, Kawanishi C, Onishi H, Nezu A, Kimura K, et al: A duplicated PLP gene causing Pelizaeus-Merzbacher disease detected by comparative multiplex PCR. *Am J Hum Genet* **59**:32, 1996.

75. Ellis D, Malcolm S: Proteolipid protein gene dosage effect in Pelizaeus-Merzbacher disease. *Nat Genet* **6**:333, 1994.

76. Harding B, Ellis D, Malcolm S: A case of Pelizaeus-Merzbacher disease showing increased dosage of the proteolipid protein gene. *Neuropathol Appl Neurobiol* 21:11, 1995.

77. Woodward K, Kendall E, Vetrie D, Malcolm S: Pelizaeus-Merzbacher disease: Identification of Xq22 proteolipid protein duplications and characterization of breakpoints by interphase FISH. *Am J Hum Genet* 63:207, 1998.

78. Willard HF, Riordan JR: Assignment of the gene for myelin proteolipid protein to the X chromosome: Implications for X-linked myelin disorders. *Science* 230:940, 1985.

79. Mattei MG, Alliel PM, Dautigny A, Passage E, Pham-Dinh D, Mattei JF, Jolles P: The gene encoding for the major brain proteolipid (PLP) maps on the q-22 band of the human X chromosome. *Hum Genet* 72:352, 1986.

80. Hudson LD, Berndt J, Puckett C, Kozak CA, Lazzarini RA: Aberrant splicing of proteolipid protein mRNA in the dysmyelinating jimpy mouse. *Proc Natl Acad Sci U S A* 84:1454, 1987.

81. Dautigny A, Mattei M.-G, Morello D, Alliel PM, Pham-Dinh D, Amar L, Arnaud D, et al: The structural gene coding for myelin-associated proteolipid protein is mutated in *jimpy* mice. *Nature* 321:867, 1986.

82. Nave KA, Bloom FE, Milner RJ: A single nucleotide difference in the gene for myelin proteolipid protein defines the jimpy mutation in mouse. *J Neurochem* 49:5665, 1987.

83. Macklin WB, Gardinier MB, King KD, Kampf K: An AG → GG transition at a splice site in the myelin proteolipid protein gene in jimpy mice results in the removal of an exon. *FEBS Lett* 223:417, 1987.

84. Koeppen AH, Ronca NA, Greenfield EA, Hans MB: Defective biosynthesis of proteolipid protein in Pelizaeus-Merzbacher disease. *Ann Neurol* 21:159, 1987.

85. Cremers FPM, Pfeiffer R, van de Pol TJR, Hofker MH, Kruse TA, Wieringa B, Ropers HH: An interstitial duplication of the X chromosome in a male allows physical fine mapping of probes from the Xq13-q22 region. *Hum Genet* 77:23, 1987.

86. Trofatter J, Dlouhy SR, DeMyer W, Conneally PM, Hodes ME: Pelizaeus-Merzbacher disease: Tight linkage to proteolipid protein gene exon variant. *Proc Natl Acad Sci U S A* 86:9427, 1989.

87. Boespflug-Tanguy O, Mimault C, Melki J, Cavagna A, Giraud G, Pham-Dinh D, Datugue B, et al: Genetic homogeneity of Pelizaeus-Merzbacher disease (PMD): Tight linkage to the proteolipoprotein (PLP) locus in 16 affected families. *Am J Hum Genet* 55:461, 1994.

88. Kobayashi H, Garcia C, Alfonso G, Marks H, Hoffman E: Molecular genetics of familial spastic paraplegia: A multitude of responsible genes. *J Neurol Sciences* 137:131, 1996.

89. Sistermans EA, de Wijs IJ, de Coo RFM, Smit LME, Menko FH, van Oost BA: A (G-to-A) mutation in the initiation codon of the proteolipid protein gene causing a relatively mild form of Pelizaeus-Merzbacher disease in a Dutch family. *Hum Genet* 97:337, 1996.

90. Nance MA, Boyadjiev S, Pratt VM, Taylor S, Hodes ME, Dlouhy SR: Adult-onset neurodegenerative disorder due to proteolipid protein gene mutation in the mother of a man with Pelizaeus-Merzbacher disease. *Neurology* 47:1333, 1996.

91. Hodes ME, DeMyer WE, Pratt VM, Edwards MK, Dlouhy SR: Girl with signs of Pelizaeus-Merzbacher disease heterozygous for a mutation in exon 2 of the proteolipid protein gene (PLP). *Am J Med Genet* 55:397, 1995.

92. Pratt VM, Keifer JR, Lühdetie J, Schleutker J, Hodes ME, Dlouhy SR: Linkage of a new mutation in the proteolipid protein (PLP) gene to Pelizaeus-Merzbacher disease (PMD) in a large Finnish kindred. *Am J Med Genet* 52:1053, 1993.

93. Hodes ME, Blank CA, Pratt VM, Morales J, Napier J, Dlouhy SR: Nonsense mutation in exon 3 of the proteolipid protein gene (PLP) in a family with an unusual form of Pelizaeus-Merzbacher disease. *Am J Med Genet* 69:121, 1997.

94. Duncan ID, Jackson KF, Hammang JP, Marren D, Hoffman R: Development of myelin mosaicism in the optic nerve of heterozygotes of the X-linked myelin-deficient (md) rat mutant. *Dev Biol* 157:336, 1993.

95. Gow A, Southwood CM, Lazzarini RA: Disrupted proteolipid protein trafficking results in oligodendrocyte apoptosis in an animal model of Pelizaeus-Merzbacher disease. *J Cell Biol* 140:925, 1998.

96. Nadon NL, Arnheiter H, Hudson LD: A combination of PLP and DM-20 transgenes promotes partial myelination in the jimpy mouse. *J Neurochem* 63:822, 1994.

97. Schneider A, Griffiths JR, Readhead C, Nave K-Å: Dominant-negative action of the *jimpy* mutation in mice complemented with an autosomal transgene for myelin proteolipid protein. *Proc Natl Acad Sci U S A* 92:4447, 1995.

98. Yang X, Skoff RP: Proteolipid protein regulates the survival and differentiation of oligodendrocytes. *J Neurosci* 17:2056, 1997.

99. Bridge PJ, D'Souza CR, Van Oost BA: A de novo Tyr$^{206\text{-Cys}}$ mutation in the proteolipid protein causes Pelizaeus-Merzbacher disease. *Am J Hum Genet* 972:183, 1991.

100. Iwaki A, Muramoto T, Iwaki T, Furumi H, Dario-deLeon ML, Tateishi J, Fukumaki Y: A missense mutation in the proteolipid protein gene responsible for Pelizaeus-Merzbacher disease in a Japanese family. *Hum Mol Genet* 2:19, 1993.

101. Pratt, VM, Naidu S, Dlouhy SR, Marks HG, Hodes ME: A novel mutation in exon 3 of the proteolipid protein gene in Pelizaeus-Merzbacher disease. *Neurology* 45:394, 1995.

102. Bridge PJ, Wilkins PJ: The role of proteolipid protein gene mutations in Pelizaeus-Merzbacher disease. *Am J Hum Genet* 51:A209 (Abst. 823), 1992.

103. Verhagen WIM, Huygen PLM, Smeets HJM, Renier WO, de Wijs I: A new proteolipid protein mutation in Pelizaeus-Merzbacher disease. *J Neurol Sci* 147:215, 1997.

104. Shine HD, Readhead C, Popko B, Hood L, Sidman RL: Morphometric analysis of normal, mutant, and transgenic CNS: Correlation of myelin basic protein expression to myelinogenesis. *J Neurochem* 58:342, 1992.

105. Lupski JR: Charcot-Marie-Tooth disease: lessons in genetic mechanisms. *Mol Med* 4:3, 1998.

106. Nadon NL, Duncan ID, Hudson LD: A point mutation in the proteolipid protein gene of the "shaking pup" interrupts oligodendrocyte development. *Development* 110:529, 1990.

107. Pearsall GB, Nadon NL, Wolf MK, Billings-Gagliardi S: Jimpy-4J mouse has a missense mutation in exon 2 of the PLP gene. *Dev Neurosci* 19(4):337, 1997.

108. Dlouhy SR, Pratt VM, Boyadjiev S, Hodes ME: Pelizaeus-Merzbacher caused by de novo mutation. *J Neuropathol Exp Neurol* 52:331, 1993.

109. Osaka H, Inoue K, Kawanishi C, Sugiyama N, Onishi H, Suzuki K, Kimura S, et al: Proteolipid protein gene analysis in Pelizaeus-Merzbacher disease [Abstract 1599]. *Am J Hum Genet* 59(4):A276, 1996.

110. Doll R, Natowicz MR, Schiffmann R, Smith FI: Molecular diagnostics for myelin proteolipid protein gene mutations in Pelizaeus-Merzbacher disease. *Am J Hum Genet* 51:161, 1992.

111. Boison D, Stoffel W: Myelin-deficient rat: A point mutation in exon III (A → C, Thr75 → Pro) of the myelin proteolipid protein causes dysmyelination and oligodendrocyte death. *EMBO J* 8:3295, 1989.

112. Simons R, Riordan JR: The myelin-deficient rat has a single base substitution in the third exon of the myelin proteolipid protein gene. *J Neurochem* 54:1079, 1990.

113. Weimbs T, Dick T, Stoffel W, Boltshauer E: A point mutation at the X-chromosomal proteolipid protein locus in Pelizaeus-Merzbacher disease leads to disruption of myelinogenesis. *Biol Chem Hoppe Seyler* 371:1175, 1990.

114. Pratt VM, Trofatter JA, Schinzel A, Dlouhy SR, Conneally PM, Hodes ME: A new mutation in the proteolipid protein (PLP) gene in a German family with Pelizaeus-Merzbacher disease. *Am J Med Genet* 38:136, 1991.

115. Strautnieks S, Rutland P, Winter RM, Baraitser M, Malcolm S: Pelizaeus-Merzbacher disease: detection of mutations Thr$^{181}$ → Pro and Leu$^{223}$ → Pro in the proteolipid protein gene and prenatal diagnosis. *Am J Hum Genet* 51:871, 1992.

116. Inoue K, Osaka H, Kawanishi C, Sugiyama N, Ishii M, Sugita K, Yamada Y, et al: Mutations in the proteolipid protein gene in Japanese families with Pelizaeus-Merzbacher disease. *Neurology* 48:283, 1997.

117. Gencic S, Abuelo D, Ambler M, Hudson LD: Pelizaeus-Merzbacher disease: An X-linked neurologic disorder of myelin metabolism with a novel mutation in the gene encoding proteolipid protein. *Am J Hum Genet* 45:435, 1989.

118. Otterbach B, Stoffel W, Ramaekers V: A novel mutation in the proteolipid protein gene leading to Pelizaeus-Merzbacher disease. *Biol Chem Hoppe Seyler* 374:75, 1993.

119. Pratt VM, Boyadjiev S, Dlouhy SR, Silver K, DerKaloustian VM, Hodes ME: Pelizaeus-Merzbacher disease in a family of Portuguese origin caused by a point mutation in exon 5 of the proteolipid protein gene. *Am J Med Genet* 55:402, 1994.

120. Pham-Dinh D, Popot JL, Boespflug-Tanguy O, Landrieu P, Deleuze JF, Boue J, Jolles P, et al: Pelizaeus-Merzbacher disease: A valine to phenylalanine point mutation in a putative extracellular loop of myelin proteolipid. *Proc Natl Acad Sci U S A* 88:7562, 1991.

121. Donnelly A, Colley A, Crimmins D, Mulley J: A novel mutation in exon 6 (F236S) of the proteolipid protein gene is associated with spastic paraplegia. *Hum Mutat* 8:384, 1996.

122. Kawanishi C, Osaka H, Owa K, Inoue K, Miyakawa T, Onishi H, Yamada Y, et al: A new missense mutation in exon 6 of the proteolipid protein gene in a patient with Pelizaeus-Merzbacher disease. *Hum Mutat* **9**:475, 1997.

123. Pratt VM, Dlouhy SR, Hodes ME: Pelizaeus-Merzbacher disease: A point mutation in exon 6 of the proteolipid protein (PLP) gene. *Clin Genet* **47**:99, 1995.

124. Pham-Dinh D, Boespflug-Tanguy O, Mimault C, Cavagna A, Giraud G, Leberre G, Lemarec B, et al: Pelizaeus-Merzbacher disease: A frameshift deletion/insertion event in the myelin proteolipid gene. *Hum Mol Genet* **4**:465, 1993.

125. Kurosawa K, Iwaki A, Miyake S, Imaizumi K, Kuroki Y, Fukamaki Y: A novel insertional mutation at exon VII of the myelin proteolipid protein gene in Pelizaeus-Merzbacher disease. *Hum Mol Genet* **2**:2187, 1993.

126. Kleindorfer DO, Dlouhy SR, Pratt VM, Jones MC, Trofatter JA, Hodes ME: In-frame deletion in the proteolipid protein gene in a family with Pelizaeus-Merzbacher disease. *Am J Med Genet* **55**:405, 1995.

127. Pratt VM, Dlouhy SR, Hodes ME: Possible cryptic splice site found in the PLP gene in a patient with Pelizaeus-Merzbacher disease [Abstract 2358]. *Am J Hum Genet* **49**:416, 1991.

128. Strautnieks S, Malcolm S: A G to T mutation at a splice site in a case of Pelizaeus-Merzbacher disease. *Hum Mol Genet* **2**:2191, 1993.

129. Brüstle O, Jones KN, Learish RD, Karram K, Choudhary K, Wiestler OD, Duncan ID, Mckay RD: Embryonic stem cell-derived glial precursors: A source of myelinating transplants. *Science* **285**:754, 1999.

# Aspartoacylase Deficiency (Canavan Disease)

*Arthur L. Beaudet*

## HISTORICAL

The disorder now identified as aspartoacylase deficiency is equivalent to the condition variously called spongy degeneration of the brain, spongy degeneration of the central nervous system in infancy, or spongy degeneration of infancy, and many publications have used the eponymic designation, Canavan disease. The first definition of this condition as a distinct clinical entity is properly credited to van Bogaert and Bertrand in 1949.[1,2] In retrospect, the first clinical description is attributed to Globus and Strauss in 1928.[3] In 1931, Canavan described an infant with prominent enlargement of the head and cerebral and cerebellar spongy degeneration under the designation "Schilder's encephalitis periaxialis diffusa."[4] Eiselsberg is credited with the recognition of the familial nature of the disorder in 1937,[5] but, like Jervis,[6,7] she described the condition as Krabbe disease. The reports of von Bogaert and Bertrand[1,2] were comprehensive and described the essential pathologic and clinical features as well as the predilection for the occurrence of the disorder in Ashkenazic infants. In a more detailed review of the historical literature,[8] Banker et al. pointed out that the Canavan eponym is hardly justified, because her report was not the first clinical description, did not recognize the familial or ethnic aspect to the disorder, and did not recognize spongy degeneration as the unique pathologic feature; the designation *aspartoacylase deficiency* may be most appropriate, but the eponym is widely used.

Unraveling of the biochemical basis of infantile spongy degeneration began with the description of urinary excretion of *N*-acetylaspartic acid (NAA) by Kvittingen et al.,[9] but aspartoacylase was reported to be normal in cultured fibroblasts; presumably the failure to demonstrate the enzyme deficiency was due to the choice of conditions for enzyme analysis. In 1987, Hagenfeldt et al. reported *N*-acetylaspartic aciduria and identified aspartoacylase deficiency,[10] but neither of these biochemical reports recognized the association with infantile spongy degeneration. Matalon et al.,[11,12] and Divry et al.[13,14] are credited with the recognition that aspartoacylase deficiency correlated with infantile spongy degeneration (Canavan disease). Kaul et al. went on to isolate a cDNA clone for human aspartoacylase and identified the common mutation in Jewish patients.[15] Matalon and colleagues have contributed extensively to observations in recent years as reviewed elsewhere.[16]

## CLINICAL FEATURES

In addition to the landmark descriptions of von Bogaert and Bertrand,[1,2] Banker and colleagues, and others have provided excellent reviews of the clinical and pathologic features of infantile spongy degeneration.[8,17-19] Ungar and Goodman reviewed cases of infantile spongy degeneration in Israel from 1965 to 1980.[20] Although infants are usually normal in the first month of life, they may exhibit poor visual fixation, irritability, and poor suck at

birth.[19] They demonstrate poor head control, poor eye contact, seizures, and abnormal muscle tone beginning in the second to fourth month, and all those with the classic phenotype are clearly neurologically abnormal before 6 months of age (Table 229-1). Some skills, such as grasping, visual attentiveness, and smiling, may be acquired and subsequently lost. Increase in head circumference is uniformly present by 6 months of age and may be associated with delayed closure of the anterior fontanelle. This correlates with a substantial increase in brain weight at necropsy, which is most conspicuous if death occurs before 3 years of age. Brain weight is closer to the normal range thereafter (Fig. 229-1).[21] Motor activity is consistently abnormal with diminished muscle tone and decreased motor activity early in life and spasticity at later times, although this transition may occur as early as 5 weeks of age or as late as 3 years of age.[8] Increased deep tendon reflexes and the presence of Babinski signs are common, and the patients progress to extreme hypertonicity with pseudobulbar palsy and decerebrate or decorticate posturing. Tonic extensor spasms are common with exaggerated opisthotonic posturing in response to stimuli. Seizures, usually generalized tonic and clonic type, occur in about half of patients; dysphagia, optic atrophy, and nystagmus are reported in a significant but lesser fraction.[20] There has been a suggestion that the phenotype may include a mild hypopigmentation,[17,20] but this finding is of uncertain significance. The occurrence of a primary intracranial teratoid/rhabdoid tumor in one child was judged to be coincidental.[22]

Occasional patients may have a somewhat later age of onset,[23] and prolonged survival can occur in some cases.[24,25] Suggestions that there might be a juvenile form of disease[26-29] require further study to determine if there are milder mutations or other modifying factors which might account for such a phenotype. Cholelithiasis has been reported in one case,[30] but this association may not be significant. Based on necropsy data,[21] it would appear that the majority of deaths are relatively evenly distributed over the first 3 years of life with some patients surviving substantially longer. The disorder is most common in the Ashkenazic population (see "Genetics and Incidence" below).

Depending on the clinical presentation, differential diagnoses might include disorders whose diagnosis should be clarified by biochemical studies as for GM1 gangliosidosis or Krabbe disease. The increased head circumference can raise the possibility of Sotos syndrome, but the neurologic progression should distinguish this disorder. Although megalencephaly also occurs in Alexander disease, the pathologic findings are distinct. Other disorders with familial megalencephaly and leukodystrophy with unknown biochemical defect are reported.[31-33] At this time, biochemical analysis for aspartoacylase deficiency or the associated *N*-acetylaspartic aciduria can be readily utilized to provide a definitive diagnosis.

### Cerebral Imaging

There are numerous reports of CT and MRI studies of the brain in aspartoacylase deficiency.[34-43] The most consistent findings are diffuse symmetric abnormalities of white matter that are sometimes quite nonuniform. The white matter disease can be seen

---

A list of standard abbreviations is located immediately preceding the index in each volume. Additional abbreviations used in this chapter include: NAA = *N*-acetylaspartic acid; NAAG = *N*-acetyl-aspartyl-glutamate.

**Table 229-1** Clinical Features of Aspartoacylase Deficiency

Normal first month of life
Poor head control and hypotonia at 2–4 months
Generalized seizures
Opisthotonic posturing
Loss of very early milestones
Increased head circumference
Leukodystrophy on MRI or CT
Hypotonia progresses to spasticity
Decerebrate or decorticate posturing late

using CT or ultrasound.[41] Many investigators have used proton magnetic resonance spectroscopy to quantitate the levels of NAA in the brain *in vivo*. Most have reported increased amounts of this compound in the brain relative to other metabolites such as choline and creatinine,[34,36–38] although some reports emphasize normal levels of NAA with reduced levels of these other metabolites.[38,39,44,45] The increase in NAA can also be quantitated in cerebrospinal fluid using magnetic resonance spectroscopy.[44] Although changes in white matter are not always present,[40] MRI studies usually show symmetric diffuse low signal intensity on T1-weighted images and high signal intensity on T2-weighted images (Fig. 229-2).

## GENETICS AND INCIDENCE

Infantile spongy degeneration due to aspartoacylase deficiency is an autosomal recessive disorder (MIM 271900). A review of cases reported from 1928 to 1977 appeared in 1979 and identified 83 cases in 48 families that were believed to meet the appropriate clinical and pathologic criteria for a diagnosis of infantile spongy degeneration.[17] Consanguinity was found in 23 percent of 48 families in one study,[17] being slightly more frequent in the non-Jewish families than in the Jewish families. Although there was a suggestion of a statistically significant difference in male:female ratio,[17] there was no difference when the Jewish and non-Jewish cases were combined, and this is unlikely to be of significance. Of the 42 families with known ethnic origin, 28 were Jewish (mostly Ashkenazic) with multiple other ethnic groups represented including German, Swiss, Austrian, Irish, Italian, French Canadian, Ojibway Indian, and Iranian (see Banker and Victor[17] for bibliography). Of 11 families identified in Israel, 7 were Ashkenazic with the others being Iraqi, Yemenite, or Spanish Moroccan.[20] There are also reports of Japanese and Turkish

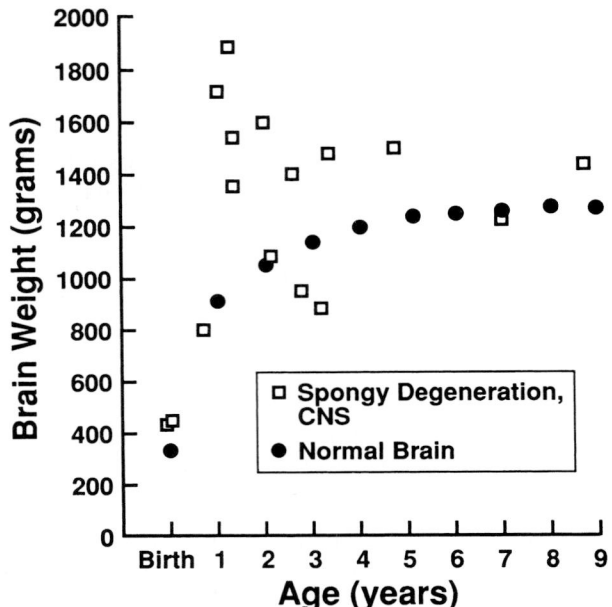

**Fig. 229-1** Brain weights in infantile spongy degeneration compared to normal mean values. (*From Adachi and Aronson.*[21] *Used with permission.*)

patients.[46–48] There is some evidence that the ancestors of Ashkenazic patients originated from eastern Poland, Lithuania, and western Ukraine,[8] but some may have come from more scattered regions in Europe.[20] Although the disease is definitely relatively rare and occurs preferentially in the Ashkenazic population, one group reported diagnosing 145 patients biochemically by 1993,[15] suggesting that the disorder may be somewhat more common than has been appreciated. In more recent years, there have been numerous reports of patients documented biochemically by the presence of *N*-acetylaspartic aciduria and/or aspartoacylase deficiency[13,23,24,30,35,37,39,40,49–56] including at least 24 patients from Saudi Arabia.[57]

## PATHOLOGY

Histopathology of the brain provided the primary diagnostic criterion for infantile spongy degeneration from the time of the classic delineation of van Bogaert and Bertrand in 1949 until the

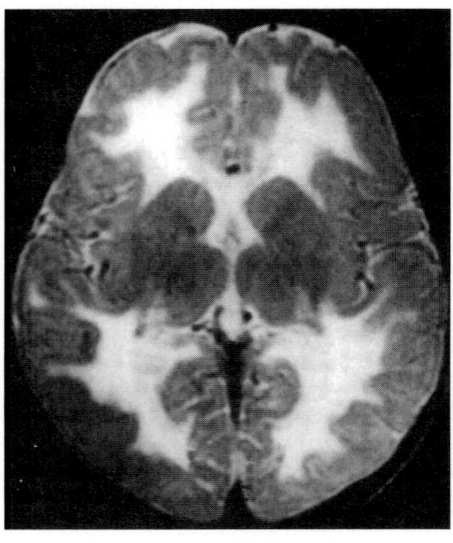

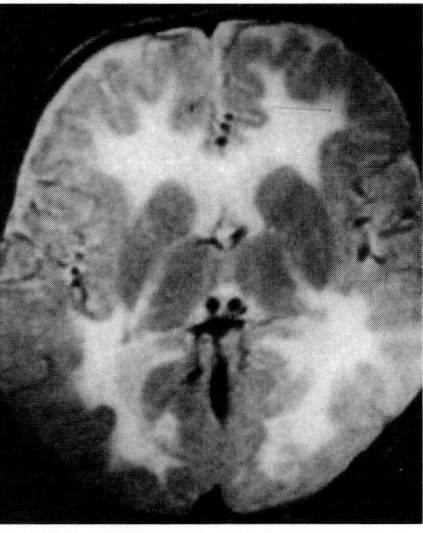

**Fig. 229-2** MRI of the brain showing severe white matter changes. *Left*: MRI (2300/80) in a 2-year-old girl showing severe changes in the subcortical white matter. *Right*: MRI (2000/80) in a 12-month-old boy also showing severe changes in the subcortical white matter. (*From Brismar.*[35] *Used with permission.*)

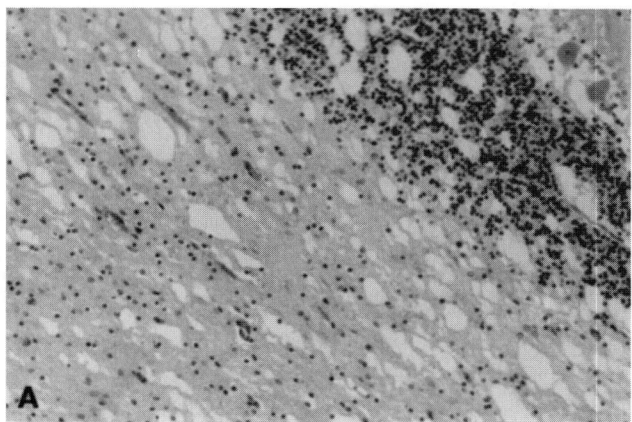

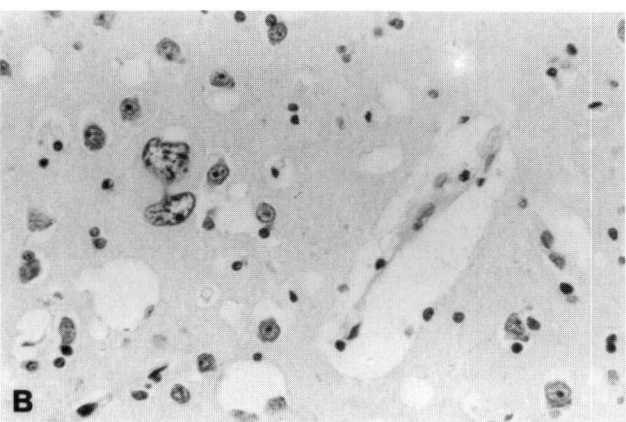

**Fig. 229-3 Histopathology showing spongy degeneration.** *Panel A:* **Cerebellar folia showing spongy degeneration. The vacuoles tend to be oriented parallel to the fibers, and are concentrated in the sub-Purkinje cell layer and in the white matter adjacent to the internal granular cell layer. (H&E × 40)** *Panel B:* **White matter showing Alzheimer type II astrocytes. The nuclei are enlarged, altered in shape and have a well-defined nuclear membrane. (H&E × 100)** *(Courtesy of Dawna Armstrong, M.D. and Hannes Vogel, M.D.)*

biochemical delineation of the disorder in the late 1980s, and detailed descriptions are available.[1,2,8,17,21] At autopsy, the white matter is characteristically soft and gelatinous. The spongy or vacuolization change (Fig. 229-3) is seen in the lower layers of the gray matter and in the subcortical white matter, with the more central white matter tending to be relatively or entirely spared. There is extensive loss of myelin, maintenance or slight increase in numbers of oligodendroglia, and a prominent increase in protoplasmic astrocytes. van Bogaert and Bertrand postulated that these changes might represent a form of chronic edema. Interestingly in the context of the newer biochemical knowledge, in 1958,[58] Wolman suggested that catabolites of low molecular value might contribute to edema formation, although he proposed that these might be breakdown products of myelin.

Adachi and colleagues performed extensive ultrastructural studies.[21,26,59] At the electron microscopic level, vacuoles are demonstrated to be within the swollen cytoplasm and processes of protoplasmic astrocytes in the cortex, and the vacuolated appearance of the white matter is primarily related to swelling of the protoplasmic astrocytes. The membrane-bound vacuoles in the cytoplasm appear to arise from the smooth portion of the endoplasmic reticulum. In the subcortical white matter, vacuoles are also found between split lamellae of the myelin spirals. The split occurs between the major dense lines of myelin. Vacuoles are thought to communicate through ruptured membranes into widened extracellular spaces. Mitochondria in astrocytes showed

elongations and contain distended and distorted cristae. Biochemically, there is marked loss of proteolipid protein and total lipids in the white matter,[60,61] but these changes are thought to be nonspecific.

## BIOCHEMISTRY

*N*-acetyl-L-aspartic acid (NAA) is a compound of particular interest because it is found only in the nervous system, because the concentration of free NAA is enormous, and because its function is almost totally enigmatic. NAA was discovered in 1956,[62] and a review of the literature published in 1989[43] provides an extensive bibliography regarding topics such as regional distribution and quantitation within the brain, species differences, changes induced by exogenous substances and treatments, synthesis, breakdown, and possible functions. The concentration of NAA is second only to glutamate in total concentration of free amino acids in mammalian brain. That concentrations of NAA can be studied *in vivo* using proton magnetic resonance spectroscopy should prove to be an important tool for understanding the clinical significance of this compound.

NAA is synthesized from acetyl-CoA and L-aspartic acid by an enzyme termed acetyl-CoA-L-aspartate *N*-acetyltransferase (EC 2.3.1.2) (Fig. 229-4).[43,63–65] The enzyme is not in the supernatant of cellular extracts and is thought to be located in a subcellular organelle, perhaps mitochondria,[66] and its distribution within the nervous system has been suggested to be similar to that of *N*-acetyl-aspartyl-glutamate (NAAG),[67] suggesting that NAA may act as a precursor for NAAG. The function of NAAG is also unclear, although there is some evidence for action on receptors of Purkinje cells.[68] Speculations regarding the function of NAA include the possibilities that the acetyl group is incorporated into brain lipids, that it might stabilize the concentration of acetyl-CoA, that it might serve as a storage form of aspartate, and that it might serve as a precursor for NAAG. NAA may function as a cofactor in conversion of lignoceric acid to cerebronic acid.[69] NAA is found in the synaptosomal fraction while NAAG is present in the mitochondrial fraction.[70] There are numerous immunohistochemical studies localizing NAA and NAAG in the nervous system,[71–73] but the function of each compound remains relatively obscure. Perhaps the development of mice with knockout mutations for the enzyme synthesizing NAA would provide further insight into the function of this compound.

Aspartoacylase was first described as a form of amino acid acylase.[74] Subsequently amino acid acylase II was found to hydrolyze NAA preferentially[75] and was designated aspartoacylase (*N*-acyl-L-aspartate amidohydrolase; EC 3.5.1.15). The enzyme hydrolyzes NAA to acetic acid and aspartic acid (Fig. 229-4). Aspartoacylase was purified from bovine brain and found to be a 55-kDa monomer with highest abundance in white matter.[76] The enzyme is variously reported to be cytosolic or membrane associated and is solubilized by detergent,[76,77] but the cDNA sequence does not suggest the existence of a leader peptide.[15]

The pathogenesis of the phenotype in aspartoacylase deficiency is unclear. Because there are many alternative sources for acetate and aspartate in the brain, it would seem unlikely that deficiency of the products of the reaction is important. Increased concentrations

**acetyl-CoA-L-aspartate *N*-acetyltransferase (EC 2.3.1.2)**

acetyl-CoA + L-aspartate → acetylaspartate + CoA-SH

**aspartoacylase (*N*-acyl-L-aspartate amidohydrolase; EC 3.5.1.15)**

acetylaspartate → L-aspartate + acetate

**Fig. 229-4 Pathways for synthesis and degradation of *N*-acetylaspartic acid.**

of NAA in tissues and fluids would suggest the possibility that NAA or related metabolites might have toxic effects. There is no explanation for the fact that most patients are asymptomatic for the first month of life and then rapidly develop symptoms, although enzymatic and metabolite abnormalities are present prenatally. Concentrations of NAA are reported to increase sixfold from birth to 20 days of age in rats,[78] but findings in humans regarding changes in concentration after birth are inconclusive.[43] It has been suggested that elevated level of NAAG may interfere with the function of the *N*-methyl-D-aspartate (NMDA) receptor.[79,80] A lengthy presentation of possible mechanisms of pathogenesis is available,[81] and it has been suggested that NAA may normally function as a component of a molecular water pump.[82]

## MOLECULAR GENETICS

Matalon and colleagues purified bovine aspartoacylase to obtain partial amino acid sequence that was used to construct primers to isolate a bovine cDNA clone.[83] The bovine cDNA was then used to isolate a human cDNA of 1435 bp with 158 bp of 5′ untranslated and 316 bp of 3′ untranslated sequence (GenBank NM 000049).[15] The human cDNA predicts a 313-amino-acid protein that is 92 percent identical to the bovine sequence. The predicted molecular mass of 36 kDa contrasts with the biochemical determination of 58 kDa for the bovine enzyme, but there are five potential phosphorylation sites and one potential *N*-glycosylation site in the human sequence. Northern blot analysis revealed transcripts of 1.44 and 5.4 kb, with intensity greatest in skeletal muscle followed by kidney and brain. Expression of the human cDNA sequence in bacteria resulted in modest levels of aspartoacylase activity. The gene for aspartoacylase (gene symbol = ASPA) was found to be comprised of 6 exons spread over 29 kb of genomic DNA,[84] and the human gene was mapped to chromosome 17p13-pter.

In the initial cloning report,[15] a single nucleotide change was found in patients with aminoacylase deficiency changing Glu at codon 285 to Ala (E285A). This mutation was found in 85 percent of 34 mutant chromosomes tested.[15] Additional mutations have been identified (Table 229-2) including mutation of Tyr at codon 231 to nonsense (Y231X), Ala at codon 305 to Glu (A305E), and a splicing mutation in intron 2 (433-2A → G).[85] Analysis of 88 disease chromosomes from Ashkenazi Jewish patients identified the mutation in all but one with E285A, Y231X, and 433-2A → G representing 83, 15, and 1 percent of the chromosomes, respectively.[85] Analysis of 40 disease chromosomes from non-Jewish families of European descent identified the A305E mutation in 24 and the E285A mutation in one with unknown mutations of 15 chromosomes. Numerous other mutations were reported since the previous edition of this chapter.[86–88] Canavan disease is not currently included in the locus specific mutation databases (http://ariel.ucs.unimelb.edu.au:80/~cotton/mdi.htm), but hopefully will be added in the future.

## DIAGNOSIS AND TREATMENT

It should be possible to suspect the diagnosis of aspartoacylase deficiency based on clinical features and cranial imaging studies. Ashkenazic ancestry is present in a substantial fraction of cases. If the disorder is suspected, a diagnosis can be confirmed by the

**Table 229-2 Common Aspartoacylase Mutations***

| Nucleotide Change | Protein Coding | Ethnicity |
|---|---|---|
| 854A → C | E285A | Ashkenazic |
| 693C → A | Y231X | Ashkenazic |
| 914C → A | A305E | European, non-Jewish |

*At least 27 less common mutations are known.[110]

demonstration of increased amounts of NAA in the urine using gas chromatography/mass spectroscopy (GC/MS)[89,90] and/or by enzyme analysis of cultured fibroblasts;[11,91] enzyme analysis of leukocytes is not reported. The mass spectra for derivitized metabolites of NAA have been published, and accurate quantitation of levels in urine, plasma, and cerebrospinal fluid have been reported using stable isotope dilution methods.[89,90] Normal ranges of NAA in urine were reported as 6.6 to 35.4 or 12.7 ± 7.8 μM/mM of creatinine in two studies with affected values typically being more than twentyfold above the upper limits of normal. Activity of aspartoacylase is readily detected in cultured skin fibroblasts with values being profoundly reduced in affected patients.[89,90] Enzyme activity has been measured spectrophotometrically as aspartic acid produced using absorbance at 340 nm to quantitate conversion of NADH to NAD in the presence of malate dehydrogenase and aspartate aminotransferase.[10,11] A sensitive radiometric assay utilizes ion exchange chromatography to quantitate the production of [³H]acetate from [³H]NAA.[91] Since the first two cases of *N*-acetylaspartic aciduria were reported without recognizing the association with infantile spongy degeneration, it seems likely that some infants will continue to be diagnosed on the basis of urinary organic acid analysis in patients with neurologic symptoms where the diagnosis of infantile spongy degeneration is not specifically being considered. For this reason, laboratories performing urinary organic acid analysis should be alert to the conditions necessary for extraction and detection of NAA and to the significance of this compound in the urine. Mutation analysis will also permit diagnosis in the majority of Jewish patients and in a significant fraction of non-Jewish patients, but biochemical studies should remain the primary basis for diagnosis or ruling out the condition.

## PRENATAL DIAGNOSIS

Prenatal diagnosis has been attempted, primarily using quantitation of NAA in amniotic fluid and measuring aspartoacylase activity in cultured amniotic fluid cells or chorionic villus samples (CVS). Early reports[57,92] have been supplanted by subsequent more extensive experience. Prenatal diagnosis using stable isotope dilution to quantitate NAA in the amniotic fluid found values within the normal range in a fetus later born and found to be healthy,[89] and retrospective analysis of amniotic fluid revealed elevation of NAA in two affected pregnancies.[93] In one report, 19 pregnancies at 1 in 4 risk were analyzed using enzyme assay on cultured CVS and amniocytes, as well as measurement of NAA in amniotic fluid;[94] 16 pregnancies were predicted to be normal and 3 were predicted to be affected. With expansion of this series, the same group found that 4 of 24 fetuses predicted to be normal were born affected.[83] One study of 17 pregnancies[95] compared quantitation of amniotic fluid NAA in four laboratories; 8 of 17 pregnancies were predicted to be affected, and biochemical or clinical data were available in 6 of these 8 to indicate a correct diagnosis. One case yielded ambiguous data, and one false negative result occurred. Enzyme analysis of cultured amniotic fluid cells is not reliable because enzyme activity is low in normal cells.[95,96] There is evidence that direct analysis of CVS is reliable for enzyme assay although cultured CVS cells are not.[97] It has been emphasized that isotope dilution methods are more reliable for quantitation of NAA and that normal values in amniotic fluid increase during gestation.[93]

Overall, the data suggest that there are modest elevations of NAA in amniotic fluid during the second trimester, but these increases are minimal by comparison to the findings in postnatal urine. Although prenatal diagnosis by measurement of amniotic fluid NAA is accurate in the majority of cases, the separation of values in affected and unaffected pregnancies is marginal, and numerous diagnostic errors have occurred. Use of isotope dilution methods and appropriate gestational controls should provide improved reliability. Levels of aspartoacylase activity in cultured CVS and cultured amniocytes are very low by comparison to cultured skin fibroblasts, and are not reliable for prenatal diagnosis. Given these problems and a growing experience with molecular diagnosis,[98–100] diagnosis by DNA analysis is far more preferable and can be used in addition to measurement of NAA in amniotic fluid. DNA diagnosis should be straightforward in cases where the mutations can be identified in the index case or parents.

## TREATMENT

There is no known treatment for aspartoacylase deficiency. It is of interest to know whether inhibitors of the enzyme that synthesizes NAA can be developed and tested for safety and efficacy in animal models. Although there are reports of attempts at somatic gene therapy,[101,102] studies are very preliminary, and success in this regard is likely to be years away.

## PREVENTION

Carrier-detection programs combined with prenatal diagnosis have led to a substantial reduction in the occurrence of Tay Sachs disease in the Ashkenazic population (see Chap. 153). With recognition that two mutations account for almost all carriers in the Ashkenazic population, it was straightforward to consider adding Canavan disease to existing heterozygote screening programs such as those for Tay Sachs disease.[103] The carrier frequency in the Ashkenazic population is reported to be 1 in 37 to 1 in 60.[16,104,105] A benign polymorphism is reported in the region of the Y231X mutation requiring distinction of the benign and pathologic mutations.[106] A committee of the American College of Obstetrics and Gynecology has recommended that molecular carrier screening be offered to Ashkenazic couples.[107] It is likely that the occurrence of live-born infants with Canavan disease in the Ashkenazic population will decline on this basis. Concern has been expressed that royalty fees may limit the utilization of carrier testing (Boston Globe, Dec. 20, 1999).

## ANIMAL MODELS

Spongy degeneration of white matter has been reported in silver foxes,[108] Hereford calves,[109] an Egyptian Mau kitten, a Silkie terrier puppy, a Samoyed puppy, and Labrador retrievers (see Hagen and Bjerkå[94] for bibliography). In cases in which adequate samples are available, it is of interest to know whether any of these animal models are associated with aspartoacylase deficiency, but no data have yet been reported. The literature implies that additional affected animals can be bred in the case of the silver foxes[108] and Hereford calves.[109] It is possible to prepare a mouse model using gene-targeting methodology.

## REFERENCES

1. van Bogaert L, Bertrand I: Sur une idiotie familiale avec dégénérescence spongieuse de nevraxe. *Acta Neurol Belg* **49**:572, 1949.
2. van Bogaert L, Bertrand I: *Spongy Degeneration of the Brain in Infancy.* Amsterdam, North Holland, 1967.
3. Globus JH, Strauss I: Progressive degenerative subcortical encephalopathy (Schilder's disease). *Arch Neurol Psychiatry* **20**:1190, 1928.
4. Canavan MM: Schilder's encephalitis periaxialis diffusa. *Arch Neurol Psychiat* **25**:299, 1931.
5. Eiselsberg F: Über frühkindliche familiäre diffuse Hirnsklerose. *Z Kinderheilk* **58**:702, 1937.
6. Jervis GA: Early infantile acute diffuse sclerosis of the brain (Krabbe's type). *Am J Dis Child* **64**:1055, 1942.
7. Jervis GA: Early infantile acute diffuse sclerosis of brain (Krabbe's disease). *Mod Probl Pediatr* **1**:781, 1954.
8. Banker BQ, Robertson JT, Victor M: Spongy degeneration of the central nervous system in infancy. *Neurology* **14**:981, 1964.
9. Kvittingen EA, Guldal G, Borsting S, Skalpe IO, Stokke O, Jellum E: N-Acetylaspartic aciduria in a child with a progressive cerebral atrophy. *Clin Chim Acta* **158**:217, 1986.
10. Hagenfeldt L, Bollgren I, Venizelos N: N-Acetylaspartic aciduria due to aspartoacylase deficiency—A new aetiology of childhood leukodystrophy. *J Inherit Metab Dis* **10**:135, 1987.
11. Matalon R, Michals K, Sebesta D, Deanching M, Gashkoff P, Casanova J: Aspartoacylase deficiency and N-acetylaspartic aciduria in patients with Canavan disease. *Am J Med Genet* **29**:463, 1988.
12. Matalon R: Reply to Drs. Divry and Mathieu. *Am J Med Genet* **32**:551, 1989.
13. Divry P, Vianey-Liaud C, Gay C, Macabeo V, Rapin F, Echenne B: N-Acetylaspartic aciduria: Report of three new cases in children with a neurological syndrome associating macrocephaly and leukodystrophy. *J Inherit Metab Dis* **11**:307, 1988.
14. Divry P, Mathieu M: Aspartoacylase deficiency and N-acetylaspartic aciduria in patients with Canavan disease. *Am J Med Genet* **32**:550, 1989.
15. Kaul R, Gao GP, Balamurugan K, Matalon R: Cloning of the human aspartoacylase cDNA and a common missense mutation in Canavan disease. *Nat Genet* **5**:118, 1993.
16. Matalon R, Michals K, Kaul R: Canavan disease: From spongy degeneration to molecular analysis. *J Pediatr* **127**:511, 1995.
17. Banker BQ, Victor M: Spongy degeneration of infancy, in Goodman RM, Motulsky AG (eds): *Genetic Diseases Among Ashkenazi Jews.* New York, Raven Press, 1979, p 201.
18. Buchanan DS, Davis RL: Spongy degeneration of the nervous system. *Neurology* **15**:207, 1965.
19. Traeger EC, Rapin I: The clinical course of Canavan disease. *Pediatr Neurol* **18**:207, 1998.
20. Ungar M, Goodman RM: Spongy degeneration of the brain in Israel: A retrospective study. *Clin Genet* **23**:23, 1983.
21. Adachi M, Aronson SM: Studies on spongy degeneration of the central nervous system (van Bogaert-Bertrand type), in Aronson SM, Volk BW (eds): *Inborn Disorders of Sphingolipid Metabolism.* Oxford, Pergamon Press, 1967, p 129.
22. Manhoff DT, Rorke LB, Yachnis AT: Primary intracranial atypical teratoid/rhabdoid tumor in a child with Canavan disease. *Pediatr Neurosurg* **22**:214, 1995.
23. von Moers A, Sperner J, Michael T, Scheffner D, Schutgens RHB: Variable course of Canavan disease in two boys with early infantile aspartoacylase deficiency. *Dev Med Child Neurol* **33**:824, 1991.
24. Zelnik N, Luder AS, Elpeleg ON, Gross-Tsur V, Amir N, Hemli JA, Fattal A, Harel S: Protracted clinical course for patients with Canavan disease. *Dev Med Child Neurol* **35**:355, 1993.
25. Zafeiriou DI, Kleijer WJ, Maroupoulos G, Anastasiou AL, Augoustidou-Savvopoulou P, Paladopoulou EE, Fagan E, Payne S: Protracted course of N-acetylaspartic aciduria in two non-Jewish siblings: Identical clinical and magnetic resonance imaging findings. *Brain Dev* **21**:205, 1999.
26. Adachi M, Volk BW: Protracted form of spongy degeneration of the central nervous system (van Bogaert and Bertrand type). *Neurology* **18**:1084, 1968.
27. Brucher JM, Dom R, Robin A: Degenerescence spongieuse juvenile du système nerve central. Ses rapports avec la maladie d'Hallervorden-Spatz et les dystrophies neuroaxonales. *Rev Neurol* **119**:425, 1968.
28. Jellinger K, Seitelberger F: Juvenile form of spongy degeneration of the CNS. *Acta Neuropathol* **13**:276, 1969.
29. Goodhue WW, Couch RD, Nakimi H: Spongy degeneration of the CNS. An instance of the rare juvenile form. *Arch Neurol* **36**:481, 1979.
30. Bakon M, Strauss S, Shental I, Elpeleg ON: Cholelithiasis in Canavan disease. *J Ultrasound Med* **12**:363, 1993.
31. Harbord MG, Harden A, Harding B, Brett EM, Baraitser M: Megalencephaly with dysmyelination, spasticity, ataxia, seizures and distinctive neurophysiological findings in two siblings. *Neuropediatrics* **21**:164, 1990.
32. Aicardi J, Boulloche J, Bourgeois M, Aicardi J: Leukoencephalopathy, megalencephaly, and mild clinical course. A recently individualized familial leukodystrophy. Report on five new cases. *J Child Neurol* **11**:349, 1996.
33. Mejaski-Bosnjak V, Besenski N, Brockmann K, Pouwels PJW, Frahm J, Hanefeld FA: Cystic leukoencephalopathy in a megaloencephalic child: Clinical and magnetic resonance imaging/magnetic resonance spectroscopy findings. *Pediatr Neurol* **16**:347, 1997.
34. Grodd W, Krägeloh-Mann I, Petersen D, Trefz FK, Harzer K: *In vivo* assessment of N-acetylaspartate in brain in spongy degeneration (Canavan's disease) by proton spectroscopy. *Lancet* **336**:437, 1990.
35. Brismar J, Brismar G, Gascon G, Ozand P: Canavan disease: CT and MR imaging of the brain. *AJNR Am J Neuroradiol* **11**:805, 1990.

36. Marks HG, Caro PA, Wang ZY, Detre JA, Bogdan AR, Gusnard DA, Zimmerman RA: Use of computed tomography, magnetic resonance imaging, and localized $^1$H magnetic resonance spectroscopy in Canavan's disease: A case report. *Ann Neurol* **30**:106, 1991.

37. Austin SJ, Connelly A, Gadian DG, Benton JS, Brett EM: Localized $^1$H NMR spectroscopy in Canavan's disease: A report of two cases. *Magn Reson Med* **19**:439, 1991.

38. Grodd W, Krägeloh-Mann I, Klose U, Sauter R: Metabolic and destructive brain disorders in children: Findings with localized proton MR spectroscopy. *Radiology* **181**:173, 1991.

39. Barker PB, Bryan RN, Kumar AJ, Naidu S: Proton NMR spectroscopy of Canavan's disease. *Neuropediatrics* **23**:263, 1992.

40. Toft PB, Geiß-Holtorff R, Rolland MO, Pryds O, Müller-Forell W, Christensen E, Lehnert W, Lou HC, Ott D, Hennig J, Henriksen O: Magnetic resonance imaging in juvenile Canavan disease. *Eur J Pediatr* **152**:750, 1993.

41. Bührer C, Bassir C, von Moers A, Sperner J, Michael T, Scheffner D, Kaufmann HJ: Cranial ultrasound findings in aspartoacylase deficiency (Canavan disease). *Pediatr Radiol* **23**:395, 1993.

42. McAdams HP, Geyer CA, Done SL, Deigh D, Mitchell M, Ghaed VN: CT and MR imaging of Canavan disease. *AJNR Am J Neuroradiol* **11**:397, 1990.

43. Birken DL, Oldendorf WH: N-Acetyl-l-aspartic acid: A literature review of a compound prominent in $^1$H-NMR spectroscopic studies of brain. *Neurosci Biobehav Rev* **13**:23, 1989.

44. Wittsack H-J, Kugel H, Roth B, Heindel W: Quantitative measurements with localized $^1$H MR spectroscopy in children with Canavan's disease. *J Magn Reson Imaging* **6**:889, 1996.

45. Blüml S: *In vivo* quantitation of cerebral metabolite concentrations using natural abundance $^{13}$C MRS at 1.5 T. *J Magn Reson* **136**:219, 1999.

46. Hamaguchi H, Nihei K, Nakamoto N, Ezoe T, Naito H, Hara M, Yokota K, Inoue Y, Matsumoto I: A case of Canavan disease: The first biochemically proven case in a Japanese girl. *Brain Dev* **15**:367, 1993.

47. Kobayashi K, Tsujino S, Ezoe T, Hamaguchi M, Nihei K: Missense mutation (I143T) in a Japanese patient with Canavan disease. *Hum Mutat Suppl* **1**:S308, 1998.

48. Rady PL, Vargas T, Tyring SK, Matalon R, Langenbeck U: Novel missense mutation (Y231C) in a Turkish patient with Canavan disease. *Am J Med Genet* **87**:273, 1999.

49. Elpeleg ON, Amir N, Barash V, Glick B, Gross-Tsur V, Shachar E, Shapira Y, Tzelnik N: Canavan disease and N-acetylaspartic aciduria. *Neuropediatrics* **20**:238, 1989.

50. Ozand PT, Gascon GG, Dhalla M: Aspartoacylase deficiency and Canavan disease in Saudi Arabia. *Am J Med Genet* **35**:266, 1990.

51. Yalaz K, Topçu M, Topaloglu H, Gürçay Ö, Özcan OE, Önol B, Renda Y: N-Acetylaspartic aciduria in Canavan disease: Another proof in two infants. *Neuropediatrics* **21**:140, 1990.

52. Michelakakis H, Giouroukos S, Divry P, Katsarou E, Rolland MO, Skardoutsou A: Canavan disease: Findings in four new cases. *J Inherit Metab Dis* **14**:267, 1991.

53. de Coo IFM, Gabreëls FJM, Renier WO, DePont JJHHM, van Haelst UJGM, Veerkamp JH, Trijbels JMF, Jaspar HHJ, Renkawek K: Canavan disease: Neuromorphological and biochemical analysis of a brain biopsy specimen. *Clin Neuropathol* **10**:73, 1991.

54. Ozand PT, Devol EB, Gascon GG: Neurometabolic diseases at a national referral center: Five years experience at the King Faisal Specialist Hospital and Research Centre. *J Child Neurol Suppl* **7**:S4, 1992.

55. Bartalini G, Margollicci M, Balestri P, Farnetani MA, Cioni M, Fois A: Biochemical diagnosis of Canavan disease. *Child Nerv Syst* **8**:468, 1992.

56. Matalon R, Kaul R, Casanova J, Michals K, Johnson A, Rapin I, Gashkoff P, Deanching M: Aspartoacylase deficiency: The enzyme defect in Canavan disease. *J Inherit Metab Dis* **12(Suppl)**:329, 1989.

57. Ozand PT, Gascon GG, Aqeel AL, Nester MJ, Feryal RR, Gleispach H, Cook JD, Odaib AAL, Leis HJ: Prenatal detection of Canavan disease. *Lancet* **337**:735, 1991.

58. Wolman M: The spongy type of diffuse sclerosis. *Brain* **81**:243, 1958.

59. Adachi M, Torii J, Schneck L, Volk BW: Electron microscopic and enzyme histochemical studies of the cerebellum in spongy degeneration (van Bogaert and Bertrand type). *Acta Neuropathol (Berl)* **20**:22, 1972.

60. Lees MB, Folch-Pi J: A study of some human brains with pathological changes, in Folch-Pi J (ed): *Chemical Pathology of the Nervous System.* Oxford, Pergamon Press, 1961, p 75.

61. Kamoshita S, Rapin I, Suzuki K: Spongy degeneration of the brain. *Neurology (Minneap)* **19**:975, 1968.

62. Tallan HH, Moore S, Stein WH: N-Acetyl-l-aspartic acid in brain. *J Biol Chem* **219**:257, 1956.

63. Knizley H Jr: The enzymatic synthesis of N-acetyl-l-aspartic acid by a water-insoluble preparation of a cat brain acetone powder. *J Biol Chem* **242**:4619, 1967.

64. Goldstein FB: Biosynthesis of N-acetyl-L-aspartic acid. *J Biol Chem* **234**:2702, 1959.

65. Goldstein FB: The enzymatic synthesis of N-acetyl-L-aspartic acid by subcellular preparations of rat brain. *J Biol Chem* **244**:4257, 1969.

66. Patel TB, Clark JB: Synthesis of N-acetyl-L-aspartate by rat brain mitochondria and its involvement in mitochondrial/cytosolic carbon transport. *Biochem J* **184**:539, 1979.

67. Truckenmiller ME, Namboodiri MAA, Brownstein MJ, Neale JH: N-Acetylation of l-aspartate in the nervous system: Differential distribution of a specific enzyme. *J Neurochem* **45**:1658, 1985.

68. Sekiguchi M, Okamoto K, Sakai Y: Excitatory action of N-acetylaspartylglutamate on Purkinje cells in guinea pig cerebellar slices: An intrasomatic study. *Brain Res* **423**:23, 1987.

69. Shigematsu H, Okamura N, Shimeno H, Kishimoto Y, Kan L, Fenselau C: Purification and characterization of the heat-stable factors essential for the conversion of lignoceric acid to cerebronic acid and glutamic acid: Identification of N-acetyl-L-aspartic acid. *J Neurochem* **40**:814, 1983.

70. Reichelt KL, Fonnum F: Subcellular localization of N-acetyl-aspartyl-glutamate, N-acetyl-glutamate and glutathione in brain. *J Neurochem* **16**:1409, 1969.

71. Moffett JR, Namboodiri MAA, Cangro CB, Neale JH: Immunohisto-chemical localization of N-acetylaspartate in rat brain. *Neuroreport* **2**:131, 1991.

72. Moffett JR, Namboodiri MAA, Neale JH: Enhanced carbodiimide fixation for immunohistochemistry: Application to the comparative distributions of N-acetylaspartylglutamate and N-acetylaspartate immunoreactivities in rat brain. *J Histol Cytochem* **41**:559, 1993.

73. Ory-Lavollée L, Blakely RD, Coyle JT: Neurochemical and immuno-cytochemical studies on the distribution of N-acetyl-aspartylglutamate and N-acetyl-aspartate in rat spinal cord and some peripheral nervous tissues. *J Neurochem* **48**:895, 1987.

74. Birnbaum SM: Aminoacylase: Amino acid acylases I and II from hog kidney. *Methods Enzymol* **2**:115, 1955.

75. Birnbaum SM, Levintow L, Kingsley RB, Greenstein JP: Specificity of amino acid acylases. *J Biol Chem* **194**:455, 1952.

76. Kaul R, Casanova J, Johnson AB, Tang P, Matalon R: Purification, characterization, and localization of aspartoacylase from bovine brain. *J Neurochem* **56**:129, 1991.

77. Goldstein FB: Amidohydrolases of brain; enzymatic hydrolysis of N-acetyl-L-aspartate and other N-acyl-L-amino acids. *J Neurochem* **26**:45, 1976.

78. Tallan HH: Studies on the distribution of N-acetyl-L-aspartic acid in brain. *J Biol Chem* **224**:41, 1957.

79. Burlina A, Skaper SD, Mazza MR, Ferrari V, Leon A, Burlina AB: N-acetylaspartylglutamate selectively inhibits neuronal responses to N-methyl-D-aspartic acid *in vitro*. *J Neurochem* **63**:1174, 1994.

80. Burlina AP, Ferrari V, Divry P, Gradowska W, Jakobs C, Bennett MJ, Sewell AC, Dionisi-Vici C, Burlina AB: N-Acetylaspartylglutamate in Canavan disease: An adverse effector? *Eur J Pediatr* **158**:406, 1999.

81. Baslow MH, Resnik TR: Canavan disease. *J Mol Neurosci* **9**:109, 1997.

82. Baslow MH: Molecular water pumps and the aetiology of Canavan disease: A case of the sorcerer's apprentice. *J Inherit Metab Dis* **22**:99, 1999.

83. Matalon R, Kaul R, Michals K: Canavan disease: Biochemical and molecular studies. *J Inherit Metab Dis* **16**:744, 1993.

84. Kaul R, Balamurugan K, Gao GP, Matalon R: Canavan disease: Genomic organization and localization of human *ASPA* to 17p13-ter and conservation of the *ASPA* gene during evolution. *Genomics* **21**:364, 1994.

85. Kaul R, Gao GP, Aloya M, Balamurugan K, Petrosky A, Michals K, Matalon R: Canavan disease: Mutations among Jewish and non-Jewish patients. *Am J Hum Genet* **55**:34, 1994.

86. Shaag A, Anikster Y, Christensen E, Glustein JZ, Fois A, Michelakakis H, Nigro F, Pronicka E, Ribes A, Zabot MT, Elpeleg ON: The molecular basis of Canavan (aspartoacylase deficiency) disease in European non-Jewish patients. *Am J Hum Genet* **57**:572, 1995.

87. Kaul R, Gao GP, Matalon R, Aloya M, Su Q, Jin M, Johnson AB, Schutgens RBH, Clarke JTR: Identification and expression of eight

novel mutations among non-Jewish patients with Canavan disease. *Am J Hum Genet* **59**:95, 1996.

88. Matalon R, Michals-Matalon K: Biochemistry and molecular biology of Canavan disease. *Neurochem Res* **24**:507, 1999.
89. Jakobs C, ten Brink HJ, Langelaar SA, Zee T, Stellaard F, Macek M, Srsnová K, Srsen S, Kleijer WJ: Stable isotope dilution analysis of *N*-acetylaspartic acid in CSF, blood, urine and amniotic fluid: Accurate postnatal diagnosis and the potential for prenatal diagnosis of Canavan disease. *J Inherit Metab Dis* **14**:653, 1991.
90. Kelley RI, Stamas JN: Quantification of *N*-acetyl-L-aspartic acid in urine by isotope dilution gas chromatography-mass spectrometry. *J Inherit Metab Dis* **15**:97, 1992.
91. Barash V, Flhor D, Morag B, Boneh A, Elpeleg ON, Gilon C: A radiometric assay for aspartoacylase activity in human fibroblasts: Application for the diagnosis of Canavan's disease. *Clin Chim Acta* **201**:175, 1991.
92. Jakobs C, ten Brink HJ, Divry P, Rolland MO: Prenatal diagnosis of Canavan disease. *Eur J Pediatr* **151**:620, 1992.
93. Kelley RI: Prenatal detection of Canavan disease by measurement of *N*-acetyl-L-aspartate in amniotic fluid. *J Inherit Metab Dis* **16**:918, 1993.
94. Matalon R, Michals K, Gashkoff P, Kaul R: Prenatal diagnosis of Canavan disease. *J Inherit Metab Dis* **15**:392, 1992.
95. Bennett MJ, Gibson KM, Sherwood WG, Divry P, Rolland MO, Elpeleg ON, Rinaldo P, Jakobs C: Reliable prenatal diagnosis of Canavan disease (aspartoacylase deficiency): Comparison of enzymatic and metabolite analysis. *J Inherit Metab Dis* **16**:831, 1993.
96. Rolland MO, Mandon G, Bernard A, Zabot MT, Mathieu M: Unreliable verification of prenatal diagnosis of Canavan disease: Aspartoacylase activity in deficient and normal fetal skin fibroblasts. *J Inherit Metab Dis* **17**:748, 1994.
97. Rolland MO, Divry P, Mandon G, Thoulon JM, Fiumara A, Mathieu M: First-trimester prenatal diagnosis of Canavan disease. *J Inherit Metab Dis* **16**:581, 1993.
98. Elpeleg ON, Shaag A, Anikster Y, Jakobs C: Prenatal detection of Canavan disease (Aspartoacylase deficiency) by DNA analysis. *J Inherit Metab Dis* **17**:664, 1994.
99. Matalon R, Kaul R, Gao GP, Michals K, Gray RGF, Bennett-Briton S, Norman A, Smith M, Jakobs C: Prenatal diagnosis for Canavan disease: The use of DNA markers. *J Inherit Metab Dis* **18**:215, 1995.
100. Besley GT, Elpeleg ON, Shaag A, Manning NJ, Jakobs C, Walter JH: Prenatal diagnosis of Canavan disease—Problems and dilemmas. *J Inherit Metab Dis* **22**:263, 1999.
101. Marshall E: New Zealand's leap into gene therapy. *Science* **271**:1489, 1996.
102. During M: Gene therapy in New Zealand. *Science* **272**:467, 1996.
103. Shuber AP, Michalowsky LA, Nass GS, Skoletsky J, Hire LM, Kotsopoulos SK, Phipps MF, Barberio DM, Klinger KW: High throughput parallel analysis of hundreds of patient samples for more than 100 mutations in multiple disease genes. *Hum Mol Genet* **6**:337, 1997.
104. Elpeleg ON, Anikster Y, Barash V, Branski D, Shaag A: The frequency of the C854 mutation in the aspartoacylase gene in Ashkenazi Jews in Israel. *Am J Hum Genet* **55**:287, 1994.
105. Kronn D, Oddoux C, Phillips J, Ostrer H: Prevalence of Canavan disease heterozygotes in the New York metropolitan Ashkenazi Jewish population. *Am J Hum Genet* **57**:1250, 1995.
106. Alford RL, DeMarchi JM, Richards CS: Frequency of a DNA polymorphism at position Y231 in the aspartoacylase gene and its impact on DNA-based carrier testing for Canavan disease in the Ashkenazi Jewish population. *Hum Mutat* **Suppl 1**:S161, 1998.
107. ACOG committee opinion. Screening for Canavan disease. Number 212, November 1998. Committee on Genetics. American College of Obstetricians and Gynecologists. *Int J Gynaecol Obstet* **65**:91, 1999.
108. Hagen G, Bjerkås I: Spongy degeneration of white matter in the central nervous system of silver foxes (*Vulpes vulpes*). *Vet Pathol* **27**:187, 1990.
109. Duffel SJ: Neuraxial oedema of Hereford calves with and without hypomyelinogenesis. *Vet Rec* **118**:95, 1986.
110. Matalon RM, Michals-Matalon K: Spongy degeneration of the brain, Canavan disease: Biochemical and molecular findings. *Front Biosci* **5**:D307, 2000.

# The Inherited Epilepsies

*Jeffrey L. Noebels*

1. *Heredity* represents the single largest etiology of the epilepsies, a common and extremely heterogeneous set of neurologic disorders defined by repeated clinical seizure episodes linked to aberrant electrical synchronization of the brain. Like cardiac arrhythmias, epileptic seizures display distinctive electrographic patterns that reflect signaling abnormalities within critical cortical networks. The seizures are due to primary molecular defects intrinsic to neurons or glia that alter membrane or synaptic excitability, or to induced excitability fluctuations when these circuits become the downstream targets of developmental or metabolic disturbances.

2. *Genetic transmission patterns* of epilepsy are both Mendelian and complex; most cases are sporadic. Currently recognized monogenic syndromes represent a small subset of all epilepsies. While some phenotypes are comprised only of seizures, in many syndromes, epilepsy is only one highly variable element of a broader clinical spectrum, because genes associated with epilepsy may be expressed in both neural and nonneural tissues.

3. *Epileptic seizures* are categorized by the extent of their cerebral involvement (partial or generalized); by the sparing or impairment of consciousness (simple or complex); and by the pattern of associated motor activity (atonic, astatic, tonic, clonic, arrest). Clinical *epilepsy syndromes* are defined by the seizure type, natural history, precipitating factors, drug sensitivity, and the presence of associated neurologic deficits. In *benign* epilepsy syndromes, the seizures resolve over time; in others, the seizure disorder may be stationary for prolonged periods, or herald the onset of even more frequent seizures, progressive neurologic deficits, or death.

4. *Molecular mechanisms* and the affected neuronal circuits differ broadly among defined seizure types and between epilepsy syndromes. Numerous gene loci have now been identified for some common seizure patterns and syndromes, many of which are recognized to comprise multiple, genetically distinct diseases. These findings indicate that inherited epilepsies reflect a large and diverse group of rare genetic disorders.

5. *Genes for epileptogenesis* include a broad range of molecules regulating brain assembly, activity, and cell death. The underlying human epilepsy syndromes discovered to date can be provisionally divided into three broad categories. The first category includes developmental cortical malformations and cellular *migration disturbances* leading to early structural changes in neural connectivity. The second category consists of dynamic *excitability defects* in neuronal ion channels, receptors, and the regulation of synaptic transmission. The third category comprises *errors of cellular homeostasis* and intermediary metabolism leading to oxidative deficiency, aberrant proteolysis, and neurode-

generation. Spontaneous mutations and targeted mutagenesis in experimental models reveal an even more extensive array of genes associated with epilepsy that affect synaptogenesis, vesicle release, and neuroplasticity.

6. *Epilepsy genes*, despite their remarkable functional diversity, represent a specific subgroup of neurogenetic disorders, because many inherited defects in the biology of neurons or glia do not lead to a seizure phenotype. Those that are not permissive for spontaneous epilepsy may lower the threshold for seizures triggered by various stimuli or other mutant alleles. Genomic comparisons of tissue from identified monogenic epilepsies with multigenic and acquired syndromes may ultimately reveal the critical molecular neuropathology required for an epileptic phenotype.

7. *Molecular neuroplasticity* triggered by the seizures themselves significantly obscures identification of the intervening neural mechanisms, and the modulating signals that determine the episodic appearance are still poorly understood. Epilepsy can result in abnormal brain development, and abnormal brain development can result in epilepsy. Because human brain tissue is typically unavailable until misleading terminal stages, serial analysis of orthologous mouse models of human disease genes will help reveal the molecular pathogenesis of most inborn errors.

8. *Specific antiepileptic pharmacology* can control, but not cure, seizure disorders. Some epilepsies are medically intractable, and the underlying brain pathology may progress with significant morbidity and shortened life span. Recent advances in clinical diagnosis, molecular genetics, and experimental genetic models have increased the early recognition and understanding of inherited epileptogenesis, and may ultimately lead to novel pharmacology designed toward prevention or reversal of the underlying defects.

The epilepsies are an ancient neurologic phenotype whose exact molecular causes have remained mysterious until the last few years of gene discovery. The disorder is common, affecting all age groups and approximately 1 percent of the population worldwide.[1] Symptomatic or acquired epilepsies comprise about one-third of all new cases of epilepsy and a majority of those at older ages. They arise as sequelae from a spectrum of acute or chronic injury to the brain, including vascular insufficiency, infection, tumor, trauma, and metabolic and drug-induced encephalopathies. Genetic disorders account for the next largest source of epilepsy, from 20 to 30 percent, and nonsyndromic, sporadic cases of "pure epilepsy" without historical or clinical evidence of brain injury account for the large remaining fraction of individuals with epilepsy of indeterminate etiology.

Over 180 known Mendelian variants share epilepsy as one expression of the inherited gene error.[2] Although these syndromes are individually rare and constitute only a fraction of all patients with seizures, the general category of gene-linked epilepsies represents the most common cause of a phenotype that ranks second only to mental retardation as the most prevalent human neurologic disorder. Seizures are the most frequent manifestation of neurologic dysfunction in the neonatal period,[3] and may go unrecognized due to immaturity of the central nervous system.[4] Because most genetic epilepsies appear early in life, they pose significant risk to normal neocortical development[5] and often signal the onset of complex neurologic syndromes. Inherited epilepsies thus represent one of the most important, yet difficult, of all seizure etiologies to accurately diagnose and treat.

## NON-MENDELIAN EPILEPSIES

Epilepsies without discernible etiology or a clear Mendelian mode of inheritance are the most frequent clinical presentation, comprising at least two-thirds of all diagnoses.[6] Whether these cases represent sporadic mutations in one or several genes, environmentally induced alterations in seizure threshold, or a combination of both is uncertain. Multiple factors, including *de novo* mutations of an extremely large pool of candidate genes, small family size, equivocal clinical seizure classification, and wide variations in the seizure type, onset, or accompanying phenotypes in related family members may all contribute to this complexity. Nonparametric linkage methods such as affected sib pair analysis, or large-scale genomic approaches involving direct evaluation of multiple candidate loci, may prove helpful in the future in isolating the genes. However, clinical ascertainment of distinctive seizure patterns among the variety of episodic phenotypes remains a major obstacle.

## DEFINITION OF EPILEPSY GENES

Epilepsy genes encode molecules capable of altering the normal development of cellular mechanisms that control synchronization and burst firing in cortical neurons. This is an empirical definition based on the observation that human and experimental inherited epilepsies arise from a broad spectrum of gene lesions that ultimately modify the biology of neuronal membranes to produce episodic instability of network firing patterns.[7]

Epilepsy is a highly specific and conditional brain excitability trait. Many anatomic lesions of the neocortex that are visible at both the cellular and macroscopic levels do not display recurrent seizures; those that do so are not electrically hyperactive at all times. No other aspect except the aberrant electrical discharge itself has yet provided an explanation for the intermittent clinical seizure patterns, or served as a valid marker for the disease. While each epilepsy mutation described to date initiates a specific loss or gain of function in the gene product, most of these genes control multiple signaling pathways within neurons, leading to protean cellular pathologies. Consequently, the most consistent phenotypic marker of an "epileptic neuron" is not cytologic, but electric: the spontaneous appearance of a giant synchronized membrane depolarization ("the paroxysmal depolarizing shift" or PDS) in intracellular recordings from neurons within an epileptic focus.[8] All genes for convulsive seizures must eventually be understood in terms of their position in the pathway that regulates this neuronal behavior in cortical networks. The lack of a characteristic morphologic signature of the lesion, and the ephemeral temporal expression of the electrocortical phenotype, make this family of neuronal membrane disorders leading to synchronized bursting an elusive defect to understand at the molecular level.

## LABORATORY CHARACTERIZATION OF CLINICAL EPILEPSY PHENOTYPES

Electroencephalography (EEG) combined with video monitoring can help establish the diagnosis of epilepsy, determine the electrocortical seizure type, and help clarify its site of origin. Epileptiform abnormalities in the EEG tracing may be focal or generalized. The main types of focal epileptiform discharges arise from the temporal, frontal, occipital, centroparietal, centrotemporal, and midline regions of the brain.[9] Detection of seizure origin is often obscured by deep or small foci, regional brain anatomy, or rapid spread of epileptiform discharges throughout the brain. Depth recordings and functional imaging are used to evaluate deeper structures. Currently recognized patterns of epileptiform discharges consist of the generalized 3 Hz spike-and-wave, slow or atypical spike-and-wave variants, paroxysmal fast or electrodecremental activity, and hypsarrhythmic (variable, high-voltage spike and slow wave) patterns. Status epilepticus, either focal or generalized, is manifested by recurrent seizure activity without interim clinical recovery. Benign epileptiform EEG variants not associated with seizures but possibly implicated as subclinical traits have also been identified, including the "14 & 6" spike bursts; small, sharp spikes; wicket waves; 6 Hz spike-and-wave discharges; and rhythmic temporal theta activity.

Anatomic and functional brain assessment using coregistered EEG, magnetic resonance imaging, and single-positron emission tomography of cerebral blood flow can help to further subcategorize seizure patterns and define specific epilepsy syndromes (Fig. 230-1).[10,11] These tools will greatly contribute to the isolation of new genetic syndromes, as well as improving the clinical staging of disease progression and response to therapy.

## BASIC MECHANISMS OF EPILEPSIES

The EEG activity of individuals with epilepsy may deviate from its normal repertoire of unsynchronized and rhythmic activity to reveal intermittent fast discharges, evidence that powerful endogenous inhibitory mechanisms are transiently unable to suppress bursting activity within the cortex. During these isolated interictal EEG "spikes," which are clinically asymptomatic if they occur infrequently, the firing pattern of single cortical neurons is invariably characterized by an extraordinarily large depolarization with repetitive firing, the paroxysmal depolarizing burst (PDS), an event that reflects a giant EPSP-like depolarization of the dendritic arbor. This neuronal pattern of sudden, *excessive depolarization* in an "epileptic neuron" has been experimentally reproduced by agents that selectively open depolarizing voltage- and ligand-gated ion channels (i.e., $Na^+$, $Ca^{++}$, and AMPA or NMDA-type glutamate receptors) or antagonize those responsible for membrane repolarization (i.e., voltage- or ligand-gated $K^+$ and $Cl^-$ channels),[12] suggesting that ion channelopathies may represent the simplest gene candidates for mutations linked with epilepsy. Indeed, voltage- and ligand-gated channels serve as primary targets for most anticonvulsants currently in use.[13] The PDS represents *abnormal synchronization* of impulse firing within an epileptic circuit, and it is useful to assume that all inherited epileptic lesions producing this discharge ultimately do so by disturbing the balance of synaptic excitation and inhibition in a distributed way that allows transient neuronal oscillations to produce sustained regenerative ictal events (Fig. 230-2).

Rhythmic firing is an innate property of normal brain. Increased neuronal synchronization can be achieved acutely by enhancing intrinsic membrane excitability in individual cells, numerically altering excitatory or inhibitory synaptic strength and timing within an appropriately connected network, or facilitating nonsynaptic (ephaptic) signaling through gap junctions or osmotic shifts in the extracellular space (Fig. 230-2). Chronic lesions that trigger cell loss, axon outgrowth, and synaptic repositioning irreversibly alter circuit structure along with more dynamic changes in transmitters, receptors, or neurotransporter function. The patterns of cellular and molecular plasticity within epileptic circuits are complex, and specific to the gene defect in question. Not all patterns of neuronal depolarization are sufficient to cause synchronous discharges, and not all discharges trigger sustained, regenerative seizures.

Repetitive EEG spiking may signal a transition to a seizure, followed by the propagation, either slowly or instantaneously, of

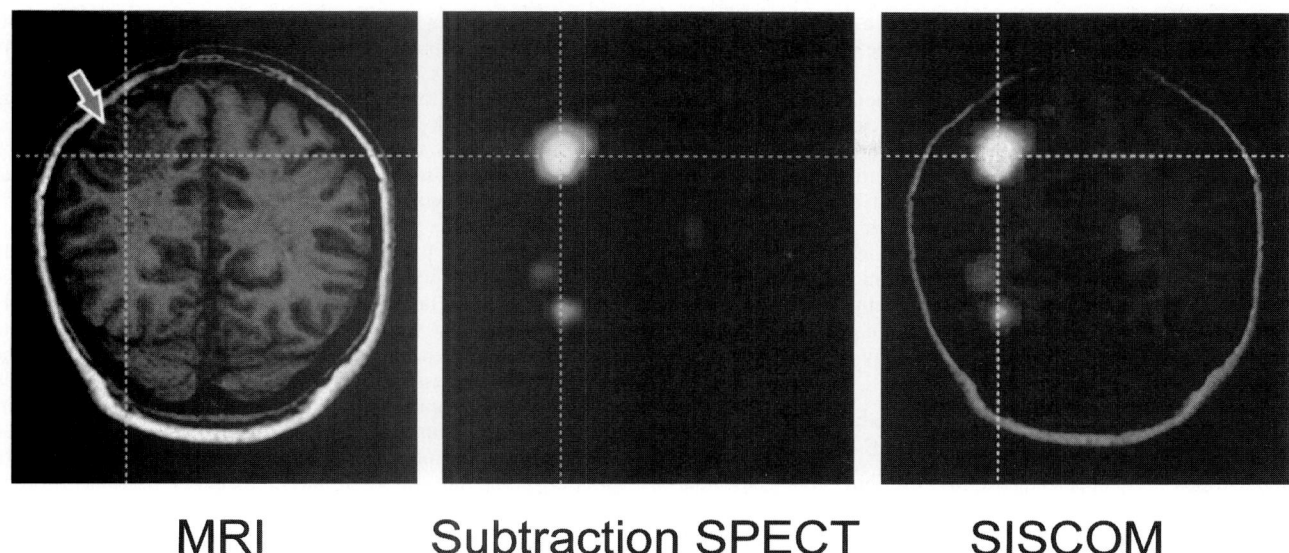

MRI          Subtraction SPECT          SISCOM

**Fig. 230-1 Coregistration** of structural MRI study of cortical dysplasia in the perirolandic region (*left*) with subtraction ictal single photon computed emission tomography (SPECT) study (*center*) yields a SISCOM image (*right*) that demonstrates the concordance between the cortical malformation and epileptic hypermetabolism and elevated blood flow. (*From G. Cascino. Used with permission.*[352])

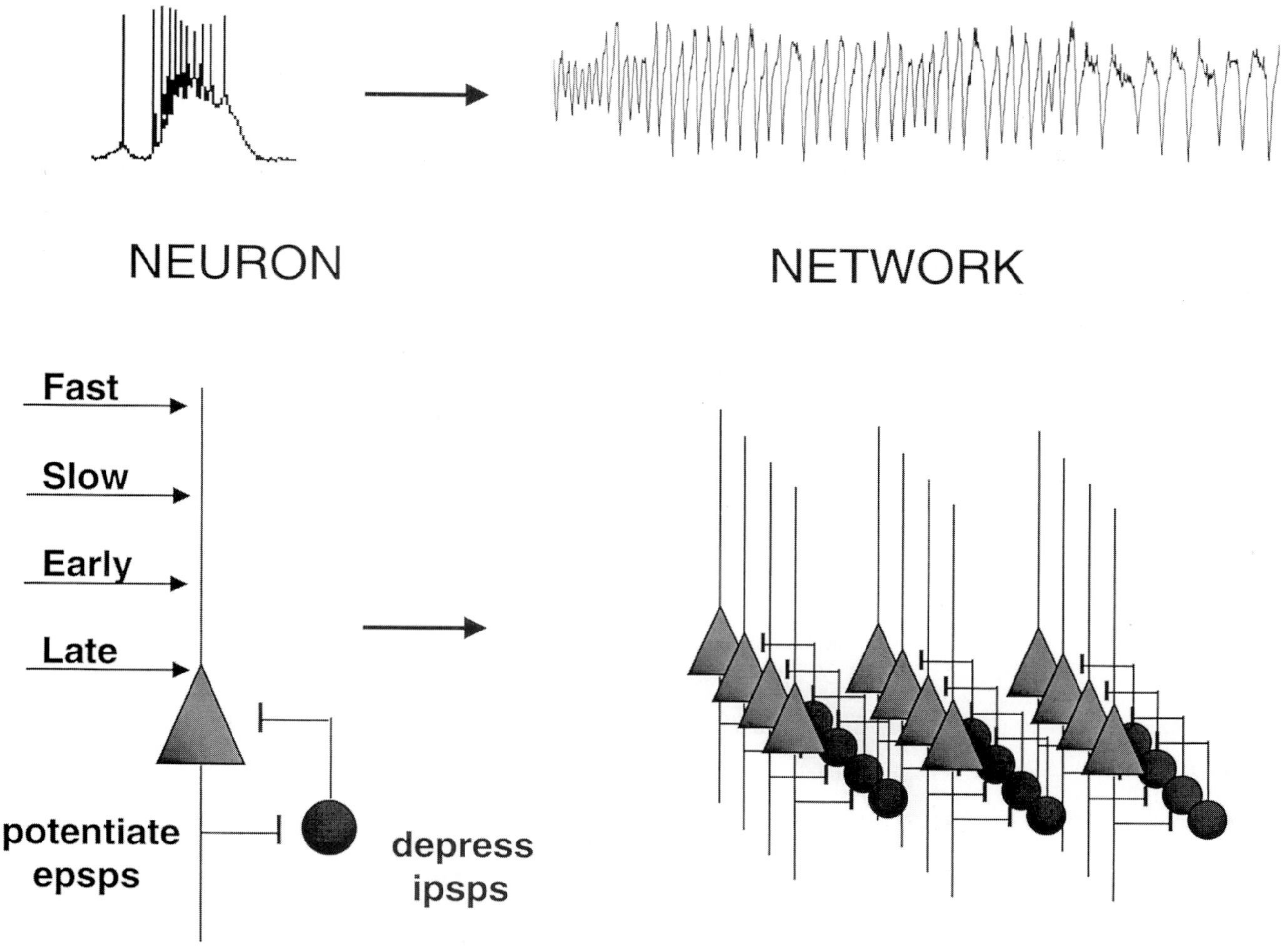

**Fig. 230-2 Cellular mechanisms** underlying abnormal bursting and cortical synchronization are complex and depend upon the expression of multiple genes. The paroxysmal depolarizing shift (PDS) (seen in intracellular recording at left above) can be initiated by direct or downstream alterations in membrane excitability molecules. Cellular bursting of this kind is modulated by the timing of incoming signals, both excitatory and inhibitory, that cause summation of postsynaptic potentials. Abnormal EEG synchronization during an epileptic seizure (right above) occurs when the connectivity of the depolarized neurons within the cortical network permits recurrent positive feedback and aberrant oscillations.

neuronal synchronization throughout the brain. The actual causes of the sudden appearance of an EEG discharge in a small neuronal population, how it overcomes powerful inhibitory control mechanisms ("surround inhibition") that normally prevent the spread of a focal seizure, and the mechanisms that eventually terminate the seizure discharge are not fully understood. It is likely that each of these steps depend on the specific inherited defect. Intrinsic brain excitability varies in different cortical subregions depending on the local cytoarchitectonics, allowing widely expressed genes to differentially alter regional seizure susceptibility. While a variety of cellular epileptogenic mechanisms have been identified by stimulating the normal brain,[14-16] few of these have been fully analyzed in genetic models of epilepsy where the same critical molecular pathways may or may not remain intact.

## THE DIVERSITY OF CANDIDATE GENES AND PATHWAYS FOR EPILEPTOGENESIS

Major strides have been made in describing the molecular mechanisms regulating bursting and synaptic excitability that underlie acute seizure episodes in the neocortex. Primary genes for seizure generation involve those that mediate or regulate depolarization and repolarization of neuronal membranes (Fig. 230-2). Principal candidate genes identified from in vivo drug phenocopy experiments and in isolated brain slices include those for voltage- and ligand-gated ion channels and transporters. Static defects in these molecules can transiently alter repetitive firing patterns in neural circuits, and reproduce the rapidly reversible electrical phenotype underlying a seizure discharge. Other heritable defects involve more complex alterations of the excitatory balance in cortical networks. These genes may act by disturbing the developmental programs underlying the determination of cell number, the migration and lamination of cortical neurons, the wiring of cortical local circuits, and the maturation or selective vulnerability of specific cell types or synapses (Fig. 230-3).

Neurogenetic analysis of the epilepsies also requires a distinction between primary lesions that favor one or a few seizures, and those that can lead to a lifelong chronic seizure disorder. Development of the chronic epileptic state, or *epileptogenesis*, is complex. This process involves, to varying degrees, the graded acquisition of cortical hyperexcitability by elevated membrane excitability; loss of inhibition; synaptic potentiation; neuronal dedifferentiation; synaptic remodeling; neuronal dropout; changes in glia; expression of novel transmitters; and altered transporter expression. The tempo of neuronal plasticity is also critical to understanding the onset of epilepsy, which may involve multiple defective developmental steps along the pathogenic trajectory from mutant gene to mature epileptic brain. In the case of genetically defined epilepsies, the problem centers on identifying how and when the gene defect renders specific circuits susceptible to epileptic synchronization at various stages of brain development.[17] This is particularly challenging when the gene is diffusely expressed throughout the nervous system, thus obscuring the actual network altered by the mutation. Reactive brain plasticity is also a critical mechanism influencing the natural history of the seizure disorder (including compensatory cellular alterations that alleviate or aggravate the condition), as well as its characteristic profile for antiepileptic therapy.

The molecular pathway to epileptogenesis is undoubtedly distinct in each genetic syndrome, and progresses in characteristic temporal patterns. Benign infantile epilepsies begin with an early onset of seizures, while other syndromes are delayed into childhood, adolescence, and adulthood. The syndromes may be stationary or progressive, and have various sequelae in the brain depending on the underlying defect, the seizure pattern and its severity, and concurrent events in brain development. These considerations reinforce the conclusion that candidate genes for epileptogenesis are likely to arise from an extremely broad spectrum of biochemical function.

## CANDIDATE GENES REVEALED BY NEUROGENETIC MODEL SYSTEMS

### Excitability Mutations in *Drosophila*

Mutations in other genomes are beginning to reveal genes for human epilepsies, both as simple causes of monogenic disorders and as complex trait loci for multigenic epilepsy. An early example was the gene for the delayed rectifier potassium channel subunit Kv1.1, deleted in the spontaneous hyperactive *Drosophila* fruit fly mutant *shaker*,[18,19] and targeted by homologous recombination in the mKv1.1 null mutant mouse with severe seizures,[20] prior to its identification as a human epilepsy gene.[21] Other voltage-gated ion channel mutations producing neuronal hyperexcitability phenotypes in the *Drosophila* nervous system, including Herg, a potassium channel underlying the human LQT syndrome of episodic cardiac arrhythmia, are under study,[22] and merit consideration as candidate epilepsy genes in human families.

### Epilepsy Mutations in the Mouse

Spontaneous and transgenic mutations in mouse models have revealed over 30 genes for epileptogenesis (Table 230-1). The genes so far identified fall into three major and interrelated functional categories. The first involves mutations of genes that contribute to brain development, in particular those known to be involved in the cell cycle, regional compartmentalization of the forebrain, and signaling molecules that play a role in the migration of cortical neuroblasts. The second category comprises genes for (a) molecules that determine membrane excitability, such as the voltage-gated ion channels; (b) transmitter release, including the genes for inhibitory peptide neurotransmitters or enzymes for GABA synthesis; and (c) vesicle proteins and neurotransporters involved in transmitter reuptake. The final category includes genes involved in various (as yet unrelated) intracellular "housekeeping" pathways involved in intermediary metabolism, protein degradation, and cellular homeostasis. These genes identify mechanisms that are also likely etiologies of inherited human seizure disorders.

## HUMAN EPILEPSY SYNDROMES WITH DEFINED GENES

Various classifications of epilepsy have been proposed, the most widely accepted being that of the ILAE in 1989, which is currently under review.[23] The major criteria that determine a syndrome are based primarily on the seizure type and brain localization, etiology, presumed pathology, precipitating factors, age of onset, severity, and natural history.

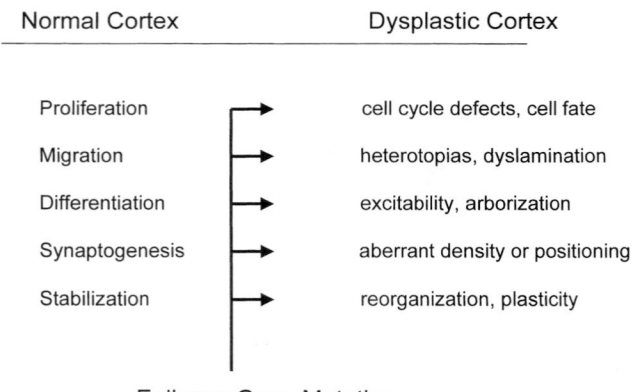

| Normal Cortex | Dysplastic Cortex |
|---|---|
| Proliferation | cell cycle defects, cell fate |
| Migration | heterotopias, dyslamination |
| Differentiation | excitability, arborization |
| Synaptogenesis | aberrant density or positioning |
| Stabilization | reorganization, plasticity |

Epilepsy Gene Mutation

**Fig. 230-3 Possible functional sites of action of mutant genes producing cortical dysplasias and developmental epilepsy.**

**Table 230-1 Gene Mutations with Spontaneous Epileptic Phenotypes in the Mouse**

| Gene | | Function |
|---|---|---|
| **Targeted disruptions** | | |
| OTX1 | | Homeodomain protein |
| NeuroD | | bhlh transcription factor |
| bmi-1 | | $Zn^{++}$ finger motif proto-oncogene |
| CBP-B | | Brain-specific DNA binding protein |
| P35 | | Cyclin-dependent kinase 5 activator |
| 5HT2c | | Serotonin receptor |
| NPY | | Neuropeptide Y |
| GABRb3 | | GABA receptor $\beta$ subunit |
| synapsin 1,2 | | Vesicle protein |
| Glyt-1 | | Glutamate transporter |
| GluRB | | Q/R editing site of glutamate receptor subunit |
| GAD65 | | Glutamate decarboxylase isozyme |
| Cam kinase II$\alpha$ | | $Ca^{++}$/calmodulin protein kinase |
| TNAP | | Nonspecific alkaline phosphatase |
| IP3 | | Inositol triphosphate receptor |
| PLC $\beta$1 | | Phospholipase C $\beta$ isozyme |
| G$\alpha$o | | G-protein $\alpha$ subunit |
| AMT | | Aspartate methyltransferase |
| Kv1.1 | | Voltage-gated, delayed rectifying $K^+$ channel |
| **Spontaneous mutations** | | |
| Girk2 | (weaver) | G-protein coupled inward rectifier $K^+$ channel |
| ROR$\alpha$ | (staggerer) | Nuclear hormone receptor |
| myoVa | (dilute-lethal) | Unconventional myosin |
| Cacn1a1 | (tottering) | Voltage-gated P/Q calcium channel $\alpha$ subunit |
| | (lethargic) | $\beta$4 subunit |
| | (stargazer) | $\gamma$2 subunit |
| | (ducky) | $\alpha$2$\delta$ subunit |
| NHE1 | (slow wave epilepsy) | Sodium/hydrogen exchanger |
| | (dilute-lethal) | Novel myosin heavy chain |
| AP3$\delta$ | (mocha) | Adaptin protein |

Individual seizure types have multiple etiologies; many that are strongly genetic will have more than one gene responsible, and these multiple loci will also likely prove to be functionally heterogeneous. Nevertheless, monogenic modes of transmission represent an increasingly recognized category of epilepsy. Seizure

disorders arising from the effects of a single gene are currently regarded as distinct diseases, while those arising from multigenic or multifactorial etiologies defy further delineation and remain classified as idiopathic. The appearance of associated neurologic deficits places many epilepsy syndromes in a nosologic overlap with those developed for mental retardation, ataxia, myoclonus, myopathies, and other inherited conditions.

In the remainder of this chapter, defined monogenic diseases where epilepsy is a major presenting clinical feature will be reviewed. The genes giving rise to the human seizure phenotypes are presented according to three main biologic categories: those currently recognizable by an anatomic defect impairing an early step in brain assembly, those directly altering intrinsic neuronal excitability molecules, and those with effects centering on the perturbation of cellular homeostasis, intracellular signaling, and metabolism. This functional categorization is only one of several possible, and the attributes are not mutually exclusive, because inborn errors of excitability or metabolism can alter early development, connectivity, or neuronal longevity, and vice versa. Indeed, the near-continuous interdependence of these three properties throughout brain development raises significant challenges to a precise neurobiologic understanding of mechanisms for epileptogenesis even once the gene has been identified. To facilitate this goal, transgenic mice are being constructed that express identical mutations in the human epilepsy genes to explore pathogenic mechanisms, to identify novel biologic targets, and to serve as biologic test systems to validate new therapy. Several such orthologous mutations have been engineered to date and are discussed below.

## DISTURBANCES OF CORTICAL DEVELOPMENT AND MIGRATION

Congenital causes of seizure disorders may begin during embryonic development of the brain, and consist of accelerated or arrested cellular division, migration, or maturation at some early stage (Table 230-2). With the advent of advanced imaging methodologies that enable in vivo ascertainment, neuronal migration disorders now appear to be a significant cause of childhood epilepsy.[24] Individuals with diffuse structural defects present clinically with seizures, mental retardation, and sensorimotor impairment, while the manifestation of more focal unilateral defects is confined to epilepsy.[25] The EEG shows continuous or frequent rhythmic epileptogenic discharges, and seizures due to migration abnormalities are often medically intractable.[26] Resection of dysplastic cortex may be necessary to control localized seizures in these cases.[27]

Migrational disturbances identified in epileptic brain range from isolated microscopic heterotopias of neurons that are found, either singly or in clusters, lying above or below their appropriate cortical lamina in the molecular layer or within subjacent or periventricular white matter,[28] to more diffuse cortical lamination

**Table 230-2 Genes for Human Cortical Malformations with Epilepsy**

| Syndrome | Chromosome | Gene Product | Function | Refs |
|---|---|---|---|---|
| Miller-Dieker lissencephaly | 17p13.3 | LIS1 | brain platelet-activating factor acetyl-hydrolase | Reine et al. 1993,[43] Hattori et al. 1994[46] |
| Subcortical band heterotopia (double cortex) | Xq22.3 | Doublecortin DCX/XLIS | novel microtubule-stabilizing kinase | Gleeson et al.,[33] des Portes[34] |
| Fukuyama muscular dystrophy | 9q31 | fukutin | novel protein | Toda et al.,[59] Kobayashi et al.[60] |
| Tuberous sclerosis | 9q34 | TSC1 hamartin | novel protein | van Slegtenhorst et al. 1997[66] |
| | 16p 13.3 | TSC2 tuberin | rapGTPase chaperone for hamartin | European Consortium 1993[67] |
| Schizencephaly | 10q26 | EMX2 | Homeodomain protein | Brunelli et al. 1996[62] |
| Bilateral periventricular nodular heterotopia | Xq28 | filamin 1 | Actin-linking phosphoprotein | Fox et al. 1998[85] |

defects, polymicrogyria, and agyria. The molecular and physiological analysis of changes in ion channels and neurotransmitter expression in these syndromes awaits the creation of appropriate mouse models of the disorders.

### Lissencephaly and Subcortical Band Heterotopia

X-linked lissencephaly and subcortical band heterotopia ("double cortex") are allelic cortical malformations mapping to human Xq22.3-Xq23 associated with arrest of migrating cerebral cortical neurons, abnormal gyration, and lamination defects.[29] Histologically, the lissencephalic cortex is divisible into four abnormal layers, with the stratum most characteristic for this malformation consisting of a broad heterotopic zone of neurons extending from the ventricle to a cell-sparse region lying beneath a simplified outer layer. The broad heterotopic zone is visible on MRI scan, and brains showing this malformation are associated with a range of cortical surface abnormalities extending from agyria to pachygyria (decreased convolutions) that define the lissencephaly spectrum. Affected patients inherit clinical epilepsy phenotypes with other disorders ranging from mild cognitive impairment to blindness, hearing loss, and profound mental retardation.[30]

In contrast, subcortical band heterotopia is characterized by a distinct band of neurons placed abnormally between the ventricle and the superficial cortical layers (Fig. 230-4). A genetic relationship between the double cortex and lissencephaly syndromes was recently confirmed.[31,32] A balanced translocation in an XLIS patient permitted the identification of a 10-kb brain-specific cDNA that encodes a novel 40-kDa protein named doublecortin *(DCX/XLIS)*.[33,34] Nine double cortex/X-linked lissencephaly families and 26 sporadic double cortex patients have been found to show independent doublecortin mutations, at least one of them a *de novo* mutation.[35,36] These studies demonstrate that the double cortex phenotype results from mutations in *DCX* in females and that lissencephaly is the male manifestation of the same genetic defect, although rare exceptions of the male double cortex phenotype are reported.[37]

Mosaicism is the likely mechanism that allows the two distinct cortical pathologies to be sex-determined manifestations of the same gene mutation. Cortical neurons are born near the ventricle and normally migrate radially to be deposited near the cortical surface. Owing to X inactivation in females, only one X chromosome is expressed in a migrating neuron. According to this model, neurons in females that inactivate the normal X chromosome and express an X with a *DCX* mutation could be arrested early in the migratory trajectory in the cortical subplate, where they reside as a subcortical band, while neurons that inactivate the mutant X and express a normal X chromosome may migrate properly to the cortical surface where they comprise the outer cortical layer. Therefore, the double cortex phenotype in females represents a functional brain mosaicism for neurons with *doublecortin* mutations. Neurons in males with *DCX* mutations all display inadequate migration, which is phenotypically expressed as the more severe X-linked lissencephaly.

The doublecortin protein encoded by *DCX* is novel and its cellular functions are beginning to be determined. Doublecortin is highly expressed during brain development, mainly in fetal neurons including precursors. It has no enzymatic activity, but is subject to phosphorylation by the protein kinase Abl, a signal transduction molecule that is also involved in neuronal migration, as revealed by the analysis of mouse mutants (see below). *DCX* closely resembles a protein containing a $Ca^{2+}$/calmodulin kinase domain, suggesting that the migration may be regulated through $Ca^{2+}$-dependent signaling.[38] Several studies have now detected a microtubule-stabilizing role.[39–41]

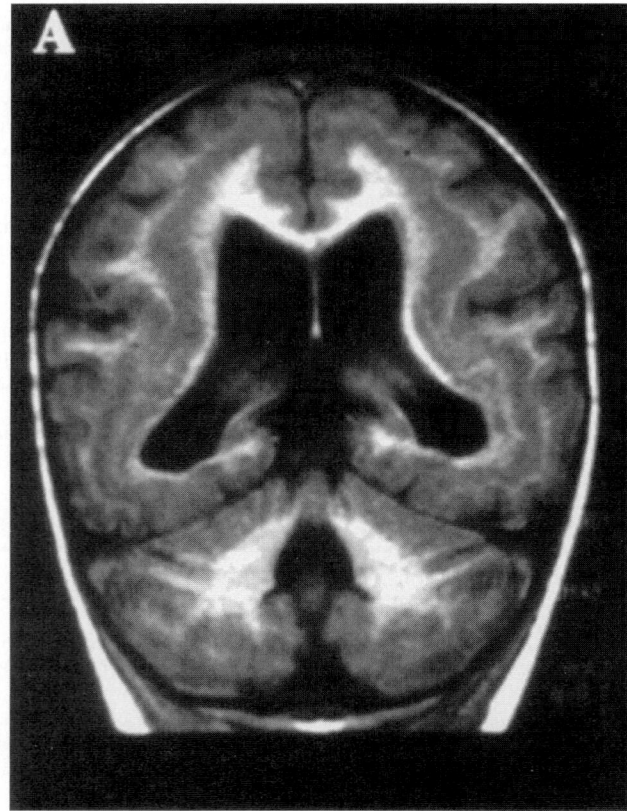
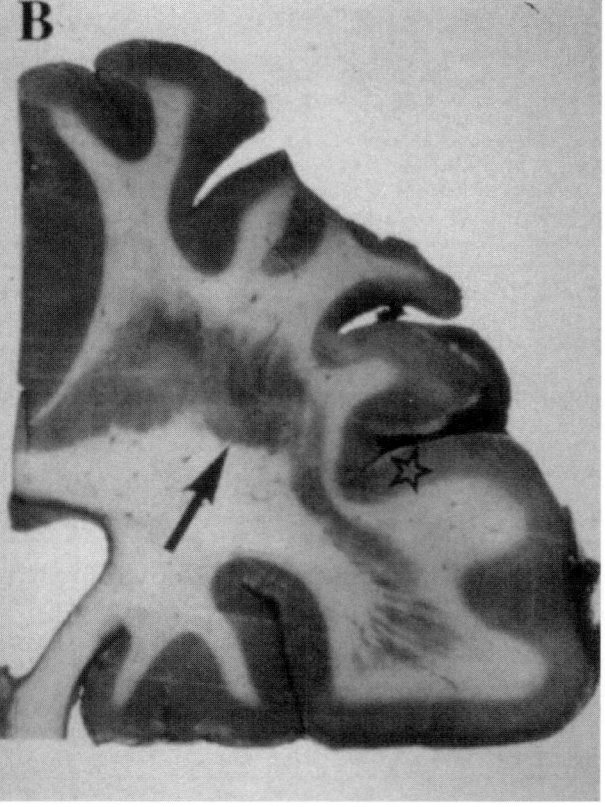

**Fig. 230-4 Cortical migrational disturbances and inherited epilepsy. The subcortical band heterotopia arising from mutation of the doublecortin gene on Xq22.3-Xq23 produces the "double cortex"** syndrome shown in an MRI (*left*) and in a pathologic specimen (*arrow, right*). (*Used with permission of C. Walsh.*[33])

## Miller-Dieker Lissencephaly

In this classical form of lissencephaly, a heterozygous deletion or mutation in *LIS1* on chromosome 17p13.3 causes the cortical malformation.[42-46] Miller-Dieker lissencephaly (MDL) results from a hemideletion of *LIS1*, which encodes a nonenzymatic subunit of a brain platelet-activating factor acetylhydrolase (PAFAH IB) strongly expressed in the fetal cortical plate.[47] *LIS1* belongs to a family of genes that have identical coding sequences (*LIS1* [chromosome 17] and *LIS2* [chromosome 2]). In the brain, *LIS1* is the more abundant gene. Fogli et al.[48] have correlated intracellular levels of *LIS1* protein with the neuroradiologic appearance of the brain in cases of MDL. Patients were found to either not make protein from the mutated *LIS1* gene or to produce a reduced level of an abnormal protein, thus confirming *LIS1* protein deficiency as a mechanism for the disorder. The protein is localized in pioneer neurons in the ventricular neuroepithelium,[49] and interacts with microtubules[50] and with signaling molecules regulating microtubule-based motors.[51] The recent production of a mouse model for *LIS1* deletions[52,53] will lead to further understanding of the role of the LIS1 protein in neuronal migration.

Specific EEG changes, including abnormally fast background activity with exceptionally high voltage that increases with age, and unusually high-voltage, sharp, slow-wave complexes, have been reported in Miller-Dieker lissencephaly.[54]

## Fukuyama Congenital Muscular Dystrophy (FCMD)

Fukuyama-type congenital muscular dystrophy is an autosomal recessive muscular dystrophy associated with a spectrum of epilepsy and severe mental retardation.[55] It is most common in the Japanese population. Neuroradiologic imaging of patients with this cortical dysplasia show thickened, cobblestone-like cortices, termed polymicrogyria, that predominantly affect the frontal lobes; approximately half show a smooth, pachygyric cortex, termed lissencephaly type II, distributed over temporal-parietal and occipital lobes.[56] The white matter is also abnormal, and cerebellar cysts and polymicrogyria are present in 90 percent of the cases. In 32 of 36 cases of FCMD, seizures with focal paroxysmal EEG discharges developed before 3 years of age. Abnormal background EEG consisting of diffuse alpha and/or abundant spindle activity and rolandic spikes was observed, and visual-evoked potentials revealed abnormal findings in the majority of cases examined.[57,58]

The FCMD gene encodes a novel 461-amino-acid protein fukutin that is not found at the sarcolemmal membrane, as are other gene products for muscular dystrophies, but may be a secreted protein.[59,60] Neither the localization nor function of fukutin in central nervous system neurons has yet been determined.

## Schizencephaly

Schizencephaly is a rare disorder of brain development characterized by a full thickness cleft, either unilateral or bilateral, within the cerebral hemispheres. The walls of the clefts are lined by polymicrogyric cortical gray matter. Portions of the cerebral hemispheres may be missing. The clinical presentation is typically characterized by mental retardation, seizures, hypotonia or spasticity, and blindness or speech defects. Using SSCP analysis, 17 sporadic patients with this anomaly were heterozygous for a mutant homeobox gene, Emx2, including two brothers that showed the same splicing mutation in the first intron despite a normal allele of the gene in both parents and two unaffected sibs.[61-64]

EMX2 is one of four vertebrate homeobox genes (EMX1, 2, and OTX1, 2) expressed in forebrain neurons and important in regionalization of the brain. EMX2 is expressed in embryonic germinal neuroepithelium in the neocortex, hippocampus, and parahippocampal cortex, and may play a role in cell proliferation and migration.[64]

## Tuberous Sclerosis

Tuberous sclerosis (TS) is an autosomal dominant disorder with a broad phenotypic spectrum that includes seizures, mental retardation, renal dysfunction, dermatologic abnormalities, and various benign and malignant tumors in the affected individuals. The disorder is caused by mutation of either the TSC1 or TSC2 tumor-suppressor genes. Approximately half of TS families show linkage to TSC1, and half to TSC2.[65] The TSC1 gene codes for hamartin,[66] a novel protein with no significant homology to TSC2, which encodes tuberin,[67] a member of the rap GTPase-activating protein (rapGAP) family for rap1 and rab5. Hamartin and tuberin interact in vivo at predicted coiled-coil domains, suggesting that both molecules function in the same complex rather than in separate molecular pathways.[68] Tuberin expression in the adult brain is limited to the olfactory bulb, brain stem nuclei, cerebellar Purkinje cells, and motor neurons in the ventral spinal cord. In contrast, rapGAP is expressed in many different cell types, but not in cerebellar Purkinje cells or spinal cord motor neurons, and there is significant expression of rapGAP in astrocytes. The restricted distribution of tuberin expression relative to rap1 and rapGAP suggests that tuberin may be a primary rap1 regulator in a subset of neurons.[69]

The neuropathologic lesion of TSC consists of highly epileptogenic foci of dysplastic cerebral cortex (tubers) containing abnormally shaped neurons and giant ("balloon") cells.[70] Mutation of the TSC genes apparently disrupts differentiation and maturation of certain neuronal precursors, and the gene products are potential regulators of cellular proliferation. The molecular pathology of TSC balloon cells has been analyzed by immunohistochemical analysis of embryonic or immature neuronal markers.[71] Antibodies to neuronal precursor proteins (nestin, Ki-67, and proliferating cell nuclear antigen) stained dysmorphic neurons and giant cells, while neurons in adjacent normal cortex were not labeled. Amplification of poly (A)+ mRNA obtained from intracellular sampling of the dysmorphic cells revealed mRNAs encoding nestin and other cell cycle markers of immature neurons. Analysis of balloon cells for the presence of nucleolar organizer regions involved in cellular proliferation using both a silver impregnation technique and an antibody for proliferating cell nuclear antigen (PCNA) expression revealed that the dysmorphic cells are unlikely to be undergoing proliferative activity.[72]

## Other Neurophakomatoses

Neurocutaneous syndromes are characterized by congenital dysplastic abnormalities involving the nervous system and skin. The most common neurocutaneous syndromes manifesting epilepsy are TSC and the Sturge Weber syndrome (SWS).[73] Unlike TSC, cerebral angiomatosis associated with SWS is not known to involve a gene with primary neuronal expression; however, the association of cerebral and cutaneous vascular hamartomas constitutes a distinct, hereditary clinicopathologic entity with autosomal dominant inheritance and variable penetrance. The clinical manifestations are visible vascular cutaneous nevi, epilepsy, cerebral hemorrhage, and calcifications, and focal neurologic deficits. One case was reported of an early infantile form of SWS associated with a four layered microgyric cortex underlying the angioma, suggesting that a complex migrational disorder can result when the lesion is expressed early in development.[74] MRI and SPECT imaging in seven cases of this early variant with seizures diagnosed in the first year of life show hyperperfusion and accelerated myelination in areas beneath the leptomeningeal angiomas.[75]

Other examples of glioneuronal malformations with histologic resemblance to tuberous sclerosis, but without extracerebral evidence of a phakomatosis, can be found in surgical specimens removed from patients with pharmacoresistant epilepsies, and their relationship to TSC1-2 gene mutations are unclear. Microsatellite and RFLP analysis of DNA extracted from these epilepsy-associated tuberous sclerosis-like malformations in brain samples from 11 patients failed to reveal TSC mutations, suggesting that these immature neuronal forms are genetically heterogeneous.[76]

Neurofibromatosis, von Hippel-Lindau disease, and other rare entities, such as epidermal nevus syndrome, are also accompanied by epilepsy, but whether the link is genetic or fortuitous remains unclear. In patients with NF1 neurofibromatosis, infantile spasms are present at varying ages.[77,78] However, structural lesions are not typically evident on imaging studies, and the clinical presentations differ from those seen in other neurocutaneous syndromes, both with respect to their positive response to steroid therapy and cognitive outcome, suggesting a benign association of the two disorders.[79]

### Bilateral Periventricular Nodular Heterotopia

Bilateral periventricular nodular heterotopia (BPNH) is a brain migration disturbance characterized by symmetric periventricular nodular masses of gray matter containing well-differentiated neurons presenting with variable clinical severity. The disorder typically presents with sporadic or familial epilepsy as the sole symptom, primarily in females, although multiple anomaly cases with MR have also been reported.[80-82] The BPNH syndrome has been mapped to chromosome Xq28 based on linkage studies in multiplex families.[83,84]

A gene for BPNH has recently been identified as filamin 1 (FLN1).[85] FLN1 encodes an actin-cross-linking phosphoprotein that transduces ligand-receptor binding into actin reorganization, and is required for cellular locomotion. FLN1 is expressed at high levels in the developing cortex, is required for neuronal migration from the ventricular zone to the cortex, and plays an essential role during embryogenesis.

Both pyramidal and local circuit neurons appear in the nodules, but no reactive gliosis is present. Unilateral nodular subcortical heterotopias can also be detected.[86] The presence of large neuronal aggregates suggests that the defect of neuronal migration could also involve overproduction of neuroblasts and/or disruption of mechanisms for naturally occurring cell death. In a series of 33 patients, partial seizures were present in over 80 percent of patients, mainly in temporoparietal-occipital areas. The interictal EEG abnormalities were typically focal and consistent with the location of the heterotopia.[87] Despite the focality of the discharge, resection of the anterior temporal lobe in medically resistant subcortical nodular heterotopia cases produces a generally unfavorable outcome, suggesting a broader effect of the gene on cortical excitability.[87-89] Glucose metabolism and perfusion studies in BPNH reveal activity similar to normal cortex.[90]

Recent neuropathologic analyses of human malformations are beginning to reveal details of the neuronal abnormalities within dysplastic circuits. Increases in the number of giant pyramidal neurons in deeper cortical layers, coupled with a decrease of calcium-binding protein, immunopositive GABAergic neurons, and abnormal synaptic terminals onto pyramidal neurons, suggest that one factor contributing to epileptogenesis may be a reduction of inhibitory inputs within the dysplastic cortex.[91] Glutamate receptor changes have also been described. In contrast to nondysplastic neurons, dysplastic neurons in epileptic brain are typically immunopositive for both NMDAR1 and NMDAR2A/B receptors, while both groups are immunoreactive to AMPA GluR2/3.[92] This pattern suggests that hyperexcitability of dysplastic cortical regions may arise in part from aberrant coassembly of NMDAR2A/B subunits with selectively expressed NMDAR1 splice variants.[93]

### Mouse Models of Cortical Dysplasia and Seizures

Mutation of genes critical for brain development now provides experimental model systems to further explore the link between cortical pattern malformations and epilepsy. The murine Otx1 homeodomain gene, which is related to orthodenticle (otd), a gene required for *Drosophila* head development, is involved in temporally and spatially regulated events during morphogenesis of the forebrain. Otx1−/− mice generated by gene targeting exhibit multiple abnormalities affecting development of temporal and perirhinal areas, the hippocampus, the mesencephalon, and the cerebellum, along with spontaneous epileptic behavior.[94] Otx1 mRNA is expressed by the precursors of deep-layer neurons within the developing cerebral ventricular zone, and in a subpopulation of neurons within cortical layers 5 and 6 during postnatal and adult life. The distinct spatial and temporal patterns suggest that Otx1 may play a role in the differentiation of neurons in the deep layers of the cerebral cortex.[95] Mutations in the human EMX2 gene produce epilepsy,[62,63] but EMX2 null mouse mutants die shortly after birth.[64] Mice lacking p35, a neuron-specific activator of cyclin-dependent kinase 5, and thus of p35/cdk5 kinase activity, display severe cortical lamination defects and suffer from seizures and sporadic adult lethality.[96] Analysis of neuronal birth dates indicates a developmental reversal of the normal lamination order of cortical neurons, such that earlier-born neurons reside in superficial layers and later-generated neurons occupy deep layers.

In contrast to these models, several mutant mice have severely disturbed cortical lamination defects without a known seizure phenotype, demonstrating that major alterations of intracortical neuronal positions are not necessarily epileptogenic. For example, the reelin gene encodes a large extracellular protein secreted by pioneer Cajal-Retzius neurons during neurodevelopment and is expressed in a subset of GABAergic inhibitory neurons in the adult cortex.[97-100] Mutations in reelin result in a severely defective cortical lamination pattern with loss of the inside-out migration pattern, but no aberrant EEG or seizure phenotype.[101] Two other recessive mouse mutants, scrambler and yotari, exhibit cortical dysplasia and arise from mutations in mdab1, a murine gene related to the *Drosophila* gene disabled (dab).[102-105] Both scrambler and yotari mice express mutated forms of mdab1 messenger RNA and loss of mDab1 protein, a phosphoprotein that may function downstream from reelin, as an intracellular adaptor in protein kinase pathways in migrating neuronal populations.[106] The absence of seizures in these mice is further evidence of the molecular specificity that determines epileptogenicity in cortical dysplasias.

### Mental Retardation Syndromes and Epilepsy

**Fragile X.** Of the five folate-sensitive fragile sites that have been analyzed at the molecular level (FRAXA, FRAXE, FRAXF, FRA16A, and FRA11B), three of the genes (FRAXA, FRAXE, and FRA11B) have been identified and are linked to clinical disorders, including epilepsy. Each of these fragile sites is associated with hypermethylated (CCG)n triplet-repeat expansions. The genes are described in detail elsewhere.[107]

Characteristic epileptiform discharges in fragile X subjects have prompted further clinical studies to investigate the correlation between FRAX mutations and a predisposition to epilepsy.[108] EEG studies of patients with an amplification in the FRM1 gene were paired with genetic analyses of FRM1 in 16 children with benign childhood epilepsy with centrotemporal spikes (BECT, Rolandic epilepsy).[109] Focal sharp waves activated by sleep were evident in 8 of 14 young (aged 4 to 8 years) male patients with a verified mutation in exon 1 of the FRM1 gene, and 6 of these patients experienced partial seizures during sleep. No epileptiform EEG abnormalities were present under the age of 4 or over the age of 8. In children with Rolandic epilepsy who were studied for fragile X mutations, 1 of the 16 children studied was found to carry a fragile X premutation, and generalized spike wave complexes were evident in a 5-year-old girl with an FRM1 premutation. These observations suggest a role for the FRM1 gene in epileptogenesis. In a recent large study of epilepsy in fragile X males, 18 percent of 192 patients had seizures, none of which began before 2 years of age. A majority showed an age-related paroxysmal EEG pattern.[110]

Hunter syndrome is a lethal, X-linked, lysosomal storage disorder caused by iduronate-2-sulphatase (IDS) deficiency.

Patients with complete deletion of the IDS locus show seizure disorders. Genotype-phenotype correlations in deletion patients reveal that epilepsy in two individuals correlates with a deletion extending proximal to the IDS locus and including part of the FMR2 locus, while nonseizure phenotypes were associated with distal deletions.[111] These data implicate FMR2 as a candidate gene for epilepsy, when mutated with IDS.

Two mouse models of fragile X mutations have been constructed.[112,113] Chronic EEG monitoring has so far failed to detect seizures or epileptiform abnormalities in either of these models on the genetic backgrounds studied (J. Noebels, D. Nelson, unpublished data).

## Phenotypic Overlap of Mental Retardation and Epilepsy

In some cases, the appearance of seizures may be the first clinical harbinger of an impending neurodevelopmental defect with broader significance. Many epilepsies overlap with mental retardation (MR) syndromes, and together these represent the two most common disease phenotypes affecting the nervous system. In a recent study of 98 mentally retarded children aged 6 to 13 years, epileptiform EEG activity was present in 91 percent, and nearly one-half had intractable seizures.[114] The coexistence of MR and seizures significantly complicates an understanding of the etiology of these two neurologic deficits in inherited syndromes, primarily because their exact onsets are often difficult to separate and ascertain. There are three major temporal variables. Epileptogenic pathology can begin at virtual any ontogenetic stage, and clinical seizures may commence immediately, or within a characteristic age range. Second, the patterns of superimposed seizure-induced neuronal injury are highly age-dependent. Finally, some epilepsies may commence as relatively subtle seizure disorders, and escape detection until later stages when the seizures become clinically significant. Thus the onsets and interactions between seizure pathophysiology and the development of cognitive dysfunction are not stationary, and may progress from prenatal life into adulthood.

The OMIM registry currently lists over 850 entries for mental retardation syndromes; only 7 percent of these include epilepsy as a phenotypic element. Less severe cognitive changes are likely to coexist with many inherited epilepsy syndromes. Effective seizure control will not always prevent the appearance of cognitive delay, indicating that seizures themselves are not necessarily causative.[115] The debate regarding whether seizures themselves directly injure the developing brain continues, and is obscured by the many different possible underlying molecular etiologies. In experimental models, seizures associated with defects in NMDA receptors that result in enhanced neuronal calcium entry,[116] or on certain genetic backgrounds where cell vulnerability is increased by the loss of molecules such as p53,[117,118] are directly excitotoxic. In contrast, seizures occurring in brain tissue with neuroprotective mechanisms intact, or where genes mediating neuronal degeneration have been crippled,[119] may show far less cell death. A severe seizure disorder is inevitably deleterious to normal learning, and the added depression of neuronal excitability by concomitant AED therapy is an ever-present confounding variable.

Understanding these relationships requires further analysis of genetically defined syndromes and their dependence on modifier genes. Many variants involving cerebral dysgenesis, MR, and epilepsy are being described clinically and pathologically, and will be of great utility in the future as the underlying mutations are identified.

## DISTURBANCES OF MEMBRANE EXCITABILITY AND NEUROTRANSMISSION

Mutation of proteins critically responsible for membrane electrogenesis, action potential generation, and the repolarization of membranes are prime candidates for endogenous bursting defects in single neurons, and hence for epilepsy. Similarly, the molecules mediating neurotransmitter release, receptor modulation, and transmitter reuptake from the synaptic cleft are key control points in network rhythmicity. A third category includes gap junction proteins and related mechanisms responsible for regulating nonsynaptic intercellular communication.

The premise that mutation of genes responsible for the action potential in excitable tissue would be lethal at fetal stages was rapidly dispelled by the discovery of ion channelopathies underlying cardiac and skeletal muscle syndromes.[120] It is now evident that central nervous system channelopathies share critical attributes, notably the expression of episodic and activity-dependent phenotypes. Alterations in membrane electrogenesis give rise to conditional neuronal spike-firing threshold alterations, abnormal network oscillations, and neurologic phenotypes ranging from seizures to episodic ataxias, migraine, and neurodegeneration. The presence of 13 genes for sodium-channel pore-forming subunits, a similar number for voltage-gated calcium channels, and over 60 known potassium-channel genes signals a rich source of primary candidate gene loci for inherited epilepsy syndromes, and secondary modifications of ion channels in epileptic tissue.[121]

### Ion Channelopathies

**Sodium Channels.** A syndrome of generalized seizures has been identified in an Australian pedigree bearing a point mutation in a transmembrane $\beta 1$ subunit of the voltage-gated sodium channel. Genotype analysis of a large (378-member) pedigree, including 42 individuals, allowed linkage to chromosome 19q13.1 in a subgroup of 26 members with complex seizure histories.[122,123] The disorder in this subgroup was autosomal dominant with reduced penetrance. The seizures were of early onset and in some cases coincided with febrile episodes, but there was no correlation with age, and the GEFS+ (generalized epilepsy with febrile seizures) disorder is not simply related to the common clinical syndrome of febrile convulsions. The latter syndrome affects 2 to 5 percent of all children under the age of 5 years and is likely to have a variety of causes, including a locus mapped to chromosome 8q13-21.[124] Interestingly, a second locus for a GEFS+ gene has been assigned to chromosome 2q21-q23,[125] and another form of febrile seizures has been localized to chromosome 2q23-24,[126] both in a region containing a cluster of four other sodium channel $\alpha$ subunits. A separate locus on chromosome 12p13 for a conditional aspect of this phenotype, periodic fevers, has also been reported,[127,128] and represents a potential candidate gene for febrile seizure interactions in susceptible families.

The linkage region identified on chromosome 19q13.1 coincides with a locus for a benign infantile convulsion syndrome.[129] Candidate gene analysis revealed a C-G transposition at nt 387 in the third exon within the voltage-gated sodium channel $\beta$ subunit SCN1B gene.[123] Single-strand conformation polymorphism analyses showed that the mutation was not present in 50 unrelated probands with febrile seizure histories. The $\alpha$ subunit of the sodium channel forms the ion selective pore, and is modulated by two auxiliary transmembrane subunits, $\beta 1$ and $\beta 2$, both widely expressed in the brain. The mutation alters a conserved cysteine residue of the $\beta 1$ subunit, thereby disrupting a predicted disulfide bridge responsible for maintaining an extracellular immunoglobulin-like fold resembling that of contactin, a neural cell adhesion molecule.[130]

The $\beta 1$ subunit is expressed in muscle and brain and interacts with multiple $\alpha$ subunits, but the precise functional alteration in the brain pathway giving rise to the seizure disorder remains to be determined. Despite the extracellular location of this mutated domain,[131] co-expression of the human mutant $\beta 1$ subunit with a rat brain Na$^+$-channel $\alpha$ subunit in *Xenopus laevis* oocytes demonstrated that the mutation reduces the normal ability of the wild-type $\beta 1$ allele to accelerate inactivation kinetics of the sodium current. The effect of the mutant $\beta 1$ subunit was generally similar to that observed in the absence of a wild-type $\beta 1$ subunit, suggesting partial loss of function. $\beta 1$ subunits may regulate the kinetics of the persistent sodium current, suggesting that mutation of this gene could raise the probability of a channel showing prolonged gating kinetics.[131] While the temperature sensitivity of this shift and its effects on channel sorting or density in cortical neurons have not been explored, the mutation appears capable of modulating sodium channel gating kinetics in a way that may favor repetitive firing and seizures. Loss of this subunit might similarly affect the cardiac sodium channel SCN5A, where mutations are linked to the cardiac long QT syndrome.[132,133] The α subunit of this cardiac channel has recently been found to be expressed in limbic regions of the brain known for a low threshold for epilepsy, suggesting that the SCN5A channel may be an additional candidate sodium-channel gene for epilepsy.[134]

Acquired alterations in sodium channel subunit composition, expression, and function are known to occur in human epilepsies[135–137] and in experimental models of inherited seizures or hypoxic brain damage,[138–140] and both primary and secondary alterations in these ion channels may be related to subsequent hyperexcitability in neurons and astrocytes.

**Potassium Ion Channels.** A dominantly inherited syndrome in newborns, benign familial neonatal convulsions (BFNC, EBN1), was mapped from a single large pedigree and localized to chromosome 20q13.2.[141] The clinical syndrome consists of brief clonic seizures beginning in the first week of life, typically remitting by 6 months of age, although some cases may last into adulthood. In two other BFNC pedigrees, a second locus (EBN2) was found on chromosome 8q24.[142–144] Both loci have now been identified. EBN1 was cloned from a small deletion that included a novel voltage-gated potassium channel, KCNQ2 on chromosome 20q13.3,[145,146] and EBN2 was found by mapping a second member of the KQT family, KCNQ3, to the chromosome 8q24 locus where missense mutations were identified in members of a large BFNC pedigree.[147]

KCNQ2 mutations in BFNC probands include a deletion, two transmembrane missense mutations, two frameshifts, and one splice-site mutation, all suggesting loss of function. Expression of the mutated channel in oocytes does not yield measurable current.[148] The KCNQ3 missense mutation lies within the critical pore region at the same conserved amino acid that is mutated in KvLQT1 (KCNQ1) in a cardiac LQT patient.

Amino acid sequence comparisons reveal that both genes show strong homology to KvLQT1, the potassium channel encoded by KCNQ1 that is associated with over 50 percent of the cases of hereditary long QT syndrome.[149] KCNQ2 and KCNQ3 are similarly distributed in brain tissue.[150] Heterologous expression of KCNQ2 or KCNQ3 elicits voltage-gated, rapidly activating K+-selective currents similar to those of KvLQT1, but the currents are not increased by coexpression with the β subunit KCNE1 (minK, IsK).[148] Recent coexpression analysis reveals that KCNQ2 and KCNQ3 may combine as heterodimers to control the inhibitory M-current, a slowly activating and deactivating membrane repolarization widely expressed in cortical and hippocampal neurons.[151] This current is modulated by cyclic AMP[150] and is named for its activation of muscarinic acetylcholinergic receptors, thereby linking cholinergic pathways to an altered potassium-dependent repolarization that underlies this age-specific epileptic syndrome.[152]

## Ion Channelopathies in Mice with Epileptic Phenotypes

**Potassium Channels.** Several K+ channel mutations are now known to produce activity-dependent neuronal repolarization defects favoring seizures. Because of the nonuniform distribution of some channel proteins within the cell, certain neuronal compartments may be particularly affected. For example, mice lacking the *shaker*-type delayed rectifier Kv1.1, a voltage-gated potassium channel α subunit that is highly expressed at presynaptic nerve terminals, display frequent spontaneous seizures.[20] In hippocampal slices from homozygous Kv1.1 null animals, the intrinsic passive properties of CA3 pyramidal cell somas are

normal. However, antidromic action potentials are recruited at lower thresholds, indicating axon terminal hyperexcitability, a known mechanism for ectopic firing and seizure spread.[153] Furthermore, stimulation of hippocampal pathways triggers synaptically mediated epileptiform bursts. These data indicate that loss of Kv1.1 protein from its normal localization in axons and terminals increases excitability and repetitive firing in neurons, with associated increased neurotransmitter release, in some cases, interestingly, of GABA.[154]

The mutant mouse *weaver* shows seizures, and the gene has been identified as Girk2, a G-protein-coupled inward rectifying potassium channel.[155] The mutation is located in the pore region of the channel and alters selectivity of the ionic currents. Girk1 and Girk2 form heteromultimers in neurons, and the expression of both is decreased in weaver brain.[156] Stimulation of inhibitory neurotransmitter receptors, such as the presynaptic gamma-aminobutyric acid type B (GABAB) receptors, activates GIRK channels, which, in turn, influence membrane excitability. The amplitude of the GABAB receptor-activated current is severely attenuated in cells isolated from both weaver and Girk2 null mutant mice, indicating a loss of synaptic inhibitory strength.[157,158] Weaver cells show defective migration, which is most clearly evident in granule cells granule in the cerebellar cortex. Deletion of the Girk2 gene reveals normal lamination; yet seizures persist, suggesting the seizure phenotype may depend more on membrane excitability changes than on the neuronal migration behavior regulated by this channel.[159] Dependence of the repolarization defect on the basal level of excitation was recently demonstrated by rescue of the migration defect in mice doubly homozygous for weaver and a deletion of the glutamate NMDA NR1-receptor gene, indicating that channelopathy phenotypes are conditionally dependent on endogenous levels of excitability.[160]

**Calcium Channels.** No genes have yet been identified for human generalized absence epilepsies, but a series of spontaneous recessive mutations in the mouse show spike-wave seizures that resemble this pattern of thalamocortical discharge,[161] and four of them encode subunits for voltage-gated neuronal calcium ion channels. The *tottering* mouse bears a point mutation in the α1A subunit, 1 of 10 known transmembrane pore-forming proteins that determine the selectivity, kinetics, and pharmacology of the channel.[162] The *lethargic* mouse encodes a truncated β4 subunit, one of four auxiliary cytoplasmic proteins that interact with the α1A channel and modulate its biophysical properties.[163] The *lethargic* mutation results in a functional null mutation of the β4 subunit, but alternative pairing ("reshuffling") of the remaining β1 to 3 subunits may partially rescue the loss of this subunit and create a complex channelopathy affecting multiple calcium-channel subtypes.[164] The *stargazer* mutation interrupts transcription of a novel transmembrane γ2 subunit that favors inactivation of calcium current.[165] Finally, mutation of the *ducky* gene results in the loss of mRNA for the α2δ subunit, a membrane-spanning subunit that potentiates current through α1 subunits.[166] The neurologic phenotypes and intervening cellular alterations in these calcium-channel subunit mutations were recently reviewed.[167]

Dominant mutations in a brain-specific P/Q-type voltage-dependent Ca2+ channel α1 subunit gene (CACNL1A4) have been identified in individuals with chromosome 19-linked hemiplegic migraine and episodic ataxia.[168,169] No clear association with epilepsy has yet been made in these families, although partial cosegregation of familial hemiplegic migraine and a benign familial infantile epileptic syndrome has been reported.[170]

## Other Genes Underlying the Spike-Wave Phenotype

Two other genes underlying the spike-wave absence epilepsy phenotype have been identified in spontaneous mouse mutants. The first locus, *slow wave epilepsy* (swe), encodes the gene for a neuronal membrane transporter, the sodium hydrogen exchanger

NHE1.[171] The mutant transcript is prematurely truncated, resulting in a functional null mutation. Young mice homozygous for the *swe* locus show generalized 3/sec spike-wave activity, infrequent tonic/clonic seizures, and ataxia. Physiological analysis of cells from the swe mutant reveals loss of function, predicting delayed pH recovery from an intracellular acid load. Downstream membrane excitability changes and synaptic transmission resulting from this defect in membrane proton transport remain to be explored.

The second locus, *mocha 2j*, encodes the $\delta$ subunit of a tetrameric adaptor protein complex AP3 expressed diffusely in brain.[172] Loss of AP3$\delta$ leads to absence of an intact AP3 complex and impaired sorting proteins destined for membrane insertion, including the zinc transporter ZNT3 that is associated with synaptic vesicles in mouse brain. Failure of normal ZNT3 sorting reduces the sequestration of zinc into neurotransmitter vesicles in neocortex and hippocampus, where its absence may affect a broad range of postsynaptic ion channels and receptors.

## Transmitter and Receptor Defects

**Autosomal Dominant Nocturnal Frontal Lobe Epilepsy.** A familial frontal lobe epilepsy syndrome (autosomal dominant nocturnal frontal lobe epilepsy, ADNFLE) has been delineated. It consists of major motor seizures while asleep. The condition was originally misdiagnosed as a sleep disorder. ADNFLE in a large Australian pedigree was mapped to a region on chromosome 20 q13.2-13.3 coinciding with the neuronal nicotinic acetylcholine receptor $\alpha 4$ subunit (CHRNA4) gene.[173] Affected family members revealed a missense mutation replacing serine with phenylalanine at nt48 in the second transmembrane domain. The mutation was found in 21 affected family members and in 4 obligate carriers, but not in 333 healthy control subjects. Seven families with sporadic cases of ADNFLE were not linked to this locus, and one other family has shown some evidence of linkage to chromosome 15q24.[174] Other mutations have since been identified.[175] Based on the sleep disorder phenotype, video-polysomnography was used in another clinical series. In more than 40 patients with nocturnal motor attacks, 30 percent showed ictal epileptiform EEG during the attacks. In five families, linkage to chromosome 15q24 was excluded, again suggesting genetic heterogeneity for this phenotype.[176] EEG and functional imaging studies reveal variable abnormalities in the frontal lobes of individuals bearing $\alpha 4$ nACHR mutations.[177]

The $\alpha 4$ nACHR is expressed in all layers of neocortex, throughout the cerebellar cortex and in other brain regions,[178] where it resides predominantly on postsynaptic membranes. Biophysical studies of the human mutation coexpressed with $\beta$ subunits in *Xenopus laevis* oocytes reveal that mutant AChR responses exhibit faster desensitization upon activation by acetylcholine, and show slower recovery from desensitization, less inward rectification, and essentially no Ca$^{2+}$ permeability compared to wild-type $\alpha 4 \beta 2$ AChRs.[179,180] In single-channel studies, wild-type $\alpha 4 \beta 2$ AChR channel currents exhibited two conductances, while mutant AChRs exhibited only one conductance of 11 pS. The net effect of the mutation is to reduce AChR function. This could result in cerebral hyperexcitability if the AChRs were an important part of inhibitory responses within cortical circuits where acetylcholine may reduce and redistribute intracortical inhibition by differentially altering spike thresholds in columnar microcircuits.[181,182]

### Transmitters and Receptors Identified in Mouse Models

**GABA.** Defects in GABA, the major inhibitory neurotransmitter in the mammalian brain, are prime candidates for inherited epilepsies. Two glutamate decarboxylase isoforms, GAD65 and GAD67, synthesize GABA. The individual roles of the two isoforms are poorly understood, but differences in saturation binding with cofactor and subcellular localization suggest that GAD65 may provide dynamic reserve pools of GABA for rapid regulation of inhibitory neurotransmission.

While mutant mice with targeted deletions of the GAD67 gene are born with developmental abnormalities and die shortly after birth,[183] GAD65−/− mice appear normal at birth, and basal GABA levels and holo-GAD activity are normal, but the pyridoxal 5' phosphate-inducible apo-enzyme reservoir is significantly decreased.[184] GAD65−/− mice develop spontaneous seizures that result in increased mortality. Fear or mild stress can precipitate the seizures, and expression of the seizure-associated immediate early gene *c-fos* reveals involvement of limbic regions of the brain. Recent evidence suggests that the critical period of plasticity and synaptogenesis by thalamocortical afferent terminals is also altered in the cortex of these mice.[185]

**NPY.** Neuropeptide Y (NPY), a 36-amino-acid transmitter distributed throughout the nervous system, is colocalized with GABA at many synapses and inhibits synaptic transmission. Seizures occur in NPY-deficient mice, and mutants are more susceptible to seizures and uncontrollable status epilepticus induced by convulsants than are wild-type mice.[186,187] In NPY null mutants, intracerebroventricular NPY infusion delivered before convulsant administration prevented death in NPY-deficient mice, suggesting a critical role for endogenous NPY in limiting seizure activity.

**GABA Receptors.** GABA receptors are pentameric complexes responsible for the majority of synaptic inhibition in the brain. Mice lacking three contiguous genes for the GABA A receptor, $\alpha 5$, $\gamma 3$, and $\beta 3$, survive poorly and show seizures, while those lacking only $\alpha 5$ and $\gamma 3$ do not show seizures.[188] Targeted deletion of the $\beta 3$ subunit of the GABA A-type receptor produces epilepsy, myoclonus, and epileptiform EEG discharges in surviving mice. The brain morphology is grossly unaffected, but the total brain GABA A-receptor density is reduced by about 50 percent.[189,190]

**Glutamate Receptors.** RNA adenosine deaminases are involved in the editing of mRNAs coding for glutamate receptor subunits, responsible for the majority of postsynaptic excitation in the central nervous system. Mice expressing an editing-incompetent allele of the glutamate B (GLURB) gene produce glutamate receptors that permit excessive calcium ion entry, resulting in an early and severe seizure disorder with extensive hippocampal cell death.[116,191]

**Glutamate Transporters.** Extracellular levels of the excitatory neurotransmitter glutamate in the nervous system are maintained by integral plasma membrane transporters that actively remove glutamate from the extracellular space. Homozygous mice deficient in GLT-1, a widely distributed astrocytic transporter responsible for the majority of glial glutamate uptake, show lethal spontaneous seizures, hippocampal neuronal loss, and increased susceptibility to acute cortical injury.[192] These effects can be attributed to elevated levels of residual extracellular glutamate. Interestingly, mice deficient in EAAC-1, a neuronal glutamate transporter expressed throughout the brain, kidney, and small intestine, develop dicarboxylic aminoaciduria but no neurodegeneration or seizure phenotype.[193]

## DISTURBANCES OF CELLULAR METABOLISM

Seizures, either isolated or repeated, and myoclonus are common to many inherited metabolic encephalopathies at some stage of their progression (Table 230-3). The seizures are usually generalized tonic/clonic, but may also have spike-wave absence components. The irregular myoclonic jerks may be segmental, or progress to involve all of the musculature. Ataxia and other motor abnormalities, including upper motor neuron spasticity and polyneuropathies, are common.

The relationship of myoclonus to epilepsy is still poorly understood, and the pathogenesis is believed to primarily involve cortical and subcortical circuitry.[194] Two forms of cortical

**Table 230-3** Epilepsy and Myoclonus in the Inherited Metabolic Encephalopathies

| Disorders | Epilepsy | Myoclonus |
|---|---|---|
| Acute intermittent porphyria | ++ | 0 |
| Alpers syndrome | +++ | ++ |
| Alexander disease | ++ | 0 |
| Bielschowsky-Jansky disease | +++ | +++ |
| Hyperglycinemia | +++ | 0 |
| Huntington chorea | ++ | 0 |
| Late infantile or juvenile G$_{M2}$-gangliosidosis | ++ | ++ |
| Juvenile neuraminidase deficiency | 0 | +++ |
| Other types of late infantile or juvenile lipidosis (Niemann-Pick, Gaucher, Austin disease, G$_{M1}$-gangliosidosis, type 2) | ++ | + |
| Late-onset intermittent amino acidopathies | ++ | 0 |
| Menkes disease | +++ | + |
| Polyunsaturated fatty acid lipidosis | + | ++ |
| Progressive familial myoclonic epilepsy, Lafora type | +++ | +++ |
| Progressive familial myoclonic epilepsies, with nonspecific neuronal generation and malignant course | +++ | +++ |
| Ramsay Hunt dyssynergia cerebellaris myoclonica | ++ | +++ |
| Spielmeyer-Vogt-Batten disease | ++ | + |

Seizures, isolated or repeated, occur occasionally in most metabolic encephalopathies. In this table, only the diseases in which epilepsy and/or myoclonus constitute a major and early feature are listed.
Modified from Adams and Lyon.[353]

myoclonus, positive and negative (where a brief silencing of cortical activity occurs), are now recognized. The presence of this readily identifiable phenotype with ataxia and dementia has facilitated clinical recognition of a distinct subset of inherited disorders, the progressive myoclonic epilepsies, and major progress in elucidating these genes has been made in the last decade.

## Progressive Myoclonic Epilepsies

The progressive myoclonus epilepsies (PMEs) are a group of molecularly distinct diseases with a similar presentation, characterized by myoclonus, tonic-clonic seizures, myoclonic seizures, and progressive neurologic dysfunction, including dementia, ataxia, and extrapyramidal signs. Six major PME syndromes are inherited as autosomal recessive traits, namely, myoclonic epilepsy and ragged-red fiber disease (MERRF), Unverricht-Lundborg (EPM1), the neuronal ceroid lipofuscinoses (NCL1-8), Gaucher disease, sialidoses, and Lafora disease. The genetic bases of 11 PME subtypes have now been determined (Table 230-4). Loss-of-function mutations have been identified in the mitochondrial tRNA (lys) gene in MERRF; the cystatin B gene in EPM1;[195,196] the palmitoyl-protein thioesterase gene in NCL-1;[197] a lysosomal peptidase gene in NCL-2;[198,199] two novel genes (*CLN3* and *CLN5*) in NCL-3 and NCL-5;[200,201] a putative transmembrane protein in NCL-8;[202] the β-glucocerebrosidase gene in Gaucher type 3;[203] the neuraminidase and galactosidase genes in sialidoses;[204,205] and laforin in Lafora disease.[206] The cellular pathogenesis of these disorders may provide general insight into mechanisms of neurodegeneration, because several of the mutations result in cell death and formation of intracellular inclusion bodies in a variety of cell types.

**Myoclonic Epilepsy and Ragged-Red Fiber Disease.** Myoclonic epilepsy and ragged-red fiber disease (MERRF) is a severe, multisystem disorder characterized by myoclonus, seizures, progressive cerebellar syndrome, muscle weakness, and the presence of ragged-red fibers in the muscle biopsy. The disorder is usually associated with point mutations, either A8344G or T8356C, in the gene encoding the mitochondrial tRNA(Lys), but mutations of the tRNA-Leu gene responsible for MELAS (mitochondrial encephalomyopathy, lactic acidosis, and strokelike episodes) and the gene for tRNA-Val are also observed.[207–209] Patients harboring these mutations carry both mutant and wild-type alleles within each cell (heteroplasmy). There is some clinical and EEG overlap between the diseases,[210,211] although SPECT measurements of cerebral perfusion are decreased in MELAS patients with ischemic episodes, but normal in MERRF patients.[212]

Although the mutation is maternally inherited, males and females are equally affected. Mutant transmitochondrial cell lines harboring a pathogenic point mutation at either A8344G or T8356C in the human tRNA(Lys) gene exhibit severe defects in respiratory chain activity, protein synthesis, and in steady state levels of mitochondrial translation products, indicating that these two different mtDNA point mutations result in near identical protein synthesis defects at the cellular level contributing to MERRF pathogenesis.[213]

More than 50 point mutations in mitochondrial DNA associated with maternally inherited or occasionally sporadic encephalomyopathies have been described.[214] These mutations produce a broad quantitative spectrum of clinical phenotypes, and some patterns relevant to pathogenesis are emerging. While all patients within the maternal lineage harbor the same mutation, the nature and severity of the symptoms vary markedly among individuals, correlating with age and the inherited mutant gene load in the individual's mitochondrial DNA.

A general paradigm for age-related decline in mitochondrial DNA diseases has been outlined, and may be a relevant basis for epileptogenesis.[215] In this model, inherited mutations inhibit the electron transport chain, damaging the mitochondrial DNA, and further reducing oxidative phosphorylation. Once oxidative phosphorylation drops below a critical threshold specific for the neuronal pathway, clinical symptoms appear. While a direct relationship between the mutation load and mitochondrial respiratory chain function has been established in muscle,[216] the correlation has been more difficult to establish in the central nervous system. For example, there are widespread decreases in cytochrome oxidase (COXII) in the MERRF brain extending beyond regions with clear cell death.[217] In another study, severely affected brain regions, including dentate nuclei, Purkinje cells, and inferior olivary nuclei were microdissected from MERRF (A-G) (nt) 8344 tRNAlys tissue and mtDNA levels were compared with unaffected regions.[218] The level of the mitochondrial tRNAlys mutation did not correlate with neuronal vulnerability in different neuronal subsets. While it appears that factors other than the simple proportion of mutant to normal mtDNA may contribute to cell survival, alterations in membrane excitability may show a more linear relationship with cell stress due to mitochondrial dysfunction. Two other pathogenic features of mitochondrial function apart from energy metabolism can be considered.[209] Along with depolarization due to membrane active transport failure, the uncoupling of mitochondrial function from intracellular calcium homeostasis and free radical generation may play a significant, but still poorly understood, role in altered excitability.

**Ceroid Lipofuscinosis.** The neuronal ceroid lipofuscinoses (NCL) comprise a set of at least eight distinct human diseases characterized by progressive visual failure, epilepsy, myoclonias, and neurodegeneration. An autofluorescent lipopigment accumulates in lysosomes of neurons and other cell types. NCLs are among the most common inherited neurodegenerative disorders of childhood and lead to premature death.[219,220]

**Table 230-4 Genes for Progressive Myoclonic Epilepsy and Neuroceroid Lipofuscinoses**

| Gene | Product | Chr | Syndrome | Age of Onset | Seizure Type | Neurological Phenotype | Refs |
|---|---|---|---|---|---|---|---|
| MERRF | tRNA-lys | MtDNA | MERRF | Child-late adult | Myoclonic seizures | Progressive seizures, ataxia, myopathy, deafness, optic atrophy | Shoffner et al. 1990[322] |
| EPM1 | Cystatin B cysteine protease inhibitor | 21q22.3 | Unverricht-Lundborg | 6–15 years | Myoclonic seizures | Progressive dementia, ataxia and seizures | Pennacchio et al. 1996[195] |
| EPM2 | Laforin novel protein tyrosine phosphatase | 6q24 | Lafora | 14 years | Myoclonic seizures | Rapidly progressive dementia, seizures, lethal | Minassian et al. 1998 |
| Sialidosis | neuraminidase | 6p21 | Gaucher | infantile | Myoclonic seizures | Cherry-red spot, myoclonus, choreoathetosis, seizures | Pshezhetsky et al. 1997[227] |
| DRPLA | Atrophin-1 | 12p12.3-p13.1 | Dentatorubral-pallidoluysian atrophy | Variable in adolescence | Myoclonic seizures | Myoclonus, epilepsy, ataxia, choreoathetosis, dementia | Onodera et al. 1995[232] |
| CLN1 (infantile) | Palmitoylprotein thioesterase | 1p32 | Santavuori-Haltia | 5–18 months | Massive myoclonus | Progressive visual loss, hypotonia, psychomotor regression, early death < 10 yrs | Vesa et al. 1995[323] |
| CLN2 (late infantile) | lysosomal pepstatin-insensitive carboxypeptidase | 11p15 | Jansky-Bielschowsky | 2–4 years | Massive myoclonus atonic, astatic seizures, atypical absences | Visual loss, early death < 15 yrs | Zhong et al. 1998[324] |
| CLN3 juvenile | Novel protein with 6TM domain | 16p12.1-11.2 | Batten/Spielmeyer-Vogt-Sjögren | 5–10 | Massive myoclonus, GTC | Visual loss, cerebellar and extrapyramidal signs, psychomotor slowing, death < 20 years | Intl. Consortium 1995[325] |
| CLN5 (variant of late infantile) | Novel protein | 13q21.1-q32 | Late infantile | 4–7 | Myoclonic epilepsy | Late onset Finnish variant of CLN1 | Savukoski et al. 1998[201] |
| CLN8 | Novel protein | 8pter-p22 | | 5–10 | Tonic-clonic seizures | Progressive epilepsy with mental retardation | Ranta et al. 1999[202] |

Five genes for the neuronal ceroid lipofuscinoses have been identified (Table 230-4). CLN1, the gene for infantile NCL (Santavuori-Haltia disease), encodes palmitoyl protein thioesterase (PPT), a lysosomal enzyme. Most patients bear the same point mutation. CLN2, the gene for the late infantile variant (Jansky-Bielschowsky disease), encodes lysosomal pepstatin-insensitive carboxypeptidase, another lysosomal enzyme, while CLN3, the gene for juvenile NCL (Batten or Spielmeyer-Vogt-Sjögren disease), and CLN5, the gene for the late onset Finnish variant of late infantile NCL, are both novel proteins.

Minor syndromes have been identified, displaying either lipopigments with classic curvilinear ultrastructure, or granular osmiophilic deposits.[220] Curvilinear storage lipopigments contain subunit C of the mitochondrial adenosine triphosphate synthase; the proteolipid pigments of the granular osmiophilic type show sphingolipid activator proteins (SAPs),[221] and the pathophysiologic significance of both are still unclear. Various pathogenetic mechanisms, including defective lipid peroxidation, abnormal dolichols and dolichol phosphates, and defects in protease inhibitors, have been proposed, but the precise mechanisms underlying the neurological deficits have not been determined.

Electrophysiological and imaging abnormalities may help to identify individuals at presymptomatic stages.[222] Brain perfusion studies with the Tc-99m-HMPAO SPECT method in patients with infantile, juvenile NCL, and late infantile Jansky-Bielschowsky variant disease reveal hypoperfusion prior to structural abnormalities seen on MRI or CT in these disorders. The typical SPECT findings at an early stage of infantile NCL are bilateral forebrain hypoperfusion, with reduction in cerebellar perfusion appearing later. Juvenile NCL patients also show hypoperfusion in regions not detected on CT. Genotype-phenotype correlations performed in patients with mutations in the CLN3 gene for juvenile NCL reveal that the onset of visual failure and epilepsy is dependent on gene dose in patients both homozygous and heterozygous for the 1.02-kb disease deletion.[223]

Two murine models of NCL have been reported, the motor neuron degeneration (mnd) mouse mapped to chromosome 8,[224] and a variant phenotype, neuronal ceroid lipofuscinosis (nclf).[202,225] Both homozygous mutants exhibit a similar phenotype, developing progressive retinal atrophy early in life and paralysis at around 9 months of age, though seizures were not reported. The nclf gene is located on chromosome 9 in a region homologous with human chromosome 15q21, where the gene for one variant of late infantile NCL, CLN6, recently was mapped.[226]

**Sialidoses.** Two genetically distinct human storage disorders are associated with either a primary or a secondary deficiency of lysosomal neuraminidase: sialidosis and galactosialidosis. Sialidoses are rare autosomal recessive heterogeneous neuronal diseases that begin from infancy. Mental retardation, seizures, progressive myoclonus, and cherry-red spots in the macula characterize sialidosis type 1, a late-infantile onset form. This form is caused by structural mutations in the neuraminidase gene.[227] Galactosialidosis involves a primary defect of a protective protein/cathepsin A (PPCA) protein that displays both cathepsin A and C-terminal deamidase activity. The inhibitor associates with $\beta$-galactosidase and neuraminidase to protect them from intralysosomal proteolysis. This form leads to a combined deficiency of neuraminidase and $\beta$-D-galactosidase. A range of storage products accumulate in lysosomes, and a spectrum of central nervous system deficits result.[228]

Electrophysiological studies of sialidoses show paroxysmal activity in the EEG, cortical myoclonus, and high-amplitude somatosensory-evoked potentials consistent with cortical hyper-excitability.[229] Young adults with sialidosis are insensitive to either light or sound but are highly sensitive to somatosensory stimulation and movement. Some patients with sialidosis may have two distinct types of myoclonus, either a stimulus-insensitive facial myoclonus without an EEG correlate, or stimulus-sensitive massive jerks associated with EEG spikes.[230] The underlying network excitability disturbances are unknown.

A mutant mouse strain bearing a point mutation in the neu-1 locus with partial deficiency of lysosomal neuraminidase has been studied, but seizures were not reported in this model.[231]

**Dentatorubral-Pallidoluysian Atrophy.** Dentatorubral-pallidoluysian atrophy (DRPLA) is an autosomal dominant neurologic disorder presenting with variable combinations of epilepsy, myoclonus, cerebellar ataxia, choreoathetosis, and dementia. An unstable expansion of a CAG repeat encoding a polyglutamine tract within a gene on chromosome 12 has been identified in DRPLA patients.[232,233] Patients with early onset of the progressive myoclonus epilepsy phenotype show large expansions, and there is a strong correlation between expansion size and the age of disease onset. A recent description of a pedigree showing autosomal recessive spastic paraplegia and mild ataxia without epilepsy, myoclonus, or dementia showed homozygosity for an intermediate size CAG repeat (40 to 41 repeats) in the DRPLA gene within affected family members,[234] while the heterozygous parents were neurologically intact. This suggests that the progressive myoclonic epilepsy is a separable element of the DRPLA syndrome that may depend on severe loss of the DRPLA gene function.

The DRPLA gene product (atrophin-1) is a neuronal cytoplasmic protein of approximately 190 kDa with unknown function, and a larger (205-kDa) protein is found in DRPLA brains.[235] In rat

brain, the homologous protein is expressed early and throughout development with wide expression in other tissues, including skeletal muscle, heart, lung, and kidney.[236] Analysis of mRNA from brain regions of DRPLA patients shows smaller sizes of CAG repeats expressed within the cerebellum, reflecting somatic mosaicism of the expanded alleles of the DRPLA gene.[232] Recent evidence demonstrates that pathologic ubiquitination of abnormal DRPLA protein complex plays a role in DRPLA pathology.[237] The abnormal proteolytic processing, nuclear localization, and protein aggregation mechanisms causing selective neuronal cell death and atrophy within the cerebellar outflow tract and basal ganglia are under active pursuit, and a mouse model expressing a full-length atrophin-1 gene is available.[238,239]

The EEG activity of patients with hereditary DRPLA reveals epileptiform patterns in the majority of those with seizures. Atypical spike-wave complexes and slow wave bursts were the most frequent patterns observed.[240] Photosensitivity was revealed in 25 percent of these patients, all of whom showed a progressive myoclonus epilepsy syndrome. Abnormal EEG background activity was evident in nearly all patients. Children with DRPLA may present with partial epilepsies,[241] but the types of seizures and EEG changes vary as the disease progresses.[242]

There is evidence of altered excitability in thalamus and brain stem of DRPLA patients. Auditory-evoked potentials show reduced or absent brain stem components and delayed latencies.[243] In addition, short latency somatosensory-evoked potentials (SEP) have prolonged central conduction time and reduced amplitude of cortical components. Two patients with onset of symptoms in the first decade had extremely enlarged flash visual-evoked potentials with shortened latency even in the absence of giant SEPs. The test could prove useful in diagnosis.[244]

A related disorder, benign adult familial myoclonus epilepsy (BAFME) is an autosomal dominant form not linked to the DRPLA gene.[245] Several forms of benign myoclonic epilepsies where a chromosomal locus has been defined include the autosomal dominant (AD) juvenile myoclonic epilepsy (JME) in chromosome 6p11, the autosomal dominant childhood absence epilepsy that evolves to JME in chromosome 1p, familial adult myoclonic epilepsy, and a JME susceptibility locus on chromosome 8. Other myoclonic epilepsy syndromes with onset in the first year of life have been reviewed.[246]

**Unverricht-Lundborg Disease.** Unverricht-Lundborg disease (EPM1) is an autosomal recessive disorder characterized by myoclonus, tonic-clonic seizures, and ataxia before the age of 16 years.[247,248] In contrast to other PMEs, EPM1 is not associated with inclusion bodies or mitochondrial defects. Progressive neurologic dysfunction, including ataxia, begins between 6 and 15 years of age, and may occur before or after the onset of seizures. Clinical severity varies both between and within families, and patients may average an IQ decline of 10 points per decade. The scant neuropathologic analysis available in ungenotyped cases reveals variable patterns of injury, ranging from widespread neurodegenerative changes to a more restricted cellular loss in the cerebellum.[249,250]

Various mutations in the cystatin B gene (stefin B) mapping to 21q22.3 have been implicated in the EPM1 phenotype, including a G $\rightarrow$ C substitution in the last nucleotide of intron 1 predicted to cause a splicing defect, and a C $\rightarrow$ T at amino acid position 68, resulting in a truncated cystatin B protein. A third mutation showing undetectable amounts of cystatin B mRNA by northern blot analysis consists of an insertion of unstable tandem dodecamer repeats in the 5' flanking promoter region of the cystatin B gene. This mutation is distinct from conventional trinucleotide repeat expansions, and may be the most common mutation in EPM1.[251-254] Reduced expression in promoter region expansion mutations may be the result of altered spacing between promoter elements.[255] There is little correlation between size and age of onset in affected individuals.[252] All mutations are predicted to result in loss of function.

Cystatin B is a member of a large class of proteins that inhibit cysteine proteases,[256] and is widely distributed within the cytosol of different cell types. The protein is a tightly binding reversible inhibitor of cathepsins B, H, L, and S, and the cysteine protease papain in vitro. However, the cathepsins are intralysosomal proteases involved in general protein catabolism.[257] The lack of cystatin B in EPM1 suggests that this disease is the result of excessive proteolysis in the cytosol, possibly explaining the absence of intracellular inclusions in this disorder.

Little regarding the pathogenesis of hyperexcitability in Unverricht-Lundborg disease is known as yet. Cortical somatosensory-evoked fields measured by magnetoencephalography are two to six times larger than in normal control subjects, but cortical auditory-evoked fields are attenuated, suggesting regional alterations in cortical area excitability.[258]

An orthologous model of Unverricht-Lundborg disease in a mouse deficient in the cystatin B gene shows a pronounced neurologic phenotype of myoclonus evident during sleep, seizures with generalized spiking EEG discharges, and progressive apoptosis of neurons, predominantly within the cerebellar granule cell layer.[259]

**Lafora Disease.** Lafora disease (LD) is an autosomal recessive disorder that typically presents in the second decade with progressive myoclonus epilepsy, intellectual decline, and death within 10 years. The metabolic error in LD results in storage of a polyglucosan in tissues including the brain, skin, and liver, and diagnosis may be made by biopsy of skin, muscle, liver, or brain. Rare forms of LD have been described with a later onset that follow a more benign course.[260,261]

Recently, a gene (EPM2A) for a novel protein, laforin, was identified by positional cloning of a candidate gene at chromosome 6q24.[262,263] The encoded protein shows a consensus amino acid sequence indicative of a protein tyrosine phosphatase (PTP) that is widely expressed in tissues. In nine LD families, six distinct point mutations were identified, and in another family, a microdeletion was identified, all co-segregating with the affected individuals.[262] Eight other loss-of-function mutations within the gene have been described.[263]

Occipital seizures and presymptomatic EEG abnormalities are seen in LD patients,[264–266] and a gradual increase in somatosensory EP amplitude is observed, leading to an early giant potential suggestive of hyperexcitability in the sensory motor cortex. Positron emission tomography studies show diffusely decreased cortical glucose metabolic rate and cerebral blood flow, and moderately lowered oxygen metabolic rate, though there is no increase in blood flow or glucose and oxygen metabolism in the sensorimotor cortex despite the presence of giant evoked potentials.[267] This suggests that the hyperexcitability is not due to any significant deficit of cortical energy metabolism.

## EPILEPSY AND DEFECTIVE PROTEIN DEGRADATION

### Angelman Syndrome

Angelman syndrome (AS) is an imprinted neurodevelopmental syndrome featuring mental retardation, seizures, and ataxia. In about 70 percent of cases, AS is caused by large de novo maternal deletions at 15q11-q13.[268] Nondeleted cases involve uniparental (paternal) disomy of chromosome 15, or imprinting mutations. Recently, truncation mutations were found in the E6-AP ubiquitin protein ligase gene (UBE3A, E6-AP) within this critical region in AS individuals who are nondeleted and who do not have uniparental disomy or imprinting defects.[269,270]

Comparisons of epilepsy phenotypes have been made among the AS mutations, including chromosome 15q11-13 deletions, uniparental disomy (UPD), methylation imprinting abnormalities,

and mutation in the UBE3A gene. These studies reveal epilepsy and characteristic EEG abnormalities, consisting of diffuse, bifrontally dominant, high-amplitude 1 to 3 Hz notched or triphasic or polyphasic slow waves, or slow and sharp waves in all genotypes.[271–274] Deletion patients had severe intractable epilepsy, most frequently with atypical absences and myoclonias, and less frequently with generalized extensor tonic seizures or flexor spasms. Epileptic spasms have been recorded in AS patients as old as 41 years.

The UBE3A ligase gene functions in the protein ubiquitination pathway. The expression of the UBE3A protein is imprinted with silencing of the paternal allele in hippocampus and cerebellum in mouse brain. Using mice with paternal UPD encompassing the UBE3A gene, in situ hybridization analysis reveals markedly reduced expression of UBE3A in Purkinje cells, hippocampal neurons, and mitral cells of the olfactory bulb in UPD mice compared to non-UPD mice, while other brain regions show little decrement in UBE3A mRNA.[275] Loss of UBE3A ligase activity in these cells is predicted to selectively impair the metabolism of specific proteins.

One protein target of UBE3A ligase activity was recently identified as the p53 tumor-suppressor gene. Jiang et al. determined that mice with maternal deficiency (m−/p+) for UBE3A show neurologic deficits resembling human AS with motor dysfunction, inducible seizures, a learning deficit, and impaired long-term potentiation (LTP) of hippocampal synapses.[276] The cytoplasmic abundance of p53 was increased in neurons from m−/p+ mice and in human AS brain tissue, demonstrating that UBE3A ligase activity normally promotes degradation of this protein. Interestingly, seizures in normal brain can induce the expression of p53, where it can be found in the nucleus of apoptotic neurons.[277,278] These initial findings suggest novel biochemical pathways for disinhibition and neuronal dysfunction in the AS nervous system.

The gene for the β3 subunit of GABA receptors lies within the AS imprinting region, although it is not known to be imprinted. A null mutant for the GABRβ3 gene shows seizures in both hetero- and homozygotes, suggesting that in some AS deletions, the loss of a GABRβ3 allele could modulate the seizure disorder caused by the UBE3A mutation.[189,190] Interestingly, Odano et al. employed an in vivo receptor mapping technique using iodine-123 iomazenil and single-photon emission tomography (SPET) to examine benzodiazepine (BZ)-receptor binding, an indirect measure of GABA-receptor density, in a patient with Angelman syndrome (AS) without a GABRβ3 deletion.[279] BZ-labeled receptor density was severely decreased in the cerebellum, and mildly decreased in the frontal and temporal cortices and basal ganglia, indicating a probable defect in GABAergic synaptic inhibitory function despite the presence of the GABRβ3 gene.

A mouse model constructed to inherit a paternal duplication of the homologous AS region has also been reported, and shows an EEG abnormality with remarkable similarity to the generalized slow delta patterns observed in AS individuals.[280]

### Presenilin-1 and Amyloidosis

In a study of 16 individuals from two families affected with early onset (<50 years) autosomal dominant familial Alzheimer disease, seizures were common and preceded by myoclonus. Serial MRIs showed progressive cortical atrophy appearing within 3 to 4 years of the onset of neurologic symptoms, and positron emission tomography studies revealed parietotemporal hypometabolism. The diagnosis of Alzheimer disease was pathologically confirmed in one individual from each family. A mutation was found at codon 139 in the presenilin-1 gene on chromosome 14, and results in a methionine to valine substitution that cosegregates with the disease.[281] A distinct Ser169Pro mutation is associated with generalized myoclonic seizures several years after the early onset (<35 years) of cognitive decline has been identified in a Spanish kindred. The mutation predicts a kink in the α-helix of the transmembrane domain of the PS1 protein that will disrupt its normal structure.[321]

Familial transthyretin (TTR) amyloidosis is a storage disorder that commonly presents with peripheral neuropathy. A kindred affected by a slowly progressive dementia, seizures, ataxia, hemiparesis, and decreased vision, but without neuropathy, was identified with TTR amyloid deposits in the leptomeninges and the brain parenchyma. This disorder is linked to a mutation substituting valine with glycine at codon 30 of the TTR gene.[282]

### L-Isoaspartate (D-Aspartate) O-Methyltransferase Deficiency

Insights into epileptogenic lesions produced by aberrant protein metabolism are also emerging from targeted gene deletion mutations in mice. Proteins containing L-asparaginyl and L-aspartyl residues are degraded by reactions that generate isomerized aspartyl derivatives and reduce biologic function. Repair of these proteins occurs by enzymatic methyl esterification of the abnormal residues. Mice deficient in L-isoaspartate (D-aspartate) O-methyltransferase, strongly expressed in normal brain, develop lethal seizures in adolescence.[283,284] L-Isoaspartate, a putative substrate, is increased ninefold in the brains of null mutants, which were enlarged after 4 weeks of age. Apical dendrites of pyramidal neurons in the cerebral cortex showed aberrant arborization and microtubules.[283] The anticonvulsant dipropylacetic acid prolonged survival but failed to prevent lethality. While the downstream molecular targets remain to be defined, this mutant model demonstrates that accumulation of potentially dysfunctional L-isoaspartyl- and D-aspartyl-containing proteins may produce a progressive epilepsy phenotype.

## OTHER GENETICALLY DEFINED EPILEPSY SYNDROMES

Two examples of inherited epilepsy relating to decreased glucose availability have been described. The first involves a defect in facilitated transport of glucose across the blood-brain barrier. Haploinsufficiency and point mutations of the glucose transporter gene GLUT1 (chromosome 1p35-p31.3) expressed in brain endothelial cells have been identified in two patients with infantile seizures, developmental delay, and microcephaly who had normal circulating blood glucose, low-to-normal cerebrospinal fluid lactate levels, but persistently low CSF glucose levels (hypoglycorrhachia).[285] This profile is consistent with defective transport of glucose into the central nervous system across the endothelial blood-brain barrier. Atypical absence seizures were common in this potentially treatable hexose deficiency syndrome.[286]

A second example involves glycogen storage disease type III (GSD-III), an autosomal recessive disease resulting from deficient glycogen debranching enzyme (GDE) activity. Analysis of the GDE gene in a hypoglycemic child with recurrent seizures who was enzyme-deficient in both liver and muscle (GSD-IIIa) revealed an insertion in the GDE cDNA (4529insA), resulting in premature truncation of the protein.[287] Other mutations have since been identified.

### Nonketotic Hyperglycinemia

Nonketotic hyperglycinemia (NKH) can be caused by inherited errors in genes encoding the glycine cleavage multienzyme system. In a large Israeli-Arab kindred with NKH, 14 children were affected, and all had seizures and respiratory failure within 2 days after birth. Enzymatic analysis revealed that T-protein activity was deficient in one liver specimen, and a missense mutation resulting in an amino acid substitution from histidine to arginine at position 42 (H42R) was identified in affected family members.[288]

### Rett Syndrome

Rett syndrome (RS) is an X-linked dominant encephalopathy of females clinically defined by autistic behavior, seizures, and decline of cognitive and motor skills early in life. The progressive disorder begins with apparently normal psychomotor development up to 18 months of age, followed by a rapid deterioration leading to severe mental retardation, autism, hand dyspraxia and handwringing movements, jerky truncal ataxia, microcephaly, and epilepsy.[289] The regressive stage is followed by apparent stability lasting through decades.[290] RS brains show cortical architectonic abnormalities of various types, including selective thinning of superficial pyramidal cell layers, dendritic spine changes, and diffuse loss of synaptic markers; but unlike partial epilepsies, no migrational disturbances are found.[291]

A gene for RS was recently identified on Xq28 that encodes methyl-CpG binding protein 2,[292,293] one of three proteins known to bind methylated DNA in a protein complex capable of repressing gene transcription.[294] In 6 of 21 sporadic RS patients, de novo mutations leading to partial or complete loss of function were identified. This defect should result in increased transcription of still unidentified neural genes normally silenced by DNA methylation.

Variants of RS have been reported, notable for partial recovery of psychomotor function with age. Partial speech and hand praxia are regained, while the autistic features persist. Epilepsy is less common in this subgroup.[295] One case with a phenotype similar to RS, including severe mental retardation, autistic behavior, inappropriate handwashing movements, and epilepsy, has been linked to a deletion of chromosome 18q21.1q22.3.[296] This case implicates a second member of the MeCP family assigned to this chromosome, or a candidate locus for an autosomal gene altered by the MeCP2 protein.

Tonic, generalized clonic, partial, absence, and myoclonic seizures are all seen in RS. In one study, nearly half of RS patients showed multiple seizure types.[297] The interictal EEG is abnormal with epileptiform discharges. Seizures may present as young as 18 months and as old as 7 years. The EEG is of additional early diagnostic value in distinguishing RS from other mental retardation syndromes.[298] Central spike-wave complexes are characteristic of RS, and easy to distinguish from the large amplitude 2 to 3 Hz frontal slowing, posterior spikes, and triphasic frontal waves of AS. RS patients also show an unusual and prominent rhythmical theta frequency (4 to 6/sec) pattern over central regions, which may be congruent with the motor dysfunction in these patients.[299] Epileptiform abnormalities over parasagittal regions are also present during all stages of sleep, although spiking is more prominent during the initial onset of stage 1 to 2 non-REM sleep.[300]

Visual- and somatosensory-evoked potentials (VEPs and SEPs) show abnormal enhancement in RS patients, although the giant responses may subside with disease progression.[301,302] Cortical hypoperfusion of varying severity is detectable at an early stage in a large proportion of patients by SPECT studies,[303] but there was no regional correlation with EEG abnormalities.

Other mapped epilepsy syndromes whose genes have not yet been defined are listed in Table 230-5.

### Hereditary Myoclonus and Hyperekplexia/Startle Disease

Myoclonic jerks and repetitive contractions or spasms may involve discharges in the frontal cortex or originate subcortically at various levels of the brain stem and spinal cord. The basic mechanisms of these discharges and their relationship to epilepsy remain poorly understood, although they may coexist with seizures and help refine the diagnostic category of various epilepsy syndromes.[304]

Along with the inherited storage disorders of PME, additional insights into mechanisms of myoclonus have emerged from both human and mouse gene identification in hereditary hyperekplexia, or startle disease. Startle disease is an autosomal dominant disorder characterized by marked neuromuscular spasticity in infancy diminishing during the first years of life, and an exaggerated myoclonic response to unexpected acoustic or tactile

**Table 230-5** Mapped Genetic Epilepsy Phenotypes with Still Unidentified Gene Mutations

| Chromosome | Phenotype | Reference |
|---|---|---|
| 1. terminal deletion (1q)(q43) | Partial motor seizures in late infancy with centrotemporal spike discharges resembling benign rolandic epilepsy | Vaughn et al., 1996[326] |
| 2. 2:4 insertional translocation (2;4)(p24;p15.3p13) | Macrocephaly, hypotonia, psychomotor retardation, multiple minor congenital anomalies, and EEG abnormalities | Asamoah et al., 1998[327] |
| 3. 2q23-q24 | Febrile seizures | Pfeiffer et al., 1999[126] |
| 4. p14.2-p12.1 | Dominant generalized epilepsy with an unusual delta EEG pattern | Zara et al., 1998[328] |
| 5. 6p21 susceptibility locus for EJM1 | Juvenile myoclonic epilepsy susceptibility locus located within or near the HLA region | Liu et al., 1995[329] Sander et al., 1998[330] |
| 6. 7q11.23 | Williams syndrome infantile spasms with interictal hypsarrhythmia | Tsao et al., 1997[331] |
| 7. 8, distal short arm: childhood progressive epilepsy | Recessive generalized tonic-clonic seizures with onset at 5–10 years and progressive MR with onset 2–5 years after the first seizures | Tahvanainen et al., 1994[332] |
| 8. 8p23; progressive epilepsy with MR (EPMR) | Recessive childhood onset epilepsy and mental retardation | Ranta et al., 1997[333] Ryan et al., 1997[334] |
| 9. 10q: partial complex epilepsy | Dominant secondarily generalized seizures with auditory prodrome | Ottman et al., 1995[335] Poza et al., 1999[336] |
| 10. Maternally derived partial duplication of 14q and deletion of proximal 15q. | Myoclonic epilepsy, mental retardation and cortical migration disorder | Iannetti et al., 1996[337] |
| 11. Duplication of the 15q11-13 region containing GABR5 and GABRB3 genes | Autism, epilepsy, ataxia | Bundey et al., 1994[338] |
| 12. 15q.14: susceptibility locus for JME | Juvenile-onset myoclonic epilepsy | Elmslie et al., 1997[339] |
| 13. 15q14 | Rolandic epilepsy with centrotemporal spikes | Neurbauer et al., 1998[340] |
| 14. 15q21-q23 | Late onset Indian variant of neuroceroid lipofuscinosis CLN1 | Sharp et al., 1997[341] |
| 15. 15q24 | Autosomal dominant nocturnal frontal lobe epilepsy | Phillips et al., 1998[342] |
| 16. 16, pericentromeric: infantile convulsions and movement disorder | Dominant benign infantile familial convulsions with paroxysmal choreoathetosis | Szepetowski et al., 1997[343] Lee et al., 1998[344] |
| 17. 16p12-p11.2 | Rolandic epilepsy, paroxysmal dystonia, and writer's cramp | Guerrini et al., 1999[345] |
| 18. 19p13.3 | Infantile febrile convulsions | Johnson et al., 1998[122] |
| 19. 19q | Benign familial infantile convulsions | Guipponi et al., 1997[129] |
| 20. Chromosome 20 ring: association with abnormal EEG and seizures | Abnormal interictal EEG pattern of rhythmic theta waves and frontotemporal seizures with generalized spike waves | Canevini et al., 1998[346] |
| 21. Trisomy 21: Down syndrome | MR, generalized tonic-clonic seizures, infantile spasms, startle-induced reflex seizures, hypotonia | Johannsen et al., 1996[347] Silva et al., 1996[348] |
| 22. 22q13 | Epilepsy and spinocerebellar ataxia | Matsuura et al., 1999[349] |
| 23. 22q11-q12 | Partial epilepsy with variable foci | Xiong et al., 1999[350] |
| 24. Xp11.4-Xp22.11 | Infantile spasms (West syndrome) | Stromme et al., 1999[351] |

stimuli in adults. Linkage analyses in several large families mapped the disorder to chromosome 5q33-q35, and point mutations in the gene encoding the $\alpha1$ subunit of the glycine receptor (GLRA1) have been identified.[305,306] Mutation analysis has not revealed a contribution of the GLRA1 gene in all affected patients,[307] suggesting that hyperekplexia-like syndromes can be caused by other genes, in particular those encoding other subunits of the functional glycine receptor complex.

The receptor for the inhibitory neurotransmitter glycine is a member of the ligand-gated ion channel receptor superfamily. Some mutations result in the substitution of leucine or glutamine for arginine 271, a charged residue located near the pore region of the channel. The effects of this mutation on glycine receptor behavior are still being analyzed. Rather than the predicted affect on chloride permeation, Rajendra et al. found no effect on the selectivity of the mutant channel; instead, they identified two hundred to four hundredfold decreases in sensitivity of the receptor to the agonist glycine.[308] Glycine-binding affinity to the receptor was reduced 50 to 100 times without altering the binding affinity of strychnine, a competitive antagonist. Analysis of a second mutation in the $\alpha1$ subunit revealed a lower glycine sensitivity than wild-type $\alpha1\beta$ receptors, a greatly reduced Hill coefficient, no change in the equilibrium constant for strychnine binding, and shorter channel openings for the $\alpha1(K276E)\beta$ mutant.[309] Therefore, mutations linked to startle disease reduce the efficacy of glycinergic inhibitory neurotransmission by reduced agonist responsiveness or impaired opening of the channel.

Measurement of cerebral function using proton MRSI in patients with hyperekplexia showed a reduction of the relative resonance intensity of neuronal markers (N-acetylaspartate choline-containing compounds, and creatine) in frontal and central regions.[310] In two individuals, EEG abnormalities in the frontal lobes were coincident with the MRSI findings, indicating the presence of frontal neuronal dysfunction, which may interact with subcortical regions to produce hyperekplexia. Autonomic responses measured by the galvanic skin response are also augmented[311] in the disorder.

### Mouse Mutants with Myoclonus

Three autosomal recessive mouse mutants show spasticity and reflex myoclonus. The *spasmodic* mouse phenotypically resembles startle disease, and is also associated with a missense mutation in GLRA1.[312] As in the human disease, glycine receptors on spasmodic neurons show reduced agonist sensitivity when expressed in vitro. The related *oscillator* mutant maps to the same GLRA1 locus as *spasmodic* and shows a frameshift mutation caused by a 7-bp microdeletion within the same gene, producing a functional null allele devoid of $\alpha 1$ polypeptide and strychnine binding.[313] Spinal glycine receptor content was significantly reduced in the $+/\mathrm{GLRA1}(spd^{ot})$ genotype, and heterozygotes showed an increased acoustic startle response consistent with haplotype insufficiency of the glycine receptor in the human condition. The *spastic* mouse displays muscular spasticity, myoclonus, and reduced GLRA levels, and bears a mutation in the gene encoding the $\beta$ subunit (GLRB) of the glycine receptor. A LINE-1 element insertion within intron 6 of GLRB results in exon skipping, and accumulation of truncated GLRB mRNA transcripts.[314,315] The phenotypes of the three disorders vary in severity. Symptoms in *oscillator* mice begin at postnatal day 11 to 14 and the mice die before 3 weeks of age, while *spastic* and *spasmodic* symptoms appear at 4 weeks of age with lessening severity in adulthood.[316] Although lethal in *oscillator* mice, a recessive null mutation (deletion of exons 1 to 6) in the GLRA1 gene has been reported in a child with exaggerated startle reflexes, demonstrating that the critical functions of the glycine-mediated inhibition in mice can be partially compensated in the human.[317]

Interestingly, tissue levels of the postsynaptic protein gephyrin are drastically reduced in the $\mathrm{Glra1}(spd^{ot})/\mathrm{Glra1}(spd^{ot})$ genotype.[318] Gephyrin is a cytoplasmic protein involved in anchoring postsynaptic glycine receptors and GABAA receptors at inhibitory synapses.[319] Sequence analysis of the gephyrin gene reveals similarity to proteins essential for activity of a molybdoenzyme cofactor. Mice deficient in the tubulin-binding gephyrin gene show that it is required both for synaptic clustering of glycine receptors in spinal cord and for molybdoenzyme activity in nonneural tissues. The gephyrin null mutant phenotype resembled that of human hyperekplexia and hereditary molybdenum cofactor deficiency, suggesting that gephyrin function may be impaired in both diseases.

Molybdenum cofactor deficiency (MoCoD) is an autosomal recessive disorder characterized by profound mental retardation and severe intractable seizures. In humans, MoCoD leads to the combined deficiency of sulfite oxidase, xanthine dehydrogenase, and aldehyde oxidase. Homozygosity mapping of two consanguineous kindreds of Israeli-Arab origin demonstrated linkage of a MoCoD gene to an 8-cM region on chromosome 6p21.3, between markers D6S1641 and D6S1672.[320] These data provide a molecular link between epilepsy, myoclonus, and inhibitory transmission at glycinergic synapses.

### CONCLUSION

Critical progress in the discovery of genes linked with human epilepsies has been made in the last decade. While the defined monogenic syndromes recognized to date account for only a minority of the large clinical population with idiopathic seizure disorders, the functional diversity of these genes provides extraordinary insight into the biologic control pathways of synchronous neuronal activity in the brain. For each molecule pinpointed by the single gene disorders, neurobiologic analysis in orthologous mouse models of the human disease will determine its effects on developing neurons, and the developmental stage when it interferes with the excitability of neural networks. An understanding of the relative contributions of each affected gene will accelerate solving the mechanisms of epileptogenesis underlying the more complex multigenic syndromes.

Seizures may arise directly out of an alteration in the defective gene signal, or out of a complex developmental cascade of molecular and cellular plasticity. These downstream pathways can be modified by multiple genes in the background, and therefore represent a source of additional targets for therapy. At present, the identification of epilepsy genes allows early and accurate diagnosis of affected individuals, exclusion of family members that are not affected, and genotypic evidence useful for family planning. In these patients, the gene will eventually help translate current symptomatic therapy of seizures into molecular strategies that effectively prevent or correct the neuronal effects of the genetic error.

### ACKNOWLEDGMENTS

The author wishes to acknowledge generous support from the National Institute of Neurological Disorders and Stroke, and The Blue Bird Circle Foundation for Pediatric Neurology.

### REFERENCES

1. Hauser WA, Hesdorfer DC: *Epilepsy: Frequency, Causes, and Consequences.* New York, Demos Press, 1990.
2. McKusick VA: *Mendelian Inheritance in Man. Catalogs of Human Genes and Genetic Disorders*, 12th ed. Baltimore, Johns Hopkins University Press, 1998.
3. Volpe JJ: *Neurology of the Newborn*, 3d ed. Philadelphia, WB Saunders, 1995.
4. Mizrahi EM: Consensus and controversy in the clinical management of neonatal seizures. *Clin Perinatol* 16:485, 1989.
5. Schwartzkroin PA, Moshe SL, Noebels JL, Swann JW (eds): *Brain Development and Epilepsy.* New York, Oxford University Press, 1995.
6. Hauser WA, Annegers JF, Rocca WA: Descriptive epidemiology of epilepsy: Contributions of population-based studies from Rochester, Minnesota. *Mayo Clin Proc* 71:576, 1996.
7. Noebels JL: Targeting epilepsy genes. *Neuron* 16:241, 1996.
8. Johnston D, Brown TH: The synaptic nature of the paroxysmal depolarizing shift in hippocampal neurons. *Ann Neurol* 16:S65, 1984.
9. Westmoreland BF: Epileptiform electroencephalographic patterns. *Mayo Clin Proc* 71:501, 1996.
10. Kuzniecky R: Magnetic resonance and functional magnetic resonance imaging: Tools for the study of human epilepsy. *Curr Opin Neurol* 10:88, 1997.
11. O'Brien TJ, So EL, Mullan BP, Hauser MF, Brinkmann BH, Bohnen NI, Hanson D, et al.: Subtraction ictal SPECT co-registered to MRI improves clinical usefulness of SPECT in localizing the surgical seizure focus. *Neurology* 50:445, 1998.
12. Gutnick MJ, Crill WE: The cortical neuron as a physiological unit, in Gutnick MJ, Mody I (eds): *The Cortical Neuron.* New York, Oxford University Press, 1995, p 33.
13. Ragsdale DS, Avoli M: Sodium channels as molecular targets for antiepileptic drugs. *Brain Res Rev* 26:16, 1998.
14. Prince DA, Connors BW: Mechanisms of interictal epileptogenesis. *Adv Neurol* 44:275, 1986.
15. Delgado-Escueta AV, Wilson WA, Olsen RW, Porter RJ (eds): *Jasper's Basic Mechanisms of the Epilepsies*, 3rd ed. Philadelphia, Lippincott-Williams and Wilkins, 1999.
16. Dichter MA: Basic mechanisms of epilepsy: Targets for therapeutic intervention. *Epilepsia* 38(Suppl 9):S2, 1997.
17. Noebels JL, Sutherland ML, Nahm WK, Di Pasquale E: Molecular and cellular plasticity in developing epileptic brain. *Cold Spring Harb Symp Quant Biol* 61:319, 1996.

18. Jan YN, Jan LY, Dennis MJ: Two mutations of synaptic transmission in *Drosophila. Proc R Soc Lond B Biol Sci* **198**:87, 1977.

19. Tempel BL, Papazian DM, Schwarz TL, Jan YN, Jan LY: Sequence of a probable potassium channel component encoded at Shaker locus of *Drosophila. Science* **237**:770, 1987.

20. Smart SL, Lopantsev V, Zhang CL, Robbins CA, Wang H, Chiu SY, Schwartzkroin PA, et al.: Deletion of the KV1.1 potassium channel causes epilepsy in mice. *Neuron* **20**:809, 1998.

21. Zuberi SM, Eunson LH, Spauschus A, De Silva R, Tolmie J, Wood NW, McWilliam RC, et al.: A novel mutation in the human voltage-gated potassium channel gene (Kv1.1) associates with episodic ataxia type 1 and sometimes with partial epilepsy. *Brain* **122**:817, 1999.

22. Pavlidis P, Tanouye MA: Seizures and failures in the giant fiber pathway of *Drosophila* bang-sensitive paralytic mutants. *J Neurosci* **15**:5810, 1995.

23. Engel J Jr: Classifications of the International League Against Epilepsy: Time for reappraisal. *Epilepsia* **39**:1014, 1998.

24. Byrd SE, Osborn RE, Bohan TP, Naidich TP: The CT and MR evaluation of migrational disorders of the brain. Part I. Lissencephaly and pachygyria. *Pediatr Radiol* **19**:151, 1989.

25. Aicardi J: Syndromic classification in the management of childhood epilepsy. *J Child Neurol* **9(Suppl 2)**:14, 1994.

26. Palmini A, Gambardella A, Andermann F, Dubeau F, da Costa JC, Olivier A, Tampieri D, et al.: Intrinsic epileptogenicity of human dysplastic cortex as suggested by corticography and surgical results. *Ann Neurol* **37**:476, 1995.

27. Guerreiro MM, Andermann F, Andermann E, Palmini A, Hwang P, Hoffman HJ, Otsubo H, et al.: Surgical treatment of epilepsy in tuberous sclerosis: strategies and results in 18 patients. *Neurology* **51**:1263, 1998.

28. Meencke HJ: Neuron density in the molecular layer of the frontal cortex in primary generalized epilepsy. *Epilepsia* **26**:450, 1985.

29. Palmini A, Andermann F, Aicardi J, Dulac O, Chaves F, Ponsot G, Pinard JM, et al.: Diffuse cortical dysplasia, or "the double cortex" syndrome: the clinical and epileptic spectrum in 10 patients. *Neurology* **41**:1656, 1991.

30. Barkovich AJ, Guerrini R, Battaglia G, Kalifa G, N'Guyen T, Parmeggiani A, Santucci M, et al.: Band heterotopia: Correlation of outcome with magnetic resonance parameters. *Ann Neurol* **36**:609, 1994.

31. des Portes V, Pinard JM, Smadja D, Motte J, Boespfng-Tanguy O, Moutard ML, Desguerre I, et al.: Dominant X linked subcortical laminar heterotopia and lissencephaly syndrome (XSCLH/LIS): Evidence for the occurrence of mutation in males and mapping of a potential locus in Xq22. *J Med Genet* **34**:177, 1997.

32. Ross ME, Allen KM, Srivastava AK, Featherstone T, Gleeson JG, Hirsch B, Harding BN, et al.: Linkage and physical mapping of X-linked lissencephaly/SBH (XLIS): A gene causing neuronal migration defects in human brain. *Hum Mol Genet* **6**:555, 1997.

33. Gleeson JG, Allen KM, Fox JW, Lamperti ED, Berkovic S, Scheffer I, Cooper EC, et al.: Doublecortin, a brain-specific gene mutated in human X-linked lissencephaly and double cortex syndrome, encodes a putative signaling protein. *Cell* **92**:63, 1998.

34. des Portes V, Pinard JM, Billuart P, Vinet MC, Koulakoff A, Carrie A, Gelot A, et al.: A novel CNS gene required for neuronal migration and involved in X-linked subcortical laminar heterotopia and lissencephaly syndrome. *Cell* **92**:51, 1998.

35. des Portes V, Francis F, Pinard JM, Desguerre I, Moutard ML, Snoeck I, Meiners LC, et al.: Doublecortin is the major gene causing X-linked subcortical laminar heterotopia. *Hum Mol Genet* **7**:1063, 1998.

36. Gleeson JG, Minnerath SR, Fox JW, Allen KM, Luo RF, Hong SE, Berg MJ, et al.: Characterization of mutations in the gene doublecortin in patients with double cortex syndrome. *Ann Neurol* **45**:146, 1999.

37. Pilz DT, Kuc J, Matsumoto N, Bodurtha J, Bernadi B, Tassinari CA, Dobyns WB, et al.: Subcortical band heterotopia in rare affected males can be caused by missense mutations in DCX (XLIS) or LIS1. *Hum Mol Genet* **8**:1757, 1999.

38. Sossey-Alaoui K, Hartung AJ, Guerrini R, Manchester DK, Posar A, Puche-Mira A, Andermann E, et al.: Human doublecortin (DCX) and the homologous gene in mouse encode a putative Ca2+-dependent signaling protein which is mutated in human X-linked neuronal migration defects. *Hum Mol Genet* **7**:1327, 1998.

39. Gleeson JG, Lin PT, Flanagan LA, Walsh CA: Doublecortin is a microtubule-associated protein and is expressed widely by migrating neurons. *Neuron* **23**:257, 1999.

40. Horesh D, Sapir T, Francis F, Wolf SG, Caspi M, Elbaum M, Chelly J, et al.: Doublecortin, a stabilizer of microtubules. *Hum Mol Genet* **8**:1599, 1999.

41. Francis F, Koulakoff A, Boucher D, Chafey P, Schaar B, Vinet MC, Friocourt G, et al.: Doublecortin is a developmentally regulated, microtubule-associated protein expressed in migrating and differentiating neurons. *Neuron* **23**:247, 1999.

42. Dobyns WB, Stratton RF, Parke JT, Greenberg F, Nussbaum RL, Ledbetter DH: Miller-Dieker syndrome: lissencephaly and monosomy 17p. *J Pediatr* **102**:552, 1983.

43. Reiner O, Carrozzo R, Shen Y, Wehnert M, Faustinella F, Dobyns WB, Caskey CT, et al.: Isolation of a Miller-Dieker lissencephaly gene containing G protein-subunit-like repeats. *Nature* **364**:717, 1993.

44. Chong SS, Pack SD, Roschke AV, Tanigami A, Carrozo R, Smith ACM, Dobyns WB, et al.: A revision of the lissencephaly and Miller-Dieker critical regions in chromosome 17p13.3. *Hum Mol Genet* **6**:147, 1997.

45. Lo Nigro C, Chong SS, Smith ACM, Dobyns WB, Carrozzo R, Ledbetter DH: Point mutations and an intragenic deletion in LIS1, the lissencephaly causative gene in isolated lissencephaly sequence and Miller-Dieker syndrome. *Hum Mol Genet* **6**:157, 1997.

46. Hattori M, Adachi H, Tsujimoto M, Arai H, Inoue K: Miller-Dieker lissencephaly gene encodes a subunit of brain platelet-activating factor acetylhydrolase. *Nature* **370**:216, 1994.

47. Reiner O, Albrecht U, Gordon M, Chianese KA, Wong C, Gal-Gerber O, Sapir T, et al.: Lissencephaly gene (LIS1) expression in the CNS suggests a role in neuronal migration. *J Neurosci* **15**:3730, 1995.

48. Fogli A, Guerrini R, Moro F, Fernandez-Alvarez E, Livet MO, Renieri A, Cioni M, et al.: Intracellular levels of the LIS1 protein correlate with clinical and neuroradiological findings in patients with classical lissencephaly. *Ann Neurol* **45**:154, 1999.

49. Clark GD, Mizuguchi M, Antalffy B, Barnes J, Armstrong D: Predominant localization of the LIS family of gene products to Cajal-Retzius cells and ventricular neuroepithelium in the developing human cortex. *J Neuropathol Exp Neurol* **56**:1044, 1997.

50. Sapir T, Elbaum M, Reiner O: Reduction of microtubule catastrophe events by LIS1, platelet-activating factor acetylhydrolase subunit. *EMBO J* **16**:6977, 1997.

51. Morris SM, Albrecht U, Reiner O, Eichele G, Yu-Lee LY: The lissencephaly gene product Lis1, a protein involved in neuronal migration, interacts with a nuclear movement protein, NudC. *Curr Biol* **8**:603, 1998.

52. Hirotsune S, Fleck MW, Gambello MJ, Bix GJ, Chen A, Clark GD, Ledbetter DH, et al.: Graded reduction of Pafah1b1 (Lis1) activity results in neuronal migration defects and early embryonic lethality. *Nat Genet* **19**:333, 1998.

53. Paylor R, Hirotsune S, Gambello MJ, Yuva-Paylor L, Crawley JN, Wynshaw-Boris A: Impaired learning and motor behavior in heterozygous Pafah1b1 (Lis1) mutant mice. *Learn Mem* **6**:521, 1999.

54. Worle H, Keimer R, Kohler B: Miller-Dieker syndrome (type I lissencephaly) with specific EEG changes. *Monatsschr Kinderheilkd* **138**:615, 1990.

55. Yoshioka M, Kuroki S: Clinical spectrum and genetic studies of Fukuyama congenital muscular dystrophy. *Am J Med Genet* **53**:245, 1994.

56. Aida N: Fukuyama congenital muscular dystrophy: a neuroradiologic review. *J Magn Reson Imaging* **8**:317, 1998.

57. Segawa M, Nomura Y, Hachimori K, Shinoyama N, Hosaka A, Mizuno Y: Fukuyama type congenital muscular dystrophy as a natural model of childhood epilepsy. *Brain Dev* **1**:113, 1979.

58. Wu L, Hirokazu O, Makiko O, Yukio F: Fukuyama type congenital muscular dystrophy with central-temporal EEG foci (rolandic spikes). *Chin Med Sci J* **8**:162, 1993.

59. Toda T, Segawa M, Nomura Y, Nonaka I, Masuda K, Ishihara T, Sakai M, et al.: Localization of a gene for Fukuyama type congenital muscular dystrophy to chromosome 9q31-33. *Nat Genet* **5**:283, 1993.

60. Kobayashi K, Nakahori Y, Miyake M, Matsumura K, Kondo-Iida E, Nomura Y, Segawa M, et al.: An ancient retrotransposal insertion causes Fukuyama-type congenital muscular dystrophy. *Nature* **394**:388, 1998.

61. Capra V, De Marco P, Moroni A, Faiella A, Brunelli S, Tortori-Donati P, Andreussi I, et al.: Schizencephaly: surgical features and new molecular genetic results. *Eur J Pediatr Surg* **1(Suppl)**:27, 1996.

62. Brunelli S, Faiella A, Capra V, Nigro V, Simeone A, Cama A, Boncinelli E: Germline mutations in the homeobox gene EMX2 in patients with severe schizencephaly. *Nat Genet* **12**:94, 1996.

63. Faiella A, Brunelli S, Granata T, D'Incerti L, Cardini R, Lenti C, Battaglia G, et al.: A number of schizencephaly patients including 2 brothers are heterozygous for germline mutations in the homeobox gene EMX2. *Eur J Hum Genet* **5**:186, 1997.

64. Yoshida M, Suda Y, Matsuo I, Miyamoto N, Takeda N, Kuratani S, Aizawa S: Emx1 and Emx2 functions in development of dorsal telencephalon. *Development* **124**:101, 1997.

65. Crino PB, Henske EP: New developments in the neurobiology of the tuberous sclerosis complex. *Neurology* **53**:1384, 1999.

66. van Slegtenhorst M, de Hoogt R, Hermans C, Nellist M, Janssen B, Verhoef S, Lindhout D, et al.: Identification of the tuberous sclerosis gene TSC1 on chromosome 9q34. *Science* **277**:805, 1997.

67. The European Chromosome 16 Tuberous Sclerosis Consortium: Identification and characterization of the tuberous sclerosis gene on chromosome 16. *Cell* **75**:1305, 1993.

68. van Slegtenhorst M, Nellist M, Nagelkerken B, Cheadle J, Snell R, van den Ouweland A, Reuser A, et al.: Interaction between hamartin and tuberin, the TSC1 and TSC2 gene products. *Hum Mol Genet* **7**:1053, 1998.

69. Geist RT, Reddy AJ, Zhang J, Gutmann DH: Expression of the tuberous sclerosis 2 gene product, tuberin, in adult and developing nervous system tissues. *Neurobiol Dis* **3**:111, 1996.

70. Vinters HV, Kerfoot C, Catania M, Emelin JK, Roper SN, DeClue JE: Tuberous sclerosis-related gene expression in normal and dysplastic brain. *Epilepsy Res* **32**:12, 1998.

71. Crino PB, Trojanowski JQ, Eberwine J: Internexin, MAP1B, and nestin in cortical dysplasia as markers of developmental maturity. *Acta Neuropathol (Berl)* **93**:619, 1997.

72. De Rosa MJ, Farrell MA, Burke MM, Secor DL, Vintners HV: An assessment of the proliferative potential of "balloon cells" in focal cortical resections performed for childhood epilepsy. *Neuropathol Appl Neurobiol* **18**:566, 1992.

73. Kotagal P, Rothner AD: Epilepsy in the setting of neurocutaneous syndromes. *Epilepsia* **34(Suppl 3)**:S71, 1993.

74. Simonati A, Colamaria V, Bricolo A, Bernardina BD, Rizzuto N: Microgyria associated with Sturge-Weber angiomatosis. *Childs Nerv Syst* **10**:392, 1994.

75. Adamsbaum C, Pinton F, Rolland Y, Chiron C, Dulac O, Kalifa G: Accelerated myelination in early Sturge-Weber syndrome: MRI-SPECT correlations. *Pediatr Radiol* **26**:759, 1996.

76. Wolf HK, Normann S, Green AJ, von Bakel I, Blumcke I, Pietsch T, Wiestler OD, et al.: Tuberous sclerosis-like lesions in epileptogenic human neocortex lack allelic loss at the TSC1 and TSC2 regions. *Acta Neuropathologica (Berl)* **93**:93, 1997.

77. Fois A, Tine A, Pavone L: Infantile spasms in patients with neurofibromatosis type 1. *Childs Nerv Syst* **10**:176, 1994.

78. Korf BR, Carrazana E, Holmes GL: Patterns of seizures observed in association with neurofibromatosis 1. *Epilepsia* **34**:616, 1993.

79. Motte J, Billard C, Fejerman N, Sfaello Z, Arroyo H, Dulac O: Neurofibromatosis type one and West syndrome: a relatively benign association. *Epilepsia* **34**:723, 1993.

80. Fink JM, Dobyns WB, Guerrini R, Hirsch BA: Identification of a duplication of Xq28 associated with bilateral periventricular nodular heterotopia. *Am J Hum Genet* **61**:379, 1997.

81. Guerrini R, Dobyns WB: Bilateral periventricular nodular heterotopia with mental retardation and frontonasal malformation. *Neurology* **51**:499, 1998.

82. Dobyns WB, Guerrini R, Czapansky-Beilman DK, Pierpont ME, Breningstall G, Yock DH Jr, Bonanni P, et al.: Bilateral periventricular nodular heterotopia with mental retardation and syndactyly in boys: A new X-linked mental retardation syndrome. *Neurology* **49**:1042, 1997.

83. Huttenlocher PR, Taravath S, Mojtahedi S: Periventricular heterotopia and epilepsy. *Neurology* **44**:51, 1994.

84. Eksioglu YZ, Scheffer IE, Cardenas P, Knoll J, DiMario F, Ramsby G, Berg M, et al.: Periventricular heterotopia: An X-linked dominant epilepsy locus causing aberrant cerebral cortical development. *Neuron* **16**:77, 1996.

85. Fox, JW, Lamperti ED, Eksioglu YZ, Hong SE, Feng Y, Graham DA, Scheffer IE, et al.: Mutations in filamin 1 prevent migration of cerebral cortical neurons in human periventricular heterotopia. *Neuron* **21**:1315, 1998.

86. Spreafico R, Pasquier B, Minotti L, Garbelli R, Kahane P, Grand S, Benabid AL, et al.: Immunocytochemical investigation on dysplastic human tissue from epileptic patients. *Epilepsy Res* **32**:34, 1998.

87. Battaglia G, Granata T, Farina L, D'Incerti L, Franceschetti S, Avanzini G: Periventricular nodular heterotopia: Epileptogenic findings. *Epilepsia* **38**:1173, 1997.

88. Dubeau F, Tampieri D, Lee N, Andermann E, Carpenter S, Leblanc R, Olivier A, et al.: Periventricular and subcortical nodular heterotopia. A study of 33 patients. *Brain* **118**:1273, 1995.

89. Li LM, Dubeau F, Andermann F, Fish DR, Watson C, Cascino GD, Berkovic SF, et al.: Periventricular nodular heterotopia and intractable temporal lobe epilepsy: Poor outcome after temporal lobe resection. *Ann Neurol* **41**:662, 1997.

90. Morioka T, Nishio S, Sasaki M, Yoshida T, Kuwabara Y, Ohta M, Fukui M: Functional imaging in periventricular nodular heterotopia with the use of FDG-PET and HMPAO-SPECT. *Neurosurg Rev* **22**:41, 1999.

91. Spreafico R, Battaglia G, Arcelli P, Andermann F, Dubeau F, Palmini A, Olivier A, et al.: Cortical dysplasia: An immunocytochemical study of three patients. *Neurology* **50**:27, 1998.

92. Babb TL, Ying Z, Hadam J, Penrod C: Glutamate receptor mechanisms in human epileptic dysplastic cortex. *Epilepsy Res* **32**:24, 1998.

93. Ying Z, Babb TL, Comair YG, Bingaman W, Bushey M, Touhalisky K: Induced expression of NMDAR2 proteins and differential expression of NMDAR1 splice variants in dysplastic neurons of human epileptic neocortex. *J Neuropathol Exp Neurol* **57**:47, 1998.

94. Acampora D, Mazan S, Avantaggiato V, Barone P, Tuorto F, Lallemand Y, Brulet P, et al.: Epilepsy and brain abnormalities in mice lacking the Otx1 gene. *Nat Genet* **14**:218, 1996.

95. Frantz GD, Weimann JM, Levin ME, McConnell SK: Otx1 and Otx2 define layers and regions in developing cerebral cortex and cerebellum. *J Neurosci* **14**:5725, 1994.

96. Chae T, Kwon YT, Bronson R, Dikkes P, Li E, Tsai LH: Mice lacking p35, a neuronal specific activator of Cdk5, display cortical lamination defects, seizures, and adult lethality. *Neuron* **18**:29, 1997.

97. D'Arcangelo G, Miao GG, Chen SC, Soares HD, Morgan JI, Curran T: A protein related to extracellular matrix proteins deleted in the mouse mutant reeler. *Nature* **374**:719, 1995.

98. Hirotsune S, Takahara T, Sasaki N, Hirose K, Yoshiki A, Ohashi T, Kusakabe M, et al.: The reeler gene encodes a protein with an EGF-like motif expressed by pioneer neurons. *Nat Genet* **10**:77, 1995.

99. Alcantara S, Ruiz M, D'Arcangelo G, Ezan F, de Lecea L, Curran T, Sotelo C, et al.: Regional and cellular patterns of reelin mRNA expression in the forebrain of the developing and adult mouse. *J Neurosci* **18**:7779, 1998.

100. D'Arcangelo G, Curran T: Reeler: New tales on an old mutant mouse. *Bioessays* **20**:235, 1998.

101. Noebels JL: Gene control of cortical excitability, in Gutnick MJ, Mody I (eds): *The Cortical Neuron*. New York, Oxford University Press, 1995, p 210.

102. Yoneshima H, Nagata E, Matsumoto M, Yamada M, Nakajima K, Miyata T, Ogawa M, et al.: A novel neurological mutant mouse, yotari, which exhibits reeler-like phenotype but expresses CR-50 antigen/reelin. *Neurosci Res* **29**:217, 1997.

103. Sheldon M, Rice DS, D'Arcangelo G, Yoneshima H, Nakajima K, Mikoshiba K, Howell BW, et al.: Scrambler and yotari disrupt the disabled gene and produce a reeler-like phenotype in mice. *Nature* **389**:730, 1997.

104. Howell BW, Hawkes R, Soriano P, Cooper J: Neuronal position in the developing brain is regulated by mouse disabled-1. *Nature* **389**:733, 1997.

105. Ware ML, Fox JW, Gonzalez JL, Davis NM, Lambert de Rouvroit C, Russo CJ, Chua SC Jr, et al.: Aberrant splicing of a mouse disabled homolog, mdab1, in the scrambler mouse. *Neuron* **19**:239, 1997.

106. Rice DS, Sheldon M, D'Arcangelo G, Nakajima K, Goldowitz D, Curran T: Disabled-1 acts downstream of reelin in a signaling pathway that controls laminar organization in the mammalian brain. *Development* **125**:3719, 1998.

107. Warren ST, Sherman SL: The fragile X syndrome. Chap. 64 this text.

108. Musumeci SA, Colognola RM, Ferri R, Gigli GL, Petrella MA, Sanfilippo S, Bergonzi P, et al.: Fragile-X syndrome: A particular epileptogenic EEG pattern. *Epilepsia* **29**:41, 1988.

109. Kluger G, Bohm I, Laub MC, Waldenmaier C: Epilepsy and fragile X gene mutations. *Pediatr Neurol* **15**:358, 1996.

110. Musumeci SA, Hagerman RJ, Ferri R, Bosco P, Dalla Bernardina B, Tassinari CA, De Sarro GB, et al.: Epilepsy and EEG findings in males with fragile X syndrome. *Epilepsia* **40**:1092, 1999.

111. Timms KM, Bondeson ML, Ansari-Lari MA, Lagerstedt K, Muzny DM, Dugan-Rocha SP, Nelson DL, et al.: Molecular and phenotypic variation in patients with severe Hunter syndrome. *Hum Mol Genet* **6**:479, 1997.

112. The Dutch-Belgian Fragile X Consortium. Fmr1 knockout mice: A model to study fragile X mental retardation. *Cell* **78**:23, 1994.

113. Warren ST, Sherman SL: The fragile X syndrome. Chap. 64 this text.

114. Steffenburg U, Hedstrom A, Lindroth A, Wiklund LM, Hagberg G, Kyllerman M: Intractable epilepsy in a population-based series of mentally retarded children. *Epilepsia* **39**:767, 1998.

115. Bourgeois BF: Antiepileptic drugs, learning, and behavior in childhood epilepsy. *Epilepsia* **39**:913, 1998.

116. Brusa R, Zimmermann F, Koh DS, Feldmeyer D, Gass P, Seeburg PH, Sprengel R: Early-onset epilepsy and postnatal lethality associated with an editing-deficient GluR-B allele in mice. *Science* **270**:1677, 1995.

117. Xiang H, Hochman DW, Saya H, Fujiwara T, Schwartzkroin PA, Morrison RS: Evidence for p53-mediated modulation of neuronal viability. *J Neurosci* **16**:6753, 1996.

118. Schauwecker PE, Steward O: Genetic determinants of susceptibility to excitotoxic cell death: Implications for gene targeting approaches. *Proc Natl Acad Sci U S A* **94**:4103, 1997.

119. Tsirka SE, Gualandris A, Amaral DG, Strickland S: Excitotoxin-induced neuronal degeneration and seizure are mediated by tissue plasminogen activator. *Nature* **377**:340,1995.

120. Ptacek L: Channelopathies: Hypo/hyperkalemia. Chap. 204 in this text.

121. Mody I: Ion channels in epilepsy. *Int Rev Neurobiol* **42**:199, 1998.

122. Johnson EW, Dubovsky J, Rich SS, O'Donovan CA, Orr HT, Anderson VE, Gil-Nagel A, et al.: Evidence for a novel gene for familial febrile convulsions, FEB2, linked to chromosome 19p in an extended family from the Midwest. *Hum Mol Genet* **7**:63, 1998.

123. Wallace RH, Wang DW, Singh R, Scheffer IE, George AL Jr, Phillips HA, Saar K, et al.: Febrile seizures and generalized epilepsy associated with a mutation in the Na⁺-channel beta1 subunit gene SCN1B. *Nat Genet* **19**:366, 1998.

124. Wallace RH, Berkovic SF, Howell RA, Sutherland GR, Mulley JC: Suggestion of a major gene for familial febrile convulsions mapping to 8q13-21. *J Med Genet* **33**:308, 1996.

125. Baulac S, Gourfinkel-An I, Picard F, Rosenberg-Bourgin M, Prud'-homme J-F, Baulac M, Brice A: A second locus for familial generalized epilepsy with febrile seizures plus maps to chromosome 2q21-q23. *Am J Hum Genet* **65**:1078, 1999.

126. Peiffer A, Thompson J, Charlier C, Otterud B, Varvil T, Pappas C, Barnitz C, et al.: A locus for febrile seizures (FEB3) maps to chromosome 2q23-24. *Ann Neurol* **46**:671, 1999.

127. McDermott MF, Ogunkolade BW, McDermott EM, Jones LC, Wan Y, Quane KA, McCarthy J, et al.: Linkage of familial Hibernian fever to chromosome 12p13. *Am J Hum Genet* **62**:1446, 1998.

128. Mulley J, Saar K, Hewitt G, Ruschendorf F, Phillips H, Colley A, Sillence D, et al.: Gene localization for an autosomal dominant familial periodic fever to 12p13. *Am J Hum Genet* **62**:884, 1998.

129. Guipponi M, Rivier F, Vigevano F, Beck C, Crespel A, Echenne B, Lucchini P, et al.: Linkage mapping of benign familial infantile convulsions (BFIC) to chromosome 19q. *Hum Mol Genet* **6**:473, 1997.

130. McCormick KA, Isom LL, Ragsdale D, Smith D, Scheuer T, Catterall WA: Molecular determinants of Na⁺ channel function in the extracellular domain of the beta1. *J Biol Chem* **273**:3954, 1998.

131. Isom LL, Scheuer T, Brownstein AB, Ragsdale DS, Murphy BJ, Catterall WA: Functional co-expression of the beta 1 and type IIA alpha subunits of sodium channels in a mammalian cell line. *J Biol Chem* **270**:3306, 1995.

132. Makita N, Shirai N, Nagashima M, Matsuoka R, Yamada Y, Tohse N, Kitabatake A: A de novo missense mutation of human cardiac Na⁺ channel exhibiting novel molecular mechanisms of long QT syndrome. *FEBS Lett* **423**:5, 1998.

133. Wang Q, Shen J, Splawski I, Atkinson D, Li Z, Robinson JL, Moss AJ, et al.: SCN5A mutations associated with an inherited cardiac arrhythmia, long QT syndrome. *Cell* **80**:805, 1995.

134. Hartmann HA, Colom LV, Sutherland ML, Noebels JL: Selective localization of cardiac SCN5A sodium channels in limbic regions of rat brain. *Nat Neurosci* **2**:593, 1999.

135. Reckziegel G, Beck H, Schramm J, Elger CE, Urban BW: Electro-physiological characterization of Na⁺ currents in acutely isolated human hippocampal dentate granule cells. *J Physiol (Lond)* **509**:139, 1998.

136. O'Connor ER, Sontheimer H, Spencer DD, de Lanerolle NC: Astrocytes from human hippocampal epileptogenic foci exhibit action potential-like. *Epilepsia* **39**:347, 1998.

137. Lombardo AJ, Kuzniecky R, Powers RE, Brown GB: Altered brain sodium channel transcript levels in human epilepsy. *Mol Brain Res* **35**:84, 1996.

138. Noebels JL, Marcom PK, Jalilian-Tehrani MH: Sodium channel density in hypomyelinated brain increased by myelin basic protein gene deletion. *Nature* **352**:431, 1991.

139. Sashihara S, Yanagihara N, Kobayashi H, Izumi F, Tsuji S, Murai Y, Mita T: Overproduction of voltage-dependent Na⁺ channels in the developing brain of genetically seizure-susceptible E1 mice. *Neuroscience* **48**:285, 1992.

140. Xia Y, Haddad GG: Voltage-sensitive Na⁺ channels increase in number in newborn rat brain after in utero hypoxia. *Brain Res* **635**:339, 1994.

141. Leppert M, Anderson VE, Quattlebaum T, Stauffer D, O'Connell P, Nakamura Y, Lalouel JM, et al.: Benign familial neonatal convulsions linked to genetic markers on chromosome 20. *Nature* **337**:647, 1989.

142. Ronen GM, Rosales TO, Connolly M, Anderson VE, Leppert M: Seizure characteristics in chromosome 20 benign familial neonatal convulsions. *Neurology* **43**:1355, 1993.

143. Lewis TB, Leach RJ, Ward K, O'Connell P, Ryan SG: Genetic heterogeneity in benign familial neonatal convulsions: Identification of a new locus on chromosome 8q. *Am J Hum Genet* **53**:670, 1993.

144. Steinlein O, Schuster V, Fischer C, Haussler M: Benign familial neonatal convulsions: Confirmation of genetic heterogeneity and further evidence for a second locus on chromosome 8q. *Hum Genet* **95**:411, 1995.

145. Singh NA, Charlier C, Stauffer D, DuPont BR, Leach RJ, Melis R, Ronen GM, et al.: A novel potassium channel gene, KCNQ2, is mutated in an inherited epilepsy of newborns. *Nat Genet* **18**:25, 1998.

146. Biervert C, Schroeder BC, Kubisch C, Berkovic SF, Propping P, Jentsch TJ, Steinlein OK: A potassium channel mutation in neonatal human epilepsy. *Science* **279**:403, 1998.

147. Charlier C, Singh NA, Ryan SG, Lewis TB, Reus BE, Leach RJ, Leppert M: A pore mutation in a novel KQT-like potassium channel gene in an idiopathic epilepsy family. *Nat Genet* **18**:53, 1998.

148. Yang WP, Levesque PC, Little WA, Conder ML, Ramakrishnan P, Neubauer MG, Blanar MA: Functional expression of two KvLQT1-related potassium channels responsible for an inherited idiopathic epilepsy. *J Biol Chem* **273**:19419, 1998.

149. Keating K, Sanguinetti MC: Long QT syndrome. Chap. 203 in this text.

150. Schroeder BC, Kubisch C, Stein V, Jentsch TJ: Moderate loss of function of cyclic-AMP-modulated KCNQ2/KCNQ3 K+ channels causes epilepsy. *Nature* **396**:687, 1998.

151. Wang H-S, Pan Z, Shi W, Brown BS, Wymore RS, Cohen IS, Dixon JE, et al.: KCNQ2 and KCNQ3 potassium channel subunits: Molecular correlates of the M-channel. *Science* **282**:1890, 1998.

152. Hamilton SE, Loose MD, Qi M, Levey AI, Hille B, McKnight GS, Idzerda RL, et al.: Disruption of the m1 receptor gene ablates muscarinic receptor-dependent M current regulation and seizure activity in mice. *Proc Natl Acad Sci U S A* **94**:13311, 1997.

153. Noebels JL, Prince DA: Development of focal seizures in cerebral cortex: Role of axon terminal bursting. *J Neurophysiol* **41**:1267, 1978.

154. Zhang CL, Messing A, Chiu SY: Specific alteration of spontaneous GABAergic inhibition in cerebellar Purkinje cells in mice lacking the potassium channel Kv1.1. *J Neurosci* **19**:2852, 1999.

155. Patil N, Cox DR, Bhat D, Faham M, Myers RM: A potassium channel mutation in weaver mice implicates membrane excitability in granule cell differentiation. *Nat Genet* **11**:126, 1995.

156. Peterson AS, Liao YJ, Jan YN, Jan LY: Heteromultimerization of G-protein-gated inwardly rectifying K⁺ channel proteins GIRK1 and GIRK2 and their altered expression in weaver brain. *J Neurosci* **16**:7137, 1996.

157. Slesinger PA, Stoffel M, Jan YN, Jan LY: Defective gamma-aminobutyric acid type B receptor-activated inwardly rectifying K⁺ currents in cerebellar granule cells isolated from weaver and Girk2 null mutant mice. *Proc Natl Acad Sci U S A* **94**:12210, 1997.

158. Jarolimek W, Baurle J, Misgeld U: Pore mutation in a G-protein-gated inwardly rectifying K⁺ channel subunit causes loss of K⁺-dependent inhibition in weaver hippocampus. *J Neurosci* **18**:4001, 1998.

159. Signorini S, Liao YJ, Duncan SA, Jan LY, Stoffel M: Normal cerebellar development but susceptibility to seizures in mice lacking G protein-coupled, inwardly rectifying K⁺ channel GIRK2. *Proc Natl Acad Sci U S A* **94**:923-7, 1997.

160. Jensen P, Surmeier DJ, Goldowitz D: Rescue of cerebellar granule cells from death in weaver NR1 double mutants. *J Neurosci* **19**:7991, 1999.

161. Noebels JL: Analysis of inherited epilepsy using single locus mutations in mice. *Fed Proc* **38**:2405, 1979.

162. Fletcher CF, Lutz CM, O'Sullivan TN, Shaughnessy JD Jr, Hawkes R, Frankel WN, Copeland NG, et al.: Absence epilepsy in tottering mutant mice is associated with calcium channel defects. *Cell* **87**:607, 1996.

163. Burgess DL, Jones JM, Meisler MH, Noebels JL: Mutation of the $Ca^{2+}$ channel beta subunit gene Cchb4 is associated with ataxia and seizures in the lethargic (lh) mouse. *Cell* **88**:385, 1997.

164. Burgess DL, Biddlecome GH, McDonough SI, Diaz, ME, Zilinski CA, Bean BP, Campbell KP, et al.: Subunit reshuffling modifies N- and P/Q-type $Ca^{2+}$ channel subunit compositions in lethargic mouse brain. *Mol Cell Neurosci* **13**:293, 1999.

165. Letts VA, Felix R, Biddlecome GH, Arikkath J, Mahaffey CL, Valenzuela A, Bartlett FS 2d, et al.: The mouse stargazer gene encodes a neuronal $Ca^{2+}$-channel gamma subunit. *Nat Genet* **19**:340, 1998.

166. Barclay J, Rees, M: Mouse models of spike-wave epilepsy. *Epilepsia* **40**(Suppl 3):17, 1999.

167. Burgess DL, Noebels JL: Voltage-dependent calcium channel mutations in neurological disease. *Ann N Y Acad Sci* **868**:199, 1999.

168. Ophoff RA, Terwindt GM, Vergouwe MN, van Eijk R, Oefner PJ, Hoffman SM, Lamerdin JE, et al.: Familial hemiplegic migraine and episodic ataxia type-2 are caused by mutations in the $Ca^{2+}$ channel gene CACNL1A4. *Cell* **87**:543, 1996.

169. Yue Q, Jen JC, Thwe MM, Nelson SF, Baloh RW: *De novo* mutation in CACNA1A caused acetazolamide-responsive episodic ataxia. *Am J Med Genet* **77**:298, 1998.

170. Terwindt GM, Ophoff RA, Lindhout D, Haan J, Halley DJ, Sandkuijl LA, Brouwer OF, et al.: Partial cosegregation of familial hemiplegic migraine and a benign familial infantile epileptic syndrome. *Epilepsia* **38**:915, 1997.

171. Cox GA, Lutz CM, Yang CL, Biemesderfer D, Bronson RT, Fu A, Aronson PS, et al.: Sodium/hydrogen exchanger gene defect in slow-wave epilepsy mutant mice. *Cell* **91**:139, 1997.

172. Kantheti P, Qiao X, Diaz ME, Peden AA, Meyer GE, Carskadon SL, Kapfhamer D, et al.: Mutation in AP-3 delta in the mocha mouse links endosomal transport to storage deficiency in platelets, melanosomes, and synaptic vesicles. *Neuron* **21**:111, 1998.

173. Steinlein OK, Mulley JC, Propping P, Wallace RH, Phillips HA, Sutherland GR, Scheffer IE, et al.: A missense mutation in the neuronal nicotinic acetylcholine receptor alpha 4 subunit is associated with autosomal dominant nocturnal frontal lobe epilepsy. *Nat Genet* **11**:201, 1995.

174. Phillips HA, Scheffer IE, Crossland KM, Bhatia KP, Fish DR, Marsden CD, Howell SJ, et al.: Autosomal dominant nocturnal frontal-lobe epilepsy: Genetic heterogeneity and evidence for a second locus at 15q24. *Am J Hum Genet* **63**:1101, 1998.

175. Hirose S, Iwata H, Akiyoshi H, Kobayashi K, Ito M, Wada K, Kaneko S, et al.: A novel mutation of CHRNA4 responsible for autosomal dominant nocturnal frontal lobe epilepsy. *Neurology* **53**:1749, 1999.

176. Oldani A, Zucconi M, Asselta R, Modugno M, Bonati MT, Dalpra L, Malcovati M, et al.: Autosomal dominant nocturnal frontal lobe epilepsy. A video-polysomnographic and genetic appraisal of 40 patients and delineation of the epileptic syndrome. *Brain* **121**:205, 1998.

177. Hayman M, Scheffer IE, Chinvarun Y, Berlangieri SU, Berkovic SF: Autosomal dominant nocturnal frontal lobe epilepsy: Demonstration of focal frontal onset and intrafamilial variation. *Neurology* **49**:969, 1997.

178. Nakayama H, Shioda S, Okuda H, Nakashima T, Nakai Y: Immunocytochemical localization of nicotinic acetylcholine receptor in rat cerebral cortex. *Mol Brain Res* **32**:321, 1995.

179. Weiland S, Witzemann V, Villarroel A, Propping P, Steinlein O: An amino acid exchange in the second transmembrane segment of a neuronal nicotinic receptor causes partial epilepsy by altering its desensitization kinetics. *FEBS Lett* **398**:91, 1996.

180. Bertrand S, Weiland S, Berkovic SF, Steinlein OK, Bertrand D: Properties of neuronal nicotinic acetylcholine receptor mutants from humans suffering from autosomal dominant nocturnal frontal lobe epilepsy. *Br J Pharmacol* **125**:751, 1998.

181. Kuryatov A, Gerzanich V, Nelson M, Olale F, Lindstrom J: Mutation causing autosomal dominant nocturnal frontal lobe epilepsy alters $Ca^{2+}$ permeability, conductance, and gating of human alpha4beta2 nicotinic acetylcholine receptors. *J Neurosci* **17**:9035, 1997.

182. Xiang Z, Huguenard JR, Prince DA: Cholinergic switching within neocortical inhibitory networks. *Science* **281**:985, 1998.

183. Condie BG, Bain G, Gottlieb DI, Capecchi MR: Cleft palate in mice with a targeted mutation in the gamma-aminobutyric acid-producing enzyme glutamic acid decarboxylase 67. *Proc Natl Acad Sci U S A* **94**:11451, 1997.

184. Kash SF, Johnson RS, Tecott LH, Noebels JL, Mayfield RD, Hanahan D, Baekkeskov S: Epilepsy in mice deficient in the 65-kDa isoform of glutamic acid decarboxylase. *Proc Natl Acad Sci U S A* **94**:14060, 1997.

185. Hensch TK, Fagiolini M, Mataga N, Stryker MP, Baekkeskov S, Kash SF: Local GABA circuit control of experience-dependent plasticity in developing visual cortex. *Science* **282**:1504, 1998.

186. Erickson JC, Clegg KE, Palmiter RD: Sensitivity to leptin and susceptibility to seizures of mice lacking neuropeptide Y. *Nature* **381**:415, 1996.

187. Baraban SC, Hollopeter G, Erickson JC, Schwartzkroin PA, Palmiter RD: Knock-out mice reveal a critical antiepileptic role for neuropeptide Y. *J Neurosci* **17**:8927, 1997.

188. Culiat CT, Stubbs LJ, Montgomery CS, Russell LB, Rinchik EM: Phenotypic consequences of deletion of the gamma 3, alpha 5, or beta 3 subunit of the type A gamma-aminobutyric acid receptor in mice. *Proc Natl Acad Sci U S A* **91**:2815, 1994.

189. Homanics GE, DeLorey TM, Firestone LL, Quinlan JJ, Handforth A, Harrison NL, Krasowski MD, et al.: Mice devoid of gamma-aminobutyrate type A receptor beta3 subunit have epilepsy, cleft palate, and hypersensitive behavior. *Proc Natl Acad Sci U S A* **94**:4143, 1997.

190. DeLorey TM, Handforth A, Anagnostaras SG, Homanics GE, Minassian BA, Asatourian A, Fanselow MS, et al.: Mice lacking the beta3 subunit of the GABAA receptor have the epilepsy phenotype and many of the behavioral characteristics of Angelman syndrome. *J Neurosci* **18**:8505, 1998.

191. Feldmeyer D, Kask K, Brusa R, Kornau HC, Kolhekar R, Rozov A, Burnashev N, et al.: Neurological dysfunctions in mice expressing different levels of the Q/R site-unedited AMPAR subunit GluR-B. *Nat Neurosci* **2**:57, 1999.

192. Tanaka K, Watase K, Manabe T, Yamada K, Watanabe M, Takahashi K, Iwama H, et al.: Epilepsy and exacerbation of brain injury in mice lacking the glutamate transporter GLT-1. *Science* **276**:1699, 1997.

193. Peghini P, Janzen J, Stoffel W: Glutamate transporter EAAC-1-deficient mice develop dicarboxylic aminoaciduria and behavioral abnormalities but no neurodegeneration. *EMBO J* **16**:3822, 1997.

194. Brown P, Day BL, Rothwell JC, Thompson PD, Marsden CD: Intrahemispheric and interhemispheric spread of cerebral cortical myoclonic activity and its relevance to epilepsy. *Brain* **114**:2333, 1991.

195. Pennacchio LA, Lehesjoki AE, Stone NE, Willour VL, Virtaneva K, Miao J, D'Amato E, et al.: Mutations in the gene encoding cystatin B in progressive myoclonus epilepsy. *Science* **271**:1731, 1996.

196. Virtaneva K, D'Amato E, Miao J, Koskiniemi M, Norio R, Avanzini G, Franceschetti S, et al.: Unstable minisatellite expansion causing recessively inherited myoclonus epilepsy, EPM1. *Nat Genet* **5**:393, 1997.

197. Mitchison HM, Hofmann SL, Becerra CH, Munroe PB, Lake BD, Crow YJ, Stephenson JB, et al.: Mutations in the palmitoyl-protein thioesterase gene (PPT; CLN1) causing juvenile neuronal ceroid lipofuscinosis with granular osmiophilic deposits. *Hum Mol Genet* **7**:291, 1998.

198. Liu CG, Sleat DE, Donnelly RJ, Lobel P: Structural organization and sequence of CLN2, the defective gene in classical late infantile neuronal ceroid lipofuscinosis. *Genomics* **50**:206, 1998.

199. Zhong N, Wisniewski KE, Hartikainen J, Ju W, Moroziewicz DN, McLendon L, Brooks SS, et al.: Two common mutations in the CLN2 gene underlie late infantile neuronal ceroid lipofuscinosis. *Clin Genet* **54**:234, 1998.

200. The International Batten Disease Consortium: Isolation of a novel gene underlying Batten disease, CLN3. *Cell* **82**:949, 1995.

201. Savukoski M, Klockars T, Holmberg V, Santavuori P, Lander ES, Peltonen L: CLN5, a novel gene encoding a putative transmembrane protein mutated in Finnish variant late infantile neuronal ceroid lipofuscinosis. *Nat Genet* **19**:286, 1998.

202. Ranta S, Zhang Y, Ross B, Lonka L, Takkunen E, Messer A, Sharp J, et al.: The neuronal ceroid lipofuscinoses in human EPMR and mnd mutant mice are associated with mutations in CLN8. *Nat Genet* **23**:233, 1999.

203. Wigderson M, Firon N, Horowitz Z, Wilder S, Frishberg Y, Reiner O, Horowitz M: Characterization of mutations in Gaucher patients by cDNA cloning. *Am J Hum Genet* **44**:365, 1989.

204. Pshezhetsky AV, Richard C, Michaud L, Igdoura S, Wang S, Elsliger MA, Qu J, et al.: Cloning, expression and chromosomal mapping of human lysosomal sialidase and characterization of mutations in sialidosis. *Nat Genet* **15**:316, 1997.

205. Mueller OT, Henry WM, Haley LL, Byers MG, Eddy RL, Shows TB: Sialidosis and galactosialidosis: Chromosomal assignment of two genes associated with neuraminidase-deficiency disorders. *Proc Natl Acad Sci U S A* **83**:1817, 1986.

206. Minassian BA, Lee JR, Herbrick JA, Huizenga J, Soder S, Mungall AJ, Dunham I, et al.: Mutations in a gene encoding a novel protein tyrosine phosphatase cause progressive myoclonus epilepsy. *Nat Genet* **20**:171, 1998.
207. Graeber MB, Muller U: Recent developments in the molecular genetics of mitochondrial disorders. *J Neurol Sci* **153**:251, 1998.
208. Tiranti V, D'Agruma L, Pareyson D, Mora M, Carrara F, Zelante L, Gasparini P, et al.: A novel mutation in the mitochondrial tRNA(Val) gene associated with a complex neurological presentation. *Ann Neurol* **43**:98, 1998.
209. Cock H, Shapira AHV: Mitochondrial DNA mutations and mitochondrial dysfunction in epilepsy. *Epilepsia* **40(Suppl 3)**:33, 1999.
210. Serra G, Piccinnu R, Tondi M, Muntoni F, Zeviani M, Mastropaolo C: Clinical and EEG findings in eleven patients affected by mitochondrial encephalomyopathy with MERRF-MELAS overlap. *Brain Dev* **18**:185, 1996.
211. Tulinius MH, Hagne I: EEG findings in children and adolescents with mitochondrial encephalomyopathies: A study of 25 cases. *Brain Dev* **13**:167, 1991.
212. Watanabe Y, Hashikawa K, Moriwaki H, Oku N, Seike Y, Kodaka R, Ono J, et al.: SPECT findings in mitochondrial encephalomyopathy. *J Nucl Med* **39**:961, 1998.
213. Masucci JP, Schon EA, King MP: Point mutations in the mitochondrial tRNA(Lys) gene: Implications for pathogenesis and mechanism. *Mol Cell Biochem* **174**:215, 1997.
214. Schon EA, Bonilla E, DiMauro S: Mitochondrial DNA mutations and pathogenesis. *J Bioenerg Biomembr* **29**:131, 1997.
215. Wallace DC, Lott MT, Shoffner JM, Ballinger S: Mitochondrial DNA mutations in epilepsy and neurological disease. *Epilepsia* **35(Suppl 1)**:S43, 1994.
216. Chinnery PF, Howell N, Lightowlers RN, Turnbull DM: Molecular pathology of MELAS and MERRF. The relationship between mutation load and clinical phenotypes. *Brain* **120**:1713, 1997.
217. Sparaco M, Schon EA, DiMauro S, Bonilla E: Myoclonic epilepsy with ragged-red fibers (MERRF): An immunohistochemical study of the brain. *Brain Pathol* **5**:125, 1995.
218. Zhou L, Chomyn A, Attardi G, Miller CA: Myoclonic epilepsy and ragged red fibers (MERRF) syndrome: Selective vulnerability of CNS neurons does not correlate with the level of mitochondrial tRNAlys mutation in individual neuronal isolates. *J Neurosci* **17**:7746, 1997.
219. Mole SE: Recent advances in the molecular genetics of the neuronal ceroid lipofuscinoses. *J Inherit Metab Dis* **19**:269, 1996.
220. Goebel HH, Sharp JD: The neuronal ceroid-lipofuscinoses. Recent advances. *Brain Pathol* **8**:151, 1998.
221. Tyynela J, Suopanki J, Santavuori P, Baumann M, Haltia M: Variant late infantile neuronal ceroid-lipofuscinosis: Pathology and biochemistry. *J Neuropathol Exp Neurol* **56**:369, 1997.
222. Liewendahl K, Vanhanen SL, Heiskala H, Raininko R, Nikkinen P, Launes J, Santavuori P: Brain perfusion SPECT abnormalities in neuronal ceroid lipofuscinoses. *Neuropediatrics* **28**:71, 1997.
223. Jarvela I, Autti T, Lamminranta S, Aberg L, Raininko R, Santavuori P: Clinical and magnetic resonance imaging findings in Batten disease: analysis of the major mutation (1.02-kb deletion). *Ann Neurol* **42**:799, 1997.
224. Cox GA, Mahaffey CL, Frankel WN: Identification of the mouse neuromuscular degeneration gene and mapping of a second site suppressor allele. *Neuron* **21**:1327, 1998.
225. Bronson RT, Donahue LR, Johnson KR, Tanner A, Lane PW, Faust JR: Neuronal ceroid lipofuscinosis (nclf), a new disorder of the mouse linked to chromosome 9. *Am J Med Genet* **77**:289, 1998.
226. Sharp JD, Wheeler RB, Lake BD, Savukoski M, Jarvela IE, Peltonen L, Gardiner RM, et al.: Loci for classical and a variant late infantile neuronal ceroid lipofuscinosis map to chromosomes 11p15 and 15q21-23. *Hum Mol Genet* **6**:591, 1997.
227. Pshezhetsky AV, Richard C, Michaud L, Igdoura S, Wang S, Elsliger MA, Qu J, et al.: Cloning, expression and chromosomal mapping of human lysosomal sialidase and characterization of mutations in sialidosis. *Nat Genet* **15**:316, 1997.
228. Okamura-Oho Y, Zhang S, Callahan JW: The biochemistry and clinical features of galactosialidosis. *Biochim Biophys Acta* **1225**:244, 1994.
229. Tobimatsu S, Fukui R, Shibasaki H, Kato M, Kuroiwa Y: Electro-physiological studies of myoclonus in sialidosis type 2. *Electroencephalogr Clin Neurophysiol* **60**:16, 1985.
230. Rapin I: Myoclonus in neuronal storage and Lafora diseases. *Adv Neurol* **43**:65, 1986.
231. Rottier RJ, Bonten E, d'Azzo A: A point mutation in the neu-1 locus causes the neuraminidase defect in the SM/J mouse. *Hum Mol Genet* **7**:313, 1998.
232. Onodera O, Oyake M, Takano H, Ikeuchi T, Igarashi S, Tsuji S: Molecular cloning of a full-length cDNA for dentatorubral-pallidoluysian atrophy and regional expressions of the expanded alleles in the CNS. *Am J Hum Genet* **57**:1050, 1995.
233. Koide R, Ikeuchi T, Onodera O, Tanaka H, Igarashi S, Endo K, Takahashi H, et al.: Unstable expansion of CAG repeat in hereditary dentatorubral-pallidoluysian atrophy (DRPLA). *Nat Genet* **6**:9, 1994.
234. Kurohara K, Kuroda Y, Maruyama H, Kawakami H, Yukitake M, Matsui M, Nakamura S: Homozygosity for an allele carrying intermediate CAG repeats in the dentatorubral-pallidoluysian atrophy (DRPLA) gene results in spastic paraplegia. *Neurology* **48**:1087, 1997.
235. Yazawa I, Nukina N, Hashida H, Goto J, Yamada M, Kanazawa I: Abnormal gene product identified in hereditary dentatorubral-pallidoluysian atrophy (DRPLA) brain. *Nat Genet* **10**:99, 1995.
236. Schmitt I, Epplen JT, Riess O: Predominant neuronal expression of the gene responsible for dentatorubral-pallidoluysian atrophy (DRPLA) in rat. *Hum Mol Genet* **4**:1619, 1995.
237. Yazawa I, Nakase H, Kurisaki H: Abnormal dentatorubral-pallidoluysian atrophy (DRPLA) protein complex is pathologically ubiquitinated in DRPLA brains. *Biochem Biophys Res Commun* **260**:133, 1999.
238. Kanazawa I: Molecular pathology of dentatorubral-pallidoluysian atrophy. *Philos Trans R Soc Lond B Biol Sci* **354**:1069, 1999.
239. Sato T, Oyake M, Nakamura K, Nakao K, Fukusima Y, Onodera O, Igarashi S, et al.: Transgenic mice harboring a full-length human mutant DRPLA gene exhibit age-dependent intergenerational and somatic instabilities of CAG repeats comparable with those in DRPLA patients. *Hum Mol Genet* **8**:99, 1999.
240. Inazuki G, Baba K, Naito H: Electroencephalographic findings of hereditary dentatorubral-pallidoluysian atrophy (DRPLA). *Jpn J Psychiatry Neurol* **43**:213, 1989.
241. Hattori H, Higuchi Y, Okuno T, Asato R, Fukumoto M, Kondo I: Early-childhood progressive myoclonus epilepsy presenting as partial seizures in dentatorubral-pallidoluysian atrophy. *Epilepsia* **38**:271, 1997.
242. Saitoh S, Momoi MY, Yamagata T, Miyao M, Suwa K: Clinical and electroencephalographic findings in juvenile type DRPLA. *Pediatr Neurol* **18**:265, 1998.
243. Miyazaki M, Hashimoto T, Nakagawa R, Yoneda Y, Tayama M, Kawano N, Murayama N, et al.: Characteristic evoked potentials in childhood-onset dentatorubral-pallidoluysian atrophy. *Brain Dev* **18**:389, 1996.
244. Kasai K, Onuma T, Kato M, Kato T, Takeya J, Sekimoto M, Watanabe K, et al.: Differences in evoked potential characteristics between DRPLA patients and patients with progressive myoclonic epilepsy: Preliminary findings indicating usefulness for differential diagnosis. *Epilepsy Res* **37**:3, 1999.
245. Kuwano A, Takakubo F, Morimoto Y, Uyama E, Uchino M, Ando M, Yasuda T, et al.: Benign adult familial myoclonus epilepsy (BAFME): An autosomal dominant form not linked to the dentatorubral pallidoluysian atrophy (DRPLA) gene. *J Med Genet* **33**:80, 1996.
246. Minassian BA, Sainz J, Delgado-Escueta AV: Genetics of myoclonic and myoclonus epilepsies. *Clin Neurosci* **3**:223, 1995-96.
247. Koskiniemi M, Donner M, Majuri H, Haltia M, Norio R: Progressive myoclonus epilepsy: A clinical and histopathological study. *Acta Neurol Scand* **50**:307, 1974.
248. Koskiniemi M, Toivakka E, Donner M: Progressive myoclonus epilepsy: Electroencephalographic findings. *Acta Neurol Scand* **50**:333, 1974.
249. Haltia M, Kristensson K, Sourander P: Neuropathological studies in three Scandinavian cases of progressive myoclonus epilepsy. *Acta Neurol Scand* **45**:63, 1969.
250. Ferro FM, Mazza S, D'Angelo C: Neuropathological study of a case of progressive familiar myoclonic epilepsy. *Riv Patol Nerv Ment* **96**:127, 1975.
251. Lafreniere RG, Rochefort DL, Chretien N, Rommens JM, Cochius JI, Kalviainen R, Nousiainen U, et al.: Unstable insertion in the 5' flanking region of the cystatin B gene is the most common mutation in progressive myoclonus epilepsy type 1, EPM1. *Nat Genet* **15**:298, 1997.
252. Virtaneva K, D'Amato E, Miao J, Koskiniemi M, Norio R, Avanzini G, Franceschetti S, et al.: Unstable minisatellite expansion causing recessively inherited myoclonus epilepsy, EPM1. *Nat Genet* **15**:393, 1997.

253. Lalioti MD, Scott HS, Buresi C, Rossier C, Bottani A, Morris MA, Malafosse A, et al.: Dodecamer repeat expansion in cystatin B gene in progressive myoclonus epilepsy. *Nature* **386**:847, 1997.

254. Lalioti MD, Scott HS, Genton P, Grid D, Ouazzani R, M'Rabet A, Ibrahim S, et al.: A PCR amplification method reveals instability of the dodecamer repeat in progressive myoclonus epilepsy (EPM1) and no correlation between the size of the repeat and age at onset. *Am J Hum Genet* **62**:842, 1998.

255. Lalioti MD, Scott HS, Antonarakis SE: Altered spacing of promoter elements due to the dodecamer repeat expansion contributes to reduced expression of the cystatin B gene in EPM1. *Hum Mol Genet* **8**:1791, 1999.

256. Turk V, Bode W: The cystatins: Protein inhibitors of cysteine proteinases. *FEBS Lett* **285**:213, 1991.

257. Bohley P, Seglen PO: Proteases and proteolysis in the lysosome. *Experientia* **48**:151, 1992.

258. Karhu J, Hari R, Paetau R, Kajola M, Mervaala E: Cortical reactivity in progressive myoclonus epilepsy. *Electroencephalogr Clin Neurophysiol* **90**:93, 1994.

259. Pennacchio LA, Bouley DM, Higgins KM, Scott MP, Noebels JL, Myers RM: Progressive ataxia, myoclonic epilepsy and cerebellar apoptosis in cystatin B-deficient mice. *Nat Genet* **20**:251, 1998.

260. Footitt DR, Quinn N, Kocen RS, Oz B, Scaravilli F: Familial Lafora body disease of late onset: report of four cases in one family and a review of the literature. *J Neurol* **244**:40, 1997.

261. Kaufman MA, Dwork AJ, Willson NJ, John S, Liu JD: Late-onset Lafora's disease with typical intraneuronal inclusions. *Neurology* **43**:1246, 1993.

262. Minassian BA, Lee JR, Herbrick JA, Huizenga J, Soder S, Mungall AJ, Dunham I, et al.: Mutations in a gene encoding a novel protein tyrosine phosphatase cause progressive myoclonus epilepsy. *Nat Genet* **20**:171, 1998.

263. Serratosa JM, Gomez-Garre P, Gallardo ME, Anta B, Beltan-Valero de Bernabe D, Lindhout D, Augustijn PB: A novel protein tyrosine phosphatase gene is mutated in progressive myoclonus epilepsy of the Lafora type (EPM2). *Hum Mol Genet* **8**:345,1999.

264. Acharya, Orizaola P, Calleja J: Progressive study of EEG and evoked potentials in Lafora disease. *Rev Neurol* **27**:81, 1998.

265. Ponsford S, Pye IF, Elliot EJ: Posterior paroxysmal discharge: An aid to early diagnosis in Lafora disease. *J R Soc Med* **86**:597, 1993.

266. Yen C, Beydoun A, Drury I: Longitudinal EEG studies in a kindred with Lafora disease. *Epilepsia* **32**:895, 1991.

267. Tsuda H, Katsumi Y, Nakamura M, Ikeda A, Fukuyama H, Kimura J, Shibasaki H: Cerebral blood flow and metabolism in Lafora disease. *Rinsho Shinkeigaku* **35**:175, 1995.

268. Williams CA, Zori RT, Hendrickson J, Stalker H, Marum T, Whidden E, Driscoll DJ, et al.: Angelman syndrome. *Curr Probl Pediatr* **25**:216, 1995.

269. Matsuura T, Sutcliffe JS, Fang P, Galjaard RJ, Jiang YH, Benton CS, Rommens JM, et al.: *De novo* truncating mutations in E6-AP ubiquitin-protein ligase gene (UBE3A) in Angelman syndrome. *Nat Genet* **15**:74,199.7

270. Kishino T, Lalande M, Wagstaff J: UBE3A/E6-AP mutations cause Angelman syndrome. *Nat Genet* **15**:70, 1997.

271. Minassian BA, DeLorey TM, Olsen RW, Philippart M, Bronstein Y, Zhang Q, Guerrini R, et al.: Angelman syndrome: Correlations between epilepsy phenotypes and genotypes. *Ann Neurol* **43**:485, 1998.

272. Laan LA, Halley DJ, den Boer AT, Hennekam RC, Renier WO, Brouwer OF: Angelman syndrome without detectable chromosome 15q11-13 anomaly: Clinical study of familial and isolated cases. *Am J Med Genet* **76**:262, 1998.

273. van den Ouweland AM, Bakker PL, Halley DJ, Catsman-Berrevoets CE: Angelman syndrome: AS phenotype correlated with specific EEG pattern may result in a high detection rate of mutations in the UBE3A gene. *J Med Genet* **36**:723, 1999.

274. Buoni S, Grosso S, Pucci L, Fois A: Diagnosis of Angelman syndrome: Clinical and EEG criteria. *Brain Dev* **21**:296, 1999.

275. Albrecht U, Sutcliffe JS, Cattanach BM, Beechey CV, Armstrong D, Eichele G, Beaudet AL: Imprinted expression of the murine Angelman syndrome gene, Ube3a, in hippocampal and Purkinje neurons. *Nat Genet* **17**:75, 1997.

276. Jiang YH, Armstrong D, Albrecht U, Atkins CM, Noebels JL, Eichele G, Sweatt JD et al.: Mutation of the Angelman ubiquitin ligase in mice causes increased cytoplasmic p53 and deficits of contextual learning and long-term potentiation. *Neuron* **21**:799, 1998.

277. Sakhi S, Sun N, Wing LL, Mehta P, Schreiber SS: Nuclear accumulation of p53 protein following kainic acid-induced seizures. *Neuroreport* **31**:493, 1996.

278. Shaffer LG, Ledbetter DH, Lupski JR: Chap. 65, this volume.

279. Odano I, Anezaki T, Ohkubo M, Yonekura Y, Onishi Y, Inuzuka T, Takahashi M, et al.: Decrease in benzodiazepine receptor binding in a patient with Angelman syndrome detected by iodine-123 iomazenil and single-photon emission tomography. *Eur J Nucl Med* **23**:598, 1996.

280. Cattanach B, Barr JA, Beechey CV, Martin J, Noebels J, Jones J: A candidate model for Angelman syndrome in the mouse. *Mamm Genome* **8**:472, 1997.

281. Fox NC, Kennedy AM, Harvey RJ, Lantos PL, Roques PK, Collinge J, Hardy J, et al.: Clinicopathological features of familial Alzheimer's disease associated with the M139V mutation in the presenilin 1 gene. Pedigree but not mutation specific age at onset provides evidence for a further genetic factor. *Brain* **120**:491, 1997.

282. Petersen RB, Goren H, Cohen M, Richardson SL, Tresser N, Lynn A, Gali M, et al.: Transthyretin amyloidosis: A new mutation associated with dementia. *Ann Neurol* **41**:307, 1997.

283. Kim E, Lowenson JD, MacLaren DC, Clarke S, Young SG: Deficiency of a protein-repair enzyme results in the accumulation of altered proteins, retardation of growth, and fatal seizures in mice. *Proc Natl Acad Sci U S A* **94**:6132, 1997.

284. Yamamoto A, Takagi H, Kitamura D, Tatsuoka H, Nakano H, Kawano H, Kuroyanagi H, et al.: Deficiency in protein L-isoaspartyl methyltransferase results in a fatal progressive epilepsy. *J Neurosci* **18**:2063, 1998.

285. Seidner G, Alvarez MG, Yeh J-I, O'Driscoll KR, Klepper J, Stump TS, Wang D, et al.: GLUT-1 deficiency syndrome caused by haploinsufficiency of the blood-brain barrier hexose carrier. *Nat Genet* **18**:188, 1998.

286. Boles RG, Seashore MR, Mitchell WG, Kollros PR, Mofidi S, Novotny EJ: Glucose transporter type 1 deficiency: A study of two cases with video-EEG. *Eur J Pediatr* **158**:978, 1999.

287. Shen J, Bao Y, Chen YT: A nonsense mutation due to a single base insertion in the 3'-coding region of glycogen debranching enzyme gene associated with a severe phenotype in a patient with glycogen storage disease type IIIa. *Hum Mutat* **9**:37, 1997.

288. Kure S, Mandel H, Rolland MO, Sakata Y, Shinka T, Drugan A, Boneh A, et al.: A missense mutation (His42Arg) in the T-protein gene from a large Israeli-Arab kindred with nonketotic hyperglycinemia. *Hum Genet* **102**:430, 1998.

289. Hagberg B, Aicardi J, Dias K, Ramos O: A progressive syndrome of autism, dementia, ataxia, and loss of purposeful hand use in girls: Rett's syndrome: Report of 35 cases. *Ann Neurol* **14**:471, 1983.

290. von Tetzchner S, Jacobsen KH, Smith L, Skjeldal OH, Heiberg A, Fagan JF: Vision, cognition and developmental characteristics of girls and women with Rett syndrome. *Dev Med Child Neurol* **38**:212, 1996.

291. Belichenko PV, Hagberg B, Dahlstrom: A Morphological study of neocortical areas in Rett syndrome. *Acta Neuropathol (Berl)* **93**:50, 1997.

292. Amir RE, Van den Veyver MW, Tran CQ, Francke U, Zoghbi H: Rett syndrome is caused by mutations in X-linked MECP2, encoding methyl-CpG-binding protein 2. *Nat Genet* **23**:185, 1999.

293. Zoghbi HY: Rett syndrome. Chap. 255 this text.

294. Hendrich B, Bird A: Identification and characterization of a family of mammalian methyl-CpG binding proteins. *Mol Cell Biol* **18**:6538, 1998.

295. Zappella M: The preserved speech variant of the Rett complex: a report of 8 cases. *Eur Child Adolesc Psychiatry* **6(Suppl 1)**:23, 1997.

296. Gustavsson P, Kimber E, Wahlstrom J, Anneren G: Monosomy 18q syndrome and atypical Rett syndrome in a girl with an interstitial deletion (18)(q21.1q22.3). *Am J Med Genet* **82**:348, 1999.

297. Nieto-Barrera M, Nieto-Jimenez M, Diaz F, Campana C, Sanchez ML, Ruiz del Portal L, Siljestrom ML: Clinical course of epileptic seizures in Rett's syndrome. *Rev Neurol* **28**:449, 1999.

298. Laan LA, Brouwer OF, Begeer CH, Zwinderman AH, Gert van Dijk J: The diagnostic value of the EEG in Angelman and Rett syndrome at a young age. *Electroencephalogr Clin Neurophysiol* **106**:404, 1998.

299. Niedermeyer E, Naidu SB, Plate C: Unusual EEG theta rhythms over central region in Rett syndrome: Considerations of the underlying dysfunction. *Clin Electroencephalogr* **28**:36, 1997.

300. Aldrich MS, Garofalo EA, Drury I: Epileptiform abnormalities during sleep in Rett syndrome. *Electroencephalogr Clin Neurophysiol* **75**:365, 1990.

301. Yamanouchi H, Kaga M, Arima M: Abnormal cortical excitability in Rett syndrome. *Pediatr Neurol* 9:202, 1993.

302. Yoshikawa H, Kaga M, Suzuki H, Sakuragawa N, Arima M: Giant somatosensory evoked potentials in the Rett syndrome. *Brain Dev* 13:36, 1991.

303. Lappalainen R, Liewendahl K, Sainio K, Nikkinen P, Riikonen RS: Brain perfusion SPECT and EEG findings in Rett syndrome. *Acta Neurol Scand* 95:44, 1997.

304. Marseille Consensus Group: Classification of progressive myoclonus epilepsies, and related disorders. *Ann Neurol* 28:113, 1990.

305. Rees MI, Andrew M, Jawad S, Owen MJ: Evidence for recessive as well as dominant forms of startle disease (hyperekplexia) caused by mutations in the alpha 1 subunit of the inhibitory glycine receptor. *Hum Mol Genet* 3:2175, 1994.

306. Shiang R, Ryan SG, Zhu YZ, Hahn AF, O'Connell P, Wasmuth JJ: Mutations in the alpha 1 subunit of the inhibitory glycine receptor cause the dominant neurologic disorder, hyperekplexia. *Nat Genet* 5:351, 1993.

307. Vergouwe MN, Tijssen MA, Shiang R, van Dijk JG, al Shahwan S, Ophoff RA, Frants RR: Hyperekplexia-like syndromes without mutations in the GLRA1 gene. *Clin Neurol Neurosurg* 99:172, 1997.

308. Rajendra S, Lynch JW, Pierce KD, French CR, Barry PH, Schofield PR: Startle disease mutations reduce the agonist sensitivity of the human inhibitory glycine receptor. *J Biol Chem* 269:18739, 1994.

309. Lewis TM, Sivilotti LG, Colquhoun D, Gardiner RM, Schoepfer R, Rees M: Properties of human glycine receptors containing the hyperekplexia mutation alpha1(K276E), expressed in *Xenopus* oocytes. *J Physiol (Lond)* 507:25, 1998.

310. Bernasconi A, Cendes F, Shoubridge EA, Andermann E, Li LM, Arnold DL, Andermann F: Spectroscopic imaging of frontal neuronal dysfunction in hyperekplexia. *Brain* 121:1507, 1998.

311. Tijssen MA, Voorkamp LM, Padberg GW, van Dijk JG: Startle responses in hereditary hyperekplexia. *Arch Neurol* 54:388, 1997.

312. Ryan SG, Buckwalter MS, Lynch JW, Handford CA, Segura L, Shiang R, Wasmuth JJ, et al.: A missense mutation in the gene encoding the alpha 1 subunit of the inhibitory glycine receptor in the spasmodic mouse. *Nat Genet* 7:131, 1994.

313. Kling C, Koch M, Saul B, Becker CM: The frameshift mutation oscillator (Glra1(spd-ot)) produces a complete loss of glycine receptor alpha1-polypeptide in mouse central nervous system. *Neuroscience* 78:411, 1997.

314. Kingsmore SF, Giros B, Suh D, Bieniarz M, Caron MG, Seldin MF: Glycine receptor beta-subunit gene mutation in spastic mouse associated with LINE-1 element insertion. *Nat Genet* 7:136, 1994.

315. Mulhardt C, Fischer M, Gass P, Simon-Chazottes D, Guenet JL, Kuhse J, Betz H, et al.: The spastic mouse: aberrant splicing of glycine receptor beta subunit mRNA caused by intronic insertion of L1 element. *Neuron* 13:1003, 1994.

316. Simon ES: Phenotypic heterogeneity and disease course in three murine strains with mutations in genes encoding for alpha 1 and beta glycine receptor subunits. *Mov Disord* 12:221, 1997.

317. Brune W, Weber RG, Saul B, von Knebel Doeberitz M, Grond-Ginsbach C, Kellerman K, Meinck HM, et al.: A GLRA1 null mutation in recessive hyperekplexia challenges the functional role of glycine receptors. *Am J Hum Genet* 58:989, 1996.

318. Feng G, Tintrup H, Kirsch J, Nichol MC, Kuhse J, Betz H, Sanes JR: Dual requirement for gephyrin in glycine receptor clustering and molybdoenzyme activity. *Science* 282:1321, 1998.

319. Kneussel M, Brandstatter JH, Laube B, Stahl S, Muller U, Betz H: Loss of postsynaptic GABAA receptor clustering in gephyrin-deficient mice. *J Neurosci* 19:9289, 1999.

320. Shalata A, Mandel H, Reiss J, Szargel R, Cohen-Akenine A, Dorche C, Zabot MT, et al.: Localization of a gene for molybdenum cofactor deficiency, on the short arm of chromosome 6, by homozygosity mapping. *Am J Hum Genet* 63:148, 1998.

321. Ezquerra M, Carnero C, Blesa R, Gelpi JL, Ballesta F, Oliva RA: Presenilin 1 mutation (Ser169Pro) associated with early-onset AD and myoclonic seizures. *Neurology* 52:566, 1999.

322. Shoffner JM, Lott MT, Lezza AM, Seibel P, Ballinger SW, Wallace DC: Myoclonic epilepsy and ragged-red fiber disease (MERRF) is associated with a mitochondrial DNA tRNA(Lys) mutation. *Cell* 61:931, 1990.

323. Vesa J, Hellsten E, Verkruyse LA, Camp LA, Rapola J, Santavuori P, Hofmann SL, et al.: Mutations in the palmitoyl protein thioesterase gene causing infantile neuronal ceroid lipofuscinosis. *Nature* 376:584, 1995.

324. Zhong N, Wisniewski KE, Hartikainen J, Ju W, Moroziewicz DN, McLendon L, Sklower-Brooks SS, et al.: Two common mutations in the CLN2 gene underlie late infantile neuronal ceroid lipofuscinosis. *Clin Genet* 54:234, 1998.

325. International Batten Disease Consortium: Isolation of a novel gene underlying Batten disease, CLN3. *Cell* 82:949, 1995.

326. Vaughn BV, Greenwood RS, Aylsworth AS, Tennison MB: Similarities of EEG and seizures in del(1q) and benign rolandic epilepsy. *Pediatr Neurol* 15:261, 1996.

327. Asamoah A, Nandi KN, Prouty L, Thurmon TF, Chen H: A case of insertional translocation involving chromosomes 2 and 4. *Clin Genet* 53:142, 1998.

328. Zara F, Labuda M, Garofalo PG, Durisotti C, Bianchi A, Castellotti B, Patel PI, et al.: Unusual EEG pattern linked to chromosome 3p in a family with idiopathic generalized epilepsy. *Neurology* 51:493, 1998.

329. Liu AW, Delgado-Escueta AV, Gee MN, Serratosa JM, Zhang QW, Alonso ME, Medina MT, et al.: Juvenile myoclonic epilepsy in chromosome 6p12-p11: locus heterogeneity and recombinations. *Am J Med Genet* 63:438, 1996.

330. Sander T, Bockenkamp B, Hildmann T, Blaszczyk R, Kretz R, Wienker TF, Volz A, et al.: Refined mapping of the epilepsy susceptibility locus EJM1 on chromosome 6. *Neurology* 49:842, 1997.

331. Tsao CY, Westman JA: Infantile spasms in two children with Williams syndrome. *Am J Med Genet* 71:54, 1997.

332. Tahvanainen E, Ranta S, Hirvasniemi A, Karila E, Leisti J, Sistonen P, Weissenbach J, et al.: The gene for a recessively inherited human childhood progressive epilepsy with mental retardation maps to the distal short arm of chromosome 8. *Proc Natl Acad Sci U S A* 91:7267, 1994.

333. Ranta S, Lehesjoki AE, de Fatima Bonaldo M, Knowles JA, Hirvasniemi A, Ross B, de Jong PJ, et al.: High-resolution mapping and transcript identification at the progressive epilepsy with mental retardation locus on chromosome 8p. *Genome Res* 9:887, 1997.

334. Ryan SG, Chance PF, Zou CH, Spinner NB, Golden JA, Smietana S: Epilepsy and mental retardation limited to females: an X-linked dominant disorder with male sparing. *Nat Genet* 17:92, 1997.

335. Ottman R, Risch N, Hauser WA, Pedley TA, Lee JH, Barker-Cummings C, Lustenberger A, et al.: Localization of a gene for partial epilepsy to chromosome 10q. *Nat Genet* 10:56, 1995.

336. Poza JJ, Saenz A, Martinez-Gil A, Cheron N, Cobo AM, Urtasun M, Marti-Masso JF, et al.: Autosomal dominant lateral temporal epilepsy: clinical and genetic study of a large Basque pedigree linked to chromosome 10q. *Ann Neurol* 45:182, 1999.

337. Iannetti P, Spalice A, Mingarelli R, Raucci U, Novelli A, Dallapiccola B: Myoclonic epilepsy, neuroblast migration disorders, and maternally derived partial duplication 14q/deletion 15q. *Ann Genet* 39:26, 1996.

338. Bundey S, Hardy C, Vickers S, Kilpatrick MW, Corbett JA: Duplication of the 15q11-13 region in a patient with autism, epilepsy and ataxia. *Dev Med Child Neurol* 36:736, 1994.

339. Elmslie FV, Rees M, Williamson MP, Kerr M, Kjeldsen MJ, Pang KA, Sundqvist A, et al.: Genetic mapping of a major susceptibility locus for juvenile myoclonic epilepsy on chromosome 15q. *Hum Mol Genet* 6:1329, 1997.

340. Neubauer BA, Fiedler B, Himmelein B, Kampfer F, Lassker U, Schwabe G, Spanier I, et al.: Centrotemporal spikes in families with rolandic epilepsy: Linkage to chromosome 15q14. *Neurology* 51:1608, 1998.

341. Sharp JD, Wheeler RB, Lake BD, Savukoski M, Jarvela IE, Peltonen L, Gardiner RM, et al.: Loci for classical and a variant late infantile neuronal ceroid lipofuscinosis map to chromosomes 11p15 and 15q21-23. *Hum Mol Genet* 6:591, 1997.

342. Phillips HA, Scheffer IE, Crossland KM, Bhatia KP, Fish DR, Marsden CD, Howell SJ, et al.: Autosomal dominant nocturnal frontal-lobe epilepsy: Genetic heterogeneity and evidence for a second locus at 15q24. *Am J Hum Genet* 63:1108, 1998.

343. Szepetowski P, Rochette JB: Familial infantile convulsions and paroxysmal choreoathetosis: A new neurological syndrome linked to the pericentromeric region of human chromosome 16. *Am J Hum Genet* 61:889, 1997.

344. Lee WL, Tay A, Ong HT, Goh LM, Monaco AP, Szepetowski P: Association of infantile convulsions with paroxysmal dyskinesias (ICCA syndrome): Confirmation of linkage to human chromosome 16p12-q12 in a Chinese family. *Hum Genet* 103:608, 1998.

345. Guerrini R, Bonanni P, Nardocci N, Parmeggiani L, Piccirilli M, De Fusco M, Aridon P, et al.: Autosomal recessive rolandic epilepsy with paroxysmal exercise-induced dystonia and writer's cramp: Delineation

of the syndrome and gene mapping to chromosome 16p12-11.2. *Ann Neurol* **45**:344, 1999.

346. Canevini MP, Sgro V, Zuffardi O, Canger R, Carrozzo R, Rossi E, Ledbetter D, et al.: Chromosome 20 ring: A chromosomal disorder associated with a particular electroclinical pattern. *Epilepsia* **39**:942, 1998.

347. Johannsen P, Christensen JE, Goldstein H, Nielsen VK, Mai J: Epilepsy in Down syndrome — Prevalence in three age groups. *Seizure* **5**:121, 1996.

348. Silva ML, Cieuta C, Guerrini R, Plouin P, Livet MO, Dulac O: Early clinical and EEG features of infantile spasms in Down syndrome. *Epilepsia* **37**:977, 1996.

349. Maatsuura T, Achari M, Khajavi M, Bachinski LL, Zoghbi HY, Ashizawa T: Mapping of the gene for a novel spinocerebellar ataxia with pure cerebellar signs and epilepsy. *Ann Neurol* **45**:407, 1999.

350. Xiong L, Labuda M, Li DS, Hudson TJ, Desbiens R, Patry G, Verret S, Langevin P, et al.: Mapping of a gene determining familial partial epilepsy with variable foci to chromosome 22q11-q12. *Am J Hum Genet* **65**:1698, 1999.

351. Stromme P, Sundet K, Mork C, Cassiman JJ, Fryns JP, Claes S: X linked mental retardation and infantile spasms in a family: New clinical data and linkage to Xp11.4-Xp22.11. *J Med Genet* **36**:374, 1999.

352. O'Brien TJ, So EL, Mullan BP, Hauser MF, Brinkmann BH, Bohnen NI, Hanson D, et al.: Subtraction ictal SPECT co-registered to MRI improves clinical usefulness of SPECT in localizing the surgical seizure focus. *Neurology* **50**:445, 1998.

353. Adams RD, Lyon G: *Neurology of Hereditary Metabolic Diseases of Children*. New York, McGraw Hill, 1982.

354. Plaster NM, Uyama E, Uchino M, Ikeda T, Flanigan KM, Kondo I, Ptacek LJ: Genetic localization of the familial adult myoclonic epilepsy (FAME) gene to chromosome 8q24. *Neurology* **53**:1180, 1999.

355. Szepetowski P, Rochette J, Berquin P, Piussian C, Lathrop GM, Monaco AP: Familial infantile convulsions and paroxysmal choreoathetosis: A new neurological syndrome linked to the pericentromeric region of human chromosome 16. *Am J Hum Genet* **61**:889, 1997.

# Spinal Muscular Atrophy

*Cristina Panozzo* ∎ *Tony Frugier*
*Carmen Cifuentes-Diaz* ∎ *Judith Melki*

Spinal muscular atrophies (SMA) are characterized by degeneration of lower motor neurons and occasionally bulbar motor neurons leading to progressive limb and trunk paralysis associated with muscular atrophy. Childhood SMA is a frequent recessive autosomal disorder and represents a common genetic cause of death in childhood. A positional cloning strategy allowed the localization and the identification of the survival of motor neuron gene (SMN). These developments have greatly improved the clinical management and family planning options of SMA patients and their parents. Furthermore, the presence or the absence of a SMN gene defect contributed to a better nosology of SMA-related diseases. The last 10 years saw major advances in the field of SMA. The function of the SMN gene product has been, at least partly, elucidated, and mouse models of SMA have been created. These advances represent starting points for designing therapeutic strategies of this devastating neurodegenerative disease for which no curative treatment is known so far.

## CLINICAL PHENOTYPES

The various types of SMA can be distinguished clinically by the distribution of weakness, by the pattern of inheritance, and by the age of onset.

### Infantile SMA

There are two different forms of infantile SMA: an acute form or type I (MIM 253300) and a more chronic form or type II (MIM 253550). Both are inherited as autosomal recessive traits.

The acute or type I SMA, first described by Werdnig[1,2] and by Hoffmann,[3] is characterized by its severe generalized muscle involvement and fatal outcome. In about one-third of cases, the disease manifests before birth by diminished fetal movements in utero or by mild contractures. In the other cases, the onset occurs at birth or within the first 6 months of life. Generalized weakness associated with areflexia is the most common clinical features. Active movements are usually confined to the fingers and toes. Fasciculations can be detected in the tongue. The face is usually spared and the infant usually has a bright, normal expression. Intercostal paralysis with severe collapse of the chest is the rule. Breathing is almost entirely diaphragmatic, the diaphragmatic muscle being spared. The extraocular movements are normal. Feeding and breathing difficulties are usually responsible for death within 2 years of age. Some studies have presented survival statistics on type I SMA indicating that all patients with an age of onset in the first 6 months of life are deceased by 2 years of age.[4,5] Another study showed a bad prognosis for patients with onset within the first 3 months of life; 50 percent died by 7 to 8 months and all were deceased before 5 years of age.[6] However, life span of many patients with early SMA onset is often better than expected.

Type II SMA is a more slowly progressive generalized disease with a variable prognosis. Infants are able to sit unsupported but none are able to stand or walk unaided. Atrophy and fasciculations of the tongue are frequent and spontaneous tremor of the fingers may be evident. Tendon reflexes are diminished or absent. Clinical progression is slow or appears even to arrest. All children will develop, if untreated, severe scoliosis and respiratory ventilation defect. Life expectancy is highly variable, ranging up to adult life in some cases.

### Juvenile and Adult SMA

In juvenile SMA or type III or Kugelberg-Welander disease (MIM 253400),[7] symptoms start from 18 months to 30 years of age. All patients are able to walk and proximal muscle weakness is progressive. Subsequently, the patients show difficulties in climbing stairs and gait becomes waddling. Muscle weakness associated with muscle atrophy is more proximal than distal. There is no evidence of sensory or upper motor neuron involvement. About one-fourth of the patients exhibit a hypertrophy of the calves, a feature similar to that observed in Duchenne or Becker muscular dystrophies.[8] Finally, adult SMA is defined by an age of onset after 20 or 30 years of age. Aside from age of onset, the diagnostic criteria are identical to the other forms of SMA.[9]

In 1991, the international SMA consortium subdivided childhood SMA into three clinical groups based on the age of onset, age of death, and the achievement of certain motor milestones (Table 231-1).[10] Clinical severity actually displays a continuous range from the severe to the mild forms of the disease.

### Investigations

Biochemical investigations of patients with proximal SMA reveal no specific abnormalities. Increased serum creatine phosphokinase (CK) activity is found in about half of the patients with type III SMA.[11] The values can be 2 to 10 times higher than the normal upper limit.

Electromyographic (EMG) investigations reveal spontaneous discharge activity in resting muscle, increased amplitude, and prolonged duration of motor unit potentials during voluntary effort. Other EMG features of severe denervation are commonly found in older patients. Although nerve conduction velocity is generally considered normal, some decrease in velocity has been demonstrated in severe cases.[12]

Histologic studies of skeletal muscle show the typical changes of denervation with small groups of atrophic muscle fibers associated with markedly hypertrophied fibers.[13,14] Small angular fibers randomly intermixed with normal-sized fibers are often observed. Atrophic fibers are arranged in groups that are usually of uniform fiber type based on the myosin ATPase reaction. This is considered as an extensive collateral reinnervation of previously denervated muscle fibers by sprouts from surviving motor neurons. In SMA type III, but not in infantile SMA (type I or II), one can observe markedly hypertrophic fibers, excessive variation in fiber size, and internal nuclei. Degenerative changes with necrosis and regenerative fibers associated with proliferative interstitial connective tissue can be observed.[14] Because these changes are

**Table 231-1 Classification of Childhood SMA**

| Designation | Symptoms (months) | Course | Death (years) |
|---|---|---|---|
| I | 0–6 | Never sit | <2 |
| II | <18 | Never stand | >2 |
| III | >18 | Stands alone | Adult |

characteristic features of primary myopathies, they have been interpreted as "pseudomyopathic" changes. In addition, these myopathic changes are usually found in patients with high serum levels of CK activity and may suggest the presence of a myopathic process secondary to neurogenic process. However, these pseudomyopathic changes are not observed in other human neurogenic diseases, which suggests that they can be specific to the molecular mechanism resulting in or associated with juvenile SMA.

The most striking neuropathologic feature found at autopsy of SMA patients is a loss of the large anterior horn cells of the spinal cord. In the remaining surviving motor neurons, a severe degree of central chromatolysis is visible. These cells appear as large ballooned cells without stored substances. Other anterior horn cells are pyknotic. In addition, there are occasional figures of neuronophagia associated with astrogliosis and the anterior roots are very small.[13]

### Differential Diagnosis

Although the signs of SMA type I, II, or III are more or less stereotyped, there are a number of conditions that must be considered by the clinician depending on the age of the patient.

**Myopathies and Miscellaneous Diseases.** Diseases with a floppy infant syndrome, including congenital myotonic dystrophy, Prader-Willi syndrome (MIM 176270), myasthenia gravis (MIM 254200), congenital myopathies, and congenital muscular dystrophy, should be considered in the differential diagnosis of infantile SMA. Proximal muscle weakness of the upper and lower limbs associated with the presence of hypertrophic calves and the high level of CK activity found in one-fourth of type III SMA patients may lead to the consideration of Becker muscular dystrophy in the differential diagnosis. The X-linked inheritance pattern of Becker muscular dystrophy distinguishes it from SMA. The EMG is the most valuable diagnostic tool for differentiating the SMA from myopathies although muscle biopsy may sometimes be required for the diagnosis.

**Other Forms of SMA.** Other forms of SMA can be differentiated from proximal SMA based on the clinical features or the mode of inheritance.

Bulbar and spinal muscular atrophy or Kennedy syndrome is an X-linked recessive disease characterized by proximal muscle weakness with onset between 20 and 40 years of age (see Chap. 161). Muscle cramps are common. Dysphagia and dysarthria, due to bulbar involvement associated with gynecomastia and testicular atrophy, are specific to the Kennedy syndrome. The diagnosis is based on the detection of expansion of a (CAG) triplet in the androgen receptor gene.[15]

Distal SMA is a peroneal muscular atrophy similar to Charcot Marie Tooth disease (CMT; MIM 601472) type I or type II (see Chap. 227). The most important feature distinguishing distal SMA from CMT is the absence of sensory signs. Distal SMA is a clinically and genetically heterogeneous disease. The age of onset of symptoms varies from early childhood to adulthood. Recessive and dominant forms are observed. Genetic linkage studies showed that distal SMA is not linked to the SMA locus on chromosome 5q.[16] Two genetic loci for distal SMA have been identified so far. The disease gene maps to chromosome 7p in a family showing a

clinical phenotype starting in the upper limbs. In the classic phenotype, the disease gene has been mapped on chromosome 12q24.[17,18] It remains to be established how frequent these loci are involved in distal SMA. No gene has been identified so far.

## CLINICAL GENETICS

SMA represents the second most common fatal recessive autosomal disorder after cystic fibrosis with an incidence of 1/6000.[19–22] Segregation analysis has shown that types I, II, and III SMA are inherited as autosomal recessive traits, although alternative hypotheses have been proposed to account for the lower-than-expected segregation ratio evident in sibships with type II SMA.[23–26] In addition, some studies have suggested that males are more frequently affected with SMA than females, particularly in type II SMA. Another feature that has not yet been clarified is the variability in clinical severity within a sibship. It has been reported that one child may be affected with type I SMA, whereas a sib may have a later onset consistent with type II, or in other families, one sib may be affected with type II, while another may have a milder form or type III. Another intriguing feature was the existence of an increased incidence in first-degree relatives of parents of affected persons.[23–26] Finally, an autosomal dominant inheritance has also been observed in both juvenile and adult form representing 2 percent of infantile and about 30 percent of adult SMA.

## MOLECULAR GENETICS

### Genomic Complexity and Instability at the SMA Locus

It was hoped that characterization of SMA at the molecular level would provide insight into its pathophysiology. By linkage analyses, types I, II, and III SMA have all been mapped to chromosome 5q11.2-13.3,[27–30] suggesting that they are allelic disorders. A high-resolution genetic map contributed to narrowing the SMA-critical region and allowed prenatal diagnosis in SMA families.[31,32] The genetic interval was cloned into a yeast artificial chromosome (YAC) contig spanning the SMA locus.[33–35] The physical map showed that the SMA gene lies within a complex genomic region containing multicopy repetitive sequences, pseudogenes, and retrotransposon-like sequences. These observations suggested that this area of the genome might be unstable. Consistent with this notion, the physical maps of the SMA region derived from cloned contigs were not consistent and determination of the physical organization of the candidate genes was difficult.

Inherited or *de novo* deletions were observed in SMA patients.[35] *De novo* rearrangements were identified using polymorphic markers (C272 identical to Ag1CA) or C212 in at least 2 percent of SMA patients.[35,36] This represented a high frequency of *de novo* rearrangements as compared with that observed in cystic fibrosis (<0.01 percent) and could be explained by the instability of the 5q13 region. The occurrence of *de novo* mutations would indicate a recurrence risk lower than the expected value of 25 percent. Additionally, germ line mosaicism has been proved in one family; this has implications for the counseling of SMA families undergoing prenatal genetic analysis.[37]

Further characterization of the SMA locus revealed a chromosomal region containing an inverted duplication, each element (about 500 kb) containing four genes: the *SMN* gene;[38] *NAIP*, the gene encoding neuronal apoptosis inhibitory protein;[39] the gene encoding p44, a subunit of the basal transcription factor TFIIH;[40,41] and the *H4F5* gene[42] (Fig. 231-1). Large-scale sequencing analysis confirmed the complexity of the region.[43]

### Identification of SMN, the SMA-Determining Gene

Detailed characterization of the smallest deletions detected in SMA patients allowed the identification and characterization of the

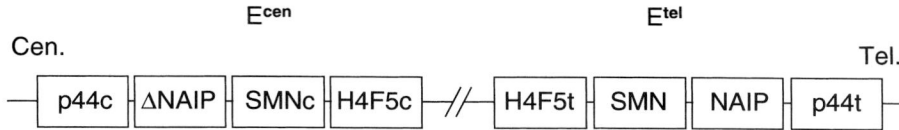

Cen.

Tel.

Fig. 231-1 Representation of the SMA locus. Abbreviations: E[cen] = centromeric element; E[tel] = telomeric element; Cen. = centromere; Tel. = Telomere.

SMN gene. The SMN gene exists in duplicate with a highly homologous copy, SMNc; both are transcribed. In the first analysis of SMA patients by Lefebvre et al., the telomeric copy of *SMN* was lacking in 98 percent of the patients; the remaining patients carried intragenic mutations.[38] The centromeric copy of *SMN* (*SMNc*) was present in all patients and absent in 5 percent of control individuals.[38] Similar results were reported in other series of SMA patients (Table 231-2).[44-51] The percentage of nondeleted patients varies in the different studies, which may in part be explained by different ascertainment of patients. The identification of additional mutations in SMA patients gave further support to the view that *SMN* is the gene responsible for causing SMA (Fig. 231-2).[44,51-56] No homozygous deletion of both *SMN* and *SMNc* genes has been reported so far, suggesting that such a genotype likely results in a nonviable fetus.

Only five nucleotides distinguish *SMN* from *SMNc* (Fig. 231-3). One of these is located in exon 7 and is responsible for the alternative splicing of exon 7 that is specific to *SMNc* transcripts[38,57,58] (Fig. 231-4). The analysis of RNA in SMA patients showed a marked increase of the transcript lacking exon 7 (SMNΔ7) as compared to the RNA pattern of control individuals suggesting that the truncated transcripts represent the major form derived from the *SMNc* gene.[38] The only difference detectable so far at the transcriptional level between *SMN* and *SMNc* is the presence of this alternatively spliced product specific to *SMNc*. Interestingly, the presence of *SMNc* gene in SMA patients is not able to compensate for *SMN* defects. Therefore, the development of the SMA phenotype is caused by two events: (a) the *SMN* gene defect, and (b) indirectly, the fact that the alternative splicing of *SMNc* exon 7 leads to a decreased amount of the full-length *SMNc* transcript. The *SMN* gene is also named *SMN1*. Similarly, the *SMNc* gene is also referred to as *SMN2*. We use the original names in this chapter.

## Genetic Diagnosis and Carrier Detection

The high frequency of *SMN* deletions in SMA patients (92.8 percent) provides a direct and accurate genetic test for diagnostic confirmation and prenatal prediction of SMA.[59,60] Homozygous deletion of *SMN* has been observed in atypical forms of SMA associated with congenital heart defects, in arthrogryposis, in some cases of congenital axonal neuropathy, and in some patients affected with adult form of SMA.[61-66] In contrast, neither deletion of the *SMN* gene nor linkage to chromosome 5q has been observed in SMA associated with diaphragmatic involvement, SMA with

olivopontocerebellar atrophy, autosomal dominant form of SMA, amyotrophic lateral sclerosis, or post-polio syndrome[67-71] (Table 231-3). Rare cases of homozygous *SMN* exon 7 deletion or conversion have been reported in asymptomatic relatives of haploidentical type II or III SMA patients.[45,72,73] Initially, these results led to the suggestion that other genes or mechanisms could produce the SMA phenotype. However, the description of additional mutations within the *SMN* gene, biochemical investigations of the SMN protein in SMA patients, and the generation of a mouse model of SMA demonstrated that the *SMN* gene is responsible for SMA. These rare exceptions actually suggest the presence of modifying gene(s) unlinked to chromosome 5q. The genomic complexity of the region and its high degree of variability hamper the ability to directly detect the SMA carriers. More recently, the development of heterozygosity test for *SMN* exon 7 deletion based on a quantitative multiplex PCR analysis had important implications for relatives of SMA patients carrying a homozygous deletion of *SMN* exon 7, spouse of carriers or SMA patients, or in patients with clinical findings consistent with SMA but without homozygous deletion of the *SMN* gene. The only limitation (false negative) of this test is due to the presence of two SMN genes per chromosome.[51,74-76]

## Phenotype-Genotype Correlation

No phenotype-genotype correlation at the *SMN* locus has been established. The genetic analyses of *SMN*, *NAIP*, and *p44* genes in large series of SMA patients revealed that large-scale deletions, including the telomeric version of these genes, are associated with type I SMA phenotype.[40,41,77,78] However, smaller rearrangements or point mutations of the *SMN* gene only can also result in a severe phenotype, suggesting that *NAIPt* and/or *p44t* deletions are not directly involved in the severity of SMA. Further analyses by Southern blot and pulsed-field gel electrophoresis of DNA of SMA revealed that the absence of *SMN* gene in type I SMA is associated with gene dosage effect, whereas no gene dosage effect was detected in type III SMA.[38,79] These observations raised the hypothesis of a gene deletion event in type I SMA and a gene conversion event that would result in an increased number of *SMNc* copies in type III SMA[38,79,80] (Fig. 231-5). However, rare cases of severe forms are also associated with an increased number of *SMNc* copies (no gene dosage effect), suggesting that other factors may influence the severity of the disease.[81] Yet, in the majority of cases, an \ increased number of *SMNc* copies correlates with milder SMA phenotypes, suggesting that the *SMNc* gene is translated into an, at least, partially functional protein and could be regarded as a modifying gene in SMA.

## BIOCHEMICAL ASPECTS

### SMN and the Spliceosomal Complex

The *SMN* gene encodes a novel protein of 294 amino acids with a molecular weight of 38 kDa that shows no significant homology to any other protein. Its function was unknown when the gene was identified. In 1996, an important step towards the molecular and cellular characterization of SMN protein was unintentionally provided by identifying proteins interacting with heterogeneous nuclear ribonucleoproteins (hnRNPs), a group of abundant nuclear proteins binding pre-mRNAs and nuclear mRNAs.[82,83] These authors used the RGG box, a consensus motif of RNA binding located at the C-terminus of the hnRNP U protein, as bait in a yeast two-hybrid screening of a HeLa cDNA library.[83] The SMN

**Table 231-2** Homozygous Deletion or Conversion of SMN Exon 7 in Different SMA Populations

| Authors | SMA patients (%) |
| --- | --- |
| Lefebvre et al. (1995, 231–38) | 226/229 (98.6) |
| Bussaglia et al. (1995, 231–44) | 50/54 (92.5) |
| Cobben et al. (1995, 231–45) | 96/103 (93.2) |
| Velasco et al. (1996, 231–46) | 53/65 (81.5) |
| Chang et al. (1995, 231–47) | 42/42 (100) |
| Rodrigues et al. (1996, 231–48) | 175/187 (93.5) |
| Capon et al. (1996, 231–49) | 117/122 (95.9) |
| Spiegel et al. (1996, 231–50) | 43/57 (75.4) |
| Wirth et al. (1999, 231–51) | 483/525 (92) |
| Total | 1285/1384 (92.8) |

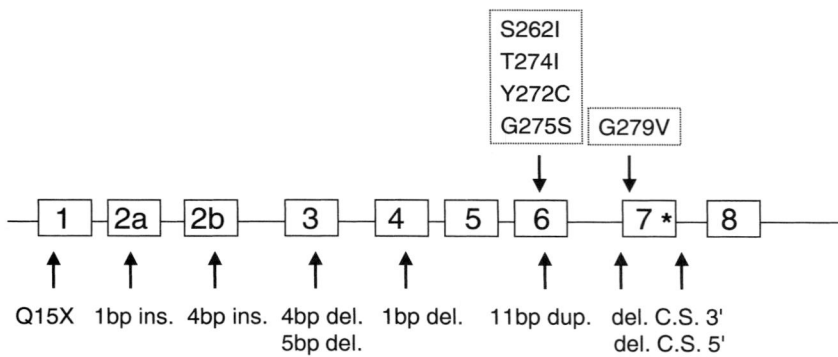

**Fig. 231-2 Intragenic mutations of the SMN gene in SMA patients.** Abbreviations: ins. = insertion; dup. = duplication; del. = deletion; C.S. = consensus splice site; (*) = stop codon.

protein was identified as partner and then used as bait in a second screen to identify SMN interacting proteins. They found that the SMN protein interacts with both the full-length SMN and the protein lacking the C-terminus corresponding to the product of the alternatively spliced *SMNc* transcript, with fibrillarin and with two novel proteins. One is called SMN interacting protein 1 (SIP1). It is a 279-amino-acid protein that shows significant homology with a yeast protein termed Brr1, which is involved in snRNP biogenesis in yeast.[83-85]

Immunofluorescence experiments using monoclonal antibodies specific for SMN detected SMN protein in both the cytoplasm and the nucleus of HeLa cells. In the nucleus, the monoclonal antibody labeled several prominent nuclear structures that are most often found adjacent to coiled bodies and that have been called "gems" for "gemini of coiled bodies."[83] Coiled bodies are highly conserved structures in evolution and are found in widely divergent organisms including plants and animals.[85] These nuclear structures, which were recently renamed Cajal bodies, are often observed near nucleoli.[86,87] Coiled bodies are known to contain small nuclear ribonucleoproteins (snRNP U1, U2, U4/U6, and U5) and several proteins, including p80-coilin and fibrillarin, but not pre-mRNAs, and are likely involved in the metabolism of small nuclear RNAs. The subcellular localization of SMN protein and its interaction with components of the spliceosomal complex suggest that SMN may have a role in RNA metabolism.

Further genetic and biochemical investigations demonstrated that the C-terminal domain (aa 242 to 278) of SMN binds specifically and directly to Sm proteins except Sm F or G, while the N-terminal domain (aa 13 to 44) of SMN binds strongly with SIP1 *in vitro* (aa 13 to 44)[85,88] (Fig. 231-6). In addition, SMN forms part of a large protein complex that contains SIP1 as well as several spliceosomal snRNP proteins, suggesting that SMN is involved in the biogenesis of spliceosomal snRNPs.[88] The biogenesis of snRNPs (U1, U2, U4, U5) is a complicated, multistep process that requires the bidirectional transport of snRNAs through the nuclear envelope.[89-92] The spliceosomal snRNAs, which are essential components of the splicing reaction, are first exported to the cytoplasm where they associate with the Sm proteins. Within the assembled Sm core domain, the 7-methyl-guanosine (m7G) cap of the snRNAs is hypermethylated and varying number of nucleotides are trimmed from the 3'-end of

several of the snRNAs. These processes are important for the nuclear import of the assembled snRNP particles.

The characterization of the SMN protein function was further refined by Pellizzoni et al.[93] They showed that a mutant *SMN* cDNA lacking the N-terminal 27 codons (SMNΔN27) transfected into mammalian cells causes reorganization of snRNPs, gems, and coiled bodies. This observation suggested that the SMN protein might have a role in splicing reaction *in vitro*. In specific conditions, *in vitro* splicing was enhanced when the reaction was preincubated with a wild-type SMN and inhibited when preincubated with SMNΔN27. Interestingly, *in vitro* splicing is unchanged by preincubation of SMN lacking the C-terminus or Y272C. These results suggest, indirectly, a loss of SMN function in these mutants. In addition, *in vitro* experiments showed that the 37-amino-acid region encoded by exon 6 and containing Y-G elements (aa 242 to 278) is required for self-association and binding for SMN to Sm proteins.[94,95] Interestingly, several missense mutations (including Y272C) in this region have been identified in SMA patients and have been shown to disrupt SMN binding to Sm proteins.[95] Sm proteins are essential components of the pre-mRNA splicing machinery. These data suggest that SMN binding to Sm proteins is defective in SMA, although this has not been demonstrated *in vivo*. The C-terminal 16 amino acids encoded by exon 7 of SMN (aa 278 to 294), which is lacking in most patients, is also required for oligomerization of SMN, although this activity is not completely abolished because a two-hybrid screen with SMN as bait identified SMNΔ7.[83,94,95] More recently, *in vivo* experiments in mutant mice carrying homozygous deletion of *Smn* exon 7 directed to neurons revealed that the truncated protein lacking the C-terminus leads to a lack of gems associated with a defect of coiling assembly into coiled bodies.[96] These data suggested that the C-terminus is required for nuclear targeting of SMN into gems, resulting in a defect in the normal pathway of gem/coiled body formation. In addition, these data support the view that coiled bodies and gems are closely related or even identical structures. Further morphologic analyses showed that SMN and SIP1 are indeed colocalized with snRNP in coiled bodies in primary culture of neurons, suggesting that gems and coiled bodies are likely the same nuclear structure.[87,97]

These data strongly support the view that the SMN protein is involved in pre-mRNA splicing machinery and has a determining role in the biogenesis of gem/coiled bodies. Despite this

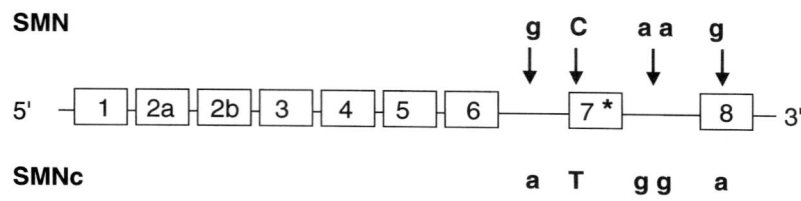

**Fig. 231-3 Nucleotide discrepancies found between *SMN* and *SMNc* genes.** (*) indicates the position of the stop codon.

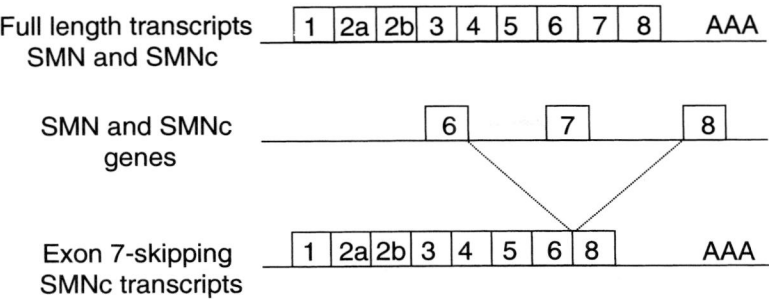

**Fig. 231-4 Differential splicing of exon 7 in *SMN* and *SMNc* transcripts.**

understanding of the SMN function, the molecular mechanism leading to SMA remains unclear. SMN is indeed ubiquitously expressed and the marked reduction of SMN in type I SMA patients is observed both in motor neurons, the target cells in SMA, and, for example, in liver, which does not show any functional defect in patients.[98] These data suggest the following hypotheses: (a) Large amounts of SMN protein may be required for particular pre-mRNA splicing reaction in motor neurons and a loss of SMN function would result in defects restricted to some RNA molecule(s); (b) SMN may have a specific function related to RNA metabolism in motor neurons through an interacting protein or RNA specific to motor neurons; and (c) SMN may have another function. A possible relationship between SMN and neuron degeneration was provided in 1997 by Iwahashi et al.[99] Using a yeast two-hybrid screen, the authors identified SMN as Bcl-2 interacting partner. This work pointed out that SMN alone has a weak antiapoptotic effect in mammalian cells, but that SMN coexpressed with Bcl-2 enhances Bcl-2 antiapoptotic activity. Furthermore, they showed that the Y272C mutant SMN exerts no synergism with Bcl-2. Further investigations on SMN and Bcl-2 interactions should help explain the involvement of SMN in the apoptotic pathway.

### Correlation between Clinical Severity and SMN Protein Level in SMA

SMN protein studies in SMA and control individuals were performed by both immunoblot and immunohistochemical analyses.[98,100] Immunoblot analyses of lymphoblastoid cell lines from controls and SMA patients demonstrated that both the *SMN* and *SMNc* genes are transcribed and translated into a protein of similar mobility. A tight correlation between the amount of protein encoded by the *SMNc* gene and the clinical manifestations of the disease was observed in a large cohort of SMA patients. In addition, the marked reduction in the amount of SMNc protein in all type I patients was not found to correlate with a large deletion involving SMN and the neighboring genes, *NAIP* or *p44*. This observation provides the first molecular basis of the clinical severity in SMA. Similar results were reported in cultured

fibroblasts.[100] SMN protein expression in human fetal tissues (liver and spinal cord) revealed a decreased amount of SMNc protein in both type I and type III SMA, the level being more reduced in severe than in mild forms of the disease.[98,100] A marked reduction of the SMN protein was also reported in postnatal spinal cord samples of type I SMA patients.[101]

Immunohistochemical analyses of the SMN protein showed that motor neurons of the spinal cord from controls have a large amount of cytoplasmic SMN protein and gems in the nucleus. The lack of or marked reduction of nuclear SMNc staining in motor neurons of type I or type III SMA patients respectively raises the question of whether gems are present in SMA.[98,100] These data demonstrated that the protein encoded by the SMNc gene is functionally active, as its level is directly correlated to the clinical severity of the disease. These results, taken together ascribe SMA to a dosage effect of SMN. The absence of the *SMN* gene without gene dosage effect in type III has been ascribed to gene conversion events replacing *SMN* by *SMNc* and resulting in an increased number of *SMNc* gene copies. The SMNc protein level could, therefore, depend on the *SMNc* copy number or the integrity of *SMNc* gene regulatory elements in SMA. Thus, characterization of SMN and SMNc at the protein level gives additional support to the view that SMNc is a modifying gene in SMA.

Further investigations have been undertaken to determine whether the differences between the two gene products are accounted for by alternative splicing of exon 7 in *SMNc* transcripts or a variable promoter activity. The analysis of the promoters of the SMN and SMNc genes show that the sequence and activity for both gene promoters are quasi-identical.[102,103] Therefore, the different levels of protein encoded by the *SMN* or *SMNc* genes are the result of either differences in regulation of gene expression or different posttranscriptional regulation. The alternative splicing of exon 7 is specific for the SMNc gene. Studying the role of this splicing event and the stability of either the *SMNc* transcripts, with or without exon 7, or the corresponding proteins, should contribute to an understanding of the regulation of *SMN* and *SMNc* gene expression.

### MOUSE MODELS OF SMA

No spontaneous murine Smn mutant has been identified so far. To gain insight into the pathogenesis of SMA and to understand the function of SMN inferred from the SMA phenotype, several strategies have been carried out.

The first approach consisted of targeted disruption of the murine *Smn* gene through homologous recombination in embryonic stem cells. Early embryonic lethality was observed in mice homozygous for the null allele, which may be explained by the absence of duplication of *Smn* in mice.[104-106] In addition, no degeneration of motor neurons was observed in heterozygous mice, suggesting that a 50 percent reduction of *Smn* gene dosage has no deleterious effects.[106]

An elegant approach was based on the production of two mouse lines, one carrying a deletion of *Smn* exon 7 produced by homologous recombination, and the other expressing the human

**Table 231-3 SMN Gene Analysis in Disorders Closely Related to SMA**

| Allelic to SMA | Nonallelic to SMA |
| --- | --- |
| Adult form of SMA (type IV)* | Amyotrophic lateral sclerosis |
| Congenital heart defect with SMA | Spinal form of CMT |
| Arthrogryposis multiplex congenita* | Diaphragmatic SMA |
| Congenital axonal neuropathy* | Post-polio syndrome |
| Congenital fiber type dysproportion* | SMA plus olivopontocerebellar hypoplasia |

*Indicates the presence of genetic heterogeneity, a subgroup being allelic to SMA.

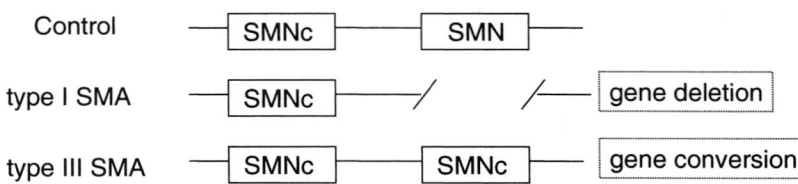

Fig. 231-5 Representation of the phenotype-genotype correlations in SMA. Only one allele is indicated.

*SMNc* gene produced by microinjection of a 115-kb genomic DNA transgene that also contains part of centromeric *NAIP* and intact *H4F5* genes[107] (Fig. 231-7A). Mice homozygous for both deletion of *Smn* exon 7 and the 115-kb *SMNc* transgene developed a variety of symptoms, including lower body weight, short and enlarged tails, edema, chronic necrosis of the tail and hindlimbs, and a variable age of survival. The most severe phenotype, called type 1, was characterized by the absence of furry hair and death before 10 days of life. Poor activity and death before 4 weeks of age characterized an intermediate phenotype (classified into type 2 group). Mice with the type 3 phenotype survived normally and are characterized by short and enlarged tails. Surprisingly, only 3 of 30 mutant mice of the type 2 phenotype developed paralysis of the hindlimbs associated with loss of motor neurons and chromatolysis of the remaining motor neurons. The different phenotypes observed within the same litter was correlated with the transgene copy number, although this requires further study. The absence of tail and hindlimbs in some mutant mice are intriguing clinical features that could be due to the potential deleterious effect of an additional copy of *NAIP*, *H4F5*, or another sequence. Fine characterization of the neuromuscular system of mutant mice will be very helpful in determining whether these mutant mice are a model for human SMA.

A similar approach was adopted by creating a mouse line carrying a transgene that contains the human *SMNc* gene only[108] (Fig. 231-7B). Mice carrying a low copy number of *SMNc* and harboring a homozygous null *Smn* allele (*Smn*−/−) develop a severe phenotype leading to death either in utero, or in the first 6 h after birth, or before 6 days of age. Crosses of (*Smn*−/−) mice with those carrying a high copy number of the *SMNc* transgene result in mice without an abnormal phenotype. Interestingly, surviving mutant mice with a low copy number of *SMNc* display abnormal motor behavior associated with a severe loss of motor neurons of the spinal cord and brain stem at the latest stage of disease. These data suggest that neuronal death is a late manifestation of the disease phenotype. In addition, the absence of abnormal phenotype in mutant mice carrying a high copy number of the *SMNc* transgene confirms that *SMNc* is able to rescue the embryonic lethality of the *Smn* knockout mice and demonstrates that an increased copy number of *SMNc* reduces the severity of the phenotype. These results are consistent with those observed in human SMA.

A different approach has been carried out by using the Cre/lox P recombination system of bacteriophage P1[96,109,110] (Fig. 231-7C). A mouse line carrying two lox P sites flanking SMN exon 7 was established through homologous recombination.

Mice heterozygous or homozygous for the lox P-flanked *Smn* exon 7 allele (*SmnF7*) appear, as expected, similar in size and morphology to wild-type mice. Cre-mediated deletion of *Smn* exon 7 directed to neurons has been achieved by crossing the SMNF7 mice with a transgenic mouse line expressing Cre recombinase in neurons, but not in skeletal muscle. Mutant mice can be easily distinguished from their control littermates by a severe motor defect that is associated with tremors, which becomes evident beginning at 2 weeks of age. Mutant mice exhibit a reduced life expectancy, dying at a mean age of 25 days. Morphologic analysis on transverse sections of several skeletal muscles revealed the presence of groups of atrophic muscle fibers and angular fibers intermixed with normal-sized fibers consistent with a skeletal muscle denervation process. A morphologic analysis on transverse semithin sections of spinal cord was performed and revealed pronounced morphologic changes of nuclei of motor neurons characterized by the presence of indentations of the nuclear membrane without significant loss of motor neurons of the anterior horns at 2 weeks of age. Interestingly, biochemical investigation revealed that the mouse *Smn* transcript lacking exon 7 is translated into a truncated protein lacking the C-terminal 15 amino acids. Immunohistochemical studies showed a pattern of Smn expression restricted to the cytoplasm of motor neurons. The lack of gems in motor neuron nuclei has been demonstrated by the absence of SIP1 labeling and is associated with a defect in the coiling assembly into coiled bodies. Therefore, this approach indicates that SMN protein lacking the C-terminus (the most common mutation found in SMA) causes a defect in nuclear targeting of SMN protein into gems, which cannot proceed further on the normal pathway of gem/coiled body formation, and thus identifies a biochemical defect in SMA. The mice produced in this experiment exhibit a motor defect related to a muscle denervation process of neurogenic origin, a constant feature found in human SMA. The morphologic changes in motor neurons occurring in response to the lack of SMN have not been reported in human SMA, suggesting they likely represent the early events of neuronal degeneration that lead later to motor neuron loss, typical of that found in autopsy material of SMA patients.[13] In addition, these data demonstrate that an SMN gene defect limited to neurons leads to a SMA phenotype *in vivo*, indicating that motor neurons are the primary site of damage in SMA.[96]

Although the generation of animal models of SMA required sophisticated strategies to avoid embryonic lethality, the different approaches provided important and complementary information. In the first strategy,[107,108] the authors demonstrated that the

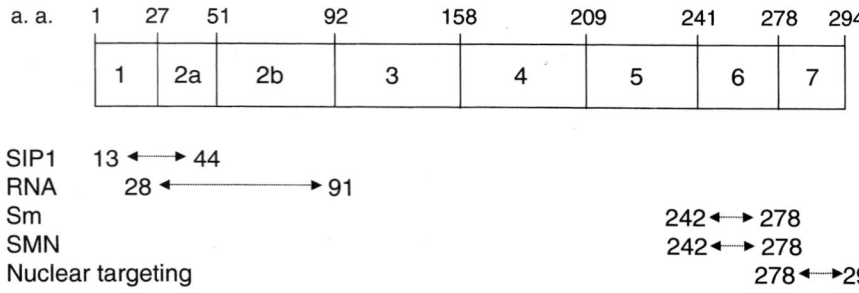

Fig. 231-6 Representation of the binding or the functional domains of the SMN protein. Amino acid numbers are shown above the SMN protein sequence. Vertical bars indicate the limits of each coding exon (1 to 7). Binding of SMN to proteins or functional domains are indicated below.

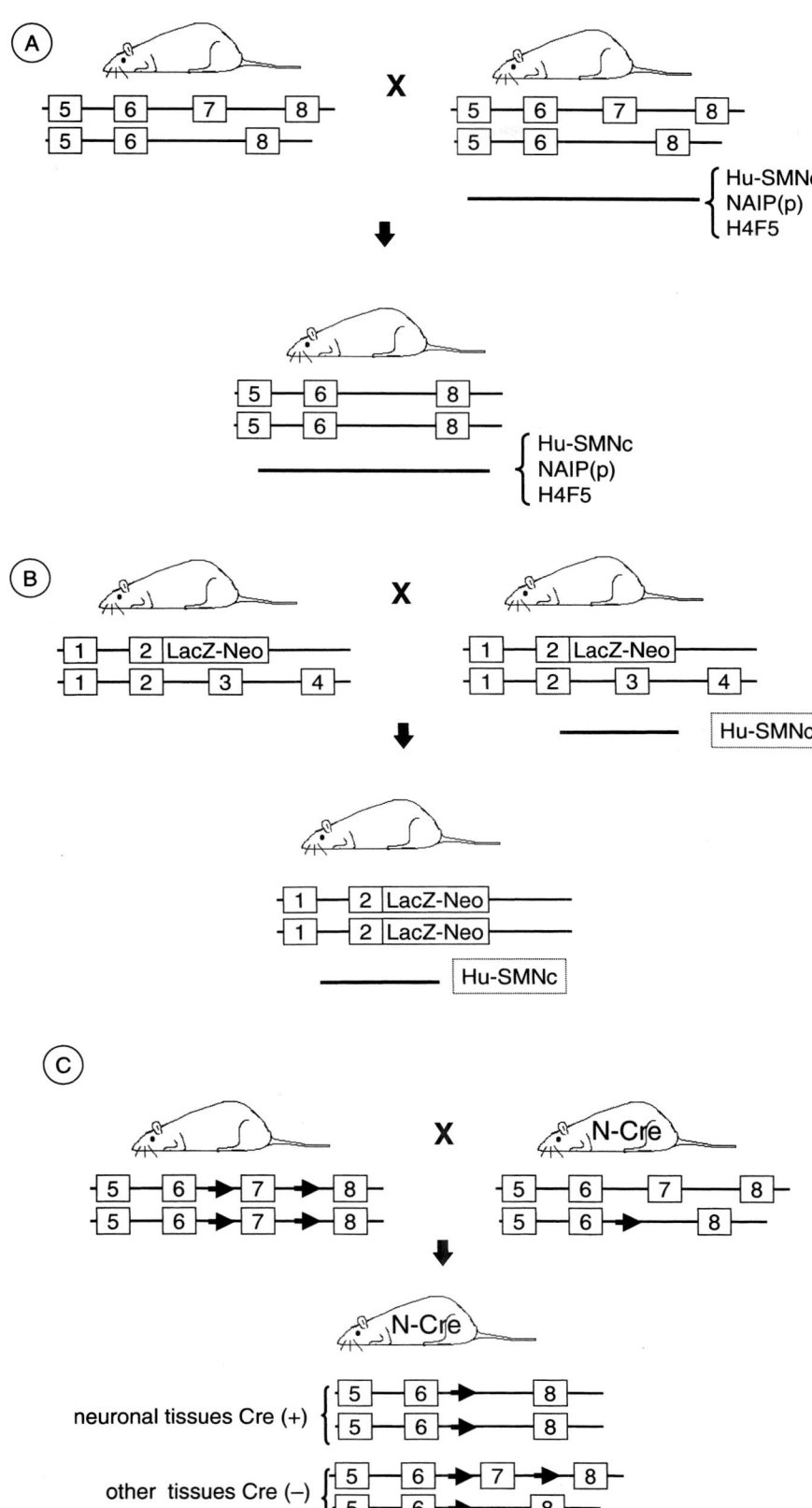

Fig. 231-7 Genetic strategies used to create a mouse model of SMA. *A*, Mutant mice carrying a heterozygous deletion of *Smn* exon 7 (*left*) have been crossed with a mouse line carrying, in addition to the heterozygous deletion of *Smn* exon 7, a 115-kb human genomic DNA transgene containing *SMNc* (Hu-SMNc), part of *NAIP* (*NAIPp*), and *H4F5* (*right*). Boxes indicate the exons and black solid line indicates the transgene. Mice carrying both the homozygous deletion of SMN exon 7 and the human transgene display abnormal phenotypes. *B*, Mutant mice carrying a heterozygous deletion of *Smn* from exon 2 (*left*) have been crossed with a mouse line carrying, in addition to the same *Smn* mutation, a human genomic DNA transgene containing *SMNc* only (Hu-SMNc, *right*). Mice carrying both the homozygous deletion of *Smn* and the human *SMNc* gene transgene display abnormal phenotypes. *C*, Mutant mice carrying two loxP sites flanking *Smn* exon 7 (*left*, SMNF7) have been crossed with a mouse line carrying, in addition to the heterozygous deletion of *Smn* exon 7 (SMN$\Delta$7), a transgene expressing the Cre recombinase in neurons (indicated by N-Cre, *right*). The mutant mice carrying the SMNF7/SMN$\Delta$7 genotype and the N-Cre transgene display an abnormal phenotype. In neuronal tissues, Cre-mediated deletion of the SMNF7 allele leads to a homozygous deletion of *Smn* exon 7 (Cre+). In nonneuronal tissues, SMNF7 remains intact because the Cre recombinase is not expressed (Cre−). LoxP sites are indicated by arrows. Human *SMNc* transgene or conditional targeting of *SMN* restricted to neurons are able to avoid early embryonic lethality.

number of human *SMNc* genes modulates the phenotypic severity of *Smn* defect in mice, a low copy number of *SMNc* associated with a severe phenotype characterized by a loss of motor neurons resembling SMA type I. The second strategy[96] provided evidence that (a) motor neurons are the primary site of damage in SMA;

(b) denervation of skeletal muscle is pronounced in the absence of motor neuron death and results in a phenotype resembling human SMA type II or III; and (c) the most frequent gene mutation found in human SMA causes a defect in nuclear targeting of SMN into gems.

These animal models are likely to become important tools for the design of therapeutic strategies to counter human SMA.

## CONCLUSIONS AND PERSPECTIVES

### From Patient to Gene

The progress in our understanding of SMA is an excellent example of synergism between medicine and molecular genetics. Careful definition of a clinical phenotype leads to a selection of homogeneous cohort of patients and their families. This, in turn, enabled a positional cloning strategy that lead to identification of the *SMN* gene and its protein product. These advances provide efficient tools to either confirm or exclude the diagnosis of the "classical" forms of the disease. More interestingly, these advances allow the investigation of SMA phenotypes associated with additional symptoms or atypical cases, including very severe or very mild forms of the disease. Based on the presence or the absence of molecular defects in *SMN*, a better nosology of SMA-related diseases has been established. These developments have greatly improved the clinical management and family-planning options of SMA patients and their parents. Molecular studies of *SMN* in children affected by type I SMA will allow predictive testing for other family members and should receive a high priority from everyone involved in the management of these lethal disorders.

### Prospects for Therapy of SMA

Currently, no primary treatment is available for SMA. The last 10 years, however, have seen major advances that should provide a foundation for developing therapeutic strategies. Some ideas based on our current understanding of SMA are as follows.

**Compensation of the *SMN* Defect by Expression of *SMNc*.** It is well established that *SMNc* expression is highly correlated with the clinical severity of the disease both in humans and, more recently, in mice. The alternative splicing of *SMNc* exon 7 leads to the production of both a full length and a truncated *SMNc* protein lacking the C-terminus (Fig. 231-4). Mice heterozygous for deletion of *Smn* exon 7 did not have an abnormal phenotype. This result argues against the hypothesis of a dominant negative effect of the truncated protein. Thus, the identification of agents able to induce SMNc gene expression may lead to attractive strategies for therapy of SMA.

Preventing exon 7 skipping in transcripts derived of the *SMNc* gene represents a related but alternative therapeutic approach. *SMN* is distinguished from *SMNc* by only five nucleotide differences (Fig. 231-4). One of these, located in exon 7, is responsible for the splicing out of exon 7 in a majority of *SMNc* transcripts and produces a transcript that encodes a protein with little or no function. Because SMA patients retain a normal *SMNc* gene, a strategy targeted at preventing *SMNc* exon 7 skipping theoretically could provide therapy for SMA.

**Identification of Incorrectly Spliced RNA Transcripts That Result from Spliceosome Malfunction.** *In vitro* biochemical investigations strongly support the view that the SMN protein has an important role in spliceosome function and pre-mRNA splicing. A logical therapeutic approach involves promoting assembly of spliceosomal components in the absence of SMN. At the current time, this approach is entirely theoretical but, as we learn more about the function of the SMN protein and its role in spliceosome assembly and processing of mRNA, this strategy may become feasible. Alternatively, identification of aberrantly spliced transcripts in the appropriate tissues, namely motor neurons, could lead to a better understanding of SMN pathophysiology. Mouse models of SMA represent important tools for this work. Comparative transcript or protein analyses of unaffected and affected spinal cord samples from these animals should contribute to the identification of RNA transcripts processed abnormally in *SMA*. Alternatively, the presence of a well-characterized RNA-processing defect in other tissues may help identify candidate RNA molecules in spinal cord. RNA molecule(s) defective in SMA may represent novel therapeutic targets to counter the disease process in SMA.

**The Molecular Pathway Resulting in Motor Neuron Degeneration.** The pathophysiology of SMA may, secondarily, involve a pathway similar to that observed in other neurodegenerative disorders. Identification of the molecules involved in these disorders could provide therapeutic targets in SMA. Neuroprotective agents or neurotrophic factors may protect neurons against toxicity or promote sprouting or survival of motor neurons. The availability of animal models will provide a system to test the efficacy of molecules with such biological properties in slowing or preventing the neurodegeneration of SMA.

The goal of prevention of neurodegeneration in SMA is both challenging and important. The observation of a severe denervation process in mouse models without marked loss of motor neurons strongly suggests that motor neuron loss is a late manifestation of the disease. Thus, there appears to be a window of therapeutic opportunity between diagnosis and loss of motor function. Conditional expression of an intact *SMN* gene at different stages of the disease in the mouse models of SMA should provide an answer to this question and will open new avenues for therapy of this devastating neurodegenerative disease.

## ACKNOWLEDGMENTS

We greatly thank Arnold Munnich, Jean Louis Mandel, Jean Frezal, and Pierre Chambon for constant support and invaluable discussions. Work in our laboratory was supported by the Institut National de la Santé et de la Recherche Médicale (INSERM), the Association Française contre les Myopathies (AFM), the Fondation pour la Recherche Médicale and Families of SMA (USA).

## REFERENCES

1. Werdnig G: Zwei fruhinfantile hereditare Falle von progressiver Muskelatrophie unter dem Bilde der Dystrophie, aber auf neurotischer Grundlage. *Arch Psychiat* **22**:437, 1891.
2. Werdnig G: Die fruhinfantile progressive spinale amyotrophie. *Arch Psychiatr* **26**:706, 1894.
3. Hoffmann J: Uber die hereditare progressive spinale muskelatrophie in kindesalter. *Muenchen Med Wschr* **47**:1649, 1900.
4. Thomas N, Dubowitz V: The natural history of type I (severe) spinal muscular atrophy. *Neuromusc Disord* **4**:497, 1994.
5. Ignatius J: The natural history of severe spinal muscular atrophy—Further evidence for clinical subtypes. *Neuromusc Disord* **4**:527, 1994.
6. Zerres K, Wirth B, Rudnik-Schoneborn: Spinal muscular atrophy-clinical and genetic correlations. *Neuromusc Disord* **7**:202, 1997.
7. Kugelberg E, Welander L: Heredofamilial juvenile muscular atrophy simulating muscular dystrophy. *Acta Neurol Psychiatr* **75**:500, 1956.
8. Bouwsma G, Vanwijngaarden: Spinal muscular atrophy and hypertrophy of the calves. *J Neurol Sci* **44**:275, 1980.
9. Pearn J, Hudgson P, Walton JN: A clinical and genetic study of spinal muscular atrophy of adult onset. *Brain* **101**:591, 1978.
10. Munsat TL: Workshop report: International SMA collaboration. *Neuromusc Disord* **1**:81, 1991.
11. Namba T, Aberfeld DC, Grob D: Chronic spinal muscular atrophy. *J Neurol Sci* **11**:401, 1970.
12. Moosa A, Dubowitz V: Motor nerve conduction velocity in spinal muscular atrophy of childhood. *Arch Dis Child* **51**:974, 1976.
13. Byers RK, Banker BQ: Infantile muscular atrophy. *Arch Neurol* **5**:140, 1961.
14. Mastaglia FL, Walton JN: Histological and histochemical changes from cases of chronic juvenile and early adult spinal muscular atrophy (the Kugelberg-Welander syndrome). *J Neurol Sci* **12**:15, 1971.
15. La Spada AR, Wilson EM, Lubahn DB, Harding AE, Fischbeck KH: Androgen receptor gene mutations in X-linked spinal muscular and bulbar muscular atrophy. *Nature* **352**:77, 1991.

16. Hanash A, Leguern E, Birouk N, Clermont O, Pouget J, Bouche P, Munnich A, et al: SMN gene analysis of the spinal form of Charcot-Marie-Tooth disease. *J Med Genet* **34**:507, 1997.

17. Christodoulou K, Kyriakides T, Hristova AH, Georgiou DM, Kalaydjieva L, Yshpekova B, Ivanova T, et al: Mapping of a distal form of spinal muscular atrophy with upper limb predominance to chromosome 7p. *Hum Mol Genet* **4**:1629, 1995.

18. Timmerman V, De Jonghe P, Simokovic S, Lofgren A, Beuten J, Nelis E, Ceuterick C, et al: Distal hereditary motor neuropathy type II (distal HMN II): Mapping of a locus to chromosome 12q24. *Hum Mol Genet* **5**:1065, 1996.

19. Roberts DF, Chavez J, Court SDM: The genetic component in child mortality. *Arch Dis Child* **45**:33, 1970.

20. Pearn J: The gene frequency of acute Werdnig-Hoffmann disease (SMA type I). A total population survey in North-East England. *J Med Genet* **10**:260, 1973.

21. Pearn J: Incidence, prevalence and gene frequency studies of chronic childhood spinal muscular atrophy. *J Med Genet* **15**:409, 1978.

22. Czeizel A, Hamula J: A Hungarian study on Werdnig-Hoffmann disease. *J Med Genet* **26**:761, 1989.

23. Hausmanowa-Petrusewicz I, Zaremba J, Borkowska J: Chronic proximal spinal muscular atrophy of childhood and adolescence: Problems of classification and genetic counselling. *J Med Genet* **22**:350, 1985.

24. Bouwsma G, Leschot NJ: Unusual pedigree patterns in seven families with spinal muscular atrophy: Further evidence for the allelic model hypothesis. *Clin Genet* **30**:145, 1986.

25. Zerres K, Stephan M, Kehren U, Grimm T: Becker's allelic model to explain unusual pedigrees with spinal muscular atrophy. *Clin Genet* **31**:276, 1987.

26. Muller B, Melki J, Burlet P, Clerget-Darpoux F: Proximal spinal muscular atrophy (SMA) types II and III in the same sibship are not caused by different alleles at the SMA locus on 5q. *Am J Hum Genet* **50**:892, 1992.

27. Bruzstowicz LM, Lehner T, Castilla LH, Penchaszadeh GK, Wilhelmsen KC, Daniels RJ, Davies KE, et al: Genetic mapping of chronic childhood-onset spinal muscular atrophy to chromosome 5q11.2-q13.3. *Nature* **344**:540, 1990.

28. Melki J, Abdelhak S, Sheth P, Bachelot MF, Burlet P, Marcadet A, Aicardi J, et al: Gene for proximal spinal muscular atrophies maps to chromosome 5q. *Nature* **344**:767, 1990.

29. Melki J, Sheth P, Abdelhak S, Burlet P, Bachelot MF, Lathrop M, Frézal J, et al: Mapping of acute (type I) spinal muscular atrophy to chromosome 5q12-q14. *Lancet* **336**:271, 1990.

30. Gilliam TC, Bruzstowicz LM, Castilla LH, Lehner T, Penchaszadeh GK, Daniels RJ, Byth BC, et al: Genetic homogeneity between acute and chronic forms of spinal muscular atrophy. *Nature* **345**:823, 1990.

31. Melki J, Abdelahak S, Burlet P, Raclin V, Kaplan J, Spiegel R, Gilgenkantz S, et al: Prenatal prediction of Werdnig-Hoffmann disease using linked polymorphic DNA probes. *J Med Genet* **29**:171, 1992.

32. Daniels RJ, Suthers GK, Morrison KE, Thomas NH, Francis MJ, Mathew CG, Loughlin S, et al: Prenatal prediction of spinal muscular atrophy. *J Med Genet* **29**:165, 1992.

33. Francis MJ, Morrisson KE, Campbell L, Grewal PK, Christodoulou Z, Daniels RJ, Monaco AP, et al: A contig of non-chimeric YACs containing the spinal muscular atrophy gene in 5q13. *Hum Mol Genet* **2**:1161, 1993.

34. Kleyn PW, Ang CH, Lien LL, Vitale E, Pan J, Ross BM, Grunn A, et al: Construction of a yeast artificial chromosome contig spanning the SMA disease gene region. *Proc Natl Acad Sci U S A* **90**:6801, 1993.

35. Melki J, Lefebvre S, Bürglen L, Burlet P, Clermont O, Millasseau P, Reboullet S: *De novo* and inherited deletions of the 5q13 region in spinal muscular atrophies. *Science* **264**:1474, 1994.

36. Wirth B, Schmidt T, Hahnen E, Rudnik-Schöneborn S, Krawczak M, Müller-Myhsok B, Schönling J, et al: *De novo* rearrangements found in 2% of index patients with spinal muscular atrophy: Mutational mechanisms, parental origin, mutation rate and implications for genetic counselling. *Am J Hum Genet* **61**:1102, 1997.

37. Campbell L, Daniels RJ, Dubowitz V, Davies KE: Maternal mosaicism for a second mutational event in a type I spinal muscular atrophy family. *Am J Hum Genet* **63**:37, 1998.

38. Lefebvre S, Bürglen L, Reboullet S, Clermont O, Burlet P, Viollet L, Benichou B, et al: Identification and characterization of a spinal muscular atrophy-determining gene. *Cell* **80**:155, 1995.

39. Roy N, Mahadevan MS, McLean M, Shutler G, Yaraghi Z, Farahani R, Baird S, et al: The gene for neuronal apoptosis inhibitor protein is partially deleted in individuals with spinal muscular atrophy. *Cell* **80**:167, 1995.

40. Bürglen L, Seroz T, Miniou P, Lefebvre S, Burlet P, Munnich A, Viegas-Pequignot E, et al: The gene encoding p44, a subunit of the transcription factor TFIIH, is involved in large-scale deletions associated with Werdnig-Hoffmann disease. *Am J Hum Genet* **60**:72, 1997.

41. Carter TA, Bönnemann CG, Wang CH, Obici S, Parano E, de Fatima Bonaldo M, Ross BM, et al: A multicopy transcription-repair gene, BTF2p44, maps to the SMA region and demonstrates SMA associated deletions. *Hum Mol Genet* **6**:229, 1997.

42. Scharf JM, Endrizzi MG, Wetter A, Huang S, Thompson TG, Zerres K, Dietrich WF, et al: Identification of a candidate modifying gene for spinal muscular atrophy by comparative genomics. *Nat Genet* **20**:83, 1998.

43. Chen Q, Baird SD, Mahadevan M, Besner-Johnston A, Farahani R, Xuan JY, Kang X, et al: Sequence of a 131-kb region of 5q13.1 containing the spinal muscular atrophy candidate genes SMN and NAIP. *Genomics* **48**:121, 1998.

44. Bussaglia E, Clermont O, Tizzano E, Lefebvre S, Bürglen L, Cruaud C, Urtizberea JA, et al: A frame-shift deletion in the survival motor neuron gene in Spanish spinal muscular atrophy patients. *Nat Genet* **11**:335, 1995.

45. Cobben JM, Van der Steege G, Grootscholten PM, de Visser M, Scheffer, H, Buys C: Deletions of the survival motor neuron gene in unaffected siblings of patients with spinal muscular atrophy. *Am J Hum Genet* **57**:805, 1995.

46. Velasco E, Valero C, Valero A, Moreno F, Hernandez-Chico C: Molecular analysis of the SMN and NAIP genes in Spanish spinal muscular atrophy (SMA) families and correlation between number of copies of cBCD541 and SMA phenotype. *Hum Mol Genet* **5**:257, 1996.

47. Chang JG, Jong YJ, Huang JM, Wang WS, Yang TY, Chang CP, Chen YJ, et al: Molecular analysis of spinal muscular atrophy in Chinese. *Am J Hum Genet* **57**:1503, 1995.

48. Rodrigues NR, Owen N, Talbot K, Patel S, Muntoni F, Ignatius J, Dubowitz, et al: Gene deletions in spinal muscular atrophy. *J Med Genet* **33**:93, 1996.

49. Capon F, Levato C, Semprini S, Pizzuti A, Merlini L, Novelli G, Dallapiccola B: Deletion analysis of SMN and NAIP genes in spinal muscular atrophy Italian families. *Muscle Nerve* **19**:378, 1996.

50. Spiegel R, Hagmann A, Boltshauser E, Moser H: Molecular genetic diagnosis and deletion analysis in Type I-III spinal muscular atrophy. *Schweiz Med Wochenschr* **126**:907, 1996.

51. Wirth B, Herz M, Wetter A, Moskau S, Hahnen E, Rudnik-Schoneborn S, Wienker T, et al: Quantitative analysis of survival motor neuron copies: Identification of subtle SMN1 mutations in patients with spinal muscular atrophy, genotype-phenotype correlation, and implications for genetic counseling. *Am J Hum Genet* **64**:1340, 1999.

52. Parsons DW, McAndrew PE, Monani UR, Mendell JR, Burghes AHM, Prior TW: An 11 base pair duplication in exon 6 of the SMN gene produces a type I spinal muscular atrophy (SMA) phenotype: Further evidence for SMN as the primary SMA-determining gene. *Hum Mol Genet* **5**:1727, 1996.

53. Brahe C, Clermont O, Zappata S, Tiziano F, Melki J, Neri G: Frameshift mutation in the survival motor neuron gene in a severe case of SMA type I. *Hum Mol Genet* **5**:1971, 1996.

54. Talbot K, Ponting CP, Theodosiou AM, Rodrigues NR, Surtees R, Mountford R, Davies KE: Missense mutation clustering in the survival motor neuron gene: A role for a conserved tyrosine and glycine rich region of the protein in RNA metabolism? *Hum Mol Genet* **6**:497, 1997.

55. Hahnen E, Schönling J, Rudnik-Schöneborn S, Raschke H, Zerres K, Wirth B: Missense mutations in exon 6 of the survival motor neuron gene in patients with spinal muscular atrophy (SMA). *Hum Mol Genet* **6**:821, 1997.

56. Bürglen L, Patel S, Dubowitz V, Melki J, Muntoni F: A novel point mutation in the SMN gene in a patient with type III spinal muscular Atrophy. *First Congress of the World Muscle Society.* London, Elsevier, S39, 1996.

57. Burglen L, Lefebvre S, Clermont O, Burlet P, Viollet L, Cruaud C, Munnich A, Melki J: Structure and organization of the human survival motor neurone gene. *Genomics* **32**:479, 1996.

58. Lorson CL, Hahnen E, Androphy EJ, Wirth B: A single nucleotide in the SMN gene regulates splicing and is responsible for spinal muscular atrophy. *Proc Natl Acad Sci U S A* **96**:6307, 1999.

59. Van der Steege G, Grootscholten PM, van der Vlies P, Draaijirs TG, Osinga J, Cobben JM, Scheffer H, et al: PCR-based DNA test to confirm clinical diagnosis of autosomal recessive spinal muscular atrophy. *Lancet* **345**:985, 1995.

60. Raclin V, Saugier-Veber P, Bürglen L, Munnich A, Melki J: *De novo* deletions in spinal muscular atrophy: Implications for genetic counselling. *J Med Genet* **34**:86,1997.

61. Bürglen L, Spiegel R, Ignatus J, Cobben JM, Landrieu P, Lefebvre S, Munnich A, et al: SMN gene deletion in variant of infantile spinal muscular atrophy. *Lancet* **346**:316, 1995.

62. Bürglen L, Amiel J, Viollet L, Lefebvre S, Burlet P, Clermont O, Raclin V, et al: SMN gene deletion in the arthrogryposis multiplex congenital-spinal muscular atrophy association. *J Clin Invest* **98**:1130, 1996.

63. Korinthenberg R, Sauer M, Ketelsen UP, Hanemann CO, Stoll G, Graf M, Baborie A, et al: Congenital axonal neuropathy caused by deletions in the spinal muscular atrophy region. *Ann Neurol* **42**:364, 1997.

64. Brahe C, Servidei S, Zappata S, Ricci E, Tonali P, Neri G: Genetic homogeneity between childhood-onset and adult-onset autosomal recessive spinal muscular atrophy. *Lancet* **346**:741, 1995.

65. Zerres K, Rudnik-Schöneborn S, Forket R, Wirth B: Genetic basis of adult onset muscular atrophy. *Lancet* **346**:1162, 1995.

66. Clermont O, Burlet P, Lefebvre S, Bürglen L, Munnich A, Melki J: SMN gene deletions in adult-onset spinal muscular atrophy. *Lancet* **346**:1712, 1995.

67. Novelli G, Capon F, Tamisari L, Grandi E, Angelini C, Guerrini P, Dallapiccola B: Neonatal spinal muscular atrophy with diaphragmatic paralysis is unlinked to 5q11.2-q13. *J Med Genet* **32**:216, 1995.

68. Rudnik-Schoneborn S, Wirth B, Rohrig D, Saule H, Zerres K: Exclusion of the gene locus for spinal muscular atrophy on chromosome 5q in a family with infantile olivopontocerebellar atrophy (OPCA) and anterior horn cell degeneration. *Neuromuscul Disord* **5**:19, 1995.

69. Kausch K, Muller CR, Grimm T, Ricker K, Rietschel M, Rudnik-Schoneborn S, Zerres K: No evidence for linkage of autosomal dominant proximal spinal muscular atrophies to chromosome 5q markers. *Hum Genet* **86**:317, 1991.

70. Jackson M, Morrison KE, Al-Chalabi A, Bakker M, Leigh PN: Analysis of chromosome 5q13 genes in amyotrophic lateral sclerosis: Homozygous NAIP deletion in a sporadic case. *Ann Neurol* **39**:796, 1996.

71. Bartholdi D, Gonzalez H, Borg C, Melki J: Absence of SMN gene deletion in post-polio syndrome. *Neuromusc Disord* **10**:99, 2000.

72. Hahnen E, Fokert R, Marke C, Rudnik-Schöneborn S, Schönling J, Zerres K, Wirth B: Molecular analysis of candidate genes on chromosome 5q13 in autosomal recessive spinal muscular atrophy: Evidence of homozygous deletions of SMN gene in unaffected individuals. *Hum Mol Genet* **4**:1927, 1995.

73. Wang CH, Xu J, Carter TA, Ross BM, Dominski MK, Bellcross CA, Penchaszadeh GK, et al: Characterization of survival motor neuron (SMNt) gene deletions in asymptomatic carriers of spinal muscular atrophy. *Hum Mol Genet* **5**:359, 1996.

74. McAndrew PE, Parsons DW, Simard LR, Rochette C, Ray PN, Mendell JR, Prior TW, et al: 22 Identification of proximal spinal muscular atrophy carriers and patients by analysis of SMNT and SMNC gene copy number. *Am J Hum Genet* **60**:1411, 1997.

75. Parsons DW, McAndrew PE, Allinson PS, Parker WD Jr, Burghes AH, Prior TW: Diagnosis of spinal muscular atrophy in an SMN non-deletion patient using a quantitative PCR screen and mutation analysis. *J Med Genet* **35**:674, 1998.

76. Schwartz M, Sorensen N, Hansen FJ, Hertz JM, Norby S, Tranebjaerg L, Skovby F: Quantification, by solid-phase minisequencing, of the telomeric and centromeric copies of the survival motor neuron gene in families with spinal muscular atrophy. *Hum Mol Genet* **6**:99, 1997.

77. Burlet P, Bürglen L, Clermont O, Lefebvre S, Viollet L, Munnich A, Melki J: Large-scale deletion of the 5q13 region are specific to Werdnig-Hoffmann disease. *J Med Genet* **33**:281, 1996.

78. Rodrigues NR, Owen N, Talbot K, Patel S, Muntoni F, Ignatius J, Dubowitz: Gene deletions in spinal muscular atrophy. *J Med Genet* **33**:93, 1996.

79. Campbell L, Potter A, Ignatius J, Dubowitz V, Davies KE: Genomic variation and gene conversion in spinal muscular atrophy: Implications for disease process and clinical phenotype. *Am J Hum Genet* **61**:40, 1997.

80. van der Steege G, Grootscholten PM, Cobben JM, Zappata S, Scheffer H, den Dunnen JT, et al: Apparent gene conversions involving the SMN gene in the region of the spinal muscular atrophy locus on chromosome 5. *Am J Hum Genet* **59**:834, 1996.

81. Talbot K, Rodrigues NR, Ignatius J, Muntoni F, Davies KE: Gene conversion at the SMN locus in autosomal recessive spinal muscular atrophy does not predict a mild phenotype. *Neuromuscul Disord* **7**:198, 1997.

82. Dreyfuss G, Matunis MJ, Piñol-Roma S, Burd CG: hnRNP proteins and biogenesis of mRNA. *Ann Rev Biochem* **62**:89, 1993.

83. Liu Q, Dreyfuss G: A novel nuclear structure containing the survival of motor neuron proteins. *EMBO J* **15**:3555, 1996.

84. Noble SM, Guthrie C: Transcriptional pulse-chase analysis reveals a role for a novel snRNP-associated protein in the manufacture of spiceosomal snRNPs. *EMBO J* **15**:4368, 1996.

85. Liu Q, Fischer U, Wang F, Dreyfuss G: The spinal muscular atrophy disease gene product, SMN, and its associated protein SIP1 are in a complex with spliceosomal snRNP proteins. *Cell* **90**:1013, 1997.

86. Gall JG, Tsvetkov A, Wu ZA, Murphy C: Is the sphere organelle coiled body a universal nuclear component? *Dev Genet* **16**:25, 1995.

87. Carvalho T, Almeida F, Calapez A, Lafarga M, Berciano MT, Carmo-Fonseca M: The spinal muscular atrophy disease gene product, SMN: A link between snRNP biogenesis and the Cajal (Coiled) body. *J Cell Biol* **147**:715, 1999.

88. Fischer U, Liu Q, Dreyfuss G: The SMN-SIP1 complex has an essential role in spliceosomal snRNP biogenesis. *Cell* **90**:1023, 1997.

89. DeRobertis EM: Nucleoplasmic segregation of proteins and RNAs. *Cell* **32**:1021, 1983.

90. Mattaj IW, Englmeier L: Nucleoplasmic transport: the soluble phase. *Annu Rev Biochem* **67**:265, 1998.

91. Neuman de Vegvar H, Dahlberg JE: Nucleocytoplasmic transport and processing of small nuclear RNA precursor. *Mol Cell Biol* **10**:3365, 1990.

92. Mattaj IW: U snRNP assembly and transport, in Birnstiel M (ed): *Structure and Function of Major and Minor Small Nuclear Ribonucleoprotein Particles.* New York, Springer-Verlag, 1988, p 100.

93. Pellizzoni L, Naoyuki K, Charroux B, Dreyfuss G: A novel function for SMN, the spinal muscular atrophy disease gene product, in pre-mRNA splicing. *Cell* **95**:615, 1998.

94. Lorson CL, Strasswimmer J, Yao JM, Baleja JD, Hahnen E, Wirth B, Le T, et al: SMN oligomerization defect correlates with spinal muscular atrophy severity. *Nat Genet* **19**:63, 1998.

95. Pellizzoni L, Charroux B, Dreyfuss G: SMN mutants of spinal muscular atrophy patients are defective in binding to snRNP proteins. *Proc Natl Acad Sci U S A* **96**:11167, 1999.

96. Frugier T, Tiziano FD, Cifuentes-Diaz C, Miniou P, Roblot N, Dierich A, Le Meur M, et al: Nuclear targeting defect of SMN lacking the C-terminus in a mouse model of spinal muscular atrophy. *Hum Mol Genet* **9**:849, 2000.

97. Gall J, Bellini M, Wu Z, Murphy C: Assembly of the nuclear transcription and processing machinery: Cajal bodies (coiled bodies) and transcriptosomes. *Mol Biol Cell* **10**:4385, 1999.

98. Lefebvre S, Burlet P, Liu Q, Bertrandy S, Clermont O, Munnich A, Dreyfuss G, et al: Correlation between severity and SMN protein level in spinal muscular atrophy. *Nat Genet* **16**:265, 1997.

99. Iwahashi H, Eguchi Y, Yasuhara N, Hanafusa T, Matsuzawa Y, Tsujimoto Y: Synergistic anti-apoptotic activity between Bcl-2 and SMN implicated in spinal muscular atrophy. *Nature* **390**:413, 1997.

100. Coovert DD, Le TT, McAndrew PE, Strasswimmer J, Crawford TO, Mendell JR, Coulson S, et al: The survival motor neuron protein in spinal muscular atrophy. *Hum Mol Genet* **6**:1205, 1997.

101. Battaglia G, Princivalle A, Forti F, Lizier C, Zeviani M: Expression of the SMN gene, the spinal muscular atrophy determining gene, in the mammalian central nervous system. *Hum Mol Genet* **6**:1961, 1997.

102. Echaniz-Laguna A, Miniou P, Bartholdi D, Melki J: The promoters of the survival motor neuron gene (SMN) and its copy (SMNc) share common regulatory elements. *Am J Hum Genet* **64**:1365, 1999.

103. Monani UR, PcPherson JD, Burghes AHM: Promoter analysis of the human centromeric and telomeric survival motor neuron genes (SMNc and SMNt). *Biochem Biophys Acta* **1445**:330, 1999.

104. Violet L, Bertrandy S, Bueno Brunialti AL, Lefebvre S, Burlet P, Clermont O, Cruaud C, et al: cDNA isolation, expression and chromosomal localization of the mouse survival motor neuron gene (Smn). *Genomics* **40**:185, 1997.

105. DiDonato CJ, Chen XN, Kerenberg JR, Nadeau JH, Simard LR: Cloning, characterization and copy number of the murine survival motor neuron gene: Homolog of the spinal muscular atrophy-determining gene. *Genome Res* **7**:339, 1997.

106. Schrank B, Götz R, Gunnersen JM, Ure JM, Toyka KV, Smith AG, Sendtner M: Inactivation of the survival motor neuron gene, a candidate gene for human spinal muscular atrophy, leads to massive cell death in early mouse embryos. *Proc Natl Acad Sci U S A* **94**:9920, 1997.

107. Hsieh-Li HM, Chang JG, Jong YJ, Wu MH, Wang NM, Tsai CH, Li H: A mouse model for spinal muscular atrophy. *Nat Genet* **24**:66, 2000.

108. Monani U.R, Sendtner M, Coovert DD, Parons WD, Andreassi C, Le TT, Jablonka S, et al: The human centromeric survival motor neuron gene (SMN2) rescues embryonic lethality in SMN −/− mice and results in a mouse with spinal muscular atrophy. *Hum Mol Genet* **9**:333, 2000.

109. Sternberg N, Hamilton D: Bacteriophage P1 site-specific recombination. I. Recombination between loxP sites. *J Mol Biol* **150**:467, 1981.

110. Sauer B, Henderson N: Site-specific DNA recombination in mammalian cells by the Cre recombinase of bacteriophage P1. *Proc Natl Acad Sci U S A* **85**:5166, 1988.

# Friedreich Ataxia and AVED

*Michel Koenig*

## CLINICAL AND PATHOLOGIC FEATURES

In 1863, Nicholaus Friedreich, Professor of Medicine in Heidelberg, described a "degenerative atrophy of the posterior columns of the spinal cord" leading to progressive ataxia, sensory loss and muscle weakness, often associated with scoliosis, foot deformity, and cardiopathy.[1,2] Not until the late 1970s were large series of patients analyzed to establish clear diagnostic criteria.[3,4] Recessive inheritance was firmly established as an essential feature of Friedreich ataxia (FRDA).[3–6] The Québec Collaborative Group identified the clinical features of typical FRDA and proposed them as diagnostic criteria.[3] They were, however, too strict for the diagnosis of early cases. Harding distinguished the early signs and symptoms from those that may not be present at the onset, but that have to manifest as the disease evolves[4] (Table 232-1). These studies, as well as more recent ones,[7,8] identified an important degree of clinical variability, both among and within the families. Atypical FRDA, including adult-onset Friedreich ataxia (LOFA)[9,10] (MIM 229300), and Friedreich ataxia with retained reflexes (FARR), a variant in which tendon reflexes in the lower limbs are preserved,[11] were recognized by genetic linkage studies to be part of the same entity. The identification of the most common FRDA mutation, an unstable hyperexpansion of a GAA triplet repeat polymorphism,[12] clarified the origin and mechanism of the clinical variations.

Onset is usually around puberty, but wide variations are observed, ranging from 2 to 50 years (mean and standard deviation are $15\pm8$ years).[13] "Typical" FRDA patients have onset before age 20.[3] Age of onset is more variable among families than within families.[4,14] Gait instability (65 percent) or generalized clumsiness (25 percent) is the usual initial symptom. Occasionally, nonneurologic manifestations, such as as scoliosis (5 percent) or cardiomyopathy (5 percent), precede the onset of ataxia.[15]

The cardinal neurologic feature of FRDA is a progressive, unremitting, mixed cerebellar-sensory ataxia. Most commonly, it begins with clumsiness in gait and frequent falls (truncal ataxia). Limb incoordination, dysmetria, and intention tremor then follow. Speech becomes slow and jerky with sudden utterances (dysarthria) within 5 years after onset.[3,4,7,8] Deep sensory loss is another cardinal manifestation of FRDA. Loss of position and vibration sense is commonly found at onset and invariably after 2 years. Perception of light touch, pain, and temperature are initially normal, but tend to decrease in most patients with advanced disease. Also a consequence of sensory axonal neuropathy, the loss of tendon reflexes, at least in the lower limbs, has been considered an obligatory feature that needs to be present at onset to establish

the diagnosis.[3,4] Extensor plantar response was also considered an obligatory sign. However, exceptions exist. Other pyramidal signs (spasticity) are usually absent, obscured by the predominant loss of tendon reflexes and decrease of muscle tone.[15] Muscle weakness is common and progressive, particularly at the lower limbs, usually affecting the proximal muscles first.[16] Atrophy of distal lower limb muscles and of small hand muscles is sometimes observed, even early in the course of the disease.[4] The most common abnormality of ocular movements in FRDA is fixation instability.[17] Ophthalmoparesis is not observed and nystagmus is uncommon. About 30 percent of the patients develop optic atrophy, with or without visual impairment, particularly in the later stages of disease.[15] Sensorineural hearing loss, more common with advanced disease, affects about 20 percent of the patients.[18,19]

Neuropathologic studies show an invariable loss of the large primary sensory neurons of the dorsal root ganglia (DRG).[20] Atrophy of the central branches of the corresponding axons causes thinning of the dorsal roots, particularly at the lumbosacral level, and atrophy of the peripheral branches causes loss of large myelinated fibers from peripheral nerves. The fine unmyelinated fibers are well preserved, and interstitial connective tissue is increased. The motor component of peripheral nerves is well preserved. Degeneration of the posterior columns of the spinal cord is the hallmark of the disease.[20] The posterior columns contain the central axonal branches of the large sensory neurons. As for the DRG, the fibers originating more caudally are more severely affected. Atrophy is also observed in the spinocerebellar tracts, the dorsal being more affected than the ventral. Clarke columns, where the spinocerebellar tracts originate, show severe loss of neurons. Therefore, the sensory systems providing information to the brain and cerebellum about the position and speed of body segments, particularly the lower limbs, are severely compromised in FRDA. Motor neurons in the ventral horns are well preserved, but the long crossed and uncrossed corticospinal motor tracts are atrophied, explaining the pyramidal signs. The pattern of atrophy of the corticospinal tracts suggests a "dying back" process.[21] In the brain stem, *trans*-synaptic degeneration can be observed in the gracile and cuneate nuclei where the dorsal column tracts terminate, and in the medial lemnisci that continue the central sensory pathway above these nuclei.[20] Sensory cranial nerves also show myelin pallor and loss of fibers. The cerebellar cortex shows only mild loss of Purkinje cells late in the disease course. This pattern of involvement contrasts with other inherited degenerative ataxias,[22] in particular with the group of early onset ataxias with retained reflexes (EOCA), where the cerebellum is much more atrophic than the cervical spinal cord. The deep cerebellar nuclei, where cerebellar efferents originate, are severely affected with marked neuronal loss and gliosis in the dentate nucleus.[20] As a consequence, the superior cerebellar pedunculi appear markedly atrophic. Other cerebral structures do not appear to be directly involved by the disease, with the exception of a loss of large pyramidal cells in the primary motor areas.

Cardiomyopathy is a frequent nonneurologic finding in FRDA. Cardiac involvement is more often observed in patients with an

A list of standard abbreviations is located immediately preceding the index in each volume. Additional abbreviations used in this chapter include: AVED = ataxia with isolated vitamin E deficiency; CMT = Charcot-Marie-Tooth disease; DRG = dorsal root ganglia; EOCA = early onset Friedreich ataxia with retained reflexes; FARR = Friedreich ataxia with retained reflexes; FRDA = Friedreich ataxia; LOFA = late onset Friedreich ataxia; MPP = mitochondrial processing peptidase; NCV = nerve conduction velocity; SAP = sensory action potential; VLCFA = very long chain fatty acids.

**Table 232-1** Compared Frequency of Clinical Signs Between Friedreich Ataxia and AVED Patients

| Clinical sign | Friedreich ataxia | | AVED |
| --- | --- | --- | --- |
| | Dürr et al.[13] % | Harding[4] % | Cavalier et al.[103] % |
| Gait and limb ataxia | 99 | 99 | 98 |
| Dysarthria | 91 | 97 | 77 (39) |
| Lower-limb areflexia | 87 | 99 | 85 (40) |
| Loss of vibratory sense | 78 | 73 | 86 |
| Extensor plantar reflexes | 79 | 89 | 58 |
| Muscle weakness in lower limb | 67 | 88 | 35 (31) |
| Head titubation | 0 | — | 37 (39) |
| Cardiomyopathy | 63 (75) | — | 19 (42) |
| Diabetes or impaired glucose tolerance | 32 (61) | 10 | 0 (16) |
| n* | 140 | 115 | 43 |

*Number of patients, unless otherwise noted (in parentheses after the corresponding frequency).

earlier age of onset. The most common complaints are shortness of breath (40 percent of patients) and palpitations (11 percent).[4] Enlargement of the heart is the typical finding, with thickening of ventricular walls and/or interventricular septum,[23,24] which is best evidenced by echocardiography.[4,25] Electrocardiographic abnormalities include widespread T-wave inversions and signs of ventricular hypertrophy.

About 10 percent of FRDA patients have diabetes mellitus, and an additional 20 percent have carbohydrate intolerance. A detailed study of glucose and insulin metabolism in FRDA patients revealed a deficiency in arginine-stimulated insulin secretion in all cases, including normotolerant individuals,[26] suggesting that beta cells are invariably affected by the primary genetic defect of FRDA. The pancreas of patients with diabetes mellitus show a loss of islet cells without sign of autoimmune inflamation.[27]

Most patients have skeletal abnormalities even in the early phase of the disease. Kyphoscoliosis affects over 85 percent of patients and may be severe in 10 percent, particularly when onset is before puberty.[3] It may cause pain and cardiorespiratory problems. Pes cavus and pes equinovarus, although found in more than 50 percent of patients, are not typical of FRDA, being even more common in other neuropathic diseases as Charcot-Marie-Tooth disease (CMT).

Electromyographic and electroneurographic studies in FRDA reveal the underlying dying-back axonal sensory neuropathy. Sensory action potentials (SAPs) in peripheral nerves are severely reduced or absent, even early in the course of the disease.[28-30] Motor and sensory nerve conduction velocities (NCVs) are within or just below the normal range, a feature that helps distinguishing an early case of FRDA from a case of demyelinating hereditary sensorimotor neuropathy, as CMT.

## DIFFERENTIAL DIAGNOSIS

FRDA may mimic other neuropathies or ataxias, particularly at the early stages of the disease when clinical presentation is not complete. The range of diseases that may overlap with FRDA depends on the age of onset. Early onset may pose the problem of differential diagnosis with ataxia telangiectasia, mitochondrial disorders, adrenoleukodystrophy, and several lysosomal storage diseases. These can be distinguished from FRDA by abnormal values of circulating α-fetoprotein and carcinoembryonic antigen, lactate, pyruvate, serum very long chain fatty acids (VLCFA),

urinary organic acids, and leukocyte and/or fibroblast lysosomal enzymes. Inherited vitamin E deficiencies have an onset range similar to FRDA. Measurement of serum vitamin E and lipoproteins will identify the cases with AVED (ataxia with isolated vitamin E deficiency, discussed below) and abetalipoproteinemia (Bassen-Kornzweig disease). Later onset will pose the problem of differential diagnosis with adrenomyeloneuropathy (elevated VLCFA), Refsum disease (elevated serum phytanic acid), CMT, which can be distinguished from FRDA by electromyography as discussed above, and dominant ataxias that have no sensory components and show cerebellar atrophy on CT scans or MRI. For all these diseases, atypical presentations exist with late onset recessive cases due to mild missense mutations or early onset dominant cases by anticipation, which adds to the difficulty of diagnosis at onset.

## PROGNOSIS AND TREATMENT

FRDA is a progressive disease that inevitably leads to increasing disability. Patients lose their ability to walk on average 15 years after onset, but variability is very large.[4,31] Early onset and left ventricular hypertrophy appear to be predictors of a faster rate of progression of the disease.[31,32] The burden of neurologic impairment, cardiomyopathy, and, occasionally, diabetes cause a shortened life expectancy.[31] Older studies found that most patients died in their thirties, but survival may be significantly prolonged with treatment of cardiac symptoms, particularly arrhythmias, by antidiabetic treatment (insulin is the eventual treatment), and by preventing and controlling complications resulting from prolonged disability. Carefully assisted patients may live several more decades. Physical therapy can help patients in dealing with their neurologic deficit. Hypotheses for future therapies based on antioxidants and iron chelators were proposed following the discovery of the defective gene.

## THE FRDA GENE

In the early 1980s, several seemingly contradictory reports suggested that anomalies of the intermediate metabolism were present in FRDA.[33] In the absence of a convincing biochemical defect, positional cloning appeared as the sole strategy to identify the Friedreich ataxia gene. The FRDA gene was localized on chromosome 9 by linkage analysis with restriction fragment length polymorphisms (RFLP) by Chamberlain's group of in 1988,[34] and localization was confirmed shortly thereafter with a second, tightly linked RFLP located in 9q13-q21.[35,36] Subsequent genetic studies indicated that FRDA is a homogenous genetic entity, located close to the initial two linked RFLPs.[37-40] The construction of a 1-Mb physical map saturated with highly polymorphic microsatellite markers[41] and analysis, in an international collaborative effort, of rare meiotic recombination events allowed us to progressively narrow down the disease locus to a final 150 kb interval,[42] excluding several genes that we and others identified in the region[43-45] (Fig. 232-1).

A novel gene was isolated in the critical interval, but the search for mutations in the protein-coding exons was initially deceiving. Only 5 of 184 unrelated patients studied had a point mutation in the heterozygous state, which is inconsistent with a recessive inheritance.[12] Search for gross alterations in the noncoding parts of the frataxin gene eventually revealed the presence in all patients of an enlarged fragment in intron 1. Sequencing showed a short GAA trinucleotide repeat, located in the middle of an Alu sequence, that is massively expanded into the 200 to 1300 repeat range, on 98 percent of the alleles of patients with typical FRDA.[12] This was unexpected, because trinucleotide expansions had previously been found only in diseases showing clinical anticipation (a feature that cannot be observed in an autosomal recessive disease such as FRDA), and involved the GC-rich triplets CGG/CCG and CAG/CTG.[46] The gene encoded a novel protein of unknown function that was named frataxin.

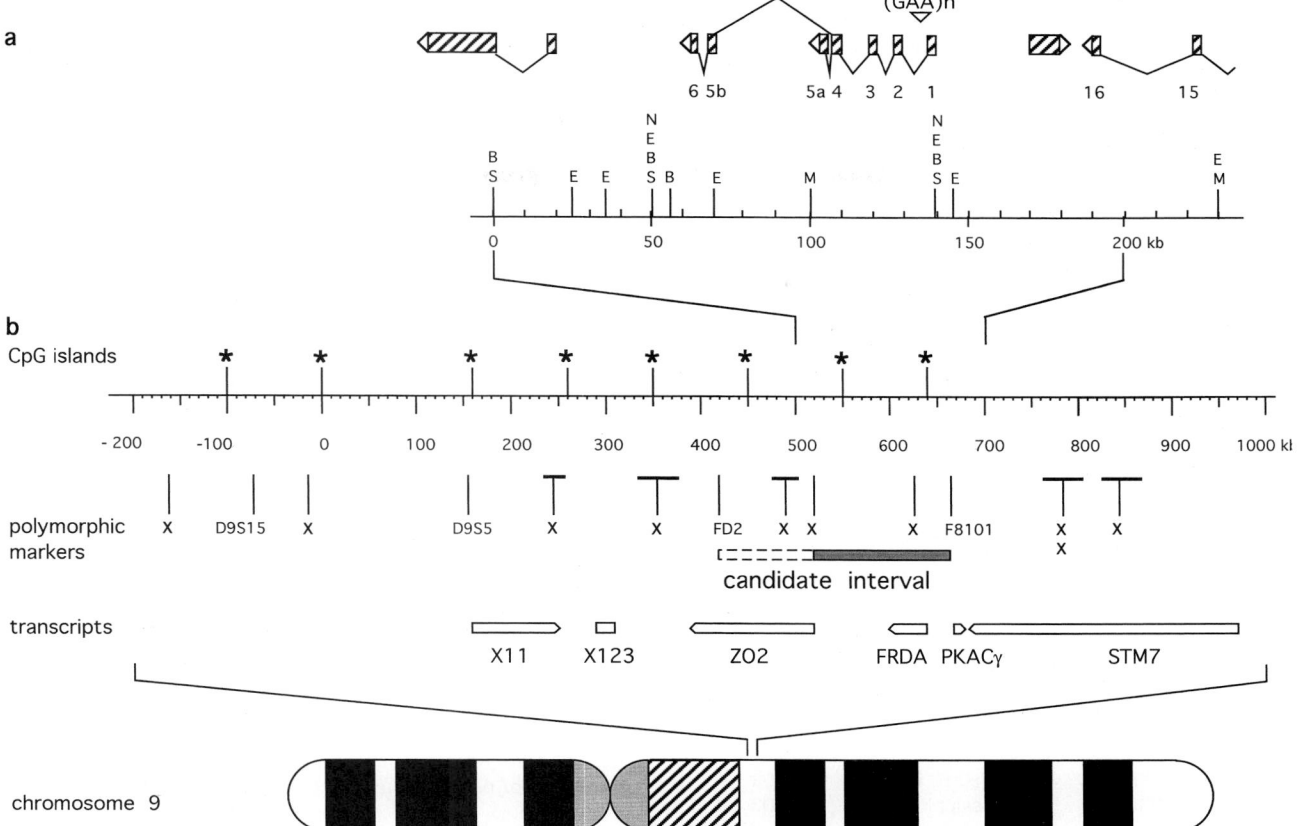

Fig. 232-1 *A*, Exon structure of the frataxin gene. (GAA)n indicates the position of the trinucleotide expansion in patients. Position of CpG islands is indicated by cluster of rare cutter enzymes. *B*, The Friedreich ataxia region on chromosome 9q13. Some polymorphic markers, that were critical to map the FRDA gene, are indicated. Other markers are indicated by Xs. The candidate region was eventually narrowed down to 240 kb between FD2 and F8101. Absence of mutations in the ZO2 gene of patients further reduced the critical interval to 150 kb (gray bar). The position of CpG islands is indicated by asterisks. A transcriptional map is shown at the bottom. Arrowheads indicate the direction of transcription, when known.

The human frataxin gene encompasses 80 kb and is composed of 7 exons, 2 of which (5b and 6) are used only in a quantitatively minor alternative transcript (Fig. 232-1). Northern blot analysis in human and mouse, RNAse protection assay, and cDNA cloning indicate that the 1.3-kb major transcript is made from 5 exons (1 to 5a). This transcript encodes a protein of 210 amino acids that has no resemblance to proteins of known function, although well-conserved homologues have been identified in the worm *C. elegans* and in the yeast (*S. cerevisiae*) from the systematic genome sequencing projects of these organisms. The claim that the exons of the frataxin gene are in fact alternative 3′ exons of the neighboring STM7 gene,[47] was subsequently negated.[48–50]

Expression of the frataxin gene was analyzed by northern blot (in human and mouse tissues) and by *in situ* hybridization (in mouse only), and correlates in part with the main sites of pathology of the disease.[12,48,51] DRG are the major sites of expression in the nervous system, from embryonic day 12 until adult life. They contain the cell bodies of all sensory nerves, receiving axons from the periphery and sending axons to the posterior columns up to the bulb. Deep sensory neuropathy and degeneration of the posterior columns appear therefore as a direct consequence of reduced frataxin level in these structures. Expression in the spinal cord is comparatively much lower, suggesting that degeneration of the spinocerebellar tracts and of the Clarke columns containing, respectively, the axons and the cell bodies (in the posterior horn) of secondary neurons projecting to the cerebellum might be secondary to degeneration of the DRG neurons. Significant frataxin expression is also observed in the granular layer of the cerebellum. Degeneration of the motor corticospinal (pyramidal) tracts might correlate with frataxin expression in mature cells of the developing forebrain,[51] although it was not detected in mouse adult cerebral cortex.[48] Expression in mouse brain is mostly restricted to the periventricular zone in embryos and to the corresponding ependymal layer in adults.[48] The frataxin gene is also expressed in nonneuronal tissues, such as heart and pancreas, which may account for hypertrophic cardiomyopathy and the increased incidence of diabetes observed in FRDA patients.[12,48] Frataxin is also prominently expressed in tissues apparently not affected by the disease, such as liver, muscle, thymus, and brown fat. All tissues highly expressing frataxin are rich in mitochondria, with brown fat, present in newborns, being particularly rich.[48] The difference between nonaffected and affected tissues may lie in the nondividing nature of the latter (neurons, cardiocytes and *β* cells of the pancreas), implying that cells are not replaced when they die. In addition, neurons and cardiocytes have an exclusive aerobic metabolism, making them more sensitive to mitochondrial defect.

## THE FRDA MUTATIONS

All FRDA patients have at least one GAA expansion mutation, most being homozygotes for the expansion. Less than 5 percent are compound heterozygotes with a point mutation in the frataxin gene on the nonexpanded chromosome.[12,52] Truncating and missense mutations are equally represented (Table 232-2), although missense mutations are only found in the second half

**Table 232-2** Mutations in Friedreich Ataxia and AVED

**Point Mutations Found in Friedreich Ataxia**

| Nucleotide change | Predicted effect on coding sequence | Geographic origin | Reference |
|---|---|---|---|
| 1A>C | incorrect initiation | USA | 52 |
| 2T>C | incorrect initiation | Sweden | 52 |
| 3G>T | incorrect initiation | Germany, Poland | 49, 128 |
| 158delC | frameshift | France | 52 |
| 158insC | frameshift | Poland-Canada | 52 |
| 317T>G | L106X | France | 12 |
| 364G>T | D122Y | Germany | 52 |
| 384 + 1G > A | exon 3 skipping | England | 129 |
| 385-2A>G | exon 4 skipping | Spain | 12 |
| 389G>T | G130V | USA, France | 52–54 |
| 460A>T | I154F | Italy | 12 |
| 467T>C | L156P | Sweden | 52 |
| 482 + 3delA | exon 4 skipping | Italy | 52 |
| 517T>G | W173G | USA, Italy | 52 |
| 545T>A | L182H | France | 52 |
| 548A>G | H183R | France | 52 |

**Mutations in the α-TTP Gene of AVED Patients**

| Exon | Nucleotide change | Effect on coding sequence | Reference* |
|---|---|---|---|
| 1 | 175C>T | R59W (R, R, R) | 103 |
| 2 | 205-1G>C | exon 2 skipping and frameshift after R68 | 103 |
| 2 | 306A>G | no change on G102 (possible splice site activation) | 103 |
| 2 | 303T>G | H101Q (H, P, P) | 124 |
| 2 | 358G>A | A120T (S, E, N) | 103 |
| 3 | 400C>T | R134X (protein truncation) | 103 |
| 3 | 421G>A | E141K (E, E, Q) | 103 |
| 3 | 486delT | frameshift after G162 | 103, 125 |
| 3 | 513insTT | frameshift after I171 | 123, 125 |
| 3 | 530AG>6 | frameshift after A176 | 123 |
| 3 | 548T>C | L183P (V, L, S) | 126 |
| 3 | 552G>A | exon 3 skipping and frameshift after T184 | 98, 115 |
| 4 | 575G>A | R192H (R, K, G) | 103, 124 |
| 4 | 661C>T | R221W (R, R, K) | 103 |
| 5 | 744delA | frameshift after E248 | 123 |

*For missense mutations, the corresponding amino acid in rat α-TTP, human cis-retinaldehyde binding protein (CRALBP) and yeast SEC14 protein, respectively, is given in parentheses.

of the protein. In most cases, point mutations are found in clinically typical FRDA patients. Two of seven missense mutations (D122Y and G130V) appear, however, to be associated with an atypical presentation associating retained knee reflexes (sometimes brisk), absence of dysarthria, moderate ataxia, slow progression, but not late onset.[52–54] The clustering of these two mutations may reflect the presence of a functionally defined domain of frataxin.

The clinical equivalence between the GAA intronic expansion and the truncating mutations suggests that the expansion acts by loss of function on frataxin. Indeed, RT-PCR and RNAse protection experiments revealed that frataxin mRNA levels are markedly decreased when compared to controls or unrelated

ataxias.[12,49,55] RNAse protection and in vitro transcription experiments suggest that the expansion act at the transcriptional level, rather than interfere with the splicing of intron 1.[55,56] Experiments using in vitro and in vivo expression systems revealed that the GAA repeat interferes with transcription in an orientation and length-dependent manner.[55,56] The interference was most pronounced in the physiological orientation, when synthesis of the GAA-rich transcript was attempted, raising the possibility that the formation of a triple-helical structure involving the transcribed GAA expansion is the basic pathologic mechanism.[57]

The direct involvement of the GAA expansion as the cause of FRDA is demonstrated by the very significant inverse correlation between the size of the smaller of the two expansions and the age of onset ($r = -0.69$ to $-0.75$; Fig. 232-2), the severity of the disease, and the risk occurrence of optional signs, such as cardiomyopathy, scoliosis, and diabetes.[13,32,58–61] These observations suggest that some frataxin is produced from alleles carrying smaller expansions in a length-dependent manner. This was confirmed using a monoclonal antibody directed against frataxin,[50] and is in agreement with the transcript analyses. The smallest pathologic expansions are in the range of 90 to 110 repeats, usually found in patients with late onset and atypical presentation of the disease,[13,62] although exceptions exist.[63] As a consequence, the molecular definition of Friedreich ataxia, based on the presence of the GAA expansion mutation, is broader than the previous clinically based definition. Carriers of small expansions (< 400 repeats) often show onset of the symptoms after age 25 or have retained tendon reflexes,[13,32,58–60] features previously considered as exclusion criteria.[4] Detection of the expansion mutation thus provides a most useful diagnostic test. The length of expansion has, however, little value for individual prognosis, given the large scattering of points along the correlation curve.

## EPIDEMIOLOGY AND EXPANSION INSTABILITY

FRDA is the most common of the hereditary ataxias in the Caucasian population. It generally accounts for half of the overall heredodegenerative ataxia cases, and for three-quarters of those with onset before age 25.[64] The disease seems to have a fairly similar prevalence of around $2 \times 10^{-5}$ in almost all studied Caucasian populations.[5,64–67] This figure was confirmed by the direct estimation of GAA expansion carriers in French and German populations at 1 in 85, including the small expansions that would result in homozygotes in LOFA or atypical FRDA.[62,63] Given the high carrier frequency, the finding of a heterozygous expansion in a Caucasian patient should lead to the search for a point mutation in the other allele or to frataxin western blot analysis, in order to confirm the involvement of the frataxin gene. FRDA families revealing a pseudo-autosomal inheritance with incomplete penetrance are not uncommon, again in relation with the high carrier frequency. No patient compound heterozygote or homozygote for two point mutations has been reported to date. This might be explained both by the very low likelihood of its occurrence (4 in 10,000 FRDA patients in the absence of consanguinity) and by the lethality associated with two mutations that totally inactivate the frataxin gene by not allowing the expression of residual frataxin levels as expansion mutations might. Therefore, the absence of the expansion almost excludes the FRDA diagnosis. FRDA is rare in Finland and among black Africans, and nonexistent in Japan (S. Tsuji, M. Watanabe, and N. Tachi, personal communications). Rare nonallelic heterogeneity may be present.[68,69]

Linkage disequilibrium studies traced back the origin of the GAA expansion mutations and clarify why FRDA appears restricted to the Caucasian population. The normal GAA repeats in the Caucasian population cluster in two classes of alleles, with about 80 percent of alleles having 8 to 12 GAAs and 17 percent having 16 to ≈34 GAAs.[62,63,70] The second class of alleles does not seem to exist in far-east Asian populations (M. Cossée and M. Pandolfo, personal communications). Linkage disequilibrium

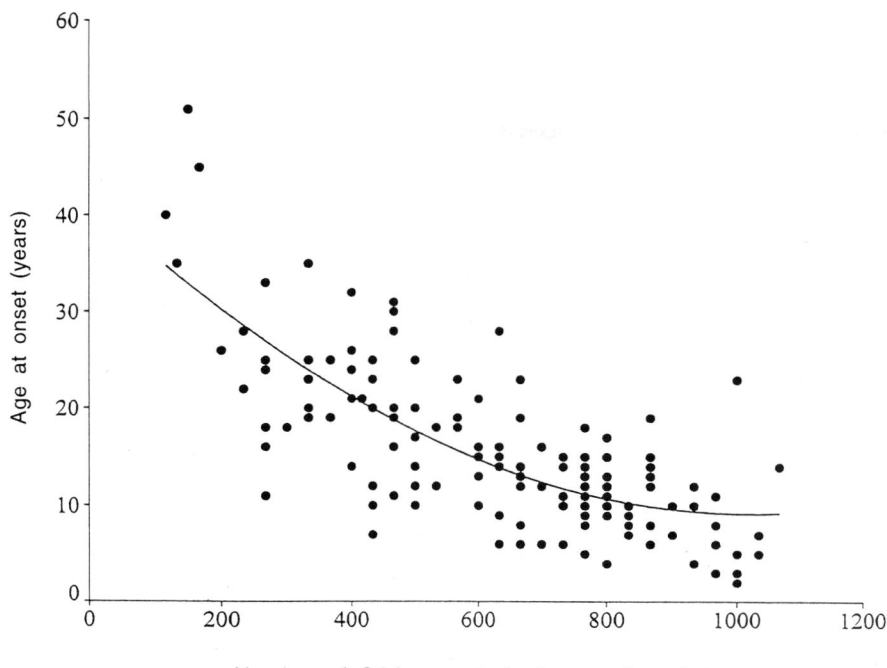

**Fig. 232-2** Example of correlation between age of onset and the number of GAA repeats in the smaller expansion alleles of FA patients.[13]

analysis demonstrated that at least 93 percent of large normal alleles (16 to 34 GAAs) originated from a single ancient founder event affecting GAA length, and that these large normal alleles are the precursors of the the expanded alleles,[62] a mechanism very similar to that proposed for myotonic dystrophy,[71] where the large normal alleles (19 to 30 CTGs) serve as a reservoir for further expansion (Fig. 232-3). As in dominant and X-linked diseases, recurrent events seem to be an important source for large expansions, because intermediate unstable alleles (premutations of 34 to 65 pure GAA) have been found in a few cases of extreme instability (changes to expansions of 300 to 630 repeats in a single generation).[62,63,70] These dramatic, single-step, size changes might represent exceptional cases selected by the occurrence of an affected child, because not all parental transmissions of a pure GAA premutation or small expansion showed dramatic instability.[62,70] Also, several very large normal alleles (from 33 to 55

triplets) were observed that contain interrupting (GAGGAA)n repeats,[62,70] which may confer stability, as in other trinucleotide repeat diseases, such as FRAXA, SCA1, and SCA2. Preliminary results on transmission of large expansions suggest that when transmitted from the father, large expansions have a tendency to contract, a result also supported by sperm analysis.[59,72] Somatic instability appears less pronounced than for myotonic dystrophy, with appearance of three expansion sizes, instead of two, in only a few patients.

## FRATAXIN LOCALIZES AT MITOCHONDRIAL MEMBRANES

A first suggestion that frataxin could be a mitochondrial protein came from phylogenetic studies. Sequence comparisons showed the presence of more distant homologues in gram-negative

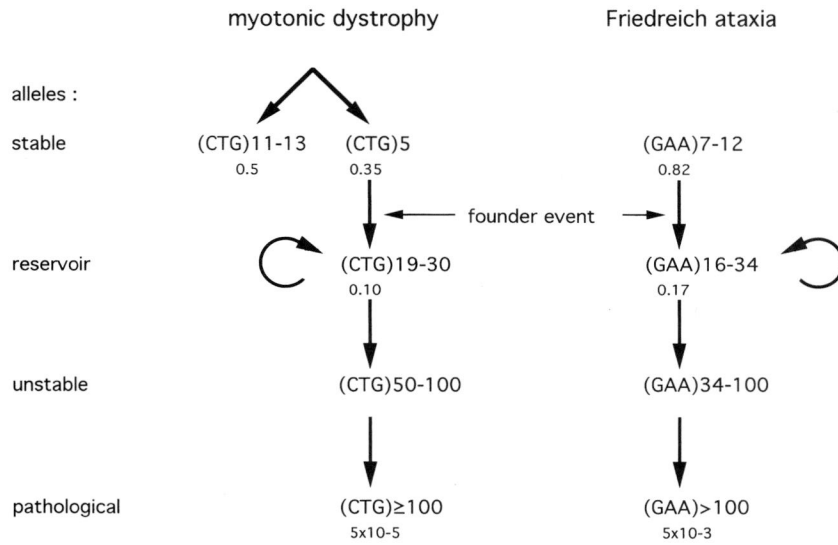

**Fig. 232-3** Compared evolution of the Friedreich ataxia GAA repeat[62] and the myotonic dystrophy CTG repeat.[71] The frequency of each class of allele is given below the length range. Polymerase slippage (circular arrow) is assumed to generate variability within the "reservoir" class.

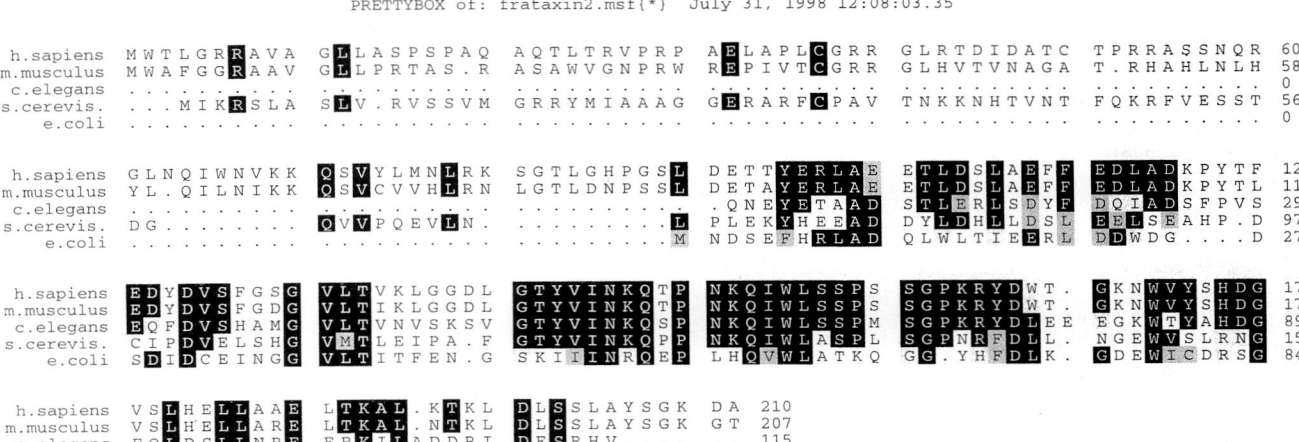

```
PRETTYBOX of: frataxin2.msf{*}  July 31, 1998 12:08:03.35

  h.sapiens  M W T L G R R A V A  G L L A S P S P A Q  A Q T L T R V P R P  A E L A P L C G R R  G L R T D I D A T C  T P R R A S S N Q R   60
m.musculus  M W A F G G R A A V  G L L P R T A S . R  A S A W V G N P R W  R E P I V T C G R R  G L H V T V N A G A  T . R H A H L N L H   58
 c.elegans  . . . . . . . . . .  . . . . . . . . . .  . . . . . . . . . .  . . . . . . . . . .  . . . . . . . . . .  . . . . . . . . . .    0
s.cerevis.  . . . M I K R S L A  S L V . R V S S V M  G R R Y M I A A A G  G E R A R F C P A V  T N K K N H T V N T  F Q K R F V E S S T   56
    e.coli  . . . . . . . . . .  . . . . . . . . . .  . . . . . . . . . .  . . . . . . . . . .  . . . . . . . . . .  . . . . . . . . . .    0

  h.sapiens  G L N Q I W N V K K  Q S V Y L M N L R K  S G T L G H P G S L  D E T T Y E R L A E  E T L D S L A E F F  E D L A D K P Y T F  120
m.musculus  Y L . Q I L N I K K  Q S V C V V H L R N  L G T L D N P S S L  D E T A Y E R L A E  E T L D S L A E F F  E D L A D K P Y T L  117
 c.elegans  . . . . . . . . . .  . . . . . . . . . .  . . . . . . . . . .  . Q N E Y E T A A D  S T L E R L S D Y F  D Q I A D S F P V S   29
s.cerevis.  D G . . . . . . . .  Q V V P Q E V L N .  . . . . . . . . . L  P L E K Y H E E A D  D Y L D H L L D S L  E E L S E A H P . D   97
    e.coli  . . . . . . . . . .  . . . . . . . . . .  . . . . . . . . . M  N D S E F H R L A D  Q L W L T I E E R L  D D W D G . . . . D   27

  h.sapiens  E D Y D V S F G S G  V L T V K L G G D L  G T Y V I N K Q T P  N K Q I W L S S P S  S G P K R Y D W T .  G K N W V Y S H D G  179
m.musculus  E D Y D V S F G D G  V L T I K L G G D L  G T Y V I N K Q T P  N K Q I W L S S P S  S G P K R Y D W T .  G K N W V Y S H D G  176
 c.elegans  E Q F D V S H A M G  V L T N V S K S V   G T Y V I N K Q S P  N K Q I W L S S P M  S G P K R Y D L E E  E G K W T Y A H D G   89
s.cerevis.  C I P D V E L S H G  V M T L E I P A . F  G T Y V I N K Q P P  N K Q I W L A S P L  S G P N R F D L L .  N G E W V S L R N G  155
    e.coli  S D I D C E I N G G  V L T I T F E N . G  S K I I I N R Q E P  L H Q V W L A T K Q  G G . Y H F D L K .  G D E W I C D R S G   84

  h.sapiens  V S L H E L L A A E  L T K A L . K T K L  D L S S L A Y S G K  D A   210
m.musculus  V S L H E L L A R E  L T K A L . N T K L  D L S S L A Y S G K  G T   207
 c.elegans  E Q L D S L L N R E  F R K I L A D D R I  D F S R H V . . . .  . .   115
s.cerevis.  T K L T D I L T E E  V E K A I S K S Q .  . . . . . . . . . .  . .   174
    e.coli  E T F W D L L E Q A  A T Q Q A G E T V S  F R . . . . . . . .  . .   106
```

Fig. 232-4 Alignment of frataxin primary sequence from various species and with the *E. coli* homologue. Note the highly conserved domain from amino acids 141 to 167 of human frataxin. The N-terminal sequence of the *C. elegans* preprotein is not yet identified.

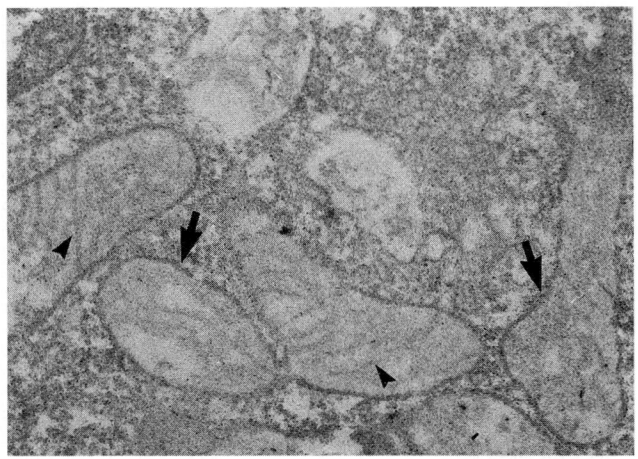

A

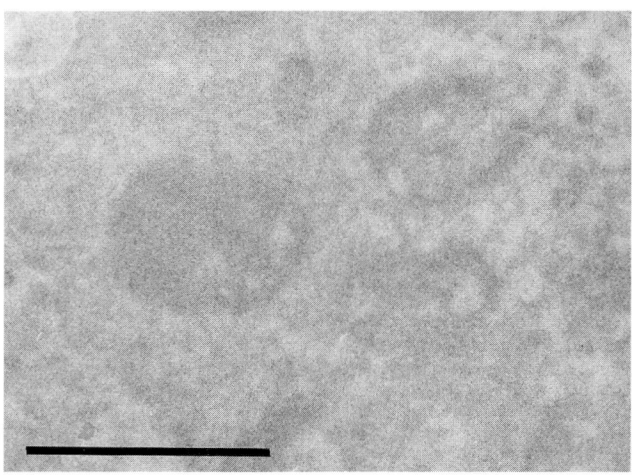

B

Fig. 232-5 Immunoelectron microscopy reveals that frataxin is associated with mitochondrial membranes in transfected HeLa cells (*courtesy of Drs V. Campuzano and C. Hindelang*). *A*, Pre-embedding MAb 1G2 peroxidase immunodetection labels the mitochondrial surrounding membranes (*arrows*) and crests (*arrow heads*). Scale bar = 1μm. *B*, Negative control without primary antibody.

(γ-purple), but not in gram-positive, bacteria,[73] suggesting that the frataxin gene might be derived from the bacterial precursor of the mitochondrial genome that shares phylogenetic ancestry with gram-negative bacteria, and that it underwent transfer to the nuclear genome. The region of sequence conservation corresponds to the second half of human frataxin and is highest for a segment between amino acids 141 and 167 (Fig. 232-4). Furthermore, computer analysis predicted a mitochondrial-targeting signal at the N-terminus of yeast and mouse frataxin, a domain that is absent in the bacterial homologues.[48] Human and yeast frataxin were directly demonstrated to be mitochondrial proteins by epitope tagging experiments and colocalization with well-established mitochondrial markers.[48,74–76] Mitochondrial localization of endogenous frataxin was demonstrated using specific monoclonal antibodies. Immunoelectron microscopy results indicate that frataxin, that has no hydrophobic transmembrane segment, is nevertheless associated with mitochondrial membranes and crests[50] (Fig. 232-5). The first 20 amino acids are sufficient to target the human frataxin to mitochondria. The targeting signal is removed during frataxin import by a two-cleavage process, resulting in an 18-kDa mature protein.[50] The two cleavage steps involve the mitochondrial processing peptidase (MPP), a dimeric protease whose β subunit binds to the N-terminus of frataxin.[77,78] However, frataxin binding and cleavage appears partially affected by disease causing missense mutations in its C-terminal moiety (G130V and I154F, Table 232-2), and maturation of the I154F mutant was reduced compared to wild-type frataxin in an *in vivo* overexpresssion system. Further investigations are needed to determine whether the maturation abnormality is related to the pathologic process in FRDA patients.

## MUTANTS OF THE YEAST FRATAXIN HOMOLOGUE

Yeast as a model organism provides a powerful system to study frataxin function. Three independent groups observed that deletion of the yeast frataxin gene, YDL120w (also called YFH1 for Yeast Frataxin Homolog), results in impaired growth on glycerol, a nonfermentable source of carbon, accumulation of mitochondria-deficient rho⁻ clones and reduced respiration.[48,74,75,79] Moreover, the mutant yeast showed a higher sensitivity to hydrogen peroxide, iron, and copper, than the wild-type strains.[74,79] The yeast frataxin gene was independently isolated as a multicopy suppressor able to rescue a yeast mutant strain unable to grow on iron-limited medium.[74] At the source of the iron sensitivity, it was found that

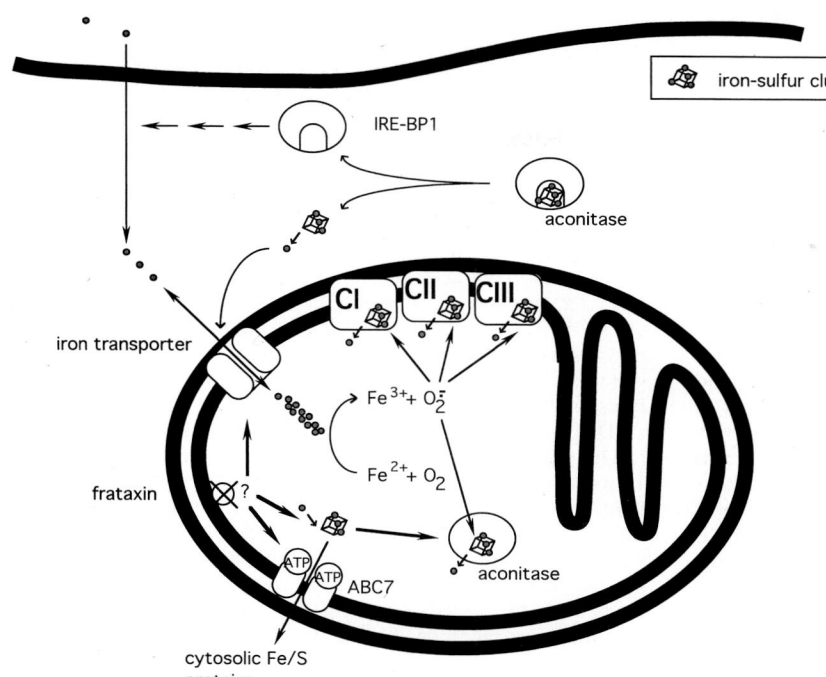

**Fig. 232-6 Molecular pathology in Friedreich ataxia.[85] Frataxin, associated with mitochondrial membranes regulates iron homeostasis in this organelle. Frataxin disruption results in inactivation of mitochondrial iron-sulfur proteins (contained in complexes I, II, and III of the oxidative phosphorylation pathway and mitochondrial aconitase) and in mitochondrial iron accumulation. Frataxin disruption results also in cytosolic iron-sulfur inactivation, as evidenced by cytosolic aconitase transformation into Iron-Responsible Element Binding Protein (IRE-BP1) by loss of the iron-sulfur cluster.**

the YFH1 (YDL120w) mutants have a mitochondrial iron content tenfold higher than the wild-type, while total iron concentration was normal.[74,79]

Two other yeast mutants that specifically accumulate iron in the mitochondria are worth a mention here. The ATM1 gene encodes a seven transmembrane ATP-binding cassette (ABC) ATPase (a putative ABC transporter), that when mutated causes mitochondrial iron accumulation at twentyfold the normal level.[80] ATM1 seems to be involved in export of iron-sulfur clusters, which are assembled in the mitochondria, because cytosolic iron-sulfur enzymes are inactivated before the mitochondrial ones and before mitochondrial iron accumulation.[81] Attempts to identify a direct functional relation between frataxin and ATM1 have failed so far. Mutants of the Ssq1 gene, encoding a low-abundance mitochondrial heat-shock 70 protein (mtHsp70), accumulate mitochondrial iron at concentrations up to fortyfold the normal level, depending on extracellular iron concentration.[82] MtHsp70 proteins act as chaperones that pull imported peptides into the mitochondrial matrix, prior to their cleavage by MPP.[83] Ssq1 mutants show partially altered frataxin second step maturation cleavage. The dramatic iron accumulation of Ssq1 mutants suggest that Ssq1 acts on the import of a cascade of proteins involved in mitochondrial iron homeostasis, a pathway that may be altered in YFH1 mutants as well.

## BIOCHEMICAL DEFECT AND TENTATIVE PATHOGENIC MODEL IN FRDA

If the function of human frataxin is similar to that of the yeast protein, this would suggest that iron accumulates in mitochondria of Friedreich ataxia patients, and could result in hypersensitivity to oxidative stress, as a consequence of the Fenton reaction ($Fe^{++}$ catalyzed production of hydroxyl radical). Indeed, iron deposits have been observed in heart myofibrils of FRDA patients.[84] Cardiomyopathy in FRDA patients could thus be a result of iron overload (as in thalassemia or in hemochromatosis) or might reflect a selective sensitivity of heart mitochondria to frataxin deficiency. Rötig et al. found selective deficiencies of the respiratory chain complexes I, II, and III, and of both mitochondrial and cytosolic aconitase activities in the heart biopsy of two patients.[85] No deficiency was found in the muscle,

fibroblasts, and lymphocytes of the same patients. The common link between all these enzymes and complexes is that they contain iron-sulfur (Fe-S) cluster in their active sites (Fig. 232-6). Selective deficiency of the iron-sulfur proteins has not been found in 60 biopsies of patients with cardiomyopathy, several of which had mitochondrial DNA mutation.[85] Iron-sulfur protein deficiency is therefore not a mere consequence of mitochondrial dysfunction but might reflect a direct consequence of frataxin deficiency prior to iron accumulation. The inactivation of a cytosolic iron-sulfur enzyme, such as cytosolic aconitase, suggests that a general iron-sulfur defect is the underlying mechanism, as is the case for the ATM1 mutant in yeast.[81] Missense mutations in ABC7, the human homologue of the ATM1 gene, cause a rare X-linked recessive disease, associating spinocerebellar ataxia and anemia.[86] The loss of cytosolic aconitase activity observed in FRDA might also reflect a decrease of cytosolic iron content, because cytosolic aconitase, also known as the iron responsive element-binding protein 1 (IRE-BP1) is switched from one function to the other by low iron concentration leading to the detachment of the iron-sulfur cluster[87] (Fig. 232-6).

Study of the biochemical defect in the yeast mutant should reveal the role of the frataxin homolog in iron homeostasis and iron-sulfur cluster biogenesis. Further biochemical analysis of appropriate target tissues may be difficult in man, and a mouse model of FRDA (by knockout of the frataxin gene) should be extremely valuable to understand the pathologic consequences of frataxin deficiency in mammalian cells and tissues. Many questions remain unsolved and particularly the cause for the relatively late onset and slow progression of the disease, as well as the specificity of neurodegeneration, while disruption of the corresponding gene in yeast results in a dramatic and rapid phenotype. It is possible that the expansion mutation does not extinguish totally frataxin expression, allowing the production of residual amount of frataxin compatible with cellular survival. Complete and conditional knockout of the mouse frataxin gene may answer this issue. It is also possible that cell types requiring frataxin during embryonic development select precursors with a shorter expansion mutation, allowing for a higher residual frataxin level. Lastly, mammalian cells, unlike yeast cells, cannot survive in the absence of oxidative phosphorylation, and may develop numerous protective pathways against free radical toxicity.

Vitamin E is one of the compounds that might compensate, in part, for loss of frataxin function.

## ATAXIA WITH ISOLATED VITAMIN E DEFICIENCY

Chronic vitamin E deficiency has been suspected for 20 years to cause a progressive neurodegenerative disease, based on studies of rats fed on low vitamin E diet and from the observation of patients with primary vitamin E deficiency[88,89] or secondary to fat malabsorption, chronic cholestasis, pancreatic insufficiency or cystic fibrosis.[90–92] Vitamin E (or its major active form α-tocopherol) is a major liposoluble antioxidant molecule, protecting biologic membranes against lipid peroxidation.[93] Accordingly, erythrocytes from isolated vitamin E patients revealed increased peroxidation sensitivity on hemolysis and evidence of lipid peroxidation.[94–98] Therefore, ataxia and neuropathy secondary to vitamin E deficiency are thought to result from reduced protection against oxidative stress caused by free radical toxicity. However, the neuronal specificity, affecting mostly large sensory neurons like in FRDA, is not explained by the ubiquitous localization of vitamin E in human tissues. Some forms of severe vitamin E deficiency are inherited diseases. One is abetalipoproteinemia (MIM 200100) with vitamin E deficiency secondary to fat malabsorption caused by mutations in the gene encoding the microsomal triglyceride transfer protein (see Chap. 115).

In ataxia with isolated vitamin E deficiency (AVED; MIM 277460), the sole and primary biochemical abnormality is very low vitamin E levels in serum. Burck and colleagues[88] described the first case of AVED in 1981. For 10 years, AVED was considered an extremely rare entity, until the discovery of an important founder clustering in North Africa.[99,100] In several instances, AVED appeared strikingly similar to FRDA (Table 232-1).[99,101,102] Despite much clinical overlap, AVED presents with a very low rate of cardiomyopathy, a higher incidence of head titubation and sometimes dystonia.[103] Retinitis pigmentosa or visual impairment can be found,[103,104] particularly in the late onset Japanese form,[105,106] a feature reminiscent of abetalipoproteinemia and Refsum disease. Peripheral neuropathy is less pronounced than in FRDA, with occasional normal[88,89,97,107–109] or moderately reduced[94,95,98,101,106,110–114] SAP, compared to the markedly decreased or absent SAP even early in FRDA. Sensory-evoked

responses are normal or subnormal in the peripheral nervous system, but abnormal centrally, when recorded at the cervical and cortical levels.[95,98,106–108,110,113,114] These features are in agreement with sensory nerve biopsies that show a normal number of total myelinated fibers with normal-to-moderate loss of large, myelinated fiber,[106,108,113,115] and with the single central nervous system pathologic study that reports moderate alteration of the DRGs but severe atrophy of the posterior columns and bulbar Goll and Burdach nuclei, and important loss of Purkinje cells in the cerebellum.[116] Peripheral nerve regeneration was frequently noted in biopsies, contrary to Friedreich ataxia nerve biopsies.[113] Vacuolar lipofuscin pigment deposits are found in muscle[88,89,101,110,111] and in the central[116] and peripheral[106,108,113,115] nervous tissues. The deposits are autofluorescent, electron-dense, membrane-bound, and phosphatase acid positive, suggesting a lysosomal origin.[88,89,101,108,110,111]

Diagnosis is made by measurement of serum vitamin E ($< 2.5$ mg/liter, often $< 1$ mg/liter, with normal values of 6 to 15 mg/liter) in the absence of fat malabsorption (normal plasma lipids) and of other liposoluble vitamins deficiency. In normal subjects, vitamin E is absorbed and secreted from the intestine into plasma in chylomicrons. The chylomicron remnants are taken up by the liver, which then selects only one stereoisomer of tocopherol (the RRR-α stereoisomer) from all the forms of vitamin E for secretion in nascent very-low-density lipoproteins (VLDL) (Fig. 232-7).[117] Other isomers and stereoisomers are eliminated, presumably through the bile. The specific transfer of vitamin E to nascent VLDL is the work of a liver-specific protein, the α-tocopherol transfer protein (α-TTP), purified and microsequenced by the group of Arai and colleagues from rat liver.[118,119] AVED patients absorb vitamin E normally, but their conservation of plasma RRR-α-tocopherol is poor due to impaired secretion of RRR-α-tocopherol in VLDL,[120,121] suggesting that α-TTP is the primary defective protein. In the absence of recycling, the entire plasma pool of vitamin E is rapidly eliminated in a little more than a day.[122]

The defective gene was localized by homozygosity mapping with the Tunisian AVED families on chromosome 8q13,[102] a region that was subsequently shown to contain the human α-TTP gene.[104] This gene is composed of 5 exons and encodes a 278-amino-acid protein that exhibits structural homologies with the

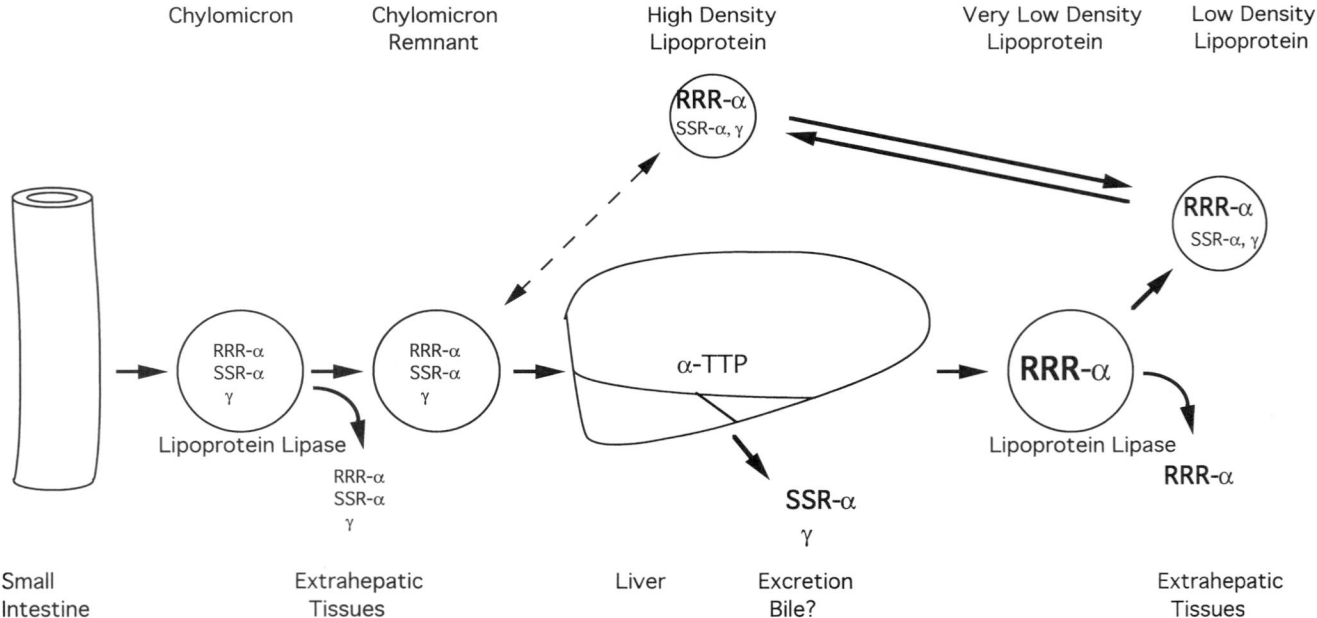

Fig. 232-7 Vitamin E transport and recycling in blood. The differential pathways of selected isomers and stereoisomers (γ, SSR-α, and RRR-α) of vitamin E are depicted.[127]

*cis*-retinaldehyde-binding protein (CRALBP, present only in the retina) and the yeast Sec14 protein, involved in phosphatidylinositol and phosphatidylcholine transfer into membranes.[104,119] Mutations are scattered throughout all five exons in AVED patients.[103,123–125] Up to now, 15 mutations have been described[98,103,115,126] (Table 232-2). The North African mutation, 744delA, results in truncation of the last 30 amino acids. Haplotype analysis has demonstrated the founder origin of the 744delA mutation.[123] Mutations 513insTT, 486delT, and R134X have been found in several unrelated European and North American families.[103] The R134X mutations might represent several recurrent changes at a CpG mutational hot spot, while the 513insTT mutations might spread from a common ancestor, as suggested by haplotype analyses.[103] The most frequent mutation in Japan is a missense change, H101Q,[106,124] which is associated with a very mild phenotype.

Early measurement of serum vitamin E in cases of recessive or sporadic ataxia is most important, as vitamin E supplementation may prevent the development of severely crippling clinical manifestations in the vitamin E deficient forms. AVED appears to be as frequent as FRDA in populations from North Africa, while it is much rarer in Western countries.[100,103] It is striking that two inherited entities, one resulting from reduced protection against free radicals (AVED) and the other resulting from increased free radical toxicity (FRDA), present with similar neurodegenerative specificities.

## ACKNOWLEDGMENTS

I wish to thank my colleagues and collaborators V. Campuzano, M. Cossée, H. Koutnikova, L. Cavalier, H. Sadoulet-Puccio, J.-L. Mandel, M. Pandolfo, L. Montermini, S. Jiralerspong, K. Ohshima, L. Cova, A. Vescovi, F. Foury, A. Rötig, P. Rustin, A. Brice, A. Durr, C. Ben Hamida, S. Belal, M. Ben Hamida, F. Hentati, K. Ouahchi, M. Arita, and H. Arai for their important contribution to the molecular unraveling of Friedreich ataxia and AVED. Research in our laboratory is supported by the Centre National de la Recherche Scientifique, the Institut National de la Santé et de la Recherche Médicale, the Association Française contre les Myopathies and the Hôpitaux Universitaires de Strasbourg and the Human Frontier Science Program.

## REFERENCES

1. Friedreich N: Uber degenerative Atrophie der spinalen Hinterstränge. *Virchows Arch Pathol Anat* **26**:391, 1863.
2. Friedreich N: Uber degenerative Atrophie der spinalen Hinterstränge. *Virchows Arch Pathol Anat* **26**:433, 1863.
3. Geoffroy G, Barbeau A, Breton G, Lemieux B, Aube M, Leger C, Bouchard JP: Clinical description and roentgenologic evaluation of patients with Friedreich ataxia. *Can J Neurol Sci* **3**:279, 1976.
4. Harding AE: Friedreich's ataxia: A clinical and genetic study of 90 families with an analysis of early diagnosis criteria and intrafamilial clustering of clinical features. *Brain* **104**:589, 1981.
5. Skre H: Friedreich's ataxia in western Norway. *Clin Genet* **7**:287, 1975.
6. Harding AE, Zilkha KJ: "Pseudo-dominant" inheritance in Friedreich's ataxia. *J Med Genet* **18**:285, 1981.
7. Filla A, De Michele G, Caruso G, Marconi R, Campanella G: Genetic data and natural history of Friedreich's disease: A study of 80 Italian patients. *J Neurol* **237**:345, 1990.
8. Muller-Felber W, Rossmanith T, Spes C, Chamberlain S, Pongratz D, Deufel T: The clinical spectrum of Friedreich's ataxia in German families showing linkage to the FRDA locus on chromosome 9. *Clin Invest* **71**:109, 1993.
9. Klockgether T, Chamberlain S, Wullner U, Fetter M, Dittmann H, Petersen D, Dichgans J: Late-onset Friedreich's ataxia. Molecular genetics, clinical neurophysiology, and magnetic resonance imaging. *Arch Neurol* **50**:803, 1993.
10. De Michele G, Filla A, Cavalcanti F, Di Maio L, Pianese L, Castaldo I, Calabrese O, et al: Late onset Friedreich's disease: Clinical features and mapping of mutation to the FRDA locus. *J Neurol Neurosurg Psychiatry* **57**:977, 1994.
11. Palau F, De Michele G, Vilchez JJ, Pandolfo M, Monros E, Cocozza S, Smeyers P, et al: Early-onset ataxia with cardiomyopathy and retained tendon reflexes maps to Friedreich's ataxia locus on chromosome 9q. *Ann Neurol* **37**:359, 1995.
12. Campuzano V, Montermini L, Moltò MD, Pianese L, Cossée M, Cavalcanti F, Monros E, et al: Friedreich ataxia: Autosomal recessive disease caused by an intronic GAA triplet repeat expansion. *Science* **271**:1423, 1996.
13. Dürr A, Cossée M, Agid Y, Campuzano V, Mignard C, Penet C, Mandel J-L, et al: Clinical and genetic abnormalities in patients with Friedreich's ataxia. *N Engl J Med* **335**:1169, 1996.
14. Winter RM, Harding AE, Baraitser M, Bravery MB: Intrafamilial correlation in Friedreich's ataxia. *Clin Genet* **20**:419, 1981.
15. Pandolfo M: Friedreich's ataxia. *Curr Neurol* **17**:47, 1997.
16. Beauchamp M, Labelle H, Duhaime M, Joncas J: Natural history of muscle weakness in Friedreich's ataxia and its relation to loss of ambulation. *Clin Orthop* **311**:270, 1995.
17. Spieker S, Schulz JB, Petersen D, Fetter M, Klockgether T, Dichgans J: Fixation instability and oculomotor abnormalities in Friedreich's ataxia. *J Neurol* **242**:517, 1995.
18. Ell J, Prasher D, Rudge P: Neuro-otological abnormalities in Friedreich's ataxia. *J Neurol Neurosurg Psychiatry* **47**:26, 1984.
19. Cassandro E, Mosca F, Sequino L, De Falco FA, Campanella G: Otoneurological findings in Friedreich's ataxia and other inherited neuropathies. *Audiology* **25**:84, 1986.
20. Oppenheimer DR, Esiri MM: Disease of the basal ganglia, cerebellum and motor neurons, in Adams JH, Corsellis JAN, Duchen LW (eds): *Greenfield's Neuropathology*, 5th ed. London, Arnold, 1992, p 1015.
21. Said G, Marion MH, Selva J, Jamet C: Hypotrophic and dying-back nerve fibers in Friedreich's ataxia. *Neurology* **36**:1292, 1986.
22. Riva A, Bradac GB: Primary cerebellar and spinocerebellar ataxia: An MRI study on 63 cases. *J Neuroradiol* **22**:71, 1995.
23. Gottdiener JS, Hawley RJ, Maron BJ, Bertorini TF, Engle WK: Characteristics of the cardiac hypertrophy in Friedreich's ataxia. *Am Heart J* **103**:525, 1982.
24. Pasternac A, Krol R, Petitclerc R, Harvey C, Andermann E, Barbeau A: Hypertrophic cardiomyopathy in Friedreich's ataxia: Symmetric or asymmetric? *Can J Neurol Sci* **7**:379, 1980.
25. Morvan D, Komajda M, Doan LD, Brice A, Isnard R, Seck A, Lechat P, et al: Cardiomyopathy in Friedreich's ataxia: A Doppler-echocardiographic study. *Eur Heart J* **13**:1393, 1992.
26. Finocchiaro G, Baio G, Micossi P, Pozza G, Di Donato S: Glucose metabolism alterations in Friedreich's ataxia. *Neurology* **38**:1292, 1988.
27. Schoenle EJ, Boltshauser EJ, Baekkeskov S, Landin Olsson M, Torresani T, von Felten A: Preclinical and manifest diabetes mellitus in young patients with Friedreich's ataxia: No evidence of immune process behind the islet cell destruction. *Diabetologia* **32**:378, 1989.
28. McLeod JG: An electrophysiological and pathological study of peripheral nerves in Friedreich's ataxia. *J Neurol Sci* **12**:333, 1971.
29. Peyronnard JM, Bouchard JP, Lapointe M: Nerve conduction studies and electromyography in Friedreich's ataxia. *Can J Neurol Sci* **3**:313, 1976.
30. Ackroyd RS, Finnegan JA, Green SH: Friedreich's ataxia. A clinical review with neurophysiological and echocardiographic findings. *Arch Dis Child* **59**:217, 1984.
31. De Michele G, Perrone F, Filla A, Mirante E, Giordano M, De Placido S, Campanella G: Age of onset, sex, and cardiomyopathy as predictors of disability and survival in Friedreich's disease: A retrospective study on 119 patients. *Neurology* **47**:1260, 1996.
32. Montermini L, Richter A, Morgan K, Justice CM, Julien D, Castelloti B, Mercier J, et al: Phenotypic variability in Friedreich ataxia: Role of the associated GAA triplet repeat expansion. *Ann Neurol* **41**:675, 1997.
33. Cedarbaum JM, Blass JP: Mitochondrial dysfunction and spinocerebellar degenerations. *Neurochem Pathol* **4**:43, 1986.
34. Chamberlain S, Shaw J, Rowland A, Wallis J, South S, Nakamura Y, von Gabain A, et al: Mapping of mutation causing Friedreich' ataxia to human chromosome 9. *Nature* **334**:248, 1988.
35. Fujita R, Agid Y, Trouillas P, Seck A, Tommasi-Davenas C, Driesel AJ, Olek K, et al: Confirmation of linkage of Friedreich ataxia to chromosome 9 and identification of a new closely linked marker. *Genomics* **4**:110, 1989.
36. Hanauer A, Chery M, Fujita R, Driesel AJ, Gilgenkrantz S, Mandel JL: The Friedreich ataxia gene is assigned to chromosome 9q13-q21 by

mapping of tightly linked markers and shows linkage disequilibrium with D9S15. *Am J Hum Genet* **46**:133, 1990.

37. Keats BJB, Ward LJ, Shaw J, Wickremasinghe A, Chamberlain S: "Acadian" and "classical" forms of Friedreich ataxia are most probable caused by mutations at the same locus. *Am J Med Genet* **33**:266, 1989.

38. Chamberlain S, Shaw J, Wallis J, Rowland A, Chow L, Farrall M, Keats B, et al: Genetic homogeneity at the Friedreich ataxia locus on chromosome 9. *Am J Hum Genet* **44**:518, 1989.

39. Fujita R, Hanauer A, Sirugo G, Heilig R, Mandel JL: Additional polymorphisms at marker loci D9S5 and D9S15 generate extended haplotypes in linkage disequilibrium with Friedreich ataxia. *Proc Natl Acad Sci U S A* **87**:1796, 1990.

40. Pandolfo M, Sirugo G, Antonelli A, Weitnauer L, Ferreti L, Leone M, Dones I, et al: Friedreich ataxia in Italian families: Genetic homogeneity and linkage disequilibrium with the marker loci D9S5 and D9S15. *Am J Hum Genet* **47**:228, 1990.

41. Rodius F, Duclos F, Wrogemann K, Le Paslier D, Ougen P, Billault A, Belal S, et al: Recombinations in individuals homozygous by descent localize the Friedreich Ataxia locus in a cloned 450-kb interval. *Am J Hum Genet* **54**:1050, 1994.

42. Montermini L, Rodius F, Pianese L, Moltò MD, Cossée M, Campuzano V, Cavalcanti F, et al: The Friedreich ataxia critical region spans a 150-kb interval on chromosome 9q13. *Am J Hum Genet* **57**:1061, 1995.

43. Duclos F, Boschert U, Sirugo G, Mandel J-L, Hen R, Koenig M: Gene in the region of the Friedreich ataxia locus encodes a putative transmembrane protein expressed in the nervous system. *Proc Natl Acad Sci U S A* **90**:109, 1993.

44. Duclos F, Rodius F, Wrogemann K, Mandel J-L, Koenig M: The Friedreich ataxia region: Characterization of two novel genes and reduction of the critical region to 300 kb. *Hum Mol Genet* **3**:909, 1994.

45. Carvajal J, Pook MA, Doudney K, Hillermann R, Wilkes D, Al-Mahdawi S, Williamson R, et al: Friedreich ataxia: A defect in signal transduction? *Hum Mol Genet* **4**:1411, 1995.

46. Paulson HL, Fischbeck KH: Trinucleotide repeats in neurogenetic disorders. *Annu Rev Neurosci* **19**:79, 1996.

47. Carvajal J, Pook MA, dos Santos M, Doudney K, Hillermann R, Minogue S, Williamson R, et al: The Friedreich's ataxia gene encodes a novel phosphatidylinositol-4-phosphate 5-kinase. *Nat Genet* **14**:157, 1996.

48. Koutnikova H, Campuzano V, Foury F, Dollé P, Cazzalini O, Koenig M: Studies of human, mouse and yeast homologues indicate a mitochondrial function for frataxin. *Nat Genet* **16**:345, 1997.

49. Cossée M, Campuzano V, Koutnikova H, Fischbeck KH, Mandel J-L, Koenig M, Bidichandani S, et al: Frataxin fracas. *Nat Genet* **15**:337, 1997.

50. Campuzano V, Montermini L, Lutz Y, Cova L, Hindelang C, Jiralerspong S, Trottier Y, et al: Frataxin is reduced in Friedreich ataxia patients and is associated with mitochondrial membranes. *Hum Mol Genet* **6**:1771, 1997.

51. Jiralerspong S, Liu Y, Montermini L, Stifani S, Pandolfo M: Frataxin shows developmentally regulated tissue-specific expression in the mouse embryo. *Neurobiol Dis* **4**:103, 1997.

52. Cossée M, Dürr A, Schmitt M, Dahl N, Trouillas P, Allinson P, Kostrzewa M, et al: Friedreich ataxia: Point mutations and clinical presentation of compound heterozygotes. *Ann Neurol* **45**:200, 1999.

53. Bidichandani S, Ashizawa T, Patel PI: Atypical Friedreich ataxia caused by compound heterozygosity for a novel missense mutation and the GAA triplet-repeat expansion. *Am J Hum Genet* **60**:1251, 1997.

54. Forrest SM, Knight M, Delatycki MB, Paris D, Williamson R, King J, Yeung L, et al: The correlation of clinical phenotype in Friedreich ataxia with the site of point mutations in the FRDA gene. *Neurogenetics* **1**:253, 1998.

55. Bidichandani S, Ashizawa T, Patel PI: The GAA triplet-repeat expansion in Friedreich ataxia interferes with transcription and may be associated with an unusual DNA structure. *Am J Hum Genet* **62**:111, 1998.

56. Ohshima K, Montermini L, Wells RD, Pandolfo M: Inhibitory effects of expanded GAA*TTC triplet repeats from intron I of the Friedreich ataxia gene on transcription and replication *in vivo*. *J Biol Chem* **273**:14588, 1998.

57. Ohshima K, Kang S, Larson JE, Wells RD: Cloning, characterization, and properties of seven triplet repeat DNA sequences. *J Biol Chem* **271**:16773, 1996.

58. Filla A, De Michele G, Cavalcanti F, Pianese L, Monticelli A, Campanella G, Cocozza S: The relationship between trinucleotide

(GAA) repeat length and clinical features in Friedreich ataxia. *Am J Hum Genet* **59**:554, 1996.

59. Monros E, Moltò MD, Martinez F, Cañizares J, Blanca J, Vilchez JJ, Prieto F, et al: Phenotype correlation and intergenerational dynamics of the Friedreich ataxia GAA trinucleotide repeat. *Am J Hum Genet* **61**:101, 1997.

60. Lamont PJ, Davis MB, Wood NW: Identification and sizing of the GAA trinucleotide repeat expansion of Friedreich's ataxia in 56 patients. Clinical and genetic correlates. *Brain* **120**:673, 1997.

61. Isnard R, Kalotka H, D,rr A, Cossèe M, Schmitt M, Pousset F, Thomas D, et al: Correlation between left ventricular hypertrophy and GAA trinucleotide repeat length in Friedreich's ataxia. *Circulation* **95**:2247, 1997.

62. Cossée M, Schmitt M, Campuzano V, Reutenauer L, Moutou C, Mandel J-L, Koenig M: Evolution of the Friedreich's ataxia trinucleotide repeat expansion: Founder effect and premutations. *Proc Natl Acad Sci U S A* **94**:7452, 1997.

63. Epplen C, Epplen JT, Frank G, Miterski B, Santos EJM, Schöls L: Differential stability of the (GAA)n tract in the Friedreich ataxia gene. *Hum Genet* **99**:834, 1997.

64. Harding AE: Classification of the hereditary ataxias and paraplegias. *Lancet* **1**:1151, 1983.

65. Romeo G, Menozzi P, Ferlini A, Fadda S, Di Donato S, Uziel G, Lucci B: Incidence of Friedreich ataxia in Italy estimated from consanguineous marriages. *Am J Hum Genet* **35**:523, 1983.

66. Leone M, Brignolio F, Rosso MG, Curtoni ES, Moroni A, Tribolo A, Schiffer D: Friedreich's ataxia: a descriptive epidemiological study in an Italian population. *Clin Genet* **38**:161, 1990.

67. Lopez-Arlandis JM, Vilchez JJ, Palau F, Sevilla T: Friedreich's ataxia: An epidemiological study in Valencia, Spain, based on consanguinity analysis. *Neuroepidemiology* **14**:14, 1995.

68. Kostrzewa M, Klockgether T, Damian MS, Müller U: Locus heterogeneity in Friedreich ataxia. *Neurogenetics* **1**:43, 1997.

69. Christodoulou K, Deymeer F, Serdaroglu P, Ozdemir C, Georgiou DM, Papadopoulou E, Zamba E, et al: Genetic heterogeneity in Friedreich's ataxia: Indication for a second locus on chromosome 9. *Am J Hum Genet* **61**:A271, 1997.

70. Montermini L, Andermann E, Richter A, Pandolfo M, Cavalcanti F, Pianese L, Iodice L, et al: The Friedreich ataxia GAA triplet repeat: Premutation and normal alleles. *Hum Mol Genet* **6**:1261, 1997.

71. Imbert G, Kretz C, Johnson K, Mandel J-L: Origin of the expansion mutation in myotonic dystrophy. *Nat Genet* **4**:72, 1993.

72. Pianese L, Cavalcanti F, De Michele G, Filla A, Campanella G, Calabrese O, Castaldo I, et al: The effect of parental gender on the GAA dynamic mutation in the FRDA gene. *Am J Hum Genet* **60**:463, 1997.

73. Gibson TJ, Koonin EV, Musco G, Pastore A, Bork P: Friedreich's ataxia protein: Bacterial homologs point to mitochondrial dysfunction. *Trends Neurosci* **19**:465, 1996.

74. Babcock M, de Silva D, Oaks R, Davis-Kaplan S, Jiralerspong S, Montermini L, Pandolfo M, et al: Regulation of mitochondrial iron accumulation by Yfh1, a putative homolog of frataxin. *Science* **276**:1709, 1997.

75. Wilson RB, Roof DM: Respiratory deficiency due to loss of mitochondrial DNA in yeast lacking the frataxin homologue. *Nat Genet* **16**:352, 1997.

76. Priller J, Scherzer CR, Faber PW, MacDonald ME, Young AB: Frataxin gene of Friedreich's ataxia is targeted to mitochondria. *Ann Neurol* **42**:265, 1997.

77. Koutnikova H, Campuzano V, Koenig M: Maturation of wild type and mutated frataxin by the mitochondrial processing peptidase. *Hum Mol Genet* **7**:1485, 1998.

78. Branda SS, Cavadini P, Adamec J, Kalousek F, Taroni F, Isaya G: Yeast and human frataxin are processed to mature form in two sequential steps by the mitochondrial processing peptidase. *J Biol Chem* **274**:22763, 1999.

79. Foury F, Cazzalini O: Deletion of the yeast homologue of the human gene associated with Friedeich's ataxia elicits iron accumulation in mitochondria. *FEBS Lett* **411**:373, 1997.

80. Kispal G, Csere P, Guiard B, Lill R: The ABC transporter Atm1p is required for mitochondrial iron homeostasis. *FEBS Lett* **418**:346, 1997.

81. Kispal G, Csere P, Prohl C, Lill R: The mitochondrial proteins Atm1p and Nfs1p are essential for biogenesis of cytosolic Fe/S proteins. *EMBO J* **18**:3981, 1999.

82. Knight SAB, Sepuri NBV, Pain D, Dancis A: Mt-Hsp70 homolog, Ssc2p, required for maturation of yeast frataxin and mitochondrial iron homeostasis. *J Biol Chem* **273**:18389, 1998.

83. Pfanner N: Mitochondrial import: Crossing the aqueous intermembrane space. *Curr Biol* **8**:R262, 1998.

84. Lamarche JB, Shapcott D, Côté M, Lemieux B: Cardiac iron deposits in Friedreich's ataxia, in Lechtenberg R (ed): *Handbook of Cerebellar Diseases*. New York, Marcel Dekker, 1993, p 453.

85. Rötig A, deLonlay P, Chretien D, Foury F, Koenig M, Sidi D, Munnich A, et al: Frataxin gene expansion causes aconitase and mitochondrial iron-sulfur protein deficiency in Friedreich ataxia. *Nat Genet* **17**:215, 1997.

86. Allikmets R, Raskind WH, Hutchinson A, Schueck ND, Dean M, Koeller DM: Mutation of a putative mitochondrial iron transporter gene (ABC7) in X-linked sideroblastic anemia and ataxia (XLSA/A). *Hum Mol Genet* **8**:743, 1999.

87. Kaptain S, Downey WE, Tang C, Philpott C, Haile D, Orloff DG, Harford JB, et al: A regulated RNA binding protein also possesses aconitase activity. *Proc Natl Acad Sci U S A* **88**:10109, 1991.

88. Burck U, Goebel HH, Kuhlendahl HD, Meier C, Goebel KM: Neuromyopathy and vitamin E deficiency in man. *Neuropediatrics* **12**:267, 1981.

89. Laplante P, Vanasse M, Michaud J, Geoffroy G, Brochu P: A progressive neurological syndrome associated with an isolated vitamin E deficiency. *Can J Neurol Sci* **11**:561, 1984.

90. Landrieu P, Said G: Peripheral neuropathy and chronic cholestasis due to paucity of interlobular bile ducts. *Arch Fr Pediatr* **37**:445, 1980.

91. Elias E, Muller DP, Scott J: Association of spinocerebellar disorders with cystic fibrosis or chronic childhood cholestasis and very low serum vitamin E. *Lancet* **2**:1319, 1981.

92. Muller DP, Lloyd JK, Wolff OH: Vitamin E and neurological function. *Lancet* **1**:225, 1983.

93. Di Mascio P, Murphy ME, Sies H: Antioxidant defense systems: The role of carotenoids, tocopherols, and thiols. *Am J Clin Nutr* **53**:194S, 1991.

94. Shorer Z, Parvari R, Bril G, Sela B-A, Moses S: Ataxia with isolated vitamin E deficiency in four siblings. *Pediatr Neurol* **15**:340, 1996.

95. Sokol RJ, Kayden HJ, Bettis DB, Traber MG, Neville H, Ringel S, Wilson WB, et al: Isolated vitamin E deficiency in the absence of fat malabsorption—Familial and sporadic cases: characterization and investigation of causes. *J Lab Clin Med* **111**:548, 1988.

96. Kohlschütter A, Hubner C, Jansen W, Lindner SG: A treatable familial neuromyopathy with vitamin E deficiency, normal absorption, and evidence of increased consumption of vitamin E. *J Inherit Metab Dis* **11**:149, 1988.

97. Amiel J, Maziere JC, Beucler I, Koenig M, Reutenauer L, Loux N, Bonnefont D, et al: Familial isolated vitamin E deficiency. Study of a multiplex family with a 5-year therapeutic followup. *J Inherit Metab Dis* **18**:333, 1995.

98. Schuelke M, Mayatepek E, Inter M, Becker M, Pfeiffer E, Speer A, Hubner C, et al: Treatment of ataxia in isolated vitamin E deficiency caused by alpha-tocopherol transfer protein deficiency. *J Pediatr* **134**:240, 1999.

99. Ben Hamida M, Belal S, Sirugo G, Ben Hamida C, Panayides K, Ioannou P, Beckmann J, et al: Friedreich's ataxia phenotype not linked to chromosome 9 and associated with selective autosomal recessive vitamin E deficiency in two inbred Tunisian families. *Neurology* **43**:2179, 1993.

100. Dorflinger N, Linder C, Ouahchi K, Gyapay G, Weissenbach J, Le Paslier D, Rigault P, et al: Ataxia with vitamin E deficiency: Refinement of genetic localisation and analysis of linkage disequilibrium using new markers in 14 families. *Am J Hum Genet* **56**:1116, 1995.

101. Stumpf DA, Sokol R, Bettis D, Neville H, Ringel S, Angelini C, Bell R: Friedreich's disease: V. Variant form with vitamin E deficiency and normal fat absorption. *Neurology* **37**:68, 1987.

102. Ben Hamida C, Dorflinger N, Belal S, Linder C, Reutenauer L, Dib C, Gyapay G, et al: Localization of Friedreich ataxia phenotype with selective vitamin E deficiency to chromosome 8q by homozygosity mapping. *Nat Genet* **5**:195, 1993.

103. Cavalier L, Ouahchi K, Kayden HJ, Di Donato S, Reutenauer L, Mandel J-L, Koenig M: Ataxia with isolated vitamin E deficiency: Heterogeneity of mutations and phenotypic variability in a large number of families. *Am J Hum Genet* **62**:301, 1998.

104. Arita M, Sato Y, Miyata A, Tanabe T, Takahashi E, Kayden HJ, Arai H, et al: Human a-tocopherol transfer protein: cDNA cloning, expression and chromosomal localisation. *Biochem J* **306**:437, 1995.

105. Yokota T, Shiojiri T, Gotoda T, Arai H: Retinitis pigmentosa and ataxia caused by a mutation in the gene for the α-tocopherol transfer protein. *N Engl J Med* **335**:1770, 1996.

106. Yokota T, Shiojiri T, Gotoda T, Arita M, Arai H, Ohga T, Kanda T, et al: Friedreich-like ataxia with retinitis pigmentosa caused by the His101Gln mutation of the α-tocopherol transfer protein gene. *Ann Neurol* **41**:826, 1997.

107. Harding AE, Matthews S, Jones S, Ellis CJ, Booth IW, Muller DP: Spinocerebellar degeneration associated with a selective defect of vitamin E absorption. *N Engl J Med* **313**:32, 1985.

108. Yokota T, Wada Y, Furukawa T, Tsukagoshi H, Uchihara T, Watabiki S: Adult-onset spinocerebellar syndrome with idiopathic vitamin E deficiency. *Ann Neurol* **22**:84, 1987.

109. Rayner RJ, Doran R, Roussounis SH: Isolated vitamin E deficiency and progressive ataxia. *Arch Dis Child* **69**:602, 1993.

110. Krendel DA, Gilchrist JM, Johnson AO, Bossen EH: Isolated deficiency of vitamin E with progressive neurologic deterioration. *Neurology* **37**:538, 1987.

111. Trabert W, Stober T, Mielke V, Siu Heck F, Schimrigk K: Isolierter Vitamin-E-Mangel. *Fortschr Neurol Psychiat* **57**:495, 1989.

112. Jackson CE, Amato AA, Barohn RJ: Isolated vitamin E deficiency. *Muscle Nerve* **19**:1161, 1996.

113. Zouari M, Feki M, Ben Hamida C, Larnaout A, Turki I, Belal S, Mebazaa A, et al: Electrophysiology and nerve biopsy: Comparative study in Friedreich's ataxia and Friedreich's ataxia phenotype with vitamin E deficiency. *Neuromuscul Disord* **8**:416, 1999.

114. Martinello F, Fardin P, Ottina M, Ricchieri GL, Koenig M, Cavalier L, Trevisan CP: Supplemental therapy in isolated vitamin E deficiency improves the peripheral neuropathy and prevents the progression of ataxia. *J Neurol Sci* **156**:177, 1998.

115. Tamaru Y, Hirano M, Kusaka H, Ito H, Imai T, Ueno S: α-Tocopherol transfer protein gene: Exon skipping of all transcripts causes ataxia. *Neurology* **49**:584, 1997.

116. Larnaout A, Belal S, Zouari M, Fki M, Ben Hamida C, Goebel HH, Ben Hamida M, et al: Friedreich's ataxia with isolated vitamin E deficiency: A neuropathological study of a Tunisian patient. *Acta Neuropathol* **93**:633, 1997.

117. Kayden HJ: The neurologic syndrome of vitamin E deficiency: A significant cause of ataxia. *Neurology* **43**:2167, 1993.

118. Sato Y, Hagiwara K, Arai H, Inoue K: Purification and characterization of the alpha-tocopherol transfer protein from rat liver. *FEBS Lett* **288**:41, 1991.

119. Sato Y, Arai H, Miyata A, Tokita S, Yamamoto K, Tanabe T, Inoue K: Primary structure of alpha-tocopherol transfer protein from rat liver. *J Biol Chem* **268**:17705, 1993.

120. Traber MG, Sokol RJ, Burton GW, Ingold KU, Papas AM, Huffaker JE, Kayden HJ: Impaired ability of patients with familial isolated vitamin E deficiency to incorporate alpha-tocopherol into lipoproteins secreted by the liver. *J Clin Invest* **85**:397, 1990.

121. Traber MG, Sokol RJ, Kohlschütter A, Yokota T, Muller DPR, Dufour R, Kayden HJ: Impaired discrimination between stereoisomers of alpha-tocopherol in patients with familial isolated vitamin E deficiency. *J Lipid Res* **34**:201, 1993.

122. Traber MG, Ramakrishnan R, Kayden HJ: Human plasma vitamin E kinetics- demonstrate rapid recycling of plasma RRR-α-tocopherol. *Proc Natl Acad Sci U S A* **91**:10005, 1994.

123. Ouahchi K, Arita M, Kayden HJ, Hentati F, Ben Hamida M, Sokol R, Arai H, et al: Ataxia with isolated vitamin E deficiency is caused by mutations in the a-tocopherol transfer protein. *Nat Genet* **9**:141, 1995.

124. Gotoda T, Arita M, Arai H, Inoue K, Yokota T, Fukuo Y, Yazaki Y, et al: Adult-onset spinocerebellar dysfunction caused by a mutation in the gene for a-tocopherol transfer protein. *N Engl J Med* **333**:1313, 1995.

125. Hentati A, Deng HX, Hung WY, Nayer M, Ahmed MS, He X, Tim R, et al: Human α-tocopherol transfer protein: Gene structure and mutations in familial vitamin E deficiency. *Neurology* **39**:295, 1996.

126. Shimohata T, Date H, Ishiguro H, Suzuki T, Takano H, Tanaka H, Tsuji S, et al: Ataxia with isolated vitamin E deficiency and retinitis pigmentosa. *Ann Neurol* **43**:273, 1998.

127. Kayden HJ, Traber MG: Transport of vitamin E in human lipoproteins, in Mino M, Nakamura H, Diplock AT, Kayden HJ (eds): *Vitamin E. Its Usefulness in Health and in Curing Diseases*. Basel, Karger, 1993, p 85.

128. Zühlke C, Laccone F, Cossée M, Kohlschütter A, Koenig M, Schwinger E: Mutation of the start codon in the FRDA1 gene: Linkage analysis of three pedigrees with the ATG to ATT transversion points to a unique common ancestor. *Hum Genet* **103**:102, 1998.

129. Doudney K, Pook MA, Al-Mahdawi S, Carvajal J, Hillermann R, Chamberlain S: A novel splice site mutation (384+1 G→A) in the Friedreich's ataxia gene. *Hum Mutat* **11**:415, 1998.

# Tuberous Sclerosis

*Julian R. Sampson*

1. Tuberous sclerosis is a multisystem hamartomatosis that is transmitted as an autosomal dominant trait with highly variable expression. Prevalence among newborns is estimated to be over 1 in 10,000 and is not thought to show significant geographic variation.
2. Frequent manifestations of tuberous sclerosis include seizures, intellectual handicap, behavioral problems, a variety of skin lesions, and renal angiomyolipomas and cysts. Cardiac rhabdomyomas and hepatic angiomas are also common, but usually asymptomatic. The lungs and endocrine system are less frequently involved. Management is directed toward the early detection and treatment of important medical and psychological complications and the provision of genetic counseling.
3. Two tuberous sclerosis-determining genes have been identified by positional cloning and are termed *TSC1* and *TSC2*. A wide range of inactivating germ line mutations occur in patients with tuberous sclerosis. Demonstration of loss of heterozygosity or intragenic mutations affecting the corresponding wild-type allele in hamartomas indicates that both genes function as Knudson-type tumor suppressors.
4. The *TSC1* and *TSC2* encoded proteins hamartin and tuberin are not homologous but interact directly with one another to form a largely cytosolic complex. Their cellular roles are not well understood.
5. The Eker rat is a naturally occurring model of *TSC2* inactivation. Its recognition has facilitated direct experimental confirmation of the tumour suppressor properties of *TSC2*. The *gigas* phenotype in *Drosophila* results from inactivating mutations of a gene orthologous to *TSC2*. Homozygous *gigas* −/− cells exhibit a phenotype of cellular hypertrophy and endoreduplication of DNA.

Tuberous sclerosis (MIM 191100, 191092), or the tuberous sclerosis complex (TSC),[1,2] is still sometimes referred to by the eponymous titles of Bourneville disease[3] or Pringle disease.[4] In the past, the now redundant neologism epiloia (epilepsy and anoia or mindlessness) was commonly applied.[5,6] TSC has protean manifestations and may be encountered in any branch of clinical medicine. Two TSC determining genes, *TSC1* and *TSC2*, were identified during the 1990s. Molecular genetic analysis of constitutional mutations in affected individuals and of somatic mutations in TSC-associated hamartomas has elucidated a tumor suppressor mechanism that underlies the phenotypic manifestations in many organs. The *TSC1* and *TSC2* genes encode novel proteins that have been termed hamartin and tuberin for which the cellular roles are largely unknown.

---

A standard list of abbreviations is located immediately preceding the index in each volume. Additional abbreviations used in this chapter include: ADKPD = autosomal dominant polycystic kidney disease; CDK = cyclin-dependent kinase; GAP = GTPase-activating protein; LAM = lymphangioleiomyomatosis; LOH = loss of heterozygosity; MEN1 = multiple endocrine neoplasia type 1; *PKD1* = polycystic kidney disease 1 gene; TSC = tuberous sclerosis; *TSC1* = tuberous sclerosis 1 gene; *TSC2* = tuberous sclerosis 2 gene.

## CLINICAL FINDINGS AND DIAGNOSIS

### Central Nervous System Manifestations

Many of the most frequent and serious complications of TSC reflect involvement of the brain. These include epilepsy in approximately 80 percent of patients, intellectual handicap in up to 50 percent, and autism and other behavioral abnormalities in over 50 percent.[7] Cortical tubers, subependymal nodules, and subependymal giant cell astrocytomas are central nervous system hallmarks of TSC[8,9] (Fig. 233-1). Abnormal white matter migration tracks, abnormalities of myelination, and cerebellar lesions similar to tubers also occur. By contrast, the spinal cord is rarely, if ever, affected. Tubers are discrete areas of loss of normal cortical architecture and, during life, are best visualized by magnetic resonance imaging. Macroscopic pathologic examination reveals a loss of gyral and sulcal modelling and microscopically there is loss of normal hexalaminar organization. A region of astrocytic gliosis may surround tubers. Characteristic cellular components are cytomegalic neurons, often with abnormally clumped chromatin, and balloon cells (Fig. 233-2).[10] Isolated regions of focal cortical dysplasia can appear indistinguishable from cortical tubers. Solitary tuber-like lesions in patients without other manifestations of TSC are, therefore, no longer considered diagnostic of TSC. Subependymal nodules are found along the surface of the lateral ventricles in the majority of patients with TSC and may affect the aqueduct or fourth ventricle. Some, particularly those adjacent to the foramen of Munro, continue to grow and are then classified as subependymal giant cell astrocytomas. If left untreated, these tumors may lead to hydrocephalus and potentially fatal neurologic complications. Subependymal nodules and subependymal giant cell astrocytomas may contain a heterogeneous mixture of polygonal, epithelioid, and spindle cells, and abnormally large cells similar to those in tubers.[9]

### Ophthalmic Manifestations

Fundal hamartomas (Fig. 233-3) are reported to occur in approximately 50 percent of patients with TSC,[11] although they are not always detected by direct ophthalmoscopy through undilated pupils. Lesions may be flat or nodular (the latter may calcify) and achromic patches affecting the retinal pigment epithelium are common.[12] Visual loss is exceptional, but may be caused by foveal involvement or by continuing growth of nodular lesions. On histopathologic examination, the nodular lesions appear similar to subependymal nodules and subependymal giant cell astrocytomas. A wide variety of nonfundal ophthalmic findings have been reported, including skin lesions affecting the lids, pigmentary abnormalities of the iris and coloboma.

### Dermatologic Manifestations

Initial clinical diagnosis of TSC often rests on the identification of skin signs (Fig. 233-4). These include angiofibromas affecting the face (previously and inaccurately termed adenoma sebaceum) and of the nail beds (subungual or periungual fibromas), fibromatous plaques of the forehead and scalp, collagenous hamartomas of the dermis termed shagreen patches, hypopigmented macules and skin tags (molluscum fibrosum pendulum).[13–15]

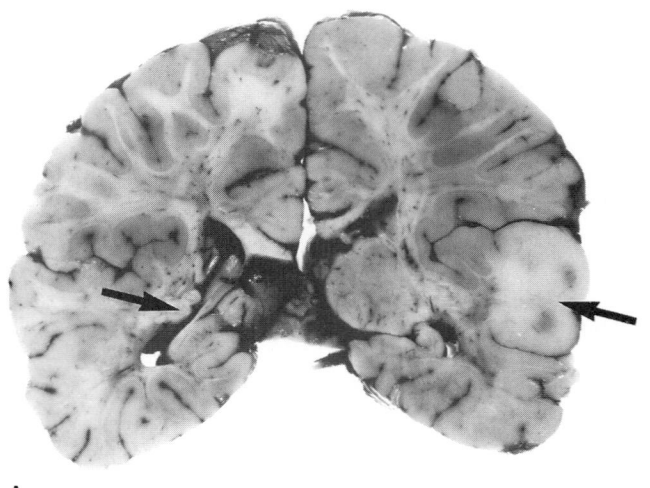

A

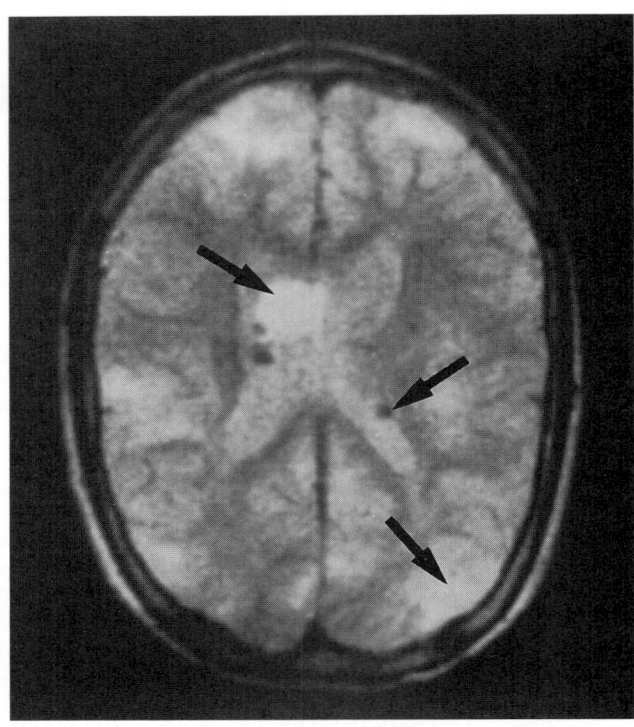

B

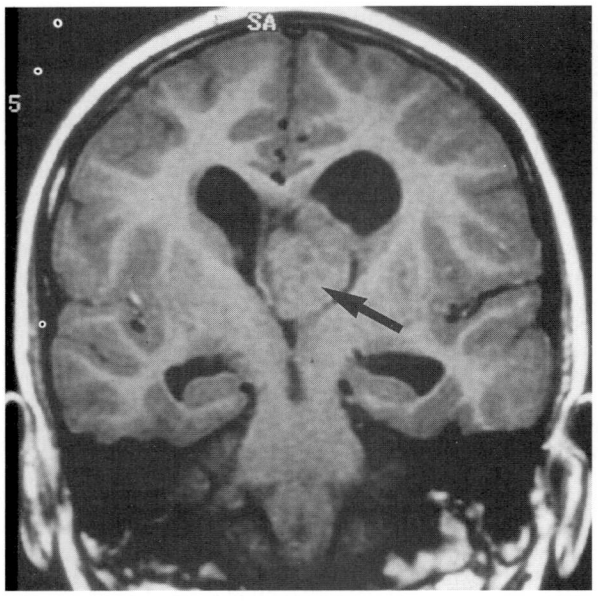

C

Fig. 233-1 Gross and magnetic nuclear resonance imaging appearances of the brain in TSC. *A,* Coronal section of postmortem brain showing multiple subependymal nodules (*left arrow*) and large cortical tuber (*right arrow*). (*Courtesy of Dr. A. Dean.*) *B,* Early generation T2-weighted magnetic resonance image of axial section of brain showing partially intraventricular hyperintense subependymal giant cell astrocytoma in the right frontal horn (*arrow on left*), hypointense subependymal nodules (*arrow*), and hyperintense cortical tubers (*arrow lower right*). *C,* T1-weighted magnetic resonance image of coronal section of brain showing nonhomogeneous isointense giant cell astrocytoma in the anterior part of the third ventricle (*arrow*) causing hydrocephalus. (*Courtesy of Dr. A. Dean.*)

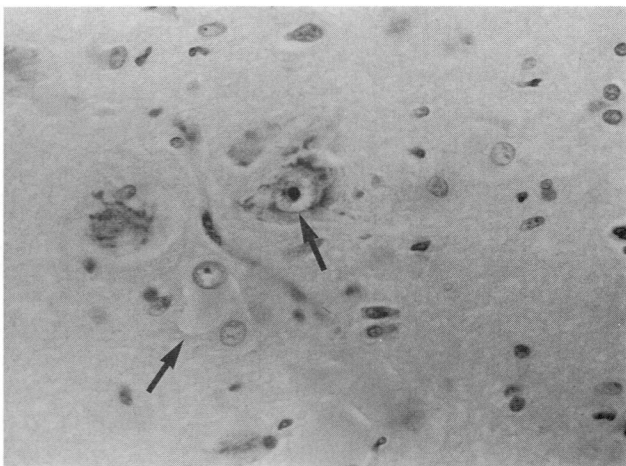

A

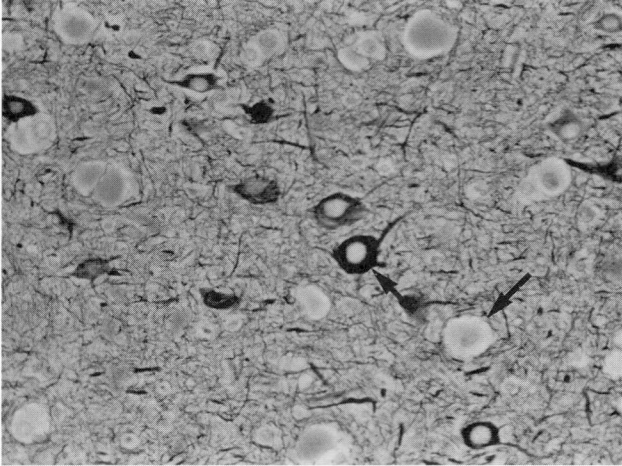

B

Fig. 233-2 Histopathologic appearances of cortical tuber. *A,* Hematoxylin and eosin-stained section showing a cytomegalic neuron (*arrow on right*) adjacent to a balloon cell (*arrow on left*). *B,* Silver-stained section showing irregular arrangement of cytomegalic neurons (dark-staining argyrophilic cytoplasm), contrasting with balloon cells (pale cytoplasm). (*Courtesy of Dr. A. Dean.*)

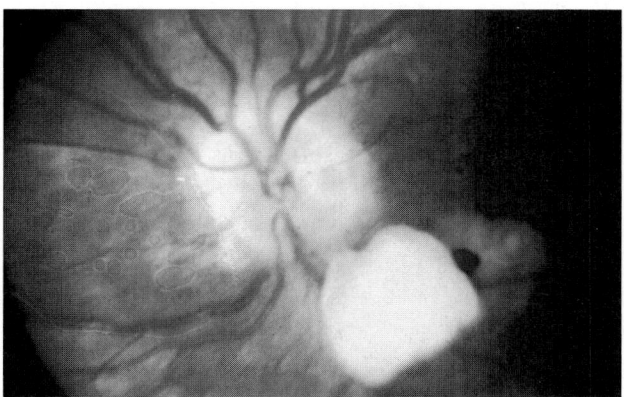

**Fig. 233-3 Large, raised (mulberry type) fundal hamartoma adjacent to optic disc.**

Hypopigmented macules, which are more readily visualized under ultraviolet (Wood's) light in fair skinned individuals, may be present in infancy, and frequently prompt consideration of TSC when observed in association with infantile spasms.[16] They are seen in most young children with TSC, but less frequently in older patients.[14] Similar macules are seen in approximately 5 percent of the normal population,[17,18] but the presence of more than three macules is considered a major diagnostic feature. Hypopigmented macules contain normal numbers of melanocytes, but show reduction in size, number, and melanization of melanosomes.[19]

Angiofibromas of the face initially develop as an angiomatous rash affecting the nasolabial folds, cheeks and chin. The rash commonly first appears at a few years of age, but may do so much later. The philtrum is relatively spared. With increasing age the

lesions increase in size and density and become more sclerotic. Angiofibromas also frequently affect the nail beds and are then referred to as ungual fibromas. Similar lesions may develop in response to trauma in normal individuals. Shagreen patches contain variable proportions of collagen, elastic tissue, smooth muscle, fat and vascular elements. They occur in many locations, but most commonly in the lumbosacral area. Soft fibromata, either pedunculated or sessile, may be found on the neck or trunk, and may be very numerous.

## Renal Manifestations

Renal complications are second only to central nervous system causes of morbidity and mortality in TSC.[20] Angiomyolipomas (Fig. 233-5) are the most frequent renal lesion, being demonstrable on ultrasound scan in 50 to 80 percent of patients by 10 years of age.[21,22] Severe or symptomatic involvement appears to be more common in females, and this may reflect hormonally promoted growth, because expression of estrogen and progesterone receptors has been demonstrated in angiomyolipomas.[23] They are usually benign growths that contain variable proportions of fat and smooth muscle and vessels that have disorganized medial smooth muscle and lack elastic laminae.[24] Hemorrhage into the retroperitoneal space or collecting system is the most frequent complication and can be life threatening.[25] Risk of hemorrhage is related to tumor size and catastrophic bleeding is very unusual from those under 3.5 cm in diameter. The rate of growth is variable[26] but occasionally rapid.[22] Massive involvement of both kidneys may be lead to renal failure.[27] When the fat content of an angiomyolipoma is low, radiologic confusion with renal cell carcinoma may occur, and even histopathologic differentiation may be difficult.[28,29] Very recently, malignant angiomyolipoma has been recognized as a distinct entity[30] (Fig. 233-6) and, like the benign counterpart, usually stains positively with HMB-45, a monoclonal antibody to melanocyte antigen gp100.

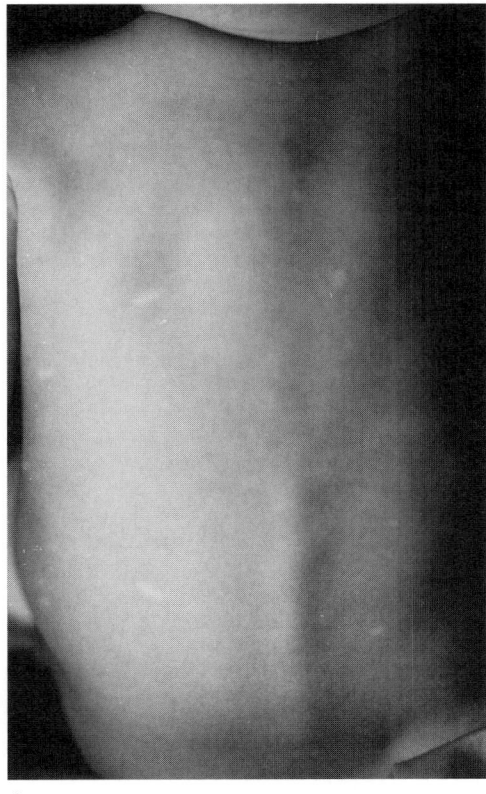

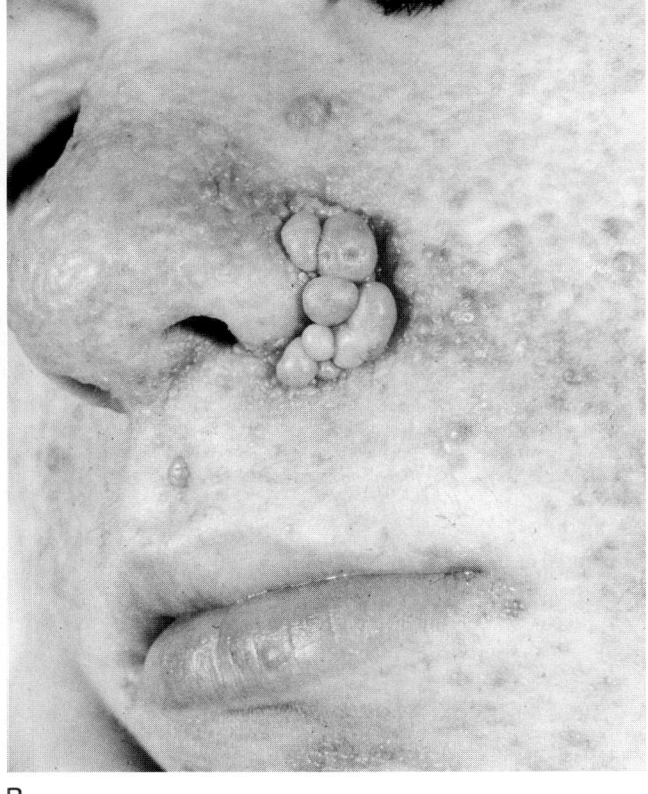

A                    B

**Fig. 233-4 Dermatologic features of tuberous sclerosis:** *A*, hypomelanotic macules; *B*, facial angiofibromas; *C*, shagreen patch; *D*, ungual fibromas; and, *E*, forehead plaque.

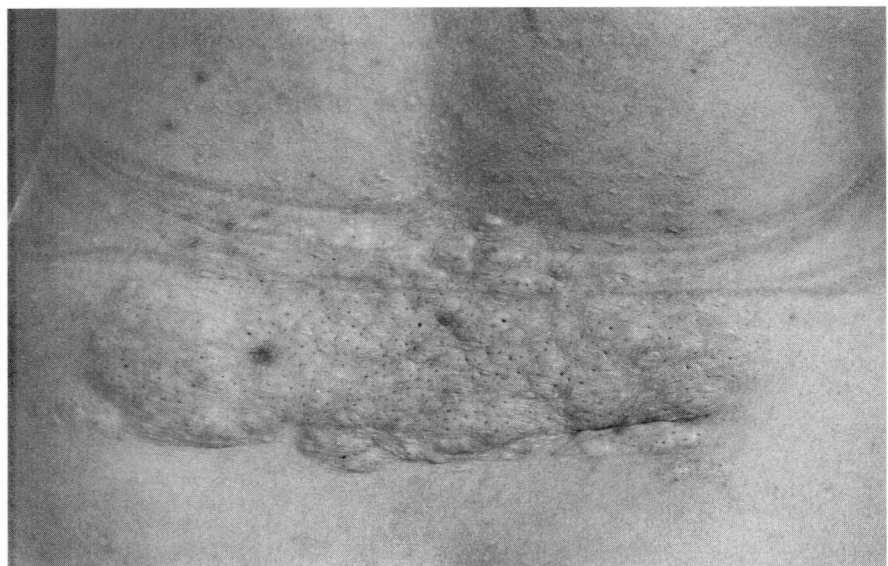

C

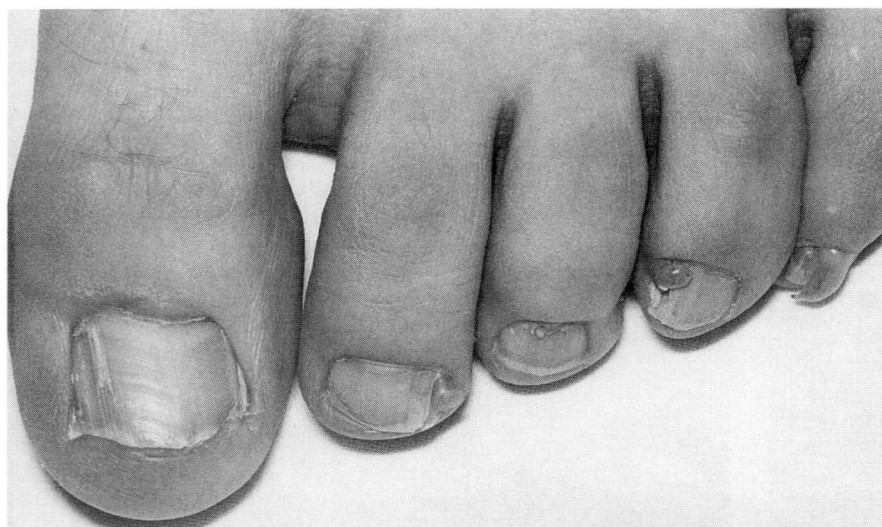

D

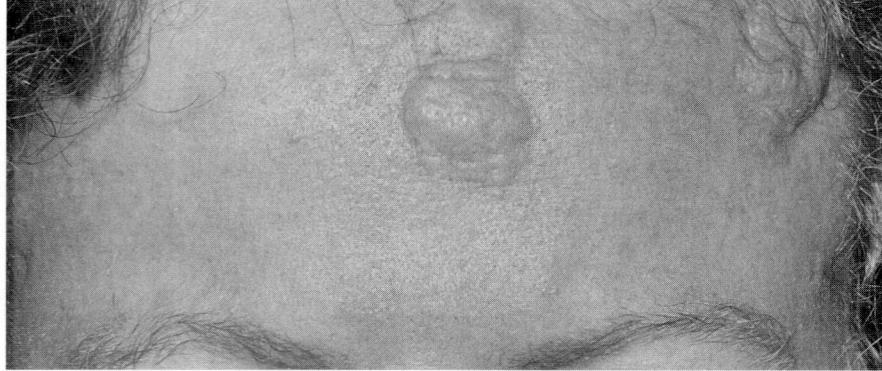

E

Fig. 233-4 (Continued)

Renal cysts are frequent in TSC, but in most patients, they are small and few in number and of no functional consequence. In a few percent of patients, the kidneys are enlarged and severely polycystic (Fig. 233-7). These cases may present antenatally, in infancy, or later. Severe hypertension and eventual progression to end stage renal failure are frequent (Fig. 233-8).[31] The cystic epithelium in TSC is hypertrophic and hyperplastic and the lining cells have strongly eosinophilic cytoplasm (Fig. 233-9).[32]

Renal cell carcinoma is infrequently seen in TSC. However, a number of reports of bilateral and multifocal renal cell carcinoma

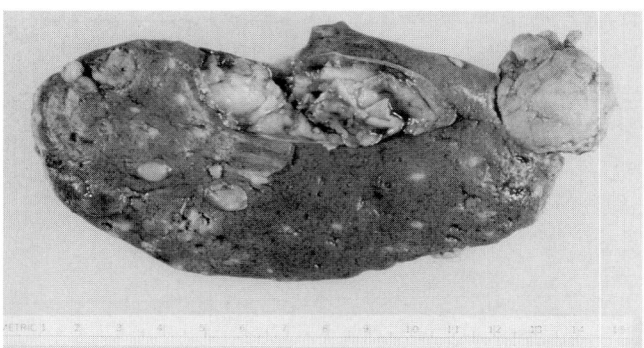

Fig. 233-5 Gross appearance of postmortem kidney specimen showing one large and innumerable small angiomyolipomas. The patient, a middle-aged female with known TSC, had died of exsanguinating hemorrhage from a ruptured angiomyolipoma in the opposite kidney. (*Courtesy of Dr. J. Bernstein.*)

with unusually early age at diagnosis are consistent with germ line *TSC1* and/or *TSC2* mutations acting as renal cell carcinoma predisposition alleles in at least some cases.[33] Immunohistochemical positivity for HMB-45 does not appear to distinguish angiomyolipoma from carcinoma in patients with TSC.[29] A number of reports also suggest a possible association between TSC and oncocytoma,[34,35] an unusual benign tumor composed of cells with abundant eosinophilic cytoplasm filled with mitochondria. However, confusion with atypical angiomyolipoma may be responsible.

## Pulmonary Manifestations

Symptomatic lung involvement by lymphangioleiomyomatosis (LAM) (Fig. 233-10) is recognized in only a small minority of patients with TSC. It occurs almost exclusively in postpubertal females. The true frequency of LAM in TSC is unknown. Lung cysts or recurrent pneumothoraces were reported in 2.6 percent of patients registered with the National Tuberous Sclerosis Association (of the United States of America) and in 2.3 percent of 338 patients with TSC who were evaluated at the Mayo Clinic in Rochester, Minnesota.[36] Presentation of LAM may be with progressive dyspnoea on exertion with or without cough and haemoptysis or acutely with pneumothorax or occasionally with chylothorax. Rate of progression is highly varaible, but the condition can persue a relentless and ultimately fatal course.[37] Although chest radiograph may be abnormal, high resolution computerised tomography of the chest is the most informative non-invasive diagnostic test and usually shows diffuse involvment of the lung parenchyma with thin walled cysts (Fig. 233-11).[36] Histopathologic examination reveals obstructive infiltration of alveolar septa, bronchioles, lymphatics and blood vessels by

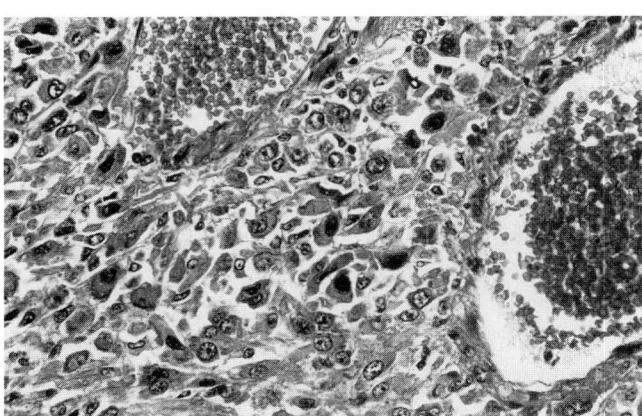

Fig. 233-6 Photomicrograph of malignant angiomyolipoma showing bizarre perivascular epithelial cells. (*Courtesy of Dr. J. Bernstein.*)

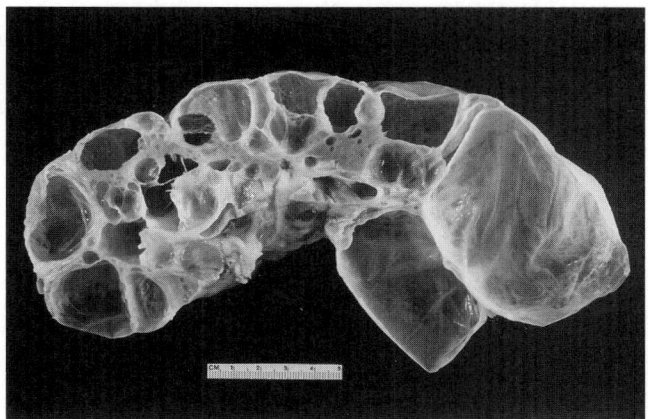

A

B

Fig. 233-7 Severely cystic kidney from an adolescent boy with TSC. Computed axial tomography, transverse section of abdomen, showing very severe polycystic kidney disease in a young child with TSC. (*Courtesy of Dr. J. Bernstein.*)

smooth muscle-like cells with eosinophilic cytoplasm (Fig. 233-12). Like their counterparts in angiomyolipomas, these cells contain vesicular structures that stain with HMB-45, distinguishing LAM from the smooth-muscle-cell infiltration associated with metastatic cystic sarcoma or benign metastasizing leiomyoma.[38] An apparently sporadic form of LAM that is often associated with extrapulmonary lymphatic involvement and with renal angiomyolipoma, but without cutaneous, brain, or other manifestations of TSC, is recognized in approximately 1 per 1,000,000 of the population.[39] The relationship to TSC has recently been clarified as somatic bi-allelic inactivation of *TSC2* and has been demonstrated in cells from some sporadic LAM cases.[39a] The children of these individuals do not appear to be at high risk of TSC or LAM.

Other lung pathologies associated with TSC are clear-cell tumor of the lung[40] and multifocal micronodular pneumocyte hyperplasia. This is a recently recognized histopathologic abnormality comprising focal proliferation of type II alveolar cells that is often associated with LAM in patients with TSC, and occasionally in those with "sporadic" LAM.[41] It does not appear to have important functional consequences.

## Cardiac Manifestations

Cardiac rhabdomyomas develop during fetal life and can be detected by echocardiography in approximately 60 to 80 percent of infants and children with TSC.[42,43] They are well-circumscribed nonencapsulated masses containing large ovoid or polygonal cells that are glycogen laden and resemble cardiac myoblasts.[44] Most infants with cardiac rhabdomyomas have TSC[43] and, in these cases, the tumors are typically multiple, ventricular in location and

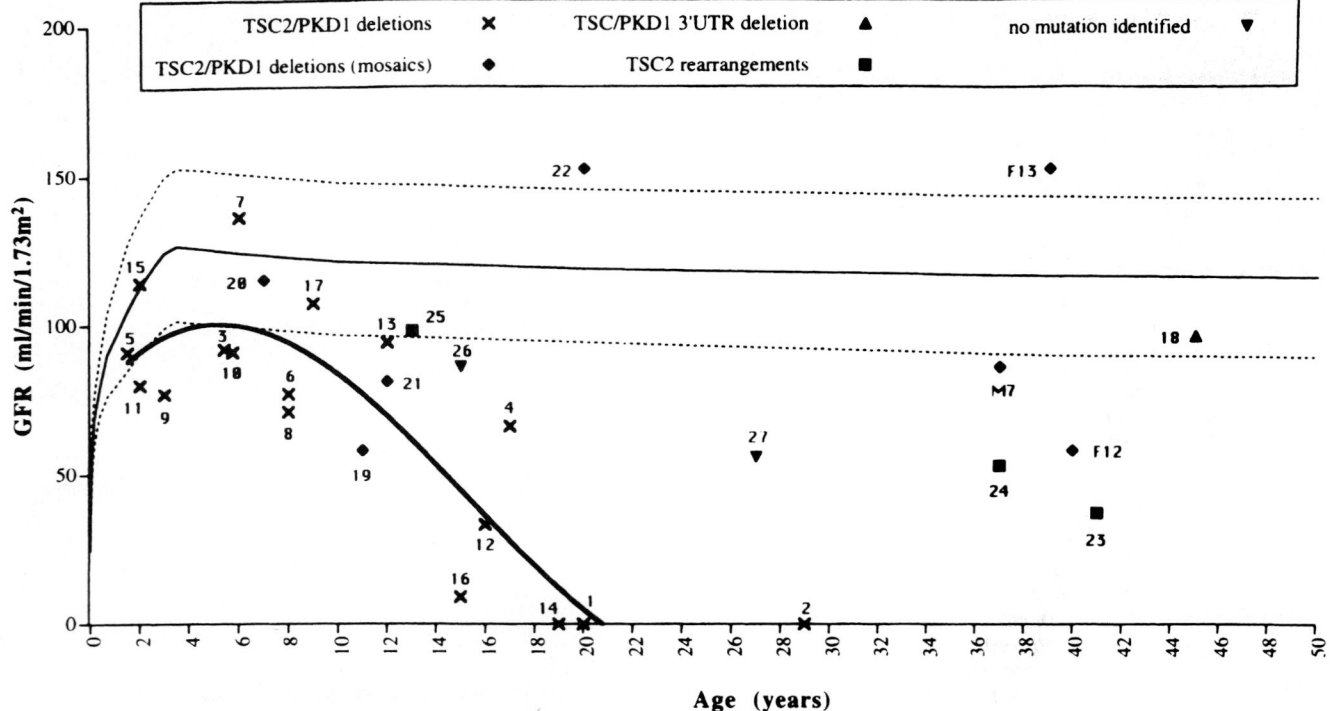

**Fig. 233-8 Cross-sectional renal function data in patients with tuberous sclerosis and polycystic kidney disease.** For each patient, the most recent estimate of glomerular filtration rate corrected for body surface area is plotted relative to a nomogram of glomerular filtration rates corrected for body surface area at different ages (mean and ± 2 SD). Three data points (M7, F12, F13) are for mildly affected adults who were mosaic for contiguous deletions of *TSC2*

and *PKD1* and who had more severely affected offspring with constitutional *TSC2* and *PKD1* deletions (cases 7, 12, and 13). The curve of best fit is for cases with apparently nonmosaic deletions involving the coding regions of *TSC2* and *PKD1* (*From Sampson JR, et al. Renal cystic disease in tuberous sclerosis: role of the polycystic kidney disease 1 gene. Am J Hum Genet 61:843, 1997. Used with permission.*)

often intramural. Routine antenatal screening for fetal abnormality using high resolution ultrasound scan is increasingly leading to unexpected prenatal detection of suspected TSC, through identification of cardiac rhabdomyomas. Ultrasound scanning of the fetal heart has also been used as a specific prenatal test in pregnancies at high risk of TSC.[45] During postnatal life the tumors involute or become relatively smaller as the heart grows.[46] The prognosis of cardiac rhabdomyomas is very good and the majority remain asymptomatic. Rarely, critically located tumors may obstruct outflow leading to cardiac failure or sudden death in the neonatal period (Fig. 233-13). Arrhythmia is the most frequent

presentation in older children and adults. Conduction abnormalities may be present in the absence of echocardiographically demonstrable rhabdomyomas.

## Involvement of Other Systems

**Vascular Involvement.** Aneurysms of the aorta and large arteries have been described, though infrequently.[47,48] Aneurysms of the intracerebral arteries have also been reported.[49]

**Skeletal Involvement.** Skeletal involvement is common,[50] but usually asymptomatic and is often identified coincidentally. Sclerosis (e.g., affecting the pelvis), periosteal new bone formation (especially in the metacarpals and metatarsals) and cystic changes are frequently seen. Bone deformity associated with localized overgrowth and rib expansion are infrequent but recognized abnormalities. Multiple pits affecting the dental enamel are frequent in TSC and are occasionally seen in the general population.[51,52]

**Endocrine Involvement.** Angiomyolipoma of the adrenal gland and papillary adenoma of the thyroid (which is otherwise extremely uncommon) have been reported a number of times in association with TSC.[53] Parathyroid hyperplasia, pancreatic islet cell tumors, and pituitary adenomas have been reported in combination with TSC.[54] This polyglandular phenotype is normally associated with multiple endocrine neoplasia type1 (MEN1). Interestingly, facial angiofibromatosis has also been reported in MEN1,[55] but the apparent overlap between the TSC and MEN1 phenotypes has not been extensively investigated.

**Other Organs.** Hepatic and splenic hemangiomas are almost always asymptomatic but may be identified by abdominal ultrasound.[56] Small and usually asymptomatic hamartomatous

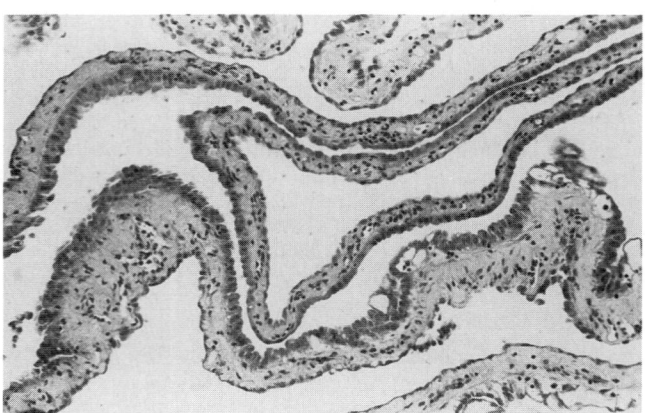

**Fig. 233-9 Renal biopsy of a cystic lesion from a young child with TSC showing attenuated septa lined with hyperplastic and hypertrophic epithelium highly characteristic of TSC.** (*Courtesy of Dr. J. Bernstein.*)

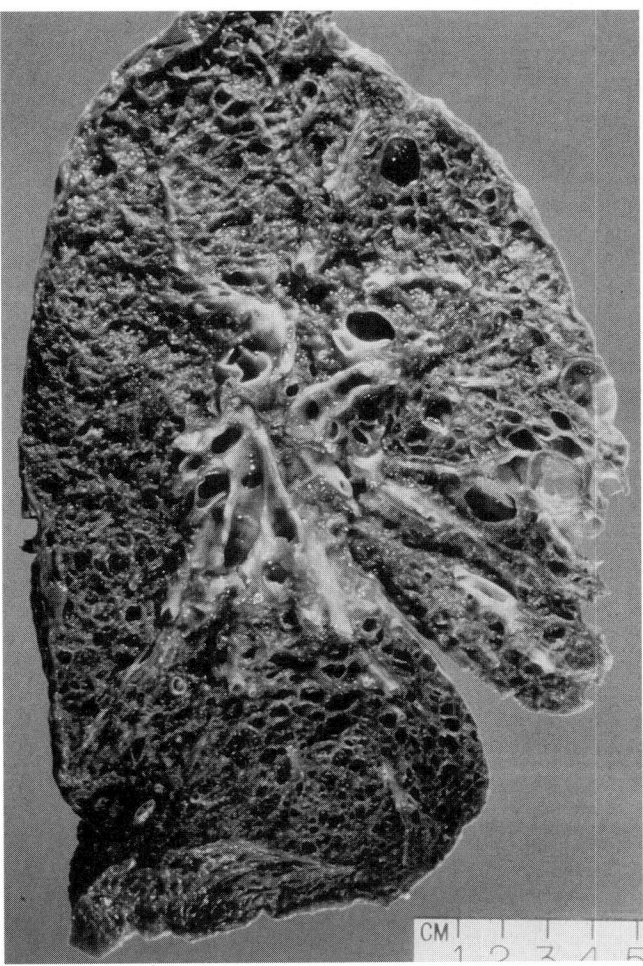

**Fig. 233-10 Cut surface of lung in advanced lymphangioleiomyomatosis showing thick and thin walled cysts. (*Courtesy of Dr. F. McCormack.*)**

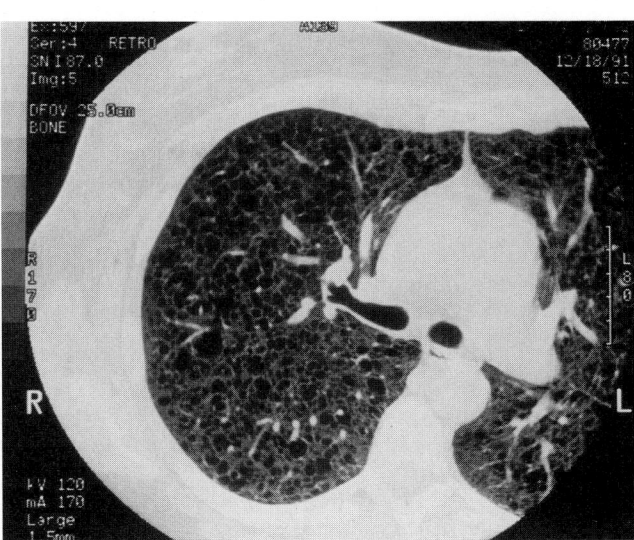

**Fig. 233-11 Computed axial tomography, transverse section of chest, showing extensive cystic pulmonary disease in tuberous sclerosis associated lymphangioleiomyomatosis. (*Courtesy of Dr. F. McCormack.*)**

polyps of the large bowel appear to be a frequent manifestation.[57] Larger hamartomatous and adenomatous polyps appear exceptional.[58]

### Clinical Diagnosis

Clinical diagnosis is based on features identified by physical examination and by radiographic and histopathologic investigation. Criteria for clinical diagnosis have been substantially revised in recent years and no single finding is now considered pathognomic of TSC.[59] Definitive diagnosis is made in the presence of specific combinations of features (Table 233-1). The evolving clinical definition reflects both an increasing awareness of overlaps with other disease phenotypes and new insights gained through molecular genetic analysis.

### EPIDEMIOLOGY

Several recent geographically based surveys in the United Kingdom and the United States have determined the minimum childhood prevalence of TSC to be 1 in 10,000 to 1 in 15,000.[60-62] However, medical ascertainment is unlikely to be complete and the true prevalence is certainly higher.[63]

TSC is transmitted as an autosomal dominant trait with very high and possibly complete penetrance.[64] Some 60 to 70 percent of cases are sporadic and appear to represent new mutations and the mutation rate has been estimated at $2.5 \times 10^{-5}$ per gamete.[60] The TSC phenotype shows extreme variability within, as well as

between, families.[65] Reports of large families in which all affected members have particularly mild disease[66] or marked renal disease[67] suggest that, despite intrafamily variability of expression, some level of genotype-phenotype correlation is likely.

### MANAGEMENT

Good management of TSC should include an initial assessment for medical complications and for developmental, psychologic, and behavioral problems at the time of diagnosis. There should be ongoing review for symptomatic and asymptomatic complications so that interventions can be introduced in a planned way whenever possible.[68] The multisystem nature of TSC can lead to fragmentation of medical care and the identification of a coordinating physician with a special interest can be very helpful. Specific multidisciplinary clinics and integrated care pathways have been developed at some centres, but at present, only a small proportion of patients have their management overseen in this way.

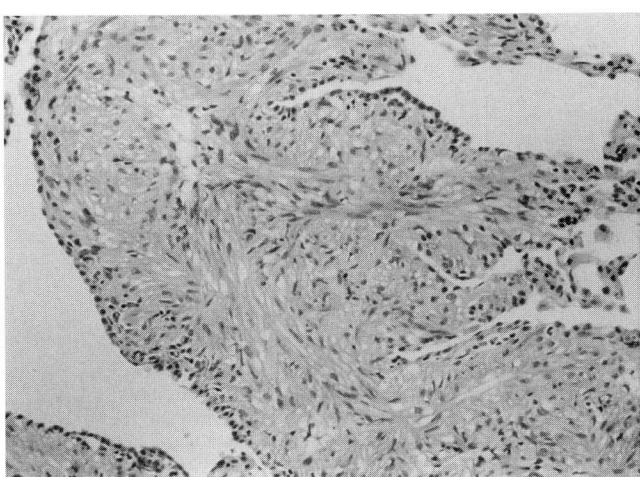

**Fig. 233-12 Photomicrograph of hematoxylin and eosin-stained lung section in lymphangioleiomyomatosis. There are characteristic, densely packed, smooth-muscle-like cells. (*Courtesy of Dr. F. McCormack.*)**

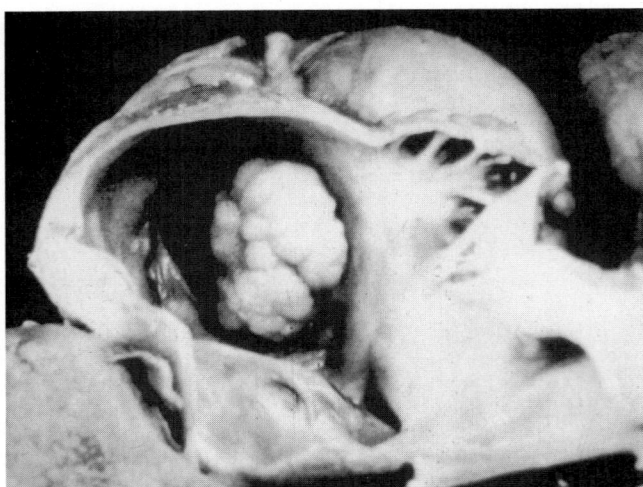

**Fig. 233-13 Postmortem appearance of large cardiac rhabdomyoma.**

### Central Nervous System

Poor outcome with regard to intellectual function is associated with early onset and intractability of seizures, and particularly with infantile spasms.[69] Urgent control of generalized seizures in the infant or young child with TSC is a priority. Vigabatrin is widely used in Europe and has proved to be the most effective drug for treatment of infantile spasms in TSC.[70,71] It has been recommended that treatment be continued for at least 3 years in patients who become seizure free. Vigabatrin has been associated with

**Table 233-1 Diagnostic Criteria for Tuberous Sclerosis**

Major features
1. Facial angiofibromas or forehead plaques
2. Nontraumatic ungual or periungual fibromas
3. > 3 hypomelanotic macules
4. Shagreen patch (connective tissue nevus)
5. Multiple retinal hamartomas
6. Cortical tuber*
7. Subependymal nodule
8. Subependymal giant cell astrocytoma
9. Cardiac rhabdomyoma
10. Lymphangioleiomyomatosis†
11. Renal angiomyolipoma†

Minor features
1. Multiple randomly distributed pits in dental enamel
2. Hamartomatous rectal polyps
3. Bone cysts‡
4. Cerebral white matter "migration tracts"*‡
5. Gingival fibromas
6. Nonrenal hamartoma‡
7. Retinal achromic patch
8. "Confetti" skin depigmentation
9. Multiple renal cysts

Definite TSC: either 2 major features or 1 major plus 2 minor features
Probable TSC: 1 major feature plus 1 minor feature
Possible TSC: Either 1 major feature of 2 or more minor features

*When cerebral cortical dysplasia and cerebral white matter migration tracts occur together, they should be counted as one feature of TSC.
†When both lymphangioleiomyomatosis and renal angiomyolipomas are present, other features of tuberous sclerosis should be present before a definite diagnosis is made.
‡Radiographic confirmation is sufficient.
Adapted from Roach, Gomez, Northrup, 1998.

development of nasal visual field defects in some cases, but this is rarely symptomatic.[72,73] Visual fields should be monitored where possible. Carbamazepine is frequently used in the treatment of focal seizures in older children and adults, but may precipitate the recurrence of infantile spasms in very young patients. Seizure control is frequently problematic in patients with TSC and, when seizures are intractable, neurosurgical assessment should be considered. Only a small minority of patients will be found to have sufficiently discrete epileptogenic foci to be good candidates for epilepsy surgery.

Giant cell astrocytomas are histologically benign but locally invasive tumors that develop in approximately 6 percent of patients, usually in childhood or early adult life. They are often located near the foramen of Munro, leading to hydrocephalus.[8,74] Recognition of raised intracranial pressure is frequently delayed in patients with intellectual disability. Some authors have suggested regular neuroradiologic surveillance,[68] but its place is not universally accepted.

### Developmental and Behavior Problems

Developmental and behavioral problems are a major concern for the families of many patients with TSC. Early recognition facilitates appropriate liaison with educational, psychologic and social agencies. Deterioration in development or behavior should prompt assessment to exclude underlying medical problems including brain tumor (subependymal giant cell astrocytoma), subclinical epilepsy, pain from renal disease, and the side effects of antiepileptic medication.

### Skin

Vascular (red) facial angiofibromas can be effectively treated using pulsed dye laser or VersaPulse laser. Argon laser treatment appears to carry a higher risk of causing hypopigmentation. Skin-resurfacing lasers (for example Ultrapulse $CO_2$ or erbium/YAG) are required for more fibrotic lesions. Surgical approaches may be considered in severe cases. Surgical excision may also be considered for forehead or scalp plaques or ungual fibromas.

### Kidneys

Regular monitoring for hypertension and one to three yearly renal ultrasound scan have been recommended as surveillance measures.[68] Renal function should be monitored in those patients with structural renal abnormalities. Large (>3.5 cm) angiomyolipomas are more likely to hemorrhage than smaller lesions,[75-77] but absolute criteria for intervention in the asymptomatic patient have not been agreed. Embolization, partial nephrectomy, or occasionally total nephrectomy may be required for bleeding from angiomyolipomas. Renal replacement therapy, including renal transplantation may be indicated in the minority of patients who reach end stage renal disease.[78,79] Those with polycystic kidney disease due to contiguous deletion of the *TSC2* and *PKD1* genes are at high risk of renal failure.[31]

### Lungs

Respiratory symptoms (particularly in the postpubertal female patient) should prompt investigation for lymphangioleiomyomatosis by computerized tomography of the chest and pulmonary function testing. Baseline computerized tomography has been suggested in early adulthood for female patients with TSC,[68] but its benefits are unproved. Referral to a respiratory physician with a special interest in this disorder is recommended for patients with suspected LAM.

### Heart

Echocardiography for the detection of cardiac rhabdomyoma may prove helpful diagnostically in the infant with suspected TSC.[68] Routine follow-up is not required in the asymptomatic patient, and surgical resection of cardiac rhabdomyomas is very rarely indicated. The possibility of arrhythmia masquerading as a seizure

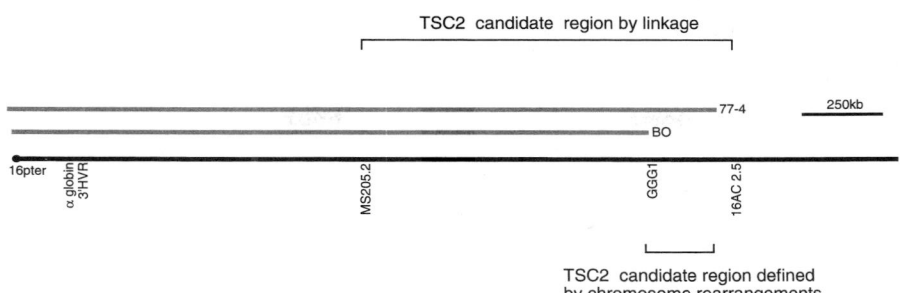

**Fig. 233-14** Rearrangements involving 16p13.3 that defined the *TSC2* candidate region. Critical meiotic recombination events in families showing linkage of TSC to 16p13 first identified a candidate region extending between the polymorphic markers MS205.2 and 16AC2.5. Deletions involving 16p13.3 in patient 77-4, who manifested the TSC phenotype, and in patient BO, who did not, defined a much smaller candidate region in which *TSC2* could be sought. (*From Sampson JR, The TSC2 gene and tuberin, in Gomez MR, Sampson JR, Holets Whittemore V (eds):* Tuberous Sclerosis Complex, *3rd ed. New York, Oxford University Press, 1999. Used with permission.*)

disorder should be considered in patients with unexplained loss of consciousness.

## Genetic Counseling and Evaluation of Family Members

The family with a member, or members, affected by TSC should be offered genetic counseling. Genetic risks, including those due to germ-line mosaicism,[80,81] need to be discussed. Assessment of family members who are concerned about their own status has traditionally included clinical and ophthalmologic examination, cranial computerized tomography or magnetic resonance imaging, and renal ultrasound scan.[82,83] Although nonpenetrance occurs rarely, if at all,[64,84,84a] genetic status can be difficult to determine, for example when one or two white macules, or an isolated renal cyst or possible angiomyolipoma are detected. Molecular genetic diagnosis can facilitate accurate genetic counseling and prenatal diagnosis for an increasing proportion of families.[85,85a]

## THE *TSC1* AND *TSC2* GENES

### Positional Cloning of the *TSC1* and *TSC2* Genes

The TSC determining genes *TSC1* and *TSC2* have been identified by positional cloning.[86,87] *TSC1* was localized to chromosome 9q34 in 1987 by linkage analysis in a modest set of families using only protein and blood group polymorphisms.[88] Evidence for locus heterogeneity was established soon afterwards[89,90] but localization of *TSC2* to 16p13.3 was only achieved in 1992 through systematic genome screening.[91] Key meiotic recombi-

nation events were identified that refined the *TSC1* and *TSC2* candidate regions to intervals of 1 to 1.5 Mb.[92–95] The approaches subsequently used to isolate the two genes differed substantially. The rapid identification of *TSC2* in 1993 was facilitated by the analysis of microscopic and submicroscopic rearrangements at 16p13.3 in a small number of critical patients. By contrast, the eventual identification of *TSC1* in 1997, followed large-scale genomic sequencing of the candidate region.

### Identification of *TSC2*

Critical positional information for *TSC2* was obtained by analysis of deletions of 16p13.3-pter in two patients, one with and one without TSC.[86] Together these rearrangements implicated a region of just 300 kb as likely to contain *TSC2* (Fig. 233-14). The region was cloned as a set of overlapping cosmids and screened for large rearrangements in a panel of 255 unrelated patients with TSC using pulsed-field gel analysis. Five deletion mutations of between 30 and more than 100 kb were detected, all involving a 120-kb area from which four genes were identified. One gene was disrupted by all five deletions, making it a strong candidate for *TSC2* (Fig. 233-15). The identification of several intragenic TSC associated deletions by conventional Southern analysis then confirmed the identify of *TSC2*.

### Characterization of *TSC2*

The *TSC2* gene comprises 41 coding exons and one 5′ untranslated exon[96,97] (GenBank L48517 to L48546). Exons 25, 26, and 31 are subject to alternative splicing.[96,98] *TSC2* encodes tuberin, a previously unknown protein, with a full-length isoform of 1807

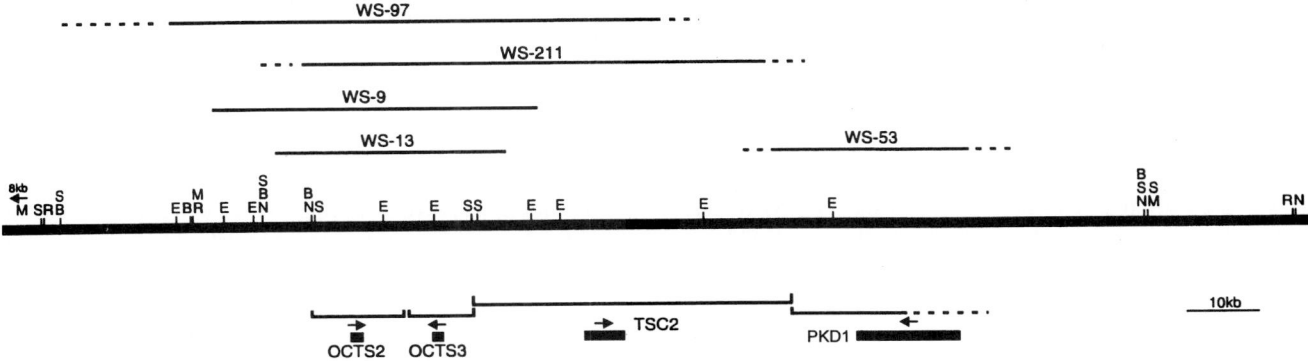

**Fig. 233-15** Deletions and genes at the *TSC2* locus. Genomic sites for the enzymes *Bss*HII (B); *Mlu*I (M); *Not*I (N); *Nru*I (R); *Sac*II (S); and a partial map of *Eco*RI (E). Sites are indicated on a physical map spanning approximately 180 kb. The genomic extents of five deletions identified by pulsed-field gel electrophoresis are shown above the map (solid lines, with dotted lines representing regions of uncertainty). The genomic extents (square brackets), transcript sizes (solid boxes) and directions of transcription (arrows) of four genes isolated from the region are shown below the map. Only one gene was disrupted by all of the deletions, implicating it as *TSC2*. Its identity was subsequently confirmed by the identification of intragenic mutations in patients with TSC.

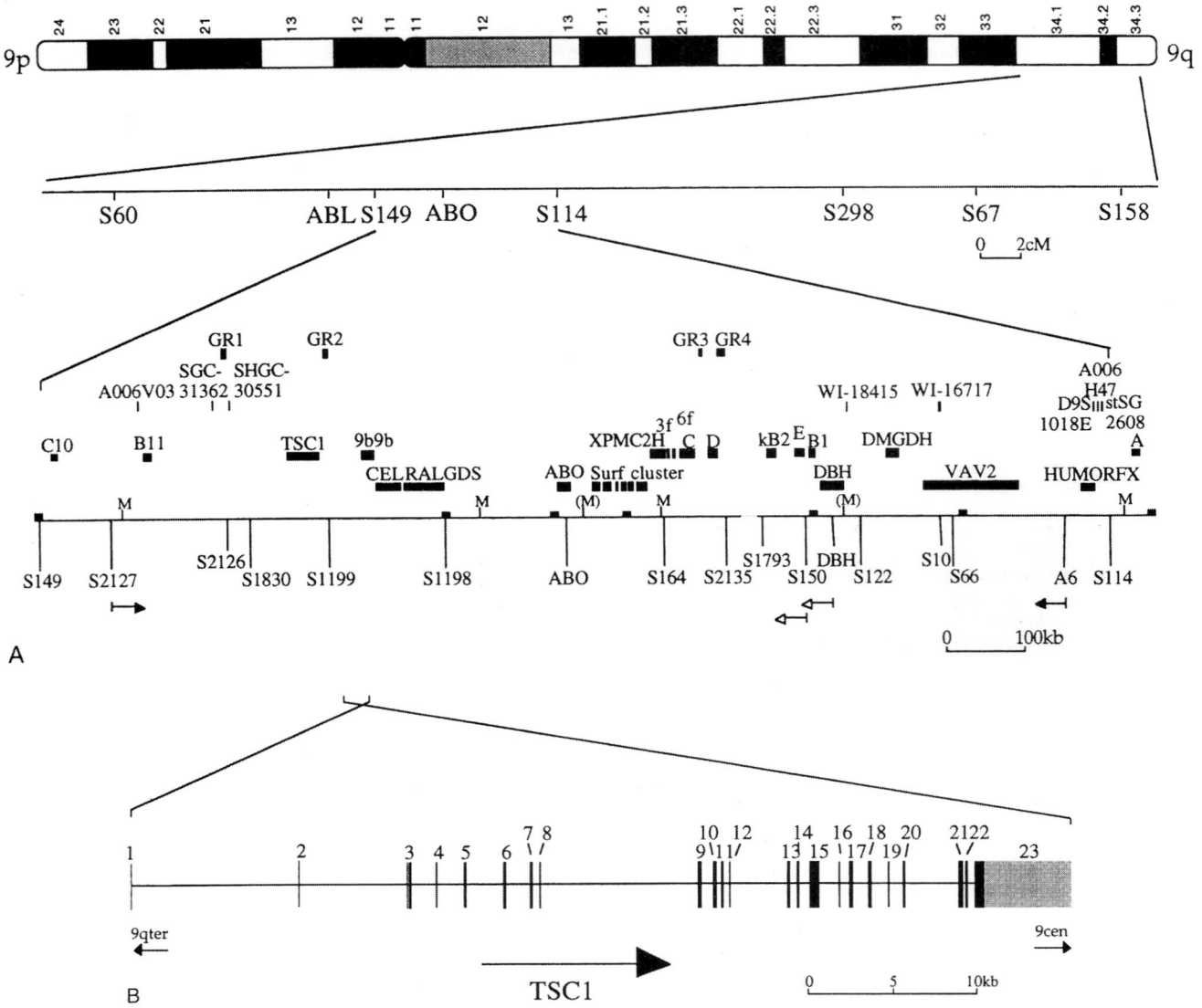

**Fig. 233-16 A:** The *TSC1* region at chromosome 9q34. The ideogram (*top*) represents a G banded metaphase chromosome 9. The genetic map (*middle*) indicates the approximate positions of marker loci and the ABO blood group (ABO) and Abelson oncogene (ABL) loci. A more detailed physical map of the candidate region (*bottom*) indicates positional information from key recombination events in affected individuals (*solid arrows*) and unaffected individuals (*open arrows*). The approximate positions of *Mlu*I sites (M, with sites that partially cut in genomic DNA in brackets) and of probes used to screen for large rearrangements in patients with TSC by pulsed-field gel electrophoresis are indicated immediately above the map (*solid boxes*). Genes previously mapped to the region, novel cDNAs isolated from the region, ESTs mapped to the region, and additional possible genes predicted by Grail analysis are represented by solid boxes at progressively higher levels. **B:** Structure of the *TSC1* gene. The distribution of exons 1 to 23 is indicated. Exons 3 through 23 include coding sequence. The large arrow indicates the direction of transcription. (*Excerpted from the TSC1 Consortium: Identification of the tuberous sclerosis gene TSC1 on chromosome 9q34,* Science *277:805, 1997. Copyright 1997 American Association for the Advancement of Science. Used with permission.*)

amino acids (198 kDa). A region spanning residues 1517 to 1674 and encoded by exons 34 through 38 has significant homology to the GTPase-activating proteins (GAPs) human rap1GAP and murine Spa1.[86,99] GAPs are negative regulators of the ras superfamily of small GTPases that play diverse roles including control of cell proliferation and differentiation, vesicular trafficking, and modulation of the cytoskeleton, suggesting a number of possible cellular mechanisms for the proposed tumor-suppressor properties of *TSC2*.

## Identification of *TSC1*

After *TSC1* was mapped to 9q34, a number of genetic linkage studies defined a 1.4-Mb candidate region, which was cloned as a series of overlapping cosmid and P1 artificial chromosome clones (Fig. 233-16). Screens for large rearrangements in patients with TSC that might have implicated a specific part of the region proved negative.[87] During efforts to identify *TSC1*, 30 genes were isolated from or mapped to the candidate region and many were investigated as positional candidates for *TSC1*, but none were shown to harbor TSC-associated mutations. Genomic sequencing of the entire candidate region was, therefore, initiated, enabling the systematic identification of exons which were then screened for TSC-associated mutations. A predicted exon that contained frameshift mutations in affected individuals was rapidly identified and shown to be part of a gene, the full sequence and genomic structure of which were determined by comparison of genomic and cDNA sequences (GenBank AC002096 and AF013168, respectively). Further analysis of the gene revealed 32 distinct mutations, confirming its identity as *TSC1*.[87]

## Characterization of *TSC1*

The *TSC1* gene contains 23 exons of which numbers 3 to 23 are coding. Hamartin, the predicted product, is a novel protein of 1164 amino acids (130 kDa).[87] It has no significant homology to tuberin or other known vertebrate proteins, but it does have significant homology to a *Schizosaccharomyces pombe*-predicted protein (GenBank Q09778). Unlike tuberin, hamartin contains no predicted GAP-related domain, but it does contain a strongly predicted coiled-coil domain (residues 730 to 965).[100]

## *TSC1* AND *TSC2* MUTATIONS

### Germ-Line Mutations of *TSC1* and *TSC2*

Both the *TSC1* and *TSC2* genes exhibit diverse mutational spectra with relatively few recurrent mutations. However, the proportions of different classes of mutations observed at the two loci are quite distinct (Fig. 233-17). Databases of mutations at the *TSC1* and *TSC2* loci include the Human Gene Mutation Database (www.uwcm.ac.uk/uwcm/mg/hgmd0.html) and a TSC gene specific database (http://expmed.bwh.harvard.edu/ts/).

*TSC1* mutations have been identified in only 15 to 20 percent of TSC probands.[64,85,101-106] Large rearrangements at the *TSC1* locus have been sought using pulsed-field gel and conventional

Southern analysis but, by contrast to the *TSC2* locus, such rearrangements appear to be very rare.[85] The vast majority of *TSC1* mutations appear to be nonsense changes, microdeletions and insertions, and splice site changes, all of which would be predicted to be truncating. Mutations are distributed throughout the coding region; the majority occurs in exons 15 through 21; mutations in exons 22 and 23 have not been reported. *TSC1* mutations are significantly underrepresented in sporadic as opposed to familial cases[85,101,107] and a lower frequency of intellectual impairment has been reported among *TSC1* than *TSC2* sporadic cases.[85,101] A lower proportion of medically ascertained sporadic *TSC1* cases and a milder phenotype in *TSC1* disease would be predicted in if both germ line and somatic mutation rates were lower at the *TSC1* locus than at the *TSC2* locus.

Comprehensive mutation analysis of *TSC2* has revealed large rearrangements including multiexon and whole-gene deletions in approximately 15 percent of cases.[85] Pathogenic missense mutations, which occur rarely, if at all, at the *TSC1* locus, account for a further 15 percent of *TSC2* mutations.[85] Some clustering is observed in exons encoding the GAP-related domain of tuberin, suggesting a critical function for this region. The remaining mutations are mainly nonsense changes, small insertions and deletions, and splice site changes, and these are distributed throughout the gene.[85,103,106,108-110]

There are a number of reports of germ line and somatic mosaicism at the *TSC1* and *TSC2* loci[80,81,111,112] and somatic mosaicism may be present in 10 percent or more of new mutation

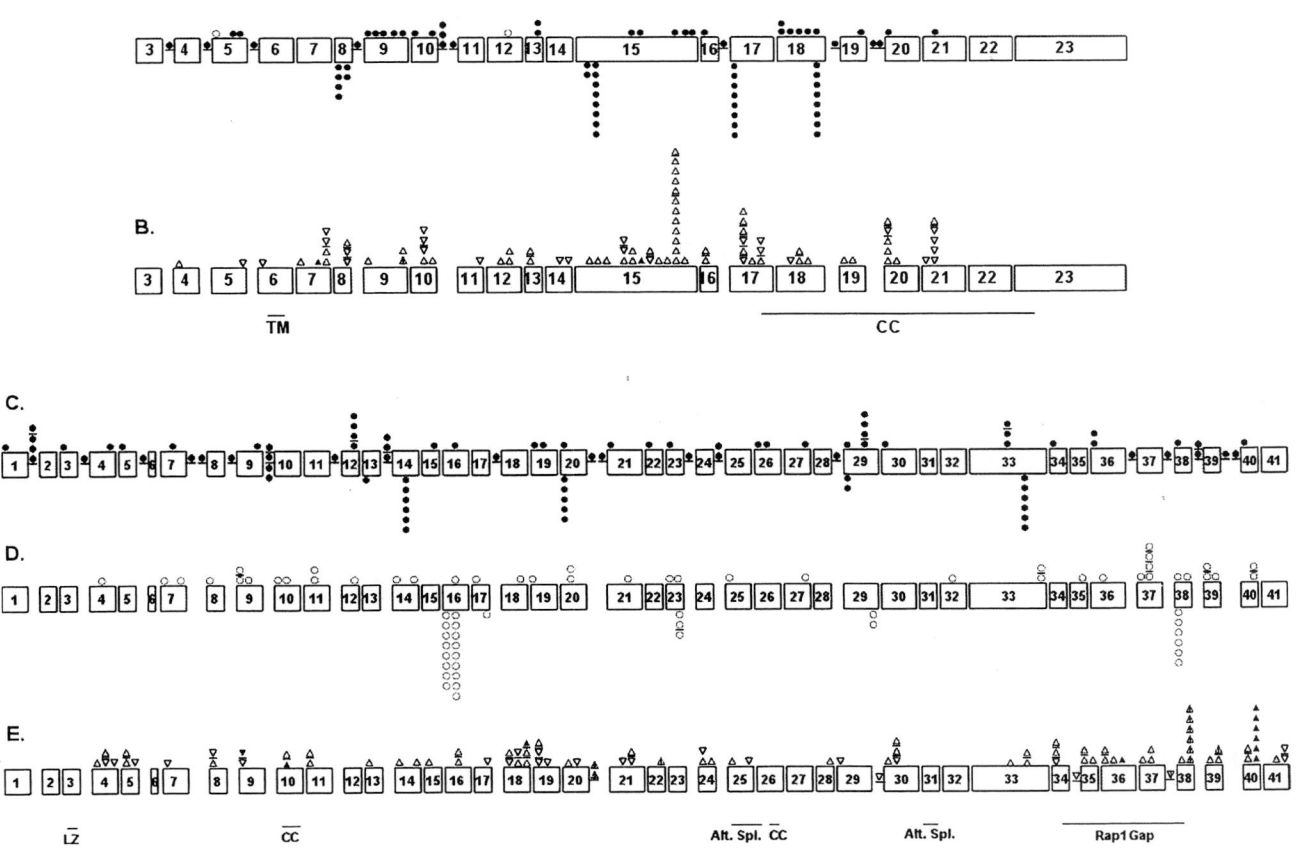

**Fig. 233-17** Germ line mutation spectra of *TSC1* and *TSC2*. In *TSC1*, mutations are binned at 40 bp/bin; in *TSC2*, mutations are binned at 60 bp/bin. A small horizontal line delimits mutations occurring at nearby positions. Partial introns are drawn when a mutation occurs in the intron. Symbols: filled circles = nonsense; filled circles with line = splicing point mutations; open circles = missense; filled triangles = in-frame indel; open triangles = frameshift indel; triangle pointing upward = deletion; triangle pointing downward = insertion. Point mutations occurring at CpG sites are drawn below the gene. Putative functional domains are shown at the bottom for each gene. *A, TSC1* point mutations. *B, TSC1* insertions and deletions. *C, TSC2* truncating point mutations. *D, TSC2* missense mutations. *E, TSC2* insertions and deletions. In addition, approximately 15 percent of mutations are whole exon, multiexon, or whole gene deletions, or other large rearrangements at the TSC2 locus (not shown). (*Courtesy of Dr. M.P. Reeve.*)

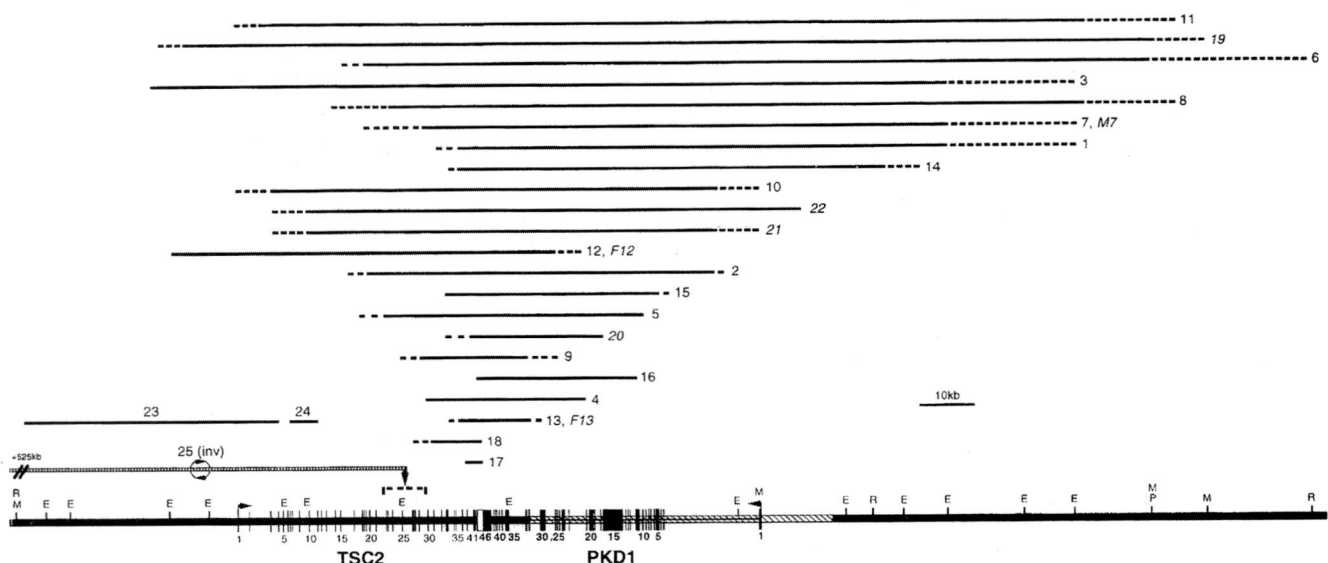

**Fig. 233-18** Deletions and an inversion at the *TSC2-PKD1* locus in patients with TSC and polycystic kidney disease. The genomic map is shown as a solid bar with restriction sites for *Eco*RI (E), *Mlu*I (M), and *Nru*I (R) indicated. The hatched region indicates part of the *PKD1* locus, which is duplicated elsewhere on chromosome 16. The locations of exons of the *PKD1* gene and *TSC2* gene are shown and the directions of transcription are arrowed. The regions of DNA deleted in TSC patients with polycystic kidney disease are shown above the map. The solid lines show the region definitely deleted and the dashed lines regions of uncertainty. Patients found to be mosaic for deletions are numbered in italics. The proximal inversion breakpoint in patient 25 is illustrated, the distal breakpoint lies ≈600 kb telomeric. The mechanisms leading to polycystic kidney disease in this patient, and in patients 23 and 24 in whom the deletions do not involve the structural *PKD1*, gene have not been determined. (*Adapted from Sampson JR, et al. Renal cystic disease in tuberous sclerosis: Role of the polycystic kidney disease 1 gene, Am J Hum Genet 61:848, 1997. Used with permission.*)

cases.[112] Low-level somatic mosaicism poses a significant challenge in molecular genetic diagnostics.[113]

## A Contiguous Gene Deletion Syndrome Involving *TSC2* and *PKD1*

The *TSC2* gene is located immediately distal to the *PKD1* gene that is mutated in autosomal dominant polycystic kidney disease (ADPKD) type 1 (see Chap. 215).[114] The genes are arranged 3′ to 3′ with their polyadenylation signals lying only 60 bp apart.[115] Deletion mutations at the locus may involve both genes and a contiguous gene deletion syndrome of TSC and severe early onset polycystic kidney disease has been defined (Fig. 233-18).[31,116] In ADPKD type 1, the onset of macroscopic renal cystic disease is usually in adult life and onset of end stage renal disease occurs at a mean age of 53 years.[117] Though well-recognized, prenatal or childhood presentation of ADPKD type 1 occurs in only 1 to 2 percent of cases.[118] By contrast, contiguous deletion of *TSC2* and *PKD1* is usually associated with early onset and severe renal cystic disease, often diagnosed in utero or shortly after birth and progression to end-stage renal failure by late childhood or early adult life occurs in a high proportion of cases.[31] In the most comprehensive study of the contiguous gene deletion syndrome so far conducted, 4 of 27 index cases were shown to be somatic mosaics as were the relatively mildly affected and secondarily ascertained parents of 3 further index cases.[31]

## Somatic Mutations in Hamartomas

Hamartomas from patients with TSC, including angiomyolipomas, rhabdomyomas, subependymal giant cell astrocytomas and angiofibromas frequently show somatic deletions in the vicinities of the TSC genes manifest as loss of heterozygosity (LOH).[119–123] These observations are consistent with the classification of both genes as Knudson-type tumor suppressors. LOH has been observed less frequently at the *TSC1* locus than at the *TSC2* locus,[124,125] as expected given the small proportion of patients with germ line *TSC1* mutations. There is little evidence for LOH in cortical tubers,[125] possibly reflecting the mixture of cell types

evident in these lesions on histopathologic examination.[8,10] Both LOH and intragenic mutation of the *TSC1* gene have been reported in TSC associated renal cell carcinoma.[87,122]

Several recent studies have assessed whether *TSC1* or *TSC2* are mutated in sporadic hamartomas or sporadic malignant tumors. LOH encompassing the *TSC2* locus at 16p13.3 has been reported in sporadic angiomyolipomas[126] and in angiomyolipomas associated with lymphangioleiomyomatosis in patients without other manifestations of TSC.[127] LOH associated with intragenic mutation of the retained allele has been reported in sporadic bladder cancer,[128] a malignancy that is not thought to be overrepresented in patients with TSC. Reduced or absent expression of tuberin has been reported to occur in approximately 30 percent of sporadic glioblastomas,[129] but in a molecular genetic study of the *TSC1* and *TSC2* genes, inactivating mutations affecting both alleles were not demonstrated at either locus in a wide range of sporadic glial and glioneuronal tumors.[130] Clarification of whether the TSC genes play significant roles in the genesis of tumors that are not usually associated with the TSC phenotype requires further investigation.

## ANIMAL MODELS

There are currently no reported animal models for *TSC1*, but rat, mouse, and *Drosophila* models carrying mutant *TSC2* alleles have been reported and have provided a valuable resource for investigating putative functions of tuberin.

### Eker Rat

The Eker rat is a naturally occurring rodent model for TSC carrying an inactivating retrotransposon insertion mutation in exon 30 of the rat *TSC2* gene.[131,132] The Eker rat was first described in 1954 when the strain was noted to develop bilateral multifocal solid and cystic renal adenomas.[133] The phenotype was shown to be transmissible as an autosomal dominant trait with embryonic lethality in the homozygote.[134–136] Numerous extrarenal manifestations of the Eker phenotype have been described, including uterine leiomyoma, splenic hemangioma, pituitary adenoma,[137] and, most recently, subependymal hamartomas analogous to those found in the human brain in TSC.[138] However, cortical tubers have not been identified. Allelic loss and intragenic mutation affecting *TSC2* have been demonstrated in tumors in the Eker rat.[139–141] More direct evidence for the tumor-suppressor properties of *TSC2* has been provided by transgenic expression of *TSC2* in the Eker rat[142] and Eker tumor cell lines.[143,144] Embryos that are homozygous for the Eker mutation die at days 10 to 12 and have disrupted neuroepithelial growth and development.[145]

### *TSC2* Knockout Mice

Mice with targeted disruption of *TSC2* have been generated and shown to express a phenotype very similar to the Eker rat.[146,147] Heterozygous mice develop solid and cystic adenomas, with or without papillary projections by 6 months of age. Renal cell carcinoma develops in 5 to 10 percent of mice by 18 months, with metastatic disease occurring in some cases. Histologically benign hepatic hemangiomas and histologically malignant but nonmetastasizing hemangiosarcomas of the limbs and tail are frequently seen. Lung adenomas also occur (in about one-third of mice) but seem to have limited growth potential and are not associated with functional deficit. There is no reported evidence for brain lesions. Homozygous mice die in midgestation (E10.5 to E12.5) and exhibit growth failure, hepatic hypoplasia, and anemia.

### The *gigas* Mutant in *Drosophila*

It has recently been demonstrated that the *Drosophila* mutant *gigas*[148] results from mutations affecting the *TSC2* homolog.[149] In tissue-specific expression systems, homozygous *gigas* eye and wing cells are hypertrophied and have been shown to contain a tenfold excess of DNA, reflecting continued rounds of DNA replication without cell division. The loss of coordination of DNA synthesis with mitosis was shown to be associated with failure of the normal degradation of cyclins A and B. In contrast to hamartomatous TSC cells in man and in mammalian models, structure and organization of *gigas* $-/-$ cells appear otherwise normal.

## ANALYSIS OF HAMARTIN AND TUBERIN

### Expression of Hamartin and Tuberin

The *TSC2* transcript is widely expressed in developing and adult human tissues[86,150–152] and in the developing nervous system, heart and kidneys in rodents.[153,154] Some tissues and organs that are not usually involved in TSC, such as spinal cord and testis, also express high levels of tuberin. Particularly high expression has been noted in the olfactory bulb, brain stem nuclei, cerebellar Purkinje cells, and motor neurons of the ventral spinal cord; the islets of Langerhans, eccrine sweat glands, and vascular endothelium of small vessels also stain intensely.[152] It is unknown whether the different isoforms of tuberin show tissue or developmental stage specific differential expression. By immuno-histochemical analysis, the expression pattern of hamartin in normal human tissues has been shown to be almost identical to that of tuberin.[155]

### Hamartin and Tuberin Interact Directly

A direct interaction between hamartin and tuberin is supported by assays using the yeast 2-hybrid system, by coimmunoprecipitation and by colocalization.[100,155] Cofractionation experiments are consistent with hamartin and tuberin forming a predominantly cytosolic complex, although a small proportion of both proteins appears to be membrane associated.[155,156] Attempts to clarify the subcellular localization of the proteins by immunofluorescence microscopy have yielded different results in different cell types. Localization of native tuberin to the Golgi was suggested by studies in a number of tumor-derived cell lines,[157] but diffuse cytoplasmic staining has been noted on overexpression in Cos

cells.[100,156] A punctate cytoplasmic distribution of hamartin has been reported both on overexpression in Cos cells and on detection of endogenous protein in cultured 293 cells.[100,155] This appears to reflect protein aggregation, rather than localization to vesicular organelles.[156] Further studies are required to determine with certainty the subcellular location(s) of hamartin and tuberin in a variety of normal cells and at different stages of the cell cycle and to relate the direct interaction between the proteins to their cellular roles and the TSC phenotype.

### *TSC1* and *TSC2* as Tumor Suppressors

LOH at the *TSC1* or *TSC2* locus in TSC-associated hamartomas[119–125] and at the *Tsc2* locus in renal and other lesions in the Eker rat[139,140] and *Tsc2* knockout mice[146,147] suggest that the genes encode tumor suppressors. Expression of a wild-type *Tsc2* transgene in cell lines derived from Eker tumors, and introduction of a wild-type *Tsc2* allele into the germ line in the Eker rat, have provided direct support for the tumor-suppressor properties of *TSC2*.[142–144] The cellular mechanisms through which hamartin and tuberin regulate cell growth are not yet fully understood.

### Possible Cellular Roles of Hamartin and Tuberin

**GTPase Activation.** A region of homology between tuberin and the GTPase-activating proteins (GAPs) rap1GAP and Spa1 was noted when the *TSC2* gene was identified[86,99] suggesting that tuberin might function as a GAP. Modest GAP activity of tuberin for rap1 and for rab5 was demonstrated biochemically,[158,159] but it is unclear whether these activities are of physiological importance.

**Endocytosis and Vesicular Trafficking.** During screens for tuberin interacting proteins, tuberin was found to interact with rabaptin, a rab5 effector, implying a role for tuberin in endocytosis.[159] The rate of fluid phase endocytosis was reduced on reintroduction of tuberin into tuberin-deficient cells. However, others have not been able to replicate these findings[156] and their relevance to TSC remains unconfirmed.

**Cell Cycle Control.** Antisense inhibition of *TSC2* expression has been reported to induce quiescent $G_0$-arrested fibroblasts to undergo CDK-dependent reentry into the cell cycle.[160] However, the apparent cytoplasmic localization of tuberin would not support a direct role in nuclear cell-cycle events. By contrast, *TSC2*$-/-$ cells from the *Drosophila* mutant *gigas* exhibit continuing DNA synthesis without cell division.[149] In cell culture, hamartin has been shown to attenuate proliferation through an effect on $G_1$ phase control.[160a]

**Neuronal Differentiation.** The central nervous system pathology of TSC implicates *TSC1* and *TSC2* in neuronal differentiation. Posttranscriptional up-regulation of tuberin expression has been observed upon induction of neuronal differentiation and antisense inhibition of tuberin appears to inhibit neuronal differentiation in culture.[161]

**Transcriptional Activation.** Possible transcriptional activation domains of tuberin have been suggested by observation of autoactivation in yeast 2-hybrid assays and CAT assays in Hela and NIH3T3 cells.[162] Others have reported that tuberin can modulate transcription mediated via steroid hormone receptor activation.[163]

**Adhesion.** Hamartin has been shown to interact with the ERM (ezrin-radixin-moesin) actin building protiens and to play a role in rho mediated cell-matrix adhesion.[164]

None of the specific cellular roles so far proposed for hamartin or tuberin have been corroborated by independent observation and a unifying hypothesis linking current observations is lacking. Several studies have, however, provided evidence for a direct interaction between these proteins,[100,155,163] indicating their participation in at least some cellular processes. The challenge is to clarify these processes and their relationship to the pathogenesis of TSC.

## REFERENCES

1. Moolten SE: Hamartial nature of tuberous sclerosis complex and its bearing on the tumour problem: Report of a case with tumour anomaly of the kidney and adenoma sebaceum. *Arch Int Med* **69**:589, 1942.
2. Caviness VS Jr: Forward, in Gomez MR, Sampson JR, Holets Whittemore V (eds): *Tuberous Sclerosis Complex*, 3rd ed. New York, Oxford University Press, 1999, p v.
3. Bournville DM: Sclerose tubereuse des circonvolutions cerebrales: Idiotie et epilepsie hemiplgique. *Arch Neurol (Paris)* **1**:81,1880.
4. Pringle JJ: A case of congenital adenoma sebaceum. *Brit J Dermatol* **2**:1, 1890.
5. Sherlock EB: *The Feeble-Minded*. London, McMillan, 1911.
6. Gunther M, Penrose LS: The genetics of epiloia. *J Genet* **31**:413, 1935.
7. Gomez MR: Natural history of cerebral tuberous sclerosis, in Gomez MR, Sampson JR, Holets Whittemore V (eds): *Tuberous Sclerosis Complex*, 3rd ed. New York, Oxford University Press, 1999, p 29.
8. Scheithauer BW, Reagan TJ: Neuropathology, in Gomez MR, Sampson JR, Holets Whittemore V (eds.): *Tuberous Sclerosis Complex*, 3rd ed. New York, Oxford University Press, 1999, p 101.
9. Hirose T, Sheithauer BW, Lopes MBS, Gerber HA, Altermatt HJ, Huckee MJ, VandenBerg SR: Tuber and subependymal giant cell astrocytoma associated with tuberous sclerosis: An immunohisto-chemical, ultrastructural, and immunoelectron microscopic study. *Acta Neuropathol* **90**:387, 1995.
10. Crino PB, Dichter MA, Trojanowski JQ, Eberwine JH: Embryonic neuronal markers in tuberous sclerosis: single cell molecular pathology. *Proc Natl Acad Sci U S A* **93**:14152, 1996.
11. Robertson DM: Ophthalmic findings, in Gomez MR, Sampson JR, Holets Whittemore V (eds): *Tuberous Sclerosis Complex*, 3rd ed. New York, Oxford University Press, 1999, p 145.
12. Northrup H, Kwiatkowski DJ, Roach ES, Dobyns WB, Lewis RA, Herman GE, Rodriguez E, et al: Evidence for genetic heterogeneity in tuberous sclerosis: One locus on chromosome 9 and at least one locus elsewhere. *Am J Hum Genet* **51**:709, 1992.
13. Webb DW, Clarke A, Osborne JP: The cutaneous features of tuberous sclerosis: A population study. *Brit J Dermatol* **135**:1, 1996.
14. Rogers RS, O'Connor WJ: Dermatologic features, in Gomez MR, Sampson JR, Holets Whittemore V (eds.): *Tuberous Sclerosis Complex*, 3rd ed. New York, Oxford University Press, 1999, p 160.
15. Fryer AE, Osborne JP, Schutt W: Forehead plaque: A presenting skin sign in tuberous sclerosis. *Arch Dis Child* **62**:292, 1987.
16. Fitzpatrick TB, Szabo G, Hori Y, Simone AA, Reed WB, Greenberg MH: White leaf-shaped macules: Earliest visible sign of tuberous sclerosis. *Arch Dermatol* **98**:1, 1968.
17. Norio R, Oksanen T, Rantanen J: Hypopigmented skin alterations resembling tuberous sclerosis in normal skin. *J Med Genet* **33**:184, 1996.
18. Vanderhooft SL, Francis JS, Pagon RA, Smith LT, Sybert VP: Prevalence of hypopigmented macules in a healthy population. *J Pediatr* **129**:355, 1996.
19. Jimbow K, Fitzpatrick TB, Szabo G, Hori Y: Congenital circum-scribed hypomelanosis: Characterisation based on electron micro-scopic study of tuberous sclerosis, nevus depigmentosus, and piebaldism. *J Invest Dermatol* **64**:50, 1977.
20. Shepherd CW, Gomez MR, Lie JT: Causes of death in patients with tuberous sclerosis. *Mayo Clin Proc* **66**:792, 1991.
21. Cook JA, Oliver K, Mueller RF, Sampson JR: A cross-sectional study of renal involvement in tuberous sclerosis. *J Med Genet* **33**:480, 1996.
22. Ewalt DE, Sheffield E, Sparagana SP, Delgada MR, Roach ES: Renal lesion growth in children with tuberous sclerosis complex. *J Urol* **160**:141, 1998.
23. Logginidou H, Ao X, Russo I, Henske EP: Frequent estrogen and progesterone receptor immunoreactivity in renal angiomyolipomas from women with pulmonary lymphangioleiomyomatosis. *Chest* **117**:25, 2000.
24. Elbe JN: Angiomyolipoma of the kidney. *Semin Diagn Pathol* **15**:21, 1998.
25. Hellstrom PA, Mehik A, Talja MT, Siniluoto TM, Perala JM, Leinonen SS: Spontaneous subcapsular or perirenal haemorrhage caused by renal tumours: A urological emergency. *Scand J Urol Nephrol* **33**:17, 1999.
26. Lemaitre L, Yann R, Dubrulle F, Claudon M, Duhamel A, Danjou P, Mazeman E: Renal angiomyolipoma: Growth followed up with CT and/or US. *Radiology* **197**:598, 1995.
27. Neumann HPH, Bruggen V, Berger DP, Herbst E, Blum U, Morgenroth A, Schollmeyer P, et al: Tuberous sclerosis complex with end stage renal failure. *Nephrol Dial Transplant* **10**:349, 1995.
28. Ohkawa M, Kadoya M, Nonomura A: Renal angiomyolipoma composed primarily of smooth muscle element: Diagnostic con-siderations. *Urol Int* **54**:230, 1995.
29. Bornsson J, Short MP, Kwiatkowski D, Henske EP: Tuberous sclerosis-associated renal cell carcinoma. Clinical, pathological and genetic features. *Am J Pathol* **149**:1201, 1996.
30. Pea M, Bonetti G, Martignoni E, Henske E, Manfrin E, Colato C, Bernstein J: Apparent renal cell carcinomas in tuberous sclerosis are heterogeneous: The identification of malignant epithelioid angio-myolipoma. *Am J Surg Pathol* **22**:180, 1998.
31. Sampson JR, Maheshwar MM, Aspinwall R, Thompson P, Cheadle JP, Ravine D, Roy S, et al: Renal cystic disease in tuberous sclerosis: Role of the polycystic kidney disease 1 gene. *Am J Hum Genet* **61**:843, 1997.
32. Bernstein J: Renal cystic disease in tuberous sclerosis complex. *Pediatr Nephrol* **7**:490, 1993.
33. Sampson JR, Patel A, Mee AD: Multifocal renal cell carcinoma in sibs from a chromosome 9 linked (TSC1) tuberous sclerosis family. *J Med Genet* **32**:848, 1995.
34. Green JAS: Renal oncocytoma and tuberous sclerosis. *S Afr Med J* **71**:47, 1987.
35. Srinivas V, Herr WH, Hajdu EO: Partial nephrectomy for a renal oncocytoma associated with tuberous sclerosis. *J Urol* **133**:263, 1985.
36. Castro M, Shepherd CW, Gomez MR, Lie JT: Pulmonary tuberous sclerosis. *Chest* **107**:189, 1995.
37. Lie JT: Pulmonary tuberous sclerosis, in Gomez MR, Sampson JR, Holets Whittemore V (eds): *Tuberous Sclerosis Complex*, 3rd ed. New York, Oxford University Press, 1999, p 207.
38. Bonetti F, Chiodera PL, Pea M, Martignoni G, Bosi F, Zamboni G, Mariuzzi GM: Transbronchial biopsy in lymphangiomyomatosis of the lung. HMB45 for diagnosis. *Am J Surg Pathol* **17**:1092, 1993.
39. Johnson S: Lymphangioleiomyomatosis: Clinical features, manage-ment and basic mechanisms. *Thorax* **54**:254, 1999.
39a. Carsillio T, Astrinidis A, Henske EP: Mutations of the TSC2 gene are a cause of sporadic pulmonary lymphangioleiomyomatosis. *Proc Natl Acad Sci USA* **97**:6085, 2000.
40. Bonetti F, Pea M, Martignoni G, Doglioni C, Zamboni G, Capelli P, Rimoni P, et al: Clear cell ("sugar") tumour of the lung is a lesion strictly related to angiomyolipoma. The concept of a family of lesions characterised by the presence of the perivascular epithelioid cell. *Pathology* **26**:230, 1994.
41. Guninee D, Singh R, Azumi N, Singh G, Przygodzki RM, Travis W, Koss M: Multifocal micronodular pneumocyte hyperplasia: A distinctive pulmonary manifestation of tuberous sclerosis. *Mod Pathol* **8**:902, 1995.
42. Smith HC, Watson GH, Patel RG, Super M: Cardiac rhabdomyomata in tuberous sclerosis: Their course and diagnostic value. *Arch Dis Child* **64**:196, 1989.
43. Webb DW, Thomas RD, Osborne JP: Cardiac rhabdomyomas and their association with tuberous sclerosis. *Arch Dis Child* **68**:367, 1993.
44. Burke AP, Virmani R: Cardiac rhabdomyoma: A clinicopathologic study. *Mod Pathol* **4**:70, 1991.
45. Crawford DC, Garrett C, Tynan M, Neville B, Allan LD: Cardiac rhabdomyomata as a marker for the antenatal detection of tuberous sclerosis. *J Med Genet* **20**:303, 1983.
46. DiMario FJ, Diana D, Leopold H, Chameides L: Evolution of cardiac rhabdomyoma in tuberous sclerosis complex. *Clin Pediatr* **26**:532, 1996.
47. van Reedt Dortland RWH, Bax NMA, Huber J: Aortic aneurysm in a 5-year-old boy with tuberous sclerosis. *J Pediatr Surg* **26**:1420, 1991.
48. Hite SH, Kuo JS, Cheng EY: Axillary artery aneurysm in tuberous sclerosis: Cross-sectional imaging findings. *Pediatr Radiol* **28**:554, 1998.
49. Beltramello A, Puppini G, Bricolo A, Andreis IA, el-Dalati G, Longa L, Polidoro S, et al: Does tuberous sclerosis complex include intracranial aneurysms? *Pediatr Radiol* **29**:206, 1999.
50. Hoffman AD: Imaging the skeleton and the great vessels, in Gomez MR, Sampson JR, Holets Whittemore V (eds): *Tuberous Sclerosis Complex*, 3rd ed. New York, Oxford University Press, 1999, p 240.

51. Mlynarczyk G: Enamel pitting: A common symptom of tuberous sclerosis. *Oral Surg Oral Med Pathol* **71**:63, 1991.
52. Sampson JR, Attwood D, Al Mughery AS, Reid JS: Pitted enamel hypoplasia in tuberous sclerosis. *Clin Genet* **42**:50, 1992.
53. Zimmermann D: The endocrine system in tuberous sclerosis complex, in Gomez MR, Sampson JR, Holets Whittemore V (eds): *Tuberous Sclerosis Complex*, 3rd ed. New York, Oxford University Press, 1999, p 218.
54. Ilgren EB, Westmoreland D: Tuberous sclerosis: Unusual associations in four cases. *J Clin Pathol* **37**:272, 1984.
55. Darling TN, Skarulis MC, Steinberg SM, Marx SJ, Spiegel AM, Turner M: Multiple facial angiomas and collagenomas in patients with multiple endocrine neoplasia type 1. *Arch Dermatol* **133**:853, 1997.
56. Jowziak S, Pedich M, Rajszys P, Michalowicz R: Incidence of hepatic hamartomas in tuberous sclerosis. *Arch Dis Child* **67**:1363, 1992.
57. Gould SR, Stewart JB, Temple IN: Rectal polyposis in tuberous sclerosis. *J Mental Defic Res* **34**:465, 1990.
58. Devroese G, Lemieux B, Masse S, Lamarche J, Herman P: Colonic hamartomas in tuberous sclerosis. *Gastroenterology* **94**:182, 1988.
59. Roach ES, Gomez MR, Northrup H: Tuberous sclerosis complex consensus conference: Revised clinical diagnostic criteria. *J Child Neurol* **13**:624, 1998.
60. Sampson JR, Scahill S, Stephenson JBP, Mann LA, Connor JM: Genetic aspects of tuberous sclerosis in the west of Scotland. *J Med Genet* **26**:28, 1989.
61. Webb DW, Fryer AE, Osborne JP: Morbidity associated with tuberous sclerosis: A population study. *Dev Med Child Neurol* **338**:146, 1996.
62. Shepherd CW, Beard CM, Gomez MR, Kurland JT, Whisnant JP: Tuberous sclerosis complex in Olmstead County, Minnesota, 1950–1989. *Arch Neurol* **48**:400, 1991.
63. O'Callaghan FJK, Shiell AW, Osborne JP, Martyn C: Prevalence of tuberous sclerosis estimated by capture-recapture analysis. *Lancet* **351**:1490, 1998.
64. Young JM, Burley MW, Jeremiah SJ, Jeganathan D, Ekong R, Osborne JP, Povey S: A mutation screen of the TSC1 gene reveals 26 protein truncating mutations and 1 splice site mutation in a panel of 79 tuberous sclerosis patients. *Ann Hum Genet* **62**:203, 1998.
65. Northrup, H, Wheless JW, Bertin TK, Lewis RA: Variability of expression in tuberous sclerosis. *J Med Genet* **30**:41, 1993.
66. Fryer AE, Osborne JP, Tan R, Siggers DC: Tuberous sclerosis: A large family with no history of seizures or mental retardation. *J Med Genet* **24**:547, 1987.
67. O'Callaghan TJ, Edwards JA, Tobin M, Mookerjee BK: Tuberous sclerosis with striking renal involvement in a family. *Arch Intern Med* **135**:1082, 1975.
68. Roach ES, DiMario FJ, Kandt RS, Northrup H: Tuberous sclerosis consensus conference: Recommendations for diagnostic evaluation. *J Child Neurol* **14**:401, 1999.
69. Shepherd CW, Houser OW, Gomez MR: MR findings in tuberous sclerosis complex and correlation with seizure development and mental impairment. *Am J Neuroradiol* **16**:149, 1995.
70. Chiron C, Dumas C, Jambaque I, Mumford J, Dulac O: Randomized trial comparing vigabatrin and hydrocortisone in infantile spasms due to tuberous sclerosis. *Epilepsy Res* **26**:389, 1997.
71. Hancock E, Osborne JP: Vigabatrin in the treatment of infantile spasms in tuberous sclerosis: Literature review. *J Child Neurol* **14**:71, 1999.
72. Sankar R, Wasterlain CG: Is the devil we know the lesser of two evils? Vigabatrin and visual fields. *Neurology* **52**:1537, 1999.
73. Vanhatalo S, Paakkonen L: Visual field constriction in children treated with vigabatrin. *Neurology* **52**:1713, 1999.
74. Crino PB, Henske EP: New developments in the neurobiology of tuberous sclerosis complex. *Neurology* **53**:1384, 1999.
75. Oesterling JE, Fishman EK, Goldman SM, Marshall FF: The management of renal angiomyolipoma. *J Urol* **135**:1121, 1986.
76. Van Baal JG, Fleury P, Brummelkamp WH: Tuberous sclerosis and the relation with renal angiomyolipoma. A genetic study on the clinical aspects. *Clin Genet* **35**:167, 1989.
77. Van Baal JG, Smits NJ, Keeman JN, Lindhout D, Verhoef S: The evolution of renal angiomyolipomas in patients with tuberous sclerosis. *J Urol* **152**:35, 1994.
78. Clarke A, Hancock E, Kingswood C, Osborne JP: End-stage renal failure in adults with the tuberous sclerosis complex. *Nephrol Dial Transplant* **14**:988, 1999.

79. Sampson JR: The kidney in tuberous sclerosis: Manifestations and molecular genetic mechanisms. *Nephrol Dial Transplant* **11(Suppl 6)**:34, 1996.
80. Yates JR, van Bakel I, Sepp T, Payne SJ, Webb DW, Nevin NC, Green AJ: Female germline mosaicism in tuberous sclerosis confirmed by molecular genetic analysis. *Hum Mol Genet* **6**:2265, 1997.
81. Rose VM, Au KS, Pollom G, Roach ES, Prashner HR, Northrup H: Germ-line mosaicism in tuberous sclerosis: How common? *Am J Hum Genet* **64**:986, 1999.
82. Fryer AE, Chalmers AH, Osborne JP: The value of investigation for genetic counselling in tuberous sclerosis. *J Med Genet* **27**:217, 1990.
83. Al Gazali LI, Arthur RJ, Lamb JT, Hammer HM, Coker TP, Hirschmann PN, Gibbs J, Meuller RF: Diagnostic and counselling difficulties using a fully comprehensive screening protocol for families at risk for tuberous sclerosis. *J Med Genet* **26**:694, 1989.
84. Webb DW, Osborne JP: Non-penetrance in tuberous sclerosis. *J Med Genet* **28**:417, 1991.
84a. Osborne JP, Jones AC, Burley MW, Jeganathan D, Young J, O'Callaghan FJ, Sampson JR, et al: Non-penetrance in tuberous sclerosis. *Lancet* **355**:1698, 2000.
85. Jones AC, Shayamsundar MM, Thomas M, Maynard J, Idziaszczyk S, Tomkins S, Sampson JR, et al: Comprehensive mutation analysis of TSC1 and TSC2 and phenotypic correlations in 150 families with tuberous sclerosis. *Am J Hum Genet* **64**:1305, 1999.
85a. Jones AC, Sampson JR, Hoogendorn B, Cohen D, Cheadle JP: Application and evaluation of denaturing HPLC for molecular genetic analysis in tuberous sclerosis. *Hum Genet* **106**:663, 2000.
86. The European Chromosome 16 Tuberous Sclerosis Consortium: Identification and characterisation of the tuberous sclerosis gene on chromosome 16. *Cell* **75**:1305, 1993.
87. The TSC1 Consortium: Identification of the tuberous sclerosis gene TSC1 on chromosome 9q34. *Science* **277**:805, 1997.
88. Fryer AE, Chalmers A, Connor JM, Fraser I, Povey S, Yates AD, Yates JRW, Osborne JP: Evidence that the gene for tuberous sclerosis is on chromosome 9. *Lancet* **i**:659, 1987.
89. Sampson JR, Yates JRW, Pirrit LA, Fleury P, Winship I, Beighton P, Connor JM: Evidence for genetic heterogeneity in tuberous sclerosis. *J Med Genet* **26**:511, 1989.
90. Connor JM, Sampson JR: Recent linkage studies in tuberous sclerosis: chromosome 9 markers. *Ann N Y Acad Sci* **615**:265, 1991.
91. Kandt RS, Haines JL, Smith M, Northrup H, Gardner RJM, Short MP, Dumars K, et al: Linkage of an important gene locus for tuberous sclerosis to a chromosome 16 marker for polycystic kidney disease. *Nat Genet* **2**:37, 1992.
92. Nellist M, Brook-Carter PT, Connor JM, Kwiatkowski DJ, Johnson P, Sampson JR: Identification of markers flanking the tuberous sclerosis locus on chromosome 9 (TSC1). *J Med Genet* **30**:224, 1993.
93. Haines JL, Short MP, Kwiatkowski DJ, Jewell A, Andermann E, Bejjani B, Yang CH, Gusella JF, Amos JA: Localisation of one gene for tuberous sclerosis within 9q32-9q34, and further evidence for heterogeneity. *Am J Hum Genet* **49**:764, 1991.
94. Au KS, Merrell J, Buckler A, Blanton SH, Northrup H: Report of a critical recombination further narrowing the TSC1 region. *J Med Genet* **33**:559, 1996.
95. Kwiatkowski DJ, Armour J, Bale AE, Fountain JW, Goudie D, Haines JL, Knowles MA, et al: Report on the second international workshop on human chromosome 9. *Cytogenet Cell Genet* **64**:94, 1993.
96. Maheshwar MM, Sandford R, Nellist M, Cheadle JP, Sgotto B, Vaudin M, Sampson JR: Comparative analysis and genomic structure of the tuberous sclerosis 2 (TSC2) gene in human and pufferfish. *Hum Mol Genet* **5**:131, 1996.
97. Kobayashi T, Urakami S, Cheadle JP, Aspinwall R, Harris P, Sampson JR, Hino O: Identification of a leader exon and a core promoter for the rat TSC2 gene and structural comparison with the human homologue. *Mamm Genome* **8**:554, 1997.
98. Xu L, Sterner C, Maheshwar M, Wilson PJ, Nellist M, Short PM, Haines JL, et al: Alternative splicing of the tuberous sclerosis 2 (TSC2) gene in human and mouse tissues. *Genomics* **27**:475, 1995.
99. Maheshwar MM, Cheadle JP, Jones AC, Myring J, Fryer AE, Harris PC, Sampson JR: The GAP related domain of tuberin, the product of the TSC2 gene, is a target for missense mutations in tuberous sclerosis. *Hum Mol Genet* **6**:1991, 1997.
100. van Slegtenhorst M, Nellist M, Nagelkerken B, Cheadle J, Snell R, van den Ouweland A, Reuser A, et al: Interaction between hamartin

and tuberin, the TSC1 and TSC2 gene products. *Hum Mol Genet* **7**:1053. 1998.

101. Jones AC, Daniells CE, Snell RG, Tachataki M, Idziaszczyk SA, Krawczak M, Sampson JR, et al: Molecular genetic and phenotypic analysis reveals differences between TSC1 and TSC2 associated familial and sporadic tuberous sclerosis. *Hum Mol Genet* **6**:2155, 1997.

102. Kwiatkowska J, Jozwiak S, Hall F, Henske E, Haines J, McNamara P, Braiser J, et al: Comprehensive analysis of the TSC1 gene: observations on frequency of mutation, associated features, and nonpenetrance. *Ann Hum Genet* **62**:277, 1998.

103. Mayer K, Ballhausen W, Rott H-D: Mutation screening of the entire coding regions of the TSC1 and the TSC2 gene with the protein truncation test (PTT) identifies frequent splicing defects. *Hum Mutat* **14**:401, 1999.

104. Ali JBM, Sepp T, Ward S, Green AJ, Yates JRW: Mutations in the TSC1 gene account for a minority of patients with tuberous sclerosis. *J Med Genet* **35**:969, 1998.

105. van Slegtenhorst M, Verhoef S, Tempelaars A, Bakker L, Wang Q, Wessels M, Bakker R, et al: Mutational spectrum of the TSC1 gene in a cohort of 225 tuberous sclerosis complex patients: No evidence for genotype-phenotype correlation. *J Med Genet* **36**:285, 1999.

106. Niida Y, Lawrence-Smith N, Banwell A, Hammer E, Lewis J, Beauchamp R, Sims K, et al: Analysis of both TSC1 and TSC2 germline mutations in 126 unrelated patients with tuberous sclerosis. *Hum Mutat* **14**:412, 1999.

107. Benit P, Kara-Mostefa A, Hadj-Rabia S, Munnich A, Bonnefont JP: Protein truncation test for screening hamartin gene mutations and report of new disease-causing mutations. *Hum Mutat* **14**:428, 1999.

108. Beauchamp RL, Banwell A, McNamara P, Jacobsen M, Higgins E, Northrup H, Short P, et al: Exon scanning of the entire TSC2 gene for germline mutations in 40 unrelated patients with tuberous sclerosis. *Hum Mutat* **12**:408, 1998.

109. Au KS, Rodriguez JA, Finch JL, Volcik KA, Roach ES, Delgado MR, Rodriguez E Jr, et al: Germ-line mutational analysis of the TSC2 gene in 90 tuberous-sclerosis patients. *Am J Hum Genet* **62**:286, 1998.

110. Gilbert JR, Guy V, Kumar A, Wolpert C, Kandt R, Aylesworth A, Roses AD, et al: Mutation and polymorphism analysis in the tuberous sclerosis 2 (TSC2) gene. *Neurogenetics* **1**:267, 1998.

111. Verhoef S, Vrtel R, van Essen TV, Bakker L, Sikkens E, Halley D, Lindhout D, et al: Somatic mosaicism and clinical variation in tuberous sclerosis complex. *Lancet* **345**:202, 1995.

112. Verhoef S, Bakker L, Tempelaars AMP, Hesseling-Janssen ALW, Mazurczak T, Jozwiak S, Fois A, et al: High rate of mosaicism in tuberous sclerosis complex. *Am J Hum Genet* **64**:1632, 1999.

113. Kwiatkowska J, Wigowska-Sowinska J, Napierala D, Slomski R, Kwiatkowski DJ: Mosaicism in tuberous sclerosis as a potential cause of the failure of molecular diagnosis. *N Engl J Med* **340**:703, 1999.

114. The European Polycystic Kidney Disease Consortium: The polycystic kidney disease 1 gene encodes a 14kb transcript and lies within a duplicated region on chromosome 16. *Cell* **77**:881, 1994.

115. Harris PC, Ward CJ, Peral B, Hughes J: Autosomal dominant polycystic kidney disease: Molecular analysis. *Hum Mol Genet* **4**:1745, 1995.

116. Brook-Carter PT, Peral B, Ward CJ, Thompson P, Hughes J, Maheshwar MM, Nellist M, et al: Deletion of the TSC2 and PKD1 genes associated with severe infantile polycystic kidney disease — A contiguous gene syndrome. *Nat Genet* **8**:328, 1994.

117. Hateboer N, v Dijk MA, Bogdanova N, Coto E, Saggar-Malik A, San Milan JL, Torra R, et al: Comparison of phenotypes of polycystic kidney disease types 1 and 2. *Lancet* **353**:103, 1999.

118. Zerres K, Rudnik-Schoneborn, S, Deget F: Childhood onset autosomal dominant polycystic kidney disease in sibs: Clinical picture and recurrence risk. *J Med Genet* **30**:583, 1993.

119. Green AJ, Smith M, Yates JRW: Loss of heterozygosity on chromosome 16p13.3 in hamartomas from tuberous sclerosis patients. *Nat Genet* **6**:193, 1994.

120. Green AJ, Johnson PH, Yates JRW: The tuberous sclerosis gene on chromosome 9q34 acts as a growth suppressor. *Hum Mol Genet* **3**:1833, 1994.

121. Carbonara C, Longa L, Grosso E, Borrone C, Garre MG, Brisigotti M, Migone M: 9q34 loss of heterozygosity in a tuberous sclerosis astrocytoma suggests a growth suppressor-like activity also for the TSC1 gene. *Hum Mol Genet* **3**:829, 1994.

122. Sepp T, Green AJ, Yates JRW: Loss of heterozygosity in tuberous sclerosis hamartomas. *J Med Genet* **33**:962, 1996.

123. Au KS, Herbert AA, Roach ES, Northrup H: Complete inactivation of the TSC2 gene leads to formation of hamartomas. *Am J Hum Genet* **65**:1790, 1999.

124. Carbonara C, Longa L, Grosso E, Mazzucco G, Borrone C, Garre ML, Brisigotti M, et al: Apparent preferential loss of heterozygosity at TSC2 over TSC1 chromosomal regions in tuberous sclerosis hamartomas. *Genes Chromosomes Cancer* **15**:18, 1996.

125. Henske EP, Scheithauer BW, Short MP, Wollmann R, Nahmias J, Hornigold N, van Slegtenhorst M, et al: Allelic loss is frequent in tuberous sclerosis kidney lesions but rare in brain lesions. *Am J Hum Genet* **59**:400, 1996.

126. Henske EP, Neumann HPH, Scheithauer BW, Herbst EW, Short MP, Kwiatkowski DJ: Loss of heterozygosity in the tuberous sclerosis (TSC2) region of chromosome band 16p13 occurs in sporadic as well as TSC-associated renal angiomyolipomas. *Genes Chromosomes Cancer* **13**:295, 1995.

127. Smolarek TA, Wessner LL, McCormack FX, Mylet JC, Menon AG, Henske EP: Evidence that lymphangiomyomatosis is caused by TSC2 mutations: Chromosome 16p13 loss of heterozygosity in angiomyolipomas and lymph nodes from women with lymphangiomyomatosis. *Am J Hum Genet* **62**:810, 1998.

128. Hornigold N, Devlin J, Davies AM, Aveyard JS, Habuchi T, Knowles MA: Mutation of the 9q34 TSC1 gene in sporadic bladder cancer. *Oncogene* **18**:2657, 1999.

129. Weinecke R, Guha A, Maize J, Heidelman R, DeClue J, Gutmann D: Reduced TSC2 RNA and protein in sporadic astrocytomas and ependymomas. *Ann Neurol* **42**:230, 1997.

130. Parry L, Maynard J, Price SA, Patel A, Whittaker-Axon S, Von Diemling A, Cheadle JP, et al: Analysis of the TSC1 and TSC2 genes in sporadic glial and glioneuronal tumours. *Am J Hum Genet* **64(Suppl 4)**:A315, 1999.

131. Kobayashi T, Hirayama Y, Kobayashi E, Kubo Y, Hino O: A germline insertion in the tuberous sclerosis (TSC2) gene gives rise to the Eker rat model of dominantly inherited cancer [published erratum appears in *Nat Genet* 9:218, 1995]. *Nat Genet* **9**:70, 1995.

132. Yeung RS, Xiao GH, Jin F, Lee WC, Testa JR, Knudson AG: Predisposition to renal carcinoma in the Eker rat is determined by germ-line mutation of the tuberous sclerosis 2 (TSC2) gene. *Proc Natl Acad Sci U S A* **91**:11413, 1994.

133. Eker R: Familial renal adenomas in Wistar rats. *Acta Path Microbiol Scand* **34**:554, 1954.

134. Eker R, Mossige J: A dominant gene for renal adenomas in the rat. *Nature* **189**:858, 1961.

135. Eker R, Mossige J, Johannessen JV, Aars H: Hereditary renal adenomas and adenocarcinomas in rats. *Diagn Histopathol* **4**:99, 1981.

136. Hino O, Mitani H, Knudson AG: Genetic predisposition to transplacentally induced renal cell carcinomas in the Eker rat. *Cancer Res* **53**:5856, 1993.

137. Everitt JI, Goldsworthy TL, Wolf DC, Walker CL: Hereditary renal cell carcinoma in the Eker rat: A rodent familial cancer syndrome. *J Urol* **148**:1932, 1992.

138. Yeung RS, Katsetos CD, Klein-Szanto A: Subependymal astrocytic hamartomas in the Eker rat model of tuberous sclerosis. *Am J Pathol* **151**:1477, 1997.

139. Yeung RS, Xiao GH, Everitt JI, Jin F, Walker CL: Allelic loss at the tuberous sclerosis 2 locus in spontaneous tumors in the Eker rat. *Mol Carcinog* **14**:28, 1995.

140. Kubo Y, Kikuchi Y, Mitani H, Kobayashi E, Kobayashi T, Hino O: Allelic loss at the tuberous sclerosis (TSC2) gene locus in spontaneous uterine leiomyosarcomas and pituitary adenomas in the Eker rat model. *Jpn J Cancer Res* **86**:828, 1995.

141. Kobayashi T, Urakami S, Hirayama Y, Yamamoto T, Nishizawa M, Takahara T, Kubo Y, Hino O: Intragenic TSC2 somatic mutations as Knudson's second hit in spontaneous and chemically induced renal carcinomas in the Eker rat model. *Jpn J Cancer Res* **88**:254, 1997.

142. Kobayashi T, Mitani H, Takahashi R, Hirabayashi M, Ueda M, Tamura H, Hino O: Transgenic rescue from embryonic lethality and renal carcinogenesis in the Eker rat model by introduction of a wild-type TSC2 gene. *Proc Natl Acad Sci U S A* **94**:3990, 1997.

143. Orimoto K, Tsuchiya H, Kobayashi T, Matsuda T, Hino O: Suppression of the neoplastic phenotype by replacement of the TSC2 gene in Eker rat renal carcinoma cells. *Biochem Biophys Res Commun* **219**:70, 1996.

144. Jin F, Wienecke R, Xiao G-H, Maize JC, DeClue J, Yeung R: Suppression of tumorigenicity by the wild-type tuberous sclerosis 2

(Tsc2) gene and its C-terminal region. *Proc Natl Acad Sci U S A* **93**:9154, 1996.

145. Rennebeck G, Kleymenova EV, Anderson R, Yeung RS, Artzt K, Walker CL: Loss of function of the tuberous sclerosis 2 tumor suppressor gene results in embryonic lethality characterized by disrupted neuroepithelial growth and development. *Proc Natl Acad Sci U S A* **95**:15629, 1998.

146. Onda H, Lueck A, Marks PW, Warren HB, Kwiatkowski DJ: TSC2(+/−) mice develop tumors in multiple sites that express gelsolin and are influenced by genetic background. *J Clin Invest* **104**:687, 1999.

147. Kobayashi T, Minowa O, Kuno J, Mitani H, Hino O, Noda T: Renal carcinogenesis, hepatic hemangiomatosis, and embryonic lethality caused by a germ-line TSC2 mutation in mice. *Cancer Res* **59**:1206, 1999.

148. Ferrus A, Garcia-Bellido A: Morphogenetic mutants detected in mitotic recombination clones. *Nature* **260**:425, 1976.

149. Ito N, Rubin G: *gigas*, a *Drosophila* homolog of tuberous sclerosis gene product-2, regulates the cell cycle. *Cell* **96**:529, 1999.

150. Geist RT, Gutmann DH: The tuberous sclerosis 2 gene is expressed at high levels in the cerebellum and developing spinal cord. *Cell Growth Differ* **6**:1477, 1995.

151. Kerfoot C, Wienecke R, Menchine M, Emelin J, Maize JC Jr, Welsh CT, Norman MG, et al: Localization of tuberous sclerosis 2 mRNA and its protein product tuberin in normal human brain and in cerebral lesions of patients with tuberous sclerosis. *Brain Pathol* **6**:367, 1996.

152. Wienecke R, Maize JC, Reed JA, de Gunzburg J, Yeung RS, DeClue JE: Expression of the TSC2 product tuberin and its target rap1 in normal human tissues. *Am J Pathol* **150**:43, 1997.

153. Olsson PG, Schofield JN, Edwards YH, Frischauf AM: Expression and differential splicing of the mouse TSC2 homolog. *Mamm Genome* **7**:212, 1996.

154. Kim KK, Pajak L, Wang H, Field LJ: Cloning, developmental expression, and evidence for alternative splicing of the murine tuberous sclerosis (TSC2) gene product. *Cell Mol Biol Res* **41**:515, 1995.

155. Plank TL, Yeung RS, Henske EP: Hamartin, the product of the tuberous sclerosis 1 (TSC1) gene, interacts with tuberin and appears to be localised to cytoplasmic vesicles. *Cancer Res* **58**:4766, 1998.

156. Nellist M, van Slegtenhorst MA, Goedbloed M, van den Ouweland AMW, Halley DJJ, van der Sluijs P: Characterization of the cytosolic tuberin-hamartin complex: Tuberin is a cytosolic chaperone for hamartin. *J Biol Chem* **274**:35647, 1999.

157. Wienecke R, Maize JC, Shoarinejad F, Vass WC, Reed J, Bonifacino JS, Resau JH, et al: Co-localization of the TSC2 product tuberin with its target Rap1 in the Golgi apparatus. *Oncogene* **13**:913, 1996.

158. Wienecke R, Konig A, DeClue JE: Identification of tuberin, the tuberous sclerosis-2 product—Tuberin possesses specific rap1GAP activity. *J Biol Chem* **270**:16409, 1995.

159. Xiao G-H, Shoarinejad F, Jin F, Golemis EA, Yeung RS: The tuberous sclerosis 2 gene product, tuberin, functions as a Rab5 GTPase activating protein (GAP) in modulating endocytosis. *J Biol Chem* **272**:6097, 1997.

160. Soucek T, Pusch O, Wienecke R, DeClue JE, Hengstschlager M: Role of the tuberous sclerosis gene-2 product in cell cycle control. *J Biol Chem* **272**:29301, 1997.

160a. Miloeuoza A, Rosner M, Nellist M, Halley D, Bernaschek G, Hengstschläger M: The TSC1 gene product, hamartin negatively regulates cell proliferation. *Hum Mol Genet* **9**:1721, 2000.

161. Soucek T, Holzl G, Bernaschek, G, Hengstschlager M: A role of the tuberous sclerosis gene-2 product during neuronal differentiation. *Oncogene* **16**:2197, 1998.

162. Tsuchiya H, Orimoto K, Kobayashi T, Hino O: Presence of potent transcriptional activation domains in the predisposing tuberous sclerosis (TSC2) gene product of the Eker rat model. *Cancer Res* **56**:429, 1996.

163. Henry KW, Yuan X, Koszewski NJ, Onda H, Kwiatkowski DJ, Noonan DJ: Tuberous sclerosis gene 2 product modulates transcription mediated by steroid hormone receptor family members. *J Biol Chem* **273**:20535, 1998.

164. Lamb RF, Roy C, Diefenbach TJ, Vitners HV, Johnson MW, Jay DG, Hall A: The TSC1 tumour suppressor hamartin regulates cell adhesion through ERM proteins and the GTPase Rho. *Nature Cell Biol* **2**:281, 2000.

# Alzheimer Disease and the Frontotemporal Dementias: Diseases with Cerebral Deposition of Fibrillar Proteins

*P.H. St George-Hyslop* ▪ *L.A. Farrer* ▪ *M. Goedert*

1. **Alzheimer disease (AD), Lewy body variant of Alzheimer disease (LBV), and the frontotemporal dementias (FTD) are a class of adult-onset neurodegenerative dementias characterized by the intracellular and/or extracellular accumulation of proteins which assemble into β-pleated sheet fibrils.**
2. **Missense mutations in the β-amyloid precursor protein (βAPP) gene on chromosome 21, in the presenilin 1 (PS1) gene on chromosome 14, and the presenilin 2 (PS2) on chromosome 1, are associated with early-onset forms of familial Alzheimer disease. Mutations in these genes result in altered processing of βAPP and the relative over-production of either all forms of the β-amyloid peptide or specific overproduction of isoforms ending at residue 42.**
3. **The ε4 (Cys112Arg) variant of apolipoprotein E (APOE) is associated in a dose-dependent fashion with increased risk for late-onset Alzheimer disease (after age 55) and with Lewy body variant of Alzheimer disease. The inheritance of one or more APOE ε4 alleles is not deterministic for AD, and the mechanism by which inheritance of one or more ε4 alleles causes AD is unclear.**
4. **Allelic association studies have identified several putative candidate genes in which nucleotide sequence variants have been associated with AD. These studies have received only partial replication, and the true role of these candidate genes in AD remains unclear.**
5. **Hyperphosphorylated forms of the microtubule-associated protein Tau are consistent neuropathologic features of AD, LDV, and FTD. Coding region and splice-site mutations in the Tau gene on chromosome 17 are associated with a subtype of frontotemporal dementia (FTDP-17). These mutations probably affect filament assembly by several different mechanisms including alterations in the sequence of microtubule binding sites and alterations in the relative abundance of longer (4 repeat) isoforms of Tau relative to shorter (3 repeat) isoforms.**
6. **The currently identified genes associated with inherited risk for these diseases represent approximately half of the probable genetic factors causing these diseases. As the**
remaining susceptibility genes are identified, they will likely contribute to a more complete understanding of the pathogenesis of these disorders.

Alzheimer disease (AD), Lewy body variant of Alzheimer disease (LBV), and the frontotemporal dementias (FTD) are the three commonest causes of adult-onset dementia and together represent a unique class of neurologic diseases (MIM 104300 (AD); 127750 (LBV); 601630 (FTD)).

These diseases are linked biochemically by virtue of the fact that each is characterized by the pathologic deposition of fibrillary proteins either in cerebral neurons (Tau protein), in the cerebral extracellular space (amyloid β-peptide), or both. As is described below, current work suggests that in AD and LBV, pathologic processing of the β-amyloid precursor protein precedes abnormal Tau processing. Conversely, in some forms of FTD, abnormal processing of Tau is the initiating event causing neurodegeneration.

These diseases typically present in mid-to-late adult life with a constellation of symptoms that reflect dysfunction and degeneration of neural cells in the cerebral cortex and other selected brain regions. The clinical symptoms of these diseases vary but include progressive defects in memory and higher cognitive functions such as performing complex learned motor tasks (apraxias) and reasoning. In FTD, the clinical syndrome can be overshadowed by behavioral disturbances (disinhibition, aggressivity, etc.) and speech disturbances (aphasia) that arise from involvement of the frontal neocortex. Similarly, the FTD symptom complex frequently includes additional features such as muscle rigidity, tremor, bradykinesia (parkinsonism), and motor neuron-induced muscle weakness (amyotrophy). In contrast, the clinical features of AD and LBV (such as recent and immediate memory deficits, and deficits in praxis, reasoning, and judgment) are those stemming from involvement of the temporal lobe, hippocampus, and the parietal association cortices, with lesser involvement of frontal lobes (until late in the disease). LBV overlaps with AD, sharing most of the clinical and neuropathologic features of AD, but being differentiated by the presence of prominent visual hallucinations, sensitivity to phenothiazine tranquilizers, and the presence of Lewy bodies in the neocortex. All three diseases display distinctive pathologic changes in the brain. In all three diseases there is prominent loss of neurons in selected cerebral cortical regions, that is, hippocampus and temporoparietal neocortices in AD and LBV (Fig. 234-1a) and frontal cortex in FTD (Fig. 234-1b).

In AD and LBV, a second prominent neuropathologic feature is a complex, fibrillar protein deposit in the extracellular space of the

A list of standard abbreviations is located immediately preceding the index in each volume. Additional abbreviations used in this chapter include: AD = Alzheimer disease; LBV = Lewy body variant of AD; FTD = frontotemporal dementia; APP = -amyloid precursor protein; A = amyloid -peptide; NPRAP = neuronal plakophillin-related armadillo protein; A2M = 2-macroglobulin.

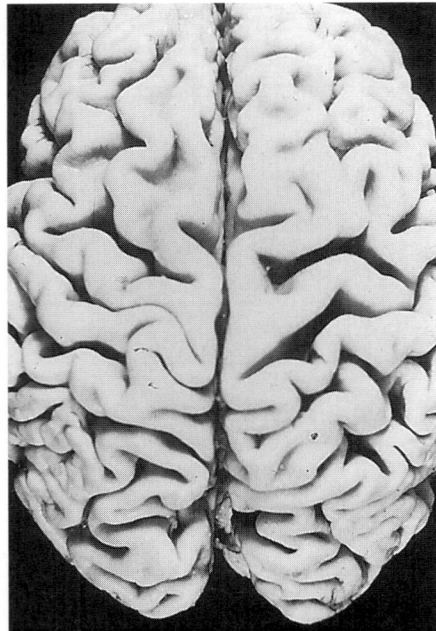

A

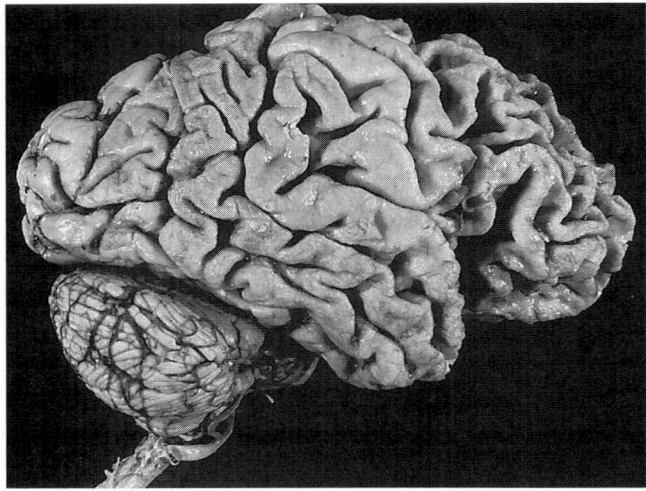

B

**Fig. 234-1 Gross pathology.** *A,* Gross pathologic specimen of human brain affected with Alzheimer disease showing massive diffuse neocortical atrophy. Note the large sulci reflecting loss of mass in the neocortical gyri. *B,* Gross pathologic specimen of a brain affected with frontotemporal dementia. Note the severe atrophy of the frontal lobe (right side).

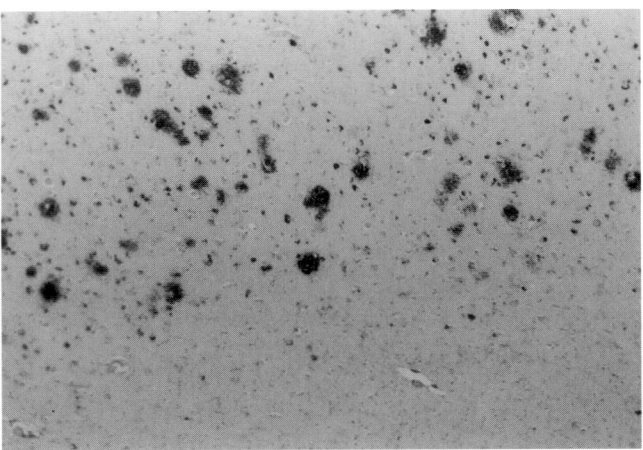

**Fig. 234-2 Microscopic extracellular pathology.** Photomicrograph of cortical tissue from a patient with Alzheimer disease stained with anti-Aβ antibodies showing the fibrillar protein deposits (spherical brown structures) in the extracellular space that have been called senile or amyloid plaques.

cerebral cortex termed senile or amyloid plaques (Fig. 234-2). These plaques contain a number of proteins including apolipoprotein E and α₁-antichymotrypsin, but the principal protein component is a 40 to 42-amino acid peptide organized into β-pleated sheet amyloid fibrils (amyloid-β-peptide or Aβ), which is derived by proteolytic cleavage of a longer precursor (β-amyloid precursor protein (βAPP)).

Finally, AD, LBV, and FTD are all characterized by the presence of intraneuronal inclusions composed of phosphorylated forms of Tau, a microtubule-associated protein. While both the biochemistry and the electron microscopic morphology of these intracellular phosphorylated Tau aggregates usually differ between AD and FTD, they appear similar at the light microscope level, where, in AD, they are termed neurofibrillary tangles (Fig. 234-3a). In some cases of FTD other intracellular inclusions can

also be seen including "motor neuron disease-like inclusions" (Tau-negative, ubiquitin positive) and tau-positive "Pick bodies" (Fig. 234-3b and Fig. 234-3c, respectively).

The overlap between AD and LBV is considerable not only in their major clinical and neuropathologic features, but also in their genetic bases (i.e., both show associations with the apolipoprotein E ε4 variant; see below). As a result, the genetics of AD and LBV are discussed together. A more detailed discussion of the clinical and neuropathologic attributes of all three diseases can be found in any standard textbook of neurology and neuropathology.

## BIOCHEMICAL GENETICS OF ALZHEIMER'S DISEASE

In the past several years, a number of genetic epidemiology studies have been undertaken on probands with AD and their families.[1-7] Cumulatively, these studies (see review in reference 6) strongly argue that the familial aggregation of AD is not due simply to the high frequency of AD in the general population. These studies suggest that the age-dependent risk and the overall lifetime risk for AD in first-degree relatives of AD probands varies from 10 to 50 percent. The most comprehensive recent study suggests an age-dependent risk curve asymptotic to a final risk of 38 percent by age 85 years.[7] The latter study, as well as several other earlier epidemiologic studies, make it difficult to assign a pure mendelian mode of transmission in the majority of AD cases. Instead, these studies imply that the majority of cases of familially clustered AD probably reflect a complex mode of transmission such as one or more common independent, but incompletely-penetrant, single autosomal gene defects; a multigenic trait; or a mode of transmission in which genetic and environmental factors interact. Nevertheless, there is a small proportion of AD cases (~10 percent) which appear to be transmitted as a pure autosomal dominant mendelian trait with age-dependent but high penetrance. Analysis of these pedigrees with molecular genetic tools has led to the discovery of at least four different genetic loci associated with inherited susceptibility to AD (MIM 104300, 104760, 104310, 104311, 600759, 602096).

### The Amyloid Precursor Protein

The first gene to be identified in association with inherited susceptibility to AD was the amyloid precursor protein gene (βAPP). The βAPP gene on chromosome 21 encodes an alternatively spliced transcript, which in its longest isoform encodes a single transmembrane spanning polypeptide of 770 amino acids (GenBank Y00264).[8-11] Alternative splicing of exon 7

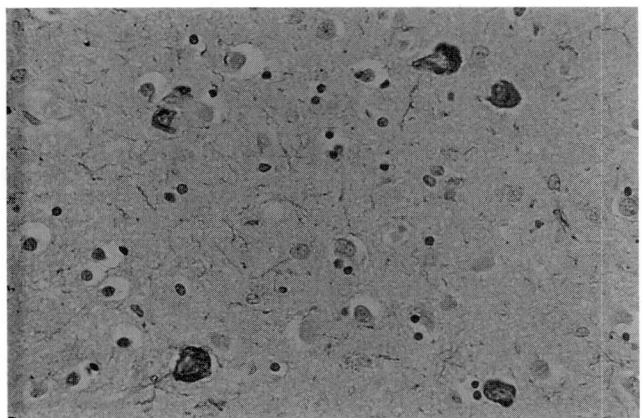

A

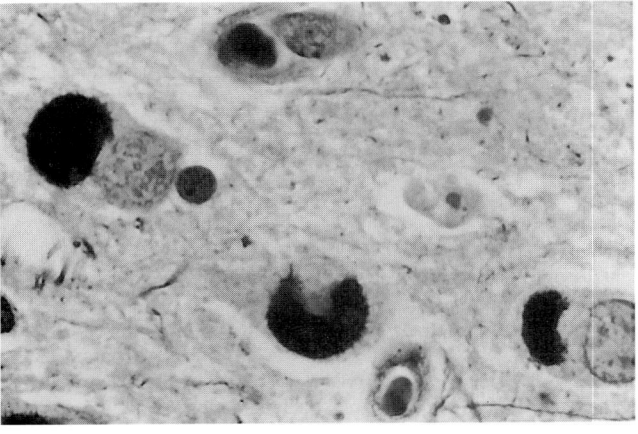

B

C

**Fig. 234-3 Microscopic intracellular pathology.** *A,* Light photomicrograph of intracellular neurofibrillary tangles (large, dark-brown structures) and extracellular neuropil threads (long, thin, light-brown structures) in a patient with Alzheimer disease immunostained with an anti-Tau antibody AT8. *B,* Tau-negative ubiquitin-positive intracellular inclusions (black structures) immunostained with an antiubiquitin antibody in granule cells of the dentate gyrus of a case of FTD. *C,* Intraneuronal Pick bodies in cortical pyramidal cells stained with Bielschowsky silver stain in a case of FTD.

(which encodes a Kunitz serine protease inhibitor protein domain), exon 8 (which encodes a sequence homologous to the ox-2 antigen), and exon 13a result in polypeptides of 695 amino acids (which are expressed predominantly in brain), and 751 and 770 amino acids (are the predominant isoforms in nonneuronal

tissues), and several other minor transcripts.[12] There have been considerable advances in the understanding of the processing of the $\beta$APP protein; they are reviewed in detail elsewhere.[13] The $\beta$APP precursor protein undergoes a series of endoproteolytic cleavages (Fig. 234-4). One of these results from the putative membrane-associated $\alpha$-secretase, which cleaves $\beta$APP within the A$\beta$ peptide domain between residues Lys$_{687}$ and Leu$_{688}$ (codon numbering of $\beta$APP$_{695}$), that is, between residues 16 and 17 of A$\beta$, and liberates the extracellular N-terminus of $\beta$APP (which was previously identified at protease nexin II, a protease inhibitor possibly involved in coagulation). This pathway is "nonamyloidogenic" because the cleavage precludes the formation of A$\beta$ peptide.

The other cleavage pathway, which occurs in part in the endosomal-lysosomal compartment, involves $\beta$- and $\gamma$-secretases, which give rise to a series of peptides that contain the 40 to 42 amino acid A$\beta$ peptide ($\beta$-secretase cleaves between Met$_{671}$ and Asp$_{672}$; $\gamma$-secretase cleaves after Ile$_{712}$, Thr$_{714}$, or Val$_{715}$ to generate A$\beta_{40}$, A$\beta_{42}$ or A$\beta_{43}$). A$\beta$ ending at residue 40 is the predominant isoform produced during normal metabolism of $\beta$APP.[14–19] Current evidence suggests that A$\beta_{40}$ is predominantly produced in endosomal-lysosomal systems.[20,21] A$\beta$ peptides ending at residue 42 or 43 (A$\beta_{42/43}$ or long-tailed A$\beta$), on the other hand, are thought to be more fibrillogenic and more neurotoxic.[19] Substantial evidence suggests that these longer isoforms may be generated at intracellular sites such as the ER and *cis*-Golgi, which, in neurons at least, are distinct from the sites of A$\beta_{40}$ synthesis,[22–24] although lipid-rich raft domains (caveolae) have also been suggested as sites of A$\beta$ generation.[25] These secretases, and especially the specific $\gamma$-secretases giving rise to the more fibrillogenic and potentially neurotoxic long-tailed A$\beta_{1–42}$, appear to play a central role in the pathogenesis of at least some of the genetic forms of AD associated with presenilin and $\beta$APP mutations, and possibly also in nongenetic forms (see below and reviews in references 13 and 26).

The function of $\beta$APP is currently unknown. Knockout of the murine $\beta$APP gene has not been illuminating because it leads only to subtle phenotypes including minor weight loss, decreased locomotion, abnormal forelimb motor activity, and minor nonspecific reactive gliosis in the cortex.[27] In vitro studies in cultured cells suggest that secreted $\beta$APP ($\beta$APP$_s$) can function as an autocrine factor stimulating cell proliferation, cell adhesion, and supporting NGF induced neurite outgrowth of PC12 cells.[28,29] Other studies have implied a role for $\beta$APP in signal transduction by association of $\beta$APP with heterotrimeric GTP-binding proteins.[30]

Several lines of evidence led to the suspicion that the $\beta$APP gene was the site of mutations associated with AD. First, patients with Down syndrome (Trisomy 21) almost invariably develop the neuropathologic attributes of AD by age 40 years (there is considerable variation in the age of onset of actual dementia, which may in part be modulated by the genotype at APOE; see below).[10,31–34] Second, the gene encoding the full-length $\beta$APP protein is located on chromosome 21.[8] Third, genetic linkage studies had shown weak but suggestive evidence for linkage of a familial AD locus on chromosome 21 near the markers D21S1/D21S11, which map near the $\beta$APP gene.[35,36] Fourth, genetic linkage and mutational studies of the $\beta$APP gene identified a Glu693Gln missense mutation of the $\beta$APP gene (codon numbering of the $\beta$APP$_{770}$ isoform) in affected and at-risk members of families with hereditary cerebral hemorrhage with amyloidosis of the Dutch type (HCHWA-D).[37]

Subsequently, direct nucleotide sequencing led to the discovery of several different missense mutations in exons 16 and 17 of the $\beta$APP gene in families with early-onset AD (Table 234-1). Some of these missense mutations are probably not pathogenic mutations either because they have also been detected in normal elderly relatives, or because they are not present in all affected members of these pedigrees. Nevertheless, the missense mutations at codon 670/671 (Swedish mutation),[38] at codon 692 (Flemish mutation),[39] at codon 716,[40] and at codon 717[41–45] seem quite clearly

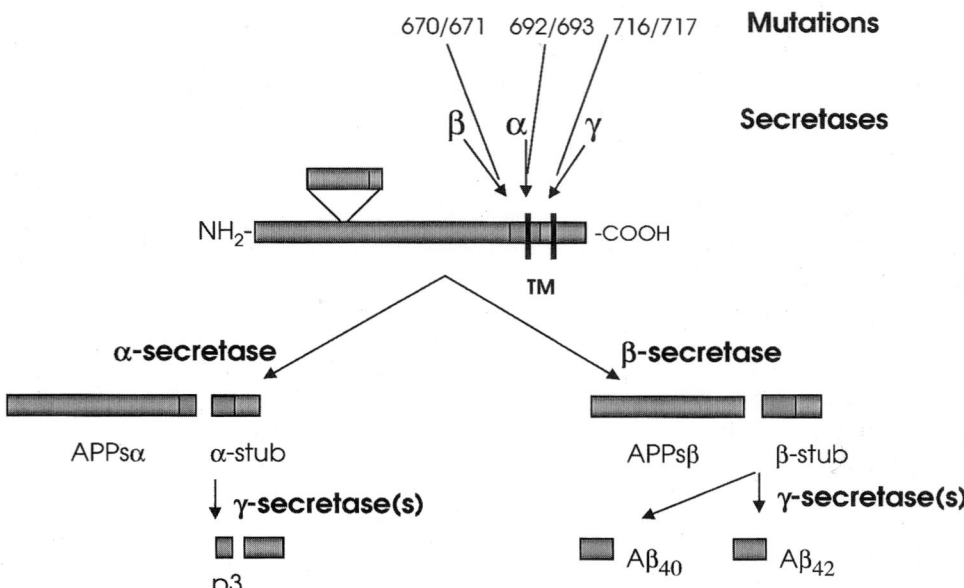

Fig. 234-4. Topology of the β-amyloid precursor protein and its principal routes of endoproteolytic cleavage.

to be pathogenic. The mutations at codon 670/671 and at codon 692 are rare, having been seen only in single families. Mutations at codon 717 on the other hand have been seen in approximately 20 unrelated pedigrees from different ethnic origins. The majority of such mutations at codon 717 were seen in Anglo-Saxon, Italian, and Japanese subjects. The reason for this aggregation is unclear because within each ethnic group there is no common haplotype of genetic markers within or surrounding the βAPP gene.[46] The absence of a conserved haplotype around the βAPP gene in βAPP$_{717}$ carriers in the same ethnic group argues against a common founder for the βAPP$_{717}$ mutation in each ethnic group as the explanation for apparent clustering in these ethnic groups.

That all of the clearly pathogenic mutations cluster close to the β-secretase site after Met$_{671}$ (K670N/M671L), α-secretase site after Lys$_{687}$ (A692G and E639Q), or γ-secretase site after Thr$_{714}$ (I716V and V717I) led to the hypothesis that these mutations might cause AD by influencing the processing of βAPP.[38] Further investigation confirmed that mutations at codons 716 and 717 led to a selective increase in the production of Aβ peptides ending at residue 42/43.[40,47–51] The K670N/M671L mutation, on the

### Table 234-1 Missense Mutations in the βAPP Gene

| Codon | Mutation | Phenotype |
|---|---|---|
| 655 | Gln → Asp | Late onset AD; no segregation |
| 670/671 | Lys-Met → Asn-Leu | FAD; increased Aβ production |
| 673 | Ala → Thr | No disease phenotype |
| 692 | Ala → Gly | FAD + cerebral haemorrhage; increased Aβ |
| 693 | Gln → Gly | Late onset AD; no segregation |
| | Gln → Gln | HCHWA-D |
| 713 | Ala → Val | Schizophrenia; no segregation |
| | Ala → Thr | AD; no segregation |
| 716 | Gln → Val | FAD |
| 717 | Val → Ile | FAD; increased long Aβ isoforms |
| | Val → Phe | FAD |
| | Val → Gly | FAD |

Adapted with permission from St George-Hyslop P: *Genetics of Alzheimer disease*, in Markesbery W, (Ed): *Neuropathology of Dementing Diseases*. London, Edward Arnold, 1997.

other hand, appears to augment the production of both Aβ$_{40}$ and Aβ$_{42/43}$.[52] The A692G mutation has a more complicated effect on βAPP processing. This mutation causes impaired α-secretase cleavage, increased heterogeneity of secreted Aβ species, and increased hydrophobicity of the Aβ.[50] The A692G mutation has clinical features that in some cases are similar to those of HCHWA-D, and that, in other cases, are more similar to AD but with somewhat subtle differences in the size of the amyloid cores.[53] The Glu693Gln mutation causes an increased propensity for Aβ to form fibrils.[54]

The relative or absolute overproduction of Aβ peptide, and in particular of Aβ$_{42}$, as an effect of βAPP mutations that leads to neurodegeneration is an attractive hypothesis. This hypothesis is supported by the observation that mutations in presenilin 1 and presenilin 2 (see below) also affect βAPP metabolism and lead to overproduction of β$_{42}$. Moreover, there is substantial evidence that Aβ$_{42}$ peptides have an enhanced propensity to fibril formation[16,18,19] and that such a conformational change is necessary to change the inert (or even marginally neurotrophic) soluble Aβ into toxic Aβ.[18,19] Multiple molecular mechanisms have been postulated to explain the neurotoxic effects of Aβ. These include induction of apoptosis by direct effects upon cell membranes, by indirect effects such as potentiation of neurotoxic effects of excitatory amino acids, oxidative stress, and increases in intracellular calcium and free radicals.[55–57] However, although the preponderance of available evidence supports the notion that presenilin mutations cause AD neurodegeneration via a mechanism involving overproduction of Aβ peptides, at least one experimental result suggests that βAPP mutations could cause apoptosis by a mechanism that is independent of Aβ peptide production. Specifically, a series of experiments has shown that, for the βAPP$_{717}$ mutations at least, the mutations are able to induce apoptosis by causing constitutive activation of the heterotrimeric GTP-binding protein, G$_0$.[58,59] Furthermore, although some βAPP and PS1/PS2 mutations are associated with overproduction of Aβ peptides, such overproduction of Aβ peptide (as opposed to increased deposition and/or decreased clearance) is not a universal feature of all cases of sporadic AD.[60]

### Apolipoprotein E

Genetic linkage studies in pedigrees with predominantly late-onset familially clustered AD provided suggestive evidence (z = +2.5 at θ = 0.00) for the existence of a second AD susceptibility locus near the markers *BCL3* and *ATP1A3,* which map to chromosome 19q12-q13 (GenBank M10065, K00396).[61] While this initial localization was both crude and tentative, Strittmatter et al. isolated proteins from the CSF that were capable of binding the Aβ peptide.[62] Microsequencing of these peptides revealed that one was apolipoprotein E (APOE).[62] The gene for APOE maps on chromosome 19q13, very close to the markers showing evidence for linkage and/or association with late-onset AD. Simultaneously, APOE was found in the senile plaques of AD, inferring that APOE may be a pathologic chaperone.[63] Together, these observations suggested that the APOE gene itself was the AD susceptibility locus.

The APOE gene in humans contains three common coding sequence polymorphisms. The most common coding sequence variant, ε3, reflects the presence of a cysteine at codon 112 and arginine at codon 158, and is present in approximately 75 percent of Caucasians. A second coding sequence variant, ε4, reflects substitution of arginine for cysteine at codon 112, and is present in approximately 15 percent of Caucasians. The third coding sequence variant, ε2, contains cysteine at codons 112 and 158, and is present in approximately 10 percent of Caucasians. Analysis of these coding sequence polymorphisms in normal control populations and in patients with AD has consistently shown that (a) there is an increase in the frequency of the ε4 allele in patients with AD (ε4 allele frequency in AD is approximately 40 percent),[64] and (b) there is a smaller reduction in the frequency of the ε2 allele (to about 2 percent in AD).[65] More significantly, there is a dose-dependent relationship between the number of copies of ε4 and the age-of-onset of AD, such that ε4/ε4 subjects have an earlier onset (mean age of onset is less than 70 years) than heterozygous ε4 subjects (mean onset of after 70 years).[66] Subjects with an ε2 allele, on the other hand, have a later onset (mean age of onset for ε2/ε3 is greater than 90 years).[65] The association between ε4 and AD has been robustly confirmed in numerous studies and in several different ethnic groups (reviewed in reference 67), and currently it seems that APOE ε4 accounts for ~ 30 to 50 percent of the genetic risk for AD in population studies. The association is weaker with advanced age of onset, and the putative protective role of the ε2 allele is less clear at younger ages of onset (where ε2 may even be associated with a more aggressive course).[68,69] Currently, the major exception to the association of APOE ε4 with AD arises from studies in African-Americans and Hispanics, which studies have generated conflicting results.[70–72] It is unclear whether these conflicting results reflect small sample sizes or whether there is a true lack of association between AD and APOE ε4 in subsets of these populations.

Although the association between APOE ε4 and AD is robust (with the possible exceptions noted above), it is not entirely specific. Observations of patients with head injury[73,74] and spontaneous intracerebral hemorrhage,[75] and of patients undergoing elective cardiac bypass surgery,[76] suggest a poorer cognitive outcome for patients with the ε4 allele. There is also evidence for synergistic effects of a history of head injury and APOE ε4 on risk for AD,[73] such that patients with APOE ε4 and a head injury have a tenfold increase in risk for AD compared to a twofold increase with APOE ε4 alone, and no increase for head injury alone. Reports of association between the ε4 allele and Creutzfeldt-Jacob disease[77] and multi-infarct dementia[78] are conflicting, although the majority of studies appear not to detect an association between ε4 and these diseases.[79,80] However, there is a confirmed association between the ε4 allele and the Lewy body variant of AD, which has an overlapping but subtly different clinical phenotype from classical AD (e.g., more frequent hallucinations and sensitivity to neuroleptics).[81]

The mechanism by which the ε4 allele is associated with an earlier onset of AD and by which the ε2 allele is associated with a later onset is unclear. As is discussed below, the genetic data (the association of AD exclusively with the ε4 allele, a protective effect for the ε2 allele, and dose-dependent relationship between the ε4 copy number and age of onset of AD) provide a strong argument

that the ε4/ε2 polymorphism is an actual biologic effector in the APOE gene. Currently, however, the possibility that the true pathogenic mutations/polymorphisms in nearby sequences are simply in linkage disequilibrium with ε4/ε2 cannot be entirely excluded (see below). Nevertheless, a large body of biochemical evidence has been accumulated to support various hypotheses on how these APOE coding sequence polymorphisms might promote/protect against AD. The most obvious hypothesis is that APOE ε4/ε2 polymorphisms might influence the production, distribution, or clearance of the Aβ peptide. This hypothesis is supported by observations that the genotype at APOE accounts for some of the variation in age-of-onset in subjects carrying the βAPP Val717Ile mutation (but not the APP_{692} mutation), suggesting a direct biochemical interaction between APOE and βAPP or its metabolic products.[82–85] Second, subjects with one or more APOE ε4 alleles have a higher Aβ peptide plaque burden than do subjects with no ε4 alleles.[86] In vitro studies suggest that delipidated APOE ε4 binds Aβ more avidly than APOE ε3.[62,87] Third, there is evidence that both APOE and Aβ may be cleared through the low-density lipoprotein-related (LRP) receptor and that APOE ε4 and the Aβ peptide may compete for clearance through the LRP receptor.[88] Finally, transgenic mice that have an intact endogenous APOE gene and that overexpress human βAPP with the Val717Phe mutant under the control of the PDGF β-subunit promoter, develop profuse deposits of extracellular Aβ by 9 months of age. In contrast, when the same transgene is expressed on an APOE^{−/−} background, there is a dramatic reduction in extracellular Aβ deposition, thus supporting the hypothetical role for APOE in sequestering extracellular Aβ.[89]

While theories attempting to explain a role for APOE ε4 mediated by alterations in brain Aβ peptide levels have received the greatest attention, there is also some biochemical evidence to suggest a relationship between APOE and neurofibrillary tangles and synaptic density. In vitro APOE isoform-specific binding experiments with Tau and MAP2 suggest that ε3 binds to both Tau and MAP2 better than the ε4 isoform.[90–92] This has led to suggestions that ε2 and ε3 may protect and sequester microtubule associated proteins better than ε4, thereby reducing the ability of Tau to bind to itself, become hyperphosphorylated, and form paired helical filaments. This is supported by the fact that neurofibrillary degeneration begins earlier in ε4 carriers than in non-ε4 carriers.[93] APOE immunoreactivity has been detected within the neuronal cytoplasm, and particularly at the base of proximal dendrites, suggesting that although APOE is not transcribed in neurons, it can be imported into neurons from extracellular sources.[94] This would place APOE in the right location for interactions with microtubule associated proteins.

Finally, there is a good correlation between the degree of clinical dementia and the decrease in synaptic density in AD as measured by both MAP2 and synaptophysin immunoreactivity.[95] It has been suggested that APOE may be involved in synaptic plasticity during regeneration and repair, and that the ε4 allele is less efficient in this role. Thus, APOE knockout mice also show an age-dependent decrease in synaptic density and spontaneous Aβ peptide aggregation within astrocytic processes.[96] Several types of neural tissue culture cells demonstrate decreased neurite outgrowth in the presence of APOE ε4 in the media rather than APOE ε3.[97,98] Perhaps, then, the APOE isoforms might differentially affect synapse formation in response to injury, learning, and aging.

In addition to the ε2/ε3/ε4 coding sequence polymorphisms, several polymorphisms have been discovered in the 5′-promoter of the APOE gene. These sequence polymorphisms have attracted interest because of preliminary data from quantitation of APOE levels in the brains, CSF, or serum of patients with AD. Data from some, but not all, studies suggest that subjects with AD have a 1.5- to threefold higher levels of APOE than do subjects with the same genotype but without AD.[99–103] Two different studies provide a potential explanation for this observation. Thus, the Th1/E47cs polymorphism[104] and homozygosity for the −491 A allele[105] are suspected to increase risk for AD independently of

APOE ε4, and to cause this increased risk for AD by altering the transcriptional activity of APOE (although direct proof of the latter in vivo remains to be obtained). A follow-up study by the original group provided supporting evidence for an effect of the Th1/E47cs T allele and a weaker effect for the −491 T allele.[106] However, several other independent studies using large sample sizes (> 88 AD patients) were unable to replicate these findings, although they did confirm that the −491 A/T polymorphism at least, is in linkage disequilibrium with the APOE ε2/ε3/ε4 polymorphism.[107,108] Another polymorphism in the intron 1 enhancer region also failed to show association with AD beyond what was anticipated through its linkage disequilibrium with the ε2/ε3/ε4 polymorphism.[109]

## Presenilin 1

After the discovery that βAPP missense mutations and the APOE polymorphisms did not account for all cases of FAD, several groups undertook a survey of the nonsex-linked chromosomes other than chromosomes 19 and 21. These studies identified a series of polymorphic markers located on chromosome 14q24.3 (D14S43, D14S71, D14S77 and D14S53) that showed robust evidence of linkage to a particularly aggressive early-onset (onset 25 to 65 years; mean 45 years) form of familial Alzheimer disease (z > 23.0 at θ = 0.01).[110–112] Subsequent genetic mapping studies narrowed the region containing this third Alzheimer susceptibility locus (AD3) to a region of approximately 10 cM between the marker D14S271 at the centromeric end and D14S53 at the telomeric end, a physical distance of approximately 7 Mb. The actual disease gene (presenilin 1) was then isolated using a positional cloning strategys,[113] and a homologue (presenilin 2) was subsequently mapped to chromosome 1 (see below).

The chromosome 14 AD3 subtype gene, presenilin 1 (PS1), is highly conserved in evolution, being present in C. elegans[114] and D. melanogaster,[115] and appears to encode a polytopic integral membrane protein (GenBank L42110). Theoretical predictions based upon Kyte-Doolittle hydrophobicity analysis suggest that there are between 5 and 10 membrane-spanning domains, that the N-terminus is acidically charged, and that there is a large hydrophilic, acidically charged loop domain between the putative sixth and seventh transmembrane domains.[113,116] Partial direct experimental support for a polytopic structure has been obtained from studies in transfected cells (see below).

The presenilin 1 gene is transcribed at low levels in many different cell types, both within the central nervous system and also in non-neurological tissues.[113] In the central nervous system, PS1 transcripts can be detected by in situ hybridization in the neocortex (especially in cortical neurons in layers II and IV), neurons of the CA1 to CA3 fields of the hippocampus, granule cell neurons of the dentate gyrus, subiculum, cerebellar Purkinje and granule cells, and deep nuclei, as well as lesser amounts in the olfactory bulb, striatum, some brainstem nuclei, and thalamus. Despite intense signals on northern blots of the corpus callosum, there is very little in situ hybridization signal detectable in oligodendrocytes in white matter.[117] However, following injury such as kanaic acid injection into cerebral white matter there is induction of significant PS1 mRNA expression in white matter.[118]

The genomic structure of the PS1 gene has been elucidated and some of the transcriptional regulatory elements have been defined.[119] Like the βAPP gene, there is evidence for alternate splicing of the PS1 transcript. Thus, there is a variably present 4-amino acid VRQS insert which arises from use of an alternate splice donor site at the 3′ end of exon 4.[119–121]

Immunoblotting and immunohistochemical studies suggest that the PS1 protein is approximately 50 kDa in size and is predominantly located within intracellular membranes in the endoplasmic reticulum, perinuclear envelope, the Golgi apparatus, and some as yet uncharacterized intracytoplasmic vesicles.[122,123] The tissue-specific expression patterns of PS1 protein largely reflect those of the mRNA.[124] Studies of the topology of PS1 suggest that the N-terminus and the residues in the TM6–TM7 loop are both located in the cytoplasm (Fig. 234-5).[122,125–127]

The orientation of the C-terminus is not yet completely resolved.[122,125–127] However, the predominance of opinion suggests that it is oriented to the cytoplasm and that the preceding hydrophobic residues either are membrane associated or represent two additional transmembrane domains (TM7 and TM8). Studies of the PS1 protein in brain tissue, as well as many other peripheral tissues, reveal that only very small amounts of the PS1 holoprotein exist within the cell at any given time.[128,129] Instead, the holoprotein is actively catabolized, possibly by at least two different proteolytic mechanisms. One of these mechanisms appears to involve the proteasome.[130] Another proteolytic mechanism involves a series of heterogeneous endoproteolytic cleavages near residue 290 within the TM6–TM7 cytoplasmic loop domain.[128,129] This endoproteolytic cleavage generates a series of N- and C-terminal heterogeneous fragments of approximately 35 kDa and 18 to 20 kDa, respectively. Remarkably, the stoichiometry of the N- and C-terminal fragments is tightly maintained on a 1:1 ratio, and the absolute abundance of the N- and C-terminal fragments is also tightly regulated such that artificial overexpression of PS1 results in only a modest increase in N- and C-terminal fragments.[128] This has led to the suggestion that

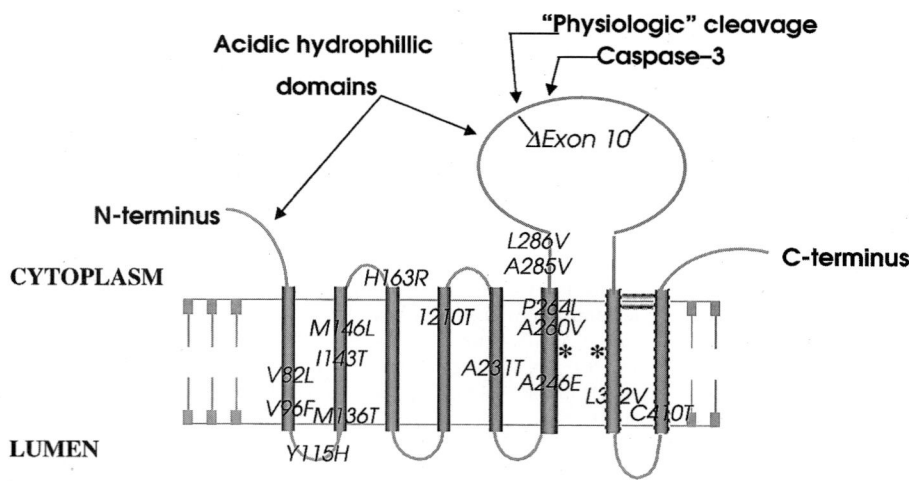

**Fig. 234-5** Putative topology of the PS1 protein showing the location of several Alzheimer disease-related mutations.

the process of endoproteolytic cleavage involves a tightly regulated saturable process.[131]

A third proteolytic mechanism acting upon the presenilin holoproteins involves members of the caspase 3 family of proteases. Activation of apoptosis by a variety of means that culminate in activation of caspase 3 results in cleavage of PS1 near residue aspartate 345 and the equivalent aspartate residue in PS2 (Asp 329).[132–134] It is currently unclear whether caspase mediated endoproteolytic cleavage of the presenilins is actively involved in the regulation of apoptotic signal pathways (preliminary data suggest an antiapoptotic effect for the C-terminal derivative of PS1 cleaved by caspase).[135] Alternatively, the presenilins might simply represent innocent bystanders that are cleaved by the caspase enzyme once apoptosis is activated. Certainly, caspase-mediated cleavage of the presenilins is not required for the effects of the presenilins on amyloidogenesis and *Notch* signaling.[134]

It is currently unclear whether the holoprotein, the endoproteolytic fragments, or both have biologic functions. However, it is clear that the native form of the holoprotein and its endoproteolytic fragments are components of high molecular weight, multimeric protein complexes. Thus, the holoprotein appears to be a component of an ~180-kDa complex that is predominantly resident within the rough endoplasmic reticulum (rER).[131,136,137] Both the N-terminal fragment (NTF) and the C-terminal fragment (CTF) appear to associate with each other as heterodimeric components of a larger (~250 kDa) multimeric protein complex that appears to be resident in the endoplasmic reticulum, Golgi apparatus, and some additional intracellular membranous domains whose identity has not been entirely clarified.[25,131,136,137] The latter may include detergent insoluble glycosphingolipid-rich domains (which have also been called lipid-rich rafts). It has been suggested that inclusion of the presenilin proteins in these high molecular weight membrane-bound complexes plays a critical role in the processing of PS1. Specifically, it has been suggested that the incorporation of the holoprotein and its subsequent endoproteolytic cleavage and incorporation into a larger complex represents a rate-limiting step in the processing pathway.[138] However, once incorporated into these high molecular weight complexes, the endoproteolytic fragments remain together with a stable 1:1 stoichiometry and with very long half-lives.[131,136,137] Holoprotein monomers that fail to get incorporated in these complexes are rapidly degraded with a half-life of less than 1 h via a proteasome-dependent mechanism.[130] It also appears likely that incorporation of the presenilin proteins and their derivatives into these complexes is necessary for the biologic activity of the presenilins.[139]

The identity of the other components of the presenilin complexes is currently under investigation. However, a combination of yeast-two-hybrid, coimmunoprecipitation, immunohistochemistry, and biochemical fractionation studies reveals that, in peripheral tissues and in brain, the presenilins associate with β-catenin, a member of the armadillo protein superfamily.[137,140] In brain, the presenilins also associate with a novel armadillo protein termed neuronal plakophillin-related armadillo protein (NPRAP) or δ-catenin.[137,140] The functional significance of the presenilin : armadillo interactions is not entirely clear because the armadillo proteins have diverse functions, ranging from a structural role in stabilization of intercellular junctions (including synapses) to intracellular transduction of receptor-mediated signals (e.g., Wnt and certain growth factors) to participation in apoptotic cell death pathways. There is evidence from some laboratories that presenilins may also directly interact with βAPP[141,142] and filamen.[143] However, not all laboratories confirm the latter results.[131] More recently, a novel, Type 1 transmembrane glycoprotein, nicastrin, has been identified as another functional component of the presenilin complexes.[332] Nicastrin is necessary for some aspects of *Notch/glp-1* signalling during embryonic development in *C. elegans*, and absence of nicastrin results in embryonic lethality. Mutations of a conserved hydrophilic domain in the N-terminus of nicastrin can significantly modulate γ-

secretase cleavage of βAPP and the production of Aβ *in vitro*. Nicastrin can bind to the C-terminal stubs of βAPP, which are derived from α-secretase cleavage (C83-βAPP) or β-secretase cleavage (C99-βAPP), the immediate precursors of Aβ. Similarly, nicastrin can bind the furin- and kuzbanian-cleaved, membrane-tethered fragments of *Notch*, which are the substrates for the signal-dependent S3-cleavage that liberates the *Notch* intracellular domain during signal transduction. Currently, it seems likely that there is a bi-directional interaction between the presenilins and nicastrin which serves to regulate the subsequent γ-secretase or S3-cleavage events.

The normative function of presenilin 1 has not yet been defined. Functional analogies have been made to the weakly homologous SPE4 protein of *C. elegans*, which is involved in maintenance of a Golgi-derived membranous organelle thought important in the partitioning of protein and cell membrane products in the maturing spermatocyte of *C. elegans*.[144] This has led to speculation that the PS1 protein might serve a similar role in protein and membrane trafficking.[113] This hypothesis is supported by two different lines of direct experimental evidence. First, ablation of functional PS1 expression by homozygous targeted disruption of the murine PS1 gene causes aberrant processing of βAPP with the failure of γ-secretase cleavage of the C-terminal stubs of βAPP derived from α-secretase or β-secretase cleavage.[145] Failure of γ-secretase cleavage results in the accumulation of uncleaved α-secretase or β-secretase stubs in a variety of intracellular loci including the endoplasmic reticulum, Golgi, and lysosomes.[145,146] A similar effect has been achieved by (artificially) mutating either of two conserved aspartate residues (D258 and D387) in putative TM domains of PS1 and PS2. Second, as described earlier, the presenilins form multimeric protein complexes with the *armadillo* protein β-catenin,[137,140] and missense mutations in PS1 and PS2 cause mistrafficking of this presenilin ligand.[147] These results suggest that PS1 might be directly involved in trafficking of βAPP, βAPP derivatives or components of the putative γ-secretase enzyme. Alternatively, PS1 might serve as an adaptor for, or an activator of γ-secretase. Finally, the loss-of-function effect caused by the artificial D258E or D387E mutations suggests that these residues may be part of the active site of a novel aspartyl protease and that PS1 is itself γ-secretase. This result, however, must be tempered with the knowledge that mutation of these aspartate residues also has a structural effect on the presenilin complexes.[333] Nevertheless, functional assays have shown that γ-secretase proteolytic activity co-purifies with presenilin 1 in a high molecular weight complex. More impressively, several transition-site analogue inhibitors of aspartyl proteases, which block γ-secretase activity, can be chemically cross-linked to the presenilins, indicating that if the presenilins are not themselves the catalytic component of γ-secretase, they are likely to be physically very close to the catalytic site within a multimeric protein complex.

Other putative roles for presenilin 1 have included a role in the regulation of intercellular signal transduction during development, in apoptosis, and possibly in intracellular calcium ion homeostasis. The former suggestion arose because null mutations in a second presenilin orthologue in *C. elegans* (*sel12*) exert a suppressor effect on abnormalities in vulva progenitor cell fate decisions induced by activated *Notch* mutants.[114] *Notch* is involved in intercellular signaling during development. SEL12 protein shows stronger amino acid sequence identity to the human presenilin proteins than does SPE4. A role for mammalian presenilins in Notch-mediated signal transduction is further supported by the fact that homozygous targeted knockout of the murine PS1 gene (using homologous recombination) causes embryonic lethality around day E13 and is associated with: (a) severe developmental defects in somite formation and axial skeleton formation; (b) the occurrence of cerebral hemorrhage; and (c) reduced *Notch* and *delta* transcription in selected cell types.[148,149] Similar phenotypes have been observed in mice with targeted knockouts of the murine *Notch1* and DLL1 genes, supporting the hypothesis that PS1 has

**Table 234-2 Missense Mutations in the Presenilin Genes**

| Codon | Location | | Mutation | Phenotype |
|---|---|---|---|---|
| | | | | PRESENILIN I |
| 79 | N-term loop | | Ala → ? | FAD, onset 64 years |
| 82 | TM1 | | Val → Leu | FAD, onset 55 years |
| 95 | TM1 | | Val → Phe | FAD |
| 115 | TM16TM2 loop | | Tyr → His | FAD, onset 37 years |
| 117 | TM16TM2 loop | | Pro → Leu | FAD, onset 28 years |
| 120 | TM16TM2 loop | | Glu → Asp | FAD, onset 48 years |
| 139 | TM2 | | Met → Thr | FAD, onset 49 years |
| 139 | TM2 | | Met → Val | FAD, onset 40 years |
| 143 | TM2 | | Ile → Thr | FAD, onset 35 years |
| 146 | TM2 | | Met → Leu | FAD, onset 45 years |
| 146 | TM2 | | Met → Val | FAD, onset 38 years |
| 146 | TM2 | | Met → Ile | FAD, onset 40 years |
| 163 | TM3 interface | | His → Arg | FAD, onset 50 years |
| 163 | TM3 interface | | His → Tyr | FAD, onset 47 years |
| 171 | TM3 | | Leu → Pro | FAD, onset 40 years |
| 209 | TM4 interface | | Gly → Val | FAD |
| 213 | TM4 interface | | Ile → Thr | FAD |
| 231 | TM5 | | Ala → Thr | FAD, onset 52 years |
| 233 | TM5 | | Met → Thr | FAD, onset 35 years |
| 235 | TM5 | | Leu → Pro | FAD, onset 32 years |
| 246 | TM6 | | Ala → Glu | FAD, onset 55 years |
| 260 | TM6 | | Ala → Val | FAD, onset 40 years |
| 263 | TM66TM7 loop | | Cys → Arg | FAD, onset 47 years |
| 264 | TM66TM7 loop | | Pro → Leu | FAD, onset 45 years |
| 267 | TM66TM7 loop | | Pro → Ser | FAD, onset 35 years |
| 280 | TM66TM7 loop | | Glu → Ala | FAD, onset 47 years |
| 280 | TM66TM7 loop | | Glu → Gly | FAD, onset 42 years |
| 285 | TM66TM7 loop | | Ala → Val | FAD, onset 50 years |
| 286 | TM66TM7 loop | | Leu → Val | FAD, onset 50 years |
| del291–319 | TM66TM7 loop | | Short loop | FAD, |
| 384 | TM66TM7 loop | | Gly → Ala | FAD, onset 35 years |
| 392 | TM66TM7 loop | | Leu → Val | FAD, onset 25–40 years |
| 410 | TM7 | | Cys → Tyr | FAD, onset 48 years |
| | | | | PRESENILIN II |
| 141 | 1 | TM2 | Asn → Ile | FAD, onset 50–65 years |
| 239 | 4 | TM5 | Met → Val | FAD, onset variable 45–84 yrs |

Adapted with permission from St George-Hyslop P: Genetics of Alzheimer disease, in Markesbery W, (Ed): *Neuropathology of Dementing Diseases.* London, Edward Arnold, 1997.

either a direct or an indirect role in intercellular signal transduction.[150] A role in the suppression of apoptosis has been suggested from studies in transfected cells. Overexpression of full-length wild-type PS1 or wild-type PS2 can cause apoptosis in transfected cells, and mutations further sensitize these cells to apoptosis, possibly through a mechanism involving heterotrimeric G-coupled proteins sensitive to pertussis toxin.[151] It is of note that mutations in βAPP are also thought to cause constitutive activation of programmed cell death pathways involving heterotrimeric G-coupled proteins.[58,59]

To date, more than 40 different mutations have been discovered in the PS1 gene (Table 234-2). The majority of these mutations are missense mutations giving rise to the substitution of a single amino acid. These mutations are predominantly located in highly conserved transmembrane domains, at or near putative membrane interfaces, or in the N-terminal hydrophobic or C-terminal hydrophobic residues of the putative TM6-TM7 loop domain. Two splicing-defect mutations have been identified. One involves a point mutation in the splice acceptor site at the 5′ end of exon 10 (in some exon numbering systems, exon 10 is labeled exon

9).[152–154] Because exon 9 and exon 11 are in-frame, this mutation allows exon 9 to be fused in-frame with exon 11, thereby removing a series of charged residues at the apex of the hydrophilic acidically-charged TM6–TM7 loop domain. Interestingly, this mutation removes residues near the endoproteolytic cleavage site at residue 290 and results in the production of increased quantities of uncleaved holoprotein, which appears to be incorporated normally in the high molecular weight ER and Golgi-resident complexes.[128,136] The second splice-site mutation arises from deletion of a G nucleotide from the splice donor site at the 3′ end of exon 5 (reference 155 and Rogaeva, unpublished). An alternate GT splice donor site four base pairs further downstream in intron 5 is used, which causes the in-frame insertion of an extra tyrosine residue within the luminal TM1–TM2 loop domain (Rogaeva et al., unpublished).

The wide scattering of missense mutations led to speculation that the effect of most of the FAD-related mutations is a gain-of-function effect.[156] This is partially borne out by two observations in PS1 knockout animals ($PS1^{-/-}$). First, these animals have a phenotype of early perinatal mortality without evidence of Alzheimer disease.[148,149] This loss-of-function phenotype in $PS1^{-/-}$ animals can be completely rescued by both wild-type and mutant PS1 transgenes.[157,158] Second, $PS1^{-/-}$ mice have a defect in βAPP processing manifest by the failure of γ-secretase cleavage and the accumulation of the C-terminal stubs of βAPP following α- and β-secretase cleavage (α- and β-stubs).[145] This defect in βAPP processing is completely reversed by both wild-type and mutant PS1 transgenes. A gain of function is imparted by the mutant transgenes because they also induce an increase in $A\beta_{42}$, which, as described below, is a consistent biochemical effect of PS1 mutations.[157,158] However, a very different perspective is provided by studies using human PS1 cDNAs in complementation assays of mutant sel12 in *C. elegans*. These studies suggest that the wild-type human PS1, but not mutant human PS1 cDNAs are able to complement the loss-of-function sel12 mutants.[159,160] The latter result argues that the human PS1 mutants may not be fully functional (but do not fully preclude a gain-of-function effect as well).

Regardless of whether PS1 (and PS2) mutations cause a gain of function or a loss of function, it seems likely that one effect is to alter the processing of βAPP by preferentially favoring the production of potentially toxic long-tailed Aβ peptides ending at residue 42 or 43.[60,161–164] Thus, fibroblasts from heterozygous carriers of PS1 mutations, various cell lines transfected with βAPP and βAPP cDNAs, as well as the brain from transgenic mice overexpressing mutant PS1 transgenes, contain or secrete increased quantities of long Aβ peptide isoforms with only a variable but minor increase in short-tailed Aβ peptides.[60,161–164] Direct measurements of Aβ peptide isoforms in the postmortem brain tissue of patients dying with PS1-linked FAD also show marked increases in the amount of long-tailed Aβ isoforms compared to control brain tissue and to brain tissue from subjects with sporadic Alzheimer disease.[165]

As with βAPP mutations, while there is a substantial body of work to suggest that defective processing of βAPP and over-production of $A\beta_{42}$ are intimately associated with PS1 mutations, evidence has also emerged that suggests that PS1 and PS2 mutations modulate cellular sensitivity to apoptosis induced by a variety of factors including staurosporine, Aβ peptide, serum withdrawal and NGF withdrawal.[118,151,166,167] Currently, these data are still evolving and the apparent paradox of a putative "apoptosis promoting effect" for the presenilins and the existence of viable transgenic mice overexpressing mutant or wild-type presenilin cDNAs, but lacking widespread apoptosis, remains to be explained.

A third way in which PS1 mutations might lead to AD is by altering the metabolism of the presenilin proteins in a manner analogous to the effects of βAPP mutations on the metabolism of βAPP holoprotein. Evidence to support this is somewhat conflicting. It is clear that the exon 10 splicing mutation does inhibit the formation of N- and C-terminal fragments.[128] This observation clearly indicates that the formation of N- and C-terminal fragments is not necessary for the genesis of AD. Interestingly, however, the mutant $PS1_{\Delta Exon 10}$ holoprotein is incorporated into the higher molecular weight complex which contains the N- and C-terminal fragments.[136] Preliminary studies of cultured cells overexpressing missense mutant presenilin cDNAs had suggested that missense mutations might also inhibit the physiological endoproteolytic cleavage events.[168] Further studies, however, have yielded conflicting results. Some studies suggest that only a subset of mutations (e.g., C410Y) inhibit endoproteolytic cleavage while others (e.g., G384A) did not.[169] Other studies of the levels of mutant presenilin proteins in the brains of transgenic mice seemed to suggest the opposite result: namely PS1 missense mutations cause an increased accumulation of physiological endoproteolytic cleavage fragments,[170] while PS2 mutations have no effect on the physiological endoproteolytic process.[171] Preliminary studies also suggest that PS2 mutations might increase the sensitivity of PS2 to caspase 3-mediated cleavage.[132] However, this was not borne out in subsequent studies in cultured cells or in homogenates of brain tissue from subjects with PS1 mutations (the levels of various PS1 derivatives were indistinguishable from controls).[172]

## Presenilin 2

During the cloning of the presenilin 1 gene on chromosome 14 a very similar sequence was identified in the public nucleotide sequence databases (GenBank L44577).[173,174] Further analysis revealed that this similar nucleotide sequence was derived from a gene on chromosome 1q42.1, and encodes a polypeptide whose open reading frame contained 448 amino acids. The sequence of this peptide showed substantial amino acid sequence identity with that of the presenilin 1 protein (overall identity approximately 60 percent), and would be predicted to have a structural organization very similar to that of PS1 protein. Within the TM domains, the amino acid sequence identity between this new gene and presenilin 1 was even higher (approximately 90 percent). However, the pattern of transcription of this novel gene was slightly different from that of presenilin 1, being expressed less homogeneously in the brain and in peripheral tissues. In fact, PS2 was maximally expressed in cardiac muscle, skeletal muscle, and pancreas. Nevertheless, when the genomic organization of this novel gene was worked out it was apparent that many of the intron-exon boundaries (especially those relating to the highly conserved transmembrane domains) were identical between this gene and presenilin 1.[119,175,176] Cumulatively, these observations suggested that this novel gene, which became known as presenilin 2,[173] was a homologue of the presenilin 1 gene on chromosome 14. Not surprisingly, the predicted topology of PS2 is similar to that of PS1, and it also forms similar but independent multimeric protein complexes which contain β-catenin.[136,137]

Mutational analyses uncovered two different missense mutations in the presenilin 2 gene in families segregating early onset forms of Alzheimer disease. The first mutation (Asn141Ile) was detected in a proportion of families of Volga German ancestry, in which the FAD locus had been independently mapped by genetic linkage studies to chromosome 1.[173,174] The second mutation (Met239Val) was discovered in an Italian pedigree.[173] However, in contrast to the frequency of presenilin 1 mutations, screening of large data sets reveal, that presenilin 2 mutations are likely to be rare.[176]

Another profound difference between the presenilin 2 mutations and those in the βAPP and PS1 gene is that the phenotype associated with PS2 mutations is much more variable.[176,177] Thus, in the vast majority of carriers, the illness begins between the ages of 35 and 65 years for PS1 mutations, and between 40 and 65 years for βAPP mutations. In contrast, the range of age-of-onset in heterozygous carriers of PS2 mutations is between 40 and 85 years of age, and there is at least one instance of apparent nonpenetrance

in an asymptomatic octogenarian transmitting the disease to affected offspring.[176,178,179] A similar, but less profound variation in age-of-onset within families segregating the βAPP V717I mutation has been ascribed to a modifying effect by the APOE gene.[82-84] Thus, carriers of the βAPP V717I mutation who have one or more ε4 alleles at APOE have an earlier onset than do heterozygous carriers of the V717I mutation who have the ε2 allele and no ε4 alleles of APOE. However, because the effect of APOE ε4 on the age-at-onset in PS2 mutations is either absent or less profound, modifier loci other than APOE probably account for much of this variation.

The relationship of the normal function of presenilin 2 to that of presenilin 1 remains unknown. Although both proteins reside within the perinuclear envelope, endoplasmic reticulum, Golgi, and some as yet uncharacterized intracytoplasmic vesicles, they appear to form distinct high molecular weight complexes,[131,137] and their tissue-specific patterns of expression are different.[173,175] Nevertheless, given the strong similarities in structure and in amino acid sequence of the respective proteins, it would seem likely that PS1 and PS2 have similar or overlapping activities. This is supported by the fact that the effect of PS2 mutations is similar to those of PS1 mutations and by the fact that the residues mutated in PS2 are conserved in PS1. Thus, PS2 mutations, like PS1 mutations, increase the secretion of long-tailed Aβ peptides.[60,164] PS2 mutations may also cause increased sensitivity to apoptosis, but it is unclear whether this is an effect independent of their ability to cause increased Aβ peptide secretion.[118,166] Finally, although $PS2^{-/-}$ mice have essentially no detectable Notch-deficient embryonic phenotype, and have apparently normal βAPP processing (in contrast to $PS1^{-/-}$ mice), double knock-out mice ($PS1^{-/-}$ and $PS2^{-/-}$) have very profound and more severe Notch-deficient embryonic phenotypes and essentially complete cessation of γ-secretase activity.[334-336] This result suggests that the activities of PS1 and PS2 are likely to be overlapping and slightly redundant.

## The Chromosome 12 Locus

The observation that presenilin 1, presenilin 2, βAPP, and APOE mutations/polymorphisms accounted for approximately half of the genetic variance of AD prompted a number of groups to undertake genome surveys to identify other susceptibility loci. Using two independent data sets of late-onset AD pedigrees (n = 16; n = 38), a novel AD locus was identified in the pericentromeric region of chromosome 12 between the markers D12S1042 and D12S390 (z = 3.5).[180] Follow-up studies in a dataset of 53 independent pedigrees confirmed the presence of an AD susceptibility gene within a larger (approximately 60-cM) region of chromosome 12 in a subset of pedigrees.[181] This latter study also indicated that pedigrees showing evidence for linkage to chromosome 12 generally had an onset after the age of 60, an unambiguous pattern of familial clustering with at least three affected family members that was independent of their APOE status. The subset of pedigrees that did not show linkage to chromosome 12 presumably reflects the presence of one or more genetic susceptibility factors elsewhere in the genome.

The identity of the chromosome 12 locus at the moment is unclear. Several candidate genes, including α2-macroglobulin (A2M), low-density lipoprotein receptor-related protein (LRP1), ARF2 and so on, map within this interval. Some of these genes (e.g., ARF3, Wnt1, plakophillin 2, ITR2) were excluded by the failure to find nucleotide sequence changes in their open reading frames that are either enriched in, or unique to, patients with the chromosome 12 form of AD. Some biochemical studies have suggested a role for A2M protein in AD (through its ability to bind Aβ and through competition with both Aβ and APOE for clearance through the LRP1 receptor). This work led to speculation that A2M might be the site of mutations associated with AD (see reference 182 for a summary). Considerable support for this concept (which links Aβ, APOE, A2M, and LRP1 in one biochemical cascade) was provided when a preliminary family-based association study detected an association between AD and an intronic insertion/deletion polymorphism at the 5'-splice site of exon 18 of A2M in a dataset of 104 pedigrees collected by the National Institute of Mental Health.[182] However, follow-up studies in a larger dataset of NIMH pedigrees (n = 142), in several datasets of independent pedigrees (> 60 pedigrees each), and in several sporadic AD case-control datasets (> 100 subjects each), failed to confirm an association between AD and this insertion/deletion polymorphism in A2M.[183] Furthermore, no biologic effect could be discerned for the A2M polymorphism.[183] Together, these results suggested that the original observation may have been an artifact. Another potential candidate gene on chromosome 12, LRP1, has also generated ambiguous results when studied using conventional allelic association (case-control) methods. Thus, the 87-bp allele of tetranucleotide repeat polymorphism in the 5'-promoter of LRP was reported to be significantly increased in late onset sporadic AD cases.[184] However, in an independent collection of French AD cases, the 87-bp allele was significantly decreased in frequency,[185] and a study of more than 130 patients with sporadic AD showed no significant association with either allele.[186] Similarly, several studies have suggested a weak, borderline statistically significant association (e.g., p < 0.01 not corrected for multiple testing) for homozygosity of the C,C allele of the C766T polymorphism in exon 3 of LRP.[187–189] However it was not significantly different from controls in several other comparable studies.[190–192]

## Other Genes

Although five different genetic loci associated with inherited susceptibility to AD are now known, several large surveys of subjects with familial Alzheimer disease have indicated that they still do not account for the disease in all pedigrees. Pedigrees lacking mutations in any of the four known AD genes and failing to cosegregate with chromosome 12 markers do not display a singular phenotype, but, instead, comprise a mix of early-onset autosomal dominant pedigrees and late-onset multiplex pedigrees. Consequently, it is likely that there are several FAD genes yet to be found. Some of these FAD loci will probably be associated with rather rare, but highly penetrant defects similar to those seen with mutations in PS1 and βAPP. Other genes may result in incompletely penetrant autosomal dominant traits like that associated with PS2. However, it is likely that a significant proportion of the remaining genes will have effects similar to that of APOE, in which the presence or absence of other genetic and environmental risk factors influences the ultimate phenotype.

Attempts to identify novel AD susceptibility genes have followed two strategies. One strategy, a continuation of the conventional positional cloning strategy, has attempted to show cosegregation of marker alleles with the disease phenotype (identity by descent) in pedigrees multiply affected by AD. These studies have assessed cosegregation using both conventional parametric lod score methods as well as newer nonparametric methods.[180,181,193] However, because these methods work best for pedigrees multiply affected with AD, increasing emphasis has been placed on the use of simple case-control studies (such as those so effectively used to discover the association between AD and APOE). More recently, the case-control method for discovering allelic associations was supplemented by novel statistical methods (family-based association methods) that enable examination of allele sharing between affected sibs compared to unaffected sibs, such as the sibship disequilibrium transmission test (SDT) and the sib-transmission disequilibrium test (S-TDT).[182,194] These family-based association methods examine the parental alleles transmitted to unaffected siblings as a source of control chromosome information that, theoretically, is better matched for ethnicity and genetic background.

The conventional case-control allelic association tests yielded positive results on a significant number of genes, many of which are plausible biochemical candidate genes. However, most of these studies have not received the same robust replication as the association between AD and the ε4 allele of APOE. As a result, it is difficult to discern whether the reported associations are true but perhaps limited to particular subsets of AD, or whether they represent statistically significant but biologically incorrect results. The possibility of biologically false positive results in allelic association studies is a well-recognized problem in human genetics, and can arise when the test and control populations are not drawn from identical genetic backgrounds (i.e., due to population stratification). Recently, in an attempt to rectify the high false positive rate for simple allelic association studies, some studies have begun to use the newer family-based association methods.[182]

A partial list of candidate genes provisionally identified as putative AD susceptibility loci includes: homozygosity for the A allele of an intronic polymorphism in $\alpha_1$-chymotrypsin;[195] 5 repeat allele of an intronic insertion-deletion polymorphism in the very-low-density lipoprotein receptor;[196] neutral coding sequence and intronic polymorphisms in low-density lipoprotein receptor-related protein;[187] homozygosity for the common "1" allele of an intronic polymorphism in presenilin 1;[197] K-variant of butyrylcholinesterase;[198] and homozygosity for the Val/Val variant of the V443I polymorphism in bleomycin hydrolase.[199] However, most of these candidate genes have not received widespread confirmation when tested in independent but comparable datasets.[107,108,200–204]

## The Mitochondrial Genome and Alzheimer Disease

The role of mitochondria in some stages of apoptosis and the slight preponderance of females with AD suggest that mutations in the mitochondrial genome might play a role in the genesis of AD. Analysis of mitochondrial DNA has led to conflicting results. Thus, heteroplasmic mutations at nucleotide 5460 in codon 331 of subunit 2 of NADH dehydrogenase-ubiquinone oxidoreductase were found in mtDNA from 10 of 19 brain samples affected by AD, but were absent in all 11 normal brain samples.[205] Follow-up studies, however, either failed to find these mutations in 14 of 14 sporadic AD patients or observed them at a lower frequency in patients with AD (4.4 percent) as compared to normal controls (8.6 percent).[206,207] A variant at position 4336 within the tRNA(Gln) gene was found in ~ 5 percent of AD patients, but only 0.7 percent of controls.[207] A variant at position 3397 that converted methionine to valine within the ND1 gene was reported in 2.7 percent of AD subjects but 0 percent of controls.[207] Again, follow-up studies yielded inconsistent results, some appearing to support the existence of mutations at position 4336 as a risk for AD,[208] others failing to find differences in the frequency of mutations at position 4336 between controls and AD affected patients.[209,210] Finally, missense mutations within the mitochondrial cytochrome oxidase genes MTCO1 and MTCO2 were proposed to be associated with late-onset AD.[211] However, follow-up studies revealed that these sequence differences actually arose from contamination of the mtDNA with nuclear DNA, and that the contaminating nuclear DNA contained these sequence differences within nuclear pseudogenes.[212]

## Role of βAPP, APOE, and the Presenilins in the Pathogenesis of "Sporadic" AD

The appearance of derivatives of βAPP, APOE,[63,86,213] and PS1 proteins[124,214] in pathologic structures in brain tissue of subjects with "sporadic" AD argues that these proteins are involved in the disease, including "sporadic" AD. The most pressing evidence for a role of these genes in sporadic AD obviously derives from the population-based studies showing an association between the ε4 allele of APOE as described above. There is some evidence to suggest that homozygosity for the more common 1 allele of an intronic polymorphism within the PS1 gene might be associated with nearly doubling of risk for late-onset "sporadic" AD.[197,215,216] However, multiple follow-up studies in several different populations have generally not confirmed this association.[204,217–220] Nevertheless, a small number of missense mutations have been observed in the PS1 gene (but not in the PS2 gene) of patients with apparently "sporadic" AD (e.g. PS1 H163R and PS2 M139K).[221-223]

## Gene Interactions in AD

A prevailing theory of the pathogenesis of AD is that the various causes of this disease affect a biochemical pathway that leads to AD and to mismetabolism of $\beta$APP with the subsequent pathologic deposition of $A\beta$ peptide. Such a single biochemical pathway hypothesis would predict the existence of interactions between the known AD susceptibility genes, a prediction for which there is now increasing evidence. Thus, the APOE genotype influences age of onset in carriers of the $\beta$APP$_{V717I}$ mutation,[82,84] but not the $\beta$APP$_{692}$ missense mutation.[85] This interaction between APOE and $\beta$APP is also evident in transgenic mice (see above).[89] There is a small degree of variation of age at onset in families with PS1 mutations and a greater degree of variation in age at onset in families segregating PS2 mutations that appears to arise from genetic modifiers, but the role of APOE is somewhat unclear.[176,177] However, clear evidence for additive effects of mutations in PS1 and $\beta$APP is provided by the analysis of $A\beta$ peptide production in transfected cells and cerebral $A\beta$ deposition in transgenic mice expressing both mutants.[164,224-226] Thus, $A\beta_{42}$ production is dramatically increased in cell lines and in the brains of transgenic mice expressing both mutant PS1 and mutant $\beta$APP cDNAs, indicating that these mutations are likely to act in different places within the same biochemical cascade.

## Transgenic Models of AD

Transgenic mice have been created in which mutant human $\beta$APP or mutant human PS1 transgenes have been overexpressed in mouse brain. The first such transgene used a spliceable human $\beta$APP transgene that carried the Val717Phe missense mutation expressed under the platelet-derived growth factor receptor $\beta$ subunit promoter.[227] This transgene produced abundant quantities of mutant $\beta$APP and resulted in the accumulation of diffuse deposits of $A\beta$ peptide in the brain and abnormal synaptic morphology at about 9 months of age, but was not associated with obvious cognitive deficits or the appearance of neurofibrillary tangles.[96,228] A second transgenic mouse overexpressing the human $\beta$APP$_{695}$ transcript containing the 670/671 missense mutation also resulted in the widespread accumulation of $A\beta$ peptide and the appearance of dysmorphic synapses and developed a very subtle behavioral deficit by about 9 months of age, although they did not show neurofibrillary pathology.[228] A third transgenic mouse overexpressing mutant human $\beta$APP was recently described, in which there is some evidence for neuronal loss and staining for abnormally phosphorylated Tau, as well as prominent extracellular $A\beta$ deposition possibly due to the higher levels of $\beta$APP expression in this line.[229] However, as in the other two lines, no neurofibrillary tangles were observed. Finally, overexpressing mutant forms of PS1 or PS2 has created several transgenic animals.[162,164] While at the time of writing, these animals are too young to develop any neuropathology, biochemical measurements show that transgenic mice with mutant presenilins have increased levels of long-tailed isoforms of $A\beta$ peptide in the brain. Interestingly, several groups have found that cross-breeding mice that overexpress mutant PS1 with mice that overexpress mutant $\beta$APP results in accelerated $A\beta$ deposition,[164,224-226] arguing that these genes act at different points within the same biochemical pathway leading to AD. One of the principal uses of transgenic murine models of Alzheimer disease is that they provide a means to rapidly test and develop new therapies for the disorder. The growing evidence that the accumulation of $A\beta$-peptide, and especially $A\beta_{42}$, assembled into oligomeric aggregates (or protofibrils), is an essential event in the pathogenesis of Alzheimer disease, has led to attempts to inhibit the production, or accelerate the removal of $A\beta$. One somewhat unexpected strategy to achieve the latter goal has been to immunize transgenic mice with $A\beta_{42}$.[337] Several groups have now shown that this results in a dramatic

reduction in the number of amyloid plaques and an improvement in the cognitive deficits of murine models of Alzheimer disease.[337-339] Significantly, the antibodies which are most effective in this regard are those directed toward fibrillar forms of $A\beta$.[338,339] Furthermore, these beneficial effects on cognition and on neuropathology can be achieved with only modest changes in $A\beta$-peptide levels in brain (presumably because protofibrillar forms of $A\beta$ are a low abundance, labile species).[339]

# BIOCHEMICAL GENETICS OF FRONTOTEMPORAL DEMENTIAS

Most cases of frontotemporal dementia are sporadic,[230,231] with a proportion being inherited. In a population study from the Netherlands, 38 percent of cases of frontotemporal dementia were found to be familial.[232] In 1994, linkage of a familial disease called disinhibition-dementia-parkinsonism-amyotrophy complex (DDPAC) to chromosome 17q21-22 was described.[233] It was followed by reports showing linkage of a number of inherited dementing diseases with preceding personality changes to the same region of chromosome 17.[234-241] In 1996, a consensus conference was held that led to the grouping of these diseases under the heading of "frontotemporal dementia and parkinsonism linked to chromosome 17" (FTDP-17).[242] At the time, disease in 13 families was considered to be definitely or probably linked to chromosome 17. Neuropathologically, some of these familial frontotemporal dementias had been shown to be characterized by an abundant filamentous pathology made of hyperphosphorylated Tau protein, similar to that observed in Alzheimer disease.[243-245] This, together with the fact that the Tau gene maps to the region of the critical interval on chromosome 17[246] made Tau a strong candidate gene. The discovery of at close to 20 different exonic and intronic mutations in the Tau gene (Fig. 234-6) in over 40 families with frontotemporal dementia shows that the Tau gene is indeed the FTDP-17 locus.[247-257]

## Tau Protein in Normal Human Brain

Tau, one of the first microtubule-associated proteins to be identified, associates with microtubules and promotes microtubule assembly in vitro (GenBank J03778).[258] Analysis of the Tau protein reveals that it is heterogeneous, existing in several different isoforms and in different states of posttranslational modification.[258-265] The isolation of cDNA clones encoding the various Tau isoforms has led to an understanding of this molecular diversity.[266-272]

All known Tau isoforms are produced from a single gene by alternative mRNA splicing. The six Tau isoforms expressed in adult human brain range from 352 to 441 amino acids in length and differ from each other by the presence or absence of three inserts.[268,269] Eleven exons (numbered 1 to 13) make up the longest human brain tau.[272] Exons 6 and 8 have not been found in human brain Tau cDNA clones, whereas exons 2, 3, and 10 are subject to alternative mRNA splicing.[268,269,272] The most striking feature of the Tau sequences is the presence of three or four tandem repeats of 31 or 32 amino acids located in the C-terminal half, each containing a characteristic Pro-Gly-Gly-Gly motif. The extra repeat of 31 amino acids (encoded by exon 10) in the isoforms with four repeats is inserted within the first repeat of the isoforms with three repeats in a way that preserves the periodic pattern. Besides being distinguished by the presence of 3 or 4 tandem repeats, some Tau isoforms contain 29 (encoded by exon 2) or 58 (encoded by exons 2 and 3) amino acid inserts located near the amino-terminus.[269] In immature human brain, only the shortest Tau isoform with three repeats is expressed.[268] The developmental shift of human Tau bands from a simple fetal to a more complex adult pattern thus involves the transition from the expression of the isoform with three repeats containing no amino-terminal inserts, to the expression of all six isoforms. Tau isoforms with a large additional insert in the amino-terminal half (encoded by exon 4A) have been described in the peripheral nervous

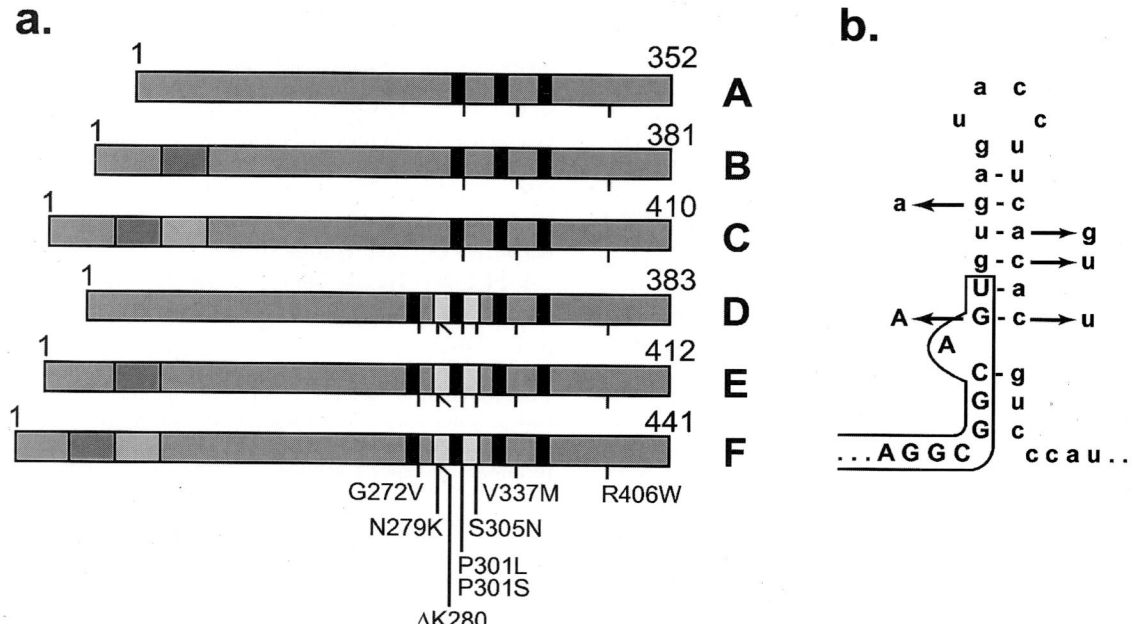

**Fig. 234-6** Mutations in the Tau gene in frontotemporal dementia and parkinsonism linked to chromosome 17 (FTDP-17). *A*, Diagram of the six Tau isoforms (A to F) that are expressed in adult human brain. [The color coded version of this figure is shown in the online version of this book]. Alternatively spliced exons are shown in red (exon 2), green (exon 3), and yellow (exon 10), with black bars indicating the microtubule-binding repeats. Nine missense mutations, three silent mutations and, one deletion mutation in the coding region are shown. They affect all six Tau isoforms, with the exception of N279K,

ΔK280, L284L, N296N, P301L, P301S, S305N, and S305S, which only affect Tau isoforms with four microtubule-binding repeats. Amino acid numbering corresponds to the 441 amino acid isoform of human brain Tau. *B*, Secondary structure representation of the stem-loop in the pre-mRNA at the exon 10-5′ intron boundary. The S305N and S305S mutations, as well as the five known intronic mutations are indicated. They all destabilize the stem-loop structure. Exon sequences are shown in capital letters and intron sequences are shown in lowercase letters.

system.[270–272] These "big Tau" proteins correspond to the 110-kDa protein expressed in peripheral ganglia.

Experiments with synthetic peptides and with Tau proteins produced by expression in *Escherichia coli* have shown that the C-terminal repeats and some adjoining sequences constitute microtubule-binding domains.[273–277] Microtubules assembled in the presence of Tau show arms projecting from the surface.[278] Tau thus consists of a C-terminal microtubule-binding domain and an amino-terminal projection domain, with the latter determining the spacing between adjacent microtubules.[279] Recombinant Tau isoforms with four repeats induce faster microtubule assembly than those with three repeats, as might be expected if one Tau molecule links a number of tubulin subunits.[280] Similar microtubule-binding domains are found in the otherwise structurally unrelated high-molecular weight microtubule-associated proteins MAP2[281] and MAP4,[282] and in PTL-1 ("protein with Tau-like repeats"), a microtubule-associated protein from the nematode *Caenorhabditis elegans*.[283] The sequencing of the genome of *Drosophilia melanogaster* has revealed the existence of a single protein with Tau-like repeats.[283a] This protein may be the ancestor of Tau, MAP2 and MAP4. A Tau-like repeat is also present in the high molecular weight MAP-homologous protein-1 (MHP1) from *Saccharomyces cerevisiae*.[284]

When individual human Tau isoforms that have been expressed in *E. coli* are mixed together, they give a characteristic set of six bands, ranging from 48 to 67 kDa in apparent molecular mass.[280] True molecular masses of the different isoforms range from 37 to 46 kDa; therefore, Tau is anomalously retarded on denaturing gels, as has been clear since the sequencing of the first Tau isoforms.[266,267] Comparison of the pattern of recombinant Tau isoforms with that of native Tau shows that the four major Tau isoforms in adult human brain correspond to isoforms with 3 and 4 repeats without amino-terminal inserts, and to isoforms with 3 and 4 repeats containing the first amino-terminal insert of 29 amino acids. Isoforms with 3 and 4 repeats with the 58-amino acid

amino-terminal insert are also found, albeit at lower levels.[280] These findings establish that the six isoforms identified by cDNA cloning account for the Tau isoforms in adult human brain, where similar levels of three-repeat and four-repeat isoforms are the norm. There exist true species differences in the expression of Tau isoforms. Immature rodent brain expresses the shortest three-repeat Tau isoform, like immature human.[268,285] However, unlike adult human brain, adult rodent brain only expresses three Tau isoforms, each with four microtubule-binding repeats.[285,286]

Tau is an abundant protein in both central and peripheral nervous systems. In brain, it is found predominantly in nerve cells, with lower levels in some glial cells. Within nerve cells, it is found mainly in axons.[287] Although Tau has been detected in some nonneuronal tissues, it is clear that it is predominantly expressed in the nervous system. The major physiological function of Tau derives from its ability to promote microtubule assembly and to bind to microtubules, which are thus stabilized. Inactivation of the Tau gene by homologous recombination leads to no overt phenotype, indicating that Tau is not an essential protein.[288]

Tau is a phosphoprotein and phosphorylation is also developmentally regulated.[289,290] Thus, Tau from developing brain is phosphorylated more than Tau from adult brain, implying selective dephosphorylation of the shortest Tau isoform during brain maturation. Tau from developing brain is phosphorylated at 15 known sites in the shortest isoform, whereas Tau from adult brain is phosphorylated at a minimum of 9 sites in the six isoforms.[290] With the exception of Ser262, which is located at the beginning of the first repeat, all the known phosphorylation sites in Tau are located outside the microtubule-binding repeat region. Phosphorylation is heterogeneous, implying that a given Tau molecule is partially phosphorylated at some, but not all, of these sites. Many of these sites are serine or threonine residues that are followed by a proline, suggesting that proline-directed protein kinases may phosphorylate Tau in normal brain. Accordingly, mitogen-activated protein kinase,[291] glycogen synthase kinase-3,[292] neuronal cdc2-like kinase,[293] and stress-activated protein kinases[294] phosphorylate Tau at many of these sites in vitro. Studies using lithium chloride as a specific inhibitor have strongly suggested that glycogen synthase kinase-3 is a Tau kinase in brain.[295,296] Tau phosphorylation by a number of protein kinases is markedly stimulated by sulfated glycosaminoglycans, such as heparin and heparan sulphate.[297-301]

The phosphorylation state of a protein is the result of a balance between protein kinase and protein phosphatase activities. Of the major phosphatase activities in a brain extract, Tau is dephosphorylated predominantly by the trimeric form of phosphatase 2A (PP2A).[302,303] The use of SV40 small t as a specific inhibitor has shown that PP2A controls the phosphorylation state of Tau in vivo.[304] Phosphorylation negatively regulates the function of Tau. Thus, the more phosphorylated Tau is, the less able it is to bind to microtubules and to promote microtubule assembly.[294,305,306] Hyperphosphorylation is an invariant feature of the filamentous Tau deposits that characterize a number of neurodegenerative diseases.

## Tau Mutations in FTDP-17

Tau mutations in FTDP-17 are either missense, silent and deletion mutations in the coding region or intronic mutations located close to the 5′ splice site of the intron following the alternatively spliced exon 10 (Fig. 234-6).

Missense mutations are located in the microtubule-binding repeat region or close to it. Mutations in exon 9 (K257T, G272V), exon 12 (V337M, and exon 13 (G389R, R406W) affect all six Tau isoforms.[247,248,257b,257e] By contrast, mutations in exon 10 (N279K, ΔK280, L284L, N296N, P301L, P301S, S305N, and S305S) only affect Tau isoforms with four microtubule-binding repeats (Fig. 234-6).[247,248,250-257a,257d,257f] Most missense mutations reduce the ability of Tau to interact with microtubules, as reflected by a marked reduction in the ability of mutated Tau proteins to promote microtubule assembly.[252,257,257b,257e,307] Mutations in exon 10 (ΔK280, P301L, and P301S) produced the largest effects, with intermediate reductions for mutations in exons 9 (K257T, G272V) and 12 (V337M), and a smaller reduction for the mutation in exon 13 (G389R and R406W) In addition, several missense mutations have been shown to promote sulphated glycosaminoglycan-induced assembly of recombinant Tau into filaments.[257e,307a,307b]

Intronic mutations are located at positions +3, +12, +13, +14, and +16, with the first nucleotide of the splice-donor site of the intron following exon 10 taken as +1 (Fig. 234-6).[248,249,255,256,257c] Secondary structure predictions have suggested the presence of an RNA stem-loop structure at the exon 10-5′ intron boundary, which is disrupted by the intronic mutations.[248,249] In addition, the +3 mutation is predicted to lead to increased binding of U1snRNA to the 5′ splice site.[249] Exon trapping has shown that the intronic mutations lead to increased splicing of exon 10.[249,308] Increased production of transcripts encoding exon 10 has also been demonstrated in brain tissue from patients with Tau intronic mutations.[248] This is reflected by a change in the ratio of three-repeat to four-repeat Tau isoforms, resulting in a net overproduction of four-repeat isoforms.[249,255,309]

The proposed existence of a stem-loop structure at the exon 10-5′ intron boundary[248,249] has been put on a firm footing with the determination of the three-dimensional structure of a 25-nucleotide-long RNA from the exon 10 5′ intron boundary (extending from positions −5 to +19) by NMR spectroscopy[308] as well as by gel mobility shift assays with purified U1snRNP and oligonucleotide-directed RNaseH cleavage experiments.[308a] The stem of this Tau exon 10 regulatory element RNA consists of a single, stable G-C base pair that is separated from a double-helix of 6 bp by an unpaired adenine. As is often the case of single nucleotide purine bulges, the unpaired adenine at position −2 does not extrude into solution, but intercalates into the double-helix. The apical loop consists of six nucleotides that adopt multiple conformations in

rapid exchange. The structure differs in several respects from two proposed representations of the stem-loop.[248,249]

The known intronic mutations of FTDP-17 are located in the upper part of the stem of the Tau exon 10 regulatory element. All five mutations reduce the thermodynamic stability of the stem-loop, but to various extents.[257c,308] The largest drop in melting temperature was observed for the +3 mutation. The +12 and +14 mutations also produced a large reduction in melting temperature, whereas the effects of the +13 and +16 mutations were smaller. Of these intronic mutations, only the +3 mutation does not lead to the formation of a G-U base pair. It leads instead to a less stable A-C pair, which explains why it has the largest destabilizing effect on the stem-loop structure. The differential reductions in stem-loop stability resulting from the intronic FTDP-17 mutations were reflected in exon-trapping experiments.[308] The +3 mutation produced the largest increase in the splicing of exon 10, followed by the +12 and +14 mutations. The effects of the +13 and +16 mutations were smaller.

These findings indicate that an intact stem-loop structure is necessary to ensure a correct ratio of three-repeat to four-repeat Tau isoforms. The stability of the stem-loop structure is likely to regulate access of the mRNA splicing machinery to the exon-intron junction. The presence of a stable stem-loop structure reduces access, but mutations in the stem-loop unmask the splice junction, leading to increased production of exon 10-containing transcripts. It follows that reduced transcription of exon 10 could be of therapeutic benefit in FTDP-17 cases with mutations in the Tau exon 10 regulatory element RNA. Single nucleotide bulges, such as the adenine at position −2, are common recognition elements of RNA-binding proteins and can be exploited as recognition points for the binding of small regulatory molecules. Thus, the aminoglycoside antibiotic neomycin has been found to bind to both wild-type and mutant Tau exon 10 regulatory element RNAs, which were stabilized as a result.[308b] Melting temperatures of the mutant regulatory elements in the presence of neomycin approached those of the wild-type sequence, suggesting a possible therapeutic avenue for cases with Tau mutations that destabilize the exon 10 regulatory element RNA.

The emerging picture is one of missense mutations that lead to a reduced ability of Tau to interact with microtubules, and of intronic mutations whose primary effects are at the RNA level, resulting in an overproduction of Tau isoforms with four microtubule-binding repeats.[310] However, two missense mutations in exon 10 deviate from this rule in that they do not lead to a reduction in the ability of Tau to promote microtubule assembly.[309,311] Instead, they increase splicing of exon 10, as is the case of the intronic mutations.[311] The same is true of the silent mutations L284L and N296N in exon 10.[257a,257f] The N279K mutation (AAT to AAG) in Tau[251] creates a purine-rich splice-enhancer sequence that explains its effects on exon trapping[311] and soluble four-repeat Tau in brain.[309] The L284L and N296N mutations disrupt exon splice silencer sequences, accounting for their effects in exon trapping experiments.[257a,257f,311a,311b] Mutations N279K, L284L, and N296N have revealed the existence of exon 10 splicing enhancer and silencer elements within the exon itself. The S305N mutation (AGT to AAT) in Tau[253] changes the last amino acid in exon 10. This sequence forms part of the stem-loop structure and the mutation produces a G to A transition at position −1. The silent mutation S305S (AGT to AGC) also forms part of the stem-loop and produces a T to C transition at position 0.[257d] It is, therefore, not surprising that the S305N and S305S mutations lead to a marked increase in the splicing of exon 10.[257d,311] Like the +3 mutation, the −1 mutation is expected to lead to increased binding of U1 snRNA to the 5′ splice site. However, this is not the case of the S305S mutation. Besides mutations in the intron following exon 10, additional pathogenic mutations may exist in other introns of the Tau gene. Thus, a G to A transition at position +33 of the intron following exon 9 has been described in a patient with familial frontotemporal dementia.[252] It disrupts one of several (A/T)GGG repeats that

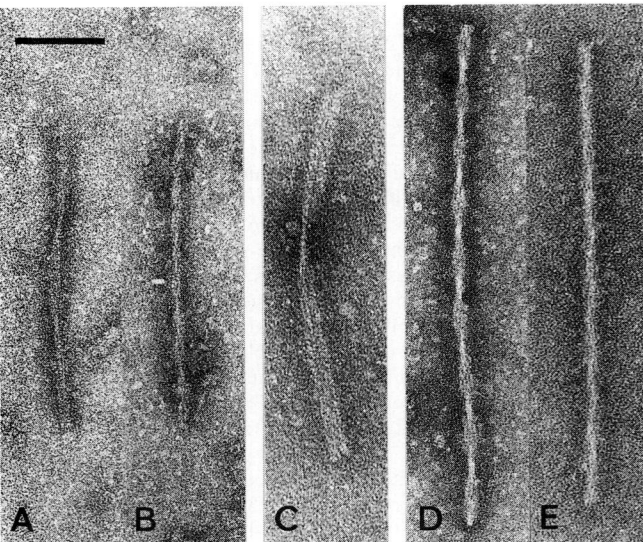

**Fig. 234-7** Tau filaments in FTDP-17. Dutch family 1 (with the P301L mutation in exon 10) is characterized by the presence of narrow twisted-ribbons (*A*) and occasional rope-like filaments (*B*). The Tau pathology is both neuronal and glial. Familial multiple-system tauopathy with presenile dementia (with the +3 nitronic mutation) is characterized by wide twisted-ribbons (*C*), which may be formed by two copies of the narrow twisted-ribbons joined across the central axis. The Tau pathology is both neuronal and glial. Seattle family A (with the V337M mutation in exon 12) is characterized by the presence of paired helical (*D*) and straight (*E*) filaments. The Tau pathology is largely neuronal. Scale bar = 100 nm.

may play a role in the regulation of the alternative splicing of exon 10.

## Neuropathology of FTDP-17

All cases of FTDP-17 examined to date show the presence of an abundant filamentous pathology made of hyperphosphorylated Tau protein. Extracellular Aβ deposits and intracellular α-synuclein deposits are not seen in the vast majority of cases. Strikingly, the morphologies of Tau filaments and their isoform compositions appear to be determined by whether Tau mutations affect mRNA splicing of exon 10, or whether they are missense mutations located inside or outside exon 10 (Fig. 234-7).[310]

Mutations in Tau that affect splicing of exon 10 lead to the formation of wide twisted-ribbon-like filaments that contain only four-repeat Tau isoforms.[244,255,256,257c] This has been shown in familial multiple system tauopathy with presenile dementia (MSTD) with the +3 intronic mutation,[249] in FTD-Kumamoto with the +12 mutation[256c] in familial progressive subcortical gliosis with the +16 mutation,[255] and in Duke family 1684 with the +16 mutation.[256] Similar results have been obtained in pallido-ponto-nigral degeneration with the N279K mutation in exon 10 whose primary effects are at the RNA level.[251,309,311,312] The same may be true of the families with the L284L, N296N, S305N, and S305S mutations in exon 10 whose primary effects are also at the RNA level.[253,257a,257d,257f,311] In all these FTDP-17 families, the Tau pathology is widespread and present in both nerve and glial cells, with an abundant glial component.

Mutations in exon 10 that do not affect mRNA splicing of Tau lead to the formation of narrow twisted-ribbons that contain four-repeat Tau isoforms, with a small amount of the most abundant three-repeat isoform.[254,313] This was shown in Dutch family 1 and in an American family, both with the P301L mutation.[248,254] Based on electron microscopy of tissue sections, the same also appears to be true of the Italian family with the P301S mutation.[257] At present, no neuropathologic information is available for the Dutch family with the ΔK280 mutation.[252] The P301L, P301S, and ΔK280 mutations all lead to a markedly reduced ability of Tau

to promote microtubule assembly.[252,257,307] This is not the case of the N279K and S305N mutations that increase splicing of exon 10[311] and whose Tau pathologies are, therefore, like those in families with intronic mutations.[253,312] In brain tissue from individuals with the P301L and P301S mutations, Tau pathology is widespread and present in both nerve cells and glial cells.[248,254,257] When compared with mutations that affect splicing of exon 10, the glial component is less pronounced. Some coding region mutations located outside exon 10 of Tau lead to the formation of PHFs and SFs that contain all six Tau isoforms.[243,314,314a] This was shown for Seattle family A with the V337M mutation in exon 12,[247] and for two families with the R406W mutation in exon 13.[248,314a] The morphologies of Tau filaments were found to be indistinguishable from those of Alzheimer's disease.[243,314a] Other coding region mutations located outside exon 10 give rise to a Tau pathology that closely resembles that of Pick's disease. This has been shown for the K257T and G272V mutations in exon 9, as well as for the G389R mutation in exon 13.[257b,257e,313] In families with coding region mutations located outside exon 10, Tau pathology is found in nerve cells, without a significant glial component.

## Pathogenesis of FTDP-17

The pathway leading from a mutation in the Tau gene to neurodegeneration is unknown. The likely primary effect of most missense mutations is a reduced ability of mutated Tau to interact with microtubules.[307,309] It may be equivalent to a partial loss of function, with resultant microtubule destabilization and deleterious effects on cellular processes, such as rapid axonal transport. However, in the case of the intronic mutations and the N279K, L284L, N296N, S305N and S305S mutations in exon 10, this appears unlikely. The net effect of these mutations is increased splicing of exon 10, leading to a change in the ratio of three-repeat to four-repeat Tau isoforms, and resulting in the overproduction of four-repeat isoforms.[248,249,251,257a,257d,257f,308,309,311] Moreover, missense mutations in exon 10 will only affect 20 to 25 percent of Tau molecules, with 75 to 80 percent of Tau being normal. Consequently, it is possible that a correct ratio of wild-type, three-repeat to four-repeat Tau is essential for the normal function of Tau in human brain. An alternative hypothesis is that a partial loss of function of Tau is necessary for setting in motion the mechanisms that ultimately lead to filament assembly. Earlier work had suggested that three-repeat and four-repeat Tau isoforms may bind to different sites on microtubules.[315] Overproduction of Tau isoforms with four repeats may result in an excess of Tau over available binding sites on microtubules, thus creating a gain of toxic function similar to that of most missense mutations, with unbound excess Tau available for assembly into filaments.[310] Besides leading to a partial loss of function phenotype, some Tau mutations may have additional effects on phosphorylation[315a] and filament assembly.[257e,307a,307b]

Where studied, pathologic Tau from FTDP-17 brain is hyperphosphorylated.[245] As known mutations in Tau do not create additional phosphorylation sites (with the possible exception of the P301S and K257T mutations), hyperphosphorylation of Tau to probably an event downstream of the primary effects of the mutations and may be a consequence of the partial loss of function. It will reinforce the effects of the mutations, because it is well established that hyperphosphorylated Tau is unable to bind to microtubules.[305,306] At present, there is no experimental evidence linking hyperphosphorylation of Tau to filament assembly, and it is unclear whether hyperphosphorylation is either necessary or sufficient for assembly. Thus, assembly of full-length hyperphosphorylated recombinant Tau into filaments has not been observed. In fact, experimental studies in vitro have shown that interactions between Tau and negatively charged sugar polymers, such as sulfated glycosaminoglycans and RNA, lead to rapid assembly into twisted and straight filaments in a phosphorylation-independent manner.[300,316–320] These studies have provided the first robust method for the assembly of synthetic filaments from full-length Tau protein.

However, the mechanisms that lead to assembly of Tau into filaments in brain remain to be discovered. It is possible that a reduced ability to interact with microtubules, which could have several different causes, is a necessary first step for filament assembly. Assembly is an energetically unfavorable, nucleation-dependent process that requires a critical concentration of Tau.[316,320] Many cells may have levels of Tau below the critical concentration. Other cells may have effective mechanisms for preventing the formation of Tau nuclei or may be able to degrade them once they have formed. Insufficient protective mechanisms and high Tau concentrations may underlie the selective degeneration of nerve cells and glial cells, which is especially striking in FTDP-17, with the characteristic, sometimes unilateral, razor-sharp demarcations between affected and unaffected areas in cerebral cortex.

The precise significance of the different filament morphologies observed in FTDP-17 is not clear. It is known that the repeat region of Tau forms the densely packed core of PHFs and SFs, with the amino- and carboxyl-terminal parts of the molecule forming a proteolytically sensitive coat. Also, for filaments assembled in vitro in the presence of sulfated glycosaminoglycans, the morphology of the filaments depends on the number of repeats in the Tau isoform used.[316] Thus, mutations in the repeat region or a change in relative amounts of three- and four-repeat isoforms could well influence filament morphology. Treatment of PHFs with acid leads to untwisted ribbon-like filaments like those seen in familial MSTD, suggesting a close similarity in packing of Tau molecules in the various structures.[244,321] The most important aspect may be the extended filamentous nature of the assemblies and the deleterious effect that this has on intracellular processes, rather than the detailed morphology of the different filaments.

## Animal Models of the Tauopathies

Transgenic mouse lines have been produced that overexpress individual wild-type three-repeat or four-repeat human Tau isoforms within nerve cells.[286,321a,321b,321c,321d] Human tau protein was expressed in the somatodendritic compartment of some nerve cells, where it was immunoreactive with a number of phosphorylation-dependent anti-tau antibodies, reminiscent of the pre-tangle stage of AD. Mice from the highest expressing lines[321b,321c,321d] showed marked axonopathy and amyotrophy, accompanied by numerous neurofilament-positive spheroids. No clear evidence of tau filaments or nerve cell loss was presented. This work has shown that the accumulation of non-filamentous human tau protein is sufficient to cause some nerve cell dysfunction. However, the pathological changes observed were much less pronounced than those found in FTDP-17.

A separate experimental system is the lamprey nervous system, where individual, identified nerve cells were injected with plasmid DNA encoding the shortest human brain tau isoform (352 amino acid isoform).[321e,321f] This resulted in the overexpression of hyperphosphorylated human tau protein in the somatodendritic compartment of nerve cells. It was accompanied by the formation of tau filaments and the degeneration of nerve cells.

The discovery of mutations in the tau gene in FTDP-17 is leading to the production of transgenic mouse lines expressing mutated human tau protein in nerve cells and glial cells. A first study reporting expression of the shortest four-repeat human tau isoform with the P301L mutation (383 amino acid isoform) has shown the formation of filaments made of hyperphosphorylated tau protein and the degeneration of affected nerve cells.[321g] Neurofibrillary tangles, axonopathy, amyotrophy, spheroids, and reactive gliosis were also present. Taken together, these findings are consistent with the view that the formation of tau filaments is a major determinant of nerve cell degeneration in the Tauopathies.

## Implications for Alzheimer Disease and Other Diseases with Tau Pathology

A major implication deriving from the work on FTDP-17 is that a normal ratio of functional Tau isoforms to microtubules appears to be essential to prevent neurodegeneration.[310] This finely tuned balance may be very sensitive to disruption, in line with the fact that a large percentage of the general population develops limited filamentous Tau pathology with ageing.[322] The new work has firmly established that the events leading to a filamentous Tau pathology or the mere presence of Tau filaments are sufficient for the degeneration of affected nerve cells and glial cells and the onset of dementia. This had long been suspected to be the case, largely because of the good correlation between neurofibrillary lesions and nerve cell degeneration in AD.

The findings in FTDP-17 may shed light on the mechanisms that lead to the filamentous Tau pathology of AD. Seattle family A has shown that a V337M mutation in the third microtubule-binding domain is sufficient to lead to a Tau pathology that is indistinguishable from that of AD in its ultrastructural and biochemical characteristics.[243,247] The same is true of the R406W mutation in the carboxyl-terminal region of Tau.[248,314a] As in AD, the Tau filaments are PHFs and SFs that consist of all six Tau isoforms.[243] The proportions of PHFs (90 to 95 percent) and SFs (5 to 10 percent) A are also identical to those found in AD. It suggests that in AD a reduced ability of Tau to interact with microtubules may also be upstream of hyperphosphorylation and filament assembly.

The presence of mutations in the amyloid precursor protein ($\beta$APP) gene in about 30 families with early onset AD has revealed a genetic lesion that leads to a filamentous Tau pathology,[41] as has the larger number of families with mutations in the presenilin genes.[113] In these families, Tau pathology must be downstream of $\beta$APP and presenilin dysfunction, but it may be the Tau pathology that eventually causes neurodegeneration. The various FTDP-17 families now show that primary lesions in Tau itself can lead to neurodegeneration. It remains to be seen whether one can generalize from these familial cases to the 20 to 25 million cases of "sporadic" AD.

Filamentous Tau deposits are also the defining neuropathologic characteristic of neurodegenerative diseases that have been subsumed under the heading of "Pick complex."[323] They include progressive supranuclear palsy, corticobasal degeneration, Pick disease, and several other diseases. The Tau pathology of progressive supranuclear palsy and corticobasal degeneration bears a striking resemblance to that of cases of FTDP-17 with mutations that destabilize the exon 10 splicing regulatory element. Thus, filamentous Tau deposits are present in both nerve cells and glial cells.[324] Moreover, Tau filaments are either straight or have the appearance of twisted ribbons, and consist only of four-repeat isoforms.[325,326] Individuals within some FTDP-17 families have presented with a diagnosis of either progressive supranuclear palsy[257d] or corticobasal degeneration.[257,257f,326,326a] The similarities with FTDP-17 suggest that progressive supranuclear palsy and corticobasal degeneration may be exon 10 splicing diseases that are caused by an overproduction of four-repeat Tau isoforms. One study has reported an increase in exon 10-containing transcripts in brainstem in progressive supranuclear palsy.[326b] It remains to be seen whether this is reflected in increased levels of soluble four-repeat tau isoforms. Although progressive supranuclear palsy is usually sporadic, several case-control studies have shown a genetic association between progressive supranuclear palsy and a GT dinucleotide repeat polymorphism located in the intron between exons 9 and 10 of the Tau gene.[327–329] In healthy Caucasians, approximately 50 percent of subjects are homozygous for the A0 allele (with 11 GT repeats). This figure is approximately 95 percent for patients with progressive supranuclear palsy.

The known alleles are thought to be in linkage disequilibrium with the disease locus, which is believed to be the Tau gene. One study has reported that corticobasal degeneration is also associated with the A0 allele of the GT dinucleotide repeat polymorphism.[329a] Mutations within additional, as yet unknown, Tau exon 10-splicing regulatory elements may thus well predispose to progressive supranuclear palsy and corticobasal degeneration:

With respect to the isoform composition of Tau filaments, Pick disease is believed to be the opposite of progressive supranuclear palsy and corticobasal degeneration has been reported that it is characterized by filaments that are made of Tau isoforms with three microtubule-binding repeats.[330,331] Although most cases of Pick disease are thought to be sporadic, the finding that mutations in exons 9 (K257T and G272V) and 13 (G389R) of Tau give rise to a clinical picture and a neuropathology that are similar to those of Pick disease indicates the relevance of FTDP-17 for understanding Pick disease.[257b,257c,313] These mutations affect all six tau isoforms and the tau filaments in cases with the K257T[257e] and G389R[257b] mutations contain three-repeat and four-repeat Tau isoforms. It appears that depending on the positions of Tau missense mutations in exons 9, 12 and 13, and perhaps the nature of these mutations, a filamentous tau pathology ensues that resembles that of either AD or Pick disease. The mechanisms underlying this exquisite specificity remain to be established.

The emerging picture is one where FTDP-17, progressive supranuclear palsy, corticobasal degeneration and Pick disease are all primary tauopathies. On clinical grounds, the P301S mutation in Tau leads to either Pick disease or corticobasal degeneration in different members of the same family.[257] Similarly, the S305S mutation leads to either FTD or progressive supranuclear palsy [257d], indicating that genetic background can influence clinical presentation. Taken together, these findings support the existence of a "Pick complex"[323] and suggest that Tau dysfunction is its pathologic substrate.

## REFERENCES

1. Heyman A, Wilkinson WE, Stafford JA, Helms MJ, Sigmon AH, Weinberg T: Alzheimer's disease: A study of epidemiological aspects. *Ann Neurol* **15**:335, 1984.
2. Rocca WA, Amaducci LA, Schoenberg BS: Epidemiology of clinically diagnosed Alzheimer's disease. *Ann Neurol* **19**:415, 1986.
3. Breitner JC, Silverman JM, Mohs RC, Davis KL: Familial aggregation in Alzheimer disease: Comparison of risk among relatives of early- and late-onset cases, and among male and female relatives in successive generations. *Neurology* **38**:207, 1988.
4. Farrer LA, Myers RH, Connor L, Cupples LA, Growdon JH: Segregation analysis reveals evidence of a major gene for Alzheimer disease. *Am J Hum Genet* **48**:1026, 1991.
5. Bergem ALM, Engedal K, Kringlen E: Twin concordance and discordance for vascular dementia and dementia of the Alzheimer type. *Neurobiol Aging* **13(Supp 1)**:66, 1992.
6. Katzman R, Kawas C: The epidemiology of dementia and Alzheimer disease, in Terry RD, Katzman R, Bick KL (eds): *Alzheimer Disease.* New York, Raven, 1994, p. 25.
7. Lautenschlager NT, Cupples LA, Rao VS, Auerbach SA, Becker R, Burke J, Chui H, Duara R, Volicer L, Waring SC, Growdon JH, Farrer LA: Risk of dementia among relatives of Alzheimer disease patients in the MIRAGE study: What is in store for the oldest old? *Neurology* **46**:641, 1996.
8. Kang J, Lemaire HG, Unterbeck A, Salbaum JM, Masters CL, Multhaup G, Beyreuther K, Müller-Hill B: The precursor of Alzheimer disease amyloid A4 protein resembles a cell surface receptor. *Nature* **325**:733, 1987.
9. Goldgaber D, Lerman MI, McBride OW: Characterization and chromosomal localization of a cDNA encoding brain amyloid of Alzheimer's disease. *Science* **235**:877, 1987.
10. Robakis NK, Lahiri DK, Brown HR, Rubenstein R, Mehta B, Wisniewski H, Goller N: Expression studies of the gene encoding the Alzheimer's disease and Down syndrome amyloid peptide, in Swann JW (ed): *Disorders of the Developing Nervous System: Changing Views on Their Origins, Diagnoses and Treatments.* New York, Alan R Liss, 1988, p 183.
11. Tanzi RE, Gusella JF, Watkins PC, Bruns GAP, St George-Hyslop PH, Van Keuren ML: Amyloid β-protein gene: cDNA, mRNA distribution and genetic linkage near the Alzheimer locus. *Science* **235**:880, 1987.
12. Kitaguchi N, Takahashi Y, Tokushima Y, Shiojiri S, Ito H: Novel precursor of Alzheimer's disease amyloid protein shows protease inhibitory activity. *Nature* **331**:530, 1988.
13. Selkoe DJ: Normal and abnormal biology of β-Amyloid Precursor Protein. *Ann Rev Neurosci* **17**:489, 1994.
14. Shoji M, Golde T, Ghiso J, Chung T, Estus S, Shaffer L, Cai X-D, McKay D, Frangione B Younkin S: Production of the Alzheimer amyloid β protein by normal proteolytic processing. *Science* **258**:126, 1992.
15. Haass C, Schlossmacher MG, Hung AY, Vigo-Pelfrey C, Mellon A, Ostaszewski BL, Lieberburg I, Koo EH, Schenk D, Teplow DB, Selkoe DJ: Amyloid β-peptide is produced by cultured cells during normal metabolism. *Nature* **359**:322, 1992.
16. Jarrett JT, Lansbury PT: Seeding, one-dimensional crystallization of amyloid: A pathogenic mechanism in Alzheimer's disease and scrapie? *Cell* **73**:1055, 1993.
17. Yankner BA, Duffy LK, Kirschner DA: Neurotrophic and neurotoxic effects of amyloid β protein: Reversal by tachykinin neuropeptides. *Science* **250**:279, 1990.
18. Pike CJ, Burdick D, Walencewicz AJ, Glabe CG, Cotman CW: Neurodegeneration induced by beta-amyloid peptides in vitro: The role of peptide assembly state. *J Neurosci* **13**:1676, 1993.
19. Lorenzo A, Yanker BA: β-amyloid neurotoxicity requires fibril formation and is inhibited by Congo red. *Proc Natl Acad Sci USA* **91**:12243, 1994.
20. Golde TE, Estus S, Younkin LH, Selkoe DJ, Younkin SG: Processing of the amyloid protein precursor to potentially amyloidogenic derivatives. *Science* **255**:728, 1992.
21. Haass C, Koo EH, Mellon A, Hung AY, Selkoe DJ: Targeting of cell surface β-amyloid precursor protein to lysosomes: Alternative processing into amyloid-bearing fragments. *Nature* **357**:500, 1992.
22. Wild-Bode C, Capell A, Yamazaki TUL, Steiner H, Ihara Y, Haass C: Intracellular generation and accumulation of amyloid beta-peptide terminating at amino acid 42. *J Biol Chem* **272**:16085, 1997.
23. Cook DG, Forman M, Sung JC, Leight S, Kolson DL, Iwatsubo Y, Lee VM-Y: Alzheimer amyloid β(1–42) peptide is generated in the endoplasmic reticulum/intermediate compartment of NT2N cells. *Nat Med* **3**:1021, 1997.
24. Hartmann T, Beiger S, Bruhl B, Tienari PJ, Ida N, Roberts G, Allsop D, Masters CL, Dotti CG, Unsicker K, Beyreuther K: Distinct sites of intracellular production for Alzheimer's disease Aβ40/42-amyloid peptides. *Nat Med* **3**:1016, 1997.
25. Lee S-J, Liyanage U, Bickel P, Xia W, Lansbury PT, Kosik K: A detergent-insoluble membrane compartment contains Aβ in vivo. *Nat Med* **4**:730, 1998.
26. Yankner BA: Mechanisms of neuronal degeneration in Alzheimer's disease. *Neuron* **16**:921, 1996.
27. Zheng H, Jiang M, Trumbauer ME, Hopkins R, Sirinathsinghji DJ, Stevens KA, Corner MW, Slunt HH, Sisodia SS, Chen HY, Van der Ploeg LH: Mice deficient for the amyloid precursor protein gene. *Ann N Y Acad Sci* **777**:421, 1996.
28. Saitoh T, Sundsmo M, Roch J-M, Kimura N, Cole G, Schubert D, Oltersdorf T, Schenk DB: Secreted form of amyloid β-protein is involved in the growth regulation of fibroblasts. *Cell* **58**:615, 1989.
29. Milward AE, Papadopoulos R, Fuller SJ, Moir RD, Small D, Beyreuther K, Masters CL: The amyloid protein precursor of Alzheimer disease is a mediator of the effects of NGF on neurite outgrowth. *Neuron* **9**:129, 1992.
30. Nishimoto I, Okamoto T, Matsuura Y, Takahashi S, Murayama Y, Ogata F: Alzheimer amyloid protein precursor complexes with brain GTP-binding protein Go. *Nature* **362**:75, 1993.
31. Wisniewski KE, Dalton AJ, McLachlan DRC, Wen GY, Wisniewski HM: Alzheimer's disease in Down's syndrome: Clinicopathologic studies. *Neurology* **17**:278, 1985.
32. Wisniewski HM, Rabe A: Discrepancy between Alzheimer type neuropathology and dementia in persons with Down's syndrome. *Ann N Y Acad Sci* **477**:247, 1986.
33. Rumble B, Retallack R, Hilbich C: Amyloid A4 protein and its precursor in Down's syndrome and Alzheimer's disease. *N Engl J Med* **320**:1446, 1989.
34. Schupf N, Kapell D, Lee JH, Zigman W, Canto B, Tycko B, Mayeux R: Onset of dementia is associated with apolipoprotein E e4 in Down syndrome. *Ann Neurol* in press, 1997.
35. St George-Hyslop PH, Haines JL, Farrer LA, van Broeckhoven C, Goate AM, Crapper-McLachlan DR, et al: Genetic linkage studies suggest that Alzheimer's disease is not a single homogeneous disorder. *Nature* **347**:194, 1991.
36. Goate A, Haynes AR, Owen MJ, Farrall M, James LA, Lai LY, Mullan M, Rossor M, Hardy J: Predisposing locus for Alzheimer disease on chr 21. *Lancet* **1**:352, 1989.

37. Levy E, Carman MD, Fernandez-Madrid IJ, Power MD, Lieberburg I, Sjoerd G, van Duinen SG, Bots G, Luyendijk W, Frangione B: Mutation of the Alzheimer's disease amyloid gene in hereditary cerebral hemorrhage — Dutch type. *Science* **248**:1124, 1990.

38. Mullan MJ, Crawford F, Axelman K, Houlden H, Lilius L, Winblad B, Lannfelt L, Hardy J: A pathogenic mutation for probable Alzheimer's disease in the APP gene at the N-terminus of $\beta$-amyloid. *Nat Genet* **1**:345, 1992.

39. Hendricks M, van Duijn CM, Cras P, Cruts M, van Hul W, Van Harskamp F, Warren A, McInnis M, Antonarakis G, Martin J-J, Hofman A, Van Broeckhoven C: Presenile dementia and cerebral hemorrhage linked to a mutation at codon 692 of the $\beta$-amyloid Precursor protein gene. *Nat Genet* **1**:218, 1992.

40. Eckman CB, Mehta ND, Crook R, Perez-Tur J, Prihar G, Pfieffer E, Graff-Radford N, Hinder P, Yager D, Zenk B, Refolo LM, Prada CM, Younkin SG, Hutton M, Hardy J: A new pathogenic mutation in the APP gene (I716V) increases the relative production of A$\beta$(42/43). *Hum Mol Genet* **6**:2087, 1997.

41. Goate AM, Chartier-Harlin M-C, Mullan M, Brown J, Crawford F, Fidani L, Guiffra L, Haynes A, Hardy JA: Segregation of a missense mutation in the amyloid precursor protein gene with familial Alzheimer disease. *Nature* **349**:704, 1991.

42. Chartier-Harlin M-C, Crawford F, Holden H, Warren A, Hughes D, Fidani L, Goate A, Rossor M, Hardy J, Mullan M: Early onset Alzheimer's disease caused by mutations at codon 717 of the $\beta$-amyloid gene. *Nature* **353**:844, 1991.

43. Murrell J, Farlow M, Ghetti B, Benson MD: A mutation in the amyloid precursor protein associated with hereditary Alzheimer's disease. *Science* **254**:97, 1991.

44. Karlinsky H, Vaula G, Haines JL, Ridgley J, Bergeron C, Mortilla M, Tupler R, Percy M, Robitaille Y, Crapper-MacLachlan DR, St George-Hyslop P: Molecular and prospective phenotypic characterization of a pedigree with familial Alzheimer disease and a missense mutation in codon 717 of the $\beta$-amyloid precursor protein (APP) gene. *Neurology* **42**:1445, 1992.

45. Naruse S, Igarashi S, Kobyashi H, Aoki K, Inuzuki I, Kaneko K, Shimizu T, Iihara K, Kojima T, Miyatake T, Tsuji S: Missense mutation (Val → Ile) in exon 17 of the amyloid precursor protein gene in Japanese Familial Alzheimer disease. *Lancet* **337**:978, 1991.

46. The French Alzheimer's Disease Study Group: No founder effect in three novel Alzheimer's disease families with APP 717 Val Ile mutation. *J Med Genet* **33**:1, 1996.

47. Citron M, Oltersdorf T, Haass C, McConlogue C, Hung AY, Seubert P, Vigo-Pelfrey C, Lieberburg I, Selkoe DJ: Mutation of the $\beta$-amyloid precursor protein in familial Alzheimer's disease increases $\beta$-protein production. *Nature* **360**:672, 1992.

48. Cai XD, Golde TE, Younkin SG: Release of excess amyloid beta protein from a mutant beta protein precursor. *Science* **259**:514, 1992.

49. Susuki N, Cheung TT, Cai X-D, Odaka A, Otvos L, Eckman C, Golde T, Younkin SG: An increased percentage of long amyloid $\beta$ protein secreted by familial amyloid $\beta$ protein precursor ($\beta$APP717) mutants. *Science* **264**:1336, 1994.

50. Haass C, Hung AY, Selkoe DJ, Teplow DB: Mutations associated with a locus for familial Alzheimer's disease result in alternative processing of amyloid $\beta$-protein precursor. *J Biol Chem* **269**:17741, 1994.

51. Haass C, Lemere C, Capell A, Citron M, Selkoe D: The Swedish mutation causes early onset Alzheimer's disease by $\beta$-secretase cleavage within the secretory pathway. *Nat Med* **1**:1291, 1995.

52. Citron M, Vigo-Pelfrey C, Teplow DB, Miller C, Schenk D, Johnston J, Winblad B, Venizeelos N, Lannfelt L, Selkoe DJ: Excessive production of amyloid $\beta$-protein by peripheral cells of symptomatic and presymptomatic patients carrying the Swedish familial Alzheimer's disease mutation. *Proc Natl Acad Sci USA* **91**:11993, 1994.

53. Cras P, Van Harskamp F, Hendriks L, Ceuterick C, van Duijn CM, Stefanko SZ, Hofman A, Kros JM, van Broeckhoven C, Martin JJ: Presenile Alzheimer's dementia characterized by amyloid angiopathy and large amyloid core type senile plaques in the APP 692 Ala → Gly mutation. *Acta Neuropathol (Berl)* **1996**:253, 1998.

54. Wisniewski T, Frangione B: Peptides homologous to the amyloid protein of Alzheimer's disease containing a glutamine for a glutamic acid substitution have accelerated amyloid fibril formation. *Biochem Biophys Res Comm* **180**:1528, 1991.

55. Arispe N, Pollard HB, Rojas E: Giant multilevel cation channels formed by Alzheimer disease amyloid $\beta$ protein in a bilayer membrane. *Proc Natl Acad Sci USA* **90**:10573, 1993.

56. Mattson MP, Cheng B, Davis D, Bryant K, Lieberburg I, Rydel R: Beta-amyloid peptides destabilize calcium homeostasis and render human cortical neurons vulnerable to excitotoxicity. *J Neurosci* **12**:376, 1992.

57. Mattson MP, Goodman Y: Different amyloidogenic peptides share a similar mechanism of neurotoxicity involving reactive oxygen species and calcium. *Brain Res* **676**:219, 1995.

58. Okamoto T, Takeda S, Murayama Y, Ogata E, Nishimoto I: Ligand-dependent G protein coupling function of amyloid transmembrane precursor. *J Biol Chem* **270**:4205, 1995.

59. Yamatsuji T, Nishimoto I: G protein-mediated neuronal DNA fragmentation induced by familial Alzheimer's disease-associated mutants of APP. *Science* **272**:1349, 1996.

60. Scheuner D, Eckman L, Jensen M, Sung X, Citron M, Suzuki N, Bird T, Hardy J, Hutton M, Lannfelt L, Selkoe D, Younkin S: Secreted amyloid-$\beta$ protein similar to that in the senile plaques of Alzheimer disease is increased in vivo by presenilin 1 and 2 and APP mutations linked to FAD. *Nat Med* **2**:864, 1996.

61. Pericak-Vance MA, Bedout JL, Gaskell PC, Roses AD: Linkage studies in Familial Alzheimer disease — evidence for chromosome 19 linkage. *Am J Hum Genet* **48**:1034, 1991.

62. Strittmatter WJ, Saunders AM, Schmechel D, Goldgaber D, Roses AD, et al: Apolipoprotein E: High-affinity binding to $\beta$/A4 amyloid and increased frequency of type 4 allele in familial Alzheimer's disease. *Proc Natl Acad Sci USA* **90**:1977, 1993.

63. Wisniewski T, Frangione B, Apolipoprotein E: A pathological chaperone protein in patients with cerebral and systemic amyloid. *Neurosci Lett* **135**:235, 1992.

64. Saunders A, Strittmatter WJ, Schmechel S, St George-Hyslop P, Pericak-Vance M, Joo SH, Rosi BL, Gusella JF, Crapper-McLachlan DR, Growden J, Alberts MJ, Hulette C, Crain B, Goldgaber D, Roses AD: Association of apolipoprotein E allele e4 with the late-onset familial and sporadic Alzheimer disease. *Neurology* **43**:1467, 1993.

65. Corder EH, Saunders AM, Risch NJ: Apolipoprotein E type 2 allele decreases the risk of late-onset Alzheimer disease. *Nat Genet* **7**:180, 1994.

66. Corder EH, Saunders AM, Srittmatter WJ, Schmechel DE, Gaskell PC, Small GW, Roses AD, Haines JL, Pericak-Vance MA: Gene dosage of apolipoprotein E type 4 allele and the risk for Alzheimer's disease in late onset families. *Science* **261**:921, 1993.

67. Roses AD: Apolipoprotein E alleles as risk factors in Alzheimer disease. *Annu Rev Med* **47**:387, 1996.

68. Rebeck GW, Perls T, West H, Sodhi P, Lipsitz LA, Hyman BT: Reduced apolipoprotein e4 allele in the oldest old Alzheimer's patients and cognitively normal individuals. *Neurology* **44**:1513, 1994.

69. Van Duijn CM, de Knijff P, Crutts M, Wehnert A, Havekes LM, Hofman A, Van Broeckhoven C: Apolipoprotein E4 allele in a population-based study of early onset Alzheimer disease. *Nat Genet* **7**:74, 1994.

70. Maestre G, Ottman R, Stern Y, Mayeux R: Apolipoprotein E and Alzheimer disease: Ethnic variation in genotype risks. *Ann Neurol* **37**:254, 1995.

71. Hendrie HC, Hall KS, Hui S: Apolipoprotein E genotypes and Alzheimer's disease in a community study of elderly African Americans. *Ann Neurol* **37**:118, 1995.

72. Tang MX, Stern Y, Marder K, Bell K, Gurland B, Lantigua R, Andrews H, Feng L, Tycko B, Mayeux R: The APOE e4 and the risk of Alzheimer disease among African Americans, whites, and Hispanics. *JAMA* **279**:751, 1998.

73. Mayeux R, Ottman R: Synergistic effects of traumatic head injury and ApoE e4 in patients with Alzheimer's disease. *Neurology* **45**:555, 1995.

74. Roses AD, Saunders AM: Head injury, amyloid $\beta$ and Alzheimer's disease. *Nat Med* **1**:603, 1995.

75. Alberts MJ, Graffagnino C: ApoE genotype and survival from intracerebral hemorrhage. *Lancet* **346**:575, 1995.

76. Newman MF, Croughwell ND: Predictors of cognitive decline after cardiac operation. *Ann Thorac Surg* **59**:1326, 1995.

77. Pickering-Brown SM, Mann DM, Owen F, Ironside JW, de Silva R, Roberts DA, Balderson DJ, Cooper PN: Allelic variations in apolipoprotein E and prion protein genotype related to plaque formation and age of onset in sporadic Creutzfeldt-Jakob disease. *Neurosci Lett* **187**:127, 1995.

78. Shimano H, Ishibashi S, Murase T, Gotohda T, Yamada N, Takahu F, Ohtomo E: Plasma apolipoproteins in patients with multi-infarct dementia. *Atherosclerosis* **79**:257, 1989.

79. Saunders AM, Schmader K, Breitner JCS, Benson D, Brown WT, Goldfarb L, Goldgaber D, Manwaring MG, Pericak-Vance M, Roses

AD: Apolipoprotein E e4 allele distribution in late onset AD and in other amyloid-forming diseases. *Lancet* **342**:710, 1993.

80. Salavatore M, Seeber AC, Nacmias B, Petraroli R, D'Assandro M, Sorbi S, Pocchiari M: Apolipoprotein E in sporadic and familial Creutzfeldt-Jakob disease. *Neurosci Lett* **199**:95, 1995.

81. Olichney JM, Hansen LA, Galasko D, Saitoh T, Hofstetter CA, Katzman R, Thal LJ: The ApoE e4 allele is associated with increased neuritic plaques and cerebral amyloid angiopathy in AD and in Lewy body variant. *Neurology* **47**:190, 1996.

82. St George-Hyslop PH, Tsuda T, Crapper-McLachlan DR, Karlinsky H, Pollen D, Lippa C: Alzheimer's disease and possible gene interaction. *Science* **263**:536, 1994.

83. Sorbi S, Nacmias B, Forleo P, Amaducci L: Epistatic effect of APP717 mutation and apolipoprotein E genotype in familial Alzheimer disease. *Ann Neurol* **38**:124, 1995.

84. Nacmias B, Latteraga S, Tulen P, Piacentini S, Bracco L, Amaducci L, Sorbi S: ApoE genotype and familial Alzheimer's disease: A possible influence on age-of-onset in APP717Val → Ile mutated families. *Neurosci Lett* **183**:1, 1995.

85. van Broeckhoven C, Backhovens H, Cruts M, Martin JJ, Crook R, Houlden H, Hardy J: APOE genotype does not modulate age of onset in families with chromosome 14 encoded Alzheimer's disease. *Neurosci Lett* **169**:179, 1994.

86. Schmechel DE, Saunders AM, Strittmatter WJ, Joo SH, Hulette C, Crain B, Goldgaber D, Roses AD: Increased vascular and plaque beta-A4 amyloid deposits in sporadic Alzheimer disease patients with apolipoprotein e4. *Proc Natl Acad Sci USA* **90**:9649, 1993.

87. Strittmatter WJ, Weisgraber KH, Huang DY, Schmechel D, Saunders AM, Roses AD: Binding of human lipoprotein E to synthetic amyloid beta peptide: Isoform-specific effects and implications for late onset AD. *Proc Natl Acad Sci USA* **90**:8098, 1993.

88. Kounnas MZ, Moir RD, Rebeck GW, Bush AI, Argaves W, Hyman BT, Strickland DK: LDL Receptor related protein, a multifunctional ApoE receptor binds secreted βAPP and mediates its degradation. *Cell* 1994.

89. Bales KR, Verina T, Dodel RC, Du Y, Altsteil L, Bender M, Hyslop P, Johnstone EM, Little SP, Cummins DJ, Piccardo P, Ghetti B, Paul SM: Lack of apolipoprotein E dramatically reduces amyloid beta-peptide deposition. *Nat Genet* **17**:254, 1997.

90. Strittmater WJ, Saunders AM, Goedert M, Weisgraber KH, Dong LM, Jakes R, Huang D, Pericak-Vance M, Schmechel D, Roses A: Isoform-specific interactions of ApoE with microtubule associated protein Tau: Implications for Alzheimer disease. *Proc Natl Acad Sci USA* **91**:11183, 1994.

91. Huang DY, Goedert M, Strittmatter W, Schmechel D, Weisgraber K, Roses AD: Isoform-specific interactions of apolipoprotein E with microtubule associated protein MAP2c: Implications for Alzheimer disease. *Neurosci Lett* **182**:55, 1995.

92. Huang DK, Weisgraber KH, Strittmatter D, Goldgaber D, Roses AD: ApoE3 binding to Tau tandem repeat I is abolished by Tau serine262 phosphorylation. *Neurosci Lett* **192**:209, 1995.

93. Ohm TG, Kirca M: Apolipoprotein E polymorphism influences not only cerebral senile plaque load but also Alzheimer type neurofibrillary degeneration. *Neuroscience* **66**:583,1995.

94. Han SH, Einstein G: Apolipoprotein E is localized to the cytoplasm of human cortical neurons: A light and electron microscopic study. *J Neuropathol Exp Neurol* **53**:535, 1994.

95. Terry RD, Masliah E,Hansen L: Structural basis of the cognitive alterations in Alzheimer disease, in Terry RD, Masliah E, Hansen L (eds): *Alzheimer Disease*. New York, Raven Press, 1994, p 179.

96. Masliah E, Mallory M: Neurodegeneration in the central nervous system of ApoE-deficient mice. *Exp Neurol* **136**:107, 1995.

97. Nathan BP, Bellosta S, Sanan DA, Weisgraber KH, Mahley RW, Pitas RE: Differential effects of apolipoproteins E3 and E4 on neuronal growth in vitro. *Science* **264**:850, 1994.

98. Nathan BP, Bellosta S: The inhibitory effect of apolipoprotein E e4 on neurite outgrowth is associated with microtubule depolymerization. *J Biol Chem* **270**:19791, 1995.

99. Taddei K, Clarnette R, Gandy SE, Martins RN: Increased plasma apolipoprotein E (APOE) levels in Alzheimer's disease. *Neurosci Lett* **223**:29, 1997.

100. Lindh M, Blomber M, Jensen M, Basun H, Lannfelt L, Engvall B, Scharnagel H, Mätz W, Wahlund LO, Cowburn RF: Cerebrospinal fluid APOE levels in Alzheimer's disease patients are increased at follow-up and show a correlation with Tau protein. *Neurosci Lett* **229**:85, 1997.

101. Slooter AJ, de Knijff P, Hofman A, Cruts M, Breteler MM, van Broeckhoven C, Havekes LM, van Duijn CM: Serum APOPE level is not increased in Alzheimer's disease: The Rotterdam Study. *Neurosci Lett* **248**:21, 1998.

102. Hahne S, Nordstedt C, Ahlin A, Nyback H: Levels of CSF APOE in patients with Alzheimer's disease and healthy controls. *Neurosci Lett* **224**:99, 1997.

103. Pirttila T, Soininen H, Heinonen O, Lehtimaki T, Bogdanovic N, Paljarvi L, Kosunen O, Winblad B, Riekkinen PS, Wisniewski HM, Mehta PD: APOE levels in brains from Alzheimer disease patients and controls. *Brain Res* **722**:71, 1996.

104. Lambert JC, Pasquier F, Cottel D, Frigard B, Amyouel P, Chartier-Harlin JC: A new polymorphism in the APOE promoter associated with risk of developing Alzheimer's disease. *Hum Mol Genet* **7**:533, 1998.

105. Bullido MJ, Artiga MJ, Recuero M, Sastre I, Garcia MA, Aldulo J, Lendon C, Han SW, Morris JC, Frank A, Vasquez J, Goate A, Valdivieso F: A polymorphism in the regulatory region of APOE associated with risk for Alzheimer's disease. *Nat Genet* **18**:69, 1998.

106. Lambert JC, Berr C, Pasquier F, Delacourte A, Frigard B, Cottel D, Perez-Tur J, Mouroux V, Mohr M, Cecyre D, Galasko D, Lendon C, Poirier J, Hardy J, Mann D, Amouyel P, Chartier-Harlin MC: Pronounced impact of the Th1/E47cs mutation compared with the −491 AT mutation on neural APOE gene expression and risk of developing Alzheimer disease. *Hum Mol Genet* **7**:1511, 1998.

107. Town T, Paris D, Fallin D, Duara R, Barker W, Gold M, Crawford F, Mullan M: The −491 A/T apolipoprotein E promoter polymorphism association with Alzheimer's disease: Independent risk and linkage disequilibrium with the known APOE polymorphism. *Neurosci Lett* **252**:95, 1998.

108. Song YQ, Rogaeva E, Premkumar S, Brindle N, Kawarai T, Orlacchio A, Yu G, Levesque G, Nishimura M, Ikeda M, Pei Y, O'Toole C, Duara R, Barker W, Sorbi S, Freedman M, Farrer L, St George-Hyslop P: Absence of association between Alzheimer disease and the −491 regulatory polymorphisms of APOE. *Neurosci Lett* **250**:189, 1998.

109. Mui S, Briggs M, Chung H, Wallace RB, Gomez-Isla T, Rebeck GW, Hyman BT: A newly identified polymorphism in the apolipoprotein E enhancer gene region is associated with Alzheimer's disease and strongly with the E4 allele. *Neurology* **47**:196, 1996.

110. Schellenberg GD, Bird TD, Wijsman EM, Orr HT, Anderson L, Nemens E, White JA, Bonnycastle L: Genetic linkage evidence for a familial Alzheimer's disease locus on chr 14. *Science* **258**:668, 1992.

111. St George-Hyslop PH, Haines J, Rogaev E, Mortilla M, Vaula G, Pericak-Vance M, Foncin J-F, Montesi M, Bruni A, Sorbi S, Rainero I, Pinessi I, Pollen D, Polinsky R, Nee L, Kennedy J, Macciardi F, Rogeava E, Liang Y, Alexandrova N, Lukiw W, Schlumpf K, Tsuda T, Farrer L, Cantu J-M, Duara R, Amaducci L, Bergamini L, Gusella J, Roses A, Crapper MacLachlan D: Genetic evidence for a novel familial Alzheimer disease gene on chromosome 14. *Nat Genet* **2**:330, 1992.

112. Van Broeckhoven C, Backhovens H, Cruts M, De Winter G, Bruyland M, Cras P, Martin J-J: Mapping of a gene predisposing to early-onset Alzheimer's disease to chromosome 14q24.3. *Nat Genet* **2**:335, 1992.

113. Sherrington R, Rogaev E, Liang Y, Rogaeva E, Levesque G, Ikeda M, Chi H, Lin C, Holman K, Tsuda T, Mar L, Fraser P, Rommens JM, St George-Hyslop P: Cloning of a gene bearing missense mutations in early onset familial Alzheimer's disease. *Nature* **375**:754, 1995.

114. Levitan D, Greenwald I: Facilitation of lin-12-mediated signalling by sel-12, a *Caenorhabditis* elegans S182 Alzheimer's disease gene. *Nature* **377**:351, 1995.

115. Boulianne G, Livne-Bar I, Humphreys JM, Rogaev E, St George-Hyslop P: Cloning and mapping of a close homologue of human presenilins in D. melanogaster. *Neuroreport* **8**:1025, 1997.

116. Doan A, Thinakaran G, Borchelt DR, et al.: Protein topology of presenilin. *Neuron* **17**:1023, 1996.

117. Lee MK, Slunt HH, Martin LJ, et al.: Expression of presenilin 1 and 2 (PS1 and PS2) in human and murine tissues. *J Neurosci* **16**:7513, 1996.

118. Cribbs DH, Chen LS, Cotman CW, LaFerla FM: Injury induces presenilin-1 gene expression in mouse brain. *Neuroreport* **7**:1773, 1996.

119. Rogaev EI, Sherrington R, Wu C, Levesque G, Liang Y, Rogaeva EA, Chi H, Ikeda M, Holman K, Lin C, Lukiw WJ, de Jong PJ, Fraser PE, Rommens JM, St George-Hyslop PH: Analysis of the 5′ sequence, genomic structure and alternative splicing of the presenilin 1 gene

associated with early onset Alzheimer's disease. *Genomics* **40**:415, 1997.

120. The Alzheimer's Disease Collaborative Group: The structure of the presenilin I gene and the identification of six mutations in early onset AD pedigrees. *Nat Genet* **11**:219, 1995.

121. Cruts M, Martin J-J, Van Broeckhoven C: Molecular genetic analysis of familial early-onset Alzheimer's disease linked to chromosome 14q24.3. *Hum Mol Genet* **4**:2363, 1995.

122. De Strooper B, Beullens M, Contreras B, Craessaerts K, Moechars D, Bollen M, Fraser P, St George-Hyslop P, Van Leuven F: Posttranslational modification, subcellular localization and membrane orientation of the Alzheimer's disease associated presenilins. *J Biol Chem* **272**:3590, 1997.

123. Walter J, Capell A, Grunberg J, Pesold B, Schindzielorz A, Prior R, Podlisny MB, Fraser P, St George-Hyslop P, Selkoe D, Haass C: The Alzheimer's disease associated presenilins are differentially phosphorylated proteins located predominantly within the endoplasmic reticulum. *Molec Med* **2**:673, 1996.

124. Uchihara T, El Hachim, HK, Duyckearts C, Foncin C, Fraser PE, Levesque L, St George-Hyslop P, Hauw JJ: Widespread immunoreactivity of presenilin in neurons of normal and Alzheimer's disease brain: Double-labeling immunohistochemical study. *Acta Neuropathol* **92**:325, 1996.

125. Lehmann S, Chiesa R, Harris DA: Evidence for a six-transmembrane domain structure for PS1. *J Biol Chem* **272**:12047, 1997.

126. Li X, Greenwald I: Membrane topology of the C. elegans sel12 presenilin. *Neuron* **17**:1015, 1996.

127. Doan A, Thinakaran G, Borchelt DR, Slunt HH, Ratovitsky T, Podlisny M, Selkoe DJ, Seeger M, Gandy SE, Price DL, Sisodia SS: Protein topology of presenilin 1. *Neuron* **17**:1023, 1996.

128. Thinakaran G, Borchelt DR, Lee MK, Slunt HH, Spitzer L, Kim G, Ratovisky T, Davenport F, Nordstedt C, Seeger M, Levey AI, Gandy SE, Jenkins NA, Copeland N, Price DL, Sisodia SS: Endoproteolysis of presenilin 1 and accumulation of processed derivatives in vivo. *Neuron* **17**:181, 1996.

129. Podlisny M, Citron M, Amarante P, Sherrington R, Weiming X, Zhang J, Diehl T, Levesque G, Fraser P, Haass C, Koo EHM, Seubert P, St George-Hyslop P, Teplow D, Selkoe DJ: Presenilin proteins undergo heterogeneous endoproteolysis between Thr291 and Ala299 and occur as stable N- and C-terminal fragments in normal brain tissue. *Neurobiol Dis* **3**:325, 1997.

130. Fraser PE, Levesque G, Yu G, Mills L, Thirwell J, Frantseva M, Carlen P, St George-Hyslop P: Presenilin 1 is actively degraded by the 26S proteasome. *Neurobiol Aging* In press 1998.

131. Thinakaran G, Regard JB, Bouton CML, Harris CL, Price DL, Borchelt DR, Sisodia SS: Stable association of the presenilin derivatives and absence of presenilin interactions with APP. *Neurobiol Dis* **4**:438, 1998.

132. Kim TW, Pettingell WH, Jung YK, Kovacs DM, Tanzi RE: Alternative cleavage of Alzheimer-associated presenilins during apoptosis by a caspase-3 family protease. *Science* **277**:373, 1997.

133. Grunberg J, Walter J, Loetscher H, Deuschle U, Jacobsen H, Haass C: Alzheimer's disease associated presenilin 1 holoprotein and its 18–20 kDa C-terminal fragment are death substrates for proteases of the caspase family. *Biochemistry* **37**:2263, 1998.

134. Brockhaus M, Grunberg J, Rohrig S, Loetscher H, Wittenburg N, Baumeister R, Jacobsen H, Haass C: Caspase-mediated cleavage is not required for the activity of presenilins in amyloidogenesis and NOTCH signalling. *Neuroreport* **9**:1481, 1998.

135. Vito P, Ghayur T, D'Adamio L: Generation of anti-apoptotic presenilin-2 polypeptides by alternate transcription, proteolysis, and caspase 3 cleavage. *J Biol Chem* **272**:28315, 1997.

136. Capell A, Grunberg J, Pesold B, Diehlmann A, Citron M, Nixon R, Beyreuther K, Selkoe DJ, Haass C: The proteolytic fragments of the Alzheimer's disease-associated presenilin-1 form heterodimers and occur as a 100–150 kDa molecular mass complex. *J Biol Chem* **273**:3205, 1998.

137. Yu G, Chen F, Levesque G, Nishimura M, Zhang D-M, Levesque L, Rogaeva E, Xu D, Liang Y, Duthie M, St George-Hyslop P, Fraser PE: The presenilin 1 protein is a component of a high molecular weight intracellular complex that contains β-catenin. *J Biol Chem* **273**:16470, 1998.

138. Thinakaran G, Harris CL, Ratovitski T, Davenport F, Slunt HH, Price DL, Borchelt DR, Sisodia, SS: Evidence that levels of presenilins (PS1 and PS2) are coordinately regulated by competition for limiting cellular factors. *J Biol Chem* **272**:28415, 1997.

139. Tomita T, Tokuhiro S, Hashimoto T, Aiba K, Saido TC, Maruyama K, Iwatsubo T: Molecular dissection of domains in mutant presenilin 2 that mediate overproduction of amyloidogenic forms of amyloid-beta-peptides. Inability of truncated forms of PS2 with FAD mutation to increase secretion of Aβ42. *J Biol Chem* **273**:21153, 1998.

140. Zhou J, Liyanage U, Medina M, Ho C, Simmons AD, Lovett M, Kosik KS: Presenilin 1 interacts with a novel member of the armadillo family. *Neuroreport* **8**:2085, 1997.

141. Weidemann A, Paliga K, Durrwang U, Czech C, Evin G, Masters CL, Beyreuther K: Formation of stable complexes between two Alzheimer's disease gene products: Presenilin-2 and β-amyloid precursor protein. *Nat Med* **3**:328, 1997.

142. Xia W, Zhang J, Perez R, Koo EH, Selkoe DJ: Interaction between amyloid precursor protein and presenilins in mammalian cells: Implications for the pathogenesis of Alzheimer disease. *Proc Natl Acad Sci USA* **94**:8208, 1997.

143. Zhang W, Han SW, McKeel DW, Goate A, Wu JY: Interaction of presenilins with the filamin family of actin binding proteins. *J Neurosci* **18**:914, 1998.

144. L'Hernault SW, LArduengo PM: Mutation of a putative sperm membrane protein in *Caenohabitis elegans* prevents sperm differentiation but not its associated meiotic divisions. *J Cell Biol* **119**:55, 1992.

145. De Strooper B, Saftig P, Craessaerts K, Vanderstichele H, Guhde G, Annaert W, Von Figura K, Van Leuven F: Deficiency of presenilin 1 inhibits the normal cleavage of amyloid precursor protein. *Nature* **391**:387, 1998.

146. Chen F, Rozmahel R, St George-Hyslop P, et al: submitted. 1998.

147. Nishimura M, Yu G, Levesque G, et al: Presenilin mutations dominantly modulate β-catenin trafficking. *Nat Med* **5**:164, 1999.

148. Shen J, Bronson RT, Chen DF, Xia W, Selkoe DS, Tonegawa S: Skeletal and CNS defects in presenilin-1 deficient mice. *Cell* **89**:629, 1997.

149. Wong PC, Zheng H, Chen H, Becher MW, Sirinathsinghji DJ, Trumbauer ME, Chen HY, Price DL, Van Der Ploeg LH, Sisodia SS: Presenilin 1 is required for Notch and Dll1 expression in the paraxial mesoderm. *Nature* **387**:288, 1997.

150. Conlon RA, Reaume AG, Rossant J: Notch1 is required for the coordinate segmentation of somites. *Development* **121**:1533, 1995.

151. Wolozin B, Iwasaki K, Vito P, Ganjei K, Lacana E, Sunderland T, Zhao B, Kusiak JW, D'Adamio L: Participation of presenilin 2 in apoptosis: Enhanced basal activity conferred by an Alzheimer mutation. *Science* **274**:1710, 1996.

152. Sato S, Kamino K, Miki T, Doi A, Li K, St George-Hyslop P, Ogihara T, Sakaki Y: Splicing mutation of presenilin 1 gene for early onset familial Alzheimer's disease. *Hum Mutat* **1**:S91, 1998.

153. Perez-Tur J, Froelich S, Prihar G, Crook R, Baker M, Duff K, Wragg M, Hardy J, Goate A, Lannfelt L, Hutton M: A mutation in Alzheimer's disease destroying a splice acceptor site in the presenilin 1 gene. *Neuroreport* **7**:297, 1996.

154. Kwok JB, Tadder K, Fisher C, Hallup M, Brooks W, Nicholson G, St George-Hyslop P, Fraser PE, Relkin N, Gandy SE, Schofield R, Martins R: Sequence analysis of presenilin genes in early-onset Alzheimer disease reveals a novel (Met233Thr) presenilin 1 mutation. *Neuroreport* **8**:1537, 1997.

155. Tysoe C, Whittaker J, Xuereb J, Cairns NJ, Cruts M, Van Broeckhoven C, Wilcock G, Rubinsztein DC: A presenilin-1 truncating mutation is present in two cases with autopsy confirmed early-onset Alzheimer disease. *Am J Hum Genet* **62**:70, 1998.

156. Van Broeckhoven C: Presenilins and Alzheimer disease. *Nat Genet* **11**:230, 1995.

157. Davis JA, Naruse S, Chen H, Eckman C, Younkin S, Price D, Borchelt DR, Sisodia S, Wong PC: An Alzheimer's disease-linked PS1 variant rescues the developmental abnormalities of PS1-deficient embryos. *Neuron* **20**:603, 1998.

158. Qian S, Jiang P, Guan X-O, Singh G, Trumbauer ME, Yu H, Chen H, Van der Ploeg LHT, Zheng H: Mutant human presenilin protects presenilin 1 null mouse against embryonic lethality and elevates Aβ1-42/43 expression. *Neuron* **20**:611, 1998.

159. Levitan D, Doyle T, Brousseau D, Lee M, Thinakaran G, Slunt H, Sisodia S, Greenwald I: Assessment of normal and mutant human presenilin function in *Caenorrhabditis elegans*. *Proc Natl Acad Sci USA* **93**:14940, 1996.

160. Baumeister R, Leimer U, Zweckbronner I, Jakubek C, Grunberg J, Haass C: Human presenilin-1, but not familial Alzheimer's disease (FAD) mutants, facilitate *Caenorhabditis elegans* Notch signalling

independently of proteolytic processing. *Genes Function* **1**:149, 1997.

161. Martins RN, Turner BA, Carroll RT, Sweeney D, Kim KS, Wisniewski HM, Blass JP, Gibson GE, Gandy SE: High levels of amyloid beta-protein from S182 (Glu246) familial Alzheimer's cells. *Neuroreport* **7**:217, 1995.

162. Duff K, Eckman C, Zehr C, Yu X, Prada CH, Perez-Tur J, Hutton M, Refolo L, Zenk B, Hardy J, Younkin S: Increased amyloid beta 42(43) in brains of mice expressing mutant presenilin 1. *Nature* **383**:710, 1996.

163. Borchelt DR, Thinakaran G, Eckman CB, Lee MK, Davenport F, Ratovitsky T, Prada CM, Kim G, Seekins S, Yager D, Slunt HH, Wang R, Seeger M, Levey AI, Gandy SE, Copeland NG, Jenkins NA, Price DL, Younkin SG, Sisodia, SS: Familial Alzheimer's disease-linked presenilin 1 variants elevate Aβ1-42/1-40 ration in vitro and in vivo. *Neuron* **17**:1005, 1996.

164. Citron M, Westaway D, Xia W, Carlson G, Diehl TS, Levesque G, Johnson-Wood K, Lee M, Seubert P, Davis A, Kholodenko D, Motter R, Sherrington R, Perry B, Yao H, Strome R, Lieberburg I, Rommens J, Kim S, Schenk D, Fraser P, St George-Hyslop P, Selkoe DJ: Mutant presenilins of Alzheimer's disease increase production of 42 residue amyloid β-protein in both transfected cells and transgenic mice. *Nat Med* **3**:67, 1997.

165. Tamaoka A, Fraser PE, Ishii K, Sahara N, Ozawa K, Ikeda M, Saunders AM, Komatsuzaki Y, Sherrington R, Levesque G, Yu G, Rogaeva E, Shoji S, Nee LE, Pollen DA, Hendriks L, Martin JJ, van Broeckhoven C, Roses AD, Farrer LA, St George-Hyslop PH, Mori H: Amyloid beta-protein isoforms in brain of subjects with PS1 linked, βAPP linked, and sporadic Alzheimer disease. *Brain Res Mol Brain Res* **56**:178, 1998.

166. Vito P, Lacana E, D'Adamio L: Interfering with apoptosis: Ca(2+)-binding protein ALG-2 and Alzheimer's disease gene ALG-3. *Science* **271**:521, 1996.

167. Gou Q, Sopher BL, Furukawa K, Pham DG, Robinson N, Martin GM, Mattson MP: Alzheimer's presenilin mutation sensitizes neural cells to apoptosis induced by trophic factor withdrawal and amyloid β-peptide: Involvement of calcium and oxyradicals. *J Neurosci* **17**:4212, 1997.

168. Mercken M, Takahashi H, Honda T, Sato,S,, Murayama M, Nakazato Y, Noguchi K, Imahori K,Takashima A: Characterization of human presenilin 1 using N-terminal specific monoclonal antibodies: Evidence that Alzheimer mutations affect proteolytic processing. *FEBS Lett* **389**:297, 1996.

169. Murayama O, Honda T, Mercken M, Murayama M, Yasutake K, Nihonmatsu N, Nakazato Y, Michel G, Song S, Sato K, Takahashi H, Takashima A: Different effects of Alzheimer-associated mutations of presenilin 1 on its processing. *Neurosci Lett* **229**:61, 1997.

170. Lee MK, Borchelt DR, Kim G, Thinakaran G, Slunt HH, Ratovitski T, Martin LJ, Kittur A, Gandy S, Levey AI, Jenkins N, Copeland N, Price DL, Sisodia SS: Hyperaccumulation of FAD-linked presenilin-1 variants in vivo. *Nat Med* **3**:756, 1997.

171. Oyama F, Sawamura N, Kobyashi K, Morishima-Kawashima M, Kuramochi T, Ito M, Tomita T, Murayama K, Saido TC, Iwatsubo T, Capell A, Walter J, Grunberg J, Ueyama Y, Haass C, Ihara Y: Mutant presenilin 2 transgenic mouse: Effect on an age-dependent increase of amyloid beta-protein 42 in the brain. *J Neurochem* **71**:313, 1998.

172. Okochi M, Ishii K, Usami M, Sahara N, Kametani F, Tanaka K, Fraser PE, Ikeda M, Saunders AM, Martin JJ, Van Broeckhoven C, St George-Hyslop P, Roses AD, Mori H: Proteolytic processing of presenilin-1 (PS1) is not associated with Alzheimer's disease with or without PS1 mutations. *FEBS Lett* **418**:162, 1997.

173. Rogaev EI, Sherrington R, Rogaeva EA, Levesque G, Ikeda M, Liang Y, Chi H, Lin C, Holman K, Tsuda T, Mar L, Sorbi S, Nacmias B, Piacentini S, Amaducci L, Chumakov I, Cohen D, Lannfelt L, Fraser PE, Rommens JM, St George-Hyslop P: Familial Alzheimer's disease in kindreds with missense mutations in a novel gene on chromosome 1 related to the Alzheimer's disease type 3 gene. *Nature* **376**:775, 1995.

174. Levy-Lahad E: A familial Alzheimer's disease locus on chromosome 1. *Science* **269**:970, 1995.

175. Levy-Lahad E, Poorkaj P, Wang K, Fu YH, Oshima J, Mulligan J, Schellenberg GD: Genomic structure and expression of STM2, the chromosome 1 familial Alzheimer disease gene. *Genomics* **34**:198, 1996.

176. Sherrington R, Froelich S, Sorbi S, Campion D, Chi H, Rogaeva EA, Levesque G, Rogaev EI, Lin C, Liang Y, Ikeda M, Mar L, Brice A, Agid Y, Percy ME, Clerget-Darpiux F, Karlinsky H, Piacentini S,

Marcon G, Nacmias B, Amaducci L, Frebourg T, Lannfelt L, Rommens JM, St George-Hyslop PH: Alzheimer's disease associated with mutations in presenilin-2 is rare and variably penetrant. *Hum Mol Genet* **5**:985, 1996.

177. Bird TD, Levy-Lehad E, Poorkaj J, Nochlin D, Sumi SM, Nemens EJ, Wijsman E, Schellenberg GD: Wide range in age of onset for chromosome 1 related familial AD. *Ann Neurol* **40**:932, 1997.

178. Bird TD: Familial Alzheimer's disease in American descendants of the Volga Germans: Probable genetic founder effect. *Ann Neurol* **23**:25, 1988.

179. Bird TD, Sumi SM, Nemens EJ, Schellenberg GD, Martin G, et al: Phenotypic heterogeneity in familial Alzheimer's disease: A study of 24 kindreds. *Ann Neurol* **25**:12, 1989.

180. Pericak-Vance MA, Bass MP, Yamaoka LH, Gaskell PC, Scott WK, Terwedow HA, Menold MM, Conneally PM, Small GW, Vance JM, Saunders AM, Roses AD, Haines JL: Complete genomic screen in late-onset familial Alzheimer disease. Evidence for a new locus on chromosome 12. *JAMA* **278**:1282, 1997.

181. Rogaeva E, Premkumar S, Song Y, Sorbi S, Brindle N, Paterson J, Duara R, Levesque G, Yu G, Nishimura M, Ikeda M, O'Toole C, Kawarai T, Jorge R, Vilano J, Bruni, A, Farrer L, St George-Hyslop P: Evidence for an Alzheimer disease susceptibility locus on chr 12, and for further locus heterogeneity. *JAMA* **280**:614, 1998.

182. Blacker D, Wilcox MA, Laird NM, Rodes L, Horvath SM, Go RCP, Perry R, Watson B, Bassett SS, McInnis MG, Albert, MS, Hyman BT, Tanzi RE: Alpha-2-macroglobulin is genetically associated with AD. *Nat Genet* **19**:357, 1998.

183. Rogaeva E, Premkumar S, Grubber J, Vance JJ, Scott W, Roses AD, Haines J, St George-Hyslop P, Farrer L, Pericak-Vance M: Re-analysis of the association of Alpha-2-macroglobulin and Alzheimer's disease. *Nat Genet* **22**:19 1999.

184. Lendon CL, Talbot CJ, Craddock NJ, Han SW, Wragg M, Morris JC, Goate AM: Genetic association studies between dementia of the Alzheimer's type and three receptors for apolipoprotein E in a Caucasian population. *Neurosci Lett* **222**:187, 1997.

185. Wavrant-DeVrieze F, Perez-Tur J, Lambert JC, Frigard B, Pasquier F, Delacourte A, Amouyel P, Hardy J, Chartier-Harlin MC: Association between the low density lipoprotein receptor-related protein (LRP) and Alzheimer's disease. *Neurosci Lett* **227**:68, 1997.

186. Clatworthy AE, Gomez-Isla T, Rebeck GW, Wallace RB, Hyman BT: Lack of association of a polymorphism in the low density lipoprotein receptor related protein gene with Alzheimer's disease. *Arch Neurol* **54**:1289, 1997.

187. Kang DE, Saitoh T, Chen X, Xia Y, Masliah E, Hansen LA, Thomas RG, Thal LJ, Katzman R: Genetic association of the low density lipoprotein receptor-related protein gene (LRP), an apolipoprotein E receptor with late onset Alzheimer's disease. *Neurology* **49**:56, 1997.

188. Kamboh MI, Ferrell RE, DeKosky ST: Genetic association studies between Alzheimer's disease and two polymorphisms in the low density lipoprotein receptor related protein gene. *Neurosci Lett* **244**:65, 1998.

189. Hollenbach E, Ackerman S, Hyman BT, Rebeck GW: Confirmation of an association between a polymorphism in Exon 3 of the low density lipoprotein receptor related protein gene and Alzheimer's disease. *Neurology* **50**:1905, 1998.

190. Fallin D, Kundtz A, Town T, Gauntlett AC, Duara R, Barker W, Crawford F, Mullan M: No association between the low density lipoprotein receptor related protein (LRP) gene and late onset Alzheimer's disease in a community based sample. *Neurosci Lett* **233**:145, 1997.

191. Baum L, Chen L, Ng HK, Chan YS, Mak YT, Woo J, Chiu HF, Pang CP: Low-density lipoprotein receptor related gene exon 3 poly-morphism association with Alzheimer disease in Chinese. *Neurosci Lett* **247**:33, 1998.

192. Woodward R, Singleton AB, Gibson AM, Edwardson JA, Morris CM: LRP gene and late onset Alzheimer's disease. *Lancet* **352**:239, 1998.

193. Kruglyak L, Daly MJ, Reeve-Daly MP, Lander ES: Parametric and non-parametric linkage analysis: A unified multipoint approach. *Am J Hum Genet* **58**:1347, 1996.

194. Spielman RS, Ewens WJ: A sibship test for linkage in the presence of association: The sib transmission/disequilibrium. *Am J Hum Genet* **62**:450, 1998.

195. Kamboh MI, Sanghera DK, Ferrell RE, DeKosky ST: ApoE e4 associated Alzheimer's disease risk is modified by alpha 1 anti-chymotrypsin polymorphism. *Nat Genet* **10**:486, 1995.

196. Okuizumi K, Onodera O, Namba Y, Ikeda K, Yamamoto T, Seki K, Ueki A, Nanko S, Tanaka H, Takahashi H, Tsuji S: Genetic

association of the very low density lipoprotein (VLDL) receptor gene with sporadic AD. *Nat Genet* **11**:207, 1995.

197. Wragg M, Hutton M, Talbot C, Busfeild F, Han SW, Lendon C, Clark RF, Morris JC, Goate A, Hardy J, Rossor M, Houlden H, Karran E, Roberts G, Craddock N: Genetic association between and intronic polymorphism in presenilin 1 gene and late onset Alzheimer disease. *Lancet* **347**:509, 1996.

198. Lehmann DJ, Johnston C, Smith AD: Synergy between the genes for butyrylcholinesterase K variant and apolipoprotein E4 in late onset confirmed Alzheimer disease. *Hum Mol Genet* **6**:1933, 1997.

199. Montoya SE, Aston CE, DeKosky ST, Kamboh MI, Lazo JS, Ferrell RE: Bleomycin hydrolase is associated with risk of sporadic Alzheimer's disease. *Nat Genet* **18**:211, 1998.

200. Haines JL, Pritchard ML, Saunders AM, Schildkraut JM, Growdon JH, Gaskell P, Farrer LA, Auerbach SA, Gusella JF, Yamaoka L, Conneally PM, Roses AD, Pericak-Vance MA: No genetic effect of alpha-1 antichymotrypsin in Alzheimer disease. *Genomics* **33**:53, 1996.

201. Brindle N, Song Y, Rogaeva E, Premkumar S, Levesque G, Yu G, Ikeda M, Nishimura M, Paterson A, Sorbi S, Duara R, Farrer L, St George-Hyslop P: Analysis of the butyrylcholinesterase gene and nearby chromosome 3 markers in Alzheimer disease and aging. *Hum Mol Genet* **7**:933, 1998.

202. Crawford F, Fallin D, Suo Z, Abdullah L, Gold M, Gauntlett A, Duara R, Mullan M: The butyrylcholinesterase gene is neither independently nor synergistically associated with late-onset AD in clinic and community based populations. *Neurosci Lett* **249**:115, 1998.

203. Farrer LA, Pericak-Vance MA, Haines JL, Rogaeva E, Song Y, McGraw WT, Premkumar E, Scott WK, Yamaoka LH, Saunders AM, Roses AD, Auerbach SA, Sorbi S, Duara R, Abraham CR, St George-Hyslop PH: Analysis of the association between Bleomycin hydrolase and Alzheimer disease in Caucasians. *Ann Neurol* **44**:808, 1998.

204. Scott WK, Growdon JH, Roses AD, Haines JL, Pericak-Vance M: Presenilin 1 polymorphism and Alzheimer disease. *Lancet* **347**:1186, 1996.

205. Lin FH, Lin R, Wisniewski HM, Hwang Y-W, Grundke-Iqbal I, Healy-Louie G, Iqbal K: Detection of point mutations in codon 331 of mitochondrial NADH dehydrogenase subunit 2 in Alzheimer's brains. *Biochem Biophys Res Commun* **182**:238, 1992.

206. Petruzella, V, Chen, X, Schon EA: Is a point mutation in mitochondrial ND2 gene associated with Alzheimer disease. *Biochem Biophys Res Commun* **186**:491, 1992.

207. Shoffner JM, Brown MD, Torroni A, Lott MT, Cabell MF, Mirra SS, Beal MF, Yang CC, Gearing M, Salvo R, Watts RL, Juncos JL, Hansen LA, Crain BJ, Fayad M, Reckford CL, Wallace DC: Mitochondrial DNA variants observed in Alzheimer disease and Parkinson disease patients. *Genomics* **17**:171, 1993.

208. Hutchin T, Cortopassi G: A mitochondrial DNA clone is associated with increased risk for Alzheimer disease. *Proc Natl Acad Sci USA* **92**:6892, 1995.

209. Tysoe C, Robinson D, Brayne C, Dening T, Paykel ES, Huppert FA, Rubinsztein DC: The tRNA(gln) 4336 mitochondrial DNA variant is not a high penetrance mutations which predisposes to dementia before the age of 76 years. *J Med Genet* **33**:1002, 1996.

210. Zsurka G, Kalman J, Csaszar A, Rasko I, Janka Z, Venetianer P: No mitochondrial haplotype was found to increase risk for Alzheimer's disease. *Biol Psychiatry* **44**:371, 1998.

211. Davis RE, Miller S, Herrnstadt C, Ghosh SS, Fahy E, Shinobu LA, Galasko D, Thal LL, Beal MF, Howell N, Parker WDJ: Mutations in mitochondrial cytochrome C oxidase genes segregate with late onset Alzheimer disease. *Proc Natl Acad Sci USA* **94**:4526, 1997.

212. Wallace DC, Stugard C, Murdock D, Schurr T, Brown MD: Ancient mtDNA sequences in the human nuclear genome: a potential source of errors in identifying pathogenic mutations. *Proc Natl Acad Sci USA* **94**:14900, 1997.

213. Wisniewski T, Lalowski M, Golabek A, Vogel T, Frangione B: Is Alzheimer's disease an ApoE amyloidosis? *Lancet* **345**:956, 1995.

214. Wisniewski T, Palha JA, Ghiso J, Frangione B: S182 protein in Alzheimer's neuritic plaques. *Lancet* **346**:1366, 1996.

215. Wang X, DeKosky ST, Wisniewski S, Aston S, Kamboh MI: Genetic association of two chromosome 14 genes (presenilin 1 and alpha-1-antichymotrypsin) with Alzheimer disease. *Ann Neurol* **44**:387, 1998.

216. Aldudo J, Bullido MJ, Frank A, Valdivieso F: Presenilin genotype (2/2) is associated with late onset Alzheimer disease in Spanish patients. *Alzheimer's Research* **3**:141, 1997.

217. Lendon CL, Myers A, Cummings A, Goate AM, St Clair D: A polymorphism in the presenilin 1 gene does not modify risk for

Alzheimer's disease in a cohort with sporadic early onset. *Neurosci Lett* **228**:212, 1997.

218. Tysoe C, Galinsky D, Robinson D, Brayne CE, Easton DF, Huppert FA, Dening T, Paykel ES, Rubinsztein DC: Analysis of alpha-1-antichymotrypsin, presenilin 1, angiotensin-converting enzyme, and methylenetetrahydrofolate reductase loci as candidates for dementia. *Am J Med Genet* **74**:207, 1997.

219. Sodeyama N, Itoh Y, Suematsu N, Matsushita M, Otomo E, Mizusawa H, Yamada M: Presenilin 1 intronic polymorphism is not associated with Alzheimer type neuropathological changes or sporadic Alzheimer's disease. *J Neurol Neurosurg Psychiatry* **64**:548, 1998.

220. Kowalska A, Wender M, Lannfelt L: Lack of association between an intronic polymorphism in the PS1 gene and sporadic late-onset Alzheimer disease in Polish patients. *Dement Geriatr Cogn Disord* **9**:137, 1998.

221. Tanahashi N, Kawakatsu S, Kaneko N, Yamanaka H, Takahashi K, Tabira T: Sequence-analysis of presenilin 1 gene mutation in Japanese Alzheimer disease patients. *Neurosci Lett* **218**:139, 1996.

222. Reznick-Wolf H, Machado J, Haroutunian V, DeMarco L, Walter GF, Goldman B, Davidson M, Johnston JA, Lannfelt L, Dani SU, Friedman E: Somatic mutations analysis of the APP and presenilin 1 and 2 genes in Alzheimer's disease brains. *J Neurogenet* **12**:55, 1998.

223. Dumanchin C, Brice A, Campion D, Hannequin D, Martin C, Moreau V, Agid Y, Martinez M, Clerget-Darpoux F, Frebourg T: De novo presenilin mutations are rare in clinically sporadic early onset Alzheimer's disease cases. *J Med Genet* **35**:672, 1998.

224. Citron M, Eckman CB, Diehl TS, Corcoran C, Ostaszewski BL, Xia W, Levesque G, St George-Hyslop P, Younkin S, Selkoe S: Additive effects of PS1 and APP mutations on secretion of the 42-residue amyloid beta-protein. *Neurobiol Dis* **5**:107, 1998.

225. Holcomb L, Gordon MN, McGowan E, Yu X, Benkovic S, Jantzen P, Wright K, Saad I, Mueller R, Morgan D, Sanders S, Zehr C, O'Campo K, Hardy J, Prada CM, Eckman C, Younkin S, Hsiao K, Duff K: Accelerated Alzheimer-type phenotype in transgenic mice carrying both mutant amyloid precursor protein and presenilin 1 transgenes. *Nat Med* **4**:97, 1998.

226. Borchelt DR, Ratovitski T, van Lare J, Lee MK, Gonzales V, Jenkins NA, Copeland NG, Price DL, Sisodia S: Accelerated amyloid deposition in brains of transgenic mice co-expressing mutant PS1 and amyloid precursor protein. *Neuron* **19**:939, 1997.

227. Games D, Adams D, Alessandrini A, Barbour R, Berthelette P, Blackwell C, Carr T, Clemens J, Donaldson T, Gillespie F, Lieberburg I, Schenk D: Alzheimer-type neuropathology in transgenic mice overexpressing V717F beta-amyloid precursor protein. *Nature* **373**:523, 1995.

228. Hsiao K, Chapman P, Nilsen S, Eckman C, Horigoya Y, Younkin S, Yang FS, Cole G: Correlative memory deficits, A$\beta$ elevation, and amyloid plaques in transgenic mice. *Science* **274**:99, 1996.

229. Calhoun MF, Wiederhold K-H, Abramowski D, Phinney A, Probst A, Sturchler-Pierrat C, Staufenbiel M, Sommer B, Jucker M: Neuron loss in APP transgenic mice. *Nature* **395**:755, 1998.

230. Brun A, Englund B, Gustafson L, Passant U, Mann DMA, Neary D, Snowden JS: The Lund and Manchester groups. Consensus statement: Clinical and neuropathological criteria for frontotemporal dementia. *J Neurol Neurosurg Psychiat* **57**:416, 1994.

231. Neary D, Snowden JS, Gustafson L, Passant U, Stuss D, Black S, Freedman M, Kertesz A, Robert PH, Albert M, Boone K, Miller BL, Cummings J, Benson DF: Frontotemporal lobar degeneration. A consensus on clinical diagnostic criteria. *Neurology* **5**:1546, 1998.

232. Stevens M, van Duijn CM, Kamphorst W, de Knijff P, Heutink P, van Gool WA, Scheltens P, Ravid R, Oostra BA, Niermeijer MF, van Swieten JC: Familial aggregation in frontotemporal dementia. *Neurology* **50**:1541, 1998.

233. Wilhelmsen KC, Lynch T, Pavlov E, Higgins M, Nygaard TG: Localization of disinhibition-dementia-parkinsonism-amyotrophy complex to 17q21-22. *Am J Hum Genet* **55**:1159, 1994.

234. Petersen RB, Tabaton M, Chen SG, Monari L, Richardson SL, Lynch T, Manetto V, Lanska DJ, Markesbery WR, Currier RD, Autilio-Gambetti L, Wilhelmsen KC, Gambetti P: Familial progressive subcortical gliosis: Presence of prions and linkage to chromosome 17. *Neurology* **45**:1062, 1995.

235. Wijker M, Wszolek ZK, Wolters ECH, Rooimans MA, Pals G, Pfeiffer RF, Lynch T, Rodnitzky RL, Wilhelmsen KC, Arwert F: Localization of the gene for rapidly progressive autosomal dominant parkinsonism and dementia with pallido-ponto-nigral degeneration to chromosome 17q21. *Hum Mol Genet* **5**:151, 1996.

236. Yamaoka LH, Welsh-Bohmer KA, Hulette CM, Gaskell PC, Murray M, Rimmler JL, Helms BR, Guerra M, Roses AD, Schmechel DE, Pericak-Vance MA: Linkage of frontotemporal dementia to chromosome 17: Clinical and neuropathological characterization of phenotype. *Am J Hum Genet* **59**:1306, 1996.

237. Heutink P, Stevens M, Rizzu P, Bakker E, Kros JM, Tibben A, Niermeijer MF, van Duijn CM, Oostra BA, van Swieten JC: Hereditary frontotemporal dementia is linked to chromosome 17q21-22: A genetic and clinicopathological study of three Dutch families. *Ann Neurol* **41**:150, 1997.

238. Froelich S, Basun H, Forsell C, Lilius L, Axelman K, Andreadis A, Lannfelt L: Mapping of a disease locus for familial rapidly progressive frontotemporal dementia to chromosome 17q21-22. *Am J Med Genet* **74**:380, 1997.

239. Bird TD, Wijsman EM, Nochlin D, Leehey M, Sumi SM, Payami H, Poorkaj P, Nemens E, Raskind M, Schellenberg GD: Chromosome 17 and hereditary dementia: Linkage studies in three non-Alzheimer families and kindreds with late-onset FAD. *Neurology* **48**:949, 1997.

240. Murrell JR, Koller D, Foroud T, Goedert M, Spillantini MG, Edenberg H, Farlow M, Ghetti B: Familial multiple system tauopathy with presenile dementia localized to chromosome 17. *Am J Hum Genet* **61**:1131, 1997.

241. Lendon CL, Lynch T, Norton J, McKeel DW, Busfield F, Craddock N, Chakraverty S, Gopalakrishnan G, Shears SD, Grimmett W, Wilhelmsen KC, Hansen L, Morris JC, Goate AM: Hereditary dysphasic disinhibition dementia. A frontotemporal dementia linked to chromosome 17q21-22. *Neurology* **50**:1546, 1998.

242. Foster NL, Wilhelmsen KC, Sima AAF, Jones MZ, D'Amato C, Gilman S, Spillantini MG, Lynch T, Mayeux RP, Gaskell PC, Hulette C, Pericak-Vance MA, Welsh-Bohmer KA, Dickson DW, Heutink P, Kros J, van Swieten JC, Arwert F, Ghetti B, Murrell JR, Lannfelt L, Hutton M, Phelps CH, Snyder DS, Oliver E, Ball MJ, Cummings JL, Miller BL, Katzman R, Reed L, Schelper RL, Lanska DJ, Brun A, Fink JK, Khul DE, Knopman DS, Wszolek Z, Miller CL, Bird, TD, Lendon C, Elechi C: Frontotemporal dementia and parkinsonism linked to chromosome 17: A consensus statement. *Ann Neurol* **41**:706, 1997.

243. Spillantini MG, Crowther RA, Goedert M: Comparative study of the neurofibrillary pathology of Alzheimer's disease and familial presenile dementia with tangles. *Acta Neuropathol* **92**:42, 1996.

244. Spillantini MG, Goedert M, Crowther RA, Murrell JR, Farlow MJ, Ghetti B: Familial multiple system tauopathy with presenile dementia: A disease with abundant neuronal and glial Tau filaments. *Proc Natl Acad Sci USA* **94**:4113, 1997.

245. Spillantini MG, Bird TD, Ghetti B: Frontotemporal dementia and parkinsonism linked to chromosome 17: A new group of tauopathies. *Brain Pathol* **8**:387, 1998.

246. Neve RL, Harris P, Kosik KS, Kurnit DM, Donlon TA: Identification of cDNA clones for the human microtubule-associated protein Tau and chromosomal localization of the genes for Tau and microtubule-associated protein 2. *Mol Brain Res* **1**:271, 1986.

247. Poorkaj P, Bird TD, Wijsman E, Nemens E, Garruto RM, Anderson L, Andreadis A, Wiederholt WC, Raskind M, Schellenberg GD: Tau is a candidate gene for chromosome 17 frontotemporal dementia. *Ann Neurol* **43**:815, 1998.

248. Hutton M, Lendon CL, Rizzu P, Baker M, Froelich S, Houlden H, Pickering-Brown S, Chakraverty S, Isaacs A, Grover A, Hackett J, Adamson J, Lincoln S, Dickson D, Davies P, Petersen RC, Stevens M, de Graaff E, Wauters E, van Baren J, Hillebrand M, Joosse M, Kwon JM, Nowotny P, Che LK, Norton J, Morris JC, Reed LA, Trojanowski JQ, Basun H, Lannfelt L, Neystat M, Fahn S, Dark F, Tannenberg T, Dodd P, Hayward N, Kwok DBJ, Schofield PR, Andreadis A, Snowden J, Craufard A, Neary D, Owen F, Oostra BA, Hardy J, Goate A, van Swieten J, Mann D, Lynch T, Heutink P: Association of missense and 5'-splice-site mutations in Tau with the inherited dementia FTDP-17. *Nature* **393**:702, 1998.

249. Spillantini MG, Murrell JR, Goedert M, Farlow MR, Klug A, Ghetti B: Mutation in the Tau gene in familial multiple system tauopathy with presenile dementia. *Proc Natl Acad Sci USA* **95**:7737, 1998.

250. Dumanchin C, Camuzat A, Campion D, Verpillat P, Hannequin D, Frebourg T, Brice A: Segregation of a missense mutation in the microtubule-associated protein Tau in familial frontotemporal dementia and parkinsonism. *Hum Mol Genet* **7**:1825, 1998.

251. Clark LN, Poorkaj P, Wszolek Z, Geschwind DH, Nasreddine ZS, Miller B, Li D, Payami H, Awert F, Markopoulou K, Andreadis A, D'Souza I, Lee VMY, Reed L, Trojanowski JQ, Zhukareva V, Bird T,

Schellenberg G, Wilhelmsen KC: Pathogenic implications of mutations in the Tau gene in pallido-ponto-nigral degeneration and related neurodegenerative disorders linked to chromosome 17. *Proc Natl Acad Sci USA* **95**:13103, 1998.

252. Rizzu P, van Swieten JC, Joosse M, Hasegawa M, Stevens M, Tibben A, Niermeijer MF, Hillebrand M, Ravid R, Oostra BA, Goedert M, van Duijn CM, Heutink P: High prevalence of mutations in the microtubule-associated protein Tau in a population study of frontotemporal dementia in the Netherlands. *Am J Hum Genet* **64**:414, 1999.

253. Iijima M, Tabira T, Poorkaj P, Schellenberg GD, Trojanowski JQ, Lee VMY, Schmidt ML, Takahashi K, Nabika T, Matsumoto T, Yamashita Y, Yoshioka S, Ishino H: A distinct familial presenile dementia with a novel missense mutation in the Tau gene. *Neuroreport* **10**:497, 1999.

254. Mirra SS, Murrell JR, Gearing M, Spillantini MG, Goedert M, Crowther RA, Levey AI, Jones R, Green J, Shoffner JM, Wainer BH, Schmidt ML, Trojanowski JQ, Ghetti B: Tau pathology in a family with dementia and a P301L mutation in tau. *J Neuropathol Exp Neurol* **58**:335, 1999.

255. Goedert M, Spillantini MG, Crowther RA, Chen SG, Parchi P, Tabaton M, Lanska DJ, Markesbery WR, Wilhelmsen KC, Dickson DW, Petersen RB, Gambetti P: Tau gene mutation in familial progressive subcortical gliosis. *Nat Med* **5**: 454, 1999

256. Hulette CM, Pericak-Vance MA, Roses AD, Schmechel DE, Yamaoka LH, Gaskell PC, Welsh-Bohmer KA, Crowther RA, Spillantini MG: Neuropathologic features of frontotemporal dementia and parkinsonism linked to chromosome 17q21-22 (FTDP-17): Duke family 1684. *J Neuropathol Exp Neurol* **58**:859, 1999.

257. Bugiani O, Murrell JR, Giaccone G, Hasegawa M, Ghigo G, Tabaton M, Morbin M, Primavera A, Carella F, Solaro C, Grisoli M, Savoiardo M, Spillantini MG, Tagliavini F, Goedert M, Ghetti B: Frontotemporal dementia and corticobasal degeneration in a family with a P301S mutation in Tau. *J Neuropathol Exp Neurol* **58**:667, 1999

257a. D'Souza I, Poorkaj P, Hong M, Nochlin D, Lee VM-Y, Bird TD, Schellenberg GD: Missense and silent tau gene mutations cause frontotemporal dementia with parkinsonism-chromosome 17 type, by affecting multiple alternative RNA splicing regulatory elements. *Proc Natl Acad Sci USA* **96**:5598, 1999.

257b. Murrell JR, Spillantini MG, Zolo P, Guazzelli M, Smith MJ, Hasegawa M, Redi F, Crowther RA, Pietrini P, Ghetti B, Goedert M: *Tau* gene mutation G389R causes a tauopathy with abundant Pick body-like inclusions and axonal deposits. *J Neuropathol Exp Neurol* **58**:1207, 1999.

257c. Yasuda M, Takamatsu J, D'Souza I, Crowther RA, Kawamata T, Hasegawa M, Hasegawa H, Spillantini MG, Tanimukai S, Poorkaj P, Varani L, Varani G, Iwatsubo T, Goedert M, Schellenberg GD, Tanaka C: A novel mutation at position +12 in the intron following exon 10 of the tau gene in familial frontotemporal dementia (FTD-Kumamoto). *Ann Neurol* **47**:422, 2000.

257d. Stanford PM, Halliday GM, Brooks WS, Kwok JBJ, Storey CE, Creasey H, Morris JGL, Fulham MJ, Schofield PR: Progressive supranuclear palsy pathology caused by a novel silent mutation in exon 10 of the *tau* gene. *Brain* **123**:880, 2000.

257e. Rizzini C, Goedert M, Hodges JR, Smith MJ, Jakes R, Hills R, Xuereb JH, Crowther RA, Spillantini MG: Tau gene mutation K257T causes a tauopathy similar to Pick's disease. *J Neuropathol Exp Neurol*, in press.

257f. Spillantini MG, Yoshida H, Rizzini C, Lantos PL, Khan N, Rossor MN, Goedert M, Brown J: A novel *Tau* mutation (N296N) in familial dementia with swollen achromatic neurons and corticobasal inclusion bodies. *Ann Neurol*, in press.

258. Weingarten MD, Lockwood AH, Hwo S-H, Kirschner MW: A protein factor essential for microtubule assembly. *Proc Natl Acad Sci USA* **72**:1858, 1975.

259. Cleveland DW, Hwo S-Y, Kirschner MW: Purification of tau, a microtubule-associated protein that induces assembly of microtubules from purified tubulin. *J Mol Biol* **116**:207, 1977.

260. Cleveland DW, Hwo S-Y, Kirschner MW: Physical and chemical properties of purified Tau factor and the role of Tau in microtubule assembly. *J Mol Biol* **116**:227, 1977.

261. Mareck A, Fellous A, Francon J, Nunez J: Changes in composition and activity of microtubule-associated proteins during development. *Nature* **284**:353, 1980.

262. Couchie D, Nunez J: Immunological characterization of microtubule-associated proteins specific for the immature brain. *FEBS Lett* **188**:331, 1985.

263. Lindwall G, Cole RD: Phosphorylation affects the ability of Tau protein to promote microtubule assembly. *J Biol Chem* **259**:5301, 1984.

264. Drubin DG, Feinstein SC, Shooter EM, Kirschner MW: Nerve growth factor-induced neurite outgrowth in PC12 cells involves the coordinate induction of microtubule assembly and assembly promoting factors. *J Cell Biol* **101**:1799, 1985.

265. Peng I, Binder LI, Black MM: Biochemical and immunological analyses of cytoskeletal domains of neurons. *J Cell Biol* **102**:252, 1986.

266. Lee G, Cowan N, Kirschner MW: The primary structure and heterogeneity of Tau protein from mouse brain. *Science* **239**:285, 1988.

267. Goedert M, Wischik CM, Crowther RA, Walker JE, Klug A: Cloning and sequencing of the cDNA encoding a core protein of the paired helical filament of Alzheimer disease. *Proc Natl Acad Sci USA* **85**:4051, 1988.

268. Goedert M, Spillantini MG, Potier MC, Ulrich J, Crowther RA: Cloning and sequencing of the cDNA encoding an isoform of microtubule-associated protein Tau containing four tandem repeats: Differential expression of Tau protein mRNAs in human brain. *EMBO J* **8**:393, 1989.

269. Goedert M, Spillantini MG, Jakes R, Rutherford D, Crowther RA: Multiple isoforms of human microtubule-associated protein tau: Sequences and localization in neurofibrillary tangles of Alzheimer's disease. *Neuron* **3**:519, 1989.

270. Goedert M, Spillantini MG, Crowther RA: Cloning of a big Tau microtubule-associated protein characteristic of the peripheral nervous system. *Proc Natl Acad Sci USA* **89**:1983, 1992.

271. Couchie D, Mavilia C, Georgieff IS, Liem RKH, Shelanski ML, Nunez J: Primary structure of high molecular weight Tau present in the peripheral nervous system. *Proc Natl Acad Sci USA* **89**:4378, 1992.

272. Andreadis A, Brown MW, Kosik KS: Structure and novel exons of the human Tau gene. *Biochemistry* **31**:10626, 1992.

273. Ennulat DJ, Liem RKH, Hashim GA, Shelanski ML: Two separate 18-amino acid domains of Tau promote the polymerization of tubulin. *J Biol Chem* **264**:5327, 1989.

274. Lee G, Rook SL: Expression of Tau protein in non-neuronal cells: Microtubule binding and stabilization. *J Cell Sci* **102**:227, 1992.

275. Butner KA, Kirschner MW: Tau protein binds to microtubules through a flexible array of distributed weak sites. *J Cell Biol* **115**:717, 1991.

276. Gustke N, Trinczek B, Biernat J, Mandelkow EM, Mandelkow E: Domains of Tau protein and interactions with microtubules. *Biochemistry* **33**:9511, 1994.

277. Goode BL, Denis PE, Panda D, Radeke MJ, Miller HP, Wilson L, Feinstein SC: Functional interactions between the proline-rich and repeat regions of Tau enhance microtubule binding and assembly. *Mol Biol Cell* **8**:353, 1997.

278. Hirokawa N, Shiomura Y, Ogabe S: Tau proteins: The molecular structure and mode of binding on microtubules. *J Cell Biol* **107**:1449, 1988.

279. Chen J, Kanai Y, Cowan N, Hirokawa N: Projection domains of MAP2 and Tau determine spacings between microtubules in dendrites and axons. *Nature* **360**:674, 1992.

280. Goedert M, Jakes R: Expression of separate isoforms of human Tau protein: Correlation with the Tau pattern in brain and effects on tubulin polymerization. *EMBO J* **9**:4225, 1990.

281. Lewis SA, Wang D, Cowan NJ: Microtubule-associated protein MAP2 shares a microtubule binding motif with Tau protein. *Science* **242**:936, 1988.

282. Aizawa H, Emori Y, Murofushi H, Kawasaki H, Sakai H, Suzuki K: Molecular cloning of a ubiquitously distributed microtubule-associated protein with $M_r$ 190,000. *J Biol Chem* **265**:13849, 1990.

283. Goedert M, Baur CP, Ahringer J, Jakes R, Hasegawa M, Spillantini MG, Smith MJ, Hill F: PTL-1, a microtubule-associated protein with Tau-like repeats from the nematode Caenorhabditis elegans. *J Cell Sci* **109**:2661, 1996.

283a. Rubin GM, Yandell MD, Wortman JR, Miklos GLG, Nelson CR, Hariharan IK, Fortini ME, Li PW, Apweiler R, Fleischmann W, Cherry JM, Henikoff S, Skupski MP, Misra S, Ashburner M, Birney E, Boguski MS, Brody T, Brokstein P, Celniker SE, Chervitz SA, Coates D, Cravchik A, Gabrielian A, Galle RF, Gelbart WM, George RA, Goldstein LSB, Gong F, Guan P, Harris NL, Hay BA, Hoskins RA, Li J, Li Z, Hynes RO, Jones SJM, Kuehl PM, Lemaitre B, Littleton JT, Morrison DK, Mungall C, O'Farrell PH, Pickeral OK,

Sue C, Vosshall LB, Zhang J, Zhao Q, Zheng XH, Zhong F, Zhong W, Gibbs R, Venter JC, Adams MD, Lewis S: Comparative genomics of the eukaryotes. *Science* **287**:2204, 2000.

284. Irminger-Finger I, Hurt E, Roebuck A, Collart MA, Edelstein SJ: *MHP1*, an essential gene in Saccharomnyces cerevisiae required for microtubule function. *J Cell Biol* **135**:1323, 1996.

285. Kosik KS, Orecchio LD, Bakalis S, Neve RL: Developmentally regulated expression of specific Tau sequences. *Neuron* **2**:1389, 1989.

286. Gštz J, Probst A, Spillantini MG, Schäfer T, Jakes R, Bürki K, Goedert M: Somatodendritic localisation and hyperphosphorylation of Tau protein in transgenic mice expressing the longest human brain Tau isoform. *EMBO J* **14**:1304, 1995.

287. Binder LI, Frankfurter A, Rebhun KI: The distribution of Tau in the mammalian central nervous system. *J Cell Biol* **101**:1771, 1985.

288. Harada A, Oguchi K, Okabe S, Kuno J, Terada S, Oshima T, Sato-Yoshitake R, Takei Y, Noda T, Hirokawa N: Altered microtubule organization in small-calibre axons of mice lacking Tau protein. *Nature* **369**:488, 1994.

289. Goedert M, Jakes R, Crowther RA, Six J, Lübke U, Vandermeeren M, Cras P, Trojanowski JQ, Lee VM-Y: The abnormal phosphorylation of Tau protein at serine 202 in Alzheimer's disease recapitulates phosphorylation during development. *Proc Natl Acad Sci USA* **90**:5066, 1993.

290. Watanabe A, Hasegawa M, Suzuki M, Takio K, Morishima-Kawashima M, Titani K, Arai T, Kosik KS, Ihara Y: In vivo phosphorylation sites in fetal and adult rat Tau. *J Biol Chem* **268**:25712, 1993.

291. Drewes G, Lichtenberg-Kraag B, Döring F, Mandelkow EM, Biernat J, Dorée M, Mandelkow E: Mitogen-activated protein (MAP) kinase transforms Tau protein into an Alzheimer-like state. *EMBO J* **11**:2131, 1992.

292. Hanger DP, Hughes K, Woodgett JR, Brion JP, Anderton BH: Glycogen synthase kinase-3 induces Alzheimer's disease-like phosphorylation of tau: generation of paired helical filament epitopes and neuronal localization of the kinase. *Neurosci Lett* **147**:58, 1992.

293. Paudel HK, Lew J, Zenobia A, Wang JH: Brain proline-directed kinase phosphorylates Tau on sites that are abnormally phosphorylated in Tau associated with Alzheimer's disease paired helical filaments. *J Biol Chem* **268**:23512, 1993.

294. Goedert M, Hasegawa M, Jakes R, Lawler S, Cuenda A, Cohen P: Phosphorylation of microtubule-associated protein Tau by stress-activated protein kinases. *FEBS Lett* **409**:57, 1997.

295. Munoz-Montado JR, Moreno FJ, Avila J, Diaz-Nido J: Lithium inhibits Alzheimer's disease-like Tau phosphorylation in neurons. *FEBS Lett* **411**:183, 1997.

296. Hong M, Chen DCR, Klein PS, Lee VM-Y: Lithium reduces Tau phosphorylation by inhibition of glycogen synthase kinase-3. *J Biol Chem* **272**:25326, 1997.

297. Mawal-Dewan M, Sen PC, Abdel-Ghany M, Shalloway D, Racker E: Phosphorylation of Tau protein by purified $p34^{cdc28}$ and a related protein kinase from neurofilaments. *J Biol Chem* **267**:19705, 1992.

298. Brandt R, Lee G, Teplow DB, Shalloway D, Abdel-Ghany M: Differential effect of phosphorylation and substrate modulation on Tau's ability to promote microtubule growth and nucleation. *J Biol Chem* **269**:11776, 1994.

299. Yang SD, Yu JS, Shiah SG, Huang JJ: Protein kinase $F_A$/glycogen synthase kinase-3α after heparin potentiation phosphorylates Tau on sites abnormally phosphorylated in Alzheimer's disease brain. *J Neurochem* **63**:1416, 1994.

300. Hasegawa M, Crowther RA, Jakes R, Goedert M: Alzheimer-like changes in microtubule-associated protein Tau induced by sulfated glycosaminoglycans. Inhibition of microtubule binding, stimulation of phosphorylation, and filament assembly depend on the degree of sulfation. *J Biol Chem* **272**:33118, 1997.

301. Qi Z, Zhu X, Goedert M, Fujita DJ, Wang JH: Effect of heparin on phosphorylation site specificity of neuronal cdc2-like kinase. *FEBS Lett* **423**:227, 1998.

302. Goedert M, Cohen ES, Jakes R, Cohen P: p42 MAP kinase phosphorylation sites in microtubule-associated protein Tau are dephosphorylated by protein phosphatase $2A_1$: Implications for Alzheimer's disease. *FEBS Lett* **312**:95, 1992.

303. Goedert M, Jakes R, Qi Z, Wang JH, Cohen P: Protein phosphatase 2A is the major enzyme in brain that dephosphorylates Tau protein phosphorylated by proline-directed protein kinases or cyclic AMP-directed protein kinase. *J Neurochem* **65**:2804, 1995.

304. Sontag E, Nunbhadki-Craig V, Lee G, Bloom GS, Mumby MC: Regulation of the phosphorylation state and microtubule-binding activity of Tau by protein phosphatase 2A. *Neuron* 17:1201, 1996.

305. Bramblett GT, Goedert M, Jakes R, Merrick SE, Trojanowski JQ, Lee VM-Y: Abnormal Tau phosphorylation at Ser$^{396}$ in Alzheimer's disease recapitulates development and contributes to reduced microtubule binding. *Neuron* 10:1989, 1993.

306. Yoshida H, Ihara Y: Tau in paired helical filament is functionally distinct from fetal Tau: Assembly incompetence of paired helical filament tau. *J Neurochem* 61:1183, 1993.

307. Hasegawa M, Smith MJ, Goedert M: Tau proteins with FTDP-17 mutations have a reduced ability to promote microtubule assembly. *FEBS Lett* 437:207, 1998.

307a. Nacharaju P, Lewis J, Easson C, Yen S, Hackettt J, Hutton M, Yen S-H: Accelerated filament formation from tau protein with specific FTDP-17 mutations. *FEBS Lett* 447:195, 1999.

307b. Goedert M, Jakes R, Crowther RA: Effects of frontotemporal dementia FTDP-17 mutations on heparin-induced assembly of tau filaments. *FEBS Lett* 450:306, 1999.

308. Varani L, Hasegawa M, Spillantini MG, Smith MJ, Murrell JR, Ghetti B, Klug A, Goedert M, Varani G: Structure of Tau exon 10 splicing regulatory element RNA and destabilization by mutations of frontotemporal dementia and parkinsonism linked to chromosome 17. *Proc Natl Acad Sci USA* 96:8229, 1999

308a. Jiang Z, Cote J, Kwon JM, Goate AM, Wu JY: Aberrant splicing of tau pre-mRNA caused by intronic mutations associated with the inherited dementia frontotemporal dementia with parkinsonism linked to chromosome 17. *Mol Cell Biol* 20:4036, 2000.

308b. Varani L, Spillantini MG, Geodest M, Varani G: Structural basis for recognition of the RNA major groove in the tau exon 10 splicing regulatory element by aminoglycoside antibiotics. *Nucl Ac Res* 28:710, 2000.

309. Hong M, Zhukareva V, Vogelsberg-Ragaglia V, Wszolek Z, Reed L, Miller BI, Geschwind DH, Bird TD, McKeel D, Goate A, Morris JC, Wilhelmsen KC, Schellenberg GD, Trojanowski JQ, Lee VM-Y: Mutation-specific functional impairments in distinct Tau isoforms of hereditary FTDP-17. *Science* 282:1914, 1998.

310. Goedert M, Crowther RA, Spillantini MG: Tau mutations cause frontotemporal dementias. *Neuron* 21:955, 1998.

311. Hasegawa M, Smith MJ, Iijima M, Tabira T, Goedert M: FTDP-17 mutations N279K and S305N in Tau produce increased splicing of exon 10. *FEBS Lett* 443:93, 1999.

311a. Grover A, Houlden H, Baker M, Adamson J, Lewis J, Prihar G, Pickering-Brown S, Duff K, Hutton M: 5' Splice site mutations in tau associated with the inherited dementia FTDP-17 affect a stem-loop structure that regulates alternative splicing of exon 10. *J Biol Chem* 274:15134, 1999.

311b. D'Souza I, Schellenberg GD: Determinants of 4-repeat tau expression. Coordination between enhancing and inhibitory splicing sequences for exon 10 inclusion. *J Biol Chem* 275:17700, 2000.

312. Reed LA, Schmidt ML, Wszolek ZK, Balin BJ, Soontornniyomkij V, Lee VM-Y, Trojanowski JQ, Schelper RL: The neuropathology of a chromosome 17-linked autosomal dominant parkinsonism and dementia ("pallido-ponto-nigral degeneration"). *J Neuropathol Exp Neurol* 57:588, 1998.

313. Spillantini MG, Crowther RA, Kamphorst W, Heutink P, van Swieten JC: Tau pathology in two Dutch families with mutations in the microtubule-binding region of Tau. *Am J Pathol* 153:1359, 1998.

314. Reed LA, Grabowski TJ, Schmidt ML, Morris JC, Goate A, Solodkin A, van Hoesen GW, Schelper RL, Talbot CJ, Wragg MA, Trojanowski JQ: Autosomal dominant dementia with widespread neurofibrillary tangles. *Ann Neurol* 42:564, 1997.

314a. Van Swieten JC, Stevens M, Rosso SM, Rizzu P, Joosse M, de Koning I, Kamphorst W, Ravid R, Spillantini MG, Niermeijer MF, Heutink P: Phenotypic variation in hereditary frontotemporal dementia with tau mutations. *Ann Neurol* 46:617, 1999.

315. Goode BL, Feinstein SC: Identification of a novel microtubule binding and assembly domain in the developmentally regulated inter-repeat region of Tau. *J Cell Biol* 124:769, 1994.

315a. Dayanandan R, Van Slegtenhorst M, Mack TGA, Ko L, Yen S-H, Leroy K, Brion JP, Anderton BH, Hutton M, Lovestone S: Mutations in tau reduce its microtubule binding properties in intact cells and affect its phosphorylation. *FEBS Lett* 446:228, 1999.

316. Goedert M, Jakes R, Spillantini MG, Hasegawa M, Smith MJ, Crowther RA: Assembly of microtubule-associated protein Tau into Alzheimer-like filaments induced by sulphated glycosaminoglycans. *Nature* 383:550, 1996.

317. Perez M, Valpuesta JM, Medina M, Montejo de Garcini E, Avila J: Polymerization of Tau into filaments in the presence of heparin: The minimal sequence required for Tau-Tau interaction. *J Neurochem* 67:1183, 1996.

318. Kampers T, Friedhoff P, Biernat J, Mandelkow EM, Mandelkow E: RNA stimulates aggregation of microtubule-associated protein Tau into Alzheimer-like paired helical filaments. *FEBS Lett* 339:344, 1996.

319. Arrasate M, Perez M, Valpuesta JM, Avila J: Role of glycosaminoglycans in determining the helicity of paired helical filaments. *Am J Pathol* 151:1115, 1997.

320. Friedhoff P, von Bergen M, Mandelkow EM, Davies P, Mandelkow E: A nucleated assembly mechanism of Alzheimer paired helical filaments. *Proc Natl Acad Sci USA* 95:15712, 1998

321. Crowther RA: Structural aspects of pathology in Alzheimer's disease. *Biochim Biophys Acta* 1096:1, 1991.

321a. Brion JP, Tremp G, Octave JN: Transgenic expression of the shortest human tau affects its compartmentalization and its phosphorylation as in the pretangle stage of Alzheimer's disease. *Am J Pathol* 154:255, 1999.

321b. Ishihara T, Hong M, Zhang B, Nakagawa Y, Lee MK, Trojanowski JQ, Lee VM-Y: Age-dependent emergence and progression of a tauopathy in transgenic mice overexpressing the shortest human tau isoform. *Neuron* 24:751, 1999.

321c. Spittaels K, Van den Haute C, Van Dorpe J, Bruynseels K, Vandezande K, Laenen I, Geerts H, Mercken M, Sciot R, Van Lommel A, Loos R, Van Leuven F: Prominent axonopathy in the brain and spinal cord of transgenic mice overexpressing four-repeat human tau protein. *Am J Pathol* 155:2153, 1999.

321d. Probst A, Götz J, Wiederhold KH, Tolnay M, Mistl C, Jaton AL, Hong M, Ishihara T, Lee VM-Y, Trojanowski JQ, Jakes R, Crowther RA, Spillantini MG, Bürki K, Goedert M: Axonopathy and amyotrophy in mice transgenic for human four-repeat tau protein. *Acta Neuropathol* 99:469, 2000.

321e. Hall GF, Yao J, Lee G: Tau overexpressed in identified lamprey neurons in situ is spatially segregated by phosphorylation state, forms hyperphosphorylated, dense aggregations and induces neurodegeneration. *Proc Natl Acad Sci USA* 94:4733, 1997.

321f. Hall GF, Chu B, Lee G, Yao J: Human tau filaments induce microtubule and synapse loss in an in vivo model of neurofibrillary degenerative disease. *J Cell Sci* 113:1373, 2000.

321g. Lewis J, McGowan E, Rockwood J, Melrose H, Nacharaju P, Van Slegtenhorst M, Gwinn-Hardy K, Murphy MP, Baker M, Yu X, Duff K, Hardy J, Corral A, Lin W-L, Yen S-H, Dickson DW, Davies P, Hutton M: Neurofibrillary tangles, amyotrophy and progressive motor disturbance in mice expressing mutant (P301L) tau protein. *Nat Genet* 25:402, 2000.

322. Braak H, Braak E: Frequency of stages of Alzheimer-related lesions in different age categories. *Neurobiol Aging* 18:35, 1997.

323. Kertesz A, Munoz D: Pick's disease, frontotemporal dementia and Pick complex. Emerging concepts. *Arch Neurol* 55:302, 1998.

324. Chin SS-M, Goldman JE: Glial inclusions in CNS degenerative diseases. *J Neuropathol Exp Neurol* 55:499, 1996.

325. Flament S, Delacourte A, Verny M, Hauw JJ, Javoy-Agid F: Abnormal Tau proteins in progressive supranuclear palsy. Similiarities and differences with the neurofibrillary degeneration of the Alzheimer type. *Acta Neuropathol* 81:591, 1991.

326. Ksiezak-Reding H, Morgan K, Mattiace LA, Davies P, Liu WK, Yen S-H, Weidenheim K, Dickson DW: Ultrastructure and biochemical composition of paired helical filaments in corticobasal degeneration. *Am J Pathol* 145:1496, 1994.

326a. Brown J, Lantos PL, Roques P, Fidani L, Rossor MN: Familial dementia with swollen achromatic neurons and corticobasal inclusion bodies: a clinical and pathological study. *J Neurol Sci* 135:21, 1996.

326b. Chambers CB, Lee JM, Troncoso JC, Reich S, Muma NA: Overexpression of four-repeat tau mRNA isoforms in progressive supranuclear palsy but not in Alzheimer's disease. *Ann Neurol* 46:325, 1999.

327. Conrad C, Andreadis A, Trojanowski JQ, Dickson DW, Kang D, Chen X, Wiederholt W, Hansen L, Masliah E, Thal LJ, Katzman R, Mia Y, Saitoh T: Genetic evidence for the involvement of Tau in progressive supranuclear palsy. *Ann Neurol* 41:277, 1997.

328. Higgins JJ, Litvan I, Pho LT, Li W, Nee LE: Progressive supranuclear palsy is in linkage disequilibrium with the Tau and not the α-synuclein gene. *Neurology* 50:270, 1998.

329. Bennett P, Bonifati V, Boniuccelli U, Colosimo C, De Mari M, Fabbrini G, Marconi R, Meco G, Nicholl DJ, Stochhi F, Venacore N,

Vieregge P, Williams AC: Direct genetic evidence for involvement of Tau in progressive supranuclear palsy. *Neurology* **51**:982, 1998.

329a. Di Maria E, Tabaton M, Vigo T, Abbruzzese G, Bellone E, Donati C, Frasson E, Marchese R, Montagna P, Munoz DG, Pramstaller PP, Zanusso G, Ajmar F, Mandich P: Corticobasal degeneration shares a common genetic background with progressive supranuclear palsy. *Ann Neurol* **47**:374, 2000.

330. Sergeant N, David JP. Lefranc D, Vermersch P, Wattez A, Delacourte A: Different distribution of phosphorylated Tau protein isoforms in Alzheimer's and Pick's diseases. *FEBS Lett* **412**:578, 1997.

331. Delacourte A, Sergeant N, Wattez A, Gauvreau D, Robitaille Y: Vulnerable neuronal subsets in Alzheimer's and Pick's disease are distinguished by their isoform distribution and phosphorylation. *Ann Neurol* **43**:193, 1998.

332. Yu G, Nishimura M, Arawaka S, Levitan D, Zhang L, Tandon A, Song Y, Rogaeva E, Chen F, Kawarai T, Supala A, Levesque L, Yu H, Yang D-S, Holmes E, Milman P, Liang Y, Zhang D-M, D-H. X, Sato C, Rogaev E, Smith M, Janus C, Zhang Y, Aebersold R, Farrer L, Sorbi S, Bruni AC, Fraser PE, St George-Hyslop PH: Nicastrin modulates presenilin-mediated *Notch/Glp1* signal transduction and betaAPP processing. *Nature* **407**:48–54, 2000.

333. Yu G, Chen F, Nishimura M, Steiner H, Tandon A, Kawarai T, Arawaka S, Supala A, Song Y-Q, Rogaeva E, Holmes E, Zhang D-M, Milman P, Fraser P, Haass C, St George-Hyslop P: Mutation of Conserved Aspartates Affect Maturation of both Aspartate-Mutant and Endogenous presenilin 1 and presenilin 2 Complexes. *J. Biol. Chem.*: in press 2000.

334. Donoviel D, Hadjantonalis AK, Ikeda M, Zheng H, St George-Hyslop P, Bernstein A: Mice lacking both presenilin genes exhibit early embryonic patterning defects. *Genes Dev.* **13**:2801 1999.

335. Zhang Z, Nadeau P, Song W, Donoviel D, Yuan M, Bernstein A, Yankner BA: Presenilins are required for gamma-secretase cleavage of beta-APP and transmembrane cleavage of Notch-1. *Nat Cell Biol* **2**:463 2000.

336. Herreman A, Serneels L, Annaert W, Collen D, Schoonjans L, De Strooper B: Total inactivation of gamma-secretase activity in presenilin-deficient embryonic stem cells. *Nat Cell Biol* **2**: 461 2000.

337. Schenk D, Barbour R, Dunn W, Gordon G, Grajeda H, Guido T, Hu K, Huang J, Johnson-Wood K, Khan K, Lieberburg I, Vasquez N, Vandervert C, Walker S, Wogulis M, Yednock T, Games D, Seubert P: Immunization with Abeta attenuates Alzheimer's Disease-like pathology in the PDAPP mouse. *Nature* **400**:173 1999.

338. Bard F, Cannon C, Barbour R, Burke RL, Games D, Grajeda H, Guido T, Hu K, Huang L, Johnson-Wood K, Khan K, Kholodenko D, Lee M, Lieberburg I, Motter R, Nguyen M, Soriano F, Vasquez N, Weiss K, Welch B, Seubert P, Schenk D, Yednock T: Peripherally administered antibodies against amyloid beta-peptide enter the central nervous system and reduce pathology in a mouse model of alzheimer disease [In Process Citation]. *Nat Med* **6**:916 2000

339. Janus C, Pearson J, McLaurin J, Mathews PM, Jiang Y, Schmidt SD, Chishti MA, Horne P, Heslin D, French J, Nixon RA, Mercken M, Fraser PE, Bergeron C, St George-Hyslop PH, Westaway D: A$\beta$-Immunization Reduces Spatial Learning Impairment And Dense Cored Amyloid Plaque Burden In An Animal Model Of Alzheimer's Disease Without Affecting Brain A$\beta$-Peptide Levels. *Nature* submitted 2000.

# EYE

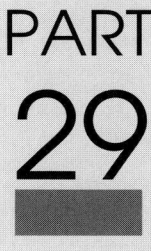

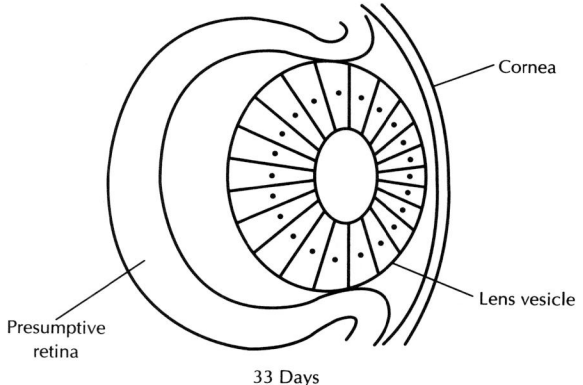

Cornea

Lens vesicle

Presumptive
retina

33 Days

# Retinitis Pigmentosa and Stationary Night Blindness

*Thaddeus P. Dryja*

1. *Retinitis pigmentosa* is the name given to a set of heritable degenerations of the retina. Patients with retinitis pigmentosa typically experience night blindness and loss of the midperipheral visual field early in the disease. As the disease progresses, the visual field is reduced to a shrinking island of central vision (called *tunnel vision*) and scattered patches of far peripheral vision. In many cases, all useful vision is lost during middle age. In advanced cases and sometimes even in early cases, the fundus oculi exhibits the following features: thin retinal vessels, a pale optic nerve head, and clumps of intraretinal pigment. Related diseases that feature progressive degeneration of the retina include cone-rod degeneration, cone degeneration, and macular degeneration. In cone-rod degeneration, there is early loss of visual acuity due to a progressive panretinal degeneration that in early stages affects cone photoreceptors more severely than rod photoreceptors. In cone degeneration, cones but not rods degenerate. In macular degeneration (see Chap. 243), cones and rods degenerate in the macula but not elsewhere in the retina. Most forms of retinitis pigmentosa and related retinal degenerations affect only the eye, although in a minority of cases the retinal degeneration is one feature of a syndrome that includes other systemic abnormalities, such as retinitis pigmentosa and deafness in Usher syndrome. In young patients with the symptom of night blindness, it is important to differentiate retinitis pigmentosa from stationary night blindness. Both diagnostic categories feature defective vision in dim light as an early symptom, but in stationary night blindness, cone photoreceptors and daytime vision do not deteriorate substantially during the patient's lifetime.

2. Measuring the retina's electrical response to flashes of light is the best way to distinguish the early stages of progressive retinal degeneration such as retinitis pigmentosa from nonprogressive retinal diseases such as stationary night blindness. This noninvasive measurement, called the *electroretinogram* (ERG), can be used to diagnose young patients with retinitis pigmentosa and many other forms of retinal degeneration even before visual symptoms or funduscopic abnormalities are apparent.

3. The visual loss in retinitis pigmentosa and related retinal degenerations corresponds to the degeneration of photoreceptor cells of the retina. Molecular genetic and biochemical studies have revealed that the defects causing these cells to die can be placed into three categories depending on the mutant gene in each case: (a) a primary biochemical defect inherent in the photoreceptor cells (the

rods, the cones, or both cell types), (b) a primary biochemical defect in neighboring retinal cells such as the retinal pigment epithelium, or (c) a peculiar sensitivity of the photoreceptors or the retinal pigment epithelium to a generalized metabolic defect. In stationary night blindness, rod photoreceptors malfunction because of defects inherent in them or perhaps in the cells they synapse with; however, the rod or cone photoreceptors do not degenerate at a rate symptomatically faster than that which accompanies normal aging.

4. Families with retinitis pigmentosa, cone-rod degeneration, cone degeneration, or stationary night blindness can demonstrate any of the known monogenic inheritance patterns: autosomal dominant, autosomal recessive, or X-linked. A syndromic form of retinitis pigmentosa, Kearns-Sayre syndrome, is transmitted with a maternal, or mitochondrial, inheritance pattern. In addition, in some families, retinitis pigmentosa is transmitted in a digenic fashion, where affected individuals are double heterozygotes for defects in both of two unlinked genes. There is nonallelic or locus heterogeneity within the categories of dominant (at least 10 loci implicated), recessive (over 22 loci), or X-linked retinitis pigmentosa (at least 3 loci). Stationary night blindness can be allelic to forms of retinitis pigmentosa.

5. Most retinitis pigmentosa genes remain unidentified. Of those which are known, some encode members of the rod phototransduction cascade (e.g., rhodopsin, the $\alpha$ or $\beta$ subunits of rod cGMP-phosphodiesterase, and the $\alpha$ subunit of the rod cGMP-gated cation channel, and arrestin). Other identified genes encode proteins important to the structure of photoreceptor outer segments (*RDS* and *ROM1*) or encode proteins with unknown function (*RPE65*, *TULP1*, *ABCR*, *RPGR*, and *RP2*). Some genes causing syndromic forms of retinal degeneration also have been identified. Examples are the genes encoding myosin VIIa causing Usher syndrome type I, a presumed extracellular matrix protein causing Usher syndrome type II, $\alpha$-tocopherol transfer protein causing retinitis pigmentosa and Friedrich-like ataxia, and phytanoyl-CoA $\alpha$-hydroxylase causing Refsum disease. The identified retinitis pigmentosa genes account for an estimated 35 to 50 percent of all cases of the disease. Forms of cone-rod degeneration are caused by mutations in the gene encoding guanylate cyclase, the transcription factor crx, or the ABCR protein of unknown function. Cone degeneration can be caused by mutations in the gene encoding guanylate cyclase activator 1A. Rod monochromacy, a form of colorblindness due to absent or nonfunctional cone photoreceptors, can be caused by mutations in the cone cGMP-gated cation channel. Mutations in the following genes encoding proteins in the

A list of standard abbreviations is located immediately preceding the index in each volume. Nonstandard abbreviations used in this chapter include: ERG = electroretinogram; TULP = tubby-like protein.

phototransduction cascade are responsible for some forms of autosomal dominant or recessive stationary night blindness: rhodopsin, the $\alpha$ subunit of rod transducin, the $\beta$ subunit of rod cGMP-phosphodiesterase, rhodopsin kinase, and rod arrestin. A form of X-linked stationary night blindness is due to mutations in an L-type calcium channel.

6. Patients with abetalipoproteinemia (MIM 200100; see Chap. 115), Refsum disease (MIM 266510; see Chap. 132), or deficiency in $\alpha$-tocopherol transfer protein can exhibit the signs and symptoms of retinitis pigmentosa as the first manifestations of disease. Because vision-saving treatments are available for these conditions, it is important to consider them in all newly diagnosed patients with retinitis pigmentosa. Also noteworthy in this regard is that at least some patients with a related hereditary retinal degeneration named *gyrate atrophy* (MIM 258870; see Chap. 83) may benefit from specifically modifying their diet. For the nonsyndromic forms of retinitis pigmentosa and for Usher syndrome, oral supplements of vitamin A have been reported to slow the rate of cone photoreceptor degeneration. No other therapy advocated to slow or stop the course of retinitis pigmentosa or related retinal degenerations has been tested in a large, double-blind clinical trial. However, a night vision scope can help to alleviate the symptom of night blindness in some patients. Also, acetazolamide has been reported to ameliorate temporarily the cystoid macular edema that reduces central vision in some cases, although this drug can have serious side effects.

## BACKGROUND

There may be well over 100 genetic loci where mutations cause hereditary retinal degeneration in humans. Some of the resulting diseases are designated *retinitis pigmentosa*, whereas others have features sufficiently distinctive to have been given separate names. It has not been possible to elaborate clinical criteria that unambiguously and consistently distinguish retinitis pigmentosa from some other forms of retinal degeneration, so the phrase *retinitis pigmentosa and allied diseases* has been used to encompass related diseases such as cone-rod dystrophy, cone dystrophy, congenital amaurosis (MIM 204000; see Chap. 237), gyrate atrophy (MIM 258870; see Chap. 83), Best disease (vitelliform macular dystrophy, MIM 153700; see Chap. 243), Stargardt juvenile macular degeneration (MIM 248200; see Chap. 244), and choroideremia (MIM 303100; see Chap. 236). This chapter will exclude lengthy discussion of those allied diseases described elsewhere in this book. Additional types of hereditary retinal dysfunction are not progressive and therefore fall outside the category of *retinal degeneration*, such as, for example, color blindness (see Chap. 238) and stationary night blindness. Stationary night blindness is covered in this chapter because some cases represent allelic variants at identified retinitis pigmentosa genes.

### Clinical Description

**Ocular Symptoms.** Retinitis pigmentosa and related retinal degenerations have visual symptoms corresponding to the location and types of photoreceptors that are dead or malfunctional. In this regard, it should be noted that most day-to-day vision is in an environment with sufficient light that normally sighted individuals perceive colors; this indicates that the vision is being mediated by cone photoreceptors. It should be remarked also that well over 90 percent of photoreceptors must be nonfunctional in a region of the retina for a scotoma (blind spot) to occur.[1] Because of these factors, young patients with retinitis pigmentosa or a related retinal degeneration may have no symptoms even though most photoreceptors have already died or are malfunctional. In particular, most or even all rod function may be absent throughout the retina,

yet a patient may not realize that he or she is night blind because rod function is ordinarily not necessary in a modern, electrically illuminated nighttime environment. A patient's subjective onset of symptoms does not indicate the onset of a retinal degeneration any more than a myocardial infarction signals the onset of cardiovascular disease. It is likely that all photoreceptor degenerations begin very early in life,[2] perhaps as soon as the photoreceptors are formed.

In typical retinitis pigmentosa, rod photoreceptors are affected more severely than cones early in the disease. A deficiency in night vision is often the first reported symptom and is due to degeneration or malfunction of rod photoreceptors throughout the retina. As the disease progresses, an absolute scotoma develops in the midperipheral visual field corresponding to regions in the midperipheral retina (an area with a high rod/cone ratio in normal retinas), where all cone photoreceptors have died as well.[3] This ring scotoma gradually enlarges so that in advanced cases only two islands of vision remain: a central island centered at the fixation point (fovea) and a rim of peripheral vision usually in the temporal field of both eyes. Photoreceptor function, measured by electroretinography (described later in this chapter) or by visual field area, is lost at an exponential rate with a half-life ranging from about 3 to 15 years in different patients.[4–7] In many patients, all vision ultimately is lost, although the age at which complete blindness occurs can vary markedly between different families and even between affected patients in the same family. The funduscopic appearance also can vary, with some patients having dense accumulations of intraretinal pigment, others none, and still others intermediate amounts. Some of the variability in the symptoms and fundus picture is a reflection of the allelic and nonallelic heterogeneity of retinitis pigmentosa and allied retinal degenerations. However, the wide range in the type and severity of disease found among patients with the same primary gene defect[8–10] indicates that secondary genetic factors or environmental factors play an important role.

Retinitis pigmentosa is sometimes referred to as *rod-cone dystrophy* or *rod-cone degeneration* because rods generally are affected earlier and more severely than cones. In patients with cone-rod dystrophy or cone-rod degeneration, on the other hand, cone photoreceptor cells have a more severe malfunction and degenerate more quickly than rods. *Cone dystrophy* or *cone degeneration* is used to describe patients in whom cone photoreceptors gradually degenerate but rods do not. Since fine visual acuity is mediated by the fovea, which contains mostly cones, patients with cone-rod dystrophy or cone dystrophy typically report loss of acuity as the first symptom. Rod monochromacy or congenital achromatopsia is a disease in which cones are either absent or nonfunctional from birth, leaving the patient with only rod function that does not substantially deteriorate over a lifetime. In macular degeneration, rod and cone photoreceptors die only in the macular region of the retina, a region that includes the fovea. Affected patients lose their central visual field and can suffer a great reduction in visual acuity, but they retain peripheral vision. Patients with stationary night blindness report no vision in dim light (i.e., light so dim that normally sighted people will not see colors). Central visual acuity may be decreased, but there is no substantial decrease in cone function during the patient's lifetime.

**Ocular Findings.** A complete ocular examination including a dilated retinal examination and the recording of electroretinograms (ERGs) is necessary for evaluating patients suspected of having retinitis pigmentosa or an allied disease. In most cases of retinitis pigmentosa, central visual acuity remains good until late in the disease.[3] Slit-lamp examination often reveals posterior subcapsular cataract, vitreous liquefaction, and vitreous cells. Early in the disease, the fundus can appear normal, although a subtle attenuation or thinning of the retinal vessels is usually present. As the disease progresses, the retinal vascular attenuation becomes more pronounced. The optic nerve head becomes pale in

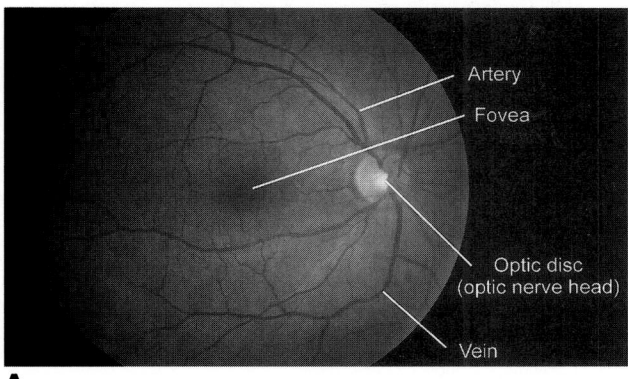

**A**

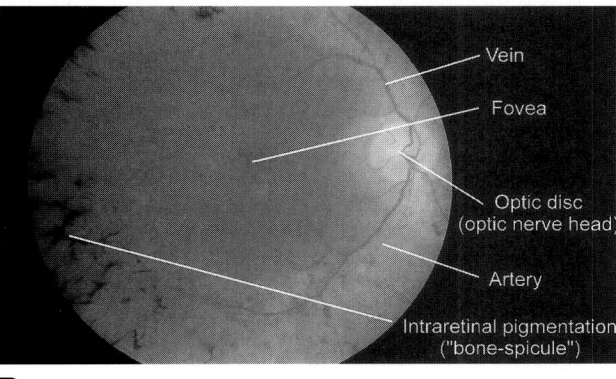

**B**

**Fig. 235-1 Normal fundus (A) and a fundus of a patient affected with retinitis pigmentosa (B). The affected fundus has thin retinal blood vessels, a pale optic nerve head, and intraretinal pigment deposits. See Color Plate 18.**

many cases.[11] In addition, clumps of intraretinal pigment, called *bone-spicule pigmentation*, appear in the midperiphery. The pattern of fundus pigmentation can vary between patients, but it is characteristically symmetric between the two eyes.[12] A classic triad of funduscopic features is characteristic of advanced cases: retinal vascular attenuation, intraretinal pigmentation, and pallor of the optic nerve head (Fig. 235-1).

Cystoid macular edema is found occasionally.[13,14] Cataract is very common.[11,15,16] Both are potentially treatable causes of reduced central vision in retinitis pigmentosa.[17,18] In about 9 percent of cases, drusen of the optic nerve head or peripapillary nerve fiber layer develop.[19] In a few percent of patients, telangiectatic retinal vessels are seen, often bilaterally, mimicking Coats disease; they respond to treatment with photocoagulation or other means.[11]

Patients with cone-rod dystrophy or cone dystrophy typically have reduced central visual acuity (e.g., 20/80 or worse) early in the disease. Funduscopy in cone-rod degeneration can show attenuated retinal vessels and disturbances of the retinal pigment epithelium such as intraretinal bone-spicule pigment deposits or thinning of the retinal pigment epithelium. Patients with cone dystrophy have a small central scotoma (a few degrees in diameter) and typically a fundus that is normal, including a vasculature of normal caliber. There may be a pigmentary disturbance in the macula.

Patients with stationary night blindness have daytime visual acuity that is normal or is slightly to moderately reduced.[20] Visual fields are full to bright stimuli. The fundus appears normal except that myopia-related abnormalities are present in those patients with moderate to high myopia, which is frequent in patients with the X-linked complete type[20] and in some elderly patients who may have a few scattered intraretinal pigment deposits in the

periphery.[21] Patients with the Oguchi form of night blindness have a normal fundus when dark-adapted, but the color of the fundus changes to a golden-brown hue when light-adapted. This is called the *Mizuo phenomenon.*[22]

**Electroretinography.** ERGs are recordings of the retina's electrical responses to flashes of light. ERGs are done noninvasively with electrodes embedded in a contact lens that rests on the cornea. One electrode rests on the cornea and the other on the inner lid; a separate "ground" electrode is pasted to the skin of the forehead or cheek. Other arrangements of electrodes can be used. The ERG is viewed on an oscilloscope screen with corneal voltage on the *y* axis and time on the *x* axis. The detected waveforms are due to the summation of electric currents occurring in a variety of retinal cell types. The response to a brief (usually less than 0.1 ms) flash of light (Fig. 235-2) is divided into components or *waves*, called the *a wave, b wave,* and *c wave* (for review, see Berson[23]). The a wave is a fast, cornea-negative response derived from electric currents generated directly by photoreceptors. The slower, cornea-positive b wave has the largest amplitude. Although it is derived from fluxes of potassium ions within and surrounding Müller cells in the inner retina,[24] it is directly dependent on functional photoreceptors, and its magnitude makes it the most convenient measure of the health of photoreceptors. The c wave, a slow, cornea-positive response, does not customarily play a major role in the diagnosis or evaluation of patients with retinitis pigmentosa.

After a normal person's eyes have adapted to darkness for at least 30 minutes, a flash of bright white light will stimulate both rods and cones to give an ERG waveform that sums the contributions of both photoreceptor types. Depending on the intensity of the flash and other factors, the normal b wave in response to a flash of bright white light is several hundred microvolts in amplitude; it can approach a millivolt in individuals with very reduced ocular pigmentation such as albinos. Conditions can be adjusted to measure rod and cone function separately. For example, a flash of blue light, if dim enough, will stimulate the

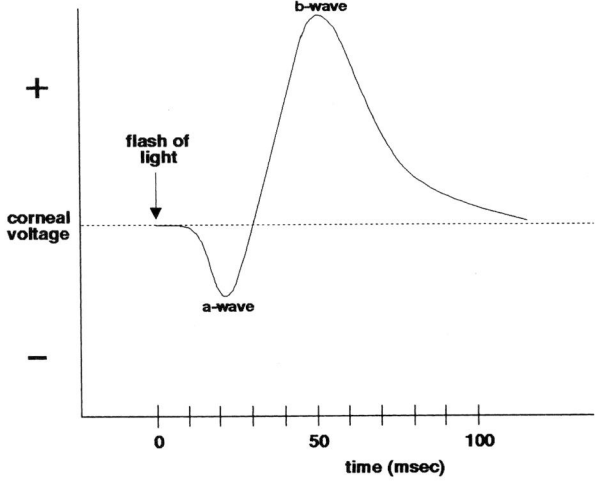

**Fig. 235-2 Schematic diagram of an ERG in response to a flash of light. The voltage (*y* axis) is measured with an electrode embedded in a contact lens resting on the cornea. A second electrode is either in the same lens or pasted to the skin around the eye; a ground electrode is also either in the lens or attached elsewhere on the head, e.g., to the forehead. The retina is exposed to a brief flash of light through a dilated pupil at time zero. The basic electrical response of the retina as an organ is a corneal-negative a wave followed by a corneal-positive b wave. A much slower, corneal-positive c wave is not shown in this figure. The time scale on the *x* axis is approximate, since the actual response times (called *implicit times*) for the a and b waves vary according to the intensity of the stimulus.**

more light-sensitive rods but not the cones. In this situation, the ERG is termed a *rod ERG*, and it will be an indicator of rod function. Cone function can be isolated by stimulating the retina with flashes of bright white light repeated 30 times per second (30 Hz). Rods are too slow to generate responses to individual flashes of light at this frequency. In a normal individual, this 30-Hz bright white flickering light generates a 30-cycle-per-second waveform called a *cone ERG* that is derived exclusively from cones and the cones' indirect stimulation of Müller cells. Other ways to record cone function through ERG are to use flashes of red light that will preferentially stimulate long-wavelength and medium-wavelength (i.e., red and green) cones but not rods or to record the ERG in response to bright flashes of light, sometimes of specific colors, after allowing a patient to adapt to a background light (the *photopic ERG*).

In the evaluation of a patient for a hereditary retinal degeneration, ERGs employ full-field flashes of light (called *Ganzfeld stimulation*) that simultaneously stimulate the entire retina. With the appropriately standardized conditions, one can reliably and reproducibly measure the magnitude and timing of the ERG. Many patients affected with retinitis pigmentosa have ERG b-wave amplitudes of less than 10 µV, so computer averaging of signals may be necessary to measure the severity of disease accurately.[25] A reduction in the amplitude of the rod and/or cone responses may be observed both in patients with a progressive retinal degeneration such as retinitis pigmentosa, cone-rod degeneration, and cone degeneration and in patients with nonprogressive retinal disease such as stationary night blindness, rod monochromacy, or self-limited sector retinitis pigmentosa.[26,27] Within a family known to have a progressive retinal degeneration, affected members have a reduction in amplitude below normal for age and a delay in response times (called *implicit times*) even early in the disease when there may be no other symptoms or signs of the disease.[2,28] Patients with stationary night blindness have reduced rod and sometimes cone ERG amplitudes, but the cone responses will have normal implicit times.[26] With few exceptions, a delay in rod or cone ERG responses even in the face of relatively high amplitudes signifies a progressive retinal degeneration. Recording the ERG at regular intervals (e.g., biannually) allows one to measure the rate of retinal degeneration,[4] making it possible to estimate the number of years of remaining vision. Also, ERGs can help in the identification of female carriers of X-linked retinitis pigmentosa, since such carriers ordinarily have subnormal responses[29,30] that are probably a reflection of a reduction in photoreceptor number or function as a consequence of lyonization.

Patients with macular degeneration such as Stargardt juvenile macular degeneration or the very prevalent age-related macular degeneration (see Chap. 243) have full-field ERG responses that are practically normal in amplitude and timing. This is so because the peripheral retina functions well in these diseases. The macula accounts for about 10 percent of the entire surface of the retina. Even if it is completely destroyed, one would expect about a 10 percent reduction in ERG amplitude, which is too small a reduction to reliably distinguish affected patients from age-matched normal controls. In contrast, patients who are moderately or severely affected with a panretinal degeneration such as retinitis pigmentosa have ERG amplitudes reduced well below 95 percent of the lower limit of the normal range; even mildly affected patients have ERG amplitudes reduced below 50 percent of the normal range. Retinal degeneration or malfunction confined to the macula can be documented objectively with specialized ERGs such as focal ERGs, where the light flashes are not Ganzfeld but are spots of light directed at the macula,[31-33] or multifocal ERGs,[34] where the light stimuli are in the form of black-and-white hexagons in a tesselated pattern with the timing of the illumination of each hexagon governed by computer software that also correlates responses with the regions of the retina that are stimulated.[35,36]

ERGs can help to differentiate specific forms of stationary night blindness. A classic categorization relies on the relative sizes of the rod a wave and rod b wave. In simple terms, patients with a normally sized or large rod a wave but a small b wave are classified as having the Schubert-Bornschein type of stationary night blindness, whereas those with a small or absent a wave have the Riggs type.[37,38] Most families with the Schubert-Bornschein type have an X-linked or autosomal recessive inheritance pattern. Some of those with the Riggs type show an autosomal dominant pattern, and these have sometimes been referred to as having the *Nougaret type*, eponymously labeled after the founder of a large family with dominant stationary night blindness originating in southern France.[39-41] However, not all Riggs-type cases with dominant inheritance have a defect in the same gene, so the name *Nougaret type* probably should be reserved for those with the same gene defect as found in the Nougaret family (see "Rod Transducin," below).

The absent rod a wave in the Riggs type of stationary night blindness is used as evidence that the physiologic defect is in the rod photoreceptors themselves,[42] whereas the presence of an a wave but reduced or absent b wave in the Schubert-Bornschein type points to a defect in the bipolar cell layer or to the synaptic connection between the rod photoreceptors and the bipolar cells. To some extent, these predictions have been substantiated by recent molecular genetic identification of some of the genes causing forms of the Riggs type of disease. As described below, defects in three rod photoreceptor-specific genes encoding members of the rod phototransduction cascade (rhodopsin,[21,43] the $\alpha$ subunit of rod transducin,[44] and the $\beta$ subunit of rod cGMP phosphodiesterase[45]) are known causes of stationary night blindness with an absent or substantially reduced rod a wave. However, the situation is a bit more complex because recent investigations have found that many patients previously categorized as having the Riggs or Nougaret type have substantial rod function but that the rods require light intensities close to or within the range at which cones also respond.[46,47] Furthermore, patients classically categorized as having the Schubert-Bornschein type can be divided into incomplete and complete forms based on whether or not partial rod function can be detected by the ERG and other methods.[20] The incomplete form appears to always be inherited as an X-linked trait, whereas the complete form may be X-linked or autosomal recessive.[20] There is recent evidence from linkage studies that the X-linked complete and incomplete forms are caused by distinct loci on Xp and that neither is allelic with known X-linked retinitis pigmentosa loci.[48]

**Pathology.** There are numerous reports of pathologic examination of eyes from patients with retinitis pigmentosa.[49-66] The earliest changes are found in the rod and cone photoreceptors (Fig. 235-3), which are reduced in number. Outer segments are absent, inner segments are reduced in size, and some photoreceptor nuclei are pyknotic. In some cases, rods are affected earlier and more severely than cones; in others, rods and cones are equally involved. Regardless of the primary gene defect and the consequent biochemical abnormality inducing photoreceptor cell death, the dying cells activate the apoptotic pathway prior to their ultimate demise.[67-70]

The later pathologic changes exhibited in the retina and in other ocular tissues are presumably a consequence of the photoreceptor degeneration and are not specific to retinitis pigmentosa. These abnormalities include degeneration of the inner nuclear layer (bipolar, amacrine, horizontal, and Müller cells) and the ganglion cell layer, especially in the retinal periphery.[66] Cataract is very common.[15,16]

There are histopathologic counterparts for each part of the funduscopic triad of retinitis pigmentosa: bone-spicule pigmentation, vascular attenuation, and pallid optic disk. The bone-spicule pigmentation is due to pigmented macrophages (thought to be metaplastic retinal epithelial cells[63]) migrating into the retina and congregating often but not exclusively around retinal vessels.[50] The retinal vessels are attenuated for two reasons. First, a reduction in the number of photoreceptors allows the chorioca-

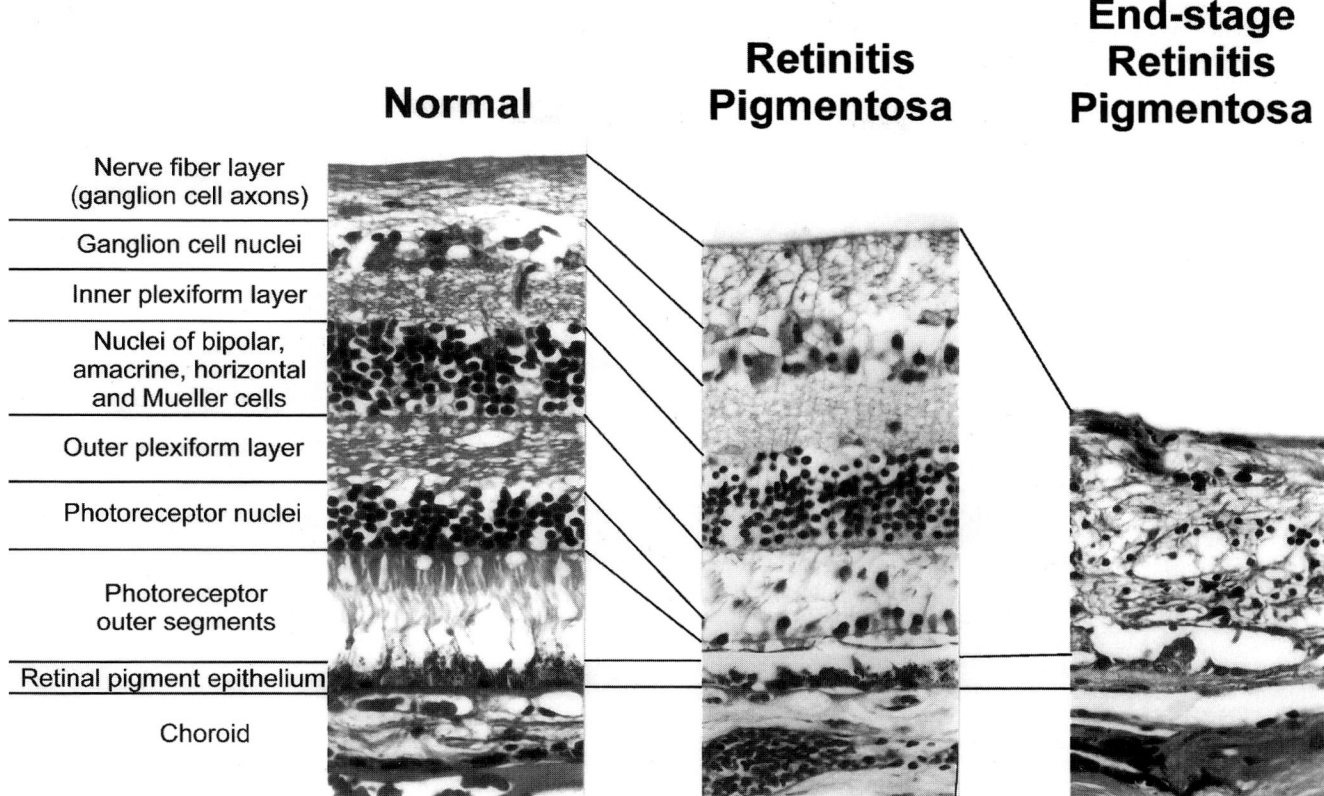

| Normal | Retinitis Pigmentosa | End-stage Retinitis Pigmentosa |

Nerve fiber layer (ganglion cell axons)

Ganglion cell nuclei

Inner plexiform layer

Nuclei of bipolar, amacrine, horizontal and Mueller cells

Outer plexiform layer

Photoreceptor nuclei

Photoreceptor outer segments

Retinal pigment epithelium

Choroid

**Fig. 235-3** Light micrographs of a normal human retina (*left*), a retina with retinitis pigmentosa (*center*), and a retina with end-stage retinitis pigmentosa (*right*). Light rays enter from the top of the figure. A photon must pass through the nerve fiber layer, ganglion cell layer, inner plexiform layer, bipolar cell layer, outer plexiform layer, and photoreceptor nuclear layer before reaching a photoreceptor outer segment, where it can interact with rod or cone opsin to initiate vision. The center panel shows histologic changes observed in eyes with early to moderately advanced retinitis pigmentosa. The photoreceptor outer segments are absent, and the number of photoreceptor nuclei is reduced. The space between the remaining photoreceptor nuclei and the retinal pigment epithelium is a processing artifact. In end-stage retinitis pigmentosa, there are no recognizable cell layers. The retina is reduced in thickness and cell number. A retina with this severe degeneration would be blind.

pillaris to supply a larger share of the retina, thereby reducing the demands on the retinal vasculature and presumably inducing autoregulatory reduction in blood flow. Second, a hyaline thickening of the retinal vessels has been observed in advanced cases examined pathologically. The pale optic disk correlates with a proliferation of glial cells in the optic nerve head. This glial proliferation extends from the disk to the posterior retina to form an epiretinal membrane.

Less well studied is the histopathology of cone degenerations. The interested reader is referred to a comprehensive textbook of eye pathology.[71] With regard to stationary night blindness, the complement of rod photoreceptors can be either normal[72] or reduced[73] in number. Some Japanese patients with Oguchi disease have photoreceptor cell degeneration similar to that seen in retinitis pigmentosa.[74-76]

## Variants of Retinitis Pigmentosa

There are many variant forms of retinitis pigmentosa distinguished by their fundus appearance or by other clinical features. Examples are retinitis pigmentosa sans pigmento (progressive photoreceptor degeneration without intraretinal pigmentation), retinitis punctata albescens (retinitis pigmentosa with small subretinal yellow deposits in the fundus), pericentral retinitis pigmentosa (pigmentary degeneration occurring circumferentially around the macula), paravenous retinitis pigmentosa (pigmentary degeneration predominantly along the major retinal vessels), clumped pigmentary retinal degeneration (retinitis pigmentosa with patches of hyperpigmented retinal pigment epithelium), unilateral retinitis pigmentosa (panretinal degeneration confined to only one eye), and

inverse retinitis pigmentosa (probably equivalent to cone degeneration or cone-rod degeneration). Gene defects for most of these variants have not been identified, and it is possible that some, like paravenous retinitis pigmentosa or unilateral retinitis pigmentosa, are not hereditary. Two other variants are discussed briefly below, retinitis pigmentosa with preserved paraarteriolar retinal pigment epithelium and sector retinitis pigmentosa.

**Retinitis Pigmentosa with Preserved Paraarteriolar Retinal Pigment Epithelium.** In this form of retinitis pigmentosa, the fundus shows bone-spicule pigmentation except in zones along the courses of the retinal arteries. This variant appears in all affected members of involved families. The responsible gene is unidentified but has been mapped to chromosome 1q31-32.1.[77-80]

**Sector Retinitis Pigmentosa.** This term refers to rare patients with scotomas in the peripheral visual field and the funduscopic appearance of retinitis pigmentosa (bone-spicule pigmentation and attenuated vessels) typically confined to the corresponding regions of the fundus, usually the inferonasal quadrant of both eyes. Outside the affected regions, the fundi show no significant photoreceptor degeneration. ERG responses are reduced in amplitude, consistent with the proportion of retinal area affected; there is no prolongation of implicit times.[26] Sector retinitis pigmentosa is sometimes dominantly inherited, but no gene defects have been reported thus far. It is difficult to envision that the disease is due to somatic mosaicism for a retinitis pigmentosa allele that affects only a portion of the fundus, since the pattern of degeneration is often symmetric between the two eyes.

Sector retinitis pigmentosa is important to recognize because it progresses slowly, if at all, and does not lead to blindness. This benign prognosis does not always apply to patients with "sectorial,"[81] "sectoral,"[82,83] or regionalized[84,85] retinitis pigmentosa, which are forms of retinitis pigmentosa that, early in their course, are more severe in certain regions (usually in the inferior fundus). Older patients with sectorial, sectoral, or regionalized retinitis pigmentosa have degeneration of the entire fundus that cannot be distinguished from typical retinitis pigmentosa. Confusingly, the term *sector retinitis pigmentosa* is not used uniformly to refer to the relatively self-limited form of retinal degeneration.

## Retinitis Pigmentosa as Part of a Multisystem Disease

In most cases, patients with retinitis pigmentosa or cone-rod degeneration have no associated systemic or extraocular abnormalities. However, there are multisystem diseases in which a retinal degeneration similar to retinitis pigmentosa or cone-rod dystrophy is a part. Although rare, the most noteworthy are diseases for which effective treatment is available to ameliorate the retinal degeneration. These are abetalipoproteinemia (MIM 200100; see Chap. 115), Refsum disease (MIM 266510; see Chap. 132), gyrate atrophy (see Chap. 83), and recessive retinitis pigmentosa and Friedrich-like ataxia due to defective α-tocopherol transfer protein.[86,87] It should be noted briefly here that patients with abetalipoproteinemia or ataxia due to defective α-tocopherol transport protein can recover retinal function after therapy with vitamin A,[88,89] or vitamin E,[90] respectively. With regard to Refsum disease, dietary modification aimed at reducing the intake of phytanic acid levels is of benefit in slowing or stopping the associated retinal degeneration.[91] Similarly, patients with gyrate atrophy appear to benefit from a diet that restricts the intake of ornithine precursors.[92]

A substantial minority patients with retinitis pigmentosa report some degree of hearing deficiency. In most of these cases, the combination of hearing loss and retinitis pigmentosa is usually inherited together as an autosomal recessive trait that is termed *Usher syndrome*. Usher syndrome has been divided into three major types according to clinical findings. In Usher syndrome type I, retinitis pigmentosa is associated with vestibular ataxia and profound congenital deafness[93–99]; in Usher syndrome type II, there is retinitis pigmentosa with partial hearing loss[100]; and in Usher syndrome type III, there is retinitis pigmentosa and progressive hearing loss.[101] Most cases of Usher syndrome type II are due to a gene on chromosome 1q41. Most cases of Usher syndrome type III are due to an unidentified gene on chromosome 3q21-24. At least six genes (on chromosomes 10q, 11p15.1, 11q13.5, 14q32, 21q21, and elsewhere[99]) can cause Usher syndrome type I, one of which encodes myosin VIIa (Table 235-1). There is a solitary family reported with a dominantly inherited syndrome of retinitis pigmentosa, hearing impairment, and subclinical myopathy caused by a mitochondrial mutation.[102]

Some other multisystem diseases in which retinal degeneration is a feature are Bardet-Biedl syndrome (recessive retinitis pigmentosa associated with polydactyly, truncal obesity, hypogonadism, short stature, and mental retardation),[103–107] dominant cerebellar ataxia with pigmentary macular dystrophy,[108–110] Batten disease (recessive neuronal ceroid lipofuscinosis; see Chap. 154),[111,112] and the syndrome of X-linked macular degeneration, congenital ataxia, and late-onset progressive myoclonic encephalopathy.[113] Retinitis pigmentosa is also a feature of Kearns-Sayre syndrome (external ophthalmoplegia, pigmentary retinal degeneration, and cardiomyopathy), due to a deletion in the mitochondrial genome[114–116] (see Chap. 105). Additional types of syndromic retinal degeneration are listed in Table 235-1.

## Prevalence of Hereditary Retinal Degeneration

Retinitis pigmentosa occurs in all races, although the incidence of the disease differs somewhat from nation to nation.[117–127] In the

**Table 235-1 Chromosome Assignments of Genes Causing Retinal Degeneration or Stationary Night Blindness**

| | |
|---|---|
| 1p32 | palmitoyl protein thioesterase (*CLN1*) |
| | Infantile neuronal ceroid-lipofuscinosis[411] |
| 1p31 | *RPE65* |
| | Recessive retinitis pigmentosa[325,326] |
| | Congenital amaurosis[324,325] |
| 1p13 | *ABCR* (ATP-binding cassette transporter of the retina) |
| | Stargardt juvenile macular degeneration[311,412] |
| | Cone-rod degeneration[314,315] |
| 1q31-32.1 | Unidentified gene |
| | Recessive retinitis pigmentosa with preserved paraarteriolar retinal pigment epithelium[77–80] |
| 1cen-q21 | Unidentified gene |
| | Dominant retinitis pigmentosa[413] |
| 1q25-q31 | Unidentified gene |
| | Age-related macular degeneration, dry type[414] |
| 1q41 | USH2A |
| | Usher syndrome type II[367] |
| 1q44 | Unidentified gene implicated in single patient with a translocation breakpoint |
| | Cone dystrophy[415] |
| 2p16 | Unidentified gene |
| | Dominant macular degeneration (Doyne honeycomb dystrophy)[416] |
| | Dominant radial drusen (malattia leventinese)[417] |
| 2p14-13 | Unidentified gene |
| | Alstrom syndrome[418] |
| 2q11 | α subunit of the cone cGMP-gated cation channel |
| | Recessive rod monochromacy[279] |
| 2q31-33 | Unidentified gene |
| | Recessive retinitis pigmentosa[419] |
| 2q24-37 | Arrestin |
| | Oguchi disease (stationary night blindness)[75,76,284] |
| | Recessive retinitis pigmentosa[75,76,83] |
| 3p21 | Rod α-transducin |
| | Dominant stationary night blindness (Nougaret form)[44] |
| 3p21.1-12 | Ataxin-7 |
| | Dominant cerebellar ataxia with pigmentary macular dystrophy[420] |
| 3p12 | Unidentified gene |
| | Bardet-Biedl syndrome[103,104] |
| 3q21-q24 | Rhodopsin |
| | Dominant retinitis pigmentosa[198,199,227,421] |
| | Recessive retinitis pigmentosa[237,240] |
| | Dominant stationary night blindness[21,43,215] |
| 3q21-25 | Unidentified gene |
| | Usher syndrome type III[368] |
| 3q21-24 | Ceruloplasmin |
| | Syndromic retinal degeneration[422] |
| 4p16.3 | β subunit of rod cGMP phosphodiesterase |
| | Recessive retinitis pigmentosa[252] |
| | Dominant stationary night blindness[45] |
| 4p14-q13 | α subunit of rod cGMP-gated channel |
| | Recessive retinitis pigmentosa[278] |
| 4q22-q24 | Microsomal triglyceride transfer protein |
| | Abetalipoproteinemia (Bassen-Kornzweig syndrome)[423] |
| 5q31.2-q34 | α subunit of rod cGMP phosphodiesterase |
| | Recessive retinitis pigmentosa[258] |
| 6p21.1 | Guanylate cyclase activator 1A |
| | Dominant cone dystrophy[302,424] |
| 6p21 | Tubby-like protein-1 (*TULP1*) |
| | Recessive retinitis pigmentosa[334,336,425] |

**Table 235-1** (*Continued*)

| | |
|---|---|
| 6p21.1-cen | *RDS* or *peripherin/RDS*<br>Dominant retinitis pigmentosa[354,355,426]<br>Dominant macular dystrophy[426]<br>Dominant retinitis punctata albescens[136]<br>Digenic retinitis pigmentosa[133] |
| 6cen-q14 | Unidentified gene<br>Recessive retinitis pigmentosa[427] |
| 6q11-15 | Unidentified gene<br>Stargardt-like dominant macular dystrophy<br>(possible allelic to cone-rod dystrophy)[428] |
| 6q13-15 | Unidentified gene (*CORD7*)<br>Dominant cone-rod dystrophy (possible allellic<br>to dominant Stargardt-like dystrophy)[429] |
| 6q14-q16.2 | Unidentified gene<br>North Carolina dominant macular dystrophy[430]<br>Dominant progressive bifocal chorioretinal<br>atrophy[431] |
| 7p21-15 | Unidentified gene<br>Dominant cystoid macular dystrophy[432–434] |
| 7p21-15 | Unidentified gene<br>Dominant retinitis pigmentosa with variable<br>expressivity[432,435,436] |
| 7q21-22 | *PEX1*<br>Infantile Refsum disease[437] |
| 7q31-32 | Unidentified gene<br>Dominant retinitis pigmentosa[438–441] |
| 8q11-21 | Unidentified gene<br>Dominant retinitis pigmentosa[442,443] |
| 8q13.1-13.3 | α-Tocopherol-transfer protein<br>Retinitis pigmentosa and Friedrich-like<br>ataxia[86,444] |
| 9q34-qter | Unidentified gene<br>Dominant retinitis pigmentosa, hearing<br>impairment, and subclinical myopathy[102] |
| 10pter-p11.2 | Phytanoyl-CoA α-hydroxylase<br>Refsum disease[445,446] |
| 10q26 | Ornithine aminotransferase<br>Gyrate atrophy[447–449] |
| 10q | Unidentified gene<br>Usher syndrome type I[93] |
| 11p15 | *CLN2* (a lysosomal protein)<br>Classical late-infantile neuronal ceroid<br>lipofuscinosis[450] |
| 11p15 | Unidentified gene<br>Helicoid peripapillary chorioretinal<br>degeneration[451,452] |
| 11p15 | Unidentified gene<br>Usher syndrome type I[94–96] |
| 11q12-13 | Bestrophin<br>Best vitelliform macular dystrophy[453] |
| 11q13 | *ROM1*<br>Digenic retinitis pigmentosa[133] |
| 11q13 | Unidentified gene<br>Bardet-Biedl syndrome[104,105] |
| 11q13.5 | myosin VIIa<br>Usher syndrome type I[97] |
| 12 | No retinal degeneration genes mapped so far |
| 13q22 | *CLN5*<br>Late infantile neuronal ceroid lipofuscinosis[454] |
| 13q34 | Unidentified gene<br>Dominant Stargardt macular dystrophy[455] |
| 13q34 | Rhodopsin kinase<br>Oguchi disease[285,286] |
| 14q32 | Unidentified gene<br>Usher syndrome type I[366] |
| 15q21-23 | Unidentified gene<br>Variant late infantile neuronal ceroid<br>lipofuscinosis[456] |

**Table 235-1** (*Continued*)

| | |
|---|---|
| 15q22 | Unidentified gene<br>Bardet-Biedl syndrome[106] |
| 15q24 | Unidentified gene<br>Tapetoretinal degeneration, mental retardation,<br>and spasticity[457] |
| 15q26 | Cellular retinaldehyde binding protein<br>Recessive retinitis punctata albescens[139] |
| 16p12.3-12.1 | Unidentified gene<br>Recessive retinitis pigmentosa[458] |
| 16p12.1 | *CLN3* (a lysosomal protein)[459]<br>Juvenile neuronal ceroid lipofuscinosis<br>(Batten or Spielmeyer-Vogt disease)[111,112] |
| 16p13 | Phosphomannomutase-2<br>Carbohydrate-deficient glycoprotein type I<br>syndrome[460,461] |
| 16q21 | Unidentified gene<br>Bardet-Biedl[104,107] |
| 17p | Unidentified gene<br>Dominant central areolar choroidal dystrophy<br>(same chromosomal region as guanylate<br>cyclase)[462] |
| 17p13-12 | Unidentified gene<br>Dominant progressive cone dystrophy[463–465] |
| 17p13.3 | Unidentified gene<br>Dominant retinitis pigmentosa[466–468] |
| 17p13.1 | Guanylate cyclase<br>Leber congenital amaurosis[295]<br>Dominant cone-rod dystrophy[297,298] |
| 17q22 | Unidentified gene<br>Dominant retinitis pigmentosa[469] |
| 18q21.1 | Unidentified gene<br>Cone-rod dystrophy (one case with deletion)[470] |
| 19q13.1-13.2 | Transcription factor crx<br>Dominant cone-rod dystrophy[339,340]<br>Congenital amaurosis[341] |
| 19q13.4 | Unidentified gene (possibly protein kinase C)[471]<br>Dominant retinitis pigmentosa with reduced<br>penetrance[135,472,473] |
| 20 | No retinal degeneration genes mapped so far |
| 21q21 | Unidentified gene<br>Usher syndrome type I[99] |
| 22qter-q13 | Tissue inhibitor of metalloproteinase-3<br>Sorsby fundus dystrophy[474] |
| Xpter-p22.33 | Unidentified gene<br>Macular degeneration, congenital ataxia, late-<br>onset progressive myoclonic encephalopathy[113] |
| Xp22.3-22.1 | *XLRS1*<br>Retinoschisis[475] |
| Xp22.13-22.11 | Unidentified gene<br>X-linked dominant retinitis pigmentosa[132] |
| Xp21.1 | *RPGR*<br>Retinitis pigmentosa[306,307,310]<br>Possibly stationary night blindness[142,143] |
| Xp11.4-11.3 | Unidentified gene<br>Complete stationary night blindness<br>(*CSNB1*)[48,144] |
| Xp11.4-11.23 | Unidentified gene<br>Retinitis pigmentosa and mental handicap[476] |
| Xp11.3 | Unidentified gene<br>Cone dystrophy[477,478] |
| Xp11.3 | RP2<br>X-linked retinitis pigmentosa[305] |
| Xp11.23 | L-type calcium channel<br>Incomplete stationary night blindness<br>(*CSNB2*)[48,145,146]<br>Possibly allelic with Åland Island eye<br>disease[48] |

*Continued on next page*

**Table 235-1** (*Continued*)

| | |
|---|---|
| Xp21 | Dystrophin |
| | Abnormal rod ERG[479,480] |
| Xq21 | Component A of Rab geranylgeranyl transferase |
| | (a Rab escort protein) |
| | Choroideremia[481–483] |
| Xq | Red/green cone opsin |
| | X-linked cone degeneration[484] |
| Xq27 | Unidentified gene |
| | X-linked progressive cone dystrophy[485] |
| Y | Unidentified gene (possibly present) |
| | Single family with apparent Y-linked retinitis |
| | pigmentosa[486] |
| | Mitochondrial genome deletion |
| | Kearns-Sayre syndrome[114–116] |

United States, it has a prevalence of around 0.02 to 0.03 percent, affecting over 50,000 people.[117,118,120] Except for age-related macular degeneration (see Chap. 243), the prevalence of the allied diseases is much lower and not as well studied. The three types of Usher syndrome together have a combined prevalence of around 5 per 100,000,[125–128] which corresponds to about 5 to 15 percent of all cases of retinitis pigmentosa. The Bardet-Biedl syndrome accounts for a few percent of the cases of retinitis pigmentosa.[127,129]

The proportions of retinitis pigmentosa patients exhibiting each inheritance pattern vary between ethnic groups. For example, the X-linked type accounts for 14 to 16 percent of families in England,[119,122] 8 percent in the United States and Ontario, Canada,[117,118,120,123] and only 1 percent in Switzerland.[121] In the state of Maine,[118] retinitis pigmentosa was found to be inherited as an autosomal dominant trait in 19 percent of affected families (43 percent of patients), as an autosomal recessive trait in 19 percent of families (20 percent of patients), and as an X-linked trait in 8 percent of families (8 percent of patients). The proportions of patients differ from the proportions of families because, for example, a family with dominant retinitis pigmentosa will have, on average, more affected individuals than a family with recessive retinitis pigmentosa. Patients with "isolated" retinitis pigmentosa, representing 46 percent of families (23 percent of patients), are defined as those with no other affected family members (simplex cases). Most of these cases probably are autosomal recessive, although some could represent new dominant or X-linked mutations. Patients with uncertain family history (e.g., adopted) are designated "undetermined" (8 percent of families; 6 percent of patients).

The prevalences of cone degeneration, cone-rod degeneration, and stationary night blindness are not known, but all are thought to be less common than retinitis pigmentosa.

### Determination of Inheritance Pattern

It is straightforward to determine the inheritance pattern in families with numerous affected members over many generations. In the majority of families with retinitis pigmentosa, however, there are only a few affected members, perhaps only one, or the family history is uncertain. In these situations, clinical findings, such as refractive error, the severity of the disease, and the age at which complete blindness occurs, can help to determine which inheritance type is most likely. For example, patients with autosomal dominant retinitis pigmentosa often retain some useful vision after age 60, whereas patients with X-linked disease usually are blind by age 45 and patients with autosomal recessive disease typically retain vision until age 60.[130] Males with X-linked retinitis pigmentosa commonly have more than 2 diopters of myopia and astigmatism with a horizontal or oblique axis of cylinder of more than 1 diopter.[130,131] Hyperopia or less than 1 diopter of myopia favors the diagnosis of dominant retinitis

pigmentosa.[130] Recording the extent of bone-spicule pigmentation in patients under age 20 is also of value, since if the pigmentation is not found in all four quadrants, it is likely that the patient has an autosomal dominant form of retinitis pigmentosa.[130] Evaluating and interpreting these parameters will not allow one to definitively diagnose a particular genetic type of retinitis pigmentosa. Nevertheless, these parameters can be helpful in genetic counseling, especially when dealing with an affected male with a negative or uncertain family history, in whom X-linked, dominant, and recessive types of retinitis pigmentosa are all possible. It is also important to note that an ophthalmologic examination coupled with ERGs can identify unaffected female carriers of X-linked retinitis pigmentosa.[29,30] Consequently, evaluation of the mother of an isolated male with retinitis pigmentosa often can determine whether he has X-linked disease. In some families with X-linked retinitis pigmentosa, female carriers are always affected, although more mildly than the males; this X-linked, semidominant inheritance pattern may be specific to a particular retinitis pigmentosa gene in Xp22.[132]

In most families with dominant retinitis pigmentosa, all carriers are affected, and even young patients without subjective visual abnormalities invariably can be shown through ophthalmic examination or ERGs to have retinal degeneration. However, in a minority of families, some obligate heterozygotes are asymptomatic and show no evidence of retinal degeneration. In some cases, these are due to a digenic inheritance pattern where affected individuals are always double heterozygotes for mutations at two unlinked loci (see discussion of the *RDS* and *ROM1* genes later in this chapter)[133,134]; heterozygotes at only one of the two loci are unaffected. In other families, notably those with retinitis pigmentosa due to an as yet unidentified gene mapping to 19q, the penetrance of the mutation appears to be governed by wild-type alleles at the same locus (or a closely linked one) inherited from the noncarrier parent.[135]

There are as yet no recognized clinical features that uniquely and unambiguously point to a specific mutation or a specific gene causing retinitis pigmentosa. However, there are some reported genotype-phenotype correlations. Rod function is absent from birth in patients with null mutations in the genes encoding essential members of the rod photoreceptor cascade, such as the $\alpha$ or $\beta$ subunits of rod cGMP phosphodiesterase or the $\alpha$ subunit of the rod cGMP-gated channel; in contrast, some patients with dominant rhodopsin mutations such as *P23H* have some rod function in youth reported subjectively and documented through objective tests such as the ERG. The fundi of some patients with mutations in the *RDS* gene or the *CRALBP* gene have subretinal flecks or deposits at the level of the retinal pigment epithelium.[10,136–139]

Many allied diseases have different inheritance patterns in different families. Cone dystrophy, cone-rod dystrophy, and stationary night blindness can each be inherited as X-linked, autosomal recessive, or autosomal dominant traits. Genes for some forms of X-linked stationary night blindness map approximately to the same regions where the *RP2* and *RP3* genes causing X-linked retinitis pigmentosa are found on Xp,[140–143] making it possible that particular alleles at these retinitis pigmentosa loci may cause stationary night blindness, much the same way that different mutations at the rhodopsin locus can cause either retinitis pigmentosa or stationary night blindness.[43] However, other data indicate that two X-linked stationary night blindness genes are in the interval between the *RP2* and *RP3* loci and are distinct from both of them.[48,144] One of these genes causes the complete form of the Schubert-Bornschein type of stationary night blindness, whereas the other, which codes for an L-type calcium channel,[145,146] causes the incomplete form.[48] A form of X-linked stationary night blindness called *Åland Island eye disease* may be allelic with X-linked incomplete stationary night blindness.[48] There is also a report of a family with apparent X-linked stationary night blindness in which female carriers but not male carriers were affected, for reasons still unknown.[147]

Categorizing patients with retinitis pigmentosa or an allied disease according to genetic type is valuable for the following reasons: One justification, of course, is to aid genetic counseling, since it is not yet possible to identify the responsible genetic defect in most patients by molecular genetic analysis. Second, because severity of retinitis pigmentosa correlates with inheritance pattern, an approximate prognosis for vision can be provided to a patient even if the precise gene defect is unknown. Third, in the event that therapies specific for particular types of retinitis pigmentosa become available, it will be advantageous to know in advance the cohort of patients who will benefit. It is also possible that future analyses of cohorts of patients with defects in the same gene may reveal clinical features specific to that set of patients.

## GENES CAUSING RETINITIS PIGMENTOSA AND ALLIED DISEASES

There is evidence from gene identifications or linkage studies for over 55 genetic loci where mutations cause nonsyndromic or syndromic retinal degeneration (see Table 235-1; for an updated listing, go to *http://www.sph.uth.tmc.edu/RetNet/*). Reports of families not showing linkage to any of the relevant chromosomal regions indicate that additional retinal degeneration genes exist. For example, a recent publication mentions three families with dominant retinitis pigmentosa not linked to any of the nine chromosomal regions known to contain dominant retinitis pigmentosa genes.[148]

At least 30 retinal degeneration genes have been identified; the rest are unidentified genes mapped by linkage analyses. Some cause types of retinal degeneration described in other chapters, such as gyrate atrophy (see Chap. 83), choroideremia (see Chap. 236), macular degeneration (see Chap. 243), congenital amaurosis (see Chap. 237), Kearns-Sayre syndrome (see Chap. 105), and abetalipoproteinemia (see Chap. 115). Only rough estimates can be gleaned from the literature regarding the proportions of cases accounted for by each of the identified genes causing nonsyndromic retinitis pigmentosa or Usher syndrome. In their totality, it is estimated that the identified genes account for about 35 to 50 percent of all cases. Below is a description of the identified genes causing nonsyndromic retinitis pigmentosa, Usher syndrome, cone-rod dystrophy, and stationary night blindness.

### Retinal Disease Caused by Defects in Genes Encoding Members of the Rod Phototransduction Cascade

**Summary of the Phototransduction Cascade.** Some of the genes so far identified as causes of hereditary retinal degeneration or malfunction normally encode proteins in the phototransduction cascade. This cascade is the biochemical pathway that mediates the light-sensing activity of photoreceptor cells (for reviews, see Stryer[149] or Hargrave and McDowell[150]). Rod phototransduction is the better studied; cone photoreceptors have similar or identical components. Below is a brief description of the rod phototransduction pathway, followed by a summary of each component's role in retinitis pigmentosa and allied diseases.

In rods, the pathway takes place in the outer segment of each rod photoreceptor. In this specialized, light-sensing region, there is a stack of about 1000 disks (Fig. 235-4), which are flattened vesicles with membranes composed of approximately equimolar amounts of protein and lipid.[151] About 80 percent of the protein in the outer segment disk membranes is rhodopsin,[152] also called *rod opsin*. Rhodopsin is one of the best-studied members of a large family of membrane-bound, seven-helix, G-protein-coupled receptors.[153] In the dark-adapted state, the protein component, called *opsin*, is covalently linked to the chromophore 11-*cis*-retinal (Fig. 235-5), a derivative of vitamin A. A photon of light interacts with the chromophore, changing its conformation to all-*trans*; this in turn induces conformational changes in rhodopsin that serve to activate it. There are about 40 million rhodopsin molecules in the disk membranes of each rod photoreceptor outer segment.[154–156]

Photoactivated rhodopsin interacts with the next member of the cascade (step 2 in Fig. 235-6), a G-protein called *transducin*. It is a heterotrimeric protein that is attached to the disk membrane through isoprenylation of its $\gamma$ subunit.[157–159] There are about one-tenth the number of transducin molecules than rhodopsin molecules residing on the disk membranes. Each photoactivated rhodopsin molecule activates a transducin molecule every 1 to 5 mseconds before it is deactivated by rhodopsin kinase and arrestin.[160]

On interaction with photoactivated rhodopsin, the $\alpha$ subunit of transducin exchanges a bound GDP moiety for GTP. The activated, GTP-bound $\beta$ subunit detaches from the $\beta$ and $\gamma$ subunits of transducin and associates with the next member of the cascade (step 3 in Fig. 235-6). This is cGMP phosphodiesterase, another heteromeric complex with active $\alpha$ and $\beta$ subunits and two inhibitory $\gamma$ subunits. The enzyme cGMP phosphodiesterase also resides on disk membranes, a location mediated through isoprenylation of the $\alpha$ and $\beta$ subunits.[161] The GTP-bound form of rod $\alpha$-transducin interacts specifically with the inhibitory $\gamma$ subunit of cGMP phosphodiesterase. There ensues a substantial increase in the activity of cGMP phosphodiesterase and a consequential fall in the concentration of cGMP in the cytoplasm. The cytoplasmic cGMP concentration controls the proportion of cGMP-gated cation channels that are open in the plasma membrane of the rod outer segment. In the dark, a few percent of the channels are open, allowing cations such as sodium and calcium to enter the cell. There is a compensatory efflux of cations mediated by two proteins, the $Na^+/Ca^2\text{-}K^+$ exchanger (also in the plasma membrane of the outer segment)[162,163] and $Na^+\text{-}K^+$ ATPase (which may be only in the rod inner segment). The flow of cations into and out of the photoreceptor outer segment produces the "dark current" that is measured through patch-clamp recordings.[164] In response to light, phosphodiesterase is activated, the concentration of cGMP is reduced, and the proportion of channels that are open will fall (step 4 in Fig. 235-6). This will cause a graded hyperpolarization of the plasma membrane because of the constant efflux of cations mediated by the $Na^+/Ca^2\text{-}K^+$ exchanger and $Na^+\text{-}K^+$ ATPase. The degree of hyperpolarization of the plasma membrane will correspond to cytoplasmic cGMP concentration, which in turn is a reflection of the amount of light that the rod is experiencing. As a neuron, the rod photoreceptor can convey the hyperpolarization in the outer segment to the synaptic region, where it decreases the amount of neurotransmitter (glutamate) released. The entire cascade is extremely sensitive in the dark-adapted rod; absorption of a single photon of light is sufficient to stimulate a human rod photoreceptor.[165]

Additional proteins shut the cascade off. Rhodopsin kinase and arrestin serve to deactivate photoactivated rhodopsin[166,167] (step 5 in Fig. 235-6). A protein called *RGS9* (regulator of G-protein signaling) stimulates the inherent GTPase activity of transducin so that it quickly returns to its inactive, GDP-bound form.[168] Guanylate cyclase activating protein (GCAP) responds to the changes in cytoplasmic calcium levels and stimulates guanylate cyclase, which in turn replenishes the reservoir of cGMP in the cytoplasm of the outer segment[169] (step 6 in Fig. 235-6).

Other components of the cascade play important roles. Calcium ions and proteins such as recoverin, phosducin, calmodulin, and protein kinase C have a role in modulating the sensitivity of rods,[170–182] but no defects in the respective genes have yet been found to cause a hereditary retinal disease. Proteins of the retinal pigment epithelium such as CRALBP and RPE65 may have a role in the conversion of the all-*trans*-retinal (produced when rhodopsin is activated) to 11-*cis*-retinal to regenerate photosensitive rhodopsin.[183–185] Additional proteins that have obscure roles in mammalian photoreceptors, such as the mammalian homologue of the *Drosophila* rdgB protein,[186] are under active investigation.[187]

**Rhodopsin.** This is the most abundant protein in outer segment disks, comprising over 80 percent of the membrane-bound protein

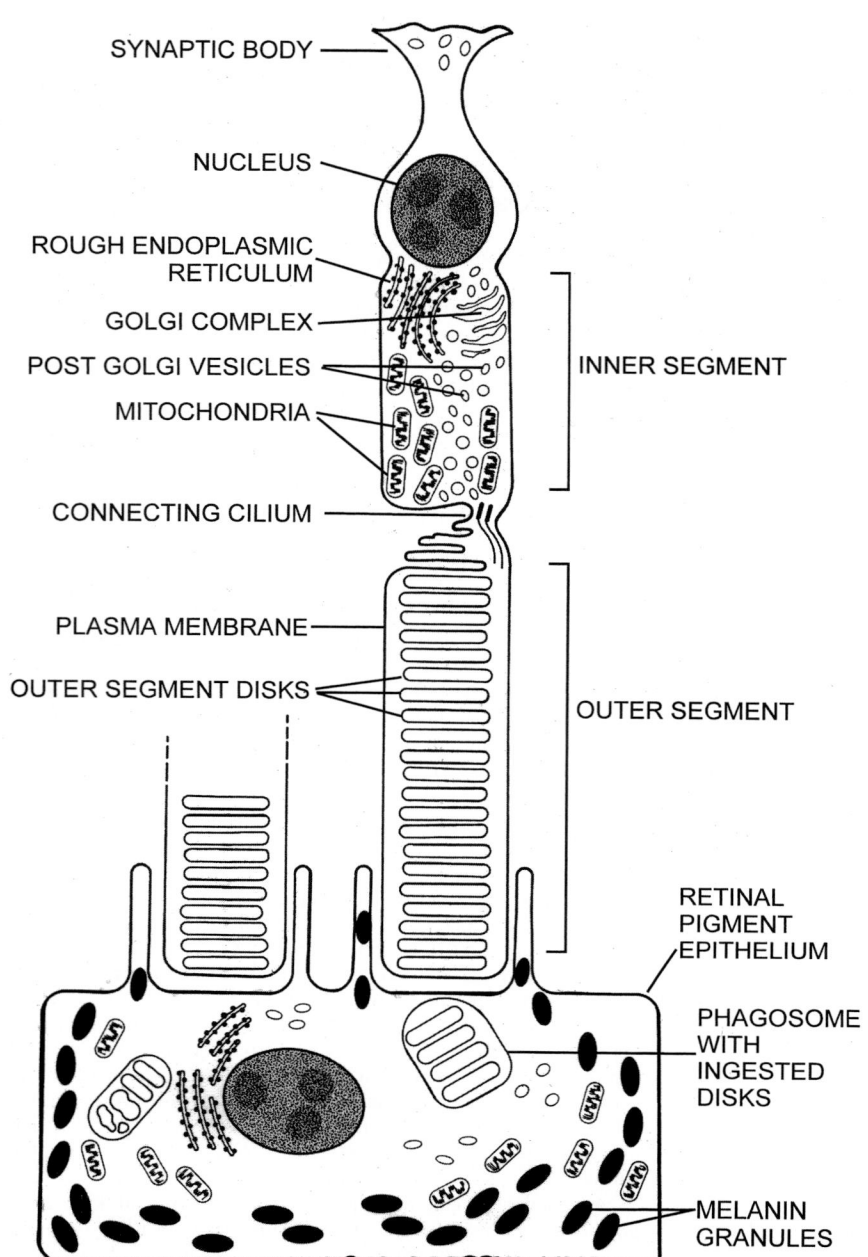

SYNAPTIC BODY

NUCLEUS

ROUGH ENDOPLASMIC RETICULUM

GOLGI COMPLEX

POST GOLGI VESICLES

MITOCHONDRIA

CONNECTING CILIUM

PLASMA MEMBRANE

OUTER SEGMENT DISKS

INNER SEGMENT

OUTER SEGMENT

RETINAL PIGMENT EPITHELIUM

PHAGOSOME WITH INGESTED DISKS

MELANIN GRANULES

**Fig. 235-4 Schematic representation of a rod photoreceptor and an adjacent retinal pigment epithelial cell. The photoreceptor cell is oriented so that its proximal end is at the top. Disks containing rhodopsin are stacked in the rod outer segment. Their molecular components, including rhodopsin, are synthesized in the inner segment and transported to the outer segment. Approximately 10 percent of the outer segment is synthesized each day, with the newly manufactured disks being the basal disks.[407,408] An equally large segment of distal outer segment is phagocytosed daily by the retinal pigment epithelium. The retinal pigment epithelium contains fragments of outer segments in phagocytotic vesicles. (Adapted from Fig. 6 in Berson et al.[8] Used by permission.)**

in the rod outer segment.[152,188] Each molecule of rhodopsin traverses a disk membrane seven times[189] (Fig. 235-7). The transmembrane domains are rich in hydrophobic amino acids. They encircle the 11-*cis*-retinal moiety,[190,191] called the *chromophore* (see Fig. 235-5), that is covalently linked to a lysine residue (Lys296) in the seventh transmembrane domain. The transmembrane domains form a molecular environment for the chromophore that tunes the peak in its absorption spectrum to 498 nm.

***Dominant Rhodopsin Mutations Causing Retinitis Pigmentosa.*** Mutations in the rhodopsin gene, on chromosome 3q21-24, are responsible for about 25 percent of cases of dominant retinitis pigmentosa in the United States and about 20 percent of cases elsewhere in the world.[192] Since about 40 percent of all patients with retinitis pigmentosa are from families with a dominant inheritance pattern,[118] one can calculate that about 8 to 10 percent of all cases of retinitis pigmentosa are due to dominant rhodopsin mutations. Over 90 different mutations have been reported[193] (see

Fig. 235-7). The most common mutation in North America is the missense allele *P23H* (an alteration of codon 23 to specify histidine instead of proline); it accounts for about 9 percent of all cases of dominant retinitis pigmentosa there.[192] This mutation has not been found on other continents.[194] Furthermore, it is in strong linkage disequilibrium with an intragenic microsatellite repeat polymorphism, indicating that the North American families probably all descend from a common ancestor who carried the *P23H* allele.[195] Similarly, with few exceptions,[196,197] each of the other dominant rhodopsin mutations has been found in a single family, suggesting that this locus has a low mutation rate. The most striking exception involves codon 347, where the mutation *P347L* appears to have arisen a number of times in Europe, North America, and Japan.[195,198–201] Only one instance of a new germ-line mutation has been documented, and this is also a *P347L* allele.[198] Still, the *P347L* mutation is responsible for only a small minority of rhodopsin-related retinitis pigmentosa cases worldwide, probably only a few percent.

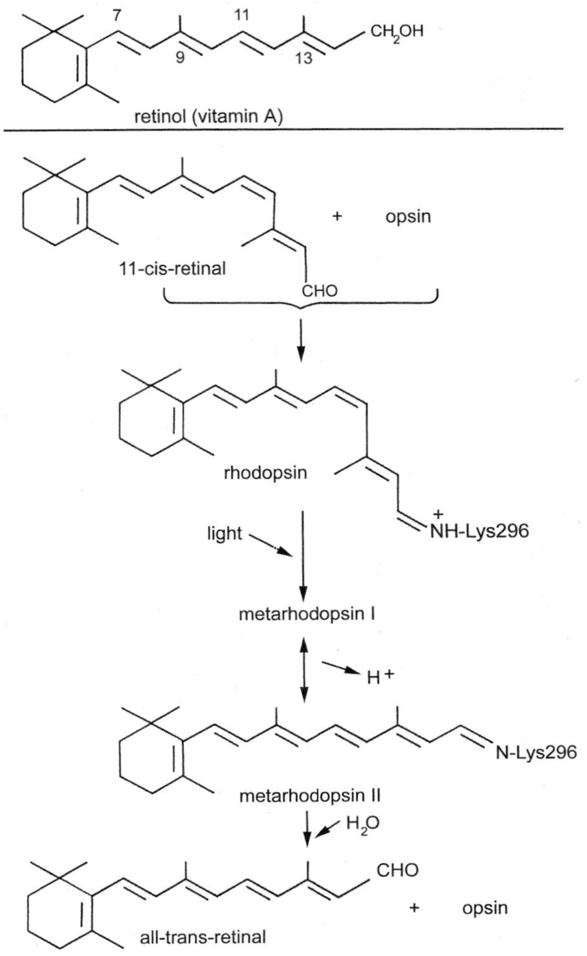

**Fig. 235-5 Chemical structures of the vitamin A derivatives that participate in the visual cycle.** The chemical structure of retinol (vitamin A) is shown at the top. Retinol is converted to the aldehyde 11-*cis*-retinal in the retinal pigment epithelium. On transport to the photoreceptor outer segments, this 11-*cis*-retinal (called the *chromophore*) forms a covalent (Schiff-base) linkage to a lysine residue at position 296 in rod opsin to produce a light-sensitive molecule. The structure of that covalent bond is represented in the middle of this figure. A photon of light will convert the 11-*cis*-retinal to all-*trans*-retinal, creating metarhodopsin I. A proton is lost from metarhodopsin I to form metarhodopsin II, which is the form of photoactivated, deprotonated opsin that can activate transducin. The all-*trans*-retinal detaches from opsin at an exponential rate with a half-life of about 4 to 7 minutes.[287-289] The opsin molecule is then able to regenerate by incorporating a new molecule of 11-*cis*-retinal. The molecule of all-*trans*-retinal must travel back to the retinal pigment epithelium to be reconverted to 11-*cis*-retinal.

*Characteristics of the Dominant Rhodopsin Mutations Causing Retinitis Pigmentosa.* Most of the dominant rhodopsin gene defects are missense mutations; a few are short in-frame deletions of a few codons or truncations or elogations of the C-terminus. Only one dominant nonsense mutation early in the reading frame has been reported.[64,202,203] Figure 235-7 shows a schematic model of rhodopsin with the amino acids affected by dominant mutations circled. Most of the mutations involve the intradiskal or transmembrane regions of the protein, with a final cluster near the C-terminus of the molecule.

Considerable effort is currently being devoted to elucidating the pathogenic properties of these mutant opsins. So far, a number of intriguing observations of some of the mutant opsins have been reported, but no common property that might explain their pathogenicity has been discovered. Since the cytoplasmic loops of rhodopsin interact with transducin,[204] and since they are rarely affected by these mutations, one may surmise that the pathogenicity of these mutant opsins is not related to an interference with phototransduction. However, it has been proposed that some of the mutant opsins may cause rod photoreceptor degeneration by constitutively activating the phototransduction cascade (i.e., regardless of whether they are exposed to light).[205] This would simulate constant exposure to light, which is a known cause of retinal degeneration, particularly in albino animals.[206,207] Support for this "equivalent light"[205] hypothesis comes from some mutants, such as *K296E*, that constitutively activate transducin in vitro.[208] However, some rhodopsin mutants that have been analyzed do not have a propensity to activate transducin in the dark.[209] Furthermore, the *K296E* allele expressed in vivo in transgenic mice does not activate the phototransduction cascade because it is constitutively phosphorylated and bound to arrestin.[210] Another piece of evidence against the equivalent light hypothesis comes from the ERG. Continuous activation of rod photoreceptors should cause a decrease in the cone implicit time in the ERG.[211] This is the opposite of what is observed in patients[28,212] and in transgenic mice[210,213] with rhodopsin mutations including the *K296E*.[214] Finally, other rhodopsin mutants (*A292E* and *G90D*) that appear to stimulate the cascade in vitro desensitize rods without causing a clinically significant retinal degeneration. They are found in patients with such a slow rate of photoreceptor degeneration that the patients are considered by some clinicians to have a form of stationary night blindness rather than retinitis pigmentosa.[21,43,215] Because of these observations, the equivalent light hypothesis is not universally accepted for explaining the pathogenicity of dominant rhodopsin mutants. The concept may be an explanation for defects in other members of the phototransduction cascade, such as the cGMP-gated channel (see below).

Another possible pathogenetic mechanism concerns structural defects induced by the mutations. Many of the affected amino acids in the intradiscal space, especially those near the cystine residues coupled by a disulfide bond between the second and third intradiscal loops, are in regions necessary for the normal three-dimensional conformation of rhodopsin and its ability to integrate within cellular membranes. Furthermore, most of the mutations affecting amino acids in the transmembrane domains replace hydrophobic residues with charged ones. These may destabilize the transmembrane domains and distort the overall structure of the protein. Based on these observations, one may conclude that a common property of the mutant opsins is an abnormality in their conformation that interferes with their synthesis in the endoplasmic reticulum, their processing by the Golgi, or their transport to or incorporation into outer segment disk membranes. The accumulation of mutant rhodopsin in the inner segments or other regions besides outer segments of rod photoreceptors could be especially detrimental because rods do not ordinarily catabolize rhodopsin (normally it is phagocytosed and catabolized by the adjacent retinal pigment epithelial cells) and because rods produce prodigious amounts of rhodopsin (almost 1 percent of the protein produced daily by the cells).

Support for this general mechanism comes from experimental studies of mutant rhodopsins expressed in vitro and in transgenic mice. When expressed in a monkey kidney cell line, some mutant rhodopsins poorly incorporate chromophore and give other indications that they are improperly folded.[209,216-219] Many of the mutants congregate in the endoplasmic reticulum rather than the plasma membrane.[216,217] And at least one of the mutants (*Q344X*) that does travel to the plasma membrane in kidney cells does not efficiently travel to outer segments when expressed in rod photoreceptors in transgenic mice.[220] Expression of various dominant rhodopsin mutants in transgenic mice or transgenic pigs causes abnormalities in the formation of outer segment disks,[221] accumulation of rhodopsin and other photoreceptor proteins in aberrant locations such as the synaptic region,[222,223] or formation of extracellular vesicles around the inner and outer

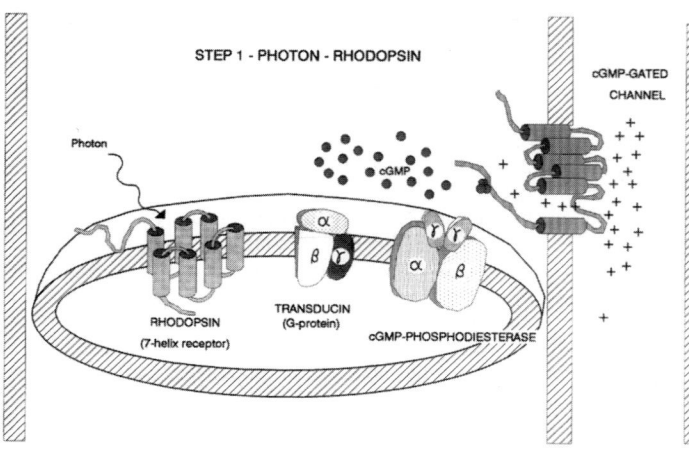

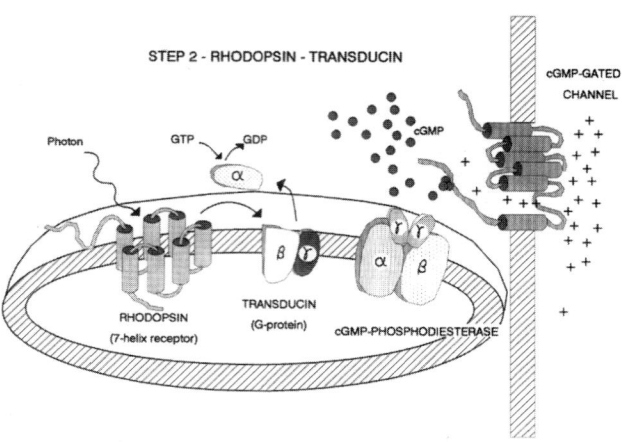

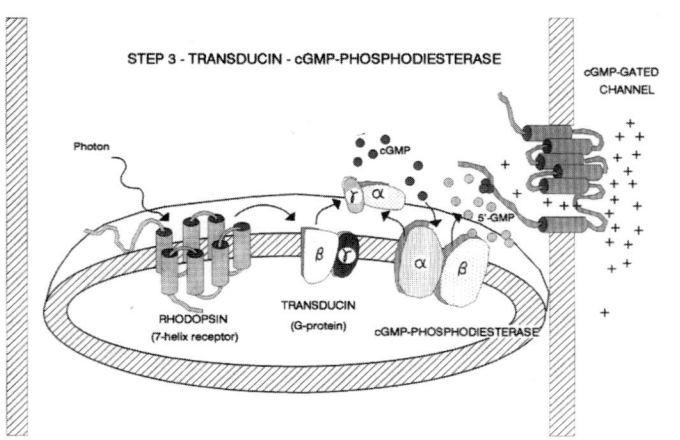

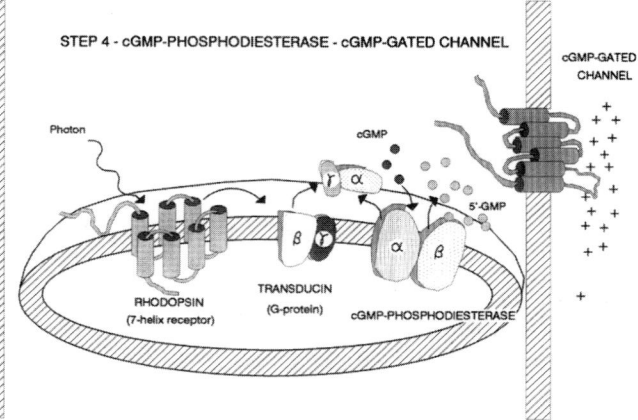

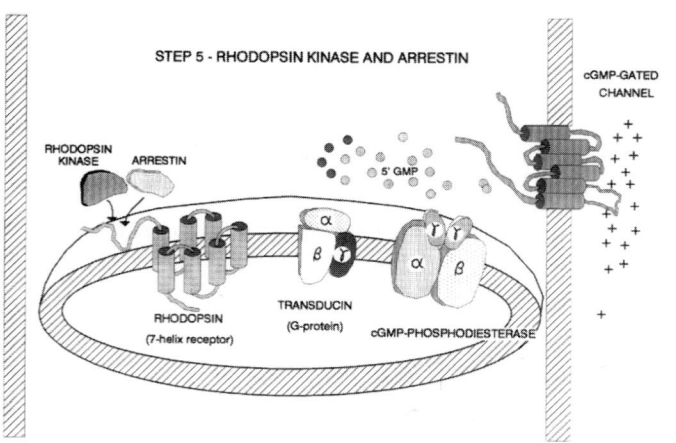

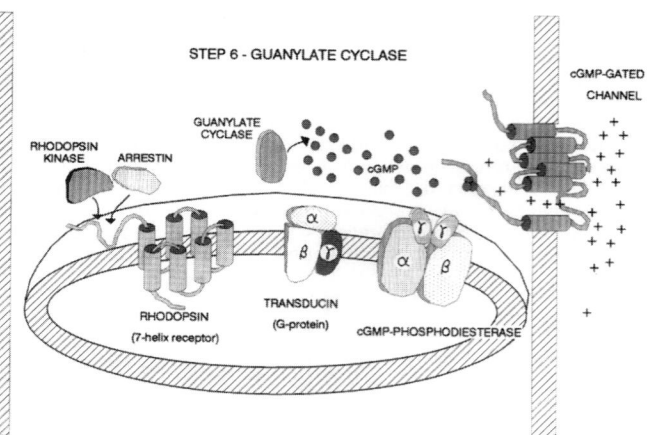

**Fig. 235-6 Phototransduction.** A schematic view of a disk in the outer segment is shown with rhodopsin, transducin, and cGMP phosphodiesterase in the disk membrane. A molecule of the cGMP-gated channel is present in the plasma membrane. In step 1, a photon of light strikes the rhodopsin molecule. In step 2, the photoactivated activated rhodopsin molecule interacts with transducin, inducing the α subunit to replace its bound GDP with a GTP moiety and to detach from the β and γ subunits. In step 3, the activated transducin α subunit interacts with the γ subunit of cGMP phosphodiesterase, thereby activating this enzyme, which reduces the level of cGMP in the cytoplasm by converting it to 5′-GMP. In step 4, the reduction in cytoplasmic cGMP causes the cGMP-gated channel to close. This hyperpolarizes the plasma membrane because the flow of cations (sodium and calcium) into the cell is reduced. In step 5, the phototransduction cascade begins its recovery phase when rhodopsin kinase phosphorylates the photoactivated rhodopsin molecule and arrestin binds to the phosphorylated rhodopsin. Once arrestin forms a complex with rhodopsin, it can no longer interact with transducin. The transducin α subunit hydrolyzes its bound GTP to form a GDP-complex (not shown) that is inactive and forms a complex with the β and γ subunits. In step 6, guanylate cyclase replenishes the cytoplasm with cGMP, and the cGMP-gated channel subsequently reopens.

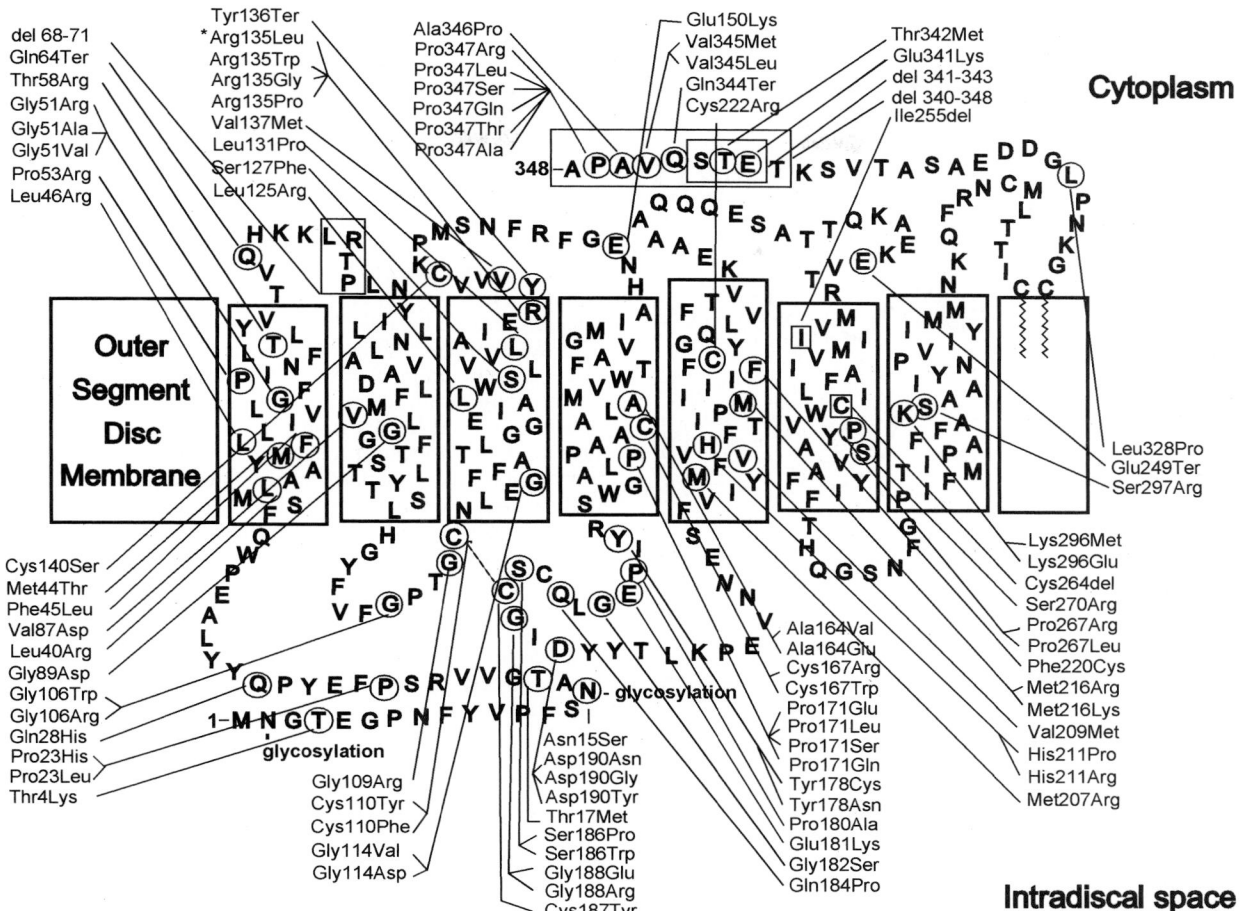

**Fig. 235-7 Model of rhodopsin using the single-letter amino acid code.** Rhodopsin has 348 amino acid residues, with the initial methionine in the intradiscal space. The peptide traverses the outer segment disk membrane seven times. Each circle denotes an amino acid that is altered by a missense mutation or nonsense mutation in at least one family with retinitis pigmentosa. All the mutations are dominant except Glu150Lys and Glu249Ter,[240,237] which are recessive. The missense mutation Arg135Leu is highlighted with an asterisk because two different DNA sequence changes producing the same missense change have been reported in separate families.[199,409] Open boxes indicate dominant mutations that are deletions of one or a few codons or frameshift deletions affecting the C-terminus. Not shown are two dominant mutations causing stationary night blindness Ala292Glu and Gly90Asp.[43,21] The circled lysine residue (K) in the seventh transmembrane domain is the one to which the chromophore 11-*cis*-retinal covalently binds; it is circled because it is the target of missense mutations in families with dominant retinitis pigmentosa.[192,410,487] The transmembrane domains to form a pocket surrounding 11-*cis*-retinal (not shown). Two asparagine-linked glycosylation sites that are present near the N-terminus in the intradiscal space are indicated.

segments[210]; all these findings may be an expected consequence of mutant rhodopsin molecules that are folded improperly. Analysis of dominant rhodopsin mutations in *Drosophila* shows not only that the mutant rhodopsin molecules are not transported to the rhabdomeres (the insect equivalent to rod outer segments) but also that they interfere with the transport of wild-type rhodopsin to the rhabdomeres.[224]

This body of evidence suggests that the mutant rhodopsins cause degeneration by interfering with protein synthesis or transport in the inner segment or the formation of outer segment disks. However, there are some observations that remain unexplained. For example, chimeric mouse retinas with some photoreceptors expressing *P347S* rhodopsin suffer degeneration of both the mutant and the wild-type photoreceptors.[225] Second, it remains a mystery why cone photoreceptors degenerate in patients with a defect in rhodopsin, a protein that is specific to rods. For that matter, it remains a mystery why cones degenerate in any form of retinitis pigmentosa due to a defect in a rod-specific gene.

***Clinical Findings in Rhodopsin-Related Dominant Retinitis Pigmentosa.*** As might be expected for defects in a rod-specific gene, rhodopsin mutations generally cause a more severe defect in rod function than in cone function in young patients, as measured by ERGs[195,196,226–229] (Fig. 235-8). In fact, one of the first reports of the more severe loss of rod ERG responses in some cases of autosomal dominant retinitis pigmentosa was based on a family now known to carry a rhodopsin mutation (*P23H*).[230] The decrease in rod ERG signal amplitudes in young patients correlates with the reduction in the amount of rhodopsin in the retina as measured by imaging fundus reflectometry.[231] Later in the disease most cones degenerate as well.

There are reports of histopathology from patients known to have one of the following defects in the rhodopsin gene: *P23H*,[8,52] *T17M*,[62] and *Q64X*.[64] In these cases there was a reduced number or absence of rods and a reduced number of cones with degenerating inner segments and absent outer segments.

The severity of the disease appears to correlate with specific mutations. In general, the severity of disease tends to be worse for mutations affecting residues in the cytoplasmic regions than in the intradiscal space, with an intermediate severity associated with mutations affecting residues in the transmembrane domains.[232] However, there is considerable intrafamilial variability,[8,9,196,228] so a rigorous analysis of visual field areas, ERG amplitudes, etc. including many affected patients with each mutation will be

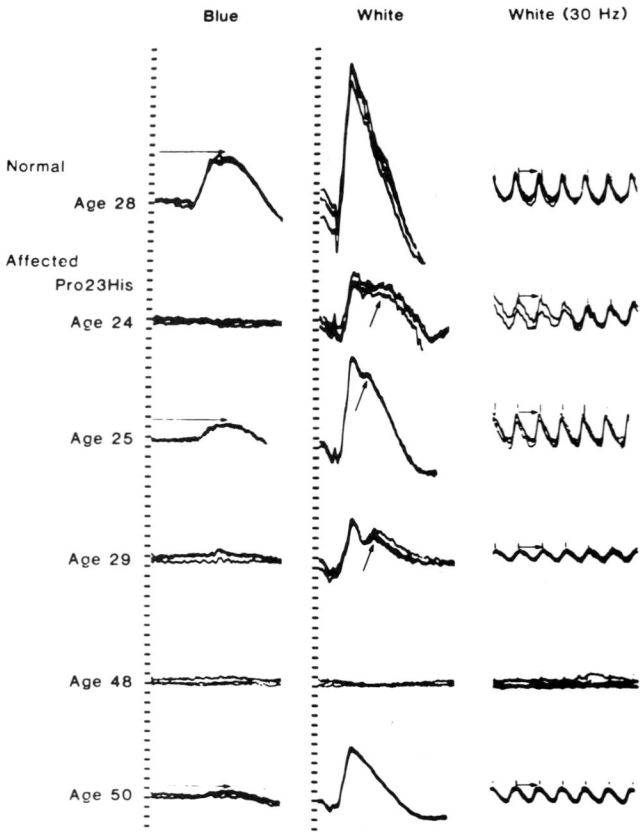

Blue     White     White (30 Hz)

Normal
Age 28

Affected
Pro23His
Age 24

Age 25

Age 29

Age 48

Age 50

**Fig. 235-8** ERGs of a normal individual (*top*) and five different patients with autosomal dominant retinitis pigmentosa due to a rhodopsin mutation (*P23H*). The tracings in the left-hand column are the responses to single flashes of blue light that is so dim that only rods are stimulated. The middle column shows the responses to bright white light flashes that stimulate both rods and cones. The right-hand column shows the responses to bright white light flashing 30 times per second; cones but not rods are able to show individual responses to light flashing at this high frequency. (In each tracing, two or three consecutive sweeps are superimposed.) Hence, going from the left to the right columns, one observes rod-isolated responses, combined rod and cone responses, and cone-isolated responses. Young patients with retinitis pigmentosa (24-, 25-, and 29-year-old patients) have dramatically reduced rod responses to dim blue light (*left column*) and reduced but biphasic responses to bright white light (*middle column*). The biphasic response is due to a delay in the response time of the rods. The arrows in the middle column point to the delayed rod-response peaks. This phenomenon is also observed in the left-hand column with the horizontal arrows that indicate rod response times. Cone responses (*right column*) are relatively normal in amplitude and timing (horizontal arrows) in the 24- and 25-year-old patients but reduced in amplitude and somewhat delayed in the 29-year-old patient. The 48-year-old patient with more advanced disease has markedly reduced rod, rod-plus-cone, and cone amplitudes. Interestingly, the 50-year-old affected patient (a sibling of the 48-year-old) has less severe degeneration, indicated here by ERG responses which, although abnormal, are clearly detectable. The calibration symbol in the lower right corner designates 50 ms horizontally and 100 mV vertically. (*From Berson et al.*[8] *Used by permission.*)

required to substantiate these clinical impressions. This sort of statistical analysis has been performed for two relatively common mutations, *P23H* and *P347L*. Patients with *P23H* have, on average, a larger ERG amplitude and patients with *P347L* have a smaller amplitude than patients with dominant retinitis pigmentosa without these mutations.[8,9] There has as yet been no prospective study of patients with rhodopsin mutations to determine if differences in severity are due to variation in the rate of

progression of the retinal degeneration, to variation in the level of photoreceptor function at birth, or to a combination of the two.

Most middle-aged patients with a dominant rhodopsin mutation show retinal degeneration and intraretinal pigmentation in all four quadrants of the fundus.[8,9,228] However, some clinicians report a preferential involvement of the inferior fundus in patients with *T17M*,[226,233] *P23H*,[82,234] *T58R*,[226,235] *G106R*,[236] or *G182S*.[233] The basis for this preferential involvement of the inferior fundus (which corresponds to the superior visual field) is unknown, although there is speculation that it is related to phototoxic effects, with the inferior fundus being exposed to and suffering from more intense overhead lighting.[82]

After exposure to bright light, rods lose their light sensitivity and require in a normal individual 20 to 40 minutes of complete darkness to regain their maximal sensitivity to light. Those patients with a dominant rhodopsin defect who retain some rod function typically take a longer time to dark-adapt. One group found that the rate of dark adaptation by rods and the time required for them to recover maximal sensitivity is allele-specific.[226,231] For example, patients with *T58R* recovered maximal sensitivity after 150 minutes in the dark, *P23H* after 3 to 6 hours, and *T17M* after 24 hours.[231]

***Recessive Rhodopsin Alleles Causing Retinitis Pigmentosa and Rod Dysfunction.*** A few recessive mutations in the rhodopsin gene have been reported. The first was found after a screen of over 100 families with recessive retinitis pigmentosa,[237] suggesting that recessive rhodopsin alleles are rare causes of retinitis pigmentosa. It was the nonsense mutation *E249X*, and it was found in the only affected member of a sibship that was the product of a consanguineous mating. Being a nonsense mutation, this allele may produce an unstable mRNA so that no mutant protein may be produced at all. If it were expressed, the mutant would be nonfunctional because it would have a truncated C-terminus and be missing the sixth and seventh transmembrane domains, including the Lys296 residue that is covalently linked to the chromophore 11-*cis*-retinal. The 29-year-old patient, who was a homozygote, had no rod function and reduced cone function detected by ERG.[237] Heterozygous carriers of this mutation (i.e., the parents and three siblings) had a slight reduction in the amplitude of the rod responses to dim flashes of light but normal rod responses to bright flashes of light. Similar ERG responses were recorded from unaffected individuals from another family without retinitis pigmentosa who were heterozygous for a different null mutation affecting the splice donor site of intron 4.[238] The findings in the unaffected heterozygote carriers of null rhodopsin alleles point to a subtle abnormality in rods predicted to have reduced amounts of rhodopsin. This phenotype may correspond to the shortened rod outer segments and very slow loss of photoreceptors found in transgenic mice heterozygous for a rhodopsin null allele.[239]

The missense mutation *E150K* was found to cosegregate with recessive retinitis pigmentosa in a consanguineous family with four affected siblings.[240] The mechanism by which this missense mutation is a recessive cause of retinitis pigmentosa remains obscure. The mutation is striking because all other missense rhodopsin mutations cause either dominant retinitis pigmentosa or dominant stationary night blindness or are nonpathogenic.

***Dominant Rhodopsin Alleles Causing Stationary Night Blindness.*** Two rhodopsin mutations have been discovered that cause stationary night blindness. Both are missense mutations (*A292E* and *G90D*), and both are dominant. The *A292E* rhodopsin, when coupled to a chromophore, produces a variant that responds normally to photons of light. However, *A292E* rhodopsin without a chromophore will still stimulate transducin, whereas wild-type opsin will not. It is documented that there normally is a constant physiologic turnover of chromophore in rod photoreceptors,[241] and it is likely that there is an interval of time when opsin is without a chromophore during this exchange. During this interval, *A292E* opsin would activate the phototransduction cascade. The length of the time *A292E* would lack a chromophore during each exchange is unknown. However, about a dozen activated opsin molecules appearing per second would be sufficient to desensitize a rod photoreceptor, based on the amount of light that is necessary to do the same in a normal subject.

The second rhodopsin mutation causing stationary night blindness, *G90D*, also has been studied experimentally, and a similar mechanism for the rod defect has been proposed. In addition, the chromophore in *G90D* rhodopsin apparently has an abnormally high rate of spontaneous isomerization (i.e., induced thermally rather than via photons). The actions of empty opsin and spontaneously isomerizing rhodopsin are equivalent to about 10 photoisomerizations per rod per second.[21] The rod desensitization is probably a consequence of the resulting constant stimulation of the phototransduction cascade like that proposed for the *A292E* rhodopsin.

Only one family has been found that segregates the *G90D* mutation.[21] Most affected members with *G90D* have normal cone ERGs. The combination of greatly reduced rod ERGs and normal cone ERGs is typical of stationary night blindness rather than the forms of retinitis pigmentosa caused by other dominant missense mutations of the rhodopsin gene. However, at least two members of the *G90D* pedigree, although asymptomatic, have reduced cone ERG amplitudes, and the older members have narrowed retinal vessels and some bone-spicule pigmentation in the fundus. Because of these signs, the phenotype caused by the *G90D* allele could be considered a very mild form of retinitis pigmentosa. However, the good subjective vision even in the elderly carriers with mild funduscopic stigmata of retinitis pigmentosa make it more practical to call the phenotype *stationary night blindness*, thereby categorizing it as a nonblinding retinal malfunction.

**Rod Transducin.** Transducin is the G-protein in photoreceptor cells that responds to photoactivated rhodopsin. It is a heterotrimeric protein; the α subunit is specific to photoreceptor cells, with rods and cones each expressing their own α subunit from separate genetic loci. The three-dimensional structure of the rod protein has been ascertained in both the GDP-bound and GTP-bound states.[242,243]

Only one pathogenic mutation has been reported in the gene encoding the α subunit of rod transducin (chromosome 3p21[244]); none has been reported as yet in the genes encoding the α subunit of cone transducin or the β or γ subunits of rod or cone transducin. The defect in rod α-transducin is the missense mutation *G38D* found as a cause of dominant stationary night blindness in one family originating in the town of Vendémian in southern France.[44] The disease is named after the affected founder, Jean Nougaret, a butcher who immigrated to the region in the seventeenth century.[39–41]

The glycine affected by the Nougaret mutation is in close proximity to the bound GTP/GDP moiety. Its strong conservation among G-proteins suggests that it has an important role in stabilizing bound GTP or facilitating the exchange of GTP for GDP. The glycine at the homologous position in distantly related ras proteins is frequently found to be mutant in a variety of cancers.[245–248] Changing this glycine in ras proteins or in the more closely related G-protein Gsα produces mutants that are overactive due to diminished inherent GTPase activity or to a reduced ability to respond to GTPase-activating proteins, called GAPs.[249] There are as yet no reports of analyses of *G38D* transducin in vitro to determine if it is also constitutively active through deranged GTPase activity or through other mechanisms. Such a functional defect would be consistent with the observed night blindness in patients with the Nougaret mutation, since constitutive activity of the mutant transducin would desensitize rod photoreceptors in a manner equivalent to constant background light. In fact, with careful measurement of dark-adaptation rates and ERGs, one can

document that rods are present and are functional in patients with the Nougaret form of night blindness. However, the rods respond only to high ambient light intensities at which cones are also sensitive.[47] This reduction in rod sensitivity and the ERG findings can be simulated in normal individuals by adapting them to light of moderate intensity.[47]

**Rod cGMP Phosphodiesterase.** Activated rod transducin will activate the next member of the phototransduction cascade, cGMP phosphodiesterase. In rods, cGMP phosphodiesterase is a tetrameric protein with enzymatically active α and β subunits and two inhibitory γ subunits. The genes encoding the α and β subunits are on chromosomes 5q31.2-34 and 4p16.3, respectively,[250,251] and encode proteins with similar sequences. Recessive, presumably null mutations in both genes have been found in patients with retinitis pigmentosa.[252–258] Roughly 2 to 4 percent of patients with recessive retinitis pigmentosa have defects in the gene encoding the β subunit[255,259]; mutations affecting the α subunit also account for a small percentage of cases.[260]

Naturally arising nonsense mutations in three animal models of retinitis pigmentosa have defects in rod cGMP phosphodiesterase. The retinal degeneration (*rd*) mouse[261] and the rod/cone dysplasia (*rcd*-1) Irish setter dog have defects in the gene encoding the β subunit,[262–264] and the Cardigan Welsh Corgi dog has a defect in the gene encoding the α subunit.[265] Before their demise, the photoreceptors in the animal models with β-subunit mutations have very high levels of cGMP,[266,267] probably as a consequence of reduced or absent basal phosphodiesterase activity.[268] These high cGMP levels are toxic.[269] This toxicity may be related to the effect of cGMP on the cGMP-gated cation channels in the plasma membrane or on other metabolic pathways. With regard to the cation channels, it should be noted that in a normal retina only a few percent of the channels are open in the dark when cGMP levels are maximal.[270] It is the closure of this small proportion of channels that hyperpolarizes the plasma membrane in the light. With abnormally high cGMP levels in retinas with no phosphodiesterase, a high proportion of cation channels should be open, presumably causing a huge and fatal influx of cations.

Patients with recessive retinitis pigmentosa due to deficient cGMP phosphodiesterase, because of either a defective α or β subunit, recall no night vision from early childhood. Their ERGs show no rod component and a markedly reduced and delayed cone component.[252,258] Their visual deterioration is a consequence of the gradual degeneration of the cone photoreceptors through mechanisms that remain obscure, especially since the rod α and β subunits of phosphodiesterase are not expressed by cones. Cones have instead a cGMP-phosphodiesterase complex composed of two identical active subunits, each called α′, and two cone-specific inhibitory γ subunits. No defects in the genes encoding these cone proteins have yet been reported in humans.

A single dominant mutation, *H258N*, has been described in the rod β-posphodiesterase gene.[45] It was found in a large Danish family with dominantly inherited stationary night blindness with clinical features very similar to those found in Nougaret night blindness due to rod trandsucin mutation (see above).[46] The biochemical mechanism for reduced rod sensitivity caused by the β-phosphodiesterase mutation is unknown, but a constitutive phosphodiesterase activity mimicking constant light exposure has been proposed.[45]

No pathogenetic defects in the gene encoding the inhibitory γ subunit of rod cGMP phosphodiesterase, assigned to chromosome 17q21.1,[271] have been discovered in humans with retinal degeneration.[272] However, knockout of the gene in transgenic mice produces a retinal degeneration with features similar to those found in the *rd* mouse, including elevated cytoplasmic cGMP levels in the degenerating retina.[273] The high cytoplasmic levels of cGMP are not expected if the function of the γ subunit is solely to inhibit the α and β subunits.

A protein that aids in the solubilization of the α-β-γ₂ phosphodiesterase complex has been discovered recently.[274]

It is named the $\delta$ subunit of rod cGMP phosphodiesterase and is encoded by a gene on chromosome 2q36.[275] This gene has not been implicated as a cause of any photoreceptor disease.

**The Rod cGMP-Gated Cation Channel.** The cGMP-gated channels in the plasma membrane of the outer segments of rod photoreceptors respond to changes in cytoplasmic cGMP. In the dark-adapted retina, cGMP levels are high, and a few percent of the cation channels are open.[270] On activation of phosphodiesterase in the light, cytoplasmic cGMP levels decrease, and the proportion of cation channels that are open decreases. This causes an increase in the polarization of the plasma membrane that is transmitted to the synaptic region of the photoreceptor, where it decreases the release of neurotransmitter.

The channels are composed of an $\alpha$ and a $\beta$ subunit encoded by genes on chromosomes 4p14-q13 and 16q13, respectively.[276,277] Null mutations in the gene encoding the $\alpha$ subunit lead to autosomal recessive retinitis pigmentosa. Only 3 families with mutations in this gene were gleaned from a set of 173 that were screened, indicating that this gene probably accounts for less than 2 percent of recessive retinitis pigmentosa cases.[278] Null mutations leading to absent functional channels may derange the physiology of rod photoreceptors by causing a presumably deleterious hyperpolarization of the plasma membrane. Affected patients report no night vision from early childhood, suggesting that the rod photoreceptors are malfunctional or degenerate before or soon after birth; cone photoreceptors degenerate later. No dominant mutations have been reported in the gene encoding the rod $\alpha$ subunit. No surveys of patients for mutations in the rod $\beta$ subunit gene have been published.

**The Cone cGMP-Gated Cation Channel.** Cone photoreceptors have a cGMP-gated cation channel encoded on chromosome 2q11 that is similar in amino acid sequence to the $\alpha$ subunit of the rod cGMP-gated cation channel. Patients with loss-of-function defects in this gene have no cone function but normal rod function, a disease called *rod monochromacy* or *achromatopsia*[279] (see Chap. 238). It is not known if the absent cone function is accompanied by degeneration of the cone photoreceptors. Rod photoreceptors function normally.

**Rhodopsin Kinase and Rod Arrestin.** These two proteins act in sequence to deactivate rhodopsin to stop the phototransduction cascade. Rhodopsin kinase recognizes photoactivated rhodopsin and phosphorylates serine and threonine residues near rhodopsin's C-terminus.[280,281] Arrestin forms a complex with phosphorylated rhodopsin, and this complex prevents further interaction of the activated rhodopsin with transducin. Rhodopsin kinase and rod arrestin are encoded by genes on chromosomes 13q34 and 2q37, respectively.[282,283]

Absence of either protein through recessive mutations causes Oguchi disease, a form of night blindness.[284-286] Rod malfunction arises because without either rhodopsin kinase or arrestin, photoactivated rhodopsin continues to activate transducin until it loses its photoisomerized chromophore, all-*trans*-retinal. After a human retina is exposed to light, photoactivated rhodopsin is regenerated with 11-*cis*-retinal according to an exponential function with a half-life of about 4 to 7 minutes.[287-289] Even if only a few percent of the 40 million rhodopsin molecules in each rod are bleached, it can take more than 2 hours for complete regeneration.[290] In the meantime, without phosphorylation and binding to arrestin, the remaining unregenerated rhodopsin molecules continue to activate the phototransduction cascade, thereby desensitizing the rods as if they were being exposed to a constant background light. In fact, patients with Oguchi disease can recover rod sensitivity after dark adaptation for a few hours.[286,290] After this time, they can see dim lights and their rod ERG response to a single flash of light will be normal in amplitude and timing. However, no ERG response to a second light flash will be recordable until another prolonged period of dark adaptation has ensued.

Rhodopsin kinase is present in cone photoreceptors as well as rod photoreceptors, and it appears that it is the G-protein-coupled receptor kinase that phosphorylates activated cone opsin. One would expect that patients with Oguchi disease due to a nonfunctional rhodopsin kinase should have a defect in cone function. In fact, a subtle abnormality in the recovery of cone function after a bleaching light was detected in a patient with Oguchi disease homozygous for a null mutation in the rhodopsin kinase gene.[286] A more severe, subjectively discernible abnormality of cone function did not occur, possibly because cones may rapidly replace isomerized chromophore, thereby decreasing the need for deactivation of cone opsin through phosphorylation and arrestin binding.

There is one other rather distinctive feature of Oguchi disease. While the color of the fundus is normal after prolonged dark adaptation, the color of the fundus changes to a dark or golden hue after a few minutes in the light. The reason for the color change, called the *Mizuo phenomenon*, is not known with certainty. Some authors speculate that it is due to elevated extracellular potassium levels generated in the retina in response to an excessive stimulation of rod photoreceptors.[291]

The few patients reported in the literature with recessive, presumably null mutations in the rhodopsin kinase gene have Oguchi disease with no signs of photoreceptor degeneration.[285,286] However, some patients with null mutations in the arrestin gene exhibit a photoreceptor degeneration similar to retinitis pigmentosa in addition to the prolonged dark adaptation and Mizuo phenomenon that are characteristic of Oguchi disease.[75,76,83] Other patients homozygous for the same mutation are reported to have Oguchi disease without retinitis pigmentosa. It remains a mystery why retinitis pigmentosa develops in some patients. Little insight into this question has come from animal models. Elimination of the function of arrestin in *Drosophila* uniformly causes a photoreceptor degeneration that depends on exposure to light.[167] A report of transgenic mice lacking arrestin did not mention fundus color or whether the photoreceptors degenerated over time.[292]

**Guanylate Cyclase.** Rod and cone photoreceptor cells make their own specific versions of most of the proteins in the phototransduction cascade. The diseases caused by defects in the rod versions that are discussed above are either rod-specific (e.g., stationary night blindness) or cause forms of retinitis pigmentosa with early loss of rod photoreceptors and later, secondary loss of cone photoreceptors. In contrast, both rods and cones seem to use the same guanylate cyclase,[293] the enzyme responsible for replacing cGMP that is lost during activation of the phototransduction cascade. Loss-of-function mutations in this gene, found on chromosome 17p13.1,[294] would be expected to affect both photoreceptor types, and discovery of patients with recessive mutations in this gene have borne out this expectation. These patients have a form of Leber congenital amaurosis.[295] The *rd* chicken, a naturally arising animal model of retinal degeneration, also has a defect in the retinal guanylate cyclase gene.[296] Dominant missense mutations also have been reported in families with cone-rod dystrophy.[297,298]

One presumes that the absence of guanylate cyclase in humans with congenital amaurosis or in the *rd* chicken strain produces extremely low levels of cGMP that fatally interfere with the physiology of rod and cone outer segments, perhaps through a greatly reduced abundance of open cGMP-gated cation channels in the plasma membrane. The dominant missense mutations causing cone-rod dystrophy are possibly hypomorphic or dominant-negative alleles inducing a phenotype less severe than congenital amaurosis.

**Guanylate Cyclase Activator 1A.** This photoreceptor protein stimulates guanylate cyclase when cytoplasmic calcium levels are low, perhaps thereby serving a role in light adaptation.[299,300] It is encoded by a gene on chromosome 6p21.1.[301] A missense change in this gene causes dominantly inherited cone dystrophy in one reported family,[302] probably by activating guanylate cyclase even when calcium concentrations are high in the dark.[303,304]

## RETINAL DISEASE CAUSED BY DEFECTS IN OTHER IDENTIFIED GENES

### X-Linked Retinitis Pigmentosa (*RPGR* and *RP2*)

There are at least three retinitis pigmentosa genes on the X chromosome. In the chronological order in which they were mapped, the loci are *RP2*, *RP3*, and *RP15*, and they are within Xp11.3, Xp21.1, and Xp22.13-22.11, respectively. The unidentified *RP15* gene is remarkable because female carriers uniformly have signs and symptoms of retinitis pigmentosa, although they have less severe disease than their affected male relatives.[132] This feature prompted its designation as an X-linked dominant trait.

A positional cloning approach was used to identify *RP2* and *RP3*.[305–307] The *RP3* gene was found first. It is now named *RPGR* (retinitis pigmentosa GTPase regulator) because of sequence similarity with the guanine nucleotide exchange factor RCC1. It is found in the Golgi complex and is expressed in many tissues including the neural retina and the retinal pigment epithelium.[306,308] Its function is unknown. Many mutations found in this gene are obviously null, such as frameshift, nonsense, and intron splice-site mutations. Mutations in *RPGR* are found in only about 20 percent of patients with X-linked retinitis pigmentosa.[309,310] This is surprising low considering that prior linkage studies pointed to the *RP3* gene as accounting for a majority of X-linked families. There is speculation that another retinitis pigmentosa gene may be nearby or that one or more unevaluated regions of the *RPGR* gene may be frequently mutant.

*RP2* was the second X-linked retinitis pigmentosa gene to be identified. It codes for an ubiquitously expressed 350-amino-acid protein with weak homology to a protein, cofactor C, important in the folding of β-tubulin.[305] The proportion of patients with X-linked retinitis pigmentosa due to mutations in this gene is unknown.

### ABCR

The *ABCR* gene, found within chromosome 1p13, was first identified as being responsible for recessively inherited Stargardt disease.[311] This is a hereditary degeneration of the macula of the retina. Affected individuals with Stargardt disease typically suffer a severe loss of central vision in adolescence and adulthood (see Chap. 243). A characteristic feature of the disease is the accumulation of large amounts of lipofuscin in retinal pigment epithelial cells. The lipofuscin interferes with the light wavelengths used for fluorescein angiography of the retina, creating what is termed the *dark choroid phenomenon*. Missense, frameshift, and splice-site mutations have been found in the *ABCR* gene in patients with Stargardt disease.[311–313,327]

Some individuals with mutations in this gene develop a panretinal degeneration that has been called retinitis pigmentosa.[314,315] However, these patients have early, severe involvement of the macula, so the term *inverse retinitis pigmentosa* or, even better, *severe cone-rod dystrophy* is preferable. The mutations found in the patients with cone-rod dystrophy were either splice-site mutations or frameshifts. It remains unknown why these mutations cause a phenotype more severe than Stargardt disease. Research into the possible role of the *ABCR* gene in age-related macular degeneration is discussed in Chap. 243.

The protein product is found in rod photoreceptor outer segments. Its function is unknown, but its similarities to ATP-binding cassette transporters,[311] its phosphorylation in light,[316] and its position in the rim region of rod outer segment disk

membranes[317–319] have prompted speculation that it has some direct or indirect role in phototransduction.

### Cellular Retinal Binding Protein (CRALBP)

CRALBP is a carrier protein for 11-*cis*-retinol and/or 11-*cis*-retinal.[320] These vitamin A-related compounds (also referred to as *retinoids*) are important to the physiology of vision, particularly because 11-*cis*-retinal forms the light-sensitive chromophore in both rhodopsin and the cone opsins. CRALBP is found in the retinal pigment epithelium and the Müller cells of the retina but not in other retinal cell types. The gene, encoded on chromosome 15q26,[321] has been found to be mutant in the affected siblings in one family with recessive retinitis pigmentosa.[139] The missense change interfered with the protein's ability to form a complex with 11-*cis*-retinal. A distinctive feature of these cases is that young patients have yellow flecks at the level of the retinal pigment epithelium seen by funduscopy (i.e., the diagnosis is retinitis punctata albescens).

### RPE65

The *RPE65* gene, mapped to chromosome 1p31,[322] encodes a nonglycosylated protein present exclusively in the cytoplasm of the retinal pigment epithelium.[184,323] Its function is not known, but there is speculation that it has a role in the synthesis or metabolism of retinoids, since its amino acid sequence shows similarities to plant dioxygenases that metabolize carotenoids.[185]

Some patients with recessive mutations of this gene have severe retinal degeneration and are blind within the first few years of life.[324,325] Others lose vision during the first two decades of life and exhibit the funduscopic features of retinitis pigmentosa.[325,326] The two categories of patients have been diagnosed as having Leber congenital amaurosis or severe retinitis pigmentosa, respectively. The difference is not likely to indicate two separate phenotypes but rather may reflect a range in severity of retinal degeneration that may correlate with residual function of one or both recessive mutant alleles. Most patients with Leber congenital amaurosis have two likely null alleles (frameshift, nonsense, or splice-site mutations), whereas those with severe retinitis pigmentosa have at least one missense allele that is likely a hypomorphic allele. Confirmation of this conjecture will await a better understanding of the function of RPE65.

The *RPE65* gene accounts for about 2 percent of cases with recessive retinitis pigmentosa and roughly 16 percent of congenital amaurosis.[325]

### TULP1

The *tubby* strain of mouse carries a naturally arising mutation causing photoreceptor degeneration, deafness, and obesity.[328–330] The responsible mouse gene was identified in 1996.[331,332] Its function remains unknown. No pathogenetic mutations have been reported to date in the human homologue of *tubby*. However, there is a family of related proteins, called *tubby-like proteins* (TULPs). One member of this family is called TULP1. It is encoded by a gene on human chromosome 6p21.3 and is expressed specifically in retina and testis.[333] Recessive mutations in the *TULP1* gene have been found in a few unrelated families with recessive retinitis pigmentosa, two of which are from the Dominican Republic.[334–336] Based on a survey of patients with recessive retinitis pigmentosa derived mostly from the United States and Canada, the *TULP1* gene appears to account for less than 1 percent of cases. The function of TULP1 in the retina is unknown.

### CRX

The human *CRX* gene, assigned to chromosome 19q13, encodes a transcription factor of the homeobox type that has a role in the development, differentiation, and maintenance of rod and cone photoreceptors.[337,338] The factor recognizes a DNA sequence found in the promoter region of many photoreceptor-specific genes such as the β subunit of rod cGMP phosphodiesterase, rod arrestin, and interphotoreceptor retinoid-binding protein. Dominant mutations in the gene cause cone-rod degeneration[339,340] or Leber congenital amaurosis.[341] It is not known why different mutations cause the different clinically defined phenotypes. The mutations appear to be comparable in that frameshifts deleting the C-terminal region can cause either phenotype. Perhaps the mutations differ only in severity, with the cases of Leber congenital amaurosis representing one extreme of cone-rod degeneration in which cones and rods degenerate within the first few months of life. The observation that the patients with Leber congenital amaurosis were isolated cases each with a heterozygous, *de novo* mutation prompted speculation that other factors in addition to the primary mutation may be required to produce that severe phenotype.[341]

## L-Type Calcium Channel

Incomplete stationary night blindness inherited as an X-linked recessive trait is due to mutations in an L-type calcium channel. The role of this protein in cellular physiology is unknown. The protein is found in photoreceptor cells and in cells of the inner nuclear layer of the retina.[145,146] The gene is within Xp11.23.

## RDS

The *RDS* gene product, also called peripherin/RDS, is a glycoprotein found in the rims of rod and cone outer segment disks.[342,343] Two converging paths led to its identification. One was the result of studies of a spontaneously arising murine model of retinitis pigmentosa, named the *rds* strain for *retinal degeneration slow*.[344] Travis et al.[345] used an mRNA subtractive hybridization technique to isolate a cDNA sequence corresponding to the wild-type allele at the murine *rds* locus. The encoded protein was predicted to contain 346 amino acid residues. The mutant *rds* allele is a null mutation caused by the insertion of a 9.2-kb extraneous murine sequence into the open reading frame.[346] Concurrently and independently, Molday et al.[347] studied a 39-kDa protein found in the peripheral (rim) region of the outer segment disks (hence the name *peripherin*) that was identified on the basis of its reaction with monoclonal antibodies. The monoclonal antibodies were used to isolate the corresponding bovine cDNA sequence.[348] Bovine RDS is also composed of 346 residues and has an amino acid sequence that is 92.5 percent identical to the murine protein,[349] a congruity that lead to the realization that the proteins were the same (with amino acid differences due to species variation).

The RDS protein exists in outer segments as a glycosylated dimer, with the two molecules linked by one or more disulfide bonds. The dimer forms a noncovalent complex with itself to form a homotetramer or, alternatively, forms a complex with a dimer of the related protein ROM1 (a protein discussed below). Both the RDS and ROM1 proteins have four hydrophobic regions each thought to traverse the disk membrane and a conserved glycosylation site in the large loop between third and fourth transmembrane domains. The precise structure of the tetrameric complex remains unknown. The complex is believed to have a role in maintaining the structure of the outer segment disks.[342,348,350]

**Dominant Peripherin/RDS Alleles Causing Retinitis Pigmentosa and Other Retinal Degenerations.** All the mutations reported in the human *RDS* gene, encoded on chromosome 6p21.1-cen,[351] are dominant, and all cause a panretinal malfunction, as evidenced by abnormalities in the full-field ERG. Most mutations have been found in patients with cone-rod dystrophy or a related disease that causes early degeneration of the macula and loss of central visual acuity. Some of these patients have subretinal deposits of a yellow or yellow-white substance that is seen by funduscopy; if so, the diagnosis has been termed *butterfly-shaped macular dystrophy, pattern dystrophy*, or *vitelliform dystrophy*. Among patients with a cone-rod degeneration or macular degeneration, there is no obvious correlation between the type of mutation and the specific diagnosis, since there are families in which different diagnoses have been given to the affected relatives

with the same mutation.[10,352,353] A minority of mutations has been found in patients with typical retinitis pigmentosa where rod function is lost first and cone function and central visual acuity later.[134,354,355] Some of the patients with this pattern of photoreceptor degeneration also have subretinal deposits early in the disease, and the diagnosis thus becomes retinitis punctata albescens.[136] Among patients with retinitis pigmentosa, the *RDS* gene accounts for about 3 to 4 percent of cases.[134]

The variably present subretinal deposits remain an enigma. By funduscopy, they appear to be within or adjacent to the retinal pigment epithelium. They have not been reported in the *rds* strain of mice, and histopathologic studies of the deposits in humans with *RDS* mutations also have not been reported.

It remains unclear why certain *RDS* mutations more severely affect cones and others more severely affect rods. It possibly could be a consequence of some residual function of the mutant allele, with those alleles causing retinitis pigmentosa being hypomorphs. This speculation springs from the observation that almost all mutations causing retinitis pigmentosa are missense mutations or short in-frame single-codon deletions. In contrast, a large fraction, perhaps 30 to 50 percent, of mutations causing cone-rod degeneration are nonsense mutations, frameshift mutations, or large deletions that are likely to be nulls.

## ROM1

The *ROM1* gene within chromosome band 11q13 was encountered first by McInnes et al.[356] during a search for genes expressed specifically in the retina. It encodes a protein that is similar to RDS in sequence and predicted structure. As discussed in the section on the *RDS* gene above, the ROM1 and RDS proteins form a tetrameric complex at the rim region of photoreceptor outer segment disk membranes,[357] and it is hypothesized that this complex may have an important role in creating the structure of the disk, possibly by promoting the bend in the disk membrane at the rim region. In view of the role of the *RDS* gene in some retinal degenerations, a number of investigations have been published searching for photoreceptor diseases that may be induced by mutations in the *ROM1* gene. Missense and frameshift mutations have been found in a handful of families with retinitis pigmentosa, but in most cases there were examples of unaffected relatives without retinal degeneration or the respective families were so small that a meaningful segregation analysis was impossible.[358–360] One missense change, *A118G*, ultimately was categorized as a nonpathogenic polymorphism found only in blacks.[134]

**Digenic Retinitis Pigmentosa.** While there is no strong evidence that defects in *ROM1* alone can cause monogenic retinitis pigmentosa or an allied disease, there are reports of families in which affected members all have defects in both *ROM1* and *RDS*. In all these families, the mutation in *RDS* is the missense change *L185P*. This mutation is found heterozygously in every affected member, but it is also found in many unaffected individuals. The factor that distinguishes affected from unaffected carriers of the *RDS-L185P* change is that the affected carriers also have a heterozygous *ROM1* mutation. In three of the reported families, the *ROM1* changes are frameshift mutations likely to produce null alleles,[133] whereas in the fourth family it is a missense change (*G113E*).[134]

The requirement for double heterozygosity creates what is called a *digenic inheritance pattern* (Fig. 235-9). Since the *RDS* and *ROM1* genes are on separate chromosomes, the mutations segregate independently. Affected individuals, who are termed *double heterozygotes*, can pass both mutations to their offspring. The resulting parent-to-child transmission mimics a dominant inheritance pattern except that the transmission ratio is 25 percent rather than 50 percent. Another distinctive feature in each family is that the disease begins in the offspring of a mating of unaffected individuals, with one parent carrying the *RDS*-L185P mutation and the other a *ROM1* mutation. Thus the first two

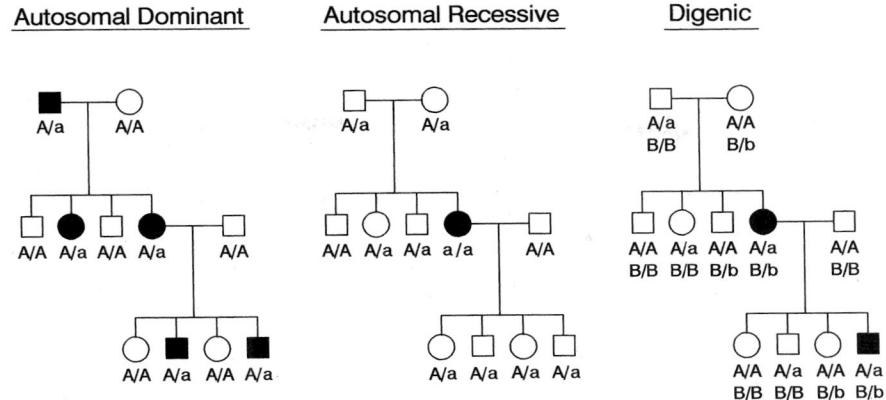

**Fig. 235-9** Comparison of autosomal dominant, autosomal recessive, and digenic inheritance in retinitis pigmentosa. The first two generations of the idealized digenic pedigree mimic the autosomal recessive pedigree because unaffected parents have affected offspring and because the ratio of affected to unaffected offspring is 25 percent. In the second to third generations of the digenic pedigree, there is direct parent-to-child transmission, similar to what is seen in the dominant pedigree, but the transmission ratio is 25 percent rather than 50 percent. These features are due to the requirement in a digenic disease that affected individuals be double heterozygotes. Uppercase letters designate wild-type alleles, and lowercase letters designate mutant alleles.

generations simulate a recessive inheritance pattern, with parents being unaffected and 25 percent of offspring being affected on average.

Studies of the *RDS* and *ROM1* mutations found in these families point to an explanation for the digenic inheritance pattern.[361] Wild-type RDS can form either a homotetrameric complex or a heterotetrameric complex consisting of two RDS and two ROM1 molecules. ROM1 is unable to form homotetramers, so wild-type photoreceptors have a mixture of homotetramers composed only of RDS molecules and heterotetamers composed of RDS plus ROM1 molecules. The mutant RDS-L185P protein is unable to form a homotetrameric complex and therefore requires ROM1 for a functional complex. According to the proposed model, as long as there are two functional *ROM1* alleles, an individual heterozygous for an *RDS-L185P* allele will have sufficient ROM1 to produce the functional complexes necessary to support photoreceptors. However, if a carrier of *RDS-L185P* has only one functional *ROM1* allele, there is a deficit of functional complexes, and photoreceptor degeneration results.

The occurrence of phenotypes in double heterozygotes of two unlinked genes has been observed in fruit flies,[362] nematodes,[363] and yeast.[364] The phenomenon is called *nonallelic noncomplementation* rather than digenic inheritance because parent-to-offspring transmission is usually not studied. Instead, the double heterozygotes are the offspring produced by mating individuals that are homozygous for mutations at different loci during experiments designed to define complementation groups. Most genes complement each other, so a cross of homozygotes for two different genes yields double heterozygotes that have the wild-type phenotype. Certain pairs of genes do not complement each other (hence the term *nonallelic noncomplementation*), and the double heterozygote offspring are affected. Like the *RDS* and *ROM1* genes, a feature shared by the noncomplementing genes in these species is that the members of each gene pair encode proteins that interact with each other, usually by forming a polymeric complex.

The term *digenic inheritance* has been applied in other instances where individuals with mutations in two different genes develop a phenotype not associated with either gene alone. The genotype showing the trait may not necessarily be double heterozygous. For example, mice develop spina bifida if they are both homozygous for a recessive *undulated* allele (a genotype that by itself causes a kinky tail) and heterozygous for a dominant *Patch* allele (which alone causes a patchy coat pattern).[365]

## MYOSIN VIIa AND OTHER GENES CAUSING USHER SYNDROME

Linkage analyses show that there are at least six different genes causing Usher syndrome type I,[93,96,97,99,366] one causing Usher syndrome type II,[367] and one causing Usher syndrome type III.[368] The unidentified Usher syndrome type I gene on chromosome 11p15 is noteworthy because alleles at nearby marker loci are the same in all affected patients, suggesting that a single mutation is responsible for all cases and that all affected individuals descend from a single ancestor who carried this mutation.[96]

The first Usher gene identified is one that causes type I disease (retinitis pigmentosa with profound congenital deafness and vestibular ataxia).[97] The gene, on chromosome 11q13.5, encodes myosin VIIa. Myosins are proteins with mechanochemical functions and are categorized into two groups, called *conventional myosins* and *unconventional myosins*.[369] The myosins in both groups have a head domain that can bind actin and move along an actin chain while hydrolyzing ATP. The groups differ in their tail domains. Conventional myosins are those with a tail structure similar to that found in myosin II, the most-well known myosin that works with actin to create motion in skeletal muscle, smooth muscle, and cardiac muscle. The tails of conventional myosins form filamentous dimers. The tails of unconventional myosins do not ordinarily form filaments. Both types are thought to be involved in the movement of cells or in the translocation of intracellular components. Myosin VIIa is an unconventional myosin.

The pathogenic mutations reported in the human myosin VIIa gene are all recessive and appear to be null mutations.[370–372] Recessive mutations of the murine homologue produces *shaker* mice with deafness and vestibular disease but no retinal degeneration.[373] The absence of retinal degeneration in the *shaker* mice may be due to differences in the retinal cell types expressing myosin VIIa. In humans the protein is in both the photoreceptors and the retinal pigment epithelium, whereas in mice it is only in the retinal pigment epithelium.[374,375] However, this explanation is not so clear-cut, since there are reports of patients with nonsyndromic deafness (i.e., without retinitis pigmentosa) due to recessive mutations in the myosin VIIa gene.[376,377] It is unknown why some recessive myosin VIIa mutations cause Usher syndrome type I and others only deafness.

The precise function of myosin VIIa is unknown. In the cochlea it is present in the inner and outer hair cells.[375,378] In human retinal pigment epithelium, it is found in the apexes of the cells, where it is necessary for the localization of melanin granules to that region.[379] In human photoreceptor cells, it is found in the connecting cilia between inner and outer segments.[380] It is also found in other human tissues such as lung, kidney, and testis,[381] where it may have no vital function, since no disease of these tissues is evident in patients with myosin VIIa mutations.

## USH2A

The Usher II gene within chromosome 1q41 accounts for about half of all cases of Usher syndrome. It codes for a protein of 1550 amino acids, including a presumed signal sequence at the N-terminus.[367] The protein has an amino acid sequence suggesting that it is an extracellular cell adhesion molecule or matrix protein. It is expressed in the retina and in other tissues. The reported pathogenic mutations are frameshifts that are likely to result in null alleles.[367]

## CARE AND THERAPY OF PATIENTS

**Limitations in Driving Motor Vehicles.** Patients with retinitis pigmentosa appear to have a higher than normal chance of having an accident while driving a motor vehicle.[382] There are anecdotal reports of patients with stationary night blindness being involved in motor vehicle accidents at night.[383] In some cases, visual function may be sufficiently compromised that a patient must be advised to drive only during the day or not to drive at all even if the vision meets legal technical requirements. Particular attention should be given to loss of peripheral vision in retinitis pigmentosa.[384] Some patients may need to be reminded that visual aides such as a night scope do not provide sufficient peripheral visual field to permit safe driving.

**Medical Therapies.** A randomized, blinded study of 601 adult patients with the common forms of retinitis pigmentosa or Usher syndrome found that an oral supplement of vitamin A palmitate (15,000 IU/d) reduced the average rate of retinal degeneration as monitored by the cone ERG.[7] The authors of this study also observed a nonstatistically significant trend suggesting that vitamin E supplements were deleterious. Based on these results, many ophthalmologists recommend that adults with retinitis pigmentosa take daily vitamin A supplements, that they avoid vitamin E supplements, and that they otherwise eat a balanced diet. Patients on this regimen should be followed periodically to be sure the vitamin A supplements do not cause liver damage, although such a side effect has only been reported in patients taking much larger doses.[385]

Oral vitamin A also has been found to ameliorate night blindness present in patients with Sorsby macular dystrophy[386] (see Chap. 243). Parenteral vitamin A is therapeutic for the retinal degeneration that develops in patients with abetalipoproteinemia[88] (see Chap. 115), and of course, parenteral or oral vitamin A cures patients with night blindness and reduced visual acuity due to dietary insufficiency of vitamin A, if given soon enough.[387] Vitamin E supplements are beneficial for patients with retinal degeneration due to a deficiency in α-tocopherol transfer protein.[90]

Carbonic anhydrase inhibitors such as acetazolamide or methazolamide have been reported to ameliorate temporarily the cystoid macular edema that reduces central vision in some patients with retinitis pigmentosa,[17,18] although this drug can have serious side effects.[388,389] A night vision scope can help to alleviate the symptom of night blindness in some patients with retinitis pigmentosa,[390] and it may be beneficial to some patients with stationary night blindness.

There are therapeutic diets for patients with gyrate atrophy (see Chap. 83) or Refsum disease (see Chap. 132).

**Reduction in Light Exposure.** There are anecdotal reports of patients claiming a noticeable decrease in their vision after exposure to bright light. Studies of animal models with hereditary retinal degeneration, such as the *RCS* rat,[391] fruit flies with a dominant rhodopsin allele,[392] or transgenic mice with a dominant rhodopsin gene defect,[393,394] indicate that decreasing light exposure slows the course of retinal degeneration. For these reasons, many ophthalmologists recommend sunglasses for patients with retinitis pigmentosa, although there is no proof that this practice is beneficial in humans. In fact, a study of two patients who wore a light-occluding contact lens unilaterally for 5 years did not experience an increase or decrease in the rate of retinal degeneration in the treated eyes.[395] However, that study included too few patients to be conclusive on this matter. Perhaps light reduction helps only patients with certain gene defects, and the two patients in the light-deprivation study did not have those defects. In this regard, it should be noted that one of those patients is now known to have digenic retinitis pigmentosa due to mutations in the *RDS* and *ROM1* genes.[134]

**Highly Speculative Therapies.** Some other proposed treatments for retinitis pigmentosa have received publicity in the popular news media but have not been studied in a controlled, blinded fashion to determine if they are beneficial, deleterious, or of no consequence. Many have not even been tested in laboratory animals to determine their safety or efficacy. Examples are intramuscular injections of a poorly described mixture including yeast RNA in Russia,[396] a series of exposures to hyperbaric oxygen in France (the details of which have not been reported in the medical literature), or an obscurely described regimen including electric stimulation, exposure of patient's blood to ozone, and ocular surgery in Cuba.[397–400] Patients who choose to take such highly supposititious therapies are urged to have pre- and post-treatment evaluations including ERGs by an unbiased ophthalmologist to determine if there is an adverse effect. With regard to the Cuban treatment, an objective evaluation of a group of patients could not discern a significant difference in retinal disease before and after treatment[397]; in addition, there is a report of patients who received this therapy who developed iatrogenic diplopia from extraocular movement disorders.[400]

**Work on Future Therapies.** There is much present-day research aimed at developing new therapies for retinitis pigmentosa. One approach is to use adenoviral vectors or other gene-transfer methods to transfer therapeutic genes to photoreceptor cells or the retinal pigment epithelium. To be therapeutic, the transferred genes could code for wild-type versions of those inactivated by recessive mutations,[401] for survival factors such as basic fibroblast growth factor,[402] for antiapoptosis factors such as bcl-x,[392,403,404] or for ribozymes that will specifically attack mutant mRNA from a dominant allele.[405] Another approach is to design and develop a electronic microchip that might stimulate either bipolar cells or ganglion cells to mimic the signals that these neurons normally produce.[406] Finally, there has been work directed at developing protocols to permit the transplantation of fragments of retina obtained from cadavers or from human fetuses. All these methods are currently beset with problems to be overcome before they can be applied to patients.

## ACKNOWLEDGMENTS

I thank members of my laboratory for careful reading of the manuscript and numerous helpful suggestions, especially T. McGee, M. Athanas, and C. Briggs, and special thanks to my close colleague E. L. Berson for many years of informal education and formal research collaboration. T. McGee and L. Mikula produced many of the figures. I also gratefully acknowledge support from NIH Grants EY08683 and EY11655 and a fellowship from the *Ministere de l'Education Nationale, de la Recherche et de la Technologie* of France. Much of this chapter was written while the author was a visiting associate professor at the Université René Descartes (Paris V) and the Hôpital Necker-Enfants Malades in Paris, France.

# REFERENCES

1. Geller AM, Sieving PA: How many cones are required to "see": Lessons from Stargardt's macular dystrophy and from modeling with degenerate photoreceptor arrays, in Hollyfield JG (ed): *Retinal Degeneration*. New York, Plenum Press, 1993, p 25.
2. Andréasson S, Ponjavic V: Full-field electroretinograms in infants with hereditary tapetoretinal degeneration. *Acta Ophthalmol Scand* **74**(suppl 219):19, 1996.
3. Sunga RN, Sloan LL: Pigmentary degeneration of the retina: Early diagnosis and natural history. *Invest Ophthalmol Vis Sci* **6**:309, 1967.
4. Berson EL, Sandberg MA, Rosner B, Birch DG, Hanson AH: Natural course of retinitis pigmentosa over a three-year interval. *Am J Ophthalmol* **99**:240, 1985.
5. Holopigian K, Greenstein V, Seiple W, Carr RE: Rates of change differ among measures of visual function in patients with retinitis pigmentosa. *Ophthalmology* **103**:398, 1996.
6. Grover S, Fishman GA, Anderson RJ, Alexander KR, Derlacki DJ: Rate of visual field loss in retinitis pigmentosa. *Ophthalmology* **104**:460, 1997.
7. Berson EL, Rosner B, Sandberg MA, Hayes KC, Nicholson BW, Weigel-DiFranco C, Willett W: A randomized trial of vitamin A and vitamin E supplementation for retinitis pigmentosa. *Arch Ophthalmol* **111**:761, 1993.
8. Berson EL, Rosner B, Sandberg MA, Dryja TP: Ocular findings in patients with autosomal dominant retinitis pigmentosa and a rhodopsin gene defect (Pro23His). *Arch Ophthalmol* **109**:92, 1991.
9. Berson EL, Rosner B, Sandberg MA, Weigel-DiFranco C, Dryja TP: Ocular findings in patients with autosomal dominant retinitis pigmentosa and rhodopsin, proline-347-leucine. *Am J Ophthalmol* **111**:614, 1991.
10. Weleber RG, Carr RE, Murphey WH, Sheffield VC, Stone EM: Phenotypic variation including retinitis pigmentosa, pattern dystrophy, and fundus flavimaculatus in a single family with a deletion of codon 153 or 154 of the peripherin/RDS gene. *Arch Ophthalmol* **111**:1531, 1993.
11. Pruett RC: Retinitis pigmentosa: Clinical observations and correlations. *Trans Am Ophthalmol Soc* **81**:693, 1983.
12. Biro I: Symmetrical development of pigmentation as a specific feature of the fundus pattern in retinitis pigmentosa. *Am J Ophthalmol* **55**:1176, 1963.
13. Newsome DA: Retinal fluorescein leakage in retinitis pigmentosa. *Am J Ophthalmol* **101**:354, 1986.
14. Ffytche TJ: Cystoid maculopathy in retinitis pigmentosa. *Trans Ophthalmol Soc UK* **92**:265, 1992.
15. Heckenlively J: The frequency of posterior subcapsular cataract in the hereditary retinal degenerations. *Am J Ophthalmol* **93**:733, 1982.
16. Fishman GA, Anderson RJ, Lourenco P: Prevalence of posterior subcapsular lens opacities in patients with retinitis pigmentosa. *Br J Ophthalmol* **69**:263, 1985.
17. Cox SN, Hay E, Bird AC: Treatment of chronic macular edema with acetazolamide. *Arch Ophthalmol* **106**:1190, 1988.
18. Fishman GA, Gilbert LD, Fiscella RG, Kimura AE, Jampol LM: Acetazolamide for treatment of chronic macular edema in retinitis pigmentosa. *Arch Ophthalmol* **107**:1445, 1989.
19. Grover S, Fishman GA, Brown J: Frequency of optic disc or parapapillary nerve fiber layer drusen in retinitis pigmentosa. *Ophthalmology* **104**:295, 1997.
20. Miyake Y, Yagasaki K, Horiguchi M, Kawase Y, Kanda T: Congenital stationary night blindness with negative electroretinogram: A new classification. *Arch Ophthalmol* **104**:1013, 1986.
21. Sieving PA, Richards JE, Naarendorp F, Bingham EL, Scott K, Alpern M: Dark-light: Model for nightblindness from the human rhodopsin Gly-90 → Asp mutation. *Proc Natl Acad Sci USA* **92**:880, 1995.
22. Bergsma DR Jr., Chen CJ: The Mizuo phenomenon in Oguchi disease. *Arch Ophthalmol* **115**:560, 1997.
23. Berson EL: Electrical phenomena in the retina, in Hart WM (ed): *Adler's Physiology of the Eye*. St Louis: Mosby, 1992, p 641.
24. Kline RP, Ripps H, Dowling JE: Generation of b-wave currents in the skate retina. *Proc Natl Acad Sci USA* **75**:5727, 1978.
25. Andreasson SOL, Sandberg MA, Berson EL: Narrow-band filtering for monitoring low-amplitude cone electroretinograms in retinitis pigmentosa. *Am J Ophthalmol* **105**:500, 1988.
26. Berson EL, Howard J: Temporal aspects of the electroretinogram in sector retinitis pigmentosa. *Arch Ophthalmol* **86**:653, 1971.
27. Berson EL: Retinitis pigmentosa. The Friedenwald Lecture. *Invest Ophthalmol Vis Sci* **34**:1659, 1993.
28. Berson EL: Retinitis pigmentosa and allied retinal diseases: Electrophysiologic findings. *Trans Am Acad Ophthalmol Otolaryngol* **81**:659, 1976.
29. Berson EL, Rosen JB, Simonoff EA: Electroretinographic testing as an aid in detection of carriers of X-chromosome-linked retinitis pigmentosa. *Am J Ophthalmol* **87**:460, 1979.
30. Fishman GA, Weinberg AB, McMahon TT: X-linked recessive retinitis pigmentosa: Clinical characteristics of carriers. *Arch Ophthalmol* **104**:1329, 1986.
31. Sandberg MA, Jacobson SG, Berson EL: Foveal cone electroretinograms in retinitis pigmentosa and juvenile macular degeneration. *Am J Ophthalmol* **88**:702, 1979.
32. Sandberg MA, Hanson AH, Berson EL: Foveal and parafoveal cone electroretinograms in juvenile macular degeneration. *Ophthalmic Paediatr Genet* **3**:83, 1983.
33. Matthews GP, Sandberg MA, Berson EL: Foveal cone electroretinograms in patients with central visual loss of unexplained etiology. *Arch Ophthalmol* **110**:1568, 1992.
34. Sutter EE, Tran D: The field topography of ERG components in man: I. The photopic luminance response. *Vision Res* **32**:433, 1992.
35. Kretschmann U, Seeliger MW, Ruether K, Usui T, Apfelstedt-Sylla E, Zrenner E: Multifocal electroretinography in patients with Stargardt's macular dystrophy. *Br J Ophthalmol* **82**:267, 1998.
36. Hood DC, Holopigian K, Greenstein V, Seiple W, Li J, Sutter EE, Carr RE: Assessment of local retinal function in patients with retinitis pigmentosa using the multi-focal ERG technique. *Vision Res* **38**:163, 1998.
37. Schubert G, Bornschein H: Beitrag zur Analyse des menschlichen Elektroretinogramms. *Ophthalmologica* **123**:396, 1952.
38. Riggs LA: Electroretinography in cases of night blindness. *Am J Ophthalmol* **38**:70, 1954.
39. Nettleship E: A history of congenital stationary night-blindness in nine consecutive generations. *Trans Ophthalmol Soc UK* **27**:269, 1907.
40. Truc H: Généalogie d'une famille héméralope depuis prés de trois siècles, 270 ans, 10 générations, 2121 membres, 135 héméralopes. *Bull Soc Ophtalmol Fr* **26**:285, 1909.
41. Dejean C, Gassenc R: Note sur la genealogie de la famille Nougaret, de Vendémian. *Bull Soc Ophtalmol Fr* **1**:96, 1949.
42. Peachey NS, Fishman GA, Kilbride PE, Alexander KR, Keehan KM, Derlacki DJ: A form of congenital stationary night blindness with apparent defect of rod phototransduction. *Invest Ophthalmol Vis Sci* **31**:237, 1990.
43. Dryja TP, Berson EL, Rao VR, Oprian DD: Heterozygous missense mutation in the rhodopsin gene as a cause of congenital stationary night blindness. *Nature Genet* **4**:280, 1993.
44. Dryja TP, Hahn LB, Reboul T, Arnaud B: Missense mutation in the gene encoding the a subunit of rod transducin in the Nougaret form of congenital stationary night blindness. *Nature Genet* **13**:358, 1996.
45. Gal A, Orth U, Baehr W, Schwinger E, Rosenberg T: Heterozygous missense mutation in the rod cGMP phosphodiesterase $\beta$-subunit gene in autosomal dominant stationary night blindness. *Nature Genet* **7**:64, 1994.
46. Rosenberg T, Gal A, Simonsen SE: ERG findings in two patients with autosomal dominant congenital stationary night blindness and His258Asn mutation of the $\beta$-subunit of rod photoreceptor cGMP-specific phosphodiesterase, in Anderson RE (ed): *Degenerative Diseases of the Retina*. New York, Plenum Press, 1995, p 377.
47. Sandberg MA, Pawlyk BS, Dan J, Arnaud B, Dryja TP, Berson EL: Rod and cone function in the Nougaret form of stationary night blindness. *Arch Ophthalmol* **116**:867, 1998.
48. Boycott KM, Pearce WG, Musarella MA, Weleber RG, Maybaum TA, Birch DG, Miyake Y, Young RSL, Bech-Hansen NT: Evidence for genetic heterogeneity in X-linked congenital stationary night blindness. *Am J Hum Genet* **62**:865, 1998.
49. Friedenwald J: Discussion of Verhoeff's observations of pathology of retinitis pigmentosa. *Arch Ophthalmol* **4**:767, 1930.
50. Verhoeff FH: Microscopic observations in a case of retinitis pigmentosa. *Arch Ophthalmol* **5**:392, 1931.
51. Cogan DG: Pathology [of retinitis pigmentosa]. *Trans Am Acad Ophthalmol Otolaryngol* **54**:629, 1950.
52. Kolb J, Gouras P: Electron microscopic observations of human retinitis pigmentosa, dominantly inherited. *Invest Ophthalmol Vis Sci* **13**:487, 1974.
53. Szamier RB, Berson EL, Klein R, Meyers S: Sex-linked retinitis pigmentosa: Ultrastructure of photoreceptors and pigment epithelium. *Invest Ophthalmol Vis Sci* **18**:145, 1979.

54. Gartner S, Henkind P: Pathology of retinitis pigmentosa. *Ophthalmology* **89**:1425, 1982.

55. Meyer KT, Heckenlively JR, Spitznas M, Foos RY: Dominant retinitis pigmentosa: A clinicopathologic correlation. *Ophthalmology* **89**:1414, 1982.

56. Szamier RB, Berson EL: Histopathologic study of an unusual form of retinitis pigmentosa. *Invest Ophthalmol Vis Sci* **22**:559, 1982.

57. Flannery JG, Farber DB, Bird AC, Bok D: Degenerative changes in a retina affected with autosomal dominant retinitis pigmentosa. *Invest Ophthalmol Vis Sci* **30**:191, 1989.

58. Milam AH, Jacobson SG: Photoreceptor rosettes with blue cone opsin immunoreactivity in retinitis pigmentosa. *Ophthalmology* **97**:1620, 1990.

59. Berson EL, Adamian M: Ultrastructural findings in an autopsy eye from a patient with Usher's syndrome type II. *Am J Ophthalmol* **114**:748, 1992.

60. To KW, Adamian M, Jakobiec FA, Berson EL: Olivopontocerebellar atrophy with retinal degeneration: An electroretinographic and histopathologic investigation. *Ophthalmology* **100**:15, 1993.

61. Brosnahan DM, Kennedy SM, Converse CA, Lee WR, Hammer HM: Pathology of hereditary retinal degeneration associated with hypobetalipoproteinemia. *Ophthalmology* **101**:38, 1994.

62. Li Z-Y, Jacobson SG, Milam AH: Autosomal dominant retinitis pigmentosa caused by the threonine-17-methionine rhodopsin mutation: Retinal histopathology and immunocytochemistry. *Exp Eye Res* **58**:397, 1994.

63. Li ZY, Possin DE, Milam AH: Histopathology of bone spicule pigmentation in retinitis pigmentosa. *Ophthalmology* **102**:805, 1995.

64. Milam AH, Li Z-Y, Cideciyan AV, Jacobson SG: Clinicopathologic effects of the Q64ter rhodopsin mutation in retinitis pigmentosa. *Invest Ophthalmol Vis Sci* **37**:753, 1996.

65. To KW, Adamian M, Jakobiec FA, Berson EL: Clinical and histopathologic findings in clumped pigmentary retinal degeneration. *Arch Ophthalmol* **114**:950, 1996.

66. Santos A, Humayun MS, De Juan E Jr., Greenburg RJ, Marsh MJ, Klock IB, Milam AH: Preservation of the inner retina in retinitis pigmentosa: A morphometric analysis. *Arch Ophthalmol* **115**:511, 1997.

67. Chang GQ, Hao Y, Wong F: Apoptosis: final common pathway of photoreceptor death in *rd, rds,* and rhodopsin mutant mice. *Neuron* **11**:595, 1993.

68. Lolley RN, Rong H, Craft CM: Linkage of photoreceptor degeneration by apoptosis with inherited defect in phototransduction. *Invest Ophthalmol Vis Sci* **35**:358, 1994.

69. Portera-Cailliau C, Sung CH, Nathans J, Adler R: Apoptotic photoreceptor cell death in mouse models of retinitis pigmentosa. *Proc Natl Acad Sci USA* **91**:974, 1994.

70. Tso MOM, Zhang C, Abler AS, Chang CJ, Wong F, Chang GQ, Lam TT: Apoptosis leads to photoreceptor degeneration in inherited retinal dystrophy of RCS rats. *Invest Ophthalmol Vis Sci* **35**:2693, 1994.

71. Green WR: Retina, in Spencer WH (ed): *Ophthalmic Pathology. An Atlas and Textbook.* Philadelphia, Saunders, 1996, p 667.

72. Vaghefi HA, Green WR, Kelley JS, Sloan LL, Hoover RE, Patz A: Correlation of clinicopatholgic findings in a patient: Congenital night blindness, branch retinal vein occlusion, cilioretinal artery, drusen of the optic nerve head, and intraretinal pigmented lesion. *Arch Ophthalmol* **96**:2097, 1978.

73. Franceschetti A, Francois J, Babel J: *Chorioretinal Heredodegenerations.* Springfield, IL, Charles C Thomas, 1963.

74. Yamanaka M: Histologic study of Oguchi's disease: Its relationship to pigmentary degeneration of the retina. *Am J Ophthalmol* **68**:19, 1969.

75. Maw M, Kumaramanickavel G, Kar B, John S, Bridges R, Denton M: Two Indian siblings with Oguchi disease are homozygous for an arrestin mutation encoding premature termination. *Hum Mutat Suppl* **1**:S317, 1998.

76. Nakazawa M, Wada Y, Tamai M: Arrestin gene mutations in autosomal recessive retinitis pigmentosa. *Arch Ophthalmol* **116**:498, 1998.

77. van den Born LI, van Soest S, van Schooneveld MJ, Riemslag FCC, de Jong PTVM, Bleeker-Wagemakers EM: Autosomal recessive retinitis pigmentosa with preserved para-arteriolar retinal pigment epithelium. *Am J Ophthalmol* **118**:430, 1994.

78. van Soest S, van den Born LI, Gal A, Farrar GJ, Bleeker-Wagemakers EM, Westerveld A, Humphries P, Sandkuijl LA, Bergen AAB: Assignment of a gene for autosomal recessive retinitis pigmentosa (*RP12*) to chromosome 1q31-q32.1 in an inbred and genetically heterogeneous disease population. *Genomics* **22**:499, 1994.

79. Leutelt J, Oehlmann R, Younus F, van den Born LI, Weber JL, Denton MJ, Mehdi SQ, Gal A: Autosomal recessive retinitis pigmentosa locus maps on chromosome 1q in a large consanguineous family from Pakistan. *Clin Genet* **47**:122, 1995.

80. van Soest S, Nijenhuis ST, van den Born LI, Bleeker-Wagemakers EM, Sharp E, Sandkuijl LA, Westerveld A, Bergen AAB: Fine mapping of the autosomal recessive retinitis pigmentosa locus (*RP12*) on chromosome 1q: Exclusion of the phosducin gene (*PDC*). *Cytogenet Cell Genet* **73**:81, 1996.

81. Sullivan LJ, Makrisk GS, Dickinson P, Mulhall LEM, App D, Forrest S, Cotton RGH, Loughnan MS: A new codon 15 rhodopsin gene mutation in autosomal dominant retinitis pigmentosa is associated with sectorial disease. *Arch Ophthalmol* **111**:1512, 1993.

82. Heckenlively JR, Rodriguez JA, Daiger SP: Autosomal dominant sectoral retinitis pigmentosa: Two families with transversion mutation in codon 23 of rhodopsin. *Arch Ophthalmol* **109**:84, 1991.

83. Nakamachi Y, Nakamura M, Fujii S, Yamamoto M, Okubo K: Oguchi disease with sectoral retinitis pigmentosa harboring adenine deletion at position 1147 in the arrestin gene. *Am J Ophthalmol* **125**:249, 1998.

84. Massof RW, Finkelstein D: Two forms of autosomal dominant primary retinitis pigmentosa. *Doc Ophthalmol* **51**:289, 1981.

85. Lyness AL, Ernst W, Quinlan MP, Clover GM, Arden GB, Carter RM, Bird AC, Parker JA: A clinical, psychophysical, and electroretinographic survey of patients with autosomal dominant retinitis pigmentosa. *Br J Ophthalmol* **69**:326, 1985.

86. Shimohara T, Date H, Ishiguro H, Suzuki T, Takano H, Tanaka H, Tsuji S, Hirota K: Ataxia with isolated vitamin E deficiency and retinitis pigmentosa. *Ann Neurol* **43**:273, 1998.

87. Yokota T, Shiojiri T, Gotoda T, Arai H: Retinitis pigmentosa and ataxia caused by a mutation in the gene for the α-tocopherol transfer protein. *New Engl J Med* **335**:1770, 1996.

88. Gouras P, Carr RE, Gunkel RD: Retinitis pigmentosa in abetalipoproteinemia: Effect of vitamin A. *Invest Ophthalmol Vis Sci* **10**:784, 1971.

89. Sperling MA, Hiles DA, Kennerdell JS: Electroretinographic responses following vitamin A therapy in abetalipoproteinemia. *Am J Ophthalmol* **73**:342, 1972.

90. Yokota T, Shiorjiri T, Gotoda T, Arita M, Arai H, Ohga T, Kanda T, Suzuki J, Imai T, Matsumoto H, Harino S, Kiyosawa M, Mizusawa H, Inoue K: Friedreich-like ataxia with retinitis pigmentosa caused by the His101Gln mutation of the α-tocopherol transfer protein gene. *Ann Neurol* **41**:826, 1997.

91. Refsum S: Heredopathia atactica polyneuritiformis. *Arch Neurol* **38**:605, 1981.

92. Kaiser-Kupfer MI, Caruso RC, Valle D: Gyrate atrophy of the choroid and retina: Long-term reduction of ornithine slows retinal degeneration. *Arch Ophthalmol* **109**:1539, 1991.

93. Wayne S, der Kaloustian VM, Schloss M, Polomeno R, Scott DA, Hejtmancik JF, Sheffield VC, Smith RJH: Localization of the Usher syndrome type ID gene (*Ush1D*) to chromosome 10. *Hum Mol Genet* **5**:1689, 1996.

94. Smith RJH, Lee EC, Kimberling WJ, Daiger SP, Pelias MZ, Keats BJB, Jay M, Bird A, Reardon W, Guest M, Ayyagari R, Hejtmancik JF: Localization of two genes for Usher syndrome type I to chromosome 11. *Genomics* **14**:995, 1992.

95. Ayyagari R, Nestorowicz A, Li Y, Chandrasekharappa S, Chinault C, van Tuinen P, Smith RJH, Hejtmancik JF, Permutt MA: Construction of a YAC contig encompassing the Usher syndrome type 1C and familial hyperinsulinism loci on chromosome 11p14-15.1. *Genome Res* **6**:504, 1996.

96. Marietta J, Walters KS, Burgess R, Ni L, Fukushima K, Moore KC, Hejtmancik JF, Smith RJH: Usher's syndrome type IC: Clinical studies and fine-mapping the disease locus. *Ann Otol Rhinol Laryngol* **106**:123, 1997.

97. Weil D, Blanchard S, Kaplan J, Guilford P, Gibson F, Walsh J, Mburu P, Valera A, Levilliers J, Weston MD, Kelley PM, Kimberling WJ, Wagenaar M, Levi-Acobas F, Larget-Piet D, Munnich A, Steel KP, Brown SDM, Petit C: Defective myosin VIIA gene responsible for Usher syndrome type Ib. *Nature* **374**:60, 1995.

98. Kaplan J, Gerber S, Bonneau D, Rozet JM, Delrieu O, Briard ML, Dollfus H, Ghazi I, Dufier JL, Frézal J, Munnich A: A gene for Usher syndrome type I (*USH1A*) maps to chromosome 14q. *Genomics* **14**:979, 1992.

99. Chaïb H, Kaplan J, Gerber S, Vincent C, Ayadi H, Slim R, Munnich A, Weissenbach J, Petit C: A newly identified locus for usher syndrome type I, *USH1E*, maps to chromosome 21q21. *Hum Mol Genet* **6**:27, 1997.

100. Kimberling WJ, Weston MD, Moller C, van Aarem A, Cremers CWRJ, Sumegi J, Ing PS, Connolly C, Martini A, Milani M, Tamayo ML, Bernal J, Greenberg J, Ayuso C: Gene mapping of Usher syndrome type IIa: Localization of the gene to a 2.1-cM segment on chromosome 1q41. *Am J Hum Genet* **56**:216, 1995.
101. Sankila EM, Pakarinen L, Kaariainen H, Aittomaki K, Karjalainen S, Sistonen P, de la Chapelle A: Assignment of an Usher syndrome type III (*USH3*) gene to chromosome 3q. *Hum Mol Genet* **4**:93, 1995.
102. Mansergh FC, Millington-Ward S, Kennan A, Kiang A-S, Humphries M, Farrar GJ, Humphries P, Kenna PF: Retinitis pigmentosa and progressive sensorineural hearing loss caused by a C12258A mutation in the mitochondrial MTTS2 gene. *Am J Hum Genet* **64**:971, 1999.
103. Sheffield VC, Carmi R, Kwitek-Black A, Rokhlina T, Nishimura D, Duyk GM, Elbedour K, Sunden SL, Stone EM: Identification of a Bardet-Biedl syndrome locus on chromosome 3 and evaluation of an efficient approach to homozygosity mapping. *Hum Mol Genet* **3**:1331, 1994.
104. Beales PL, Warner AM, Hitman GA, Thakker R, Flinter FA: Bardet-Biedl syndrome: A molecular and phenotypic study of 18 families. *J Med Genet* **34**:92, 1997.
105. Leppert M, Baird L, Anderson KL, Otterud B, Lupski JR, Lewis RA: Bardet-Biedl syndrome is linked to DNA markers on chromosome 11q and is genetically heterogeneous. *Nature Genet* **7**:108, 1994.
106. Carmi R, Rokhlina T, Kwitek-Black AE, Elbedour K, Nishimura D, Stone EM, Sheffield VC: Use of a DNA pooling strategy to identify a human obesity syndrome locus on chromosome 15. *Hum Mol Genet* **4**:9, 1995.
107. Kwitek-Black AE, Carmi R, Duyk GM, Buetow KH, Elbedour K, Parvari R, Yandava CN, Stone EM, Sheffield VC: Linkage of Bardet-Biedl syndrome to chromosome 16q and evidence for non-allelic genetic heterogeneity. *Nature Genet* **5**:392, 1993.
108. Benomar A, Krols L, Stevanin G, Cancel G, LeGuern E, David G, Ouhabi H, Martin JJ, Durr A, Zaim A, Ravise N, Busque C, Penet C, van Regemorter N, Weissenbach J, Yahyaoui M, Chkili T, Agid Y, van Broeckhoven C, Brice A: The gene for autosomal dominant cerebellar ataxia with pigmentary macular dystrophy maps to chromosome 3p12-p21.1. *Nature Genet* **10**:84, 1995.
109. Gouw LG, Kaplan CD, Haines JH, Digre KB, Rutledge SL, Matilla A, Leppert M, Zoghbi HY, Ptacek LJ: Retinal degeneration characterizes a spinocerebellar ataxia mapping to chromosome 3p. *Nature Genet* **10**:89, 1995.
110. Holmberg M, Johansson J, Forsgren L, Heijbel J, Sandgren O, Holmgren G: Localization of autosomal dominant cerebellar ataxia associated with retinal degeneration and anticipation to chromosome 3p12-p21.1. *Hum Mol Genet* **4**:1441, 1995.
111. Gardiner M, Sandford A, Deadman M, Poulton J, Cookson W, Reeders S, Jokiaho I, Peltonen L, Eiberg H, Julier C: Batten disease (Spielmeyer-Vogt disease, juvenile onset neuronal ceroid-lipofuscinosis) gene (*CLN3*) maps to human chromosome 16. *Genomics* **8**:387, 1990.
112. Lerner TJ, Boustany R-MN, Anderson JW, D'Arigo KL, Schlumpf K, Buckler AJ, Gusella JF, Haines JL, Kremmidiotis G, Lensink IL, Sutherland GR, Callen DF, Taschner PEM, de Vos N, van Ommen G-JB, Breuning MH, Doggett NA, Meincke LJ, Liu Z-Y, Goodwin LA, Tesmer JG, Mitchison HM, O'Rawe AM, Munroe PB, Jarvela IE, Gardiner RM, Mole SE: Isolation of a novel gene underlying Batten disease, *CLN3*. *Cell* **82**:949, 1995.
113. Des Portes V, Bachner L, Brüls T, Beldjord C, Billuart P, Soufir N, Bienvenu T, Vinet MC, Malaspina E, Marchiani V, Bertini E, Kahn A, Franzoni E, Chelly J: X-linked neurodegenerative syndrome with congenital ataxia, late-onset progressive myoclonic encephalopathy and selective macular degeneration, linked to Xp22.33-pter. *Am J Med Genet* **64**:69, 1996.
114. Zeviani M, Moraes CT, DiMauro S, Nakase H, Bonilla E, Schon EA, Rowland LP: Deletions of mitochondrial DNA in Kearns-Sayre syndrome. *Neurology* **38**:1339, 1988.
115. Lestienne P, Ponsot G: Kearns-Sayre syndrome with muscle mitochondrial DNA deletion. *Lancet* **1**:885, 1988.
116. Moraes CT, DiMauro S, Zeviani M, Lombes A, Shanske S, Miranda AF, Nakase H, Bonilla E, Werneck LC, Servidei S, Nonaka I, Koga Y, Spiro AJ, Brownell AKW, Schmidt B, Schotland DL, Zupanc M, DeVivo DC, Schon EA, Rowland LP: Mitochondrial DNA deletions in progressive external ophthalmoplegia and Kearns-Sayre syndrome. *New Engl J Med* **320**:1293, 1989.
117. Boughman JA, Conneally PM, Nance WE: Population studies of retinitis pigmentosa. *Am J Hum Genet* **32**:223, 1980.
118. Bunker CH, Berson EL, Bromley WC, Hayes RP, Roderick TH: Prevalence of retinitis pigmentosa in Maine. *Am J Ophthalmol* **97**:357, 1984.
119. Jay M: On the heredity of retinitis pigmentosa. *Br J Ophthalmol* **66**:405, 1982.
120. Fishman GA: Retinitis pigmentosa: Genetic percentages. *Arch Ophthalmol* **96**:822, 1978.
121. Ammann F, Klein D, Bohringer HR: Resultats preliminaires d'une enquete sur la frequence et la distribution geographique des degenerescences tapeto-retiniennes en suisse (etude de cinq cantons). *J Genet Hum* **10**:99, 1961.
122. Bundey S, Crews SJ: A study of retinitis pigmentosa in the city of Birmingham: II Clinical and genetic heterogeneity. *J Med Genet* **21**:421, 1984.
123. Macrae WG: Retinitis pigmentosa in Ontario: A survey. *Birth Defects* **18**:175, 1982.
124. Nájera C, Millán JM, Beneyto M, Prieto F: Epidemiology of retinitis pigmentosa in the Valencian community (Spain). *Genet Epidemiol* **12**:37, 1995.
125. Hope CI, Bundey S, Proops D, Fielder AR: Usher syndrome in the city of Birmingham: Prevalence and clinical classification. *Br J Ophthalmol* **81**:46, 1997.
126. Rosenberg T, Haim M, Hauch A-M, Parving A: The prevalence of Usher syndrome and other retinal dystrophy-hearing impairment associations. *Clin Genet* **51**:314, 1997.
127. Haim M: Prevalence of retinitis pigmentosa and allied disorders in Denmark: II. Systemic involvement and age at onset. *Acta Ophthalmol* **70**:417, 1992.
128. Boughman JA, Vernon M, Shaver KA: Usher syndrome: definition and estimate of prevalence from two high-risk populations. *J Chron Dis* **36**:595, 1983.
129. Klein D, Ammann F: The syndrome of Laurence-Moon-Bardet-Biedl and allied diseases in Switzerland: Clinical, genetic, and epidemiologic studies. *J Neurol Sci* **9**:479, 1969.
130. Berson EL, Rosner B, Simonoff E: Risk factors for genetic typing and detection in retinitis pigmentosa. *Am J Ophthalmol* **89**:763, 1980.
131. Fishman GA, Farber MD, Derlacki DJ: X-linked retinitis pigmentosa: Profile of clinical findings. *Arch Ophthalmol* **106**:369, 1988.
132. McGuire RE, Sullivan LS, Blanton SH, Church MW, Heckenlively JR, Daiger SP: X-linked dominant cone-rod degeneration: Linkage mapping of a new locus for retinitis pigmentosa (*RP15*) to Xp22.13-p22.11. *Am J Hum Genet* **57**:87, 1995.
133. Kajiwara K, Berson EL, Dryja TP: Digenic retinitis pigmentosa due to mutations at the unlinked *peripherin/RDS* and *ROM1* loci. *Science* **264**:1604, 1994.
134. Dryja TP, Hahn LB, Kajiwara K, Berson EL: Dominant and digenic mutations in the *peripherin/RDS* and *ROM1* genes in retinitis pigmentosa. *Invest Ophthalmol Vis Sci* **38**:1972, 1997.
135. McGee TL, Devoto M, Ott J, Berson EL, Dryja TP: Evidence that the penetrance of mutations at the *RP11* locus causing dominant retinitis pigmentosa is influenced by a gene linked to the homologous *RP11* allele. *Am J Hum Genet* **61**:1059, 1997.
136. Kajiwara K, Sandberg MA, Berson EL, Dryja TP: A null mutation in the human *peripherin/RDS* gene in a family with autosomal dominant retinitis punctata albescens. *Nature Genet* **3**:208, 1993.
137. Meins M, Gruning G, Blankenagel A, Krastel H, Reck B, Fuchs S, Schwinger E, Gal A: Heterozygous "null allele" mutation in the human *peripherin/RDS* gene. *Hum Mol Genet* **2**:2181, 1993.
138. Nichols BE, Sheffield VC, Vandenburgh K, Drack AV, Kimura AE, Stone EM: Butterfly-shaped pigment dystrophy of the fovea caused by a point mutation in codon 167 of the *RDS* gene. *Nature Genet* **3**:202, 1993.
139. Maw MA, Kennedy B, Knight A, Bridges R, Roth KE, Mani EJ, Mukkadan JK, Nancarrow D, Crabb JW, Denton MJ: Mutation of the gene encoding cellular retinaldehyde-binding protein in autosomal recessive retinitis pigmentosa. *Nature Genet* **17**:198, 1997.
140. Gal A, Schinzel A, Orth U, Fraser NA, Mollica F, Craig IW, Kruse T, Machler M, Neugebauer M, Bleeker-Wagemakers LM: Gene of X-chromosomal congenital stationary night blindness is closely linked to DXS7 on Xp. *Hum Genet* **81**:315, 1989.
141. Musarella MA, Weleber RG, Murphey WH, Young RSL, Anson-Cartwright L, Mets M, Kraft SP, Polemeno R, Litt M, Worton RG: Assignment of the gene for complete X-linked congenital stationary night blindness (*CSNB1*) to Xp11.3. *Genomics* **5**:727, 1989.
142. Bergen AAB, Ten Brink JB, Riemslag F, Schuurman EJM, Tijmes N: Localization of a novel X-linked congenital stationary night blindness locus: Close linkage to the RP3 type retinitis pigmentosa gene region. *Hum Mol Genet* **4**:931, 1995.
143. Bergen AAB, Ten Brink JB, Riemslag F, Schuurman EJM, Meire F, Tijmes M, de Jong PTVM: Conclusive evidence for a distinct

congenital stationary night blindness locus in Xp21.1. *J Med Genet* **33**:869, 1996.

144. Hardcastle AJ, David-Gray ZK, Jay M, Bird AC, Bhattacharya SS: Localization of CSNBS (*CSNB4*) between the retinitis pigmentosa loci *RP2* and *RP3* on proximal Xp. *Invest Ophthalmol Vis Sci* **38**:2750, 1997.

145. Strom TM, Nyakatura G, Apfelstedt-Sylla E, Hellebrand H, Lorenz B, Weber BHF, Wutz K, Gutwillinger N, Rüther K, Drescher B, Sauer C, Zrenner E, Meitinger T, Rosenthal A, Meindl A: An L-type calcium-channel gene mutated in incomplete X-linked congenital stationary night blindness. *Nature Genet* **19**:260, 1998.

146. Bech-Hansen NT, Naylor MJ, Maybaum TA, Pearce WG, Koop B, Fishman GA, Mets M, Musarella MA, Boycott KM: Loss-of-function mutations in a calcium-channel α1-subunit gene in Xp11.23 cause incomplete X-linked congenital stationary night blindness. *Nature Genet* **19**:264, 1998.

147. Ruttum MS, Lewandowski MF, Bateman JB: Affected females in X-linked congenital stationary night blindness. *Ophthalmology* **99**:747, 1992.

148. Inglehearn CF, Tarttelin EE, Plant C, Peacock RE, Al-Maghtheh M, Vithana E, Bird AC, Bhattacharya SS: A linkage survey of 20 dominant retinitis pigmentosa families: Frequencies of the nine known loci and evidence for further heterogeneity. *J Med Genet* **35**:1, 1998.

149. Stryer L: The molecules of visual excitation. *Sci Am* **257**:42, 1987.

150. Hargrave PA, McDowell JH: Rhodopsin and phototransduction: A model system for G protein-linked receptors. *FASEB J* **6**:2323, 1992.

151. Fliesler SJ, Anderson RE: Chemistry and metabolism of lipids in the vertebrate retina. *Prog Lipid Res* **22**:79, 1983.

152. Papermaster DS, Dreyer WJ: Rhodopsin content in the outer segment membranes of bovine and frog retinal rods. *Biochemistry* **13**:2438, 1974.

153. Applebury ML, Hargrave PA: Molecular biology of the visual pigments. *Vision Res* **12**:1881, 1986.

154. Fulton AB, Dodge J, Schremser JL, Armstrong A, Lanier F, Dawson WW, Williams TP: The quantity of rhodopsin in human eyes. *Curr Eye Res* **9**:1211, 1990.

155. van Kuijk FJGM, Lewis JW, Buck P, Parker KR, Kliger DS: Spectrophotometric quantitation of rhodopsin in human retina. *Invest Ophthalmol Vis Sci* **32**:1962, 1991.

156. Missotten PL: Etude des batonnets de la retine humaine au microscope electronique. *Ophthalmologica* **140**:200, 1960.

157. Fukada Y, Takao T, Ohguro H, Yoshizawa T, Akino T, Shimonishi Y: Farnesylated gamma-subunit of photoreceptor G protein indispensable for GTP-binding. *Nature* **346**:658, 1990.

158. Lai RK, Perez-Sala D, Canada FJ, Rando RR: The gamma subunit of transducin is farnesylated. *Proc Natl Acad Sci USA* **87**:7673, 1990.

159. Bigay J, Faurobert E, Franco M, Chabre M: Roles of lipid modifications of transducin subunits in their GDP-dependent association and membrane binding. *Biochemistry* **33**:14081, 1994.

160. Bownds MD, Arshavsky VY: What are the mechanisms of photoreceptor adaptation? *Behav Brain Sci* **18**:415, 1995.

161. Qin N, Pittler SJ, Baehr W: In vitro isoprenylation and membrane association of mouse rod photoreceptor cGMP phosphodiesterase alpha and beta subunits expressed in bacteria. *J Biol Chem* **267**:8458, 1992.

162. Cervetto L, Lagnado L, Perry RJ, Robinson DW, McNaughton PA: Extrusion of calcium from rod outer segments is driven by both sodium and potassium gradients. *Nature* **337**:740, 1989.

163. Kim TSY, Reid DM, Molday RS: Structure-function relationships and localization of the Na/Ca-K exchanger in rod photoreceptors. *J Biol Chem* **273**:16561, 1998.

164. Demontis GC, Ratto GM, Bisti S, Cervetto L: Effect of blocking the $Na^+/K^+$ATPase on $Ca^{2+}$ extrusion and light adaptation in mammalian retinal rods. *Biophys J* **69**:439, 1995.

165. Hecht S, Schlaer S, Pirenne MH: Energy, quanta, and vision. *J Gen Physiol* **25**:819, 1942.

166. Palczewski K, Rispoli G, Detwiler PB: The influence of arrestin (48K protein) and rhodopsin kinase on visual transduction. *Neuron* **8**:117, 1992.

167. Dolph PJ, Ranganathan R, Colley NJ, Hardy RW, Socolich M, Zuker CS: Arrestin function in inactivation of G protein-coupled receptor rhodopsin in vivo. *Science* **260**:1910, 1993.

168. Snow BE, Antonio L, Suggs S, Siderovski DP: Cloning of a retinally abundant regulator of G-protein signaling (*RGS-r/RGS16*): genomic structure and chromosomal localization of the human gene. *Gene* **206**:247, 1998.

169. Koch KW, Stryer L: Highly cooperative feedback control of retinal rod guanylate cyclase by calcium ions. *Nature* **334**:64, 1988.

170. Klenchin VA, Calvert PD, Bownds MD: Inhibition of rhodopsin kinase by recoverin: Further evidence for a negative feedback system in phototransduction. *J Biol Chem* **270**:16147, 1995.

171. Chen C-K, Inglese J, Lefkowitz RJ, Hurley JB: $Ca^{2+}$-dependent interaction of recoverin with rhodopsin kinase. *J Biol Chem* **270**:18060, 1995.

172. Polans A, Baehr W, Palczewski K: Turned on by $Ca^2$! The physiology and pathology of $Ca^{2+}$-binding proteins in the retina. *Trends Neurosci* **19**:547, 1996.

173. Sanada K, Shimizu F, Kameyama K, Haga K, Haga T, Fukada Y: Calcium-bound recoverin targets rhodopsin kinase to membranes to inhibit rhodopsin phosphorylation. *FEBS Lett* **384**:227, 1996.

174. Bauer PH, Muller S, Puzicha M, Pippig S, Obermaier B, Helmreich EJM, Lohse MJ: Phosducin is a protein kinase A-regulated G-protein regulator. *Nature* **358**:73, 1992.

175. Wilkins JF, Bitensky MW, Willardson BM: Regulation of the kinetics of phosducin phosphorylation in retinal rods. *J Biol Chem* **271**:19232, 1996.

176. Newton AC, Williams DS: Rhodopsin is the major in situ substrate of protein kinase C in rod outer segments of photoreceptors. *J Biol Chem* **268**:18181, 1993.

177. Udovichenko IP, Cunnick J, Gonzalez K, Takemoto DJ: The visual transduction and the phosphoinositide system: a link. *Cell Signal* **6**:601, 1994.

178. Udovichenko IP, Cunnick J, Gonzalez K, Yakhnin A, Takemoto DJ: Protein kinase C in rod outer segments: Effects of phosphorylation of the phosphodiesterase inhibitory subunit. *Biochem J* **317**:291, 1996.

179. Greene NM, Williams DS, Newton AC: Kinetics and localization of the phosphorylation of rhodopsin by protein kinase C. *J Biol Chem* **270**:6710, 1995.

180. Udovichenko IP, Newton AC, Williams DS: Contribution of protein kinase C to the phosphorylation of rhodopsin in intact retinas. *J Biol Chem* **272**:7952, 1997.

181. Grunwald ME, Yu WP, Yu HH, Yau KW: Identification of a domain on the β-subunit of the rod cGMP-gated cation channel that mediates inhibition by calcium-calmodulin. *J Biol Chem* **273**:9148, 1998.

182. Weitz D, Zoche M, Müller F, Beyermann M, Körschen HG, Kaupp UB, Koch KW: Calmodulin controls the rod photoreceptor CNG channel through an unconventional binding site in the N-terminus of the β-subunit. *EMBO J* **17**:2273, 1998.

183. Saari JC, Bredberg DL, Noy N: Control of substrate flow at a branch in the visual cycle. *Biochemistry* **33**:3106, 1994.

184. Tsilou E, Hamel CP, Yu S, Redmond TM: RPE65, the major retinal pigment epithelium microsomal membrane protein, associates with phospholipid liposomes. *Arch Biochem Biophys* **346**:21, 1997.

185. Tan BC, Schwartz SH, Zeevaart JAD, McCarty DR: Genetic control of abscisic acid biosynthesis in maize. *Proc Natl Acad Sci USA* **94**:12235, 1997.

186. Chang JHT, Milligan S, Li YY, Chew CE, Wiggs J, Copeland NG, Jenkins NA, Campochiaro PA, Hyde DR, Zack DJ: Mammalian homologue of *Drosophila* retinal degeneration *B* rescues the mutant fly phenotype. *J Neurosci* **17**:5881, 1997.

187. Palczewski K: Is vertebrate phototransduction solved? New insights into the molecular mechanism of phototransduction. *Invest Ophthalmol Vis Sci* **35**:3577, 1994.

188. Daemen FJM: Vertebrate rod outer segment membranes. *Biochim Biophys Acta* **300**:255, 1973.

189. Mirzadegan T, Liu RSH: Probing the visual pigment rhodopsin and its analogues by molecular modeling analysis and computer graphics, in Osborne NN, Chader GJ (eds): *Retinal Research*, Vol 11. Oxford, England, Pergamon Press, 1991, p 57.

190. Davies A, Schertler GFX, Gowan BE, Saibil HR: Projection structure of an invertebrate rhodopsin. *J Struct Biol* **117**:36, 1996.

191. Unger VM, Hargrave PA, Baldwin JM, Schertler GFX: Arrangement of rhodopsin transmembrane α-helices. *Nature* **389**:203, 1997.

192. Vaithinathan R, Berson EL, Dryja TP: Further screening of the rhodopsin gene in patients with autosomal dominant retinitis pigmentosa. *Genomics* **21**:461, 1994.

193. Daiger SP, Sullivan LA, Rodriguez JA: Correlation of phenotype with genotype in inherited retinal degeneration. *Behav Brain Sci* **18**:452, 1995.

194. Farrar GJ, Kenna P, Redmond R, McWilliam P, Bradley DG, Humphries MM, Sharp EM, Inglehearn CF, Bashir R, Jay M, Watty A, Ludwig M, Schinzel A, Samanns C, Gal A, Bhattacharya S, Humphries P: Autosomal dominant retinitis pigmentosa: absence of

the rhodopsin proline-histidine substitution (codon 23) in pedigrees from Europe. *Am J Hum Genet* **47**:941, 1990.

195. Dryja TP, McGee TL, Hahn LB, Cowley GS, Olsson JE, Reichel E, Sandberg MA, Berson EL: Mutations within the rhodopsin gene in patients with autosomal dominant retinitis pigmentosa. *New Engl J Med* **323**:1302, 1990.

196. Richards JE, Kuo CY, Boehnke M, Sieving PA: Rhodopsin Thr58Arg mutation in a family with autosomal dominant retinitis pigmentosa. *Ophthalmology* **98**:1797, 1991.

197. Artlich A, Horn M, Lorenz B, Bhattacharya S, Gal A: Recurrent 3-bp deletion at codon 255/256 of the rhodopsin gene in a German pedigree with autosomal dominant retinitis pigmentosa. *Am J Hum Genet* **50**:876, 1992.

198. Dryja TP, Hahn LB, Cowley GS, McGee TL, Berson EL: Mutation spectrum of the rhodopsin gene among patients with autosomal dominant retinitis pigmentosa. *Proc Natl Acad Sci USA* **88**:9370, 1991.

199. Sung CH, Davenport CM, Hennessey JC, Maumenee IH, Jacobson SG, Heckenlively JR, Nowakowski R, Fishman G, Gouras P, Nathans J: Rhodopsin mutations in autosomal dominant retinitis pigmentosa. *Proc Natl Acad Sci USA* **88**:6481, 1991.

200. Fujiki K, Hotta Y, Hayakawa M, Sakuma H, Shiono T, Noro M, Sakuma T, Tamai M, Hikiji K, Kawaguchi R, Hoshi A, Nakajima A, Kanai A: Point mutations of rhodopsin gene found in Japanese families with autosomal dominant retinitis pigmentosa (ADRP). *Jpn J Hum Genet* **37**:125, 1992.

201. Inglehearn CF, Keen TJ, Bashir R, Jay M, Fitzke F, Bird AC, Crombie A, Bhattacharya S: A completed screen for mutations of the rhodopsin gene in a panel of patients with autosomal dominant retinitis pigmentosa. *Hum Mol Genet* **1**:41, 1992.

202. Macke JP, Davenport CM, Jacobson SG, Hennessey JC, Gonzalez-Fernandez F, Conway BP, Heckenlively J, Palmer R, Maumenee IH, Sieving P, Gouras P, Good W, Nathans J: Identification of novel rhodopsin mutations responsible for retinitis pigmentosa: Implications for the structure and function of rhodopsin. *Am J Hum Genet* **53**:80, 1993.

203. Jacobson SG, Kemp CM, Cideciyan AV, Macke JP, Sung CH, Nathans J: Phenotypes of stop codon and splice site rhodopsin mutations causing retinitis pigmentosa. *Invest Ophthalmol Vis Sci* **35**:2521, 1994.

204. Konig B, Arendt A, McDowell JH, Kahlert M, Hargrave PA, Hofmann KP: Three cytoplasmic loops of rhodopsin interact with transducin. *Proc Natl Acad Sci USA* **86**:6878, 1989.

205. Lisman J, Fain G: Support for the equivalent light hypothesis for RP. *Nature Med* **1**:1254, 1995.

206. Kuwabara T: Retinal recovery from exposure to light. *Am J Ophthalmol* **70**:187, 1970.

207. Cicerone CM: Cones survive rods in the light-damaged eye of the albino rat. *Science* **194**:1183, 1976.

208. Robinson PR, Cohen GB, Zhukovsky EA, Oprian DD: Constitutively active mutants of rhodopsin. *Neuron* **9**:719, 1992.

209. Min KC, Zvyaga TA, Cypess AM, Sakmar TP: Characterization of mutant rhodopsins responsible for autosomal dominant retinitis pigmentosa. *J Biol Chem* **268**:9400, 1993.

210. Li T, Snyder WK, Olsson JE, Dryja TP: Transgenic mice carrying the dominant rhodopsin mutation *P347S*: Evidence for defective vectorial transport of rhodopsin to the outer segments. *Proc Natl Acad Sci USA* **93**:14176, 1996.

211. Sandberg MA, Berson EL, Effron MH: Rod-cone interaction in the distal human retina. *Science* **212**:829, 1981.

212. Berson EL: Ocular findings in a form of retinitis pigmentosa with a rhodopsin gene defect. *Trans Am Ophthalmol Soc* **88**:355, 1990.

213. Goto Y, Peachey NS, Ripps H, Naash MI: Functional abnormalities in transgenic mice expressing a mutant rhodopsin gene. *Invest Ophthalmol Vis Sci* **36**:62, 1995.

214. Li T, Franson WK, Gordon JW, Berson EL, Dryja TP: Constitutive activation of phototransduction by K296E opsin is not a cause of photoreceptor degeneration. *Proc Natl Acad Sci USA* **92**:3551, 1995.

215. Rao VR, Cohen GB, Oprian DD: Rhodopsin mutation G90D and a molecular mechanism for congenital night blindness. *Nature* **367**:639, 1994.

216. Sung CH, Schneider BG, Agarwal N, Papermaster DS, Nathans J: Functional heterogeneity of mutant rhodopsins responsible for autosomal dominant retinitis pigmentosa. *Proc Natl Acad Sci USA* **88**:8840, 1991.

217. Sung CH, Davenport CM, Nathans J: Rhodopsin mutations responsible for autosomal dominant retinitis pigmentosa: Clustering of functional classes along the polypeptide chain. *J Biol Chem* **268**:26645, 1993.

218. Liu X, Garriga P, Khorana HG: Structure and function in rhodopsin: Correct folding and misfolding in two point mutants in the intradiscal domain of rhodopsin identified in retinitis pigmentosa. *Proc Natl Acad Sci USA* **93**:4554, 1996.

219. Kaushal S, Khorana HG: Structure and function in rhodopsin: 7. Point mutations associated with autosomal dominant retinitis pigmentosa. *Biochemistry* **33**:6121, 1994.

220. Sung CH, Makino C, Baylor D, Nathans J: A rhodopsin gene mutation responsible for autosomal dominant retinitis pigmentosa results in a protein that is defective in localization to the photoreceptor outer segment. *J Neurosci* **14**:5818, 1994.

221. Liu XR, Wu TH, Stowe S, Matsushita A, Arikawa K, Naash MI, Williams DS: Defective phototransductive disk membrane morphogenesis in transgenic mice expressing opsin with a mutated N-terminal domain. *J Cell Sci* **110**:2589, 1997.

222. Roof DJ, Adamian M, Hayes A: Rhodopsin accumulation at abnormal sites in retinas of mice with a human P23H rhodopsin transgene. *Invest Ophthalmol Vis Sci* **35**:4049, 1994.

223. Li ZY, Wong F, Chang JH, Possin DE, Hao Y, Petters RM, Milam AH: Rhodopsin transgenic pigs as a model for human retinitis pigmentosa. *Invest Ophthalmol Vis Sci* **39**:808, 1998.

224. Colley NJ, Cassill JA, Baker EK, Zuker CS: Defective intracellular transport is the molecular basis of rhodopsin-dependent dominant retinal degeneration. *Proc Natl Acad Sci USA* **92**:3070, 1995.

225. Huang PC, Gaitan AE, Hao Y, Petters RM, Wong F: Cellular interactions implicated in the mechanism of photoreceptor degeneration in transgenic mice expressing a mutant rhodopsin gene. *Proc Natl Acad Sci USA* **90**:8484, 1993.

226. Jacobson SG, Kemp CM, Sung CH, Nathans J: Retinal function and rhodopsin levels in autosomal dominant retinitis pigmentosa with rhodopsin mutations. *Am J Ophthalmol* **112**:256, 1991.

227. Dryja TP, McGee TL, Reichel E, Hahn LB, Cowley GS, Yandell DW, Sandberg MA, Berson EL: A point mutation of the rhodopsin gene in one form of retinitis pigmentosa. *Nature* **343**:364, 1990.

228. Berson EL, Sandberg MA, Dryja TP: Autosomal dominant retinitis pigmentosa with rhodopsin, valine-345-methionine. *Trans Am Ophthalmol Soc* **89**:117, 1991.

229. Apfelstedt-Sylla E, Kunisch M, Horn M, Rüther K, Gerding H, Gal A, Zrenner E: Ocular findings in a family with autosomal dominant retinitis pigmentosa and a frameshift mutation altering the carboxyl terminal sequence of rhodopsin. *Br J Ophthalmol* **77**:495, 1993.

230. Berson EL, Gouras P, Gunkel RD: Rod responses in retinitis pigmentosa, dominantly inherited. *Arch Ophthalmol* **80**:58, 1968.

231. Kemp CM, Jacobson SG, Roman AJ, Sung CH, Nathans J: Abnormal rod dark adaptation in autosomal dominant retinitis pigmentosa with proline-23-histidine rhodopsin mutation. *Am J Ophthalmol* **113**:165, 1992.

232. Sandberg MA, Weigel-DiFranco C, Dryja TP, Berson EL: Clinical expression correlates with location of rhodopsin mutation in dominant retinitis pigmentosa. *Invest Ophthalmol Vis Sci* **36**:1934, 1995.

233. Fishman GA, Stone EM, Sheffield VC, Gilbert LD, Kimura AE: Ocular findings associated with rhodopsin gene codon 17 and codon 182 transition mutations in dominant retinitis pigmentosa. *Arch Ophthalmol* **110**:54, 1992.

234. Stone EM, Kimura AE, Nichols BE, Khadivi P, Fishman GA, Sheffield VC: Regional distribution of retinal degeneration in patients with the proline to histidine mutation in codon 23 of the rhodopsin gene. *Ophthalmology* **98**:1806, 1991.

235. Fishman GA, Stone EM, Gilbert LD, Kenna P, Sheffield VC: Ocular findings associated with a rhodopsin gene codon 58 transversion mutation in autosomal dominant retinitis pigmentosa. *Arch Ophthalmol* **109**:1387, 1991.

236. Fishman GA, Stone EM, Gilbert LD, Sheffield VC: Ocular findings associated with a rhodopsin gene codon 106 mutation: Glycine-to-arginine change in autosomal dominant retintis pigmentosa. *Arch Ophthalmol* **110**:646, 1992.

237. Rosenfeld PJ, Cowley GS, McGee TL, Sandberg MA, Berson EL, Dryja TP: A null mutation in the rhodopsin gene causes rod photoreceptor dysfunction and autosomal recessive retinitis pigmentosa. *Nature Genet* **1**:209, 1992.

238. Rosenfeld PJ, Hahn LB, Sandberg MA, Dryja TP, Berson EL: Low incidence of retinitis pigmentosa among heterozygous carriers of a specific rhodopsin splice site mutation. *Invest Ophthalmol Vis Sci* **36**:2186, 1995.

239. Humphries MM, Rancourt D, Farrar GJ, Kenna P, Hazel M, Bush RA, Sieving PA, Sheils DM, McNally N, Creighton P, Erven A, Boros A,

Gulya K, Capecchi MR, Humphries P: Retinopathy induced in mice by targeted disruption of the rhodopsin gene. *Nature Genet* **15**:216, 1997.

240. Kumaramanickavel G, Maw M, Denton MJ, John S, Srikumari CRS, Orth U, Oehlmann R, Gal A: Missense rhodopsin mutation in a family with recessive RP. *Nature Genet* **8**:10, 1994.

241. Defoe DM, Bok D: Rhodopsin chromophore exchanges among opsin molecules in the dark. *Invest Ophthalmol Vis Sci* **24**:1211, 1983.

242. Noel JP, Hamm HE, Sigler PB: The 2.2 A crystal structure of transducin-α complexed with GTP-gamma-S. *Nature* **366**:654, 1993.

243. Lambright DG, Noel JP, Hamm HE, Sigler PB: Structural determinants for activation of the α-subunit of a heterotrimeric G protein. *Nature* **369**:621, 1994.

244. Wilkie TM, Gilbert DJ, Olsen AS, Chen XN, Amatruda TT, Korenberg JR, Trask BJ, de Jong P, Reed RR, Simon MI, Jenkins NA, Copeland NG: Evolution of the mammalian G protein alpha subunit multigene family. *Nature Genet* **1**:85, 1992.

245. Reddy EP, Reynolds RK, Santos E, Barbacid M: A point mutation is responsible for the acquisition of transforming properties by the T24 human bladder carcinoma oncogene. *Nature* **300**:149, 1982.

246. Tabin CJ, Bradley SM, Bargmann CI, Weinberg RA, Papageorge AG, Scolnick EM, Dhar R, Lowy DR, Chang EH: Mechanism of activation of a human oncogene. *Nature* **300**:143, 1982.

247. Santos E, Reddy EP, Pulciani S, Feldmann RJ, Barbacid M: Spontaneous activation of a human proto-oncogene. *Proc Natl Acad Sci USA* **80**:4679, 1983.

248. Saez R, Chan AM-L, Miki T, Aaronson SA: Oncogenic activation of human R-*ras* by point mutations analogous to those of prototype H-*ras* oncogenes. *Oncogene* **9**:2977, 1994.

249. Graziano MP, Gilman AG: Synthesis in *Escherichia coli* of GTPase-deficient mutants of Gsα. *J Biol Chem* **264**:15475, 1989.

250. Pittler SJ, Baehr W, Wasmuth JJ, McConnell DG, Champagne MS, van Tuinen P, Ledbetter D, Davis RL: Molecular characterization of human and bovine rod photoreceptor cGMP phosphodiesterase alpha-subunit and chromosomal localization of the human gene. *Genomics* **6**:272, 1990.

251. Weber B, Riess O, Hutchinson G, Collins C, Lin B, Kowbel D, Andrew S, Schappert K, Hayden MR: Genomic organization and complete sequence of the human gene encoding the beta subunit of the cGMP phosphodiesterase and its localization to 4p16.3. *Nucl Acids Res* **19**:6263, 1991.

252. McLaughlin ME, Sandberg MA, Berson EL, Dryja TP: Recessive mutations in the gene encoding the β-subunit of rod phosphodiesterase in patients with retinitis pigmentosa. *Nature Genet* **4**:130, 1993.

253. Bayés M, Giordano M, Balcells S, Grinberg D, Vilageliu L, Martinez I, Ayuso C, Benitez J, Ramos-Arroyo MA, Chivelet P, Solans T, Valverde D, Amselem S, Goossens M, Baiget M, Gonzalez-Duarte R, Besmond C: Homozygous tandem duplication within the gene encoding the β-subunit of rod phosphodiesterase as a cause of autosomal recessive retinitis pigmentosa. *Hum Mutat* **5**:228, 1995.

254. Danciger M, Blaney J, Gao YQ, Zhao DY, Heckenlively JR, Jacobson SG, Farber DB: Mutations in the *PDE6B* gene in autosomal recessive retinitis pigmentosa. *Genomics* **30**:1, 1995.

255. McLaughlin ME, Ehrhart TL, Berson EL, Dryja TP: Mutation spectrum of the gene encoding the β subunit of rod phosphodiesterase among patients with autosomal recessive retinitis pigmentosa. *Proc Natl Acad Sci USA* **92**:3249, 1995.

256. Valverde D, Solans T, Grinberg D, Balcells S, Vilageliu L, Bayés M, Chivelet P, Besmond C, Goossens M, González-Duarte R, Baiget M: A novel mutation in exon 17 of the β-subunit of rod phosphodiesterase in two RP sisters of a consanguineous family. *Hum Genet* **97**:35, 1996.

257. Saga M, Mashima Y, Akeo K, Kudoh J, Oguchi Y, Shimizu N: A novel homozygous Ile535Asn mutation in the rod cGMP phosphodiesterase β-subunit gene in two brothers of a Japanese family with autosomal recessive retinitis pigmentosa. *Curr Eye Res* **17**:332, 1998.

258. Huang SH, Pittler SJ, Huang X, Oliveira L, Berson EL, Dryja TP: Autosomal recessive retinitis pigmentosa caused by mutations in the α subunit of rod cGMP phosphodiesterase. *Nature Genet* **11**:468, 1995.

259. Veske A, Orth U, Rüther K, Zrenner E, Rosenberg T, Baehr W, Gal A: Mutations in the gene for the β-subunit of rod photoreceptor cGMP-specific phosphodiesterase (PDEB) in patients with retinal dystrophies and dysfunctions, in Anderson RE (ed): *Degenerative Diseases of the Retina*. New York, Plenum Press, 1995, p 313.

260. Meins M, Janecke A, Marschke C, Denton MJ, Kumaramanickavel G, Pittler S, Gal A: Mutations in PDE6A, the gene encoding the α-subunit of rod photoreceptor cGMP-specific phosphodiesterase, are rare in autosomal recessive retinitis pigmentosa, in LaVail MM, Hollyfield JG,

Anderson RE (eds): *Degenerative Retinal Diseases*. New York, Plenum Press, 1997, p 237.

261. Pittler SJ, Baehr W: Identification of a nonsense mutation in the rod photoreceptor cGMP phosphodiesterase beta-subunit gene of the *rd* mouse. *Proc Natl Acad Sci USA* **88**:8322, 1991.

262. Suber ML, Pittler SJ, Qin N, Wright GC, Holcombe V, Lee RH, Craft CM, Lolley RN, Baehr W, Hurwitz RL: Irish setter dogs affected with rod/cone dysplasia contain a nonsense mutation in the rod cGMP phosphodiesterase beta-subunit gene. *Proc Natl Acad Sci USA* **90**:3968, 1993.

263. Clements PJM, Gregory CY, Peterson-Jones SM, Sargan DR, Bhattacharya SS: Confirmation of the rod cGMP phosphodiesterase beta subunit (*PDEβ*) nonsense mutation in affected *rcd*-1 Irish setters in the UK and development of a diagnostic test. *Curr Eye Res* **12**:861, 1993.

264. Ray K, Baldwin VJ, Acland GM, Blanton SH, Aguirre GD: Cosegregation of codon 807 mutation of the canine rod cGMP phosphodiesterase beta gene and *rcd1*. *Invest Ophthalmol Vis Sci* **35**:4291, 1994.

265. Petersen-Jones SM, Entz D, Sargan DR: Mutation linked to cGMP-phosphodiesterase alpha gene causes generalised progressive retinal atrophy in the Cardigan Welsh Corgi (abstract). *Invest Ophthalmol Vis Sci* **39**:S880, 1998.

266. Farber DB, Lolley RN: Cyclic guanosine monophosphate: elevation in degenerating photoreceptor cells of the C3H mouse retina. *Science* **186**:449, 1974.

267. Aguirre G, Farber D, Lolley R, O'Brien P, Alligood J, Fletcher RT, Chader G: Retinal degenerations in the dog: III. Abnormal cyclic nucleotide metabolism in rod-cone dysplasia. *Exp Eye Res* **35**:625, 1982.

268. Schmidt SY, Lolley RN: Cyclic-nucleotide phosphodiesterase. *J Cell Biol* **57**:117, 1973.

269. Lolley RN, Farber DB, Rayborn ME, Hollyfield JG: Cyclic GMP accumulation causes degeneration of photoreceptor cells: Simulation of an inherited disease. *Science* **196**:664, 1977.

270. Nakatani K, Yau KW: Guanosine 3',5'-cyclic monophosphate-activated conductance studied in a truncated rod outer segment of the toad. *J Physiol (Lond)* **395**:731, 1988.

271. Tuteja N, Danciger M, Klisak I, Tuteja R, Inana G, Mohandas T, Sparkes RS, Farber DB: Isolation and characterization of cDNA encoding the gamma-subunit of cGMP phosphodiesterase in human retina. *Gene* **88**:227, 1990.

272. Hahn LB, Berson EL, Dryja TP: Evaluation of the gene encoding the gamma subunit of rod phosphodiesterase in retinitis pigmentosa. *Invest Ophthalmol Vis Sci* **35**:1077, 1994.

273. Tsang SH, Gouras P, Yamashita CK, Kjeldbye H, Fisher J, Farber DB, Goff SP: Retinal degeneration in mice lacking the gamma subunit of the rod cGMP phosphodiesterase. *Science* **272**:1026, 1996.

274. Florio SK, Prusti RK, Beavo JA: Solubilization of membrane-bound rod phosphodiesterase by the rod phosphodiesterase recombinant δ subunit. *J Biol Chem* **271**:24036, 1996.

275. Ershova G, Derré J, Chételin S, Nancy V, Berger R, Kaplan J, Munnich A, De Gunzburg J: cDNA sequence, genomic organization and mapping of *PDE6D*, the human gene encoding the delta subunit of the cGMP phosphodiesterase of retinal rod cells to chromosome 2q36. *Cytogenet Cell Genet* **79**:139, 1997.

276. Pittler SJ, Lee AK, Altherr MR, Howard TA, Seldin MF, Hurwitz RL, Wasmuth JJ, Baehr W: Primary structure and chromosomal localization of human and mouse rod photoreceptor cGMP-gated cation channel. *J Biol Chem* **267**:6257, 1992.

277. Ardell MD, Aragon I, Oliveira L, Porche GE, Burke E, Pittler SJ: The β subunit of human rod photoreceptor cGMP-gated cation channel is generated from a complex transcription unit. *FEBS Lett* **389**:213, 1996.

278. Dryja TP, Finn JT, Peng Y-W, McGee TL, Berson EL, Yau K-W: Mutations in the gene encoding the α subunit of the rod cGMP-gated channel in autosomal recessive retinitis pigmentosa. *Proc Natl Acad Sci USA* **92**:10177, 1995.

279. Kohl S, Marx T, Giddings I, Jägle H, Jacobson SG, Apfelstedt-Sylla E, Zrenner E, Sharpe LT, Wissinger B: Total colourblindness is caused by mutations in the gene encoding the α-subunit of the cone photoreceptor cGMP-gated cation channel. *Nature Genet* **19**:257, 1998.

280. Ohguro H, Van Hooser JP, Milam AH, Palczewski K: Rhodopsin phosphorylation and dephosphorylation in vivo. *J Biol Chem* **270**:14259, 1995.

281. Zhao X, Palczewski K, Ohguro H: Mechanism of rhodopsin phosphorylation. *Biophys Chem* **56**:183, 1995.

282. Khani SC, Abitbol M, Yamamoto S, Maravic-Magovcevic I, Dryja TP: Characterization and chromosomal localization of the gene for human rhodopsin kinase. *Genomics* **35**:571, 1996.

283. Calabrese G, Sallese M, Stornaiuolo A, Stuppia L, Palka G, de Blasi A: Chromosome mapping of the human arrestin (*SAG*), β-arrestin 2 (*ARRB2*), and β-adrenergic receptor kinase 2 (*ADRBK2*) genes. *Genomics* **23**:286, 1994.

284. Fuchs S, Nakazawa M, Maw M, Tamai M, Oguchi Y, Gal A: A homozygous 1-base pair deletion in the arrestin gene is a frequent cause of Oguchi disease in Japanese. *Nature Genet* **10**:360, 1995.

285. Yamamoto S, Sippel KC, Berson EL, Dryja TP: Defects in the rhodopsin kinase gene in patients with the Oguchi form of stationary night blindness. *Nature Genet* **15**:175, 1997.

286. Cideciyan AV, Zhao XY, Nielsen L, Khani SC, Jacobson SG, Palczewski K: Null mutation in the rhodopsin kinase gene slows recovery kinetics of rod and cone phototransduction in man. *Proc Natl Acad Sci USA* **95**:328, 1998.

287. Rushton WAH, Campbell FW, Hagins WA, Brindley GS: The bleaching and regeneration of rhodopsin in the living eye of the albino rabbit and of man. *Optic Acta* **1**:183, 1955.

288. Rushton WAH: Dark adaptation and the regeneration of rhodopsin. *J Physiol* **156**:166, 1961.

289. Ripps H, Weale RA: Rhodopsin regeneration in man. *Nature* **222**:775, 1969.

290. Carr RE, Ripps H: Rhodopsin kinetics and rod adaptation in Oguchi's disease. *Invest Ophthalmol Vis Sci* **6**:426, 1967.

291. de Jong PTVM, Zrenner E, van Meel GJ, Keunen JEE, van Norren D: Mizuo phenomenon in X-linked retinoschisis. *Arch Ophthalmol* **109**:1104, 1991.

292. Xu J, Dodd RL, Makino CL, Simon MI, Baylor DA, Chen J: Prolonged photoresponses in transgenic mouse rods lacking arrestin. *Nature* **389**:505, 1997.

293. Liu X, Seno K, Nishizawa Y, Hayashi F, Yamazaki A, Matsumoto H, Wakabayashi T, Usukura J: Ultrastructural localization of retinal guanylate cyclase in human and monkey retinas. *Exp Eye Res* **59**:761, 1994.

294. Oliveira L, Miniou P, Viegas-Pequignot E, Rozet J-M, Dollfus H, Pittler SJ: Human retinal guanylate cyclase (*GUC2D*) maps to chromosome 17p13.1. *Genomics* **22**:478, 1994.

295. Perrault I, Rozet JM, Calvas P, Gerber S, Camuzat A, Dollfus H, Châtelin S, Souied E, Ghazi I, Leowski C, Bonnemaison M, Le Paslier D, Frézal J, Dufier J-L, Pittler S, Munnich A, Kaplan J: Retinal-specific guanylate cyclase gene mutations in Leber's congenital amaurosis. *Nature Genet* **14**:461, 1996.

296. Semple-Rowland SL, Lee NR, Van Hooser JP, Palczewski K, Baehr W: A null mutation in the photoreceptor guanylate cyclase gene causes the retinal degeneration chicken phenotype. *Proc Natl Acad Sci USA* **95**:1271, 1998.

297. Kelsell RE, Gregory-Evans K, Payne AM, Perrault I, Kaplan J, Yang RB, Garbers DL, Bird AC, Moore AT, Hunt DM: Mutations in the retinal guanylate cyclase (*RETGC-1*) gene in dominant cone-rod dystrophy. *Hum Mol Genet* **7**:1179, 1998.

298. Perrault I, Rozet J-M, Gerber S, Kelsell RE, Souied E, Cabot A, Hunt DM, Munnich A, Kaplan J: A *retGC-1* mutation in autosomal dominant cone-rod dystrophy. *Am J Hum Genet* **63**:651, 1998.

299. Palczewski K, Subbaraya I, Gorczyca WA, Helekar BS, Ruiz CC, Ohguro H, Huang J, Zhao X, Crabb JW, Johnson RS, Walsh KA, Gray-Keller MP, Detwiler PB, Baehr W: Molecular cloning and characterization of retinal photoreceptor guanylyl cyclase-activating protein. *Neuron* **13**:395, 1994.

300. Dizhoor AM, Hurley JB: Inactivation of EF-hands makes GCAP-2 (p24) a constitutive activator of photoreceptor guanylyl cyclase by preventing a $Ca^{2+}$-induced "activator-to-inhibitor" transition. *J Biol Chem* **271**:19346, 1996.

301. Subbaraya I, Ruiz CC, Helekar BS, Zhao X, Gorczyca W, Pettenati MJ, Rao PN, Palczewski K, Baehr W: Molecular characterization of human and mouse photoreceptor guanylate cyclase activating protein (GCAP) and chromosomal localization of the human gene. *J Biol Chem* **269**:31080, 1994.

302. Payne AM, Downes SM, Bessant DAR, Taylor R, Holder GE, Warren MJ, Bird AC, Bhattacharya SS: A mutation in guanylate cyclase activator 1A (*GUCA1A*) in an autosomal dominant cone dystrophy pedigree mapping to a new locus on chromosome 6p21.1. *Hum Mol Genet* **7**:273, 1998.

303. Dizhoor AM, Boikov SG, Olshevskaya EV: Constitutive activation of photoreceptor guanylate cyclase by Y99C mutant of GCAP-1. *J Biol Chem* **273**:17311, 1998.

304. Sokal I, Li N, Surgucheva I, Warren MJ, Payne AM, Bhattacharya SS, Baehr W, Palczewski K: GCAP1(Y99C) mutant is constitutively active in autosomal dominant cone dystrophy. *Mol Cell* **2**:129, 1998.

305. Schwahn U, Lenzner S, Dong J, Feil S, Hinzmann B, Van Duijnhoven G, Kirschner R, Hemberger M, Bergen AAB, Rosenberg T, Pinckers AJLG, Fundele R, Rosenthal A, Cremers FPM, Ropers HH, Berger W: Positional cloning of the gene for X-linked retinitis pigmentosa 2. *Nature Genet* **19**:327, 1998.

306. Meindl A, Dry K, Herrmann K, Manson F, Ciccodicola A, Edgar A, Carvalho MRS, Achatz H, Hellebrand H, Lennon A, Migliaccio C, Porter K, Zrenner E, Bird A, Jay M, Lorenz B, Wittwer B, D'Urso M, Meitinger T, Wright A: A gene (*RPGR*) with homology to the RCC1 guanine nucleotide exchange factor is mutated in X-linked retinitis pigmentosa (RP3). *Nature Genet* **13**:35, 1996.

307. Roepman R, Van Duijnhoven G, Rosenberg T, Pinckers AJLG, Bleeker-Wagemakers LM, Bergen AAB, Post J, Beck A, Reinhardt R, Ropers HH, Cremers FPM, Berger W: Positional cloning of the gene for X-linked retinitis pigmetosa 3: Homology with the guanine-nucleotide exchange factor RCC1. *Hum Mol Genet* **5**:1035, 1996.

308. Yan D, Swain PK, Breuer D, Tucker RM, Wu WP, Fujita R, Rehemtulla A, Burke D, Swaroop A: Biochemical characterization and subcellular localization of the mouse retinitis pigmentosa GTPase regulator (mRpgr). *J Biol Chem* **273**:19656, 1998.

309. Fujita R, Buraczynska M, Gieser L, Wu WP, Forsythe P, Abrahamson M, Jacobson SG, Sieving PA, Andréasson S, Swaroop A: Analysis of the *RPGR* gene in 11 pedigrees with the retinitis pigmentosa type 3 genotype: Paucity of mutations in the coding region but splice defects in two families. *Am J Hum Genet* **61**:571, 1997.

310. Buraczynska M, Wu W, Fujita R, Buraczynska K, Phelps E, Andréasson S, Bennett J, Birch DG, Fishman GA, Hoffman DR, Inana G, Jacobson SG, Musarella MA, Sieving PA, Swaroop A: Spectrum of mutations in the *RPGR* gene that are identified in 20 percent of families with X-linked retinitis pigmentosa. *Am J Hum Genet* **61**:1287, 1997.

311. Allikmets R, Singh N, Sun H, Shroyer NF, Hutchinson A, Chidambaram A, Gerrard B, Baird L, Stauffer D, Peiffer A, Rattner A, Smallwood P, Li Y, Anderson KL, Lewis RA, Nathans J, Leppert M, Dean M, Lupski JR: A photoreceptor cell-specific ATP-binding transporter gene (*ABCR*) is mutated in recessive Stargardt macular dystrophy. *Nature Genet* **15**:236, 1997.

312. Allikmets R, Wasserman WW, Hutchinson A, Smallwood P, Nathans J, Rogan PK, Schneider TD, Dean M: Organization of the *ABCR* gene: Analysis of promoter and splice junction sequences. *Gene* **215**:111, 1998.

313. Gerber S, Rozet JM, van de Pol TJR, Hoyng CB, Munnich A, Blankenagel A, Kaplan J, Cremers FPM: Complete exon-intron structure of the retina-specific ATP binding transporter gene (*ABCR*) allows the identification of novel mutations underlying Stargardt disease. *Genomics* **48**:139, 1998.

314. Martínez-Mir A, Paloma E, Allikmets R, Ayuso C, del Rio T, Dean M, Vilageliu L, Gonzàlez-Duarte R, Balcells S: Retinitis pigmentosa caused by a homozygous mutation in the Stargardt disease gene *ABCR*. *Nature Genet* **18**:11, 1998.

315. Cremers FPM, van de Pol DJR, Van Driel M, Den Hollander AI, Van Haren FJJ, Knoers NVAM, Tijmes N, Bergen AAB, Rohrschneider K, Blankenagel A, Pinckers AJLG, Deutman AF, Hoyng CB: Autosomal recessive retinitis pigmentosa and cone-rod dystrophy caused by splice site mutations in the Stargardt's disease gene *ABCR*. *Hum Mol Genet* **7**:355, 1998.

316. Thomson JL, Brzeski H, Dunbar B, Forrester JV, Fothergill JE, Converse CA: Photoreceptor rim protein: Partial sequences of cDNA show a high degree of similarity to ABC transporters. *Curr Eye Res* **16**:741, 1997.

317. Illing M, Molday LL, Molday RS: The 220-kDa Rim protein of retinal rod outer segments is a member of the ABC transporter superfamily. *J Biol Chem* **272**:10303, 1997.

318. Sun H, Nathans J: Stargardt's ABCR is localized to the disc membrane of retinal rod outer segments. *Nature Genet* **17**:15, 1997.

319. Azarian SM, Travis GH: The photoreceptor rim protein is an ABC transporter encoded by the gene for recessive Stargardt's disease (*ABCR*). *FEBS Lett* **409**:247, 1997.

320. Crabb JW, Carlson A, Chen Y, Goldflam S, Intres R, West KA, Hulmes JD, Kapron JT, Luck LA, Horwitz J, Bok D: Structural and functional characterization of recombinant human cellular retinaldehyde-binding protein. *Protein Sci* **7**:746, 1998.

321. Intres R, Goldflam S, Cook JR, Crabb JW: Molecular cloning and structural analysis of the human gene encoding cellular retinaldehyde-binding protein. *J Biol Chem* **269**:25411, 1994.

322. Hamel CP, Jenkins NA, Gilbert DJ, Copeland NG, Redmond TM: The gene for the retinal pigment epithelium-specific protein RPE65 is localized to human 1p31 and mouse 3. *Genomics* **20**:509, 1994.

323. Hamel CP, Tsilou E, Harris E, Pfeffer BA, Hooks JJ, Detrick B, Redmond TM: A developmentally regulated microsomal protein specific for the pigment epithelium of the vertebrate retina. *J Neurosci Res* **34**:414, 1993.

324. Marlhens F, Bareil C, Griffoin JM, Zrenner E, Amalric P, Eliaou C, Liu SY, Harris E, Redmond TM, Arnaud B, Claustres M, Hamel CP: Mutations in *RPE65* cause Leber's congenital amaurosis. *Nature Genet* **17**:139, 1997.

325. Morimura H, Fishman GA, Grover SA, Fulton AB, Berson EL, Dryja TP: Mutations in the RPE65 gene in patients with autosomal recessive retinitis pigmentosa or Leber congenital amaurosis. *Proc Natl Acad Sci USA* **95**:3088, 1998.

326. Gu SM, Thompson DA, Srikumari CRS, Lorenz B, Finckh U, Nicoletti A, Murthy KR, Rathmann M, Kumaramanickavel G, Denton MJ, Gal A: Mutations in *RPE65* cause autosomal recessive childhood-onset severe retinal dystrophy. *Nature Genet* **17**:194, 1997.

327. Nasonkin I, Illing M, Koehler MR, Schmid M, Molday RS, Weber BHF: Mapping of the rod photoreceptor ABC transporter (ABCR) to 1p21-p22.1 and identification of novel mutations in Stargardt's disease. *Hum Genet* **102**:21, 1998.

328. Coleman DL, Eicher EM: Fat (*fat*) and tubby (*tub*): Two autosomal recessive mutations causing obesity syndromes in the mouse. *J Hered* **81**:424, 1990.

329. Heckenlively JR, Chang B, Erway LC, Peng C, Hawes NL, Hageman GS, Roderick TH: Mouse model for Usher syndrome: Linkage mapping suggests homology to Usher type I reported at human chromosome 11p15. *Proc Natl Acad Sci USA* **92**:11100, 1995.

330. Ohlemiller KK, Hughes RM, Mosinger-Ogilvie J, Speck JD, Grosof DH, Silverman MS: Cochlear and retinal degeneration in the tubby mouse. *Neuroreport* **6**:845, 1995.

331. Kleyn PW, Fan W, Kovats SG, Lee JJ, Pulido JC, Wu Y, Berkemeier LR, Misumi DJ, Holmgren L, Charlat O, Woolf EA, Tayber O, Brody T, Shu P, Hawkins F, Kennedy B, Baldini L, Ebeling C, Alperin GD, Deeds J, Lakey ND, Culpepper J, Chen H, Glücksmann-Kuis MA: Identification and characterization of the mouse obesity gene *tubby*: A member of a novel gene family. *Cell* **85**:281, 1996.

332. Noben-Trauth K, Naggert JK, North MA, Nishina PM: A candidate gene for the mouse mutation *tubby*. *Nature* **380**:534, 1996.

333. North MA, Naggert JK, Yan Y, Noben-Trauth K, Nishina PM: Molecular characterization of *TUB, TULP1*, and *TULP2*, members of the novel *tubby* gene family and their possible relation to ocular diseases. *Proc Natl Acad Sci USA* **94**:3128, 1997.

334. Hagstrom SA, North MA, Nishina PM, Berson EL, Dryja TP: Recessive mutations in the gene encoding the tubby-like protein TULP1 in patients with retinitis pigmentosa. *Nature Genet* **18**:174, 1998.

335. Banerjee P, Kleyn PW, Knowles JA, Lewis CA, Ross BM, Kovats SG, Lee JJ, Penchaszadeh GK, Ott J, Jacobson SG, Gilliam TC: *TULP1* mutation in two extended Dominican kindreds with autosomal recessive retinitis pigmentosa (*RP14*). *Nature Genet* **18**:177, 1998.

336. Gu SM, Lennon A, Li Y, Lorenz B, Fossarello M, North M, Gal A, Wright A: Tubby-like protein-1 mutations in autosomal recessive retinitis pigmentosa. *Lancet* **351**:1103, 1998.

337. Furukawa T, Morrow EM, Cepko CL: Crx, a novel *otx*-like homeobox gene, shows photoreceptor-specific expression and regulates photoreceptor differentiation. *Cell* **91**:531, 1997.

338. Chen SM, Wang QL, Nie ZQ, Sun H, Lennon G, Copeland NG, Gilbert DJ, Jenkins NA, Zack DJ: Crx, a novel Otx-like paired-homeodomain protein, binds to and transactivates photoreceptor cell-specific genes. *Neuron* **19**:1017, 1997.

339. Freund CL, Gregory-Evans CY, Furukawa T, Papaioannou M, Looser J, Ploder L, Bellingham J, Ng D, Herbrick JAS, Duncan A, Scherer SW, Tsui LC, Loutradis-Anagnostou A, Jacobson SG, Cepko CL, Bhattacharya SS, McInnes RR: Cone-rod dystrophy due to mutations in a novel photoreceptor-specific homeobox gene (*CRX*) essential for maintenance of the photoreceptor. *Cell* **91**:543, 1997.

340. Swain PK, Chen SM, Wang QL, Affatigato LM, Coats CL, Brady KD, Fishman GA, Jacobson SG, Swaroop A, Stone E, Sieving PA, Zack DJ: Mutations in the cone-rod homeobox gene are associated with the cone-rod dystrophy photoreceptor degeneration. *Neuron* **19**:1329, 1997.

341. Freund CL, Wang QL, Chen SM, Muskat BL, Wiles CD, Sheffield VC, Jacobson SG, McInnes RR, Zack DJ, Stone EM: De novo mutations in the *CRX* homeobox gene associated with Leber congenital amaurosis. *Nature Genet* **18**:311, 1998.

342. Arikawa K, Molday LL, Molday RS, Williams DS: Localization of peripherin/rds in the disk membranes of cone and rod photoreceptors: Relationship to disk membrane morphogenesis and retinal degeneration. *J Cell Biol* **116**:659, 1992.

343. Moritz OL, Molday RS: Molecular cloning, membrane topology, and localization of bovine rom-1 in rod and cone photoreceptor cells. *Invest Ophthalmol Vis Sci* **37**:352, 1996.

344. van Nie R, Ivanyi D, Demant P: A new H-2 linked mutation, *rds*, causing retinal degeneration in the mouse. *Tissue Antigens* **12**:106, 1978.

345. Travis GH, Brennan MB, Danielson PE, Kozak CA, Sutcliffe JG: Identification of a photoreceptor-specific mRNA encoded by the gene responsible for *retinal degeneration slow (rds)*. *Nature* **338**:70, 1989.

346. Ma J, Norton JC, Allen AC, Burns JB, Hasel KW, Burns JL, Sutcliffe JG, Travis GH: *Retinal degeneration slow (rds)* in mouse results from simple insertion of a *t* haplotype-specific element into protein-coding exon II. *Genomics* **28**:212, 1995.

347. Molday RS, Hicks D, Molday L: Peripherin: A rim-specific membrane protein of rod outer segment discs. *Invest Ophthalmol Vis Sci* **28**:50, 1987.

348. Connell GJ, Molday RS: Molecular cloning, primary structure, and orientation of the vertebrate photoreceptor cell protein peripherin in the rod outer segment disk membrane. *Biochemistry* **29**:4691, 1990.

349. Connell G, Bascom R, Molday L, Reid D, McInnes RR, Molday RS: Photoreceptor peripherin is the normal product of the gene responsible for retinal degeneration in the *rds* mouse. *Proc Natl Acad Sci USA* **88**:723, 1991.

350. Travis GH, Sutcliffe JG, Bok D: The *retinal degeneration slow (rds)* gene product is a photoreceptor disc membrane-associated glycoprotein. *Neuron* **6**:61, 1991.

351. Travis GH, Christerson L, Danielson PE, Klisak I, Sparkes RS, Hahn LB, Dryja TP, Sutcliffe JG: The human retinal degeneration slow (*RDS*) gene: Chromosomal assignment and structure of the mRNA. *Genomics* **10**:733, 1991.

352. Apfelstedt-Sylla E, Theischen M, Rüther K, Wedemann H, Gal A, Zrenner E: Extensive intrafamilial and interfamilial phenotypic variation among patients with autosomal dominant retinal dystrophy and mutations in the human *RDS/peripherin* gene. *Br J Ophthalmol* **79**:28, 1995.

353. Kohl S, Christ-Adler M, Apfelstedt-Sylla E, Kellner U, Eckstein A, Zrenner E, Wissinger B: *RDS/peripherin* gene mutations are frequent causes of central retinal dystrophies. *J Med Genet* **34**:620, 1997.

354. Farrar GJ, Kenna P, Jordan SA, Rajendra KS, Humphries MM, Sharp EM, Sheils DM, Humphries P: A three-base-pair deletion in the peripherin-RDS gene in one form of retinitis pigmentosa. *Nature* **354**:478, 1991.

355. Kajiwara K, Hahn LB, Mukai S, Travis GH, Berson EL, Dryja TP: Mutations in the human retinal degeneration slow gene in autosomal dominant retinitis pigmentosa. *Nature* **354**:480, 1991.

356. Bascom RA, Manara S, Collins L, Molday RS, Kalnins VI, McInnes RR: Cloning of the cDNA for a novel photoreceptor membrane protein (rom-1) identifies a disk rim protein family implicated in human retinopathies. *Neuron* **8**:1171, 1992.

357. Goldberg AFX, Molday RS: Subunit composition of the peripherin/rds-rom-1 disk rim complex from rod photoreceptors: Hydrodynamic evidence for a tetrameric quaternary structure. *Biochemistry* **35**:6144, 1996.

358. Bascom RA, Liu L, Heckenlively JR, Stone EM, McInnes RR: Mutation analysis of the *ROM1* gene in retinitis pigmentosa. *Hum Mol Genet* **4**:1895, 1995.

359. Sakuma H, Inana G, Murakami A, Yajima T, Weleber RG, Murphey WH, Gass JDM, Hotta Y, Hayakawa M, Fujiki K, Gao YQ, Danciger M, Farber D, Cideciyan AV, Jacobson SG: A heterozygous putative null mutation in *ROM1* without a mutation in peripherin/RDS in a family with retinitis pigmentosa. *Genomics* **27**:384, 1995.

360. Martínez-Mir A, Vilela C, Bayés M, Valverde D, Dain L, Beneyto M, Marco M, Baiget M, Grinberg D, Balcells S, Gonzàlez-Duarte R, Vilageliu L: Putative association of a mutant *ROM1* allele with retinitis pigmentosa. *Hum Genet* **99**:827, 1997.

361. Goldberg AFX, Molday RS: Defective subunit assembly underlies a digenic form of retinitis pigmentosa linked to mutations in peripherin *rds* and *rom-1*. *Proc Natl Acad Sci USA* **93**:13726, 1996.

362. Hays TS, Deuring R, Robertson B, Prout M, Fuller MT: Interacting proteins identified by genetic interactions: A missense mutation in alpha-tubulin fails to complement alleles of the testis-specific beta-tubulin gene of *Drosophila melanogaster*. *Mol Cell Biol* **9**:875, 1989.

363. Kusch M, Edgar RS: Genetic studies of unusual loci that affect body shape of the nematode *Caenorhabditis elegans* and may code for cuticle structural proteins. *Genetics* **113**:621, 1986.

364. Stearns T, Botstein D: Unlinked noncomplementation: Isolation of new conditional-lethal mutations in each of the tubulin genes of *Saccharomyces cerevisiae*. *Genetics* **119**:249, 1988.

365. Helwig U, Imai K, Schmahl W, Thomas BE, Varnum DS, Nadeau JH, Balling R: Interaction between *undulated* and *Patch* leads to an extreme form of spina bifida in double-mutant mice. *Nature Genet* **11**:60, 1995.

366. Larget-Piet D, Gerber S, Bonneau D, Rozet JM, Marc S, Ghazi I, Dufier JL, David A, Bitoun P, Weissenbach J, Munnich A, Kaplan J: Genetic heterogeneity of Usher syndrome type I in French families. *Genomics* **21**:138, 1994.

367. Eudy JD, Weston MD, Yao S, Hoover DM, Rehm HL, Ma-Edmonds M, Yan D, Ahmad I, Cheng JJ, Ayuso C, Cremers C, Davenport S, Moller C, Talmadge CB, Beisel KW, Tamayo M, Morton CC, Swaroop A, Kimberling WJ, Sumegi J: Mutation of a gene encoding a protein with extracellular matrix motifs in Usher syndrome type IIa. *Science* **280**:1753, 1998.

368. Joensuu T, Blanco G, Pakarinen L, Sistonen P, Kaariainen H, Brown S, de la Chapelle A, Sankila EM: Refined mapping of the usher syndrome type III locus on chromosome 3, exclusion of candidate genes, and identification of the putative mouse homologous region. *Genomics* **38**:255, 1996.

369. Cheney RE, Mooseker MS: Unconventional myosins. *Curr Opin Cell Biol* **4**:27, 1992.

370. Weston MD, Kelley PM, Overbeck LD, Wagenaar M, Orten DJ, Hasson T, Chen ZY, Corey D, Mooseker M, Sumegi J, Cremers C, Möller C, Jacobson SG, Gorin MB, Kimberling WJ: Myosin VIIA mutation screening in 189 Usher syndrome type 1 patients. *Am J Hum Genet* **59**:1074, 1996.

371. Adato A, Weil D, Kalinski H, Pel-Or Y, Ayadi H, Petit C, Korostishevsky M, Bonne-Tamir B: Mutation profile of all 49 exons of the human myosin VIIA gene, and haplotype analysis, in Usher 1B families from diverse origins. *Am J Hum Genet* **61**:813, 1997.

372. Lévy G, Levi-Acobas F, Blanchard S, Gerber S, Larget-Piet D, Chenal V, Liu XZ, Newton V, Steel KP, Brown SDM, Munnich A, Kaplan J, Petit C, Weil D: Myosin VIIA gene: Heterogeneity of the mutations responsible for Usher syndrome type IB. *Hum Mol Genet* **6**:111, 1997.

373. Gibson F, Walsh J, Mburu P, Varela A, Brown KA, Antonio M, Beisel KW, Steel KP, Brown SDM: A type VII myosin encoded by the mouse deafness gene *shaker-1*. *Nature* **374**:62, 1995.

374. El-Amraoui A, Sahly I, Picaud S, Sahel J, Abitbol M, Petit C: Human Usher 1B mouse *shaker-1*: The retinal phenotype discrepancy explained by the presence/absence of myosin VIIA in the photoreceptor cells. *Hum Mol Genet* **5**:1171, 1996.

375. Weil D, Lévy G, Sahly I, Lévi-Acobas F, Blanchard S, El-Amraoui A, Crozet F, Philippe H, Abitbol M, Petit C: Human myosin VIIA responsible for the Usher 1B syndrome: A predicted membrane-associated motor protein expressed in developing sensory epithelia. *Proc Natl Acad Sci USA* **93**:3232, 1996.

376. Liu X-Z, Walsh J, Mburu P, Kendrick-Jones J, Cope MJTV, Steel KP, Brown SDM: Mutations in the myosin VIIa gene cause non-syndromic recessive deafness. *Nature Genet* **16**:188, 1995.

377. Weil D, Küssel P, Blanchard S, Lévy G, Levi-Acobas F, Drira M, Ayadi H, Petit C: The autosomal recessive isolated deafness, *DFNB2*, and the Usher 1B syndrome are allelic defects of the myosin-VIIA gene. *Nature Genet* **16**:191, 1997.

378. Hasson T, Heintzelman MB, Santos-Sacchi J, Corey DP, Mooseker MS: Expression in cochlea and retina of myosin VIIa, the gene product defective in Usher syndrome type 1B. *Proc Natl Acad Sci USA* **92**:9815, 1995.

379. Liu X, Ondek B, Williams DS: Mutant myosin VIIa causes defective melanosome distribution in the RPE of *shaker-1* mice. *Nature Genet* **19**:117, 1998.

380. Liu XR, Vansant G, Udovichenko IP, Wolfrum U, Williams DS: Myosin VIIa, the product of the Usher 1B syndrome gene, is concentrated in the connecting cilia of photoreceptor cells. *Cell Motil Cytoskel* **37**:240, 1997.

381. Self T, Mahony M, Fleming J, Walsh J, Brown SDM, Steel KP: *Shaker-1* mutations reveal roles for myosin VIIA in both development and function of cochlear hair cells. *Development* **125**:557, 1998.

382. Szlyk JP, Alexander KR, Severing K, Fishman GA: Assessment of driving performance in patients with retinitis pigmentosa. *Arch Ophthalmol* **110**:1709, 1992.

383. Armington JC, Schwab GJ: Electroretinogram in nyctalopia. *Arch Ophthalmol* **52**:725, 1954.

384. Szlyk JP, Fishman GA, Master SP, Alexander KR: Peripheral vision screening for driving in retinitis pigmentosa patients. *Ophthalmology* **98**:612, 1991.

385. Herbert V: Toxicity of 25,000 IU vitamin A supplements in "health" food users. *Am J Clin Nutr* **36**:185, 1982.

386. Jacobson SG, Cideciyan AV, Regunath G, Rodriguez FJ, Vandenburgh K, Sheffield VC, Stone EM: Night blindness in Sorsby's fundus dystrophy reversed by vitamin A. *Nature Genet* **11**:27, 1995.

387. Panozzo G, Babighian S, Bonora A: Association of xerophthalmia, flecked retina, and pseudotumor cerebri caused by hypovitaminosis A. *Am J Ophthalmol* **125**:708, 1998.

388. Fishman GA, Glenn AM, Gilbert LD: Rebound of macular edema with continued use of methazolamide in patients with retinitis pigmentosa. *Arch Ophthalmol* **111**:1640, 1993.

389. Greenstein VC, Holopigian K, Siderides E, Seiple W, Carr RE: The effects of acetazolamide on visual function in retinitis pigmentosa. *Invest Ophthalmol Vis Sci* **34**:269, 1993.

390. Berson EL, Mehaffey L, Rabin AR: A night vision pocketscope for patients with retinitis pigmentosa. *Arch Ophthalmol* **91**:495, 1974.

391. LaVail MM, Battelle B-A: Influence of eye pigmentation and light deprivation on inherited retinal dystrophy in the rat. *Exp Eye Res* **21**:167, 1975.

392. Davidson FF, Steller H: Blocking apoptosis prevents blindness *Drosophila* retinal degeneration mutants. *Nature* **391**:587, 1998.

393. Naash ML, Peachey NS, Li Z-Y, Gryczan CC, Goto Y, Blanks J, Milam A, Ripps H: Light-induced acceleration of photoreceptor degeneration in transgenic mice expressing mutant rhodopsin. *Invest Ophthalmol Vis Sci* **37**:775, 1996.

394. Wang M, Lam TT, Tso MOM, Naash MI: Expression of a mutant opsin gene increases the susceptibility of the retina to light damage. *Vis Neurosci* **14**:55, 1997.

395. Berson EL: Light deprivation and retinitis pigmentosa. *Vision Res* **20**:1179, 1980.

396. Katznelson LA, Khoroshilova-Maslova IP, Eliseyeva RF: A new method of treatment of retinitis pigmentosa/pigmentary abiotrophy. *Ann Ophthalmol* **22**:167, 1990.

397. Berson EL, Remulla JFC, Rosner B: Evaluation of patients with retinitis pigmentosa receiving electric stimulation, ozonated blood, and ocular surgery in Cuba. *Arch Ophthalmol* **114**:560, 1996.

398. Peláez O: Evaluation of patients with retinitis pigmentosa receiving electric stimulation, ozonated blood, and ocular surgery in Cuba. *Arch Ophthalmol* **115**:133, 1997.

399. Berson EL, Remulla JFC, Rosner B, Sandberg MA, Weigel-DiFranco C: Evaluation of patients with retinitis pigmentosa receiving electric stimulation, ozonated blood, and ocular surgery in Cuba: Reply. *Arch Ophthalmol* **115**:133, 1997.

400. Gerding H: Evaluation of patients with retinitis pigmentosa receiving electric stimulation, ozonated bleed, and ocular surgery in Cuba. *Arch Ophthalmol* **115**:1215, 1997.

401. Bennett J, Tanabe T, Sun DX, Zeng Y, Kjeldbye H, Gouras P, Maguire AM: Photoreceptor cell rescue in retinal degeneration (*rd*) mice by in vivo gene therapy. *Nature Med* **2**:649, 1996.

402. LaVail MM, Unoki K, Yasumura D, Matthes MT, Yancopoulos GD, Steinberg RH: Multiple growth factors, cytokines, and neurotrophins rescue photoreceptors from the damaging effects of constant light. *Proc Natl Acad Sci USA* **89**:11249, 1992.

403. Chen J, Flannery JG, LaVail MM, Steinberg RH, Xu J, Simon MI: bcl-2 overexpression reduces apoptotic photoreceptor cell death in three different retinal degenerations. *Proc Natl Acad Sci USA* **93**:7042, 1996.

404. Joseph RM, Li T: Overexpression of bcl-2 and bcl-XL transgenes and photoreceptor degeneration. *Invest Ophthalmol Vis Sci* **37**:2434, 1996.

405. Drenser KA, Timmers AM, Hauswirth WW, Lewin AS: Ribozyme-targeted destruction of RNA associated with autosomal-dominant retinitis pigmentosa. *Invest Ophthalmol Vis Sci* **39**:681, 1998.

406. Zrenner E, Miliczek KD, Gabel VP, Graf HG, Guenther E, Haemmerle H, Hoefflinger B, Kohler K, Nisch W, Schubert M, Stett A, Weiss S: The development of subretinal microphotodiodes for replacement of degenerated photoreceptors. *Ophthalmic Res* **29**:269, 1997.

407. Young RW: The renewal of photoreceptor cell outer segments. *J Cell Biol* **33**:61, 1967.

408. Young RW: Visual cells and the concept of renewal. *Invest Ophthalmol Vis Sci* **15**:700, 1976.

409. Andreasson S, Ehinger B, Abrahamson M, Fex G: A six generation family with autosomal dominant retinitis pigmentosa and a rhodopsin gene mutation (arginine-135-leucine). *Ophthalmic Paediatr Genet* **13**:145, 1992.

410. Keen TJ, Inglehearn CF, Lester DH, Bashir R, Jay M, Bird AC, Jay B, Bhattacharya SS: Autosomal dominant retinitis pigmentosa: Four new mutations in rhodopsin, one of them in the retinal attachment site. *Genomics* **11**:199, 1991.

411. Vesa J, Hellsten E, Verkruyse LA, Camp LA, Rapola J, Santavuori P, Hofmann SL, Peltonen L: Mutations in the palmitoyl protein thioesterase gene causing infantile neuronal ceroid lipofuscinosis. *Nature* **376**:584, 1995.

412. Kaplan J, Gerber S, Larget-Piet D, Rozet JM, Dollfus H, Dufier JL, Odent S, Postel-Vinay A, Janin N, Briard ML, Frézal J, Munnich A: A gene for Stargardt's disease (fundus flavimaculatus) maps to the short arm of chromosome 1. *Nature Genet* **5**:308, 1993.

413. Xu SY, Rosenberg T, Gal A: Refined genetic mapping of autosomal dominant retinitis pigmentosa locus *RP18* reduces the critical region to 2 cM between *D1S442* and *D1S2858* on chromosome 1q. *Hum Genet* **102**:493, 1998.

414. Klein ML, Schultz DW, Edwards A, Matise TC, Rust K, Berselli CB, Trzupek K, Weleber RG, Ott J, Wirtz MK, Acott TS: Age-related macular degeneration: Clinical features in a large family and linkage to chromosome 1q. *Arch Ophthalmol* **116**:1082, 1998.

415. Tranebjaerg L, Sjo O, Warburg M: Retinal cone dysfunction and mental retardation associated with a de novo balanced translocation 1:6(q44;q27). *Ophthalmic Paediatr Genet* **7**:167, 1986.

416. Gregory CY, Evans K, Wijesuriya SD, Kermani S, Jay MR, Plant C, Cox N, Bird AC, Bhattacharya SS: The gene responsible for autosomal dominant Doyne's honeycomb retinal dystrophy (*DHRD*) maps to chromosome 2p16. *Hum Mol Genet* **5**:1055, 1996.

417. Héon E, Piguet B, Munier F, Sneed SR, Morgan CM, Forni S, Pescia G, Schorderet D, Taylor CM, Streb LM, Wiles CD, Nishimura DY, Sheffield VC, Stone EM: Linkage of autosomal dominant radial drusen (malattia leventinese) to chromosome 2p16-21. *Arch Ophthalmol* **114**:193, 1996.

418. Collin GB, Marshall JD, Cardon LR, Nishina PM: Homozygosity mapping at Alstrom syndrome to chromosome 2p. *Hum Mol Genet* **6**:213, 1997.

419. Bayés M, Goldaracena B, Martínez-Mir A, Iragui-Madoz MI, Solans T, Chivelet P, Bussaglia E, Ramos-Arroyo MA, Baiget M, Vilageliu L, Balcells S, Gonzàlez-Duarte R, Grinberg D: A new autosomal recessive retinitis pigmentosa locus maps on chromosome 2q31-q33. *J Med Genet* **35**:141, 1998.

420. David G, Abbas N, Stevanin G, Durr A, Yvert G, Cancel G, Weber C, Imbert G, Saudou F, Antoniou E, Drabkin H, Gemmill R, Giunti P, Benomar A, Wood N, Ruberg M, Agid Y, Mandel JL, Brice A: Cloning of the *SCA7* gene reveals a highly unstable CAG repeat expansion. *Nature Genet* **17**:65, 1997.

421. Sheffield VC, Fishman GA, Beck JS, Kimura AE, Stone EM: Identification of novel rhodopsin mutations associated with retinitis pigmentosa by GC-clamped denaturing gradient gel electrophoresis. *Am J Hum Genet* **49**:699, 1991.

422. Yamaguchi K, Takahashi S, Kawanami T, Kato T, Sasaki H: Retinal degeneration in hereditary ceruloplasmin deficiency. *Ophthalmologica* **212**:11, 1998.

423. Narcisi TME, Shoulders CC, Chester SA, Read J, Brett DJ, Harrison GB, Grantham TT, Fox MF, Povey S, De Bruin TWA, Erkelens DW, Muller DPR, Lloyd JK, Scott J: Mutations of the microsomal triglyceride-transfer-protein gene in abetalipoproteinemia. *Am J Hum Genet* **57**:1298, 1995.

424. Harada T, Harada C, Watanabe M, Inoue Y, Sakagawa T, Nakayama N, Sasaki S, Okuyama S, Watase K, Wada K, Tanaka K: Functions of the two glutamate transporters GLAST and GLT-1 in the retina. *Proc Natl Acad Sci USA* **95**:4663, 1998.

425. Kerrison JB, Koenekoop RK, Arnould VJ, Zee D, Maumenee IH: Clinical features of autosomal dominant congenital nystagmus linked to chromosome 6p12. *Am J Ophthalmol* **125**:64, 1998.

426. Wells J, Wroblewski J, Keen J, Inglehearn C, Jubb C, Eckstein A, Jay M, Arden G, Bhattacharya S, Fitzke F, Bird A: Mutations in the human retinal degeneration slow (*RDS*) gene can cause either retinitis pigmentosa or macular dystrophy. *Nature Genet* **3**:213, 1993.

427. Ruiz A, Borrego S, Marcos I, Antiñolo G: A major locus for autosomal recessive retinitis pigmentosa on 6q, determined by homozygosity mapping of chromosomal regions that contain gamma-aminobutyric acid receptor clusters. *Am J Hum Genet* **62**:1452, 1998.

428. Stone EM, Nichols BE, Kimura AE, Weingeist TA, Drack A, Sheffield VC: Clinical features of a Stargardt-like dominant progressive macular dystrophy with genetic linkage to chromosome 6q. *Arch Ophthalmol* **112**:765, 1994.

429. Kelsell RE, Gregory-Evans K, Gregory-Evans CY, Holder GE, Jay MR, Weber BHF, Moore AT, Bird AC, Hunt DM: Localization of a gene (*CORD7*) for a dominant cone-rod dystrophy to chromosome 6q. *Am J Hum Genet* **63**:274, 1998.

430. Small KW, Weber JL, Roses AD, Pericak-Vance MA: North Carolina macular dystrophy maps to chromosome 6. *Genomics* **13**:681, 1992.

431. Kelsell RE, Godley BF, Evans K, Tiffin PAC, Gregory CY, Plant C, Moore AT, Bird AC, Hunt DM: Localization of the gene for progressive bifocal chorioretinal atrophy (*PBCRA*) to chromosome 6q. *Hum Mol Genet* **4**:1653, 1995.

432. Inglehearn CF, Carter SA, Keen TJ, Lindsey J, Stephenson AM, Bashir R, Al-Maghtheh M, Moore AT, Jay M, Bird AC, Bhattacharya SS: A new locus for autosomal dominant retinitis pigmentosa on 7p. *Nature Genet* **4**:51, 1993.

433. Kremer H, Pinckers A, van dem Helm B, Deutman AF, Ropers HH, Mariman ECM: Localization of the gene for dominant cystic macular dystrophy on chromosome 7p. *Hum Mol Genet* **3**:299, 1994.

434. Inglehearn C, Keen TJ, Al-Maghtheh M, Bhattacharya S: Loci for autosomal dominant retinitis pigmentosa and dominant cystoid macular dystrophy on chromosome 7p are not allelic. *Am J Hum Genet* **55**:581, 1994.

435. Inglehearn CF, Keen TJ, Al-Maghtheh M, Gregory CY, Jay MR, Moore AT, Bird AC, Bhattacharya SS: Further refinement of the location for autosomal dominant retinitis pigmentosa on chromosome 7p (*RP9*). *Am J Hum Genet* **54**:675, 1994.

436. Kim RY, Fitzke FW, Moore AT, Jay M, Inglehearn C, Arden GB, Bhattacharya SS, Bird AC: Autosomal dominant retinitis pigmentosa mapping to chromosome 7p exhibits variable expression. *Br J Ophthalmol* **79**:23, 1995.

437. Rueber BE, Germain-Lee E, Collins CS, Morrell JC, Ameritunga R, Moser HW, Valle D, Gould SJ: Mutations in *PEX1* are the most common cause of perixisome biogenesis disorders. *Nature Genet* **17**:445, 1997.

438. Jordan SA, Farrar GJ, Kenna P, Humphries MM, Sheils DM, Kumar-Singh R, Sharp EM, Soriano N, Ayuso C, Benitez J, Humphries P: Localization of an autosomal dominant retinitis pigmentosa gene to chromosome 7q. *Nature Genet* **4**:54, 1993.

439. Millán JM, Martínez F, Vilela C, Beneyto M, Prieto F, Nájera C: An autosomal dominant retinitis pigmentosa family with close linkage to *D7S480* on 7q. *Hum Genet* **96**:216, 1995.

440. McGuire RE, Jordan SA, Braden VV, Bouffard GG, Humphries P, Green ED, Daiger SP: Mapping the RP10 locus for autosomal dominant retinitis pigmentosa on 7q: Refined genetic positioning and localization within a well-defined YAC contig. *Genome Res* **6**:255, 1996.

441. Mohamed Z, Bell C, Hammer HM, Converse CA, Esakowitz L, Haites NE: Linkage of a medium sized Scottish autosomal dominant retinitis pigmentosa family to chromosome 7q. *J Med Genet* **33**:714, 1996.

442. Blanton SH, Heckenlively JR, Cottingham AW, Friedman J, Sadler LA, Wagner M, Friedman LH, Daiger SP: Linkage mapping of autosomal dominant retinitis pigmentosa (RP1) to the pericentric region of human chromosome 8. *Genomics* **11**:857, 1991.

443. Xu SY, Denton M, Sullivan L, Daiger SP, Gal A: Genetic mapping of RP1 on 8q11-q21 in an Australian family with autosomal dominant retinitis pigmentosa reduces the critical region to 4 cM between *D8S601* and *D8S285*. *Hum Genet* **98**:741, 1996.

444. Gotoda T, Arita M, Arai H, Inoue K, Yokota T, Fukuo Y, Yazaki Y, Yamada N: Adult-onset spinocerebellar dysfunction caused by a mutation in the gene for the α-tocopherol-transfer protein. *New Engl J Med* **333**:1313, 1995.

445. Mihalik SJ, Morrell JC, Kim D, Sacksteder KA, Watkins PA, Gould SJ: Identification of *PAHX*, a Refsum disease gene. *Nature Genet* **17**:185, 1997.

446. Jansen GA, Ofman R, Ferdinandusse S, Ijlst L, Muijsers AO, Skjeldal OH, Stokke O, Jakobs C, Besley GTN, Wraith JE, Wanders RJA: Refsum disease is caused by mutations in the phytanoyl-CoA hydroxylase gene. *Nature Genet* **17**:190, 1997.

447. Mitchell G, Brody L, Looney J, Steel G, Suchanek M, Dowling C, Der Kaloustian V, Kaiser-Kupfer M, Valle D: An initiator codon mutation in ornithine-δ-aminotransferase causing gyrate atrophy. *J Clin Invest* **81**:630, 1988.

448. Inana G, Hotta Y, Zintz C, Takki K, Weleber RG, Kennaway NG, Nakayasu K, Nakajima A, Shiono T: Expression defect of ornithine aminotransferase gene in gyrate atrophy. *Invest Ophthalmol Vis Sci* **29**:1001, 1988.

449. Ramesh V, McClatchey AI, Ramesh N, Benoit LA, Berson EL, Shih VE, Gusella JF: Molecular basis of ornithine aminotransferase deficiency in B$_6$-responsive and -nonresponsive forms of gyrate atrophy. *Proc Natl Acad Sci USA* **85**:3777, 1988.

450. Sleat DE, Donnelly RJ, Lackland H, Liu C-G, Sohar I, Pullarkat RK, Lobel P: Association of mutations in a lysosomal protein with classical late-infantile neuronal ceroid lipofuscinosis. *Science* **277**:1802, 1997.

451. Fossdal R, Magnusson L, Weber JL, Jensson O: Mapping the locus of atrophia areata, a helicoid peripapillary chorioretinal degeneration with autosomal dominant inheritance, to chromosome 11p15. *Hum Mol Genet* **4**:479, 1995.

452. Eysteinsson T, Jónasson F, Jónsson V, Bird AC: Helicoidal peripapillary chorioretinal degeneration: electrophysiology and psychophysics in 17 patients. *Br J Ophthalmol* **82**:280, 1998.

453. Petrukhin K, Koisti MJ, Bakall B, Li W, Xie G, Marknell T, Sandgren O, Forsman K, Holmgren G, Andreasson S, Vujic M, Bergen AAB, McGarty-Dugan V, Figueroa D, Austin CP, Metzker ML, Caskey CT, Wadelius C: Identification of the gene responsible for Best macular dystrophy. *Nature Genet* **19**:241, 1998.

454. Savukoski M, Klockars T, Holmberg V, Santavuori P, Lander ES, Peltonen L: *CLN5*, a novel gene encoding a putative transmembrane protein mutated in Finnish variant late infantile neuronal ceroid lipofuscinosis. *Nature Genet* **19**:286, 1998.

455. Zhang K, Bither PP, Park R, Donoso LA, Seidman JG, Seidman CE: A dominant Stargardt's macular dystrophy locus maps to chromosome 13q34. *Arch Ophthalmol* **112**:759, 1994.

456. Sharp JD, Wheeler RB, Lake BD, Savukoski M, Jarvela IE, Peltonen L, Gardiner RM, Williams RE: Loci for classical and a variant late infantile neuronal ceroid lipofuscinosis map to chromosomes 11p15 and 15q21-23. *Hum Mol Genet* **6**:591, 1997.

457. Mitchell SJ, McHale DP, Campbell DA, Lench NJ, Mueller RF, Bundey SE, Markham AF: A syndrome of severe mental retardation, spasticity, and tapetoretinal degeneration linked to chromosome 15q24. *Am J Hum Genet* **62**:1070, 1998.

458. Finckh U, Xu SY, Kumaramanickavel G, Schürmann M, Mukkadan JK, Fernandez ST, John S, Weber JL, Denton MJ, Gal A: Homozygosity mapping of autosomal recessive retinitis pigmentosa locus (*RP22*) on chromosome 16p12.1-p12.3. *Genomics* **48**:341, 1998.

459. Järvelä I, Sainio M, Rantamäki T, Olkkonen VM, Carpén O, Peltonen L, Jalanko A: Biosynthesis and intracellular targeting of the CLN3 protein defective in Batten disease. *Hum Mol Genet* **7**:85, 1998.

460. Matthijs G, Schollen E, Pardon E, Veiga-Da-Cunha M, Jaeken J, Cassiman JJ, Van Schaftingen E: Mutations in *PMMM2*, a phospho-mannomutase gene on chromosome 16p13, in carbohydrate-deficient glycoprotein type I syndrome. *Nature Genet* **16**:88, 1997.

461. Matthijs G, Schollen E, Van Schaftingen E, Cassiman J-J, Jaeken J: Lack of homozygotes for the most frequent disease allele in carbohydrate-deficient glycoprotein syndrome type IA. *Am J Hum Genet* **62**:542, 1998.

462. Lotery AJ, Ennis KT, Silvestri G, Nicholl S, McGibbon D, Collins AD, Hughes AE: Localisation of a gene for central areolar choroidal dystrophy to chromosome 17p. *Hum Mol Genet* **5**:705, 1996.

463. Balciuniene J, Johansson K, Sandgren O, Wachtmeister L, Holmgren G, Forsman K: A gene for autosomal dominant progressive cone dystrophy (*CORD5*) maps to chromosome 17p12-p13. *Genomics* **30**:281, 1995.

464. Small KW, Syrquin M, Mullen L, Gehrs K: Mapping of autosomal dominant cone degeneration to chromosome 17p. *Am J Ophthalmol* **121**:13, 1996.

465. Kelsell RE, Evens K, Gregory CY, Moore AT, Bird AC, Hunt DM: Localisation of a gene for dominant cone-rod dystrophy (*CORD6*) to chromosome 17p. *Hum Mol Genet* **6**:597, 1997.

466. Goliath R, Shugart Y, Janssens P, Weissenbach J, Beighton P, Ramasar R, Greenberg J: Fine localization of the locus for autosomal dominant retinitis pigmentosa on chromosome 17p. *Am J Hum Genet* **57**:962, 1995.

467. Kojis TL, Heinzmann C, Flodman P, Ngo JT, Sparkes RS, Spence MA, Bateman JB, Heckenlively JR: Map refinement of locus *RP13* to

468. Tarttelin EE, Plant C, Wissenbach J, Bird AC, Bhattacharya SS, Inglehearn CF: A new family linked to the *RP13* locus for autosomal dominant retinitis pigmentosa on distal 17p. *J Med Genet* **33**:518, 1996.

469. Bardien S, Ramesar R, Bhattacharya S, Greenberg J: Retinitis pigmentosa locus on 17q (RP17): Fine localization to 17q22 and exclusion of the *PDEG* and *TIMP2* genes. *Hum Genet* **101**:13, 1997.

470. Warburg M, Sjo O, Tranebjaerg L, Fledelius HC: Deletion mapping of a retinal cone-rod dystrophy: Assignment to 18q211. *Am J Med Genet* **39**:288, 1991.

471. Al-Maghtheh M, Vithana EN, Inglehearn CF, Moore T, Bird AC, Bhattacharya SS: Segregation of a *PRKCG* mutation in two RP11 families. *Am J Hum Genet* **62**:1248, 1998.

472. Al-Maghtheh M, Inglehearn CF, Keen TJ, Evans K, Moore AT, Jay M, Bird AC, Bhattacharya SS: Identification of a sixth locus for autosomal dominant retinitis pigmentosa on chromosome 19. *Hum Mol Genet* **3**:351, 1994.

473. Xu SY, Nakazawa M, Tamai M, Gal A: Autosomal dominant retinitis pigmentosa locus on chromosome 19q in a Japanese family. *J Med Genet* **32**:915, 1995.

474. Weber BHF, Vogt G, Pruett RC, Stöhr H, Felbor U: Mutations in the tissue inhibitor of metalloproteinases-3 (TIMP3) in patients with Sorsby's fundus dystrophy. *Nature Genet* **8**:352, 1994.

475. Sauer CG, Gehrig A, Warneke-Wittstock R, Marquardt A, Ewing CC, Gibson A, Lorenz B, Jurklies B, Weber BHF: Positional cloning of the gene associated with X-linked juvenile retinoschisis. *Nature Genet* **17**:164, 1997.

476. Aldred MA, Dry KL, Knight-Jones EB, Hardwick LJ, Teague PW, Lester DH, Brown J, Spowart G, Carothers AD, Raeburn JA, Bird AC, Fielder AR, Wright AF: Genetic analysis of a kindred with X-linked mental handicap and retinitis pigmentosa. *Am J Hum Genet* **55**:916, 1994.

477. Hong HK, Ferrell RE, Gorin MB: Clinical diversity and chromosomal localization of X-linked cone dystrophy (*COD1*). *Am J Hum Genet* **55**:1173, 1994.

478. Seymour AB, Dash-Modi A, O'Connell JR, Shaffer-Gordon M, Mah TS, Stefko ST, Nagaraja R, Brown J, Kimura AE, Ferrell RE, Gorin MB: Linkage analysis of X-linked cone-rod dystrophy: Localization to Xp11.4 and definition of a locus distinct from *RP2* and *RP3*. *Am J Hum Genet* **62**:122, 1998.

479. Cibis GW, Fitzgerald KM, Harris DJ, Rothberg PG, Rupani M: The effects of dystrophin gene mutations on the ERG in mice and humans. *Invest Ophthalmol Vis Sci* **34**:3646, 1993.

480. Sigesmund DA, Weleber RG, Pillers DAM, Westall CA, Panton CM, Powell BR, Heon E, Murphey WH, Musarella MA, Ray PN: Characterization of the ocular phenotype of Duchenne and Becker muscular dystrophy. *Ophthalmology* **101**:856, 1994.

481. Seabra MC, Brown MS, Slaughter CA, Sudhof TC, Goldstein JL: Purification of component A of Rab geranylgeranyl transferase: Possible identity with the choroideremia gene product. *Cell* **70**:1049, 1992.

482. Andres DA, Seabra MC, Brown MS, Armstrong SA, Smeland TE, Cremers FPM, Goldstein JL: cDNA cloning of component A of Rab geranylgeranyl transferase and demonstration of its role as a Rab escort protein. *Cell* **73**:1091, 1993.

483. Seabra MC, Brown MS, Goldstein JL: Retinal degeneration in choroideremia: Deficiency of Rab geranylgeranyl transferase. *Science* **259**:377, 1993.

484. Reichel E, Bruce AM, Sandberg MA, Berson EL: An electroretino-graphic and molecular genetic study of X-linked cone degeneration. *Am J Ophthalmol* **108**:540, 1989.

485. Bergen AAB, Pinckers AJLG: Localization of a novel X-linked progressive cone dystrophy gene to Xq27: Evidence for genetic heterogeneity. *Am J Hum Genet* **60**:1468, 1997.

486. Zhao G-Y, Hu D-N, Xia H-X, Xia Z-C: Y-linked inheritance in a 4-generation family with retinitis pigmentosa. *Ophthalmic Genet* **16**:75, 1995.

487. Sullivan JM, Scott KM, Falls HF, Richards JE, Sieving PA: A novel rhodopsin mutation at the retinal binding site (Lys-296-Met) in ADRP. *Invest Ophthalmol Vis Sci* **35**(Suppl):1149, 1994.

# Choroideremia

*Frans P. M. Cremers* ▪ *Hans-Hilger Ropers*

1. Choroideremia (CHM) is a progressive degeneration of the retinal pigment epithelium, choroid, and retina that is inherited in an X-chromosomal recessive fashion.

2. Usually, night blindness is the first clinical sign, and it already may be present in early childhood and is followed by visual loss. Typically, the central vision is not affected until late in the disease. Many patients are blind by age 45, but the course of the disease is very variable.

3. These symptoms are paralleled by loss of the choroidal vessels and depigmentation of the fundus, which are most prominent in the midperiphery, whereas the macular region is conspicuously spared. In the end stage of the disorder, the fundus is of scleral whiteness, choroidal vessels are absent except for possible remnants in the macular region, and retinal vessels are sometimes attenuated.

4. With an estimated incidence of 1 in 100,000, CHM is regarded as a rare disorder. However, in contrast to many other retinopathies, there is only one gene involved in CHM, which renders mutations in the *CHM* gene a relatively frequent cause of blindness.

5. Linkage studies and clinical findings in males with X-chromosomal deletions have assigned the *CHM* gene (MIM 303100) to Xq21, and subsequent molecular studies have led to its isolation by means of positional cloning strategies. The *CHM* gene encodes an mRNA of approximately 6.0 kb and a protein of 653 amino acids. Microdeletions, translocations, and a variety of small mutations in patients with classic CHM have established that dysfunction of this gene is the fundamental cause of CHM.

6. In the western European population, roughly 25 percent of patients with CHM have deletions encompassing part of the *CHM* gene. Frameshift, stop codon, and splice-site mutations have been observed in approximately 50 percent of patients. Invariably, *CHM* gene mutations result in the absence or truncation of the protein.

7. Sequence comparisons revealed that the product of the *CHM* gene is identical to a subunit of the heterotrimeric Rab geranylgeranyl transferase (GGT). Thus the CHM protein, also called REP-1 (Rab escort protein-1), plays an indispensable role in the prenylation of Rab GTPases.

8. A closely related but intronless gene, choroideremia-like (*CHML/REP-2*) (MIM 118825), has been isolated. The *CHML/REP-2* gene maps to human chromosome 1q42-qter. Like *CHM/REP-1*, *CHML/REP-2* is ubiquitously expressed, and in Rab GGTase assays, REP-1 and REP-2 have largely overlapping substrate specificities.

9. Recently, a novel member of the Rab GTPase family, Rab27, has been isolated from lymphoblastoid cells that is prenylated much more efficiently by REP-1 than by REP-2. Rab27 is highly, but not uniquely, expressed in the rat eye, particularly in the retinal pigment epithelium (RPE) and choroid. Since these tissues are generally believed to be involved in the degenerative process, underprenylation of Rab27 may explain why in humans, clinical features of CHM are confined to the eye.

10. In the mouse, targeted inactivation of the *chm/rep-1* gene causes early embryonic lethality if the defective gene is transmitted maternally. Chimeric males and their heterozygous offspring are viable but show patchy loss of the photoreceptor cell layer. Thus generation of an animal model for CHM may be possible if the embryonic lethality can be overcome.

Choroideremia (CHM) (MIM 303100) belongs to a large and heterogeneous group of genetic disorders that are characterized by progressive degeneration of the retina and the choroid. These disorders can be inherited in an autosomal dominant, autosomal recessive, or X-linked fashion. CHM, like at least two different forms of retinitis pigmentosa, is an X-linked disorder that almost exclusively affects males. A precise clinical description of this disorder was published 120 years ago, but it took 70 years to establish its progressive nature and its mode of inheritance. Presymptomatic diagnosis and carrier detection in families became possible in the mid-1980s when close linkage with DNA markers was found. These studies and subsequent molecular analyses of microdeletions encompassing the Xq21 band were instrumental for the isolation of the *CHM* gene on the basis of its known chromosomal location. Sequence comparisons have shown that the *CHM* gene encodes a subunit of Rab geranylgeranyl transferase and is indispensable for prenylation of Rab GTPases. The *CHM* gene is ubiquitously expressed, and it is not clear yet why mutations in this gene give rise to an eye-specific disorder. So far the generation of an animal model for CHM has failed because targeted inactivation of the mouse *chm/rep-1* gene resulted in embryonic lethality.

## HISTORY AND CLINICAL ASPECTS

CHM was first described by Mauthner in 1872,[1] who coined this name because he thought that the condition reflected the congenital absence of the choroid. Despite some earlier suggestions that CHM might be a progressive disorder,[2,3] Bedell[4] was the first to conclude, after thorough review of the literature and on the basis of own observations, that CHM may be defined "as a condition in which the choroid disappears . . . in a definite uniform manner." Several authors provided further evidence for progression of this disease,[5,6] which was widely accepted after the description of a large Canadian family by McCulloch and McCulloch.[7] The concept of CHM as an X-linked disorder with full manifestation in males and minor clinical signs in female carriers was independently worked out by Waardenburg[8] and

A list of standard abbreviations is located immediately preceding the index in each volume. Nonstandard abbreviations used in this chapter include CHM = choroideremia; RPE = retinal pigment epithelium; ERG = electroretinogram; EOG = electrooculogram; RP = retinitis pigmentosa.

Goedbloed[9] on the basis of literature studies and their own observations. Apart from the studies of the McCullochs[7,10] and a detailed survey of Sorsby et al.,[11] several other large studies such as those of Kurstjens,[12] Krill,[13] and Kärnä[14] have further contributed to the clinical definition of CHM.

Night blindness is usually the first clinical sign of the disorder, and most patients report to have been night-blind since their early childhood.[4,14–16] Less frequently, night blindness remains unnoticed before patients are 20 years old.[11,15,17,18] Occasionally, it may not be present before the midthirties[10,12] or beyond.[19]

Usually, first signs of visual loss involve the midperiphery. Central vision frequently is preserved until the end stage of the disorder, and often there is also residual vision in the periphery. However, visual fields can vary considerably, even between the two eyes of one patient, and may appear as annular scotomas, tunnel vision, or visual fields of irregular shape. In his study of 45 patients, Kurstjens[12] observed large blind spots and reduced equatorial sensitivity, equatorial scotomas, annular scotomas, and central and peripheral temporal remnants as the most frequent findings.

Moderate myopia is more common among patients with CHM than in the normal population. As shown by McCulloch and McCulloch,[7] Kurstjens,[12] and in particular by Kärnä[14] in his large and detailed study, the myopia is progressive and correlated with the course of the disease. Repeatedly, disorders of color vision also have been observed.[15,20,21] Jaeger and Grützner[22] reported on disturbances in the blue-green range of the spectrum that were correlated with the severity of the disorder. In several patients, these changes resembled protanopia, whereas in others, deuteranopic changes were reported. Additional anomalies included punctiform and fibrillary opacities in the vitreous body.[1,7,12] Infrequently, cataract also was present and was mostly of the subcapsular type.[12,23,24]

### Clinical Diagnosis

According to Krill,[13] the fundus changes can be divided into three stages, the first of which consists of pigmentary stippling and fine atrophy of the retinal pigment epithelium (RPE) of the posterior and equatorial parts of the fundus. These findings resemble those seen in female carriers (see below). In the first stage, there is also focal atrophy of the choriocapillary layer and atrophy of the larger choroidal vessels around the optic disc and in the equatorial area. Choroidal vascular atrophy is preceded by depigmentation of the fundus, which reflects the degeneration of the RPE.

In the second stage, the atrophy of the choroid and RPE spreads from the midperiphery inward and from the disc outward. Usually, choroidal vessels of all sizes are involved, but in some cases, only the choroidal capillaries are damaged. The choroidal vessels of the macula are not affected, and pigmentary mottling is no longer seen except in the far periphery. In the third stage of the disorder, atrophy of the choroidal vessels is almost complete except in the far periphery, in the macula, and sometimes near the optic disc. The fundus is yellowish white or greenish white, and attenuation of the retinal vessels may occur at this stage (Fig. 236-1).

The rate and degree of the atrophy vary, even within families.[25,26] For example, McCulloch and McCulloch[7] described a completely white fundus in a 7-year-old patient, whereas, on the other hand, changes were very slight in a 45-year-old patient. Not infrequently, conspicuous first-stage changes were found in boys aged between 1 and 4 years.[7,12,17,18]

Abnormal light and dark adaptation are other early signs of the disorder.[12,18,21,27,28] On dark adaptation testing, elevated rod final thresholds are observed, and usually, rod adaptation is disturbed earlier or more profoundly than cone adaptation. Changes generally are correlated with the degree of retinal degeneration.[15,24,25]

Electroretinographic signs involve both the scotopic and the photopic components. Usually, however, the degeneration follows a rod-cone pattern with reduced rod responses and normal or reduced cone responses.[12,14,29,30] Scotopic responses even may

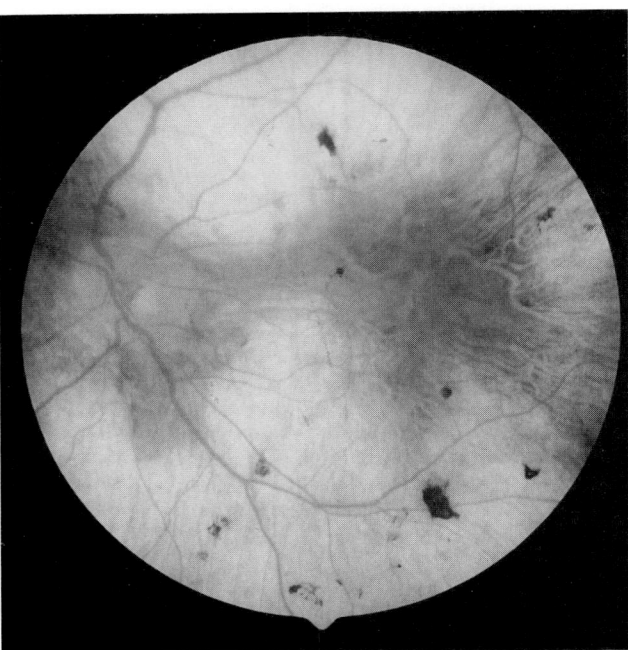

**Fig. 236-1** Fundus of a CHM patient with a deletion of exons 1 and 2 (patient 1167, see Fig. 236-3) at age 30. Note the severe atrophy of the choroid and RPE affecting the entire fundus except for the macular region and the area surrounding the optic disc. At this stage, retinal arteries are still spared. See Color Plate 19.

disappear totally before the photopic responses become disturbed.[12,20] At the terminal stage, the electroretinogram (ERG) is no longer recordable.[14,25] In the great majority of patients examined, the electrooculogram (EOG) was abnormal,[12,31,32] although a patient with an extinguished ERG but a normal EOG has been described.[33] In contrast, Krill[13] thought that abnormal ERGs are mostly preceded by changes in the EOG.

Early changes of the choroidal vessels, including capillaries, can be detected by fluorescein angiography. Depending on the severity of the disorder, choroidal capillaries can be absent over large areas,[10,16,34,35] and these changes can precede ophthalmoscopic signs considerably.[13] Usually, there is macular hyperfluorescence, which is due to degeneration of the RPE.[31] In general, changes seen on fluorescein angiography are more extensive than expected from ophthalmoscopic findings.

So far histologic examination of the eyes of CHM patients has been confined to far advanced cases. Absence of the RPE, the choroid, and the photoreceptor outer segments was seen with varying degrees of preservation in the macular region. McCulloch[36] reported on thickened and hyalinized choroidal vessels, but these findings were not confirmed by others. In a patient studied by Grützner and Vogel,[37] proliferation of the RPE was seen, and a considerable part of the retina was substituted by glial tissue. Gliosis of the inner parts of the retina, doubling of the basal membrane of the RPE, and thickening of Bruch's membrane were observed by Ghosh and McCulloch.[38]

### Clinical Findings in Female Carriers

Female carriers are mostly asymptomatic. Few have minor signs of the disorder, and serious vision impairment is rare.[39–42] Berson et al.[43] found ERG abnormalities in 4 of 26 heterozygous females, but 25 of 26 had conspicuous fundus abnormalities such as pigment changes in the periphery closely resembling the fine mottling that is characteristic of initial stages of the disease in males. Histopathologic findings have been reported for 4 cases. The first case was unremarkable.[13] In two other female carriers from the same family investigated by Ghosh et al.[44] and MacDonald et al.,[45] the RPE was found to be irregular in thickness and pigmentation. Areas of marked atrophy involving both the RPE and photoreceptors were bordered by areas with normal photoreceptors. The choriocapillaris and Bruch's membrane appeared normal. Scanning microscopy of the retina of one carrier female revealed pleomorphic RPE cells and loss of polygonal structure and villi.[45] No specific changes in the photoreceptors were found in the latter study. These findings indicate that in the RPE, disruption of the active fluid transport from the retina to the choroid and the delivery of nutrients to the retina may be important in the disease process.

As in males, fundus changes in carrier females are progressive, beginning in the midperiphery and leading to degeneration of the RPE and the choroid, often including the area surrounding the optic disc. Later on, there are numerous white dots scattered throughout the retina, and with increasing age, sclerosis of the choroid is seen. While in general the severity of fundus changes in female carriers is correlated with their age, fundus changes in young heterozygotes may be far more severe than in their carrier mothers.[11,13] Variable cellular mosaicism resulting from random inactivation of one of the two X chromosomes in cells of the early female embryo[46] may be a major cause of the varying clinical manifestation of CHM in female carriers, but it is of note that in males the clinical picture and the course of the disease are also very variable. Severe manifestation of the disease in females can result from skewed X-inactivation, homozygosity, or disruption of the *CHM* gene by X-autosome translocations. In females with reciprocal X-autosome translocations, X-chromosome inactivation is nonrandom; usually the normal X is preferentially inactivated, whereas both translocation fragments remain active. Therefore, in line with analogous observations in Duchenne muscular dystrophy, clinical signs of CHM in females with *de novo* X-autosomal translocations suggested that chromosome breakage had disrupted the only active copy of the *CHM* gene. This has been confirmed by subsequent molecular analyses.

## Other Disorders Associated with CHM and Differential Diagnosis

Apart from a variety of ocular symptoms that are interpreted as direct or indirect manifestations of the fundamental defect, association of CHM with various other diseases has been reported. Sensorineural hearing loss was found in 10 of the patients studied by McCulloch and McCulloch[7] and in 1 of Scobee's patients.[6] One of the patients of Dachevzkaya and Polonsky[47] was mute, and Murdoch[16] described a patient with congenital hearing loss. CHM also has been described in combination with dwarfism,[48] but the absence of night blindness in this patient and of fundus changes in the mother render the diagnosis of CHM in this case rather unlikely. CHM-like symptoms also have been observed in a family with a complex, apparently X-linked disorder including anhidrotic ectodermal dysplasia, skeletal abnormalities, and mental retardation[49] and in patients with chorioretinopathy and pituitary dysfunction.[50,51] CHM also was diagnosed in a 33-year-old man with leukoencephalopathy and arylsulfatase A pseudodeficiency,[52] as well as in two brothers with hereditary motor neuropathy.[53] In another CHM case, the patient also suffered from a pinealoma.[54] The molecular relationship, if any, between these disorders and CHM has not yet been clarified, but in the family described by Van den Bosch,[49] both a deletion and an inversion disrupting the *CHM* and anhidrotic ectodermal dysplasia genes have been excluded (H van Bokhoven, JAJM van den Hurk, HH Ropers, FPM Cremers, unpublished observation, 1998). In contrast, deletions on the proximal long arm of the X chromosome have been identified as the primary defect in a variety of patients with CHM, mental retardation, deafness, and other features. As discussed below, molecular characterization of these deletions and the above-mentioned X-autosome translocations in female patients has been instrumental for fine mapping of the *CHM* gene and, eventually, its isolation by positional cloning.

The differential diagnosis of CHM includes gyrate atrophy (MIM 258870; see Chap. 83), which clinically may be almost identical with CHM. Apart from characteristic circular lesions seen in the fundus of most patients with gyrate atrophy, distinguishing features are the mode of inheritance, which for gyrate atrophy is autosomal recessive, and the elevated plasma ornithine level in these patients, which is due to a defect in the enzyme ornithine aminotransferase.[55,56] In early stages of the disease, CHM is sometimes indistinguishable from X-chromosomal recessive retinitis pigmentosa (RP) (MIM 602772), but in these patients, follow-up studies and examination of affected relatives will establish the diagnosis.[57] Nevertheless, in a large American family with Italian ancestry, the male proband was diagnosed by an experienced retina specialist at the ages of 3 and 15 years as having X-linked RP. Obligate carriers, however, demonstrated radially oriented clumping of the RPE, which is characteristic of CHM. Haplotype analysis of X-chromosomal markers excluded linkage of the gene defect with markers from the *XRP2* and *XRP3* regions on the short arm of the X chromosome and showed cosegregation with markers *pJ59* and *DXS1002* situated close to the *CHM* gene at Xq21.[58] An A → T transversion in exon 14 of the *CHM* gene was found that leads to a C-terminal 99-amino-acid truncation of the predicted CHM protein. This result shows that *CHM* mutations could be involved in other so-called XRP families. Not infrequently, autosomal dominant RP (see Chap. 235) is diagnosed in female CHM carriers because of similar funduscopic findings. In contrast to the situation in autosomal dominant RP, in which funduscopic changes are accompanied by alterations of the ERG and narrowed visual fields, ERG and visual fields are normal in most CHM carriers.[14,57] Other similar diseases include Bietti crystalline retinal dystrophy[59] (MIM 210370) and acquired retina damage due to thioridazine toxicity.[60] Ocular symptoms similar to CHM also have been seen in patients with mitochondrial myopathies.[57,61]

## CLONING OF THE *CHM* GENE

### Genetic and Physical Mapping

**Linkage Studies.** Early genetic linkage studies excluded a location of the *CHM* gene close to the Xg blood group on the distal short arm and the color blindness locus near Xqter.[14,62-64] Only in 1985, linkage studies with DNA markers were successful. In three informative families studied by Nussbaum *et al.*,[65,66] no recombinants were detected between *CHM* and *DXYS1*, a polymorphic marker located in the Xq21 band. Subsequent studies refined the location to an interval between *DXYS1* and *DXS72*.[67-74] These findings have been confirmed by clinical and molecular analyses in patients with deletions involving part of Xq21, as discussed below.

**Contiguous Gene Syndromes.** The first deletion spanning part of the Xq21 band was described by Tabor *et al.*[75] in a male with cleft lip and palate, agenesis of the corpus callosum, and severe mental retardation (MR) (Fig. 236-2, patient NP). After the discovery of linkage between *DXYS1* and the *CHM* locus,[66] ophthalmologic reexamination revealed fundus changes characteristic of CHM in its early stage. The patient's mother and sister, who were both heterozygous for the deletion, were diagnosed as being carriers of CHM. Moreover, the deletion was shown to span the *DXYS1* locus, thereby corroborating its linkage with CHM.[69,76,77] Since then, several other males with cytogenetically detectable Xq21 deletions have been described, and it has become apparent that their phenotypes almost invariably include CHM, deafness with a temporal bone defect (DFN3), and "unspecific" MR[76-89] (see Fig. 236-2). Detailed genotype-phenotype comparisons revealed that the DFN3 and MR loci resided in interval 2 (see Fig. 236-2), whereas the *CHM* gene mapped to interval 3 defined by the DNA loci *DXS95*, *DXS165*, and *DXS233*.[83] Apart from CHM, DFN3 and cleft lip and palate (CPX; MIM 303400) had been described as separate genetic entities segregating in families, and linkage studies had assigned these disorders to Xq13-q22 (DFN3)[90,91] and

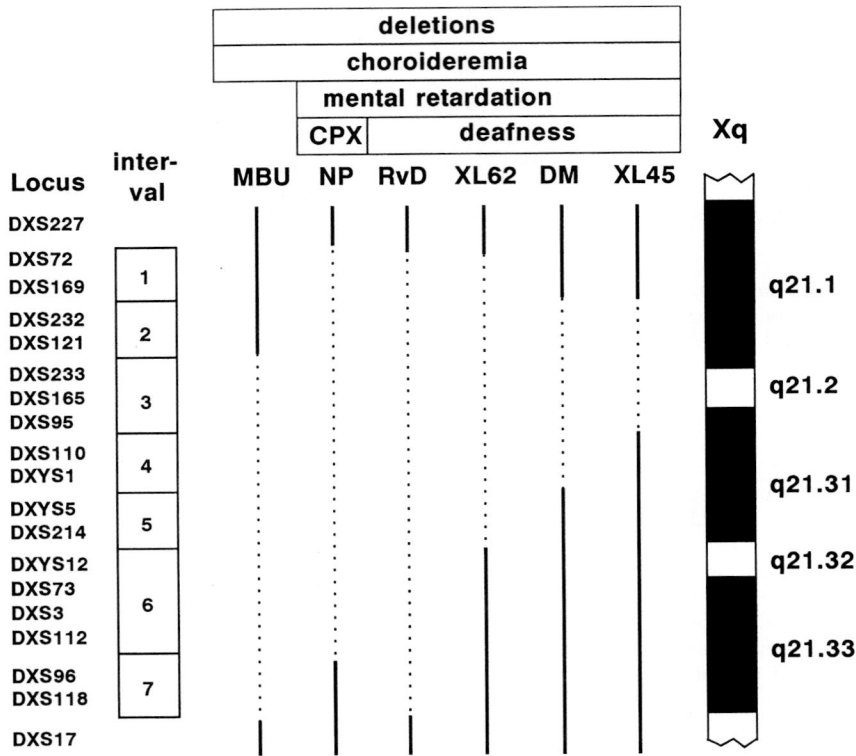

Fig. 236-2 Deletion interval map of the Xq21 region. The DNA probes used in Southern analysis are indicated at the left. Deleted chromosomal segments are indicated by stippled lines. Intervals and banding pattern are not drawn to scale. (*Adapted from Cremers et al.*[83] *Used by permission of Genomics.*)

Xq21.1-q21.31 (CPX).[92–95] The gene underlying DFN3, *POU3F4*, was isolated based on its absence in patients with classic DFN3 in a region just proximal to the CHM critical region.[96]

## Physical Fine Mapping

**Deletions Associated with Classic CHM.** Further refinement of the localization was achieved when Cremers *et al.*[97] extended their search for deletions to patients with classic, i.e., nonsyndromic, CHM. With one of the probes from interval 3, p1bD5 (locus *DXS165*), two deletions could be found in a series of eight unrelated CHM patients[97] (Fig. 236-3, patients 3.5 and 7.6). Generation of additional probes in the vicinity of the *DXS165* locus by preparative field inversion gel electrophoresis, cloning of deletion end points, and chromosome jumping[98–101] led to the detection of additional deletions that ranged in size between a few kilobases to more than 10 Mb[102,103] (see Fig. 236-3).

**X-Autosome Translocations.** Molecular analyses of the breakpoints on the X chromosome in two females with balanced X;7 and X;13 translocations and CHM[41,42] have corroborated the results of deletion mapping. In addition to CHM, both females showed primary amenorrhea, which is a common feature in X-autosome translocations involving the proximal Xq.[104] In both translocations, the breakpoints on the X chromosome were situated in band Xq21.2. Cremers *et al.*[105] could position the breakpoint of the X;13 translocation in the center of the region defined by deletion mapping as the site of the *CHM* gene (see Fig. 236-3). These results were confirmed by Merry *et al.*[99,106] The X;7 translocation breakpoint was found to be located in the 5′ part of the *CHM* gene (see "Isolation of the *CHM* Gene," below).

## Isolation of the *CHM* Gene

Employing two clones from the critical region for CHM-pJ11 and pJ60 (see Fig. 236-3) — human genomic DNA phage clones were isolated spanning a region of 45 kb. Single- and low-copy probes subsequently were tested for evolutionary conservation by

hybridization to Southern blots containing DNA from several vertebrates. Screening a human retinal cDNA library[107] with a probe that showed sequence conservation in several vertebrates, including mouse and chicken, resulted in the isolation of overlapping cDNA clones.[108] Subsequent rescreening of this and other cDNA libraries with DNA probes from the 5′ and 3′ ends of the consensus cDNA enabled isolation of the full-length cDNA sequence.[106,108,109] The cDNA contains an open reading frame (ORF) of 1959 bp coding for 653 amino acids (Fig. 236-4). The *CHM* gene consists of 15 exons spanning a genomic region of 100 to 150 kb.[109] In both affected females with X-autosome translocations, the *CHM* gene was found to be disrupted. The X;13 breakpoint is situated between exons 12 and 13, and the X;7 breakpoint lies between exons 3 and 4[102,109] (see Fig. 236-4).

## MUTATION SPECTRUM AND DIAGNOSTIC ASPECTS

### Microdeletions

Employing polymerase chain reaction (PCR) primers flanking each exon, 80 apparently unrelated CHM patients from Germany, the Netherlands, Denmark, Finland, and other European countries were screened for deletions. Approximately 25 percent of the CHM patients show deletions encompassing one or several exons. Only 3 of 18 deletions are intragenic, whereas the others extend beyond the gene (see Fig. 236-3). The largest deletions found extend distally and include more than 10 Mb of DNA.[102,103] It is remarkable that Merry *et al.*[106] have not found a single functionally relevant structural rearrangement of the *CHM* gene in 34 American CHM patients. The marked discrepancy between these studies may be explained by founder effects resulting in a low number of different mutations in the American population. It is noteworthy in this context that even within the United States the incidence of CHM may show significant geographic differences. On the West Coast, it is considered the most frequent form of retinal degeneration,[57] whereas in New England, CHM seems to

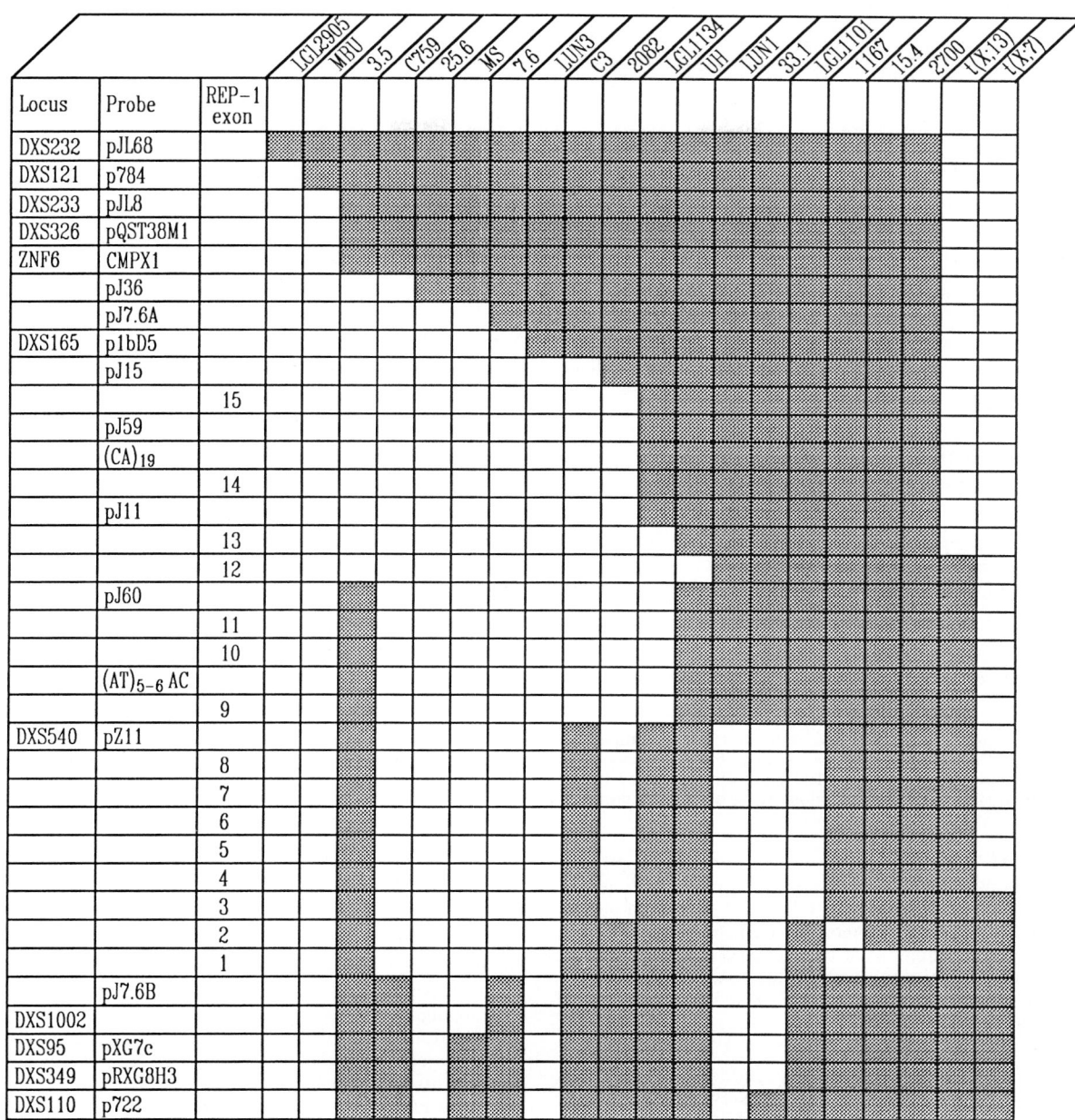

**Fig. 236-3** Deletion map of the *CHM* locus and location of *CHM* exons at Xq21.2. Nondeleted segments are given as gray boxes. (*From Van den Hurk et al.*[103] *Used by permission of Human Mutation.*)

be much rarer than X-linked RP (E Berson, personal communication, Boston, 1995). Strong founder effects also have been detected on CHM mutation screening in northern Finland.[110]

### Point Mutations and Small Insertions/Deletions

Employing the polymerase chain reaction single-strand conformation polymorphism (PCR-SSCP) technique,[111] small mutations were found in approximately 50 percent of patients. All mutations except one are predicted to result in the loss of function of the *CHM* gene; i.e., they result in premature termination of translation[54,58,103,110,112–119] (Table 236-1). In one case, a possible missense mutation (*Q471L*) was found,[120] but analysis of lymphoblastoid cells derived from that patient revealed the absence of the CHM protein (M Seabra, personal communication, London, 1998). The mutant nucleotide is positioned in the 5′ splice site of exon 11 and results in the skipping of exon 11 and truncation of the CHM protein.[121] Sankila *et al.*[110] were able to show that most

patients in the Salla region of northern Finland carry the same mutation-an insertion into the 5′ splice site downstream of exon 13-that gives rise to aberrant splicing. By genealogic studies, this mutation could be traced back to a founder couple born 13 generations ago. Mutation screening so far has failed to detect a common defect in the *CHM* gene; one mutation—a deletion of the tetranucleotide TGTT in exon 13—was encountered in three apparently unrelated families from Denmark,[113] southern Germany,[112] and France.[122] It is of note that in the normal *CHM* gene, the TGTT tetranucleotide is present in tandem, which may render this sequence particularly prone to mutation, e.g., by polymerase slippage during replication. The *R267X* (829C>T; see Table 236-1) mutation was found in two unrelated CHM patients.[103,116]

Given the fact that all *CHM* mutations lead to an inactive or absent CHM protein, the absence of a correlation between the clinical severity and the genotypic changes is not surprising. So far there is no clear explanation for the conspicuous intrafamilial

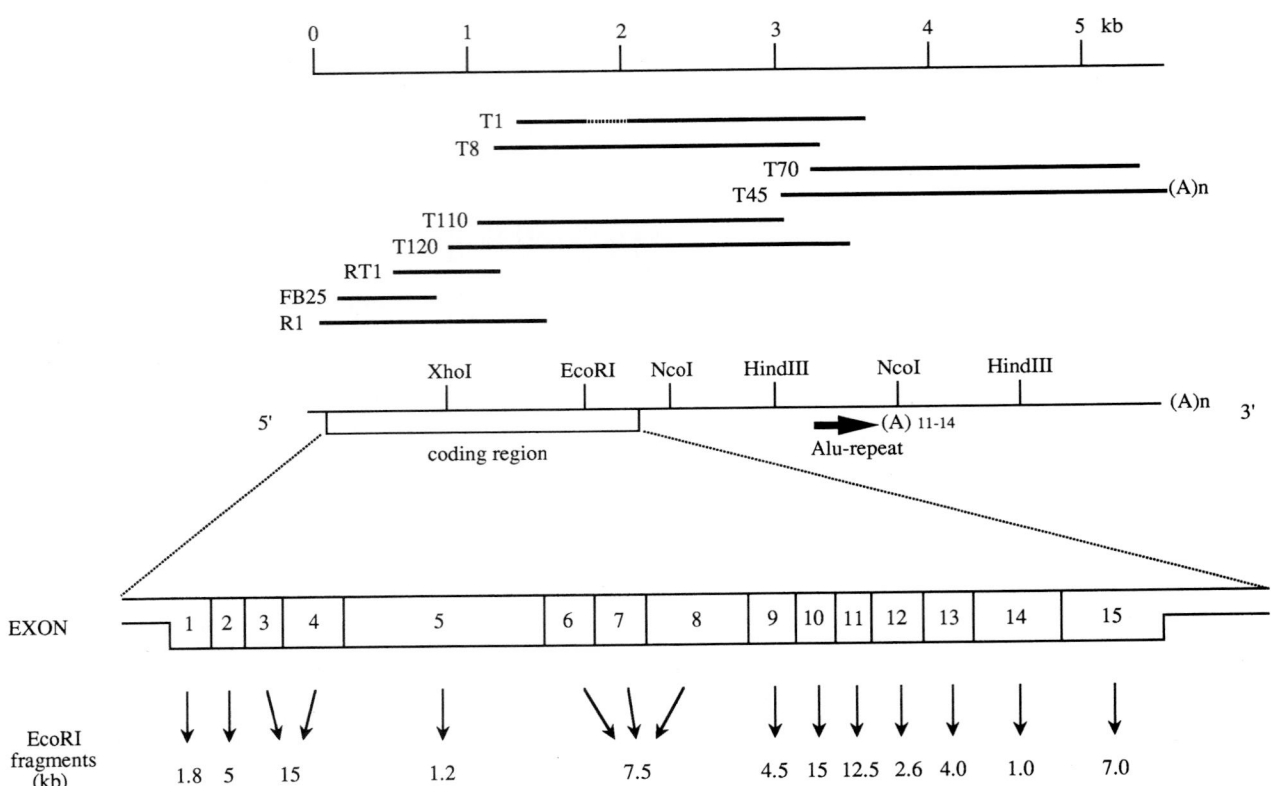

**Fig. 236-4 cDNA map of the *CHM* gene.** Schematic representation of the overlapping cDNA clones corresponding to the *CHM* gene with the restriction map given at the top. The open reading frame (ORF) encodes a polypeptide of 653 amino acids. At the bottom: Exon/exon structure and corresponding genomic EcoRI fragments. (*Adapted from Van Bokhoven et al.*[109] *Used by permission of Human Molecular Genetics.*)

variability of CHM, but it is conceivable that its clinical picture and course are modulated by the recently discovered *CHML* gene, which is structurally very similar to *CHM* (see "Isolation of the Human *CHM*-like Gene on Chromosome 1," below). It is striking that no missense mutations have been observed yet. This may indicate that (most) missense mutations are functionally neutral, give rise to a different phenotype, or are lethal in human early embryonic development.

### Molecular Diagnosis

New mutations in CHM are rare, and in most cases, the disorder is familial. Deletions involving one or several *CHM* exons can be readily identified by exon PCR. PCR-SSCP analysis of individual exons reveals another 50 percent of the mutations. The apparent absence of mutations in approximately 25 percent of CHM patients may be explained by the fact that SSCP analysis only reveals 80 percent of the mutations[123] and that the promoter region was not analyzed. Since the gene is cloned, direct sequencing of exons carrying known familial mutations was performed routinely using DNA extracted from chorionic villi of at-risk male fetuses.[124,125]

Since all mutations identified thus far result in truncation of the CHM protein, and because the *CHM* gene is expressed ubiquitously, the protein truncation test (PTT) is particularly useful to identify mutations. Beaufrère *et al.*[116,121] employed the PTT test by amplifying three overlapping segments of the cDNA from lymphoblast RNA and performing *in vitro* transcription/translation. In this way, they identified protein-truncating mutations in each of six CHM families. One of the main advantages of the PTT test is that splice-site mutations located outside the canonical splice donor and acceptor sites are also detected. Apart from these direct methods, a large variety of closely linked flanking and intragenic markers are available for the indirect diagnosis of this disorder.[126–128]

### ISOLATION OF THE HUMAN *CHM*-LIKE GENE ON CHROMOSOME 1

An autosomal homologue of the human *CHM* gene was isolated by Cremers *et al.*[129] in the course of experiments aiming at the cloning of the 5' end of the *CHM* cDNA. When a fetal brain cDNA library was probed with a murine *chm* cDNA clone, four partly overlapping recombinant phages were identified whose sequences differed from those of the human *CHM* cDNA consensus. The consensus cDNA of this *CHM*-like (*CHML*) gene encodes 656 amino acids. Alignment of this sequence with the human *CHM* consensus cDNA revealed 76 percent amino acid identity and 95 percent similarity. The human *CHML* gene contains no introns and is believed to have arisen through retrotransposition of the *CHM* gene. The human *CHML* gene was mapped to 1q42-qter using human rodent cell hybrids.[130] In the mouse, the *chml* gene was mapped to chromosome 1, approximately 5.4 cM distal to D1Mit15 and 18.3 cM proximal to D1Mit17 by analysis of interspecific backcross mice.[131] Northern and western blot analyses have shown that both CHM and CHML are ubiquitously expressed in humans and rats.[108,132] Thus far no immunohistochemical data have been obtained to shed further light on the (sub)cellular location of these proteins.

### BIOCHEMICAL FUNCTION OF THE *CHM* GENE

#### The CHM Protein Is a Rab Escort Protein

Through a protein sequence homology search, similarity was identified between the CHM/REP and Rab GDP dissociation inhibitor (GDI) proteins[129,133] and between these proteins and the N-terminal flavin adenine dinucleotide (FAD)/nicotinamide adenine dinucleotide (NAD)-binding motif found in several bacterial dehydrogenases.[134] Independently, the crystal structure of the

**Table 236-1** Nucleotide Substitutions and Small Insertions/Deletions in the *CHM/REP-1* Gene

| Location | Mutation* | Effect | References |
|---|---|---|---|
| **Nonsense Mutations** | | | |
| EX5 | 346C > T | G106X | 115 |
| EX5 | 559G > T | E177X | 116 |
| EX6 | 829C > T | R267X | 103,116 |
| EX7 | 907C > T | R293X | 102 |
| Ex8 | 1030C > T | G334X | 103 |
| EX8 | 1162insAAT | Y378X | 115 |
| EX9 | 1248C > A | C406X | 115 |
| EX11 | 1388CC > G | S453X | 112 |
| EX12 | 1501G > T | E491X | 112 |
| EX12 | 1514C > A | S495X | 112 |
| EX12 | 1527C > A | C499X | 113 |
| EX14 | 1693A > T | R555X | 58 |
| EX14 | 1703C > G | S558X | 114 |
| **Frameshift Mutations** | | | |
| EX4 | 323delT | Frameshift | 116 |
| EX5 | 555delAG | Frameshift | 102 |
| EX5 | 610insA | Frameshift | 102 |
| EX6 | 779delA | Frameshift | 103 |
| EX8 | 1183insC | Frameshift | 102 |
| EX10 | 1313delTC | Frameshift | 116 |
| EX11 | 1393delG | Frameshift | 115 |
| EX12 | 1476delA | Frameshift | 112 |
| EX13 | 1608A > CC | Frameshift | 54 |
| EX13 | 1614delTGTT | Frameshift | 112,113,122 |
| EX14 | 1680delTT | Frameshift | 113 |
| **Splice-Site Mutations** | | | |
| IVS9 | 1274IVS + 1G > A | 5′ Splice signal | 103 |
| IVS10 | 1379IVS + 2insGGT | Aberrant splicing | 103 |
| EX11 | 1442A > T | 5′ Splice signal; G-471L | 120 |
| IVS12 | 1541IVS-2A > G | Aberrant splicing | 113 |
| IVS13 | 1639IVS + 2insT | Aberrant splicing | 110 |
| IVS13 | 1639IVS + 3A > C | Aberrant splicing | 119 |
| IVS14 | 1801IVS-1G > A | 3′ Splice signal | 103 |

*The nucleotide positions correspond to the sequence published by van Bokhoven et al.[109]

bovine α-isoform of Rab GDI revealed a striking tertiary resemblance to a FAD-binding domain found in monooxygenases and oxidases.[135] The functional role of the predicted FAD/NAD-binding domain in the CHM/REP proteins, as well as its significance in the pathogenesis of CHM, remains unclear.

Seabra *et al.*[136,137] discovered striking similarities between amino acid sequences of REP-1, a newly isolated subunit of a geranylgeranyl transferase from rat brain, and the deduced product of the human *CHM* gene. Subsequent cloning of the rat cDNA confirmed homology to the human *CHM* cDNA.[138] Prenyl modification of Rab proteins is a prerequisite for membrane anchoring, where Rab GTPases have important roles as regulators of protein trafficking. The CHM/REP-1 protein binds the unprenylated Rabs and presents them to the α and β subunits of Rab geranylgeranyl transferase (Rab GGTase) (Fig. 236-5). After prenylation, the CHM/REP-1 protein escorts the Rabs to an as yet unknown acceptor molecule.[138,139] Thereafter, the CHM/REP-1 protein dissociates from the Rab and engages in another round of prenylation. In yeast, both the α/β catalytic component of RabGGTase (encoded by the *MAD2* and *BET2* genes) and REP (encoded by the *MRS6/MSI4* gene) are essential for cell viability.[140–145] It is likely that complete loss of REP activity would be lethal in humans too. CHM patients show markedly decreased but still detectable Rab GGTase activity,[137] even when the *CHM/REP-1* gene is deleted, suggesting that residual activity

is due to partial compensation by another gene. Indeed, biochemical studies with recombinant proteins have shown that the homologous gene CHML/REP-2 can substitute for *CHM/REP-1* in the prenylation of various Rab proteins.[146] It has been hypothesized that in choroid and retina, CHML/REP-2 cannot fully compensate the loss of CHM/REP-1. This may be explained by different specificities of these proteins for Rab substrates that are expressed in the retina. Recently, evidence supporting this view has been presented.[147] A novel Rab protein, designated Rab27, is not prenylated in lymphoblastoid cells from CHM patients, whereas other Rabs are modified properly. In rats, Rab27 is expressed at high levels in the RPE and the choroid, generally believed to be involved in the early phase of the degenerative process. In CHM cells, a small proportion of Rab27 is found membrane-associated, presumably because Rab27 can be prenylated by CHML/REP-2 at low efficiency.[147] This may explain the slow progression of the disease.

## DISRUPTION OF THE *CHM* GENE IS MALE LETHAL IN MOUSE EMBRYOS

To study the pathogenesis in more detail and to construct an experimental system for gene-replacement studies, attempts were made to develop a mouse model by gene targeting.[148] A genomic segment of the mouse *chm/rep-1* gene encompassing exons 6, 7, and 8 was isolated, and a neomycine gene was inserted into exon 8, thereby disrupting the open reading frame. This construct was electroporated into embryonic stem (ES) cells, and after proper selection, two clones were recovered in which the construct carrying the neomycine gene had replaced the corresponding endogenous *chm/rep-1* gene sequences by homologous recombination. Both ES clones were injected into blastocysts, which were implanted in pseudopregnant mice. Several chimeras were born, males of which were mated to C57BL/6 female mice. Among the offspring, six female mice showed the agouti coat color indicative of germ-line transmission of the *CHM* mutation. Breeding of these heterozygous female mice with C57BL/6 male mice only resulted in offspring carrying normal *chm/rep-1* alleles. To investigate the possibility that this was due to early embryonic selection, blastocysts were investigated for the presence of the mutant allele. Employing nested PCR, one male and two female blastocysts out of nine blastocysts studied were shown to carry the mutated *chm/rep-1* gene. Thus it appears that disruption of the *chm/rep-1* gene causes embryonic lethality in males; in females, it is lethal if the mutated *chm/rep-1* allele is present on the maternal X Chromosome but not if present on the paternal X chromosome. A plausible explanation for this observation would be that in mice expression of the *chm/rep-1* gene is required for the development or function of extraembryonic membranes. It has been documented extensively that in female mouse embryos the paternal X chromosome is preferentially inactivated in extra-embryonic tissues.[149,150] As a result, in female embryo's that inherit the mutated X from their mother, the *chm/rep-1* gene is functionally absent in extraembryonic tissues because the wild-type gene on the paternal X chromosome is inactive. In contrast, female embryos carrying the targeted *chm/rep-1* gene on their paternal X chromosome would be healthy because this X chromosome is physiologically inactive; the only active *chm/rep-1* gene is the wild-type one on the maternal X chromosome.

To study possible effects of the CHM mutation on the function and structure of the eye, heterozygote females and chimeras were investigated employing electroretinographic and histologic techniques. Compared with control mice, chimeras showed variable b-wave amplitudes, some of which were reduced by 70 percent compared with average values of four control groups and displayed marked loss of the photoreceptor cell layer in large areas of the fundus. In these regions, the RPE apparently was intact and lined with ganglion cells. Heterozygote female mice merely showed a reduced number of photoreceptor cell nuclei but no significant b-wave alterations.

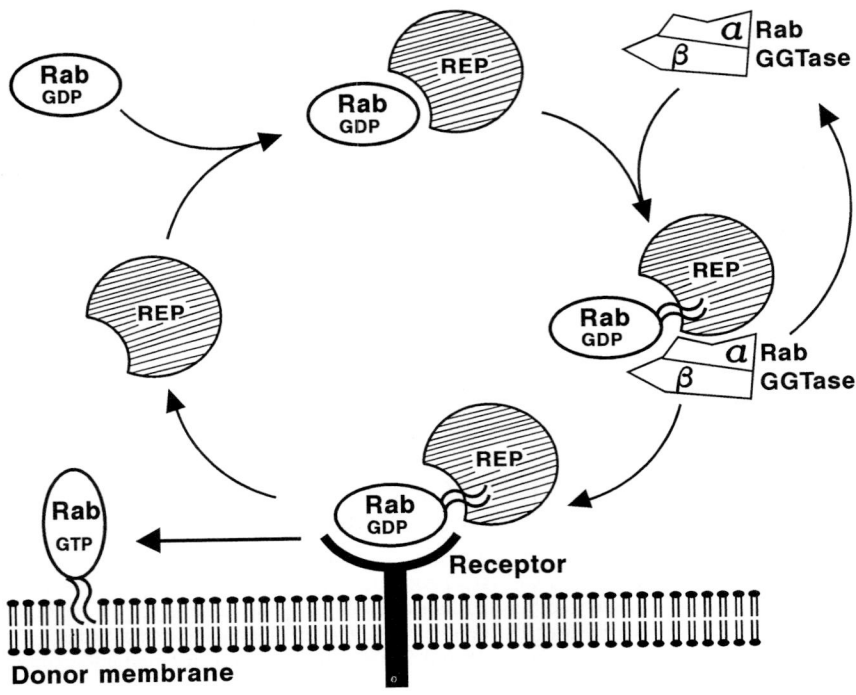

**Fig. 236-5** Model depicting the cycling of REP. REP binds a GDP-bound Rab and presents it to the catalytic Rab GGT$\alpha/\beta$ subunits. Upon geranylgeranylation, Rab GGT dissociates and the REP-Rab complex moves to a putative receptor which facilitates attachment of the prenylated Rab to the donor membrane.

These findings suggest that mutant male mice may be a useful model for CHM in humans if only they would survive. Provided that placental dysfunction is the only cause of the embryonic lethality, it may be possible to rescue these mice by introduction of a *CHM/REP-1* transgene controlled by a placenta-specific promoter or by generating mice with "conditional knockouts." Such experiments are in progress.

## ACKNOWLEDGMENTS

We thank J. A. J. M. van den Hurk for her help in collecting all data on CHM mutations and for critically reading this manuscript. The choroideremia research is supported by the Netherlands Organization for Scientific Research (NWO).

## REFERENCES

1. Mauthner H: Ein Fall von Chorioideremia. *Ber Naturw-med Ver Insbruck* **2**:191, 1872.
2. Pöllot W: Atypische Chorioretinitis pigmentosa hereditaria. *Graefes Arch Ophthalmol* **80**:379, 1912.
3. Usher CH: Choroideremia. *Trans Ophthalmol Soc UK* **55**:164, 1935.
4. Bedell AJ: Choroideremia. *Arch Ophthalmol* **17**:444, 1937.
5. Schutzbach M: Uber erbliche Aderhaut-Netzhaut-erkrankung. *Graefes Arch Ophthalmol* **138**:315, 1938.
6. Scobee R: Choroideremia: The nature of the condition and case reports. *Am J Ophthalmol* **26**:1135, 1943.
7. McCulloch C, McCulloch RJP: A hereditary and clinical study of choroideremia. *Trans Am Acad Ophthalmol Otolaryngol* **52**:160, 1948.
8. Waardenburg PJ: Chorioideremie als Erbmerkmal. *Acta Ophthalmol* **20**:235, 1942.
9. Goedbloed J: Mode of inheritance in choroideremia. *Ophthalmologica* **104**:308, 1942.
10. McCulloch JC: Choroideremia: A clinical and pathologic review. *Trans Am Ophthalmol Soc* **67**:142, 1969.
11. Sorsby A, Franceschetti A, Joseph R, Davey JB: Choroideremia: Clinical and genetic aspects. *Br J Ophthalmol* **36**:547, 1952.
12. Kurstjens JH: Choroideremia and gyrate atrophy of the choroid and retina. *Doc Ophthalmol* **19**:1, 1965.
13. Krill AE: *Krill's Hereditary Retinal and Choroidal Diseases, Vol II: Clinical Characteristics.* Hagerstown, MD, Harper & Row, 1977, p 976.
14. Kärnä J: Choroideremia: A clinical and genetic study of 84 Finnish patients and 126 female carriers. *Acta Ophthalmol* **176**(suppl):1, 1986.
15. François J: Choroideremia (progressive chorioretinal degeneration). *Int Ophthalmol Clin* **8**:949, 1968.
16. Murdoch JL: Choroideremia. *Birth Defects* **7**:196, 1971.
17. Shapiro I, Gorlin RJ: X-linked choroidal sclerosis. A stage of choroideremia. *Minn Med* **57**:259, 1974.
18. Hammerstein W, Bischof G, Leide E: Chorioideremie im Kindesalter. *Klin Monatsbl Augenheilkd* **174**:599, 1979.
19. Magder H: Choroideremia: Report of a case. *Arch Ophthalmol* **33**:468, 1945.
20. Pameyer JK, Waardenburg PJ, Henkes HE: Choroideremia. *Br J Ophthalmol* **44**:724, 1960.
21. Rubin ML, Fishman RS, McKay RA: Choroideremia: Study of a family and literature review. *Arch Ophthalmol* **76**:563, 1966.
22. Jaeger W, Grützner P: Der Funktionsverfall bei progressiver tapeto-chorioidaler Degeneration (Chorioideremie). *Ophthalmologica* **143**:305, 1962.
23. Spear D, Stephens FE: Choroideremia, its inheritance in a family. *Trans Pacif Coast Oto-Ophthalmol Soc* **33**:215, 1952.
24. Takki K: Differential diagnosis between the primary total choroidal vascular atrophies. *Br J Ophthalmol* **58**:24, 1974.
25. Sieving PA, Niffenegger JH, Berson JL: Electroretinographic findings in selected pedigrees with choroideremia. *Am J Ophthalmol* **101**:361, 1986.
26. Ponjavic V, Abrahamson M, Andréasson S, van Bokhoven H, Cremers FPM, Ehinger B, Fex G: Phenotype variations within a choroideremia family lacking the entire *CHM* gene. *Ophthalmic Genet* **16**:143, 1995.
27. Jacobson J, Stephens G: Hereditary choroidoretinal degeneration: Study of a family including electroretinography and adaptometry. *Arch Ophthalmol* **67**:321, 1962.
28. Noble KG, Carr RE, Siegel IM: Fluorescein angiography of the hereditary choroidal dystrophies. *Br J Ophthalmol* **61**:43, 1977.
29. Waardenburg PJ: Observations in choroideremia and in the female carrier of the disease. *Acta 18th Cong Ophthalmol Belge* **2**:1578, 1958.
30. Franceschetti A, François J, Babel L: *Les Héredodégénérescences Chorio-rétiniennes.* Paris, Masson, 1963.
31. Krill AE, Archer D: Classification of the choroidal atrophies. *Am J Ophthalmol* **72**:562, 1971.
32. François J, de Bradendere J, Stockmans L: Choroidéremie (Dégénérescence chorio-rétinienne progressive). *Bull Soc Belge Ophthalmol* **146**:384, 1967.
33. Schmöger E, Busch I, Lukassek B: Histologischer Beitrag zur Chorioideremie. *Ophthalmologica* **166**:144, 1973.
34. Fouanon C: *La choroidérémie.* Thesis, Universite de Nantes, 1971.

35. Krill AE, Newell FW, Chishti MI: Fluorescein studies in diseases affecting the retinal pigment epithelium. *Am J Ophthalmol* **66**:470, 1968.

36. McCulloch JC: The pathological findings in two cases of choroideremia. *Trans Am Acad Ophthalmol Otolaryngol* **50**:565, 1950.

37. Grützner P, Vogel MH: Klinischer Verlauf und histologischer Befund bei progressiver tapeto-chorioidealer Degeneration (Chorioideremia). *Klin Monatsbl Augenheilkd* **162**:206, 1973.

38. Ghosh M, McCulloch JC: Pathological findings from two cases of choroideremia. *Can J Ophthalmol* **15**:147, 1980.

39. Fraser GRF, Friedmann AI: Choroideremia in a female. *Br Med J* **2**:732, 1968.

40. Harris GS, Miller JR: Choroideremia: Visual defects in a heterozygote. *Arch Ophthalmol* **80**:423, 1968.

41. Kaplan J, Gilgenkrantz S, Dufier JL, Frézal J: Choroideremia and ovarian dysgenesis associated with an X;7 *de novo* balanced translocation. Human Gene Mapping 10: Tenth International Workshop on Human Gene Mapping. *Cytogenet Cell Genet* **51**:1022, 1989.

42. Siu VM, Gonder JR, Jung JH, Sergovich FR, Flintoff WF: Choroideremia associated with an X-autosomal translocation. *Hum Genet* **84**:459, 1990.

43. Berson EL, Rosner JB, Simonoff EA: Electroretinographic testing as an aid in detection of carriers of X-chromosome-linked retinitis pigmentosa. *Am J Ophthalmol* **87**:460, 1979.

44. Ghosh M, McCulloch C, Parker JA: Pathological study in a female carrier of choroideremia. *Can J Ophthalmol* **23**:181, 1988.

45. MacDonald IM, Chen MH, Addison DJ, Mielke BW, Nesslinger NJ: Histopathology of the retinal pigment epithelium of a female carrier of choroideremia. *Can J Ophthalmol* **32**:329, 1997.

46. Lyon MF: Sex chromatin and gene action in the mammalian X-chromosome. *Am J Hum Genet* **14**:135, 1962.

47. Dachevzkaya NP, Polonsky BZ: Two cases of choroideremia. *Vestn Oftalmol* **83**:89, 1970.

48. Valk LEM, Binkhorst PG: A case of familial dwarfism with choroideremia, myopia, posterior polar cataract, and zonular cataract. *Ophthalmologica* **132**:299, 1956.

49. van den Bosch J: A new syndrome in three generations of a Dutch family. *Ophthalmologica* **137**:422, 1959.

50. Judisch GF, Lowry RB, Hanson JW, McGillivary BC: Chorioretinopathy and pituitary dysfunction: The CPD syndrome. *Arch Ophthalmol* **99**:253, 1981.

51. Menon RK, Ball WS, Sperling MA: Choroideremia and hypopituitarism: An association. *Am J Med Genet* **34**:511, 1989.

52. Matsuyama W, Kuriyama M, Nakagawa M, Kanazawa H, Takenaga S, Ijichi S, Osame M: Choroideremia with leukoencephalopathy and arylsulfatase A pseudodeficiency. *J Neurol Sci* **138**:161, 1996.

53. Kawata A, Hayashi H, Yoshida H, Kanda T, Tanabe H: Two siblings of distal hereditary motor neuropathy with choroideremia. *Clin Neurol* **30**:1010, 1990.

54. Hotta Y, Fujiki K, Hayakawa M, Kohno N, Kitagawa H, Doi R, Kanai A: A hemizygous A to CC base change of the *CHM* gene causing choroideremia associated with pinealoma. *Graefes Arch Clin Exp Ophthalmol* **235**:653, 1997.

55. Trijbels JMF, Sengers RCA, Bakkeren JAJM, de Kort AFM, Deutman AF: L-Ornithine-ketoacid-transferase deficiency in cultured fibroblasts of a patient with hyperornithinemia and gyrate atrophy of the choroid and retina. *Clin Chim Acta* **79**:371, 1977.

56. O'Donnel JJ, Sandman RP, Martin SR: Gyrate atrophy of the retina: Inborn error of l-ornithine:2-oxoacid aminotransferase. *Science* **200**:200, 1978.

57. Heckenlively JR, Bird AC: Choroideremia, in Heckenlively JR (ed): *Retinitis Pigmentosa*. Philadelphia, Lippincott, 1988, p 176.

58. Forsythe P, Maguire A, Fujite R, Moen C, Swaroop A, Bennett J: A carboxy-terminal truncation of 99 amino acids resulting from a novel mutation (Arg555 → stop) in the *CHM* gene leads to choroideremia. *Exp Eye Res* **64**:487, 1997.

59. Welch RB: Bietti's tapetoretinal degeneration with marginal corneal dystrophy: Crystalline retinopathy. *Trans Am Ophthalmol Soc* **75**:164, 1977.

60. Meredith TA, Aaberg TM, Willerson WD: Progressive chorioretinopathy after receiving thioridazine. *Arch Ophthalmol* **96**:1172, 1978.

61. Herzberg NH, van Schooneveld MJ, Bleeker-Wagemakers EM, Zwart R, Cremers FPM, van der Knaap MS, Bolhuis PA, et al: Kearns-Sayre syndrome with a phenocopy of choroideremia instead of pigmentary retinopathy. *Neurology* **43**:218, 1993.

62. Other A: Choroideremia and the Xg blood group. *Acta Ophthalmol* **46**:79, 1968.

63. Bell AG, McCulloch JC: Choroideremia and the Xg locus: Another look for linkage. *Clin Genet* **2**:239, 1971.

64. Eriksson AW, Eskola MR, Forsius HR, Frants RR, Kärnä J, Sanger R: X-chromosomal intermediate chorioideremia and uveal coloboma in a family: Interrelation and linkage studies. *Clin Genet* **10**:355, 1976.

65. Lewis RA, Nussbaum RL, Ferrell R: Mapping X-linked ophthalmic diseases: Provisional assignment of the locus for choroideremia to Xq13-q24. *Ophthalmology* **92**:800, 1985.

66. Nussbaum RL, Lewis RA, Lesko JG, Ferrell R: Choroideremia is linked to the restriction fragment length polymorphism *DXYS1* at Xq13-21. *Am J Hum Genet* **37**:473, 1985.

67. Sankila E-M, de la Chapelle A, Kärnä J, Forsius H, Frants R, Eriksson A: Choroideremia: Close linkage to *DXYS1* and *DXYS12* demonstrated by segregation analysis and historical-genealogical evidence. *Clin Genet* **31**:315, 1987.

68. Jay M, Wright AF, Clayton JF, Deans M, Dempster M, Bhattacharya SS, Jay B: A genetic linkage study of choroideremia. *Ophthalmic Paediatr Genet* **7**:201, 1986.

69. Schwartz M, Rosenberg T, Niebuhr E, Lundsteen C, Sardemann H, Andersen O, Yang H-M, et al: Choroideremia: Further evidence for assignment of the locus to Xq13-Xq21. *Hum Genet* **74**:449, 1986.

70. Lesko JG, Lewis RA, Nussbaum RL: Multipoint linkage analysis of loci in the proximal long arm of the human X chromosome: Application to mapping the choroideremia locus. *Am J Hum Genet* **40**:303, 1987.

71. MacDonald IM, Sandre RM, Wong P, Hunter AGW, Tenniswood MPR: Linkage relationships of X-linked choroideremia to *DXYS1* and *DXS3*. *Hum Genet* **77**:233, 1987.

72. Sankila E-M, Lehner T, Eriksson AW, Forsius H, Kärnä J, Page D, Ott J, et al: Haplotype and multipoint linkage analysis in Finnish choroideremia families. *Hum Genet* **84**:66, 1989.

73. Wright AF, Nussbaum RL, Bhattacharya SS, Jay M, Lesko JG, Evans HJ, Jay B: Linkage studies and deletion screening in choroideremia. *J Med Genet* **27**:496, 1990.

74. Sankila E-M, Sistonen P, Cremers FPM, de la Chapelle A: Choroideremia: Linkage analysis with physically mapped close DNA-markers. *Hum Genet* **87**:348, 1991.

75. Tabor A, Andersen O, Lundsteen C, Niebuhr E, Sardemann H: Interstitial deletion in the "critical region" of the long arm of the X chromosome in a mentally retarded boy and his normal mother. *Hum Genet* **64**:196, 1983.

76. Rosenberg T, Schwartz M, Niebuhr E, Yang H-M, Sardemann H, Andersen O, Lundsteen C: Choroideremia in interstitial deletion of the X chromosome. *Ophthalmic Paediatr Genet* **7**:205, 1986.

77. Rosenberg T, Niebuhr E, Yang H-M, Parving A, Schwartz M: Choroideremia, congenital deafness and mental retardation in a family with an X chromosomal deletion. *Ophthalmic Paediatr Genet* **8**:139, 1987.

78. Ayazi S: Choroideremia, obesity and congenital deafness. *Am J Ophthalmol* **92**:63, 1981.

79. Hodgson SV, Robertson ME, Fear CN, Goodship J, Malcolm S, Jay B, Bobrow M, et al: Prenatal diagnosis of X-linked choroideremia with mental retardation, associated with a cytologically detectable X-chromosome deletion. *Hum Genet* **75**:286, 1987.

80. Nussbaum RL, Lesko JG, Lewis RA, Ledbetter SA, Ledbetter DH: Isolation of anonymous DNA sequences from within a submicroscopic X chromosomal deletion in a patient with choroideremia, deafness, and mental retardation. *Proc Natl Acad Sci USA* **84**:6521, 1987.

81. Cremers FPM, van de Pol TJR, Wieringa B, Hofker MH, Pearson PL, Pfeiffer RA, Mikkelsen M, et al: Molecular analysis of male-viable deletions and duplications allows ordering of 52 DNA probes on proximal Xq. *Am J Hum Genet* **43**:452, 1988.

82. Schwartz M, Yang H-M, Niebuhr E, Rosenberg T, Page DC: Regional localization of polymorphic DNA loci on the proximal long arm of the X chromosome using deletions associated with choroideremia. *Hum Genet* **78**:156, 1988.

83. Cremers FPM, van de Pol TJR, Diergaarde PJ, Wieringa B, Nussbaum RL, Schwartz M, Ropers H-H: Physical fine mapping of the choroideremia locus using Xq21 deletions associated with complex syndromes. *Genomics* **4**:41, 1989.

84. Yang H-M, Lund T, Niebuhr E, N(rby S, Schwartz M, Shen L: Exclusion mapping of 12 X-linked disease loci and 10 DNA probes from the long arm of the X-chromosome. *Clin Genet* **38**:94, 1990.

85. Yang H-M, Lund T, Niebuhr E, N(rby S, Schwartz M, Shen L: A deletion panel of the long arm of the X chromosome: Subregional localization of 22 DNA probes. *Hum Genet* **85**:25, 1990.

86. Wells S, Mould S, Robins D, Robinson D, Jacobs P: Molecular and cytogenetic analysis of a familial microdeletion of Xq. *J Med Genet* **28**:163, 1991.

87. Bach I, Robinson D, Thomas N, Ropers H-H, Cremers FPM: Physical fine mapping of genes underlying X-linked deafness and non fra(X)-X-linked mental retardation at Xq21. *Hum Genet* **89**:620, 1992.

88. Reardon W, Roberts S, Phelps PD, Thomas NS, Beck L, Issac R, Hughes HE: Phenotypic evidence for a common pathogenesis in X-linked deafness pedigrees and in Xq13-q21 deletion related deafness. *Am J Med Genet* **44**:513, 1992.

89. Kandpal G, Jacob ANK, Kandpal RP: Transcribed sequences encoded in the region involved in contiguous deletion syndrome that comprises X-linked stapes fixation and deafness. *Somat Cell Mol Genet* **22**:511, 1996.

90. Brunner HG, van Bennekom CA, Lambermon EMM, Oei TL, Cremers CWRJ, Wieringa B, Ropers H-H: The gene for X-linked progressive mixed deafness with perilymphatic gusher during stapes surgery (*DFN3*) is linked to PGK. *Hum Genet* **80**:337, 1988.

91. Wallis C, Ballo R, Wallis G, Beighton P, Goldblatt J: X-linked mixed deafness with stapes fixation in a Mauritian kindred: Linkage to Xq probe pDP34. *Genomics* **3**:299, 1988.

92. Moore GE, Ivens A, Chambers J, Farrall M, Williamson R, Page DC, Bjornsson A, et al: Linkage of an X-chromosome cleft palate gene. *Nature* **326**:91, 1987.

93. Gorski SM, Adams KJ, Birch PH, Friedman JM, Goodfellow PJ: The gene responsible for X-linked cleft palate (*CPX*) in a British Columbia native kindred is localized between *PGK1* and *DXYS1*. *Am J Hum Genet* **50**:1129, 1992.

94. Gorski SM, Adams KJ, Birch PH, Chodirker BN, Greenberg CR, Goodfellow PJ: Linkage analysis of X-linked cleft palate and ankyloglossia in Manitoba Mennonite and British Columbia native kindreds. *Hum Genet* **94**:141, 1994.

95. Forbes SA, Brennan L, Richardson M, Coffey A, Cole CG, Gregory SG, Bentley DR, et al: Refined mapping and YAC contig construction of the X-linked cleft palate and ankyloglossia locus (*CPX*) including the proximal X-Y homology breakpoint within Xq21.3. *Genomics* **31**:36, 1996.

96. de Kok YJM, van der Maarel SM, Bitner-Glindzicz M, Huber I, Monaco AP, Malcolm S, Pembrey ME, et al: Association between X-linked mixed deafness and mutations in the POU domain gene *POU3F4*. *Science* **267**:685, 1995.

97. Cremers FPM, Brunsmann F, van de Pol TJR, Pawlowitzki IH, Paulsen K, Wieringa B, Ropers H-H: Deletion of the *DXS165* locus in patients with classical choroideremia. *Clin Genet* **32**:421, 1987.

98. van de Pol TJR, Cremers FPM, Brohet RM, Wieringa B, Ropers H-H: Derivation of clones from the choroideremia locus by preparative field inversion gel electrophoresis. *Nucl Acids Res* **18**:725, 1990.

99. Merry DE, Lesko JG, Siu V, Flintoff WF, Collins F, Lewis RA, Nussbaum RL: *DXS165* detects a translocation breakpoint in a woman with choroideremia and a *de novo* X;13 translocation. *Genomics* **6**:609, 1990.

100. Cremers FPM, Sankila E-M, Brunsmann F, Jay M, Jay B, Wright A, Pinckers AJLG, et al: Deletions in patients with classical choroideremia vary in size from 45 kb to several megabases. *Am J Hum Genet* **47**:622, 1990.

101. Cremers FPM, Brunsmann F, Berger W, van Kerkhoff EPM, van de Pol TJR, Wieringa B, Pawlowitzki IH, et al: Cloning of the breakpoints of a deletion associated with choroideremia. *Hum Genet* **86**:61, 1990.

102. van Bokhoven H, Schwartz M, Andréasson S, van den Hurk JAJM, Bogerd L, Jay M, Rüther K, et al: Mutation spectrum in the *CHM* gene of Danish and Swedish choroideremia patients. *Hum Mol Genet* **3**:1047, 1994.

103. van den Hurk JAJM, Schwartz M, van Bokhoven H, van de Pol TJR, Bogerd L, Pinckers AJLG, Bleeker-Wagemakers EM, et al: Molecular basis of choroideremia (*CHM*): Mutations involving the Rab escort protein-1 (*REP-1*) gene. *Hum Mutat* **9**:110, 1997.

104. Teboul M, Mujica P, Chery M, Leotard B, Gilgenkrantz S: Translocations X-autosomes équilibrées et retard mental: Contribution à la cartographie des retards mentaux liés à l'X (à l'exclusion de L'X-FRA). *J Genet Hum* **37**:179, 1989.

105. Cremers FPM, van de Pol TJR, Wieringa B, Collins FS, Sankila E-M, Siu VM, Flintoff WF, et al: Chromosomal jumping from the *DXS165* locus allows molecular characterization of four microdeletions and a de novo chromosome X/13 translocation associated with choroideremia. *Proc Natl Acad Sci USA* **86**:7510, 1989.

106. Merry DE, Jänne PA, Landers JE, Lewis RA, Nussbaum RL: Isolation of a candidate gene for choroideremia. *Proc Natl Acad Sci USA* **89**:2135, 1992.

107. Nathans J, Thomas D, Hogness DS: Molecular genetics of human color vision: The genes encoding blue, green, and red pigments. *Science* **232**:193, 1986.

108. Cremers FPM, van de Pol TJR, van Kerkhoff EPM, Wieringa B, Ropers H-H: Cloning of a gene that is rearranged in patients with choroideraemia. *Nature* **347**:674, 1990.

109. van Bokhoven H, van den Hurk JAJM, Bogerd L, Philippe C, Gilgenkrantz S, de Jong P, Ropers H-H, et al: Cloning and characterization of the human choroideremia gene. *Hum Mol Genet* **3**:1041, 1994.

110. Sankila E-M, Tolvanen R, van den Hurk JAJM, Cremers FPM, de la Chapelle A: Aberrant splicing of the *CHM* gene is a significant cause of choroideremia. *Nature Genet* **1**:109, 1992.

111. Orita M, Iwahana H, Kanazawa H, Hayashi K, Sekiya T: Detection of polymorphisms of human DNA by gel electrophoresis as single-strand conformation polymorphisms. *Proc Natl Acad Sci USA* **86**:2766, 1989.

112. van den Hurk JAJM, van de Pol TJR, Molloy CM, Brunsmann F, Rüther K, Zrenner E, Pinckers AJLG, et al: Detection and characterization of point mutations in the choroideremia candidate gene by PCR-SSCP analysis and direct DNA sequencing. *Am J Hum Genet* **50**:1195, 1992.

113. Schwartz M, Rosenberg T, van den Hurk JAJM, van de Pol TJR, Cremers FPM: Identification of mutations in Danish choroideremia families. *Hum Mutat* **2**:43, 1993.

114. Beaufrère L, Tuffery S, Hamel C, Arnaud B, Demaille J, Claustres M: A novel mutation (S558X) causing choroideremia. *Hum Mutat* **8**:395, 1996.

115. Nesslinger N, Mitchell G, Strasberg P, MacDonald IM: Mutation analysis in Canadian families with choroideremia. *Ophthalmic Genet* **17**:47, 1996.

116. Beaufrère L, Tuffery S, Hamel C, Bareil C, Arnaud B, Demaille J, Claustres M: The Protein truncation test (PTT) as a method of detection for choroideremia mutations. *Exp Eye Res* **65**:849, 1997.

117. Beaufrère L, Tuffery S, Hamel C, Bareil C, Arnaud B, Demaille J, Claustres M: Diagnostic génétique rapide des femmes conductrices apparentées à des sujets atteints de choroïdérémie. *J Fr Ophtalmol* **20**:534, 1997.

118. Nesslinger N, Horrocks S, Ray PN, Strasberg P, MacDonald IM: A 3-base-pair insertional mutation in the choroideremia gene. *Hum Mutat* Suppl 1:S38, 1998.

119. Beaufrère L, Rieu S, Hache J-C, Dumur V, Claustres M, Tuffery S: Altered rep-1 expression due to substitution at position +3 of the IVS13 splice-donor site of the choroideremia (*CHM*) gene. *Curr Eye Res* **17**:726, 1998.

120. Donnelly P, Menet H, Fouanon C, Herbert O, Moisan JP, Le Roux MG, Pascal O: Missense mutation in the choroideremia gene. *Hum Mol Genet* **3**:1017, 1994.

121. Beaufrère L, Girardet A, Arnaud B, Claustres M, Tuffery S: Mise au point d'un test diagnostique de la choroïdérémie: Le test de troncation des protéines (PTT). *J Fr Ophtalmol* **21**:345, 1998.

122. Pascal O, Donnelly P, Fouanon C, Herbert O, Le Roux MG, Moisan JP: A new (old) deletion in the choroideremia gene. *Hum Mol Genet* **2**:1489, 1993.

123. Michaud J, Brody LC, Steel G, Fontaine G, Martin LS, Valle D, Mitchell G: Strand-separating conformational polymorphism analysis: Efficacy of detection of point mutations in the human ornithine d-aminotransferase gene. *Genomics* **13**:389, 1992.

124. van den Hurk JAJM, van Zandvoort PM, Brunsmann F, Pawlowitzki IH, Holzgreve W, Szabo P, Cremers FPM, et al: Prenatal exclusion of choroideremia. *Am J Med Genet* **44**:822, 1992.

125. Schwartz M, Rosenberg T: Prenatal diagnosis of choroideremia. *Acta Ophthalmol Scand* **74**:33, 1996.

126. van Bokhoven H, van Genderen C, Ropers H-H, Cremers FPM: Dinucleotide repeat polymorphism within the choroideremia gene at Xq21.2. *Hum Mol Genet* **3**:1446, 1994.

127. van Bokhoven H, van den Hurk JAJM, Bogerd L, van de Pol TJR, Ropers H-H, Cremers FPM: A highly polymorphic microsatellite marker located within the choroideremia gene. *Ophthalmic Genet* **17**:119, 1996.

128. Philippe C, Arnould C, Sloan F, van Bokhoven H, van der Velde-Visser SD, Chery M, Ropers H-H, et al: A high resolution interval map of the q21 region of the human X chromosome. *Genomics* **27**:539, 1995.

129. Cremers FPM, Molloy CM, van de Pol TJR, van den Hurk JAJM, Bach I, Geurts van Kessel AHM, Ropers H-H: An autosomal homologue of

the choroideremia gene colocalizes with the Usher syndrome type II locus on the distal part of chromosome 1q. *Hum Mol Genet* **1**:71, 1992.

130. van Bokhoven H, van Genderen C, Molloy CM, van de Pol TJR, Cremers CWRJ, van Aarem A, Schwartz M, et al: Mapping of the choroideremia-like (*CHML*) gene at 1q42-qter and mutation analysis in patients with Usher syndrome type II. *Genomics* **19**:385, 1994.

131. Barbosa MDFS, Johnson SA, Achey K, Gutierrez MJ, Wakeland EK, Kingsmore SF: Genetic mapping of the choroideremia-like rab escort protein-2 gene on mouse chromosome 1. *Mammalian Genome* **6**:488, 1995.

132. Desnoyers L, Anant J, Seabra M: Geranylgeranylation of Rab proteins. *Biochem Soc Trans* **24**:699, 1998.

133. Fodor E, Lee RT, O'Donnell JJ: Analysis of choroideraemia gene. *Nature* **351**:614, 1991.

134. Koonin EV: Human choroideremia protein contains a FAD-binding domain. *Nature Genet* **12**:237, 1996.

135. Schalk I, Zeng K, Wu S-K, Stura EA, Matteson J, Huang M, Tandon A, et al: Structure and mutational analysis of Rab GDP-dissociation inhibitor. *Nature* **381**:42, 1996.

136. Seabra MC, Brown MS, Slaughter CA, Südhof TC, Goldstein JL: Purification of component A of Rab geranylgeranyl transferase: Possible identity with the choroideremia gene product. *Cell* **70**:1049, 1992.

137. Seabra MC, Brown MS, Goldstein JL: Retinal degeneration in choroideremia: Deficiency of Rab geranylgeranyl transferase. *Science* **259**:377, 1993.

138. Andres DA, Seabra MC, Brown MS, Armstrong SA, Smeland TE, Cremers FPM, Goldstein JL: cDNA cloning of component A of Rab geranylgeranyl transferase and demonstration of its role as a Rab escort protein. *Cell* **73**:1091, 1993.

139. Alexandrov K, Horiuchi H, Steele-Mortimer O, Seabra MC, Zerial M: Rab escort protein-1 is a multifunctional protein that accompanies newly prenylated rab proteins to their target membranes. *EMBO J* **13**:5262, 1994.

140. Waldherr M, Ragnini A, Schweyen RJ, Boguski MS: MRS6: Yeast homologue of the choroideraemia gene. *Nature Genet* **3**:193, 1993.

141. Jiang Y, Rossi G, Ferro-Novick S: Bet2p and Mad2p are components of a prenyltransferase that adds geranylgeranyl onto Ypt1p and Sec4p. *Nature* **366**:84, 1993.

142. Jiang Y, Ferro-Novick S: Identification of yeast component A: Reconstitution of the geranylgeranyltransferase that modifies Ypt1p and Sec4p. *Proc Natl Acad Sci USA* **91**:4377, 1994.

143. Benito-Moreno RM, Miaczynska M, Bauer BE, Schweyen RJ, Ragnini A: Mrs6p, the yeast homologue of the mammalian choroideraemia protein: Immunological evidence for its function as the Ypt1p Rab escort protein. *Curr Genet* **27**:23, 1994.

144. Fujimura K, Tanaka K, Nakano A, Toh-e A: The *Saccharomyces cerevisiae MSI4* gene encodes the yeast counterpart of component A of Rab geranylgeranyltransferase. *J Biol Chem* **269**:9205, 1994.

145. Ragnini A, Teply R, Waldherr M, Voskova A, Schweyen RJ: The yeast protein Mrs6p, a homologue of the rabGDI and human choroideraemia proteins, affects cytoplasmic and mitochondrial functions. *Curr Genet* **26**:308, 1994.

146. Cremers FPM, Armstrong SA, Seabra MC, Brown MS, Goldstein JL: REP-2, a Rab escort protein encoded by the choroideremia-like gene. *J Biol Chem* **269**:2111, 1994.

147. Seabra MC, Ho YK, Anant JS: Deficient geranylgeranylation of Ram/Rab27 in choroideremia. *J Biol Chem* **270**:24420, 1995.

148. van den Hurk JAJM, Hendriks W, van de Pol TJR, Oerlemans F, Jaissle G, Rüther K, Kohler K, et al: Mouse choroideremia gene mutation causes photoreceptor cell degeneration and is not transmitted through the female germline. *Hum Mol Genet* **6**:851, 1997.

149. Tagaki N, Sasaki M: Preferential inactivation of the paternally derived X chromosome in the extraembryonic membranes of the mouse. *Nature* **256**:640, 1975.

150. West JD, Frels WI, Chapman VM, Papaioannou VE: Preferential expression of the maternally derived X chromosome in the mouse yolk sac. *Cell* **12**:873, 1977.

# Leber Congenital Amaurosis

*Josseline Kaplan* ■ *Jean-Michel Rozet*
*Isabelle Perrault* ■ *Arnold Munnich*

1. **Leber congenital amaurosis (LCA) (MIM 204000) is characterized by severe or complete loss of visual function apparent early in infancy with failure to follow visual stimuli, nystagmus, and roving eye movements. Affected individuals have an extinguished electroretinogram and eventually develop abnormalities of the ocular fundus including a pigmentary retinopathy. Although many LCA patients have no additional abnormalities, in some there is associated mental retardation. LCA is inherited as an autosomal recessive trait. Aside from helping the patient adapt to life with no visual function, there is no treatment.**
2. **The LCA phenotype is genetically heterogeneous, with mutations in at least three genes causing the disorder. LCA1 maps to 17p13 and encodes retGC-1, a photoreceptor-specific guanylate cyclase. LCA2 maps to 1p31 and encodes RPE65, a 61-kDa retinal pigment epithelium (RPE)-specific microsomal protein. Mutations at this locus also have been shown to cause childhood-onset severe retinal dystrophy (CSRD). LCA3 maps to 19q13.3 and encodes CRX, a homeodomain transcription factor that is a positive activator of several photoreceptor-specific genes.**
3. **Animal models of LCA include the *rd/rd* chick, in which blindness precedes photoreceptor degeneration. The responsible gene (*GC1*) encodes a guanylate cyclase with 61 percent amino acid identity to mammalian guanylate cyclase 1, and a deletion/insertion mutant allele has been identified in the *rd/rd* chick. Additionally, a mouse model with targeted disruption of the murine guanylate cyclase gene (*GCE*) has been produced. These mice exhibit an early loss of the cone ERG followed later by loss of the rod ERG. Finally, a mouse model with targeted disruption of the *RPE65* gene has been produced. These animals have a severely abnormal dark-adapted ERG and subtle morphologic abnormalities of the photoreceptor outer segments.**

## BACKGROUND

Originally described by Leber in 1869, Leber congenital amaurosis (LCA) is an autosomal recessive disease distinct from other retinal dystrophies and responsible for congenital blindness.[1] The diagnosis is usually made at birth or during the first months of life in an infant with total blindness or greatly impaired vision, normal fundus, and an extinguished electroretinogram (ERG).[2] This condition, the most early and severe of all inherited retinopathies, was largely unrecognized until two population studies from Sweden[3] and Holland[4] revealed that it is not uncommon. Indeed, LCA accounts for at least 5 percent of all retinal dystrophies and probably much more in countries with a high rate of consanguinity.[5,6] Genetic heterogeneity in LCA has long been suspected since the report by Waardenburg of normal children born to affected parents.[7] LCA is either isolated or associated with various extraocular abnormalities, including renal dysplasia (Senior-Loken syndrome, MIM 266900), vermis agenesia (Joubert syndrome, MIM 213300), and inherited metabolic diseases, i.e., hyperthreoninemia[8] and peroxisomal disorders.[9] These latter associations most likely represent distinct clinical and genetic entities and will not be covered in this chapter.

Until 1996, little was known regarding the pathophysiology of LCA, but the disease was considered to be a consequence of either impaired development or extremely early degeneration of photoreceptors.[10] The identification of photoreceptor-specific guanylate cyclase gene mutations in LCA strongly suggests that the photoactivated transduction cascade is severely impaired in this disease.[11]

## CLINICAL PHENOTYPE

The infant with LCA is usually blind at birth, but frequently this feature is recognized later (2–3 months), when parents note that the child does not follow objects or light. Yet there is a certain degree of clinical heterogeneity in isolated LCA. In most cases, visual acuity is only consistent with finger counting, whereas a few patients have an initially preserved vision, with visual acuity occasionally reaching 6/60 to 6/30 (J Kaplan, unpublished data). Most patients have severe photophobia from birth, and some display early night blindness (J Kaplan, unpublished data).

The recognition of severe visual impairment is based on pendular nystagmus, roving eye movements, absent ocular pursuit, and eye poking (digitoocular sign of Franceschetti).[13] Ophthalmologic examination reveals that the fundus is normal initially, a feature that contrasts with a nonrecordable ERG and emphasizes the early and dramatic impairment of both cone and rod photoreceptor cells. After several years, fundus abnormalities appear, namely, salt-and-pepper pigmentation, bone corpuscular pigment, attenuation of retinal vessels, atrophy of the retinal pigment epithelium (RPE) and choriocapillaris, and occasionally, multiple irregular yellowish white flecks deep in the peripheral and midperipheral retina.[14,15] Although visual acuity, visual fields, and ERG tend to remain constant, the fundus changes are progressive, as observed in late-onset retinitis pigmentosa (RP). In addition, keratoconus may develop.[16] Hypermetropia is a quasi-constant feature, possibly resulting in a shortened axial length of the globe.[17] Finally, it is important to realize that psychomotor retardation may be associated with LCA. It is not clear whether LCA with neurologic abnormalities is genetically distinct from isolated LCA. However, this is unlikely because several families segregate both isolated LCA and LCA with mental retardation or neurologic symptoms.[18,19] It is possible that neurologic and behavioral problems may be secondary to early congenital blindness.

## PATHOLOGY

Until now, little was known regarding the pathophysiology of the disease, and only few pathologic examinations were available. Electron microscopy of eyes from an 18-month-old affected

A list of standard abbreviations is located immediately preceding the index in each volume. Nonstandard abbreviations used in this chapter include: LCA = Leber congenital amaurosis; ERG = electroretinogram; RPE = retinal pigment epithelium; CSRD = childhood-onset severe retinal dystrophy; RP = retinitis pigmentosa.

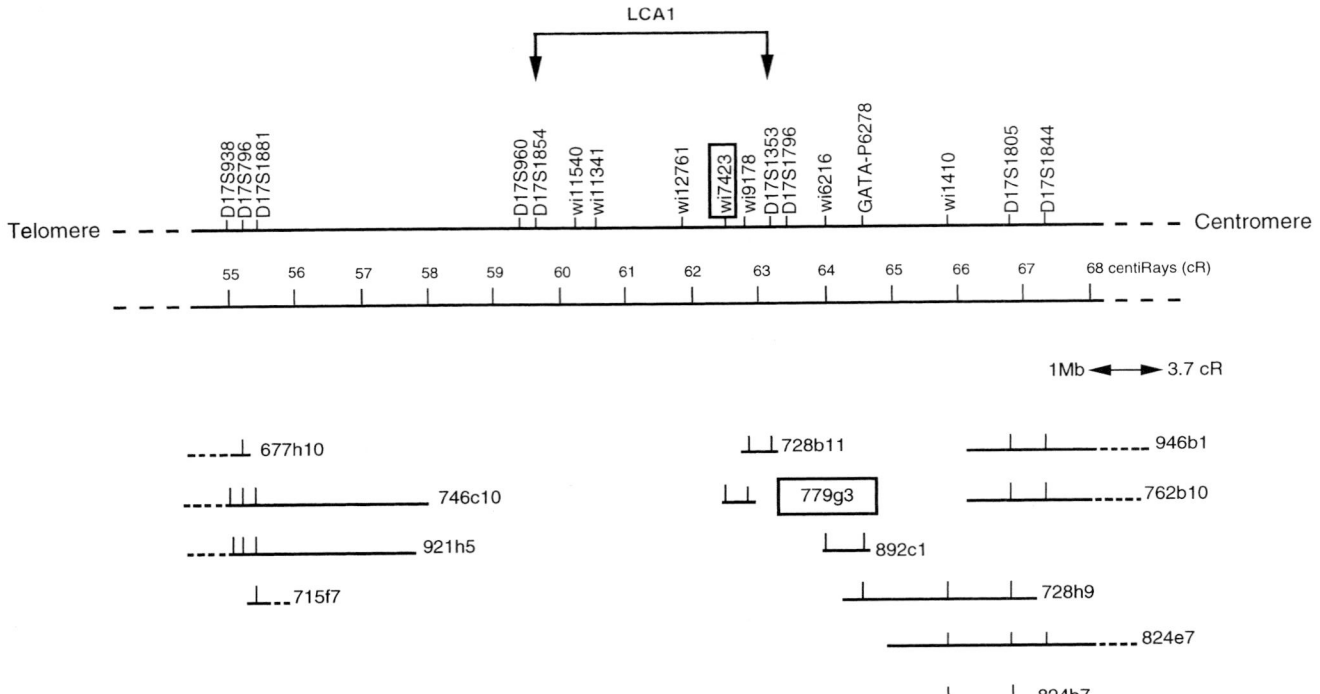

**Fig. 237-1** Genetic and radiation hybrid map of the chromosome 17p13.1 region spanning the *LCA1* locus. The positions of ESTs on YAC clones of the region are indicated by vertical dashes.

Japanese girl showed distinctive changes in the outer retinal layers and choroid, whereas the inner retinal layers were nearly normal.[10] Characteristic early lesions were apparently due to deposits of pieces of outer segments and apical processes of RPE cells and macrophages. These findings suggest that maturation and differentiation of both photoreceptor and RPE cells are impaired in the disease. Studying the eyes of a 6-month-old LCA baby with neurologic involvement also revealed apparently normal inner segments but shortened and abnormal outer segments.[20]

## MAPPING *LCA1* AND EVIDENCE FOR GENETIC HETEROGENEITY

### Linkage Studies

In 1993, Dollfus et al.[18] ascertained 15 unrelated multiplex families affected with LCA. They generated an exclusion map of the genome starting from chromosome 17, since a major gene of the visual transduction cascade in photoreceptor cells, the cGMP phosphodiesterase $\gamma$ subunit (cGMP-PDE$\gamma$), maps to its long arm. A positive Lod score value for probe LEW101 at the *D17S40* locus was found in 9 of 15 informative pedigrees ($Z_{max} = 2.32$ at $\theta = 0.05$). Yet subsequent linkage analyses using highly polymorphic microsatellite DNA markers of the Genethon database showed no significant linkage for any of the markers on the long arm and proximal short arm of chromosome 17.

Subsequently, an analysis of polymorphic markers of the short arm of chromosome 17 showed significant linkage at the *D17S1353* locus ($Z_{max} = 5.14$ at $\theta = 0.15$).[19] When the families were split into two groups, based on their ethnic origin, the presence of a gene for LCA on 17p was confirmed by both homozygosity mapping and linkage analyses in five families of Maghrebian origin (four consanguineous), whereas negative results were found in 10 families of French ancestry. Haplotype analyses supported the placement of the disease gene (*LCA1*) between loci *D17S796* and *D17S786*. In 1996, extending their panel of multiplex families, Camuzat et al.[21] confirmed the genetic

heterogeneity of LCA and refined the mapping of *LCA1* to a 1-cM region on chromosome 17p13.1 between markers *D17S938* and *D17S1353*.[21] Based on three key recombinants, Perrault et al.[11] were able to reduce the genetic interval encompassing the disease gene to a critical region of less than 1 cM between loci *D17S1353* and *D17S1854* (Fig. 237-1).

### Physical Mapping

Starting from the flanking markers *D17S1854* and *D17S1353*, Perrault et al.[11] ordered 12 yeast artificial chromosome (YAC) clones on chromosome 17p13.1 using expressed sequence tags (ESTs) and sequence tagged sites (STSs) of the region[11] (see Fig. 237-1). None of the candidate genes expressed in the retina and located on chromosome 17 mapped to these YACs, namely, recoverin,[22] $\beta$-arrestin 2,[23] phosphatidylinositol transfer protein,[24] and pigment epithelium-derived factor gene.[25] Interestingly, EST WI7423 corresponding to the human photoreceptor-specific guanylate cyclase gene (*retGC-1*, also called *GUC2D*), catalyzing the conversion of GTP to cyclic $3',5'$-guanosine monophosphate (cGMP) and located on chromosome 17p13.1,[26] was found to map to YAC 779g3 (see Fig. 237-1). Therefore, *retGC-1* was regarded as an excellent candidate gene by both position and function.

## IDENTIFICATION OF *LCA1*

The organization of the human *retGC-1* gene was unknown, but the sequence of the human cDNA[27] and the organization of the mouse gene *GCE* had been reported.[28] *GCE* (16 kb) contains 20 exons and maps to mouse chromosome 11 in a region with conservation of synteny to human chromosome 17p13.1. Based on the genomic organization of the mouse gene, Perrault et al.[11] derived the exon-intron boundaries of the human gene. The human *retGC-1* gene (16 kb) contains 20 exons and is highly similar to its mouse counterpart (87 percent amino acid identity). The coding sequence of *retGC-1* was screened for point mutations by direct sequence analysis of genomic DNA of LCA patients belonging to eight families linked to chromosome 17p13.[20] Homozygosity for a

(a)                                        (b)

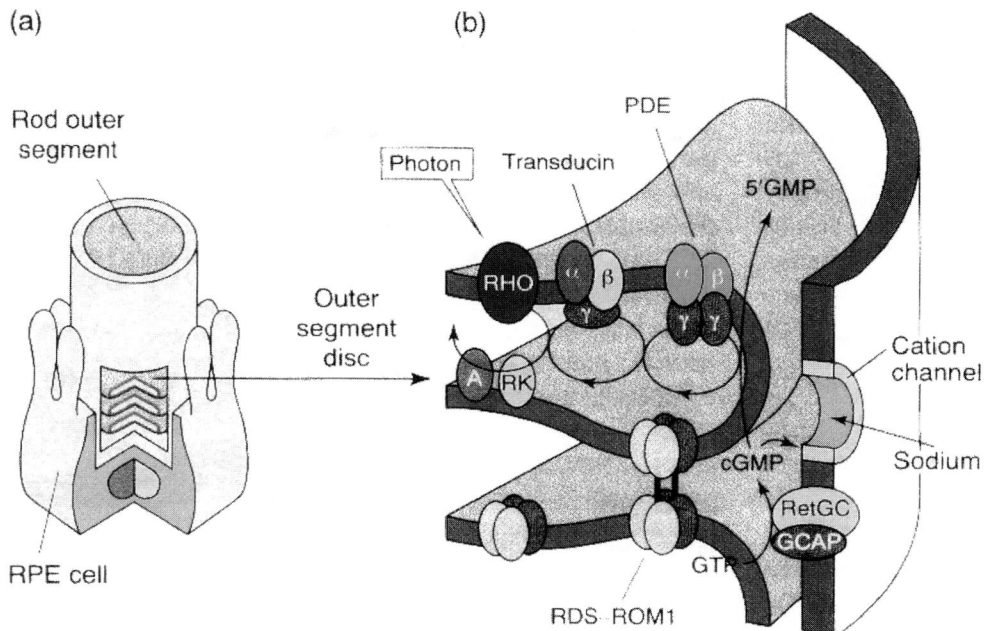

**Fig. 237-2 (A)** A rod photoreceptor-retinal pigment epithelial complex and **(B)** rod outer-segment discs. The phototransduction pathway: Incident light (photon) photoactivates rhodopsin (RHO), which initiates a cascade reaction involving transducin and phosphodiesterase (PDE). This leads to a relative decrease in intracellular cGMP, closure of sodium channels, and cell hyperpolarization. In the recovery process of photoreceptors, the photoactivated transduction cascade is abolished, and the level of cGMP concentration in photoreceptors is restored to the dark level by the conversion of GTP to 3′,5′-cGMP catalyzed by the guanylate cyclase (RetGC). Regeneration of rhodopsin involves arrestin (A) and rhodopsin kinase (RK). RDS-ROM1 interaction is involved in maintaining rod outer-segment structural integrity. Abbreviations: GCAP, guanylate cyclase activating protein; RDS-ROM1, retinal degeneration slow, rod outer-segment membrane protein. See Color Plate 20. (**Used with permission from Gregory-Evans K, Bhattacharya SS: Clinical blindness: Current concepts in the pathogenesis of human outer retinal dystrophies. Trends Genet 3:103, 1998.**)

missense mutation in exon 8 at nucleotide 1767 (T → C), changing a phenylalanine into a serine, was found in all affected siblings of two consanguineous Arab-Algerian families.[11] Moreover, in a Jewish Sefardi family of Tunisian origin, homozygosity for a single base pair deletion (delC) was found in exon 2 at bp 460, resulting in a premature translation termination at codon 165. Similarly, in an Arab family of Tunisian origin, a homozygous single base pair deletion in exon 2 was observed at bp 693 (delC) that resulted in a premature translation termination at codon 215. The two frameshift mutations are predicted to result in the complete absence of both catalytic and kinase-like domains of the protein.

In 1998, Perrault et al. extended their panel of LCA families to a total of 40 and found 18 different mutations in 20 families originating from various countries around the world (particularly Mediterranean countries). Among these 18 mutations, 5 were homozygous frameshift mutations, 2 were splice-site changes (1 homozygous), and 11 were missense mutations (5 homozygous, unpublished data). It is worth noting that the mutations identified in LCA families were scattered throughout the coding sequence of the *retGC-1* gene, except exons 11 to 13, which are involved in the dimerization of the RETGC protein[29,30] (Fig. 237-2). Interestingly, Kelsell et al.[31] mapped a gene for progressive autosomal dominant cone-rod dystrophy (*CORD6*) to the genetic interval encompassing *LCA1* on chromosome 17p13. Subsequently, Kelsell et al.[32] and Perrault et al.[33] independently showed that the disease resulted from heterozygosity for mutations in exon 13 of the *retGC-1* gene and speculated that in cone-rod dystrophy, mutations of this exon might exert a dominant negative effect, hindering the dimerization of the normal counterpart.

## FUNCTION OF RETGC-1

Two major forms of guanylate cyclase have been recognized, a membrane-bound and a soluble form.[34] The membrane guanylate cyclases are composed of large single subunits consisting of (1) an extracellular ligand-binding N-terminal domain, (2) a transmembrane domain, (3) an internal protein kinase homology region, and (4) a C-terminal catalytic domain.[35] Two photoreceptor-specific membrane retinal guanylyl cyclases (retGC-1 and retGC-2) have been identified so far[27,36] and found to form homodimers in preference to heterodimers.[37] These cyclases belong to a new guanylate cyclase subfamily different from the peptide receptor guanylate cyclase family. Indeed, photoreceptor guanylate cyclase is not activated by natriuretic peptides but by retinal-specific activators (GCAPs).[38] GCAPs are $Ca^{2+}$-binding proteins of the calmodulin gene family that contain four EF hand $Ca^{2+}$-binding motifs.[39] To date, two GCAPs have been identified in human retinas (GCAP1 and GCAP2).[40,41] Both GCAPs have been shown to activate retGC-1 in the presence of a low $Ca^{2+}$ concentration, a regulatory mechanism that leads to accelerated synthesis of cGMP, the internal messenger of phototransduction, after photobleaching. Electron microscopy and immunocytochemical studies using anti-retGC1 antibodies have shown that retGC-1 is found predominantly in the outer segments of cones, suggesting that the high retGC-1 activity in cones may be responsible for the rapid recovery of cGMP concentration to the dark level.[42]

Photoreceptor cells normally convert light energy into an electrical signal through a transduction process that consists of an enzymatic cascade. In the excitation process of both rod and cone photoreceptors, photoactivated rhodopsin stimulates cGMP phosphodiesterase through GTP/GDP exchange on transducin, a retinal G protein, resulting in the hydrolysis of cGMP and the closure of cGMP-gated cation channels with hyperpolarization of the plasma membrane[43,44] (Fig. 237-3). Indeed, following illumination, the entry of $Ca^{2+}$ through the cGMP-gated channel stops, but its export by the exchanger continues. Consequently, the cytosolic level of $Ca^{2+}$ drops (from about 500 to 50 nM), stimulating the production of guanylate cyclase.[38] In the recovery process of photoreceptors, the photoactivated transduction cascade

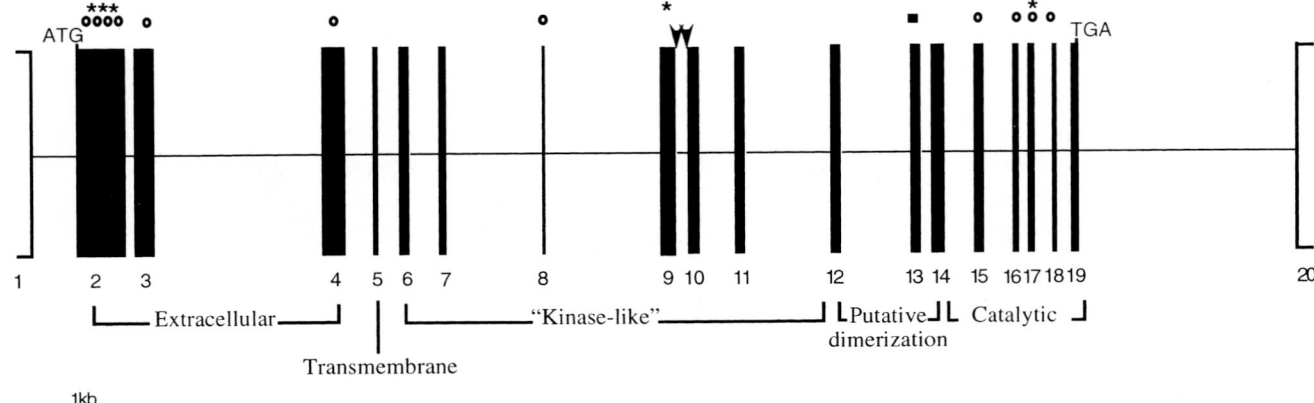

**Fig. 237-3** Structure of the human *retGC-1* gene and positions of mutations identifed in *LCA1* and *CORD6* patients. Exons are indicated by boxes with numbers. The extracellular domain is encoded by exons 2 to 4, and exon 5 corresponds to the transmembrane domain. The kinase-like and cyclase catalytic domains are encoded by exons 6 to 12 and 14 to 19, respectively. The putative dimerization domain is encoded by exon 12 to 14. The position of missense, frameshift, and splice mutations identified in *LCA1* are indicated by dots, asterisks, and arrows, respectively, whereas the dark square shows the position of mutations detected in *CORD6*.

is abolished, and the level of cGMP concentration in photoreceptors is restored to the dark level by the conversion of GTP to 3′,5′-cGMP catalyzed by the guanylate cyclase (see Fig. 237-3). Newly synthesized cGMP reopens the channels to restore the dark state, and both $Ca^{2+}$ and $Na^+$ enter the photoreceptor outer segment through cGMP-gated channels.[45]

The discovery of missense and frameshift *retGC-1* mutations suggests that cGMP production in photoreceptor cells is abolished in LCA.[11] Consequently, the excitation process of rod and cone photoreceptors is markedly impaired due to consistent closure of cGMP-gated cation channels, with hyperpolarization of the plasma membrane. The cGMP concentration in photoreceptor cells cannot be restored to the dark level, leading to a situation equivalent to consistent light exposure during photoreceptor development. This hypothesis is consistent with the histologic findings observed in previous reports (see "Pathology," above).

## IDENTIFICATION OF *LCA2*

### Mutation Screening of *RPE65* in LCA Patients

In 1997, Marlhens et al.[46] surveyed the *RPE65* gene for mutations in two LCA patients aged 20 and 13 years. *RPE65* encodes a specific RPE microsomal protein. They found compound heterozygosity for two alleles: a deletion of an adenine at cDNA position 1067 in a stretch of consecutive adenine residues and a T → C transition at cDNA position 700 in a CpG site, resulting in a nonsense mutation (*R234X*). These mutations were inherited from the clinically unaffected mother and father, respectively.

### Structure and Function of *RPE65*

The RPE is a simple monolayer located immediately below the outer segments of the photoreceptors. It is involved in many aspects of outer retinal metabolism that are essential to the continued maintenance of the photoreceptor cells, including functions such as the retinoid visual cycle and photoreceptor outer segment disk phagocytosis and recycling. In 1993, Hamel et al.[47] characterized and cloned the unique RPE-specific microsomal protein RPE65, whose function is conserved across vertebrate species and therefore whose gene is regarded as a candidate gene for hereditary retinal disorders involving RPE. In 1994, Hamel et al.[48] mapped *RPE65* to 1p31 in humans and to the distal portion of chromosome 3 in mouse.

In 1995, Nicoletti et al.[49] identified the product of the *RPE65* gene as a 61-kDa protein abundant in RPE. They confirmed the

assignment of *RPE65* to 1p31 and showed it spans over 20 kb of genomic DNA. A single transcript of approximately 2.9 kb is present in human RPE and not detected in other tissues. The deduced 533-amino-acid sequence has 98.7 percent similarity to the bovine protein but shows no significant similarity to any other entry in the databases. Expression of the protein appears to depend on the presence of environmental factors, since the corresponding transcripts are rapidly lost from RPE cells established in culture. Nicoletti et al.[49] suggested that down-regulation may occur posttranscriptionally, since AU-rich elements (proposed to target RNA for rapid degradation) are present throughout the 3′ untranslated region. The tissue-specific expression, high abundance, evolutionary conservation, developmental regulation, and sequence of the 3′ untranslated region suggest that the 61-kDa protein is the product of a functionally important gene whose expression is tightly regulated. Recently, Hamel et al.[50] proposed that RPE65 could be the isomerase catalyzing the conversion of all-*trans*-retinyl-ester to 11-*cis*-retinol in the RPE (Fig. 237-4).

### *RPE65* versus *retGC-1* Gene Mutations in LCA: One or Two Diseases?

In 1997, Gu et al.[51] reported mutations of the *RPE65* gene in five unrelated families affected with autosomal recessive childhood-onset severe retinal dystrophy (CSRD), clinically different from LCA. Very recently, Morimura et al.[52] studied 45 LCA families and identified 9 different *RPE65* mutations in 7 unrelated patients, confirming the first report of Marlhens et al.[46] and suggesting that some cases of LCA may represent the extreme end of a spectrum of diseases classified as retinal dystrophies. In fact, Perrault et al. recently studied a panel of 54 LCA families and found *retGC-1* mutations in 20 and 4 *RPE65* mutations in 4 (unpublished data). Subsequently, the clinical history of the probands was revisited extensively, allowing the authors to establish unexpected genotype-phenotype correlations among the so-called LCA patients.[29] Their results suggest that *RPE65* mutations are responsible for a severe congenital progressive retinal dystrophy similar to but different from the congenital stationary blindness caused by *retGC-1* mutations.

## *CRX*, A THIRD GENE IMPLICATED IN LCA (*LCA3*)?

### Structure and Function of *CRX*

In 1997, Freund et al.[53] described a cone-rod homeobox-containing gene (*CRX*) encoding a 299-amino-acid protein with a

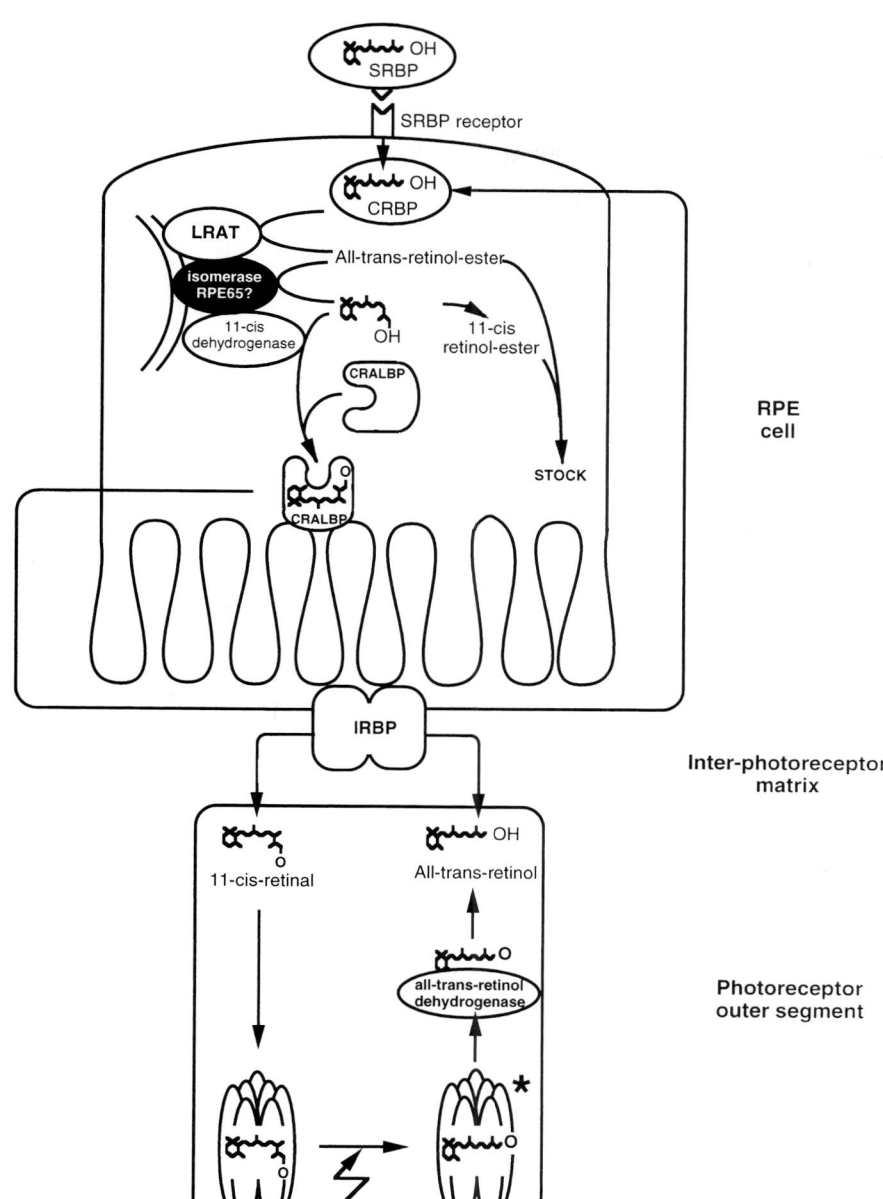

RPE
cell

Inter-photoreceptor
matrix

Photoreceptor
outer segment

**Fig. 237-4 Transport and metabolism of vitamin A.** All-*trans*-retinol (vitamin A) is transported from blood to the RPE by the serum retinol-binding protein (SRBP). The all-*trans*-retinol associated with the cytosolic retinoid-binding protein (CRBP) is esterified in the retinal pigment epithelium by lecithin retinol acyl transferase (LRAT) to produce an all-*trans*-retinyl ester. This ester is directly transformed into 11-*cis*-retinol by an isomerohydrolase enzyme (RPE65?) in a process that couples the negative free energy of hydrolysis of the acyl ester to the formation of the strained 11-*cis*-retinoid. This last molecule is transported by the cellular retinaldehyde-binding protein (CRALBP) and transformed to 11-*cis*-retinal by the 11-*cis* dehydrogenase. The interphotoreceptor retinoid-binding protein (IRBP) shuttles retinoids between the retinal pigment epithelium and the rod outer segment.

predicted mass of 32 kDa, similar to that of the human OTX1 and OTX2 homeodomain proteins. The *CRX* homeodomain is located near the N-terminus at residues 39 to 99 and belongs to the prd class. The other domains of the CRX protein include a WSP motif and a OTX tail. The *CRX* gene maps to 19q13.3 and expresses an abundant 4.5-kb transcript in retina but not in any other of 10 tissues or cells tested.[53] Simultaneously, Furukawa et al.[54] isolated the mouse *CRX* gene from mouse retina. CRX binds and transactivates the sequence TAATCC/A, which is found in the promoters of several photoreceptor-specific genes, including the opsin genes from many species. Furukawa et al.[54] showed in mouse that CRX expression is restricted to developing and mature photoreceptor cells, but overexpression of CRX in cultured rod cells increased the frequency of clones containing rod photoreceptors exclusively and reduced that of clones containing amacrine interneurons and Müller glial cells. In addition, presumptive photoreceptor cells expressing a dominant-negative form of CRX failed to form proper photoreceptor outer segments

and terminals. The authors concluded that CRX is a photoreceptor-specific transcription factor that plays a crucial role in the differentiation of photoreceptor cells.[54] Very recently, it has been demonstrated that CRX transactivates the rhodopsin promotor as well as other photoreceptor-specific genes synergistically with a second photoreceptor transcription factor, neural retina leucine (NRL) zipper.[55]

## Mutation Screening of *CRX* in LCA

Considering that CRX is essential for photoreceptor maintenance and that dominant-negative *CRX* mutants hampered outer segment biogenesis in developing retina, Freund et al.[56] surveyed the *CRX* gene for mutations in LCA patients. They identified two heterozygote *de novo* deletions in *CRX:* a 2-bp deletion at the E168 codon and a 1-bp deletion at the G217 codon in two unrelated LCA patients. Both deletions caused frameshifts, and the predicted proteins lacked the conserved C-terminus. The E168del2bp mutant had lost an AG dinucleotide from the GAG codon for the eleventh residue within the conserved 13-amino-acid WSP motif. Even if the mRNA containing this premature stop codon was stable, 45 percent of the protein would be lost and replaced with a new C-terminus of 4 amino acids (VPFA). The G217del1bp mutant was due to the deletion of a G nucleotide, again within a short conserved sequence, and the protein would lack 25 percent of the C-terminus with one additional amino acid (alanine) encoded after the frameshift. Both deletions would abolish the OTX tail.[56] Recently, McInnes et al.[55] showed that *CRX* mutations lead to a decreased synergy with neural retina leucine. Surprisingly, the E168del2bp mutation occurred in the same codon as a mutation found in an autosomal dominant cone-rod dystrophy (*CORD2*) family,[53] raising the question of whether the second *CRX* mutation in LCA patients is in a nonscreened region of the gene or the second *CRX* allele in these LCA patients is a hypomorphic allele that is relatively common in the general population. A parent carrying an allele with modest functional consequences would be unaffected. Paired with either of the deletion alleles reported here, however, a hypomorphic allele would reduce CRX function below a critical threshold and cause LCA. Alternatively, LCA in these families could result from digenic inheritance. In this case, the second mutation would be in a second gene, hitherto unidentified, whose protein product would interact with CRX. The argument of a hypomorphic allele can be extended to the digenic model. In this instance, a *CRX* deletion allele would be paired with a hypomorphic allele at another locus, encoding a polymorphic variant protein that interacts less effectively with CRX. Again, such a combination would reduce CRX function below a critical threshold to lead to disease.

## ANIMAL MODELS OF LCA

### The *rd/rd* Chicken

In the retinal degenerate (*rd*) chicken, a model for recessively inherited retinal degeneration, blindness precedes photoreceptor degeneration in the retina. The first degenerative changes appear in both rod and cone outer segments approximately 7 to 10 days after hatching. By 8 months of age, only a few degenerating cone cells remain in the outer retina.[57,58] The RPE shows pathologic changes only after the photoreceptor cells have begun to degenerate.[59] The absence of both scotopic and photopic ERGs at hatch suggested failure of the phototransduction mechanism in this model.[57] The *rd* chicken therefore was regarded as an excellent animal model for LCA. In 1998, after identifying *retGC-1* mutations in LCA patients, Semple-Rowland et al.[60] showed that the levels of cGMP in developing and predegenerate *rd/rd* photoreceptors are only 10 to 20 percent of those present in age-matched controls. They subsequently isolated the chicken *GC1* gene. Comparisons of the predicted chicken *GC1* amino acid sequence with their human,[27] bovine,[61] rat,[62] and mouse[28] counterparts revealed that chicken *GC1* is 62 percent identical to mammalian *GC1* and that the domain structures are identical. Half the chicken *GC1* cDNAs harbor a unique 87-bp nucleotide sequence encoding 29 amino acids located between the membrane and putative kinase domains.[60] This splice variant has not been identified in rat retina[60] or in human macular/peripheral retina (J Kaplan, unpublished data), suggesting that it may be unique to avian species. Most interestingly, a deletion of the *GC1* cDNA was found in *rd/rd* chicken retina. Sequence analyses revealed that exons 4 to 7 were replaced by an 81-bp fragment in inverse orientation[60] (Fig. 237-5). This deletion/insertion preserved the reading frame of the transcript. The mutant GC1 protein lacked the membrane-spanning domain and flanking regions essential for proper folding and enzyme activity.

### Characterization of a *GCE* Knockout Mouse

In 1998, Birch et al.[63] produced a mouse model lacking the *GCE* gene. In *GCE*$^{-/-}$ mice, the most striking abnormality was the 98

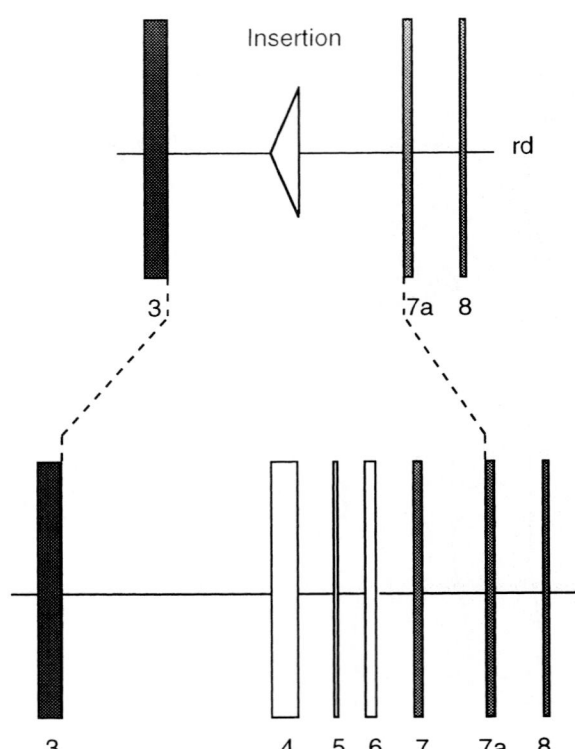

**Fig. 237-5** Model of the *rd* gene defect based on the sequences of *rd/rd* cDNA clones. The splice variant found in both normal and *rd/rd* chicken *GC1* tarnscripts is represented as a unique putative exon (X7A). The 81-bp sequence insert replacing exons 4 to 7 in the *rd/rd* transcripts is indicated by an arrowhead.

percent reduction in cone ERG activity at 3 to 5 weeks of age and the complete absence of detectable cone ERG activity in mice over 12 weeks old. An early loss or a failure of cones to develop was confirmed by histologic analyses. The maximum rod photoresponse amplitude was 70 percent lower than normal at 3 to 5 weeks despite normal histologic appearance of rods and was 92 percent lower by 26 weeks with mild histologic alterations. These findings suggested that loss of *GCE* activity leads to an early and profound loss of cone function in *GCE*$^{-/-}$ mouse, as it is observed in *LCA1* patients (J Kaplan, unpublished data).

### Characterization of a *RPE65* Knockout Mouse

In 1998, Redmond et al.[64] produced a mouse genetic model lacking the *RPE65* gene. No changes in RPE morphology were noted in 7-week-old +/− or −/− animals, nor was there any loss of photoreceptor nuclei. However, in the −/− animals, subtle changes were seen in photoreceptor outer segments by light microscopy. By electron microscopy, the disks were slightly disorganized and not as tightly packed as in the +/+ and +/− controls. In contrast, the dark-adapted ERG of *RPE65*$^{-/-}$ mice was severely abnormal compared with the +/− and +/+ littermates, whereas the light-adapted ERG of *RPE65*$^{-/-}$ mice were normal (similar to +/+ animals).[64] These findings could be related to the natural history of the disease in LCA patients harboring mutations in the *RPE65* gene and suggest that RPE65 is essential for vision but not for outer segment morphogenesis. The *RPE65* knockout mouse model hopefully will clarify the role of RPE65 in the development and function of the RPE/photoreceptor complex and provide a model system for the study of both LCA2 and autosomal recessive CSRD in which *RPE65* mutations have been recognized.

# ADDENDUM

## AIPL1, A FOURTH GENE IMPLICATED IN LCA (LCA5)

### Structure and Function of AIPL1

In 2000, Sohocki et al.[65] described in arylhydrocarbon receptor interacting protein-like (AIPL1) encoding a 384-amino-acid protein with a predicted mass of 44 kDa, similar to arylhydrocarbon receptor interacting protein (AIP), a member of the FK506-binding protein (FABP) family. The AIPL1 protein sequence includes three tetratricopeptide repeats (TPR), a 34-amino-acid motif found in proteins with nuclear transport or protein chaperone activity. *In situ* hybridization indicated expression in rat and mouse pineal gland and a high level of expression in adult mouse retina throughout the outer molecular layer and photoreceptor inner segments, and no expression in the cornea. It is worth noting that the AIPL1 gene maps to 17p13.1, only 2.5 Mb distal to the retGC-1 gene. The genomic structure of the AIPL1 gene has been reported; AIPL1 consists of six coding exons and five introns.[65]

### Mutation Screening of AIPL1 in LCA

Due to the proximity of AIPL1 and retGC1, linkage mapping may not distinguish between the two genes. Further, it is possible that LCA patients who are identical by descent (IBD) at one locus are also IBD at the other. Therefore, both AIPL1 and retGC-1 should be screened for mutations in families whose LCA locus maps to 17p13. In a Pakistani family in which LCA mapped to 17p13.1, Sohocki et al.[65] demonstrated homozygosity for a nonsense mutation, R278X. In addition to this original LCA family, they found disease-causing mutation of the AIPL1 gene in three of fourteen LCA families not tested previously for linkage. More recently, Perrault et al.[66] screened 130 LCA families and found six different mutations in eight families.

## OTHER LCA LOCI

In addition to the four identified LCA genes, two other disease causing genes have been localized on human chromosome: LCA4 on chromosome 14q24 in a single consanguineous family originating from Saudi Arabia,[67] and LCA6 on chromosome 6q11-q16 in a consanguineous family from Switzerland who emigrated to Pennsylvania and who belongs to the Old River Brethren community.[68]

## REFERENCES

1. Leber T: Uber retinitis pigmentosa and angeborene amaurose. *Graefes Arch Klin Exp Ophthalmol* **15**:13, 1869.
2. Franceschetti A, Dieterle P: L'importance diagnostique de l'électro-rétinogramme dans les dégénérescences tapéto-rétiniennes avec rétrécissement du champ visuel et héméralopie. *Conf Neurol* **14**:184, 1954.
3. Alstrom CH, Olson O: Heredo-retinopathia congenitalis monohydrida recessiva autosomalis. *Hereditas* **43**:1, 1957.
4. Schappert-Kimmijser J, Henkes HE, van de Bosch J: Amaurosis congenita (Leber). *Arch Ophthalmol* **61**:211, 1959.
5. Foxman SG, Heckenlively JR, Batemen BJ, Wirstschaffer JD: Classification of congenital and early-onset retinitis pigmentosa. *Arch Ophthalmol* **103**:1502, 1985.
6. Kaplan J, Bonneau D, Frézal J, Munnich A, Dufier JL: Clinical and genetic heterogeneity in retinitis pigmentosa. *Hum Genet* **85**:635, 1990.
7. Waardenburg PJ, Schappert-Kimmijser J: On various recessive biotypes of Leber congenital amaurosis. *Acta Ophthalmol (Copenh)* **41**:317, 1963.
8. Hayasaka S, Hara S, Mizuno K, Narisawa K, Tada K: Leber congenital amaurosis associated with hyperthreoninemia. *Am J Ophthalmol* **101**:475, 1986.
9. Ek J, Kase BF, Reith A, Bjorkhem I, Pedersen JI: Peroxisomal dysfunction in boy with neurologic symptoms and amaurosis (Leber disease): Clinical and biochemical findings similar to those observed in Zellweger syndrome. *J Pediatr* **108**:19, 1986.
10. Mizuno K, Takei Y, Sears ML, Peterson WS, Carr RE, Jampol LM: Leber congenital amaurosis. *Am J Ophthalmol* **83**:32, 1967.
11. Perrault I, Rozet JM, Calvas P, Gerber S, Camuzat A, Dollfus H, Chatelin S, Souied E, Ghazi I, Leowski C, Bonnemaison M, Le Paslier D, Frezal J, Dufier JL, Pittler S, Munnich A, Kaplan J: Retinal-specific guanylate cyclase gene mutations in Leber congenital amaurosis. *Nat Genet* **14**:461, 1996.
12. Traboulsi EI, Maumenee IH: Photoaversion in Leber congenital amaurosis. *Ophthalmic Genet* **16**:27, 1995.
13. Franceschetti A, Forni S: Dégénérescence Tapéto-rétinienne (type Leber) avec aspect marbré du fond d'oeil périphérique. *Ophthalmologica* **135**:610, 1958.
14. Edwards WC, Price WD, MacDonald R: Congenital amaurosis of retinal origin (Leber). *Am J Ophthalmol* **72**:724, 1971.
15. Chew E, Deutman A, Pinckers A, Dekerk A: Yellowish flecks in Leber congenital amaurosis. *Br J Ophthalmol* **68**:727, 1984.
16. Karel I: Keratoconus in congenital diffuse tapetoretinal degeneration. *Ophthalmologica* **155**:8, 1968.
17. Wagner RS, Caputo AR, Nelson LB, Zanoni D: High hyperopia in Leber congenital amaurosis. *Arch Ophthalmol* **103**:1507, 1985.
18. Dollfus H, Rozet JM, Delrieu O, Vignal A, Ghazi I, Dufier JL, Mattei MG, Weissenbach J, Frezal J, Kaplan J, Munnich A: Clinical and genetic heterogeneity of Leber congenital amaurosis, in Hollyfield JG, Anderson KE, La Vail MM (eds): *Retinal Degeneration*. New York, Plenum Press, 1993, pp 143-152.
19. Camuzat A, Dollfus H, Rozet JM, Gerber S, Bonneau D, Bonnemaison M, Briard ML, Dufier JL, Ghazi I, Leowski C, Weissenbach J, Frezal J, Munnich A, Kaplan J: A gene for Leber congenital amaurosis maps to chromosome 17p. *Hum Mol Genet* **8**:1447, 1995.
20. Noble KC, Carr RE: Leber congenital amaurosis: A retrospective study of 33 cases and a histopathological study of one case. *Arch Ophthalmol* **96**:818, 1978.
21. Camuzat A, Rozet JM, Dollfus H, Gerber S, Perrault I, Weissenbach J, Munnich A, Kaplan J: Evidence of genetic heterogeneity of Leber congenital amaurosis (LCA) and mapping of *LCA1* to chromosome 17p13. *Hum Genet* **97**:798, 1996.
22. Murakami A, Yajima T, Inana G: Isolation of human retinal genes: Recoverin cDNA and gene. *Biochem Biophys Res Commun* **187**:234, 1992.
23. Calabres G, Sallese M, Stornaiuolo A, Stuppia L, Palka G, De Blasi A: Chromosome mapping of the human arrestin (*SAG*), β-arrestin 2 (*ARRB2*), and β-adrenergic receptor kinase 2 (*ADRBK2*) genes. *Genomics* **23**:286, 1994
24. Fitzgibbon J, Pilz A, Gayther S, Appukuttan B, Dulai KS, Delhanty JD, Helmkamp GM Jr, Yarbrough LR, Hunt DM: Localization of the gene encoding human phosphatidylinositol transfert protein (*PITPN*) to 17p13.3 a gene showing homology to *Drosophila* retinal degeneration B gene (*rdgB*). *Cytogenet Cell Genet* **67**:205, 1994.
25. Tombran-Tink J, Pawar H, Swaroop A, Rodriguez I, Chader GJ: Localization of the gene for pigment epithelium derived factor (PEDF) to chromosome 17p13.1 and expression in cultured human retinoblastoma cells. *Genomics* **19**:266, 1994.
26. Oliveira L, Miniou P, Viegas-Pequignot E, Rozet JM, Dollfus H, Pittler SJ: Human retianl guanylate cyclase (*GUC2D*) maps to chromosome 17p13.1. *Genomics* **22**:478, 1994.
27. Shyjan AW, de Sauvage FJ, Gillett NA, Goeddel DV, Lowe DG: Molecular cloning of a retina-specific membrane guanylyl cyclase. *Neuron* **9**(4):727, 1992.
28. Yang RB, Fulle HJ, Garbers DL: Chromosomal localization and genomic organization of genes encoding guanylyl cyclase receptors expressed in olfactory sensory neurons and retina. *Genomics* **31**:367, 1996.
29. Perrault I, Rozet JM, Gerber S, Souied E, Cabot A, Munnich A, Kaplan J: A retinal-specific guanylate cyclase gene (*retGC-1*) mutation in autosomal dominant cone-rod dystrophy (*CORD6*). *Exp Eye Res* **67**:A891, 1998.
30. Laura RP, Dizhoor AM, Hurley JB: The membrane guanylyl cyclase, retinal guanylyl cyclase-1, is activated through its intracellular domain. *J Biol Chem* **271**:11646, 1996.
31. Kelsell ER, Evans K, Gregory YC, Moore TA, Bird CA, Hunt MD: Localisation of a gene for dominant cone-rod dystrophy (*CORD6*) to chromosome 17p. *Hum Mol Genet* **4**:597, 1997.
32. Kelsell RE, Gregory-Evans K, Payne AM, Perrault I, Kaplan J, Yang RB, Garbers DL, Bird AC, Moore AT, Hunt DM: Dominant cone-rod dystrophy caused by mutations of the retinal guanylate cyclase (*retGC-1*) gene. *Hum Mol Genet* **7**:1179, 1998.

5954 PART 29 / EYE

33. Perrault I, Rozet JM, Gerber S, Kelsell RE, Souied E, Cabot A, Hunt DM, Munnich A, Kaplan J: A *retGC-1* mutation in autosomal dominant cone-rod dystrophy. *Am J Hum Genet* **63**:651, 1998.

34. Yuen PST, Garbers DL: Guanylyl cyclase receptors. *Annu Rev Neurosci* **15**:193, 1992.

35. Garbers DL, Lowe DG: Guanylyl cyclase receptors. *J Biol Chem* **269**:30741, 1994.

36. Lowe DG, Dizhoor AM, Liu K, Gu Q, Spencer M, Laura R, Lu L, Hurley JB: Cloning and expression of a second photoreceptor-specific membrane retina guanylyl cyclase (retGC), retGC-2. *Proc Natl Acad Sci USA* **92**:5535, 1995.

37. Yang RB, Garbers DL: Two eye guanylyl cyclases are expressed in the same photoreceptor cells and form homomers in preference to heteromers. *J Biol Chem* **272**:13738, 1997.

38. Dizhoor AM, Lowe DG, Olshevskaya EU, Laura RP, Hurley JB: The human photoreceptor membrane guanylate cyclase is present in outer segments and is regulated by calcium and soluble activator. *Neuron* **12**:1345, 1994.

39. Dizhour AM, Hurley JB: Inactivation of EF-hands makes GCAP-2 (p24) a constitutive activator of photoreceptor guanylyl cyclase by preventing a $Ca^2$-induced "activator-to-inhibitor" transition. *J Biol Chem* **32**:19346, 1996.

40. Subbaraya I, Ruiz CC, Helekar BS, Zhao X, Gorczyca WA, Pettenati MJ, Rao PN, Palczewski K, Baehr W: Molecular characterization of human and mouse photoreceptor guanylate cyclase-activating protein (GCAP) and chromosomal localization of the human gene. *J Biol Chem* **269**:31080, 1994.

41. Dizhoor AM, Olshevskaya EV, Henzel WJ, Wong SC, Stults JT, Ankoudinova I, Hurley JB: Cloning, sequencing and expression of a 24-kDa $Ca^{2+}$-binding protein activating photoreceptor guanyly cyclase. *J Biol Chem* **270**:25200, 1995.

42. Liu X, Seno K, Nishizawa Y, Hayashi F, Yamazaki A, Matsumoto H, Wakabayashi T, Usukura J: Ultrastructural localization of retinal guanylate cyclase in human and monkey retinas. *Exp Eye Res* **59**:761, 1994.

43. Chabre M, Deterre P: Molecular mechanism of visual phototransduction. *Eur J Biochem* **179**:255, 1989.

44. Gregory-Evans K, Bhattacharya SS: Clinical blindness: Current concepts in the pathogenesis of human outer retinal dystrophies. *Trends Genet* **3**:103, 1998.

45. Lolley RN, Lee RH: Cyclic GMP and photoreceptor function. *FASEB J* **4**:3001, 1990.

46. Marlhens F, Bareil C, Griffoin, JM, Zrenner E, Amalric P, Eliaou C, Liu SY, Harris E, Redmond TM, Arnaud B, Claustres M, Hamel CP: Mutations in *RPE65* cause Leber congenital amaurosis. *Nature Genet* **17**:139, 1997.

47. Hamel CP, Tsilou E, Pfeffer BA, Hooks JJ, Detrick B, Redmond TM: Molecular cloning and expression of RPE65, a novel retinal pigment epithelium-specific microsomal protein that is post-transcriptionally regulated in vitro. *J Biol Chem* **268**:15751, 1993.

48. Hamel CP, Jenkins NA, Gilbert DJ, Copeland NG, Redmond TM: The gene for the retinal pigment epithelium-specific protein RPE65 is localized to human 1p31 and mouse 3. *Genomics* **20**:509, 1994.

49. Nicoletti A, Wong DJ, Kawase K, Gibson LH, Yang-Feng TL, Richards JE, Thompson DA: Molecular characterization of the human gene encoding an abundant 61-kDa protein specific to the retinal pigment epithelium. *Hum Mol Genet* **4**:641, 1995.

50. Hamel CP, Marlhens F, Griffoin JM, Bariel B, Claustres M, Arnaud B: Different mutations in *RPE65* are associated with variability in the severity of retinal dystrophies. *Exp Eye Res* **67**:A893, 1998.

51. Gu S, Thompson DA, Srikumari CRS, Lorenz B, Finckh U, Nicoletti A, Murthy KR, Rathmann M, Kumaramanickavel G, Denton MJ, Gal A: Mutations in *RPE65* cause autosomal recessive childhood-onset severe retinal dystrophy. *Nature Genet* **17**:194, 1997.

52. Morimura H, Fishman GA, Grover SA, Fulton AB, Berson EL, Dryja TP: Mutations in the *RPE65* gene in patients with autosomal recessive retinitis pigmentosa or Leber congenital amaurosis. *Proc Natl Acad Sci USA* **95**:3088, 1998.

53. Freund CL, Gregory-Evans CY, Furukawa T, Papaioannou M, Looser J, Ploder L, Bellingham J, Ng D, Herbrick JA, Duncan A, Scherer SW, Tsui LC, Loutradis-Anagnostou A, Jacobson SG, Cepko CL, Bhattacharya SS, McInnes RR: Cone-rod dystrophy due to mutations in a novel photoreceptor-specific homeobox gene (*CRX*) essential for maintenance of the photoreceptor. *Cell* **91**:543, 1997.

54. Furukawa T, Morrow EM, Cepko CL: Crx, a novel *otx*-like homeobox gene, shows photoreceptor-specific expression and regulates photoreceptor differentiation. *Cell* **91**:531, 1997.

55. McInnes RR, Freund CL, Chen S, Wang OL, Ploder L, Jacobson SG, Zack DJ, Stone EM: *De novo* mutations in the *CRX* homeobox gene associated with Leber congenital amaurosis (LCA). *Exp Eye Res* **67**:A81, 1998.

56. Freund CL, Wang QL, Chen S, Muskat BL, Wiles CD, Sheffield VC, Jacobson SG, McInnes RR, Zack DJ, Stone EM: *De novo* mutations in the *CRX* homeobox gene associated with Leber congenital amaurosis. *Nature Genet* **18**:311, 1998.

57. Ulshafer RJ, Allen C, Dawson WW, Wolf ED: Hereditary retinal degeneration in the Rhode Island Red chicken: I. Histology and ERG. *Exp Eye Res* **39**:125, 1984.

58. Ulshafer RJ, Allen CB: Hereditary retinal degeneration in the Rhode Island Red chicken: Ultrastructural analysis. *Exp Eye Res* **40**:865, 1985.

59. Ulshafer RJ, Allen CB: Ultrastructural changes in the retinal pigment epithelium of congenitally blind chickens. *Curr Eye Res* **4**:1009, 1985.

60. Semple-Rowland SL, Lee NR, Van Hooser JP, Palczewski K, Baehr W: A null mutation in the photoreceptor guanylate cyclase gene causes the retinal degeneration chicken phenotype. *Proc Natl Acad Sci USA* **95**:1271, 1998.

61. Goraczniak RM, Duda T, Sitaramayya A, Sharma RK: Structural and functional characterization of the rod outer segment membrane guanylate cyclase. *Biochem J* **302**:455, 1994.

62. Yang RB, Foster DC, Garbers DL, Fulle HJ: Two membrane forms of guanylyl cyclase found in the eye. *Proc Natl Acad Sci USA* **92**:602, 1995.

63. Birsh DG, Yang RB, Garbers DL: Detectable responses to light in guanylyl cyclase (GC-E) deficient mice. *Invest Ophthalmol Vis Sci* **4**:A2992, 1998.

64. Redmond M, Yu S, Lee E, Bok D, Hamasaki D, Pfeifer K: Characterization of a *RPE65* knockout mouse: A model for Leber congenital amaurosis type II. *Invest Ophthalmol Vis Sci* **4**:A2994, 1998.

65. Sohocki MM, Bowne SJ, Sullivan LS, Blackshaw S, Cepko CL, Payne AM, Bhattacharya SS, Khaliqs Mehdi SQ, Birch DG, Harrison WR, Elder FFB, Heckenlively JR, Daiger SP: Mutations in a new photoreceptor-pineal gene on 17p cause Leber congenital amaurosis. *Nature Genet* **24**:79, 2000.

66. Perrault I, Rozet JM, Gerber S, Ducroq D, Ghazi I, Leowski C, Souied E, Dufier JL, Munnich A, Kaplan J: Extensive screening for disease causing genes and several candidate genes in 130 LCA families affected with Leber congential amaurosis. *Invest Ophthalmol Vis Sci* **41**:A496, 2000.

67. Stockton DW, Lewis RA, Abboud EB, Al-Rajhi A, Jabak M, Anderson KL, Lupski JR: A novel locus for Leber congenital amaurosis on chromosome 14q24. *Hum Genet* **103**:328, 1998.

68. Dharmaraj S, Li Y, Robitaille JM, Silva E, Zhu D, Mitchell TM, Maltby LP, Baffoe-Bonnie AB, Maumenee IH: A novel locus for Leber congenital amaurosis maps to chromosome 6q. *Am J Hum Genet* **66**:319, 2000.

# Color Vision and Its Genetic Defects

## Arno G. Motulsky ■ Samir S. Deeb

1. Color vision has intrigued scientists for several hundred years. Red-green color vision defects are common and among the first recognized X-linked traits. The molecular genetics of the visual pigments mediating normal and defective color vision have been elucidated and provide the basis for an understanding of the genetic basis of normal and abnormal color vision.

2. The retina is a displaced part of the brain and includes four different photoreceptors: rods containing rhodopsin and cones containing photopigments sensitive to either blue (short-wave), green (middle-wave), or red (long-wave). Normal color vision is trichromatic and is subserved by these three cone pigments. Rhodopsin is used for dim-light vision, whereas the various cone photopigments mediate vision in bright light and color vision. The photopigments have characteristic absorption maxima with wide regions of overlap. The four human visual pigments are similar in their amino acid sequences and are members of the heptahelical transmembrane receptor family that includes olfactory receptors. The red and green pigments differ by at most 15 amino acids. Differences at three residues (180, 277, and 285) largely account for spectral differences between these pigments.

3. The autosomal genes for rhodopsin and the blue pigment are located at chromosome 3q21–24 and 7q31.3–q32, respectively. The red-green pigment gene complex maps to a subterminal site on the long arm of the X chromosome (Xq28) linked to the loci for adrenoleukodystrophy, glucose-6-phosphate deficiency, and hemophilia. The red-green gene arrays are composed of a single red pigment gene (six exons) and one or more green pigment genes (six exons) located downstream (3′) of the red gene. About 25 percent of male Caucasians have a single green pigment gene, whereas the rest have two, three, or more green pigment genes. Almost half of Japanese and African-American males only have a single green pigment gene. The high homology of the red and green opsin genes (including introns) predisposes to unequal crossover and accounts for the numerical polymorphism. Gene expression studies suggest that only the two most proximal among several pigment genes are expressed in the retina. The ratio of red to green pigment mRNAs in human retinas varies widely (1–10, with a mode of 4).

4. Illegitimate recombination between the red and green pigment genes causes deletions or the formation of hybrid genes and explains the genetic basis of the majority of color vision defects. The deletion of green pigment genes leaves a single red pigment gene that is characteristically associated with deuteranopia (G⁻). Affected individuals are dichromatic because they completely lack functional green cones. The finding of severe trichromatic deuteranomaly (G′) in a few individuals with this genetic makeup remains unexplained.

5. Exon 5 (which includes two residues that account for two-thirds of the spectral difference between the red and green pigments) plays a major role in spectral tuning. The recombinational exchange of exon 5 produces hybrid pigments with large spectral shifts and corresponding effects on color vision.

6. 5′ Green–red 3′ hybrid genes with or without additional green genes usually are associated with deuteranomaly — a milder type of color vision defect with a red-shifted absorption maximum for the green pigment. Individuals with 5′ green–red 3′ hybrid genes who have normal color vision carry the variant gene in a more downstream location of the gene array, where it is not expressed.

7. 5′ Red–green 3′ fusion genes are always associated with protan abnormalities (R⁻ or R′). Those who have a single hybrid gene only are always protanopic (R⁻) and are therefore dichromats. Those who have additional normal green genes are either protanopic (R⁻) or protanomalous (R′) (i.e., a milder defect with slightly green-shifted absorption maximum of the red pigment) depending on whether Ala (protanopia) or Ser (protanomaly) is present at position 180 of the hybrid pigment.

8. A rare cause of red-green color vision defect (1/64 among color-defective males) is a point mutation of a critical cysteine residue of the green pigment (C203R).

9. A single-amino-acid polymorphism (serine/alanine) at position 180 of the X-linked red pigment gene occurs in different ethnic groups. Serine occupies this position in 64 percent of Caucasians, 80 percent of African-Americans, and 84 percent of Japanese. Individuals with with normal color vision (who have the serine variant) perceive red color as a deeper red than those who have alanine at position 180, as shown by color matching. The Ser/Ala polymorphism also affects the spectral sensitivities of various hybrid genes.

10. Tritan or blue pigment abnormalities are caused by missense mutations in the blue pigment gene and are transmitted (some with incomplete penetrance) as autosomal dominant traits.

A list of standard abbreviations is located immediately preceding the index in each volume. Nonstandard abbreviations used in this chapter include: GP6D = glucose-6-phosphate dehydrogenase; ERG = electroretinography; LCR = locus control region; BCM = blue cone monochromacy.

11. The detection of color vision is often based on plate tests that require color discrimination of shapes or numbers. The standard test for detection of subtypes of color vision defects is quantitative anomaloscopy using color matching.

12. Subjective color perception is most severely compromised in dichromats (i.e., in deuteranopes and particularly in protanopes), who cannot discriminate between colors in the red-green region of the spectrum. More subtle abnormalities are seen in trichromatic subjects with deuteranomaly and protanomaly, whose color discrimination capacities are weakened but not absent. Tasks requiring practical color discrimination may be performed adequately even by some fairly severely affected persons who test as abnormal on various color vision test systems such as color plate tests.

13. Blue cone monochromacy is a rare disease that manifests as complete functional absence of red and green cone function. It can be caused by deletion of a critical regulatory element upstream (5′) of the red-green gene complex that is required for expression of both the red and the green gene(s). Alternate causes involve point mutations of a single red-green hybrid gene that completely abolishes its function. The C203R mutation is frequently involved.

14. Complete achromatopsia, or red monochromacy, is another rare disease that involves complete functional absence of red, green, and blue cone function. A number of mutants with gene encoding the $\alpha$ subunit of cone c-AMP-gated cation channels have been implicated in this disorder.

15. Deuteranomaly is the most common defect in Caucasian populations (4–5 percent). The other defects (protanopia, protanomaly, deuteranopia) have frequencies of about 1 percent each. The frequency of color vision defects in most other populations is lower, ranging around 3 to 4 percent among Japanese and those of African descent, and is largely accounted for by fewer deuteranomalous individuals. The relatively high frequency of human color vision defects mainly results from unequal crossover between the highly homologous red and green pigment genes in this multigene complex. The high frequency of deuteranomalous individuals is unexplained. The role of selection to explain population differences in deuteranomaly remains undefined.

16. Female heterozygotes for the X-linked color vision defects are common in Caucasians (about 15 percent) and usually do not manifest color vision defects. Compound transheterozygotes for protan and deutan defects have normal color vision. Compound transheterozygotes for protanomaly/protanopia as well as those for deuteranomaly/deuteranopia will manifest with the milder of the two defects (i.e., anomaly), as expected on molecular grounds.

17. There is a high frequency (19 percent) of green-red fusion genes among African-Americans that are not expressed as color vision defects. About one-third of Africans have a phenotypically silent polymorphism manifesting as a shortened red pigment gene that resembles the normal (shortened) green pigment gene by lacking a block of three Alu repeat elements. This homology may predispose to more illegitimate recombination and possibly explain the higher frequency of green-red fusion genes in this population.

18. The evolution of the color vision gene complex has been elucidated. Rhodopsin was the first product of the undifferentiated ancestral gene (800 million years ago). Three hundred million years later, the blue gene developed from the single middle-wave gene, and only 30 million years ago, the red and green genes diverged from each other. Further duplication of the green pigment genes then occurred.

Color vision as a natural phenomenon has intrigued scientists for several hundred years.[1] Severe defects in red-green color vision have been known for about 200 years[2,3] and milder anomalies for over 100 years. Pedigrees of "color blindness" extending over several generations were reported[4] long before the rediscovery of Mendel's laws. Very early in the history of human genetics, the American pioneer of fruitfly genetics, Wilson[5] in 1911, suggested X-linked recessive inheritance as the explanation for the transmission of "color blindness." Color blindness therefore represents one of the first human traits shown to follow Mendelian inheritance. When hemophilia also was shown to be an X-linked trait, mapping of the hemophilia and color-blindness genes was undertaken by classic linkage methods in families where both genes segregated.[6] Failure of recombination between these traits suggested close linkage of their genes. Family studies also mapped the glucose-6-phosphate dehydrogenase (G6PD) locus as tightly linked to the red-green color vision locus,[7] and the very close proximity of these three genes was demonstrated by physical mapping.[8].

Color vision has helped to establish the field of human visual psychophysics—a subfield of physiologic psychology that, among other phenomena, studies the detailed physiology and psychology of human color vision.[9] These investigations are not only interesting and important in their own right but may provide clues to other sensory phenomena in human neurobiology.

The elucidation of the molecular bases of normal and abnormal color vision pigments has revolutionized ongoing studies in this field.[10,11] Unlike elsewhere in the human central nervous system, where sophisticated gene-phenotype comparisons are not yet feasible, fundamental studies on gene structure and function can now be correlated with psychophysical observations or tests that assess the phenotype of color vision and its abnormalities quantitatively. Slight differences in red color perception among "normal" human individuals that had been discovered earlier by psychophysical methods[12-17] now can be related to a frequent genetic polymorphism of the red visual pigment gene caused by a single-amino-acid substitution.[18] It is likely that similar phenomena exist elsewhere in the human nervous system to explain slight differences in perception between human individuals.

After the molecular biology of the photopigments underlying normal red-green and blue color vision was elucidated, various genotype-phenotype correlations in color vision defects emerged and are the topic of ongoing research in molecular biology and psychophysics.[19] While recent advances have provided a good comprehension of the biology and genetics of the visual pigments, the neurobiology of color perception involving the neural pathways of the brain is less well understood. A full understanding of color vision in all its aspects therefore requires much additional work. This chapter will be concerned largely with the biology and pathology of cone photoreceptors, their pigments, and the resulting color vision abnormalities. Ongoing work on rhodopsin and other vision-related proteins and their mutations has explained the cause of a significant proportion of cases of retinitis pigmentosa and is covered elsewhere in this book (see Chap. 235).

## COLOR AND COLOR VISION[20-23]

The scientific study of color started with the observation of the color spectrum by Newton over 300 years ago.[24] Sunlight or white light refracted by a glass prism could be split into a series or a rainbow of colors. Newton suggested that any particular color was characterized by its degree of "refrangibility," or wavelength, in modern terms. Light at each angle of refraction had a characteristic color ranging from violet for the most refracted rays over blue, green, yellow, orange, and red to the other end of the color spectrum. We know now that visible colors represent the range of electromagnetic radiation extending from about 400 nm (violet) to

700 nm (1 nm = 1 billionth of a meter, or $10^{-9}$ m). Visible radiation of a particular wavelength (monochromatic light) under well-defined conditions has a characteristic color for observers with normal color vision.

Most naturally occurring colors or hues may be produced by mixing combinations of monochromatic light of different wavelengths. Newton already noticed this phenomenon in that the human eye could not distinguish between a mixture of red and green light and the sensation produced by pure yellow light that had a refractive index intermediate between red and green.

During the nineteenth century, the trichromatic theory of color perception was developed.[25-27] It was shown that lights of three different wavelengths or primaries were sufficient to produce lights of any perceived hue and brightness. Most colors can be matched by a mixture of three primary lights. Each trio of primary lights has to include a long-wave, an intermediate-wave, and a short-wave light. Equal portions of these lights produce the perception of white. Color vision, therefore, was shown to be a system with only three perceptual dimensions.

The retina[28] is a part of the brain that has been displaced to the eye during embryonic development and, unlike other brain structures, can be viewed directly by an ophthalmoscope. Light is absorbed by specialized retinal neurons known as *photoreceptors*. The resulting signals are processed to the lateral geniculate nucleus and from there to the visual cortex of the brain. The normal human eye has four types of photoreceptors: rods and three classes of cones. Rods contain rhodopsin, have a maximal sensitivity at about 500 nm (blue-green region of the spectrum), and mediate vision in dim light (scotopic vision). No color is perceived under scotopic conditions, and all colors appear grayish white. Rods are more numerous than cones and are more frequent in the periphery of the retina. The biologic substrates of the three primary lights that mediate color vision are the retinal cones. In conformance with the trichromatic theory, a variety of psychophysical approaches suggested that there are three types of cone, each containing a different visual pigment. Direct proof of the existence of three classes of photoreceptors came from microspectrophotometric measurements that were capable of determining the absorbance of single photoreceptor cells in the retina.[29-33] Three different but overlapping spectral sensitivity curves were obtained (Fig. 238-1). The blue, or short-wave, sensitive pigment

($\lambda_{max}$ = 420 nm) had only a small degree of overlap with the middle-wave (green) and long-wave (red) pigment that had absorption maxima differing by only about 30 nm. Both green and red cones are active across most of the spectrum, but particularly between 450 and 650 nm.

The maximal sensitivities of long-wave sensitive (LWS), middle-wave sensitive (MWS), and short-wave sensitive (SWS) cones are at approximately 560, 530, and 420 nm, respectively. These cones are sometimes referred to as *red* (long-wave), *green* (middle-wave), and *blue* (short-wave) *cones*. Although useful for characterization of the receptors and their pigments, the terms *blue, green,* and *red* are misnomers because the spectrum of each is spread over a considerable range and they overlap with each other, as well as with the spectrum of rhodopsin (see Fig. 238-1). Cones are differentiated morphologically from rods by the tapered shape of their outer segment. Each cone contains only a single type of photopigment that is operative under lighted (photopic) conditions.

A small area of the retina — the fovea — is centrally located on the visual axis of the eye. It is about 0.3 mm in diameter and contains about 10,000 cones. The fovea has no rods and very few blue cones and has evolved as a specialized organ of high acuity and of red-green color vision.

The photoreceptors are located in the outermost layer of the retina and are overlaid by a pigmented epithelial layer that absorbs strong light and prevents backscatter of light. There are about twice as many "red" cones as "green" cones in the human retina, with considerable variation between individuals.[34-38] The similarity of red and green cones (see below) precludes their direct measurement, and quantitation requires indirect psychophysical methodology. The number of blue cones can be assessed directly by immunocytochemical staining. They comprise 10 to 20 percent of the total number of red or green cones.[39] The various visual pigment molecules are concentrated in the outer segments of the photoreceptors and are comprised of about 1000 to 2000 transverse disks containing about $10^9$ photopigment molecules (Fig. 238-2A).

## MOLECULAR BIOLOGY OF VISUAL PIGMENTS

The four human visual pigments — rhodopsin and the blue, red, and green pigments — are composed of a protein moiety, called *opsin*, that is covalently linked to the chromophore 11-*cis*-retinal via a protonated Schiff base formed between the aldehyde group of retinal and the ε-amino group of a highly conserved lysine residue.[40] A characteristic topographic motif of this family of photoreceptors is the heptahelical transmembrane bundle within which the chromophore is held[41] (see Fig. 238-2A, 2B). Despite having an identical chromophore, these pigments have very different absorption spectra. Therefore, differences in spectral characteristics of the photopigments are dictated by the interaction of amino acid side chains at key positions with the chromophore. Residues within the membrane bilayer that interact directly with the chromophore retinal, as well as those which indirectly influence the structure of the pocket within which the chromophore is embedded, are likely to play important roles in tuning the absorption spectrum of the photopigment. For example, amino acids at positions 180, 277, and 285 (see Fig. 238-2B) contribute the majority of the spectral difference between the red and green photopigments. The transmembrane segments are believed to be largely α-helical in character.[42] The visual pigments belong to an evolutionarily related superfamily of heptahelical transmembrane receptors that includes the adrenergic, serotonergic, dopaminergic, muscarinic, and olfactory chemoreceptors (Fig. 238-3) (see also ref. 43 for review).

In addition to the heptahelical structural motifs, members of this superfamily share many features of the process of cellular signal transduction. The absorption of a single photon of light causes the isomerization of the retinal chromophore of photopigments from the 11-*cis* to the all-*trans* configuration (see

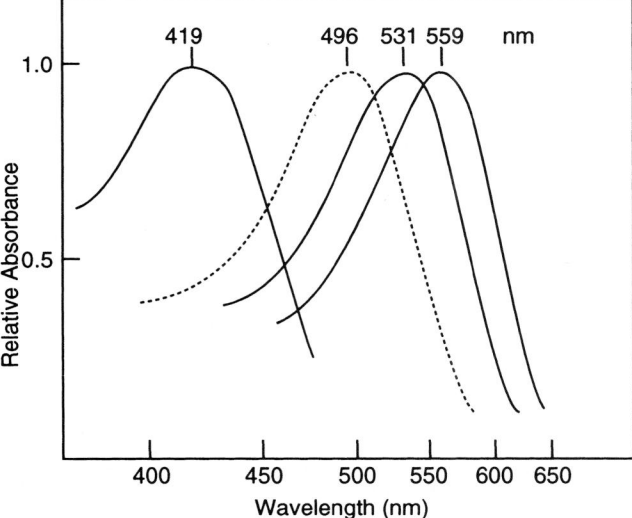

**Fig. 238-1 Absorption spectra of the four human photoreceptors. The dotted line is for rhodopsin, and the solid lines are for the blue ($\lambda_{max}$ = 419 nm), the green ($\lambda_{max}$ = 531 nm), and the red ($\lambda_{max}$ = 559 nm) cones. These curves are based on microspectrophotometric measurements of individual cones from human retinas. (Adapted with permission from Dartnall et al.[31])**

A. Cone outer segment

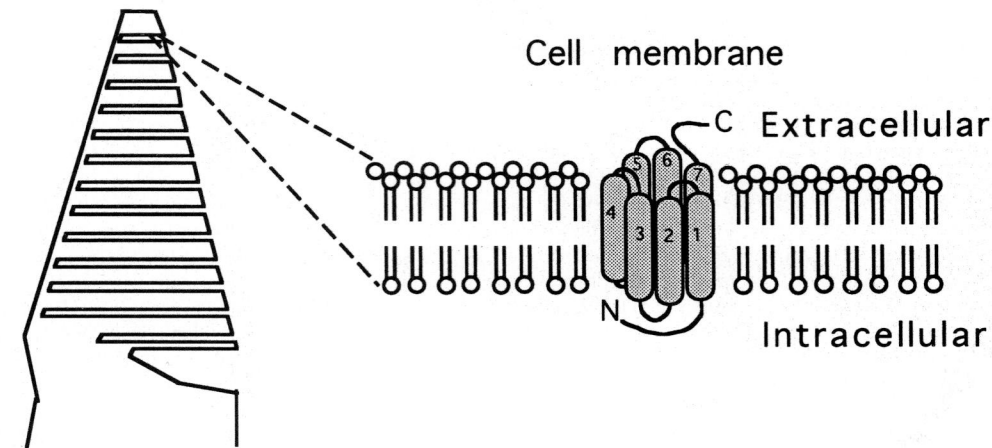

B.

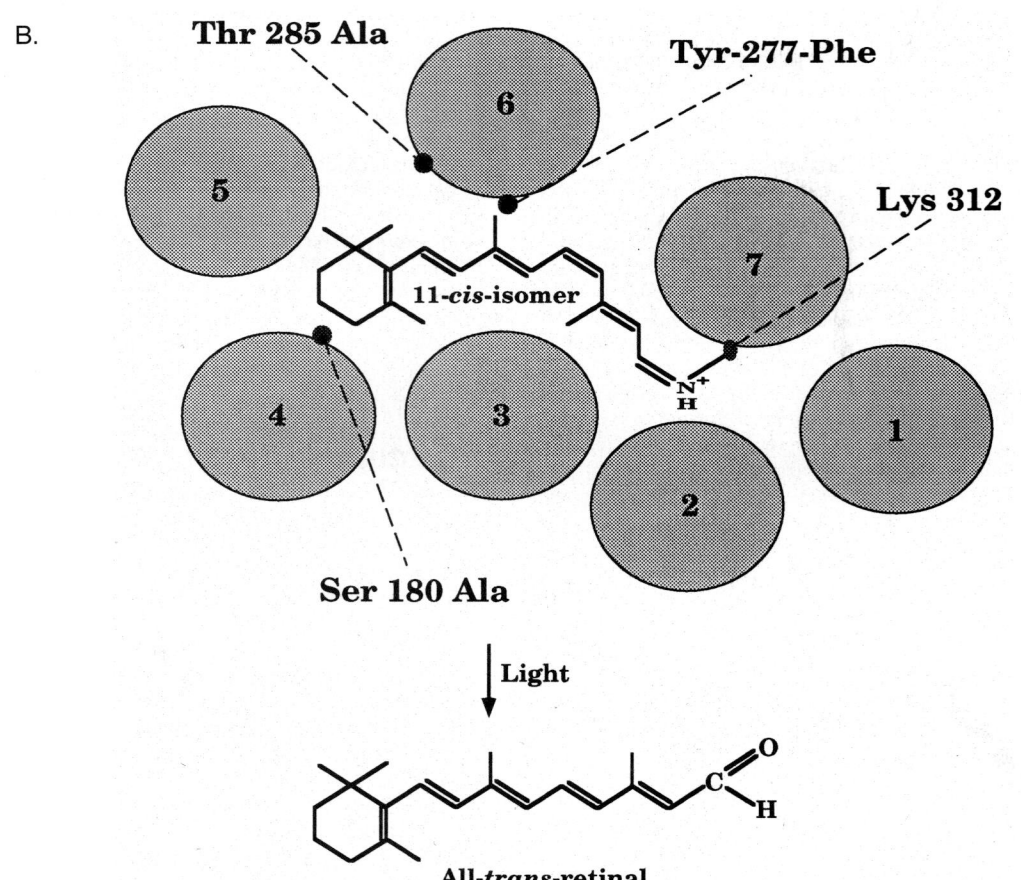

**Fig. 238-2** (*A*) Diagram of a cone photoreceptor outer segment showing the invaginated plasma membrane that is packed with photopigment molecules. An enlarged segment of the plasma membrane bilayer within which is embedded a photopigment molecule. Each photopigment consists of seven α-helices that traverse the plasma membrane (indicated by bars connecting open circles) to form a bundle that holds the chromophore 11-*cis*-retinal. The α-helices are linked by extracellular and intracellular amino acid loops as indicated. N and C represent the N- and C-termini of the opsin molecule, respectively. (*B*) Top view of a photopigment showing the arrangement of the seven helices around the chromophore retinal. Retinal is covalently linked to the opsin by forming a Schiff base with lysine at position 312. Shown are locations of the three amino acid residues that interact with the chromophore and contribute the majority of the spectral difference between the red (amino acid on left of residue number) and green (amino acid on right) pigments. For example, at position 285, the red opsin has Thr, whereas the green opsin has Ala. The absorption of light of the appropriate wavelength by the photopigment causes a cis-to-trans isomerization of the chromophore, which is the primary event in visual excitation. This isomerization induces a conformational change in the opsin that triggers the activation of transducin and the rest of the signal transduction cascade culminating in hyperpolarization of the membrane and generation of a nerve impulse. All-*trans*-retinal is hydrolyzed from the opsin and diffuses away. It is then isomerized into 11-*cis*-retinal, which associates with opsin to form the photopigment.

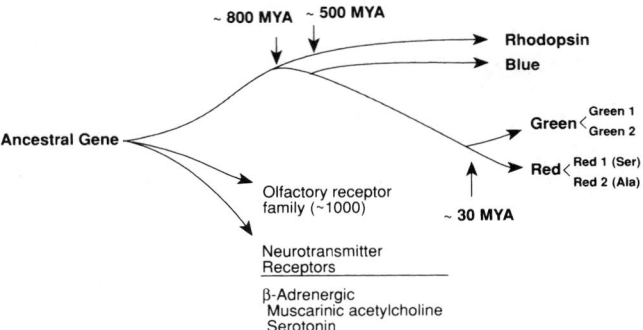

**Fig. 238-3 Evolution of the superfamily of heptahelical G-protein-coupled receptors.** A chronology for the evolutionary relationships among members of the human opsin gene family. (MYA, million years ago.) The terms *blue*, *green*, and *red* refer to the corresponding visual pigments. *Green 1* and *green 2* refer to the green pigment duplication (and further multiplication of the green pigment genes). *Red 1* (Ser) and *red 2* (Ala) refer to the common Ser/Ala polymorphism[18] affecting the human red pigment genes.

Fig. 238-2*B*). This isomerization results in the formation of a conformationally activated intermediate of the photopigment that triggers the signal-amplification cascade.[44–46] The first step in this cascade involves activation of transducin (a G-protein), which, in turn, activates a cGMP phosphodiesterase. The resulting decrease in cGMP levels triggers closure of cGMP-gated membrane cation channels and hyperpolarization of the photoreceptor cell.

The four human photopigments share varying degrees of sequence similarity. Pairwise comparisons of amino acid sequences are depicted in Fig. 238-4.[10] The red and green photopigments are far more closely related to each other (96

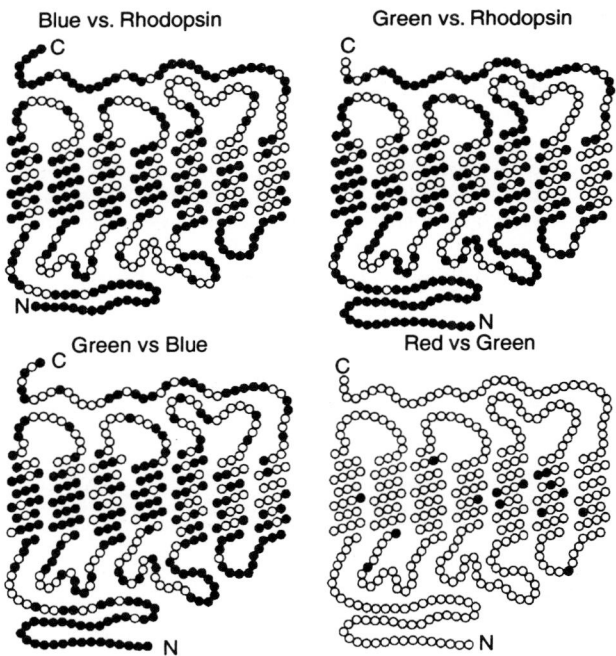

**Fig. 238-4 Amino acid sequence identities among the human visual pigments.** The secondary structures of the opsins with the seven α-helical segments that span the plasma membrane are shown. The N-terminal ends (N) are exposed at the luminal surface of the disk membrane, whereas the C-terminal ends (C) are exposed at the cytoplasmic surface. Sequence identities are indicated by open circles and differences by filled circles. Note the remarkable identity of the red and green pigments as contrasted with comparisons of the other pigments. (*Adapted with permission from Nathans et al.*[10])

percent amino acid sequence identity) than any other pair of pigments (40–45 percent identity), reflecting the more recent duplication of the ancestral red and green pigment gene (see Fig. 238-3). This is in agreement with the observation that humans and Old World monkeys possess both red and green photopigment, whereas most New World monkeys have a single polymorphic long-wavelength photopigment.[47–49] Recently, Jacobs et al.[50] showed that one genus of New World monkeys (*Alouatta*, the howler monkey) has two X-linked photopigment genes, probably due to an independent gene duplication. Males and females of this genus have full trichromatic color vision.

It has been estimated that the common ancestor of the three human color vision genes diverged from that of rhodopsin about 800 million years ago (MYA), the green and red pigment genes diverged from the blue about 500 MYA, and the red and green pigment genes diverged from each other about 30 MYA[10,51–53] (see "Evolution," below).

Differences in amino acid residues, especially those at positions within the membrane bilayer that allow interaction with retinal, are likely to underlie differences in spectral characteristics among the photopigments. The absorption spectra of the blue-, red-, and green-sensitive photopigments that are involved in color vision are shown in Fig. 238-1. These spectra were determined by microspectrophotometry of individual human cone cells[31] and show absorption maxima at approximately 420, 530, and 560 nm for the blue, red, and green cone pigments, respectively. Neural comparisons of quantal catches by the three cone classes give the sensation of color. The ratio between quantal catches by the three photoreceptors, which varies with wavelength of light (see Fig. 238-1), is interpreted by the brain as a color along the spectrum. The fourth pigment, rhodopsin, which is found in the rod-shaped photoreceptors and mediates vision in dim light, absorbs maximally at approximately 495 nm. The human red and green color vision pigments absorb light of longer wavelength than rhodopsin and the blue pigments. This shift to longer wavelengths during evolution of the visual pigments is likely to have resulted from acquisition by the red and green pigments of a chloride ion–binding site. Wang et al.[54] showed that a large red shift results from binding of chloride ion to the human red and green pigments and identified two residues, His at position 197 and Lys at position 200, to be critical for this binding. These two residues are conserved in all long-wave cone pigments and are absent in all rhodopsins and short-wave cone pigments. The absorption maxima of the in vitro–synthesized photopigments are in good agreement with the maxima determined by microspectrophotometry.[55–57] The red and green photopigments differ in at most 15 of a total of 364 amino acid residues (see Fig. 238-4). The presence of hydroxyl-bearing versus nonpolar residues constitues the difference at 7 of these 15 positions, all of which lie within one turn of the helix of the location of the retinylidene group of the chromophore.[58] All other amino acid differences do not involve significant changes in polarity and therefore are unlikely to influence spectral sensitivity of the pigments.

Two types of evidence support the hypothesis that spectral tuning could result from the substitution of polar for nonpolar residues. One is derived from relating differences in amino acid sequence to spectral characteristics of the middle- to long-wave visual pigments of humans and Old and New World monkeys. The results indicated that spectral tuning of these pigments depends on the presence of hydroxyl-bearing versus nonpolar residues at positions 180, 277, 285,[59] and 233.[60,61] Another line of evidence comes from experiments involving site-directed mutagenesis and expression in tissue culture cells of sequence variants of the human red and green photopigments. The two reconstituted red pigment variants bearing Ser or Ala at position 180 were shown to differ in their wavelength of maximal absorption by 5 nm (Ser at 180 = 557 nm; Ala at 180 = 552 nm), as determined by photobleaching difference absorption spectroscopy.[62] The absorption characteristics of other in vitro–expressed pigments[62,63] (see also below) indicated that the spectral difference between red and green photopigments is determined by only 7 amino acid residues at positions 116, 180, 230, 233, 277, 285, and 309. In agreement with earlier results, positions 180 (Ser versus Ala), 277 (Tyr versus Phe), and 285 (Thr versus Ala) (see Fig. 238-2B) accounted for the majority of the 31-nm spectral difference (5, 7, and 14 nm, respectively) between the red and green pigments. This conclusion is further supported by in vitro spectral studies on bovine rhodopsin that involved mutagenesis of the residues equivalent to positions 180, 277, and 285 of the red and green opsins.[64]

The recent cloning and characterization of the genes that encode the photopigment apoproteins (opsins) largely has been due to the pioneering work of Nathans and collaborators. Based on partial amino acid sequence data, they first isolated and characterized cDNA and genomic clones of rhodopsin.[65] Using low-stringency hybridization, a bovine probe subsequently was used to isolate clones of human rhodopsin[65] and the blue, green, and red opsin genes.[10] Furthermore, cDNA probes containing coding sequences of bovine rhodopsin detected (using Southern blot hybridization) homologous sequences of other photopigment genes in DNA of a variety of vertebrate and invertebrate organisms,[66] indicating the high degee of sequence conservation among members of this family of genes.

A comparison of the intron/exon organization of some members of the photopigment gene family is given in Fig. 238-5. The rhodopsin and blue pigment genes are located at 3q21–24 and 7q31.3–q32, respectively, and have remarkably similar organization characterized by five exons encoding polypeptides of 348 amino acids. On the other hand, the red and green pigment genes, which are located in close proximity to each other on the X chromosome (Xq28), are almost identical in structure. Both the red and green pigment genes have six instead of five exons and encode proteins that are 364 amino acid residues in length. Exon 1 of the red and green pigment genes has no homologue in the rhodopsin and blue pigment genes.

The green pigment gene in all humans studied is 1.28 kb shorter than the red pigment gene due to a deletion in intron 1. The identical deletion in the red pigment gene has been observed as a polymorphic trait among one-third of African-Americans (frequency of short red, 0.35) but is much rarer among Japanese (0.02) and Europeans (<0.01).[67] The difference in length of intron 1 between the "long" red on the one hand and the "short" red and green pigment genes on the other was shown to be due to the presence of three Alu repeat elements plus 328 bp of unique sequence DNA.[68] This block containing the three Alu elements was not found in intron 1 of the red or green pigment genes of the Old World monkeys and orangutans but was present in intron 1 of both the red and green pigment genes of gorillas and chimpanzees. The nucleotide sequence and the estimated ages of the three Alu elements suggest that their insertion occurred sequentially in the Old World monkey lineage prior to duplication of the single ancestral X chromosome–linked pigment gene. After gene duplication, deletion of the entire block containing the Alu

elements from the green pigment gene created the "short" intron 1 variant. Gene conversion between the highly homologous red and green pigment genes may have generated the "short" intron 1 of the red pigment gene.

The red and green pigment genes are arranged in a head-to-tail tandem array comprised of one red pigment gene 5′ of one or more green pigment genes, as determined by Southern blot hybridization, pulsed-field electrophoresis, and restriction enzyme analysis of genomic cosmid clones.[8,10,11,67] The red-green gene complex on the long arm of the X chromosome (q28) is located approximately 250 kb telomeric to the adrenoleukodystrophy gene[69] and approximately 800 to 1000 kb centromeric from the G6PD and coagulation factor VIII (F8C) loci.[8] A study in families of homosexual men suggested the presence of a gene (or genes) in the Xq28 region that influences at least one subtype of male sexual orientation.[70] The exact position and nature of this putative gene (or genes) is not known.

The number of green pigment genes is polymorphic and varies in frequency distribution among males of different ethnic origin, as shown in Table 238-1.[67,71] The observed direct relationship between frequency of green pigment genes and frequency of red-green color vision defects in these three ethnic groups is intriguing. Nathans et al.[11] proposed unequal recombination in the red-green pigment intergenic region (approximately 15 kb in length) as a mechanism of altering copy number of the green pigment gene (Fig. 238-6). A larger number of green opsin genes per array may lead to a higher probability of unequal recombination.

The question of whether all the green opsin genes are expressed in the retina was addressed by (1) determining spectral luminous efficiency (a measure of the relative numbers of red and green cones) as a function of the number of green opsin genes in the array in a group of 26 males who have normal color vision and (2) detection of the mRNA products of the red and green pigment genes in postmortem male retinas.[72] The results of the first approach indicated that spectral luminous efficiency is not correlated with the number of green pigment gene copies in an array and support the hypothesis (see below) that only one green opsin gene is expressed in the retina (Lindsey et al., unpublished observations from our group, 1993). The results from the second approach, described in detail below, also support the preceding hypothesis.

The relative representation of the red- and green-sensitive cones in the human retina has been determined by a number of investigators. Psychophysical and electrophysiologic studies indicated that (1) there are more red than green cones in the normal human retina and (2) the red-green ratio varies from 0.33 to 9, with an average value of about 2.[34,36,38,73,74] A narrower range of ratios (1.46–2.36) was observed by Cicerone and Nerger.[37] Microspectrophotometric measurements on seven eyes of individuals with normal color vision gave an average red-to-green cone ratio in the foveal region of 1.39.[75] All these studies used small,

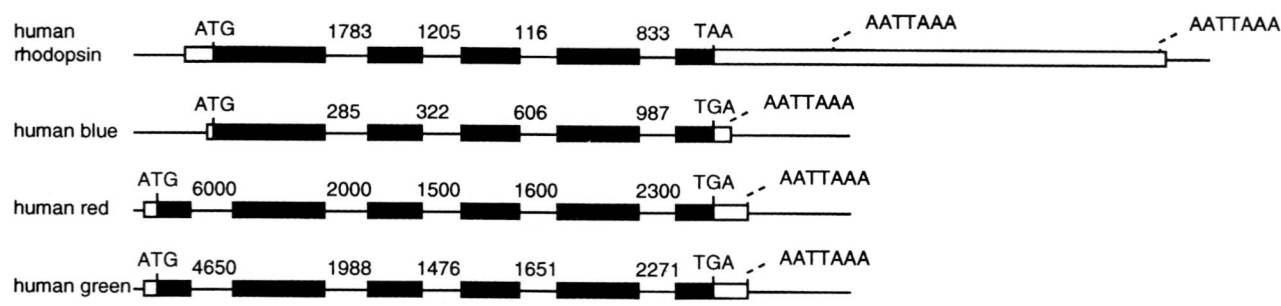

**Fig. 238-5** Comparison of the structure of the human visual pigment genes. Coding sequences of the genes are denoted by boxes and noncoding regions by lines (not to scale). Open boxes represent untranslated regions, and filled boxes denote the coding regions. The length of introns in number of base pairs is shown. Also indicated are the initiation and termination codons and the polyadenylation signal sequences. (*Adapted with permission from Applebury and Hargrave.*[120])

**Table 238-1** Green Pigment Gene in Different Populations with "Normal" Molecular Genotypes (Excluding Individuals with Deletions or Fusion Genes)

| Population (Males) | n | Number of Green Pigment Genes | | | |
|---|---|---|---|---|---|
| | | 1 | 2 | 3 | ≥4 |
| African-American | 81 | 0.42* | 0.42 | 0.10 | 0.06 |
| Japanese | 97 | 0.48 | 0.31 | 0.15 | 0.05 |
| Caucasian | 113 | 0.22 | 0.51 | 0.19 | 0.08 |

*Proportion of green genes: Caucasian versus African-Americans, $\chi^2 = 8.79$, $p < 0.01$; Caucasian versus Japanese, $\chi^2 = 16.08$, $p < 0.001$; African-Americans versus Japanese, $\chi^2 = 0.74$, $p > 0.3$.
SOURCE: Data from Drummond = Borg et al.[71]

centrally located test fields, and therefore, the observed ratios were representative of the foveal region.

Yamaguchi et al.[72] determined the ratio of expressed red to green retinal mRNA in 51 unselected postmortem male retinas. The ratio varied widely (1–10, with a mode of 4) and was not correlated with that of red to green pigment genes. One explanation for the discrepancy between these results on cone ratios derived from mRNA analysis and the foveal ratio of about 2 may be that this ratio is higher in the peripheral retina than in the fovea. Since only about 10 percent of the cones are located in the fovea, the ratios obtained by the Yamasuchi et al.[72] studies came from whole retinal mRNA and represent largely extrafoveal cones. On the other hand, estimates of red-to-green cone ratios (average of 2, with a range of 0.67–9.0) obtained on 16 subjects with normal color vision by flicker photometric electroretinography (ERG) were similar using either small or very large test fields,[34] suggesting that the red-to-green cone ratio does not change significantly throughout the retina. This conclusion is consistent with results from psychophysical methods indicating that the red-to-green cone ratio does not change with retinal eccentricity.[76,77] (See Addendum 1 and 2.)

The distribution of red and green photoreceptors in the nonhuman primate retina was shown to be random.[78,79] In humans, Gowdy and Cicerone,[80] using hyperacuity performances for two-color normal observers, showed more red than green cones

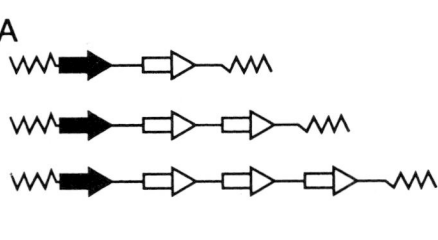

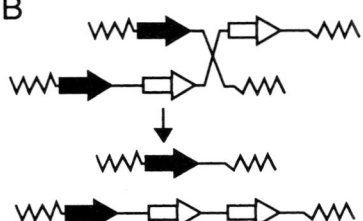

**Fig. 238-6** Polymorphism in the number of green opsin genes. (*A*) Diagram of the X-linked red-green gene arrays that differ in the number of green opsin genes. Filled arrows denote red opsin genes, and open arrows denote green opsin genes. Straight lines represent intergenic regions, and wavy lines represent regions that flank the gene complex. (*B*) Unequal recombination within intergenic regions as a mechanism of generating polymorphism in the number of green opsin genes in an array.

in the central fovea with random arrangement. (See Addendum 1 and 2)

## COLOR VISION DEFECTS

Color vision defects have been recognized for almost 200 years. The famous chemist Dalton reported his own color vision defect to the Manchester Literary and Philosophical Society in 1794.[2] Dalton reported that an "image which others call red appears to me as little more than a shade or defect of light." Orange, yellow, and green appeared to him as different shades of yellow. Color vision defects are sometimes referred to as *daltonism*. A recent study of Dalton's DNA from his preserved eyes indicated that he was a deuteranope lacking the green (middle-wave) pigment[81] (see below).

Red-green color vision defects are a group of X-linked abnormalities that are common in the male European population (8 percent).[82–84] Several types of color vision defects exist[82–84] (Table 238-2). When the color-sensitive receptors for either the long-wave pigment (red) or the middle-wave pigment (green) are completely absent, color vision is dichromatic rather than trichromatic. Such individuals have only two, instead of the normal three, visual pigments (i.e., either green and blue or red and blue, but not green, red, and blue). Depending on whether long-wave (red) or middle-wave (green) pigment is absent, dichromats are classified as *deuteranopes*, who lack functional cones with green pigment (G⁻), or *protanopes*, who lack cones with red visual pigment (R⁻). The complete lack of the respective visual pigments in dichromats was proven first by microspectrophotometry that failed to detect absorption of the characteristic wavelength for the red pigment in protanopes (R⁻) and for the green pigment in deuteranopes (G⁻).[31,32,78,85] The frequency of these traits in the Caucasian population ranges around 1 percent for protanopia as well as for deuteranopia. Molecular studies demonstrate complete absence of the green visual pigments in deuteranopes, whereas protanopia has been associated with red-green fusion genes that have the characteristics of normal green pigment.[11,19]

The other X-linked color vision anomalies are associated with trichromatic color vision and are known as *deuteranomaly* (G′) and *protanomaly* (R′)[82] (see Table 238-2). In these defects, all three visual pigments are present, but microspectrophotometric measurements showed displacement of the green and red pigment spectral sensitivity curves in deuteranomaly and protanomaly, respectively, and suggested the presence of visual pigments with altered spectral characteristics.[86–88] Deuteranomalous and protanomalous subjects thus were assumed to carry variant visual pigments. Molecular studies indicated the presence of green-red fusion genes in deuteranomaly (G′)[11,19] and red-green fusion genes in protanomaly (R′).[11,19] However, a few deuteranomalous individuals had a complete absence of green pigment genes.[19] Current molecular methodology has been unsuccessful in differentiating protanopes from protanomalous individuals, since both have red-green fusion genes (see below for details). Furthermore, green-red fusion genes are not infrequently found in persons with normal color vision[19,67,71] but presumably are located in downstream locations where they are not expressed (see below).

Considerable variation in the severity of the trichromatic abnormalities (protanomaly and deuteranomaly) has been observed.[82,83] Some scientists have divided the various trichromatic anomalies into mild, moderate, and severe deuteranomaly or protanomaly.[89] It would be expected that a given subtype of defect generally would express with a similar degree of severity in all affected male members of a family who carry the same mutation. However, intrafamilial variability of color vision defects has been observed occasionally as in other examples of identical mutations of a variety of human genetic diseases. Further work to relate the molecular lesion to the severity of the defect needs to be done. The frequency of deuteranomaly in Europeans ranges between 4 and 5 percent, whereas the frequency of protanomaly is around 1 percent (see ref. 82).

**Table 238-2** Classification of Common Color Vision Defects

| Type | Inheritance | Frequency (Europeans) | Type of Color Vision | Vision Defect |
|------|-------------|----------------------|----------------------|---------------|
| **Red-green defects** | | | | |
| Protanopia (R⁻) | X-linked recessive | ~1% | Dichromatic | Severe red-green color confusion |
| Deuteranopia (G⁻) | X-linked recessive | ~1% | Dichromatic | Moderate to severe red-green color confusion |
| Protanomaly (R') | X-linked recessive | ~1% | Trichromatic | Mild red-green color confusion |
| Deuteranomaly (G') | X-linked recessive | ~4–5% | Trichromatic | Mild red-green color confusion |
| **Blue-yellow defects** | | | | |
| Tritanopia* | Autosomal dominant | 1 in 500 (or fewer) (?) | Dichromatic* | Blue-yellow color confusion |
| Tritanomaly* | Autosomal dominant | ? | Trichromatic* | Mild blue-yellow color confusion |

*Distinction between tritanopia and tritanomaly not fully clarified.

Abnormalities affecting the blue- or short-wave-sensitive pigment are known as *tritanopia*.[90] (The origin of the terms *protan*, *deutan*, and *tritan* is derived from the Greek and refers to the first, second, and third variants of color defect.) The differentation of tritanopia from tritanomaly is not as clear for the green-red defects. Tritanopia defects are much rarer than deutan or protan abnormalities but have been estimated to occur as frequently as 1 in 500 individuals.[91] Tritanopic individuals have problems with the perception of blue color. The defect is inherited as an autosomal dominant trait, as might be expected by the location of the blue pigment gene of chromosome 7. The molecular basis of tritan abnormalities are missense mutations, and three different amino acid substitutions (see below) have been observed.[92,93] Variability in expression has been noticed in several pedigrees. In fact, some individuals with the characteristic amino acid substitution did not manifest with the phenotypic color vision defect.[92]

Unlike the amino acid substitutions of rhodopsin that often are associated with rod degeneration leading to autosomal dominant retinitis pigmentosa (see Chap. 235), there are no other ophthalmologic or clinical consequences associated with the various deutan, protan, and tritan types of color vision defects. Visual acuity is unaffected. The color vision defects are expressed early in life[94] and remain constant throughout the life span.

## Phenotypic Detection of Color Vision Defects[82,95,96]

**Color Chart Tests.** A large number of different tests have been devised for the detection of color vision anomalies. Most of these have not been standardized and are not in general use. Therefore, they will not be discussed here. The tests discussed below are most useful for detection of genetic color vision defects.

Pseudoisochromatic plates are used widely for screening of color vision defects. The figures to be discriminated on these plates appear in shades of different chromatic quality. These tests use patterns of variously colored printed dots that usually are shaped as numbers. The subject is asked to read or trace a shape or number. The charts are so designed that persons with color vision defects will either miss shapes or numbers and/or will see different shapes than persons with normal color vision. The most widely used variety are the Ishihara (Japan) charts and the American Optical H-R-R (Hardy-Rand-Ritter) polychromatic plates. Illumination should be standardized at diffused daylight during testing (100-W blue daylight bulb or MacBeth easel lamp), since various pigments in the charts may vary in gloss, giving clues to a color-defective person. Ordinary tungsten bulbs may allow deuteranomalous persons to read test charts correctly. Ishihara charts have had the most use. Distinction between deutan and protan abnormalities is usually possible, but no definite reliance for subclassification should be placed on the charts' results because severe anomalous trichromats often cannot be differentiated from dichromats.

Ishihara charts do not detect tritanopia, whereas the H-R-R charts will. When color vision abnormalities are found on chart testing, anomaloscopy (see below) usually is done in genetic studies to confirm the type of color vision defect.

**Color Arrangement Tests.** The Farnsworth-Munsell 100 Hue Test[97] has been used widely to evaluate chromatic discrimination loss. In this test, a series of 85 color chips is arranged in their natural order of hue. Each chip has an appropriate number on its back that refers to its order in the series. Depending on the mistakes made, a standardized score is calculated and recorded on a special chart. Characteristic patterns for protans, deutans, and tritans are obtained, but differentiation between protanomaly and protanopia is difficult.

**Anomaloscopy.** Anomaloscopy has been used widely and is based on color matching. Lord Rayleigh devised a simple test system to classify individuals with red-green color vision abnormalities. The observer views a pure yellow light (589–590 nm) on one-half of a screen, while the other half of the screen projects a mixture of red (650 nm) and green (545–550 nm) lights. The brightness or intensity of the yellow light, as well as the proportion of the green and red lights, are adjusted by the subject until both hemifields appear identical in color and brightness. Under the color condition of the Rayleigh match, color detection by the short-wave-sensitive or blue-pigment cones is negligible. The most frequently used instrument is the Nagel anomaloscope. The range of accepted matches of mixtures of green and red light against yellow is recorded, as is the midpoint of such matches. Figure 238-7 shows typical findings for normal and various color-defective persons.

Normal individuals accept matches in a narrow range. Dichromats such as protanopic and deuteranopic subjects will match yellow with any and all ratios of red and green, including red and green alone. Thus any sufficiently bright red-green mixture will produce a match. Dichromatic deuteranopes require much more yellow to match pure red than dichromatic protanopes, who need only a small amount of yellow to match the red field, which they perceive as of low intensity.

Protanomalous subjects produce match ranges that are shifted to the red side of the spectrum, whereas the matches of deuteranomalous subjects are displaced to the green. Subjects with severe deuteranomaly and severe protanomaly tend to have quite wide characteristically displaced match ranges, whereas those with milder anomalous defects have narrower match ranges.

Most large-scale investigations of color vision defects start with assessment of color vision by plate test followed by anomaloscopy only among those individuals who fail the test. Anomaloscopic findings in a given individual are constant and do not change. As might be expected, anomaloscopic results of different affected family members usually but not always are similar. The viewing angle conventionally is 2°. With larger viewing angles, most protanopes are classified as protanomalous, and some deuteranopes as deuteranomalous.

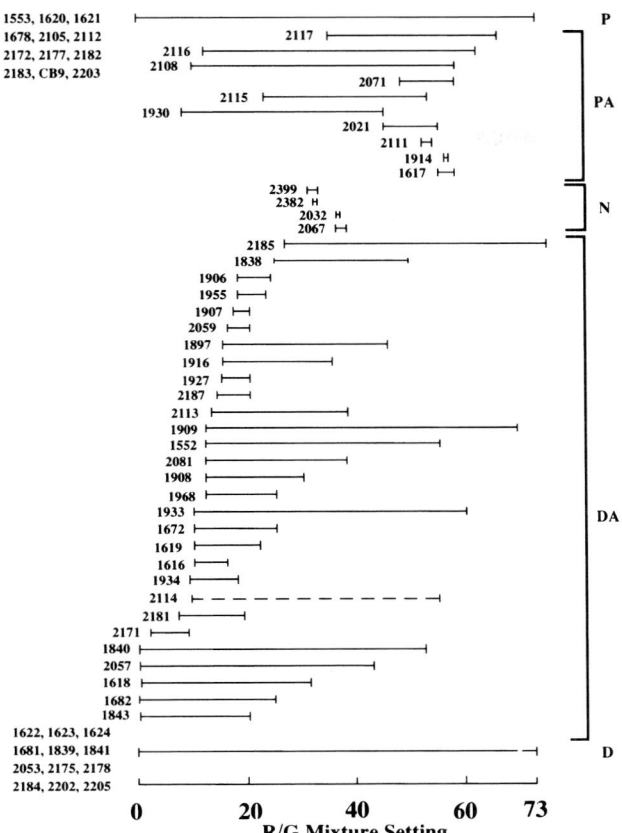

**Fig. 238-7** Anomaloscopic Rayleigh match ranges of protan, deutan, and normal male individuals. Each horizontal line represents the range of mixtures of red and green lights that the observer could not distinguish from the standard yellow light. Identification numbers shown next to the horizontal lines refer to subjects of a large study.[19] Subject 2114 (- - - -) had a variable and unreliable match range. P, Protanopic; PA, protanomaly; D, deuteranopia; DA, deuteranomaly; N, normal. (*Used with permission from Deeb et al.[19]*)

**Electroretinography.[98]** An objective assessment of color vision may be possible with ERG. All other test measurements are based on the observer's subjective perception of color. In ERG, a corneal electrode placed on an anesthetized dilated eye records the retinal response to standardized flashes of light. Because of the somewhat invasive nature of the test, no extensive experience of the various benign genetic color vision defects has as yet been reported. However, color vision defects characterized as deutan (36 subjects) and protan (32 subjects) (with no indication of the proportion of dichromats and trichromats) could be discriminated by the log ratio of the sensitivity at short (480-nm) and long (620-nm) wavelengths (sensitivity quotient).[99] Female carrier detection was particularly successful for deutan carriers and less so for protan heterozygotes.[99]

## Color Perception and Color Defects: Practical Implications[100]

Color vision defects affect perceptions of color. A large proportion of the population, therefore, lives in a different perceptual world than those with normal color vision. Normal trichromatic color vision helps to define objects in complex multicolored settings, as can be observed by comparing a colored photograph with a black-and-white rendering of the same scene. The color perception of color-defective observers has been studied in a few individuals who for unknown reasons were color defective in one eye only. One otherwise healthy young woman was deuteranopic in the left eye and color normal in the right eye (see ref. 82). Her color-vision-defective eye had only three color sensations—gray, yellow, and blue—and lacked any green and red sensations. Her normal eye gave normal color vision. In a film showing the color world of this woman (MN8246, Color Vision Deficiency, Research Division, Bureau Medicine and Surgery, Department of the Navy, Washington), a room furnished entirely from gray, blue, and yellow materials had the same color appearance to her defective eye as similar objects covering the entire range of colors, including red and green. Color perception of the usual deuteranopes conforms to this general pattern. Dichromatic protanopia appears as a more severe defect than deuteranopia. Protanopes confuse not only red, yellow, and green, like deuteranopes, but also deep red, dark brown, or even black and have particular problems with red color perception. A ripe red fruit may be considered black by a protanope.

Color perception differences in anomalous trichromats are more subtle than in dichromats. Green and red are not absent but appear weakened in intensity. Deuteranomaly is considered to be the mildest anomaly. More subtle differences in color perception are seen in individuals who either have an alanine (62 percent) or a serine (38 percent) at position 180 of the red pigment gene. Those with 180 serine (~62 percent) perceive a deeper red than those who have serine at this position. Based on Hardy-Weinberg statistics, it is expected that about 47 percent of Caucasian women are heterozygotes for both the 180 alanine and 180 serine variant. Due to X inactivation, about half the cones in most women will have alanine at position 180, and the other half have serine at that site. Such women have four types of cones—blue, green, and two types of red cones—and might have tetrachromatic vision. Further tests need to be done to determine whether such females have superior color discrimination under certain conditions as compared with trichromats.

Color-vision-defective persons, including dichromats, usually have no problem with the naming of colors. Apparently there are enough differences in color sensation to allow the denotation of the appropriate color as taught by parents and teachers.

It has been claimed by anecdotal evidence that color-defective observers can see through colored patterns that deceive normal observers.[101] This advantage would be useful under military conditions and could have played a role in the evolution of color vision.[102] Dichromats, in fact, perform better than normal trichromats under experimental conditions where texture was camouflaged by color.[103] No anomalous trichromats were tested in this study. A recent study showed that color-blind individuals have a lower threshold for light perception than color-normal individuals.[104] This would give color-blind individuals a selective advantage under low light conditions.

X-linked red-green color vision defects are cardinal examples of common genetic traits that have been used for some time to exclude applicants from a variety of industrial, marine, air, rail, and military occupations that require the ability to distinguish colors. A genetic condition per se is not reason for occupational discrimination unless such a trait makes its carriers unable to carry out a job-related task. Occupational exclusion, however, is appropriate if an affected employee's work places others at physical risk. There is no consensus as to whether the risk of physical harm to the affected individual alone is sufficient reason for job exclusion. Some would leave such decisions to the affected person, particularly if the possible damage is uncertain or may only occur in the distant future. The problems in applying these rules in a fair manner to defects of color vision comes from difficulties in interpreting abnormal color vision tests. Thus, when actual tasks requiring color discrimination instead of various artificial testing systems such as plate tests are used, many color-defective persons may perform adequately.[105,106] The validity of rigid color vision standards for occupational selection, therefore, has been questioned (see ref. 107). Cole[108] suggested variable standards for the many different occupations that require color discrimination. It has been suggested that the specifications for practical testing and its rigor should be based on the probability, severity, and socioeconomic consequences of adverse reactions that may be caused by difficulties with color discrimination.

In general, deuteranopic and protanopic dichromats perform more poorly on color discrimination than those with anomalous trichromacy. Most, but not all, dichromats have difficulties in selection of colored articles and materials, including foods. No studies have shown that color vision defects have been the cause of aircraft accidents.[109] On self-reporting and under conditions of confidentiality, 49 percent of dichromats reported color confusion at traffic lights, 33 percent found it difficult to distinguish traffic lights from street lighting, and 22 percent had difficulty detecting rear brake lights.[110] It is therefore noteworthy that rear-end collisions, particularly under conditions of poor visibility, were slightly more common among protan drivers, who have more problems with perception of red rear warning lights.[111] However, there is general agreement in most jurisdictions that nonprofessional automobile drivers with color vision defects should have no driving restrictions. Nevertheless, some observers are impressed with the data suggesting that color-deficient drivers have significant difficulties.[112] These authors suggest shape and not just color coding of traffic lights as well as counseling color-defective drivers to exert caution at intersections and advising protans to double the usually recommended distance that separates their vehicle from the car ahead.

## Molecular Genetics of Color Vision Defects

**Red-Green Color Vision Defects.** Nathans and collaborators isolated and sequenced the genes that specify the three opsins responsible for normal color vision[10] and showed how these genes are different in individuals with red-green color vision defects.[11] Based on their study of 25 red-green color-deficient males, they concluded that, in the majority of cases, color vision defects result from unequal recombination between the highly homologous red and green pigment genes (98 percent identity in DNA sequence of exons, introns, and 3′ flanking regions). Such events lead to deletions of the green pigment genes (see Fig. 238-6) or to the formation of full-length hybrid genes consisting of portions of both red and green pigment genes (Fig. 238-8). With few exceptions, the deletion of green pigment genes was associated with deuteranopia (G⁻R⁺), 5′ green-red hybrid genes with deuteranomaly (G′R⁺), and 5′ red-green hybrids with either protanopia (R⁻G⁺) or protanomaly (R′G⁺). An interesting observation was that some males had normal green and red pigment genes in addition to the hybrids and yet tested as deutans.

Determination of the gross structure of the red and green pigment gene arrays in males was made by quantitative Southern blot analysis, taking advantage of differences in length of DNA fragments generated from the red and green opsin genes on digestion with the restriction enzymes EcoRI, BamHI, and RsaI. Figure 238-9 shows autoradiographs of Southern blots of genomic

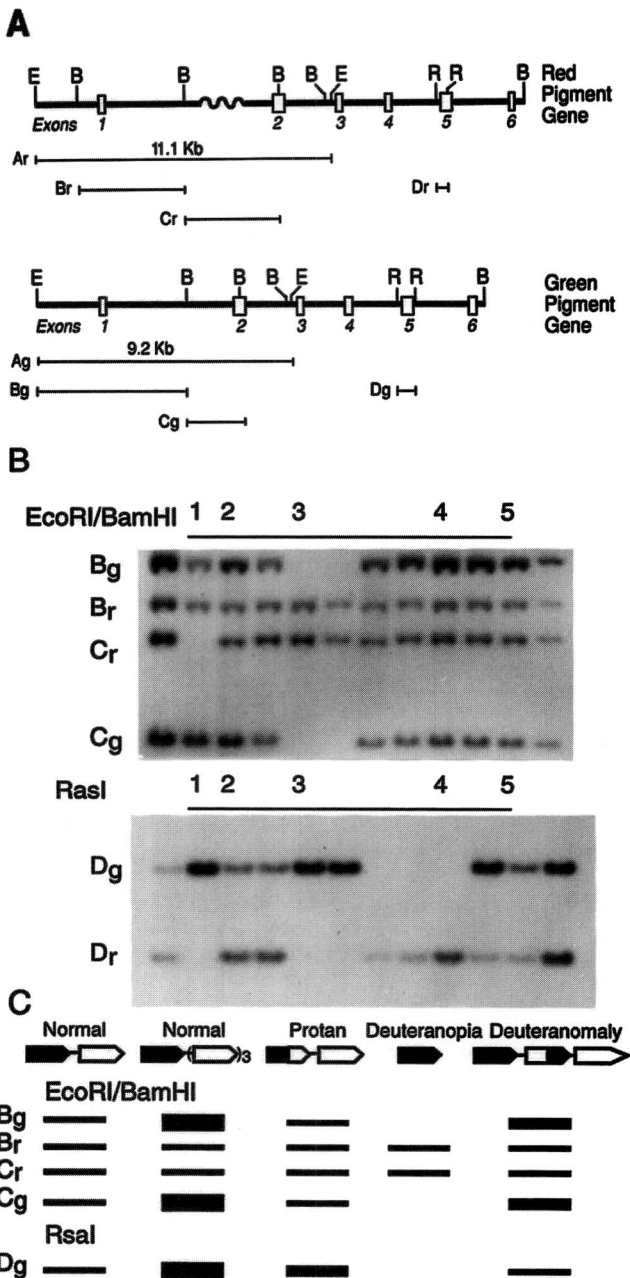

**Fig. 238-9** Southern blot analysis of the X-linked red-green gene locus. (*A*) Partial restriction maps of the red and green pigment genes. E, *Eco*RI; B, *Bam*HI; R, *Rsa*I. Open boxes denote the six exons. The restriction fragments A–D used in distinguishing red from green-specific sequences are shown below the genes. The A–C fragments derived from the red opsin gene (Ar, Br, Cr) are longer than those derived from the green gene (Ag, Bg, Cg) due to a 1.5-kb insertion in the first intron (*wavy line*). The absence of a *Rsa*I site in the green opsin exon 5 accounts for the larger Rsal fragment of the green opsin gene (Dg). (*Adapted with permission from Nathans et al.*[11]) (*B*) Autoradiograph of Southern blots of genomic DNA samples from males with normal and defective color vision digested with either a combination of EcoRI and BamHI or Rsal. The EcoRI-BamHI fragments (B and C) were detected by hybridization to a 350-bp cDNA probe encompassing exon 1 and part of exon 2, whereas the D fragments were detected by a 400-bp genomic probe from the 3′ end of intron 4 of the green opsin gene.[11] Typical examples of Southern blot patterns were selected. Lane 1: An individual with protanopia who has a single red-green hybrid gene with the C and D fragments of the red gene replaced by the corresponding fragments of the green pigment gene. Lane 2:

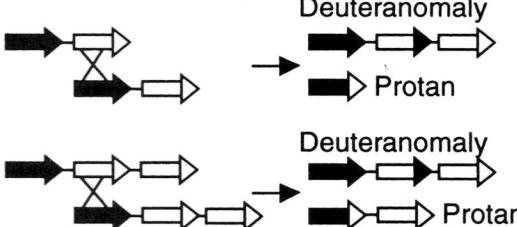

**Fig. 238-8** Generation of red-green hybrid genes. Unequal recombination between the highly homologous red and green opsin genes generates 5′ red-green hybrids typically found in individuals with the protan class of color vision defects (protanopia and protanomaly) and 5′ green-red hybrid genes found among individuals with deuteranomaly. Filled arrows denote red gene sequences, and open arrows represent green opsin gene sequences. (*Used with permission from Drummond-Borg et al.*[71])

DNA isolated from males with normal and defective color vision together with the deduced genotypes.[11]

The following important and interesting questions were raised: Is the point of fusion in red-green hybrid genes correlated with the severity of the color vision defect? Which amino acid residues contribute significantly to the difference in absorption characteristics between the red and green opsins? Are all genes in the red-green cluster equally expressed?

These questions were addressed by studying the relationship between genotype and phenotype among males who had normal color vision and others who had defective red-green color vision.[19] In addition to the use of quantitative Southern blot analysis to detect deletions and hybrid red-green opsin genes, amplifications by the polymerase chain reaction (PCR) and single-strand conformation polymorphism (SSCP) were used to determine the approximate points of recombination in hybrid genes. Recombination between the red and green opsin genes would be expected to occur more frequently in introns than in exons, since introns are, on average, 10 times longer and are as homologous as exons in this gene complex.[8,10,11,113] Evidence supporting this expectation was provided by analysis of hybrid genes of 64 individuals with defective color vision (see below and ref. 19). Recombinations in introns 1 and 4 could be assigned with certainty, whereas those in introns 2 and 3 could not be differentiated because the sequence of exon 3 of the red is not always different from that of the green opsin gene.[10,19,114] Recombinations in intron 1 would convert one pigment gene to the other (i.e., green to red), whereas those occuring in intron 5 would have no effect because exons 1 and 6 in the red and green opsin genes have identical sequences. Recombinations in exons 2, 3, and 4 would be expected to result in hybrid genes (5′ green-red or 5′ red-green) that encode six corresponding chimeric pigments with maximal sensitivities distributed between those of the normal red and green pigments (530–560 nm). These six hybrid genes (3′ red-green and 3′ green-red) are shown in Figure 238-10. However, since there are two common alleles of the red opsin gene that differ by having either Ala or Ser at position 180[18] and by approximately 4 to 5 nm in absorption maxima,[62] nine instead of six common types of hybrid opsin genes would be expected to exist in the population. Merbs and Nathans[56] examined photobleaching difference spectra of in vitro–produced red-green hybrids commonly found in the population and showed that amino acid residues in exons 2, 3, 4, and 5 that differ between the red and green pigments produce varying degrees of spectral shifts (see Fig. 238-10).

In a study of 64 red-green color-defective Caucasian males, the great majority of defects were associated with either deletion of the green opsin gene or the formation of 5′ red-green or 5′ green-red full-length hybrid genes.[19] The results, described below, were

**Fig. 238-10** Spectral characteristics of the hybrid visual pigments commonly found among individuals with defective color vision. The right-hand column shows the exon composition of the six possible hybrid genes resulting from unequal recombination between the red and green opsin genes occurring in introns 2, 3, and 4. Filled and open boxes denote red and green gene exons, respectively. Hybrid opsins would not be formed as a result of recombinations in introns 1 and 5, since the sequences of exons 1 and 6 are identical in the two pigment genes. The normal red and green opsin genes are included for comparison. The left-hand column gives the designations for each hybrid pigment. For example, R3G4 denotes a 5′ red-green hybrid with the first three exons derived from the red gene and the last three exons from the green gene. Note that whenever exon 3 of a hybrid is derived from the red opsin gene, two forms of the hybrid are possible depending on whether Ser or Ala is found at position 180 in exon 3. The $\lambda_{max}$ values were determined from photobleaching difference absorption spectra of recombinant pigments expressed in tissue culture cells transfected with cDNA clones encoding the various hybrid opsins.[56]

basically in agreement with those obtained in the earlier study of 25 subjects by Nathans et al.[11]

**Protan Subjects.** Twenty-three (36 percent) of 64 color-deficient males[19] were protans, and their anomaloscopic Rayleigh match ranges are given in Fig. 238-7. Figure 238-11 shows the observed gene arrays, points of fusion, and class of protan defect [protanopic (P) or protanomalous (PA)] for the same subjects. The gene arrays of all protans were characterized by the presence of 5′ red-green hybrid opsin genes instead of the normal red opsin gene. In all cases, the intron of fusion was upstream of exon 5, thus indicating that exon 5 is critical in establishing the spectral characteristics of a normal red pigment. The replacement of exon 5 of the red opsin gene with that of the green opsin produced a hybrid pigment that was sufficiently greenlike in its spectral properties that the subjects performed as protans. The significant role of exon 5 of the red opsin gene was somewhat predicted, since it contains two of the three amino acid residues (at positions 277 and 285) thought to be mainly responsible for the difference in spectral properties between the red and green photopigments (see Fig. 238-12).

The relationship between structure of the pigment and its spectral properties as determined by ERG was investigated in a protanope who had a 5′ red-green hybrid gene in which the point of fusion was in intron 3.[115] The absorption spectrum of the pigment encoded by this hybrid gene (which encoded Ala at position 180) was very similar to that of the green pigment, suggesting that sequence differences in exons 2 and 3 contribute little to the difference in absorption between the red and green

**(Fig 238-9 caption continued)**
A deuteranomalous individual who has normal red pigment gene and a green-red hybrid pigment gene (see diagram in part *C*). Lane 3: An individual with deuteranopia who has only a normal red gene (see diagram in part *C*). Lane 4: A deuteranomalous individual with a gene array comprised of normal red and green as well as a green red hybrid pigment genes. Lane 5: An individual with normal color vision who has multiple green pigment genes. The unmarked lanes show patterns similar to those described above. (*C*) Diagrammatic representation of Southern blot patterns for males with normal and defective color vision. The color vision phenotypes and the structure of the red-green gene arrays associated with the EcoRI-BamHI, and RsaI Southern blot patterns are shown above the Southern blot. Filled and open arrows denote red and green gene sequences, respectively. The width of the solid lines representing restriction fragments reflects the relative quantity of DNA that is quantified by densitometry. In protanomaly and protanopia (protan), the Dr fragment is missing, indicating loss of the 3′ portion of the red pigment gene, while the 5′ portion of the green gene is present. In deuteranopia, Bg, Cg, and Dg fragments are missing, indicating complete deletion of the green pigment gene. In deuteranomaly, the relative proportions of fragments is shifted, indicating the presence of green-red hybrid genes.

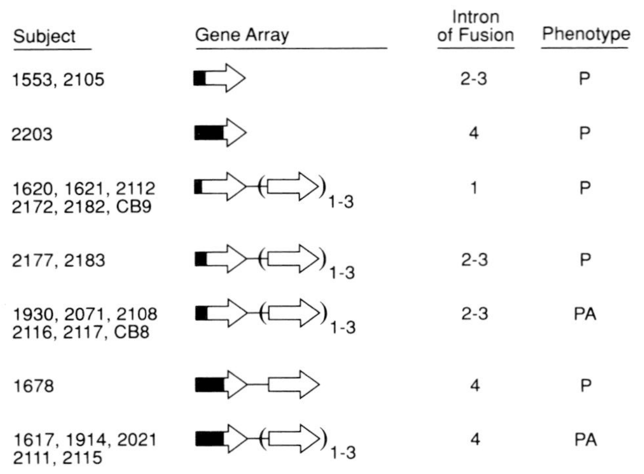

| Subject | Gene Array | Intron of Fusion | Phenotype |
|---------|-----------|------------------|-----------|
| 1553, 2105 | | 2-3 | P |
| 2203 | | 4 | P |
| 1620, 1621, 2112 2172, 2182, CB9 | ⟩₁₋₃ | 1 | P |
| 2177, 2183 | ⟩₁₋₃ | 2-3 | P |
| 1930, 2071, 2108 2116, 2117, CB8 | ⟩₁₋₃ | 2-3 | PA |
| 1678 | | 4 | P |
| 1617, 1914, 2021 2111, 2115 | ⟩₁₋₃ | 4 | PA |

**Fig. 238-11 Red-green color vision–pigment gene arrays found in males with protan color vision defects. Hybrid pigment genes consist of 5′ red opsin gene sequences (*filled arrows*) followed by green opsin gene sequences (*open arrows*). The subscript numbers 1–3 refers to the number of normal green opsin genes present, including subjects with 1, 2, or 3 green pigment genes. The color vision phenotype, as determined by anomaloscopy, is indicated as P, protanopia; PA, protanomaly. The assignment of intron of the fusion in hybrid genes was made on the basis of results of Southern blot analysis, PCR amplification, and sequencing of exons.[19] The uncertainty in assigning the fusion point to introns 2 or 3 results from the presence of polymorphisms in exon 3, the alleles of which are shared by the red and green opsin genes; 2–3 therefore indicates fusion points in either intron 2 or 3. (*Used with permission from Deeb et al.[19]*)**

photopigments. These results are consistent with those obtained by measuring bleaching difference spectra of in vitro–produced types of red-green hybrid genes.[56] They showed that the exchange of exon 5 sequences resulted in a major spectral shift in $\lambda_{max}$

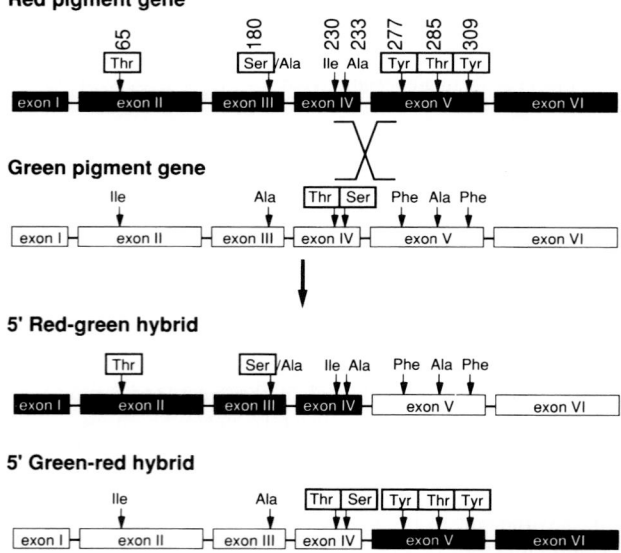

**Fig. 238-12 The importance of exon 5 in determining spectral sensitivities of hybrid pigments. The positions at which the red and green opsins differ by the presence of hydroxyl-bearing (*boxed*) versus nonpolar amino acid residues are shown. Recombination in intron 4 results in the exchange of three of these residues, two of which have been shown to account for the major difference in $\lambda_{max}$ between the normal red and green pigments. The red-green hybrid is as observed in protan subject 2203 of Fig. 238-11, and the green-red hybrid is as observed in deutan subject 1682 of Fig. 238-13. (*Used with permission from Deeb et al.[19]*)**

(15–20 nm), whereas differences in exons 2 to 4 appeared to have smaller effects (see Fig. 238-10).

Subjects who had *only* the red-green hybrid gene in their arrays test as protanopes regardless of the point of fusion, whereas those who had one or more normal green opsin genes in addition to the hybrid gene test as either protanopic or protanomalous. The distribution of match ranges was quite similar for subjects with either intron 2–3 or 4 fusions. The Ser/Ala polymorphism at position 180 in the red opsin appears to underlie the preceding discrepancy between genotype and phenotype. In a study of 19 protan subjects[116] who had one 5′ red-geen opsin gene as well as one or more normal green opsin gene, protanopes and protanomalous subjects could be differentiated (with one exception) on the basis of whether Ser or Ala was present at position 180 of the red portion of the hybrid gene, respectively. The presence of Ser encoded a hybrid pigment that differed by 5 nm in $\lambda_{max}$ from that of the normal green opsin, and this was associated with protanomaly. When Ala was present at position 180 of the hybrid, there was no difference in $\lambda_{max}$, and the subject were protanopic (see above and Fig. 238-13).

**Deutan Subjects.** The Rayleigh match ranges (see Fig. 238-7) of 41 of 64 color-deficient males placed them in the deutan series.[19] The gene arrays and estimated points of fusion for 40 of these deutans are shown in Fig. 238-14. One of the deuteranomalous subjects had a grossly normal gene array but had a point mutation in the green opsin gene (see below). All deutans had a normal red opsin gene, and all subjects (except the individual with the point mutation) had major gene rearrangements that could be detected by Southern blot analysis and/or gene-specific PCR amplification across intron 4.

***Gene Deletions.*** Thirteen of the 41 deutans were shown to completely lack green opsin gene sequences. Ten of the 13 subjects were classified by anomaloscopy as deuteranopes as expected, since they have only one red opsin gene. Surprisingly, the remaining 3 tested as severe deuteranomalous trichromats. Since they have only a red opsin gene, they should be completely unable to discriminate the red and green lights from the yellow standard light in the anomaloscope, yet they can do so. The pattern of a single red opsin gene in a deuteranomalous subject also has been observed in a previous study.[11]

***Simple Hybrid Genes.*** Twenty-five of the 41 deutans had gene arrays characterized by the presence of one or more full-length 5′ green-red hybrid opsin genes in addition to a normal red opsin gene (see Fig. 238-14). In 18 of these subjects, one or more normal green opsin genes were found in addition to the normal red and hybrid genes. Except for two subjects who tested as deuteranopic (dichromats), these gene arrays were associated with deuteranomaly. In one of the deuteranopes (subject 1907), and most likely in the other (subject 1681), the points of fusion in their hybrid genes

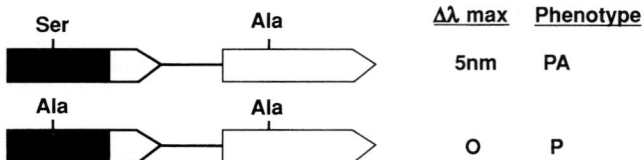

| | | Δλ max | Phenotype |
|---|---|--------|-----------|
| **Ser** | **Ala** | 5nm | PA |
| **Ala** | **Ala** | O | P |

**Fig. 238-13 The Ser/Ala polymorphism in the red opsin gene plays a role in determining protan subtypes. Diagrams of X-linked gene arrays each composed of a red-green hybrid gene (fusion in intron 4) and a normal green opsin gene. The hybrid gene with Ser at position 180 differs by 5 nm in $\lambda_{max}$ ($\Delta\lambda_{max}$) from the normal green opsin. A difference in $\lambda_{max}$ of this magnitude makes for protanomaly (PA), since trichromacy is preserved by this anomalous red-green pigment. In contrast, the Ala-containing hybrid has the same $\lambda_{max}$ as the normal green pigment, making the carrier a protanopic (P) dichromat.**

| Subject | Gene Array | Intron of Fusion | Phenotype |
|---|---|---|---|
| 1622, 1623, 1839<br>1841, 2053, 2175<br>2178, 2184, 2202<br>2205 | | N/A | D |
| 1897, 1933, 2185 | | N/A | DA |
| 1624 | | 1 | D |
| 1907 | | 2-3 | DA |
| 1682, 1934, 1955<br>1968, 1908 | | 4 | DA |
| 1681 | | 1-3 | D |
| 1552, 1618, 1619<br>1843, 1916, 2057<br>2059, 2113, 2114<br>2181, 2187 | | 1-3 | DA |
| 1616, 1672<br>2081, 2171 | | 4 | DA |
| 1840, 1906 | | 1-3 | DA |
| 1838, 1927 | | 1-3 & 4 | DA |

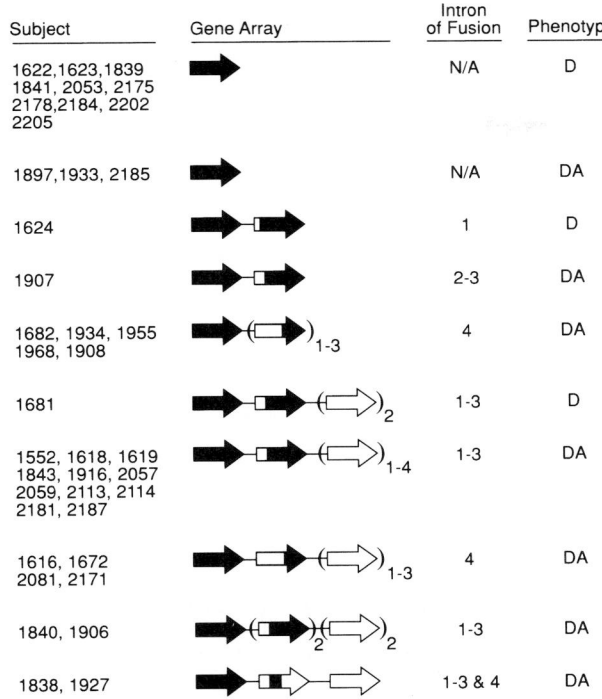

**Fig. 238-14** Color vision gene arrays found in subjects with deutan color vision defects. Explanations concerning the gene arrays are given in the legend to Fig. 238-13. D, deuteranopia; DA, deuteranomaly. Note that 3 of 13 individuals who had only a single red opsin gene unexpectedly tested as anomalous trichromats (deuteranomalous) instead of dichromats (deuteranopic). Furthermore, individual 1681 who had normal red and green opsin genes in addition to a green-red hybrid gene tested as a deuteranope, suggesting that the two normal green opsin genes are not expressed. N/A, not applicable. (*Used with permission from Deeb et al.[19]*)

were in intron 1, causing the expected deuteranopia. The fusion points in all the other deuteranomalous subjects were located in introns 2 to 4.

As seen in the protan subjects, 5′ green-red hybrid genes that resulted from a crossover in intron 4 (i.e., exchanged exons 5 and 6) encoded a pigment that was essentially redlike in absorption spectrum.

The presence of more than one hybrid gene in the array does not seem to be associated with a more severe color vision defect. Neither does the presence in arrays of normal green opsin genes in addition to normal red and hybrid genes. One explanation for these observations is that not all the opsin genes in an array are expressed in the retina (see below).

***Double Fusion Genes.*** Deuteranomaly in two subjects (1838 and 1927) was associated with a novel type of hybrid gene (5′ green-red-green) in which a central segment encompassing exon 4 and possibly exon 3 was exchanged between the red and green opsin genes, presumably due to a double crossover or a gene conversion event. In these cases, the two hydroxyl-bearing residues at positions 230 and 233 in exon 4 of the green opsin gene were replaced by Ile and Ala, respectively, suggesting a role for one or both of these amino acids in determining spectral sensitivities of the photopigments. The results of Merbs and Nathans[56] support this hypothesis. They showed that amino acid differences in either exon 3 or 4 could produce a spectral shift of 4 nm (see Fig. 238-10).

***A Point Mutation in a Single Case of Deuteranomaly.*** The gene array of one of the subjects (CB 1909) with severe deuteranomaly (match range of 12–68) had no gross rearrangements. Examina-

tion of the coding sequences of his red and green opsin genes revealed that all three of his green opsin genes had a C → T transition at nucleotide 648 that translates to the substitution of Arg for Cys at position 203.[117] Screening of 63 other color-defective subjects known to have major gene rearrangements revealed another deuteranomalous individual (CB 1843) who carried the same mutation in one of his three green opsin genes. The same C203R mutation had been observed in 16 unrelated families with blue cone monochromacy.[118,119] In these cases, the mutation was in the green segments of 5′ red-green hybrid genes. These results suggest that the C203R mutant allele of the green opsin gene may be common in the general population. Indeed, the same mutation also was found in a green gene of 1 of 65 male subjects with normal color vision. The Cys residue is highly conserved among all visual pigments studied so far, as well as among other seven-transmembrane-segment receptors, such as the adrenergic, muscarinic, dopaminergic, and serotonergic receptors.[43,120]

The Cys 203 residue is believed to form a disulfide bridge with Cys 126, thus covalently linking the first and second extracellular loops of the opsins. Results of in vitro mutagenesis studies showed that the corresponding cysteine residues in bovine rhodopsin (residues 110 and 187) and in the hamster beta-adrenergic receptor (residues 106 and 187) are essential for function of these proteins.[121,122] Therefore, the C203R mutation is very likely to abolish function of the green-sensitive photoreceptor. Furthermore, in analogy with the mutant rhodopsin alleles associated with autosomal dominant retinitis pigmentosa,[123,124] this mutation may predispose to certain X-linked cone dystrophies as a result of accumulation of the abnormal protein. A sequence rearrangement in the red opsin gene has been found to cosegregate in one family with X-linked progressive cone degeneration.[125]

***Synopsis.*** Based on analysis of at least 90 males with red-green color vision defects,[11,19,126] inter- and intragenic recombinations between the red and green opsin genes, which result in green opsin gene deletions or shuffling of exons between the two genes, account for all but the one case of color vision defect, found to be due to a C203R mutation. Exon 5 plays a major role in spectral tuning, since it contains three of the seven residues that distinguish red from green opsins. Molecular analysis of the red and green opsin genes could classify subjects into either the protan or deutan series. Although certain trends were evident, the genotype at the level of coding sequence occasionally was not correlated with the color vision phenotype within the protan and deutan series. Nagel anomaloscopy may not provide a sufficiently accurate quantitative assessment of ability of red-green color-deficient subjects to discriminate color.[13] Alternatively, severity of color deficiency may not be a function of the sequence of hybrid pigments only. Postreceptoral neural factors[127,128] and variation in the amount of pigment synthesized or in the ratio of red to green cones[129] were proposed to account for variation in color discrimination. Position-dependent expression of genes of the red-green locus explains why the more distal location of hybrid genes and mutant green opsin genes in addition to normal red and green opsin genes does not result in altered color vision.

**Selective Expression among Multiple Green Opsin Genes: Only One Gene Is Expressed.** The frequency of 5′ green-red hybrid genes was observed to be higher than the reported frequency of color vision defects among Caucasian and especially among African-American males[67,71] (see below), suggesting that such hybrid genes may not always lead to color vision defects. This was proven to be the case by showing that 4 of 129 Caucasian males with anomaloscopically determined normal color vision had a 5′ green-red hybrid gene in addition to normal red and green opsin genes.[19] In addition, a male with normal color vision was found to have the C203R mutation in one of his five green opsin genes,[117] and another (subject 1681 in Fig. 238-14), who had a green-red hybrid opsin gene in addition to normal red and green opsin genes, tested as deuteranope, indicating that his normal green opsin genes were nonfunctional.[19]

The hypothesis that not all opsin genes in an array are expressed in the retina was advanced to explain these observations. Green opsin gene sequences in genomic DNA were compared with the corresponding mRNA sequences expressed in postmortem retinal tissues. Advantage was taken of a relatively common but silent polymorphism (A versus C at the third position of codon 283) in exon 5 of the green opsin gene.[130] The two alleles can be differentiated by PCR amplification of exon 5 followed by SSCP analysis or digestion with EcoO109_1. Results of such a comparison in 10 male subjects who had two or more green opsin genes in their genomic DNA clearly showed that when the two alleles of exon 5 were present, only one was represented in expressed retinal mRNA,[130] indicating the expression of only a single green opsin gene. In addition to the expression of a single green opsin gene, retinal RNA from the same individuals contained a single red opsin-encoding mRNA sequence.

In another set of 51 unselected postmortem retinas, three male donors of unknown color vision status had gene arrays comprised of one red, one 5′ green–red 3′ hybrid and one normal green pigment genes. We found that the expressed mRNA transcripts were encoded by the normal red and the 5′ green–red 3′ hybrid but not by the normal green pigment gene and therefore presumably reflected deuteranomalous color vision. The other two retina specimens expressed the normal red and green pigment genes but not the green-red hybrid and presumably had normal color vision.[72] In another study, the lack of expression of green pigment genes carried by deutan subjects was confirmed.[131] Regardless of the presence or absence of hybrid genes, it generally was observed that the red pigment gene, which occupies the most proximal position in the array, was expressed at a higher level (fourfold) than the green pigment gene.[72] This was confirmed in a subsequent study.[131] These results are consistent with those of molecular and ERG studies by our group on deutans who carry normal red and green and a 5′ green–red 3′ hybrid gene.[132] In all seven subjects studied, the green pigment was undetectable by ERG spectral sensitivity measurements.

Neitz and Neitz[133] suggested that a large proportion of males with normal color vision have a large number of red and green pigment genes with at least two expressed red pigment genes as well as at least two expressed green pigment genes. Extensive data using Southern blot analysis,[19,114,130] PCR-based methodologies,[72] as well as pulsed-field gel electrophoresis (which is a more direct method of estimating the total number of genes in an array from its length)[134] are most consistent with a much lower average number (mean of 2) of genes in the array and with the presence of only a single red pigment gene. Furthermore, in arrays that contain more than one green pigment gene, only one is expressed in the retina.[130] (See Addendum 3).

The model illustrated in Fig. 238-15 was proposed[130] to explain such selective expression of one of a set of green opsin genes in an array. In this model, a locus control region (LCR) regulates expression of the opsin genes of the array in a position-dependent manner. Thus, in red cones, the LCR forms a stable, transcriptionally active complex with the red opsin promoter, whereas in green cones, the LCR forms a complex with the proximal green opsin promoter. Active complexes between the LCR and green opsin promoters located downstream of the proximal green opsin promoter are much less favored. We therefore suggest that only the most proximal green pigment gene is expressed in an array of several green pigment genes that may include 5′ green-red hybrid pigment genes. (See Addendum 4).

The concept of an LCR was first suggested for the regulatory sequences 5′ upstream of the beta-globin gene locus. The globin LCR was shown to be essential for developmental switching of expression from fetal to adult globin genes and indicated that the order of the genes comprising this locus is important for such a transcriptional switch.[135–138] Evidence for an LCR at the red-

## A. Expression in red cones

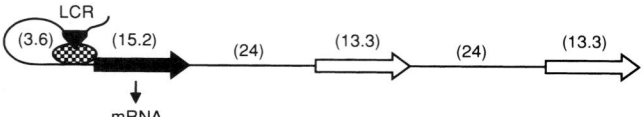

## B. Expression in green cones

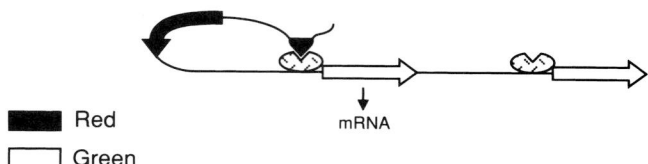

■ Red
□ Green

**Fig. 238-15 Model for selective expression in the X-linked red-green gene complex. Numbers denote length in kilobase pairs. (A) Red cone-specific gene transcription occurs as a result of stable coupling (mediated by DNA-binding proteins) of the LCR to the red gene promoter. (B) The LCR preferentially and stably couples to the proximal green opsin gene promoter and turns on its expression. Distal green opsin promoters are not activated presumably due to the low probability of coupling to the LCR. (Adapted with permission from Winderickx et al.[130])**

green opsin locus has been provided by Nathans et al.,[118] who found that, in some instances, blue cone monochromacy, a disorder in which *both* red and green cone functions are absent, is associated with deletion of a regulatory sequence located 3.8 to 4.3 kb upstream of the transcription-initiation site of the red opsin gene and 43 kb upstream of the proximal green opsin gene. They subsequently showed that a region between −3.1 and −3.7 kb of the red opsin gene is required for cone-specific expression of the beta-galactosidase reporter gene in transgenic mice.[139]

**Blue Cone Monochromacy.** Blue cone monochromacy (BCM) (MIM 303700), also referred to as Pi₁ monochromacy or *X-linked incomplete achromatopsia*,[100] is an extremely rare disorder ( < 1 in 100,000) in which both red and green cone sensitivities are absent. The physiologic functions of both rods and blue cones are preserved. Significant linkage of BCM to the red-green pigment gene locus was established by analysis of RFLP alleles at the two DNA markers, *DXS15* and *DXS52*.[140] This led Nathans et al.[118] to analyze the red-green locus in individuals with BCM. Their studies on 38 families with BCM have uncovered two mechanisms for generating this phenotype (reviewed in ref. 119). The first, found in 14 families, involved deletions (587 bp to 55 kb) that included a regulatory sequence located approximately 3.4 kb 5′ upstream of the transcription-initiation site of the red opsin gene. In some of these individuals, the red and green opsin genes were unaffected, whereas in others, the deletions extended into the red opsin gene. This regulatory region, referred to as an LCR (see above), was shown, in transgenic mice, to be essential for directing expression of the β-galactosidase reporter gene to both long- and short-wavelength-sensitive cones in the mouse retina.[139] The second mechanism of generating BCM, found in 20 families, involved unequal homologous recombination between the green and red opsin genes that reduced the gene array to only a single red or a 5′ red-green hybrid gene. In 16 of these families, the green opsin portion of the hybrid gene had a C203R substitution, which apparently rendered the encoded hybrid opsin nonfunctional. Evidence that the C203R substitution encodes a nonfunctional photopigment was provided by Kazmi et al.,[141] who expressed a recombinant human M-pigment carrying this mutation in cultured cells. The expressed opsin was misfolded, retained in the endoplasmic reticulum, and defective in interaction with the chromophore and activation of transducin. Furthermore, disruption of the same disulfide bond due to a mutation (C187Y) in rhodopsin caused early and severe autosomal dominant retinitis pigmentosa in one family.[142] The same C203R mutation was found to be relatively common (2 percent) in the green opsin genes of Caucasian males[117] but may not always be expressed because of its distal position in the array (see below). Progressive central retinal dystrophy has been reported in some patients with BCM,[118] indicating that cone degeneration may result from the accumulation of an abnormally assembled photopigment in analogy with the mutations in rhodopsin found to underlie autosomal dominant retinitis pigmentosa.[123] In one kindred, BCM was shown to be due to the presence of the inactivating C203R mutation in exon 4 of both the red-green-red hybrid gene and the green pigment gene carried on the X chromosome of affected males.[143] It is interesting to note that funduscopy in two older affected males in this family revealed atrophy of the retinal pigment epithelium and the chorionic choriocapillaris layer in the macula.

Other than the common C203R mutation, Nathans and colleagues observed two other photopigment inactivating substitutions associated with BCM: R247ter and P307L. Furthermore, a Danish male patient with BCM was found to have a single red pigment gene in which exon 4 is deleted and no green pigment genes.[144] The deletion alters the translational reading frame and creates a stop codon. The encoded defective protein is predicted to lack the three C-terminal transmembrane helices of the red pigment. Defective red pigment gene function in the absence of green pigment genes caused BCM.

**Tritanopia.** Tritanopia (MIM 190900) is a rare autosomal dominant[91] disorder characterized by selective loss of blue-sensitive photoreceptor function and greatly diminished or absent chromatic discrimination in the blue region of the spectrum. A survey in the Netherlands indicates that its frequency in the population may be as high as 1 in 500.[145] Three missense mutations in the gene encoding the blue pigment opsin, located at 7q31.3–q32,[10] have been shown to cause tritanopia: G79R in two Japanese subjects, S214P in two Caucasian subjects, and P264S in three Caucasian subjects.[92,93] The three mutant alleles cosegregate with tritanopia in an autosomal dominant fashion, but incomplete penetrance was observed in association with the G79R substitution. The mutations affect residues located in the second, fifth, and sixth transmembrane α-helical segments of the blue pigment opsin. The dominant mode of inheritance suggests that accumulation of a defective opsin within photoreceptors causes either loss of function or cell death, reminiscent of mutations in the rhodopsin and peripherin genes that cause a subset of autosomal dominant retinitis pigmentosa. Tritanopia also has been observed in association with some disorders of vision such as autosomal dominant juvenile optic atrophy.[146,147]

**Complete Achromatopsia.** Complete achromatopsia or rod monochromacy (MIM 216900) is a rare autosomal recessive trait characterized by total loss of color vision, photophobia, nystagmus, and loss of visual acuity. A locus for complete achromatopsia has been mapped to 2q11.[148] A candidate gene (CNGA3), encoding the α-subunit of the cone photoreceptor cGMP-gated cation channel, had been mapped to the same region.[149] This channel plays a critical role in the light-triggered signal-transduction cascade in all three classes of cones leading to hyperpolarization of the photoreceptor membrane. Kohl et al.[150] reported the presence of missense mutations in CNGA3 in five families with complete achromatopsia. (See Addendum 5).

## A Single Amino Acid Polymorphism Explains Variation In Normal Color Vision

Subtle variations in color perception in the red-green region of the spectrum have been observed among individuals considered to have normal color vision. Rayleigh color matches of male subjects

with normal color vision fell into two main groups[17,18,151–153] and suggested a difference of several nanometers in the red pigment absorption spectra. Females with normal color vision show a third and larger group with intermediate values of match midpoints.[17] A similar, independently described Rayleigh match variability in families suggested transmission by X-linked inheritance.[16] These observations pointed to the presence of two common alleles of the red pigment gene. Assuming the occurrence of X-chromosome inactivation, females who are heterozygous for such a polymorphism would be expected to have patches of cones containing either one or the other of the pigment forms and therefore would show a color match distribution intermediate between those of the two homozygotes.

The subtle differences in color matching observed among individuals with normal color vision (as well as among deuteranopic dichromats, who have only a red opsin gene) have been suggested to be a reflection of small variations in the absorption maxima of the red or green photopigments.[12–15,154]

A common single-amino-acid polymorphism (62 percent Ser, 38 percent Ala) at residue 180 of the red photopigment was discovered in the Caucasian population.[18] Fifty Caucasian males with normal color vision were tested for the hypothesis that the two major groups in the distribution of color matching could be explained by the preceding Ser/Ala polymorphism. The frequency distributions of Rayleigh match midpoints and of the deduced amino acid sequence of the red photopigment (Fig. 238-16) show that higher sensitivity to red light (i.e., requirement of less red in the mixture of red and green to match the standard yellow light) was highly correlated with the presence of Ser at position 180.[18] These males therefore have a different perception of red light than those having the alanine allele at this site. Females having both the Ala and Ser alleles would be expected to have two types of red photoreceptors due to X-chromosome inactivation and thus may have tetrachromatic vision. This is analogous to the situation in New Word monkeys, who have only a single X-chromosome-encoded middle–long-wavelength pigment gene with several alleles, where females heterozygous for two alleles of this gene achieve trichromacy and males and homozygous females test as dichromats.[49] The frequency of the Ser/Ala polymorphism among African-Americans is 80/20 percent (S. Deeb, unpublished observation, 1993), and among Japanese it is 84/16 percent.[155]

The importance of the presence of Ser or Ala at position 180 in spectral tuning of photopigments had been deduced already from studies of the visual pigments of Old and New World monkeys.[59] A difference of 6 nm was observed between the peaks of maximal sensitivity (562 nm for Ser-containing pigments and 556 nm for Ala-containing pigments, as determined by ERG of the pigments of two tamarin monkeys that differed in sequence by only Ser versus Ala at position 180. The results of Merbs and Nathans[62] of direct determination of the bleaching difference absorption spectra of human red pigments (expressed in tissue culture cells transfected with complementary DNA clones) that differed in sequence by Ser versus Ala at position 180 were thus in good agreement with the ERG results in the monkeys (557 and 552 nm for the Ser- and Ala-containing reconstituted pigments, respectively), as well as with the human color matching data. These results support the finding that the Ser/Ala polymorphism at position 180 of the red pigment underlies the observed variation in red-green color vision among people with normal color vision.

Other amino acid polymorphisms have been observed in both the red (eight sites) and green (five sites) opsin genes. These polymorphisms give rise in the general population to 15 and 18 different green and red opsins, respectively. Nine of these polymorphisms are located in exon 3. Alleles of these polymorphisms are shared between the red and green opsin genes, suggesting a history of relatively frequent gene conversion or unequal recombination, mainly localized to exon 3, during the evolution of the two lineages.[114]

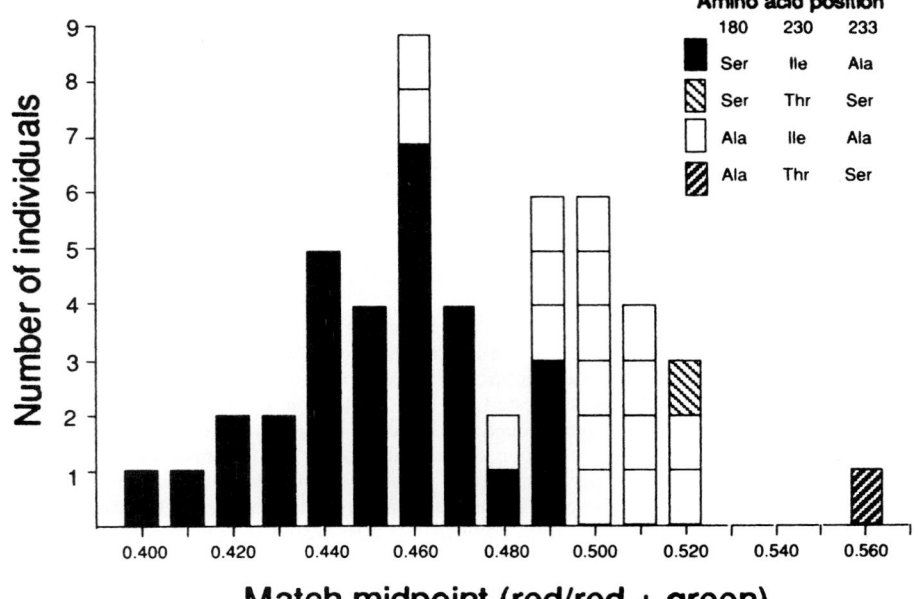

Fig. 238-16 Correlation of the Rayleigh match midpoint (center of match range) with the presence of serine or alanine at position 180 of the red photopigment. The 50 subjects were Caucasian males who tested as having normal color vision. Determination of color matches was made by measuring the proportion of red in a mixture of red and green lights that was perceived to match a standard yellow light. The presence of serine at position 180 correlates with higher sensitivity to red light (i.e., less red light is used to mix with green light to match the standard yellow light). Two individuals who had Thr and Ser instead of Ile and Ala at positions 230 and 233, respectively, required more red light in the mixture in comparison with others with the same amino acid at position 180. (*Used with permission from Winderickx et al.*[18])

## Heterozygosity and Homozygosity among Females with X-Linked Color Vision Defects

Because of the high frequency of X-linked color vision defects among males, there will be a large number of female heterozygotes for these genes in the population. Among males, the gene frequency and trait frequency of an X-linked trait (p) are identical. Males have either have (p) or do not have (q) the X-linked trait under study. The expected frequency of female heterozygotes and homozygotes can be calculated by the Hardy-Weinberg law, where 2pq will be the number of heterozygotes and $q^2$ the number of affected homozygotes. Homozygotes will be defective in color vision similar to affected males. The number of female heterozygotes (2pq) for each of the defective color vision categories is about twice the number of defective color vision male hemizygotes. Since the total frequency of color vision defects among European populations is 8 percent (p), about 15 to 16 percent (2pq) of the female population will be heterozygotes for one or another red-green color vision defect. The majority of such heterozygotes (7–10 percent) are heterozygotes for deuteranomaly, since this abnormality is the most frequent defect.

Occasional heterozygotes who express phenotypic color vision defects may have a single X chromosome such as in Turner syndrome or may come from the small proportion of females with extremely skewed X-inactivation who by chance have inactivated most of their normal X chromosome and thus express the mutant X chromosome.[156,157] Skewed X-inactivation appears to be more common in one member of identical female twin pairs,[158] and six pairs of heterozygote female identical twins discordant for color vision have been reported.[159-163] The expected skewed inactivation of one X chromosome has been demonstrated directly in one of the twin pairs.[158] Furthermore, two of five Dionne identical quintuplet girls were color blind,[161] as was one of three identical triplet Japanese girls.[164]

The population frequency of skewed X chromosome inactivation was investigated among 400 unselected pairs of Caucasian identical female twins who included about 60 heterozygotes for red-green color vision defects (~15 percent of 400 unselected females are expected to be carriers of red-green color vision defects). Discordant X chromosome inactivation with one twin being defective in color vision and the other having normal color vision was observed in only two twin pairs, suggesting a low population frequency (~3 percent) of the skewed inactivation

phenomenon in identical female twins (unpublished observations by the Seattle group, 1998).

As expected by the X-inactivation hypothesis, heterozygotes are mosaics for normal and abnormal color vision in their retinas. Thus, by shining a very narrow beam of red or green light into the retinas of female heterozygotes for X-linked color vision defects, patches of defective color perception were found.[165,166] In other experiments, heterozygotes made more errors than controls when asked to identify the color of briefly presented stimuli under conditions that did not allow any eye movement.[167]

These findings are consistent with earlier data that mild abnormalities of color vision often can be detected on psychophysical testing where groups of heterozygotes are compared with normal controls.[82,100,168] Such minor deviations have been observed with pseudoisochromatic plate reading, anomaloscopy, and tests that assessed hue and saturation discrimination.[100] The so-called Schmidt sign is the most obvious abnormality and can be elicited by many different psychophysical techniques. It is found in protan heterozygotes. The defect consists of a reduction in the relative luminous efficiency curve compared with that in normal and affected hemizygotes.[169] Similar findings have been observed in the relative spectral luminous efficiency function of deutan heterozygotes and consisted of a lessened sensitivity at short wavelengths.[169]

ERG has been successful in identifying a fairly large number of both protan and deutan heterozygotes by the ratio of sensitivity at short (480-nm) and long (620-nm) wavelengths for the rapid off response.[99]

The molecular abnormalities in heterozygotes reflect those observed in males with color vision defects. Molecular methodology that depends on Southern blots of various restriction fragments of the red and green pigment gene usually does not allow molecular detection of heterozygotes. However, when family studies are done and affected fathers and brothers are tested by the appropriate techniques, molecular genotypes of females can be determined.[126] Detection of female carriers of protan defects can be made by PCR amplification without knowledge of the status of family members.[170] Amplification is carried out using a forward primer that is specific for the red pigment gene promoter, with a reverse primer in intron 5 that is common to both red and green pigment genes. The amplification of a segment that contains a green pigment exon 5 would indicate that the female is a carrier of a gene array containing a

5′ red–green 3′ hybrid gene in the most proximal position. Such a gene array is characteristic for protanopia and protanomaly.

Compound heterozygotes for protan and deutan defects will be observed. The most frequent compound type are females with a deuteranomaly allele on one X chromosome and an allele for one of the other color vision defects (deuteranopia, protanopia, or protanomaly) on the other. Compound heterozygotes for both deuteranomaly and deuteranopia will manifest with deuteranomaly,[82,100] as expected from the molecular findings, since a deleted green pigment gene is not expressed, whereas a visual pigment with somewhat abnormal sensitivity such as a green-red fusion gene in deuteranomaly will manifest. Similarly, protanope/protanomalous heterozygotes manifest with protanomaly, demonstrating that, among protans, the mild phenotype also is dominant over the more severe one.

In contrast, compound heterozygotes for both a deutan and protan defect will *not* present with color vision defects.[83,100] This finding is not surprising, since normal alleles for red and green pigments are present in addition to the defects in both the protan and deutan genes. Such females, therefore, are functionally heterozygotes for both the deutan and the protan genes and therefore will have normal color vision. Compound heterozygosity for protanopia/deuteranomaly and protanomaly/deuteranomaly was studied in one large family by molecular techniques and showed no color vision abnormalities.[126]

With a population frequency of 1 percent for protanopia, protanomaly, and deuteranopia each and 5 percent for deuteranomaly among Caucasians, the expected frequency of homozygotes with defective color vision ($p^2$) for protanopia, protanomaly, and deuteranopia is approximately 1 in 10,000 for each of these categories (total 3 in 10,000) and 1 in 400 for deuteranomaly homozygotes. The total frequency of color vision defects among female homozygotes is less than the squared number of the male frequency ($p^2 = 0.0064$), since compound heterozygotes for protan and deutan defects are phenotypically normal.

## POPULATION STUDIES

The frequency of color vision defects among populations of European origin ranges around 8 percent.[82,100] A large number of individuals (several thousand) have been tested by anomaloscopy in many different studies. The results are very similar, in that 50 to 60 percent of the different color vision defects are caused by deuteranomaly, so between 4 and 5 percent of the male population has this defect (see ref. 71). The frequencies of the other defects, protanopia, protanomaly, and deuteranopia, all range around 1 percent or slightly more. Generally, on the rare occasions when anomaloscopy is done on all test subjects, the frequency of color vision defects appears slightly higher than that detected in studies that rely on initial plate testing followed by anomaloscopy only on those who test as abnormal. Because of the more complex procedures involved in anomaloscopy, studies on non-European populations, except for the Japanese, have not been done frequently. Color vision defects were found less frequently in practically all other populations as compared with Europeans. Among Chinese and Japanese, the frequency of all color vision defects combined together is around 4 to 6 percent,[67,74,82,155,171] whereas somewhat lower frequencies (4 percent or less) have been found among populations of African origin.[82,172,173] The lower frequencies among non-Europeans are largely caused by fewer deuteranomalous individuals.[174] Deuteranopia is seen in frequencies of 1 to 2 percent in practically all populations, whereas protanopia occurs somewhat less frequently (0.2–1.2 percent). The *combined* frequency of the severe dichromatic defects in both European and non-European populations everywhere varies between 1 to 3.5 percent.[175]

### Molecular Population Studies

Molecular investigations of color vision genes among population groups have not been done extensively. In the first study among U.S. males of European origin,[71] more molecular abnormalities were found than expected by the frequency of color vision anomalies. Thus, among 134 males who were not phenotypically tested, 21 (15.7 percent) showed molecular abnormalities of the red or green color vision genes. Two of 134 (1.5 percent) had a deletion of the green pigment gene and presumably were deuteranopes. Six (4.4 percent) had red-green fusion genes, presumably associated with protanopia or protanomaly. Nine (6.7 percent) had green-red fusion genes, and another 4 (5.2 percent) had findings suggestive of double crossovers (green-red-green). In a later study of 129 U.S. white males, 4 individuals with green-red fusion genes and *normal* color vision, as assessed by anomaloscopy, were found.[19] The higher frequency of green-red hybrid genes as compared with the lower frequency of color vision defects is explained by nonexpression of these hybrid genes when located in a more distal position in the green pigment gene array (see above).

Red-green hybrid genes appear to be expressed as protan defects. While the duplication of green but not of red pigment genes can be explained by the fact that green pigment genes, unlike the red pigment genes, are flanked by 24 kb of almost identical intergenic DNA that favors illegitimate recombination, the higher frequency of green-red pigment genes compared with red-green hybrids cannot be explained on this basis. The ratio of green-red and red-green hybrid genes is expected to be 1:1 because the reciprocal product of a green-red fusion gene will be a red-green fusion gene if the underlying mechanism is recombination (see Fig. 238-8). In a study of 102 African-American males whose phenotypic color vision was unknown, 20 (19.6 percent) were found to have green-red fusion genes.[67] A single green pigment gene deletion and no red-green fusion genes (protans) were detected in this sample. However, no less than 36 (35 percent) individuals had a polymorphism consisting of a shortened (1.5-kb) red pigment gene involving intron 1. This polymorphism, which also was seen in a small percentage of Caucasians and Japanese, had no effect on color vision — an expected effect because it did not involve any coding sequence. The high frequency of green-red fusion genes (19.6 percent) among African-Americans was much higher than the expected frequency of deuteranomaly observed in various population samples of African origin (1–2 percent). Whether the visual pigment gene pattern in Africans is such that more such green-red fusion genes are located in a distal position of the green pigment gene complex and therefore are not expressed requires further study.

The polymorphism associated with the shortened red pigment gene may predispose to a higher frequency of unequal crossovers between the red and green pigment gene.[67] This shortened red pigment gene resembles a green pigment gene in that both the polymorphic red and the normal green pigment gene lack the 1.5-kb intervening sequence seen in the normal red pigment gene. Illegitimate pairing between these more similar shortened genes therefore may cause a higher frequency of fusion genes. Thus 8 of 57 (14 percent) of those with the standard red pigment gene had green-red fusion genes, whereas 33 percent (12 of 36) of those with the polymorphic shortened red pigment gene had green-red fusion genes. The polymorphic red pigment gene had a similar frequency among individuals with the common polymorphisms G6PD A+ and A−, suggesting no allelic association or linkage disequilibrium of the shortened red pigment genes and the closely linked G6PD locus.[67] It is therefore not likely that this red pigment gene polymorphism owes its existence to selection of the G6PD A+ and A− type (although more data on G6PD A− are required to be certain). Furthermore, no correlation between G6PD and color vision defects has been observed.[176]

Molecular analysis was performed on the red and green pigment gene arrays of 203 Japanese-American males from the Seattle area (of nonadmixed Japanese ancestry) who were not studied for color vision status.[67,155] Gene arrays that are usually associated with color vision deficiencies (deletion of the green and green-red hybrid genes) were detected in approximately 5 percent of these individuals, which is nearly the same as the frequency of color vision defects in Japanese males in Japan. Therefore, the majority of green-red hybrid genes carried by Japanese males appear to be associated with defective color vision. This is consistent with the observation that gene arrays of Japanese contain relatively few green pigment genes (42 percent of Japanese have a single green pigment gene). Thus a hybrid gene in such arrays would have a high probability of expression in the retina. The higher frequency of green-red hybrid genes than would be expected from the frequency of phenotypic color vision defects among Caucasian males may be due to the presence of a higher average number of green pigment genes per array (only 22 percent carry one green pigment gene), making it less likely for a green-red hybrid gene to be expressed. While these findings may explain the Japanese-Caucasian differences, the high frequency of unexpressed green-red fusion genes among African-Americans remains unexplained.

All the polymorphisms that were detected among the Japanese had been observed among Caucasians and African-Americans. However, compared with Caucasians, the Japanese population was more uniform with respect to the number of different haplotypes (60 percent having the same haplotype) of the red pigment gene. This difference is largely due to the lower degree of the S180A polymorphism among Japanese.

### Selection in Color Vision Defects?

Since the frequency of all types of color vision defects is increased among modern Europeans as compared with other populations, it was reasoned that color vision defects, regardless of type, were strongly selected against in "primitive habitats."[177,178] It was reasoned that the introduction of agriculture relaxed selection pressure and color vision defects became more common to account for current high frequencies among Europeans. The principal problem with this hypothesis is its failure to consider the different subtypes of color vision defects.[175] The frequencies of dichromats appear fairly similar in developed populations and those under development (see above). Even allowing for misdiagnosis in field studies where anomaloscopic studies were not done, the detection of the more severely affected dichromats is fairly certain on plate tests, so the finding of similar frequencies of dichromacy in all populations seems rather firm.

In view of the higher frequency of deuteranomaly in Europeans, selection may have been operative on this trait, but the nature of selection is difficult to define. Heterozygote women for deuteranomaly may be expected to be tetrachromatic because X-inactivation would render them mosaics for slightly abnormal as well as for normal green pigment genes in addition to having normal blue and red visual pigment. Possibly, such a tetrachromatic state in females, as well as hemizygosity for deuteranomaly, may have provided a selective advantage that has now disappeared. Why protanomalous women would not have such an advantage, however, is not clear. Cruz-Coke[179] suggested that women heterozygotes for color vision defects are more fertile. However, Mollon et al.[180] were unable to show any differences between heterozygotes and normal individuals when considering the time period between either marriage and birth of the first child or discontinuation of contraception and beginning of pregnancy. In any case, the most important reason for the relatively high frequency of the various red-green color vision defects appears to be the multigene structure of the color vision gene array that allows relatively frequent recombination with the formation of fusion genes and deletions.

## EVOLUTION OF TRICHROMATIC COLOR VISION IN PRIMATES[53]

The evolution of the visual pigment genes is fairly clear.[53] An ancestral gene coded for the precursor gene of a variety of related protein molecules known as the *G-protein-coupled receptors*. These receptors are also known as *heptahelical receptors* (crossing

the membrane seven times) and include beta-adrenergic receptors, serotonin receptors, muscarinic acetylcholine, and S-K receptors. The ancestral visual pigment is part of this family. Some 800 million years ago, the ancestral visual pigment diverged into the rod pigment rhodopsin and the yet undifferentiated cone pigment gene. Some 500 million years ago, a short-wavelength-sensitive gene, or blue pigment gene, and a single middle-wavelength or green-red pigment, gene diverged from each other (see Fig. 238-2). This ancient system of short- (blue) and long-wavelength (green-red) signals probably was shared by all diurnal animals. About 30 to 40 million years ago and after separation of the New World from the Old World lineages, the single green-red pigment gene duplicated. The two copies of the gene diverged in sequence to give rise to the green (middle-wave) and red (long-wave) pigment genes to provide trichromatic color vision, which is shared by most humans and Old World monkeys. Thus most New World monkeys have a single X-chromosome-linked photopigment gene encoding a red-green pigment. In these species, all males have dichromatic color vision. Several alleles of the single red-green pigment gene that encode photopigments with different absorption maxima were discovered in several species of New World monkeys. Females that carry any two of these alleles were shown to have trichromatic color vision.[49] Jacobs et al.[50] showed that one genus of new word monkeys (*Alouatta*, the howler monkey) has two X-linked photopigment genes. Males and females of this genus have full trichromatic color vision. Comparison of the sequences of the red and green pigments of such howler monkeys and those of Old and New World monkeys indicated that the gene duplication in the howler monkey occurred after the split between New and Old World lineages and is more recent that the duplication of the Old World primate gene.[181] Furthermore, the duplication in the howler monkey was the result of unequal recombination between two alleles of the ancestral gene that encoded pigments with different spectral sensitivities.[181]

The red and green photopigments of eight species of fruit-eating Old World monkeys that inhabit different regions of Africa and Asia exhibit relatively homogeneous $\lambda_{max}$ values (a 5-nm variation in both pigments) of 556 and 535 nm, respectively, as determined by microspectrophotometry.[182] Thus their color vision is predicted to be very similar to that of humans. The coding sequence and deduced amino acid sequence of the red and green pigment genes of the chimpanzee, gorilla, and orangutan were highly homologous to the equivalent human pigments.[183] None of the amino acid differences occurred at sites known to influence pigment absorption characteristics. Therefore, the absorption maxima of the red and green photopigments of the apes were predicted to be within less than 2 nm of the corresponding human pigments and indicated that color vision in these primates was very similar, if not identical, to that in humans. In this study, 14 within-species DNA sequence polymorphisms also were detected. Interestingly, 6 of these polymorphisms had been observed among humans, suggesting that they predated the evolution of higher primates. Alleles at these polymorphic sites are often shared between red and green pigment genes. The average synonymous rate of sequence divergence between these pigment genes was approximately one-tenth that estimated for other proteins of higher primates. The high degree of homology and juxtaposition of these two genes on the X chromosome have promoted relatively frequent homologous recombination/gene conversion that led to sequence homogenization. However, natural selection has operated to maintain the degree of separation in $\lambda_{max}$ between the red and green pigments for optimal chromatic discrimination. This represents a unique case of molecular coevolution of two homologous genes that functionally interact at the behavioral level. It has been proposed that a selective advantage of trichromatic color vision is the ability to detect colored fruits against a background of green foliage. This suggests that the spectral characteristics of the red and green visual pigments had coevolved with the reflectance chromaticities of the natural environment in order to maximize the difference between the signals from a particular fruit and the surrounding foliage. Regan et al.[182] provided support for this hypothesis by showing that spectral tuning of the red and green cones of the trichromatic fruit-eating red howler monkey *Alouatta seniculus* is optimal for detecting yellow and orange fruits eaten by these monkeys under natural conditions of the rain forest.

## ADDENDUM

### 1. Red/green (R/G) cone ratios in the living human eye[185,186]

High-resolution imaging of the living human retina was accomplished using a high-magnification fundus camera equipped with adaptive optics that minimized corneal and lens aberrations. In one man, selected because of unusual green-sensitivity as determined by electroretinography, the R/G cone ratio was 1.15. In another randomly selected male subject, the R/G ratio was 3.79. Cones appeared randomly arranged in both subjects.

### 2. Red/green (R/G) cone pigment ratios in retinas of Old World monkeys[187]

The red:green cone ratio and distribution were investigated by mRNA and electrophysiologic measurements in the retina. The mRNA red/green ratio in the whole retina ranged from 0.6 to 7.0 (mean: 1.6 st. dev. 0.56; $n = 26$). This ratio did not change with eccentricity up to 9 mm (approximately 45 degrees), but was 30% greater in the temporal retina compared with the nasal retina. mRNA R/G ratios were in good agreement with R/G cone ratios in the same retinas as inferred from electrophysiologic measurements. Both the mRNA and electrophysiologic measures, therefore, reflect the relative number of red and \ green cones.

### 3. Direct visual resolution of gene copy number in the human photopigment gene array[188,189]

Fluorescent *in situ* hybridization allowed direct visualization of complete visual pigment gene arrays on single extended fibers of the X-chromosome. Using this novel technique, the number of genes per array in males was found to be identical to that measured by pulsed-field electrophoresis[134] in the same men. An average number of three genes per array was obtained by both of these direct methods, confirming earlier estimates with less direct techniques.[71,72]

### 4. Position of the green-red hybrid gene in the visual pigment gene array determines color-vision phenotype[190]

The crucial role of the specific location of a given in the visual pigment gene complex for determining color vision phenotype was demonstrated in men who carried three pigment genes: red gene, green gene, and green-red hybrid gene.[190] Such men on phenotypic testing were either deutans ($n = 12$) or had normal color vision ($n = 5$). Using long-range amplification by PCR allowed sequencing and positional assignment of the second and third gene of the array (the first gene always being the red gene). The red-green hybrid gene of all 12 color deficient deutans was always in the second position, whereas the red-green hybrid gene in the fiver men with normal color vision was in the third or terminal position. Thus, only the first two genes of the array are expressed in the retina. This was further confirmed by studying mRNA expression *in vitro* in fiver postmortein retinas where premortein color vision status was unknown. These retinas had three pigment genes, including one green-red hybrid gene. Only genes occupying the first (red gene) and the second position (green or green-red hybrid genes) were expressed as mRNA. Therefore, only genes in the first two positions of the color vision pigment array were expressed, whereas those in more distal positions were largely silent. However, unequal recombination events could rearrange the hybrid genes to the more proximal position resulting in their expression.

### 5. Complete achromatopsia

A second locus for recessive complete achromatopsia was identified at chromosome 8q 21–22 among the Pingelapese islanders of Micronesia,[191,192] who have a high incidence of this disorder. A unique Pingelap missense mutation and several mutations at this locus in other affected families were found in *CNGB3*, a new gene that encodes the $\beta$-subunit of the cone cyclic nucleotide (cGMP)-gated cation channel. Both the $\alpha$- and $\beta$-subunits of the cGMP-gated channel therefore are essential for phototransduction in all three classes of cone.

## REFERENCES

1. Gouras P: The history of colour vision, in Gouras P (ed): *Vision and Visual Dysfunctions*. Boca Raton, CRC Press, 1992, p 1.
2. Dalton J: Extraordinary facts relating to the vision of colours, with observations. *Mem Lit Philos Soc Lond* **5**:28, 1798.
3. Emery AEH: John Dalton (1766–1844). *J Med Genet* **25**:422, 1988.
4. Horner JF: Die Erblichkeit des Daltonismus. *Amtl Ber Verwalt Med Kantons Zurich* 108, 1876.
5. Wilson EB: The sex chromosomes. *Arch Mikrosk Anat Enwicklungsmech* **77**:249, 1911.
6. Bell J, Haldane JBS: The linkage between the genes for colour-blindness and haemophilia in man. *Proc R Soc Lond [B]* **123**:119, 1937.
7. Porter IH, Schulze J, McKusick VA: Linkage between G6PD-deficiency and colour blindness. *Nature* **193**:503, 1962.
8. Feil R, Aubourg P, Heilig R, Mandel JL: A 195-kb cosmid walk encompassing the human Xq28 color vision pigment genes. *Genomics* **6**:367, 1990.
9. Boynton RM: *Human Color Vision*. New York, Holt, Rinehard, Winston, 1979.
10. Nathans J, Thomas D, Hogness DS: Molecular genetics of human color vision: The genes encoding blue, green and red pigments. *Science* **232**:193, 1986.
11. Nathans J, Piantanida TP, Eddy RL, Shows TB, Hogness DS: Molecular genetics of inherited variation in human color vision. *Science* **232**:203, 1986.
12. Stiles WS, Burch JM: Colour-matching investigation: Final report (1958). *Optica Acta* **6**:1, 1959.
13. Alpern M, Wake T: Cone pigments in human deutan color vision defects. *J Physiol* **266**:595, 1977.
14. Alpern M, Pugh EN Jr: Variation in the acrtion spectrum of erythrolabe among deuteranopes. *J Physiol* **266**:613, 1977.
15. Alpern M, Moeller J: The red and green visual pigments of deuteranomalous trichromacy. *J Physiol* **266**:647, 1977.
16. Waaler GHM: Heredity of two types of colour normal vision. *Nature* **215**:406, 1967.
17. Neitz J, Jacobs GH: Polymorphism of the long-wavelength cone in normal human color vision. *Nature* **323**:623, 1986.
18. Winderickx J, Lindsey DT, Sanocki E, Teller DY, Motulsky AG, Deeb SS: Polymorphism in red photopigment underlies variation in colour matching. *Nature* **356**:431, 1992.
19. Deeb SS, Lindsey DT, Hibiya Y, Sanocki E, Winderickx J, Teller DY, Motulsky AG: Genotype-phenotype relationships in human red/green color vision defects: Molecular and psychophysical studies. *Am J Hum Genet* **51**:687, 1992.
20. Teller DY: Color vision, in Dulbecco R (ed): *Encyclopedia of Human Biology*. San Diego, Academic Press, 1991, p 575.
21. Cornsweet TN: *Visual Perception*. New York, Academic Press, 1970.
22. Lennie P, D'Zmura M: Mechanisms of color vision. *CRC Crit Rev Neurobiol* **3**:333, 1988.
23. Mollon JD, Sharpe LT (eds): *Colour Vision: Physiology and Psychophysics*. London, Academic Press, 1983.
24. Newton I: New theory about light and colours. *Phil Trans R Soc Lond* **80**:3075, 1671.
25. Young T: On the theory of light and colors. *Phil Trans R Soc Lond* **92**:20, 1802.
26. Maxwell JC: On colour vision. *Proc R Inst Great Britain* **6**:260, 1872.
27. Helmholtz HLF von: On the theory of compound colours. *Philsophical Magazine (Series 4)* **4**:519, 1852.
28. Dowling JE: *The Retina: An Approachable Part of the Brain*. Cambridge, MA, Harvard University Press, 1987.
29. Brown PK, Wald G: Visual pigments in single rods and cones of the human retina. *Science* **144**:45, 1964.

30. MacNichol EF, Levine JS, Mansfield RJW, et al: Microspectrophotometry of visual pigments in primate photoreceptors, in Mollon JD, Sharpe LT (eds): *Colour Vision: Physiology and Phychophysics*. London, Academic Press, 1983, p 13.

31. Dartnall HJA, Bowmaker JK, Mollon JD: Human visual pigments: Microspectrophotometric results from the eyes of seven persons. *Proc R Soc Lond [B]* **220**:115, 1983.

32. Rushton WAH: The Newton lecture: The chemical basis of colour vision and colour blindness. *Nature* **206**:1087, 1965.

33. Bowmaker JK, Astell S, Hung DM, Mollon JD: Photosensitive and photostable pigments in the retinae of Old World monkeys. *J Exp Biol* **55**:1, 1991.

34. Jacobs GH, Neitz J: Electrophysiological estimates of individual variation in the L/M cone ratio, in Drum B (ed): *Colour Vision Deficiencies XI*. The Netherlands, Kluwer Academic Publishers, 1993, p 107.

35. Rushton WAH, Baker HD: Red/green sensitivity in normal vision. *Vision Res* **4**:75, 1964.

36. Vimal RLP, Pokorny J, Smith VC, Shevell SK: Foveal cone thresholds. *Vision Res* **29**:61, 1989.

37. Cicerone CM, Nerger JL: The relative numbers of long-wavelength-sensitive and middle-wavelength-sensitive cones in the human fovea centralis. *Vision Res* **19**:115, 1989.

38. Wesner MF, Pokorny J, Shevell SK, Smith VC: Foveal cone detection statistics in color normals and dichromats. *Vision Res* **31**:1021, 1991.

39. Curcio CA, Allen KA, Sloan KR, Lerea CL, Hurley JB, Klock IB, Milam AH: Distribution and morphology of human cone photoreceptors stained with anti-blue opsin. *J Comp Neurol* **312**:610, 1991.

40. Wang JH, McDowell JH, Hargrave P: Site of attachment of 11-*cis*-retinal in bovine rhodopsin. *Biochemistry* **19**:5111, 1980.

41. Caron MC, Lefkowitz RJ: Model systems for the study of seven-transmembrane-segment receptors. *Annu Rev Biochem* **60**:653, 1991.

42. Henderson R: The purple membrane from *Halobacterium holobium*. *Annu Rev Biophys Bioengng* **6**:87, 1977.

43. Dohlman G, Thorner J, Caron M, Lefkowitz R: Model systems for the study of seven-transmembrane-segment receptors. *Annu Rev Biochem* **60**:653, 1991.

44. Fung BK-K, Hurley JB, Stryer L: Flow of information in the light-triggered cyclic nucleotide cascade of vision. *Proc Natl Acad Sci USA* **78**:152, 1981.

45. Fung BK-K, Stryer L: Photolyzed rhodopsin catalyzes the exchange of GTP for bound GDP in retinal rold outer segments. *Proc Natl Acad Sci USA* **77**:2500, 1980.

46. Stryer L: Visual excitation and recovery. *J Biol Chem* **266**:1071, 1991.

47. Jacobs GH: Within-species variation in visual capacity among squirrel monkeys (*Saimiri sciureus*): Sensitivity difference. *Vision Res* **23**:239, 1983.

48. Jacobs GH: Within-species variation in visual capacity among squirrel monkeys (*Saimiri sciureus*): Colour vision. *Vision Res* **24**:1267, 1984.

49. Jacobs GH, Neitz J: Inheritance of color vision in New World monkey (*Saimiri sciureus*). *Proc Natl Acad Sci USA* **84**:2545, 1987.

50. Jacobs GH, Neitz M, Deegan E, Neitz J: Trichromatic color vision among New World monkeys. *Nature* **382**:156, 1996.

51. Yokoyama S, Yokoyama R: Molecular evolution of human visual pigment genes. *Mol Biol Evol* **6**:186, 1989.

52. Mollon JD, Jordan G: Eine evolutionare Interpretation des menschlichen Farbensehen. *Die Farbe* **35/36**:139, 1988.

53. Bowmaker JK: The evolution of vertebrate visual pigments and photoreceptors, in Cronly-Dillon JR, Gregory RL (eds): *Vision and Visual Dysfunction*, Vol 2: *Evolution of Eye and Visual Systems*. London, Macmillan, 1991, p 63.

54. Wang Z, Asenjo AB, Oprian DD: Identification of the Cl-binding site in the human red and green color vision pigments. *Biochemistry* **32**:2125, 1993.

55. Nathans J, Weitz CJ, Agarwal N, Nir I, Papermaster DS: Production of bovine rhodopsin by mammalian cell lines expressing cloned cDNA: Spectrophotometry and subcellular localization. *Vision Res* **29**:907, 1989.

56. Merbs SL, Nathans J: Absorption spectra of the red-green and green-red hybrid pigments of anomalous color vision. *Science* **258**:464, 1992.

57. Oprian DD, Asenjo AB, Lee N, Pelletier SL: Design, chemical synthesis, and expression of genes for the three human color vision pigments. *Biochemistry* **30**:11367, 1991.

58. Kosower EM: Assignment of groups responsible for the "opsin shift" and light absorptions of rhodopsin and red, green, and blue iodopsins (cone pigments). *Proc Natl Acad Sci USA* **85**:1076, 1988.

59. Neitz M, Neitz J, Jacobs GH: Spectral tuning of pigments underlying red-green color vision. *Science* **252**:971, 1991.

60. Williams AJ, Hunt DM, Bowmaker JK, Mollon JD: The polymorphic pigments of the marmoset: spectral tuning and genetic basis. *EMBO J* **1**:2039, 1992.

61. Ibbotson RE, Hunt DM, Bowmaker JK, Mollon JD: Sequence divergence and copy number of the middle- and long-wave photopigments in Old World monkeys. *Proc R Soc Lond [B]* **247**:145, 1992.

62. Merbs SL, Nathans J: Absorption spectra of human cone pigments. *Nature* **356**:433, 1992.

63. Asenjo AB, Rim J, Oprian DD: Molecular determinants of human red/green color discrimination. *Neuron* **12**:1131, 1994.

64. Chan T, Lee M, Sakmar TP: Introduction of hydroxyl-bearing amino acids causes bathochromic spectral shifts in rhodopsin. *J Biol Chem* **267**:9478, 1992.

65. Nathans J, Hogness DS: Isolation, sequence analysis, and intron-exon arrangement of the gene encoding bovine rhodopsin. *Cell* **34**:807, 1983.

66. Martin RL, Wood C, Baehr W, Applebury ML: Visual pigment homologies revealed by DNA hybridization. *Science* **232**:1266, 1986.

67. Jorgensen AL, Deeb S, Motulsky AG: Molecular genetics of X-chromosome-linked color vision among populations of African and Japanese ancestry: High frequency of a shortened red pigment gene among Afro-Americans. *Proc Natl Acad Sci USA* **87**:6512, 1990.

68. Meagher M, Jorgensen AL, Deeb SS: Sequence and evolutionary history of the length polymorphism in intron 1 of the human red photopigment gene. *J Mol Evol* **43**:622, 1996.

69. Mosser J, Douar AM, Sarde CO, Kioschis P, Feil R, Moser H, Poustka AM, et al: Putative X-linked adrenoleukodystrophy gene shares unexpected homology with ABC transporters. *Nature* **361**:726, 1993.

70. Hamer DH, Hu S, Magnuson VL, Hu N, Pattatucci AML: A linkage between DNA markers on the X-chromosome and male sexual orientation. *Science* **261**:321, 1993.

71. Drummond-Borg M, Deeb S, Motulsky AG: Molecular patterns of X-chromosome-linked color vision genes among 134 men of European ancestry. *Proc Natl Acad Sci USA* **86**:983, 1989.

72. Yamaguchi T, Motulsky AG, Deeb SS: Visual pigment gene structure and expression in human retinae. *Hum Mol Genet* **6**:981, 1997.

73. de Vries HL: The heredity of the relative numbers of red and green receptors in the human eye. *Genetica* **24**:199, 1947.

74. Ichikawa H, Akio M: Genetic studies on defective color vision in junior high school students. *Mod Prob Ophthalmol* **13**:265, 1974.

75. Dartnall HJA, Bowmaker JK, Mollon JD: Human visual pigments: Microspectrophotometric results from the eyes of seven persons. *Proc R Soc Lond [B]* **220**:115, 1993.

76. Nerge JL, Cicerone CM: The ratio of L cones to M cones in the human parafoveal retina. *Vision Res* **32**:879, 1992.

77. Cicerone CM, Otake S: Color-opponent sites: Individual variability and changes with retinal eccentricity. *Investig Ophthalmol Vis Sci Suppl* **38**:2130, 1997.

78. Mollon JD, Bowmaker JK, Dartnall HJA, et al: Microspectrophotometric and psychophysical results fro the same deuteranopic observer, in Verriest G (ed): *Colour Vision Deficiencies VII*. The Netherlands, Dr W. Junk, 1984, p 303.

79. Packer OS, Williams DR, Bensinger DG: Photopigment transmittance imaging of the primate photoreceptor mosaic. *J Neurosci* **16**:2251, 1996.

80. Gowdy PD, Cicerone CM: The spatial arrangement of the L and M cones in the central fovea of the living human eye. *Vision Res* **38**:2575, 1998.

81. Hunt DM, Dulai KS, Bowmaker JK, Mollon JD: The chemistry of John Dalton's color blindness. *Science* **267**:984, 1995.

82. Kalmus H: *Diagnosis and Genetics of Defective Colour Vision*. Oxford, England, Pergamon Press, 1965.

83. Piantanida T: Genetics of inherited colour vision deficiencies, in Foster DH (ed): *Inherited and Acquired Colour Vision Deficiencies*. Boca Raton, FL, CRC Press, 1991, p 88.

84. Jaeger W: Genetics of congenital colour deficiencies, in Autrum VH, Jung R, Loewenstein D, McKay M, Teuber HL (eds): *Handbook of Sensory Physiology*. Heidelberg, Springer-Verlag, 1972, p 625.

85. Rushton WAH: A foveal pigment in the deuteranope. *J Physiol (Lond)* **176**:24, 1965.

86. Rushton WAH, Powell DS, White KD: Pigments in anomalous trichromats. *Vision Res* **13**:2017, 1973.

87. Piantanida T, Sperling H: Isolation of a third chromatic mechanism in the deuteranomalous observer. *Vision Res* **13**:2049, 1973.

88. Piantanida TP, Sperling HG: Isolation of a third chromatic mechanism in the protanomalous observer. *Vision Res* **13**:2033, 1973.

89. Francois J: *Heredity in Opthalmology.* St Louis, Mosby, 1961.

90. Wright WD: The characteristics of tritanopia. *J Opt Soc Am* **42**:509, 1952.

91. Went LN, Pronk N: The genetics of tritan distrubances. *Hum Genet* **69**:255, 1985.

92. Weitz CJ, Miyake Y, Shinzato K, Montag E, Zrenner E, Went LN, Nathans J: Human tritanopia associated with two amino acid substitutions in the blue sensitive opsin. *Am J Hum Genet* **50**:496, 1992.

93. Weitz CJ, Went LN, Nathans J: Human tritanopia associated with a third amino acid substitution in the blue-sensitive visual pigment. *Am J Hum Genet* **51**:444, 1992.

94. Knoblauch K, Bieber ML, Werner JS: M- and L-cones in early infancy: I. VEP responses to receptor-isolating stimuli at 4- and 8- weeks of age. *Vision Res* **38**:1753, 1998.

95. Birch J, Chisholm IA, Kinnear P, et al: Clinical testing methods, in Pokorny J, Smith VC, Verriest G, Pinckers AJLG (eds): *Congenital and Acquired Color Vision Defects.* New York, Grune & Stratton, 1979, p 83.

96. Anonymous: NRC Report: Procedures for testing color vision. Report of Working Group 41. Washington, DC, NRC-NAS, 1981 (*http://www.ul.cs.cmu.edu/books/color-vision/color.htm*).

97. Farnsworth D: *Farnsworth-Munsell 100 Hue Test for the Examination of Color Discrimination Manual.* Baltimore, Munsell Color Co., 1957.

98. Berson EL: Electrical phenomena in the retina, in Moses RA (ed): *Adler's Physiology of the Eye: Clinical Application.* St Louis, Mosby, 1975, p 453.

99. Hanazaki H, Tanabe J, Kawasaki K: Electroretinographic findings in congenital red-green color deficiency, in Ohta Y (ed): *Color Vision Deficiencies.* Berkeley, Kugler and Ghedini, 1990, p 71.

100. Pokorny J, Smith VC, Verriest G: Congenital color defects, in Pokorny J, Smith VC, Verriest G, Pinckers AJLG (eds): *Congenital and Acquired Color Vision Defects.* New York, Grune and Stratton, 1979, p 183.

101. Judd DB: Color blindness and the detection of camouflage. *Science* **97**:544, 1943.

102. Adam A: A further query on color blindness and natural selection. *Soc Biol* **16**:197, 1969.

103. Morgon MJ, Adam A, Mollon JD: Dichromats detect colour camouflaged objects that are not detected by trichomats. *Proc R Soc Lond [B]* **248**:291, 1992.

104. Verhulst S, Maes FW: Scotopic vision in colour-blinds. *Vision Res* **38**:3387, 1998.

105. Kuyk TK, Veres JG III, Lahey MA, Clark DJ: The ability of protan color defectives to perform color-dependent air traffic control tasks. *Am J Optom Physiol Opt* **63**:582, 1986.

106. Kuyk TK, Veres JG, Lahey MA, Clark DJ: Ability of deutan color defectives to perform simulated air traffic control tasks. *Am J Optom Physiol Opt* **64**:2, 1987.

107. Vingrys AJ, Cole BL: Are standards of colour vision in the transport industries justified? *Ophthalmol Physiol Opt* **8**:1257, 1988.

108. Cole B: Does defective colour vision really matter? in Drum B (ed): *Colour Vision Deficiencies XI.* The Netherlands, Kluwer Academic Publishers, 1993, p 67.

109. Webb N: Color-vision testing for airline pilots. *JAMA* **258**:841, 1987.

110. Steward JM, Cole BL: What do color vision defectives say about everyday tasks? *Optom Vis Sci* **66**:288, 1989.

111. Verriest G, Neubauer O, Marre M, et al: New investigations on the relationships between congenital colour vision defects and road traffic safety, in Verriest G (ed): *Colour Vision Deficiencies,* Vol V. Bristol, Hilger, 1980, p 331.

112. Whillans MG, Allen MJ: Color defective drivers and safety. *Optom Vis Sci* **69**:463, 1992.

113. Vollrath D, Nathans J, Davis RW: Tandem array of huma visual pigment genes at Xq28. *Science* **240**:1669, 1988.

114. Windericks J, Battisti L, Hibiya Y, Motulsky AG, Deeb SS: Haplotype diversity in the human red and green opsin genes: Evidence for frequent sequence exchange in exon 3. *Hum Mol Genet* **2**:1413, 1993.

115. Neitz J, Neitz M, Jacobs GH: Analysis of fusion gene and encoded photopigment of colour-blind humans. *Nature* **342**:679, 1989.

116. Deeb SS, Windericks J, Motulsky AG: Correlation between Rayleigh match range in protans and deutans and the difference in $\lambda_{max}$ between hybrid and normal pigments, in Drum B (ed): *Documenta Ophthalmologica Proceedings Series 57: Color Vision Deficiencies XII.*

Dordrecht, The Netherlands, Kluwer Academic Publishers, 1995, p. 119.

117. Winderickx J, Sanocki E, Lindsey DT, Teller DY, Motulsky AG, Deeb SS: Defective colour vision associated with a missense mutation in the human green visual pigment gene. *Nature Genet* **1**:251, 1992.

118. Nathans J, Davenport CM, Maumenee IH, Heijtmancik JF, Litt M, Loverien E, Weleber R, et al: Molecular genetics of blue cone monochromacy. *Science* **245**:831, 1990.

119. Nathans J, Merbs SL, Sung CH, Weitz CJ, Wang Y: Molecular genetics of human visual pigments. *Annu Rev Genet* **26**:403, 1992.

120. Applebury M, Hargrave PA: Molecular biology of the visual pigments. *Vision Res* **26**:1881, 1986.

121. Karnik SS, Sakmar TP, Chen HB, Khorana HG: Cysteine residues 110 and 187 are essential for the formation of correct structure in bovine rhodopsin. *Proc Natl Acad Sci USA* **85**:8459, 1988.

122. Dixon RAF, Sigal IS, Candelore MR, Register RB, Scattergood W, Rands E, Strader CD: Structural features required for ligand binding to the β-adrenergic receptor. *EMBO J* **6**:3269, 1987.

123. Dryja TP, McGee TL, Hahn LB, Cowley GS, Ollson JE, Reichel E, Sandberg MA, et al: Mutations within the rhodopsin gene in patients with autosomal dominant retinitis pigmentosa. *New Engl J Med* **323**:1302, 1990.

124. Tnglehearn CF, Keen TJ, Bashir R, Jay M, Fitzke F, Bird AC, Crombie A, et al: A completed screen for mutations of the rhodopsin gene in a panel of patients with autosomal dominant retinitis pigmentosa. *Hum Mol Genet* **1**:41, 1992.

125. Reichel E, Bruce AM, Sandberg MA, Berson EL: An electroretinographic and molecular genetic study of X-linked cone degeneration. *Am J Ophthalmol* **108**:540, 1989.

126. Drummond-Borg M, Deeb S, Motulsky AG: Molecular basis of abnormal red-green color vision: A family with three types of color vision defects. *Am J Hum Genet* **43**:675, 1988.

127. Hurvich LM: Color vision deficiencies, in Jameson D, Hurvich LM (eds): *Handbook of Sensory Physiology.* Berlin, Springer-Verlag, 1972, p 581.

128. Nagy AL, Purl KF: Color discrimination and neural coding in color vision deficients. *Vision Res* **27**:483, 1987.

129. Pokorny J, Smith VC: The functional nature of polymorphism of human color vision, in Anonymous (ed): *Frontiers of Visual Sciences: Proceedings of a 1985 Symposium.* Washington, National Academy Press, 1987, p 150.

130. Winderickx J, Battisti L, Motulsky AG, Deeb SS, Adam A: Selective expression of the human X-linked green opsin genes. *Proc Natl Acad Sci USA* **89**:9710, 1992.

131. Sjoberg SA, Neitz M, Balding S, Neitz J: L-cone pigments genes expressed in normal colour vision. *Vision Res* **38**:3213, 1998.

132. Crognale MA, Teller DY, Motulsky AG, Deeb SS: Severity of color vision defects: Electroretinographic (ERG), molecular and behavioral studies. *Vision Res* **38**:3213, 1998.

133. Neitz M, Neitz J: Numbers and ratios of visual pigment genes for normal red-green color vision. *Science* **267**:1013, 1995.

134. Macke JP, Nathans J: Individual variation in size of the human red and green visual pigment gene array. *Invest Ophthalmol Vis Sci* **38**:1040, 1997.

135. Behringer RR, Ryan TM, Palmiter RD, Brinster RL, Townes TM: Human d to β-globin gene switching in transgenic mice. *Genes Dev* **4**:380, 1990.

136. Enver T, Raich N, Ebens AJ, Papyannopoulou T, Constantini F, Stamatoyannopoulos G: Developmental regulation of human fetal-to-adult globin gene switching in transgenic mice. *Nature* **344**:309, 1990.

137. Stamatoyannopoulos G: Human hemoglobin switching. *Science* **252**:383, 1991.

138. Hanscombe O, Whyatt D, Fraser P, Yannoutsos N, Greaves D, Dillon N, Grosveld F: Importance of globin gene order to correct developmental expression. *Genes Dev* **5**:1387, 1991.

139. Wang Y, Macke JP, Merbs SL, Zack D, Klaunberg B, Bennet J, Gearhart J, et al: A locus control region adjacent to the human red and green visual pigment genes. *Neuron* **9**:429, 1992.

140. Lewis RA, Holcomb JD, Bromley WC, Wilson MC, Roderick TH, Hejtmancik JF: Mapping X-linked ophthalmic diseases: III. Provisional assignment of the locus for blue cone monochromacy to Xq28. *Arch Ophthalmol* **105**:1055, 1987.

141. Kazmi MA, Sakmar TP, Ostrer H: Mutation of a conserved cysteine in the X-linked cone opsin causes color vision deficiencies by disrupting protein folding and stability. *Invest Ophthalmol Vis Sci* **38**:1047, 1997.

142. Richards JE, Scott KM, Sieving PA: Disruption of conserved rhodopsin disulfide bond by Cys187Tyr mutation causes early and severe

autosomal dominant retinitis pigmentosa. *Ophthalmology* **102**:669, 1995.

143. Reyniers E, Van Thienen MN, Meire F, De Boulle K, Devries K, Kestelijn P, Willems PJ: Gene conversion between red and defective green opsin gene in blue cone monochromacy. *Genomics* **29**:323, 1995.

144. Ladekjaer-Mikkelsen AS, Rosenberg T, Jorgensen AL: A new mechanism in blue cone monochromatism. *Hum Genet* **98**:403, 1996

145. Van Heel L, Went LN, Van Norren D: Frequency of tritan disturbances in a population study. *Color Vision Defic* **5**:256, 1980.

146. Krill AE, Smith VC, Pokorny J: Further studies supporting the identity of congenital tritanopia and hereditary dominant optic atrophy. *Invest Ophthalmol* **10**:45, 1971.

147. Miyake Y, Yagasaki K, Ichikawa H: Differential diagnosis of congenital tritanopia and dominantly inherited juvenile optic atrophy. *Arch Ophthalmol* **103**:496, 1985.

148. Arbour NC, Zlotogora J, Knowlton RG, Merin S, Rosenmann A, Kanis AB, Rokhlina T, et al: Homozygosity mapping of achromatopsia to chromosome 2 using DNA pooling. *Hum Mol Genet* **6**:689, 1997.

149. Yu WP, Grunwald ME, Yau KW: Molecular cloning, functional expression and chromosomal localization of a human homolog of the cyclic nucleotide-gated ion channel of retinal cone photoreceptors. *FEBS Lett* **393**:211, 1996.

150. Kohl S, Marx T, Giddings I, Jagle H, Jacobson SG, Apfelsted-Sylla E, Zrenner E, et al: Total color blindness is caused by mutations in the gene encoding the α-subunit of the cone photoreceptor cGMP-gated channel. *Nature Genet* **19**:257, 1998.

151. Eisner A, MacLeod DIA: Flicker photometric study of chromatic adaptation: Selective suppression of cone inputs by colored backgrounds. *J Opt Soc Am* **71**:705, 1981.

152. Elsner AE, Burns SA: Classes of color normal observers. *J Opt Soc Am* **4**:123, 1987.

153. Neitz J, Jacobs GH: Polymorphism in normal huma color vision and its mechanism. *Vision Res* **30**:621, 1990.

154. Alpern MJ: Lack of uniformity in colour matching. *J Physiol* **288**:85, 1979.

155. Deeb SS, Alvarez A, Malkki M, Motulsky AG: Molecular patterns and sequence polymorphisms in the red and green visual pigment genes of Japanese men. *Hum Genet* **95**:501, 1995.

156. Lascari AD, Hoak JC, Taylor JC: Christmas disease in a girl. *Am J Dis Child* **117**:585, 1969.

157. Ingerslev J, Schwartz M, Lamm LU, Kruse TA, Bukh A, Stenberg S: Female haemophilia A in a family with seeming extreme bidirectional lyonization tendency: Abnormal premature X-chromasome inactivation? *Clin Genet* **35**:41, 1989.

158. Jorgensen AL, Philip J, Raskind WH, Matsushita M, Christensen B, Dreyer V, Motulsky AG: Different patterns of X inactivation in MZ twins discordant for red-green color-vision deficiency. *Am J Hum Genet* **51**:291, 1992.

159. Nettleship E: Some unusual pedigrees of color blindness. *Trans Ophthalmol Soc UK* **32**:309, 1912.

160. Stocks P, Karn MN: A biometric investigation of twins and their brothers and sisters. *Ann Eugen* **5**:17, 1933.

161. Walls GL: Peculiar color blindness in peculiar people. *AMA Arch Ophthalmol* **62**:41, 1959.

162. Kourlischer L, Zanen J, Meunier A: *La theorie de Lyon peut-elle expliquer la desparite exceptionnellment observee de la perception coloree chez des jumelles univitellines? Comptes-rendues du 1er Congres International de Neuro-Ophtalmologie.* Basel, Karger, 1968.

163. Philip J, Vogelius-Anderson CH, Dreyer V, Freiesleben E, Gurtler H, Hauge M, Kissmeyer-Nielsen F, et al: Color vision deficiency in one of two presumably monozygotic twins with secondary amenorhoea. *Ann Hum Genet* **33**:185, 1969.

164. Yokota A, Shin Y, Kimura J, et al: Congenital deuteranomaly in one of three MZ triplets, in Ohta Y (ed): *Color Vision Deficiencies VIII.* Tokyo, Kuguler Ghedini, 1990, p 199.

165. Born G, Grutzner P, Hemminger H: Evidenz fur eine Mosaikstruktur der Netzhaut bei Konduktorinnen fur dichromasie. *Hum Genet* **32**:189, 1976.

166. Grutzner P, Born G, Hemminger HJ: Colored stimuli within the central visual field of carriers of dichromatism. *Mod Prob Ophthalmol* **17**:147, 1976.

167. Cohn SA, Emmerich DS, Carlson EA: Differences in the responses of heterozygous carriers of colorblindness and normal controls to briefly presented stimuli. *Vision Res* **29**:255, 1989.

168. Jordan G, Mollon JD: A study of women heterozygous for colour deficiencies. *Vision Res* **33**:1495, 1993.

169. Verriest G: Chromaticity discrimination in protan and deutan heterozygotes. *Farbe* **21**:7, 1972.

170. Kainz PM, Neitz M, Neitz J: Molecular detection of female carriers of protan defects. *Vision Res* **38**:3365, 1998.

171. Nemoto H, Murao M: A genetic studies of colorblindness. *Jpn J Hum Genet* **6**:165, 1961.

172. Crooks KBM: Further observations on color blindness among Negroes with genealogic and geographic notes. *Hum Biol* **8**:451, 1936.

173. Adam A: Colorblindness in Africa. *Metabol Pediatr Opthalmol* **5**:181, 1981.

174. Adam A: Polymorphisms of red-green vision among populations of the tropics, in Roberts DF, De Stefano GF (eds): *Genetic Variation and Its Maintenance.* Cambridge, England, Cambridge University Press, 1986, p 245.

175. Adam A: A call for re-examination of the selection-relaxation theory, in Ahuja YR, Neel JV (eds): *Genetic Microdifferentiation in Human and Other Animal Populations.* Dehli, India, Indian Anthropological Association, 1985, p 181.

176. Filippi G, Rinaldi A, Palmarino R, Seravalli E, Siniscalco M: Linkage disequilibrium for two X-linked genes in Sardinia and its bearing on the statistical mapping of the human X chromosome. *Genetics* **86**:199, 1977.

177. Post RH: Population differences in red and green colour vision deficiency: Review and query on selection relaxation. *Eugen Q* **9**:131, 1962.

178. Post RH: Possible cases of relaxed selection in civilized populations. *Humangenetik* **13**:253, 1971.

179. Cruz-Coke R, Varela A: Inheritance of alcoholism: Its association with color blindness. *Lancet* **2**(7476):1282, 1966.

180. Mollon JD: On the origins of polymorphisms, in Committee on Vision (ed): *Frontiers of Visual Science.* Washington, National Academy Press, 1987.

181. Hunt DM, Dulai KS, Cowing JA, Julliot C, Mollon JD, Bowmaker JK, Li WH, et al: Molecular evolution of trichromacy in primates. *Vision Res* **38**:3299, 1998.

182. Regan BC, Julliot C, Simmen B, Vienot F, Charles-Domique P, Mollon JD: Frugivory and color vision in *Alouatta seniculus*, a trichromatic platyrrhine monkey. *Vision Res* **38**:3321, 1998.

183. Deeb S, Jorgensen AL, Battisti L, Iwasaki L, Motulsky AG: Sequence divergence of the red and green visual pigments in the great apes and humans. *Proc Natl Acad Sci USA* **91**:7262, 1998.

184. Mollon J: Mixing genes and mixing colors. *Curr Biol* **3**:82, 1993.

185. Roorda A, Williams DR: The arrangement of the three cone classes in the living human eye. *Nature* **397**:320, 1999.

186. Williams DR, Roorda A: The trichromatic come mosaic in the human eye. In Gegenfurtner KR, Sharpe LT (eds): *Color vision: from Genes to Perception.* Cambridge, UK, Cambridge University Press, 1999, p. 113.

187. Deeb SS, Diller LC, Williams DR, Dacey DM: Interindividual and topographical variation of L:M cone ratios in monkey retinas. *J Opt Soc Am A Opt Image Sci Vis* **17**:538, 2000.

188. Wolf S, Sharpe LT, Schmidt HJ, Knau H, et al.: Direct visual resolution of gene copy number in the human photopigment gene array. *Invest Ophthalmol Vis Sci* **40**:1585, 1999.

189. Sharpe LT, Stockman A, Jägle H, Nathans J: Opsin genes, cone photopigments, color vision, and color blindness. In Gegenfurtner KR, Sharpe LT (eds): *Color Vision: from Genes to Perception.* Cambridge, UK, Cambridge University Press, 1999, p. 3.

190. Hayashi T, Motulsky AG, Deeb SS: Position of a "green-red" hybrid gene in the visual pigment gene array determines colour-vision phenotype. *Nat Genet* **22**:90, 1999.

191. Winick JD, Blundell ML, Galke BL, Salam AA, Leal SM, Karayiorgou M: Homozygosity mapping of the Achromatopsia locus in the Pingelapese. *Am J Hum Genet* **64**:1679–1685, 1999.

192. Sundin O, Yang J-M, Li Y, Zhu Z, Hurd JN, Mitchell TN, Silva ED, Maumenee IH: Genetic basis of total colour blindness among the Pingelapese islanders. *Nat Genet* **5**:289, 2000.

# Norrie Disease

*Wolfgang Berger* ■ *Hans-Hilger Ropers*

1. **Norrie disease (ND) (MIM 310600) is a severe form of congenital blindness characterized by degenerative and proliferative changes in the neuroretina and vitreous followed by progressive atrophy of the eyes.**
2. **Leukokoria, due to retrolental structures and retinal detachment, can be recognized shortly after birth. Other ocular hallmarks of ND are persistent hyperplastic primary vitreous, hyaloid vessels, shallow anterior chamber, and vitreoretinal hemorrhages.**
3. **One-third of patients are mentally retarded and develop sensorineural deafness. Occasionally, other clinical features are seen, including hypogonadism and microcephaly, some of which may be due to defects extending to neighboring genes.**
4. **The disease is inherited as an X-linked recessive trait. Male-to-male transmission has been excluded, and carrier females are usually healthy.**
5. **Linkage and deletion mapping studies have assigned the *ND* locus to a 600-kb segment of the Xp11.3-p11.4 interval and paved the way for its isolation by positional cloning.**
6. **The gene encodes a 133-amino-acid polypeptide with an N-terminal signal sequence and a C-terminal cysteine-knot motif. It shows homology with proteins involved in cell interaction and differentiation processes. Computer modeling and expression studies suggest the formation of homodimers via the C-terminal Cys-knot.**
7. **So far mutations have been described in more than 90 patients with ND. Missense mutations are the most frequent (50 percent), followed by deletions (15–20 percent) and nonsense mutations (13 percent). Mutations in this gene can give rise to three clinically distinct phenotypes, i.e., ND, exudative vitreoretinopathy (EVR) (MIM 143200), and retinopathy of prematurity (ROP).**
8. **A mouse mutant lacking the N-terminal portion of the *ND* gene was generated by gene targeting. Mutant mice show histologic and pyhsiologic changes in the innermost layers of the retina, including the ganglion and nerve fiber layers.**

Norrie disease (ND) (OMIM 310600) is a severe X-linked recessive form of congenital blindness characterized by progressive atrophy of the eye and a variety of other ocular symptoms. At least one-third of patients are mentally retarded and develop hearing loss later in life. Linkage studies assigned the underlying gene defect to the proximal short arm of the X chromosome, just proximal to the genes for the monoamine oxidases A and B. The *ND* gene was isolated by positional cloning, and mutations have been described in more than 90 patients worldwide. Mutations in the *ND* gene also have been found in patients with exudative vitreoretinopathy (EVR) (MIM 143200) and retinopathy of prematurity (ROP), two clinically distinct phenotypes characterized by abnormal retinal vascularization, vitreoretinal hemorrhages, and retinal detachment. In ND, too, the severity of the

disease and its clinical course can vary widely, even among members of the same family. Mutation screening is facilitated by the small size of the *ND* gene, and reliable molecular diagnosis is possible.

The function of the *ND* gene is not yet known in detail, but protein homologies, computer modeling data, first biochemical analyses, and histologic examination of a mouse mutant suggest that the protein acts as an extracellular growth factor in the inner retina, possibly playing a role in the vascularization of the neuronal layers.

## CLINICAL CONSIDERATIONS

In 1961, Mette Warburg reported a Danish family with 7 affected males in four generations suffering from congenital blindness and pseudotumour of the retina.[1] In 5 of these patients, deafness developed later in life, and 4 were mentally handicapped. A literature survey revealed 48 similar cases in 9 families. Warburg named this disease after another Danish ophthalmologist, Gordon Norrie, who had described a similar condition in 1927. All 9 families reviewed by Warburg showed X-chromosomal recessive transmission but variable clinical manifestations of the disease.[2–4]

### The Ocular Phenotype

Bilateral leukokoria, caused by retrolental membranes and detachment of the retina, is one of the earliest findings in ND and can be recognized soon after birth. In the course of the disease, the eyes shrink and become atrophic (hence *atrophia bulborum hereditaria*, another designation of the disease). Other ocular manifestations include cataract, shallow anterior chamber, anterior and posterior synechiae, retrolental fibrovascular tissue, vitreoretinal hemorrhages, retinal folding and detachment, bilateral and congenital pseudotumor of the retina (pseudoglioma), and hyperplasia of the retinal pigment epithelium.[5–7] Alterations in the vitreous body are reminiscent of remnants of hyaloid vessels and a persistent primary vitreous.[6] In some cases, a marked dilatation of iris vessels has been observed. Histologic sections from patients show attenuation and disorganization of the nuclear layers of the retina with rosettes comprised of photoreceptor and bipolar cells,[8] a severely decreased number of ganglion cells,[8,9] and dislocation of some of the residual ganglion cells to the inner plexiform layer.[9] Abnormal retinal fibrovascularization, large areas of hemorrhages, and subretinal exudates also were described.[10,11]

Most of the published histologic data concern rather advanced stages of the disease. They were obtained from eyes enucleated in early childhood on suspicion of retinoblastoma. There is one report in the literature on the histology of the retina in an 11-week-old fetus at risk.[12] Development of the retinal pigment epithelium and stratification of the retina were considered normal, with an intact nerve fiber layer and neuroblasts differentiating into inner and outer layers. Posterior to the neuroblastic layer was a zone of photoreceptor proliferation without outer-segment formation. Increased glial cell proliferation was not found either in the retina or in the optic nerve. In addition, the primary vitreous was normally vascularized. These data suggest that early prenatal development is normal and that first signs of the disease do not

---

A list of standard abbreviations is located immediately preceding the index in each volume. Nonstandard abbreviations used in this chapter include: ND = Norrie disease; EVR = exudative vitreoretinopathy; ROP = retinopathy of prematurity.

develop before gestational week 11. However, the molecular diagnosis in this patient was only based on segregation of closely linked DNA markers, and there is no direct molecular proof that this fetus was really affected. Morphologic and histologic data from patients with established *ND* gene mutations are available from three independent reports. The first was obtained from an enucleated eye of a simplex case at 2 months of age.[13] The ocular manifestations include a wrinkled posterior lens capsule, elongated ciliary processes with proliferation of ciliary epithelium cells, large retrolental blood vessels (most likely presenting remnants of the hyaloid artery), and a detached hemorrhagic and gliotic retina containing rosettes as a feature of retinal dysplasia.

The second case, a specimen obtained during vitreoretinal surgery of a 6-month-old boy, displays complete detachment of the incoherently vascularized retina in the right eye and less advanced intraocular changes in the left eye, where detachment and membrane formation were limited to the posterior pole.[9] There was no evidence of persisting hyaloid blood vessels. The detached retina showed a severe reduction in the number of retinal ganglion cells. The inner nuclear layer showed striking disorganization and hypoplasia. Only a few blood vessels were visible. Outer nuclear and photoreceptor cell layers revealed only minor morphologic changes with rosette-like structures; extensive fibrovascular proliferation was seen in the vitreous.

The third depiction of histologic characteristics in ND was obtained from an enucleated eye at 1 month after birth.[14] Histologic examination demonstrated a totally detached dysplastic retina with rosettes. There also was evidence of gliosis but no abnormal vascularization.

**Mental Retardation and Deafness.** At least one-third of patients are mentally retarded and develop sensorineural deafness later in life. Many studies have shown that mental retardation and progressive sensorineural hearing loss can be highly variable, even within one family. Among 35 affected males from six families from Sweden and Denmark studied by Warburg,[4] 20 showed mental retardation. Of these, 9 were severely mentally retarded, whereas 11 showed a moderate deficiency. Eleven of 35 patients had progressive hearing loss, ranging from total deafness to minor hearing impairment which could be treated with hearing aids. Another study reported 10 affected males in three generations of a family from Egypt.[15] Two of the affected males showed profound deafness, and 3 patients were moderately hard of hearing.

Histologic data were obtained from the ear of a 77-year-old affected male from a family with 7 affected individuals in four generations.[16] The propositus had been blind shortly after birth and had shown developmental delay. At 12 years of age, his IQ was 50. Impaired hearing was first noticed at the age of 30 years. Audiometric testing at the age of 75 years revealed profound sensorineural hearing loss. Vestibular function was normal in this patient. Severe degeneration of the hair cells in the organ of Corti was observed, which was most prominent in the basal turn. In addition, the tectorial membrane and stria vascularis exhibited severe degenerative changes in both ears. A marked loss of spiral ganglion cells was found, and deposits of collageneous fibrous tissue were seen between the remaining spiral ganglion cells. The fibrosis was particularly pronounced around some blood vessels within Rosenthal's canal. Histologic examination of the brain did not reveal specific alterations.[16]

Recent studies have shown that ocular symptoms, mental retardation, and deafness are pleiotropic effects of mutations in a single gene (see below).

## Pathogenic Mechanisms Leading to ND

Concerning the primary defect and early pathogenetic events, two different hypotheses have been put forward:

1. An early neuroectodermal defect may lead to premature arrest in retinal development with associated malformations in the primary and secondary vitreous.[3] According to this model, changes in the retina are primary. Consequently, development of the secondary vitreous (which originates exclusively from the retina) fails. This leads to proliferation of the primary vitreous, which fills the interior of the eye, and subsequently, the eye becomes atrophic. Alterations in the brain and ear, leading to mental deterioration and sensorineural hearing loss, also can be explained by a defect in neuroectodermal development.

2. Abnormal vascular proliferation may result in the formation of retrolental membranes and masses, thereby producing tractional forces that separate the developing retina from the retinal pigment epithelium.[12] This may then lead to secondary retinal dysplasia.

## Atypical and Syndromic Forms of ND

ND patients have been described with very complex phenotypes. Moreira-Filho and Neustein presented a presumptive new variant of ND in a Brazilian Negro sibship with six affected males.[17] In addition to the characteristic ocular stigmata, all patients were microcephalic, and two of them had cryptorchidism and absent pubic and axillary hair. Microcephaly also was diagnosed in several patients of an Egyptian family with ND.[15] In addition, some patients displayed short distal phalanges of the thumbs as well as sexual impotence by age 30 in three cases. Microcephaly, hypogonadism, growth retardation, and immunodeficiency were found in a patient reported by Gal et al.[18] Additional ND cases with an atypical clinical course including growth and developmental delays as well as gonadal hypoplasia have been described (Table 239-1). Frequently, submicroscopic interstitial deletions of the proximal short arm of the X chromosome were found in these patients, suggesting that these complex phenotypes are due to the involvement of adjacent genes.

## Differential Diagnosis

The spectrum of diseases that show one or more of the ocular hallmarks of ND include retinoblastoma, persistent hyperplastic primary vitreous (PHPV), familial EVR, retinal dysplasia of Reese, Coat's disease, and X-linked juvenile retinoschisis (XLRS). In the vast majority of the patients, differential diagnosis is possible on clinical grounds alone or by a combination of clinical examination and DNA analysis. In contrast to ND, leukokoria associated with a persistent hyperplastic primary vitreous is usually unilateral and is not inherited in an X-linked recessive fashion.[19] Retinal dysplasia of Reese is often associated with severe extraocular malformations of the head, lung, heart, urogenital system, or skeleton and leads to death usually within the first year of life. ND, ROP, and familial EVR can be distinguished from retinoblastoma and XLRS by mutation analysis in the respective genes. ROP is characterized by abnormal retinal vascularization and neovascularization, retinal traction, falciform folding, and detachment. Clinical manifestations in exudative vitreoretinopathy comprise defective vascularization of the retina, retinal folding and detachment, and vitreoretinal hemorrhages. In both ROP and familial EVR, mutations in the *ND* gene have been detected (see below), but neither of the diseases is associated with mental deficiency nor hearing impairment. Infants with ND frequently are diagnosed as having retinoblastoma, which also can occur bilaterally. Retinoblastoma is due to mutations in a tumor-suppressor gene that was cloned in 1986.[20] Likewise, the gene for XLRS has been isolated recently, and mutation detection is possible in more than 90 percent of patients.[21,22]

# GENETICS OF ND

## Genetic and Physical Mapping of the *ND* Locus

The hereditary nature of the disease and its X-chromosomal mode of inheritance have been amply documented. Family studies

**Table 239-1** Extraocular Symptoms in ND Patients with Complex Phenotypes

| Clinical Symptoms | Chromosomal Rearrangement | Reference |
|---|---|---|
| Hypogonadism | Not examined | 67 |
| Microcephaly, intrafamilial variability of hypogonadism (bilateral cryptorchidism, absent pubic and axillary hair) | Not examined | 17 |
| General hypotonia, abnormal EEG, cleft lip, high-arched palate | t(X;10) | 41 |
| Microcephaly, short thumbs, intrafamilial variability of sexual impotence at age > 30 | Not examined | 15 |
| Microcephaly, immunodeficiency, growth retardation, hypogonadism | del(DXS7, MAOA, MAOB, ND) | 18,36 |
| Growth retardation, microcephaly, hypogonadism, seizures but normal EEG, severe developmental retardation | del DXS7 | 68 |
| Developmental delay, hampered in walking, cannot speak, self-abusive behavior | del(DXS77, DXS7) | 69 |
| Several developmental delays, microcephaly, small stature, hypotnia | del (MAOA, MAOB, ND exon 3) | 36,38 |
| Gonadal hypoplasia, scarce pubic hair | inv(ND exon 2) | 36; WB, unpublished data |

revealed (1) the absence of male-to-male transmission, (2) that, in general, women are not affected, and (3) that, in pedigrees, all affected males are related through their mothers. In 1985, tight linkage of the *ND* gene with *DXS7*, a DNA marker from the proximal short arm of the X chromosome, established its assignment to the Xp11.4-p11.3 interval.[23,24] Shortly thereafter, *DXS7* was found to be deleted in several patients with ND. In most of these patients, the genes for the monoamine oxidases A and B (*MAOA* and *MAOB*) were deleted as well[18,25–30] (see Table 239-1). MAOA and MAOB are both involved in the degradation of biogenic amine neurotransmitters and play important neurophysiologic roles that render their genes promising candidate genes for ND. Soon it became clear, however, that MAOA and MAOB activities are normal in most patients with ND, indicating that *MAO* gene defects do not play a role in this disease.[31] This was corroborated by the finding that mutations in the *MAOA* gene give rise to behavioral changes but do not cause abnormalities of the eye.[32–34] The identification of a recombination event separating *DXS7* and *ND*[35] and detailed characterization of microdeletions assigned the *ND* locus to a small chromosome segment proximal to *DXS7* and the *MAO* genes.[36–38]

## Positional Cloning of the *ND* Gene

A yeast artificial chromosome (YAC) clone was isolated and subcloned to generate a cosmid contig encompassing the relevant Xp segment.[36] Individual clones from this contig were used to screen ND patients for additional microdeletions by Southern blot analysis. In this way, several deletions were identified varying in size between two and several hundred kilobases. Some of the deletions did not overlap; therefore, DNA sequences separating these deletions had to contain at least part of the *ND* gene (Fig. 239-1). Genomic clones from the relevant interval were used to screen cDNA libraries from fetal brain and adult retinal tissue. This led to identification of expressed sequences corresponding to a 1.8-kb transcript in RNA from brain and retina and, eventually, to isolation of cDNA clones spanning the entire gene.[36,37] The gene is not expressed in adult heart, spleen, lung, liver, skeletal muscle, and testis, as shown by Northern blot analysis. Sequence analysis revealed an open reading frame of 133 amino acids. With the cDNA as probe, deletions were detected in almost 20 percent of patients, which rendered this gene a strong candidate for *ND*.[36,37]

Characterization of its genomic structure and subsequent mutation analysis provided conclusive evidence for its causative role in ND. Exon-intron boundaries were determined by sequencing of genomic DNA fragments that hybridized to the complementary DNA. The coding sequence was shown to be interrupted by two introns of 15 and 9 kb, and the 3 exons consist of 209, 381, and 1245 bp, respectively. The translation start codon is in exon 2.[39,40]

## Mutation Spectrum in Patients and Genotype-Phenotype Correlations

Since isolation of the gene in 1992, a large number of mutations have been described. Their spectrum includes a translocation,[41] an inversion,[42] several deletions,[36,37,43] and more than 70 point mutations. The majority of the point mutations represent missense (47) and nonsense (12) mutations (Table 239-2 and Fig. 239-2). Frameshift and splice-site mutations were observed in 9 and 4 patients, respectively.[9,39,44–46]

Mutations in the *ND* gene also were detected in patients with X-linked recessive and sporadic familial EVR and advanced ROP (stages 4B and 5) (for references, see Table 239-1). In general, mutations at position 121 give rise to a less severe phenotype, characterized by mild ND, familial EVR, or ROP.[47–49] While this holds true for Arg → Trp mutations, Arg → Gln mutations at the same position have been found in patients with mild and classic ND, as in 11 affected males from a Spanish family who were born blind and presented with the full-blown picture of ND.[50] Similarly, a Lys → Asn mutation at position 58 can lead to classic ND but also to familial EVR.[48,50]

Intrafamilial variability of the ocular phenotype was reported in a large Polish pedigree with 12 affected males, all but one presenting with the characteristic ocular symptoms.[51] The only exception was a 40-year-old male who had the same *ND* gene mutation as all other patients in this family (A63D). In this patient, vision was partially preserved until his fifth decade. Slit-lamp biomicroscopy revealed remnants of a persistent primary vitreous and hyaloid artery, and on angiography, the peripheral retina was shown to be avascular. Partially preserved vision was reported in a few other patients but is very rare. Detailed clinical examination of patients with defined molecular defects also has revealed that mental retardation and deafness, which occur in at least one-third of patients, are pleiotropic effects of mutations in the *ND* gene.[39,44] The fact that the same mutation can give rise to quite different phenotypes suggests the involvement of additional genetic or environmental factors in the pathogenesis of this disorder.

Venous insufficiency was shown to cosegregate with ND in 15 affected males from a large Costa Rican family with a missense mutation L61F in the *ND* gene.[52] This may indicate that venous insufficiency is another pleiotropic effect of *ND* gene mutations or

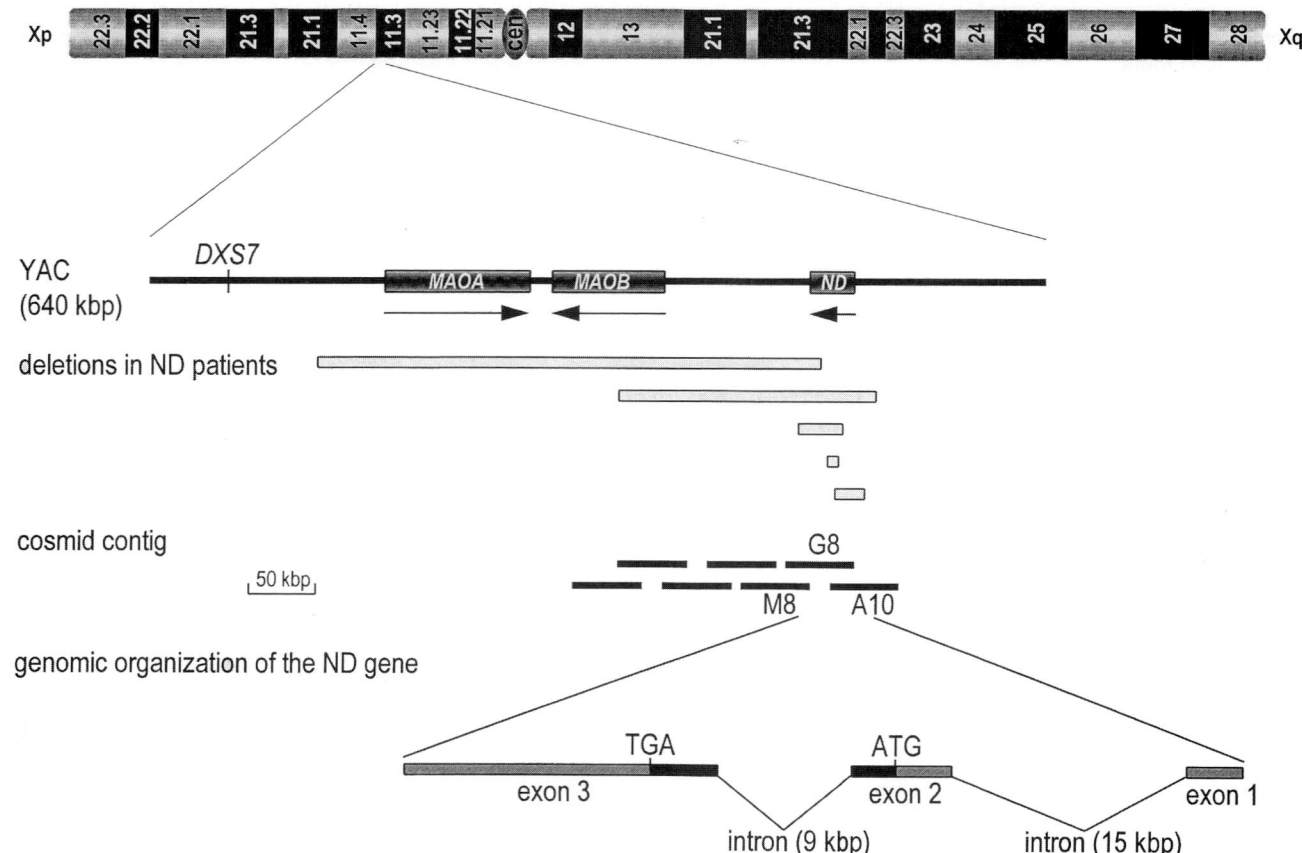

**Fig. 239-1** Schematic drawing of the human X chromosome and physical map the Xp interval carrying the *ND* gene. A 640-kb yeast artificial chromosome (YAC) clone was isolated containing *DXS7* and the *MAO* genes, which had been shown previously to flank the *ND* locus. A cosmid contig was constructed in the respective region, and several clones from this contig (A10, G8, and M8) detected small deletions in ND patients (*open bars*). The cosmids were then used for isolation of complementary DNA clones, and alignment of cDNA and genomic sequence data established the exon-intron structure of the *ND* gene. The gene consists of three exons interrupted by two introns of 15 and 9 kb, respectively. The open reading frame (ORF) is contained entirely within exons 2 and 3 and codes for a polypeptide of 133 amino acids (*black bars*). The orientation of the genes is indicated by arrows below the boxes representing the *ND* and *MAO* genes.

point to a second unrelated gene defect that is closely linked to the *ND* locus.

## FUNCTIONAL ROLE OF THE *ND* GENE

### The ND Protein Sequence Homologies and Three-Dimensional Structure

Analysis of the ND protein defined two characteristic domains: a signal peptide of 24 residues at the N-terminus, suggesting that this protein is secreted, and a cysteine-rich C-terminal domain.[40,53] Database searches have identified homologies of this cysteine-rich domain with mucins, the *Drosophila* slit protein, von Willebrand factor, and the growth factor-binding proteins Cef-10 and Cyr61.[40,43] Mucin proteins represent highly glycosylated extracellular proteins present in mucosal fluids and are primarily responsible for their gel-like character.[54] The homology extends from the first cysteine residue of the ND protein at position 39 to the very C-terminal end (see Fig. 239-2). Transient expression of in vitro-mutated mucin molecules in COS-7 cells revealed a function of this Cys-rich C-terminal domain in dimerization of the protein.[55]

In *Drosophila*, the slit protein is expressed in a subset of glial cells along the midline of the developing central nervous system.[56] Down-regulation of slit leads to disruption of the developing midline cells and the commissural axon pathway. Slit is thought to

be an extracellular protein involved in interactions between midline glial cells, their extracellular environment, and the commissural axons crossing the midline.

The von Willebrand protein is a coagulation factor, and its C-terminal Cys-rich domain, which displays homology with the ND polypeptide, is responsible for dimerization.[57]

The growth factor-binding protein Cyr61 was shown recently to trigger migration of endothelial cells, angiogenesis, and tumor growth.[58] Cef-10, another protein showing homology with the C-terminal Cys-rich domain of the ND protein, can be considered a chicken orthologue of Cyr61 (89 percent protein sequence identity and 92 percent similarity).[59] Cyr61 belongs to a family of connective tissue growth factors that show an overall identity of 30 to 38 percent with insulin-like growth factor-binding proteins (IGFBPs) at the N-terminus.[60] The protein induces chemotactic endothelial cell migration through the $\alpha_v\beta_3$-integrin-mediated pathway, and in the rat, it was shown that Cyr61 is capable of inducing corneal neovascularization in vivo.[58]

Transfection of COS-7 cells with different constructs encoding the ND protein, as well as mutant alleles, has provided a first clue to its biochemical function.[61] These studies showed that the ND protein is secreted and forms dimers and oligomers that are associated with the extracellular matrix. Crosslinking experiments revealed that the dimers constitute an important structural unit of the oligomers. Oligomerization, but not dimerization, was abolished by replacing the cysteine residue at position 95 by an

**Table 239-2 Missense and Nonsense Mutation in the *ND* Gene**

| Codon | Phenotype | Exchange | Reference |
|-------|-----------|----------|-----------|
| 1 | ND | Met, Arg | 44 |
| 1 | ND | Met, Val | 70 |
| 1 | ND | Met, Val | 70 |
| 1 | ND | Met, Val | 46 |
| 13 | ND | Leu, Arg | 71 |
| 29 | ND | Ser, Stop | 40 |
| 39 | ND | Cys, Arg | 14 |
| 41 | EVR, sporadic | Arg, Lys | 48 |
| 42 | Familial EVR | His, Arg | 48 |
| 44 | ND | Tyr, Cys | 40 |
| 57 | ND | Ser, Stop | 39 |
| 58 | ND | Lys, Asn | 50 |
| 58 | EVR, sporadic | Lys, Asn | 48 |
| 60 | ND | Val, Glu | 40 |
| 61 | ND | Leu, Phe | 39 |
| 61 | ND and venous insufficiency | Leu, Phe | 52 |
| 61 | ND | Leu, Pro | 44 |
| 63 | ND | Ala, Asp | 44 |
| 65 | ND | Cys, Tyr | 72 |
| 65 | ND | Cys, Trp | 44 |
| 69 | ND, female carrier | Cys, Ser | 73 |
| 73 | ND | Ser, Stop | 74 |
| 74 | ND | Arg, Cys | 39 |
| 74 | ND | Arg, Cys | 45 |
| 75 | ND | Ser, Cys | 39 |
| 90 | ND | Arg, Pro | 39 |
| 95 | ND | Cys, Arg | 75 |
| 96 | ND | Cys, Tyr | 39 |
| 96 | ND | Cys, Tyr | 40 |
| 101 | Mild ND | Ser, Phe | 74 |
| 104 | Mild ND | Lys, Gln | 76 |
| 105 | ND | Ala, Thr | 77 |
| 108 | ROP | Leu, Pro | 49 |
| 109 | ND | Arg, Stop | 78 |
| 109 | ND | Arg, Stop | 44 |
| 109 | ND | Arg, Stop | 44 |
| 109 | ND | Arg, Stop | 62 |
| 110 | ND | Cys, Stop | 39 |
| 110 | ND | Cys, Stop | 39 |
| 110 | ND | Cys, Arg | 45 |
| 110 | Familial EVR | Cys, Gly | 77 |
| 120 | EVR, sporadic | Tyr, Cys | 48 |
| 121 | ND | Arg, Gln | 50 |
| 121 | Mild ND | Arg, Gln | 76 |
| 121 | Familial EVR | Arg, Leu | 79 |
| 121 | Familial EVR | Arg, Leu | 62 |
| 121 | Mild ND | Arg, Trp | 76 |
| 121 | Familial EVR, mild ND | Arg, Trp | 78 |
| 121 | Familial EVR | Arg, Trp | 80 |
| 121 | ROP | Arg, Trp | 49 |
| 121 | ROP | Arg, Trp | 49 |
| 121 | ROP | Arg, Trp | 49 |
| 123 | ND | Ile, Asn | 44 |
| 123 | ND | Ile, Asn | 44 |
| 124 | Familial EVR | Leu, Phe | 81 |
| 126 | ND | Cys, Stop | 45 |
| 126 | ND | Cys, Stop | 78 |
| 126 | ND | Cys, Ser | 46 |
| 128 | ND | Cys, Stop | 82 |
| 128 | ND | Cys, Stop | 44 |

alanine. Two additional mutations, introduced by site-directed mutagenesis (V60E and R121Q), show a decrease in the amount of extracellular protein compared with the intracellular level, inversely to the wild-type construct. These data suggest that these altered proteins are aberrantly secreted. Decreased extracellular protein levels and additional structural alterations in the mutant protein may be responsible for the disease phenotype.

Molecular modeling of the *ND* gene product predicts a tertiary structure very similar to that of transforming growth factor $\beta$ and put it into a family of growth factors containing a cysteine-knot motif.[53] The computer analysis also predicts the formation of dimers, which is in good agreement with experimental data obtained from transient expression of the ND protein, the submaxillary mucin, and their experimentally altered isoforms.[55,61]

It is noteworthy in this context that female as well as male offspring of *ND* gene mutation carriers can develop peripheral inner retinal vascular abnormalities reminiscent of regressed ROP. Similar alterations were found in carrier females, but offspring of affected males did not show peripheral retinopathy.[62] These observations suggest a role of the protein in vasculogenesis rather than neuroectodermal development. Mintz-Hittner et al.[62] speculated that the mutated ND protein may have a transplacental effect on normal vascularization of the inner retina.

## Cloning of the Mouse Orthologue and Generation of an Animal Model for ND

The human cDNA was used to isolate the homologous transcript of the mouse from a brain cDNA library. The gene was shown to be X-linked in the mouse and to consist of three exons.[63,64] It encodes a polypeptide of 131 amino acids, and sequence comparison between mouse and human proteins revealed 94 percent identity. Tissue-specific expression was analyzed by RNA *in situ* hybridization. High expression levels were found in the inner nuclear layer and the ganglion cell layer of the retina, in Purkinje cells of the cerebellum, and in the mitral and sensory cell layers of the olfactory epithelia 2 weeks after birth.[63] In contrast, no transcript was detected in the ear, gonads, kidney, liver, lung, spleen, gut, and tongue of 4- to 6-month-old mice.

The wild-type *ND* gene was inactivated in mouse embryonic stem (ES) cells by homologous recombination of a targeting construct replacing the coding portion of exon 2 by a neomycin cassette, which removes 56 amino acid residues from the N-terminus of the ND protein (Fig. 239-3A). Similar mutations, e.g., exon 2 deletions, have been observed in ND patients.[40,43] ES cells carrying the inactivated gene copy were injected into blastocysts, and embryos were transferred to pseudopregnant carrier mothers. This gave rise to chimeric male offspring that transmitted the mutation through their germ line. Heterozygous female offspring of these males were mated with wild-type males, which resulted in hemizygous mutant mice. Macroscopically, eyes were normally developed, and ocular atrophy was not observed until age 2 years and 3 months (W Berger, unpublished results, 1999). Hemizygous mutant males as well as carrier females were analyzed by ophthalmologic, morphologic, and electrophysiologic means.

## Histologic and Electrophysiologic Characterization of the Retina in Mutant Mice

Initial ophthalmologic examination in mutant animals was performed by slit-lamp biomicroscopy 3 weeks after birth.[63] Precipitate-like structures were observed in the vitreous body that were absent in wild-type animals. Histologic data were obtained from mouse eyes enucleated between 4 and 26 weeks after birth. The most prominent finding was the presence of blood vessels in the posterior vitreal chamber surrounded by fibrous tissue in all eyes examined.[63,65] Another conspicuous abnormality was a general disorganization of the retinal ganglion cell layer in hemizygous mutant animals (see Fig. 239-3C,D). Some of the nuclei from the ganglion cell layer seemed to migrate into the inner plexiform layer, whereas the ganglion cell layer was found to be completely disorganized. Changes involving the outer and inner nuclear layers as well as the outer plexiform layer and outer segments of the photoreceptor cells showed a patchy distribution.

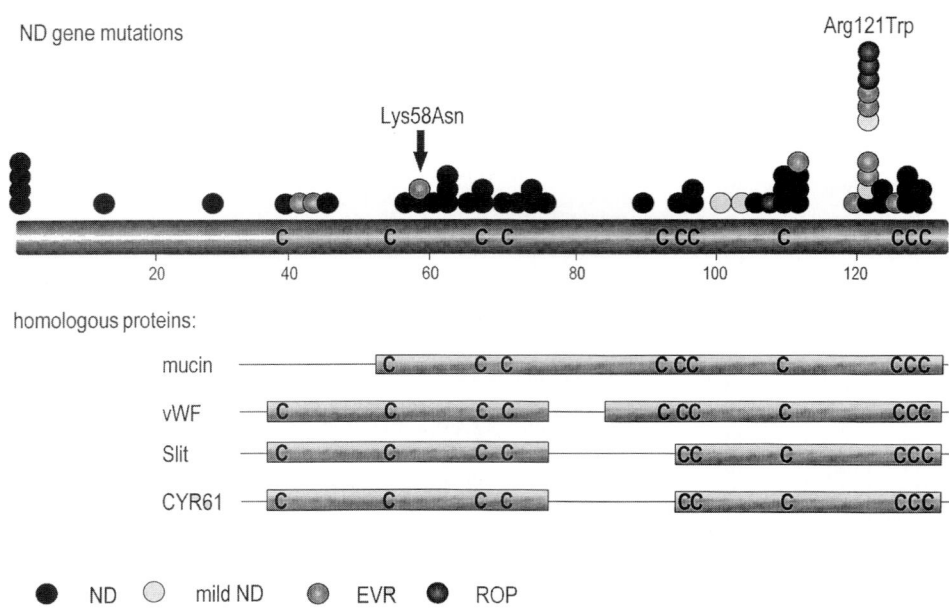

Fig. 239-2 Missense and nonsense mutations in the ND protein leading to classic and mild ND, EVR, and ROP. The positions of altered amino acids are indicated by dots above the ND protein. A scale is given below. A K58N mutation was reported in two different families, leading to ND or familial EVR, respectively. Another missense mutation, R121W, was shown in patients with ROP, familial EVR, or mild ND. The cysteine residues forming the Cys-knot motif are indicated for ND and homologous proteins including mucin, von Willebrand factor (vWF), *slit*, and Cyr61. Gaps remaining after alignment are represented by the thin black lines.

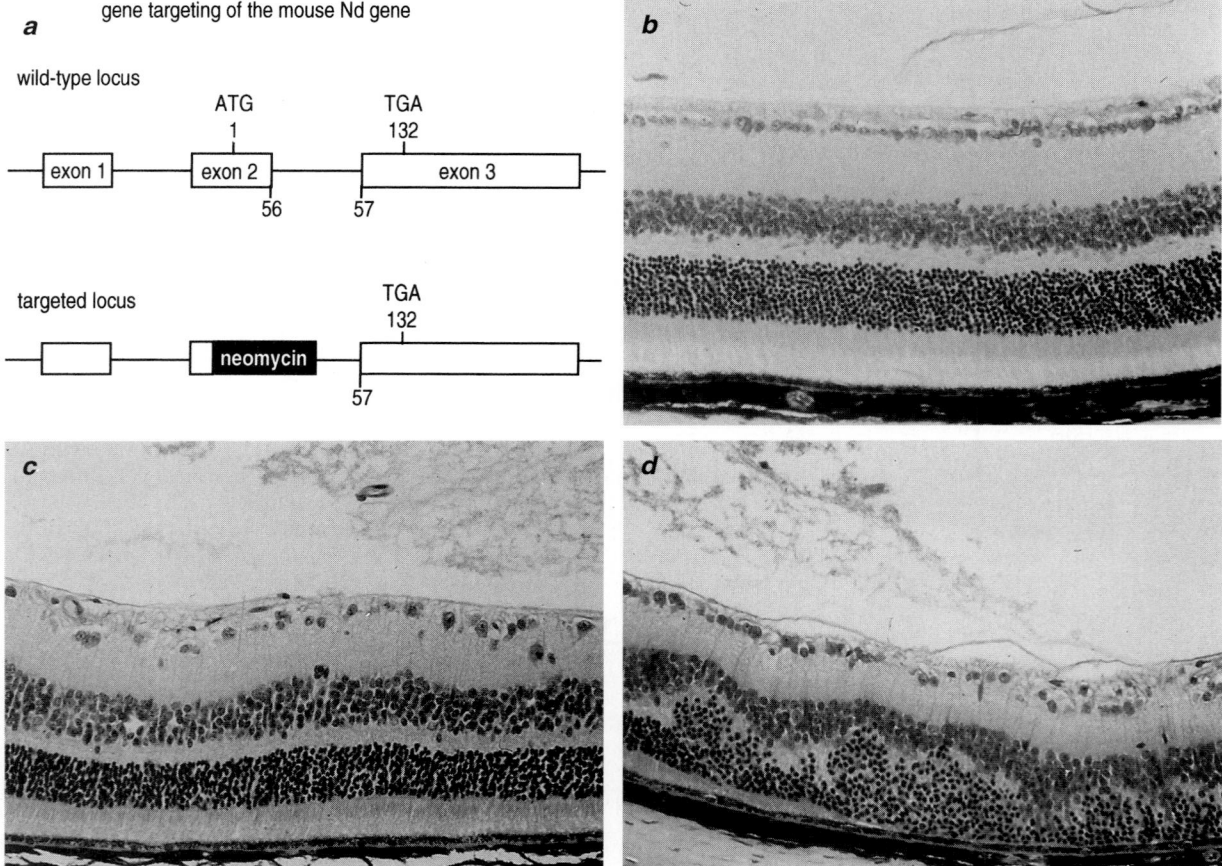

Fig. 239-3 Partial replacement of exon 2 of the mouse *Nd* gene by gene targeting (*A*) and histologic findings in wild-type (*B*) and mutant retinas (*C*,*D*). (*A*) The targeting construct replaces the protein coding part of exon 2 with a neomycin cassette yielding a truncated protein that lacks the 56 N-terminal amino acids. (*B*) Eosin-stained 5-μm section of a wild-type mouse retina. The different layers are indicated on the right: vitreous body (VB), ganglion cell layer (GCL), inner plexiform layer (IPL), inner nuclear layer (INL), outer plexiform layer (OPL), outer nuclear layer (ONL), photoreceptor outer segments (OS), and the retina pigment epithelium (RPE). (*C*) Mildly affected area from a retina of a mutant mouse. The picture shows vascularized material within the posterior vitreous and conspicuous dysgenesis of ganglion cell nuclei. Some of these cells seem to migrate in the inner plexiform layer. The distal retinal layers slightly undulate but otherwise are inconspicuous. (*D*) A severely affected region from the retina of a mutant animal. In the outer retinal layers, OPL and the outer segments of the photoreceptor cells have disappeared, whereas vitreal changes and ganglion cell disorganization are similar to the more mildly affected segment of the retina.

In severely affected areas, the outer plexiform layer and the outer segments of the photoreceptors disappeared, and hyperpigmentation of the retinal pigment epithelium was seen. Otherwise, the retina was normally differentiated, and there was no evidence of progression of the disease in older animals. In mutant mice, alterations in the vitreous are considerably milder than in patients with ND, but the retinal histology bears striking similarities, in particular the dysgenesis of the ganglion cell layer and focal changes in the outer nuclear and photoreceptor layers.[8,9]

In ND mice, the vascular system of the retina also was examined.[65] At postnatal day 9 of normal mouse development, hyaloid vessels become atrophic, and the inner retinal vessels start to sprout. At this developmental stage, inactivation of the *ND* gene does not lead to dramatic qualitative and quantitative changes. In contrast, vascular changes were observed at postnatal day 14. The outer layers of the neuroretina (OPL, outer plexiform layer; ONL, outer nuclear layer; INL, inner nuclear layer; IPL, inner plexiform layer) show an almost complete lack of blood vessels except for the main branches of the retinal artery. In contrast, the number of blood vessels in the ganglion and nerve fiber layers is increased, possibly due to neovascularization processes or remnants of hyaloid vessels incorporated in the inner limiting membrane. In mutant animals older than 20 days, fenestration in retinal vessels occurs. Moreover, penetration of vessels through the inner limiting membrane, as well as persistence of hyaloid vessels, has been observed in the vitreous of gene-targeted mice older than 20 days. Most prominent morphologic changes were found in retinal cell layers, which showed elevated expression of the *ND* gene 14 days after birth.[63]

Electroretinograms (ERGs) of hemizygous mutant mice displayed a severe loss of the b wave, leading to a negatively shaped scotopic ERG and a marked reduction in oscillatory potentials.[66] The a wave was normal at low-flashlight intensities and showed a moderate loss of amplitude with brighter flashes. Scanning laser ophthalmoscopy revealed snowflake-like opacities in the posterior part of the vitreous, located predominantly at the central portions. Moreover, retinal vessels were dislocated to the vitreal chamber, and some had a bulb-like appearance. Retinal pigment epithelium alterations included pigment mottling in most parts of the retina that could be better seen in the periphery. These data suggest a more severe defect of the inner retina (containing neural and glial cells) and relatively mild symptoms in the outer retina (containing photoreceptor cells) and the pigment epithelium. In heterozygous females, ERG analyses and laser scanning ophthalmoscopy did not show significant pathologic changes.

## Possible Pathogenic Mechanisms

The ND protein may have an important function in vascularization of the inner retina through sprouting of small blood vessels from the main branches of the retinal artery. This hypothesis is supported by (1) histologic findings in patients with ND and allelic disorders, (2) observations in a mouse mutant carrying an inactive *ND* gene, (3) angiographic findings in offspring of gene mutation carriers, and (4) homology of the ND protein to Cyr61, a growth factor associated with the extracellular matrix that induces corneal neovascularization.

Biochemical analyses involving transient expression of the ND protein in COS-7 cells suggest that it forms dimers or oligomers that are associated with the extracellular matrix when released from cells of the inner retina (possibly via integrin-mediated binding). The matrix-bound form may then trigger migration of endothelial cells and sprouting of blood vessels leading to a normally vascularized retina. When the *ND* gene is not expressed, vascularization cannot occur, and ganglion cells as well as other neurons start to degenerate. This degeneration leads to glial cell proliferation, seen as a massive gliosis in patients with ND. Due to these primary alterations in the neuroretina, the secondary vitreous fails to develop, and the primary vitreous (as well as hyaloid vessels) persists. This explains the vitreal pathology seen in patients. In agreement with the model proposed by Warburg,[3]

these changes therefore are considered to be secondary effects. Additional ocular symptoms affecting the lens, iris, and cornea may be tertiary consequences.

Alternatively, the function of the ND protein could involve the maintenance and/or differentiation of ganglion or glial cells. Further data on the biochemical characterization of the ND protein and detailed examination of the mouse model are needed to clarify the precise function of the *ND* gene. In particular, histologic and pathophysiologic examination of the ears and brain of ND mice may reveal alterations in these organs that would render these animals particularly suitable models for studying the molecular pathogenesis of ND. Additional clues to the function of this gene can be expected from ongoing experiments aimed at identifying additional players in the molecular pathway involving the *ND* gene. Characterization of these genes and their products also may provide an explanation for the clinical variability in ND that is not due to genetic variation in the *ND* gene itself.

***Note added in proof.*** Recently, another disease phenotype, designated Coats disease, was shown to be associated with a mutation in the Norrie disease gene. Coats disease is characterized by unilateral abnormal development of the retinal vasculature (retinal telangiectasis). Analysis of the retinae of 9 affected males demonstrated a somatic mutation in one of them (C96w). The same DNA sequence exchange was identified in a female with unilateral Coats disease who had a son with Norrie disease. Both mother and son carried the mutation in their germline, and it was speculated that unilateral disease in the female carrier is due to nonrandom X-inactivation in the affected eye or a somatic mutation that inactivates the second, normal allele,

## REFERENCES

1. Warburg M: Norrie's disease: A new hereditary bilateral pseudotumour of the retina. *Acta Ophthalmol* **39**:757–772, 1961.
2. Warburg M: Norrie's disease (atrofia bulborum hereditaria). *Acta Ophthalmol* **41**:134–146, 1963.
3. Warburg M: Norrie's disease: A congenital progressive oculo-acoustico-cerebral degeneration. *Acta Ophthalmol* **89**(suppl.):1–147, 1966.
4. Warburg M: Norrie's disease. *J Ment Defic Res* **12**:247–251, 1968.
5. Townes PL, Roca PD: Norrie's disease (hereditary oculo-acoustic-cerebral degeneration): Report of a United States family. *Am J Ophthalmol* **76**:797–803, 1973.
6. Warburg M: Norrie's disease: Differential diagnosis and treatment. *Acta Ophthalmol* **53**:217–236, 1975.
7. Johnston SS, Hanna JE, Nevin NC, Bryars JH: Norrie's disease. *Birth Defects* **18**:729–738, 1982.
8. Apple DJ, Fishman GA, Goldberg MF: Ocular histopathology of Norrie's disease. *Am J Ophthalmol* **78**:196–203, 1974.
9. Schroeder B, Hesse L, Brück W, Gal A: Histopathological and immunohistochemical findings associated with a null mutation in the Norrie disease gene. *Ophthalmic Genet* **18**:71–77, 1997.
10. Enyedi LB, de Juan E, Gaitan A: Ultrastructural study of Norrie's disease. *Am J Ophthalmol* **111**:439–445, 1991.
11. Saini JS, Sharma A, Pillai P, Mohan K: Norries disease. *Ind J Ophthalmol* **40**:24–26, 1992.
12. Parsons MA, Curtis D, Blank CE, Hughes HN, McCartney CE: The ocular pathology of Norrie disease in a fetus of 11 weeks gestational age. *Graefes Arch Clin Exp Ophthalmol* **230**:248–251, 1992.
13. Chynn EW, Walton DS, Hahn LB, Dryja TP: Norrie disease: Diagnosis of a simplex case by DNA analysis. *Arch Ophthalmol* **114**:1136–1138, 1996.
14. Joos KM, Kimura AE, Vandenburgh K, Bartley JA, Stone EM: Ocular findings associated with a Cys39Arg mutation in the Norrie disease gene. *Arch Ophthalmol* **112**:1574–1579, 1994.
15. Hafez M, El-Tahhan H, Abdalla A, Ibrahim Z, Tawfik A, El-Desoky M: A presumptive new presentation of Norrie's disease. *Egypt J Genet Cytol* **11**:213–225, 1982.
16. Nadol JB, Eavey RD, Liberfarb RM, Merchant SN, Williams R, Climenhager D, Albert DM: Histopathology of the ears, eyes, and brain in Norrie's disease (oculoacousticocerebral degeneration). *Am J Otolaryngol* **11**:112–124, 1990.
17. Moreira-Filho CA, Neustein I: A presumptive new variant of Norrie's disease. *J Med Genet* **16**:125–128, 1979.

18. Gal A, Wieringa B, Smeets DFCM, Bleeker-Wagemakers L, Ropers HH: Submicroscopic interstitial deletion of the X chromosome explains a complex genetic syndrome dominated by Norrie disease. *Cytogenet Cell Genet* **42**:219–224, 1986.

19. LaRussa F, Wesson MD: Norrie's disease vs. PHPV: One family's dilemma. *J Am Optom Assoc* **63**:404–408, 1992.

20. Lee WH, Bookstein R, Hong F, Young LJ, Shew JY, Lee EY: Human retinoblastoma susceptibility gene: Cloning, identification, and sequence. *Science* **235**:1394–1399, 1986.

21. Sauer CG, Gehrig A, Warnecke-Wittstock R, Marquardt A, Ewing CC, Gibson A, Lorenz B, et al: Positional cloning of the gene associated with X-linked juvenile retinoschisis. *Nature Genet* **17**:164–170, 1997.

22. The Retinoschisis Consortium: Functional implications of the spectrum of mutations found in 234 cases with X-linked juvenile retinoschisis (XLRS). *Hum Mol Genet* **7**:1185–1192, 1998.

23. Bleeker-Wagemakers LM, Friedrich U, Gal A, Wienker TF, Warburg M, Ropers HH: Close linkage between Norrie disease, a cloned DNA sequence from the proximal short arm, and the centromere of the X chromosome. *Hum Genet* **71**:211–214, 1985.

24. Gal A, Stolzenberger C, Wienker T, Wieacker P, Ropers HH, Friedrich U, Bleeker-Wagemakers L, et al: Norrie's disease: Close linkage with genetic markers from the proximal short arm of the X chromosome. *Clin Genet* **27**:282–283, 1985.

25. de la Chapelle A, Sankila E-M, Lindlöf M, Aula P, Norio R: Norrie disease caused by a gene deletion allowing carrier detection and prenatal diagnosis. *Clin Genet* **28**:317–320, 1985.

26. Sims KB, de la Chapelle A, Norio R, Sankila E-M, Hsu Y-PP, Rinehart WB, Correy TJ, et al: Monoamine oxidase deficiency in males with an X chromosome deletion. *Neuron* **2**:1069–1076, 1989.

27. Diergaarde PJ, Wieringa B, Bleeker-Wagemakers EM, Sims KB, Breakefield XO, Ropers HH: Physical fine-mapping of a deletion spanning the Norrie gene. *Hum Genet* **84**:22–26, 1989.

28. Lan NC, Heinzmann C, Gal A, Klisak I, Orth U, Lai E, Grimsby J, et al: Human monoamine oxidase A and B genes map to Xp11.23 and are deleted in a patient with Norrie disease. *Genomics* **4**:552–559, 1989.

29. Murphy DL, Sims KB, Karoum F, de la Chapelle A, Norio R, Sankila E-M, Breakefield XO: Marked amine and amine metabolite changes in Norrie disease patients with an X-chromosomal deletion affecting monoamine oxidase. *J Neurochem* **54**:242–247, 1990.

30. Collins FA, Murphy DL, Reiss AL, Sims KB, Lewis JG, Freund L, Karoum F, et al: Clinical, biochemical, and neuropsychiatric evaluation of a patient with a contiguous gene syndrome due to a microdeletion Xp11.3 including the Norrie disease locus and monoamine oxidase (MAOA and MAOB) genes. *Am J Med Genet* **42**:127–134, 1992.

31. Sims KB, Ozelius L, Corey T, Rinehart WB, Liberfarb R, Haines J, Chen WJ, et al: Norrie disease gene is distinct from the monoamine oxidase genes. *Am J Hum Genet* **45**:424–434, 1989.

32. Brunner HG, Breakefield XO, Ropers HH, van Oost BA: Abnormal behavior associated with a point mutation in the structural gene for monoamine oxidase A. *Science* **262**:578–580, 1993.

33. Cases O, Seif I, Grimsby J, Gaspar P, Chen K, Pournin S, Muller U, et al: Aggressive behavior and altered amounts of brain serotonin and norepinephrine in mice lacking MAOA. *Science* **268**:1763–1766, 1998.

34. Lenders JWM, Eisenhofer G, Abeling NGGM, Berger W, Murphy DL, Konings CH, Wagemakers LMB, et al: Specific genetic deficiencies of the A and B isoenzymes of monoamine oxidase are characterized by distinct neurochemical and clinical phenotypes. *J Clin Invest* **97**:1010–1019, 1996.

35. Katayama S, Wohlferd M, Golbus MS: First demonstration of recombination between the gene for Norrie disease and probe L1.28. *Am J Med Genet* **30**:967–970, 1988.

36. Berger W, Meindl A, van de Pol TJR, Cremers FPM, Ropers HH, Dörner C, Monaco A, et al: Isolation of a candidate gene for Norrie disease by positional cloning. *Nature Genet* **1**:199–203, 1992.

37. Chen Z-Y, Hendriks RW, Jobling MA, Powell JF, Breakefield XO, Sims KB, Craig IW: Isolation and characterization of a candidate gene for Norrie disease. *Nature Genet* **1**:204–208, 1992.

38. Sims KB, Lebo RV, Benson G, Shalish C, Schuback D, Chen Z-Y, Bruns G, et al: The Norrie disease gene maps to a 150 kbp region on chromosome Xp11.3. *Hum Mol Genet* **1**:83–89, 1992.

39. Berger W, van de Pol D, Warburg M, Gal A, Bleeker-Wagemakers L, de Silva H, Meindl A, et al: Mutations in the candidate gene for Norrie disease. *Hum Mol Genet* **1**:461–465, 1992.

40. Meindl A, Berger W, Meitinger T, van de Pol D, Achatz H, Dörner C, Haasemann M, et al: Norrie disease is caused by mutations in an extracellular protein resembling C-terminal globular domain of mucins. *Nature Genet* **2**:139–143, 1992.

41. Ohba N, Yamashita T: Primary vitreoretinal dysplasia resembling Norrie disease in a female: Association with X/autosome chromosomal translocation. *Br J Ophthalmol* **70**:64–71, 1986.

42. Pettenati MJ, Rao PN, Weaver JRG, Thomas IT, McMahan MR: Inversion (X)(p11.4q22) associated with Norrie disease in a four generation family. *Am J Med Genet* **45**:577–580, 1993.

43. Chen Z-Y, Battinelli EM, Hendriks RW, Powell JF, Middleton-Price H, Sims KB, Breakefield XO, et al: Norrie disease gene: characterization of deletions and possible function. *Genomics* **16**:533–535, 1993.

44. Schuback DE, Chen Z-Y, Craig IW, Breakefield XO, Sims KB: Mutations in the Norrie disease gene. *Hum Mutat* **5**:285–292, 1995.

45. Fuchs S, Pol Dvd, Beudt U, Kellner U, Meire F, Berger W, Gal A: Three novel and two recurrent mutations of the Norrie disease gene in patients with Norrie syndrome. *Hum Mutat* **8**:85–88, 1996.

46. Gal A, Veske A, Jojart G, Grammatico B, Huber B, Gu S, del Porto G, et al: Norrie-Warburg syndrome: Two novel mutations in patients with classical clinical phenotype. *Acta Ophthalmol Scand* **74**:13–16, 1996.

47. Meindl A, Lorenz B, Achatz H, Hellebrand H, Schmitzvalckenberg P, Meitinger T: Missense mutations in the ndp gene in patients with a less severe course of norrie disease. *Hum Mol Genet* **4**:489–490, 1995.

48. Shastry BS, Hejtmancik JF, Trese MT: Identification of novel missense mutations in the Norrie disease gene associated with one X-linked and four sporadic cases of familial exudative vitreoretinopathy. *Hum Mutat* **9**:396–401, 1997.

49. Shastry BS, Pendergast SD, Hartzer MK, Liu X, Trese MT: Identification of missense mutations in the Norrie disease gene associated with advanced retinopathy of prematurity. *Arch Ophthalmol* **115**:651–655, 1997.

50. Fuentes J-J, Volpini V, Fernández-Toral F, Coto E, Estivill X: Identification of two new missense mutations (K58N and R121Q) in the Norrie disease (ND) gene in two Spanish families. *Hum Mol Genet* **2**:1953–1955, 1993.

51. Zaremba J, Feil S, Juszko J, Myga W, van Duijnhoven G, Berger W: Intrafamilial variability of the ocular phenotype in a Polish family with a missense mutation (A63D) in the Norrie disease gene. *Ophthalmic Genet* **19**:157–164, 1998.

52. Rehm HL, Gutiérrez-Espeleta GA, Garcia R, Jiménez G, Khetarpal U, Priest JM, Sims KB, et al: Norrie disease gene mutation in a large Costa Rican kindred with a novel phenotype including venous insufficiency. *Hum Mutat* **9**:402–408, 1997.

53. Meitinger T, Meindl A, Bork P, Rost B, Sander C, Haasemann M, Murken J: Molecular modelling of the Norrie disease protein predicts a cystine knot growth factor tertiary structure. *Nature Genet* **5**:376–380, 1993.

54. Shimizu Y, Shaw S: Mucins in the mainstream. *Nature* **366**:630–631, 1993.

55. Perez-Vilar J, Hill RL: The carboxyl-terminal 90 residues of porcine submaxillary mucin are sufficient for forming disulfide-bonded dimers. *J Biol Chem* **273**:6982–6988, 1998.

56. Rothberg JM, Jacobs JR, Goodman CS, Artavanis-Tsakonas S: Slit: An extracellular protein necessary for development of midline glia and commissural axon pathways contains both EGF and LRR domains. *Genes Dev* **4**:2169–2187, 1990.

57. Voorberg J, Fontijn R, Calafat J, Janssen H, van Mourik JA, Pannekoek H: Assembly and routing of von Willebrand factor variants: the requirements for disulphide-linked dimerization reside within the carboxy-terminal 151 amino acids. *J Cell Biol* **113**:195–205, 1991.

58. Babic AM, Kireeva ML, Kolesnikova TV, Lau LF: CYR61, a product of a growth factor-inducible immediate early gene, promotes angiogenesis and tumor growth. *Proc Natl Acad Sci USA* **95**:6355–6360, 1998.

59. Bradham DM, Igarashi A, Potter RL, Grotendorst GR: Connective tissue growth factor: A cysteine-rich mitogen secreted by human vascular endothelial cells is related to the src-induced immediate early gene product CEF-10. *J Cell Biol* **114**:1285–1294, 1991.

60. Kim H-S, Nagalla S-R, Oh Y, Wilson E, Roberts CTJ, Rosenfeld RG: Identification of a family of low-affinity insulin-like growth factor binding proteins (IGFBPs): characterization of connective tissue growth factor as a member of the IGFBP superfamily. *Proc Natl Acad Sci USA* **94**:12981–12986, 1997.

61. Perez-Vilar J, Hill R-L: Norrie disease protein (Norrin) forms disulfide-linked oligomers associated with the extracellular matrix. *J Biol Chem* **272**:33410–33415, 1997.

62. Mintz-Hittner HA, Ferrel RE, Sims KB, Fernandez KM, Gemmell BS, Satriano DR, Caster J, et al: Peripheral retinopathy in offspring of carriers of Norrie disease gene mutations: Possible transplacental effect of abnormal norrin. *Ophthalmology* **103**:2128–2134, 1996.

63. Berger W, v.d.Pol D, Bächner D, Oerlemans F, Winkens H, Hameister H, Wieringa B, et al: An animal model for Norrie disease (ND): Gene targeting of the mouse ND gene. *Hum Mol Genet* **5**:51–59, 1996.

64. Battinelli EM, Boyd Y, Craig IW, Breakefield XO, Chen Z-Y: Characterization and mapping of the mouse NDP (Norrie disease) locus (*Ndp*). *Mamm Genome* **7**:93–97, 1996.

65. Richter M, Gottanka J, May CA, Welge-Lüssen U, Berger W, Lütjen-Drecoll E: Retinal vasculature changes in Norrie disease mice. *Invest Ophthalmol Vis Sci* **39**:2450–2457, 1998.

66. Ruether K, van de Pol D, Jaissle G, Berger W, Tornow RP, Zrenner E: Retinoschisislike alterations in the mouse eye due to gene targeting of the Norrie dieseease (ND) gene. *Invest Ophthalmol Vis Sci* **38**:710–718, 1997.

67. Nance WE, Hara S, Hansen A, Elliott J, Lewis M, Chown B: Genetic linkage studies in a Negro kindred with Norrie's disease. *Am J Hum Genet* **21**:423–429, 1969.

68. Donnai D, Mountford RC, Read AP: Norrie disease resulting from a gene deletion: Clinical features and DNA studies. *J Med Genet* **25**:73–78, 1988.

69. Zhu D, Antonarakis SE, Schmeckpeper BJ, Diergaarde PJ, Greb AE, Maumenee IH: Microdeletion in the X-chromosome and prenatal diagnosis in a family with Norrie disease. *Am J Med Genet* **33**:485–488, 1989.

70. Isashiki Y, Ohba N, Yanagita T, Hokita N, Doi N, Nakagawa M, Ozawa M, et al: Novel mutation at the initiation codon in the norrie disease gene in two japanese families. *Hum Genet* **95**:105–108, 1995.

71. Fuchs S, Xu SY, Caballero M, Salcedo M, La O A, Wedemann H, Gal A: A missense point mutation (Leu13Arg) of the Norrie disease gene in a large Cuban kindred with Norrie disease. *Hum Mol Genet* **3**:655–656, 1994.

72. Strasberg P, Liede HA, Stein T, Warren I, Sutherland J, Ray PN: A novel mutation in the Norrie disease gene predicted to disrupt the cystine knot growth factor motif. *Hum Mol Genet* **4**:2179–2180, 1995.

73. Chen Z-Y, Battinelli EM, Woodruff G, Young I, Breakefield XO, Craig IW: Characterization of a mutation within the NDP gene in a family with a manifesting female carrier. *Hum Mol Genet* **2**:1727–1729, 1993.

74. Walker JL, Dixon J, Fenton CR, Hungerford J, Lynch SA, Stenhouses SA, Christian A, et al: Two new mutations in exon 3 of the NDP gene: S73X and S101F associated with severe and less severe ocular phenotype, respectively. *Hum Mutat* **9**:53–56, 1997.

75. Isashiki Y, Ohba N, Yanagita T, Hokita N, Hotta Y, Hayakawa M, Fujiki K, et al: Mutations in the Norrie disease gene: A new mutation in a Japanese family. *Br J Ophthalmol* **79**:703–704, 1995.

76. Meindl A, Lorenz B, Achatz H, Hellebrand H, Schmitz-Valckenberg P, Meitinger T: Missense mutations in the *NDP* gene in patients with a less severe course of Norrie disease. *Hum Mol Genet* **4**:489–490, 1995.

77. Torrente I, Mangino M, Gennarelli M, Novelli G, Giannotti A, Vadalà A, Dallapiccola B: Two new missense mutations (A105T and C110G) in the Norrin gene in two Italian families with Norrie disease and familial exudative vitreoretinopathy. *Am J Med Genet* **72**:242–244, 1997.

78. Kellner U, Fuchs S, Bornfeld N, Foerster MH, Gal A: Ocular phenotypes associated with two mutations (R121W, C126X) in the Norrie disease gene. *Ophthalmic Genet* **17**:67–74, 1996.

79. Johnson K, Mintz-Hittner HA, Conley YP, Ferrell RE: X-linked exudative vitreoretinopathy caused by an arginine to leucine substitution (R121L) in the Norrie disease protein. *Clin Genet* **50**:113–115, 1996.

80. Shastry BS, Hejtmancik JF, Plager DA, Hartzer MK, Trese MT: Linkage and candidate gene analysis of X-linked familial exudative vitreoretinopathy. *Genomics* **27**:341–344, 1995.

81. Chen Z-Y, Battinelli EM, Fielder A, Bundey S, Sims K, Breakfield XO, Craig IW: A mutation in the Norrie disease gene (*NDP*) associated with X-linked familial exudative vitreoretinopathy. *Nature Genet* **5**:180–183, 1993.

82. Wong F, Goldberg MF, Hao Y: Identification of a nonsense mutation at codon 128 of the Norrie's disease gene in a male infant. *Arch Ophthalmol* **111**:1553–1557, 1993.

83. Black CGM, Perveen R, Bonshek R, Cahill M, Layton-Smith J, Lloyd IC, McLeod D: Coats' disease of the retina (unilateral retinal telangiectasis) caused by somatic mutation in the NDP gene: A role for norrin in retinal angiogenesis. *Hum Mol Genet* **8**:2031–2035, 1993.

# Transcription Factors in Eye Disease and Ocular Development

D. Jonathan Horsford ▪ Isabel Hanson ▪ Carol Freund
Roderick R. McInnes ▪ Veronica van Heyningen

1. The regulation of cell division, growth, migration, programmed death, and differentiation, necessary for the development of tissues and organs, requires the ordered activation and silencing of thousands of genes in a spatially and temporally controlled manner. Many of these developmental processes are controlled by tissue-specific transcription factors. In addition, the maintenance of the differentiated state is often regulated by the same transcription factors required for formation of the mature cell. Mutations in 10 human (Table 240-1) transcription factor genes have been shown to disrupt mammalian eye development or maintenance. Mutations in an additional 18 mouse transcription factor genes have also been found to be associated with developmental abnormalities of the eye (Table 240-2). Human eye phenotypes (Table 240-1) can involve one or more ocular structures. Developmental anomalies that affect many parts of the eye are termed panocular defects, whereas other abnormalities may be restricted to the anterior segment, posterior segment, or the differentiation or maintenance of photoreceptors.

2. Panocular defects are broad phenotypes that arise by at least two different general mechanisms. The first, best illustrated by heterozygous mutations in the paired/homeobox gene PAX6, reflects the fact that the gene is expressed in and required for the normal development and/or maintenance of all regions of the developing eye: both neural and pigmented retina, iris, lens, and surface ectoderm (Fig. 240-2). Thus, PAX6 mutations cause panocular disease in the sense that many different parts of the eye may be affected, although in many patients only one region is predominantly abnormal. The second mechanism by which panocular defects arise reflects the fact that a gene expressed in one region of the developing eye may nevertheless be essential, via secondary physiological processes, for the normal development of other ocular structures. This mechanism is illustrated by the abnormalities that result from mutations in the CHX10 homeobox gene because, at least in the two patients identified to date, the eye is small and many structures are abnormal, even though the developmental expression of CHX10 in the eye is restricted solely to the progenitor cells of the neuroretina.

3. PAX6, mapping to chromosome 11p13, is a transcription factor with both a paired- and a homeodomain. It is mutated in aniridia and related anomalies. Most aniridia mutations lead to premature protein truncations, and haploinsufficiency. Cases classified as aniridia always have severe iris hypoplasia and usually one or more of the following features: foveal/macular hypoplasia, cataracts, glaucoma, and corneal limbal insufficiency, making this a panocular and progressive developmental disease. More infrequently (<10 percent of cases analyzed) missense mutations are seen. Foveal hypoplasia, Peters anomaly, corectopia and cataracts have been observed in these amino acid substitution cases. These "variant" phenotypes usually have less severe or no iris involvement. The universal involvement of PAX6 in the development of the eye in species ranging from Drosophila to humans serves as a paradigm for wide-ranging evolutionary conservation of key developmental regulators. This concept allows us to use a broad range of model organisms to understand gene function and define interacting developmental pathways. Although there is no reduction in eye size in aniridia, the heterozygous null mouse Small eye mutant is a good model for the human disease spectrum. Eye development is sensitive to PAX6 gene dosage, because either an increase or a decrease in dosage results in eye defects in mouse. Loss-of-function mutations caused by chromosomal rearrangements well outside the transcribed region of the gene (position effects) have suggested a requirement for long distance control of PAX6, as well as for FKHL7 and PITX2. PAX6 is expressed in the forebrain, cerebellum, neural tube, olfactory system, and the pancreas, but its heterozygous phenotype is confined to the eye, although the mouse homozygous loss of function phenotype reflects more fully the broad expression spectrum.

4. CHX10 is a paired-like homeodomain protein with a homolog in C. elegans and with vertebrate orthologs and homologs. CHX10 and proteins related to it also share a second conserved motif, of 55 amino acids, the CVC

A list of standard abbreviations is located immediately preceding the index in each volume. Additional abbreviations used in this chapter include: ADCC = autosomal dominant congenital cataract; adRP = autosomal dominant retinitis pigmentosa; AROA = autosomal recessive ocular albinism; ASMD = anterior segment mesenchymal dysgenesis; CRD = cone rod dystrophy; CVC = a 55-amino-acid domain found in certain homeodomain proteins expressed in the developing eye or other neurosensory organs; IGD = iridogoniodysgenesis; LCA = Leber's congenital amaurosis; ORF = open reading frame; OS = outer segment; POAG = primary open-angle glaucoma; RP = retinitis pigmentosa; RPE = retinal pigment epithelium; SHH = Sonic hedgehog; SOD = septo-optic dysplasia; WS = Waardenburg syndrome; WS2A = Waardenburg syndrome type 2A; YAC = yeast artificial chromosome.

domain, of unknown function. CHX10 regulates neuronal development, particularly the proliferation of progenitor cells and the formation of interneurons. Homozygous putative null mutations of the human *CHX10* homeobox gene, which maps to 14q24.3, affect only the eye, resulting in blindness with microphthalmia and cataracts; in mice, null mutations cause an orthologous phenotype. During eye development, the expression of mouse *Chx10* is restricted to neuroretinal progenitor cells. Differentiation of progenitors into the cells of the adult retina is associated with a restriction of *Chx10* expression to the cells of the inner nuclear layer, the highest level of expression being in bipolar cells, the major retinal interneurons. Mice homozygous for the *Chx10 or* null allele have other major phenotypes in addition to small eyes and cataracts: absence of the optic nerve (ganglion cell axons are present but do not exit the eye) and a hypocellular retina in which there is a complete absence of detectable bipolar cells. The two human mutations (R200Q and R200P) dramatically reduce or abate binding of the mutant proteins to CHX10 target sequences. The human and mouse severe loss-of-function phenotypes are remarkably similar, although the human patients have abnormalities of the iris, but optic nerves are present. The discovery of human *CHX10* mutations was due to the prior characterization of the mouse mutant. This experience highlights, as is the case for many of the genes discussed in this chapter, the power of mouse models to contribute to the knowledge of human disease.

5. Anterior segment defects, affecting primarily the anterior chamber, iris, lens, cornea, and trabecular network, are phenotypically varied, and result from mutations in a number of different transcription factor genes: *FKHL7*, *PITX2*, *PITX3*, and *MITF*. Similar phenotypes result from mutations at different loci, and there is a phenotypic overlap with some *PAX6* missense mutations. In many cases, there is within-family and even left/right eye phenotypic variation.

6. Missense mutations, protein truncations and deletions/translocations of the *FKHL7* (forkhead-like) gene, on chromosome 6p25, result in a spectrum of autosomal dominant anterior segment eye phenotypes. The *FKHL7* DNA binding domain has a winged-helix configuration. Once more, the genetic mechanism is haploinsufficiency. The phenotypes can be categorized as Axenfeld Rieger anomaly, with iridogoniodysgenesis and posterior embryotoxon often associated with glaucoma. Somewhat surprisingly, a mutation in the mouse *FKHL7*-orthologous gene, now called *Foxc1* was originally defined at the neonatally lethal *congenital hydrocephalus* locus. The homozygous mutant phenotype reflects the broader gene expression in neural crest and mesodermal (lateral and paraxial) cells. Affected tissues include the heart and multiple skeletal defects as well as the eye. Detailed analysis of heterozygous mice, a possible model system for human disease, reveals failure of the cornea to separate from the lens (reminiscent of Peters anomaly) with aberrant development of the inner corneal mesenchymal layer.

7. Mutations in the paired/bicoid-like homeodomain gene *PITX2*, at 4q25, result in the anterior segment disorders of Rieger syndrome and iridogonial dysgenesis syndrome. These autosomal dominant disorders are due to *PITX2* haploinsufficiency which affects ocular mesenchymal cells during eye development and are also seen in a mouse with targeted disruptions of *Pitx2*. *PITX2* mutants also have associated tooth and umbilical anomalies, hallmarks of Rieger and iridogoniodysgenesis syndromes. Hetero-

zygotes for the mouse-targeted *Pitx2* disruption mirror the human phenotype with corectopia, iris anomalies, and tooth malocclusion. This haploinsufficiency reflects only part of the expression pattern: in mesenchyme around the eye, Rathke's pouch, dental lamina, limbs, and mesentry. Homozygous loss-of-function animals die at midgestation with heart defects, reflecting the role of *Pitx2* in laterality determination.

8. *PITX3*, mapping to chromosome 10q25, is closely related to *PITX2*. The two reported protein truncation mutations have been associated with autosomal dominant anterior segment mesenchymal dysgenesis and with inherited congenital cataract. Once more, the heterozygous loss-of-function phenotype reflects only part of the expression pattern in the lens, ocular, and periocular mesenchyme, and in mesenchyme of the tongue, and tooth primordia, as well as those forming head muscles and condensing around vertebrae and sternum; additionally prominent developing central nervous system expression is seen in Rathke's pouch and the midbrain. No mouse model has been reported.

9. Autosomal dominant Waardenburg syndrome type 2A (WS2A) is associated with mutations in *MITF*, a bHLH-leucine zipper transcription factor gene expressed predominantly in developing pigment cells and neural crest cells. Patients present with hypo- or heterochromic irides due to defective migration of neural crest cells into the iris during eye development. The nonocular phenotypes include abnormalities in skin and hair pigmentation and hearing loss. MITF maps to 3p14.1-p12.3. The discovery of the microphthalmic mouse harboring *Mitf* mutations led to the link between *MITF* and WS2A. An important finding in the homozygous *Mitf* mouse is the presence of severe eye defects (microphthalmia and retinal degeneration) due to an increase in the proliferation of retinal pigment epithelial cells, demonstrating a critical role for *Mitf* in the division and differentiation of these retinal cells.

10. Posterior segment defects affect only the retina and optic nerve region of the eye. These include optic nerve defects due to mutations in *PAX2* and *HESX1*, and abnormalities in photoreceptor differentiation or maintenance due to mutations in *CRX* and *NRL*.

11. *PAX2*, a member of the *PAX* gene family that maps to 10q24, is mutated in a proportion of renal coloboma syndrome cases. Mutations documented so far are all in the N-terminal DNA-binding regions of the gene, mostly leading to premature protein truncations and haploinsufficiency. The phenotype in this syndrome is highly variable with optic disc colobomas and vesicoureteral reflux, sometimes leading to renal failure, as the most severe manifestations. Intrafamilial variation has revealed some subclinical eye and kidney abnormalities. Occasional deafness, reflecting in part the expression pattern of *PAX2*, has been noted. Mouse *PAX2* models are available: the phenotypes of heterozygous *Krd* deletion, targeted knockouts and the *Pax2^Neu* truncation mutation, all mirror the human phenotype. Abnormalities in the neonatally lethal homozygous mice mirror more closely the expression pattern: in the developing brain, with eventual restriction to the midbrain-hindbrain boundary, spinal cord, ventral optic vesicle, optic vesicle, and developing kidney and ureter. *PAX2* is also present and implicated in eye development in *Drosophila*.

12. The paired-like homeobox gene *HESX1* is mutated in one case of autosomal recessive septo-optic dysplasia with

additional brain and pituitary defects. A similar phenotype is seen in the mouse model. *HESX1* maps to 3p21.1-p21.2. Mouse *Hesx1* is briefly expressed in early midline tissue, which induces neural tissue that will ultimately form anterior head structures. In addition, *Hesx1* is expressed in the developing pituitary gland.

13. Mutations in two genes, *CRX* and *NRL*, affect photoreceptor differentiation or maintenance. *CRX*, the cone-rod homeobox gene, regulates the expression of many genes encoding photoreceptor OS proteins, particularly rhodopsin and the cone opsins. *CRX* is a homeobox gene of the paired-like class that is expressed only in rod and cone photoreceptors and in the pineal gland. The gene maps to 19q13.3. Mutations in *CRX* are found in some patients with the early onset disorder Lebers congenital amaurosis (LCA) (both autosomal dominant and recessive forms), in which the photoreceptors either do not form or degenerate early, as well as the later onset retinal degeneration, autosomal dominant cone rod dystrophy (CRD). Very similar mutations are present in both types of patients, and all are likely to be null or other severe loss of function alleles. Comparison of the retinal phenotypes in LCA and CRD patients with *CRX* mutations indicate that they are part of a phenotypic spectrum, the severity of the phenotype being determined primarily by factors other than the *CRX* mutation itself. In mice homozygous for a targeted deletion of *Crx* the photoreceptors are born, but they fail to form outer segments and eventually degenerate. Thus, the CRX protein is required for the differentiation and maintenance of mammalian rod and cone photoreceptors.

14. At least one mutation in the *NRL* gene, which encodes a basic leucine zipper protein expressed in postmitotic retinal and neuronal cells, results in autosomal dominant retinitis pigmentosa (RP). The gene maps to 14q11.1-q11.2, and one RP family whose disease also maps to this region, has a gain-of-function mutation (S50T) within the conserved transactivation domain of the protein. *In vitro* studies indicate that this substitution increases the transactivation by CRX of rhodopsin, one of the CRX target genes. Thus, increased expression of rhodopsin may occur in affected individuals and be responsible for the photoreceptor degeneration. These findings demonstrate that *NRL* is essential for the viability of human photoreceptors.

# INTRODUCTION

## Genetic Disease and the Developing Eye

Eye disease is common in the human population, and developmental eye anomalies generally present in childhood;[1] congenital blindness, the majority of which is genetic in the developed world, occurs in these populations at a frequency of 0.2 to 0.3 per 10,000 live births.[2,3] In a 1985 survey of McKusick's *Mendelian Inheritance in Man*,[4] the eye was involved in 27 percent of the 2811 phenotypes recorded, making it the fourth most common system affected by genetic disease in man. Both positional cloning and the candidate gene approach[5,6] have led to the identification of genes associated with developmental eye anomalies. At a conservative estimate more than 200 human loci for genetic ocular disease have been mapped (www.ncbi.nlm.nih.gov/omim/ ;www.gdb.org/), including those for developmental eye defects — with or without the involvement of other tissues. More than 100 mouse eye mutants have also been mapped (www.informatics. jax.org/). In both species, many other phenotypically defined inherited eye disorders remain to be assigned to loci.

The high frequency of inherited ocular disease in humans is due to two factors: (a) the eye is not essential for viability, and (b) mutations affecting the eye often lead to readily detectable phenotypes or to significant dysfunction requiring clinical attention. The genes found to be associated with abnormalities in eye formation have given insight into both normal development and the pathology caused by mutation. Mutations in transcription factor genes, the focus of this chapter, are also responsible for developmental defects in many other organ systems,[7,8] as well as many forms of cancer. Mutations in 10 human (Table 240-1) transcription factor genes have been shown to disrupt mammalian eye development or maintenance. Mutations in an additional 18 mouse transcription factor genes have also been shown to be associated with developmental abnormalities of the eye (Table 240-2). In contrast, the environmental cues and signaling events required for the formation of the eye are largely unknown, and to date, no disorders affecting the development of the human eye alone have been shown to result from mutations in signaling molecule genes.

## The Developmental Anatomy of the Human Eye and Retina

The gross structure of the human eye is shown in Fig. 240-1. This remarkable sensory organ develops from the embryonic forebrain in a series of distinct morphologic stages (Fig. 240-2), which are described in Table 240-3. The pattern of gene expression during eye development is generally reported in terms of these stages; Table 240-4 summarizes current knowledge of the periods of transcription factor gene expression in mouse. Surface ectoderm, neural ectoderm, neural crest-derived mesenchyme, and mesodermal mesenchyme all contribute to the development of the vertebrate eye. Documenting the stages of human eye development is hampered by the difficulty of obtaining human embryonic and fetal material for analysis; nevertheless, information has been gathered from the series of embryos in the Carnegie Institute's collection.[9,10] This information was readily supplemented by the study of eye development in model organisms, where the vertebrate eye is more accessible, both *in utero* in mammals, but particularly *in ovo* in the chick and in amphibians and fishes. Thus, much is known about the developmental anatomy of the mouse eye,[11,12] and considerable information on lens induction and retinal development comes from this species, as well as other vertebrates.[13–17] Important comparisons have also been made with the compound eye of the fruit fly *Drosophila*.[18] Unexpectedly, mutations at many *Drosophila* loci have provided essential information on genes whose homologues have been discovered to play a key role in vertebrate eye development.[19–22]

## Early Development of the Anterior Segment

The cornea in front and the lens at the back bound the anterior segment. The iris, composed partly of neuroepithelium, projects into this space, which is filled with the aqueous humor. The trabecular meshwork is a sieve-like network of cells forming the iridocorneal junction (or anterior angle) of the eye. In the normal eye, aqueous humor, produced by the ciliary bodies in the posterior chamber, fills the space between the cornea and lens, bathing the iris. The aqueous humor maintains an even pressure within the healthy eye, by a balance of continual secretion and drainage through the trabecular network. Increased intraocular pressure, as well as other anomalies that affect the optic nerve-head, may lead to glaucoma.

The developing anterior segment receives a major contribution from cells of the neural crest mesenchyme which immigrate in three waves into the space between the surface ectoderm and the optic cup following formation and separation of the lens vesicle.[23,24] The anterior epithelial layer of the cornea is formed from the surface ectoderm but the posterior stromal layers and endothelium are derived from the migrating neural crest cells which arrive at around 7 to 8 weeks' gestation (mouse E12 to E13).[9,10,24] The posterior epithelial layer of the iris forms from

**Table 240-1 Inherited Eye Diseases in Human and Mouse Due to Mutations in Transcription Factor Genes**

| Gene | Protein | Function | Disease | Inheritance | Genetic mechanisms | Phenotypes |
|------|---------|----------|---------|-------------|-------------------|------------|
| **Panocular Diseases** | | | | | | |
| *PAX6* | Dual DNA binding: Paired box & Homeodomain of paired-like class | Required for (i) surface ectoderm induction to form lens and all subsequent development of dual layered retina, iris, and cornea (ii) development of forebrain, cerebellum, nasal structures, and pancreas | Aniridia | A.D. | Haploinsufficiency for most classical aniridias. Some variant aniridias associated with rare dominant missense mutations. | ***Human*** Aniridia (partial or complete absence of the iris), accompanied by foveal or optic nerve hypoplasia, cataract, glaucoma and corneal dystrophy, nystagmus ***Mouse*** Heterozygotes: small eye, cataract, iris hypoplasia, lens-cornea adhesions. Homozygotes: neonatal lethal with anophthalmia, rudimentary nasal structures and forebrain plus cerebellar anomalies, pancreatic anomalies |
| *CHX10* | Homeodomain of paired-like class | Required for (i) proliferation of neuroretinal progenitor cells and (ii) development, differentiation, or maintenance of bipolar cells | Micropthalmia | A.R. | Loss of function alleles | ***Human*** Microphthalmia, cataracts, iris coloboma, and blindness ***Mouse*** Homozygotes: microphthalmia, optic nerve aplasia, and cataracts |
| **Anterior Segment Defects** | | | | | | |
| *MITF* | A basic helix-loop-helix, leucine zipper transcription factor | (i) In human and mouse, regulates genes in melanin synthesis pathway (ii) In mice, required for normal eye growth and to prevent hyperproliferation of the RPE; mechanisms unknown | Waardenburg syndrome type 2 (see Chap. 244 for other Waardenburg syndromes) | A.D. | Haploinsufficiency | ***Human*** Iris pigment defects, hearing loss, white forelock ***Mouse*** Heterozygotes: minor eye and skin pigment defects Homozygotes: small eye, with hyperproliferation of RPE, defects in various other pigment cell types |
| *FKHL7* | Forkhead winged helix domain—binds to DNA as monomer | (i) Required for normal development of cornea and iris, and for pressure control—neural crest and paraxial mesoderm (ii) Homozygotes die perinatally with hemorrhagic hydrocephalus and skeletal defects | Axenfeld-Rieger anomaly | A.D. | Haploinsufficiency | ***Human*** Major: iridogoniodysgenesis, posterior embryotoxon Minor: glaucoma, iris hypoplasia, polycoria and/or corectopia ***Mouse*** Homozygotes: iris hypoplasia, corneal defects, unfused eyelids Heterozygotes: anterior segment defects including defects of the trabecular meshwork and Schlemm's canal |

| Gene | Class | Function/Expression | Disorder | Inheritance | Mechanism | Phenotype |
|---|---|---|---|---|---|---|
| PITX2 | Homeodomain—bicoid-like in paired-like class | Required for development of ocular mesenchyme, maxillary and mandibular epithelia, and the umbilicus. Also expressed in developing pituitary and involved in determination of laterality. | Rieger syndrome, iridogonial dysgenesis syndrome | A.D. | Haploinsufficiency | **Human** Rieger anomaly and dental hypoplasia, facial dysmorphism, and umbilical abnormalities **Mouse** Homozygote: optic nerve coloboma, absence of ocular muscles Heterozygote: corectopia, iris abnormalities |
| PITX3 | Homeodomain—bicoid-like in paired-like class | Expression in developing lens placode and maturing lens. Involved in mesencephalic dopaminergic dopaminergic system development. Expressed in tongue, incisors, and mesenchyme around sternum, vertebrae, and head muscles. | Anterior segment mesenchymal dysgenesis; congenital cataract | A.D. | Haploinsufficiency | **Human** Defects in all tissues of anterior eye chamber |

### Posterior Segment Defects

| Gene | Class | Function/Expression | Disorder | Inheritance | Mechanism | Phenotype |
|---|---|---|---|---|---|---|
| PAX2 | Paired domain, conserved octapeptide motif and partial homeodomain | Expression in developing optic cup narrowed to just optic stalk, particularly the retinal fissure. Expression in kidney and otic vesicle. | Renal coloboma syndrome | A.D. | Haploinsufficiency | **Human** Optic nerve coloboma, renal hypoplasia, vesicoureteral reflux, occasional deafness **Mouse** Homozygotes: globe colobomata, optic nerve defects, and absence of optic chiasm Heterozygotes: optic nerve coloboma |
| HESX1 | Homeodomain of paired-like class | Required for forebrain, optic vesicle nasal placode, and pituitary development | Septo-optic dysplasia | A.R. | One allele known, with a severe loss of function | **Human** Optic disc hypoplasia, midline brain abnormalities, pituitary hormone defects, and septum pellucidum absence |

### Abnormalities of Photoreceptor Differentiation or Maintenance

| Gene | Class | Function/Expression | Disorder | Inheritance | Mechanism | Phenotype |
|---|---|---|---|---|---|---|
| CRX | Homeodomain protein of the paired-like class | Morphogenesis and maintenance of the photoreceptor outer segment (OS). Transactivation of the expression of rhodopsin and other OS proteins. | Cone rod dystrophy | A.D. | Haploinsufficiency. Some alleles may be dominant negative. | **Human** Degeneration of cone, then rod, photoreceptors **Mouse** Homozygotes: lack of photoreceptor outer segments and circadian rhythm abnormalities |
| CRX | As above | As above | Lebers congenital amaurosis | A.D. / A.R. | Haploinsufficiency or dominant negative alleles / Loss-of-function alleles | **Human** Congenital absence of functional photoreceptors, or early photoreceptor degeneration |
| NRL | A basic motif/leucine zipper domain protein | A cotransactivator, with CRX, of rhodopsin expression. Otherwise, unknown. | Retinitis pigmentosa | A.D. | One mutant allele known—gain of function allele, which increases transactivation of rhodopsin | **Human** Rod photoreceptor degeneration |

**Table 240-2** Mouse Eye Phenotypes Due to Loss-of-Function Mutations in Transcription Factors

| Gene | Protein | Mutation type | Loss-of-function eye phenotype (homozygote phenotypes except where stated) | Human mapping | References |
|---|---|---|---|---|---|
| Gli3 | Zinc finger | $Gli3^{xt}$ 80kb deletion $Gli3^{xt-J}$: deletion of 3' end of coding | Embryo: variable, normal eyes to eye development arrest at E9.5 | 7p13 | 72–74 |
| Hes1 | Basic helix-loop-helix | Targeted deletion | Embryo: premature retinal cell differentiation, increases in amacrine and rod cells, bipolar cell death | 3q28-3q29 | 75, 76 |
| Hfhbf1 (human FKHL1) | Forkhead winged helix domain | Targeted deletion | Embryo: ventrally rotated eyes, defects in nasal retina, loss of ventral eye structures, and replacement with retinal tissue | 14q11-13 | 77–79 |
| Lhx2 | Homeodomain protein of the LIM class | Targeted deletion | Embryo: eye development halts at E9.5 Adult: anopthhalmia | 9q33-q34 | 80, Unigene: www.ncbi.nlm. nih.gov/UniGene/ |
| Mash1 | Basic helix-loop-helix | Targeted deletion | Embryo: delay in retinal cell differentiation, decrease in bipolar cells, increase in Muller cells | 12q22-q23 | 81–83 |
| NeuroD | Basic helix-loop-helix | Targeted deletion | Embryo: defects in rate of differentiation, and amounts of various retinal cell types | 2q32 | 84, 85 |
| Otx1 | Homeodomain protein of the orthodenticle class | Targeted deletion | Adult: iris reduction, absence of lachrymal and Harderian glands, ciliary bodies | 2p13 | 86, 87 |
| Otx2 | Homeodomain protein of the orthodenticle class | Targeted deletion | Homozygous embryo: severe head defects Heterozygous embryo: variable, micro- and anophthalmia, defects in iris, ocular muscles, cornea, lens, changes in neuroretina and RPE layers | 14q21-q22 | 87–90 |
| Pou4f2 | Homeodomain protein of the POU class | Targeted deletion | Adult: loss of 70% of ganglion cells, requirement for Brn3b in early differentiation of postmitotic retinal ganglion cell precursors | 4q31.2 | 91–94 |
| Prox1 | Homeodomain protein | Targeted deletion | Homozygous embryo: decrease in lens fibre elongation, increase in lens cell proliferation, defects in lens cell differentiation | 1q32.2-q32.3 | 95, 96 |
| Edr | Polycomb Group | Targeted deletion | Embryo: variable, unilateral and bilateral micro- and anophthalmia, optic cup hypoplasia | | 97 |
| Rar α, β, γ | Steroid hormone receptor | Targeted deletion | α—See Rxrb β—Retrolenticular membrane defects γ—See Rxrb | α—9q34 β—6p21.3 γ—1q22-q23 | Review [98,99–103] Mapping: see OMIM |
| Rax | Homeodomain protein of the paired-like class | Targeted deletion | Adult: anophthalmia Embryo: Eye development halts at E9.0 | | 15 |
| Rxr α, β, γ | Steroid hormone receptor | Targeted deletion | α—Ventral eye defects only: cornea, retina, anterior chamber, optic nerve coloboma β—Essential when combined with other Rar or Rxr alleles: defects in eyelids, cornea, anterior chamber, conjunctiva, lens (fibres, retrolenticular membrane, ventral rotation), retina (coloboma of retina and optic nerve, dysplasia, ventral defects) | α—17Q21 β—3P24.3 γ—12q13 | See RAR references |
| Vax1 | Homeodomain protein of the empty spiracles class | Targeted deletion | Adult: optic nerve coloboma and optic nerve dysgenesis Embryo: defects in optic stalk and optic nerve formation and differentiation | 10q26.1 | 104, 105 |

A targeted deletion is also known as a knockout mouse. The loss-of-function is further characterized as to the genotype and whether the eye defects are seen during embryogenesis or in an adult mouse. References describe the phenotype as well as human mapping data.

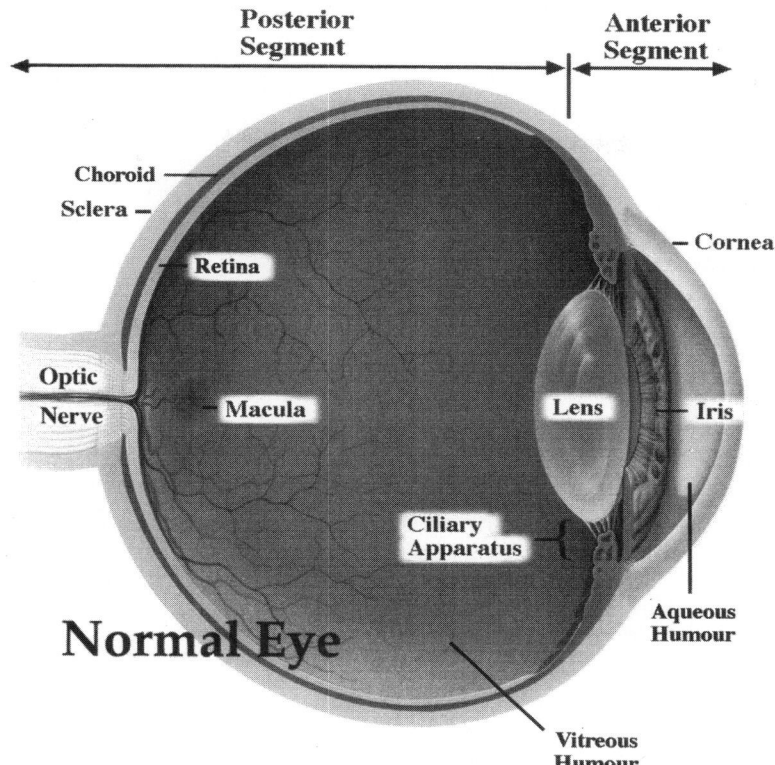

**Fig. 240-1 A schematic of a human adult eye.** The adult eye can be subdivided into two major domains: the anterior and posterior eye. The anterior segment includes the tissues shown on the right, moving from distal to proximal, the cornea, aqueous humour, iris, and lens. The lens is attached to the globe of the eye via the ciliary muscles and trabecular meshwork, which are derived from the ciliary body. The ciliary muscles and trabecular meshwork comprise the ciliary apparatus. The trabecular meshwork regulates the intraocular pressure of the eye by regulating fluid movement between the anterior and posterior regions of the eye. The posterior segment is made up of the most proximal parts of the eye. These include the retina proper and the back of the eye where the optic nerve exits. On the outside of the globe is the sclera, which adds rigidity to the eye. Internal to this layer is the choroid, which is made up largely of blood vessels. The innermost tissue is the retina, which contains two major types of cells: an external layer one cell thick, the retinal pigment epithelium (RPE), and an internal, multilayered neuroretina. The globe is filled with the vitreous humor. Light enters the eye through the transparent cornea, through the pupil in the center of the iris, and is focused on the back of the neuroretina by the lens (see Fig. 240-2 for a photograph of the neuroretina). Light scatter is reduced by the retinal pigment epithelium. Photons are captured by the photoreceptors located at the outside of the neuroretina adjacent to the RPE, and the energy is transduced to electric signals. The signal is passed through interneurons of the retina to the ganglion cells at the inner part of the neuroretina. The axons of ganglion cells exit the eye at the optic disc and fasciculate to form the optic nerve which travels to the optic centres of the brain. The human eye contains a specialized region of the neuroretina called the fovea or macula, where cone photoreceptors are concentrated. Light is focused on the fovea, and the high cone number results in high acuity vision. (*Figure modified from Timothy J. Peters and Co. Inc. Copyright 1994 by Tim Peters and Company, Inc., Peapack, NJ, USA. Used with permission.*)

forward growth of the bilayered rim of the optic cup whereas the anterior stromal layer is formed from neural crest mesenchyme. The neural crest in this region also forms a vascular layer across the front of the lens called the prepupillary membrane. This later involutes to leave a clear central pupil and the relatively avascular collarette of the iris, but remnants of this tissue may remain in some individuals as so-called persistent pupillary strands which are seen as pale fine fibrous threads crossing the pupil in front of the lens. The trabecular meshwork is formed exclusively from neural crest cells. Development of the iris and trabecular meshwork takes place in several stages and is completed relatively late in gestation (eighth month in humans, E18 mice). Normal development of the iris is dependent on complete closure of the optic fissure at about 6 weeks (E12 to E12.5).

## Posterior Eye Development

The basic structure of the posterior part of the eye is established during the major phase of ocular organogenesis (up to E11 in mouse, 33 days of gestation in humans;) (Fig. 240-1, Fig. 240-2, and Table 240-3).[9–12,24] During this time, the optic vesicle grows out from the prosencephalon and induces lens formation from the overlying surface ectoderm. As the lens vesicle buds off from the surface ectoderm, the optic vesicle invaginates to form the bilayered optic cup with a channel, called the choroidal fissure, running along the ventral side. At the same time the optic stalk, which maintains the connection between the optic cup and the forebrain, undergoes involution along its ventral side to form the optic groove; the optic groove is continuous with the choroidal fissure. As soon as this major phase of morphogenesis is complete, the individual layers of the eye begin to assume the characteristics of their mature structures. The inner layer of the optic cup — the future neural retina — undergoes extensive proliferation to generate retinal precursor cells (see "Retinal Development" below). At the same time, the outer layer of the optic cup — the future pigmented retinal epithelium — is relatively inactive in terms of cell division, but begins to express pigment. The hyaloid artery enters the space between the retina and the lens — the future vitreous cavity — through the choroidal fissure and forms the blood supply to the posterior part of the developing lens. Mesenchymal cells also enter the cavity and differentiate into phagocytes and fibroblasts of the primary vitreous, the latter of which will secrete the collagenous matrix of the mature vitreous.

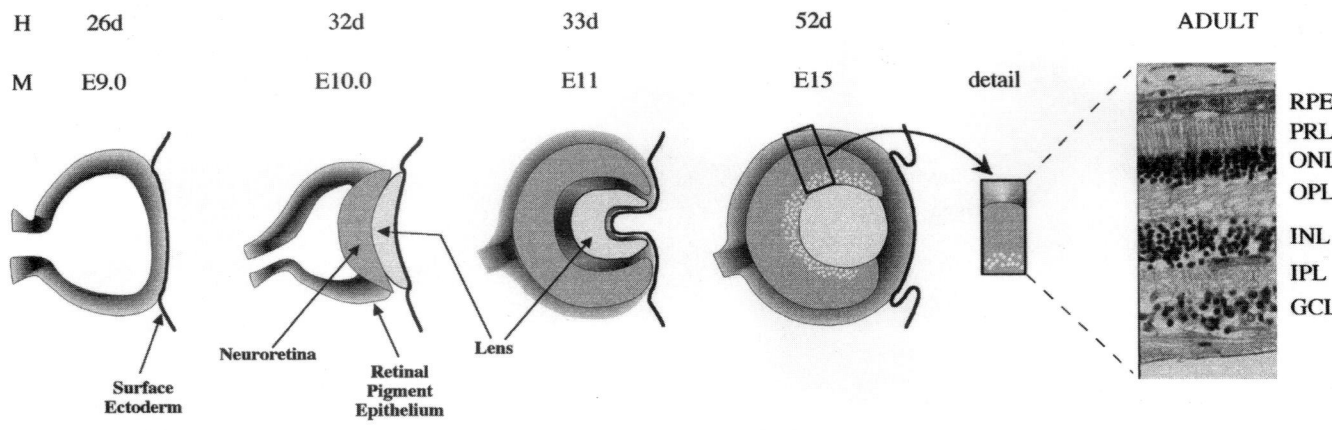

Fig. 240-2 A schematic presentation of early stages of mouse and human eye development, and their chronology during embryogenesis. Human eye development is described in more detail in Table 240-3. The emphasis is on the morphogenesis of the eye cup and lens, and the development of the neuroretina and the retinal pigment epithelium (RPE). Three major stages are emphasized: the optic vesicle stage, the lens placode stage, and the optic cup stage. The first morphologic manifestation of mammalian eye development is the evagination of the embryonic forebrain to form the optic pit. This evagination becomes a lateral diverticulation of the forebrain, the optic vesicle. As the optic vesicle approaches the overlying surface ectoderm, it induces the formation of the lens placode, which later invaginates and pinches off to form the lens vesicle and, eventually, the lens. The cells of the lens vesicle nearest the optic cup differentiate into elongated lens fibers, while the lateral cells, closest to the surface ectoderm, remain as a monolayer. The invagination of the optic vesicle creates the two-layered optic cup, an outside layer which give rise to the RPE, and an inner layer of progenitor cells, which go on to develop into the neuroretina. The iris develops from the peripheral edge of the optic cup, from a cell layer continuous with the neuroretina. The cornea develops from a layer of overlying ectoderm. In the depiction of an E11.5 retina, some visibly differentiating cells are illustrated; the majority of the first differentiating cells one can detect are ganglion cells. In the adult retina, the nucleus of each cell type is situated in one of three nuclear layers; two plexiform layers containing the processes of retinal cells separate the nuclear layers. The photoreceptor and ganglion cell layers contain those two respective cell types. The inner nuclear layer contains the cell bodies of four major cell types: horizontal cells, bipolar cells, amacrine cells, and Müller cells. The photo is of a human retina, stained with hematoxylin and eosin. PRL = photoreceptor layer; ONL = outer nuclear layer; OPL = outer plexiform layer; INL = inner nuclear layer; IPL = inner plexiform layer; GCL = ganglion cell layer. (*Modified from Figure 1 of Freund et al.*[5] *Used with permission.*)

By E12.5 to E13 in mouse (44 days in humans) the neural layer of the optic cup is organized into two major cellular layers, the outer neuroblastic layer (adjacent to the pigment layer) and the inner neuroblastic layer. Nerve fibers from the inner neuroblastic layer begin to extend into the optic stalk, which will give rise to the optic nerve. The optic stalk soon becomes completely filled with nerve fibers. Shortly afterward, the lips of the choroidal fissure fuse together, enclosing the blood vessels within the eye. Condensation of mesenchymal cells occurs around the optic cup, giving rise to the sclera. In the later stages of prenatal development, the most dramatic changes are seen in the neural retina, which undergoes extensive differentiation to generate the many neural cell types. In mouse and man, retinal development continues after birth.

### Retinal Development

Because mutations in several transcription factor genes have been shown to affect the proliferation and/or differentiation of the neuroretina, some description of retinal development is required (reviewed in references 13, 25, and 26). Development of the neuroretina is first characterized by the proliferation of progenitor cells (Fig. 240-2). The mitotic progenitor cells of the neuroretina are multipotent: each appears to have the potential to form any of the six major classes of mature retinal neurons (photoreceptors, bipolar, horizontal, interplexiform, amacrine, and ganglion cells), as well as Müller cells, a type of glial cell. The neuroretinal progenitor cells first begin to leave the cell cycle at E10.5 in mouse[27] (human stage 14 to 32 days), and therefore, as indicated in Fig. 240-2, some retinal progenitors continue to proliferate, while others are differentiating into mature neurons. Each retinal cell type is born within a developmental interval characteristic of that cell; ganglion cells, for example, are amongst the first born retinal neurons in mouse ("born" referring to the day a cell becomes postmitotic), and bipolar cells amongst the last. The timing and mechanisms of the commitment of a retinal progenitor

to become a specific cell type are largely unknown, but it appears that progenitors are competent to become committed to a specific fate only after they exit the mitotic cycle. The commitment of a competent postmitotic progenitor cell to a specific cell fate is controlled by signals from the microenvironment.[13,26,28]

### Eye Evolution and Development

Charles Darwin perceived the eye as an "organ of extreme perfection and complication"—a challenging system to fit into his theory of evolution. Darwin's theory postulates that evolution takes place by gradual change while maintaining constant functionality of all essential components. It is unlikely, therefore, that eyes built to the radically different plans observed in different phyla, can have evolved sequentially.[29,30] It is now considered probable that eyes as sophisticated image-forming organs have evolved independently, presumably incorporating some common ancestral cell type, 40 or more times in different phyla.[31,32] Molecular techniques reveal that a series of conserved homologous genes play a major role in ocular development and function, in the diverse phyla studied, from worms to man.[20,33–35] These findings suggest that ancestral groups of coadapted genes, with a central role in sensory-neural cell development, have evolved together to create a primitive photosensitive cell type that has been used repeatedly to build different types of eyes.[36] This concept is echoed throughout evolutionary developmental biology.[37]

## AN OVERVIEW OF TRANSCRIPTION FACTORS IN DEVELOPMENT

The regulation of development is one of the most complex of biologic processes, and our understanding of the molecular mechanisms for exerting developmental control is still rudimentary. To achieve the precise pattern of cell division, growth,

**Table 240-3** A Comparison of the Timing of Eye Development Stages During the Embryonic Period Between Human and Mouse

| Developmental events | Human | Mouse |
|---|---|---|
| Optic evagination of neural ectoderm at the optic sulcus. | stage 11, 14 somites ~24 days postovulation | E8.5 |
| Optic vesicle touches surface ectoderm; both thicken; optic vesicle is covered by and surface ectoderm is lined by a basement membrane. | stage 13, 30+ somites ~28 days postovulation | E9.5 |
| Early invagination of the lens placode; delineation of the choroid fissure. | stage 14 ~32 days postovulation | E10 |
| Lens pit closed, lens vesicle formed, lens surrounded by capsule and early primary lens fibers appear. Restored surface ectoderm overlying lens is presumptive anterior surface of cornea. Double layered optic cup begins to express pigment in the outer layer. The neural retina consists of 5–6 rows of cells. | stage 15 ~33 days postovulation | E11 |
| Pentagonal optic cup around the developing lens, still with large lens vesicle. Perilental blood vessels visible. Retinal pigment becoming clearly visible. Edges of the optic fissure are in contact. | stage 16 ~37 days postovulation | E11.5 |
| Lens fibers thickening and encroaching on lens cavity, eventually making vesicle cresent shaped. Internal neuroblastic layer of the retina seen as cells migrate from the primary zone, starting in the region of the future macula. Optic fissure nearly closed, but optic stalk still has lumen communicating with diencephalon. | stage 17 ~41 days postovulation | E12-12.5 |
| Cell migration has formed the internal neuroblastic layer throughout the retina. Cavity of lens vesicle becoming obliterated by primary lens fibers. Characteristic arch of posterior lens nuclei seen in thickened primary lens fibers. Mesenchyme has begun to invade the region between the surface epithelium and surface ectoderm; formation of the posterior corneal epithelium begins (mesothelium of the anterior chamber). | stage 18 44 days postovulation | E12.5-13 |
| Optic nerve still slender, with fibres reaching only short distance beyond retina. Lips of retinal fissure temporarily everted near optic stalk. Neural crest-derived mesenchyme begin to condense around optic cup to form the sclera. Posterior epithelium of cornea distinguishable. | stage 19 47–48 days postovulation | E13.5 |
| Nerve fibers become visible in retina. Lumen of optic stalk becoming obliterated. Lens cavity obliterated, lens suture begins to form. Cornea has anterior and posterior epithelium with an intervening acellular layer. Crystallins and other lens proteins begin to form. | stage 20 50–51 days postovulation | E14.5 |
| Hyaloid groove visible at the bulbar end of optic nerve. Some nerve-fibers arriving at the brain, with the optic tract reaching the site of the lateral geniculate body. | stage 21 52 days postovulation | E15 |
| Mesenchyme surrounding optic nerve forms sheath. Scleral condensation is now definite. Bergemeister's papilla discernible surrounding the exit of the hyaloid artery from optic nerve. Pupillary membrane and anterior develop. | stage 22 54 days postovulation | E16.5 |
| A vascular canal is present in the optic nerve. Basement membrane of anterior epithelium formed. Retina now has pigmented layer, external limiting membrane, proliferative zone, external neuroblastic, transient fiber layer, internal neuroblastic and nerve fiber layer and internal limiting membrane. 2° vitreous body and 2° lens fibers forming. | stage 23 56–57 days postovulation | E17-17.5 |

Human details from O'Rahilly et al.,[9] O'Rahilly and Muller,[10] and Bron et al.,[24] and the sometimes difficult-to-make mouse comparisons from Pei and Rhodin[11] and Kaufman.[12]

migration, programmed cell death, and differentiation necessary to create a complex organism requires the ordered activation and silencing of thousands of genes in a spatially and temporally controlled manner. The constantly and permanently changing environment of a developing cell distinguishes developmental regulation from virtually all other types of biologic control.

The cornerstones of developmental regulation are the signaling events within and between cells, and the competence of cells to produce and respond to signals.[38,39] Transcription factors are *trans*-acting proteins that affect the rate of RNA synthesis of target genes by specific interactions with DNA and/or other proteins.[8] The silencing and activation of downstream genes that is necessary for developmental regulation is achieved mainly by tissue-specific transcription factors whose expression is temporally and spatially restricted. Transcription factors usually act through multiprotein complexes that include both ubiquitously expressed general factors required for RNA polymerase activity and other tissue-specific factors.[8] Tissue-specific transcription factors may act as transcriptional activators or repressors, or, depending on the

context, have either effect;[40] sometimes both mechanisms are elicited by different protein isoforms derived from the same gene under different cellular conditions.[41,42] Ultimately, tissue-specific transcription factors mediate the control of transcriptional switching required to execute developmental programs that culminate in mature tissues and organs.

## Identification of Transcription Factors

Transcription factors are identified by their association with other transcription regulatory proteins in functional assays, by the effect of mutations in the genes encoding them, or, perhaps most often, by their possession of domains found in previously defined transcription factors, including those encoded by genes characterized in other organisms such as *Drosophila*. These domains include, for example, DNA-binding domains such as homeodomains, zinc fingers, POU, and LIM, and paired domains.[5,7] Novel motifs emerge as sequence comparisons are made increasingly frequently in the genome era.[20,43,44] As implied by this ability to categorize them, transcription factors belong to

**Table 240-4 Transcription Factors Expressed in the Developing Mammalian Eye**

**Time of Eye Expression**

Time axis markers: E8.5, E11.5, E14.5, E17.5, P0, Adult

| Transcription Factor | Notable Sites of Eye Expression | Reference |
|---|---|---|
| Rax (prd-1 HB) | E7.5: anterior neural plate, proliferating retina | 15, 104 |
| Lhx2 (LIM HB) | optic pit, retina, INL, glial cells in optic stalk | 80, 105 |
| Pax6 (prd HB) | neuroretina, lens, cornea | 106–109 |
| Rar-α,β,γ (steroid receptor) | α—widely expressed, β—similar to α, retrolenticular membrane, γ—low levels | 110–112 |
| Six3 (HB) | neuroretina, lens, optic stalk, adult retina, RPE | 34, 48 |
| Erbal2§ (steroid receptor) | widely expressed | 113 |
| Vax1 (ems HB) | optic vesicle, disk, stalk | 105, 114 |
| Mitf (bHLH, ZIP) | optic vesicle, RPE, ciliary body | 115–118 |
| Tlx§ (steroid receptor) | optic vesicle, stalk, cup, nerve, GCL | 119 |
| Prox1 (HB) | optic vesicle, neuroretina, lens | 49, 95 |
| Pax2 (prd HB) | optic vesicle, cup, stalk, nerve | 106, 120–122 |
| Msx1 (msh HB) | neuroretina, nasal ciliary body | 123 |
| Msx2 (msh HB) | neuroretina, surface epithelium | 123 |
| Chx10 (CVC HB) | neuroretina, INL | 67, 124 |
| Atoh3§ (bHLH) | neuroretina, INL | 125, 125 |
| Mash1 (bHLH) | proliferating cells, presumptive INL, GCL | 81, 127 |
| Gbx2 (HB) | optic vesicle | 128 |
| Hfhbf2§ (WH) | temporal optic stalk and neuroretina | 129 |
| Gli,2,3 (Zn F) | Gli-outer retina 2,3-optic stalk, lens | 130 |
| Sox 1,2 (HMG) | 1—lens 2—presumptive lens | 16, 131, 132 |
| Eya1,2,3 (eya) | retina, lens, RPE, other eye structures | 20 |
| Dach (Dachbox) | eye mesenchyme, neuroretina | 44, 133 |
| Slu (Zn F) | lens | 134 |
| Erbal3§ (nuclear receptor) | neuroretina, ONL, optic stalk, nerve | 135, 136 |
| Otx1 (otd HB) | non-neural eye structures, iris | 137, 138 |
| Otx2 (otd HB) | neuroretina and other eye structures | 137, 138 |
| Pitx3 (prd-1 HB) | lens | 139, 140 |
| Hfhbf1§ (WH) | nasal optic stalk and neuroretina | 129 |
| Hes1 (bHLH) | retinal mitotic cells until P10 | 75 |

*(Continued to next page)*

**Table 240-4** (Continued)

| Gene (motif) | Expression timeline | Expression location | References |
|---|---|---|---|
| *RPF-1* (POU IV) | ▬▬▬▬▬ | neuroretina, GCL, amacrine | 141 |
| *Neurod* (bHLH) | ▬▬▬▬▬ | differentiating neurons, adult retina | 84, 142 |
| *Dlx1,2* (dl1 HB) | •••▬▬••• | 1, 2 have similar retina expression, 1 more abundant | 128, 143 |
| *Hmx1,2,3*§ (hmx HB) | •••▬▬••• | optic vesicle, optic cup | 144, 145 |
| *Twist* (bHLH) | ▬▬▬▬ | eye mesenchyme, cornea, eyelids | 146 |
| *Foxc1*§ (WH) | ▬▬▬▬ | eye mesenchyme, cornea, eyelids | 147 |
| *Atoh4*§ (bHLH) | ▬▬▬••• | optic vesicle, neuroretina | 148 |
| *Pitx2*§ (prd-1 HD) | •••▬•••   •••▬ | eye mesenchyme | 139, 149 |
| *Aprop1*§ (nuclear receptor) | •••▬••• | optic cup, vesicle, stalk | 114, 136 |
| *ROR β*§ (nuclear receptor) | ▬▬▬▬ | neuroretina, INL, CGL | 150 |
| *Atoh5*§ (HLH) | ▬▬▬▬ | proliferating neuroretinal cells | 151 |
| *Nhlh1*§ (HLH) | •••▬▬••• | sensory layer of optic cup | 152 |
| *Gsh-1* (HB) | •••▬▬••• | optic stalk | 153 |
| *Crx* (prd-1 HB) | ▬▬▬▬ | photoreceptors | 154 |
| *Titf1, Nkx2-2*§ (NK1 HB) | •••▬▬••• | optic recess, retina | 155, 156 |
| *Rxr-α,β,γ* (steroid receptor) | ▬▬••• | α,β—diffuse   γ—neuroblastic retina | 157 |
| *Nrl* (bZIP) | ▬▬▬▬ | all postmitotic retinal cells | 158, 159 |
| *Cutl1*⁷§ (cut HB) | •••▬▬••• | neuroretina | 160 |
| *Png1*§ (Zn F) | •••▬▬••• | GCL | 161 |
| *Pou4f1,2,3*§ (POU IV HB) | ▬ ▬ ▬ ▬ ▬ | GCL precursors, 1 more abundant | 92–94, 162–166 |
| *Emx1,2* (ems HB) | •••▬▬••• | neuroretina, lens | 137, 167 |
| *Mid1*§ (Zn F) | •••▬•••▬••• | lens | 168 |
| *Hes5* (bHLH) | •••▬▬ | high until P6, ONL | 169 |
| *Isl1* (LIM HB) | •••▬ | INL, GCL | 170 |
| *Six2,5* (HB) | •••▬ | INL, ONL, GCL and RPE | 48 |

Genes expressed earliest are listed first (as determined in mouse or rat). The increasingly shaded line denotes the progression of eye development: E8.5 is embryonic day 8.5, P0 denotes postnatal day 0. A line that ends between P0 and Adult indicates that expression ends during postnatal development. Dots indicate that expression has not been determined or not reported precisely. A dashed line indicates varied reports of expression. The transcription factor motif associated with each gene is indicated: homeobox (HB) and their accompanying class (prd, prd-1, ems, hmx (NK), msh, otd, dll, cut, POU, CVC, LIM); winged helix motif (WH); (basic) helix-loop-helix domain ((b)HLH); zinc-finger motif (Zn F); high mobility group protein (HMG); leucine zipper motif (ZIP) steroid receptors and novel domains (eya, dachbox). Genetic nomenclature is from the Mouse Genome Database (www.informatics.jax.org/). Abbreviations: GCL = ganglion cell layer; ONL = outer nuclear layer; INL = inner nuclear layer; RPE = retinal pigmented epithelium.
§Accepted gene symbols: *Lhx2* = LIM homeobox protein 2, was *LH-2*;

*Erbal2* = avian erythroblastic leukemia viral (v-erb-a), oncogene homolog-like 2 (was *EAR2* and a COUP-TF family members); Tlx = Tailless; *Atoh3,4,5* = Atonal homologue 3, 4, 5 (was Math3,4a,5); *Hfhbfl,2* = HNF-3/forkhead, brain factor 1,2; *Erbal3* = avian erythroblastic leukemia viral (v-erb-a) oncogene homolog-like 3 (was *EAR3/COUP-TFI*); Hmx1 = H6 homeobox 1; Hmx2 (was *Nkx-5.2*), Hmx3 (was *Nkx-5.1*); *Foxcl* = Forkhead box C1 (was Mf1); *Pitx2* = paired-like homeodomain transcription factor 2 (was *Rieg*); *Aporp1* = apolipoprotein regulatory protein 1 (was *COUP-TFII/ ARP-1*); *Nhlh1* = Nescient helix loop helix 1 (was *NSCL*); *Titf1* = thyroid transcription factor (was *TTF-1, Nkx2-1*); *Nkx2-2* = NK2 transcription factor 2; *Cutl1* = cut homeobox-like 1 (Was *mClox, Phox2*); *Png1* = postmitotic neural gene-1; *Pou4f1,2,3* = POU class IV factor 1,2,3 (was Brn-3a, -3b,-3c); *Mid1* = Midline 1; *RORβ* = retinoid-related orphan receptor β.
Modified from Table 2 of Freund et al.[5] Used by permission of *Human Molecular Genetics* and Oxford University Press.

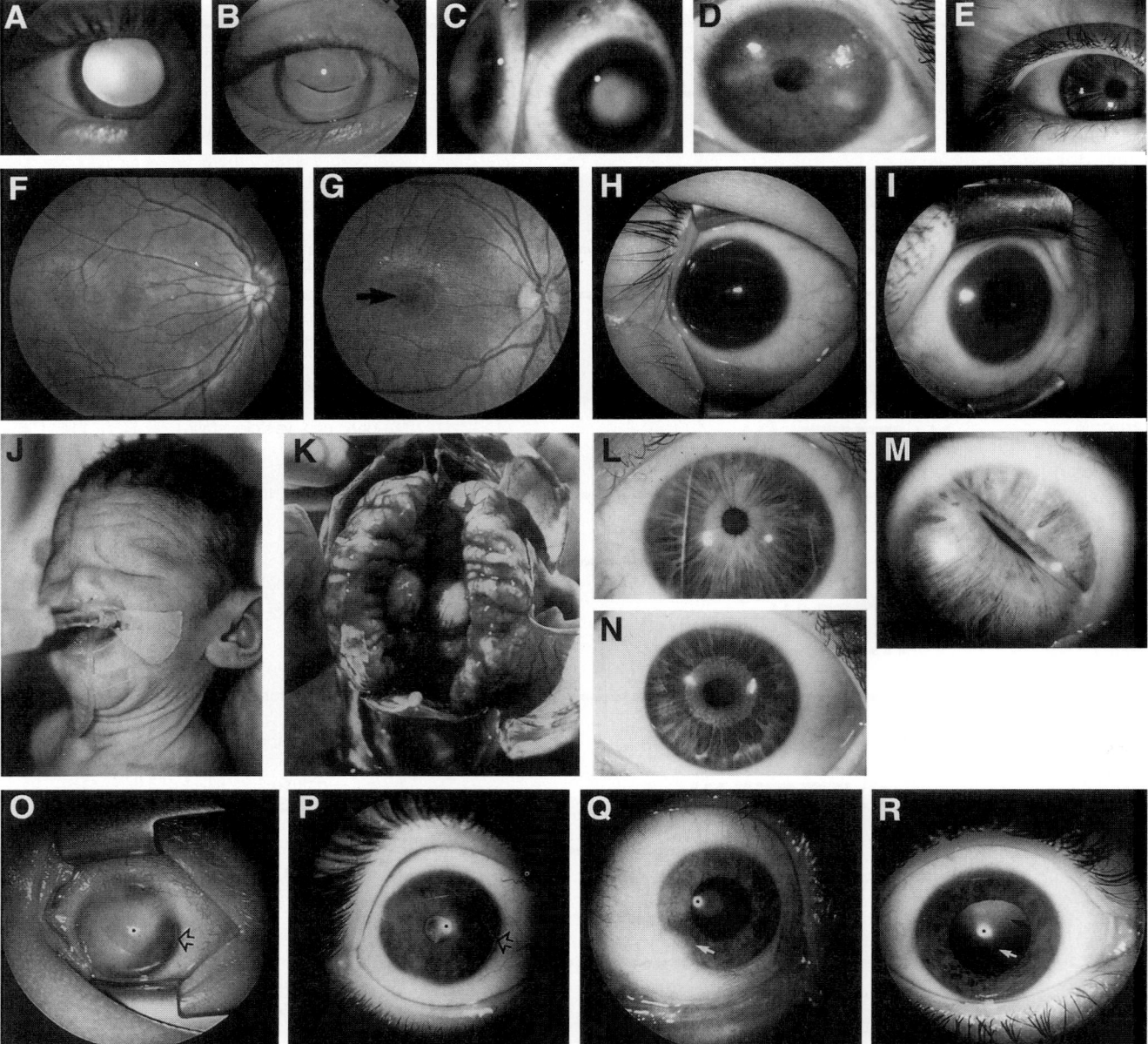

Fig. 240-3 Phenotypic variability of *PAX6* mutations and phenotypic overlap with mutations at other loci. *A*, Virtual absence of iris in classical aniridia. The red reflex from the retina is seen in this undilated eye. (*From S. Day: Developmental abnormalities of the anterior segment. 23, Fig. 23.14, in Taylor D (ed): Pediatric Ophthalmology, 2nd ed., Boston, Blackwell Scientific 1990. Used with permission.*) The mutation has not been defined in this individual. *B*, The same patient 6 years later, with subluxation of the lens, presence of cataract and glaucoma, illustrating the progressive nature of this developmental eye anomaly. (*From S. Day: Developmental abnormalities of the anterior segment. 23, Fig. 23.14, in Taylor D (ed): Pediatric Ophthalmology, 2nd ed., Boston, Blackwell Scientific 1990. Used with permission.*) *C*, Gonioscopic view of Peters anomaly case with R26G *PAX6* mutation.[199] The lens corneal adhesion is seen with posterior embryotoxon. (*From Holmstrom et al.[200] Used with permission.*) *D*, Autosomal dominant keratitis with intron 10 splice-acceptor site mutation −2 AT. (*From Mirzayans et al.[201] Used with permission.*) *E*, Corectopia and iris hypoplasia with absent collarette, mild corneal limbal dystrophy, and hypoplasia of the optic nerve and macula in patient with V126D *PAX6* paired-box mutation. (*From Hanson et al.[202] Used with permission.*) *F*, Isolated foveal hypoplasia in case with R128C *PAX6* paired-box mutation. (*From Azuma et al.[203] Used with permission.*) *G*, Normal right fundus showing the darker fovea with no blood vessels encroaching on it. (*From Azuma et al.[203] Used with permission.*) *H*, Apparently normal iris of case with foveal hypoplasia (*G*). (*From Azuma et al.[203] Used with permission.*) *I*, Uveal ectropion, invasion of the cornea by conjunctival epithelium, posterior embryotoxon in case with missense mutation Q422R in the most C-terminal amino acid of *PAX6*. (*From Azuma and Yamada.[204] Used with permission.*) *J*, Facial features of the *PAX6* compound heterozygous neonate carrying two different *PAX6* mutations with anophthalmia, fused eyelids, choanal atresia, and microcephaly. The infant died at day 8 postpartum. (*From Glaser et al.[188] Used with permission.*) *K*, The severe brain malformations in compound heterozygote neonate (shown in J), were revealed at autopsy. (*From Glaser et al.[188] Used with permission.*) *L*, Member of autosomal dominant Axenfeld-Rieger anomaly family[205] with S82T *FKHL7* mutation.[206] Marked iris stromal hypoplasia and corectopia are accompanied by prominent displacement of the Schwalbe line (the white line) detached from the cornea and crossing the anterior chamber. (*From Gould et al.[205] Used with permission.*) *M*, Slit-lamp photograph of hypoplastic iris revealing the pupillary sphincter muscle and distorted iris (corectopia) in a familial Rieger syndrome case with W133X *PITX2* mutation. Posterior embryotoxon and an anteriorly displaced Schwalbe line are also seen. Affected individuals also have tooth anomalies and failure of normal umbilical skin involution. (*From Semina et al.[207] Used with permission.*) *N*, Iris stroma hypoplasia and distinct pupillary sphincter muscle in a case of familial iridogoniodysgenesis syndrome (IGDS) with an R70H mutation in the homeobox domain

recognizable families and subfamilies that have been highly conserved through evolution.

## Conserved Gene Cassettes

Interacting groups of transcription-factor molecules have recently been described as "gene cassettes,"[36] because their components are coadapted to work together in multimeric complexes and they have been utilized as a group when new species evolve. Evolutionary divergence among members of such groups is constrained by the need for continuing interactions.[45] Members of such gene cassettes stand out as exceptionally highly conserved across large evolutionary distances. The *PAX6* gene, with a pivotal role in eye development, is a key example of stringent conservation across many phyla, with a greater than 93 percent amino acid identity throughout its length among vertebrates, and showing more than 90 percent homeodomain and 73 percent paired-domain identity to the nematode worm *Caenorhabditis elegans*.[46,47]

Several other genes implicated in eye disease and eye development also show a very high degree of conservation from fruit flies to humans (e.g., Kawakami et al.[48]). This conserved homology has made possible a two-way traffic: flies to mammals for the eye genes *sine oculis* and *eyes absent*,[34,49,50] and mammals to flies for the *Pax2* and *Rx* genes[21,51] in gene identification, both at the practical nucleic acid screening level and also by sequence database searching.[43] Six homologous descendants of *Drosophila sine oculis*,[22,48,52,53] four of *eyes absent*,[20,54] and one of *dachshund*[44] have so far been identified in mammals, and, in several cases, shown to be expressed during early eye development. These genes have also been shown to interact physically and genetically in *Drosophila* eye development[55,56] and may therefore also interact in fulfilling similar functions in vertebrates eye formation, including humans. The significance of finding such high degrees of conservation both at sequence and functional levels, lies in the possibility of exploring gene interactions relevant to human development and disease, in simpler, more experimentally amenable organisms like *Drosophila* or even *C. elegans*.

Because gene cassettes define groups of transcription factors that function together in regulating development, it seems likely that the *cis*-regulatory DNA target sequences to which the factors bind may also be conserved and utilized in a modular combinatorial manner. The identification of these sequences is at a very early stage in vertebrates. Examples of how such sequences are used in development is provided by other organisms, for example in the modular regulation of two sea urchin genes[57,58] (discussed by Roush[59]).

## The Biologic Functions of Transcription Factors in Development

During development transcription factors have four general roles. First, they may induce the cells in which they are expressed to produce signals that modify the microenvironment, thereby influencing the developmental program of neighboring cells, or, in an autocrine fashion, of themselves. A second role is to make cells competent to respond to appropriate environmental stimuli.

Third, because of the changes in gene expression and cell responsiveness that they initiate, transcription factors ultimately regulate the changes in the biology of cells that underlie development. These changes include cell division, growth, migration, programmed cell death, and the conferring of identity on a cell or a region of the embryo. In this last role, transcription factors inform cells about their location in the developing embryo, and "tell" cells what kind of cells they should be.[39,60,61] In both invertebrates and vertebrates, one well-known example of such regional specification occurs in the development of axial structures, which are defined by the particular combination of one class of homeobox genes—the *Hox* genes—expressed by cells in each region of the axis. The specific combination of *Hox* genes required for the formation of a particular region is referred to as the *Hox code* of that region.[62,63] Consequently, the combination of transcription factors expressed by a cell in a particular environment is termed its transcription factor code. Finally, transcription factors establish the programs of cell-specific gene expression that define the differentiated phenotype of the cell.

**Maintenance of the Differentiated State.** Transcription factor genes active in development are often also expressed in mature tissues, where they are essential to the maintenance of the differentiated state.[8,64,65] This principle is well illustrated in the eye. Several genes shown to be associated with developmental eye defects, including, for example, *PAX6*, *CHX10*, and *CRX*, continue to be expressed in the adult eye,[66–68] and at least in the case of the retinal gene *CRX*, loss of function leads to loss of the differentiated phenotype and cell death.[69–71] A requirement for ongoing expression of some genes in differentiated tissues may also underlie the presently unexplained progressive components of many developmental eye anomalies, such as the limbal stem cell deficiency leading to corneal opacification that occurs in some patients with aniridia due to mutations in *PAX6*. Thus, in addition to the demonstrated roles of *CRX* and *NRL* in photoreceptor degenerations (see "Photoreceptor Differentiation and Maintenance"), other eye-expressed transcription factors are likely to be implicated in later-onset diseases.

## CATEGORIES OF DEVELOPMENTAL EYE DISEASE

A variety of human eye disease phenotypes result from mutations in transcription factor genes (Table 240-1), and these phenotypes can involve one or more ocular structures. Grossly, the adult human eye can be partitioned into anterior and posterior segments (Fig. 240-1). The anterior segment comprises the cornea, sclera, iris, trabecular network, and lens, as well as the aqueous humor-containing anterior chamber that these structures enclose. The posterior segment consists of the choroid enclosing the retina, and the vitreous humor, which is in contact with the posterior lens.

## PANOCULAR DISEASES

Developmental anomalies that affect many parts of the eye may be described as panocular defects, which are broad phenotypes that arise by at least two different general mechanisms. The first, best illustrated by heterozygous mutations in the homeobox gene *PAX6*, reflects the fact that the gene is expressed in and required for the normal development and/or maintenance of all regions of the developing eye: both neural and pigmented retina, iris, lens, and surface ectoderm (Fig. 240-2). Thus, although aniridia is frequently described as an anterior segment anomaly, it is more accurately classified as a panocular disorder[171] because the iris anomaly is frequently accompanied by cataracts and glaucoma and by corneal and retinal abnormalities (Fig. 240-3). Not surprisingly, homozygous loss of *PAX6* gene function leads to complete absence of eye development (Fig. 240-3).

The second mechanism by which panocular defects arise is illustrated by the abnormalities that result from mutations in the *CHX10* homeobox gene. These mutations are global in their

**(Figure 240-3 Continued)** of *PITX2*. (*From Kulak et al.*[208] *Used with permission.*) O, Member of anterior segment mesenchymal dysgenesis (ASMD) family[209] with a 17-bp insertion into the *PITX3* gene, leading to premature protein truncation showing central corneal leucoma with iris adhesion and cataract. (*From Semina et al.*[140] *Used with permission.*) P, Member of ASMD family in *N*: dense cataractous lens overshadows a translucent central corneal leucoma. (*From Semina et al.*[140] *Used with permission.*) Q, Member of ASMD family in *N*: dense cataractous lens overshadows a dense peripheral corneal leucoma with an iris adhesion. (*From Semina et al.*[140] *Used with permission.*) R, Member of ASMD family in *N*: small corneal and lens opacities might escape detection without the family history and slit-lamp observation. (*From Semina et al.*[140] *Used with permission.*)

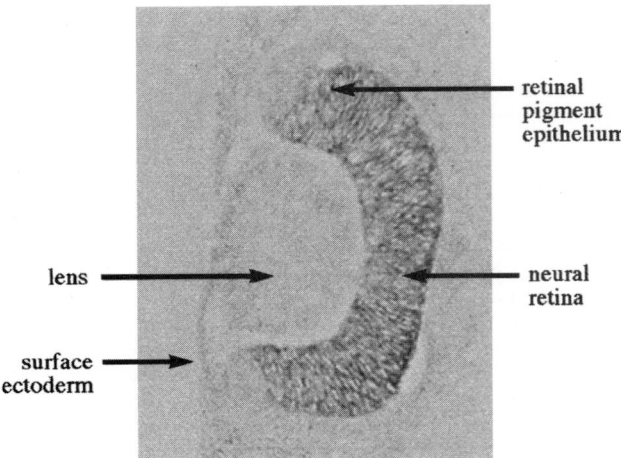

lens

surface
ectoderm

retinal
pigment
epithelium

neural
retina

**Fig. 240-4** *Chx10* expression in the developing mouse eye. *In situ* hybridization of an E10.5 transverse section through a mouse eye probed with *Chx10* RNA. The probe is DIG (digoxigenin)-labeled RNA. *Chx10* expression is seen as dark staining. *Chx10* is present solely in the developing neuroretina (central layer) at this stage, and has never been detected in the developing lens (far right layer) or RPE (layer just to the right of the neuroretina).[173] At this stage, the RPE is unpigmented, and as it is unstained with *Chx10* message, it is hard to identify in this image. Thus, the panocular phenotype that results in both human and mouse from *CHX10* mutations is due to primary neuroretinal defects that affect the development of the entire eye. The panocular phenotypes that result from mutations in *PAX6* or *CHX10* result from different pathophysiological mechanisms.

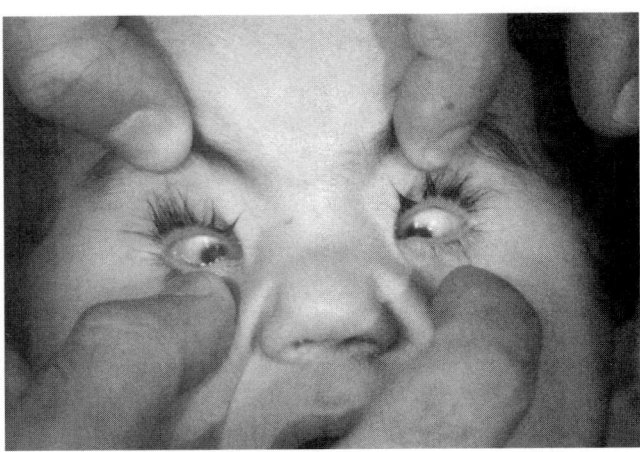

**Fig. 240-5** Null mutations in *CHX10* cause microphthalmia. The photograph illustrates the microphthalmia of an individual who is homozygous for the R200Q mutation in *CHX10*. (*From Horsford et al.*[173] *Used with permission.*) The patient also has cataracts and iris coloboma.

effects, even though the developmental expression of *CHX10* in the eye is restricted to one cell type, the progenitor cells of the neuroretina (Fig. 240-4). Patients with homozygous loss of *CHX10* function have microphthalmia (Fig. 240-5) and cataracts, and are blind, presumably due to their having thin hypocellular retinas that lack bipolar interneurons (see "Mutations in the Mouse *Chx10* Gene and Microphthalmia" below). This complex phenotype indicates that the loss of *CHX10* function in neuroretinal progenitors during development leads to secondary defects in other regions of the eye that do not express *CHX10*, but which are, nevertheless, dependent on the activities of *CHX10*-dependent signals produced by the neuroretinal progenitors.

## Aniridia Caused by *PAX6* Mutations

Aniridia (MIM 106200) is chiefly characterized by congenital absence of the iris. Typically, a small iris stump is present but it can often only be viewed with a gonioscope.[174] Associated anomalies can include foveal hypoplasia, optic nerve hypoplasia and progressive corneal dystrophy, cataract, and glaucoma.[171] Many cases of aniridia are sporadic (with no prior family history) but most show clear autosomal dominant inheritance with very high penetrance, although the phenotype can be extremely variable.[175]

Aniridia was the first human developmental eye abnormality for which a gene was identified. This gene, *PAX6*, plays a fundamental role in ocular and sensory development in a variety of organisms and has been studied intensively.

**Gene Identification.** The aniridia gene was localized to 11p13 through analysis of the deleted chromosomes of individuals with a rare contiguous gene syndrome: Wilms tumor, aniridia, genitourinary anomalies and mental retardation (WAGR syndrome, MIM 194072). Both *WT1*, the Wilms tumor predisposition gene, and *PAX6*, the aniridia gene, were isolated by positional cloning from the deletion interval.[46,172] Intragenic *PAX6* mutations were soon identified in familial and sporadic aniridia patients.[176,177]

Although the majority of sporadic cases are caused by intragenic *PAX6* mutations—with no associated increase in the risk of Wilms tumor—the possibility of a WAGR deletion must be borne in mind whenever a new sporadic case is identified. In such cases, molecular cytogenetic testing by chromosomal fluorescence *in situ* hybridization (FISH) is indicated to check the integrity of the *WT1-PAX6* interval.[178,179] Any deletion patient should be monitored appropriately, usually by renal ultrasound scans, for tumor development.

*PAX6* **Gene and Protein Structure: Conservation.** The transcribed exons and introns of the genomic *PAX6* gene cover approximately 25 kb, for which full-sequence is available. The gene consists of 14 exons, with the translation start site in exon 4;[177] exon 5a is subject to alternative splicing. *PAX6* is a member of the *Pax* gene family, encoding a protein of 422 amino acids including a 128-amino-acid DNA-binding motif—the paired domain—originally identified in the *Drosophila* segmentation gene *paired*. In common with many other *Pax* genes, *PAX6* also encodes a second DNA-binding domain called a paired-type homeodomain. The paired domain is subdivided into N-terminal and C-terminal subdomains, each resembling a homeodomain. The paired domain and paired-type homeodomain both mediate protein-DNA interactions.[180-182] The PAX6 protein thus contains three homeodomain-like DNA-binding modules, which together have the capacity to interact with many tens of base pairs of DNA. Extensive biochemical and biophysical studies of PAX5, PAX6, PAX3, and *Drosophila* paired proteins reveal a complex interplay between the closely juxtaposed modules.[180-186] In PAX6, the potential for protein/DNA interaction is further extended by an alternatively spliced 14-amino-acid peptide in the N-terminal paired subdomain whose inclusion affects target sequence recognition.[183,187] It seems likely that the PAX6 protein is capable of binding a range of target sequences, with alternative splicing capable of modulating the target specificity. The C-terminal third of the protein is rich in serine, proline, and threonine, and has *trans*-activating properties through interaction with general transcription factors to bring about activation of target genes once the appropriate DNA elements have been bound.[177,188]

The complete PAX6 protein sequence is highly conserved across vertebrates (see *PAX6* "Lessons from Model Systems" below), while the paired- and homeodomains are around 90 percent amino acid identical from *Homo sapiens* to *Drosophila* and *C. elegans*.[35]

**Regulation of Downstream Target Genes.** Although it has been possible to assign likely functional roles to the different domains of the PAX6 protein, we are a long way from understanding exactly how PAX6 locates its targets within the enormous complexity of genomic DNA, and how it interacts with the many other protein molecules that make up the transcriptional complex. To date only a few putative PAX6 binding sites have been identified; these include the promoters of genes for crystallins,[189,190] cell adhesion molecules L1 and NCAM,[191,192] glucagon and insulin,[193] and *PAX6* itself in quail.[194] Given the complex expression pattern of *PAX6* (see "*PAX6* Gene Expression" below), the transcriptional targets and cofactors of PAX6 protein are likely to be many and varied. Definition of the full-spectrum of physiologically relevant transcription-factor target genes remains a fundamentally important, but as yet elusive, task for developmental and molecular biologists. Recent demonstration[195] of ectopic *Pax6* expression in *Xenopus* leading to ectopic eye formation, also revealed induction of additional homeobox eye marker genes *Otx2*, *Six3*, and *Rx/Rax*, although there is no suggestion that these genes are direct targets of Pax6 protein.

***PAX6* Gene Expression.** Detailed gene expression has been studied most intensively in the developing mouse,[66,109] although expression in the developing human eye has also been examined.[172,196] The observed *PAX6* expression in all layers of the developing eye (Fig. 240-6) is highly consistent with the panocular nature of aniridia. *PAX6* is first expressed in the developing prosencephalon from E8 in mouse gestation. The *PAX6*-positive domain narrows as the optic placode is defined and the optic vesicle evaginates to meet the surface ectoderm, at which stage expression is also induced in the surface ectoderm, which, in turn, invaginates to form the *PAX6*-positive lens placode. Both the prospective pigment epithelium and the neural retina, which comprise the double-layered early optic cup, express *PAX6*. Subsequently, retinal expression is confined to the ganglion and amacrine cells of the developing neural retina. The nasal placodes, and subsequently the olfactory bulb and nasal epithelium, are *PAX6*-positive. There is strong expression in the developing

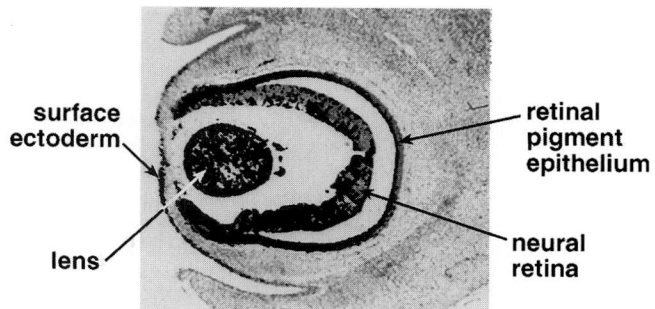

**Fig. 240-6 Expression pattern of *PAX6* in the developing human eye.** *PAX6* expression is revealed by radioactive RNA *in situ* hybridization in a section through the eye of a 49-day-old human fetus. Silver grains (seen as black signal) are seen in all major surface ectoderm and neuroectoderm derived structures: (from left) corneal precursor surface ectoderm, lens, neural retina, and retinal pigment epithelium (RPE). RPE expression is decaying by this stage and some of the signal results from light scattering by the pigment granules, but RPE *PAX6* expression is seen clearly at early stages in albino mice. (*From Ton et al.[172] Used with permission.*) This broad eye expression helps to explain the panocular nature of *PAX6*-associated disease.

telencephalon: in the cortex, thalamus, pituitary, and pineal. From about E13 parts of the cerebellar system develop from *PAX6*-positive rhombic lip derivatives in the rhombencephalon. Four precerebellar nuclei and the granule cells of the cerebellum all express *PAX6* strongly.[197] In the neural tube, PAX6-positive cells give rise to subsets of motor neurons and interneurons.[198] Finally, the alpha and beta cells of the pancreas express *PAX6*.

***PAX6* Mutations.** Nearly 200 mutations in the *PAX6* gene have now been reported. These have been archived in the Human *PAX6* Mutation Database[210] (www.hgu.mrc.ac.uk/Softdata/PAX6/). The spectrum of intragenic PAX6 mutations is summarized diagrammatically in Fig. 240-7.

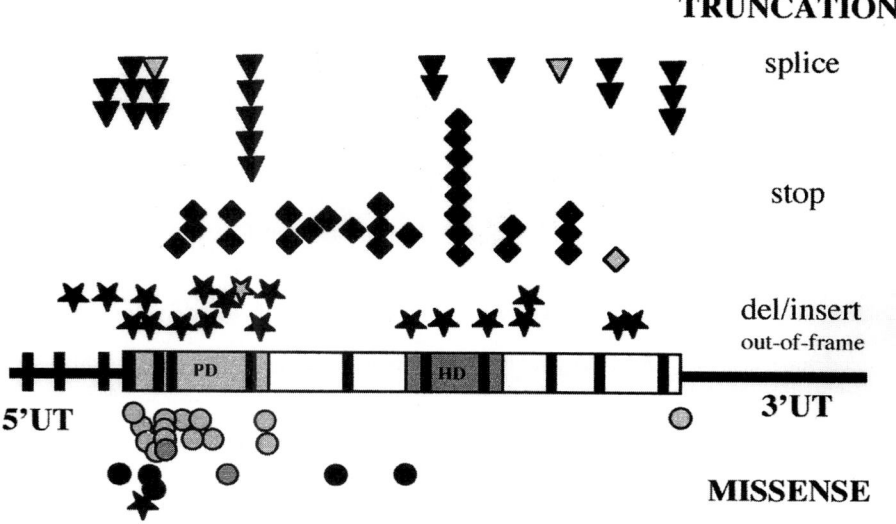

**Fig. 240-7 Representation of the majority of *PAX6* mutations reported by September 1999.** Regularly updated information may be found at www.hgu.mrc.ac.uk/Softdata/PAX6/. Most mutations defined in patients reported as standard "aniridia" cases lead to premature protein truncation, through direct stop codon mutations (black diamond) and deletions/insertions (black star) or splice errors (black triangle), which lead to out-of-frame changes. A few of the premature truncation changes are found in cases with familial cataracts without reported iris changes (stippled symbols), and in one case, anterior keratitis (hatched triangle). Many missense mutations, still mostly confined to the paired box lead, to variant phenotypes related to aniridia (gray circle) (see Table 240-5). A few missense mutations are associated with aniridia (black circle). Two missense mutations are apparently associated with syndromic phenotypes (horizontal striped circle), while a missense change in the final amino acid before the stop codon leads to a distinct corneal phenotype.

**Protein Truncation Mutations in the Human *PAX6* Gene Cause Aniridia.** The vast majority of reported *PAX6* mutations are in classical aniridia patients. In general, each familial or sporadic case of aniridia is caused by a different *PAX6* mutation, necessitating screening of the whole gene to identify the alteration. A small number of mutations have been reported independently more than once; these almost always occur at CpG dinucleotides, which are well-known "hot spots" for single nucleotide substitutions.[47] New (sporadic) mutations go on to be inherited in dominant fashion in subsequent generations. It is now apparent that the *PAX6* mutation spectrum in aniridia patients is highly biased.[46,47] Nearly all aniridia patients have mutations predicted to cause premature truncation of the PAX6 protein: nonsense (stop codon) changes, splice mutations, and small frameshifting insertions or deletions. The phenotype of individuals with such intragenic mutations is generally indistinguishable from that of patients with a deletion of the entire *PAX6* gene. The vast majority of these mutations are essentially null alleles from which the protein product, if any, has little or no normal function. Therefore, aniridia can be classified as a haploinsufficiency disease. A rare compound heterozygote for two different *PAX6* mutations has been reported with anophthalmia, hypoplastic nasal structures, and severe brain anomalies (Fig. 240-3). The mother had aniridia as a result of a classical paired-domain protein truncation; the father had familial cataracts caused by a chain termination in the transactivation domain, near the C-terminus of PAX6, with some predicted residual gene activity.[188] This case is strongly reminiscent of the Small-eye mouse homozygote phenotype (see "Mouse Small-eye Phenotype Caused by *Pax6* Mutations" below).

Relatively few *PAX6* missense mutations have been identified so far, and while some are associated with aniridia, most lead to different eye phenotypes (Table 240-5).

Classical aniridia is thus associated at high frequency with readily identifiable *PAX6* mutations.[47,202] In contrast, no *PAX6* mutations could be demonstrated[211] in Gillespie syndrome (MIM 206700), which is described as aniridia associated with cerebellar hypoplasia and some degree of mental retardation. The eye phenotype, without lens and corneal opacities, is considered distinct from classical isolated aniridia cases.[212] A t(X;11) translocation with an 11p12 breakpoint was recently reported in a case with Gillespie syndrome.[213]

**Aniridia Associated with Long-Range Disruption of the *PAX6* Locus.** Although the vast majority of aniridia patients have intragenic *PAX6* mutations that are predicted to lead to a 50 percent reduction of functional protein product, a small number of aniridia patients have an intact *PAX6* gene associated with chromosomal breakpoints 30 to 130 kb beyond the 3' end of the *PAX6* gene.[214] Similar phenomena, sometimes described as position effects,[215,216] have also been observed for *FKHL7* (see "*FKHL7* Gene and Protein Structures; Conservation" below) in a patient with glaucoma[217] and for *RIEG/PITX2* (see "*PITX2* Gene Identification" below) in a patient with Rieger syndrome.[218] The existence of such mutations tells us that, in these cases at least, intact long-range genomic organization needs to be maintained for correct gene expression. The molecular mechanisms at play here are still being unraveled, but the concept of their existence is important to bear in mind whenever any sort of gene replacement therapy is contemplated.

Additionally, loss-of-function changes outside the gene transcription unit serve as a reminder that loss-of-function mutations may be produced by other upstream, downstream, and intronic changes that are generally not searched for in most mutation screening programs.

**Missense Mutations in the Human *PAX6* Gene Associated with Peters Anomaly and Other Phenotypes.** Peters anomaly is generally classified as an anterior segment anomaly. However, a report of a patient with features of both Peters anomaly and aniridia suggested that there may be a common underlying mechanism in some cases.[219] Analysis of the ocular defects in adult Small-eye mice (heterozygous for a mutation in the *Pax6* gene) revealed a small percentage of eyes with corneal opacification and adhesions between the lens and the posterior surface of the cornea, reminiscent of Peters anomaly.[199] Thus, both the human eye disease literature and careful examination of the mouse model system for aniridia (see "Mouse Small-eye Phenotype Caused by *Pax6* Mutations" below) suggested the possibility of an etiologic relationship between aniridia and Peters anomaly. In one sporadic case of Peters anomaly, the patient had an interstitial deletion of chromosome 11 encompassing *PAX6*, the aniridia gene.[199] This suggested that *PAX6* haploinsufficiency could result in a Peters-like phenotype in a small proportion of mice and humans, alternative to the "typical" loss of function phenotype (aniridia). *PAX6* missense mutations have also been found in two familial cases of Peters anomaly, one in a girl whose mother and brother had features more typical of Riegers' anomaly,[199] and one in a woman whose daughter had features more typical of aniridia.[220] It should be noted that *PAX6* mutations are by no means a common cause of Peters anomaly; in one cohort of 15 cases, no *PAX6* mutations were found.[221]

The observation of Peters anomaly associated *PAX6* mutations also suggested that similar mutations might be implicated in phenotypes generally classified as distinct from classical aniridia. *PAX6* mutations have now been found in cases of neonatal cataract and corneal pannus,[188] ectopia pupillae with juvenile cataract and glaucoma,[183] dominantly inherited keratitis,[201] isolated foveal hypoplasia,[203] uveal ectropion,[204] congenital nystagmus with cataract,[202] and ectopia pupillae.[202] Interestingly, many of the mutations associated with these non-aniridia phenotypes are missense mutations, mostly located in the paired box (see Table 240-5 and Fig. 240-7). Owing to the modular nature of paired domain function, it seems likely that amino acid substitutions interfere with binding of the PAX6 protein to some targets but not others, thus affecting some aspects of eye development more severely than others, and ultimately resulting in different phenotypes.[202] Recently, a novel missense mutation, in the alternatively spliced exon 5a, was found in three independent cases.[222] The phenotypes included Peters anomaly, Axenfeld anomaly, and cataracts.

Figure 240-7 depicts the spectrum of *PAX6* mutations diagrammatically. The phenotypic spectrum associated with *PAX6* mutations is illustrated in Fig. 240-3, which also seeks to show the overlap in phenotype between *PAX6*-associated anomalies and those resulting from mutations at other loci, which are mutated in various anterior segment anomalies.

### Lessons from Model Systems

*Mouse Small-eye Phenotype Caused by Pax6 Mutations.* The mouse ortholog of *PAX6* was isolated at the same time as the human and found to map in the vicinity of a classical mouse mutation called Small eye (*Sey*).[109] *Sey* is semidominant with heterozygotes having microphthalmia, while homozygotes have anophthalmia, arhinia, and brain abnormalities,[227,228] and die soon after birth. Analysis of the *Pax6* gene in mice carrying two independent *Sey* alleles (*Sey^Ed* and *Sey^Neu*) revealed mutations, predicted to truncate the Pax6 protein, in both cases.[228] The phenotype of homozygous *Sey* mice correlates well with the expression pattern of *Pax6* during embryogenesis.[109] In *Sey* homozygotes, the optic vesicles develop from the neural ectoderm, but lens induction fails, and the eye structures then degenerate.[110]

Although the most obvious consequence of heterozygous *Pax6* mutation in mice is a reduction in ocular globe size (in contrast to human aniridia patients, who have normal eye size), closer examination of *Sey/+* mice revealed eye anomalies strikingly similar to those observed in aniridia patients.[199] The observation that a proportion of genetically identical *Sey/+* mice had adhesion of the anterior surface of the lens to the posterior surface of the cornea, highly reminiscent of Peters anomaly, suggested the

**Table 240-5** Missense Mutation Phenotypic Spectrum

| Mutation | Phenotype | Genetics | Reference |
|---|---|---|---|
| M1K | total aniridia, intermediate nystagmus, lens ectopia, late cataract, mild corneal dystrophy, glaucoma | familial | 223 |
| N17S & I29V | bilateral aniridia, cataract, foveal hypoplasia, nystagmus | sporadic | 224 |
| G18W | iris hypoplasia, cataract, optic nerve hypoplasia, secondary glaucoma; mother: Peters anomaly | familial | 220 |
| R26G | Peters anomaly and Rieger-like anomaly, posterior embrytoxon (anterior segment malformation) | familial | 199 |
| A33P | "partial aniridia," some iris remnants, cataract | familial | 202 |
| I42S | r. stromal hypoplasia and atypical coloboma, l circumpupillary aplasia, neonatal cataract and nystagmus, hypoplastic optic nerve head and fovea, late corneal vascularization | familial | 223 |
| S43P | aniridia, cataracts, nystagmus, bilateral microcornea, reduced axial length, mild peripheral corneal vascularization | sporadic | 202 |
| R44Q | aniridia, cataract, nystagmus, foveal hypoplasia | sporadic | 224 |
| (V7D): alternative splice exon | l. corneal opacity and iridocorneal adhesion (Peters anomaly) and microphthalmos, r. corneal opacity, sclerocornea, posterior embryotoxon and foveal hypoplasia | familial | 222 |
| (V7D): alternative splice exon | nystagmus, microcornea, peripheral iridocorneal adhesion (Axenfeld anomaly), bilateral foveal hypoplasia | sporadic | 222 |
| (V7D): alternative splice exon | bilateral congenital corneal opacity and cataract high myopia, nystagmus, subnormal electroencephalogram bilaterally; adehesion of cervical bones, vascular anomaly in brain stem | sporadic syndromic | 222 |
| (V7D): alternative splice exon | nystagmus and bilateral congenital cataracts | sporadic | 222 |
| V53L | circumpupillary iris aplasia, moderate photophobia, normal optic nervehead, preserved foveal reflexes, early nystagmus disappeared | familial | 223 |
| T63P | stromal hypoplasia, ectopia pupillae, intermediate nystagmus, lens ectopia, mild corneal dystophy, glaucoma in twenties. Anterior chamber angles wide, fibrous mass partially obscuring trabecular meshwork | familial | 223 |
| G64V | normal looking irides, cataract, nystagmus (both congenital), foveal hypoplasia, tilted optic discs, corneal vascularization | familial | 202 |
| A78E & R208E | stromal hypoplasia, eccentric pupil, mild nystagmus, early cataract (two mutations in different alleles) | familial | 223 |
| 187R | aniridia, microcephaly, developmental delay syndromic | sporadic | 225 |
| V126D | iris hypoplasia, circumpupillary aplasia (absent collarette), ectopia pupillae, mild limbal corneal dystrophy, optic nerve hypoplasia, macular hypoplasia | new mutation, syndromic father mosaic | 202 |
| R128C | isolated foveal hypoplasia | familial | 203 |
| Q178H | aniridia, cataract, optic nerve hypoplasia | familial | 224 |
| R208W | aniridia (no follow-up details) | familial | 226 |
| Q422R | uveal ectropion, invasion of cornea by conjunctival epithellium, posterior embryotoxon | sporadic | 204 |

Description of phenotypes associated with each reported *PAX6* missense mutation (see Fig. 240-3); clear lines = aniridia; pale gray lines = variant phenotypes distinct from classical aniridia; dark gray lines = syndromic disease with additional noneye phenotypes.

possible involvement of *PAX6* mutations in this phenotype (see "Missense Mutations in the Human *PAX6* Gene Associated with Peters Anomaly and other Phenotypes" above).

The functional conservation of PAX6 was highlighted by the generation of transgenic mice carrying the human *PAX6* gene on a large YAC (yeast artificial chromosome) clone.[229] The transgene was able to correct the phenotype of *Sey* mutants, including homozygotes that would otherwise have died. The importance of correct *PAX6* dosage for normal development was also underlined by the finding that mice carrying multiple copies of the transgene on a normal background had developmental eye anomalies, typified by microphthalmia.[229]

The *Sey* mouse has given valuable phenotypic clues about the involvement of *PAX6* mutation in human ocular anomalies, but it has also illuminated the role of *Pax6* in neural development, which may be the archetypal function of the this gene. *Pax6* is essential for normal organization of the embryonic forebrain,[230,231] for migration of cortical neuronal precursors,[232] and for specifying neuronal identity in the hindbrain, particularly in the cerebellum[197] and cervical spinal cord.[198] *Pax6* homozygous mutant mice also have defective pancreatic development and do not produce glucagon.[193,233] This spectrum of anomalies closely reflects the *PAX6* expression pattern. It is not clear why haploinsufficiency leads only to an eye phenotype.

***PAX6 in Other Vertebrates.*** The *PAX6* gene has been isolated and studied in a large number of vertebrates, many of which have distinct different advantages for the study of gene function in development. Thus early functional analysis of *PAX6* in the rat,[234] in zebrafish,[235] in birds — both chick[198,236] and quail[194] — and in *Xenopus*,[237] have contributed greatly to our understanding of *PAX6* gene function. Study of the quail gene has provided insight into alternative promoter usage and *PAX6* autoregulation.[238] Ready manipulation in zebrafish has permitted analysis of the signaling pathways, revealing that Sonic hedgehog (SHH) down-regulates *PAX6* expression and up-regulates *PAX2* expression in the development of the optic nerve (see also "*PAX2* in Zebrafish" below). Recently, work in the adult bovine eye, which is large enough for detailed dissection, has permitted analysis of alternative splice form expression.[239] The widespread interest in *PAX6* function in so many species has also made possible extensive genomic sequence comparison,[240] which may ultimately reveal the presence of important control elements outside the translated and transcribed regions.[241] As far as amino acid sequence is concerned, *PAX6* is one of the most highly conserved proteins known, with 93 to 100 percent amino acid identity among vertebrates.

***PAX6 in Invertebrates: A Master Gene for Eye Development?*** A major advance in the *PAX6* story was made with the discovery of a *Drosophila* ortholog (with >90 percent amino acid identity in both paired- and homeodomains) at the *eyeless* (*ey*) locus.[19] This gene is also essential for eye development; flies carrying two mutant alleles of *ey* have reduced or absent compound eye structures. In addition, if either *ey* or one of the vertebrate *Pax6* homologs is artificially expressed in non-eye imaginal discs, it can induce the development of compound eyes in ectopic sites such as the legs and antennae.[242] This led to the suggestion that *PAX6* is a "master gene" for eye development throughout phylogeny, capable of imposing an ocular fate on early, undifferentiated tissue.[243,244] The reported formation of small ectopic eyes in *Xenopus* in response to injection of *XPax6* mRNA at the 16-cell stage,[195] provides a strong parallel to eyeless function in *Drosophila*. These experiments highlighted the potential for functional conservation of genes separated by hundreds of millions of years of evolution and opened up new discussion on the evolutionary origins of ocular structures and the archetypal role of PAX6. [30,243,244] It seems likely that PAX6 had a role in the specification of neuronal or sensory structures long before the phylogenetic advent of vision. At some stage, a primitive light-sensitive cell appeared under the control of PAX6 but it is unclear at what level PAX6 might have been involved with this event. There is evidence in *Drosophila* that eyeless protein directly controls the expression of rhodopsin which would provide a fundamental link between PAX6 and visual function;[245] however, *PAX6* is not expressed in the photoreceptors of vertebrates or in a subset of *Amphioxus* photoreceptors.[246] Once the fundamental link was established between control (by PAX6), directly or indirectly, of essential visual proteins (e.g., rhodopsin) it is likely that the subsequent elaboration of light sensitive cells into an organ recognizable as an eye occurred repeatedly, thus explaining the enormous diversity of eye structures in extant species.[31,32] It is debatable whether this type of stepwise evolution of visual systems would be described as mono- or polyphyletic.[244] One complication in drawing parallels between *Drosophila* and vertebrates is that *Drosophila* has two additional *PAX6*-like genes, twin of *eyeless* (*toy*) and *eye gone* (*eyg*).[247,248] Because there is conspicuous absence of evidence for additional *PAX6* genes in higher organisms, *Drosophila* may have taken advantage of gene duplication to generate transcriptional diversity, which in vertebrates is achieved through highly complex transcriptional control at a single locus. Nevertheless, the similarities between *Drosophila* and vertebrate *Pax6* gene function are striking. There is recent evidence for some degree of functional conservation between *Drosophila* and mouse extragenic regulatory domains for *eyeless* and *Pax6* expression.[18]

*PAX6* has also been isolated from sea urchin, squid, ribbonworm, nematode, and flatworm (reviewed in reference 35). Recent papers on ancestral *PAX6*-related genes in coral,[249] hydra, and jellyfish[250] have contributed to the concept of *PAX6* as a key gene in early sensorineural development. The proposed existence of co-evolving gene cassettes (see "Introduction" above) suggests that ancestral homologs should exist for a number of the interacting proteins which have been defined predominantly in *Drosophila*, where eye development has been most extensively studied.

**Conclusions.** PAX6 serves as a paradigm for studying the role of transcription factors in disease. Like many major developmental regulator genes, it shows a high degree of evolutionary conservation at both the sequence and functional levels. Once it was identified as a disease-associated gene, much functional information could be gained from gathering data on human mutation-associated phenotypes. However, the high degree of conservation among vertebrate species and with *PAX6* genes in other phyla, can contribute very significantly to our understanding of the broader role of PAX6 in ocular and neural development. Human disease phenotypes associated with *PAX6* mutation may also be better understood through the investigation of gene function in more tractable organisms. Any possible improvements in disease management, because several of the eye phenotypes elicited by *PAX6* mutation are progressive, will also have to be explored initially in model systems.

## Microphthalmia Due to Mutations in the *CHX10* Homeobox Gene

Microphthalmia (MIM 309700), a clinically and genetically heterogeneous group of disorders characterized by a small globe of the eye , occurs with a prevalence rate of 1.7 per 10,000. Historically the phenotype of microphthalmia (small eye) was clinically distinct from anophthalmia (absence of an eye). Microphthalmia is now considered part of a phenotypic spectrum from the most extreme form, anophthalmia (MIM 206900), to various degrees of microphthalmia.[251] Microphthalmia is often seen with other ocular phenotypes or systemic phenotypes. If the eye is small but otherwise normal, the condition is referred to as nanophthalmia (MIM 600165). Microphthalmia can occur as an isolated finding, or in association with other ocular (Fig. 240-5) or systemic phenotypes. Autosomal dominant, autosomal recessive and X-linked patterns of inheritance have been described. Six microphthalmia/anophthalmia loci have been identified, two are

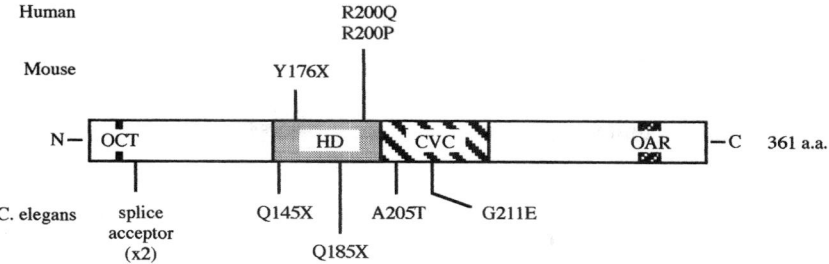

**Fig. 240-8 Mutations in *CHX10* cause microphthalmia in human and mouse.** Mutations in the *CHX10* gene presented on a schematic of the CHX10 protein, including the paired-like homeodomain (HD), CVC domain (CVC), octapeptide (OCT), and the OAR domain (OAR). The mouse *ocular retardation (or^J* allele) mutation is shown above, along with the two human mutations. All three mutations are homozygous in affected individuals.[67,173] Mutations in the *C. elegans ceh-10* gene are shown below, including hypomorphic splice mutations and severe nonsense and missense mutations in the homeodomain and CVC domain.[260]

X-linked (microphthalmia at Xp22.31;[252] anophthalmia at Xq27-q28[253]), two are autosomal dominant (nanophthalmia at 11p;[254] microphthalmia at 16p13.3[255]), and two are autosomal recessive (microphthalmia at 14q32;[256] microphthalmia at 14q24.3[257]). In addition, sporadic microphthalmia has also been reported.[258] Microphthalmia is often seen with other ocular phenotypes, most notably cataracts, anterior chamber defects, and colobomas. *CHX10* is the only identified gene that is mutated in human microphthalmia.

**Gene Identification.** The human *CHX10* gene was first identified in a screen for genes which are expressed abundantly in adult retina and which are highly conserved in mammals.[124] Subsequently, the mouse *Chx10* ortholog was cloned and mapped to distal mouse chromosome 12. The mouse gene mapped very closely to the locus for a mouse small eye phenotype called *ocular retardation (or)*, which was first identified in 1962.[259] One *or* allele, the recessive *J* allele identified at the Jackson laboratory (*or^J*), was found to carry a premature nonsense mutation (Tyr176Stop) that generated a true null[67] ("see Mutations in the Mouse *Chx10* Gene and Microphthalmia"). The major observable phenotype of the *or^J/or^J* mouse (the *Chx10^{-/-}* mouse) is microphthalmia. The discovery of the association between mutations in the mouse *Chx10* gene and ocular retardation ultimately led to the identification of mutations in the human *CHX10* gene in patients with isolated (i.e., nonsyndromic) autosomal recessive microphthalmia (see "Mutations in the Human *CHX10* Gene Cause Microphthalmia").

**CHX10 Protein Structure and Conservation.** The *CHX10* gene encodes a homeodomain transcription factor with several domains in addition to the homeodomain (Fig. 240-8). The homeodomain is of the *paired-like* class and is further subclassified by having a glutamine at position 50 (Q50), a critical residue in the DNA recognition helix. Alignment of the CHX10 protein and a *C. elegans* homolog, ceh-10, led to the recognition of a second conserved region in both proteins, the CVC domain, which is situated immediately C-terminal to the homeodomain. The CVC domain was named after the first three proteins in which it was found, ceh-10, Vsx1, and Chx10.[261,262] To date, the 55-amino-acid CVC domain has been reported only in proteins that (a) also contain a homeodomain and (b) are expressed in the developing eye or other neurosensory organs. The juxtaposition of the CVC domain to the homeodomain suggests that the CVC domain may also bind to DNA and possibly modify CHX10 binding by the homeodomain. Alternatively, the CVC domain may mediate protein-protein interactions with other transcription factors. Missense mutations have been identified in the CVC domain of the *C. elegans ceh-10* gene, and these mutations generate phenotypes identical to early nonsense mutations in *ceh-10*, demonstrating that the CVC domain is critical for ceh-10 function. A third motif in the CHX10 protein is the 14-amino-acid

C-terminal OAR domain, which is also found in several other *paired-like* homeodomain proteins such as Rx/Rax[106] and members of the PITX family. The function of the OAR domain is unknown. Like many other *paired-like* homeodomain proteins, CHX10 also contains an octapeptide motif (FGIQEILG) near the amino terminus. However the CHX10 octapeptide is diverged from the more conventional sequence (HSIDGILG) found in other *paired-like* homeodomain transcription factors.[61]

The CHX10 protein has been conserved throughout evolution. The mouse protein is 99 percent identical to human CHX10,[124] the chick ortholog is 86 percent identical,[263] the zebra fish ortholog (also called Alx) is 81 percent identical,[264] a goldfish homolog (also called Vsx-2) is 70 percent identical,[265] and a second goldfish Chx10 homolog, Vsx-1, is 65 percent identical. Although the *C. elegans* homolog ceh-10 is only 40 percent identical overall, it is 82 percent identical in the homeodomain and 74 percent identical in the CVC domain.[266]

**Chx10 Expression in Mouse.** In the developing and mature eye, *Chx10* is expressed solely in the retina. *Chx10* expression is present in retinal neuroblasts throughout mouse development, as well as in a subset of cells in the mature retina.[124] The *Chx10* mRNA is first detected at E9.5, in the presumptive neuroretina of the optic vesicle. The transcript continues to be expressed in apparently all proliferating retinal progenitor cells (Fig. 240-4), but in adult retina, the *Chx10* mRNA and protein are restricted to cells of the inner nuclear layer, where expression is strongest in bipolar cells and less in amacrine cells. *Chx10* is also expressed in other regions of the developing embryo, most notably the ventral hindbrain and spinal cord. In particular, Chx10 is a marker in the spinal cord for differentiated V2 interneurons in the developing chick.[198] The expression patterns of the vertebrate *Chx10* orthologs and homologs are highly homologous: transcripts are detected first in proliferating neuroretinal cells, and subsequently, in differentiated interneurons. Similarly, the *ceh-10* gene is expressed in neurosensory cells, including AIY interneurons.[266] In summary, CHX10 and its related proteins are found in interneurons in various parts of the vertebrate or *C. elegans* nervous system: bipolar interneurons in the vertebrate eye, V2 cells in the vertebrate spinal cord, and AIY interneurons in the nematode.

**Regulation of Downstream Target Genes by CHX10.** To date, no downstream target genes of CHX10 have been identified, although a homeobox gene, *ceh-23*, may be downstream of ceh-10 in *C. elegans*, because *ceh-10* mutants do not express *ceh-23*.[260] However, insight into potential biologic functions regulated by CHX10 was obtained by the discovery that, at least *in vitro*, CHX10 acts as a repressor at promoters containing the so-called P3 DNA-binding site: TAAT(N)₃ATTA.[267] Interestingly, the octapeptide of other *paired-like* homeodomain proteins has been shown to mediate transcriptional repression both *in vitro* and *in vivo*.[268,269]

**Table 240-6** The Phenotypes of Mice and Humans with Null Mutations in the CHX10 Gene Are Virtually Identical

|  | Type of Mutation | Microphthalmia | Cataracts | Optic nerve aplasia | Iris coloboma |
|---|---|---|---|---|---|
| Mouse | Nonsense, null | Yes | Yes | Yes | Abnormal iris |
| Human | Missense, null | Yes | Yes | Optic nerve present | yes |

The mouse phenotype described is that of the homozygous or[J] mouse,[67] while the human phenotype is that of a proband homozygous for the R200Q mutation.[173]

A second important step in determining the function of CHX10 was using PCR-based oligonucleotide selection to identify the DNA sequence to which the CHX10 protein prefers to bind *in vitro*. The consensus sequence to which CHX10 preferentially binds was an octanucleotide, TAATTAGC.[173] Unexpectedly, this binding site is very different from that of other *paired-like* homeodomain proteins, which preferentially bind a P3 site[270] such as the one referred to above.

**Mutations in the Human *CHX10* Gene Cause Microphthalmia.** The association between mutations in the human *CHX10* gene and autosomal recessive isolated (i.e., nonsyndromic) microphthalmia was first made in 1999, when a small inbred Turkish family was examined for homozygosity for markers near or within candidate genes for human microphthalmia or anophthalmia. Cosegregation was detected between the microphthalmia phenotype and a series of DNA markers flanking the *CHX10* gene on 14q24.3.[173] The human *CHX10* gene was a strong candidate for recessive microphthalmia because of the mouse ocular retardation phenotype. The proband, who was blind, was not only microphthalmic (Fig. 240-5), but also had congenital cataracts and iris coloboma (Table 240-6). The proband and other affected members of the family were found homozygous for a missense mutation, R200Q, in the DNA-recognition helix of the homeodomain.[173] A second microphthalmic proband, also the offspring of consanguineous unaffected parents, was discovered to be homozygous for a different missense mutation in the R200 codon (R200P) (Fig. 240-8). None of the individuals with mutations in the *CHX10* gene had any extraocular abnormality. In particular, no neurologic dysfunction of the spinal cord was evident, indicating that, although the *CHX10* gene is expressed in the mature and developing hindbrain and spinal cord, it is apparently not an essential gene in these parts of the nervous system.

The R200 residue is at position 53 of the homeodomain, a position occupied by arginine in 344 of 346 homeodomains reported in one survey.[61] The R200Q substitution was therefore predicted to be a null allele, because this arginine normally contacts the phosphate backbone of the DNA by a hydrogen bond and a nonhydrogen electrostatic bond.[182] As predicted, the substitution of a basic (arginine) for a uncharged (glutamine or proline) residue at this position was found to impair the binding of the CHX10 protein to its octanucleotide recognition sequence (Fig. 240-9).

**Lessons from Model Systems**
*Mutations in the Mouse* Chx10 *Gene and Microphthalmia.* As with the human *CHX10* mutations, the microphthalmic phenotype of the $Chx10^{-/-}$ (or[J]) mouse is also caused by a null mutation (Y176X) in the gene.[67] The resulting complete loss of *Chx10* function leads to abnormalities in both the developing and mature retina. In the developing eye, there is a pronounced reduction in the proliferative capacity of retinal progenitor cells, whereas in the mature retina there is a specific absence of bipolar interneurons. The decrease in the size of the entire developing eye is detectable as early as E11.5. Because *Chx10* is expressed only in the developing neuroretinal progenitor cells, the small eye must be due in some way, to the loss of *Chx10* function in the developing neuroretina.[67,272] The adult retina of the mutant mouse is thin, hypocellular, and moderately disorganized. In addition, the mice have optic nerve aplasia (ganglion cell axons are present but they

do not exit the eye) and cataracts. Apart from the above-mentioned absence of detectable bipolar interneurons, all of the other major cell types of the mature retina are present. The failure to produce mature bipolar cells is consistent with the fact that the highest level of *Chx10* expression in the mature retina is in these cells.[124] Interestingly, although *Chx10* is expressed in other types of neurons in the inner nuclear layer, these other cells — including horizontal cells, Müller cells, and amacrine cells — are

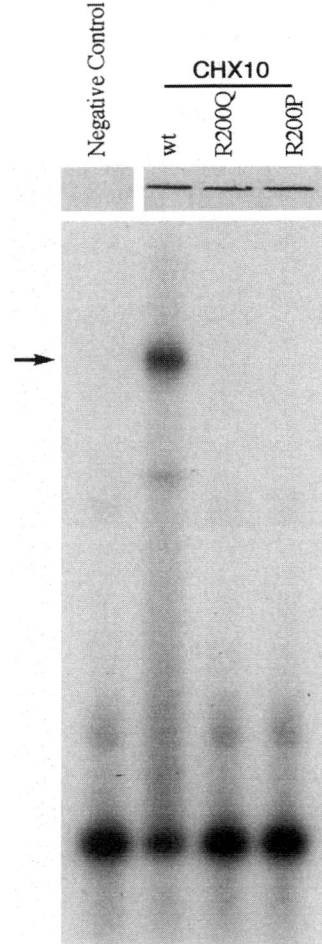

**Fig. 240-9** The wild-type CHX10 protein binds preferentially to the octanucleotide TAATTAGC. The CHX10 proteins with mutations (R200Q or R200P) associated with microphthalmia had grossly reduced binding to the oligonucleotide. *Lane 1:* Negative control (no CHX10 DNA). *Lane 2:* Wild-type CHX10 protein and the octanucleotide, showing the normal band shift associated with binding. *Lanes 3 and 4:* Neither the R200Q or R200P CHX10 protein manifest appreciable binding to the octanucleotide, indicating that they have a complete or near-complete loss of CHX10 function. Above the band shift lanes is a western blot probed with anti-c-myc to detect myc-tagged human CHX10 protein. Similar amounts of CHX10 protein are in each protein extract.

nevertheless present in the mutant. Thus, *Chx10* regulates both the proliferation of the retinal progenitor cells as well as the specification, differentiation, or maintenance of bipolar cells.

***Lessons from the Mouse Model.*** The power of mouse genetics to contribute to the understanding of human eye disease genes is exemplified by the role of the *ocular retardation* mouse in the identification of human *CHX10* mutations in patients with isolated microphthalmia. The phenotypes of humans and mice with homozygous null allele mutations in the respective *CHX10* genes are essentially orthologous (see Table 240-6).

This conservation of function is particularly notable because mutations in other genes that cause microphthalmia in mouse, such as heterozygous mutations in *Pax6* and homozygous mutations in *Mitf*, are not associated with microphthalmia in humans (although mutations in these human genes are associated with *other* eye phenotypes, as discussed in other sections of this chapter). The biologic basis of the species difference in the effect of mutations in some microphthalmia genes and not others is unclear, but its elucidation is likely to provide insight into important regulatory events in mammalian eye development. A second unexpected consequence of the loss of *Chx10* function, in both human and mouse, is the presence of cataracts. Disruption of lens development or maintenance would not have been predicted from the expression pattern of *Chx10*, because neither the mRNA nor protein has been seen in the developing lens.[273] The lens abnormalities suggest, consequently, that *Chx10*-dependent signal(s) from the retina are required for normal lens formation. These signals may also be the mediators of the small eye phenotype that affects the overall size of the eye.

***CHX10 in Zebrafish and* C. elegans.** The functional conservation of the CHX10 protein extends beyond the near-identical mouse and human eye phenotypes. In the zebrafish, *Chx10* antisense oligonucleotides incubated with developing embryos generated eye defects very similar to those seen in the microphthalmic mouse and human.[264] These included microphthalmia, changes in the shape of the globe, disorganized or absent retina, and RPE malformation. In *C. elegans*, *ceh-10* is necessary for neuronal differentiation and migration.[260] Hypomorphic *ceh-10* mutations have migration defects in canal-associated neurons (CAN cells), producing a withered tail. Nonsense mutations in the homeodomain of *ceh-10* are larval lethal and lead to loss of differentiated AIY interneurons. The AIY cells are still present, yet do not express *ceh-23*. As mentioned above, point mutations in the CVC domain of *ceh-10* result in the same phenotype as nonsense mutations. Consequently, (a) these CVC-domain amino acids are necessary for CVC function, and (b) the CVC domain is critical for the overall function of ceh-10.

**Conclusions.** In summary, all of the above findings establish that the *CHX10* homeobox gene is essential for the normal development of the human eye. *CHX10* functions in eye development to regulate proliferation of neuroretinal progenitor cells, and the development or maintenance of bipolar cells. In addition, if *CHX10* function is lost from neuroretinal progenitor cells, the growth of the whole eye is impaired, causing microphthalmia. The similarity between the human, mouse, and zebrafish *CHX10* null or loss-of-function phenotypes indicates that the function of the CHX10 protein is virtually orthologous in vertebrates.

## ANTERIOR SEGMENT ANOMALIES

Following the major stages of morphogenesis illustrated in Fig. 240-2, ocular tissues undergo an extensive phase of maturation to achieve the diverse and highly specialized structures of the adult eye (Fig. 240-1). The anterior part of the optic cup and the presumptive cornea undergo cell proliferation, differentiation and migration to form the anterior segment, comprising such functionally diverse tissues as the posterior layers of the cornea,

the iris and the trabecular meshwork. Molecular mechanisms underlying these complex processes are poorly understood. Identification of mutant genes in humans and mice with developmental abnormalities affecting these structures has proved to be the most successful approach to identifying transcription factors that play a key role in anterior segment development.

### Categories of Anterior Segment Anomalies: Phenotypic and Genetic Heterogeneity

Anterior segment anomalies have been broadly divided into those thought to result from abnormal development of the cornea: Peters anomaly (MIM 604229), sclerocornea, congenital endothelial dystrophy, and anterior staphyloma; and those thought to result from abnormal development of the angle and the iris: posterior embryotoxon, Axenfeld anomaly, Rieger anomaly, and iridogonio-iodysgenesis (MIM 137600 and MIM 601631)[274] and Waardenburg syndrome. In fact, the distinction between these two classes is frequently blurred and there are reported cases in which the two eyes of one patient, or individuals within a single family, display anomalies from both classes.[200,219] The clinical presentation of these eye diseases has been described in detail (e.g., Taylor[1]). From a genetic point of view it is more helpful to view these disorders as a spectrum of anterior segment dysgeneses in which there is often no clear genotype-phenotype correlation; indeed there is considerable overlap of the phenotypes elicited by mutations at different loci (see Fig. 240-3). The observed genetic heterogeneity underlines the need for flexibility in classifying this whole group of disorders.

### Phenotypic and Genetic Heterogeneity

**Axenfeld-Rieger Anomaly.** Axenfeld and Rieger anomalies are related developmental disorders of the anterior chamber, associated with iridogoniodysgenesis: abnormalities of the iris stroma, trabecular meshwork, and cornea. They are usually bilateral, mostly with autosomal dominant inheritance. About half of all cases are associated with glaucoma, which has major manifestations in the posterior segment where optic disk cupping causes gradual loss of vision. Axenfeld anomaly is typically characterized by posterior embryotoxon—a prominent, anteriorly positioned Schwalbe line[1,24]—with multiple processes between the iris and Schwalbe line. Rieger anomaly includes the features of Axenfeld anomaly with the addition of iris hypoplasia, polycoria (multiple pupils) and/or corectopia (displaced pupil).[174] The distinction between Axenfeld anomaly and Rieger anomaly is often blurred, particularly when differently affected individuals are found in one family, so the two are often classified together as a single entity known as Axenfeld-Rieger anomaly.

**Rieger Syndrome.** Rieger syndrome is a dominantly inherited condition[275] involving malformations of the eyes, teeth, and skin (MIM 180500; MIM 601499). It is chiefly characterized by Rieger anomaly (see "Axenfeld-Rieger Anomaly" above) with dental hypoplasia (reduction in the size and number of teeth) and often maxillary hypoplasia resulting in a characteristic facial appearance. Failure of umbilical skin involution is frequently seen.[1,174] Occasional isolated growth insufficiency and cardiac defects are additional features. Two loci have been linked to this syndrome, one at 4q25[276] for which a gene has been identified (see "*PITX2*: The Rieger Syndrome Gene at 4q25," below). Rieger syndrome is no exception to the general rule of genetic heterogeneity in disorders involving anterior segment abnormalities. A large Rieger syndrome pedigree was tested for linkage to 4q25 but no association was found. Further analysis of this family provided evidence for a second locus at 13q14 (MIM 601499),[277] where a member of the forkhead family, *FKHR*, maps (see "*FKHL7* in Iridogonial Dysgenesis, Glaucoma, and Axenfeld-Rieger Anomaly" below).

**Iridogoniodysgenesis.** Iridogoniodysgenesis (IGD) is defined by abnormalities of the iridocorneal angle and the anterior stromal layer of the iris. IGD patients suffer from raised intraocular pressure from an early age, resulting in juvenile glaucoma. IGD may occur as an isolated entity (iridogoniodysgenesis anomaly, IGDA) or with systemic defects (iridogoniodysgenesis syndrome, IGDS). IGDA or *IRID1* (MIM 601631) has been mapped to the 6p25 region[278,279] (see "*FKHL7* in Iridogonial Dysgenesis, Glaucoma, and Axenfeld-Rieger Anomaly" below). IGDS or *IRID2* (MIM 137600) has been mapped to 4q25.[280] The map location and phenotypic similarity with Rieger syndrome suggested the possibility that this family was a variant Rieger syndrome case.

**Peters Anomaly.** Peters anomaly is a congenital ocular abnormality involving the presence of a central corneal opacity with defects in the underlying corneal endothelium.[274] There may be adhesions between the corneal defect and either the iris collarette or the lens. Commonly associated ocular anomalies include glaucoma and cataract.

Most cases of Peters anomaly appear to be sporadic, but a few well-documented familial cases, usually with autosomal dominant inheritance, are also found. Affected relatives of an individual with Peters anomaly may display other anterior segment disorders such as Rieger anomaly or sclerocornea.[200] Such intrafamilial heterogeneity again emphasizes the difficulties in classifying anterior segment disorders. In two such cases, *PAX6* mutations were identified (see "Missense Mutations in the Human *PAX6* Gene Associated with Peters Anomaly and Other Phenotypes," above), but, as discussed, most Peters anomaly cases show no *PAX6* mutation.[221] A *PITX2* splice mutation has been reported in one case with Peters anomaly in one eye.[281]

Some cases of Peters anomaly are associated with systemic abnormalities. One well-characterized association is with short-limb dwarfism, called Peters Plus syndrome (MIM 261540). The absence of vertical transmission of Peters Plus syndrome, coupled with the incidence of consanguinity, suggests recessive inheritance.[282]

**Anterior Segment Mesenchymal Dysgenesis.** Anterior segment mesenchymal dysgenesis (MIM 107250) is a general term used to describe some families in which no single specific anomaly predominates. The eye phenotype involves all tissues of the anterior chamber, implying abnormalities in all three waves of neural crest migration or of the ectodermally derived structures of the optic cup, lens, and cornea.[209]

Following linkage studies and candidate gene approaches, several transcription factor genes have been identified that harbor disease-causing mutations in an overlapping spectrum of anterior segment anomalies.

**Waardenburg Syndrome (WS).** WS is an autosomal dominant disorder characterized by pigment defects of the eye, hair, and skin and by hearing loss. The eye phenotype is hypopigmented or heterochromatic irides. Mutations in the transcription factor gene *MITF* result in a subset of WS2 patients, termed Waardenburg syndrome type 2. In a later section (see "Human Mutations in *MITF* Cause Waardenburg Syndrome Type 2" below), we review the relationship between mutations in the *MITF* gene and WS2, and the essential role of the MITF transcription factor in mammalian eye development, as illustrated by the severe eye defects present in the homozygous *Mitf* mutant mouse.

### *FKHL7* in Iridogonial Dysgenesis, Glaucoma, and Axenfeld-Rieger Anomaly

*Gene Identification.* Studies to uncover genes involved in predisposition to early onset glaucoma associated with developmental anomalies of the iris and iridocorneal angle, resulted in identification of a major locus, *IRID1* (MIM 601631), at chromosome 6p25. Linkage analyses of families with iridogoniodysgenesis anomaly,[278,279] Axenfeld-Rieger anomaly,[205] familial glaucoma iridogoniodysplasia,[283] and familial glaucoma with goniodysgenesis[206] have all implicated involvement of a locus at 6p25.

Chromosomal rearrangements involving 6p25 in patients with anterior segment malformations provided further evidence for the role of *IRID1* in normal eye development.[217] Candidate genes within the *IRID1* region were identified through cloning of the chromosomal breakpoint from an individual carrying a balanced t(6;13) translocation associated with multiple congenital anomalies including glaucoma. Two genes were found nearby, one of which, *FKHL7* (previously known as *FREAC-3*), is a member of a family of transcriptional regulators related to the *Drosophila* developmental gene *forkhead*. Four families predominantly affected by Axenfeld-Rieger anomaly were found to have point mutations in *FKHL7*.[217] In an independent study, *FKHL7* was analyzed in a large patient panel and found to be mutated in three patients classified as having Axenfeld-Rieger anomaly.[206] Although there is considerable phenotypic variability,[217] *FKHL7* mutations appear to occur mainly in patients or families with a primary diagnosis of Axenfeld-Rieger anomaly, and the presence of an abnormal Schwalbe line may be an important indicator suggesting an underlying *FKHL7* mutation. Deletion of the *FKHL7* gene is also likely to account for the anterior segment phenotype of patients with monosomy of this 6p region.[284] As with *PAX6*, all available evidence suggests that the ocular anomalies are the consequence of *FKHL7* haploinsufficiency. The *FKHL7* phenotype has now been extended to a case of glaucoma with heart anomalies and deafness, reflecting even more closely the expression pattern of this gene.[285]

Extensive analysis of *FKHL7* failed to reveal any mutation in four other *IRID1*-linked families, all of which show phenotypes more characteristic of iridogoniodysgenesis anomaly than Axenfeld-Rieger anomaly.[206] In one of these families, *FKHL7* involvement was excluded through segregation analysis of an informative polymorphism. Thus, it seems likely that *IRID1* is a complex locus and that there is at least one other gene in this region which, when mutated, can predispose to iridogonial dysgenesis/glaucoma. A second forkhead-like gene was recently identified in this chromosomal region[286] and in the homologous mouse region.[287] In addition a deletion case of anterior segment anomaly where *FKHL7* is not included in the deletion has been reported.[288]

*FKHL7 Gene and Protein Structure; Conservation.* *FKHL7* is a member of the winged-helix/forkhead-like gene family (see Fig. 240-10). This extensive family is implicated in developmental control of many tissues, often in response to signaling by members of the TGF/BMP family. *FKHL7* transcript sizes are 3.0 and 3.9 kb in most of the expressing tissues, with an additional 3.4 kb mRNA present in kidney.[217] Length variation may be produced by polyadenylation site variation. A single coding exon, showing 89 percent nucleotide and 92 percent amino acid identity with the mouse ortholog *Foxc1/ Mf1*, comprises the genomic gene. The coding region occupies 1659 bp, encoding 553 amino acids.[206] The conserved DNA-binding forkhead domain, that places *FKHL7* into its gene family, extends from amino acid 69 to amino acid 178. This domain is generally described as a winged-helix domain, a variant of the helix-turn-helix motif with two additional loops (the wings) on the C-terminal side of the main HTH region. Monomeric DNA binding is effected by the recognition alpha-helix intruding into the major groove of the DNA, while the loops provide additional backbone contacts.[289]

More distant extragenic elements are probably involved in control of *FKHL7* expression, because the translocation breakpoint in a primary congenital glaucoma patient (with additional multiple congenital anomalies) carrying a balanced t(6;13)(p25.3;q22.3) translocation (missing only 11 bp of chromosome 6 sequence) lies about 25 kb outside the *FKHL7* transcription unit.[217] As several *FKHL7* point mutations have been identified in anterior segment anomaly cases,[217] *FKHL7* is clearly implicated in this phenotype. Its loss of function is presumably elicited by position effect mechanisms similar to those observed for *PAX6*.[214,216] However, the intragenic disruption of the

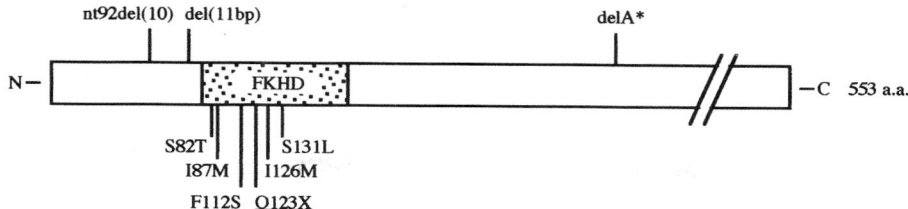

**Fig. 240-10** Mutations in *FKHL7/Foxc1* in Axenfeld-Rieger anomaly. Mutations in the *FKHL7* gene presented on a schematic of the FKHL7 protein, including the forkhead domain (FKHD). Above the proteins schematic are deletions; below are missense or nonsense muta-tions. The mutation associated with the congenital hydrocephalus (ch) mouse is underlined. The starred mutation is a deletion of an alanine in an alanine tract that was found in a patient with primary open-angle glaucoma.[147,206,217,285]

neighboring gene, *GMDS*, with strong homology to *GDP mannose 4,6-dehydratase*, or a gene deletion on chromosome 13, may account for the additional more severe anomalies in this translocation patient.[217]

***Regulation of Downstream Target Genes.*** Very little is known about the genes under the direct regulatory control of FKHL7. *In vitro* binding selection experiments on random oligonucleotide target sequences have defined a shared core sequence of (RTAAAYA) for all *FREAC* family genes.[289] At the same time, domain-swap experiments implied that gene-specific binding differences at flanking sites result from sequence differences in neighboring protein subregions. More detailed analysis of the forkhead protein-nucleic acid interaction suggested that protein binding leads to an 80° to 90° DNA bending.[289]

Specific downstream targets have not yet been defined. Analysis of the *Mf1* mutant mouse (see "A Mouse Model for FKHL7-Associated Glaucoma," below)[290] suggests that components of cell-cell adhesion systems may be regulated by this forkhead gene. The epithelial tight-junction protein zona occludens, ZO-1, is almost completely absent in the developing cornea of homozygous mutant mice, but is perhaps unlikely to be a direct target of FKHL7 regulation, as there is some residual expression. In contrast, the expression of *Pitx2* is unaltered in *Mf1*[−/−] mice, implying strongly that this gene which is mutated in some anterior segment anomalies, is not directly regulated by FKHL7.

***FKHL7 Gene Expression.*** During mouse development (E7.5 to E9.5), cells of two distinct origins express *FKHL7/Mf1*:[291] neural crest cells and mesoderm cells, both paraxial and lateral. When assessed by northern blot studies using fetal and adult mouse polyA RNAs, the expression pattern is seen to be broad.[147,217,289,290] Early studies suggested the absence of adult expression. However, subsequent analysis, including study of the lacZ knockout mice, which share the phenotypic spectrum of the natural congenital hydrocephalus mutant (see "A Mouse Model for FKHL7-Associated Glaucoma," below), reveals wide-ranging expression. High-level expression is seen in the eye and the kidney,[217] particularly in mesodermal derivatives such as the periocular mesenchyme.[147,206]

***FKHL7 Mutations.*** Several disease-associated intragenic muta-tions in *FKHL7* have been identified; they are depicted in Fig. 240-10. An 11-bp early deletion, leading to predicted protein termination N-terminal to the winged helix domain, was identified in two brothers with glaucoma, one with Rieger anomaly, the other with iris hypoplasia; their father, carrying the same mutation had only isolated posterior embryotoxon.[217] Three missense muta-tions, all within the third helix of the winged helix domain were identified in three further small families: S131L in a mother and daughter with Rieger anomaly and glaucoma; I126M in a father and son with Axenfeld anomaly; and in a three-generation family, F112S was associated with Axenfeld anomaly in two affected individuals and Rieger anomaly in two others.[217] Independent analysis in families and sporadic cases with iridogonial dysgenesis

or Axenfeld-Rieger anomaly[206] also revealed three disease-causing mutations (a 10-bp early truncating deletion, S82T, and I87M) all in Axenfeld-Rieger anomaly cases. Additional poly-morphism, for numbers of repeated glycine (codon GGC) residues at two different sites C-terminal to the winged helix domain, were also observed in this study. The mouse *ch* mutation (see "A Mouse Model for *FKHL7*-Associated Glaucoma," below and reference 147) was shown to be a premature truncation at Q123X, in the winged helix domain. It remains to be seen whether *FKHL7* mutations C-terminal to the winged helix domain also cause anterior segment anomalies. It is clear, however, that a number of phenotypically similar cases that map to this chromosomal region have not revealed *FKHL7* mutations and, in some cases, *FKHL7* seems to have been excluded as a candidate gene (see *FKHL7* "Gene Identification" above). However, in these cases the possibility of long range derangement of *FKHL7* expression must be excluded, as there is evidence that such mechanisms can lead to disease.[206,285]

A preliminary report has described an FKHL7 frameshift mutation in a family with Rieger anomaly, sensorineural hearing loss, and atrial septal defect.[285] The same report also mentions an individual with primary open angle glaucoma (POAG) showing in frame deletion of three alanine residues in a poly-alanine tract in the C-terminal region—a variant not seen in 384 controls.

***A Mouse Model for FKHL7-Associated Glaucoma.*** Naturally occurring and targeted mutations of *Mf1*, the original name for the mouse *FKHL7* ortholog, now renamed *Foxc1*, are responsible for the classical congenital hydrocephalus (*ch*) phenotype in mice.[147] Like *Pax6*, *Mf1* mutations exhibit clear dosage effects: homo-zygous *ch*[−/−] mice have hydrocephalus, ocular anomalies, and multiple skeletal defects, while heterozygotes have anterior segment anomalies including defects of the trabecular meshwork and Schlemm's canal.[206] The *ch*[+/−] mouse promises to be a valuable animal model for glaucoma, and provides a fascinating example of a classical mouse mutant which was thought to be recessive but is now known to be semidominant following reexamination in the light of *FKHL7* identification as a human disease gene. Recent detailed phenotypic analysis[290] revealed that in mice, the major eye anomaly is associated with failure of the cornea to separate from the lens, which is the result of the aberrant development of the mesenchymally derived inner corneal endothelial layer.

The much more severe, neonatally lethal, phenotype of homozygous congenital hydrocephalus mice is not generally seen in the human population. The spectrum of anomalies seen in these mice, does however, illustrate more clearly the expression pattern of the gene.[147]

## *PITX2*: The Rieger Syndrome Gene at 4q25
***Gene Identification.*** The Rieger syndrome gene was identified using a classical approach combining linkage analysis in well-characterized families and definition of chromosomal abnormal-ities in rare individuals with cytogenetic rearrangements. Linkage studies of three Rieger syndrome families revealed a tight

association with markers mapping to 4q25.[276] The critical region was further defined by physical mapping, which utilized two Rieger syndrome-associated translocation breakpoints shown to be 50 kb apart, spanned by a cosmid contig. One of these cosmids was shown to include *PITX2*, a gene possessing a paired-type homeobox, one of three closely-related pituitary homeobox genes, related to that of the *Drosophila* developmental gene *bicoid*, with a lysine residue at amino acid 50 in the homeodomain.[207]

The breakpoints, positioned about 15 kb upstream and 50 kb downstream of the 18-kb genomic gene, apparently cause the phenotype by position effects.[216] An additional translocation break 90 kb upstream of the gene has also been reported, suggesting a requirement for intact long-range *cis*-control of *PITX2* expression.[218]

*PITX2* was also isolated several times independently of its role in Rieger syndrome: as a key downstream modulator of left-right asymmetry (reviewed in references 292 and 293); as a homeodomain-bearing pituitary developmental regulator;[149] and as a target of trithorax regulation modulated in human acute leukemia.[294]

***PITX2 Gene and Protein Structure, Conservation.*** The human gene, transcribed from telomeric to centromeric direction, consists of four exons that encode a 2125-bp transcript.[207] The 813-bp open reading frame spans from exon 2 to 4, with the homeodomain encoded mostly by exon 3 but terminating in exon 4. The predicted protein product comprises 271 amino acids, with the homeodomain extending from residues 39 to 98. Alternative splicing with additional intron-exon complexity has been recognized in the mouse, producing a larger 317-amino-acid product. A third isoform, also differing from other products in the N-terminal region, is produced by alternative promoter usage.[149] Greater than 99 percent amino acid sequence identity is observed between the human and mouse proteins. In addition, 97 percent nucleotide sequence identity, with probable functional significance, is seen over a 270-bp region in the 3′ untranslated region of the mRNA. Orthologs from a number of vertebrate species have been identified, including the prevertebrate cephalochordate *Branchiostoma*. In addition, homologs are also found in *Drosophila* and *C. elegans*. The availability of these model systems should make functional analysis easier.

***Regulation of Downstream Genes.*** The *PITX2* downstream target genes are not yet defined. Identifying physiologically relevant targets of DNA-binding developmental regulators is one of the toughest goals to fulfill. There is a suggestion that the early acting homeobox gene *Hesx1* may be a target because in homozygous *Pitx2* knockout mice, *Hesx1* expression is abolished in the early E12.5 pituitary.[149] In terms of its function in laterality determination, *Pitx2* acts downstream of other asymmetry genes such as *Shh*, *nodal*, and *lefty*, *iv*, and *inv*, but there is no evidence for direct target relationships.

The PITX2 protein can bind the defined target sequence for *Drosophila* bicoid. Functional analysis of wild-type and mutant PITX2 proteins using electrophoretic mobility shift assays, protein binding, and transient transfection assays revealed impaired activity and instability of mutant proteins carrying amino acid substitutions found in Rieger syndrome patients.[296]

***PITX2 Gene Expression.*** In keeping with the Rieger syndrome phenotype, *PITX2* expression was originally observed by whole-mount *in situ* hybridization in 11-day mouse embryos in the mesenchyme around the eye, Rathke's pouch, in the dental lamina, limb mesenchyme, the dorsal mesentery, and the vitelline and umbilical vessels.[207] Further analysis is summarized by Yost,[293] where the asymmetric *Pitx2* expression is discussed, describing broadly that *Pitx2* expression is bilateral in the cephalic mesoderm and pituitary precursors, but on the left side of lateral-plate mesoderm structures, and of the cardiac tube and gut. Expression patterns are altered in mouse laterality mutants. Conversely, ectopic expression of *Pitx2* in the right lateral-plate mesoderm

alters looping of the heart and gut and isomerizes body rotation in developing chick and *Xenopus* where these experiments can be performed (reviewed in reference 292).

***PITX2 Mutations.*** The first intragenic point mutations in *PITX2* were described in two sporadic and four familial cases in which all three cardinal signs of Rieger syndrome were present in at least one family member. The mutations (Fig. 240-11) were L54Q, W133X, and two splice-site mutations in the families, and two further missense mutations, T68P and R91P for the sporadic cases. Subsequently, a PITX2 missense mutation, R70H, was identified in a family with iridogonial dysgenesis syndrome (iris hypoplasia, iridocorneal angle defects, and glaucoma, as well as maxillary hypoplasia, dental anomalies, inguinal hernia, and hypospadias).[208] Autosomal dominant iris hypoplasia with glaucoma was associated in one family with an R46W missense change.[295]

A *PITX2* mutation has also been described in association with Peters anomaly.[281] The child in this case had systemic features of Rieger's syndrome and typical features of Rieger's anomaly in the left eye; the right eye, however, showed the characteristic central corneal opacification of Peters anomaly (see "Peters Anomaly" above). A similar combination of ocular phenotypes (Rieger-like in one eye, Peters-like in the other) has been described in association with a *PAX6* mutation.[199] Clearly, careful evaluation of systemic defects can help in assessing the likelihood of *PAX6* or *PITX2* involvement.

***Mouse Model for PITX2 Loss of Function.*** Several groups have generated mice with *Pitx2* intragenic deletions by gene targeting in ES cells.[297–299] Homozygous total loss-of-function animals die in utero at E13.5 to E14.5, probably as a result of abnormal heart development, but the normal rightward looping of the heart tube and gut is unaltered, although there is right isomerization of the lung. Careful further examination of these null mutants at or before E13.5 reveals optic nerve coloboma, absence of ocular muscles, failure of ventral body wall closure, maxillary defects, and tooth anomalies, as well as arrest of pituitary development. A less severe phenotype, with death of the homozygotes at E18.5, is observed where a partial loss-of-function allele was created by insertion of the LoxP site-flanked selectable marker into an intron which gave rise to an allele with altered splicing characteristics.[297] Examination of the heterozygotes from this line, and from the null allele, revealed some of the features typical of Rieger syndrome: corectopia and iris anomalies, as well as malocclusion of teeth.[297]

### PITX3 in Anterior Segment Anomalies
**Gene Identification.** The mouse homolog, *Pitx3*, was identified through screening a mouse cDNA library with a *Pitx2* homeobox probe.[139] Initial studies revealed early expression in the develop-

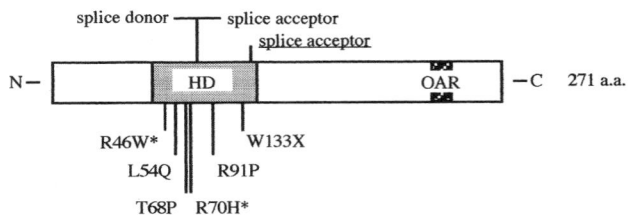

**Fig. 240-11** Mutations in *PITX2* are associated with Rieger syndrome, iridogoniodysgenesis syndrome, and Peters anomaly.[207,208,281,295] Mutations in the *PITX2* gene presented on a schematic of the PITX2 protein, including the homeodomain (HD) and OAR domain. Splice-site mutations are shown above, while missense and nonsense mutations are shown below the schematic. All the mutations are associated with Rieger syndrome except *, which is associated with iridogoniodysgenesis syndrome, and the underlined mutation, which is mutated in an individual with Peters anomaly.

ing eye, particularly in the lens which was interesting in view of the chromosomal localization of *Pitx3* on mouse chromosome 19, in the region of the mouse locus *aphakia* associated with maldevelopment of the lens and reduced eye size in homozygotes. Early studies, however, revealed no *Pitx3* coding region mutations in aphakia mice.[139] The human homolog *PITX3* was subsequently isolated and mapped to chromosome 10q25, the conserved synteny region for the mouse chromosome 19 locus.[140] No human eye disease phenotype had been previously assigned to this region, necessitating a less focused search for possible disease associations.[140]

***PITX3 Gene, Protein Structure and Conservation.*** Like *PITX2*, the *PITX3* gene consists of four exons, the first of which is predicted to be entirely noncoding. Intron positioning is identical to that of *PITX2* and *PITX1*, with the homeodomain spanning from exon 3 to exon 4. A region of very high GC content (80 percent) is found upstream of the first methionine. There is strong amino acid similarity among PITX family members throughout the protein, but in the homeodomain mouse Pitx3 shows 100 percent and 97 percent identity with mouse Pitx2 and Pitx1, respectively.[139] A highly conserved 14-amino-acid motif, the OAR domain, is present C-terminal of the homeodomain in PITX3, as well as in other paired-type homeobox proteins.

***Pitx3 Gene Expression.*** *In situ* hybridization studies[139] provided detailed information on eye expression at various stages in development. Strong expression was seen in the equatorial (bow) regions of the lens at E11, and throughout the lens by E15. The eye muscles and eyelid also express *Pitx3* at E15. Subsequently, more detailed analysis[140] revealed strong expression in the midbrain region, tongue, and incisor primordia, and in the condensing mesenchyme around the sternum and vertebrae, and in the head muscles. In the rat, expression in the dopaminergic neurons of the mesencephalic region was documented.[300]

***Regulation of Downstream Genes.*** No downstream target genes have so far been identified for the *Pitx/PITX* gene family, despite their involvement in eye disease.

***Human Mutations in PITX3.*** Four families with various developmental eye anomalies were analyzed for linkage with the *PITX3* chromosomal region. One anterior segment mesenchymal dysgenesis (ASMD) family showed tight linkage to polymorphic markers flanking *PITX3*. ASMD cases have malformations involving each of the three mesenchymal neural crest migrations (Table 240-4), making *PITX3* a likely candidate gene based on expression pattern. In addition, mindful of the phenotype/genotype heterogeneity observed in developmental eye disease, 80 samples from familial cases with Rieger syndrome, isolated anterior segment malformations, Axenfeld and Rieger anomalies with other associated systemic abnormalities and some familial cases of congenital cataracts, were screened for *PITX3* mutations. So far, mutations have been documented in two cases (Fig. 240-12). First, a 17-bp insertion, into a region where an 11-bp repeat is duplicated, has been identified in a family with ASMD syndrome,

leading to quite a long region of out-of-frame change before termination.[140] The second mutation, a S13N missense change in an autosomal dominant congenital cataract (ADCC) mother and son, was documented as a *de novo* change when the mother's parents were shown to have only wild-type sequence.[140]

**Conclusions.** All the anterior segment anomalies described here are caused by loss of function of one copy of a gene (haploinsufficiency). In each case, that gene has many other crucial functions in development, implied by the extensive nonocular expression pattern and demonstrated by the homozygous loss of function phenotype in animal models (e.g., neuronal development, *PAX6*; left-right asymmetry, *PITX2*; brain and skeletal development, *FKHL7*).

A recurring theme is the extreme phenotypic variability that occurs in these disorders, sometimes even between the two genetically identical eyes of a single individual carrying one mutation. This variability probably reflects the dependence of normal eye development on the precise dosage of these genes, and the fact that a molecular defect in the early stages of anterior segment development may not have an entirely predictable and reproducible outcome given the enormous complexity of the subsequent tissue interactions that must take place. In a single individual, the phenotypic outcome may depend on the precise number of transcripts from a gene at some critical stage. Between individuals, the activity of other genes may ameliorate or exacerbate the shortfall in the mutated gene. From a genetic perspective, remember that there is generally no simple genotype-phenotype correlation. From a clinical perspective, knowledge of the underlying mutation may be useful in deciding what clinical strategies to take; there may be increased risks associated with some surgical interventions due to the reduced regenerative power of tissues carrying certain mutations.

The phenotypic overlap between patients with mutations in *PAX6*, *PITX3*, *PITX2*, and *FKHL7* must point to functional interrelationships between these proteins. The ectodermally derived (*PAX6*-expressing) structures of the optic cup, the lens, and the presumptive cornea must communicate through cell-surface markers and secreted signaling proteins with the incoming neural crest-derived mesenchyme (*PITX2*-, *PITX3*-, and *FKHL7*-expressing). The stage is set for a more detailed understanding of how these genes act to coordinate the multiple tissue interactions of the anterior segment.

## Waardenburg Syndrome

Waardenburg syndrome (WS) is a phenotype characterized principally by auditory and pigmentary abnormalities. The characteristic eye pigmentation defects of WS (Table 240-7, Fig. 240-13) are hypopigmented or heterochromatic irides and occasionally, hypopigmented fundi.[301,302] The major nonocular phenotypes of WS include defects of pigmentation of the skin or hair (particularly a white forelock) and hearing loss. The underlying cause of these diverse phenotypes is a disruption in the development, migration, or differentiation of melanocytes and neural crest cells. Four types of WS have been distinguished by clinical and molecular criteria and found to result from mutations in at least five different genes (Table 240-7).[302–304] Additional WS genes remain to be identified because mutations in the five known WS genes do not account for all patients. WS is discussed comprehensively in Chap. 244. Only a brief overview is presented here, with particular attention to the associated eye defects.

**MITF.** Waardenburg syndrome type 1 (WS1) is a dominantly inherited condition due to mutations in the transcription factor gene *PAX3*.[302] Affected patients show the canonical pigmentary defects of WS in addition to a craniofacial defect, dystopia canthorum (outward displacement of the inner canthi of the eyes). WS2, caused by mutations in *MITF*, is also dominant, but can be distinguished from WS1 by the absence of dystopia canthorum. WS3 patients resemble those with WS1 except that, by definition,

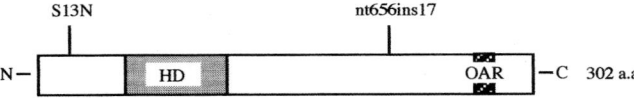

**Fig. 240-12 Mutations in *PITX3* are associated with anterior segment mesenchymal dysgenesis.[140] Mutations in the *PITX3* gene presented on a schematic of the PITX3 protein, including the homeodomain (HD) and OAR domain. The N13S missense mutation is associated with autosomal-dominant congenital cataracts. The 17-nucleotide insertion is present in a family with ASMD and cataracts.**

**Table 240-7** The Four Types of Waardenburg Syndrome and Their Associated Genes

| WS type | OMIM number | Associated genes | Inheritance | Eye phenotype | Other phenotypes |
|---|---|---|---|---|---|
| 1 | 193500 | PAX3 | Dominant | Iris pigment defects | Hearing loss, white forelock and dystopia canthorum |
| 2A | 193500 | MITF (15 %) | Dominant | Iris pigment defects | Hearing loss, white forelock |
| 2B | | Unknown gene(s) (85%) | Dominant | Iris pigment defects | Hearing loss, white forelock |
| 3 | 148820 | PAX3 | Recessive and dominant | Iris pigment defects | Hearing loss, white forelock, dystopia canthorum and limb defects |
| 4 | 277580 | SOX10 | Dominant | Iris pigment defects | Hearing loss, white forelock and Hirschsprung disease |
| | 277580 | EDN3, EDNRB | Recessive | Iris pigment defects | Hearing loss, white forelock and Hirschsprung disease |

See text for references. Table adapted from Read;[302] see also Chap. 244.

WS3 patients also have limb defects. Like WS1, WS3 is also the result of mutations in *PAX3* although both recessive and dominant inheritance of WS3 have been identified. WS4 patients have classic WS pigmentary defects and no dystopia canthorum, but their phenotype includes Hirschsprung disease. When WS4 is dominantly inherited, mutations have been found in the putative transcription factor *SOX10*. In contrast, patients with recessive WS4 have been discovered to have defects in either the gene encoding the *Endothelin 3* (*EDN3*) ligand, or one of its receptors, *EDNRB*. Mouse models for all four Waardenburg syndromes have been identified (WS1 and 3: *Splotch* mouse (*Pax3*);[305] WS2: *microphthalmia* mouse (*Mitf*);[116,306] WS4: *Dom* mouse (*Sox10*),[307] *lethal-spotting* mouse (*Edn3*),[302] and *piebald-lethal* mouse (*Ednrb*)[302]).

The differences in the WS phenotypes may be due to the cells affected.[302] WS2 appears to result from defects in melanocytes of neural crest origin fated to become auditory and pigmentary cells. However, WS1, 2, and 3 appear to be the consequence of abnormalities in melanocytes as well as other neural crest cells. Neural crest cells are involved in the development of various tissues including facial bones and limb muscles, accounting for the more complex phenotypes of WS1, 2, and 3.

**Waardenburg Syndrome Type 2A.** Although mutations in the *MITF* gene are associated with WS2, they are responsible for only

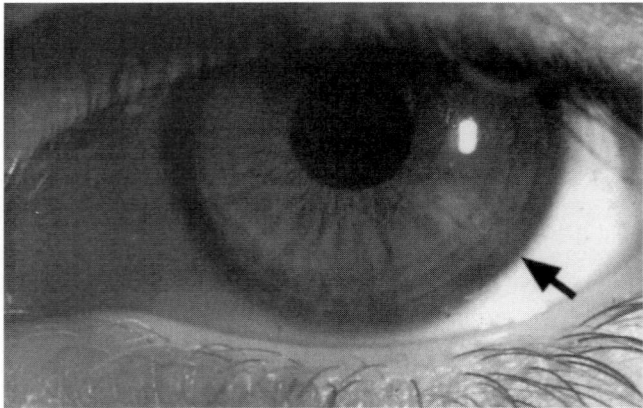

Fig. 240-13 Photograph of the iris of a patient with a hypopigmented iris and thin iris stroma. This patient was not demonstrated as having WS2 or an *MITF* mutation, but the phenotype of the iris and white forelock suggest WS2. The arrowhead identifies the hypopigmented radial section of the left iris. See Chap. 244 for photographs of patients with identified Waardenburg syndrome. (*Photograph kindly provided by Isabelle Russell-Eggitt, Great Ormond Street Hospital for Children, London, England.*)

15 percent of cases, and consequently at least one other gene, presently unidentified, is associated with WS2;[302,308] WS2 patients with *MITF* mutations are classified as having WS2A. In this chapter, we examine in particular the role of the *MITF* gene (associated with one form of WS, type 2A) in eye development, because *MITF* is the only one of the WS-associated genes known to be expressed in the developing eye.[116,118] The *MITF* gene encodes a basic helix-loop-helix, leucine-zipper transcription factor, which is of fundamental importance to mammalian eye development, because homozygous mutations in the mouse *Mitf* gene are associated with severe developmental eye defects. These defects extend well-beyond the abnormalities in iris pigmentation (hypopigmented or heterochromatic irides) found in patients with all types of WS, including type 2. The iris phenotypes are thought to originate in abnormalities in the neural crest cells that migrate into the iris, rather than in cells that originate in the developing eye per se. The homozygous *Mitf* mouse eye abnormalities include a small eye and retinal degeneration due to hyperproliferation of the (RPE) cells.

**Gene Identification.** In 1993, mutations in the mouse *Mitf* gene were found to be associated with a classic semidominant mouse mutant, microphthalmia (*mi*).[116,306] This discovery led to the cloning of the human *MITF* gene from a melanocyte cDNA library. The mouse *Mitf* gene is located on chromosome 6, 40 cM from the centromere.[309] Human *MITF* maps to chromosome 3p14.1-p12.3.[310] Two WS2 families were also mapped to proximal 3p, in the region of *MITF*,[311] suggesting *MITF* as a WS2 candidate gene. This candidacy was supported by the similarity of the auditory and pigmentary phenotype of WS2 patients and the microphthalmic (*mi*) mouse. WS2 patients were found to carry *MITF* mutations (see "Human Mutations in *MITF* Cause Waardenburg Syndrome Type 2," below).[308] Spontaneous *Mitf* mutations have also been identified in hamster,[312,313] quail,[314] and rats.[313]

**MITF Protein Structure and Conservation.** The microphthalmia basic helix-loop-helix transcription factor contains a leucine-zipper domain, a motif that, in other proteins, mediates protein-protein interactions (Fig. 240-14).[317,318] The human and mouse MITF proteins are 94 percent identical overall, with 100 percent identity in the bHLH domain.[116,306,310] In addition, the leucines of the leucine zipper, as well as the spacing between them, are perfectly conserved. The MITF polypeptide is similar to the bHLH-ZIP proteins TFEB, TFEC, and TFE3.[319] Each of these three related proteins, which together with MITF make up the small MiT protein family, has been shown to heterodimerize both with MITF and with one another, each combination having a different DNA-binding affinity. TFEB and TFE3 are expressed ubiquitously, while TFEC is tissue-restricted in its expression; apart from MITF, no other member of the MiT family has been shown to have a role in development.

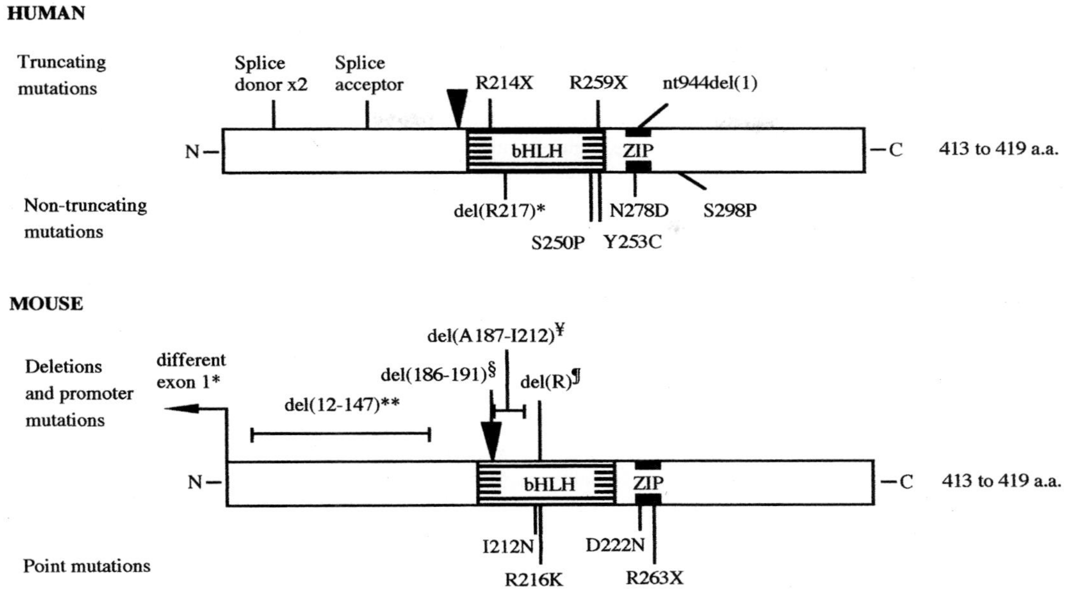

**HUMAN**

Truncating
mutations

Splice donor x2    Splice acceptor        R214X    R259X    nt944del(1)

N —— [ bHLH  ZIP ] —— C    413 to 419 a.a.

Non-truncating
mutations

del(R217)*        N278D    S298P

S250P  Y253C

**MOUSE**

Deletions
and promoter
mutations

different
exon 1*

del(A187-I212)¥

del(186-191)§   del(R)𝕁

del(12-147)**

N —— [ bHLH  ZIP ] —— C    413 to 419 a.a.

I212N    D222N

Point mutations

R216K    R263X

**Fig. 240-14** Mutations in the human *MITF* gene presented above a schematic of the MITF protein, a basic helix-loop-helix, leucine-zipper transcription factor. Truncating mutations are shown above; nontruncating mutations are shown below. All the mutations shown are associated with WS2 except *, which is associated with the Tietze-Smith syndrome (see text). The insertion point for the 18-bp alternatively spliced exon is shown above the schematic (*arrowead*). A stop codon is abbreviated as an X. (*Adapted from Read.*[302] *Used with permission.*) Mutations in the mouse *Mitf* gene presented below a schematic of the MITF protein. Deletions and promoter mutations are shown above, point mutations below. All mutations are alleles associated with the *microphthalmic* mouse. *The *red-eyed white* allele is a deletion of upstream sequences resulting in cryptic splicing and a novel N-terminal peptide. **An intragenic deletion. §A small deletion disrupts splicing and removes the alternatively spliced exon in the *spotted* allele which has no homozygous phenotype, but is associated with a microphthalmic phenotype only when present with another *Mitf* allele in a compound hetero-zygote. ¥A small deletion in the basic domain, 3′ to the alternatively spliced exon. 𝕁One arginine, exact position unknown, is deleted from the basic domain. (*Figure compiled using data from Steingrimsson et al.*[315] *and Moore.*[316])

In addition to the potential modulation of MITF activity through the formation of various heterodimers, differential splicing produces multiple MITF isoforms. In mouse, there are three alternatives of exon 1, each generating different proteins at the N-terminus,[315,320,321] one specifically present in melanocytes, another in the heart, and a third isoform that is specific to the RPE. Another alternative splice event occurs within intron 5, resulting in two isoforms that either include or omit six amino acids immediately N-terminal to the bHLH domain.[116] The splice form with the six-amino-acid insert has slightly higher DNA-binding affinity.[319] MITF is regulated by MAP kinase phosphorylation, part of the Steel/Kit pathway in melanocytes.[322] This phosphorylation event increases the transactivation of the *MITF* downstream gene, *tyrosinase* (see Fig. 240-15).

**Mitf Expression.** *Mitf* expression in the developing mouse eye has been characterized extensively.[116–118,320] The transcript is first detected at E9.5 in the whole-optic vesicle, but by E10.5 expression is reduced to the presumptive RPE, where it continues to be detected until E16.5. *Mitf* is also expressed in the developing

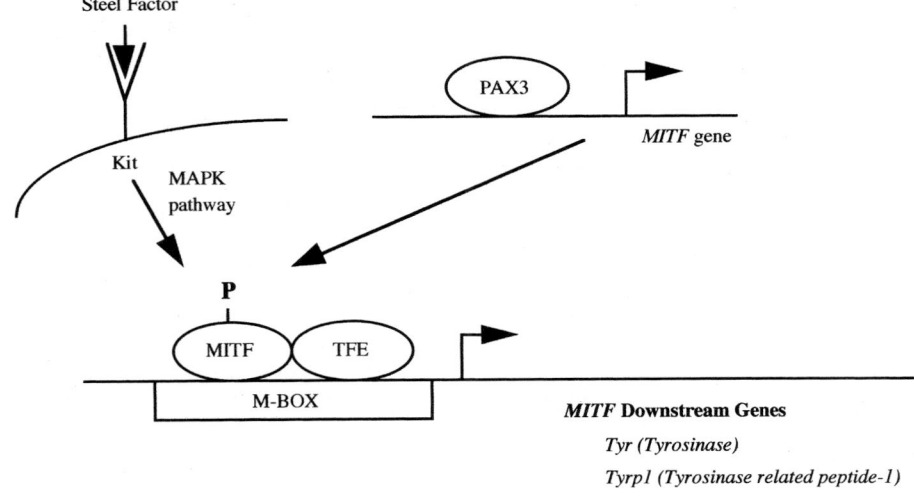

Steel Factor

PAX3

*MITF* gene

Kit    MAPK
pathway

**P**

MITF   TFE

M-BOX

*MITF* **Downstream Genes**

*Tyr (Tyrosinase)*

*Tyrp1 (Tyrosinase related peptide-1)*

*Dct (DOPAchrome tautomerase)*

*Kit (tyrosine kinase receptor)*

**Fig. 240-15** The MITF protein has been positioned in various biochemical and genetic pathways. The MITF protein has been shown in melanoma cell lines to be phosphorylated by the MAP kinase pathway in response to Steel factor. This phosphorylation event increases the ability of MITF to trans-activate one of its downstream targets, the major pigmentation gene *Tyr*. MITF may also transactivate *Tyrp1*, *Dct*, and *Kit*. All four promoters (*Tyr*, *Tyrp1*, *Dct*, and *Kit*) contain an MITF binding site called the M-box. MITF functions by heterodimerizing with proteins of the TFE family. PAX3 protein binds to an *MITF* promoter construct *in vitro*, producing a significant increase in the transcription of the *MITF* gene in melanoma cells. See text for details and references.

neural crest, specific cells surrounding the otic vesicle (the presumptive inner ear structure), and hair follicles. This pattern is consistent with the disruption of normal auditory intermediate cells of the stria vascularis and pigment cell formation in WS2.[323] Adult mice, and cells lines derived from the corresponding tissues, express *Mitf* in heart, lung, uterus, skin, mast cells, and melanocytes.[116] The phenotype associated with heterozygous WS2 mutations is milder than the homozygous phenotype observed for most recessive mouse *mi* alleles, where affected tissues include the eye—particularly the retina—the inner ear, coat pigment, mast cells, and osteoclasts.[316,324] RPE and forebrain melanocytes are of distinct origin, and the latter appear to be unaffected in individuals heterozygous for *MITF* mutations (in both humans and mice), while RPE melanocytes are very abnormal in mice homozygous for *Mitf* mutations.

**Regulation of the *MITF* Gene and Target Genes of the MITF Protein.** MITF is a transcriptional activator that interacts with other proteins to regulate the expression of downstream genes by binding to a conserved 11-bp DNA element: the M box (core sequence: CATGTG).[319] The three major pigmentation enzyme genes—*Tyrosinase (Tyr)*, *Tyrosinase related peptide 1 (Tyrp1)*, and *Dopachrome tautomerase (Dct)*, previously known as *Tyrosinase related peptide 2 (Tyrp2)*—all contain an M-box in their promoters. Although there is no evidence for *in vitro* binding of MITF to the human *Tyrosinase* promoter, MITF does activate transcription from this promoter in expression assays.[325,326] There is also evidence for MITF regulation of *Tyrp1* and *Dct*, as well as the *Kit* gene (cytokine receptor).[117,327,328] Mitf also interacts with the retinoblastoma and CBP/p300 protein *in vitro*.[329,330]

The MITF protein has been positioned in a number of biochemical pathways (Fig. 240-15): as a target of phosphorylation from the Steel/Kit/MAP kinase pathway,[322] directly downstream of PAX3,[331] and upstream of pigmentation enzyme genes.[319] PAX3 up-regulates the expression of *MITF in vitro* and mutant PAX3 proteins associated with WS1 fail to transactivate *MITF*.[331] The *PAX3* transactivation of *MITF* is consistent with the similar auditory-pigmentary phenotypes observed in WS1 (due to mutations in *PAX3*) and WS2 (due to mutations in *MITF*).

*Effects of MITF Activity In Vivo.* In tissue culture model systems, MITF is required for the determination of RPE cell fate and for the down-regulation of cell proliferation. Ectopic *MITF* expression converts NIH 3T3 fibroblasts into cells with features of melanocytes,[332] including characteristic morphology and the expression of *MITF* downstream proteins. RPE cells expressing mutant *Mitf* undergo increased proliferation, and lose their pigmented phenotype; ectopic *Mitf* can rescue both of these changes.[314] MITF also appears to negatively regulate *PAX6* expression in both chick and quail, although it is not known whether this regulation is direct.[314,320] The ectopic *PAX6* expression may be causal in the loss of an RPE phenotype and gain of neuroretina-like features in RPE cells.

**Human Mutations in *MITF* Cause Waardenburg Syndrome Type 2.** As of 1997, 11 human *MITF* mutations had been identified in association with WS2[302,308,333] (Fig. 240-14). *MITF* mutations associated with WS2 include truncating mutations predicted to be loss-of-function null alleles (splice mutations, nonsense changes, and frameshift deletions), and nontruncating changes that may or may not be loss-of-function mutations (a three-nucleotide deletion and missense mutations). One *MITF* mutation was also found in a family with autosomal dominant Tietz-Smith syndrome (MIM 103500), of which the major phenotypes are albinism and complete nerve deafness.[334] Given that MITF functions in several biochemical pathways, the remaining, as yet unidentified genes in these pathways may be mutated in WS2 (Fig. 240-15). In contrast to the mouse no recessive disease-causing mutations in the human *MITF* gene have been identified to date, but this may be due in part to ascertainment

bias in human populations that are largely outbred with low mutant gene frequency.

Recently digenic inheritance involving *MITF* was identified,[335] highlighting the role of *MITF* as a genetic modifier locus. Two families with both WS2 and autosomal recessive ocular albinism (AROA) were shown to (a) harbor a heterozygous mutation in *MITF* (a one-nucleotide deletion in exon 8) and (b) to be either heterozygous or homozygous for a *TYR* polymorphism (R402Q) that by itself is nondeleterious. Thus, *MITF* appears to act as a modifier locus of the *TYR* phenotype, consistent with MITF being a transcriptional regulator of *TYR*. These findings illustrate an important principle of medical genetics: transcription factor variants that regulate a polymorphic gene product can increase the clinical heterogeneity of a disease.

**Mouse Mutations in *Mitf* Cause Microphthalmia.** To date, 21 alleles of *Mitf* have been shown to produce the microphthalmic (*mi*) mouse phenotype[118,316] (Fig. 240-14). A diversity of mutations has been shown to cause both semidominant and autosomal recessive disease. *Mitf* mutations affect the cells in which the protein is developmentally expressed (see "Mitf Expression," above).[117,316] The most severe phenotypic manifestations occur with alleles in which the DNA-binding domain is altered. The range of phenotypic characteristics includes microphthalmia, retinal degeneration, osteoporosis, an inner ear defect with possible hearing loss, pigmentation abnormalities, reduced mast cell numbers, and neural crest cell defects. A major feature of the severe eye phenotype is hyperplasia of the RPE, indicating that Mitf normally represses RPE cell proliferation. The RPE proliferation leads to defects in the choroidal fissure.[324] The expression of *Tyr* and *Tyrp1* is undetectable in *Mitf* mutant RPE cells, which may also contribute to the RPE cell abnormalities.[117] Progressive retinal degeneration is seen with some alleles, and is probably due to defects in RPE cell function;[118,316] a normal RPE is essential for the maintenance of the mammalian photoreceptor.[336]

**Lessons from the Mouse Model.** The study of the microphthalmic mouse has made several major contributions to the understanding of the role of the *MITF* gene in human disease. Identification of the mouse *Mitf* gene[116,306] and analysis of the microphthalmic mouse led to the discovery of the association between mutations in human *MITF* gene and the human disease Waardenburg syndrome type 2A.[302,308] Subsequently, analysis of *Mitf/MITF* mutations in mouse and humans has highlighted major unexpected differences in the genetic mechanisms at this locus in the two species.

A striking example is the contrast in the pattern of inheritance and phenotype resulting from two near-identical nonsense mutations, R263X in mouse and R259X in human, both of which occur just N-terminal to the leucine zipper motif.[319,337] The R263X allele is fully recessive in mouse, while the human R259X allele is autosomal dominant. The homozygous R263X mouse (*cloudy eyes* allele) has microphthalmia, reduced eye pigmentation, and cataracts.[316] In contrast, human heterozygotes for the R259X allele have Waardenburg syndrome type 2A, which is not associated with cataracts.

Additional complexity in the effect of the same mutation in the two species is shown by the different heterozygous phenotypes that occur in carriers of the R217Δ allele. In human carriers, the allele causes autosomal dominant Tietz Syndrome, which is similar to WS2A except that the patients also have albinism and complete nerve deafness.[333] In contrast, R217Δ is semidominant in mice, their hearing is normal, and they have only a small depigmented skin splotch.[116,324]

Finally, molecular evidence of mutations in MITF/Mitf protein supports different genetic mechanisms between mouse and human. In the mouse, *in vitro* studies suggest that these semidominant alleles are dominant negatives that disrupt the basic DNA-binding

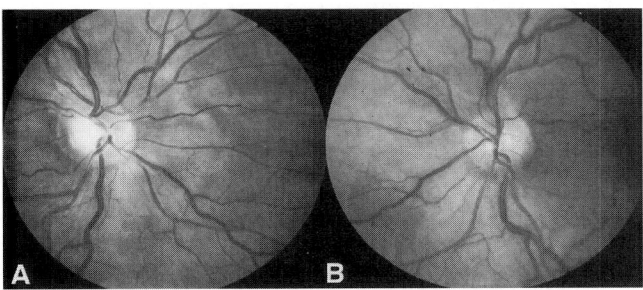

**Fig. 240-16** Eye phenotype associated with *PAX2* mutations. Right and left optic disc of patient with heterozygous G76S *PAX2* mutation. (*Photograph and patient details kindly provided by Dr. Anita Leys, Leuven, Belgium.*) Left disc nearly normal, but with unusual vascular pattern; abnormal right disc slightly enlarged and with an optic pit and anomalous vascular pattern. Proteinuria detected at age 11 years, led to renal insufficiency with end-stage renal failure at age 22 years in this individual. Affected family members all had papillorenal syndrome and mild eye phenotypes.[341] *PAX2* loss-of-function mutations often give rise to more severe optic disk anomalies including coloboma.[340]

domain.[319] In contrast, human *MITF* alleles that result in autosomal dominant WS2 are likely to be due to haploinsufficiency.[333,337] These examples suggest that humans are either more sensitive than mice to *MITF* gene dosage effects, or that there are substantial differences in the effects of modifier genes in the two species.

In contrast to the mouse, the Syrian hamster has dominant *Mitf* mutations that lead to haploinsufficiency.[116,312] The hamster phenotype is similar to humans with WS2 pigment defects, and heavy hearing loss is present in heterozygotes. Thus, the hamster may be a better model for WS2 than the mouse. Because no humans with homozygous *MITF* mutations have been identified, either the result is in embryonic lethality or a phenotype that has not yet been identified.

## POSTERIOR EYE DEFECTS

### Renal-Coloboma Syndrome

Renal-coloboma syndrome (MIM 120330) is a rare, dominantly inherited syndrome typically featuring optic nerve coloboma a crater-like excavation of the optic disc (Fig. 240-16), renal hypoplasia, and vesicoureteral reflux (regurgitation of urine from the bladder to the kidneys). A major feature of renal-coloboma syndrome is extreme phenotypic variability. Some affected individuals have subclinical renal anomalies, while others have end-stage renal failure in childhood; similarly, some patients have profound visual handicap while others have optic disc anomalies

so mild that they are only detectable by detailed ophthalmologic examination.[338-341] The fact that many patients have more subtle defects of the optic papilla rather than overt colobomata has lead to the suggestion that "papillorenal syndrome" may be a more suitable name for this disorder.[341] In some cases, sensorineural deafness is present.[340] This is consistent with the PAX2 expression pattern.

**Gene Identification.** The *Pax2* gene was originally identified in the mouse as part of a study to characterize vertebrate genes related to a key *Drosophila* developmental gene called *paired*. Genomic and cDNA libraries were screened with probes from *paired*, resulting in the identification of a mouse gene called *Pax1*; probes from *Pax1* were used, in turn, to isolate other members of the family including *Pax2*.[342,343] Nine ammalian *Pax* genes are now known, all of which, like *Drosophila paired*, encode a 128-amino-acid DNA-binding motif called a paired domain.[344,345] Orthologous *Pax2* genes have also been isolated in man,[346] *Xenopus*,[347] and zebrafish. The zebrafish genome contains two *Pax2*-like genes, *Pax2.1* (formerly *Pax[zf-b]*) and *Pax2.2*.[348-350] The human *PAX2* locus consists of 12 exons spread over 70 kb[351] and maps to 10q22.1-q24.3.[346] Mouse *Pax2* maps to the homologous genomic region on chromosome 19.[343,352]

*PAX2* **Protein Structure and Conservation.** The vertebrate *Pax2* proteins contain a paired domain of 128 amino acids, an octapeptide motif located 40 amino acids C-terminal of the paired domain, and a truncated form of the paired-type homeodomain consisting only of the first alpha-helix (Fig. 240-17).[342,346,348] The major protein isoform is 393 amino acids in humans, 392 in mice, and 391 in zebrafish (Pax2.1). However, it is clear that multiple alternative mRNA splice forms exist in all species examined so far, with 12 splice variants observed in zebrafish.[342,346-348,350,353] The consequence of alternative splicing for PAX2 protein function remains to be investigated in detail, but it is potentially a powerful mechanism by which PAX2 function could be modulated during development. A major splice variant in both mouse and man involves the inclusion of a 69-bp exon, which results in the insertion of an additional 23 amino acids into the protein between the octapeptide and the truncated homeodomain. The protein products generated by this splice variant have been detected on western blots of mouse embryonic tissues and human Wilms tumors.[353]

When the amino acid sequences of the PAX proteins are compared, PAX2 falls into a discrete subclass with PAX8 and PAX5. These three paralogous proteins are closely related in sequence and share the same overall structure, with a paired domain, octapeptide, and truncated homeodomain.[343-345] The high degree of conservation suggests that genes of the *PAX2/5/8* subclass diverged relatively recently, around the time of the vertebrate radiation, and, indeed, it appears that the primitive chordate *Amphioxus* has a single gene of this class, termed

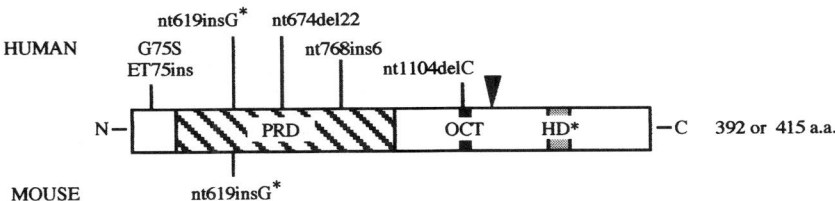

**Fig. 240-17** Mutations in human *PAX2* are associated with renal-coloboma syndrome.[338-341,358] *Mutations in the PAX2 gene presented on a schematic of the PAX2 protein, including a partial homeodomain (HD\*), a paired domain (PRD), and an octapeptide (OCT). Above the schematic are human mutations; below are mouse mutations. \*The nt619insG has been reported in six* independent families/individuals, as well as the *Pax2^Neu* mouse.[359] Two other mutations have been identified in *PAX2*—a dinucleotide insertion (2G) and a six-nucleotide deletion—but their exact locations are unpublished. The 23-amino-acid alternatively spliced exon (*arrowhead*) has been identified in kidney only.[353]

*AmphiPax2/5/8*.[354] The archetypal *Pax2/5/8* gene, however, is undoubtedly ancient in origin, and has been detected in sea urchin, *Drosophila, C. elegans*, and, sponge, hydra, and jellyfish.[250,355,356]

The PAX2 protein contains a well-characterized DNA binding motif, the paired domain, and has DNA-binding activity.[353] Of the PAX2/5/8 subclass the PAX5 paired domain has been studied in most detail, with a detailed biochemical analysis of the amino acids necessary to determine DNA-binding specificity.[180] The structure and function of the paired domain is discussed in more detail in the section on PAX6 above (see "*PAX6* Gene and Protein Structure; Conservation"). Evidence is emerging that paired domains of the PAX2/5/8 subclass may interact with proteins as well as DNA; the beta hairpin at the N-terminus of the paired domain has been shown to interact with members of the Ets family.[357]

***PAX2* Expression.** In common with other members of the *Pax* gene family, *Pax2* has a spatially and temporally complex expression pattern.[344,345] Major domains of expression include the central nervous system, eye, ear, and kidney, where *Pax2* expression is consistently initiated shortly after the onset of organogenesis and is then dynamically modulated as subsequent phases of differentiation occur.

*Pax2* is expressed in the developing spinal cord and developing brain. In the developing nervous system, *Pax2* is first expressed at E7.5 in a domain extending from the prospective forebrain to the prospective hindbrain.[360] By E9.5, *Pax2* expression in the brain is restricted to the midbrain-hindbrain boundary, where it overlaps with the expression of *Pax5* and *Pax8*.[66,120] *Pax2* is also expressed in a lateromedial domain along the length of the developing spinal cord.[120,344]

In the eye, *Pax2* is initially expressed at E9 in the ventral half of the optic vesicle. At E10, it is expressed in the ventral part of the optic cup. By E11, Pax2 expression in the optic cup is restricted to the lips of the optic fissure, but there is now strong expression in the optic stalk. At later stages, *Pax2* is expressed in the optic stalk and optic disc, and in a small subset of retinal cells.[120,360]

In the developing ear, *Pax2* expression commences at E9 in the otic vesicle. At later stages, *Pax2* expression is restricted ventrally to the region that will give rise to the saccule and cochlea (the auditory portion of the inner ear).[120,360]

*Pax2* is expressed throughout kidney development.[342,345,353,361] In the pronephros (E9 to E10), *Pax2* is detected in the pronephric tubules, nephric duct, nephric cord, and Wolffian duct. In the mesonephros (E11 to E12), *Pax2* is expressed in the mesonephric tubules. In the early metanephros, *Pax2* is expressed in the ureter and developing collecting ducts and in the mesenchymal condensations around the ureteric branches. *Pax2* continues to be expressed in the differentiating regions of the metanephric kidney (E13 onwards), but expression gradually declines as the structures mature.

Once *Pax2* was identified as a marker for early kidney development in mouse, the human *PAX2* gene immediately became a focus of interest in terms of a possible relationship with the Wilms' tumor gene, *WT1*. Wilms' tumor is a pediatric nephroblastoma that can be caused by *WT1* mutations, and the *WT1* gene itself is expressed in the developing urogenital system.[362] Human *PAX2* was found to be expressed in the embryonic kidney and in Wilms' tumors;[346,353] however, no link has yet been established between *PAX2* mutation and predisposition to Wilms' tumor.

**Regulation of Downstream Genes.** In common with PAX6, the DNA targets of the PAX2 protein are poorly characterized to date. Two potential target genes, *WT1* and *Engrailed2*, were identified based on their expression patterns overlapping that of *PAX2*.

Based on the coexpression of *PAX2* and *WT1* during fetal kidney development, the ability of PAX2 protein to transactivate the *WT1* promoter was tested by cotransfection of appropriate expression and reporter constructs into cultured cells.[363,364]

Specific regions of the *WT1* promoter were found to function in this assay. There may be a reciprocal interaction between *WT1* and *PAX2*, because the WT1 protein was found to repress expression from the *PAX2* promoter in transfection experiments.[365]

The expression pattern of the *En2* gene overlaps with that of *Pax2* at the midbrain-hindbrain boundary. An enhancer fragment upstream of the *En2* promoter was found to direct reporter gene expression to the midbrain-hindbrain boundary in transgenic mice. The enhancer contains two binding sites for the Pax2/5/8 subclass of proteins. When these binding sites were disrupted, no reporter gene expression was detected at the midbrain-hindbrain boundary.[366] In addition, *En2* expression was greatly reduced in *Pax2^Neu* homozygous embryos.[356]

**Human Mutations in *PAX2* Cause Renal-Coloboma Syndrome.** With kidney defects frequently resulting in end-stage renal failure, and extensive phenotypic variability confounding accurate diagnoses, there were no sufficiently large well-characterized renal-coloboma syndrome families available for linkage studies, so it was not possible to determine a genomic map position for this disorder. *PAX2* was deduced as a likely candidate gene on the basis of the known expression pattern in the developing mouse embryo and the phenotype of a heterozygous mouse *Pax2* deletion mutant called *Krd* (see "Mouse Mutations in *Pax2* Cause Kidney and Retinal Defects" below). *PAX2* mutation screening was undertaken in renal-coloboma syndrome patients, and heterozygous mutations were initially found in two different families (Fig. 240-17). Both mutations were predicted to truncate the PAX2 protein.[338,339] Subsequent studies have further delineated the syndrome and have emphasized the phenotypic variability, even between individuals carrying the same mutation.[340,341] In some affected individuals, the phenotypic spectrum extends to hearing loss and microcephaly, while in others the kidney or ocular phenotype alone had come to attention.

Ocular defects range from visually debilitating optic nerve colobomata with associated myopia, nystagmus, and strabismus to very mild optic disc anomalies, sometimes evident only as an unusual pattern of retinal blood vessels with no apparent consequences for visual function.[339,341] One of the most frequently seen mutations, including that seen in a recently described mouse ENU mutant,[359] is insertion of an extra nucleotide into a homoguanine tract taking the protein out of frame and leading to premature truncation. Recently, contraction of the same homoguanine tract by a single nucleotide was seen in a mother and daughter with relatively mild eye and kidney phenotypes.[367] Even where the mutations are identical, the outcome of any given *PAX2* mutation seems highly susceptible to the influence of genetic modifiers and stochastic factors during early development. A child with renal-coloboma syndrome, carrying the more frequent homoguanine tract insertion, was also found to have Chiari I malformation, a severe brain anomaly.[364] In another report, a child with sporadic renal-coloboma syndrome was found to have a *de novo* chromosomal translocation t(10;13) breaking within the *PAX2* gene at 10q24.3-25.1.[368] Given the extreme phenotypic variation of the syndrome, it might be predicted that a proportion of individuals with isolated ocular defects or isolated kidney defects within the renal-coloboma syndrome spectrum may carry *PAX2* mutations. There is a report of a *PAX2* mutation in association with isolated renal hypoplasia,[355] but it seems from other studies that *PAX2* mutation is not a common cause of isolated ocular colobomata or isolated vesicoureteral reflux.[369,370]

*PAX2* mutations are archived on the Web in the Human PAX2 Allelic Variant Database (www.hgu.mrc.ac.uk/Softdata/PAX2/). Taking all the mutation data together, renal-coloboma syndrome seems to result from loss of function of one copy of the *PAX2* gene. Thus *PAX2* provides another example — along with *PAX6, PAX3, PITX2, PITX3, MITF*, and *FKHL7* (see elsewhere in this chapter) — of a gene in which haploinsufficiency leads to dominantly inherited congenital malformations with extensive phenotypic variability. Normal human development is clearly critically dependent on the correct dosage of these genes.

## Pax2 in Model Systems

### Mouse Mutations in Pax2 Cause Kidney and Retinal Defects.
The consequence of Pax2 mutation for mammalian development was first revealed by the Krd mouse. The Krd (kidney and retinal defects) mutation, generated by insertional transgenesis, is a deletion that spans approximately 7 cM on chromosome 19 and encompasses the Pax2 gene.[371] Despite the relatively large size of the deletion, the phenotypic anomalies in heterozygous animals, including developmental defects of the kidneys and the retina, seem to result mainly from Pax2 haploinsufficiency.[372] The heterozygous Krd phenotype has been studied in great detail to ascertain the effect of a reduction of Pax2 dosage on development of the mouse eye.[372] In $Krd^{+/-}$ embryos, the choroidal fissure forms (and later fuses) normally in the optic cup, but the optic groove fails to form, leading to abnormalities of optic stalk and optic disc development. In adult mice, the consequences of this are seen as broadening and cupping of the optic disc and abnormalities throughout the neural retina, including thinning of all the neural layers. Electroretinograms were indicative of abnormal photoreceptor and bipolar cell function.[373]

The consequence of homozygous loss of Pax2 function cannot be studied in Krd mutants because $Krd^{-/-}$ embryos die early in gestation, most likely as a result of loss of function of all the genes within the deletion. The effects of complete loss of Pax2 function have been addressed in the Pax2 knockout mouse $Pax2^{-/-}$. In newborn $Pax2^{-/-}$ mice, the kidneys, ureters, and genital tracts were absent,[361] and the eyes had complete colobomata of the globes.[360] In addition, the optic chiasm was absent, with all the optic neurons projecting ipsilaterally. In the ear, the cochlea and spinal ganglion were absent. Homozygous embryos had exencephaly because of failure of fusion of the neural folds in the midbrain region.[360] Heterozygous $Pax2^{+/-}$ mice showed renal and ocular defects very similar to those previously observed in $Krd^{+/-}$ mice, and in mice heterozygous for a spontaneously occurring allele called $Pax2^{Neu}$.[359] $Pax2^{Neu}$ carries a single nucleotide insertion in the Pax2 coding region in exactly the same position as five patients with renal-coloboma syndrome. Although the optic, otic, and renal malformations in $Pax2^{Neu}$ mice were similar to those in $Pax2^{-/-}$ mice, the brain phenotype was less severe due to a genetic background effect, and allowed more detailed analysis of the morphologic defects and altered expression pattern of other genes. The midbrain-hindbrain region and cerebellum were both completely absent in homozygous $Pax2^{Neu}$ embryos. The expression of En2, normally found in the midbrain-hindbrain boundary, was almost completely absent.[359]

### Lessons from the Mouse Model.
The embryonic expression pattern of Pax2 and the phenotype of Krd heterozygotes were critical in implicating the human PAX2 gene in renal-coloboma syndrome.[339] This provides an excellent example of the way in which an animal model can give invaluable clues about the role of a gene in human disease in the complete absence of any human mapping information. Comparison of the ocular phenotype in heterozygous and homozygous mutant mice has also given insights into the etiology of coloboma: Pax2 is essential for formation of the optic groove but not the choroidal fissure; it is essential, however, for fusion of the choroidal fissure.[359,360,372] Intriguingly, there is a difference in the level of Pax2 activity required for these two processes: heterozygous animals display optic nerve colobomata because the optic groove never forms; the choroidal fissure meanwhile fuses normally. Homozygous animals have complete colobomata of the globes, in addition to the optic nerve defects, because the choroidal fissure never fuses. The Pax2 mutant mice have again emphasized the key role of Pax genes in mammalian development.

### PAX2 in Zebrafish.
The effects of Pax2 mutation on development have also been extensively studied in the experimentally tractable zebrafish. Zebrafish have two Pax2-like genes, Pax2.1 (previously pax[zf-b]) and Pax2.2.[349,350] The Pax2.1 gene most closely resembles human and mouse Pax2 in expression pattern and genomic organization. Mutations of Pax2.1 result in a phenotype called no isthmus (noi), characterized by defective development of the optic nerve, optic chiasm, and the midbrain-hindbrain boundary.[350,374] Defective midbrain-hindbrain development is also seen if Pax2.1 function is inactivated by antibodies.[375] Examination of midbrain-hindbrain organization in a series of noi alleles has begun to clarify the relationship between Pax2.1 and other transcriptional regulators and signaling molecules encoded by eng2, eng3, wnt1, fgf8, and her5.[350] noi mutants have also shown that Pax2.1 is essential for expression of Pax5 and Pax8 in the midbrain-hindbrain boundary.[349]

Further insights into the regulation of ocular Pax gene expression has come from study of the zebrafish mutant cyclops (cyc), which carries a mutation in ndr2, a nodal-related gene of the TGFβ superfamily, and displays severe developmental abnormalities of the midline including cyclopia.[376] In the cyc mutant, Pax2.1 expression is dramatically down-regulated, while Pax6 is up-regulated, implying a role for midline signaling in the normal partitioning of the eye primordia and reciprocal activation of Pax genes therein.[235] When another midline signal Sonic hedgehog (shh) is experimentally overexpressed in zebrafish embryos, the domain of Pax2.1 expression is expanded and that of Pax6 diminished, with a consequent increase in the amount of optic stalk-like tissue and a decrease in retinal tissue.[235] In this way, signaling molecules linking Pax2 and Pax6 expression can be identified, and their role in eye development explored.

### Pax2 in Invertebrates.
Pax2 joins the growing list of genes that are expressed in the visual systems of both vertebrates and invertebrates. The classic Drosophila eye development mutant sparkling (spa) carries a mutation in D-Pax2, the fly ortholog of vertebrate PAX2.[21] Unlike its vertebrate counterpart, spa is expressed after the main morphogenetic events of eye development, playing a role in the differentiation of cone and pigment cells. D-Pax2 mutations are also responsible for the failure of sensory bristle development in the Drosophila mutant shaven (sv).[377,378] During bristle formation, D-Pax2 expression is controlled by the Notch signaling pathway. Many developmental parallels will likely be drawn as the regulators, DNA targets, and interacting cofactors of PAX2 and D-Pax2 emerge.

Mutations in a PAX2/5/8-like gene also underlie the egl-38 phenotype in C. elegans.[379] egl-38 was initially identified during a screen for animals with defective male tail development; in hermaphrodites, the same mutation prevents normal egg laying. In both cases, specific cells fail to achieve their normal identity, duplicating the fate of neighboring cells instead.

### Conclusion.
As more haploinsufficient genes are uncovered (see Table 240-1), a major theme is emerging of extreme, and often deceptive, phenotypic variability. PAX2 is no exception; although only a small number of individuals with PAX2 mutations have so far been described, the variability in presentation of individuals with renal-coloboma syndrome is remarkable. The clear message is that thorough systemic examination is essential for the accurate diagnosis of renal-coloboma syndrome, and should lead to the ascertainment of many more cases that may have been overlooked due to atypical presentation.

The PAX2 story provides an excellent example of the power of animal models to link a gene with a "candidate disease." The expression pattern of Pax2 in normal mouse embryos and the phenotype of $Krd^{+/-}$ mice together provided compelling evidence for a role of human PAX2 in renal-coloboma syndrome, which role was subsequently confirmed by mutation analysis.

The key role PAX2 plays in organogenesis is emphasized by PAX2-expressing structures being deficient or completely absent in

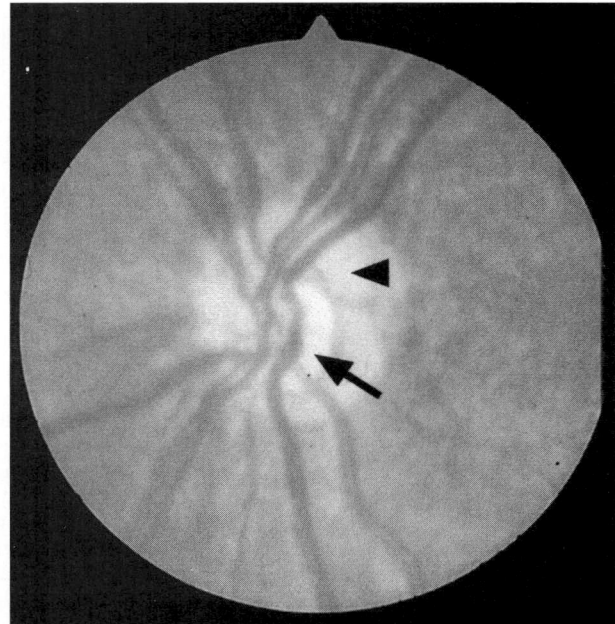

Fig. 240-18 The ocular phenotype of a patient with septo-optic dysplasia. The photograph shows the back of the retina of a child highlighting the optic nerve hypoplasia. The central light tissue, indicated with the arrow, is the optic nerve tissue. The surrounding area, with the arrowhead, represents "double-ring sign" and does not contain optic nerve tissue. This patient has not been tested for a *HESX1* mutation. (*Photograph kindly provided by Dr. Alex Levin, Hospital for Sick Children, Toronto, Canada.*)

loss-of-function mutants (human, mouse, zebra fish, or *Drosophila*). It is clear from a variety of systems that *PAX2* expression is intimately related to that of other transcriptional regulators—including other PAX proteins—and a range of signaling molecules. The future challenge is to understand at the molecular level how *PAX2* gene expression is initiated and how the PAX2 protein coordinates the expression of downstream target genes.

## Septo-Optic Dysplasia

Septo-optic dysplasia (MIM 182230) is a systemic disorder with an eye phenotype of hypoplastic optic discs with a double margin (Fig. 240-18). In addition, patients have defects of the brain: an absent septum pellucidum and midline brain abnormalities, such as agenesis of the corpus callosum and hypoplasia of the cerebellum, and hypoplasia of the pituitary gland resulting in hormone deficiency (growth hormone only or a number of pituitary hormones).[380–383] Most cases of septo-optic dysplasia (SOD) are sporadic, but a few familial cases have been reported with autosomal recessive inheritance.[384,385] *HESX1* is the only gene that has yet been identified to be mutated in SOD.

**The *HESX1* Gene.** The *HESX1* gene encodes a homeodomain protein that is expressed very early in the developing mouse embryo as well as in the pituitary gland (see "*Hsx1* Expression," below). A homozygous missense mutation in the homeobox of *HESX1* causes septo-optic dysplasia in one family.[386] A *Hesx1*-targeted null allele mouse has varying penetrance, with homozygous mice presenting defects of the brain, pituitary gland, and eye.

**Gene Identification.** *Hesx1* was first identified in the mouse as an ES cell homeobox gene.[387] It was mapped to mouse chromosome 14 A3-B.[388] Later studies showed strong developmental expression in the developing pituitary gland (Rathke's pouch, so it was named Rathke's pouch homeobox gene, *Rpx*[389]). A targeted

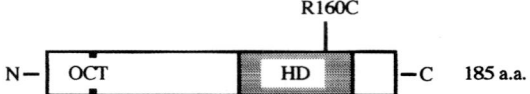

Fig. 240-19 Mutations in *HESX1* cause septo-optic dysplasia. The mutation in the *HESX1* gene presented on a schematic of the HESX1 protein, including a homeodomain (HD) and an octapeptide (OCT). Patients with SOD are homozygous for this missense mutation.[386]

deletion mouse was generated and the major phenotypes were micro- or anophthalmia, forebrain defects, midline defects of the brain, bifurcation of Rathke's pouch, and pituitary dysplasia.[386] Many of these phenotypic features are also observed in SOD patients, prompting a screen to find mutations in *HESX1* in human SOD individuals. The human *HESX1* was cloned and mapped chromosome 3p21.1-p21.2.[386] A homozygous missense mutation in *HESX1* in one consanguineous SOD family was identified.

**HESX1 Protein Structure and Conservation.** Two protein motifs are recognized in the 185 amino acids of HESX1, including a homeodomain and an octapeptide (Fig. 240-19). The homeodomain is located in the C-terminal half of the protein and is of the *paired-like* class. Near the N-terminus is an octapeptide (FSIE-HILG), a conserved eight-amino-acid motif that is proposed to play a role in transcriptional repression by paired-like homeodomain proteins.[268,269] The mouse *Hesx1* was cloned and shares 95 percent identity in the homeodomain and 81 percent overall identity with human *HESX1*.[386,387,389] There is a 3'UTR splice variant of the mouse *Hesx1* gene, although the significance of the splice event is not known.[390]

**Hesx1 Expression.** The *Hesx1* transcription factor is expressed in the developing head regions during embryogenesis and is essential for development of anterior midline central nervous system structures and the pituitary. Examination of the time course and abundance of *Hesx1* transcripts was studied in mouse development.[389] *In situ* analysis first detects expression during early gastrulation, although it may begin even earlier. Expression is consistently detected in midline tissue that is postulated to induce anterior head structures. By E8.5, expression is detected in the prosencephalon, oral ectoderm, and a nearby area of rostral foregut endoderm. By E9 to E9.5, expression is further restricted to Rathke's pouch, which forms part of the pituitary. Within the pituitary, expression is extinguished as cells differentiate, and no further expression is detected after E14.5. Expression analysis in the developing eye was unfortunately not explicitly reported.

**Regulation of Downstream Genes.** *Hesx1* is similar in sequence to a number of pituitary homeobox genes, including *Prop-1*, *Pit-1*, and the *Pitx* genes. Prop-1 is a homeodomain protein with a Q at position 9 of the third helix of the homeodomain and binds DNA at a P3 palindromic site: TAAT(N)$_3$ATTA.[391] Because Prop-1 and Hesx1 are both homeodomain proteins that share similar spatiotemporal expression patterns (developing pituitary), interactions between the two proteins upon binding to a P3 site was examined. The two proteins bind as a heterodimer, and in transcription assays, Hesx1 antagonizes activation by Prop-1 *in vitro*. HESX1 can also bind to the P3 oligonucleotide alone, although it was not reported if this was as a monomer or dimer[386].

**Human Mutations in *HESX1* Cause Septo-Optic Dysplasia.** The observed similarity between the mouse phenotype and the presentation of humans with SOD stimulated a *HESX1* mutation screen in patients with SOD and related phenotypes.[386] One extensive consanguineous pedigree was found to be segregating a point mutation in *HESX1* (Fig. 240-19). Two sibs with agenesis of the corpus callosum and panhypopituitarism (the same patients originally described in reference 385) are homozygous for a mutation within the homeodomain. The single base change alters codon 160, replacing a conserved arginine with a cysteine in the protein (R160C). An arginine residue at this position (R53) in a *paired-like* homeodomain is known from crystal structures to contact the DNA backbone.[270,392] Consistent with the suggested importance of this contact, electromobility shift assays demonstrated that the mutant HESX1 protein does not bind to its known consensus sequence.[386] Heterozygotes (nine in this family) for the R160C mutation do not display any of the features of SOD, as might be expected from the low frequency of affected heterozygotes in mice. A second *HESX1* point mutation (N125S) was also observed in the eighteenth residue of the homeodomain in a patient with sporadic pituitary hypoplasia. Because the proband was heterozygous for the mutation and because the mutation was also found in unaffected family members, the authors concluded that it was unlikely that N125S was responsible for the patient's phenotype. However, given the phenotypic variation observed in mice heterozygous and homozygous for a null allele, the relationship of this homeodomain mutation to disease is still uncertain.

**Mouse Mutations in *Hesx1* Cause Septo-Optic Dysplasia.** Disruption of the mouse *Hesx1* gene revealed homozygous mutant SOD phenotypes.[386] The earliest defects were observed at E8.5. All homozygous mutant embryos have a reduced amount of forebrain tissue and no optic vesicles. However, the defects fell into two very different classes: (a) mice with severe defects that are neonatal lethal; the pups are born with an overall small head, short nose, and micro- or anophthalmia; and (b) mice that are less deformed and often have only unilateral eye defects; although some die before weaning, members of this group can survive to adulthood and reproduce. The second milder phenotype of unilateral micro- or anophthalmia and less severe craniofacial dysplasia is also found in approximately 1 percent of heterozygotes. Although the phenotypic expression in homozygotes was variable, the consistent features involving the eyes include craniofacial dysplasia and anophthalmia or microphthalmia. Defects outside of the eye region include forebrain midline defects and absence of the septum pellucidum. The *Hesx1* eye phenotype may therefore be due to (a) eye-specific expression that has not yet been identified, or (b) earlier defects in presumptive eye tissues where *Hesx1* is expressed. This information will be critical in understanding the role of *HESX1* in eye development and disease.

**Lessons from the Mouse Model.** The *Hesx1* story again emphasizes the ability of mouse genetics to make links between human diseases and the genes that cause them. In addition, the mouse model offers insight into the genetics of *Hesx1* and SOD. For example given the evidence of the occasional penetrance of the phenotype in heterozygous mutant mice, it is conceivable that heterozygous mutations in families can cause mild SOD, as illustrated by the family with the N125S mutation.

**Conclusions.** In summary, a continuing search for mutations in *HESX1* in both familial and sporadic cases of SOD is warranted. In addition, further assessment of the role of *Hesx1* in mouse optic development, including detailed analysis of *Hesx1* expression in the eye, is needed to understand the eye phenotype that results from loss of *Hesx1* function.

## Photoreceptor Differentiation and Maintenance

The two types of photoreceptors, rods and cones, are named for the shape of their respective specialized light-sensing organelles, the outer segments (OSs). Rhodopsin, the light sensitive pigment that traps photons, is found in the OS. In humans, rods constitute 95 percent of the photoreceptors and mediate peripheral vision and vision in dim light. Although only 5 percent of photoreceptors are cones, they are spatially arranged to provide visual acuity and color vision, and are highly concentrated in the macula. Inherited photoreceptor diseases, of which the majority are degenerative, result in a wide range of clinical phenotypes depending, amongst other factors, on whether rods or cones are predominantly affected in the initial phases of the disease.

In this section, we discuss photoreceptor diseases associated with mutations in two transcription factor genes: *CRX*, the cone-rod homeobox gene, and *NRL*, the neural retina leucine zipper gene (Table 240-1). The CRX protein regulates the expression of many genes encoding photoreceptor OS proteins, including rhodopsin. NRL is a cotransactivator with CRX in the regulation of rhodopsin expression, and probably of other OS proteins as well.

**Structure and Function of the Rod Photoreceptor Outer Segment.** The *CRX* and *NRL* genes are required for the maintenance of the OS of the photoreceptor. The finger-like OS of rod photoreceptors is a specialized cilium composed of a plasma membrane surrounding a stack, in primates, of approximately 1000 lipid membranous disks[393] (Fig. 240-20). A major feature of photoreceptor biology is that the disks in the OS turn over, in primates, at a rate of about 10 percent per day, presumably to prevent the accumulation of light damage. Disk morphogenesis

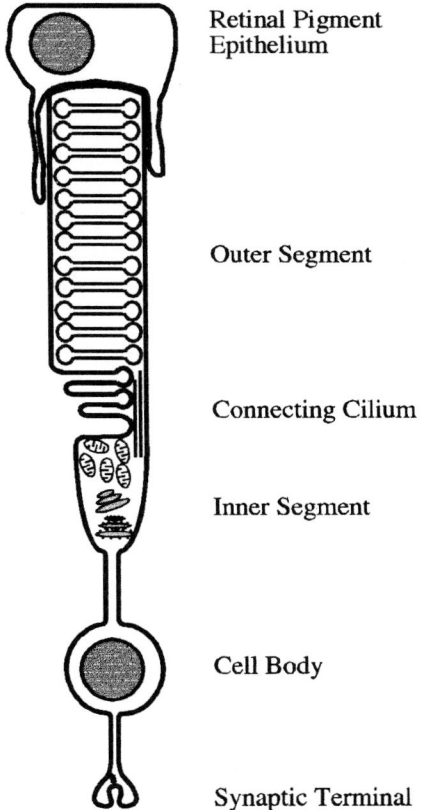

**Fig. 240-20** A schematic of the structure of a vertebrate photoreceptor. Each cell may be divided structurally and functionally into four separate domains. The synaptic terminal contacts the secondary neurons of the retina that comprise the inner nuclear layer (INL). The cell body contains the photoreceptor nucleus and is located within the outer nuclear layer (ONL) of the retina. The photoreceptor inner segment (IS) contains the majority of the photoreceptor metabolic machinery, including the ER-Golgi complex and the mitochondria. Connected to the inner segment by a thin cilium is the outer segment (OS), which contains a well-organized array of flat, membranous disks. These OS disks are the site of light absorption in the cell, and contain the molecules needed to convert light into a biochemical signal.

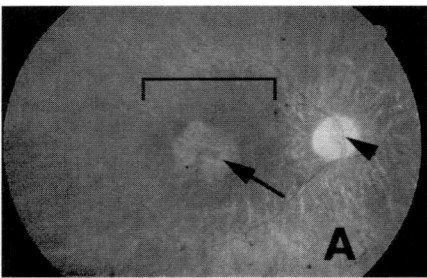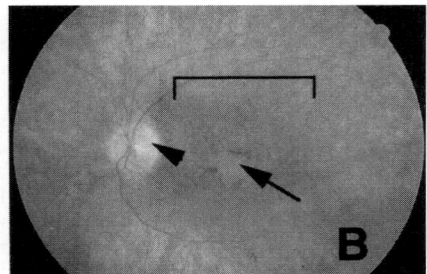

**Fig. 240-21** Fundus photographs of diseases from *CRX* mutations illustrating similar atrophic macular lesions, more preserved RPE surrounding the macula, and peripheral pigmentary degeneration. *A* is from an adCRD patient at age 50 (heterozygous for the E168del1nt *CRX* mutation). *B* is from an LCA patient at age 22 (heterozygous for the E168del1nt *CRX* mutation). Both retinas show atrophic macular lesions (*arrow*), and the mid- and far periphery (*bracket, above*) show depigmentation, bone spiculelike pigment, and chorioretinal atrophy. The retinal vessels are also attenuated. An arrowhead indicates optic nerve tissue. (*Figures kindly provided by Samuel Jacobson, Scheie Eye Institute, Philadelphia, PA.*)

occurs at the base of each OS, whereas disk shedding is due to phagocytosis by the retinal pigment epithelial cells of the disks at the tips of each OS. Rhodopsin, the most abundant OS protein, is embedded in the disk membrane. Other proteins of the phototransduction cascade, such as transducin, arrestin, and phosphodiesterase are also present in the OS, either associated with the membrane or in the cytoplasm (see Chap. 235).

**Disorders of Photoreceptor Development Due to Mutations in Transcription Factor Genes.** Failure of the development, differentiation, or maintenance of the photoreceptor is associated with loss of vision and often, complete blindness; the OS is commonly the site of the primary pathology. In some congenitally blind infants, there is an absence of functional photoreceptors; the cells may not form at all, or, in other instances, they form, but fail to develop OSs, as occurs in mice with a complete loss of function of the *Crx* gene[394] (see "Mutations in the *CRX* Gene Associated with Cone-Rod Dystrophy and Leber Congenital Amaurosis," below). Congenital blindness due to any of these abnormalities is called Leber congenital amaurosis (LCA).[395–398] Affected newborns or infants have little or no retinal photoreceptor function, as demonstrated by an electroretinogram (ERG). To date, three LCA genes have been identified, and LCA type III (MIM 602225, MIM 204000) is the result of mutations in *CRX*[71,399,400] (Fig. 240-21B). LCA is generally autosomal recessive, but both recessive and dominant mutations in the *CRX* gene have been reported (see "Mutations in the *CRX* Gene Associated with Cone-Rod Dystrophy and Leber Congenital Amaurosis," below). LCA is reviewed in Chap. 237.

**Disorders of Photoreceptor Maintenance Due to Mutations in Transcription Factor Genes.** In some patients with photoreceptor disease, the development of the cells and their OSs has been entirely normal, and the defect is an inability to maintain either the structure or function of the OS. The failure of photoreceptor maintenance leads to degeneration of rods or cones, or both, and gives rise to a range of disorders including, in the case of mutations in the *CRX* and *NRL* genes, cone rod dystrophy and retinitis pigmentosa, respectively.

Cone rod dystrophy (CRD) is initially characterized by the death of cones, with central visual loss, poor color vision, and diminished visual acuity. As the disease progresses, rods also die and peripheral as well as night vision are lost.[401–403] The disease is genetically heterogeneous, with autosomal dominant, autosomal recessive, and X-linked forms,[404] and several CRD genes have been identified (see Chap. 235). Mutations in *CRX* are responsible for dominant disease at the CORD2 locus (MIM 120970; see Fig. 240-21A).

Retinitis pigmentosa (RP) due to mutations in *NRL* are discussed below (see "A Human Mutation in *NRL* Causes Autosomal Dominant RP (adRP))," following the review of the

*CRX* gene. Other inherited retinal degenerations are reviewed in Chaps. 237 and 243.

***Identification, Overall Function, and Mapping of the CRX Gene.*** The *CRX* gene was cloned by three groups employing different strategies aimed at identifying retinal transcription factors.[69,154,405] *CRX* is the only transcription factor gene known to be photoreceptor-specific in its expression.[69,154,405] It is required for the maintenance of mature, differentiated rods and cones. Recent studies of mice with targeted *Crx* mutations confirm that the gene is essential for the biogenesis of the photoreceptor OS[394] (see "The Role of CRX in Regulating Photoreceptor Development and Gene Expression" below), but there is no strong evidence to indicate that it plays a significant role in photoreceptor development, and mice with a complete loss of *Crx* function form photoreceptors (although without outer segments.[394] The human gene maps to chromosome 19q13.3, within the genetic interval containing the CORD2 cone rod dystrophy locus.[69,405] This localization led to discovery of *CRX* mutations in a subset of patients with CRD.[69–71] The mouse ortholog maps to the proximal region of mouse chromosome 7.[405]

***CRX Gene Structure and Expression Pattern.*** The 897-bp open reading frame of *CRX* is encoded in three exons, an organization conserved in the two most closely related homeobox genes, *OTX1* and *OTX2*.[69,70] There is also an additional 5' exon, containing untranslated sequence that has not yet been defined.[70] The gene encodes a 299-amino-acid homeodomain protein with a predicted molecular weight of 32.3 kDa, although the apparent mass on immunoblots is 39 kDa.[405] *Crx* expression is first detected in the developing mouse retina at E12.5,[154,405] a time at which cone photoreceptors begin to differentiate. Subsequently, the gene is expressed continuously in developing photoreceptors, with maximal expression levels during rod differentiation. *CRX* is also abundantly expressed in the pineal gland, an organ that expresses many genes that encode proteins of the phototransduction pathway.

***Conservation of the CRX Protein.*** The CRX protein is highly conserved between human and mouse (97 percent amino acid identity), and between human and cow (96 percent identity); between all three species, the homeodomain is 100 percent conserved.[69,154,405] The *paired-like* homeodomain of CRX is 88 percent and 86 percent identical to the homeodomains of OTX1 and OTX2, respectively, and 85 percent identical to that of the *Drosophila* orthodenticle protein,[406] which is required for the development of ocelli, light-sensitive organs of the fruit fly. Outside the homeodomain, the overall identity between CRX and OTX1 or OTX2 is low (29 percent and 33 percent, respectively), apart from two short amino acid motifs of unknown function, the 13-amino-acid WSP motif (residues 158 to 170; ATVSIWSPASESP),

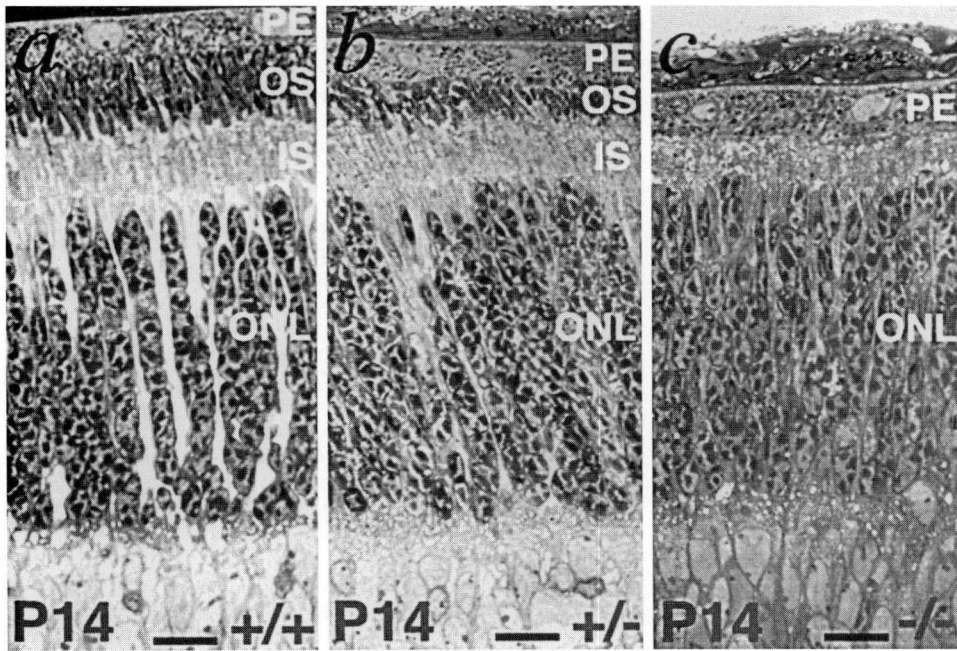

**Fig. 240-22 Histologic sections from *Crx* mutant mice.[394] Retinal sections from mice 14 days after birth (P14) shows that in wild-type mice (*a*), the outer segments appear normal. In heterozygous *Crx*[+/−] mice (*b*), the outer segments are somewhat short, and in the homozygous *Crx* mutant mice (*c*), the outer segments are absent. (*Figure kindly provided by Takahisa Furukawa and Connie Cepko, Harvard Medical School, Cambridge, MA.*)**

and the 12-amino-acid OTX-tail at the C-terminus (residues 284 to 295). CRX has one OTX-tail motif, whereas OTX1 and OTX2 each have two.

***Regulation of Photoreceptor Gene Expression by CRX.*** The CRX protein binds to a consensus sequence (C or T)TAATCC, or a variant, TAATCA, found upstream of several genes encoding proteins of the photoreceptor OS, including rhodopsin, inter-photoreceptor-binding protein (IRBP), the red, green, and blue cone opsins, and arrestin.[154,405] The CRX consensus binding site is, therefore, very similar to the OTX1 and OTX2 consensus site: TAATC(C or T). Mutation analysis identified critical residues for CRX binding in the bovine rhodopsin promoter at the Ret 1 site: GAAGCCAATTAAGCCCCTCGTT; and Ret 4 site: CAGCCGG-GAGCTTAGGGAGGG. The critical residues are underlined and are located at −132 to −127 bp for Ret 1 and at −51 to −46 for Ret 4.[405]

***The Role of CRX in Regulating Photoreceptor Development and Gene Expression.*** Three different approaches have established that the *CRX* gene is required for both the morphogenesis of the OS and for the maintenance of mammalian photoreceptor viability. First, using retroviral gene transfer into differentiating rat photoreceptors, Cepko and colleagues demonstrated that neuro-retinal progenitors carrying a dominant negative *CRX* allele developed into photoreceptors, but that these cells lacked OSs.[154] Second, and correspondingly, mutations in the human *CRX* gene

have been associated with little or no photoreceptor function early in life (i.e., LCA; see the next section).[71,399,400] Furthermore, mutations in the *CRX* gene may also lead to cone-rod dystrophy, indicating that *CRX* is required for the maintenance of both rod and cone photoreceptors.[69–71] Finally, and most directly, although mice carrying gene-targeted *Crx* alleles develop normal numbers of rod and cone photoreceptors (indicating that the gene appears to have no role in cell fate decisions), they fail to form OSs, and manifest photoreceptor degeneration[394] (Fig. 240-22).

The *Crx*[−/−] mice also provided critical insight into the role of the CRX protein in the regulation of photoreceptor gene expression, and unexpectedly, the results were not entirely concordant with the predictions made on the basis of the *in vitro* DNA binding and transcription assays referred to above. Of the promoters activated *in vitro* by CRX, and of those that contain CRX binding elements or Ret1 sites, the expression of rhodopsin, recoverin, the cone opsins, rod transducin, and arrestin are all reduced in the retina of *Crx*[−/−] animals.[394] Unexpectedly, the expression of *IRBP* is normal in the absence of CRX, indicating that *IRBP*, as well as other photoreceptor genes are regulated by other, as yet unknown, transcription factors. A summary of photoreceptor gene expression in *Crx*[−/−] mice is presented in Table 240-8.

***Mutations in the CRX Gene Associated with Cone-Rod Dystrophy and Leber Congenital Amaurosis.*** CRX mutations were found to cosegregate with the disease at 19q13.3 in several

**Table 240-8 The Abundance of Photoreceptor Gene Transcripts in the Retina of Crx[−/−] Mice Compared to Wild-Type Mice at Postnatal Day 10[394]**

| Greatly reduced | Slightly reduced | Up-regulated | Unchanged |
|---|---|---|---|
| rhodopsin | cone transducin | cone cGMP-gated channel | IRBP |
| blue cone opsin | rod PDE-$\beta$ | neuroD | ROM1 |
| red/green cone opsin | cone PDE-$\alpha$ | | rhodopsin kinase |
| rod transducin $\alpha$ | rod cGMP-gated channel | | |
| cone arrestin | rod arrestin | | |
| recoverin | peripherin | | |
| | ABCR | | |

Table kindly provided by Takahisa Furukawa and Connie Cepko, Harvard Medical School, Cambridge, MA

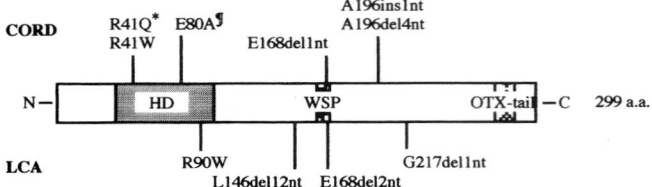

**Fig. 240-23** Mutations in human *CRX* are associated with both CRD and LCA. Mutations in the *CRX* gene presented on a schematic of the CRX protein, including a paired-like homeodomain (HD), a WSP motif, and an OTX-tail. Mutations associated with dominant CRD are shown above the figure; LCA-associated mutations are shown below. The *R41Q mutation has been reported twice. ¶The E80A mutation has been independently identified in two families.

CRD families.[69–71] The *CRX* mutations associated with CRD are summarized in Fig. 240-23. The demonstration that *CRX* mutations lead to a retinal degeneration affecting both rods and cones led to a search for mutations in other photoreceptor disorders.[71,399] LCA was a particularly strong candidate phenotype because mouse photoreceptor cells that expressed the dominant negative CRX protein did not form outer segments or synaptic terminals,[154] defects that would be expected to cause congenital blindness due to a failure to form functional photoreceptors. *CRX* mutations in LCA have been identified by several groups[71,399,400] (Fig. 240-23).

***Similar CRX Mutations in LCA and CRD.*** Inspection of the *CRX* disease-causing alleles shown in Fig. 240-23 reveals that very similar mutations are associated with both the early onset phenotype LCA and the later onset disorder CRD. In both disorders, the mutations fall into two broad groups, missense mutations in highly conserved residues, largely in the homeodomain, and mutations that are predicted to truncate the protein prematurely. The homeodomain substitutions are likely to impair the ability of the mutant CRX protein to bind DNA, a prediction that was confirmed by *in vitro* binding studies for the R41W mutation associated with CRD,[70] and by *in vitro* and *in vivo* studies of DNA binding and transactivation of rhodopsin expression for the R90W mutation associated with LCA.[400]

The premature truncation mutations are all predicted to result in loss of the conserved OTX-tail of CRX (Fig. 240-23), although these mutations may also destabilize the protein. All of the known *CRX* mutations are likely to cause haploinsufficiency, but is also possible that those which allow the synthesis of a stable mutant protein, particularly the missense mutations in the homeodomain, generate dominant negative proteins that still interact with other proteins in the transcription complex, thereby preventing those proteins from participating in effective transcription complexes.[69]

***Similar Retinal Phenotypes in LCA and CRD Due to CRX Mutations.*** To compare the phenotypes resulting from mutations that are likely to have comparable effects on the *CRX* gene, CRD and LCA patients with similar deletions were examined by a single physician.[407] Shared phenotypic features were identified in three members of a family with CRD, who carry the E168Δ1bp mutation, and two individual LCA patients with either the E168Δ2bp or the G217Δ1bp mutation. Initially, all these subjects had central visual loss with malfunction of both rods and cones throughout the retina, but the rate of disease progression differed substantially. The CRD patients noted visual disturbances, including reduced night vision and declining acuity beginning in childhood, progressing over decades to severe central and peripheral vision loss. In contrast, both LCA patients had severe visual abnormalities, including undetectable or subnormal ERGs, within the first year of life. The similar appearance of the fundus of one of the CRD patients and one of the LCA patients is shown in Fig. 240-21. Thus, the common features of disease expression in

these patients reflect their near-identical molecular etiology.[407] The basis of the difference in the rate of disease progression is unclear, but seems likely to be due to the effect of modifier genes. Variable phenotypic expression due to nearly identical mutations is also found with the *PAX6* gene[47] and many other retinal degeneration genes, such as *RDS* (RetNet[404]).

Interestingly, the R90W substitution (Fig. 240-23) associated with recessive LCA manifests a gene dosage effect.[400] The proband had a typical LCA phenotype with severe and nearly complete loss of vision and reduced ERG amplitudes (by 98 percent) from birth, and extensive pigmentary changes in the fundus. Both parents and an older sibling were heterozygous for the R90W mutation, and although they were relatively asymptomatic, the parents had clinical findings consistent with mild CRD, including color vision defects and ERG abnormalities of the cones and macular rods.

***The Pathogenesis of Disease Due to Mutations in the CRX Gene.*** As a major regulator of the expression of many OS transcripts, particularly rhodopsin (Table 240-8), CRX is critical for OS biogenesis and disk renewal. Although the mechanisms by which *CRX* mutations lead to photoreceptor death are unknown, the failure to generate or maintain normal OSs is the basic cellular abnormality. This point is most directly demonstrated by the absence of OSs and the photoreceptor death that occurs in *Crx* gene-targeted mice,[394] phenotypes that are also likely to be found in patients with LCA who are born with little or no photoreceptor function (see "Mutations in the *CRX* Gene Associated with Cone-Rod Dystrophy and Leber Congenital Amaurosis" above). CRD is likely to be due to the failure to maintain the morphogenesis of new disks in the OS per se, or to the reduced expression of one or more of the OS proteins. One major consequence of the loss of *CRX* function is the reduction in the expression of rhodopsin. As shown by mice with only a single functional rhodopsin allele (*Rho*[+/−] mice), reduced rhodopsin expression leads to OS disorganization, shorter OSs, and a reduction in photoreceptor cell number; the photoreceptors of mice with a complete absence of rhodopsin expression die.[408]

***Inheritance Patterns of Disease Due to CRX Mutations.*** In all families identified to date with CRD due to *CRX* mutations, the disease has had a dominant pattern of inheritance.[69–71] In contrast, two modes of inheritance have been identified for LCA due to *CRX* mutations. One recessive LCA pedigree segregated a homozygous mutation in *CRX*, and upon close examination of the heterozygous and apparently unaffected parents, signs of mild CRD were detected.[400] In contrast, a *CRX* mutation was found in a seven-generation pedigree[71] in which LCA is clearly inherited as a dominant trait. In addition, in two small families with single affected members, each proband carried an allele with a *de novo* *CRX* mutation, and the disease is therefore apparently dominant.[399]

**Retinitis Pigmentosa (RP) Associated with a Mutation in the *NRL* Gene.** RP is a clinically and genetically heterogeneous disorder reviewed thoroughly in Chap. 235. The primary phenotypic features include progressive vision loss usually beginning with night blindness and loss of peripheral visual fields, reflecting the degeneration of rod photoreceptors; central vision loss occurs later, as the cones die. A rare cause of autosomal dominant RP results from a failure of photoreceptor maintenance due to a mutation of the *NRL* gene.[409] To date, this mutation is the only known association between *NRL* and disease.

***The Identification of the NRL Gene and Protein.*** The *NRL* gene was initially identified using a subtraction cloning strategy for genes expressed specifically in the retina.[158] The 681-bp open reading frame of the *NRL* gene encodes a 237-amino-acid transcription factor with a basic motif/leucine zipper domain (see Fig. 240-24). The protein is similar to that of the Jun and Fos

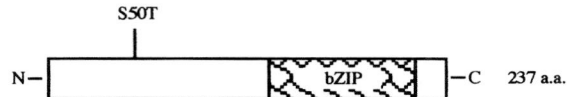

**Fig. 240-24** A mutation in *NRL* is associated with autosomal dominant retinitis pigmentosa. The mutation in the *NRL* gene is presented on a schematic of the NRL protein, including the basic leucine zipper (bZIP). The only identified mutation in *NRL* is in an RP patient.[409]

oncoprotein family, with particularly strong resemblance to v-maf protein, an avian retroviral oncoprotein.[158] Like these relatives, NRL is able to form homo- and heterodimers, and binds to an AP1-like DNA sequence.[410] The basic motif and leucine zipper of NRL in the C-terminal third, place NRL in the bZIP protein family. The N-terminal third of NRL contains a proline-serine-rich region that is the putative transactivation domain. The protein is highly conserved between human and mouse with 90 percent overall amino acid identity. The amino acid sequences of the proline-serine-rich domain, the basic motif, and leucine zipper domain are identical in human and mouse.[411] The *NRL* gene maps to human chromosome 14q11.1-q11.2[412] and to chromosome 14 in the mouse.[257]

***NRL Gene Structure and Expression Pattern.*** The *NRL* gene is organized into three exons and the ORF is contained entirely within the second and third exons. There are three transcripts (2.7 kb, 2.0 kb, and 1.3 kb) expressed from this gene, with differing polyadenylation sites.[411,413] The earliest developmental expression of *Nrl* in the mouse retina is detected at E13.5,[159] and coincides with the cells becoming postmitotic. *Nrl* is also expressed throughout the embryonic nervous system in a pattern suggesting that it is present only in postmitotic neurons. Postnatally, *Nrl* expression in the brain and spinal cord diminishes, but it remains strong in all three layers of the adult retina.

***Regulation of Photoreceptor Gene Expression by NRL.*** Proteins of the bZIP family can bind to DNA as heterodimers or homodimers. Studies of NRL show that it can bind to variants of the AP-1 site, and can heterodimerize with Fos or Jun *in vitro*.[410,414] NRL homodimers bind a palindromic sequence $TGC(N)_{6-7}GCA$ called the NRE (NRL responsive element).[415] The human rhodopsin promoter contains a variant NRE,[416] and NRL is a component of the protein complex that binds to this site.[417] *In vitro*, NRL is able to regulate expression of reporter genes from plasmids that contain the NRE. The NRE and one of the CRX binding sites (Ret 4) are adjacent to one another in the rhodopsin promoters of human, mouse, and bovine, and NRL and CRX act synergistically in activating the expression of rhodopsin: coexpression of NRL and CRX activates expression 115-fold from a construct bearing the rhodopsin promoter.[405] Discovery of this interaction is an important step in defining the network of transcription factors that regulate photoreceptor gene maintenance.

***A Human Mutation in NRL Causes Autosomal Dominant RP (adRP).*** As a transcription factor highly expressed in the adult retina, the *NRL* gene has been extensively examined for mutations in patients with photoreceptor diseases including adRP, autosomal recessive RP and LCA. An initial survey of the *NRL* gene and rhodopsin NRE in 53 patients revealed only a nonpathogenic polymorphic C to T nucleotide change in the 5′ upstream region of the *NRL* gene of a patient with adRP.[418] Subsequently, *NRL* was suggested as a candidate gene for adRP when full genome linkage analysis of a large pedigree discovered linkage at 14q11.

Sequencing *NRL* from affected members of this family showed a TCA to ACA codon change that replaced a serine with a threonine at position 50 (S50T) of the protein[409] (see Fig. 240-23). This residue falls within the conserved transactivation domain in exon 2 and is a serine in all Maf proteins that contain a

transactivation domain. Unexpectedly, the mutant protein alone has increased ability to activate expression from the rhodopsin promoter and in assays that included CRX as a synergistic activator, tenfold less NRL was required for half-maximal activation, although at saturating amounts of NRL, the level of transactivation was the same for either the wild-type or mutant NRL. The pathogenic mechanism of this missense substitution may arise from overexpression of OS proteins, particularly rhodopsin.[409] This hypothesis is supported by the fact that overexpression of rhodopsin in animal models causes photoreceptor cell death.[419] The widespread expression of *Nrl* in early mouse embryonic stages suggests that a null mutation of human *NRL* may be embryonic lethal.

## THE FUTURE OF EYE DEVELOPMENT RESEARCH

Elucidation of the regulatory mechanisms that underlie mammalian eye and retinal development will be a demanding task. However, the human and mouse genome projects, together with knowledge of eye development in other organisms, including flies,[43,420,421] will ultimately make it possible to understand how the eye is made and maintained. For example, the increasing number of targeted genes in mice is likely to be highly informative about eye development, yet this is a vastly underutilized resource: of the 72 transcription factors presently known to be expressed in the mammalian eye, mouse mutants (targeted alleles or spontaneous mutations) exist for 36, yet the eye was apparently not examined in 11 of these animals.[422] In the coming years, the main goals of basic and applied research in eye development will be (a) to identify all of the regulatory molecules that control human eye formation and to determine their relationship to genetic eye diseases, (b) to understand the function of these molecules, as well as the relationships between them (i.e., which gene controls what other genes, and when), and (c) with respect to the retina in particular, to identify and characterize the retinal stem cells and progenitor cells which give rise the mature retina.

In the long-term, the medical benefits of this work will be enormous. First, it will be possible to make specific molecular diagnoses in many patients with congenital eye defects, and to provide their families with accurate genetic counseling. Second, and in the longer term, it may be possible to prevent the retinal cell death associated with genes such as *CRX* and *NRL*, which are necessary for photoreceptor maintenance; this aim should be achievable using gene therapy or pharmacologic approaches. Finally, knowledge of stem cells and progenitor cells, again particularly of the retina, but also in the cornea, is likely to make feasible the replacement of damaged tissue.

## REFERENCES

1. Taylor D: *Pediatric Opthalmology*, 2nd ed. Cambridge, MA, Blackwell Scientific Publications, 1997.
2. Williamson WD, Desmond MM, Andrew LP, Hicks RN: Visually impaired infants in the 1980s. A survey of etiologic factors and additional handicapping conditions in a school population. *Clin Pediatr* **26**:241, 1987.
3. Robinson GC, Jan JE, Kinnis C: Congenital ocular blindness in children, 1945 to 1984. *Am J Dis Child* **141**:1321, 1987.
4. Costa T, Scriver CR, Childs B: The effect of Mendelian disease on human health: A measurement. *Am J Med Genet* **21**:231, 1985.
5. Freund C, Horsford DJ, McInnes RR: Transcription factor genes and the developing eye: A genetic perspective. *Hum Mol Genet* **5**:1471, 1996.
6. van Heyningen V: Developmental eye disease—a genome era paradigm. *Clin Genet* **54**:272, 1998.
7. Engelkamp D, van Heyningen V: Transcription factors in disease. *Curr Opin Dev Biol* **6**:334, 1996.
8. Semenza GL: *Transcription Factors and Human Disease*. New York, Oxford University Press, 1998.
9. O'Rahily R: The timing and sequence of events in the development of the human endocrine system during the embryonic period proper. *Anat Embryol (Berl)* **166**:439, 1983.

10. O'Rahily R, Muller F: *Developmental stages in human embryos.* Washington, DC, Carnegie Institution, 1987.

11. Pei YF, Rhodin JA: The prenatal development of the mouse eye. *Anat Rec* **168**:105, 1970.

12. Kaufman M: *The Atlas of Mouse Development.* Toronto, Harcourt Brace Jovanovich, 1992.

13. Cepko C, Austin C, Yang X, Alexiades M, Ezzeddine D: Cell fate determination in the vertebrate retina. *Proc Natl Acad Sci U S A* **93**:589, 1996.

14. Tomarev SI: *Pax-6, eyes absent,* and *Prox 1* in eye development. *Int J Dev Biol* **41**:835, 1997.

15. Mathers PH, Grinberg A, Mahon KA, Jamrich M: The *Rx* homeobox gene is essential for vertebrate eye development. *Nature* **387**:603, 1997.

16. Nishiguchi S, Wood H, Kondoh H, Lovell-Badge R, Episkopou V: *Sox1* directly regulates the?γ-crystallin genes and is essential for lens development in mice. *Genes Dev* **12**:776, 1998.

17. Zygar CA, Cook TL, Grainger RMJ: Gene activation during early stages of lens induction in *Xenopus. Development* **125**:3509, 1998.

18. Xu XP, Zhang Z, Heaney S, Yoon A, Michelson AM, Maas RL: Regulation of *PAX6* expression is conserved between mice and flies. *Development* **126**:383, 1999.

19. Quiring R, Walldorf U, Kloter U, Gehring WJ: Homology of the *eyeless* gene of *Drosophila* to the *small eye* gene in mice and aniridia in humans. *Science* **265**:785, 1994.

20. Xu P-X, Woo I, Beier DR, Maas RL: Mouse *Eya* homologues of the *Drosophila eyes absent* gene require *Pax6* for expression in lens and nasal placoDE. *Development* **124**:219, 1997.

21. Fu W, Noll M: The *Pax2* homolog sparkling is required for development of cone and pigment cells in the *Drosophila* eye. *Genes Dev* **11**:2066, 1997.

22. Toy J, Yang JM, Leppert GS, Sundin OH: The *optx2* homeobox gene is expressed in early precursors of the eye and activates retina-specific genes. *Proc Natl Acad Sci U S A* **95**:10643, 1998.

23. Johnston MC, Noden DM, Hazelton RD, Coulombre JL, Coulombre AJ: Origins of avian ocular and periocular tissues. *Exp Eye Res* **29**:27, 1979.

24. Bron AJ, Tripathi RC, Tripathi BJ: *Wolff's Anatomy of the Eye and Orbit.* London, Chapman and Hall, 1997.

25. Harris WA, Perron M: Molecular recapitulation: The growth of the vertebrate retina. *Int J Dev Biol* **42**:299, 1998.

26. Cepko CL: The roles of intrinsic and extrinsic cues and bHLH genes in the determination of retinal cell fates. *Curr Opin Neurobiol* **9**:37, 1999.

27. Young R: Cell differentiation in the retina of the mouse. *Anat Rec* **212**:199, 1985.

28. Belliveau MJ, Cepko CL: Extrinsic and intrinsic factors control the genesis of amacrine and cone cells in the rat retina. *Development* **126**:555, 1999.

29. Nilsson DE: Eye ancestry: Old genes for new eyes. *Curr Biol* **6**:39, 1996.

30. Harris WA: Pax-6: Where to be conserved is not conservative. *Proc Natl Acad Sci U S A* **94**:2098, 1997.

31. Salvini-Plawen L, Mayr E: *On the Evolution of Photoreceptors and Eyes.* New York, Plenum, 1977.

32. Dawkins R: *Climbing Mount Improbable.* London, Viking, 1996.

33. Bonini NM, Bui QT, Gray-Board GL, Warrick J: The *Drosophila eyes absent* gene directs ectopic eye formation in a pathway conserved between flies and vertebrates. *Development* **124**:4819, 1997.

34. Oliver G, Mailhos A, Wehr R, Copeland NG, Jenkins R, Gruss P: *Six3,* a murine homolgue of the *sine oculis* gene, demarcates the most anterior border of the developing neural plate and is expressed during eye development. *Development* **121**:4045, 1995.

35. Callaerts P, Halder G, Gehring WJ: *PAX-6* in development and evolution. *Annu Rev Neurosci* **20**:483, 1997.

36. Desplan C: Eye development: Governed by a dictator or a junta? *Cell* **91**:861, 1997.

37. Holland PW: The future of evolutionary developmental biology. *Nature* **402**:C41, 1999.

38. Gilbert S: *Developmental Biology.* Sunderland, MA, Sinauer Associates, 1997.

39. Wolpert L: *Principles of Development.* New York, Oxford University Press, 1998.

40. Sauer F, Jackle H: Dimerization and the control of transcription by Kruppel. *Nature* **364**:454, 1993.

41. Biesecker LG: Strike three for *GLI3. Nat Genet* **17**:259, 1997.

42. Aza-Blanc P, Kornberg TB: Ci: A complex transducer of the hedgehog signal. *Trends Genet* **15**:458, 1999.

43. Banfi S, Borsani G, Bulfone A, Ballabio A: *Drosophila*-related expressed sequences. *Hum Mol Genet* **6**:1745, 1997.

44. Hammond KL, Hanson IM, Brown AG, Lettice LA, Hill RE: Mammalian and *Drosophila dachshund* genes are related to the *Ski* proto-oncogene and are expressed in eye and limb. *Mech Dev* **74**:121, 1998.

45. Hartwell LH, Hopfield JJ, Leibler S, Murray AW: From molecular to modular cell biology. *Nature* **402**:C47, 1999.

46. Hanson I, van Heyningen V: *Pax6:* More than meets the eye. *Trends Genet* **11**:268, 1995.

47. Prosser J, van Heyningen V: *PAX6* mutations reviewed. *Hum Mutat* **11**:93, 1998.

48. Kawakami K, Ohto H, Takizawa T, Saito T: Identification and expression of *six* family genes in mouse retina. *FEBS Lett* **393**:259, 1996.

49. Oliver G, Sosa-Pineda B, Geisendorf S, Spana EP, Doe CQ, Gruss P: *Prox 1,* a prospero-related homeobox gene expressed during mouse development. *Mech Dev* **44**:3, 1993.

50. Zimmerman JE, Bui QT, Steingrimsson E, Nagle DL, Fu W, Genin A, Spinner RB, et al: Cloning and characterization of two vertebrate homologs of the *Drosophila eyes absent* gene. *Genome Res* **7**:128, 1997.

51. Eggert T, Hauck B, Hildebrandt R, Gehring WJ, Walldorf U: Isolation of a Drosophila homolog of the vertebrate homeobox gene Rx and its possible role in brain and eye development. *Proc Natl Acad Sci U S A* **95**:2343, 1998.

52. Boucher CA, Carey R, Edwards YH, Siciliano MJ, Johnson KJ: Cloning of the human *SIX1* gene and its assignment to chromosome 14. *Genomics* **33**:140, 1996.

53. Heath SK, Carne S, Hoyle C, Johnson KJ, Wells DJ: Characterisation of expression of *mDMAHP,* a homeodomain-encoding gene at the murine DM locus. *Hum Mol Genet* **6**:651, 1997.

54. Duncan MK, Kos L, Jenkins RA, Gilbert DJ, Copeland RG, Tomarev SI: Eyes absent: A gene family found in several metazoan phyla [Published erratum appears in *Mamm Genome* 1997;8(11):877]. *Mamm Genome* **8**:479, 1997.

55. Pignoni F, Hu B, Zavitz KH, Xiao J, Garrity PA, Zipursky SL: The eye-specification proteins so and eya form a complex and regualte multiple steps in *Drosophila* eye development. *Cell* **91**:881, 1997.

56. Chen R, Amoui M, Zhang Z, Mardon G: Dachshund and eyes absent proteins form a complex and function synergistically to induce ectopic eye development in *Drosophila. Cell* **91**:893, 1997.

57. Yuh CH, Moore JG, Davidson EH: Quantitative functional interrelations within the cis-regulatory system of the *S. purpuratus Endo16* gene. *Development* **122**:4045, 1996.

58. Kirchhamer CV, Davidson EH: Spatial and temporal information processing in the sea urchin embryo: Modular and intramodular organization of the *CyIIIa* gene *cis*-regulatory system. *Development* **122**:333, 1996.

59. Roush W: "Smart" genes use many cues to set cell fate. *Science* **272**:652, 1996.

60. Awgulewitsch A, Utset MF, Hart CP, McGinnis W, Ruddle FH: Spatial restriction in expression of a mouse homeo box locus within the central nervous system. *Nature* **320**:328, 1986.

61. Duboule D: *Guidebook to the Homeobox Genes.* Toronto, Oxford University Press, 1994.

62. Hunt P, Krumlauf R: Deciphering the Hox code: Clues to patterning branchial regions of the head. *Cell* **66**:1075, 1991.

63. Kessel M, Gruss P: Homeotic transformations of murine vertebrae and concomitant alteration of Hox codes induced by retinoic acid. *Cell* **67**:89, 1991.

64. Blau HM: Differentiation requires continuous active control. *Ann Rev Bioch* **61**:1213, 1992.

65. Dahmane R, Lee J, Robins P, Heller P, Ruiz I, Altaba A: Activation of the transcription factor Gli1 and the Sonic hedgehog signalling pathway in skin tumours [Published erratum appears in *Nature* 390(6659):536, 1997]. *Nature* **389**:876, 1997.

66. Stoykova A, Gruss P: Roles of *Pax*-genes in developing and adult brain as suggested by expression patterns. *J Neurosci* **14**:1395, 1994.

67. Burmeister M, Novak J, Liang M-Y, Basu S, Ploder L, Hawes RO, Vidgen D, et al: *Ocular retardation* mouse caused by *Chx10* homeobox null allele: Impaired retinal progenitor proliferation and bipolar cell differentiation. *Nat Genet* **12**:376, 1996.

68. Hanson I, van Heyningen V: Unpublished data.

69. Freund CL, Gregory-Evans CY, Furukawa T, Papaioannou M, Looser J, Ploder L, Bellingham J, et al: Cone-rod dystrophy due to mutations in a novel photoreceptor-specific homeobox gene (CRX) essential for maintenance of the photoreceptor. *Cell* **91**:543, 1997.

70. Swain PK, Chen S, Wang QL, Affatigato LM, Coats CL, Brady KD, Fishman GA, et al: Mutations in the cone-rod homeobox gene are associated with the cone-rod dystrophy photoreceptor degeneration. *Neuron* **19**:1329, 1997.

71. Sohocki MM, Sullivan LS, Mintz-Hittner HA, Birch D, Heckenlively JR, Freund CL, McInnes RR, et al: A range of clinical phenotypes associated with mutations in CRX, a photoreceptor transcription factor gene. *Am J Hum Genet* **63**:1307, 1998.

72. Franz T, Besecke A: The development of the eye in homozygotes of the mouse mutant *extra-toes. Anat Embryol* **184**:355, 1991.

73. Hui CC, Joyner AL: A mouse model of Greig cephalopolysyndactyly syndrome: The *extra-toes^J* mutation contains an intragenic deletion of the *Gli3* gene. *Nat Genet* **3**:241, 1993.

74. Ruppert J, Vogelstein B, Arheden K, Kinzler K: *GLI3* encodes a 190-kilodalton protein with multiple regions of GLI similarity. *Mol Cell Biol* **10**:5408, 1990.

75. Tomita K, Ishibashi M, Nakahara K, Ang-S, Nakanishi S, Guillemot F, Kageyama R: Mammalian *hairy* and enhancer of *Split homolog 1* regulates differentiation of retinal neurons and is essential for eye morphogenesis. *Neuron* **16**:723, 1996.

76. Feder JN, Li L, Jan LY, Jan YN: Genomic cloning and chromosomal localization of *HRY*, the human homolog to the *Drosophila* segmentation gene, hairy. *Genomics* **20**:56, 1994.

77. Xuan S, Baptista C, Balas G, Tao W, Soares V, Lai E: Winged helix trancription factor BF-1 is essential for the development of the cerebral hemispheres. *Neuron* **14**:1141, 1995.

78. Kastury K, Li J, Druck T, Su H, Vogt PK, Croce CM, Huebner K: The human homologue of the retroviral oncogene *qin* maps to chromosome 14q13. *Proc Natl Acad Sci U S A* **91**:3616, 1994.

79. Huh S, Hatini V, Marcus RC, Li SC, Lai E: Dorsal-ventral patterning defects in the eye of BF-1-deficient mice associated with a restricted loss of *shh* expression. *Dev Biol* **211**:53, 1999.

80. Porter FD, Drago J, Xu Y, Cheema SS, Wassif C, Huang S-P, LeeE, et al: *Lhx2*, a LIM homeobox gene, is required for eye, forebrain, and definitive erythrocyte development. *Development* **124**:2935, 1997.

81. Tomita K, Nakanishi S, Guillemot F, Kageyama R: *Mash1* promotes neuronal differentiation in the retina. *Genes Cells* **1**:765, 1996.

82. Renault B, Lieman J, Ward D, Krauter K, Kucherlapati R: Localization of the human achaete-scute homolog gene (ASCL1) distal to phenylalanine hydroxylase (PAH) and proximal to tumor rejection antigen (TRA1) on chromosome 12q22-q23. *Genomics* **30**:81, 1995.

83. Twells R, Weiming X, Ball D, Allotey R, Williamson R, Chamberlain S: Exclusion of the neuronal *nitric oxide synthase* gene and the human *achaete-scute homologue 1* gene as candidate loci for spinal cerebellar ataxia. *Am J Hum Genet* **56**:336, 1995.

84. Morrow EM, Furukawa T, Lee JE, Cepko CL: *Neuro D* regulates multiple functions in the developing neural retina in rodent. *Development* **126**:23, 1999.

85. Tamimi R, Steingrimsson E, Copeland RG, Dyer-Montgomery K, Lee JE, Hernandez R, Jenkins RA, et al: The *NEUROD* gene maps to human chromosome 2q32 and mouse chromosome 2. *Genomics* **34**:418, 1996.

86. Acampora D, Mazan S, Avantaggiato V, Barone P, Tuorto F, Lallemand Y, Brulet P, et al: Epilepsy and brain abnormalities in mice lacking the *Otx1* gene. *Nat Genet* **14**:218, 1996.

87. Kastury K, Druck T, Huebner K, Barletta C, Acampora D, Simeone A, Faiella A, et al: Chromosome locations of human *EMX* and *OTX* genes. *Genomics* **22**:41, 1994.

88. Ang SL, Jin O, Rhinn M, Daigle R, Stevenson L, Rossant J: A targeted mouse *Otx2* mutation leads to severe defects in gastrulation and formation of axial mesoderm and to deletion of rostral brain. *Development* **122**:243, 1996.

89. Matsuo I, Kuratani S, Kimura C, Takeda R, Aizawa S: Mouse *Otx2* functions in the formation and patterning of rostral head. *Genes Dev* **9**:2646, 1995.

90. Acampora D, Mazan S, Lallemand Y, Avantaggiato V, Maury M, Simeone A, Brulet P: Forebrain and midbrain regions are deleted in *Otx2^{-/-}* mutants due to a defective anterior neuroectoderm specification during gastrulation. *Development* **121**:3279, 1995.

91. Xiang M, Zhou L, Peng Y, Byers M, Eddy R, Shows T, Nathans J: The gene for Brn-3b: A POU domain protein in retinal ganglion cells is assigned to the q31.2 region of chromosome 4 [Abstract]. *Human Genome Mapping Workshop 93*:7, 1993.

92. Gan L, Xiang M, Zhou L, Wagner DS, Klein WH, Nathans J: POU domain factor Brn-3b is required for the development of a large set of retinal ganglion cells. *Proc Natl Acad Sci U S A* **93**:3920, 1996.

93. Erkman L, McEvilly RJ, Luo L, Ryan AK, Hooshmand F, O'Connell SM, Keithley EM, et al: Role of transcription factors Brn-3.1 and Brn-3.2 in auditory and visual system development. *Nature* **381**:603, 1996.

94. Xiang M: Requirement for Brn3b in early differentiation of postmitotic retinal ganglion cell precursors. *Dev Biol* **197**:155, 1998.

95. Wigle JT, Chowdhury K, Gruss P, Oliver G: *Prox1* function is crucial for mouse lens-fibre elongation. *Nat Genet* **21**:318, 1999.

96. Zinovieva RD, Duncan MK, Johnson TR., Torres R, Polymeropoulos MH, Tomarev SI: Structure and chromosomal localization of the human homeobox gene *Prox 1. Genomics* **35**:517, 1996.

97. Takihara Y, Tomotsune D, Shirai M, Katoh-Fukui Y, Nishii K, Motaleb MA, Nomura M, et al: Targeted disruption of the mouse homologue of the *Drosophila polyhomeotic* gene leads to altered anteroposterior patterning and neural crest defects. *Development* **124**:3673, 1997.

98. Kastner P, Mark M, Chambon P: Nonsteroid nuclear receptors: What are genetic studies telling us about their role in real life? *Cell* **83**:859, 1995.

99. Lohnes D, Mark M, Mendelsohn C, Dolle P, Dierich A, Gorry P, Gansmuller A, et al: Function of the retinoic acid receptors (RARs) during development (I) Craniofacial and skeletal abnormalities in RAR double mutants. *Development* **120**:2723, 1994.

100. Mendelsohn C, Lohnes D, Decimo D, Lufkin T, LeMeur M, Chambon P, Mark M: Function of the retinoic acid receptors (RARs) during development (II). Multiple abnormalities at various stages of organogenesis in RAR double mutants. *Development* **120**:2749, 1994.

101. Kastner P, Grondona JM, Mark M, Gansmuller A, LeMeur M, Decino D, Vonesch J-L, et al: Genetic analysis of RXRα developmental function: Convergence of RXR and RAR signaling pathways in heart and eye morphogenesis. *Cell* **78**:987, 1994.

102. Ghyselinck RB, Dupe V, Dierick A, Messaddeq R, Garnier J-M, Rochette-Egly C, Chambon P, et al: Role of the retinoic acid receptor beta (RARβ) during mouse development. *Int J Dev Biol* **41**:425, 1997.

103. Grondona JM, Kastner P, Gansmuller A, Decimo D, Chambon P, Mark M: Retinal dysplasia and degeneration in RARβ2/RARγ2 compound mutant mice. *Development* **122**:2173, 1996.

104. Hallonet M, Hollemann T, Pieler T, Gruss P: *Vax1*, a novel homeobox-containing gene, directs development of the basal forebrain and visual system. *Genes Dev* **13**:3106, 1999.

105. Barbieri AM, Lupo G, Bulfone A, Andreazzoli M, Mariani M, Fougerousse F, Consalez GG, et al: A homeobox gene, *vax2*, controls the patterning of the eye dorsoventral axis. *Proc Natl Acad Sci U S A* **96**:10729, 1999.

106. Furukawa T, Kozak CA Cepko CL: *Rax*, a novel paired-type homeobox gene, shows expression in the anterior neural fold and developing retina. *Proc Natl Acad Sci U S A* **94**:3088, 1997.

107. Xu Y, Baldassare M, Fisher P, Rathbun G, Oltz EM, Yancopoulos GD, Jessell TM, et al: *LH-2*: A LIM/homeodomain gene expressed in developing lymphocytes and neural cells. *Proc Natl Acad Sci U S A* **90**:227, 1993.

108. Chalepakis G, Stoykova A, Wijnholds J, Tremblay P, Gruss P: Pax: Gene regulators in the developing nervous system. *J Neurobiol* **24**:1367, 1993.

109. Walther C, Gruss P: *Pax-6*, a murine paired-box gene, is expressed in the developing CNS. *Development* **113**:1435, 1991.

110. Grindley JC, Davidson DR, Hill RE: The role of *Pax-6* in eye and nasal development. *Development* **121**:1433, 1995.

111. Koromo BM, Yang J-M, Sundin OH: The *Pax-6* homeobox gene is expressed throughout the corneal and conjunctival epithelia. *Invest Ophthalmol Vis Sci* **38**:108, 1997.

112. Dolle P, Ruberte E, Leroy P, Morriss-Kay G, Chambon P: Retinoic acid receptors and cellular retinoid binding proteins. *Development* **110**:1133, 1990.

113. Ruberte E, Dolle P, Krust A, Zelent A, Morriss-Kay G, Chambon P: Specific spatial and temporal distribution of retinoic acid receptor gamma transcripts during mouse embryogenesis. *Development* **108**:213, 1990.

114. Jonk L, de Jonge M, Pals C, Wissink S, Vervaart J, Schoorlemmer J, Kruijer W: Cloning and expression during development of three murine members of the COUP family of nuclear orphan receptors. *Mech Dev* **47**:81, 1994.

115. Hallonet M, Hollemann T, Wehr R, Jenkins RA, Copeland RG, Pieler T, Gruss P: *Vax1* is a novel homeobox-containing gene expressed in the developing anterior ventral forebrain. *Development* **125**:2599, 1998.

116. Hodgkinson CA, Moore KJ, Nakayama A, Steingrinsson E, Copeland RG, Jenkins RA, Arnheiter H: Mutations at the mouse *microphthalmia* locus are associated with defects in a gene encoding a novel basic-helix-loop-helix-zipper protein. *Cell* **74**:395, 1993.

117. Nakayama A, Nguyen M-TT, Chen CC, Opdecamp K, Hodgkinson CA, Arnheiter H: Mutations in *microphthalmia*, the mouse homolog of the human deafness gene *MITF*, affect neuroepithelial and neural crest-derived melanocytes differently. *Mech Dev* **70**:155, 1998.

118. Bora R, Conway SJ, Liang H, Smith SB: Transient overexpression of the *Microphthalmia* gene in the eyes of *microphthalmia vitiligo* mutant mice. *Dev Dyn* **213**:283, 1998.

119. Monaghan AP, Grau E, Bock D, Schutz G: The mouse homolog of the orphan nuclear receptor *tailless* is expressed in the developing forebrain. *Development* **121**:839, 1995.

120. Nornes H, Dressler G, Knapik E, Deutsch U, Gruss P: Spatially and temporally restricted expression of *Pax2* during mouse neurogenesis. *Development* **109**:797, 1990.

121. Puschel AW, Westerfield M, Dressler GR: Comparative analysis of *Pax-2* protein distributions during neurulation in mice and zebra fish. *Mech Dev* **38**:197, 1992.

122. Rowitch D, McMahon A: *Pax-2* expression in the murine neural plate precedes and encompasses the expression domains of *Wnt-1* and *En-1*. *Mech Dev* **52**:3, 1995.

123. Monaghan A, Davidson D, Sime C, Graham E, Baldock R, Bhattacharya S, Hill R: The *Msh*-like homeobox genes define domains in the developing vertebrate eye. *Development* **112**:1053, 1991.

124. Liu ISC, Chen J, Ploder L, Vidgen D, van der Kooy D, Kalnins VI, McInnes RR: Developmental expression of a novel murine homeobox gene (*Chx10*): Evidence for roles in determination of the neuroretina and inner nuclear layer. *Neuron* **13**:377, 1994.

125. Takebayashi K, Takahashi S, Nakanishi S, Asashima M, Kageyama R: Conversion of ectoderm into a neural fate by *ATH-3*, a vertebrate basic helix-loop-helix gene homolgous to *Drosophila* proneural gene *atonal*. *EMBO J* **16**:384, 1997.

126. Tsuda H, Takebayashi K, Nakanishi S, Kageyama R: Structure and promoter analysis of *Math3* gene, a mouse homolog of *Drosophila* proneural gene *atonal*. *J Biol Chem* **11**:6327, 1998.

127. Guillemot FJA: Dynamic expression of the murine Achaete-Scute homologue *Mash-1* in the developing nervous system. *Mech Dev* **42**:171, 1993.

128. Bulfone A, Puelles L, Porteus M, Frohman M, Martin G, Rubenstein J: Spatially restricted expression of *Dlx-1*, *Dlx-2* (*Tes-1*), *Gbx-2*, and *Wnt-3* in the embryonic day 12.5 mouse forebrain defines potential transverse and longitudinal segmental boundaries. *J Neurosci* **13**:3155, 1993.

129. Hatini V, Tao W, Lai E: Expression of winged helix genes, *BF-1* and *BF-2*, define adjacent domains within the developing forebrain and retina. *J Neurobiol* **25**:1293, 1994.

130. Hui CC, Slusarski D, Platt KA, Holmgren R, Joyner AL: Expression of three mouse homologs of the *Drosophila* segment polarity gene *cubitus interruptus*, *Gli*, *Gli-2*, and *Gli-3*, in ectoderm- and mesoderm-derived tissues suggests multiple roles during postimplantation development. *Dev Biol* **162**:402, 1994.

131. Kamachi Y, Sockanathan S, Liu Q, Breitman M, Lovell-Badge R, Kondoh H: Involvement of SOX proteins in lens-specific activation of crystallin genes. *EMBO J* **14**:3510, 1995.

132. Kamachi Y, Uchikawa M, Collignon J, Lovell-Badge R, Kondoh H: Involvement of Sox1, 2 and 3 in the early and subsequent molecular events of lens induction. *Development* **125**:2521, 1998.

133. Caubit X, Thangarajah R, Theil T, Wirth J, Nothwang HG, Ruther U, Krauss S: Mouse Dac, a novel nuclear factor with homology to *Drosophila* dachshund shows a dynamic expression in the neural crest, the eye, the neocortex, and the limb bud. *Dev Dyn* **214**:66, 1999.

134. Sefton M, Sanchez S, Nieto MA: Conserved and divergent roles for members of the *Snail* family of transcription factors in the chick and mouse embryo. *Development* **125**:3111, 1998.

135. Lu X, Salbert G, Pfahl M: An evolutionary conserved COUP-TF binding element in a neural-specific gene and *COUP-TF* expression patterns support a major role for COUP-TF in neural development. *Mol. Endocrinol.* **8**:1774, 1994.

136. Qiu Y, Cooney A, Kuratani S, DeMayo F, Tsai S, Tsai M-J: Spatiotemporal expression patterns of chicken ovalbumin upstream promoter-transcription factors in the developing mouse central nervous system: Evidence for a role in segmental patterning of the diencephalon. *Proc Natl Acad Sci U S A* **91**:4451, 1994.

137. Simeone A, Acampora D, Gulisano M, Stornaiuolo A, Boncinelli E: Nested expression domains of four homeobox genes in developing rostral brain. *Nature* **358**:687, 1992.

138. Simeone A, Acampora D, Mallamaci A, Stornaiuolo A, D'Apice MR, Nigro V, Boncinelli E: A vertebrate gene related to *orthodenticle* contains a homeodomain of the bicoid class and demarcates anterior neuroectoderm in the gastrulating mouse embryo. *EMBO J* **12**:2735, 1993.

139. Semina E, V, Reiter RS, Murray JC: Isolation of a new homeobox gene belonging to the *Pitx/Rieg* family: Expression during lens development and mapping to the *aphakia* region on mouse chromosome 19. *Hum Mol Genet* **6**:2109, 1997.

140. Semina EV, Ferell RE, Mintz-Hittner HA, Bitoun P, Alward WL, Reiter RS, Funkhauser C, et al: A novel homeobox gene *PITX3* is mutated in families with autosomal dominant cataracts and ASMD. *Nat Genet* **19**:167, 1998.

141. Zhou H, Yoshioka T, Nathans J: Retina-derived POU-domain factor-1: A complex POU-domain gene implicated in the development of retinal ganglion and amacrine cells. *J Neurosci* **16**:2261, 1996.

142. Lee JE, Hollenberg SM, Snider L, Turner DL, Lipnick R, Weintraub H: Conversion of *Xenopus* ectoderm into neurons by NeuroD, a basic helix-loop-helix protein. *Science* **268**:836, 1995.

143. Dolle P, Price M, Duboule D: Expression of the murine *Dlx-1* homeobox gene during facial, ocular and limb development. *Differentiation* **49**:93, 1992.

144. Bober E, Baum C, Braun T, Hans-Henning A: A novel NK-related mouse homeobox gene: Expression in central and peripheral nervous structures during embryonic development. *Dev Biol* **162**:288, 1994.

145. Wang W, van de Water T, Lufkin T: Inner ear and maternal reproductive defects in mice lakcing the Hmx3 homeobox gene. *Development* **125**:621, 1998.

146. Bourgeois P, Bolcato-Bellemin A-L, Danse J-M, Blocj-Zupan A, Yoshiba K, Stoetzel C, Perrin-Schmitt F: The variable expressivity and incomplete penetrance of the *twist*-null heterozygous mouse phenotype resemble those of human Saethre-Chotzen syndrome. *Hum Mol Genet* **7**:945, 1998.

147. Kume T, Deng KY, Winfrey V, Gould DB, Walter MA, Hogan BL: The forkhead/winged helix gene *Mf1* is disrupted in the pleiotropic mouse mutation congenital hydrocephalus. *Cell* **93**:985, 1998.

148. Gradwohl G, Fode C, Guillemot F: Restricted expression of a novel murine *atonal*-related bHLH protein in undifferentiated neural precursors. *Dev Biol* **180**:227, 1996.

149. Gage PJ, Camper SA: Pituitary homeobox 2, a novel member of the bicoid-related family of homeobox genes, is a potential regulator of anterior structure formation. *Hum Mol Genet* **6**:457, 1997.

150. Chow L, Levine EM, Reh TA: The nuclear receptor transcription factor, retinoid-related orphan receptor beta, regulates retinal progenitor proliferation. *Mech Dev* **77**:149, 1998.

151. Brown RL, Kanekar S, Vetter ML, Tucker PK, Gemza DL, Glaser T: Math5 encodes a murine basic helix-loop-helix transcription factor expressed during early stages of retinal neurogenesis. *Development* **125**:4821, 1998.

152. Begley CG, Lipkowitz S, Gobel V, Mahon KA, Bertness V, Green AR, Gough NM, et al: Molecular characterization of *NSCL*, a gene encoding a helix-loop-helix protein expressed in the developing nervous system. *Proc Natl Acad Sci U S A* **89**:38, 1992.

153. Valerius M, Li H, Stock J, Weinstein M, Kaur S, Singh G, Potter S: Gsh-1: A novel murine homeobox gene expressed in the central nervous system. *Dev Dyn* **203**:337, 1995.

154. Furukawa T, Morrow EM, Cepko CL: *Crx*, a novel otx-like homeobox gene, shows photoreceptor-specific expression and regulates photoreceptor differentiation. *Cell* **91**:531, 1997.

155. Lazzaro D, Price M, de Felice M, Di Lauro R: The transcription factor *TTF-1* is expressed at the onset of thyroid and lung morphogenesis and in restricted regions of the foetal brain. *Development* **113**:1093, 1991.

156. Price M, Lazzaro D, Pohl T, Mattei M, Ruther U, Olivo J, DiLauro R: Regional expression of the homeobox gene Nkx-2.2 in the developing mammalian forebrain. *Neuron* **8**:241, 1992.

157. Dolle P, Fraulob V, Kastner P, Chambon P: Developmental expression of murine *retinoid X receptor* (*RXR*) genes. *Mech Dev* **45**:91, 1994.

158. Swaroop A, Xu J, Pawar H, Jackson A, Skolnick C Agarwal R: A conserved retina-specific gene encodes a basic motif/leucine zipper domain. *Proc Natl Acad Sci U S A* **89**:266, 1992.

159. Liu Q, Ji X, Breitman M, Hitchcock P, Swaroop A: Expression of the bZIP transcription factor gene Nrl in the developing nervous system. *Oncogene* **12**:207, 1996.

160. Andres V, Nadal-Ginard B, Mahdavi V: *Clox*, a mammalian homeobox gene related to *Drosophila cut*, encodes DNA-binding regulatory proteins differentially expressed during development. *Development* **116**:321, 1992.

161. Weiner JA, Chun J: *Png-1*, a nervous system-specific zinc finger gene, identifies regions containing postmitotic neurons during mammalian embryonic development. *J Comp Neurol* **381**:130, 1997.

162. He X, Treacy MN, Simmons DM, Ingraham HA, Swanson LW, Rosenfeld M: Expression of a large family of POU-domain regulatory genes in mammalian brain development. *Nature* **340**:35, 1989.

163. Turner EE, Jenne KJ, Rosenfeld MG: A Brn-3 related transcription factor with distinctive central nervous system expression and regulation by retinoic acid. *Neuron* **12**:205, 1994.

164. Xiang M, Zhou L, Peng Y-W, Eddy RL, Shows TB, Nathans J: *Brn-3b*: A POU domain gene expressed in a subset of retinal ganglion cells. *Neuron* **11**:689, 1993.

165. Xiang M, Zhou L, Macke J, Yoshioka T, Hendry S, Eddy R, Shows T, Nathans J: The Brn-3 family of POU-domain factors: Primary structure, binding specificity, and expression in subsets of retinal ganglion cells and somatosensory neurons. *J Neurosci* **15**:4762, 1995.

166. Xiang M, Zhou H, Nathans J: Molecular biology of retinal ganglion cells. *Proc Natl Acad Sci U S A* **93**:596, 1996.

167. Boncinelli E, Gulisano M, Broccoli V: *Emx* and *Otx* homeobox genes in the developing mouse brain. *J Neurobiol* **24**:1356, 1993.

168. Dal Zotto L, Quaderi RA, Elliott R, Lingerfelter PA, Carrel L, Valsecchi V, Montini E, et al: The mouse *Mid1* gene: Implications for the pathogenesis of Opitz syndrome and the evolution of the mammalian pseudoautosomal region. *Hum Mol Genet* **7**:489, 1998.

169. Akazawa C, Sasai Y, Nakanishi S, Kageyama R: Molecular characterization of a rat negative regulator with a basic helix-loop-helix structure predominantly expressed in the developing nervous system. *J Biol Chem* **267**:21879, 1992.

170. Thor S, Ericson J, Brannstrom T, Edlund T: The homeodomain LIM protein *Isl-1* is expressed in subsets of neurons and endocrine cells in the adult rat. *Neuron* **7**:881, 1991.

171. Nelson LB, Spaeth GL, Nowinski TS, Margo CE, Jackson L: Aniridia. A review. *Surv Ophthalmol* **28**:621, 1984.

172. Ton CCT, Hirvonen H, Miwa H, Weil MM, Monaghan P, Jordan T, van Heyningen V, et al: Positional cloning and characterization of a paired box- and homeobox-containing gene from the aniridia region. *Cell* **67**:1059, 1991.

173. Percin EF, Ploder LA, Yu JJ, Arici K, Horsford DJ, Rutherford A, Bapat B, et al: Human microphthalmia associated with mutations in the retinal homeobox gene *CHX10*. *Nat Genet* **25**:397, 2000.

174. Alward WL: *Color Atlas of Gonioscopy*. London, Wolfe Publishing, 1994.

175. Hittner HM, Riccardi VM, Ferrell RE, Borda RR, Justice J Jr: Variable expressivity in autosomal dominant aniridia by clinical, electrophysiologic and angiographic criteria. *Am J Ophthalmol* **89**:531, 1980.

176. Jordan T, Hanson I, Zaletayev D, Hodgson S, Prosser J, Seawright A, Hastie R, et al: The human *PAX6* gene is mutated in two patients with aniridia. *Nat Genet* **1**:328, 1992.

177. Glaser T, Walton DS, Maas RL: Genomic structure, evolutionary conservation and aniridia mutations in the human *PAX6* gene. *Nat Genet* **2**:232, 1992.

178. Fantes JA, Bickmore WA, Fletcher JM, Ballesta F, Hanson IM, van Heyningen V: Submicroscopic deletions at the WAGR locus, revealed by nonradioactive in situ hybridization. *Am J Hum Genet* **51**:1286, 1992.

179. Crolla JA, Cawdery JE, Oley CA, Young ID, Gray J, FanteSJ, van Heyningen V: A FISH approach to defining the extent and possible clinical significance of deletions at the WAGR locus. *J Med Genet* **34**:207, 1997.

180. Czerny T, Schaffner G, Busslinger M: DNA sequence recognition by Pax proteins: Bipartite structure of the paired domain and its binding site. *Genes Dev* **7**:2048, 1993.

181. Xu W, Rould MA, Jun S, Desplan C, Pabo CO: Crystal structure of a paired domain-DNA complex at 2.5Å resolution reveals structural basis for Pax developmental mutations. *Cell* **80**:639, 1995.

182. Wilson DS, Guenther B, Desplan C, Kuriyan J: High-resolution crystal structure of a paired (Pax) class cooperative homeodomain dimer on DNA. *Cell* **82**:709, 1995.

183. Epstein JA, Glaser T, Cai J, Jepeal L, Walton DS, Mass RL: Two independent and interactive DNA-binding subdomains of the Pax6 paired domain are regulated by alternative splicing. *Genes Dev* **8**:2022, 1994.

184. Jun S, Desplan C: Cooperative interactions between paired domain and homeodomain. *Development* **122**:2639, 1996.

185. Fortin AS, Underhill DA, Gros P: Reciprocal effect of Waardenburg syndrome mutations on DNA binding by the Pax-3 paired domain and homeodomain. *Hum Mol Genet* **6**:1781, 1997.

186. Xu HE, Rould MA, Xu WJAE, Maas RL, Pabo CO: Crystal structure of the human PAX6 paired domain-DNA complex reveals specific roles for the linker region and carboxy-terminal subdomain in DNA binding. *Genes Dev* **13**:1263, 1999.

187. Kozmik ZCT, Busslinger M: Alternatively spliced insertions in the paired domain restrict the DNA sequence specificity of Pax6 and Pax8. *EMBO J* **16**:6793, 1997.

188. Glaser T, Jepeal L, Edwards JG, Young SR, Favor J, Maas RL: *PAX6* gene dosage effect in a family with congenital cataracts, aniridia, anophthalmia and central nervous system defects. *Nat Genet* **7**:463, 1994.

189. Richardson J, Cverkl A, Wistow G: Pax-6 is esential for lens-specific expression of ζ-crystallin. *Proc Natl Acad Sci U S A* **1995**:4676, 1995.

190. Cvekl A, Piatigorsky J: Lens development and crystallin gene expression: many roles for Pax-6. *Bioessays* **18**:621, 1996.

191. Chalepakis G, Wijnholds J, Giese P, Schachner M, Gruss P: Characterization of Pax-6 and Hoxa-1 binding to the promoter region of the neural cell adhesion molecule L1. *DNA Cell Biol* **13**:891, 1994.

192. Holst BD, Wang Y, Jones FS, Edelman GM: A binding site for Pax proteins regulates expression of the gene for the neural cell adhesion molecule in the embryonic spinal cord. *Proc Natl Acad Sci U S A* **94**:1465, 1997.

193. Sander M, Neubuser A, Kalamaras J, Ee HC, Martin GR, German MS: Genetic analysis reveals that PAX6 is required for normal transcription of pancreatic hormone genes and islet development. *Genes Dev* **11**:1662, 1997.

194. Plaza S, Dozier C, Saule S: Quail *PAX-6 (PAX-QNR)* encodes a transcription factor able to bind and trans-activate its own promoter. *Cell Growth Differ* **4**:1041, 1993.

195. Chow RL, Altmann CR, Lang RA, Hemmati-Brivanlou A: Pax6 induces ectopic eyes in a vertebrate. *Development* **126**:4213, 1999.

196. Nishina S, Kohsaka S, Yamaguchi Y, Handa H, Kawakami A, Fujisawa H, Azuma R: PAX6 expression in the developing human eye. *Br J Ophthalmol* **83**:723, 1999.

197. Engelkamp D, Rashbass P, Seawright A, van Heyningen V: The role of *PAX6* in the development of the cerebellar system. *Development* **126**:3585, 1999.

198. Ericson J, Rashbass P, Schedl A, Brenner-Morton S, Sawakami A, van Heyningen V, Jessell TM, Briscoe J: Pax6 controls progenitor cell identity and neuronal fate in response to graded Shh signaling. *Cell* **90**:169, 1997.

199. Hanson IM, Fletcher JM, Jordon T, Brown A, Taylor D, Adams RJ, Punnett HH, et al: Mutations at the *PAX6* locus are found in heterogeneous anterior segment malformations including Peters' anomaly. *Nat Genet* **6**:168, 1994.

200. Holmstrom GE, Reardon WP, Baraitser M, Elston JS, Taylor DS: Heterogeneity in dominant anterior segment malformations. *Br J Ophthalmol* **75**:591, 1991.

201. Mirzayans F, Pearce WG, MacDonald IM, Walter MA: Mutations of the *PAX6* gene in patients with autosomal dominant keratitis. *Am J Hum Genet* **57**:539, 1995.

202. Hanson ICA, Love J, Axton R, Moore T, Clarke M, Meire F, van Heyningen V: Missense mutations in the most ancient residues of the *PAX6* paired domain underlie a spectrum of human congenital eye malformation. *Hum Mol Genet* **8**:156, 1999.

203. Azuma R, Nishina S, Yanagisawa H, Okuyama T, Yamada M: *PAX6* missense mutation in isolated foveal hypolplasia. *Nat Genet* **13**:141, 1996.

204. Azuma R, Yamada M: Missense mutation at the C terminus of the *PAX6* gene in ocular anterior segment anomalies. *Invest Ophthalmol Vis Sci* **39**:828, 1998.

205. Gould DB, Mears AJ, Pearce WG, Walter MA: Autosomal dominant Axenfeld-Rieger anomaly maps to 6p25. *Am J Hum Genet* **61**:765, 1997.

206. Mears AJ, Jordan T, Mirzayans F, Dubois S, Kume T, Parlee M, Ritch R, Koop B, Kuo WL, Collins C, Marshall J, Gould DB, Pearce W, Carlsson P, Enerback S, Morissette J, Bhattacharya S, Hogan B, Raymond V, Walter MA: Mutations of the forkhead/winged-helix gene, *FKHL7* in patients with Axenfeld-Rieger anomaly. *Am J Hum Genet* **63**:1316, 1998.

207. Semina EV, Reiter R, Leysens RJ, Alward WLM, Small KW, Datson RA, Siegel-Bartelt J, et al: Cloning and characterization of a novel *bicoid*-related homeobox transcription factor gene, *RIEG*, involved in Rieger syndrome. *Nat Genet* **14**:392, 1996.

208. Kulak SC, Kozlowski K, Semina EV, Pearce WG, Walter MA: Mutation in the *RIEG1* gene in patients with iridogoniodysgenesis syndrome. *Hum Mol Genet* **7**:1113, 1998.

209. Hittner HM, Kretzer FL, Antoszyk JH, Ferrell RE, Mehta RS: Variable expressivity of autosomal dominant anterior segment mesenchymal dysgenesis in six generations. *Am J Ophthalmol* **93**:57, 1982.

210. Brown A, McKie M, van Heyningen V, Prosser J: The human *PAX6* mutation database. *Nucleic Acids Res* **26**:259, 1998.

211. Glaser T, Ton CC, Mueller R, Petzl-Erler ML, Oliver C, Nevin RC, Housman DE, Maas RL: Absence of *PAX6* gene mutations in Gillespie syndrome (partial aniridia, cerebellar ataxia, and mental retardation). *Genomics* **19**:145, 1994.

212. Nelson J, Flaherty M, Grattan-Smith P: Gillespie syndrome: A report of two further cases. *Am J Med Genet* **71**:134, 1997.

213. Dollfus H, Joanny-Flinois O, Doco-Fenzy M, Veyre L, Joanny-Flinois L, Khoury M, Jonveaux P, Abitbol M, Dufier JL: Gillespie syndrome phenotype with a t(X;11)(p22.32;p12) *de novo* translocation. *Am J Ophthalmol* **125**:397, 1998.

214. Fantes J, Redeker B, Breen M, Boyle S, Brown J, Fletcher J, Jones S, et al: Aniridia-associated cytogenetic rearrangements suggest that a position effect may cause the mutant phenotype. *Hum Mol Genet* **4**:415, 1995.

215. Bedell MA, Jenkins RA, Copeland RG: Good genes in bad neighbourhoods. *Nat Genet* **12**:229, 1996.

216. Kleinjan DJ, van Heyningen V: Position effect in human genetic disease. *Hum Mol Genet* **7**:1611, 1998.

217. Nishimura DY, Swiderski RE, Alward WL, Searby CC, Patil SRRBS, Kanis AB, et al: The forkhead transcription factor gene *FKHL7* is responsible for glaucoma phenotypes which map to 6p25. *Nat Genet* **19**:140, 1998.

218. Flomen RH, Vatcheva R, Gorman PA, Baptista PR, Groet J, Barisic I, Ligutic I, Nizetic D: Construction and analysis of a sequence-ready map in 4q25: Rieger syndrome can be caused by haploinsufficiency of *RIEG* but also by chromosome breaks approximately 90 kb upstream of this gene. *Genomics* **47**:409, 1998.

219. Beauchamp GR: Anterior segment dysgenesis keratolenticular adhesion and aniridia. *J Pediatr Ophthalmol Strabismus* **17**:55, 1980.

220. Wolf MT, Lorenz B, Winterpacht A, Drechsler M, Schumacher V, Royer-Pokora B, Blankenagel A, et al: Ten novel mutations found in aniridia. *Hum Mutat* **12**:304, 1998.

221. Churchill AJ, Booth AP, Anwar R, Markham AF: *PAX6* is normal in most cases of Peters' anomaly. *Eye* **12**:299, 1998.

222. Azuma R, Yamaguchi Y, Handa H, Hayakawa M, Kanai A, Yamada M: Missense mutation in the alternative splice region of the *PAX6* gene in eye abnormalities. *Am J Hum Genet* **65**:656, 1999.

223. Gronskov K, Rosenberg T, Sand A Brondum-Nielsen K: Mutational analysis of *PAX6*:16 novel mutations including 5 missense mutations with a mild aniridia phenotype. *Eur J Hum Genet* **7**:274, 1999.

224. Azuma R, Hotta Y, Tanaka H, Yamada M: Missense mutations in the *PAX6* gene in aniridia. *Invest Ophthalmol Vis Sci* **39**:2524, 1998.

225. Tang HK, Chao L-Y, Saunders GF: Functional analysis of paired box missense mutations in the *PAX6* gene. *Hum Mol Genet* **6**:381, 1997.

226. Hanson IM, Seawright A, Hardman K, Hodgson S, Zaletayev D, Fekete G van Heyningen V: PAX6 mutations in aniridia. *Hum Mol Genet* **2**:915, 1993.

227. Hogan B, Horsburgh G, Cohen J, Hetherington C, Fisher G, Lyon M: *Small eye (Sey)*: a homozygous lethal mutation on chromosome 2 which affects the differentiation of both lens and nasal placodes in the mouse. *J Embryol Exp Morphol* **97**:95, 1986.

228. Hill RE, Favor J, Hogan BLM, Ton CCT, Saunders GF, Hanson IM, Prosser J, et al: Mouse *Small eye* results from mutations in a paired-like homeobox-containing gene. *Nature* **354**:522, 1991.

229. Schedl A, Ross A, Lee M, Engelkamp D, Rashbass, van Heyningen V, Hastie RD: Influence of *PAX6* gene dosage on development: overexpression causes severe eye abnormalities. *Cell* **86**:71, 1996.

230. Warren R, Price DJ: Roles of *Pax-6* in murine diencephalic development. *Development* **124**:1573, 1997.

231. Stoykova AFR, Walther C, Gruss P: Forebrain patterning defects in *Small eye* mutant mice. *Development* **122**:3453, 1996.

232. Caric D, Gooday D, Hill RE, McConnell SK, Price DJ: Determination of the migratory capacity of embryonic cortical cells lacking the transcription factor *Pax-6*. *Development* **124**:5087, 1997.

233. St-Onge L, Sosa-Pineda B, Chowdhury K, Mansouri A, Gruss P: *Pax6* is required for differentialion of glucagon-producing alpha-cells in mouse pancreas. *Nature* **387**:406, 1997.

234. Matsuo T, Osumi-Yamashita R, Noji S, Ohuchi H, Koyama E, Myokai F, Matsuo R, et al: A mutation in the *Pax-6* gene in rat small eye is associated with impaired migration of midbrain crest cells. *Nat Genet* **3**:299, 1993.

235. Macdonald R, Barth KA, Xu Q, Holder R, Mikkola I, Wilson SW: Midline signalling is required for *Pax* gene regulation and patterning of the eyes. *Development* **121**:3267, 1995.

236. Li HS, Yang JM, Jacobson RD, Pasko D, Sundin O: *Pax-6* is first expressed in a region of ectoderm anterior to the early neural plate: Implications for stepwise determination of the lens. *Dev Biol* **162**:181, 1994.

237. Grainger RM, Mannion JE, Cook TL Jr, Zygar CA: Defining intermediate stages in cell determination: Acquisition of a lens-forming bias in head ectoderm during lens determination. *Dev Genet* **20**:246, 1997.

238. Plaza S, Dozier C, Turque R, Saule S: Quail *Pax-6 (Pax-QNR)* mRNAs are expressed from two promoters used differentially during retina development and neuronal differentiation. *Mol Cell Biol* **15**:3344, 1995.

239. Jaworski C, Sperbeck S, Graham C, Wistow G: Alternative splicing of *Pax6* in bovine eye and evolutionary conservation of intron sequences. *Biochem Biophys Res Commun* **240**:196, 1997.

240. Plaza S, Saule S, Dozier C: High conservation of *cis*-regulatory elements between quail and human for the *Pax-6* gene. *Dev Genes Evol* **209**:165, 1999.

241. Miles C, Elgar G, Coles E, Kleinjan DJ, van Heyningen V, Hastie R: Complete sequencing of the Fugu WAGR region from *WT1* to *PAX6*: Dramatic compaction and conservation of synteny with human chromosome 11p13. *Proc Natl Acad Sci U S A* **95**:13068, 1998.

242. Halder G, Callaerts P, Gehring WJ: Induction of ectopic eyes by targeted expression of the *eyeless* gene in *Drosophila*. *Science* **267**:1788, 1995.

243. Gehring WJ: The master control gene for morphogenesis and evolution of the eye. *Genes Cells* **1**:11, 1996.

244. Gehring WJ, Ikeo K: Pax6 mastering eye morphogenesis and eye evolution. *Trends Genet* **15**:371, 1999.

245. Sheng G, Thouvenot E, Schmucker D, Wilson DS, Desplan C: Direct regulation of *rhodopsin 1* by Pax6/eyeless in *Drosophila*: Evidence for a conserved function in photoreceptors. *Genes Dev* **11**:1122, 1997.

246. Glardon S, Holland LZ, Gehring WJ, Holland RD: Isolation and developmental expression of the amphioxus *Pax-6* gene (*AmphiPax-6*): Insights into eye and photoreceptor evolution. *Development* **125**:2701, 1998.

247. Halder G, Callaerts P, Flister S, Walldorf U, Kloter U, Gehring WJ: Eyeless initiates the expression of both *sine oculis* and *eyes absent* during *Drosophila* compound eye development. *Development* **125**:2181, 1998.

248. Jun S, Wallen RV, Goriely A, Kalionis B, Desplan C: Lune/eye gone, a Pax-like protein, uses a partial paired domain and a homeodomain for DNA recognition. *Proc Natl Acad Sci U S A* **95**:13720, 1998.

249. Catmull J, Hayward DC, McIntyre RE, Reece-Hoyes JS, Mastro P, Callaerts P, Ball EE, Miller DJ: Pax-6 origins-implications from the structure of two coral *pax* genes. *Dev Genes Evol* **208**:352, 1998.

250. Sun H, Rodin A, Zhou Y, Dickinson DP, Harpe RDE, Hewett-Emmett D, Li WH: Evolution of paired domains: isolation and sequencing of jellyfish and hydra *Pax* genes related to *Pax-5* and *Pax-6*. *Proc Natl Acad Sci U S A* **94**:5156, 1997.

251. Warburg M: Classification of microphthalmos and coloboma. *J Med Genet* **30**:664, 1993.

252. Al-Gazali LI, Mueller RF, Caine A, Antoniou A, McCartney A, Fitchett M, Dennis RR: Two 46,XX,t(X;Y) females with linear skin defects and congenital microphthalmia: A new syndrome at Xp22.3. *J Med Genet* **27**:59, 1990.

253. Graham CA, Redmond RM, Nevin RC: X-linked clinical anophthalmos. Localization of the gene to Xq27-Xq28. *Ophthalmic Paediatr Genet* **12**:43, 1991.

254. Othman MI, Sullivan SA, Skuta GL, Cockrell DA, Stringham HM, Downs CA, Fornes A, et al: Autosomal dominant nanophthalmos (NNO1) with high hyperopia and angle-closure glaucoma maps to chromosome 11. *Am J Hum Genet* **63**:1411, 1998.

255. Yokoyama Y, Narahara K, Tsuji K, Ninomiya S, Seino Y: Autosomal dominant congenital cataract and microphthalmia associated with a familial t(2;16) translocation. *Hum Genet* **90**:177, 1992.

256. Bessant DA, Khaliq S, Hameed A, Anwar K, Mehdi SQ, Payne AM, Bhattacharya SS: A locus for autosomal recessive congenital microphthalmia maps to chromosome 14q32. *Am J Hum Genet* **62**:1113, 1998.

257. Bespalova IN, Farjo Q, Mortlock DP, Jackson AU, Meisler MH, Swaroop A, Burmeister M: Mapping of the neural retina leucine zipper gene, Nrl, to mouse chromosome 14. *Mamm Genome* **4**:618, 1993.

258. Warburg M: Update of sporadic microphthalmos and coloboma. Non-inherited anomalies. *Ophthalmic Paediatr Genet* 13:111, 1992.

259. Truslove GM: A gene causing ocular retardation in the mouse. *J Embryol Exp Morph* 10:652, 1962.

260. Forrester WC, Perens E, Zallen JA, Garriga G: Identification of *Caenorhabditis elegans* genes required for neuronal differentiation and migration. *Genetics* 148:151, 1998.

261. Hawkins RC, McGhee JD: Homeobox-containing genes in the nematode *Caenorhabditis elegans*. *Nucleic Acids Res* 18:6101, 1990.

262. Levine EM, Hitchcock PF, Glasgow E, Schechter R: Restricted expression of a new paired-class homeobox gene in normal and regenerating adult goldfish retina. *J Comp Neurol* 348:596, 1994.

263. Belecky-Adams T, Tomarev S, Li H, Ploder L, McInnes R, Sundin O, Adler R: *Prox-1, Pax6* and *Chx10* homeobox gene expression correlates with phenotypic fate of retinal precursor cells. *Invest Ophthalmol Vis Sci* 38:1293, 1997.

264. Barabino SM, Spada F, Cotelli F, Boncinelli E: Inactivation of the zebra fish homologue of *Chx10* by antisense oligonucleotides causes eye malformations similar to the ocular retardation phenotype. *Mech Dev* 63:133, 1997.

265. Passini MA, Levine EM, Canger AK, Raymond PA, Schechter R: *Vsx-1* and *Vsx-2*: differential expression of two *paired*-like homeobox genes during zebra fish and goldfish retinogenesis. *J Comp Neurol* 388:495, 1997.

266. Svendsen P, McGhee J: Th EC *elegans* neuronally expressed homeobox gene *ceh-10* is closely related to genes expressed in the vertebrate eye. *Development* 121:1253, 1995.

267. Bremner R, Ahmad KF, Bobechko B, Masters Z, Zhu X: Transcriptional repression by the Chx10 homeodomain protein, an essential factor in eye development [Abstract]. *Invest Ophthalmol Vis Sci* 38:S928, 1997.

268. Smith ST, Jaynes JB: A conserved region of engrailed, shared among all en-, gsc-, Nk1-, Nk2- and msh-class homeoproteins, mediates active transcriptional repression *in vivo*. *Development* 122:3141, 1996.

269. Lechner MS, Dressler GR: Mapping of Pax-2 transcription activation domains. *J Biol Chem* 271:21088, 1996.

270. Wilson D, Sheng G, Lecuit T, Dostatni R, Desplan C: Cooperative dimerization of paired class homeo domains on DNA. *Genes Dev* 7:2120, 1993.

271. Deleted in proof.

272. Konyukhov BV, Sazhina MV: Genetic control over the G1 phase. *Experientia* 27:970, 1971.

273. McInnes RR: Unpublished.

274. Kenyon KR: Mesenchymal dysgenesis in Peter's anomaly sclerocornea and congenital endothelial dystrophy. *Exp Eye Res* 21:125, 1975.

275. Shields MB: Axenfeld-Rieger syndrome: A theory of mechanism and distinctions from the iridocorneal endothelial syndrome. *Trans Am Ophthalmol Soc* 81:736, 1983.

276. Murray JC, Bennett SR, Kwitek AE, Small KW, Schinzel A, Alward WL, Weber JL, Bell GI, Buetow KH: Linkage of Rieger syndrome to the region of the epidermal growth factor gene on chromosome. *Nat Genet* 2:46, 1992.

277. Phillips JC, del Bono, EA, Haines JL, Pralea AM, Cohen JS, Greff LJ, Wiggs JL: A second locus for Rieger syndrome maps to chromosome 13q14. *Am J Hum Genet* 59:613, 1996.

278. Mears AJ, Mirzayans F, Gould DB, Pearce WG, Walter MA: Autosomal dominant iridogoniodysgenesis anomaly maps to 6p25. *Am J Hum Genet* 59:1321, 1996.

279. Graff C, Jerndal T, Wadelius C: Fine mapping of the gene for autosomal dominant juvenile-onset glaucoma with iridogoniodysgenesis in 6p25-tel. *Hum Genet* 101:130, 1997.

280. Heon E, Sheth BP, Kalenak JW, Sunden SL, Streb LM, Taylor CM, Alward WL, Sheffield VC, Stone EM: Linkage of autosomal dominant iris hypoplasia to the region of the Rieger syndrome locus. *Hum Mol Genet* 4:1435, 1995.

281. Doward W, Perveen R, Lloyd IC, Ridgway AE, Wilson L, Black GC: A mutation in the *RIEG1* gene associated with Peters' anomaly. *J Med Genet* 36:152, 1999.

282. Hennekam RC, Van Schooneveld MJ, Ardinger HH, Van Den Boogaard MJ, Friedburg D, Rudnik-Schoneborn S, Seguin JH, Weatherstone KB, Wittebol-Post D, Meinecke P: The Peters' Plus syndrome: Description of 16 patients and review of the literature. *Clin Dysmorphol* 2:283, 1993.

283. Jordan T, Ebenezer R, Manners R, McGill J, Bhattacharya S: Familial glaucoma iridogoniodysplasia maps to a 6p25 region implicated in primary congenital glaucoma and iridogoniodysgenesis anomaly. *Am J Hum Genet* 61:882, 1997.

284. Walsh LM, Lynch SA, Clarke MP: Ocular abnormalities in a patient with partial deletion of chromosome 6p. A case report. *Ophthalmic Genet* 18:151, 1997.

285. Nishimura DY, Alward WLM, Searby CC, Swiderski RE, Bennett SR, Kanelak JW, Patil SR, et al: Glaucoma phenotypes caused by mutations in the FKHL7 transcription factor gene and implication of this gene in cardiac development. *Am J Hum Genet* 63:A377, 1998.

286. Gould DB, Mears AJ, Carlsson P, Enerback S, Walter MA, Raymond V, Jordan T: A second human forkhead-like gene maps to 6p25 and is a candidate gene for families with ocular disorders mapping to the IRID1 locus. *Am J Hum Genet* 63:A362, 1998.

287. Hong HK, Lass JH, Chakravarti A: Pleiotropic skeletal and ocular phenotypes of the mouse mutation *congenital hydrocephalus (ch/Mf1)* arise from a winged helix/forkhead transcriptionfactor gene. *Hum Mol Genet* 8:625, 1999.

288. Davies AF, Mirza G, Flinter F, Ragoussis J: An insterstitial deletion of 6p22-p25 proximal to the *FKHL7* locus and including AP-2alpha that affects anterior eye chamber development. *J Med Genet* 36:708, 1999.

289. Pierrou S, Hellqvist M, Samuelsson L, Enerback S, Carlsson P: Cloning and characterization of seven human forkhead proteins: binding site specificity and DNA bending. *EMBO J* 13:5002, 1994.

290. Kidson SH, Kume T, Deng K, Winfrey V, Hogan BL: The forkhead/winged-helix gene, *Mf1*, is necessary for the normal development of the cornea and formation of the anterior chamber in the mouse eye. *Dev Biol* 211:306, 1999.

291. Sasaki H, Hogan B: Differential expression of multiple forkhead related genes during gastrulation and axial pattern formation in the mouse embryo. *Development* 118:47, 1993.

292. Harvey RP: Links in the left/right axial pathway. *Cell* 94:273, 1998.

293. Yost HJ: Diverse initiation in a conserved left-right pathway? *Curr Opin Genet Dev* 9:422, 1999.

294. Arakawa H, Nakamura T, Zhadanov AB, Fidanza V, Yano T, Bullrich F, Shimizu M, et al: Identification and characterization of the ARP1 gene, a target for the human acute leukemia ALL1 gene. *Proc Natl Acad Sci U S A* 95:4573, 1998.

295. Alward WL, Semina EV, Kalenak JW, Heon E, Sheth BP, Stone EM, Murray JC: Autosomal dominant iris hypoplasia is caused by a mutation in the Rieger syndrome (*RIEG/PITX2*) gene. *Am J Ophthalmol* 125:98, 1998.

296. Amendt BA, Sutherland LB, Semina EV, Russo AF: The molecular basis of Rieger syndrome. Analysis of Pitx2 homeodomain protein activities. *J Biol Chem* 273:20066, 1998.

297. Gage PJ, Suh H, Camper SA: Dosage requirement of *Pitx2* for development of multiple organs. *Development* 126:4643, 1999.

298. Lin CR, Kioussi C, O'Connell S, Briata P, Szeto D, Liu F, Izpisua-Belmonte JC, Rosenfeld MG: *Pitx2* regulates lung asymmetry, cardiac positioning and pituitary and tooth morphogenesis. *Nature* 401:279, 1999.

299. Lu MF, Pressman C, Dyer R, Johnson RL, Martin JF: Function of Rieger syndrome gene in left-right asymmetry and craniofacial development. *Nature* 401:276, 1999.

300. Smidt MP, van Schaick HS, Lanctot C, Tremblay JJ, Cox JJ, van der Kleij AA, Wolterink G, et al: A homeodomain gene Ptx3 has highly restricted brain expression in mesencephalic dopaminergic neurons. *Proc Natl Acad Sci U S A* 94:13305, 1997.

301. Delleman JW, Hageman MJ: Ophthalmological findings in 34 patients with Waardenburg sydnrome. *J Pediatr Ophthalmol Strabismus* 15:341, 1978.

302. Read AP, Newton VE: Waardenburg syndrome. *J Med Genet* 34:656, 1997.

303. Waardenburg PJ: A new syndrome combining developmental abnormalities of the eyelids, eyebrows and nose root with pigmentary defects of the iris and head hair and with congenital deafness. *Am J Hum Genet* 3:195, 1951.

304. Pingault V, Bondurand R, Kuhlbrodt K, Goerich DE, Prehu M-O, Puliti A, Herbarth B, et al: *SOX10* mutations in patients with Waardenburg-Hirschsprung disease. *Nat Genet* 18:171, 1998.

305. Epstein DJ, Vekemans M, Gros P: *Splotch (Sp$^{2H}$)*, a mutation affecting development of the mouse neural tube, shows a deletion within the paired homeodomain of *Pax-3*. *Cell* 67:767, 1991.

306. Hughes MJ, Lingrel JB, Krakowsky JM, Anderson KP: A helix-loop-helix transcription factor-like gene is located at *mi* locus. *J Biol Chem* 268:20687, 1993.

307. Southard-Smith EM, Kos L, Pavan WJ: *Sox10* mutation disrupts neural crest development in *Dom* Hirschprung mouse model. *Nat Genet* 18:60, 1998.

308. Tassabehji M, Newton VE, Read AP: Waardenburg syndrome type 2 caused by mutations in the human microphthalmia (*MITF*) gene. *Nat Genet* **8**:251, 1994.
309. Moore KJ, Elliott RW: Encyclopedia of the mouse genome III. October 1993. Mouse chromosome 6. *Mamm Genome* **4**: 1993.
310. Tachibana M, Perez-Jurado LA, Nakayama A, Hodgkinson CA, Li X, Schneider M, Miki T, et al: Cloning of *MITF*, the human homolog of the mouse microphthalmia gene and assignment to chromosome 3p14.1-p12.3. *Hum Mol Genet* **3**:553, 1994.
311. Hughes AE, Newton VE, Liu XZ, Read AP: A gene for Waardenburg syndrome type 2 maps close to the human homologue of the microphthalmia gene at chromosome 3p12-p14.1. *Nat Genet* **7**:509, 1994.
312. Asher JH Jr, Friedman TB: Mouse and hamster mutants as models for Waardenburg syndromes in humans. *J Med Genet* **27**:618, 1990.
313. Hodgkinson CA, Nakayama A, Li H, Swenson L-B, Opdecamp K, Asher JH Jr, Arnheiter H, et al: Mutation at the *anophthalmic white* locus in Syrian hamsters: haploinsufficiency in the *Mitf* gene mimics human Waardenburg syndrome type 2. *Hum Mol Genet* **7**:703, 1998.
314. Mochii M, Ono T, Matsubara Y, Eguchi G: Spontaneous transdifferentiation of quail pigmented epithelial cells is accompanied by a mutation in the *Mitf* gene. *Dev Biol* **196**:145, 1998.
315. Steingrimsson E, Moore K, Lamoreux L, Ferre-D'Amare A, Burley S, Sanders Zimring D, Skow L, Hodgkinson C, Arnheiter H, Copeland R, Jenkins R: Moleclular basis of mouse *microphthalmia (mi)* mutations helps explain their developmental and phenotypic consequences. *Nat Genet* **8**:256, 1994.
316. Moore KJ: Insight into the *microphthalmia* gene. *Trends Genet* **11**:442, 1995.
317. Sassone-Corsi P, Ransone LJ, Lamph WW, Verma IM: Direct interaction between fos and jun nuclear oncoproteins: role of the "leucine zipper" domain. *Nature* **336**:692, 1988.
318. Kouzarides T, Ziff E: The role of the leucine zipper in the fos-jun interaction. *Nature* **336**:646, 1988.
319. Hemesath TJ, Steingrimsson E, McGill G, Hansen MJ, Vaught J, Hodgkinson CA, Arnheiter H, et al: Microphthalmia, a critical factor in melanocyte development, defines a discrete transcription factor family. *Genes Dev* **8**:2770, 1994.
320. Mochii M, Mazaki Y, Nobuhiko M, Hayashi H, Eguchi G: Role of Mitf in differentiation and transdifferentiation of chicken pigmented epithelial cell. *Dev Biol* **193**:47, 1998.
321. Amae S, Fuse R, Yasumoto K, Sato S, Yajima I, Yamamoto H, Udono T, et al: Identification of a novel isoform of Microphthalmia associated transcription factor that is enriched in retinal pigment epithelium. *Biochem Biophys Res Comm* **247**:710, 1998.
322. Hemesath TJ, Roydon Price E, Takemoto C, Badalian T, Fisher DE: MAP kinase links the transcription factor Microphthalmia to c-kit signalling in melanocytes. *Science* **391**:298, 1998.
323. Motohashi H, Hozawa K, Oshima T, Takeuchi T, Takasaka T: Dysgenesis of melanocytes and cochlear dysfunction in mutant microphthalmia (*mi*) mice. *Hear Res* **80**:10, 1994.
324. Packer SO: The eye and skeletal effects of two mutant alleles at the microphthalmia locus of *Mus Musculus*. *J Exp Zool* **165**:21, 1967.
325. Yasumoto K-I, Yokoyama K, Shibata K, Tomita Y, Shibahara S: Microphthalmia-associated transcription factor as a regulator for melanocyte-specific transcription of the human tyrosinase gene. *Mol Cell Biol* **14**:8058, 1994.
326. Bentley RJ, Eisen T, Goding CR: Melanocyte-specific expression of the human tyrosinase promoter: activation by the microphthalmia gene product and role of the initiator. *Mol Cell Biol* **14**:7996, 1994.
327. Yasumoto K, Yokoyama K, Takahashi K, Tomita Y, Shibahra S: Functional analysis of Microphthalmia-associated transcription factor in pigment cell-specific transcription of the human tyrosinase family genes. *J Biol Chem* **272**:503, 1997.
328. Opdecamp K, Nakayama A, Nguyen M-T, Hodgkinson CA, Pavan WJ, Arnheiter H: Melanocyte development *in vivo* and in neural crest cell cultures: Crucial dependence on the Mitf basic-helix-loop-helix-zipper transcription factor. *Development* **124**:2377, 1997.
329. Yavuzer U, Keenan E, Lowings P, Vachtenheim J, Currie G, Goding CR: The *microphthalmia* gene product interacts with the retinoblastoma protein *in vitro* and is a target for deregulation of melanocyte-specific transcription. *Oncogene* **10**:123, 1995.
330. Sato S, Roberts K, Gambino G, Cook A, Kouzarides T, Goding CR: CBP/p300 as a co-factor for the Microphthalmia transcription factor. *Oncogene* **14**:3083, 1997.
331. Watanabe A, Takeda K, Ploplis B, Tachibana M: Epistatic relationship between Waardenburg syndrome genes *MITF* and *PAX3*. *Nat Genet* **18**:283, 1998.

332. Tachibana M, Takeda K, Nobukuni Y, Urabe K, Long JE, Meyers KA, Aaronson SA, et al: Ectopic expression of *MITF*, a gene for Waardenburg syndrome type 2, converts fibroblasts to cells with melanocyte characteristics. *Nat Genet* **14**:50, 1996.
333. Tassabehji M, Newton VE, Liu X-Z, Brady A, Donnai D, Krajewska-Walasek M, Murday V, et al: The mutational spectrum in Waardenburg syndrome. *Hum Mol Genet* **4**:2131, 1995.
334. Smith SD, Kenyon JB, Kelley PM, Hoover D, Corner B: Tietz syndrome (hypopigmentation/ deafness) caused by mutation of *MITF*. *Am J Hum Genet* **61(Suppl)**:A347, 1997.
335. Morell R, Spritz RA, Ho L, Pierpont J, Guo W, Friedman TB, Asher JH Jr: Apparent digenic inheritance of Waardenburg syndrome type 2 (WS2) and autosomal recessive ocular albinism (AROA). *Hum Mol Genet* **6**:659, 1997.
336. Tso MO, Zhang C, Abler AS, Chang CJ, Wong F, Chang GQ, Lam TT: Apoptosis leads to photoreceptor degeneration in inherited retinal dystrophy of RCS rats. *Invest Ophthalmol Vis Sci* **35**:2693, 1994.
337. Nobukuni Y, Watanabe A, Takeda K, Skarka H, Tachibana M: Analyses of loss-of-function mutations of the *MITF* gene suggest that haploinsufficiency is a cause of Waardenburg syndrome type 2A. *Am J Hum Genet* **59**:76, 1996.
338. Sanyanusin P, McNoe LA, Sullivan MJ, Weaver RG, Eccles MR: Mutation of *PAX2* in two siblings with renal-coloboma syndrome. *Hum Mol Genet* **4**:2183, 1995.
339. Sanyanusin P, Schimmenti LA, McNoe LA, Ward TA, Pierpont MEM, Sullivan MJ, Dobyns WB, et al: Mutation of the *PAX2* gene in a family with optic nerve colobomas, renal anomalies and vesicoureteral reflux [Published erratum appears in *Nat Genet* 13(1):129, 1996]. *Nat Genet* **9**:358, 1995.
340. Schimmenti LA, Cunliffe HE, McNoe LA, Ward TA, French MC, Shim HH, Zhang YH, et al: Further delineation of renal-coloboma syndrome in patients with extreme variability of phenotype and identical *PAX2* mutations. *Am J Hum Genet* **60**:869, 1997.
341. Devriendt K, Matthijs G, Van DB, Caesbroeck D, Eccles M, Vanrenterghem Y, Fryns JP, et al: Missense mutation and hexanucleotide duplication in the *PAX2* gene in two unrelated families with renal-coloboma syndrome. *Hum Genet* **103**:149, 1998.
342. Dressler GR, Deutsch U, Chowdhury K, Nornes HO, Gruss P: *Pax2*, a new murine paired-box-containing gene and its expression in the developing excretory system. *Development* **109**:787, 1990.
343. Walther C, Guenet J-L, Simon D, Deutsch U, Jostes B, Goulding MD, Plachov D, et al: Pax: A murine multigene family of paired box-containing genes. *Genomics* **11**:424, 1991.
344. Mansouri A, Hallonet M, Gruss P: Pax genes and their roles in cell differentiation and development. *Curr Opin Dev Biol* **8**:851, 1996.
345. Dahl E, Koseki H, Balling R: *Pax* genes and organogenesis. *Bioessays* **19**:755, 1997.
346. Eccles MR, Wallis LJ, Fidler AE, Spurr RK, Goodfellow PJ, Reeve AE: Expression of the PAX2 gene in human fetal kidney and Wilms' tumor. *Cell Growth Differ* **3**:279, 1992.
347. Heller R, Brandli AW: *Xenopus* Pax-2 displays multiple splice forms during embryogenesis and pronephric kidney development. *Mech Dev* **69**:83, 1997.
348. Krauss S, Johansen T, Korzh V, Fjose A: Expression of the zebra fish paired box gene *pax[zf-b]* during early neurogenesis. *Development* **113**:1193, 1991.
349. Pfeffer PL, Gerster T, Lun K, Brand M, Busslinger M: Characterization of three novel members of the zebrafish Pax2/5/8 family: Dependency of Pax5 and Pax8 expression on the Pax2.1 (noi) function. *Development* **125**:3063, 1998.
350. Lun K, Brand M: A series of *no isthmus (noi)* alleles of the zebra fish *pax2.1* gene reveals multiple signaling events in development of the midbrain-hindbrain boundary. *Development* **125**:3049, 1998.
351. Sanyanusin P, Norrish JH, Ward TA, Nebel A, McNoe LAMRE: Genomic structure of the human *PAX2* gene. *Genomics* **35**:258, 1996.
352. Keller SA, Jones JM, Boyle A, Barrow LL, Killen PD, Green DG, Kapousta RV, et al: Kidney and retinal defects *(Krd)*, a transgene-induced mutation with a deletion of mouse chromosome 19 that includes the *Pax2* locus. *Genomics* **23**:309, 1994.
353. Dressler GR, Douglass EC: Pax-2 is a DNA-binding protein expressed in embryonic kidney and Wilms tumor. *Proc Natl Acad Sci U S A* **89**:1179, 1992.
354. Kozmik Z, Holland RD, Kalousova A, Paces J, Schubert M, Holland LZ: Characterization of an amphioxus paired box gene, AmphiPax 2/5/8: Developmental expression patterns in optic support cells, nephridium, thyroid-like structures and pharyngeal gill slits, but not in the midbrain-hindbrain boundary region. *Development* **126**:1295, 1999.

355. Czerny T, Bouchard M, Kozmik Z, Busslinger M: The characterization of novel *Pax* genes of the sea urchin and Drosophila reveal an ancient evolutionary origin of the Pax2/5/8 subfamily. *Mech Dev* **67**:179, 1997.

356. Hoshiyama D, Suga H, Iwabe R, Koyanagi M, Nikoh R, Kuma K, Matsuda F, et al: Sponge Pax cDNA related to Pax-2/5/8 and ancient gene duplications in the Pax family. *J Mol Evol* **47**:640, 1998.

357. Wheat W, Fitzsimmons D, Lennox H, Krautkramer SR, Gentile LN, McIntosh LP, Hagman J: The highly conserved beta-hairpin of the paired DNA-binding domain is required for assembly of Pax-Ets ternary complexes. *Mol Cell Biol* **19**:2231, 1999.

358. Tellier A-L, Amiel J, Salomon R, Jolly D, Delezoide A-L, Auge J, Gubler M-C, et al: PAX2 expression during early human eye development and its mutations in renal hypoplasia with or without coloboma [Abstract]. *Am J Hum Genet* **63(Suppl)**:A7, 1998.

359. Favor J, Sandulache R, Neuhauser-Klaus A, Pretsch W, Chatterjee B, Senft E, Wurst W, et al: The mouse *Pax2(Neu)* mutation is identical to a human *PAX2* mutation in a family with renal-coloboma syndrome and results in developmental defects of the brain, ear eye, and kidney. *Proc Natl Acad Sci U S A* **93**:13870, 1996.

360. Torres M, Gomez-Pardo E Gruss P: *Pax2* contributes to inner ear patterning and optic nerve trajectory. *Development* **122**:3381, 1996.

361. Torres M, Gomez-Pardo E, Dressler G, Gruss P: *Pax-2* contols multiple steps of urogenital development. *Development* **121**:4057, 1995.

362. Pritchard-Jones K, Fleming S, Davidson D, Bickmore W, Porteous D, Gosden C, Bard J, et al: The candidate Wilms' tumour gene is involved in genitourinary development. *Nature* **346**:194, 1990.

363. Dehbi M, Ghahremani M, Lechner M, Dressler G, Pelletier J: The paired-box transcription factor PAX2 positively modulates expression of the Wilms' tumor suppressor gene (WT1). *Oncogene* **13**:447, 1996.

364. McConnell MJ, Cunliffe HE, Chua LJ, Ward TA, Eccles MR: Differential regulation of the human Wilms tumour suppressor gene (*WT1*) promoter by two isoforms of PAX2. *Oncogene* **14**:2689, 1997.

365. Stayner CK, Cunliffe HE, Ward TA, Eccles MR: Cloning and characterization of the human *PAX2* promoter. *J Biol Chem* **273**:25472, 1998.

366. Song D-L, Chalepakis G, Gruss P, Joyner AL: Two Pax-binding sites are required for early embryonic brain expression of an Engrailed-2 transgene. *Development* **122**:627, 1996.

367. Schimmenti LA, Shim HH, Wirtschafter JD, Panzarino VA, Kashtan CE, Kirkpatrick SJ, Wargowski DS, et al: Homonucleotide expansion and contraction mutations of *PAX2* and inclusion of Chiari 1 malformation as part of Renal-Coloboma syndrome. *Hum Mutat* **14**:369, 1999.

368. Narahara K, BakerE, Ito S, Yokoyama Y, Yu S, Hewitt D, Sutherland GR, et al: Localisation of a 10q breakpoint within the *PAX2* gene in a patient with a *de novo* t(10;13) translocation and optic nerve coloboma-renal disease. *J Med Genet* **34**:213, 1997.

369. Choi KL, McNoe LA, French MC, Guilford PJ, Eccles MR: Absence of *PAX2* gene mutations in patients with primary familial vesicoureteric reflux. *J Med Genet* **35**:338, 1998.

370. Cunliffe HE, McNoe LA, Ward TA, Devriendt K, Brunner HG, Eccles MR: The prevalence of PAX2 mutations in patients with isolated colobomas or colobomas associated with urogenital anomalies. *J Med Genet* **35**:806, 1998.

371. Kelley MW, Turner JK, Reh TA: Retinoic acid promotes differentiation of photoreceptors *in vitro*. *Development* **120**:2091, 1994.

372. Otteson DC, Shelden E, Jones JM, Kameoka J, Hitchcock PF: *Pax2* expression and retinal morphogenesis in the normal and *Krd* mouse. *Dev Biol* **193**:209, 1998.

373. Green DG, Kapousta-Bruneau RV, Hitchcock PF, Keller SA: Electrophysiology and density of retinal neurons in mice with a mutation that includes the *Pax2* locus. *Invest Ophthalmol Vis Sci* **38**:919, 1997.

374. Macdonald R, Scholes J, Strahle U, Brennan C, Holder R, Brand M, Wilson SW: The Pax protein Noi is required for commissural axon pathway formation in the rostral forebrain. *Development* **124**:2397, 1997.

375. Krauss S, Maden M, Holder R, Wilson SW: Zebra fish *pax[b]* is involved in the formation of the midbrain-hindbrain boundary. *Nature* **360**:87, 1992.

376. Rebagliati MR, Toyama R, Haffter P, Dawid IB: *Cyclops* encodes a nodal-related factor involved in midline signaling. *Proc Natl Acad Sci U S A* **95**: 1998.

377. Fu W, Hong D, Frei E, Noll M: *shaven* and *sparkling* are mutations in separate enhancers of the *Drosophila* Pax2 homolog. *Development* **125**:2943, 1998.

378. Kavaler J, Fu W, Duan H, Noll M, Posakony JW: An essential role for the *Drosophila* Pax2 homolog in the differentiation of adult sensory organs. *Development* **126**:2261, 1999.

379. Chamberlin H, Palmer RE, Newman AP, Sternberg PW, Baillie DL, Thomas JH: The PAX gene *egl-38* mediates developmental patterning in *Caenorhabditis elegans*. *Development* **124**:3919, 1997.

380. Hoyt WF, Kaplan SL, Grumbach MM, Glaser JS: Septo-optic dysplasia and pituitary dwarfism. *Lancet* **1**:893, 1970.

381. Brook CG, Sanders MD, Hoare RD: Septo-optic dysplasia. *BMJ* **3**:811, 1972.

382. Rush JA, Bajandas FJ: Septo-optic dysplasia (de Morsier syndrome). *Am J Ophthalmol* **86**:202, 1978.

383. Willnow S, Kiess W, Butenandt O, Dorr HG, Enders A, Strasser-Vogel B, Egger J, et al: Endocrine disorders in septo-optic dysplasia (De Morsier syndrome) — Evaluation and follow up of 18 patients. *Eur J Pediatr* **155**:179, 1996.

384. Benner JD, Preslan MW, Gratz E, Joslyn J, Schwartz M, Kelman S: Septo-optic dysplasia in two siblings. *Am J Ophthal* **109**:632, 1990.

385. Wales JKH, Quarrell OWJ: Evidence for possible Mendelian inheritance of septo-optic dysplasia. *Acta Paediatr* **85**:391, 1996.

386. Dattani MT, Martinez-Barbera J-P, Thomas PQ, Brickman JM, Gupta R, Martensson I-L, Toresson H, et al: Mutations in the homeobox gene HESX1/Hesx1 associated with septo-optic dysplasia in human and mouse. *Nat Genet* **19**:125, 1998.

387. Thomas PQ, Rathjen PD: *HES-1*, a novel homeobox gene expressed by murine embryonic stem cells, identifies a new class of homeobox genes. *Nucleic Acids Res* **20**:5840, 1992.

388. Webb GC, Thomas PQ, Ford JH, Rathjen PD: *Hesx1*, a homeobox gene expressed by murine embryonic stem cells, maps to mouse chromosome 14, bands A3-B. *Genomics* **18**:464, 1993.

389. Hermesz E, Mackem S, Mahon KA: *Rpx*: A novel anterior-restricted homeobox gene progressively activated in the prechordal plate, anterior neural plate and Rathke's pouch of the mouse embryo. *Development* **122**:41, 1996.

390. Thomas PQ, Johnson BV, Rathjen J, Rathjen PD: Sequence, genomic organization, and expression of the novel homeobox gene *Hesx1*. *J Biol Chem* **270**:3869, 1995.

391. Sornson MW, Wu W, Dasen JS, Flynn SE, Norman DJ, O'Connell SM, Gukovsky I, et al: Pituitary lineage determination by the *Prophet of Pit-1* homeodomain factor defective in Ames dwarfism. *Nature* **384**:327, 1996.

392. Kissinger CR, Liu BS, Martin-Blanco E, Kornberg TB, Pabo CO: Crystal structure of an engrailed homeodomain-DNA complex at 2.8Å resolution: A framework for understanding homeodomain-DNA interactions. *Cell* **63**:579, 1990.

393. Young RW: Shedding of discs from rod outer segments in the rhesus monkey. *J Ultrastruct Res* **34**:190, 1971.

394. Furukawa T, Morrow EM, Li T, Davis FC, Cepko CL: Retinopathy and attenuated circadian entrainment in Crx-deficient mice. *Nat Genet* **23**:466, 1999.

395. Foxman SG, Heckenlively JR, Bateman B, Wirtschafter JD: Classification of congenital and early onset retinitis pigmentosa. *Arch Ophthalmol* **103**:1502, 1985.

396. Noble KG, Carr RE: Leber's congenital amaurosis: A retrospective study of 33 cases and a histopathological study of one case. *Arch Ophthalmol* **96**:818, 1978.

397. Fulton AB, Hansen RM, Mayer DL: Vision in Leber congenital amaurosis. *Arch Ophthalmol* **114**:698, 1996.

398. Heher KL, Traboulsi EI, Maumenee IH: The natural history of Leber's congenital amaurosis. *Ophthalmology* **99**:241, 1992.

399. Freund CL, Wang, Q-L, Chen S, Muskat BL, Wiles CD, Sheffield VC, Jacobson SG, et al: De Novo mutations in the *CRX* homeobox gene associated with Leber congenital amaurosis. *Nat Genet* **18**:311, 1998.

400. Swaroop A, Wang QL, Wu W, Cook J, Coats C, Xu S, Chen S, et al: Leber congenital amaurosis caused by a homozygous mutation (R90W) in the homeodomain of the retinal transcription factor CRX: Direct evidence for the involvement of CRX in the development of photoreceptor function. *Hum Mol Genet* **8**:299, 1999.

401. Evans K, Duvall-Young J, Fitzke FW, Arden GB, Bhattacharya SS, Bird AC: Chromosome 19q cone-rod retinal dystrophy: ocular phenotype. *Arch. Ophthalmol.* **113**:195, 1995.

402. Szylyk JP, Fishman GA, Alexander KR, Peachey RS, Derlacki DJ: Clinical subtypes of cone-rod dystrophy. *Arch Ophthalmol* **111**:781, 1993.

403. Yagasaki K, Jacobson SG: Cone-rod dystrophy: Phenotypic diversity by retinal function testing. *Arch Ophthalmol* **107**:701, 1989.

404. Bird AC: Retinal photoreceptor dystrophies: Ll. Edward Jackson memorial lecture. *Am J Ophthalmol* **119**:543, 1995.

405. Chen S, Wang QL, Nie Z, Sun H, Lennon G, Copeland RG, Gilbert DJ, et al: Crx, a novel Otx-like paired-homeodomain protein, binds to and transactivates photoreceptor cell-specific genes. *Neuron* **19**:1017, 1997.

406. Finkelstein R, Smouse D, Capaci TM, Spradling AC, Perrimon R: The *orthodenticle* gene encodes a novel homeodomain protein involved in the development of Drosophila nervous system and ocellar visual structures. *Genes Dev* **4**:1516, 1990.

407. Jacobson SG, Cideciyan AV, Huang Y, Hanna DB, Freund CL, Affatigato LM, Carr RE, et al: Retinal degenerations with truncation mutations in the cone-rod homeobox (*CRX*) gene. *Invest Ophthalmol Vis Sci* **39**:2417, 1998.

408. Humphries MM, Rancourt D, Farrar GJ, Kenna P, Hazel M, Bush RA, Sieving PA, et al: Retinopathy induced in mice by targeted disruption of the rhodopsin gene. *Nat Genet* **15**:216, 1997.

409. Bessant DA, Payne AM, Mitton KP, Wang QL, Swain PK, Plant C, Bird AC, et al: A mutation in NRL is associated with autosomal dominant retinitis pigmentosa. *Nat Genet* **21**:355, 1999.

410. Kerppola TK, Curran T: Maf and Nrl can bind to AP-1 sites and form heterodimers with Fos and Jun. *Oncogene* **9**:675, 1994.

411. Farjo Q, Jackson AU, Xu J, Gryzenia M, Skolnick C, Agarwal R, Swaroop A: Molecular characterization of the murine neural retina leucine zipper gene, NRL. *Genomics* **18**:216, 1993.

412. Yang-Feng TL, Swaroop A: Neural retina-specific leucine zipper gene NRL (D14S46E) maps to human chromosome 14q11.1-q11.2. *Genomics* **14**:491, 1992.

413. He L, Campbell ML, Srivastava D, Blocker YS, Harris JR, Swaroop A, Fox DA: Spatial and temporal expression of AP-1 responsive rod photoreceptor genes and bZIP transcription factors during development of the rat retina. *Mol Vis* **4**:32, 1998.

414. Kataoka K, Makoto R, Nishizawa M: Maf nuclear oncoprotein recognizes sequences related to an AP-1 site and forms heterodimers with both Fos and Jun. *Mol Cell Biol* **14**:700, 1994.

415. Kerppola TK, Curran T: A conserved region adjacent to the basic domain is required for recognition of an extended DNA binding site by Maf/Nrl family proteins. *Oncogene* **9**:3149, 1994.

416. Nathans J, Hogness DS: Isolation and nucleotide sequence of the gene encoding human rhodopsin. *Proc Natl Acad Sci U S A* **81**:4851, 1984.

417. Rehemtulla A, Warwar R, Kumar R, Ji X, Zack DJ, Swaroop A: Thebasic motif-leucine zipper transcription factor Nrl can positively regulate rhodopsin gene expression. *Proc Natl Acad Sci U S A* **93**:191, 1996.

418. Farjo Q, Jackson A, Pieke-Dahl S, Scott K, Kimberling WJ, Sieving PA, Richards JE, et al: Human bZIP transcription factor gene NRL: Structure, genomic sequence, and fine linkage mapping at 14q11.2 and negative mutation analysis in patients with retinal degeneration. *Genomics* **45**:395, 1997.

419. Olsson JE, Gordon JW, Pawlyk BS, Roof D, Hayes A, Molday RS, Mukai S, et al: Transgenic mice with a rhodopsin mutation (Pro23His): A mouse model of autosomal dominant retinitis pigmentosa. *Neuron* **9**:815, 1992.

420. Kumar J, Moses K: Transcription factors in eye development: A gorgeous mosaic? *Genes Dev* **11**:2023, 1997.

421. Treisman J: A conserved blueprint for the eye. *Bioessays* **21**:843, 1999.

422. Horsford DJ, McInnes RR: Personal communication.

# Molecular Biology and Inherited Disorders of the Eye Lens

## J. F. Hejtmancik ■ M. I. Kaiser ■ Joram Piatigorsky

1. Cells of the eye lens are derived from the surface ectoderm and consist of a single cell type which, as they differentiate into fiber cells, lose their protein synthetic capabilities. In addition to cytoskeletal and membrane components, lens cells contain large amounts of structural proteins called *crystallins*. Because proteins in the lens nucleus cannot be replaced, they must be stable in the face of oxidative and ultraviolet insults.

2. Lens crystallins, which are structural proteins contributing to lens transparency, comprise more than 90 percent of the soluble protein. Lenses of most species contain α-, β-, and γ-crystallins, also called *ubiquitous crystallins*. α-Crystallins are heat-shock proteins also found in a variety of nonlens tissues. In addition to their refractive roles, the α-crystallins serve as molecular chaperones to prevent protein aggregation resulting from oxidative stress and thus protect the lens from cataract. The β- and γ-crystallins belong to a superfamily with the microbial stress proteins.

3. In addition to the ubiquitous crystallins, there are also proteins called *taxon-specific crystallins*, which occur at a high concentration in the lens but are present only in selected species. Many of the taxon-specific crystallins function as enzymes in nonlens tissues, where they are expressed at low concentrations. These enzyme crystallins seem to have arisen by a process called *gene sharing*, in which a single gene may acquire more than one function in several tissues.

4. One requirement for a protein to function as a crystallin is the ability for it to be expressed at high levels in the lens. Transcriptional regulation, which is accomplished through a complex combination of cis and trans regulatory elements, appears to be very important for the high expression of crystallins in the lens.

5. Lens transparency also requires maintenance of a reduced state to minimize oxidative damage to crystallins and other proteins over their long lifetimes. To do this, the lens uses multiple mechanisms. The glutathione redox cycle is especially important. In addition, osmotic balance is critical for lens transparency, and the lens accomplishes this by a combination of active transport by the anterior cuboidal epithelia and an extensive array of communicating channels connecting lens fiber cells.

6. Animal models for human cataracts have contributed a great deal to our knowledge of this disease. They show that mutations in genes encoding lens crystallins, including βB2-crystallin, γ-crystallins, and ζ-crystallin, and proteins necessary for cellular homeostasis, especially intercellular communication and membrane proteins, including MP26 and MP19, can lead to cataracts. In addition, mice in which homologous recombination has been used to inactivate a number of genes including αA-crystallin, osteonectin, connexin43, and connexin46, develop cataract.

7. In humans, many genes appear to be able to cause cataracts. Linkage studies have implicated multiple loci in cataractogenesis, and mutations in candidate genes at linked loci, including αC-crystallin, αD-crystallin, βB2-crystallin, βA3-crystallin, αA-crystallin, phakinen, MIP, connexin46, and connexin50, have been associated with human cataracts. In addition, cataracts can occur as part of many inherited and chromosomal syndromes.

The eye lens transmits and focuses light onto the retina. Containing perhaps the highest concentration of proteins found in any tissue, the lens has been studied intensively for over a century. In 1833, Sir David Brewster deduced the fine structure of the cod lens, calculating that it contained 5 million fiber cells, each 4.8 mm, using only a candle and a finely ruled steel bar.[1] Study of lens biochemistry began in 1894 when Mörner described the high concentrations of heterogeneous structural proteins now known as *crystallins*.[2] A cataract locus was among the first autosomal loci to be mapped.[3] Thus the lens has served as a model system for the advancement of developmental and structural biology, as well as playing an important role in inherited diseases.

## BIOLOGY OF THE LENS

At birth, the human lens weighs about 65 mg, increasing to about 160 mg in the first decade of life and to about 250 mg by 90 years of age.[4] In the crystallin lens, the proteins may reach 60 percent of the total tissue weight.[5]

### Development

The human lens can first be detected at 3 to 4 weeks of gestation, in the 4-mm embryo.[6] It is derived from surface ectoderm that begins to thicken and forms the lens placode; then it invaginates toward the developing optic cup to form the lens pit. The lens pit closes, and the resulting lens vesicle is pinched off from surface ectoderm.[6] Cells along the posterior layer of the optic vesicle elongate to fill the vesicle by the seventh week of development and become primary fiber cells. These eventually will become the embryonic lens nucleus (the central nonnucleated fiber cells),[6] while the remaining cells become the cuboidal anterior epithelium, some of which will divide and differentiate to become secondary fibers[7] (Fig. 241-1). While the developmental control of lens

A list of standard abbreviations is located immediately preceding the index in each volume. Nonstandard abbreviations used in this chapter include: GFAP = glialfibrillary acidic protein.

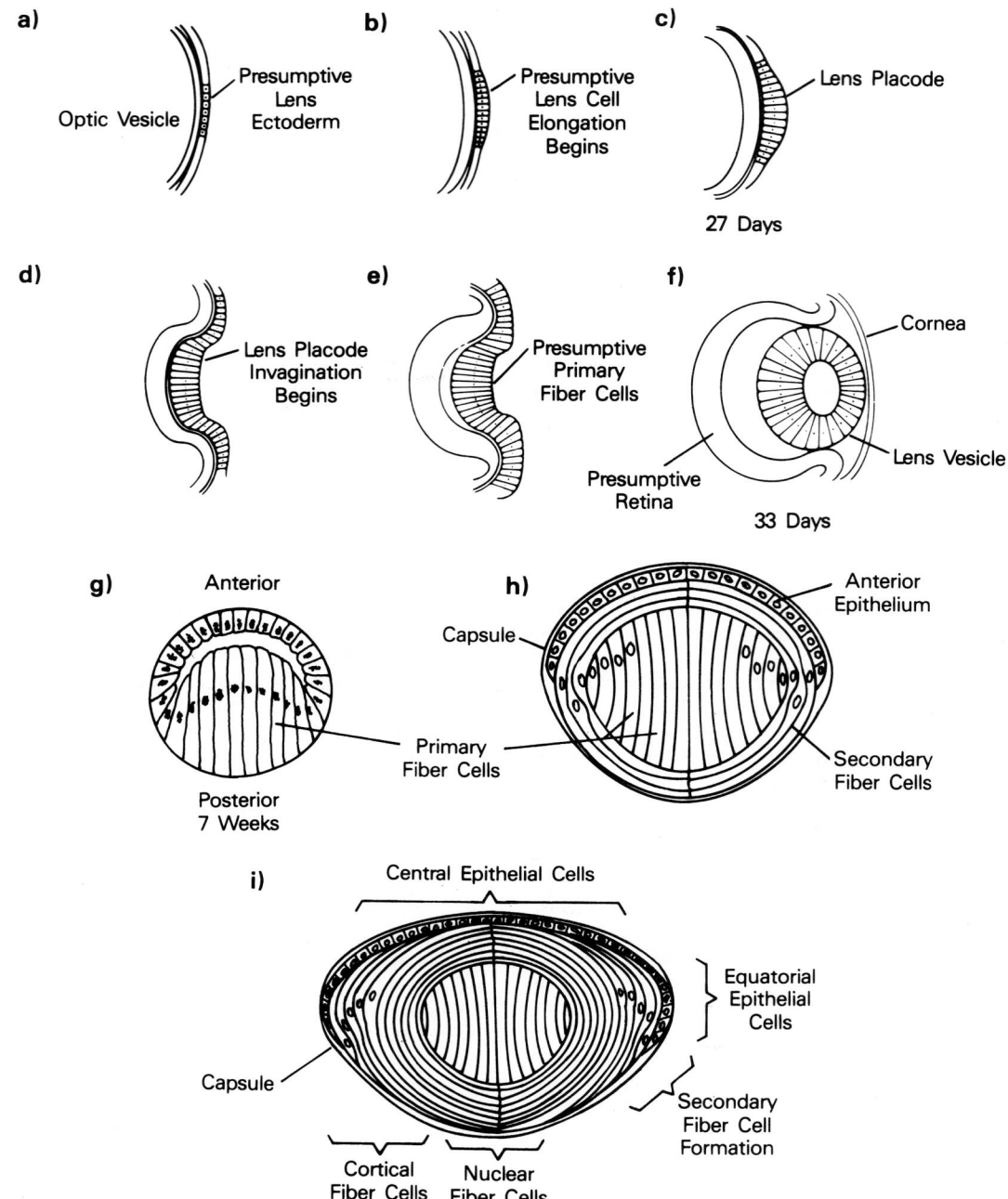

**Fig. 241-1 Development and structure of the crystallin lens. Some parts of this figure are adapted from Fig. 1 of Piatigorsky,[14] indicating the conservation of developmental processes in the eye lens.**

differentiation is just beginning to be understood, *Pax-6* seems to be essential for lens development from the earliest stages,[8–11] and *six3*, a vertebrate homologue of the *Drosophila* sine-oculis gene, can induce lens formation as well.[12] Targeted deletion of *Sox1* results in microphthalmia and cataract with failure of lens fiber cells to elongate.[13]

The lens is surrounded by a collagenous capsule throughout life. The basal poles of the epithelial cells face anteriorly, resting on this capsule, whereas those of the fiber cells face posteriorly.[7] The epithelial cells are connected by gap junctions,[15] allowing exchange of low-molecular-weight metabolites and ions, but have few or no tight junctions (zonula occludens) that would seal the extracellular spaces to low-molecular-weight proteins and ions.[16,17] Ultrastructurally, anterior cuboidal epithelial cells are

rich in organelles and contain large amounts of actin, myosin, vimentin, microtubules, spectrin, and α-actinin, presumably to stabilize them during accommodation.[18–20] Both the anterior epithelial cells and fiber cells contain large amounts of crystallins.

Fiber cells make up the bulk of the lens. Nucleated fiber cells form a highly ordered concentric shell around the nonnucleated central fiber cells that make up the lens nucleus. There is little extracellular space between the fiber cells, which have many interdigitations.[7,21] Adjacent fiber cells are connected by many junctional complexes, which allow for passage of metabolites between cells.[19,20] The major soluble components of fiber cells are the lens crystallins, which make up about 90 percent of the water-soluble protein, and cytoskeletal components, including actin, myosin, vimentin, α-actinin, and microtubules.[22]

The lens has a single cell type that follows a regular developmental pattern throughout life, resulting in the lens architecture described earlier with a single layer of anterior epithelial cells overlaying the fiber cells wrapped onionlike around the lens nucleus.[21] There is a germinative zone just anterior to the equator, where most mitotic division occurs. The cells then move laterally toward the equator, where the anterior epithelial cells begin to form secondary fibers. The density of organelles, including the mitochondria, Golgi bodies, and both rough and smooth endoplasmic reticulum, decreases in differentiating lens fiber cells. As the cells elongate, they move toward the lens nucleus, inserting anteriorly beneath the cuboidal epithelial cells and posteriorly below the posterior capsule. During this process, it seems clear that transcriptional control plays a significant role in the differential synthesis of lens crystallins (see ref. [23]). The distribution of the $\beta$-crystallins in chickens[24,25] and the $\beta$- and $\gamma$-crystallins in rats[26,27] provides examples of the spatial and temporal control of crystallin gene expression during lens development.

The lens is surrounded by a transparent basement membrane called the *lens capsule*[28] that contributes to shaping the lens during accommodation.[29,30] The major components of the lens capsule are type IV collagen, laminin, entactin, heparin sulfate proteoglycan, and fibronectin.[31,32] The capsule has a uniform parallel alignment of filaments of varying thickness.[32] The lens capsule is produced anteriorly by the cuboidal epithelium and posteriorly by the fiber cells.[28] Growth of the capsule is slower at the posterior surface, where it remains thinner. In humans, the capsule is first detectable at 5 to 6 weeks of gestation[6] and continues to thicken throughout life.[30]

## Aging

The lens is susceptible to damage with aging because its cells cannot be replaced in this encapsulated tissue and its proteins cannot turn over in the nonnucleated fiber cells. Not only does this result in a decrease in function of the normal aged lens, but it also sets the stage for development of senescent cataract in individuals with additional environmental insult or genetic proclivity. As the lens ages, vacuoles and multilamellar bodies appear between fiber cells, and occasionally, the fiber plasma membrane is disrupted.[33] Most of the elaborate cytoskeletal structure of the lens cells disappears with aging,[34] and by the fifth decade, the ability to accommodate is essentially lost.[35,36] There is a decrease in transparency of the normal lens with aging so that the intensity of light reaching the retina is reduced by about tenfold by 80 years of age.[37]

Enzymatic activity in the lens tends to decrease with age and to be lower in the central cells of the lens nucleus than in the cortical and anterior epithelial cells.[38] As the lens ages, the Na+ and Ca2+ concentrations rise, reflecting an increase in lens permeability or a decrease in pumping efficiency.[37] The crystallins also show age-related changes. There is an increase in high-molecular-weight aggregates and water-insoluble protein between 10 and 50 years of age, especially in the $\alpha$-crystallins but also in the $\beta$- and $\gamma$-crystallins.[39,40] There is also partial degradation of $\beta$-crystallins, membranes, and enzymes. An example is the nonenzymatic cleavage of $\alpha$A-crystallin between Asn 101 and Glu 102.[41] With aging, both the N- and C-terminal arms of half the intrinsic membrane protein (MP26) molecules undergo proteolysis to form MP22.[42] The lens contains neutral proteinase, also called the *multicatalytic-proteinase complex*, that preferentially degrades oxidized proteins,[43] leucine aminopeptidase,[44] calpains,[45] and the protease cofactor ubiquitin,[46] whose activation increases after oxidative stress.[47] The activity of these proteinases is controlled by inhibitors that appear to be concentrated at the periphery of the lens.

Aging also leads to covalent modifications of crystallins and other lens proteins, including an increase in disulfide bridges, deamidation of asparagine and glutamine residues,[44] and racemization of aspartic acid residues.[48] An aspartate residue in $\alpha$A-crystallin appears especially susceptible because it easily forms a succinimide intermediate.[49] This may be associated with the nonenzymatic cleavage of $\alpha$-crystallin mentioned earlier. Phosphorylation of lens proteins also occurs.[41,50] Nonenzymatic glycosylation (glycation) occurs, especially of the $\varepsilon$-amino groups of lysine.[51] Through the Maillard reaction, the glycation products can result in increased pigmentation, nontryptophan fluorescence, and nondisulfide covalent crosslinks.[52] Lens proteins also can undergo carbamylation, which can induce cataract,[53] and may be the mechanism for the association of cataract with chronic diarrhea and uremia.[54] $\gamma$-Crystallins, and especially $\gamma$S-crystallin, are particularly susceptible to degradation and modification in age-dependent and other cataracts, largely being degraded to low-molecular-weight peptides by increased proteolysis in the cataractous lens.[44,55-58]

## Transparency

The main functions of the lens are to transmit and focus light on the retina. In fact, about 80 percent of the refraction is performed by the cornea, and the lens serves to fine-tune the focusing onto the retina. The young human lens is colorless, although a gradual increase in yellow pigmentation occurs with age.[59] The lens transmits very little light below 390 nm but transmits light with wavelengths up to 1200 nm efficiently. This is well above the limit of visual perception (about 720 nm). Lens transparency results from tight packing of the proteins, resulting in a constant refractive index over distances approximating the wavelength of light.[60,61] As the proteins are diluted to concentrations below 450 mg/ml, light scattering by lens proteins actually increases.[62,63] In addition, there is a gradual increase in the refractive index of the human lens from the cortex (1.38, 73–80 percent $H_2O$) to the nucleus (1.41, 68 percent $H_2O$), where there is an enrichment of tightly packed $\gamma$-crystallins.

## MOLECULAR BIOLOGY OF THE LENS CRYSTALLINS

Crystallins make up more than 90 percent of the water-soluble protein and are critical to lens function. They are most simply defined as proteins that are found in high concentration in the lens, fulfilling a structural role for transparency and refraction.[5] In 1894, Mörner first separated bovine lens proteins into three soluble fractions and one insoluble fraction.[2] The soluble fractions comprised the $\alpha$-, $\beta$-, and $\gamma$-crystallins found in all vertebrate lenses. In the mature human lens, $\alpha$-crystallin makes up 40 percent; $\beta$-crystallin, 35 percent; and $\gamma$-crystallin, 25 percent of total crystallin protein. The $\beta$- and $\gamma$-crystallins show sequence and tertiary structure homology and form the $\beta\gamma$ superfamily (see below).

### $\alpha$-Crystallins

The $\alpha$-crystallins are products of two similar genes, $\alpha$A and $\alpha$B. Human $\alpha$A- and $\alpha$B-crystallins have a 57 percent sequence similarity,[64-66] with $\alpha$A-crystallin containing 173 and $\alpha$B-crystallin 175 residues. Circular dichroism studies suggest that in solution, $\alpha$-crystallins have a predominantly $\beta$-sheet structure.[67] Native $\alpha$-crystallins exist in the lens as globular aggregates ranging from 300 to 1200 kDa. Two models have been proposed to explain $\alpha$-crystallin quaternary structure. The first suggests that the $\alpha$-crystallin monomers are arranged in three concentric layers with $\alpha$A-crystallin innermost and mixtures of $\alpha$A- and $\alpha$B-crystallins in the outer two layers.[68] A second model proposes that the $\alpha$-crystallin aggregate behaves as a protein micelle.[69,70] The latter model seems more likely now, since it can be shown that $\alpha$A and $\alpha$B occupy equivalent and dynamic positions in the aggregate, with subunit exchange occurring easily.[70-73] Cryoelectron microscopy has shown that recombinant $\alpha$B-crystallin has a hollow central core surrounded by a protein shell with variable monomer packing.[74] Although $\alpha$A-, $\alpha$B-, and even $\alpha$A$_{ins}$-crystallins appear to occupy equivalent positions in the $\alpha$-crystallin aggregate,[70,71] they are expressed in different tissues, have radically different effects in knockout mice,[75,76] and differ in their phosphorylation,[77,78] structural properties,[79] and chaperone functions,[79] suggesting that each fulfills a unique role in the lens

α-Crystallins undergo both cAMP-dependent[50,80] and CAMP-independent[77,78] phosphorylation. α-Crystallins are also dephosphorylated by an enzyme related to calcineurin that is found in lens epithelial cells and at a low level in fiber cells.[81] The biologic functions of α-crystallin phosphorylation are not known. Phosphorylation does not seem to influence the chaperone activity[82] or the inhibitory effect on in vitro assembly of glial fibrillary acidic protein and vimentin[83] of α-crystallin. Phosphorylation of α-crystallin does, however, stabilize actin filaments and prevent their depolymerization by cytochalasin.[84] The phosphorylation of αB-crystallin is stimulated by stress, including hydrogen peroxide treatment of cultured lenses[82] and heat treatment of heart and diaphragm muscle.[85] Although speculative, it is possible that phosphorylation or palmitoylation[86] of α-crystallin may modulate its association with cell membranes[87] or cytoskeletal elements[88] or may be involved in signal transduction. Phosphorylation of α-crystallins has been reviewed recently.[89]

The α-crystallins are highly conserved through evolution. For example, the average rate of evolutionary change in αA-crystallin is a low 3 replacements per 100 residues per 100 million years.[90] α-Crystallins are evolutionarily related to the small heat-shock proteins of *Drosophila*, with especially close homology in the C-terminal half.[91] There is also similarity between α-crystallins and the egg antigen P40 from *Schistosoma mansoni*.[92] Thus α-crystallins probably originated from and are members of the small heat-shock protein family.[5,93] Rodents[94–96] and some other mammals[97] have a second αA-crystallin protein containing an extra internal peptide as the result of alternative RNA splicing. The internal peptide (between amino acids 63 and 64 of the αA-crystallin chain) is encoded in a separate exon called the *insert exon*.[98] The αA_ins-polypeptide is interchangeable with the αA- and αB-polypeptides in the α-crystallin aggregate.[70] Humans do not have the αA_ins-crystallin because the insert exon in the αA-crystallin gene is not used and has been inactivated by deletion of a base pair, becoming a *pseudoexon*.[99]

The α-crystallins are not lens-specific. αB-Crystallin is found in heart, lung, brain, skeletal muscle, kidney, and retina, although at lower levels than in the lens.[100,101] In the heart, αB-crystallin is found in aggregates of 400 to 650 kDa.[102] In skeletal muscle it accumulates in response to stretching.[103] The brains of patients with Alexander disease accumulate αB-crystallin,[104] as do the brains of scrapie-infected hamsters.[105] αB-Crystallin is also relatively abundant in fibroblasts from patients with Werner syndrome.[106] αB-Crystallin is inducible by both heat[107] and osmotic shock[108] in cultured cells. αA-Crystallin has been detected immunologically at low levels in many tissues and at moderate levels in spleen and thymus.[109] In the subterranean mole rat, which has nonfunctional eyes, αA-crystallin has undergone less evolutionary drift than might be expected, presumably because of a nonlens function, although its evolutionary rate is faster in the mole rat than in species that require lens transparency for vision.[110]

Both αA- and αB-crystallin can function as molecular chaperones, in that they can protect both αβ- and α-crystallins and enzymes from thermal aggregation, although they do not cycle these proteins in the manner of true chaperones.[111,112] The chaperone function of the α-crystallins should serve to protect lens proteins from denaturing with age and probably explains their presence in nonlenticular tissues. The chaperone function of αB-crystallin is modulated by the products of common metabolic pathways such as pantethine and glutathione[113] and can be enhanced by ATP.[114] It involves the C-terminal domain of the protein.[115] The chaperone activity of α-crystallin appears to involve structural transitions resulting in the appropriate placement of hydrophobic surfaces within a multimeric molten globular state.[116] Whatever the mechanism, the chaperone function of the α-crystallins should serve to protect against cataractogenesis by

reducing the aggregation of partially denatured proteins that accumulate within the lens during aging. In addition to its chaperone ability, α-crystallin possesses autokinase activity.[77] Thus the α-crystallins can be considered as members of the enzyme-crystallins and may be involved in metabolic pathways important for the development, maintenance, or pathology of the lens and other tissues.

The structure of the duplicated αA- and αB-crystallin genes is highly conserved in all animals studied so far, except for the αA-crystallin insert exon, which is absent from some species.[5,98,117] There are three exons in both the αA- and αB-crystallin genes. When present, the insert exon of the αA gene is situated between exons 1 and 2.[95,98] The first exon codes for a twice-repeated 30-amino-acid motif, and the second and third exons contain sequences homologous to the small heat-shock proteins.[91,118] The human αA-crystallin gene maps to chromosome 21[95] and the αB-crystallin gene to chromosome 11.[119] Transcriptional activity of the αA-crystallin promoter has been studied extensively.[120] Sequences between bases −366 and +46 can initiate transcription of foreign genes introduced into transfected cells[121] and transgenic mice in a lens-specific fashion,[121,122] with bases −88 to +46 being critical.[123]

## βγ-Crystallins

The β- and γ-crystallins are antigenically distinct but are members of a related βγ-crystallin superfamily, as determined by sequence similarities of 30 percent in aligned regions[124] and by the tertiary structure of their central globular domains.[125,126] They show distinct behavior in terms of their developmental expression and the tendency of the β-crystallins to associate into macromolecular complexes.

## γ-Crystallins

The γ-crystallins have a molecular mass of about 21 kDa and show the highest symmetry of any crystallized protein, which may contribute to their high stability in the lens.[127,128] The first crystallin structure to be solved by high-resolution x-ray crystallography was γB-crystallin.[127,128] The 174 amino acids are arranged into four repeated segments called *Greek key motifs*. Each Greek key motif consists of an extremely stable, torqued β-pleated sheet resembling the characteristic pattern found on classical Greek pottery.[127] The first and second motifs are in the N-terminal domain, and the third and fourth motifs are in the C-terminal domain of the protein (Fig. 241-2). More recently, the structures of γD-, γE-, and γF-crystallin have been solved.[129,130] Their structures are similar to that of γB-crystallin.

The γ-crystallins accumulate specifically in the lens fibers and are the predominant crystallins in the lens nucleus, which maintains the highest protein concentration and is the hardest (most dehydrated) section of the lens. The γ-crystallins are abundant in almost all mammals, including humans, and species with hard lenses (such as fish and rodents) that lack the accommodative powers of the softer lenses found in birds and reptiles. Birds and reptiles, as well as other selected species throughout the vertebrates, use other proteins as their major crystallins in the lens nucleus (see below). Thus γ-crystallins appear especially adapted for high-density molecular packing.[129] γ-Crystallins can be subdivided into two groups: γABC- and γDEF-crystallins.[131,132] Proteins in the latter group have higher critical temperatures for phase separation and are largely responsible for the occurrence of the *cold cataract*,[133] a reversible opacity that occurs on cooling of the lens. This difference may relate to the use of more aminoaromatic interactions in the third motif of the high Tc proteins or a higher Arg/Lys ratio and histidine content.[130]

βγ-Crystallins appear distantly related to protein S, a sporulation-specific protein of the bacteria *Myxococcus xanthus*, to spherulin 3a of the slime mold *Physarum polycephalum*,[134] to CRBG-GEOCY of the sponge *Geodia cydonium*,[135] and to *A1M1*, a tumor-suppressor gene.[136] A computer-generated model of

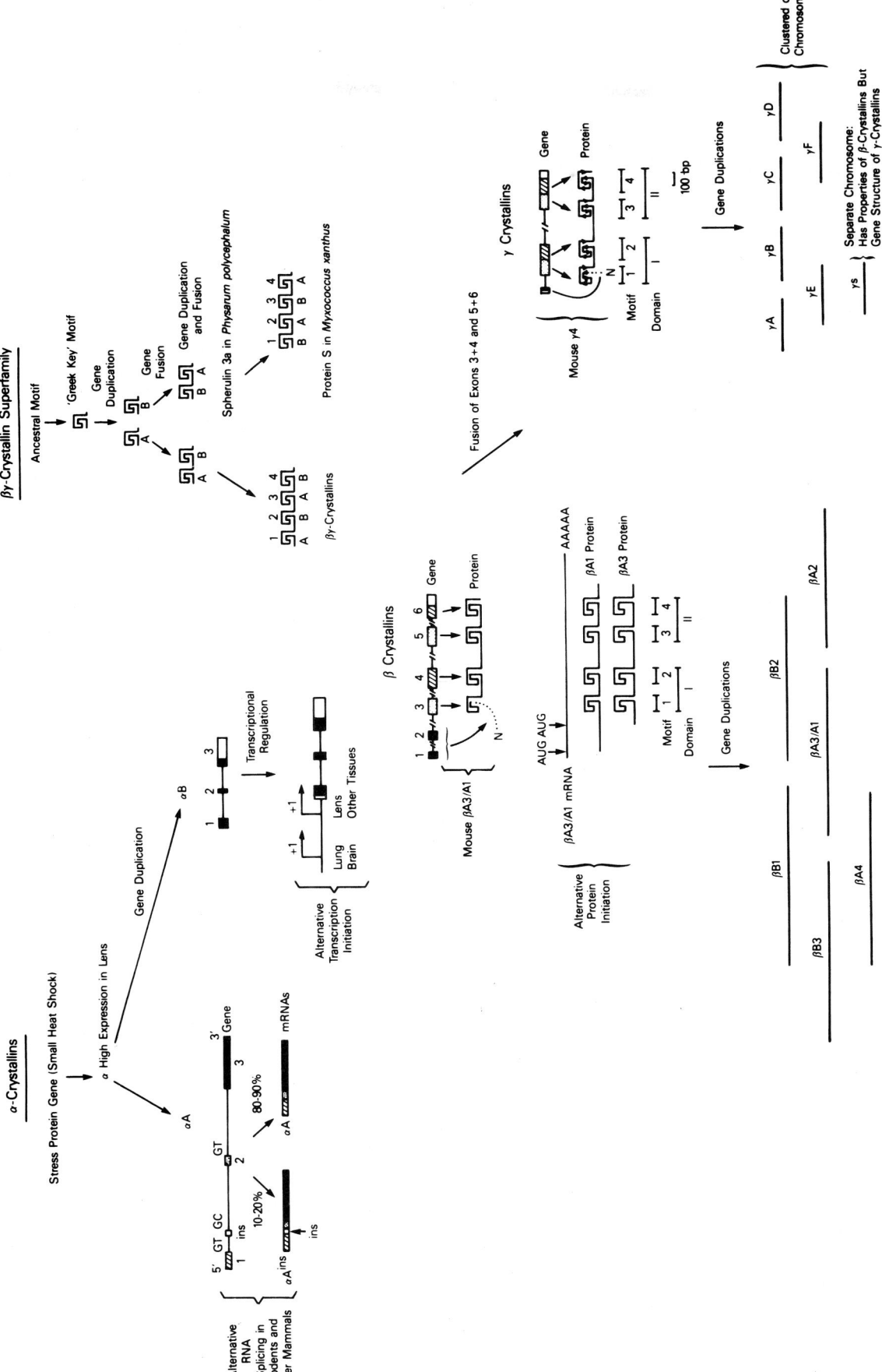

**Fig. 241-2 Evolution of the ubiquitous α-, β-, and γ-crystallins and their structure. Details are described in the text. The α-crystallins are related to heat-shock proteins; the β- and γ-crystallins form a superfamily related to stress proteins.**

spherulin 3a suggests that it can fold into two Greek key motifs. This would make it similar to a single domain of γ-crystallin, suggesting that evolution of the βγ-crystallin superfamily originated from an ancestral gene coding for a single Greek key motif which, through successive gene duplication and fusion, gave rise to the complete βγ-crystallin structure. This is consistent with the ability of the recombinant isolated C-terminal domain to form a stable dimer.[137] The order of the motifs is reversed in spherulin 3a relative to the βγ-crystallins. Protein S shows the typical fourfold repeated Greek key motifs, but as with spherulin 3a, the order of the motifs is the reverse of that in the βγ-crystallins, suggesting that divergence of these genes occurred before the initial fusion of the first two primitive motifs into a domain structure[138] (see Fig. 241-2). These microbial proteins can be induced by physiologic stresses such as osmotic stress,[134] providing a functional parallel to the α-crystallins and some taxon-specific crystallins (see below).

All γ-crystallin genes have three exons (see Fig. 241-2). The first exon encodes the 5′ noncoding region and the first three amino acids, the second exon encodes the first (N-terminal) domain consisting of the first and second Greek key motifs, and the third exon encodes the second (C-terminal) domain consisting of Greek key motifs three and four.[139,140] Six functional γ-crystallin genes have been identified in rats.[126] By contrast, only three γ-crystallin polypeptides have been identified in humans, with γE and γF being pseudogenes.[141] γC- and γD-crystallins are the primary human γ-crystallins; γA is expressed at lower levels.[142,143] The promoters of the γ-crystallins appear to be lens-specific when used in combination with reporter genes (see below)[144–147] and are activated by retinoid signaling[148,149] and by the transcription factor SOX1[13] as described below.

γS-crystallin (formerly called βs) represents a link between the β- and γ-crystallins.[150–153] Many physical and chemical properties of the γS protein resemble those of β-crystallins. γS-Crystallin is slightly larger than most γ-crystallins, having 177 residues including an N-terminal arm like the β-crystallins.[151] It also has a lower isoelectric point than most γ-crystallins, as do the β-crystallins. Moreover, in contrast to the N-termini of the other γ-crystallins, γS has a blocked N-terminus, again like the β-crystallins. In humans, the γS-crystallin gene is on chromosome 3,[154] whereas all other γ-crystallin genes are clustered on chromosome 2q33-35.[155–157] Finally, γS-crystallin is expressed later in development than the other γ-crystallins, particularly in the adult, when expression of other γ-crystallins is low or has ceased.[158] Also, γS-crystallin is expressed in birds and reptiles.[159,160] However, in contrast to the β-crystallins and like the other γ-crystallins, γS-crystallin exists in solution as a monomeric protein. It is especially important that the gene structure of γS-crystallin has three exons,[151,152] making it similar to the other γ-crystallins and distinctly different from the β-crystallins, which have six exons.[5,126]

## β-Crystallins

β-Crystallins are divided into two groups, with the βA2-, βA1/A3-, and βA4-crystallins having lower isoelectric points than the βB1-, βB2-, and βB3-crystallins.[126] The lower isoelectric group is referred to as *acidic* and the higher isoelectric group as *basic*, although the isoelectric points of both are slightly above neutral. Each is encoded by a separate gene, except for the βA3- and βA1-polypeptides, which originate from separate AUG translation initiation codons on the same mRNA[5] (see Fig. 146-2). The β-crystallin polypeptides range in size from about 23 to 32 kDa. Globular domains of β-crystallins have about 45 to 60 percent sequence similarity with each other and about 30 percent sequence similarity with globular domains of γ-crystallins.[5,161,162] The N- and C-terminal arms are much less well conserved than the globular core, usually showing about 30 percent sequence similarity to the arms of orthologous β-crystallins.[161–163] Basic β-crystallins have both N- and C-terminal arms, whereas acidic β-crystallins have only N-terminal arms. The primary structures of

many β-crystallins from cows, mice, rats, chickens, frogs, and humans have been deduced from cDNA sequences.[164] Human βA3/A1-crystallin has more than 90 percent identity with its bovine and mouse homologues.[165] The β-crystallins may undergo posttranslational modification, including proteolytic cleavage of βB1,[166] phosphorylation of βB2 and βB3,[167,168] and glycosylation of βB1.[169]

The β-crystallins associate preferentially in a paired fashion, acidic with basic into dimers of about 50 kDa, and then in a more complex fashion into larger aggregates of 150 to 200 kDa.[170] The crystal structure of βB2-crystallin has been solved to 2.1 Å resolution.[171] This β-crystallin has an extended interchain domain. The widely separated N- and C-terminal domains of one β-crystallin polypeptide are paired in an antiparallel fashion with the C- and N-terminal domains of a second β-crystallin polypeptide. In the γ-crystallins, this connecting peptide folds back on itself so that the two domains of a single molecule pair with each other.[172] Higher oligomerization of β-crystallins appears to occur by association of dimers and may require at least one protein with an N-terminal extension.[166,170] Site-specific mutagenesis has been used to substitute the γ2-crystallin connecting peptide into murine βA3-crystallin and, conversely, part of the βB2-crystallin connecting peptide into γ2-crystallin without any effect on association in either case.[173,174] Similar techniques have been used to show that although the N-terminal arm is not essential for dimerization of βA3-crystallin, it greatly facilitates association.[175] However, removal of N- and C-terminal arms of rat βB2-crystallin,[176] mutation of the specific sequence or deletion of part of the N- or C-terminal arms of chick βB1-crystallin, or deletion of the 17 amino acids differentiating rat βA3- from βA1-crystallin[177] did not alter its association properties.

β-Crystallin genes have six exons, the first one coding for the N-terminal extension and the next four for the four Greek key motifs (see Fig. 241-2). The C-terminal arm is also encoded by the sixth exon.[126,161,165,178,179] The exons encoding the first and third motifs and second and fourth motifs show especially high homology, suggesting that an intermediate step in evolution of the βγ-crystallin superfamily may have been a two-motif structure that was then reduplicated and underwent a second fusion event to create the present βγ-crystallin core structure[180] (see Fig. 241-2). In contrast to the γ-crystallins, the βA3/A1- and βA2-crystallin genes are dispersed in the species examined: Human βA3/A1 is on chromosome 17 and human βA2-crystallin is on chromosome 2 near the γ-crystallin cluster.[126,181,182] However, βB1-, βB2-, and βB3-crystalin and a pseudogene, ΨβB2-crystallin, are linked on chromosome 22,[183] representing a β-crystallin gene cluster (Table 241-1).

In a fashion similar to the α-crystallins, both the β- and γ-crystallins have been shown to be expressed in nonlens tissue. β-Crystallin mRNAs and peptides have been detected in a variety of nonlens tissues including chicken retina, cornea, brain, and kidney[184] and mouse[185,186] and cat[185,187] retina. Four γ-crystallins and βA4-crystallin were detected in nonlens tissues at various stages of *Xenopus* development.[188,189] γS-Crystallin expression has been detected in the retina and cornea of adult cow eyes and the retinas of 1-month-old mice.[190] Nonlens expression of the βγ-crystallins suggests that they may have nonrefractive functions as do the α crystallins. While this is unclear, βB2-crystallin does appear to have autokinase activity.[187]

## Taxon-Specific Crystallins

Taxon-specific crystallins are proteins that occur in the lens at a high concentration (usually 10 percent or more of the protein) but are found only in one or, more generally, a few species.[5] Many taxon-specific crystallins appear to have arisen by a process called *gene sharing*, in which a single gene product acquires an additional function without duplication, often retaining its original function in nonlens tissues.[93,191–193] When a single gene product is used for two separate functions, it becomes subject to double evolutionary selection. Gene sharing implies that a mutation in a

**Table 241-1 Chromosomal Locations of Human Ubiquitous Crystallin Genes**

| Crystallin | Chromosome |
|---|---|
| αA-Crystallin | 21q22.3 |
| αB-Crystallin | 11q22.3-q23.1 |
| βA1/A3-Crystallin | 17q11.1-q12 |
| βA2-Crystallin | 2q34-q36 |
| β-Crystallin cluster | |
| βA4-Crystallin* | 22q11.2-q12.1 |
| βB1-Crystallin* | 22q11.2-q12.1 |
| βB2-Crystallin* | 22q11.2-q12.1 |
| βB3-Crystallin* | 22q11.2-q12.1 |
| ΨβB2-Crystallin | 22q11.2-q12.1 |
| γ-Crystallin cluster | |
| γA-Crystallin† | 2q33-q35 |
| γB-Crystallin† | 2q33-q35 |
| γC-Crystallin† | 2q33-q35 |
| γD-Crystallin† | 2q33-q35 |
| ΨγE-Crystallin† | 2q33-q35 |
| ΨγF-Crystallin† | 2q33-q35 |
| ΨγG-Crystallin† | 2q33-q35 |
| γs-Crystallin | 3pter |

*Closely linked.
†Closely linked.

regulatory sequence resulting in a change in gene expression may lead to a new function for the encoded protein before or even without gene duplication and without loss of its original function. Gene duplication and specialization of function for one of the two proteins may occur later, as appears to have happened with the δ- and α-crystallins.[192] These potential evolutionary schemes are shown in Fig. 241-3.

The occurrence of gene sharing begs the question of what criteria exist for a protein to serve as a crystallin. Amazingly, almost all the known taxon-specific crystallins are either active metabolic enzymes or inactive derivatives clearly related to enzymes (Table 241-2). Thus they are generally known as *enzyme-crystallins*. Crystallins in the lens nucleus cannot be renewed during the lifetime of the individual and so must be extremely stable. Even though many proteins can serve refractive roles as crystallins, the α- and βγ-crystallins seem to be preferred, at least in vertebrates. A comparative study of the thermal stability of crystallins in four vertebrate classes indicates that the taxon-specific crystallins tend to be more labile than the ubiquitous crystallins.[194] Interestingly, many of the crystallins are related to stress proteins or detoxification enzymes[93,134,192] (see Table 241-1). In addition to being derived from detoxification enzymes, many enzyme-crystallins can bind pyridine nucleotides (NADH or NADPH), elevating the concentration of these compounds in the lens.[195,196] It has been suggested that these elevated nucleotides may stabilize the enzyme-crystallins; alternatively, they may combat oxidative stress by affecting the redox cycle in vivo or act as near-ultraviolet filters.[196] This suggests that crystallins may have been selected not only for their ability to satisfy the optical requirements for refraction but also for their ability to protect the transparent lens from long-term deterioration due to physiologic insults throughout life. Since many proteins appear able to satisfy the requirements for optical transparency, the ability of a gene to be expressed at high levels in the lens may be a particularly important criterion for recruitment as a lens crystallin.[197]

Argininosuccinate lyase/δ-crystallin, a major enzyme-crystallin confined to bird and reptile lenses, is perhaps the most intensively studied taxon-specific crystallin.[198,199] The original argininosuccinate lyase gene has been duplicated, with one copy (δ2) continuing to code for argininosuccinate lyase and the second (δ1) evolving to code for an enzymatically inactive but highly similar crystallin.[200-202] Crystallographic analyses of turkey δ1-crystallin[203] and duck mutant argininosuccinate lyase/δ2-crystallin[204] have shown a remarkable similarity between the enzymatically inactive δ1- and the active δ2-crystallin polypeptides. These studies have suggested that small structural differences in domain 1 (of three domains) in the N-terminal tail

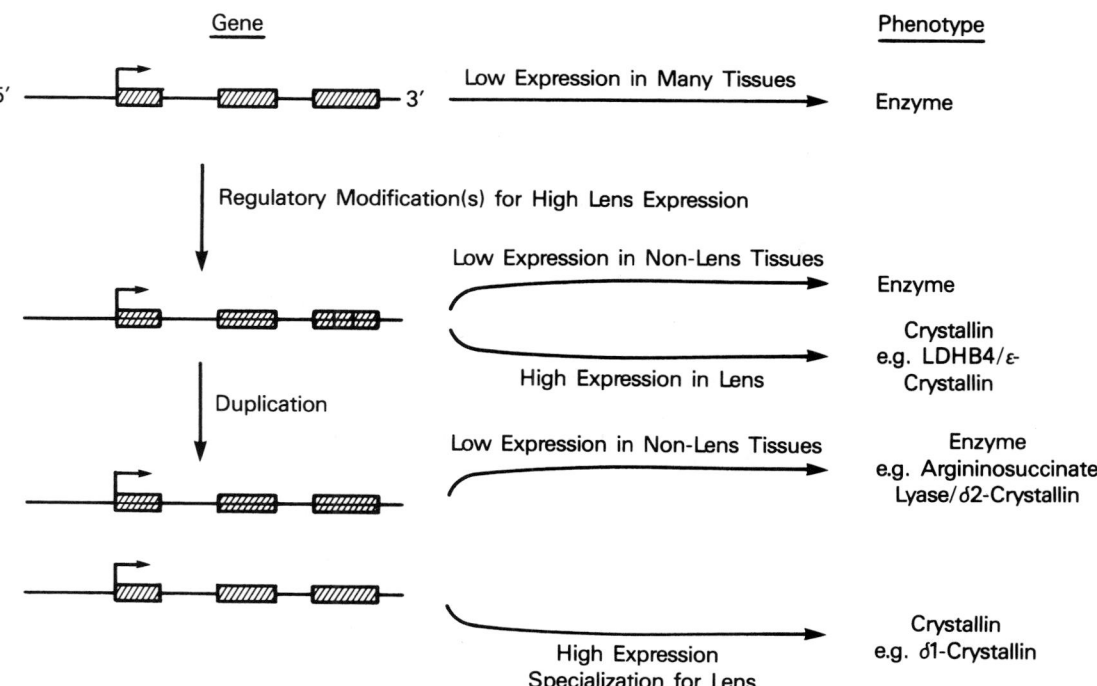

**Fig. 241-3** General evolutionary scheme for taxon-specific crystallins. High expression in the lens may occur without gene duplication or may be followed by gene duplication.

**Table 241-2** Summary of Lens Crystallin Gene Families

| Distribution | Crystallin | (Related) or Identical |
|---|---|---|
| | $\alpha$ | (Small heat-shock proteins) |
| | | (*Schistosoma mansoni* antigen p40) |
| | | $\alpha$ has nonlens expression |
| Represented in all vertebrates | | (*Myxococcus xanthus* protein S) |
| | $\beta$ | (*Physarum polycephalum* spherulin 3a) |
| | $\gamma$ | (EDSP) |
| | | (A1M1) |
| | | Some $\beta$s have nonlens expression |
| | $\delta1$ | (Argininocuccinate lyase) |
| Birds and reptiles | $\delta2$ | Argininosuccinate lyase |
| | $\epsilon$ | Lactate dehydrogenase B |
| | $\zeta$ | (NADPH:quinone reductase) |
| | $\pi$ | Glyceraldehyde-3-phosphate dehydrogenase |
| | $\iota$ | (Cellular retinol-binding protein) |
| Some mammals | $\eta$ | Cytoplasmic aldehyde dehydrogenase |
| | $\lambda$ | (Hydroxyacyl CoA dehydrogenase) |
| | $\mu$ | (Ornithine cyclodeaminase) |
| Many species | $\tau$ | $\alpha$-Enolase |
| Frogs | $\rho$ | (NADPH-dependent reductases) |
| | SL11/LOPS4 | Glutathione-S-transferase |
| Cephalopods | S | (Glutathione S-transferase) |
| | $\Omega$/L | (Aldehyde dehydrogenase) |
| Jellyfish | J | (Novel proteins) |

and the amino acid 76–91 loop are responsible for the loss of catalytic activity in the specialized $\delta1$-crystallin protein and that the loss of enzymatic activity in $\delta1$-crystallin is due to its inability to bind substrate.

In other enzyme crystallins, no gene duplication has occurred, and the same gene codes for both the enzyme and the refractive lens crystallin. For example, $\epsilon$-crystallin is identical to lactate dehydrogenase B4 (LDHB4).[205,206] Purified duck $\epsilon$-crystallin has a specific activity at least 70 percent of that of purified LDHB4 enzyme from the heart. LDHB4/$\epsilon$-crystallin comprises 10 percent of duck lens protein, far beyond that needed for enzymatic activity. $\zeta$-Crystallin in the guinea pig is another enzyme-crystallin that is encoded in a single-copy gene. It is structurally related to the alcohol dehydrogenases[207] and has quinone oxidoreductase activity.[208] $\zeta$-Crystallin is one of the enzyme-crystallins that binds reduced nucleotides and is associated with high levels of these cofactors in the lens, possibly providing some protection against oxidative stress.[195] $\eta$-Crystallin of elephant shrews[209] is an interesting case of an enzyme, cytosolic aldehyde dehydrogenase 1 (ALDH1), that has undergone gene duplication, with the two daughter genes following different expression patterns. One of the genes, ALDH1/$\eta$-crystallin, became highly specialized for lens expression and also was collaterally recruited to be the major form of ALDH1 present in other eye tissues. The other daughter gene, ALDH-nl (for nonlens), is the predominant form of ALDH1 expressed in the liver of the elephant shrew.[210] ALDH1/$\eta$-crystallin has retinaldehyde dehydrogenase activity. Some enzyme-crystallins appear enzymatically inactive and have not been associated with a specific, enzymatically active daughter

gene with a different expression pattern. Two examples are $\lambda$-crystallin/hydroxyl CoA dehydrogenase in rabbits[211] and $\rho$-crystallin/NADPH-dependent reductase in frogs.[212] To date, related enzymes have been identified for all taxon-specific crystallins except the J1-crystallins in the jellyfish lens.[213] Recent reviews of enzyme-crystallins are available.[193,213]

## Crystallin Gene Regulation

The refractive properties of the lens depend on concentrations and distributions of crystallins within the lens, which in turn depend on the precise temporal and spatial regulation of crystallin gene expression. There is a gradient of refractive index increasing from the periphery to the center of the lens that correlates with an increasing concentration and varying composition of crystallins.[61] Thus the optical properties of the lens depend on the pattern of crystallin gene expression.

Developmental studies correlating crystallin expression with their mRNAs[14,23,25–27,214,214] and experiments with transgenic mice[123,145,146,215–217] have provided convincing evidence that transcriptional controls play a major role in the preferential expression of crystallin genes in the lens. Deletion and site-specific mutagenesis experiments have identified a number of different cis elements and enhancers used by crystallin genes for high expression in the lens.[120] Examples of cis-acting DNA sequences involved in lens expression include those for mouse $\alpha$A-[121,218–221] and $\alpha$B-,[222–225] chicken $\beta$B1-[226] and $\beta$A3A1-,[227] mouse[147,228–230] and rat[229] $\gamma$-, chicken $\delta1$-[200,231–234] and $\delta2$-[200,232] and guinea pig $\zeta$-crystallin[235] genes. In general, the high preferential expression of the crystallin genes in the lens occurs by an interaction of sequences governing lens specificity, with enhancer sequences responsible for the amount of transcription that takes place.

In addition to using multiple cis-regulatory sequences for lens expression, the present evidence suggests a corresponding diversity of trans-acting regulatory proteins. DNA-protein complexes generally observed in electrophoretic gel mobility shift experiments using crystallin regulatory sequences form with nuclear proteins derived from many tissues,[197] suggesting that ubiquitous transcription factors play an important role in crystallin gene expression. An example is $\alpha$A-CRYBP1, a putative transcription factor implicated in the control of the mouse $\alpha$A-crystallin gene (Fig. 241-4). The $\alpha$A-CRYBP1 mRNA is found in many tissues.[218] The sequence motif to which the protein binds is present in many genes and is similar to that which binds transcription factors belonging to the NF-kB/dorsal/rel family.[236] It is possible that the $\alpha$A-CRYBP1 binding protein is modified in a tissue-specific fashion, leading to a form of the protein used for preferential expression of the $\alpha$A-crystallin gene in the lens. Quantitative aspects also can be a consideration. For example, an oligonucleotide containing a single copy of the $\alpha$A-CRYBP1 gene sequence increases expression of a *Herpes simplex* thymidine kinase (tk) promoter/CAT fusion gene selectively in transfected mouse lens epithelial cells transformed with the T-antigen of SV40.[237] Multiple copies of the same sequence decrease its lens-cell preference.[237]

One of the major questions of crystallin gene expression concerns the basis for preferred, or in some cases specific, function in the lens. The diversity of sequences that control lens-specific expression in transgenic mice has frustrated early attempts to define one or more regulatory elements that are responsible for the high activity of many different crystallin genes in the lens. Recently, however, a few transcription factors that have widespread roles for directing the expression of crystallin genes to the lens have been identified. Interestingly, these transcription factors also have very important general developmental roles.

PAX-6, a protein that binds DNA via specialized structural motifs called *paired* and *homeodomains*, has been shown to be one of several[238] fundamental transcription factors for the development of eyes of both vertebrates and invertebrates.[239,240] Indeed, the importance of PAX-6 for eye development was found initially as a mutation responsible for aniridia in humans[241] and *small eye*

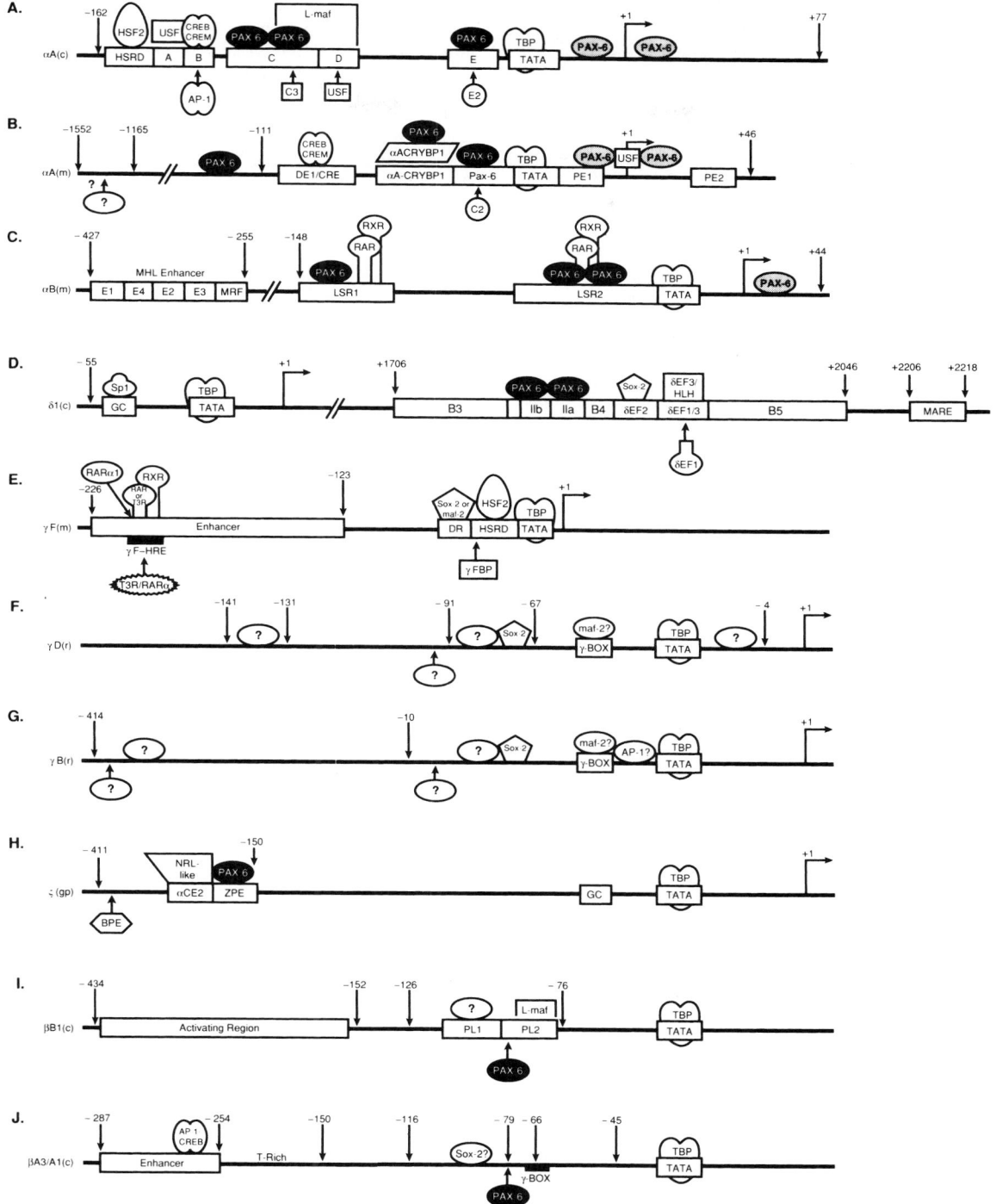

**Fig. 241-4** Diagrammatic representation of regulatory sequences associated with crystallin genes. Note that each gene has a different arrangement of elements, yet all are expressed either specifically or highly preferentially in the lens. DNA regions that bind trans-acting factors are shown in boxes, and activators (repressors) are shown above (under) the boxes, respectively. Most but not all of the PAX-6 binding sites have been tested in transfection experiments. The PAX-6 proteins whose sites have not been confirmed functionally are shaded more lightly. (*A*) Chicken αA-crystallin 5′ flanking region.[247] The αCE2[591] sequence binds L-MAF and is present in numerous crystallin genes.[255] Proteins C3 and E2 are undefined and have only been detected in gel shift assays.[247] (*B*) Mouse αA-crystallin 5′ flanking region.[219] The non-tissue-specific protein C2 binds the PAX-6 site, as does PAX-6 (*C*) Mouse αB-crystallin 5′ flanking region, which contains a muscle-heart-lens (MHL) enhancer,[223,259] as well as lens-specific regions (LSR1 and LSR2).[222,224,251] E4 is a heart-specific serum response factor-like protein-binding site, and MRF (muscle regulatory factor) binds MyoD-family members. (*D*) Chicken δ1-crystallin 5′ flanking and the enhancer in the third intron.[231,233,234,248,253] Activator δEF3 (a helix-loop-helix, HLH, protein) competes for binding with the repressor δEF1. (*E*) Mouse γF-crystallin 5′ flanking region.[148,149,228,230,253] (*F*) Rat γD-crystallin 5′ flanking region.[254] (*G*) Rat γB-crystallin 5′ flanking region.[254] (*H*) Guinea pig ζ-crystallin 5′ flanking region.[235,256] (*I*) Chicken βB1-crystallin 5′ flanking region.[215,226] (*J*) Chicken βA3/A1-crystallin 5′ flanking region.[216,227] (*Adapted with permission from Cvekl and Piatigorsky.[250]*)

in mice.[242] Later, the eyeless mutation in *Drosophila* was shown to be due to defective expression of the *Pax-6* gene.[243] Most remarkably, the *Pax-6* genes of *Drosophila*, mouse,[8] squid,[244] and ascidians[245] are able to induce ectopic eyes when expressed in imaginal discs that normally would give rise to the wing, leg, or antenna in the developing fly. *Pax-6* also can induce a lens when expressed ectopically in the ectoderm of *Xenopus* embryos.[246] In addition to this early developmental role, transfected *Pax-6* can activate the mouse[219] and chicken[247] αA-, mouse αB-,[224] chicken δ1-[248] and guinea pig ζ-crystallin[235] promoters (see Fig. 241-4). Interestingly, *Pax-6* also represses the chicken βB1-crystallin promoter by competition for the same sequence that binds a different, still undefined positive factor.[249,250] *Pax-6* and crystallin gene expression has been reviewed recently.[250]

The retinoic acid receptors (RARS) also have important roles for eye development and can activate several crystallin genes, as indicated in Fig. 241-4. Retinoid signaling was first linked with activation of the mouse γF-crystallin gene by RAR/RXR binding to a novel retinoic acid response element (γF-HRE).[148] This regulation is complex inasmuch as γF-HRE is activated by T₃R/RXR as well as RAR/RXR occupancy at the same site.[149] RARβ/RXRβ also has been shown to activate the mouse αB-crystallin promoter in cotransfection experiments by binding, along with PAX-6,[224] to the lens-specific control elements LSR1 and LSR2.[251] The chicken δ1-crystallin enhancer, located in the third intron of the gene,[234] is also activated by RARβ in contransfection experiments in the presence of retinoic acid.[232] Since the binding site for the retinoic acid receptors on the δ1-crystallin enhancer is not known, it remains possible that retinoid activation is indirect in this case. It is interesting to note that in parallel experiments, neither PAX-6 nor RARβ activated the chicken δ2-crystallin/argininosuccinate lyase enhancer,[232] consistent with the fact that this gene has a relatively low expression in the chicken lens.

SOX is another group of transcription factors that have critical roles in activating crystallin genes in the lens (see Fig. 241-4). SOX family members are related to SRY (a testis-determining protein) and have characteristic HMG boxes for DNA binding. SOX1 and 2, members of the B subfamily of these proteins,[252] can activate the chicken γ1- and mouse γF-crystallin genes[253] and the rat γB- and γD-crystallin genes.[254] The SOX proteins are expressed in numerous tissues, including the eye and central nervous system. Recently, it has been shown that mice lacking the *Sox1* gene have small eyes with opaque lenses.[13] All the γ-crystallins are downregulated and lens fiber cell elongation is impaired in these SOX1-deficient lenses. By contrast, expression of α- and β-crystallins appeared normal in *Sox1* null mice. SOX1 binds directly to a promoter sequence that is conserved in all the mouse γ-crystallin genes. Thus the SOX transcription factors appear to have a critical role in the expression of the γ-crystallin genes in mice and the δ-crystallin genes in chickens.

MAF proteins are additional transcription factors that make an important contribution to the expression of crystallin genes in the lens. The MAF proteins are grouped into large and small subclasses of bZIP proteins. A recent report has shown that L-MAF, related to the large subfamily of proteins that includes MAFB, c-MAF, and NRL, is lens-specific in chicken embryos and can activate the chicken αA-crystallin promoter by binding to an enhancer sequence called αCE2.[255] αCE2 contains a core half-site of MAF response elements (MAREs) found in other genes.[221] Other crystallin promoters (mouse αA- and γF-, chicken βB1-, and guinea pig ζ-crystallin) also have αCE2-like (MARE) sequences that can be activated in cotransfection experiments by binding MAF family members.[255,256] Although L-MAF has not been found in the rat lens, *maf-1* and *maf-2* mRNAs are temporally and spatially regulated in the lens during development, suggestive of putative roles in crystallin gene regulation.[257] Neither *maf-1* (primarily in the lens epithelia) nor *maf-2* (primarily in the lens fibers) are lens-specific; both are found in numerous tissues. The rat γD-crystallin promoter was activated approximately twofold by cotransfection with *maf-2* but not with *maf-1*.[254] Like the other

transcription factors that can activate crystallin gene expression, the MAF proteins appear to have important roles in the early development of the lens. *L-maf* is expressed already at the lens placode stage of development and can induce lens differentiation when transfected into cultured cells or when expressed ectopically in chicken embryos.[255]

In addition to being positively activated, the crystallin genes are also subject to negative regulation, as indicated by the factors shown below the genes in Fig. 241-4. Indeed, silencing of gene expression appears to play an important role in the temporal and spatial regulation of crystallin gene expression. One example is the repression of chicken βB1-crystallin promoter activity by PAX-6 mentioned earlier.[249] Composite element B of the chicken αA-crystallin promoter is an earlier example of crystallin gene repression. This cis-control element is activated by a member of the CREB/CREM family of transcription factors in the lens and is suppressed by an AP-1 family member (JunD or Fra2) in fibroblasts.[247] The regulated expression of the six rat γ-crystallin genes involves the phased appearances of transcription factors that activate followed by factors that repress promoter activity during lens fiber cell differentiation.[254] δEF1 is not confined to the lens and probably contributes to the suppression of δ1-crystallin in nonlenticular tissues.[233] BPE is a recent example of a putative silencer, not yet cloned, of the guinea pig ζ-crystallin that represses expression in the brain and thus contributes to lens specificity.[256] The rat βB2-crystallin gene is a particularly complex and interesting example of the interplay between at least two silencers in the promoter and first intron. These cooperate to create an enhancer that contributes to the lens-preferred and developmentally regulated expression of the gene.[258]

As discussed earlier, crystallins have been recruited from ubiquitously expressed proteins with nonrefractive functions and, in many cases, continue to be expressed outside the lens, performing their original roles. Thus these multifunctional crystallin genes are under complex developmental regulation in nonlens tissues as well as in the lens. αB-Crystallin has been studied most extensively with respect to nonlens expression. An enhancer that elevates gene expression in skeletal muscle, heart, lung, and other tissues, as well as in the lens, has been identified upstream of the lens-specific control regions.[259] One of the enhancer elements (αBE4, called E4 in Fig. 241-4) binds a protein immunologically related to serum response factor (SRF) and appears to confer heart-specific expression,[223] whereas another element (MRF) interacts with MyoD family members for expression in skeletal muscle.[259] The enhancer elements of αBE1, αBE2, and αBE3 (called E1, E2, and E3 in Fig. 241-4) bind unidentified proteins not yet cloned that appear to be critical for activation of the enhancer. The PAX-6 and retinoic acid receptor interactions with the proximal, lens-specific control elements LSR1 and LSR2 of the αB-crystallin promoter were described earlier.[224,251] Thus the regulated expression of the αB-crystallin gene in different tissues is governed by the interactions of shared and tissue-specific transcription factors. In addition to its constitutive expression driven by transcriptional regulation,[217] the αB-crystallin gene in different tissues is also induced by heat and other stresses[107,108] and is overexpressed in a number of systemic diseases, especially neurologic disorders.[260] The molecular mechanisms involved for induction and overexpression of the αB-crystallin gene are not yet known. It is likely that the overexpression of αB-crystallin in pathologic states is a protective response against physiologic stress.

The experiments described earlier and diagrammed in Fig. 241-4 portray the dynamism of evolution at the level of gene regulation. Clearly, the expression and function of crystallin genes did not originate in and are not limited to the lens. One of the most fascinating and important aspects of crystallin gene regulation is that the evolutionary events that led to the high expression of these multifunctional genes in the lens were intimately associated with the origin of a new function for the encoded proteins, namely, refraction. It follows that abnormal expression of these genes may affect both lens and nonlens tissues and, conversely, that defects involving the nonrefractive functions of crystallins or crystallin gene regulatory factors may cause lens abnormalities. An example of the medical importance of crystallin gene regulation is the activation of the human γE-crystallin pseudogene promoter by mutations surrounding the TATA box as a cause of the Coppock-like cataract.[261] Thus understanding crystallin gene regulation has far-reaching implications directly touching on evolution, development, gene expression, and disease.

## Membrane Proteins

Approximately 2 percent of lens proteins are membrane-associated and have molecular masses ranging from 10 to over 250 kDa. Some are components of the cytoskeletal structure, such as N-cadherin, a 135-kDa intrinsic membrane protein that may be involved in cell-cell adhesion.[262] The calpactins are extrinsic membrane proteins attached to the membrane through calcium and are probably involved in membrane-cytoskeleton interactions.[19,20] Neural cell adhesion molecule 2 (NCAM 2) has been implicated in cell adhesion and contributes to the appropriate arrangement of gap junctions in developing lens fiber cells.[263] Other membrane proteins are enzymes including glyceraldehyde-3-phosphate dehydrogenase and other glycolytic enzymes on the endoplasmic reticulum[264] and a variety of ATPases. There are also intrinsic membrane proteins specific to lens fiber cells whose function remains unknown, e.g., a 17- to 19-kDa protein.[265] A number of these proteins have been implicated in cataracts, either in humans or in natural or engineered animal models (see "Cataracts," below).

The best studied and most abundant membrane protein of the lens is intrinsic membrane protein 26 (MP26, MIP). MP26 is a lens-specific single polypeptide with a molecular mass of 28,200 kDa (263 residues) that comprises about 50 percent of the lens membrane protein.[19,20,266] Circular dichroism studies show that about half of MP26 forms a helix. The amino acid sequence has been deduced from a cloned MP26 cDNA.[267] MP26 exists as a tetramer.[268] A model has been constructed that suggests that MP26 forms α-helical coils that traverse the membrane six times. The C- and N-termini are both on the cytoplasmic side, consistent with a possible role for MP26 as a junctional protein.[267] MP26 is a member of the aquaporin (AQP) family, which transport small molecules such as water and glycerol.[269,270] The crystal structure of AQP1 has been solved and shows an in-plane, intramolecular twofold axis of symmetry located in the hydrophobic core of the membrane bilayer. The AQP1 monomer is composed of six membrane-spanning, tilted α-helices that form a barrel that encloses a water-selective channel.[271] The genes for both AQP2 and MP26 are on chromosome 12q13.[272]

Transfection of a human MP26 promoter/CAT fusion gene into embryonic chicken lens epithelial cells has demonstrated the ability of the MP26 gene regulatory sequences to function in lens cells.[273] Electron microscopic immunocytochemistry demonstrates MP26 in junctional complexes of lens fiber cell plasma membranes but not in the anterior lens epithelia or nonlens cell membranes.[274,275] It occurs in thin (11 to 13 nm) junctions in single membranes, as well as between cells, so that it may form channels to the extracellular space rather than intercellular channels, as do the connexins. MP26 also can form channels permeable to ions and other small molecules in liposomes and artificial membrane systems.[276–279] It has been suggested that MP26 may bind calmodulin.[280] MP26 is a substrate of endogenous protein kinase,[268,281] raising the possibility that metabolic control of its structure has functional significance. In addition, MP26 is palmitoylated, as is its degradation product MP22.[86]

## Gap Junction Proteins

The lens is avascular and must depend on intercellular junctions for nutrition and cell-to-cell communication. The thick, 16- to 17-nm junctions appear to be the lens equivalent of gap junctions found in other tissues and may contain connexins in homomeric or heteromeric combinations.[282] Lens junctions contain the intrinsic membrane protein connexin50, also called *MP70* or *gap membrane channel protein alpha8* (Gja8), which is a member of the connexin gene family.[282–284] Connexin50 is most prevalent in outer cortical fibers, where it undergoes age-related degradation to MP38, which remains in the functional gap junctions.[285] It is also phosphorylated by a specific membrane-associated kinase.[286,287] Connexin50 is encoded by a single exon on chromosome 1q21.1, as are connexin37 and connexin40.[288,289]

## Cytoskeletal Proteins

Many cytoskeletal proteins found in the lens are common to other tissues, including actin, ankyrin, myosin, vimentin, spectrin, and α-actinin. It is likely that a complex network of proteins immediately below the cell membrane similar to that in erythrocytes[290] contributes to the maintenance of the shape of differentiating fiber cells of the lens cortex. α- and β-Tubulins are components of microtubules, which are arrayed lengthwise in the peripheral cytoplasm in cortical fiber cells and are rare in nuclear fiber cells and epithelial cells.[291] Microtubules may contribute to the maintenance of the elongated shape of fiber cells and may be involved in the interkinetic migration of the nuclei in dividing lens epithelial cells.[292]

Actin filaments are closely associated with lens cell membranes[293,294] and may play a role in accommodation.[21,295,296] Nonmuscle β- and γ-actins are found in lens microfilaments, also called *thin filaments*.[297] Actin filaments are associated with cell membranes and may interact with intercellular junctions.[298,299] Tropomodulin and α-actinin interact with actin in microfilaments, especially in elongating cortical fibers.[300,301]

Vimentin, which usually occurs in mesenchymally derived cells, forms the intermediate filament in lens cells.[302] It can be highly phosphorylated.[303] These 10-nm filaments can occur as extrinsic membrane proteins but are found more commonly in the cytoplasm.[18] Vimentin-containing intermediate filaments occurs primarily in epithelial cells. While some vimentin is expressed in superficial cortical cells, vimentin-containing filaments are replaced by CP49 filaments deeper in the cortex.[304] Vimentin expression increases approximately threefold during embryonic chicken lens development and then decreases after hatching.[305] Transfection experiments have shown that vimentin gene expression is controlled by a complex set of positive and negative cis-regulatory 5' flanking sequences.[305,306] Glial fibrillary acidic protein (GFAP), an intermediate-filament protein usually seen in cells of neurectodermal origin, is also expressed in lens anterior epithelial cells and disappears on differentiation to fiber cells.[307,308] While the developmental pattern of these vimentin and GFAPs suggest that their disappearance is related to fiber cell differentiation, their specific roles remain unknown.

Other cytoskeletal proteins appear to be unique to the lens.[22,309,310] The beaded filament consists of a 7- to 9-nm backbone filament with 12- to 15-nm globular protein particles spaced along it.[19] The central filament contains CP-115 (also called *filensin*), and the globular beads contain CP-115 as well as CP-49 (also called *phakinin*).[309,311,312] Both these proteins are highly divergent members of the intermediate-filament family.[313] As mentioned earlier, beaded filaments emerge in the differentiating fiber cells as vimentin-containing intermediate filaments disappear.[304] There are excellent reviews available of lens membrane and cytoskeletal proteins and their biochemistry.[18,314,315]

There is an emerging role for α-crystallins in assembly, maintenance, and remodeling of the cytoskeleton. CP-49 and CP-115 copolymerize in vitro to form 10-nm fibers similar to intermediate filaments.[311,316] These proteins will not assemble with vimentin, and assembly is inhibited when the vimentin rod or tail domain is substituted for that of CP-115.[317] However, when they assemble in the presence of α-crystallin, a structure similar to a beaded chain is formed.[316] In addition, α-crystallins inhibit the in vitro assembly of both GFAP and vimentin in an ATP-dependent

**Table 241-3** Lens Metabolism

| Pathway | % Glucose Used | Additional Importance |
|---|---|---|
| Anaerobic glycolysis | 78% | — |
| Pentose phosphate | 14% | Pentoses for NADPH |
| Sorbitol pathway | 5% | Sugar cataract formation |
| Citric acid cycle | 3% | Limited to epithelial cells |

manner,[83] shifting these proteins from formed filaments to the soluble pool. Finally, both α-crystallin knockout mice and human mutations suggest that interactions between α-crystallins and the cytoskeleton are important for both muscle and lens function (see below).

## LENS METABOLISM

### Energy Metabolism

In general, metabolic pathways of the lens are similar to those of other tissues.[318,319] However, the avascular nature of the lens, which receives the vast majority of its nutrients from the aqueous humor,[320] and the gradual loss of intracellular organelles from differentiating fiber cells place specific constraints on lens metabolism. Use of various metabolic pathways for energy production in the whole lens is summarized in Table 241-3. Most of the glucose metabolized in the lens is handled by anaerobic glycolysis. The citric acid cycle is active only in the anterior epithelial cells, which still contain mitochondria. This pathway produces about 20 to 30 percent of the total ATP in the lens, even though only about 3 percent of the glucose passes through this cycle.[321,322] The lens can maintain adequate ion balance, high-energy phosphate levels, and protein synthesis in the absence of oxygen, but exposure of the lens to iodoacetate, an inhibitor of 3-phosphoglyceraldehyde dehydrogenase of the Embden-Meyerhof pathway results in swelling, ionic changes, and cataracts.[323,324] Stimulation of the pentose phosphate pathway occurs when cultured lenses are exposed to oxidative stress induced by hydrogen peroxide[325–327] or hyperbaric oxygen,[328] apparently acting through an increase in hexokinase activity.

It has been suggested that aldose reductase may increase sorbitol in the lens to protect against daily diet- and disease-related changes in aqueous humor osmolality,[329] in a fashion similar to sorbitol action in the renal medulla.[330,331] The osmotic hypothesis suggests a common pathogenic mechanism in the cataracts resulting from diabetes mellitus or galactosemia. Aldose reductase reduces glucose to sorbitol and galactose (more readily) to galactitol.[332] While sorbitol is metabolized by sorbitol dehydrogenase, galactitol is not, perhaps making it a more damaging molecule. The increase in intracellular fluid in response to these polyols results in lens swelling, increased membrane permeability, electrolyte abnormalities, and metabolic dysfunction.[333–335] Polyol accumulation has been demonstrated to cause cataracts in transgenic mice expressing the aldose reductase gene in the lens.[336] Although the human lens contains significantly less aldose reductase activity than that of the commonly studied rat, in vitro cultured human lenses from diabetic patients accumulate higher levels of polyols than those from nondiabetic subjects, and the accumulation is inhibited by aldose reductase inhibitors.[337] Thus, while the mechanism of sugar cataract is controversial,[338] the hope that inhibition of aldose reductase may inhibit polyol accumulation, osmotic damage, and cataract in humans with abnormalities in sugar metabolism is currently being tested.[319]

### Maintenance of a Reduced State

A major threat to lens transparency lies in the accumulation of oxidative damage to the crystallins and other molecules over an individual's lifetime. It has been suggested that oxidative stress also may mediate damage from other insults, such as that from ultraviolet light.[339] Since peroxides are generated in fiber and anterior epithelial cells, the average concentration of $H_2O_2$ is 30 mM in the normal human eye, and it can be much higher in patients with cataracts.[340] The lens responds to this stress by accumulating reducing agents, especially glutathione, which is the most abundant low-molecular-weight thiol in aerobic organisms. There is a gradient of glutathione concentration in the lens, with the highest concentration in the anterior epithelium, next in the cortical regions, and lowest in the nucleus.[341] In the normal lens the cortical glutathione level is not age-dependent.[342] Lens glutathione presumably acts as a sulfhydryl buffer for maintaining protein thiols in a reduced state and protecting against oxidative damage to other residues.

The lens uses both the glutathione redox cycle and catalase for the detoxification of $H_2O_2$.[343] Catalase is confined to peroxisomes by histochemical localization,[344] but enzymes of the glutathione redox cycle (glutathione reductase and peroxidase) are distributed throughout the cytoplasm. The mercapturic acid pathway using glutathione-S-transferase is also important in protecting the lens from oxidative damage.[345] However, glutathione reductase is the main enzyme maintaining glutathione in a reduced state in the lens,[44] and individuals with homozygous deletions of glutathione-S-transferase M are not at increased risk for cataracts.[346] It is interesting that the major crystallins in cephalopods are closely related to glutathione-S-transferase.[199,347] The effectiveness of these reducing pathways results in only 2 to 5 percent of lens glutathione existing in the oxidized form under normal conditions. Recent studies using cell lines, inhibitors of catalase and glutathione reductase, transgenic mice overexpresing glutathione peroxidase, and glutathione peroxidase null mice have shown that these oxidative defense systems operate together and show considerable redundancy, so lesions in one may be compensated by the activity of the other enzymatic pathways.[348,349] Efforts are underway to use peroxidases as anticataract agents by protecting the lens for oxidative stress.[350]

### Osmoregulation

Osmoregulation occurs by active transport, with $Na^+,K^+$-dependent ATPase exchanging sodium out of the lens for potassium into the lens. Most of the $Na^+,K^+$-dependent ATPase is in the anterior epithelium, but some is also found in the anterior cortex and fiber membranes around suture systems.[16,351] The cations are followed by passive diffusion of chloride and water.[352] Cytochemistry has indicated that $Na^+,K^+$-ATPase is localized to the apicolateral membranes of the anterior epithelial cells.[353,354] Because the lens capsule is slightly permeable to both sodium and potassium and most transport is by the anterior epithelium, there is a concentration gradient anterior to posterior for potassium and posterior to anterior for sodium.[355] $Na^+,K^+$-dependent ATPase can be induced in lens epithelial cells but not fiber cells by increased membrane permeability from amphotericin B treatment.[356] $Ca^{2+}$-ATPase also occurs in the lens, with the highest specific activity in the anterior epithelium, but the bulk of activity is in the cortical lens fibers. This results in the lens having a lower $Ca^{2+}$ concentration than the aqueous or vitreous humor.[357,358] $Ca^{2+}$-ATPase activity is decreased in membranes isolated from cataractous lenses.[359]

The movement of different macromolecules is controlled in various ways by the lens. The lens capsule is the first barrier for diffusion. Horseradish peroxidase (molecular weight, 40,000) can penetrate the lens capsule, whereas ferritin (molecular weight, 500,000) cannot.[16] The capsule is penetrable by low-molecular-weight crystallins but not by higher molecular weight α-crystallin.[360] Low-molecular-weight proteins such as horseradish peroxidase and dyes also readily penetrate the anterior epithelial layer.[15] However, passage of metabolites between the epithelial cells and fiber cells is probably through endocytotic processes rather than through the few gap junctions found connecting them.[7,16,361] The fiber cells are connected by extensive communicating channels, as shown by dye injection[17,362] and electrophysiologic studies.[363,364] Sugar transport in the lens closely resembles that seen in muscle and blood cells.[365,366]

## MOLECULAR BIOLOGY OF CATARACTS

*Cataract*, defined here as a lens opacity, can have multiple causes and generally is associated with breakdown of the lens micro-architecture.[33,34,367] Vacuole formation will cause large fluctuations in density and hence abrupt changes in the index of refraction, resulting in light scattering. Light scattering and opacity will occur if there is a significant amount of high-molecular-weight protein aggregates 1000 Å or more in size.[368,369] The short-range ordered packing of the crystallins is important in this regard; crystallins must exist in a homogeneous phase. A number of biochemical or physical insults can cause phase separation into protein-rich and protein-poor regions within the lens fibers, resulting in light scattering.[368–374] The physical basis of lens transparency is beyond the scope of this chapter and has been reviewed elsewhere.[60,368–370]

### Animal Models

Since cataractogenesis is a complex process accompanied by numerous secondary changes, animal models may provide useful information for delineating the causes of senescent and other cataracts. Hereditary cataracts in rodents have been especially useful in this regard.[375]

The Philly mouse displays an autosomal dominant cataract in which there is a deficiency of βB2-crystallin polypeptide.[376,377] βB2-crystallin mRNA has a deletion of 12 nucleotides, resulting in a 4-amino-acid deletion in the encoded protein. It has been hypothesized that this causes aberrant folding of the protein and that cataract formation occurs as a result of the molecular instability of this crystallin.[378,379]

Guinea pig strain 13/N has an autosomal dominant cataract more severe in homozygotes than in heterozygotes.[380,381] A peculiarity of the guinea pig and other hystricomorphic mammals is that ζ-crystallin is a major crystallin found in the lens.[382] In the heterozygous 13/N guinea pig, levels of ζ-crystallin are reduced, and an abnormal smaller protein is present. This is due to a mutation in a splice site resulting in a loss of an entire exon during RNA processing, with consequent deletion of 34 amino acids in the protein.[383] It is not clear whether the molecular lesion in guinea pig strain 13/N results in a cataract by destabilizing ζ-crystallin or destroying an enzymatic activity. However, both the Philly mouse and guinea pig 13/N cataracts suggest that appropriate concentrations of stable crystallins are critical for maintenance of lens transparency.

A number of additional models suggest that some metabolic lesions also can cause cataracts. The Nakano mouse has autosomal recessive cataracts mapping to chromosome 16 and showing reduced synthesis of the α- and β-crystallins.[384,385] This is probably due to an increase in the $Na^+/K^+$ ratio occurring because of inhibition of the sodium-potassium pump.[335,386] The Fraser mouse, which displays an autosomal dominant cataract, shows preferential loss of γ-crystallins and their mRNAs.[387,388] However, the gene causing this cataract segregates independently of the γ-crystallin gene cluster.[389] It resides on chromosome 10 and has been suggested to be allelic with the mouse lens opacity gene (*LOP*).[390] The eye lens obsolescence (*ELO*) mouse cataract shows preferential reduction in γ-crystallin mRNAs.[391] The *ELO* locus is on chromosome 1 near the γ-crystallin gene cluster, although a recombination event has been documented between the cataract and the γ-crystallin genes.[391] In addition, many other animal cataract models have been described phenotypically but not characterized molecularly.[392] An interesting cataract develops in the Emory mouse after several months of life, possibly modeling senescent cataracts in humans.[393] A series of mutations of the γ-crystallins in mice suggests that these genes can cause cataracts through altering lens development as well as

by virtue of their structural role in maintaining lens transparency.[394]

### Genetically Engineered Animal Models

Transgenic mice provide an extremely powerful tool for the study of lens transparency.[395] In practice, creation of cataractous transgenic mouse lines is facilitated by the lens being readily examined for transparency, providing a rapid and efficient means to screen for phenotypic effects of transgenic insertions. Most cataracts in transgenic mice are associated with abnormalities of lens development, especially uncontrolled growth, toxic ablation of specific lens cells, or immune destruction of the lens. Lens abnormalities have been caused in transgenic mice using a variety of strategies. Expression of diphtheria toxin or ricin under the control of a lens-specific γ-crystallin or α-crystallin promoter, respectively, has caused ablations within the lens.[144,396] Synthesis of granulocyte-macrophage colony-stimulating factor (a leukocytic chemotactic factor) in transgenic mice resulted in inflammatory destruction of lens cells and cataract formation.[397] Transgenic mice with vimentin overexpressed in lens cells also have cataracts, probably due to developmental aberration.[398] In addition, there are a number of genetically engineered mouse models with cataracts resulting from abnormalities of development,[399–401] immunity,[397,402,403] growth,[404–406] the cytoskeleton,[398,407,408] membrane transport,[409] lens crystallins,[75] or proteolysis of lens proteins.[410]

In addition to transgenic expression of normal or modified proteins, disrupted expression of a protein normally found in the lens has been shown to cause cataracts. Lack of αA-crystallin expression causes cataracts in which inclusion bodies in central lens fiber cells contain αB-crystallin.[75] Osteonectin is a secreted glycoprotein that binds type IV collagen and other intercellular matrix components in the lens and elsewhere. Disruption of osteonectin expression results in cataract with vacuolization of differentiating fiber cells and rupture of the lens capsule but no obvious nonlens pathology.[411] Absence of connexin46[412] results in nuclear cataracts associated with proteolysis of crystallins, absence of connexin50 gives ocular abnormalities including cataract,[413] and absence of normal connexin43 expression results in changes consistent with early cataractogenesis.[414] Similarly, the absence of γ-crystallins in *Sox1* null mice leads to cataract.[13] These engineered cataract models emphasize the importance of the crystallins, cytoskeleton, and intercellular matrix for lens transparency.

## HUMAN CATARACTS

### Definition

In the most general sense, *cataract* is defined as any opacity in the lens. For clinical diagnostic purposes, however, the characteristics of a cataract must be defined precisely. Opacities that are the natural result of biologic aging must be distinguished from those which are secondary to pathologic processes related to environmental, nutritional, or genetic factors or those which occur as a consequence of systemic disease. With aging, random flecklike opacities in the cortex of the lens may be detected by slit-lamp biomicroscopy in normal individuals, usually beginning by the third decade of life. Age-related changes in the color and clarity of the lens also occur.[415–418] A clinically useful classification scheme must distinguish these changes of normal aging from specific pathologic opacities. Rigorous clinical classification is particularly important because cataracts are an obvious and diagnostic phenotypic feature for many inherited disorders (Table 241-4).

### Classification

Characteristics used for diagnostic classification of human cataracts include age of onset, location, size, pattern, number, shape, density, progression, and severity in terms of interfering with visual acuity or function. Defined by age at onset, a *congenital* or *infantile cataract* is visible within the first year of

**Table 241-4** Inherited Syndromes Associated with Cataracts

| Syndrome | Reference |
|---|---|
| **Primarily Ocular Syndromes** | |
| **Autosomal dominant** | |
| Aniridia | 419 |
| Anterior segment mesenchymal dysgenesis | 420 |
| Cornea guttata | 421 |
| Granular corneal dystrophy | 422 |
| Familial exudative vitreoretinopathy | 423 |
| Foveal hypoplasia | 424 |
| Hyaloideoretinal degeneration of Wagner | 425 |
| Hyperferritinemia with congenital cataracts | 426 |
| Iris pigment layer cleavage | 427 |
| Mesenchymal dysgenesis of the anterior segment | 428 |
| Microcornea | 429 |
| Microphthalmia | 430 |
| Persistent hyperplastic pupillary membrane | 431 |
| Retinitis pigmentosa | 432, 433 |
| Snowflake vitreoretinal degeneration | 434 |
| Vitreoretinochoroidopathy | 435 |
| **Autosomal recessive** | |
| Amyloid corneal dystrophy | 436 |
| Cone-rod degeneration | 432 |
| Choroideremia | 432 |
| Favre hyaloideoretinal degeneration | 437 |
| Leber congenital amaurosis type I | 438 |
| Microphthalmia and nystagmus | 439 |
| Retinitis pigmentosa | 432, 433 |
| **X-linked** | |
| Microcornea and slight microphthalmia | 430 |
| Norrie disease | 440 |
| Nystagmus | 441 |
| Retinitis pigmentosa | 442 |
| **Other Genetic Syndromes Associated with Cataracts** | |
| **Autosomal dominant** | |
| Aberrant oral frenula and growth retardation | 443 |
| Cerebellar ataxia, deafness, and dementia | 444 |
| Chondrodysplasia punctata | 445 |
| Clouston syndrome | 441 |
| Cochleosaccular degeneration | 446 |
| Congenital lactose intolerance | 447 |
| Desmin-related myopathy | 448 |
| Dwarfism with stiff joints and ocular abnormalities | 449 |
| Esophageal and vulval leiomyomatosis with nephropathy* | 450 |
| Fechtner syndrome | 441 |
| Flynn-Aird syndrome* | 451 |
| Hallermann-Streiff syndrome (new mutation) | 452 |
| Hereditary mucoepithelial dysplasia | 453 |
| Histiocytic dermatoarthritis | 454 |
| Incontinentia pigmenti (autosomal dominant new mutation) | 455 |
| Long-chain 3-hydroxyacyl CoA dehydrogenase deficiency | 456 |

**Table 241-4** (*Continued*)

| Syndrome | Reference |
|---|---|
| Metatropic dwarfism type II (Kniest disease) | 457 |
| Kyrle disease (follicular keratosis) | 458 |
| Mitochondrial myopathy (two types) | 459, 460 |
| Marshall syndrome | 461 |
| Multiple epiphyseal dysplasia with myopia and conductive deafness* | 462 |
| Myotonic dystrophy | 463 |
| Nail-patella syndrome | 464 |
| Neurofibromatosis type II | 465 |
| Oculodentodigital syndrome | 441 |
| Optic atrophy and neurologic disorder | 466 |
| Osteopathica striata and deafness | 460 |
| Paronychia congenita syndrome | 441 |
| Progeria syndrome (autosomal dominant new mutation) | 467 |
| Schprintzen velocardiofacial syndrome | 468 |
| Sorbitol dehydrogenase | 469 |
| Split-hand and congenital nystagmus | 470 |
| Stickler syndrome | 471 |
| Trichomegaly | 472 |
| **Autosomal recessive** | |
| Absence leg deficiency* | 473 |
| Agenesis of the corpus callosum, combined immunodeficiency, and hypopigmentation* | 474 |
| Axonal encephalopathy with necrotizing myopathy and cardiomyopathy* | 475 |
| Bardet-Biedl syndrome | 476 |
| Cataract, microcephaly, failure to thrive, and kyphoscoliosis (CAMFAK) syndrome | 441 |
| Cardiomyopathy | 477 |
| Cerebral cholesterinosis (cerebrotendinous xanthomatosis) | 478 |
| Cerebrooculofacioskeletal (COFS) syndrome | 479 |
| Chondrodysplasia punctata | 445 |
| Cockayne syndrome | 480 |
| Congenital ichthyosis | 481 |
| Crome syndrome* | 482 |
| Dysequilibrium syndrome | 483 |
| Galactosemia (kinase and transferase) | 484 |
| Glutathione reductase deficiency | 485 |
| Gyrate atrophy | 486 |
| Hallermann-Streiff syndrome | 487 |
| Hard-E syndrome | 488 |
| Homocysteinuria | 489 |
| Hypertrophic neuropathy* | 490 |
| Hypogonadism* | 491 |
| Osteogenesis imperfecta with microcephaly* | 492 |
| Mannosidosis | 493 |
| Majewski syndrome | 494 |
| Marinesco-Sjögren syndrome | 495 |
| Martsolf syndrome | 496 |
| Mevalonic aciduria | 497 |
| Myopathy and hypogonadism* | 498 |
| Nathalie syndrome* | 499 |
| Neu-Laxova syndrome | 500 |
| Neuraminidase deficiency | 501 |
| Neutral lipid storage disease | 502 |
| Pellagra-like syndrome* | 503 |
| Phenylketonuria | 504 |
| Polycystic kidney and congenital blindness | 505 |

**Table 241-4** (Continued)

| Syndrome | Reference |
| --- | --- |
| Preus oculocerebral hypopigmentation syndrome | 506 |
| Refsum syndrome | 507 |
| Roberts-SC phocomelia syndrome | 508 |
| Rothmund Thomson syndrome | 509 |
| Schwartz-Jampel syndrome | 508 |
| Short stature, mental retardation, and ocular abnormalities* | 510 |
| Smith-Lemli-Opitz syndrome | 511 |
| Tachycardia, hypertension, microphthalmos, and hyperglycinuria* | 512 |
| Toriello microcephalic primordial dwarfism* | 513 |
| Usher syndrome | 514 |
| Werner syndrome | 515 |
| Wilson disease | 516 |
| Zellweger syndrome | 507 |
| **X-linked** | |
| Albright hereditary osteodystrophy | 517 |
| Alport syndrome | 518 |
| Fabry disease | 519 |
| Glucose-6-phosphate dehydrogenase deficiency | 520 |
| Incontinentia pigmenti | 521 |
| Lenz dysplasia | 522 |
| Lowe syndrome | 523 |
| Nance-Horan syndrome | 524 |
| Pigmentary retinopathy and mental retardation | 525 |
| Renal tubular acidosis II | 526 |
| X-linked dominant chondrodysplasia punctata | 527 |
| **Chromosome anomalies** | |
| Trisomy 10q | 508 |
| Trisomy 13 | 508 |
| Trisomy 18 | 508 |
| 18p- | 508 |
| 18q- | 508 |
| Trisomy 20p | 508 |
| Trisomy 21 | 508 |
| XO syndrome | 508 |

*This syndrome has been described in a single kindred.

NOTE: Although references are given in which the cataracts found in the preceding syndromes are described, useful clinical summaries of most of these syndromes are found in Smith[508] or McKusick.[441] In some cases, no single best source was obvious, and the summary in Smith or McKusick is given as the primary reference.

life, a *juvenile cataract* occurs within the first decade of life, a *presenile cataract* occurs before the age of 45 years, and the *senile* or *age-related cataract* occurs thereafter. The age of onset of a cataract does not necessarily indicate its etiology. Congenital cataracts may be hereditary or secondary to a noxious intrauterine event. Cataracts associated with a systemic or genetic disease may not occur until the second or third decade (e.g., cataracts associated with retinitis pigmentosa). Even age-related cataracts, thought to be due to multiple insults accumulated over many years, have a genetic component, making certain individuals more vulnerable to the environmental insults.

Location is a reproducible and reliable criterion by which to classify cataracts and chart their progression. Several classification

systems have been developed based on the anatomic location of the opacity, i.e., involving the nucleus, the posterior capsule, the cortex, or mixed (combinations of the former). All these systems depend on the use of slit-lamp biomicroscopy and examination through a dilated pupil. These classification systems include the LOCS II system (lens opacity classification system),[528] the Wisconsin system,[529] the Hopkins system,[530] and the Oxford system.[531] These classifications have focused primarily on acquired rather than congenital cataract. Documentation may be made either clinically by comparing the slit-lamp biomicroscopic appearance with a set of standard photographs or by direct comparison of photographs of the affected lens using slit-lamp and retroillumination photography with standard photographs (LOCS II). These techniques for the most part have been used for research studies but can be adapted to determine the presence and progression of lens opacities in a clinical setting.

In an attempt to deal with congenital cataract, Merin has proposed a system based on morphologic classification. Accordingly, the cataract is classified as total (mature), polar (anterior or posterior), zonular (nuclear, lamellar, sutural), and capsular or membranous.[532]

Since lens development follows a well-documented timed sequence, the location of a lens opacity provides information about the time at which the pathologic process intervened, thereby aiding in determining the etiology. Nuclear opacities from the most central region outward denote cataract formation occurring at the time of the development of that portion of the involved lens nucleus—embryonic (first 3 months), fetal (third to eighth month), infantile (after birth), or adult. Since the lens fibers are laid down constantly throughout life, lens opacities that develop postnatally appear in the cortex as cortical opacities or appear just beneath the posterior lens capsule as subcapsular opacities, e.g., cataracts caused by topical steroid drugs and radiation. Polar opacities involve either the anterior or posterior pole of the lens and may include the posterior subcapsular lens cortex extending to the lens capsule. When both anterior and posterior poles are involved, the term *bipolar* is used. Zonular or lamellar cataracts affect the lens fibers, which are formed at the same time, resulting in a shell-like opacity at the level at which the fibers were laid down. The regions on which the lens fibers converge are referred to as the *Y sutures*, visible by slit-lamp biomicroscopy as an upright Y anteriorly and an inverted Y posteriorly. Theories of cataract development[533] suggest that abnormalities in lens-fiber development or maturation may lead to a predisposition to cataract development later in life. This is supported by examples in animals (the Philly mouse) and in humans (gyrate atrophy)[486] (see Chap. 83).

Size, pattern, shape, and density of lens opacities are determined in part by etiology, location, the ongoing process of cataractogenesis, and other, unknown, influences. Microdots and cortical flecks may be insignificant if few in number and random in location, but if the number exceeds 25 per quadrant[534,535] with a specific distribution such as the radial pattern in the Lowe carrier,[536,537] their clinical significance becomes apparent. Other examples include the cortical cataract in neurofibromatosis type 2[465,538] or the metachromasia seen in myotonic dystrophy patients.[463]

## Hereditary Cataract

The frequency of hereditary cataracts in humans is not precisely known but has been estimated to be between 8.3 and 25 percent of congenital cataracts.[539,540] Hereditary cataracts include cases in which only the lens is involved, or the lens opacity may be associated with other ocular anomalies such as microphthalmia, aniridia, other anterior chamber developmental anomalies, retinal degenerations, chromosomal abnormalities, and multisystem genetic disorders such as Lowe syndrome and neurofibromatosis type 2. In some cases this distinction is not clear. Inherited cataracts may be isolated in some individuals and associated with additional findings in others, as in the developmental abnormality anterior segment mesenchymal dysgenesis, resulting from abnormalities in the *PITX3* gene.[420] The recently described hyperferritinemia-cataract syndrome (MIM 600886) is an autosomal dominant trait with early-onset bilateral cataracts caused by systemic overexpression of the ferritin L-chain.[541]

Hereditary cataract may be classified by the mode of inheritance, with all Mendelian inheritance patterns being described. Autosomal dominant congenital cataracts are the most frequent. Phenotypically identical cataracts have been localized to different genetic loci and may have different inheritance patterns (see below), whereas phenotypically variable cataracts can be found in a single large family.[542] Linkage analysis is a powerful tool to sort out the different genetic loci that can cause human cataracts.

## Linkage Analysis of Cataracts

Eleven cataract loci currently have been identified by linkage analysis, and genetic heterogeneity has been demonstrated for a variety of specific cataract phenotypes (Table 241-5). Sequence changes in candidate genes in many of the mapped loci show association with cataracts and are absent from control populations. All the proposed mutations cause a nonconservative change in the amino acid sequence of the protein that would be predicted to have a significant effect on its structure and function. In addition, many of the candidate genes cause cataracts when mutated or absent in natural or engineered animal models.

Aberrations in connexins have been implicated in two forms of inherited human cataract. The autosomal dominant lamellar (central pulverulent) cataract (CAE) originally described by Nettleship and Ogilvie in 1906[543] was linked to the Duffy locus on chromosome 1q21-q25 by Renwick and Lawler[3] and has been associated with a C to T transition in codon 88 of connexin50 (GJA8) by Shiels et al.[544] This mutation results in substitution of a serine for a highly conserved proline residue. A zonular pulverulent cataract has been localized to chromosome 13 near the connexin46 (gap junction α3) gene by Mackay et al.[545] It was shown to be associated with an A to G transition at nucleotide 188 of this gene, resulting in a nonconservative N63S substitution in the first extracellular loop (E1), which mediates intermembrane coupling of connexin hexamers to form gap-junction channels.[546] A second family with punctate cataracts mapping to the same region were shown to have a C inserted at nucleotide 1137 resulting in a frameshift with substitution of 87 aberrant and apparently random amino acids for the 31 amino acids of the normal C-terminus. Disruption of connexin46 and connexin50 is predicted to result in defects in membrane targeting and junctional permeability. Absence of mutations similar to those described here in connexin46 and connexin50 have been associated with cataracts in mice.[412,413]

Mutations in the βγ-crystallins also have been implicated in human cataracts. The Coppock-like genes encoding cataract have been linked to the region of the γ-crystallin gene cluster in one large family with an LOD score of 7.58 and no recombinations ($\theta = 0$).[547] This cataract is thought to be caused by activated expression of the normally unexpressed ωγE-crystallin pseudogene, which is truncated at the end of the first motif.[261] A single β-crystallin motif would be structurally unstable, and expression of the truncated first motif may result in high phase separation.[143] Cataracts from three additional families also map to this region.[548–550] A locus for nuclear lamellar cataract with sutural opacities has been mapped to chromosome 17q11-q12[551] and is associated with a splice mutation in the third exon of βA3A1-crystallin.[552] This is predicted to cause truncation of the mutant βA3-crystallin after the first Greek key motif, producing an unstable peptide similar to that seen with the Coppock-like cataract. Autosomal dominant congenital cataracts in a second family map to a wide but overlapping region of chromosome 17.[553] Autosomal dominant congenital cerulean cataracts show linkage with markers on chromosome 22q and are associated with a chain-termination mutation in βB2-crystallin at the beginning of exon 6, which would result in absence of the fourth Greek key motif.[554]

As suggested by animal models, mutant or absent α-crystallins also have been associated with inherited cataracts. An autosomal dominant congenital zonular nuclear cataract that can progress to include cortical and posterior subcapsular opacities in adults maps to the αA-crystallin region on chromosome 21q22.3.[555] These are associated with a sequence change in αA-crystallin substituting a cysteine for an arginine (R120C) that is invariant in α-crystallins throughout mammals and in chickens and frogs as well. The precise mechanism through which this alteration may cause cataracts has yet to be determined. When this arginine is changed to glycine in αB-crystallin (R120G), it forms large aggregates with desmin in smooth muscle cells, causing a severe myopathy associated with cataracts.[448] This is reminiscent of the behavior of αB-crystallin in αA-crystallin knockout mice,[75] whereas αB-crystallin knockout mice develop a late-onset fatal myopathy without cataracts.[76]

Cataracts at a number of mapped loci have not yet been associated with sequence changes in candidate genes. The Volkmann cataract, which has variable progressive central and zonular nuclear and sutural morphology, has been mapped to chromosome 1p36,[556] and a second family has cataracts cosegregating with the Evans phenotype in the same chromosomal region.[557] A morphologically distinct posterior polar cataract also maps to the same region.[558] Whether these represent one or several loci is not yet clear. A zonular autosomal dominant cataract initially studied by Marner has been linked to haptoglobin.[559,560]

### Table 241-5 Human Cataract Loci Identified by Linkage Analysis

| Locus | Chromosome | Candidate | MIM |
|---|---|---|---|
| *CCV* (Volkmann) | 1p36 | | 115665 |
| *CPP* (posterior polar) | 1p34-p36 | | 116600 |
| *CAE1* (CZP1, Duffy-linked) | 1q21-q25 | Connexin50 (GJA8) | 116200 |
| *CCL* (Coppock-like) | 2q33-q35 | γC-Crystallin | 123660 |
| *CACA* (aculeiform) | 2q33-q35 | γD-Crystallin | 115700 |
| *BFSP2* (nuclear and sutural) | 3q21-3q22 | BFSP2 phakinen | 603212 |
| *ADC* (Polymorphic lamellar) | 12q12-12q14 | MIP | 154050 |
| *CZP* | 13 | Connexin46 (GJA3) | 601885 |
| *CAM* (Marner) | 16q22 | Near haptoglobin | 116800 |
| *CTAA2* (anterior polar) | 17p13 | | 601202 |
| *CCZS* (zonular sutural) | 17q11-q12 | βA3-Crystallin | 600881 |
| *CCA1* (cerulean, blue dot) | 17q24 | | 115660 |
| *CRYAA, ARG116CYS* | 21q22.3 | αA-Crystallin | 123580.001 |
| *CCA2* (cerulean, blue dot) | 22q | βB2-Crystallin | 601547 |

An autosomal dominant total congenital cataract also has shown probable linkage (LOD score of 2.1 at $\theta = 0.1$) to haptoglobin, suggesting that these loci may be allelic.[561] A locus for an autosomal dominant congenital anterior polar cataract lies on chromosome 17p13.[562] Finally, a locus for autosomal dominant nuclear and cortical cerulean congenital cataracts maps to chromosome 17q24.[563]

While most studies have been of dominant cataracts, an interesting autosomal recessive congenital cataract has been associated with "i" phenotype on chromosome 9q21 in 17 of 18 Japanese individuals[564] and some Caucasians.[565] Linkage analysis has been carried out on this locus in four Japanese families, giving an LOD score of 3.4 at $\theta = 0$.[566]

**Chromosome Abnormalities and Complex Syndromes Associated with Cataracts.** Chromosomal abnormalities can suggest chromosomal locations of genes that can cause cataracts when their structure or expression is disrupted. Isolated congenital total cataracts have occurred in a father and son with a translocation, t(3;4)(p26.2.;p15).[567] Isolated congenital anterior polar cataracts have occurred in four family members with a balanced translocation, t(2:14)(p25;q24).[568] A balanced translocation, t(2:16)(p22.3;p13.3), was coinherited with congenital cataracts and microphthalmia in four members of another family.[569] In addition, cataracts have been associated with unbalanced chromosomal rearrangements,[570-572] and with trisomy of chromosomes 13, 18, 21, and 20p, as well as 18p-, 18q-, and XO syndrome, as listed in Table 241-4. These patients, of course, also have additional abnormalities. These studies emphasize the genetic heterogeneity of autosomal dominant congenital cataracts indicated by linkage analysis. While the number of known cataract loci has increased dramatically in the last few years, as many as 30 that can cause autosomal dominant cataracts have been estimated to exist in humans,[573] so much work remains to be done in understanding inherited congenital cataracts.

Cataracts also occur in association with a variety of multiple malformation syndromes listed in Table 241-4. In some cases, this association appears to be the result of truly pleiotropic effects of a single gene, whereas in others the cataracts appear to be secondary to pathology occurring primarily in the retina or ciliary body. Conversely, these cataracts also can be accompanied by additional lens pathology such as microphakia, coloboma, or abnormal positioning of the lens. As might be expected, cataracts frequently are associated with diseases resulting in marked involvement of the retina, choroid, or portions of anterior chamber structures. In addition, cataracts frequently occur with skin diseases such as epidermal dystrophies and a variety of bone and cartilage dysplasias. Inherited syndromes and diseases with which cataracts are associated are summarized in Table 241-4. Many of these diseases have been studied or mapped extensively, especially on the X chromosome.

**Abnormalities of Lens Size, Shape, and Position Associated with Cataracts.** Coloboma of the lens, which may be associated with coloboma of the uvea (choroid, ciliary body, iris), is a congenital anomaly that may show an asymmetry of the lens with a peripheral flattening of indentation and loss of zonules usually in the six o'clock position. Associated cataractous changes are not uncommon. Coloboma of the lens has been seen in Stickler (MIM 108300) and Marfan (MIM 154700) syndromes.[574,575] *Microspherophakia* refers to a small spherical lens that produces a high lenticular myopia due to the shape of the lens. Frequently these lenses can be subluxated with a displacement into the anterior chamber, resulting in a pupillary block (obstruction of the pupil by the lens) causing an acute onset of elevated intraocular pressure. Frequently these lenses become cataractous. The Weill-Marchesani syndrome (MIM 277600) is a rare example of microspherophakia, associated with short stature, brachycephaly, prognathism, and peg-shaped teeth.[576]

Lentiglobus and lenticonus are abnormalities of the shape of the lens associated with localized axial deformities of contour of the anterior or posterior surface of the lens. *Lentiglobus* usually refers to spherical bulging of the anterior surface, whereas *lenticonus* refers to conical changes usually of the posterior surface. Both create a central thickening and hence a high myopia. Posterior lentiglobus most frequently occurs as a unilateral condition and frequently is associated with a localized lens opacity. Anterior lenticonus occurrs in about 25 percent of patients with Alport syndrome (MIM 104200), a larger number than those with cataracts.[577]

Abnormal positions of the lens can occur, either with a partial dislocation, or subluxation, which may be due to weakened, stretched, or broken zonules. Signs and symptoms pathognomonic of these conditions are iridodonesis (tremulous iris movement), astigmatism, and occasionally, monocular diplopia. Complications include pupillary block, chorioretinal damage, or an ocular inflammatory (uveitic) response. Genetic diseases associated with subluxation of the lens include Marfan syndrome,[578] in which the lens is usually dislocated up and outward, and homocystinuria,[579] in which the lens is usually dislocated downward. Nonspecific dislocation can occur in the Weill-Marchesani syndrome,[580] Lowe syndrome,[523] and other rare conditions, such as sulfite oxidase deficiency[581] (MIM 272300) and some forms of primordial dwarfism. Marfan syndrome, Weill-Marchesani syndrome, and autosomal dominant ectopia lentis can be caused by a defect in the fibrillin gene on chromosome 15 (15q21.1).[580,582]

## Evaluation

In addition to diagnostic considerations, evaluation of cataract includes a careful assessment of its effect on visual acuity and visual function. The first assessment in small children (0–3 years of age) may be done by observation-fixing, following, and covering of the alternative eyes to determine response (covering the eye with good vision will create a more fretful, objecting, crying child). More accurate assessment involves specialized testing by visually evoked cortical responses, preferential looking, or the forced-choice method.[583,584] With older children, subjective tests, including identification of the illiterate E or Allen cards (picture-differentiating tests), are used. Finally, once the alphabet is learned, conventional acuity testing by a logEDTRS or Snellen chart may be used.

Cataracts may be visualized in a variety of ways. On examination with a handlight, a cataract may present as a white pupillary opacity (leukocoria). Direct ophthalmoscopy is useful with the principle that if the examiner can see the optic nerve and macula, the patient can probably see out. Focusing on the optic nerve and macula, a hazy view of the posterior pole may indicate opacification in the visual axis and serve as an estimate of how poorly the patient may see. Nonetheless, the definitive description of a lens opacity depends on a slit-lamp biomicroscopic examination through a widely dilated pupil, allowing for direct illumination and retroillumination with appropriate magnification to visualize the lens opacity and define its clinical features. Photographs are useful to document the features and progression of the cataract.

## Differential Diagnosis and Diagnostic Tests

The differential diagnosis of a hereditary cataract includes several considerations. First, prenatal insults including viral or other infectious diseases may have associated cataracts. Rubella directly involves the lens, whereas other infectious agents produce ocular inflammation (uveitis) with secondary cataracts. The latter include toxoplasmosis, mumps, measles, influenza, chickenpox, herpes simplex, herpes zoster, cytomegalovirus, and echovirus type 3, all of which can be screened for by TORCH titers. Additionally, patients with congenital infections often have some nonocular involvement that may include rash, hepatitis, thrombocytopenia, microcephaly, intracerebral calcifications, and/or sensorineural deafness. Second, developmental abnormalities in premature or dysmature patients may cause cataracts. These may be associated with low birth weight, birth anoxia, and/or CNS involvement with seizures, cerebral palsy or hemiplegia, or retinopathy of prematurity. Third, perinatal-postnatal problems such as hyperglycemia and hypocalcemia may cause cataracts. These are associated with signs of diabetes or tetany, respectively, and can be screened for by routine clinical chemistries. Fourth, cataracts may occur in association with other ocular abnormalities including anterior chamber abnormalities, e.g., Reiger syndrome (MIM 180500), primary hyperplastic vitreous (MIM 257910), aniridia (MIM 106200), microophthalmia, or retinopathies such as retinal dysplasia (MIM 312550) or Norrie disease (MIM 310600). Fifth, there are many multisystem syndromes associated with cataracts (see Table 241-4). These can be evaluated by clinical examination, chromosome analysis, and specific blood and urine chemistries.

## Treatment

Proper management of cataracts includes early diagnosis with prompt evaluation to identify etiology when possible. In some instances, e.g., galactosemia (see Chap. 72), rapid diagnosis and treatment may permit recovery of the lens to a normal state of clarity. Determination of the extent of compromise in visual acuity also is important. If visual function is significantly impaired, surgery may be required. The type of surgery, the use of intraocular lenses, and special procedures such as fitting cataract lenses and epikeratophakia are beyond the scope of this chapter.

Studies in kittens[585] and nonhuman primates[586,587] show that unequal input into cortical neurons due to unilateral form deprivation results in more severe visual deficits than does bilateral deprivation. Thus ophthalmic surgeons generally consider a unilateral, dense, congenital cataract to be a surgical emergency, whereas bilateral dense cataracts can be scheduled in a more routine fashion. Usual practice suggests that limited dense cataracts can be operated successfully in the first weeks of life, whereas bilateral cataracts can be operated successfully up to 3 months of age. With prompt surgery, the visual prognosis is better for bilateral as compared with unilateral cases and in less dense cataracts as compared with total opacities. When congenital cataracts are associated with other ocular abnormalities and/or systemic disease, a poorer visual outcome often results.[587–589] Lastly, it should be emphasized that communication between clinicians, therapists, and teachers, combined with counseling of patients, is very important in the treatment of young cataract patients and their families.[590]

## REFERENCES

1. Brewster D: On the anatomical and optical structure of the crystalline lens of animals, particularly that of cod. *Phil Trans R Soc Lond A* **123**:323, 1833.
2. Morner CT: Untersuchungender protein-substanzen in den lichtbrechenden Medien des Auges. *Hoppe-Seylers Z Physiol Chem* **18**:61, 1894.
3. Renwick JH, Lawler SD: Probable linkage between a congenital cataract locus and the Duffy blood group locus. *Ann Hum Genet* **27**:67, 1963.
4. Harding JJ, Rixon KC, Marriott FHC: Men have heavier lenses than women of the same age. *Exp Eye Res* **25**:651, 1977.
5. Wistow GJ, Piatigorsky J: Lens crystallins: The evolution and expression of proteins for a highly specialized tissue. *Annu Rev Biochem* **57**:479, 1988.
6. Mann I: *The Development of the Human Eye*. New York, Grune and Stratton, 1964.
7. Kuzak JR: Embryology and anatomy of the lens, in Tasman W, Jaeger EA (eds): *Duane's Clinical Ophthalmology*. Philadelphia, Lippincott, 1990, p 1.
8. Halder G, Callaerts P, Gehring WJ: Induction of ectopic eyes by targeted expression of the eyeless gene in *Drosophila*. *Science* **267**:1788, 1995.
9. Hanson I, van Heyningen V: *Pax6*: More than meets the eye. *Trends Genet* **11**:268, 1995.
10. Walther C, Gruss P: *Pax-6*, a murine paired box gene, is expressed in the developing CNS. *Development* **113**:1435, 1991.
11. Fujiwara M, Uchida T, Osumi-Yamashita N, Eto K: Uchida rat (rSey): A new mutant rat with craniofacial abnormalities resembling those of the mouse Sey mutant. *Differentiation* **57**:31, 1994.
12. Oliver G, Loosli F, Koster R, Wittbrodt J, Gruss P: Ectopic lens induction in fish in response to the murine homeobox gene *Six3*. *Mech Dev* **60**:233, 1996.
13. Nishiguchi S, Wood H, Kondoh H, Lovell-Badge R, Episkopou V: *Sox1* directly regulates the gamma-crystallin genes and is essential for lens development in mice. *Genes Dev* **12**:776, 1998.
14. Piatigorsky J: Lens differentiation in vertebrates: A review of cellular and molecular features. *Differentiation* **19**:134, 1981.
15. Goodenough DA, Dick JSB, Lyons JE: Lens metabolic cooperation: A study of mouse lens transport and permeability visualized with freeze-substitution autoradiography and electron microscopy. *J Cell Biol* **86**:576, 1980.
16. Gorthy WC, Snavely MR, Berrong ND: Some aspects of transport and digestion in the lens of the normal young adult rat. *Exp Eye Res* **12**:112, 1971.
17. Rae JL, Stacey T: Lanthanum and procion yellow as extracellular markers in the crystalline lens of the rat. *Exp Eye Res* **28**:1, 1979.
18. Ramaekers FCS, Bloemendal H: Cytoskeletal and contractile structures in lens cell differentiation, in Bloemendal H (ed): *Molecular and Cellular Biology of the Eye Lens*. New York, Wiley, 1981, p 85.
19. Benedetti L, Dunia I, Ramaekers FCS, Kibbelaar MA: Lenticular plasma membranes and cytoskeleton, in Bloemendal H (ed): *Molecular and Cellular Biology of the Eye Lens*. New York, Wiley, 1981, p 137.
20. Alcala H, Maisel H: Biochemistry of lens plasma membranes and cytoskeleton, in Maisel H (ed): *The Ocular Lens*. New York, Marcel Dekker, 1985, p 169.
21. Rafferty NS: Lens morphology, in Maisel H (ed): *The Ocular Lens*. New York, Marcel Dekker, 1985, p 1.
22. Ireland M, Maisel H: A family of lens fiber cell specific proteins. *Lens Eye Tox Res* **6**:623, 1989.
23. Piatigorsky J: Gene expression and genetic engineering in the lens. Friedenwald lecture. *Invest Ophthalmol Vis Sci* **28**:9, 1987.
24. Ostrer H, Beebe DC, Piatigorsky J: Beta-crystallin mRNAs: Differential distribution in the developing chicken lens. *Dev Biol* **86**:403, 1981.
25. Hejtmancik JF, Beebe DC, Ostrer H, Piatigorsky J: Delta- and beta-crystallin mRNA levels in the embryonic and posthatched chicken lens: Temporal and spatial changes during development. *Dev Biol* **109**:72, 1985.
26. Van Leen RW, Van Roozendaal KEP, Lubsen NH, Schoenmakers JG: Differential expression of crystallin genes during development of the rat eye lens. *Dev Biol* **120**:457, 1987.
27. Aarts HJ, Lubsen NH, Schoenmakers JG: Crystallin gene expression during rat lens development. *Eur J Biochem* **183**:31, 1989.
28. Young RW, Ocumpaugh DE: Autoradiographic studies on the growth and development of the lens capsule in the rat. *Invest Ophthalmol Vis Sci* **5**:583, 1966.
29. Koretz JF, Handelman GH: How the human eye focuses. *Sci Am* **256**:92, 1988.
30. Fisher RF, Pettet BE: The postnatal growth of the capsule of the human crystalline lens. *J Anat* **112**:207, 1972.
31. Parmigiani C, McAvoy J: Localisation of laminin and fibronectin during rat lens morphogenesis. *Differentiation* **28**:53, 1986.
32. Cammarata PR, Cantu-Crouch D, Oakford L, Morrill A: Macromolecular organization of the bovine lens capsule. *Tissue Cell* **18**:83, 1986.
33. Vrensen G, Kappelhof J, Willikens B: Aging of the human lens. *Lens Eye Tox Res* **7**:1, 1990.
34. Kuszak JR, Deutsch TA, Brown HG: Anatomy of aged and senile cataractous lenses, in Albert D, Jacobiec F (eds): *Principles and Practice of Ophthalmology: Basic Sciences*. Philadelphia, Saunders, 1994, p 82.
35. Koretz JF, Kaufman PL, Neider MW, Goeckner PA: Accommodation and presbyopia in the human eye — aging of the anterior segment. *Vis Res* **29**:1685, 1989.
36. Davson H: *Physiology of the Eye*. New York, Pergaman Press, 1990.
37. Sample PA, Esterson FD, Weinreb RN, Boynton RM: The aging lens: In vivo assessment of light absorption in 84 human eyes. *Invest Ophthalmol Vis Sci* **8**:1306, 1988.
38. Hockwin O, Ohrloff C: The eye in the elderly: Lens, in Platt D (ed): *Geriatrics*. Berlin, Springer-Verlag, 1984, p 373.

39. Roy D, Spector A: Absence of low-molecular weight alpha-crystallin in nuclear region of old human lens. *Proc Natl Acad Sci USA* **73**:3484, 1976.

40. McFall-Ngai MJ, Ding L-L, Takemoto LJ, Horwitz J: Spatial and temporal mapping of the age-related changes in human lens crystallins. *Exp Eye Res* **41**:745, 1985.

41. Voorter CE, De Haard-Hoekman WA, Roersma ES, Meyer HE, Bloemendal H, de Jong WW: The in vivo phosphorylation sites of bovine alpha B-crystallin. *FEBS Lett* **259**:50, 1989.

42. Horwitz J, Wong MM: Peptide mapping by limited proteolysis in sodium dodecyl sulfate of the main intrinsic polypeptides isolated from human and bovine lens plasma membranes. *Biochim Biophys Acta* **622**:134, 1980.

43. Wagner BJ, Margolis JW, Garland D, Roseman JE: Bovine lens neutral proteinase preferentially hydrolyses oxidatively modified glutamine synthetase. *Exp Eye Res* **43**:1141, 1986.

44. Harding JJ, Crabbe MJC: The lens: Development, proteins, metabolism and cataract, in Davson H (ed): *The Eye*, Vol. IB, 3. Orlando, FL, Academic Press, 1984, p 207.

45. David LL, Shearer TR: Purification of calpain II from rat lens and determination of endogenous substrates. *Exp Eye Res* **42**:227, 1986.

46. Jahngen JH, Lipman RD, Eisenhauer DA, Jahngen EG Jr, Taylor A: Aging and cellular maturation cause changes in ubiquitin-eye lens protein conjugates. *Arch Biochem Biophys* **276**:32, 1990.

47. Shang F, Gong X, Taylor A: Activity of ubiquitin-dependent pathway in response to oxidative stress: Ubiquitin-activating enzyme is transiently up-regulated. *J Biol Chem* **272**:23086, 1997.

48. Masters PM, Bada JL, Zigler JS Jr: Aspartic acid racemisation in the human lens during ageing and in cataract formation. *Nature* **268**:71, 1977.

49. Groenen PJTA, van den IjPR, Voorter CE, Bloemendal H, de Jong WW: Site-specific racemization in ageing alpha A-crystallin. *FEBS Lett* **269**:109, 1990.

50. Spector A, Chiesa R, Sredy J, Garner W: cAMP-dependent phosphorylation of bovine lens alpha-crystallin. *Proc Natl Acad Sci USA* **82**:4712, 1985.

51. Garlick RL, Mazer JS, Chylack LT Jr, Tung WH, Bunn HF: Nonenzymatic glycation of human lens crystallin: Effect of aging and diabetes mellitus. *J Clin Invest* **74**:1742, 1984.

52. Augusteyn RC: Distribution of flourescence in the human cataractous lens. *Ophthalmic Res* **7**:217, 1975.

53. Harding JJ: Possible causes of the unfolding of proteins in cataract and a new hypothesis to explain the high prevalence of cataract in some countries, in Regnault F, Hockwin O, Courtois Y (eds): *Aging of the Lens*. Amsterdam, Elsevier, 1980.

54. Harding JJ, Rixon KC: Carbamylation of lens proteins: A possible factor in cataractogenesis in some tropical countries. *Exp Eye Res* **31**:567, 1980.

55. Straatsma BR, Horwitz J, Takemoto LJ, Lightfoot DO, Ding LL: Clinicobiochemical correlations in aging-related human cataract. *Am J Ophthalmol* **97**:457, 1984.

56. Takemoto L, Straatsma BR, Horwitz J: Immunochemical characterization of the major low molecular weight polypeptide (10K) from human cataractous lenses. *Exp Eye Res* **48**:261, 1989.

57. Takemoto LJ, Hansen JS, Zigler JS, Horwitz J: Characterization of polypeptides from human nuclear cataracts by Western blot analysis. *Exp Eye Res* **40**:205, 1985.

58. David LL, Shearer TR: Role of proteolysis in lenses: A review. *Lens Eye Tox Res* **6**:725, 1989.

59. Lerman S: *Radiant Energy and the Eye*. New York, Macmillan, 1980.

60. Benedek GB: Theory of transparency of the eye. *Appl Optics* **10**:459, 1971.

61. Delaye M, Tardieu A: Short-range order of crystallin proteins accounts for eye lens transparency. *Nature* **302**:415, 1983.

62. Bettelheim FA, Siew EL: Effect of changes in concentration upon lens turbidity as predicted by the random fluctuation theory. *Biophys J* **41**:29, 1983.

63. Delaye M, Gromiec A: Mutual diffusion of crystallin proteins at finite concentrations: A light scattering study. *Biopolymers* **22**:1203, 1983.

64. de Jong WW, Terwindt EC, Bloemendal H: The amino acid sequence of the chain of human alpha-crystallin. *FEBS Lett* **58**:310, 1975.

65. Kramps JA, deMan BM, de Jong WW: The primary structure of the B₂ chain of human alpha-crystallin. *FEBS Lett* **74**:82, 1977.

66. van der Ouderaa FJ, de Jong WW, Hilderink A, Bloemendal H: The amino acid sequence of the alphaB₂ chain of bovine alpha-crystallin. *Eur J Biochem* **49**:157, 1974.

67. Horwitz J: Some properties of the low molecular weight alpha-crystallin from normal human lens: Comparison with bovine lens. *Exp Eye Res* **19**:49, 1974.

68. Tardieu A, Laporte D, Licinio P, Krop B, Delaye M: Calf lens alpha-crystallin quarternary structure: A three-layer model. *J Mol Biol* **192**:711, 1986.

69. Augusteyn RC, Koretz JF: A possible structure for alpha-crystallin. *FEBS Lett* **222**:1, 1987.

70. Thomson JA, Augusteyn RC: On the structure of alpha-crystallin: Construction of hybrid molecules and homopolymers. *Biochim Biophys Acta* **994**:246, 1989.

71. Hendriks W, Weetink H, Voorter CE, Sanders J, Bloemendal H, de Jong WW: The alternative splicing product alpha Aⁱⁿˢ-crystallin is structurally equivalent to alpha A and alpha B subunits in the rat alpha-crystallin aggregate. *Biochim Biophys Acta* **1037**:58, 1990.

72. Bova MP, Ding LL, Horwitz J, Fung BK: Subunit exchange of alpha A-crystallin. *J Biol Chem* **272**:29511, 1997.

73. Sun TX, Liang JN: Intermolecular exchange and stabilization of recombinant human alphaA- and alphaB-crystallin. *J Biol Chem* **273**:286, 1998.

74. Haley DA, Horwitz J, Stewart PL: The small heat-shock protein, alphaB-crystallin, has a variable quaternary structure. *J Mol Biol* **277**:27, 1998.

75. Brady JP, Garland D, Duglas-Tabor Y, Robison WG Jr, Groome A, Wawrousek EF: Targeted disruption of the mouse alpha A-crystallin gene induces cataract and cytoplasmic inclusion bodies containing the small heat shock protein alpha B-crystallin. *Proc Natl Acad Sci USA* **94**:884, 1997.

76. Wawrousek EF, Brady JP: AlphaB-crystallin gene knockout mice develop a severe, fatal phenotype late in life. *Invest Ophthalmol Vis Sci* **39**:S523, 1998.

77. Kantorow M, Piatigorsky J: Alpha-crystallin/small heat shock protein has autokinase activity. *Proc Natl Acad Sci USA* **91**:3112, 1994.

78. Kantorow M, Horwitz J, van Boekel MA, de Jong WW, Piatigorsky J: Conversion from oligomers to tetramers enhances autophosphorylation by lens alpha A-crystallin: Specificity between alpha A- and alpha B-crystallin subunits. *J Biol Chem* **270**:17215, 1995.

79. Sun TX, Das BK, Liang JJ: Conformational and functional differences between recombinant human lens alphaA-and alphaB-crystallin. *J Biol Chem* **272**:6220, 1997.

80. Voorter CE, Mulders JW, Bloemendal H, de Jong WW: Some aspects of the phosphorylation of alpha-crystallin A. *Eur J Biochem* **160**:203, 1986.

81. Chiesa R, Spector A: The dephosphorylation of lens alpha-crystallin A chain. *Biochem Biophys Res Commun* **162**:1494, 1989.

82. Wang K, Ma W, Spector A: Phosphorylation of alpha-crystallin in rat lenses is stimulated by H2O2 but phosphorylation has no effect on chaperone activity. *Exp Eye Res* **61**:115, 1995.

83. Nicholl ID, Quinlan RA: Chaperone activity of alpha-crystallins modulates intermediate filament assembly. *EMBO J* **13**:945, 1994.

84. Wang K, Spector A: Alpha-crystallin stabilizes actin filaments and prevents cytochalasin-induced depolymerization in a phosphorylation-dependent manner. *Eur J Biochem* **242**:56, 1996.

85. Ito H, Okamoto K, Nakayama H, Isobe T, Kato K: Phosphorylation of alphaB-crystallin in response to various types of stress. *J Biol Chem* **272**:29934, 1997.

86. Manenti S, Dunia I, Benedetti EL: Fatty acid acylation of lens fiber plasma membrane proteins: MP26 and alpha-crystallin are palmitoylated. *FEBS Lett* **262**:356, 1990.

87. Mulders JWM, Stokkermans J, Leunissen JAM, Benedetti EL, Bloemendal H, de Jong WW: Interaction of alpha-crystallin with lens plasma membranes: Affinity for MP26. *Eur J Biochem* **152**:721, 1985.

88. Lasser A, Balazs EA: Biochemical and fine structure studies on the water-insoluble components of the calf lens. *Exp Eye Res* **13**:292, 1972.

89. Kantorow M, Piatigorsky J: Phosphorylation of αA- and αB-crystallin. *Int J Biol Macromol* **22**:307, 1998.

90. de Jong WW, Gleaves JT, Boulter D: Evolutionary changes of alpha-crystallin and the phylogeny of mammalian orders. *J Mol Evol* **10**:123, 1977.

91. Ingolia TD, Craig EA: Four small *Drosophila* heat shock proteins are related to each other and to mammalian alpha-crystallin. *Proc Natl Acad Sci USA* **79**:2360, 1982.

92. Nene V, Dunne DW, Johnson KS, Taylor DW, Cordingley JS: Sequence and expression of a major egg antigen from *Schistosoma mansoni*: Homologies to heat shock proteins and alpha-crystallins. *Mol Biochem Parasitol* **21**:179, 1986.

93. de Jong WW, Hendriks W, Mulders JW, Bloemendal H: Evolution of eye lens crystallins: The stress connection. *Trends Biochem Sci* **14**:365, 1989.

94. Cohen LH, Westerhuis LW, de Jong WW, Bloemendal H: Rat alpha-crystallin A chain with an insertion of 22 residues. *Eur J Biochem* **89**:259, 1978.

95. van den Heuvel R, Hendriks W, Quax W, Bloemendal H: Complete structure of the hamster alphaA-crystallin gene: Reflection of an evolutionary history by means of exon shuffling. *J Mol Biol* **185**:273, 1985.

96. Cohen LH, Westerhuis LW, Smits DP, Bloemendal H: Two structurally closely related polypeptides encoded by 14-S mRNA isolated from rat lens. *Eur J Biochem* **89**:251, 1978.

97. Hendriks W, Sanders J, de Leij L, Ramaekers F, Bloemendal H, de Jong W: Monoclonal antibodies reveal evolutionary conservation of alternative splicing of the alphaA-crystallin primary transcript. *Eur J Biochem* **174**:133, 1988.

98. King CR, Piatigorsky J: Alternative RNA splicing of the murine alpha A-crystallin gene: Protein-coding information within an intron. *Cell* **32**:707, 1983.

99. Jaworski CJ, Piatigorsky J: A pseudo-exon in the functional human alpha A-crystallin gene. *Nature* **337**:752, 1989.

100. Bhat SP, Nagineni CN: Alpha B subunit of lens-specific protein alpha-crystallin is in other ocular and non-ocular tissues. *Biochem Biophys Res Commun* **158**:319, 1989.

101. Dubin RA, Wawrousek EF, Piatigorsky J: Expression of the murine alpha B-crystallin gene is not restricted to the lens. *Mol Cell Biol* **9**:1083, 1989.

102. Bhat SP, Horwitz J, Srinivasan A, Ding L: AlphaB-crystallin exists as an independent protein in the heart and in the lens. *Eur J Biochem* **202**:775, 1991.

103. Atomi Y, Yamada S, Nishida T: Early changes of alpha B-crystallin mRNA in rat skeletal muscle to mechanical tension and denervation. *Biochem Biophys Res Commun* **181**:1323, 1991.

104. Iwaki T, Kume-Iwaki A, Liem RK, Goldman JE: Alpha B-crystallin is expressed in non-lenticular tissues and accumulates in Alexander's disease brain. *Cell* **57**:71, 1989.

105. Duguid JR, Bohmont CW, Liu NG, Tourtellotte WW: Changes in brain gene expression shared by scrapie and Alzheimer disease. *Proc Natl Acad Sci USA* **86**:7260, 1989.

106. Murano S, Thweatt R, Shmookler Reis RJ, Jones RA, Moerman EJ, Goldstein S: Diverse gene sequences are overexpressed in Werner syndrome fibroblasts undergoing premature replicative senescence. *Mol Cell Biol* **11**:3905, 1991.

107. Klemenz R, Frohli E, Steiger RH, Schafer R, Aoyama A: Alpha B-crystallin is a small heat shock protein. *Proc Natl Acad Sci USA* **88**:3652, 1991.

108. Dasgupta S, Hohman TC, Carper D: Hypertonic stress induces alpha B-crystallin expression. *Exp Eye Res* **54**:461, 1992.

109. Kato K, Shinohara H, Kurobe N, Goto S, Inaguma Y, Ohshima K: Immunoreactive alphaA-crystallin in rat non-lenticular tissues detected with a sensitive immunoassay method. *Biochim Biophys Acta* **1080**:173, 1991.

110. Hendriks W, Leunissen J, Nevo E, Bloemendal H, de Jong WW: The lens protein alpha A-crystallin of the blind mole rat, *Spalax ehrenbergi*: Evolutionary change and functional constraints. *Proc Natl Acad Sci USA* **84**:5320, 1987.

111. Horwitz J, Huang QL, Ding L, Bova MP: Lens alpha-crystallin: Chaperone-like properties. *Methods Enzymol* **290**:365, 1998.

112. Horwitz J: Alpha-crystallin can function as a molecular chaperone. *Proc Natl Acad Sci USA* **89**:10449, 1992.

113. Clark JI, Huang QL: Modulation of the chaperone-like activity of bovine alpha-crystallin. *Proc Natl Acad Sci USA* **93**:15185, 1996.

114. Muchowski PJ, Clark JI: ATP-enhanced molecular chaperone functions of the small heat shock protein human alphaB crystallin. *Proc Natl Acad Sci USA* **95**:1004, 1998.

115. Muchowski PJ, Bassuk JA, Lubsen NH, Clark JI: Human alphaB-crystallin: Small heat shock protein and molecular chaperone. *J Biol Chem* **272**:2578, 1997.

116. Raman B, Rao CM: Chaperone-like activity and temperature-induced structural changes of alpha-crystallin. *J Biol Chem* **272**:23559, 1997.

117. Thompson MA, Hawkins JW, Piatigorsky J: Complete nucleotide sequence of the chicken alpha A-crystallin gene and its 5′ flanking region. *Gene* **56**:173, 1987.

118. Wistow G: Domain structure and evolution in alpha-crystallins and small heat-shock proteins. *FEBS Lett* **181**:1, 1985.

119. Brakenhoff RH, Guerts van Kessel AH, Oldenburg M, Wijnen JT, Bloemendal H, Meera Khan P, Schoenmakers JG: Human alpha B-crystallin (*CRYA2*) gene mapped to chromosome 11q12–q23. *Hum Genet* **85**:237, 1990.

120. Piatigorsky J, Zelenka PS: Transcriptional regulation of crystallin genes: Cis elements, transfactors and signal transduction systems in the lens, in Wasserman PW (ed): *Advances in Developmental Biochemistry*, Vol 1 Greenwich, CT, JAI Press, 1992, p 211.

121. Chepelinsky AB, King CR, Zelenka PS, Piatigorsky J: Lens-specific expression of the chloramphenicol acetyltransferase gene promoted by 5′ flanking sequences of the murine alpha A-crystallin gene in explanted chicken lens epithelia. *Proc Natl Acad Sci USA* **82**:2334, 1985.

122. Overbeek PA, Chepelinsky AB, Khillan JS, Piatigorsky J, Westphal H: Lens-specific expression and developmental regulation of the bacterial chloramphenicol acetyltransferase gene driven by the murine alphaA-crystallin promoter in transgenic mice. *Proc Natl Acad Sci USA* **82**:7815, 1985.

123. Wawrousek EF, Chepelinsky AB, McDermott JB, Piatigorsky J: Regulation of the murine alpha A-crystallin promoter in transgenic mice. *Dev Biol* **137**:68, 1990.

124. Driessen HP, Herbrink P, Bloemendal H, de Jong WW: Primary structure of the bovine beta-crystallin Bp chain: Internal duplication and homology with gamma-crystallin. *Eur J Biochem* **121**:83, 1981.

125. Wistow G, Slingsby C, Blundell T, Driessen H, de Jong W, Bloemendal H: Eye-lens proteins: The three-dimensional structure of beta-crystallin predicted from monomeric gamma-crystallin. *FEBS Lett* **133**:9, 1981.

126. Lubsen NH, Aarts HJM, Schoenmakers JGG: The evolution of lenticular proteins: the beta- and gamma-crystallin supergene family. *Prog Biophys Mol Biol* **51**:47, 1988.

127. Blundell T, Lindley P, Miller L, Moss D, Slingsby C, Tickle I, Turnell B, Wistow G: The molecular structure and stability of the eye lens: X-ray analysis of gamma-crystallin II. *Nature* **289**:771, 1981.

128. Wistow GJ, Turnell B, Summers L, Slingsby C, Moss D, Miller L, Lindley P, Blundell T: X-ray analysis of the eye lens protein gamma-II crystallin at 1s.9 A resolution. *J Mol Biol* **170**:175, 1983.

129. White HE, Driessen HPC, Slingsby C, Moss DS, Lindley PF: Packing interactions in the eye lens: Structural analysis, internal symmetry and lattice interactions of bovine gamma IVa-crystallin. *J Mol Biol* **207**:217, 1989.

130. Norledge BV, Hay RE, Bateman OA, Slingsby C, Driessen HP: Towards a molecular understanding of phase separation in the lens: A comparison of the x-ray structures of two high Tc gamma-crystallins, gammaE and gammaF, with two low Tc gamma-crystallins, gammaB and gammaD. *Exp Eye Res* **65**:609, 1997.

131. Siezen RJ, Wu E, Kaplan ED, Thomson JA, Benedek GB: Rat lens gamma-crystallins: Characterization of the six gene products and their spatial and temporal distribution resulting from differential synthesis. *J Mol Biol* **199**:475, 1988.

132. Broide ML, Berland CR, Pande J, Ogun OO, Benedek GB: Binary-liquid phase separation of lens protein solutions. *Proc Natl Acad Sci USA* **88**:5660, 1991.

133. Tanaka T, Benedek GB: Observation of protein diffusivity in intact human and bovine lenses with application to cataract. *Invest Ophthalmol* **14**:449, 1975.

134. Wistow G: Evolution of a protein superfamily: Relationships between vertebrate lens crystallins and microorganism dormancy proteins. *J Mol Evol* **30**:140, 1990.

135. Krasko A, Muller IM, Muller WE: Evolutionary relationships of the metazoan beta gamma-crystallins, including that from the marine sponge *Geodia cydonium*. *Proc R Soc Lond B Biol Sci* **264**:1077, 1991.

136. Ray ME, Wistow G, Su YA, Meltzer PS, Trent JM: A1M1, a novel non-lens member of the beta-gamma-crystallin superfamily associated with the control of tumorigenicity in human malignant melanoma. *Proc Natl Acad Sci USA* **94**:3229, 1997.

137. Norledge BV, Mayr EM, Glockshuber R, Bateman OA, Slingsby C, Jaenicke R, Driessen HP: The x-ray structures of two mutant crystallin domains shed light on the evolution of multidomain proteins. *Nature Struct Biol* **3**:267, 1996.

138. Wistow G, Summers L, Blundell T: *Myxococcus xanthus* spore coat protein S may have a similar structure to vertebrate lens beta gamma-crystallins. *Nature* **315**:771, 1985.

139. Moormann RJM, den Dunnen JT, Mulleners L, Andreoli P, Bloemendal H, Schoenmakers JGG: Strict co-linearity of genetic and protein folding domains in an intragenically duplicated rat lens gamma-crystallin gene. *J Mol Biol* **171**:353, 1983.

140. Lok S, Tsui LC, Shinohara T, Piatigorsky J, Gold R, Breitman M: Analysis of the mouse gamma-crystallin gene family: Assignment of multiple cDNAs to discrete genomic sequences and characterization of a representative gene. *Nucl Acids Res* **12**:4517, 1984.

141. Meakin SO, Du RP, Tsui LC, Breitman ML: Gamma-crystallins of the human eye lens: Expression analysis of five members of the gene family. *Mol Cell Biol* **7**:2671, 1987.

142. Russell P, Meakin SO, Hohman TC, Tsui LC, Breitman ML: Relationship between proteins encoded by three human gamma-crystallin genes and distinct polypeptides in the eye lens. *Mol Cell Biol* **7**:3320, 1987.

143. Siezen RJ, Thomson JA, Kaplan ED, Benedek GB: Human lens gamma-crystallin: Isolation, identification, and characterization of the expressed gene products. *Proc Natl Acad Sci USA* **84**:6088, 1987.

144. Breitman ML, Clapoff S, Rossant J, Tsui LC, Glode LM, Maxwell IH, Bernstein A: Genetic ablation: Targeted expression of a toxin gene causes microphthalmia in transgenic mice. *Science* **238**:1563, 1987.

145. Lok S, Breitman ML, Chepelinsky AB, Piatigorsky J, Gold RJ, Tsui LC: Lens-specific promoter activity of a mouse gamma-crystallin gene. *Mol Cell Biol* **5**:2221, 1985.

146. Goring DR, Rossant J, Clapoff S, Brietman ML, Tsui LC: In situ detection of beta-galactosidase in lenses of transgenic mice with a gamma-crystallin/*lacZ* gene. *Science* **235**:456, 1987.

147. Lok S, Stevens W, Breitman ML, Tsui LC: Multiple regulatory elements of the murine gamma 2-crystallin promoter. *Nucl Acids Res* **17**:3563, 1989.

148. Tini M, Otulakowski G, Breitman ML, Tsui LC, Giguère V: An everted repeat mediates retinoic acid induction of the gamma F-crystallin gene: Evidence of a direct role for retinoids in lens development. *Genes Dev* **7**:295, 1993.

149. Tini M, Fraser RA, Giguere V: Functional interactions between retinoic acid receptor-related orphan nuclear receptor (ROR alpha) and the retinoic acid receptors in the regulation of the gamma F-crystallin promoter. *J Biol Chem* **270**:20156, 1995.

150. van Dam AF: Purification and composition studies of betaS-crystallin. *Exp Eye Res* **5**:255, 1966.

151. Quax-Jeuken Y, Driessen H, Leunissen J, Quax W, de Jong W, Bloemendal H: BetaS-crystallin: Structure and evolution of a distinct member of the beta gamma-superfamily. *EMBO J* **4**:2597, 1985.

152. van Rens GL, Raats JM, Driessen HP, Oldenburg M, Wijnen JT, Khan PM, de Jong WW, Bloemendal H: Structure of the bovine eye lens gamma s-crystallin gene (formerly beta s). *Gene* **78**:225, 1989.

153. Zigler JS Jr, Russell P, Horwitz J, Reddy VN, Kinoshita JH: Further studies on low molecular weight crystallins: Relationship between the bovine beta s, the human 24 kD protein and the gamma-crystallins. *Curr Eye Res* **5**:395, 1986.

154. Wijnen JT, Oldenburg M, Bloemendal H, Meera-Khan P: GS(gamma-S)-crystallin (CRYGS) assignment to chromosome 3. *Cytogenet Cell Genet* **51**:1108, 1989.

155. Willard HF, Meakin SO, Tsui LC, Breitman ML: Assignment of human gamma crystallin multigene family to chromosome 2. *Somat Cell Mol Genet* **11**:511, 1985.

156. den Dunnen JT, Jongbloed RJE, Geurts van Kessel AHM, Schoenmakers JGG: Human lens gamma-crystallin sequences are located in the p12-qter region of chromosome 2. *Hum Genet* **70**:217, 1985.

157. Shiloh Y, Donlon T, Bruns G, Breitman ML, Tsui LC: Assignment of the human gamma-crystallin gene cluster (*CRYG*) to the long arm of chromosome 2, region q33–36. *Hum Genet* **73**:17, 1986.

158. Slingsby C, Croft LR: Developmental changes in the low molecular weight proteins of the bovine lens. *Exp Eye Res* **17**:369, 1973.

159. McDevitt DS, Croft LR: On the existence of gamma-crystallin in the bird lens. *Exp Eye Res* **25**:473, 1977.

160. van Rens GL, de Jong WW, Bloemendal H: One member of the gamma-crystallin gene family, gamma s, is expressed in birds (letter). *Exp Eye Res* **53**:135, 1991.

161. Peterson CA, Piatigorsky J: Preferential conservation of the globular domains of the beta A3/A1-crystallin polypeptide of the chicken eye lens. *Gene* **45**:139, 1986.

162. Hejtmancik JF, Thompson MA, Wistow G, Piatigorsky J: cDNA and deduced protein sequence for the beta B1-crystallin polypeptide of the chicken lens: Conservation of the PAPA sequence. *J Biol Chem* **261**:982, 1986.

163. Berbers GAM, Hoekman WA, Bloemendal H, de Jong WW, Kleinschmidt T, Braunitzer G: Homology between the primary structures of the major bovine beta-crystallin chains. *Eur J Biochem* **139**:467, 1984.

164. Bloemendal H, de Jong WW: Lens proteins and their genes. *Prog Nucl Acid Res Mol Biol* **41**:259, 1991.

165. Hogg D, Tsui LC, Gorin M, Breitman ML: Characterization of the human beta-crystallin gene Hu beta A3/A1 reveals ancestral relationships among the beta gamma- crystallin superfamily. *J Biol Chem* **261**:12420, 1986.

166. Berbers GAM, Hoekman WA, Bloemendal H, de Jong WW, Kleinschmidt T, Braunitzer G: Proline- and alanine-rich N-terminal extension of the basic bovine beta-crystallin B1 chains. *FEBS Lett* **161**:225, 1983.

167. Kleiman NJ, Chiesa R, Kolks MA, Spector A: Phosphorylation of beta-crystallin B2 (beta Bp) in the bovine lens. *J Biol Chem* **263**:14978, 1988.

168. Voorter CE, Bloemendal H, de Jong WW: In vitro and in vivo phosphorylation of chicken beta B3-crystallin. *Curr Eye Res* **8**:459, 1989.

169. Wistow G, Roquemore E, Kim HS: Anomalous behavior of beta B1-crystallin subunits from avian lenses. *Curr Eye Res* **10**:313, 1991.

170. Slingsby C, Bateman OA: Qartenary interactions in eye lens beta-crystallins: Basic and acidic subunits of beta-crystallins favor heterologous association. *Biochemistry* **29**:6592, 1990.

171. Bax B, Lapatto R, Nalini V, Driessen H, Lindley PF, Mahadevan D, Blundell TL, Slingsby C: X-ray analysis of beta B2-crystallin and evolution of oligomeric lens proteins. *Nature* **347**:776, 1990.

172. Wistow G, Turnell B, Summers L, Slingsby C, Moss D, Miller L, Lindley P, Blundell T: X-ray analysis of the eye lens protein gamma-II crystallin at 1.9 Å resolution. *J Mol Biol* **170**:175, 1983.

173. Mayr EM, Jaenicke R, Glockshuber R: Domain interactions and connecting peptides in lens crystallins. *J Mol Biol* **235**:84, 1994.

174. Hope JN, Chen H-C, Hejtmancik JF: Aggregation of betaA3-crystallin is independent of the specific sequence of the domain connecting peptide. *J Biol Chem* **269**:21141, 1994.

175. Hope JN, Chen HC, Hejtmancik JF: BetaA3/A1-crystallin association: Role of the amino-terminal arm. *Protein Eng* **7**:445, 1994.

176. Kroone RC, Elliott GS, Ferszt A, Slingsby C, Lubsen NH, Schoenmakers JGG: The role of the sequence extensions in beta-crystallin assembly. *Protein Eng* **7**:1395, 1994.

177. Werten PJL, Carver JA, Jaenicke R, de Jong WW: The elusive role of the N-terminal extension of betaA3- and betaA1-crystallin. *Protein Eng* **9**:1021, 1996.

178. Inana G, Piatigorsky J, Norman B, Slingsby C, Blundell T: Gene and protein structure of a beta-crystallin polypeptide in murine lens: Relationship of exons and structural motifs. *Nature* **302**:310, 1983.

179. den Dunnen JT, Moormann RJM, Lubsen NH, Schoenmakers JGG: Intron insertions and deletions in the beta/gamma-crystallin gene family: The rat betaB1 gene. *Proc Natl Acad Sci USA* **83**:2855, 1986.

180. Moormann RJM, den Dunnen JT, Bloemendal H, Schoenmakers JGG: Extensive intragenic sequence homology in two distinct rat lens gamma-crystallin cDNAs suggests duplications of a primordial gene. *Proc Natl Acad Sci USA* **79**:6876, 1982.

181. Hogg D, Gorin MB, Heinzmann C, Zollman S, Mohandas T, Klisak I, Sparkes RS, Breitman M, Tsui LC, Horwitz J: Nucleotide sequence for the cDNA of the bovine beta B2 crystallin and assignment of the orthologous human locus to chromosome 22. *Curr Eye Res* **6**:1335, 1987.

182. Sparkes RS, Mohandas T, Heinzmann C, Gorin MB, Zollman S, Horwitz J: Assignment of a human beta-crystallin gene to 17cen-q23. *Hum Genet* **74**:133, 1986.

183. Aarts HJM, den Dunnen JT, Lubsen NH, Schoenmakers JGG: Linkage between the beta B2 and beta B3 crystallin genes in man and rat: a remnant of an ancient beta-crystallin gene cluster. *Gene* **59**:127, 1987.

184. Head MW, Peter A, Clayton RM: Evidence for the extralenticular expression of members of the beta-crystallin gene family in the chick and a comparison with delta-crystallin during differentiation and transdifferentiation. *Differentiation* **48**:147, 1991.

185. Head MW, Sedowofia K, Clayton RM: Beta B2-crystallin in the mammalian retina. *Exp Eye Res* **61**:423, 1995.

186. Dirks RP, van GS, KrUse JJ, Jorissen L, Lubsen NH: Extralenticular expression of the rodent betaB2-crystallin gene. *Exp Eye REs* **66**:267, 1998.

187. Kantorow M, Horwitz J, Sergeev YV, Hejtmancik JF, and Piatigorsky J: Extralenticular expression cAMP-dependent kinase phosphorylation and autophosphorlyation of betaB2-crystallin. *Invest Ophthalmol Vis Sci* **38**:S205, 1997.

188. Smolich BD, Tarkington SK, Saha MS, Grainger RM: *Xenopus* gamma-crystallin gene expression: Evidence that the gamma-crystallin gene family is transcribed in lens and nonlens tissues. *Mol Cell Biol* **14**:1355, 1994.

189. Brunekreef GA, van GS, Destree OH, Lubsen NH: Extralenticular expression of *Xenopus laevis* alpha-, beta-, and gamma-crystallin genes. *Invest Ophthalmol Vis Sci* **38**:2764, 1997.

190. Sinha D, Esumi N, Jaworski C, Kozak CA, Pierce E, Wistow G: Cloning and mapping the mouse *Crygs* gene and non-lens expression of gammaS-crystallin. *Mol Vis* **4**:8, 1998.

191. Piatigorsky J, Wistow GJ: Enzyme/crystallins: Gene sharing as an evolutionary strategy. *Cell* **57**:197, 1989.

192. Piatigorsky J, Wistow GJ: The recruitment of crystallins: New functions precede gene duplication. *Science* **252**:1078, 1991.

193. Piatigorsky J: Gene sharing in lens and cornea: Facts and implications. *Prog Ret Eye Res*, **17**:145, 1998.

194. McFall-Ngai MJ, Horwitz J: A comparative study of the thermal stability of the vertebrate eye lens: Antarctic ice fish to the desert iguana. *Exp Eye Res* **50**:703, 1990.

195. Rao CM, Zigler JS Jr: Levels of reduced pyridine nucleotides and lens photodamage. *Photochem Photobiol* **56**:523, 1992.

196. Zigler JS Jr, Rao PV: Enzyme/crystallins and extremely high pyridine nucleotide levels in the lens. *FASEB J* **5**:223, 1991.

197. Piatigorsky J: Lens crystallins: Innovation associated with changes in gene regulation. *J Biol Chem* **267**:4277, 1992.

198. Piatigorsky J: Delta crystallins and their nucleic acids. *Mol Cell Biochem* **59**:33, 1984.

199. Wistow G, Piatigorsky J: Recruitment of enzymes as lens structural proteins. *Science* **236**:1554, 1987.

200. Thomas G, Zelenka PS, Cuthbertson RA, Norman BL, Piatigorsky J: Differential expression of the two delta-crystallin/argeninosuccinate lyase genes in the lens, heart and brain of the chicken embryo. *New Biol* **2**:903, 1990.

201. Kondoh H, Araki I, Yasuda K, Matsubasa T, Mori M: Expression of the chicken "delta 2-crystallin" gene in mouse cells: Evidence for encoding of argininosuccinate lyase. *Gene* **99**:267, 1991.

202. Piatigorsky J, Horwitz J: Characterization and enzyme activity of argininosuccinate lyase/delta-crystallin of the embryonic duck lens. *Biochim Biophys Acta* **1295**:158, 1996.

203. Simpson A, Bateman O, Driessen H, Lindley P, Moss D, Mylvaganam S, Narebor E, Slingsby C: The structure of avian eye lens delta-crystallin reveals a new fold for a superfamily of oligomeric enzymes (see comments) [published erratum appears in *Nature Struct Biol* **1**(11):831, 1994]. *Nature Struct Biol* **1**:724, 1994.

204. Abu-Abed M, Turner MA, Vallee F, Simpson A, Slingsby C, Howell PL: Structural comparison of the enzymatically active and inactive forms of delta crystallin and the role of histidine 91. *Biochemistry* **36**:14012, 1997.

205. Wistow GJ, Mulders JWM, de Jong WW: The enzyme lactate dehydrogenase as a structural protein in avian and crocodilian lenses. *Nature* **326**:622, 1987.

206. Hendriks W, Mulders JW, Bibby MA, Slingsby C, Bloemendal H, de Jong WW: Duck lens epsilon-crystallin and lactate dehydrogenase B4 are identical: A single-copy gene product with two distinct functions. *Proc Natl Acad Sci USA* **85**:7114, 1988.

207. Borras T, Persson B, Jornvall H: Eye lens zeta-crystallin relationships to the family of "long-chain" alcohol/polyol dehydrogenases: Protein trimming and conservation of stable parts. *Biochemistry* **28**:6133, 1989.

208. Rao PV, Zigler JS Jr: Zeta-crystallin from guinea pig lens is capable of functioning catalytically as an oxidoreductase. *Arch Biochem Biophys* **284**:181, 1991.

209. Wistow G, Kim H: Lens protein expression in mammals: Taxon-specificity and the recruitment of crystallins. *J Mol Evol* **32**:262, 1991.

210. Graham C, Hodin J, Wistow G: A retinaldehyde dehydrogenase as a structural protein in a mammalian eye lens: Gene recruitment of eta-crystallin. *J Biol Chem* **271**:15623, 1996.

211. Mulders JW, Hendriks W, Blankesteijn WM, Bloemendal H, de Jong WW: Lambda-crystallin, a major rabbit lens protein, is related to hydroxyacyl-coenzyme A dehydrogenases. *J Biol Chem* **263**:15462, 1988.

212. Carper D, Nishimura C, Shinohara T, Dietzschold B, Wistow G, Craft C, Kador P, Kinoshita JH: Aldose reductase and rho-crystallin belong to the same protein superfamily as aldehyde reductase. *FEBS Lett* **220**:209, 1987.

213. Tomarev SI, Piatigorsky J: Lens crystallins of invertebrates—diversity and recruitment from detoxification enzymes and novel proteins. *Eur J Biochem* **235**:449, 1996.

214. Van Leen RW, Breuer ML, Lubsen NH, Schoenmakers JG: Developmental expression of crystallin genes: In situ hybridization reveals a differential localization of specific mRNAs. *Dev Biol* **123**:338, 1987.

215. Duncan MK, Li X, Ogino H, Yasuda K, Piatigorsky J: Developmental regulation of the chicken beta B1-crystallin promoter in transgenic mice. *Mech Dev* **57**:79, 1996.

216. McDermott JB, Cvekl A, Piatigorsky J: Lens-specific expression of a chicken beta A3/A1-crystallin promoter fragment in transgenic mice. *Biochem Biophys Res Commun* **221**:559, 1996.

217. Haynes JI2, Duncan MK, Piatigorsky J: Spatial and temporal activity of the alpha B-crystallin/small heat shock protein gene promoter in transgenic mice. *Dev Dyn* **207**:75, 1996.

218. Nakamura T, Donovan DM, Hamada K, Sax CM, Norman B, Flanagan JR, Ozato K, Westphal H, Piatigorsky J: Regulation of the mouse alpha A-crystallin gene: Isolation of a cDNA encoding a protein that binds to a cis sequence motif shared with the major histocompatibility complex class I gene and other genes. *Mol Cell Biol* **10**:3700, 1990.

219. Cvekl A, Kashanchi F, Sax CM, Brady J, Piatigorsky J: Transcriptional regulation of the mouse alphaA-crystallin gene: Activation dependent on a cyclic AMP-responsive element (DE1/CRE) and a Pax-6-binding site. *Mol Cell Biol* **15**:653, 1995.

220. Sax CM, Iiagan JG, Haynes JI: Lens-preferred activity of the −1809/+46 mouse alpha A-crystallin promoter in stably integrated chromatin. *Biochim Biophys Acta* **1305**:49, 1996.

221. Matsuo I, Yasuda K: The cooperative interaction between two motifs of an enhancer element of the chicken alpha A-crystallin gene, alpha CE1 and alpha CE2, confers lens-specific expression. *Nucl Acids Res* **20**:3701, 1992.

222. Gopal-Srivastava R, Piatigorsky J: Identification of a lens-specific regulatory region (LSR) of the murine alpha B-crystallin gene. *Nucl Acids Res* **22**:1281, 1994.

223. Gopal-Srivastava R, Haynes JI 2, Piatigorsky J: Regulation of the murine alpha B-crystallin/small heat shock protein gene in cardiac muscle. *Mol Cell Biol* **15**:7081, 1995.

224. Gopal-Srivastava R, Cvekl A, Piatigorsky J: Pax-6 and alphaB-crystallin/small heat shock protein gene regulation in the murine lens: Interaction with the lens-specific regions, LSR1 and LSR2. *J Biol Chem* **271**:23029, 1996.

225. Haynes JI, Gopal-Srivastava R, Piatigorsky J: Alpha B-crystallin TATA sequence mutations: Lens-preference for the proximal TATA box and the distal TATA-like sequence in transgenic mice. *Biochem Biophys Res Commun* **241**:407, 1997.

226. Roth HJ, Das GC, Piatigorsky J: Chicken betaB1-crystallin gene expression: Presence of conserved functional polyoma enhancer-like and octomer binding-like promoter elements found in non-lens genes. *Mol Cell Biol* **11**:1488, 1991.

227. McDermott JB, Cvekl A, Piatigorsky J: A complex enhancer of the chicken beta A3/A1-crystallin gene depends on an AP-1-CRE element for activity. *Invest Ophthalmol Vis Sci* **38**:951, 1997.

228. Liu QR, Tini M, Tsui LC, Breitman ML: Interaction of a lens cell transcription factor with the proximal domain of the mouse gamma F-crystallin promoter. *Mol Cell Biol* **11**:1531, 1991.

229. Peek R, van der Logt P, Lubsen NH, Schoenmakers JG: Tissue- and species-specific promoter elements of rat gamma-crystallin genes. *Nucl Acids Res* **18**:1189, 1990.

230. Yu CC-K, Tsui L-C, Breitman ML: Homologous and heterologous enhancers modulate spatial expression but not cell-type specificity of the murine gamma-crystallin promoter. *Development* **110**:131, 1990.

231. Goto K, Okada TS, Kondoh H: Functional cooperation of lens-specific and nonspecific elements in the delta 1-crystallin enhancer. *Mol Cell Biol* **10**:958, 1990.

232. Li X, Cvekl A, Bassnett S, Piatigorsky J: Lens-preferred activity of chicken delta1- and delta2-crystallin enhancers in transgenic mice and evidence for retinoic acid-responsive regulation of the delta1-crystallin gene. *Dev Genet* **20**:258, 1997.

233. Funahashi J, Sekido R, Murai K, Kamachi Y, Kondoh H: Delta-crystallin enhancer binding protein delta EF1 is a zinc finger-homeodomain protein implicated in postgastrulation embryogenesis. *Development* **119**:433, 1993.

234. Hayashi S, Goto K, Okada TS, Kondoh H: Lens-specific enhancer in the third intron regulates expression of the chicken delta1-crystallin gene. *Genes Dev* **1**:818, 1987.

235. Richardson J, Cvekl A, Wistow G: Pax-6 is essential for lens-specific expression of zeta-crystallin. *Proc Natl Acad Sci USA* **92**:4676, 1995.

236. Gilmore TD: NF-kappa B, KBF1, dorsal, and related matters. *Cell* **62**:841, 1990.

237. Sax CM, Klement JF, Piatigorsky J: Species-specific lens activation of the thymidine kinase promoter by a single copy of the mouse alpha A-CRYBP1 site and loss of tissue specificity by multimerization. *Mol Cell Biol* **10**:6813, 1990.

238. Desplan C: Eye development: Governed by a dictator or a junta? (comment). *Cell* 91:861, 1997.
239. Callaerts P, Halder G, Gehring WJ: PAX-6 in development and evolution. *Annu Rev Neurosci* 20:483, 1997.
240. Macdonald R, Wilson SW: Pax proteins and eye development. *Curr Opin Neurobiol* 6:49, 1996.
241. Ton CC, Hirvonen H, Miwa H, Weil MM, Monaghan P, Jordan T, van HV, Hastie ND, Meijers-Heijboer H, Drechsler M: Positional cloning and characterization of a paired box- and homeobox-containing gene from the aniridia region. *Cell* 67:1059, 1991.
242. Hill RE, Favor J, Hogan BL, Ton CC, Saunders GF, Hanson IM, Prosser J, Jordan T, Hastie ND, van Heyningen V: Mouse small eye results from mutations in a paired-like homeobox-containing gene [published erratum appears in *Nature* 355(6362):750, 1992]. *Nature* 354:522, 1991.
243. Quiring R, Walldorf U, Kloter U, Gehring WJ: Homology of the eyeless gene of *Drosophila* to the small eye gene in mice and aniridia in humans (see comments). *Science* 265:785, 1994.
244. Tomarev SI, Callaerts P, Kos L, Zinovieva R, Halder G, Gehring W, Piatigorsky J: Squid *Pax-6* and eye development. *Proc Natl Acad Sci USA* 94:2421, 1997.
245. Glardon S, Callaerts P, Halder G, Gehring WJ: Conservation of *Pax-6* in a lower chordate, the ascidian *Phallusia mammillata*. *Development* 124:817, 1997.
246. Altmann CR, Chow RL, Lang RA, Hemmati-Brivanlou A: Lens induction by Pax-6 in *Xenopus laevis*. *Dev Biol* 185:119, 1997.
247. Cvekl A, Sax CM, Bresnick EH, Piatigorsky J: Complex array of positive and negative elements regulates the chicken alphaA-crystallin gene: Involvement of Pax-6, USF, CREB and/or CREM, and AP-1 proteins. *Mol Cell Biol* 14:7363, 1994.
248. Cvekl A, Sax CM, Li X, McDermott JB, Piatigorsky J: Pax-6 and lens-specific transcription of the chicken delta 1-crystallin gene. *Proc Natl Acad Sci USA* 92:4681, 1995.
249. Duncan MK, Haynes JI 2, Cvekl A, Piatigorsky J: Dual roles for Pax-6: A transcriptional repressor of lens fiber cell specific beta-crystallin genes. *Mol Cell Biol* 18:5579, 1998.
250. Cvekl A and Piatigorsky J: Lens development and crystallin gene expression: Many roles for Pax-6. *Bioessays* 18:621, 1996.
251. Gopal-Srivastava R, Cvekl A, Piatigorsky J: Involvement of retinoic acid/retinoid receptors in the regulation of murine αB-crystallin/small heat shock protein gene expression in the lens. *J Biol Chem* 273:17954, 1998.
252. Collignon J, Sockanathan S, Hacker A, Cohen-Tannoudji M, Norris D, Rastan S, Stevanovic M, Goodfellow PN, Lovell-Badge R: A comparison of the properties of *Sox-3* with *Sry* and two related genes, *Sox-1* and *Sox-2*. *Development* 122:509, 1996.
253. Kamachi Y, Sockanathan S, Liu Q, Breitman M, Lovell-Badge R, Kondoh H: Involvement of SOX proteins in lens-specific activation of crystallin genes. *EMBO J* 14:3510, 1995.
254. Klok EJ, Van Genesen ST, Civil A, Schoenmakers JG, Lubsen NH: Regulation of expression within a gene family: The case of the rat gammaB- and gammaD-crystallin promoters. *J Biol Chem* 273:17206, 1998.
255. Ogino H, Yasuda K: Induction of lens differentiation by activation of a bZIP transcription factor, L-Maf. *Science* 280:115, 1998.
256. Sharon-Friling R, Richardson J, Sperbeck S, Lee D, Rauchman M, Maas R, Swaroop A, Wistow G: Lens-specific gene recruitment of zeta-crystallin through Pax6, Nrl-Maf, and brain suppressor sites. *Mol Cell Biol* 18:2067, 1998.
257. Yoshida K, Imaki J, Koyama Y, Harada T, Shinmei Y, Oishi C, Matsushima-Hibiya Y, Matsuda A, Nishi S, Matsuda H, Sakai M: Differential expression of *maf*-1 and *maf*-2 genes in the developing rat lens. *Invest Ophthalmol Vis Sci* 38:2679, 1997.
258. Dirks RP, Kraft HJ, Van Genesen ST, Klok EJ, Pfundt R, Schoenmakers JG, Lubsen NH: The cooperation between two silencers creates an enhancer element that controls both the lens-preferred and the differentiation stage-specific expression of the rat beta B2-crystallin gene. *Eur J Biochem* 239:23, 1996.
259. Dubin RA, Gopal-Srivastava R, Wawrousek EF, Piatigorsky J: Expression of the murine alphaB-crystallin gene in lens and skeletal muscle: Identification of a muscle-preferred enhancer. *Mol Cell Biol* 11:4340, 1991.
260. Sax CM, Piatigorsky J: Expression of the alpha-crystallin/small heat shock protein/molecular chaperone genes in the lens and other tissues. *Adv Enzymol* 69: 155, 1994.
261. Brakenhoff RH, Henskens HAM, van Rossum MWPC, Lubsen NH, Schoenmakers JGG: Activation of the gammaE-crystallin pseudogene in the human hereditary Coppock-like cataract. *Hum Mol Genet* 3:279, 1994.
262. Atreya PL, Barnes J, Katar M, Alcala J, Maisel H: *N*-Cadherin of the human lens. *Curr Eye Res* 8:947, 1989.
263. Watanabe M, Kobayashi H, Rutishauser U, Katar M, Alcala J, Maisel H: NCAM in the differentiation of embryonic lens tissue. *Dev Biol* 135:414, 1989.
264. Xu KY, Becker LC: Ultrastructural localization of glycolytic enzymes on sarcoplasmic reticulum vesicles. *J Histochem Cytochem* 46:419, 1998.
265. Mulders JW, Voorter CE, Lamers C, De Haard-Hoekman WA, Montecucco C, van de VeWJ, Bloemendal H, de Jong WW: MP17, a fiber-specific intrinsic membrane protein from mammalian eye lens. *Curr Eye Res* 7:207, 1988.
266. Chepelinsky AB: The MIP transmembrane channel gene family, in Peracchia C (ed): *Handbook of Membrane Channels: Molecular and Cellular Physiology*. New York, Academic Press, 1994, p 413.
267. Gorin MB, Yancey SB, Cline J, Revel JP, Horwitz J: The major intrinsic protein (MIP) of the bovine lens fiber membrane: Characterization and structure based on cDNA cloning. *Cell* 39:49, 1984.
268. Schey KL, Fowler JG, Schwartz JC, Busman M, Dillon J, Crouch RK: Complete map and identification of the phosphorylation site of bovine lens major intrinsic protein. *Invest Ophthalmol Vis Sci* 38:2508, 1997.
269. Park JH, Saier MH Jr: Phylogenetic characterization of the MIP family of transmembrane channel proteins. *J Membr Biol* 153:171, 1996.
270. Yang B, Verkman AS: Water and glycerol permeabilities of aquaporins 1–5 and MIP determined quantitatively by expression of epitope-tagged constructs in *Xenopus* oocytes. *J Biol Chem* 272:16140, 1997.
271. Cheng A, van HA, Yeager M, Verkman AS, Mitra AK: Three-dimensional organization of a human water channel. *Nature* 387:627, 1997.
272. Saito F, Sasaki S, Chepelinsky AB, Fushimi K, Marumo F, Ikeuchi T: Human AQP2 and MIP genes, two members of the MIP family, map within chromosome band 12q13 on the basis of two-color FISH. *Cytogenet Cell Genet* 68:45, 1995.
273. Pisano MM, Chepelinsky AB: Genomic cloning and complete nucleotide sequence of the human gene encoding the major intrinsic protein (MIP) of the lens. *Gene* 11:981, 1991.
274. Zampighi GA, Gall JE, Ehring GR, Simon SA: The structural organization and protein compositions of lens fiber junctions. *J Cell Biol* 108:2255, 1989.
275. FitzGerald PG, Bok D, Horwitz J: Immunocytochemical localization of the main intrinsic polypeptide (MIP) in ultrathin frozen sections of rat lens. *J Cell Biol* 97:1491, 1983.
276. Gooden MM, Rintoul DA, Takehana M, Takemoto L: Major intrinsic polypeptide (MIP 26K) from lens membrane: Reconstitution into vesicles and inhibition of channel forming activity by peptide antiserum. *Biochem Biophys Res Commun* 128:993, 1985.
277. Peracchia C, Girsch SJ: Permeability and gating of lens gap junction channels incorporated into liposomes. *Curr Eye Res* 4:431, 1985.
278. Zampighi GA, Hall JE, Kreman M: Purified lens junctional protein forms channels in planner lipid films. *Proc Natl Acad Sci USA* 82:8468, 1985.
279. Ehring GR, Zampighi G, Horwitz J, Bok D, Hall JE: Properties of channels reconstituted from the major intrinsic protein of lens membranes. *J Gen Physiol* 96:631, 1990.
280. Louis CF, Hogan P, Visco L, Strasburg G: Identity of the calmodulin-binding proteins in bovine lens plasma membranes. *Exp Eye Res* 50:495, 1990.
281. Garland D, Russell P: Phosphorylation of lens fiber cell membrane proteins. *Proc Natl Acad Sci USA* 82:653, 1985.
282. Jiang JX, Goodenough DA: Heteromeric connexons in lens gap junction channels. *Proc Natl Acad Sci USA* 93:1287, 1996.
283. Kistler J, Christie D, Bullivant S: Homologies between gap junction proteins in lens, heart and liver. *Nature* 331:721, 1988.
284. Gruijters WT, Kistler J, Bullivant S, Goodenough DA: Immunolocalization of MP70 in lens fiber 16–17-nm intercellular junctions. *J Cell Biol* 104:565, 1987.
285. Kistler J, Schaller J, Sigrist H: MP38 contains the membrane-embedded domain of the lens fiber gap junction protein MP70. *J Biol Chem* 265:13357, 1990.
286. Arneson ML, Cheng HL, Louis CF: Characterization of the ovine-lens plasma-membrane protein-kinase substrates. *Eur J Biochem* 234:670, 1995.
287. Berthoud VM, Beyer EC, Kurata WE, Lau AF, Lampe PD: The gap-junction protein connexin56 is phosphorylated in the intracellular loop and the carboxy-terminal region. *Eur J Biochem* 244:89, 1997.

288. Church RL, Wang JH, Steele E: The human lens intrinsic membrane protein MP70 (*Cx50*) gene: Clonal analysis and chromosome mapping [published erratum appears in *Curr Eye Res* 14(10):979, 1995]. *Curr Eye Res* **14**:215, 1995.

289. Geyer DD, Church RL, Steele ECJ, Heinzmann C, Kojis TL, Klisak I, Sparkes RS, Bateman JB: Regional mapping of the human MP70 (*Cx50*; connexin50) gene by fluorescence in situ hybridization to 1q21s.1. *Mol Vis* **3**:13, 1997.

290. Allen DP, Low PS, Dola A, Maisel H: Band 3 and ankyrin homologues are present in eye lens: Evidence for all major erythrocyte membrane components in same non-erythroid cell. *Biochem Biophys Res Commun* **149**:266, 1987.

291. Kuwabara T: Microtubules in the lens. *Arch Ophthalmol* **79**:189, 1968.

292. Piatigorsky J: Lens cell elongation in vitro and microtubules. *Ann NY Acad Sci* **253**:333, 1975.

293. Rafferty NS, Scholz DL, Goldberg M, Lewyckyj M: Immunocyto-chemical evidence for an actin-myosin system in lens epithelial cells. *Exp Eye Res* **51**:591, 1990.

294. Ireland M, Lieska N, Maisel H: Lens actin: Purification and localization. *Exp Eye Res* **37**:393, 1983.

295. Kibbelaar MA, Ramaekers FC, Ringens PJ, Selten-Versteegen AM, Poels LG, Jap PH, van Rossum AL, Feltkamp TE, Bloemendal H: Is actin in eye lens a possible factor in visual accomodation. *Nature* **285**:506, 1980.

296. Rafferty NS, Scholz DL: Comparative study of actin filament patterns in lens epithelial cells: Are these determined by the mechanisms of lens accommodation. *Curr Eye Res* **8**:569, 1989.

297. Alcala J, Maisel H: Biochemistry of lens plasma membranes and cytoskeleton, in Maisel H (ed): *The Ocular Lens: Structure, Function and Pathology.* New York, Marcel Dekker, 1985.

298. Kam Z, Volberg T, Geiger B: Mapping of adherens junction components using microscopic resonance energy transfer imaging. *J Cell Sci* **108**:1051, 1995.

299. Lo WK, Mills A, Kuck JF: Actin filament bundles are associated with fiber gap junctions in the primate lens. *Exp Eye Res* **58**:189, 1994.

300. Sussman MA, McAvoy JW, Rudisill M, Swanson B, Lyons GE, Kedes L, Blanks J: Lens tropomodulin: Developmental expression during differentiation. *Exp Eye Res* **63**:223, 1996.

301. Lo WK, Shaw AP, Wen XJ: Actin filament bundles in cortical fiber cells of the rat lens. *Exp Eye Res* **65**:691, 1997.

302. Ramaekers FC, Osborn M, Schimid E, Weber K, Bloemendal H, Franke WW: Identification of the cytoskeletal proteins in lens-forming cells, a special epitheloid cell type. *Exp Cell Res* **127**:309, 1980.

303. Sredy J, Roy D, Spector A: Identification of two of the major phosphorylated polypeptides of the bovine lens utilizing a lens cAMP-dependent protein kinase system. *Curr Eye Res* **3**:1423, 1984.

304. Sandilands A, Prescott AR, Carter JM, Hutcheson AM, Quinlan RA, Richards J, FitzGerald PG: Vimentin and CP49/filensin form distinct networks in the lens which are independently modulated during lens fibre cell differentiation. *J Cell Sci* **108**:1397, 1995.

305. Sax CM, Farrell FX, Zehner ZE, Piatigorsky J: Regulation of vimentin gene expression in the ocular lens. *Dev Biol* **139**:56, 1990.

306. Krimpenfort PJ, Schaart G, Peiper FR, Ramaekers FC, Cuypers HT, van den Heuvel RM, Vree Egberts WT, can Eyrs GJ, Berns A, Bloemendal H: Tissue-specific expression of a vimentin-desmin hybrid gene in transgenic mice. *EMBO J* **7**:941, 1988.

307. Hatfield JS, Skoff RP, Maisel H, Eng L, Bigner DD: The lens epithelium contains glial fibrillary acidic protein (GFAP). *J Neuroimmunol* **8**:347, 1985.

308. Boyer S, Maunoury R, Gomes D, de Nechaud B, Hill AM, Dupouey P: Expression of glial fibrillary acidic protein and vimentin in mouse lens epithelial cells during development in vivo and during proliferation and differentiation in vitro: Comparison with the developmental appearance of GFAP in the mouse central nervous system. *J Neurosci Res* **27**:55, 1990.

309. FitzGerald PG, Gottlieb W: The M*r*115 kD fiber cell-specific protein is a component of the lens cytoskeleton. *Curr Eye Res* **8**:801, 1989.

310. FitzGerald PG, Casselman J: Discrimination between the lens fiber cell 114 kD cytoskeletal protein and alpha-actinin. *Curr Eye Res* **9**:873, 1990.

311. Goulielmos G, Gounari F, Remington S, Muller S, Haner M, Aebi U, Georgatos SD: Filensin and phakinin form a novel type of beaded intermediate filaments and coassemble *de novo* in cultured cells. *J Cell Biol* **132**:643, 1996.

312. Ireland M, Maisel H: Phosphorylation of chick lens proteins. *Curr Eye Res* **3**:961, 1984.

313. Hess JF, Casselman JT, FitzGerald PG: Gene structure and cDNA sequence identify the beaded filament protein CP49 as a highly divergent type I intermediate filament protein. *J Biol Chem* **271**:6729, 1996.

314. Mathias RT, Rae JL: Transport properties of the lens. *Am J Physiol* **249**:C181, 1985.

315. Georgatos SD, Gounari F, Goulielmos G, Aebi U: To bead or not to bead? Lens-specific intermediate filaments revisited. *J Cell Sci* **110**:2629, 1997.

316. Carter JM, Hutcheson AM, Quinlan RA: In vitro studies on the assembly properties of the lens proteins CP49, CP115: Coassembly with alpha-crystallin but not with vimentin. *Exp Eye Res* **60**:181, 1995.

317. Goulielmos G, Remington S, Schwesinger F, Georgatos SD, Gounari F: Contributions of the structural domains of filensin in polymer formation and filament distribution. *J Cell Sci* **109**:447, 1996.

318. Cheng H-M, Chylack LT: Lens metabolism, in Maisel H (ed): *The Ocular Lens.* New York, Marcel Dekker, 1985, p 223.

319. Kador PF: Biochemistry of the lens: Intermediary metabolism and sugar cataract formation, in Albert DM, Jacobiec FA, Dowling JE, Raviola E (eds): *Principles and Practice of Ophthalmology: Basic Sciences.* Philadelphia, Saunders, 1994, p 146.

320. Reddy VN: Dynamics of transport systems in the eyes. Friedenwald lecture. *Invest Ophthalmol Vis Sci* **18**:1000, 1979.

321. Trayhurn P, Van Heyningen R: The role of respiration in the energy metabolism of the bovine lens. *Biochem J* **129**:507, 1972.

322. Hockwin O, Blum G, Korte I, Murata T, Radetzki W, Rast F: Studies on the citric acid cycle and its portion of glucose breakdown by calf and bovine lenses in vitro. *Ophthalmic Res* **2**:143, 1971.

323. Kinoshita JH, Merola LO: The utilization of pyruvate and its conversion to glutamate in calf lens. *Exp Eye Res* **1**:53, 1961.

324. Aviram A, Schalitt M, Kassem N, Groen JJ: Glucose utilization, glutathione, potassium and sodium content of isolated bovine lens. *Clin Chim Acta* **14**:442, 1966.

325. Giblin FJ, Nies DE, Reddy VN: Stimulation of the hexose monophosphate shunt in rabbit lens in response to oxidation by glutathione. *Exp Eye Res* **33**:289, 1981.

326. Giblin FJ, McCready JP, Reddan JR, Dziedzic DC, Reddy VN: Detoxification of $H_2O_2$ by cultured rabbit lens epithelial cells: Participation of the glutathione redox cycle. *Exp Eye Res* **40**:827, 1985.

327. Cheng HM, Aguiar E, Ford JJ, Kelleher P, Lam DM: Proton NMR spectroscopy of glucose consumption by cultured lens epithelial cells. *J Ocul Pharmacol* **2**:319, 1986.

328. Giblin FJ, Schrimscher L, Chakrapani B, Reddy VN: Exposure of rabbit lens to hyperbaric oxygen in vitro: Regional effects on GSH level. *Invest Ophthalmol Vis Sci* **29**:1312, 1988.

329. Seland JH, Chylack LT Jr: Acute glucose-derived osmotic stress in rabbit lenses. *Acta Ophthalmol (Copenh)* **64**:533, 1986.

330. Burg MB, Kador PF: Sorbitol, osmoregulation, and the complications of diabetes. *J Clin Invest* **81**:635, 1988.

331. Chylack LT Jr, Tung W, Harding R: Sorbitol production in the lens: A means of counteracting glucose-derived osmotic stress [published erratum appears in *Ophthalmic Res* 19(6):365, 1987]. *Ophthalmic Res* **18**:313, 1986.

332. Kinoshita JH: Cataracts in galactosemia: The Jonas Friedenwald memorial lecture. *Invest Ophthalmol* **4**:786, 1965.

333. Kador PF, Kinoshita JH: Diabetic and galactosaemic cataracts. *Ciba Found Symp* **106**:110, 1984.

334. Kinoshita JH, Fukushi S, Kador P, Merola LO: Aldose reductase in diabetic complications of the eye. *Metabolism* **28**:462, 1979.

335. Piatigorsky J: Intracellular ions, protein metabolism, and cataract formation. *Curr Topics Eye Res* **3**:1, 1980.

336. Lee AY, Chung SK, Chung SS: Demonstration that polyol accumulation is responsible for diabetic cataract by the use of transgenic mice expressing the aldose reductase gene in the lens. *Proc Natl Acad Sci USA* **92**:2780, 1995.

337. Chylack LT Jr, Henriques HF, Cheng HM, Tung WH: Efficacy of Alrestatin, an aldose reductase inhibitor, in human diabetic and nondiabetic lenses. *Ophthalmology* **86**:1579, 1979.

338. Crabbe MJ, Goode D: Aldose reductase: A window to the treatment of diabetic complications? *Prog Retin Eye Res* **17**:313, 1998.

339. Dillon J: UV-B as a pro-aging and pro-cataract factor. *Doc Ophthalmol* **88**:339, 1994.

340. Spector A, Garner WH: Hydrogen peroxide and human cataract. *Exp Eye Res* **33**:673, 1981.

341. Reddy VN: Glutathione and its function in the lens — an overview. *Exp Eye Res* **50**:771, 1990.

342. Pau H, Graf P, Sies H: Glutathione levels in human lens: Regional distribution in different forms of cataract. *Exp Eye Res* **50**:17, 1990.

343. Giblin FJ, Reddan JR, Schrimscher L, Dziedzic DC, Reddy VN: The relative roles of the glutathione redox cycle and catalase in the detoxification of H₂O₂ by cultured rabbit lens epithelial cells. *Exp Eye Res* **50**:795, 1990.

344. Mancini MA, Unaker NJ, Giblin FJ, Reddan JR: Histochemical localization of catalase in cultured lens epithelial cells. *Ophthalmic Res* **21**:369, 1989.

345. Awasthi YC, Saneto RP, Srivastava SK: Purification and properties of bovine lens glutathione-*S*-transferase. *Exp Eye Res* **30**:29, 1980.

346. Alberti G, Oguni M, Podgor M, Sperduto RD, Tomarev S, Grassi C, Williams S, Kaiser-Kupfer M, Maraini G, Hejtmancik JF: Glutathione-*S*-transferase M1 genotype and age-related cataracts: Lack of association in an Italian population. *Invest Ophthalmol Vis Sci* **37**:1167, 1996.

347. Tomarev SI, Zinovieva RD: Squid major lens polypeptides are homologous to glutathione-*S*-transferases subunits. *Nature* **336**:86, 1988.

348. Spector A, Yang Y, Ho YS, Magnenat JL, Wang RR, Ma W, Li WC: Variation in cellular glutathione peroxidase activity in lens epithelial cells, transgenics and knockouts does not significantly change the response to H₂O₂ stress. *Exp Eye Res* **62**:521, 1996.

349. Spector A, Ma W, Wang RR, Yang Y, Ho YS: The contribution of GSH peroxidase-1, catalase and GSH to the degradation of H₂O₂ by the mouse lens. *Exp Eye Res* **64**:477, 1997.

350. Spector A, Ma W, Wang RR, Kleiman NJ: Microperoxidases catalytically degrade reactive oxygen species and may be anti-cataract agents. *Exp Eye Res* **65**:457, 1997.

351. Neville MC, Paterson CA, Hamilton PM: Evidence for two sodium pumps in the crystalline lens of the rabbit eye. *Exp Eye Res* **27**:637, 1978.

352. Kinsey VE, Reddy DVN: Studies on the crystallin lens. *Invest Ophthalmol* **4**:104, 1965.

353. Unakar NJ, Tsui JY: Sodium-potassium-dependent ATPase I: Cytochemical localization in normal and cataractous rat lenses. *Invest Ophthalmol Vis Sci* **19**:630, 1980.

354. Palva M, Palkama A: Electronmicroscopical, histochemical and biochemical findings on the Na-ATPase activity in the epithelium of the rat lens. *Exp Eye Res* **22**:229, 1976.

355. Paterson CA: Distribution and movement of ions in the ocular lens. *Doc Ophthalmol* **31**:1, 1976.

356. Delamere NA, Dean WL, Stidam JM, Moseley AE: Differential expression of sodium pump catalytic subunits in the lens epithelium and fibers. *Ophthalmic Res* **28**(suppl 1):73, 1996.

357. Hightower KR, Leverenz V, Reddy VN: Calcium transport in the lens. *Invest Ophthalmol Vis Sci* **19**:1059, 1980.

358. Borchman D, Paterson CA Delamere N: Ca⁺²-ATPase activity in the rabbit and bovine lens. *Curr Eye Res* **8**:1049, 1989.

359. Paterson CA, Zeng J, Husseini Z, Borchman D, Delamere NA, Garland D, Jimenez-Asensio J: Calcium ATPase activity and membrane structure in clear and cataractous human lenses. *Curr Eye Res* **16**:333, 1997.

360. Francois H, Rabaey M: Permeability of the lens capsule for the lens proteins. *Arch Ophthalmol* **36**:837, 1958.

361. Brown HG, Pappas GD, Ireland ME, Kuszak JR: Ultrastructural biochemical and immunologic evidence of receptor-mediated endocytosis in the crystalline lens. *Invest Ophthalmol Vis Sci* **31**:2579, 1990.

362. Rae JL: The movement of procion dye in the crystalline lens. *Invest Ophthalmol* **13**:147, 1974.

363. Duncan G, Jacob TJC: The lens as a physiochemical system in the eye, in Davson H (ed): *The Eye*. New York, Academic Press, 1984, p 159.

364. Rae JL, Mathias RT: The physiology of the lens, in Maisel H (ed): *The Ocular Lens*. New York, Marcel Dekker, 1985, p 93.

365. Kern HL, Ho CK: Localization and specificity of the transport system for sugars in the calf lens. *Exp Eye Res* **15**:751, 1973.

366. Patterson JW: A review of glucose transport in the lens. *Invest Ophthalmol* **4**:667, 1965.

367. Harding CV, Maisel H, Chylack LT: The structure of the human cataractous lens, in Maisel H (ed): *The Ocular Lens*. New York, Marcel Dekker, 1985, p 405.

368. Benedek GB, Chylack LT, Libondi T, Magnante P, Pennett M: Quantitative detection of the molecular changes associated with early cararactogenesis in the living human lens using quasielastic light scattering. *Curr Eye Res* **6**:1421, 1987.

369. Bettelheim FA: Physical basis of lens transparency, in Maisel H (ed): *The Ocular Lens*. New York, Marcil Dekker, 1985, p 265.

370. Benedek GB, Clark JI, Serrallach EU, Young CY, Mengel T, Sauke A, Bagg A, Benedek K: Light scattering and reversible cataracts in calf and human lens. *Phil Trans R Soc Lond A* **293**:329, 1979.

371. Clark JI, Benedek GB: Phase diagram for cell cytoplasm from the calf lens. *Biochem Biophys Res Commun* **95**:482, 1980.

372. Tanaka T, Ishimoto C, Chylack LT Jr: Phase separation of a protein-water mixture in cold cataract in the young rat lens. *Science* **197**:1010, 1977.

373. Delaye M, Clark JI, Benedek GB: Identification of scattering elements responsible for lens opacification in cold cataracts. *Biophys J* **37**:647, 1982.

374. Clark JI, Carper D: Phase separation in lens cytoplasm is genetically linked to cataract formation in the Philly mouse. *Proc Natl Acad Sci USA* **84**:122, 1987.

375. Smith RS, Sundberg JP, Linder CC: Mouse mutations as models for studying cataracts. *Pathobiology* **65**:146, 1997.

376. Kador PF, Fukui HN, Fukushi S, Jernigan HM Jr, Kinoshita JH: Philly mouse: A new model of hereditary cataract. *Exp Eye Res* **30**:59, 1980.

377. Carper D: Deficiency of functional messenger RNA for a developmentally regulated beta-crystallin polypeptide in a hereditary cataract. *Science* **217**:463, 1982.

378. Nakamura M, Russell P, Carper DA, Inana G, Kinoshita JH: Alteration of a developmentally regulated, heat-stable polypeptide in the lens of the Philly mouse: Implications for cataract formation. *J Biol Chem* **263**:19218, 1988.

379. Chambers C, Russell P: Deletion mutation in an eye lens beta-crystallin: An animal model for inherited cataract. *J Biol Chem* **266**:6742, 1991.

380. Amsbaugh DF, Stone SH: Autosomal dominant congenital nuclear cataracts in strain 13/N guinea pigs. *J Hered* **75**:55, 1984.

381. Huang QL, Du XY, Stone SH, Amsbaugh DF, Datiles M, Hu TS, Zigler JS Jr: Association of hereditary cataracts in strain 13/N guinea-pigs with mutation of the gene for zeta-crystallin. *Exp Eye Res* **50**:317, 1990.

382. Huang QL, Russell P, Stone SH, Zigler JS Jr: Zeta-crystallin, a novel lens protein from the guinea pig. *Curr Eye Res* **6**:725, 1987.

383. Rodriguez IR, Gonzalez P, Zigler JS Jr, Borras T: A guineq-pig hereditary cataract contains a splice-site deletion in a crystallin gene. *Biochim Biophys Acta* **1180**:44, 1992.

384. Hiai H, Kato S, Horiuchi Y, Shimada R, Tsuruyama T, Watanabe T, Matsuzawa A: Mapping of nakano cataract gene nct on mouse chromosome 16. *Genomics* **50**:119, 1998.

385. Kobayashi S, Kasuya M, Itoi M: Changes in lens proteins induced at the early stage of cataractogenesis in cac (Nakano) mice. *Exp Eye Res* **49**:553, 1989.

386. Fukui HN, Merola LO, Kinoshita JH: A possible cataractogenic factor in the Nakano mouse lens. *Exp Eye Res* **26**:477, 1978.

387. Garber AT, Winkler C, Shinohara T, King CR, Inana G, Piatigorsky J, Gold RJ: Selective loss of a family of gene transcripts in a hereditary murine cataract. *Science* **227**:74, 1985.

388. Kuliszewski M, Rupert J, Gold R: The ontogeny of gamma-crystallin mRNAs in CatFraser mice. *Genet Res* **52**:45, 1988.

389. Rupert JL, Kuliszewki M, Tsui LC, Breitman ML, Gold RJ: The murine cataractogenic mutation, *Cat Fraser*, segregates independently of the gamma crystallin genes. *Genet Res* **51**:23, 1988.

390. Muggelton-Harris AL, Festing MFW, Hall M: A gene location for the inheritance of the cataract Fraser (*CATFr*) mouse congenital cataract. *Gen Res Camb* **49**:235, 1987.

391. Quinlan P, Oda S, Breitman ML, Tsui LC: The mouse eye lens obsolescence (*Elo*) mutant: Studies on crystallin gene expression and linkage analysis between the mutant locus and the gamma-crystallin genes. *Genes Dev* **1**:637, 1987.

392. Zigler JS Jr: Animal models for the study of maturity-onset and hereditary cataract. *Exp Eye Res* **50**:651, 1990.

393. Kuck JF: Late onset hereditary cataract of the Emory mouse: A model for human senile cataract. *Exp Eye Res* **50**:659, 1990.

394. Graw J: Cataract mutations as a tool for developmental geneticists. *Ophthalmic Res* **28**(suppl 1):8, 1996.

395. Gotz W: Transgenic models for eye malformations. *Ophthalmic Genet* **16**:85, 1995.

396. Landel CP, Zhao J, Bok D, Evans GA: Lens-specific expression of recombinant ricin induces developmental defects in the eyes of transgenic mice. *Genes Dev* **2**:1168, 1988.

397. Lang RA, Metcalf D, Cuthbertson RA, Lyons I, Stanley E, Kelso A, Kannourakis G, Williamson DJ, Klintworth GK, Gonda TJ, Dunn AR: Transgenic mice expressing a hemopoetic growth factor gene (GM-CSF) develop accumulations of macrophages, blindness, and a fatal syndrome of tissue damage. *Cell* **51**:675, 1987.

398. Capetanaki Y, Smith S, Heath JP: Overexpression of the vimentin gene in transgenic mice inhibits normal lens cell differentiation. *J Cell Biol* **109**:1653, 1989.

399. Srinivasan Y, Lovicu FJ, Overbeek PA: Lens-specific expression of transforming growth factor beta 1 in transgenic mice causes anterior subcapsular cataracts. *J Clin Invest* **101**:625, 1998.

400. Martin WD, Egan RM, Stevens JL, Woodward JG: Lens-specific expression of a major histocompatibility complex class I molecule disrupts normal lens development and induces cataracts in transgenic mice. *Invest Ophthalmol Vis Sci* **36**:1144, 1995.

401. Perez-Castro AV, Tran VT, Nguyen-Huu MC: Defective lens fiber differentiation and pancreatic tumorigenesis caused by ectopic expression of the cellular retinoic acid-binding protein I. *Development* **119**:363, 1993.

402. Geiger K, Howes E, Gallina M, Huang XJ, Travis GH, Sarvetnick N: Transgenic mice expressing IFN-gamma in the retina develop inflammation of the eye and photoreceptor loss. *Invest Ophthalmol Vis Sci* **35**:2667, 1994.

403. Egwuagu CE, Sztein J, Chan CC, Reid W, Mahdi R, Nussenblatt RB, Chepelinsky AB: Ectopic expression of gamma interferon in the eyes of transgenic mice induces ocular pathology and MHC class II gene expression. *Invest Ophthalmol Vis Sci* **35**:332, 1994.

404. Mahon KA, Chepelinsky AB, Khillan JS, Overbeek PA, Piatigorsky J, Westphal H: Oncogenesis of the lens in transgenic mice. *Science* **235**:1622, 1987.

405. Eva A, Graziani G, Zannini M, Merin LM, Khillan JS, Overbeek PA: Dominant dysplasia of the lens in transgenic mice expressing the dbl oncogene. *New Biol* **3**:158, 1991.

406. Griep AE, Herber R, Jeon S, Lohse JK, Dubielzig RR, Lambert PF: Tumorigenicity by human papillomavirus type 16 E6 and E7 in transgenic mice correlates with alterations in epithelial cell growth and differentiation. *J Virol* **67**:1373, 1993.

407. Bloemendal H, Raats JM, Pieper FR, Benedetti EL, Dunia I: Transgenic mice carrying chimeric or mutated type III intermediate filament (*IF*) genes. *Cell Mol Life Sci* **53**:1, 1997.

408. Dunia I, Pieper F, Manenti S, van dK, Devilliers G, Benedetti EL, Bloemendal H: Plasma membrane-cytoskeleton damage in eye lenses of transgenic mice expressing desmin. *Eur J Cell Biol* **53**:59, 1990.

409. Dunia I, Smit JJ, van der Valk MA, Bloemendal H, Borst P, Benedetti EL: Human multidrug resistance 3-P-glycoprotein expression in transgenic mice induces lens membrane alterations leading to cataract. *J Cell Biol* **132**:701, 1996.

410. Mitton KP, Kamiya T, Tumminia SJ, Russell P: Cysteine protease activated by expression of HIV-1 protease in transgenic mices. MIP26 (aquaporin-0) cleavage and cataract formation in vivo and ex vivo. *J Biol Chem* **271**:31803, 1996.

411. Gilmour DT, Lyon GJ, Carlton MB, Sanes JR, Cunningham JM, Anderson JR, Hogan BL, Evans MJ, Colledge WH: Mice deficient for the secreted glycoprotein SPARC/osteonectin/BM40 develop normally but show severe age-onset cataract formation and disruption of the lens. *EMBO J* **17**:1860, 1998.

412. Gong X, Li E, Klier G, Huang Q, Wu Y, Lei H, Kumar NM, Horwitz J, Gilula NB: Disruption of alpha3-connexin gene leads to proteolysis and cataractogenesis in mice. *Cell* **91**:833, 1997.

413. White TW, Goodenough D A: Ocular abnormalities in connexin50 knockout mice. *Mol Biol Cell* **8**:93, 1997.

414. Gao Y, Spray DC: Structural changes in lenses of mice lacking the gap junction protein connexin43. *Invest Ophthalmol Vis Sci* **39**:1198, 1998.

415. Datiles MB, Kinoshita JH: Pathogenesis of cataracts, in Tasman W, Jaeger EA (eds): *Duane's Clinical Ophthalmology.* Philadelphia, Lippincott, 1991.

416. Young R: *Age-Related Cataract.* New York, Oxford University Press, 1991.

417. Weekers R, Delmarcelle Y, Luyckx-Bacus J, Collignon J: Morphological changes of the lens with age and cataract, in *The Human Lens — In Relation to Cataract: Ciba Foundation 19* (new series). Amsterdam, Elservier Scientific Publications, 1973, p 24.

418. Weale RA: Physical changes due to age and cataract, in Duncan G (ed): *Mechanism of Cataract Formation in the Human Lens.* New York, Academic Press, 1981, p 47.

419. Elsas FJ, Maumenee IH, Kenyon KR, Yoder F: Familial aniridia with preserved ocular function. *Am J Ophthalmol* **83**:718, 1977.

420. Semina EV, Ferrell RE, Mintz-Hittner HA, Bitoun P, Alward WL, Reiter RS, Funkhauser C, Daack-Hirsch S, Murray JC: A novel homeobox gene *PITX3* is mutated in families with autosomal-dominant cataracts and ASMD. *Nature Genet* **19**:167, 1998.

421. Traboulsi EI, Weinberg RJ: Familial congenital cornea guttata with anterior polar cataracts. *Am J Ophthalmol* **108**:123, 1989.

422. Moller HU: Granular corneal dystrophy Groenouw type I: Clinical aspects and treatment. *Acta Ophthalmol* **68**:384, 1990.

423. Gitter KA, Rothschild H, Waltman DD, Scott B, Azar P: Dominantly inherited peripheral retinal neovascuoarization. *Arch Ophthalmol* **96**:1601, 1978.

424. O'Donnell FE, Pappas HR: Autosomal dominant foveal hypoplasia and presenile cataracts: A new syndrome. *Arch Ophthalmol* **100**:279, 1982.

425. Alexander RL, Shea M: Wagner's disease. *Arch Ophthalmol* **74**:310, 1965.

426. Beaumont C, Leneuve P, Devaux I, Scoazec JY, Berthier M, Loiseau MN, Grandchamp B, Bonneau D: Mutation in the iron responsive element of the L-ferritin mRNA in a family with dominant hyper-ferritinaemia and cataract. *Nature Genet* **11**:444, 1995.

427. Kafer O: Dominant vererbte Spaltung des Pigmentblattes von Iris und Ciliarkoepfer mit consekutiver Microphakie, Ectopia lentis und Cataract. *Graefes Arch Klin Exp Ophthalmol* **202**:133, 1977.

428. Hittner HM, Kretzer FL, Antoszyk JH, Ferrell RE, Mehta RS: Variable expressivity of autosomal dominant anterior segment mesenchymal dysgenesis in six generations. *Am J Ophthalmol* **93**:57, 1982.

429. Friedmann MW, Wright ES: Hereditary microcornea and cataract in 5 generations. *Am J Ophthalmol* **35**:1017, 1952.

430. Capella JA, Kaufman HE, Lill FJ, Cooper G: Hereditary cataracts and microphthalmia. *Am J Ophthalmol* **56**:454, 1963.

431. Cassady JR, Light A: Familial persistent pupillary membranes. *Arch Ophthalmol* **58**:438, 1957.

432. Heckenlively J: The frequency of posterior subcapsular cataract in the hereditary retinal degenerations. *Am J Ophthalmol* **93**:733, 1982.

433. Berson EL, Rosner B, Simonoff E: Risk factors for genetic typing and detection in retinitis pigmentosa. *Am J Ophthalmol* **89**:763, 1980.

434. Hirose T, Lee KY, Schepens CL: Snowflake degeneration in hereditary vitreoretinal degeneration. *Am J Ophthalmol* **77**:143, 1974.

435. Kaufman SJ, Goldberg MF, Orth DH, Fishman GA, Tessler H, Mizuno K: Autosomal dominant vitreoretinochoroidopathy. *Arch Ophthalmol* **100**:272, 1982.

436. Stock EL, Kielar RA: Primary familial amyloidosis of the cornea. *Am J Ophthalmol* **82**:266, 1976.

437. Favre M: A propos de deux cas de degenerescence hyaloideoretinienne: Two cases of hyaloidretinal degeneration. *Ophthalmologica* **135**:604, 1958.

438. Alstrom CH: Heredo-retinopathia congenitalis monohybrida recessiva autosomalis: A genetical statistical study in clinical collaboration with Olof Olson. *Hereditas* **43**:1, 1957.

439. Temtamy SA, Shalash BA: Genetic heterogeneity of the syndrome: Microophthalmos with congenital cataract. *Birth Defects* **10**(4):292, 1974.

440. Warburg M: Norrie's disease: A new hereditary bilateral pseudotumour of the retina. *Arch Ophthalmol* **39**:757, 1961.

441. *Mendelian Inheritance in Man.* Baltimore, Johns Hopkins University Press, 1992 (also online at http://www3.ncbi.nlm.nih.gov/Omim/searchomim.html).

442. Heck AF: Presumptive X-linked intermediate transmission of retinal degenerations: Variations and coincidental occurrence with ataxia in a large family. *Arch Ophthalmol* **70**:143, 1963.

443. Wellesley D, Carman P, French N, Goldblatt J: Cataracts, aberrant oral frenula, and growth retardation: A new autosomal dominant syndrome. *Am J Med Genet* **40**:341, 1991.

444. Stromgen E, Dalby A, Dalby MA, Ranheim B: Cataracts, deafness, cerebellar ataxia, psychosis, and dementia—a new syndrome. *Acta Neurol Scand* **43**(suppl.):261, 1970.

445. Spranger JW, Opitz JM, Bidder U: Heterogeneity of chondrodysplasia punctata. *Humangenetik* **11**:190, 1971.

446. Nadol JB Jr, Burgess B: Cochleosaccular degeneration of the inner ear and progressive cataracts inherited as an autosomal dominant trait. *Laryngoscope* **92**:1028, 1982.

447. Russo G, Mollica F, Mazzone D, Santonocito B: Congenital lactose intolerance of gastrogenic origin associated with cataracts. *Acta Paediatr Scand* **63**:457, 1974.

448. Vicart P, Caron A, Guicheney P, Li Z, Prevost M-C, Faure A, Chateau D, Chapon F, Tome F, Dupret J-M, Paulin D, Fardeau M: A missense mutation in the B-crystallin chaperone gene causes a desmin-related myopathy. *Nature Genet* **20**:92, 1998.

449. Moore WT, Federman DD: Familial dwarfism and stiff joints. *Arch Intern Med* **115**:398, 1965.

450. Cochat P, Guibaud P, Garcia-Torres R, Roussel B, Guarner B, Larbre F: Diffuse leiomyomatosis in Alport syndrome. *Pediatrics* **113**:339, 1988.

451. Flynn P, Aird RB: A neuroectodermal syndrome of dominant inheritance. *J Neurol Sci* **2**:161, 1965.

452. Francois J: A new syndrome: dyscephalia with bird face and dental anomalies, nanism, hypotrichosis, cutaneous atrophy, microphthalmia, and congenital cataract. *Arch Ophthalmol* **60**:842, 1958.

453. Witkopf CJ, White JG, King RA, Dahl MV, Young WG, Dauk JJ: Hereditary mucoepithelial dysplasia: A disease apparently of desmosome and gap junction formation. *Am J Hum Genet* **31**:414, 1979.

454. Zayid I, Farraj S: Familial histiocytic dermatoarthritis: A new syndrome. *Am J Med* **54**:793, 1973.

455. Carney RG: Incontinentia pigmenti: A world statistical analysis. *Arch Dermatol* **112**:535, 1976.

456. Tyni T, Kivela T, Lappi M, Summanen P, Nikoskelainen E, Pihko H: Ophthalmologic findings in long-chain 3-hydroxyacyl-CoA dehydrogenase deficiency caused by the G1528C mutation: A new type of hereditary metabolic chorioretinopathy. *Ophthalmology* **105**:810, 1998.

457. Kniest W, Leiber B: Kniest's syndrome. *Monatsschr Kinderheilkd* **125**:970, 1977.

458. Tessler HH, Apple DJ, Goldberg MF: Ocular findings in a kindred with Kyrle disease. *Arch Ophthalmol* **90**:278, 1973.

459. Pepin B, Mikol J, Goldstein B, Aron JJ, Lebuisson DA: Familial mitochondrial myopathy with cataract. *J Neurol Sci* **45**:191, 1980.

460. Walker BA: Osteopathia striata with cataracts and deafness. *Birth Defects* **4**:295, 1969.

461. Marshall D: Ectodermal dysplasia: Report of a kindred with ocular abnormalities and hearing defect. *Am J Ophthalmol* **45**:143, 1958.

462. Beighton P, Goldberg L, Op't Hof J: Dominant inheritance of multiple epiphyseal dysplasia, myopia and deafness. *Clin Genet* **14**:173, 1978.

463. Ashizawa T, Hejtmancik JF, Liu J, Perryman MB, Epstein HF, Koch DD: Diagnostic value of ophthalmologic findings in myotonic dystrophy: Comparison with risks calculated by haplotype analysis of closely linked restriction fragment length polymorphisms. *Am J Med Genet* **42**:55, 1992.

464. Quintanilla E, Rodrigo A, Temino MA, Ayesa C, Olivares C: Nail-patella syndrome with ocular involvement: Study of 5 generations. *Actas Dermosifiliogr* **72**:415, 1981.

465. Kaiser-Kupfer MI, Freidlin V, Datiles MB, Edwards PA, Sherman JL, Parry D, McCain LM, Eldridge R: The association of posterior capsular lens opacities with bilateral acoustic neuromas in patients with neurofibromatosis type 2. *Arch Ophthalmol* **107**:541, 1989.

466. Garcin R, Delthil S, Man HX, Chimenes H: Sur une affection heredo-familiale associant cataracte, atrophie optique, signes extra-pyramidaux et certains stigmates de la maladie de Friedreichs. (Sa position nosologique par rapport au syndrome de Behr, au syndrome de Marinesco-Sjogren et a la maladie de Friedreich avec signes oculaires). *Rev Neurol* **104**:373, 1961.

467. DeBusk FL: The Hutchinson-Gilford progeria syndrome. *J Pediatr* **80**:697, 1972.

468. Shprintzen RJ, Wang F, Goldberg R, Marion R: The expanded velocardiofacial syndrome (VCF): Additional features of the most common clefting syndrome. *Am J Hum Genet* **37**:A77, 1985.

469. Vaca G, Ibarra B, Bracamontes M, Garcia-Cruz D, Sanchez-Corona J, Medina C, Wunsch C, Gonzalez-Quiroga G, Cantu JM: Red blood cell sorbitol dehydrogenase deficiency in a family with cataracts. *Hum Genet* **61**:338, 1982.

470. Neugebauer H: Spalthand und fus mit familiarer besonderheit. *Z Orthop* **95**:500, 1962.

471. Seery CM, Pruett RC, Liberfarb RM, Cohen BZ: Distinctive cataract in the Stickler syndrome. *Am J Ophthalmol* **110**:143, 1990.

472. Goldstein JH, Hutt AE: Trichomegaly, cataract, and hereditary spherocytosis in two siblings. *Am J Ophthalmol* **73**:333, 1972.

473. McKusick VA, Weilbaecher RG, Gragg GW: Recessive inheritance of a congenital malformation syndrome. *JAMA* **204**:113, 1968.

474. Dionisi Vici C, Sabetta G, Gambarara M, Vigevano F, Vertini E, Boldrini R, Parisi SG, Quinti I, Aiuti F, Fiorilli M: Agenesis of the corpus callosum, combined immunodeficiency, bilateral cataract, and hypopigmentation in two brothers. *Am J Med Genet* **29**:1, 1988.

475. Lyon G, Arita F, Le Galloudec E, Vallee L, Misson J-P, Ferriere G: A disorder of axonal development, necrotizing myopathy, cardiomyopathy, and cataracts: A new familial disease. *Ann Neurol* **27**:193, 1990.

476. Riise R: Visual function in Laurence-Moon-Bardet-Biedl syndrome. *Acta Ophthalmol Suppl (Copenh)* **182**:128, 1987.

477. Sengers RCA, ter Haar BGA, Trijbels JMF, Willems JL, Daniels O, Stadhouders AM: Congenital cataract and mitochondrial myopathy of skeletal and heart muscle associated with lactic acidosis after exercise. *J Pediatr* **86**:873, 1975.

478. Seland JH, Slagsvold JE: The ultrastructure of lens and iris in cerebrotendinous xanthomatosis. *Acta Ophthalmol* **55**:201, 1977.

479. Grizzard WS, O'Donnell JJ, Carey JC: The cerebrooculofacioskeletal syndrome. *Am J Ophthalmol* **89**:293, 1980.

480. Pearce WG: Ocular and genetic features of Cockayne's syndrome. *Can J Ophthalmol* **7**:435, 1972.

481. Pinkerton OD: Cataract associated with congenital ichthyosis. *Arch Ophthalmol* **60**:393, 1958.

482. Crome L, Duckett S, Franklin AW: Congenital cataracts, renal tubular necrosis and encephalopathy in two sisters. *Arch Dis Child* **38**:505, 1963.

483. Sanner G: The dysequilibrium syndrome: A genetic study. *Neuropadiatrie* **4**:403, 1973.

484. Gitzelmann R: Hereditary galactokinase deficiency, a newly recognized cause of juvenile cataracts. *Pediatr Res* **1**:14, 1967.

485. Loos H, Roos D, Weening R, Houwerzijl J: Familial deficiency of glutathione reductase in human blood cells. *Blood* **48**:53, 1976.

486. Kaiser-Kupfer MI, Kuwabara T, Uga S, Takki K, Valle D: Cataract in gyrate atrophy clinical and morphological studies. *Invest Ophthalmol Vis Sci* **24**:432, 1983.

487. Caspersen I, Warburg M: Hallermann-Streiff syndrome. *Acta Ophthalmol* **46**:358, 1968.

488. Pagon RA, Clarren SK, Milam DF Jr, Hendrickson AE: Autosomal recessive eye and brain anomalies: Warburg syndrome. *J Pediatr* **102**:542, 1983.

489. Spaeth GL, Barber GW: Homocystinurias. Its ocular manifestations. *J Pediatr Ophthalmol* **3**:42, 1966.

490. Gold GN, Hogenhuis LAH: Hypertrophic interstitial neuropathy and cataracts. *Neurology* **18**:526, 1968.

491. Lubinsky MS: Cataracts and testicular failure in three brothers. *Am J Med Genet* **16**:149, 1983.

492. Buyse M, Bull MJ: A syndrome of osteogenesis imperfecta, microcephaly, and cataracts. *Birth Defects* **14**(6B):95, 1978.

493. Arbisser AI, Murhree AL, Garcia CA, Howell RR: Ocular findings in mannosidosis. *Am J Ophthalmol* **82**:465, 1976.

494. Chess J, Albert DM: Ocular pathology of the Majewski syndrome. *Br J Ophthalmol* **66**:736, 1982.

495. Herva R, von Wendt L, von Wendt G, Saukkonen AL, Leisti J: A syndrome with juvenile cataract, cerebellar atrophy, mental retardation and myopathy. *Neuropediatrics* **18**:164, 1987.

496. Martsolf JT, Hunter AGW, Haworth JC: Severe mental retardation, cataracts, short stature and primary hypogonadism in two brothers. *Am J Med Genet* **1**:291, 1978.

497. Hoffmann G, Gibson KM, Brandt IK, Bader PI, Wappner RS, Sweetman L: Mevalonic aciduria — an inborn error of cholesterol and nonsterol isoprene biosynthesis. *New Engl J Med* **314**:1610, 1986.

498. Lundberg PO: Hereditary myopathy, oligophrenia, cataract, skeletal abnormalities and hypergonadotropic hypogonadism: A new syndrome. *Acta Genet Med Gemellol* **23**:245, 1974.

499. Cremers CWRJ, ter Haar BGA, Van Rens TJG: The Nathalie syndrome: A new hereditary syndrome. *Clin Genet* **8**:330, 1975.

500. Neu RL, Kajii T, Gardner LI, Nagyfy SF: A lethal syndrome of microcephaly with multiple congenital anomalies in three siblings. *Pediatrics* **47**:610, 1971.

501. Thomas PK, Abrams JD, Swallow D, Stewart G: Sialidosis type I: Cherry red spot-myoclonus syndrome with sialidase deficiency and altered electrophoretic mobility of some enzymes known to be glycoproteins: Is. Clinical findings. *J Neurol Neurosurg Psychiatm* **42**:873, 1979.

502. Williams ML, Koch TK, O'Donnell JJ, frost PH, Epstein LB, Grizzard WS, Epstein CJ: Ichthyosis and neutral lipid storage disease. *Am J Med Genet* **20**:711, 1985.

503. Salih MAM, Bender DA, McCreanor GM: Lethal familial pellagra-like skin lesion associated with neurologic and developmental impairment and the development of cataracts. *Pediatrics* **76**:787, 1985.

504. Kwashima H, Kawano M, Masaki A, Sato T: Three cases of untreated classical PKU: A report on cataracts and brain calcification. *Am J Med Genet* **29**:89, 1988.

505. Fairly KF, Leighton PW, Kincaid-Smith P: Familial visual defects associated with polycystic kidney and medullary sponge kidney. *Br Med J* **1**:1060, 1963.

506. Preus M, Fraser FC, Wigglesworth JW: An oculocerebral hypopigmentation syndrome. *J Genet Hum* **31**:323, 1983.

507. Folz SJ, Trobe JD: The peroxisome and the eye. *Surv Ophthalmol* **35**:353, 1991.

508. Jones KL: *Smith's Recognizable Patterns of Human Malformation*. Philadelphia, Saunders, 1988.

509. Rothmund A: Uber Cataracte in Verbindung mit einer eigenthuemlichen Hautdegeneration. *Graefes Arch Klin Exp Ophthalmol* 14:159, 1868.

510. Mollica F, Pavone L, Antener I: Short stature, mental retardation and ocular alterations in three siblings. *Helv Paediatr Acta* 27:463, 1972.

511. Cotlier E, Rice P: Cataracts in the Smith-Lemli-Opitz syndrome. *Am J Ophthalmol* 72:955, 1971.

512. Adams CW, Nance WE: Persistent tachycardia, paroxysmal hypertension, and seizures: Association with hyperglycinuria, dominantly inherited microphthalmia, and cataracts. *JAMA* 202:525, 1967.

513. Toriello HV, Horton WA, Oostendorp A, Waterman DF, Higgins JV: An apparently new syndrome of microcephalic primordial dwarfism and cataracts. *Am J Med Genet* 25:1, 1986.

514. Hallgren B: Retinitis pigmentosa combined with congenital deafness: With vestibulocerebellar ataxia and mental abnormality in a proportion of cases. *Acta Psychiat Neurol Scand* 34(suppl. 138):9, 1959.

515. Epstein CJ, Martin GM, Schultz AL, Motulsky AG: Werner's syndrome: A review of its symptomatology, natural history, pathologic features, genetics and relationship to the natural aging process. *Medicine* 45:177, 1966.

516. Tso MO, Fine BS, Thorpe HE: Kayser-Fleischer ring and associated cataract in Wilson's disease. *Am J Ophthalmol* 79:479, 1975.

517. Fitch N: Albright's hereditary osteodystrophy: A review. *Am J Med Genet* 11:11, 1982.

518. Arnott EJ, Crawford MD, Toghill PJ: Anterior lenticonus and Alport's syndrome. *Br J Ophthalmol* 30:390, 1966.

519. Scher NA, Letson RD, Desnick RJ: The ocular manifestations in Fabry's disease. *Arch Ophthalmol* 97:671, 1979.

520. Orzalesi N, Sorcinelli R, Guiso G: Increased incidence of cataracts in male subjects deficient in glucose-6-phosphate dehydrogenase. *Arch Ophthalmol* 99:69, 1981.

521. Carney RG: Incontinentia pigmenti, a world statistical analysis. *Arch Dermatol* 112:535, 1976.

522. Herrmann H and Opitz JM: The Lenz microphthalmia syndrome. *Birth Defects* 5(2):138, 1969.

523. Wadelius C, Fagerholm P, Pettersson U, Anneren G: Lowe oculocerebrorenal syndrome: DNA based linkage of the gene to X124-q26, using tightly linked flanking markers and the correlation to lens examination in carrier diagnosis. *Am J Hum Genet* 44:241, 1989.

524. Nance WE, Warburg M, Bixler D, Helveston EM: Congenital X-linked cataract, dental anomalies and brachymetacarpalia. *Birth Defects* 10(4):285, 1974.

525. Mirhosseini SA, Holmes LB, Walton DS: Syndrome of pigmentary retinal degeneration, cataract, microcephaly, and severe mental retardation. *J Med Genet* 9:193, 1972.

526. Winsnes A, Monn E, Stokke O, Feyling T: Congenital persistent proximal type real tubular acidosis in two brothers. *Acta Paediatr Scand* 68:861, 1979.

527. Happle R: Cataracts as a marker of genetic heterogeneity in chondrodysplasia punctata. *Clin Genet* 19:64, 1981.

528. Chylack LT, Leske MC, McCarthy D, Khu T, Dashwagi T, Sperduto R: Lens opacities classification system II (LOCS II). *Arch Ophthalmol* 107:991, 1989.

529. Klein BEK, Klein R, Linton KLP, Magli YL, Neider MW: Assessment of cataracts from photography in the Beaver Dam eye study. *Ophthalmology* 97:1428, 1990.

530. Taylor HR, West SK: The clinical grading of lens opacities. *Aust NZ J Ophthalmol* 17:81, 1989.

531. Sparrow J, Bron A, Brown N, Ayliff W, Hall A: The Oxford clinical cataract classification and grading system. *Int Ophthalmol* 9:207, 1986.

532. Merin S: Congenital cataracts, in Goldberg MF (ed): *Genetic and Metabolic Eye Disease.* Boston, Little, Brown, 1974, p 337.

533. Kuszak JR: Embryology and anatomy of the lens, in Tasman W, Jaeger EA (eds): *Duane's Clinical Ophthalmology.* Philadelphia, Lippincott, 1990.

534. Holmes LB, McGowan BL, Efron ML: Lowe's syndrome: A search for the carrier state. *Pediatrics* 44:358, 1969.

535. Brown N, Gardner RJ: Lowe syndrome: Identification of the carrier state. *Birth Defects* 12(6):579, 1976.

536. Delleman JW, Bleeker-Wapemakers EM, van Veleen AWC: Opacities of the lens indicating carrier status in the oculocerebrorenal (Lowe) syndrome. *J Pediatr Ophthalmol* 14:205, 1976.

537. Cibis GW, Waeltermann JM, Whitcraft CT, Tripathi RC, Harris DJ: Lenticular opacities in carriers of Lowe's syndrome. *Ophthalmology* 93:1041, 1986.

538. Pearson-Webb MA, Kaiser-Kupfer MI, Eldridge R: Eye findings in bilateral acoustic (central) neurofibromatosis: Association with presenile lens opacities and cataracts but absence of Lisch nodules. *New Engl J Med* 315:1553, 1986.

539. Francois J: Genetics of cataract. *Ophthalmologica* 184:61, 1982.

540. Merin S, Crawford JS: The etiology of congenital cataracts: A survey of 386 cases. *Can J Ophthalmol* 6:178, 1971.

541. Levi S, Girelli D, Perrone F, Pasti M, Beaumont C, Corrocher R, Albertini A, Arosio P: Analysis of ferritins in lymphoblastoid cell lines and in the lens of subjects with hereditary hyperferritinemia-cataract syndrome. *Blood* 91:4180, 1998.

542. Hejtmancik JF: The genetics of cataract: Our vision becomes clearer. *Am J Hum Genet* 62:520, 1998.

543. Nettleship E, Ogilvie FM: A peculiar form of hereditary congenital cataract. *Trans Ophthal Soc UK* 26:191, 1906.

544. Shiels A, Mackay D, Ionides A, Berry V, Moore A, Bhattacharya S: A missense mutation in the human connexin50 gene (*GJA8*) underlies autosomal dominant "zonular pulverulent" cataract, on chromosome 1q. *Am J Hum Genet* 62:526, 1998.

545. Mackay D, Ionides A, Berry V, Moore A, Bhattacharya S, Shiels A: A new locus for dominant "zonular pulverulent" cataract, on chromosome 13. *Am J Hum Genet* 60:1474, 1997.

546. Mackay D, Ionides A, Kibar Z, Rouleau G, Berry V, Moore A, Shiels A, Bhattacharya S: Connexin46 mutations in autosomal dominent congenital cataract. *Am J Hum Genet* 64:1357, 1999.

547. Lubsen NH, Renwick JH, Tsui LC, Breitman ML, Schoenmakers JG: A locus for a human hereditary cataract is closely linked to the gamma-crystallin gene family. *Proc Natl Acad Sci USA* 84:489, 1987.

548. Rogaev EI, Rogaeva EA, Korovaitseva GI, Farrar LA, Petrin AN, Keryanov SA, Turaeva S, Chumakov I, St. George-Hyslop P, Ginter EK: Linkage of polymorphic congenital cataract to the gamma-crystallin gene locus on human chromosome 2q33–35. *Hum Mol Genet* 5:699, 1997.

549. Ayyagari R, Padma T, Murty JS, Basti S, Rao GN, Scott MH, Wozencraft L, Kaiser-Kupfer M, Hejtmancik JF: Localization of genes for autosomal dominant congenital cataracts to chromosomes 2 and 17. *Am J Hum Genet* 55:A 180, 1997.

550. Heon E, Munier F, Tsilfidis C, Liu S: Mapping of congenital aculeiform cataract to chromosome 2q33. *Invest Ophthalmol Vis Sci* 38:S934, 1997.

551. Padma T, Ayyagari R, Murty JS, Basti S, Fletcher T, Rao GN, Kaiser-Kupfer M, Hejtmancik JF: Autosomal dominant zonular cataract with sutural opacities localized to chromosome 17q11-12. *Am J Hum Genet* 57:840, 1995.

552. Kannabiran C, Basti S, Balasubramanian D, Majumdar K, Rao GN, Kaiser-Kupfer M, Hejtmancik JF: Autosomal dominant zonular cataract with sutural opacities: Result of a splice site mutation. *Invest Ophthalmol Vis Sci* 39:S418, 1998.

553. Geyer DD, Johannes M, Masser DS, Flodman P, Spence MA, Clancy K, Walter NAR, Sikela JM, Bateman JB: Identification of a novel locus for autosomal dominant congenital cataract on chromosome 17q. *Invest Ophthalmol Vis Sci* 39:S419, 1998.

554. Litt M, Carrero-Valenzuela R, LaMorticella DM, Schultz DW, Mitchell TN, Kramer P, Maumenee IH: Autosomal dominant cerulean cataract is associated with a chain termination mutation in the human beta-crystallin gene *CRYBB2*. *Hum Mol Genet* 6:665, 1997.

555. Litt M, Kramer P, LaMorticella DM, Murphey W, Lovrien EW, Weleber RG: Autosomal dominant congenital cataract associated with a missense mutation in the human alpha crystallin gene *CRYAA*. *Hum Mol Genet* 7:471, 1998.

556. Eiberg H, Lund AM, Warburg M, Rosenberg T: Assignment of congenital cataract Volkmann type (*CCV*) to chromosome 1p36. *Hum Genet* 96:33, 1995.

557. Huang CH, Chen Y, Reid M, Ghosh S: Genetic recombination at the human RH locus: A family study of the red-cell Evans phenotype reveals a transfer of exons 2–6 from the *RHD* to the *RHCE* gene. *Am J Hum Genet* 59:825, 1996.

558. Ionides AC, Berry V, Mackay DS, Moore AT, Bhattacharya SS, Shiels A: A locus for autosomal dominant posterior polar cataract on chromosome 1p. *Hum Mol Genet* 6:47, 1997.

559. Eiberg H, Nielsen LS, Klausen J, Dahlen M, Kristensen M, Bisgaard ML, Moller N, Mohr J: Linkage between serum cholinesterase 2 (CHE2) and gamma- crystallin gene cluster (*CRYG*): Assignment to chromosome 2. *Clin Genet* 35:313, 1989.

560. Marner E, Rosenberg T, Eiberg H: Autosomal dominant congenital cataract: Morphology and genetic mapping. *Acta Ophthalmol* 67:151, 1989.

561. Richards J, Maumenee IH, Rowe S, Lourien EW: Congenital cataract possibly linked to haptoglobin. *Cytogenet Cell Genet* 37:570, 1984.

562. Berry V, Ionides AC, Moore AT, Plant C, Bhattacharya SS, Shiels A: A locus for autosomal dominant anterior polar cataract on chromosome 17p. *Hum Mol Genet* **5**:415, 1996.

563. Armitage MM, Kivlin JD, Ferrell RE: A progressive early onset cataract gene maps to human chromosome 17q24. *Nature Genet* **9**:37, 1995.

564. Ogata H, Okubo Y, Akabane T: Phenotype i associated with congenital cataract in Japanese. *Transfusion* **19**:166, 1979.

565. Macdonald EB, Douglas R, Harden PA: A Caucasian family with the i phenotype and congenital cataracts. *Vox Sang* **44**:322, 1983.

566. Yamaguchi H, Okubo Y, Tanaka M: A note on possible close linkage between the li blood locus and a congenital cataract locus. *Proc Jpn Acad* **48**:625, 1972.

567. Reese PD, Tuck-Miller CM, Maumenee IH: Autosomal dominant congenital cataract associated with chromosomal translocation [t(3;4)(p26.2;p15)]. *Arch Ophthalmol* **105**:1382, 1987.

568. Moross T, Vaithilingam SS, Styles S, Gardner HA: Autosomal dominant anterior polar cataracts associated with a familial 2;14 translocation. *J Med Genet* **21**:52, 1984.

569. Yokoyama Y, Narahara K, Tsuji K, Nonomiya S, Seino Y: Autosomal dominant congenital cataract and microphthalmia associated with a familial t(2; 16) translocation. *Hum Genet* **90**:177, 1992.

570. Monaghan KG, Van DD, Wiktor A, Feldman GL: Cytogenetic and clinical findings in a patient with a deletion of 16q23s.1: First report of bilateral cataracts and a 16q deletion. *Am J Med Genet* **73**:180, 1997.

571. Rubin SE, Nelson LB, Pletcher BA: Anterior polar cataract in two sisters with an unbalanced 3;18 chromosomal translocation. *Am J Ophthalmol* **117**:512, 1994.

572. Petit P, Devriendt K, Vermeesch JR, De CP, Fryns JP: Unusual de novo t(13;15)(q12.1;p13) translocation leading to complex mosaicism including jumping translocation. *Ann Genet* **41**:22, 1998.

573. Ehling UH: Genetic risk assessment. *Annu Rev Genet* **25**:255, 1991.

574. Schlote T, Volker M, Knorr M, Thiel HJ: Lens coloboma and lens dislocation in Stickler (Marshall) syndrome. *Klin Monatsbl Augenheilkd* **210**:227, 1997.

575. Mehrotra AS, Solanki N, Sabharwal KK: Bilateral coloboma of lens in Marfan's syndrome. *Ind J Ophthalmol* **33**:201, 1985.

576. Jensen AD, Cross HE, Paton D: Ocular complications in the Weill-Marchesani syndrome. *Am J Ophthalmol* **77**:261, 1974.

577. Colville DJ, Savige J: Alport syndrome: A review of the ocular manifestations. *Ophthalmic Genet* **18**:161, 1997.

578. Mir S, Wheatley HM, Hussels IE, Whittum-Hudson JA, Traboulsi EI: A comparative histologic study of the fibrillin microfibrillar system in the lens capsule of normal subjects and subjects with Marfan syndrome. *Invest Ophthalmol Vis Sci* **39**:84, 1998.

579. Mudd SH, Skovby F, Levy HL, Pettigrew KD, Wilcken B, Pyeritz RE, Andria G, Boers GH, Bromberg IL, Cerone R: The natural history of homocystinuria due to cystathionine beta-synthase deficiency. *Am J Hum Genet* **37**:1, 1985.

580. Wirtz MK, Samples JR, Kramer PL, Rust K, Yount J, Acott TS, Koler RD, Cisler J, Jahed A, Gorlin RJ, Godfrey M: Weill-Marchesani syndrome—possible linkage of the autosomal dominant form to 15q21.1. *Am J Med Genet* **65**:68, 1996.

581. Goh A, Lim KW: Sulphite oxidase deficiency—a report of two siblings. *Singapore Med J* **38**:391, 1997.

582. Tsipouras P, Del Mastro R, Sarfarazi M, Lee B, Vitale E, Child AH, Godfrey M, Devereux RB, Hewett D, Steinmann B, Viljoen D, Sykes B, Kilpatrick M, Ramirez F: Genetic linkage of the Marfan syndrome, ectopia lentis, and congenital contractural arachnodactyly to the fibrillin genes on chromosomes 15 and 5. *New Engl J Med* **326**:906, 1992.

583. Dobson V, Teller DY: Visual acuity in human infants: A review and comparison of behavioral and electrophysiological studies. *Vision Res* **18**:1469, 1978.

584. Atkinson J, Braddick O: Assessment of visual acuity in infancy and early childhood. *Acta Ophthalmol Suppl (Copenh)* **157**:18, 1983.

585. Weisel TN, Hubel DH: Comparison of the effects of unilateral and bilateral eyelid closure on cortical responses in kittens. *J Neurophysiol* **28**:1029, 1965.

586. Harwerth RS, Smith EL 3, Paul AD, Crawford ML, von Noorden GK: Functional effects of bilateral form deprivation in monkeys. *Invest Ophthalmol Vis Sci* **32**:2311, 1991.

587. Robb RM, Mayer DL, Moore BD: Results of early treatment of unilateral congenital cataracts. *J Pediatr Ophthalmol Strabismus* **24**:178, 1987.

588. Nelson LB: Diagnosis and management of cataracts in infancy and childhood. *Ophthalmic Surg* **15**:688, 1984.

589. Gelbart SS, Hoyt CS, Jastrebski G, Marg E: Long-term visual results in bilateral congenital cataracts. *Am J Ophthalmol* **93**:615, 1982.

590. Burns EC, Jones RB: Long term management of congenital cataracts. *Arch Dis Child* **60**:322, 1985.

591. Matsuo I, Yasuda K: The cooperative interaction between two motifs of an enhancer element of the chicken alpha A-crystallin gene, alpha CE1 and alpha CE2, confers lens-specific expression. *Nucl Acids Res* **20**:3701, 1992.

# The Glaucomas

*Val C. Sheffield* ■ *Wallace L. M. Alward* ■ *Edwin M. Stone*

1. The glaucomas are a heterogeneous group of diseases that result in death of the optic nerve. Together, these disorders are the leading cause of irreversible blindness in the world. The glaucomas are categorized into open-angle, closed-angle, and congenital glaucoma based on the mechanism by which aqueous outflow is impeded in the anterior chamber of the eye. Primary open-angle glaucoma (POAG) accounts for the vast majority of glaucoma cases. Major risk factors for development of this disorder are age, race, elevated intraocular pressure, and family history. Genetic mapping studies have resulted in the identification of five POAG loci. A subset of POAG cases occurs at a young age and is known as juvenile onset primary open-angle glaucoma (JOAG, MIM 137750). This disorder was mapped to and shown to be caused by mutations in a gene (GLC1A, MIM 137750) that codes for a 504-amino acid protein known as myocilin. Mutations in the GLC1A gene have been shown to account for nearly all cases of autosomal dominant JOAG, and 3 to 4 percent of cases of adult onset POAG. Glaucoma caused by GLC1A mutations is inherited as an autosomal dominant disorder with high penetrance and variable expressivity.

2. Normal tension glaucoma is a subtype of POAG that is defined by the presence of glaucomatous optic nerve changes and visual field loss in patients with normal intraocular pressure. This disorder is thought to occur because of polygenic or multifactorial inheritance. A locus (GLC1E) for this disorder has been reported on chromosome 10p14-p15 based on study of a single pedigree.

3. Pigmentary glaucoma (MIM 600510) is a form of open-angle glaucoma characterized by the presence of dense black pigment in the trabecular meshwork of the eye. The formation of glaucoma in patients with this disorder is thought to be secondary to the dispersion of melanosomes from the iris into the aqueous humor, and subsequently into the trabecular meshwork. Two loci thought to cause autosomal dominant inheritance of pigmentary glaucoma have been reported.

4. Exfoliative glaucoma is a common form of open-angle glaucoma in which increased intraocular pressure is secondary to deposition of a fibrillar material throughout the anterior segment of the eye. This disorder is a disease of the elderly. It has a high incidence in some populations, including Scandinavians and Navajo Indians. No genetic loci have been identified for this disorder.

5. Corticosteroids have been well documented as inducing elevated intraocular pressure in some patients. Susceptibility to steroid-induced glaucoma appears to have genetic components.

6. Closed-angle glaucoma is characterized by impedance of aqueous humor outflow secondary to the iris being displaced over the trabecular meshwork. This disorder can develop suddenly and, unlike other forms of glaucoma, results in recognizable symptoms including nausea, vomiting, headache, and severe eye pain.

7. The developmental glaucomas result from an abnormality of the iridocorneal angle present at birth that results in decrease aqueous outflow and increased intraocular pressure. The developmental glaucomas can occur as an isolated ocular abnormality, in which case it is known as primary congenital glaucoma (PCG), or they can occur in conjunction with a variety of other ocular and/or extraocular abnormalities. Primary congenital glaucoma has an incidence of about 1 in 10,000 live births. Many cases of PCG appear to be inherited as autosomal recessive traits. Two PCG loci have been reported. Recently, mutations in the CYP1B1 gene on chromosome 2 have been shown to cause PCG.

8. A number of abnormalities involving the anterior segment of the eye, including Rieger anomaly (MIM 180500), Axenfeld anomaly, and iris hypoplasia (MIM 137600), are associated with glaucoma. When extraocular findings, including dental hypoplasia and umbilical abnormalities, occur with these anterior chamber abnormalities, the disorder is known as Axenfeld-Rieger syndrome (MIM 601631). Axenfeld-Rieger syndrome is an autosomal dominant disorder, which is caused by a mutation in the PITX2/RIEG1 homeobox gene on chromosome 4q. A second Axenfeld-Rieger Syndrome locus has been reported on chromosome 13.

9. Several congenital glaucoma-related phenotypes transmitted in an autosomal dominant manner have been mapped to chromosome 6p25. These phenotypes include Rieger anomaly, Axenfeld anomaly, and iridogoniodysgenesis (MIM 601631). These disorders are caused by mutations in the FKHL7 gene. A number of other genetic eye disorders can lead to congenital glaucoma, including Peter's anomaly (MIM 106210), aniridia, and posterior polymorphous corneal dystrophy (MIM 122000).

10. Current methods of screening for glaucoma are inadequate. Identification of genes involved in glaucoma will lead to molecular screening methods that should reduce the incidence of blindness resulting from glaucoma. A careful family history should be obtained from patients with glaucoma, and genetic counseling should be made available.

## INTRODUCTION

Glaucoma is an optic neuropathy in which the axons, vessels, and supporting structures of the optic nerve are gradually lost. This, combined with backbowing of the collagenous latticework through which the axons exit the eye, gives rise to the excavation or "cupping" of the optic nerve head that is visible ophthalmo-

A list of standard abbreviations is located immediately preceding the index in each volume. Additional abbreviations used in this chapter include: JOAG, juvenile open angle glaucoma; PCG, primary congenital glaucoma; POAG, primary open angle glaucoma; TIGR, trabecular meshwork-induced glucocorticoid response protein.

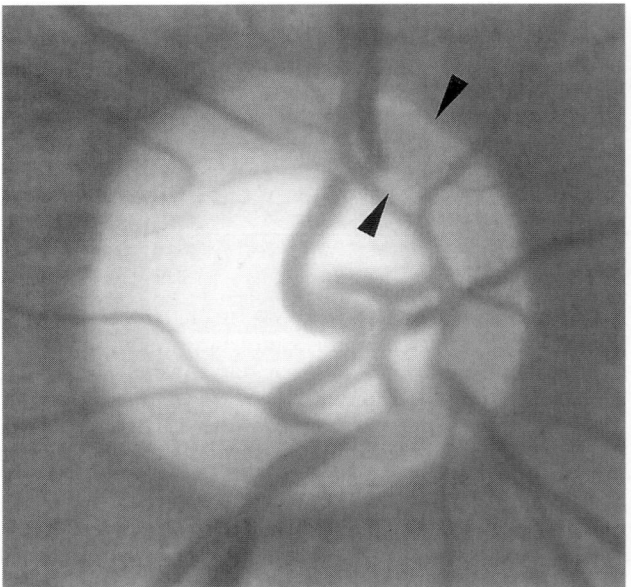

A

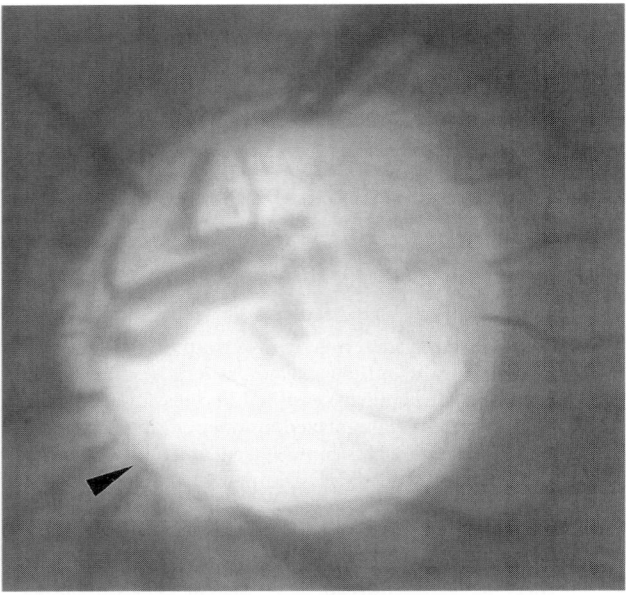

B

Fig. 242-1 Optic nerves of a patient with unilateral glaucoma. The right optic nerve (left frame) has an intact rim of nerve tissue (between the arrows). The left optic nerve (right frame) has lost virtually all of the neural rim, note how the vessels turn abruptly and are lost from view in the deep cup that extends to the periphery of the disc (arrow).

scopically (Fig. 242-1). When sufficient optic nerve head tissue is lost, visual function is affected, first by a loss of peripheral vision (Fig. 242-2), and ultimately by a loss of central visual acuity.

Glaucoma is the leading cause of irreversible blindness in the world. It is estimated that 66.8 million persons have glaucoma and of these, 6.7 million are blind.[1] In the United States, glaucoma is the second leading cause of permanent blindness and the leading cause among Americans with African ancestry.[2]

An elevated intraocular pressure is found in most patients with glaucoma, but is not required for the diagnosis. Many patients have an elevated intraocular pressure without ever developing glaucomatous optic nerve head damage. These patients are considered to have ocular hypertension and are at increased risk for developing glaucoma at a later date. At the other extreme are patients who have typical glaucomatous optic neuropathy with visual field loss but who have never had a documented elevated intraocular pressure. These patients are considered to have normal tension glaucoma, a subtype of primary open-angle glaucoma.

To understand the classification of glaucoma, it is helpful to understand the basics of aqueous humor dynamics. Because the cornea and the lens are transparent, they must be avascular. Therefore, these structures have a circulation system composed of a clear aqueous humor. The aqueous is created by the epithelium that covers the ciliary body, circulates around the lens, through the pupil, and throughout the anterior chamber, and, ultimately, is drained through the trabecular meshwork into the venous system (Fig. 242-3). Elevated intraocular pressure is due to an inadequate outflow of aqueous humor from the eye. The glaucomas are categorized into three broad categories based on the mechanism by which aqueous outflow is impeded: open-angle, closed-angle, and congenital. Each of these broad categories is further subdivided into primary and secondary causes. The glaucomas for which there is information regarding chromosomal linkage or gene identification are listed in Table 242-1.

## OPEN-ANGLE GLAUCOMAS

The open-angle glaucomas are characterized by the presence of a wide angle between the cornea and the iris that allows for unimpeded outflow of aqueous and for unobstructed visualization of the trabecular meshwork by gonioscopy.

### Primary Open-Angle Glaucoma

**Clinical Phenotype.** In patients with primary open-angle glaucoma (POAG), the iridocorneal angle is open and appears entirely normal with no evidence of excessive pigmentation or other structural changes. POAG is by far the most common form of glaucoma in the United States.

**Diagnosis.** Diagnosis of POAG is based on elevated intraocular pressure, the presence of cupping of the optic nerve head demonstrated by ophthalmoscopy, and loss of peripheral vision in an optic nerve-related pattern.

**Risk Factors.** The four major risk factors for the development of POAG are age, race, elevated intraocular pressure, and family history.[2] POAG is uncommon before the age of 40, and when diagnosed before age 40, the disorder is considered a separate subcategory of glaucoma known as JOAG. The prevalence of glaucoma increases with age, and in some studies, advanced age is a more important risk factor than elevated intraocular pressure.[2,3] In the United States, patients of African heritage develop glaucoma earlier and have a more severe form of the disease. African-Americans have four to five times the prevalence of glaucoma than European-Americans.[4] Elevated intraocular pressure, while not absolutely required for the diagnosis of glaucoma, is a major risk factor for its development.[5] The majority of patients with POAG have an elevated intraocular pressure. The higher the intraocular pressure, the greater the risk of developing glaucoma. Patients with a positive family history of POAG are at an increased risk of developing the disease.[6–8]

Other risk factors for the development of glaucoma are minor and more variable, and include myopia, diabetes mellitus, and cardiovascular disease.[2]

**Genetics and Molecular Biology.** Although the suggestion that some cases of POAG are inherited was first made over 150 years ago,[9,10] acceptance of POAG as an inherited disease became widespread only after a number of glaucoma disease loci were successfully identified. Prior to these molecular studies, the familial nature of POAG was supported mainly by epidemiologic studies, reports of concordance in twins, and reports of families in which the disorder segregated in a Mendelian fashion. Formal

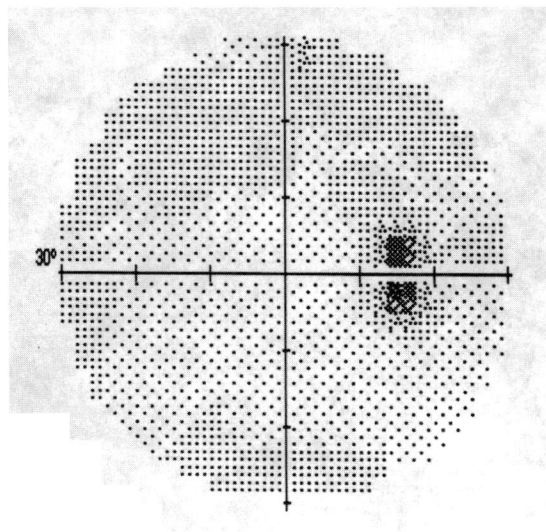

A

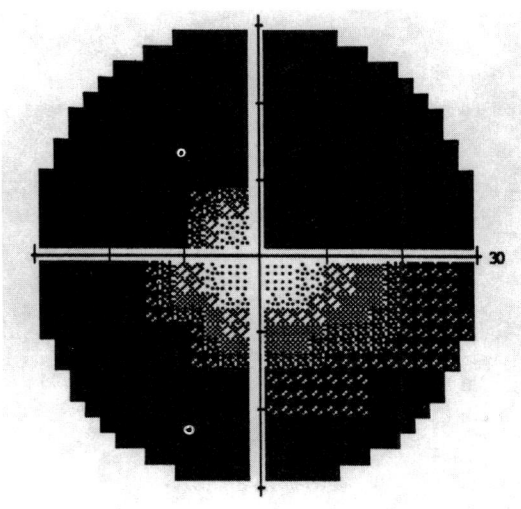

B

**Fig. 242-2. Automated visual fields. Frame A is the visual field of a patient without ocular disease. The black spot is the normal blind spot and represents the optic nerve, which is not covered by retina. Frame B is the visual field of a patient with advanced glaucomatous loss that is represented by the black and dark gray areas.**

Factors associated with glaucoma, such as intraocular pressure,[8,26] outflow facility,[27] cup-to-disc ratio,[28,29] and hypertensive response to corticosteroids,[30] have all been shown to have a heritable component.

A number of different loci involved in POAG have been identified, clearly demonstrating it is genetically heterogeneous. By convention, each locus has been given the prefix designation "GLC" referring to glaucoma, followed by the number "1," which refers to the open-angle subtype of glaucoma. Finally, each locus has been given a letter designation (i.e., A, B, C, etc.) which refers to the order in which the loci were identified. Sheffield et al. reported the first genetic linkage of a POAG locus to chromosome 1 with a large autosomal dominant pedigree consisting of 22 individuals affected with JOAG.[31] This locus, designated GLC1A, is linked to the disease in almost all pedigrees with juvenile-onset glaucoma,[32–34] and to some pedigrees that display a range of phenotypes from ocular hypertension to POAG with an onset after the age of 40 years.[35] Efforts to fine map the disease locus resulted in the narrowing of the candidate interval.[36] As discussed more fully below, the gene responsible for GLC1A glaucoma was recently identified.[37]

Stoilova et al. mapped a locus for adult-onset POAG to 2cen-q13. This locus is designated GLC1B.[38] The clinical characteristics of the families mapping to the GLC1B locus include autosomal dominant inheritance, low to moderate intraocular pressure, onset in the fifth decade of life, and good response to medical treatment.[38] Wirtz et al. used a single large pedigree to map a third autosomal dominant POAG locus (GLC1C) to chromosome 3q21 to 3q24.[39] To date, other families mapping to this locus have not been reported. Sarfarazi and coworkers recently reported the mapping of two additional adult-onset glaucoma loci (GLC1D and GLC1E) to chromosomes 8 and 10.[40,41] The genes causing GLC1B through GLC1E glaucoma have yet to be identified.

The majority of cases of POAG are thought to be the result of multifactorial inheritance, although some studies have suggested that POAG is inherited as an autosomal dominant with reduced penetrance.[42] A number of studies using affected pedigree member and affected sib pair study designs are ongoing but have not yet yielded any new statistically established loci. An alternative approach for identifying POAG genes that is likely to be fruitful is the use of mouse models. John and coworkers recently reported strain differences in intraocular pressure between inbred mouse strains.[43] Crosses between these strains should allow mapping of loci controlling intraocular pressure.

Using a combination of positional cloning and candidate gene screening, Stone et al. identified a gene on the long arm of chromosome 1 that causes most cases of autosomal dominant JOAG. The gene was initially mapped to a 23 cM interval on chromosome 1.[37] The interval was narrowed to about 1 cM using several extended pedigrees and comparison of haplotypes between affected kindreds. A physical map of the interval was constructed, and genes mapping to the narrowed interval were considered to be candidates and were screened for mutations.[36,37] Initial identification of the GLC1A gene was based on mutation identification in extended pedigrees segregating juvenile-onset disease. Later, screening of unrelated probands with adult-onset POAG revealed GLC1A sequence variation that was significantly greater than that present in controls, further supporting GLC1A as an important glaucoma-causing gene.[37] A follow-up study of 716 primarily Caucasian patients with adult-onset POAG and 596 ethnically matched controls identified 16 probable disease-causing mutations.[44] These mutations accounted for 4.6 percent of the glaucoma cases in probands. The most common mutation, Gln368ter, was found to account for almost half of the cases. The age at which the diagnosis was made in patients with GLC1A mutations ranged from 8 years to 77 years. The Q368ter mutation is associated with a significantly later age of onset (range 36 to 77 years; average age = 59 years) compared to the other reported mutations.[44] These data demonstrate that adult-onset glaucoma can be inherited as an autosomal dominant

segregation analyses have not been reported. Several studies reported a high incidence of glaucoma among individuals with a family history.[6,8,11–13] In these studies, prevalence rates were reported to be five- to twentyfold higher in individuals with a first-degree relative with glaucoma as compared to the general population. Variations in these studies can be attributed to population differences and differences in study design. Twin studies also support a genetic component of glaucoma, although no large twin studies (i.e., with statistically significant data) have been reported .[14] Case reports of twins showing both concordance[14–18] and discordance[14,19,20] for POAG have been reported, suggesting that both genetic and nongenetic factors play a role in this form of glaucoma. Numerous extended kindreds in which glaucoma segregates in a Mendelian manner (both autosomal dominant and autosomal recessive) have been reported.[21–25] Such families are perhaps the strongest evidence that glaucoma is heritable. The percentage of cases of POAG that are classified as hereditary in the literature ranges from 5 percent to 50 percent.[2]

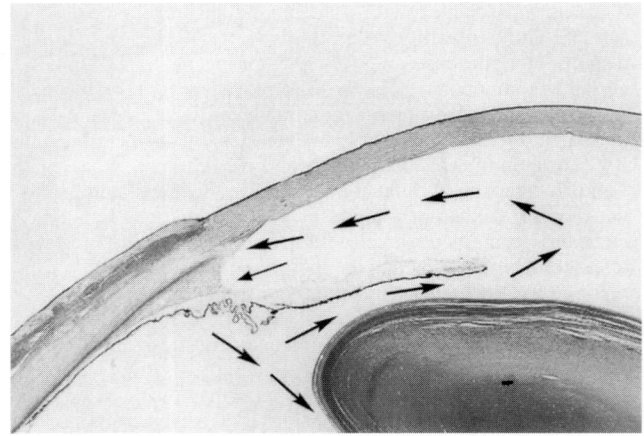

**Fig. 242-3. Anterior segment circulation. The left frame shows the parts of the anterior chamber. The right frame shows the route of aqueous flow. The aqueous is made in the ciliary body and flows around the lens, through the pupil, and throughout the anterior** chamber, ultimately exiting through the trabecular meshwork. A smaller amount (about 10 percent) leaves via the uveoscleral pathway through the ciliary body face. (*From Alward, WLM. N Eng J Med 339:1298, 1998.*[44] *Used with permission.*)

disorder. Due to the late onset of the disease in some cases, a positive family history may not be apparent. Morissette et al. recently reported a sequence variant (K423E) in the GLC1A gene, found in a large extended kindred, which appears to cause disease when found in the heterozygous state, but not in the homozygous state.[45]

The GLC1A gene encodes a 504-amino acid protein referred to initially as the trabecular meshwork-induced glucocorticoid

**Table 242-1 The Inheritance of Diseases Commonly Associated with Glaucoma**

| Disease (MIM#) | Chromosome Location | Ref. | Gene (MIM#) | Ref. |
|---|---|---|---|---|
| OPEN ANGLE GLAUCOMAS | | | | |
| Primary | | | | |
| Primary open angle | | | | |
| GLC1A (137750) | 1q23-25 | 31 | GLC1A/myocilin (601652) | 37 |
| GLC1B (137760) | 2cen-q13 | 38 | | |
| GLC1C (601682) | 3q21-24 | 39 | | |
| GLC1D | 8p23 | 40 | | |
| GLC1E | 10p15-14 | 41 | | |
| Juvenile open angle (137750) | 1q23-25 | 37 | GLC1A/myocilin (601652) | 37 |
| Normal tension | 10p15-14 | 41 | | |
| Associated with syndrome | | | | |
| Nail patella syndrome (161200) | 9q34 | 150 | LMX1B (602575) | 150 |
| Secondary | | | | |
| Pigmentary (600510) | 7q35-36 | 62 | | |
| | 18q11-21 | 61 | | |
| DEVELOPMENTAL | | | | |
| Primary | | | | |
| Primary congenital | | | | |
| GLC3A (231300) | 2p21 | 105 | CYP1B1 (601771) | 113 |
| GLC3B (600975) | 1p36 | 106 | | |
| | 6p25 | 107 | FKHL7 (601090) | 107 |
| Associated with syndrome | | | | |
| Aniridia(106210) | 11p13 | 138 | PAX6 (106210) | 135 |
| Anterior segment mesenchymal dysgenesis (107250) | 10q25 | 127 | PITX3 (602669) | 127 |
| Axenfeld-Rieger's anomaly (601631) | 6p25 | 111 | FKHL7 (601090) | 107 |
| Ectopia Lentis (simple) (129600) | 154q21 | 151 | FBN1/fibrillin (134797) | 151 |
| Iridogoniodysgenesis (601631) | 6p25 | 128 | | |
| Iris hypoplasia (137600) | 4q25 | 125 | RIEG1 (PITX2) (601542) | 126 |
| Lowe's syndrome (309000) | Xq25 | 152 | OCRL-1 (309000) | 153 |
| Marfan syndrome (154700) | 154q21 | 154 | FBN1/fibrillin (134797) | 155 |
| Neurofibromatosis I (162200) | 17q11 | 156 | NF1/neurofibromin (162200) | 157 |
| Peters' anomaly (106210) | 11p13 | 132 | PAX6 (106210) | 132 |
| Posterior polymorphous corneal dystrophy (122000) | 20q11 | 146 | | |
| Riegers' syndrome | | | | |
| Type 1 (RIEG1) (180500) | 4q25 | 122 | RIEG1 (PITX2) (601542) | 123 |
| Type 2 (RIEG2) (601499) | 13q14 | 124 | | |

MIM = Mendelian Inheritance in Man. This table lists diseases that have glaucoma as a major feature and for which at least one genetic locus has been identified. There are many rare syndromes that have glaucoma as a minor component; these are not included in this list. The latter are reviewed in Johnson et al.[158]

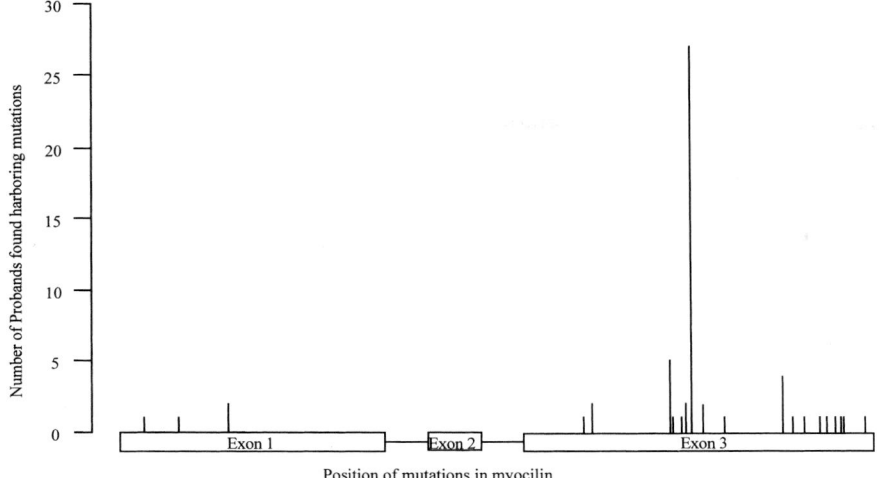

Fig. 242-4. Diagram of the GLC1A structural gene with three exons. Most disease-causing mutations are in exon 3.

response protein (TIGR). Upon the recommendation of the Human Genome Organization Nomenclature Committee, the protein is now officially referred to as myocilin. This protein has a molecular mass of 57 kDa and is expressed in a wide range of tissues.[46,47] Myocilin has an aminoterminal hydrophobic region, a domain displaying 25 percent homology with myocin heavy chain, and an olfactomedin-like domain at the C-terminus. In addition, a leucine zipper-like motif with a leucine at every seventh position is found between amino acids 117 to 169. Arginine residues are found at every eleventh position from amino acid 125 to amino acid 169. The normal role of myocilin and the mechanism by which mutations in this gene cause glaucoma are not yet known. The gene consists of three exons. Of interest is that nearly all glaucoma-associated mutations in this gene are in exon three (Fig. 242-4), which suggests that alterations elsewhere in the gene only rarely cause glaucoma. The mechanism by which GLC1A mutations cause increased intraocular pressure and glaucoma has not yet been demonstrated.

**Treatment.** The optic neuropathy of glaucoma cannot be treated directly at the present time. Treatment is, therefore, directed at the one major risk factor that can be altered, elevated intraocular pressure. Intraocular pressure is usually lowered by one or more topical medications, which include $\beta$-adrenergic antagonists, prostaglandin analogs, adrenergic agonists, carbonic anhydrase inhibitors, and cholinergic agonists. These medications either decrease aqueous humor production or increase aqueous humor outflow. Oral carbonic anhydrase inhibitors can be used to decrease aqueous humor production, but these agents have been almost completely replaced by topical drugs that have fewer systemic side effects. If the intraocular pressure is not adequately controlled with medications, argon laser can be applied to the trabecular meshwork to increase aqueous outflow. This procedure, called argon laser trabeculoplasty, decreases intraocular pressure in about 80 percent of patients, but the effect may be lost after a few years.[48] If medical and laser therapy fails to control intraocular pressure, a new route of aqueous egress can be created surgically in the form of a trabeculectomy or by insertion of a drainage tube (a seton or valve).

Lowering intraocular pressure has been shown to slow glaucomatous damage and to protect the optic nerve head from further damage.[49,50]

## Normal-Tension Glaucoma

**Clinical Phenotype.** Normal tension glaucoma is a subtype of primary open-angle glaucoma. It is arbitrarily defined as glaucomatous optic neuropathy and visual field loss in a patient whose intraocular pressure has never been recorded above the normal range (up to 21 mm Hg). It is felt that the optic nerve head damage in normal-tension glaucoma may have a more vascular etiology than the nerve head damage that occurs in high-pressure glaucomas.

**Diagnosis.** Normal-tension glaucoma is associated with a normal appearing anterior segment. The trabecular meshwork is readily visualized on gonioscopy and appears normal. The optic nerve head cupping tends to be more focal than that seen in high-pressure glaucoma and is more likely to selectively involve the inferotemporal and superotemporal portions of the optic nerve head. The visual fields show optic nerve-related field loss. When compared with high-pressure glaucomas the visual field loss is more central and denser.

**Risk Factors.** Patients with normal-tension glaucoma are on average much older than patients with POAG. They are also more likely than the general population to have a history of vasospastic disease such as migraine headache[51] or Raynaud's phenomenon.[52] There is evidence that patients with progressive normal-tension glaucoma may have impaired circulation to the optic nerve head associated with nocturnal systemic hypotension.[53]

**Genetics and Molecular Biology.** There have been few genetic studies of normal-tension glaucoma. Evidence that normal-tension glaucoma has a genetic component is based on prevalence differences between races and populations, as well as the segregation of normal-tension glaucoma as an autosomal dominant disorder in a few reported kindreds.[54] The prevalence of normal-tension glaucoma in Japan is reported to exceed 2 percent of the population over the age of 40, much greater than the prevalence seen in the United States.[55] Like POAG, normal-tension glaucoma is likely to be a genetically heterogeneous disorder. In most cases of normal-tension glaucoma, there is not a strong family history, the lack of which suggests either polygenic or multifactorial inheritance.

Sarfarazi et al. recently reported the identification of a locus (GLC1E) on chromosome 10p14-p15 in a large British family with a phenotype consistent with normal-tension glaucoma.[41] The maximum lod score when an "affected only" analysis was performed was 3.57 at D10S506. A maximum lod score of 10 at a recombination fraction of zero was observed at marker D10S1216 when unaffected individuals were also included in the analysis. No genes involved in this form of glaucoma have yet been identified. The existence of the normal-tension glaucoma entity stresses the important concept that glaucoma is not simply a disorder of increased intraocular pressure, but that factors involved in susceptibility and resistance to ganglion cell death also play a role.

**Treatment.** Like POAG, the treatment of normal tension glaucoma is directed at lowering intraocular pressure. A large collaborative randomized trial studying the benefits and risks of treating normal-tension glaucoma has shown that a 30 percent reduction of intraocular pressure slows the progression this disease.[56] Some researchers have suggested that oral calcium channel blockers be used to improve optic nerve head blood flow.[57] There is concern that the systemic hypotension induced by these medications may be detrimental to the optic nerve head.[53]

## Pigmentary Glaucoma

**Clinical Phenotype.** Pigmentary glaucoma (MIM 600510) is a form of "secondary" open-angle glaucoma in which the trabecular meshwork is visible on gonioscopy but is filled with dense black pigment. The pigment originates from the posterior surface of the iris.[58] The mechanism of pigment dispersion syndrome appears to be the following. First, during a blink, aqueous is expressed from the posterior chamber into the anterior chamber of the eye. In susceptible eyes, this excess aqueous in the anterior chamber pushes the iris posteriorly. This posterior bowing of the iris brings the pigment epithelium of the iris into contact with the lens zonules.[59] Abrasion of the zonules against the pigment epithelium causes the epithelium to be disrupted, dispersing melanosomes into the aqueous humor.[58] This pigment is then deposited in several areas. A vertical stripe of pigment is deposited on the corneal endothelium (Krukenberg spindle). Pigment can also be deposited over the anterior surface of the iris as well as at the junction of the posterior lens capsule and zonules. It is the deposition of pigment granules in the trabecular meshwork that can lead to an elevated intraocular pressure and, ultimately, to glaucoma. If all of the signs of pigment dispersion and deposition are present but there is no glaucoma, the disorder is called pigment dispersion syndrome. When glaucoma ensues, it is called pigmentary glaucoma.

**Diagnosis.** The diagnosis of pigmentary glaucoma is made by recognizing the deposition of pigment on the cornea, anterior iris, trabecular meshwork, and the lens-zonule interface. In addition, on retroillumination there are transillumination defects visible in the iris where light shines through areas that have lost their pigmented epithelium.

**Risk Factors.** Pigment dispersion syndrome is most commonly seen in Caucasians; it is rare in other races.[60] It is a disease that is more frequently seen in myopic individuals and is uncommon in patients who are not myopic.[60] It is a disease that occurs earlier in life than most glaucomas, being most common in persons between the ages of 20 and 40 years.[60] Men and women appear to have equal rates of pigment dispersion, but men are more likely to develop glaucoma and, when they do, to develop glaucoma at a younger age.[60]

**Genetics and Molecular Biology.** Evidence that pigment dispersion syndrome is genetic is limited to studies of a few extended pedigrees in which it appears to be inherited as an autosomal dominant disorder.[61,62] Most cases of pigment dispersion appear to be isolated. Three autosomal dominant pigment dispersion pedigrees were used to map a locus on chromosome 7q35-q36.[62] A single pedigree yielded a maximum 2-point lod score of 5.72 at a recombination fraction of zero.[62] A second locus was recently reported to map to chromosome 18q11-q21 with a maximum lod score of 3.3 (theta = 0) in a single pedigree.[61]

**Treatment.** Pigmentary glaucoma is treated like POAG. There is some theoretical advantage to using cholinergic agonists because of their ability to reverse the iris backbowing and to stop the dispersion of pigment.[63] Laser trabeculoplasty also works well because the marked trabecular pigmentation absorbs the laser energy well.[64] More recently, laser iridotomies have been performed in selected patients to eliminate the iris backbowing and to prevent the iris pigment from being abraded.[65]

## Exfoliative Glaucoma

Exfoliative glaucoma (also called pseudoexfoliative or glaucoma capsulare) is a common form of secondary glaucoma in which a fibrillar material is deposited throughout the anterior segment of the eye, as well as in tissues throughout the body. Elevated intraocular pressure results from physical blockage of the trabecular meshwork and damage to trabecular endothelial cells.

**Clinical Phenotype.** Exfoliation is a disease of the elderly. These patients are typically older than patients with POAG. They have somewhat more marked elevation of the intraocular pressure and that may be more difficult to control. Exfoliative glaucoma is frequently unilateral or markedly asymmetrical.

**Diagnosis.** In exfoliation syndrome, there is a deposition of fibrillar material throughout the anterior segment of the eye. This is deposited as a ground-glass-appearing coating on the anterior lens capsule. The chaffing of the iris against the lens causes the material to be worn off in the zone of iris-lens touch, creating a bull's-eye pattern on the anterior lens capsule. The material that is rubbed free can appear as flaky debris at the pupillary margin. The pigment epithelium of the iris is rubbed away near the pupil and creates transillumination defects in the iris. In the iridocorneal angle, the trabecular meshwork is heavily pigmented. The exfoliative material is found throughout the body, although it appears to cause pathology in the eye alone.[66,67]

**Risk Factors.** Exfoliation syndrome is most common among the elderly.[68] It clusters in populations but is found to some degree in most populations. It is the most common cause of glaucoma in Scandinavian countries.[69] It is not seen in Eskimos but is found in up to 38 percent of Navajo Indians.[70,71] Women are more likely to develop exfoliative glaucoma than men, but this may in part be due to an increased life span.[72]

**Genetics.** Gifford described a father and son with exfoliative glaucoma.[73] No large pedigrees have been reported. There are some pedigrees that contain members with both exfoliative and POAG.[74] This observation, coupled with the variation in disease prevalence among different populations, is consistent with a role for genetic factors in the pathogenesis of this disease.

**Treatment.** Exfoliative glaucoma is treated in the same way as POAG. It is more likely to be poorly controlled by medical means and require surgical intervention. Laser trabeculoplasty can be quite effective in patients with exfoliation syndrome.[75]

## Steroid-Induced Glaucoma

It is well-established that many eyes will mount an ocular hypertensive response to corticosteroids.[76,77] The response can be low, intermediate, or high,

**Clinical Phenotype.** Elevated intraocular pressure is found weeks to months after initiation of corticosteroid therapy. The response is greatest when the corticosteroids are administered topically or injected into the tissues surrounding the eye. There is also some elevation in intraocular pressure noted with oral, dermatological, and inhaled corticosteroids. The elevated intraocular pressure is not associated with any visible structural change in the eye.

**Diagnosis.** Careful follow-up is critical in patients placed on chronic corticosteroids. The intraocular pressure rise generally takes a few weeks to occur, but can be seen at any time from a few days to many months following the initiation of therapy.

**Risk Factors.** Patients with primary open-angle glaucoma[77] and their relatives[78] are at high risk of demonstrating an elevated intraocular pressure when treated with corticosteroids.

**Genetics.** Based on steroid challenges to families, Becker and Armaly suggested that corticosteroid responsiveness was inherited through a single recessive gene.[78,79] Other authors have questioned the single-gene theory.[80-82]

**Treatment.** When possible, the corticosteroids are discontinued or reduced. If the corticosteroids cannot be reduced, then the patient is treated like a patient with primary open-angle glaucoma.

## CLOSED-ANGLE GLAUCOMAS

Closed-angle glaucomas are characterized by the presence of iris over the trabecular meshwork, which impedes aqueous humor outflow. Gonioscopy reveals the iris as displaced forward obscuring the meshwork. Angle closure can develop suddenly, and when it does, it causes a very dramatic clinical picture characterized by elevation of intraocular pressure to very high levels (60mm Hg and above), nausea, vomiting, headache, and severe eye pain. Angle closure can also develop intermittently or chronically with a gradual adherence of the iris to the trabecular meshwork and permanent closure of the trabecular meshwork.

### Primary Pupillary Block

Primary pupillary block is a special form of closed-angle glaucoma that appears to develop without a precipitating cause. There is abnormal contact between the iris and the lens at the pupil. Aqueous humor becomes trapped behind the iris and drives the iris forward, over the trabecular meshwork (Fig. 242-5).

**Diagnosis.** The diagnosis of closed-angle glaucoma is made based by gonioscopic examination of the iridocorneal angle.

**Risk Factors.** Angle-closure glaucoma typically develops in elderly patients whose lenses are usually thicker than those of younger patients. It is also much more common among patients who have a hyperopic (farsighted) refractive error. Hyperopic eyes are smaller than normal, and all of the structures are more tightly packed, leading to contact between the iris and the anterior lens capsule.

**Genetics.** Prevalence rates of angle-closure glaucoma vary dramatically among different populations.[83] For example, the incidence in Caucasians over the age of 40 is reported to be less than 0.2 percent,[84-86] whereas the frequency in Eskimos is reported to be 20 to 40 times higher.[87-90] The incidence among Asians is also reported to be several fold higher than in Caucasians[91,92] Although population frequency differences could be due to environmental factors, genetic differences are likely to play a role. The chief factor is reported to be the structure of the anterior chamber of the eye with those at risk for angle-closure

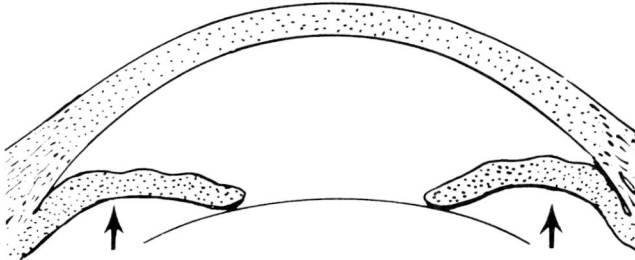

**Fig. 242-5. Mechanism of angle closure due to pupillary block. A relative seal forms between the iris and lens trapping aqueous humor behind the iris and driving the iris forward onto the trabecular meshwork. The angle formed by the iris and cornea closes. Compare this to the open angle in Fig. 242-1. (*From Alward, WLM. Color Atlas of Gonioscopy, St. Louis, CV Mosby, 1994. Used with permission.*)**

glaucoma having shallower anterior chamber depths (see Congdon et al.[83] for review). Factors determining the anterior chamber depth and axial eye length are likely to be genetic.[93,94] There are no reported genetic loci involved in angle-closure glaucoma, nor are there loci reported to control anterior chamber depth.

**Treatment.** The treatment of primary pupillary block angle closure is to create a new pathway for the posterior chamber fluid to flow into the anterior chamber by creating a laser opening through the iris, which is called an iridotomy, that interrupts the pupillary block.[95] If a patient has narrow angles without glaucoma or is diagnosed early in the course of angle closure, laser treatment is curative. Ideally, patients at risk for angle closure will be diagnosed by gonioscopy prior to having an acute attack and before any loss of vision. If a patient has long-standing disease, there may be adherence of the iris to the trabecular meshwork or chronic damage to the trabecular meshwork such that the intraocular pressure remains elevated. These patients are treated with medications; if medical therapy failed, they would undergo trabeculectomy.

## DEVELOPMENTAL GLAUCOMAS

An anatomic abnormality in the iridocorneal angle at birth ultimately leads to decreased aqueous outflow and increased intraocular pressure resulting in glaucoma. Developmental glaucomas can occur as an isolated entity with no other ocular abnormalities, in which case it is called primary congenital glaucoma (PCG). Glaucoma can also be associated with a host of ocular and systemic defects. Infants and children—like adults—can also develop secondary glaucomas from inflammation, neovascularization, aphakia, and other processes.

### Primary Congenital Glaucoma

In patients with PCG, the iridocorneal angle does not fully develop and has an immature or fetal appearance on gonioscopy. The iris has an anterior insertion into the trabecular meshwork and the beams of the trabecular meshwork are thickened.[96]

**Diagnosis.** PCG is usually diagnosed in the first few months of life. Eighty percent of cases are diagnosed by 1 year of age. The parents generally note that the child is very light-sensitive with resultant blepharospasm and tearing. Pressure-induced clouding of the normally clear cornea diffracts light and makes the eyes very sensitive to any bright environment. In addition, the parents may note that the child's eyes are larger than normal. This is especially obvious in unilateral cases.

On examination, the patients have large eyes with large corneas. The corneas have Haab's striae, which are cracks through Descemet's membrane. On gonioscopy, the iridocorneal angle is immature and poorly developed. The patients are typically myopic due to the long axial eye length. As in all glaucomas, the optic nerve demonstrates cupping. In children, unlike adults, there is potential for marked reversal of optic nerve head cupping once the intraocular pressure is normalized. The intraocular pressure is elevated; however, intraocular pressure is difficult to measure in young patients.

**Genetics and Molecular Biology.** Congenital glaucoma is an uncommon disease, affecting about 1 in 10,000 live births.[97] Although some cases of PCG are sporadic, evidence indicates that many cases are genetic. An autosomal recessive mode of inheritance has been clearly demonstrated in some families.[98-100] Furthermore, an increased incidence of congenital glaucoma in offspring of consanguineous marriages is evident, further supporting an autosomal recessive mode of inheritance.[101] Reports in the literature suggest that PCG is familial in 10 to 40 percent of cases.[97,102-104] This is likely to be an underestimation, particularly in consanguineous families and populations in which inbreeding is common.

Loci involved in congenital glaucoma have been identified by genetic mapping as well as by analysis of individuals with chromosome anomalies and congenital glaucoma. Sarfarazi et al. identified the first congenital glaucoma locus (GLC3A on chromosome 2p21) by using genetic linkage mapping in several families of Turkish ancestry.[105] A second locus (GLC3B), on chromosome 1p21, was identified later.[106] In addition to these genetically mapped loci, several loci have been implicated based on the identification of chromosome anomalies in patients with congenital glaucoma. Loci for which at least two independent cases suggest involvement in congenital glaucoma include chromosome 6p25 (balanced translocation and deletion),[107] 11q (partial deletions of 11q and 11q-syndrome),[108] and chromosome 9p24-9pter (deletions).[109] Several congenital glaucoma-related phenotypes have been reported to map to chromosome 6p25 using genetic linkage analysis in extended pedigrees showing autosomal dominant segregation.[107,110–112]

Recently, Stoilov et al. identified the disease-causing gene in the locus on chromosome 2p21.[113] Candidate genes within the genetic interval were screened and three different truncating mutations were identified in the cytochrome P4501B1 (CYP1B1) gene.[113] Congenital glaucoma cases caused by mutations in the CYP1B1 gene are inherited as an autosomal recessive disorder, and are likely due to loss of function of CYP1B1 activity. Cytochrome p450 enzymes are a large multigene family of mixed function mono-oxidases. The exact mechanism of disease caused by loss of function of CYP1B1 is not known, although it has been speculated that CYP1B1 participates in the metabolism of a yet unidentified biologically active molecule that is important in eye development. Numerous CYP1B1 mutations have now been identified in a variety of different populations, indicating that mutations in this gene are be the most common cause of congenital glaucoma.[113–115]

Recently, Nishimura et al. isolated the chromosomal breakpoints from a congential glaucoma patient with a balanced translocation involving chromosome 6p25 and 13q13.[107] The chromosome 6p25 breakpoint in this patient was near a forkhead transcription factor gene, FKHL7.[107] This gene was shown to be deleted in a second congenital glaucoma patient with a small deletion involving 6p25. These data suggested that FKHL7 is involved in some cases of congenital glaucoma. Further work demonstrated that mutations in the FKHL7 gene can cause congenital glaucoma with associated anterior segment defects.[107] FKHL7 is more fully discussed in the following section.

**Treatment.** PCG is treated surgically. The thickened and compacted trabecular meshwork beams are lysed with a small knife passed across the anterior chamber (goniotomy) or with an instrument that is threaded into Schlemm's canal and rotated to break into the anterior chamber (trabeculotomy).[116] Medical therapy for congenital glaucoma is used to treat patients whose intraocular pressures do not adequately respond to surgical treatment. Topical medical therapy is more dangerous in children than adults because the drop dosage required for a response is typically the same as that for adults, yet with a much smaller blood volume, the risk of systemic toxicity is much greater.

### Axenfeld-Rieger Syndrome

Axenfeld-Rieger syndrome (MIM 601631) is a term that is used to refer to a group of conditions that share many phenotypic features including posterior embryotoxon, Axenfeld anomaly, Rieger anomaly, and Rieger syndrome (MIM 180500). These conditions are also referred to as "anterior segment mesenchymal dysgenesis" (MIM 107250)[117] although the origin of the cells in the anterior chamber appears to be neural crest and not mesenchyme.[118]

**Clinical Phenotype.** On slit-lamp examination, patients typically have an anteriorly displaced Schwalbe's line that allows the anterior border of the trabecular meshwork to be visible through the peripheral cornea. When this is seen, the patient is considered to have posterior embryotoxon. Posterior embryotoxon, while a component of all of the conditions in the Axenfeld-Rieger family of diseases, is by itself a normal variant not associated with glaucoma. If the patient with posterior embryotoxon also has strands of iris connecting the peripheral iris to the posterior embryotoxon, the patient is said to have Axenfeld anomaly. Patients with Axenfeld anomaly and associated hypoplasia of the iris are said to have Rieger anomaly. The changes in the iris can be subtle or very striking, including extra pupils or distorted and displaced pupils. If a patient has the ocular signs of Rieger anomaly and, in addition, has extraocular signs of maxillary hypoplasia, hypertelorism, hypodontia, microdontia, and/or redundant periumbilical skin, the patient is said to have Rieger's syndrome. In Axenfeld's anomaly, Rieger's anomaly, and Rieger's syndrome, glaucoma develops in about 50 percent of cases. The onset may be in infancy, but generally develops somewhat later in life.[119]

**Genetics and Molecular Biology.** Considerable progress has been made toward understanding the molecular genetics of Axenfeld-Rieger syndrome. Rieger recognized that this disorder was transmitted as an autosomal dominant disease with variable expressivity.[120,121] Heterogeneity was suggested by the association of several different cytogenetic abnormalities with this phenotype.[122] The most frequent cytogenetic abnormalities in patients with Rieger syndrome involve chromosome 4, which fact contributed to the initial genetic linkage mapping of this disease to 4q[122] as well as to the subsequent identification of the responsible gene.[123] Locus heterogeneity of Rieger syndrome is supported by the identification of a second Rieger syndrome locus (RIEG2) on chromosome 13q14 by linkage analysis in a single large pedigree.[124] This family had 11 affected patients, 9 of whom reportedly had evidence of glaucoma. Ten of the affected individuals had other systemic abnormalities including dental anomalies, cranial facial dysmorphism, hydrocephalus, cryptorchidism, hearing defects, kidney abnormalities, and congenital heart defects. These patients differ from classic Rieger syndrome in that none were demonstrated to have redundant periumbilical skin. The gene causing RIEG2 has not been identified.

Semina et al.[123] used two translocations at 4q25 in patients with Rieger syndrome to identify the gene (PITX2/RIEG1) causing 4q-linked Rieger syndrome. The PITX2/RIEG1 gene belongs to a new class of homeobox genes. There are four exons, with the first exon consisting of noncoding sequence while the homeobox sequence is encoded by exons 3 and 4. Several disease-causing mutations of PITX2/RIEG1 have been identified in this gene.[123] The gene appears to account for the majority of cases of classic Rieger syndrome with anterior chamber defects of the eye, dental hypoplasia, and umbilical anomalies. Heon et al. demonstrated that the RIEG1 locus is linked to an iris hypoplasia phenotype in a single large pedigree.[125] A mutation in the PITX2/RIEG1 gene has been identified in this family, indicating that this gene can cause iris hypoplasia in the absence of other features of Rieger syndrome.[126]

Another member of the PITX/RIEG homeobox gene family, PITX3, was recently identified and shown to be expressed in the anterior segment of the eye.[127] Mutations in this gene were found in two families with autosomal-dominant cataracts and anterior segment defects, including corneal clouding.[127]

Several congenital glaucoma-related phenotypes transmitted in an autosomal dominant fashion have been shown to map to chromosome 6p25 with genetic linkage studies in extended families. These phenotypes include Rieger anomaly,[111] Axenfeld anomaly,[111] and iridogoniodysgenesis.[128] The families reported to link to chromosome 6p25 do not appear to have the classic systemic features of Rieger syndrome (dental and umbilical anomalies) but have anterior segment defects which overlap those found in Rieger syndrome. Nishimura et al. identified a gene that is mutated in some patients with 6p-linked anterior segment abnormalities by cloning the translocation breakpoint in a patient with congenital glaucoma.[107] Mutations in this forkhead transcription factor gene (*FKHL7*) have been identified in probands and families with a wide range of eye phenotypes, including Rieger anomaly, Axenfeld anomaly, iris hypoplasia, and posterior embryotoxin with and without congenital glaucoma.[107] The mouse homologue of *FKHL7* designated MF1, is expressed abundantly in the developing mouse embryo as well as a number of adult tissues. Homozygous null MF1 mice die at birth with hydrocephalus, eye defects, and multiple skeletal abnormalities.[129] The classic mouse mutant, congenital hydrocephalus, is the result of a frameshift mutation in the mouse homologue of the FKHL7 gene which leads to a protein truncation prior to the DNA-binding domain. The mouse phenotype, as well as reports of human patients with systemic abnormalities associated with anterior chamber defects suggest that human FKHL7 mutations could result in systemic phenotypes including hydrocephalus, deafness, kidney defects and congenital heart defects. Some evidence for congenital heart defects in patients with FKHL7 mutations is accumulating.[107]

**Treatment.** Axenfeld-Rieger syndrome is treated much like PCG if it occurs early in life; if it occurs later in life, it is treated like primary open-angle glaucoma.

## Peters Anomaly

Peters anomaly (MIM 106210) is a very rare condition that is sometimes classified with the Axenfeld-Rieger family of diseases. In Peters anomaly, the central portion of the cornea fails to develop properly. There is no Descemet's membrane and no endothelium. The cornea, therefore, has a central opacity that is the hallmark of Peters anomaly. Roughly 50 percent of patients with Peters anomaly develop glaucoma.[130,131]

One patient with Peters anomaly was found to have a mutation in the PAX6 gene.[132]

## Aniridia

In the majority of patients with aniridia (MIM 106210), there is no visible iris by slit-lamp examination. The name is somewhat of a misnomer in that gonioscopic examination does demonstrate a small stump of iris. Glaucoma develops when this small stump of iris is pulled over the trabecular meshwork by fine adhesions between the iris and the cornea.

**Diagnosis.** There are a number of ocular features of aniridia. The most striking is the apparent lack of iris in most patients. With time, the cornea becomes vascularized and opaque, a condition termed pannus. The lenses frequently develop cataractous changes. The most serious associated ocular finding is hypoplasia of the fovea, which leads to decreased central vision. Nystagmus develops in patients who have very poor vision from early in life. In those patients, there is usually foveal hypoplasia and the prognosis for vision better than 20/200 is poor. Aniridia can also be associated with a host of systemic abnormalities including mental retardation and genitourinary abnormalities. The most important abnormality to recognize in association with aniridia is Wilms tumor, which is seen in patients who have sporadic cases of aniridia.[133]

**Genetics and Molecular Biology.** Aniridia can occur as either an isolated defect or in association with systemic abnormalities. Deletions involving chromosome 11p13 can result in the well-studied contiguous gene syndrome consisting of Wilms' tumor, aniridia, genitourinary abnormalities, and mental retardation (WAGR syndrome).[133,134] The *PAX6* gene, one of a family of paired box transcription factor genes, causes the aniridia component of WAGR syndrome.[135–137] Balanced translocations involving 11p13 can lead to isolated aniridia.[138]

Familial aniridia is an autosomal dominant disease. A locus on chromosome 2p was initially mapped in 1980 and designated AN1.[139] The locus on chromosome 11 was therefore named AN2. More recent evidence indicates that there is probably not an aniridia locus on chromosome 2p.[140] The vast majority of cases of aniridia have been show to be due to mutations in the *PAX6* gene on chromosome 11p. Numerous mutations in the *PAX6* gene have been identified and phenotypes caused by mutations in this gene have been expanded to include Peters anomaly, cataracts with corneal dystrophy (resulting from compound heterozygosity of the *PAX6* gene), foveal hypoplasia, and keratitis.[132,141–143] Mutations in the mouse *pax6* homologue cause an aniridia-like phenotype in the mouse called small eye (sey).[144] Approximately one-third of *PAX6*-related cases of aniridia result from new mutations, the remaining cases result from an inherited mutation in this gene.[137]

**Treatment.** The treatment of aniridia depends on the age at diagnosis. If there is some open angle and the patient is quite young, then goniotomy or trabeculotomy can be employed to reestablish the iridocorneal angle.[145] If the patient is somewhat older, treatment could be undertaken with medical therapy or with the adult-type surgeries of trabeculectomy or seton operations.

## Posterior Polymorphous Corneal Dystrophy

Posterior polymorphous corneal dystrophy (MIM 122000) is an uncommon disorder of the corneal endothelium in which the endothelium takes on epithelial-like characteristics. The abnormal endothelium can grow across the iridocorneal angle and pull the iris up over the angle, leading to a secondary synechial angle closure.

**Clinical Phenotype.** Patients with posterior polymorphous corneal dystrophy have abnormal corneas in which the normally smooth and clear endothelial layer is marred by blisters and lines of epithelial-like cells.

**Diagnosis.** The diagnosis is made by slit-lamp examination of the cornea and the corneal endothelium. On gonioscopy the iridocorneal angle is often closed by bands of iris tissue that have become adherent to the cornea.

**Genetics and Molecular Biology.** Posterior polymorphous corneal dystrophy is an autosomal-dominant disease. A locus for this disorder was shown to map to chromosome 20 in a large pedigree consisting of 21 affected individuals.[146] A related disorder, congenital endothelial corneal dystrophy, was shown to map to the same interval on chromosome 20, suggesting that these disorders may be allelic.[147]

# POPULATION SCREENING AND GENETIC COUNSELING

## Population Screening

Screening for glaucoma has proved difficult. It has been performed using intraocular pressure, optic nerve head examination, and visual field testing. Elevated intraocular pressure is the easiest risk factor to detect, but, unfortunately, has very poor sensitivity and specificity.[148] Up to one-half of glaucoma patients will have normal intraocular pressures at the time of a screening encounter. On the other hand, the vast majority of patients whose pressures are slightly elevated never develop glaucoma. Thus, a screening test based on intraocular pressure has unacceptably low sensitivity and specificity. One can adjust the definition of an abnormal pressure to increase the sensitivity. Unfortunately, however, if the intraocular pressure threshold is lowered to increase the sensitivity of the test, then the specificity becomes extremely low. Conversely, if the pressure level required for a failed screening is made high then the sensitivity is very poor.[148] Optic nerve head screening is hampered because it requires a skilled examiner, or photographic or other imaging technologies that are expensive.[148,149] Visual field testing is expensive, time-consuming, and has a marked learning curve.[148,149] Thus, to date there is no single, good screening test for glaucoma. The hope is that molecular genetics will provide such a screen once the genes that cause the vast majority of glaucomas are known.

When one considers factors that are important in deciding on the utility of population screening for a given genetic disease, population screening for mutations in the GLC1A gene is intriguing. First, glaucoma is an insidious disease that causes no symptoms until late in its course and is difficult even for experienced clinicians to diagnose in its early stages. Second, if untreated, the disorder results in blindness. Third, effective treatment for the disease that can preserve vision in most patients is currently available. Finally, although the GLC1A gene accounts for only a subset of all glaucoma, enough is known about sequence variations in the gene and the predicted phenotype resulting from those mutations, that a sensitive and specific test could be designed.

## Genetic Counseling

Until recently, genetic counseling was seldom offered to patients and families with glaucoma. It is now clear that at least a subset of cases of adult-onset glaucoma is inherited as an autosomal dominant disorder, and nearly all cases of juvenile glaucoma for which there is a family history are caused by mutations in a single gene (GLC1A).[37] Mutation analysis in the CYP1B1 gene in congenital glaucoma patients from a variety of populations indicates that mutations in this gene account for a large portion of congenital glaucoma, and that congenital glaucoma caused by mutations in this gene is inherited as an autosomal recessive disease.[113] Based on the above new information, a careful family history should be taken for all glaucoma patients, and genetic testing should be strongly considered in those with a family history of glaucoma.

Most at-risk individuals should have a thorough eye examination at about age 40. This examination should include intraocular pressure measurements and careful optic nerve head examination, looking for signs of glaucoma. Follow-up examinations should be performed every few years. For individuals with a family history of adult onset glaucoma, repeat examinations should be performed every year. If there is a family history of early onset glaucoma (before age 40), screening examinations should begin earlier in life. In the future, it may be feasible to base the age at which to begin screening examinations on genotypic information, although this is not currently possible. Therefore, the age should be guided by the earliest known age of onset in the family. For patients with a family history of glaucoma and/or known mutations, it is helpful to obtain baseline optic nerve head photographs against which to compare the nerve appearance in future examinations. This permits the earliest possible recognition of change. Baseline and intermittent visual field examinations are also useful in patients at high risk, particularly if the optic nerve head appearance in not completely normal.

## REFERENCES

1. Quigley HA: Number of people with glaucoma worldwide. *Br J Ophthalmol* **80**:389, 1996.
2. Leske MC: The epidemiology of open-angle glaucoma: A review. *Am J Epidemiol* **118**:166, 1983.
3. Armaly MF: Lessons to be learned from the Collaborative Glaucoma Study. *Surv Ophthalmol* **25**:139, 1980.
4. Tielsch JM, Sommer A, Katz J, Royall RM, Quigley HA, Javitt J: Racial variations in the prevalence of primary open-angle glaucoma. *JAMA* **266**:369, 1991.
5. Sommer A: Intraocular pressure and glaucoma [Editorial]. *Am J Ophthalmol* **107**:186, 1989.
6. Kellerman L, Posner A: The value of heredity in the detection and study of glaucoma. *Am J Ophthalmol* **40**:681, 1955.
7. Tielsch JM, Katz J, Sommer A, Quigley HA, Javitt JC: Family history and risk of primary open angle glaucoma — The Baltimore Eye Survey. *Arch Ophthalmol* **112**:69, 1994.
8. Becker B, Kolker AE, Roth FD: Glaucoma family study. *Am J Ophthalmol* **50**:557, 1960.
9. Benedict TWG: *Abhaundlungen zus dem Gebiete der Augenheilkunde.* Breslau: L. Freunde, 1842.
10. von Arlt CG: *Die krankeiten des auges für praktische Ärzte.* Prague, 1853.
11. François J: Genetics and primary open-angle glaucoma. *Am J Ophthalmol* **61**:652, 1966.
12. Jay B, Paterson G: The genetics of simple glaucoma. *Trans Ophthalmol Soc UK* **90**:161, 1970.
13. Paterson G: A nine-year follow-up of studies on first-degree relatives of patients with glaucoma simplex. *Trans Ophthalmol Soc UK* **90**:515, 1970.
14. Teikari JM, Airaksinen PJ, Kaprio J, Koskenvuo M: Primary open-angle glaucoma in 2 monozygotic twin pairs. *Acta Ophthalmol (Copenh)* **65**:607, 1987.
15. Kurten H, Halle S: Ein 81 jahriges, eineiiges zwillings-bruderpaar. *Arch Rassen Gessell Biol* **28**:38, 1934.
16. Westerland KE: *Clinical and Genetic Studies on the Primary Glaucoma Diseases.* Copenhagen: Busck, 1947.
17. Biró I: Notes on the heredity of glaucoma. *Ophthalmologica* **98**:43, 1939.
18. Agarwal LP, Mohan M, Malik SR, Gupta AK: Glaucoma in twins. *All India Ophthalmol Soc* **12**:132, 1964.
19. Glees M, Ried A: Beitrag zur frage der Erblichke it des glaukoms. *Graefes Arch Clin Exp Ophthalmol* **142**:495, 1941.
20. Shikunova RN: Two pairs of twins with hereditary signs of simple open angle glaucoma. *Vestn Oftalmol* **185**:87, 1972.
21. Courtney RH, Hill EH: Hereditary juvenile glaucoma simplex. *JAMA* **97**:1602, 1931.
22. Crombie AL, Cullen JF: Hereditary glaucoma: Occurrence in five generations of an Edinburgh family. *Br J Ophthalmol* **48**:143, 1964.
23. Harris D: The inheritance of glaucoma — A pedigree of familial glaucoma. *Am J Ophthalmol* **60**:91, 1965.
24. Stokes WH: Hereditary primary glaucoma. *Arch Ophthalmol* **24**:885, 1940.
25. Beiguelman B, Prado D: Recessive juvenile glaucoma. *J Genet Hum* **12**:53, 1963.
26. Armaly MF: The genetic determination of ocular pressure in the normal eye. *Arch Ophthalmol* **78**:187, 1967.
27. Armaly MF, Monstavicius BF, Sayegh RE: Ocular pressure and aqueous outflow facility in siblings. *Arch Ophthalmol* **80**:354, 1968.
28. Armaly MF: Genetic determination of cup/disc ratio of the optic nerve. *Arch Ophthalmol* **78**:35, 1967.
29. Bengtsson B: The inheritance and development of cup and disc diameters. *Acta Ophthalmol* **58**:733, 1980.
30. Armaly MF: Inheritance of dexamethasone hypertension and glaucoma. *Arch Ophthalmol* **77**:747, 1967.
31. Sheffield VC, Stone EM, Alward WLM, Drack AV, Johnson AT, Streb LM, Nichols BE: Genetic linkage of familial open angle glaucoma to chromosome 1q21-q31. *Nat Genet* **4**:47, 1993.
32. Richards JE, Lichter PR, Boehnke ML, Uro J, Torrez D, Wong D, Johnson AT: Mapping of a gene for autosomal dominant juvenile-onset primary open-angle glaucoma to chromosome 1q. *Am J Hum Genet* **54**:62, 1994.
33. Wiggs JL, Haines JL, Paglinauan C, Fine A, Sporn C, Lou D: Genetic linkage of autosomal dominant juvenile glaucoma to 1q21-q31 in three affected pedigrees. *Genomics* **21**:299, 1994.
34. Graff C, Urbak SF, Jerndal T, Wadelius C: Confirmation of linkage to 1q21-31 in a Danish autosomal dominant juvenile-onset glaucoma family and evidence of genetic heterogeneity. *Hum Genet* **96**:285, 1995.
35. Morissette J, Côté G, Anctil J-L, Plante M, Amyot M, Héon E, Trope G, Weissenbach J, Raymond V: A common gene for juvenile and adult-onset primary open-angle glaucomas confined to chromosome 1q. *Am J Hum Genet* **56**:1431, 1995.
36. Sunden SLF, Alward WLM, Nichols BE, Rokhlina TR, Nystuen A, Stone EM, Sheffield VC: Fine mapping of the autosomal dominant juvenile open angle glaucoma (GLC1A) region and evaluation of candidate genes. *Genome Res* **6**:862, 1996.
37. Stone EM, Fingert JH, Alward WLM, Nguyen TD, Polansky JR, Sunden SLF, Nishimura D, Clark AF, Nystuen A, Nichols BE, Mackey DA, Ritch R, Kalenak JW, Craven ER, Sheffield VC: Identification of a gene that causes primary open angle glaucoma. *Science* **275**:668, 1997.
38. Stoilova D, Child A, Trifan OC, Crick RP, Coakes RL, Sarfarazi M: Localization of a locus (GLC1B) for adult-onset primary open angle glaucoma to the 2cen-q13 region. *Genomics* **36**:142, 1996.

39. Wirtz MK, Samples JR, Kramer PL, Rust K, Topinka JR, Yount J, Koler RD, Acott TS: Mapping a gene for adult-onset primary open-angle glaucoma to chromosome 3q [see comments]. *Am J Hum Genet* **60**:296, 1997.

40. Trifan OC, Traboulsi EI, Stoilova D, Alozie I, Nguyen R, Raja S, Sarfarazi M: A third locus (GLC1D) for adult-onset primary open-angle glaucoma maps to the 8q23 region. *Am J Ophthalmol* **126**:17, 1998.

41. Sarfarazi M, Child A, Stoilova D, Brice G, Desai T, Trifan OC, Poinoosawmy D, Crick RP: Localization of the fourth locus (GLC1E) for adult-onset primary open-angle glaucoma to the 10p15-p14 region. *Am J Hum Genet* **62**:641, 1998.

42. François J, Heintz-De Bree C: Personal research on the heredity of chronic simple (open-angle) glaucoma. *Am J Ophthalmol* **62**:1067, 1966.

43. John SW, Hagaman JR, MacTaggart TE, Peng L, Smithes O: Intraocular pressure in inbred mouse strains. *Invest Ophthalmol Vis Sci* **38**:249, 1997.

44. Alward WL, Fingert JH, Coote MA, Johnson AT, Lerner SF, Junqua D, Durcan FJ, McCartney PJ, Mackey DA, Sheffield VC, Stone EM: Clinical features associated with mutations in the chromosome 1 open-angle glaucoma gene (GLC1A). *N Engl J Med* **338**:1022, 1998.

45. Morissette J, Clepet C, Moisan S, Dubois S, Winstall E, Vermeeren D, Nguyen TD, Polansky JR, Cote G, Anctil JL, Amyot M, Plante M, Falardeau P, Raymond V: Homozygotes carrying an autosomal dominant TIGR mutation do not manifest glaucoma [Letter]. *Nat Genet* **19**:319, 1998.

46. Fingert JH, Ying L, Swiderski RE, Nystuen AM, Arbour NC, Alward WLM, Sheffield VC, Stone EM: Characterization and comparison of the human and mouse GLC1A glaucoma genes. *Genome Res* **8**:377, 1998.

47. Kubota R, Noda S, Wang Y, Minoshima S, Asakawa S, Kudoh J, Mashima Y, Oguchi Y, Shimizu N: A novel myosin-like protein (myocilin) expressed in the connecting cilium of the photoreceptor: Molecular cloning, tissue expression, and chromosomal mapping. *Genomics* **41**:360, 1997.

48. Spaeth GL, Baez KA: Argon laser trabeculoplasty controls one third of cases of progressive, uncontrolled, open angle glaucoma for 5 years. *Arch Ophthalmol* **110**:491, 1992.

49. Epstein DL, Krug JH, Hertzmark E, Remis LL, Edelstein DJ: A long-term clinical trial of timolol therapy versus no treatment in the management of glaucoma suspects. *Ophthalmology* **96**:1460, 1989.

50. Kass MA, Gordon MO, Hoff MR, Parkinson JM, Allan E K, Hart WH, Becker B: Topical timolol administration reduces the incidence of glaucomatous damage in ocular hypertensive individuals. *Arch Ophthalmol* **107**:1590, 1989.

51. Phelps CD, Corbett JJ: Migraine and low-tension glaucoma. A case-control study. *Invest Ophthalmol Vis Sci* **26**:1105, 1985.

52. Gasser P, Flammer J, Guthauser U, Mahler F: Do vasospasms provoke ocular diseases? *Angiology* **41**:213, 1990.

53. Hayreh SS, Zimmerman MB, Podhajsky P, Alward WLM: Nocturnal arterial hypotension and its role in optic nerve head and ocular ischemic disorders. *Am J Ophthalmol* **117**:603, 1994.

54. Bennett SR, Alward WLM, Folberg R: An autosomal dominant form of low-tension glaucoma. *Am J Ophthalmol* **108**:238, 1989.

55. Levene RZ: Low-tension glaucoma: A critical review and new material. *Surv Ophthalmol* **24**:621, 1980.

56. Collaborative Normal-Tension Glaucoma Study Group: Comparison of glaucomatous progression between untreated patients with normal-tension glaucoma and patients with therapeutically reduced intraocular pressures. *Am J Ophthalmol* **126**:487, 1998.

57. Netland PA, Chaturvedi N, Dreyer EB: Calcium channel blockers in the management of low-tension and open-angle glaucoma. *Am J Ophthalmol* **115**:608, 1993.

58. Campbell DG: Pigmentary dispersion and glaucoma: A new theory. *Arch Ophthalmol* **97**:1667, 1979.

59. Liebmann JM, Tello C, Chew SJ, Cohen H, Ritch R: Prevention of blinking alters iris configuration in pigment dispersion syndrome and in normal eyes. *Ophthalmology* **102**:446, 1995.

60. Farrar SM, Shields MB, Miller KN, Stoup CM: Risk factors for the development and severity of glaucoma in the pigment dispersion syndrome. *Am J Ophthalmol* **108**:223, 1989.

61. Andersen JS, Parrish R, Greenfield D, DelBono EA, Haines JL, Wiggs JL: A second locus for the pigment dispersion syndrome and pigmentary glaucoma maps to 18q11-q21. *Am J Hum Genet* **63**:A279, 1998.

62. Andersen JS, Pralea AM, DelBono EA, Haines JL, Gorin MB, Schuman JS, Mattox CG, Wiggs JL: A gene responsible for the pigment dispersion syndrome maps to chromosome 7q35-q36 [see comments]. *Arch Ophthalmol* **115**:384, 1997.

63. Haynes WL, Johnson AT, Alward WLM: Inhibition of exercise-induced pigment dispersion in a patient with pigmentary dispersion syndrome. *Am J Ophthalmol* **109**:601, 1990.

64. Lunde MW: Argon laser trabeculoplasty in pigmentary dispersion syndrome with glaucoma. *Am J Ophthalmol* **96**:721, 1983.

65. Karickhoff JR: Pigmentary dispersion syndrome and pigmentary glaucoma: A new mechanism concept, a new treatment, and a new technique [see comments]. *Ophthalmic Surg* **23**:269, 1992.

66. Streeten B, Dark A, Wallace R, Li Z-Y, Hoepner J: Pseudoexfoliative fibrillopathy in the skin of patients with ocular pseudoexfoliation. *Am J Ophthalmol* **110**:490, 1990.

67. Streeten BW, Li Z-Y, Wallace RN, Eagle RC, Keshgegian AA: Pseudoexfoliative fibrillopathy in visceral organs of a patient with pseudoexfoliation syndrome. *Arch Ophthalmol* **110**:1757, 1992.

68. Aasved H: Mass screening for fibrillopathia epitheliocapsularis, so-called senile exfoliation or pseudoexfoliation of the anterior lens capsule. *Acta Ophthalmol* **49**:334, 1971.

69. Ringvold A, Blika S, Elsas T, Guldahl J, Brevik T, Hesstvedt P, Hoff K, Hoisen H, Kjorsvik S, Rossvold I: The middle-Norway eye-screening study. II. Prevalence of simple and capsular glaucoma. *Acta Ophthalmol (Copenh)* **69**:273, 1991.

70. Faulkner HW: Pseudo-exfoliation of the lens among the Navajo Indians. *Am J Ophthalmol* **72**:206, 1971.

71. Forsius H: Prevalence of pseudoexfoliation of the lens in Finns, Lapps, Icelanders, Eskimos, and Russians. *Trans Ophthalmol Soc U K* **99**:296, 1979.

72. Kozart DM, Yanoff M: Intraocular pressure status in 100 consecutive patients with exfoliation syndrome. *Ophthalmology* **89**:214, 1982.

73. Gifford H Jr: A clinical and pathologic study of exfoliation of the lens capsule. *From the Department of Ophthalmology, College of Medicine, University of Nebraska Presented at the 93rd annual meeting of the American Ophthalmology Society*, Hot Springs, Virginia, June 1957. 508, 1958.

74. Jerndal T, Svedbergh B: Goniodysgenesis in exfoliation glaucoma. *Adv Ophthalmol* **35**:45, 1978.

75. Logan P, Burke E, Joyce PD, Eustace P: Laser trabeculoplasty in the pseudo-exfoliation syndrome. *Trans Ophthalmol Soc UK* **103**:586, 1983.

76. Becker B, Mills DW: Corticosteroids and intraocular pressure. *Arch Ophthalmol* **70**:500, 1963.

77. Armaly MF: Effects of corticosterids on intraocular pressure and fluid dynamics. II. The effects of dexamethasone in the glaucomatous eye. *Arch Ophthalmol* **70**:492, 1963.

78. Armaly M: The heritable nature of dexamethasone-induced ocular hypertension. *Arch Ophthalmol* **75**:32, 1966.

79. Becker B, Hahn KA: Topical corticosteroids and heredity in primary open-angle glaucoma. *Am J Ophthalmol* **57**:543, 1964.

80. François J: Corticosteroid glaucoma. *Ann Ophthalmol* **9**:1075, 1977.

81. François J, Heintz-De Bree C, Tripathi RC: The cortisone test and the heredity of primary open-angle glaucoma. *Am J Ophthalmol* **62**:844, 1966.

82. Schwartz JT, Reuling FH, Feinleibm M, Garrison RJ, Collie DJ: Twin heritability study of the corticosteroid response. *Trans Am Acad Ophthalmol Otolaryngol* **77**:126, 1973.

83. Congdon N, Wang F, Tielsch JM: Issues in the epidemiology and population-based screening of primary angle-closure glaucoma. *Surv Ophthalmol* **36**:411, 1992.

84. Bankes JL, Perkins ES, Tsolakis S, Wright JE: Bedford glaucoma survey. *BMJ* **1**:791, 1968.

85. Bengtsson B: The prevalence of glaucoma. *Br J Ophthalmol* **65**:46, 1981.

86. Hollows FC, Graham PA: Intra-ocular pressure, glaucoma, and glaucoma suspects in a defined population. *Br J Ophthalmol* **50**:570, 1966.

87. Alsbirk PH: Primary angle-closure glaucoma: Oculometry, epidemiology, and genetics in a high-risk population. *Acta Ophthalmol* **54**:5, 1976.

88. Cox JE: Angle closure among the Alaskan Eskimos. *Glaucoma* **6**:135, 1984.

89. Drance SM: Angle closure among Canadian Eskimos. *Arctic Ophthalmol Forum* **8**:252, 1973.

90. Van Rens GHMB, Arkell SS, Charlton W, Doesburg W: Primary angle closure glaucoma among Alaskan Eskimos. *Doc Ophthalmol* **70**:265, 1988.

91. Lim ASM: Primary angle closure glaucoma in Singapore. *Aust J Ophthalmol* **7**:23, 1979.

92. Hung PT: Aetiology and mechanism of primary angle closure glaucoma. *Asian Pac J Ophthalmol* **2**:82, 1990.

93. Tomlinson A, Leighton DA: Ocular dimensions in the heredity of angle-closure glaucoma. *Br J Ophthalmol* **57**:475, 1973.

94. Lowe R: Primary angle-closure glaucoma family histories and anterior chamber depths. *Br J Ophthalmol* **48**:191, 1964.

95. Perkins ES: Laser iridotomy. *BMJ* **2**:580, 1970.

96. Broughton WL, Fine BS, Zimmerman LE: Congenital glaucoma associated with a chromosomal defect—a histologic study. *Arch Ophthalmol* **99**:481, 1981.

97. DeLuise VP, Anderson DR: Primary infantile glaucoma (congenital glaucoma). *Surv Ophthalmol* **28**:1, 1983.

98. Gencik A, Genciková A, Gerinec A: Genetic heterogeneity of congenital glaucoma. *Clin Genet* **17**:241, 1980.

99. Genciková A, Gencik A: Congenital glaucoma in gypsies from Slovakia. *Hum Genet* **32**:270, 1982.

100. Hafez M, Moustafa EE, Mokpel TH, Settein S, El-Serogy H: Evidence of HLA-linked susceptibility gene(s) in primary congenital glaucoma. *Dis Markers* **8**:191, 1990.

101. Turacli ME, Aktan SG, Sayli BS, Akarsu N: Therapeutical and genetical aspects of congenital glaucomas. *Int Ophthalmol* **16**:359, 1992.

102. Bonaïti C, Demenais F, Briard M-L, Feingold J: Consanguinity in multifactorial inheritance: Application to data on congenital glaucoma. *Hum Hered* **28**:361, 1978.

103. Demenais F, Bonaiti C, Briard M-L, Feingold J, Frézal J: Congenital glaucoma: Genetic models. *Hum Genet* **46**:305, 1979.

104. Demenais F: Further analysis of familial transmission of congenital glaucoma. *Am J Hum Genet* **35**:1156, 1983.

105. Sarfarazi M, Akarsu AN, Hossain A, Turacli ME, Aktan SG, Barsoum-Homsy M, Chevrette L, Sayli BS: Assignment of a locus (GLC3A) for primary congenital glaucoma (buphthalmos) to 2p21 and evidence of genetic heterogeneity. *Genomics* **30**:171, 1995.

106. Akarsu AN, Turacli ME, Aktan SG, Barsoum-Homsy M, Chevrette L, Sayli BS, Sarfarazi M: A second locus (GLC3B) for primary congenital glaucoma (Buphthalmos) maps to the 1p36 region. *Hum Mol Genet* **5**:1199, 1996.

107. Nishimura DY, Swiderski RE, Alward WL, Searby CC, Patil SR, Bennet SR, Kanis AB, Gastier JM, Stone EM, Sheffield VC: The forkhead transcription factor gene FKHL7 is responsible for glaucoma phenotypes which map to 6p25. *Nat Genet* **19**:140, 1998.

108. Ishida Y, Watanabe N, Ishihara Y, Matsuda H: The 11q syndrome with mosaic partial deletion of 11q. *Acta Paediatr Jpn* **34**:592, 1992.

109. Verbraak FD, Pogany K, Pilon JW, Mooy CM, de France HF, Hennekam RC, Bleeker-Wagemakers EM: Congenital glaucoma in a child with partial 1q duplication and 9p deletion. *Ophthalmic Paediatr Genet* **13**:165, 1992.

110. Walter MA, Mirzayans F, Mears AJ, Hickey K, Pearce WG: Autosomal-dominant iridogoniodysgenesis and Axenfeld-Rieger syndrome are genetically distinct. *Ophthalmology* **103**:1907, 1996.

111. Gould DB, Mears AJ, Pearce WG, Walter MA: Autosomal dominant Axenfeld-Rieger anomaly maps to 6p25 [Letter]. *Am J Hum Genet* **61**:765, 1997.

112. Jordan T, Ebenezer N, Manners R, McGill J, Bhattacharya S: Familial glaucoma iridogoniodysplasia maps to a 6p25 region implicated in primary glaucoma and iridogoniodysgenesis anomaly. *Am J Hum Genet* **61**:882, 1997.

113. Stoilov I, Akarsu AN, Sarfarazi M: Identification of three different truncating mutations in cytochrome P4501B1 (CYP1B1) as the principal cause of primary congenital glaucoma (Buphthalmos) in families linked to the GLC3A locus on chromosome 2p21. *Hum Mol Genet* **6**:641, 1997.

114. Stoilov I, Akarsu AN, Alozie I, Child A, Barsoum-Homsy M, Turacli ME, Or M, Lewis RA, Ozdemir N, Brice G, Aktan SG, Chevrette L, Coca-Prados M, Sarfarazi M: Sequence analysis and homology modeling suggest that primary congenital glaucoma on 2p21 results from mutations disrupting either the hinge region or the conserved core structures of cytochrome P4501B1. *Am J Hum Genet* **62**:573, 1998.

115. Bejjani BA, Lewis RA, Tomey KF, Anderson KL, Dueker DK, Jabak M, Astle WF, Otterud B, Leppert M, Lupski JR: Mutations in CYP1B1, the gene for cytochrome P4501B1, are the predominant cause of primary congenital glaucoma in Saudi Arabia. *Am J Hum Genet* **62**:325, 1998.

116. Anderson DR: Trabeculotomy compared to goniotomy for glaucoma in children. *Ophthalmology* **90**:805, 1983.

117. Ferrell RE, Hittner HM, Kretzer FL, Antoszyk JH: Anterior segment mesenchymal dysgenesis: Probable linkage to the MNS blood group on chromosome 4. *Am J Hum Genet* **34**:245, 1982.

118. Shields MB: Axenfeld-Rieger syndrome: a theory of mechanism and distinctions from the iridocorneal endothelial syndrome. *Trans Am Ophthalmol Soc* **81**:736, 1983.

119. Shields MB, Buckley E, Klintworth GK, Thresher R: Axenfeld-Rieger syndrome. A spectrum of developmental disorders. *Surv Ophthalmol* **29**:387, 1985.

120. Rieger H: Erbfragen in der augenheilkunde. *Graefes Arch Clin Exp Ophthalmol* **143**:277, 1941.

121. Rieger H: Dysgenesis mesodermalis corneae et iridis. *Z Augenheilk* **86**:333, 1935.

122. Murray JC, Bennett SR, Kwitek AE, Small KW, Schinzel A, Alward WLM, Weber JL, Bell GI, Buetow KH: Linkage of Rieger syndrome to the region of the epidermal growth factor gene on chromosome 4. *Nat Genet* **2**:46, 1992.

123. Semina EV, Reiter R, Leysens NJ, Alward WLM, Small KW, Datson NA, Siegel-Bartelt J, Bierke-Nelson D, Bitoun P, Zabel BU, Carey JC, Murray JC: Cloning and characterization of a novel biocide-related homeobox transcription factor gene, RGS, involved in Rieger syndrome. *Nat Genet* **14**:392, 1996.

124. Phillips JC, del Bono EA, Haines JL, Pralea AM, Cohen JS, Greff LJ, Wiggs JL: A second locus for Rieger syndrome maps to chromosome 13q14. *Am J Hum Genet* **59**:613, 1996.

125. Heon E, Sheth B, Kalenak J, Sunden S, Streb L, Taylor C, Alward W, Sheffield V, Stone E: Linkage of autosomal dominant iris hypoplasia to the region of the Rieger syndrome locus (4q25). *Hum Mol Genet* **4**:1435, 1995.

126. Alward WLM, Semina EV, Kalenak JW, Heon E, Sheth BP, Stone EM, Murray JC: Autosomal dominant iris hypoplasia is caused by a mutation in the Rieger syndrome (RIEG/PITX2) gene. *Am J Ophthalmol* **125**:98, 1998.

127. Semina EV, Ferrell RE, Mintz-Hittner HA, Bitoun P, Alward WL, Reiter RS, Funkhauser C, Daack-Hirsch S, Murray JC: A novel homeobox gene PITX3 is mutated in families with autosomal-dominant cataracts and ASMD. *Nat Genet* **19**:167, 1998.

128. Mears AJ, Mirzayans F, Gould DB, Pearce WG, Walter MA: Autosomal dominant iridogoniodysgenesis anomaly maps to 6p25. *Am J Hum Genet* **59**:1321, 1996.

129. Kume T, Deng KY, Winfrey V, Gould DB, Walter MA, Hogan BL: The forkhead/winged helix gene Mf1 is disrupted in the pleiotropic mouse mutation congenital hydrocephalus. *Cell* **93**:985, 1998.

130. Waring GOd, Bourne WM, Edelhauser HF, Kenyon KR: The corneal endothelium. Normal and pathologic structure and function. *Ophthalmology* **89**:531, 1982.

131. Kenyon KR: Mesenchymal dysgenesis in Peter's anomaly, sclerocornea and congenital endothelial dystrophy. *Exp Eye Res* **21**:125, 1975.

132. Hanson IM, Fletcher JM, Jordan T, Brown A, Taylor D, Adams RJ, Punnett HH, van Heyningen V: Mutations at the PAX6 locus are found in heterogeneous anterior segment malformations including Peters' anomaly. *Nat Genet* **6**:168, 1994.

133. Miller RW, Fraumeni JF, Manning MD: Association of Wilms' tumor with aniridia, hemihypertrophy, and other congenital malformations. *N Engl J Med* **270**:922, 1964.

134. Riccardi VM, Sujansky E, Smith AC, Francke U: Chromosomal imbalance in the Aniridia-Wilms' tumor association: 11p interstitial deletion. *Pediatrics* **61**:604, 1978.

135. Ton CCT, Hirvonen H, Miwa H, Weil MM, Monaghan P, Jordan T, van Heyningen V, Hastie ND, Meijers-Heijboer H, Drechsler M, Brigitte R-P, Collins F, Anand S, Strong LC, Saunders GF: Positional cloning and characterization of a paired box- and homeobox-containing gene from the aniridia region. *Cell* **67**:1059, 1991.

136. Hanson IM, Seawright A, Hardman K, Hodgson S, Zaletayev D, Fekete G, van Heyningen V: PAX6 mutations in aniridia. *Hum Mol Genet* **7**:915, 1993.

137. Hanson I, Van Heyningen V: Pax6: More than meets the eye. *Trends Genet* **11**:268, 1995.

138. Simola KO, Knuutila S, Kaitila I, Pirkola A, Pohja P: Familial aniridia and translocation t(4;11)(q22;p13) without Wilms' tumor. *Hum Genet* **63**:158, 1983.

139. Ferrell RE, Chakravarti A, Hittner HM, Riccardi VM: Autosomal dominant aniridia: Probable linkage to acid phosphatase-1 locus on chromosome 2. *Proc Natl Acad Sci U S A* **77**:1580, 1980.

140. Lyons LA, Martha A, Mintz-Hittner HA, Saunders GF, Ferrell RE: Resolution of the two loci for autosomal dominant aniridia, AN1 and AN2, to a single locus on chromosome 11p13. *Genomics* **13**:925, 1992.

141. Mirzayans F, Pearce WG, MacDonald IM, Walter MA: Mutation of the PAX6 gene in patients with autosomal dominant keratitis. *Am J Hum Genet* **57**:539, 1995.

142. Azuma N, Nishina S, Yanagisawa H, Okuyama T, Yamada M: PAX6 missense mutation in isolated foveal hypoplasia [Letter]. *Nat Genet* **13**:141, 1996.

143. Prosser J, van Heyningen V: PAX6 mutations reviewed. *Hum Mutat* **11**:93, 1998.

144. Ton CCT, Miwa H, Saunders GF: Small eye (Sey): Cloning and characterization of the murine homolog of the human aniridia gene. *Genomics* **13**:251, 1992.

145. Walton DS: Aniridic glaucoma: The results of gonio-surgery to prevent and treat this problem. *Trans Am Ophthalmol Soc* **84**:59, 1986.

146. Heon E, Mathers WD, Alward WLM, Weisenthal R, Sunden S, Fishbaugh J, Taylor C, Krachmer J, Sheffield VC, Stone EM: Linkage of posterior polymorphous corneal dystrophy to 20q11. *Hum Mol Genet* **4**:485, 1995.

147. Toma NM, Ebenezer ND, Inglehearn CF, Plant C, Ficker LA, Bhattacharya SS: Linkage of congenital hereditary endothelial dystrophy to chromosome 20. *Hum Mol Genet* **4**:2395, 1995.

148. Tielsch JM: Screening for glaucoma: a continuing dilemma, in Ball SF, Franklin RM (eds): *Transactions of the New Orleans Academy of Ophthalmology*. Amsterdam: Keigler, 1993, pp 1–11.

149. Quigley HA: Current and future approaches to glaucoma screening. *J Glaucoma* **7**:210, 1998.

150. Lichter PR, Richards JE, Downs CA, Stringham HM, Boehnke M, Farley FA: Cosegregation of open-angle glaucoma and the nail-patella syndrome. *Am J Ophthalmol* **124**:506, 1997.

151. Edwards MJ, Challinor CJ, Colley PW, Roberts J, Partington MW, Hollway GE, Kozman HM, Mulley JC: Clinical and linkage study of a large family with simple ectopia lentis linked to FBN1. *Am J Med Genet* **53**:65, 1994.

152. Streiff EB, Straub W, Golay L: Les manifestations oculaires du syndrome de Lowe. *Ophthalmologica* **135**:632, 1958.

153. Attree O, Olivos IM, Okabe I, Bailey LC, Nelson DL, Lewis RA, McInnes RR, Nussbaum RL: The Lowe's oculocerebrorenal syndrome gene encodes a protein highly homologous to inositol polyphosphate-5-phosphatase. *Nature* **358**:239, 1992.

154. Kainulainen K, Pulkkinen L, Savolainen A, Kaitila I, Peltonen L: Location on chromosome 15 of the gene defect causing Marfan syndrome. *N Engl J Med* **323**:935, 1990.

155. Haefliger IO, Flammer J: Fluctuation of the differential light threshold at the border of absolute scotomas — Comparison between glaucomatous visual field defects and blind spots. *Ophthalmology* **98**:1529, 1991.

156. Barker D, Wright E, Nguyen K, Cannon L, Fain P, Goldgar D, Bishop DT, Carey J, Baty B, Kivlin J, et al.: Gene for von Recklinghausen neurofibromatosis is in the pericentromeric region of chromosome 17. *Science* **236**:1100, 1987.

157. Gutmann DH, Collins FS: The neurofibromatosis type 1 gene and its protein product, neurofibromin. *Neuron* **10**:335, 1993.

158. Johnson AT, Alward WLM, Sheffield VC, Stone EM: Genetics and glaucoma, in Ritch R, Shields MB, Krupin T, (eds): *The Glaucomas*. St. Louis, CV Mosby, 1996, pp 39–54.

# Inherited Macular Dystrophies and Susceptibility to Degeneration

*Richard Alan Lewis* ▪ *Rando Allikmets* ▪ *James R. Lupski*

1. **The genes for four different inherited macular dystrophies were recently identified. These include Best vitelliform dystrophy, Doyne honeycomb retinal dystrophy (also known as malattia leventinese), Sorsby macular dystrophy, and Stargardt disease. The first three are autosomal dominant clinical disorders; Stargardt macular dystrophy is an autosomal recessive trait.**
2. **The gene for Best disease, *VMD2*, encodes bestrophin which is a tetraspan transmembrane protein of unknown function. Both the Doyne (*EFEMP1*) and Sorsby (*TIMP-3*) genes encode extracellular matrix proteins. The Stargardt macular dystrophy gene, *ABCR*, encodes an ATP-binding cassette transporter that appears to transport retinaldehyde or a derivative across the rim of the photoreceptor disc membrane, possibly out of the rod outer segment disc to the cytosol of the rod photoreceptor. Each of the four genes is expressed in the retina; *VMD2* is expressed specially in RPE and *ABCR* expressed exclusively in the photoreptor cells.**
3. **Mutations of *VMD2*, *EFEMP1*, and *TIMP3* are associated with their respective macular dystrophies. However, homozygous and compound heterozygous mutations of *ABCR* are associated with a plethora of retinal phenotypes including: Fundus Flavimaculatus, Stargardt disease, combined cone-rod dystrophy, and retinitis pigmentosa (RP19). Some heterozygous *ABCR* mutations may be associated with a multifactorial disorder, Age-Related Maculopathy.**

The human eye is an extraordinarily complex organ comprised of numerous tissues derived from all three embryologic layers. Thus, it is not surprising that the eye is a common site of manifestations of genetic disease, both single gene and multifactorial disorders. Indeed, a casual search through the major catalogs of hereditary disorders suggests that at least 25 percent of all human disorders either affect the eye primarily or involve ocular structures with distinctive or characteristic manifestations. The eye was the location for the first modern description of an hereditary disorder (colorblindness),[1,2] the target of the first modern textbook of genetics,[3] the source of the first mathematical modeling of an oncogene requiring two mutational events (retinoblastoma),[4] the site of first isolation of a human oncogene (retinoblastoma),[5] and the target of the first prenatal prediction of a cancer phenotype (retinoblastoma).[6]

Modern molecular technology has revolutionized the field of genetic eye research, beginning with the mapping of two different forms of X-linked retinitis pigmentosa in 1984 and 1985.[7,8] The most common genetic eye diseases encountered clinically, and those that have been studied most extensively, are disorders of the retina and RPE, caused by defects in the structure or function of the photoreceptors or the RPE itself. For simplicity, retinal dystrophies have been classified into two types, those that primarily or initially affect the peripheral vision, such as retinitis pigmentosa (RP), and those that primarily affect central vision, the macular area. (In this chapter, the macular area means the zone of the retina visible with an ophthalmoscope between the major temporal vascular arcades extending from the optic disc, or roughly a circular region centered on the point of fixation extending to the edge of the optic nerve, vertically to the arcades, and roughly an equal distance temporally. This corresponds approximately to the central 15 to 20 degrees of visual field. The fovea, or the central 5 to 7 degrees of visual field, is approximately the same size as the optic disc and is definable by a fine elliptical light reflection (long axis horizontal) surrounding the point of central fixation.) Central retinal dystrophies can be divided into those that primarily affect the fovea or macula, termed "macular dystrophies," and those that may start centrally and progress peripherally, such as combined cone-and-rod dystrophies. Macular dystrophies characteristically affect central visual acuity early in life, and peripheral vision is retained substantially longer and often indefinitely.

In the United States, at least 50 percent of all forms of diminished central vision are inherited.[9,10] Several genetic disorders appear to affect the eye almost exclusively and foveal function most of all. For this chapter, we have selected a few single-gene disorders that appear at relatively young ages, whose genes have been cloned, and whose dysfunctions provide models for Age-Related Maculopathy (ARM), another later onset disorder.

To maintain consistency in nomenclature and compatibility of this discussion within the broader field of postnatal genetically determined defects, we have adhered to narrow definitions of two

A list of standard abbreviations is located immediately preceding the index in each volume. Additional abbreviations used in this chapter include: *ABCR*, ABCR = ATP-binding cassette transporter retina-specific gene and protein; AMD = age-related macular degeneration; ARM = Age-Related Maculopathy; BMD = Best macular dystrophy; DHRD = Doyne honeycomb retinal dystrophy; *EFEMP1*, EFEMP1 = EGF (epidermal growth factor)-containing fibrillin-like extracellular matrix protein 1 gene and protein; EOG = electro-oculogram; ERG = electroretinogram; FF = Fundus Flavimaculatus; RmP = rim protein; RP = retinitis pigmentosa; RPE = retinal pigment epithelium; SFD = Sorsby fundus dystrophy; STGD = Stargardt macular dystrophy; STR = short-tandem repeat; *TIMP3* = tissue inhibitor of metalloproteinases-3; *VMD2* = vitelliform macular dystrophy gene.

differing concepts, "dystrophy" and "degeneration." "Dystrophy" derives from two Greek words, dys- ($\delta\upsilon\sigma$-), a prefix whose meaning is opposite to that of eu- ($\varepsilon\upsilon$-, meaning "well"), that is, of "un-" or "mis-," and in the combined form, dys- implies "bad" or "unlucky," thus, either destroying the good sense of the word to which it is attached or increasing its bad sense; and trophé ($\tau\rho\omega\phi\eta$), meaning "nourishment," "food," "maintenance," or "nurture." Thus, the concept of dystrophy suggests defective nutrition, a primary, bilateral, genetic disorder with distinct histopathologic and clinicopathologic features. Historically, the term dystrophy has applied to genetically determined or hereditary, localized inborn errors of metabolism, that are bilateral and symmetric in paired organs, and classically axial, with reference to ophthalmic disorders, involving vision early, and typically avascular with slow progression.[11-13] Dystrophies thus appear in specific cells in otherwise normal tissues, and, by expansion, imply a genetic determination such that all cells manufacturing the abnormal gene product ultimately express variant morphology or function.

By contrast, the term "degeneration" originates from Latin and derives ultimately from "de-" meaning "down" or "from," and "genus, generis," the "race," "stock," or "kind". Degeneration, therefore, represents a deterioration, a sinking from a higher to a lower level or type, worsening its (previously normal) physical qualities. Degenerations may be either monocular or binocular but are necessarily a secondary phenomenon, resulting from prior insult in otherwise mature tissues. Consequently, degenerations are secondary to age, trauma, inflammation, or some other alteration or degradation of initially normal tissues. They may be unilateral but, if bilateral, are asymmetric, classically peripheral, or eccentric, tend to involve vision later in life, and frequently are associated with vascularization.[13] Distinctively, affections related to aging are usually not considered dystrophies, presumably because in the past, no one expected the occurrence of preprogrammed changes in genetic expression later in life. We avoid the application of the term dystrophy to the aging process by itself, unless there is a clear association with a genetically determined, bilateral, and symmetric event.[14,15] Ultimately, of course, these concepts may merge, except for the intrinsic vascularization, because there are single-gene models for poliosis in young adults, premature cataracts in Werner syndrome, and "macular degeneration" in individuals with mutations in the peripherin gene.[16]

This chapter focuses on the clinical manifestations and molecular genetics of four inherited macular dystrophies (Table 243-1): Best vitelliform dystrophy, Doyne honeycomb retinal dystrophy, Sorsby fundus dystrophy, and Stargardt macular dystrophy; and the multifactorial disorder Age-Related Maculopathy (ARM) (Fig. 243-1).

**Table 243-1 Clinical Manifestations of Inherited Macular Dystrophies**

| | Clinical | ERG | EOG | Fluorescein angiography |
|---|---|---|---|---|
| Best | egg yolk cyst | nml | abn | — |
| Doyne | radial drusen honeycomb | ns | ns | window defects |
| Sorsby | central retinal lesion chorioretinal atrophy (night vision impairment) | — | — | — |
| Stargardt | yellow pisciform flecks ns = nonspecific | ns | ns | • dark choroid • "bulls-eye maculopathy" |

Key: nml = normal; abn = abnormal; ns = nonspecific

# BEST VITELLIFORM DYSTROPHY (MIM 153700)

## Alternative Names

Best disease, central exudative detachment of the retina, hereditary macular (pseudo-) cysts, and vitelliform (vitelliruptive, vitelline) macular degeneration.

## Minimal Diagnostic Criteria

Best vitelliform macular dystrophy is an autosomal dominant dystrophy of the retinal pigment epithelium, characterized by a distinctive, if not pathognomonic, "egg yolk cyst" in the foveal area, which must be present in at least one member of the family under investigation. It is associated with the concurrence of a normal ERG (electroretinogram) and an abnormal light peak/dark trough ratio on an EOG (electro-oculogram).

## History

In 1905, Best published observations of a family of 59 individuals, 8 of whom had a "congenital" macular dystrophy, equally affecting males and females.[17] He described "foveal changes which consisted of red, round, sharply defined foci that closely resembled the cicatrix of central chorioretinitis." Several plates from his manuscript clearly show different stages of the disease, including the classic vitelliform lesion, a shallow secondary macular detachment with pseudohypopyon, and a disciform scar in the fovea. (A pseudohypopyon occurs when the yellow lipofuscin-like material stored in the "egg yolk" breaks forward into the subretinal space and settles inferiorly, like the keel of a boat.) A similar family was described by Falls in 1949 and amplified in 1969, in which 10 individuals were affected over 4 successive generations and in which the youngest (age 3 years) identifiable person demonstrated a circular foveal lesion.[18] All families with this disease in its various manifestations are compatible with an autosomal dominant mode of transmission, many of which have clear evidence of male-to-male transmission.

## Genetics and Demographics

Best vitelliform dystrophy is an autosomal dominant trait with wide phenotypic variability in expression of the ophthalmoscopic lesions, both in the fovea and in the extrafoveal retina. However, in families in which the abnormally low EOG light peak/dark trough ratio is a distinguishing marker, all members of the family bearing the gene can be identified by electrophysiologic testing when they are old enough to cooperate. The frequency of Best vitelliform dystrophy is unknown. Best's family was of German origin, and most reported families arise from Western Europe, Scandinavia, and the United States; it has been noted in many other populations.

## Natural History and Visual Function

Children at risk for this disorder are born typically with the appearance of normal fundi. Although the characteristic ophthalmoscopic pathology with an intact "egg yolk" in the fovea is rarely present in the first several years of life, it begins to evolve between the ages of 4 and 10 years[19] (Fig. 243-1A). Schoolage and teenage children, as well as adults, may complain of blurred vision, uncorrectable poor central acuity, or metamorphopsia, depending on the evolution of their retinal pathology. More than three-fourths of patients retain visual acuity equal or better than 20/40 in at least one eye, despite what may occasionally be dramatic ophthalmoscopic changes in the fovea. However, some older individuals may demonstrate loss of visual acuity over time and develop complex atrophic and disciform lesions in the fovea which results in loss of visual acuity to less than 20/70 and as poor as 20/400.[20,21]

## Ophthalmoscopy

Numerous classifications of the appearance and staging of the foveal pathology have been published.[18,22,23] Each of these is as yet imperfect and incomplete, because they typically do not

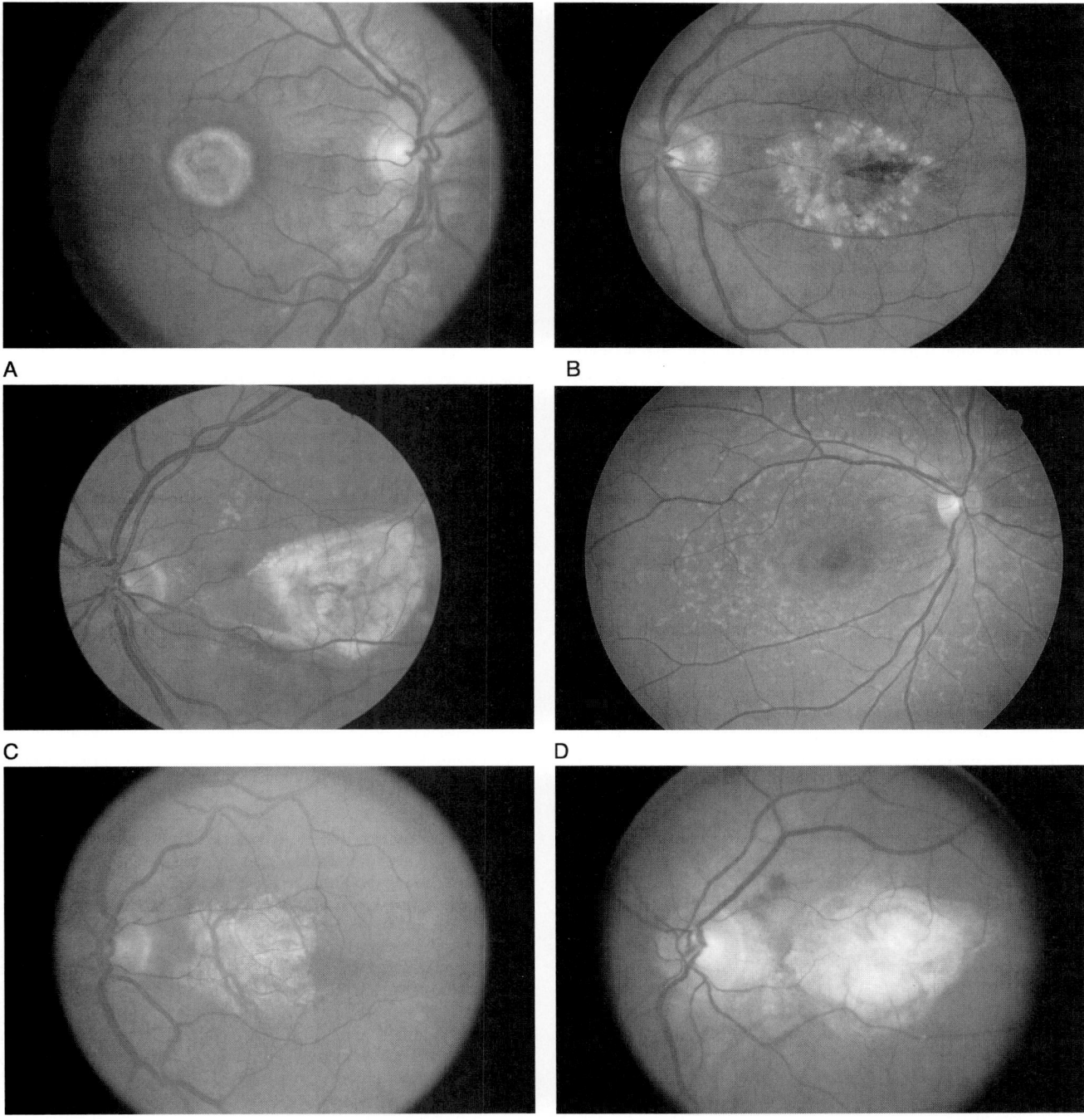

**Fig. 243-1 Clinical manifestations of macular dystrophy and degeneration. *A*, Best disease.** The right macula of a 12-year-old boy with a typical "egg yolk" accumulation. Corrected visual acuity is 20/30. Note the normal optic disc, retinal vasculature, and surrounding pigment epithelium. ***B*, Doyne honeycomb dystrophy.** The left macula of a 45-year-old woman of Swiss-German ancestry who first noted visual distortion at age 27 years. Corrected visual acuity is 20/100. Note the densely packed drusen-like bodies centrally with associated pigment disruption, surrounded by tiny drusen in a radial array. ***C*, Sorsby fundus dystrophy.** The left macula of a 39-year-old engineer with end-stage disciform macular scarring that began at age 36 years. Two sisters, his mother, and his maternal grandmother each developed disciform macular degeneration before age 40 years. ***D*, Stargardt disease/Fundus Flavimaculatus.** The right fundus of a 17-year-old female with slowly progressive loss of central vision over 4 years, now 20/100 in each eye. Note the slight temporal pallor of the optic disc, the fine, sandy atrophy of the pigment epithelium in the fovea, and a myriad of flecks, some circular, some coalescent in short chains inside and just outside the major vascular arcade. ***E*, Age-Related Maculopathy.** Geography atrophy: The left macula of a 68-year-old shows a sharply marginated thinning of the retinal pigment epithelium, enhancing visualization of the large choroidal vessels and the deeper sclera. ***F*, Age-Related Maculopathy.** Disciform degeneration: The left macula of a 72-year-old with a healed white "fibrous" central scar in the shape of a "disc" under the retina. See Color Plate 21.

account for both the central and peripheral changes that may occur in any one individual, and because they are not predictive. In most infants and young children, the macula is normal at birth, although some individuals are described as having foveal hypoplasia as

judged by the absence of a normal neuroepithelial light reflex (foveal light reflex). This may be identical with the "carrier state", rarely described in older adults who demonstrate the genetic potential to transmit the disease to their offspring, but who themselves have no visible vitelliform ophthalmoscopic pathology and yet have an abnormal light peak/dark trough ratio on EOG.

The earliest visible pathology, sometimes termed the previtelliform stage, shows a subtle yellow fine pigment disturbance often with a "speckled" appearance in the pigment epithelium under the central fovea. Rarely, a subtle blocking defect and occasionally a window defect on fluorescein angiography may be present at this time.[19]

By the second half of the first decade of life, and occasionally later, a yellow-orange "cyst" evolves, simulating an intact egg yolk, centered in and under the umbo, and involving up to 1 disc diameter in size of the RPE. Although usually bilateral and symmetric, asymmetries in both extent and size have been documented. This vitelliform cyst may occasionally remain intact into middle age with little disturbance in visual function, and most of these patients retain visual acuity better than 20/50 in the involved eye.[20]

This intact vitelliform cyst may then atrophy and flatten, giving the appearance of a "scrambled egg," often with slight to moderate reduction in visual acuity. It may also be associated with a secondary retinal detachment and layering of the yellow material as a pseudohypopyon in front of the RPE and behind the serous detachment of the sensory retina. This lipofuscin-like yellow material will change orientation with head position and is compatible with good visual acuity. In the evolution of the pseudo-hypopyon stage, various events may transpire. Reabsorption of the yellow material may leave an indistinct area of pigment epithelium atrophy, occasionally as large as several disc diameters, yellow to orange in color, with visibility of the choroidal vasculature. Alternatively, a subretinal neovascular membrane may invade the defective pigment epithelium even in the first decade of life, and ultimately evolve to a fibrous white disciform scar. Remarkably, many individuals with these disciform lesions retain paradoxically good visual acuity, sometimes in the 20/30 to 20/50 range. Finally, central foveal pigment epithelial and choroidal atrophy, resembling geographic atrophy of the RPE or central areolar choroidal sclerosis, may occur in middle-aged and older individuals. Subretinal and subpigment epithelial hemorrhage with reactive hypertrophic pigment proliferation may intervene at any of these stages.[24]

Some patients manifest extrafoveal vitelliform lesions varying in size from large drusen to a disc-diameter in size eccentric to the fovea, singly or multiply, unilaterally or bilaterally. Rarely, pseudohypopyons and eccentric disciform scars may occur in these extrafoveal lesions as well. Occasionally, the retinal phenotype does not appear.[25]

Because of the wide variability in phenotypic manifestation, a clinician must be constantly cognizant of the natural history of the disease and the disparity between fundus appearance and visual function. The physician must examine, or arrange to have examined, other family members at risk for different stages of the disease. When "atypical" or unusual manifestations occur in an older individual of a family, the retinal findings in the younger family member, especially the typical vitelliform formation, will permit a precise diagnosis.

## Associated Ocular Features

Characteristically, patients with Best vitelliform dystrophy are hypermetropic (farsighted), with no other expected ocular anomalies. Because of the hypermetropia, both accommodative and partially accommodative esotropia and other forms of strabismus have been documented, including anisometropic amblyopia. Rarely, exudative macular detachment has been reported. Nonocular events do not occur.

## Diagnostic Procedures

The standard range of psychophysiologic and electrophysiologic studies are normal, except EOG and fluorescein angiography. The majority of patients have normal color perception, dark adaptation, and visual fields (except for central scotomata).

The electroretinogram when performed by standard techniques is usually normal. However, there is a definite and consistent change in the EOG. Indeed, the disparity between the presence of a normal ERG and a distinctly abnormal light peak/dark trough ratio (Arden ratio) on electro-oculography is a defining diagnostic criterion for this disorder. Only butterfly pigment epithelial dystrophy of the fovea shares this disparity of a normal ERG with pathologic alteration in the EOG.[22] When the lipofuscin-like material is present, either in an intact vitelliform foveal cyst or an extrafoveal vitelliform or drusen-like lesion, blocked fluorescence is expected on a fluorescein angiogram; no late leakage into these cysts is seen. However, if the cyst evolves into a pseudohypopyon, or if there is partial reabsorption of the lipofuscin or other pigment epithelial atrophy, then transmission or window defects may occur where the lipofuscin is missing and the pigment epithelium disrupted or atrophic. In the presence of a subretinal neovascular membrane in an evolving disciform lesion, fluorescein angiography will also define the limits of the subretinal neovascularization.

# DOYNE HONEYCOMB RETINAL DYSTROPHY (MIM 126600)

## Alternate Names

Autosomal dominant radial macular drusen, dominant radial macular drusen, hyaline tapeto-retinal degeneration (honeycomb/colloid degeneration), Holthouse-Batten-Tay macular degeneration, Malattia Leventinese.

## Minimal Diagnostic Criteria

Doyne honeycomb retinal dystrophy (DHRD) is the eponym for a group of hereditary ocular disorders characterized by the appearance of ophthalmoscopically distinct lesions in the fovea and macula beginning in the second half of the first decade of life into the second decade of life. A diffuse "granite-like" appearance with small- to medium-sized, highly uniform drusen in the foveal area, sometimes with smaller lesions with radial and linear distribution outside the fovea cluster centrally, and additional lesions are localized near the edge of the optic nerve, both temporally and nasally.

## History

Although various forms of this disorder were described as early as 1875 by Hutchinson and Tay, the best description of this macular and peripapillary disorder was presented by Klainguti in 1932 in his summary to the Swiss Ophthalmological Society of three family trees and three isolated cases with a distinctive tapetoretinal dystrophy.[26,27] Variously called retinitis circinata and subsequently retinitis airolensis (from the name of the village Airolo), and finally malattia leventinese, this disorder is most frequently found among individuals who live in the Leventine Valley or who have ancestral origin in the Tessin Canton of Switzerland, extending southward into northern Italy. Some individuals were reported by Vogt as early as 1925 and in multiple studies thereafter between 1940 and 1955.[28] Many families emigrated from this area to France and England, thus creating independent descriptions of a highly symmetric foveal disease.

## Genetics and Demographics

DHRD is an autosomal dominant trait with wide phenotypic variability in expression of the ophthalmoscopic lesions, both in the fovea and the extrafoveal retina. However, most families can be traced to origins in the Leventine Valley in central southern Switzerland and northern Italy. The genetic locus for this disorder has been assigned to chromosome 2p16.[29,30] The frequency of DHRD is unknown. Although the historically important family was Swiss, families of German, English, Belgian, and North American ancestry have been reported.

## Natural History and Visual Function

The phenotype of DHRD begins with "fine" and "hard" drusen in the central and nasal fovea in the last half of the second decade of life. Most individuals with the disease develop extensive radial, macular, and peripapillary drusen, and subsequent pigment epithelial atrophy, pigment migration, and visual loss during the fourth and fifth decades of life.[30,31] Some individuals may develop an "abortive" form, in which large subretinal drusen occur adjacent to the optic disc without central macular and radial drusen. These individuals seldom have visual impairment.

## Ophthalmoscopy

Varying descriptions of the retinal pathology have been characterized by different authors, depending on access to individual families and the age at first examination. In the earliest stages, small, fine, punctiform white, well-demarcated, drusen-like bodies cluster in the macular region and sometimes around the optic disc. The fine small nature of these lesions is slightly reminiscent of fundus albipunctatus, but there is no pigment proliferation, and visual acuity, visual fields, and night vision are normal.

Toward the age of 30 to 40 years, the drusen become larger and denser in the papillomacular bundle, found around the optic disc and along the major arcades, often arranged irregularly simulating a "honeycomb." The ophthalmoscopic appearance of a gray-white mosaic, often with pigment proliferation localized in the fovea and adjacent to the disc, which results in loss of visual acuity (Fig. 243-1B). In the later stages, atrophy of the RPE and consequent loss of the drusen, with a geographic atrophy in the posterior pole with residual pigment clumps and advanced sclerosis of the choroidal vessels, remains.[28,31,32]

## Diagnostic Procedures

In the early stages, standard psychophysiologic and electrophysiologic studies are normal. Rarely, aberrations in the electroretinogram and the electro-oculogram have been documented, but these are nonspecific and noncharacterizing.

Retinal fluorescein angiography will show window defects corresponding with the drusen, atrophic window defects in the area of geographic atrophy, and blocked fluorescence in the areas of reactive hyperpigmentation. There are no other associated ocular features or anomalies.

## SORSBY FUNDUS DYSTROPHY (MIM 136900)

### Alternative Names

Sorsby pseudoinflammatory macular dystrophy, pseudoinflammatory chorioretinal degeneration of the posterior pole, and hereditary hemorrhagic macular dystrophy.

### Minimal Diagnostic Criteria

Sorsby pseudoinflammatory macular dystrophy is a fundus dystrophy that becomes manifest in the fourth and fifth decades of life, originally associated with "a central retinal lesion showing oedema, haemorrhage, and exudates developing into generalized choroidal atrophy with massive pigment proliferation."[33,34] Although originally described in four (or possibly five) English families, the disorder has been described in several other populations. Often, small drusen-like bodies, sometimes called "colloid bodies," evolve into pigment epithelial atrophy well before the disciform disease begins. In addition, peripheral reticular and pigmentary clumping develops prior to and associated with subretinal neovascularization, both in the macular area and in the retinal periphery.[35,36] Mild deutan color anomalies have been reported in some families; subjective complaints of night vision impairment have been associated with alterations in dark adaptation.[37] The development of both macular and extramacular disciform degeneration, both bilateral and multiple in one eye, is a strong clue (in the absence of other systemic disease) to this diagnosis.

### History

In 1940 and 1949, Sorsby described five families with a fundus dystrophy characterized by dominant inheritance with complete penetrance, loss of central vision from disciform macular degeneration, and progressive atrophy of the peripheral retina and choroid with eccentric disciform disease and pigment clumping and proliferation. Subsequent studies of these same families and similar families documented mild peripheral "albinotic" fundus lesions, extensive hyaline bodies in the RPE varying from punctate yellow to white spots, including those extending around the nasal side of the optic nerve, which may either hypofluoresce or hyperfluoresce in the early stages of fluorescein angiography.[36,38]

### Genetics and Demographics

Sorsby pseudoinflammatory macular dystrophy is an autosomal dominant trait with wide phenotypic varibility in expression and an age-dependent penetrance. The initial lesions appear as drusen or colloid bodies, very small and disseminated throughout the entire posterior pole, and classically symptomless. Typically, in the third and fourth decades of life, subretinal neovacularization in the macular area may evolve into classic disciform scars. Eccentric disciform degeneration is an expected event. No affected individual in families with this disorder escapes visual loss in the fourth decade.

### Ophthalmoscopy

The earliest visible pathology is scattered microdrusen in the foveal area, in an otherwise normal-appearing RPE. Later, exudative macular degeneration and disciform disease evolves toward widespread chorioretinal atrophy, encompassing the macular areas and the retinal periphery (Fig. 243-1C). Much of this simulates disciform macular degeneration associated with drusen in the aging population, but the onset of central visual impairment is typically in the third and fourth decades. A family whose detailed history involves progressive degeneration of the posterior pole transmitted through multiple generations should be considered highly suspect for this disorder. Progressive chorioretinal atrophy, pigment proliferation and migration, and eccentric disciform disease complete the picture.[34,35,38-40]

### Associated Ocular Features

Characteristically, individuals and families with Sorsby pseudoinflammatory macular dystrophy have some complaints about night visual impairment and occasional complaints of color vision distortion, but no other ocular anomalies are expected. Supplemental vitamin A therapy may bolster photoreceptor function and moderate the associated nightblindness.[41]

## STARGARDT MACULAR DYSTROPHY (MIM 248200)

### Alternative Names

Stargardt disease, Fundus Flavimaculatus, juvenile cone dystrophy, and juvenile macular degeneration.

### Minimal Diagnostic Criteria

Stargardt disease (STGD) is an autosomal recessive dystrophy of the central fovea, characterized by a classically juvenile to adolescent onset of a "bull's-eye" maculopathy, reasonably rapid and progressive loss of central vision, color vision, and discriminate fine vision, with mild temporal pallor of the optic nerve. A substantial fraction of patients will develop yellow "flecks" in the RPE in the perifoveal or equatorial retina over two decades after the onset of central visual impairment.

### History

In 1909, Stargardt described seven children in two families with a bilateral progressive macular dystrophy, becoming visually symptomatic between the ages of 8 and 16 years.[42] Since his original description, the age of onset has been lowered to as young age 3 to 4 years, and upward into the fifth and sixth decades.

Independently, in 1962, Francescetti described a similar disorder in family isolates from Switzerland, emphasizing the distribution of yellow flecks and naming the condition Fundus Flavimaculatus (FF).[43] With the introduction of fluorescein angiography, the characteristic "dark choroid" became an additional distinguishing feature of each phenotype from other causes of "cone dystrophies" with bull's-eye-type maculopathy. The confusion as to whether STGD and FF represented independent disorders or the same condition with differential expression was resolved once the disorders were mapped to the same region of human chromosome 1 and after different mutations of the same gene with different ages of onset were defined at a molecular level (see "Clinical Spectrum of *ABCR* Mutations" and reference [94]).

### Genetics and Demographics

Stargardt disease is a bilateral progressive retinal dystrophy that has occurred in almost every population in the world. Moderate variations in the age of onset and the extent of perifoveal and peripheral flecks have influenced the clinical interpretation. Stargardt disease is accepted as a single-gene autosomal recessive disorder, despite considerable intrafamilial and interfamilial heterogeneity in age of onset and retinal manifestations.[44–47]

A few families have been reported with a similar phenotype and a dominant pattern of transmission, but most of these families either do not show the same onset and progression of disease, or they lack the dark choroid.[48–51] Thus, they have been labeled as dominant Stargardt disease, although it would be preferable to retain the eponym solely for the classic pattern of inheritance since Stargardt himself described the recessive form.

### Natural History and Visual Function

A diminution in visual acuity variously described as "haze" or "blur" is usually the symptom that brings patients to medical attention. Visual acuity at presentation may vary from as good as 20/20 to as bad as < 20/200, depending on the age of onset and duration of disease (and thus, patient age). However, progressive deterioration in the first decade of disease is more severe with earlier onset than later onset.[52] Typically, adolescent and adult individuals with Stargardt disease tend to be to two diopters more myopic than the mean spherical equivalent of the normal population.[53] Color-vision testing suggests a mild protan deficiency, but various patterns become progressively more severe as visual acuity deteriorates. In the most advanced cases, severe dyschromatopsia or near achromatopsia is an outcome.[54] Visual field examination reveals a central scotoma; some peripheral field constriction may occur. Considerable confusion has evolved from electrophysiological testing, and numerous articles demonstrate mild to moderate abnormalities particularly in the photopic component of the electroretinogram and a consequent reduction in the light peak/dark trough ratio of the electro-oculogram.[55] However, these procedures are nonspecific and nondiagnostic by themselves. Similarly, dark adaptation final thresholds are elevated frequently.[56] Short-term supplemental vitamin A therapy does not provide objective improvement of dark adaptation, and, based on current pathophysiological models, may be harmful.[57]

### Ophthalmoscopy

Various schemata have been devised to describe the ophthalmoscopic manifestations of this condition. None of them is flawless. In no case is the macular area completely normal. Early in the evolution of the disease, there is a flattening of the foveal light reflex and loss of the umbo with a fine granularity in the retinal pigment epithelium centrally. Fluorescein angiography at this stage may suggest only a faint bull's-eye transmission defect and the more characteristic dark choroid feature. Over time, the pigment epithelial change becomes more dramatic, sometimes described as "beaten metal" or "snail slime," and resembles the granular reflection of oblique sunlight on the side of a salt lick.[46,47]

A wreath of pigment epithelial yellow flecks, long axis circumferential to the fovea, may appear in the posterior pole as the bull's-eye become more apparent. Flecks in the midretinal periphery evolve into a reticular pattern, again with a broad circumferential or wreath-like appearance (Fig. 243-1D). Over time, the individual yellow flecks atrophy at their margins with a granular or cocoa-powder pigment speckling, often times with a brownish discoloration in the center, best viewed by proximal scatter illumination with a contact lens and slit-lamp biomicroscope.[58,59]

Eventually, diffuse geographic atrophy of the fovea, granular depigmentation of the midretinal pigment epithelium, and, in some instances, peculiar metaplastic pigment patches at the level of the pigment epithelium may appear. Occasional cases of dramatic zonal or geographic hyperpigmented metaplasia of the pigment epithelium occur either spontaneously or after minimal blunt trauma.[60–62] Disciform macular degeneration is a rare outcome.[63,64]

### Diagnostic Procedures

As mentioned, electrophysiologic studies are nonspecific and give varying responses. Therefore, they are not useful either to identify or to confirm the diagnosis, because none of the procedures is diagnostic.

The most consistent diagnostic finding occurs in fluorescein angiography, where the absence of choroidal visualization through the nearly normal-appearing pigment epithelium is the hallmark. The central bull's-eye macular atrophy provides a window (transmission) defect, which evolves into a sharply marginated defect as geographic atrophy occurs in the first few decades of the disease.[65]

In the early stages, the pigment epithelial yellow-orange flecks may be invisible or hypofluorescent, but as they atrophy, they also have a marginal halo window defect and a central hypofluorescent-blocking defect. A zone of pigment epithelium between one quarter and one half disc diameter wide surrounding the optic nerve is spared almost invariably. The flecks do not invade the far retina anterior to the equator. The pigment epithelium there may persist in showing the dark choroid, even after extensive atrophy of the posterior pigment epithelium evolves.[46,47,66]

### Associated Ocular Features

The most common "associated" feature is a pigmentary proliferation at the level of the pigment epithelium, different from true retinitis pigmentosa. No other ocular or systemic manifestations occur with Stargardt disease or Fundus Flavimaculatus. However, systemic argyrosis (a cutaneous discoloration caused by silver) has been reported to cause a dark choroid on fluorescein angiography.[67]

## AGE-RELATED MACULOPATHY (ARM) (MIM 603075)

### Alternative Names

Age-Related Macular degeneration (AMD), choroidal neovascularization, drusen, disciform macular degeneration, geographic atrophy of the retinal pigment epithelium, and serous and hemorrhagic detachments of the retinal pigment epithelium.

### Minimal Diagnostic Criteria

Age-Related Maculopathy (ARM) is a degenerative disorder affecting the macula or central visual area and characterized clinically by the appearance of drusen and pigmentary abnormalities in the retinal pigment epithelium and retina in the early stages, followed by either geographic atrophy of the pigment epithelium, or choroidal neovascular membrane, or pigment epithelial detachment, and ultimately fibrous or disciform scarring of the macula in the late stages.

Although numerous schemata for classification have been devised, including an International Classification and Grading

System, none has achieved universal acceptance.[68–70] Drusen, historically called colloid bodies or hyaline bodies, appear in the retinal pigment epithelium as small whitish-yellow dots of varying size, typically after age 50 years. Ophthalmoscopically, they tend to calcify over time, evolve minute pigmentary changes, and may become confluent. Some investigators distinguish between drusen that are large in appearance and uniform on their borders ("hard") or indistinct ("soft") beginning among people who are at least age 50 years and older.[68,71,72] Some ophthalmologists do not consider the presence of indistinct drusen or reticular drusen as clear evidence of early macular degeneration, unless they definitively affect vision.[73–76] As a result, historic prevalence rates and incidence rates of ARM in the population vary widely with whether the reports are clinic-based or population-based and whether single or multiple observers are involved in the description of the individuals studied.[70,77–79]

## Natural History and Visual Function

The later stages of ARM are recognized universally to be associated with moderate to severe loss of vision. Geographic atrophy is considered a "dry" form of late ARM, while serous or hemorrhagic pigment epithelial detachments and choroidal neovascular membranes and disciform scars are classically referred to as "wet" or "exudative" forms of ARM (72, 80).

**Geographic Atrophy.** Geographic atrophy is deemed present when at least 150 to 200 microns of well-demarcated, hypopigmented, atrophic pigment epithelium is present, often with choroidal vessels visible. These zones seem to arise from areas of regressing or atrophic drusen and occasionally after the flattening or spontaneous collapse of a serous (or hemorrhagic) detachment of the retinal pigment epithelium (Fig. 243-1E).

**Choroidal Neovascularization.** Choroidal neovascularization is the ingrowth of new choroidal vessels into the subretinal or subpigment epithelial space through breaks in Bruch's membrane. A definitive segregation between these two can be made classically only on fluorescein angiography, sometimes augmented by indocyanine green angiography.

**Disciform Scar.** The end stage of subretinal neovascularization is a fibrovascular scar that destroys the outer neuroepithelial retina and pigment epithelium, lying between the choroid and retina. Disciform scars vary widely in appearance, color, and extent, depending on their size, the duration and age of the lesion, and the presence and the amount of subretinal blood, exudates, and exudative detachment of the sensory retina with overlying cystoid degeneration (Fig. 243-1F).

## Prevalence

Estimates of prevalence of ARM range significantly between populations and even within the same population. Some of these differences are based on the selected definition(s) of ARM. Age differences, genetic differences, and demographic characteristics of the population may substantially influence individual risk rates to develop ARM.[70,77,79,81–83]

The prevalence of later stages of ARM (both geographic atrophy and disciform disease) increase significantly with age in all populations and studies performed. For example, in the United States, individuals age 75 years and older have a prevalence rate of late ARM of approximately 8 percent.[75,79,80]

## Incidence

Few population-based studies have monitored the appearance of new forms of ARM over time. The best studies in the United States cover the defined population in the Beaver Dam region of Wisconsin and yield a 5-year incidence of the later stages of ARM of about 1 percent (segregated approximately as 0.6 percent of the population for disciform disease in at least one eye, and approximately 0.3 percent of geographic atrophy in at least one eye).[79]

## Genetics

Many epidemiologic surveys support a familial influence on ARM.[73,84–87] Historically, one large case-control study of family records suggested that a positive family history of ARM was the strongest predictor of its reoccurrence, assuming at least one family member (parent or sibling) was affected, when compared to a family in which there was no history of ARM in another family member.[88] Other clinic-based surveys have demonstrated a statistically increased risk of ARM among first-degree relatives (parents and sibs) of individuals over age 40 years with ARM compared to those over age 40 with no ARM.[86]

Several twin studies also confirm a high concordance rate of ARM among monozygotic twins and a lower concordance among dizygotic twins, suggesting genetic predispositions to macular degeneration.[89–93] Recently, identification of the *ABCR* gene as causative of the classic recessive form of Stargardt disease led to an investigation of family relatives for other features of macular degeneration. Retrospective information suggests that at least 20 percent of Stargardt families have parents or grandparents (old enough to be in the risk range) with various forms of ARM.[94]

## Ophthalmoscopy

Geographic atrophy of the retinal pigment epithelium (GARPE) is the advanced form of "dry" or atrophic macular degeneration. It appears to be responsible for about 20 percent of severe loss of central vision and legal blindness, but a much larger percentage of moderate visual impairment among individuals over age 55 years in the United States.

Antecedent to the development of geographic atrophy, drusen of various types, both soft, hard, and calcific, are present and evolve to become so extensive that the macular drusen resorb and atrophy of the pigment epithelium remains. Fluorescein angiography generally shows sharply marginated hyperfluorescence corresponding closely to the area of pigment epithelial thinning in the ophthalmoscopic and photographic examinations.[72,80]

## Disciform Macular Degeneration

Neovascular or disciform macular degeneration occurs when neovascularization arises from the choriocapillaris and breaks through the Bruch's membrane into the subpigment epithelial and subretinal space. The fibrovascular tissue proliferates within and under Bruch's membrane, perhaps elevating it, and ultimately breaks further into the subretinal space. This creates an irregular elevation of the pigment epithelium or a brownish-gray to gray-green discoloration beneath the sensory retina, often associated with subretinal fluid, subretinal or intraretinal blood, and exudate on the margin or within the detachment. The fluorescein angiographic appearance of choroidal neovascularization associated with ARM is considerably variable, as mentioned earlier. Two basic angiographic patterns, classic and occult, have been recognized by various investigators.

Classic subretinal neovascular membranes fluoresce brightly in the early stage of the angiogram, at the time of choroidal and early arterial perfusion, sometimes associated with a well-defined, lacy, or fishnet type of abnormal subretinal capillary vessels, much larger than retinal capillaries. Thus, the boundary or extent of these new vessels can be readily determined in the early phases of the angiogram. Because these neovascular fronds lack tight endothelial junctions, increasing fluorescence and leakage from these vessels evolve in the mid- and late stages of the angiogram, becoming increasingly intense, and thereby blurring the boundary of the neovascular membrane compared to the earlier frames and then leaking into the overlying secondary retinal detachment.

Occult neovascularization occurs in a variety of angiographic situations that do not conform to the classic definition. Some of these may occur in association with "fibrovascular pigment epithelial detachment" or indistinct late phase leakage, in which a neovascular net cannot be identified.

## Therapy

At the moment, there is no known or proposed effective therapy of any sort for the atrophic stage of macular degeneration (GARPE). Various theoretical approaches, including supplemental micronutrients and vitamins, are under clinical trial, but as of this writing, nothing has been proven to be effective or beneficial in slowing or altering the natural history of this manifestation.[95]

For the "wet" type of macular degeneration, various interventions have been explored by major clinical trials. Since the 1970s, laser photocoagulation has been recognized as potentially beneficial in the treatment of some subretinal neovascular membranes. Subsequently, the Macular Photocoagulation Studies defined clinical benefit compared to the natural history of disease for neovascular membranes that were outside the foveal avascular zone, on the margin of the foveal avascular zone, and within the subfoveal space. However, various treatment regimens yielded significant visual impairment directly related to the treatment itself, and therefore, laser treatment is considered for neovascular membranes only when they meet eligibility criteria from these proven studies. Eyes with exudative macular-degeneration not meeting Macular Photocoagulation Studies eligibility criteria should be observed or preferably enrolled in well-designed, prospective, randomized clinical trials evaluating a novel but promising treatment approach compared to accepted treatment protocols and to a comparative natural history cohort.[95]

## MOLECULAR GENETICS OF MACULAR DEGENERATION

Four genes have been identified that when mutated convey a macular dystrophy phenotype (Table 243-2). The gene causing Best disease *VMD2* encodes bestrophin, a tetraspan transmembrane protein of unknown function. Both the Doyne (*EFEMP1*) and Sorsby (*TIMP3*) genes encode extracellular matrix proteins. The function of EFEMP1, the EGF-containing fibrillin-like extracellular matrix protein 1, is unknown, while tissue inhibitor of metalloproteinase-3 (TIMP3) is one of three known proteins that inhibit matrix metalloproteinases. The Stargardt macular dystrophy gene, *ABCR*, encodes an ATP-binding cassette transporter that appears to transport a key chemical component of the visual cycle across the rim of the photoreceptor disc membrane in the outer segments. Each of the four genes is expressed in the retina; *VMD2* specifically expressed in the RPE, and *ABCR* is exclusively expressed in photoreceptors.

### VMD2 (GenBank NM 004183)

The gene for Best vitelliform macular dystrophy (BMD) (MIM 153700) was mapped to 11q13[96] (Table 243-2). This location was confirmed in multiple populations and the genetic interval refined.[97–101] Interestingly, haplotype analysis identified a 37-year-old male who appeared to represent nonpenetrance.[102] Physical mapping identified several genes in the genetic interval.[103] Independently, two groups identified the *VMD2* gene, which is mutated in Best disease.

In one study, meiotic recombination mapping in a single large Swedish pedigree narrowed the Best locus to ≈800 kb. Sequence scanning of shotgun libraries prepared from nine PAC clones detected a high degree of similarity with a retina-specific human cDNA. The gene contained 11 exons and appeared to span at least 16 kb of genomic sequence.[104] The 1755-bp open reading frame predicted a 585-amino-acid protein of 68 kDa with homology to the RFP (Arg-Phe-Pro) protein family. The protein was named bestrophin to acknowledge that mutations within the gene result in Best macular dystrophy.[104]

Five missense amino acid substitutions were identified in bestrophin among six independent families, including both a W93C mutation that segregated with meiotic recombinants in the Swedish family and a Y227N alteration in a Dutch kindred. This latter mutation has also been described elsewhere.[104,105] The *VMD2* gene is expressed selectively in the RPE of the adult mouse and human eye; the only other identified expression was in the Sertoli cells of the mouse testis. Neither the function of bestrophin nor that of any related RFP family members can be inferred from the amino acid sequence. However, based upon the known BMD pathology, including the abnormal accumulation of lipofuscin in RPE cells associated with progressive macular degeneration, Petrukhin et al.[104] suggested that bestrophin may mediate the transport or the metabolism of an essential component of lipofuscin granules. Considering a correlation between the expression pattern of human *VMD2* and its rodent homologue and the tissue distribution of the long chain fatty acid docosahexanoic acid (DHA), bestrophin might be involved in either the transport or the metabolism of polyunsaturated fatty acids in the human retina.[104] Interestingly, the *VMD2* gene overlaps in a tail-to-tail manner with another gene. The *VMD2* gene contains a 174-bp region of antisense sequence complementary to the 3' UTR of the brain-specific form of ferritin heavy-chain mRNA.[104] Oxidative decomposition of polyunsaturated fatty acids in the retina can be catalyzed by ferrous iron,[106] and iron-induced damage to the outer segments results in the accumulation of lipofuscin granules in RPE cells.[107]

In an independent study, a physical map consisting of YAC[108] and PAC[109] contigs in combination with gene identification approaches[103,110] isolated several genes in the candidate interval. Northern blot analysis showed that one of these nine novel genes was expressed exclusively in the RPE as a single 2.4-kb transcript.[105] The corresponding gene, *VMD2*, contained 11 exons in an open reading frame of 1755 bp predicting a 585-amino-acid protein of 67.7 kDa. Ten missense amino acid mutations and 1 amino acid deletion mutation were identified in 12 other families with Best disease, and the alterations cosegregated with the disease.[105]

As mentioned above, the 3' UTR of *VMD2* mRNA contains a region of antisense complementary to the 3' end of the brain-

**Table 243-2** Inherited Macular Dystrophy

| Disease | Inheritance | MIM | Genome location | Gene | Protein |
|---------|-------------|-----|-----------------|------|---------|
| Best | AD | 153700 | 11q13 | VMD2 | bestrophin |
| Doyne | AD | 126600 | 2p16 | EFEMP1 | EGF-containing fibrillin-like extracellular matrix protein 1 |
| Sorsby | AD | 136900 | 22q12.1-q13.2 | TIMP3 | tissue inhibitor of metalloproteinase-3 |
| Stargardt | AR | 248200 | 1q21-p22.1 | ABCR | ABCR or rim protein |

specific form of ferritin mRNA. Ferritin is an iron-storage protein that is important in the prevention of the deleterious oxidation of the ferrous form of iron within cells. The antisense regulation of ferritin and/or bestrophin expression might contribute to the pathogenesis of other forms of macular degeneration.[105]

Mutation analysis of the VMD2 gene in 13 other families segregating Best macular dystrophy identified 7 distinct mutations in 9 families.[111] These included a novel frameshift mutation (1574delCA), the first to be identified in the 3' one-third of the gene, and two missense amino acid substitutions (W93C and R218C) reported previously.[104,105] Three of the seven families in which a VMD2 mutation was confirmed showed a nonpenetrant individual; one of these three families segregated the R28C alteration and two families segregated the E300D mutation.[111] However, in 4 of 13 families no disease-associated alterations were detected.

Similarly, an independent study detected 15 different missense mutations in 19 of 22 families with BMD.[112] In both VMD2 mutation detection studies, the identified missense amino acid substitutions appeared to cluster in certain regions of the protein. Five mutations—G299E, E300D, D301E, F3055, and T3071—lie close to one another, suggesting that this region of the protein may also have an important function.[111,112] This domain might be exposed to the outer surface of the protein because it is highly negatively charged and may be involved in binding a positively charged molecule such as a ligand substrate.[111] All currently identified variants VMD2 are displayed on the VMD2 mutation database Web site (www.uni-wuerzburg.de/human-genetics/vmd2.html).

## EFEMP1 (GenBank NM 004105)

The gene for Doyne honeycomb retinal dystrophy (MIM 126600) was mapped to 2p16[113,114] (Table 243-2). Refined genetic mapping and physical analysis narrowed the region to 3 Mb.[115] A positional candidate approach identified a gene, EFEMP1, in which a single amino acid substitution (R345W) segregated with Malattia Leventinese or DHRD.[116]

Thirty-three families including 131 affected individuals were genotyped with 19 STR markers from the critical interval.[116] Haplotype sharing in 23 Swiss families who were believed for geographic reasons to share a common ancestor revealed a smaller interval. After physical mapping for verification of the genetic map and evaluation of candidate genes, six genes were screened for coding sequence alterations. Three genes were present in retinal cDNA libraries and mapping within the narrowest genetic interval. After genomic structure characterization, these genes were screened in a large cohort of families segregating either Doyne honeycomb retinal dystrophy or Malattia Leventinese. A mutation in the EFEMP1 gene, a C > T transition predicting a R345W missense amino acid substitution, was identified in 161 of the 162 patients tested, while no alteration was found in 477 control unaffected individuals or in 494 unrelated patients with AMD.[116] The one patient from one discordant family was found, on reexamination, to have a phenotype more consistent with AMD. One patient was shown to be homozygous for the R345W mutation; that patient's phenotype was similar to that observed in the heterozygous state, suggesting a true dominant allele.[116] Thus, a single amino acid substitution causes all known cases of DHRD. This may represent a founder effect or potentially a hypermutable base.

The EFEMP1 gene was originally isolated through differential screening of a cDNA library constructed from a patient with Werner syndrome.[117] It was previously mapped to 2p16.[118,119] The gene encoded the protein S1-5, which was found to be over-expressed in senescent fibroblasts and induced by growth arrest of young cells through depletion. The protein belongs to the family of extracellular matrix glycoprotein known as fibrillins and contains multiple EGF (epidermal growth factors) modules. A related family member EFEMP2 was recently mapped to chromosome

11q13,[119] a gene-rich region that also contains the major locus for Bardet-Biedl syndrome, BBS1.[120]

## TIMP3 (GenBank NM 000362)

The gene for Sorsby fundus dystrophy (MIM 136900) was initially mapped to chromosome 22q13[121] (Table 243-2). This same genomic region contained the gene for tissue inhibitor of metalloproteinases-3, TIMP3, which was known to play a pivotal role in remodeling the extracellular matrix. As a positional candidate gene, TIMP3 was screened for mutations in two families segregating Sorsby fundus dystrophy.[122] Two mutations, S181C and W168C, introduce an additional cysteine residue in the C-terminal region of the mature protein.[122]

The tissue inhibitors of metalloproteinases (TIMPs) are a group of zinc-binding endopeptidases involved in the degradation of the extracellular matrix. TIMP3 encodes a 188-amino-acid mature polypeptide with a 23-residue signal peptide.[123,124] The nucleotide sequence and deduced translational product of the TIMP3 cDNA are highly similar to the TIMP1 and TIMP2 gene products, including 12 conserved cysteine residues at the same relative position. TIMP3 is encoded by 5 exons extending over approximately 55 kb of genomic DNA.[125] TIMP3 localizes to the extracellular matrix in both its glycosylated and unglycosylated forms.[126] The NH2-terminal domain is responsible for the metalloproteinase inhibitor activity while the C-terminal domain is important for mediating the specific functions of the molecule.

The finding of the TIMP3 mutation in Sorsby fundus dystrophy focused attention on the metabolism of the extracellular matrix and its control in other macular dystrophies.[122] A comparison of amino acid sequences of TIMP1, 2, and 3 demonstrates 12 conserved cysteine residues at the same relative position that are implicated in the correct protein folding by forming 6 intrachain disulfide bonds.[122] The finding of different mutations resulting in changes to cysteine in two original families with Sorsby fundus dystrophy suggests that intramolecular disulfide bond formation may prevent proper folding of the three-dimensional proteins.[122] Interestingly, two other Sorsby associated TIMP3 mutations, one in a German-Czech family S156C[127] and the other in a Finnish family G166C,[128] resulted in amino acid substitutions to cysteine. Sixteen families with Sorsby have been reported to segregate a S156C mutation,[129,130] of which 15 were from diverse parts of the British Isles.[128]

## ABCR (GenBank NM 000350)

The gene for Stargardt macular dystrophy (MIM 248200) was mapped initially to 1p21-p13 in eight French kindreds.[131] Four additional families with what was deemed a later onset macular dystrophy were shown to link to the same region, thus supporting by genetic analysis the long-held clinical suspicion that these phenotypes represented allelic variants of the same mutant gene.[132]

In a large study of 47 families, mostly North American outbred kindreds, Anderson et al. confirmed linkage of STGD to 1p markers with a lod score of 32.7 and demonstrated the genetic homogeneity of this disorder.[133] Twenty-two disease chromosomes showed informative crossover events between the disease locus and flanking polymorphic markers, thus refining the STGD locus to a 4-cM interval. Haplotype analysis identified four cases of nonpenetrant offspring, each of whom carried two STGD alleles identical with an affected sibling.[133]

Physical analysis with an STS content mapping approach delineated a YAC contig containing STGD-linked markers that spanned approximately 31 cM and completely encompassed the 4-cM critical interval delineated by historic recombinants. This landmark mapping approach yielded a physical map that excluded the positional candidate genes such as RPE65 and the α-subunit of cone transducin.[133] The ABCR gene was mapped to the YAC contig encompassing the genetic (4-cM) critical interval.[134]

The ABC (ATP-binding cassette) superfamily includes genes whose products are transmembrane proteins involved in

**Table 243-3** Inherited Human Disease Associated with Mutations in ABC Transporters

| Disease | MIM | Gene |
| --- | --- | --- |
| Cystic fibrosis; CBAVD | 219700 | Cystic fibrosis transmembrane conductance regulator (CFTR) |
| Adrenoleukodystrophy | 300100 | ALD |
| Persistent hyperinsulinemic hypoglycemia of infancy (PHHI) | 601820 | Sulfonylurea receptor (SUR) |
| Progressive familial intrahepatic cholestasis (PFIC2) | 601847 | Bile salt export pump (BSEP) |
| PFIC3 | 602347 | Multidrug-resistant (MDR3); P-glycoprotein 3 (PGY3) |
| Dubin-Johnson syndrome; hyperbilirubinemia II | 237500 | Canalicular multispecific organic anion transporter (CMOAT;MRP2) |
| HLA class I deficiency | 170260 | Transporter associated with antigen processing (TAP2) |
| STGD1, RP19, arCRD, AMD | 248200 | ABCR |
| Tangier, Familial HDL deficiency | 205400 | ABC1 |
| Pseudoxanthoma elasticum (PXE) | 264800 | ABCC6 |

energy-dependent transport of a wide spectrum of substrates across membranes.[135,136] Many diseases caused by mutations in members of this superfamily result in defects in the transport of specific substrates (Table 243-3).[137–147] ABCR is expressed in the retina and encodes an ATP-binding cassette (ABC) transporter gene, thus making ABCR an excellent positional candidate for STGD. Indeed, both compound heterozygote and homozygote ABCR mutations were identified in STGD patients.[133] A high percentage of missense mutations was observed, implying that most STGD patients have at least one allele that retains partial function.[134]

The ABCR gene includes 50 coding exons that spans a genomic region of approximately 150 kb.[148–150] The open reading frame of 6819 bp encodes a predicted 2273-amino-acid protein of approximately 220 kDa.[134] The ABCR mRNA is specific to the retina and approximately 8 kb in length.[134] The ABCR protein localizes to the disc membrane of the outer segments of the photoreceptors.[151,151a] ABCR is identical to Rim protein.[151–153] Rim protein was initially purified from frog and bovine rod outer segments and shown to be localized to the rims of the disc.[154,155] It comprises approximately 1 to 3 percent of the rod outer segment membrane proteins and binds nucleotides.[156] The estimated mole ratio of ABCR to rhodopsin is approximately 1:120.[151]

**Function of ABCR.** Retinaldehyde (retinal) stimulates ATP hydrolysis by purified and reconstituted ABCR, suggesting that ABCR may transport retinal in an energy-dependent (ATP) manner.[157] All-trans-retinal stimulates the ATPase activity of ABCR, three to fourfold with a half-maximal effect at 10 to 15 μM. Both 11-cis and 13-cis retinal show similar activity; by contrast, among 37 structurally diverse nonretinoid compounds studied, including 9 previously characterized substrates or sensitizers of another ABC transporter P-glycoprotein, only 4 show significant ATPase stimulation when tested at 20 μM.[157] The dose-response curves of these four compounds indicate multiple binding sites or interactions with ABCR. Thus, these data suggest that retinoids, and most likely retinal, are the natural substrate for transport by ABCR in rod outer segments.[157]

The knockout mouse orthologue of ABCR, abcr, has been constructed.[158] Homozygous mice lacking abcr show delayed dark adaptation, increased all-trans-retinal following light exposure, elevated phosphatidylethanolamine (PE) in outer segments, accumulation of the protonated Schiff base complex of all-trans-retinal and PE (N-retinylidene-PE), and deposition of a major lipofuscin fluorophore (N-retinylidene-N-retinylethanolamine or A2-E) in RPE.[158] These data suggest that ABCR functions as an outwardly directed flippase for N-retinylidene-PE.[158] A model for ABCR function, photoreceptor degeneration, and visual loss in the ABCR-mediated diseases has been proposed as a three-step process: (a) protonated N-retinylidene-PE accumulates in the outer segments due to loss of the flippase activity; (b) isomers of A2-E build up in the RPE lysosomes resulting in progressively impaired digestion of phagocytosed photoreceptor outer segments and ultimate dissolution of cellular membranes; and (c) photoreceptors die due to loss of RPE support functions.[158a]

The observations of increasing ATPase activity of reconstituted ABCR in the presence of all-trans-retinal was explained by the flippase model in the following way: The increase in ATPase activity was seen only when ABCR was reconstituted in the presence of PE. Thus, it was suggested that all-trans-retinal reacted with PE to form N-retinylidene-PE, the substrate for the ABCR flippase.[157,158]

**Clinical Spectrum of ABCR Mutations.** Both clinical and genetic studies suggested that Stargardt disease and late-onset FF are part of the same clinical spectrum. Indeed, ABCR mutations were identified in early onset STGD, as well as late onset FF.[94,134,159–162] Late-onset disease appears to correlate with milder mutant ABCR alleles.[94,160] It has been noted that most STGD-associated ABCR mutant alleles were missense mutations[134] and that there is no instance of STGD that had two apparent null alleles, suggesting retention of partial function of at least one mutant allele.[134] Indeed three groups have reported that null alleles at the ABCR locus are associated with a more severe clinical phenotype similar to retinitis pigmentosa.[163–165] In fact, ABCR double-null mutations are responsible for the RP19 locus.[166] A fourth retinal dystrophy phenotype, a severe combined cone-rod dystrophy, has also been associated with specific combinations of ABCR mutant alleles.[164] In fact, ABCR mutations account for 80% of cone-rod dystrophy families in one study.[164a] Some pedigrees segregate both STGD and retinitis pigmentosa,[94,165] or both RP19 and cone-rod dystrophy,[164] depending upon the paired combinations of ABCR mutant alleles in the nuclear families.

A large genotype/phenotype analysis identified ABCR mutations and correlated the age-of-onset of 150 families with STGD. Interestingly, in a pseudodominant STGD family, sibs with

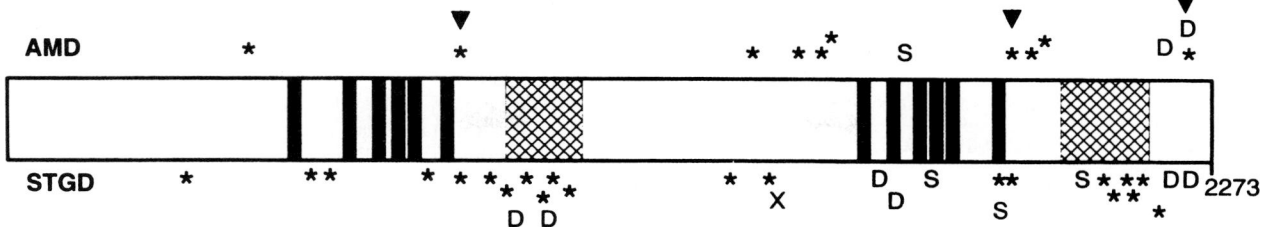

Fig. 243-2 Diagram of the *ABCR* gene with STGD and AMD alterations. Transmembrane domains predicted by hydropathy plot are shown as black bars, and the ATP-binding domains are shown as hatched bars below. Arrows indicate alterations identified in both STGD1 and AMD patients shown mutations; D = deletions; S = splice donor site mutations; X = stop codon-generating mutation. The number at the right signifies the last codon.

identical compound heterozygous mutations were concordant for the half-decade of onset of visual symptoms.[94] These observations suggested that the selected combination of specific *ABCR* mutant alleles determines the age at onset of this disease phenotype.[94] Analysis of 53 families in which both *ABCR* mutant alleles were identified enabled a correlation between the position in the ABCR protein of the combination of mutant alleles and age-of-onset of the disease. These genotype/phenotype correlations suggested that missense amino acid substitutions located in the N-terminal one-third of ABCR seem to be associated with earlier onset of disease and may represent misfolding alleles.[94]

The study of 40 Western European patients with Stargardt disease identified one mutation, 2588G > C, in 15 of 40 (37.5 percent) patients.[161] This mutation shows linkage disequilibrium with a rare polymorphism, 2828G > A, suggesting a founder effect. Interestingly, the 2588 G > C mutation not only causes a substitution of an alanine for glycine at amino acid residue 863 (G863A), but also affects the splicing at the 3′ splice site 3 bp downstream in exon 17.[161] Thus, the resulting mutant ABCR proteins either lack Gly863 or contain the missense mutation G863A. The authors hypothesized that this 2588G > C alteration was a mild mutation that causes STGD only in combination with another severe *ABCR* mutation. This concept was supported by the observation that the accompanying *ABCR* mutations in at least 5 of 8 STGD patients were potentially null (severe) and that a combination of two mild (G863A) mutations was not observed among 68 STGD patients.[161] This linkage disequilibrium has been confirmed independently in a North American population of mostly European descent.[167]

Another striking observation about mutations at the *ABCR* locus was the high frequency of complex alleles, that is, more than one mutation on a single disease chromosome.[94] In 10 (7 percent) of the 150 European-American families, 2 different mutations were identified on a single chromosome, resulting in several different complex alleles.[94] These data emphasize the importance of segregation analysis of all *ABCR* variants in families with STGD.[94] The frequency of *ABCR* complex alleles is similar to that reported with another ABC transporter, the gene *CFTR* responsible for cystic fibrosis.[168]

**ABCR Heterozygous Mutations and Susceptibility to AMD.** Given the several phenotypic similarities between STGD and ARM, including the accumulation of drusen in and under the RPE and the frequent progressive atrophy of the macular RPE, the hypothesis that some ABCR alterations may be associated with AMD was tested.[169] The 50 coding exons of *ABCR* were screened in 167 unrelated AMD patients and 220 racially matched population controls. The cohort consisted of 96 AMD patients from Boston and 71 from Utah. Thirty-three patients (20 percent) had wet AMD and 80 percent had the dry form. Thirteen different AMD-associated alterations in *ABCR* were detected among 26 AMD patients (16 percent).[169] Most were missense mutations, but two changes were deletions representing frameshifts and one was

at a splice donor site.[169] The AMD-associated alterations were scattered throughout the coding sequence of *ABCR*, although more were located toward the 3′ end.[169] Interestingly, most were missense mutations located outside of conserved functional domains such as the ATP-binding cassette regions[169] (Fig. 243-2). Among the Utah and Boston AMD patients, similar fractions of variants in AMD patients were observed (13 of 71 and 13 of 96, respectively). Furthermore, there was a similar distribution of the common mutant alleles G1961E (2 and 4) or D2177N (5 and 2) among the two cohorts. Interestingly, three AMD-associated *ABCR* variants[169] had been identified previously in families with STGD (R1898H, G1961E, 6519del11).[134] Subsequently, four other AMD-associated *ABCR* mutations (E471K, R1129L, 5196+1 G > A, and L1970F) were identified in unrelated STGD families.[94,169] More impressively, 21 percent of 145 STGD families report a positive family history of AMD in the ancestral lineage of direct descent to the STGD-affected sibship.[94]

These findings suggest a model that predicts that some hypomorphic alleles, when present in the heterozygous state, result in phenotypic effects after prolonged periods of malfunction (>65 years). These deleterious consequences result from the cumulative effects of diminished transport of a critically important molecule. The buildup of a potentially toxic byproduct could also further exacerbate the disease. Based on the identification of heterozygous *ABCR* variants in AMD patients compared with controls, it was concluded that some mutations that cause recessive STGD might enhance susceptibility to AMD in the heterozygous state.[169] We have never found more than one AMD-associated variant chromosome in *ABCR* or in any AMD proband, which is consistent with a dominant susceptibility locus.[169] One prediction of this model is that those grandparents in STGD families who are heterozygous for an *ABCR* mutation may be susceptible to AMD. Evidence to support this prediction was published recently.[170,171]

This concept of phenotypic effects for heterozygous mutant alleles of genes responsible for recessive diseases is not novel. In fact, several published examples of susceptibility to multifactorial disease are associated with heterozygous mutations in a gene responsible for a recessive disease phenotype (Table 243-4).[172-178] One example of an association between a monogenic disorder and a multifactorial disease is familial hypercholesterolemia (FH).[172] Homozygotes for mutations in the gene encoding the LDL receptor develop extremely high serum-LDL levels and typically die of myocardial infarction as young adults. Heterozygotes develop moderately high LDL levels and manifest a multifactorial disorder, coronary artery disease, in their fourth or fifth decades.[172] Cystic fibrosis is a common recessive disorder characterized by meconium ileus, pulmonary infection, and pancreatic insufficiency. Heterozygotes for mutation in *CFTR*, possibly the best-studied eukaryotic ABC-transporter gene, show an increased prevalence of chronic pancreatitis.[173,174] Thus, in each of the examples listed in Table 243-4, heterozygous mutations in the causative single gene disease predispose the carrier individuals to

**Table 243-4 Recessive Disorders with Heterozygote Predisposition to Multifactorial Disease**

| Monogenic disease | MIM | Gene | Multifactorial disease |
|---|---|---|---|
| Familial hypercholesterolemia | 143890 | LDLR | Coronary artery disease |
| Cystic fibrosis | 219700 | CFTR | Pancreatic insufficiency |
| Ataxia-telangiectasia | 208900 | ATM | Breast cancer |
| $\alpha_1$-Antitrypsin deficiency | 107400 | AAT | Chronic obstructive lung disease |
| Hyperlipoproteinemia | 238600 | LPL | Ischemic heart disease |
| Stargardt disease | 248200 | ABCR | Age-related macular degeneration |

express a multifactorial trait, whereas homozygous or compound heterozygous mutations in the same gene cause a classically recessive disorder, usually with an earlier onset and more definitive clinical phenotype.

The finding that heterozygous mutations in *ABCR* are associated with AMD created substantial excitement as the first substantive clue to a genetic and biologic causation of AMD, but also some controversy. Initially, two letters questioned the selection of patients and controls, as well as the statistical analysis.[179,180] However, both further studies and additional statistical analysis of the original controls confirmed the initial interpretation.[181]

Three studies have provided additional data on allelic variation of *ABCR* in AMD.[182–184] Each claims to reject an association between alterations in the *ABCR* gene and AMD, but, unfortunately, none of these reports reproduces the original study. Problems with replication are (a) patient selection and (b) efficiency of mutation detection. In all three studies, the patient population was enriched for individuals with the neovascular, or wet, form of AMD. For example, Stone et al. studied a cadre of individuals that purportedly contained 60 percent of patients with wet AMD, while the fraction of all 167 subjects in the original report[169] who had wet AMD was 20 percent and those with dry AMD was 80 percent, closely resembling the proportion of the two forms of AMD in the general population. Thus, their report[182] sustains the initial conclusion that variants of *ABCR* are rare in wet AMD.[169] Similarly, a Japanese study[183] included 87.5 percent of its 80 patients with the wet form of the disease, and an independent American study reported 80 percent of all patients with disciform disease.[184]

To make a statement about the lack of sequence variants in a gene in a cohort of patients, one must assure that the mutation scanning method employed will detect the substantial majority of all sequence changes. Regrettably, this was not true in all these studies.[182–184] For *ABCR*, a valid standard for the efficiency of mutation screening is the fraction of mutations found in STGD patients, because *ABCR* is the gene exclusively responsible for classic recessive STGD.[134] Stone et al. found *ABCR* mutations in a mere 19 percent of STGD chromosomes (82 of 430; Table 2 of reference 182), while two other studies found *ABCR* mutations in 57 percent[94] or 62 percent[162] of STGD chromosomes. Furthermore, Stone et al. did not find any double-mutant chromosomes or complex alleles in their cadre of STGD patients, which have been reported at 7 percent of STGD chromosomes.[94] Thus, the mutation detection rate even for STGD[162,182] is much lower when compared to other laboratories.[94,162] Similarly, in another laboratory, mutation detection was performed on only 20 percent of the coding exons and no noncoding regions.[183] A third group[184] did

not find even the numerous common *ABCR* polymorphisms identified by multiple European and American laboratories,[134,161,182] thus rendering the presented results effectively uninterpretable.

To investigate further the heuristic observation that heterozygous *ABCR* mutations may confer increased risk to AMD,[169] the two most common AMD-associated *ABCR* alterations, G1961E and D2177N, were sought in a large collaborative study among 15 different centers in North America and Europe.[185] These two mutations alone were screened in 1218 unrelated AMD patients of Caucasian origin and 1258 reportedly unaffected unrelated individuals as controls. These two abnormal sequence changes were found in one allele of *ABCR* in 40 AMD patients ($\approx$3.4 percent) and 13 controls ($\approx$0.9 percent); a statistically significant difference ($P < 0.0001$).[185] The results remain significant ($P < 0.0001$) on the independent sample even after exclusion of the data from the previous pilot study.[169] In AMD, the 4 percent frequency of these two mutations alone, G1961E and D2177N ($\approx$4 percent), is a significant fraction in the context of a complex disorder. For comparison, 4 percent is greater than the frequency of all reported myocillin variants (2 to 4 percent) in 1703 glaucoma patients from 5 different populations.[186] Furthermore, the myocillin mutations are heterozygous in a dominant disease, and thus may represent either later onset or variability of expression of the autosomal dominant juvenile-onset open-angle glaucoma.[186]

**A Model for *ABCR* in Retinal Dystrophy and Degeneration.** Based on the findings of homozygous and compound heterozygous mutations of ABCR in STGD, FF, cone-rod dystrophy, RP19, and the finding of heterozygous *ABCR* mutations in AMD, a model of ABCR function has been derived.[94,169,181,187] In this model (Fig. 243-3), the severity of the retinal dystrophy is inversely proportional to the residual ABCR activity. Severe mutations in both *ABCR* alleles result in complete loss of ABCR activity (two null alleles) and cause a retinitis pigmentosa phenotype. Two hypomorphic mutations, or a combination of a hypomorphic mutation with a null allele, can result in FF or STGD. A single, mild, heterozygous *ABCR* mutation acting over a prolonged time

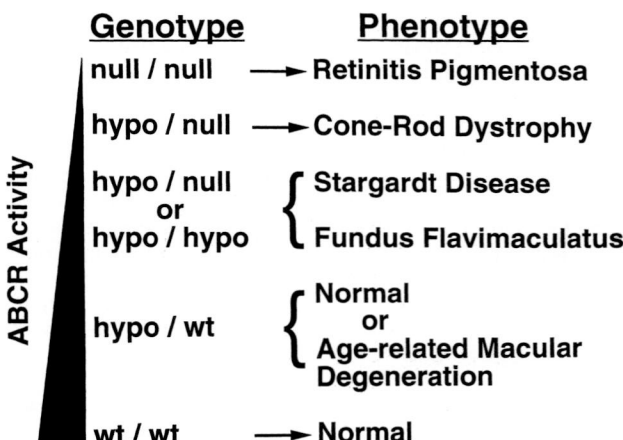

**Fig. 243-3 Phenotypes associated with *ABCR* mutations.** At left, ABCR activity is represented by the filled triangle and depicts decreasing activity towards the top. Genotypes are denoted for both chromosomes. Null denotes mutations that lead to no functional protein products including frameshift, nonsense, and some splice and missense mutations. Hypo denotes hypomorphic alleles including most missense and splice mutations and some C-terminal frameshift and nonsense mutations. WT denotes wild-type or normal alleles. Arrows indicate association between genotypes and phenotypes; the bracket indicates that Stargardt disease and Fundus Flavimaculatus may be caused by either of the indicated genotypes.

may enhance a susceptibility to AMD. This dominant suscept-ibility may result in AMD, if the proper interaction and exposure to environmental influences occur.[187a]

## CONCLUSIONS

Four different genes encoding proteins representing different molecular pathways are responsible for clinically distinct inherited macular dystrophies. Mutations in *VMD2*, *TIMP3* , and *EFEMP1* are responsible for Best, Sorsby, and Doyne diseases respectively. However, sequence variants in these genes have not been shown to occur with the multifactorial disorder age-related macular degeneration.[116,188–190]

The *ABCR* gene has been linked directly to the visual cycle. Its protein product ABCR, a photoreceptor ATP-binding cassette transporter, has been shown to transport retinal or a derivative thereof. Compound heterozygous and homozygous mutations in *ABCR* are responsible for a broad range of retinal dystrophic phenotypes including a late onset disorder FF, an earlier onset STGD, and a severe form of RP. Thus, ABCR is likely to be responsible for a substantial amount of retinal pathology.[94,161,170] The finding that some heterozygous *ABCR* mutations are associated with the multifactorial disorder AMD[134,185] suggests an even more prominent role for *ABCR* in visual impairment. Further therapies for AMD could be directed at improving the transport function of ABCR or at blocking the accumulation of toxic products that result directly from impaired transport by ABCR.[187a]

Recently, an explosion in new information about genes has involved a variety of physiological processes in the human eye and, therefore, the defects in these genes lead to many disease phenotypes. Studies of the *in vivo* function of single genes and their protein products will help to decipher the causes of multifactorial complex phenotypes.

## REFERENCES

1. Hunt DM, Dulai KS, Bowmaker JK, Mollon JD: The chemistry of John Dalton's color blindness. *Science* **267**:984, 1995.
2. Dalton J: The lecture by Dalton was delivered on 31 October 1794. *Mem Man Lit Philos Soc 5:28*, 1798. Reprinted in the *Edinb J Sci* **5**:88, 1831.
3. Waardenburg PJ: *Das menschliche Auge und seine Erbanlagen.* The Hague, Netherlands Martinus Nijhoff, 1932.
4. Knudson AG Jr: Mutation and cancer: Statistical study of retino-blastoma. *Proc Natl Acad Sci U S A* **68**:820, 1971.
5. Friend SH, Bernards R, Rogelj S, Weinberg RA, Rapaport JM, Albert DM, Dryja TP: A human DNA segment with properties of the gene that predisposes to retinoblastoma and osteosarcoma. *Nature* **323**:643, 1986.
6. Cavenee WK, Murphree AL, Shull MM, Benedict WF, Sparks RS, Kock E, Nordenskjold M: Prediction of familial predisposition to retinoblastoma. *N Engl J Med* **314**:1201, 1986.
7. Bhattacharya SS, Wright AF, Clayton JF, Price WH, Phillips CI, McKeown CME, Jay M, et al: Close genetic linkage between X-linked retinitis pigmentosa and a restriction fragment length polymorphism identified by recombinant DNA probe L1.28. *Nature* **309**:253, 1984.
8. Nussbaum RL, Lewis RA, Lesko JG, Ferrell R: Mapping X-linked ophthalmic diseases: II. Linkage relationship of X-linked retinitis pigmentosa to X chromosomal short arm markers. *Hum Genet* **70**:45, 1985.
9. Fraser GR, Friedmann AI: *The Causes of Blindness in Children.* Baltimore, MD, Johns Hopkins University Press, 1967.
10. Jan JE, Freeman RD, Scott EP: *Visual Impairment in Children and Adolescents.* New York, Grune and Stratton, 1977.
11. Duke-Elder SS, Leigh AG: Corneal degenerations, dystrophies and pigmentations, in Duke-Elder SS (ed): *System of Ophthalmology.* London, Henry Kimpton, 1965, p 863.
12. Waring IGO, Rodrigues MM, Laibson PR: Corneal dystrophies. I. Dystrophies of the epithelium, Bowman's layer and stroma. *Surv Ophthalmol* **23**:71, 1978.
13. Duke-Elder SS, Dobree JH: Diseases of the retina, in Duke-Elder SS (ed): *System of Opthalmology.* London, Henry Kimpton, 1967, p 528.
14. Deutman AF: The Hereditary dystrophies of the posterior pole of the eye, in Deutman AF (ed): *Assen, The Netherlands,* Koninklijke Van Gorcum, 1971, 1;16.
15. Warburg M, Møller HU: Dystrophy: A revised definition. *J Med Genet* **26**:769, 1989.
16. Marshall J: The ageing retina: Physiology or pathology. *Eye* **1**:282, 1987.
17. Best F: Ueber eine hereditare Maculaaffektion. *Z Augenheilkd* **13**:199, 1905.
18. Falls HF: The polymorphous manifestations of Best's disease (vitelliform eruptive disease of the retina). *Trans Am Ophthalmol Soc* **67**:265, 1969.
19. Maloney WF, Robertson DM, Duboff SM: Hereditary vitelliform macular degeneration. *Arch Ophthalmol* **95**:979, 1977.
20. Mohler CW, Fine SL: Long-term evaluation of patients with Best's vitelliform dystrophy. *Ophthalmology* **88**:688, 1980.
21. Fishman GA, Baca W, Alexander KR, Derlacki DJ, Glenn AM, Viana M: Visual acuity in patients with Best vitelliform macular dystrophy. *Ophthalmology* **100**:1665, 1993.
22. Deutman AF: Vitelliform dystrophy of the fovea, in Deutman AF (ed): *The Hereditary Dystrophies of the Posterior Pole of the Eye.* Assen, The Netherlands, Koninklijke Van Gorcum, 1971, p 198.
23. Noble KG, Scher BM, Carr RE: Polymorphous presentations in vitelliform macular dystrophy: Subretinal neovascularisation and central choroidal atrophy. *Br J Ophthalmol* **62**:561, 1978.
24. Lewis RA: Juvenile hereditary macular dystrophies, in Newsome DA (ed): *Retinal Dystrophies and Degenerations.* New York, Raven Press, 1988, p 115.
25. Weber BHF, Stöhr H, Walker D: A case of nonpenetrance in Best's disease. *Am J Ophthalmol* **118**:398, 1994.
26. Doyne RW: A peculiar condition of choroiditis occurring in several members of the same family. *Trans Ophthal Soc UK* **19**:71, 1899.
27. Klainguti R: Die Tapeto-retinal degeneration im Kanton Tessin. *Klin Monatsbl Augenheilkd* **89**:253, 1932.
28. Franceschetti A, François J, Babel J: *Chorioretinal Heredodegenera-tions.* Springfield, IL, Charles C. Thomas, 1974, p 384.
29. Héon E, Piguet B, Munier F, Sneed SR, Morgan CM, Forni S, Pescia G, et al: Linkage of autosomal dominant radial drusen (Malattia Leventinese) to chromosome 2p16-21. *Ophthalmic Mol Genet* **114**:193, 1996.
30. Edwards AO, Klein ML, Berselli CB, Hejtmancik JF, Rust K, Wirtz MK, Weleber RG, et al: Malattia Leventinese: Refinement of the genetic locus and phenotypic variability in autosomal dominant macular drusen. *Am J Ophthalmol* **126**:417, 1998.
31. Deutman AF: Dominant drusen of Bruch's membrane, in Deutman AF (ed): *The Hereditary Dystrophies of the Posterior Pole of the Eye* Assen, The Netherlands, Van Gorcum, 1971, p 366.
32. Evans K, Gregory CY, Wijesuriya SD, Kermani S, Jay MR, Plant C, Bird AC: Assessment of the phenotypic range seen in Doyne honeycomb retinal dystrophy. *Arch Ophthalmol* **115**:904, 1997.
33. Sorsby A: The dystrophies of the macula. *Brit J Ophthalmol* **24**:469, 1940.
34. Sorsby A, Joll-Mason ME: A fundus dystrophy with unusual features. *Brit J Ophthalmol* **33**:67, 1949.
35. Hoskin A, Sehmi K, Bird AC: Sorsby's pseudoinflammatory macular dystrophy. *Br J Ophthalmol* **65**:859, 1981.
36. Polkinghorne PJ, Malcolm RC, Berninger T, Lyness AL, Sehmi K, Bird AC: Sorsby's fundus dystrophy. *Ophthalmology* **96**:1763, 1989.
37. Hamilton WK, Ewing CC, Ives EJ, Carruthers JD: Sorsby's fundus dystrophy. *Ophthalmology* **96**:1755, 1989.
38. Babel J, Cabernard E, Klein D, Korol S, Kräuchi H, Schafroth P: Pseudo-inflammatory chorioretinal degeneration of the posterior pole. *Graefes Arch Clin Exp Ophthalmol* **219**:236, 1982.
39. Dreyer RF, Hidayat AA: Pseudoinflammatory macular dystrophy. *Am J Ophthalmol* **106**:154, 1988.
40. Capon MRC, Marshall J, Krafft JI, Alexander RA, Hiscott PS, Bird AC: Sorsby's fundus dystrophy: A light and electron microscopic study. *Ophthalmology* **96**:1769, 1989.
41. Jacobson SG, Cideciyan AV, Regunath G, Rodriguez FJ, Vanden-burgh K, Sheffield VC, Stone EM: Night blindness in Sorsby's fundus dystrophy reversed by vitamin A. *Nat Genet* **11**:27, 1995.
42. Stargardt K: Über familiäre, progressive degeneration in der maculagegend des auges. *Albrecht von Graefes Archiv fur Ophthal-mologie* **71**:534, 1909.
43. Franceschetti A: Über tapeto-retinale degenerationen im Kindesalter, in von Sautter H (eds): *Entwicklung und Fortschritt in der Augen-heilkunde.* Stuttgart, Germany, Ferdinand Enke Verlag, 1963, p 107.

44. François P, Turut P, Puech B, Hache J-C: Maladie de Stargardt et Fundus Flavimaculatus. *Arch Ophtalmol (Paris)* **35**:817, 1975.

45. Hadden OB, Gass JDM: Fundus flavimaculatus and Stargardt's disease. *Am J Ophthalmol* **82**:527, 1976.

46. Fishman GA: Fundus flavimaculatus: A clinical classification. *Arch Ophthalmol* **94**:2061, 1976.

47. Noble KG, Carr RE: Stargardt's disease and Fundus Flavimaculatus. *Arch Ophthalmol* **97**:1281, 1979.

48. Cibis GW, Morey M, Harris DJ: Dominantly inherited macular dystrophy with flecks (Stargardt). *Arch Ophthalmol* **98**:1785, 1980.

49. Zhang K, Bither PP, Park R, Donoso LA, Seidman JG, Seidman CE: A dominant Stargardt's macular dystrophy locus maps to chromosome 13q34. *Arch Ophthalmol* **112**:759, 1994.

50. Stone EM, Nichols BE, Kimura AE, Weingeist TA, Drack A, Sheffield VC: Clinical features of a Stargardt-like dominant progressive macular dystrophy with genetic linkage to chromosome 6q. *Arch Ophthalmol* **112**:765, 1994.

51. Kniazeva M, Chiang MF, Morgan B, Anduze AL, Zack DJ, Zhang K: A new locus for autosomal dominant Stargardt-like disease maps to chromosome 4. *Am J Hum Genet* **64**:1394, 1999.

52. Fishman GA, Farber M, Patel BS, Derlacki DJ: Visual acuity loss in patients with Stargardt's macular dystrophy. *Ophthalmology* **94**:809, 1987.

53. Doka DS, Fishman GA, Anderson RJ: Refractive errors in patients with Fundus Flavimaculatus. *Br J Ophthalmol* **66**:227, 1982.

54. Klein BA, Krill AE: Fundus flavimaculatus: Clinical, functional, and histopathologic observations. *Am J Ophthalmol* **64**:3, 1967.

55. Fishman GA, Young RSL, Schall SP, Vasques VA: Electro-oculogram testing in Fundus Flavimaculatus. *Arch Ophthalmol* **97**:1896, 1979.

56. Fishman GA, Farbman JS, Alexander KR: Delayed rod dark adaptation in patients with Stargardt's disease. *Ophthalmology* **98**:957, 1991.

57. Glenn AM, Fishman GA, Gilbert LD, Derlacki DJ: Effect of vitamin A treatment on the prolongation of dark adaptation in Stargardt's dystrophy. *Retina* **14**:27, 1994.

58. Gelisken O, DeLaey JJ: A clinical review of Stargardt's disease and/or Fundus Flavimaculatus with follow-up. *Int Ophthalmol* **8**:225, 1985.

59. Armstrong JD, Meyer D, Xu S, Elfervig JL: Long-term follow-up of Stargardt's disease and Fundus Flavimaculatus. *Ophthalmology* **105**:448, 1998.

60. De Laey JJ, Verougstraete C: Hyperlipofuscinosis and subretinal fibrosis in Stargardt's disease. *Retina* **15**:399, 1995.

61. Ober RR, Limstrom SA, Simon RM: Traumatic retinopathy in Stargardt's disease. *Retina* **17**:251, 1996.

62. Gass JDM, Hummer J: Focal retinal pigment epithelial dysplasia associated with Fundus Flavimaculatus. *Retina* **19**:297, 1999.

63. Klein R, Lewis RA, Myers SM, Myers FL: Subretinal neovascularization associated with Fundus Flavimaculatus. *Arch Ophthalmol* **96**:2954, 1978.

64. Leveille AS, Morse PH, Burch JV: Fundus flavimaculatus and subretinal neovascularization. *Ann Ophthalmol* **14**:331, 1982.

65. Bonnin P, Passot M, Triolaire-Cotten M-T: Le signe du silence choroïdien dans les dégénérscences tapéto-rétiniennes posterieures, in De Laey JJ (ed): *International Symposium on Fluorescein Angiography.* The Hague, Dr. W. Junk bv Publishers, 1976, p 461.

66. Ernest JT, Krill AE: Fluorescein studies in Fundus Flavimaculatus and drusen. *Am J Ophthalmol* **62**:1, 1966.

67. Cohen SY, Quentel G, Egasse D, Cadot M, Ingster-Moati I, Coscas GJ: The dark choroid in systemic argyrosis. *Retina* **13**:312, 1993.

68. Klein R, Davis MD, Magli YL, Segal P, Klein BEK, Hubbard L: The Wisconsin age-related maculopathy grading system. *Ophthalmology* **98**:1128, 1991.

69. Bird AC, Bressler NM, Bressler SB, Chisholm IH, Coscas G, Davis MD, de Jong PTVM, et al: An international classification and grading system for age-related maculopathy and age-related macular degeneration. *Surv Ophthalmol* **39**:367, 1995.

70. Vingerling JR, Dielemans I, Hofman A, Grobbee DE, Hijmering M, Kramer CFL, de Jong PTVM: The prevalence of age-related maculopathy in the Rotterdam study. *Ophthalmology* **102**:205, 1995.

71. Sarks SH: Drusen and their relationship to senile macular degeneration. *Aust J Ophthalmol* **8**:117, 1980.

72. Gass JDM: Drusen and disciform macular detachment and degeneration. *Arch Ophthalmol* **90**:206, 1973.

73. Smiddy WE, Fine SL: Prognosis of patients with bilateral macular drusen. *Ophthalmology* **91**:271, 1984.

74. Pauleikhoff D, Barondes MJ, Minassian D, Chisholm IH, Bird AC: Drusen as risk factors in age-related macular disease. *Am J Ophthalmol* **109**:38, 1990.

75. Arnold JJ, Sarks SH, Killingsworth MC, Sarks JP: Reticular pseudodrusen: A risk factor in age-related maculopathy. *Retina* **15**:183, 1995.

76. Curcio CA, Millican L: Basal linear deposit and large drusen are specific for early age-related maculopathy. *Arch Ophthalmol* **117**:329, 1999.

77. Klein R, Klein B, Linton KLP: Prevalence of age-related maculopathy. *Ophthalmology* **99**:933, 1992.

78. Holz FG, Wolfensberger TJ, Piguet B, Gross-Jendroska M, Wells JA, Minassian DC, Chisholm IH, et al: Bilateral macular drusen in age-related macular degeneration: Prognosis and risk factors. *Ophthalmology* **101**:1522, 1994.

79. Klein R, Klein BEK, Jensen SC, Meuer SM: The five-year incidence and progression of age-related maculopathy: The Beaver Dam Eye Study. *Ophthalmology* **104**:7, 1997.

80. Bressler NM, Bressler SB, Fine SL: Age-related macular degeneration. *Surv Ophthalmol* **32**:375, 1988.

81. Gregor Z, Joffe L: Senile macular changes in the black African. *Br J Ophthalmol* **62**:547, 1978.

82. Klein R, Rowland ML, Harris MI: Racial/ethnic differences in age-related maculopathy. *Ophthalmology* **102**:371, 1995.

83. Lim JI, Kwok A, Wilson DK: Symptomatic age-related macular degeneration in Asian patients. *Retina* **18**:435, 1998.

84. Heiba IM, Elston RC, Klein BEK, Klein R: Sibling correlations and segregation analysis of age-related maculopathy: The Beaver Dam Eye Study. *Genet Epidemiol* **11**:51, 1994.

85. Piguet B, Wells JA, Palmvang IB, Wormald R, Chisholm IH, Bird AC: Age-related Bruch's membrane change: A clinical study of the relative role of hereditary and environment. *Br J Ophthalmol* **77**:400, 1993.

86. Seddon JM, Ajani UA, Mitchell BD: Familial aggregation of age-related maculopathy. *Am J Ophthalmol* **123**:199, 1997.

87. Klein ML, Schultz DW, Edwards A, Matise TC, Rust K, Berselli CB, Trzupek K, et al: Age-related macular degeneration: Clinical features in a large family and linkage to chromosome 1q. *Arch Ophthalmol* **116**:1082, 1998.

88. Hyman LG, Lilienfeld AM, Ferris FL, Fine SL: Senile macular degeneration: A case-control study. *Am J Epidemiol* **118**:213, 1983.

89. Melrose MA, Magargal LE, Lucier AC: Identical twins with subretinal neovascularization complicating senile macular degeneration. *Ophthalmic Surg* **16**:648, 1985.

90. Meyers SM, Zachary AA: Monozygotic twins with age-related macular degeneration. *Arch Ophthalmol* **106**:651, 1988.

91. Dosso AA, Bovet J: Monozygotic twin brothers with age-related macular degeneration. *Ophthalmologica* **205**:24, 1992.

92. Klein ML, Mauldin WM, Stoumbos VD: Hereditary and age-related macular degeneration. *Arch Ophthalmol* **112**:932, 1994.

93. Meyers SM, Greene T, Gutman FA: A twin study of age-related macular degeneration. *Am J Ophthalmol* **120**:757, 1995.

94. Lewis RA, Shroyer NF, Singh N, Allikmets R, Hutchinson A, Li Y, Lupski JR, et al: Genotype/phenotype analysis of a photoreceptor-specific ABC transporter gene, *ABCR*, in Stargardt disease. *Am J Hum Genet* **64**:422, 1999.

95. Berger JW, Fine SL: Laser treatment for choroidal neovascularization, in Berger JW, Fine SL, Maguire MG (eds): *Age-Related Macular Degeneration.* St. Louis, CV Mosby, 1999, p 279.

96. Stone EM, Nichols BE, Streb LM, Kimura AE, Sheffield VC: Genetic linkage of vitelliform macular degeneration (Best's disease) to chromosome 11q13. *Nat Genet* **1**:246, 1992.

97. Forsman K, Graff C, Nordstrom S, Johansson K, Westermark E, Lundgren E, Gustavson K-H, et al: The gene for Best's macular dystrophy is located at 11q13 in a Swedish family. *Clin Genet* **42**:156, 1992.

98. Weber BHF, Walker D, Muller B, Mar L: Best's vitelliform dystrophy (VMD2) maps between D11S903 and PYGM: No evidence for locus heterogeneity. *Genomics* **20**:267, 1994.

99. Hou Y-C, Richards JE, Bingham EL, Pawar H, Scott K, Segal M, Lunetta KL, et al: Linkage study of Best's vitelliform macular dystrophy (VMD2) in a large North American family. *Hum Hered* **46**:211, 1996.

100. Graff C, Eriksson A, Forsman K, Sandgren O, Holmgren G, Wadelius C: Refined genetic localization of the Best disease gene in 11q13 and physical mapping of linked markers on radiation hybrids. *Hum Genet* **101**:263, 1997.

101. Nichols BE, Bascom R, Litt M, McInnes R, Sheffield VC, Stone EM: Refining the locus for Best vitelliform macular dystrophy and mutation analysis of the candidate gene *ROM1*. *Am J Hum Genet* **54**:95, 1994.
102. Weber BHF, Walker D, Muller B: Molecular evidence for non-penetrance in Best's disease. *J Med Genet* **31**:388, 1994.
103. Stöhr H, Marquardt A, Rivera A, Cooper PR, Nowak NJ, Shows TB, Gerhard DS, et al: A gene map of the Best's vitelliform macular dystrophy region in chromosome 11q12-q13.1. *Genome Res* **8**:48, 1998.
104. Petrukhin K, Koisti MJ, Bakall B, Li W, Xie G, Marknell T, Sandgren O, et al: Identification of the gene responsible for Best macular dystrophy. *Nat Genet* **19**:241, 1998.
105. Marquardt A, Stöhr H, Passmore LA, Krämer F, Rivera A, Weber BHF: Mutations in a novel gene, *VMD2*, encoding a protein of unknown properties cause juvenile-onset vitelliform macular dystrophy (Best's disease). *Hum Mol Genet* **7**:1517, 1998.
106. Katz ML, Stientjes HJ, Gao CL, Christianson JS: Iron-induced accumulation of ipofuscin-like fluorescent pigment in the retinal pigment epithelium. *Invest Ophthalmol Vis Sci* **34**:3161, 1993.
107. Katz ML, Christianson JS, Gao CL, Handelman GJ: Iron-induced fluorescence in the retina: Dependence on vitamin A. *Invest Ophthalmol Vis Sci* **35**:3613, 1994.
108. Qin S, Nowak NJ, Zhang J, Sait SNJ, Mayers PG, Higgins MJ, Cheng Y, et al: A high-resolution map of chromosome 11. *Proc Natl Acad Sci U S A* **93**:3149, 1996.
109. Cooper P, Nowak NJ, Higgins MJ, Simpson SA, Stöhr H, Marquardt A, Weber BHF, et al: A sequence ready high resolution physical map of the Best's macular dystrophy gene region in 11q12-13. *Genomics* **41**:185, 1997.
110. Cooper PR, Nowak NJ, Higgins MJ, Church DM, Shows TB: Transcript mapping of the human chromosome 11q12-q13.1 gene-rich region identifies several newly described conserved genes. *Genomics* **49**:419, 1998.
111. Caldwell GM, Kakuk LE, Griesinger IB, Simpson SA, Nowak NJ, Small KW, Maumenee IH, et al: Bestrophin gene mutations in patients with best Vitelliform macular dystrophy. *Genomics* **58**:98, 1999.
112. Bakall B, Marknell T, Ingvast S, Koisti MJ, Sandgren O, Li W, Bergen AA, et al: The mutation spectrum of the bestrophin protein-functional implications. *Hum Genet* **104**:383, 1999.
113. Gregory CY, Evans K, Wijesuriya SD, Kermani S, Jay MR, Plant C, Cox N, et al: The gene responsible for autosomal dominant Doyne's honeycomb retinal dystrophy (DHRD) maps to chromosome 2p16. *Hum Mol Genet* **5**:1055, 1996.
114. Heon E, Piguet B, Munier F, Sneed SR, Morgan CM, Forni S, Pescia G, et al: Linkage of autosomal dominant radial drusen (Malattia Leventinese) to chromosome 2p16-21. *Arch Ophthalmol* **114**:193, 1996.
115. Kermani S, Gregory-Evans K, Tarttelin EE, Bellingham J, Plant C, Bird AC, Fox M, et al: Refined genetic and physical positioning of the gene for Doyne honeycomb retinal dystrophy (DHRD). *Hum Genet* **104**:77, 1999.
116. Stone EM, Lotery AJ, Munier FL, Héon E, Piguet B, Guymer RH, Vandenburgh K, et al: A single *EFEMP1* mutation associated with both Malattia Leventinese and Doyne honeycomb retinal dystrophy. *Nat Genet* **22**:199, 1999.
117. Lecka-Czernik B, Lumpkin CKJ, Goldstein S: An overexpressed gene transcript in senescent and quiescent human fibroblasts encoding a novel protein in the epidermal growth factor-like repeat family stimulates DNA synthesis. *Mol Cell Biol* **15**:120, 1995.
118. Ikegawa S, Toda T, Okui K, Nakamura Y: Structure and chromosomal assignment of the human S1-5 gene (FBNL) that is highly homologous to fibrillin. *Genomics* **35**:590, 1996.
119. Katsanis N, Venable S, Smith JR, Lupski JR: Isolation of a paralog of the Doyne honeycomb retinal dystrophy gene from the Bardet-Biedl 1 critical region. *Hum Genet* **106**:66, 2000.
120. Leppert M, Baird L, Anderson KL, Otterud B, Lupski JR, Lewis RA: Bardet-Biedl syndrome is linked to DNA markers on chromosome 11q and is genetically heterogeneous. *Nat Genet* **7**:108, 1994.
121. Weber BHF, Vogt G, Wolz W, Ives EJ, Ewing CC: Sorsby's fundus dystrophy is genetically linked to chromosome 22q13-qter. *Nat Genet* **7**:158, 1994.
122. Weber BHF, Vogt G, Pruett RC, Stöhr H, Felbor U: Mutations in the tissue inhibitor of metalloproteinases-3 (TIMP3) in patients with Sorsby's fundus dystrophy. *Nat Genet* **8**:352, 1994.
123. Apte SS, Mattei M-G, Olsen BR: Cloning of the cDNA encoding human tissue inhibitor of metalloproteinases-3 (TIMP-3) and mapping of the TIMP3 gene to chromosome 22. *Genomics* **19**:86, 1994.
124. Wilde CG, Hawkins PR, Coleman RT, Levine WB, Delegeane AM, Okamoto PM, Ito LY, et al: Cloning and characterization of human tissue inhibitor of metalloproteinases-3. *DNA Cell Biol* **13**:711, 1994.
125. Stöhr H, Roomp K, Felbor U, Weber BHF: Genomic organization of the human tissue inhibitor of metalloproteinases-3 (TIMP3). *Genome Res* **5**:483, 1995.
126. Langton KP, Barker MD, McKie N: Localization of the functional domains of human tissue inhibitor of metalloproteinases-3 and the effects of a Sorsby's fundus dystrophy mutation. *J Biol Chem* **273**:16778, 1998.
127. Felbor U, Stohr H, Amann T, Schonherr U, Weber BHF: A novel Ser156Cys mutation in the tissue inhibitor of metalloproteinase-3 (TIMP3) in Sorsby's fundus dystrophy with unusual clinical features. *Hum Mol Genet* **4**:2415, 1995.
128. Felbor U, Suvanto EA, Forsius HR, Eriksson AW, Weber BHF: Autosomal recessive Sorsby fundus dystrophy revisited: molecular evidence for dominant inheritance. *Am J Hum Genet* **60**:57, 1997.
129. Wijesuriya SD, Evans K, Jay MR, Davison C, Weber BHF, Bird AC, Bhattacharya SS, et al: Sorsby's fundus dystrophy in the British Isles: Demonstration of a striking founder effect by microsatellite-generated haplotypes. *Genome Res* **6**:92, 1996.
130. Carrero-Valenzuela RD, Klein ML, Weleber RG, Murphey WH, Litt M: Sorsby fundus dystrophy: A family with the ser181cys mutation of the tissue inhibitor of metalloproteinases 3. *Arch Ophthalmol* **114**:737, 1996.
131. Kaplan J, Gerber S, Larget-Piet D, Rozet J-M, Dollfus H, Dufier J-L, Odent S, et al: A gene for Stargardt's disease (*Fundus Flavimaculatus*) maps to the short arm of chromosome 1. *Nat Genet* **5**:308, 1993.
132. Gerber S, Rozet J-M, Bonneau D, Souied E, Camuzat A, Dufier J-L, Amalric P, et al: A gene for late-onset Fundus Flavimaculatus with macular dystrophy maps to chromosome 1p13. *Am J Hum Genet* **56**:396, 1995.
133. Anderson KL, Baird L, Lewis RA, Chinault AC, Otterud B, Leppert M, Lupski JR: A YAC contig encompassing the recessive Stargardt disease gene (*STGD*) on chromosome 1p. *Am J Hum Genet* **57**:1351, 1995.
134. Allikmets R, Singh N, Sun H, Shroyer NF, Hutchinson A, Chidambaram A, Gerrard B, et al: A photoreceptor cell-specific ATP-binding transporter gene (*ABCR*) is mutated in recessive Stargardt macular dystrophy (Erratum published in *Nat Genet* 17:22). *Nat Genet* **15**:236, 1997.
135. Dean M, Allikmets R: Evolution of ATP-binding cassette transporter genes. *Curr Opin Genet Dev* **5**:779, 1995.
136. Allikmets R, Gerrard B, Hutchinson A, Dean M: Characterization of the human ABC superfamily: isolation and mapping of 21 new genes using the Expressed Sequence Tags database. *Hum Mol Genet* **5**:1649, 1996.
137. Riordan JR, Rommens JM, Kerem B, Alon N, Rozmahel R, Grezelczak Z, Zielenski J, et al: Identification of the cystic fibrosis gene: cloning and characterization of complementary DNA. *Science* **245**:1066, 1989.
138. Mosser J, Douar AM, Sarde CO, Kioschis P, Feil R, Moser H, Poustka AM, et al: Putative X-linked adrenoleukodystrophy gene shares unexpected homology with ABC transporters. *Nature* **361**:726, 1993.
139. Thomas PM, Cote GJ, Wohllk N, Haddad B, Mathew PM, Rabl W, Aguilar-Bryan L, et al: Mutations in the sulfonylurea receptor gene in familial persistent hyperinsulinemic hypoglycemia of infancy. *Science* **268**:426, 1995.
140. Shimozawa N, Tsukamoto T, Suzuki Y, Orii T, Shirayoshi Y, Mori T, Fujiki Y: A human gene responsible for Zellweger syndrome that affects peroxisome assembly. *Science* **255**:1132, 1992.
141. de la Salle H, Hanau D, Fricker D, Urlacher A, Kelly A, Salamero J, Powis SH, et al: Homozygous human TAP peptide transporter mutation in HLA class I deficiency. *Science* **265**:237, 1994.
142. Strautnieks SS, Bull LN, Knisely AS, Kocoshis SA, Dahl N, Arnell H, Sokal E, et al: A gene encoding a liver-specific ABC transporter is mutated in progressive familial intrahepatic cholestasis. *Nat Genet* **20**:233, 1998.
143. De Vree JML, Jacquemin E, Sturm E, Cresteil D, Bosma PJ, Aten J, Deleuze J-F, et al: Mutations in the *MDR3* gene cause progressive familial intrahepatic cholestasis. *Proc Natl Acad Sci U S A* **95**:282, 1998.
144. Wada M, Toh S, Taniguchi K, Nakamura T, Uchiumi T, Kohno K, Yoshida I, et al: Mutations in the canalicular multispecific organic anion transporter (*cMOAT*) gene, a novel ABC transporter, in patients with hyperbilirubinemia II/Dubin-Johnson syndrome. *Hum Mol Genet* **7**:203, 1998.

145. Books-Wilson A, Marcil M, Clee SM, Zhang L-H, Roomp K, van Dam M, Yu L, et al: Mutations in *ABC1* in Tangier disease and familial high-density lipoprotein deficiency. *Nat Genet* 22:336, 1999.

146. Bodzioch M, Orsó E, Klucken J, Langmann T, Böttcher A, Diederich W, Drobnik W, et al: The gene encoding ATP-binding cassette transporter 1 is mutated in Tangier disease. *Nat Genet* 22:347, 1999.

147. Rust S, Rosier M, Funke H, Real J, Amoura Z, Piette J-C, Deleuze J-F, et al: Tangier disease is caused by mutations in the gene encoding ATP-binding cassette transporter 1. *Nat Genet* 22:352, 1999.

148. Allikmets R, Wasserman WW, Hutchinson A, Smallwood P, Nathans J, Rogan PK, Schneider TD, et al: Organization of the *ABCR* gene: Analysis of promoter and splice junction sequences. *Gene* 215:111, 1998.

149. Azarian SM, Megarity CF, Weng J, Horvath DH, Travis GH: The human photoreceptor rim protein gene (*ABCR*): Genomic structure and primer set information for mutation analysis. *Hum Genet* 102:699, 1998.

150. Gerber S, Rozet JM, van de Pol TJR, Hoyng CB, Munnich A, Blankenagel A, Kaplan J, et al: Complete exon-intron structure of the retina-specific ATP binding transporter gene (*ABCR*) allows the identification of novel mutations underlying Stargardt disease. *Genomics* 48:139, 1998.

151. Sun H, Nathans J: Stargardt's *ABCR* is localized to the disc membrane of retinal rod outer segments. *Nat Genet* 17:15, 1997.

151a. Molday LL, Rabin AR, Molday RS: ABCR expression in foveal cone photoreceptors and its role in Stargardt macular dystrophy. *Nat Genet* 25:257, 2000.

152. Illing M, Molday LL, Molday RS: The 280-kDa rim protein of retinal rod outer segments is a member of the ABC transporter superfamily. *J Biol Chem* 272:10303, 1997.

153. Azarian SM, Travis GH: The photoreceptor rim protein is an ABC transporter encoded by the gene for recessive Stargardt's disease. *FEBS Lett* 409:247, 1997.

154. Papermaster DS, Converse CA, Zorn M: Biosynthetic and immuno-chemical characterization of a large protein in frog and cattle rod out segment membranes. *Exp Eye Res* 23:105, 1976.

155. Papermaster DS, Schneider BG, Zorn MA, Kraehenbuhl JP: Immunocytochemical localization of a large intrinsic membrane protein to the incisures and margins of frog rod outer segment disks. *Cell Biol* 78:415, 1978.

156. Shuster TA, Nagy AK, Farber DB: Nucleotide binding to the rod outer segment rim protein. *Exp Eye Res* 46:647, 1988.

157. Sun H, Molday RS, Nathans J: Retinal stimulates ATP hydrolysis by purified and reconstituted ABCR, the photoreceptor-specific ATP-binding cassette transporter responsible for Stargardt disease. *J Biol Chem* 274:8269, 1999.

158. Weng J, Mata NL, Azarian SM, Tzekov RT, Birch DG, Travis GH: Insights into the function of rim protein in photoreceptors and etiology of Stargardt's disease from the phenotype in *abcr* knockout mice. *Cell* 98:13, 1999.

158a. Mata NL, Weng J, Travis GH: Biosynthesis of a major lipofuscin fluorophore in mice and humans with ABCR-mediated retinal and macular degeneration. *Proc Natl Acad Sci USA* 97:7154, 2000.

159. Nasokin I, Illing M, Koehler MR, Schmid M, Molday RS, Weber BHF: Mapping of the rod photoreceptor ABC transporter (ABCR) to 1p21-p22.1 and identification of novel mutations in Stargardt's disease. *Hum Genet* 102:21, 1998.

160. Rozet J-M, Gerber S, Souied E, Perrault I, Châtelin S, Ghazi I, Leowski C, et al: Spectrum of *ABCR* gene mutations in autosomal recessive macular dystrophies. *Eur J Hum Genet* 6:291, 1998.

161. Maugeri A, van Driel MA, van de Pol DJR, Klevering BJ, van Haren FJJ, Tijmes N, Bergen AAB, et al: The 2588G → C mutation in the *ABCR* gene is a mild frequent founder mutation in the western European population and allows the classification of *ABCR* mutations in patients with Stargardt disease. *Am J Hum Genet* 64:1024, 1999.

162. Fishman GA, Stone EM, Grover S, Derlacki DJ, Haines HL, Hockey RR: Variation of clinical expression in patients with Stargardt dystrophy and sequence variations in the *ABCR* gene. *Arch Ophthalmol* 117:504, 1999.

163. Martinez-Mir A, Paloma E, Allikmets R, Ayuso C, del Rio T, Dean M, Vilageliu L, et al: Retinitis pigmentosa caused by a homozygous mutation in the Stargardt disease gene *ABCR*. *Nat Genet* 18:11, 1998.

164. Cremers FPM, van de Pol DJR, vanDriel M, den Hollander AI, van Haren FJJ, Knoers NVAM, Tijmes N, et al: Autosomal recessive retinitis pigmentosa and cone-rod dystrophy caused by splice site mutations in the Stargardt's disease gene *ABCR*. *Hum Mol Genet* 7:355, 1998.

164a. Maugeri A, Klevering BJ, Rohrschneider K, Blankenagel A, Brunner HG, Deutman AF, Hoyng CB, Cremers FPM: Mutations in the ABCR 4 (ABCR) gene are the major cause of autosomal recessive cone-rod dystrophy. *Am J Hum Genet* 67:960, 2000.

165. Rozet J-M, Gerber S, Ghazi I, Perrault I, Ducroq D, Souied E, Cabot A, et al: Mutations of the retinal specific ATP binding transporter gene (*ABCR*) in a single family segregating both autosomal recessive retinitis pigmentosa RP19 and Stargardt disease: evidence of clinical heterogeneity at this locus. *J Med Genet* 36:447, 1999.

166. Martinez-Mir A, Bayes M, Vilageliu L, Grinberg D, Ayuso C, del Rio T, Garcia-Sandoval B, et al: A new locus for autosomal recessive retinitis pigmentosa (RP19) maps to 1p13-1p21. *Genomics* 40:142, 1997.

167. Shroyer NF, Lewis RA, Lupski JR: Complex inheritance of *ABCR* mutations in Stargardt disease: Linkage disequilibrium, complex alleles and pseudodominance. *Hum Genet* 106:244, 2000.

168. Zielenski J, Tsui L-C: Cystic fibrosis: Genotypic and phenotypic variations. *Ann Rev Genet* 29:777, 1995.

169. Allikmets R, Shroyer NF, Singh N, Seddon JM, Lewis RA, Bernstein P, Peiffer A, et al: Mutation of the Stargardt disease gene (*ABCR*) in age-related macular degeneration. *Science* 277:1805, 1997.

170. Shroyer NF, Lewis RA, Allikmets R, Singh N, Dean M, Leppert M, Lupski JR: The rod photoreceptor ATP-binding cassette transporter gene, *ABCR*, and retinal disease: From monogenic to multifactorial. *Vision Res* 39:2537, 1999.

171. Souied EH, Ducroq D, Gerber S, Ghazi I, Rozet J-M, Perrault I, Munnich A, et al: Age-related macular degeneration in grandparents of patients with Stargardt disease: Genetic study. *Am J Ophthalmol* 128:173, 1999.

172. Goldstein JL, Brown MS: Familial hypercholesterolemia: Identification of a defect in the regulation of 3-hydroxy-3-methylglutaryl coenzyme A reductase activity associated with overproduction of cholesterol. *Proc Natl Acad Sci U S A* 70:2804, 1973.

173. Sharer N, Schwarz M, Malone G, Howarth A, Painter J, Super M, Braganza J: Mutations of the cystic fibrosis gene in patients with chronic pancreatitis. *N Engl J Med* 339:645, 1998.

174. Cohn JA, Friedman KJ, Noone PG, Knowles MR, Silverman LM, Jowell PS: Relation between mutations of the cystic fibrosis gene and idiopathic pancreatitis. *N Engl J Med* 339:653, 1999.

175. Athma P, Rappaport R, Swift M: Molecular genotyping shows that ataxia-telangiectasia heterozygotes are predisposed to breast cancer. *Cancer Genet Cytogenet* 92:130, 1996.

176. Heim RA, Lench NJ, Swift M: Heterozygous manifestations in four autosomal recessive human cancer-prone syndromes: Ataxia telangiectasia, xeroderma pigmentosum, Fanconi anemia, and Bloom syndrome. *Mutat Res* 284:25, 1992.

177. Poller W, Meisen C, Olek K: DNA polymorphisms of the $\alpha_1$-antitrypsin gene region in patients with chronic obstructive pulmonary disease. *Eur J Clin Invest* 20:1, 1990.

178. Wittrup HH, Tybjæg-Hansen A, Abildgaard S, Steffensen R, Schnohr P, Nordestgaard BG: A common substitution (Asn291Ser) in lipoprotein lipase is associated with increased risk of ischemic heart disease. *J Clin Invest* 99:1606, 1997.

179. Dryja TP, Briggs CE, Berson EL, Rosenfeld PJ, Abitbol M: *ABCR* gene and age-related macular degeneration. *Science* 279:1107a, 1998.

180. Klaver CW, Assink JM, Bergen AAB, van Duijn CM: *ABCR* gene and age-related macular degeneration. *Science* 279:1107a, 1998.

181. Dean M, Allikmet R, Shroyer NF, Lupski JR, Lewis RA, Leppert M, Bernstein PS, et al: *ABCR* gene and age-related macular degeneration. *Science* 279:1107a, 1998.

182. Stone EM, Webster AR, Vandenburgh K, Streb LM, Hockey RR, Lotery AJ, Sheffield VC: Allelic variation in *ABCR* associated with Stargardt disease but not age-related macular degeneration. *Nat Genet* 20:328, 1998.

183. Kuroiwa S, Kojima H, Kikuchi T, Yoshimura N: ATP binding cassette transporter retina genotypes and age-related macular degeneration: an analysis on exudative non-familial Japanese patients. *Br J Ophthalmol* 83:613, 1999.

184. De La Paz MA, Guy VK, Abou-Donia S, Heinis R, Bracken B, Vance JM, Gilbert JR, et al: Analysis of the Stargardt disease gene (*ABCR*) in age-related macular degeneration. *Ophthalmology* 106:1531, 1999.

185. Allikmets R and the International ABCR Screening Consortium: Further evidence of an association of the ABCR alleles with age-related macular degeneration. *Am J Hum Genet* **67**:487, 2000.

186. Fingert JH, Héon E, Leibmann JM, Yamamoto T, Craig JE, Rait J, Kawase K, et al: Analysis of myocillin mutations in 1703 glaucoma patients from five different populations. *Hum Mol Genet* **8**:899, 1999.

187. van Driel MA, Maugeri A, Klevering BJ, Hoyng CB, Cremers FPM: *ABCR* unites what ophthalmologists divide(s). *Ophthalmic Genet* **9**:117, 1998.

187a. Lewis RA, Lupski JR: Macular degeneration: The emerging genetics. *Hospital Practice* **35**:41, 2000.

188. Allikmets R, Seddon JM, Bernstein PS, Hutchinson A, Atkinson A, Sharma S, Gerrard B, et al: Evaluation of the Best disease gene in patients with age-related macular degeneration and other maculopathies. *Hum Genet* **104**:449, 1999.

189. De La Paz MA, Pericak-Vance MA, Lennon F, Haines JL, Seddon JM: Exclusion of *TIMP3* as a candidate locus in age-related macular degeneration. *Invest Ophthalmol Vis Sci* **38**:1060, 1997.

190. Felbor U, Doepner D, Schneider U, Zrenner E, Weber BHF: Evaluation of the gene encoding the tissue inhibitor of metalloproteinases-3 in various maculopathies. *Invest Ophthal Vis Sci* **38**:1054, 1997.

# MULTISYSTEM INBORN ERRORS OF DEVELOPMENT

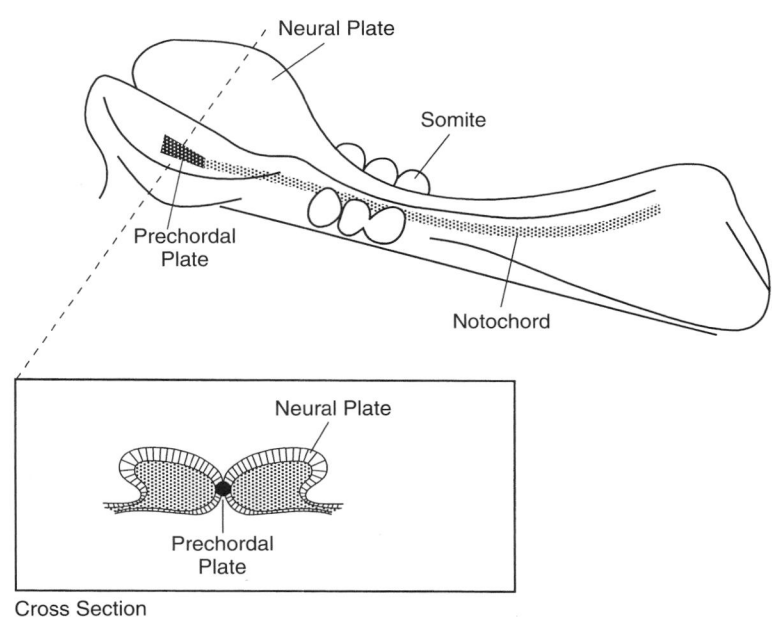

Neural Plate

Somite

Prechordal Plate

Notochord

Neural Plate

Prechordal Plate

Cross Section

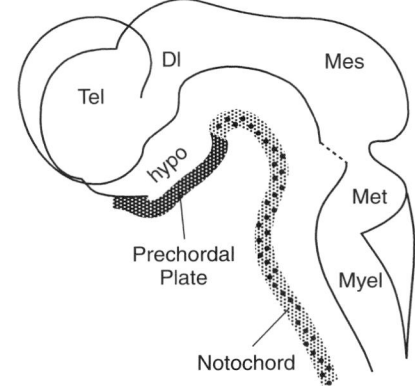

Tel

Di

Mes

hypo

Met

Myel

Prechordal Plate

Notochord

# Waardenburg Syndrome

*Andrew P. Read*

1. Waardenburg syndrome is a clinical label attached to a heterogeneous set of auditory-pigmentary syndromes, the primary cause of which is a patchy lack of melanocytes in the hair, eyes, skin, and stria vascularis. The syndrome is classified into four subtypes. Type 1, with dystopia canthorum, is caused by mutations in the *PAX3* gene (OMIM 193500). Type 2, without dystopia, is heterogeneous; a proportion is caused by changes in the *MITF* gene (OMIM 193510). Type 3, resembling type 1 but with additional contractures or hypoplasia of the upper limb joints and muscles, is a rare variant presentation of type 1 (OMIM 148820). Type 4, with Hirschsprung disease, is heterogeneous, being caused by mutations in the *EDN3*, *EDNRB*, *SOX10*, or other unidentified genes (OMIM 277580). All forms are inherited as autosomal dominant characters, except for the type 4, caused by mutations in *EDN3* or *EDNRB*, which are recessive. The hearing loss in all forms is congenital, sensorineural, and nonprogressive. There are no specific treatments, and management is symptomatic.

2. The classic description of the syndrome was given by Waardenburg in 1951; the name of David Klein is sometimes attached to the syndrome in recognition of his description of a severely affected patient at about the same time. The prevalence is about 1 in 40,000, or 1 to 2 percent of congenitally deaf people.

3. Waardenburg syndrome is an example of an auditory-pigmentary syndrome. Related syndromes are known in many mammals and particularly in mice. The mouse mutants fall into the cochleosaccular group of Steel, which has as immediate cause a physical absence of melanocytes from areas of the hair, eye, skin, and stria vascularis. Without melanocytes in the stria vascularis, no endocochlear potential is generated, and there is no hearing. All melanocytes except those of the retinal pigment epithelium derive from the embryonic neural crest. Waardenburg syndrome types 1, 3, and 4 are neurocristopathies, affecting more than one neural crest derivative. Type 2 appears to be melanocyte-specific.

4. Formal diagnostic criteria are shown in Table 244-2. Waardenburg syndrome is variable between and within families, and the penetrance of the major signs is tabulated in Table 244-3. Many complications have been described, but most are of uncertain status. Cleft lip or palate and neural tube defects are rare complications of type 1 WS.

5. Dystopia canthorum must be established by measuring the inner canthal, interpupillary, and outer canthal distances and calculating the W index according to the formula in Fig. 244-4. If the W value, averaged across all affected family members, is greater than 1.95, a diagnosis of type 1

WS may be made. Type 1 WS is a distinctive and fairly homogeneous entity; none of the other types forms a single distinct genetic entity.

6. Mouse models exist for each subtype of Waardenburg syndrome: *Splotch* for type 1 and type 3, *microphthalmia* for type 2, and *piebald-lethal*, *lethal-spotted*, and *Dominant megacolon* for type 4. These models were important aids to identifying the human genes.

7. Type 1 WS was mapped to 2q35 and type 2 to 3p12-p14.3 by family linkage studies, and positional candidate genes were identified. Type 3 WS patients are either heterozygous or homozygous for mutations in the type 1 gene. The three genes identified in type 4 were identified from mouse candidate genes with only limited human mapping work.

8. Type 1 WS is caused by haploinsufficiency due to loss-of-function mutations in the *PAX3* gene. This gene encodes a transcription factor that is active in the early embryo, and the human mutations affect the two DNA-binding domains of the protein, the paired domain and homeodomain. Most mutations are private to particular families. Identifying a mutation does not allow the nature or severity of the syndrome in an individual to be predicted. Two homozygotes have been described. One was a fetus with lethal neural tube defects; the other was a child without a neural tube defect and with generally normal development apart from very severe type 3 WS.

9. *MITF* mutations are seen in about 10 percent of patients with type 2 WS. The *MITF* gene encodes a transcription factor that is believed to be a master gene for melanocyte differentiation. Most mutations cause loss of function, and the symptoms are caused by haploinsufficiency. In two families with *MITF* mutations, a more severe and consistent dominant albinism-deafness phenotype (Tietz-Smith syndrome) is probably the result of a dominant-negative effect.

10. Type 4 WS is very rare and heterogeneous. A few patients have been shown to be homozygous for loss-of-function mutations in the *EDN3* or *EDNRB* genes, encoding endothelin-3 and its receptor. In heterozygotes, these mutations appear as low-penetrance Hirschsprung disease genes. A few patients have been found who are heterozygous for mutations in the *SOX10* transcription-factor gene. In the mouse, homozygosity for *SOX10* deficiency is lethal.

11. Identifying the genes and pathways involved in the different types of Waardenburg syndrome casts light on the normal processes of neural crest differentiation. Different downstream targets of *PAX3* action show differential sensitivity to reduced dosage levels of PAX3 protein. *PAX3* controls development of limb muscles through *MyoD* and *Met*; when this fails, the result is type 3 WS. *PAX3* also controls the expression of *MITF*. *MITF* is probably the master gene for melanocyte development, which explains the very similar melanocyte defects in type 1 and type 2 WS.

---

A list of standard abbreviations is located immediately preceding the index in each volume. Nonstandard abbreviations used in this chapter include: WS = Waardenburg syndrome; WS1 = Waardenburg syndrome type 1; WS2 = Waardenburg syndrome type 2; WS3 = Waardenburg syndrome type 3; WS4 = Waardenburg syndrome type 4.

**Table 244-1** The Four Types of Waardenburg Syndrome

| Type | MIM No. | Inheritance* | Distinguishing Feature | Comments |
|------|---------|-------------|------------------------|----------|
| 1 | 193500 | Ad | Dystopia canthorum, W > 1.95 | Nearly all have *PAX3* mutations |
| 2 | 193510 | Ad | No dystopia | Heterogeneous; 10% have *MITF* mutations |
| 3 (Klein-Waardenburg) | 148820 | Ad (most cases sporadic) | Hypoplasia of limb muscles; contractures of elbows, fingers | Variant presentation of WS1; mostly *PAX3* heterozygotes; some may be homozygotes |
| 4 (Shah-Waardenburg) | 277580 | Ar or Ad | Hirschsprung disease | Heterogeneous; includes homozygotes for *EDN3* or *EDNRB* mutations and heterozygotes for *SOX10* mutations |

*Ar, autosomal recessive; Ad, autosomal dominant.

12. **The symptoms of Waardenburg syndrome are nonprogressive, and treatment is symptomatic. When a mutation has been defined, it is possible to predict prenatally whether a fetus will carry the mutation but not how severely it will be affected. Supplements of folate in pregnancy probably are advisable where the fetus is at risk for type 1 WS (to prevent neural tube defects).***

Today we associate the name of Petrus Waardenburg with the prototypic human auditory-pigmentary syndrome, but Waardenburg was an ophthalmologist by training, and his interest was first aroused by the eye malformations of his patients. His first published patient, presented to a meeting of the Dutch Ophthalmological Society on December 14, 1947, was a man with "dystopia punctorum lacrimarum, blepharophimosis, and partial iris atrophy."[1] He also was deaf-mute, but Waardenburg apparently did not at the time make the connection; he mentioned a report of twins with the same eye abnormality who were "coincidentally" also deaf-mute. The following year, while Waardenburg was visiting Geneva, David Klein showed him a 10-year-old girl who also had dystopia canthorum but with a remarkably severe auditory-pigmentary syndrome. Realizing that coincidences were multiplying, Waardenburg was prompted to undertake a systematic search among 1050 inmates of five Dutch institutions for the deaf. His results, published in a monumental paper in the *American Journal of Human Genetics* in 1951,[2] defined the syndrome now named after him. Arias in 1971 distinguished type 1 and type 2 Waardenburg syndrome (WS)[3]; Waardenburg's work applies mainly to type 1 Waardenburg syndrome (WS1). Certain very rare cases with additional features have been labeled type 3 Waardenburg syndrome (WS3) and type 4 Waardenburg syndrome (WS4), as described below.

Waardenburg[2] estimated the prevalence of his syndrome as 1 in 42,000, or 1.43 percent of the congenitally deaf, whereas Fraser[4] reported 2.12 to 3.01 per 100,000 from his study of 2355 deaf children. These estimates do not distinguish WS1 from type 2 Waardenburg syndrome (WS2)—WS3 and WS4 are both exceedingly rare—but probably underestimate the frequency of gene carriers who have normal hearing.

## AUDITORY-PIGMENTARY SYNDROMES IN MAN AND ANIMALS

The combination of pigmentary disturbances and hearing loss had been well known in a variety of mammals since long before Waardenburg's paper. In his *Origin of the Species*, Charles Darwin commented on the fact that white cats with blue eyes are often deaf

and puzzled over the connection. The association of white spotting (or white fur) and deafness is known in cats, dogs, mink, horses, and cattle,[5] and especially in mice, where many different mutants show hearing loss with white spotting, pigmentary dilution, or totally white coat (reviewed in ref. 6). A list of mouse mutants with hearing loss is maintained by Steel[6,7] as a resource to suggest possible positional candidates for human deafness genes. The mice are commonly classified into three groups: morphogenetic (abnormal structure of the bony labyrinth or membranes), neuroepithelial (failure of a grossly normal cochlea to transduce sound—potential homologues of human nonsyndromic deafness genes), and cochleosaccular (with a primary defect of the stria vascularis).[6] It is the cochleosaccular class that is associated with pigmentary disturbance. Histologic examination shows that the white skin lacks melanocytes (distinguishing these cases from albinos, where melanocytes are present but are unable to synthesize melanin). The connection with deafness arises from an as yet unexplained requirement for melanocytes in the stria vascularis of the inner ear. Melanin is not needed for this function—albinos have normal hearing but in the absence of melanocytes, the stria is abnormally thin, the correct ionic composition of the endolymph is not maintained, no endocochlear potential is generated, and later in development Reissner's membrane collapses, leading to destruction of the organ of Corti.[8,9]

With the exception of the melanocytes in the retinal pigment epithelium, which derive from the neuroectoderm of the embryonic optic vesicle, all melanocytes of the body originate in the embryonic neural crest. Thus absence of melanocytes could be due to a failure of differentiation in the neural crest, a failure of melanoblasts to migrate, or a failure of proliferation, terminal differentiation, or survival of melanocytes in their final location. Usually the melanocyte deficiency in auditory-pigmentary syndromes is patchy, but sometimes a general dilution of pigmentation is seen, perhaps suggesting limited terminal proliferation of melanocytes. Countless genes must be involved in these processes, and so the genetics of auditory-pigmentary syndromes is likely to be complex. A distinction may be made usefully between those syndromes where only melanocytes are involved and those where there is a broader malfunction of the embryonic neural crest.

The clinical label of WS has been applied to a heterogeneous collection of auditory-pigmentary syndromes-Waardenburg's core group plus anything similar that does not clearly fit under any other label. Four subclasses of WS are commonly recognized (Table 244-1). Of these, WS1 is a discrete, well-defined genetic entity, WS2 as currently defined is common but highly heterogeneous, WS3 is a rare variant of WS1, and WS4 is a rare but heterogeneous group. WS2 appears melanocyte-specific, whereas WS1, WS3, and WS4 show a wider neurocristopathy. Not all pigmentary abnormalities are classified as WS. Patchy but extensive depigmentation without hearing loss is labeled as *piebaldism* and is for the most part genetically distinct from WS, being caused by loss-of-function mutations in the *KIT* oncogene[10]; uniform dilution of pigmentation with hearing loss is usually described as *Tietz-Smith syndrome* or *albinism-deafness*.

---

*GENBANK accession numbers: human: *PAX3*-U12263, X15043, X15252, X15253, U12262, U12260, U12258, U12259 (exons 1-8, respectively); *MITF*-Z29678; *EDN3*-J05081; *EDNRB*-L06623; SOX10-AJ001183; mouse: *Pax-3*-X59358; *Mi*-U16322; *Edn3*-U32330; *Ednrb*-U32329; *Sox10*-AF047043. Mutation database: There is no specific Waardenburg mutation database at present. The Human Mutation Database (*http://www.uwcm.ac.uk/uwcm/mg/hgmd0.html*) finds *PAX3*, *MITF*, and *EDN3* mutations queried with "Waardenburg."

**Table 244-2** Diagnostic Criteria for Waardenburg Syndrome Types 1 and 2 as Proposed by the Waardenburg Consortium[14]

To be counted as affected, an individual must have two major or one major plus two minor criteria from the following list:

**Major criteria**
- Congenital sensorineural hearing loss
- Pigmentary disturbances of iris
  (a) Complete heterochromia iridum, two eyes of different color
  (b) Partial or segmental heterochromia; segments of blue or brown pigmentation in one or both eyes
  (c) Hypoplastic blue eyes, characteristic brilliant blue in both eyes
- Hair hypopigmentation, white forelock
- Dystopia canthorum, W > 1.95 averaged over affected family members (this was modified from the original proposal of W > 2.07 in the light of experience)
- Affected first degree relative

**Minor criteria**
- Congenital leukoderma, several areas of hypopigmented skin
- Synophyrys or medial eyebrow flare
- Broad and high nasal root
- Hypoplasia of alae nasi
- Premature greying of hair, scalp hair predominantly white before age 30

For WS2, we suggest (see text) that it may be useful to set a more stringent criterion: To be classified as affected, a person should show two major features and have a first-degree relative who also shows two major features.

In some cases this is allelic with one form of WS (see below). Other rare syndromes including auditory and pigmentary features can be found in the OMIM catalogue[11] and in the book by Gorlin, Toriello, and Cohen.[12] One of these rare syndromes, craniofacial-deafness-hand syndrome (MIM 122880) is allelic to WS1.[13]

## CLINICAL PHENOTYPES

The features of WS were classified by the Waardenburg Consortium into major, minor, and rare, and diagnostic criteria were drawn up, as shown in Table 244-2.[14] Table 244-3 shows the frequency of major and minor features in patients personally examined by Prof. Valerie Newton and Dr. X. Z. Liu in Manchester, with figures from the literature for comparison.[15] The phenotype is very variable even within a family, as illustrated in Fig. 244-1 for WS1 and Fig. 244-2 for WS2. Figure 244-3 shows typical facial appearances.

### Hearing Loss

The hearing loss in WS is of a sensorineural type and is congenital and normally nonprogressive. It can be unilateral or bilateral and is variable between and within families. A profound bilateral loss is the most common type, particularly in WS1. After removal of the probands (who had mostly been referred to the audiologic clinic) 52 percent of the WS1 and 78 percent of WS2 patients examined in Manchester (see Table 244-3) had hearing loss[15]; in an earlier series,[16] the figures were 69 and 87 percent. Hageman and Delleman[17] reported only 25 and 50 percent, respectively, but probably counted milder cases as unaffected. Newton et al.[18] reported audiologic findings on 64 WS children under age 16. Of the 24 with WS1, 14 had bilateral symmetric loss, all greater than 100 dB, and 2 had unilateral or asymmetric loss. Of the 40 with WS2, 24 had bilateral symmetric loss (2, 21–40 dB; 4, 41–60 dB; 3, 81–100 dB; and 15, >100 dB), 6 were bilateral asymmetric, and 4 unilateral.

### Eye Color

Heterochromia can be complete, with two differently colored pupils, typically one blue and one brown, or segmental, where sharply demarcated sectors of different colors are present in an eye. Hypoplastic blue eyes were seen in 15 percent of our WS1 series[15] and are particularly striking in people from dark-skinned races, who would be expected to have brown eyes. In our experience, they are less common in WS2 (3 of 81 cases). They are commonly associated with profound hearing loss.

### Hair Color

The classic WS patient has a white forelock, and this was seen in 48 percent of WS1 and 28 percent of WS2 patients in the Manchester series.[15] The forelock can vary in size from a few hairs to a clump, and it may be present at birth and then disappear or may appear later, typically in the teens. Early graying (defined by the Waardenburg Consortium[14] as scalp hair predominantly white before age 30) is common. Besides the classic white forelock, a bizarre range of other hair pigmentary abnormalities has been reported, including red and black forelocks and backlocks of various colors. Patients often dye their hair to hide a forelock.

### Skin Pigmentation

White skin patches are frequent in WS1 (37 percent in our series) but less so in WS2. Patients with extensive depigmentation but no dystopia canthorum may have piebaldism, with possible mutation in the *KIT* gene[10] rather than WS. Carriers of *KIT* mutations usually have normal hearing, but there is one report of a child with a *KIT* mutation who has extensive depigmentation and profound sensorineural hearing loss.[19] Relatively few WS2 patients have been tested for *KIT* mutations.

### Other Complications

A long list of complications of WS can be found in the literature (summarized by Da Silva[20]). The problem when counseling families with WS is to distinguish among four categories:

- Genuine rare complications of WS1 such as the limb problems of WS3
- Genuine rare complications of WS2 (these need to be considered separately, since WS1 and WS2 are genetically quite distinct)

**Table 244-3** Penetrance (%) of Clinical Features of Type 1 and Type 2 Waardenburg Syndrome

| Type | Source | n | SNHL | Hetl | HypE | WF | EG | Skin | HNR | Eyb |
|------|--------|-----|------|------|------|----|----|------|-----|-----|
| WS1 | Liu et al. | 60 | 58 | 15 | 15 | 48 | 38 | 36 | 100 | 63 |
| | Literature | 210 | 57 | 31 | 18 | 43 | 23 | 30 | 52 | 70 |
| WS2 | Liu et al. | 81 | 78 | 42 | 3 | 23 | 30 | 5 | 0 | 7 |
| | Literature | 43 | 77 | 54 | 23 | 16 | 14 | 12 | 14 | 7 |

NOTE: SNHL, sensorineural hearing loss; Hetl, heterochromia irides; HypE, hypoplastic blue eyes; WF, white forelock; EG, early greying; Skin, white skin patches; HNR, high nasal root; Eyb, medial eyebrow flare.
SOURCE: Data from Liu et al.[15]

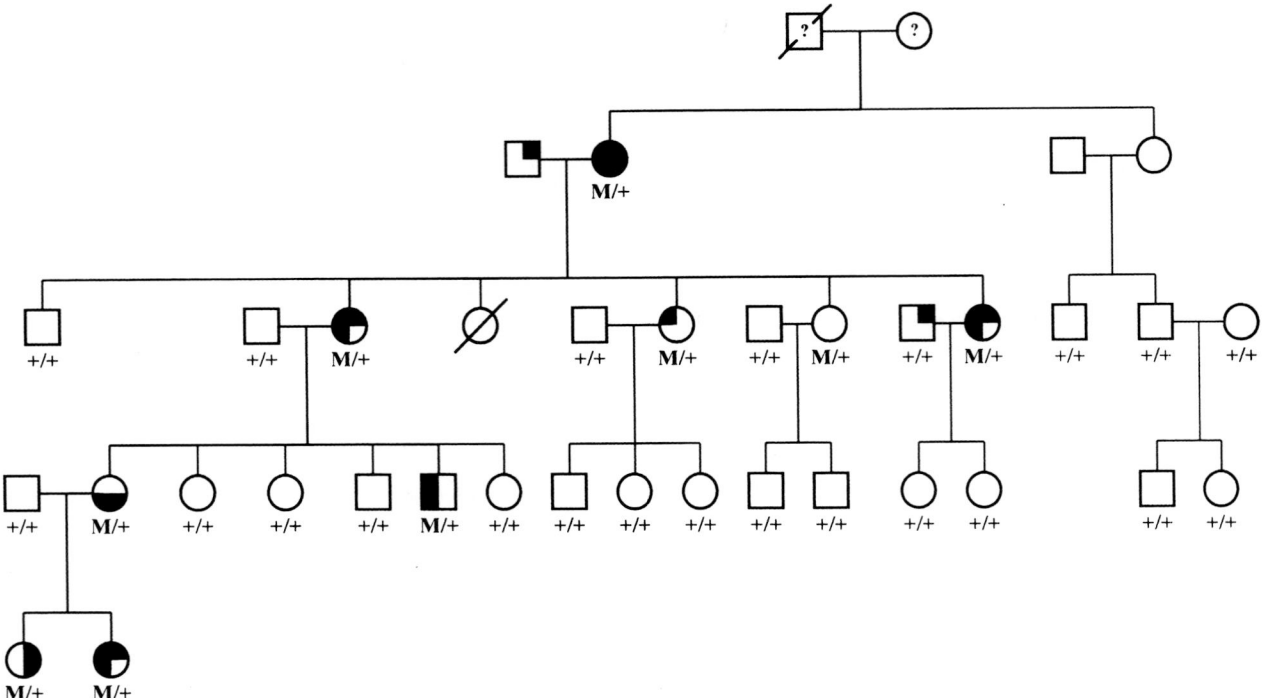

**Fig. 244-1 Within-family variability of WS1. All individuals labeled M/+ carry the *PAX3* mutation Q254X and have dystopia canthorum. *Upper right quadrant*: Sensorineural hearing loss. *Lower right*:** Heterochromia. *Lower left*: White forelock. *Upper left*: Other manifestation (early graying, hypoplastic blue eyes, white skin patches, etc.).

- Reported complications that were purely coincidental findings
- Reported complications in patients with neurocristopathies or other conditions that were described as WS but are really separate syndromes

In the study of Liu et al.,[15] other abnormalities were reported in 25 of 270 WS1 patients: cleft lip/palate (6), severe myopia (5), Sprengel shoulder (3), lipomas (3), spina bifida (2), cardiac defect (2), mental retardation (2), Raynaud's sign (1), and hypothyroidism (1). Nine of these were from the Manchester data and 16 from

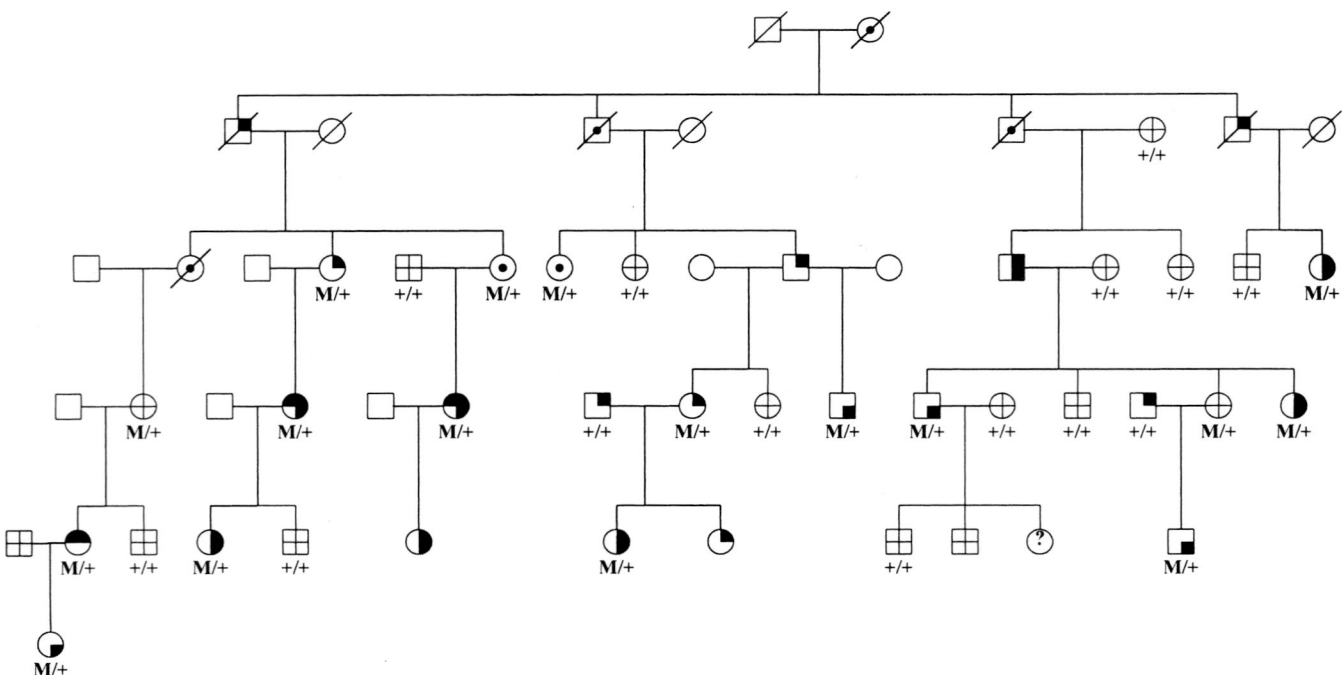

**Fig. 244-2 Within-family variability of WS2. All individuals labeled M/+ carry a mutation abolishing the exon 1 splice donor site in the *MITF* gene. None has dystopia canthorum. *Upper right quadrant*:** Sensorineural hearing loss. *Lower right*: Heterochromia. *Lower left*: White forelock. *Upper left*: Other manifestation (early graying, hypoplastic blue eyes, white skin patches, etc.).

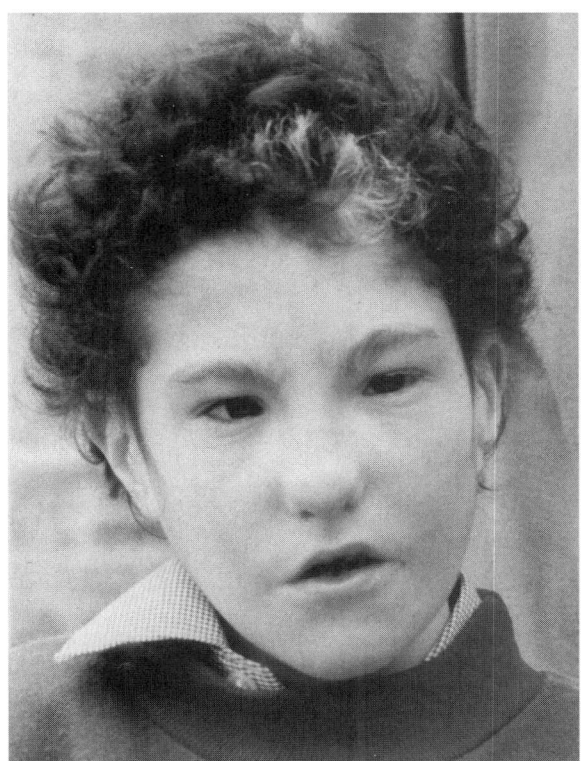

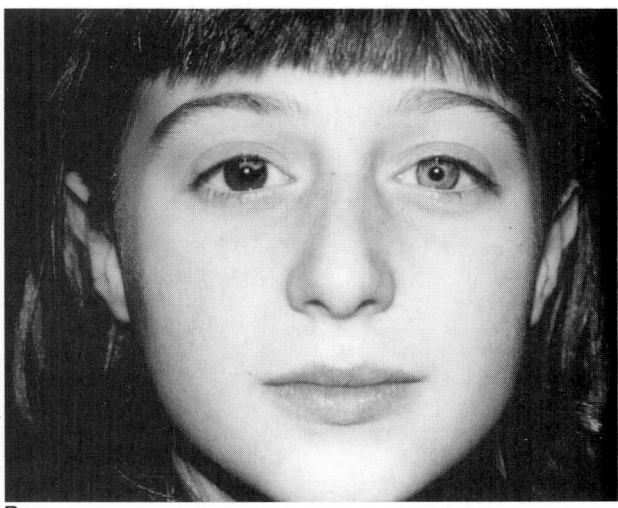

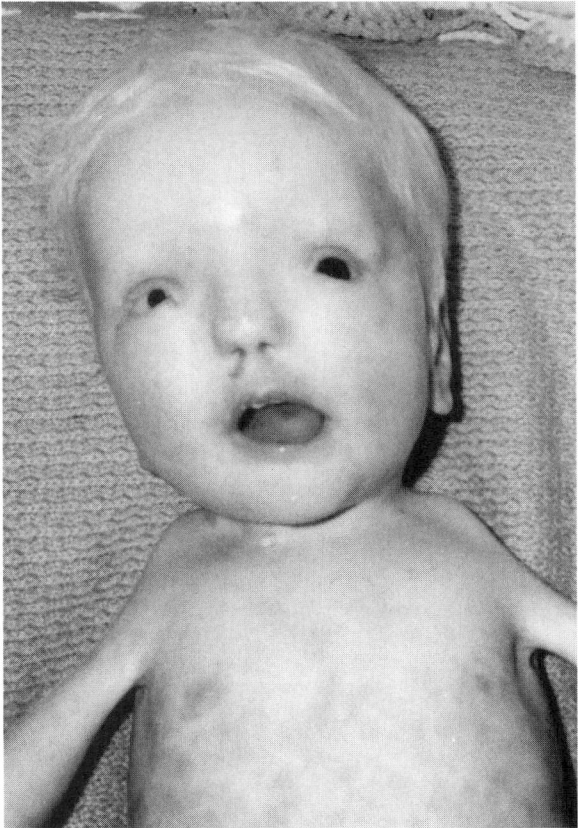

**Fig. 244-3 Typical facial appearances of WS. (*A*) Heterozygote for WS1. Note the dystopia canthorum, medial eyebrow flaring, typical nose, and white forelock. There is unilateral sensorineural hearing loss. This boy has a complete deletion of the *PAX3* gene. (*B*) Heterozygote for WS2. Note the normal build of the face, with heterochromia (left eye blue, right eye brown with a blue segment). There is a bilateral 45-dB hearing loss. She has a splice-site mutation of the *MITF* gene. (C) Homozygote for WS1. Note the extreme dystopia, extensive depigmentation, and severe amyoplasia. There is profound bilateral hearing loss. This child is homozygous for the *PAX3* mutation S84F; pictures of him as a baby were published by Zlotogora et al.[27] (*Photo courtesy of Dr. Joel Zlotogora.*)**

the literature. There is a small but definite risk of neural tube defects with WS1, probably preventable by folate supplementation in pregnancy,[21] and probably also a risk of cleft palate. Hirschsprung disease does not seem to be significantly more frequent among families with WS1; the well-known Waardenburg-Hirschsprung association is via the genetically distinct WS4 syndromes (which, however, may be reported as WS2 with Hirschsprung disease). Studies of *Splotch* mice suggest that heart defects may be a risk in WS1, and there are a few reports of such problems.

The defining criteria of WS2 are melanocyte-specific, and one might expect few effects on other systems. However, most early reports of complications of WS do not distinguish between type 1

and type 2, so it is difficult to assess the range of complications specific to type 2. In the study of Liu et al.,[15] other abnormalities were recorded in only 2 of 124 WS2 patients, both Hirschsprung cases from the literature. Restricting ourselves to families with known *MITF* mutations (and as mentioned below, although there are not many families, some of them are extremely large), there is no evidence of significant complications. One couple in the Australian family (see below) had four of their five children affected by Hirschsprung disease (one singleton and all three of triplets produced after in vitro fertilization; E. Haan, personal communication, 1995), but there are no other cases elsewhere in that extensive pedigree, and it is not known whether the affected children carried the mutation.

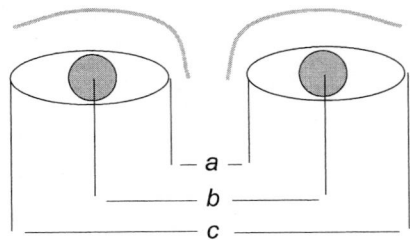

Procedure:

1.  Measure a, b, c in mm using a rigid ruler held against the face.

2.  Calculate X = (2a-0.2119c-3.909) / c

3.  Calculate Y = (2a-0.2479b-3.909) / b

4.  Calculate W = X + Y + a/b

**Fig. 244-4 Definition of the W index. The formula is best set up on a spreadsheet to allow easy calculation. The criterion for WS1 is that W (averaged across all affected family members) should be greater than 1.95.**

## CLINICAL SUBTYPES OF WS

### Type 1 Waardenburg Syndrome (OMIM 193500)

The distinguishing feature of WS1 is dystopia canthorum, which is present in 99 percent of patients.[3,22] Together with dystopia, there is typically a broad, high nasal root. Synophyrys of the eyebrows is common, although, of course, this is also quite common in the general population. It is often disguised by plucking.

For reliable diagnosis, dystopia needs to be assessed by calculating the W index from the inner canthal, interpupillary, and outer canthal measurements rather than relying on clinical impression. The necessary formula is shown in Fig. 244-4. The rather bizarre numbers stem from a discriminant analysis. The importance of measuring the eyes and calculating the W index was demonstrated in the linkage studies performed by the Waardenburg Consortium. In the initial study,[14] only 45 percent of "WS1" families as defined by report of "hypertelorism," "wide-spaced eyes," or dystopia, mapped to 2q35. However, when the classification was based on explicitly measured W values,[23] all families linked to 2q had a mean W of affected members of 2.03 or greater, and all unlinked families had a mean W of 1.87 or less (Fig. 244-5). The previously accepted threshold value of W of 2.07 or greater misclassified one family that had in fact earlier been

reported as an example of a WS2 family with a *PAX3* mutation[24] but is now seen as a WS1 family.

Thus, for a diagnosis of WS1, the average W value of all affected people in the family should be 1.95 or more. If the average W is less than 1.95, the diagnosis is WS2. Within a family, the degree of dystopia can vary, and an occasional individual may fall the wrong side of the threshold, as illustrated in Fig. 244-5. Inevitably, the attempt to define a threshold value of a continuous variable will not be 100 percent successful, and the definitive criterion for WS1 should be demonstration of a *PAX3* mutation.

### Type 2 Waardenburg Syndrome (OMIM 193510)

In 1971, Arias[3] pointed out that dystopia canthorum was not a universal feature of WS; in some families all affected people had dystopia, whereas in others none did. He defined WS without dystopia as type 2. While the Waardenburg Consortium diagnostic criteria (see Table 244-2) work well for WS1, they seem less satisfactory for WS2. A single individual who is deaf and has a white forelock or heterochromia fits the criteria for WS2, but extended type 2 families with many affected individuals are uncommon. On the other hand, we see many families where, perhaps, a woman with a white forelock has a deaf child or a sister with heterochromia. Evidently these are families where a

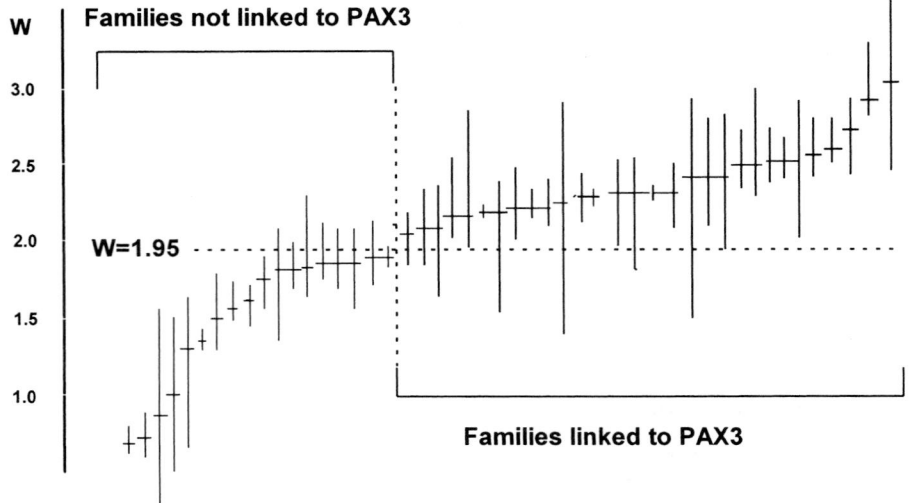

**Fig. 244-5 Classification of WS families according to W index and *PAX3* linkage. Each vertical line represents a family and shows the maximum and minimum W values among affected individuals in the family. The cross-bar shows the average W value of affected people within each family. All families showing linkage to the *PAX3* locus on chromosome 2q35 (WS1 families) have the average W > 1.95, whereas all unlinked families (WS2 families) have the average W < 1.95. However, for individuals, the ranges overlap. (*Data from the Waardenburg Consortium.*[23])**

polygenic or low-penetrance dominant tendency to neural crest or melanocyte malfunction exists. They may or may not qualify as WS2 families, depending on whether or not one individual happens to show two major features. We have investigated many of these "penumbra" families for mutations in the *PAX3*, *MITF*, *EDNRB*, and *EDN3* genes, with uniformly negative results. Our families with *MITF* mutations have a much more unambiguous history of WS. Probably for guiding mutation screening, a better criterion of WS2 may be that a person should show two major features, as defined in Table 244-2, and have a first-degree relative who also shows two major features.

When comparing the penetrances of the various features of WS2 with those for WS1 in Table 244-3, it is important to remember that a person can be diagnosed as having WS1 if he or she has only dystopia and an affected relative, whereas, without dystopia as a guide, a diagnosis of WS2 cannot be made unless the patient has hearing loss or a pigmentary anomaly plus an affected relative. This probably accounts for the rather higher frequency of hearing loss recorded in the WS2 patients.

The relative frequency of the two types has been reported very differently by different authors. Waardenburg's great paper[2] had reported dystopia in 159 of 161 subjects, but this high proportion is a result of bias of ascertainment — Waardenburg was always especially interested in the eye malformation of his syndrome. Arias and Mota[22] and Hageman and Dellemann[17] thought type 2 was more common than type 1. In our own clinical referral population, ascertained through deaf probands and not a systematic population sample, families that meet the diagnostic criteria in Table 244-2 for WS2 substantially outnumber those that meet the criteria for WS1. However, when patients rather than families are counted, the picture changes. As discussed earlier, unambiguously dominant classic WS2 in a large extended family is rare.

Figure 244-2 shows part of our largest family and illustrates the range of phenotypes. This family is especially interesting because it is probably a branch of the huge Australian family mentioned in OMIM. Both carry the same mutation in the *MITF* gene, and both can be traced back to the Ayrshire area of southwest Scotland. A very large "Ayrshire family" with inherited deafness was described by James Kerr Love, honorary aurist to the Glasgow Deaf and Dumb Institution in 1896,[25] with branches having emigrated to Australia and America. We have found the same mutation in another large British family with ill-defined Scottish ancestry. It is tempting to speculate that a significant proportion of classic WS2 patients on three continents may be part of one vast extended family.

## Waardenburg-Klein or Type 3 Waardenburg Syndrome (OMIM 148820)

In August 1947, some months before Waardenburg presented his first patient at a meeting in the Netherlands, David Klein had presented a patient to the Swiss Society of Genetics in Geneva. This 10-year-old girl had a severely disabling amyoplasia-like condition affecting her arms and shoulders, with absence of muscles, joint contractures, axillary webs, and camptodactyly of all fingers, in addition to dystopia canthorum, profound bilateral hearing loss, and extensive depigmentation of her skin, hair, and eyes; for photographs and a historical description, see Klein.[26] It was after seeing this patient in 1948 that Waardenburg was moved to begin his systematic investigation. In his paper,[2] Waardenburg speculated that she might be homozygous for his syndrome. This question has recently been resolved (see below). The patient strikingly resembles a proven WS1 homozygote described by Zlotogora et al.[27] and illustrated in Fig. 244-3, but Klein[26] describes her parents as normal and nonconsanguineous. Klein's patient was so different from the patients Waardenburg investigated later in the Netherlands that he came to doubt her relevance to his syndrome, a view that gave rise to some ill feeling.

Subsequently, the label *Klein-Waardenburg syndrome* or *WS3* was applied to rare patients with the combination of typical WS

and hypoplasia or contractures of the limb muscles or joints. Details of the early reports are well summarized by Goodman et al.[28] With the exception of Zlotogora's patient mentioned earlier, all reported WS3 patients are much less severely affected than Klein's patient. In only one case[28] does WS3 recur within a family. The proband in this family had dystopia canthorum (W = 2.25) and decreased hearing in his right ear. His pigmentation was normal, but his mother reported that he had a small white forelock as a child. His arms were hypoplastic with decreased muscle mass, limitation of movement at both elbows, no movement of his wrists, and flexion contractures of all fingers. His sister had dystopia (W = 2.28), normal pigmentation, but moderate hypoplasia of her hand muscles and flexion contractures of her fingers. Her clinical picture was complicated by microcephaly, severe mental retardation, and spastic paraplegia, presumed unrelated to her WS.[28] A later report[29] described the two children of the proband who both have WS facial features together with bilateral flexion contractures of the fingers.

All other reported cases of WS3 are either sporadic[26,30] or have relatives with typical WS1.[26,31] Molecular analysis has revealed that several WS3 patients, including those in the family reported by Goodman et al.[28] and Sheffer and Zlotogora[29] and the family of Wieacker,[31] are heterozygous for *PAX3* mutations.[32,33] Thus it appears that the label WS3 has been applied to at least three classes of patients:

1. Patients heterozygous for a *PAX3* mutation that normally does not affect limb development but that for some reason has produced more severe effects in this particular case (the family of Marx in ref. 26; family WS.105 in ref. 33). Since *PAX3* is known to control expression of MyoD in limb buds (see below), it is not surprising that mutations occasionally should affect limb development.
2. Patients with a *PAX3* mutation that regularly affects limb development in heterozygotes (the family of Goodman and Sheffer; see ref. 29).
3. Patients homozygous for *PAX3* mutations (although note that most homozygotes are expected to have lethal neural tube defects; see below): the patients of Zlotogora et al.[27] (see Fig. 244-3) and maybe Klein.[26]

As far as we are aware, the combination of WS2 with WS3-like limb abnormalities (i.e., WS3 without dystopia canthorum) has not been described.

## Shah-Waardenburg or Type 4 Waardenburg Syndrome (OMIM 277580)

The rare patients having a combination of hearing loss, pigmentary abnormalities, and Hirschsprung disease are described as having *Shah-Waardenburg syndrome* or WS4. Enteric neurons, like melanocytes, are neural crest derivatives, and this combination of effects is presumably the result of defects in a population of pluripotent neural crest cells in the embryo or in a regulatory mechanism used by several lineages.

In 1962, Shah et al.[34] described 12 babies that had white forelocks and Hirschsprung disease, born to five Indian families. A pigmentary anomaly of the eyes also was mentioned ("isochromia irides, light brown irides with mosaic pattern"), but this was said to be "a common inherited condition in our population." It is not clear whether any had dystopia canthorum, and all the babies died before their hearing could be tested. Later, Omenn and McKusick[35] described six cases in four pedigrees. Two were said to have dystopia, and a third had "typical Waardenburg syndrome," but eye measurements were not reported. One pedigree was clearly dominant, the others each have only a single case of complete WS4, but in two cases relatives had hearing loss or hypopigmentation of the hair or a raised inner canthal distance.

These initial reports left open the question whether Hirschsprung disease is an occasional complication of typical WS1 and/ or WS2 or whether there exist one or more unitary and distinctive

**Table 244-4** *Pax-3* Mutations in the *Splotch* Mouse, a Model for Type 1 Waardenburg Syndrome

| Allele | Features | PAX-3 Mutation | Reference |
|---|---|---|---|
| Sp (Splotch) | Heterozygotes: white belly spot; normal hearing; dystopia on certain genetic backgrounds Homozygotes: as Sp²ᴴ | 3′ end of intron 3 CTTTTCTCCAG to CTTTCGTGTG (splice acceptor site is underlined) | 42 |
| Spʳ (Splotch-retarded) | Heterozygotes: as Sp, but also growth retarded. Homozygotes: preimplantation lethal | Large chromosomal deletion, ca. 14 cM, including whole of Pax-3 | 43 |
| Sp²ᴴ | Heterozygotes: as Sp Homozygotes: All have lethal neural tube defects; 60% die at E13.5–14.5 from heart defects | Deletion of 32 basepairs within the homeodomain | 44 |
| Spᵈ (Splotch-delayed) | Heterozygotes: as Sp Homozygotes: as Sp, but survive longer | Point mutation G42R in the paired domain | 45 |

Mendelian WS4 syndromes. Recent molecular studies have greatly clarified the position. Hirschsprung disease is rare among patients with *PAX3* mutations, probably no more common than in the general population, and conversely, patients with *RET* mutations (that can cause Hirschsprung disease) are not at increased risk of hearing loss (M Seri, personal communication, 1997). Three separate genetic defects have been identified that can produce a WS-Hirschsprung disease phenotype, as described below (recessive in the case of endothelin-3 and endothelin receptor B, dominant with *SOX10* mutations), in each case with quite variable expression. In addition, some patients with as yet undefined molecular defects have neurocristopathies that fall into the WS4 spectrum.

## MOUSE MODELS OF WS

Each subtype of WS has a murine homologue: *Splotch* (*Sp*) for WS1 and WS3; *microphthalmia* (*mi*) for WS2; and *piebald-lethal* (*s¹*), *lethal spotted* (*ls*), and *Dominant megacolon* (*Dom*) for the different forms of WS4.

### Splotch, a Model for WS1

*Sp* mice have been studied extensively as a model for human neural tube defects.[36] Almost all homozygous embryos have lethal neural tube defects[36] and defective development of limb muscles.[37] Interestingly, they show defective folate handling, and the neural tube defects can be rescued at least partially with folate supplementation.[21] About half of all the homozygous embryos die at E14 with severe heart malformations strikingly similar to those of Di George syndrome.[38,39] Heterozygous *Sp/+* mice appear normal except for a white belly splotch. A broad snout, corresponding to the dystopia of WS1, is recognizable on some genetic backgrounds,[40] but they have normal hearing.[41] The mutations in most of the known *Splotch* alleles have been characterized (Table 244-4).

### Microphthalmia, a Model for WS2

Despite the name, *mi* mutations primarily affect pigmentation. For a review of mutations at this locus, see Moore.[46] Over a dozen alleles are known, some recessive and others dominant. Heterozygotes are either unaffected or show spotting and/or dilution of coat color. Homozygotes have white coats, together with varying combinations of abnormalities of the eye (microphthalmia, sometimes retinal degeneration, or cataracts), inner ear, skeleton

(delayed eruption of incisors and later, osteopetrosis), and a deficiency of mast cells and natural killer (NK) cells. The *vitiligo* (*miᵛⁱᵗ*) homozygote shows progressive depigmentation of the coat, reminiscent of the early graying seen in many WS2 patients. Some alleles modify the effects of others, a particularly striking example being the *spotted* (*miˢᵖ*) allele that produces no effect in *miˢᵖ/+* or *miˢᵖ/miˢᵖ* mice but does produce a phenotype in compound heterozygotes such as *miˢᵖ/Miʷʰ*.

The *mi* gene was cloned by two groups, taking advantage of fortuitous transgene insertions that generated new mutant alleles.[47,48] Most of the mutations have now been defined. Table 244-5 gives some examples. The molecular pathology is considered below.

### Lethal spotting, piebald lethal, and Dominant megacolon, Models for WS4

Three mouse mutants have white spotting plus megacolon (Hirschsprung disease). The *piebald* (*s*) mouse has a mild mutation that causes white spotting in 20 percent of homozygotes, but homozygotes for a severe allele, *piebald-lethal* (*s¹*), are almost completely white (but retain melanocytes in the retinal pigment epithelium) and always have megacolon.[51] The *lethal spotting* (*ls*) mouse again shows white spotting and megacolon in homozygotes.[51] Mice heterozygous for the *Dominant megacolon* (*Dom*) mutation show a phenotype in heterozygotes similar to *s¹/s¹* or *ls/ls* homozygotes, whereas *Dom/Dom* homozygotes are embryonic lethal.[52]

All three mutants were candidate homologues for human Hirschsprung disease or WS4, and programs were mounted to clone the underlying genes. Unexpectedly, a targeted knockout of the endothelin receptor B gene *Ednrb* turned out to have identified the *piebald* (*s*) gene.[53] Targeted disruption of the gene for the Ednrb ligand then identified the *lethal spotting* gene as the endothelin 3 (*Edn3*) gene.[54] *Dom* was identified as the *SOX10* gene by positional cloning.[55,56]

## MAPPING AND IDENTIFICATION OF WS GENES

### WS1 and PAX3

An early report of possible linkage of WS1 and ABO blood group[57] has not been confirmed. A number of possible candidate locations were suggested on the basis of phenotypic resemblance to mouse mutants,[58] but the decisive clue came from the report by

**Table 244-5** Examples of *mi* Gene Mutations in the *microphthalmia* Mouse, a Model for Type 2 Waardenburg Syndrome

| Allele | Phenotype | Mutation |
|---|---|---|
| *mi* | Heterozygotes: white head spot Homozygotes: white coat, hearing loss, microphthalmia, osteopetrosis, reduced mast cells | In-frame deletion of 3 basepairs del(R214) |
| *Mi^or* (Oak Ridge) | Heterozygotes: diluted pigment plus white spot on head (like white forelock) Homozygotes: white coat, microphthalmia, osteopetrosis | Missense mutation R216K in basic region |
| *Mi^b* (brownish) | Heterozygotes: dilution of color but no spots Homozygotes: white coat; normal-sized eyes | Missense mutation G244D in helix 2 of HLH domain |
| *Mi^wh* (white) | Heterozygotes: diluted pigment plus white spots; inner ear defect Homozygotes: white coat, reduced eye size, inner ear defects, reduced mast cells | Missense mutation I212N in basic region |
| *mi^ce* (cloudy eyes) | Heterozygotes: normal Homozygotes: white coat, reduced eye size, inner ear defect, cataracts | Nonsense mutation R263X after helix 2 of HLH domain |
| *mi^vit* (vitiligo) | Heterozygotes: normal Homozygotes: initial spotting, progressive depigmentation with retinal degeneration | Missense mutation D222N in helix 1 of HLH domain |
| *mi^sp* (spotted) | Heterozygotes: normal Homozygotes: normal Double heterozygotes with *mi*, *Mi^wh*, etc. show modified pigmentation | Insertion of 1 nucleotide, causing a shift in the relative proportions of two differentially spliced *mi* transcripts |

SOURCE: Data from refs. 49 and 50. Many other mutant *mi* alleles have been described.

Ishikiriyama et al.[59] in 1989 of a Japanese child with *de novo* WS1 and an inversion, inv(2)(q35;q37.3). Linkage was quickly established ($\hat{z} = 4.76$ at $\theta$ 0.023)[60] between WS1 and an RFLP in the placental alkaline phosphatase gene *ALPP*, believed at the time to map to 2q37 but subsequently shown to map to 2q35-q36. Collaborative studies by the Waardenburg Consortium showed that, provided careful attention was paid to measuring the W index, all informative families with WS1 showed linkage to 2q

markers, whereas no WS2 families did.[23] The distal part of human chromosome 2q has well-preserved homology with proximal chromosome 1 in the mouse. This led Foy et al.[60] to suggest that *Splotch* was the mouse homologue of WS1, a suggestion confirmed when the genes underlying both phenotypes were cloned.

The mouse *Pax-3* gene was known to map in the general region of *Splotch* on chromosome 1 and, because of its pattern of expression in the embryonic neural crest, was a good candidate for *Splotch*. Similarly, once human linkage analysis had shown that WS1 was the likely human homologue of *Splotch*,[60] the human *PAX3* gene became a strong candidate for the WS1 gene. Mutation screening was performed independently and simultaneously in the mouse and humans. Part of the human *Pax-3* homologue had been isolated by Burri et al.[61] under the name *HUP2*. Mutations were quickly found in mouse by the Montreal group[42,44,45] and in humans independently by Baldwin et al.[62] and ourselves.[63] At the time this attracted considerable interest because WS1 was the first human disease shown to be caused by inherited mutations in a homeobox gene.

## Other WS Loci

Mapping of WS2 was more difficult. Since the syndrome is defined negatively, by the absence of dystopia, it seemed likely that it would be heterogeneous, and in addition, very few WS2 families are suitable for analysis. Most families are small, and without dystopia, there is no reliable guide to affection status; individuals with minimal signs or with coincidental hearing loss are likely to be misclassified. The *microphthalmia* mouse had long been recognized as a good candidate homologue of WS2,[58] but poor conservation of human-mouse synteny around the *mi* locus on mouse chromosome 6 prevented successful prediction of the corresponding location in humans. Genes closely linked to *mi* have human homologues at 3p25-p26 (*Raf-1*, *Il5r*), 3q21-q24 (*Rho*), and 10q11 (*Ret*), but markers from these loci showed no linkage to WS2 (M Tassabehji and AP Read, unpublished data, 1992).

One very large family was available in Manchester that was suitable for a full genome search (Fig. 244-2 shows part of the pedigree), and using this family, Hughes et al.[64] showed linkage to several microsatellite markers at 3p12-p14, particularly *D3S1261* ($\hat{z} = 6.48$ at zero recombination). Meanwhile, Tachibana et al.[65] had isolated *MITF* (microphthalmia-associated transcription factor), the human homologue of the mouse *mi* gene, and mapped it by fluorescence in situ hybridisation to 3p14. This made *MITF* a compelling candidate for 3p-linked WS2, and mutations were found quickly.[66] It is still not known what proportion of WS2 families map to this location, although the low success rate of *MITF* mutation screening (see below) suggests that it is a small minority, maybe 10 to 15 percent. No other WS2 locus has yet been defined.

With both the 2q and the 3p linkages, work proceeded rapidly from initial linkage to identification of the disease gene, so in neither case has a detailed genetic map around the disease locus been defined by studies within affected families. WS3, as described earlier, is almost never familial and is not suitable for linkage studies. For WS4, again, most cases are sporadic, but an initial location on 13q22 was defined in a single very large and complex Mennonite family.[67] The suspicion that 13q included a neurocristopathy locus was reinforced by several case reports of patients with 13q deletions who had either Hirschsprung disease[68–70] or WS2.[71] In the Mennonite family, the pattern of inheritance was complex, with both recessive and autosomal dominant inheritance with reduced penetrance being possible, and evidently more than one Hirschsprung disease-susceptibility gene is segregating in the family. Thus precise localization of the 13q gene by linkage analysis was difficult but fortunately was rendered unnecessary when identification of *Ednrb* as the gene underlying the mouse *piebald-lethal* mutant (see above) suggested a strong positional candidate. This was confirmed when a mutation was demonstrated in the human *EDNRB* gene in the Mennonite family.[72] The other WS4 genes, *EDN3* and *SOX10*, were defined by mutation analysis of candidate genes without human mapping work.

## MOLECULAR PATHOLOGY OF WS: *PAX3* AND WS1

### Structure and Function of *PAX3*

*PAX3* is one of a family of nine human *PAX* genes, defined by the presence of a paired box (Table 244-6). The paired box, a 128-amino-acid DNA-binding domain, is so called because it was originally recognized in the *Drosophila* gene *paired* (*prd*).[73] Some members of the *PAX* gene family also contain a homeobox. Within the *PAX* family, *PAX3* and *PAX7* are closely related, as are *PAX2*, *PAX5* and *PAX8*, and *PAX1* and *PAX9*. *PAX3*, *PAX4*, *PAX6*, and *PAX7* have a complete homeobox, *PAX2*, *PAX5*, and *PAX8* have a truncated homeobox that is unlikely to be functional, whereas *PAX1* and *PAX9* completely lack a homeobox. Family members are dispersed to different chromosomal locations, and each has a mouse homologue. Study of naturally occurring human and mouse mutants and mouse knockouts has shown that loss-of-function mutations at each of the nine loci have significant effects on embryonic development, at least in homozygotes and often in heterozygotes. For general reviews of *PAX* genes, see refs 74-76.

The mouse *Pax-3* sequence[90] predicted a protein containing both a paired domain and a homeodomain. Burri's original *HUP2* sequence[61] contained only the paired box of the human *PAX3*. A complete human cDNA sequence was obtained by Hoth et al.[32] The human gene extends over approximately 100 kb of genomic DNA[91] and has been localized by FISH to the boundary of 2q35 and 2q36.[92] Exon-intron boundaries were defined and polymerase chain reaction (PCR) primers designed to amplify each exon

from genomic DNA,[32,33,93] and recently, the 3' structure has been characterized. The human *PAX3* gene has 10 exons, with the paired box in exons 2 to 4 and the homeobox in exons 5 and 6 (Fig. 244-6).

Alternative splice forms of *PAX3* have been reported. Tsukamoto et al.[94] reported amplifying two novel transcripts from adult human tissues. One transcript reads through from exon 4 into intron 4 and is predicted to encode an extra 19 amino acids from the intron 4 sequence until a stop codon is reached. A second transcript uses a cryptic acceptor site within intron 4 to splice a novel small exon containing an in-frame stop codon onto the normal exon 1 to 4 product. There is also differential splicing of the 3' end of the transcript. Barber (see ref 142 and TD Barber personal communication 1997) has shown that most transcripts use a donor splice site located within exon 8 as originally defined,[32] leading to skipping of the last 6 amino acids of exon 8 and incorporation of 32 new amino acids encoded by two new 3' exons. No differential functions have been ascribed to any of these variants. The variants described by Tsukamoto et al.[94] lack a homeobox and closely resemble the predicted transcripts from some apparently nonfunctional *PAX3* mutants (see below). A possibly functional differential splice event occurs at the start of exon 3 in mouse *Pax-3*.[95] Two alternative splice acceptor sites lead to the presence or absence of glutamine-108, and these two forms differ in their binding to some oligonucleotide targets. The published sequences of most other paired-domain proteins do not contain this glutamine (see the alignments in ref. 96).

All PAX proteins are DNA-binding transcription factors that are expressed in the early embryo, mostly in the developing nervous system. Related paired-domain proteins exist in many other organisms. As with all transcription factors, identifying the upstream regulators and downstream targets has proved difficult. In vitro studies have attempted to define the target DNA sequences

**Table 244-6** The *PAX* Gene Family

| Gene | Loss-of-Function Phenotype in Mouse | Reference | Human Map Location | Loss-of-function Phenotype in Humans | Reference |
|---|---|---|---|---|---|
| *PAX1/Pax-1* | *Undulated*[a]: −/−: vertebral abnormalities etc | 77 | 20p11 | ? | |
| *PAX2/Pax-2* | −/−[b]: renal agenesis, eye and brain abnormalities | 78 | 10q25 | +/−: vesicoureteral reflux, optic neuroma | 86 |
| *PAX3/Pax-3* | *Splotch*[a]: +/−: pigmentary changes −/−: neural tube defects etc | 36−45 | 2q35 | +/−: Waardenburg syndrome type 1 and type 3 | |
| *PAX4/Pax-4* | −/−[b]: absence of pancreatic β-cells | 79 | 7q31.3 | ? | |
| *PAX5/Pax-5* | −/−[b]: Block of B-cell differentiation, altered patterning of midbrain | 80 | 9p13 | ? | |
| *PAX6/Pax-6* | −/−: *Small eye*[a]: defects of eyes and nose | 81, 82 | 11p13 | +/−: aniridia, Peter anomaly | 87, 88 |
| *PAX7/Pax-7* | −/−[b]: malformations of face and cephalic neural crest derivatives | 83 | 1p36 | ? | |
| *PAX8/Pax-8* | −/−[b]: absence of follicular cells of thyroid | 84 | 2q12 | +/−: thyroid agenesis | 89 |
| *PAX9/Pax-9* | −/−[b]: no thymus or parathyroids; limb and skeletal abnormalities; arrest of tooch development | 85 | 14q12 | ? | |

NOTE: +/−: phenotype of heterozygote, −/−: phenotype of homozygote. For fuller descriptions of phenotypes, see refs. 74−76 and individual references cited.
[a]Naturally occurring mouse mutant
[b]Mouse knockout

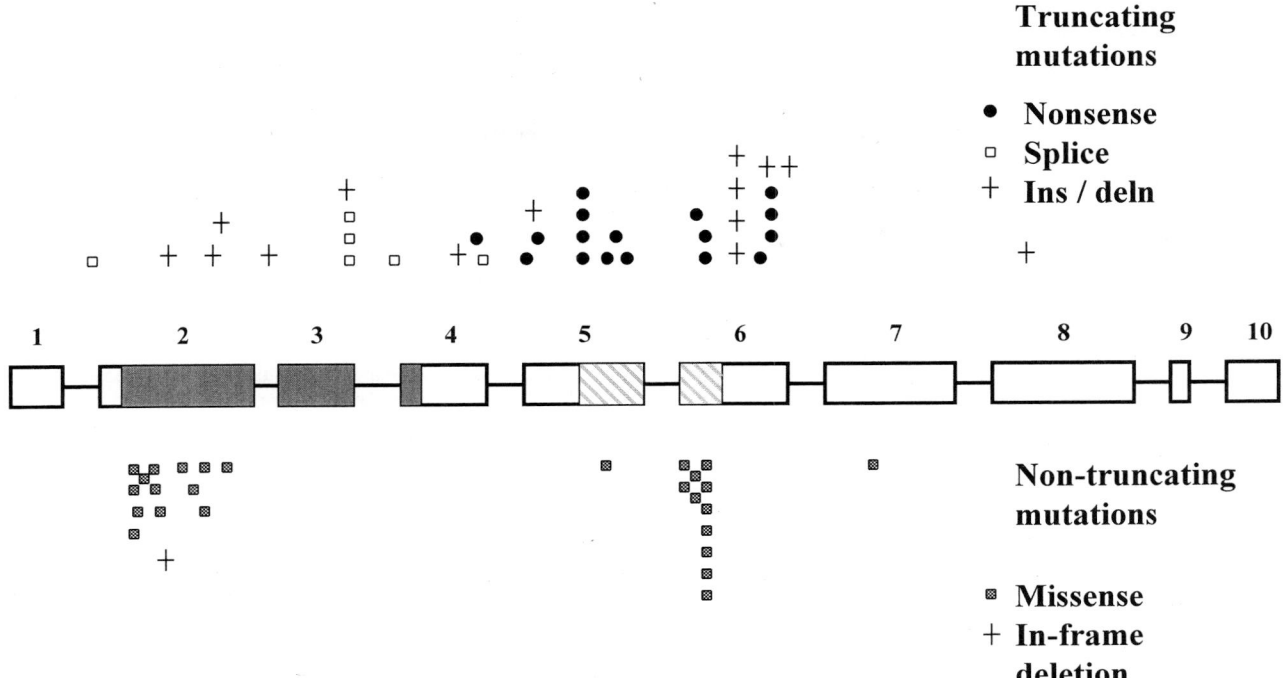

Fig. 244-6 *PAX3* gene structure and mutations. The gene comprises 10 exons; the paired box in exons 2 to 4 and the homeobox in exons 5 to 6 are marked. The distribution of truncating (frameshifting insertions or deletions, splice-site, and nonsense) mutations and nontruncating (in-frame deletion and missense) mutations are shown. Note that missense mutations causing WS are almost entirely confined to the 5′ part of the paired box and the 3′ part of the homeobox.

bound by PAX proteins. A poorly conserved set of sequences has been identified that bind isolated paired domains, but how far these identify natural targets of PAX proteins is unclear. One starting point is the e5 sequence from the *Drosophila even-skipped* gene, which is known to bind prd protein, as a target; however, there is no evidence of interaction between *paired* and *even-skipped* in the intact *Drosophila*. Systematic mutation of e5 nucleotides suggested a consensus Pax recognition sequence of GTTCC.[97] Alternatively, the Selex procedure[98] can be used to select from a random mixture of oligonucleotides those which bind paired domains. Protein-DNA complexes are precipitated, the bound oligonucleotides are amplified, and these are used in further rounds of selection. In this way, a consensus binding sequence TTCACGC(A/T)T(G/C)ANT(G/T)(A/C) was identified for the PAX2 and PAX6 paired domains.[98] This sequence is similar but not identical to known natural targets of PAX5 and PAX8. A similar exercise for the PAX3 paired domain suggested a sequence CGTCACG(G/C)TT.[99] For the homeodomain, a core sequence TAATN$_{2-3}$ATTA is recognized by PAX homeodomains.[100]

Most studies of in vitro binding have suggested that it is primarily the N-terminal part of the paired domain that makes the specific DNA contacts, and analysis of mutations (see below) supports this. However, more recently, evidence has accumulated that the C-terminal part also may be important.[101] There is also evidence that the paired and homeodomains bind cooperatively, because PAX3 proteins with mutations in the homeodomain show diminished binding by the paired domain to its target.[102]

All binding assays suffer from the problem that they can only define the sequences with the tightest binding, which may well not be the natural targets. Transcription factors that control important developmental switches need a very finely balanced affinity for their targets so that they can bind in some circumstances and not in others. It may well be that the sequence with the strongest affinity for the protein would not fulfill that requirement (just as hemoglobins with too high an oxygen affinity

cause oxygen transport to malfunction). Additionally, cell transfection assays suffer from the uncontrollable and often unnaturally high levels of expression achieved. The alternative is to try to identify natural downstream targets by genetic analysis. Here the main problem is to distinguish direct from indirect effects. In the case of *PAX3*, *MITF, Met*, and *MyoD* have been identified as targets. These have very interesting implications that are discussed below.

Having bound its DNA target, PAX3 protein must cause some action, and there is evidence that the C-terminal 78 amino acids of the protein, which are rich in proline, serine, and threonine, can activate transcription of a reporter gene located downstream of a PAX3-binding sequence.[103] Curiously, the N-terminal 90 amino acids, including the 5′ part of the paired domain, strongly inhibit transcription of target constructs in vitro.[103] Recently, evidence has emerged of protein-protein interactions involving the homeodomain of PAX3.[104]

## Mutation Analysis of *PAX3*

Mutations have been found in most parts of the *PAX3* gene, with the notable exception of the 3′ end downstream of the homeobox. Point mutations include missense, nonsense, and splice-site mutations and numerous frameshifting small deletions and insertions. Several patients have complete deletion of the gene. Most mutations are private, but a few recur. Six families have missense mutations of arginine-271, and four have the nonsense mutation R223X; both mutations affect the mutable CpG dinucleotide. A further four families have an insertion of an extra guanine into a run of six guanines [variously called 874ins(G) or 880ins(G)]; this is likely due to slipped-strand mispairing, a known hotspot mechanism. There is also at least one common expressed polymorphism, T315K,[93] that occasionally has been mistaken for a pathogenic mutation.

Figure 244-6 and Table 244-7 show the *PAX3* mutations described to date. Two interesting features emerge from this collection. First, with only rare exceptions (see below), deletions,

**Table 244-7** *PAX3* Mutations

| Mutation | Exon and Position | Phenotype | Reference |
|---|---|---|---|
| **Deletion/disruption of gene** | | | |
| del(2)(q34q36.2) | | WS1, growth retardation, mental retardation | 93 |
| del(2)(q**) | | WS3 | 30 |
| del(2)(q35−q36.1) | | WS1; below average intelligence | 105 |
| del(2)(q35q36.2) | | WS3+spina bifida (2 cases) | 106 |
| inv(2)(q35q37.3) | | WS1 | 59 |
| **Truncating mutations** | | | |
| 86−2 A → G | E2 | WS1 | 107 |
| 191del(17) | E2 | WS1 | 33 |
| 266del(14) | E2 | WS1 | 108 |
| 288del(1) | E2 | WS1 | 24 |
| **del(16) | E2? | WS3 | Unpub. |
| 358del(G) | E3 | WS1 | 33 |
| 364del(5) | E3 | WS1 | 33 |
| 451+1 G → T | E3 | WS1 | 93 |
| 451+1 G → A | E3 | WS1 | 109 |
| 451+2 T → G | E3 | WS1 | Unpub. |
| 452−2 A → G | E4 | WS1 | 93 |
| 556del(2) | E4 | WS1 | 24 |
| R195X | E4 | WS1 | Unpub. |
| A196T | E4 | WS1 | 33 |
| 596del(5) | E5 | WS1+spina bifida | 112 |
| Q200X | E5 | WS1 | 111 |
| S201X | E5 | BU4 | 111 |
| R223X | E5 | WS1 (4 families) | Unpub. 111 |
| E235X | E5 | BU8 | 111 |
| E251X | E5 | WS1 | 33 |
| Q254X | E5 | WS1 | 33 |
| W266X | E6 | WS1 | Unpub. |
| W274X | E6 | WS1 (2 families) | 33 |
| 874ins(G) | E6 | WS1 (4 families) | 33,111 |
| 916del(C) | E6 | WS3 | 33 |
| Y305X | E6 | WS1 | Unpub. |
| Y312X | E6 | WS1 | Unpub. |
| Q313X | E6 | WS1 (2 families) | Unpub., 111 |
| 954del(1) | E6 | WS1 | 111 |
| 1185ins(TGA) | E8 | WS1 | 111 |
| **Missense and other nontruncating mutations** | | | |
| F45L | E2 PB-N | WS1 | 93 |
| N47H | E2 PB-N | WS3 | 32 |
| N47K | E2 PB-N | Craniofacial-deafness-hand | 13 |
| P50L | E2 PB-N | WS1 | 62 |
| R56C | E2 PB-N | WS1 | Unpub. |
| R56L | E2 PB-N | WS1 | 32 |
| V60M | E2 PB-N | WS1 | 111 |
| M62R | E2 PB-N | WS1 | Unpub. |
| 185del(18) | E2 PB-N | WS1 | 63 |
| V78M | E2 PB-N | WS1 | 33 |
| G81A | E2 PB-N | WS1 | 24 |
| S84F | E2 PB-N | WS1 and homozygote | 27 |
| K85E | E2 PB-N | WS1 | 111 |
| G99D | E2 PB-N | WS1 | 93 |
| F238S | E5 | WS1 | 111 |
| V265F | E6 HD-H3 | WS1 | 110 |

**Table 244-7** (Continued)

| Mutation | Exon and Position | Phenotype | Reference |
|---|---|---|---|
| W266C | E6 HD-H3 | WS1 | 33 |
| N269L | E6 HD-H3 | WS1+homozygote | Unpub. |
| R270L | E6 HD-H3 | WS1 | Unpub. |
| R270C | E6 HD-H3 | WS1 | 33 |
| R271C | E6 HD-H3 | WS1 (3 families) | 33, unpub. |
| R271G | E6 HD-H3 | WS1 | 110 |
| R271H | E6 HD-H3 | WS1 (2 families) | 33 |
| S342G | E7 | WS1 | unpub |

NOTE: Location of mutations: PB-N: N-terminal part of paired domain. HD-H3: 3rd helix of homeodomain. Unpub., M Tassabehji & AP Read, unpublished data.

nonsense mutations, and missense mutations all produce substantially the same (variable) WS1 phenotype. This points strongly to haploinsufficiency as the molecular mechanism underlying WS1. Second, while nonsense and frameshifting mutations are distributed through most of the gene sequence, missense mutations are almost entirely confined to two regions, the 5′ part of the paired box in exon 2 and the third helix of the homeodomain in exon 6. These regions have been identified in x-ray crystallography studies of related proteins as making the main protein-DNA contacts,[96,114,115] and in fact, the known sites of missense mutations coincide precisely with residues that make important contacts. In vitro studies by electrophoretic mobility shift analysis have confirmed that several of the missense mutants encode proteins with defective DNA binding.[102]

One apparent exception to the rule that missense mutations affect highly conserved amino acids that make crucial DNA contacts is the mutation A196T (see Table 244-7). This affects a nonconserved amino acid with no known function in the PAX3 protein. However, looking at the DNA sequence, we see that the mutation is a G → A transversion affecting the 3′ end nucleotide of exon 4. The 3′ end nucleotide of most exons is usually G, and in other genes its replacement by A leads to missplicing.[116] Thus probably A196T is a splicing mutation. Another questionable mutation is S342G, the only missense mutation we have found in the 3′ part of the gene. Whether it is pathogenic or just a rare nonpathogenic variant is not known.

It is interesting to note that no missense mutations have been found in codons 186 to 193 in exon 4. These encode the octapeptide HSIDGILS that is a conserved feature of many *PAX* genes. No function has been ascribed to this octapeptide, and the absence of missense mutations suggests that it may not be vital for the normal function of *PAX3*. Similarly, missense mutations have not been seen in the C-terminal transactivation domain (with the possible exception of S342G described earlier). Possibly these sequences have a less dosage-sensitive function than the DNA-binding sequences, so there is no phenotype in heterozygotes. Any function is likely to be downstream of the DNA-binding function because homozygous *Sp/Sp* mice with no functional Pax-3 protein generally have a similar phenotype to *Sp^d/Sp^d* mice with the octapeptide and transactivation domain intact. It would be interesting to see mice with targeted point mutations in these domains.

### Genotype-Phenotype Correlations

WS1 is very variable, and one naturally asks whether there is any correlation between clinical features and type of mutation. Families often ask what the risk would be of hearing loss if they had a mutation-bearing child but are usually not concerned about the pigmentary features. Given the wide variability within families, any genotype-phenotype correlation must be weak. However, careful statistical analysis by the Waardenburg Consortium[117] suggests that pigmentary effects are stronger with mutations that delete the homeodomain than with missense mutations or deletions that include the paired domain. Unfortunately, no significant predictor of hearing loss was found. Our own small study (unpublished) of neural tube defects in WS1 again shows no predictor. For example, a small family in which three people have WS1 with spina bifida occulta[118] has the same mutation, R271C, as two larger families in which there are no neural tube defects.

One exception to the lack of genotype-phenotype correlation concerns replacements of asparagine-47 of PAX3. A small family with N47H is the only known example of familial WS3[29,32] (see above), suggesting that the mutation has a more severe effect than other loss-of-function mutations. A second family has a striking lack of nasal cartilage, leading to an unusual phenotype described as craniofacial-deafness-hand syndrome (OMIM 122880).[13] The appearance is really quite different from typical WS1, but the affected people have a *PAX3* mutation, N47K. This family is the only example of a *PAX3* mutation causing a different condition from WS1 (apart from the role of *PAX3-FKHR* gene fusions in rhabdomyosarcoma,[119] which are gain-of-function mutations, unlike the loss-of-function mutations causing WS). DNA-binding studies provide some support for the view that there is something special about asparagine-47. Like many paired-domain mutations, N47H abolishes binding to a paired target, but uniquely, it also increases binding by the homeodomain to a homeodomain-specific oligonucleotide.[102]

### PAX3 Homozygotes

Mice homozygous for *Splotch* mutations have lethal defects (see above), and in view of the frequency of deaf-deaf marriages, this is a risk to be borne in mind for humans. Thus it was a considerable surprise when Zlotogora et al.[27] showed that a severely affected child born to consanguineous affected Arab-Israeli parents was homozygous for the mutation S84F. The child (see Fig. 244-3) had severe WS3 features, including white hair and eyebrows; depigmented skin; extreme dystopia canthorum (W > 3); rigidity of shoulders, elbows, and wrists; severe muscle wasting of the shoulders, pectoral region, and upper limbs; and severe bilateral hearing loss-but no neural defect. He is apparently mentally normal though severely disabled by his joint contractures. It is tempting to speculate that S84F is a particularly mild mutation, but the parents had typical WS1. A further similarly affected child is reported to have been born in another branch of the family but died soon after birth.

Recently Bottani and colleagues (see ref. 142) have shown that Klein's original patient[26] is a compound heterozygote for two *PAX3* mutations, G99S/R270C. The parental origin of these mutations is unknown. A very different homozygous phenotype is shown by the fetus conceived through incest between a French Gypsy brother and sister each with typical WS1.[120] The fetus was aborted because of anencephaly seen on ultrasound scan. On examination, it showed many similarities to *Sp/Sp* mouse fetuses. The fetus was exencephalic, the neck was very short and webbed, all four limbs had severe joint restriction with major webs, and there was complete disorganization of the spine, as well as many internal malformations. DNA analysis showed that both parents carried the homeodomain missense mutation N269L, and the fetus was homozygous[33] (M Tassabehji and AP Read, unpublished data, 1997).

## MOLECULAR PATHOLOGY OF WS: *MITF* AND WS2

### Structure and Function of *MITF*

Once the human *MITF* cDNA had been isolated,[65] exon-intron boundaries were defined by sequencing clones from vectorette libraries and PCR primers designed to amplify each exon.[66] The genomic structure is similar to mouse *mi*, with the coding sequence contained in nine exons (Fig. 244-7). At least in the mouse, an alternative promoter and 5′ exon are used in the heart, and there are two alternative starts for exon 6, separated by 18 nucleotides, giving isoforms with or without the six amino acids TACIFP just upstream of the basic domain.[49]

*MITF* encodes a member of the well-known basic helix-loop-helix leucine zipper (bHLH-ZIP) protein family. These proteins form homo- or heterodimers through their HLH and ZIP domains, and the dimers bind DNA through their basic domains. The DNA targets of bHLH-ZIP proteins have a consensus core sequence (the E-box) CANNTG. A specific target of *mi*, the M-box (AGT-CATGTGCT), has been identified in the promoter region of several melanocyte-specific genes such as tyrosinase and tyrosinase-related protein 1.[122] Cotransfection experiments show that mi protein activates transcription from promoters containing an *M*-box.[121] It has been suggested that *mi* may be a master gene for melanocyte differentiation, and in support of this, mouse 3T3 fibroblast cells take on a melanocyte-like appearance when transfected with *mi* and start to express tyrosinase and TRP1.[123] As discussed below, it has been shown recently that expression of *MITF* is controlled by *PAX3*.[124]

**Mutation Analysis of *MITF*.** Relatively few families have so far proved to carry *MITF* mutations. The mutations found to date, all in heterozygous form, include missense, nonsense, and splice-site point mutations (Table 244-8). The missense mutations mostly affect residues in the known functional domains, such as N278D, which places a polar amino acid in the mating face of the leucine zipper. An interesting family was reported by Morell et al.[126] An *MITF* mutation, 944del(1), caused WS2 in a family. A sequence variant in the tyrosinase gene, R402Q, also was segregating in the family. This variant is a common polymorphism that encodes an enzyme with reduced catalytic activity. When present in isolation, it has no phenotypic effect, but in compound heterozygotes with a mutant *TYR* allele, it produces an autosomal recessive ocular albinism. Individuals in the family who had just the tyrosinase variant were normal, as expected, but when they had both the *MITF* mutation and the tyrosinase variant, they had WS2 plus ocular albinism.

**Genotype-Phenotype Correlations.** *Mi* is one of the few loci where at the moment the molecular pathology is richer in the mouse than in humans. Many mutant alleles are known in the mouse, some of which are recessive and others semidominant, and some compound heterozygotes show allelic interactions (see Table 244-5). In humans, all the known alleles are manifest in heterozygotes — probably in the mouse they would be classed as semidominant because no doubt homozygotes, if we ever saw them, would be much more dramatically affected. Heterozygous mice, when affected at all, usually show spotting of the coat to varying degrees or occasionally uniform dilution of pigmentation (in *Mi^b^/+* mice, for example). No hearing loss is reported for heterozygous mice, although homozygotes for several alleles including *mi*, *Mi^wh^*, and *mi^ce^* are affected.[46] As with *Splotch* mice, humans are evidently more sensitive to hearing loss, but otherwise, the phenotypic range in humans is rather similar to that in heterozygous mice, with variable pigmentary disturbances. The range of phenotypes in homozygous mice is quite wide, including microophthalmia, osteopetrosis, and defective mast cell function. We have tested individuals with various candidate severe recessive syndromes, such as the Yemenite deaf-blind-hypopigmentation syndrome or black locks-albinism-deafness syndrome,[12] but have so far failed to discover any *MITF* homozygotes. A deaf and depigmented patient described by Hultén et al.[129] is certainly homozygous for some pigmentary defect, but more probably *KIT* than *MITF*.

Because mi protein binds its DNA target as a dimer, mutant forms that can dimerize but then prevent the dimer from binding DNA can show dominant-negative effects. Thus it is predicted that null alleles and mutants affecting the HLH-ZIP dimerization

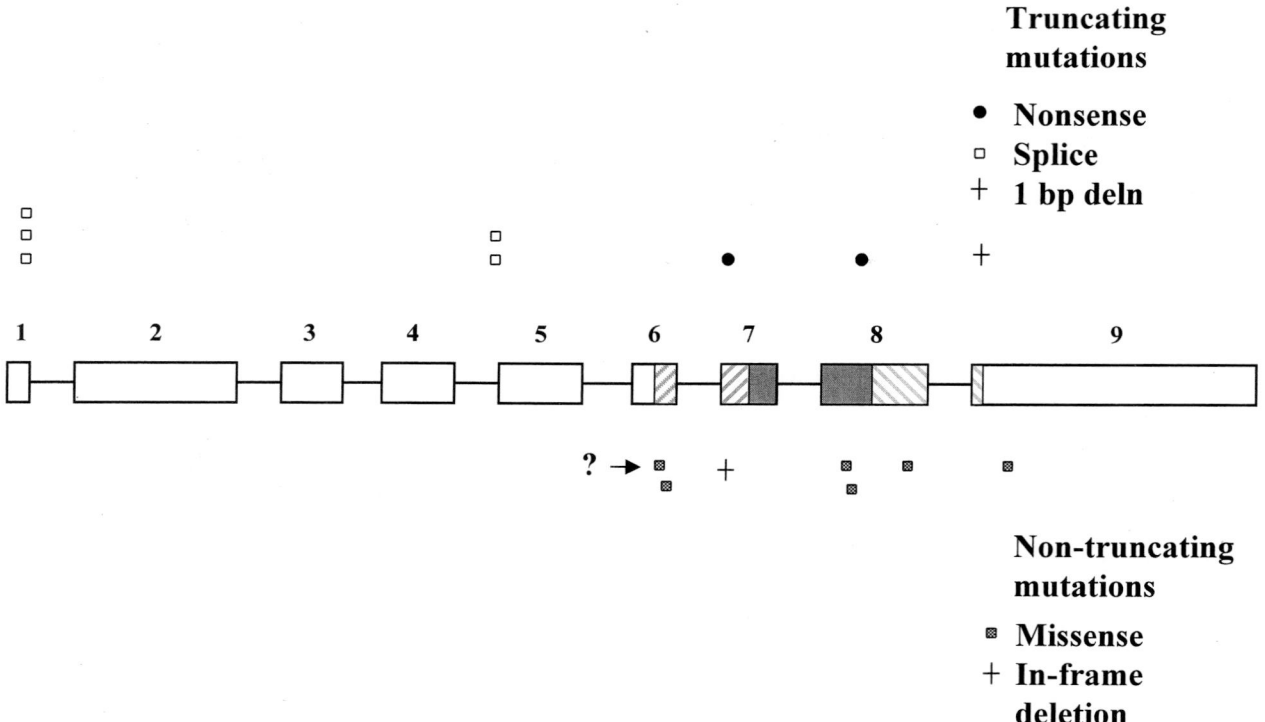

Fig. 244-7 *MITF* gene structure and mutations. The gene comprises 9 exons; the basic DNA-binding domain in exons 6 and 7, and the helix-loop-helix and leucine zipper dimerization domains in exons 7 and 8 and 8 and 9 are marked. The distribution of truncating (a 1-bp deletion and several splice-site and nonsense mutations) and nontruncating (an in-frame deletion and several missense) mutations are shown. The question mark indicates that R203K, an amino-acid substitution found in an affected person, may not be pathogenic because it does not track with WS2 in the family.

domains would be either recessive, or dominant if there is haploinsufficiency, whereas mutants affecting the DNA-binding basic domain have the potential to be dominant via a dominant-negative effect. These predictions have been tested in gel mobility assays in vitro.[122,130] The products of four basic-domain mutants *mi*, *Mi^{wh}*, *Mi^{or}*, and *mi^{ew}* not only failed to bind their DNA target but also interfered with binding of the wild-type protein. In vivo, however, only two of the four alleles show a significant phenotype in heterozygotes. The likely cause is failure of the *mi* and *mi^{ew}* products to localize to the cell nucleus[130]; probably the basic domain also contains the nuclear localization signal. At least one HLH-domain mutant, *Mi^b*, also shows defective DNA binding,[50] reminding us that dividing a linear diagram of the amino acid sequence into a series of neatly defined domains does not necessarily reflect the three-dimensional reality.

The activity of mi protein is regulated by phosphorylation of serines, at least in part through the Erk-2 protein kinase, which in turn is regulated by the *KIT* oncogene.[131] This may be the mechanism through which *KIT* mutations produce piebaldism. One WS2 mutation, S298P, replaces a serine that is a target for phosphorylation (see ref 143 & M. Tachibana personal communication 1997), in this case almost certainly by a mechanism independent of the KIT/Erk-2 system. Other complications in the molecular pathology of *mi* mutants include the possible role of heterodimers (mi protein forms heterodimers with the closely related bHLH-ZIP proteins TFEB, TFEC, and TFE3[122]) and possible differential functions of the isoforms produced by use of alternative splice acceptors at the start of exon 6. The only molecular effect of the *mi^{sp}* mutant is to prevent use of one of these sites,[49] but the mutation has a phenotype (see Table 244-5).

In humans, mutations in *MITF* can produce two different phenotypes in heterozygotes. The majority of mutations cause the relatively mild and variable WS2 syndrome. These mutations include splice-site mutants that are presumably null alleles and HLH or zipper mutants that are likely to be defective in dimerization, as well as the phosphorylation-defective S298P mutation. In two families, however, *MITF* mutations produced a much more severe and consistent phenotype. We found the del(R214) mutation in a mother and son.[127] The mother was congenitally deaf, and she had blue eyes, red hair, which went gray at age 16, and generalized skin hypopigmentation with numerous

**Table 244-8** *MITF* Mutations

| Mutation | Exon and Position | Phenotype | Reference |
|---|---|---|---|
| **Truncating mutations** | | | |
| 153+1 G → A | E1 splice donor | WS2 (3 families) | 66, 33, unpub. |
| 562−2 A → C | E5 splice acceptor | WS2 (2 families) | 66, unpub. |
| R214X | E7 Basic | WS2 | 125 |
| R259X | E8 HLH | WS2 | 127 |
| 944del(A) | E8 Zip | WS2 | 126 |
| **Missense and other nontruncating mutations** | | | |
| R203K | E6 Basic | WS2 or nonpathogenic | 33 |
| N207K | E6 Basic | Tietz | 128 |
| Del(R214) | E7 Basic | Tietz | 127 |
| S250P | E8 (HLH helix 2) | WS2 | 33 |
| Y253C | E8 | WS2 | Unpub. |
| N278D | E8 Zip | WS2 | 33 |
| S298P | E9 | WS2 | 33 |

Location of mutations: HLH: helix-loop-helix domain. Unpub: M Tassabehji & APR, unpublished data.

orange freckles. Her baby son was deaf, had auburn hair, blue eyes (at 18 months), and generalized hypopigmentation. Deafness with uniform pigmentary dilution rather than patchy depigmentation is labeled *Tietz-Smith syndrome* (OMIM 103500). This syndrome was described originally by Tietz[132] in a six-generation family where 14 people showed profound sensorineural hearing loss and uniform pigmentary dilution (partial albinism), except for the irides, which were blue with no nystagmus or photophobia. Recently, this family was shown to carry the basic domain mutation N207K in *MITF*.[128] It was reported that there was also a "CG to GC transversion adjacent to the splice junction" in exon 5.

Clearly, the *MITF* mutations in Tietz families are having a different, more severe, and more consistent effect in heterozygotes than the *MITF* mutations seen in WS2 families, and it seems likely that they do this through a dominant-negative effect. Del(R214) is identical to the original mouse *mi* mutation. As mentioned earlier, the mouse mi protein shows a dominant-negative effect in vitro, but the effect was limited in the cells studied because the mutant protein localized poorly (but partially) to the nucleus. We have tested several other families with a Tietz phenotype and not found other *MITF* mutations.

Comparing those WS2 families with known *MITF* mutations with those where no mutation was found, no clear clinical difference emerges. All the *MITF* families have classic and clearly inherited WS2, apart from those with Tietz-Smith syndrome; we have not found *MITF* mutations in any of the many "WS2 penumbra" cases tested. The incidence of hearing loss is high in *MITF* families but not dramatically higher than in other WS2 families.

### EDNRB, EDN3, and SOX10 in WS4

As described earlier, WS4, or Shah-Waardenburg syndrome, was a clinical label given to a probably highly heterogeneous group of patients who had Hirschsprung disease with deafness and/or pigmentary disturbances. Research on the mouse mutants, *piebald-lethal*, *lethal spotted*, and *Dominant megacolon* led to identification of mutations in the *EDNRB*, *EDN3*, and *SOX10* genes in a small number of patients (Table 244-9). (See Chap. 251 for other details of Hirschsprung disease.)

Endothelins are a family of three peptide hormones (endothelin-1, -2, and -3) that act through two transmembrane receptors (A and B), mainly in the control of vascular tone. The system is of considerable interest as a drug target, and mouse knockouts of all five genes have been produced. Unexpectedly, the *ednrb* and *edn3* knockouts identified the *piebald-lethal* ($s^l$) and *lethal spotted* (*ls*) loci, respectively. The phenotype of both these mutants was megacolon with spotting of the coat. The precise role of the endothelin system in neural crest function has yet to be defined.

*EDNRB* maps to 13q22 in humans, a location already known through chromosomal deletions to affect neural crest development and to which a WS4-like phenotype had been mapped in one family (see above). Puffenberger et al.[72] identified an *EDNRB* mutation, W276C, in affected family members. Many other patients with isolated Hirschsprung disease and some with WS2 or WS4 have been tested for *EDNRB* mutations, and a few have proved positive.

*EDN3* maps to 20q13. The locus encodes a large inactive precursor, preproendothelin 3, from which the active 21-amino-acid peptide (ET3) is released by proteolytic cleavage. Although there was no prior linkage evidence in humans for a neurocristo-pathy locus at this location, there is a case report[133] of a child with a balanced *de novo* 7;20 translocation with features of WS4. Again, testing a range of patients revealed heterozygous *EDN3* mutations in a few patients with isolated Hirschsprung disease. One family reported by Hofstra et al.[135] is particularly interesting (Fig. 244-8). The two affected children were homozygous for the C159F mutation in *EDN3* and had classic WS4 with total colonic aganglionosis, profound bilateral hearing loss, hypoplastic blue eyes (in Pakistani children), and pigmentary disturbances. The

parents, who were first cousins, were phenotypically normal but both heterozygous for C159F. Five first-degree relatives of the parents had hearing loss (2), pigmentary disorders (2), and pigmentary disorder plus hypoplastic blue eyes (1). That part of the pedigree looks remarkably like the "WS2 penumbra" families discussed earlier. Nevertheless, we have tested many such families for mutations in *EDNRB* and *EDN3* with uniformly negative results.

The *Sox10* gene underlying the *Dominant megacolon* (*Dom*) mouse mutant was isolated recently by positional cloning by two groups.[55,56] It encodes a member of the SOX family of transcription factors, characterized by the presence of a highly conserved HMG domain that is believed to bind double-stranded DNA and bend it, creating sites for other DNA-binding proteins to act. A human *SOX10* cDNA was isolated by screening a brain cDNA library with a rat *sox10* cDNA probe, and the genomic structure was established mainly by database searching. Primers were designed to amplify each exon, and genomic DNA samples from a range of patients were analyzed. No mutations were found in 34 patients with uncomplicated Hirschsprung disease, but mutations were found in four families with a WS4 phenotype.[138] Three of the mutations are truncating, and the fourth inserts two amino acids within the HMG domain.

### Genotype-Phenotype Relationships

Genotype-phenotype relationships are not at all straightforward with *EDNRB* or *EDN3* mutations, but a WS4 phenotype is most likely to be seen in homozygotes, and in this respect, they fit the original definition of Shah-Waardenburg syndrome as recessive. In the Mennonite family studied by Puffenberger et al.,[72] rather than simply determining a WS4 phenotype, the *EDNRB* mutation W276C behaved as one component of a polygenic determinant. Hirschsprung disease was seen in 17 of 23 W276C homozygotes and 17 of 82 heterozygotes but also 5 of 45 people homozygous for the normal allele. Some people homozygous for the mutation were deaf or had a white forelock without Hirschsprung disease, some had Hirschsprung disease without any WS features, and some had varying combinations of both.

*SOX10* mutations are dominant, although since many will be *de novo* and no doubt cases of parental mosaicism eventually will be found, these families can appear recessive. Expression is variable; in the only familial case reported,[138] a woman and her two children had the frameshifting mutation 1076del(GA). Both children had WS4 with Hirschsprung disease, but the mother showed only deafness and a white forelock. Unlike *EDNRB* and *EDN3*, *SOX10* mutations do not appear, on the present limited evidence, to be found in patients with uncomplicated Hirschsprung disease.

It is unlikely that mutations in these three genes are the only cause of WS4. Although rare, WS4 is probably highly heterogeneous. Phenotypes falling within the general definition of WS4 may result from any number of rather generalized disturbances of early neural crest function.

## WS AND DEVELOPMENT OF THE NEURAL CREST

A major reason for studying WS is to cast light on differentiation of the neural crest in the early embryo, and through the work described earlier, parts of the picture are starting to come together (Figs. 244-9 and 244-10). The subtypes of WS show the effects of different levels of PAX3 dosage and of disturbance of neural crest development at different stages.

*PAX3* is dosage-sensitive, as befits a gene and product that control a developmental switch (see Fig. 244-9). The effective dosage depends not only on the function of the *PAX3* gene but also on the genes determining the products that interact with PAX3 protein — a slight deficiency on one side may be compensated by increased efficiency on the other, within limits set by the developmental program. Development of the facial bones is especially sensitive to reduced *PAX3* dosage, and dystopia

**Table 244-9** Mutations in the *EDN3, EDNRB,* and *SOX10* Genes Associated with Type 4 Waardenburg Syndrome

| Mutation | Exon and Position | Phenotype | Reference |
|---|---|---|---|
| **EDN3 mutations** | | | |
| C159F (homozygous) | E3 (downstream of ET-3 sequence) | Total colonic aganglionosis, bilateral profound hearing loss, hypoplastic blue eyes | 135 |
| 262GC → T (homozygous) | E2 (frameshift upstream of ET-3 sequence) | Total colonic aganglionosis, bilateral hearing loss, pale blue eyes, white skin patches | 136 |
| **EDNRB mutations** | | | |
| W276C (homozygous) | E4 | Variable: HSCR and/or WS2 (see text) | 72 |
| A183G (homozygous) | E2 (3rd trans-membrane domain) | HSCR, deaf, white forelock, heterochromia | 134 |
| **SOX10 mutations** | | | |
| E189X (heterozygous) | E4 (3′ of HMG domain) | Short-segment HSCR, bilateral profound hearing loss, white hair, blue eyes, depigmented skin patches | 138 |
| Y83X (heterozygous) | E3 (5′ of HMG domain) | HSCR, profound bilateral hearing loss, fair hair, blue eyes. | 138 |
| 482ins(6) (heterozygous) | E4 (in-frame insertion within HMG box) | Short segment HSCR, deaf | 138 |
| 1076del(GA) (heterozygous) | E5 (frameshifting deletion 3′ of HMG box) | Variable; see text | 138 |

NOTE: Mutations in *EDN3* and *EDNRB* are more commonly seen in patients with uncomplicated Hirschsprung disease; see Chakravarti[137] and Chap. 251 of work for more details.

canthorum is a near-universal consequence of haploinsufficiency for *PAX3*. Melanocyte development is somewhat less sensitive, and so pigmentary problems and hearing loss appear rather variably in people with a half-dose of PAX3 protein. Limb defects generally appear only at dosage levels below 50 percent, although occasional heterozygotes for normal loss-of-function alleles show some minimal limb problems, and carriers of mutations affecting asparagine-47 appear to suffer stronger effects. Finally, at very low levels of PAX3 function, neural tube defects are seen.

PAX3 protein controls a number of genes, of which *MITF*, *MET*, and *MyoD* are particularly interesting here. Tachibana's group[124] showed that PAX3 controls expression of *MITF*. The *MITF* promoter contains the sequence ATTAATACTACTGCAAC. The underlined elements are proposed consensus-binding sequences for the PAX3 homeodomain and paired domain, respectively. Gel retardation assays and cell transfection studies showed that PAX3 (but not the P50L, R271G, or W266C mutant forms of PAX3) binds to this sequence in vitro and activates

transcription in HeLa or melanoma cells of a reporter gene placed downstream of this part of the *MITF* promoter. This is likely to be the route through which the *PAX3* locus influences melanocyte differentiation.

Epstein et al.[99] showed that the *met* gene is specifically activated by *Pax-3*. Like *MITF*, the *met* promoter contains a *Pax-3* binding site and activates transcription of a downstream reporter gene when coexpressed with *Pax-3*. *Met* encodes a tyrosine kinase that is a receptor for hepatocyte growth factor/scatter factor and is required for limb muscle development in mouse embryos. In *Splotch* mice, *met* expression in the somites is largely abolished, and this prevents migration of myoblasts into the limb buds. Probably independently of this, *Pax-3* regulates the activity of the master muscle differentiation gene, *MyoD*.[139] *Pax-3* has thus emerged as a key regulator of skeletal muscle development that is both necessary and sufficient to activate *MyoD* expression and to initiate the myogenic program in cells.[139] These interactions explain the limb defects in WS3 and *Splotch* mice.

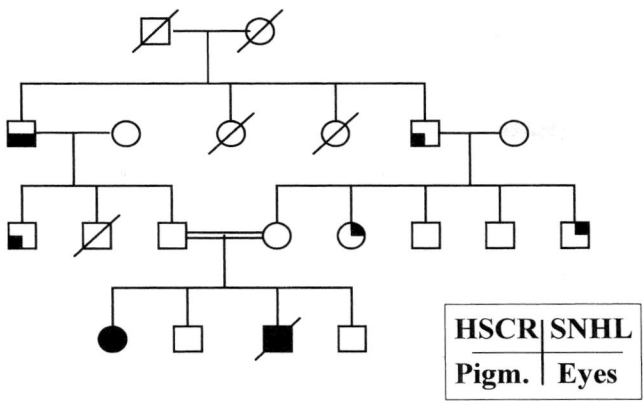

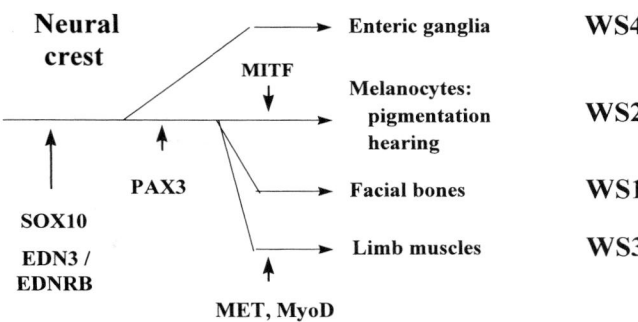

Fig. 244-10 Role of genes described in this chapter in neural crest differentiation and relationship to the various subtypes of WS.

Fig. 244-8 A Pakistani family with two children with WS-Hirschsprung disease who are homozygous for the *EDN3* mutation C159F. Note the five relatives with hearing loss or pigmentary abnormalities of the hair and/or eyes, thus resembling the "WS2 penumbra" families described in the text. (*Used with permission from Hofstra et al.*[135]) HSCR, Hirschsprung disease, SNHL, sensorineural hearing loss.

The WS4 genes (*SOX10* and *EDN3/EDNRB*) are required in lineages ancestral to both enteric neurons and melanocytes. Whether they affect a single pluripotent lineage or whether two different neural crest lineages both depend on function of these genes remains to be discovered. *MITF*, by contrast, appears in the context of WS as a melanocyte-specific gene stimulating expression of genes such as tyrosinase and tyrosinase-related protein 1, whose promoters contain the M-box sequence. Loss of function mutations in *MITF* cause WS2, and dominant-negative mutations cause Tietz-Smith syndrome.

Note, however, that as usual in development, all the findings cannot be fit onto a single linear pathway. Although *SOX10* is shown in Fig. 244-10 acting upstream of *PAX3*, the lineages affected by mutations in the two genes overlap only partially. The few patients so far described with *SOX10* (or *EDN3/EDNRB*) mutations did not have dystopia canthorum, a near-universal

feature of people with *PAX3* mutations, nor did they have limb defects. *MITF* in the figure appears as a melanocyte-specific downstream effector of *PAX3*, which is certainly one of its roles, but the range of phenotypes seen in *mi* mice (including mast cell defects, delayed dental eruption, and osteopetrosis) shows that *mi* also has other functions that are probably not controlled by *PAX3*. One of the major themes to emerge from studies of embryogenesis over the past two decades is that development is controlled by combinatorial actions of gene networks, not by single linear pathways, and the content of this chapter well illustrates this theme.

## MANAGEMENT AND TREATMENT

Hearing loss is the only general problem in WS1 or WS2, although occasional patients are troubled by the dystopia, which can be unsightly if pronounced. The hearing loss is sensorineural and not necessarily symmetric. Normally, it is nonprogressive (despite a few counterexamples), and management depends on the severity.

Prenatal diagnosis is possible for cases with a known mutation but is rarely requested. Patients thinking of the possibility need to understand that molecular analysis can predict whether a fetus carries the mutation but not how severely it will be affected. Gene therapy is a theoretical possibility but seems unlikely because the defects of WS arise so early in embryonic development. However, the hearing loss is secondary, caused by failure to maintain the correct ionic composition of the endolymph, and may in principle be preventable. Bosher and Hallpike[140] reported that hearing loss appears postnatally in deaf white cats.

Although the risk of neural tube defects is low, folate supplementation in pregnancy probably is advisable where the fetus is at risk of WS1, since *Splotch* mice show defective handling of folate, and their neural tube defects are folate-responsive.[21]

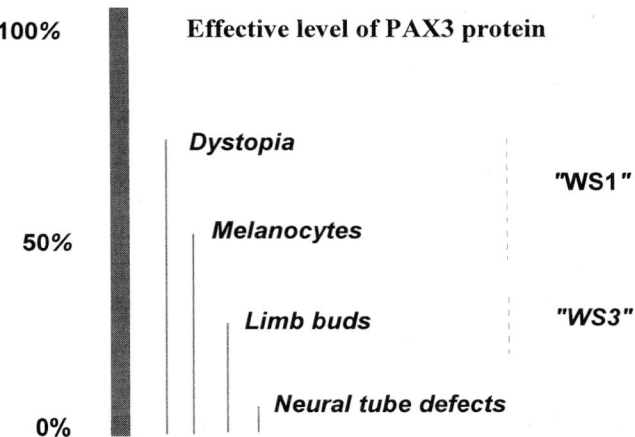

Fig. 244-9 PAX3 dosage effects. The features of WS1 and WS3 are caused by inadequate levels of the *PAX3* gene product. The effective level of PAX3 protein depends on the *PAX3* gene dosage, on the biologic activity of any mutant PAX3 protein, and on variations in the cellular systems that respond to PAX3 signaling. Dystopia canthorum is always seen when *PAX3* gene dosage is reduced; melanocyte defects are common in people with 50 percent dosage but variable and not universal. Limb defects (WS3) are uncommon in heterozygotes and may reflect abnormal activity of particular mutant proteins or inefficient PAX3 response systems. Neural tube defects are seen only in homozygotes and then not always.

## REFERENCES

1. Waardenburg PJ: Dystopia punctorum lachrimarum, blepharophimosis en partiele irisatrophie bij een doofstomme. *Ned Tschr Geneesk* **92**:3463, 1948.
2. Waardenburg PJ: A new syndrome combining developmental anomalies of the eyelids, eyebrows and nose root with pigmentary defects of the iris and head hair and with congenital deafness. *Am J Hum Genet* **3**:195, 1951.
3. Arias S: Genetic heterogeneity in the Waardenburg syndrome. *Birth Defects* **7**:87, 1971.
4. Fraser GR: *The Causes of Profound Deafness in Childhood.* Baltimore, Johns Hopkins University Press, 1976.
5. Steel KP, Bock GR: Hereditary inner-ear abnormalities in animals. *Arch Otolaryngol* **109**:22, 1983.
6. Steel KP: Inherited hearing defects in mice. *Annu Rev Genet* **29**:675, 1995.
7. Accessible through the Hereditary Hearing Loss Homepage at *http://dnalab-www.uia.ac.be/dnalab/hhh*.
8. Steel KP, Barkway C, Bock GR: Strial dysfunction in mice with cochleo-saccular abnormalities. *Hearing Res* **27**:11, 1987.

9. Steel KP, Barkway C: Another role for melanocytes: Their importance for normal stria vascularis development in the mammalian inner ear. *Development* **107**:453, 1989.

10. Giebel LB, Spritz RA: Mutation of the *KIT* (mast/stem cell growth factor receptor) proto-oncogene in human piebaldism. *Proc Natl Acad Sci USA* **88**:8696, 1991.

11. Online Mendelian Inheritance in Man *http://www3.ncbi.nlm.nih.gov/Omim/*.

12. Gorlin RJ, Toriello HV, Cohen MM: *Hereditary Hearing Loss and its Syndromes*. Oxford, England: Oxford University Press, 1995.

13. Asher JH Jr, Sommer A, Morrell R, Friedman TB: Missense mutation in the paired domain of *PAX3* causes craniofacial-deafness-hand syndrome. *Hum Mutat* **7**:30, 1996.

14. Farrer LA, Grundfast KM, Amos J, Arnos KS, Asher JH, Beighton P, Diehl SR, et al: Waardenburg syndrome (WS) type 1 is caused by defects at multiple loci, one of which is near ALPP on chromosome 2: First report of the WS Consortium. *Am J Hum Genet* **50**:902, 1992.

15. Liu XZ, Newton VE, Read AP: Waardenburg syndrome type 2: Phenotypic findings and diagnostic criteria. *Am J Med Genet* **55**:95, 1995.

16. Newton VE: Hearing loss and Waardenburg syndrome: Implications for genetic counselling. *J Laryngol Otol* **104**:97, 1990.

17. Hageman M, Delleman J: Heterogeneity in Waardenburg syndrome. *Am J Hum Genet* **29**:468, 1977.

18. Newton VE, Liu XZ, Read AP: The association of sensorineural hearing loss and pigmentation abnormalities in Waardenburg syndrome. *J Audiol Med* **3**:69, 1994.

19. Spritz RA, Beighton P. Piebaldism with deafness: Molecular evidence for an expanded syndrome. *Am J Med Genet* **75**:101, 1998.

20. Da-Silva EO: Waardenburg I syndrome: A clinical and genetic study of two large Brazilian kindreds, and literature review. *Am J Med Genet* **40**:65, 1991.

21. Fleming A, Copp AJ: Embryonic folate metabolism and mouse neural tube defects. *Science* **280**:2107, 1998.

22. Arias S, Mota M: Apparent non-penetrance for dystopia in Waardenburg syndrome type 1 with some hints on the diagnosis of dystopia canthorum. *J Genet Hum* **26**:101, 1978.

23. Farrer LA, Arnos KS, Asher JH, Baldwin CT, Diehl SR, Friedman TB, Greenberg J, et al.: Locus heterogeneity for Waardenburg syndrome is predictive of clinical subtypes. *Am J Hum Genet* **55**:728, 1994.

24. Tassabehji M, Read AP, Newton VE, Patton M, Gruss P, Harris R, Strachan T: Mutations in the *PAX3* gene causing Waardenburg syndrome type 1 and type 2. *Nature Genet* **3**:26, 1993.

25. Love JK: *Deaf Mutism: A Clinical and Pathological Study*. Glasgow, James MacLehose & Sons, 1896.

26. Klein D: Historical background and evidence for dominant inheritance of the Klein-Waardenburg syndrome (type III). *Am J Med Genet* **14**:231, 1983.

27. Zlotogora J, Lerer I, Bar-David S, Ergaz Z, Abielovich D: Homozygosity for Waardenburg syndrome. *Am J Hum Genet* **56**:1173, 1995.

28. Goodman RM, Lewinthal I, Solomon A, Klein D: Upper limb involvement in the Klein-Waardenburg syndrome. *Am J Hum Genet* **11**:425, 1982.

29. Sheffer R, Zlotogora J: Autosomal dominant inheritance of Klein-Waardenburg syndrome. *Am J Med Genet* **42**:320, 1992.

30. Pasteris NG, Trask BJ, Sheldon S, Gorski JL: Discordant phenotypes of two overlapping deletions involving the *PAX3* gene on chromosome 2q35. *Hum Mol Genet* **2**:953, 1993.

31. Wieacker P: Waardenburg-syndrome Typ 1 und Typ 3 (Klein-Waardenburg Syndrom) in der gleichen Familie. *Med Genet* **6**:236, 1994.

32. Hoth CF, Milunsky A, Lipsky N, Sheffer R, Clarren SK, Baldwin CT: Mutations in the paired domain of the human *PAX3* gene cause Klein-Waardenburg syndrome (WS-III) as well as Waardenburg syndrome type 1 (WS-1). *Am J Hum Genet* **52**:455, 1993.

33. Tassabehji M, Newton VE, Liu XZ, Brady A, Donnai D, Krajewska-Walasek M, Murday V, et al.: The mutational spectrum in Waardenburg syndrome. *Hum Mol Genet* **4**:2131, 1995.

34. Shah KN, Dalal SJ, Sheth PN, Joshi NC, Ambani LM: White forelock, pigmentary disorder of the irides and long segment Hirschsprung disease: Possible variant of Waardenburg syndrome. *J Pediatr* **99**:432, 1981.

35. Omenn GS, McKusick VA: The association of Waardenburg syndrome and Hirschsprung megacolon. *Am J Med Genet* **3**:217, 1979.

36. Moase CE, Trasler DG: Splotch locus mouse mutants: model for neural tube defects and Waardenburg syndrome type 1 in humans. *J Med Genet* **29**:145, 1992.

37. Franz T, Kothary R, Surani MAH, Halata Z, Grim M: The *Splotch* mutation interferes with muscle development in the limbs. *Anat Embryol* **187**:153, 1993.

38. Franz T: Persistent truncus arteriosus in the *Splotch* mouse. *Anat Embryol* **180**:457, 1989.

39. Conway SJ, Henderson DJ, Kirby ML, Anderson RH, Copp AJ: Development of a lethal congenital heart defect in the *splotch* (*Pax3*) mutant mouse. *Cardiovasc Res* **36**:163, 1997.

40. Asher JH Jr, Harrison RW, Morell R, Carey ML, Friedman TB: Effects of *PAX3* modifier genes on craniofacial morphology, pigmentation and viability: A murine model of Waardenburg syndrome variation. *Genomics* **34**:285, 1996.

41. Steel KP, Smith RJH: Normal hearing in *Splotch* (*Sp/+*), the mouse homologue of Waardenburg syndrome type 1. *Nature Genet* **2**:75, 1992.

42. Epstein DJ, Vogan KJ, Trasler DG, Gros P: A mutation within intron 3 of the *PAX3* gene produces aberrantly spliced mRNA transcripts in the splotch (*Sp*) mouse mutant. *Proc Natl Acad Sci USA* **90**:532, 1993.

43. Epstein DJ, Malo D, Vekemans M, Gros P: Molecular characterization of a deletion encompassing the *Splotch* mutation on mouse chromosome 1. *Genomics* **10**:89, 1991.

44. Epstein DJ, Vekemans M, Gros P: *Splotch* (*Sp2H*), a mutation affecting development of the mouse neural tube, shows a deletion within the paired homeodomain of *Pax-3*. *Cell* **67**:767, 1991.

45. Vogan KJ, Epstein DJ, Trasler DG, Gros P: The *Splotch-delayed* (*Sp^d*) mouse mutant carries a point mutation within the paired box of the *Pax-3* gene. *Genomics* **17**:364, 1993.

46. Moore KJ: Insight into the *microphthalmia* gene. *Trends Genet* **11**:442, 1995.

47. Hodgkinson CA, Moore KJ, Nakayama A, Steingrimsson E, Copeland NG, Jenkins NA, Arnheiter H: Mutations at the mouse *microphthalmia* locus are associated with defects in a gene encoding a novel basic-helix-loop-helix-zipper protein. *Cell* **74**:395, 1993.

48. Hughes MJ, Lingrel JB, Krakowsky JM, Anderson KP: A helix-loop-helix transcription factor-like gene is located at the *mi* locus. *J Biol Chem* **268**:20687, 1993.

49. Steingrimsson E, Moore KJ, Lamoreux ML, Ferré-D'Amaré AR, Burley SK, Sanders Zimring DC, Skow LC, et al.: Molecular basis of mouse *microphthalmia* (*mi*) mutations helps explain their developmental and phenotypic consequences. *Nature Genet* **8**:256, 1994.

50. Steingrimsson E, Nii A, Fisher DE, Ferré-D'Amaré AR, McCormick RJ, Russell LB, Burley SK, et al.: The semidominant *Mi^b* mutation identifies a role for the HLH domain in DNA binding in addition to its role in protein dimerization. *EMBO J* **15**:6280, 1996.

51. Lane PW: Association of megacolon with two recessive spotting genes in the mouse. *J Hered* **57**:29, 1966.

52. Lane PW, Liu HM: Association of megacolon with a new dominant spotting gene (*Dom*) in the mouse. *J Hered* **75**:435, 1984.

53. Hosoda K, Hammer RE, Richardson JA, Baynash AG, Cheung JC, Giaid A, Yanagisawa M: Targeted and natural (piebald-lethal) mutations of endothelin-B receptor gene produce megacolon associated with spotted coat color in mice. *Cell* **79**:1267, 1994.

54. Baynash AG, Hosoda K, Giaid A, Richardson JA, Emoto N, Hammer RE, Yanagisawa M: Interaction of endothelin-3 with endothelin-B receptor is essential for development of epidermal melanocytes and enteric neurons. *Cell* **79**:1277, 1994.

55. Southard-Smith EM, Kos L, Pavan WJ: *Sox10* mutation disrupts neural crest development in *Dom* Hirschsprung mouse model. *Nature Genet* **18**:60, 1998.

56. Herbarth B, Pingault V, Bondurand N, Kuhlbrodt K, Hermans-Borgmeyer I, Puliti A, Lemort N, et al.: Mutation of the *Sry*-related *Sox10* gene in dominant megacolon, a mouse model for human Hirschsprung disease. *Proc Natl Acad Sci USA* **95**:5161, 1998.

57. Simpson JL, Falk CT, Morillo-Cucci G, Allen FHJ, German J: Analysis for possible linkage between the loci for the Waardenburg syndrome and various blood group and serological traits. *Humangenetik* **23**:45, 1974.

58. Asher JH, Friedman TB: Mouse and hamster mutants as models for Waardenburg syndrome in humans. *J Med Genet* **27**:618, 1990.

59. Ishikiriyama S, Tonoki H, Shibuya Y, Chin S, Harada N, Abe K, Niikawa N: Waardenburg syndrome type I in a child with *de novo* inversion (2) (q35q37.3). *Am J Med Genet* **33**:505, 1989.

60. Foy C, Newton VE, Wellesley D, Harris R, Read AP: Assignment of WS1 locus to human 2q37 and possible homology between Waarden-

burg syndrome and the *Splotch* mouse. *Am J Hum Genet* **46**:1017, 1990.

61. Burri M, Tromvoukis Y, Bopp D, Frigerio G, Noll M: Conservation of the paired domain in metazoans and its structure in three isolated human genes. *EMBO J* **8**:1183, 1989.

62. Baldwin CT, Hoth CF, Amos JA, da-Silva EO, Milunsky A: An exonic mutation in the *HuP2* paired domain gene causes Waardenburg's syndrome. *Nature* **355**:637, 1992.

63. Tassabehji M, Read AP, Newton VE, Harris R, Balling R, Gruss P, Strachan T: Waardenburg syndrome patients have mutations in the human homologue of the *Pax-3* paired box gene. *Nature* **355**:635, 1992.

64. Hughes A, Newton VE, Liu XZ, Read AP: A gene for Waardenburg syndrome type 2 maps close to the human homologue of the *microphthalmia* gene at chromosome 3p12-p14.1. *Nature Genet* **7**:509, 1994.

65. Tachibana M, Perez-Jurado LA, Nakayama A, Hodgkinson CA, Li X, Schneider M, Miki T, et al: Cloning of *MITF*, the human homologue of the mouse *microphthalmia* gene and assignment to chromosome 3p14.1-p12.3. *Hum Mol Genet* **3**:553, 1994.

66. Tassabehji M, Newton VE, Read AP: *MITF* gene mutations causing type 2 Waardenburg syndrome. *Nature Genet* **8**:251, 1994.

67. Puffenberger EG, Kauffman ER, Bolk S, Matise TC, Washington SS, Angrist M, Weissenbach J, et al: Identity-by-descent and association mapping of a recessive gene for Hirschsprung disease on human chromosome 13q22. *Hum Mol Genet* **3**:1217, 1994.

68. Kiss P, Osztovics M: Association of 13q deletion and Hirschsprung disease. *J Med Genet* **26**:793, 1989.

69. Lamont MA, Fitchett M, Dennis NR: Insterstitial deletion of distal 13q associated with Hirschsprung disease. *J Med Genet* **26**:100, 1989.

70. Bottani A, Xie Y, Binkert F, Schinzel A: A case of Hirschsprung disease with a chromosome 13 microdeletion, del(13) (q32.3q33.2): Potential mapping of one disease locus. *Hum Genet* **87**:748, 1991.

71. Van Camp G, Van Thienen MN, Handig I, Van Roy B, Rao VS, Milunsky A, Read AP, et al: Chromosome 13q deletion with Waardenburg syndrome: Further evidence for a gene involved in neural crest function on 13q. *J Med Genet* **32**:531, 1995.

72. Puffenberger EG, Hosoda K, Washington SS, Nakao K, deWit D, Yanagisawa M, Chakravarti A: A missense mutation of the endothelin-B receptor gene in multigenic Hirschsprung's disease. *Cell* **79**:1257, 1994.

73. Bopp D, Burri M, Baumgartner S, Frigiero G, Noll M: Conservation of a large protein domain in the segmentation gene *paired* and in functionally related genes of *Drosophila*. *Cell* **47**:1033, 1986.

74. Strachan T, Read AP: *PAX* genes. *Curr Opin Genet Dev* **4**:427, 1994.

75. Mansouri A, Hallonet M, Gruss P: *PAX* genes and their roles in cell differentiation and development. *Curr Opin Cell Biol* **8**:851, 1996.

76. Dahl E, Koseki H, Balling R: *PAX* genes and organogenesis. *Bioessays* **19**:755, 1997.

77. Balling R, Deutsch U, Gruss P: *Undulated*, a mutation affecting the development of the mouse skeleton, has a point mutation in the paired box of *Pax-1*. *Cell* **55**:531, 1988.

78. Torres M, Gomez-Pardo E, Dressler GR, Gruss P: *Pax-2* controls multiple steps of urogenital development. *Development* **121**:4057, 1995.

79. Sosa-Pineda B, Chowdhury K, Torres M, Oliver G, Gruss P: The *Pax-4* gene is essential for differentiation of insulin-producing beta cells in the mammalian pancreas. *Nature* **386**:399, 1997.

80. Urbanek P, Wang ZQ, Fetka I, Wagner EF, Busslinger M: Complete block of early B-cell differentiation and altered patterning of the posterior midbrain in mice lacking Pax5/BSAP. *Cell* **79**:901, 1994.

81. Hill RE, Favor J, Hogan BLM, Ton CCT, Saunders GF, Hanson IM, Prosser J, Jordan T, Hastie ND, van Heyningen V: Mouse small eye results from mutations in a paired-like homeobox-containing gene. *Nature* **354**:522, 1991.

82. Ton CCT, Miwa H, Saunders GF: Small eye (*SEY*): Cloning and characterization of the murine homolog of the human *Aniridia* gene. *Genomics* **13**:251, 1992.

83. Mansouri A, Stoykova A, Torres M, Gruss P: Dysgenesis of cephalic neural crest derivatives in *Pax7-/-* mutant mice. *Development* **122**:831, 1996.

84. Mansouri A, Chowdhury K, Gruss P: Follicular cells of the thyroid gland require *Pax8* gene function. *Nature Genet* **19**:87, 1998.

85. Peters H, Neubuser A, Kratochwil K, Balling R: *Pax9*-deficient mice lack pharyngeal pouch derivatives and teeth and exhibit craniofacial and limb abnormalities. *Genes Dev* **12**:2735, 1998.

86. Sanyanusin P, Schimmenti LA, McNoe TA, Ward TA, Pierpont ME, Sullivan MJ, Dobyns WB, et al: Mutation of the *PAX2* gene in a family with optic nerve colobomas, renal anomalies and vesicoureteral reflux. *Nature Genet* **13**:129, 1996.

87. Jordan T, Hanson I, Zaletayev D, Hodgson S, Prosser J, Seawright A, Hastie N, van Heyningen V: The human *PAX6* gene is mutated in two patients with aniridia. *Nature Genet* **1**:328, 1992.

88. Hanson I, Fletcher JM, Jordan T, Brown A, Taylor D, Adams RJ, Punnett HH, Van Heyningen V: Mutations at the *PAX6* locus are found in heterogeneous anterior segment malformations including Peters' anomaly. *Nature Genet* **6**:168, 1994.

89. Macchia PE, Lapi P, Krude H, Pirro MT, Missero C, Chiovato L, Souabni A, et al: *PAX8* mutations associated with congenital hypothyroidism caused by thyroid dysgenesis. *Nature Genet* **19**:83, 1998.

90. Goulding MD, Chalepakis G, Deutsch U, Erselius JR, Gruss P: Pax-3, a novel murine DNA-binding protein expressed during early neurogenesis. *EMBO J* **10**:1135, 1991.

91. Macina R, Barr F, Galili N, Reithman H: Genomic organization of the human *PAX3* gene: DNA sequence analysis of the region disrupted in alveolar rhabdomyosarcoma. *Genomics* **26**:1, 1995.

92. Lu-Kuo J, Ward DC, Spritz RA: Fluorescence in situ hybridization mapping of 25 markers on distal human chromosome 2q surrounding the human Waardenburg syndrome type 1 (WS1) locus (*PAX3* gene). *Genomics* **16**:173, 1993.

93. Tassabehji M, Newton VE, Leverton K, Turnbull K, Seemanova E, Kunze J, Sperling K, et al: *PAX3* gene structure and mutations: close analogies between Waardenburg syndrome type 1 and the *Splotch* mouse. *Hum Mol Genet* **3**:1069, 1994.

94. Tsukamoto K, Nakamura Y, Niikawa N: Isolation of two isoforms of the *PAX3* gene transcripts and their tissue-specific alternative expression in human adult tissues. *Hum Genet* **93**:270, 1994.

95. Vogan KJ, Underhill DA, Gros P: An alternative splicing event in the *Pax-3* paired domain identifies the linker region as a key determinant of paired domain DNA-binding activity. *Mol Cell Biol* **16**:6677, 1996.

96. Xu W, Rould MA, Jun S, Desplan C, Pabo CO: Crystal structure of a paired domain-DNA complex at 2.5 Å resolution reveals structural basis for *Pax* developmental mutations. *Cell* **80**:639, 1995.

97. Chalepakis G, Fritsch R, Fickenscher H, Deutsch U, Goulding M, Gruss P: The molecular basis of the *undulated/Pax-1* mutation. *Cell* **67**:767, 1991.

98. Epstein JA, Cai J, Glaser T, Jepeal L, Maas R: Identification of a *Pax* paired domain recognition sequence and evidence for DNA-dependent conformational changes. *J Biol Chem* **269**:8355, 1994.

99. Epstein JA, Shapiro DN, Cheng J, Lam PYP, Maas RL: Pax3 modulates expression of the c-Met receptor during limb muscle development. *Proc Natl Acad Sci USA* **93**:4213, 1996.

100. Wilson D, Sheng G, Lecuit T, Dostatni N, Desplan C: Co-operative dimerization of paired class homeodomains on DNA. *Genes Dev* **7**:2120, 1993.

101. Vogan KJ, Gros P: The C-terminal subdomain makes an important contribution to the DNA binding activity of the *Pax-3* paired domain. *J Biol Chem* **272**:28289, 1997.

102. Fortin AS, Underhill DA, Gros P: Reciprocal effect of Waardenburg syndrome mutations on DNA binding by the *Pax-3* paired domain and homeodomain. *Hum Mol Genet* **6**:1781, 1997.

103. Chalepakis G, Jones FS, Edelman GM, Gruss P: *Pax-3* contains domains for transcription activation and transcription inhibition. *Proc Natl Acad Sci USA* **91**:12745, 1994.

104. Magnaghi P, Roberts C, Lorain S, Lipinski M, Scambler PJ: *HIRA*, a mammalian homologue of *Saccharomyces cerevisiae* transcriptional co-repressors, interacts with Pax3. *Nature Genet* **20**:74, 1998

105. Wu B-L, Milunsky A, Wyandt H, Hoth C, Baldwin C, Skare J: In situ hybridisation applied to Waardenburg syndrome. *Cytogenet Cell Genet* **63**:29, 1993.

106. Nye JS, Balkin N, Lucas H, Knepper PA, McLone DG, Charrow J: Myelomeningocele and Waardenburg syndrome (type 3) in patients with interstitial deletions of 2q35 and the *PAX3* gene: Possible digenicinheritance of a neural tube defect. *Am J Med Genet* **75**:401, 1998.

107. Attaie A, Kim E, Wilcox ER, Lalwani AK: A splice-site mutation affecting the paired box of *PAX3* in a three generation family with Waardenburg syndrome type I (WS1). *Mol Cell Probes* **11**:233, 1997.

108. Morell R, Friedman TB, Moeljopawiro S, Hartono, Soewito, Asher JH: A frameshift mutation in the HuP2 paired domain of the probable

human homologue of murine Pax-3 is responsible for Waardenburg syndrome type 1 in an Indonesian family. *Hum Mol Genet* **1**:243, 1992.

109. Butt J, Greenberg J, Winship I, Sellars S, Beighton P, Ramesar R: A splice junction mutation in PAX3 causes Waardenburg syndrome in a South African family. *Hum Mol Genet* **3**:197, 1994.

110. Lalwani AK, Brister JR, Fex J, Grundfast KM, Ploplis B, San Agustin TB, Wilcox ER: Further elucidation of the genomic structure of *PAX3*, and identification of two different point mutations within the *PAX3* homeobox that cause Waardenburg syndrome type 1 in two families. *Am J Hum Genet* **56**:75, 1995.

111. Baldwin CT, Hoth CF, Macina RA, Milunsky A: Mutations in PAX3 that cause Waardenburg syndrome type 1: Ten new mutations and review of the literature. *Am J Med Genet* **58**:115, 1995.

112. Hol FA, Hamel BC, Geurds MP, Mullaart RA, Barr FG, Macina RA, Mariman EC: A frameshift mutation in the gene for PAX3 in a girl with spina bifida and mild signs of Waardenburg syndrome. *J Med Genet* **32**:52, 1995.

113. Morell R, Carey ML, Lalwani AK, Friedman TB, Asher JH: Three mutations in the paired homeodomain of PAX3 that cause Waardenburg syndrome type 1. *Hum Hered* **47**:38, 1997.

114. Gehring WJ, Qian YK, Billeter M, Furukubo-Tokunaga K, Schier AF, Resendez-Perez D, Affolter M, et al: Homeodomain-DNA recognition. *Cell* **78**:211, 1994.

115. Wilson DS, Guenther B, Desplan C, Kuriyan J: High resolution crystal structure of a paired (*Pax*) class cooperative homeodomain dimer on DNA. *Cell* **82**:709, 1995.

116. Cooper DN, Krawczak M: *Human Gene Mutation.* Oxford, England: Bios Scientific Publishers, 1993.

117. DeStefano AL, Cupples LA, Arnos KS, Asher JH, Baldwin CT, Blanton S, Carey ML, et al: Correlation between Waardenburg syndrome phenotype and genotype in a population of individuals with identified *PAX3* mutations. *Hum Genet* **102**:499, 1998.

118. Kromberg JGR, Krause A: Waardenburg syndrome and spina bifida. *Am J Med Genet* **45**:536, 1993.

119. Galili N, Davies RJ, Fredericks WJ, Mukhopadhyay S, Rauscher FJ, Emanuel BS, Rovera G, et al: Fusion of a fork head domain gene to *PAX3* in the solid tumour alveolar rhabdomyosarcoma. *Nature Genet* **5**:230, 1993.

120. Aymé S, Philip N: Possible homozygous Waardenburg syndrome in a fetus with exencephaly. *Am J Med Genet* **59**:263, 1995.

121. Lowings P, Yavuzer U, Goding CR: Positive and negative elements regulate a melanocyte-specific promoter. *Mol Cell Biol* **12**:3653, 1992.

122. Hemesath TJ, Steingrimsson E, McGill G, Hansen M, Vaught J, Hodgkinson CA, Arnheiter H, et al: Microphthalmia, a critical factor in melanocyte development, defines a discrete transcription factor family. *Genes Dev* **8**:2770, 1994.

123. Tachibana M, Takeda K, Nobokuni Y, Urabe K, Long JE, Meyers KA, Aaronson SA, et al: Ectopic expression of *MITF*, a gene for Waardenburg syndrome type 2, converts fibroblasts to cells with melanocyte characteristics. *Nature Genet* **14**:50, 1996.

124. Watanebe A, Takeda K, Ploplis B, Tachibana M: Epistatic relationship between Waardenburg syndrome genes *MITF* and *PAX3*. *Nature Genet* **18**:283, 1998.

125. Nobokuni Y, Watanebe A, Takeda K, Skarka H, Tachibana M: Analyses of loss-of-function mutations of the MITF gene suggest that haploinsufficiency is a cause of Waardenburg syndrome type 2a. *Am J Hum Genet* **59**:76, 1996.

126. Morell R, Spritz RA, Ho L, Pierpont J, Guo W, Friedman TB, Asher JH: Apparent digenic inheritance of Waardenburg syndrome type 2 (WS2) and autosomal recessive ocular albinism (AROA). *Hum Mol Genet* **6**:659, 1997.

127. Amiel J, Watkin PM, Tassabehji M, Read AP, Winter RM: Mutation of the *MITF* gene in albinism-deafness syndrome (Tietz syndrome). *Clin Dysmorphol* **7**:17, 1998.

128. Smith SD, Kenyon JB, Kelley PM, Hoover D, Comer B: Tietz syndrome (hypopigmentation/deafness) caused by mutation of *MITF* (abstract). *Am J Hum Genet* **61**(suppl.):A347, 1997.

129. Hultén M, Honeyman MM, Mayne AJ, Tarlow MJ: Homozygosity in piebald trait. *J Med Genet* **24**:568, 1987.

130. Takebayash K, Chida K, Tsukamoto I, Morii E, Munakata H, Arnheiter H, Kuroki T, et al: The recessive phenotype displayed by a dominant negative microphthalmia-associated transcription factor mutant is a result of impaired nuclear localization potential. *Mol Cell Biol* **16**:1203, 1996.

131. Hemesath TM, Roydon-Price E, Takemoto C, Badalian T, Fisher DE: MAP kinase links the transcription factor *Microphthalmia* to c-*Kit* signalling in melanocytes. *Nature* **391**:298, 1998.

132. Tietz W: A syndrome of deaf-mutism associated with albinism showing dominant autosomal inheritance. *Am J Hum Genet* **15**:259, 1963.

133. Hood OJ, Doyle M, Hebert AA, Oelberg DG: Association of Waardenburg syndrome type II and a *de novo* balanced 7;20 translocation. *Dysmorphol Clin Genet* **3**:122, 1989.

134. Attié T, Till M, Pelet A, Amiel J, Edery P, Boutrand L, Munnich A, et al: Mutation of the endothelin-receptor B gene in Waardenburg-Hirschsprung disease. *Hum Mol Genet* **4**:2407, 1995.

135. Hofstra RM, Osinga J, Tan-Sindhunata G, Wu Y, Kamsteeg EJ, Stulp RP, van Ravenswaaij-Arts C, et al: A homozygous mutation in the endothelin-3 gene associated with a combined Waardenburg type 2 and Hirschsprung phenotype (Shah-Waardenburg syndrome). *Nature Genet* **12**:445, 1996.

136. Edery P, Attié T, Amiel J, Pelet A, Eng C, Hofstra RFM, Martelli H, et al: Mutation of the endothelin-3 gene in the Waardenburg-Hirschsprung disease (Shah-Waardenburg syndrome). *Nature Genet* **12**:442, 1996.

137. Chakravarti A: Endothelin receptor-mediated signaling in Hirschsprung disease. *Hum Mol Genet* **5**:303, 1996.

138. Pingault V, Bondurand N, Kuhlbrodt K, Goerich D, Prehu M-O, Legius E, Matthijs G, et al: *SOX10* mutations in patients with Waardenburg-Hirschsprung disease. *Nature Genet* **18**:171, 1998.

139. Rawls A, Olson EN: MyoD meets its maker. *Cell* **89**:5, 1997.

140. Bosher SK, Hallpike CS: Observations on the histogenesis of the inner ear degeneration of the deaf white cat and its possible relationship to the aetiology of certain unexplained varieties of human congenital deafness. *J Laryngol* **80**:222, 1966.

141. Bottani A, Antonarakis SE, Blouin JL: *PAX3* missense mutations (G99S and R270C) in the original patient descrbed with Klein-Waardenburg (WS3) syndrome. *Am J Hum Genet* **65**(suppl):A143, 1999.

142. Barber TD, Baber MC, Cloutier TE, Friedman TB: PAX3 gene strucure, alternative splicing and evolution. *Gene* **237**:311, 1999.

143. Takeda K, Takemoto C, Kobayashi I, Watanebe A, Nobokuni Y, Fisher DE, Tachibana M: Ser298 of MITF, a mutation site in Waardenburg syndrome type 2 is a phosphorylation site with functional significance. *Hum Mol Genet* **9**:125, 2000.

# Craniosynostosis Syndromes

*Maximilian Muenke* ■ *Andrew O.M. Wilkie*

1. Craniosynostosis, the premature fusion of one or several sutures of the skull, is one of the commonest craniofacial anomalies at birth with a prevalence of 1 in 2100 to 3000. The shape of the skull is altered depending on which of the sutures are fused prematurely.

2. The etiology of craniosynostosis is heterogeneous. Isolated occurrence with unknown etiology is common, mostly affecting the sagittal suture. Syndromic craniosynostosis has been described in over 100 syndromes which have been delineated based on the suture involvement (most commonly the coronal sutures), craniofacial anomalies, associated limb and other organ system involvement, and inheritance pattern (autosomal dominant and recessive, and X-linked). The clinical features of 27 of the most distinct and important clinical entities associated with craniosynostosis are tabulated.

3. The classical craniosynostosis syndromes are inherited in an autosomal dominant fashion and include Apert (MIM 101200), Pfeiffer (MIM 101600), Saethre-Chotzen (MIM 101400), and Crouzon (MIM 123500) syndromes. They were originally described as separate clinical entities with Apert and sporadic Pfeiffer syndrome generally tending to be more severe than Crouzon and Saethre-Chotzen syndrome.

4. Recently, the molecular bases of these classical disorders, a new common craniosynostosis syndrome (Muenke syndrome (MIM 134394)), and several of the rare craniosynostosis syndromes have been identified. Pfeiffer syndrome is heterogeneous and due to heterozygous mutations in fibroblast growth factor receptor (FGFR) genes 1 and 2. Heterozygous mutations in *FGFR2* also cause Apert, Crouzon, Jackson-Weiss (MIM 123150), and Beare-Stevenson (MIM 123790) syndromes. Muenke syndrome was newly defined by a specific mutation in *FGFR3*, which corresponds to an amino acid substitution equivalent to one change in Apert syndrome in *FGFR2* and in Pfeiffer syndrome in *FGFR1*. Crouzon syndrome with acanthosis nigricans is due to a mutation in *FGFR3*. Cytogenetic deletions and translocations involving 7p21.1 and various heterozygous mutations in the *TWIST* gene, which maps to this region, cause Saethre-Chotzen syndrome. A missense mutation of the fibrillin-1 (*FBN1*) gene was identified in a single patient with Shprintzen-Goldberg syndrome (MIM 182212), which is probably genetically heterozygous. Lastly, a specific heterozygous mutation in the *MSX2* gene, which has only been observed in a single family, causes Boston-type craniosynostosis (MIM 123101), the first craniosynostosis syndrome in which the genetic etiology was identified.

5. The diagnosis of craniosynostosis syndromes is by clinical examination aided by radiographic imaging of the skull, hands, and feet. Mutation analysis has enabled refinement of this classification by highlighting the etiologic similarities of some disorders (for example, Crouzon and Pfeiffer syndromes due to mutations of *FGFR2*), whilst clinically similar phenotypes can result from mutations in different genes (for example *FGFR3* and *TWIST*). Molecular analysis also enables the identification of mildly affected carrier parents as well as early prenatal diagnosis.

6. Treatment consists of craniofacial surgery and neurosurgery, and surgical correction of anomalies of the hands and feet. Anomalies in other organ systems (e.g., respiratory difficulties and others) are treated system by system.

7. The pattern of mutations in *FGFR1*, *FGFR2*, and *FGFR3*, which encode related transmembrane receptor tyrosine kinase proteins, is highly nonrandom. The majority of the craniosynostosis mutations are clustered around the third extracellular immunoglobulin-like domain and are missense substitutions. The recurrent nucleotide transversions causing Apert and Muenke syndromes have the highest mutation rates for transversions currently known in the human genome.

8. Functional studies suggest that these FGFR mutations are activating. Three major mechanisms of activation have been described. The first results in increased affinity for fibroblast growth factors (FGFs), the FGFR ligands. The second is FGF independent and promotes covalent or noncovalent receptor dimerization, which is required for activation. Finally, ectopic expression of alternative FGFR splice forms may confer the cell with novel ligand-binding properties.

9. A second important cause of craniosynostosis is heterozygous mutations in TWIST, a transcription factor. In contrast to the FGFR mutations, TWIST mutations appear to result in functional haploinsufficiency and so a wider range of molecular lesions is observed including intragenic mutations, large deletions, and translocations occurring up to 250 kb away from the gene.

10. Growth of the skull and maintenance of suture patency represent a balance between cell division and differentiation. Craniosynostosis mutations provide a genetic means to identify some of the proteins that play a critical role in

---

A list of standard abbreviations is located immediately preceding the index in each volume. Additional abbreviations used in this chapter include: *Alu* = common repetitive sequence in human DNA; b-HLH = basic helix-loop-helix; DFR1 = *Drosophila* gene orthologue of FGFR; FGF = fibroblast growth factor; FGFR = fibroblast growth factor receptor; MAPK = mitogen-activated protein kinase; Miz1 = (Msx-interacting-zinc finger) transcription factor; *msh* = muscle segment homeobox gene of *Drosophila*; *MSX2/Msx2* = human/mouse gene symbols for the MSH (*Drosophila*) homeobox homolog 2; PTB = phosphotyrosine binding; SH2 = Src homology 2; *TWIST/Twist* = human/mouse gene symbols for a transcription factor originally named in *Drosophila*.

suture development. This provides a platform for ongoing work to understand the processes of suture biogenesis and the pathophysiology of craniosynostosis mutations.

## INTRODUCTION

### Terminology

Craniosynostosis or craniostenosis is the premature fusion of one or several sutures of the calvaria leading to an abnormal shape of the skull. The major sutures of the calvaria include the coronal, lambdoid, and squamosal, all of which are paired (Fig. 245-1A). The sagittal and the metopic sutures are single (Fig. 245-1A). At birth, these sutures are open and the nonmidline sutures overlap slightly (Fig. 245-1B). Depending on which of the sutures are fused prematurely, the skull can develop a characteristic shape. Simple synostosis of the coronal sutures leads to brachycephaly or short-headedness; variant head shapes include acrocephaly and oxycephaly (pointed head), or turricephaly (tower-shaped head). Unilateral coronal synostosis gives rise to anterior plagiocephaly,

which is associated with asymmetry of the face and skull (Fig. 245-1C). Dolichocephaly, or long-headedness, is seen in premature fusion of the sagittal suture. A variant is scaphocephaly (keel-shaped head) (Fig. 245-1C). Trigonocephaly or triangular-shaped head results from premature closure of the metopic suture. Posterior plagiocephaly is sometimes caused by unilateral fusion of the lambdoid suture but is more commonly nonsynostotic and related to abnormal mechanical forces.[2a] Compound synostosis, that is, two or more sutures are involved, can lead to complex head shapes including cloverleaf ("Kleeblattschädel") malformation.[3]

### Classification

Various classifications of craniosynostosis have been applied over the years, one of them using the anatomic nomenclature depending on which suture is involved (see "Terminology" above). This descriptive classification is used in cases of isolated craniosynostosis, which do not fit into any of the known craniosynostosis syndromes. A clinical classification based on the craniofacial findings, anomalies in other organ systems, and pedigree

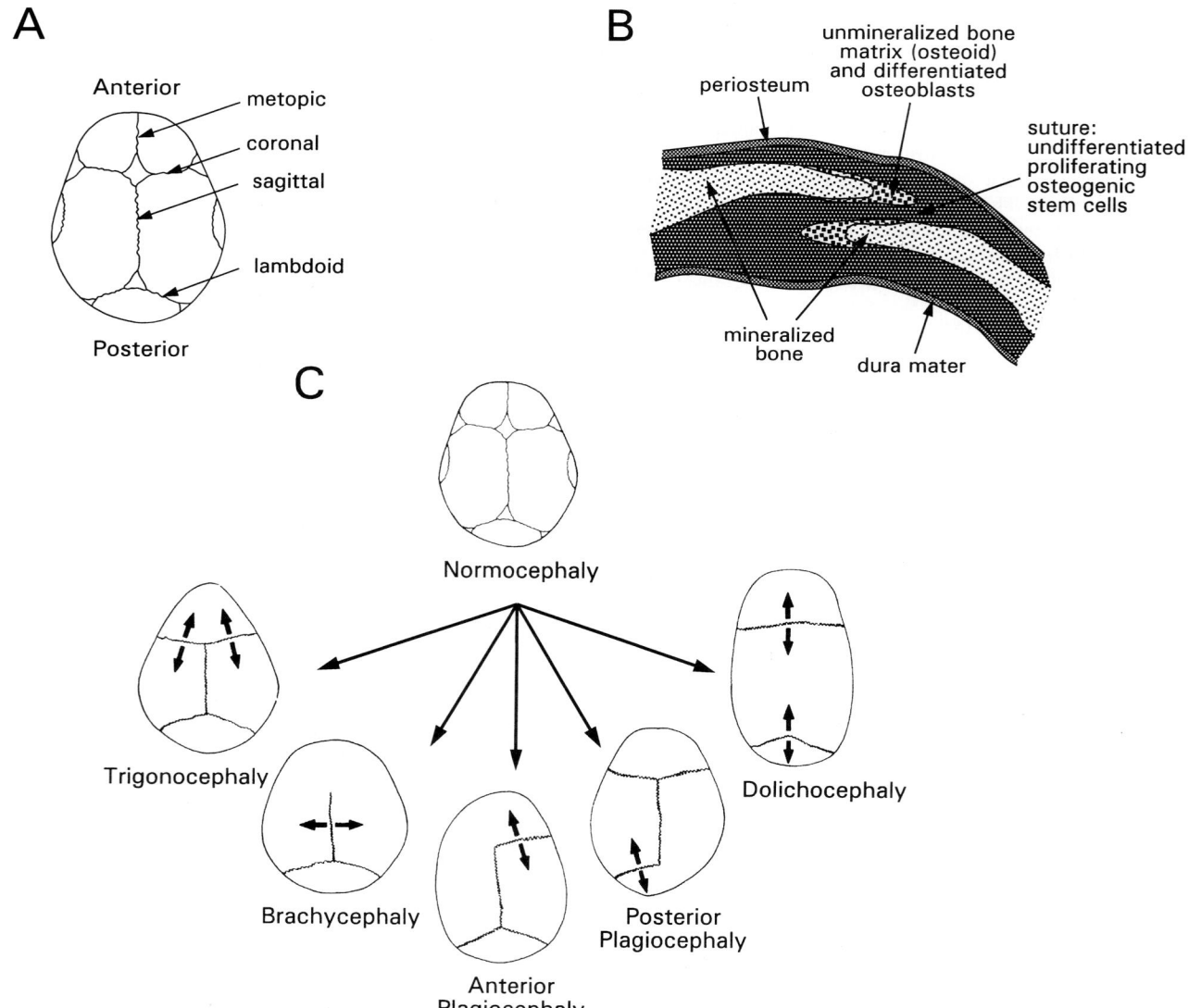

Fig. 245-1 Diagram of the sutures of the skull. *A,* Superior view of the normal infant skull. The anterior fontanelle is bordered by the metopic, coronal, and sagittal sutures, and the posterior fontanelle is bordered by the sagittal and the lambdoid sutures. *B,* Cross-section through the coronal suture. The skull bones overlap slightly. In craniosynostosis, the narrow space separating the bones is obliterated. (Modified from Wilkie[1]). *C,* Premature fusion of the sutures leads to an abnormal head shape. Compensatory expansion (arrows) occurs particularly at neighboring unfused sutures. (*Modified from Cohen and MacLean.*[2])

information has been used to describe well-known ("classical") and rare monogenic craniosynostosis syndromes. Over 100 such syndromes are known.[2] The more common ones are listed in Table 245-1. The recent identification of mutations, especially in the fibroblast growth factor receptor (FGFR) genes, provides new insight into the clinical classification. The clinical findings in craniosynostosis syndromes with an identified gene defect(s) are described in the text below.

## Frequency

The most accurate surveys of the frequency of craniosynostosis among live-born infants suggest a prevalence of 1 in 2100 to 1 in 3000.[10,11,30,31,34] The most common craniosynostosis syndromes include Apert (4.5 percent of all cases with craniosynostosis), Saethre-Chotzen (4.5 percent), Crouzon (4.5 percent), and Muenke syndrome (approximately 8 percent). Autosomal recessive craniosynostosis syndromes are not common (Table 245-1). Craniofrontonasal syndrome is the most common X-linked craniosynostosis syndrome.

## CLINICAL FINDINGS

### Apert Syndrome

Apert syndrome (MIM 101200) was first described in 1906[35] with numerous subsequent clinical reports (for recent reviews see references 36 to 41). It is characterized by craniosynostosis (brachycephaly), midface hypoplasia, broad thumbs and great toes, symmetric syndactyly of the hands and feet, and other anomalies (Fig. 245-2). Inheritance pattern is autosomal dominant in the few families with parent-to-child transmission. Germ line mosaicism was proposed in an unaffected couple who had two children with Apert syndrome,[42] although this has not been confirmed at a molecular level. The great majority ($\sim$98 percent) of Apert syndrome cases are sporadic. The de novo occurrence was clinically correlated with increased paternal age.[43] The exclusive paternal origin of new mutations in Apert syndrome has been demonstrated at a molecular level.[44] The birth prevalence, estimated as 1 in 65,000 to 1 in 80,000 newborns, is high among the craniosynostosis syndromes (4.5 percent of all cases with craniosynostosis).[45,46]

Clinical findings in Apert syndrome tend to be more severe and affect more organ systems than in most cases of the other common craniosynostosis syndromes. The skull malformations include turribrachycephaly with a disproportionately high cranium with frontal bossing and occasional asymmetry. The anterior fontanelle is extremely wide open at birth extending from the root of the nose to the posterior fontanelle. This midline calvarial defect closes completely only during the third year of life. Other anomalies of the skull include a malformed and often asymmetric cranial base and very short anterior fossa.

Facial anomalies consist of hypertelorism with downslanting palpebral fissures and exorbitism (Fig. 245-2). Strabismus is common, as are myopia, hyperopia, astigmatism, and dissociated eye movements.[47] The midface is hypoplastic with relative mandibular prognathism. The nasal bridge is depressed, the shape of the nose beaked. The palate can be highly arched, often with a median furrow or cleft of the soft palate, and the uvula can be bifid. Dental anomalies (malocclusion, delayed or ectopic eruption of teeth) are common.[48] Significant hearing loss is seen in some individuals.

Central nervous system findings include anomalies of the corpus callosum, septum pellucidum, or limbic structures; hypoplasia of the cerebral white matter and heterotopic gray matter; megalencephaly; and/or ventriculomegaly.[37] Progressive hydrocephalus is present in only a minority of the patients with ventriculomegaly.[49] Intelligence is variable and ranges from normal (40 to 50 percent) to mild and moderate mental retardation[50] (for a more detailed discussion see "Complications of Craniosynostosis" below).

Hands and feet are syndactylous, which is characteristic for Apert syndrome, and differ from other craniosynostosis syndromes (Figs. 245-2 and 245-3; references 51 to 53) except Philadelphia type craniosynostosis (Table 245-1). In the hand, the central three digits are always syndactylous with a broad thumb and part of the fifth finger separate (type 1 according to the classification by Upton).[51] In the "mitten-hand" deformity, the fifth finger is part of the syndactylous mass (type 2), and fusion of all digits ("rosebud") is seen in type 3. Syndactyly of the feet may involve the three lateral digits (type 1), digits 2 to 5 (type 2), or all digits (type 3). Fusion of digits is associated with fusion of the corresponding nails.

The thumbs and great toes are broad and deviate away from the other digits. Incomplete postaxial polydactyly of the hands and preaxial polydactyly of the feet may be present.[51,54,55] Other limb anomalies include limited mobility at the glenohumeral joint, which worsens with growth, moderate shortening of the humerus, and limitation of elbow extension.[39] Progressive synostosis of the bones in the hands, feet, and cervical spine is common. Fusions of the cervical vertebrae are present in 68 percent of patients with Apert syndrome, C5-C6 fusion being the most common.[56]

Skin findings include acneiform eruption in more than 70 percent of patients. Other cutaneous manifestations are common and include skin dimples at the shoulders, elbows, and knuckles; hyperhidrosis; hyperkeratoses; hypopigmentation; and nail infections.[40] Low-frequency anomalies in the cardiovascular, respiratory, gastrointestinal, and genitourinary systems are reviewed elsewhere.[38]

The majority of patients with Apert syndrome have one of two specific heterozygous mutations in the FGFR2 gene (S252W or P253R) (Table 245-2).[57] Genotype-phenotype comparison found no convincing difference in the prevalence of most malformations in Apert syndrome with the following exceptions: Cleft palate was significantly more common in patients with the S252W mutation, whereas syndactyly of both hands and feet was more severe with the P253R mutation.[53,57a] Cleft palate in Apert syndrome reflects a more generalized disturbance in growth of the craniofacial skeleton, which suggests that two clinical subtypes of Apert syndrome may be recognized, one with more severe craniofacial features but milder syndactyly, the other with severe syndactyly but relatively milder craniofacial problems (see "Reappraisal of the Clinical Classification of Craniosynostosis" below).

### Beare-Stevenson Syndrome

Beare-Stevenson syndrome or cutis gyrata syndrome of Beare and Stevenson (MIM 123790) was first described in 1969.[87] Beare-Stevenson syndrome is a rare sporadic condition with early demise, with only nine published cases.[82,87–92] Characteristic clinical findings include the corrugated skin furrows (cutis gyrata), which affect the scalp, forehead, face, neck, trunk, hands, and feet, and acanthosis nigricans. Other skin anomalies include skin tags and an enlarged umbilical stump. Craniosynostosis can be severe, and was present in four of six cases, with cloverleaf skull in three of these four cases.[2] Additional findings in some cases include hypertelorism, broad nasal bridge, ear defects, cleft palate, hypodontia, choanal atresia, bifid scrotum, anogenital anomalies, and coccygeal eversion.

All reported cases have been sporadic, with an increased paternal age in some. Heterozygous mutations of FGFR2, S372C and Y375C, have been described (Table 245-2), whereas some patients did not have mutations in these regions, suggesting further genetic heterogeneity.[82,92]

### Boston-Type Craniosynostosis

Craniosynostosis Boston type (MIM 123101) was described in a single large family with 19 affected individuals in three generations and autosomal dominant inheritance of craniosynostosis.[93] This disorder has complete penetrance but variable expressivity with regards to craniofacial anomalies, ranging from fronto-orbital recession with normal midface in adults and frontal

**Table 245-1 Clinical and Molecular Findings in Patients with Craniosynostosis Syndromes**

| Syndrome/MIM | Craniofacial Findings | Extremities | Additional Findings | Genetic Etiology | References |
|---|---|---|---|---|---|
| Antley-Bixler syndrome 207410 | Brachycephaly, severe midface hypoplasia | Humeroradial synostosis, femoral bowing, long palms and fingers | Choanal stenosis, genital anomalies | Autosomal recessive but clinically similar cases may have heterozygous *FGFR2* mutations | 4, 5 |
| Apert syndrome 101200 | Acrocephaly with wide open fontanelle at birth, hypertelorism, shallow orbits, midface hypoplasia, narrow palate, occasionally cleft palate | Syndactyly of hands and feet including fusion of bony structures, broad thumbs and great toes | Variable mental retardation, corpus callosum anomalies, ventricular dilatation, fused cervical vertebrae | Autosomal dominant, usually sporadic, rarely familial, mutations in *FGFR2* S252W and P253R (and others, see Table 245-2) | see text |
| Baller-Gerold syndrome 218600 | Oxycephaly, trigononcephaly | Absent or hypoplastic radius, thumb, and carpal and metacarpal bones, short and curved ulna | Vertebral and rib anomalies, short stature, mental retardation | Genetic heterogeneity, autosomal recessive | 6, 7 |
| Beare-Stevenson syndrome 123790 | Varying degrees of craniosynostosis with cloverleaf skull in some | | Cutis gyrata; acanthosis nigricans; umbilical, genital, and anal anomalies | Usually sporadic, mutations in *FGFR2* S372C, Y375C | see text |
| Boston-type craniosynostosis 123101 | Variable, nondiagnostic craniosynostosis with supraorbital recession | | Seizures, poor vision | Autosomal dominant in one large family with mutation in *MSX2* P148H | see text |
| Carpenter syndrome 201000 | Acrocephaly, hypertelorism | Preaxial polydactyly, syndactyly, brachydactyly | Mental retardation | Autosomal recessive | 8, 9 |
| Coronal craniosynostosis | Bilateral or unilateral craniosynostosis | | | Sporadic or autosomal dominant (14%); bicoronal synostosis more often familial than unicoronal synostosis | 10, 11 |
| Cranioectodermal dysplasia 218330 | Dolichocephaly, sparse hair | Rhizomelic limb shortening, brachydactyly, cutaneous syndactyly | Eye and dental anomalies, short thorax | Autosomal recessive | 12 |
| Craniofrontonasal syndrome 304110 | Brachycephaly, plagiocephaly, hypertelorism, grooved nasal tip, facial asymmetry, novel phenotypic pattern; more severe in females than in males | Broad first toes, syndactyly, longitudinally grooved fingernails | Wiry hair, clavicular/scapular anomalies | Most common X-linked craniosynostosis syndrome with gene locus in Xp22 | 13, 14 |
| Craniomicromelic syndrome 602558 | Coronal craniosynostosis, micrognathia exorbitism | Intrauterine growth retardation, shortness of all limbs | Absent or hypoplastic gallbladder, hypoplastic ileum, lungs, fallopian tubes | Rare lethal autosomal recessive condition | 15 |
| Crouzon syndrome 123500 | Shallow orbits, exorbitism, hypertelorism, strabismus, hypoplastic maxilla with relative mandibular prognathism | Limbs appear normal, but mild radiologic abnormalities are frequent | Occasionally conductive hearing loss, mental retardation | Autosomal dominant, mutations in *FGFR2*, predominantly exons JgIIIa and JgIIIc (see Table 245-2) | see text |

| Syndrome | Craniofacial features | Limb features | Other features | Inheritance/molecular | References |
|---|---|---|---|---|---|
| Crouzon with acanthosis nigricans 134934.0011 | Similar to Crouzon syndrome, cementomas of jaw | | Acanthosis nigricans, melanocytic nevi | Rare, sporadic, mutation in FGFR3, A391E | see text |
| Dubowitz syndrome 223370 | Microcephaly, short palpebral fissures, micrognathia | | Short stature, mental retardation in some, genital, anorectal anomalies | Autosomal recessive, chromosomal instability | 16, 17 |
| Greig cephalopolysyndactyly 175700 | Frontal bossing, broad nasal root, hypertelorism, craniosynostosis in <5% | Polysyndactyly, broad thumbs, broad great toes | | Autosomal dominant, deletions and translocations in 7p13 interrupting GLI3, mutations in GLI3 | 18, 19 |
| Jackson-Weiss syndrome 123150 | Variable craniofacial anomalies with midface hypoplasia | Normal thumbs, broad great toes, syndactyly and bony fusions in feet | | Autosomal dominant inheritance in one enormous family with FGFR2 A344G mutation | see text |
| Jacobsen syndrome 147791 | Metopic synostosis with trigonocephaly, hypertelorism, ptosis of eyelids, low nasal bridge | | Mild to moderate psychomotor retardation, cardiac defects, thrombocytopenia | De novo cytogenetic deletions: del(11)(q23.3 -> qter) | 20–22 |
| Lambdoid craniosynostosis 600775 | Posterior plagiocephaly, occipital flattening, frontal bossing | | | Sporadic, rare, occasionally autosomal dominant | 2a, 23 |
| Metopic craniosynostosis 190440 | Trigonocephaly | | | Sporadic, autosomal dominant in two 3-generation families | 22, 24 |
| Muenke syndrome 134394.0014, 602849 | Variable findings including bilateral or unilateral coronal synostosis, macrocephaly, midface hypoplasia | Variable brachydactyly, broad great toes in some, characteristic radiographic findings | Normal height, sensorineural hearing loss and mental retardation in some patients | Autosomal dominant, mutation in FGFR3, P250R, appears to be one of the most common craniosynostosis syndromes and includes Adelaide type craniosynostosis | see text |
| Opitz C syndrome 211750 | Trigonocephaly with prominent metopic crest, microcephaly, typical facial appearance | Syndactyly, polydactyly in some | Severe mental retardation, midline brain anomalies, heart defects, genitourinary anomalies | Sporadic, some familial cases with autosomal recessive inheritance, genetically heterogeneous, multiple chromosomal anomalies | 25, 26 |
| Osteoglophonic dwarfism 166250 | Craniosynostosis of varying degrees including cloverleaf skull, depressed nasal bridge, frontal bossing, prognathism | | Rhizomelic dwarfism, "hollowed-out" metaphyses | Autosomal dominant, although mostly sporadic | 27, 28 |
| Pfeiffer syndrome 101600 | Brachycephaly, acrocephaly, hypertelorism, shallow orbits, exorbitism, flat midface, cloverleaf skull in sporadic cases | Broad thumbs and great toes which are medially deviated, variable cutaneous syndactyly | Occasionally conductive hearing loss, radiohumeral synostosis, mental retardation, variable visceral anomalies | Autosomal dominant, both sporadic and familial, mutations in FGFR1 P252R and FGFR2, exons IgIIIa and IgIIIc (see Table 245-2) | see text |

(Continued on next page)

**Table 245-1** (*Continued*)

| Syndrome/MIM | Craniofacial Findings | Extremities | Additional Findings | Genetic Etiology | References |
|---|---|---|---|---|---|
| Philadelphia syndrome 601222 | Sagittal craniosynostosis | Mitten-like syndactyly (similar to Apert syndrome), no bony syndactyly | Normal intelligence | Autosomal dominant inheritance in a 5-generation family | 29 |
| Sagittal craniosynostosis 123100 | Scaphocephaly, dolichocephaly, oxycephaly | | | Usually sporadic and nongenetic, some autosomal dominant families | 30, 31 |
| Saethre-Chotzen syndrome 101400 | Variable brachycephaly with maxillary hypoplasia, low frontal hairline, shallow orbits, hypertelorism, strabismus, small ears with prominent ear crus | Mild cutaneous syndactyly, broad great toes in valgus position, contractures of elbows and knees | | Autosomal dominant with mutations in *TWIST* (see Table 245-2); due to phenotypic overlap to Muenke syndrome mutation in *FGFR3*, P250R in some | see text |
| Shprintzen-Goldberg craniosynostosis 182212 | Severe exophthalmos, midface hypoplasia | Arachnodactyly, camptodactyly | Generalized connective tissue disorder, skeletal anomalies, obstructive apnea, developmental delay | Heterogeneous, autosomal dominant, *FBN1* (fibrillin-1) C1223Y mutation | see text |
| Thanatophoric dysplasia 187600 | Cloverleaf skull | Severe growth deficiency with short limbs and curvature of the long bones | Multiple skeletal anomalies, perinatal death due to severe respiratory compromise | Sporadic, mutations in *FGFR3* R248C, S249C, G370C, S371C, Y373C, K650E, and others | 32, 33 |

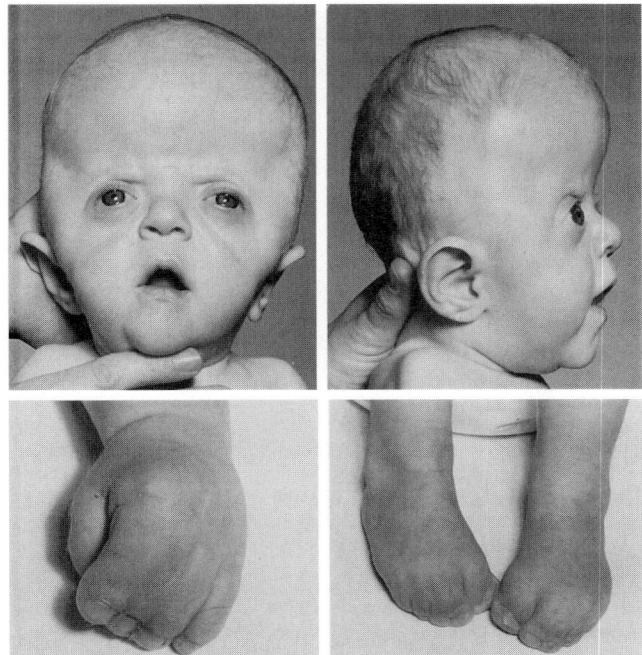

**Fig. 245-2 Craniofacial and limb anomalies in Apert syndrome. Severe turribrachycephaly with exorbitism and midfacial hypoplasia. Fingers 2 to 4 are fused, as are toes 2 to 5.**

bossing in infants, to cloverleaf skull deformity in two cases. Associated findings included headaches, poor vision due to myopia or hyperopia, and seizures. A cleft of the soft palate and a triphalangeal thumb were seen in one affected individual each. Hands and feet were generally normal, as was intelligence. A heterozygous mutation in the homeobox gene MSX2 (P148H) located at chromosome 5q34-q35 was shown in the affected individuals in this family.[94,95] To date, no other family with Boston syndrome has been identified; mutations of MSX2 more commonly cause parietal foramina without craniosynostosis.[95a]

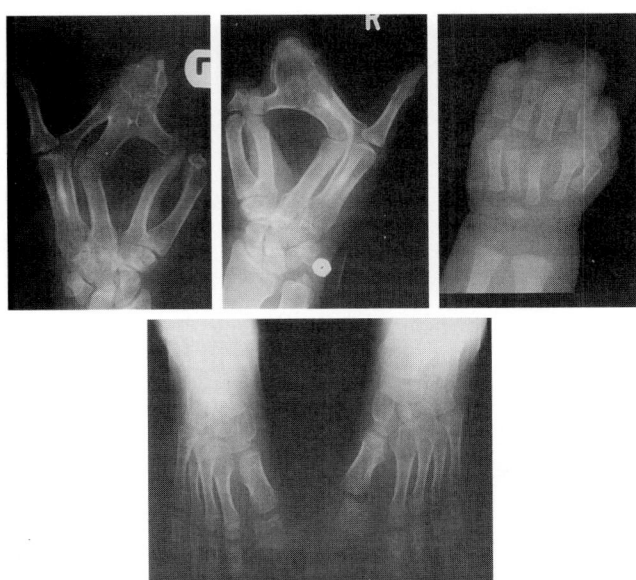

**Fig. 245-3 Hand and foot radiographs in Apert syndrome. Transverse and longitudinal osseous fusions of digits 2 to 4 (top left, middle) and longitudinal fusions of proximal and middle phalanges, without transverse fusions, in a different patient. Broad and shortened first toes (bottom).**

## Crouzon Syndrome

Crouzon syndrome (MIM 123500) was first described in 1912;[96] there have been numerous reports since then (for review see references 2 and 97). It is characterized by coronal or multiple suture synostosis with maxillary hypoplasia, a prominent beaked nose, shallow orbits, and exorbitism (Fig. 245-4).[49,98] Crouzon syndrome has an autosomal dominant mode of inheritance with high penetrance and moderate variability of the clinical findings. Approximately half of the cases are familial; the other half are new mutations with evidence of advanced paternal age. In cases with FGFR2 mutations, exclusive paternal origin of the mutations has been demonstrated.[98a] Crouzon syndrome is one of the most common craniosynostosis syndromes, having a birth prevalence of 1 in 65,000 newborns (approximately 4.5 percent of all craniosynostosis cases).[99]

Clinical findings include brachycephaly, but also scaphocephaly and trigonocephaly.[100] In one large family, the proband had a cloverleaf skull, several sibs had classic Crouzon syndrome, and several relatives had exorbitism and midface hypoplasia without craniosynostosis.[101] Intelligence is usually normal. Seizures are infrequent. Brain anomalies, for example agenesis of the corpus callosum, are rare whereas progressive hydrocephalus, which may be associated with herniation of the cerebellar tonsils is not uncommon.[49,102,103] Syringomyelia is a rare but important association.[49]

Hypertelorism and external strabismus are common. Other ophthalmologic findings may include poor vision, optic atrophy, nystagmus, and exposure conjunctivitis and keratitis.[104] Mild to moderate hearing deficit is present in half of the cases. Hypoplastic maxilla and relative prognathism is common. Cervical spine fusions are common (30 percent), mostly involving C2-C3,[105,106] and calcification of the stylohyoid ligament occurs in 50 percent of patients.[107] Hands and feet are clinically normal, although minor differences were noted on metacarpophalangeal profile patterns.[108–110] Airway obstruction and/or visceral anomalies are rare compared with Apert and Pfeiffer syndromes.[107,111]

Linkage studies have mapped Crouzon syndrome to chromosome 10q25-q26,[112] and numerous heterozygous mutations were identified in FGFR2 (see Table 245-2).

## Crouzon Syndrome with Acanthosis Nigricans

Although Crouzon syndrome was first reported in 1912, Crouzon syndrome with acanthosis nigricans was first mentioned in 1948 (for a review, see reference 113). Several cases were published in the mid-1980s and recently with the identification of a consistent heterozygous mutation (A391E) in FGFR3.[84,114,115] This is recognized as a distinct clinical and molecular entity (MIM 134934.0011). Acanthosis nigricans associated with Crouzon syndrome is rare. It is usually reported in females with an early onset of skin findings including hyperpigmentation, hyperkeratosis, and melanocytic nevi. Verrucous hyperplasia develops predominantly in flexural areas such as the axillae, but also in the neck, face (perioral, periorbital, nasolabial areas), chest, and abdomen. Craniofacial anomalies are similar to those in Crouzon syndrome and include brachycephaly due to coronal synostosis, hypertelorism, downslanting of the palpebral fissures, and ocular proptosis. Additional anomalies have been described in some patients: choanal atresia, cemental dysplasia of both jaws (cementomas), hydrocephalus, hypoplasia of the foramen magnum, scoliosis, and spinal stenosis with paresthesia of the lower limbs.

## Jackson-Weiss Syndrome

Jackson-Weiss syndrome (MIM 123150) was first reported in 1976[116] in a large Amish kindred, in which 88 affected individuals were personally examined and another 50 were reliably reported to be affected. Inheritance is autosomal dominant with high penetrance and variability in expression. Craniosynostosis with midface hypoplasia, frontal prominence, and foot anomalies with

**Table 245-2 FGFR Mutations Identified in Craniosynostosis**

| Gene | Mutation* | Codon change | Phenotype[†] | N[‡] | Reference[§] |
|---|---|---|---|---|---|
| FGFR1 | P252R | CCT → CGT | P | 13 | 58 |
| FGFR2[¶] | Y105C | TAT → TGT | C | 2 | 59 |
| | S252W | TCG → TGG | A,P | 262 | 57 |
| | S252F | TCG → TTT | A | 2 | 60 |
| | S252L | TCG → TTG | N,C | 1 | 60 |
| | S252F,P253S | TCG → TTC | P | 1 | 60 |
| | | CCT → TCT | | | |
| | P253R | CCT → CGT | A | 128 | 57 |
| | S267P | TCC → CCC | P,C,AB,S | 4 | 61 |
| | G268-269ins | 803-804ins3 | C | 1 | 62 |
| | VV269-270Δ | 804-809del | S | 1 | 63 |
| | F276V | TTT → GTT | P,C | 6 | 64 |
| | C278F | TGC → TTC | C,P,J | 18 | 61 |
| | Y281C | TAC → TGC | C | 1 | Wilkie, unpublished |
| | HIQ287-289Δ | 858-866del | C | 1 | 61 |
| | I288M, | 864-881del | P | 1 | 65 |
| | QWIKHV289-294Δ | | | | |
| | Q289P | CAG → CCG | C,J | 3 | 61 |
| | W290R | TGG → CGG | C | 3 | 61 |
| | W290G | TGG → GGG | C | 2 | 66 |
| | W290C | TGG → TGC | P,AB | 5 | 67 |
| | W290C | TGG → TGT | P | 5 | 68 |
| | K292E | AAG → GAG | C | 1 | 69 |
| | Y301C | TAC → TGC | C | 1 | 64 |
| | | 940-3−4insAlu** | A | 1 | 70 |
| | | 940-3T → G** | P | 1 | 71 |
| | | 940-2A → G** | P,A | 9 | 72 |
| | | 940-2A → T** | P | 2 | 73 |
| | | 940-1G → C** | P | 2 | 74 |
| | | 940-1G → A** | P | 2 | 65 |
| | | 940-946del 7insACC** | P | 1 | 74a |
| | A314S | GCC → TCC | P | 4 | 71 |
| | A315S | GCC → TCC | U | 2 | Wilkie, unpublished |
| | D321A | GAC → GCC | P | 4 | 72 |
| | Y328C | TAT → TGT | C | 1 | 75 |
| | N331I | AAT → ATT | C | 1 | 76 |
| | A337P | GCT → CCT | C | 1 | 77 |
| | DAims337-338 | 1011-1012ins6 | C | 1 | 76 |
| | G338R | GGG → CGG | C | 3 | 78 |
| | G338E | GGG → GAG | C | 2 | 59 |
| | Y340H | TAT → CAT | C | 6 | 79 |
| | Y340C | TAT → TGT | P | 3 | 65 |
| | T341P | ACG → CCG | P | 3 | 80 |
| | C342Y | TGC → TAC | C,P | 28 | 79 |
| | C342R | TGC → CGC | P,C,J,AB | 29 | 79 |
| | C342F | TGC → TTC | C | 3 | 61 |
| | C342S | TGC → TCC | P,C,J | 8 | 78 |
| | C342S | TGC → AGC | P,C,J | 7 | 79 |
| | C342S | TGC → TCT | P | 1 | 65 |
| | C342W | TGC → TGG | C,P | 9 | 66 |
| | C342G | TGC → GGC | P | 2 | 65 |
| | A344A | GCG → GCA** | C,U | 10 | 79 |
| | A344G | GCG → GGG | J,C | 2 | 75 |
| | A344P | GCG → CCG | P | 1 | 62 |
| | S347C | TCT → TGT | C | 9 | 75 |
| | | 1041-1042insAlu** | A | 1 | 70 |
| | S351C | TCC → TGC | P,U,AB | 18 | 59 |
| | S354C | TCT → TGT | C | 8 | 79 |
| | A355V | GCA → GTA | C | 1 | 80a |
| | WLT356-358Δ | 1066-1074del | C | 1 | 76 |
| | L357S | TTG → TCG | C | 1 | 81 |
| | V359F | GTT → TTT | C,P | 1 | 62 |
| | | 1084-1085ins6** | P | 1 | 62 |
| | | 1084+3A → G** | P | 2 | 65 |
| | S372C | TCC → TGC | BS | 1 | 82 |
| | Y375C | TAC → TGC | BS | 3 | 82 |

**Table 245-2** (*Continued*)

| Gene | Mutation* | Codon change | Phenotype[†] | N[‡] | Reference[§] |
|------|-----------|--------------|-----------|------|-----------|
| | G384R | GGG → AGG | U | 1 | 59 |
| FGFR3 | P250R | CCG → CGG | M | 123 | 83 |
| | A391E | GCG → GAG | C-A | 12 | 84 |

* Notation for mutations follows Antonarakis et al.[85]
† Syndrome abbreviations: A-Apert; AB-Antley-Bixler; BS-Beare-Stevenson; C-Crouzon; C-A-Crouzon/acanthosis nigricans; J-Jackson-Weiss; M-Muenke syndrome; N-normal phenotype; P-Pfeiffer syndrome; S-Saethre-Chotzen; U-unclassified.
‡ Number of unrelated individuals. Includes unpublished data from the authors' laboratories.
§ Earliest reference to the mutation is given.
¶ Amino acid and nucleotide numbering based on Dionne et al.[86] Nucleotide numbering starts at initiator Met codon (nucleotide 180 in original sequence). In FGFR2, nucleotides 749-939 encode the JgIIIa exon and 940-1084 encode the JgIIIc exon.
** Effect on splicing proven or presumed.

various cutaneous syndactylies and varying degrees of medially deviated and enlarged great toes characterize Jackson-Weiss syndrome. Thumbs are normal in all cases except one with fusion of the phalanges, and only one individual was reported with webbing of the fingers. Some affected individuals had no craniofacial anomalies on clinical and radiographic exam. Intelligence is normal. The variability of clinical findings is so marked that with the exception of Apert syndrome the entire spectrum of acrocephalosyndactylies was seen in the reported family.[116] Because of the lack of thumb anomalies in Jackson-Weiss syndrome, several families with craniosynostosis and foot anomalies have been assigned this diagnosis,[117,118,132] but were later found to have mutations in FGFR1 and FGFR3, respectively, different from the FGFR2 A344G alteration identified in the original family.[75] There is also overlap between the Jackson-Weiss phenotype and phenotypes associated with different mutations of FGFR2, leading to further confusion (see "Reappraisal of the Clinical Classification of Craniosynostosis" below). In our opinion, the diagnosis of Jackson-Weiss syndrome in sporadic cases or small families is likely to cause more confusion than enlightenment. We therefore propose that the designation Jackson-Weiss syndrome be reserved for the original large family until a new nomenclature for the acrocephalosyndactylies, combining clinical and molecular data, is agreed on.

## Muenke Syndrome

Muenke syndrome (MIM 134934.0014 and 602849), which has also been called Muenke craniosynostosis or FGFR3-associated coronal synostosis, was first described in 1996 in sporadic cases and autosomal-dominant families with a unique point mutation in FGFR3 (P250R).[83,119] Penetrance is incomplete. The phenotypic spectrum is so variable that patients with this specific mutation previously had been diagnosed as Pfeiffer, Saethre-Chotzen, Crouzon syndromes,[63,83,119–122] as well as Jackson-Weiss syndrome,[118] Adelaide-type craniosynostosis,[123] Ventruto syndrome,[124] nonsyndromic craniosynostosis,[83,119] and brachydactyly associated craniosynostosis.[125,126]

The birth prevalence of Muenke syndrome has not been accurately determined, but one study suggests 1 in 30,000.[126] Based on a comparison to other craniosynostosis syndromes, it appears that the mutation associated with this syndrome is common in sporadic or familial patients with uni- or bicoronal synostosis whose findings do not fit into any of the classic craniosynostosis syndromes. The mutation rate is estimated to be one of the highest in the human genome and comparable with that of achondroplasia (1138G → A in *FGFR3*; see Chap. 210) and Apert syndrome (755C → G in *FGFR2*; discussed in this chapter).[126]

Clinical findings in over 60 patients from more than 20 unrelated families include bi- or unicoronal synostosis (67 percent), midface hypoplasia (59 percent), downslanting palpebral fissures (50 percent), and ptosis (27 percent) (Fig. 245-5).[119] In cases with bicoronal synostosis, bulging of the temporal fossae may give a wide-face appearance.[127] However, some mutation carriers do not show any signs of craniosynostosis, having only macrocephaly (6 percent) or even normal head size.[119,128,129] In a prospective study, this specific *FGFR3* mutation was identified in 4 of 37 affected individuals with unicoronal synostosis only, some cases of which were previously attributed to intrauterine constraint.[128] Moloney et al.[126] and Reardon et al.[121] have also described anterior plagiocephaly.

Sensorineural hearing loss is seen in some (37 percent), as is developmental delay (37 percent). In another study, mental retardation was noted in four of nine patients with this mutation.[121] The extreme phenotypic variability is emphasized by a five-generation family in which the P250R mutation in *FGFR3* segregates with moderate congenital bilateral sensorineural deafness and low penetrance of craniosynostosis.[130] Lajeunie et al.[127] reported a greater severity of phenotype in females than males.

Hand anomalies are found in some, but not all, affected individuals and include brachydactyly (30 percent) and clinodactyly (42 percent) with characteristic radiographic findings, such as thimble-like middle phalanges (60 percent), coned epiphyses (75 percent), and carpal fusions (13 percent) (Figs. 245-5 and 245-6).

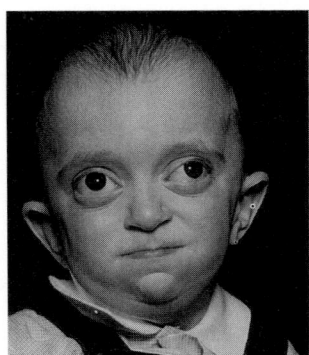
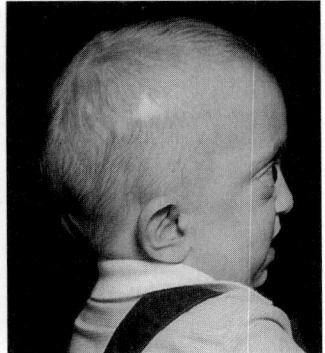
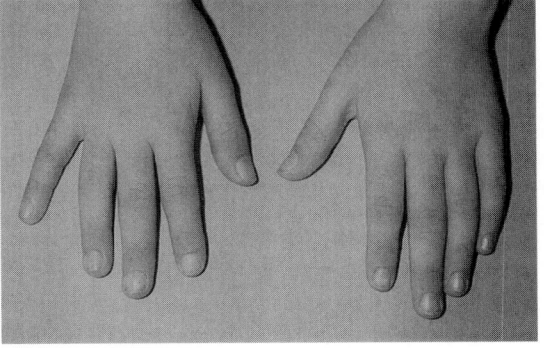

**Fig. 245-4** Craniofacial anomalies in Crouzon syndrome. Note midfacial hypoplasia, exorbitism, and beaked nose. Hands appear normal.

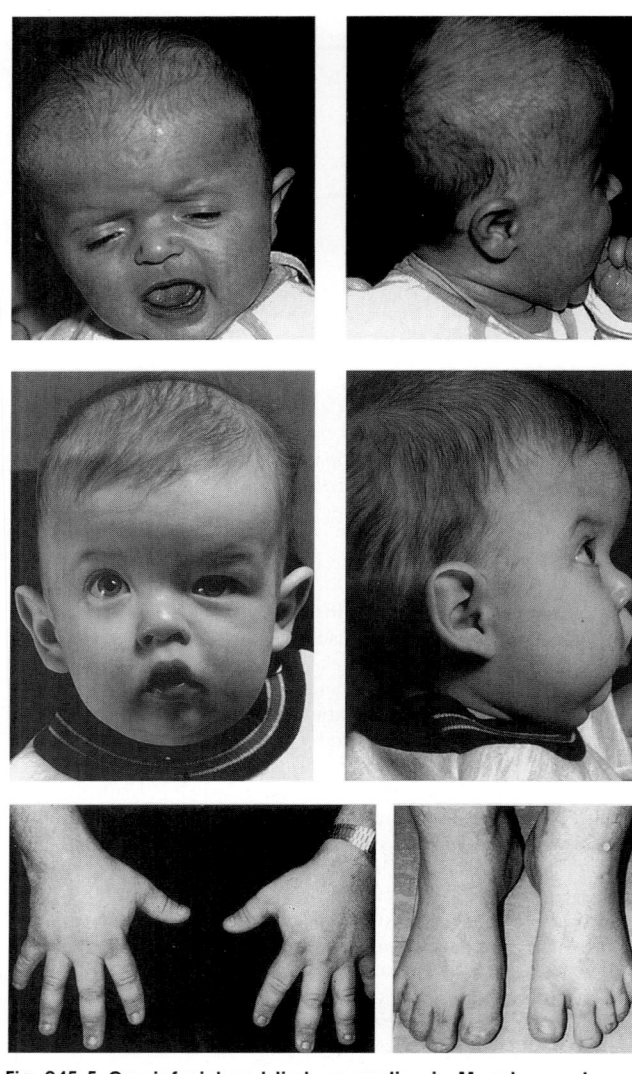

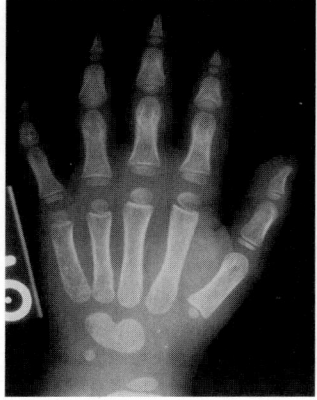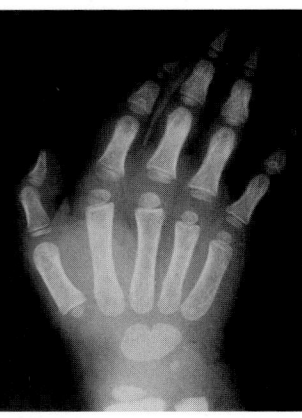

**Fig. 245-6 Radiographs of hands in Muenke syndrome. Brachydactyly with short thimble-like middle phalanges of the second through fifth fingers and fusion of the capitate and hamate bones of the wrists.**

**Fig. 245-5 Craniofacial and limb anomalies in Muenke syndrome. Note symmetric facial appearance due to bicoronal synostosis (in upper panel) and plagiocephaly due to unilateral coronal synostosis (in middle panel). Mild brachydactyly of hands and feet (in lower panel). (*From Muenke et al.*[119] *Used by permission of American Journal of Human Genetics*).**

Some patients have broad halluces (26 percent) that are not deviated. Radiologic findings in the feet include short, broad middle phalanges (13 percent), coned epiphyses (86 percent), and calcaneocuboid fusions (35 percent). Height is normal, in contrast to *FGFR3*-associated dwarfism syndromes.

## Pfeiffer Syndrome

Pfeiffer syndrome (MIM 101600) was first described in 1964[131] in a three-generation family with autosomal-dominant inheritance. Craniosynostosis, broad thumbs, and broad great toes characterize it. Numerous familial cases have been described since the original report (see reviews in references 132 and 133). Penetrance is complete; expressivity is variable. In addition to familial occurrence, sporadic cases due to new mutations are well known. These commonly have a more severe phenotype. The birth prevalence of Pfeiffer syndrome is not known, but it is clearly less common than Apert, Crouzon, Muenke, and Saethre-Chotzen syndromes.

Clinical subtypes of Pfeiffer syndrome were proposed before the underlying etiology was known.[132] Classic Pfeiffer syndrome, or type 1, has the best prognosis and is compatible with a normal life span and normal intelligence in most cases. In contrast,

Pfeiffer syndrome types 2 and 3 have a higher risk for neurodevelopmental problems and reduced life expectancy.[68,134–142] Both types are sporadic, and findings are more severe, including severe ocular proptosis and elbow ankylosis. Type 2 has a cloverleaf skull in contrast to type 3. Exceptions with a more favorable prognosis have been reported.[139]

Linkage studies in families with Pfeiffer syndrome demonstrated genetic heterogeneity with loci on chromosomes 8p11.2[58,143] and 10q25-q26,[71] with mutations in the genes coding for the fibroblast growth factor receptors 1 and 2 (*FGFR1*, *FGFR2*), respectively (see "FGFR Mutations in Craniosynostosis" below). Pfeiffer syndrome type 1 has been reported with mutations in *FGFR1* and *FGFR2*, whereas patients with types 2 and 3 have mutations in *FGFR2* only (Table 245-2). Several large families that were considered to have some findings consistent with Pfeiffer syndrome were excluded from either of these two regions, but mapped to chromosome 4p16 and were later demonstrated to have Muenke syndrome.[83,119]

Craniofacial features in Pfeiffer syndrome are variable and secondary to synostosis mostly involving the coronal sutures.[144,145] Findings include a turribrachycephalic skull, midface hypoplasia with relative mandibular prognathism, beaked nose, low nasal bridge, hypertelorism, downslanting palpebral fissures, exorbitism, strabismus, highly arched palate, and crowded teeth (Figs. 245-7 and 245-8).

Intelligence is usually normal, although mental deficiency has been observed, particularly in sporadic cases. Rare central nervous system anomalies include large ventricles, hydrocephalus, Arnold-Chiari malformation, and seizures.[148]

Anomalies of the hands and feet differ from any other craniosynostosis syndrome.[73,149,150] Characteristically, the thumbs and great toes are broad and deviated away from the other digits (Figs. 245-7, 245-8, 245-9, and 245-10). However, the thumbs may be of normal width, which may lead to doubt whether a diagnosis of Jackson-Weiss or Pfeiffer syndrome should be made. We suggest that, unless part of the large Amish kindred, it creates less confusion if such cases are labeled as Pfeiffer syndrome. Brachydactyly is often present, as is partial soft tissue syndactyly of the fingers and toes. Radiographic findings of the hands include malformed and fused phalanges of the thumbs, short middle phalanges (brachymesophalangy) of the second and fifth fingers with complete absence in severe cases, symphalangism (complete osseous fusion of proximal, middle, and distal phalanges which occurs over several years), and occasional fusion of the proximal ends of metacarpals 4 and 5. The distal phalanx of the great toe is broad, and the proximal phalanx is malformed. Broad and short first metatarsals and fusion of carpal and tarsal bones have been described.

Additional manifestations may include cloverleaf skull (type 2 Pfeiffer syndrome), fusions of cervical and lumbar

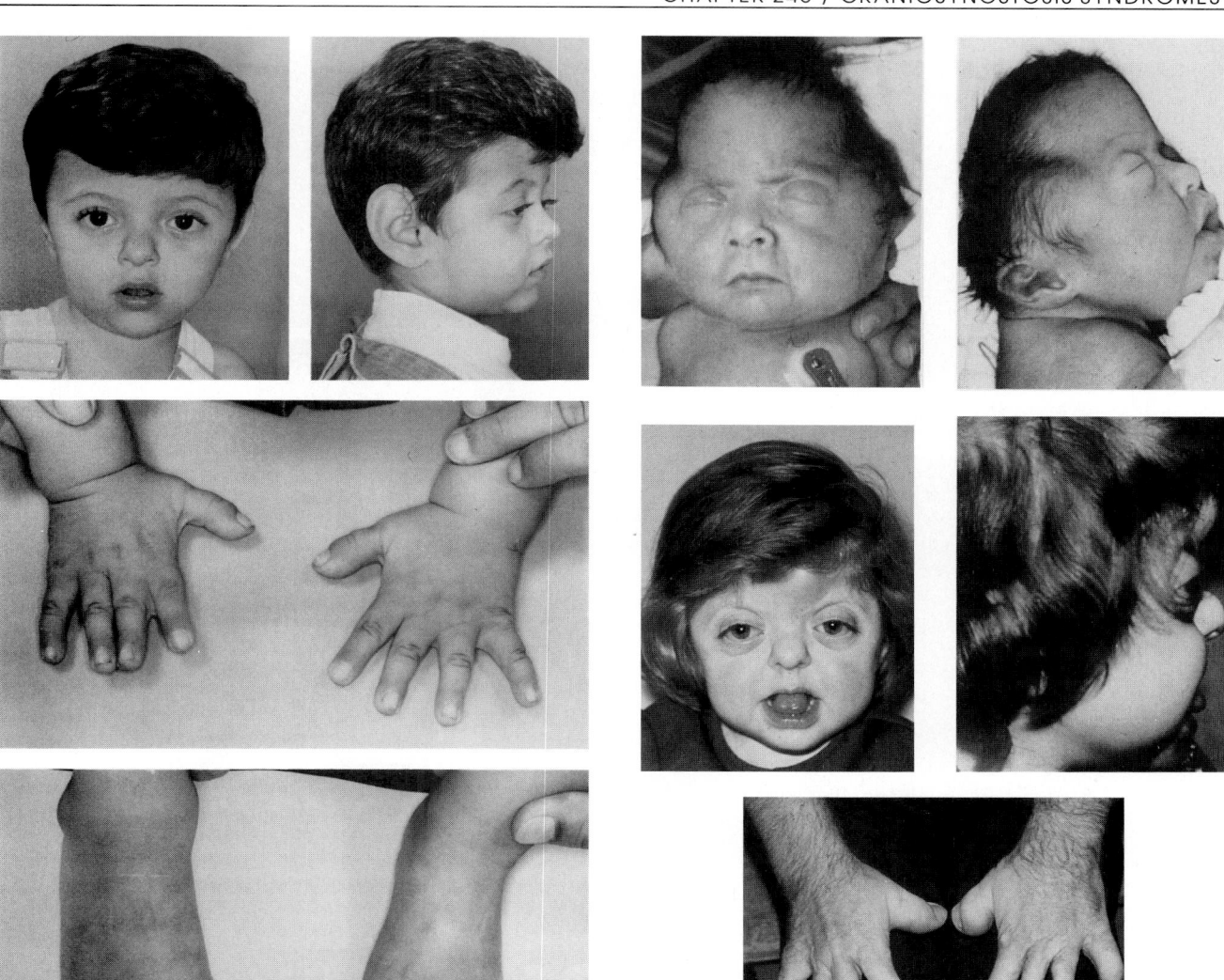

**Fig. 245-7 Mild craniofacial and limb anomalies in Pfeiffer syndrome due to *FGFR1* mutation. Brachycephaly with hypertelorism. Partial cutaneous syndactyly of fingers and toes. Note broad, medially deviated great toes. (*From Schell et al.*[146] *Used by permission of Brazilian Journal of Dysmorphology and Speech-Hearing Disorders.*)**

**Fig. 245-8 Craniofacial and limb anomalies in Pfeiffer syndrome due to *FGFR2* mutation. Cloverleaf skull with exorbitism and severe midface hypoplasia in sporadic Pfeiffer syndrome (in upper panel). Brachycephaly with hypertelorism, downslanting palpebral fissures and midface hypoplasia in familial Pfeiffer syndrome. Broad thumbs and symphalangism of all fingers. (*From Schell et al.*[71] *and Muenke et al.*[147] *Used by permission of Human Molecular Genetics and Humana Press, respectively*).**

vertebrae,[145,151] sacrococcygeal eversion,[142] cubitus valgus, synostosis of the radiohumeral and ulnar-humeral joints, shortened humerus, abnormalities of the pelvis, coxa valga, and talipes equinovarus. Abnormalities affecting other organ systems are of low frequency and include hearing loss,[152] optic nerve hypoplasia, iris coloboma,[153] choanal stenosis/atresia, bifid uvula, tracheal stenosis,[154] supernumerary teeth, gingival hypertrophy, widely spaced nipples, intestinal malrotation,[137] anal atresia or malpositioned anus,[155] pyloric stenosis, umbilical hernia, cryptorchidism, and bifid scrotum.[156]

## PFEIFFER SYNDROME CAUSED BY *FGFR1* OR *FGFR2* MUTATIONS

Prior to the finding that Pfeiffer syndrome is a genetically heterogeneous disorder linked to *FGFR1* on chromosome 8p11.2 and *FGFR2* on chromosome 10q26,[58,71,72,80,143] Pfeiffer syndrome

was considered one clinical entity. The majority of large families with Pfeiffer syndrome that have been studied by linkage and mutation analysis could be assigned to either *FGFR1* or *FGFR2*. The FGFR1 P252R mutation was identified in multiple affected individuals from unrelated families and in sporadic cases[58,62,71,77,117,146,157] (Muenke, unpublished). The phenotype in individuals with the FGFR1 P252R mutation, although somewhat variable even among affected members of the same family, is consistently milder than that of Pfeiffer syndrome due to different *FGFR2* mutations (Figs. 245-7 and 245-8).

In contrast, clinical findings in Pfeiffer syndrome due to *FGFR2* mutations are consistently more severe (Figs. 245-8 and 245-10). The original family[131] and a two-generation family with seven affected members[71] were linked to chromosome 10q25-q26 markers but were negative when sequenced for *FGFR2* exons JgIIIa and JgIIIc (Muenke, unpublished) and FGF8,[158] but presumably carry an *FGFR2* mutation outside the JgIIIa and

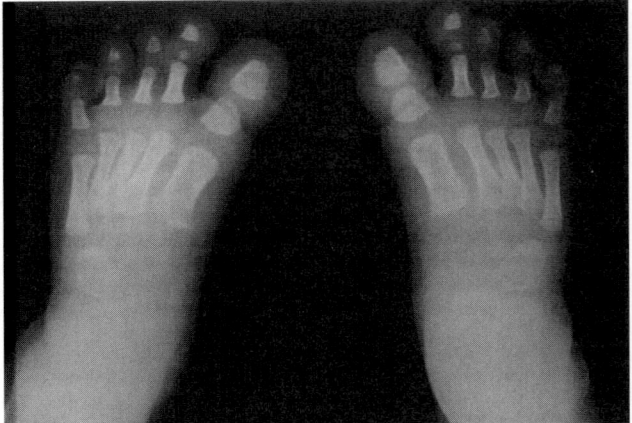

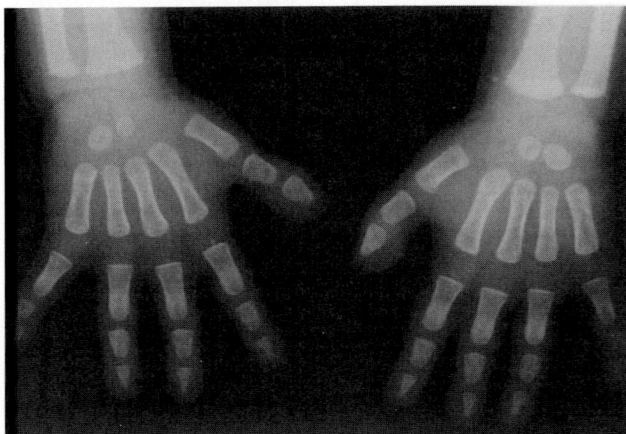

Fig. 245-9 Radiographs of hands and feet in Pfeiffer syndrome with *FGFR1* mutation. Mild brachydactyly and mildly broad thumbs and broad medially deviated great toes (same patient as Fig. 245-7).

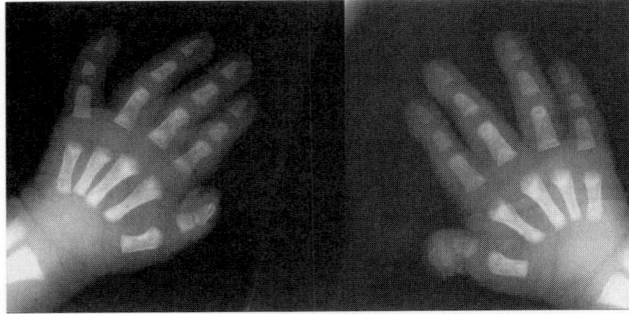

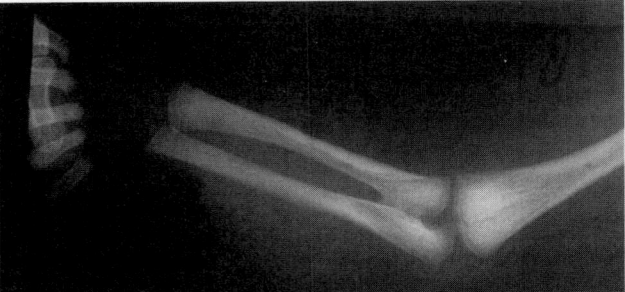

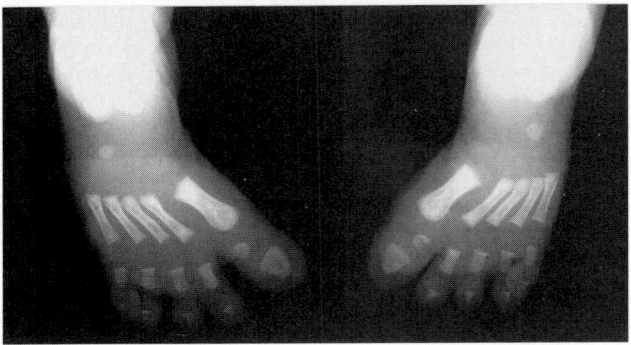

Fig. 245-10 Radiographs of hands, elbow, and feet in sporadic Pfeiffer syndrome *FGFR2* mutation. Brachydactyly of hands and feet. Abnormally broad proximal phalanges of thumb and great toe. Radioulnar and early humeroulnar fusion of elbow.

JgIIIc exons. Pfeiffer syndrome families with known *FGFR2* JgIIIa and JgIIIc mutations have been reported.[62,71,72,146,159] The clinical findings in these families consist of characteristic craniofacial and limb anomalies in "classic" Pfeiffer syndrome, which are more severe than those seen due to FGFR1 P252R mutation.

All sporadic cases of Pfeiffer syndrome with severe clinical findings, including cloverleaf skull (Fig. 245-11),[62,67,68,71,72,74,80,140–142,160] had *FGFR2* mutations.

## Saethre-Chotzen Syndrome

Saethre-Chotzen syndrome (MIM 101400) was first described in 1931.[161,162] It is characterized by brachycephaly, low frontal hairline, facial asymmetry, ptosis of the eyelids, a flat midface, and a thin, pointed nose (Fig. 245-12; see review references 163, 164, and 164a). Inheritance is autosomal dominant. Penetrance is incomplete, and expressivity is variable. Saethre-Chotzen syndrome is among the more frequent syndromes with an estimated birth prevalence of 1 in 65,000, although this may be an overestimate due to the inadvertent inclusion of cases of Muenke syndrome.

Clinical findings are variable even within the same family (Fig. 245-12). Brachycephaly due to coronal synostosis is present in most but not all cases; the time of onset and degree is variable. Frequently, plagiocephaly and facial asymmetry are present. A low-set frontal hairline is common. Ptosis of the eyelids is common, as are hypertelorism and strabismus. The nose is prominent, frequently long and pointed. Deviation of the nasal septum is common. Maxillary hypoplasia and relative mandibular prognathism is present. The palate is often narrow and highly arched. Clefting of the palate is occasional. Other oral findings include malocclusion and supernumerary teeth.[165] Ears are small and posteriorly rotated, and have a long and prominent ear crus.

Limb anomalies may include brachydactyly and partial cutaneous syndactyly frequently between fingers 2 and 3 (Fig. 245-12). Partial cutaneous syndactyly between toes 2 and 3 has been reported. The great toes can be broad and deviated towards the other toes. This may be associated with transverse duplication of the hallux, a phenotypic variant sometimes termed Robinow-Sorauf syndrome (MIM 180750) which has been shown to be an allelic variant.[165a] Other skeletal anomalies include defects of the cervical and lumbar spine, and contractures of the elbows (rarely radioulnar synostosis) and knees (see review reference 164). Occasionally, associated neurologic and psychiatric symptoms can be present.[166–168] Because of the extremely variable and overlapping phenotypes, Saethre-Chotzen and Muenke syndrome have been confused with one another.[63,119] Furthermore, some clinical findings in Saethre-Chotzen syndrome are seen in patients with craniofrontonasal syndrome (Table 245-1), from which it needs to be differentiated.

The genetic etiology of Saethre-Chotzen syndrome is different from other classic craniosynostosis syndromes and involves cytogenetic deletions, translocations, and heterozygous mutations in the *TWIST* gene at chromosome 7p21.1 (Tables 245-3 and 245-4). Patients with large deletions are more likely to have mild to moderate mental retardation[170] (see "TWIST Mutations" below).

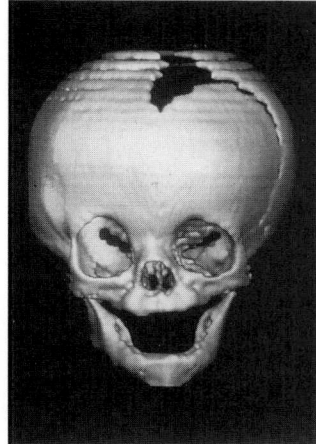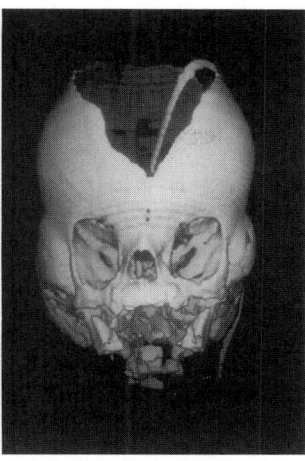

**Fig. 245-11** Three-dimensional CT scans in craniosynostosis syndromes. Plagiocephaly with facial asymmetry in a newborn with Muenke syndrome due to right unicoronal and metopic suture fusion (left). Severe synostosis of multiple sutures leading to cloverleaf skull and extremely wide open fontanelle in a newborn with sporadic Pfeiffer syndrome and FGFR2 (S351C) mutation (right).

## Shprintzen-Goldberg Syndrome

Shprintzen-Goldberg syndrome, also known as Shprintzen-Goldberg craniosynostosis syndrome or Marfanoid craniosynostosis syndrome (MIM 182212), was first described in 1982 in two unrelated boys.[177] Since the initial report, a total of 20 unrelated males and females have been described with craniosynostosis, distinct skeletal anomalies, and Marfan-like phenotype.[178–184] Dolichocephaly associated with fusion of the metopic or sagittal sutures is common (for review see reference 180). A large anterior fontanelle may not close until the second to fourth year of life. Additional craniofacial findings include shallow orbits with exophthalmos, low-set ears, maxillary and mandibular hypoplasia, and pseudocleft of the palate. Ectopia lentis has been described in only one patient.[184] Skeletal and connective tissue findings include 13 pairs of ribs, vertebral anomalies, arachnodactyly and camptodactyly, thorax anomalies (pectus carinatum or excavatum), obstructive apnea, cardiac anomalies including dilated aortic root and aortic dissection, multiple abdominal hernias, hyperelastic skin, and infantile hypotonia. Neurologic findings include developmental delay and mental retardation in some, and hydrocephalus in others.[178] Rare anomalies have been described: cloverleaf skull, ptosis, choanal atresia, atlantoaxial dislocation, intestinal malrotation, anteriorly placed anus, and hypospadias. With the exception of one family with Shprintzen-Goldberg syndrome,[178] all other reported cases were sporadic.

Shprintzen-Goldberg syndrome is probably genetically heterogeneous. Only one mutation has been substantiated to date — a de novo heterozygous mutation (C1223Y) in the fibrillin-1 (FBN1) gene of the single patient manifesting ectopia lentis.[184] A P1148A substitution, which was identified in another patient with Shprintzen-Goldberg syndrome, was subsequently found in unrelated controls and considered to be a benign variant.[185,185a]

## Complications of Craniosynostosis

Severe cases of craniosynostosis cause very complex distortions of the cranial anatomy and are associated with diverse complications, including raised intracranial pressure, hydrocephalus, cerebellar tonsillar herniation, deafness, visual problems, cleft palate, choanal atresia, dental malocclusion, respiratory problems, psychosocial difficulties, mental retardation, and death.[186] In cases of syndromic craniosynostosis caused by a single gene mutation, it can be difficult to distinguish which features arise as primary consequences of the mutation, and which are secondary to the craniosynostosis. This is an important practical issue because

surgery may reverse some of the secondary consequences of craniosynostosis, but does not alter the underlying biology of the disorder.

A particular question is whether surgery can influence mental outcome. There are many potentially reversible factors that contribute to mental retardation. An inverse relationship between raised intracranial pressure and IQ has been demonstrated.[187] Progressive hydrocephalus, associated with chronic tonsillar herniation, occurs frequently in Crouzon syndrome (12 of 22 patients).[148,188] Craniosynostosis may cause localized differences in cerebral perfusion, which normalize after surgery.[189,190,190a] Upper airway obstruction may lead to obstructive sleep apnea.[142,191,192] Diminished sensory input, especially of hearing and vision,[193] and psychosocial problems, can contribute to poor development. In addition, however, FGFs and their receptors are widely expressed in neural tissue[194] and FGFR mutations are often associated with intrinsic brain abnormalities. In Apert syndrome, for example, a wide variety of central nervous system abnormalities has been documented.[37] Magnetic resonance imaging of 60 Apert patients revealed corpus callosum abnormalities in 30 percent, hydrocephalus (mostly nonprogressive) in 43 percent, and agenesis or cavum septum pellucidum in 55 percent. Average IQ was 62 (range 10 to 114), and the three most important prognostic

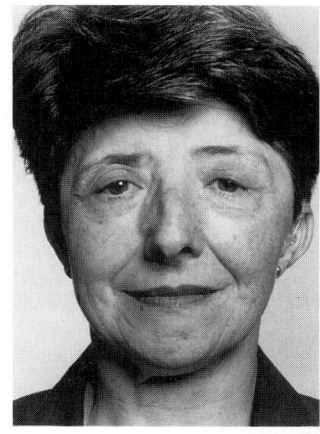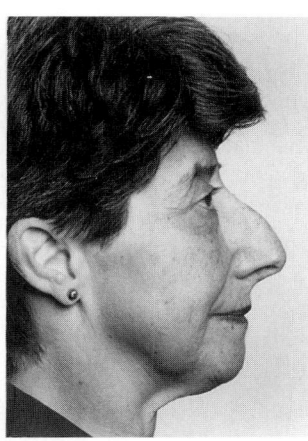

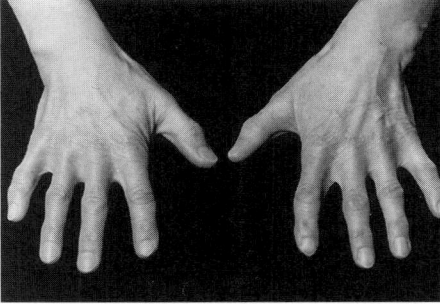

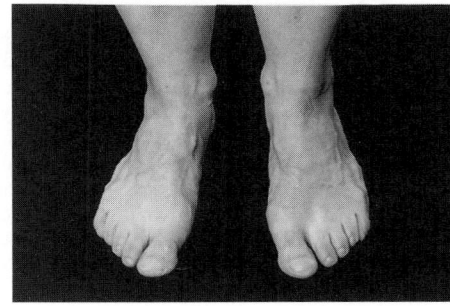

**Fig. 245-12** Mild craniofacial and limb anomalies in Saethre-Chotzen syndrome. Brachycephaly with ptosis of the eyelids, low-set hairline, and mild midface hypoplasia. Note the prominent ear crus. Mild cutaneous syndactyly between some fingers and toes.

factors for satisfactory developmental progress were operation at < 1 year, a normal septum pellucidum, and rearing in the home environment.[195] This study illustrates the mixture of treatable and untreatable factors in craniosynostosis.

## PRENATAL DIAGNOSIS OF CRANIOSYNOSTOSIS

Craniosynostosis arises relatively late during embryogenesis. In the human, ossification of the skull, which occurs directly in membrane overlying the developing brain, initiates around the ninth week of gestation. The sutures form along the lines of apposition of the spreading bone fronts, which does not occur until 15 to 20 weeks.[196] The consequence is that craniosynostosis cannot reliably be detected in low-risk pregnancies by routine ultrasound scanning at this gestation, although later on, the effects on skull shape may become obvious in severe cases.

The prenatal diagnosis of craniosynostosis by ultrasound scanning, mostly early in the third trimester, has been described in several case reports. The severity of these cases has varied from cloverleaf skull with stillbirth[197] to relatively minor deformities associated with operable craniosynostosis and a good prognosis.[198] Careful examination of the limbs is important in all cases where craniosynostosis is suspected. This may suggest specific syndromic diagnoses such as Apert,[199,200] Pfeiffer,[201] or Crouzon syndrome.[202]

Given the high proportion of new mutations, the identification of the molecular basis of craniosynostosis is likely to have a relatively minor impact on prenatal diagnosis. To date the only reports of molecular genetic prenatal diagnoses of fetuses at 50 percent risk concern single families with Crouzon and Apert syndromes.[203,204] Molecular analysis has been used to confirm a diagnosis of Apert syndrome that was suspected on ultrasound.[205] Probably the most common application of molecular genetics has been to check that the unborn sib of an individual with a de novo FGFR2 mutation does not also carry the same mutation.[206] This approach eliminates the possibility of recurrence due to germ line mosaicism, but caution is recommended in prenatal counseling before embarking on invasive diagnostic testing. Although a few possible cases of germ line mosaicism were reported in the premolecular literature,[42] none has yet been confirmed at the molecular level and it seems likely that germ line mosaicism is rare in FGFR mutations,[44,98a,207] with a recurrence risk of less than 1 percent. When this is the sole indication for prenatal diagnosis, procedures such as chorionic villus sampling that are associated with a potentially higher risk should be viewed with caution.

## DIAGNOSIS

The diagnosis in patients with premature fusion of one or several the sutures of the skull is usually made by a physical examination, frequently in the newborn period. Patients are brought to medical attention because of the abnormal shape of the skull. In cases of plagiocephaly, distinction from nonsynostotic causes is essential.[2a] A careful craniofacial examination will include an assessment of the shape of the skull and face, a test for movement of the calvarial bones, observation for the presence or absence of sutural ridging and fontanelles, and, in cases of plagiocephaly, observation of the positions of the ears relative to the shape of the front and back of the head. A dysmorphology exam is required to detect associated findings, such as midfacial hypoplasia, abnormal position of the eyes (e.g., hypertelorism and/or exorbitism), an abnormal shape of the nose, cleft palate, position, size and shape of ears, anomalies of the hands and feet, and other skeletal anomalies (for review see reference 2).

Plain skull radiographs and three-dimensional CT scans are used to document prematurely fused sutures and craniofacial dysmorphism (Fig. 245-11) (see review reference 208). Associated increased intracranial pressure may be suspected on radiologic, ophthalmologic, or neurologic examination, but requires intracranial pressure monitoring for confirmation. Radiographs of the

hands and feet, are indicated to detect syndrome-specific anomalies (for review see above and references 209 and 210). Dermatologic consultation with histologic examination of the skin can document such findings as acanthosis nigricans. Clinical findings for specific craniosynostosis syndromes are described in detail in the previous sections and in Table 245-1.

## MANAGEMENT

A multidisciplinary team approach is required for the management of the craniofacial, audiologic, ocular, oral, dental, skeletal, limb, and skin anomalies. Members of this team include pediatricians, geneticists, craniofacial, maxillofacial, and neurosurgeons, orthodontists, ophthalmologists, audiologists, speech therapists, psychologists, and others. Management is symptomatic, counseling for parents is critical, and psychosocial support is often indicated. Craniofacial surgery often requires a staged approach to reconstruction.[2] Recommended timing and number of procedures varies between different craniofacial centers, and depends on the severity of the deformities. Simple sagittal synostosis is best treated early, by strip craniectomy before 6 months of age, whereas the primary cranio-orbital surgery in infants with either Apert (Fig. 245-13), Pfeiffer, or Crouzon (Fig. 245-13) syndromes is preferentially performed at 6 to 12 months. A repeat craniotomy may be planned in early childhood. Surgical management of total midface hypoplasia, that is, total midface advancement, is performed in 5- to 7-year-old children, whereas surgical management of malocclusion is done at ages 14 to 16 years in females and 16 to 18 years in males (see reviews references 211 to 220). Increasing use is being made of distraction osteogenesis for these later procedures.[220a]

## MOLECULAR PATHOLOGY OF CRANIOSYNOSTOSIS: MUTATIONS IN *MSX2*, *FGFR1*, *FGFR2*, *FGFR3* AND *TWIST* GENES

### MSX2 Mutation in a Single Family with Craniosynostosis, Boston Type

Genetic linkage of craniosynostosis, Boston type to distal chromosome 5q was demonstrated in 1993.[94] About the same

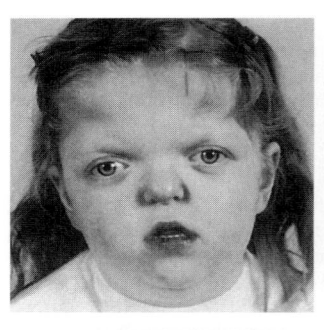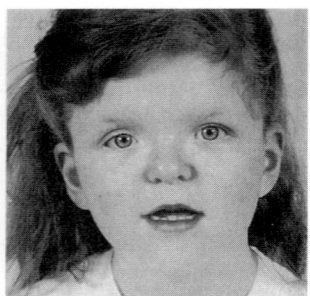
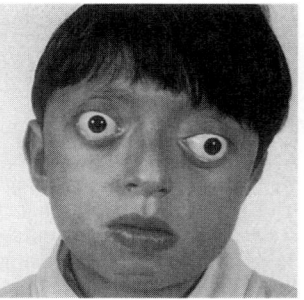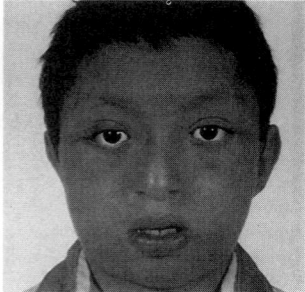

**Fig. 245-13** Craniofacial surgery in craniosynostosis syndromes. Pre- and postoperative findings in Apert (top) and Crouzon syndrome (bottom). (*From Posnick.*[211] *Used with permission from Neurosurgery Clinics of North America.*)

time, the *MSX2* gene (GenBank numbers for cDNA: d89377; gDNA: 122498, 122499) was localized to 5q34-q35, which shortly afterwards led to the demonstration in this family of the first genetic lesion causing craniosynostosis, a heterozygous P148H (CCC → CAC) mutation of MSX2.[95] This was also the first homeobox gene mutation to be described in any human disorder. Paradoxically, no further mutations in this gene have been described in craniosynostosis. The *MSX2* mutation is, therefore, of historical and academic interest, but appears to be only a minor contributor to the pathogenesis of craniosynostosis.

The P148H substitution occurs at position 7 of the highly conserved homeodomain, which is involved in both DNA and protein interactions. A target DNA binding site in the *osteocalcin* gene has been identified, and MSX2 suppresses the *osteocalcin* promoter in calvarial osteoblasts (see review reference 221). Binding studies of wild-type and mutant proteins to a known target DNA sequence using DNA mobility shift assays show that the mutant exhibits enhanced stability of DNA binding due to a reduced rate of dissociation of the complex; sequence specificity of DNA binding was not altered.[314] A yeast two-hybrid screen using MSX2 as bait identified a novel mouse protein — miz1 — that is capable of binding specifically to msx2. Moreover, the P148H mutation was shown to enhance the cooperative interaction between msx2 and miz1.[222] This unusual gain-of-function mechanism may explain why this is a rare cause of craniosynostosis, as homeodomain mutations more commonly result in loss of function.[223] Indeed, loss-of-function mutations of MSX2 have recently been described in a different calvarial phenotype, familial parietal foromina (MIM 168500).[95a] The developmental pathology of the MSX2 mutation is discussed in the section on insights into cranial suture biology.

## Structure and Function of Fibroblast Growth Factor Receptors (FGFRs)

Mutations of the fibroblast growth factor receptors (FGFRs) account for 15 to 20 percent of all cases of craniosynostosis. FGFRs are transmembrane-receptor tyrosine-kinase proteins, the principal function of which is to bind fibroblast growth factors (FGFs) and transduce signals in the cell. Ten different FGFs have been well characterized, but further family members are rapidly being identified, and at least 19 FGF-like proteins are known.[224,225,225a] It is well-established, however, that the FGFRs are encoded by four paralogous genes in the human, which are located on chromosomes 8p11.2 (*FGFR1*) gene (GenBank number for cDNA: x52833), 10q26 (*FGFR2*) (GenBank number for

cDNA: x52832), 4p16.3 (*FGFR3*) (GenBank numbers for cDNA: m58051 and gDNA: 178720 to 178738 inclusive), and 5q35.1-qter (*FGFR4*). All four FGFRs share the same general structure with three extracellular immunoglobulin (Ig)-like domains, a single transmembrane segment and a split tyrosine kinase domain (Fig. 245-14). Amino acid identity of human FGFRs is 64 to 74 percent for the extracellular domain and 72 to 85 percent for the kinase domain, and sequence comparison indicates that FGFR4 is the most diverged member of the family.[226] Heparan sulphate proteoglycans are an important cofactor for FGF binding which occurs in a 2:2 FGF:FGFR stoichiometry.[227] FGF binding involves contacts with both the IgII and IgIII domains (Fig. 245-14), the relative importance of these contacts varying with different FGFs.[229–232] X-ray crystal structures have been determined for FGF1 and FGF2,[233] the FGF1/FGF2-heparin complex,[234,235] the extracellular region of FGFR1 bound to FGF2,[235a] and the kinase domain of FGFR1.[236] The Ig-like domains of FGFRs most closely resemble the I-set and have been modeled on the structure of telokin.[237] The quaternary FGF:FGFR complex leads to (*trans*-) autophosphorylation of intracellular tyrosine residues (seven in FGFR1).[228,236,238] This results in stimulation of intrinsic protein tyrosine kinase activity, and to binding by proteins containing Src homology 2 (SH2) and phosphotyrosine binding (PTB) domains.[239,240] Major consequences include activation of the RAS/mitogen-activated protein kinase (MAPK) pathway and phosphatidylinositol hydrolysis.[241,241a]

The genes encoding the *FGFR* paralogues comprise approximately 20 exons[242–247,247a] and are modular in structure, enabling different domains to be joined by alternative splicing. All FGFRs are subject to extremely complex patterns of splicing, including forms that lack the first Ig-like domain, soluble forms comprising the first one or two Ig-like domains only, and intracellular forms that lack the transmembrane domain (see reviews references 245 and 248). Of particular relevance to the pathophysiology of craniosynostosis is the obligatory alternative splicing of the second half of the IgIII domain in FGFR1, FGFR2, and FGFR3, but not FGFR4.[242,249] This creates isoforms with distinct FGF binding characteristics,[250] as illustrated for FGFR2 (Fig. 245-15).

FGFRs are widely expressed but show complex expression patterns specific to particular tissues, stages, and splice forms.[252–256] This includes several examples where expression of different FGFRs or alternative FGFR splice forms appear mutually exclusive but occurs either in neighboring cells or sequentially in time, indicating that switching of FGFR expression may play an important role in differentiation. Additionally,

## Receptor Monomers          Receptor Dimerization

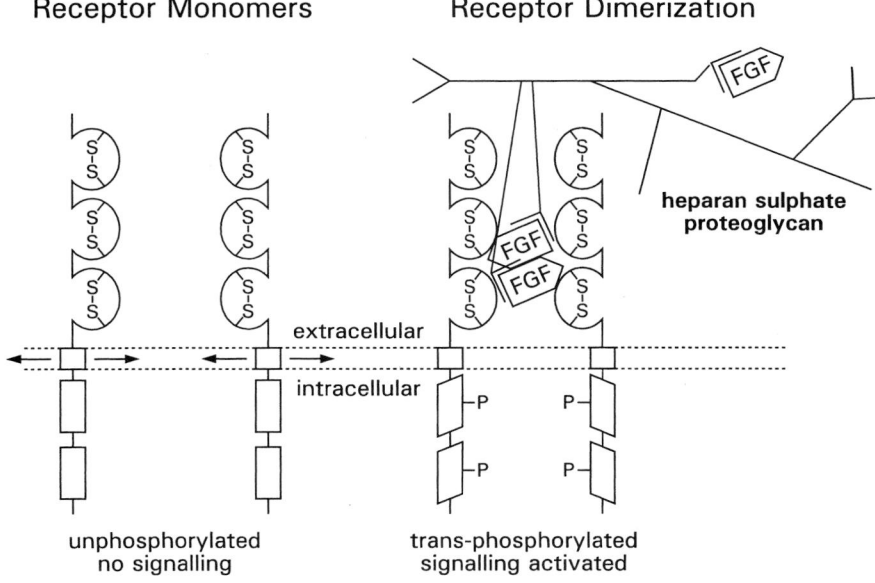

extracellular

intracellular

unphosphorylated
no signalling

trans-phosphorylated
signalling activated

heparan sulphate
proteoglycan

**Fig. 245-14 Structure and function of FGFRs.** On the left, the FGFR protein is depicted passing through the plane of the cell membrane (parallel dotted lines), with the extracellular side uppermost. Note the three disulfide-linked (-S-S-) immunoglobulin-like domains, the transmembrane domain (small rectangle), and intracellular split tyrosine-kinase domains (larger rectangles). On the right, a productive signaling complex is shown. This comprises a tetramer containing two FGF and two FGFR molecules, with contacts to heparan sulfate proteoglycan. Formation of the FGF/FGFR complex promotes transphosphorylation by the tyrosine kinase domains, leading to an altered conformation.[227,228]

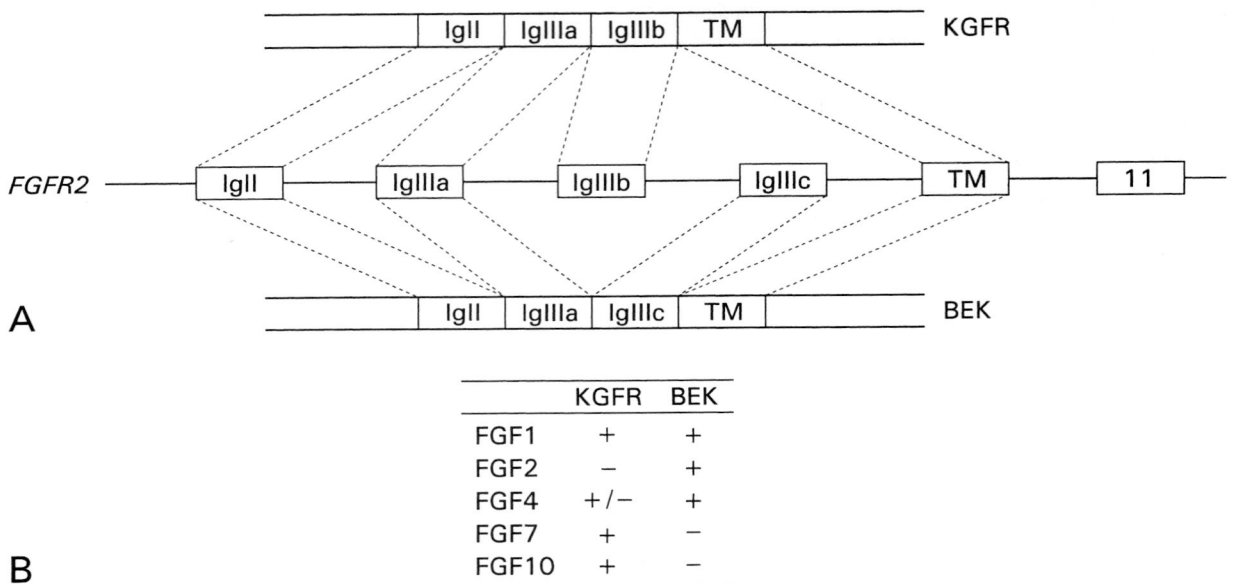

| | KGFR | BEK |
|------|------|------|
| FGF1 | + | + |
| FGF2 | − | + |
| FGF4 | +/− | + |
| FGF7 | + | − |
| FGF10 | + | − |

**Fig. 245-15 Alternative splicing of *FGFR2*. *A*, The gene structure of *FGFR2* includes alternatively spliced exons JgIIIb and JgIIIc (center). Use of exon JgIIIb generates the keratinocyte growth factor receptor** (*KGFR*) isoform, whereas use of exon JgIIIc generates the *BEK* (from "bacterially expressed kinase") isoform. *B*, Binding of the two isoforms to selected FGFs.[250,251]

complexity of signaling may be increased by formation of heterodimers when different FGFRs are expressed simultaneously.[238,257] The FGFR pathway has been implicated in a variety of cellular processes, including mitogenesis, differentiation, apoptosis, migration, and pattern formation.[258] Both FGFR1 and FGFR2 play critical roles in early embryogenesis, as demonstrated by the lethality of mice homozygous for null mutations, attributable respectively to defects of mesodermal patterning[259,260] and trophectoderm function.[261] Later functions of FGFR1 and FGFR2 have been explored genetically in the mouse by analysis of chimeras and targeted insertion of specific mutant alleles by homologous recombination. Chimera analysis has revealed a role for FGFR1 in migration through the primitive streak, with mutant cells behaving in a cell-autonomous fashion.[262,263] Additional mutations have demonstrated a critical role for FGFR2 in limb induction,[251] and for FGFR1 in limb patterning.[263,264] Homozygotes for *Fgfr3* null mutations are viable, but exhibit increased length of the vertebral column and long bones as well as deafness.[265,266] Homozygotes for *Fgfr4* are normal.[266a] In all cases, mice heterozygous for *Fgfr* null mutations are normal.

## FGFR Mutations in Craniosynostosis

Mutations of *FGFR2* were initially identified in Crouzon syndrome in 1994.[79] A candidate gene approach was used after linkage had been established to chromosome 10q in Crouzon and Jackson-Weiss and Antley-Bixler syndromes.[112,267] Further *FGFR* mutations were identified in several other craniosynostosis disorders shortly afterwards. To date, heterozygous mutations of *FGFR1*, *-2* and *-3* have been identified in seven distinct craniosynostosis syndromes. These are mild Pfeiffer syndrome (*FGFR1*); Apert, Crouzon, mild and severe Pfeiffer, and Beare-Stevenson syndromes (*FGFR2*); and Muenke syndrome and Crouzon syndrome with acanthosis nigricans (*FGFR3*). In addition, *FGFR2* mutations have been identified in some more nonspecific craniosynostosis phenotypes including Jackson-Weiss and Antley-Bixler syndromes. The mutations are summarized in Table 245-2 and the distribution of FGFR2 mutations is illustrated in Fig. 245-16. Several striking patterns are evident.

**Recurrent Nature of Mutations.** The great majority of the mutations are missense, with a few small insertions, deletions, or combined insertion/deletions, all of which remain in-frame. Additional categories are acceptor and donor splice-site mutations of exon JgIIIc and two *Alu* element insertions. The mutations vary greatly in frequency, with some being highly recurrent. The C → G nucleotide substitutions encoding the P250R mutation in FGFR3 and the S252W mutation in FGFR2 represent the most common transversions known in the human genome, with frequencies per haploid genome estimated as $8 \times 10^{-6}$ and $5 \times 10^{-6}$, respectively.[44,126] In Apert syndrome, the two common mutations were exclusively paternal in origin in 57 of 57 cases, and exhibited a significant paternal age effect.[44] Similar findings have been reported in Crouzon and Pfeiffer syndromes due to *FGFR2* mutations.[98a]

**Allelic Mutations in Different Syndromes.** As mentioned above, mutations of *FGFR2* and *FGFR3* have been associated with more than one craniosynostosis syndrome. The observation that dominantly inherited, allelic missense mutations cause distinct phenotypes suggests distinct, gain-of-function mechanisms (see "Pathophysiology of FGFR Mutations in Craniosynostosis" below). In the case of *FGFR3*, this is reinforced by the presence of further missense mutations in the syndromes of hypochondroplasia, achondroplasia, thanatophoric dysplasia, and SADDAN (severe achondroplasia with developmental delay and acanthosis nigricans) syndrome (see review reference 268; see Chap. 210). Craniosynostosis is rare in these latter disorders except in the case of thanatophoric dysplasia (Table 245-1).

**Mutations at Identical Positions of FGFR Paralogues.** These are observed in several regions of the molecule. The most notable example concerns a Ser-Pro dipeptide in the IgII-IgIII linker, part of a sequence of 16 amino acids conserved between the 4 human FGFRs (other examples occur in the juxtatransmembrane and transmembrane regions).[1] Mutations of proline to arginine in this linker cause Pfeiffer syndrome in FGFR1,[58] Apert syndrome in FGFR2,[57] and Muenke syndrome in FGFR3[83] (Fig. 245-17). This mutation was not found in FGFR4 when over 100 patients with craniosynostosis of unknown etiology were screened.[269] In addition, Apert syndrome is frequently caused by mutations in FGFR2 of the adjacent serine residue to tryptophan,[57] yet no corresponding mutation has been described in FGFR1 or FGFR3. This is readily explained by the sequence of the serine codon

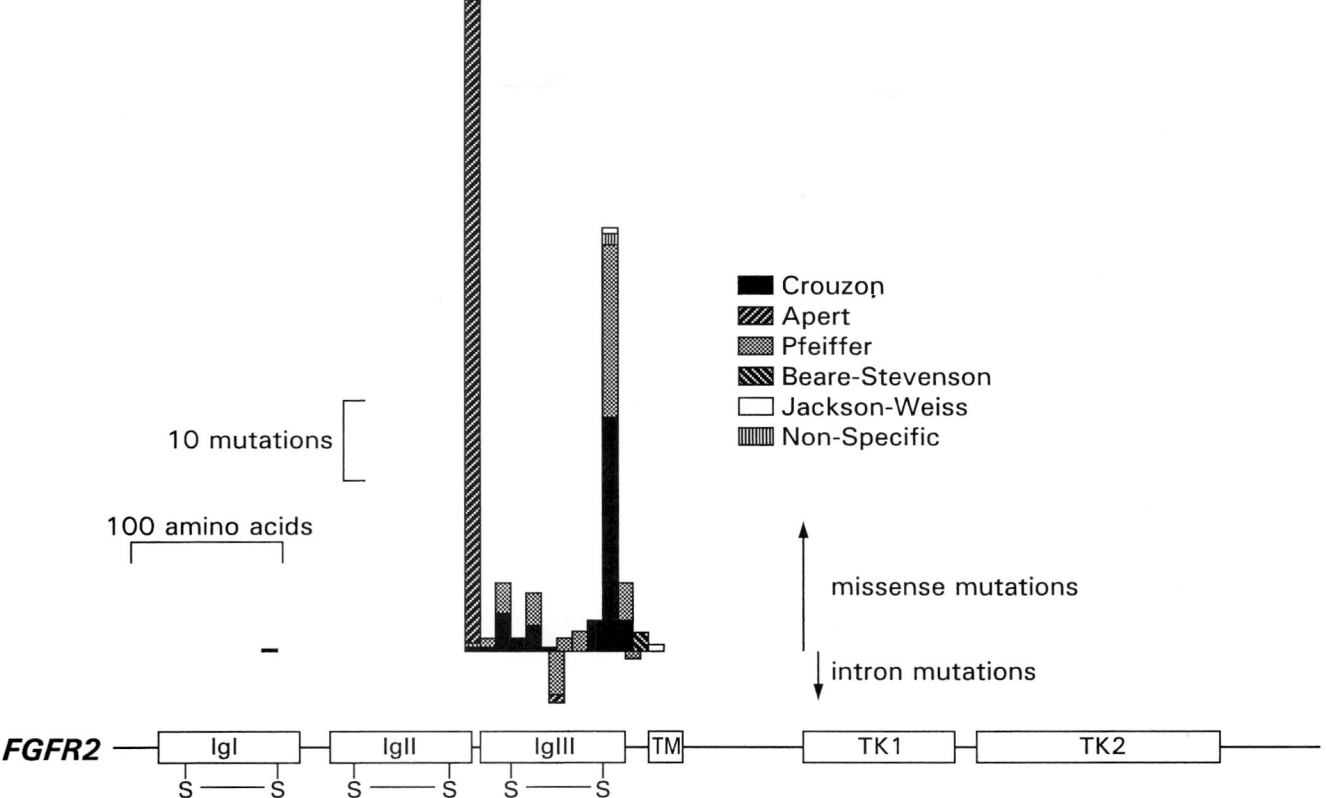

**Fig. 245-16 Distribution of FGFR2 mutations in craniosynostosis syndromes.** The histogram shows the number of mutations in independent patients observed for different syndromes, calculated at 10 amino acid intervals. The upward bars show missense mutations and the downward bars show splice site mutations. Scale is reduced ~3.7-fold for the common Apert mutations. Abbreviations: IgI, IgII, IgIII-immunoglobulin-like domains I, II, III; TM-transmembrane domain; TK1, TK2-tyrosine-kinase domains.

triplet, which differs between the *FGFR* genes (Fig. 245-17). Only in the case of *FGFR2* can the Ser codon (TCG) be mutated to the single Trp codon (TGG) by a single nucleotide substitution.

Three other rare mutations of the Ser-Pro dipeptide in the IgII-IgIII linker of FGFR2 have been described, with phenotypes ranging from normal through to Apert syndrome[60] (Fig. 245-18). This further underlines the functional importance of these residues and the specific mechanisms of action of particular missense mutations (see "Pathophysiology of FGFR Mutations in Craniosynostosis" below).

**Many Ig Domain Mutations of FGFR2 Create or Destroy a Cysteine Residue.** The highest peaks of mutation frequency in each half of the IgIII domain (Fig. 245-16) correspond exactly to the positions of the pair of disulfide bonded cysteine residues in this domain. The Cys342 residue represents a particular mutation hotspot, accounting for ~36 percent of all IgIII mutations. The six amino acid substitutions that can arise by mutating one nucleotide of the TGC codon have all been observed, a situation which is probably unprecedented in human genetics. Moreover, approximately 20 percent of mutations at noncysteine residues within IgIII are substitutions to cysteine (Table 245-2). Generation of an odd number of cysteines (one or three) in IgIII leads to intermolecular covalent dimerization (see "Pathophysiology of FGFR Mutations in Craniosynostosis" below).

**Splicing Mutations of *FGFR2*.** Although the great majority of FGFR mutations are missense, several mutations of IgIIIc have been demonstrated, or are presumed, to alter splicing of the IgIIIc exon. These fall into two categories. First, a cryptic donor splice-site (GCGGgtaatt) exists within exon JgIIIc. Activation of this site may occur either by a G → A transition of the site itself (GCAGgtaatt), which generates the apparently synonymous substitution A344A (Table 245-2) but in addition conforms better to the consensus donor site,[270,271] or by mutation of the normal donor splice-site at the end of the JgIIIc exon.[62] In both cases, use of the cryptic site generates an in-frame JgIIIc exon product that lacks 17 amino acids at its C-terminal end (Fig. 245-19). This probably disrupts IgIII structure in a fashion analogous to noncysteine mutations in IgIII.[272] Second, mutations of the 3′ (acceptor) splice site at the start of the JgIIIc exon lead to partial switching of splicing to the JgIIIb exon upstream, driving ectopic expression of the distinct KGFR splice form. This is predicted to confer the cell with novel ligand binding

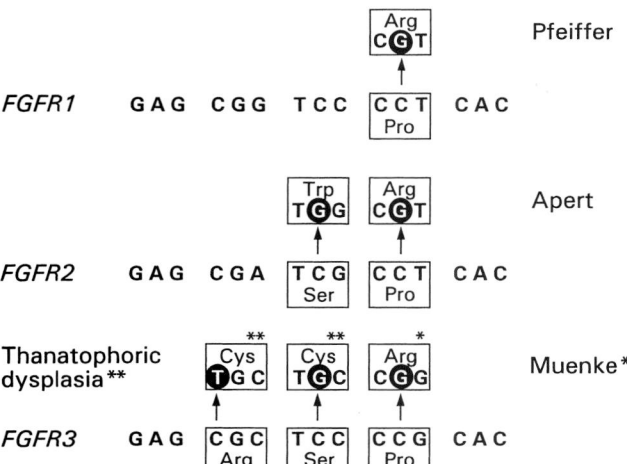

**Fig. 245-17 Distinct craniosynostosis syndromes caused by frequent mutations of the IgII-IgIII linker of the FGFR1, FGFR2 and FGFR3 paralogues.** (*Modified from Muenke et al.*[147])

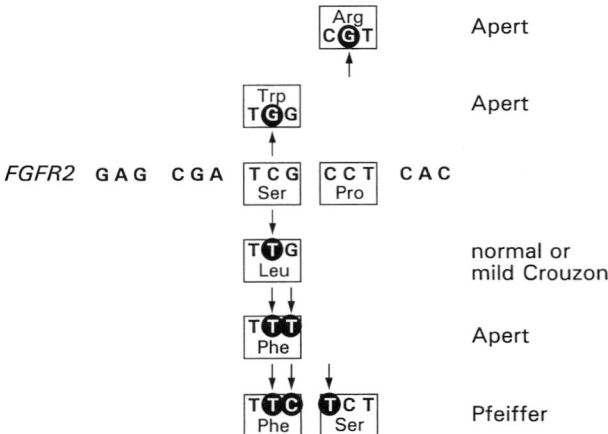

**Fig. 245-18 Frequent and rare mutations of the IgII-IgIII linker of FGFR2.** In addition to the two common mutations (S252W, P253R) causing Apert syndrome, three rare mutations with phenotypes ranging from normal to Apert syndrome have been described.[60]

characteristics (Fig. 245-15), representing a further mechanism for gain-of-function.[70]

## Reappraisal of the Clinical Classification of Craniosynostosis

Although in general, the correlation between clinical phenotype and molecular pathogenesis has proved good, identification of FGFR mutations has provided several new insights into clinical classification (see also the earlier sections on individual clinical syndromes).

**Pfeiffer Syndrome is Clinically and Genetically Heterogeneous.** Patients with the P252R mutation in FGFR1[58] usually have a mild phenotype, type 1 according to the classification of Cohen,[132] and this mutation is frequently familial. In contrast, FGFR2 mutations are associated with a wide spectrum of severity encompassing types 1, 2, and 3 of Cohen's[132] classification.[71,146] Some correlation exists between severity of different FGFR2 mutations. A tendency towards pansynostosis/cloverleaf skull and involvement of other organ systems was noted with the W290C and S351C mutations,[5a,59,67,68,70,73,81,140,142,273] whereas digital

anomalies are commonly more severe with IgIIIc acceptor splice-site mutations.[70,73]

**Apert Syndrome Shows Clinical and Allelic Heterogeneity.** Two mutations of FGFR2, S252W and P253R, account for ~99 percent of Apert syndrome mutations in a ratio of approximately 2:1.[57,70] In two studies, comparison of patients with the two different mutations showed a higher frequency of cleft palate and tendency towards more severe craniofacial malformations with the S252W mutation, but more severe syndactyly with the P253R mutation.[53,57a] This suggests that distinct mechanisms are responsible for the craniofacial and limb abnormalities of Apert syndrome. Although the other published study did not report significant correlations,[274] this was based on a smaller sample size and there appeared to be a systematic bias in the classification of syndactyly.[53]

**Crouzon, Jackson-Weiss, and Pfeiffer Syndromes with Mutations of FGFR2 Represent a Graded Continuum of Severity.** As described above, Crouzon syndrome is classically associated with clinically normal hands and feet, whereas in Pfeiffer syndrome, the thumbs and halluces are broad. However, both "rules" are subject to ambiguity because radiologic examination of the hands and feet in Crouzon syndrome often reveals subtle abnormalities,[108–110] and no consensus exists on whether patients who have "normal" thumbs but broad halluces should be labeled as Pfeiffer or Jackson-Weiss syndrome.[275,276] This has led to much confusion in the literature and led some authors to exaggerate the significance of their findings, by giving previously identified phenotypes a different name.[277] The pattern of FGFR2 mutations in these syndromes indicates that these disorders form a clinical continuum. The main value of maintaining Jackson-Weiss syndrome as a distinct nosologic entity is that the original, enormous pedigree illustrates the wide range of phenotypic variability attributable to the same FGFR2 mutation.[75,116] This provides the best evidence that factors in addition to the mutated FGFR2 allele contribute to the phenotypic picture.

**The P250R Mutation in FGFR3 Defines a New Craniosynostosis Syndrome.** As discussed above, patients who turn out to have this mutation were previously labeled with a wide variety of diagnoses (see Muenke syndrome above). Most common were either nonsyndromic coronal craniosynostosis or Saethre-Chotzen syndrome, but diagnoses of Crouzon and Pfeiffer syndromes were

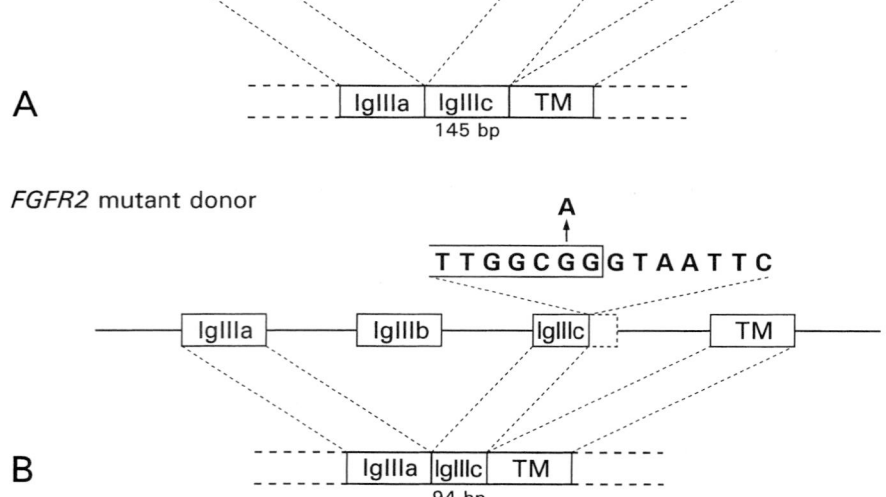

Normal *FGFR2* (BEK isoform) splicing

A

*FGFR2* mutant donor

B

**Fig. 245-19 A synonymous G → A nucleotide substitution creates a donor splice-site within *FGFR2* exon IIIc.** *A*, Normal splicing of the 145-bp IIIc *B*, Creation of the novel donor splice-site leads to preferential splicing of an isoform lacking the C-terminal 17 amino acids of the exon.[270,271]

not infrequent and several "private" syndromes had also been suggested.[119,121,124,126] This provides an excellent example of how identification of a specific mutation, and hence the correct lumping of affected individuals, allows the clinical characteristics of a "new" syndrome to emerge. The term Muenke syndrome has been suggested for this disorder (MIM 602849).

**Atypical Craniosynostosis Phenotypes and FGFR2 Mutations.** Several patients with atypical or nonspecific phenotypes have been reported to harbor FGFR2 mutations. The most important of these is the A344A mutation, which creates a donor splice-site (see "Splicing Mutations of *FGFR2*" above). This was originally described in Crouzon syndrome,[79] but may also present a nonspecific phenotype.[278] It is one of the more common FGFR2 mutations and needs to be carefully excluded. Other atypical phenotypes associated with FGFR2 mutations have been described.[5a,59,63,273] Most interesting amongst these is the only described mutation of the transmembrane domain.[59] This G384R substitution in FGFR2 differs in position by only two amino acids from the common G380R substitution of FGFR3 in achondroplasia (see Chap. 210).

### Phenotypes of Somatic Mutation of FGFRs: Epidermal Nevi and Neoplasia

A single case of somatic mutation of FGFR2 was described in a physically normal 14-year-old male with severe acne affecting one arm. A S252W mutation identical to that in Apert syndrome was detected in the affected skin, but not in the normal skin or blood of this individual.[279] It is possible that FGFR mutations contribute to other epidermal nevi or epidermal nevus syndromes.

Several of the FGFs were originally discovered because of inappropriate expression in tumor cell lines and abnormal FGFRs have also been identified in tumor cells.[280,281] Surprisingly, none of the germ line FGFR mutations is known to be associated with an increased risk of neoplasia, but further epidemiologic studies are warranted. Chimeric fusion proteins resulting from chromosome translocations involving the *FGFR1* and *FGFR3* genes have been described in stem cell myeloproliferative disorder and multiple myeloma respectively.[282-286] Additionally, some of the *FGFR3* fusions contained point mutations identified in thanatophoric dysplasia,[285,286] and the same spectrum of mutations has been observed in human bladder and cervix carcinomas.[286a] Similar processes may affect the *FGFR2* gene.

### Pathophysiology of FGFR Mutations in Craniosynostosis

**IgII-IgIII Linker Mutations.** The effects of the Apert FGFR2 mutations S252W and P253R on ligand binding to the IgIIIc domain splice form have been investigated in vitro[287] (see Table 245-5). Enhanced affinity for certain FGF ligands (most marked for FGF2), manifested as a reduced dissociation constant from the receptor, was demonstrated for both Apert mutations compared to wild-type, whereas binding to the phenotypically mild or silent mutation S252L was indistinguishable from normal. Consistent but less clear cut results were obtained using a *Xenopus* oocyte assay.[288] Specific bulky substitutions in this linker may increase its rigidity, altering the relative orientation of the IgII and IgIII domains to mimic the effects of ligand binding. This mechanism is therefore ligand-dependent and would lead to activation of signaling under conditions where availability of ligand was limiting. This provides a broad explanation for the differences in phenotype arising from linker region mutations of FGFR2 and FGFR3 compared to mutations that act by ligand-independent processes (see next section).

**IgIII Domain Mutations.** Three general categories of mutation may be recognized: those that destroy a cysteine, those that create a cysteine, and those that do not affect the number of cysteine residues (Table 245-5). In the most complete study of these mutations to date,[272,291] the capability of various mutations to transform NIH 3T3 cells was examined in FGFR2/Neu chimeric

receptor molecules. Strong transforming capability was restricted to mutations of the IgIII domain. Mutations of the cysteine residues (C278F, C342Y), a mutation to cysteine (S354C) and selected noncysteine mutations (W290G, Y340H, T341P) were strongly transforming, but if both cysteine residues were substituted, no activity resulted (S354C was not included in this latter part of the investigation). This suggests that the pathologic effect of both cysteine and noncysteine mutations requires the presence of an unpaired cysteine, which would be available to form an intermolecular disulfide bridge with another mutant molecule. Supporting this, dimeric receptor species were observed under nonreducing conditions only for those mutants showing transforming activity, after transfecting *FGFR2* mutants into COS-1 cells. These dimeric species exhibited strong phosphorylation and binding to antiphosphotyrosine antibody.

These data suggest that covalent dimerization of two mutant FGFR2 molecules leads to a constitutively activated receptor dimer. Broadly similar conclusions have been reached by other groups using a variety of experimental approaches.[288-290] Importantly, this mechanism is ligand independent, in contrast to the IgII-IgIII linker mutations. Indeed many IgIII domain mutations abolish FGF binding.[287,288,290] This may be of little consequence in the heterozygote, but in the homozygote, this loss of function is likely to cause embryonic lethality.

**Exon IIIc Acceptor Splice-Site Mutations.** A distinct gain-of-function mechanism was suggested by the identification of two Apert patients with *Alu* insertion mutations, one within the IgIIIc exon, the other within the upstream intron.[70] Investigation of RNA expression in fibroblasts from the patient with the latter mutation demonstrated ectopic expression of the IgIIIb splice form (KGFR) in fibroblasts, a cell that normally exhibits exclusive IgIIIc expression. Ectopic KGFR expression would extend the ligand sensitivity of the cell to include FGF7 and FGF10. A similar but lesser degree of ectopic KGFR expression was observed in fibroblasts from two patients with Pfeiffer syndrome and point mutations ($940-2A \rightarrow G$, $940-2A \rightarrow T$) of the IgIIIc acceptor splice site.[70] The effect correlates with the severity of limb malformations (syndactyly and broadening of digit 1) in these patients, but the explanation for the associated craniosynostosis is uncertain.

**Other FGFR Mutations.** Studies of the gain-of-function mechanisms of craniosynostosis mutations have focused on the IgII-IgIII linker region and the IgIII domain. No specific studies of the rare FGFR2 mutations in Beare-Stevenson syndrome (S372C and Y375C) or the transmembrane mutation G384R have been reported, although an artificially constructed C382R mutation was reported to cause constitutive activation, possibly by promoting hydrogen bonding between transmembrane domains[292] (Table 245-5). Several studies of analogous mutations of FGFR3 have been reported (see reference 268 and Chap. 210). The Crouzon-acanthosis nigricans FGFR3 mutation A391E may stabilize the formation of a FGFR2/mutant FGFR3 heterodimer, although evidence to support this has not yet been published.[268]

### Mutations of *TWIST* in Saethre-Chotzen Syndrome

Heterozygous mutations of the human orthologue of the *Drosophila twist* gene were first described in Saethre-Chotzen syndrome by two groups in 1997.[172,173] Saethre-Chotzen syndrome was mapped to distal chromosome 7p in 1992;[293] cytogenetically visible deletions of this region are frequently associated with craniosynostosis.[294] Identification of mutations in human *TWIST* (GenBank numbers for cDNA: u80998 and gDNA: y81071) was based on information from the mouse orthologue. One group predicted the location of the human gene from the map of conserved mouse-human synteny,[172] the other mapped the human *TWIST* gene to chromosome 7p21 and noted similarity of the phenotype of mice heterozygous for *twist* null mutations to Saethre-Chotzen syndrome.[173,295,296]

**Table 245-3** Intragenic mutations of *TWIST*

| Amino acid change* | Codon change* | Number of cases | Reference† |
|---|---|---|---|
| G61X | GGA → TGA | 1 | 169 |
| E65X | GAG → TAG | 3 | 169 |
| K77S+46aa‡ | 230delA;232T → C | 1 | 170 |
| S93G+198aa‡ | 272-273ins10 | 1 | 171 |
| GAGGGGG92-93ins | 276-277dup21 | 1 | 171 |
| Y103X | 308-309insA | 2 | 172 |
| Y103X | TAC → TAA | 2 | 173 |
| Y103X | TAC → TAG | 5 | 63 |
| E104X | GAG → TAG | 2 | 174 |
| N114D | AAC → GAG | 1 | 174a |
| R116W | CGG → TGG | 1 | 63 |
| R118C | CGC → TGC | 1 | J. Bonaventura, unpublished |
| R118H | CGC → CAC | 2 | 169 |
| R118H+167aa‡ | 353-360del8 | 1 | 174 |
| Q119P | CAG → CCG | 1 | 172 |
| R120P | CGC → CCC | 1 | 171 |
| Q122X | CAG → TAG | 1 | 63 |
| S123X | TCG → TAG | 1 | 173 |
| S123W | TCG → TGG | 1 | 170 |
| E126X | GAG → TAG | 4 | 173 |
| A129P | GCC → CCC | 1 | J. Bonaventura, unpublished |
| A129R + 159aa‡ | 384-385insC | 1 | 63 |
| L131P | CTG → CCG | 1 | 173 |
| R132P | CGG → CCG | 1 | 63 |
| I134M | ATC → ATG | 1 | 169 |
| AALRKII135-136ins | 405-406dup21 | 1 | 172 |
| P136L | CCC → CTC | 2 | 170 |
| P139S | CCC → TCC | 1 | 63 |
| KIIPTLP139-140ins | 416-417dup21 | 6 | 172, 173 |
| KIIPTLP139-140ins | 417-418dup21 | 2 | 173 |
| S140X | 418-419dup21 | 1 | 169 |
| IIPTLPS140-141ins | 420-421dup21 | 1 | 169 |
| D141Y | GAC → TAC | 2 | 63 |
| D141G | GAC → GGC | 1 | 169 |
| D141G+155aa‡ | 423-424ins25 | 1 | 174 |
| S144R | AGC → CGC | 2 | 174 |
| K145E | AAG → GAG | 1 | 174 |
| K145G + 135aa‡ | 433-455del23 | 1 | 172 |
| K145N | AAG → AAC | 1 | 169 |
| T148A | ACC → GCC | 1 | 171 |
| T148N | ACC → AAC | 1 | 175 |
| L149F | CTC → TTC | 1 | 63 |
| A152V | GCG → GTG | 1 | 63 |
| R153+135aa‡ | 460-461insA | 1 | 165a |
| R154G | AGG → GGG | 1 | 169 |
| Y155X | 465-469del5 | 1 | 174 |
| F158L | TTC → CTC | 1 | Wilkie, unpublished |
| L159F | CTC → TTC | 1 | 174 |
| Y160X | TAC → TAG | 1 | 171 |
| Q161X | CAG → TAG | 1 | 174 |
| Q161R+56aa‡ | 481delC | 1 | Wilkie, unpublished |
| A162V+54aa‡ | 485-488delTCCT | 1 | Wilkie, unpublished |
| L163F+54aa‡ | 487delC | 1 | 174 |
| E181X | GAG → TAG | 1 | 176 |

* Amino acid and nucleotide numbering based on Howard et al.[72]
† Only the first reference is given. Functional polypeptide domains of *TWIST*: basic region, 102 to 121; helix1, 122 to 137; loop, 138 to 152; helix 2, 153 to 165.
‡ Number of amino acids following frameshift.

Mammalian orthologues of the *twist* gene, originally identified in *Drosophila* were first isolated by low stringency hybridization.[297] There is only a single *TWIST/twist* gene in human/mouse, although additional related genes exist such as *dermo-1*.[298] Mammalian *TWIST* genes are much smaller (202 amino acids in human)[172] than the *Drosophila* counterpart (490 amino acids), and the major region of homology is the 57-amino acid basic helix-loop-helix (b-HLH) domain. Comparison of the *Drosophila* and human b-HLH segments shows 82 percent amino acid conservation overall, and 100 percent conservation in the basic and loop regions.[299] The HLH motif is characteristic of a large family of transcriptional proteins, the prototypes being E12 and E47.[300] The

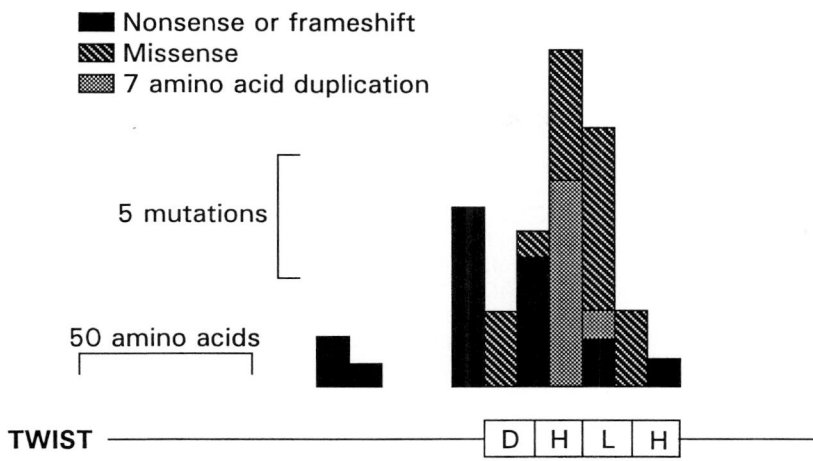

**Fig. 245-20 Intragenic mutations of TWIST in craniosynostosis. Frequency of different categories of mutation is shown at 10 amino acid intervals, with respect to the positions of the DNA binding (D), helix (H), and loop (L) domains.**

HLH segment is required for homo- or heterodimerization with partner proteins, which is necessary for DNA binding by the basic region to a specific DNA sequence (E box). HLH proteins may inhibit transcriptional activation by other family members by forming nonproductive heterodimers.[301]

Intragenic mutations of *TWIST* identified in Saethre-Chotzen syndrome are summarized in Table 245-3 and illustrated in Fig. 245-20. These fall into three major categories: nonsense and frameshift mutations that cause premature truncation of the normal protein sequence and disrupt its gross structure; missense mutations localized within the b-HLH motif; and recurrent 21-bp duplications at the end of helix 1 and in the loop region. In addition, several microdeletions of *TWIST* at or below the limit of conventional cytogenetic resolution have been described (Table 245-4). These comprise one small (~3 kb) and two large (3 to 10 Mb) interstitial deletions and two additional large deletions associated with apparently balanced chromosome translocations. Patients with large deletions are more likely to have mild to moderate mental retardation, suggesting that monosomy of contiguous genes in chromosome 7p21.1 affects neurodevelopment.[170] Finally, several additional chromosome translocations have been identified that do not appear physically to disrupt *TWIST* (Table 245-4); in the four documented cases, the breakpoint lies telomeric (3′) to *TWIST*, between 5 kb and 250 kb away.[303,304] Presumably, these exert a position effect on the gene as speculated for other diseases in which associated translocations do not physically disrupt the causative gene.[305]

The majority of these mutations are consistent with a haploinsufficiency mechanism of disease. These include the complete deletions and truncations, as well as the missense mutations and duplications in the HLH domain, which are predicted to prevent dimerization. However, the missense mutations in the DNA-binding domain might be expected to abrogate DNA binding without affecting dimerization, and hence exert a dominant negative effect.[301] Although plausible, the phenotype of the patients with these mutations does not appear to be more severe than in other cases, which does not support this mechanism and suggests that TWIST is physiologically active principally as a heterodimer. Indeed, to date no convincing genotype-phenotype correlation has been reported for intragenic *TWIST* mutations.

The recurrent 21-bp duplications represent a relatively unusual category of mutations in human molecular pathology. Five distinct duplication mutations have been described within a stretch of 16 bp, two of them occurring in multiple independent patients. Four are predicted to encode duplications of seven amino acids, but the remaining mutation introduces a stop codon and hence is truncating. This pattern of mutations favors a DNA-mediated origin for these mutations, rather than functional selection. Consistent with this, two perfect copies and one imperfect copy of a 6-bp repeat occur at consecutive 21-bp intervals in the *TWIST* gene, suggesting that the mutations arise by mispairing during DNA replication or unequal crossing over[169] (Fig. 245-21).

**Function of *twist* During Development.** In *Drosophila*, *twist* plays a critical role as a mesoderm inducer in gastrulation and expression persists during myogenesis.[306] In mice, *twist* expression is also mesodermal, although it is not required for gastrulation. RNA expression is first observed at embryonic day 7, but no protein is detectable until day 8.[307] The protein distribution in slightly later embryos reflects fairly closely the phenotype of mice homozygous for a *twist*-null mutation, which die at embryonic day 11.5 and exhibit open neural tube defects, absence of the limb apical ectodermal ridge, and abnormalities of the branchial arches and somites.[308] The phenotype of heterozygous *twist*-null mice is described in the next section.

## INSIGHTS INTO CRANIAL SUTURE BIOLOGY

The developmental biology of cranial sutures has been little studied until recently, but, as the sutures are anatomically simple, this is a relatively tractable system. Figure 245-1B is a cross-section through the coronal suture. The key developmental questions are: Why do the sutures form where they do? and How they are maintained? Craniosynostosis represents a failure of the second process, and the mutations identified give evidence of some of the critical genes involved in cranial suture maintenance. In *Drosophila*, an *FGFR* orthologue, *DFR1*, acts downstream of

**Table 245-4 Deletions and Translocations Involving *TWIST***

| Karyotype | Associated *TWIST* Deletion.? | Reference* |
|---|---|---|
| 46,XX | 2.9 kb | 170 |
| 46,del(7)(p21.1) | 3.5–5.6 Mb | 170 |
| 46,del(7)(p21.1) | 5.5–10.2 Mb | 170 |
| 46,t(7;8)(p21;q13) | >11.6 Mb | 170 |
| 46,t(2;7)(p23;p22) | >1.4 Mb | 302 |
| 46,t(7;10)(p21.2;q21.2) | translocation 70–250-kb telomeric | 169 |
| 46,t(7;18)(p21.2;q23) | translocation 70–250-kb telomeric | 169 |
| 46,t(2;7)(q21.1;p21.2) | translocation 70–250-kb telomeric | 169 |
| 46,t(5;7)(p15.3;p21.2) | ? | 169 |
| 46,t(6;7)(q16.2;p15.3) | 518-bp deletion, 5-kb telomeric | 303 |

*Only the most recent reference is given.

**Table 245-5** Functional Studies of Gain-of-Function in FGFR/Craniosynostosis Mutations

| Mechanism | Type of mutation | Mutations studied | Reference |
|---|---|---|---|
| Reduced dissociation of ligand | IgII-IgIII linker mutation | P252R (FGFR1) | 288 |
| | | S252W, P253R (FGFR2) | 287 |
| Covalent cross-linking of Cys | Loss of cysteine | C342Y (FGFR2) | 289 |
| | | C278F (FGFR2) | 288 |
| | | C342Y, C342R, C342S | 272 |
| | | C342Y (FGFR2) | 290 |
| | | C278F, C342Y (FGFR2) | 291 |
| | Gain of cysteine | S354C (FGFR2) | 272 |
| | Disruption of IgIII domain structure | Y340H, A344A (FGFR2) | 272 |
| | | W290G, T341P (FGFR2) | 291 |
| Ectopic expression of KGFR | IgIIIc acceptor splice-site mutation | 950-3–4ins*Alu*, 950-2A → G,T (FGFR2) | 70 |
| Transmembrane hydrogen bonding | Neutral → charged mutation | C382R/D, V392R (FGFR2) | 292 |
| | | A391E (FGFR3) | 268 |

*twist* in mesodermal differentiation[309] and mesodermal expression of *msh*, the *MSX2* orthologue, begins later in myogenesis and is abolished in *twist* mutations.[310,311] This raises the possibility that aspects of mesoderm formation in *Drosophila* and biogenesis of the cranial suture (a mesodermal structure) in vertebrates involve a conserved developmental pathway. However, the relative positions of *MSX2*, *FGFR*, and *TWIST* in the pathway of vertebrate cranial suture development are not yet certain.

## MSX2

Expression of *Msx2* was demonstrated in membranous bones of the calvarium and adjacent mesenchymal cells at mouse embryonic day 15.5. Shortly after birth (day 3), expression is concentrated in the sutural region and corresponds in position to the osteogenic front.[95] Later on, expression in the sagittal suture diminishes markedly and disappears completely from the dura mater.[312] Attempts to replicate the phenotype of Boston type craniosynostosis by introducing transgenic copies of *MSX2* (wild-type or P148H mutant) into mice have led to variable results. In one case, the mice were viable but a proportion (27 to 71 percent) developed premature cranial suture fusion; this was interpreted as showing that an elevated dose of MSX2 protein (normal or mutant) in the suture causes craniosynostosis.[313,314] In the other study, the mice died around birth with severe craniofacial malformations (small jaw, clefts of the face or secondary palate, exencephaly), but with no evidence of craniosynostosis.[315] These differences in phenotype are not understood but presumably relate to differences in the size of construct, nature of promoter, and copy number of integrated transgene in the two experiments. In neither case were consistent differences found between mice carrying the normal and mutant versions of the gene, indicating that the gain of function conferred by the P148H mutation is relatively weak. A further study, in which an Msx2 minigene was transgenically overexpressed in mouse cranial sutures using a specific promoter element, resulted in an increased number of proliferative osteoblastic cells in the osteogenic front.[316] Msx2 may play a

dual role in osteogenesis, both enhancing early osteogenic differentiation, but also inhibiting the terminal stages.

## FGF/FGFR Signaling

Experiments using fetal and newborn rat calvaria show that underlying dura mater is required both to specify the position and maintain the undifferentiated state of the suture.[312,317,318] This corroborates surgical observations that following removal of the entire calvarium, the skull regenerates with the sutures in an anatomically correct position. The osteoinhibitory activity has been attributed to a soluble heparin-binding factor, possibly FGF,[319] although there is better evidence implicating TGF$\beta$3.[319a] Several studies have demonstrated expression of FGFs and FGFRs at the mRNA level in the mouse cranial sutures.[312,320,321,321a] In mouse embryos, placement of an FGF2-soaked, heparin coated bead over the coronal suture resulted in down-regulation of *Fgfr2* and up-regulation of *osteopontin*, a marker of early osteogenic differentiation.[320,321a] A new suture-like structure was formed around the bead (Fig. 245-22). Expression of *Fgf2* was observed in the rat posterior frontal suture at the time of suture fusion.[321] A mouse model of Crouzon syndrome, *Bulgy-eye (Bey)*, has a retrovirus inserted in the intergenic region between the tandem *Fgf3* and *Fgf4* genes. Transcript analysis demonstrated much higher expression levels for both genes in the cranial sutures of *Bey* compared with wild-type mice.[322]

In the human, histologic examination of 19- to 28-week human fetuses with Apert syndrome due to defined *FGFR2* mutations showed increased calcified bone matrix and stronger alkaline phosphatase staining of cells in the subperiosteal area compared to controls, indicating increased maturation of preosteoblast cells. In culture, these cells showed normal growth, but increased bone differentiation markers including alkaline phosphatase and osteocalcin and produced aggregates containing abundant mineralized matrix.[323] These and similar observations[323a,323b] are consistent with the mouse studies above. A seemingly paradoxical result is that measurement of FGFR2 protein in the cranial sutures

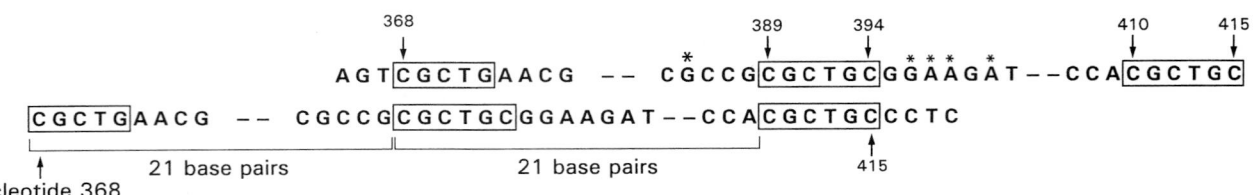

**Fig. 245-21** Possible misalignment of *TWIST* sequences from nucleotides 368 to 389/415 due to overlap of CGCTG(C) repeats, spaced 21 bp apart. \*-positions at which duplication start points have been observed. (*From Rose et al.*[169] *Used by permission of Human Molecular Genetics.*)

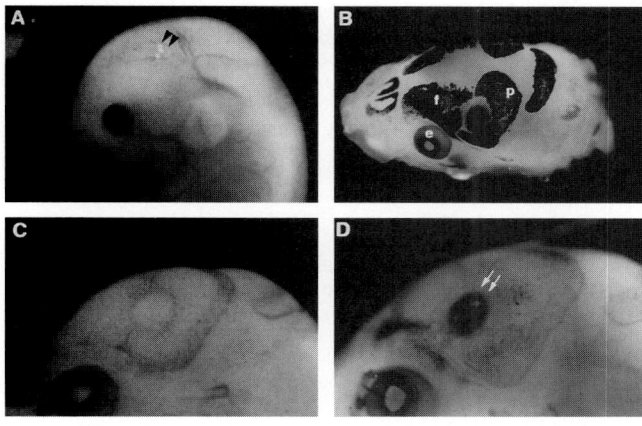

**Fig. 245-22 Artificial creation of a suture using an FGF2-soaked bead; implantation of beads onto the embryonic day 15 mouse coronal suture by ex utero surgery. *A*, Appearance of the head immediately after implantation of beads (arrowheads). *B–D*, Whole-mount in situ hybridization for *osteopontin* (a marker of preosteogenic differentiation) (*B*), *Fgfr2* (*C*) and both messages (*D*), 48 hr after bead implantation. The suture line was obliterated under the bead, but there is evidence of a new circular suture-like structure surrounding the bead. (*From Iseki et al.[320] Used by permission of Development.*)**

of Crouzon and Apert patients showed reduced levels of immunoreactivity.[324,325] This is likely to be a consequence of excessive signaling through the FGF/FGFR pathway causing down-regulation of FGFR. Several experimental systems have demonstrated this feedback loop.[326,327]

The picture that emerges from these studies suggests that FGF/FGFR signaling has different consequences at different signaling intensities. Low-intensity tonic signaling, possibly controlled by dura mater, stimulates sustained cell proliferation, prevents preosteoblast differentiation, and hence maintains the suture. Higher-intensity signaling causes suture differentiation and FGFR2 down-regulation, and is consistent with activating mechanisms for FGFR2 mutations (see "Pathophysiology of FGFR Mutations in Craniosynostosis" above). A potential therapeutic application is suggested by a report that FGF2-impregnated gelatin hydrogels stimulate bone regeneration of skull defects in rabbits.[328]

### TWIST

The phenotype of mice heterozygous for a *twist*-null mutation has been reported in detail.[296] Some of the physical abnormalities are strikingly similar to those of Saethre-Chotzen syndrome and include broadening or duplication of the first digit and altered dimensions of the skull. The phenotype shows marked sensitivity to genetic background and interesting variations in detail, with some bones advanced in growth and others delayed. For example, the *twist*-null heterozygous mice exhibit larger parietal and interparietal bones with smaller sutural spaces, yet ossification of the supraoccipital bone is delayed; this might reflect the differing embryologic origin (neurocranium versus chondrocranium respectively) of these bones.[296]

Analysis of *Twist* expression in mouse embryos demonstrated transcripts in the undifferentiated messenchymal cells of the developing cranial suture, before initiation of osteogenesis.[328a] This observation and the close parallel between *twist*-null heterozygote mice and humans with Saethre-Chotzen syndrome suggest that *TWIST* lies in a dosage-sensitive pathway controlling the differentiation of sutural mesenchymal cells into definitive osteoblasts. Haploinsufficency of *TWIST* may tip the balance of cell fate towards differentiation, causing craniosynostosis.[301] Conversely, duplication of chromosome band 7p21 in humans has been associated with unusually large, late closing fontanelles in several patients,[329] and in one case, the *TWIST* gene was shown

to be present in three copies,[330] suggesting that excessive TWIST protein maintains the bones of the neurocranium in a relatively immature state.

### REFERENCES

1. Wilkie AOM: Craniosynostosis: Genes and mechanisms. *Hum Mol Genet* **6**:1647, 1997.
2. Cohen MM Jr, MacLean RE (eds): *Craniosynostosis: Diagnosis, Evaluation, and Management.* New York, Oxford University Press, 2000.
2a. Wilkie AOM: Epidemiology and genetics of craniosynostosis. *Am J Med Genet* **90**:82, 2000.
3. Chumas PD, Cinalli G, Arnaud E, Marchac D, Renier D: Classification of previously unclassified cases of craniosynostosis. *J Neurosurg* **86**:177, 1997.
4. Hassell S, Butler MG: Antley-Bixler syndrome: A report of a patient and review of literature. *Clin Genet* **46**:372, 1994.
5. Crisponi G, Porcu C, Piu ME: Antley-Bixler syndrome: Case report and review of the literature. *Clin Dysmorph* **6**:61, 1997.
5a. Reardon W, Smith A, Honour JW, Hindmarsh P, Das D, Rumsby G, Nelson I, et al: Evidence for digenic inheritance in some cases of Antley-Bixler syndrome? *J Med Genet* **37**:26, 2000.
6. Lin AE, McPherson E, Nwokoro NA, Clemens M, Losken HW, Mulvihill JJ: Further delineation of the Baller-Gerold syndrome. *Am J Med Genet* **45**:519, 1993.
7. Ramos Fuentes FJ, Nicholson L, Scott CI Jr: Phenotypic variability in the Baller-Gerold syndrome — Report of a mildly affected patient and review of the literature. *Eur J Pediatr* **153**:483, 1994.
8. Robinson LK, James HE, Mubarak SJ, Allen EJ, Jones KL: Carpenter syndrome: Natural history and clinical spectrum. *Am J Med Genet* **20**:461, 1985.
9. Cohen DM, Green JG, Miller J, Gorlin RJ, Reed JA: Acrocephalo-polysyndactyly type II- Carpenter syndrome: Clinical spectrum and an attempt at unification with Goodman and Summitt syndromes. *Am J Med Genet* **28**:311, 1987.
10. Lajeunie E, Le Merrer M, Bonaiti-Pellie C, Marchac D, Renier D: Genetic study of nonsyndromic coronal craniosynostosis. *Am J Med Genet* **55**:500, 1995.
11. Hunter AGW, Rudd NL: Craniosynostosis. II. Coronal synostosis: Its familial characteristics and associated clinical findings in 109 patients lacking bilateral polysyndactyly or syndactyly. *Teratology* **15**:301, 1977.
12. Amar MJA, Sutphen R, Kousseff BG: Expanded phenotype of cranioectodermal dysplasia (Sensenbrenner syndrome). *Am J Med Genet* **70**:349, 1997.
13. Saavedra D, Richieri-Costa A, Guion-Almeida MI, Cohen MM Jr: Craniofrontonasal syndrome: Study of 41 patients. *Am J Med Genet* **61**:147, 1996.
14. Feldman GJ, Ward DE, Lajeunie-Renier E, Saavedra D, Robin NH, Proud V, Robb LJ, et al: A novel phenotypic pattern in X-linked inheritance: Craniofrontonasal syndrome maps to Xp22. *Hum Mol Genet* **6**:1937, 1997.
15. Barr M, Heidelberger KP, Comstock CH: Craniomicromelic syndrome: A newly recognized lethal condition with craniosynostosis, distinct facial anomalies, short limbs, and intrauterine growth retardation. *Am J Med Genet* **58**:348, 1995.
16. Thuret I, Michel G, Philip N, Hairion D, Capodario A-M, Perrimond H: Chromosomal instability in two siblings with Dubowitz syndrome. *Br J Haematol* **78**:124, 1991.
17. Hansen KE, Kirkpatrick SJ, Laxova R: Dubowitz syndrome: long-term follow-up of an original patient. *Am J Med Genet* **55**:161, 1995.
18. Vortkamp A, Gessler M, Grzeschik KH: GLI3 zinc-finger gene interrupted by translocations in Greig syndrome families. *Nature* **352**:539, 1991.
19. Wild A, Kalff-Suske M, Vortkamp A, Bornholdt D, König R, Grzeschik K-H: Point mutations in human GL13 cause Greig syndrome. *Hum Mol Genet* **6**:1979, 1997.
20. Penny LA, Dell'Aquila M, Jones MC, Bergoffen J, Cunniff C, Fryns JP, Grace E, et al: Clinical and molecular characterization of patients with distal 11q deletions. *Am J Hum Genet* **56**:676, 1995.
21. Lewanda AF, Morsey S, Reid CS, Jabs EW: Two craniosynostotic patients with 11q deletions and review of 48 cases. *Am J Med Genet* **59**:193, 1995.
22. Lajeunie E, Le Merrer M, Marchac D, Renier D: Syndromal and nonsyndromal primary trigonocephaly: Analysis of a series of 237 patients. *Am J Med Genet* **75**:211, 1998.

23. Fryburg JS, Hwang V, Lin KY: Recurrent lambdoid synostosis within two families. *Am J Med Genet* **58**:262, 1995.

24. Hennekam RCM, Van den Boogaard MJ: Autosomal dominant craniosynostosis of the sutura metopica. *Clin Genet* **38**:374, 1990.

25. Zampino G, DiRocco CD, Butera G, Balducci F, Colosimo C, Torrioli MG, Mastroiacovo P: Opitz C trigonocephaly syndrome and midline brain anomalies. *Am J Med Genet* **73**:484, 1997.

26. Omran H, Hildebrandt F, Korinthenberg R, Brandis M: Probable Opitz trigonocephaly C syndrome with medulloblastoma. *Am J Med Genet* **69**:395, 1997.

27. Kelley RI, Borns PF, Nichols D, Zackai EH: Osteoglophonic dwarfism in two generations. *J Med Genet* **20**:436, 1983.

28. Beighton P: Osteoglophonic dysplasia. *J Med Genet* **26**:572, 1989.

29. Robin NH, Segel B, Carpenter G, Muenke M: Craniosynostosis, Philadelphia type: A new autosomal dominant syndrome with sagittal craniosynostosis and syndactyly of the fingers and toes. *Am J Med Genet* **62**:184, 1996.

30. Hunter AGW, Rudd NL: Craniosynostosis. 1. Sagittal synostosis; its genetics and associated clinical findings in 214 patients who lacked involvement of the coronal suture(s). *Teratology* **14**:185, 1976.

31. Lajeunie E, Le Meffer M, Bonaiti-Pellie C, Marchac D, Renier D: Genetic study of scaphocephaly. *Am J Med Genet* **62**:282, 1996.

32. Tavormina PL, Shiang R, Thompson LM, Zhu YZ, Wilkin DJ, Lachman RS, Wilcox WR, et al: Thanatophoric dysplasia (types I and II) caused by distinct mutations in fibroblast growth factor receptor 3. *Nat Genet* **9**:321, 1995.

33. Wilcox WR, Tavormina PL, Krakow D, Kitoh H, Lachman RS, Wasmuth JJ, Thompson LM, et al: Molecular, radiologic, and histopathologic correlations in thanatophoric dysplasia. *Am J Med Genet* **78**:274, 1998.

34. Chung CS, Myrianthopoulos NC: Factors affecting risks of congenital malformations. I. Analysis of epidemiologic factors in congenital malformations. Report from the Collaborative Perinatal Project. *Birth Defects* **11**:1, 1975.

35. Apert E: De l'Acrocephalosyndactylie. *Bull Soc Med Hôp Paris* **23**:1310, 1906.

36. Cohen MM Jr, Kreiborg S: Suture formation, premature sutural fusion, and suture default zones in Apert syndrome. *Am J Med Genet* **62**:339, 1996.

37. Cohen MM Jr, Kreiborg S: The central nervous system in the Apert syndrome. *Am J Med Genet* **35**:36, 1990.

38. Cohen MM Jr, Kreiborg S: Visceral anomalies in the Apert syndrome. *Am J Med Genet* **45**:758, 1993.

39. Cohen MM Jr, Kreiborg S: Skeletal abnormalities in the Apert syndrome. *Am J Med Genet* **47**:624, 1993.

40. Cohen MM Jr, Kreiborg S: Cutaneous manifestations of Apert syndrome. *Am J Med Genet* **58**:94, 1995.

41. Upton J, Zuker RM: Apert syndrome. *Clin Plast Surg* **18**:1, 1991.

42. Allanson JE: Germinal mosaicism in Apert syndrome. *Clin Genet* **29**:429, 1986.

43. Erickson JD, Cohen MM Jr: A study of parental age effects on the occurrence of fresh mutations for the Apert syndrome. *Ann Hum Genet* **38**:89, 1974.

44. Moloney DM, Slaney SF, Oldridge M, Wall SA, Sahlin P, Stenman G, Wilkie AOM: Exclusive paternal origin of new mutations in Apert syndrome. *Nat Genet* **13**:48, 1996.

45. Cohen MM Jr, Kreiborg S, Lammer EJ, Cordero JF, Mastroiacovo P, Erickson JD, Roeper P, et al: Birth prevalence study of the Apert syndrome. *Am J Med Genet* **42**:655, 1992.

46. Tolarova MM, Harris JA, Ordway DE, Vargervik K: Birth prevalence, mutation rate, sex ratio, parents' age, and ethnicity in Apert syndrome. *Am J Med Genet* **72**:394, 1997.

47. Cheng H, Burdon MA, Shun-Shin GA, Czypionka S: Dissociated eye movements in craniosynostosis: A hypothesis revived. *Br J Opthalmol* **77**:563, 1993.

48. Kaloust S, Ishii K, Vargervik K: Dental development in Apert syndrome. *Cleft Palate Craniofac J* **34**:117, 1997.

49. Cinalli G, Renier D, Sebag G, Sainte-Rose C, Arnaud E, Pierre-Kahn A: Chronic tonsillar herniation in Crouzon's and Apert's syndromes: The role of premature synostosis of the lambdoid suture. *J Neurosurg* **83**:575, 1995.

50. Patton MA, Goodship J, Hayward R, Lansdown R: Intellectual development in Apert's syndrome: A long-term follow up of 29 patients. *J Med Genet* **25**:164, 1988.

51. Upton J: Classification and pathologic anatomy of limb anomalies. *Clin Plast Surg* **18**:321, 1991.

52. Collins ED, Marsh JL, Vannier MW, Gilula LA: Spatial dysmorphology of the foot in Apert syndrome: Three-dimensional computed tomography. *Cleft Palate Craniofac J* **32**:255, 1995.

53. Slaney SF, Oldridge M, Hurst JA, Morriss-Kay GM, Hall CM, Poole MD, Wilkie AOM: Differential effects of FGFR2 mutations on syndactyly and cleft palate in Apert syndrome. *Am J Hum Genet* **58**:923, 1996.

54. Lefort G, Sarda P, Humeau C, Rieu D: Apert syndrome with partial preaxial polydactyly. *Genet Couns* **3**:107, 1992.

55. Anderson PJ, Hall R, Smith PJ: Finger duplication in Apert's syndrome. *J Hand Surg* **5**:649, 1996.

56. Thompson DN, Slaney SF, Hall CM, Shaw D, Jones BM, Hayward RD: Congenital cervical spinal fusion: a study in Apert syndrome. *Pediatr Neurosurg* **25**:20, 1996.

57. Wilkie AOM, Slaney SF, Oldridge M, Poole MD, Ashworth GJ, Hockley AD, Hayward RD, et al: Apert syndrome results from localized mutations of *FGFR2* and is allelic with Crouzon syndrome. *Nat Genet* **9**:165, 1995.

57a. Lajeunie E, Cameron R, El Ghouzzi V, de Parseval N, Journeau P, Gonzales M, Delezoide A-L, et al: Clinical variability in patients with Apert's syndrome. *J Neurosurg* **90**:443, 1999.

58. Muenke M, Schell U, Hehr A, Robin NH, Losken HW, Schinzel A, Pulleyn LJ, et al: A common mutation in the fibroblast growth factor receptor 1 gene in Pfeiffer syndrome. *Nat Genet* **8**:269, 1994.

59. Pulleyn LJ, Reardon W, Wilkes D, Rutland P, Jones BM, Hayward R, Hall CM, et al: Spectrum of craniosynostosis phenotypes associated with novel mutations at the fibroblast growth factor receptor 2 locus. *Eur J Hum Genet* **4**:283, 1996.

60. Oldridge M, Lunt PW, Zackai EH, McDonald-McGinn DM, Muenke M, Moloney DM, Twigg SR, et al: Genotype-phenotype correlation for nucleotide substitutions in the IgII-IgIII linker of *FGFR2*. *Hum Mol Genet* **6**:137, 1997.

61. Oldridge M, Wilkie AOM, Slaney SF, Poole MD, Pulleyn LJ, Rutland P, Hockley AD, et al: Mutations in the third immunoglobulin domain of the fibroblast growth factor receptor-2 gene in Crouzon syndrome. *Hum Mol Genet* **4**:1077, 1995.

62. Meyers GA, Day D, Goldberg R, Daentl DL, Przylepa KA, Abrams LJ, Graham JM Jr, et al: FGFR2 exon IIIa and IIIc mutations in Crouzon, Jackson-Weiss, and Pfeiffer syndromes: Evidence for missense changes, insertions, and a deletion due to alternative RNA splicing. *Am J Hum Genet* **58**:491, 1996.

63. Paznekas WA, Cunningham ML, Howard TD, Kof BR, Lipson MH, Grix AW, Feingold M, et al: Genetic heterogeneity of Saethre-Chotzen syndrome, due to TWIST and FGFR mutations. *Am J Hum Genet* **62**:1370, 1998.

64. Steinberger D, Vriend G, Mulliken JB, Müller U: The mutations in FGFR2-associated craniosynostoses are clustered in five structural elements of immunoglobulin-like domain III of the receptor. *Hum Genet* **102**:145, 1998.

65. Cornejo-Roldan L, Roessler E, Muenke M: Analysis of the mutational spectrum of the *FGFR2* gene in Pfeiffer syndrome. *Hum Genet* **104**:425, 1999.

66. Park WJ, Meyers GA, Li X, Theda C, Day D, Orlow SJ, Jones MC, et al: Novel FGFR2 mutations in Crouzon and Jackson-Weiss syndromes show allelic heterogeneity and phenotypic variability. *Hum Mol Genet* **4**:1229, 1995.

67. Tartaglia M, Valeri S, Velardi F, Di Rocco C, Battaglia PA: Trp290Cys mutation in exon IIIa of the fibroblast growth factor receptor 2 (FGFR2) gene is associated with Pfeiffer syndrome. *Hum Genet* **99**:602, 1997.

68. Schaefer F, Anderson C, Can B, Say B: Novel mutation in the FGFR2 gene at the same codon as the Crouzon syndrome mutations in a severe Pfeiffer syndrome type 2 case. *Am J Med Genet* **75**:252, 1998.

69. Steinberger D, Collmann H, Schmalenberger B, Müller U: A novel mutation (a886g) in exon 5 of FGFR2 in members of a family with Crouzon phenotype and plagiocephaly. *J Med Genet* **34**:420, 1997.

70. Oldridge M, Zackai EH, McDonald-McGinn DM, Iskei S, Morriss-Kay GM, Twigg SR, Johnson D, et al: *De novo Alu* element insertions in *FGFR2* identify a distinct pathological basis for Apert syndrome. *Am J Hum Genet* **64**:446, 1999.

71. Schell U, Hehr A, Feldman GJ, Robin NH, Zackai EH, de Die-Smulders C, Viskochil DH, et al: Mutations in FGFR1 and FGFR2 cause familial and sporadic Pfeiffer syndrome. *Hum Mol Genet* **4**:323, 1995.

72. Lajeunie E, Ma HW, Bonaventure J, Munnich A, Le Merrer M, Renier D: *FGFR2* mutations in Pfeiffer syndrome. *Nat Genet* 9:108, 1995.

73. Anderson PJ, Hall CM, Evans RD, Jones BM, Hayward RD: The feet in Pfeiffer's syndrome. *J Craniofac Surg* 9:83, 1998.

74. Hollway GE, Suthers GK, Haan EA, Thompson E, David DJ, Gecz J, Nulley JC: Mutation detection in *FGFR2* craniosynostosis syndromes. *Hum Genet* 99:251, 1997.

74a. Chun KM, Teebi A, Kennedy S, Forrest CR, Pay PN: Graduated strategy for the molecular diagnosis of craniosynostosis syndromes. *Am J Hum Genet* 65(Suppl):A289, 1999.

75. Jabs EW, Li X, Scott AF, Meyers G, Chen W, Eccles M, Mao J, et al: Jackson-Weiss and Crouzon syndromes are allelic with mutations in fibroblast growth factor 2. *Nat Genet* 8:275, 1994.

76. Steinberger D, Mulliken JB, Müller U: Crouzon syndrome: Previously unrecognized deletion, duplication, and point mutation within FGFR2 gene. *Hum Mut* 8:386-390, 1996.

77. Passos-Bueno MR, Sertié AL, Richieri-Costa A, Alonso LG, Zatz M, Alonso N, Brunoni, et al: Description of a new mutation and characterization of *FGFR1*, *FGFR2* and *FGFR3* mutations among Brazilian patients with syndromic craniosynostoses. *Am J Med Genet* 78:237, 1998.

78. Gorry MC, Preston RA, White GJ, Zhang Y, Singhal VK, Losken HW, Parker MG, et al: Crouzon syndrome: Mutations in two splice forms of *FGFR2* and a common point mutation shared with Jackson-Weiss syndrome. *Hum Mol Genet* 4:1387, 1995.

79. Reardon W, Winter RM, Rutland P, Pulleyn LJ, Jones BM, Malcolm S: Mutations in the fibroblast growth factor receptor 2 gene cause Crouzon syndrome. *Nat Genet* 8:98, 1994.

80. Rutland P, Pulleyn LI, Reardon W, Baraister M, Hayward R, Jones B, Malcolm S, et al: Identical mutations in the FGFR2 gene cause both Pfeiffer and Crouzon syndrome phenotypes *Nat Genet* 9:173, 1995.

80a. Manchester DK, Allen JK, Handler M, Schaefer FV: Novel FGFR2 mutation associated with a partial Apert syndrome phenotype. *Am J Hum Genet* 65(Suppl):A477, 1999.

81. Hertz JM, Juncker I, Molhave B, Sunde L, Christensen L, Østergaard JR, Kjeldssen M, et al: Mutations in the FGFR2-gene in Crouzon syndrome. *Eur J Hum Genet* 5(Supp 1):155, 1997.

82. Przylepa KA, Paznekas W, Zhang M, Golabi M, Bias W, Bamshad MJ, Carey JC, et al: Fibroblast growth factor receptor 2 mutations in Beare-Stevenson cutis gyrata syndrome. *Nat Genet* 13:492, 1996.

83. Bellus GA, Gaudenz K, Zackai EH, Clarke LA, Szabo J, Francomano CA, Muenke M: Identical mutations in three different fibroblast growth factor receptor genes in autosomal dominant craniosynostosis syndromes. *Nat Genet* 14:174, 1996.

84. Meyers GA, Orlow SJ, Munro IR, Przylepa KA, Jabs EW: Fibroblast growth factor receptor 3 (*FGFR3*) transmembrane mutation in Crouzon syndrome with acanthosis nigricans. *Nat Genet* 11:462, 1995.

85. Antonarakis SE, Nomenclature Working Group: Recommendations for a nomenclature system for human gene mutations. *Hum Mutat* 11:1, 1998.

86. Dionne CA, Crumley G, Bellot F, Kaplow JM, Searfoss G, Ruta M, Burgess WH, et al: Cloning and expression of two distinct high-affinity receptors cross-reacting with acidic and basic fibroblast growth factors. *EMBO J* 9:2685, 1990.

87. Beare JM, Dodge JA, Nevin NC: Cutis gyratum, acanthosis nigricans and other congenital anomalies: A new syndrome. *Br J Derm* 81:241, 1969.

88. Stevenson RE, Ferlauto GJ, Taylor HA: Cutis gyratum and acanthosis nigricans associated with other anomalies: A distinctive syndrome. *J Pediatr* 92:950, 1978.

89. Hall BD, Cadle RG, Golabi M, Morris CA, Cohen MM Jr: Beare-Stevenson cutis gyrata syndrome. *Am J Med Genet* 44:82, 1992.

90. Andrews JM, Martins DMFS, Ramos RR, Ferreira LM: A severe case of Beare-Stevenson syndrome and associated congenital deformities. *Br J Plast Surg* 46:443, 1993.

91. Bratanic B, Praprotnik M, Novosel-Sever M: Congenital craniofacial dysostosis and cutis gyratum: The Beare-Stevenson syndrome. *Eur J Pediatr* 153:184, 1994.

92. Krepelová A, Baxová A, Clada P, Plavka R, Kapras J: FGFR2 gene mutation (Tyr375Cys) in a new case of Beare-Stevenson syndrome. *Am J Med Genet* 76:362, 1998.

93. Warman ML, Mulliken JB, Hayward PG, Müller U: Newly recognized autosomal dominant disorder with craniosynostosis. *Am J Med Genet* 46:444, 1993.

94. Müller U, Warman ML, Mulliken JB, Weber JL: Assignment of a gene locus involved in craniosynostosis to chromosome 5qter. *Hum Mol Genet* 2:119, 1993.

95. Jabs EW, Müller U, Li X, Ma L, Luo W, Hayworth IS, Klisak I, et al: A mutation in the homeodomain of the human *MSX2* gene in a family affected with autosomal dominant craniosynostosis. *Cell* 75:443, 1993.

95a. Wilkie AOM, Tang A, Elanko N, Walsh S, Twigg SRF, Hurst JA, Chrzanowska K, et al: Mutations of the homeobox gene MSX2 cause symmetric parietal foramina: contrasting effects of loss and gain of function mutations for skull development. *Am J Hum Genet* 65(Suppl):A47, 1999

96. Crouzon O: Dysotose cranio-faciale héréditaire. *Bull Mem Soc Med Hop* 33:545, 1912.

97. Gorlin RJ, Cohen MM Jr, Levin LS: *Syndromes of the Head and Neck. Oxford Monographs on Medical Genetics no. 19*, 3rd ed. New York, Oxford University Press, 1990.

98. Cutting C, Dean D, Bookstein FL, Haddad B, Khorramabadi D, Zonneveld FW, McCarthy JG: A three-dimensional smooth surface analysis of untreated Crouzon's syndrome in the adult. *J Craniofac Surg* 6:444, 1995.

98a. Glaser RL, Jiang W, Boyadjiev SA, Tran AK, Zachary AA, Johnson D, Walsh S, et al: Paternal origin of FGFR2 mutations in sporadic cases of Crouzon and Pfeiffer syndromes. *Am J Hum Genet* 66:768, 2000.

99. Cohen MM Jr, Kreiborg S: Birth prevalence studies of the Crouzon syndrome: Comparison of direct and indirect methods. *Clin Genet* 41:12, 1992.

100. Murdoch-Kinch CA, Bixler D, Ward RE: Cephalometric analysis of families with dominantly inherited Crouzon syndrome: An aid to diagnosis in family studies. *Am J Med Genet* 77:405, 1998.

101. Rohatgi M: Cloverleaf skull, a severe form of Crouzon's syndrome: A new concept in etiology. *Acta Neurochir* 108:45, 1991.

102. Hanieh A, Sheen R, David DJ: Hydrocephalus in Crouzon's syndrome. *Childs Nerv Syst* 5:188, 1989.

103. Proudman TW, Clark BE, Moore MH, Abbott AH, David DJ: Central nervous system imaging in Crouzon's syndrome. *J Craniofac Surg* 6:401, 1995.

104. Perlman JM, Zaidman GW: Bilateral keratoconus in Crouzon's syndrome. *Cornea* 13:80, 1994.

105. Kreiborg A, Barr M Jr, Cohen MM Jr: Cervical spine in the Apert syndrome. *Am J Med Genet* 43:704, 1992.

106. Anderson PJ, Hall CM, Evans RD, Harkness WJ, Hayward RD, Jones BM: The cervical spine in Crouzon syndrome. *Spine* 22:402,1997.

107. Proudman TW, Moore MH, Abbott AH, David DJ: Noncraniofacial manifestations of Crouzon's disease. *J Craniofac Surg* 5:218, 1994.

108. Murdoch-Kinch CA, Ward RE: Metacarpophalangeal analysis in Crouzon syndrome: Additional evidence for phenotypic convergence with the acrocephalosyndactyly syndromes. *Am J Med Genet* 73:61, 1997.

109. Anderson PJ, Hall CM, Evans RD, Jones BM, Hayward RD: Hand anomalies in Crouzon syndrome. *Skeletal Radiol* 26:113, 1997.

110. Anderson PJ, Hall CM, Evans RD, Jones BM, Hayward RD: The feet in Crouzon syndrome. *J Craniofac Genet Dev Biol* 17:43, 1997.

111. Sirotnak J, Brodsky L, Pizzuto M: Airway obstruction in the Crouzon syndrome: Case report and review of the literature. *Int J Pediatr Otorhinolaryngol* 31:235, 1995.

112. Preston RA, Post JC, Keats BJB, Aston CE, Ferrell RE, Priest J, Nouri N, et al: A gene for Crouzon craniofacial dysostosis maps to the long arm of chromosome 10. *Nat Genet* 7:149, 1994.

113. Gorlin RJ: Fibroblast growth factors, their receptors and receptor disorders. *J Craniomaxillofac Surg* 25:69, 1997.

114. Superti-Furga A, Locher ML, Steinlin M, et al: Crouzon syndrome with acanthosis nigricans, spinal stenosis and desmo-osteoblastomas: Pleiotropic effects of the FGFR3 Ala391Glu mutation. *J Craniomaxillofac Surg* 24(Suppl):112, 1996.

115. Wilkes D, Rutland P, Pulleyn LJ, Reardon W, Moss C, Ellis JP, Winter RM, et al: A recurrent mutation, ala391glu, in the transmembrane region of FGFR3 causes Crouzon syndrome and acanthosis nigricans. *J Med Genet* 33:744, 1996.

116. Jackson CE, Weiss L, Reynolds WA, Forman TF, Peterson JA: Craniosynostosis, midfacial hypoplasia, and foot abnormalities: An autosomal dominant phenotype in a large Amish kindred. *J Pediatr* 88:963, 1976.

117. Baraitser M, Bowen-Bravery M, Saldana-Garcia P: Pitfalls of genetic counselling in Pfeiffer's syndrome. *J Med Genet* 17:250, 1980.

118. Ades LC, Mulley J C, Senga IP, Morris LL, David DJ, Haan EA: Jackson-Weiss syndrome: Clinical and radiological findings in a large kindred and exclusion of the gene from 7p2l and 5qter. *Am J Med Genet* **51**:121, 1994.

119. Muenke M, Gripp KW, McDonald-McGinn DM, Gaudenz K, Whitaker LA, Bartlett SP, Markowitz RI, et al: A unique point mutation in the fibroblast growth factor receptor 3 gene (*FGFR3*) defines a new craniosynostosis syndrome. *Am J Hum Genet* **60**:555, 1997.

120. von Gernet S, Schuffenhauer S, Golla A, Lichtner P, Balg S, Muhlbauer W, Murken J, et al: Craniosynostosis suggestive of Saethre-Chotzen syndrome: Clinical description of a large kindred and exclusion of candidate regions on 7p. *Am J Med Genet* **63**:177, 1996.

121. Reardon W, Wilkes D, Rutland P, Pulleyn LJ, Malcolm S, Dean JC, Evans RD, et al: Craniosynostosis associated with FGFR3 pro250arg mutation results in a range of clinical presentations including unisutural sporadic craniosynostosis. *J Med Genet* **34**:632, 1997.

122. Golla A, Lichtner P, von Gernet S, Winterpacht A, Fairley J, Murken J, Schuffenhauer S: Phenotypic expression of the fibroblast growth factor receptor 3 (FGFR3) mutation P250R in a large craniosynostosis family. *J Med Genet* **34**:683, 1997.

123. Hollway GE, Phillips HA, Ades LC, Haan EA, Mulley JC: Localization of craniosynostosis Adelaide type to 4p16. *Hum Mol Genet* **4**:681, 1995.

124. Graham JM Jr, Braddock SR, Mortier GR, Lachman R, Van Dop C, Jabs EW: Syndrome of coronal craniosynostosis with brachydactyly and carpal/tarsal coalition due to Pro250Arg mutation in FGFR3 gene. *Am J Med Genet* **77**:322, 1998.

125. Glass IA, Chapman S, Hockley AD: A distinct autosomal dominant craniosynostosis-brachydactyly syndrome. *Clin Dysmorphol* **3**:215, 1994.

126. Moloney DM, Wall SA, Ashworth GJ, Oldridge M, Glass IA, Francomano CA, Muenke M, et al: Prevalence of Pro250Arg mutation of fibroblast growth factor receptor 3 in coronal craniosynostosis. *Lancet* **349**:1059, 1997.

127. Lajeunie E, El Ghouzzi V, Le Merrer M, Munnich A, Bonaventure J, Renier D: Sex-related expressivity of the phenotype in coronal craniosynostosis caused by the recurrent P250R FGFR3 mutation. *J Med Genet* **36**:9, 1999.

128. Gripp KW, McDonald-McGinn DM, Gaudenz K, Whitaker LA, Bartlett SP, Glatt PM, Cassileth LB, et al: Identification of a genetic cause for isolated unilateral coronal synostosis: A unique mutation in fibroblast growth factor receptor 3. *J Pediatr* **132**:714, 1998.

129. Robin NH, Scott JA, Cohen AR, Goldstein JA: Nonpenetrance in FGFR3-associated coronal synostosis syndrome. *Am J Med Genet* **80**:296, 1998.

130. Hollway GE, Suthers GK, Battese KM, Turner AM, David DJ, Mulley JC: Deafness due to pro250-to-arg mutation of FGFR3. *Lancet* **351**:877, 1998.

131. Pfeiffer RA: Dominant erbliche Akrocephalosyndaktylie. *Z Kinderheilk* **90**:301, 1964.

132. Cohen MM Jr: Pfeiffer syndrome update, clinical subtypes, and guidelines for differential diagnosis. *Am J Med Genet* **45**:300, 1993.

133. Moore MH, Cantrell SB, Trott JA, David DJ: Pfeiffer syndrome: A clinical review. *Cleft Palate Craniofac J* **32**:62, 1995.

134. Kroczek RA, Muehlbauer W, Zimmerman I: Cloverleaf skull associated with Pfeiffer syndrome pathology and management. *Eur J Pediatr* **145**:442, 1986.

135. Kreiborg S, Cohen MM Jr: A severe case of Pfeiffer syndrome associated with stub thumb on the maternal side of the family. *J Craniofacial Genet Dev Biol* **13**:73, 1993.

136. Soekarman D, Fryns JP: Pfeiffer acrocephaly syndrome in mother and son with cloverleaf skull anomaly in the child. *Genet Couns* **4**:88, 1993.

137. Barone CM, Marion R, Shanske A, Argamaso RV, Shprintzen RJ: Craniofacial limb and abdominal anomalies in a distinct syndrome relation to the spectrum of Pfeiffer syndrome type 3. *Am J Med Genet* **45**:745, 1993.

138. Kerr NC, Wilroy RS Jr, Kaufman RA: Pfeiffer syndrome with normal thumbs. *Am J Med Genet* **66**:138,1996.

139. Robin NH, Scott JA, Arnold JE, Goldstein JA, Shilling BB, Marion RW, Cohen MM Jr: Favorable prognosis for children with Pfeiffer syndrome types 2 and 3: Implications for classification. *Am J Med Genet* **75**:240, 1998.

140. Gripp KW, Stolle CA, McDonald-McGinn DM, Markowitz RI, Bartlett SP, Katowitz JA, Muenke M, et al: Phenotype of the fibroblast growth factor receptor 2 Ser351Cys mutation: Pfeiffer syndrome type III. *Am J Med Genet* **78**:356, 1998.

141. Plomp AS, Hamel BCJ, Cobben JM, Verloes A, Offermans JP, Lajeunie E, Fryns JP, et al: Pfeiffer syndrome type 2: Further delineation and review of the literature. *Am J Med Genet* **75**:245, 1998.

142. Cornejo-Roldan L, Roessler E, Zackai EH, Muenke M: Phenotype-genotype correlation in Pfeiffer syndrome caused by *FGFR2* mutations (in preparation).

143. Robin NH, Feldman GJ, Mitchell HF, Lorenz P, Wilroy RS, Zackai EH, Allanson JE, et al: Linkage of Pfeiffer syndrome to chromosome 8 centromere and evidence for genetic heterogeneity. *Hum Mol Genet* **3**:2153, 1994.

144. Moore MH, Lodge ML, Clark BE: The infant skull in Pfeiffer's syndrome. *J Craniofac Surg* **6**:483, 1995.

145. Moore MH, Lodge ML, Clark BE: Spinal anomalies in Pfeiffer's syndrome. *Cleft Palate Craniofac J* **32**:251, 1995.

146. Schell U, Richieri-Costa A, Muenke M: Genotype-phenotype correlation in two patients with familial Pfeiffer syndrome. *Braz J Dysmorphol Speech Hearing Disorders* **1**:5, 1997.

147. Muenke M, Francomano CA, Cohen MM Jr, Jabs EW: Principles of molecular medicine, in Jameson JL (ed): *Fibroblast Growth Factor Receptor Related Skeletal Disorders: Craniosynostosis and Dwarfism Syndromes*. Vol 114. Humana Press, 1998, p 1029.

148. Cinalli G, Sainte-Rose C, Kollar EM, Zerah M, Brunelle F, Chumas P, Arnaud E, et al: Hydrocephalus and craniosynostosis. *J Neurosurg* **88**:209, 1998.

149. Anderson PJ, Hall CM, Smith PJ, Evans RD, Hayward RD, Jones BM: The hands in Pfeiffer's syndrome. *J Hand Surg* **22**:537, 1997.

150. Kissel CG, Goodman EF, Boffeli TJ: Pfeiffer syndrome: A syndrome of acrocephalosyndactyly. *J Foot Surgery* **31**:149,1992.

151. Anderson PJ, Hall CM, Evans RD, Jones BM, Harkness W, Hayward RD: Cervical spine in Pfeiffer's syndrome. *J Craniofac Surg* **7**:275, 1996a.

152. Vallino-Napoli LD: Audiologic and otologic characteristics of Pfeiffer syndrome. *Cleft Palate Craniofac J* **33**:524, 1996.

153. Jones MR, De Sa LCF, Good WV: Atypical iris colobomata and Pfeiffer syndrome. *J Pediatr Ophthal Strabismus* **30**:266, 1993.

154. Stone P, Trevenen CL, Mitchell I, Rudd N: Congenital tracheal stenosis in Pfeiffer syndrome. *Clin Genet* **38**: 145,1990.

155. Ohashi H, Nishimoto H, Nishimura J, Sato M, Imaizumi S, Aihara T, Fukushima Y: Anorectal anomaly in Pfeiffer syndrome. *Clin Dysmorphol* **2**:28, 1993.

156. Goldfisher ER, Cromie WJ: Bilateral suprarenal cryptorchidism in a patient with the Pfeiffer syndrome. *J Urology* **158**:597, 1997.

157. Zippel H, Schüler KH: Dominant vererbte Akrozephalosyndaktylie (ACS). *Fortschr Röntgenstr* **110**:234, 1969.

158. Yoshiura K, Leysens NJ, Chang J, Ward D, Murray JC, Muenke M: Genomic structure, sequence, and mapping of human FGF8, with exclusion of its role in craniosynostosis/limb defect syndromes. *Am J Hum Genet* **72**:354, 1997.

159. Saldino RM, Steinbach HL, Epstein CJ: Familial acrocephalosyndactyly (Pfeiffer syndrome). *Am J Roentgenol* **116**:609, 1972.

160. Mathijssen IMJ, Vaandrager JM, Hoogeboom AJM, Hesseling-Janssen ALW, Van den Ouweland AMW: Pfeiffer's syndrome resulting from an S351C mutation in the fibroblast growth factor receptor-2 gene. *J Craniofac Surg* **9**:207, 1998.

161. Saethre H: Ein Beitrag zum Turmschaedelproblem. (Pathogenese, Erblichkeit und Symptomatologie.) *Nervenheilkd* **117**:533, 1931.

162. Chotzen F: Eine eigenartige familiäre Entwicklungsstörung. (Akrocephalosyndaktylie, Dysostosis craniofacialis und Hypertelorismus.) *Monatsschr Kinderheilkd* **55**:97, 1932.

163. Ferri J, Seiler C, Piot B, Marcier J: The Saethre-Chotzen syndrome: Report on 17 cases. *Revue de Stomatologie et de Chirurgie Maxillo Faciale* **94**:290, 1993.

164. Reardon W, Winter RM: Saethre-Chotzen syndrome. *J Med Genet* **31**:393, 1994.

164a. Pantke OA, Cohen MM Jr., Witkop CJ Jr., Feingold M, Schaumann B, Pantke HC, Gorlin RJ: The Saethre-Chotzen Syndrome. *Birth Defects: Original Article Series* **XI**:190, 1975.

165. Goho C: Dental findings in Saethre-Chotzen syndrome (acrocephalosyndactyly type II): Report of case. *ASDC J Dent Child* **65**:136, 1998.

165a. Kunz J, Hundler M, Fritz B: Identification of a frameshift mutation in the gene *TWIST* in a family affected with Robinow-Sorauf syndrome. *J Med Genet* **36**:650, 1999.

166. Thompson EM, Baraitser M, Hayward RD: Parietal foramina in Saethre-Chotzen syndrome. *J Med Genet* 21:369, 1984.

167. Fehlow P, Froehlich B, Miosge W, Otto W, Walther F: Saethre-Chotzen syndrome and associated neurological and psychiatric symptoms. *Fortschr Neurol Psychiatr* 60:66, 1992.

168. Mazzone D, Carpinato C, Di Pietro F: The Saethre-Chotzen syndrome (acrocephalosyndactyly type III). Clinical, genetic and neuropsychiatric features. *Giornale di Neuropsichiatria dell'Eta Evolutiva* 16:155, 1996.

169. Rose CSP, Patel P, Reardon W, Malcolm S, Winter RM: The *TWIST* gene, although not disrupted in Saethre-Chotzen patients with apparently balanced translocations of 7p21, is mutated in familial and sporadic cases. *Hum Mol Genet* 6:1369, 1997.

170. Johnson D, Horsley SW, Moloney DM, Oldridge M, Twigg SR, Walsh S, Barrow M, et al: A comprehensive screen for *TWIST* mutations in patients with craniosynostosis identifies a new microdeletion syndrome of chromosome band 7p21.1. *Am J Hum Genet* 63:1282, 1998.

171. Kasparcova V, Stolle CA, Gripp KW, Celle L, McDonald-McGinn D, Bartlett S, Whitaker L, et al: Molecular analysis of patients with Saethre-Chotzen syndrome: Novel mutations and polymorphisms in the *TWIST* gene. *Am J Hum Genet* 63(Supp):A367, 1998.

172. Howard TD, Paznekas WA, Green ED, Chiang LC, Ma N, Ortiz de Luna RI, Garcia Delgado C, et al: Mutations in *TWIST*, a basic helix-loop-helix transcription factor, in Saethre-Chotzen syndrome. *Nat Genet* 15:36, 1997.

173. El Ghouzzi V, Le Merrer M, Perrin-Schmitt F, Lajeunie E, Benit P, Renier D, Bourgeois P, et al: Mutations of the *TWIST* gene in the Saethre-Chotzen syndrome. *Nat Genet* 15:42, 1997.

174. El Ghouzzi V, Lajeunie E, LeMerrer M, Cormier-Daire V, Renier D, Munnich A, Bonaventure J: Mutations within or upstream of the basic helix-loop-helix domain of the *TWIST* gene are specific to Saethre-Chotzen syndrome. *Eur J Hum Genet* 7:27, 1999.

174a. Carbonara C, Sbaiz L, Genitori L, Peretta P, Mussa F, Nurisso C, Restagno G, et al: A novel N114D TWIST mutation in a Crouzon-like patient. *Am J Hum Genet* 65(Suppl): A144, 1999.

175. Ray PN, Siegel-Bartelt J, Chun K: A unique mutation in *TWIST* causes Saethre-Chotzen syndrome. *Am J Hum Genet* 61:A344, 1997.

176. Gripp KW, Stolle CA, Celle L, McDonald-McGinn DM, Whitaker LA, Zackai EH: *TWIST* gene mutation in a patient with radial aplasia and craniosynostosis: Further evidence for the heterogeneity of Baller-Gerold syndrome. *Am J Med Genet* 82:170, 1999.

177. Shprintzen RJ, Goldberg RB: A recurrent pattern syndrome of craniosynostosis associated with arachnodactyly and abdominal hernias. *Craniofac Genet Dev Biol* 2:65, 1982.

178. Ades LC, Morris LL, Power RG, Wilson M, Haan EA, Bateman JF, Milewicz DM, et al: Distinct skeletal abnormalities in four girls with Shprintzen-Goldberg syndrome. *Am J Med Genet* 57:565, 1995.

179. Furlong J, Kurczynski TW, Hennessy JR: New marfanoid syndrome with craniosynostosis. *Am J Med Genet* 26:599, 1987.

180. Greally MT, Carey JC, Milewicz DM, Hudgins L, Goldberg RB, Shprintzen RJ, Cousineau AJ, et al: Shprintzen-Goldberg syndrome: A clinical analysis. *Am J Med Genet* 76:202, 1998.

181. Hassed S, Shewmake K, Teo C, Curtis M, Cunniff C: Shprintzen-Goldberg syndrome with osteopenia and progressive hydrocephalus. *Am J Med Genet* 70:450, 1997.

182. Saal HM, Bulas DI, Allen JF, Vezina LG, Walton D, Rosenbaum KN: Patient with craniosynostosis and marfanoid phenotype (Shprintzen-Goldberg syndrome) and cloverleaf skull. *Am J Med Genet* 57:573, 1995.

183. Shah AM, Chattopadhyay A, Kher A, Bharucha BA, Karapurkar AP: Craniosynostosis with Marfan syndrome, hand and foot anomalies. *Clin Dysmorph* 5:263, 1996.

184. Sood S, Eldadah ZA, Krause W L, McIntosh I, Dietz HC: Mutation in fibrillin-I and the Marfanoid-craniosynostosis (Shprintzen-Goldberg) syndrome. *Nat Genet* 12:209, 1996.

185. Schrijver I, Liu W, Francke U: The pathogenicity of the pro1148ala substitution in the FBN1 gene: Causing or predisposing to Marfan syndrome and aortic aneurysm, or clinically innocent? *Hum Genet* 99:607, 1997.

185a. Wang M, Mathews KR, Imaizumi K, Beiraghi S, Blumberg B, Scheuner M, Graham JM Jr., et al: P1148A in fibrillin-1 is not a mutation anymore. *Nat Genet* 15:12, 1997.

186. Gosain AK, McCarthy JG, Wisoff JH: Morbidity associated with increased pressure in Apert and Pfeiffer syndromes: The need for long-term evaluation. *Plast Reconstr Surg* 97:292, 1996.

187. Renier D, Sainte-Rose C, Marchac D, Hirsch JF: Intracranial pressure in craniostenosis. *J Neurosurg* 57:370, 1982.

188. Francis PM, Beals S, Rekate HL, Pittman HW, Manwaring K, Reiff J: Chronic tonsillar herniation and Crouzon's syndrome. *Pediatr Neurosurg* 18:202, 1992.

189. Sen A, Dougal P, Padhy AK, Bhattacharya A, Kumar R, Bal C, Bajpai M, et al: Technetium-99m-HMPAO SPECT cerebral blood flow study in children with craniosynostosis. *J Nucl Med* 36:394, 1995.

190. David LR, Wilson JA, Watson NE, Argenta LC: Cerebral perfusion defects secondary to simple craniosynostosis. *J Craniofac Surg* 7:177, 1996.

190a. David LR, Genecov DG, Camastra AA, Wilson JA, Argenta LC: Positron emission tomography studies confirm the need for early surgical intervention in patients with single-suture craniosynostosis. *J Craniofac Surg* 10:38, 1999.

191. Gonsalez S, Hayward R, Jones B, Lane R: Upper airway obstruction and raised intracranial pressure in children with craniosynostosis. *Eur Respir J* 10:367, 1997.

192. Hui S, Wing YK, Kew J, Chan YL, Abdullah V, Fok TF: Obstructive sleep apnea syndrome in a family with Crouzon's syndrome. *Sleep* 21:298, 1998.

193. Stavrou P, Sgouros S, Willshaw HE, Goldin JH, Hockley AD, Wake MJC: Visual failure caused by raised intracranial pressure in craniosynostosis. *Childs Nerv Syst* 13:64, 1997.

194. Eckenstein FP: Fibroblast growth factors in the nervous system. *J Neurobiol* 25:1467, 1994.

195. Renier D, Arnaud E, Cinalli G, Sebag G, Zerah M, Marchac D: Prognosis for mental function in Apert's syndrome. *J Neurosurg* 85:66, 1996.

196. Shapiro R, Robinson F: The Embryogenesis of the Human Skull. *An Anatomic and Radiographic Atlas*. Cambridge, MA, Harvard University Press, 1980.

197. Martinelli P, Paladini D, D'Armiento M, Scarano G: Prenatal diagnosis of cloverleaf skull in the subtype 2 Pfeiffer syndrome. *Clin Dysmorphol* 6:89, 1997.

198. van der Ham LI, Cohen-Overbeek TE, Paz Y, Geuze HD, Vermeij-Keers C: The ultrasonic detection of an isolated craniosynostosis. *Prenat Diag* 15:1189, 1995.

199. Hill LM, Thomas ML, Peterson CS: The ultrasonic detection of Apert syndrome. *J Ultrasound Med* 6:601, 1987.

200. Kaufmann K, Baldinger S, Pratt I: Ultrasound detection of Apert syndrome: A case report and literature review. *Am J Perinatol* 14:427, 1997.

201. Hill LM, Grzybek PC: Sonographic findings with Pfeiffer syndrome. *Prenatal Diagn* 14:47, 1994.

202. Gollin YG, Abuhamad AZ, Inati MN, Shaffer WK, Copel JA, Hobbins HC: Sonographic appearance of craniofacial dysostosis (Crouzon syndrome) in the second trimester. *J Ultrasound Med* 12:625, 1993.

203. Schwartz M, Kreiborg S, Skovby F: First-trimester prenatal diagnosis of Crouzon syndrome. *Prenat Diagn* 16:155, 1996.

204. Chang CC, Tsai FJ, Tsai HD, Tsai CH, Hseih YY, Lee CC, Yang TC, et al: Prenatal diagnosis of Apert syndrome. *Prenat Diag* 18:621, 1998.

205. Filkins K, Russo JF, Boehmer S, Camous M, Przylepa KA, Jiang W, Jabs EW: Prenatal ultrasonographic and molecular diagnosis of Apert syndrome. *Prenat Diag* 17:1081, 1997.

206. Osada H, Ishii J, Sekiya JS: Prenatal molecular diagnosis for Apert syndrome. *Int J Gynaecol Obstet* 55:171, 1996.

207. Zlotogora J: Germ line mosaicism. *Hum Genet* 102:381, 1998.

208. Vanier ML: Radiologic evaluation of craniosynostosis, Chap 12, in Cohen MM Jr, MacLean RE (eds): *Craniosynostosis: Diagnosis, Evaluation, and Management*. 2000.

209. Poznanski AK: *The Hand in Radiologic Diagnosis: With Gamuts and Pattern Profiles*, 2d ed. Philadelphia, WB Saunders, 1984.

210. Temtamy SA, McKusick VA: The genetics of hand malformations. *Birth Defects Orig Artic Ser* 14:1, 1978.

211. Posnick JC: Craniofacial Dysostosis. Staging of reconstruction and management of the midface deformity. *Neurosurg Clin N Am* 2:683, 1991.

212. Bauer B, Habal M, Persing J, Marsh J, Ousterhout D, Salyer K, Stahl S, et al: Guidelines for care, treatment, and outcome of patients with craniosynostosis. *J Craniofac Surg* 5:72, 1994.

213. David DJ, Sheen R: Surgical correction of Crouzon syndrome. *Plast Reconstr Surg* 85:344, 1990.

214. Martinez-Perez D, Vander Woude DL, Barnes PD, Scott RM, Mulliken JB: Jugular foraminal stenosis in Crouzon syndrome. *Pediatr Neurosurg* 25:252, 1996.

215. Moore MH, David DJ: Fronto-orbital advancement for Apert syndrome in infancy—Why? *Asian J Surg* **20**:19, 1997.

216. Polley JW, Figueroa AA: Commentary on midface advancement by bone distraction on treatment of cleft deformities and on distraction osteogenesis and its application to the midface and bony orbit in the craniosynostosis syndromes. *J Craniofac Surg* **9**:119, 1998.

217. Posnick JC, Lin KY, Jhawar BJ, Armstrong D: Crouzon syndrome: Quantitative assessment of presenting deformity and surgical results based on CT scans. *Plast Reconstr Surg* **92**:1027, 1993.

218. Stelnicki EJ, Vanderwall K, Harrison MR, Longaker MT, Kaban LB, Hoffman WY: The in utero correction of unilateral coronal craniosynostosis. *Plast Reconstr Surg* **101**:287, 1998.

219. Sun P, Shin JH, Persing JA, Hemmy DC: Management of the ventricular shunt in posterior deformities of the skull in craniosynostosis. *J Craniofac Surg* **8**:38, 1997.

220. Zuker RM, Cleland HJ, Haswell T: Syndactyly correction of the hand in Apert syndrome. *Clin Plast Surg* **18**:357, 1991.

220a. Mehrara BJ, Longaker MT: New developments in craniofacial surgery research. *Cleft Palate Craniofac J* **36**:377, 1999.

221. Newberry EP, Latifi T, Battaile JT, Towler DA: Structure-function analysis of Msx2-mediated transcriptional suppression. *Biochemistry* **36**:10451, 1997.

222. Wu L, Wu H, Ma L, Sangiorgi F, Wu N, Bell JR, Lyons GE, et al: Mizl, a novel zinc finger transcription factor that interacts with Msx2 and enhances its affinity for DNA. *Mech Dev* **65**:3, 1997.

223. Engelkamp D, van Heyningen V: Transcription factors in disease. *Curr Opin Genet Dev* **6**:334, 1996.

224. Hu MCT, Qiu WR, Wang YP, Hill D, Ring BD, Scully S, Bolon B et al: FGF-18, a novel member of the fibroblast growth factor receptor family, stimulates hepatic and intestinal proliferation. *Mol Cell Biol* **18**:6063, 1998.

225. Ohbayashi N, Hoshikawa M, Kimura S, Yamasaki M, Fukui S, Itoh N: Structure and expression of mRNA encoding a novel fibroblast growth factor, FGF-18, an apical ectodermal factor. *Development* **273**:18161, 1998.

225a. Xie M-H, Holcomb I, Deuel B, Dowd P, Huang A, Vagts A, Foster J, et al: FGF-19, a novel fibroblast growth factor with unique specificity for FGFR4. *Cytokine* **11**:729, 1999.

226. Coulier F, Pontarotti P, Roubin R, Hartung H, Goldfarb M, Birnbaum D: Of worms and men: An evolutionary perspective on the fibroblast growth factor (FGF) and FGF receptor families. *J Mol Evol* **44**:43, 1997.

227. Spivak-Kroizman T, Lemmon MA, Dikic I, Ladbury JE, Pinchasi D, Huang J, Jaye M, et al: Heparin-induced oligomerization of FGF molecules is responsible for FGF receptor dimerization, activation, and cell proliferation. *Cell* **79**:1015, 1994.

228. Mohammadi M, Dikic I, Sorokin A, Burgess WH, Jaye M, Schlessinger J: Identification of six novel autophosphorylation sites on fibroblast growth factor receptor 1 and elucidation of their importance in receptor activation and signal transduction. *Mol Cell Biol* **16**:977, 1996.

229. Zimmer Y, Givol D, Yayon A: Multiple structural elements determine ligand binding of fibroblast growth factor receptors. Evidence that both Ig domain 2 and 3 define receptor specificity. *J Biol Chem* **268**:7899, 1993.

230. Cheon H-G, LaRochelle WJ, Bottaro DP, Burgess WH, Aaronson SA: High-affinity binding sites for related fibroblast growth factor ligands reside within different receptor immunoglobulin-like domains. *Proc Natl Acad Sci U S A* **91**:989, 1994.

231. Gray TE, Eisenstein M, Shimon T, Givol D, Yayon A: Molecular modeling based mutagenesis defines ligand binding and specificity determining regions of fibroblast growth factor receptors. *Biochemistry* **34**:10325, 1995.

232. Wang F, Kan M, Xu J, Yan G, McKeehan WL: Ligand-specific structural domains in the fibroblast growth factor receptor. *J Biol Chem* **270**: 10222, 1995.

233. Zhu X, Komiya H, Chirino A, Faham S, Fox GM, Arakawa T, Hsu BT, et al: Three-dimensional structures of acidic and basic fibroblast growth factors. *Science* **251**:90, 1991.

234. Faham S, Hileman RE, Fromm JR, Linhardt RJ, Rees DC: Heparin structure and interactions with basic fibroblast growth factor. *Science* **271**:1116, 1996.

235. DiGabriele AD, Lax I, Chen DI, Svahn CM, Jaye M, Schlessinger J, Hendrickson WA: Structure of a heparin-linked biologically active dimer of fibroblast growth factor. *Nature* **393**:812, 1998.

235a. Plotnikov AN, Schlessinger J, Hubbard SR, Mohammadi M: Structural basis for FGF receptor dimerization and activation. *Cell* **98**:641, 1999.

236. Mohammadi M, Schlessinger J, Hubbard SR: Structure of the FGF receptor tyrosine kinase domain reveals a novel autoinhibitory mechanism. *Cell* **86**:577, 1996.

237. Bateman A, Chothia C: Outline structures for the extracellular domains of the fibroblast growth factor receptors. *Nat Struct Biol* **2**:1068, 1995.

238. Bellot F, Crumley G, Kaplow JM, Schlessinger J, Jaye M, Dionne CA: Ligand-induced transphosphorylation between different FGF receptors. *EMBO J* **10**:2849, 1991.

239. Kavanaugh WM, Williams LT: An alternative to SH2 domains for binding tyrosine-phosphorylated proteins. *Science* **266**:1862, 1994.

240. Kouhara H, Hadari YR, Spivak-Kroizman T, Schilling J, Bar-Sagi D, Lax I, Schlessinger J: A lipid-anchored Grb2-binding protein that links FGF-receptor activation to the Ras/MAPK signaling pathway. *Cell* **89**:693, 1997.

241. Marshall CJ: Specificity of receptor tyrosine kinase signaling: Transient versus sustained extracellular signal-regulated kinase activation. *Cell* **80**:179, 1995.

241a. Vojtek AB, Der CJ: Increasing complexity of the Ras signaling pathway. *J Biol Chem* **273**:19925, 1998.

242. Johnson DE, Lu J, Chen H, Werner S, Williams LT: The human fibroblast growth factor receptor genes: A common structural arrangement underlies the mechanisms for generating receptor forms that differ in their third immunoglobulin domain. *Mol Cell Biol* **11**:4627, 1991.

243. Perez-Castro AV, Wilson J, Altherr MR: Genomic organization of the mouse fibroblast growth factor receptor 3 (*Fgfr3*) gene. *Genomics* **30**:157, 1995.

244. Perez-Castro AV, Wilson J, Altherr MR: Genomic organization of the human fibroblast growth factor receptor 3 (*FGFR3*) gene and comparative sequence analysis with the mouse *Fgfr3* gene. *Genomics* **41**:10, 1997.

245. Twigg SRF, Burns HD, Oldridge M, Heath JK, Wilkie AOM: Conserved use of a non-canonical 5′ splice site (/GA) in alternative splicing by fibroblast growth factor receptors 1, 2 and 3. *Hum Mol Genet* **7**:685, 1998.

246. Wüchner C, Hilbert K, Zabel B, Winterpacht A: Human fibroblast growth factor receptor 3 gene (FGFR3): Genomic sequence and primer set information for gene analysis. *Hum Genet* **100**:215, 1997.

247. Kostrzewa M, Müller U: Genomic structure and complete sequence of the human FGFR4 gene. *Mamm Genome* **9**:131, 1998.

247a. Zhang Y, Gorry MC, Post JC, Ehrlich GD: Genomic organization of the human fibroblast growth factor receptor 2 (*FGFR2*) gene and comparative analysis of the human *FGFR* gene family. *Gene* **230**:69, 1999.

248. Johnson DE, Williams LT: Structural and functional diversity in the FGF receptor multigene family. *Adv Cancer Res* **60**:1, 1993.

249. Chellaiah AT, McEwen DG, Werner S, Xu J, Ornitz DM: Fibroblast growth factor receptor (FGFR) 3. Alternative splicing in immunoglobin-like domain III creates a receptor highly specific for acidic FGF/FGF-1. *J Biol Chem* **269**:11620, 1994.

250. Ornitz DM, Xu J, Colvin JS, McEwen DG, MacArthur CA, Coulier F, Gao G, et al: Receptor specificity of the fibroblast growth factor family. *J Biol Chem* **271**:15292, 1996.

251. Xu X, Weinstein M, Li C, Naski M, Cohen RI, Ornitz DM, Leder P, et al: Fibroblast growth factor receptor 2 (FGFR2)-mediated reciprocal regulation loop between FGF8 and FGF10 is essential for limb induction. *Development* **125**:753, 1998.

252. Peters KG, Werner S, Chen G, Williams LT: Two FGF receptor genes are differentially expressed in epithelial and mesenchymal tissues during limb formation and organogenesis in the mouse. *Development* **114**:233, 1992.

253. Orr-Urtreger A, Bedford MT, Burakova T, Arman E, Zimmer Y, Yayon A, Givol D, et al: Developmental localization of the splicing alternatives of fibroblast growth factor receptor-2 (FGFR2). *Dev Biol* **158**:475, 1993.

254. Orr-Urtreger A, Givol D, Yayon A, Yarden Y, Lonai P: Developmental expression of two murine fibroblast growth factor receptors, *flg* and *bek*. *Development* **113**:1419, 1991.

255. Wüchner C, Nordqvist ACS, Winterpacht A, Zabel B, Schalling M: Developmental expression of splicing variants of fibroblast growth factor receptor 3 (FGFR3) in mouse. *Int J Dev Biol* **40**:1185, 1996.

256. Delezoide AL, Benoist-Lasselin C, Legeai-Mallet L, Le Merrer M, Munnich A, Vekemans M, Bonaventure J: Spatio-temporal expression

of FGFR 1, 2 and 3 genes during human embryo-fetal ossification. *Mech Dev* **77**:19, 1998.

257. Shi E, Kan M, Xu J, Wang F, Hou J, McKeehan WL: Control of fibroblast growth factor receptor kinase signal transduction by heterodimerization of combinatorial splice variants. *Mol Cell Biol* **13**:3907, 1993.

258. Goldfarb M: Functions of fibroblast growth factors in vertebrate development. *Cytokine Growth Factor Rev* **7**:311, 1996.

259. Yamaguchi TP, Harpal K, Henkemeyer M, Rossant J: *fgfr-1* is required for embryonic growth and mesodermal patterning during mouse gastrulation. *Genes Dev* **8**:3032, 1994.

260. Deng CX, Wynshaw-Boris A, Shen MM, Daugherty C, Ornitz DM, Leder P: Murine FGFR-1 is required for early postimplantation growth and axial organization. *Genes Dev* **8**:3045, 1994.

261. Arman E, Haffner-Krausz R, Chen Y, Heath JK, Lonai P: Targeted disruption of fibroblast growth factor (FGF) receptor 2 suggests a role for FGF signaling in pregastrulation mammalian development. *Proc Natl Acad Sci U S A* **95**:5082, 1998.

262. Ciruna BG, Schwartz L, Harpal K, Yamaguchi TP, Rossant J: Chimeric analysis of fibroblast growth factor receptor-1 (Fgfr1) function: a role for FGFR1 in morphogenetic movement through the primitive streak. *Development* **124**:2829, 1997.

263. Deng C, Bedford M, Li C, Xu X, Yang X, Dunmore J, Leder P: Fibroblast growth factor receptor-1 (FGFR-1) is essential for normal neural tube and limb development. *Dev Biol* **185**:42, 1997.

264. Partanen J, Schwartz L, Rossant J: Opposite phenotypes of hypomorphic and Y766 phosphorylation site mutations reveal a function for Fgfr1 in anteroposterior patterning of mouse embryos. *Genes Dev* **12**:2332, 1998.

265. Deng C, Wynshaw-Boris A, Zhou F, Kuo A, Leder P: Fibroblast growth factor receptor 3 is a negative regulator of bone growth. *Cell* **84**: 911, 1996.

266. Colvin JS, Bohne BA, Harding GW, McEwen DG, Ornitz DM: Skeletal overgrowth and deafness in mice lacking fibroblast growth factor receptor 3. *Nat Genet* **12**:390, 1996.

266a. Weinstein M, Xu X, Ohyama K, Deng C-X: FGFR-3 and FGFR-4 function cooperatively to direct alveogenesis in the murine lung. *Development* **125**:3615, 1998.

267. Li X, Lewanda AF, Eluma F, Jerald H, Choi H, Alzoie I, Proukakis C, et al: Two craniosynostotic syndrome loci, Crouzon and Jackson-Weiss, map to chromosome 10q23-q26. *Genomics* **22**:418, 1994.

268. Webster MK, Donoghue DJ: FGFR activation in skeletal disorders: too much of a good thing. *Trends Genet* **13**:178, 1997.

269. Gaudenz K, Roessler E, Vainikka S, Alitalo K, Muenke M: Analysis of patients with various craniosynostosis syndromes for Pro246Arg mutation in FGFR4. *Mol Genet Metab* **64**:76, 1998.

270. Li X, Park WJ, Pyeritz RE, Jabs EW: Effect of splicing of a silent FGFR2 mutation in Crouzon syndrome. *Nat Genet* **9**:232, 1995.

271. Del Gatto F, Breathnach R: A Crouzon syndrome synonymous mutation activates a 5′ splice site within the IIIC exon of the FGFR2 gene. *Genomics* **27**:558, 1995.

272. Galvin BD, Hart KC, Meyer AN, Webster MK, Donoghue DJ: Constitutive receptor activation by Crouzon syndrome mutations in fibroblast growth factor receptor (FGFR)2 and FGFR2/Neu chimeras. *Proc Natl Acad Sci U S A* **93**:7894, 1996.

273. Chun K, Siegel-Bartelt J, Chitayat D, Phillips J, Ray PN: FGFR2 mutation associated with clinical manifestations consistent with Antley-Bixler syndrome. *Am J Med Genet* **77**:219, 1998.

274. Park WJ, Theda C, Maestri NE, Meyers GA, Fryburg JS, Dufresne C, Cohen MM Jr, et al: Analysis of phenotypic features and FGFR2 mutations in Apert syndrome. *Am J Hum Genet* **57**:321, 1995.

275. Winter RM, Reardon W: Lumpers, splitters, and FGFRs. *Am J Med Genet* **63**:501, 1996.

276. Cohen MM Jr: A matter of reading English. *Am J Med Genet* **63**:503, 1996.

277. Tartaglia M, Di Rocco C, Lajeunie E, Valeri S, Velardi F, Battaglia PA: Jackson-Weiss syndrome: Identification of two novel FGFR2 missense mutations shared with Crouzon and Pfeiffer craniosynostotic disorders. *Hum Genet* **101**:47, 1997.

278. Steinberger D, Reinhartz T, Unsöld R, Müller U: FGFR2 mutation in clinically nonclassifiable autosomal dominant craniosynostosis with pronounced phenotypic variation. *Am J Med Genet* **66**:81, 1996.

279. Munro CS, Wilkie AOM: Epidermal mosaicism producing localised acne: Somatic mutation in *FGFR2*. *Lancet* **352**:704, 1998.

280. Hattori Y, Odagiri H, Nakatani H, Miyagawa K, Naito K, Sakamoto H, Katoh O, et al: K-*sam*, an amplified gene in stomach cancer, is a member of the heparin-binding growth factor receptor genes. *Proc Natl Acad Sci U S A* **87**:5983, 1990.

281. Lorenzi MV, Horii Y, Yamanaka R, Sakaguchi K, Miki T: *FRAG1*, a gene that potently activates fibroblast growth factor receptor by C-terminal fusion through chromosomal rearrangement. *Proc Natl Acad Sci U S A* **93**:8956, 1996.

282. Xiao S, Nalabolu SR, Aster JC, Ma J, Abruzzo L, Jaffe ES, Stone R, et al: *FGFR1* is fused with a novel zinc-finger gene, *ZNF198*, in the t(8;13) leukaemia/lymphoma syndrome. *Nat Genet* **18**:84, 1998.

283. Smedley D, Hamoudi R, Clark J, Warren W, Abdul-Rauf M, Somers G, Venter D, et al: The t(8;13)(p11;q11-12) rearrangement associated with an atypical myeloproliferative disorder fuses the fibroblast growth factor receptor 1 gene to a novel gene *RAMP*. *Hum Mol Genet* **7**:637, 1998.

284. Popovici C, Adélaïde J, Ollendorff V, Chaffanet M, Guasch G, Jacrot M, Leroux D, et al: Fibroblast growth factor receptor 1 is fused to FIM in stem-cell myeloproliferative disorder with t(8;13)(p12;q12). *Proc Natl Acad Sci U S A* **95**:5712, 1998.

285. Chesi M, Nardini E, Brents LA, Schröck E, Ried T, Kuehl WM, Bergsagel PL: Frequent translocation t(4;14)(p16.3;q32.3) in multiple myeloma is associated with increased expression and activating mutations of fibroblast growth factor receptor 3. *Nat Genet* **16**:260, 1997.

286. Richelda R, Ronchetti D, Baldini L, Cro L, Viggiano L, Marzella R, Rocchi M, et al: A novel chromosomal translocation t(4;14) (p16.3;q32) in multiple myeloma involves the fibroblast growth-factor receptor 3 gene. *Blood* **90**:4062, 1997.

286a. Cappellen D, De Oliveira C, Ricol D, Gil Diez de Medina S, Bourdin J, Sastre-Garau X, Chopin D, et al: Frequent activating mutations of FGFR3 in human bladder and cervix carcinomas. *Nat Genet* **23**:18, 1999.

287. Anderson J, Burns HD, Enriquez-Harris P, Wilkie AOM, Heath JK: Apert syndrome mutations in fibroblast growth factor receptor 2 exhibit increased affinity for FGF ligand. *Hum Mol Genet* **7**:1475, 1998.

288. Neilson KM, Friesel R: Ligand-independent activation of fibroblast growth factor receptors by point mutations in the extracellular, transmembrane, and kinase domains. *J Biol Chem* **271**:25049, 1996.

289. Neilson KM, Friesel RE: Constitutive activation of fibroblast growth factor receptor-2 by a point mutation associated with Crouzon syndrome. *J Biol Chem* **270**:26037, 1995.

290. Mangasarian K, Li Y, Mansukhani A, Basilico C: Mutation associated with Crouzon syndrome causes ligand-independent dimerization and activation of FGF receptor-2. *J Cell Physiol* **172**:117, 1997.

291. Robertson SC, Meyer AN, Hart KC, Galvin BD, Webster MK, Donoghue DJ: Activating mutations in the extracellular domain of the fibroblast growth factor receptor 2 function by disruption of the disulfide bond in the third immunoglobulin-like domain. *Proc Natl Acad Sci U S A* **95**:4567, 1998.

292. Li Y, Mangasarian K, Mansukhani A, Basilico C: Activation of FGF receptors by mutations in the transmembrane domain. *Oncogene* **14**:1397, 1997.

293. Brueton LA, van Herwerden L, Chotai KA, Winter RM: The mapping of a gene for craniosynostosis: Evidence for linkage of the Saethre-Chotzen syndrome to distal chromosome 7p. *J Med Genet* **29**:681, 1992.

294. Chotai KA, Brueton LA, van Herwerden L, Garrett C, Hinkel GK, Schinzel A, Mueller RF, et al: Six cases of 7p deletion: Clinical, cytogenetic and molecular studies. *Am J Med Genet* **51**:270, 1994.

295. Bourgeois P, Stoetzel C, Bolcato-Bellemin A-L, Mattéi M-G, Perrin-Schmitt F: The human *H-twist* gene is located at 7p21 and encodes a b-HLH protein which is 96% similar to its murine counterpart. *Mamm Genome* **7**:915, 1996.

296. Bourgeois P, Bolcato-Bellemin AL, Danse JM, Bloch-Zupan A, Yoshiba K, Stoetzel C, Perrin-Schmitt F: The variable expressivity and incomplete penetrance of the *twist*-null heterozygous mouse phenotype resemble those of human Saethre-Chotzen syndrome. *Hum Mol Genet* **7**:945, 1998.

297. Wolf C, Thisse C, Stoetzel C, Thisse B, Gerlinger P, Perrin-Schmitt F: The *M-twist* gene of *Mus* is expressed in subsets of mesodermal cells and is closely related to the *Xenopus X-twi* and the *Drosophila twist* genes. *Dev Biol* **143**:363, 1991.

298. Li L, Cserjesi P, Olson EN: Dermo-1: a novel twist-related b-HLH protein expressed in the developing dermis. *Dev Biol* **172**:280, 1995.

299. Wang SM, Coljee VW, Pignolo RJ, Rotenberg MO, Cristofalo VJ, Sierra F: Cloning of the human *twist* gene: Its expression is retained in adult mesodermally-derived tissues. *Gene* **187**:83, 1997.

300. Massari ME, Murre C: Helix-loop-helix proteins: Regulators of transcription in eucaryotic organisms. *Mol Cell Biol* **20:**429, 2000.

301. Rose CSP, Malcolm S: A TWIST in development. *Trends Genet* **13:**384, 1997.

302. Lewanda AF, Green ED, Weissenbach J, Jerald H, Taylor E, Summar ML, Phillips JA 3rd, et al: Evidence that the Saethre-Chotzen syndrome locus lies between D7S664 and D7S507, by genetic analysis and detection of a microdeletion in a patient. *Am J Hum Genet* **55:**1195, 1994.

303. Krebs I, Weis I, Hudler M, Rommens JM, Roth H, Scherer SW, Tsui LC, et al: Translocation breakpoint maps to 5 kb 3' from *TWIST* in a patient affected with Saethre-Chotzen syndrome. *Hum Mol Genet* **6:**1079, 1997.

304. Patel P, Reardon W, Malcolm S, Winter RM: Translocation breakpoints mapped approximately 70–250 Kb from the TWIST gene in three patients with Saethre-Chotzen syndrome. *J Med Genet* **35(Supp):** S78, 1998.

305. Bedell MA, Jenkins NA, Copeland NG: Good genes in bad neighbourhoods. *Nat Genet* **12:**229, 1996.

306. Baylies MK, Bate M: *twist*: A myogenic switch in *Drosophila*. *Science* **272:**1481, 1996.

307. Gitelman I: Twist protein in mouse embryogenesis. *Dev Biol* **189:**205, 1997.

308. Chen ZF, Behringer RR: *twist* is required in head mesenchyme for cranial neural tube morphogenesis. *Genes Dev* **9:**686, 1995.

309. Shishido E, Higashijima S, Emori Y, Saigo K: Two FGF-receptor homologues of *Drosophila*: One is expressed in mesodermal primordium in early embryos. *Development* **117:**751, 1993.

310. Lord PCW, Lin M-H, Hales KH, Storti RV: Normal expression and the effects of ectopic expression of the *Drosophila muscle segment homeobox (msh)* gene suggest a role in differentiation and patterning of embryonic muscles. *Dev Biol* **171:**627, 1995.

311. D'Alessio M, Frasch M: *msh* may play a conserved role in dorsoventral patterning of the neuroectoderm and mesoderm. *Mech Dev* **58:**217, 1996.

312. Kim H-J, Rice DPC, Kettunen PJ, Thesleff I: FGF-, BMP- and Shh-mediated signalling pathways in the regulation of cranial suture morphogenesis and calvarial bone development. *Development* **125:**1241, 1998.

313. Liu YH, Kundu R, Wu L, Luo W, Ignelzi MA Jr, Snead ML, Maxson RE Jr: Premature suture closure and ectopic cranial bone in mice expressing Msx2 transgenes in the developing skull. *Proc Natl Acad Sci U S A* **92:**6137, 1995.

314. Ma L, Golden S, Wu L, Maxson R: The molecular basis of Boston-type craniosynostosis: The Pro148-His mutation in the N-terminal arm of the *MSX2* homeodomain stabilizes DNA binding without altering nucleotide sequence preferences. *Hum Mol Genet* **5:**1915, 1996.

315. Winograd J, Reilly MP, Roe R, Lutz J, Laughner E, Xu X, Hu L, et al: Perinatal lethality and multiple craniofacial malformations in *MSX2* transgenic mice. *Hum Mol Genet* **6:**369, 1997.

316. Liu YH, Tang Z, Kundu RK, Wu L, Luo W, Zhu D, Sangiorgi F, et al: *Msx2* gene dosage influences the number of proliferative osteogenic cells in growth centers of the developing murine skull: A possible mechanism for *MSX2*-mediated craniosynostosis. *Dev Biol* **205:**260, 1999.

317. Opperman LA, Sweeney TM, Redmon J, Persing JA, Ogle RC: Tissue interactions with underlying dura inhibit osseous obliteration of developing cranial sutures. *Dev Dynam* **198:**312, 1993.

318. Levine JP, Bradley JP, Roth DA, McCarthy JG, Longaker MT: Studies in cranial suture biology: Regional dura mater determines overlying suture biology. *Plastic Reconstr Surg* **101:**1441, 1998.

319. Opperman LA, Passarelli RW, Nolen AA, Gampper TJ, Lin KYK, Ogle RC: Dura mater secretes soluble heparin-binding factors required for cranial suture morphogenesis. *In Vitro Cell Dev Biol* **32:**627, 1996.

319a. Opperman LA, Chhabra A, Cho RW, Ogle RC: Cranial obliteration is induced by removal of transforming growth factor (TGH)-$\beta$3 activity and prevented by removal of TGF-$\beta$2 activity from fetal rat calvaria in vitro. *J Craniofac Genet Dev Biol* **19:**164, 1999.

320. Iseki S, Wilkie AOM, Heath JK, Ishimaru T, Eto K, Morriss-Kay GM: *Fgfr2* and *osteopontin* domains in the developing skull vault are mutually exclusive and can be altered by locally applied FGF2. *Development* **124:**3375, 1997.

321. Most D, Levine JP, Chang J, Sung J, McCarthy JG, Schendel SA, Longaker MT: Studies in cranial suture biology: Up-regulation of transforming growth factor-$\beta$1 and basic fibroblast growth factor mRNA correlates with posterior frontal cranial suture fusion in the rat. *Plastic Reconstr Surg* **101:**1431, 1998.

321a. Iseki S, Wilkie AOM, Morriss-Kay GM: *Fgfr1* and *Fgfr2* have distinct differentiation- and proliferation-related roles in the developing mouse skull vault. *Development* **126:**5611, 1999.

322. Carlton MBL, Colledge WH, Evans MJ: Crouzon-like craniofacial dysmorphology in the mouse is caused by an insertional mutation at the *Fgf3/Fgf4* locus. *Dev Dynam* **21:**242, 1998.

323. Lomri A, Lemonnier J, Hott M, de Parseval N, Lajeunie E, Munnich A, Renier D, et al: Increased calvaria cell differentiation and bone matrix formation induced by fibroblast growth factor receptor 2 mutations in Apert syndrome. *J Clin* **101:**1310, 1998.

323a. Fragale A, Tartaglia M, Bernardini S, Di Stasi AMM, Di Rocco C, Velardi F, Teti A, et al: Decreased proliferation and altered differentiation in osteoblasts from genetically and clinically distinct craniosynostotic disorders. *Am J Pathol* **154:**1465, 1999.

323b. Locci P, Baroni T, Pezzetti F, Lilli C, Marinucci L, Martinese D, Becchetti E, et al: Differential in vitro phenotype pattern, transforming growth factor-b$_1$ activity and mRNA expression of transforming growth factor-b$_1$ in Apert osteoblasts. *Cell Tissue Res* **297:**475, 1999.

324. Bresnick S, Schendel S: Crouzon's disease correlates with low fibroblastic growth factor receptor activity in stenosed cranial sutures. *J Craniofac Surg* **6:**245, 1995.

325. Bresnick S, Schendel S: Apert's syndrome correlates with low fibroblast growth factor receptor activity in stenosed cranial sutures. *J Craniofac Surg* **9:**92, 1998.

326. Yayon A, Klagsbrun M: Autocrine transformation by chimeric signal peptide-basic fibroblast growth factor: Reversal of suramin. *Proc Natl Acad Sci U S A* **87:**5346, 1990.

327. Moscatelli D: Autocrine downregulation of fibroblast growth factor receptors in F9 teratocarcinoma cells. *J Cell Physiol* **160:**555, 1994.

328. Yamada K, Tabata Y, Yamamoto K, Miyamoto S, Nagata I, Kikuchi H, Ikada Y: Potential efficacy of basic fibroblast growth factor incorporated in biodegradable hydrogels for skull bone regeneration. *J Neurosurg* **86:**871, 1997.

328a. Johnson D, Iseki S, Wilkie AOM, Morriss-Kay GM: Expression patterns of Twist and FGFR1, -2 and -3 in the developing mouse coronal suggest a key role for Twist in suture initiation and biogenesis. *Mech. Dev* **91:**341, 2000.

329. Caiulo A, Bardoni B, Camerino G, Guioli S, Minelli A, Piantanida M, Crosato F, et al: Cytogenetic and molecular analysis of an unbalanced translocation (X;7)(q28;p15) in a dysmorphic girl. *Hum Genet* **84:**51, 1989.

330. Stankiewicz P, Baldermann C, Thiele E, et al: The TWIST gene is triplicated in trisomy 7p syndrome. *Eur J Hum Genet* **6:**61, 1998.

# Treacher Collins Syndrome

*Karen L. Marsh* ∎ *Michael J. Dixon*

1. Treacher Collins syndrome (TCS) (OMIM 154500) is a disorder of craniofacial development that is inherited in an autosomal dominant fashion and occurs with an incidence of approximately 1 in 50,000 live births. Forty percent of patients have a previous family history, whereas in 60 percent of patients the syndrome is thought to arise as a result of a *de novo* mutation.
2. TCS is characterized by abnormalities of the external ears, conductive hearing loss, lateral downward sloping of the palpebral fissures, cleft palate, and hypoplasia of the mandible and zygomatic complex. These features often are bilaterally symmetrical in nature. A marked variation in phenotype is observed both within and between families.
3. In the absence of a candidate gene or appropriate mouse model for the disorder, the mutated gene causing TCS (*TCOF1*) was isolated by positional cloning strategies. So far, approximately 70, mainly family-specific, mutations have been identified within the gene, which maps to chromosome 5q32-q33.1. The majority of these mutations introduce a premature termination codon.
4. Since database sequence comparisons failed to reveal any strong homology, little was known about the precise function of the protein, treacle, encoded by *TCOF1*. Recent work on the expression of treacle suggests that it is a member of a family of nucleolar phosphoproteins and, as such, may be involved in shuttling proteins between the nucleus and the cytoplasm.

## CLINICAL FEATURES

Treacher Collins syndrome (TCS) (OMIM 154500) is named after the ophthalmologist E. Treacher Collins, who first described the essential components of the syndrome in 1900.[1] The first extensive description of the condition was produced by Franceschetti and Klein, who used the term *mandibulofacial dysostosis* to describe the facial appearance.[2] TCS is the most common mandibulofacial dysostosis disorder, affecting approximately 1 in 50,000 live births, and is inherited in an autosomal dominant manner. Although the disease is thought to be highly penetrant, there is marked variation in phenotype, ranging from perinatal death due to a compromised airway to features that are so mild that it is difficult to make an unequivocal diagnosis on clinical grounds alone. The main criteria used in the diagnosis of TCS include bilaterally symmetrical midface hypoplasia (89 percent), downward slanting of the palpebral fissures (89 percent), colobomas (notching) of the lower eyelids with sparse eyelashes (69 percent), cleft palate (28 percent), micrognathia (underdevelopment of the lower jaw, 78 percent), microtia (underdevelopment or absence of pinna, 77 percent), and other deformities of the external ears, which often lead to conductive hearing loss (50 percent).[3] The typical facial appearance is depicted in Fig. 246-1.

---

A list of standard abbreviations is located immediately preceding the index in each volume. Nonstandard abbreviations used in this chapter include: TCS = Treacher Collins syndrome; STRPs = short tandem repeat polymorphisms; UTR = untranslated region.

## DIAGNOSIS AND TREATMENT

In patients with complete expression of the syndrome, TCS can be diagnosed easily on the basis of the clinical appearance, as described earlier. However, if individuals are only mildly affected, diagnosis can be difficult, and additional information may be obtained from radiologic examination.[4] Prior to identification of the gene causing TCS, the main source of information on whether or not an unborn child was affected came from prenatal ultrasonography and fetoscopy. Ultrasonography is carried out by an experienced radiologist who can visualize the face and determine whether any features of TCS are present.[5-7] It is not always possible to assess the true severity of the disorder at this stage. Thus failure to recognize any abnormalities cannot be used as proof that the fetus is unaffected. The technique of fetoscopy[8] has evolved with miniaturization of the optical device by using fiberoptics technology. The procedure enables examination of the fetus after 11 weeks of gestation and is performed transabdominally in the amniotic fluid.[9] However, there is an associated risk of fetal mortality (approximately 2 percent), which is acceptable for the majority of patients with a high recurrence risk.[10]

Most children with TCS require corrective surgery at some point during their growing years. These operations often continue into early adulthood, when facial skeletal growth is completed. The surgical procedures for TCS fall into two major categories: those involving the upper face (ears, eyes, and cheeks) and those involving the lower face (upper/lower jaws and chin). Often the first surgical procedure is to close clefts of the eyelids during infancy, by transposition and advancement of a superior palpebral flap.[11] For those individuals with malformed ears, bone-anchored hearing aids and artificial pinnae are preferable to surgical reconstruction.[12] Elongation of the jaw also can begin at an early age. Bone grafts often are required during facial surgery, although the relatively new technique of bone distraction has been employed to lengthen the jaw in the treatment of some patients with obstructive sleep apnea.[13] This involves making a surgical cut across the child's mandible, slowly drawing apart the two pieces of bone, and filling the intervening gap with new bone. However, only certain children are suitable candidates for this procedure, which, as yet, has not been subject to any long-term studies.

## EMBRYOLOGY

The tissues affected in TCS arise during early embryonic development from the first and second branchial/pharyngeal arches. Mesenchyme involved in formation of the head region is derived from paraxial and lateral plate mesoderm, neural crest, and ectodermal placodes. Neural crest cells originate in the dorsal and lateral neural tube and migrate ventrally into the branchial arches and rostrally around the forebrain and optic cup into the facial region, where they differentiate into a range of tissues appropriate to that locality. Cells from ectodermal placodes, along with those from the neural crest, form neurons of the fifth, seventh, ninth, and tenth cranial sensory ganglia.

There is some evidence, from work on animal models assessing the effects of retinoids on development, to support the theory that neural crest cells are involved in the pathogenesis of facial abnormalities. Treatment of mice and rats with large doses of vitamin A

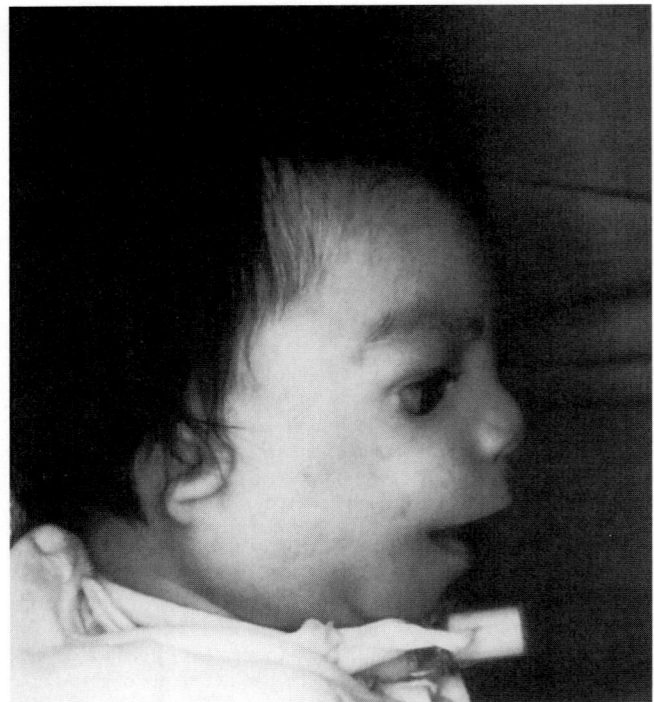

A

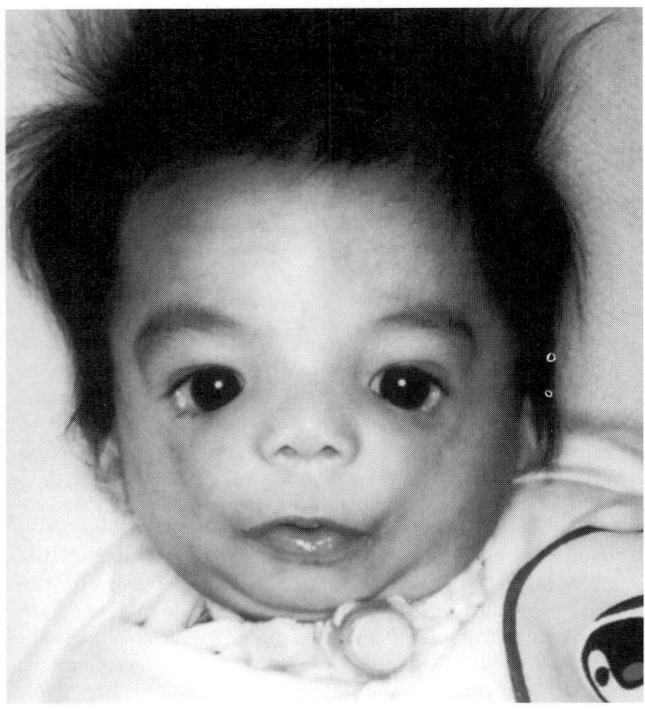

B

**Fig. 246-1 Clinical features of a child with TCS. (*A*) Lateral view to show hypoplasia of mandible and zygomatic complex and severe anomalies of the external ear. (*B*) Frontal view to show down-** slanting palpebral fissures, colobomas of the lower eyelids, and a paucity of lid lashes. The features show bilateral symmetry.

resulted in a range of features similar to those of TCS.[14,15] On this basis, it has been proposed that TCS may result from abnormal neural crest cell migration, anomalies in the extracellular matrix,[16] or improper cellular differentiation during development. Although a study by Wiley et al.[17] (1983), involving exposure of hamster embryos to *trans*-retinoic acid, also seemed to lend support to the involvement of neural crest cells, reevaluation of these results, together with more recent work, has suggested that both cells derived from the neural crest and from the ectodermal placodes are involved in the development of mandibulofacial dysostosis.[18]

## MAPPING OF THE TCS LOCUS AND ISOLATION OF THE *TCOF1* GENE

In the absence of a candidate gene or an animal model for the disorder, positional cloning strategies were used to isolate the gene mutated in TCS. The TCS locus (*TCOF1*) was mapped initially to human chromosome 5q31-q34 using restriction fragment length polymorphisms (RFLPs).[19] Due to the low informativeness of the majority of such RFLPs and the relative shortage of large families, subsequent linkage studies used the highly informative short tandem repeat polymorphisms (STRPs).[20,21] This permitted refinement of the localization to 5q32-q33.1 and establishment of markers closely flanking the disease locus.[22] To define more accurately the genetic distance between these markers and to extend a high-resolution genetic map of 5q31-q33 to include additional markers, 15 loci were mapped through the Centre d'Etude du Polymorphisme Humain reference pedigrees.[23] The resulting genetic map encompassed 29 cM on the sex-averaged map.[24] To integrate the genetic map with a physical map of the region, 13 loci from 5q31-q33, including six genes, were used to construct a radiation hybrid (RH) map. Since eight of the loci were common to both maps, this permitted their combination. Since the markers on the combined genetic linkage and RH map were formatted for the polymerase chain reaction (PCR), they facilitated the creation of yeast artificial chromosome (YAC) and cosmid contigs across the *TCOF1* critical region.[25,26] Closure of the YAC

contig confirmed the order of loci surrounding *TCOF1* as cen-*RPS14-DS519-ANX6-SPARC*-tel. A rare-cutter restriction map was constructed of those YACs covering the critical region. This map confirmed the overlaps predicted from the STS content of the various clones and resulted in identification of a large number of potential HTF islands within the critical region. The highest densities of rare-cutter restriction sites were found to be in the 150-kb interval immediately adjacent to the proximal flanking marker and in the 150-kb interval distal to *ANX6*.[26] Isolation of an STRP from a cosmid containing the 3′ untranslated region (UTR) of the *ANX6* locus,[27] and its use in genotyping recombinant individuals, excluded this locus from a causative role in the pathogenesis of TCS and permitted reduction of the candidate region to 450 kb between *RSP14* and *ANX6*.[28] Seventeen cosmids isolated from this region subsequently were grouped into three separate contigs, which spanned approximately 390 kb.

In order to isolate genes that could be screened for TCS-specific mutations, a combination of exon amplification and cDNA library screening was used to create a transcript map of the candidate region.[28] A total of 120 exon clones were isolated and found to represent 47 unique, single-copy sequences. Four exons were found to correspond to portions of the heparan sulfate *N*-deacetylase/*N*-sulfotransferase gene (*HSST*).[29,30] This enzyme catalyzes both the *N*-deacetylation and *N*-sulfation of glucosamine residues in heparan sulfate (HS).[31] As a result of expression studies in which an antibody to the *N*-sulfate domain of HS stained the outline of neural crest cells, specific regions of the brain, and mesenchymal tissues of the head and limbs,[32] *HSST* was considered to be a candidate for *TCOF1*. Nevertheless, screening of the 14 exons of *HSST* failed to reveal a single disease-specific mutation in any of the 33 TCS families tested.[30] However, identification of a dinucleotide repeat polymorphism in the 3′ UTR of *HSST*, and its subsequent use in segregation analysis, resulted in identification of overlapping recombination events in two, unrelated affected individuals. Since only the distal recombination event occurred in a large family that was linked independently to chromosome 5q31.3-q32, the cosmid contig was extended

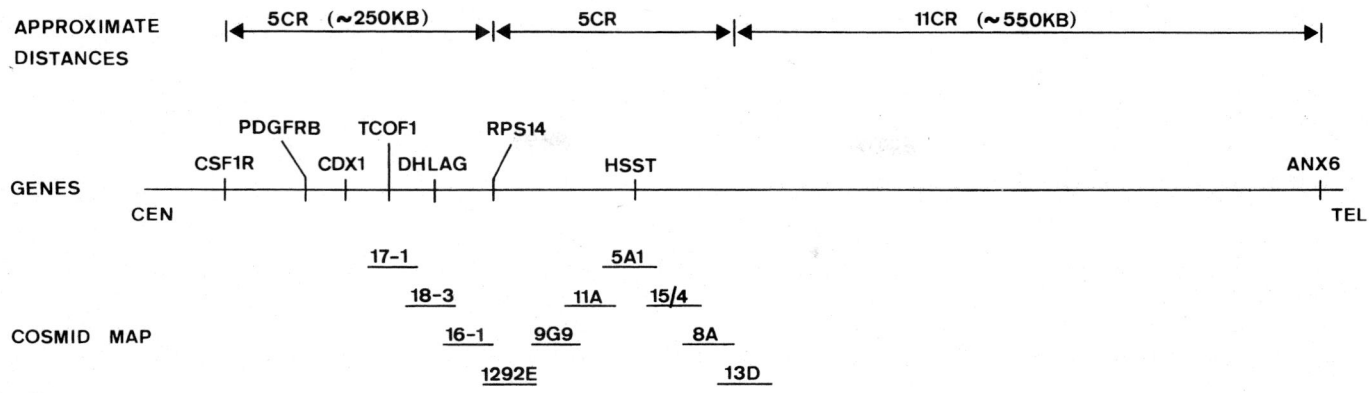

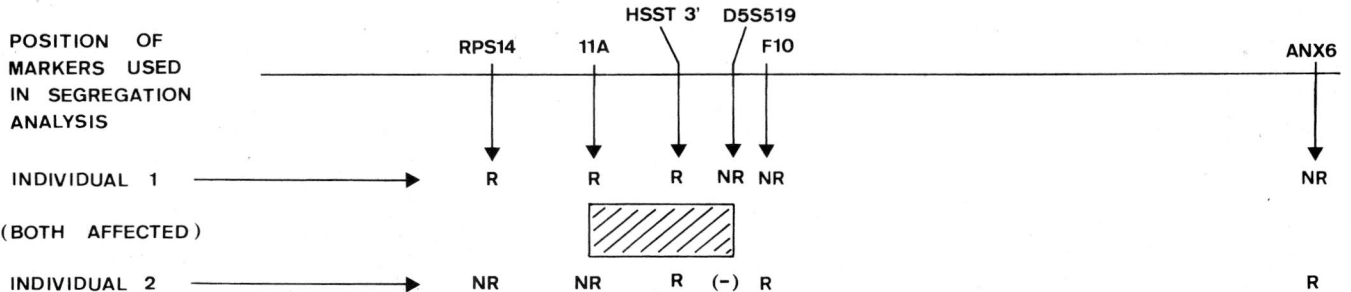

**Fig. 246-2** Schematic diagram of the region surrounding *TCOF1* to show the relative positions of the genes in the region and the positions of the STRP markers used in fine genetic mapping. The maximum area of overlapping recombination is shaded. NR, nonrecombinant; R, recombinant; (−), uninformative meiosis.

proximally to include the region defined by a recombination event at *CSF1R* that had been identified in a second large family that showed evidence of linkage to 5q.[25] As part of the attempts to extend the transcript map proximally, a previously unidentified gene, which maps proximal to *RPS14*, was isolated[33] (Fig. 246-2). Evidence that the gene for TCS indeed had been cloned positionally came from screening of this gene for mutations. Five unrelated affected individuals were found to possess mutations, all of which were predicted to cause frameshifts resulting in the creation of a premature termination codon. This gene, *TCOF1*, contains an open reading frame of 4233 bp encompassed by 26 exons, which encodes a low-complexity 144-kDa protein named *treacle*. Northern analysis indicated that *TCOF1* is expressed in a variety of fetal and adult tissues. Therefore, it is likely that the gene plays a different role during early embryogenesis from any role it may have subsequently in tissue homeostasis.

Further mutational analysis of individuals affected with TCS has revealed over 70 mainly family-specific mutations occurring along the length of the gene sequence. A majority of these mutations, in common with those identified originally, lead to the introduction of a premature termination codon. These would likely result in a reduction in mRNA levels from the mutant sequence due to nonsense-mediated mRNA degradation.[34] Several mutations, including nt4135 del(GAAAA), a 5-bp deletion toward the 3′ end of *TCOF1*, have been found in a number of unrelated families, with significant variation both within and between families. In line with these observations, it is thought that TCS is caused by haploinsufficiency.

## IMPLICATIONS FOR DIAGNOSIS

Identification of the gene involved in TCS has important implications for prenatal diagnosis. Chorionic villus samples can be analyzed at around the twelfth week of pregnancy, much earlier than any information can be gained from ultrasound imaging (≈18

weeks). Previously, diagnostic predictions could be made on the basis of linked STRPs in families showing significant evidence of linkage to 5q31.3-q32.[35] More recently, in light of identification of *TCOF1*, these predictions are now more reliable, since the presence or absence of a particular mutation can be assessed. Genetic counseling of families with TCS is complicated by allelic heterogeneity. Hence the specific mutation must be identified first within a family before any counseling or prenatal diagnosis can be carried out. Since this may require all exons to be studied, it can be a time-consuming process. In addition, even if the fetus is found to carry the disease-causing mutation, no conclusions can be drawn about the severity with which the child will be affected. Therefore, parents may opt to delay any decision making until ultrasound can be used to provide further information on the extent of the abnormalities. However, for those cases in which the fetus does not carry the mutation, parents can be reassured that their child will be unaffected.

The isolation of *TCOF1* also makes possible postnatal diagnosis of individuals who are so mildly affected as to make clinical diagnosis difficult. This is also useful for counseling apparently unaffected parents of a child in whom TCS is thought to have arisen as a result of *de novo* mutation, since it has been observed that only 40 percent of TCS patients have a family history.[36] Older paternal age has been suggested as a factor in sporadic, fresh mutational cases of several autosomal dominant disorders, including achondroplasia and Apert syndrome.[37,38] In addition, an increased mean paternal age also was evident for TCS.[39] The precise reason for this is unknown, although it could be attributed to an increased chance of gene replication errors occurring in the male germ line with advancing age.

## IS TCS HETEROGENEOUS?

All large TCS families detailed in the literature have been shown to be linked to chromosome 5q, but most families are not sufficiently large to generate a significant lod score when analyzed independently. Therefore, the possibility of locus heterogeneity in TCS cannot be ruled out. In addition, there are some affected individuals who show linkage to chromosome 5q for whom a mutation in *TCOF1* has not been identified. This may be due to limitations of the methods of detection or because a second gene is involved.

## ISOLATION OF THE MURINE HOMOLOGUE, *Tcof1*

In order to study the spatiotemporal distribution of the gene during development, the murine homologue of *TCOF1*, *Tcof1*, has been isolated recently.[40] The gene maps to the central region of murine chromosome 18, a region with conservation of synteny with human chromosome 5q21-q33, and has 74.3 percent identity with the human sequence at the nucleotide level. At the amino acid level, the sequences display 61.5 percent identity and 71.7 percent similarity. Despite this relatively low level of conservation, supportive evidence that *Tcof1* is the true orthologue of *TCOF1* comes from the fact that *Tcof1* shows no recombination with the Ia-associated invariant chain gene (*Ii*).[40,41] The *Ii* gene is the murine orthologue of the human *DHLAG* gene, which is immediately distal to *TCOF1*.

Comparison of both murine and human sequences identified conserved motifs likely to be of functional significance. RT-PCR analysis indicated that *Tcof1* is expressed in a range of murine adult and embryonic tissues, which is consistent with those expression data generated by northern analysis of the human gene.[33] Whole-mount in situ hybridization experiments on mouse embryos revealed that *Tcof1* was expressed at different levels throughout all the embryonic ages examined. The earliest expression observed was in day 8 embryos, with most intense staining in the developing first branchial arch, which ultimately will give rise to the mandible and maxilla. Of particular interest is the region of increased expression on the crests of the neural folds, immediately rostral to their point of fusion. This may coincide with a signaling event associated with fusion of the neural folds or migration of neural crest cells in the unfused region. As development progresses, expression appears to be downregulated, returning to background levels by day 10. Analysis of *Tcof1* expression, as determined by northern blot hybridization of embryonic and adult tissues, indicated that levels are still elevated at day 11, gradually decreasing from day 15 to 17.[41] These results are consistent with a fundamental role for *Tcof1* in the development of the craniofacial complex, with peak expression occurring at a time when critical morphogenetic events are taking place, including the formation and fusion of the branchial arches with the rest of the developing face.

The mouse mutant shaker-with-syndactylism, *sy*, a recessive radiation-induced mutation, has been mapped to this broad region of the genome. Characteristics of this mutation include abnormalities of the inner ear resulting in deafness, syndactylism, and defects of ossification involving the whole skeleton.[42] Other than displaying deafness, which is caused by malformation of the inner ear rather than middle ear anomalies, the *sy* homozygous mutant phenotype bears little resemblance to that of TCS, so it is unlikely that *sy* represents a mutation in the *Tcof1* gene.[41] In addition, it is interesting to note that the first arch mouse mutant, *far*, can display either bilateral or unilateral features depending on the genetic background on which the same mutation is placed.[43] Despite the fact that this mutation is not in *Tcof1*, this type of effect is reminiscent of the variable phenotype observed between different TCS family members carrying the same mutation. There is, at present, lack of a suitable mouse model for TCS. It will be important to make such a model for mandibulofacial dysostosis to allow developmental and genetic studies that are not possible in humans.

## POSSIBLE FUNCTION OF THE PROTEIN TREACLE

Following identification of *TCOF1*, only limited information was obtained from database searches. Analysis using the BLAST programs[44] revealed that the encoded protein, treacle, shows weak similarity to a family of nucleolar phosphoproteins[45,46] that have been shown to shuttle between the nucleus and the cytoplasm.[47] This included *Xenopus laevis* nucleolar phosphoprotein ($p = 4.2e^9$)[48] and nucleolar phosphoprotein 140 ($p = 2.6e^8$).[47] Nevertheless, a series of repeated units, consisting of clusters of acidic amino acids separated by stretches of basic residues, was identified within both human and murine treacle. These units were found to be encoded by individual exons, and although their function is unclear, each cluster of acidic amino acids contains a number of potential sites for casein kinase II phosphorylation,[49] suggesting that phosphorylation is important for the correct function of the protein. The homology between the nucleolar phosphoproteins and human/murine treacle appears to be greatest at these motifs. Also in common with the nucleolar phosphoproteins, treacle is a low-complexity protein, with a major part being made up of the five amino acids serine, alanine, lysine, proline, and glutamic acid. An additional feature of the protein is a lysine-rich region, which encodes a number of potential nuclear localization signals (NLSs). These sequences are essential for the transport of proteins into the nucleus. Although no single consensus sequence has emerged, NLSs are usually short, up to 12 amino acids long, and they contain a high proportion of positively charged amino acids.[50] Within treacle, the potential NLSs, which are located toward the C-terminus, are of the consensus K-K/R-X-R/K.[51]

## LOCALIZATION OF TREACLE

Polyclonal antibodies raised against the N-terminus of the treacle protein were used in a series of immunocytochemical experiments to determine the subcellular localization of treacle.[52] The protein was found in the nucleolus, which further strengthened the assumption that treacle had some features in common with the nucleolar phosphoproteins. Additional confirmatory evidence was obtained by creating a fusion protein between treacle and green fluorescent protein, which also was found to localize to the nucleolus (Fig. 246-3*A, B*). Interestingly, fusion proteins lacking putative nuclear localization signals were shown to localize to nonnuclear compartments of the cell. Parallel studies using the murine *Tcof1* sequence confirmed these observations. In addition, site-directed mutagenesis was used to recreate mutations observed in individuals with TCS [Q36X, E93X, and nt405 del(TG)]. These mutations all resulted in a premature termination codon, which was expected to result in a truncated protein lacking the nuclear localization signals normally found at the C-terminus. These proteins also were mislocalized within the cell (see Fig. 246-3*C, D*), further supporting the hypothesis that, in common with the nucleolar phosphoproteins, an integral part of treacle's function involves shuttling between the nucleolus and the cytoplasm.

## POSSIBLE MECHANISM

The nucleolus is the site of ribosome biogenesis. Although rRNA transcription, rRNA processing, and ribosome assembly have been clearly established as major functions of the nucleolus,[53] recent work suggests that the nucleolus participates in many other aspects of gene expression as well, including processing of some mRNAs and tRNA precursors.[54] At present, the precise mechanism by which disruption of treacle leads to the pathogenesis of TCS is unknown. It is interesting to speculate on the possible mechanism by which haploinsufficiency of a widely expressed protein could cause the features restricted to the face. Perfect protein synthesis is a prerequisite in embryogenesis, where each cell has an absolute requirement for a sufficient supply of proteins and organelles. It is possible, therefore, that treacle is involved in ribosome assembly and functions at a critical, rate-limiting step during development, when high levels of translational activity are essential. Any reduction in the maximum synthesis rate of treacle would likely be deleterious, leading to the morphologic defects observed in TCS. This type of mechanism has been observed in *Drosophila Minute*

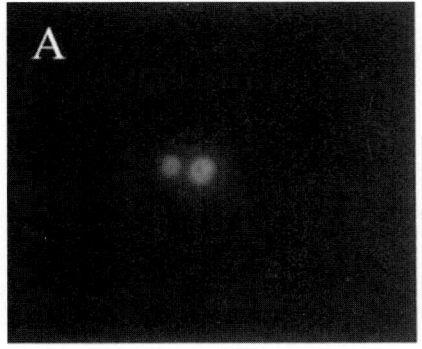
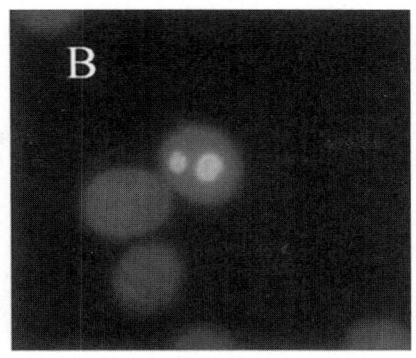
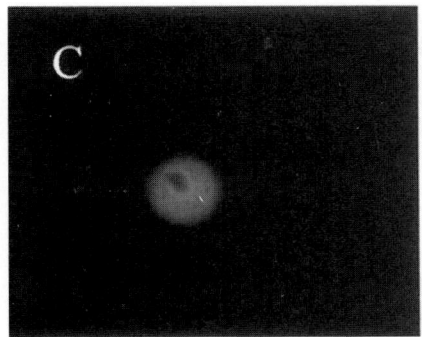
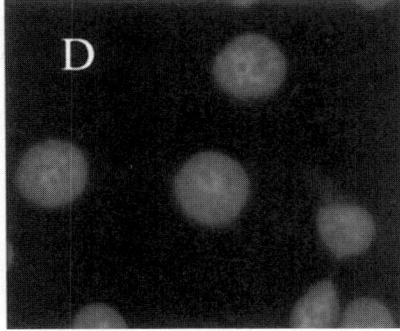

**Fig. 246-3 Localization of GFP-fusion proteins following electroporation and expression in COS-1 cells. (A) Full-length human treacle protein when tagged to GFP was visible in the nucleolus but rarely in the cytoplasm. (B) Dual staining with DAPI, to define the nuclei, confirms that treacle is localized to the nucleolus. In contrast, fusion proteins produced from constructs containing mutations are absent from the nucleolus (C, D).**

mutants, which can arise due to mutations resulting in haploinsufficiency of ribosomal proteins.[55] *Minute* strains are homozygous lethal, but heterozygotes display particular characteristics, including shortened antennae, short and sparse bristles, slow development, and female sterility, which are compatible with faulty protein synthesis.

Alternatively, treacle may interact with or shuttle proteins important for craniofacial embryogenesis. Such proteins also will be important in explaining the extremely variable phenotype that is observed between individuals even with the same mutation. Other reasons for a lack of genotype-phenotype correlations for TCS may include environmental influences or the effects of different genetic backgrounds.

TCS is the first Mendelian disorder caused by aberrant expression of a nucleolar protein. Further work is underway to determine the precise mechanisms underlying the pathogenesis of this disease.

## ADDENDUM

Recently, to investigate the developmental mechanism underlying TCS, the murine orthologue, *Tcof1*, has been inactivated by gene targeting. Heterozygous *Tcof1* mice die neonatally as a result of severe craniofacial anomalies that include agenesis of the nasal passages, abnormal development of the maxilla, acrania, exencephaly and anophthalmia. This phenotype was found to be caused by increased cell death in the neuroepithelium of the prefusion neural folds that results in a decrease in migratory neural crest cells.[56]

## REFERENCES

1. Treacher Collins E: Cases with symmetrical congenital notches in the outer part of each lid and defective development of the malar bones. *Trans Ophthalmol Soc UK* **20**:190, 1900.
2. Franceschetti A, Klein D: Mandibulo-facial dysostosis: New hereditary syndrome. *Acta Ophthalmol* **27**:143, 1949.
3. Marres HA, Cremers CW, Dixon MJ, Huygen PL, Joosten FB: The Treacher Collins syndrome: A clinical, radiological, and genetic linkage study on two pedigrees. *Arch Otolaryngol Head Neck Surg* **121**:509, 1995.
4. Dixon MJ, Haan E, Baker E, David D, McKenzie N, Williamson R, Mulley JC, et al: Association of Treacher Collins syndrome and translocation 6p21.31/16p13.11: Exclusion of the locus from these candidate regions. *Am J Hum Genet* **48**:274, 1991.
5. Meizner I, Carmi R, Katz M: Prenatal ultrasonic diagnosis of mandibulofacial dysostosis (Treacher Collins syndrome). *J Clin Ultrasound* **19**:124, 1991.
6. Milligan DA, Harlass FE, Duff P, Kopelman JN: Recurrence of Treacher Collins syndrome with sonographic findings. *Milit Med* **159**:250, 1994.
7. Cohen J, Ghezzi F, Goncalves L, Fuentes JD, Paulyson KJ, Sherer DM: Prenatal sonographic diagnosis of Treacher Collins syndrome: A case and review of the literature. *Am J Perinatol* **12**:416, 1995.
8. Nicolaides KH, Johansson D, Donnai D, Rodeck CH: Prenatal diagnosis of mandibulofacial dysostosis. *Prenat Diagn* **4**:201, 1984.
9. Ville Y, Khalil A, Homphray T, Moscoso G: Diagnostic embryoscopy and fetoscopy in the first trimester of pregnancy. *Prenat Diagn* **17**:1237, 1997.
10. Rodeck CH, Nicolaides KH: Fetoscopy and fetal tissue sampling. *Br Med Bull* **39**:332, 1983.
11. Roddi R, Vaandrager JM, van der Meulen JC: Treacher Collins syndrome: Early surgical treatment of orbitomalar malformations. *J Craniofac Surg* **6**:211, 1995.
12. Marres HA, Cremers CW, Marres EH: Treacher-Collins syndrome: Management of major and minor anomalies of the ear. *Rev Laryngol Otol Rhinol (Bord)* **116**:105, 1995.
13. Cohen SR, Simms C, Burstein FD: Mandibular distraction osteogenesis in the treatment of upper airway obstruction in children with craniofacial deformities. *Plast Reconstr Surg* **101**:312, 1998.
14. Kalter H: The teratogenic effects of hypervitaminosis A upon the face and mouth of inbred mice. *Ann NY Acad Sci* **85**:42, 1960.
15. Poswillo D: Otomandibular deformity: Pathogenesis as a guide to reconstruction. *J Maxillofac Surg* **2**:64, 1974.
16. Herring SW, Rowlatt UF, Pruzansky S: Anatomical abnormalities in mandibulofacial dysostosis. *Am J Med Genet* **3**:225, 1979.
17. Wiley MJ, Cauwenbergs P, Taylor IM: Effects of retinoic acid on the development of the facial skeleton in hamsters: Early changes involving cranial neural crest cells. *Acta Anat* **116**:180, 1983.

18. Sulik KK, Johnston MC, Smiley SJ, Speight HS, Jarvis BE: Mandibulofacial dysostosis (Treacher Collins syndrome): A new proposal for its pathogenesis. *Am J Med Genet* **27**:359, 1987.

19. Dixon MJ, Read AP, Donnai D, Colley A, Dixon J, Williamson R: The gene for Treacher Collins syndrome maps to the long arm of chromosome 5. *Am J Hum Genet* **49**:17, 1991.

20. Jabs EW, Li X, Coss CA, Taylor EW, Meyers DA, Weber JL: Mapping the Treacher Collins syndrome locus to 5q31.3-q33.3. *Genomics* **11**:193, 1991.

21. Dixon MJ, Dixon J, Raskova D, Le Beau MM, Williamson R, Klinger K, Landes GM: Genetic and physical mapping of the Treacher Collins syndrome locus: Refinement of the localisation to chromosome 5q32-q33.2. *Hum Mol Genet* **1**:249, 1992.

22. Dixon MJ, Dixon J, Houseal T, Bhatt M, Ward DC, Klinger K, Landes GM: Narrowing the position of the Treacher Collins syndrome locus to a small interval between three new microsatellite markers at 5q32-q33.1. *Am J Hum Genet* **52**:907, 1993.

23. Dausset J, Cann H, Cohen D, Lathrop M, Lalouel J, White R: Centre d'Etude du Polymorphisme Humain (CEPH): Collaborative genetic mapping of the human genome. *Genomics* **6**:575, 1990.

24. Loftus SK, Edwards SJ, Scherpbier-Heddema T, Buetow, KH, Wasmuth JJ, Dixon M: A combined genetic and radiation hybrid map surrounding the Treacher Collins syndrome locus on chromosome 5q. *Hum Mol Genet* **2**:1785, 1993.

25. Jabs EW, Li X, Lovett M, et al: Genetic and physical mapping of the Treacher Collins syndrome locus with respect to loci in the chromosome 5q3 region. *Genomics* **18**:7, 1993.

26. Dixon J, Gladwin AJ, Loftus SK, et al: A yeast artificial chromosome contig encompassing the Treacher Collins syndrome critical region at 5q31.3-q32. *Am J Hum Genet* **55**:372, 1994.

27. Crompton MR, Owens RJ, Totty NF, Moss SE, Waterfield MD, Crumpton MJ: Primary structure of the human membrane associated $Ca^{2+}$ binding protein p68: A novel member of a protein family. *EMBO J* **7**:21, 1988.

28. Loftus SK, Dixon J, Koprivnikar K, Dixon MJ, Wasmuth JJ: Transcriptional map of the Treacher Collins candidate gene region. *Genome Res* **6**:26, 1996.

29. Dixon J, Loftus SK, Gladwin AJ, Scambler PJ, Wasmuth JJ, Dixon MJ: Cloning of the human heparan sulfate-*N*-deacetylase/*N*-sulfotransferase gene from the Treacher Collins syndrome candidate region at 5q32-q33.1. *Genomics* **26**:239, 1995.

30. Gladwin AJ, Dixon J, Loftus SK, Wasmuth JJ, Dixon MJ: Genomic organisation of the human heparan sulfate-*N*-deacetylase/*N*-sulfotransferase gene: Exclusion from a causative role in the pathogenesis of Treacher Collins syndrome. *Genomics* **32**:471, 1996.

31. Wei Z, Sweidler SJ, Ishihara M, Orellana A, Hirschberg CB: A single protein catalyses both *N*-deacetylation and *N*-sulfation during the biosynthesis of heparan sulfate. *Proc Natl Acad Sci USA* **90**:3885, 1993.

32. David G, Bai XM, Van Der Schueren B, Cassiman JJ, Van Den Berghe H: Developmental changes in heparan sulfate expression: In situ detection with Mabs. *J Cell Biol* **119**:961, 1992.

33. The Treacher Collins Syndrome Collaborative Group: Positional cloning of a gene involved in the pathogenesis of Treacher Collins syndrome. *Nature Genet* **12**:130, 1996.

34. McIntosh I, Hamosh A, Dietz HC: Nonsense mutations and diminished mRNA levels. *Nature Genet* **4**:219, 1993.

35. Edwards SJ, Fowlie A, Cust MP, Liu DTY, Young ID, Dixon MJ: Prenatal diagnosis in Treacher Collins syndrome using combined genetic linkage analysis and ultrasound imaging. *J Med Genet* **33**:603, 1996.

36. Connor JM, Ferguson-Smith, MA: *Essential Medical Genetics*. Oxford, England, Blackwell Scientific, 1988.

37. Moloney DM, Slaney SF, Oldridge M, Wall SA, Sahlin PAC, Stenman G, Wilkie AO: Exclusive paternal origin of new mutations in Apert syndrome. *Nature Genet* **13**:48, 1996.

38. Tolarova MM, Harris JA, Ordway DE, Vargervik K: Birth prevalence, mutation rate, sex ratio, parents' age, and ethnicity in Apert syndrome. *Am J Med Genet* **72**:394, 1997.

39. Jones KL, Smith DW, Sedgwick Harvey MA, Hall BD, Quan L: Older paternal age and fresh gene mutation: Data on additional disorders. *J Pediatr* **86**:84, 1975.

40. Dixon J, Hovanes K, Shiang R, Dixon MJ: Sequence analysis, identification of evolutionary conserved motifs and expression analysis of murine *Tcof1* provide further evidence for a potential function for the gene and its human homologue, *TCOF1*. *Hum Mol Genet* **6**:727, 1997.

41. Paznekas WA, Zhang N, Gridley T, Jabs EW: Mouse *Tcof1* is expressed widely, has motifs conserved in nucleolar phosphoproteins, and maps to chromosome 18. *Biochem Biophys Res Commun* **238**:1, 1997.

42. Deol MS: The development of the inner ear in mice homozygous for shaker-with-syndactylism. *J Embryol Exp Morphol* **11**:493, 1963.

43. Juriloff DM, Harris MJ, Froster-Iskenius U: Hemifacial deficiency induced by a shift in dominance of the mouse mutation *far*: A possible genetic model for hemifacial microsomia. *J Craniofac Dev Biol* **7**:27, 1987.

44. Altschul SF, Gish W, Miller W, Myer EW, Lipman DJ: Basic local alignment search tool. *J Mol Biol* **215**:403, 1990.

45. Dixon J, Edwards SJ, Anderson I, Brass A, Scambler PJ, Dixon MJ: Identification of the complete coding sequence and genomic organisation of the Treacher Collins syndrome gene. *Genome Res* **7**:223, 1997.

46. Wise CA, Chiang LC, Paznekas WA, Sharma M, Musy MM, Ashley JA, Lovett M, Jabs EW: *TCOF1* encodes a putative nucleolar phosphoprotein that exhibits mutations in Treacher Collins syndrome throughout its coding region. *Proc Natl Acad Sci USA* **94**:3110, 1997.

47. Meier UT, Blobel G: Nopp140 shuttles on tracks between nucleolus and cytoplasm. *Cell* **70**:127, 1992.

48. Cairns C, McStay B: Identification and cDNA cloning of a *Xenopus* nucleolar phosphoprotein, xNopp180, that is the homologue of the rat nucleolar protein, Nopp140. *J Cell Sci* **108**:3339, 1995.

49. Kuenzal EA, Mulligan JA, Sommercorn J, Krebs EG: Substrate specificity determinants for casein kinase II as deduced from studies with synthetic peptides. *J Biol Chem* **262**:9136, 1987.

50. Dingwall C, Laskey R: Nuclear targeting sequences: A consensus? *TIBS* **16**:478, 1991.

51. Chelsky D, Ralph R, Jonak G: Sequence requirements for synthetic peptide-mediated translocation to the nucleus. *Mol Cell Biol* **9**:2487, 1989.

52. Marsh KL, Dixon J, Dixon MJ: Mutations in the Treacher Collins syndrome gene lead to mislocalisation of the nucleolar protein treacle. *Hum Mol Genet* **7**:1795, 1998.

53. Scheer U, Benavente R: Functional and dynamic aspects of the mammalian nucleolus. *Bioessays* **12**:14, 1990.

54. Pederson T: The plurifunctional nucleolus. *Nucl Acids Res* **26**:3871, 1998.

55. Saeboe-Larssen S, Lyamouri M, Merriam J, Oksvold MP, Lambertsson A: Ribosomal protein insufficiency and the minute syndrome in *Drosophila*: A dose-response relationship. *Genetics* **148**:1215, 1998.

56. Dixon J, Brakebusch C, Fässler R, Dixon MJ: Increased levels of apoptosis in the prefusion neural folds underlie the craniofacial disorder, Treacher Collins syndrome. *Hum Mol Genet* **9**:1473, 2000.

# Aarskog-Scott Syndrome

*Jerome L. Gorski*

1. **Aarskog-Scott syndrome, or faciogenital dysplasia (FGDY), is an inherited disorder characterized by a distinguishing set of craniofacial and skeletal anomalies, disproportionate short stature, and urogenital malformations.**
2. **X-linked recessive and autosomal dominant inheritance patterns have been described in FGDY, indicating the presence of genetic heterogeneity. Linkage mapping and positional cloning efforts in the proximal short arm of the X chromosome (Xp11.21) led to the isolation of the gene involved in the X-linked Aarskog-Scott syndrome (*FGD1*).**
3. **In addition to a chromosomal translocation breakpoint, two different single-base insertional frameshift mutations in the *FGD1* gene have been identified in patients with familial Aarskog-Scott syndrome.**
4. ***FGD1* encodes a guanine nucleotide exchange factor (GEF) that specifically activates Cdc42, a member of the Rho (Ras homology) family of the p21 GTPases. By activating Cdc42, FGD1 protein stimulates fibroblasts to form filopodia, cytoskeletal elements involved in cellular signaling, adhesion, and migration. Through Cdc42, FGD1 protein also activates the c-Jun N-terminal kinase (JNK) signaling cascade, a pathway that regulates cell growth, apoptosis, and cellular differentiation.**
5. ***FGD1* contains additional motifs commonly associated with signaling proteins, including a pleckstrin homology (PH) domain, an evolutionarily conserved phosphatidylinositol-3-phosphate-binding FYVE domain, and two potential Src-homology 3 (SH3) binding sites. These additional domains may function to regulate the activity and/or location of the FGD1 protein.**
6. **Within the developing mouse skeleton, FGD1 protein is expressed in precartilaginous mesenchymal condensations, the perichondrium and periostium, proliferating chondrocytes, and osteoblasts. These results suggest that FGD1 signaling may play a role in the biology of several different skeletal cell types including mesenchymal prechondrocytes, chondrocytes, and osteoblasts. The characterization of the spatiotemporal pattern of FGD1 expression in mouse embryos has provided important clues to the understanding of the pathogenesis of Aarskog-Scott syndrome.**
7. **It appears likely that the primary defect in Aarskog-Scott syndrome is an abnormality of FGD1/Cdc42 signaling resulting in anomalous embryonic development and abnormal endochondral and intramembranous bone formation.**

---

A list of standard abbreviations is located immediately preceding the index in each volume. Additional abbreviations used in this chapter include: FGDY = faciogenital dysplasia (Aarskog-Scott) syndrome; YAC = yeast artificial chromosome; RhoGEF = Ras homologous gene guanine nucleotide exchange factor; GEF = guanine nucleotide exchange factor; JNK/SAPK = c-Jun N-terminal kinase/stress-activated protein kinase; PH = pleckstrin homology domain; SH3 = Src-homology 3 domain; PtdIns(3)P = phosphatidylinositol-3-phosphate; ORF = open reading frame; MAPK = mitogen-activated protein kinase.

## CLINICAL FEATURES, DIAGNOSIS, AND THERAPY

In 1970, Dagfinn Aarskog observed the association of disproportionate short stature and certain anomalies of the face, hands, feet, and genitalia in seven males from two generations of the same family.[1] A year later, Scott reported three brothers with similar features.[2] Since these initial reports, well over 100 cases of Aarskog-Scott syndrome, or faciogenital dysplasia (FGDY), have been published.[3,4] Two reports of similarly affected brothers with osteochondritis dissecans and facial anomalies had been made earlier.[6,7] Aarskog observed that the inheritance of this condition was compatible with an X-linked recessive disorder.[1] Most families segregating this disorder have displayed an apparent X-linked recessive pattern of inheritance.[3] However, the observation that several pedigrees demonstrated apparent male-to-male transmission has suggested an autosomal dominant form of FGDY.[8,9] Therefore, genetic heterogeneity is probable.

### Physical Features of the Disorder

The Aarskog-Scott syndrome phenotype consists of a characteristic set of facial and skeletal anomalies, disproportionate short stature, and urogenital malformations. The cardinal features of this disorder are summarized in Table 247-1 and are illustrated in Fig. 247-1. The face is typically round and the forehead broad with ridging of the metopic suture. Facial features typically consist of widely spaced eyes (hypertelorism), ptosis, down-slanting palpebral fissures, and a short, upturned (anteverted) nose. The philtrum is commonly long, and the maxilla is typically hypoplastic. A number of external ear anomalies have been described, including low-set ears, posteriorly rotated auricles, and thickened, overfolded helices.[1–5] Impaired growth is the major manifestation of the disease. Although birth growth parameters were normal in most reported cases, growth retardation usually becomes apparent during the first few years of life, and affected males rarely exceed 160 cm in height.[3–5] Stature is disproportionate, and the distal extremities are most severely shortened. Isolated growth hormone deficiency has been reported in a significant number of patients.[3,5,10]

Hands and feet are broad and short (see Fig. 247-1). Interphalangeal joints are typically hypermobile, and fifth digit clinodactyly is common. However, camptodactyly and contractures of the interphalangeal joints also have been observed.[1–5] The feet are short, broad, and flat with splayed, bulbous toes; metatarsus adductus also has been observed.[3–5] The majority of affected males have a pectus excavatum and inguinal hernias. The umbilicus is protuberant and protruding. Affected males commonly have a variety of urogenital anomalies. Typically, the scrotal folds extend ventrally around the base of the penis to form what resembles a shawl; the scrotum commonly appears bifid[1–5] (see Fig. 247-1). Cryptorchidism is common, and penile hypospadias also has been reported. Typically, relative to affected males, the phenotype of obligate female heterozygotes is mild and limited to relatively short stature and a subtler form of the characteristic craniofacial anomalies.[3,4] Affected males and obligate carrier females both appear to have normal fertility.[4]

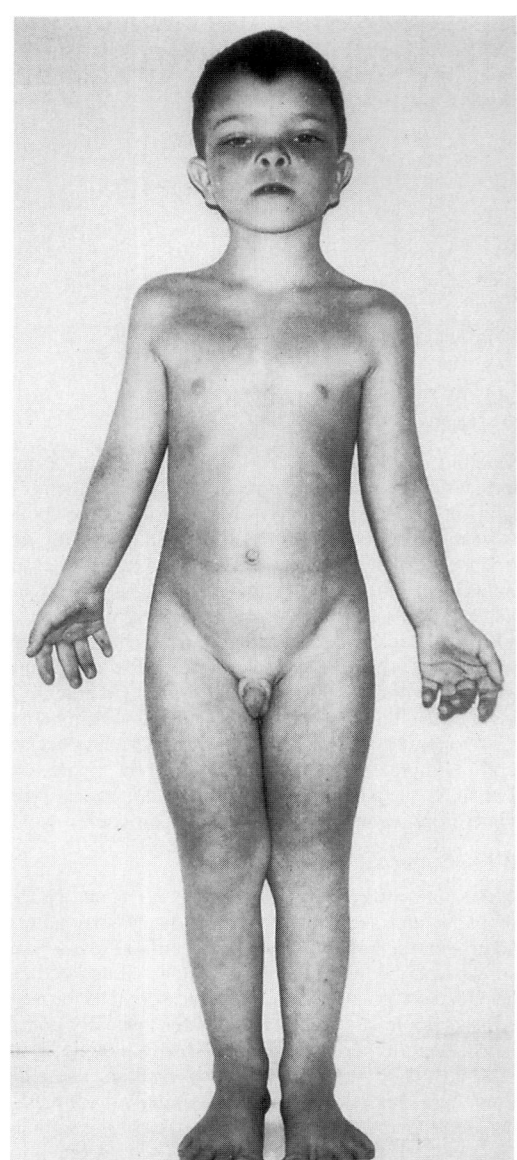

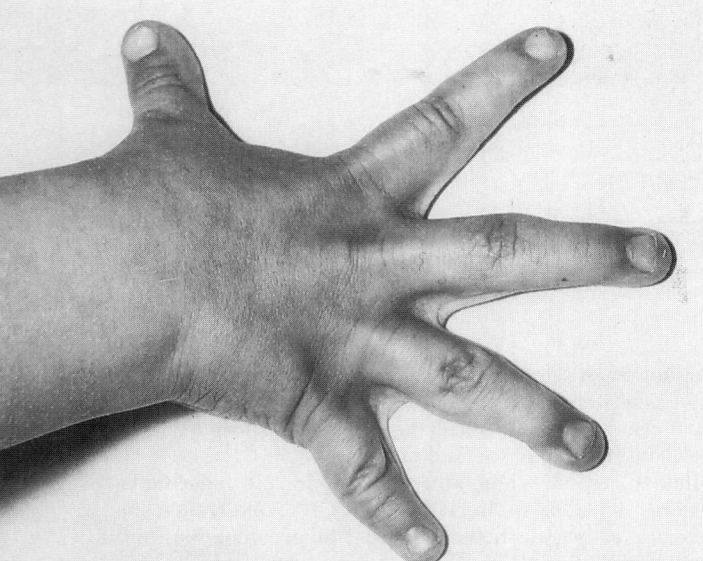

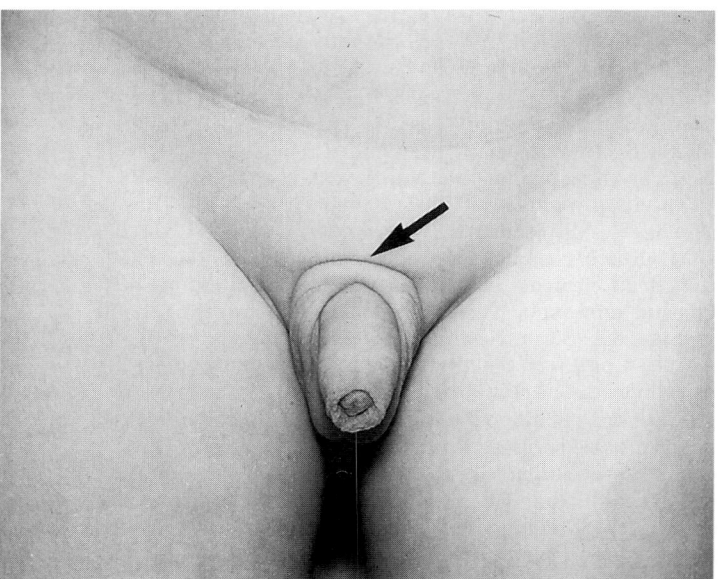

**Fig. 247-1** A male child with Aarskog-Scott syndrome illustrates the characteristic craniofacial, skeletal, and urogenital features. Facial features are characterized by a broad forehead and a widow's peak, hypertelorism, down-sloping palpebral fissures, bilateral ptosis of the upper eyelids, midface hypoplasia with a depressed nasal bridge, an anteverted nose, and low-set ears. Stature is short and disproportionate with shortened distal extremities; hands and feet are short and broad. Hand shows short phalanges, soft tissue syndactyly between the digits, camptodactyly of the fourth and fifth digits, and fifth-digit clinodactyly. The shawl scrotum is indicated (*arrow*). Consequential to scrotal folds joining ventrally over the base of the penis, an abnormal penoscrotal configuration is present. Bilateral inguinal herniorraphy scars are present. (*Courtesy of D. Aarskog, University of Bergen. Adapted from Gorski.[5] Used with permission of Humana Press.*)

The characteristic facial features are less apparent and more subtle in affected adult males.[11]

Although mild to moderate mental retardation and attention deficit disorder have been described in some affected males,[11] they do not appear to be consistent features.[3–5] Some affected males have been noted to have ophthalmoplegia and large corneal size.[3,12] Others have been observed to have enamel hypoplasia and a "col" deformity of the anterior mandible.[13] Congenitally missing teeth or delays in dental eruption also have been reported.[1,3] Affected males occasionally have a cleft lip and palate.[3] Congenital heart defects including atrial septal defects, ventricular septal defects, aortic valvular stenosis, and pulmonary valvular stenosis have been reported.[1,14] Affected males with Hirschsprungs disease, midgut malrotation, and dolichomegasig-moid also have been reported.[15,16] Some males have a single palmar crease or distally placed axial triradii.[3,4]

Radiographic abnormalities typically are limited to those observed in the cervical spine and distal extremities. These abnormalities are summarized in Table 247-1. About half the affected males have a cervical spine abnormality such as spina bifida occulta, odontoid hypoplasia, fused cervical vertebrae, and ligamentous laxity with subluxation.[3–5] Radiographic abnormalities of the hands and feet commonly consist of shortened digits, hypoplasia of the terminal phalanges, clinodactyly, fusion of the middle and distal phalanges, and retarded bone maturation.[3–5] Additional radiographic abnormalities include maxillary hypoplasia, osteochondritis dissecans, additional pairs of ribs and other segmentation anomalies, and calcified intervertebral disks.[17]

**Table 247-1** Clinical and Radiographic Features Associated with Aarskog-Scott Syndrome

| Anatomic Region or System | Clinical Features |
|---|---|
| Craniofacial | Broad forehead, abnormally formed ears, hypertelorism, down-slanted palpebral fissures, ptosis, maxillary hypoplasia, hypodontia, malocclusion (cleft lip and palate, enamel hypoplasia)* |
| Musculoskeletal | Disproportionate short stature, distally shortened limbs, brachydactyly, pectus excavatum, soft tissue syndactyly of the digits, joint hypermobility, camptodactyly, clinodactyly, broad feet, inguinal hernias (single palmar crease, abnormal dermatoglyphics) |
| Urogenital | Shawl and bifid scrotum, cryptorchidism (hypospadias) |
| Miscellaneous | Strabismus, growth hormone deficiency (mild to moderate mental retardation, attention deficit disorder, congenital heart defects) |
| Radiographic | Spina bifida occulta, odontoid hypoplasia, cervical vertebral defects, cervical ligamentous laxity, calcified intervertebral disks, additional ribs, hypoplastic phalanges, retarded bone age (osteochondritis) |

*Items in parentheses are less commonly observed.

SOURCE: From Gorski[5] used with permission of Humana Press.

## Differential Diagnosis

Several other inherited conditions, including Noonan syndrome, Robinow syndrome, and Leopard syndrome, share clinical features with Aarskog-Scott syndrome; shared features include short stature, hypertelorism, and cryptorchidism. Pseudohypoparathyroidism and hydantoin embryopathy also share several physical features with Aarskog-Scott syndrome. However, the combination of distinctive radiographic abnormalities, the characteristic pattern of craniofacial abnormalities, disproportionate short stature, shortening of the distal extremities, and characteristic unique urogenital anomalies typically distinguish Aarskog-Scott syndrome from other conditions. Among families segregating the common inherited form of Aarskog-Scott syndrome, an observed X-linked pattern of inheritance provides additional clinical confirmation.

## Therapy

Evaluations are directed toward the identification and treatment of associated medical problems and congenital malformations. Affected infants should be evaluated to identify congenital heart defects. Common structural malformations such as cryptorchidism, hypospadias, and inguinal hernias should be identified and referred to the appropriate pediatric subspecialist for surgical correction. An ophthalmologic evaluation should be performed to identify associated ocular abnormalities such as strabismus. Because of the associated problems of cervical spine instability, particular care should be taken to support an affected infant's head and to avoid head and cervical spine trauma. Radiographic studies should be performed to identify children with odontoid hypoplasia and/or cervical spine ligamentous laxity. Children with joint contractures, soft tissue syndactyly, and cervical spine anomalies should be referred to the appropriate pediatric subspecialist for surgical correction and to physical therapy for continued treatment. Children with hypodontia and malocclusion should be

referred to a pediatric dentist for care. Endocrinologic evaluations should be performed to identify children with an isolated deficiency of growth hormone. At this time, no controlled studies have been performed to assess the benefits and risks of supplemental growth hormone to Aarskog-Scott syndrome patients without isolated growth hormone deficiency.

## GENETICS

Pedigree analysis of families segregating Aarskog-Scott syndrome strongly suggests that it is typically inherited in an X-linked recessive fashion.[3,4] Infrequent reports also indicate the presence of a clinically indistinguishable autosomal dominant form of Aarskog-Scott syndrome.[8,9] X-linked inheritance is strongly supported by the male preponderance of affected individuals and the complete expression in males versus partial expression in females in the same family. However, among families segregating the X-linked form of Aarskog-Scott syndrome, clinical analysis shows relatively wide phenotypic variability between affected siblings and between affected individuals of different generations.[4,18] To date, there are no genetic mapping data on the autosomally inherited forms of FGDY. However, an individual with a multiple congenital anomaly syndrome similar to Aarskog-Scott syndrome was found to have a partial duplication of the short arm of chromosome 2.[19] This chromosomal rearrangement may be causally associated with an Aarskog-Scott syndrome phenotype and therefore may pinpoint a location for an autosomal gene involved in FGDY.

The observation that in the majority of families identified, Aarskog-Scott syndrome appeared to segregate as an X-linked recessive gene was further supported by the finding of a reciprocal X;8 chromosome translocation in a family with complete male and female disease expression.[20] The observation that the mother and son both displayed all the major features of FGDY and that, in the affected female, the translocated X chromosome was active in the majority of cells examined suggested that the translocation breakpoint directly interrupted the FGDY disease gene. This observation led to the first tentative chromosomal assignment of the X-linked FGDY gene to the pericentric region of the X chromosome. In keeping with this hypothesis, genetic linkage studies mapped the X-linked FGDY locus to the pericentric region of the X chromosome.[21,22] A reanalysis of the FGDY-specific X;8 translocation breakpoint further localized the X chromosomal breakpoint, and the putative FGDY disease gene, to the proximal short arm of the X chromosome within region Xp11.21.[23] Physical mapping studies further localized the FGDY-specific breakpoint to an estimated 350-kb region within Xp11.21.[23,24] This localization of the FGDY gene was consistent with genetic linkage data.[21,22]

## FGD1, THE X-LINKED AARSKOG-SCOTT SYNDROME GENE

The FGDY-specific X;8 translocation breakpoint within the Xp11.21 region was used as a molecular signpost to positionally clone the X-linked Aarskog-Scott syndrome gene. Molecular characterization of the FGDY-specific translocation breakpoint permitted construction of a physical map of the translocation breakpoint region and assignment of the FGDY locus to a specific interval within this map.[25] DNA markers flanking the disease-specific breakpoint were used to assemble a regional yeast artificial chromosome (YAC) contig of the breakpoint region. DNA clones derived from this contig were used to identify regional transcripts including the FGD1 cDNA[25] (Fig. 247-2). A number of lines of evidence indicated that FGD1 was the gene responsible for X-linked FGDY: (1) FGD1 mapped to Xp11.21, the region known to contain the FGDY disease locus, (2) the FGD1 gene was directly disrupted by the FGDY-specific t(X;8) breakpoint, (3) an insertional mutation, predicted to result in a severely abbreviated and nonfunctional FGD1 protein, segregated with the phenotype in an affected FGDY family, and (4) FGD1

## Xp11.21

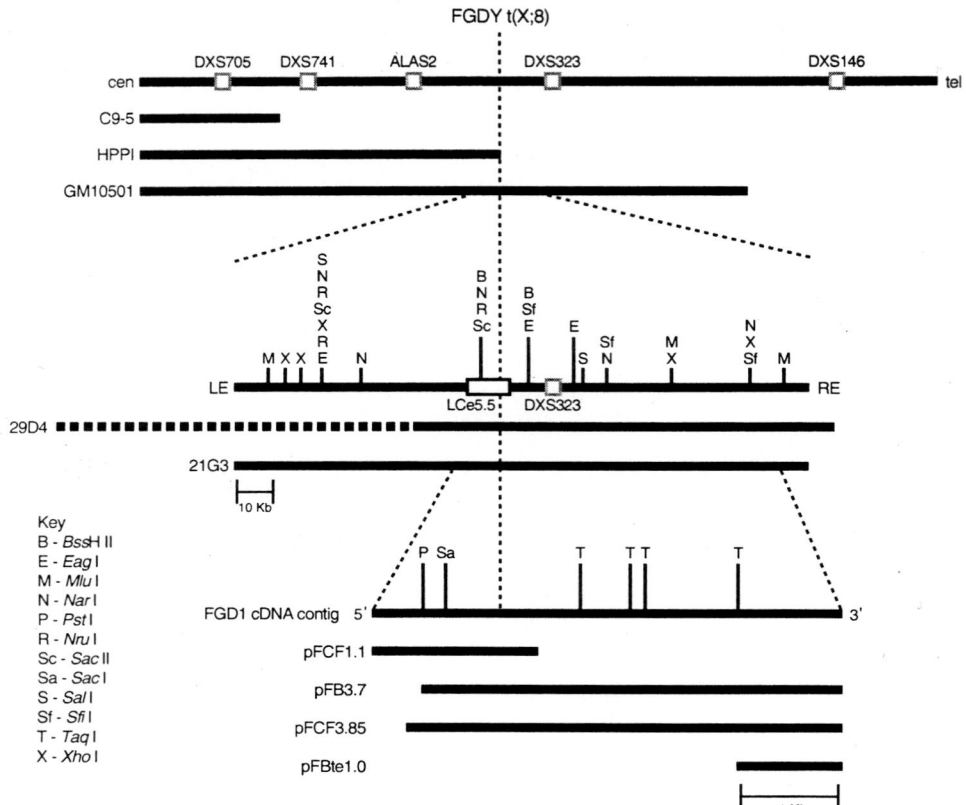

**Fig. 247-2** A schematic representation of the Aarskog-Scott syndrome region within Xp11.21 showing the *FGD1* gene positional cloning strategy. The FGDY-specific X;8 translocation breakpoint was mapped to the region between loci *ALAS2* and *DXS323*;[23] *locus order was determined previously.*[24] Bars indicate the relative X chromosome content of somatic cell hybrid lines used to map DNA markers to specific intervals within the Xp11.21 region; all bars extend to Xqter.[24,26] A detailed composite long-range restriction map of the FGDY breakpoint region derived from YAC clones *21G3* and *29D4* is shown below; bars indicate the relative clone content. LE and RE indicate the left and right ends of clone *21G3*, respectively; the interrupted bar indicates a chimeric clone segment. A composite restriction map of the *FGD1* cDNA is shown below the YAC diagram; bars indicate individual clone content. (*From Pasteris et al.*[25] *Used with permission of* Cell.)

mRNA was expressed in tissues involved in the disease phenotype, including fetal craniofacial bones.[25]

### FGD1 Encodes a Rho Guanine Nucleotide Exchange Protein

An analysis of the *FGD1* gene sequence provided insights into FGDY pathogenesis. The gene encodes a 761-amino-acid protein that displays strong evolutionary conservation. *Fgd1*, the mouse *FGD1* homologue, is 95 percent identical to *FGD1*.[26] A *Caenorhabditis elegans FGD1* homologue also has been identified.[27] Comparative sequence analysis suggested that *FGD1* encoded a guanine nucleotide exchange factor, or activator, for a member of the Rho family of p21 GTPases.[25] The Rho GTPases form a subgroup of the Ras superfamily of 20- to 30-kDa GTP-binding proteins. As a group, Rho proteins have been shown to play crucial roles in a wide spectrum of cellular functions including regulation of the actin cytoskeleton, membrane trafficking and vesicular transport, transcriptional regulation, cell growth control, and embryonic morphogenesis.[28] At least 10 mammalian Rho-like GTPases are known: RhoA, -B, -C, -D, and -E; Rac1 and -2; RacE; Cdc42, and TC10.[28] Sequence analysis shows that the Rho proteins from various species are conserved in structure and are about 50 percent homologous to each other.

Rho GTPases function as molecular switches, cycling between an inactive GDP-bound state and an active GTP-bound state. Rho guanine nucleotide exchange factors (RhoGEFs), including FGD1, constitute a rapidly growing family of diverse proteins that activate the GTPase Ras-like family of Rho proteins by catalyzing the exchange of bound GDP for free GTP. As shown schematically in Fig. 247-3, the ratio of the two states of a Rho GTPase is regulated by the opposing effects of guanine nucleotide exchange factors (GEFs), which catalyze the exchange of bound GDP for GTP, and the GTPase-activating proteins (GAPs), which increase the

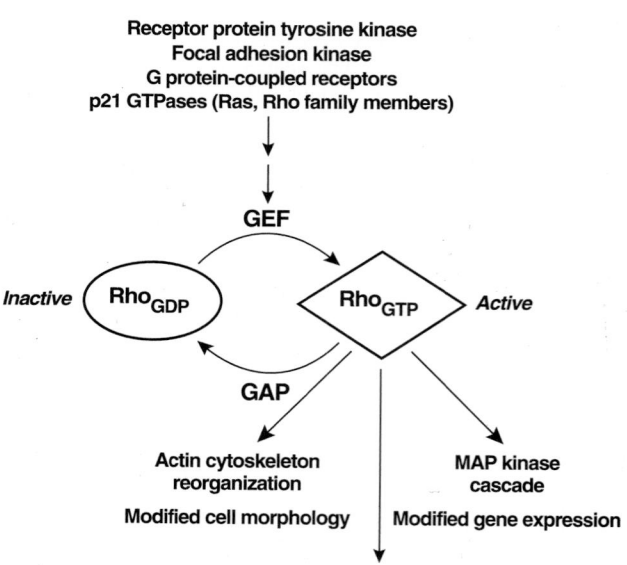

**Fig. 247-3** RhoGEFs activate a Rho protein GTPase by catalyzing the exchange of GDP for GTP. A variety of stimuli lead to the activation of Rho protein family members via RhoGEFs, including the p21 GTPase Ras, receptor protein tyrosine kinases, and G protein-coupled receptors.[28] Activated Rho leads to modified cell morphology by a reorganization of the actin cytoskeleton, a modulation of gene transcription by the activation of MAPK cascade, and the sequential activation of other Rho family member proteins. RhoGAP facilitates the hydrolysis of GTP and Rho protein inactivation. (*From Gorski.*[5] *Used with permission of Humana Press.*)

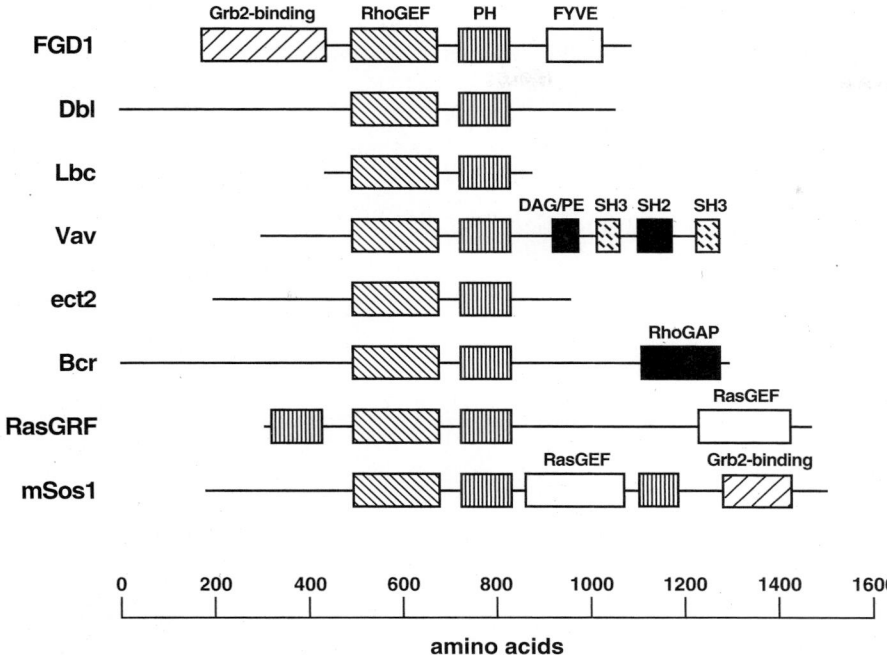

FGD1

Dbl

Lbc

Vav

ect2

Bcr

RasGRF

mSos1

Grb2-binding    RhoGEF    PH    FYVE

DAG/PE  SH3  SH2  SH3

RhoGAP

RasGEF

RasGEF    Grb2-binding

0    200    400    600    800    1000    1200    1400    1600

**amino acids**

Fig. 247-4 A schematic representation of the molecular structure of the FGD1 protein compared with other RhoGEF proteins. Structural domains are drawn approximately to scale. FGD1 contains at least four distinct domains including a RhoGEF domain and a PH domain, motifs common to all RhoGEF family members.[30] FGD1 also contains a cysteine-rich FYVE domain, a PtdIns(3)P-binding domain, and a putative SH3-binding (Grb2-binding) region. Vav contains SH3, Src-homology 2 (SH2), and a putative diacylglycerol/ phorbol ester-binding (DAG/PE) zinc butterfly motif. Bcr contains a Rho GTPase activator protein (RhoGAP) domain. RasGRF and mSos1 contain a Ras guanine nucleotide exchange factor (RasGEF) domain. (*Adapted from Gorski.[5] Used with permission of Humana Press.*)

intrinsic rate of hydrolysis of bound GTP.[29] At least 20 different RhoGEFs are known.[30] The structural organization of several RhoGEFs is shown in Fig. 247-4. Like FGD1, all RhoGEF family members contain a 200-amino-acid RhoGEF domain. A comparison of RhoGEF domain sequences from various species shows that they are conserved in primary structure and are 25 to 30 percent homologous.[30] Dbl, the prototype RhoGEF, was isolated originally by its ability to induce focus formation and tumorigenicity when expressed in NIH-3T3 cells.[31] Lbc, ect2, and most of the isolated RhoGEFs also were isolated by virtue of their transforming capability through gene transfer experiments.[30] In contrast, RhoGEFs including Cdc24, Bcr, mSos1, RasGRF, and Vav were identified by their role in cell growth regulation.[30] The recognition that Dbl contained a 29 percent sequence identity with the *Saccharomyces cerevisiae* cell division cycle protein Cdc24, a known yeast Cdc42 activator, provided the first clue that Dbl was a RhoGEF.[32] Biochemical analysis showed that Dbl was able to catalyze the release of GDP from the human homologue of Cdc42. Deletion analysis showed that the Dbl RhoGEF domain was essential and sufficient for the Cdc42 exchange activity and Dbl oncogenicity.[32–34] It remains to be determined as to how the RhoGEF domain catalyzes the exchange of GDP for GTP. For the RasGEF Son of sevenless (Sos), structural studies indicate that Sos catalyzes GDP-GTP exchange by binding to Ras to alter the structure of its nucleotide switch regions, thereby reducing the affinity of the Ras molecule for GDP.[35] However, among GEFs with a known molecular structure (i.e., Sos and ARNO, the GEF for the Arf small GTPase), although the GEF domains are primarily composed of α-helixes, the three-dimensional structure of ARNO does not resemble that of a RasGEF.[36,37] These results imply that the structural mechanisms of nucleotide exchange may differ among GEF proteins.

Cellular microinjection experiments and biochemical studies show that FGD1 is a specific activator for the p21 GTPase Cdc42.[38,39] Studies showed that the FGD1 GEF domain specifically complexed to Cdc42 but that it did not bind to other Rho proteins.[38] In addition, in a reconstituted in vitro system, the FGD1 GEF domain stimulated [³H]GDP dissociation from and [³⁵S]GTP binding to Cdc42.[38] When microinjected into cultured cells, the FGD1 GEF domain induced fibroblasts to form filopodia, actin-associated membrane complexes generated by activated Cdc42 (Fig. 247-5). Studies showed that the FGD1 GEF domain

specifically interacted with the Cdc42 protein and that FGD1-dependent filopodia formation was blocked by complexing Cdc42 to other Cdc42-binding proteins.[39] In FGD1-expressing fibroblasts, c-Jun N-terminal kinase/stress-activated protein kinase (JNK/SAPK) activity was stimulated in a manner similar to that obtained with constitutively activated Cdc42.[38,39] In addition, like constitutively expressed Cdc42, FGD1 stimulated the S6 kinase signaling cascade[38] and stimulated the passage of fibroblasts through the G₁ phase of the cell cycle.[39] Together these results showed that FGD1 is a specific Cdc42 activator and a component of the Cdc42 signaling pathway.

Immediately adjacent to the RhoGEF domain, all RhoGEF proteins, including FGD1, contain a region of sequence homology of approximately 120 amino acids termed the *pleckstrin homology (PH) domain*[25] (see Fig. 247-4). This domain was first identified as a duplicated and conserved domain in the protein pleckstrin, the major substrate of protein kinase C in platelets.[40] PH domains form a diverse family of signaling domains.[41] Some PH domains have been shown to bind to the second messenger molecule phosphatidylinositol-4,5-bisphosphate.[42] Alternatively, other PH domains have been shown to bind to the βγ-subunits of the G-proteins[43] or to proteins containing a phosphotyrosine binding (PTB) domain.[44] No specific ligand has yet to be identified for the PH domain associated with the RhoGEF family of proteins. However, in the absence of an identified ligand, the PH domain has been shown to be essential for proper cellular localization of RhoGEF proteins.[45]

A comparative analysis of FGD1 showed that it contained at least two additional conserved signaling motifs that potentially could regulate the localization and/or activity of the Cdc42GEF domain. First, the FGD1 N-terminal proline-rich region was found to contain at least two putative Src-homology 3 (SH3) domain binding sites that exhibited strong similarity to the functionally significant regions of several proteins with demonstrated SH3 domain binding, including mSos1, a RasGEF known to bind to the SH3 domain of Grb2.[25] SH3 domains have been shown to specifically bind short (9- to 10-amino-acid) proline-rich structurally conserved motifs.[46–48] Grb2, a component of the Ras signaling pathway, was shown to selectively bind to the proline-rich motifs of the mSos1 protein to form a link in a signal-transduction pathway that functionally ties tyrosine kinase receptors to Ras.[46,48] Among the identified Ras and RhoGEF

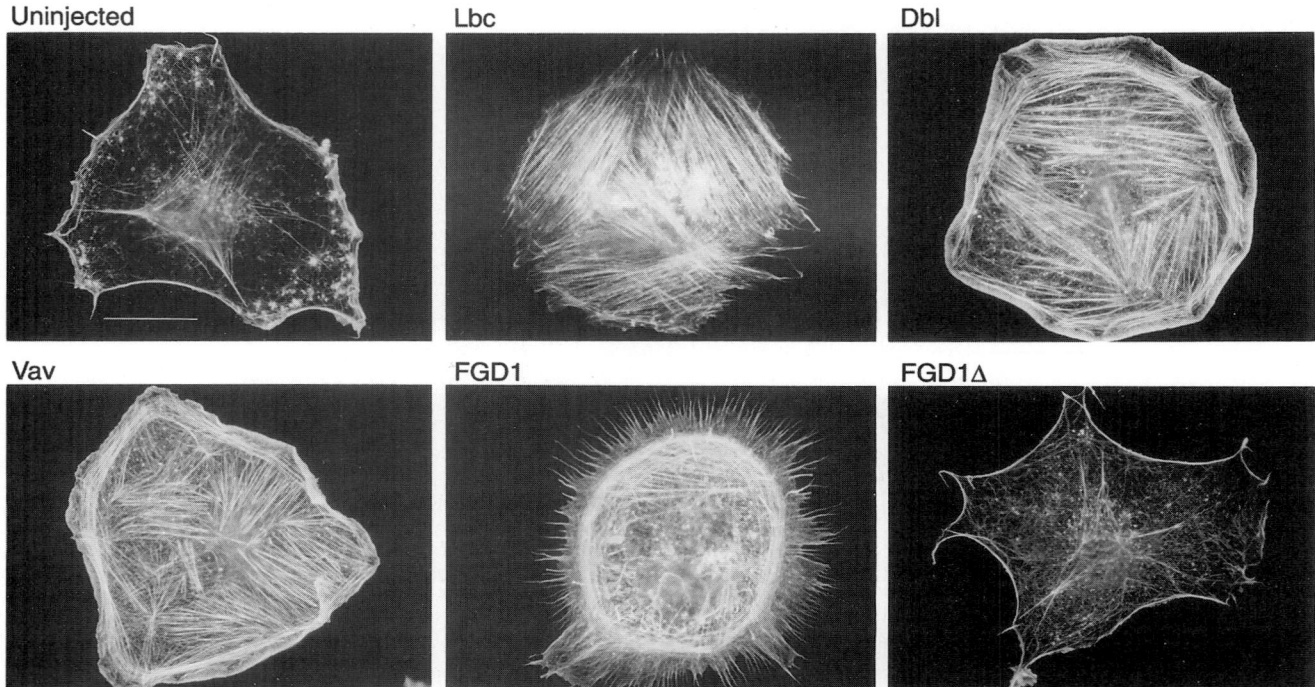

**Fig. 247-5 Fibroblasts microinjected with RhoGEF expression constructs showing the promotion of actin polymerization through the activation of different Rho proteins. FGD1, Dbl, Lbc, and Vav promote the polymerization of actin in quiescent cells; serum-starved Swiss 3T3 cells were microinjected with plasmid DNA encoding epitope-tagged RhoGEF proteins.[39] FGD1 stimulates the formation of filopodia (activation of Cdc42). In contrast, Dbl and Vav stimulate the formation of lamellipodia (activation of Rac), and Lbc stimulates the formation of actin stress fibers (activation of Rho). A construct containing an alternatively spliced form of FGD1 that lacks 36 amino acids near the N-terminal end of the GEF domain, FGD1Δ, fails to stimulate filopodial formation. Actin cytoskeletal structures in cells expressing the protein constructs were visualized with TRITC-conjugated phalloidin. Scale bar in *A* represents 20 μm and refers to all panels. (*From Olsen et al.[39] Used with permission of Current Biology.*)**

family members, mSos1 is unique in containing an SH3-, or Grb2-, binding domain. The identification of a putative proline-rich SH3-binding domain in FGD1 infers that, like Sos, the location and/or activity of the FGD1 protein may be modified by proteins containing an SH3 domain. Second, immediately downstream from the PH domain, FGD1 was found to contain a cysteine-rich evolutionarily conserved zinc-finger motif, termed the *FYVE domain*[25] (see Fig. 247-4).

At least 30 different proteins of yeast, nematode, plant, insect, and mammalian origin have been found to contain this domain.[49] Most of the proteins containing the FYVE domain are known to be involved in membrane trafficking, including the yeast vacuolar sorting proteins Vac1p[50] and Vps27p,[51] the yeast phophatidylin-ositol-4-phosphate-5-kinase Fab1,[52] and the mammalian ATPase Hrs-2.[53] Recent results have illuminated the role the FYVE domain plays in cellular signaling. Stenmark and coworkers have shown that the FYVE domains of both EEA1, a mammalian early endosomal protein, and Hrs-2 selectively bind to phosphatidyli-nositol-3-phosphate [PtdIns(3)P] and that this binding is necessary for the proteins to localize to the early endosomal membranes.[49,54] Similar studies showed that Vac1p and Vps27 also selectively bind to PtdIns(3)P.[55] The observation that the predicted FGD1 sequence contains an EEA1-like FYVE domain suggests that the FGD1 protein is likely to bind to and interact with phosphatidylinositol second-messenger molecules. Therefore, it is likely that the FGD1 protein interacts with or is regulated by the components of multiple signal-transduction pathways.

## FGD1 EXPRESSION STUDIES

A characterization of the spatiotemporal pattern of FGD1 expression has provided important clues to the understanding of

the molecular pathogenesis of Aarskog-Scott syndrome. Northern blot analyses of poly(A)+mRNA showed that the *FGD1* 4.4-kb transcript was developmentally regulated and predominantly expressed in human fetal tissues including fetal heart, brain, lung, and kidney.[25] The mouse *FGD1* homologue, *Fgd1*, was isolated to facilitate an analysis of the developmental spatiotemporal expression pattern of this gene.[26] The entire coding region of the *Fgd1* transcript was sequenced; this analysis showed that the *Fgd1* transcript contained a 2880-nucleotide open reading frame (ORF) that was predicted to encode a protein of 960 amino acids, one residue shorter than the human homologue.[26] Comparative sequence analysis showed that the mouse and human *FGD1* sequences were highly conserved. Compared with FGD1, the *Fgd1* 5′ untranslated region, ORF, and 3′ untranslated region were 95, 92, and 75 percent identical to the *FGD1* nucleotide sequence, respectively; the predicted amino acid sequences of the mouse and human *FGD1* cDNAs were 94 percent identical.[26]

To delineate the spatiotemporal pattern of *Fgd1* expression, RNA *in situ* hybridization studies were performed in mouse embryos using the *Fgd1* cDNA as probe. Fgd1 mRNA was predominantly expressed within the skeletal elements of the mouse embryo.[56] During vertebrate embryogenesis, the formation of the skeleton is genetically regulated to ensure the formation of the correct number, shape, and size of individual skeletal elements.[57] Skeletal elements are formed initially as mesenchymal templates that are later replaced by bone tissue in the process known as *endochondral ossification*. This process begins with the aggregation of undifferentiated mesenchymal cells. Later, cells in the core of the condensations differentiate into chondrocytes, and the spindle-shaped cells at the perimeter form a sheath around the cartilage, the perichondrium.[57,58] In e14.5 mouse embryos, Fgd1 is detected within multiple mesenchymal condensations including

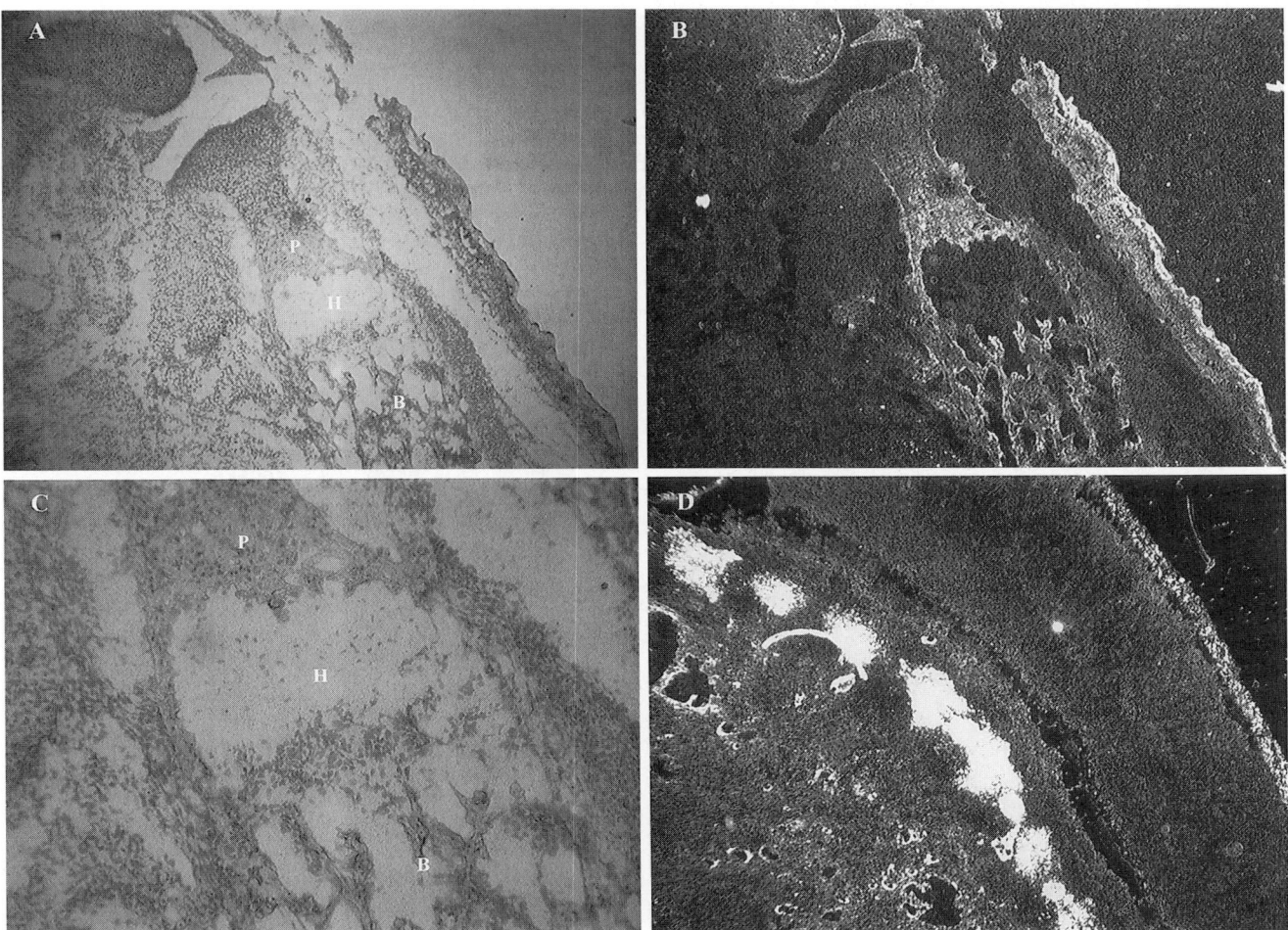

**Fig. 247-6** Expression of the mouse *Fgd1* gene during mouse skeletal development. Bright-field (*A, C*) and dark-field (*B, D*) photomicrographs of sagittal sections through the caudal region of a newborn mouse pup (*A-C*) and the caudal region of e14.5 embryo (*D*). The low-power photomicrograph in *B* shows that the *Fgd1* antisense probe detects expression in proliferating chondrocytes, cells lining the bony trabeculae, the perichondrium, and chondrocytes lining the synovial space. The bright-field low-power and high-power magnification of this section are also shown (*A* and *C*, respectively); P denotes proliferating chondrocytes, H denotes hypertrophic chondrocytes, and B denotes bony trabeculae. *D* shows that an *Fgd1* antisense probe detects expression in precartilaginous mesenchymal condensations in the caudal vertebrae in an e14.5 mouse embryo. Fgd1 expression is also detected in the squamous epithelium (*B* and *D*).

vertebral condensations (Fig. 247-6*D*), elements involved in the FGDY phenotype.

During endochondral ossification, skeletal elements elongate by chondrocyte proliferation and extracellular matrix deposition.[57] Shortly after the condensations form, chondrocytes in the central region cease proliferation, become hypertrophic, and alter their extracellular matrix. These changes in the extracellular matrix allow blood vessels to invade the hypertrophic cartilage from the perichondrium. Bone marrow cells and osteoblasts appear in association with the vascularization and replace the cartilage with bone (ossification). Final skeletal shapes result from a combination of partial cell loss (apoptosis), fusion of adjacent condensations, and a coordinated resorption and deposition of bone by osteoclasts and osteoblasts.[57,58] In newborn mouse pups, Fgd1 is detected in proliferating chondrocytes but is notably absent from hypertrophic chondrocytes (see Fig. 247-6*B*). At this developmental stage, Fgd1 is also expressed in osteoblast cells and in the perichondrium and periostium of intramembranous and endochondral skeletal elements.[56] These results suggest that FGD1/Cdc42 signaling may play a variety of roles in skeletal formation, including the formation of mesenchymal condensations and chondrocyte and osteoblast cell differentiation.

## THE MOLECULAR BASIS OF X-LINKED AARSKOG-SCOTT SYNDROME

A study of over 25 unrelated cases of X-linked FGDY failed to show evidence of a deletion in *FGD1*.[25] However, others have reported a male with Aarskog-Scott syndrome and hematologic abnormalities suggestive of X-linked sideroblastic anemia.[59] *FGD1* and the gene for erythroid delta-aminolevulinate synthase (*ALAS2*), which is responsible for X-linked sideroblastic anemia,[60] were mapped to a 350-kb interval within Xp11.21.[24] These results suggest that the previously described male may have had FGDY and sideroblastic anemia on the basis of a contiguous gene syndrome as the result of a deletion involving both *FGD1* and *ALAS2*. Unfortunately, the death of the previously described male precludes confirmation of this hypothesis. Together, these results suggest that deletions involving the *FGD1* locus may occur but that deletions do not appear to play a common role in the generation of *FGD1* mutations.

Mutation detection strategies required a detailed characterization of the *FGD1* gene structure. Structural analyses show that the *FGD1* gene is comprised of 18 exons that span 51 kb of genomic DNA within region Xp11.21.[61] The structure of the *FGD1* gene is

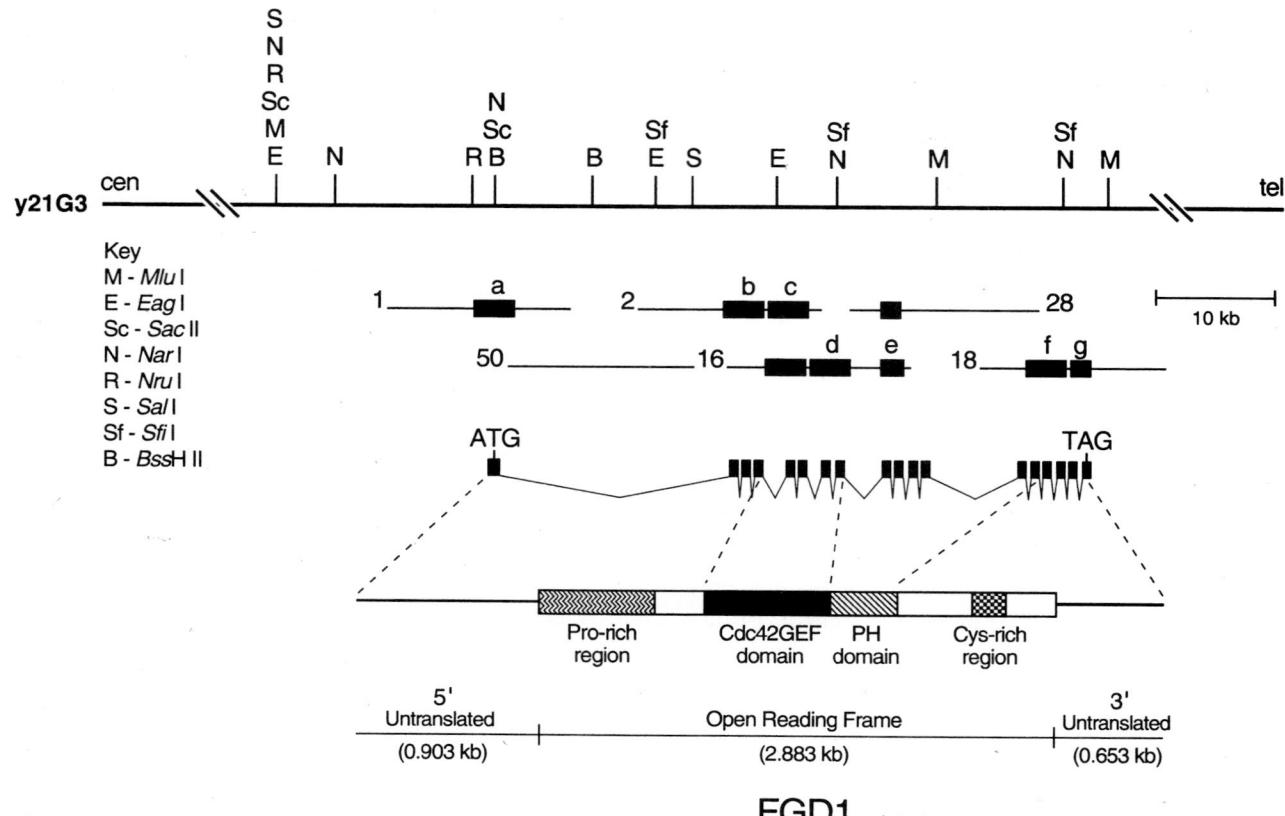

**FGD1**

**Fig. 247-7** A schematic diagram shows the genomic organization of the *FGD1* gene. A restriction map of a segment of YAC clone *21G3* is shown at the top of the figure showing the orientation of the clone relative to the centromere (cen) and telomere (tel) of the short arm of the X chromosome. A minimal tile contig of lambda bacteriophage clones derived from *21G3* (phage clones 1, 50, 2, 16, 28, and 18) is shown below the restriction map. The relative positions of exon-containing *Taq*I genomic fragments (fragments a–g) are indicated within the constructed phage contig. The genomic organization of the *FGD1* gene is shown schematically at the bottom of the figure; the relative position of each exon is illustrated. The structure of the *FGD1* transcript is shown schematically at the bottom of the figure. Exons 1–4 encode a proline-rich region and potential SH3 binding domains, exons 5–8 encode a Cdc42GEF domain, exons 9-14 encode a PH domain, and exons 15–17 encode a cysteine-rich FYVE domain. (*From Pasteris et al.*[61] *Used with permission of Genomics.*)

shown schematically in Fig. 247-7. RNase protection and primer extension studies show that the *FGD1* gene has multiple transcriptional starts and that the primary start site is located 903 bp upstream of the ATG translation-initiation codon. Sequence analysis of the 5′ region of the *FGD1* gene indicates that the FGD1 promoter lacks canonical CAAT and TATA boxes, a result consistent with the detection of multiple transcription start sites. Sequence analysis shows that all *FGD1* exon-intron splice sites conform to the AG/GT rule.[61] The first *FGD1* exon is the largest and 1210 bp in size; it contains a 903-bp 5′ untranslated region, the putative ATG start codon, and 307 bp of the ORF. The last exon is 956 bp in size and contains the TAG translation-termination site and a 651-bp 3′ untranslated region. The remaining exons range from 31 to 442 bp in size.[61] Intron sizes were determined directly by sequencing or by exon-exon PCR amplification of genomic DNA. To facilitate an analysis of FGDY patient DNA and the identification of *FGD1* mutations, at least 100 bp of flanking intronic sequence was determined for each *FGD1* intron.[61] Sequence and cDNA PCR amplification analyses showed that *FGD1* transcripts are alternatively spliced. A comparative analysis of *FGD1* cDNAs showed that, relative to clones derived from fetal craniofacial bones, cDNAs derived from fetal brain contain an alternatively spliced sixth exon that effectively removes nucleotides 2095 to 2202 of the full-length *FGD1* transcript.[61] DNA sequence analysis predicted that the alternative *FGD1* transcript encodes an abbreviated FGD1 protein that lacks 36 amino acid residues of the N-terminal Cdc42GEF

domain. Microinjection studies show that in contrast to the full-length GEF domain, the *FGD1* GEF domain containing the alternatively spliced sixth exon fails to activate Cdc42[39] (see Fig. 247-5). PCR amplification studies show that the alternatively spliced *FGD1* transcript is present in a limited number of tissues including placenta and brain.[61] However, the functional significance of the alternatively spliced transcript remains to be determined.

Although a limited number of *FGD1* mutations have been identified to date, each of the identified mutations was unique, and a high degree of mutation heterogeneity was identified. The FGDY-specific X;8 chromosome translocation was shown to result in a reciprocal translocation disrupting the first exon of the *FGD1* gene within the ORF; no detectable deletion of the *FGD1* locus was identified.[25] Two insertional *FGD1* mutations have been identified within families segregating X-linked FGDY; both are predicted to result in a premature truncation of the FGD1 protein. The first involved the insertion of an additional guanine residue at nucleotide 2122 within exon 7[25] (Fig. 247-8). Dagfinn Aarskog has shown that the insertion of a cytosine residue at nucleotide 1249 is the *FGD1* mutation segregating in the originally reported Aarskog syndrome family.[62] All these mutations are predicted to result in null *FGD1* alleles and a complete loss of FGD1 function. Others have reported an *FGD1* missense mutation involving a guanine-to-adenosine transition at nucleotide 2296 resulting in a change of amino acid residue 522 from arginine to histidine.[63] This mutation is predicted to change a strongly conserved region

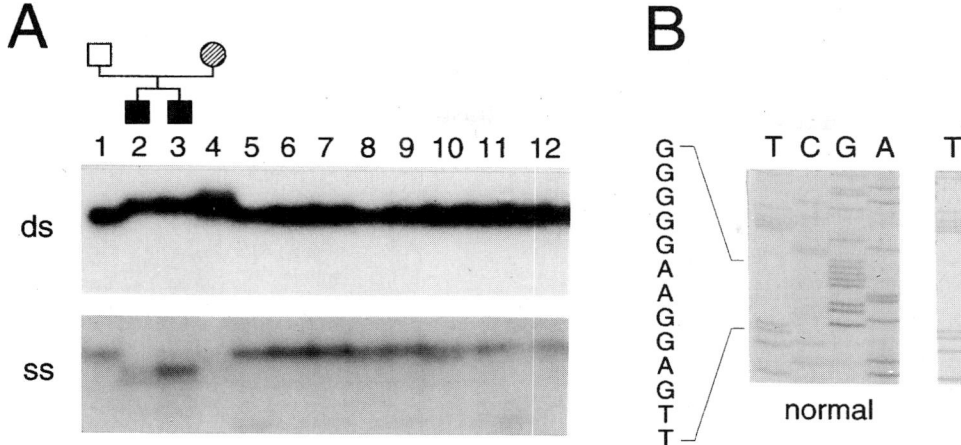

**Fig. 247-8 Single-stranded conformational polymorphism (SSCP) analysis detects an *FGD1* mutation in an Aarskog-Scott syndrome patient. (A) Double-stranded (ds) and single-stranded (ss) exon 7 *FGD1* PCR amplification products are shown. Lanes 1–4 contain products derived from members of a family segregating Aarskog-Scott syndrome; products of the normal father, the obligate carrier mother, and the two affected brothers (TS and CS) are in lanes 1, 4, 2, and 3, respectively. Lane 5 contains the products of a normal male;** lanes 6-10 contain the products of unrelated Aarskog-Scott patients; and lanes 11 and 12 contain products derived from cDNA and genomic DNA clones, respectively. **(B) Sequence analysis of the products amplified from a normal male and the Aarskog-Scott syndrome affected male CS. Compared with the normal sequence, the product of CS has an additional guanine residue, indicated by a star, inserted at nucleotide 2122, resulting in a frameshift mutation. (From Pasteris et al.[25] Used with permission of Cell.)**

of the RhoGEF domain, a change likely to result in a complete loss of function. To date, all *FGD1* mutations are predicted to result in the loss of function of the FGD1 Cdc42GEF domain.

Based on these studies, molecular diagnosis can now be offered to families with X-linked FGDY in which a specific mutation has been identified. In families in which a mutation has not yet been identified, male individuals can be tested for deletions by Southern blotting, using *FGD1* cDNA as a probe before proceeding to sequence-based mutation detection. Patients with FGDY displaying complex phenotypes should undergo chromosome analysis, and their DNA should be tested with *FGD1* and other Xp11.21 DNA markers to detect a contiguous gene syndrome. For X-linked FGDY patients without detectable deletions, a direct analysis of the *FGD1* gene should be performed using primers designed to PCR amplify *FGD1* exons to directly sequence amplified male FGDY DNA.

## MOLECULAR PATHOPHYSIOLOGY OF AARSKOG-SCOTT SYNDROME

Identified *FGD1* mutations are predicted to result in null *FGD1* alleles and loss of FGD1 function; therefore, a constitutive loss of FGD1 Cdc42GEF activity appears to result in the FGDY phenotype. In *S. cerevisiae*, *S. pombe*, *Drosophila melanogaster*, and *C. elegans*, the loss of RhoGEF activity is functionally equivalent to loss of the target Rho protein.[29] Although in vitro biochemical studies suggest that FGD1 is but one of at least several Cdc42 activators,[30,39] it is logical to hypothesize that within cells expressing the *FGD1* gene, *FGD1* mutations will alter or perturb the Cdc42 signaling pathway. Therefore, it is likely that an examination of the molecular biology of Cdc42 and the other Rho proteins will illuminate the biologic role of FGD1 signaling in human morphogenesis.

### Rho GTPases and Regulation of the Actin Cytoskeleton

The ability of eukaryotic cells to maintain or modify their shape and their degree of attachment to a substratum in response to extracellular signals is largely dependent on the organization and rearrangements of the actin cytoskeleton.[64] Regulated changes in the actin cytoskeleton are required for cellular differentiation, cell motility, cell-cell interactions, and tissue morphogenesis. The eukaryotic actin cytoskeleton is composed of actin filaments and specific actin-associated proteins.[65–67] Filamentous actin is generally organized into one of several characteristic structures; these structures and their biologic functions are listed in Table 247-2. Filopodia are thin, motile, finger-like protrusions of long actin filaments that form at the cell periphery; they play an initiating role in changing cell shape and migration. Filopodia provide critical cell-cell contacts for osteocytes.[68] Studies also show that filopodia serve an important sensory function in both migrating fibroblasts[67,69] and neural growth cones.[70] For example, stimulation of a single filopodium can result in the reorientation of an entire growth cone.[71] Lamellipodia are thin protrusive actin sheets located at the edges of motile cells. Actin stress fibers are composed of bundles of actin filaments that traverse the cell; they are linked to the extracellular matrix through focal adhesions.

Rho proteins play a critical role in regulation of the actin cytoskeleton. Rho proteins (and their activators) regulate cell shape, adhesion, and migration, properties critical to tissue morphogenesis. When constitutively active forms are expressed in cells, Rho proteins elicit distinctive actin-associated membrane complexes. Rac stimulates the formation of lamellipodia and cell ruffles, and Rho stimulates the formation of focal adhesions and cortical stress fibers.[72–74] In contrast, activated Cdc42 stimulates the formation of filopodia, or microspikes.[75,76] Furthermore, experiments show that Rho proteins are sequentially activated in a hierarchical cascade: Cdc42 activates Rac, which in turn activates Rho[75] (Fig. 247-9). However, it remains to be determined how the Rho activation cascade is regulated.

### Rho GTPases and Transcriptional Regulation

Mammalian Rho proteins also regulate mitogen-activated protein kinase (MAPK) signaling cascades.[77] Kinases belonging to the MAPK family are used throughout evolution to control cellular responses to external signals such as growth factors, inductive signals, and nutrient status; MAPKs have received particular attention because many of these kinases translocate to the cell nucleus to modulate the action of transcription factors.[78] Recent studies show that Cdc42 and Rac activate the JNK/SAPK MAPK cascade.[79,80] In contrast to the p42/44 MAPKs typically activated by Ras, the JNKs are poorly activated by mitogens but strongly

**Table 247-2** Rho Proteins Involved in the Regulation of the Actin Cytoskeleton

| Rho Protein | Actin Complex Type | Biologic Function | Associated Proteins* |
|---|---|---|---|
| Cdc42 | Filopodia | Cell morphology | Vinculin, fimbrin, talin PTK, α-actinin, ERM |
| Rac | Lamellipodia | Cell movement | Talin, fimbrin, integrin, PTK, α-actinin, ERM |
| Rho | Focal adhesion | Cell adhesion | Integrin, vinculin, talin, PTK, FAK, tensin, paxillin, zyxin, ERM, α-actinin |
| Rho | Cortical stress fiber | Cell morphology | Fodrin-spectrin, ankyrin, PTK, adhesion molecules |

*Known to comprise an actin-associated membrane complex; PTK, protein tyrosine kinase; FAK, focal adhesion kinase; ERM, ezrin, radixin, and moesin.

SOURCE: Adapted from Gorski.[5] Used with permission of Humana Press.

activated by inflammatory cytokines, tumor necrosis factor-α (TNF-α), interleukin-1β (IL-1β), and a diverse array of cellular stressors such as ultraviolet and ionizing radiation and heat shock.[81] Cdc42 appears to activate this cascade through the GTP-dependent activation of the serine/threonine kinases MLK3 and MEKK4.[82–85] In contrast, Rho is required for modulating gene transcription through the serum response factor.[86] JNK phosphorylates the N-terminus of c-Jun and other transcription factors such as ATF-2 and TCF/Elk1. The c-Fos protein interacts with c-Jun to form the AP-1 transcription factor; c-Jun also interacts with ATF-2 and other members of the ATF family to form additional transcription factors.[78] JNK modifies the AP-1 transcription factor

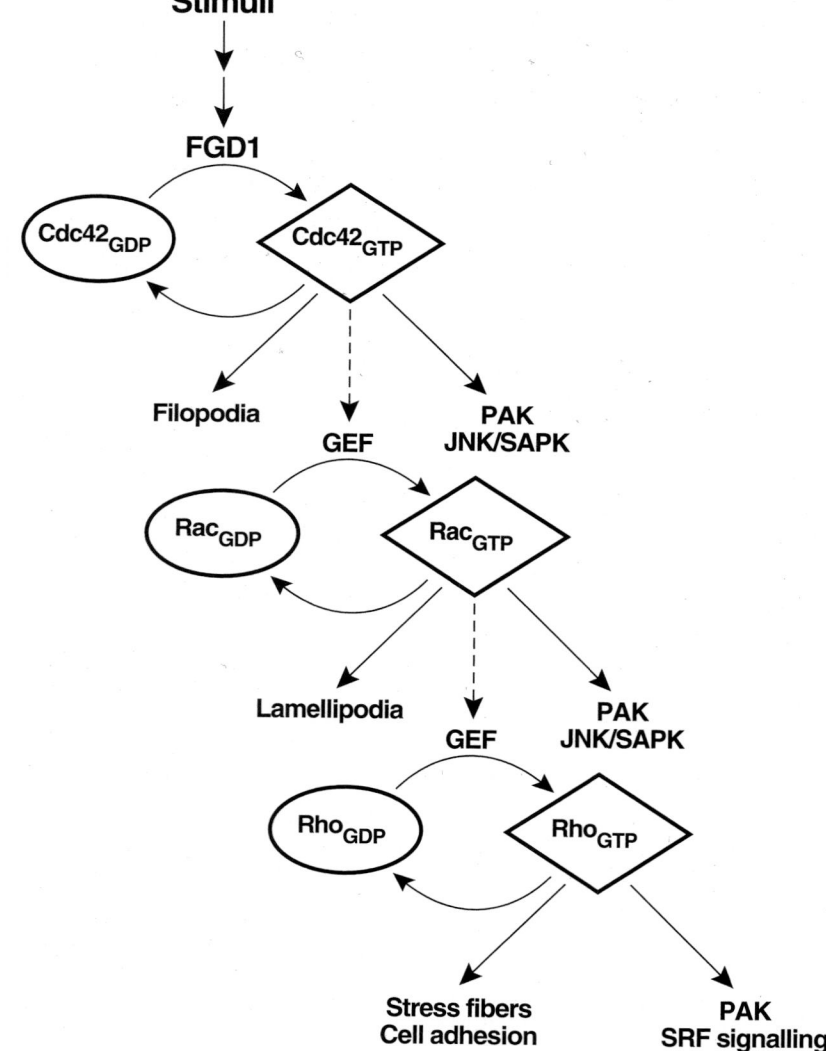

Fig. 247-9 Rho protein family members are activated in a hierarchical cascade. The activation of Cdc42 by FGD1 leads to the sequential activation of Rac and Rho.[39] Activated Cdc42 results in the formation of filopodia, whereas activated Rac leads to the formation of lamellipodia; activated Rho results in the formation of actin stress fibers and focal adhesions. Cdc42 and Rac activate the JNK/SAPK MAPK cascade via the Ser/Thr kinase PAK; Rho is required for signaling via PAK to modulate gene transcription through the serum response factor (SRF). (*Adapted from Gorski.[5] Used with permission of Humana Press.*)

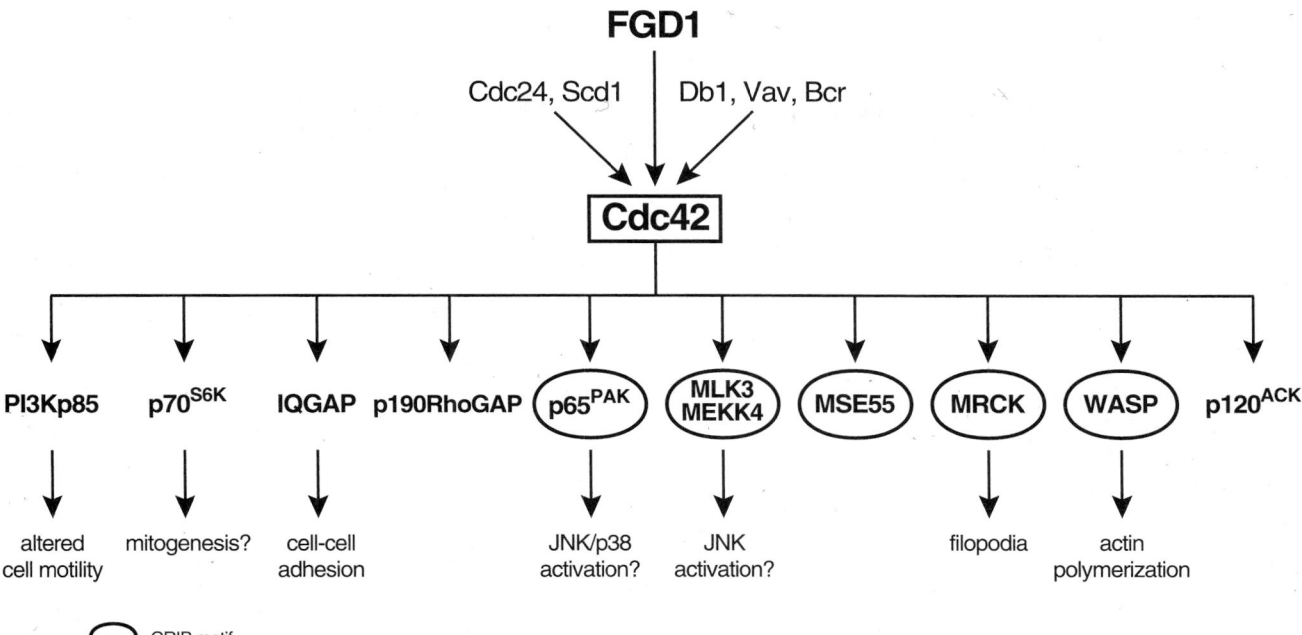

**Fig. 247-10** A variety of proteins interact with Cdc42. Biochemical in vitro studies show that a number of different RhoGEFs activate Cdc42, including FGD1, Cdc24, and the *S. pombe* homologue Scd1, Dbl, Vav, and Bcr.[30] Cdc42 interacts with a variety of targets and potential effector proteins (see text). Ovals indicate those proteins which interact with Cdc42 via a Cdc42/Rac interactive binding (CRIB) motif.[86]

through phosphorylation of c-Jun; furthermore, JNK phosphorylation of TCF/Elk1 also may enhance or modify AP-1 activation. Many types of cellular stress, including genotoxic stress, activate AP-1. Altering the tightly regulated activity of AP-1 may cause a variety of cellular abnormalities such as oncogenic transformation or apoptosis.[78]

In addition to the MLK3 and MEKK4 kinases, Cdc42 has been shown to interact with a diversity of proteins (Fig. 247-10). Some of these proteins have been shown to interact with Cdc42 through an evolutionarily conserved 18-amino-acid motif termed a *Cdc42/ Rac interactive binding (CRIB) domain*.[87] In addition to the kinases MLK3 and MEKK4, several other proteins interact with Cdc42 via a CRIB domain, including the mammalian proteins MSE55 and MRCK,[87] the actin-associated protein that is defective in Wiskott-Aldrich syndrome (WASP),[88] and the family of serine/ threonine p21-Cdc42/Rac-activated kinases termed *PAKs*.[89,90] Cdc42 also interacts with a variety of proteins that do not contain a CRIB motif, such as the 85-kDa regulatory subunit of mammalian phosphatidylinositol-3 kinase and the 190-kDa Rho GTPase-activating protein p190RhoGAP.[28] Cdc42 binds to IQGAP, a protein that contains a calmodulin-binding domain and plays a role in mediating cell-cell adhesion.[91] In addition, Cdc42 binds to and activates the 70-kDa S6 kinase, a kinase involved in cell cycle regulation.[92] Cdc42 also binds to and is inhibited by a nonreceptor tyrosine kinase termed *activated Cdc42Hs-associated kinase* (ACK).[93] However, within a given cell, it remains to be determined how many of the known Cdc42-interacting proteins are expressed and how the many potential Cdc42 interactions are regulated.

## Rho GTPases and Embryonic Development

Several lines of evidence indicate that Rho signal transduction is critical to metazoan embryogenesis. In *Drosophila, Cdc42* and *Rac1* dominant-negative mutations result in a variety of developmental defects including anomalies in the axonal and dendritic outgrowth of peripheral neurons and abnormal myoblast fusion.[94] *Cdc42* and *Rac1* mutations result in distinct phenotypes during the development of the fruit fly, results suggesting that different Rho proteins play distinct roles during development. *Cdc42* also has

been shown to play a critical role in the dorsal closure of the epidermis during fly development, a process in which the lateral epidermal cells migrate over the amnioserosa of the developing embryo to join at the dorsal midline.[95,96] The expression of dominant-negative *Cdc42* and *Rac1* alleles in a subset of imaginal disk epithelial cells has shown that these mutants have specific and nonoverlapping roles in disk development. Within these cells, Cdc42 controls epithelial cell shape changes by modulating the actin cytoskeleton during pupal and larval development.[97] In addition, Cdc42 has been shown to play an important role in wing development in the regulation of actin processes involved in the formation of epithelial wing hairs.[98] Cdc42 is also required for multiple processes during fly oogenesis including the actin-dependent transfer of nurse cell cytoplasm into the oocyte.[94] Not suprisingly, *Drosophila* RhoGEF mutations also have been associated with the regulation of cell morphology and a variety of developmental abnormalities during gastrulation.[99,100] In *C. elegans*, RhoGEF mutations have been shown to result in abnormal skeletal muscle differentiation,[101] and Rho GTPase mutations have been show to result in neuronal migration abnormalities.[102] Few experiments have been performed to study the developmental significance of Rho signal transduction in vertebrates. However, the observation that transgenic mice carrying dominant-negative *Rac* mutations have developmental defects in neurogenesis similar to those observed in *Drosophila* suggests that Rho signaling plays a critical role in mammalian morphogenesis.[103]

*FGD1* mutations could alter morphogenesis in at least two ways. Since FGD1 stimulates Cdc42 to activate the JNK/SAPK MAPK cascade, consequential to *FGD1* mutations, diminished Cdc42 activity could alter JNK/SAPK activity and critically change patterns of gene transcription. Alternatively, since FGD1 stimulates Cdc42 to modify cellular form, as a result of FGD1 mutations, diminished Cdc42 activity could alter cellular morphology. Since the actin cytoskeleton regulates cell shape, adhesion, and migration, altered patterns of cellular morphology are likely to play a critical role in skeletogenesis. Additional studies will be necessary to determine how *FGD1* mutations perturb human morphogenesis.

## ACKNOWLEDGMENTS

We thank Dr. A. Hall for the photomicrograph of the microinjection studies and Drs. D. Aarskog, C. Hou, and Z. Liu for discussions and communicating information prior to publication. This work is supported, in part, by the March of Dimes-Birth Defects Foundation Basic Sciences Grant 1-93-0326 and National Institutes of Health Grant HD34446 to JLG.

## REFERENCES

1. Aarskog D: A familial syndrome of short stature associated with facial dysplasia and genital anomalies. *J Pediatr* **77**:856, 1970.
2. Scott CI: Unusual facies, joint hypermobility, genital anomaly and short stature: A new dysmorphic syndrome. *Birth Defects* **7**(6):240, 1971.
3. Gorlin RJ, Cohen MM, Levin LS: *Syndromes of the Head and Neck*, 3d ed. New York, Oxford University Press, 1990.
4. Porteous MEM, Goudie DR: Aarskog syndrome. *J Med Genet* **28**:44, 1991.
5. Gorski JL: Aarskog-Scott syndrome, in L Jameson (ed): *Principles of Molecular Medicine*, Totowa, NJ, Humana Press, 1998, p 1039.
6. Hanley WB, McKusick V, Barranci FT: Osteochondritis dissecans and associated malformations in two brothers. *J Bone Joint Surg* **44A**:925, 1967.
7. Ainley RG: Hypertelorism (Greig's syndrome): A case report. *J Pediatr Ophthalmol* **5**:148, 1968.
8. Grier RE, Farrington FH, Kendig R, Mamunes P: Autosomal dominant inheritance of the Aarskog syndrome. *Am J Med Genet* **15**:39, 1983.
9. van de Vooren MJ, Niermeijer MF, Hoogeboom JM: The Aarskog syndrome in a large family, suggestive for autosomal dominant inheritance. *Clin Genet* **24**:439, 1983.
10. Kodama M, Fujimoto S, Namikawa T, Matsuda I: Aarskog syndrome with isolated growth hormone deficiency. *Eur J Pediatr* **135**:273, 1981.
11. Fryns J-P: Aarskog syndrome: The changing phenotype with age. *Am J Med Genet* **43**:420, 1992.
12. Kirkham TH, Milot J, Berman P: Ophthalmic manifestations of Aarskog (facial-digital-genital) syndrome. *Am J Ophthalmol* **79**:441, 1975.
13. Melnick M, Shields ED: Aarskog syndrome: New oral-facial findings. *Clin Genet* **9**:20, 1976.
14. Fernandez I, Tsukahara M, Mito H, Yoshii H, Uchida M, Matsuo K, Kajii T: Congenital heart defects in Aarskog syndrome. *Am J Med Genet* **50**:318, 1994.
15. Hassinger DD, Mulvihill JJ, Chandler JB: Aarskog syndrome with Hirschsprung's disease, midgut malrotation, and dental anomalies. *J Med Genet* **17**:235, 1980.
16. Fryns J-P: Dolichomegasigmoid in Aarskog syndrome. *Am J Med Genet* **45**:122, 1993.
17. Taybi H: *Radiology of Syndromes and Metabolic Disorders*, 2d ed. Chicago, Year Book Medical Publishers, 1983.
18. Teebi AS, Rucquoi JK, Meyn MS: Aarskog syndrome: Report of a family with review and discussion of nosology. *Am J Med Genet* **46**:501, 1993.
19. Fryns J-P, Kleczkowska A, Kenis H, Decock P, van den Berghe H: Partial duplication of the short arm of chromosome 2 [dup(2)(p13–p21)] associated with mental retardation and an Aarskog-like phenotype. *Ann Genet* **32**:174, 1989.
20. Bawle E, Tyrkus M, Lipman S, Bozimowski D: Aarskog syndrome: Full male and female expression associated with an X-autosome translocation. *Am J Med Genet* **17**:595, 1984.
21. Porteous MEM, Curtis A, Lindsay S, Williams O, Goudie D, Kamakari S, Bhattacharya SS: The gene for Aarskog syndrome is located between DXS255 and DXS566 (Xp11.2-Xq13). *Genomics* **14**:298, 1992.
22. Stevenson RE, May M, Arena JF, Millar EA, Scott CI Jr, Schroer RJ, Simensen RJ, et al.: Aarskog-Scott syndrome: Confirmation of linkage to the pericentric region of the X chromosome. *Am J Med Genet* **52**:339, 1994.
23. Glover TW, Verga V, Rafael J, Gorski JL, Bawle E, Higgins JV: Translocation breakpoint in Aarskog syndrome maps to Xp11.21 between ALAS2 and DXS323. *Hum Mol Genet* **10**:1717, 1993.
24. Gorski JL, Boehnke M, Reyner EL, Burright EN: A radiation hybrid map of the proximal short arm of the human X chromosome spanning incontinentia pigmenti 1 (IP1) translocation breakpoints. *Genomics* **14**:657, 1992.
25. Pasteris NG, Cadle A, Logie LJ, Porteous MEM, Schwartz CE, Stevenson RE, Glover TW, et al.: Isolation and characterization of the faciogenital dysplasia (Aarskog-Scott syndrome) gene: A putative rho/rac guanine nucleotide exchange factor. *Cell* **79**:669, 1994.
26. Pasteris NG, de Gouyon B, Cadle AB, Campbell K, Herman GE, Gorski JL: Cloning and regional localization of the mouse faciogenital dysplasia (*Fgd1*) gene. *Mam Genome* **6**:658, 1995.
27. Hieter P, Boguski M: Functional genomics: It's all how you read it. *Science* **278**:601, 1997.
28. Van Aelst L, D'Souza-Schorey C: Rho GTPases and signaling networks. *Genes Dev* **11**:2295, 1997.
29. Boguski MS, McCormick F: Proteins regulating *Ras* and its relatives. *Nature* **366**:643, 1993.
30. Cerione RA, Zheng Y: The *Dbl* family of oncogenes. *Curr Opin Cell Biol* **8**:216, 1996.
31. Eva A, Aaronson SA: Isolation of a new human oncogene from a diffuse B-cell lymphoma. *Nature* **316**:273, 1985.
32. Ron D, Zannini M, Lewis M, Wickner RB, Hunt LT, Graziani G, Tronick SR, et al.: A region of proto-*dbl* essential for its transforming activity shows sequence similarity to a yeast cell cycle gene, *CDC24*, and the human breakpoint cluster gene, *bcr*. *New Biol* **3**:372, 1991.
33. Hart MJ, Eva A, Evans T, Aaronson SA, Cerione RA: Catalysis of guanine nucleotide exchange on the CDC42Hs protein by the *dbl* oncogene product. *Nature* **354**:311, 1991.
34. Hart MJ, Eva A, Zangrilli D, Aaronson SA, Evans T, Cerione RA, Zheng Y: Cellular transformation and guanine nucleotide exchange activity are catalyzed by a common domain on the *Dbl* oncogene product. *J Biol Chem* **269**:62, 1994.
35. Boriack-Sjodin PA, Margarit SM, Bar-Sagi D, Kuriyan J: The structural basis of the activation of *Ras* by Sos. *Nature* **394**:337, 1998.
36. Cherfils J, Menetrey J, Mathieu M, Le Bras G, Robineau S, Beraud-Dufour S, Antonny B, et al.: Structure of the Sec7 domain of the Arf exchange factor ARNO. *Nature* **392**:101, 1998.
37. Mossessova E, Gulbis JM, Goldberg J: Structure of the guanine nucleotide exchange factor Sec7 domain of human ARNO and analysis of the interaction with Arf GTPase. *Cell* **92**:415, 1998.
38. Zheng Y, Fischer DJ, Tigyi, G, Pasteris NG, Gorski JL, Xu Y: The faciogenital dysplasia gene product FGD1 functions as a Cdc42Hs-specific guanine-nucleotide exchange factor. *J Biol Chem* **271**:33169, 1996.
39. Olsen MF, Pasteris NG, Gorski JL, Hall A: Faciogenital dysplasia protein (FGD1) and Vav, two related proteins required for normal embryonic development, are upstream regulators of Rho GTPases. *Curr Biol* **6**:1628, 1996.
40. Mayer BJ, Ren R, Clark KL, Baltimore D: A putative modular domain present in diverse signaling proteins. *Cell* **73**:629, 1993.
41. Lemmon MA, Ferguson KM, Schlessinger J: PH domains: Diverse sequences with a common fold recruit signaling molecules to the cell surface. *Cell* **85**:621, 1996.
42. Harlan JE, Hajduk PJ, Yoon HS, Fesik SW: Pleckstrin homology domains bind to phosphatidylinositol-4,5-biphosphate. *Nature* **371**:168, 1994.
43. Touhara K, Inglese J, Pitcher JA, Shaw G, Lefkowitz RJ: Binding of G protein beta gamma-subunits to pleckstrin homology domains. *J Biol Chem* **269**:10217, 1994.
44. Kavanaugh WM, Turck CW, Williams LT: PTB domain binding to signaling proteins through a sequence motif containing phosphotyrosine. *Science* **268**:1177, 1995.
45. Zheng Y, Zangrilli D, Cerione RA, Eva A: The pleckstrin homology domain mediates transformation by oncogenic *dbl* through specific intracellular targeting. *J Biol Chem* **271**:19017, 1996.
46. Li N, Batzer A, Daly R, Yajnik V, Skolnik E, Chardin P, Bar-Sagi D, et al.: Guanine-nucleotide-releasing factor hSos1 binds to Grb2 and links receptor tyrosine kinases to Ras signaling. *Nature* **363**:85, 1993.
47. Ren R, Mayer BJ, Cicchetti P, Baltimore D: Identification of a ten-amino acid proline-rich SH3 binding site. *Science* **259**:1157, 1993.
48. Rozakis-Adcock M, Fernley R, Wade J, Pawson T, Bowtell D: The SH2 and SH3 domains of mammalian Grb2 couple the EGF receptor to the Ras activator mSos1. *Nature* **363**:83, 1993.
49. Gaullier J-M, Simonsen A, D'Arrigo A, Bremnes B, Stenmark H: FYVE fingers bind PtdIns(3)P. *Nature* **394**:432, 1998.
50. Weisman LS, Wickner W: Molecular characterization of *VAC1*, a gene required for vacuole inheritance and vacuole protein sorting. *J Biol Chem* **267**:618, 1992.
51. Piper RC, Cooper AA, Yang H, Stevens TH: VPS27 controls vacuolar and endocytic traffic through a prevacuolar compartment in *Saccharomyces cerevisiae*. *J Cell Biol* **131**:603, 1995.

52. Yamamoto A, DeWald DB, Boronenkov IV, Anderson RA, Emr SD, Koshland D: Novel PI(4)P 5-kinase homologue, Fab1p, essential for normal vacuole function and morphology in yeast. *Mol Biol Cell* **6**:525, 1995.
53. Bean AJ, Seifert R, Chen YA, Sacks R, Scheller RH: Hrs-2 is an ATPase implicated in calcium-regulated secretion. *Nature* **385**:826, 1997.
54. Simonsen A, Lippe R, Christoforidis S, Gaullier J-M, Brech A, Callaghan J, Toh B-H, et al.: EEA1 links PI(3)K function to Rab5 regulation of endosome fusion. *Nature* **394**:494, 1998.
55. Burd CG, Emr SD: Phosphatidylinositol(3)-phosphate signaling mediated by specific binding to RING FYVE domains. *Mol Cell* **2**:157, 1998.
56. Gorski JL, Estrada L, Hu C, Liu Z: Skeletal-specific expression of *Fgd1* during bone formation and skeletal defects in faciogenital dysplasia (FGDY; Aarskog syndrome). *Dev Dyn* **218**:573, 2000.
57. Erlebacher A, Filvaroff EH, Gitelman SE, Derynck R: Toward a molecular understanding of skeletal development. *Cell* **80**:371, 1995.
58. Hall BK, Miyake T: The membranous skeleton: The role of cell condensations in vertebrate skeletogenesis. *Anat Embryol* **186**:107, 1992.
59. Escobar V, Weaver DD: Aarskog syndrome: New findings and genetic analysis. *JAMA* **240**:2638, 1978.
60. Cotter PD, Willard HF, Gorski JL, Bishop DF: Assignment of human erythroid delta-aminolevulinate synthase (ALAS2) to a distal subregion of band Xp11.21 by PCR analysis of somatic cell hybrids containing X;autosome translocations. *Genomics* **13**:211, 1992.
61. Pasteris NG, Buckler JM, Cadle AB, Gorski JL: Genomic organization of the faciogenital dysplasia (*FGD1*; Aarskog syndrome) gene. *Genomics* **43**:390, 1997.
62. Boman H, Knappskog PM, Aarskog D: *FGD1* mutation 1249 ins C in the original Aarskog syndrome family. (In preparation).
63. Neri G, May M, Cappa M, Steindl K, Schwartz C: Second mutation found in the *FGD1* gene causing the Aarskog syndrome. *Am J Hum Genet* **61**:A1998, 1997.
64. Bard J: *Morphogenesis: The Cellular and Developmental Processes of Developmental Anatomy.* Cambridge, England, Cambridge University Press, 1990.
65. Stossel TP: On the crawling of animal cells. *Science* **260**:1086, 1993.
66. Small JV: Lamellipodia architecture: Actin filament turnover and the lateral flow of actin filaments during motility. *Semin Cell Biol* **5**:157, 1994.
67. Zigmond SH: Signal transduction and actin filament organization. *Curr Opin Cell Biol* **8**:66, 1996.
68. Nijweide PJ, Burger EH, Nulend JK, Van der Plas A: The osteocyte, in Bilezikian JP, Raisz LG, Rodan GA (eds): *Principles of Bone Biology.* Boston, Academic Press, 1996.
69. Albrecht-Buehler G: Filopodia of spreading 3T3 cells. *J Cell Biol* **69**:275, 1976.
70. Hynes RO, Lander AD: Contact and adhesive specificities in the associations, migrations, and targeting of cells and axons. *Cell* **68**:303, 1992.
71. O'Connor TP, Duerr JS, Bentley D: Pioneer growth cone steering decisions mediated by single filopodial contacts in situ. *J Neurosci* **10**:3935, 1990.
72. Ridley AJ, Hall A: The small GTP-binding protein rho regulates the assembly of focal adhesions and actin stress fibers in response to growth factors. *Cell* **70**:389, 1992.
73. Ridley AJ, Paterson HF, Johnston CL, Diekmann D, Hall A: The small GTP-binding protein rac regulates growth factor-induced membrane ruffling. *Cell* **70**:401, 1992.
74. Ridley AJ, Hall A: Signal transduction pathways regulating Rho-mediated stress fiber formation: requirement for a tyrosine kinase. *EMBO J* **13**:2600, 1994.
75. Nobes CD, Hall A: Rho, Rac, and Cdc42 GTPases regulate the assembly of multimolecular focal complexes associated with actin stress fibers, lamellipodia, and filopodia. *Cell* **81**:53, 1995.
76. Kozma R, Ahmed S, Best A, Lim L: The Ras-related protein Cdc42 and bradykinin promote formation of peripheral actin microspikes and filopodia in Swiss 3T3 fibroblasts. *Mol Cell Biol* **15**:1942, 1995.
77. Vojtek AB, Cooper JA: Rho family members: Activators of MAP kinase cascades. *Cell* **82**:527, 1995.
78. Treisman R: Regulation of transcription by MAP kinase cascades. *Curr Opin Cell Biol* **8**:205, 1996.
79. Coso OA, Chiariello M, Yu J-C, Teranoto H, Crespo P, Xu N, et al.: The small GTP-binding proteins Rac1 and Cdc42 regulate the activity of the JNK/SAPK signaling pathway. *Cell* **81**:1137, 1995.
80. Minden A, Lin A, Claret F-X, Abo A, Karin M: Selective activation of the JNK signaling cascade and c-Jun transcriptional activity by the small GTPases Rac and Cdc42Hs. *Cell* **81**:1147, 1995.
81. Kyriakis JM, Avruch J: Protein kinase cascades activated by stress and inflammatory cytokines. *Bioessays* **18**:567, 1996.
82. Gallo KA, Mark MR, Scadden DT, Wang Z, Gu Q, Godowski PJ: Identification and characterization of SPRK, a novel Src-homology 3 domain-containing proline-rich kinase with serine/threonine kinase activity. *J Biol Chem* **269**:15092, 1994.
83. Teramoto H, Coso OA, Miyata H, Igishi T, Miki T, Gutkind JS: Signaling from the small GTP-binding proteins Rac1 and Cdc42 to the c-Jun N-terminal kinase/stress activated protein kinase pathway: A role for mixed lineage kinase 3/protein-tyrosine kinase 1, a novel member of the mixed lineage kinase family. *J Biol Chem* **271**:27225, 1996.
84. Tibbles LA, Ing YL, Kiefer F, Chan J, Iscove N, Woodgett JR, Lassam NJ: MLK3 activates the SAPK/JNK and p38/RK pathways via SEK1 and MKK3/6. *EMBO J* **15**:7026, 1996.
85. Gerwins P, Blank JL, Johnson GL: Cloning of a novel mitogen-activated protein kinase kinase kinase, MEKK4, that selectively regulates the c-Jun amino terminal kinase pathway. *J Biol Chem* **272**:8288, 1997.
86. Hill CS, Wynne J, Treisman R: The Rho family GTPases RhoA, Rac1, and Cdc42Hs regulate transcriptional activation by SRF. *Cell* 81:1159, 1995.
87. Burbelo PD, Dreschel D, Hall A: A conserved binding motif defines numerous candidate target proteins for both Cdc42 and Rac GTPases. *J Biol Chem* **270**:29071, 1995.
88. Symons M, Derry JM, Karlak B, Jiang S, Lemahieu V, Mccormick F, Francke U, Abo A: Wiskott-Aldrich syndrome protein, a novel effector for the GTPase Cdc42Hs, is implicated in actin polymerization. *Cell* **84**:723, 1996.
89. Manser E, Leung T, Salihuddin H, Zhao Z, Lim L: A brain serine/threonine protein kinase activated by Cdc42 and Rac1. *Nature* **367**:40, 1994.
90. Manser E, Chong C, Zhao Z, Leung T, Michaels G, Hall C, Lim L: Molecular cloning of a new member of the p21-Cdc42/Rac-activated kinase (PAK) family. *J Biol Chem* **270**:25070, 1995.
91. Kuroda S, Fukata M, Nakagawa M, Fujii K, Nakamura T, Ookubo T, Izawa I, et al.: Role of IQGAP1, a target of the small GTPases Cdc42 and Rac1, in regulation of E-cadherin-mediated cell-cell adhesion. *Science* **281**:832, 1998.
92. Chou M, Blenis J: The 70 kD S6 kinase complexes with and is activated by the Rho family G proteins Cdc42 and Rac1. *Cell* **85**:573, 1996.
93. Manser E, Leung T, Salihuddin H, Tan L, Lim L: A non-receptor tyrosine kinase that inhibits the GTPase activity of p21cdc42. *Nature* **363**:364, 1993.
94. Luo L, Liao YJ, Jan LY, Jan YN: Distinct morphogenetic functions of similar small GTPases: *Drosophila* Drac1 is involved in axonal outgrowth and myoblast fusion. *Genes Dev* **8**:1787, 1994.
95. Riesgo-Escovar JR, Jenni M, Fritz A, Hafen E: The *Drosophila* Jun-N-terminal kinase is required for cell morphogenesis but not for DJun-dependent cell fate specification in the eye. *Genes Dev* **10**:2759, 1996.
96. Glise B, Noselli S: Coupling of Jun amino-terminal kinase and decapentaplegic signaling pathways in *Drosophila* morphogenesis. *Genes Dev* **11**:1738, 1997.
97. Eaton S, Auvinen P, Lou L, Jan YN, Simons K: CDC42 and Rac1 control different actin-dependent processes in the *Drosophila* wing disc epithelium. *J Cell Biol* **131**:151, 1995.
98. Eaton S, Wepf R, Simons K: Roles for Rac1 and CDC42 in planar polarization and hair outgrowth in the wing of *Drosophila*. *J Cell Biol* **135**:1277, 1996.
99. Barrett K, Leptin M, Settleman J: The Rho GTPase and a putative RhoGEF mediate a signaling pathway for the cell shape changes in *Drosophila* gastrulation. *Cell* **91**:905, 1997.
100. Hacker U, Perrimon N: DRhoGEF2 encodes a member of the *Dbl* family of oncogenes and controls cell shape changes during gastrulation in *Drosophila*. *Genes Dev* **12**:274, 1998.
101. Benian GM, Tinley TL, Tang X, Borodovsky M: The *Caenorhabditis elegans* gene *unc-89*, required for muscle M-line assembly, encodes a giant modular protein composed of Ig and signal transduction domains. *J Cell Biol* **32**:835, 1996.
102. Zipkin ID, Kindt RM, Kenyon CJ: Role of a new Rho family member in cell migration and axon guidance in *C. elegans*. *Cell* **90**:883, 1997.
103. Luo L, Hensch TK, Ackerman L, Barbel S, Jan LY, Jan YN: Different effects of the Rac GTPase on Purkinje cell axons and dendritic trunks and spines. *Nature* **379**:837, 1996.

# 248

# Rubinstein-Taybi Syndrome

Fred Petrij ■ Rachel H. Giles

Martijn H. Breuning ■ Raoul C.M. Hennekam

1. The Rubinstein-Taybi syndrome (RTS) is a well-defined syndrome with a characteristic face, broad thumbs, broad big toes, and mental retardation as its major clinical hallmarks. RTS is generally a *de novo*-occurring autosomal dominant trait. The empirical recurrence risk for a couple with a previous child with RTS is as low as 0.1 percent. If, however, a person with RTS is able to reproduce, the recurrence risk could be as high as 50 percent. Birth prevalence is 1 in 100,000 to 125,000. RTS has been described in populations of many different ancestries, but the number of reports on non-Caucasian patients is low.

2. The main clinical features of the syndrome are abnormalities of the face, thumbs, and big toes, as well as growth and mental retardation. The facial appearance is striking: microcephaly, downslanting palpebral fissures, broad nasal bridge, beaked nose with the nasal septum extending below the alae, highly arched palate, and mild micrognathia. Broad thumbs and broad big toes are present in almost all cases. Terminal broadening of the phalanges of the fingers, persistent fetal pads, clinodactyly of the fifth finger, overlapping of the toes, and angulation deformities of the thumbs and halluces can also be present. There is a marked growth retardation with poor weight gain during infancy, often replaced by being overweight in later childhood. Global mental deficiency is characteristic with an average IQ between 35 and 50. Short attention span, poor coordination, and sudden mood changes characterize the behavior of RTS patients. Other findings may include eye anomalies (nasolacrimal duct obstruction, ptosis of eyelids, congenital or juvenile glaucoma, and refractive errors), specific dental anomalies (talon cusps of the permanent incisors), a variety of congenital heart defects, and skin anomalies (supernumerary nipples, nevus flammeus, hirsutism, and keloid formation). The clinical history often shows feeding problems and recurrent conjunctivitis in the neonatal period, respiratory problems in the first decade, and life-long constipation. In general, RTS patients are in good health. Although an increased risk for different types of tumors is known, life expectancy seems to be normal.

3. The diagnosis is based on the clinical presentation. Combined cytogenetic and molecular investigations of the CREB-binding protein (CBP) gene area on chromosome 16p13.3 can confirm the diagnosis in 15 to 20 percent of the cases. Gross chromosomal rearrangements such as translocations and inversions are rarely found, whereas microdeletions occur in approximately 10 percent of cases. Point mutations in the *CBP* gene leading to premature translation-termination are reported as well. Heterogeneity is expected, but no reports on involvement of other genes have yet been published.

4. The CREB-binding protein functions as a transcriptional cofactor by forming a physical bridge between the different components of the transcription machinery. It also functions as a potent histone acetyltransferase, making the DNA accessible to transcription factors. Furthermore, it is a mediator of different signaling pathways and participates in basic cellular functions such as DNA repair, cell growth, cell differentiation, apoptosis, and tumor suppression. CBP is at the center of multiple signal transduction pathways and thereby regulates the expression of many genes.

5. Animal models and biochemical evidence suggest that RTS is caused by haploinsufficiency of CBP during fetal development. The exact developmental pathways affected by reduced levels of CBP are unknown. Until the in vivo functionality of CBP is better defined, there is no available treatment for RTS.

## HISTORICAL BACKGROUND

In 1957, three Greek orthopedic surgeons, John Michail, John Matsoukas, and Stamatis Theodorou, described in the French orthopedic journal *Revue d'Orthopedie*, a 7-year-old boy as "a new case of congenital malformations of the thumbs absolutely symmetrical."[1] Other characteristics that the boy featured were "mental deficiency and physical underdevelopment, conical face with long Cyrano-type nose, muscular hypotonia with platypodia, funnel chest, cryptorchidism, and spindle-legs slightly turgid."

In that same year, U.S. pediatrician Jack Rubinstein investigated a 3.5-year-old girl with similar findings in his newly opened Cincinnati Center for Developmental Disorders.[2] In the next 2 years, he recognized 2 other children as probably having the same syndrome. In 1961, pediatric radiologist Hooshang Taybi of Oklahoma sent information, photographs, and x-rays from an additional child to Dr. Rubinstein. Three other children were diagnosed shortly thereafter. Two children with possibly the same entity were sent to Dr. Rubinstein and Dr. Taybi (see Fig. 248-1) by Dr. W.C. Marshal of London. They were at that time dismissed from the study because their thumbs were not radially deviated. Rubinstein and Taybi,[3] who were unaware of the paper by Michail and coworkers, reported in the *American Journal of Diseases of Children* that the seven children might have a new mental retardation syndrome. Matsoukas drew attention to the earlier paper in 1973,[4] and Rubinstein acknowledged their "bibliographic certificate of birth of the syndrome" shortly thereafter.[5] Warkany[6] finalized the discussion about the entity's name; as already dubbed in 1964 by Coffin et al.[7] and Job et al.,[8] the entity was named the Rubinstein-Taybi syndrome (RTS).

## EPIDEMIOLOGY

### Prevalence

Rubinstein-Taybi syndrome is an infrequent disorder. Rubinstein[9] found 11 cases out of 2937 new patients in his Diagnostic Clinic for the Mentally Retarded in Cincinnati, giving a frequency in this population of 1 in 267. Berg et al.[10] found 3 cases in 1600 institutionalized persons in the U.K., a frequency of 1 in 533. Coffin[11] reported 5 cases in 3600 institutionalized persons in

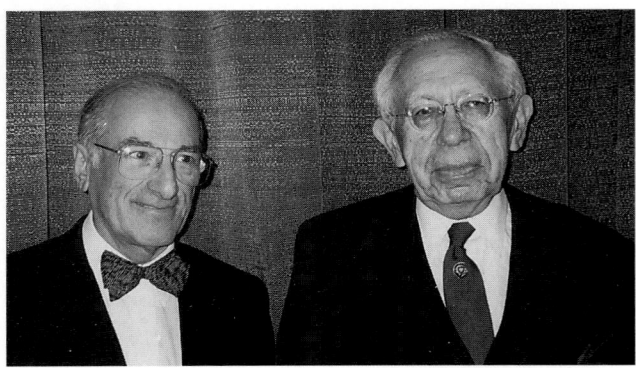

**Fig. 248-1 Hooshang Taybi and Jack H. Rubinstein at the second International Family Conference on RTS, July 1998, Cincinnati, Ohio, USA (*photo: F. Petrij*).**

California, a frequency of 1 in 720. Simpson and Brissenden[12] found 1 case per 300 institutionalized persons in Canada, and calculated a population frequency of about 1 in 300,000. As several patients proved to have a different diagnosis at careful follow-up,[13] these figures are no longer usable. Hennekam et al.[14] estimated a birth prevalence of 1/100,000 to 125,000 in the Netherlands. This figure has proved to be correct for the Netherlands in the period 1988–1998 (Hennekam, unpublished data).

### Ethnic Differences

The syndrome has been observed in Caucasians as well as in people of Asian and African background.[2,14] The number of non-Caucasian patients is low. It remains uncertain whether socio-economic bias, a publication bias, or a true lower incidence causes this. A less marked expression in non-Caucasians, which would make the diagnosis more difficult, does not seem to be the explanation, as the expression of the syndrome in all ethnic groups seems similar (reference 15; Hennekam, unpublished data).

### Mortality Data

There is no well-documented review of the life expectancy or causes of death in the syndrome. Rubinstein[2] mentioned that of the 571 individuals known to him at that time, 44 had died. Mean age at the time of reporting was 4.5 years, ranging from 1 day to 62 years old.[2,14] In a Dutch-American study, the mean ages at reporting were 8.1 years (U.S.A.) and 18.1 years (the Nether-lands), respectively.[14] In 1998, 74 patients were known in the Netherlands, of whom 5 had died in the period 1984–1998: one boy at age 2 weeks because of a congenital heart defect; another boy at 11 years because of intracranial bleeding due to idiopathic thrombocytopenic purpura; a 43-year-old man of pneumonia; a 57-year-old woman of unknown reasons; and a 68-year-old man of a fat embolus after a traumatic fracture of his upper leg (Hennekam, unpublished data). Respiratory tract infections and congenital heart defects are suggested to be the most common causes of death in infants and children.[14] Because malignancies appear to be more frequent in patients with Rubinstein-Taybi syndrome as compared to the general population,[16] this may be a more frequent cause of death. The natural history has otherwise been well documented.[17,18]

## CLINICAL MANIFESTATIONS

### Growth

Length, weight, and head circumference at birth are between the 25th and 50th percentiles.[2,19] Average birth length is 49 cm, with a range of 43.9 to 53.3 cm. Average birth weight is 3.1 kg, with a range of 2.05 to 4.28 kg. Mean head circumference is 34.2 cm

(males) and 32.2 cm (females), with a range of 29 to 38 cm.[19] Poor weight gain during infancy is typical.[19] In a study of serial measurements of 95 patients, it was found that males often become overweight for their height during childhood, while females are overweight during adolescence.[19] Several of the patients were noted to have vigorous appetites in late childhood or early adolescence. There are no clues indicating a thyroid malfunction to explain this phenomenon.[20] Values for final height attainment are 153.1 cm for males and 146.7 cm for females.[19] Mean head circumference at adulthood is 54.7 cm (males) and 52.4 cm (females). Endocrine studies showing a growth hormone deficiency have never been reported.

### Performance and Central Nervous System

Global mental deficiency is characteristic of RTS.[21] The average IQ is reported as 51 (range: 33 to 72; $n = 37$)[18] or 36 (range: 25 to 79; $n = 40$).[21] The latter is comparable to values found in older studies of small cohorts.[9,22] The higher values in the first study are probably caused by a different study design and a biased patient sample.[21] The performance IQ is generally higher than the verbal IQ.[18,21] At an older age, the full-scale IQ becomes somewhat lower, which is explained by measurement of the different abilities at different ages; for example, deficits in concept formation and more complex language tasks carry more weight in the tests with increasing age.[21] The IQ decline is not caused by a mental deterioration.

Affected individuals tend to be loving, friendly, and easy to get along with, although maladaptive behavior has also been noted. Their temperament remains friendly throughout life, although less so with increasing age.[21] A specific behavioral phenotype has been described,[21] consisting of a short attention span, poor coordination, sudden mood changes, and a preference for being alone. Persistence is low. Crowds or too much noise are especially avoided.[18,21] In adolescence and at an older age, a significant number of patients demonstrate daytime sleepiness.

Despite the high frequency of oral anatomic abnormalities, speech mechanisms and articulation are little impaired. The voice quality may be nasal or highly pitched, and some patients have a rapid speech rhythm. Their vocabulary is small and in agreement with the general IQ.[21] Despite their limited verbal abilities, their communication skills are good.

Electroencephalographic abnormalities or seizures have been noted in about two-thirds or one-fourth of patients, respectively.[2,17,18,23,24] Other major anomalies such as absence or hypoplasia of the callosal body,[2,7,25–29] Dandy-Walker anomaly,[30,31] hydrocephaly,[2] arrhinencephaly,[32] and myelinization defects[29] have been occasionally described. In the Netherlands, several patients are known to have migraines, sometimes starting as early as during childhood (Hennekam, unpublished observations).

### Craniofacial Features

Table 248-1 lists the medical problems associated with RTS.[33] The facial appearance is striking, with microcephaly; prominent forehead; downslanting palpebral fissures; epicanthal folds; strabismus; broad nasal bridge; beaked nose with the nasal septum extending below the alae; highly arched palate; and mild micrognathia. The features are recognizable in the newborn. Allanson[34] and Hennekam[17,35] have studied facial changes that occur over time. Grimacing or an unusual smile has been observed almost universally. Other findings may include long eyelashes; nasolacrimal duct obstruction; ptosis of eyelids; congenital or juvenile glaucoma; refractive error; and minor abnormalities in the shape, position, and degree of rotation of the ears.[2,3,17,22,24,31,36–43] Low-frequency abnormalities include bifid uvula;[7,23,44–47] submucosal palatal cleft;[46,48–52] bifid tongue;[39,53–56] macroglossia;[57,58] short lingual frenum;[57,59] natal teeth;[60] and thin upper lip.[45]

Talon cusps (markedly enlarged cingulum on maxillary incisor teeth) have been observed in over 90 percent of the patients'

**Table 248-1** Medical Problems in the Rubinstein-Taybi Syndrome[33]

| Feature | Percentage (*n* = 95) |
|---|---|
| Pregnancy | |
|   Gestational length | 39.9 week (range 32–44 weeks) |
|   Polyhydramnios | 30 |
| Infancy history | |
|   Respiratory problems | 51 |
|   Feeding problems | 80 |
|   Constipation | 71 |
|   Poor weight gain | 80 |
| Medical history | |
|   Visual problems | 84 |
|     Strabismus | 58 |
|     Refractive error | 41 |
|     Astigmatism | 18 |
|     Other | 4 |
|   Cataracts | 7 |
|   Glaucoma | 8 |
|   Coloboma | 5 |
|   Tear duct obstruction | 39 |
|   Ptosis | 45 |
|   Hearing loss | 24 |
|   Frequent middle ear infections | 60 |
|   Congenital heart defects | 32 |
|     PDA | 13 |
|     VSD | 12 |
|     ASD | 10 |
|     Coarctation | 3 |
|     Pulmonic stenosis | 2 |
|   Urinary tract infection | 22 |
|   Keloids or hypertrophic scarring | 25 |
|   Severe constipation | 44 |
|   Epilepsy | 23 |

permanent dentition.[45,61,62] Talon cusps are generally only very infrequently found, except in persons of Chinese descent.[63] As talon cusps are also only rarely found in patients with other syndromes,[45] the finding of a talon cusp is a strong clue for the RTS diagnosis. Cephalometric studies[64] showed a shortening of the facial height and depth, cranial base length, a marked decrease in size of the mandible, and a steep cranial base. For several dimensions, a change with age was found. The correlation between most patients was high, although this was less so in the younger patients. Objective evaluation of craniofacial structures[65] showed an equally remarkable concordance of patterns, with children under age 4 years showing some differences.

## Hands and Feet

Broad thumbs and big toes were present in almost all reported cases.[2,17,18] The terminal phalanges of the fingers tend to be broad, too. Persistent fetal pads are common.[17] Clinodactyly of the fifth fingers and overlapping of the toes are present in more than half the patients. Angulation deformities of the thumbs and halluces, together with abnormally shaped proximal phalanges, occur in about 35 percent of patients.[2,17,18,66] Abnormally shaped first metatarsals and duplication of the proximal or distal phalanx of the halluces have also been reported. Rarely noted have been postaxial polydactyly of the feet, partial cutaneous syndactyly involving the toes, and absence of the distal phalanx of the hallux.[2,3,7,17,18,22,38,67] There are no patients with confirmed RTS that have a preaxial polydactyly. The metacarpophalangeal pattern profile may be specific[68] with mild shortening of the third medial phalanx, marked shortening of the first distal phalanx, relatively normal length of the metacarpals, and in patients with a radially deviated thumb, a very short first proximal phalanx. Not all patients show this pattern, however, and in a single patient the profile may change from the specific pattern to a nonspecific pattern.[68]

Alterations in the frequency of various fingerprint patterns have been observed, but the findings have been inconsistent.[2,3,22,23,69–71]

## Skeletal System

Growth retardation and delayed bone age are common. A large anterior fontanel or delay in its closure, large foramen magnum, and parietal foramina have been reported in several patients. Other skeletal anomalies include pectus excavatum; other sternal abnormalities; rib defects; scoliosis; kyphosis; lordosis; spina bifida; flat acetabular angles; slipped capital femoral epiphysis;[72] flaring of ilia; and notched ischia.[2,17] Rubinstein,[2] Robson,[73] and Hennekam[17] have discussed other low-frequency anomalies.

The gait is commonly stiff and sometimes waddling. This may be caused by instability of the pelvis (Hennekam, unpublished observations). In general, lax ligaments, an increased fracture frequency, and hyperextensible joints have also been noted,[2,17] all pointing to a connective tissue disturbance in the syndrome. Patellar dislocation can be burdensome.[17,74,75] Several pubertal patients have severe and prolonged aseptic hip joint inflammations.[33] A tethered cord has been described,[76] but remains uncommon.

## Genitourinary System

Incomplete or delayed descent of the testes has been reported in almost all male patients. Anomalies of the urinary tract may include duplication of the kidney and ureter, renal agenesis, nephrotic syndrome, and other abnormalities.[17,77–79] Urinary tract infections occur in approximately 20 to 25 percent of patients.[17,18] Angulated penis and hypospadias have been rarely noted.[2,17]

## Malignancies

An increased tumor risk has been recognized.[16] The reported tumors include nasopharyngeal rhabdomyosarcoma;[80] intraspinal neurilemoma;[54] pheochromocytoma;[81] meningioma;[17,82] other brain tumors;[14,83–86] pilomatrixoma;[87,88] and acute leukemia.[89] Keloids or hypertrophic scarring has been described in several cases.[17,18,49,51,90,91] The localization of keloids is unremarkable; that is, they form on the upper part of the back, and on the chest, shoulders, and upper arms. Sometimes only minimal trauma such as a bee sting or rubbing by the clothes may instigate keloid formation. The patient shown in Fig. 248-2 has keloids over the sternum and the left scapula.

## Other Physical Findings

A variety of congenital heart defects has been found in about 35 percent of all patients,[2,17,18,56,92] the most common being patent ductus arteriosus and atrial or ventricular septal defects. Abnormal lung lobulation, supernumerary nipples, nevus flammeus of the forehead, nape, or back, and hirsutism (see Fig. 248-2) have been reported.[2,7,17,18,38,93] Although feeding problems are very common in the neonatal period, gastroesophageal reflux[94] is found only occasionally. Compression of the esophagus due to a vascular sling has been reported.[95] A megacolon[17,24] has been found and is probably a complication of severe constipation. Other rare complications are thymus hypoplasia;[32] IgA deficiency;[17,96,97] hyperinsulinemia;[98] bifid uterus and menstruation problems;[99] agenesis of the gallbladder;[100,101] branchial arch anomalies;[17] and congenital fusion of the eyelids (ankyloblepharon filiforme adnatum).[17,18]

Obstructive sleep apnea may cause considerable problems.[17,102] This may be caused by the combination of a narrow palate, micrognathia, hypotonia, and easy collapsibility of the laryngeal walls.[17] In one patient, these complaints necessitated a tracheostomy. In several patients, the easy collapsibility of the laryngeal walls caused problems at intubation. In a single report,

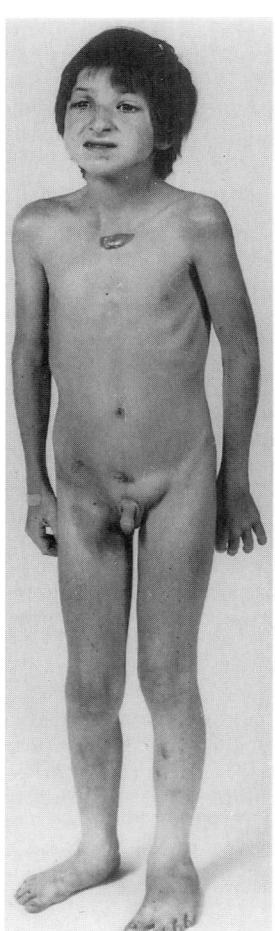 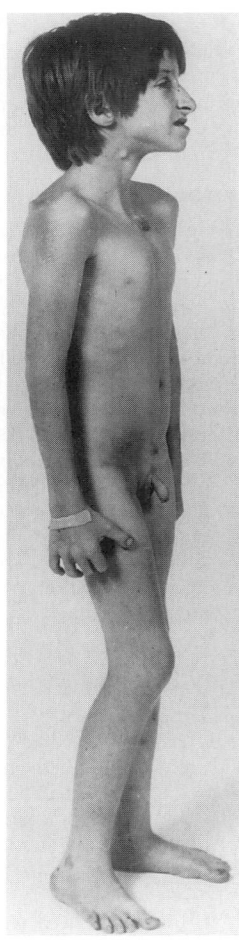 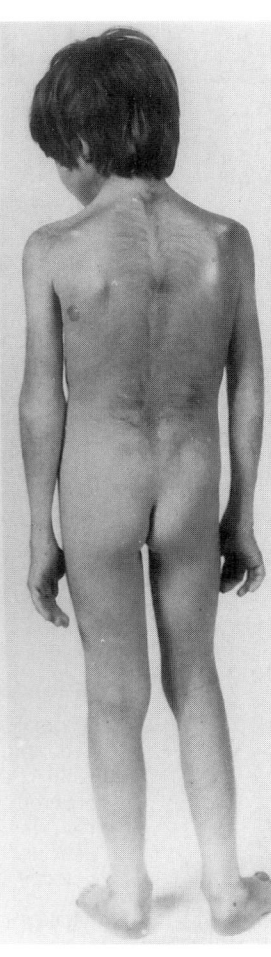

**Fig. 248-2** A 10-year-old boy with RTS. Several of the main RTS features can be seen: typical face with downslanting palpebral fissures; broad nasal bridge; beaked nose and nasal septum below alae; broad thumbs and broad big toes; several keloids (e.g., over the sternum and the left scapula); left inguinal hernia; and hirsutism.

cardiac arrhythmias after administration of a neuromuscular blocking agent (succinylcholine) were described.[103]

## Differential Diagnosis

Although many components of the syndrome may occur as isolated findings or as features of various other syndromes, the overall pattern of anomalies is sufficiently distinctive to permit diagnosis in most instances.[2,14,33] Differential diagnosis can be a problem in the newborn period. Occasionally, some cases of RTS have been confused with De Lange syndrome,[104] Saethre-Chotzen syndrome,[105] or with trisomy 13.[106] The facial features show some resemblance to the Floating-Harbor syndrome and the Gorlin-Chaudry-Moss syndrome.[33] Broad thumbs may be observed in Apert and Pfeiffer syndromes[33] and short thumbs and fingers are seen in Type D brachydactyly and Greig syndrome. A male fetus with anencephaly and a beaked nose, bifid thumbs, and hypoplastic genitalia, thought to resemble the syndrome, was found to have an interstitial deletion of chromosome 7q22.[107] Sharma et al.[108] reported on a father and daughter with a brachydactyly and conspicuous facial features, but the type of brachydactyly was completely different from the type found in Rubinstein-Taybi syndrome, and their development was normal. Three siblings have been described with faintly similar facial features and a very long hallux but other features such as congenital anodontia, almost complete absence of hair, and pigmentation anomalies allow differentiation.[109] Collins et al.[110] described a girl with a Rubinstein-Taybi–like syndrome that differed in the macrocephaly, absence of the low-hanging columellae or typical oral symptoms, normal growth, and normal width of the thumbs. Three sisters from South Africa have been described[111] with a profound mental retardation, microcephaly, short stature, and brachydactyly,

but the facial features were sufficiently different to separate the disorder. Cotsirilos et al.[112] reported a mother and two sibs affected with a Rubinstein-Taybi–like disorder. Six other relatives of the mother were reported to have broad thumbs and halluces. Grix et al.[113] described two sibs with mental retardation, growth delay, microcephaly, and broad thumbs who differed in the hypertonia, bulbous nasal tip, cleft palate, and prominent alveolar ridges. The family with broad thumbs and mental deficiency reported by Robinow[114] probably represents yet another separate entity.

## GENETICS

The Rubinstein-Taybi syndrome is generally a *de novo* occurring autosomal dominant trait. If a person with RTS is able to reproduce, the recurrence risk could be as high as 50 percent, assuming that chromosome anomalies or mutations do not increase the risk for spontaneous abortion.

### Recurrence of RTS

RTS patients seldom reproduce. Only four cases have been reported in the literature. Rohmer et al.[115] described an affected woman who delivered a premature but otherwise healthy and unaffected infant. In three other cases, women likely to be affected with RTS had a child with the syndrome.[116,117,184] In all three cases, the children clearly had more pronounced dysmorphic features and were more mentally retarded than their mothers. The diagnosis in the mothers would have been difficult without the more pronounced phenotype of their children. The fact that all three mothers were able to reproduce is probably related to their relatively mild phenotypes. The mild phenotype can be explained by the variability of the syndrome or could be caused by a somatic mosaicism. Molecular analyses on mother and child were not conclusive. All mothers had at least one unaffected child.[117,118,184]

In 1990, Hennekam et al.[14] re-evaluated all familial cases reported in the literature. Of all reported familial occurrences, only one was regarded as probably genuine. Johnson[93] described an affected brother and sister and, although the boy had a less typical facial "gestalt," the diagnosis seems likely in both children. It was calculated that the empirical recurrence risk is 0.1 percent.[14] For various reasons, the other multigenerational examples of presumed RTS were difficult to confirm.

## Mapping RTS to Chromosome 16p13.3

In 1991, Imaizumi and Kuroki[119] observed a sporadic patient with a *de novo* reciprocal translocation t(2;16)(p13.3;p13.3). Shortly thereafter, Tommerup et al.[120] found an apparently balanced *de novo* reciprocal translocation, t(7;16)(q34;p13.3). For the first time two cases were consistent for one of their breakpoints, namely 16p13.3. All 10 previously reported chromosomal rearrangements, reviewed by Hennekam et al.,[14] were inconsistent with each other. In the same year Lacombe et al.[121] provided confirmation for the assignment of RTS to 16p13.3 by reporting a *de novo* pericentric inversion of one chromosome 16— inv(16)(p13.3;q13).

## Refined Localization of the RTS Locus Between N2 (D16S138) and RT1 (D16S237)

Breuning et al.[122] reported another t(16;20) and investigated the 16p13.3 region by using two-color fluorescence *in situ* hybridization (FISH). The rank order of approximately 80 chromosome 16p cosmids was determined. The breakpoints of the t(2;16) and the t(7;16) mapped between the cosmids N2 (D16S138) and RT1 (D16S237). In the years that followed, an additional four gross of chromosomal rearrangements involving 16p13.3 were discovered. They are summarized in Table 248-2.

In a study analyzing 24 RTS patients with the N2 and RT1 probes, Breuning et al.[122] demonstrated that the RT1 signal was missing from one chromosome 16 in six patients. In five of these patients, the parents were available for FISH studies; none of them showed a deletion of RT1, indicating a *de novo* rearrangement. Hence, they found submicroscopic interstitial deletions within 16p13.3 in one-fourth of the patients. This percentage of microdeletions may have been an overestimation due to small numbers, however. An inventory of all RTS microdeletions published since then[122–127,183] shows that the 16p microdeletion frequency in RTS is more likely to be around 10 percent (see Table 248-3). Clinical features were essentially the same in patients with or without detectable deletions, with the possible exception of microcephaly, angulation of thumbs and halluces, and partial duplication of halluces.[128]

Using molecular markers, Hennekam et al.[128] found a copy of chromosome 16 from both parents in all 19 RTS patients studied, excluding uniparental disomy as a common RTS causative mechanism.

**Table 248-3** Reported RT1 Microdeletion Frequency

| Authors | Year | Patients studied | RT1 microdeletion | % |
|---|---|---|---|---|
| Breuning et al.[122] | 1993 | 24 | 6 | 25 |
| Masuno et al.[124] | 1994 | 25 | 1 | 4 |
| MacGaughran et al.[125] | 1996 | 16 | 2 | 12.5 |
| Wallerstein et al.[126] | 1997 | 64 | 7 | 11 |
| Taine et al.[127] | 1998 | 30 | 3 | 10 |
| Petrij et al.[183] | 2000 | 171 | 14 | 8 |
| Total | | 330 | 33 | 10 |

## Cloning the Region Between N2 and RT1

Chromosomal rearrangements have been repeatedly shown to facilitate the mapping of genes responsible for diseases. In addition to the constitutional rearrangements seen in RTS, the region between N2 and RT1 is also home to somatic chromosomal rearrangements leading to leukemia.[123,129,130] Because Breuning et al.[122] had demonstrated that the chromosomal breakpoints leading to these diseases both map to the area between N2 and RT1, Petrij and Giles embarked upon cloning, respectively, the gene for the Rubinstein-Taybi syndrome and the gene for the acute myeloid leukemia (AML) associated with the translocation t(8;16)(p11;p13.3).[131] The t(8;16) is a somatic rearrangement associated with acute myelogenous leukemia subtype M4/M5. AML patients observed with this translocation often exhibit erythrophagocytosis and generally have a poor prognosis (reviewed in Velloso et al.[132]).

Cosmids containing the N2 and RT1 locus were used as starting points for a classical positional cloning effort, which involved cosmid walking in a chromosome-16-specific cosmid library; use of STS markers; inter-alu PCR amplification; identification of YACs, BACs, and PACs; and subcloning of YACs into cosmids. FISH checked all YACs for integrity and location. Cosmid overlap was evaluated by Southern blot hybridization with both the cosmid in question and potential neighbor cosmids as probes. In cases of unclear cosmid overlap, additional restriction enzymes were used to clarify the restriction map, and fiber FISH was performed for confirmation. FISH checked most cosmids for signal near the telomere of chromosome 16p. Fiber FISH was also used in determining the relative position of subcontigs, orientation, and size of gaps. In this way, 1.2 Mb of genomic DNA around N2 and RT1 was cloned.[130]

Within this cloned area, 12/13 RTS/t(8;16)-AML breakpoints are restricted to 15 to 20 kb (Fig. 248-3). This clustering of RTS/t(8;16)-AML breakpoints may be explained by a predisposition in this area to chromosomal rearrangements. A part of the breakpoint region, the area just telomeric of cosmid RT166 (Fig. 248-3), is unstable in cosmids and YACs. Multiple attempts to isolate this DNA fragment in fosmid, PAC, or BAC libraries failed. Fiber FISH experiments using flanking cosmids (RT203

**Table 248-2** Translocations and Pericentric Inversions Reported in RTS

| Chromosomal rearrangement | | Year | References |
|---|---|---|---|
| t(2;16)(JAP) | (p13.3;p13.3) | 1991 | Imaizumi and Kuroki[119] |
| t(7;16) | (q34;p13.3) | 1992 | Tommerup et al.[120] |
| inv(16)(FRA) | (p13.3;q13) | 1992 | Lacombe et al.[121] |
| inv(16)(NOR) | unknown | 1993/95 | Breuning et al.[122]; Petrij et al.[123] |
| t(16;20) | (p;q) | 1995 | Petrij et al.[123] |
| t(2;16)(NL) | (q36.3;p13.3) | 1995 | Petrij et al.[123] |
| t(1;16) | (p34.1;p13.2) | 1997 | Wallerstein et al.[126] |
| t(16;Y) | unknown | 1998 | Blough, personal communication |

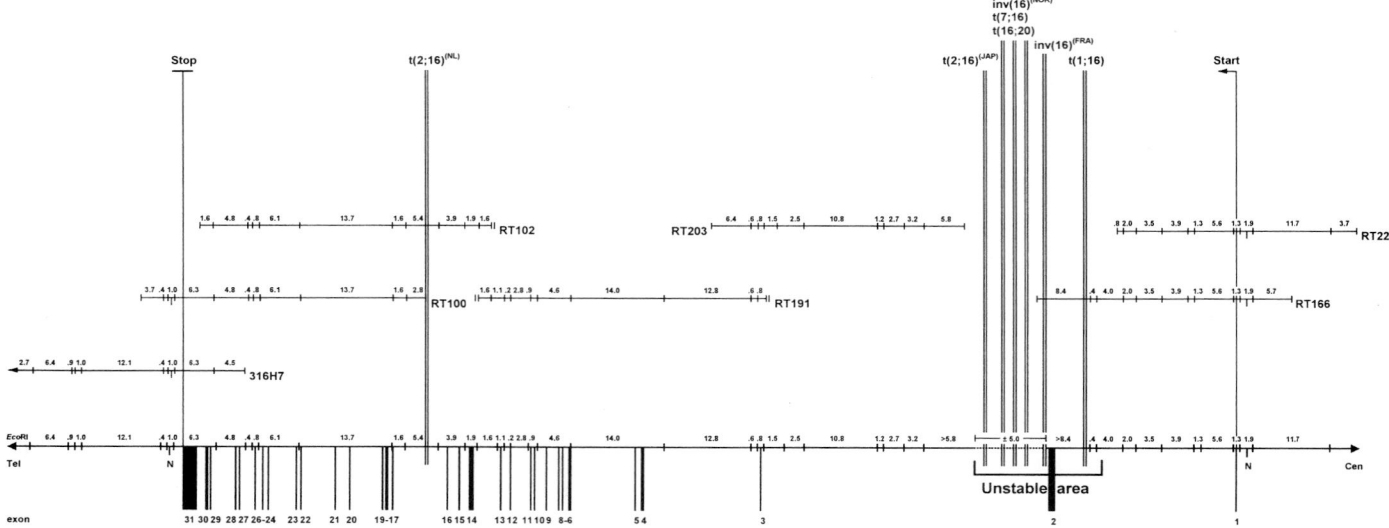

**Fig. 248-3 Distribution of RTS gross chromosomal rearrangements. Seven RTS translocation and inversion cases (the 5 t(8;16)-AML breakpoints are not depicted) and their distribution over the human _CBP_ gene area, depicted in a refined _Eco_RI/_Not_I restriction map.** RT1, RT100, RT102, RT191, RT203, and RT166 are cosmids. Vertical lines crossing a horizontal line indicate _Eco_RI restriction sites. Numbers above the DNA line are _Eco_RI fragment sizes. N = _Not_I

and RT166) and restriction mapping showed that this apparently unclonable area is approximately 5 kb in size.[130] Characterization of this region suggests that it contains certain elements conferring genomic instability, which may participate in translocation mechanisms. Sequencing this breakpoint cluster region will hopefully suggest an explanation for these phenomena.

The RTS t(2;16)[(NL)] breakpoint maps approximately 100 kb more telomeric than the breakpoint cluster, which indicates that the RTS gene is spread over a large stretch of genomic DNA (>100 kb).[123,130,184]

### Cloning the _CBP_ Gene

A set of _Pst_I subclones was isolated from cosmid RT1, one of which showed conservation with DNA from several species (zoo blot). This 288-bp _Pst_I subclone was used to screen a human fetal brain cDNA library. This method resulted in a cDNA clone (cRT0) which contained an open reading frame of 573 bp (encoding 191 amino acids) and a 3′ untranslated region (UTR) with a 19-bp poly-A tail. The open reading frame of this cDNA showed 92 percent DNA homology with murine _Cbp_.[123,130,133]

Chrivia et al.[133] discovered CBP in the mouse in 1993 as a transcriptional coactivator. The protein was named after its interaction with the cyclic-AMP-regulated enhancer binding (CREB) protein. Although officially the gene is named _CREBBP_ (CRE binding binding protein gene), it is generally referred to by its shorter acronym _CBP_. CBP and its chromosome 22 homolog p300[134,135] have been found to function as transcriptional coactivators by forming a physical bridge between the different components of the transcription machinery, as well as potent histone acetyltransferases by making the DNA accessible to transcription factors. They are mediators of different signaling pathways and participants in basic cellular functions such as DNA repair, cell growth, cell differentiation, apoptosis, and tumor suppression. In other words, CBP and p300 are at the center of multiple signal transduction pathways and thereby regulate the expression of many genes (reviewed by Giles[130,136]). It seemed that Petrij et al.[123] had found the human homolog of _CBP_. Further analyses and mutation detection of RTS patient material had to prove whether mutations in _CBP_ indeed lead to RTS.

Additional 3′ sequences were retrieved by using clone cRT0 for "cDNA walking." On the other end of the gene, a 5′ _CBP_ cDNA clone was retrieved from a human Graves disease thyroid

expression cDNA library.[123,133] An uncloned section between 5′ and 3′ cDNA sequences was analyzed by sequencing RT-PCR products of random amplified cDNA of several control individuals. The combination of 5′, 3′, and RT-PCR sequences resulted in a full-length human _CBP_ cDNA sequence of 7329 bp (GenBank accession no. 85962). Based on these data, human _CBP_ was calculated to encode a 265-kDa protein of 2442 amino acids. By hybridizing several different parts of the murine _CBP_ to the human cosmid contig, it was established that the human _CBP_ gene stretches over 159 kb of genomic DNA, from its start codon in cosmid RT166 to its termination codon in cosmid RT1 (Fig. 248-3). Human _CBP_ is, therefore, transcriptionally oriented from centromere to telomere.[130] The gene consists of 31 transcribed exons (Fig. 248-3) (ref. 183 and Doggett, unpublished data).

### Chromosomal Rearrangements Involving _CBP_

The positions of seven of the eight known RTS translocations and inversions were determined by FISH, fiber FISH, and Southern blot analysis and were squarely placed within the human _CBP_ gene area (Fig. 248-3). To determine whether this was also true for the RTS microdeletions, it was necessary to estimate the extent of these deletions. We used cosmids from the physical mapping effort as probes for FISH experiments on material from 21 RTS patients with microdeletions. In a nondeletion individual, each cosmid tested gives two distinct signals, one from each chromosome 16. However, when the genomic area corresponding to one or more of these cosmids is deleted, only one signal, from the unaffected chromosome 16, is observed. Using this method, we measured the deleted areas in RTS patients, which ranged from 50 to >650 kb, and noted that all deletions affected at least some part of the _CBP_ gene (Fig. 248-4).[183]

The RT1 cosmid, initially used by many laboratories for microdeletion screening, contains much of the 3′ end of human _CBP_. However, 5′ microdeletions would not be detected using RT1 alone. Ideally, five cosmids (RT100, RT102, RT191, RT203, and RT166) should be used to detect all submicroscopic deletions in patients with a clinical picture of RTS.[183,185] Except for the ~5 kb uncloned area between RT203 and RT166, these five cosmids cover the whole human _CBP_ gene (159 kb). Because of instability, RT1 was replaced by RT100, which also covers the 3′ end of the human _CBP_ gene (Fig. 248-3).

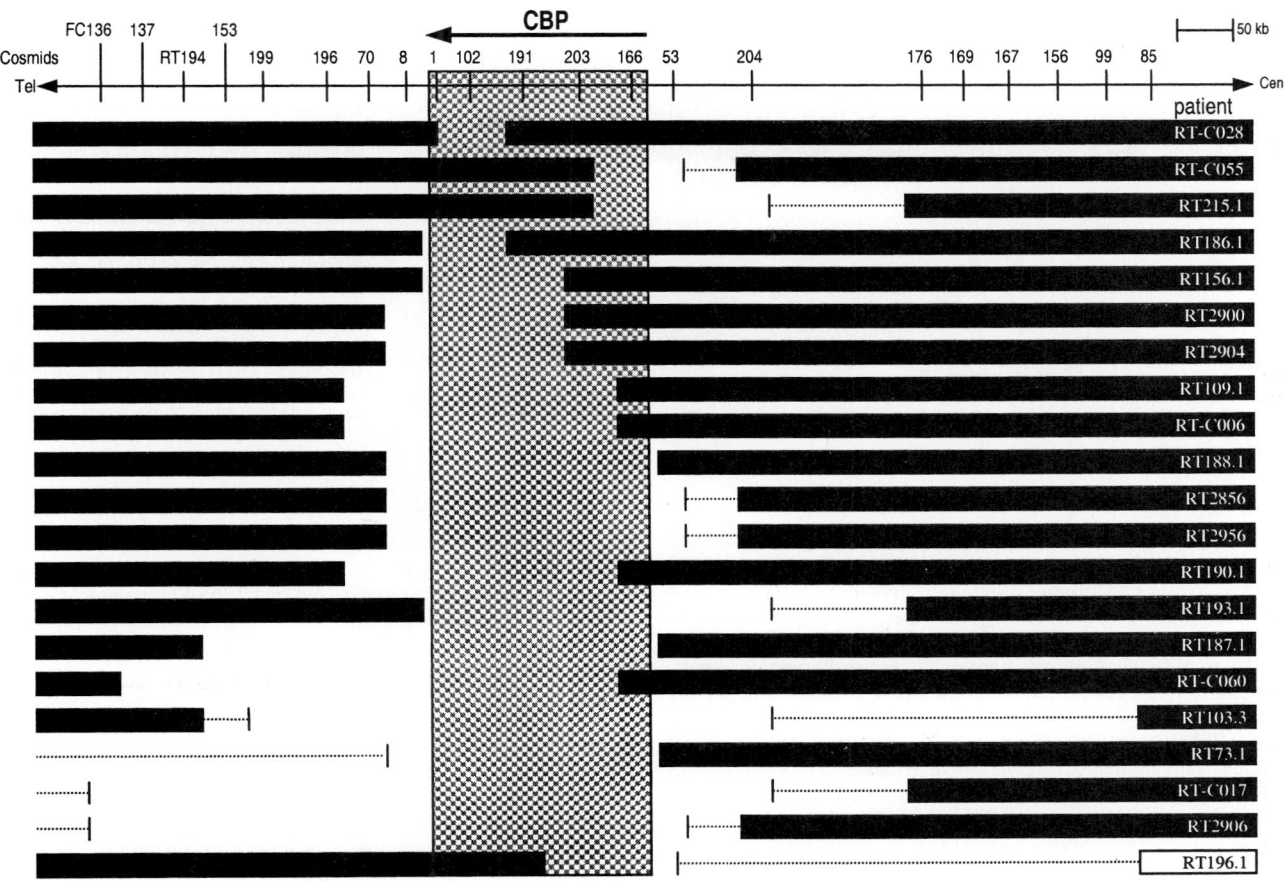

**Fig. 248-4** Representation of 21 RTS microdeletions. Black bars represent the undeleted DNA. Dashed lines represent uncloned or untested areas.

Shortly after the discovery of *CBP*'s disruption in several RTS cases, Giles et al.[129] demonstrated that the *CBP* gene was also disrupted in three t(8;16)-AML patients. Later, Borrow et al.[137] reported the fusion of *CBP* with the *MOZ* (monocytic leukemia zinc finger) gene on chromosome 8. Recently, t(11;16), another leukemia-associated somatic translocation, was described. Unlike the t(8;16)-AML, the t(11;16) is not confined to AML. It has also been observed in chronic myeloid leukemia and myelodysplastic syndrome, and is almost never *de novo*, but arises after anticancer treatment. In this case, the *MLL* (mixed lineage leukemia) gene was found to be the fusion partner of *CBP*.[138–140] CBP is thus implicated in leukemia as well as embryonic development.

### *CBP* Point Mutations in RTS

Translocations, inversions, and microdeletions certainly indicated that the *CBP* gene was disrupted in these RTS patients. Whether disrupting *CBP* causes RTS was still not fully proven; a second gene, contained within *CBP*'s introns, could still be involved. The next step was to look for more subtle mutations within the *CBP* gene of RTS patients without rearrangements. Petrij et al.[123] used the protein truncation test (PTT)[141] to look for translation-terminating mutations in such patients. They analyzed the first 1.2 kb of *CBP* in 16 RTS patients. Two of these patients harbored mutations resulting in a truncated protein product (Fig. 248-5). Sequence analyses confirmed these results (Fig. 248-6). In both patients, a codon for glutamine was changed into a stop codon by a C to T substitution (nt 406 and nt 1069, respectively). Both patients had classical RTS phenotypes; one is shown in Fig. 248-2. In this case, the mutation destroyed a *Pvu*II restriction site. This site was found to be present in both chromosomes of the parents, indicating a *de novo* mutation.

Although data indicate that these kinds of point mutations do not occur often in RTS,[183] they do show that mutations in *CBP*, and not some other gene in the area, indeed cause RTS. No reports on screening for small in-frame deletions or missense mutations are published to date. The majority of RTS cases remains unexplained. Other mechanisms that could lead to reduced CBP production, such as splice-site mutations, promoter mutations, mutations within a possible locus control region, or mutations leading to defective protein processing, cannot be excluded as causative mechanisms for RTS.

### Haploinsufficiency

The occurrence of point mutations in a single gene implies that RTS is not caused by a contiguous gene syndrome in which the deletion of several adjacent genes causes a composite set of abnormalities, as had been previously proposed. Several of the microdeletions remove the entire *CBP* gene (Fig. 248-4), which makes a dominant negative model unlikely as well. A haploinsufficiency model, in which two functional copies of the gene are required to produce sufficient product for normal development, seems to be a more likely explanation for the RTS phenotype.[142] Accordingly, recent mouse knockout experiments showed that loss of one mouse *Cbp* allele is sufficient to cause skeletal malformations.[143]

Levels of CBP may be particularly crucial at certain stages of embryonic development, explaining the RTS phenotype. Although there is a somewhat increased neoplasia frequency in RTS patients,[16] haploinsufficiency of CBP does not appear to have pathophysiological consequences after birth. It should be noted that haploinsufficiency of CBP does not lead to leukemia. CBP's oncogenic role in AML is due to its participation in a fusion transcript.

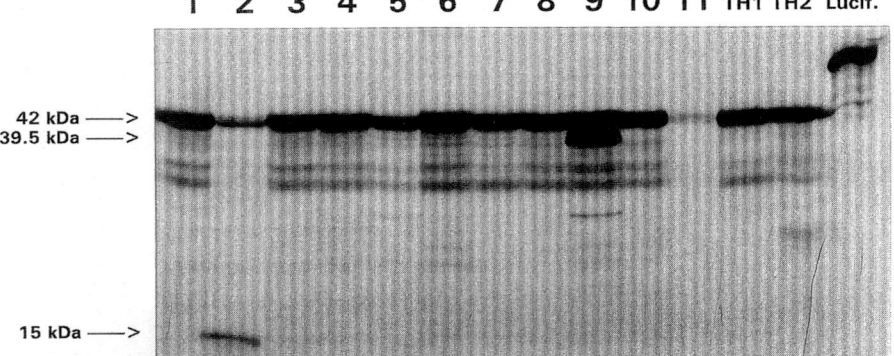

Fig. 248-5 Truncated CBP proteins in two patients with RTS. The protein truncation test (PTT) was performed on the first 1.2 kb of the human *CBP* cDNA. Patient samples 2 and 9 show a truncated protein of 15 and 39.5 kDa, respectively (normal is 42 kDa). Patient 9 is shown in Fig. 248-2. On this autoradiogram, 11 patients are depicted. Lanes marked TH are the control individuals, whereas the luciferase lane contains a control for the translation reaction. (*Reprinted with permission from Nature.*[123] *Copyright 1995; used by permission of Macmillan Magazines Limited.*)

## Heterogeneity

The relationship between a single mutated gene and the constellation of symptoms seen in RTS can be explained by CBP's role as transcriptional coactivator. Because CBP is involved in the regulation of many other genes, the polymorphic nature of these genes could amplify the variability of clinical manifestations as seen in RTS. The above mentioned mouse knockout experiments show that genetic background plays a major role in the variability of the phenotype.

It is likely that specific missense mutations in functional domains of the human *CBP* gene can also cause RTS. That only 15 to 20 percent of CBP mutations have been found to date (either by karyotyping and FISH or by PTT) and that RTS is a syndrome with a highly variable phenotype, suggest that both missense mutations in *CBP* and mutations in other genes could play a role in the etiology of RTS.

CBP is closely related to p300, discovered as a nuclear target of the adenovirus E1A oncoprotein, which maps to chromosome 22q13.[134,135] The 80 to 85 percent of RTS cases that are not caused by *CBP* nonsense mutations or gross chromosome 16 rearrangements should be tested for mutations in these genes.

## CBP FUNCTION

To understand how insufficient levels of CBP cause the Rubinstein-Taybi syndrome, a certain amount of biochemistry must be introduced. CBP is a large (265-kDa) nuclear protein involved in transcription.[133,147,148] CBP seems to be highly expressed in essentially all tissue types, but this issue has not been studied in much detail. Although no data suggest that it physically attaches to DNA itself, CBP provides a molecular bridge between transcription factors that bind to specific DNA sequences (particularly in the promoters of genes) and the complex of proteins that is required for all transcription (termed the "basal transcription machinery"). In many respects, CBP's bridging functions could be seen as creating additional levels of regulation in transcription as an adaptor, or integrator, of multiple transcription signals.

The CBP mutations catalogued to date all result in defective protein production. In approximately half of the RTS patients manifesting microdeletions, the 5′ end of the gene is deleted. In these patients, it is very likely that only the unaffected allele is capable of producing any CBP. In other patients, however, deletions and/or other rearrangements affect the *CBP* gene further

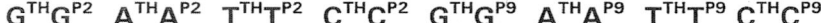

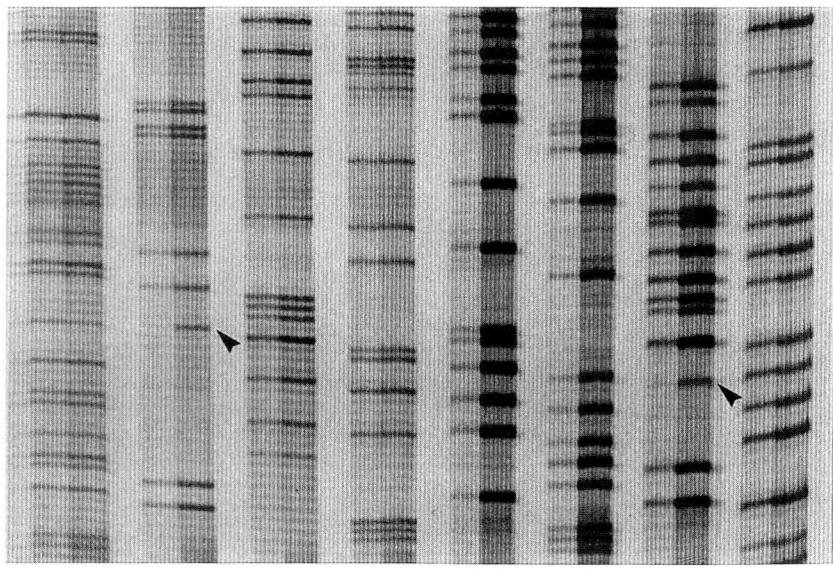

Fig. 248-6 Point mutations of *CBP* in two RTS patients. Sequence analysis of RT-PCR products from the two patients presenting a truncated protein in the PTT (Fig. 248-5). The double lanes of G, A, T, and C represent the sequences of a control individual (TH) and a patient, respectively. In the case of patient 2, sequence analysis was performed in a reversed orientation. The extra adenine (indicated by an arrowhead) represents a thymine in the 5′ to 3′ orientation, leading to the exchange of a glutamine codon with that of a stop codon. In the case of patient 9, the extra thymine (indicated by an arrowhead) leads to a similar mutation as in patient 2. (*Reprinted with permission from Nature.*[123] *Copyright 1995; used by permission of Macmillan Magazines Limited.*)

```
AA   128   Ser Ser Ala Pro Ser Leu Pro Lys Gln Ala Ala Ser Thr Ser Gly Pro   143
bp   382   TCT TCA GCC CCC AGC CTG CCT AAA CAG GCA GCC AGC ACC TCT GGG CCC   429
                                          ↓
PATIENT    Ser Ser Ala Pro Ser Leu Pro Lys ***
Nr.2       TCT TCA GCC CCC AGC CTG CCT AAA TAG    bp 406: C→T = Glutamine → Stop


AA   352   Lys Leu Ile Gln Gln Gln Leu Val Leu Leu Leu His Ala His Lys Cys   367
bp   1054  AAA CTG ATA CAG CAG CAG CTG GTT CTA CTG CTT CAT GCT CAT AAG TGT   1101
                                      ↓
PATIENT    Lys Leu Ile Gln Gln ***
Nr.9       AAA CTG ATA CAG CAG TAG    bp 1069: C→T = Glutamine → Stop
```

**Fig. 248-6a (part 2)** Representation of the point mutations of patients 2 and 9 (Fig. 248-5).

downstream. Although it is doubtful that all of these patients produce stable truncated *CBP* mRNA, in at least one patient, with a reciprocal t(2;16) translocation, stable but truncated mRNA and protein are produced.[184]

## Predicted Structure

The DNA sequence of murine *CBP*[133] indicated that CBP contains several functional motifs. Elucidation of the human *CBP* sequence[130] confirmed that these putative domains are also present in humans. As shown in Fig. 248-7, CBP was predicted to contain four putative zinc-finger domains, a bromodomain, and a large glutamine-rich region. These domains are often represented in transcriptional regulators. Although CBP was originally identified as a cofactor for the transcription factor CREB, sequence comparison to other known proteins soon established that CBP was closely related to the adenovirus E1A-associated 300-kDa protein (p300).[135,149] p300 was initially identified as a target for E1A repression, and was observed to stimulate S-phase entry of quiescent cells (reviewed in Moran[150]). Functional studies soon established that CBP and p300 are almost indistinguishable in various signal-dependent transcription pathways as well as in cell cycle regulation mechanisms (reviewed in Shikama et al.[151]). Despite their remarkable similarity in vitro, two lines of evidence suggest that CBP and p300 are not physiologically interchangeable. First, chromosomal rearrangements in confirmed RTS patients consistently involve the *CBP* locus on chromosome 16p13.3, whereas no rearrangements of the *p300* locus, at chromosome 22q13, have been reported to date. Second, inactivating mutations of one murine *Cbp* allele successfully reproduces many aspects of the RTS phenotype in mice, while the hemizygously mutated *p300* mouse displays no dysmorphic features[152] (see "Animal Models" below). Although distinct roles in retinoic acid-induced differentiation have been recently reported,[153] CBP and p300 are often lumped under one name, where researchers fail to discriminate between the two proteins.

## CBP Is a Transcriptional Adaptor/Integrator

The cyclic adenosine monophosphate (cAMP)-regulated transcriptional pathway is one of the better understood cascades influencing transcriptional activation, and so happens to be the pathway by which CBP was originally identified. It is, however, just one of many pathways in which CBP is thought to be a critical factor. CBP makes contact with and integrates the functions of C/EBP, c-Fos, chromatin, c-Jun, c-Myb, CREB, CDK2/cyclin E, E1A, E2F, NFκB, nuclear hormone receptors, p53, SRC-1, TBP, and TFIIB, just to name a few.[151] It should be noted that although CBP generally functions as a transcriptional coactivator, it is suspected to act as a repressor of transcription in conjunction with the transcription factor YY1.[154] For our purposes, however, we focus on CBP's ability to activate transcription. In this paradigm, external cellular signals (e.g., hormones, growth factors, and neurotransmitters) produce conformational changes in their receptors, which stimulate a cascade of events leading to the specific activation of a subset of genes. With the exception of CREB, and the lineage-restricted transcription factor Microphthalmia (Mi), phosphorylation is not required before binding CBP.[133,155]

A fascinating aspect of CBP in transcriptional regulation is its ability to establish cross talk between separate signaling cascades, often called signal integration (Fig. 248-8). Several groups have proposed that CBP acts as a toggle switch between multiple transduction pathways that antagonize each other by virtue of their demand for CBP. The competition for rate-limiting concentrations of CBP was originally observed between the transcription factor known as AP-1 and nuclear receptor hormones.[156] Subsequently, similar relationships were observed between the AP-1 and JAK/STAT pathways,[158] and between nuclear receptor hormones and E2F.[159] In vitro overexpression of CBP neutralizes the negative cross talk in all of these cases, suggesting that sequestration of CBP functions as a selective valve determining which set of genes is expressed. A few studies have also demonstrated that CBP can also

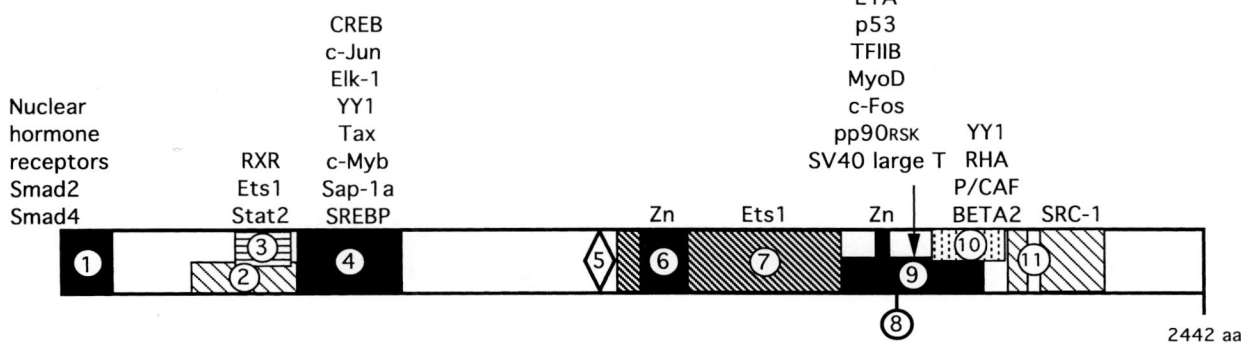

**Fig. 248-7 Representation of the human CBP molecule.** Functional domains are numbered as follows: (1) nuclear receptor binding domain; (2) N-terminal transactivation domain; (3) first cysteine/histidine-rich region; (4) CREB-binding domain; (5) bromodomain; (6) second cysteine/hystidine-rich region; (7) histone acetyltransferase domain; (8) protein kinase A phosphorylation site; (9) E1A-binding domain; (10) glutamine-rich region; (11) C-terminal transactivation site. Proteins interacting with specific domains of CBP are shown above the molecule.

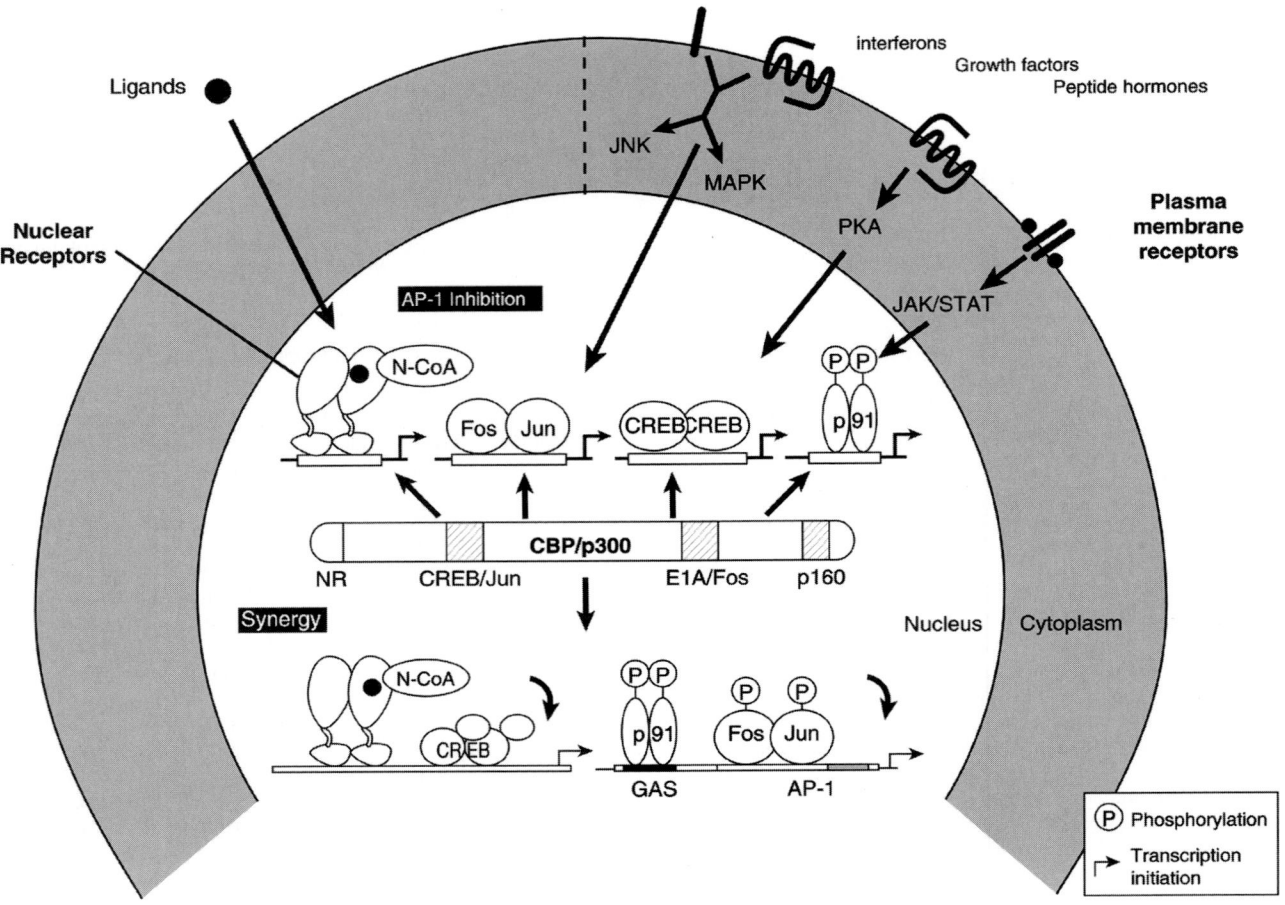

**Fig. 248-8 CBP and p300 can act as integrators of multiple signal transduction pathways. CBP and p300 serve as essential co-activator proteins for several classes of regulated transcription factors. As a result, competition for CBP and p300 may serve as a mechanism for antagonistic interactions between signaling pathways at some promoters (depicted above the molecule). (*From Glass et al.[157] Copyright 1997; used by permission of Current Biology Ltd.*)**

participate in positive cross talk between pathways. Ligand-dependent transactivation by nuclear receptor hormones is synergistically potentiated by the hematopoietic factor p45/NF-E2.[160] Once again, overexpression of CBP abolishes the synergism between these two factors, implying that the mechanism for this relationship relies on the simultaneous binding of both factors to CBP.

### CBP in Cell Cycle Control

Several lines of evidence suggest that CBP is a negative regulator of the cell cycle. CBP phosphorylation levels change during the cell cycle and hyperphosphorylation has been observed during mitosis.[161] Additionally, multiple studies show that the adenovirus oncoprotein E1A must bind CBP to achieve oncogenic transformation.[135,149] Mutated E1A oncoproteins that cannot bind members of the retinoblastoma protein (RB1) family but that retain CBP binding are able to activate G1 gene expression and entry into S phase in primary rodent cells,[162–164] indicating that CBP normally represses the G1-S phase transition. Collectively, these data point to CBP as an important suppressing element in cell cycle control.

### CBP Modifies Chromatin

DNA is supported by a protein scaffold of chromatin. The principal repeat unit of chromatin is the nucleosome, which consists of an octamer of histones, two each of H2A, H2B, H3, and H4, supporting 1.75 turns of DNA, or 146 bp of DNA. Nucleosomes are potent repressors of transcription, presumably by physically interfering with the binding of transcription factors (reviewed in Brownell et al.,[165] Montminy,[166] and Roth et al.[167]). A central question in eukaryotic transcription is how transcription factors gain access to the DNA tightly wound in chromatin. Targeted histone acetylation is thought to neutralize the positive charge of the histones and relax the interaction between histones and the negatively charged DNA.

CBP is one of few human proteins with intrinsic histone acetyltransferase (HAT) activity[168,169] (Table 248-4). Interestingly, several of the other proteins exhibiting HAT activity, such as p/CAF (p300/CBP-associated protein), SRC-1, and ACTR, bind CBP, and share CBP's function as a nuclear receptor coactivator. Most researchers believe that these cofactors act in concert with each other and with specific transcription factors to expose the promoters of genes (Fig. 248-9). Very recent evidence directly relates the recruitment of HAT complexes by transcription factors to the activation of transcription, asserting the importance of cofactors in the regulation of genes.[170]

### CBP and Cancer

As a protein involved in cell cycle control, CBP seems a likely candidate for mutations in cancer. As described earlier in this chapter (see "Chromosomal Rearrangements Involving *CBP*", the gene encoding CBP is the target of translocations in hematologic malignancies. Furthermore, RTS patients have an increased predisposition to certain types of cancer.[17] The higher prevalence of cancer in RTS patients fits the "two-hit" model for tumor

**Table 248-4** Known Human Histone Acetyltransferases (HATs)

| HAT | Interacting proteins | Histones modified |
|---|---|---|
| HAT A (hGCN5) | ADA2, ADA3, other ADAs? | H3, H4 |
| P/CAF | CBP/p300, TP53, and SRC-1 | H3, H4 |
| CBP/p300 | CREB, JUN, TP53, P/CAF, etc. (see ref. 151) | H2A, H2B, H3, H4 |
| TAF$_{II}$230/250 | TFIID subunit | H3, H4 |
| SRC-1 | CBP, p300, nuclear receptors, P/CAF, TBP | H3, H4 |
| ACTR | CBP, p300, nuclear receptors, P/CAF, TBP | H3, H4 |

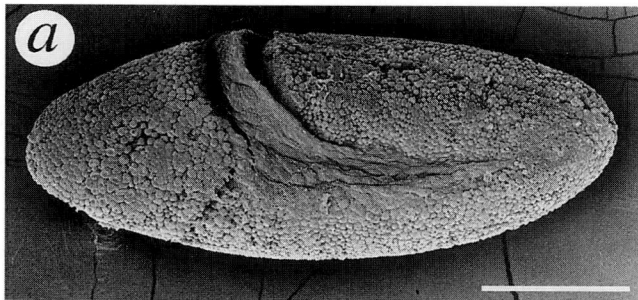

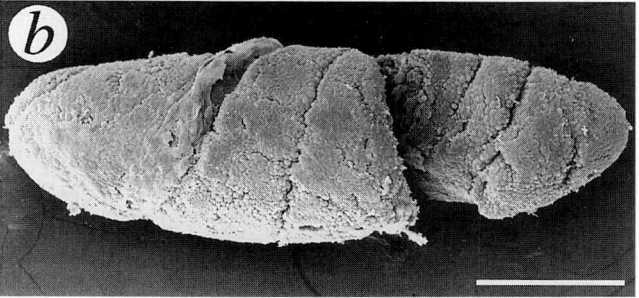

**Fig. 248-10** *Drosophila* CBP mutation experiments: (a) stage 9 wild-type control embryo; (b) late-stage 10 hemizygous CBP mutant embryo. (*Reprinted with permission from* Nature Genetics.[176] *Copyright 1997; used by permission of Macmillan Magazines Limited.*)

suppressor proteins as proposed by Knudson.[171] Accordingly, preliminary data suggest that the unaffected CBP allele is mutated in RTS patient tumors and keloids (Giles, unpublished data). Likewise, mice heterozygous for the *cbp* knock-out have a marked predisposition for hematologic tumors in which their second *cbp* allele has acquired a mutation.[186] Examination of the unaffected allele in leukemic cells with translocations affecting *CBP* should also elucidate CBP's role as a tumor suppressor. Interestingly, biallelic mutations in regions of the p300 gene that show strong homology with *CBP* have been reported in gastric, colorectal, and epithelial tumors,[172,187] suggesting that CBP may likewise function as a tumor-suppressor protein.

## CBP in Development

As evidenced by its role in RTS, normal levels of CBP are critical for the normal development of the human fetus. However, RTS does not constitute the only physiological evidence for CBP's role in the pattern formation of limb development. The hedgehog (hh) signaling pathway is an important determinant in pattern formation (reviewed in Hammerschmidt[173]). One component in *Drosophila* hh signaling is the transcription factor Cubitus interruptus (Ci), homologous to the human Gli family of zinc-finger proteins.[174] Using mutants of the *Drosophila CBP* (*dCBP*) gene, Akimaru et al. demonstrated that dCBP is a coactivator of Ci and is critical for anterior-posterior patterning in *Drosophila* embryos.[175] In a later study, the same dCBP mutants were used to link dCBP to the Dorsal-dependent expression of the *twist* gene,

indicating that dCBP is a cofactor for Dorsal[176] (Fig. 248-10). Interestingly, the mammalian ortholog of Dorsal is NF$\kappa$B, which uses CBP as an intermediary to interact with the cyclin-dependent kinases.[177,178]

These two studies in *Drosophila* suggest a biochemical link between RTS and two other human malformation syndromes. Truncating mutations of one copy of the *GLI3* gene, a human ortholog of the *Drosophila Ci*, causes the Grieg cephalosyndactyly syndrome, which is similar to RTS in limb and craniofacial dysmorphisms.[179] Because the hedgehog is known to be a critical pathway in developmental pattern formation, one could speculate that in both RTS and Grieg cephalosyndactyly syndrome, decreased hh signaling results in the overlapping developmental disturbances.

A second disease, even more analogous to RTS than Grieg syndrome, is the Saethre-Chotzen syndrome. This entity may

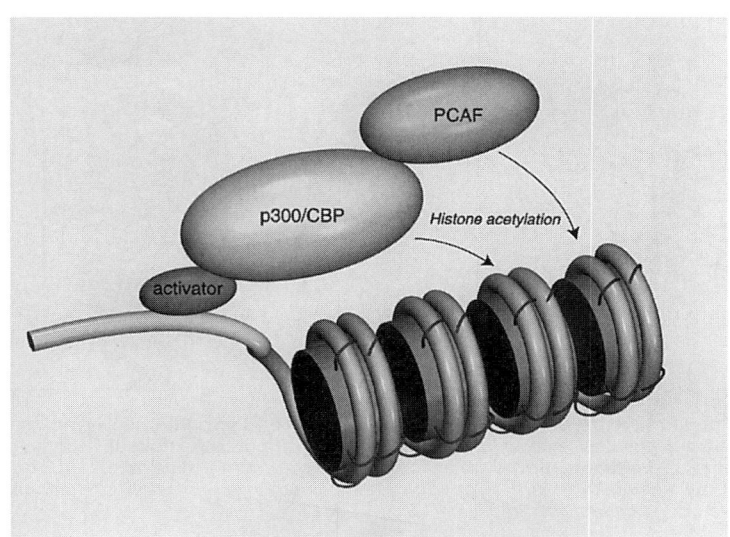

**Fig. 248-9** Model of CBP and p300's histone acetyltransferase function. CBP and p300 are thought to recruit additional acetyltransferases, for example, p300/CBP-associated factor (PCAF) (see Table 248-4), to alter or disrupt the normal repressive function of chromatin. (*From Ogryzko et al.*[168] *Copyright 1996; used by permission of Cell Press.*)

strongly resemble RTS, particularly in digit dysmorphism, to the extent that a Saethre-Chotzen patient was incorrectly diagnosed as having RTS for years by an experienced clinician.[105] Remarkably, the Saethre-Chotzen syndrome is caused by haploinsufficiency of the human *TWIST* gene product.[180,181] Because the *Drosophila* Dorsal protein recruits dCBP to initiate transcription of *twist*, it seems likely that haploinsufficiency of human CBP would influence the expression of *TWIST*, thereby resulting in a developmental disturbance common to both RTS and the Saethre-Chotzen syndrome.

### Animal Models

Recent advances in the understanding of in vivo function of CBP have largely stemmed from the use of animal models. CBP does not appear to have an ortholog in yeast, although two CBP orthologs were reported in the *C. elegans* genome.[135] The *Drosophila* ortholog of CBP (dCBP) possesses all of the protein interaction motifs and appears to function in a similar fashion as its human counterpart.[175,176]

Targeted disruption of the *Cbp* gene in mice has revealed interesting parallels. First, mice lacking a single *Cbp* allele manifest various skeletal abnormalities including delayed ossification, a large anterior fontanel, and abnormal ossification of the sternum, xiphoid process, and axial bone[143] (Fig. 248-11). These manifestations resemble many of those seen in human RTS patients.[17,143] When *Cbp* is homozygously knocked out, the mice do not survive past 9 to 11 days of gestation.[143,182] Examination of these embryos reveals that they have neural tube closure defects.[182] Heterozygous p300 inactivation, on the other hand, has no visible effect in the mutant mice that survive birth. However, up to 55 percent of the heterozygous mice die in utero, depending on the genetic background. Mice homozygous for p300 inactivating mutations strongly resemble *Cbp* knockout mice, and die after 9 to 11 days of gestation.[182] Remarkably, crossing the *Cbp* and *p300* heterozygous mutants produced double hetero-

**Table 248-5** The Combined Dose of CBP/p300 is Critical for Mouse Development

| CBP | p300 | Phenotype | Reference |
|-----|------|-----------|-----------|
| ++ | ++ | Normal | — |
| +− | ++ | Skeletal abnormalities | 146 |
| −− | ++ | Embryonic lethal | 146,182 |
| ++ | +− | Reduced viability | 182 |
| ++ | −− | Embryonic lethal | 182 |
| +− | +− | Embryonic lethal | 182 |

zygous *Cbp/p300* mutant embryos, which died *in utero* and otherwise shared phenotypic similarities to both *Cbp* and *p300* homozygous mutants. These results suggest that CBP and p300 exert common embryonal survival functions and that the combined dose of CBP and p300 is critical for mouse embryonic development (Table 248-5).

### Etiology of RTS

Animal models and biochemical evidence suggest that RTS is caused by haploinsufficiency of CBP during fetal development. However, much work must still be done to determine exactly which pathways require CBP in vivo. These data will provide important advances in the understanding of developmental regulation and cell cycle control. Until the in vivo functionality of CBP is better defined, there is no available treatment for RTS.

### ACKNOWLEDGMENTS

The authors would like to thank Ruthann I. Blough and Norman Doggett for sharing unpublished data.

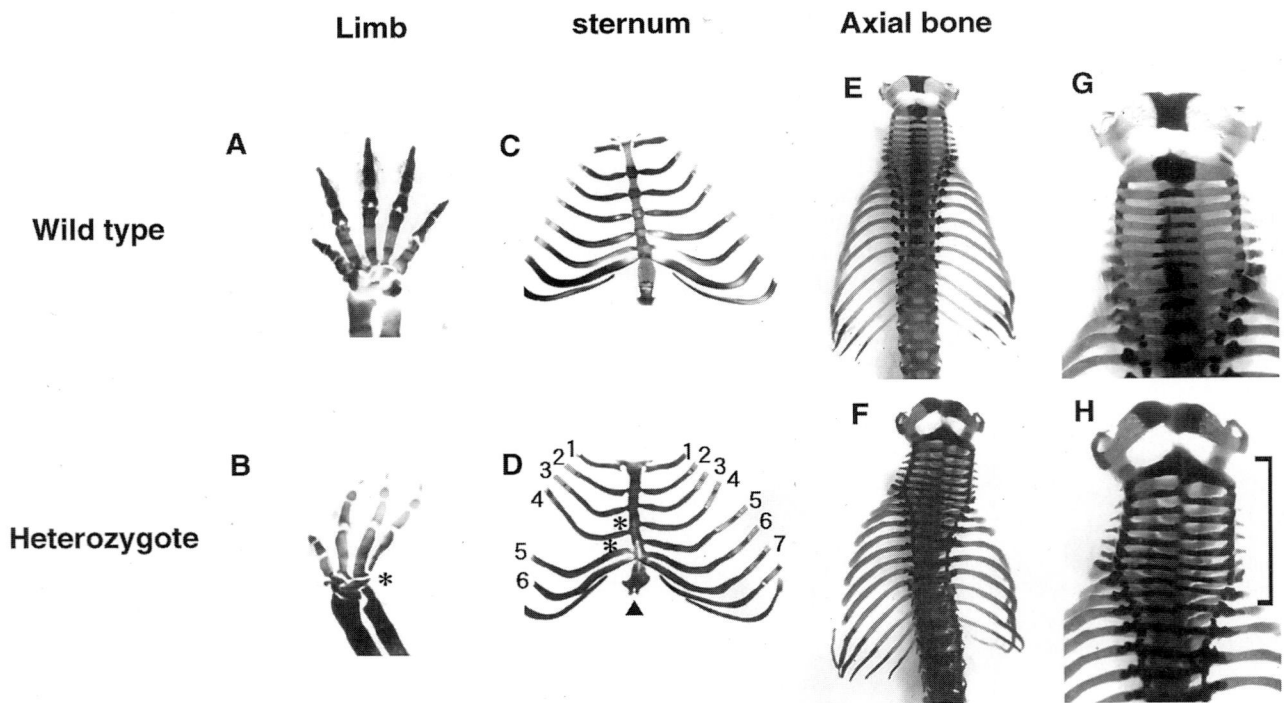

**Limb    sternum    Axial bone**

**Wild type** A C E G

**Heterozygote** B D F H

**Fig. 248-11** Severe abnormalities in *Cbp* heterozygous mice. Bone and cartilage stained specimens of the right forelimbs and sternums of a wild-type (A and C) and a *Cbp* heterozygote (B and D) mouse. Oligodactyly and misalignment of rib pairs can be observed (*). Only six ribs can be seen on the right side. Dorsal view of the vertebrae of a wild-type (E and G) and a heterozygote (F and H). In the heterozygote, the presence of 10 ribs on the right side, 14 ribs on the left side, asymmetric cervical vertebrae, extra split thoracic vertebrae, and scoliosis were observed. See Color Plate 22. (*From Tanaka et al.*[143] *Copyright 1997; used by permission of National Academy of Sciences U.S.A.*)

## REFERENCES

1. Michael J, Matsoukas J, Theodorou S: Pouce bot arque en forte abduction-extension et autres symptomes concomitants. *Rev Chir Orthop* **43**:142, 1957.
2. Rubinstein JH: Broad thumb-hallux (Rubinstein-Taybi) syndrome 1957–1988. *Am J Med Genet* **6(Suppl)**:3, 1990.
3. Rubinstein JH, Taybi H: Broad thumbs and toes and facial abnormalities. *Am J Dis Child* **105**:588, 1963.
4. Matsoukas J: Fatherhood of the so-called Rubinstein-Taybi syndrome. *Am J Dis Child* **126**:860, 1973.
5. Rubinstein JH: Fatherhood of the so-called Rubinstein-Taybi syndrome. *Am J Dis Child* **128**:424, 1974.
6. Warkany J: Difficulties of classifications and terminology of syndromes of multiple congenital anomalies. *Am J Dis Child* **128**:424, 1974.
7. Coffin GS: Brachydactyly, peculiar facies, and mental retardation. *Am J Dis Child* **108**:351, 1964.
8. Job JC, Rossier A, de Grandprey J: Etudes sur les nanismes constitutionnels. II. Le syndrome de Rubinstein et Taybi. *Ann Pédiatr* **11**:646, 1964.
9. Rubinstein JH: The broad thumbs syndrome—Progress report 1968. *Birth Defects Orig Artic Ser* **5**:25, 1969.
10. Berg JM, Smith GF, Ridler MAC, Dutton G, Green EA, Richards BW: On the association of broad thumbs and first toes with other physical peculiarities and mental retardation. *J Ment Defic Res* **10**:204, 1966.
11. Coffin GS: A syndrome of retarded development. *Am J Dis Child* **115**:698, 1968.
12. Simpson NE, Brissenden JE: The Rubinstein-Taybi syndrome. *Am J Hum Genet* **25**:225, 1973.
13. Partington MW: Rubinstein-Taybi syndrome: A follow-up study. *Am J Med Genet* **6(Suppl)**:65, 1990.
14. Hennekam RCM, Stevens CA, Van de Kamp JJP: Etiology and recurrence risk in Rubinstein-Taybi syndrome. *Am J Med Genet* **6(Suppl)**:56, 1990.
15. Char F: Rubinstein-Taybi syndrome in blacks. Follow-up from infancy to late childhood. *Proc Greenwood Genet Ctr* **8**:135, 1989.
16. Miller RW, Rubinstein JH: Tumors in Rubinstein-Taybi syndrome. *Am J Med Genet* **56**:112, 1995.
17. Hennekam RCM, Van den Boogaard MJ, Sibbles BJ, Van Spijker HG: Rubinstein-Taybi syndrome in the Netherlands. *Am J Med Genet* **6(Suppl)**:17, 1990.
18. Stevens CA, Carey JC, Blackburn BL: Rubinstein-Taybi syndrome: A natural history study. *Am J Med Genet* **6(Suppl)**:30, 1990.
19. Stevens CA, Hennekam RCM, Blackburn BL: Growth in the Rubinstein-Taybi syndrome. *Am J Med Genet* **6(Suppl)**:51, 1990.
20. Olson DP, Koenig RJ: Thyroid function in Rubinstein-Taybi syndrome. *J Clin Endocrin Metabol* **82**:3264, 1997.
21. Hennekam RCM, Baselier ACA, Beyaert E, Bos A, Blok JB, Jansma HBM, Thorbecke-Nilsen VV, et al.: Psychological and speech studies in Rubinstein-Taybi syndrome. *Am J Ment Retard* **96**:645, 1992.
22. Filippi G: The Rubinstein-Taybi syndrome: Report of 7 cases. *Clin Genet* **3**:303, 1972.
23. Robinson GC, Miller JR, Cook EG, Tischler B: Broad thumbs and toes and mental retardation: Unusual dermatoglyphic observations in two individuals. *Am J Dis Child* **111**:287, 1966.
24. Guion-Almeida ML, Richieri-Costa A: Callosal agenesis, iris coloboma and megacolon in a Brazilian boy with Rubinstein-Taybi syndrome. *Am J Med Genet* **43**:929, 1992.
25. Lamy M, Jammet ML, Ajjan N, Alibert L, Boulesteix J: Le syndrome de Rubinstein-Taybi. *Arch Fr Pediatr* **24**:472, 1967.
26. True CW, Rubinstein JH: Pathological findings in a case of the Rubinstein-Taybi syndrome, Symposium 10: Rubinstein-Taybi syndrome, in Richards BW (ed): *Proceedings, First Congress of the International Association for the Scientific Study of Mental Deficiency.* Montpellier, France, 1967, p 613.
27. Neuhauser G, Schulze H: Das Rubinstein-Taybi Syndrom. *Ztsch Kinderhlkd* **103**:90, 1968.
28. Fukunaga N, Suda S, Ebihara Y, Laovoravit N, Laovoravit M: Rubinstein-Taybi syndrome: A case report. *Acta Path Jpn* **19**:501, 1969.
29. Pogacar S, Nora NF: Neuropathology of the Rubinstein-Taybi syndrome. *J Neuropath Exp Neurol* **34**:110, 1975.
30. Barson AJ: Rubinstein-Taybi syndrome. *Arch Dis Child* **49**:495, 1974.
31. Bonioli E, Bellini C, Di Stefano A, Taccone A, Pesce MA: Dandy-Walker malformation and eye coloboma in a Rubinstein-Taybi phenotype. *Am J Hum Genet* **43**:A40, 1988.
32. Kimura H, Ito Y, Koda Y, Hase Y: Rubinstein-Taybi syndrome with thymic hypoplasia. *Am J Med Genet* **46**:293, 1993.
33. Gorlin RJ, Cohen MM Jr, Hennekam RCM: *Syndromes of the Head and Neck,* 4th ed. New York, Oxford Medical Press, (in press).
34. Allanson JE: Rubinstein-Taybi syndrome: The changing face. *Am J Med Genet* **6(Suppl)**:38, 1990.
35. Hennekam RCM: Rubinstein-Taybi syndrome: A history in pictures. *Clin Dysmorphol* **2**:87, 1993.
36. Blanck MF, Braun-Vallon S, Guillaumat ML: Deux cas de nanisme constitutionnel (syndrome de Rubinstein et Taybi) avec glaucome. *Bull Soc Opht Fr* **68**:173, 1968.
37. Klein D, Rubinstein JH, Ammann F: Caracteristiques neuro-ophtalmologiques du syndrome des "pouces larges" de Rubinstein-Taybi. A propos d'un cas meconnu. *Oto Neuro Oph* **44**:373, 1972.
38. Buchinger G, Ströder J: Rubinstein-Taybi-Syndrom bei wahrscheinlich eineiigen Zwillingen und drei weiteren Kindern. *Klin Padiatr* **185**:296, 1973.
39. Levy NS: Juvenile glaucoma in the Rubinstein-Taybi syndrome. *J Pediatr Ophthalmol* **13**:141, 1976.
40. Behrens-Baumann W: Augensymptome beim Rubinstein-Taybi-Syndrom. *Klin Monatsbl Augenheilkd* **171**:126, 1977.
41. Nelson ME, Talbot JF: Keratoglobus in the Rubinstein-Taybi syndrome. *Br J Opthalmol* **73**:385, 1989.
42. Fujisawa K, Kinoshita K, Tawara A, Inomata H: A case of Rubinstein-Taybi syndrome with goniodysgenetic glaucoma. *Acta Soc Ophthal Jpn* **94**:693, 1990.
43. Marcus-Harel T, Silverstone BZ, Seelenfreund M, Schurr D, Berson D: Retinal detachment with high myopia in the Rubinstein-Taybi syndrome. *Metab Pediatr Syst Ophthalmol* **14**:31, 1991.
44. Salmon MA: The Rubinstein-Taybi syndrome: A report of two cases. *Arch Dis Child* **43**:102, 1968.
45. Hennekam RCM, Van Doorne JM: Oral aspects of Rubinstein-Taybi syndrome. *Am J Med Genet* **6(Suppl)**:42, 1990.
46. McDonagh BJ: Syndrome of Rubinstein and Taybi. *J Irish Med Assoc* **61**:273, 1968.
47. Gravinghoff J, Tost M: Das Rubinstein-Taybi Syndrom. Ein Beitrag zum Problem der Determinationsperiode. *Monatsschr Kinderheilkd* **118**:479, 1970.
48. Verma IC: Rubinstein-Taybi syndrome. Case report. *Indian J Pediatr* **7**:672, 1970.
49. Rohlfing B, Lewis K, Singleton EB: Rubinstein-Taybi syndrome. *Am J Dis Child* **121**:71, 1971.
50. Rossolini V, Burroni M, Perrotta F: A proposito di altri due casi di sindrome di Rubinstein-Taybi. *Rev Neuropsychiatr Infant* **201**:201:445, 1978.
51. Selmanowitz VJ, Stiller MJ: Rubinstein-Taybi syndrome: Cutaneous manifestations and colossal keloids. *Arch Dermatol* **117**:504, 1981.
52. Musumeci SA, Colognola RM, Ferri R, Gigli GL, Bergonzi P: Un caso di syndrome di Rubinstein-Taybi (con epilessia e consanguineita dei genitori). *Boll Lega Ital Epil* **45/46**:153, 1984.
53. Rett A, Kahlich-Koenner DM, Madl W: Klinische und anthropologische Untersuchungen zum Rubinstein-Taybi Syndrom. *Wien Med Wochenschr* **19/20**:378, 1969.
54. Russell NA, Hoffman HJ, Bain HW: Intraspinal neurilemoma in association with the Rubinstein-Taybi syndrome. *Pediatrics* **47**:444, 1971.
55. Sehabiague J: *A propos d'une observation associant un syndrome de Rubinstein et Taybi a une triade de Fallot.* Thesis, Bordeaux, France, 1977, p 202.
56. Sautarel M, Choussat A, Sandler B, Bui-Authier F, Guiter F, Sehabiague J, Abadie D: Syndrome de Rubinstein-Taybi associe a une triade de Fallot. *Pediatrie* **33**:593, 1978.
57. Jeliu G, Saint-Rome G: Le syndrome de Rubinstein-Taybi. A propos d'une observation. *Union Med Can* **96**:22, 1967.
58. Nespoli L, Botelli A: Sindrome di Rubinstein-Taybi e sua delimitazione diagnostica. *Minerva Pediatr* **27**:1724, 1975.
59. Gotts EE, Liemohn WP: Behavioral characteristics of three children with the broad thumb-hallux (Rubinstein-Taybi) syndrome. *Biol Psychiatr* **12**:413, 1977.
60. Sinnette C, Odeku EL: Rubinstein-Taybi syndrome. The first case in an African child and the first case recognized at birth. *Clin Pediatr* **7**:488, 1968.
61. Gardner DG, Girgis SS: Talon cusps: A dental anomaly in the Rubinstein-Taybi syndrome. *Oral Surg* **47**:519, 1979.
62. Kinirons MJ: Oral aspects of Rubinstein-Taybi syndrome. *Br Dent J* **154**:46, 1983.
63. Davis PJ, Brook AH: The presentation of talon cusps: Diagnosis, clinical features, associations, and possible etiology. *Br Dent J* **160**:84, 1986.

64. Hennekam RCM, Van Den Boogaard MJ, Van Doorne JM: A cephalometric study in Rubinstein-Taybi syndrome. *J Craniofac Genet Devel Biol* **11**:33, 1991.

65. Allanson JE, Hennekam RCM: Rubinstein-Taybi syndrome: Objective evaluation of craniofacial structure. *Am J Med Genet* **71**:414, 1997.

66. Wood VE, Rubinstein JH: Surgical treatment of the thumb in the Rubinstein-Taybi syndrome. *J Hand Surg* **12**:166, 1987.

67. Taybi H, Rubinstein JH: Broad thumbs and toes, and unusual facial features: A probable mental retardation syndrome. *Am J Roentgenol* **93**:362, 1965.

68. Hennekam RCM, Van Den Boogaard MJ, Dijkstra PF, Van De Kamp JJP: Metacarpophalangeal pattern profile analysis in Rubinstein-Taybi syndrome. *Am J Med Genet* **6(Suppl)**:48, 1990.

69. Giroux J, Miller JR: Dermatoglyphics of the broad thumb and great toe syndrome. *Am J Dis Child* **113**:207, 1967.

70. Herrmann J, Opitz JM: Dermatoglyphic studies in a Rubinstein-Taybi patient, her unaffected dizygous twin sister and other relatives. *Birth Defects* **5**:22, 1969.

71. Atasu M: Dermatoglyphic findings in Rubinstein-Taybi syndrome. *J Ment Defic Res* **23**:111, 1979.

72. Bonioli E, Bellini C, Senes FM, Palmieri A, Di Stadio M, Pinelli G: Slipped capital femoral epiphysis associated with Rubinstein-Taybi syndrome. *Clin Genet* **44**:79, 1993.

73. Robson MJ, Brown LM, Sharrard WJW: Cervical spondylolisthesis and other skeletal abnormalities in Rubinstein-Taybi syndrome. *J Bone Joint Surg* **62**:297, 1980.

74. Moran R, Calthorpe D, McGoldrick F, Fogarty E, Dowling F: Congenital dislocation of the patella in Rubinstein-Taybi syndrome. *Irish Med J* **86**:34, 1993.

75. Stevens CA: Patellar dislocation in Rubinstein-Taybi syndrome. *Am J Med Genet* **72**:188, 1997.

76. Rosenbaum KN, Johnson DL, Fitz CR, McCullough DC: Tethered cord in Rubinstein-Taybi syndrome. *Am J Hum Genet* **47(Suppl)**:A75, 1990.

77. Verger P, Guillard JM, Sandler B, Ducros E: Syndrome de Rubinstein-Taybi et lithiase renale. *Rev Pédiatr* **4**:233, 1967.

78. Tanphaichitr P, Mekanandha V, Kotchbhakdi N: A case of Rubinstein-Taybi syndrome associated with nephrotic syndrome. *J Med Assoc Thai* **62**:44, 1979.

79. Giannotti P, Aragona F, Di Candio G, De Angelis M: Rubinstein-Taybi syndrome: a clinical case with a rare association with malformation uropathy. *Minerva Urol* **35**:175, 1983.

80. Sobel RA, Woerner S: Rubinstein-Taybi syndrome and nasopharyngeal rhabdomyosarcoma. *J Pediatr* **99**:1000, 1981.

81. Bonioli E, Bellini C: Rubinstein-Taybi syndrome and pheochromocytoma. *Am J Med Genet* **44**:386, 1992.

82. Bilir BM, Bilir N, Wilson GN: Intracranial angioblastic meningioma and an aged appearance in a woman with Rubinstein-Taybi syndrome. *Am J Med Genet* **6(Suppl)**:69, 1990.

83. Evans G, Burnell L, Cambell R, Gattamaneni HR, Birch J: Congenital anomalies and genetic syndromes in 1973 cases of medulloblastoma. *Med Pediatr Oncol* **21**:433, 1993.

84. Skousen GJ, Wardinsky T, Chenaille P: Medulloblastoma in patients with Rubinstein-Taybi syndrome. *Am J Med Genet* **66**:367, 1996.

85. D'Cruz CA, Karmazin N, Johal JS, Halligan G, Faerber EN: Malignant neoplasms in two patients with Rubinstein-Taybi syndrome. *Pediatr Pathol* **13**:102, 1993.

86. Lannering B, Marky I, Nordborg C: Brain tumors in childhood and adolescence in West Sweden 1970–1984. *Cancer* **66**:604, 1990.

87. Cambiaghi S, Ermacora E, Brusasco A, Canzi L, Caputo R: Multiple pilomatrixomas in Rubinstein-Taybi syndrome: A case report. *Pediatr Dermatol* **11**:21, 1994.

88. Masuno M, Imaizumi K, Ishii T, Kuroki Y, Baba N, Tanaka Y: Pilomatrixomas in Rubinstein-Taybi syndrome. *Am J Med Genet* **77**:81, 1998.

89. Jonas DM, Heilbron DC, Ablin AR: Rubinstein-Taybi syndrome and acute leukemia. *J Pediatr* **92**:851, 1978.

90. Goodfellow A, Emmerson RW, Calvert HT: Rubinstein-Taybi syndrome and spontaneous keloids. *Clin Exp Dermatol* **5**:369, 1980.

91. Sammartino A, Cerbella R, Lembo G, Federico A, Loffredo L: Syndrome de Rubinstein-Taybi à chéloïdes multiples. *J Franc Opthalmol* **9**:725, 1986.

92. Stevens CA, Bhakta MG: Cardiac abnormalities in the Rubinstein-Taybi syndrome. *Am J Med Genet* **59**:346, 1995.

93. Johnson CF: Broad thumbs and broad great toes with facial abnormalities and mental retardation. *J Pediatr* **68**:942, 1966.

94. Grunow JE: Gastroesophageal reflux in Rubinstein-Taybi syndrome. *J Pediatr Gastroenterol Nutr* **1**:273, 1982.

95. Shashi V, Fryburg JS: Vascular ring leading to tracheoesophageal compression in a patient with Rubinstein-Taybi syndrome. *Clin Genet* **48**:324, 1995.

96. Say B, Miller GC, Barber N, Grogg S: Association of birth defects and immunodeficiency. *Pediatrics* **94**:849, 1979.

97. Fragoso F, Ramos-Zepeda R, Vaca G, Hernandez A, Gonzalez-Quiroga G, Olivares N, Cantu JM: Deficiencies of cell immunity and mild intermittent hyperaminoacidemia in a patient with the Rubinstein-Taybi syndrome. *Acta Paediatr Scand* **69**:123, 1980.

98. Wyatt D: Transient hypoglycemia with hyperinsulinemia in a newborn infant with Rubinstein-Taybi syndrome. *Am J Med Genet* **37**:103, 1990.

99. Lahlou B, Carrier C: Ménométrorragies et bifidité utérine dans un cas du syndrome du "pouce en spatule." *Rev Internat Ped* **14**:5, 1971.

100. Barson AJ: Rubinstein-Taybi syndrome. *Arch Dis Child* **49**:495, 1974.

101. Martin-Gomez R, Sarmiento-Robles C, Ibanez Delgado F, Marin Morales JA, Marrero CS, Gallardo GPA: Agenesia de vesícula biliar y cístico como malformación associada en un síndrome de Rubinstein-Taybi. *Rev Esp Enf Ap Digest* **68**:357, 1985.

102. Zucconi M, Ferini-Strambi L, Erminio C, Pestalozza G, Smirne S: Obstructive sleep apnea in the Rubinstein-Taybi syndrome. *Respiration* **60**:127, 1993.

103. Stirt JA: Anesthetic problems in Rubinstein-Taybi syndrome. *Anesth Analg (Cleve)* **60**:534, 1981.

104. Kroth H: Cornelia de Lange-Syndrom I bei Zwillingen. *Arch Kinderheilkd* **173**:273, 1966.

105. Lowry RB: Overlap between Rubinstein-Taybi and Saethre-Chotzen syndromes: A case report. *Am J Med Genet* **6(Suppl)**:73, 1990.

106. Wilson MG: Rubinstein-Taybi and D trisomy syndromes. *J Pediatr* **73**:404, 1968.

107. Stevenson RE, Phelan MC, Stanislovitis P, Klinger K, Schwartz CE: Interstitial deletion of 7q22 in a fetus with anencephaly. *Proc Greenwood Genet Ctr* **8**:56, 1989.

108. Sharma AK, Haldar A, Phadke SR, Agarwal SS: Preaxial brachydactyly with abduction of thumbs and hallux varus: A distinct entity. *Am J Med Genet* **49**:274, 1994.

109. Tuomaala P, Haapanen E: Three siblings with similar anomalies in the eyes, bones and skin. *Arch Ophthalmol* **46**:365, 1968.

110. Collins OD, Sakati NA, Nyhan WL: Case report 15. *Syndr Ident* **2**:11, 1974.

111. Viljoen DL, Kallis J, Voges S, Marais AS, Van Vuuren I: An apparently new mental retardation syndrome in three elderly sisters. *Clin Genet* **40**:6, 1991.

112. Cotsirilos P, Taylor JC, Matalon R: Dominant inheritance of a syndrome similar to Rubinstein-Taybi. *Am J Med Genet* **26**:85, 1987.

113. Grix A, Blankenship W, Peterson R, Hall B: A new familial syndrome with craniofacial abnormalities, osseous defects and mental retardation. *Birth Defects* **11**:107, 1975.

114. Robinow M: A familial syndrome of mental deficiency and broad thumbs. *Birth Defects* **5**:42, 1969.

115. Rohmer F, Collard M, Bapst J, Micheletti G: Encephalopathies infantiles et dysmorphies complexes. Un cas de Rubinstein-Taybi. *Rev Oto-Neuro-Ophtalmol* **42**:306, 1970.

116. Hennekam RCM, Lommen EJP, Strengers JCM, Van Spijker HG, Jansen-Kokx TMG: Rubinstein-Taybi syndrome in a mother and son. *Eur J Pediatr* **148**:439, 1989.

117. Marion RW, Garcia DM, Karasik JB: Apparent dominant transmission of the Rubinstein-Taybi syndrome. *Am J Med Genet* **46**:284, 1993.

118. Marion RW: Personal communication, 1996.

119. Imaizumi K, Kuroki Y: Rubinstein-Taybi syndrome with de novo reciprocal translocation t(2;16)(p13.3;p13.3). *Am J Med Genet* **38**:636, 1991.

120. Tommerup N, van der Hagen CB, Heiberg A: Tentative assignment of a locus for Rubinstein-Taybi syndrome to 16p13.3 by a de novo reciprocal translocation, t(7;16)(q34;p13.3). *Am J Med Genet* **44**:237, 1992.

121. Lacombe D, Saura R, Taine L, Battin J: Confirmation of assignment of a locus for Rubinstein-Taybi syndrome gene to 16p13.3. *Am J Med Genet* **44**:126, 1992.

122. Breuning MH, Dauwerse HG, Fugazza G, Saris JJ, Spruit L, Wijnen H, Tommerup N, et al.: Rubinstein-Taybi syndrome caused by submicroscopic deletions within 16p13.3. *Am J Hum Genet* **52**:249, 1993.

123. Petrij F, Giles RH, Dauwerse JG, Saris JJ, Hennekam RCM, Masuno M., Tommerup N, et al.: Rubinstein-Taybi Syndrome is caused by

mutations in the transcriptional co-activator CBP. *Nature* **376**:348, 1995.

124. Masuno M, Imaizumi K, Kurosawa K, Makita Y, Petrij F, Dauwerse HG, Breuning MH, et al.: Submicroscopic deletion of chromosome region 16p13.3 in a Japanese patient with Rubinstein-Taybi syndrome. *Am J Med Genet* **53**:352, 1994.

125. MacGaughran JM, Gaunt L, Dore J, Petrij F, Dauwerse HG, Donnai D: Rubinstein-Taybi syndrome with deletions of FISH probe RT1 at 16p13.3: Two UK patients. *J Med Genet* **53**:352, 1996.

126. Wallerstein R, Anderson CE, Hay B, Gupta P, Gibas L, Ansari K, Cowchock FS, et al.: Submicroscopic deletions at 16p13.3 in Rubinstein-Taybi syndrome: Frequency and clinical manifestations in a North American population. *J Med Genet* **34**:203, 1997.

127. Taine L, Goizet C, Wen ZQ, Petrij F, Breuning MH, Ayme S, Saura R, et al.: Submicroscopic deletion of chromosome 16p13.3 in patients with Rubinstein-Taybi syndrome. *Am J Med Genet* **78**:267, 1998.

128. Hennekam RCM, Tilanus M, Hamel BCJ, Voshart-van Heeren H, Mariman ECM, van Beersum SEC, van den Boogaard MJH, et al.: Deletion at chromosome 16p13.3 as a cause of Rubinstein-Taybi syndrome: Clinical aspects. *Am J Hum Genet* **52**:255, 1993.

129. Giles RH, Petrij F, Dauwerse JG, van der Reijden BA, Beverstock GC, Hagemeijer A, Breuning MH: The translocation t(8;16) in ANLL M4/M5 disrupts the CBP gene on chromosome 16. *Blood* **86(Suppl)**:35, 1995.

130. Giles RH, Petrij F, Dauwerse HG, den Hollander AI, Lushnikova T, van Ommen GJ, Goodman RH, et al.: Construction of a 1.2-Mb contig surrounding, and molecular analysis of, the human CREB-binding protein (CBP/CREBBP) gene on chromosome 16p13.3. *Genomics* **42**:96, 1997.

131. Wessels JW, Mollevanger P, Dauwerse JG, Cluitmans FH, Breuning MH, Beverstock GC: Two distinct loci on the short arm of chromosome 16 are involved in myeloid leukemia. *Blood* **77**:1555, 1991.

132. Velloso ERP, Mecucci C, Michaux L, van Orshoven A, Stul M, Boogaerts M, Bosly A, et al.: Translocation t(8;16)(p11;p13) in acute nonlymphocytic leukemia: Report on two new cases and review of the literature. *Leuk Lymphoma* **21**:137, 1996.

133. Chrivia JC, Kwok RPS, Lamb N, Haglwara M, Montimny MR, Goodman RH: Phosphorylated CREB binds specifically to the nuclear protein CBP. *Nature* **365**:855, 1993.

134. Eckner R, Ewen ME, Newsome D, Gerdes M, DeCaprio JA, Bentley Lawrence J, Livingston DM: Molecular cloning and functional analysis of the adenovirus E1A-associated 300-kD protein (p300) reveals a protein with properties of a transcriptional adaptor. *Genes Dev* **8**:869, 1994.

135. Lundblad JR, Kwok RPS, Laurance ME, Harter ML, Goodman RH: Adenoviral E1A-associated protein p300 as a functional homologue of the transcriptional co-activator CBP. *Nature* **374**:85, 1995.

136. Giles RH: *Mutations of the CBP gene in human disease.* PhD Thesis. Leiden, Leiden University, 1998.

137. Borrow J, Stanton VP Jr, Andresen JM, Becher R, Behm FG, Chaganti RSK, Civin CI, et al.: The translocation t(8;16)(p11;p13) of acute myeloid leukemia fuses a putative acetyl transferase to the CREB-binding protein. *Nat Genet* **14**:33, 1996.

138. Rowley JD, Reshmi S, Sobulo O, Musvee T, Anastasi J, Raimondi S, Schneider NR, et al.: All patients with the t(11;16)(q23;p13.3) that involves MLL and CBP have treatment-related hematologic disorders. *Blood* **90**:535, 1997.

139. Sobulo OM, Borrow J, Tomek R, Reshmi S, Harden A, Schlegelberger B, Housman D, et al.: MLL is fused to CBP, a histone acetyltransferase, in therapy-related acute myeloid leukemia with a t(11;16)(q23;p13.3). *Proc Natl Acad Sci U S A* **94**:8732, 1997.

140. Taki T, Sako M, Tsuchida M, Hayashi Y: The t(11;16)(q23;p13) translocation in myelodysplastic syndrome fuses the MLL gene to the CBP gene. *Blood* **89**:3945, 1997.

141. Roest PAM, Roberts RG, Sugino S, van Ommen GJB, den Dunnen JT: Protein truncation test (PTT) for rapid detection of translation-terminating mutations. *Hum Mol Genet* **2**:1719, 1993.

142. Petrij F, Giles RH, Dorsman JC, Dauwerse JG, van Ommen GJB, Peters DJM, Breuning MH: Haploinsufficiency of CBP leads to the Rubinstein-Taybi Syndrome. *Am J Hum Genet* **59(Suppl)**:A142, 1996.

143. Tanaka Y, Naruse I, Maekawa T, Masuya H, Shiroishi T, Ishii S: Abnormal skeletal patterning in embryos lacking a single Cbp allele: A partial similarity with Rubinstein-Taybi syndrome. *Proc Natl Acad Sci U S A* **94**:10215, 1997.

144. Dallas PB, Yaciuk P, Moran E: Characterization of monoclonal antibodies raised against p300: Both p300 and CBP are present in intracellular TBP complexes. *J Virol* **71**:1726,1997.

145. Dallas PB, Cheney IW, Liao DW, Bowrin V, Byam W, Pacchione S, Kobayashi R, et al.: p300/CREB binding protein-related protein p270 is a component of mammalian SWI/SNF complexes. *Mol Cell Biol* **18**:3596, 1998.

146. Barbeau D, Charbonneau R, Whalen SG, Bayley ST, Branton PE: Functional interactions within adenovirus E1A protein complexes. *Oncogene* **9**:359, 1994.

147. Kwok RPS, Lundblad JR, Chrivia JC, Richards JP, Bächinger HP, Brennan RG, Roberts SGE, et al.: Nuclear protein CBP is a coactivator for the transcription factor CREB. *Nature* **370**:223, 1994.

148. Arias J, Alberts AS, Brindle P, Claret FX, Smeal T, Karin M, Feramisco J, et al.: Activation of cAMP and mitogen responsive genes relies on a common nuclear factor. *Nature* **370**:226, 1994.

149. Arany Z, Newsome D, Oldread E, Livingston DM, Eckner R: A family of transcriptional adaptor proteins targeted by the E1A oncoprotein. *Nature* **374**:81, 1995.

150. Moran E: DNA tumor virus transforming proteins and the cell cycle. *Curr Opin Genet Dev* **3**:63, 1993.

151. Shikama N, Lyon J, La Thangue NB: The p300/CBP family: Integrating signals with transcription factors and chromatin. *Trends Cell Biol* **7**:230, 1997.

152. Giles RH: CBP/p300 transgenic mice. *Trends Genet* **14**:214, 1998.

153. Kawasaki H, Eckner R, Yao T-S, Taira K, Chiu R, Livingston DM, Yokoyama KK: Distinct roles of the co-activators p300 and CBP in retinoic-acid-induced F9-cell differentiation. *Nature* **393**:284, 1998.

154. Lee J-S, Galvin KM, See RH, Eckner R, Livingston D, Moran E, Shi Y: Relief of YY1 transcriptional repression by adenovirus E1A is mediated by E1A-associated protein p300. *Genes Dev* **9**:1188, 1995.

155. Price ER, Ding HF, Badalian T, Bhattacharya S, Takemoto C, Yao TP, et al.: Lineage-specific signaling in melanocytes, c-Kit stimulation recruits p300/CBP to microphthalmia. *J Biol Chem* **273**:17983, 1998.

156. Kamei Y, Xu L, Heinzel T, Torchia J, Kurokawa R, Gloss B, Lin S-C, et al.: A CBP integrator complex mediates transcriptional activation and AP-1 inhibition by nuclear receptors. *Cell* **85**:403, 1996.

157. Glass CK, Rose DW, Rosenfeld MG: Nuclear receptor coactivators. *Curr Opin Cell Biol* **9**:222, 1997.

158. Horvai AE, Xu L, Korzus E, Brard G, Kalafus D, Mullen TM, et al.: Nuclear integration of JAK/Stat and Ras/AP-1 signaling by CBP and p300. *Proc Natl Acad Sci U S A* **94**:1074, 1997.

159. Costa SL, Pratt MAC, McBurney MW: E2F inhibits transcriptional activation by the retinoic acid receptor. *Cell Growth Differ* **7**:1479, 1996.

160. Cheng X, Reginato MJ, Andrews NC, Lazar MA: The transcriptional integrator CREB-binding protein mediates positive cross-talk between nuclear hormone receptors and the hematopoietic bZIP protein p45/NF-E2. *Mol Cell Biol* **17**:1407, 1997.

161. Yaciuk P, Moran E: Analysis with specific polyclonal antiserum indicates that the E1A-associated 300-kDa product is a stable nuclear phosphoprotein that undergoes cell-cycle specific modification. *Mol Cell Biol* **11**:5389, 1991.

162. Wang H-GH, Rikatake Y, Carter MC, Yaciuk P, Abraham SE, Brad Z, Moran E: Identification of specific adenovirus E1A amino-terminal residues critical to the binding of cellular proteins and to the control of cell growth. *J Virol* **10**:476, 1993.

163. Missero C, Calautti E, Eckner R, Chin J, Tsai H, Livingston DM, Dotto GP: Involvement of the cell-cycle inhibitor Cip1/WAF1 and the E1A-associated p300 protein in terminal differentiation. *Proc Natl Acad Sci U S A* **92**:5451, 1995.

164. Howe JA, Mymryk JS, Egan C, Branton PE, Bayley ST: Retinoblastoma growth suppressor and a 300-kilodalton protein both appear to regulate cellular DNA synthesis. *Proc Natl Acad Sci U S A* **87**:5883, 1990.

165. Brownell JE, Allis CD: Special HATs for special occasions: Linking histone acetylation to chromatin assembly and gene activation. *Curr Opin Genet Dev* **6**:176, 1996.

166. Montminy M: Something new to hang your HAT on. *Nature* **387**:654, 1997.

167. Roth SY, Allis CD: Histone acetylation and chromosome assembly: A single escort, multiple dances? *Cell* **87**:5, 1996.

168. Ogryzko VV, Schiltz RL, Russanova V, Howard BH, Nakatani Y: The transcriptional coactivators p300 and CBP are histone acetyltransferases. *Cell* **87**:953, 1996.

169. Bannister AJ, Kouzarides T: The CBP co-activator is a histone acetyltransferase. *Nature* **384**:641, 1996.

170. Utley RT, Ikeda K, Grant PA, Cote J, Steger DJ, Eberharter A, John S, et al.: Transcriptional activators direct histone acetyltransferase complexes to nucleosomes. *Nature* **394**:498, 1998.

171. Knudson AG: Mutation and cancer: Statistical study of retinoblastoma. *Proc Natl Acad Sci U S A* **68**:820, 1971.

172. Muraoka M, Konishi M, Kikuchi-Yanoshita R, Tanaka K, Shitara N, Chong JM, Iwama T, et al.: p300 gene alterations in colorectal and gastric carcinomas. *Oncogene* **12**:1565, 1996.

173. Hammerschmidt M, Brook A, McMahon AP: The world according to *hedgehog*. *Trends Genet* **13**:14, 1997.

174. Domínguez M, Brunner M, Hafen E, Basler K: Sending and receiving the hedgehog signal: Control by the *Drosophila* Gli protein Cubitus interruptus. *Science* **272**:1621, 1996.

175. Akimaru H, Chen Y, Dai P, Hou D-X, Nonaka M, Smolik SM, Armstrong S, et al.: *Drosophila* CBP is a co-activator of *cubitus interruptus* in *hedgehog* signalling. *Nature* **386**:735, 1997.

176. Akimaru H, Hou D-X, Ishii S: *Drosophila* CBP is required for *dorsal*-dependent *twist* gene expression. *Nat Genet* **17**:211, 1997.

177. Perkins NE, Felzien LK, Betts JC, Leung K, Beach DH, Nabel GJ: Regulation of NF-κB by cyclin-dependent kinases associated with the p300 coactivator. *Science* **275**:523, 1997.

178. Gerritsen ME, Williams AJ, Neish AS, Moore S, Shi Y, Collins T: CREB-binding protein/p300 are transcriptional coactivators of p65. *Proc Natl Acad Sci U S A* **94**:2927, 1997.

179. Vortkamp A, Gessler M, Grzechik K-H: GLI3 zinc-finger gene interrupted by translocations in Grieg syndrome families. *Nature* **352**:539, 1991.

180. El Ghouzzi V, Le Merrer M, Perrin-Schmitt F, Lajeunie E, Benit P, Renier D, Bourgeois P, et al.: Mutations of the *TWIST* gene in the Saethre-Chotzen syndrome. *Nat Genet* **15**:42, 1997.

181. Howard TD, Paznekas WA, Green ED, Chiang LC, Ma N, Ortiz De Luna RI, Garcia Delgado C, et al.: Mutations in *TWIST*, a basic helix-loop-helix transcription factor, in Saethre-Chotzen syndrome. *Nat Genet* **15**:36, 1997.

182. Yao TP, Oh SP, Fuchs M, Zhou ND, Ch'ng LE, Newsome D, Bronson RD, et al.: Gene dosage-dependent embryonic development and proliferation defects in mice lacking the transcriptional integrator p300. *Cell* **93**:361, 1998.

183. Petrij F, Dauwerse JG, Blough RI, Giles RH, van der Smagt JJ, Wallerstein R, Maaswinkel-Mooy PD, et al.: Diagnostic analysis of the Rubinstein-Taybi syndrome: five cosmids should be used for micro-deletion detection and low number of protein truncating mutations. *J Med Genet* **37**:168, 2000.

184. Petrij F, Dorsman JC, Dauwerse HG, Giles RH, Peeters T, Hennekam RCM, Breuning MH, et al.: Rubinstein-Taybi syndrome caused by a *de novo* reciprocal translocation t(2;16)(q36.3;p13.3). *Am J Med Genet* **92**:47, 2000.

185. Blough RI, Petrij F, Dauwerse JG, Milatovich-Cherry A, Weiss L, Saal HM, Rubinstein JH: Variation in microdeletions of the cyclic AMP-responsive element-binding protein gene at chromosome band 16p13.3 in the Rubinstein-Taybi syndrome. *Am J Med Genet* **90**:29, 2000.

186. Kung AL, Rebel VI, Bronson RT, Ch'ng LE, Sieff CA, Livingston DM, Yao TP: Gene dose-dependent control of hematopoiesis and hemato-logic tumor suppression by CBP. *Genes Dev* **14**:272, 2000.

187. Gayther SA, Batley SJ, Linger L, Bannister A, Thorpe K, Chin S-F, Daigo Y, et al.: Mutations truncating the EP300 acetylase in human cancers. *Nat Genet* **24**:300, 2000.

# Smith-Lemli-Opitz Syndrome

*Richard I. Kelley* ▪ *Raoul C. M. Hennekam*

Although cholesterol metabolism has been one of the most intensely studied metabolic pathways in humans, for many years the only known primary defect of the cholesterol biosynthetic pathway was mevalonic aciduria, a rare autosomal recessive deficiency of mevalonate kinase associated with developmental delays, craniofacial dysmorphism, and a variety of systemic and metabolic abnormalities (Chap. 93). However, in 1993, a second defect of cholesterol synthesis, a deficiency of 7-dehydrocholesterol reductase (DHCR7), was found to be the apparent cause of the RSH/Smith-Lemli-Opitz syndrome (SLOS), a relatively common autosomal-recessive multiple-malformation syndrome. Patients with both mild and severe forms of SLOS had markedly increased levels of 7-dehydrocholesterol (7DHC) and decreased levels of cholesterol. The finding 5 years later of disabling mutations in the DHCR7 gene in patients with SLOS confirmed SLOS as the second defect of cholesterol biosynthesis and the first affecting sterol metabolism per se.

The discovery of the biochemical cause of SLOS and the subsequent redefinition of SLOS as an inborn error of cholesterol metabolism has led not only to successful treatment of affected patients, but also to the recognition of the important role of cholesterol in vertebrate embryogenesis. Moreover, the discovery at about the same time that cholesterol is directly involved in the hedgehog embryonic signaling pathway suggested an important link between embryogenesis and the abnormal metabolism in SLOS. No less important has been the recognition of the critical role that cholesterol plays in the expression of the abnormal behaviors that characterize SLOS.

## HISTORY OF SMITH-LEMLI-OPITZ SYNDROME

Smith-Lemli-Opitz syndrome was first described as a coherent multiple malformation syndrome in 1964[1] in a report of three patients with a distinctive facial appearance and the common abnormalities of global developmental delays, microcephaly, broad alveolar ridges, hypospadias, a characteristic dermatoglyphic pattern, and severe feeding disorder. A more complete delineation of SLOS was presented in 1969 as the "RSH syndrome," a non-descriptive acronym of the first letters of the original patients' surnames.[2] The description of many new cases of SLOS over the next 20 years expanded the known characteristics of the syndrome to include midline cleft palate, cataracts, postaxial polydactyly, heart defects, and a variety of central nervous system defects (Table 249-1).[2–11] Many affected children died in the first year from failure to thrive and infections, but many others survived to adulthood. Somewhat later, several authors described patients with a lethal syndrome that resembled SLOS, so-called "type II SLOS."[12–16] These children had many of the "external" anomalies of SLOS, but died in the newborn period from severe internal malformations, including pulmonary hypoplasia, complex congenital heart disease, renal hypoplasia or agenesis, and Hirschsprung disease. In addition, some 46,XY males had severe hypogenitalism or female-appearing external genitalia. In all informative families, segregation of either form of SLOS was consistent with autosomal recessive inheritance,[2,12] and the severity of malformations and degree of mental retardation was usually similar in sibs.

Although SLOS proved to be a relatively common syndrome with estimates of incidence ranging from 1 in 40,000 to 1 in 20,000 births,[17,18] the genetic cause of the disorder was not suspected for many years. However, by the mid-1980s, a number of abnormalities of steroid and cholesterol metabolism in SLOS had been reported. In part, the search for defects of steroid metabolism had been prompted by the sexual ambiguity common in the more severely affected males, and by the finding of enlarged, lipid-depleted adrenal glands in some patients.[19] The steroid abnormalities included aberrant patterns of steroid sulfates in plasma and urine,[20] low basal and stimulated levels of testosterone, hypocholesterolemia,[12] and low maternal estriol levels in mid and late gestation.[19] However, the primary defect remained unknown until Natowicz and Evans[21] found that a patient with a relatively severe form of SLOS had essentially undetectable levels of normal urinary bile acids. An analysis of that patient's plasma sterols led to the discovery by Tint and colleagues[22] that, in addition to a low plasma cholesterol level, the patient had a more than 1000-fold increase in the plasma level of 7-dehydrocholesterol (cholesta-5,7-dien-3$\beta$-ol; "7DHC"), the immediate precursor of cholesterol in the Kandutsch-Russell biosynthetic pathway.[23] The finding of the same biochemical abnormality in additional patients with a clinical diagnosis of SLOS confirmed the sterol abnormality as a principal characteristic of SLOS.[24] Although 7DHC represented the major abnormal sterol in plasma of most SLOS patients, large amounts of two other diene isomers of 7DHC — isodehydrocholesterol (cholesta-6,8-dien-3$\beta$-ol) and 8-dehydrocholesterol (cholesta-5,8(9)-dien-3$\beta$-ol) — were also found, forming a distinctive pattern of plasma diene sterols.[24] The same diene sterol pattern subsequently was found in most patients with both classical SLOS and the more severe type II SLOS, as well as in patients with variant syndromes that could not be assigned the diagnosis of SLOS on clinical grounds alone.[25] Enzymatic support for the apparent cause of the distinctive sterol pattern — a deficiency of microsomal DHCR7 — was soon provided.[26,27] Although initial evidence suggested that the human gene for SLOS was located at 7q32.1,[28] the human DHCR7 was later cloned and localized to chromosome 11q12-13 by Moebius et al.,[29] who shortly afterward reported apparently disabling mutations of DHCR7 in 13 patients with SLOS. Mutations in DHCR7 in three additional SLOS patients by others[30,31] confirmed abnormal function of DHCR7 as the cause of most cases of SLOS.

## CLINICAL SYNDROME

### Incidence

Lowry and Yong[17] made the earliest estimate of the incidence of SLOS. They found an incidence in British Columbia between 1964 and 1971 of 1 in 40,000 births, indicating a carrier frequency of 1

**Table 249-1** Clinical Characteristics of Smith-Lemli-Opitz Syndrome

| More than 50% of patients | 10 to 50% of patients |
|---|---|
| Mental retardation ($>$95%) | Cataracts |
| Microcephaly ($>$90%) | Postaxial polydactyly |
| Hypotonia | Cardiac defect |
| Epicanthal folds | Sexual ambiguity |
| Blepharoptosis | Prenatal growth retardation |
| Low set, abnormal pinnae | Renal cystic dysplasia |
| Cleft palate | Cholestatic liver disease |
| Broad maxillary alveolar ridges | Adrenal hyperplasia |
| Small tongue | Abnormal pulmonary lobation |
| Micrognathia | Hirschsprung disease |
| Hypospadias* | Equinovarus deformity |
| Cryptorchidism* | Pyloric stenosis |
| Syndactyly of toes 2 & 3 ($>$90%) | |
| Postnatal growth retardation | |

* Greater than 50% of 46,XY patients

**Table 249-2** Finding in 167 Clinically Diagnosed Cases of Smith-Lemli-Opitz Syndrome Compared with 151 Biochemically Confirmed Cases

| Finding | Clinically diagnosed (167) (%) | Biochemically confirmed (151) (%) |
|---|---|---|
| Mental retardaton | 97 | 95 |
| Postnatal growth retardaton | 85 | 80 |
| Microcephaly | 80 | 83 |
| Structural brain anomalies | 60 | 36 |
| Ptosis | 69 | 68 |
| Cataract | 23 | 22 |
| Anteverted nares | 90 | 77 |
| Cleft palate* | 51 | 47 |
| Congenital heart defect | 50 | 54 |
| Abnormal lung lobation | 40 | 45 |
| Pyloric stenosis | 15 | 14 |
| Colonic aganglionosis | 12 | 17 |
| Renal anomalies | 40 | 43 |
| Genital anomalies | 74 | 64 |
| 2-3 Toe syndactyly | 85 | 95 |
| Polydactyly† | 52 | 48 |

*Includes cleft soft palate, submucous cleft, and cleft uvula
†Includes postaxial polydactyly of hand(s) and/or foot

percent. The incidence increased to 1 in 20,000 births when suspected but less definite cases were included. A similar study in New England found an incidence of 1 in 30,000 births. In contrast to these relatively high incidences based exclusively on clinical diagnosis, the incidence of SLOS diagnosed biochemically in similar populations appears to be lower. For example, between the two laboratories that performed approximately 90 percent of biochemical testing for SLOS in the United States between 1993 and 1998, approximately 40 new cases per year were diagnosed, or less than 1 in 60,000 births (Kelley and Tint, unpublished data). Similarly low estimates of 1 in 80,000 to 100,000 births in the Netherlands (Hennekam et al., unpublished data) and 1 in 60,000 newborns in the United Kingdom[32] have been made. Even lower incidences were reported by Tsukahara et al.[33] They found only 2 of 31 clinically diagnosed cases in Japan had abnormal 7DHC metabolism. The number of reported cases with African ancestry is also low.[25,34] Although there remains some uncertainty about the absolute incidence of SLOS in some countries, there clearly are strikingly different incidences among various ethnic groups. Both heterozygote advantage and founder effect have been suggested to explain the much higher incidence of SLOS among those of European descent.

## Clinical Overview

Most literature reports about SLOS describe only a single patient or a small number of patients. There are a few exceptions in which 10 or more cases are described, notably Opitz et al.,[2] Cherstvoy et al.,[9] Bene et al.,[35] Curry et al.,[12] Cunniff et al.,[25] and Ryan et al.[32] Furthermore, several excellent reviews in the older literature exist.[10,15,36] A tabulation of the major clinical features of patients who were described with sufficient detail in the literature is provided in Table 249-2. A comparison of the most common characteristics of patients ascertained by clinical versus biochemical diagnosis shows remarkably similar frequencies of the physical anomalies. Only structural brain anomalies and anomalies of the genitalia are somewhat more common in the clinically diagnosed group, otherwise the percentages show a remarkable similarity.

Prior to the recognition of the biochemical cause of SLOS, several authors suggested that there might be two forms of SLOS, which were distinguishable by the severity of physical anomalies and their clinical course.[12,13,37] "Type I" was the original, classical syndrome, and "type II" was a more severe entity, usually lethal in the early months of life and associated with severe internal anomalies and markedly abnormal male genitalia. Curry et al.[12] cautiously suggested that types I and II might differ genetically, whereas others thought support for a genetic

difference to be weak.[38] To address this question, Bialer et al.[15] devised a scoring system to measure the clinical severity of SLOS and analyzed the distribution of anomalies. Upon scoring 122 reported patients from literature, they found a unimodal distribution of the scores for various anomalies, which was interpreted as evidence for a continuum of severity in SLOS and against a genetic distinction between SLOS types I and II. A similar continuum of severity was found by Cunniff et al.[25] and Ryan et al.[32] in their series of biochemically confirmed cases. Both the original scoring system of Bialer et al. and a revised scoring system wherein malformation in embryologically separate organ systems are weighted equally (Kelley and Hennekam, unpublished) show strong correlations with various biochemical parameters. Subsequent molecular genetic studies confirmed that the differences in severity between SLOS types I and II are explained by the severity of the responsible mutations (see "Enzymology and Molecular Genetics" below). However, this does not preclude the existence of genetic heterogeneity in SLOS, as suggested by the cases of Anderson et al.[39]

## Differential Diagnosis of Smith-Lemli-Opitz Syndrome

Many papers describe patients with a clinical phenotype resembling SLOS, especially before the era of biochemical diagnosis. In the German literature, the designations Ullrich-Feichtiger syndrome[40] or Typus Rostockiensis,[41] a multiple congenital anomalies syndrome with facial anomalies, polydactyly, and hypospadias, probably describe severe forms of SLOS.[42] Among clinical diagnoses that have been proven or suspected to include cases of SLOS are the acrodysgenital syndrome,[37,43,44] Gardner-Silengo-Wachtel syndrome (OMIM 231060),[45,46] and holoprosencephaly-polydactyly (pseudotrisomy 13) syndrome (OMIM 264480).[47] However, the predominance in the Gardner-Silengo-Wachtel syndrome of conotruncal malformations and in holoprosencephaly-polydactyly syndrome of gonadal dysgenesis, both uncommon abnormalities in SLOS, suggests that some of these biochemically unconfirmed patients do not have SLOS. Among diagnoses that have been incorrectly assigned to patients with SLOS are Noonan syndrome (OMIM 163950), Zellweger syndrome (OMIM 214100), alpha-thalassemia-mental retardation syndrome (OMIM 301040), and Opitz syndrome

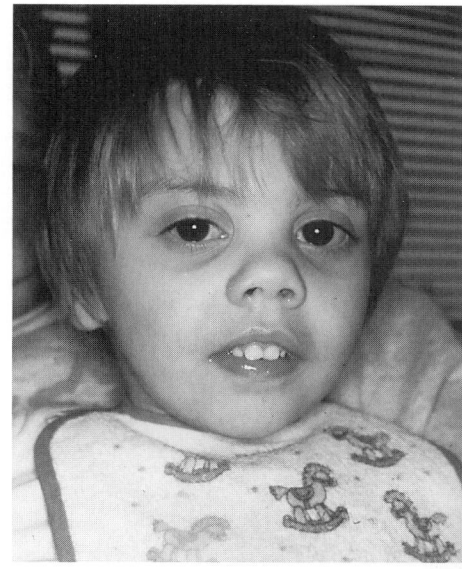
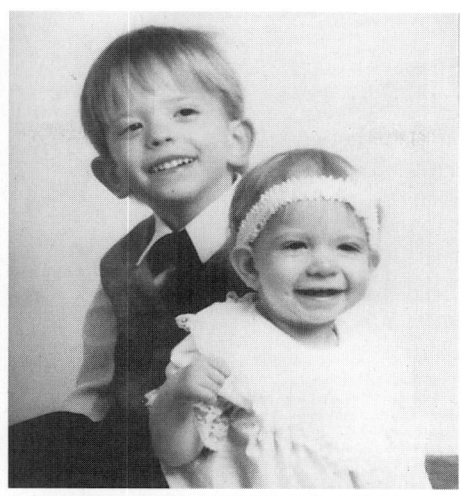
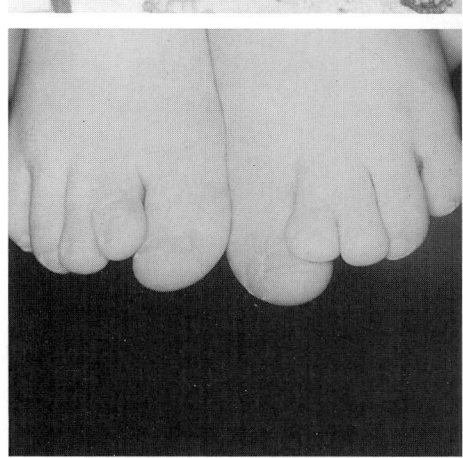
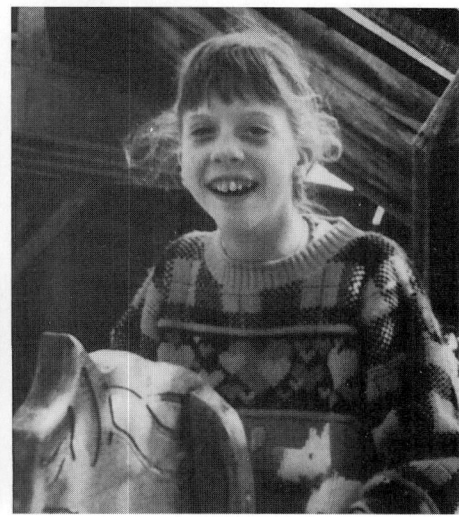

**Fig. 249-1A Smith-Lemli-Opitz syndrome. Upper left: 3 year old with cleft palate and (lower left) characteristic Y-shaped syndactyly of toes 2 and 3. Upper right: 3-year-old boy and his 8-month-old sister with near normal cholestrol levels, mildly increased 7-dehydrocholesterol levels (20–40 µg/ml), and unusually mild physical characteristics of Smith-Lemli-Opitz syndrome. Note the low-set ears and mild ptosis evident in the 3-year-old boy. Lower right: 12 year old with typical facial characteristics of classical Smith-Lemli-Opitz syndrome.**

(OMIM 145410, 300000). Other disorders that resemble SLOS, but less so, are Meckel syndrome (OMIM 249000), hydrolethalus syndrome (OMIM 236680), Pallister-Hall syndrome (OMIM 146510), and orofaciodigital syndrome type VI (OMIM 277170).[12,13,42,48,49]

## Craniofacial Characteristics

The "SLOS-face" is highly characteristic of the syndrome and easily recognized in most patients.[32,50] The most salient features are microcephaly, bitemporal narrowing, ptosis, a short nasal root, anteverted nares, and a small chin (Fig. 249-1). Two other almost universal characteristics are congenital microcephaly and ptosis, often asymmetric or unilateral. Although a prominent metopic ridge can often be palpated, true craniosynostosis is uncommon.[2] Other less frequent anomalies include hypertelorism, epicanthal folds, congenital, and occasionally postnatal, cataracts, strabismus,[11,51–53] glaucoma,[2,12] optic atrophy,[2,12,52] and microphthalmia.[5,25] The nasal bridge can be flat or high, often with a striking capillary hemangioma extending across the glabella. The degree of anteversion of the nares decreases with age but remains distinct in some adults.[32,54]

The ears often appear low set and posteriorly rotated, but are otherwise unremarkable. Congenital sensorineural hearing deficits may affect as many as 10 percent of patients, but many more severely affected children are not tested. The philtrum is long, as can be expected in shortening of the nose. Cleft lip has been reported in SLOS;[13,55,56] however, in patients with abnormal cholesterol metabolism, only the "midline" type of cleft associated with the holoprosencephaly sequence is present.[57] In some patients, the mouth is large, which, combined with frequent micrognathia, gives a distinctive appearance.[54] More severe micrognathia, including the classic Pierre Robin sequence, is not rare in SLOS. The neck can appear short, and excessive skin folds or nuchal edema are common, especially prenatally.[58]

The oral anomalies of SLOS are diagnostically important. The palate usually is highly arched, often with a midline cleft of the uvula, soft palate, or hard palate. In addition, the alveolar ridges typically are abnormally broad and conspicuously ridged. The tongue can be small with redundant sublingual tissue[12] or sublingual cysts[13,37] in the more severely affected children; rarely, the tongue is bifid.[32] Crowding and widely spaced incisors are not uncommon, and oligodontia and polydontia,[51] enamel hypoplasia,[10] and premature tooth eruption[59] have been reported. Pharyngeal abnormalities have included a small larynx[13] and small vocal cords with a subglottic shelf of excess fibrocartilaginous tissue.[12]

## Central Nervous System

The structural brain abnormalities of SLOS have been reviewed by Garcia et al.,[60] Cherstvoy et al.,[61] and Marion et al.[62] In addition to microcephaly, which is almost universal in SLOS, common abnormalities include enlarged ventricles,[2,12] hypoplasia or aplasia of the corpus callosum, and hypoplastic frontal lobes.[9,12,32] Cerebellar hypoplasia, sometimes with severe hypoplasia or aplasia of the vermis, is also not uncommon.[51,62,63] Various forms of the holoprosencephaly sequence occur in approximately 5

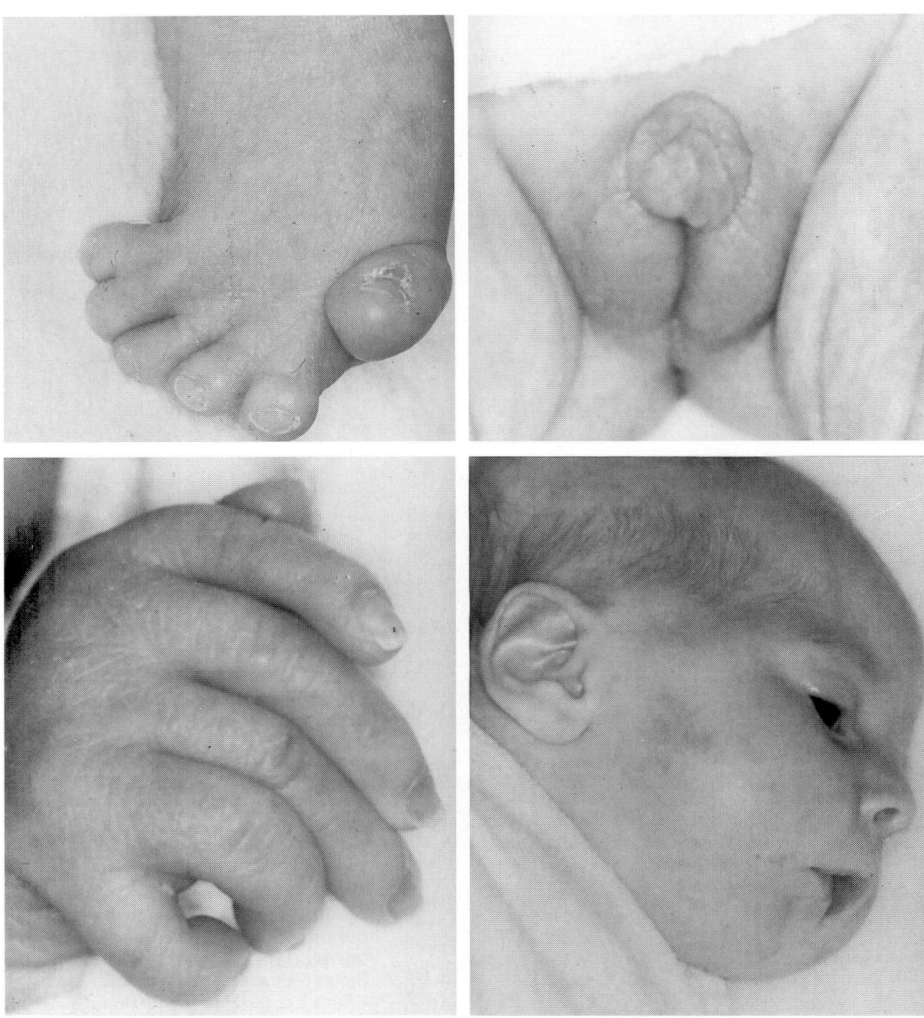

**Fig. 249-1B** Smith-Lemli-Opitz syndrome. Severely affected 46,XY patients with ambiguous genitalia (upper right), low cholesterol level of 15.3 mg/dl, and a 7-dehydrocholesterol level of 138 µg/ml). Note the complete postaxial (ulnar side) polydactyly of the hand and the striking polysyndactyly of the foot with a greatly shortened first metatarsal. The view of the face illustrates the low-set ear, severe micrognathia, and hypotonia.

percent of patients.[5,13,19,57] On histologic examination of the brain, the most important findings are disturbed cerebral neuronal migration, dysplasia of the medial olivary nuclei, and ectopic Purkinje cells.[9,51] Several authors[54] reported maturational abnormalities of the white matter, but these are not common. Although seizures are not uncommonly reported in the SLOS literature, they are uncommon in biochemically proven cases of SLOS, and may not be significantly more frequent than expected.[2,32,64]

### Skeletal Anomalies

The skeletal anomalies have been reviewed in detail.[10,15,25,32,61] Bilateral or unilateral postaxial polydactyly can be present in the hands, or, less commonly, the feet, or both. However, preaxial polydactyly has not been reported in a biochemically proven case. The thumb is generally short and proximally placed and the first metacarpals and thenar eminences are typically hypoplastic.[2,65] Other unusual digital abnormalities include ectrodactyly, mono-dactyly, and oligodactyly; radial agenesis; brachydactyly; absent middle phalanx of the second finger; radial or ulnar deviation of fingers; clinodactyly; camptodactyly; and syndactylies (between fingers 3 and 4 or 4 and 5).[2,10,12,56,66,67] Rhizomelic and mesomelic limb shortness and, more rarely, "chondrodysplasia punctata" occur in SLOS, but a true chondrodystrophy is not found.[12,13,16,32,61] Dermatoglyphics in SLOS are distinctive in having increased number of whorls on the fingertips.[2,10] One of the most consistently present anomalies of SLOS is the distinctive Y-shaped cutaneous syndactyly of the second and third toe, which has been reported in up to 99 percent of biochemically proven

cases.[25,32] Postaxial polydactyly of the feet is common in severe SLOS, and sometimes takes the form of polysyndactyly with a "windswept" foot deformity. Other lower-limb abnormalities include club foot, varus or valgus foot deformities, short first toes, and hip dislocations.[9,12,32,37] Occasionally, reported skeletal abnormalities include dense base of the skull,[37] scoliosis,[17,64] kyphosis,[17,68] ovoid vertebrae,[69] cervical ribs, thin ribs,[43,69] and missing ribs.[68] Although epiphyseal stippling (chondrodysplasia punctata) has been reported in a few cases,[1,38,69] such stippling has been found in only one biochemically confirmed case.[70]

### Genital Anomalies

The genitalia in male SLOS patients range from normal to apparent complete sex reversal.[12,13,14,15,59,71] Classically, hypospadias varies from coronal to perineoscrotal hypospadias, although the latter is uncommon except in the biochemically most severely affected cases. Cryptorchidism is common, but even with severely malformed genitalia, the testes often are easily palpated in the scrotum, which is sometimes bifid. Müllerian duct derivatives usually are absent in 46,XY males, as expected, but blind-ending vaginas, rudimentary or bicornuate uteri, and persistent cloacae have been described.[12,13,15,37,72,73] The gonads vary from normal testes to ovotestes to normal ovaries. In females, the external genitalia may appear normal or there may be distinct hypoplasia of the labia majora and minora. There are also single reports of premature thelarche and high serum-prolactin levels in a 15-month-old girl with SLOS[74] and a malignant germ-cell tumor with a contralateral streak gonad in another female.[75] Menstrual function is often irregular but otherwise normal in most SLOS adolescent females and adults, except for somewhat later menarche. One adolescent girl with SLOS and borderline intelligence gave birth to an apparently normal daughter.[17]

## Cardiovascular Anomalies

Robinson et al.,[7] Johnson,[10] and, most extensively, Lin et al.[76] have reviewed the cardiac anomalies of SLOS. Almost half of SLOS patients have a congenital heart defect; if only biochemically confirmed patients are considered, however, this percentage is somewhat lower.[25,32,76] There is a strong predominance of endocardial cushion defects and the hypoplastic left heart sequence, whereas conotruncal defects are uncommon. The five most prevalent defects found in a study of 95 biochemically confirmed cases of SLOS were: atrioventricular canal (25 percent), secundum atrial septal defect (20 percent), patent ductus arteriosus (18 percent), and membranous ventricular septal defect (10 percent).[76] Although Lin et al. hypothesized that the abnormal development of the extracellular matrix may be the cause of both the cardiac defects and the absence of ganglion cells in the bowel wall (Hirschsprung disease), abnormal development of the neural crest, which contributes substantially to the endocardial cushions, could explain both the cardiac defects and abnormal intestinal ganglion cells. In addition to structural heart defects, there is a substantially increased frequency of pulmonary hypertension in the newborn period and persistent systemic hypertension postnatally, but limited largely to patients with especially low cholesterol levels and possibly related to the abnormal steroid metabolism of these patients.[64,68,77]

## Renal and Adrenal Anomalies

Approximately one-fourth of patients with biochemically confirmed SLOS have renal anomalies,[13,32] most commonly renal hypoplasia or aplasia,[10,12,13,32,55,78] renal cortical cysts,[9,12,32] hydronephrosis,[9,32,59,79] renal ectopia,[1,9,37] ureteral duplication,[37,59] or persistent fetal lobation.[15,32,37] A number of cases with the oligohydramnios sequence caused by bilateral aplasia or other renal causes of severely diminished urinary output have been described.[12,13,78] The bladder and ureters may be hypoplastic, probably secondary to renal hypoplasia or aplasia.

Both adrenal hyperplasia[12,19] and adrenal hypoplasia[13] have been reported in SLOS, but growth and shape of the adrenals appear to be normal in most patients.[13] Histologic studies of hyperplastic SLOS adrenal glands[19] typically show deficient cortical lipid, which, in normal fetal adrenals, contains much cholesterol. Postnatal studies of adrenal function in children with SLOS have shown either normal function[80] or, in several biochemically severely affected children, decreased steroid synthesis.[81]

## Pulmonary Anomalies

Abnormal pulmonary lobation and pulmonary hypoplasia are common in the more severely affected cases of SLOS and are common causes of death in such patients.[9,12,13,37,72] As expected, pulmonary hypoplasia is also common in SLOS patients with the oligohydramnios sequence secondary to renal aplasia.[12,13] Anomalies of the laryngeal and tracheal cartilages are common even among patients with mild forms of SLOS. Serious complications have resulted from difficulties with emergent or elective intubation because of marked tracheal narrowing and other abnormalities of the laryngeal and tracheal structures[63] (Kelley, unpublished observations).

## Gastrointestinal Anomalies

Pyloric stenosis is a prominent clinical problem noted in the original description of SLOS and in many subsequent case reports.[1,2,32,82] Pyloric stenosis in SLOS has the usual characteristics of pyloric stenosis in otherwise normal children, but vomiting and other feeding problems commonly persist after surgical repair, in part due to apparent abnormalities of intestinal

motility. In the more severe cases, intestinal aganglionosis occurs, either as short segment disease or as extensive involvement of the upper and lower intestinal tract.[12,70,83,84] Even among SLOS patients lacking histologic evidence of intestinal aganglionosis, intestinal dysmotility is common, especially in the first year. However, whereas pyloric stenosis historically has been reported in up to 25 percent of SLOS patients, it is now uncommon in SLOS patients treated with supplementary cholesterol starting shortly after birth.

A small number of SLOS patients have had the unusual finding of dysplasia or aplasia of the gallbladder[12,32] or gallstones in infancy or later childhood.[12,64] More common, however, is transient or, more rarely, lethal cholestatic liver disease.[12,32,85,86] Histologically, iron pigment in liver cells is increased.[72,86] Although lipidosis is not commonly associated with SLOS, diffuse lipid storage was reported by Parnes et al.,[87] and Porter et al.[88] recently described impaired intracellular trafficking of LDL in SLOS fibroblasts.

Pancreatic islet cell hyperplasia has been reported frequently in severe SLOS.[9,12,19,37,72] The histology in these cases features nesidioblastosis and reduced quantities of somatostatin.[19,89] Other abdominal malformations that are less frequently reported include intestinal malrotations,[9,12,32] absence of the diaphragm or diaphragmatic hernia,[9,55] polysplenia and asplenia,[9] anal stenosis or atresia,[9,13,71] and Meckel's diverticulum.[2,7]

## Other Anomalies and Clinical Problems

Involuted[86] and hypoplastic thymus[84] and absent parathyroids[12] have been found. Among the more common dermatologic and hair abnormalities are hypopigmented hair,[2,90] mild to extreme skin photosensitivity in more than half of patients,[32] hyperhidrosis of the palms,[91] marked cutis marmorata,[84] and eczema.[32] Widely spaced nipples are mentioned repeatedly. There are two reports of excessive muscle rigidity after halothane anesthesia, but diagnostically elevated creatine kinase levels were not documented.[92,93]

## Natural History

The neonatal period and infancy are almost invariably associated with feeding problems including weak or abnormal suck, swallowing difficulties, vomiting, and lack of interest in feeding. Oral tactile defensiveness and failure of progression to textured foods in later months is also characteristic of the SLOS infant. As a result, more than 50 percent of patients require nasogastric tube feedings, often progressing to gastrostomy feeding for several years. As expected, patients with a cleft palate and a small mandible (Pierre Robin sequence) have the most severe feeding problems. Although gastroesophageal reflux is a common problem in patients with SLOS, such reflux is often caused by a failure to recognize that the children have congenitally small stomachs and primary intestinal dysmotility. Pyloric stenosis also is much more common in SLOS cases when compared to incidence in the general population.[76,82] Lin et al.[76] found pyloric stenosis in 7 percent of biochemically confirmed cases and in 11 percent of literature cases, but both figures may be underestimates.

Severe hypotonia is essentially universal in SLOS during infancy. Although the hypotonia is partly central in origin, congenital muscle hypoplasia also contributes. However, during the second year, muscle mass and tone improve and muscle strength and tone are typically normal in older children with SLOS. In later childhood, increased muscle tone is common and can lead to joint and skeletal problems in nonambulatory children. Such hypertonia appears to be extrapyramidal rather than spastic.

**Growth.** Failure to thrive is almost universally diagnosed in children with SLOS, but the diagnosis is incorrect more often than not. Infants with SLOS are small for gestational age and most continue to grow below the third percentile despite adequate caloric intake, indicating a fundamental, genetic hypotrophy as the basis of the growth retardation. Weight gain can be poor in the first

2 years because of feeding and GI motility problems, but most children with SLOS have normal linear and weight growth velocities in later years. Similarly, head circumference is proportionally the smallest measurement at birth and usually increases proportionally with other measurements postnatally. Although almost all SLOS children are small for their age, a formal study of the natural history of growth in SLOS has not been undertaken. Whereas most measurements for classical SLOS fall between −1 and −5 standard deviations (SD), measurements as low as −8 to −10 SD occur in more severely affected patients. With a few exceptions at the extremes, final adult height and head circumference are between 2 and 5 SD below normal.[12,13,32,94] In several published series, final height in adults was between 143 and 170 cm.[32,54,95] However, these figures are for patients with classic type I SLOS. Size at birth and growth of patients with more severe biochemical abnormalities, more of whom now survive with cholesterol treatment, are substantially less than in classic SLOS.

**Infections.** During both infancy and childhood, children with SLOS appear to have an increased rate of infections. Although many of the infections are otitis media, skin infections and pneumonias also seem to occur more often. However, despite the frequency of reflux in children with SLOS, aspiration pneumonia is surprisingly uncommon, most likely because the children's exaggerated gag reflux provides excellent airway protection. Except for a single report of abnormal monocyte oxidative metabolism,[96] no specific primary immune disturbances have been described in SLOS. However, death from sudden, overwhelming infection is not rare in SLOS, suggesting a fundamental abnormality in immune defenses or, possibly, adrenal function.[81] Apart from the high frequency of milk and soya protein allergy[68] and possibly an increased frequency of reactive airway disease, other allergies, or immunologic diseases such as eczema, thyroiditis, or arthritis, do not seem to be common in SLOS.

**Development.** With few exceptions, global psychomotor retardation is characteristic of SLOS. Although, historically, most patients have been described as severely mentally retarded (IQ 20 to 40), such apparently poor development in part reflected difficulties in testing. The average SLOS child is very sociable, has much better receptive than expressive language, and may be surprisingly mechanically adept for their degree of retardation. Because of their poor expressive language, routine developmental testing, unless performed by an expert, often underestimates the cognitive abilities of SLOS children. Gross motor development is typically more severely delayed than fine motor development, but children with SLOS usually learn to walk between 2 and 4 years of age. With the availability of biochemical testing and the recognition of many more mildly affected SLOS children, the known developmental spectrum has widened significantly. Approximately 10 percent of children with biochemically diagnosed SLOS have development in the mildly retarded range (IQ 50 to 70). A few patients with normal or borderline normal development have been described,[17,32] and it is likely that the number of patients with borderline and normal intelligence will increase, largely because biochemical testing now allows the identification of heretofore undiagnosable patients with minimal disease.

**Behavioral Abnormalities.** Excessive sleeping and poor responsiveness are common in the first few months of life. However, hours of shrill screeching or inconsolable screaming, especially at night and early in the morning, are major behavioral characteristics of SLOS later in infancy.[10,32] Other patients appear hypersensitive to all visual and auditory stimuli and must be kept in quiet, dark rooms. Ryan et al.[32] drew attention to the strikingly diminished amount of sleep in early childhood, which they found in 70 percent of their patients, some of whom slept only 2 or 3 hours at night. Although this abnormal sleeping pattern may gradually improve with age, adult SLOS patients with similar sleep problems are known. Many patients, even those with very mild clinical disease, may show self-injurious and aggressive behaviors. Most characteristic above the age of 3 years are forceful hyperarching, with or without head banging, and arm and hand biting. Aggressiveness, manifested most often as abrupt striking out, is seen when the children are frustrated. Marked tactile hypersensitivity of the hands and feet is also seen in more than 50 percent of patients. Common behavioral abnormalities that fall within the spectrum of autism include hand-flapping, abnormal obsessions, rigidity and insistence on routine, and poor visual contact. Despite these many behavioral problems, most parents describe their children as loving, affectionate, and happy.[2,32]

**Prenatal Losses and Postnatal Life Expectancy.** Although some investigators have suggested that there is an increased rate of spontaneous abortion in families with SLOS, Ryan et al.,[32] in the only systematic study of prenatal losses, found 39 propositi, 51 healthy sibs, 16 spontaneous abortions, and 7 elective terminations among 43 sibships with 113 known conceptions. Although these data do not support the hypothesis[10,18] that there is a substantially increased rate of spontaneous abortions in SLOS families, such may still obtain in families with more severely affected children, because severe cardiac or renal abnormalities have been known to lead to mid-trimester intrauterine demise of SLOS fetuses. The low 17 percent segregation ratio found in one large series[10] could also be explained by the inclusion of a proportion of genetically different disorders because the diagnoses were made clinically.

Although there are no recent figures for life expectancy in SLOS, Johnson[10] found that 27 percent of cases in her series died before 2 years of age. However, an analysis of the causes of death was not provided. As ascertainment of SLOS, even in the era of biochemical diagnosis, has been incomplete, the exact percentage of cases with early lethality remains uncertain. Clearly, however, life expectancy in SLOS is determined largely by the severity of the internal malformations and the quality of general supportive care and not by an intrinsic degenerative process.

## NORMAL STEROL BIOSYNTHESIS

Sterols are essential cellular components in both plant and animal kingdoms. They are synthesized by a complex series of reactions beginning with 3-hydroxy-3-methylglutaryl(HMG)-CoA and ending with the 30-carbon precursor of all other sterols, lanosterol (4,4′,14-trimethylcholesta-8(9),24-dien-3$\beta$-ol) (Fig.249-2). Although many of the steps in the synthesis of lanosterol are localized to the endoplasmic reticulum, some of the required enzymes are now known to be partially or exclusively localized to peroxisomes.[97,98] The first reaction, the reduction of HMG-CoA to mevalonic acid, the six-carbon acid alcohol, is catalyzed by HMG-CoA reductase, which is generally accepted as the principal rate-determining step of cholesterol biosynthesis.[99] The cytoplasmic pool of HMG-CoA that flows through mevalonic acid to sterol synthesis is physiologically distinct from the intramitochondrial pool of HMG-CoA, which has a central role in ketogenesis and the catabolism of leucine. Microsomal HMG-CoA is synthesized from the condensation of acetyl-CoA with acetoacetyl-CoA, which itself is made from two acetyl-CoA molecules via the action of acetoacetyl-CoA synthase. The coordinated transcriptional regulation of HMG-CoA reductase, acetoacetyl-CoA synthase, and the plasma membrane LDL receptor assures the maintenance of a stable cellular pool of cholesterol from both intracellular and extracellular sources.[99]

Cholesterol, a 27-carbon, monounsaturated sterol, is synthesized from lanosterol by a series of oxidations, reductions, and demethylations that, again, are mostly limited to the endoplasmic reticulum. As shown in Fig. 249-2, the multiple substrate specificities of some sterol-metabolizing enzymes suggest possible, if not actual, alternate pathways for synthesis of cholesterol. Although textbooks often indicate that desmosterol (cholesta-5,

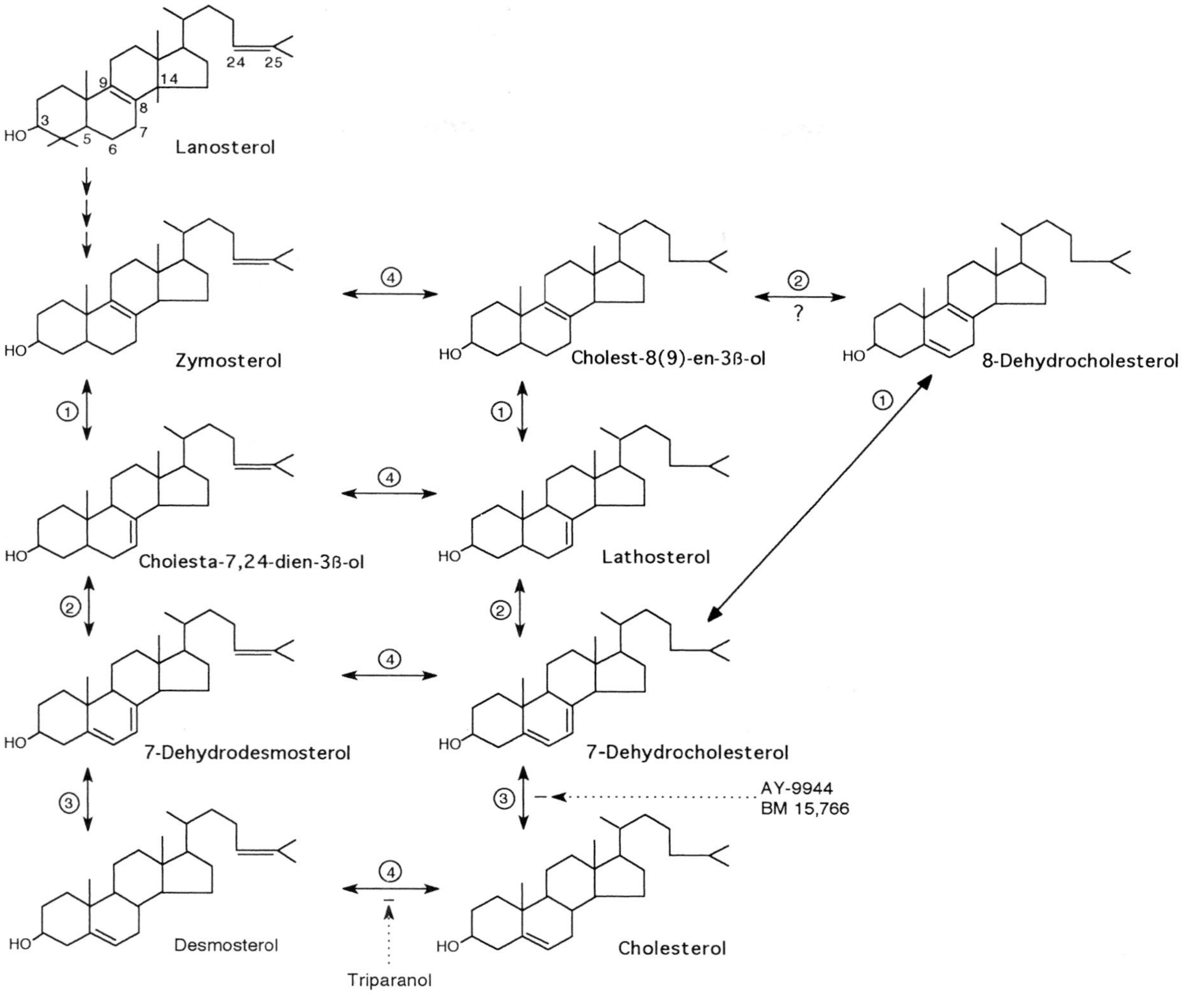

**Fig. 249-2 Enzymatic steps and major 27-carbon sterol intermediates comprising the pathway of cholesterol biosynthesis distal to the removal of 3 methyl groups (C4, C4′, C14) from the first sterol, lanosterol. The denoted enzymatic steps are: *1*, 3β-hydroxysteroid-Δ⁸,Δ⁷-isomerase (EC 5.3.3.5); *2*, 3β-hydroxysteroid-Δ⁵-desaturase** **(lathosterol dehydrogenase, EC 1.3.3.2); *3*, 3β-hydroxysteroid-Δ⁷-reductase (DHCR7, EC 1.3.1.21) inhibited by AY-9944 and BM 15,766; and *4*, 3β-hydroxysteroid-Δ²⁴-reductase (desmosterol reductase), inhibited by triparanol.**

24-dien-3β-ol) is the penultimate sterol of this series of reactions, the finding of markedly increased levels of 7DHC and almost no 7-dehydrodesmosterol in patients with SLOS suggests that the principal route of cholesterol biosynthesis in man may be the Kandutsch-Russell pathway,[23] in which the terminal sterol sequence is lathosterol to 7DHC to cholesterol. Nevertheless, the relative abundance of desmosterol in neuronal tissues, the testes, and breast milk[100–102] suggests that desmosterol may be the penultimate sterol in some tissues. Other evidence that the Kandutsch-Russell pathway is the principal pathway for most human sterol synthesis has been mostly indirect, such as the observation that the level of lathosterol (cholest-7-en-3β-ol) correlates well with the intrinsic rate of cholesterol biosynthesis.[103]

Prior to its discovery as the marker metabolite of SLOS, 7DHC was known as a minor constituent of plasma and solid tissues. In 1991, Axelson reported that 7DHC and two other diene sterols, isodehydrocholesterol (cholesta-6,8-dien-3β-ol), and 8-dehydrocholesterol (cholesta-5,8(9)-dien-3β-ol), exist in normal plasma in relatively constant proportions, most likely because of a chemical equilibrium.[104] 7DHC was found to be increased up to threefold in conditions associated with increased loss of bile acids, for example, ileal resection, and, therefore, increased cholesterol synthesis. Similarly, plasma and tissue levels of 7DHC are

increased in other conditions wherein cholesterol synthesis is markedly increased, such as familial hypercholesterolemia and cerebrotendinous xanthomatosis (Chap. 123). 7DHC also has special physiological importance as the precursor of vitamin $D_3$ via photic conversion of 7DHC to previtamin $D_3$ in skin. To what extent 7DHC enters other cholesterol metabolizing pathways in normal individuals, such as adrenal steroid and hepatic bile acid biosynthesis, is not completely understood. However, there is evidence that substantial amounts of 7DHC may be metabolized by these pathways[20,21,77] and may contribute to some of the prenatal and postnatal pathology of SLOS, such as cholestatic liver disease[86] and abnormal sexual differentiation.[20]

The enzyme that converts 7DHC to cholesterol, 3β-hydroxysteroid-Δ⁷-reductase (DHCR7; EC 1.3.1.21), is a microsomal membrane-bound enzyme with a mass of 55 kDa. DHCR7 has been purified to near homogeneity and some of its enzymatic characteristics described.[26,27,105] The gene for DHCR7 was localized to 11q12-3, cloned, and sequenced in 1997 by Moebius and colleagues,[29] who also showed that the human DHCR7 enzyme has strong homology with DHCR7s of both unicellular and multicellular eukaryotes as well as homology with 3β-hydroxysteroid-Δ¹⁴-reductases (DHCR14). In addition to requiring NADPH as a cofactor, DHCR7 activity is augmented by sterol carrier protein 2 (SCP2) and inhibited by a variety of synthetic compounds, such as AY-9944, BM 15,766, and, possibly, ligands of the sigma class.[29] DHCR7 and DHCR14 also have substantial homology with the lamin B receptor, a nuclear protein with a sterol-binding domain with intrinsic $\Delta^{14}$-reductase activity.[29,106]

Whereas the early steps of cholesterol biosynthesis are well characterized at the DNA, RNA, and protein levels, the individual enzymes, cofactors, carrier proteins, and intracellular transport steps involved in the conversion of lanosterol to cholesterol are poorly understood. Although all steps of cholesterol synthesis in mammals were once thought to take place in the endoplasmic reticulum, recent studies by Krisans and colleagues established that the second enzyme of the pathway, mevalonate kinase, and other enzymes required for the conversion of mevalonate phosphate to farnesol pyrophosphate are exclusively or largely localized to peroxisomes.[98] SCP2, a possible cofactor for DHCR7 and an apparent carrier protein for intracellular sterol transport, also appears to be targeted to and processed by peroxisomes.[107] In contrast, subcellular localization studies by Krisans and coworkers[108-110] showed that synthesis of squalene, a nonsterol precursor of lanosterol, by squalene synthase occurs exclusively in the endoplasmic reticulum.[111] Although there is evidence that peroxisomes may harbor all the enzymes necessary for the conversion of lanosterol to cholesterol,[112] the relative role of these and other peroxisomal enzymes in overall cholesterol biosynthesis and homeostasis is unclear. However, the observations that patients with Zellweger syndrome, who have defective peroxisomal assembly, have markedly depressed serum cholesterol levels[113] and that Zellweger cells in vitro have depressed rates of cholesterol synthesis[97] suggest an important role of peroxisomes in cholesterol biosynthesis.

Another important but poorly understood aspect of cholesterol biosynthesis is the complex intracellular trafficking of cholesterol. As shown by Lange et al.,[114] zymosterol (Fig. 249-2), an obligatory intermediate in the synthesis of cholesterol, appears to move from the endoplasmic reticulum to the plasma membrane and then back to the microsomal fraction of the cell where the final conversion to cholesterol occurs. The plasma membrane is the largest reservoir of free cholesterol in the cell and also interacts with exogenous cholesterol either as free cholesterol or in cholesterol-containing lipoprotein particles. Thus, the plasma membrane serves an important role in the regulation of cholesterol uptake by the cell, but how and why this apparently homogeneous pool of unesterified cholesterol interacts with zymosterol and other intermediates of cholesterol biosynthesis is not clear. There are also other pathways of intracellular transport that are important in cellular cholesterol homeostasis, because a genetic disruption of one of these pathways appears to be the cause of the lipid storage in type C Niemann-Pick disease.[115,116] Understanding intracellular trafficking and regulation of cholesterol uptake, as well as de novo cholesterol synthesis, may be important to understanding the cellular pathology of SLOS because the low total sterol levels in SLOS suggest feedback inhibition of de novo sterol synthesis at one or more levels of this complex cellular synthetic machinery.

Cholesterol is one of many different "isoprenoid" derivatives synthesized by the same initial series of microsomal and peroxisomal reactions. Other important isoprenoid derivatives whose synthesis may be influenced by changes in cholesterol metabolism include dolichols (membrane glycosylation), coenzyme Q (mitochondrial respiratory chain), heme, isopentenyladenine (tRNA), and protein isoprenoid substituents such as in Ras proteins.[117] Because the synthetic pathways of these biologically important nonsterols diverge from the cholesterol biosynthetic pathway at many different levels, the entire isoprenoid/sterol synthetic pathway is under complex, multilevel regulation to assure that, for example, a dietary excess of cholesterol does not lead to critical down-regulation of the synthesis of nonsterol metabolites in the pathway.[99] In addition, the coordinate regulation of the levels of proteins for de novo cholesterol synthesis (HMG-CoA synthase; HMG-CoA reductase) and cellular uptake

of cholesterol (low-density lipoprotein) contributes to the stability of cellular sterol levels.

## PRENATAL AND POSTNATAL STEROL PHYSIOLOGY

Of special importance to understanding the prenatal and postnatal sterol physiology of SLOS are data indicating that, in contrast to many other small metabolites, very little cholesterol for human fetal growth after the first trimester is transported to the fetus from the mother; instead, it must be synthesized by the fetus.[118,119] The apparent minimal supply of cholesterol to the fetus by the maternal circulation is best illustrated by severely affected newborns with SLOS who have plasma cholesterol levels as low as 1 mg/dl at birth, barely 2 percent of the normal newborn cholesterol level.[25] Similarly, cholesterol is deficient in all tissues of newborns with SLOS, with the most severe deficiency occurring in the brain.[120] Both in later fetal life and after birth, most, if not all, cholesterol in the brain is synthesized locally, not transported from blood lipoproteins, which appear to be taken up by most other fetal tissues.[118,121,122] However, recent molecular biologic studies have delineated maternal LDL and embryonic LDL receptors as components of a cholesterol delivery system for the early neuroepithelium, which is operant during the embryonic period in the first trimester.[123,124] The fundamental importance of this system in brain development is supported by the discovery[124] that transgenic mice lacking megalin (gp330), an LDL receptor in the embryonic neuroepithelium, develop holoprosencephaly, an early embryonic malformation sequence that has been linked to cholesterol metabolism at several levels.[57,125,126] In megalin-deficient mice, the normal uptake of maternal LDL cholesterol by the developing neuroepithelium in the first 2 months of gestation is blocked.[124] Thus, whereas delivery of cholesterol to the fetus after full development of the placenta may be minimal, critical aspects of embryonic tissue differentiation may be sensitive to maternal blood cholesterol and LDL levels.

Although most cholesterol in tissues serves as a major structural lipid of membranes, some cholesterol also enters pathways for bile acid and steroid hormone synthesis. Steroid hormones play an important role in embryonic, fetal, and postnatal sexual differentiation, and deficiencies of estrogenic and androgenic steroid synthesis can impair the formation of both male and female internal and external genitalia (Chap. 129). The consequences of defects of bile acid synthesis in syndromes other than SLOS can be largely postnatal, as in cerebrotendinous xanthomatosis, or prenatal, as in several different primary defects of bile acid biosynthesis associated with congenital cholestatic liver disease (Chap. 123) and in Zellweger syndrome, in which oxidation of the cholesterol side chain is deficient. Another fate of fetal cholesterol is the synthesis of estriol by combined action of the fetal adrenals and the placenta. Although unconjugated estriol transferred to the mother is believed to have a role in maintenance of the pregnancy, the physiological action of this sterol is unclear. In retrospect, the observation that mothers of SLOS children have low estriol levels during pregnancy[19] was an important clue to the nature of the primary biochemical defect in SLOS. Another unexpected recently discovered role of cholesterol is as a covalently bound element of active hedgehog proteins, a family of embryonic signaling proteins that may be important targets of the abnormal sterol metabolism of SLOS.[57,126,127]

## BIOCHEMISTRY

The plasma sample from the original SLOS patient studied by Tint et al.[24] showed a pattern of sterols that, except for variations in overall concentration, has been reproduced in essentially all patients with a clinical diagnosis of SLOS and abnormal cholesterol biosynthesis. As shown in Fig. 249-3, the largest abnormal peak in most samples is 7-dehydrocholesterol (cholesta-5,7-dien-3$\beta$-ol), which, as shown by Axelson,[104] is a combined

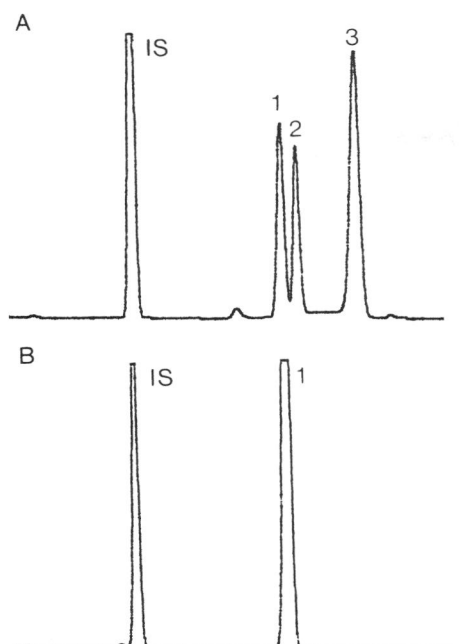

Fig. 249-3 Gas chromatographic flame-ionization profiles on 5 percent phenylmethylsilicone of sterol extracts of plasma from a child with classical Smith-Lemli-Opitz syndrome (*A*) and from a normal child (*B*). The ordinate is the detector response in arbitrary units and the abscissa elution time. The identified sterols are: IS, internal standard (epi-coprostanol); 1, cholesterol; 2, 8-dehydrocholesterol 3, combined peak of isodehydrocholesterol (cholesta-6,8-dien-3β-ol) and 7-dehydrocholesterol.

peak of 7DHC and isodehydrocholesterol (cholesta-6,8-dien-3β-ol; isoDHC). These two difficult-to-separate diene sterols appear to be in chemical equilibrium in approximately equal amounts. Almost all clinical studies of SLOS report this combined peak of diene sterols as 7DHC alone. A third diene sterol, 8-dehydrocholesterol (cholesta-5,8-dien-3β-ol; 8DHC), is normally present at about 75 percent of the amount of the combined peak of 7DHC and isoDHC. In any one patient, the level of 8DHC in plasma varies over time less than does the level of 7DHC, suggesting that 8DHC may be in a more stable metabolic pool that has a slow rate of interconversion with 7DHC. For example, when a dietary change stimulates an SLOS patient to grow, the level of 7DHC

often rises rapidly as a result of net increased *de novo* sterol synthesis, whereas that of 8DHC rises much more slowly, taking many weeks to reach a new level. Similarly, when SLOS fibroblasts or lymphoblasts are grown in cholesterol-depleted medium, 7DHC and isoDHC accumulate first, followed by a slow, time-dependent increase in 8DHC, suggesting that 7DHC is slowly converted to 8DHC.[27] A much faster rate of apparent conversion of 7DHC to 8DHC may occur in SLOS liver microsomes,[27] possibly because of the larger amount of sterol-$\Delta^8,\Delta^7$-isomerase in liver (Fig. 249-2).[128] A minor sterol, peak III in the initial report of Tint et al.,[24] was later identified as 19-nor-5,7,9(10)-cholestatrien-3β-ol,[129] and shown to be an artifact caused by thermal degradation of 8DHC.[130] However, De Fabiani et al.[131] identified in SLOS plasma small amounts of a related trienol, cholesta-5,7,9(11)-trien-3β-ol, using mild liquid chromatographic conditions, and proposed that it arises in vivo via a hydroperoxy byproduct of 7DHC, 7-hydroperoxy-cholesta-5,8-dien-3β-ol, which is present in trace amounts in SLOS plasma. What role, if any, these diene and triene sterols play in the abnormal embryogenesis or postnatal problems of SLOS is uncertain.

As in most genetic metabolic syndromes, there is a wide range of biochemical severity in patients with a clinical diagnosis of SLOS and abnormally increased levels of 7DHC. As Fig. 249-4 shows, some patients have had cholesterol levels as low as 1 mg/dl, whereas approximately 15 percent of patients have had normal cholesterol levels at diagnosis despite often substantially increased levels of 7DHC. Indeed, the availability of a biochemical test for SLOS, a syndrome diagnosed prior to 1993 by clinical criteria alone, has led to an expansion of the recognized clinical phenotype to include patients with no discrete malformations and normal or near normal intelligence as well as severely malformed fetuses that die *in utero* without a clinical diagnosis. When diagnosis of SLOS by the measurement of plasma 7DHC levels first became available, many patients with a clinical diagnosis of SLOS were found to have normal sterol metabolism.[25] However, almost all patients whose diagnosis of SLOS was made by an experienced dysmorphologist have had increased plasma levels of 7DHC.

Despite the apparently negligible transfer of cholesterol from the mother to the fetus, the most severely affected SLOS patients have measurable cholesterol levels at birth, typically 5 to 20 mg/dl.[25,120] Moreover, initial rates of cholesterol synthesis in cultured fibroblasts from patients who are predicted based on their mutations to have no DHCR7 activity may be as high as 50 percent of all sterols. Thus, there may be another genetic source of DHCR7 activity or a pathway of cholesterol synthesis not requiring DHCR7. The most likely source of such activity is the peroxisome, which has an essential role in the early steps of

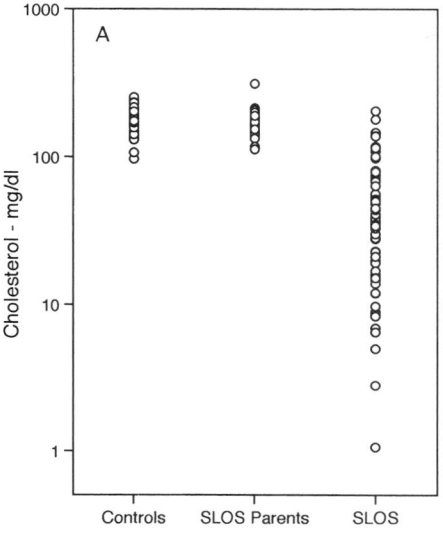

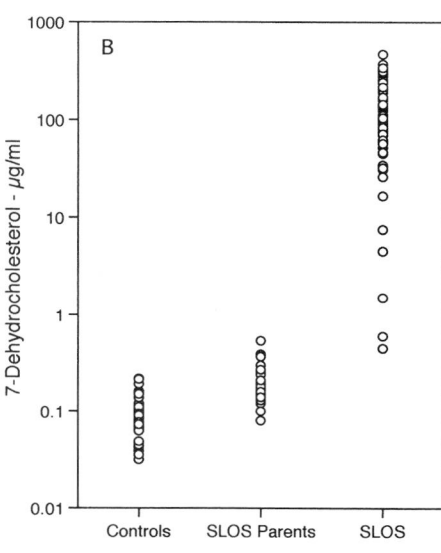

Fig. 249-4 Distribution of (*A*) plasma cholesterol and (*B*) plasma 7-dehydrocholesterol levels of Smith-Lemli-Opitz syndrome patients (N = 73) and their parents (N = 33).

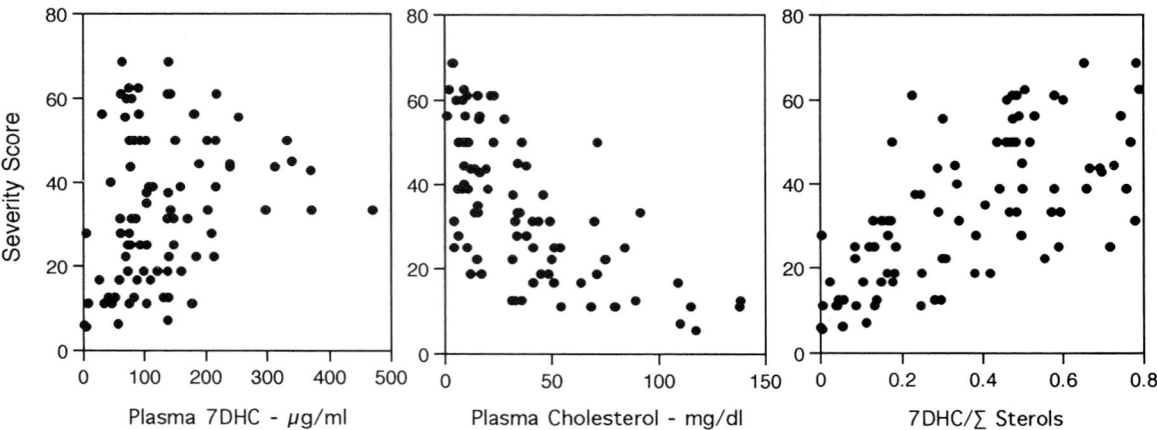

**Fig. 249-5 Distribution of clinical severity vs. plasma sterol levels and ratios in patients with Smith-Lemli-Opitz syndrome.**

cholesterol biosynthesis,[98,109,110] and which is suspected by some of having the ability to synthesize cholesterol from lanosterol.[112] Because 8DHC is abundant in SLOS tissues and can be synthesized without DHCR7, there may be a minor pathway of cholesterol biosynthesis wherein the 8(9) double bond of 8DHC is directly reduced (see Fig. 249-2).

Although the initial studies of sterol biochemistry in SLOS showed that there was a correlation between clinical and biochemical severity, the best correlation was not with the level of 7DHC, as might be expected for a primary metabolic disorder. Instead, clinical severity has correlated best with the level of cholesterol (inversely) or with 7DHC (or the sum of all dehydrosterols) expressed as a fraction of total sterols (Fig. 249-5).[25] The dehydrosterol fraction better expresses the systemic sterol abnormality than absolute blood sterol levels, which are subject to wide variations both acutely (infections, other stress reactions) and genetically (lipoprotein genotype). Although type II SLOS was delineated in 1987 as a disorder possibly genetically distinct from classic (type I) SLOS,[12] essentially all patients with a secure clinical diagnosis of type II SLOS had the same sterol profile initially reported in type I patients.[25] Compared as a group to classic SLOS, patients with multiple internal anomalies and early death have much lower total sterol levels and higher 7DHC/sterol ratios.[25,132] Although Tint et al.[132] suggested that essentially all SLOS patients with cholesterol levels lower than 10 mg/dl die at birth or in the first few months, death in SLOS is caused largely by specific visceral malformations rather than some postnatal biochemical consequence of the abnormal sterol levels. SLOS patients with cholesterol levels less than 10 mg/dl at diagnosis who are long-time survivors are not rare and usually are distinguished by a lack of major internal anomalies despite the biochemical severity measured in plasma. The finding that, with very few exceptions, siblings with SLOS have similar plasma levels of 7DHC and cholesterol and equally similar degrees of clinical severity supports the genetic basis of the differences in biochemical and clinical severity.[25] Indeed, subsequent studies of *DHCR7* mutations have shown a strong correlation between the predicted enzymatic effect of a patients' particular mutations and the clinical phenotype (see below).

As expected for an autosomal recessive disorder, the parents of SLOS patients have no or minimal physiological signs of abnormal sterol metabolism. When 7DHC is measured by sensitive mass fragmentometry, parents of SLOS patients are found to have plasma 7DHC levels with a mean that is about twice normal.[133] However, in their lymphoblasts, greater than 90 percent of SLOS parents have abnormally increased 7DHC to cholesterol ratios when the cells are cultured in cholesterol-depleted medium.[39] Although there are no obvious adverse clinical consequences of mildly abnormal 7DHC metabolism in hetero-

zygotes, no systematic survey for minor anomalies such as cleft palate, 2-3 toe syndactyly, or pyloric stenosis in unaffected SLOS family members has been done.

An interesting group of SLOS patients includes those with normal plasma cholesterol levels and mildly or minimally increased 7DHC levels.[25] Despite normal cholesterol levels at birth, almost all of these patients are microcephalic and developmentally delayed and may have any of the common nonvisceral malformations of SLOS. Although a few of these patients have plasma sterol profiles indistinguishable from those of some SLOS heterozygotes, when their fibroblasts or lymphoblasts are subcultured into lipid-depleted culture medium, the cellular concentration of 7DHC rises to levels as high as those of classic SLOS, typically 50 to 100 percent of the level of cholesterol.[39] In contrast, the cells of SLOS parents accumulate 7DHC only to 1 or 2 percent of cholesterol, as compared to less than 0.3 percent for control cells.[39,133] Unlike classic SLOS, however, when the cultured cells of mildly affected SLOS patients reach saturation density, the accumulated 7DHC often converts to cholesterol within a few days,[39] presumably reflecting higher residual enzyme activity.[134] This marked rise in the level of 7DHC in lipid-depleted cultured cells of SLOS patients with very mild plasma sterol abnormalities may reflect better the sterol metabolism of rapidly growing embryonic cells and may explain the presence of major malformations in SLOS children with almost normal plasma sterol levels. This observation also emphasizes the need to undertake physiological, enzymatic, or mutational studies in patients suspected of having SLOS but whose plasma sterol levels are normal or equivocally abnormal.

When lymphoblasts or fibroblasts from SLOS patients are grown in culture, sterol profiles are similar to those of plasma, except for the generally lower 8DHC/7DHC ratios and for the accumulation, especially in fibroblasts, of precursors of 7DHC, such as lathosterol and cholest-8(9)-en-3β-ol. To see these abnormalities, however, growth of cells in cholesterol-depleted medium using lipid-depleted fetal calf serum is essential. Repeated passage of some SLOS cell lines in normal, LDL-containing medium can suppress completely the diagnostic elevation of 7DHC.[133] Early studies with normal cultured skin fibroblasts and relatively specific inhibitors of DHCR7, such as AY-9944 and BM 15,766, produced SLOS-like profiles of diene sterols.[105,135] Such cell studies are simpler and more reproducible in lymphoblasts, because fibroblasts often have attachment problems when grown in cholesterol-depleted culture medium. This growth problem is even greater in cultured villus cells or amniocytes.[78,133] For this reason, direct sterol analysis of a chorionic villus sample (CVS) or amniotic fluid rather than sterol quantification in cultured amniocytes or cultured villus cells is preferred for biochemical prenatal diagnosis of SLOS.

The systemic nature of the biochemical defect in SLOS should be evident from the finding of very similar sterol profiles in all tissues, although there is relatively little information published on specific tissue sterol levels in SLOS. In one study,[120] the level of cholesterol in solid tissues of two severely affected children ranged between 5 and 20 percent of controls. However, in another affected infant whose plasma sterol level was less than half of normal, the total sterol level (7DHC + isoDHC + 8DHC + cholesterol) in solid tissues was normal. In most tissues of two midtrimester SLOS fetuses,[136,137] diene sterols constituted more than 75 percent of the sterols with the highest fractional ratio (> 0.90) occurring in the brain. In another case of a severely affected newborn infant,[86] cholesterol constituted only approximately 20 percent of sterols of the brain. The same infant had LDL receptor densities in various tissues, including the brain, that were substantially increased, suggesting that the abnormally low plasma total sterol levels found in most SLOS patients may partly reflect increased LDL sterol uptake from plasma, not just decreased total sterol synthesis. The fact that, apart from malformations and specific tissue abnormalities such as adrenal lipid depletion, the histology of SLOS is largely normal indicates that 7DHC and 8DHC can replace cholesterol as a structural membrane lipid.

There is as yet little known about the abnormal biochemistry of bile acids in SLOS. Although the paucity of normal bile acids and the presence of apparent abnormal bile acid species in the urine of a patient with SLOS[21] led to the discovery of abnormal sterol biosynthesis in SLOS, only a few studies since that discovery have examined bile acids in SLOS. In the original study of bile acids in SLOS,[21] a severe deficiency or absence of normal cholenoates was found in the affected patients. Several apparently abnormal compounds were presumptively identified as possible 7-dehydro forms of normal bile acid species. Patient #1 of Natowicz and Evans[21] was later studied by Tint et al.[24] and found also to have absent normal bile acids in stool, but two less severely affected patients had substantial amounts of fecal bile acids. Although bile acids are assumed to be important for efficient absorption of many fats and lipids, including cholesterol, few SLOS patients have had clinical or laboratory evidence of fat malabsorption.

Except for occasional case studies that report adrenal or gonadal steroid levels, or that mention low maternal unconjugated estriol levels,[19,78,79,138] there have been very few studies of steroid metabolism in SLOS. One of the earliest studies to suggest sterol or steroid abnormalities in SLOS[20] described abnormally high levels of DHEA sulfate and abnormally low levels of testosterone in two newborns with features of SLOS. In contrast, two older SLOS children (30 months and 5 years) were found to have abnormally low levels of DHEA sulfate. The same authors also found several immunologically and chromatographically defined steroid species that appeared to be monounsaturated relative to their expected molecular weights. In retrospect, they probably were 7-dehydro variants of the normal steroids. Reports of testosterone levels in SLOS patients include both low and normal values, with normal to mildly increased levels of FSH and LH in some, but the anecdotal and usually uncontrolled nature of these studies precludes an informed understanding of sex steroid metabolism in SLOS. Moreover, the high frequency of hypogenitalism in SLOS is not sufficient evidence to implicate inadequate steroid production or physiological sterol effects *in utero*. For example, the persistence of Müllerian remnants in some of the more severely affected SLOS patients[15] suggests defective genital morphogenesis unrelated to steroid hormone levels, possibly mediated through sterol-related dysfunction of the embryonic signaling protein, Desert hedgehog, in genital tissues.[139] More recently, Shackleton et al.[77] found that 7DHC enters and is metabolized in most basic steroid synthetic pathways, such that 7-dehydro homologs of most common urinary steroids can be found. The production of these abnormal fetal steroids is sufficiently great that SLOS in a fetus may be diagnosable by the measurement of 7-dehydro steroids in maternal urine at midgestation.[140]

## ENZYMOLOGY AND MOLECULAR GENETICS

The finding of hypocholesterolemia and markedly increased levels of 7DHC in patients with SLOS immediately focused attention on 7-dehydrocholesterol reductase ($3\beta$-hydroxysteroid-$\Delta^7$-reductase; EC 1.3.1.21; DHCR7) as a candidate deficient enzyme causing this disorder. Additional evidence for deficient DHCR7 activity causing SLOS was provided by earlier biochemical studies of AY-9944, a relatively specific inhibitor of DHCR7, which when given to mice and rats produced plasma sterols profiles essentially identical to those of patients with SLOS. Moreover, fetuses of pregnant rats treated with AY-9944 developed skeletal and craniofacial malformations similar to those of SLOS.[141,142] Other drugs that inhibit distal steps of cholesterol biosynthesis also produced SLOS-like malformations, suggesting that the cholesterol-lowering action of these drugs rather than a toxic drug byproduct was the principal teratogenic factor.[143–145]

The enzymatic conversion of 7DHC to cholesterol was first demonstrated in 1961 by Schroepfer and Frantz,[146] who showed that DHCR7 was a typical NADPH-dependent microsomal reductase. However, prior to the renewal of interest in DHCR7 because of SLOS, DHCR7 had been little studied at either a structural or DNA level, and when it was studied, it was mostly in lower organisms.[147] The first radioactive assays of DHCR7 activity in SLOS[26,27] showed that fibroblasts and liver microsomes of SLOS patients converted 7DHC to cholesterol at a rate less than 10 percent of normal. Fibroblasts of patients with the most severe forms of SLOS had significantly lower DHCR7 activities (mean 2 percent of controls) than fibroblasts of patients with milder forms of SLOS (mean 7 percent of controls). The same group found similarly reduced *DHCR7* activities using a nonradioactive assay of DHCR7 activity in which the fungal sterol, ergosterol (ergosta-5,7,22-trien-$3\beta$-ol), is converted to brassicasterol (ergosta-5,22-dien-$3\beta$-ol).[134] They also showed that fibroblasts of SLOS parents had intermediate levels of DHCR7 activity (mean 67 percent of controls), consistent with the autosomal recessive inheritance of the disorder.

At the time of the discovery of DHCR7 deficiency in SLOS, the chromosomal location of *DHCR7* was unknown. However, attention soon turned to 7q32.1, because two unrelated SLOS patients were known to have *de novo* balanced translocations at that position.[28] However, further genetic study of this region[148] and of one of the patients[149] showed that the breakpoint interrupted not *DHCR7* or another gene associated with sterol metabolism but, instead, the human metabotropic glutamate receptor 8 (*GRM8*), which is not known to have a role in DHCR7 activity or cholesterol biosynthesis in general. At about the same time, Moebius et al.[29] reported their cloning and mapping of a human microsomal *DHCR7* gene to chromosomal location 11q12-13. Interestingly, *DHCR7* was first cloned not as a gene for a sterol-metabolizing enzyme, but as a candidate gene for a "sigma-type" drug-binding protein.[150] Only after complete sequencing was the gene found to have strong homology with *DHCR7* from *Arabidopsis thaliana*. Within months, the same laboratory identified mutations in *DHCR7* in all 13 patients with classic SLOS whom they studied.[151] Two other groups working independently confirmed that patients with SLOS had apparently disabling mutations in *DHCR7*.[30,31]

The 2957-bp cDNA for the human *DHCR7* gene has an open reading frame of 1425 bp, which codes for a protein with 475 amino acid residues and a calculated mass of 54.5 kDa.[29] The gene, which spans 14 kb of genomic DNA, is organized into 9 exons and, by hydropathy plot, has between 6 and 9 transmembrane $\Delta$-helices. In addition to having a high degree of homology with *DHCR7* of *Arabidopsis thaliana*, the human *DHCR7* has substantial homology with the genes encoding sterol $\Delta14$-reductases across phyla and with the gene encoding the human

Distribution of *DHCR7* Mutations in Smith-Lemli-Opitz Syndrome

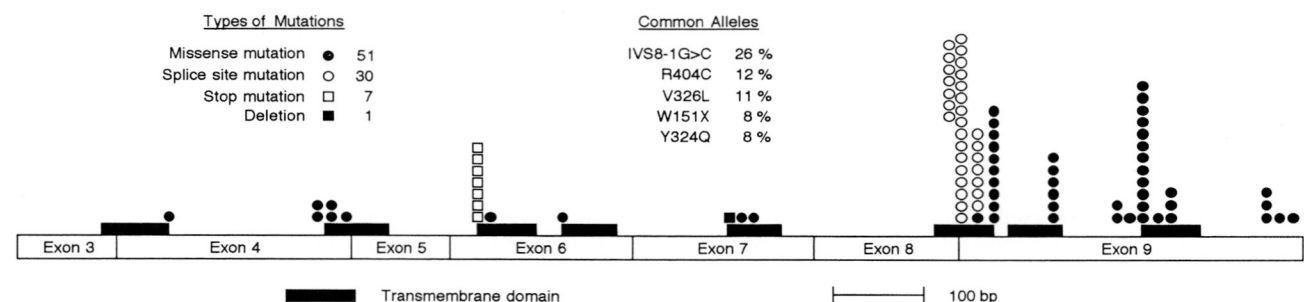

**Fig. 249-6 Distribution of SLOS mutations of 3β-hydroxysteroid-Δ⁷-reductase (DHCR7) in patients with Smith-Lemli-Opitz syndrome. (Adapted from reference 152.)**

lamin B receptor, a nuclear inner membrane protein with intrinsic sterol Δ14-reductase activity but unknown function in nuclear or cholesterol synthesizing systems.[29,106] Among the 26 alleles studied by Fitzky et al., only one example of IVS8-1G > C, a splice-site mutation that creates a 134-bp insertion between exons 8 and 9, was found.[151] However, study of a cohort of North American patients with largely European and Hispanic ancestry showed that the IVS8-1G > C mutation constituted 26 percent of SLOS alleles, and that several other alleles — R404C (12 percent), V326L (11 percent), W151X (8 percent), Y324Q (8 percent) — also occurred at relatively high frequencies.[152] Collectively, the five most common mutations accounted for two-thirds of the mutant alleles. Although these high frequencies may have evolved because of a special heterozygote advantage afforded by the particular mutations, more likely it was a combination of founder effect with a heterozygote advantage that encouraged the persistence of these mutations and of diverse missense mutations. As would be predicted in a model of heterozygote advantage, such as increased synthesis of vitamin D by heterozygotes, the most common mutations give rise to more severe enzymatic defects than the less common mutations. There is as yet no correlation between individual mutations and their effects on the sterol vitamin D and steroid metabolism in heterozygotes. Such information, however, may provide evidence for increased vitamin D levels as a possible heterozygote advantage, because evidence from European paleopathologic studies indicates that rickets was a common pediatric disease. As anticipated from biochemical studies, the most severely affected patients are either homozygotes or compound heterozygotes for mutations shown or predicted to produce no or severely reduced DHCR7 activity.[152] In contrast, most classic type I SLOS patients are compound heterozygotes for the IVS8-1G > C splice-site mutation and a second missense mutation associated with residual enzyme activity. Patients with very mild clinical and biochemical phenotypes most often are compound heterozygotes for two unique or uncommon missense mutations.[152]

## EMBRYOLOGY

The discovery of an abnormality of cholesterol biosynthesis as the cause of SLOS has led to an intense evaluation of the role of cholesterol metabolism in the abnormal morphogenesis of SLOS. Although children with the only other previously known defect of cholesterol biosynthesis, mevalonic aciduria, are dysmorphic and growth retarded,[153] there was no expectation that other defects of cholesterol biosynthesis would be associated with a severe multiple-malformation syndrome. However, earlier clinical observations and laboratory studies had suggested abnormalities in cholesterol synthesis[12] or steroid metabolism[19,20] in SLOS. Moreover, more than 20 years earlier, Roux and colleagues had

shown that inhibitors of enzymes of the distal cholesterol biosynthetic pathway, including DHCR7, caused holoprosencephaly, microcephaly, pituitary agenesis, limb defects, and genital anomalies in the pups of exposed pregnant rats or mice.[141,154] The same group also showed that feeding cholesterol to the pregnant, treated rats substantially limited or blocked the teratogenic effects of AY-9944, an inhibitor of DHCR7.[155] Prior to 1993, holoprosencephaly, a failure of normal bilobar development of the forebrain, had been reported in only one SLOS patient.[19] However, using an increased 7DHC level as a diagnostic marker, holoprosencephaly of variable severity has been found to occur in about 5 percent of patients with SLOS.[25,57] Despite the apparent etiologic relationship between abnormal cholesterol metabolism and holoprosencephaly, the mechanism by which abnormal sterol metabolism caused these severe embryologic effects remained obscure until several important related discoveries in the mid 1990s. Most important was the discovery[127] that targeted disruption in mice of Sonic hedgehog (Shh), an embryonic signaling protein, causes not only holoprosencephaly, but also distal limb defects and other skeletal anomalies. The same group showed that covalent addition of cholesterol to Shh was an essential part of the "autoprocessing" of Shh,[126,156] wherein precursor Shh protein in the presence of cholesterol cleaves itself into a nonsignaling COOH-terminal half and a mature, cholesterol-substituted, N-terminal half, Shh-N. Shh-N appears to possess all Shh signaling activity, which in vertebrates includes patterning of development in the ventral forebrain and limb buds.

Although the covalently attached cholesterol moiety is not essential for intrinsic signaling activity of Shh-N, it appears to have a role in the attachment and localization of Shh-N to cell membranes.[126] The homologous signaling proteins, "Desert hedgehog" and "Indian hedgehog," appear to have similar signaling roles in, respectively, genital and skeletal development, both important sites of malformation in SLOS.[157,158] Another link between these malformations and hedgehog proteins was made by Roessler et al.,[125] who found that heterozygosity for mutations in *SHH*, the 7q36-linked gene encoding SHH in humans, causes autosomal dominant holoprosencephaly. Other evidence that cholesterol plays an important role in embryonic forebrain development comes from the findings that targeted disruption of the gene for megalin, an important component of a system for delivery of maternal LDL cholesterol to the embryonic neuro-epithelium, caused holoprosencephaly,[124] and that possibly related central nervous system malformations occur in mice with targeted disruption of the gene encoding apolipoprotein B, another component of the embryonic cholesterol delivery system.[123]

This convergence of holoprosencephaly, SLOS, Shh, and cholesterol metabolism focused attention on the possibility that the covalent attachment of cholesterol to Shh-N and related hedgehog proteins is the link between the abnormal cholesterol metabolism of SLOS and abnormal morphogenesis in SLOS. However, Cooper et al.[159] showed that autoprocessing of hedgehog is not impaired when cholesterol in the reaction medium is replaced with 7DHC or many other 27-carbon sterols. Additional in vitro studies with AY-9944 and other teratogens that cause SLOS-like malformations in rats strongly suggested that the defect in Shh signaling resides in the target tissue and not the Shh-N signal itself.[159] There also appeared to be little correlation between the quantitative effect of the sterol synthesis inhibitor, jervine, and related compounds on cholesterol biosynthesis either in the chick embryo test system or cultured human fibroblasts (R. Kelley, M. Cooper, and P. Beachy, unpublished). However, because all the known plant teratogens of the jervine class also impair intracellular cholesterol transport, and because Patched, a putative hedgehog receptor,[160–162] contains a sterol-sensing domain,[161] there are other possible levels at which the sterol defect of SLOS may cause impaired signaling of Shh. Another possible site of action is the lamin B receptor, which has both sterol-14-reductase and a binding site structure similar to that of DHCR7.[29,106]

Shh is just one of several similarly functioning hedgehog proteins that may interact with Patched in a sterol-sensitive manner. Thus, it is possible that impaired signaling activities of Desert hedgehog[157] and Indian hedgehog[158] also play a role in SLOS in the abnormal morphogenesis of tissues that are not targets of Shh signaling. For example, although steroid abnormalities are often presumed to be the cause of the hypogenitalism of SLOS, the persistence of Müllerian remnants in some severely affected SLOS males[15] could be explained by inadequate signaling of Desert hedgehog, which is prominently expressed in Sertoli cells, the source of Müllerian inhibitory factor.[157]

Despite the attractiveness of and experimental support for the role of impaired hedgehog signaling in SLOS morphogenesis, other less specific disturbances could also contribute to the abnormal morphogenesis of SLOS. Cholesterol is severely deficient in all tissues of first trimester fetuses with 7DHC and related cholesterol precursors typically constituting 75 percent or more of fetal sterols.[78,163,164] Such a severe disturbance in membrane sterol composition may affect developmental processes that involve cell-cell interactions, as was suggested by Sulik and colleagues in their recent studies with the SLOS-mimicking teratogen, BM 15,776.[144] Even in tissue culture, SLOS fibroblasts interact abnormally with themselves and with the growth surface.[78,133] Moreover, whereas the AY-9944-treated rats studied by Roux et al. had only a few SLOS-like malformations,[141,154] the treatment of genetically cholesterol-deficient mice with a similar inhibitor, BM 15,766, led to more severe malformations and a much better phenocopy of SLOS[165] than provided by BM 15,766 alone, suggesting that in vivo a deficiency of cholesterol itself does have a contributory role in the abnormal embryologic signaling of SLOS.

Although many details of Shh function and its exact relationship to the malformations of SLOS remain to be elucidated, evidence indicates that many of the malformations of SLOS may stem from impaired hedgehog function and its downstream effects on the expression of homeobox genes. In this respect, SLOS may be one of the best examples of a "metabolic malformation" syndrome. However, among metabolic diseases that adversely affect embryonic and fetal development, SLOS may be an exception. This is because most of the many genetically characterized multiple congenital anomaly syndromes, that is, disturbances of the body plan, have not been disorders of intermediary metabolism but, instead, have been mutations of homeobox genes and other transcriptional regulators. Even the severe and diverse prenatal metabolic disturbances of Zellweger syndrome have few effects on the embryonic body plan. Thus, SLOS may be an atypical metabolic malformation syndrome, because its abnormal sterol biochemistry appears to disrupt the action of embryonic signaling pathways and, thereby, mimics

the effects of mutations in homeobox genes and their regulatory genes.

## BIOCHEMICAL DIAGNOSIS

### Diagnostic Methods

Although plasma or serum are the samples of choice for biochemical diagnosis of SLOS, almost any body tissue or fluid can be used to measure 7DHC.[24,25,27,120,133,166] Because approximately 10 percent of patients with SLOS have normal serum cholesterol levels at any age, including at birth, the blood cholesterol level cannot be used as a screening test for SLOS. Moreover, because 8DHC and 7DHC react as cholesterol in cholesterol oxidase assay methods, hospital laboratories may report a normal "cholesterol" level when more than half of the sterols are 7DHC and 8DHC. In a few affected children, the level of 7DHC may be normal or equivocally increased, but the 8DHC level is usually distinctly abnormal. In rare cases, where the levels of 7DHC and 8DHC are normal or fall in the heterozygote range (up to 0.8 µg/ml), either DHCR7 mutational testing, DHCR7 enzymatic assay, or analysis of sterol biosynthesis in cultured cells must be undertaken.[133,134,167] Under conditions of maximal growth stimulation in cholesterol-depleted cultured medium, lymphoblasts from patients with mild biochemical variants of SLOS still develop markedly increased levels of 7DHC. Similar studies can be done in cultured skin fibroblasts but take longer and are more difficult because of poor attachment of SLOS fibroblasts.

Not uncommonly, there is a need to make a retrospective biochemical diagnosis of SLOS in a child for whom there may be remaining stored tissue or laboratory samples. Samples commonly used for retrospective biochemical diagnosis of SLOS include archived plasma and serum samples, Guthrie newborn screening cards, frozen or formalin-preserved autopsy tissues, and amniotic fluids. Recovering sufficient sterol for diagnosis from formalin-preserved tissue stored more than a few months is not assured but is usually successful. Because 7DHC and 8DHC are oxygen-sensitive, diagnostic levels of 7DHC and 8DHC may be lost from inadequately sealed frozen or refrigerated samples. A loss of about 1 percent per day of 7DHC and 8DHC is typical for serum samples stored at room temperature. However, diagnoses using formalin-preserved tissues or refrigerated Guthrie cards as old as 5 years have been made.

There are a number of methods for measuring dehydrocholesterols in clinical samples and cultured cells.[24,133] Most rely on simple solvent extraction of sterols and gas chromatography (GC) on a variety of liquid phases, with more polar matrices providing superior separation of cholesterol from the dehydrosterols. In general, an abnormally increased level of 7DHC can be detected in at least 95 percent of patients with SLOS using GC and a flame ionization detector. However, for some of the biochemically least severely affected patients and some older more typical SLOS patients on high cholesterol diets, more sensitive selected-ion GC/mass fragmentometry must be used.[133] Because of the light absorptive characteristics of a conjugate diene such as 7DHC, colorimetric methods—either direct or following HPLC separation—are also available for laboratories not equipped with GC.[166,168] Although a method for fast atom bombardment mass spectrometric measurement of 7DHC/cholesterol ratios has not been developed, matrix-assisted laser-desorption time-of-flight (MALD-TOF) secondary ion mass fragmentometry can diagnose SLOS by measuring 7DHC/cholesterol ratios in Guthrie card blood spots.[169] However, MALD-TOF may not be practical for routine screening, because mildly affected patients not identified by clinical criteria commonly have 7DHC/cholesterol ratios below the limit of detection by the published method.

### Other Causes of Increased Levels of 7DHC

As a primary intermediate in the Kandutsch-Russell pathway for cholesterol biosynthesis, 7DHC exists in human tissues at a relatively constant ratio to cholesterol. Thus, in common forms of hypercholesterolemia such as familial hypercholesterolemia due to abnormalities of LDL metabolism, the absolute level of 7DHC may be increased, but the ratio relative to cholesterol is usually normal. However, in other conditions where there is marked up-regulation of cholesterol biosynthesis, such as cerebrotendinous xanthomatosis, 7DHC may be increased ten- to twentyfold, but the presence of similarly increased levels of other sterol precursors and cholestanol clearly establish the correct diagnosis. Thus, it is important that all plasma sterols be measured to avoid mis-diagnosis. Another cause of mildly increased levels of 7DHC is treatment with haloperidol, which has a high affinity for DHCR7. Because DHCR7 is a member of the sigma class of drug-binding proteins,[29] it is likely that other drugs of this class will cause increased levels of 7DHC through inhibition of DHCR7. More importantly, however, such drugs may have particularly adverse effects on patients with SLOS, who have already markedly limited activities of DHCR7 (R. Kelley, unpublished).

### Prenatal Diagnosis

Prenatal diagnosis of SLOS has been accomplished in many pregnancies both retrospectively and prospectively. As reported by several authors,[13,78,138] one of the early signs of an SLOS fetus is an abnormally low maternal serum level of unconjugated estriol (MSuE3), a fetal sterol product measured as part of the midgestational "triple marker" test used to screen for neural tube defects, Down syndrome, and trisomy 18. Other elements of the triple screen — chorionic gonadotropin and α-fetoprotein — are also mildly depressed in some SLOS pregnancies. A number of affected fetuses have also been identified by the discovery of suggestive fetal abnormalities such as nuchal edema, micro-cephaly, cleft palate, polydactyly, cystic kidneys, ambiguous genitalia, or a 46,XY karyotype in a phenotypically female fetus.

The level of 7DHC in the amniotic fluid of affected pregnancies is typically increased more than five hundredfold.[78] In some fluids from affected pregnancies, the level of cholesterol is abnormally low, whereas in others the level is surprisingly normal. Direct analysis of the sterol composition of chorionic villi at age 10 weeks also appears to be a reliable method for diagnosis of SLOS, although the relative increase in the 7DHC/cholesterol ratio is not as great as it is in amniotic fluid.[78] Theoretically, it is possible that a biochemically mildly affected SLOS fetus may have villus tissue with only an equivocally increased 7DHC/cholesterol ratio. Nevertheless, the initial experience with more than 100 pregnan-cies at risk for SLOS has yielded no false negatives and no false positives.[78] Despite the feasibility of prenatal diagnosis by molecular testing of villus tissue or amniocytes, the simplicity and accuracy of biochemical testing obviates the need for molecular analysis except, perhaps, in a rare case with ambiguous biochemical results. Although cultured amniocytes can also yield diagnostically increased levels of 7DHC, because both normal and mutant amniocytes grow poorly in the absence of cholesterol, achieving sufficient growth of amniocytes without complete suppression of the biochemical defect by cholesterol in the culture medium can be difficult. For similar reasons, and because of the poor growth of SLOS cells in tissue culture, there is little role for enzymatic assay of DHCR7 for prenatal diagnosis of SLOS.

The study of the prenatal sterol biochemistry of SLOS has yielded interesting, diagnostically useful information for counsel-ing pregnancies without a known prior risk for SLOS. As shown by Kratz and Kelley,[78] there is a modest correlation between the amniotic fluid 7DHC levels (expressed as a percent of total sterols) and the physical severity score of the affected fetus. More striking, however, is a strong inverse correlation of MSuE3 and the SLOS physical severity score. In a study of 14 monitored pregnancies, all 6 SLOS fetuses with severity scores less than 40 had MSuE3 values > 0.3 multiples of the median (MoM), whereas all but one of 8 fetuses with severity scores greater than 40 had MoMs < 0.3.[78] Because some SLOS fetuses are first identified by a low MSuE3 value, such a correlation helps predict outcome. Moreover,

as shown in one pregnancy,[140] the measurement of derivatives of estriol and 7-dehydroestriol in maternal midgestational urine may offer a noninvasive method for prenatal diagnosis of SLOS.

## CLINICAL MANAGEMENT

For 30 years following its original description, SLOS could be treated only supportively. The most common management problems were pyloric stenosis, nonspecific gastrointestinal dysmotility, feeding disorders, and severe developmental delays. Other common problems were frequent infections, complications of structural heart disease, Hirschsprung disease, and failure to thrive. Excessive irritability and sleeplessness also were char-acteristic of SLOS at all ages. As reported in a number of larger patient series, mortality in the first few years was between 25 and 50 percent, with death occurring most often in the newborn period from complications of visceral malformations.[2,10] With the recognition and treatment of the deficiency of cholesterol bio-synthesis in SLOS, however, the medical and developmental outcome of patients has changed the frequency and management of these problems substantially.

The estimated daily synthetic need for cholesterol during infancy is 30 to 40 mg/kg/day, based on isotopic analysis of newly synthesized cholesterol following infusion of deuterium water.[170,171] In adults, the daily synthetic requirement decreases to approximately 10 mg/kg/day, or between 500 and 900 mg/day in the average adult. This daily requirement is usually met by a combination of dietary cholesterol and *de novo* synthesis, balanced in a highly regulated manner. That the near elimination of cholesterol from infant formulas has not been followed by obvious deleterious effects on infant health or major changes in the average cholesterol levels of infants indicates the capacity for endogenous cholesterol biosynthesis in growing children. Studies of cholester-ol metabolism and nutrition in infants also indicate that younger infants fed cholesterol may be able to absorb their entire daily cholesterol requirement.[170] Thus, if basic regulation of cholesterol biosynthesis is normal in SLOS children, then there is reason to believe that a child with SLOS may be able to absorb sufficient dietary cholesterol to down-regulate endogenous sterol synthesis and therefore limit significantly the *de novo* production of 7DHC. For this reason, children with SLOS are routinely supplemented with dietary cholesterol with the expectation that blood cholesterol levels will rise to normal at the same time that the abnormal accumulation of 7DHC is eliminated. A complete biochemical "cure" by such therapy requires that dietary cholesterol be distributed to all cellular and tissue compartments. However, this does not appear to occur because cholesterol in the central nervous system appears to be synthesized locally and cannot be transported across the blood-brain barrier.[122] Even if cholesterol could reach brain cells and myelin, cognitive performance might not improve because the mental retardation of SLOS appears to reflect more the embryologic micrencephaly and more subtle abnormalities of cerebral neuronal development than an existing deficit of cholesterol or "disturbance" caused by 7DHC.

Although human breast milk has a high concentration of cholesterol — up to 120 mg/liter[172] — even this amount supplies less than the minimum daily cholesterol requirement of a child with SLOS, not including the large systemic deficit of cholesterol that most SLOS infants and children have at the time of diagnosis. Moreover, the hypotonia and poor suck of most SLOS neonates and older infant makes continued nutrition with breast milk throughout the first year very uncommon. Thus, for only the biochemically mildest children does supplemental cholesterol appear to be able correct the synthetic deficit, returning the level of 7DHC to the normal range, and that usually only during times of comparatively low growth velocities, such as between ages 3 and 10 years and after puberty. The higher growth velocities of children during early infancy and puberty and their greater need for cholesterol at those times further reduce the percentage of the daily cholesterol requirement that can be provided in the diet.

Common drains on cholesterol reserves in SLOS children also include infections and other systemic stress, which cause increased steroid synthesis from cholesterol, and diarrheal illnesses, during which many grams of cholesterol-derived bile acids and cholesterol present in the enterohepatic circulation can be lost in the stool. Thus, supplying purified cholesterol or a highly concentrated natural source of cholesterol to children with SLOS is critical to the success of their metabolic management.

Initial treatment protocols for SLOS provided 50 mg/kg/day cholesterol, either in natural form (eggs, cream, liver, meats, and meat-based formulas) or as purified food-grade cholesterol, with or without supplements of bile acids (cholic acid, chenodeoxycholic acid, or ursodeoxycholic acid).[173–175] For substantially growth-retarded children, treatment with cholesterol supplements is sometimes followed by striking increases in the rate of growth for several months until more appropriate weight and height percentiles are reached. Such rapid growth has occurred with combined cholesterol and bile acid supplementation, as well as with cholesterol supplementation alone. In later years of these experimental treatment protocols, increasingly higher doses of cholesterol were often given, sometimes up to 300 mg/kg/day, when there was relatively little change in a patient's blood sterol levels. Paradoxically, when SLOS children enter a growth spurt from better nutrition, cholesterol levels typically fall and 7DHC levels rise substantially despite marked clinical improvement. This transient rise in the level of 7DHC may reflect the well-known direct relationship between caloric intake and cholesterol synthesis. Although the early treatment changes in plasma sterol levels usually do not reflect the obvious clinical benefits of cholesterol supplementation, all but the most severely affected children usually show a substantial increase in the level of cholesterol over a period of years and a corresponding fall in the levels of 8DHC and 7DHC. Preliminary data from one treatment protocol indicated little difference between the clinical or biochemical effects of giving cholesterol to infant and young SLOS children at dosages of 50 versus 150 mg/kg/day (R. Kelley, unpublished data). However, there were statistically significant improvements when comparing behavior scores before and during cholesterol supplementation (R. Kelley and E. Tierney, unpublished data). More striking and more rapid changes in blood sterol levels were reported in a rat model of SLOS created by treating rats with BM 15,766, a relatively specific inhibitor of DHCR7.[176] The study examined the effects of cholic acid and lovastatin, an HMG-CoA reductase inhibitor, on the blood sterol levels and found that cholic acid had little effect. However, when the rats were given lovastatin plus cholesterol, the anticipated fall in 7DHC levels was prevented rather than enhanced. Because of the lack of definitive evidence that 7DHC is toxic, and because of the concern that HMG-CoA reductase inhibitors might limit the synthesis of other critical isoprenoid compounds, HMG-CoA reductase inhibitors are not currently used in the routine treatment of SLOS. Moreover, the observation that, within a cohort of SLOS children with equally low plasma cholesterol levels, children with the highest 7DHC levels have lower severity scores suggests that, at least in some biochemical or structural roles, 7DHC may function like cholesterol. Based on SLOS animal models[176] and on the lack of obvious clinical or biochemical benefit of bile acids in SLOS, recent SLOS treatment protocols have not included bile acid supplements. Because bile acids may down-regulate tissue levels of LDL receptors, the more rapid rise in plasma cholesterol levels and the persistently high levels of 7DHC in bile-acid supplemented patients may reflect impaired tissue uptake of sterols rather than enhanced intestinal absorption of cholesterol.[176]

In addition to the biochemical and physical changes that follow the initiation of cholesterol replacement therapy, there has also been a number of striking behavioral changes. Young children with SLOS have a distinctive behavioral phenotype, which includes irritability, sleeplessness, and sensory hypersensitivity, especially auditory and tactile. Upon treatment with supplementary cholesterol, irritability and sleep disorders may improve within days or weeks, whereas tactile hypersensitivities, especially of the hands and feet, take longer to ameliorate. Typically, all of these behaviors return when cholesterol supplementation is stopped. The behavioral improvement does not appear to correlate with any specific change in the plasma sterol profile, and even children with normal or near normal plasma cholesterol levels often show similar behavioral changes when given cholesterol supplements. After infancy, many SLOS patients develop behaviors such as rocking, finger flicking, object twirling, gaze avoidance, and various obsessions that often meet criteria for the diagnosis of autistic disorder, and which typically improve or resolve with cholesterol treatment. Insofar as 7DHC enters essentially all steroid synthetic pathways, and because dietary cholesterol alters the ratio of normal to 7-dehydrosteroids,[77,140] it is possible that the supplemental cholesterol competes more directly with 7DHC in endocrine tissues in the initial steps of steroid synthesis.

Cholesterol has been provided to SLOS infants in children in the form of cooked egg yolk, special meat-based formulas, as oil suspensions, and as aqueous suspensions.[64,173,174] All forms of cholesterol appear to be beneficial, but detailed comparisons of their efficacy in large cohorts of SLOS patients have not been undertaken. When SLOS children are hospitalized for surgery or acute medical problems and cholesterol cannot be given enterally, cholesterol in the form of LDL-containing fresh frozen plasma can have striking beneficial effects, especially for treatment of acute infections and for improved wound healing (R. Kelley, unpublished observations). Apparently, the normal depression of LDL cholesterol that occurs in normal infants at such times lowers essential stress reserves of cholesterol even further in SLOS children.

The problems of SLOS children that arise from their malformations are many and frequently require surgical correction and intensive supportive medical care. In addition to Hirschsprung disease, which may affect up to 15 percent of patients with SLOS, there is a high incidence of other structural and functional gastrointestinal problems, including microgastria, pyloric stenosis, malrotation, absent gallbladder, gastroesophageal reflux, severe colic, and dysfunctional swallowing. A large proportion of even less severely affected patients requires gavage or gastrostomy feeding for many months or years after birth. Historically, fundoplications are frequently done, but frequently are unsuccessful in treating SLOS children with gastroesophageal reflux. In most instances, gastroesophageal reflux is caused not by intrinsically abnormal gastroesophageal function, but by severe protein allergy or simple overfeeding from ill-advised attempts to make these children, who have genetic short stature, grow faster. Such problems, combined with intrinsic intestinal dysmotility, make feeding management of SLOS children extremely difficult. However, for most children, surgical intervention can be avoided with an understanding of the factors that contribute to the feeding problems. Particularly important to recognize is that up to 50 percent of SLOS children develop eosinophilic gastroenteritis or other signs of severe gastrointestinal protein allergy and require feeding with elemental formulas for many months. Indeed, the availability of such formulas and the careful management of the intestinal motility problems have all but eliminated the need for fundoplications in SLOS children. Also important in the management of nutrition of SLOS children is the recognition that there is intrinsic muscle hypoplasia in the early years. As a result, "normal" weight percentiles for SLOS infants and young children are typically 1 to 2 standard deviations less than their length percentiles. Maintaining these proportions, and thereby limiting adipose tissue, also makes more cholesterol available to important nonadipose tissues. An uncommon but sometimes severe nutritional problem in SLOS is idiopathic hypermetabolism, which most often occurs between ages 1 and 3 years. SLOS children who develop this unexplained problem may require up to 200 kcal/kg/day to maintain body weight. Because of the complicating factors of microgastria and intestinal dysmotility, such children often do not gain weight for many months, but do not otherwise seem to suffer. Tests for endocrine abnormalities or intestinal malabsorption have been normal in such cases, but signs of hypermetabolism such as warm skin and tachycardia are often noted.

Although many SLOS patients have almost a complete deficiency of normal bile acids (as determined by urinary bile acid analysis), fat malabsorption and deficiencies of fat-soluble vitamins are uncommon in SLOS. Several of the most severely affected patients developed progressive cholestatic liver disease from which they eventually succumbed.[86] Cholestatic liver disease has occurred in the absence of peripheral hyperalimentation, but when present becomes rapidly worse with hyperalimentation. However, treatment with ursodeoxycholic acid can lead to a reversal of the hyperbilirubinemia and cholestatic liver disease in some SLOS patients.

As in many other syndromes associated with weakness and hypotonia, children with SLOS have frequent respiratory and ear infections. Although many children with SLOS have GE reflux, aspiration pneumonia is relatively uncommon, possibly because SLOS children also have hypersensitive gag reflexes that protect their airways. Thus, although there may be a somewhat increased risk of aspiration when GI reflux is severe, reflux alone is not an indication for fundoplication in SLOS, but should be evaluated as indicated above and treated aggressively medically. In more severely affected infants, pulmonary hypoplasia and associated pulmonary hypertension are common causes of death.

Despite persistently low cholesterol levels in most SLOS children, clinical evidence of steroid hormone deficiency is surprisingly uncommon and has been reported in only a few children with unusually low blood cholesterol levels.[81] Among these children, the most common finding is a mild to moderate deficiency of aldosterone synthesis, usually evident by hyponatremia with hyperkalemia during the added endocrine stress of an infection. Glucocorticoid response to infection or ACTH can also be subnormal.[81] However, for most SLOS children with only moderately decreased cholesterol levels, glucocorticoid production appears to be normal and corticosteroid supplements during infections or perioperatively are usually not needed.

Photosensitivity, apparently caused by the increased levels of 7DHC in skin, is a common problem in SLOS children exposed to the sun or even just bright light; it is easily remedied by standard sunblocking creams. Without sunblocking agents, severe erythema and pain can occur within minutes of direct sun exposure. Interestingly, although 7DHC is the precursor of vitamin D, there have been no reports of skeletal or other abnormalities attributable to hypervitaminosis D, presumably because of tight regulation of the synthesis of the ultimate calciferol, 1,25-dihydroxyvitamin D (calcitriol).

## REFERENCES

1. Smith DW, Lemli L, Opitz JM: A newly recognized syndrome of multiple congenital anomalies. *J Pediatr* **64**:210, 1964.
2. Opitz JM, Zellweger H, Shannon WR, Ptacek LJ: The RSH syndrome, in Bergsma D (ed): *The First Conference on the Clinical Delineation of Birth Defects. Part II: Malformation Syndromes.* New York: The National Foundation-March of Dimes, BD:OAS V(2), 1969, p 43.
3. Fine RN, Gwinn JL, Young EF: Smith-Lemli-Opitz syndrome. Radiologic and postmortem findings. *Am J Dis Child* **115**:483, 1968.
4. Finley SC, Finley WH, Monsky DB: Cataracts in a girl with features of the Smith-Lemli-Opitz syndrome. *J Pediatr* **75**:706, 1969.
5. Kaufman R, Alcala H, Sly H, Hartmann A: Brain malformations in Smith-Lemli-Opitz syndrome. *Am J Hum Genet* **26**:47A, 1974.
6. Cotlier E, Rice P: Cataracts in the Smith-Lemli-Opitz syndrome. *Am J Ophthalmol* **72**:955, 1971.
7. Robinson CD, Perry LW, Barlee A, Mella GW: Smith-Lemli-Opitz syndrome with cardiovascular abnormality. *Pediatrics* **47**:844, 1971.
8. Dallaire L: Syndrome of retardation with urogenital and skeletal anomalies (Smith-Lemli-Opitz syndrome): Clinical features and mode of inheritance. *J Med Genet* **6**:113, 1969.
9. Cherstvoy ED, Lazjuk GI, Lurie IW, Nedzved MK, Usoev SS: The pathological anatomy of the Smith-Lemli-Opitz syndrome. *Clin Genet* **7**:382, 1975.
10. Johnson VP: Smith-Lemli-Opitz syndrome: Review and report of two affected siblings. *Z Kinderheilkd* **119**:221, 1975.
11. Gold JD, Pfaffenbach DD: Ocular abnormalities in the Smith-Lemli-Opitz syndrome. *J Ped Ophthalmol* **12**:228, 1975.
12. Curry CJ, Carey JC, Holland JS, Chopra D, Fineman R, Golabi M, Sherman S, et al.: Smith-Lemli-Opitz syndrome-type II: Multiple congenital anomalies with male pseudohermaphroditism and frequent early lethality. *Am J Med Genet* **26**:45, 1987.
13. Donnai D, Young ID, Owen WG, Clark SA, Miller PF, Knox WF: The lethal multiple congenital anomaly syndrome of polydactyly, sex reversal, renal hypoplasia, and unilobular lungs. *J Med Genet* **23**:64, 1986.
14. Scarbrough PR, Huddleston K, Finley SC: An additional case of Smith-Lemli-Opitz syndrome in a 46,XY infant with female external genitalia. *J Med Genet* **23**:174, 1986.
15. Bialer MG, Penchaszadeh VB, Kahn E, Libes R, Krigsman G, Lesser ML: Female external genitalia and müllerian duct derivatives in a 46,XY infant with the Smith-Lemli-Opitz syndrome. *Am J Med Genet* **28**:723, 1987.
16. Belmont JW, Hawkins E, Hejtmancik JF, Greenberg F: Two cases of severe lethal Smith-Lemli-Opitz syndrome. *Am J Med Genet* **26**:65, 1987.
17. Lowry RB, Yong SL: Borderline normal intelligence in the Smith-Lemli-Opitz (RSH) syndrome. *Am J Med Genet* **5**:137, 1980.
18. Opitz JM: RSH/SLO ("Smith-Lemli-Opitz") syndrome: Historical, genetic, and developmental considerations. *Am J Med Genet* **50**:344, 1994.
19. McKeever PA, Young ID: Smith-Lemli-Opitz syndrome II: A disorder of the fetal adrenals? *J Med Genet* **27**:465, 1990.
20. Chasalow FI, Blethen SL, Taysi K: Possible abnormalities of steroid secretion in children with Smith-Lemli-Opitz syndrome and their parents. *Steroids* **46**:827, 1985.
21. Natowicz MR, Evans JE: Abnormal bile acids in the Smith-Lemli-Opitz syndrome. *Am J Med Genet* **50**:364, 1994.
22. Irons M, Elias ER, Salen G, Tint GS, Batta AK: Defective cholesterol biosynthesis in Smith-Lemli-Opitz syndrome [Letter]. *Lancet* **341**:1414, 1993.
23. Kandutsch AA, Russell AE: Preputial gland tumor sterols. III. A metabolic pathway from lanosterol to cholesterol. *J Biol Chem* **235**:2256, 1960.
24. Tint GS, Irons M, Elias ER, Batta AK, Frieden R, Chen TS, Salen G: Defective cholesterol biosynthesis associated with the Smith-Lemli-Opitz syndrome. *N Engl J Med* **330**:107, 1994.
25. Cunniff C, Kratz LE, Moser A, Natowicz MR, Kelley RI: Clinical and biochemical spectrum of patients with RSH/Smith-Lemli-Opitz syndrome and abnormal cholesterol metabolism. *Am J Med Genet* **68**:263, 1997.
26. Shefer S, Salen G, Batta AK, Tint GS, Irons M, Elias ER: Reduced 7-dehydrocholesterol reductase activity in Smith-Lemli-Opitz syndrome. *Am J Med Genet* **50**:326, 1994.
27. Shefer S, Salen G, Batta AK, Honda A, Tint GS, Irons M, Elias ER, et al.: Markedly inhibited 7-dehydrocholesterol-delta 7-reductase activity in liver microsomes from Smith-Lemli-Opitz homozygotes. *J Clin Invest* **96**:1779, 1995.
28. Alley TL, Gray BA, Lee SH, Scherer SW, Tsui LC, Tint GS, Williams CA, et al.: Identification of a yeast artificial chromosome clone spanning a translocation breakpoint at 7q32.1 in a Smith-Lemli-Opitz syndrome patient. *Am J Hum Genet* **56**:1411, 1995.
29. Moebius FF, Fitzky BU, Lee JN, Paik YK, Glossmann H: Molecular cloning and expression of the human delta7-sterol reductase. *Proc Natl Acad Sci U S A* **95**:1899, 1998.
30. Wassif CA, Maslen C, Kachilele-Linjewile S, Lin D, Linck LM, Connor WE, Steiner RD, et al.: Mutations in the human sterol delta 7-reductase gene at 11q12-13 cause Smith-Lemli-Opitz syndrome. *Am J Hum Genet* **63**:55, 1998.
31. Waterham HR, Wijburg FA, Hennekam RC, Vreken P, Poll-The BT, Dorland L, Duran M, et al.: Smith-Lemli-Opitz syndrome is caused by mutations in the 7-dehydrocholesterol reductase gene. *Am J Hum Genet* **63**:329, 1998.
32. Ryan AK, Bartlett K, Clayton P, Eaton S, Mills L, Donnai D, Winter RM, et al.: Smith-Lemli-Opitz syndrome: A variable clinical and biochemical phenotype. *J Med Genet* **35**:558, 1998.
33. Tsukahara M, Fujisawa K, Yamamoto K, Hasui M, Saito C, Yamamaka T, Honda A, et al.: Smith-Lemli-Opitz syndrome in Japan [Letter; Comment]. *Am J Med Genet* **75**:118, 1998.

34. Hanissian AS, Summitt RL: Smith-Lemli-Opitz syndrome in a negro child. *J Pediatr* **74**:303, 1969.

35. Bene M, Duca D, Ioan D, Maximilian C: The Smith-Lemli-Opitz syndrome: Ten new observations. *Acta Med Auxol* **12**:5, 1980.

36. Cruveiller J, Msika S, Lafourcade J: Nanisme de Smith-Lemli-Opitz: À propos de quatre observations. Revue de la littérature. *Sem Hop (France)* **53**:843, 1977.

37. Le Merrer M, Briard ML, Girard S, Mulliez N, Moraine C, Inibert MC: Lethal acrodysgenital dwarfism: A severe lethal condition resembling Smith-Lemli-Opitz syndrome. *J Med Genet* **25**:88, 1988.

38. Meinecke P, Blunck W, Rodewald A: Smith-Lemli-Opitz syndrome. *Am J Med Genet* **28**:735, 1987.

39. Anderson AJ, Stephan MJ, Walker WO, Kelley RI: Variant RSH/Smith-Lemli-Opitz syndrome with atypical sterol metabolism. *Am J Med Genet* **78**:413, 1998.

40. Kunze J: Das Ullrich-Feichtiger-Syndrom. *Archiv Kinderheilkunde* **179**:182, 1969.

41. Hovels O, Mullereisert F: Der "Typhus Rostockiensis" als charakteristisches Kombinationsbild multipler Missbildungen (Polydaktylie, Hypospadie, Kryptorchismus, und Mikrognathie). *Z Kinderheikunde* **77**:454, 1955.

42. Lowry RB, Miller JR, MacLean JR: Micrognathia, polydactyly, and cleft palate. *J Pediatr* **72**:859, 1968.

43. Le Merrer M: Acrodysgenital dwarfism or Smith-Lemli-Opitz type II syndrome [Letter]. *Clin Genet* **40**:252, 1991.

44. Cormier-Daire V, Wolf C, Munnich A, Le Merrer M, Nivelon A, Bonneau D, Journel H, et al.: Abnormal cholesterol biosynthesis in the Smith-Lemli-Opitz and the lethal acrodysgenital syndromes. *Eur J Pediatr* **155**:656, 1996.

45. Silengo M, Kaufman RL, Kissane J: A 46,XY infant with uterus, dysgenetic gonads and multiple anomalies. *Humangenetik* **25**:65, 1974.

46. Greenberg F, Gresik MV, Carpenter RJ, Law SW, Hoffman LP, Ledbetter DH: The Gardner-Silengo-Wachtel or genito-palato-cardiac syndrome: Male pseudohermaphroditism with micrognathia, cleft palate, and conotruncal cardiac defect. *Am J Med Genet* **26**:59, 1987.

47. Verloes A, Ayme S, Gambarelli D, Gonzales M, Le Merrer M, Mulliez N, Philip N, et al.: Holoprosencephaly-polydactyly ("pseudotrisomy 13") syndrome: A syndrome with features of hydrolethalus and Smith-Lemli-Opitz syndromes. A collaborative multicentre study [Review; 34 references]. *J Med Genet* **28**:297, 1991.

48. Hennekam RC, van Noort G, de la Fuente AA: Familial holoprosencephaly, heart defects, and polydactyly. *Am J Med Genet* **41**:258, 1991.

49. Verloes A, Gillerot Y, Langhendries JP, Fryns JP, Koulischer L: Variability versus heterogeneity in syndromal hypothalamic hamartoblastoma and related disorders: Review and delineation of the cerebroacro-visceral early lethality (CAVE) multiplex syndrome. *Am J Med Genet* **43**:669, 1992.

50. Nowaczyk MJ, Whelan DT, Hill RE: Smith-Lemli-Opitz syndrome: Phenotypic extreme with minimal clinical findings. *Am J Med Genet* **78**:419, 1998.

51. Fierro M, Martinez AJ, Harbison JW, Hay SH: Smith-Lemli-Opitz syndrome: Neuropathological and ophthalmological observations. *Dev Med Child Neurol* **19**:57, 1977.

52. Kretzer FL, Hittner HM, Mehta RS: Ocular manifestations of the Smith-Lemli-Opitz syndrome. *Arch Ophthalmol* **99**:2000, 1981.

53. Bardelli AM, Lasorella G, Barberi L, Vanni M: Ocular manifestations in Kniest syndrome, Smith-Lemli-Opitz syndrome, Hallermann-Streiff-Francois syndrome, Rubinstein-Taybi syndrome and median cleft face syndrome. *Ophthalmic Paediatr Genet* **6**:343, 1985.

54. de Die-Smulders C, Fryns JP: Smith-Lemli-Opitz syndrome: The changing phenotype with age. *Genet Couns* **3**:77, 1992.

55. Stewart FJ, Nevin NC, Dornan JC: Prenatal diagnosis of Smith-Lemli-Opitz syndrome. *Am J Med Genet* **56**:286, 1995.

56. Worthington S, Goldblatt J: Smith-Lemli-Opitz syndrome: Further delineation of the phenotype. *Clin Dysmorphol* **6**:263, 1997.

57. Kelley RL, Roessler E, Hennekam RC, Feldman GL, Kosaki K, Jones MC, Palumbos JC, et al.: Holoprosencephaly in RSH/Smith-Lemli-Opitz syndrome: Does abnormal cholesterol metabolism affect the function of Sonic Hedgehog? *Am J Med Genet* **66**:478, 1996.

58. Hyett JA, Clayton PT, Moscoso G, Nicolaides KH: Increased first trimester nuchal translucency as a prenatal manifestation of Smith-Lemli-Opitz syndrome. *Am J Med Genet* **58**:374, 1995.

59. Joseph DB, Uehling DT, Gilbert E, Laxova R: Genitourinary abnormalities associated with the Smith-Lemli-Opitz syndrome. *J Urol* **137**:719, 1987.

60. Garcia CA, McGarry PA, Voirol M, Duncan C: Neurological involvement in the Smith-Lemli-Opitz syndrome: Clinical and neuropathological findings. *Dev Med Child Neurol* **15**:48, 1973.

61. Cherstvoy ED, Lazjuk GI, Ostrovskaya TI, Shved IA, Kravtzova GI, Lurie IW, Gerasimovich AI: The Smith-Lemli-Opitz syndrome. A detailed pathological study as a clue to an etiological heterogeneity. *Virchows Arch A Pathol Anat Histopathol* **404**:413, 1984.

62. Marion RW, Alvarez LA, Marans ZS, Lantos G, Chitayat D: Computed tomography of the brain in the Smith-Lemli-Opitz syndrome. *J Child Neurol* **2**:198, 1987.

63. Rutledge JC, Friedman JM, Harrod MJ, Currarino G, Wright CG, Pinckney L, Chen H: A "new" lethal multiple congenital anomaly syndrome: Joint contractures, cerebellar hypoplasia, renal hypoplasia, urogenital anomalies, tongue cysts, shortness of limbs, eye abnormalities, defects of the heart, gallbladder agenesis, and ear malformations. *Am J Med Genet* **19**:255, 1984.

64. Nwokoro NA, Mulvihill JJ: Cholesterol and bile acid replacement therapy in children and adults with Smith-Lemli-Opitz (SLO/RSH) syndrome. *Am J Med Genet* **68**:315, 1997.

65. Pinsky L, DiGeorge AM: A familial syndrome of facial and skeletal anomalies associated with genital abnormality in the male and normal genitals in the female. *J Pediatr* **66**:1049, 1965.

66. Singer LP, Marion RW, Li JK: Limb deficiency in an infant with Smith-Lemli-Opitz syndrome. *Am J Med Genet* **32**:380, 1989.

67. de Jong G, Kirby PA, Muller LM: RSH (Smith-Lemli-Opitz) syndrome: "Severe" phenotype with ectrodactyly. *Am J Med Genet* **75**:283, 1998.

68. Irons M, Elias ER, Tint GS, Salen G, Frieden R, Buie TM, Ampola M: Abnormal cholesterol metabolism in the Smith-Lemli-Opitz syndrome: Report of clinical and biochemical findings in four patients and treatment in one patient. *Am J Med Genet* **50**:347, 1994.

69. Herman TE, Siegel MJ, Lee BC, Dowton SB: Smith-Lemli-Opitz syndrome type II: Report of a case with additional radiographic findings. *Pediatr Radiol* **23**:37, 1993.

70. Wallace M, Zori RT, Alley T, Whidden E, Gray BA, Williams CA: Smith-Lemli-Opitz syndrome in a female with a de novo, balanced translocation involving 7q32: Probable disruption of an SLOS gene. *Am J Med Genet* **50**:368, 1994.

71. Dallaire L, Fraser FC: The Smith-Lemli-Opitz syndrome of retardation, urogenital and skeletal anomalies in siblings. *Birth Defects: OAS*, **V**(2), 180, 1969.

72. Kohler HG: Brief clinical report: Familial neonatally lethal syndrome of hypoplastic left heart, absent pulmonary lobation, polydactyly, and talipes, probably Smith-Lemli-Opitz (RSH) syndrome. *Am J Med Genet* **14**:423, 1983.

73. Patterson K, Toomey KE, Chandra RS: Hirschsprung disease in a 46,XY phenotypic infant girl with Smith-Lemli-Opitz syndrome. *J Pediatr* **103**:425, 1983.

74. Calvani M, Tirasacchi V, Toscano V, Bellussi A, Fortuna C: Early thelarche and hyperprolactinemia in the Smith-Lemli-Opitz syndrome. *Minerva Pediatr* **31**:1721, 1979.

75. Patsner B, Mann WJ, Chumas J: Malignant mixed germ cell tumor of the ovary in a young woman with Smith-Lemli-Opitz syndrome. *Gynecol Oncol* **33**:386, 1989.

76. Lin AE, Ardinger HH, Ardinger RH Jr, Cunniff C, Kelley RI: Cardiovascular malformations in Smith-Lemli-Opitz syndrome. *Am J Med Genet* **68**:270, 1997.

77. Shackleton CHL, Roitman E, Kelley RI: Neonatal urinary steroids in Smith-Lemli-Opitz syndrome associated with 7-dehydrocholesterol reductase deficiency. *Steroids* **64**:481, 1999.

78. Kratz LE, Kelley RI: Prenatal diagnosis of the RSH/Smith-Lemli-Opitz syndrome. *Am J Med Genet* **82**:376, 1999.

79. Rossiter JP, Hofman KJ, Kelley RI: Smith-Lemli-Opitz syndrome: Prenatal diagnosis by quantification of cholesterol precursors in amniotic fluid. *Am J Med Genet* **56**:272, 1995.

80. Pankau R, Partsch CJ, Funda J, Sippell WG: Hypothalamic-pituitary-gonadal function in two infants with Smith-Lemli-Opitz syndrome. *Am J Med Genet* **43**:513, 1992.

81. Andersson HC, Frentz J, Martinez JE, Tuck-Muller CM, Bellizaire J: Adrenal insufficiency in Smith-Lemli-Opitz syndrome. *Am J Med Genet* **82**:382, 1999.

82. Schechter R, Torfs CP, Bateson TF: The epidemiology of infantile hypertrophic pyloric stenosis. *Paediatr Perinat Epidemiol* **11**:407, 1997.

83. Kim EH, Boutwell WC: Smith-Lemli-Opitz syndrome associated with Hirschsprung disease, 46,XY female karyotype, and total anomalous pulmonary venous drainage. *J Pediatr* **106**:861, 1985.

84. Zizka J, Maresova J, Kerekes Z, Nozicka Z, Juttnerova V, Balicek P: Intestinal aganglionosis in the Smith-Lemli-Opitz syndrome. *Acta Paediatr Scand* 72:141, 1983.

85. Karsten J, Kosztolanyi G: Smith-Lemli-Opitz syndrome in siblings. *Acta Paediatr Hung* 32:127, 1992.

86. Ness GC, Lopez D, Borrego O, Gilbert-Barness E: Increased expression of low-density lipoprotein receptors in a Smith-Lemli-Opitz infant with elevated bilirubin levels. *Am J Med Genet* 68:294, 1997.

87. Parnes S, Hunter AG, Jimenez C, Carpenter BF, MacDonald I: Apparent Smith-Lemli-Opitz syndrome in a child with a previously undescribed form of mucolipidosis not involving the neurons. *Am J Med Genet* 35:397, 1990.

88. Porter FD, Wassif CA, Tsokos M, Steiner RD: Impaired intracellular LDL cholesterol metabolism in Smith-Lemli-Opitz syndrome fibroblasts. In preparation.

89. Lachman MF, Wright Y, Whiteman DA, Herson V, Greenstein RM: Brief clinical report: A 46,XY phenotypic female with Smith-Lemli-Opitz syndrome. *Clin Genet* 39:136, 1991.

90. Kenis H, Hustinx TW: A familial syndrome of mental retardation in association with multiple congenital anomalies resembling the syndrome of Smith-Lemli-Opitz. *Maandschr Kindergeneeskd* 35:37, 1967.

91. Tzouvelekis G, Antoniades K, Batma A, Nanas C: Smith-Lemli-Opitz syndrome in female, monozygotic twins. *Clin Genet* 40:229, 1991.

92. Mizushima A, Satoyoshi M: Unusual responses of muscular rigidity and hypothermia to halothane and succinylcholine: A case report of Smith-Lemli-Opitz (SLO) syndrome. *Masui* 37:1118, 1988.

93. Petersen WC, Crouch ER Jr: Anesthesia-induced rigidity, unrelated to succinylcholine, associated with Smith-Lemli-Opitz syndrome and malignant hyperthermia. *Anest Analg* 80:606, 1995.

94. Nwokoro NA, Kelley RI: Clinical, biochemical, and developmental spectrum of adults with Smith-Lemli-Opitz syndrome. In preparation.

95. Pauli RM, Williams MS, Josephson KD, Tint GS: Smith-Lemli-Opitz syndrome: Thirty-year follow-up of "S" of "RSH" syndrome. *Am J Med Genet* 68:260, 1997.

96. Zahle Ostergaard G, Nielsen H, Friis B: Defective monocyte oxidative metabolism in a child with Smith-Lemli-Opitz syndrome. *Europ J Pediatr* 151:291, 1992.

97. Hodge VJ, Gould SJ, Subramani S, Moser HW, Krisans SK: Normal cholesterol synthesis in human cells requires functional peroxisomes. *Biochem Biophys Res Commun* 181:537, 1991.

98. Stamellos KD, Shackelford JE, Tanaka RD, Krisans SK: Mevalonate kinase is localized in rat liver peroxisomes. *J Biol Chem* 267:5560, 1992.

99. Brown MS, Goldstein JL: Multivalent feedback regulation of HMG-CoA reductase, a control mechanism coordinating isoprenoid synthesis and cell growth. *J Lipid Res* 21:505, 1980.

100. Clark RM, Fey MB, Jensen RG, Hill DW: Desmosterol in human milk. *Lipids* 18:264, 1983.

101. Bourre JM, Clement M, Gerard D, Chaudiere J: Alterations of cholesterol synthesis precursors (7-dehydrocholesterol, 7-dehydrodesmosterol, desmosterol) in dysmyelinating neurological mutant mouse (quaking, shiverer and trembler) in the PNS and the CNS. *Biochim Biophys Acta* 1004:387, 1989.

102. Lin DS, Connor WE, Wolf DP, Neuringer M, Hachey DL: Unique lipids of primate spermatozoa: Desmosterol and docosahexaenoic acid. *J Lipid Res* 34:491, 1993.

103. Kempen HJM, Glatz JFC, Gevers-Leuven JA, van der Voort HA, Katan MB: Serum lathosterol is an indicator of whole-body cholesterol synthesis in humans. *J Lipid Res* 29:1149, 1988.

104. Axelson M: Occurrence of isomeric dehydrocholesterols in human plasma. *J Lipid Res* 32:1441, 1991.

105. Honda A, Shefer S, Salen G, Xu G, Batta AK, Tint GS, Honda M, et al: Regulation of the last two enzymatic reactions in cholesterol biosynthesis in rats: Effects of BM 15,766, cholesterol, cholic acid, lovastatin, and their combinations. *Hepatology* 24:435, 1996.

106. Silve S, Dupuy PH, Ferrara P, Loison G: Human lamin B receptor exhibits sterol C14-reductase activity in *Saccharomyces cerevisiae*. *Biochim Biophys Acta* 1392:233, 1998.

107. Keller GA, Scallen TJ, Clarke D, Maher PA, Krisans SK, Singer SJ: Subcellular localization of sterol carrier protein-2 in rat hepatocytes: Its primary localization to peroxisomes. *J Cell Biol* 108:1353, 1989.

108. Biardi L, Sreedhar A, Zokaei A, Vartak NB, Bozeat RL, Shackelford JE, Keller GA, et al.: Mevalonate kinase is predominantly localized in

peroxisomes and is defective in patients with peroxisome deficiency disorders. *J Biol Chem* 269:1197, 1994.

109. Biardi L, Krisans SK: Compartmentalization of cholesterol biosynthesis. Conversion of mevalonate to farnesyl diphosphate occurs in the peroxisomes. *J Biol Chem* 271:1784, 1996.

110. Krisans SK: The role of peroxisomes in cholesterol metabolism. *Am J Respir Cell Mol Biol* 7:358, 1992.

111. Stamellos KD, Shackelford JE, Shechter I, Jiang G, Conrad D, Keller GA, Krisans SK: Subcellular localization of squalene synthase in rat hepatic cells. Biochemical and immunochemical evidence. *J Biol Chem* 268:12825, 1993.

112. Appelkvist EL, Reinhart M, Fischer R, Billheimer J, Dallner G: Presence of individual enzymes of cholesterol biosynthesis in rat liver peroxisomes. *Arch Biochem Biophys* 282:318, 1990.

113. Kelley RI: Review: The cerebrohepatorenal syndrome of Zellweger, morphologic and metabolic aspects. *Am J Med Genet* 16:503, 1983.

114. Lange Y, Echevarria F, Steck TL: Movement of zymosterol, a precursor of cholesterol, among three membranes in human fibroblasts. *J Biol Chem* 266:21439, 1991.

115. Dahl NK, Daunais MA, Liscum L: A second complementation class of cholesterol transport mutants with a variant Niemann-Pick type C phenotype. *J Lipid Res* 35:1839, 1994.

116. Liscum L, Klansek JJ: Niemann-Pick disease type C. *Curr Opin Lipidol* 9:131, 1998.

117. Kato K, Cox AD, Hisaka MM, Graham SM, Buss JE, Der CJ: Isoprenoid addition to Ras protein is the critical modification for its membrane association and transforming activity. *Proc Natl Acad Sci U S A* 89:6403, 1992.

118. Carr BR, Simpson ER: Cholesterol synthesis in human fetal tissues. *J Clin Endocrin Metab* 55:447, 1982.

119. Bellknap WM, Dietschy JM: Sterol synthesis and low-density lipoprotein clearance in vivo in the pregnant rat, placenta, and fetus. *J Clin Invest* 82:2077, 1988.

120. Tint GS, Seller M, Hughes-Benzie R, Batta AK, Shefer S, Genest D, Irons M, et al.: Markedly increased tissue concentrations of 7-dehydrocholesterol combined with low levels of cholesterol are characteristic of the Smith-Lemli-Opitz syndrome. *J Lipid Res* 36:89, 1995.

121. Partridge WM, Mietus LJ: Palmitate and cholesterol transport through the blood-brain barrier. *J Neurochem* 34:463, 1980.

122. Morell P, Jurevics H: Origin of cholesterol in myelin. *Neurochem Res* 21:463, 1996.

123. Farese RV Jr, Ruland SL, Flynn LM, Stokowski RP, Young SG: Knockout of the mouse apolipoprotein B gene results in embryonic lethality in homozygotes and protection against diet-induced hypercholesterolemia in heterozygotes. *Proc Natl Acad Sci U S A* 92:1774, 1995.

124. Willnow TE, Hilpert J, Armstrong SA, Rohlmann A, Hammer RE, Burns DK, Herz J: Defective forebrain development in mice lacking gp330/megalin. *Proc Natl Acad Sci U S A* 93:8460, 1996.

125. Roessler E, Belloni E, Gaudenz K, Jay P, Berta P, Scherer SW, Tsui L, et al.: Mutations in the human *Sonic Hedgehog* gene cause holoprosencephaly. *Nat Genet* 14:357, 1996.

126. Porter JA, Young KE, Beachy PA: Cholesterol modification of Hedgehog signaling proteins in animal development. *Science* 274:255, 1996.

127. Chiang C, Litingtung Y, Lee E, Young KE, Corden JL, Westphal H, Beachy PA: Cyclopia and defective axial patterning in mice lacking Sonic hedgehog gene function. *Nature* 383:407, 1996.

128. Silve S, Dupuy PH, Labit-Lebouteiller C, Kaghad M, Chalon P, Rahier A, Taton M, et al.: Emopamil-binding protein, a mammalian protein that binds a series of structurally diverse neuroprotective agents, exhibits delta8-delta7 sterol isomerase activity in yeast. *J Biol Chem* 271:22434, 1996.

129. Batta AK, Salen G, Tint GS, Shefer S: Identification of 19-nor-5,7,9(10)-cholestatrien-3 beta-ol in patients with Smith-Lemli-Opitz syndrome. *J Lipid Res* 36:2413, 1995.

130. Ruan B, Shey J, Gerst N, Wilson WK, Schroepfer GJ Jr: Silver ion high pressure liquid chromatography provides unprecedented separation of sterols: Application to the enzymatic formation of cholesta-5,8-dien-3 beta-ol. *Proc Natl Acad Sci U S A* 93:11603, 1996.

131. De Fabiani E, Caruso D, Cavaleri M, Galli Kienle M, Galli G: Cholesta-5,7,9(11)-trien-3 beta-ol found in plasma of patients with Smith-Lemli-Opitz syndrome indicates formation of sterol hydroperoxide. *J Lipid Res* 37:2280, 1996.

132. Tint GS, Salen G, Batta AK, Shefer S, Irons M, Elias ER, Abuelo DN, et al.: Correlation of severity and outcome with plasma sterol levels

in variants of the Smith-Lemli-Opitz syndrome. *J Pediatr* **127**:82, 1995.

133. Kelley RI: Diagnosis of Smith-Lemli-Opitz syndrome by gas chromatography/mass spectrometry of 7-dehydrocholesterol in plasma, amniotic fluid and cultured skin fibroblasts. *Clin Chim Acta* **236**:45, 1995.

134. Honda M, Tint GS, Honda A, Batta AK, Chen TS, Shefer S, Salen G: Measurement of 3 beta-hydroxysteroid delta 7-reductase activity in cultured skin fibroblasts utilizing ergosterol as a substrate: A new method for the diagnosis of the Smith-Lemli-Opitz syndrome. *J Lipid Res* **37**:2433, 1996.

135. Xu G, Salen G, Shefer S, Ness GC, Chen TS, Zhao Z, Tint GS: Reproducing abnormal cholesterol biosynthesis as seen in the Smith-Lemli-Opitz syndrome by inhibiting the conversion of 7-dehydrocholesterol to cholesterol in rats. *J Clin Invest* **95**:76, 1995.

136. McGaughran JM, Clayton PT, Mills KA, Rimmer S, Moore L, Donnai D: Prenatal diagnosis of Smith-Lemli-Opitz syndrome. *Am J Med Genet* **56**:269, 1995.

137. Salen G, Tint GS, Xu G, Batta AK, Irons M, Elias ER: Abnormal cholesterol biosynthesis in the Smith-Lemli-Opitz syndrome. *Ital J Gastroenterol* **27**:506, 1995.

138. Abuelo DN, Tint GS, Kelley R, Batta AK, Shefer S, Salen G: Prenatal detection of the cholesterol biosynthetic defect in the Smith-Lemli-Opitz syndrome by the analysis of amniotic fluid sterols. *Am J Med Genet* **56**:281, 1995.

139. Kelley RI: RSH/Smith-Lemli-Opitz syndrome: Mutations and metabolic morphogenesis. *Am J Hum Genet* **63**:322, 1998.

140. Shackleton CH, Roitman E, Kratz LE, Kelley RI: Equine type estrogens produced by a pregnant woman carrying a Smith-Lemli-Opitz syndrome fetus. *J Clin Endocrinol Metab* **84**:1157, 1999.

141. Roux C, Aubry MM: Action tératogène chez le rat d'un inhibiteur de la synthèse du cholesterol, le AY 9944. *C R Soc Biol* **160**:1353, 1966.

142. Roux C, Horvath C, Dupuis R: Teratogenic action and embryo lethality of AY 9944R. Prevention by a hypercholesterolemia-provoking diet. *Teratology* **19**:35, 1979.

143. Roux C, Dupuis R, Horvath C, Giroud A: Interpretation of isolated agenesis of the pituitary. *Teratology* **19**:39, 1979.

144. DeHart DB, Lanoue L, Tint GS, Sulik KK: A rodent model of Smith-Lemli-Opitz syndrome; BM 15,766 induced teratogenesis. *Am J Med Genet* **68**:329, 1997.

145. Kolf-Clauw M, Chevy F, Siliart B, Wolf C, Mulliez N, Roux C: Cholesterol biosynthesis inhibited by BM15,766 induces holoprosencephaly in the rat. *Teratology* **56**:188, 1997.

146. Schroepfer GJ, Jr., Frantz ID: Conversion of delta7-cholestenol-4-C14 and 7-dehydrocholesterol-4-C14 to cholesterol. *J Biol Chem* **236**:3137, 1961.

147. Lecain E, Chenivesse X, Spagnoli R, Pompon D: Cloning by metabolic interference in yeast and enzymatic characterization of Arabidopsis thaliana sterol delta 7-reductase. *J Biol Chem* **271**:10866, 1996.

148. Scherer SW, Soder S, Duvoisin RM, Huizenga JJ, Tsui LC: The human metabotropic glutamate receptor 8 (GRM8) gene: A disproportionately large gene located at 7q31.3-q32.1. *Genomics* **44**:232, 1997.

149. Alley TL, Scherer SW, Huizenga JJ, Tsui LC, Wallace MR: Physical mapping of the chromosome 7 breakpoint region in an SLOS patient with t(7;20) (q32.1;q13.2). *Am J Med Genet* **68**:279, 1997.

150. Moebius FF, Striessnig J, Glossmann H: The mysteries of sigma receptors: New family members reveal a role in cholesterol synthesis [Review]. *Trends Pharmacol Sci* **18**:67, 1997.

151. Fitzky BU, Witsch-Baumgartner M, Erdel M, Lee JN, Paik YK, Glossmann H, Utermann G, et al: Mutations in the delta7-sterol reductase gene in patients with the Smith-Lemli-Opitz syndrome. *Proc Natl Acad Sci U S A* **95**:8181, 1998.

152. Witsch-Baumgartner M, Fitzky BU, Ogorelkova M, Kraft HG, Moebius FF, Glossmann H, Seedorf U, et al.: Mutational spectrum in the Delta7-sterol reductase gene and genotype-phenotype correlation in 84 patients with Smith-Lemli-Opitz syndrome. *Am J Hum Genet* **66**:402, 2000.

153. Hoffmann G, Gibson KM, Brandt IK, Bader PI, Wappner RS, Sweetman L: Mevalonic aciduria — An inborn error of cholesterol and non-sterol isoprene biosynthesis. *N Engl J Med* **314**:1610, 1986.

154. Roux C, Dupuis R, Horvath C, Talbot JN: Teratogenic effect of an inhibitor of cholesterol synthesis (AY 9944) in rats: Correlation with maternal cholesterolemia. *J Nutr* **110**:2310, 1980.

155. Barbu V, Roux C, Lambert D, Dupuis R, Gardette J, Maziere JC, Maziere C, et al.: Cholesterol prevents the teratogenic action of AY 9944: Importance of the timing of cholesterol supplementation to rats. *J Nutr* **118**:774, 1988.

156. Porter JA, von Kessler DP, Ekker SC, Young KE, Lee JJ, Moses K, Beachy PA: The product of *hedgehog* autoproteolytic cleavage active in local and long-range signalling. *Nature* **374**:363, 1995.

157. Bitgood MJ, Shen L, McMahon AP: Sertoli cell signaling by Desert hedgehog regulates the male germline. *Curr Biol* **6**:298, 1996.

158. Iwasaki M, Le AX, Helms JA: Expression of Indian hedgehog, bone morphogenetic protein 6 and gli during skeletal morphogenesis. *Mech Dev* **69**:197, 1997.

159. Cooper MK, Porter JA, Young KA, Beachy PA: Plant-derived and synthetic teratogens inhibit the ability of target tissues to respond to Sonic hedgehog signaling. *Science (USA)* **280**:1603, 1998.

160. Ingham PW, Taylor AM, Nakano Y: Role of the Drosophila patched gene in positional signalling. *Nature* **353**:184, 1991.

161. Stone DM, Hynes M, Armanini M, Swanson TA, Gu Q, Johnson RL, Scott MP, et al.: The tumour-suppressor gene patched encodes a candidate receptor for Sonic hedgehog. *Nature* **384**:129, 1996.

162. Goodrich LV, Milenkovic L, Higgins KM, Scott MP: Altered neural cell fates and medulloblastoma in mouse patched mutants. *Science* **277**:1109, 1997.

163. Mills K, Mandel H, Montemagno R, Soothill P, Gershoni-Baruch R, Clayton PT: First trimester prenatal diagnosis of Smith-Lemli-Opitz syndrome (7-dehydrocholesterol reductase deficiency). *Pediatr Res* **39**:816, 1996.

164. Sharp P, Haan E, Fletcher JM, Khong TY, Carey WF: First-trimester diagnosis of Smith-Lemli-Opitz syndrome. *Prenat Diagn* **17**:355, 1997.

165. Lanoue L, Dehart DB, Hinsdale ME, Maeda N, Tint GS, Sulik KK: Limb, genital, CNS, and facial malformations result from gene/environment-induced cholesterol deficiency: Further evidence for a link to sonic hedgehog. *Am J Med Genet* **73**:24, 1997.

166. Ruan B, Gerst N, Emmons GT, Shey J, Schroepfer GJ Jr: Sterol synthesis. A timely look at the capabilities of conventional and silver ion high performance liquid chromatography for the separation of C27 sterols related to cholesterol biosynthesis. *J Lipid Res* **38**:2615, 1997.

167. Honda A, Tint GS, Salen G, Kelley RI, Honda M, Batta AK, Chen TS, et al.: Sterol concentrations in cultured Smith-Lemli-Opitz syndrome skin fibroblasts: Diagnosis of a biochemically atypical case of the syndrome. *Am J Med Genet* **68**:282, 1997.

168. Honda A, Batta AK, Salen G, Tint GS, Chen TS, Shefer S: Screening for abnormal cholesterol biosynthesis in the Smith-Lemli-Opitz syndrome: Rapid determination of plasma 7-dehydrocholesterol by ultraviolet spectrometry. *Am J Med Genet* **68**:288, 1997.

169. Zimmerman PA, Hercules DM, Naylor EW: Direct analysis of filter paper blood specimens for identification of Smith-Lemli-Opitz syndrome using time-of-flight secondary ion mass spectrometry. *Am J Med Genet* **68**:300, 1997.

170. Cruz MLA, Wong WW, Mimouni F, Hachey DL, Setchell KDR, Klein PD, Tsang RC: Effects of infant nutrition on cholesterol synthesis rates. *Pediatr Res* **35**:135, 1994.

171. Jones JH: Regulation of cholesterol biosynthesis by diet in humans. *Am J Clin Nutr* **66**:438, 1997.

172. Jensen RG: The lipids in human milk. *Prog Lipid Res* **35**:53, 1996.

173. Elias ER, Irons MB, Hurley AD, Tint GS, Salen G: Clinical effects of cholesterol supplementation in six patients with the Smith-Lemli-Opitz syndrome (SLOS). *Am J Med Genet* **68**:305, 1997.

174. Irons M, Elias ER, Abuelo D, Bull MJ, Greene CL, Johnson VP, Keppen L, et al.: Treatment of Smith-Lemli-Opitz syndrome: Results of a multicenter trial. *Am J Med Genet* **68**:311, 1997.

175. Ullrich K, Koch HG, Meschede D, Flotmann U, Seedorf U: Smith-Lemli-Opitz syndrome: Treatment with cholesterol and bile acids [Letter]. *Neuropediatrics* **27**:111, 1996.

176. Xu G, Salen G, Shefer S, Ness GC, Chen TS, Zhao Z, Salen L, et al.: Treatment of the cholesterol biosynthetic defect in Smith-Lemli-Opitz syndrome reproduced in rats by BM 15,766. *Gastroenterology* **109**:1301, 1995.

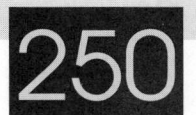

# Holoprosencephaly

*Maximilian Muenke* ■ *Philip A. Beachy*

1. Holoprosencephaly (HPE) is a structural anomaly of the developing brain in which the forebrain fails to divide into two separate hemispheres and ventricles. HPE is the most common brain defect in humans with a prevalence of 1 in 250 during early embryogenesis and 1 in 10,000 to 1 in 20,000 at birth.

2. Our understanding of the pathogenesis of HPE derives largely from the study of animal models. Embryologically, HPE is associated with a loss or failure to develop midline structures of the ventral forebrain and of the face. The resulting apposition or fusion of structures that normally develop in lateral positions gives rise to the characteristic features of HPE. Internally, these features include the defining characteristic of HPE, an undivided forebrain. Externally, severe HPE is associated with development of a cyclopic eye, resulting in superior displacement of a fused, proboscis-like nasal structure.

3. The prechordal plate mesendoderm has emerged as a structure required for induction of ventral forebrain in the overlying neural plate, and for subdivision of the eye field. Surgical, teratologic, or genetic perturbations of the prechordal plate, particularly at or before early gastrulation, are associated with HPE.

4. Genetic studies originating in *Drosophila* and extending to mice and humans have identified Sonic hedgehog, a member of the Hedgehog family of secreted signaling proteins, as a critical signal produced in the prechordal plate and required for induction of ventral forebrain structures from the overlying neural plate. Mouse embryos homozygous for *Sonic hedgehog* mutations display the features of severe HPE, and humans with heterozygous *SHH* mutations have clinical findings of HPE with variable expressivity and penetrance. Loss of *Shh* signaling may also contribute to defects in midline facial development because *Shh* is also expressed in the processes that give rise to midline facial structures. Mutation of other Shh pathway components has also been associated with ventral forebrain deficits in animal models.

5. Several plant-derived and synthetic teratogens are known to specifically block the ability of cells to respond to Shh signaling. The mechanism of this effect is not known, but these agents all appear to affect cellular cholesterol homeostasis. In addition, certain mutations in mice or humans that perturb cholesterol homeostasis cause or increase the incidence of HPE.

6. Studies in the mouse and in the zebra fish have also implicated the signaling pathway headed by *nodal* and/or related members of the TGF-β family of secreted signaling proteins as playing a critical role in prechordal mesoderm formation, migration, and signaling to the overlying prosencephalic plate.

7. The processes of ventral forebrain and midline facial development represent a particularly sensitive target for genetic or environmental perturbations. HPE can also result from combinations of distinct insults that are mild and that alone do not cause HPE. These factors together may account for the high incidence of HPE in human embryos, and for the large number of autosomal dominant human syndromes associated with HPE. In addition, the increased severity produced by a combination of genetic and possibly environmental insults may account for the high degree of variability of HPE observed within kindreds.

8. The clinical spectrum of central nervous system anomalies ranges from alobar HPE (absent interhemispheric fissure) to semilobar (midline separation only posteriorly) and lobar HPE (complete separation of the ventricles but continuity across the cortex). Accompanying facial anomalies may include anophthalmia, cyclopia, extreme hypotelorism, a single nostril nose and/or midface hypoplasia with cleft lip and/or palate.

9. Diagnosis can be done prenatally by ultrasound examination at 16 weeks of gestation or at birth by physical exam and confirmed by brain scan (CAT or MRI).

10. Treatment is done system by system and may include anticonvulsive therapy for seizures, alternative feeding methods (e.g., tube feedings), surgical management of hydrocephaly (ventriculoperitoneal shunt) and closure of clefts of lip and palate.

11. The etiology is extremely heterogeneous with environmental (e.g., maternal diabetes) and genetic factors known to cause HPE. Familial HPE has been described with autosomal dominant, autosomal recessive, and X-linked inheritance. HPE is part of many genetic syndromes: Smith-Lemli-Opitz syndrome is one of the more common ones. Lastly, cytogenetic anomalies are present in 25 to 50 percent of newborn infants with HPE. Nonrandom structural chromosomal anomalies predict at last 12 different HPE loci. To date, cytogenetic deletions and translocations have helped to define the minimal critical regions for HPE loci on chromosomes 7q36, 13q32, 2p21, 18p11.3, 21q22.3, and others.

12. The human *Sonic Hedgehog* (*SHH*) gene in 7q36 was the first HPE gene to be identified. Heterozygous deletions, nonsense, frameshift, and missense mutations in *SHH* predict a loss-of-function mechanism as one cause for HPE in humans. To date, *SHH* mutations have been found to cause HPE in 30 to 40 percent of families with autosomal dominant transmission of HPE based on structural

A list of standard abbreviations is located immediately preceding the index in each volume. Additional abbreviations used in this chapter include: AD = autosomal dominant; AR = autosomal recessive; CAT = computed axial tomography; HPE = holoprosencephaly; MCR = minimal critical region; MIHF = middle interhemispheric fusion; MRI = magnetic resonance imaging; PHS = Pallister-Hall syndrome; *PTC* = human Patched gene; RTS = Rubenstein-Taybi syndrome; *SHH* = human Sonic Hedgehog gene; SLOS = Smith-Lemli-Opitz syndrome; *SMO* = human Smoothened gene; *TGIF* = human gene for TG-interacting factor.

anomalies, whereas the detection rate in sporadic cases is low (<5 percent). Heterozygous insertions and deletions leading to frameshifts, nonsense mutations, and expansion of an alanine repeat of the human *ZIC2* gene in 13q32 have been found in HPE patients. Furthermore, heterozygous deletions and missense mutations in the homeodomain of the *SIX3* gene in 2p21 are associated with HPE. Lastly, heterozygous deletions and missense mutations of the gene coding for TG-interacting factor (TGIF) in 18p11.3 cause HPE.

13. The phenotype of individuals with *SHH, SIX3* or *TGIF* mutations is extremely variable ranging from alobar HPE and cyclopia to clinically normal mutation carriers even within the same family. In contrast, preliminary data suggest that carriers of *ZIC2* mutations have normal or only mildly dysmorphic facial findings despite severe central nervous system anomalies.

14. Future directions include studies to better define the milder end of the clinical spectrum in infants and older children with HPE in an attempt to design better therapies. On a molecular level, the long-term goal is to identify additional HPE genes and to analyze the interactions of multiple gene products and/or environmental factors in an attempt to elucidate the underlying mechanisms that contribute to the wide variability of the HPE spectrum.

## INTRODUCTION AND DEVELOPMENTAL PATHWAYS

### Terminology

Cyclopia has been known since ancient times. The Cyclopes, one-eyed giants who lived as shepherds on the coast of Sicily, were described in detail in Homer's *The Odyssey*.[1] In addition to Greek mythology, cyclopia was mentioned in writings of the early Romans. It was not until the late eighteenth and early nineteenth centuries that accurate descriptions of cyclopia in humans appeared in the scientific literature.[2] The connection between cyclopia and malformations of the central nervous system was first pointed out by Kundrat[3] and termed "arhinencephaly" to emphasize the involvement of the olfactory bulbs and tracts. Yakovlev[4] more specifically termed this malformation complex "holotelencephaly" to describe the failure of the telencephalon (endbrain) to divide into two separate cerebral hemispheres and ventricles. The term holoprosencephaly was proposed by DeMyer and Zeman[5] to emphasize the involvement of both components of the forebrain, the telencephalon and the diencephalon.

Holoprosencephaly (HPE) is characterized by a defect in the midline of the embryonic forebrain due to failure of growth and/or segmentation of the anterior end of the neural tube.[2,6,7] Pathologic studies classify the associated brain and facial malformations into three categories reflecting graded degrees of malformation, although the abnormalities form a continuous spectrum of severity. In the most severe type, alobar HPE, there is no separation of the cerebral hemispheres and there is a single ventricle. In semilobar HPE, the interhemispheric fissure is present only posteriorly, with fusion of the left and right frontal and parietal lobes. Lobar HPE, the mildest form, is characterized by separation of most of the cerebral hemispheres and lateral ventricles. However, there is fusion of the most rostral aspect of the telencephalon, the frontal lobes, especially ventrally. Frequently, these central nervous system anomalies are accompanied by craniofacial anomalies; they are rarely accompanied by anomalies of the limbs and internal organs.

### Epidemiology

The frequency of HPE is as high as 1 in 250 during early embryogenesis.[8] The live birth prevalence is estimated to be 1 in 10,000 to 1 in 20,000 live births.[9–12] However, these figures at birth may underestimate the true prevalence because some children with mild facial features might not have been diagnosed with HPE. Among those cases with an identified anatomic type, approximately 64 percent had alobar HPE, 24 percent had semilobar, and 12 percent had lobar holoprosencephaly.[11,12] When limited to those with cytogenetically normal chromosomes, the distribution among anatomic subtypes is similar (63 percent alobar, 28 percent semilobar, 9 percent lobar). Nearly twice as many live births with HPE are females as compared with males, and females more frequently have severe facial malformations. There is no known maternal or paternal age effect.

### Pathogenesis of HPE — Animal Models

Much of what we know about the pathogenesis of HPE derives from observations in animals, in which detailed descriptions of cyclopia date at least as far back as the seventeenth century. In *Records of the Colony and Plantation of New Haven from 1638 to 1648*, a cyclopic pig born in 1641 was said to have "but one eye in the middle of the face." Above the eye "a thing of flesh grew forth and hung downe...like a mans intrum' of gen'ation" (quoted in reference[13]). The accuracy evident in this description did not extend to the subsequent judgment that birth of the pig was caused by cross-species fertility, resulting in the trial and execution of an unfortunate one-eyed servant with a cataract in his defective eye.

Embryologically, HPE can be traced to varying degrees of loss or disruption in the development of ventral forebrain and midline facial structures. In normal development, the optic vesicles evaginate from the lateral walls of the forebrain, at locations separated by the developing structures of the ventral forebrain. In severe HPE, ventral forebrain structures are absent and the optic primordia consequently develop as a single unpaired evagination from the floor of the forebrain. The resulting cyclopic eye protrudes into the developing face, thus displacing the fused nasal structures superiorly and accounting for the appearance and placement of the eye and proboscis (Fig. 250-1).

Beginning in the late nineteenth century, experimental embryologists learned to induce cyclopia in diverse vertebrate species by subjecting embryos to treatment with radiation, heat, cold, hypoxia, salts, alcohols and other solvents, alkali, vitamin A, and certain plant alkaloids and synthetic compounds.[13–17] A feature common to all of these treatments was their application during early gastrulation. The most incisive early experiments were surgical manipulations carried out in the early twentieth century in amphibians by Otto Mangold,[18] husband of the well-known Hilde Mangold,[19] and Howard Adelmann.[14,15] These workers independently demonstrated that loss or removal of prechordal plate mesoderm (also known as prechordal mesodo-derm; see Fig. 250-2) caused cyclopia and a failure in formation of structures such as the chiasmatic plate and optic stalks. The prechordal plate thus was postulated to supply an influence essential for induction of ventral forebrain structures and for bilateral subdivision of an otherwise continuous eye field within the overlying prosencephalic plate.[14,15] Consistent with this view, salt and alcohol treatments that induce cyclopia in amphibians and fish have been associated with defects in forward migration of prechordal plate mesoderm so that it fails to assume its normal position under the medial prosencephalic plate.[20–22]

In recent years, the critical role of the prechordal mesendoderm has been confirmed with the use of molecular markers such as *Nkx2.1*, a homeobox gene whose expression is largely restricted to the medial aspects of the prosencephalic neural plate and whose function is required for the development of this region into the hypothalamus.[23–29] In transplantation or explant culture experiments with mouse and chick embryos, the prechordal mesendoderm is required for normal expression and can induce ectopic expression of the *Nkx2.1* marker.[27,29] In chick and amphibian embryos, molecular markers of retinal fates such as *Pax6* and *ET*, which are expressed initially in a continuous pattern across the anteromedial prosencephalic plate, require the presence of prechordal mesendoderm for later subdivision into bilateral

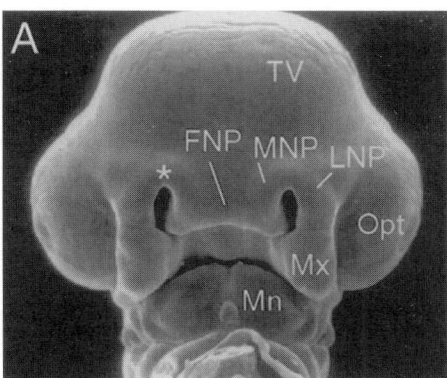
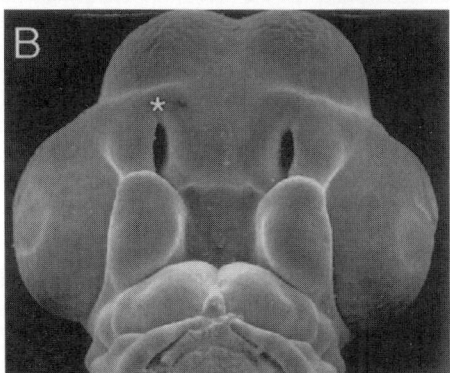
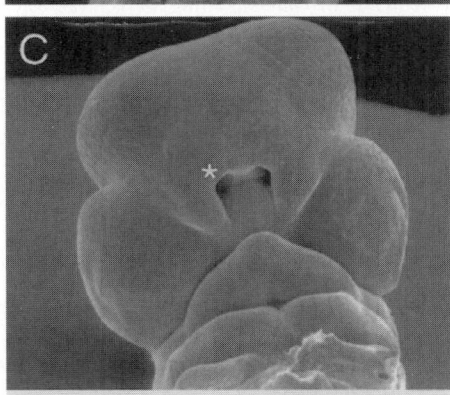
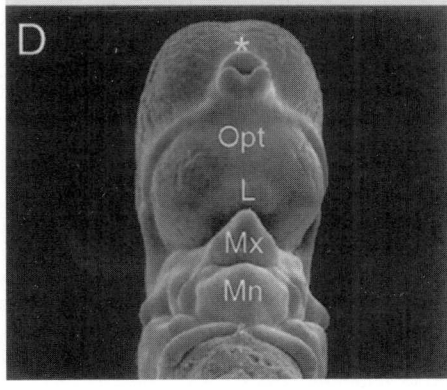

**Fig. 250-1 Loss of midline facial and forebrain structures in an animal model of holoprosencephaly.** Chick embryos treated at early gastrulation with the teratogen jervine are arranged in order of progressively more severe effects. Jervine (see Fig. 250-5) is a plant-derived compound that specifically inhibits the *Sonic hedgehog* pathway. The effects range from normal development in an untreated embryo (*A*) to partial loss of the frontonasal process and partial fusion of lateral structures (*B, C*) to complete loss of the frontonasal process and near perfect fusion at the midline of the mandibular and maxillary processes as well as the optic vesicles and lens (cyclopia), resulting in a superiorly directed displacement

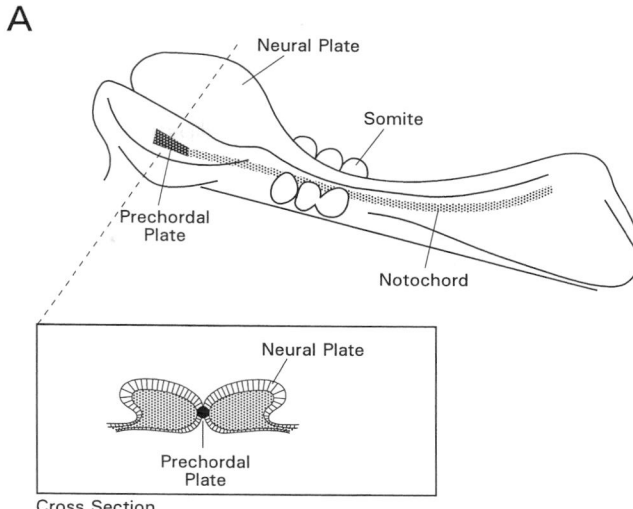
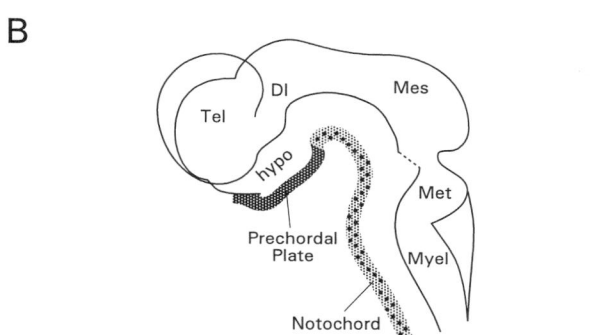

**Fig. 250-2 Prechordal plate mesendoderm underlies the embryonic ventral forebrain.** *A*, Prechordal plate mesendoderm is located beneath the midline of the neural plate at the level of the forebrain, analogous to the location of the notochord at more caudal levels of the neural plate. The inset shows a cross-section through the neural plate at the level of the forebrain. *B*, Diagram showing the relationship of the prechordal plate to the structures of the brain. Abbreviations: hypo = hypothalamus; Tel = telencephalon; Dl = diencephalon; Mes = mesencephalon; Met = metencephalon; Myel = myelencephalon. (*Modified from Rubenstein and Beachy.*[363] *Used with permission.*)

domains of expression.[29,30] In addition, mutations in several genes in the zebra fish that disrupt the prechordal mesendoderm also cause defects in ventral forebrain and eye development[31–34] (discussed in "Other Factors Involved in Ventral Forebrain Patterning" below).

The importance of prechordal mesendoderm notwithstanding, later disturbances of the prosencephalic neural plate also can cause HPE. In the chick, for example, late exposure to high concentrations of the growth factors BMP4 and BMP5[35] (see "Other Factors Involved in Ventral Forebrain Patterning" below) produces cyclopia and HPE by inducing abnormal cell death in the ventral forebrain. Cyclopia in chicks also has been produced by surgical excision of a portion of the prospective telencephalon and

of the fused olfactory pits (*D*). The forebrain is also reduced in size as ventral midline structures are lost and the telencephalic vesicles fuse to form a single midline vesicle. Abbreviations denote the optic vesicle (Opt), telencephalic vesicle (TV), frontonasal, mediolateral, and lateral nasal processes (FNP, MLP, and LNP), the olfactory pit (*), the lens primordium (L), and the maxillary and mandibular processes (Mx and Mn). (*Figure courtesy of Dr. Michael Cooper; modified from Cooper et al.*[177] *Used with permission.*)

diencephalon at the six to seven somite stage, after the process of ventral forebrain induction has begun.[36] In addition, HPE in animals, and probably also in humans, can be caused by environmental insults or genetic defects that primarily affect the ability of the neural plate to respond to signals from the prechordal mesendoderm. Some of these effects are discussed in the section "Cholesterol and Holoprosencephaly" below.

## Sonic Hedgehog Signaling and Midline Patterning of the Face and Ventral Forebrain

Induction and patterning of ventral forebrain structures by the subjacent prechordal mesendoderm implies a role for extracellular signals. The secreted signaling protein encoded by *Sonic hedgehog* (*Shh*) is expressed throughout the axial mesendoderm, including the prechordal plate.[29,37] The *hedgehog* gene was identified and isolated in *Drosophila*,[38–42] where it functions in patterning of embryonic segments and of many other tissues and structures (reviewed in reference [43]). In vertebrates, *hedgehog* homologues constitute a multigene family of which *Sonic hedgehog* is the best studied; other family members in mammals function in growth and patterning of endochondral bone (Indian hedgehog)[44–46] and of the testis (Desert hedgehog).[47] Loss of *Shh* function in *Shh−/−* mouse embryos is associated with a loss of ventral structures and cell fates throughout the neuraxis, including an extreme form of HPE at rostral levels.[48] *Shh−/−* embryos then display an absence of ventral forebrain structures and an undivided eye field, resulting in cyclopia with an overlying proboscis; the remainder of the forebrain, which expresses markers characteristic of dorsal telencephalon, develops as a single, undivided vesicle.

The phenotype of *Shh−/−* embryos indicates that the Shh protein constitutes or contributes to the signal from prechordal mesendoderm that is responsible for the induction of ventral forebrain and subdivision of the eye field. The absence of this signal results in cyclopia and alobar development of the forebrain. In addition, Shh is expressed in several epithelial components of the craniofacial primordia, including most prominently in the inferior border of the frontonasal process and in the maxillary processes.[49] By analogy to the role of Shh in limb development, Shh expression in craniofacial primordia may play an essential role in the outgrowth and patterning of these structures. Fusion of the olfactory pits to produce the proboscis seen in *Shh−/−* mice may relate to a failure of the frontonasal process to develop adequately, thus resulting in a failure to separate the olfactory pits. Similarly, defects in outgrowth of the maxillary processes may underlie the clefting of the upper lip associated with HPE. Retinoic acid treatment can suppress the expression of *Shh* in these craniofacial processes, and this may partly account for the similarities between craniofacial abnormalities induced by retinoids and those associated with HPE.[49]

Following initial expression in the axial mesendoderm, the *Shh* gene is expressed in medial neural plate and in the ventral neural tube (reviewed in reference[50]). This expression within the neuroepithelium is dependent on signals from the axial mesendoderm, and likely controls later aspects of ventral patterning and differentiation. Within the forebrain, following subdivision of the eye field, *Shh* appears to play a further role in patterning of the eye. Ectopic expression of *Shh* induces properties of the proximal optic vesicles (such as *Pax2* gene expression, normally restricted to the optic stalk region of each optic vesicle), and represses properties of the distal optic vesicles (such as expression of the genes *Pax6* and *ET*).[30,51,52] Conversely, loss of signaling, either by mutation of *Shh* or through removal of the prechordal mesendoderm, causes a decrease in *Pax2* expression[48,49] and a failure to repress *Pax6* expression in the midline.[29,30,48,49] These observations suggest that *Shh* has an initial role in signaling from the prechordal mesendoderm and later from the midline of the forebrain, thus contributing both to subdivision of the eye field and to later induction of the chiasm and optic stalk regions. Such a secondary patterning role for *Shh* signaling is consistent with the observation that the cyclopic eye of *Shh−/−* embryos consists primarily of

pigmented retinal epithelium, and lacks most other eye tissues (i.e., neural retina, optic stalk, and optic chiasmatic plate).[48] A similar loss of eye tissues is also observed in other severe cases of experimentally induced cyclopia,[14,15] and is consistent with a failure to induce *Shh* expression in the medial prosencephalic plate.

As described below, loss-of-function mutations at the human *Shh* locus are associated with an autosomal dominant form of HPE[53,54] that is less severe than that seen in the *Shh−/−* mouse. Human *Shh* function thus is haploinsufficient (i.e., requiring normal function of both alleles); this apparent increase in dosage sensitivity relative to the mouse may relate to the larger size and longer period of development of the human forebrain and facial primordia. Homozygous mutations at the human locus have not been characterized, and heterozygotes apparently do not display deficits in ventral derivatives of the more caudal neural tube, nor in the many other tissues affected in *Shh−/−* mouse embryos. The fact that heterozygous *Shh* mutations affect midline facial and ventral forebrain structures more severely than other tissues and structures suggests that the forebrain and face may constitute particularly sensitive indicators of genetic deficits in midline signaling pathways. Because of this heightened sensitivity, it might be predicted that other genes with roles in ventral forebrain and midline facial development might likewise function in a dosage-sensitive manner. The nonlethal phenotypes and dominant patterns of inheritance associated with such mutations should facilitate their detection and study in human pedigrees, suggesting that human HPE constitutes a clinical entity particularly amenable to study by genetic approaches.

The involvement of *Shh* signaling in ventral forebrain and midline facial development suggests that genetic or environmental perturbations of *Shh* protein production or of signaling pathway components also may cause HPE. It is pertinent, therefore, to review our understanding of the molecules and events in Hedgehog protein signaling. We consider first Hedgehog protein biogenesis and then consider the reception and transduction of the signal in target cells.

## Hedgehog Protein Biogenesis

Biogenesis of Hedgehog proteins (reviewed in reference[55]) has been worked out primarily for the *Drosophila* protein, but very likely applies to Hedgehog proteins from all species. Following cleavage of an N-terminal signal sequence upon entry into the secretory pathway, the Hh protein undergoes an autoprocessing reaction that involves internal cleavage between Gly-Cys residues that form part of an absolutely conserved Gly-Cys-Phe tripeptide (Fig. 250-3).[56,57] The N-terminal product of this cleavage receives a covalent cholesteryl adduct[58] and is the species active in signaling[52,57,59–64] (see Fig. 250-3). The cholesteryl moiety restricts spatial deployment of the mature signal via insertion into the lipid bilayer of the cell membrane, thus influencing the pattern of cellular responses in developing tissues. Constructs encoding Hedgehog proteins truncated at the normal site of internal cleavage produce proteins active in signaling, but studies in *Drosophila* have demonstrated that such proteins are not appropriately restricted spatially in their signaling activity, and therefore cause gross mispatterning and lethality in embryos.[65] Thus, the autoprocessing reaction is required to release the active signal from precursor and to specify the spatial distributions of this signal within developing tissues.

The C-terminal domain of the Hh precursor mediates the autoprocessing reaction and has no known additional function. The reaction proceeds by two sequential nucleophilic displacements, the first a rearrangement to replace the main chain peptide linkage between Gly-Cys with a thioester involving the Cys side chain.[58,65] In the second step, this thioester intermediate yields to an ester linkage produced by nucleophilic attack by the hydroxyl oxygen of cholesterol. Sequence analysis, mechanistic studies, and crystallographic structures reveal a striking similarity between the Hh autoprocessing domain and the intein portion of

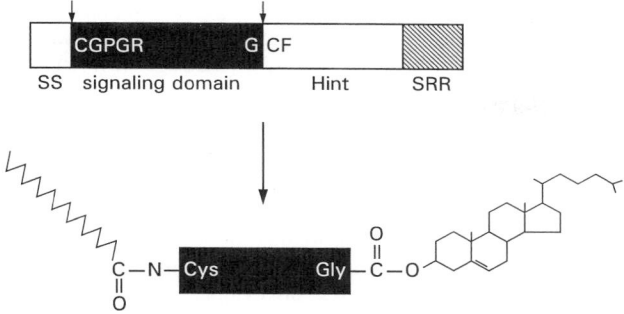

**Fig. 250-3 Autoprocessing and lipid modification of the Sonic hedgehog signaling protein.** Following cleavage of the signal sequence, Sonic hedgehog (Shh) undergoes an autoprocessing reaction that results in cleavage between Gly and Cys of a conserved Gly-Cys-Phe (GCF) tripeptide, with concerted attachment of cholesterol in an ester linkage to the C-terminus of the N-terminal cleavage product. The C-terminal portion of the precursor, consisting of a thioester-generating module (Hint) and a sterol-recognition region (SRR), is responsible for initiating and carrying out the autoprocessing reaction. The N-terminal product, which is responsible for all signaling activity, can also be modified by addition of palmitate in an amide linkage to the Cys of a conserved Cys-Gly-Pro-Gly-Arg (CGPGR) at the N-terminus of the processed protein. See text for further discussion. Abbreviations: SS = signal sequence; Hint = Hint processing domain module found in Hedgehog proteins and inteins, and involved in formation of a thioester intermediate; SRR = sterol-recognition module of the processing domain.

self-splicing proteins.[66] In addition, several families of nematode proteins also contain sequences related to the Hh autoprocessing domain. These proteins all contain a Hint module (for Hedgehog, Intein; Fig. 250-3) capable of directing the formation of an ester intermediate, with the final outcome of the reaction determined by the ultimate disposition of this common intermediate. In the Hedgehog protein, the intermediate is directed toward esterification of cholesterol by sequences C-terminal to the Hint module. These C-terminal sequences (SRR, for sterol recognition region; Fig. 250-3) are required for the second nucleophilic displacement, and presumably act to bind cholesterol and to position it appropriately for this reaction.

A second lipophilic modification of the Hedgehog protein recently was found to occur in at least some cultured cell lines on a fraction of the N-terminal signaling domain of Shh.[67] This additional modifying adduct is a fatty acid, usually palmitate, in an amide linkage with the amine of the N-terminal cysteine that is exposed by signal sequence cleavage. This Cys residue is the first of a pentapeptide, CGPGR (Fig. 250-3), that is widely conserved among species, suggesting the possibility that this conserved sequence and others nearby may be an important determinant for the palmitoylation reaction. The fatty acylation is proposed to occur via a thioester intermediate involving the side chain of the N-terminal cysteine, followed by a rearrangement to form the amide. The occurrence of this modification appears to depend largely on prior cholesterol modification because palmitoylation is much reduced when the Shh protein is produced from a truncated construct. In at least some cultured cell systems, the presence of a lipophilic modification appears to enhance activity of the Shh N-terminal signaling domain.

Missense mutations in the *Drosophila hh* gene can be divided into two classes.[57] The first class of mutations affects N-terminal coding sequences without affecting the ability of the protein to undergo processing, and these mutations presumably affect either the secretion or the activity of the signaling domain. The second class of mutations is C-terminal alterations that affect processing. Missense mutations in the human *SHH* gene associated with HPE also can be classified in this manner, with effects either on the N-terminal signaling domain or on the C-terminal processing domain.[54,68–70]

Finally, the *Drosophila* gene *oroshigane* (*oro*), is required for normal operation of the Hh signaling pathway and has been shown genetically to function upstream of Ptc and presumably other components of the Hh signal transduction machinery.[71] This genetic localization suggests that the *oro* gene product may play a role in the processing or secretion of the Hh protein. Isolation and characterization of the *oro* gene and of its product should yield insights into its function and provide a foundation for determining whether similar molecules function in human Hedgehog signaling pathways and might be mutated in HPE.

## Hedgehog Signal Transduction

Because our understanding of mammalian Hedgehog signal transduction pathways is less complete, extensive *Drosophila* studies will serve as the major point of reference and the reader is referred to several recent reviews for references and details[72,73] (Fig. 250-4). Information from human and other vertebrate systems is presented as available. The first components considered are two polytopic transmembrane proteins, Patched (Ptc)[74,75] and Smoothened (Smo),[76,77] that are proposed to function as Hh receptor components. The Ptc protein is thought to contain 12 transmembrane spans and is a negative regulator of the Hh signaling pathway in target tissues.[78] Smo on the other hand acts

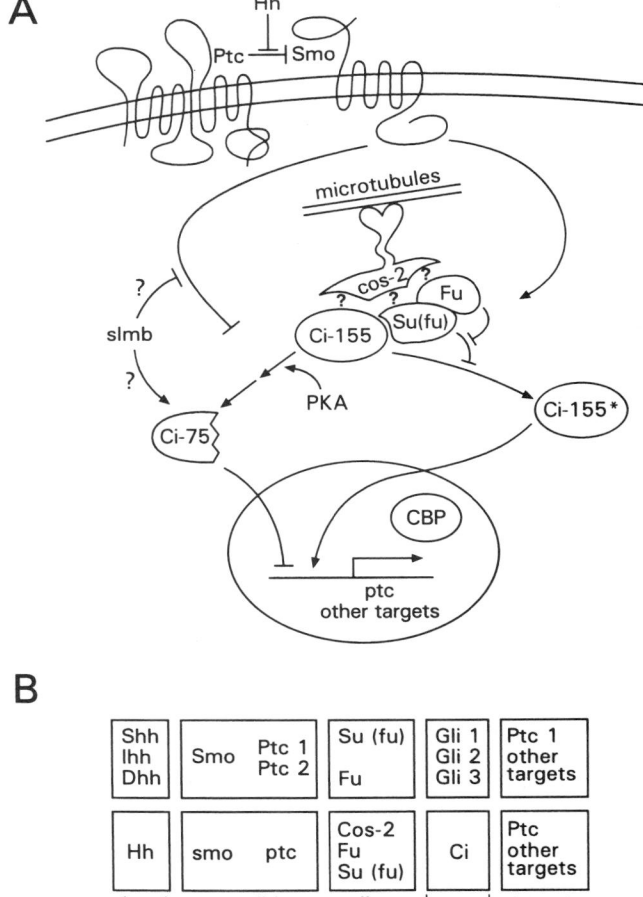

**Fig. 250-4 Model for reception and transduction of the Hedgehog signal in *Drosophila*.** *A*, The activities and relationships between Hedgehog pathway components in *Drosophila* as deduced from genetic and biochemical studies. See text for discussion and abbreviations. *B*, Mammalian homologues (*top row*) are known for all of the *Drosophila* components of the Hedgehog pathway (*bottom row*) with the exception of Costal-2 (Cos-2).

positively in the pathway and is proposed to contain seven transmembrane spans, thus resembling members of the receptor family coupled to heterotrimeric GTP binding proteins.[76,77] The genetic evidence from *Drosophila* indicates that Ptc inhibits the pathway by blocking the action of Smo and that Hh activates the pathway by releasing Ptc inhibition of Smo.[78,79] Thus, the pathway is activated in cells lacking Ptc function, even without stimulation by the Hh signal; but pathway activation requires the activity of Smo, regardless of whether this activation is caused by Hh stimulation or by loss of Ptc.[76,77] Ptc has, in addition to its cell autonomous regulatory role within target cells, a second genetically separable role in sequestering Hh protein and preventing its movement within tissues to other adjacent cells.[80]

A single vertebrate homologue of *smo*[81] and two homologues of *ptc*, *Ptc1* and *Ptc2*,[82–88] have been identified. In mice lacking function of *Ptc1*, targets of Shh signaling are ectopically activated,[89] thus indicating that Ptc1 is of major importance in regulating Shh signaling. A particularly illuminating source of information about the function of these proteins in humans has been the genetics of tumors such as basal cell carcinoma (BCC), medulloblastoma, and rhabdomyosarcoma.[86,90,91] These tumors are associated with inappropriate activation of the SHH signaling pathway and thus might be considered the antithetical twins of HPE, which is associated with a loss of pathway activity. Somatic loss of *PTC1* activity is associated with about one-third of BCC[90] and about one-tenth of medulloblastoma in humans.[86,90,92–94] These and other tumors of the type associated with pathway activation occur at high frequency in patients with Gorlin syndrome (also called BCNS, basal cell nevus syndrome, or NBCC, nevoid Basal Cell carcinoma)[95,96] a heritable condition associated with numerous developmental anomalies and caused by heterozygosity at the human *PTC1* locus.[86,90] BCC also has been found associated with particular mutations in human *SMO*;[93,97,98] these *SMO* mutations appear to activate the Shh pathway by producing constitutively activated forms of the Smo protein.[97,99] Misexpression of *Shh* in the epidermis of mice causes a condition much like human BCC,[100–102] and there is also a report of a possible dominant activating mutation in *Shh* itself.[102] These findings are consistent with genetic studies of Ptc and Smo in *Drosphila*, and support the idea that Hh pathways function similarly in flies and humans.

Additional biochemical studies have provided evidence for physical interactions of mammalian Hh proteins with mammalian Ptc proteins.[81,99,103,104] The affinity of Shh and of a series of mutated Shh protein variants for Ptc correlates tightly with the signaling potency of these Shh proteins in neural plate explant assays, strongly suggesting that the Shh/Ptc interaction is a critical event in signaling.[105] The Shh/Ptc interaction also may play a role in sequestration of the Shh protein to prevent its diffusion in tissues, as indicated by genetic studies in *Drosophila*.[106] Evidence also has been presented for a physical interaction between mammalian Smo and Ptc proteins, and this interaction has been proposed as the basis for Ptc suppression of pathway activity.[81,99,103] Although binding of Shh to Ptc has been proposed to activate the pathway by blocking the Ptc inhibition of Smo, the Ptc/Smo interaction apparently is maintained upon Shh protein binding to Ptc.[81] Thus, it remains to be demonstrated how the Ptc/Smo interaction might suppress pathway activity and how Shh binding to Ptc could affect this suppression. One additional component, Hip (Hedgehog interacting protein), has no known counterpart in *Drosophila*, and appears to interact with Hedgehog proteins and to suppress signaling when ectopically expressed at high levels.[107]

In *Drosophila*, the major transcriptional effector of the Hh signaling pathway is cubitus interruptus (Ci), a 155-kDa zinc finger-containing protein predominantly found in a microtubule associated complex with several other protein components.[108,109] In addition to the full length Ci protein (Ci155), these components include: (a) Costal-2 (Cos-2), a kinesin-related protein that may anchor the complex to the microtubules;[108,109] (b) Fused (Fu), a

putative serine/threonine kinase;[110,111] and (c) probably also Suppressor of Fused Su(Fu), a novel protein that appears to interact physically with Ci and with Fu.[112] The five zinc fingers of Ci are in the N-terminal half of the protein; the C-terminal portion contains transcriptional activation functions, including a region that interacts with CRB (CREB binding protein),[113] a transcriptional coactivator containing histone acetyl transferase activity.[114] The C-terminal portion also contains a region involved in cytoplasmic localization of the protein,[115] which functions as a nuclear export signal.[116] Operation of the nuclear export machinery appears to help maintain the unstimulated state of the pathway by promoting an exclusively cytoplasmic localization of Ci155.[116]

In the absence of Hh stimulation, a significant proportion of the Ci protein is found as a 75-kDa N-terminal fragment (Ci75) that includes the DNA-binding zinc finger region.[115] Ci75 lacks transcriptional activation and cytoplasmic localization functions present in the C-terminal portion of Ci155 and therefore is localized predominantly in the nucleus, where it acts as a repressor of Hh targets.[115,117,118] Processing of Ci155 to Ci75 is dependent on the action of cyclic AMP-dependent kinase (PKA),[119] and Ci155 is a phosphoprotein in vivo.[116] The block of processing associated with loss of PKA function causes inappropriate activation of the Hh pathway.[120–124] Processing to Ci75 also is blocked by mutation of four predicted PKA phosphorylation sites in the C-terminal domain of Ci155,[125] and the Ci protein can be phosphorylated by PKA in vitro,[125,126] suggesting that Ci is a direct target of PKA activity. Formation of Ci75 and maintenance of pathway suppression is similarly dependent on the action of Slimb, a protein likely to be involved in the targeting of ubiquitin conjugation,[119] but it is unclear whether the target of Slimb action is Ci itself[119] or another component functioning upstream of Ci.[127]

Hh protein stimulation blocks processing of Ci155 to Ci75,[115] thus lifting repression by the Ci75 protein. In addition, Hh stimulation causes a significant increase in the nuclear import and nuclear concentration of Ci155.[116] Although this nuclear Ci155 remains a small proportion of the total, it likely is responsible for transcriptional activation of Hh targets. The mechanism of regulation of nuclear transport is not yet known, although Hh stimulation appears to cause the dissociation of the Ci multiprotein complex from the microtubules,[108] and Cos-2 appears to contribute to a cytoplasmic anchoring activity.[116] Genetic studies also suggest that Hh stimulation induces formation of a transcriptionally active state of Ci155, a transition opposed by the action of Su(fu) and facilitated by a negative effect of Fu on Su(fu).[128] Both Cos-2 and Fu appear to be phosphorylated upon Hh stimulation,[108,129] but the significance of these events in signal transduction is not known.

Several observations suggest that transduction of Hh signals in mammals is similar to that in *Drosophila*. First, as in *Drosophila*, transcription of the mammalian *Ptc1* gene appears to be universally activated by Hh signaling in mammals and other vertebrates,[81,84,86] and this may serve as a mechanism for feedback regulation of the signaling pathway. Second, many of the components downstream of Smo and Ptc have counterparts in mammals. Thus, although a vertebrate counterpart to Cos-2 has not yet been reported, the expression pattern of a possible Fu homologue has been described,[103] mouse and human Su(fu) homologues have been reported,[130–132] and the Gli proteins (Gli1, Gli2, and Gli3) are the homologues of *Drosophila* Ci (see below for discussion of the Gli family). Third, it has been demonstrated in numerous vertebrate settings that pharmacologic or genetic manipulations of PKA activity influence Shh pathway activity, with an increase in cAMP and/or PKA activity causing a suppression of the pathway.[63,64,84,133–135] Finally, it has been demonstrated that elevated levels of cyclic AMP stimulate Gli2 and Gli3 protein phosphorylation in mammals and, at least in the case of Gli3, that such phosphorylation induces cleavage to produce a transcriptional repressor similar in structure and activity to Ci75.[136]

The Gli proteins are the mammalian homologues of *Drosophila* Ci and appear to be major transcriptional effectors of the Shh pathway. The *Gli1* gene is curious in its behavior because, although its function is not essential in the mouse,[137,138] it is strongly transcriptionally activated in response to Shh signaling.[139–143] In addition, ectopic expression of Gli1 mimics many aspects of ectopic Shh expression.[140,141,144] Mouse mutations affecting Gli2 and Gli3 produce phenotypes consistent with transcriptional regulatory roles in the Shh pathway[137,138,145] and in the zebra fish, ventral forebrain defects are associated with mutations that affect Gli2.[146] The phenotypes of combined mutations affecting Gli2 and Gli3 proteins in the mouse do not fully account for the phenotype of the *Shh−/−* mouse,[48,138,139,145] thus suggesting that other transcriptional effectors may play a role in Shh signal transduction. Indeed, some evidence has been presented for an as yet unidentified transcriptional effector of Shh signaling that is not a member of the Gli family, and this study also presented evidence for a positive role for an unidentified phosphatase in signaling.[147]

In *Drosophila*, the Hh signal appears to be transduced largely through posttranscriptional regulation of the Ci protein. Given the nonessential nature of Gli1 protein function in the mouse, transduction of the Shh signal could be mediated largely through Gli2 and Gli3, perhaps by a posttranscriptional mechanism similar to that of Ci. In this view, the role of augmented Gli1 gene transcription in response to Shh signaling could be to consolidate a high level of Shh pathway activation. Interestingly, several human syndromes (Pallister-Hall syndrome, PHS; postaxial polydactyly, type A, PAP-A) are associated with autosomal dominant mutations that prematurely truncate the Gli3 open reading frame, thus, presumably, producing N-terminal truncated proteins that contain the zinc finger region.[148–151] These syndromes produce a number of malformations that could be interpreted as suppression of the Shh pathway, including HPE.[151–153] These data suggest that truncated Gli proteins containing the zinc finger region could function in repression of mammalian Hh pathway targets, like the Ci75 repressor in *Drosophila*, and at least Gli3 has been shown to undergo processing similar to that of Ci.[136] One further possible parallel between *Drosophila* and mammalian pathways is highlighted by Rubinstein-Taybi syndrome (RTS), which is associated with agenesis of the corpus callosum and other neural and nonneuronal defects that could relate to a reduction in activity of Hedgehog pathways. RTS is caused by mutations affecting human CREB binding protein (CBP).[154] CBP in *Drosophila* appears to be a coactivator for Ci,[113] and the RTS defects suggest that CBP also could be a cofactor for human Gli proteins.

Given the apparent similarities between *Drosophila* and mammalian Hedgehog signal transduction pathways, even with our current incomplete understanding, it is to be expected that future genetic studies of HPE will identify mutations in human genes homologous to those already known to function in the *Drosophila* Hh signaling pathway. These mutations could reduce or inactivate the function of proteins that function positively in the pathway, or alternatively might enhance or deregulate the functions of proteins that function negatively in the pathway. Given the extreme sensitivity of ventral forebrain and midline facial development to perturbations in the Shh pathway, it is also possible that human genetic studies will help identify previously unrecognized Hh signaling pathway components.

## Other Factors Involved in Ventral Forebrain Patterning

A series of zebra fish mutations have been identified that disrupt the prechordal mesendoderm and display defects in ventral forebrain and eye development.[31–34] Two of these mutations, *knypek* and *trilobite*, appear to perturb the migration and normal position of prechordal mesendoderm cells under the midline of the ventral forebrain;[32] the severity of ventral forebrain defects in these mutations has been correlated with the distance between *Shh* expressing cells and the midline of the ventral forebrain.

The genes associated with two other zebra fish mutations that disrupt the prechordal mesendoderm, *oep* (*one-eyed pinhead*) and *cyclops* (*cyc*), have been isolated and found to encode extracellular signaling proteins that function in a common pathway. The *oep* gene encodes a membrane-associated epidermal growth factor-related protein whose loss disrupts prechordal plate mesendoderm and results in ventral forebrain deficits and cyclopia.[34,155,156] The function of *oep* is required for extracellular signaling by the product of *cyclops*,[157] which is a member of the TGF-β family of secreted protein signals.[158–160] Zebra fish mutants in the *cyclops* locus display ventral deficits throughout the neural tube, including an absence of floor plate in the spinal cord, cyclopia, and an absence of ventral forebrain structures, including all neural progenitors that normally express Shh. Expression of the normal oep protein is required within tissues that are targets for cyc protein signaling, indicating a cell autonomous requirement for function of the membrane-associated oep protein. But widespread misexpression either of the membrane-bound or of a secreted form of the oep protein can rescue the cyclopia and other forebrain defects associated with the *oep* mutation, thus demonstrating that oep protein expression need not be restricted and that it functions in a permissive, not instructive, manner in prechordal mesendoderm formation and signaling. The oep protein thus appears to be required to make cells competent to respond to the cyc signal.[157]

The closest previously identified relative of the *cyclops* gene is another member of the TGF-β family, the *nodal* gene.[158–160] Mice lacking *nodal* function display extreme defects in early gastrulation, and no mesoderm is formed.[161,162] The phenotype of *cyclops* on its own is considerably less severe than that of *nodal*, however, when combined with mutations that affect a second *nodal*-related zebra fish gene, *squint*, severe effects on early gastrulation also are observed.[158] These two zebra fish genes thus have at least partially redundant functions with regard to early gastrulation. Gene duplication and subdivision of function has been observed in the zebra fish in other instances, as indicated, for example, by the existence of three *hedgehog* genes that are expressed in midline axial tissues (instead of only one *Shh* in mammals). The function of mouse *nodal* in ventral forebrain patterning thus was not initially detected because of the failure of *nodal* mutant embryos to progress beyond early gastrulation. Consistent with such an interpretation, mouse embryos heterozygous for the *nodal* mutation and for a mutation in *Smad2* display a range of defects, including ventral forebrain deficits and cyclopia with an overlying proboscis.[163] The Smad2 protein is a cytoplasmic component that translocates to the nucleus and helps activate target gene expression in response to TGF-β signals. The *trans*-heterozygous mutant combination may produce a sufficiently mild deficit in signaling as to permit the early events of gastrulation, while disrupting the later signaling activities that in the fish are revealed by the *cyclops* mutation. Consistent with this interpretation, the zebra fish Smad2 protein also appears to function in the oep/cyc pathway.[157]

The mouse *nodal Smad2 trans*-heterozygote is illustrative of several principles that may be useful in considering human HPE. The first is that ventral forebrain and midline facial development may be particularly sensitive to mild environmental or genetic insults. Thus, in the *trans*-heterozygous mouse, HPE is produced by milder genetic insults in a particular pathway than those required to produce a severe effect on early gastrulation. This sensitivity of midline face and brain structures may also account for the widespread pattern of dominant inheritance of HPE in general and, in particular, for HPE associated with *Shh* mutations (see below). A second principle emerging from this *trans*-heterozygote is that HPE apparently can be produced by a combination of genetic insults that individually do not produce HPE. Such interactions between genetic insults or possibly between genetic and environmental insults may help account for the variability of HPE segregating with known lesions, as occurs in HPE associated with *Shh* mutations. In addition, these types of interactions may help explain the low penetrance of HPE in association with genetic diseases such as SLO (Smith-Lemli-Opitz Syndrome, see below) where HPE is found in ≈5 percent of patients.[164]

A second TGFβ family member, BMP7, is expressed throughout the axial mesoderm, including prechordal mesendoderm, and has been implicated in the induction of ventral forebrain in conjunction with Shh.[22,165] The secreted protein chordin, which is expressed in the notochord, antagonizes the action of BMP7 and appears to block the inappropriate induction of ventral forebrain fates at more caudal locations.[165] Genetic analysis of BMP7 in mouse embryogenesis is complicated by the presence of other related TGFβ family members that are expressed in overlapping patterns and that may compensate functionally in BMP7 mutant mice.[166,167] Recent studies also demonstrate that localized forebrain exposure to high levels of BMP4 and BMP5 at later stages of development can cause cyclopia and other malformations associated with HPE.[35] This effect is mediated by apoptosis of cells in the ventral forebrain after their initial specification and thus is of unknown relevance to normal development or HPE in humans.

## Cholesterol and Holoprosencephaly

As was first appreciated more than 30 years ago, HPE can be induced experimentally by treatment of pregnant rats with synthetic compounds, such as triparanol, AY9944, and BM15.766, that inhibit late-acting enzymes in cholesterol biosynthesis.[168-172] These compounds cause accumulation of desmosterol (triparanol) or of 7-dehydrocholesterol (AY9944 and BM15.766), which are the immediate precursors in alternate biosynthetic routes to cholesterol. Other compounds capable of inducing HPE are a group of plant alkaloids that include cyclopamine and jervine, from the genus *Veratrum*. These compounds were identified about 30 years ago following outbreaks of cyclopia in flocks of sheep pastured in mountain meadows where *Veratrum* species grow.[173-176] Cyclopamine and jervine are closely related to each other and steroidal in structure (see Fig. 250-5). Jervine inhibits cholesterol biosynthesis and causes accumulation of abnormally high levels of a sterol that likely is a biosynthetic precursor to cholesterol.[55]

Both of these classes of compounds have been shown to inhibit Shh signaling specifically, with little or no effect on other signaling pathways.[55,177,178] Surprisingly, in light of the critical role of cholesterol in the biogenesis of Hh proteins (see above), these compounds appear not to affect processing of the Shh protein;

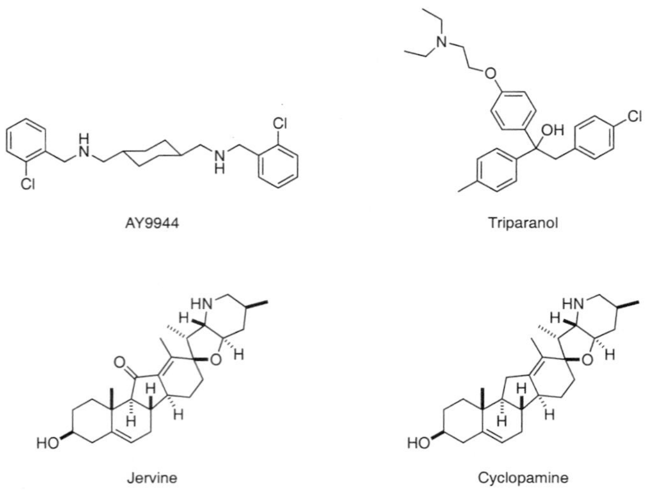

**Fig. 250-5 Teratogens that inhibit Sonic hedgehog signaling. Cyclopamine and jervine are found in plants of the species *Veratrum*. AY9944 and triparanol are synthetic compounds that have been characterized as inhibitors of distal steps of cholesterol biosynthesis.**

instead, they inhibit the ability of target tissues to respond to the Shh signal. The mechanism of this effect is not yet understood, but several points are worth noting. First, the inhibition of Shh response appears not to be due to a general reduction in cholesterol levels, because inhibitors of cholesterol synthesis that specifically act on 3-hydroxy-3-methylglutaryl-coenzyme A (HMG-CoA) reductase do not inhibit Shh signaling. Second, one of the teratogenic compounds, AY9944, has been characterized as inhibiting esterification of plasma membrane cholesterol, which requires transport of cholesterol from the plasma membrane to the endoplasmic reticulum.[179] These effects on transport and esterification require higher concentrations than those sufficient for specific inhibition of 7-dehydrocholesterol reductase. Similar levels are required for inhibition of Shh signaling and thus, AY9944 may inhibit signaling by generally affecting intracellular sterol transport and homeostasis rather than by simply blocking a biosynthetic enzyme.[177,179] Preliminary studies of the other compounds also suggest similar effects on transport.[177]

Certain genetic perturbations linked to HPE provide a further indication that sterol homeostasis plays a critical role in induction and patterning of the ventral forebrain. Mice lacking function of the endocytic receptor megalin, a member of the low-density lipoprotein (LDL) receptor family, consistently display defects in ventral forebrain development.[180] In humans, Smith-Lemli-Opitz syndrome (SLOS) is a recessive genetic disease caused by mutations in the gene encoding 7-dehydrocholesterol reductase,[181,182] the same enzyme inhibited by AY 9944[R] and BM 15.766. SLOS is characterized by numerous developmental defects including microcephaly, pituitary agenesis, limb and genital abnormalities, and defects of the heart, kidneys, and pancreas.[183-188] Approximately 5 percent of SLOS patients display signs of HPE, with malformations that tend toward the milder end of the spectrum.[164]

Although the mechanisms by which a loss of megalin function in mice or SLOS in humans can cause HPE or increase its incidence is not clear, a common feature shared by these genetic perturbations with HPE-inducing drug treatments is an effect on sterol homeostasis. The megalin receptor can bind and internalize various ligands, including LDL.[189] This receptor is highly expressed on the apical surfaces of embryonic neuroectoderm and neuroepithelium at the stage of development when ventral forebrain structures are induced, and thus may be involved in normal sterol uptake within the developing forebrain.[180,190] SLOS patients have abnormally low serum cholesterol levels and accumulate 7-dehydrocholesterol, and SLOS embryos thus are likely to experience sterol abnormalities during the stage when ventral forebrain structures are induced, thus also potentially affecting the response to Shh signaling. A possible explanation for the incomplete penetrance of HPE in SLOS patients may be supplementation via placental exchange from heterozygous mothers with largely normal sterol metabolism. The effects of these genetic perturbations of sterol homeostasis and the sterol homeostasis effects of HPE-inducing drug treatments together suggest that there may be a link between sterol homeostasis and the ability of cells to respond to Shh stimulation. Many tissues respond in a proliferative fashion to Shh stimulation,[63,191,192] and the role of such a link could be to modulate Shh-induced proliferative responses according to a meaningful index of cellular health and metabolic state. Cholesterol homeostasis may provide such an index and thus may serve as a checkpoint for Shh-induced cell responses, including proliferation.

If sterol homeostasis indeed is the common primary target of these genetic lesions and of the drug treatments, an interesting, but as yet unanswered, question is what components within the Shh signaling pathway serve as targets for these perturbations. It was noted recently that the Patched protein (Ptc), which controls the response to Shh in responding tissues (see above), contains a sterol-sensing domain (SSD).[193,194] The SSDs of two other proteins, HMG-CoA reductase and SCAP (SREBP cleavage-activating protein) confer differential responses to high and low levels of intracellular sterols,[195–197] and a third SSD-containing protein, NPC1 (encoded by the Niemann-Pick C1 disease gene) is proposed to function in intracellular sterol transport.[193,194] Although the mechanistic role of Ptc in Shh pathway regulation in target tissues is not known, the presence of a putative sterol-responsive domain suggested that it may mediate the effects of genetic and drug-induced perturbations of sterol homeostasis. Recent studies have demonstrated, however, that action of the plant alkaloids is independent of Ptc1.[197a] These plant teratogens instead appear to inhibit activity of Smoothened by a mechanism not yet known, but which might be affected by cellular membrane composition or by transport phenomena that also play a role in sterol homeostasis.

## HOLOPROSENCEPHALY IN HUMANS

### Central Nervous System Anomalies

The basic anomalies in HPE involve the brain and often the face. However, extracephalic features do occur and are detailed elsewhere.[13,198,199] The primary brain malformations consist of incomplete cleavage of the forebrain (prosencephalon) into right and left hemispheres, into telencephalon and diencephalon, and into olfactory and optic bulbs and tracts (for review see references 2, 6, and 7). In the most severe form, a single brain ventricle is present without any evidence of an interhemispheric fissure (alobar HPE, Fig. 250-6A). In semilobar HPE (Fig. 250-6B), an interhemispheric fissure separates the brain only posteriorly. In lobar HPE, right and left ventricles are completely separated; some continuity across the cortex may be retained. The spectrum of brain malformations in HPE extends from most to least severe in unbroken continuity.[20] Other findings of the central nervous system may include anomalies of midline structures such as undivided thalami, absent corpus callosum (MIM 217990),[201] callosal dysgenesis,[202–204] absent or hypoplastic olfactory bulbs and tracts (arhinencephaly), and optic bulbs and tracts. All of these latter defects may occur as part of the HPE spectrum, as isolated anomalies, or as part of various genetic entities. Rare central nervous system anomalies in combination include HPE include Dandy-Walker malformation,[205] extracerebral cyst,[206] neuronal migration anomalies,[207] retinoblastoma,[208,209] middle interhemispheric fusion,[210] abnormal circle of Willis,[211] and caudal dysgenesis.[212,213]

Recently, a variant of semilobar holoprosencephaly, known as middle interhemispheric fusion (MIHF), has been recognized as a result of improvements in magnetic resonance imaging techniques.[210] In this entity, the interhemispheric fissure is formed frontally and occipitally, while the posterior frontal and parietal regions of the brain remain fused across the midline, with normal separation and normal development of the base of the forebrain. The brain is nearly normal in the regions anterior and posterior to the fusion. In the initial three patients described, aside from interhemispheric fusion, the anterior falx cerebri was found to be hypoplastic. The corpus callosum was poorly formed and the choroid plexus was absent at the level of the fusion of the cerebral hemispheres. It is one of the only conditions in which the genu and splenium of the corpus collosum appear normal in the absence of the body. The sylvian fissures are typically more vertically oriented in MIHF and may be continuous across the midline. Subsequently, other children with this variant of semilobar HPE have been identified. The anomalies may include findings characteristic of the more severe end of HPE such as dorsal cyst (believed to be a dorsal extension of the third ventricle and almost always present when there is thalamic fusion), and complete thalamic fusion. Because the diencephalon is separated from the telencephalon the term syntelencephaly has been used to describe this variant.[210] In one patient with MIHF, a *ZIC2* mutation was identified (Brown and Muenke, unpublished).

The MIHF variant is associated with a higher incidence of migrational anomalies including heterotopias which may line the

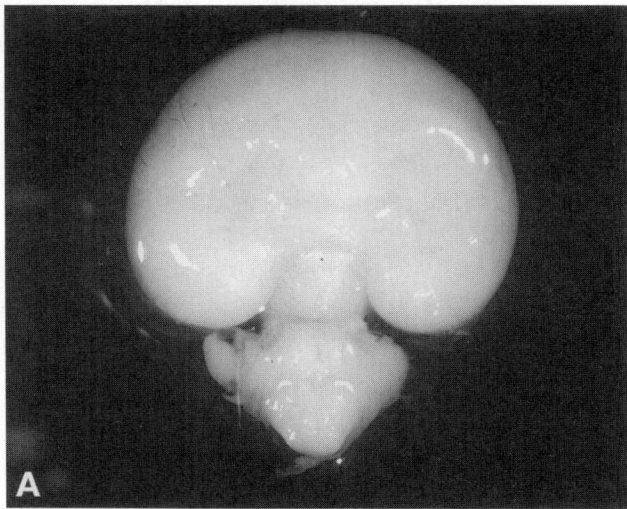

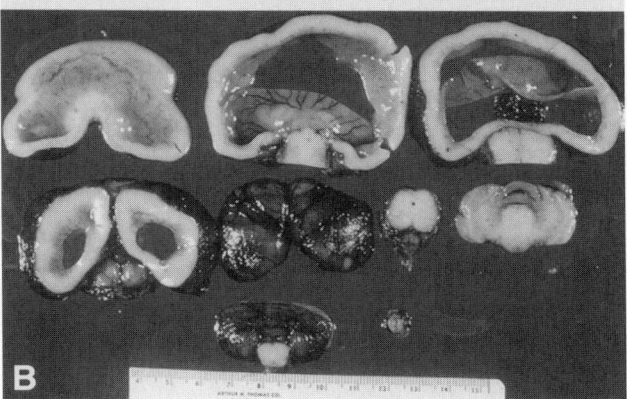

**Fig. 250-6 Brain anomalies in holoprosencephaly. *A*, Alobar HPE of the forebrain without any identifiable midline structures in an 18-week gestation male fetus with triploidy. *B*, Semilobar HPE with an incomplete interhemispheric fissure posteriorly (*lower right*) in a 30-week gestation male fetus with synophthalmia, a proboscis above the fused eye, and a deletion for chromosome 18p. Same as Fig. 250-7C. (*From Muenke et al.[364] Used by permission.*)**

wall of the holoventricle or involve the cortical regions. The basic mechanism underlying this form of HPE is not known but may involve decreased migration of mesenchyme to the middle portion of the midline telencephalon which is required for the normal formation of mid portions of the face, anterior skullbase, and anterior portion of the falx cerebri.[210a]

### Facial Anomalies

The brain malformations in HPE are frequently accompanied by facial anomalies. DeMyer[214] proposed five different facial types in HPE in which "the face predicts the brain." (I) Cyclopia: single eye or partially divided eye in singe orbit with proboscis (nose-like structure) above the eye (Fig. 250-7A to C). (II) Ethmocephaly: extreme hypotelorism but separate orbits with proboscis between the eyes (Fig. 250-7D). (III) Cebocephaly: hypotelorism with single-nostril nose (Fig. 250-7E and F). (IV) Median cleft lip with hypotelorism and flat nose (Fig. 250-7G to J). (V) Bilateral cleft of lip with median process representing the philtrum-premaxilla anlage, hypotelorism, and flat nose. Facial types I, II, and III occur in infants with alobar HPE, IV usually occurs with alobar HPE, and V occurs with alobar, or more commonly semilobar or lobar HPE. Characteristic facial features are seen in approximately 80 percent of children with severe HPE, whereas the remainder have nondiagnostic mildly dysmorphic facies[198] (see "Genes in Holoprosencephaly in Humans" below).

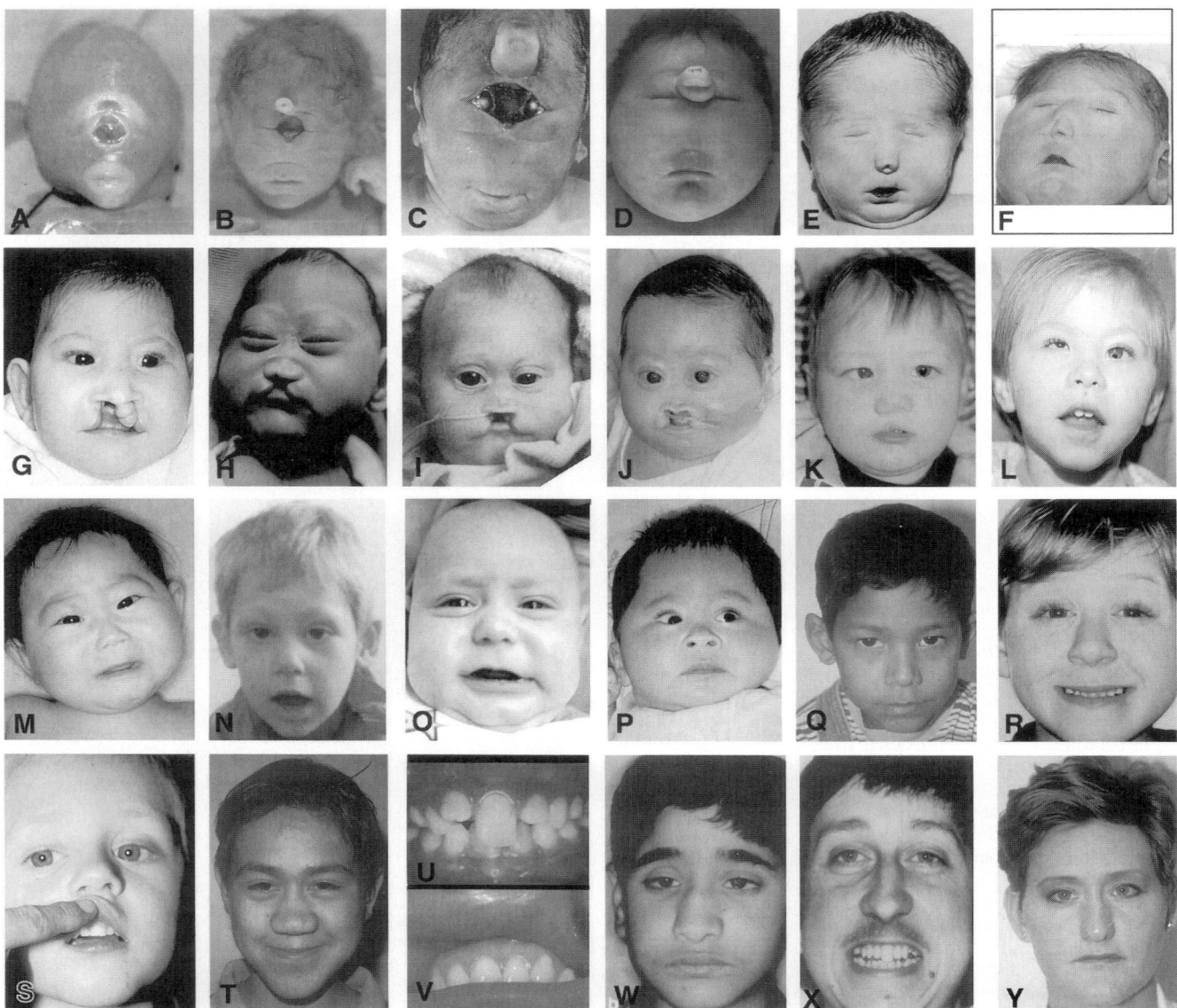

Fig. 250-7 Facial findings in holoprosencephaly and the HPE spectrum. *A,* Cyclopia with cleft palate and absent nasal structure in a 16-week gestation fetus with alobar HPE and del(2)(p21-p22.1), which is deleted for *SIX3. B,* Cyclopia with proboscis above the fused eye in a 28-week gestation fetus with alobar HPE and del(2)(p21-p23). *C,* Synophthalmia with proboscis in a 30-week gestation fetus with del(18p) who is deleted for *TGIF.* Same as in Fig. 250-6*B*). *D,* Ethmocephaly, two closely spaced but separated eyes, and a nose-like structure between the eyes in an infant of a diabetic mother. *E* and *F,* Cebocephaly, ocular hypotelorism, down-slanting palpebral fissures, and a blind-ended, single nostril in two newborn infants with alobar HPE. The etiology of HPE is unknown in (*E*). A *SHH* mutation is segregating with HPE in the family of (*F*). *G* to *K* Various clefts of the lips and/or palate in infants with HPE. *G,* Microcephaly, midface hypoplasia with absence of the nasal bones and bilateral cleft lip and palate, and mental retardation, without any identifiable structural brain anomalies in a female with *SIX3* mutation. *H,* Microcephaly, midface hypoplasia with absence of the nasal bones, and midline cleft lip and palate in a female with semilobar HPE and *TGIF* mutation. *I,* Microcephaly, midface hypoplasia with absence of the nasal bones, and bilateral cleft lip and palate in a female with semilobar HPE as part of Smith-Lemli-Opitz syndrome, characteristic biochemical defect in cholesterol metabolism, and mutation in the gene coding for 7-dehydrocholesterol reductase. *J,* Midface hypoplasia with absence of the nasal bones and bilateral cleft lip and palate, in a female with semilobar HPE, diabetes insipidus, *SHH* mutation, and deletion for *TGIF* due to a cytogenetic deletion, del(18p). *K,* Microcephaly, ocular hypotelorism, bilateral inferior iris colobomata, repaired right-sided cleft lip and palate, developmental delay, and normal brain MRI in a male with *SHH* mutation. *L,* Microcephaly, micro-ophthalmia, coloboma, and a small median philtrum pit in a female with semilobar HPE and *SIX3* mutation (same as in Fig. 250-8*E* and *F*). *M,* Microcephaly, flat nasal

bridge in a female with semilobar HPE, diabetes insipidus, short stature, and mutations in two genes: *SHH* and *ZIC2. N,* Ocular hypotelorism and only mildly dysmorphic face in a male with a *ZIC2* mutation. *O,* Microcephaly and a mildly dysmorphic face in a female with alobar HPE, profound developmental delay, and *ZIC2* mutation. *P,* Ocular hypotelorism and only mildly dysmorphic face in a female with alobar HPE and a *ZIC2* mutation (same as in Fig. 250-8 *A* to *D*). *Q,* Microcephaly and hypoplastic philtrum in a male with lobar HPE and *SHH* mutation (son of individual in *Y*; one sib had alobar HPE). *R,* Microcephaly, hypotelorism, and single central upper incisor, development delay, and a normal brain scan in a male who is deleted for *TGIF* due to a ring r(18) chromosome and del(18p). *S,* Single central incisor and developmental delay in a male with *SIX3* mutation. Three sibs had alobar HPE and the same *SIX3* mutation. *T,* Microcephaly, ocular hypotelorism, flat nose with no palpable cartilage, midface and philtrum hypoplasia, normal intelligence, and normal brain MRI in a male with *SHH* mutation (two sibs had alobar HPE). *U,* Typical single maxillary incisor and absent superior labial frenulum in a male with HPE microsigns (same as in *W*). *V,* Absent superior labial frenulum and repaired single central incisor in a female with HPE microsigns (same as in *Y*). *W,* HPE microsigns including single central incisor and ocular coloboma on the left eye in a male with above-normal intelligence whose mother has anosmia. *X,* Ocular hypotelorism, microcephaly, single incisor, and normal intelligence in a male with a *SHH* mutation. Two of his children had alobar HPE and the same *SHH* mutation. *Y,* Female with ocular hypotelorism and a single central incisor who has two children with HPE. All three have an *SHH* mutation. (*From Schell et al.[277] (A); Muenke et al.[274] (B); Muenke et al.[364] (C); Muenke[260] (D, E, H); Ardinger and Bartley[251] (F); Wallis et al.[261] (G, L, S); Kelley et al.[164] (I); Nanni et al.[69] (J, K, M, Q, T, V, Y); Brown et al.[262] (N, O, P); Overhauser et al.[320] (R); Ming and Muenke[285] (U, W); and Johnson[365] (X). Used by permission.*)

Additional craniofacial anomalies can occur as part of the HPE spectrum, although each of the following features has been observed as an isolated defect or as part of a different entity. Microcephaly is common and is occasionally part of the autosomal dominant HPE spectrum.[215] Macrocephaly is occasionally present due to accompanying hydrocephaly. Eye anomalies include anophthalmia, microphthalmia (Fig. 250-7L),[216] various degrees of hypotelorism (Fig. 250-7) but also hypertelorism, and coloboma involving various eye structures (Fig. 250-7L and W).[217] Malformations of the nose may range from complete absence (Fig. 250-7A), proboscis (Fig. 250-7B to D), flat nose without any nasal bones, agenesis of the nasal cartilage (Fig. 250-7T),[218] or nasal pyriform aperture stenosis[219–222] to well-formed nose with absent or impaired sense of smell. In addition to various midline and lateral clefts, midline palatal ridge and other palatal anomalies,[223] bifid uvula, and/or a single central upper incisor may occur in HPE.[224,225] Although the latter is nonspecific by itself, it is seen in HPE and occurs as a striking microform in autosomal dominant HPE (Fig. 250-7U). Absence of the superior labial frenulum (Fig. 250-7U and V) is another diagnostic sign in patients with the HPE spectrum.[226]

The spectrum of facial anomalies begins with cyclopia and extends in unbroken sequence to the normal face as seen in unaffected carriers of autosomal dominant HPE. The extremely variable phenotypic expression occurs not only in sporadic HPE, but within different affected members of the same family.[227,228] In contrast to this continuous aspect of HPE, qualitative distinctions and discontinuities, discussed elsewhere,[199] are crucial for genetic counseling, as well as for molecular studies.

Although most of the individuals with normal brain imaging and an HPE microform have normal intelligence, a minority has developmental delay, and this may be considered an additional microform. Furthermore, some obligate carriers in autosomal dominant pedigrees of HPE do not exhibit any clinical abnormalities, but they are still at risk for having a child with HPE.[228] Thus, recurrence risk counseling should be cautious in any individual with a family history of HPE.

## Complications of Holoprosencephaly

Developmental delay is present in virtually all affected individuals with central nervous system anomalies, although the degree of delay is variable, usually correlating with the severity of the brain malformation. Many patients on the severe end of HPE remain nonambulatory with rudimentary motor skills and lack of language, while those with less severe involvement have milder delays. True cognitive assessment may be difficult in this population and is hampered by the significant motor handicaps (spasticity, dystonia, chorea) seen in many patients, when traditional testing batteries that rely heavily on language and motor skills are used. Strategies to evaluate cognitive status of patients with HPE that do not rely on language or motor skills are being evaluated. Seizures are common, and hydrocephalus can occur. Motor handicaps may consist of truncal hypotonia with axial hypertonia. Many children have additional extrapyramidal features such as dystonia or choreiform movements of the extremities. Hypothalamic and brain stem dysfunction may lead to instability of temperature, heart rate, respiration, and swallowing difficulties. Pituitary dysgenesis in HPE[229] is manifested by endocrinologic abnormalities such as adrenal hypoplasia, diabetes insipidus,[230] hypogonadism, and thyroid hypoplasia. Feeding problems (sometimes requiring gastrostomy tubes), erratic sleep patterns, excessive intestinal gas/colic, irritability, and constipation frequently occur.[231] Aspiration pneumonias can be a complication of poor coordination of swallowing.

## Survival

There is a common perception that children with HPE do not survive beyond early infancy. While this may be frequently true for the most severely affected patients, a significant proportion of affected children can survive past 12 months. There is an inverse relationship between severity of facial phenotype and survival length among patients with normal chromosomes. While individuals with cyclopia or ethmocephaly generally do not survive beyond 1 week, those with less severe facial phenotypes may have a significantly more prolonged survival.[11] Approximately one-half of the children with alobar HPE will die before the age of 4 to 5 months, and 20 percent will live past the first year of life.[231] Among individuals with isolated semilobar or lobar HPE without significant malformations of other organ systems, more than 50 percent are alive at the age of 12 months.[12,231] Almost all of the survivors have apparently normal vision and hearing, smile, and demonstrate memory.[231]

## Prenatal Diagnosis of Holoprosencephaly

Holoprosencephaly can, in cases of alobar HPE, be diagnosed by prenatal ultrasound examination by 16 weeks of gestation.[232–238] Milder degrees of HPE, such as semilobar or lobar HPE, cannot reliably be detected. The prenatal findings of HPE are usually followed up by a high-resolution ultrasound exam to determine the presence of additional structural anomalies (e.g., clefting, abnormal cardiac, limb, and other findings).[239–243] An amniocentesis is recommended to determine the fetal karyotype, because 25 to 50 percent of infants with HPE have chromosome abnormalities (see "Cytogenetic Anomalies in HPE" below). Based on ultrasound and cytogenetic findings, an informed decision can be made regarding the management of the pregnancy, delivery, and postnatal care.

## Diagnosis

In the absence of a family history with multiple relatives who have HPE (see "Familial Holoprosencephaly" below), the diagnosis of HPE is most frequently made during the newborn period. Facial findings characteristic for HPE ("The face predicts the brain;"[214] see "Facial Anomalies" above) will alert the neonatologist to obtain subspecialty consults from clinical genetics and neurology, and occasionally from ophthalmology and cardiology. Imaging of the brain by CAT or MRI scan (Fig. 250-8) will confirm the suspected diagnosis of HPE, define its severity (alobar, semilobar, or lobar HPE) and associated central nervous system anomalies (such as hydrocephaly and others).[244–248] The workup for a newborn infant with HPE includes a detailed dysmorphology exam to rule out genetic syndromes that occasionally are associated with HPE (see "Holoprosencephaly in Syndromes" below). A prenatal history is crucial to identify potential teratogens, as is a detailed family history with emphasis on pregnancy losses, deaths in the neonatal period, or relatives with abnormal craniofacial findings and/or development delays. A brief physical exam of the parents is recommended to rule out HPE microsigns in otherwise clinically normal individuals. Cytogenetic analysis is crucial in every newborn with HPE. Chromosome analysis of the parents is recommended only if the infant has an abnormal karyotype. In selected cases, measurement of cholesterol and 7-dehydrocholesterol (and possibly other metabolites of cholesterol biosynthesis) are indicated in infants with HPE who have clinical findings consistent with the Smith-Lemli-Opitz syndrome (see Chap. 249). Currently, mutation analysis of several genes known to cause HPE (*SHH*, *ZIC2*, *SIX3*, and *TGIF*) is done in a few laboratories on a research basis only (see "Genetic Bases of Holoprosencephaly in Humans" below). Identification of the underlying etiology for HPE, such as a specific genetic syndrome with known Mendelian inheritance, a disease-causing mutation, a defect in cholesterol biosynthesis, or a cytogenetic anomaly, may aid in a more specific prognosis and/or recurrence risk counseling.

Infants with no or only mild dysmorphic facial findings and either mild or intermediate brain anomalies may not come to immediate attention during the newborn period. HPE may be diagnosed only later during the first year of life as part of a workup for developmental delay and/or failure-to-thrive.

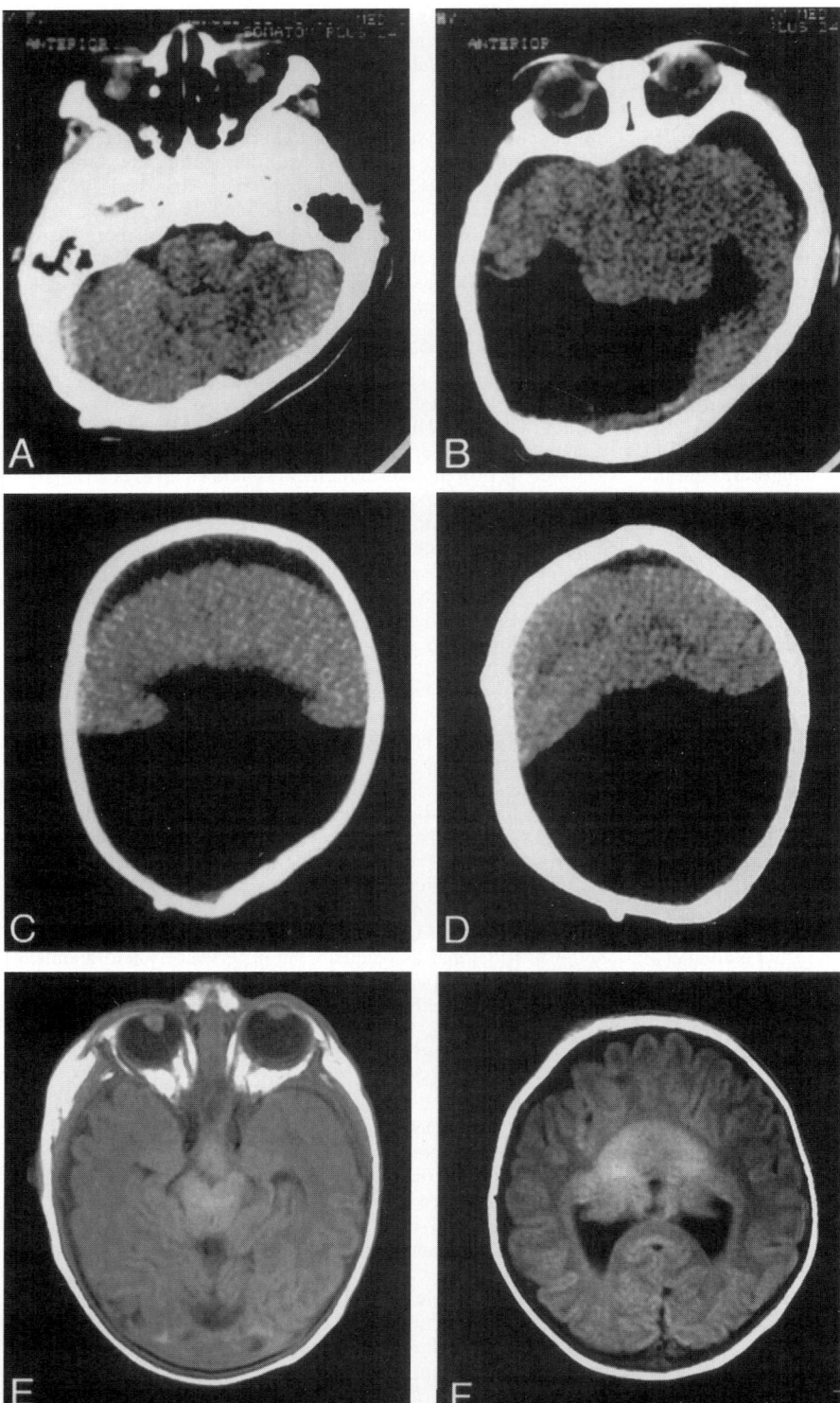

Fig. 250-8 Brain imaging in holoprosencephaly. *A* to *D*, Nonenhanced computed axial tomographic (CAT) images of the head in a child with alobar HPE and *ZIC2* mutation (same patient as in Fig. 250-7*P*). The CAT scan shows fused thalami, a fused band of brain anteriorly and a large posterior cyst consistent with alobar HPE. *E* to *F*, Magnetic resonance image (MRI) of the head of a patient with semilobar HPE and *SIX3* mutation (same patient as in Fig. 250-7*L*). Micro-ophthalmia of the right eye with triangular deformed lens with strand attaching to the lens which is consistent with persistent hyperplastic primary vitreous (PHPV) (in *E*). The anterior half of the cerebral hemispheres are fused, and the posterior half are separated by an interhemispheric fissure (in *F*) consistent with semilobar HPE. (*From Brown et al.,*[262] *and Wallis et al.*[261] *Used by permission.*)

## Management

As the clinical findings of the brain and associated anomalies in individuals vary considerably, so does the treatment. Thus, the results of an expeditious workup during the first days of life are crucial for management and prognosis. Treatment is system by system, symptomatic, and supportive. Care of a child with HPE and diabetes insipidus may include careful monitoring of fluid and electrolyte intake. Hormone replacement therapy has been

successful in some children with pituitary dysfunction. Anticonvulsive therapies can help decrease the frequency and intensity of seizures. Feeding difficulties and failure-to-thrive can be addressed by alternative feeding methods. Surgical intervention by placing a gastrostomy tube may be of help to children (and parents), when feeding becomes too difficult (i.e., long duration of feedings or severe swallowing problems). Vomiting and gastroesophageal reflux can be alleviated by a fundoplication, frequently performed at the time of the gastrostomy.

Additional surgical treatment may include the placement of a ventriculoperitoneal shunt to decrease excess cerebrospinal fluid in children with HPE and hydrocephalus. In older children, surgical repairs for various clefts of the lip and palate may be indicated.[249,250]

Children with HPE may benefit from physical, occupational, and speech therapies to include nonverbal communication and oral motor assessment/therapy. This should be individualized to the child's needs. Many children may also benefit from the use of medications to decrease spasticity and/or dystonia with the goal of improving functional outcome from improved posture/sitting in a wheelchair to enhanced, purposeful reaching and/or hand movement. Medications such as baclofen or the anticholinergic, trihexyphenidyl chloride (Artane) have allowed some children improved functional outcome.

A major aspect of the treatment is the support and counseling of the parents of a child with HPE. This includes professional help from a team of pediatricians, clinical geneticists, genetic counselors, social workers, and others. A network of health care professionals specializing in the diagnosis and care of children with HPE is organized through the Carter Centers for Brain Research in Holoprosencephaly and Related Malformations. In addition, numerous parents' support groups exist, which provide support through meeting other families, parent letters, and Web sites.

## Etiology: Teratogens and Genetic Factors

HPE is etiologically extremely heterogeneous with both environmental and genetic causes. Its formation may depend on an interaction of both genetic and environmental factors in at least some cases. There is anecdotal evidence for the role of several teratogens in HPE (ethanol,[251] retinoic acid,[252] cytomegalovirus infection,[253] anticonvulsants,[254,255] sulfasalazine,[256] maternal low-calorie weight reducing diet,[257] maternal hypocholesterolemia (Kelley and Muenke, unpublished) and many others). To date, only maternal diabetes has an epidemiologically established increased risk of HPE. The approximate risk for HPE to infants of diabetic mothers is 1 percent, which is a two hundredfold increase over the general population.[258]

Evidence for genetic causes of HPE as well as for its heterogeneity comes from (a) familial occurrence of HPE, (b) known genetic syndromes or associations with HPE, and (c) nonrandom chromosome anomalies in patients with HPE.

## Familial Holoprosencephaly

Familial instances of nonsyndromic HPE with normal chromosomes provide evidence for a genetic basis of HPE. Pedigrees have been described that support autosomal dominant (MIM 142945), autosomal recessive (MIM236100), and possibly X-linked (MIM 306990) inheritance (reviewed in references 198, 227, 259, and 260). The clinical variability can be quite striking within a single pedigree. Individuals with the full range of HPE, microforms, and even clinically normal individuals have been shown to be carriers of the abnormal gene.[54,68-70,227,261] Thus, phenotypically normal carriers are at risk of having children with HPE. Although precise genotype-phenotype correlations have not yet been performed in families with a known mutation in an HPE gene, the penetrance in autosomal dominant HPE is estimated to be 70 percent.[198] For an obligate carrier of autosomal dominant HPE, the risk for severe HPE is 16 to 21 percent, the risk for a less severe form or a microform is 13 to 14 percent, and the total risk for some clinical effect is 29 to 35 percent.[198]

Reported pedigrees with clinically unaffected parents and multiple affected sibs suggest autosomal recessive inheritance.[198,259] In addition, there are multiple examples of consanguinity, supporting the concept of autosomal recessive inheritance. However, because abnormal HPE genes are not fully penetrant and because there is the possibility of germ line mosaicism, some of these cases may actually be autosomal dominant. This could be demonstrated for all known HPE genes, *SHH, ZIC2, SIX3,* and *TGIF*.[54,68-70,222,261-263] Thus, the true

inheritance pattern of these pedigrees will be determined by molecular analysis once the genes responsible for HPE in these kindreds are identified.

## Holoprosencephaly in Syndromes

HPE can also be seen in several defined multiple malformation syndromes. It is estimated that approximately 18 to 25 percent of HPE cases have a recognizable monogenic syndrome.[11,12] There are at least 25 different conditions in which HPE has been described as an occasional finding, although the majority of these disorders are rare. In the "pseudotrisomy 13 syndrome" (MIM 264480) affected individuals have a normal karyotype, and HPE occurs with polydactyly.[264,265] Some characteristics commonly seen in trisomy 13, such as scalp defects, overlapping fingers, and nail hypoplasia, are not generally associated with "pseudotrisomy 13 syndrome."[266] HPE is associated with SLOS (MIM 270400),[164,267] and can occur in a small fraction of cases of PHS (MIM 146510), Meckel syndrome, RTS (MIM 180849), Kallmann syndrome (MIM 147950, 244200, 308700), and velocardiofacial syndrome (MIM192430) (reviewed in reference 2). HPE has been reported in association with other abnormalities in the Genoa syndrome (with craniosynostosis) (MIM 601370);[268] Lambotte syndrome (with microcephaly, prenatal growth retardation, hypertelorism) (MIM 245552);[265] hydrolethalus syndrome (with hydrocephalus, polydactyly, and other anomalies) (MIM 236680));[269] Martin syndrome (with clubfoot, spinal anomalies);[270] Steinfeld syndrome (with congenital heart disease, absent gallbladder, renal dysplasia, radial defects) (MIM 184705);[271] and with caudal dysgenesis,[213] with facial clefts and brachial amelia (MIM 601357),[272] with ectrodactyly and hypertelorism,[273] with microtia-anotia (MIM 600674), and other anomalies (reviewed in reference [13]).

The molecular defect has been identified in three of these disorders: SLOS, PHS, and RTS. It is of interest that the underlying bases in these three disorders can plausibly be connected to the Hedgehog signaling pathway. SLOS is a multiple congenital anomaly (microcephaly, characteristic facial findings, hypospadias, hypotonia, mental retardation) with autosomal recessive transmission. Four percent of SLOS cases are associated with some findings of the HPE spectrum.[164] The cause for SLOS is a biochemical block of the last step in cholesterol biosynthesis (see Chap. 249). The formation of cholesterol from 7-dehydrocholesterol (7-DHC) is blocked due to the altered enzyme, 7-dehydrocholesterol reductase, resulting in low cholesterol and a thousandfold increased 7-DHC. This block is similar to the one caused by AY9944 which has been shown to cause HPE by blocking Shh signaling in the animal model (see "Cholesterol and Holoprosencephaly" above).

PHS, a multiple congenital anomaly (hypothalamic hamartoblastoma, hypopituitarism, imperforate anus, and postaxial polydactyly) with autosomal dominant transmission in which HPE has occasionally been described, is caused by mutations in the *GLI3* gene.[148] These mutations predict premature truncation of the zinc finger-containing portion of the GLI3 protein and are suggestive of a suppression of the SHH pathway (see "Hedgehog Signal Transduction" above).

RTS is a multiple congenital anomaly with mutations in the *CBP* gene.[154] In *Drosophila*, CBP appears to be necessary for Ci activation. Furthermore, based on the RTS defects in humans, CBP appears to be a crucial cofactor for GLI proteins. Thus, the defects in PHS and RTS can potentially be explained by a reduction in activity of the SHH signaling pathway (see Hedgehog signal transduction above).

## Cytogenetic Anomalies in HPE

Chromosomal anomalies first reported in HPE involved trisomies of the D- and E-group chromosomes, that is, trisomy 13 and 18, and triploidies. Early reports of structural chromosome anomalies included those of deletions of 18p and 13q as well as ring chromosomes 13. Only with the introduction of chromosome banding in the early 1970s could these anomalies of a D-group (chromosome 13) and E-group (chromosome 18) chromosome be unequivocally determined and the extent of the deleted or duplicated chromosome material more precisely defined. To date, there have been case reports of patients with HPE and rearrangements involving virtually any chromosome, although only a limited number of chromosomal regions have been shown to be nonrandomly involved in HPE (Fig. 250-9; for references of individual case reports see the following reviews: 6, 259, 260, 274, and 275). Estimates of the frequency of chromosomal abnormalities in live births with HPE ranges from 24 percent[12] to 45 percent.[11] Although HPE has been seen in association with a large number of different chromosomal anomalies, certain chromosomal regions display recurrent involvement. In HPE patients with chromosomal anomalies, the most frequent ones involve chromosomes 13 and 18. HPE, in particular arhinencephaly, is seen in about 70 percent of the patients with trisomy 13, which has a birth prevalence of 1:5000. In addition to trisomy 13, there are numerous case reports of HPE with duplications or deletions of different regions on 13q and ring chromosomes 13. Deletions of 18p are observed in infants with this craniofacial malformation complex. HPE, in particular defects of the corpus callosum, have been reported in trisomy 18. Triploidy is yet another numerical chromosome anomaly in which HPE is seen.

Although accurate birth prevalence figures are not available, the order of frequency of nonrandom structural cytogenetic anomalies in HPE is from highest to lowest (in one author's [M.M.] experience): deletions or duplications involving various regions of 13q, del(18p), del(7)(q36), dup(3)(p24-pter), del(2)(p21), and del(21)(q22.3). All of the above chromosomal regions have been involved in the *de novo* rearrangements in sporadic HPE. In addition, balanced chromosomal translocations or other cytogenetically balanced rearrangements in a phenotypically normal parent have resulted in unbalanced chromosome complements of affected members mimicking familial HPE. Interestingly, the relative frequency of HPE varies with different cytogenetic anomalies. HPE is always present when chromosomal region 2p21 is deleted. In contrast, only half of the patients with del(7)(q36) have HPE, 10 percent with del(18p), and even less with del(21)(q22.3) (Muenke, unpublished observation).

Based on recurrent chromosomal rearrangements, it was hypothesized that these chromosomal regions may contain genes critical for normal brain development, and abnormalities in these genes could result in HPE (Muenke, 1989). At the Human Gene Mapping 11 conference, four genes which may play a role in HPE were designated:[276] *HPE1* at 21q22.3 (MIM 236100), *HPE2* at 2p21 (MIM157170), *HPE3* at 7q36 (MIM 142945), and *HPE4* at 18p (MIM142946). Based on nonrandom cytogenetic rearrangements, at least 12 chromosomal regions on 11 chromosomes may contain genes involved with HPE (Fig. 250-9).[275] The following additional chromosomal region are nonrandomly

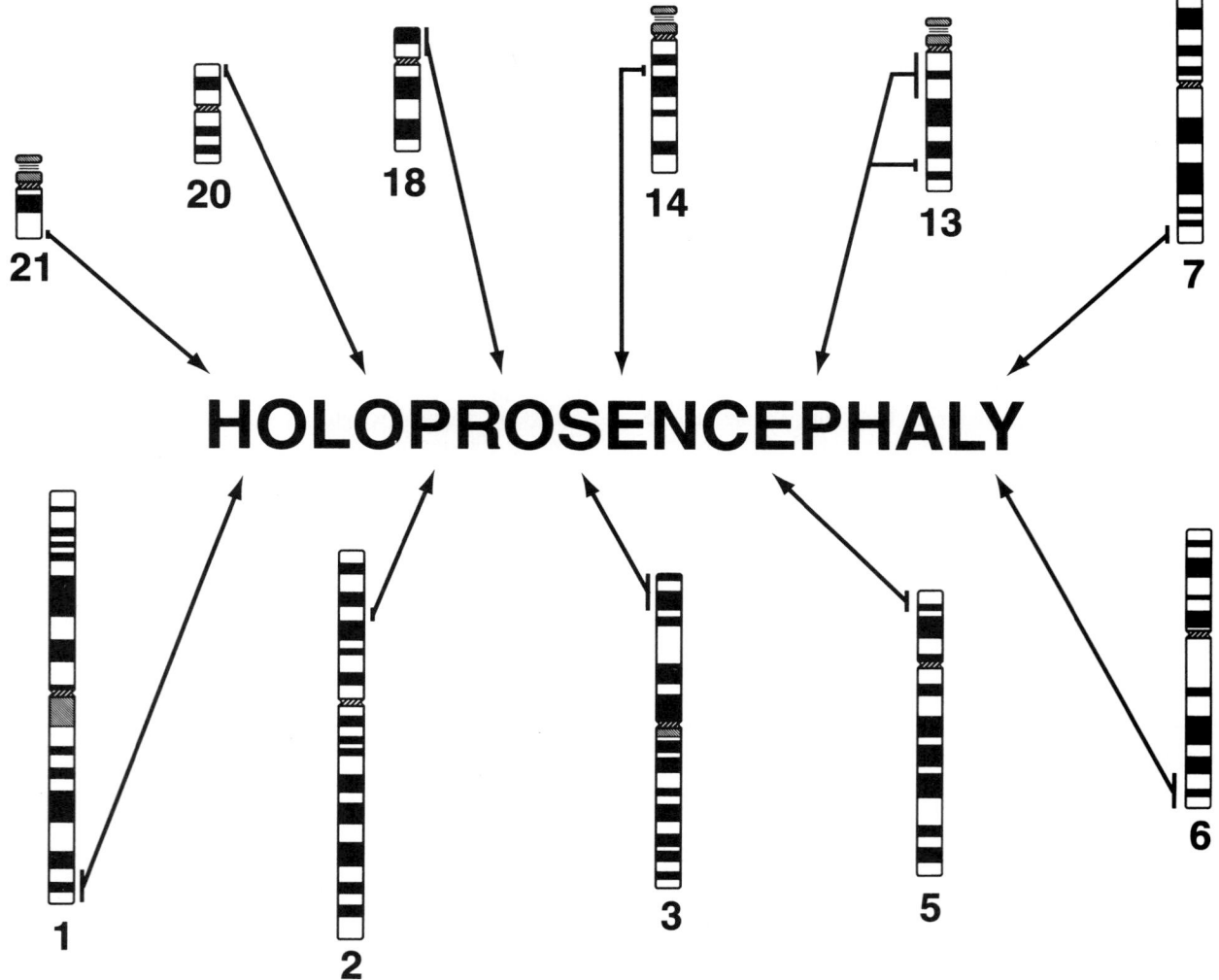

Fig. 250-9 Cytogenetic anomalies in holoprosencephaly. At least 12 human chromosomal regions have been implicated in the pathogenesis of HPE based on structural anomalies. With the exception of one region on 3p, which is duplicated, all other chromosomal regions shown here are deleted in HPE. (*From Roessler and Muenke.*[275] *Used by permission.*)

associated with HPE (proposed HPE locus designations are in parenthesis): 13q32 (*HPE5*), 3p24-pter (*HPE6*), 13q12-q14 (*HPE7*), 14q13 (*HPE8*), 20p13 (*HPE9*), 1q42-qter (*HPE10*), 5p (*HPE11*), and 6q26-qter (*HPE12*).[275]

Clinically, there is significant variation in phenotype even among individuals with the similar cytogenetic deletion.[277] Individuals with HPE due to a cytogenetic abnormality are more likely to have other organ system involvement.[12] Within the same degree of craniofacial abnormality or pathologic type of HPE, the features occurring in cytogenetically normal vs. abnormal individuals are indistinguishable.

**Position Effect in HPE.** Numerical and structural chromosome anomalies are common causes for HPE in humans (see above). Cytogenetically "balanced" translocations with breakpoints in the minimal critical region of HPE loci (*HPE1* to *HPE12*) are rare, but were critical in the identification of HPE genes. One example is a family in which a balanced t(7;9)(q36;q34) translocation segregated with the HPE carrier status.[278,279] This and other translocation breakpoints were hypothesized to cause HPE by disrupting the putative HPE gene in 7q36. However, none of the translocation breakpoints in 7q36 disrupted the *Sonic Hedgehog* (*SHH*) gene, but occurred 15 to 265 kb 5′ to the coding region of *SHH*.[53] Similarly, balanced translocations and inversions in 2p21 have been associated with HPE,[277] where the respective breakpoints do not disrupt the *SIX3* gene in 2p21 but are located within 120 to 200 kb 5′ to the coding region of *SIX3*.[261] These translocation breakpoints in 7q36 and 2p21, respectively, may cause HPE by exerting a "position" effect on *SHH* or *SIX3*, as has been shown for at least 10 disease-causing genes, including *GLI3*, *TWIST*, *SOX9*, and *PAX6* (for review see references 280 and 281). A position effect is defined as a change in the position of the gene relative to its normal chromosomal environment, but not associated with a disruption, deletion, or mutation within the gene itself. They may affect regulatory elements acting in *cis* on the expression of the gene, such as the promoter or enhancer/silencer elements, or affect the local heterochromatin configuration or locus control regions, thus altering expression. To date, all cases of proposed position effect as cause for human diseases are either in genes that are haploinsufficient or located on the X-chromosome. Thus, a position effect is only seen when reduced expression from one allele causes an altered phenotype.[281] Whether or not HPE-associated translocation breakpoints in the *HPE8* locus in 14q13 (282) and in *HPE9* in 20p13 (Muenke, unpublished observation) are coincidental or cause HPE by disrupting putative HPE genes or by exerting a position effect remains to be seen.

## Genes in Human Holoprosencephaly

***Sonic Hedgehog* Is *HPE3*.** The first HPE gene identified by positional candidate gene approach was *Sonic Hedgehog* (*SHH*) (GenBank NM 0001193 (cDNA); AC002484 (genomic DNA)). HPE has been described in many individuals with various cytogenetic deletions involving 7q36 (reviewed in references 259, 260, and 274). An HPE minimal critical region within 7q36, designated *HPE3*, was described on a molecular level.[283,284] Furthermore, most, but not all, families with autosomal dominant HPE were linked to DNA markers from this same region in 7q36.[228] The identity of *HPE3* with *SHH* was postulated on the basis of its position with respect to four key translocation breakpoints[53,284] and proved to be the gene on the basis of mutations detected initially in 10 unrelated families with autosomal dominant HPE (AD).[54,68] To date, 27 unrelated families have been reported with HPE and *SHH* mutations (Fig. 250-10).[54,68–70]

Combining the data from three studies in one laboratory[54,68,69] mutations in *SHH* accounted for 13 of 77 (17 percent) of the clinical familial HPE cases and for 10 of 267 (3.7 percent) of the sporadic cases. Therefore, *SHH* mutations were present in 23 of 344 (6.7 percent) of HPE patients. Using broad criteria for

inclusion as an AD pedigree, including features that are present to a significant degree in the general population (e.g., microcephaly, hypotelorism, mental retardation), the frequency of *SHH* mutations in AD pedigrees was 22 percent (10 of 45). When inclusion criteria for an AD pedigree were limited to structural anomalies (e.g., anosmia, corpus callosum agenesis in association with HPE, cleft lip and palate, single central incisor), the frequency of *SHH* mutations was 10 of 27 (37 percent). The finding of *SHH* mutations in only a minority of the total cohort of HPE patients underscores the significant etiologic heterogeneity of this condition. These figures should be considered estimates because functional effects of many of these mutations have not yet been studied.

Interestingly, mutational analysis of the clinically unaffected parents provided evidence for phenotypically normal mutation carriers. This emphasizes that clinically normal parents of a child with HPE may have some risk of carrying a *SHH* gene mutation, making counseling for recurrence risk more challenging. In addition, germ line mosaicism was suggested by the fact that in several families two sibs had the same *SHH* mutation, but neither parent carried the mutation.[69] No specific genotype/phenotype correlation according to type or location of the mutations in *SHH* is observed. As demonstrated by several of the pedigrees, the phenotype of carriers of a *SHH* mutation within a single family can vary from alobar HPE to clinically normal individuals.[285] Based on known domains in the hh family of proteins, we can speculate about the effects of the mutations observed in HPE patients. First, the association of chromosomal deletions that include *SHH* with HPE is consistent with a loss of SHH function.[284] Mutations could affect either the SHH-N signaling region, leading to alterations in biologic activity, or interfere with the processing reaction by affecting SHH-C, because an intact precursor molecule has little patterning activity.[56,57,61,62] Of the eight mutations predicted to cause premature termination of the SHH protein, five cause truncation within SHH-N and three cause truncation within SHH-C (Fig. 250-10). Numerous missense mutations throughout the entire coding region of SHH were observed in HPE patients (Fig. 250-10). Their functional significance is currently being analyzed.

Given the great intrafamilial clinical variability in kindreds carrying a *SHH* mutation, we speculate that other genes acting in the same or different developmental pathways might act as modifiers for the expression of the HPE spectrum. Interestingly, three HPE patients were identified with a *SHH* mutation who also had an alteration in a second gene which acts in brain development.[69] The G290N change in *SHH* was present in a patient who also had a mutation predicting an extension of an alanine repeat in exon 2 of *ZIC2*. Second, a P424A change in SHH was noted in both a child (Fig. 250-7J) who was deleted for 18pter and the putative *HPE4* gene *TGIF*,[69,222] and her mother who carried a balanced translocation involving chromosome 18. The third example is a 9-bp deletion in *SHH* (378 to 380del) in a child with HPE who also showed a missense mutation (T151A) in *TGIF*.[69,222]

In addition to potential modifier genes, environmental factors may also modulate the clinical expression of HPE.[153] The importance of cholesterol in normal SHH function[55,58,177] suggests that cholesterol levels in utero may contribute to the variable phenotype of HPE caused by *SHH* mutations (see "Cholesterol and Holoprosencephaly" above).

**Other HPE Genes in the Shh Signaling Pathway.** As detailed above (see "Hedgehog Signal Transduction"), Patched (PTC) (GenBank U43148 (cDNA)) and Smoothened (SMO) (GenBank U84401 (cDNA); AF114821.1 (genomic DNA)) are considered to be the first two components of the Hedgehog pathway. A variety of *PTC* mutations, most of which are predicted to result in protein truncation, have been detected in patients with nevoid basal cell carcinoma syndrome (NBCCS),[86,90,286] in sporadic medulloblastomas/primitive neuroectodermal tumors,[287,288] in breast carcinoma,[288] in meningioma,[288] esophageal squamous cell carcinoma,[289]

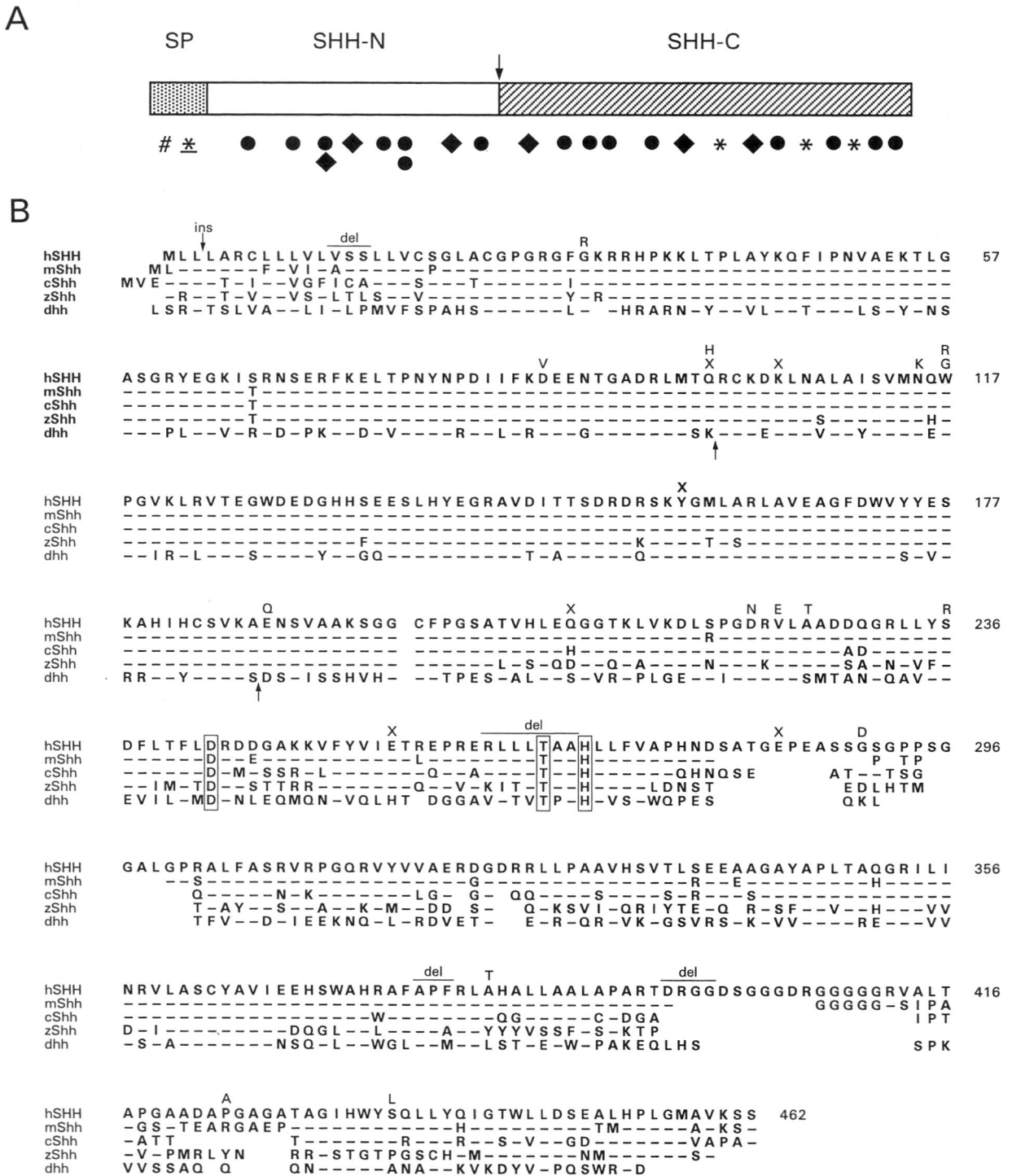

Fig. 250-10 *SHH* mutations spectrum in holoprosencephaly. *A*, The mutations are evenly distributed between the coding regions. SHH-N = signaling domain; SHH-C = autocatalytic cleavage and cholesterol transferase domain; SP = signal peptide, removed after translation; arrow = cleavage/cholesterol addition; # = insertion; * = deletion with frameshift; * = deletion without frameshift; black diamonds = nonsense mutations; black circles = missense mutations. *B*, Amino acid sequence alignment for human Sonic Hedgehog (hSHH), mouse Sonic Hedgehog (mShh), chicken Sonic Hedgehog (cShh), zebra fish Sonic Hedgehog (zShh), and *Drosophila* Hedgehog (dhh). The locations of the predicted amino acid changes in HPE patients are shown above the human SHH amino acid (data are from references 54 and 68 to 70). The positions of amino acid identity between species are indicated (−). Arrows indicate the position of the exons 1, 2, and 3, and a gap is introduced in the protein sequence to mark the position of the autocatalytic cleavage between Gly197 and Cys198 of the human protein. The residues essential for hh autoprocessing activity in Drosophila are boxed. (*Modified from Nanni et al.[69] Used by permission.*)

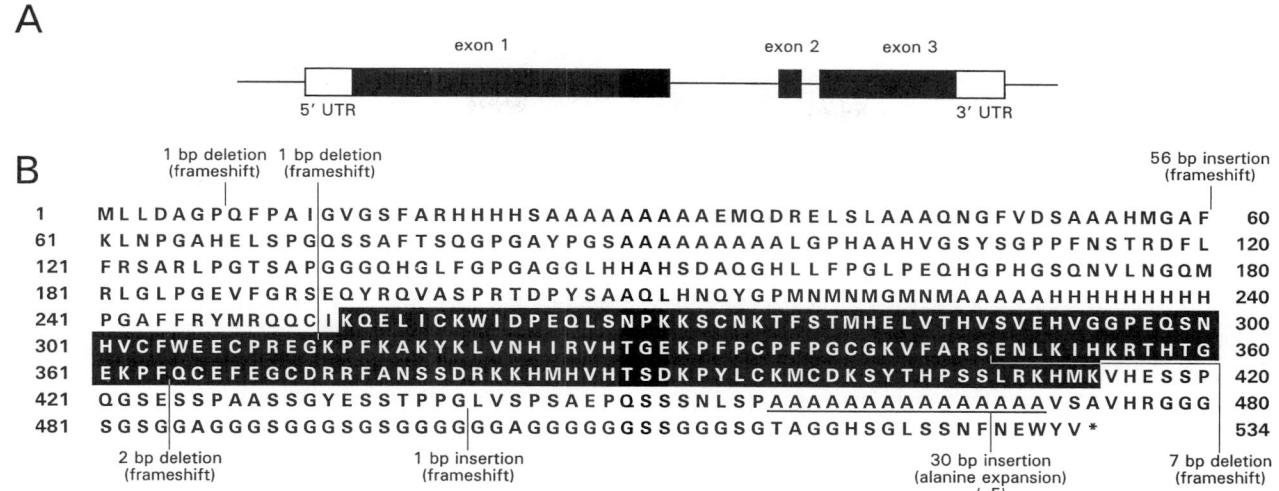

Fig. 250-11 *ZIC2* mutation spectrum in holoprosencephaly. Heterozygous mutations in *ZIC2* in HPE fall into two categories: insertions or deletions leading to frameshift and alanine expansion by insertion of 30 bp. (*Modified from Brown et al.*[262] *Used by permission.*)

and trichoepitheliomas, another type of skin tumor.[290] In contrast, HPE is known to be caused by loss of function of SHH and decreased signaling through the SHH pathway. Thus, HPE-associated mutations in PTC would be predicted to be missense mutations that alter SHH signaling. Similarly, loss-of-function of SMO or one of the cubitus interruptus homologs, the GLI proteins potentially could lead to HPE. To date, four HPE-associated missense mutations have been identified in *PTC*, two in the extracellular loops that may be required for SHH binding, and two in intracellular loops, in a region that may be involved in PTC-SMO interaction.[291] Mutational analysis of *SMO*, *GLI1*, and *GLI2* in DNA samples are in progress. To date, no HPE-associated mutations have been identified in *SMO* (Ming and Muenke, unpublished observations). DNA sequence changes predicting amino acid substitutions have been identified in *GLI1* (GenBank NM 005269 (cDNA)) and *GLI2* (GenBank NM 005270 (cDNA)), although its significance is not yet known (Roessler, Du, and Muenke, unpublished observations).

***ZIC2* Is *HPE5*.** The second gene identified in HPE is *ZIC2* (GenBank AF104902 (cDNA)), which maps to the *HPE5* minimal critical region in 13q32.[292] ZIC2 is a member of a family of proteins that includes the *Drosophila odd-paired* gene (*opa*)[293–296] and the zebra fish gene *odd-paired like* (*opl*),[297] which contain zinc finger-DNA-binding motifs of specificity very closely related to that of the Gli proteins. In *Drosophila*, the *opa* gene appears to affect the expression of targets of *hh* signaling,[293] and its expression of Zic2 in dorso/ventrally restricted stripes within mammalian neuroepithelium, including the ventral midline of the neural tube,[24] suggests that it may have a role in mediating the response to Shh signaling. In the mouse expression of *Zic2* begins during gastrulation and, later during development, is in the dorsal neural tube, eye, and distal limb.[298]

Heterozygous *ZIC2* mutations were identified in nine unrelated HPE patients. With the exception of one family, a father who appears to be a somatic mosaic and two affected children with *ZIC2* mutation, all other cases appear to be sporadic.[262,263] These mutations fall into two categories: (a) small insertions or deletions (1 to 56 bp) lead to frameshifts and stop codons predicting ZIC2 protein truncations; (b) insertion of 30 bp expands the alanine tract from normally 15 to 25 alanine residues (Fig. 250-11). The first group of mutations predicts a loss of function of one of the *ZIC2* alleles, similar to deletions of *ZIC2* in individuals with del(13)(q32). Haploinsufficiency of *ZIC2* as cause for HPE is also seen for *SHH*, *SIX3*, and *TGIF*. Expansion of the alanine tract has not yet been described for any other HPE gene, although they

occur in several homeodomain transcription factors.[299–305] Polyalanine tracts appear to cause at least three developmental disorders: polysyndactyly in humans (HOXD13)[303,306] and in the mouse (Hoxd13),[304] cleidocranial dysplasia (CBFA1),[305] and oculopharyngeal muscular dystrophy (PABP2).[307]

Preliminary clinical studies in HPE patients with *ZIC2* mutations are interesting and the results are different from those with *SHH*, *SIX3*, or *TGIF* mutations. Despite severe central nervous system anomalies consistent with HPE, the facial findings do not reflect the severity of the brain malformation (Fig. 250-7*M* to *P*). All HPE patients with *ZIC2* mutations studied to date have only mildly dysmorphic facial features including hypotelorism, flat nasal bridge, mild flattening of the midface, and microcephaly (Fig. 250-7*M* to *P*). Structural anomalies of the midface such as cyclopia, ethmocephaly, cebocephaly, premaxillary agenesis, and clefting have not been associated with *ZIC2* mutations. Thus, some of the cases with *ZIC2* mutations may contribute to the 20 percent of HPE individuals, where the face does not predict the brain.

***SIX3* Is *HPE2*.** The third HPE gene identified by positional candidate gene approach is *SIX3* (GenBank NM 005413.1 (cDNA); AF092047 (genomic DNA)), which maps to the *HPE2* locus on human chromosome 2p21.[261,277] The *HPE2* locus was characterized as a 1-Mb interval in 2p21 defined by a set of six overlapping deletions and three clustered translocations in HPE patients.[277] The mouse *Six3* gene mapped to a region on mouse chromosome 17 that is syntenic to human chromosome 2p21.[308] The vertebrate *Six3* genes have been shown to participate in midline forebrain and eye formation in several organisms.[308–311] *Six-3* message is present in the rostral, anterior region of the neural plate, optic recess, developing retina, and midline ventral forebrain.[308,312] The *SIX/so* family of transcription factors form a distantly related subclass of homeobox-containing genes that are further characterized by the presence of a contiguous homology domain, the SIX domain, which is also thought to participate in transcriptional activation.[312] Vertebrate *SIX3* genes have been shown to participate in midline forebrain and eye formation in several organisms[312] and have been isolated from chicken,[313] *Xenopus*,[314] medaka,[315] and zebra fish.[316] Sequence comparisons show extensive homology within the homeodomain in vertebrates (Fig. 250-12) and confirm that *SIX3* genes are more closely related to the recently described *Drosophila* gene *optix* than they are to *sine oculis*.[317] The *optix* gene is also crucial in the development of the visual system in the fly.

The human *SIX3* gene was analyzed as *HPE2* candidate based on the fact that it was the only known gene in the minimal critical

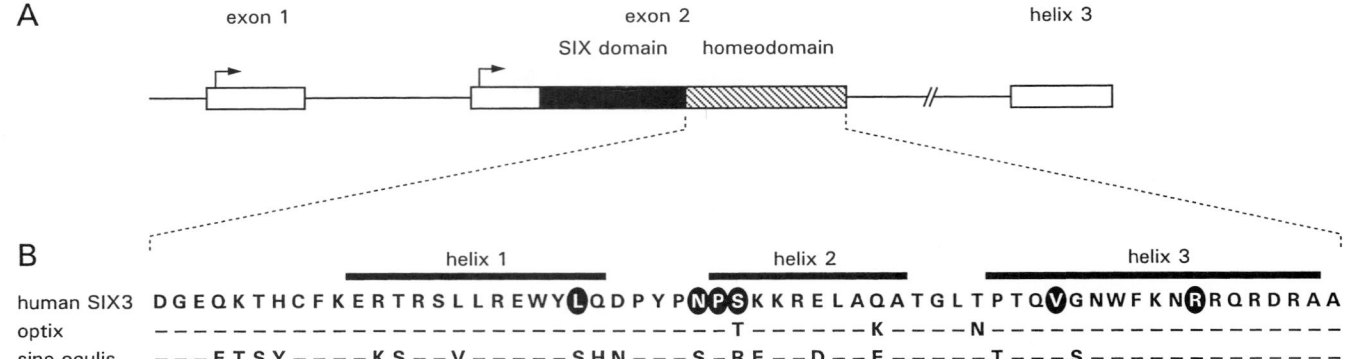

**Fig. 250-12** *SIX3 mutation spectrum in holoprosencephaly. SIX3 genomic structure and homeodomain. A,* The genomic structure is represented with the arrows indicating two potential initiation sites in exon 1 and exon 2, respectively. The SIX domain is black and the homeodomain is stippled. *B,* The 60-amino-acid homeodomain is depicted with an alignment of the Six3 amino acid sequences with respect to optix and sine oculis. Positions of identity are indicated (−). It is of interest to note that the entire amino acid sequence of the Six3 homeodomains in the mouse, chick, frog, and zebra fish are identical to the human one. (*Modified from Wallis et al.[261] Used by permission.*)

region in this interval with the correct spatial and temporal expression pattern to participate in a gastrulation-stage patterning process resulting in HPE. Four heterozygous mutations in the homeodomain of *SIX3* were identified in unrelated HPE patients in a screening of approximately 300 HPE patients,[261] including a 9-bp deletion and three missense mutations (Fig. 250-12).

These four mutations in the *SIX3* homeodomain, cytogenetic deletions of 2p21 involving the deletion of one *SIX3* allele,[277] and HPE-associated translocation breakpoints in measurable distance (up to 120 to 200 kb) from the 5′ end of the *SIX3* coding sequence (see "Cytogenetic Anomalies in HPE: Position Effect in HPE" above), are compatible with a mechanism of haploinsufficiency/loss-of-function of *SIX3* as a cause for HPE.

Mutations in *SIX3* in HPE are rare (4 in 300 HPE patients). They occur in both sporadic and familial HPE. Similar to mutations in *SHH*, the phenotypic spectrum in individuals with *SIX3* mutations is extremely variable and ranges from alobar HPE to normal mutation carrier in the same family.[261,318] Other HPE children with different *SIX3* mutations have varying findings: alobar HPE with cleft lip and palate in the 9-bp deletion,[319] semilobar HPE with micro-ophthalmia and iris coloboma consistent with the role described for SIX3 in eye development (*de novo SIX3* R257P); typical HPE face with microcephaly, bilateral cleft lip and palate, and mental retardation, but without any detectable structure central nervous system anomalies or brain scan (*de novo SIX3* L226V).

***TGIF Is HPE4.*** Based on the findings that HPE is frequently associated with various deletions involving chromosome 18p, the *HPE4* minimal region was described in 18p11.3.[320] The gene coding for TG-interacting factor (*TGIF*) (GenBank NM 003244 (cDNA)) maps to 18p[321] and was considered an *HPE4* gene candidate based on its chromosomal location in 18p, its expression pattern, and the fact that it modulates the TGFβ pathway (Fig. 250-13) components of which have been shown to be involved in HPE in animal models (see "Other Factors Involved in Ventral Forebrain Patterning" above).

TGIF is an atypical homeodomain protein that is localized in the nucleus. TGIF has been shown to act *in vitro* as a co-repressor of the MSAD2 protein by forming a complex with SMAD2/SMAD4 and recruiting histone deacetylases to the complex.[322,323] This repressive action of TGIF is in direct competition with transcriptional activators that also bind the SMAD2/SMAD4 complex to recruit histone acetylases and activate transcription. Thus, the competition between repressors such as TGIF and activators determines the magnitude of the response to TGFβ-like signals.

Interestingly, the TGIF protein was initially identified as a nuclear factor capable of binding to the retinoic acid RXR binding

site of the cellular retinol binding protein II promoter (CRBPII RXRE).[324] TGIF and RXR compete for binding to the promoter element by sterically hindering binding to overlapping sequences within the RXRE.[325] Thus, TGIF is also of interest as a repressor of retinoic acid-regulated gene transcription. Mutations in *TGIF* could potentially lead to loss of function as a repressor resulting in overactivity for retinoic acid-regulating genes, simulating the effect of excessive retinoic acid exposure. Prenatal retinoic acid exposure in mice and humans has been shown to cause abnormalities within the HPE spectrum.[252,326–328] Furthermore, a close interrelation between the Shh and retinoic acid pathways has been demonstrated in the chick embryo.[49,191,329,330] In addition, teratogens such as retinoic acid are known to modulate the phenotypes of mutations in the TGFβ signaling pathway.[331] While the function of TGIF as a repressor of TGFβ signaling and retinoic acid signaling is not yet completely understood, preliminary evidence suggests that TGIF plays a role in the pathogenesis of HPE.

To date, four heterozygous missense mutations in *TGIF* have been identified in patients with HPE.[222] These mutations predict amino acid substitutions in the N-terminal transcription-repression domain, the homeodomain between helix 1 and 2 in the Smad interacting domain. As summarized in Fig. 250-13, one of the mutations (P63R), which lies within the homeodomain, appears to

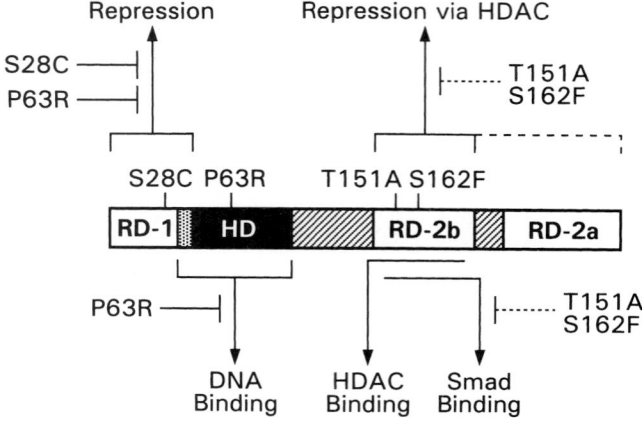

**Fig. 250-13** *TGIF mutation spectrum in holoprosencephaly.* Representation of the domain structure of TGIF is shown. The positions of the four HPE mutations are indicated with the TGIF functions they affect. HD indicates homeodomain. RD-1, RD-2a, and RD-2b represent N-terminal and C-terminal repression domains. HDAC = histone deacetylases. (*Modified from Gripp et al.[222] Used by permission.*)

**Table 250-1** Summary of Known and Potential Molecular Mechanisms of Holoprosencephaly

| Genetic factors | | Functions | Reference |
|---|---|---|---|
| **Drosophila** | **Vertebrate** | | |
| hh | Shh | Secreted signaling factor involved in embryonic patterning | 38 |
| | | mouse mutants have HPE phenotype | 48 |
| | | SHH mutations cause HPE | 54, 68–70 |
| ptc | Ptc | transmembrane protein, Shh receptor | 81, 347 |
| | | PTC mutations in human HPE | 153 |
| smo | Smo | transmembrane protein that interacts with ptc | 76, 77, 350 |
| | Hip | transmembrane protein interacts with all vertebrate hedgehogs | 107 |
| | | may negatively regulate vertebrate hedgehog signaling | |
| ci | Gli family | zinc finger transcription factor, mediates hh signaling | 118 |
| | | ectopic Gli1 activates HNF-3$\beta$, Ptc, and Shh | 140, 142 |
| | | Gli2 mouse mutants have HPE microsigns | 350 |
| | | Gli3 is associated with human disease | 148–151 |
| | HNF-3$\beta$ | transcription factor, required for the development of axial structures | 338, 339 |
| | | regulates Shh with goosecold | 340 |
| | | expressed in the head process and floor plate of the neural tube | 337 |
| | | contains Gli binding site in its enhancer | 142 |
| dpp | BMP2/4 | TGF$\beta$ family secreted protein; target of hh signaling | 351 |
| | | dpp regulates so and eya expression | 352 |
| | | dpp negatively regulates opa expression | 296 |
| | | BMP4 antagonizes opl expression | 297 |
| | | ectopic BMP4 or 5 in chick results in HPE phenotype | 35 |
| | nodal | TGF$\beta$ signaling factor; mutations cause cyclopia in animal models | 163, 353 |
| | oep | extracellular membrane associated ligand required for nodal signaling | 156 |
| | | mutations cause cyclopia in zebrafish | 157 |
| | TGF$\beta$-like | transduce TGF$\beta$ family signals by phosphorylating Smads | 354, 355 |
| | Receptors | activin receptor IB rescues oep phenotype | 157 |
| mad | Smad | mediate TGFb-like signals from cell surface to nucleus | 356 |
| | | Smad2/nodal heterozygous mouse mutants have cyclopia | 163 |
| | | rescues oep phenotype | 157 |
| | TGF | homeodomain protein that interacts with Smad2 | 322, 323 |
| | | Binds CRBPII promotor and competes with RXR for binding sites | 324 |
| | | TGIF mutations in human HPE | 222 |
| | cerberus | secreted factor that specifies anterior CNS properties | 341 |
| | | binds and represses nodal, BMP, and Wnt | 342 |
| opa | Zic family | zinc finger transcription factor, required for en and wg activity | 293 |
| | | ZIC2 mutations cause HPE | 262 |
| so/optix | six family | homeoprotein important for eye and forebrain development | 308, 309, 317, 357, 358 |
| | | so interacts with eya | 359 |
| | | SIX3 mutations cause HPE | 261 |
| | Dkk-1 | secreted protein required for head formation; Wnt against expressed in Spemann organizer and prechordal plate antibody inhibition of Dkk-1 results in microcephaly and cyclopia | 335, 336 |
| wg | Wnt family | secreted segment polarity gene activated by hh signaling | 360 |
| | floating head | homeobox gene Not, mutants lack prechordal plate | 343 |
| | | synergistic with cyclops in midline development | 344 |
| | masterblind | required for anterior structures and floating head expression | 31, 345 |
| | bozozok | homeoprotein required for forebrain specification may be downstream of Wnt and upstream of TGF$\beta$ signaling | 346 |
| **Other factors** | | | |
| Cholesterol | | may be required for proper spatial restriction of Shh signaling | 58, 65 |
| | | inhibitors of cholesterol synthesis in mice result in HPE phenotypes | 171, 361, 362 |
| | | mutations in cholesterol synthesis genes may result in human HPE | 164 |
| | | inhibitors of cholesterol synthesis inhibit Shh signaling | 177 |
| | | megalin mutations in mice lead to HPE phenotype | 180 |
| Retinoic acid | | high doses inhibit Shh and Ptc expression in craniofacial primordia | 49 |
| | | ectopic treatment induces Shh in the limb bud | 329 |
| | | acts synergistically with Activin RIIB mutation on vertebral patterning | 331 |
| | | Prenatal exposure can cause CNS abnormalities consistent with HPE | 252, 326–328 |

Modified from Wallis and Muenke.[347]

affect both DNA binding and transcriptional repression via the N-terminal, HDAC-independent domain of TGIF. The S28C mutation, which is within a minimal region containing the N-terminal repression domain, decreases the activity of this domain. The other two mutations lie within a region that is required for TGIF interaction with both Smad2 and HDAC. Only subtle defects were detected in interactions with these proteins or on transcriptional repression by this domain (Fig. 250-13). These results provide evidence that the *TGIF* mutations observed in HPE patients impair different activities of TGIF and suggest that reduction of TGIF activity can influence the developmental program and lead to HPE by altering Nodal/TGFβ signaling.

**HPE1 Maps to 21q22.3.** A minority of patients with cytogenetic deletion of 21q22.3 have some clinical findings consistent with the diagnosis of HPE. Based on these patients, this locus was designated HPE1,[276] and an *HPE1* minimal critical region was defined on a molecular level.[332] There could be several reasons for the low frequency of HPE in del(21)(q22.3): (a) the occurrence of HPE and cytogenetic deletion are coincidental; (b) in addition to loss-of-function of one gene from within the deleted region, loss-of-function of a second gene in the same pathway is required to cause HPE (e.g., the phenotype of mice that are double-heterozygous for null alleles in both nodal and Smad2 is consistent with cyclopia in over half of the embryos);[163] and (c) deletion of one gene in 21q22.3 and a mutation in the same gene on the other allele consistent with autosomal recessive inheritance. A gene that

fits this latter category is lanosterol synthase (LS). LS is an enzyme that is crucial for the first committed step in cholesterol biosynthesis. It maps to chromosome 21q22.3[333] and the *HPE1* MCR.[332] Based on its map position and its crucial role in the cholesterol pathway (see "Cholesterol and Holoprosencephaly" above), LS was analyzed as a candidate gene for *HPE1*. Its genomic structure was determined as a 22-exon gene and mutation analysis was performed in HPE patients with del(21)(q22.3) in whom one copy of the LS gene was deleted. Missense mutations were identified in the coding regions of LS; functional studies in yeast, however, did not provide evidence that these mutations alter the cholesterol pathway and are involved in HPE.[334]

**Additional HPE Candidate Genes.** With such complex pathways implicated in HPE pathogenesis, there are other genes to be considered. Candidates include factors important in forebrain development or establishing dorsal-ventral patterning of the forebrain. Some of the more relevant ones to HPE include: *Dickkopf-1 (dkk-1)*,[335,336] *HNF-3β*,[142,337–340] *cerberus (cer)*,[341,342] *floating head (flh)*,[343,344] *masterblind (mbl)*,[31,345] *bozozok (boz)*,[346] and genes that contribute to cholesterol biosynthesis. Some of these genes were identified in zebra fish and are involved in the formation of the prechordal plate, notochord, and/or neural tube. Associations with some of these genes in the nodal/TGFβ pathway have been established, making them even more interesting as candidate genes. Their proposed functions and expression patterns are summarized in Table 250-1.

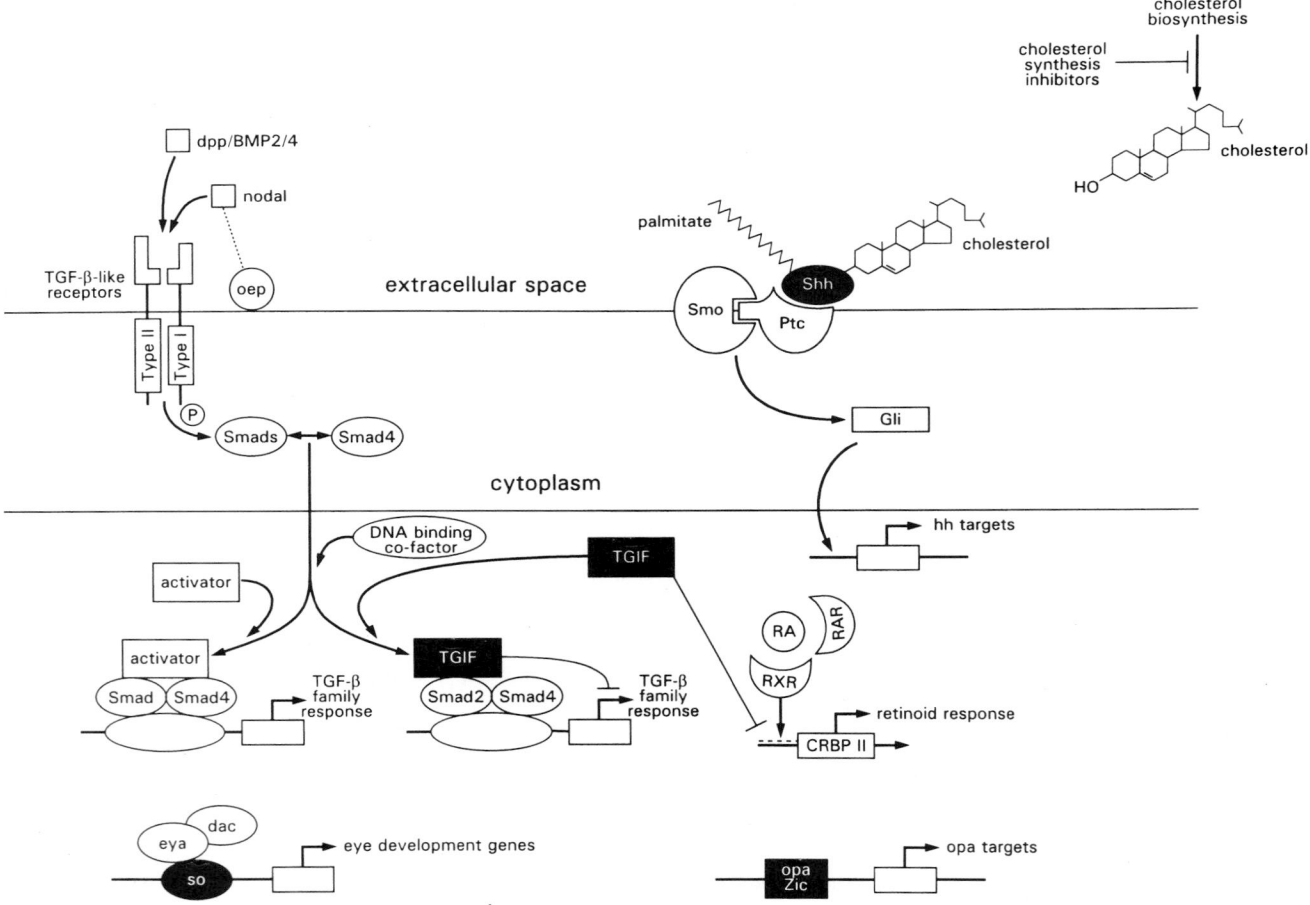

**Fig. 250-14 Association of holoprosencephaly with abnormal function of signaling pathways and cholesterol biosynthesis and of opa/ZIC2 and so/SIX3 transcription factors.** Some aspects of the interactions are speculative because not all of the links have been explicitly demonstrated experimentally and many of the links are only suggestive. In addition, results have been synthesized from several species, and each part of the pathway may not have been shown for all species. To date, the following genes (highlighted) have been implicated in HPE in humans: *SHH, ZIC2, SIX3,* and *TGIF.* For details see text. (*Modified from Wallis and Muenke.*[347] *Used by permission.*)

# FUTURE DIRECTIONS

A better understanding of the underlying mechanisms of normal and abnormal brain morphogenesis has mainly been derived from the studies of various animal models. Cloning and analysis of genes in *Drosophila*, zebra fish, and the mouse has helped identify all currently known HPE genes by a positional candidate approach. Although mutations in *SHH, ZIC2, SIX3,* and *TGIF* can result in HPE, alterations in these genes account only for a minority of both familial and sporadic instances of HPE. Thus, the search for additional HPE genes continues. The focus will be on HPE candidate genes with at least one of the following characteristics: (a) genes that map to the minimal critical regions of HPE loci, *HPE1-12* (Fig. 250-9); (b) genes that, when altered, cause HPE in animal models (Table 250-1); (c) components of signaling pathways such as SHH, retinoic acid, Nodal/TGFβ, and others (Fig. 250-14); (d) ancillary components that may be involved in transcription regulation including transcription factors such as opa/ZIC2 or so/SIX3; (e) components of the pathway of cholesterol biosynthesis and metabolism; and (f) factors important in establishing dorsal-ventral patterning of the forebrain. As the genetic factors involved in HPE are further identified, the complex relationships between these genes will be better appreciated. Elucidating how genetic and environmental influences interact to cause HPE will provide an understanding of the basis for the variation in phenotype and possibly even suggest interventions to improve outcome. Continued studies on the basis of HPE will improve our understanding of HPE on clinical, genetic, and molecular levels, and provide a powerful tool for elucidating normal forebrain development in humans.

# REFERENCES

1. Mandelbaum A: *The Odyssey of Homer, Book IX.* Berkeley, University of California Press, 1990, p 171.
2. Siebert JR, Cohen MM Jr, Sulik KK, Shaw C-M, Lemire RJ: *Holoprosencephaly. An Overview and Atlas of Cases.* New York, Wiley-Liss Publication, 1990.
3. Kundrat H: *Arhinencephalie als typische Art von Missbildung.* Graz, Von Leuschner und Lubinsky Verlag, 1882.
4. Yakovlev PI: Pathoarchitectonic studies of cerebral malformations. III. Arhinencephalies (holotelencephalies). *J Neuropath Exp Neurol* **18**:22, 1959.
5. DeMyer W, Zeman W: Alobar holoprosencephaly (arhinencephaly) with median cleft lip and palate: Clinical electroencephalographic and nosologic considerations. *Confin Neurol (Basel)* **23**:1, 1963.
6. Norman MG, McGillivray B, Kalousek DK, Hill A, Poskitt J, Norman MG (ed): Holoprosencephaly: Defects of the mediobasal prosencephalon, in *Congenital Malformations of the Brain: Pathological, Embryological, Clinical, Radiological and Genetic Aspects.* New York, Oxford University Press, 1995, p 187.
7. Golden JA: Holoprosencephaly: A defect in brain patterning. *J Neuropath Exp Neurol* **57**:1991, 1998.
8. Matsunaga E, Shiota K: Holoprosencephaly in human embryos: Epidemiologic studies of 150 cases. *Teratology* **16**:261, 1977.
9. Roach E, DeMeyer W, Conneally PM, Palmer C, Merritt AD: Holoprosencephaly: Birth data, genetic and demographic analyses of 30 families. *Birth Defects* **11**:294, 1977.
10. Urioste M, Valcarcel E, Gomez MA, Pinel I, Garcia de Leon R, Diaz de Bustamante A, Tebar R, et al: Holoprosencephaly and trisomy 21 in a child born to a nondiabetic mother. *Am J Med Genet* **30**:925, 1988.
11. Croen LA, Shaw GM, Lammer EJ: Holoprosencephaly: Epidemiologic and clinical characteristics of a California population. *Am J Med Genet.* **64**:465, 1996.
12. Olsen CL, Hughes JP, Youngblood LG, Sharpe-Stimac M: The epidemiology of holoprosencephaly and phenotypic characteristics of affected children: New York State, 1984-1989. *Am J Med Genet* **73**:217, 1997.
13. Cohen MM Jr, Sulik KK: Perspectives on holoprosencephaly. Part II. Central nervous system, craniofacial anatomy, syndrome commentary, diagnostic approach, and experimental studies. *J Craniofac Genet Dev Biol* **12**:196, 1992.
14. Adelmann HB: The problem of cyclopia. *Quart Rev Biol* **11**:116, 1936.
15. Adelmann HB: The problem of cyclopia. *Quart Rev Biol* **11**:284, 1936.
16. Rogers KT: Experimental production of perfect cyclopia in the chick by means of LiCl, with a survey of the literature on cyclopia produced experimentally by various means. *Dev Biol* **8**:129, 1963.
17. Keeler RF: Cyclopamine and related steroidal alkaloid teratogens: their occurrence, structural relationship, and biological effects. *Lipids* **10**:708, 1978.
18. Mangold O: Das Determinationsproblem. III. Das Wirbeltierauge in der Entwicklung und Regeneration. *Ergeb d Biol* **7**:193, 1931.
19. Spemann H, Mangold H: Induction of embryonic primordia by implantation of organizers from a different species, in Willier BH, Oppenheimer JM (eds): *Foundations of Experimental Embryology.* New York, Hafner, 1924, p 144.
20. Blader P, Strahle U: Casting an eye over cyclopia. *Nature* **395**:112, 1998.
21. Blader P, Strahle U: Ethanol impairs migration of the prechordal plate in the zebrafish embryo. *Dev Biol* **201**:185, 1998.
22. Holtfreter J, Hamburger V: Progressive differentiation, in Willyer DHWP, Hamburger B (eds): *Embryogenesis.* Philadelphia, WB Saunders, 1955, p 230.
23. Dale JK, Vesque C, Lints TJ, Sampath TK, Furley A, Dodd J, Placzek M: Cooperation of BMP7 and SHH in the induction of forebrain ventral midline cells by prechordal mesoderm. *Cell* **90**:257, 1997.
24. Ericson J, Muhr J, Piaczek M, Lints T, Jessell TM, Edlund T: Sonic Hedgehog induces the differentiation of ventral forebrain neurons: A common signal for ventral patterning within the neural tube. *Cell* **81**:747, 1995.
25. Foley AC, Storey KG, Stern CD: The prechordal region lacks neural inducing ability, but can confer anterior character to more posterior neuroepithelium. *Development* **124**:2983, 1997.
26. Kimura S, Hara Y, Pineau T, Fernandez-Salguero P, Fox CH, Ward JM, Gonzalez FJ: The T/ebp null mouse: Thyroid-specific enhancer-binding protein is essential for the organogenesis of the thyroid, lung, ventral forebrain, and pituitary. *Genes Devel* **10**:60, 1996.
27. Pera E, Kessel M: Patterning of the chick forebrain anlage by the prechordal plate. *Development* **124**:4153, 1997.
28. Qiu M, Shimamura K, Sussel L, Chen S, Rubenstein JLR: Control of anteroposterior and dorsoventral domains of Nkx6.1 gene expression relative to Nkx genes during vertebrate CNS development. *Mech Dev* **72**:77, 1998.
29. Shimamura K, Rubenstein JLR: Inductive interactions direct early regionalization of the mouse forebrain. *Development* **124**:2709, 1997.
30. Li HS, Tierney C, Wen L, Wu JY, Rao Y: A single morphogenetic field gives rise to two retina primordia under the influence of the prechordal plate. *Development* **124**:603, 1997.
31. Heisenberg CP, Brand M, Jiang YJ, Warga RM, Beuchle D, van Eeden FJ, Furutani-Seiki M, et al: Genes involved in forebrain development in the zebrafish, Danio rerio. *Development* **123**:191, 1996.
32. Marlow F, Zwartkruis F, Malicki J, Neuhauss SC, Abbas L, Weaver M, Driever W, et al: Functional interactions of genes mediating convergent extension, knypek and trilobite, during the partitioning of the eye primordium in zebrafish. *Dev Biol* **203**:382, 1998.
33. Schier AF, Neuhauss SCF, Harvey M, Malicki J, Solnica-Krezel L, Stainier DYR, et al: Mutations affecting the development of the embryonic zebrafish brain. *Development* **123**:165, 1996.
34. Schier AF, Neuhauss SC, Helde KA, Talbot WS, Driever W: The one-eyed pinhead gene functions in mesoderm and endoderm formation in zebrafish and interacts with no tail. *Development* **124**:327, 1997.
35. Golden JA, Bracilovic A, McFadden KA, Beesley JS, Rubenstein JLR, Grinspan JB: Ectopic bone morphogenetic proteins 5 and 4 in the chicken forebrain lead to cyclopia and holoprosencephaly. *Proc Natl Acad Sci U S A* **96**:2439, 1999.
36. Rogers KT: Experimental production of perfect cyclopia by removal of the telencephalon and reversal of bilateralization in somite-stage chicks. *Am J Anat* **115**:487, 1964.
37. Echelard Y, Epstein DJ, St.-Jacques B, Shen L, Mohler J, McMahon JA, and McMahon AP: Sonic hedgehog, a member of a family of putative signaling molecules, is implicated in the regulation of CNS polarity. *Cell* **75**:1417, 1993.
38. Nüsslein-Volhard C, Wieschaus E: Mutations affecting segment number and polarity in *Drosophila. Nature* **287**:795, 1980.
39. Lee JJ, von Kessler DP, Parks S, Beachy PA: Secretion and localized transcription suggest a role in positional signaling for products of the segmentation gene hedgehog. *Cell* **71**:33, 1992.

40. Mohler J, Vani K: Molecular organization and embryonic expression of the hedgehog gene involved in cell-cell communication in segmental patterning of Drosophila. *Development* **115**:957, 1992.

41. Tabata T, Eaton S, Kornberg TB: The *Drosophila hedgehog* gene is expressed specifically in posterior compartment cells and is a target of *engrailed* regulation. *Genes Dev* **6**:2635, 1992.

42. Tashiro S, Michiue T, Higashijima S, Zenno S, Ishimaru S, Takahashi, F, Orihara, M, et al: Structure and expression of *hedgehog*, a *Drosophila* segment-polarity gene required for cell-cell communication. *Gene* **124**:183, 1993.

43. Hammerschmidt M, Brook A, McMahon AP: The world according to hedgehog. *Trends Genet* **13**:14, 1997.

44. Chuang PT, McMahon AP: Vertebrate hedgehog signaling modulated by induction of a Hedgehog-binding protein. *Nature* **397**:617, 1999.

45. Nakamura T, Aikawa T, Iwamoto-Enomoto M, Iwamoto M, Higuchi Y, Pacifici M, Kinto N, et al: Induction of osteogenic differentiation by hedgehog proteins. *Biochem Biophys Res Commun* **237**:465, 1997.

46. Lanske B, Karaplis AC, Lee K, Luz A, Vortkamp A, Pirro A, Karperien M, et al: PTH/PTHrP receptor in early development and Indian hedgehog-regulated bone growth. *Science* **273**:663, 1996.

47. Bitgood MJ, Shen L, McMahon AP: Sertoli cell signaling by Desert hedgehog regulates the male germline. *Curr Biol* **6**:298, 1996.

48. Chiang C, Litingtung Y, Lee E, Young KE, Corden J L, Westphal H, Beachy PA: Cyclopia and defective axial patterning in mice lacking Sonic hedgehog gene function. *Nature* **383**:407, 1996.

49. Helms JA, Kim CH, Hu D, Minkoff R, Thaller C, Eichele G: Sonic hedgehog participates in craniofacial morphogenesis and is down-regulated by teratogenic doses of retinoic acid. *Dev Biol* **187**:25, 1997.

50. Tanabe Y, Jessell TM: Diversity and pattern in the developing spinal cord. *Science* **274**:1115, 1996.

51. MacDonald R, Barth KA, Xu Q, Holder N, Mikkola I, Wilson W: Midline signalling is required for Pax gene regulation and patterning of the eyes. *Development* **121**:3267, 1995.

52. Ekker SC, Ungar AR, Greenstein P, von Kessler DP, Porter JA, Moon RT, Beachy PA: Patterning activities of vertebrate hedgehog proteins in the developing eye and brain. *Curr Biol* **5**:944, 1995.

53. Belloni E, Muenke M, Roessler E, Traverso G, Siegel-Bartelt J, Frumkin A, Mitchell HF, et al: Identification of Sonic Hedgehog as a candidate gene responsible for holoprosencephaly. *Nat Genet* **14**:353, 1996.

54. Roessler E, Belloni E, Gaudenz K, Jay P, Berta P, Scherer SW, Tsui LC, et al: Mutations in the human Sonic Hedgehog gene cause holoprosencephaly. *Nat Genet* **14**:357, 1996.

55. Beachy PA, Cooper MK, Young KE, von Kessler DP, Park W-J, Tanaka Hall TM, Leahy DJ, et al: Multiple roles of cholesterol in Hedgehog protein biogenesis and signaling. *Cold Spring Harb Symp Quant Biol* **62**:191, 1997.

56. Lee JJ, Ekker SC, von Kessler DP, Porter JA, Sun BI, Beachy PA: Autoproteolysis in hedgehog protein biogenesis. *Science* **266**:1528, 1994.

57. Porter JA, von Kessler DP, Ekker SC, Young KE, Lee JJ, Moses K, Beachy PA: The product of hedgehog autoproteolytic cleavage is active in local and long-range signaling. *Nature* **374**:363, 1995.

58. Porter JA, Young KE, Beachy PA: Cholesterol modification of Hedgehog signaling proteins in animal development. *Science* **274**:255, 1996.

59. LÂpez-Martínez A, Chang DT, Chiang C, Porter JA, Ros MA, Simandl BK, Beachy PA, et al: Limb-patterning activity and restricted posterior localization of the amino-terminal product of sonic hedgehog cleavage. *Curr Biol* **5**:791, 1995.

60. Lai C-J, Ekker SC, Beachy PA, Moon RT: Patterning of the neural ectoderm of *Xenopus laevis* by the amino-terminal product of hedgehog autoproteolytic cleavage. *Development* **121**:2349, 1995.

61. Roelink H, Porter JA, Chiang C, Tanabe Y, Chang DT, Beachy PA, Jessell TM: Floor plate and motor neuron induction by different concentrations of the amino-terminal cleavage product of Sonic hedgehog autoproteolysis. *Cell* **81**:445, 1995.

62. Marti E, Bumcrot DA, Takada R, McMahon AP: Requirement of the 19K form of sonic hedgehog for induction of distinct ventral cell types in CNS explants. *Nature* **375**:322, 1995.

63. Fan CM, Porter J.A, Chiang C, Chang D T, Beachy PA, Tessier-Lavigne M: Long-range sclerotome induction by Sonic Hedgehog: Direct role of the amino-terminal cleavage product and modulation by the cyclic AMP signaling pathway. *Cell* **81**:457, 1995.

64. Hynes M, Porter JA, Chiang C, Chang D, Tessier-Lavigne M, Beachy PA, Rosenthal A: Induction of midbrain dopaminergic neurons by Sonic Hedgehog. *Neuron* **15**:35, 1995.

65. Porter JA, Ekker SC, Park W-J, von Kessler DP, Young KE, Chen C-H, Ma Y, et al: Hedgehog patterning activity: Role of lipophilic modification mediated by the carboxy-terminal autoprocessing domain. *Cell* **86**:21, 1996.

66. Hall TMT, Porter JA, Young KE, Koonin EV, Beachy PA, Leahy DJ: Crystal structure of a Hedgehog autoprocessing domain: Conservation of structure, sequence, and cleavage mechanism between Hedgehog and self-splicing proteins. *Cell* **91**:85, 1997.

67. Pepinsky RB, Zeng C, Wen D, Rayhorn P, Baker DP, Williams KP, Bixler SA, et al: Identification of a palmitic acid-modified form of human Sonic hedgehog. *J Biol Chem* **273**:14037, 1998.

68. Roessler E, Belloni E, Gaudenz K, Vargas F, Scherer SW, Tsui L-C, Muenke M: Mutations in the carboxy-terminal domain of the sonic hedgehog gene cause holoprosencephaly. *Hum Mol Genet* **6**:1847, 1997.

69. Nanni L, Ming JE, Bocian M, Steinhaus K, Bianchi DW, de Die-Smulders de C, Gianotti A, et al: The mutational spectrum of the *Sonic Hedgehog* gene in holoprosencephaly: *SHH* mutations cause a significant proportion of autosomal dominant holoprosencephaly. *Hum Mol Genet* **8**:2479, 1999.

70. Odent S, Attié-Bitach T, Blayau M, Mathieu M, Augé J, Delezoïde AL, Le Gall JY, et al: Expression of the *Sonic hedgehog* (SHH) gene during early human development and phenotypic expression of new mutations causing holoprosencephaly. *Hum Mol Genet* **8**:1683, 1999.

71. Epps JL, Jones JB, Tanda S: Oroshigane, a new segment polarity gene of *Drosophila melanogaster*, functions in hedgehog signal transduction. *Genetics* **145**:1041, 1997.

72. Goodrich LV, Scott MP: Hedgehog and patched in neural development and disease. *Neuron* **21**:1243, 1998.

73. Ingham PW: Transducing hedgehog: The story so far. *EMBO J* **17**:3505, 1998.

74. Hooper JE, Scott MP: The Drosophila patched gene encodes a putative membrane protein required for segmental patterning. *Cell* **59**:751, 1989.

75. Nakano Y, Guerrero I, Hidalgo A, Taylor A, Whittle JR, Ingham PW: A protein with several possible membrane-spanning domains encoded by the *Drosophila* segment polarity gene patched. *Nature* **341**:508, 1989.

76. Alcedo J, Ayzenzon M, Von Ohlen T, Noll M, Hooper JE: The *Drosophila* smoothened gene encodes a seven-pass membrane protein, a putative receptor for the Hedgehog signal. *Cell* **86**:221, 1996.

77. van den Heuvel M, Ingham PW: Smoothened encodes a receptor-like serpentine protein required for hedgehog signaling. *Nature* **382**:547, 1996.

78. Ingham PW, Taylor AM, Nakano Y: Role of the *Drosophila* patched gene in positional signalling. *Nature* **353**:184, 1991.

79. Ingham PW: Localized hedgehog activity controls spatial limits of wingless transcription in the Drosophila embryo. *Nature* **366**:560, 1993.

80. Chen Y, Struhl G: Dual roles for patched in sequestering and transducing hedgehog. *Cell* **87**:553, 1996.

81. Stone DM, Hynes M, Armanini M, Swanson TA, Gu Q, Johnson RL, Scott MP, et al: The tumor-suppressor gene patched encodes a candidate receptor for sonic hedgehog. *Nature* **384**:129, 1996.

82. Goodrich LV, Johnson RL, Milenkovic L, McMahon JA, Scott MP: Conservation of the hedgehog/patched signaling pathway from flies to mice: Induction of a mouse Patched gene by Hedgehog. *Genes Dev* **10**:301, 1996.

83. Marigo V, Scott MP, Johnson RL, Goodrich LV, Tabin CJ: Conservation in hedgehog signaling: Induction of a chicken patched homolog by Sonic hedgehog in the developing limb. *Development* **122**:1225, 1996.

84. Concordet JP, Lewis KE, Moore JW, Goodrich LV, Johnson RL, Scott MP, Ingham PW: Spatial regulation of a zebrafish patched homologue reflects the roles of sonic hedgehog and protein kinaseA in neural tube and somite patterning. *Development* **122**:2835, 1996.

85. Hahn H, Christiansend J, Wicking C, Zaphiropoulos PG, Chidambaram A, Gerrard B, Vorechovsky I, et al: A mammalian patched homolog is expressed in target tissues of sonic hedgehog and maps to a region associated with developmental abnormalities. *J Biol Chem* **271**:12125, 1996b.

86. Johnson RL, Rothman AL, Xie J, Goodrich LV, Bare JW, Bonifas JM, Quinn AG, et al: Human homolog of patched, a candidate gene for the basal cell nevus syndrome. *Science* **272**:1668, 1996.

87. Takabatake T, Ogawa M, Takahashi TC, Mizuno M, Okamoto M, Takeshima K: Hedgehog and patched gene expression in adult ocular tissues. *FEBS Lett* **410**:485, 1997.

88. Motoyama J, Takabatake T, Takeshima K, Hui CC: *PTCH2*, a second mouse Patched gene is co-expressed with Sonic hedgehog. *Nat Genet* **18**:104, 1998.

89. Goodrich LV, Milenkovic L, Higgins KM, Scott MP: Altered neural cell fates and medulloblastoma on mouse patched mutants. *Science* **277**:1109, 1997.

90. Hahn H, Wicking C, Zaphiropoulos PG, Gailani MP, Shanley S, Chidambaram A, Vorechovsky I, et al: Mutations of the human homolog of *Drosophila* patched in the nevoid basal cell carcinoma syndrome. *Cell* **85**:841, 1996a.

91. Hahn H, Wojnowski L, Zimmer AM, Hall J, Miller G, Zimmer A: Rhabdomyosarcomas and radiation hypersensitivity in a mouse model of Gorlin syndrome. *Nat Med* **4**:619, 1998.

92. Gailani M, Stahle-Backdahl M, Leffell D, Glynn M, Zaphiropoulos P, Pressman C, Unden A, et al: The role of the human homologue of *Drosophila* patched in sporadic basal cell carcinomas. *Nat Genet* **14**:78, 1996.

93. Reifenberger J, Wolter M, Weber RG, Megahed M, Ruzicka T, Lichter P, Reifenberger G: Missense mutations in SMOH in sporadic basal cell carcinomas of the skin and primitive neuroectodermal tumors of the central nervous system. *Cancer Res* **58**:1798, 1998.

94. Wolter M, Reifenberger J, Sommer C, Ruzicka T, Reifenberger G: Mutations in the human homologue of the Drosophila segment polarity gene patched (PTCH) in sporadic basal cell carcinomas of the skin and primitive neuroectodermal tumors of the central nervous system. *Cancer Res* **57**:2581, 1997.

95. Gorlin R: Nevoid basal-cell carcinoma syndrome. *Medicine* **66**:98, 1987.

96. Kimonis VE, Goldstein AM, Pastakia B, Yang ML, Kase R, DiGiovanna JJ, Bale AE, et al: Clinical manifestations in 105 persons with nevoid basal cell carcinoma syndrome. *Am J Med Genet* **69**:299, 1997.

97. Xie J, Murone M, Luoh S-M, Ryan A, Gu Q, Zhang C, Bonifas JM, et al: Activating Smoothened mutations in sporadic basal-cell carcinoma. *Nature* **391**:90, 1998.

98. Lam CW, Xie J, To KF, Ng HK, Lee KC, Yuen NW, Lim PL, et al: A frequent activated smoothened mutation in sporadic basal cell carcinomas. *Oncogene* **18**:833, 1999.

99. Murone M, Rosenthal A, de Sauvage FJ: Sonic hedgehog signaling by the patched-smoothened receptor complex. *Curr Biol* **9**:76, 1999.

100. Dahmane N, Lee J, Robins P, Heller P, Ruiz I, Altaba A: Activation of the transcription factor Gli1 and the sonic hedgehog signaling pathway in skin tumors. *Nature* **389**:876, 1997.

101. Fan H, Oro AE, Scott MP, Khavari PA: Induction of basal cell carcinoma features in transgenic human skin expressing Sonic Hedgehog. *Nat Med* **3**:788, 1997.

102. Oro AE, Higgins KM, Hu Z, Bonifas JM, Epstein EH Jr, Scott MP: Basal cell carcinomas in mice overexpressing sonic hedgehog. *Science* **276**:817, 1997.

103. Carpenter D, Stone DM, Brush J, Ryan A, Armanini M, Frantz G, Rosenthal A, et al: Characterization of two patched receptors for the vertebrate hedgehog protein family. *Proc Natl Acad Sci U S A* **95**:13630, 1998.

104. Marigo V, Davey RA, Zuo V, Cunningham JM, Tabin CJ: Biochemical evidence that patched in the hedgehog receptor. *Nature* **384**:176, 1996.

105. Fuse N, Maiti T, Wang B, Porter JA, Tanaka Hall TM, Leahy DJ, Beachy PA: Sonic hedgehog protein signals not as a hydrolytic enzyme but as an apparent ligand for Patched. *Proc Natl Acad Sci U S A* **96**:11049, 1999.

106. Chen Y, Struhl G: Dual roles for patched in sequestering and transducing hedgehog. *Cell* **87**:553, 1996.

107. Chuang PT, McMahon AP: Vertebrate Hedgehog signaling modulated by induction of a Hedgehog-binding protein. *Nature* **397**:617, 1999.

108. Robbins DJ, Nybakken KE, Kobajshi R, Sisson JC, Bishop JM, Therond PP: Hedgehog elicits signal transduction by means of a large complex containing the Kinesin-related protein costal2. *Cell* **90**:225, 1997.

109. Sisson JC, Ho KS, Suyama K, Scott MP: Costal2, a novel kinesin-related protein in the hedgehog signaling pathway. *Cell* **90**:235, 1997.

110. Thérond P, Busson D, Guillemet E, Limbourg-Bouchon B, Preat T, Terracol R, Tricoire H, et al: Molecular organisation and expression pattern of the segment polarity gene fused of *Drosophila* melanogaster. *Mech Dev* **44**:65, 1993.

111. Thérond P, Alves G, Limbourg-Bouchon B, Tricoire H, Guillemet E, Brissard-Zahraoui J, Lamour-Isnard C, et al: Functional domains of fused, a serine-threonine kinase required for signaling in Drosophila. *Genetics* **142**:1181, 1996.

112. Monnier V, Dussillol F, Alves G, Lamour-Isnard C, Plessis A: Suppressor of fused links fused and cubitus interruptus on the hedgehog signalling pathway. *Curr Biol* **8**:583, 1998.

113. Akimaru H, Chen Y, Dai P, Hou DX, Nonaka M, Smolik SM, Armstrong S, et al: Drosophila CBP is a co-activator of cubitus interruptus in hedgehog signalling. *Nature* **386**:735, 1997.

114. Bannister AJ, Kouzarides T: The CBP co-activator is a histone acetyltransferase. *Nature* **384**:641, 1996.

115. Aza-Blanc P, Ramirez-Weber F-A, Laget M-P, Schwartz C, Kornberg TB: Proteolysis that is inhibited by hedgehog targets cubitus interruptus protein to the nucleus and converts it to a repressor. *Cell* **89**:1043, 1997.

116. Chen CH, von Kessler DP, Park W, Wang B, Ma Y, Beachy PA: Nuclear trafficking of cubitus interruptus in the transcriptional regulation of Hedgehog target gene expression. *Cell* **98**:305, 1999.

117. Hepker J, Wang QT, Motzny CK, Holmgren R, Orenic TV: *Drosophila* cubitus interruptus forms a negative feedback loop with patched and regulates expression of Hedgehog target genes. *Development* **124**:549, 1997.

118. Alexandre C, Jacinto A, Ingham W: Transcriptional activation of hedgehog target genes in Drosophila is mediated directly by the cubitus interruptus protein, a member of the GLI family of zinc finger DNA-binding proteins. *Genes Dev* **10**:2003, 1996.

119. Jiang J, Struhl G: Regulation of the hedgehog and wingless signalling pathways by the F-box/WD40-repeat protein Slimb. *Nature* **391**:493, 1998.

120. Jiang J, Struhl G: Protein kinase A and hedgehog signaling in *Drosophila* limb development. *Cell* **80**:563, 1995.

121. Lepage T, Cohen SM, Diaz-Benjumea FJ, Parkhurst SM: Signal transduction by cAMP-dependent protein kinase A in *Drosophila* limb patterning. *Nature* **373**:711, 1995.

122. Li W, Ohlmeyer J, Lane M, Kalderon D: Function of protein kinase A in hedgehog signal transduction and *Drosophila* imaginal disc development. *Cell* **80**:553, 1995.

123. Pan D, Rubin GM: cAMP-dependent protein kinase and hedgehog act antagonistically in regulating decapentaplegic transcription in *Drosophila* imaginal discs. *Cell* **80**:543, 1995.

124. Ohlmeyer JT, Kalderon D: Dual pathways for induction of wingless expression by protein kinase A and Hedgehog in *Drosophila* embryos. *Genes Dev* **11**:2250, 1997.

125. Chen Y, Gallaher N, Goodman R, Smolik S: Protein kinase A directly regulates the activity and proteolysis of cubitus interruptus. *Proc Natl Acad Sci U S A* **95**:2349, 1998.

126. Chen Y, Cardinaux JR, Goodman RH, Smolik SM: Mutants of cubitus interruptus that are independent of PKA regulation are independent of hedgehog signaling. *Development* **126**:3607, 1999.

127. Theodosiou NA, Zhang S, Wang WY, Xu T: Slimb coordinates wg and dpp expression in the dorsal-ventral and anterior-posterior axes during limb development. *Development* **125**:3411, 1998.

128. Ohlmeyer JT, Kalderon D: Hedgehog stimulates maturation of cubitus interruptus into a labile transcriptional activator. *Nature* **396**:749, 1998.

129. Thérond PP, Knight JD, Kornberg TB, Bishop JM: Phosphorylation of the fused protein kinase in response to signaling from hedgehog. *Proc Nat Acad Sci* **93**:4224, 1996.

130. Ding Q, Fukami, S, Meng X, Nishizaki Y, Zhang X, Sasaki H, Dlugosz A, et al: Mouse suppressor of fused is a negative regulator of sonic hedgehog signaling and alters the subcellular distribution of gli1. *Curr Biol* **9**:1119, 1999.

131. Kogerman P, Grimm T, Kogerman L, Krause D, Unden AB, Sandstedt B, Toftgard R, et al: Mammalian suppressor-of-fused modulates nuclear-cytoplasmic shuttling of GLI-1. *Nat Cell Biol* **1**:312, 1999.

132. Pearse RV 2d, Collier LS, Scott MP, Tabin CJ: Vertebrate homologs of *Drosophila* suppressor of fused interact with the gli family of transcriptional regulators. *Dev Biol* **212**:323, 1999.

133. Epstein DJ, Marti E, Scott MP, McMahon AP: Antagonizing cAMP-dependent protein kinase A in the dorsal CNS activates a conserved Sonic hedgehog signaling pathway. *Development* **122**:2885, 1996.

134. Hammerschmidt M, Bitgood MJ, McMahon AP: Protein kinase A is a common negative regulator of Hedgehog signaling in the vertebrate embryo. *Genes Dev* **10**:647, 1996.

135. Ungar AR, Moon RT: Inhibition of protein kinase A phenocopies ectopic expression of hedgehog in the CNS of wild-type and cyclops mutant embryos. *Dev Biol* **178**:186, 1996.

136. Wang B, Falon JF, Beachy PA: Hedgehog-regulated processing of Gli3 produces an anterior/posterior represso gradient in the developing vertebrate limb. *Cell* **100**:423, 2000.

137. Ding Q, Motoyama J, Gasca S, Mo R, Sasaki H, Rossant J, Hui CC: Diminished Sonic hedgehog signaling and lack of floor plate differentiation in Gli2 mutant mice. *Development* **125**:2533, 1998.

138. Matise MP, Epstein DJ, Park HL, Platt KA, Joyner AL: Gli2 is required for induction of floor plate and adjacent cells, but not most ventral neurons in the mouse central nervous system. *Development* **125**:2759, 1998.

139. Vortkamp A, Lee K, Lanske B, Segre GV, Kronenberg HM, Tabin CJ: Regulation of rate of cartilage differentiation by Indian hedgehog and PTH-related protein. *Science* **273**:613, 1996.

140. Hynes M, Stone D, Dowd M, Pitts-Meek S, Goddard A, Gurney A, Rosenthal A: Control of cell pattern in the neural tube by the zinc finger transcription factor and oncogene Gli-1. *Neuron* **19**:15, 1997.

141. Lee JJ, Platt KA, Censullo P, Ruiz I Altaba AR: Gli1 is a target of Sonic Hedgehog that induces ventral neural tube development. *Development* **124**:2537, 1997.

142. Sasaki H, Hui C-C, Nakafuku M, Kondoh H: A binding site for Gli proteins is essential for HNF3β floor plate enhancer activity in transgenics and can respond to Shh *in vitro*. *Development* **124**:1313, 1997.

143. Ruiz i Altaba A: Combinatorial Gli gene function in floor plate and neuronal inductions by sonic hedgehog. *Development* **125**:2203, 1998.

144. Marigo V, Johnson RL, Vortkamp A, Tabin CJ: Sonic hedgehog differentially regulates expression of GLI and GLI3 during limb development. *Developmental Biology* **180**:273, 1996.

145. Mo R, Freer AM, Zinyk DL, Crackower MA, Michaud J, Heng HH-Q, Chik KW, et al: Specific and redundant functions of Gli2 and Gli3 zinc finger genes in skeletal patterning and development. *Development* **124**:113, 1997.

146. Karlstrom RO, Talbot WS, Schier AF: Comparative synteny cloning of zebra fish you-too: Mutations in the Hedgehog target gli2 affect ventral forebrain development. *Genes Dev* **13**:388, 1999.

147. Krishnan V, Pereira FA, Qiu Y, Chen C-H, Beachy PA, Tsai SY, Tsai M-J: Sonic hedgehog induced expression of COUP-TFII is mediated by a protein phosphatase. *Science* **278**:1947, 1997.

148. Kang S, Graham JM, Haskins-Olney A, Biesecker LG: Gli3 frame-shift mutations cause autosomal dominant Pallister-Hall syndrome. *Nat Genet* **15**:266, 1997.

149. Radhakrishna U, Wild A, Grzeschik K-H, Antonarakis SE: Mutation in GLI3 in postaxial polydactyly type A. *Nat Genet* **15**:269, 1997.

150. Wild A, Kalff-Suske M, Vortkamp A, Bornholdt D, König R, Grzeschik KH: Point mutations in human GLI3 cause Greig syndrome. *Hum Mol Genet* **6**:1979, 1998.

151. Biesecker LG: Strike three for GLI3. *Nat Genet* **15**:259, 1997.

152. Biesecker LG, Graham JM Jr: Pallister-Hall syndrome. *J Med Genet* **33**:585, 1996.

153. Ming JE, Roessler E, Muenke M: Human developmental disorders and the sonic hedgehog pathway. *Mol Med Today* **4**:343, 1998.

154. Petrij F, Giles RH, Dauwerse HG, Saris JJ, Hennekam RC, Masuno M, Tommerup N, et al: Rubinstein-Taybi syndrome caused by mutations in the transcriptional co-activator CBP. *Nature* **376**:348, 1995.

155. Strahle U, Jesuthasan S, Blader P, Garcia-Villalba P, Hatta K, Ingham PW: One-eyed pinhead is required for development of the ventral midline of the zebra fish (Danio rerio) neural tube. *Genes Funct* **1**:131, 1997.

156. Zhang J, Talbot WS, Schier AF: Positional cloning identifies zebra fish one-eyed pinhead as a permissive EGF-related ligand required during gastrulation. *Cell* **92**:241, 1998.

157. Gritsman K, Zhang J, Cheng S, Heckscher E, Talbot WS, Schier AF: The EGF-CFC protein one-eyed pinhead is essential for nodal signaling. *Cell* **97**:121, 1999.

158. Feldman B, Gates MA, Egan ES, Dougan ST, Rennebeck G, Sirotkin HI, Schier AF, et al: Zebra fish organizer development and germ-layer formation require nodal-related signals. *Nature* **395**:181, 1998.

159. Rebagliati MR, Toyama R, Fricke C, Haffter P, Dawid IB: Zebrafish nodal-related genes are implicated in axial patterning and establishing left-right asymmetry. *Dev Biol* **199**:261, 1998.

160. Sampath K, Rubinstein AL, Cheng AM, Liang JO, Fekany K, Solnica-Krezel L, Korzh V, et al: Induction of the zebra fish ventral brain and floorplate requires cyclops/nodal signalling. *Nature* **395**:185, 1998.

161. Conlon FL, Lyons KM, Takaesu N, Barth KS, Kispert A, Herrmann B, Robertson EJ: A primary requirement for nodal in the formation and maintenance of the primitive streak in the mouse. *Development* **120**:1919, 1994.

162. Zhou X, Sasaki H, Lowe L, Hogan BL, Kuehn MR: Nodal is a novel TGF-beta-like gene expressed in the mouse node during gastrulation. *Nature* **361**:543, 1993.

163. Nomura M, Li E: Smad2 role in mesoderm formation, left-right patterning and craniofacial development. *Nature* **393**:786, 1998.

164. Kelley RI, Roessler E, Hennekam RCM, Feldman GI, Kosaki K, Jones MC, Palumbos JC, et al: Holoprosencephaly in RSH/Smith-Lemli-Opitz syndrome: does abnormal cholesterol metabolism affect the function of sonic hedgehog? *Am J Med Genet* **66**:478, 1996.

165. Dale K, Sattar N, Heemskerk J, Clarke JD, Placzek M, Dodd J: Differential patterning of ventral midline cells by axial mesoderm is regulated by BMP7 and chordin. *Development* **126**:397, 1999.

166. Dudley AT, Robertson EJ: Overlapping expression domains of bone morphogenetic protein family members potentially account for limited tissue defects in BMP7 deficient embryos. *Dev Dyn* **208**:349, 1997.

167. Jena N, Martin-Seisdedos C, McCue P, Croce CM: BMP7 null mutation in mice: Developmental defects in skeleton, kidney, and eye. *Exp Cell Res* **230**:28, 1997.

168. Dehart DB, Lanoue L, Tint GS, Sulik KK: Pathogenesis of malformations in a rodent model for Smith-Lemli-Opitz Syndrome. *Am J Med Genet* **68**:328, 1997.

169. Roux C: Action teratogene du triparanol chez l'animal. *Arch Franc Pediatr* **21**:451, 1964.

170. Roux C: Action teratogene chez le rat d'un inhibiteur de la synthese du cholesterol, le AY9944. *C R Soc Biol* **160**:1353, 1966.

171. Roux C, Horvath C, Dupuis R: Teratogenic action and embryo lethality of AY 9944. Prevention by a hypercholesterolemia-provoking diet. *Teratology* **19**:35, 1979.

172. Kolf-Clauw M, Chevy F, Sillart B, Citadelle D, Roux C: Inhibition of 7-dedyrocholesterol reductase by the teratogen AY9944: A rat model for Smith-Lemli-Opitz syndrome. *Teratology* **54**:115, 1996.

173. Binns W, Thacker EJ, James LF, Huffman WT: A congenital cyclopian-type malformation in lambs. *J Am Vet Med Assoc* **134**:180, 1959.

174. Binns W, James LF, Shupe JL, Everett G: A congenital cyclopian-type malformation in lambs induced by maternal ingestion of a range plant, Veratrum californicum. *Am J Vet Res* **24**:1164, 1963.

175. Binns W, James LF, Keeler RF, Balls L: Effects of teratogenic agents in range plants. *Cancer Res* **28**:2323, 1968.

176. Keeler RF, Binns W: Teratogenic compounds of Veratrum californicum (Durand): V. Comparison of cyclopian effects of steroidal alkaloids from the plant and structurally related compounds from other sources. *Teratology* **1**:5,1968.

177. Cooper MK, Porter JA, Young KE, Beachy PA: Plant-derived and synthetic teratogens inhibit the ability of target tissues to respond to Sonic hedgehog signaling. *Science* **280**:1603, 1998.

178. Incardona JP, Gaffield W, Kapur RP, Roelink H: The teratogenic Veratrum alkaloid cyclopamine inhibits sonic hedgehog signal transduction. *Development* **125**:3553, 1998.

179. Yoshikawa H: Effects of drugs on cholesterol esterification in normal and Niemann-Pick type C fibroblasts: AY-9944, other cationic amphiphilic drugs and DMSO. *Brain Dev* **13**:115, 1991.

180. Willnow TE, Hilpert J, Armstrong SA, Rohlmann A, Jammer RE, Burns DK, Herz J: Defective forebrain development in mice lacking gp330/megalin. *Proc Natl Acad Sci U S A* **93**:8460, 1996.

181. Fitzky B, Witsch-Baumgartner M, Erdel M, Lee J, Paik Y, Glossmann H, Utermann G, et al: Mutations in the Delta7-sterol reductase gene in patients with the Smith-Lemli-Opitz syndrome. *Proc Natl Acad Sci U S A* **95**:8181, 1998.

182. Wassif C, Maslen C, Kachilele-Linjewile S, Lin D, Linck L, Connor W, Steiner R, et al: Mutations in the human sterol delta7-reductase gene at 11q12-13 cause Smith-Lemli-Opitz syndrome. *Am J Hum Genet* **63**:55, 1998.

183. Smith DW, Lemli L, Opitz JM: A newly recognized syndrome of multiple congenital anomalies. *J Ped* **64**:210, 1964.

184. Opitz JM, Zellweger H, Shannon WR, Ptacek LJ: The RSH syndrome, in Bergsma, D (ed): *The First Conference on the Clinical Delineation of Birth Defects. Part II: Malformation Syndromes*. New York, The National Foundation March of Dimes, 1969, p 43.

185. Opitz J: RSH/SLO ("Smith-Lemli-Opitz") syndrome: Historical, genetic, and developmental considerations. *Am J Med Genet* 50:344, 1994.

186. Salen G, Shefer S, Batta AK, Tint GS, Xu G, Honda A, Irons M, et al: Abnormal cholesterol biosynthesis in the Smith-Lemli-Opitz syndrome. *J Lipid Res* 37:1169, 1996.

187. Irons M, Elias ER, Salen G, Tint GS, Batta AK: Defective cholesterol biosynthesis in Smith-Lemli-Opitz syndrome. *Lancet* 341:1414, 1993.

188. Tint OS, Irons M, Elias ER, Batta AK, Frieden R, Chen TS, Salen G: Defective cholesterol biosynthesis associated with the Smith-Lemli-Opitz syndrome. *N Engl J Med* 330:107, 1994.

189. Stefansson S, Chappell DA, Argraves KM, Strickland DK, Argraves WS: Glycoprotein 330/low-density lipoprotein receptor-related protein-2 mediates endocytosis of low-density lipoproteins via interaction with apolipoprotein B100. *J Biol Chem* 270:19417, 1995.

190. Hertz J, Willnow TE, Farese RV: Cholesterol, hedgehog and embryogenesis. *Nat Genet* 15:123, 1997.

191. Riddle RD, Johnson RL, Laufer E, Tabin CJ: Sonic hedgehog mediates the polarizing activity of the ZPA. *Cell* 75:1401, 1993.

192. Ericson J, Morton S, Kawakami A, Roelink H, Jessell TM: Two critical periods of sonic hedgehog signaling required for the specification of motor neuron identity. *Cell* 87:661, 1996.

193. Carstea ED Morris JA, Coleman KG, Loftus SK, Zhang D, Cummings C, Gu J, et al: Niemann-Pick C1 disease gene: Homology to mediators of cholesterol homeostasis. *Science* 277:228, 1997.

194. Loftus SK, Morris JA, Carstea ED, Gu JZ, Cummings C, Brown A, Ellison J, et al: Murine model of Niemann-Pick C disease: Mutation in a cholesterol homeostasis gene. *Science* 277:232, 1997.

195. Gil G, Faust JR, Chin DJ, Goldstein JL, Brown MS: Membrane-bound domain of HMG CoA reductase is required for sterol-enhanced degradation of the enzyme. *Cell* 41:249, 1985.

196. Hua X, Nohturfft A, Goldstein JL, Brown MS: Sterol resistance in CHO cells traced to point mutation in SREBP cleavage-activating protein. *Cell* 87:415, 1996.

197. Nohturfft A, Brown M, Goldstein J: Sterols regulate processing of carbohydrate chains of wild-type SREBP cleavage-activating protein (SCAP), but not sterol-resistant mutants Y298CorD443N. *Proc Natl Acad Sci U S A* 95:12848, 1998.

197a. Taipale J, Cooper MK, Chen JK, Wang B, Mann RK, Milenkovic L, Scott MP, Beachy PA: Effects of oncogenic mutations in Smoothened and Patched can be reversed by cyclopamine. *Nature* 406:1005, 2000.

198. Cohen MM Jr: Perspectives on holoprosencephaly, Part I. Epidemiology, genetics, and syndromology. *Teratology* 40:211, 1989.

199. Cohen MM Jr: Perspectives on holoprosencephaly, Part III. Spectra, distinctions, continuities, and discontinuities. *Am J Med Genet* 34:271, 1989.

200. DeMyer W: Holoprosencephaly (cyclopia-arhinencephaly), in Vinken PJ, Bruyn GW (eds): *Handbook of Clinical Neurology*. Amsterdam, North-Holland, 1977, p 431.

201. Jellinger K, Gross H, Kaltenbäck E, Grisold W: Holoprosencephaly and agenesis of the corpus callosum: Frequency of associated malformations. *Acta Neuropathol* 55:1, 1981.

202. Barkovich AJ: Apparent atypical callosal dysgenesis: analysis of MR findings in six cases and their relationship to holoprosencephaly. *AJNR Am J Neuroradiol* 11:333, 1990.

203. Sener RN: Anterior callosal agenesis in mild, lobar holoprosencephaly. *Pediatr Radiol* 25:385, 1995.

204. Rubenstein D, Cajade-Law AG, Youngman V, Hise JM, Baganz M: The development of the corpus callosum in semilobar and lobar holoprosencephaly. *Pediatr Radiol* 26:839, 1996.

205. Kurokawa Y, Tsuchita H, Sohma T, Kitami K, Takeda T, Hattori H: Holoprosencephaly with Dandy-Walker cyst: Rare coexistence of two major malformations. *Childs Nerv Syst* 6:51, 1990.

206. Rössing R, Friede RL: Holoprosencephaly with retroprosencephalic extracerebral cyst. *Dev Med Child Neurol* 34:164, 1992.

207. Takahashi S, Miyamoto A, Oki J, Saino T, Inyaku F: Alobar holoprosencephaly with diabetes insipidus and neuronal migration disorder. *Pediatr Radiol* 13:175, 1995.

208. Desai VN, Shields CL, Shields JA, Donoso LA, Wagner RS: Retinoblastoma associated with holoprosencephaly. *Am J Ophthalmol* 109:355, 1990.

209. Van Overbeeke JJ, Hillen B, Verneij-Keers CHR: The arterial pattern at the base of arhinencephalic and holoprosencephalic brains. *J Anat* 185:51, 1994.

210. Barkovich JA, Quint DJ: Middle interhemispheric fusion: An unusual variant of holoprosencephaly. *AJNR Am J Neuroradiol* 14:431, 1993.

210a. Mann SS, Naidich TP, Towbin BB, Doundoulakis SH: Imaging of postnatal maturation of the skull base. *Neuroimaging Clin N Am* 10:1, 2000.

211. Arnold WH, Sperber GH, Machin GA: Anatomy of the circle of Willis in three cases of human fetal synophthalmic holoprosencephaly. *Ann Anat* 178:553, 1996.

212. O'Rahilly R, Müller F: Interpretation of some median anomalies as illustrated by cyclopia and symmelia. *Teratology* 40:409, 1989.

213. Martínez-Frías ML, Bermejo E, García A, Galán E, Prieto L: Holoprosencephaly associated with caudal dysgenesis: A clinical-epidemiological analysis. *Am J Med Genet* 53:46, 1994.

214. DeMyer W, Zeman W, Palmer CG: The face predicts the brain: Diagnostic significance of median facial anomalies for holoprosencephaly (arhinencephaly). *Pediatrics* 34:256, 1963.

215. Ardinger HH, Bartley JA: Microcephaly in familial holoprosencephaly. *J Craniofac* 8:53, 1988.

216. Artman HG, Boyden E: Microphthalmia with single central incisor and hypopituitarism. *J Med Genet* 27:192, 1990.

217. Liberfarb RM, Abdo OP, Pruett RC: Ocular coloboma associated with a solitary maxillary central incisor and growth failure: manifestations of holoprosencephaly. *Ann Ophthal* 19:226, 1987.

218. Hennekam RCM, Van Noort D, de la Fuente FA, Norbruis OF: Agenesis of the nasal septal cartilage: Another sign in autosomal dominant holoprosencephaly. *Am J Med Genet* 39:121, 1991.

219. Arlis H, Ward RF: Congenital nasal pyriform aperture stenosis. Isolated abnormality vs developmental field defect. *Arch Otolaryngol Head Neck Surg* 118:989, 1992.

220. Hui Y, Friedberg J, Crysdale WS: Congenital nasal pyriform aperture stenosis as a presenting feature of holoprosencephaly. *Intl J Pediatr Otorhinolaryngol* 31:263, 1995.

221. Lo FS, Lee YJ, Lin SP, Shen EY, Huang JK, Lee KS: Solitary maxillary central incisor and congenital nasal pyriform aperture stenosis. *Eur J Pediatr* 157:39, 1998.

222. Gripp KW, Wotton D, Edwards MC, Roessler E, Ades L, Meinecke P, Richieri-Costa A, et al: Mutations in TGIF cause holoprosencephaly and link Nodal signaling to human neural axis determination. *Nat Genet* 25:205, 2000.

223. Kjær I, Keeling J, Russell B, Daugaard-Jensen J, Hansen BF: Palate structure in human holoprosencephaly correlates with the facial malformation and demonstrates a new palatal developmental field. *Am J Med Genet* 73:387, 1997.

224. Berry SA, Pierpoint ME, Gorlin RJ: Single central incisor in familial holoprosencephaly. *J Pediatr* 104:877, 1984.

225. Hattori H, Okuno T, Momoi K, Kataoka K, Mikawa H, Shiota K: Single central maxillary incisor and holoprosencephaly. *Am J Med Genet* 28:483, 1987.

226. Martin RA, Jones KL: Absence of the superior labial frenulum in holoprosencephaly: A new diagnostic sign. *J Pediatr* 133:150, 1998.

227. Collins AL, Lunt PW, Garrett C, Dennis NR: Holoprosencephaly: A family showing dominant inheritance and variable expression. *J Med Genet* 30:36, 1993.

228. Muenke M, Gurrieri F, Bay C, Yi DH, Collins AL, Johnson VP, Hennekam RCM, et al: Linkage of a human malformation, familial holoprosencephaly, to chromosome 7 and evidence for genetic heterogeneity. *Proc Nat Acad Sci U S A* 91:8102, 1994.

229. Romshe CA, Sotos JF: Hypothalamic-pituitary dysfunction in siblings of patients with holoprosencephaly. *J Pediatr* 83:1088, 1973.

230. Hasegawa Y, Hasegawa T, Yokoyama T, Kotoh S, Tsuchiya Y: Holoprosencephaly associated with diabetes insipidus and syndrome of inappropriate secretion of antidiuretic hormone. *J Pediatr* 117:756, 1990.

231. Barr M Jr, Cohen MM Jr: Holoprosencephaly survival and performance. *Am J Med Genet* 89:116, 1999.

232. Cayea PD, Balcar I, Alberti O Jr, Jones TB: Prenatal diagnosis of semilobar holoprosencephaly. *AJR Am J Roentgenol* 142:401, 1984.

233. Nyberg DA, Mack LA, Bronstein A, Hirsch J, Pagon RA: Holoprosencephaly: Prenatal sonographic diagnosis. *AJR Am J Roentgenol* 149:1051, 1987.

234. Tomà P, Costa A, Magnano GM, Cariati M, Lituania M: Holoprosencephaly: Prenatal diagnosis by sonography and magnetic resonance imaging. *Prenat Diagn* **10**:429, 1990.

235. Bronshtein M, Wiener Z: Early transvaginal sonographic diagnosis of alobar holoprosencephaly. *Prenat Diagn* **11**:459, 1991.

236. Trout T, Budorick NE, Pretorius DH, McGahan JP: Significance of orbital measurements in the fetus. *J Ultrasound Med* **13**:937, 1994.

237. van Zalen-Sprock R, van Vugt JMG, van der Harten HJ, Nieuwint AWM, van Geijn HP: First trimester diagnosis of cyclopia and holoprosencephaly. *J Ultrasound Med* **14**:631, 1995.

238. Stagiannis KD, Sepulveda W, Bower S: Early prenatal diagnosis of holoprosencephaly: The value of transvaginal ultrasonography. *Eur J Obstet Gynecol Reprod Biol* **61**:175, 1995.

239. Berry SM, Gosden C, Snijders RJM, Nicolaides KH: Fetal holoprosencephaly: Associated malformations and chromosomal defects. *Fetal Diagn Ther* **5**:92, 1990.

240. Wilson RD, Chitayat D, McGillivray BC: Fetal ultrasound abnormalities: correlation with fetal karyotype, autopsy findings, and postnatal outcome—Five year perspective study. *Am J Med Genet* **44**:586, 1992.

241. Pretorius DH, Nelson TR: Fetal face visualization using three-dimensional ultrasonography. *J Ultrasound Med* **14**:349, 1995.

242. Genbruch U, Baschat AA, Reusche E, Wallner SJ, Greiwe M: First trimester diagnosis of holoprosencephaly with a Dandy-Walker malformation by transvaginal ultrasonography. *J Ultrasound Med* **14**:619, 1995.

243. Sonigo PC, Rypens FF, Carteret M, Delezoide AL, Brunelle FO: MR imaging of fetal cerebral anomalies. *Pediatr Radiol* **28**:212, 1998.

244. Altman NR, Altman DH, Sheldon JJ, Laborgne J: Holoprosencephaly classified by computed tomography. *AJNR Am J Neuroradiol* **5**:433, 1984.

245. McGahan JP, Nyberg DA, Mack LA: Sonography of facial features of alobar and semilobar holoprosencephaly. *AJR Am J Roentgenol* **154**:143, 1990.

246. Derakhshan I, Sabouri-Deylami M, Lofti J: Holoprosencephaly: Computerized tomographic and pneumographic findings with anatomic correlation. *Arch Neurol* **37**:55, 1980.

247. Barkovich JA, Maroldo TV: Magnetic resonance imaging of normal and abnormal brain development. *Top Magn Reson Imaging* **5**:96, 1993.

248. Liu DPC, Burrowes DM, Qureshi MN: Cyclopia: Craniofacial appearance on MR and three-dimensional CT. *AJNR Am J Neuroradiol* **18**:543, 1997.

249. Elias DL, Kawamoto HK, Wilson LF: Holoprosencephaly and midline facial anomalies: Redefining classification and management. *Plast Reconstr Surg* **90**:951, 1992.

250. Pensler JM, Giese S, Charrow J: Surgical treatment of patients with lobar holoprosencephaly: A personal note. *J Craniofac Surg* **4**:2, 1993.

251. Ronen GM, Andrews WL: Holoprosencephaly as a possible embryonic alcohol effect. *Am J Med Genet* **40**:151, 1991.

252. Lammer E, Chen D, Hoar R, Agnish N, Benk P, Braun J, Curry C, et al: Retinoic acid embryopathy. *N Engl J Med* **313**:837, 1985.

253. Byrne PJ, Silver MM, Gilbert JM, Cadera W, Tanswell AK: Cyclopia and congenital cytomegalovirus infection. *Am J Hum Genet* **28**:61, 1987.

254. Kotzot D, Weigl J, Huk W, Rott HD: Hydantoin syndrome with holoprosencephaly: A possible rare teratogenic effect. *Teratology* **48**:15, 1993.

255. Rosa F: Holoprosencephaly and antiepileptic exposures. *Teratology* **51**:230, 1995.

256. Koyama N, Komori S, Bessho T, Koyama K, Hiraumi Y, Maeda Y: Holoprosencephaly in a fetus with maternal medication of sulfasalazine in early gestation. *Clin Exp Obst Gyn* **22**:147, 1985.

257. Ronen GM: Holoprosencephaly and maternal low-calorie weight-reducing diet. *Am J Med Genet* **42**:139, 1992.

258. Barr M Jr, Hanson JW, Currey K, Sharp S, Toriello H, Schmickel RD, Wilson GA: Holoprosencephaly in infants of diabetic mothers. *J Pediatr* **102**:565, 1983.

259. Muenke M: Clinical, cytogenetic, and molecular approaches to the genetic heterogeneity of holoprosencephaly. *Am J Med Genet* **34**:237, 1989.

260. Muenke M: Holoprosencephaly as a genetic model for normal craniofacial development. *Sem Dev Biol* **5**:293, 1994.

261. Wallis DE, Roessler E, Hehr U, Nanni L, Wiltshire T, Richieri-Costa A, Gillessen-Kaesbach G, et al: Mutations in the homeodomain of the human *SIX3* gene cause holoprosencephaly. *Nat Genet* **22**:196, 1999.

262. Brown SA, Warburton D, Brown LY, Yu CY, Roeder ER, Stengel-Rutkowski S, Hennekam RC, et al: Holoprosencephaly due to mutations in ZIC2, a homologue of *Drosophila* odd-paired. *Nat Genet* **20**:180, 1998.

263. Brown SA, Brown LY, Yu CY, Warburton D, Muenke M: ZIC2, a human homologue of *odd-paired*, is in the 13q32 critical region and mutations are associated with holoprosencephaly. *Am J Hum Genet* **63**:A8, 1998.

264. Young ID, Madders DJ: Unknown syndrome: Holoprosencephaly, congenital heart defects, and polydactyly. *J Med Genet* **24**:714, 1987.

265. Verloes A, Aymé S, Gambarelli D, Gonzales M, Le Merrer M, Mulliez N, Philip N, et al: Holoprosencephaly-polydactyly ("pseudotrisomy 13") syndrome: A syndrome with features of hydrolethalus and Smith-Lemli-Opitz syndromes. A collaborative multicentre study. *J Med Genet* **28**:297, 1991.

266. Boles RG, Teebi AS, Neilson KA, Meyn MS: Pseudo-trisomy 13 syndrome with upper limb shortness and radial hypoplasia. *Am J Med Genet* **44**:638, 1992.

267. Cunniff C, Kelley RI, Krantz IE, Moser AE, Natowicz MR: The clinical and biochemical spectrum of patients with Smith-Lemli-Opitz syndrome and abnormal cholesterol metabolism. *Am J Med Genet* **68**:263, 1997.

268. Camera G, Lituania M, Cohen MM Jr: Holoprosencephaly and primary craniosynostosis: The Genoa syndrome. *Am J Med Genet* **47**:1161, 1993.

269. Bachman H, Clark RD, Salahi W: Holoprosencephaly and polydactyly: A possible expression of the hydrolethalus syndrome. *J Med Genet* **27**:50, 1990.

270. Morse RP, Rawnsley E, Sargent SK, Graham JM Jr: Prenatal diagnosis of a new syndrome: Holoprosencephaly with hypokinesia. *Prenat Diagn* **7**:631, 1987.

271. Steinfeld HJ: Case report 81: Holoprosencephaly and visceral defects with familial limb abnormalities. *Syndr Id* **8**:1, 1982.

272. Thomas M, Donnai D: Bilateral brachial amelia with facial clefts and holoprosencephaly. *Clin Dysmorph* **3**:266, 1994.

273. Hartsfield JK, Bixler D, DeMeyer WE: Syndrome identification case report 119. Hypertelorism associated with holoprosencephaly and ectrodactyly. *J Clin Dysmorphol* **2**:27, 1984.

274. Muenke M, Emanuel BS, Zackai EH: Holoprosencephaly: Association with interstitial deletion of 2p and review of the literature. *Am J Med Genet* **30**:29, 1988.

275. Roessler E, Muenke M: Holoprosencephaly: A paradigm for the complex genetics of brain development. *J Inherit Metab Dis* **21**:481, 1998.

276. Frézal J, Schinzel A: Report of the committee on clinical disorders, chromosome aberrations, and uniparental disomy. *Cytogenet Cell Genet* **58**:986, 1991.

277. Schell U, Wienberg J, Köhler A, Bray-Ward P, Ward DE, Wilson WG, Allen WP, et al: Molecular characterization of breakpoints in patients with holoprosencephaly and definition of the HPE2 critical region 2p21. *Hum Mol Genet* **5**:223, 1996.

278. Krauss CM, Liptak KJ, Aggerwai A, Robinson D: Inheritance and phenotypic expression of a t(7;9)(q36;q34)mat. *Am J Med Genet* **34**:514, 1988.

279. Hatziioannou AG, Krauss CM, Lewis MB, Halazonetis TD: Familial holoprosencephaly associated with a translocation breakpoint at chromosomal position 7q36. *Am J Med Genet* **40**:201, 1991.

280. Bedell MA, Jenkins NA, Copeland NG: Good genes in bad neighbourhoods. *Nat Genet* **12**:229, 1996.

281. Kleinjan D-J, Heyningen VV: Position effect in human genetic disease. *Hum Mol Genet* **7**:1611, 1998.

282. Kamnasaran D, Muenke M, O'Brien PCM, Ferguson-Smith MA, Cox DW: Agenesis of the corpus callosum associated with chromosome (4;14) translocation. *Am J Hum Genet* **65**:A277, 1999.

283. Gurrieri F, Trask BJ, van den Engh G, Krauss CM, Schinzel A, Pettenati MJ, Schindler D, et al: Physical mapping of the holoprosencephaly critical region of 7q36. *Nat Genet* **3**:247, 1993.

284. Roessler E, Ward DE, Gaudenz K, Belloni E, Scherer SW, Donnai D, Siegel-Bartelt J, et al: Cytogenetic rearrangements involving the loss of the sonic hedgehog gene at 7q36 cause holoprosencephaly. *Hum Genet* **100**:172, 1997.

285. Ming JE, Muenke M: Holoprosencephaly: from Homer to Hedgehog. *Clin Genet* **53**:155, 1998.

286. Chidambatam A, Goldstein AM, Gailani MR, Gerrard B, Bale SJ, DiGiovanna JJ, Bale A, et al: Mutations in the human homologue of the *Drosophila* patched gene in Caucasian and African-American Nevoid basal cell carcinoma syndrome patients. *Cancer Res* **56**:4599, 1996.

287. Raffel C, et al: Sporadic medulloblastomas contain *PTCH* mutations. *Cancer Res* **57**:842, 1997.

288. Xie J, Johnson RL, Zhang X, Bare JW, Waldman FM, Cogen PH, Menon AG, et al: Mutations of the PATCHED gene in several types of sporadic extracutaneous tumors. *Cancer Res* **57**:2369, 1997.

289. Maesawa C, Tamura G, Iwaya T, Ogasawara S, Ishida K, Sato N, Nishizuka S, et al: Mutations in the human homologue of the *Drosophila Patched* gene in esophageal squamous cell carcinoma. *Genes Chromosomes Cancer* **21**:276, 1998.

290. Vorechovsky I, Unden AB, Sandstedt B, Torfgard R, Stahle-Backdahl M: Trichoepitheliomas contain somatic mutations in the over-expressed *PTCH* gene: Support for a gatekeeper mechanism in skin tumorigenesis. *Cancer Res* **57**:4677, 1997.

291. Ming JE, Kaupas ME, Roessler E, Brunner HG, Nance WE, Stratton RF, Sujansky E, et al: Mutations of Patched in holoprosencephaly. *Am J Hum Genet* **63**:A27, 1998.

292. Brown S, Russo J, Chitayat D, Warburton D: The 13q-syndrome: The molecular definition of a critical deletion region in band 13q32. *Am J Hum Genet* **57**:859, 1998.

293. Benedyk MJ, Mullen JR, DiNardo S: Odd-paired: A zinc finger pair-rule protein required for the timely activation of engrailed and wingless in *Drosophila* embryos. *Genes Dev* **8**:105, 1994.

294. Aruga J, Nagai T, Tukuyama T, Hayashizaki Y, Okazaki Y, Chapman VM, Mikoshiba K: The mouse *Zic* gene family: Homologues of the Drosophila gene *odd-paired*. *J Biol Chem* **271**:1043, 1996.

295. Aruga J, Hayashizaki Y, Okazaki Y, Chapman VM, Mikoshiba K: Identification and characterization of *Zic4*, a new member of the mouse *Zic* gene family. *Gene* **172**:291, 1996.

296. Cimbora DM, Sakonju S: *Drosophila* midgut morphogenesis requires the function of segmentation gene *odd-paired*. *Dev Biol* **169**:580, 1995.

297. Grinblat Y, Gamse J, Patel M, Sive H: Determination of the zebra fish forebrain: Induction and patterning. *Development* **125**:4403, 1998.

298. Nagai T, Aruga J, Takada S, Gunther T, Sporle R, Schugart K, Mikoshiba K: The expression of the mouse Zic1, Zic2, and Zic3 gene suggests an essential role for Zic genes in body pattern formation. *Dev Biol* **182**:299, 1997.

299. Licht JD, Grossel MJ, Figge J, Hansen UM: *Drosophila* Kruppel protein is a transcriptional repressor. *Nature* **346**:76, 1990.

300. Bossone SA, Asselin C, Patel AJ, Marcu KB: MAZ, a zinc finger protein, binds to c-MYC and 2 gene sequences regulating transcriptional initiation and termination. *Proc Natl Acad Sci U S A* **89**:7452, 1992.

301. Han K, Manley JL: Functional domains of the *Drosophila* engrailed protein. *EMBO J* **12**:2723, 1992.

302. Han K, Manley JL: Transcriptional repression by the *Drosophila* even-skipped protein: Definition of a minimal repression domain. *Genes Dev* **7**:491, 1993.

303. Goodman FR, Mundlos S, Muragaki Y, Donnai D, Giovannucci-Uzielli MI, Lapi E, Majewski F, et al: Synpolydactyly phenotypes correlate with size of expansions in HOXD13 polyalanine tract. *Proc Natl Acad Sci U S A* **94**:7458, 1997.

304. Johnson KR, Sweet HO, Donahue LR, Ward-Bailey P, Bronson RT, Davisson MT: A new spontaneous mouse mutation of Hoxd13 with a polyalanine expansion and phenotype similar to human synpolydactyly. *Hum Mol Genet* **7**:1033, 1998.

305. Mundlos S, Otto F, Mulliken JB, Aylsworth AS, Albright S, Lindhout D, Cole WG, et al: Mutations involving the transcription factor CBFA1 cause cleidocranial dysplasia. *Cell* **89**:773, 1997.

306. Akarsu AN, Stoilov I, Yilmaz E, Sayli BS, Sarfarazi M: Genomic structure of *HOXD13* gene: A nine polyalanine duplication causes synpolydactyly in two unrelated families. *Hum Mol Genet* **5**:945, 1996.

307. Brais B, Bouchard JP, Xie YG, Rochefort DI, Chretien N, Tome FM, Lafreniere, et al: Short GCG expansions in the PABP2 gene cause oculopharyngeal muscular dystrophy. *Nat Genet* **18**:164, 1998.

308. Oliver G, Mailhos A, Wehr R, Copeland NG, Jenkins NA, Gruss P: Six3, a murine homolog of the sine oculus gene, demarcates the most anterior border of the developing neural plate and is expressed during eye development. *Development* **121**:4045, 1995.

309. Oliver G, Loosli F, Koster R, Wittbrodt J, Gruss P: Ectopic lens induction fish in response to the murine homeobox gene *Six3*. *Mech Dev* **60**:233, 1996.

310. Kobayashi M, Toyama R, Takada H, Dawid IB, Kawakami K: Overexpression of the forebrain-specific homeobox gene Six3 induces rostral forebrain enlargement in zebrafish. *Development* **125**:2973, 1998.

311. Loosli F, Winkler S, Wittbrodt J: *Six3* overexpression initiates the formation of ectopic retina. *Genes Dev* **13**:649, 1999.

312. Kawakami K, Ohto H, Takizawa T, Saito T: Identification and expression of Six family genes in mouse retina. *FEBS Lett* **393**:259, 1996.

313. Bovolenta P, Mallamaci A, Boncinelli E: Cloning and characterization of two chick homeobox genes, members of the *Six/sine oculis* family, expressed during eye development. *Int J Dev Biol* **1(Suppl)**:738, 1996.

314. Zubes ME, Perron M, Bang A, Jolt CD, Harris WA: Molecular cloning and expression analysis of the homeobox gene *Six3* in *Xenopus laevis*. *Dev Biol* **186**:314, 1997.

315. Loosli F, Koster RW, Carl M, Crone A, Wittbrodt J: *Six3*, a medaka homologue of the *Drosophila* homeobox gene *Sine oculis* is expressed in the anterior embryonic shield and the developing eye. *Mech Dev* **74**:150, 1998.

316. Seo HC, Drivenes O, Ellingsen S, Fjose A: Expression of two zebra fish homologues of the murine *Six3* gene demarcates the initial eye primordia. *Mech Dev* **73**:45, 1998.

317. Toy J, Yang J-M, Leppert GS, Sundin OH: The *Optx2* homeobox gene is expressed in early precursors of the eye and activates retina-specific genes. *Proc Natl Acad Sci U S A* **95**:10643, 1998.

318. Gillessen-Kaesbach, G: Familial holoprosencephaly: Further example of autosomal recessive inheritance. *Birth Defects* **30**:251, 1996.

319. Nanni L, Croen LA, Lammer EJ, Muenke M: Holoprosencephaly: Molecular study of a California population. *Am J Med Genet* **90**:315, 2000.

320. Overhauser J, Mitchell HF, Zackai EH, Tick DB, Rojas K, Muenke M: Physical mapping of the holoprosencephaly critical region in 18p11.3. *Am J Hum Genet* **57**:1080, 1995.

321. Edwards MC, Liegeois N, Horecka J, DePinho RA, G.F. Sprague J, Tyers M, Elledge SJ: Human CPR (cell cycle progression restoration) genes impart in a far-phenotype on yeast cells. *Genetics* **147**:1063, 1997.

322. Massagué J: TGF-$\beta$ signal transduction. *Ann Rev Biochem* **67**:753, 1998.

323. Wotton D, Lo RS, Lee S, Massagué J: A Smad transcriptional corepressor. *Cell* **97**:29, 1999.

324. Bertolino E, Reimund B, Wildt-Perinic, Clerc RG: A novel homeobox protein which recognizes a TGT core and functionally interferes with a retinoid-responsive motif. *J Biol Chem* **270**:31178, 1995.

325. Bertolino E, Wildt S, Richards G, Clerc RG: Expression of a novel murine homeobox gene in the developing cerebellar external granular layer during its proliferation. *Dev Dyn* **205**:410, 1996.

326. Webster WS, Johnston MC, Lammer EJ, Sulik K: Isoretinoin embryopathy and the cranial neural crest: An in vivo and in vitro study. *J Craniofac Genet* **6**:211, 1986.

327. Sulik KK, Cook CS, Webster WS: Teratogens and craniofacial malformations: Relationships to cell death. *Development* **103**:213, 1988.

328. Sulik KK, Dehart DB, Rogers JM, Chernoff N: Teratogenicity of low doses of all-trans retinoic acid in presomite mouse embryos. *Teratology* **51**:398, 1995.

329. Helms JA, Thaller C, Eichele G: Relationship between retinoic acid and sonic hedgehog, two polarizing signals in the chick wing bud. *Development* **120**:3267, 1994.

330. Hu D, Helms JA: The role of Shh in normal and abnormal craniofacial morphogenesis. *Development* **125**:4873, 1999.

331. Oh SP, Li E: The signaling pathway mediated by the type IIB activin receptor controls axial patterning and lateral asymmetry in the mouse. *Genes Dev* **11**:1812, 1997.

332. Muenke M, Bone LJ, Mitchell HF, Hart I, Walton K, Hall-Johnson K, Ippel EF, et al: Physical mapping of the holoprosencephaly critical region in 21q22.3, exclusion of SIM2 as a candidate gene for holoprosencephaly, and mapping of SIM2 to a region of chromosome 21 important for down syndrome. *Am J Hum Genet* **57**:1074, 1995.

333. Young M, Chen H, Lalioti MD, Antonarakis SE: The human lanosterol synthase gene maps to chromosome 21q22.3. *Hum Genet* **97**:620, 1996.

334. Roessler E, Mittaz L, Du Y, Scott HS, Chang J, Rossier C, Guipponi M, et al: Structure of the human lanosterol synthase gene and its analysis as a candidate for holoprosencephaly. *Hum Genet* **105**:489, 1999.

335. Glinka A, Wu W, Delius H, Monaghan AP, Blumenstock C, Niehrs C: Dickkopf-1 is a member of a new family of secreted proteins and functions in head induction. *Nature* 391:357, 1998.

336. Roessler E, Du Y, Glinka A, Dutra A, Niehrs C, Muenke M: The genomic structure, chromosomal localization, and analysis of the human *DKK1* head inducer gene as a candidate for holoprosencephaly. *Cytogenet Cell Genet* 89:220, 2000.

337. Ruiz i Altaba A, Prezioso VR, Darnell JE, Jessel TM: Sequential expression of *HNF-3α* and *HNF-3β* by embryonic organizing centers: the dorsal lip/node, notocord, and floor plate. *Mech Dev* 44:91, 1993.

338. Ang S-L, Rossant J: HNF-3β is essential for node and notocord formation in mouse development. *Cell* 78:561, 1994.

339. Weinstein DC, Ruiz i Altaba A, Chen WS, Hoodless P, Prezioso VR, Jessel TM, Darnell JE Jr: The winged-helix transcription factor HNF-3 beta is required for notocord development in the mouse embryo. *Cell* 78:575, 1994.

340. Filosa S, Rivera-Perez JA, Gomez AP, Gansmuller A, Sasaki H, Behringer RR, Ang SL: Goosecoid and HNF-3β genetically interact to regulate neural tube patterning during mouse embryogenesis. *Development* 124:2843, 1997.

341. Bouwmeester T, Kim S, Sasai Y, Lu B, De Robertis EM: Cerberus is a head-inducing secreted factor expressed in the anterior endoderm of the Spemann organizer. *Nature* 382:595, 1996.

342. Piccolo S, Agius E, Leyns L, Bhattacharyya S, Grunz H, Bouwmeester T, De Robertis EM: The head inducer Cerberus is a multifunctional antagonist of Nodal, BMP, and Wnt signals. *Nature* 397:707, 1999.

343. Talbot WS, Trevarrow B, Halpern ME, Melby AE, Farr G, Postlethwait JH, Jowett T, Kimmel CB, Kimelman D: A homeobox gene essential for zebra fish notocord development. *Nature* 378:150, 1995.

344. Halpern ME, Hatta K, Amacher SL, Talbot WS, Yan Y-L, Thisse B, Thisse C, Postlethwait JH, Kimmel CB: Genetic interactions in zebra fish midline development. *Dev Biol* 187:154, 1997.

345. Masai I, Heisenberg CP, Barth KA, Macdonald R, Adamek S, Wilson SW: *Floating head* and *masterblind* regulate neuronal patterning in the roof of the forebrain. *Neuron* 18:43, 1997.

346. Fekany K, Yamanaka Y, Leung T, Sirotkin HI, Topczewski J, Gates MA, Hibi M, et al: The zebra fish bozozok locus encodes Dharma, a homeoprotein essential for induction of gastrula organizer and dorsoanterior embryonic structures. *Development* 126:1427, 1999.

347. Wallis DE, Muenke M: Molecular mechanisms of holoprosencephaly. *Mol Genet Metab* 66:126, 1999.

348. Tabin CJ, McMahon AP: Recent advances in hedgehog signaling. *Trends Cell Biol* 7:442, 1997.

349. Alcedo J, Noll M: Hedgehog and its patched-smoothened receptor complex: A novel signaling mechanism at the cell surface. *Biol Chem* 37:583, 1997.

350. Hardcastle Z, Mo R, Hui C-C, Sharpe PT: The Shh pathway in tooth development: Defects in *Gli2* and *Gli3* mutants. *Development* 125:2803, 1998.

351. Heberlein U, Wolff T, Rubin GM: The TGF beta homolog *dpp* and the segment polarity gene *hedgehog* are required for propagation of a morphogenetic wave in the *Drosophila* retina. *Cell* 75:913, 1993.

352. Chen R, Amoui M, Zhang Z: Dachshund and eyes absent proteins form a complex and function synergistically to induce ectopic eye development in *Drosophila*. *Cell* 91:893, 1997.

353. Hatta K, Kimmel CB, Ho RK, Walker C: The cyclops mutation blocks specification of the floor plate of the zebra fish nervous system. *Nature* 350:339, 1991.

354. Kingsley DM: The TGF-β superfamily: New members, new receptors, and new genetic tests of function in different organisms. *Genes Dev* 8:133, 1994.

355. Whitman M: Smads and early developmental signaling by the TGFβ superfamily. *Genes Dev* 12:2445, 1998.

356. Heldin C-H, Miyazono K, Dijke PT: TGF-β signalling from cell membrane to nucleus through SMAD proteins. *Nature* 390:465, 1997.

357. Cheyette BNR, Green PJ, Martin K, Garren H, Hartenstein V, Zipursky SL: The *Drosophila sine oculis* locus encodes a homeodomain-containing protein required for the development of the entire visual system. *Neuron* 12:977, 1994.

358. Serikaku MA, O'Tousa JE: *Sine oculis* is a homeobox gene required for *Drosophila* visual system development. *Genetics* 138:1137, 1994.

359. Pignoni F, Hu B, Zavitz KH, Xiao J, Garrity PA, Zipursky SL: The eye-specification proteins So and Eya form a complex and regulate multiple steps in *Drosophila* eye development. *Cell* 91:881, 1997.

360. Forbes AJ, Nakano Y, Taylor AM, Ingham PW: Genetic analysis of hedgehog signaling in the *Drosophila* embryo. *Development* 1:15, , 1993.

361. Repetto M, Maziere JC, Citadelle D, Dupuis R, Meier M, Biade S, Quiec D, et al: Teratogenic effect of the cholesterol synthesis inhibitor AY 9944 on rat embryos *in vitro*. *Teratology* 42:611, 1990.

362. Lanoue L, Dehart DB, Hinsdale ME, Maeda N, Tint GS, Sulik KK: Limb, Genital, CNS, and facial malformations result from gene/environment-induced cholesterol deficiency: Further evidence for a link to Sonic Hedgehog. *Am J Med Genet* 73:24, 1997.

363. Rubenstein JLR, Beachy PA: Patterning of the embryonic forebrain. *Curr Opin Neurobiol* 8:18, 1998.

364. Muenke M, Page DC, Brown LG, Armson BA, Zackai EH, Mennuti MT, Emanuel BS: Molecular detection of a 45, X holoprosencephalic male. *Hum Genet* 80:219, 1988.

365. Johnson V: Holoprosencephaly: A developmental field defect. *Am J Med Genet* 34:58, 1989.

# Hirschsprung Disease

*Aravinda Chakravarti* ■ *Stanislas Lyonnet*

1. Hirschsprung disease (HSCR), or congenital aganglionosis, is defined by the absence of intramural ganglion cells in the myenteric and submucosal plexuses of the gastrointestinal (GI) tract. The disorder is classified into long-segment (L-HSCR: aganglionosis of the splenic flexure and beyond), colon-segment (aganglionosis of the descending colon), and short-segment (aganglionosis of the sigmoid colon and more distal regions) forms; a minority of patients have total colonic aganglionosis (TCA). The diagnosis of HSCR occurs in the neonatal period at a median age of 7.5 days. Clinical symptoms in neonates are variable and commonly include severe constipation, abdominal distension, and failure to pass meconium. Generally, diagnosis involves suction rectal biopsy, but full-thickness biopsy is necessary for differential diagnosis. Contemporary surgical treatment, placement of the bowel with normal peristalsis at the anus to eliminate the tonic contraction of the internal sphincter, has led to excellent prognosis and a normal life span in >75 percent of patients. Nevertheless, enterocolitis and chronic constipation remain as long-tern complications in many patients.

2. HSCR is a neurocristopathy or a disorder of neural crest (NC) cells. The NC is a transient and multipotent embryonic structure that gives rise to neuronal, endocrine and paraendocrine, craniofacial and conotruncal heart, and pigmentary tissues. In particular, the enteric nervous system (ENS) is formed from the craniocaudal migration of vagal-derived NC cells during weeks 5 to 12 of gestation. The embryologic development of the ENS is genetically programmed and known to depend on several proteins which determine and facilitate the orderly migration, proliferation, differentiation, and survival of NC cells in the walls of the GI tract to form the myenteric and submucosal plexuses. The details of ENS development explain phenotypic features of HSCR as well as its association with other syndromes involving the NC.

3. The population incidence is ≈1/5000 live births with sex-ratio 3:1 male:female; however, there is considerable population variation in both incidence and sex-ratio and

other patient characteristics. Among all cases, 18 percent have L-HSCR and 7 percent have TCA. In 70 percent of patients HSCR occurs as an isolated trait, 12 percent have a recognized chromosomal abnormality and 18 percent multiple congenital anomalies. The most common (>90 percent) chromosomal abnormality is trisomy 21, but multiple deletions of segments of chromosomes 2, 10, 13, and 17 have been noted. The congenital anomalies, beyond those associated with trisomy 21, common to HSCR include atresia or stenosis of the GI tract, polydactyly, cleft palate, cardiac septal defects, and craniofacial anomalies, defects that are explainable from NC biology. A critical finding is the higher frequency of multiple anomalies in familial (39 percent) than in isolated (21 percent) cases, suggesting underdiagnosis of specific features in the HSCR patient and warranting careful phenotypic assessment of each patient irrespective of family history. No known environmental factor has been associated with HSCR, which largely appears to be a genetic defect in NC-derived tissues.

4. Family history studies have established the recurrence risks of HSCR to be ≈3 percent and ≈17 percent for S-HSCR and L-HSCR, respectively, corresponding to heritability of ≈100 percent for either form. The increasing survival of surgically repaired patients have led to the identification of numerous multiplex families and parent-offspring transmissions. Genetic modeling has shown L-HSCR and colonic-HSCR to be inherited as rare autosomal dominant traits with low penetrance and with a substantial fraction of sporadic cases; S-HSCR is inherited as either a recessive trait with very low penetrance and minimal sporadic cases or has multifactorial inheritance. The segregation of HSCR with features of Waardenburg syndrome (Shah-Waardenburg syndrome) also shows dominant inheritance with lower penetrance of aganglionosis than the Waardenburg features. In all analyses, the penetrance of the putative gene mutants is greater in males than in females.

5. Specific genes involved in HSCR have been identified by linkage studies, positional cloning, and mutation analysis of candidate genes. In humans, five genes (the receptor tyrosine kinase *RET*, its ligand *GDNF*, the G-protein-coupled receptor *EDNRB*, its ligand *EDN3*, and the transcriptional regulator *SOX10*) have been shown to harbor multiple mutations in HSCR. In addition, the alternative *RET* ligand *NTN* and the endothelin-processing enzyme *ECE1* have single mutations in HSCR. Rare mutations in *EDN3*, *RET*, or *GDNF* are also associated with congenital central hypoventilation syndrome (CCHS). The large majority of mutations in HSCR have been recognized in *RET*, which is also the gene mutant in multiple endocrine neoplasia type 2 (MEN2). Interestingly, HSCR *RET* mutations are loss-of-function alleles, while MEN2 *RET* variants are activating mutations. The genetic features of all mutations detected show that mutations in

A list of standard abbreviations is located immediately preceding the index in each volume. Additional abbreviations used in this chapter include: CCHS = congenital central hypoventilation syndrome; *EDN3* = endothelin 3 gene; *EDNRB* = endothelin type B receptor gene; ENS = enteric nervous system; *GDNF* = glial cell line-derived neurotrophic factor gene; HSCR = Hirschsprung disease; MEN2 = multiple endocrine neoplasia type 2; NC = neural crest; *RET* = receptor tyrosine kinase proto-oncogene; *SOX10* = SOX family transcription regulator gene type 10; WS4 = Waardunberg syndrome, type 4 (also called Shah-Waardenburg syndrome).

A search for Hirschsprung disease in OMIM under the symbol HSCR reveals 12 entries covering both phenotypes and the specific genes involved. The phenotypes refer to HSCR1 (MIM 142623), largely comprising *RET* gene mutations; HSCR2 (MIM 600155), comprising *EDNRB* gene mutations; HSCR3 (MIM 600156), comprising a modifier on chromosome 21; and, congenital failure of autonomic control (MIM 209880). GenBank accession numbers: *RET*—AL022344, X12949, X15262, AJ243297; *GDNF*—L19063; *EDNRB*—D90402, AL139002; *EDN3*—J05081, AL035250; *SOX10*—AJ001183, AL031587; *NTN*—U78110; *ECE-1*—D43698, AL031005.

the *RET* pathway are haploinsufficient and HSCR occurs in mutation heterozygotes; mutations in the *EDNRB* pathway are hypomorphic and pleitropic because HSCR occurs in mutation heterozygotes, but Shah-Waardenburg syndrome occurs in mutation homozygotes. Mutations in *SOX10* are haploinsufficient and pleitropic because Shah-Waardenburg syndrome occurs in mutation heterozygotes. All mutations identified show greater penetrance in males than in females, are detected with greater frequency in L- than in S-HSCR, and in familial than in sporadic cases. However, mutations are seldom identified in more than 30 percent of HSCR cases. These studies establish the roles of *RET* and *EDNRB* signaling and *SOX10* regulation as necessary for normal ENS development.

6. Mouse models of aganglionosis and megacolon have been critical to the identification of human HSCR genes and in understanding ENS development. Homozygotes for null mutations in *Ret*, *Gdnf*, *Ednrb*, and *Edn3*, and heterozygotes for a null *Sox10* mutation, demonstrate aganglionosis in the mouse. Moreover, homozygotes for null mutations in *Ece1*, *A-raf*, *Ncx*, *Hoxa4*, and *Dlx2* also show aganglionosis in the mouse. These models emphasize the critical genes that determine ENS innervation but depart from the human phenotype in that none of them display reduced sex-dependent penetrance and none, except *Sox10*, show aganglionosis in heterozygotes.

7. Genotype-phenotype correlation in either L-HSCR or S-HSCR is very poor and is compounded by the reduced sex-dependent penetrance. Rare families in which the existence of multiple known mutations can explain trait segregation has led to the search for common modifying genes in HSCR. Recent studies show the segregation of a modifier on human chromosome 9q31 in L-HSCR families known to harbor a *RET* mutation; specifically, segregation of the 9q31 locus was restricted to families having atypical or noncoding mutations. In addition, in S-HSCR the segregation of three loci at 3p21, 10q11, and 19q12 appear to be both necessary and sufficient for explaining HSCR segregation and incidence. The susceptibility factor at 10q11 is *RET*, but typical coding sequence mutations could be identified in only 40 percent of linked families. The majority of HSCR is oligogenic, involves *RET* in almost all cases, but involves atypical noncoding variants.

8. HSCR is frequently found in association with many other neurocristopathy syndromes, such as Waardenburg and other pigmentary syndromes, CCHS, MEN2, and with neural tube defects. Additional significant associations include the Goldberg-Shprintzen syndrome and numerous others involving distal limb anomalies. These associations can be explained from our current knowledge of NC cell development and suggests an intrinsic defect, inherited or sporadic, of NC cells. HSCR is occasionally observed in patients with Bardet-Biedl syndrome, Smith-Lemli-Opitz syndrome types 1 and 2, and cartilage hair hypoplasia, which, being monogenic, suggests that some genes in common may predispose to both traits. The majority of the other common HSCR associations are chromosomal abnormalities, which suggests the action of dosage sensitive genes lying within the affected genomic segment. These syndromic associations reveal common development pathways affecting the NC and its derivatives and suggest specific candidate genes for HSCR.

9. The significant clinical and genetic knowledge in HSCR suggests that genetic counseling of patients and their families should utilize the known variation in recurrence risk by proband gender, consultand gender, segment length

involved, familiality and association with other disorders. Current data suggests that counseling for Shah-Waardenburg syndrome may follow standards for monogenic disorders, while patients with *RET* exon 10 and 11 mutations (at residues also mutant in MEN2) warrant further testing to ascertain predisposition to neuroendocrine tumors. The emerging evidence for the centrality of *RET*, in perhaps all HSCR cases, and oligogenic inheritance may allow family specific risks to be estimated in the near future.

Hirschsprung disease (HSCR), or aganglionic megacolon, is a congenital malformation characterized by the absence of the enteric ganglia along a variable length of the intestine. The disorder was first reported by the Danish pediatrician Harald Hirschsprung (1830-1916) in two unrelated boys treated until 7 and 11 months of age for severe constipation and abdominal distension resulting in congenital megacolon; he noted that "the sigmoid and descending colon were considerably dilated while the rectum was not."[1] The origin of HSCR was debated for a long time and it was not until the 1940s that the absence of intramural ganglion cells of the myenteric and submucosal plexuses (Auerbach's and Meissner's plexuses, respectively) of a segment of the large intestine was shown to be disease causing.[2] In 1948, Swenson and Bill[3] accomplished a major breakthrough by demonstrating that the affected segment was not the more proximal dilated colon; rather, it was the apparently normal distal segment that showed abnormal innervation and no peristaltic movement. Accordingly, they developed a surgical procedure, in which the aganglionic segment of the bowel is resected by an abdomino-anal pull-through.[4] This previously fatal disorder became surgically treatable and the survival of patients uncovered familial transmission of HSCR. In the last 50 years, progress in HSCR has occurred in four main areas: (a) development of reliable and simple methods of diagnosis from rectal suction biopsies using histochemical staining for acetylcholinesterase (AchE);[5] (b) development of new surgical approaches and supportive care with drastic decrease in mortality and morbidity;[6] (c) establishment of HSCR as an enteric nervous system (ENS) developmental anomaly; and (d) elucidation of the genetic causes of HSCR.

HSCR is the most common (1/5000 live births) genetic form of functional intestinal obstruction in neonates and children and stands as a model genetic disorder with complex patterns of inheritance. Developmentally, the disorder is a neurocristopathy and is characterized by the absence of a single cell-lineage originating from the neural crest (NC).

The clinical phenotype of HSCR is highly variable and occurs in association with numerous syndromes related to NC cell defects. Although Mendelian segregation of some forms of HSCR is known, the majority of patients are probably the result of oligogenic inheritance. Mutations in multiple genes participating in the receptor tyrosine kinase *RET*, endothelin type B receptor (*EDNRB*), and the transcriptional regulator *SOX10* pathways have clarified the molecular basis of HSCR. In addition, naturally occurring and targeted deletion mouse mutations in these and related genes, functional studies of gene mutations, and embryologic studies of enteric development, have been crucial in understanding the biology of this common birth defect. The genetic epidemiology of the various forms of HSCR and molecular genetics of identified genes emphasize the "multifactorial" nature of the phenotype, and provide new approaches to the genetic counseling of HSCR.

## PHENOTYPE, DIAGNOSIS AND TREATMENT

### Definition and Pathology

HSCR is defined by the absence of innervation of the distal bowel beginning with, and including, the internal anal sphincter (constant inferior limit) and extending proximally to variable lengths so that the upper limit is highly heterogeneous. The lack of an ENS in the distal segment leads to an increase in the number and size of nerve bundles and trunks in the myenteric plexuses; thus, a marked increase in cholinesterase activity, resulting from cholinergic activity in the hypertrophied nerve bundles, is observed. The clinical symptoms of HSCR, resulting directly or indirectly from the absence of ganglion cells in the affected bowel, are: (a) absence of peristalsis in the aganglionic segment; (b) absence of inhibitory neurons (including nitric oxide and VIP neurons) with permanent contraction of the abnormal bowel;[7] (c) lack of parasympathetic input with a decreased relaxation of the intestinal sphincter; (d) unopposed sympathetic activity increasing intestinal tone; (e) loss of the recto-sphincteric reflex that requires a normally innervated bowel; and (f) involvement of the nonneural intestinal microenvironment, namely, glial proteins, interstitial cells of Cajal,[8] smooth-muscle cells, and basal laminae.[9] Three other associated features might occur in a patient: a gradual process of dilatation and hypertrophy of the proximal normal bowel; perforation of the bowel; and enterocolitis.

## Classification

The classification of HSCR is according to the length of the aganglionic segment (Fig. 251-1). While the terminal portion of the rectum is always affected and the upper limit is highly variable, patients fall into two general categories: short-segment HSCR (S-HSCR: 67 to 82 percent of cases) in which aganglionosis is below the upper sigmoid, and long-segment HSCR (L-HSCR: 15 to 25 percent cases) in which aganglionosis extends beyond the splenic flexure. Patients with aganglionosis in the descending colon are variously referred to as colonic-segment HSCR, or even S- or L-HSCR. A less common (3 to 8 percent of cases) HSCR variety is total colonic aganglionosis (TCA) in which the entire colon and the terminal portion of the ileum is involved.[10] Three rare HSCR variants have been reported: (a) ultra-short segment HSCR involving the distal rectum below the pelvic floor and the anus, proximal to the normal aganglionic zone (2 cm above the pectinate line);[11] (b) total intestinal HSCR when the whole bowel is involved; and (c) suspended HSCR in which a portion of the colon is aganglionic above a normal distal segment. The last category has been reported in very few cases and is controversial.

## Clinical Presentation

The diagnosis of HSCR is currently usually made in the newborn period and in patients who are term-born (4 to 8 percent prematurity) and of normal birth weight. However, the clinical presentation of HSCR still depends on the patients' age.[12] In 41 to 64 percent of patients, age at diagnosis is below 1 month. When noncomplicated, HSCR presents as a syndrome of neonatal intestinal obstruction with these features: (a) abdominal distension, although it might not be an early feature (30 to 90 percent); (b) vomiting (18 to 67 percent), with occasional bile, or blood staining; (c) failure to pass meconium within the first 48 h of life; and (d) diarrhea and abdominal distension that is relieved by rectal stimulation or enemas. Critically, the failure to pass meconium is the first, and sometimes the sole, but near constant symptom leading to HSCR diagnosis in more than 60 percent of patients. However, this can be absent or missed, so that some patients are diagnosed later in infancy and, sometimes it appears only in adults with a severe constipation. A specific symptom, useful in HSCR clinical diagnosis, is the vacuity of the rectal ampulla with explosive passage of flatus and meconium or feces when a rectal examination is performed. Children with TCA may not present a full-blown acute intestinal obstruction syndrome and may have poor abdominal distension. The diagnosis of HSCR should also be considered in any infant with unexplained perforation of the caecum or appendix, although this is a rare complication ( < 5 percent), and in any neonates presenting with enterocolitis, which is often associated with sepsis. Beyond the neonatal period, the

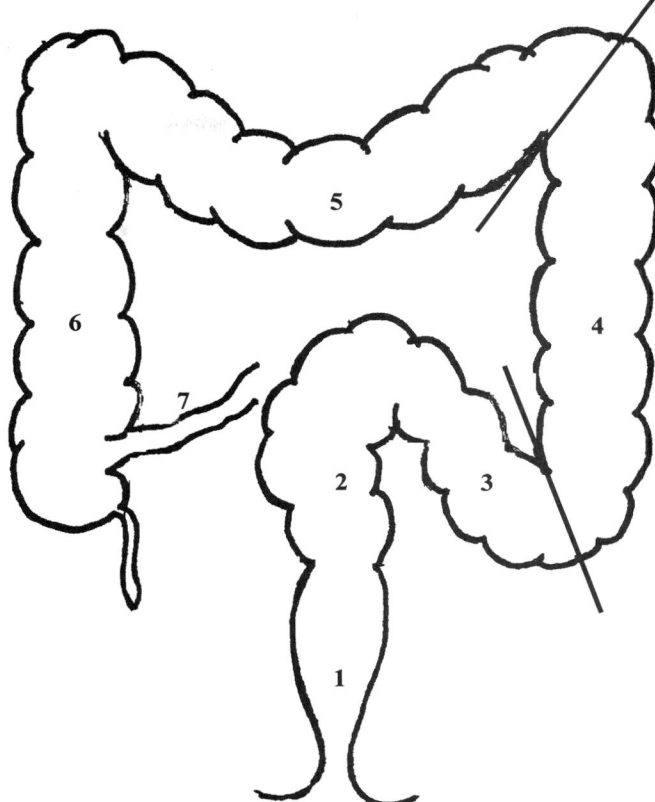

**Fig. 251-1 Classification of Hirschsprung disease by extent of aganglionosis (1 to 3: short-segment HSCR; 4: colonic-segment HSCR; 5 to 6: long-segment HSCR; the bars represent points of transition in classification. In some studies, segment 4 may be classified as either S- or L-HSCR).**

prominent clinical features at presentation include constipation (68 percent), chronic although variable abdominal distension (64 percent), vomiting (37 percent), and a history of delayed passage of meconium (40 percent). Constipation is the most common presenting symptom in older children and adults; usually, patients with late diagnosis of HSCR[13,14] have had previous evidence of gastrointestinal dysfunction, malnutrition, or failure to thrive.

## Diagnostic Investigations

**Radiology.** Plain abdominal X-ray shows a distended small bowel and proximal colon, with an empty rectum. Sometimes signs of occlusion are found with fluid levels and multiple loops of distended small bowel. A characteristic image of dilated proximal colon with the HSCR cone narrowing toward the nondistended distal gut is rather rare. Ultrasound is of a very limited value for prenatal diagnosis of HSCR.[15]

**Barium Enema.** Barium enema shows a small rectum with uncoordinated contractions, a transition zone where the narrow aganglionic bowel joins the dilated ganglionic bowel, and a delayed barium evacuation on a plain x-ray taken later. Interestingly, there may be no transition zone in TCA, while the colon looks small and appears shortened.[10,16] Barium enema is diagnostic in 80 to 92 percent of newborns with HSCR.[17]

**Anorectal Manometry.** These studies show abnormal patterns in HSCR with a characteristic absence of relaxation of the internal sphincter, which normally responds to rectal distension.[18] The abnormality of the reflex is so characteristic that anorectal manometry has often been used to diagnose HSCR in centers with special experience, with low false positive and false negative rates (5 to 25 percent, respectively). Because the normal rectoenteric reflex is not present before day 12 after birth, most diagnostic errors made are in the newborn period.[19]

**Suction Rectal Biopsy.** A sampling of submucosal plexus, which can be made with no anesthesia and few complications, is reliable in making the diagnosis of HSCR.[20,21] Because the level of aganglionosis is the same in both the submucous and myenteric plexuses, it is possible to make the diagnosis of HSCR by studying the more superficial submucosal plexuses only. In HSCR, the regular neural network of submucosal plexuses is absent and replaced by hypertrophic nerves that accompany blood vessels into the bowel wall. The hypertrophic nerves are responsible for increased acetylcholinesterase staining in the aganglionic bowel.[22] Diagnosis by suction rectal biopsy is 75 to 97 percent accurate when interpreted by an experienced pathologist.

**Full-Thickness Rectal Biopsy.** Full-thickness rectal biopsy is regarded as the "gold standard" for HSCR diagnosis but requires general anesthesia and experience in the interpretation. In particular, the very short aganglionic segment above the anal valves can be misleading. Therefore, specimens should be taken 1 to 2 cm above the anal valves in infants and at 3 to 4 cm above the anal valves in older children. Even in cases where laparotomy is indicated on clinical and radiologic findings, rectal biopsy is preferable to an extramucosal biopsy taken from the colon because the latter may have normal ganglia. The difficulty in recognizing the proximal limit of the aganglionic segment at laparotomy may require serial extramucosal biopsy along the colon with further examination of frozen sections.

### Differential Diagnosis

In the newborn with abdominal distension and failure to pass meconium, other causes of intestinal obstruction should be considered, namely: lower ileal and colonic atresia that is occasionally associated with HSCR; meconium plug syndrome; meconium ileus resulting from cystic fibrosis; intestinal malrotation or duplication; and small left colon syndrome. Other disorders, with possible functional intestinal obstruction, that should be considered are maternal infection, maternal intoxication, and hypothyroidism.

Some ENS anomalies, with functional bowel obstruction, show very similar, if not identical, presenting symptoms to those of HSCR. Although these conditions are far less common, they are still difficult to distinguish from HSCR.[23] These anomalies can be grouped as chronic intestinal pseudo-obstruction syndromes with a variable spectrum of pathologic features, including intestinal neuronal dysplasia; hypoganglionosis; immature ganglia; absent argyrophil plexuses; internal sphincter achalasia; and smooth muscle anomalies.[24] Chronic intestinal pseudo-obstruction syndromes can be divided into myopathic and neuropathic forms, the latter including the microcolon-megacystis-intestinal hypoperistalsis syndrome. While the recto-anal inhibitory reflex may be normal in these disorders, a full-thickness rectal biopsy is necessary for differential diagnosis.[25] Interestingly, some of these disorders have been excluded as being major HSCR disease loci.[26,27]

### Treatment and Prognosis

The general principle for surgical treatment of HSCR is to place the bowel with normal peristalsis at the anus and to eliminate the tonic contraction of the internal sphincter. A series of operative approaches have been developed since the initial breakthrough techniques of Swenson,[28] such as the Duhamel, Lester-Martin, and Soave procedures.[29,30] The general rules about these abdominoperineal operations include careful preoperative management with correction of dehydration, antibiotic therapy, nasogastric aspiration, and intestinal decompression, as well as the use of extemporaneous serial biopsies to demonstrate ganglion cells in the pulled down segment in an attempt to define the transition zone between ganglionic and aganglionic segments.

For many years, HSCR patients required a colostomy at the time of diagnosis to allow the proximal bowel to recover from the dilated state. Because diagnosis is now made earlier, a primary one-stage procedure is possible. Recent innovations in HSCR surgery are the use of minimally invasive procedures and laparoscopic techniques.[31] However, the treatment of children with long segment or TCA is still very difficult.[10,16,32]

The short-term complications of surgery include fistula of the anastomosis, which is usually revealed by sepsis and intestinal ileus, stenosis of the anastomosis, which is usually secondary to ischemia or minimal fistula, and enterocolitis. Enterocolitis is still the most frequent postoperative complication (15 percent) and the most significant cause of morbidity and mortality in children with HSCR.[33,34] Despite extensive clinical and experimental studies, the cause of enterocolitis in HSCR is still unknown, but may involve microbial, immunologic, and mechanical factors. A late diagnosis of HSCR and the length of the aganglionic segment do not seem to play a major role.[32] Mortality in HSCR has significantly decreased from 19 percent in the 1960s to 6 percent or less in the 1980s, indicating that it is still a life-threatening malformation, although with increasingly better prognosis.[35,36,37] The mortality in HSCR may be related to enterocolitis, sepsis, and postoperative perforation,[38] or be caused by the associated malformations. In isolated HSCR, the length of the aganglionic segment, late diagnosis, and the development of enterocolitis are the most significant factors of poor prognosis. In the long-term, more than 75 percent of HSCR patients are now cured by the initial surgical treatment.[39] However, there are long-term complications including chronic constipation (10 to 15 percent), either functional with hypertony of the internal sphincter or secondary to a too proximal anastomosis, and soiling.

## NEURAL CREST AND ENTERIC NERVOUS SYSTEM DEVELOPMENT

HSCR results from a failure of neural crest (NC) cells to migrate, proliferate, differentiate, or survive in the walls of the gastrointestinal tract to form the submucosal and myenteric plexuses. The earlier the cessation of migration, the longer the aganglionic segment, which explains why the lower rectum is the most frequently affected site. This could be related to either intrinsic abnormal properties of enteric neuroblasts or to the intestinal microenvironment. Hence, the understanding of the molecular and cellular bases of HSCR can be obtained from investigations of normal ENS development in both animal models and humans. In particular, the ENS is completely derived from the NC lineage.[40] Thus, the pattern of involvement of tissues and organs, completely or partly derived from NC cells, provide the clinician with a guide for syndrome delineation and suggestion of the genes involved in HSCR.

### Neural Crest Cell Biology (adapted from ref. 41)

The neural crest is a discrete, transient, and multipotent embryonic structure that comprises only a few cells appearing at the junction of neural and epidermal ectoderm in the neural folds of the neurula-stage embryo.[41] The NC forms according to a rostrocaudal gradient along the body axis. It releases free moving mesenchymal-like cells that follow migration routes at precise times of development, towards target embryonic sites where they settle and differentiate. The formation of NC derivatives exemplifies two crucial features in developmental biology. First, the generation of diversity is astonishing because the number of cell types known to arise from the NC is very large, as is the number of tissues and organs to which the NC contributes directly or provides the necessary environment for the development of other cell types. Second, the regulated migratory behavior of embryonic cells requires signals for induction of the lateral ridges of the closing neuroepithelium (neural folds) to facilitate the epithelio-mesenchymal transition. These processes result in migratory properties with dramatic changes in cell-cell and cell-matrix interactions, and the breakdown of the basal lamina, for migration along definite pathways, the cessation of migration, and then undergoing terminal differentiation once the target organ or tissue has been reached. While the developmental details are unknown, the accumulating data shows the following features.[41]

1. Single mammalian NC cells are pluripotent. They generate multipotent progeny cells indicating that they are capable of self-renewal and may be regarded as stem cells.
2. While most NC cells exhibit various degrees of pluripotency during migration, some clonal progeny are already committed to a single fate, as shown by antigenic markers not uniformly expressed by migrating NC cells. In particular, some neuronal precursors may be specified early in NC development, suggesting that NC derivatives are generated through progressive restriction of developmental potential.
3. NC cell migration is channeled both by permissive contact-mediated guidance and by specific chemorepellant molecules with effects either by diffusion or cell contact.
4. The ultimate phenotypic choice made by a progeny of pluripotent NC stem cells, at a given site of differentiation, results from a combination of extrinsic factors of the microenvironment and cell-intrinsic properties that modify its responsiveness to the external influences. The former has been documented by disruption of neurotrophic growth factors and receptors genes that result in deficiencies of selected subsets of NC-derived cells. Both the pathway of migration and the pattern of the ENS are imposed on crest cells as they leave the neural primordium by surrounding tissues and are not dependent on intrinsic properties regionally distributed along the neuraxis. Thus, truncal NC cells transplanted at the vagal level colonizes the gut and differentiate into enteric ganglia in which neurons synthesize acetylcholine rather than catecholamines, as specified by their normal fate, exemplifying the striking difference between the actual fate of NC cells and their developmental potential. The only exception is the restricted ability of cranial crests to form some of the complex structures of the branchial arch-derived facial skeleton, suggesting that these NC cells may have some positional information and commitment.

The biology of the NC has been derived from research on amphibian, avian, and mammalian (mouse) embryos. The experimental procedures used have relied on two principles: (a) extirpation or *in situ* destruction of the NC, where the source of NC cells, the neural folds, are removed prior to crest cell emigration and their fate inferred from observed deficiencies; and (b) differential identification of NC cells during ontogeny, providing detailed information on the migration process, fate, molecular characteristics, and phenotypes of migrating cells, homing sites, and derivatives. These studies were enabled by intrinsic and extrinsic markers. The intrinsic cytologic and molecular markers used were: (a) staining properties of cytoplasmic inclusions, cell size, or the nucleus, which are the basis of recognition of NC cells after isotopic and isochronic graft experiments between avian species (quail-chick chimaeras);[41] (b) enzymes such as acetylcholinesterase, tyrosine hydroxylase, or dopamine $\beta$ hydroxylase; (c) epitopes such as HNK-1, an antibody against a cell-surface glycolipid-labeling premigratory, and some postmigratory, NC cells; (d) transcription factors such as SLUG and MASH expressed in NC cells;[42] and (e) growth factor receptors including *EDNRB*, PDGFR$\alpha$, *RET*,[43] or the low-affinity neurotrophin receptor p75. The extrinsic markers applied to premigratory NC precursor cells to study their migration include direct lipophilic dye-labeling of cells without transplantation[44] and retroviral labeling of crest cells prior to NC cell migration.[45,46]

## Neural Crest Cell-Derived Tissues and Organs

The NC-derived tissues and organs belong to four main categories whose developmental fates are relevant to HSCR because they are defective in some syndromic associations of HSCR (Table 251-1). These categories are:

1. Neuronal tissues, including the anterior peripheral nervous system, both parasympathetic and sympathetic neurons, the spinal ganglia, sensorineurons, as well as the accompanying satellite, glial, and Schwann cells. The occurrence of autonomic nervous system anomalies, such as congenital central hypoventilation syndrome (CCHS), could be regarded as the result of a single injury on NC migration in HSCR patients.
2. Endocrine and paraendocrine tissues such as the thyroid C cells, adrenal medulla, and the connective tissue of the parathyroid and thymus. The cells producing adrenaline have long been recognized as NC derivatives at the truncal level. Interestingly, patients with the combination of HSCR and MEN2 syndromes exhibit both congenital malformations due to abnormal migration of NC towards the ENS and late-onset abnormal control of cell proliferation resulting in tumor predisposition for the adrenal- and calcitonin-producing cells.
3. Conotruncal region of the heart and craniofacial skeleton, which are regarded as mesoectodermal derivatives and include cartilage, smooth muscle, skeletal, adipose, connective, and muscular tissues. The frequent occurrence of dysmorphic features and cardiac anomalies in children with HSCR could be related to mutations with a pleiotropic effect during NC development.

**Table 251-1** Components of the Peripheral Nervous System and Other Cell Types Affected in Hirschsprung Disease (HSCR) and Neurocristopathies That Include HSCR

| | Peripheral nervous system | | | | Endocrine and paraendocrine cells | | | Pigment cells | Craniofacial mesectoderm, conotruncal heart |
| | SG | Autonomous nervous system | | | Carotid cells | Thyroid C-cells | Adrenal medulla | | |
| | | S | PS | ENS | | | | | |
|---|---|---|---|---|---|---|---|---|---|
| HSCR | | | | + | | | | | |
| WS4 | | | | + | | | | + | + |
| MEN2 | | | | + | | + | + | | |
| CCHS + HSCR | + | | + | + | + | | | | |
| YDBHS | | | | + | | | | + | + |
| BADS | | | | + | | | | + | + |

ABBREVIATIONS: SG = sensory ganglia; S = sympathetic neurons; PS = parasympathetic neurons; ENS = enteric nervous system; WS4 = Shah-Waardenburg syndrome or Waardenburg syndrome type 4; MEN2 = multiple endocrine neoplasia type 2; CCHS = congenital central hypoventilation syndrome; YDBHS = Yemenite deaf-blind hypopigmentation syndrome; BADS = black locks-albinism-deafness syndrome.

4. Pigment cells that are largely derived from the NC except those of the retina and those derived from the optic cup (the pigment of the choroid coat and outer iris has an NC origin). These data explain the importance of animal models with pigmentary anomalies, such as the dominant spotting and steel mutants, ascribed to mutation of a tyrosine kinase receptor (Kit) and its ligand (Steel factor), respectively. Direct associations between pigmentary and ENS defects, relevant to HSCR, are observed in the spotting mutants piebald lethal (s^l), lethal spotting (ls), and dominant megacolon (Dom), which have mutations in the endothelin-signaling pathway (EDNRB and EDN3) and the SOX10 transcription factor, respectively (see "Animal Models" below).

## Development of the Enteric Nervous System

**Enteric Nervous System.** The ENS belongs to the autonomic nervous system. It is composed of a large number of interconnected ganglia organized in two concentric rings throughout the gut wall: the outer myenteric plexus (Auerbach plexus) and the inner submucosal plexus (Meissner plexus). Functionally, the neurons of the ENS are divided into three types: sensorineurons that detect information from the gut, interneurons that process the sensory information, and motor neurons that provide motor innervation to smooth muscles regulating the contractility of the gut and the secretary activity of glands. The ENS should be regarded as an independent branch of the peripheral nervous system because: (a) ENS is the largest and the most extensive component of the peripheral nervous system containing more neurons (≈100 million) than the spinal cord; (b) a diversity of motor and sensorineurons coexist; (c) an intraganglion network and multiple interganglion and interplexus connections exist; (d) unique combinations of neurotransmitters or neuropeptides characterizing excitatory and inhibitory motor neurons are expressed; and, importantly, (e) the ENS is able to mediate reflex activity in the absence of central nervous system input with local reflex circuits integrating information on dilatation of the gut wall, muscle contractility, and secretion. Thus, both functionally, and developmentally, ENS is truly autonomic.

In the human, the formation of the ENS arises by craniocaudal migration of NC cells to the anal end of the rectum during the fifth to twelfth week of gestation.[47] Studies on avian embryos demonstrate that the ENS arises mainly from two independent contributions of the neural tube. First, presumptive enteric ganglioblasts emigrate from the dorsal part of the vagal neural tube, corresponding to somites 1 to 7, and follow a ventral migratory pathway entering the mesenchyme of the foregut via the posterior branchial arches. This contrasts with the lateral pathway that is traversed by melanocyte progenitors. These vagal-derived NC cells are then found in the developing pharyngeal gut, caudal branchial arches, and along the long axis of the gut, progressively colonizing the esophagus, the pre- and postumbilical intestine up to the colorectal region. These cells first form the myenteric plexuses outside the circular muscle layer; the mesenchymally derived longitudinal muscle layer forms later. The submucosal plexus is then formed by neuroblasts migrating from the myenteric plexus, across the circular muscle layer, into the submucosa. Short segment ablation experiments have shown that NC emigrating from different regions of the vagal neural tube can differ in their ability to colonize specific regions of the bowel. Indeed, innervation in the hindgut, which is more often affected in HSCR, is specifically dependent on NC at the level of somites 3 to 5.[48]

The pioneering studies by Nicole Le Douarin have shown that, in addition to the vagal region, NC cells emigrating from the sacral neural tube, posterior to somite 28, migrate into the gut, and contribute to the formation of the post umbilical ENS.[40,49] Although several studies have challenged these data,[50,51] they are now well established, and a reconciling hypothesis is that the correct migration or differentiation of the sacral NC in the hindgut is likely to require the previous presence of vagal NC-derived

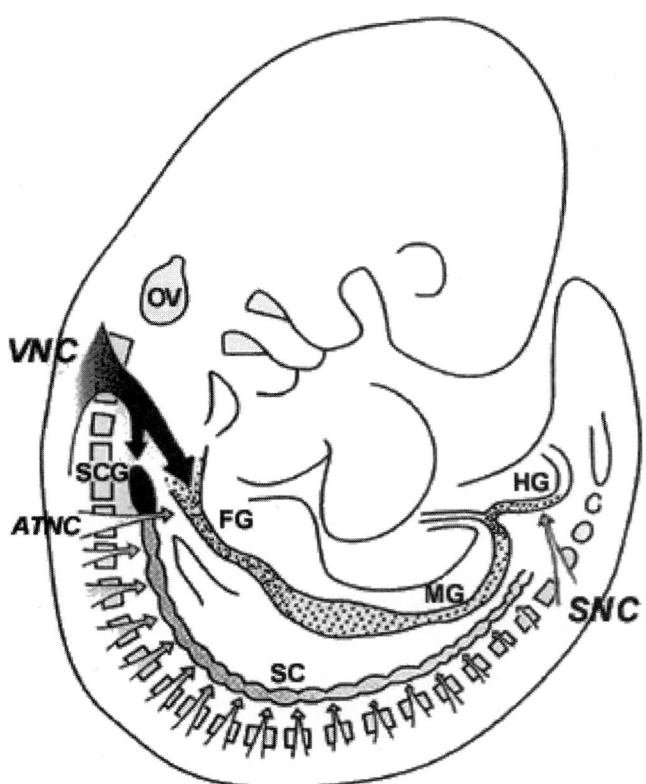

**Fig. 251-2 Representation of the derivatives of the neural crest in the mouse embryonic enteric nervous system with independent contributions originating from the vagal neural crest (VNC, somites 1 to 5), the anterior trunk neural crest (ATNC, somites 6 and 7), as well as the sacral neural crest (SNC, posterior to somite 24). The sympathoenteric (dotted) and sympathoadrenal (gray) lineages are shown. The otic vesicle (OV), superior cervical ganglia (SCG), foregut (FG), midgut (MG), and hindgut (HG) are indicated. (*Redrawn from Durbec et al.[55] and Natarajan et al.[56] with permission of V. Pachnis, National Institute for Medical Research, Mill Hill, UK.*)**

cells.[52] Recent data suggests that, in the hindgut, the submucosal ganglia derived from the vagal crest form first, and that cells emigrating from these ganglia reach the outer myenteric ganglia by migrating along blood vessels.

In mammalian embryos, the ENS is also derived from both cranial (vagal) and sacral NC (Fig. 251-2).[53] While the innervation of the foregut is contributed to by the whole anterior vagal region of the neuraxis (somites 1 to 7), the innervation of the midgut and hindgut derives from the anterior vagal area only (somite levels 1 to 5).[54] The sacral NC of mammalian embryos also contributes to the formation of the ENS, colonizes the dorsal site of the colorectum and subsequently extends to more ventral regions of the hindgut. The expression of RET in pre-enteric NC has shed some light on two complementary contributions of the vagal NC to the sympato-enteric and sympato-adrenal lineages of the peripheral nervous system, respectively.[55,56] Indeed, the vagal NC (somites 1 to 5) of the hindbrain is a RET-dependent lineage that populates both the entire gut and the superior cervical ganglion,[57] while the RET-independent sympato-adrenal lineage originates from the trunk NC (somite levels 6 and 7) and populates the foregut as well as the ganglia of the sympathetic chain, posterior to the superior cervical ganglia. Thus, while the foregut is populated by both sympato-enteric and sympato-adrenal derivatives, the midgut and hindgut receive contributions only from the sympato-enteric lineage (Fig. 251-2). These data suggest a close relationship between sympato-adrenal and enteric precursors and are relevant to the most common location of aganglionosis in HSCR.

Several critical issues regarding ENS development remain unanswered: What controls the caudal migration of enteric neuroblasts? Do they migrate along a caudally moving gradient or by cell division only? How do different subpopulations of enteric NC cells (vagal, truncal, sacral) migrate in apparently opposite directions within the same microenvironment? What stops cell migration? Why does the sacral NC fail to compensate the absence of vagal NC cells in aganglionic megacolon?

**Proteins Affecting Enteric Nervous System Development.** It is clear from the previous review that normal development of the ENS is dependent on the complex coordination of multiple processes. The developmental failure of any aspect during neuroblast formation can then manifest as megacolon in animals and as HSCR in humans.[57,58] The details of ENS development can then suggest candidate factors that are compromised in HSCR, a number of which have been studied in both the ganglionic and aganglionic bowel. These include differentiation factors for enteric neurons such as neurotrophin 3 or NGF;[59] proliferation factors such as endothelin 3[60] and its receptor;[61] factors involved in the epithelio-mesenchymal interaction such as the Ret tyrosine kinase and its ligands *GDNF* and neurturin;[62–64] extrinsic factors[65] contributing to cell-cell interaction[66] or interaction of cells with the extracellular matrix,[67] neurofilament peptides,[68] or laminin;[69] neurochemical and endocrine substances such as nitric oxide;[70] transcription factors such as *SOX10* or MASH 1; growth factors of the TGF$\beta$ family including the BMPs; and homeobox proteins such as HOX-A and MSX that likely act in the development of the intestine.

## Neurocristopathies

Bolande coined the term neurocristopathy for syndromes or tumors involving NC cells.[71] A neurocristopathy can arise following the defect at any stage of NC cell development from the emergence of the neural tube, migration, proliferation, differentiation, growth, or survival. Indeed, a common embryonic NC origin can provide the basis for an explanation of syndromes comprising anomalies of the peripheral nervous system, pigmentary, craniofacial, conotruncal heart, and adrenal medulla, and be regarded as a single embryonic field (Table 251-1). This was substantiated by clinical observations and by biological demonstration that NC cells share many common characteristics (origin, multipotentiality, migratory ability, differentiation potential).

Neurocristopathies are divided into tumors, malformations, single anomalies, and complex syndromes with multifocal association. The most frequent isolated tumors derived from NC cells are neuroblastomas (peripheral nervous system as the tissue of origin), schwannoma (Schwann cells), pheochromocytoma (chromaffin cells of the adrenal medulla), and medullary thyroid carcinoma (calcitonin producing C-cells of the thyroid). These tumor cells overexpress metabolic pathways with unregulated production of polypeptide hormones such as calcitonin, catecholamine hormones, and their derivatives. Complex tumor predisposition syndromes include neurofibromatoses and the multiple endocrine neoplasia syndromes. Isolated malformations of NC origin include cleft lip with or without palate, branchial arch syndrome, and isolated conotruncal heart defects, but the most prominent example is HSCR.[72] Finally, syndromes involving multiple anomalies of NC-derived cells are illustrated by the Waardenburg, DiGeorge, Haddad, and CHARGE syndromes.

## EPIDEMIOLOGY OF HIRSCHSPRUNG DISEASE

The major epidemiologic features of HSCR as a sex-modified multifactorial congenital trait with a population incidence of 1/5,000 live births, have usually been described in the context of genetic studies.[73] These observations may be biased in favor of familial cases and not representative of all HSCR cases.

Recent epidemiologic studies have, however, clarified the major features.

## Incidence, Sex-Ratio, and Variation of Segment Length

Clinical and pathologic improvements have made the diagnosis of HSCR highly specific. Consequently, a remarkable decline in the age at which HSCR is diagnosed has been observed. In a survey of 487 probands born prior to 1977, 79 percent, 13 percent, and 8 percent were diagnosed at ages < 1 year, 1 to 2 years and > 2 years, respectively; a small number of cases escaped detection until adolescence, and rare individuals, with a mild phenotype, were identified in adulthood only (unpublished data from reference 74). In contrast, recent surveys, based on births between 1983 and 1997, show a median age at diagnosis of 7.5 days with the majority being diagnosed at day 4.[75] Hospital discharge records and neonatal surveys can, thus, accurately identify the majority of cases.

Three epidemiologic surveys in Baltimore County, MD, during the period 1969-1977,[76] the Province of British Columbia, Canada, during the period 1964-1982,[77] and in California during the period 1983-1997,[75] have defined the incidence of HSCR based on a near-complete ascertainment of cases. The incidence, expressed as the number of cases per 10,000 live births, was estimated at 1.4 among "non-whites" and 2.3 in "whites" in Baltimore,[76] and 2.3 overall in British Columbia.[77] Surveys by the California Birth Defects Monitoring Program[75] are more instructive because they are the largest and most recent study and have classified individuals by ethnicity; the incidence varies significantly with Caucasians, African-Americans, Hispanics, and Asians having rates of 1.5, 2.1, 1.0, and 2.8 per 10,000 live births, respectively. Consequently, the assumed incidence of 1/5000 live births may be taken as a "representative" value. HSCR has long been known to exhibit a sex bias with a preponderance of males.[73] The California study showed significant variation in the sex ratio as well, with male:female ratios of 3.3, 3.4, 3.0, and 4.4 among Caucasians, African-Americans, Hispanics, and Asians, respectively, with a high correlation between increasing sex ratio and increasing incidence. These data suggest that rates of HSCR are more variable across human populations in males, than in females.

Long-segment HSCR (L-HSCR) is classically defined as aganglionosis including and beyond the splenic flexure, the remaining cases being classified as short-segment HSCR (S-HSCR), based on the differences in embryonic origin of these two segments of the gut[74] (Fig. 251-1). However, some investigators have classified patients with aganglionosis up to the descending colon as either L- or S-HSCR;[78–80] these patients are classified as colonic-segment HSCR.[74] Using the splenic flexure as the boundary, Torfs[75] showed that segment length was reported in 89 percent of cases and that among these, the frequency of L-HSCR was 18 percent, in accordance with previous genetic studies.[73,74,78–80] Importantly, ≈7 percent of all cases had TCA. Some studies[76] have noted an increased frequency of L-HSCR among "non-white" populations but this finding is not universal.[75] Importantly, the most significant feature correlated with segment length is the sex ratio, because the male:female rate is much higher for S-HSCR (4.2 to 4.4) than for L-HSCR (1.2 to 1.9).[74,75] The causes of these various differences are unclear but are likely to include both genetic and environmental factors.

## Association with Malformations

In ≈70 percent of patients, HSCR occurs as an isolated trait, ≈12 percent have a recognized chromosomal abnormality, and ≈18 percent have multiple congenital anomalies including recognized syndromes[75,81] (see "Syndromes and Associated Anomalies" below). The most common (>90 percent) chromosomal abnormality in HSCR is trisomy 21 (Down syndrome), reported in 2 to 10 percent of all cases ascertained.[73,75–77,79–81] Interestingly, these trisomy 21-HSCR cases are overwhelmingly (85 percent) males with L-HSCR,[81] but the reason for this enrichment is unknown.

Because the incidence of trisomy 21 is ≈0.15 percent in most populations, the 2 to 10 percent incidence among HSCR is equivalent to a relative risk of 13 to 67. Consequently, yet unknown dosage-sensitive genes on human chromosome 21 are a specific risk factor for HSCR. The second most frequent chromosomal abnormalities in HSCR include deletions of specific segments of the long arms of chromosomes 10[82,83] and 13,[84-88] which are the sites of the major genes for HSCR, namely, *RET* and *EDNRB*, respectively. In addition, multiple cases of deletion and duplication of chromosome 17q21-23 were recently noted.[89] Other chromosomal abnormalities observed in individual patients are described in a later section (see "Syndromes and Associated Anomalies").

Aganglionosis is one part of a constellation of congenital anomalies observed in a significant (18 percent) number of HSCR patients, excluding those with Down syndrome. Many of these associations, occur at a frequency above that dictated by chance, and are described in a later section (see "Syndromes and Associated Anomalies"). These entities, frequently familial, are increasingly being documented as the consequence of mutations in single genes so that HSCR is one of several pleiotropic effects of a gene mutation. There are, in addition, many other phenotypes of multifactorial origin, themselves parts of numerous syndromes, which occur with increased frequency among HSCR cases. The latter include gastrointestinal anomalies such as atresia or stenosis of the colon, rectum, or anal canal, cleft palate, polydactyly, and cardiac septal defects not associated with Down syndrome. The British Columbia survey[77] estimated these associations to occur with relative risks of 113, 14, 10, and 6, respectively. Recent studies have also shown a 12 percent frequency of craniofacial anomalies among HSCR patients with multiple anomalies (Chakravarti and Lyonnet, unpublished data).[81,90] Other isolated anomalies are rare and described in "Syndromes and Associated Anomalies" below. It is clear that associated anomalies are more frequently reported for familial (39 percent) than isolated (21 percent) cases, strongly suggesting underdiagnosis of specific associated features, including among monogenic syndromes.[81] Consequently, a careful phenotypic assessment by a trained dysmorphologist is warranted for each HSCR patient irrespective of family history. This may be a significant explanation of the variability in phenotypic findings across studies.

### Etiologic Hypotheses

The clinical phenotype of HSCR, and its association with other congenital anomalies and syndromes, is largely the result of developmental anomalies in NC cells and their derivatives or occur during development of the intestinal wall or its inter-action with enteric neuroblasts. The genes involved in HSCR (see "Molecular Genetics of Hirschsprung Disease" below) suggest intrinsic defects in enteric ganglion cells so that HSCR is a developmental neurocristopathy. The effect of the environment is small in HSCR and no specific factors have been identified to date. Other biologic mechanisms have been suggested as etiologic factors in HSCR. First, some have argued that HSCR is an autoimmune disorder;[91] however, no HLA associations have been detected so far. Second, a number of authors have suggested a vascular etiology for HSCR.[92,93] This hypothesis arises from the presence of fibromuscular dysplasia in the arteries of the gastrointestinal tract in > 30 percent of HSCR patients.[94] Although fibromuscular dysplasia is associated with ischemia, it is unclear whether this might be a cause or an effect. Under this hypothesis, segmental aganglionosis, which is very rare, would be more common in HSCR.

### Environmental Factors

Early genetic studies suggested that HSCR was a multifactorial trait and that environmental factors were likely to be important.[73] It is well known that families, consistent with the segregation of a dominant gene mutation, harbor clinically unaffected obligate carriers,[73,78,79] and that monozygotic twins can be discordant for

HSCR.[95] These findings urged a search for environmental factors, and in a case-control study, maternal hyperthermia was identified as an etiologic factor.[96] Mothers of HSCR patients were more likely than mothers of controls to have a history of fever or of being overheated (strenuous exercise, regular sauna use). Although this finding may be buttressed by animal studies that show that hyperthermia inhibits cell division and increases neuronal cell death, a second study failed to replicate this finding.[97] Indeed, it is unlikely that environmental factors play a major role in HSCR. A recent study demonstrates that of 13 twin pairs none of the co-twins of the index cases were affected,[75] suggesting that the discordance of the clinical phenotype may arise from the twinning process itself. A recent molecular analysis of one family demonstrated the transmission of an HSCR mutation by each of a pair of discordant monozygotic twins to their affected off-spring.[90] Consequently, stochastic mutant gene expression is an equally likely explanation of the failure of disease penetrance in HSCR.[98] In the majority of HSCR cases, the segregation of multiple unlinked disease determinants is a major explanation for failure of disease penetrance in specific individuals[90] (Chakravarti and Lyonnet, unpublished data).

## FORMAL GENETICS OF HIRSCHSPRUNG DISEASE

Familial transmission of HSCR had been noted in rare circum-stances, but the chief impediment to early genetic studies was the poor survival of HSCR patients. HSCR was effectively a lethal disorder before the establishment of modern surgical procedures. The improving survival of patients in recent times and the observation of transmission of HSCR to the offspring of surgically corrected patients prompted new studies of the role of heredity.

### Familiality

In the 1960s, genetic studies demonstrated that HSCR was familial and that recurrence risks to relatives of cases were much higher than that in the general population.[73,78] These studies emphasized the role of genes in HSCR, but failed to identify Mendelian patterns of inheritance. The recurrence risk to relatives was shown to depend on both the sex of the index case and the relative considered. Consequently, HSCR was assumed to be a sex-modified multifactorial disorder.

The familiality of HSCR was examined in detail in the sibs of patients and shown to vary by extent of aganglionosis: the recurrence risks to sibs of S-HSCR (aganglionosis below the splenic flexure) probands varied from 1.5 percent to 3.3 percent (119 to 318 sibs examined) while risks to sibs of L-HSCR probands varied from 2.9 percent to 17.6 percent (17 to 68 sibs examined).[73,78,80] Consistent with the features of a multifactorial trait, risks to relatives of female probands were higher than to those of male probands, and risks to male relatives were higher than risks to female relatives. Although the recurrence risks are small on an absolute scale, compared to the population incidence they are extraordinarily high. Specifically, assuming a population incidence of 1/5000 live births, the minimum and maximum risks of 1.5 percent and 17.6 percent correspond to relative risks of 75 and 880, respectively. Consequently, the effect of genes on HSCR recurrence is significant.

The literature described many cases of parent-offspring transmission of HSCR from surgically treated patients.[99,100] These families emphasized the role of genetic factors but could not distinguish between multifactorial inheritance in all families and autosomal dominant inheritance with reduced penetrance in some families. Evidence for the latter hypothesis arose from the identification of six multicase families with both L- and S-HSCR.[73,74,78,79] A number of multicase families described prior to the 1990s showed an intrafamilial association of HSCR with other anomalies, including ventricular septal defects, type D brachy-dactyly, bilateral double big toes, Waardenburg syndrome, and multiple endocrine neoplasia type 2.[101-104] The modes of inheritance in these families were variously described as

**Table 251-2 Genetic Epidemiologic Features of Hirschsprung Disease**

| | Long-segment HSCR | Colonic-segment HSCR | Short-segment HSCR |
|---|---|---|---|
| % Probands | 10 | 9 | 81 |
| Sex ratio (male:female) | 1.9 | 1.6 | 5.5 |
| Genetic model | Dominant | Dominant | Multifactorial or recessive |
| Penetrance (%) male:female | 66:51 | 37:29 | 17:4 |
| Sporadics (%) male:female | 41:13 | 39:21 | 4:0 |
| Recurrence risk to sibs (%) | 17 | 6 | 2 |

autosomal dominant or recessive. These families, and additional multiplex families with yet other phenotypic associations described during the past decade (see "Syndromes and Associated Anomalies" below), clarify that HSCR can occur as a syndromic form, can have high recurrence risks in specific families, and follows Mendelian patterns of inheritance, albeit with reduced penetrance. Nevertheless, the common wisdom in the 1980s classified HSCR as a multifactorial disorder in the majority of cases.[80]

## Models of Gene Segregation

To objectively quantify the role of heredity in HSCR, Badner and colleagues[74] performed a detailed segregation analysis of HSCR. These authors studied the family histories of 487 probands, assessed both by questionnaire and through medical, surgical, and pathology records. Of the studied histories, 218 probands (212 families) were ascertained in Pittsburgh, 207 probands (203 families) were ascertained by Carter and colleagues in London,[73,99] and 62 probands (62 families) were ascertained by Passarge in Cincinnati.[78,79] The importance of these data was the application of uniform classifications on all affected and the near-complete ascertainment of all first-degree relatives.

The 487 probands had a sex ratio of 3.9 and an overall recurrence risk of 4 percent to their 979 sibs. When the extent of aganglionosis was considered, the sex ratio decreased (varying between 1.3 and 7.2) and the recurrence risk to sibs increased (varying between 0 percent and 55 percent) as aganglionosis extended from the rectum to the ileum and beyond. On classifying patients as L-HSCR (splenic flexure and beyond) and S-HSCR, which comprised 11 percent and 89 percent of probands, respectively, the sex ratio and sib recurrence risks were 1.9 and 17 percent (97 sibs) and 4.4 and 3 percent (847 sibs). In addition, the data suggested considerable recurrence risk (6 percent) to sibs of those probands whose aganglionosis extended into the descending colon; these probands comprised 9 percent of all index cases and had a sex ratio of 1.6. Consequently, Badner and colleagues[74] considered three classes of HSCR: long-segment HSCR (11 percent of probands), colonic-segment HSCR (9 percent of probands) and rectosigmoid (89 percent of probands) (Fig. 251-1). Classically, the last two categories are considered as S-HSCR.

The familial patterns of HSCR were first evaluated by estimating the heritability of HSCR and considering the sex of both the proband and the proband's sibs, by L-HSCR and S-HSCR. Within L-HSCR, heritability was 100 percent and the recurrence risks varied between 9 percent (sisters of female probands) and 33 percent (brothers of female probands); within S-HSCR, heritability was between 80 percent and 95 percent, and the recurrence risks varied between 1 percent (sisters of male probands) and 5 percent (brothers of either proband). These observations demonstrated that HSCR is consistent with genetic segregation in all cases and that classifications by gender and extent of aganglionosis may reveal genetic heterogeneity since they are associated with specific patterns of risk.

Segregation analysis was then used to assess mode of inheritance in each of three categories[74] (Table 251-2). For long-segment HSCR the most parsimonious model was segregation of a rare ($\approx$0.001 percent) dominant allele; the existence of new mutations in 15 percent of HSCR cases was likely. Importantly, penetrance was intermediate (66 percent in males; 51 percent in females) and a substantial number of cases (41 percent in males; 13 percent in females) were likely to be sporadics, that is, the occurrence of HSCR in wild-type homozygotes at the imputed dominant locus. The existence of sporadics can be explained by new mutations, genetic effects at unlinked loci and environmental factors. For colonic-segment HSCR, the most parsimonious model was also the segregation of a rare ($\approx$0.002 percent) dominant allele; the existence of new mutations in HSCR was unlikely. The penetrance was lower than that for L-HSCR (37 percent in males; 29 percent in females) and a substantial number of cases (39 percent in males; 21 percent in females) were likely to be sporadics. Importantly, for the most common rectosigmoid-segment HSCR the most parsimonious models were either multifactorial inheritance with 87 percent heritability among offspring or the segregation of a common (4 percent) recessive gene; the existence of new mutations in HSCR was unlikely. The penetrance was low for the recessive model (17 percent in males; 4 percent in females) and only a small fraction of cases (4 percent in males; 0 percent in females) were likely to be sporadics. These analyses were not the result of arbitrary classifications of HSCR families into three discrete extents of aganglionosis, because reanalysis of the data by considering aganglionosis in eight segments of the gastrointestinal tract, between the rectum and the ileum, did not alter the findings.[105]

These studies established the genetic features of HSCR and emphasized four cardinal aspects of HSCR inheritance: (a) the primary role of genetic segregation in almost all HSCR cases; (b) genetic heterogeneity of HSCR (dominant, recessive, and/or multifactorial forms) by extent of aganglionosis; (c) reduced penetrance for dominant forms of HSCR; and (d) the existence of new mutations (Table 251-2). The two most enigmatic features of HSCR genetics appeared to be the greatly reduced penetrance of the imputed dominant forms of the disorder and the existence of sporadic forms even when the overall heritability is 100 percent. One hypothesis to reconcile these results is the existence of common modifier alleles in dominant HSCR forms and oligogenic, rather than multifactorial, inheritance. Segregation analysis is not an effective tool to test these hypotheses, which are best reevaluated pending gene identification.

Segregation analysis also clarified the apparently inconsistent findings of the most frequently noted association of HSCR with pigmentary (hypopigmentation, white forelock, isochromic irides) anomalies and congenital deafness.[106–109,110] This constellation, Shah-Waardenburg syndrome or Waardenburg syndrome type 4 (WS4), is considered to be an autosomal recessive trait. However, statistical analysis[111] of existing family data shows dominant inheritance for both traits; high penetrance (93 percent) for the pigmentary anomalies and deafness but low penetrance (45 percent) for HSCR. These results suggest that the two features

**Table 251-3** Molecular Genetic and Phenotypic Features of the Major and Minor Genes for HSCR in Humans

| Gene | Map location | Number of mutations | Phenotype in mutant | | % Penetrance |
| | | | Homozygotes | Heterozygotes | |
|---|---|---|---|---|---|
| *RET* | 10q11 | 89 | unobserved | HSCR | 51–72 |
| *GDNF* | 5p13 | 5 | unobserved | HSCR | ? |
| *EDNRB* | 13q22 | 15 | HSCR* | HSCR | 8–85 |
| *EDN3* | 20q13 | 2 | HSCR* | HSCR | ? |
| *SOX10* | 22q13 | 6 | unobserved | HSCR* | >80 |
| *NTN* | 19p13 | 1 | unobserved | HSCR | ? |
| *ECE-1* | 1p36 | 1 | unobserved | HSCR† | ? |

*Shah-Waardenburg syndrome (WS4).
†Cardiac defects, craniofacial abnormalities, dysmorphic features.

in WS4 are pleiotropic effects of a single gene, at least in some families, and that consanguinity can produce a more severe phenotype in the homozygote. The genes identified in HSCR have confirmed this thesis.

## MOLECULAR GENETICS OF HIRSCHSPRUNG DISEASE

The clarification of inheritance types in HSCR has led to the mapping and identification of specific mutant genes in HSCR. To date, multiple mutations in five genes encoding two receptor-ligand pairs (the receptor tyrosine kinase *RET* and its ligand glial cell line-derived neurotrophic factor (*GDNF*); the G-protein-coupled endothelin type B receptor (*EDNRB*) and its ligand endothelin-3 (*EDN3*)) and the transcription factor *SOX10* have been identified in HSCR patients. Importantly, *RET* is central to HSCR genesis and misregulation of this tyrosine kinase may be common in all forms of HSCR.

### *RET* Receptor Tyrosine Kinase Pathway

Two critical observations, the co-occurrence of HSCR with multiple endocrine neoplasia type 2 (MEN2), which maps to proximal human chromosome 10q,[112] and deletions of this same region in HSCR patients,[82,113] prompted genetic mapping in HSCR families using chromosome 10 markers. These studies, in multigenerational families segregating HSCR as an incompletely penetrant autosomal dominant disorder, led to the definitive identification of a susceptibility locus on the proximal long arm of human chromosome 10 near the genetic marker D10S176 and the proto-oncogene *RET*.[114,115] These results proved the monogenic basis of HSCR (at least in some families), the reduced penetrance of the 10q mutations in most families, and the likely genetic heterogeneity of HSCR.

Mutations in *RET* were first identified in MEN2A, which is an autosomal dominant cancer syndrome characterized by tumors of cells derived from the neural crest[116,117] (see "Syndromes and Associated Anomalies" below). Moreover, the targeted disruption of the *Ret* gene in the mouse displayed a complete lack of enteric ganglia along the intestinal tract, together with renal agenesis or severe dysgenesis[118] (see "Mouse Models of Hirschsprung Disease" below). These findings led to the identification of nonsense and missense mutations in *RET* in multiple HSCR families.[119,120] Subsequently, *RET* mutations have been identified in a variety of neuroendocrine tumors, including MEN2B[121,122] and familial/sporadic cases of medullary thyroid carcinoma (MTC).[116,117,123–125] Thus, germ line *RET* mutations can cause four distinct clinical disorders (HSCR, MEN2A, MEN2B, MTC), and in addition is rearranged in ≈20 percent of papillary thyroid carcinomas.[126]

The frequency of *RET* mutations detected in different studies varies between 10 and 50 percent,[119,120,127–129] and is dependent

on patient characteristics. Specifically, samples enriched for patients from large families or sporadic L-HSCR yields higher *RET* mutation frequency,[127,128] and in one study, the detection rate for L-HSCR cases was 75 percent.[129] Indeed, *RET* mutations are more common in L-HSCR (57 percent) than in S-HSCR (32 percent) patients. Mutations are also more common in familial (49 percent) than in sporadic (35 percent) cases.[128] These studies demonstrated that a substantial fraction (16 percent) of sporadic cases were new mutations as predicted by segregation analysis[130] (Table 251-2). The mutation detection studies also led to a direct evaluation of disease penetrance in mutation carriers, with males showing incomplete yet greater penetrance (72 percent) than females (51 percent), as suggested by segregation analysis (Tables 251-2 and 251-3). These results were remarkable because *RET* mutations recapitulated almost all properties of HSCR inheritance[74] and dispelled the view that mutations in *RET* would explain only a small fraction of syndromic HSCR families.

*RET* is a 1114-residue transmembrane protein with a signal peptide, a putative extracellular ligand-binding domain, an extracellular cadherin-like domain, a cysteine-rich region, a transmembrane region, and a conserved intracellular catalytic domain typical of other growth factor receptors such as the EGF (epidermal growth factor) receptor. To date, 89 unique mutations (missense, small insertions, and deletions) have been identified in HSCR patients and families; protein polymorphisms detected during mutation screening are also indicated (Fig. 251-3). Unlike the mouse, human patients with *RET* mutations rarely have renal abnormalities; in fact, the majority of cases with *RET* mutations have HSCR as an isolated trait (Table 251-3). The *RET* mutations identified in HSCR are unique and occur throughout the gene (protein). This is in contrast to MEN2A, in which mutations occur in a cluster of six cysteines (exon 10: residues 609, 611, 618, and 620; exon 11: residues 630 and 634),[116,117,123–125] and MEN2B, which is uniquely associated with an M918T mutation.[121,122] Intriguingly, some HSCR mutations, in families both with and without MEN2A, occur at the same cysteines as those involved in MEN2A (Fig. 251-3). The reasons for this overlap are unclear but the overlap suggests that these HSCR patients may be at risk for neuroendocrine tumors.[127]

*RET* is expressed in the developing central and peripheral nervous system (sensory, autonomic, and enteric ganglia) and the excretory system, and thus explains the null phenotype in the mouse and aganglionosis in human patients[118] (see "Mouse Models of Hirschsprung Disease" below). Biochemical studies have shown that *RET* mutations in MEN2 are activating mutations that constitutively dimerize the receptor leading to transformation.[131] while those in HSCR are inactivating mutations that lead to misfolding or failure to transport the protein to the cell surface.[132–135] The identification of HSCR patients with *RET* deletions[82,113] argues for haploinsufficiency and that 50 percent of wild-type *RET* is insufficient for normal enteric development in the

a)

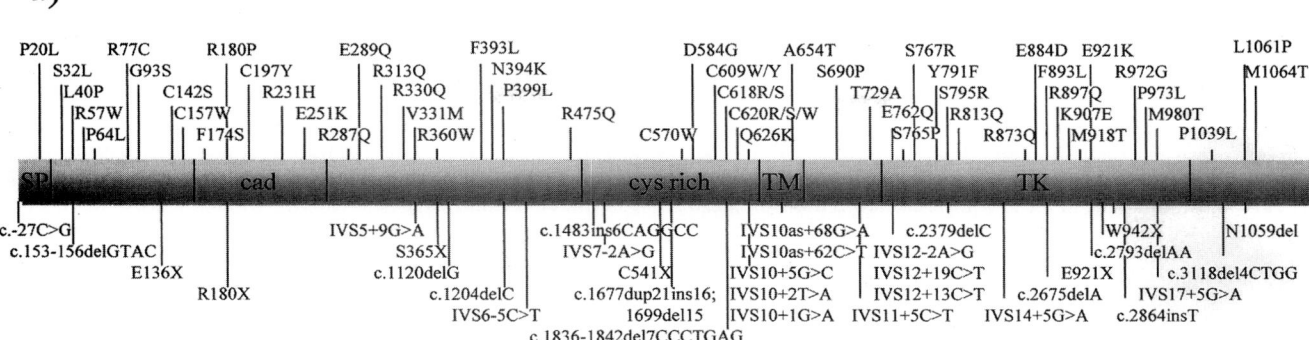

b)

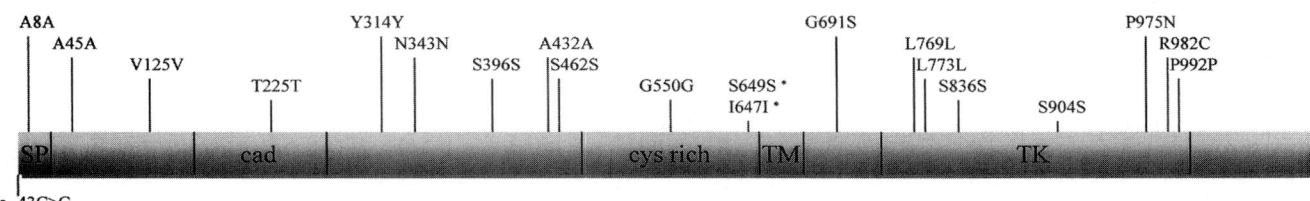

**Fig. 251-3** Representation of the *RET* protein with identified structural and functional domains (SP = signal peptide; cad = cadherin-like; cys-rich = cysteine-rich; TM = transmembrane segment; TK = tyrosine kinase domain). *A*, HSCR mutations (missense changes are indicated above the figure; nonsense, insertions, and deletions are indicated below the figure). *B*, *RET* protein polymorphisms (c.−43c > G is located in the 5′UTR; * private variants known to alter mRNA splicing[90,195]).

human. Consequently, the finding of MEN2A/MTC mutations in HSCR is enigmatic and argues against a simple activating versus inactivating model of gene action.[136]

The importance of *RET* signaling in the ENS led to the investigation of functionally related genes as HSCR candidates. Glial cell line-derived neurotrophic factor (*GDNF*) is a TGF-β-related 211-residue protein that can activate *RET* in cell culture,[137,138] is proteolytically cleaved to a 134-residue mature peptide that exists as a homodimer, and is a survival factor for many types of neurons including enteric ganglia.[139] Importantly, *GDNF* is strongly expressed early in murine development in the gut and kidney mesenchyme, and in gut smooth muscle.[140] This pattern explains the renal agenesis and lack of enteric ganglia throughout the intestinal tract of *GDNF* knockout mice, analogous to *RET* knockout mice[141–143] (see "Mouse Models of Hirschsprung Disease" below). *GDNF* mutations have been observed in five patients to date and are a rare (< 5 percent) cause of HSCR[144–146] (Table 251-3). Moreover, *GDNF* mutations are unlikely to lead to HSCR directly because four of the five patients have additional contributory factors, such as *RET* mutations and trisomy 21.

*GDNF*, being a TGF-β-related protein, is an unusual *RET* ligand because other family members activate serine-threonine kinases rather than receptor tyrosine kinases. Moreover, *GDNF* activates *RET* only in the presence of a novel glycosylphosphatidylinositol (GPI)-linked co-receptor GFRA1.[147,148] Thus, the *RET* signaling complex, requiring both a receptor tyrosine kinase and an extracellular accessory component, behaves similarly to cytokine receptor complexes.[149] No mutations in *GFRA1* have been discovered despite a careful search for variants in HSCR patients.[150,151] Currently, four structurally related GPI-linked co-receptors, *GFRA1-4*, and four related soluble growth factors, *GDNF*, neurturin (*NTN*), persephin (*PSPN*), and artemin, have been identified.[152] Specific combinations of these proteins are necessary for development and maintenance of both central and peripheral neurons, and all can signal through *RET*. Of these, one

family with a putative *NTN* mutation, in conjunction with a *RET* mutation, was identified.[153] Like *GDNF*, *NTN* does not appear to have a major effect on HSCR and probably can only exert its mutational effect in conjunction with other disruptions of *RET* signaling.

Intracellular signal transduction through *RET* occurs through the adaptor protein GRB10,[154] which also interacts with the insulin receptor and insulin-like growth factor receptor.[155] GRB10 consists of an SH2-domain at the C-terminus and has a 100-residue pleckstrin homology domain that is known to interact with components of cellular signaling and cytoskeleton organization.[156] Importantly, *GRB10* shows striking identity to the *C. elegans* gene *mig-10*, which affects anterior-posterior neuronal migration and the development of excretory canals.[157] However, no mutations in *GRB10* have been discovered despite a careful search for variants in HSCR patients.[158]

## Endothelin Type B Receptor Pathway

The ascertainment of multiple cases of HSCR within an inbred, Old Order Mennonite community raised the possibility of identifying recessive genes for aganglionosis.[109] Phenotypic examination of this kindred demonstrated that the majority of affected individuals had HSCR only, although some individuals had, in addition, features of Shah-Waardenburg syndrome (hypopigmentation, white forelock, bicolored irides, sensorineural deafness) or Down syndrome.[109,159] The kindred had significant inbreeding, yet the disorder did not segregate as a recessive trait. Similar to other HSCR forms, the recurrence risk was ≈8 percent with a 2:1 sex ratio. Genealogic analysis demonstrated that all patients could be traced to a single common ancestral couple 8 to 12 generations earlier. Consequently, a search for genomic segments common to all affected individuals identified a susceptibility locus on chromosome 13q22, and a likely modifier on chromosome 21q22.[159] Consistent with this finding is the recognition that several HSCR patients, with additional anomalies of NC cells, had *de novo* interstitial deletions of the long arm of chromosome 13[84–88] (see "Syndromes and Associated Anomalies" below). Comparative mapping suggested that the 13q22 gene was orthologous to the mouse mutation *piebald-lethal*, a murine model of aganglionosis[160] (see "Mouse Models of Hirschsprung Disease" below).

The targeted deletion of the mouse endothelin type B receptor (*Ednrb*) produced an autosomal recessive phenotype of white spotting and megacolon, bringing to light the critical role of endothelins in enteric development.[161] These authors showed that *piebald-lethal* was allelic to the knockout and arose from an *Ednrb* mutation. Based on these results, Puffenberger et al.[160] mapped the human *EDNRB* gene to chromosome 13q22 and demonstrated a missense mutation (W276C) in the Mennonite kindred. The discovery of additional mutations in *EDNRB* in other HSCR families clarified that the Mennonite mutation was not a rare explanation of aganglionosis.[26,162–164]

The Mennonite variant (W276C) was a hypomorphic mutation that did not decrease cell-surface expression or affect ligand binding appreciably, but that did reduce the signal transduction capacity; moreover, it had unusual genetic properties.[160] First, mutant homozygotes (CC) had greater penetrance than did heterozygotes (WC), but wild-type homozygotes (WW) were clinically affected as well. Second, penetrance was greater in males than in females; in males, penetrance was 85 percent, 33 percent, and 13 percent in CC, WC, and WW individuals, respectively; in females, penetrance was 60 percent, 8 percent, and 9 percent in CC, WC, and WW individuals, respectively (Table 251-3). Third, the mutation was pleiotropic because defects in epidermal melanocytes were observed in mutant homozygotes only. Thus, the sensitivity of different tissues (melanocytes versus enteric neurons) to varying levels of *EDNRB* is different. These features explained the complex pattern of inheritance and emphasized the requirement of additional genes in the HSCR phenotype, even in the genetically isolated Mennonite population.[160]

Mutation detection studies in non-inbred patients with HSCR alone identified mutant heterozygotes only, in both isolated and familial HSCR, but *de novo* mutations were not observed.[26,163,164] A mutant homozygote was observed in an inbred union and had phenotypes similar to Mennonite homozygotes.[162] Overall, *EDNRB* mutations are a small fraction of HSCR unless patients have features of WS4.[130] Importantly, and unlike *RET* mutations, *EDNRB* variants are associated largely with S-HSCR, although Mennonite patients can be either L-HSCR or S-HSCR. Penetrance in heterozygotes is incomplete but quantitative estimates are not possible for the non-inbred cases given the limited data. Genetically, the occurrence of heterozygous *EDNRB* deletions in HSCR patients[163] suggest haploinsufficiency as the cause of HSCR, analogous to *RET*. Consequently, the finding of an HSCR patient with retinoblastoma, harboring a large cytogenetic deletion spanning 13q14 to 13q22, in whom *EDNRB* is not deleted, suggests that proximal genomic rearrangements may inactivate *EDNRB*, and may be one reason why mutations within this gene are not more common.[130]

The endothelin type B receptor (EDNRB) and the structurally related type A receptor (EDNRA) are G-protein coupled heptahelical proteins that transduce signals from 21-residue potent vasoconstrictors termed endothelins (EDN1, -2, -3).[165,166] Signals that stimulate G-protein-coupled receptors produce downstream signals that often converge on controlling the concentration of cytoplasmic $Ca^{2+}$, triggering contraction and secretion in many cell types. EDNRB is a 442-residue protein expressed in many tissues, particularly in the myenteric plexus, mucosal layer, ganglia, and blood vessels of the submucosa of the colon;[167,168] the expression pattern explains the phenotype of both the mouse and the human mutations. Although, biochemically EDNRB accepts all three endothelin isopeptide ligands, the identity of the autosomal recessive spotting and aganglionosis phenotype of a targeted deletion of *Edn3* with that of *Ednrb*[169] suggests that the *EDNRB*'s physiological ligand is *EDN3*.

Baynash et al.[169] showed that the naturally occurring mouse aganglionosis mutation *lethal-spotting* harbors a mutation in *Edn3*. This observation prompted a search for *EDN3* mutations in humans: two mutations (C159F; c.262delGCinsT) have been observed, each in homozygous form, in patients with WS4.[170,171] In one of these families,[170] mutant heterozygotes were either unaffected or had mild pigmentary anomalies, as did other untested family members. Interestingly, one heterozygote for a *EDN3* frameshift mutation was identified in a patient with congenital central hypoventilation syndrome (CCHS); these patients have possible defects in the neural system concerned with the autonomic control of respiration located in the medulla and pons of the brain stem.[172] CCHS is found in association with HSCR, but this patient had chronic constipation with no documented aganglionosis. If confirmed in other families, the sensitivity of different tissues (melanocytes versus enteric neurons versus brain stem) to varying levels of *EDN3* is possibly different than that for *EDNRB*. Targeted deletions in the mouse of other genes in this pathway have led to additional insights of HSCR-related phenotypes. Thus, the *Edn1* knockout homozygous mouse does not have aganglionosis but has craniofacial abnormalities and abnormal development of the outflow tract of the heart, thymus, and thyroid; the heterozygote has elevated blood pressure.[173,174] Biologically active endothelins are proteolytically cleaved from preproendothelins by two related membrane-bound metalloproteases; one of these genes, endothelin-converting enzyme 1 (*Ece1*), processes both *Edn1* and *Edn3*. Interestingly, *Ece1* knockout homozygotes have craniofacial defects, cardiac abnormalities, lack enteric ganglia in the terminal colon, and harbor features of both *Edn1* and *Edn3* mutations.[175] A search for mutations in a patient with a rare skip-lesion HSCR, cardiac defects, craniofacial abnormalities, and additional dysmorphic features identified a R742C change in *ECE1* with reduced enzyme activity.[176]

## SOX10 Transcription Regulator

Mutations in the endothelin pathway have confirmed that mutant homozygotes, but not heterozygotes, have features of Shah-Waardenburg syndrome (WS4). However, family studies have concluded that other WS4 patients should be heterozygotes for rare mutations. This is analogous to a *de novo* mouse model of coal-color spotting and aganglionosis (*Dom*) in which heterozygotes have regional deficiencies of neural crest-derived enteric ganglia and homozygotes are embryonic lethal.[177] The *Dom* gene is *Sox10*, and is related to the Sry-type HMG box family of transcription factors.[178,179] *Sox10* is expressed in melanocytes and enteric ganglia, but expression of both *Sox10* and *Ednrb* are disrupted in mutant embryos with loss of neural crest derivatives by apoptosis. Subsequently, six heterozygous mutations in human *SOX10*, in both familial and sporadic patients with Shah-Waardenburg syndrome, have been identified;[180,181] *de novo* changes were also discovered. All six mutations identified appear to disrupt the *SOX10* gene and are likely to lead to a loss-of-function allele, so that HSCR would result from haploinsufficiency. Although the data are limited, the penetrance of the mutations appears to be high, although in one family, sibs sharing a mutation are discordant for aganglionosis.[181] Thus, *SOX10* mutations may represent a substantial fraction of WS4 patients, but are unlikely to be a major cause of HSCR alone.

It is unknown whether the reduced expression of *Ednrb* in the *Dom* mouse arises from a direct effect of *Sox10* or are indirect effects on a common subset of enteric ganglia.[178] If the effects are indirect then a third pathway is compromised in HSCR patients. Interestingly, other genes do modify *Sox10* expression in the mouse, both in melanocytes[178] and in enteric ganglia (William J. Pavan, personal communication, 2000). The identification of these genes will provide new candidates for HSCR analysis.

The "major" genes in HSCR, defined as those with multiple mutations, are *RET*, *GDNF*, *EDNRB*, *EDN3*, and *SOX10*. The minor "genes" involved are *NTN* and *ECE1*. These discoveries

**Table 251-4** Molecular Genetic and Phenotypic Features of Known Mouse Models of Aganglionosis and Congenital Megacolon

| Mouse gene | Mutation* | Mouse phenotype | | | | Human gene location |
|---|---|---|---|---|---|---|
| | | Aganglionosis/ megacolon† | Renal agenesis | Coat spotting | Craniofacial defects | |
| Ece1 | KO | S | − | + | + | 1p36 |
| Edn3 | KO, ls | S | − | + | − | 20q13 |
| Ednrb | KO, s^l | S | − | + | − | 13q22 |
| Gdnf | KO | L | + | − | − | 5p13 |
| Ret | KO | L | + | − | − | 10q11 |
| Sox10 | Dom | C | − | + | − | 22q13 |
| A-Raf | KO | M | − | − | − | Xp11 |
| Ncx | KO | S | − | − | − | 2p13 |
| Hoxa4 | KO | M | − | − | − | 7p15-p14 |
| Dlx2 | KO | S | − | − | + | 2q32 |

*ls = lethal spotting; s^l = piebald lethal; Dom = Dominant megacolon; KO = knockout.
†S = short-segment disease; C = colonic-segment disease; L = long-segment disease; M = megacolon

have elucidated the major features of the HSCR phenotype and its transmission, and are summarized in Table 251-3. Specifically, for the major genes (a) HSCR is genetically heterogeneous and due to mutations in distinct pathways; (b) most HSCR patients harbor heterozygote *RET* mutations; (c) endothelin pathway mutations lead to HSCR in heterozygotes but WS4 in homozygotes; (d) WS4 patients are frequently heterozygous for *SOX10* mutations. Overall, where the data are substantial enough to warrant a conclusion, mutation penetrance is far less than 100 percent and unequal in males and females. All of these features suggest that modification of the mutational effect in the known genes, by stochastic or epigenetic factors, or by other genes, is a distinct possibility.[130]

## MOUSE MODELS OF HIRSCHSPRUNG DISEASE

Mouse models of HSCR have been central to the identification and functional analysis of human HSCR genes (see Table 251-4). As outlined in the previous sections, spontaneous mutations in *Ednrb*,[161] *Edn3*,[169] and *Sox10*,[178] and more recent targeted disruptions of *Ret*,[118] *Gdnf*,[141–143] *Ednrb*,[161] and *Edn3*,[169] result in marked enteric aganglionosis (Table 251-4). These strains are now widely used in the examination of developmental defects associated with human HSCR and emphasize the genetic basis of NC defects.

### Ret Receptor Tyrosine Kinase Pathway

Developmental studies in mice deficient in *Ret* or *Gdnf* have demonstrated a role for these proteins in the survival and correct migration of enteric neuroblasts.[43,141–143,182–185] The majority of neurons and glia of the ENS emigrate from the vagal neural crest and migrate along a predetermined path to innervate the entire length of the gut.[173] *Ret* and its ligand *Gdnf* are expressed in certain neural crest derived populations and in the gut mesenchyme, respectively. Recent protein binding studies[147,148] have also identified the novel GPI-linked protein Gfra1 as the accessory molecule mediating *Ret:Gdnf* interaction.[138]

Homozygous null mutations of mouse *Ret* and *Gdnf* result in total intestinal aganglionosis.[118,141–143] These mice develop to term and die within the first 24 h postpartum;[118,141–143] they also exhibit pyloric stenosis, dilated proximal intestine, renal agenesis, and an empty bladder. Milk accumulates in the stomach of *Ret* null mice, unable to progress from the stomach to the intestine.[118] Likewise, *Gdnf* null mice demonstrate peristaltic failure, which correlates with their lack of enteric ganglia.[141–143] *Gdnf* null mice demonstrate some enteric innervation in the esophagus and stomach wall at embryonic day 12.5 (E12.5) but these neurons are absent in mice examined at birth.[143] Thus, some enteric

neurons can develop in the absence of *Gdnf*, but they are subsequently lost later in development.

Mice deficient in either *Ret* or *Gdnf* also demonstrate renal agenesis due to a lack of induction of the ureteric bud.[118,141–143] Metanephric kidney develops at E11 when the ureteric bud branches from the Wolffian duct into the metanephric blastema, and is triggered by inductive signals from blastemal cells.[186] Thus, these genes play an important role in the epithelial-mesenchymal interaction of ureteric bud induction in kidney development.[43,140–143,183] *Ret* is expressed in the ureteric bud and mediates transduction of a mesenchyme-derived signal (*Gdnf*), which stimulates formation, growth, and branching of the ureteric bud.[140] Null mice demonstrate a normal Wolffian duct but no ureteric bud and, consequently, no kidney. A number of these studies[118,141] have also reported that *Ret* and *Gdnf* heterozygote animals occasionally demonstrate unilateral or bilateral renal agenesis, suggesting that the role of *Gdnf* in development may be dose dependent.

These studies demonstrate that *Ret* and *Gdnf* are essential components of the signal transduction pathway required for enteric neuron development and renal organogenesis. However, the *Ret* and *Gdnf* null phenotypes are not identical.[139] *Ret* null mice only lack enteric innervation below the stomach,[118] whereas *Gdnf* null mice lack enteric neurons below the midesophagus.[141–143] Superior cervical ganglia are completely absent in *Ret* null mice, but numbers of these ganglia are only 30 percent reduced in *Gdnf*-deficient mice. These differences may reflect differences in genetic background or functional redundancy in the ligand:receptor relationship.[139]

### Ednrb Receptor Pathway

Naturally occurring and targeted mutations demonstrate that the *Ednrb*-mediated pathway is an essential component of ENS development (Table 251-4). It has been suggested that *Ednrb* signaling is further required at or before melanoblast proliferation and migration.[187,188] *Ednrb* accepts the ligands EDN1, -2, and -3 with equal affinity.[189] However, *Edn3* null mice[169] demonstrate a markedly similar phenotype to *Ednrb* null mice.[161] Mice harboring mutations in either gene exhibit autosomal recessive megacolon, aganglionosis, and white spotting. Spontaneous mutations in *Ednrb* and *Edn3* are responsible for the phenotypes known as *piebald-lethal*[161] (s^l) and *lethal spotting*[169] (ls). Mice deficient in these proteins innervate the foregut and distal small intestine appropriately, but enteric neuroblasts fail to colonize the distal large intestine.[161,169] They exhibit a narrowing of the intestine preceded by a gross distension of the lower bowel. The position and length of the transitional region of the distended and spastic regions vary between animals.[161,169] The hypomorphic *Ednrb* mutation, *piebald* (*Ednrb*[s/s]), exhibits hypopigmentation defects with variable penetrance but does not exhibit megacolon or aganglionosis. This strain is a recognized model of WS4.[190]

The above studies imply that Edn3 is the functionally relevant ligand for Ednrb; however, there are differences between the null phenotypes of *Ednrb* and *Edn3*. *Ednrb* knockout and piebald-lethal (*s*[l]) mice are almost completely white, yet mice deficient in Edn3 (*Edn3*[−/−] and *ls*)[169] are pigmented over 20 to 30 percent of their bodies. *Ednrb*-deficient mice do not survive to mate, yet 15 percent of *Edn3*-deficient mice survive into adulthood. *Edn1* and/ or *Edn2* may partially compensate for the absence of *Edn3*.[161,169] It is now known that lethal-spotting (*ls*) mice harbor a missense mutation in *Edn3*, which abolishes processing of big-Edn3 by the endothelin-converting enzyme-1 (*Ece1*).[169] Ece1 catalyzes the proteolytic activation of big-Edn1 and big-Edn3 to endothelins 1 and 3, respectively. Targeted disruption of *Ece1*[175] also results in enteric aganglionosis, craniofacial, and cardiac abnormalities.[175] These developmental abnormalities reflect the phenotype observed in *Edn1*[−/−] null animals.[173]

In an endeavor to identify the critical expression period for the receptor, a recent study generated mice with tetracycline-inducible expression of *Ednrb*.[188] These authors demonstrate that Ednrb-mediated signaling is required between E10 and E12.5, for the initiation and correct migration of melanoblasts and enteric neuroblasts.[188] This report proposes a role for Ednrb in the initiation of emigration of melanoblasts and suggests that this is consistent with its proposed role in maintaining a pool of enteric neuroblasts.[185]

### Sox10 Transcription Regulator

Mice homozygous for the dominant megacolon (*Dom*) mutation are embryonic lethal, but heterozygous mice exhibit a white belly spot, white head spot, white feet, and regional deficiencies in distal colon ENS, resulting in megacolon[177,191] (Table 251-4). *Dom* is known to be a consequence of a frameshift mutation in the mouse *Sox10* gene,[178,179] which encodes an architectural transcription factor. The Sox 10[Dom] mutation leaves the DNA binding domains intact but disrupts the transcription transactivation domain.[178,179,181] *Ednrb* transcripts are completely absent in *Sox10*[Dom/Dom] mice, and are dramatically reduced in *Sox 10*[Dom/+] mice. The decrease in *Ednrb* expression cannot fully account for the observed neural crest defect[178] as *Ednrb*[s-l/s-l] mice can survive to weaning, whereas *Sox10*[Dom/Dom] mice die in utero.[177] *Sox10*[Dom/Dom] mice demonstrate retarded colonization of the entire gut from E11 onwards, which contrasts with the spatially restricted deficiencies of *Ednrb*[s-l/s-l] mice (E12.5 onwards).[191,192]

The white spotting and megacolon observed in *Sox10*[Dom/+] mice exhibits strain dependence.[177–179,181] Consequently, *Sox10*[Dom/+] mice are now recognized as a more relevant model of WS4 than *Ednrb*[s/s] mice because they mimic the variable penetrance of aganglionosis seen in human patients. One recent study generated congenic lines[181] in an endeavor to identify the modifying locus involved.[181] The implicated locus lies on mouse chromosome 10 and is tightly linked to a locus associated with modification of the piebald (*Ednrb*[s/s]) phenotype.[181] The identification of downstream targets for *Sox10* and genes whose products modify the severity of *Sox10*[Dom] neurocristopathies will provide insight into the genetic regulation of neural crest-derived populations.

### Interaction Between Ret and Ednrb

Ret and Ednrb act through two well-established signal-transduction pathways considered biochemically independent. Recent reports, however, suggest that G-protein-coupled receptors (GPCR:Ednrb) and receptor tyrosine kinases (RTK:Ret) are parallel, synergistic and may engage in "crosstalk."[182,193,194] Such crosstalk may be mediated by modifiers. It is noteworthy that a recent study[195] reported the identification of an HSCR patient who was heterozygous for weak hypomorphic mutations within

both *RET* and *EDNRB*: each parent was heterozygous for one mutation, yet neither parent was affected. This infers a direct genetic, if not biochemical, interaction between the pathways. Each of the mouse models harbors a mutation in one gene, in isolation. Compound heterozygotes, carrying mutations in genes involved in both GPCR and RTK pathways, may further aid our understanding of the relationship between them.

### Mouse Megacolon Models

A number of recent gene-targeting studies have reported phenotypes that include varying degrees of megacolon (Table 251-4). These include *Hoxa4*[196] (homeobox family member), *Ncx*[197] (Hox11 homeobox family member), *A-Raf*[198] (Raf protein kinase family member), and *Dlx2*[199] (distal-less 2 homeobox family member). These models demonstrate abnormal development of the ENS manifested in a spectrum of intestinal aganglionosis, inappropriate innervation, or aberrant peristaltic contraction. *A-Raf* null mice also demonstrate neurologic abnormalities such as tremor, limb rigidity, and distinct stress responses.[198] *Dlx2*[−/−] mice also exhibit craniofacial abnormalities.[199] No mutation, within any of these genes, has yet been identified in HSCR patients, but they remain important models of the biology of megacolon.

### Human HSCR and Mouse Models

The pathways and genes contributing to normal enteric development can be summarized as shown in Fig. 251-4. Despite this advance, the mouse models, which carry mutations in known HSCR genes, demonstrate three distinct discrepancies with human disease. First, aganglionosis is restricted to the homozygous null genotypes in *Ret*, *Gdnf*, *Ednrb*, and *Edn3*, and to the heterozygous null genotype in *Sox10*. Human HSCR patients are only heterozygotes for mutations within *RET*, *GDNF*, *EDNRB*, *EDN3*, and *SOX10*. Patients, homozygous for mutation within *EDNRB* and *EDN3*, have the Shah-Waardenburg phenotype with pigmentation anomalies similar to the mouse. Second, full phenotypic penetrance is observed in most mouse models. The human mutations display reduced penetrance whenever this can be accurately measured (Table 251-3) and is associated with significant intra- and interfamilial variation. Third, phenotypic expression in the mouse demonstrates no sex bias, whereas human mutations in the same genes result in a twofold higher frequency of expression in males as compared to females.

The genotypic and phenotypic differences between human HSCR and the corresponding mouse models are to be expected. First, the mouse mutations are observed in the context of a homogenous genome; the human genome is highly variable, even within families. Phenotypic expression is therefore likely to be sensitive to the influence of genetic background. Second, most of the mouse models result from homozygous null mutations. The majority of human HSCR patients carry heterozygous mutations, even when these mutations result in complete loss of function. Many known human mutations are weak hypomorphic changes and are neither necessary nor sufficient for the HSCR pathology. This aspect leads to the conclusion that human disease may be multigenic.[90,228] Third, there may be intrinsic differences between mice and humans in enteric development. It is likely that these three factors account, at least in part, for the variable phenotypic expression, reduced penetrance, and complex patterns of inheritance observed in human HSCR.

## MULTIGENIC INHERITANCE OF HIRSCHSPRUNG DISEASE

Despite knowledge of the embryology of HSCR (Table 251-1), human genes involved (Table 251-3), and mouse models of megacolon and aganglionosis (Table 251-4), there is a significant gap in our knowledge or interpretation of the available data because overall genotype-phenotype correlations in HSCR are very poor (Table 251-2). Newer investigations suggest that the

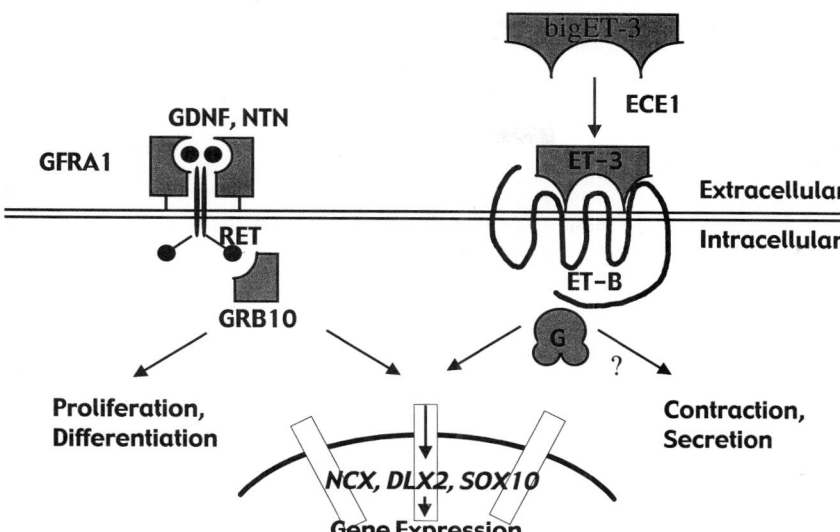

**Fig. 251-4 Genes and biochemical pathways critical to normal enteric development in the human and mouse.**

reason for the poor correlation is that the majority of HSCR cases arise from the effects of multiple susceptibility genes.

## Modifying Genes in HSCR

As noted earlier, three persistent findings in human HSCR are the significantly reduced penetrance of mutant genotypes, sex-difference in expression and penetrance variation by extent of aganglionosis. Genetic and epigenetic modification of known mutations is an attractive thesis to explain these findings. In a number of families, *GDNF* and *NTN* mutations are insufficient to explain clinical expression because these co-occur with additional *RET* mutations or trisomy 21.[144,145,153] Moreover, even in the relatively genetically homogeneous Mennonite population, non-random associations between HSCR and *RET* are observed, over and above the *EDNRB* mutations, suggesting the action of both *RET* and *EDNRB* jointly in disease expression.[130] These data suggest the centrality of *RET* in HSCR genesis and that multiple genes may be required to modulate clinical expression.

Multilocus segregation of a disorder is compatible with either (a) association of a disorder with multiple genes and genetic (locus) heterogeneity, where mutations in any one of several genes are sufficient for phenotypic expression independently of genetic background, or (b) multigenic or multifactorial inheritance resulting from the cumulative effects of multiple mutations that are sensitive to an individual's genetic background. To clarify these hypotheses, our laboratories have performed linkage analysis of 12 HSCR families with three or more affected individuals in two or more generations.[90] These families were largely representative of L-HSCR cases. As expected, linkage to the *RET* locus was demonstrated in all but one family. Extensive mutational analyses identified six missense and nonsense *RET* mutations at residues highly conserved in evolution. Two additional families had sequence alterations that likely affect normal splicing, while the remaining three linked families harbored no coding sequence variation despite being *RET*-linked. Molecular analysis of one of the splice variants showed partial usage so that *RET* expression is at >50 percent levels. Interestingly, these families showed linkage to a novel locus on chromosome 9q31, but this evidence was restricted to the six families without the missense and nonsense *RET* mutations. We conclude that in some HSCR families the *RET* mutations are severe and haploinsufficiency leads to phenotypic expression directly. On the other hand, in many other families, *RET* mutations are hypomorphic and represent weak alleles, which compromise, but do not abrogate, *RET* expression, and thus require the action of yet other mutations (at the 9q31 locus) to result in clinical expression of aganglionosis.[90] In retinoblastoma, alleles

that lead to partial loss of function are frequently incompletely penetrant.[200,201] These results emphasize the role of *RET* in HSCR and postulates that the 9q31 gene may be a modifier of *RET* expression. This 9q31 gene may be identical to the gene mutant in Riley-Day syndrome (MIM 223900; familial dysautonomia), a hereditary neuropathy resulting from a loss of subsets of autonomic neurons.

## Multigenic Inheritance of S-HSCR

The major HSCR features have mainly emerged from studies of L-HSCR and syndromic cases; our understanding of the molecular genetics of the most common form of HSCR, nonsyndromic S-HSCR, is still poor. For example, the precise role of *RET* in S-HSCR is unknown because mutation detection studies have searched coding sequences and not provided independent linkage evidence of its role based on mapping. Segregation analysis has suggested that S-HSCR and L-HSCR differ both with respect to the number of segregating genes and the penetrance of associated mutations, but whether the same genes are involved or not is unclear (Table 251-2). To test these hypotheses, we have recently performed a genome-wide mapping study in 49 nuclear families ascertained through S-HSCR probands (Chakravarti and Lyonnet, unpublished data). This analysis clearly shows that genetic effects at three loci, on human chromosomes 3p21, 10q11, and 19q12, are both necessary and sufficient to explain the incidence and sib recurrence risk of HSCR. Interestingly, none of the known candidate genes for HSCR (Table 251-4, Fig. 251-4) made any substantial contribution to disease risk. The estimated effects of mutations, expressed as the degree to which disease risk is increased at the 3p21, 10q11, and 19q12 loci, were 4.2-fold, 8.3-fold, and 5.0-fold, respectively; the estimated frequencies of susceptibility alleles at these three loci were 4 percent, 1 percent, and 5 percent, respectively. Genetic modeling showed clear evidence of multiplicative risk across loci, so that most affected individuals are heterozygous at all three loci (Chakravarti and Lyonnet, unpublished data). Consequently, typical of that expected for a complex genetic trait, S-HSCR can be explained by the multiplicative interaction of three loci with relatively common susceptibility alleles.

This last study demonstrated two additional effects that begin to unravel the complex nature of HSCR. First, the 10q11 factor is *RET* since coding sequence mutations could be identified in 40 percent of *RET*-linked families; these mutations are nonrandomly distributed largely in the extracellular domain. The mutation frequency is in agreement with previous studies,[128] but the large (88 percent of families) involvement of *RET* in S-HSCR evident from linkage analysis is not reflected in the mutation studies. Evidently, the majority of *RET* mutations are noncoding. Second, marker analysis showed a significant difference in the origin of *RET* alleles, but not those at chromosomes 3p21 and 19q12, with 78 percent of cases being maternally derived. This parent-of-origin effect may be a critical explanation of the sex difference in disease expression. Once again, the involvement of *RET*, even in the most common S-HSCR, proves its central role in all forms of HSCR, and suggests that the yet unknown 3p21 and 19q12 genes are *RET*-dependent modifiers (Chakravarti and Lyonnet, unpublished data).

## SYNDROMES AND ASSOCIATED ANOMALIES

The high rate of additional congenital anomalies in HSCR patients raises several important issues as outlined here:[78,202]

1. No constant pattern is observed and many anomalies are distantly related to the gastrointestinal tract and include distal limb, sensorineural, skin, central nervous system, cardiac, and kidney malformations.
2. Syndrome delineation of known or novel entities, including HSCR, is a key question because it has implications for disease prognosis. Indeed, because the overall prognosis of HSCR is good, the developmental outcome of a patient might be much more dependent on a syndromic diagnosis or an associated malformation.
3. While genetic issues in isolated HSCR (sporadic or familial) are discussed later, the diagnosis of syndromic forms might significantly modify genetic counseling, sometimes raising the recurrence risk to sibs as high as that observed in monogenic disorders, because many of the syndromes of HSCR and associated features have underlying Mendelian inheritance (Table 251-5).
4. Many of the associated features in HSCR patients suggest screening of candidate genes for mutations based on a common embryologic mechanism. This is particularly true for the

**Table 251-5** Non-neurocristopathy Syndromes Associated with Hirschsprung Disease

| | Syndromes | MIM # | Key features | References |
|---|---|---|---|---|
| HSCR always present | Goldberg-Shprintzen | 235730 | Cleft palate, hypotonia, mental retardation, facial dysmorphism | 233 |
| | HSCR with limb anomalies | 235740 | Polydactyly, unilateral renal agenesis, hypertelorism, deafness | 237 |
| | | 235750 | Postaxial polydactyly, ventricular septal defect | 101 |
| | | 235760 | Hypoplasia of distal phalanges and nails, dysmorphic features | 238 |
| | | 604211 | Preaxial polydactyly, heart defect, laryngeal anomalies | 239 |
| | | 306980 | Brachydactyly type D | 103 |
| | BRESEK syndrome | – | Brain abnormalities, retardation, ectodermal dysplasia, skeletal malformation, ear/eye anomalies, kidney dysplasia | 240 |
| HSCR occasionally associated | Bardet-Biedl syndrome | 209900 | Pigmentary retinopathy, obesity, hypogenitalism, mild mental retardation, postaxial polydactyly | 241, 242 |
| | Kauffman-McKusick | 236700 | Hydrometrocolpos, postaxial polydactyly, congenital heart defect | 243 |
| | Smith-Lemli-Opitz | 270400 | Growth retardation, microcephaly, mental retardation, hypospadias, 2–3 toes syndactyly, dysmorphic features | 246 |
| | Cartilage-hair hypoplasia | 250250 | Short-limb dwarfism, metaphyseal dysplasia, immunodeficiency | 247 |
| HSCR rarely associated | Fukuyama congenital muscular dystrophy | 253800 | Muscular dystrophy, polymicrogyria, hydrocephalus, MR, seizures | 248 |
| | Clayton-Smith | 258840 | Dysmorphic features, hypoplastic toes and nails, ichthyosis | 250 |
| | Kaplan | 304100 | Agenesis of corpus callosum, adducted thumbs, ptosis, muscle weakness | 251 |
| | Okamoto | 308840 | Hydrocephalus, cleft palate, corpus callosum agenesis, familial dysautonomia | 252, 254, 255 |
| Miscellaneous associations | Pallister-Hall (CAVE) | 146510 | Imperforate anus, postaxial or mesoaxial polydactyly, hypopituitarism, cleft larynx, hypothalamic hamartoblastoma | 244 |
| | Fryns | 229850 | | |
| | Aarskog | 100050 | | |
| | Jeune asphyxiating thoracic dystrophia | 208500 | | |
| | Frontonasal dysplasia | 136760 | | |
| | Osteopetrosis | | | |
| | Goldenhar | 164210 | | |
| | Lesch-Nyhan | 308000 | | |
| | Rubinstein-Taybi | 180849 | | |
| | Toriello-Carey | 217980 | | |
| | SEMDJL | 271640 | | |

anomalies related to an abnormal development of NC-derived cells. Syndrome delineation is thus a crucial step in order to propose pathogenic mechanisms for one or more subtypes of HSCR based on the precise ascertainment of associated features.

## Neurocristopathy Syndromes

The various syndromes associated with HSCR are summarized in Table 251-5, and classified as associated neurocristopathies, syndromes with HSCR as a mandatory feature, occasional association in well-known entities, and rare or miscellaneous observations.

**Waardenburg Syndrome (WS) and Related Pigmentary Syndromes.** This is a multiple congenital anomaly with white forelock, sometimes more extensive depigmentation of the skin or premature greying, heterochromia irides (sometimes only hypoplastic irides), sensorineural deafness resulting from anomaly of the organ of Corti,[203] lateral displacement of inner canthi (which defines type 1 (WS1) as opposed to WS2, WS3, or WS4), and other dysmorphic features including synophrys, high nasal bridge, and thick eyebrows. Occasional findings are true hypertelorism (10 percent), cleft lip and palate (2 to 3 percent) and congenital heart, usually septal, defects. The combination of HSCR with WS has been observed in a number of sporadic and familial cases and families reported as Shah-Waardenburg syndrome (WS4) (MIM 277580).[106,108,111,204] The vast majority, if not all, patients with WS4 show no dystopia cantorum suggesting that WS4 can be regarded as the combination of WS2 with HSCR. While dominant mutations of the *PAX3* and the *MITF* genes have been reported in WS1, WS2, or Tietze syndrome (MIM 103500), respectively, WS4 patients may be homozygous for mutations of the endothelin pathway[159,160,162,171,170,205,206] or heterozygous for *SOX10* mutations[180] (see "Molecular Genetics of Hirschsprung Disease" above). A general observation in these families is that there is a lower penetrance of HSCR as compared pigment anomalies,[207] which might explain the observation of WS without HSCR in patients with deletion of 13q21-q31, including the *EDNRB* gene.

Several patients with WS and HSCR present with central nervous system involvement including seizures, ataxia, and demyelinating peripheral and central neuropathies.[208] These patients carry heterozygous *SOX10* gain-of-function mutations.[209,210] Accordingly, progressive cerebral involvement with mental retardation, seizures, ataxia, or any neurodegenerative symptoms in an HSCR patient should prompt a search for demyelinating features on brain MRI.

Four other pigment-related syndromes are known. First, two families with Yemenite Deaf-Blind-Hypopigmentation syndrome (MIM 601706) were reported with severe early hearing loss, patchy hypo- and hyperpigmentation, microcornea, coloboma of the iris or choroidea, and nystagmus. In one of these families, a *SOX10* mutation was reported, suggesting that this syndrome may be genetically heterogeneous.[211] Second, the Black Locks-Albinism-Deafness syndrome (BADS, MIM 227010) is an autosomal recessive trait in which the hair and skin are congenitally white except for clusters of black hair occurring in locks;[212] profound congenital sensorineural deafness and brown macules are associated with no retinal pigment and subsequent nystagmus. Colonic HSCR extending to the small intestine has been reported in one BADS patient. Third, aganglionic megacolon has been reported with familial piebaldism (MIM 172800).[107,213] Fourth, HSCR and profound congenital deafness has been reported with no WS features.[110] Nevertheless, it is suggested that HSCR patients with isolated sensorineural deafness should be tested for mutations of the genes responsible for WS4.

**Congenital Central Hypoventilation Syndrome (CCHS).** Commonly termed Ondine's curse, CCHS (MIM 209880) is a primary congenital alveolar hypoventilation resulting from failure of autonomic control.[214] It is a rare life-threatening condition with abnormal ventilatory response to hypoxia and hypercapnia. CCHS patients often manifest a broader spectrum of symptoms resulting from dysfunction of the autonomous nervous system, such as, esophageal motility abnormalities, reduced control of heart rate, ocular manifestations (pupillary anomalies, convergence insufficiency, strabismus, insufficient tears), profuse sweating, decreased basal body temperature, and decreased perception of discomfort or anxiety. Isolated CCHS is regarded as a polygenic disorder, but a major locus may be involved. The overall sib recurrence risk is 5 percent and few CCHS multicase families are known. Rare mutations of the *RET* or endothelin signaling pathways have been suggested in some patients.[172,215-217]

Autopsy findings of decreased muscarinic receptor binding in the central nucleus, as well as the occasional occurrence of neuroblastoma and ganglioneuroma, suggests that CCHS is a neurocristopathy. The combination of CCHS with HSCR (Haddad syndrome, MIM 209880[218,219]), reported in ≈14 percent of CCHS patients, lends further support to the idea that this phenotype arises from a defect of migration or differentiation of NC cells. In the vast majority of CCHS-HSCR patients, aganglionosis is of the long-segment form, including TCA, with an equal sex ratio as opposed to what is observed in isolated HSCR. It has been suggested that CCHS is more severe when associated with HSCR, so that the prognosis of patients with CCHS-HSCR is poor.[220]

**Multiple Endocrine Neoplasia Type 2 (MEN2).** The MEN2 syndromes are autosomal dominant cancer predisposition syndromes subdivided into three types: familial medullary thyroid carcinoma (FMTC), MEN type 2A (MEN2A), and MEN type 2B (MEN2B). MEN2A is characterized by hyperplasia of the calcitonin-producing parafollicular cells of the thyroid with subsequent neoplastic progression to medullary thyroid carcinoma (MTC), pheochromocytoma (25 percent of cases), and hyperplasia of the parathyroid (50 percent). In addition to these features, individuals with MEN2B present with oral neuromas, marfanoid habitus, and hyperganglionosis of the hindgut, which contrasts with the absence of enteric ganglia cells in HSCR, although the clinical presentation might be similar with functional intestinal obstruction syndromes. The penetrance of MEN2 is age-related and although only about 70 percent of MEN2A gene carriers will present with MTC by the age of 70 years, the precursor lesion, namely C-cell hyperplasia, is detectable in almost all carriers by endocrine testing (pentagastrin test) prior to 40 years of age. As outlined earlier, missense mutations of the *RET* gene have been identified in MEN2A, MEN2B, and FMTC.

Only FMTC and MEN2A have been associated with HSCR in several families thus far.[102] It is worth noting that these families harbor a germ line *RET* mutation of the MEN2A or FMTC type, namely a missense mutation at either codon 618 or 620, resulting in the replacement of a cysteine by an arginine residue in most cases.[124,221-225] Clinically, individuals with HSCR may be screened for *RET* exon 10 and 11 mutations to rule out predisposition to MEN2A and associated tumors.[226,227] Association of HSCR with MEN2B is questionable and mutation of the MEN2B type (point mutation M918T) has not been found in a patient with HSCR. Occasionally, patients with L-HSCR have been reported with isolated NC-derived tumors such as neuroblastoma, ganglioneuroblastoma, and pheochromocytoma.[228-230]

**Other Neurocristopathies and Neural Tube Defects.** HSCR has been occasionally diagnosed in patients with other NC defects but with no familial or molecular evidence for a significant association, namely, cleft lip with or without cleft palate, neural tube defects (myelomeningocele),[231] and neurofibromatosis type I, although the latter combination is questionable on histologic grounds.[232]

## Syndromes with HSCR as a Significant Association

**Goldberg-Shprintzen Syndrome.** The Goldberg-Shprintzen syndrome (MIM 235730) is a rare, multiple congenital anomalies-mental retardation syndrome combining HSCR, cleft palate, hypotonia, mental retardation, and facial dysmorphic features (hypertelorism, prominent nose, synophrys, sparse hair).[233] Eleven patients have been reported so far and autosomal recessive inheritance is suggested but not proven.[234] CT scan or MRI investigations of the brain may show a ventricular dilation and irregular density of white matter suggesting a neuronal migration defect. The observations of HSCR with microcephaly, iris coloboma, cleft palate, and mental retardation may be related to this syndrome.[235,236]

**HSCR with Distal Limb Anomalies.** A series of rare syndromes with HSCR and distal limb anomalies (polydactyly or hypoplasia) have been reported. These syndromes are: (a) HSCR with polydactyly, unilateral renal agenesis, hypertelorism, and congenital deafness in sibs, suggesting autosomal recessive inheritance (MIM 235740);[237] (b) HSCR, postaxial polydactyly, and ventricular septal defects in two sibs with normal mental development in a surviving sib (MIM 235750);[101] (c) HSCR, hypoplasia of the distal phalanges and nails, and mild dysmorphic features (low-set ears with abnormal helices, up-slanting palpebral fissures, and loose skin)[238] in the offspring of a first-cousin union (MIM 235760) with additional anomalies (hydronephrosis, imperforated anus, and inguinal hernia) in at least one sib; (d) HSCR with heart defect, preaxial polydactyly, and laryngeal anomalies (short epiglottis) in a brother and a sister, both with mild developmental delay, with unaffected parents and possible recessive inheritance (MIM 604211);[239] (e) HSCR with brachydactyly type D in several males of a two-generation family with type D brachydactyly (short distal phalanges of the thumbs and first toes) (MIM 306980);[103] (f) HSCR with macrocephaly, brachydactyly, and spinal defects in a male child with thoracic and lumbar vertebrae anomalies; (g) one patient with BRESEK syndrome, an acronym for brain abnormalities (hydrocephalus), retardation, ectodermal dysplasia (including alopecia and hyperkeratosis with normal sweating), skeletal malformation (including polydactyly, hemivertebrae, and scoliosis), ear/eye anomalies (low-set and prominent ears with hearing loss, microphthalmia) and kidney dysplasia with unilateral agenesis.[240]

## Syndromes with HSCR as an Occasional Finding

HSCR has been occasionally diagnosed in three syndromes or groups of syndromes that are important to recognize for both prognosis and suggestion of candidate genes for ENS development.

**Bardet-Biedl Syndrome.** Laurence Moon Bardet-Biedl syndrome (MIM 209900) is an autosomal recessive condition characterized by pigmentary retinopathy with early macular involvement, obesity, hypogenitalism, mild mental retardation and postaxial polydactyly of hands and feet;[241,242] renal involvement is common (90 percent) including cysts, renal cortical loss, or reduced ability to concentrate urine. Cardiac defects or cardiomyopathy have been reported in some patients. Bardet-Biedl syndrome is genetically heterogeneous because at least four loci have been mapped to chromosomes 16q, 11q, 3p, and 15q. There are strong clinical overlaps between this syndrome and Kauffman-McKusick syndrome (MIM 236700), another rare autosomal recessive disorder characterized by hydrometrocolpos resulting from a transverse vaginal membrane, postaxial polydactyly, and congenital heart disease. In addition, there might be an imperforate anus, urogenital sinus, malrotation of the gut, and, in Kauffman-McKusick syndrome, syndactyly. HSCR has been reported in 10 percent of cases.[243] Mutation of a gene encoding a putative chaperonin has been recently reported for the Kauffman-McKusick syndrome.[279] Some overlap is also suggested between the previous two conditions and Pallister-Hall ano-cerebro digital

syndrome or cerebro-acro-visceral-early lethality (CAVE) multiplex syndrome, an autosomal dominant condition that includes imperforate anus, postaxial or (more characteristically) mesoaxial polydactyly, hypopituitarism, cleft larynx or bifid epiglottis, and a characteristic but not pathognomonic hypothalamic hamartoblastoma. However, thus far, it seems that HSCR has been reported in only one Pallister-Hall syndrome case.[244] Patients with Pallister-Hall syndrome may have mutations in the *GLI3* gene.

**Smith-Lemli-Opitz Syndromes Types 1 and 2 (MIM 270400).** Smith-Lemli-Opitz (SLO) is a rare autosomal recessive condition characterized by pre- and postnatal growth retardation and microcephaly, mental retardation, hypospadias with hypoplastic scrotum, syndactyly between toes 2 and 3, and dysmorphic features (ptosis, anteverted nostrils with micrognathia). Postaxial polydactyly with ambiguous external genitalia, cleft palate, cardiac malformation and cerebral anomalies have been observed in the severe lethal form (SLO2 or lethal acrodysgenital dwarfism).[245] SLO is the first multiple congenital malformation syndrome resulting from metabolic deficiency of cholesterol synthesis with mutation of the 7-dehydro-cholesterol reductase (DHCR7 gene on chromosome 11q12-q13). While HSCR has been observed in a significant number of severe SLO patients,[246] cholesterol metabolism has not yet been studied in isolated (or syndromic) HSCR patients.

**Cartilage-Hair Hypoplasia (CHH, Metaphyseal Dysplasia).** This skeletal dysplasia (MIM 250250) was first recognized in the Old Order Amish community. It has these features: metaphyseal dysplasia with short-limb dwarfism; fine, sparse, and blond hair; transient macrocytic anemia; and immunodeficiency. HSCR is a significantly associated feature (8/108 cases).[247] CHH is an autosomal recessive condition whose gene has been mapped to chromosome 9p13. It is suggested that the round inferior femoral epiphysis dysplasia (Holmgren-Connor syndrome, MIM 211120) is allelic to cartilage-hair hypoplasia, especially as HSCR has been reported in this condition as well.

**Rare Associations.** HSCR has been reported in a number of rare disorders and this rarity makes it difficult to decide whether or not these associations are significant (Table 251-5). These rare disorders include:

1. Syndromes with muscular dystrophy: congenital muscular dystrophy of the Fukuyama type including muscle, eye, and brain involvement and with similarities to Walker-Warburg and cerebro-oculo muscular syndromes;[248] and multicore myopathy;[249]
2. Syndromes with dermatologic findings: Clayton-Smith syndrome with dysmorphic features, digital abnormalities (hypoplastic toes and nails), deafness, and ichthyosis;[250] and Dermotrichic syndrome characterized by alopecia, ichthyosis, mental retardation, and seizures with an X-linked recessive pattern of inheritance, and perhaps allelic to the ichthyosis follicularis-atrichia-photophobia syndrome;
3. Syndromes with central nervous system anomalies: the X-linked recessive Kaplan syndrome of agenesis of corpus callosum with adducted thumbs, ptosis, and muscle weakness of the shoulder girdle (MIM 304100)[251] that may be allelic to hydrocephalus with HSCR and cleft palate reported with a L1CAM gene mutation;[252] other reports of HSCR patients with corpus callosum agenesis either in Toriello-Carey or related syndromes;[253,254] and microcephaly with mental retardation, abnormal CT scan, dysmorphic features, and heart defect[236] that may be related to Goldberg-Shprintzen syndrome.[233,235]

Other rare associations include the finding of HSCR with familial dysautonomia,[255] Fryns, Aarskog, Jeune asphyxiating thoracic dystrophia, frontonasal dysplasia, osteopetrosis, Goldenhar, Lesch-Nyhan, Rubinstein-Taybi, spondyloepimetaphyseal dysplasia with joint laxity (SEMDJL, MIM 271640), persistent

Mullerian duct syndromes, and asplenia with cardiovascular anomaly. Some of these combinations undoubtedly have arisen by chance.

## Chromosomal Anomalies

Associations of HSCR with chromosomal anomalies are important because they allow the mapping of genes whose haploinsufficiency or overexpression could predispose to HSCR.

**Trisomy 21 (Down Syndrome).** The association of HSCR and Down syndrome has long been recognized[256] and has been described earlier (see "Epidemiology of Hirschsprung Disease" above). The association suggests that overexpression or imbalanced expression of genes on chromosome 21 may predispose to HSCR. Most affected children have S-HSCR with a strikingly unbalanced sex ratio of 5.5 to 10.5 male:female. Histologic assessment for typical HSCR is important in Down syndrome patients, especially as simple constipation or related intestinal phenotypes, such as intestinal neuronal dysplasia, have been reported.[257] Down syndrome patients with HSCR have free trisomy 21 with few exceptions. Linkage studies have suggested that the 21q22 band may contain a modifier gene for HSCR in a Mennonite kindred, but this finding has not been confirmed in other studies.[159] Hitherto, only mutations in *RET*, *EDNRB*, and *GDNF*, the genes that predispose to HSCR, have been found in patients with Down syndrome and HSCR.[145,258]

**Deletion Syndromes.** A number of chromosomal interstitial deletions has been reported in combination with HSCR, some of them clearly indicating the locus for one of the several genes predisposing to this congenital malformation. These include: (a) deletion of 2q22-23 with short neck, microcephaly, agenesis of the corpus callosum, short stature, and suggesting a contiguous gene deletion syndrome involving a locus for HSCR;[259,260] (b) deletion 2p syndrome;[261] (c) deletion of chromosome 10q11.2 observed in multiple patients with isolated L-HSCR or TCA, which led to the mapping of the first gene (*RET*) for HSCR;[82,262] (d) deletion of chromosome 13q22.1-32.1 with dysmorphic features, mental retardation, and S-HSCR, which led to the mapping of the second gene (*EDNRB*) for HSCR;[85,87,263] (e) deletion of chromosome 22q11.2 reported in one HSCR patient with DiGeorge syndrome features.[264]

**Rare Associations.** Some findings such as cat-eye syndrome (supernumerary dicentric chromosome 22q),[265,266] mosaic trisomy 8, XXY chromosomal constitution, partial duplication of chromosome 2q, translocations,[267] tetrasomy 9p, 20p deletion,[268] and deletion/duplications of 17q21-q23,[89] have been also observed.

## Isolated Anomalies

A wide spectrum of additional isolated anomalies among HSCR cases, found in a number of studies with incidence between 5 percent and 30 percent, are important to outline.[76–78,269–272] These anomalies associated with HSCR can be divided into (a) regional anomalies occurring secondary to local bowel dilatation, such as renal obstruction, and (b) nonrandom anomalies that are not secondary to a cascade of events, occurring in other systems or, more distantly, in the gastrointestinal tract.

**Associated Regional Anomalies.** Megalonephrosis, hydronephrosis, and megalocystis could result from obstruction caused by a dilated bowel segment. Along these lines, colonic, rectal, and anal atresia or stenosis have been mentioned possibly resulting from secondary dilatation of the bowel in utero.[273,274]

**Associated Nonregional Anomalies.** Most isolated anomalies associated with HSCR are found in these areas: (a) cardiovascular defects, mostly atrioseptal or ventriculoseptal defects, found in up to 5 percent of cases with HSCR on excluding Down syndrome patients; (b) renal hypoplasia or agenesis;[275] (c) genital anomalies up to 2 to 3 percent, including hypospadias or hypoplastic scrotum; (d) nonregional gastrointestinal malformations such as Meckel diverticulum, pyloric stenosis,[254,276] single umbilical artery, inguinal hernia, or small bowel atresia;[277] (d) skeletal and limb anomalies such as polydactyly; (e) sensorineural defects such as deafness that should prompt recognition of syndromic variants of HSCR such as WS4 and related syndromes; (f) autonomic dysfunction;[176,278] and (g) isolated dysmorphic features.

Depending on the study, and whether a careful dysmorphologic examination with echographic surveys and skeletal x-ray was performed or not, the frequency of nonregional anomalies in HSCR may be as high as 23 percent. These observations should prompt clinicians to carefully assess anomalies within the following grid: dysmorphologic examination, cardiac echographic survey, urogenital echographic survey, skeletal x-ray, blood karyotype whenever one additional symptom is observed, and, eventually, brain imaging by CT scan or MRI.

## GENETIC COUNSELING AND TESTING IN HSCR

HSCR has classically been considered as a sex-modified multifactorial disorder and genetic counseling has involved assigning an overall risk of 4 percent to sibs and other first-degree relatives of a proband. Many HSCR cases are associated with known syndromes. In these cases, genetic counseling is more dependent on the prognosis of the patient with these association than on the recurrence of HSCR. In isolated HSCR, with the demonstration of variation in recurrence risk by sex of proband and consultand, and by extent of aganglionosis, more precise risk tailored to individual family structures can be provided and is warranted (Table 251-6). The success in identifying specific genes for various syndromic and nonsyndromic forms of HSCR suggests that mutation detection in familial cases may be warranted. However, except for Shah-Waardenburg syndrome (WS4), the penetrance of single-gene mutations is much less than 100 percent so that their utility to a family is questionable. Consequently, genetic testing in HSCR is performed on a research basis and currently not considered for clinical evaluation of risks. However, because some patients with isolated HSCR have *RET* exon 10 and 11 mutations that are identical to those observed in MEN2A patients (see "Molecular Genetics of Hirschsprung Disease" above), they may warrant

**Table 251-6** Percent Recurrent Risk of Hirschsprung Disease by Proband and Consultand Gender and Extent of Aganglionosis

| Consultand | Long-segment HSCR | | Colonic-segment HSCR | | Short-segment HSCR | |
|---|---|---|---|---|---|---|
| | Male | Female | Male | Female | Male | Female |
| Sib of affected male | 11 | 8 | 10 | 7 | 4 | 1 |
| Sib of affected female | 23 | 18 | 13 | 10 | 6 | 2 |
| Offspring of affected male | 18 | 13 | 11 | 9 | ~0 | ~0 |
| Offspring of affected female | 28 | 22 | 15 | 11 | ~0 | ~0 |

further testing to ascertain whether they are predisposed to neuroendocrine tumors. Recent studies emphasize oligogenic inheritance of HSCR with the identification of a specific role for *RET* and additional loci at 3p21, 9q31, and 19q12, and precise determinations of risk increase (4.2-, 5.0-, or 8.3-fold). These studies theoretically make possible molecular testing in familial cases and estimation of the recurrence risk increase to siblings. Although this approach is untested, regarding utility to HSCR families, it remains as a new scientific approach to accurate family specific genetic counseling.

## ACKNOWLEDGMENTS

We are deeply indebted to the many members of numerous HSCR families across the world, the American Pseudo-obstruction & Hirschsprung Disease Society, Inc., and the French HSCR Consortium for sharing information, donating tissue samples, and making the scientific work in our laboratories possible. We gratefully acknowledge the members of our research groups, past and present, for their enduring contributions, but particularly, Minerva Carrasquillo, Jennifer Scott, Anna Pelet, Rémi Salomon, Jeanne Amiel, and Andrew McCallion for assistance in preparation of this review.

## REFERENCES

1. Hirschsprung H: Stuhlträgheit neugeborener infolge von dilatation und hypertrophic des colons. *Jb Kinderheilk* **27**:1, 1888.
2. Whitehouse F, Kernohan J: Myenteric plexuses in congenital megacolon; Study of 11 cases. *Arch Int Med* **82**:75, 1948.
3. Swenson O, Bill A: Resection of rectum and rectosigmoid with preservation of sphincter for benign spastic lesions producing megacolon, an experimental study. *Surgery* **24**:212, 1948.
4. Swenson O: Early history of the therapy of Hirschsprung's disease: Facts and personal observations over 50 years. *J Pediatr Surg* **31**:1003, 1996.
5. Meier-Ruge, W, Lutterbeck, PM, Herzog, B, Morger R, Moser R, Scharli A: Acetylcholinesterase activity in suction biopsies of the rectum in the diagnosis of Hirschsprung's disease. *J Pediatr Surg* **7**:11, 1972.
6. Pellerin, D: Hirschsprung disease. *Ann Gastroenterol Hepatol* **28**:99, 1992.
7. Milla, PJ: Intestinal motility during ontogeny and intestinal pseudo-obstruction in children. *Pediatr Clin North Am* **43**:511, 1996.
8. Vanderwinden JM, Rumessen JJ, Liu, H, Descamps, D, De Laet, MH, Vanderhaeghen JJ: Interstitial cells of Cajal in human colon and in Hirschsprung's disease. *Gastroenterology* **111**:901, 1996.
9. Wedel T, Holschneider AM, Krammer HJ: Ultrastructural features of nerve fascicles and basal lamina abnormalities in Hirschsprung's disease. *Eur J Pediatr Surg* **9**:75, 1999.
10. Nihoul-Fékété C, Ricour C, Martelli H Jacob SL, Pellerin D: Total colonic aganglionosis (with or without ileal involvement): A review of 27 cases. *J Pediatr Surg* **21**:251, 1986.
11. Neilson IR, Yazbeck S: Ultrashort Hirschsprung's disease: Myth or reality. *J Pediatr Surg* **25**:1135, 1990.
12. Klein M, Burd R: Hirschsprung's disease, in Wyllie RY, Ams JS (eds): *Pediatric Gastrointestinal Diseases*. Philadelphia, WB Saunders, 1999, p 489.
13. Parc R, Berrod JL, Tussiot J, Loygue J: Megacolon in adults. Apropos of 76 cases. *Ann Gastroenterol Hepatol (Paris)* **20**:133, 1984.
14. Crocker NL, Messmer JM: Adult Hirschsprung's disease. *Clin Radiol* **44**:257, 1991.
15. Vermesh M, Mayden KL, Confino E, Giglia RV, Gleicher N: Prenatal sonographic diagnosis of Hirschsprung's disease. *J Ultrasound Med* **5**:37, 1986.
16. Jasonni V, Martucciello G: Total colonic aganglionosis. *Semin Pediatr Surg* **7**:174, 1998.
17. Taxman TL, Yulish BS, Rothstein FC: How useful is the barium enema in the diagnosis of infantile Hirschsprung's disease? *Am J Dis Child* **140**:881, 1986.
18. Emir H, Akman M, Sarimurat N, Kilic N, Erdogan E, Soylet Y: Anorectal manometry during the neonatal period: Its specificity in the diagnosis of Hirschsprung's disease. *Eur J Pediatr Surg* **9**:101, 1999.
19. Lopez-Alonso M, Ribas J, Hernandez A, Anguita FA, Gomez de Terreros I, Martinez-Caro A: Efficiency of the anorectal manometry for

20. Noblett HR: A rectal suction biopsy tube for use in the diagnosis of Hirschsprung's disease. *J Pediatr Surg* **4**:406, 1969.
21. Kurer MH, Lawson JO, Pambakian H: Suction biopsy in Hirschsprung's disease. *Arch Dis Child* **61**:83, 1986.
22. Bonham JR, Dale G, Scott DJ, Wagget J: Acetylcholinesterase activity in rectal biopsies: an assessment of its diagnostic value in Hirschsprung's disease [Letter]. *J Pediatr Gastroenterol Nutr* **7**:298, 1988.
23. Faure C, Goulet O, Ategbo S, Breton A, Tounian P, Ginies JL, Roquelaure B, et al: Chronic intestinal pseudoobstruction syndrome: Clinical analysis outcome, and prognosis in 105 children. French-speaking group of pediatric gastroenterology. *Dig Dis Sci* **44**:953, 1999.
24. Puri P, Wester T: Intestinal neuronal dysplasia. *Semin Pediatr Surg* **7**:181, 1998.
25. Scharli AF, Meier-Ruge W: Localized and disseminated forms of neuronal intestinal dysplasia mimicking Hirschsprung's disease. *J Pediatr Surg* **16**:164, 1981.
26. Auricchio A, Brancolini V, Casari G, Milla PJ, Smith VV, Devoto M, Ballabio A: The locus for a novel syndromic form of neuronal intestinal pseudoobstruction maps to Xq28. *Am J Hum Genet* **58**:743, 1996.
27. Barone V, Weber D, Luo Y, Brancolini V, Devoto M, Romeo G: Exclusion of linkage between *RET* and neuronal intestinal dysplasia type B. *Am J Med Genet* **62**:195, 1996.
28. Sherman JO, Snyder ME, Weitzman JJ, Jona JZ, Gillis DA, O'Donnell B, Carcassonne M, et al: A 40-year multinational retrospective study of 880 Swenson procedures. *J Pediatr Surg* **24**:833, 1989.
29. Soave F: Hirschsprung's disease. Technique and results of Soave's operation. *Br J Surg* **53**:1023, 1966.
30. Newbern WR: Hirschsprung's disease—The Duhamel modification. *Am J Gastroenterol* **47**:61, 1967.
31. Albanese CT Jennings RW, Smith B, Bratton B, Harrison MR: Perineal one-stage pull-through for Hirschsprung's disease. *J Pediatr Surg* **34**:377, 1999.
32. Tsuji H, Spitz L, Kiely EM, Drake DP, Pierro A: Management and long-term follow-up of infants with total colonic aganglionosis. *J Pediatr Surg* **34**:158, 1999.
33. Elhalaby, EA, Teitelbaum, DH, Coran AG, Heidelberger, KP: Enterocolitis associated with Hirschsprung's disease: A clinical histopathological correlative study. *J Pediatr Surg* **30**:1023, 1995.
34. Hackam DJ, Filler RM, Pearl RH: Enterocolitis after the surgical treatment of Hirschsprung's disease: Risk factors and financial impact [Comments]. *J Pediatr Surg* **33**:830, 1998.
35. Rescorla F, Morrison A, Engles D, West K, Grosfeld J: Hirshsprung's disease. Evaluation of mortality and long-term function in 260 cases. *Arch Surg* **127**:934, 1992.
36. Bourdelat D, Vrsansky P, Pages R, Duhamel B: Duhamel operation 40 years after: A multicentric study. *Eur J Pediatr Surg* **7**:70, 1997.
37. Reding R, de Ville de Goyet J, Gosseye S, Clapuyt P, Sokal E, Buts JP, Gibbs P, et al: Hirschsprung's disease: A 20-year experience. *J Pediatr Surg* **32**:1221, 1997.
38. Yanchar NL, Soucy P: Long-term outcome after Hirschsprung's disease: Patients' perspectives. *J Pediatr Surg* **34**:1152, 1999.
39. Moore SW, Albertyn R, Cywes S: Clinical outcome and long-term quality of life after surgical correction of Hirschsprung's disease. *J Pediatr Surg* **31**:1496, 1996.
40. Le Douarin N, Teillet M: The migration of neural crest cells to the wall of the digestive tract in avian embryo. *J Embryol Exp Morphol* **30**:31, 1973.
41. Le Douarin N, Kalcheim C: *The Neural Crest.* Cambridge, UK, Cambridge University Press, 1999.
42. Guillemot F, Lo LC, Johnson JE, Auerbach A, Anderson DJ, Joyner AL: Mammalian achaete-scute homolog 1 is required for the early development of olfactory and autonomic neurons. *Cell* **75**:463, 1993.
43. Pachnis V, Mankoo B, Costantini F: Expression of the *c-ret* proto-oncogene during mouse embryogenesis. *Development* **119**:1005, 1993.
44. Serbedzija GN, Burgan, S, Fraser SE, Bronner-Fraser M: Vital dye labelling demonstrates a sacral neural crest contribution to the enteric nervous system of chick and mouse embryos. *Development* **111**:857, 1991.
45. Kapur R, Yost, C, Palmiter R: A transgenic model for studying development of the enteric nervous system in normal and aganglionic mice. *Development* **116**:167, 1992.

46. Gershon MD: II. Disorders of enteric neuronal development: Insights from transgenic mice. *Am J Physiol* **277**:G262, 1999.

47. Taraviras S, Pachnis V: Development of the mammalian enteric nervous system. *Curr Opin Genet Dev* **9**:321, 1999.

48. Meijers JH, van der Sanden MP, Tibboel, D, van der Kamp AW, Luider TM, Molenaar JC: Colonization characteristics of enteric neural crest cells: Embryological aspects of Hirschsprung's disease. *J Pediatr Surg* **27**:811, 1992.

49. Dupin, E, Sextier-Sainte-Claire Deville F, Nataf V, Le Douarin NM: The ontogeny of the neural crest. *C R Acad Sci III* **316**:1062, 1993.

50. Peters-van der Sanden MJ, Kirby ML, Gittenberger-de Groot A, Tibboel D, Mulder MP, Meijers JC: Ablation of various regions within the avian vagal neural crest has differential effects on ganglion formation in the fore-, mid-, and hindgut. *Dev Dyn* **196**:183, 1993.

51. Newgreen DF, Southwell B, Hartley L, Allan IJ: Migration of enteric neural crest cells in relation to growth of the gut in avian embryos. *Acta Anat (Basel)* **157**:105, 1996.

52. Burns AJ, Douarin NM: The sacral neural crest contributes neurons and glia to the post- umbilical gut: Spatiotemporal analysis of the development of the enteric nervous system. *Development* **125**:4335, 1998.

53. Pachnis V, Durbec P, Taraviras S, Grigoriou M, Natarajan D: III. Role Of the *RET* signal transduction pathway in development of the mammalian enteric nervous system. *Am J Physiol* **275**:G183, 1998.

54. Taraviras S, Marcos-Gutierrez CV, Durbec P, Jani H, Grigoriou M, Sukumaran M, Wang LC, et al: Signaling by the *RET* receptor tyrosine kinase and its role in the development of the mammalian enteric nervous system. *Development* **126**:2785, 1999.

55. Durbec P, Larsson-Blomberg L, Schuchardt A, Costantini F, Pachnis V: Common origin and developmental dependance on c-ret of subsets of enteric and sympathetic neuroblasts. *Development* **122**:349, 1996.

56. Natarajan D, Pachnis V: Development of the enteric nervous system, in Sanderson IR, Walker WA (eds): *Development of the Gastrointestinal Tract*. Hamilton, Ontario, B. C. Decker, 1999, p 197.

57. Gershon MD: V. Genes, lineages, and tissue interactions in the development of the enteric nervous system. *Am J Physiol* **275**:G869, 1998.

58. Natarajan D, Grigoriou M, Marcos-Gutierrez CV, Atkins C, Pachnis V: Multipotential progenitors of the mammalian enteric nervous system capable of colonising aganglionic bowel in organ culture. *Development* **126**:157, 1999.

59. Kobayashi H, Hirakawa H, O'Brian DS, Puri P: Nerve growth factor receptor staining of suction biopsies in the diagnosis of Hirschsprung's disease. *J Pediatr Surg* **29**:1224, 1994.

60. Lahav R, Dupin E, Lecoin L, Glavieux C, Champeval D, Ziller C, Le Douarin NM: Endothelin 3 selectively promotes survival and proliferation of neural crest-derived glial and melanocytic precursors *in vitro*. *Proc Natl Acad Sci U S A* **95**:14214, 1998.

61. Oue T, Puri P: Altered endothelin-3 and endothelin-B receptor mRNA expression in Hirschsprung's disease. *J Pediatr Surg* **34**:1257, 1999.

62. Martucciello G, Favre A, Takahashi M, Jasonni V: Immunohistochemical localization of *RET* protein in Hirschsprung's disease. *J Pediatr Surg* **30**:433, 1995.

63. Attie-Bitach T, Abitbol M, Gerard M, Delezoide AL, Auge J, Pelet A, Amiel J, et al: Expression of the *RET* proto-oncogene in human embryos. *Am J Med Genet* **80**:481, 1998.

64. Ohshiro K, Puri P: Reduced glial cell line-derived neurotrophic factor level in aganglionic bowel in Hirschsprung's disease. *J Pediatr Surg* **33**:904, 1998.

65. Gershon MD, Tennyson VM: Microenvironmental factors in the normal and abnormal development of the enteric nervous system. *Prog Clin Biol Res* **373**:257, 1991.

66. Ikawa H, Kawano H, Takeda Y, Masuyama H, Watanabe K, Endo M, Yokoyama J, et al: Impaired expression of neural cell adhesion molecule L1 in the extrinsic nerve fibers in Hirschsprung's disease. *J Pediatr Surg* **32**:542, 1997.

67. Parikh DH, Tam PK Van Velzen D, Edgar D: The extracellular matrix components, tenascin and fibronectin, in Hirschsprung's disease: An immunohistochemical study. *J Pediatr Surg* **29**:1302, 1994.

68. Larsson LT, Sundler F: Neuronal markers in Hirschsprung's disease with special reference to neuropeptides. *Acta Histochem Suppl* **38**:115, 1990.

69. Parikh DH, Tam PK, Van Velzen D, Edgar D: Abnormalities in the distribution of laminin and collagen type IV in Hirschsprung's disease. *Gastroenterology* **102**:1236, 1992.

70. Vanderwinden JM, De Laet MH, Schiffmann SN, Mailleux P, Lowenstein CJ, Snyder SH, Vanderhaeghen JJ: Nitric oxide synthase distribution in the enteric nervous system of Hirschsprung's disease. *Gastroenterology* **105**:969, 1993.

71. Bolande R: The neurocristopathies; A unifying concept of disease arising in neural crest maldevelopment. *Hum Pathol* **5**:409, 1973.

72. Bolande RP: Hirschsprung's disease, aganglionic or hypoganglionic megacolon. Animal model: aganglionic megacolon in piebald and spotted mutant mouse strains. *Am J Pathol* **79**:189, 1975.

73. Bodian M, Carter C: A family study of Hirschsprung disease. *Ann Hum Genet* **26**:261, 1963.

74. Badner JA, Sieber WK, Garver KL, Chakravarti A: A genetic study of Hirschsprung disease. *Am J Hum Genet* **46**:568, 1990.

75. Torfs CP: An epidemiological study of Hirschsprung disease in a multiracial California population, in *The Third International Meeting: Hirschsprung Disease and Related Neurocristophathies*. Evian, France, 1998.

76. Goldberg EL: An epidemiological study of Hirschsprung's disease. *Int J Epidemiol* **13**:479, 1984.

77. Spouge D, Baird PA: Hirschsprung disease in a large birth cohort. *Teratology* **32**:171, 1985.

78. Passarge E: The genetics of Hirschsprung's disease. Evidence for heterogeneous etiology and a study of sixty-three families. *N Engl J Med* **276**:138, 1967.

79. Passarge E: Spontaneous chromosomal instability. *Humangenetik* **16**:151, 1972.

80. Garver KL, Law JC, Garver B: Hirschsprung disease: A genetic study. *Clin Genet* **28**:503, 1985.

81. Brooks AS, Breuning MH, Meijers C: Spectrum of phenotypes associated with Hirschsprung disease: An evaluation of 239 patients from a single institution, in *The Third International Meeting: Hirschsprung Disease and Related Neurocristophathies*. Evian, France, 1998.

82. Martucciello G, Bicocchi M, Dodero P, Lerone M, Silengo Cirillo M, Puliti A, Gimelli G, et al: Total colonic aganglionosis associated with interstitial deletion of the long arm of chromosome 10. *Pediatr Surg Int* **7**:308, 1992.

83. Puliti A, Covone AE, Bicocchi MP, Bolino A, Lerone M, Martucciello G, Jasonni V, et al: Deleted and normal chromosome 10 homologs from a patient with Hirschsprung disease isolated in two cell hybrids through enrichment by immunomagnetic selection. *Cytogenet Cell Genet* **63**:102, 1993.

84. Kiss P, Osztovics M: Association of 13q deletion and Hirschsprung's disease. *J Med Genet* **26**:793, 1989.

85. Lamont MA, Fitchett M, Dennis NR: Interstitial deletion of distal 13q associated with Hirschsprung's disease [Comments]. *J Med Genet* **26**:100, 1989.

86. Sparkes R, Sparkes MC, Kalina RE, Pagon RA, Salk DJ, Disteche CM: Separation of Retinoblastoma and esterase D loci in a patient with sporadic retinoblastoma and Del (13)(q14.1q22.3). *Hum Genet* **68**:258, 1984.

87. Bottani A, Xie YG, Binkert F, Schinzel A: A case of Hirschsprung disease with a chromosome 13 microdeletion, del(13)(q32.3q33.2): Potential mapping of one disease locus. *Hum Genet* **87**:748, 1991.

88. Van Camp G, Van Thienen MN, Handig I, Van Roy B, Rao VS, Milunsky A, Read AP, et al: Chromosome 13q deletion with Waardenburg syndrome: Further evidence for a gene involved in neural crest function on 13q. *J Med Genet* **32**:531, 1995.

89. Brewer C, Holloway S, Zawalnyski, P, Schinzel A, FitzPatrick, D: A chromosomal duplication map of malformations: Regions of suspected haplo- and triplolethality — and tolerance of segmental aneuploidy — in humans. *Am J Hum Genet* **64**:1702, 1999.

90. Bolk S, Pelet A, Hofstra RM, Angrist M, Salomon R, Croaker D, Buys CH, et al: A human model for multigenic inheritance: Phenotypic expression in Hirschsprung disease requires both the *RET* gene and a new 9q31 locus [Citation]. *Proc Natl Acad Sci U S A* **97**:268, 2000.

91. Kogan J, Wentzel J, Roberts DF, Scott JE: HLA antigens in Hirschsprung's disease. *Tissue Antigens* **25**:79, 1985.

92. Earlam R: A vascular cause for Hirschsprung's disease? *Gastroenterology* **88**:1274, 1985.

93. Taguchi T, Tanaka K, Ikeda K: A vascular cause of Hirschsprung's disease? *Gastroenterology* **89**:701, 1985.

94. Taguchi T, Tanaka K, Ikeda K: Fibromuscular dysplasia of arteries in Hirschsprung's disease? *Gastroenterology* **88**:1099, 1985.

95. Siplovich L, Carmi R, Bar-Ziv J, Karplus M, Mares AJ: Discordant Hirschsprung's disease in monozygotic twins. *J Pediatr Surg* **18**:639, 1983.

96. Lipson A: Hirschsprung disease in the offspring of mothers exposed to hyperthermia during pregnancy. *Am J Med Genet* **29**:117, 1988.

97. Larsson L Okmian L, Kristoffersson U: No correlation between hyperthermia during pregnancy and Hirschsprung disease in the offspring. *Am J Med Genet* **32**:260, 1989.

98. Kurnit D, Layton WM, Matthyse S: Genetics, chance and morphogenesis. *Am J Hum Genet* **41**:979, 1987.

99. Carter C, Evans K, Hickman V: Children of those treated surgically for Hirschsprung's disease. *J Med Genet* **18**:87, 1981.

100. Carmi R, Hawley P, Wood JW, Gerald PS: Hirschsprung disease in progeny of affected individuals: A case report and review of the literature. *Birth Defects Orig Artic Ser* **18**:187, 1982.

101. Laurence KM, Prosser R, Rocker I, Pearson JF, Richard C: Hirschsprung's disease associated with congenital heart malformation, broad big toes, and ulnar polydactyly in sibs: A case for fetoscopy. *J Med Genet* **12**:334, 1975.

102. Verdy M, Weber AM, Roy CC, Morin CL, Cadotte M, Brochu P: Hirschsprung's disease in a family with multiple endocrine neoplasia type 2. *J Pediatr Gastroenterol Nutr* **1**:603, 1982.

103. Reynolds JF, Barber JC, Alford BA, Chandler JG, Kelly TE: Familial Hirschsprung's disease and type D brachydactyly: A report of four affected males in two generations. *Pediatrics* **71**:246, 1983.

104. Lipson AH, Harvey J: Three-generation transmission of Hirschsprung's disease. *Clin Genet* **32**:175, 1987.

105. Badner JA: *A Genetic Study of Hirschsprung Disease* [Dissertation]. Pittsburgh, University of Pittsburgh, 1988.

106. Omenn GS, McKusick VA: The association of Waardenburg syndrome and Hirschsprung megacolon. *Am J Med Genet* **3**:217, 1979.

107. Mahakrishnan A, Srinivasan MS: Piebaldness with Hirschsprung's disease. *Arch Dermatol* **116**:1102, 1980.

108. Shah KN, Dalal SJ, Desai MP, Sheth PN, Joshi NC, Ambani LM: White forelock, pigmentary disorder of irides, and long segment Hirschsprung disease: Possible variant of Waardenburg syndrome. *J Pediatr* **99**:432, 1981.

109. Cohen IT, Gadd MA: Hirschsprung's disease in a kindred: A possible clue to the genetics of the disease. *J Pediatr Surg* **17**:632, 1982.

110. Weinberg AG, Currarino G, Besserman AM: Hirschsprung's disease and congenital deafness. Familial association. *Hum Genet* **38**:157, 1977.

111. Badner JA, Chakravarti A: Waardenburg syndrome and Hirschsprung disease: Evidence for pleiotropic effects of a single dominant gene. *Am J Med Genet* **35**:100, 1990.

112. Simpson N, Kidd KK, Goodfellow PJ, McDermid H, Myers S, Kidd JR, Jackson CE, Duncan AM, Farrer LA, Brasch K, et al: Assignment of multiple endocrine neoplasia type 2A to chromosome 10 by linkage. *Nature* **328**:528, 1987.

113. Luo Y, Ceccherini I, Pasini B, Matera I, Bicocchi MP, Barone V, Bocciardi R, et al: Close linkage with the *RET* proto-oncogene and boundaries of deletion mutations in autosomal dominant Hirschsprung disease. *Hum Mol Genet* **2**:1803, 1993.

114. Lyonnet S, Bolino A, Pelet A, Abel L, Nihoul-Fekete C, Briard ML, Mok-Siu V, et al: A gene for Hirschsprung disease maps to the proximal long arm of chromosome 10. *Nat Genet* **4**:346, 1993.

115. Angrist M, Kauffman E, Slaugenhaupt SA, Matise TC, Puffenberger EG, Washington SS, Lipson A, et al: A gene for Hirschsprung disease (megacolon) in the pericentromeric region of human chromosome 10. *Nat Genet* **4**:351, 1993.

116. Mulligan L, Kwok JB, Healey CS, Elsdon MJ, Eng C, Gardner E, Love DR, Mole SE, Moore JK, Papi L, et al: Germ-line mutations of the *RET* proto-oncogene in multiple endocrine neoplasia type 2A. *Nature* **363**:458, 1993.

117. Donis-Keller H, Dou S, Chi D, Carlson KM, Toshima, K, Lairmore TC, Howe JR, Moley JF, Goodfellow P, Wells SA Jr: Mutations in the *RET* proto-oncogene are associated with MEN 2A and FMTC. *Hum Mol Genet* **2**:851, 1993.

118. Schuchardt A, D'Agati V, Larsson-Blomberg L, Costantini F, Pachnis V: Defects in the kidney and enteric nervous system of mice lacking the tyrosine kinase receptor Ret. *Nature* **367**:380, 1994.

119. Edery P, Lyonnet S, Mulligan LM, Pelet A, Dow E, Abel L, Holder S, et al: Mutations of the *RET* proto-oncogene in Hirschsprung's disease. *Nature* **367**:378, 1994.

120. Romeo G, Ronchetto P, Luo Y, Barone V, Seri M, Ceccherini I, Pasini B, et al: Point mutations affecting the tyrosine kinase domain of the *RET* proto-oncogene in Hirschsprung's disease [Comments]. *Nature* **367**:377, 1994.

121. Hofstra R, Landsvater RM, Ceccherini I, Stulp RP, Stelwagen T, Luo Y, Pasini B, Hoppener JW, van Amstel HK, Romeo G, et al: A mutation in the *RET* proto-oncogene associated with multiple endocrine neoplasia type 2B and sporadic medullary thyroid carcinoma. *Nature* **367**:375, 1994.

122. Carlson K, Dou S, Chi,D,, Scavarda N, Toshima K, Jackson CE, Wells SA Jr, Goodfellow PJ, Donis-Keller H: Single missense mutation in the tyrosine kinase catalytic domain of the *RET* proto-oncogene is associated with multiple endocrine neoplasia type 2B. *Proc Natl Acad Sci U S A* **15**:1579, 1994.

123. Mulligan L, Eng C, Healey CS, Clayton D, Kwok JB, Gardner E, Ponder MA, Frilling A Jackson CE, Lehnert H, et al: Specific mutations of the *RET* proto-oncogene are related to disease phenotype in MEN 2A and FMTC. *Nat Genet* **6**:70, 1994.

124. Mulligan LM, Eng C, Attie T, Lyonnet S, Marsh DJ, Hyland VJ, Robinson BG, et al: Diverse phenotypes associated with exon 10 mutations of the *RET* proto-oncogene. *Hum Mol Genet* **3**:2163, 1994.

125. Eng C, Smith DP, Mulligan LM, Nagai MA, Healey CS, Ponder MA, Gardner E, et al: Point mutation within the tyrosine kinase domain of the *RET* proto-oncogene in multiple endocrine neoplasia type 2B and related sporadic tumours [Erratum published in *Hum Mol Genet* 3(4):686, 1994]. *Hum Mol Genet* **3**:237, 1994.

126. Jhiang S, Mazzaferri EL: The ret/PTC oncogene in papillary thyroid carcinoma. *J Lab Clin Med* **123**:331, 1994.

127. Angrist M, Bolk S, Thiel B, Puffenberger EG, Hofstra RM, Buys CH, Cass DT, et al: Mutation analysis of the *RET* receptor tyrosine kinase in Hirschsprung disease. *Hum Mol Genet* **4**:821, 1995.

128. Attie T, Pelet A, Edery P, Eng C, Mulligan LM, Amiel J, Boutrand L, et al: Diversity of *RET* proto-oncogene mutations in familial and sporadic Hirschsprung disease. *Hum Mol Genet* **4**:1381, 1995.

129. Seri M, Yin L, Barone V, Bolino A, Celli I, Bocciardi R, Pasini B, et al: Frequency of *RET* mutations in long- and short-segment Hirschsprung disease. *Hum Mutat* **9**:243, 1997.

130. Chakravarti A: Endothelin receptor-mediated signaling in Hirschsprung disease. *Hum Mol Genet* **5**:303, 1996.

131. Santoro M, Carlomagno F, Romano A, Bottaro DP, Dathan NA, Grieco M, Fusco A, Vecchio G, Matoskova B, Kraus MH: Activation of *RET* as a dominant transforming gene by germline mutations of MEN2A and MEN2B. *Science* **267**:381, 1995.

132. Pasini B, Borrello MG, Greco A, Bongarzone I, Luo Y, Mondellini P, Alberti L, et al: Loss of function effect of *RET* mutations causing Hirschsprung disease. *Nat Genet* **10**:35, 1995.

133. Iwashita T, Murakami H, Asai N, Takahashi M: Mechanism of ret dysfunction by Hirschsprung mutations affecting its extracellular domain. *Hum Mol Genet* **5**:1577, 1996.

134. Carlomagno F, De Vita, G, Berlingieri MT, de Franciscis V, Melillo RM, Colantuoni V, Kraus MH, et al: Molecular heterogeneity of *RET* loss of function in Hirschsprung's disease. *EMBO J* **15**:2717, 1996.

135. Pelet A, Geneste O, Edery P, Pasini A, Chappuis S, Atti T, Munnich A, et al: Various mechanisms cause *RET*-mediated signaling defects in Hirschsprung's disease. *J Clin Invest* **101**:1415, 1998.

136. Takahashi M, Iwashita T, Santoro M, Lyonnet S, Lenoir GM, Billaud M: Co-segregation of MEN2 and Hirschsprung's disease: The same mutation of *RET* with both gain and loss-of-function [Letter]? *Hum Mutat* **13**:331, 1999.

137. Durbec P, Marcos-Gutierrez C, Kilkenny C, Grigoriou M, Wartiowaara K, Suvanto P, Smith P, et al: Glial cell line-Derived Neurotrophic factor signaling through the Ret receptor tyrosine kinase. *Nature* **381**:789, 1996.

138. Trupp M, Arenas E, Fainzilber M, Nilsson AS, Sieber BA, Grigoriou M, Kilkenny C, Salazar-Grueso E, Pachnis V, Arumae U: Functional receptor for GDNF encoded by the c-ret proto-oncogene. *Nature* **381**:785, 1996.

139. Robertson K, Mason I: The *GDNF-RET* signaling partnership. *Trends Genet* **13**:1, 1997.

140. Hellmich H, Kos L, Cho ES, Mahon KA, Zimmer A: Embryonic expression of glial cell-line derived neurotrophic factor (GDNF) suggests multiple developmental roles in neural differentiation and epithelial-mesenchymal. *Mech Dev* **54**:95, 1996.

141. Moore M, Klain R, Farinas I, Sauer H, Armanini M, Phillips H, Reichart L, et al: Renal and neuronal abnormalities in mice lacking GDNF. *Nature* **382**:76, 1996.

142. Pichel J, Shen L, Hui S, Granholm A, Drago J, Grinberg A, Lee E, et al: Defects in enteric innervation and kidney development in mice lacking GDNF. *Nature* **382**:73, 1996.

143. Sanchez M, Silos-Santiago I, Frisen J, He B, Lira S, Barbacid M: Renal agenesis and the absence of enteric neurons in mice lacking GDNF. *Nature* **382**:70, 1996.

144. Angrist M, Bolk S, Halushka M, Lapchak PA, Chakravarti A: Germline mutations in glial cell line-derived neurotrophic factor

(GDNF) and *RET* in a Hirschsprung disease patient. *Nat Genet* **14**:341, 1996.

145. Salomon R, Attie T, Pelet A, Bidaud C, Eng C, Amiel J, Sarnacki S, et al: Germline mutations of the *RET* ligand *GDNF* are not sufficient to cause Hirschsprung disease. *Nat Genet* **14**:345, 1996.

146. Ivanchuk SM, Myers SM, Eng C, Mulligan LM: De novo mutation of *GDNF*, ligand for the *RET*/GDNFR-alpha receptor complex, in Hirschsprung disease. *Hum Mol Genet* **5**:2023, 1996.

147. Jing S, Wen D, Yu Y, Holst PL, Luo Y, Fang M, Tamir R, Antonio L, Hu Z, Cupples R, Louis JC, Hu S, Altrock BW, Fox GM: GDNF-induced activation of the *RET* protein tyrosine kinase is mediated by GDNFR-alpha, a novel receptor for *GDNF*. *Cell* **85**:1113, 1996.

148. Treanor J, Goodman L, de Sauvage F, Stone D, Poulsen K, Beck C, Gray C, et al: Characterization of a multicomponent receptor for *GDNF*. *Nature* **382**:80, 1996.

149. Lindsay R, Yancopoulos GD: GDNF in a bind with known orphan: Accessory implicated in new twist. *Neuron* **17**:571, 1996.

150. Angrist M, Jing S, Bolk S, Bentley K, Nallasamy S, Halushka M, Fox GM, et al: Human GFRA1: cloning, mapping, genomic structure, and evaluation as a candidate gene for Hirschsprung disease susceptibility. *Genomics* **48**:354, 1998.

151. Myers SM, Salomon R, Goessling A, Pelet A, Eng C, von Deimling A, Lyonnet S, et al: Investigation of germline GFR alpha-1 mutations in Hirschsprung disease. *J Med Genet* **36**:217, 1999.

152. Baloh R, Gorodinsky A, Golden J, Tansey M, Keck C, Popescu N, Johnson EJ, et al: GFRalpha3 is an orphan member of the *GDNF*/neurturin/persephin receptor family. *Proc Natl Acad Sci U S A* **95**:5801, 1998.

153. Doray B, Salomon R, Amiel J, Pelet A, Touraine R, Billaud M, Attie T, Bachy B, Munnich A, Lyonnet S: Mutation of the *RET* ligand, neurturin, supports multigenic inheritance in Hirschsprung disease. *Hum Mol Genet* **7**:1449, 1998.

154. Pandey A, Duan H, Di Fiore PP, Dixit VM: The Ret receptor protein tyrosine kinase associates with the SH2-containing adapter protein Grb10. *J Biol Chem* **270**:461, 1995.

155. Morrione A, Valentinis B, Resnicoff M, Xu Sq, Baserga R: The role of mGrb10alpha in insulin-like growth factor I-mediated growth. *J Biol Chem* **272**:26382, 1997.

156. Margolis B: The GRB family of SH2 domain proteins. *Prog Biophys Mol Biol* **62**:223, 1994.

157. Manser J, Roonprapunt C, Margolis B: C. elegans cell migration gene mig-10 shares similarities with a family of SH2 domain proteins and acts cell nonautonomously in excretory canal development. *Dev Biol* **184**:150, 1997.

158. Angrist M, Bolk S, Bentley K, Nallasamy S, Halushka MK, Chakravarti A: Genomic structure of the gene for the SH2 and pleckstrin homology domain-containing protein GRB10 and evaluation of its role in Hirschsprung disease. *Oncogene* **17**:3065, 1998.

159. Puffenberger EG, Kauffman ER, Bolk S, Matise TC, Washington SS, Angrist M, Weissenbach J, et al: Identity-by-descent and association mapping of a recessive gene for Hirschsprung disease on human chromosome 13q22. *Hum Mol Genet* **3**:1217, 1994.

160. Puffenberger EG, Hosoda K, Washington SS, Nakao K, deWit D, Yanagisawa M, Chakravart A: A missense mutation of the endothelin-B receptor gene in multigenic Hirschsprung's disease. *Cell* **79**:1257, 1994.

161. Hosoda K, Hammer RE, Richardson JA, Baynash AG, Cheung JC, Giaid A, Yanagisawa M: Targeted and natural (piebald-lethal) mutations of endothelin-B receptor gene produce megacolon associated with spotted coat color in mice. *Cell* **79**:1267, 1994.

162. Attie T, Till M, Pelet A, Amiel J, Edery P, Boutrand L, Munnich A, et al: Mutation of the endothelin-receptor B gene in Waardenburg-Hirschsprung disease. *Hum Mol Genet* **4**:2407, 1995.

163. Amiel J, Attie T Jan D, Pelet A, Edery P, Bidaud C, Lacombe D, et al: Heterozygous endothelin receptor B (EDNRB) mutations in isolated Hirschsprung disease. *Hum Mol Genet* **5**:355, 1996.

164. Kusafuka T, Wang Y, Puri P: Novel mutations of the endothelin-B receptor gene in isolated patients with Hirschsprung's disease. *Hum Mol Genet* **5**:347, 1996.

165. Inoue A, Yanagisawa M, Kimura S, Kasuya Y, Miyauchi T, Goto K, Masaki T: The human endothelin family: Three structurally and pharmacologically distinct isopeptides predicted by three separate genes. *Proc Natl Acad Sci U S A* **86**:2863, 1989.

166. Sakurai T, Yanagisawa M, Masaki T: Molecular characterization of endothelin receptors. *Trends Pharmacol Sci* **13**:103, 1992.

167. Inagaki H, Bishop AE, Escrig C, Wharton J, Allen-Mersh TG, Polak JM: Localization of endothelin-like immunoreactivity and endothelin binding sites in human colon. *Gastroenterology* **101**:47, 1991.

168. Sakamoto A, Yanagisawa M, Sakurai T, Takuwa Y, Yanagisawa H, Masaki T: Cloning and functional expression of human cDNA for the ETB endothelin receptor. *Biochem Biophys Res Commun* **178**:656, 1991.

169. Baynash AG, Hosoda K, Giaid A, Richardson JA, Emoto N, Hammer RE, Yanagisawa M: Interaction of endothelin-3 with endothelin-B receptor is essential for development of epidermal melanocytes and enteric neurons. *Cell* **79**:1277, 1994.

170. Hofstra RM, Osinga J, Tan-Sindhunata G, Wu Y, Kamsteeg EJ, Stulp RP, van Ravenswaaij-Arts C, et al: A homozygous mutation in the endothelin-3 gene associated with a combined Waardenburg type 2 and Hirschsprung phenotype (Shah-Waardenburg syndrome). *Nat Genet* **12**:445, 1996.

171. Edery P, Attie T, Amiel J, Pelet A, Eng C, Hofstra RM, Martelli H, et al: Mutation of the endothelin-3 gene in the Waardenburg-Hirschsprung disease (Shah-Waardenburg syndrome). *Nat Genet* **12**:442, 1996.

172. Bolk S, Angrist M, Schwartz S, Silvestri JM, Weese-Mayer DE, Chakravarti A: Congenital central hypoventilation syndrome: Mutation analysis of the receptor tyrosine kinase *RET*. *Am J Med Genet* **63**:603, 1996.

173. Kurihara Y, Kurihara H, Suzuki H, Kodama T, Maemura K, Nagai R, Oda H, Kuwaki T, Cao WH, Kamada N: Elevated blood pressure and craniofacial abnormalities in mice deficient in endothelin-1. *Nature* **368**:703, 1994.

174. Kurihara, Y, Kurihara, H Maemura, K, Kuwaki, T, Kumada, M, Yazaki, Y: Impaired development of the thyroid and thymus in endothelin-1 knockout mice. *J Cardiovasc Pharmacol* **26(Suppl 3)**:S13, 1995.

175. Yanagisawa H, Yanagisawa M, Kapur RP, Richardson JA, Williams SC, Clouthier DE, de Wit D, Emoto N, Hammer RE: Dual genetic pathways of endothelin-mediated intercellular signaling revealed by targeted disruption of endothelin converting enzyme-1 gene. *Development* **125**:825, 1998.

176. Hofstra RM, Valdenaire O, Arch E Osinga J, Kroes H, Loffler BM, Hamosh A, et al: A loss-of-function mutation in the endothelin-converting enzyme 1 (ECE- 1) associated with Hirschsprung disease, cardiac defects, and autonomic dysfunction [Letter]. *Am J Hum Genet* **64**:304, 1999.

177. Lane PW, Liu HM: Association of megacolon with a new dominant spotting gene (Dom) in the mouse. *J Hered* **75**:435, 1984.

178. Southard-Smith EM, Kos L, Pavan WJ: Sox10 mutation disrupts neural crest development in Dom Hirschsprung mouse model. *Nat Genet* **18**:60, 1998.

179. Herbarth B, Pingault V, Bondurand N, Kuhlbrodt K, Hermans-Borgmeyer I, Puliti A, Lemort N, et al: Mutation of the Sry-related Sox10 gene in Dominant megacolon, a mouse model for human Hirschsprung disease. *Proc Natl Acad Sci U S A* **95**:5161, 1998.

180. Pingault V, Bondurand N, Kuhlbrodt, K, Goerich, DE, Prehu MO, Puliti A, Herbarth B, et al: SOX10 mutations in patients with Waardenburg-Hirschsprung disease. *Nat Genet* **18**:171, 1998.

181. Southard-Smith EM, Angrist M, Ellison JS, Agarwala R, Baxevanis AD, Chakravarti A, Pavan WJ: The Sox10(Dom) mouse: Modeling the genetic variation of Waardenburg-Shah (WS4) syndrome. *Genome Res* **9**:215, 1999.

182. Prenzel N, Zwick E, Daub H, Leserer M, Abraham R, Wallasch C, Ullrich A: EGF receptor transactivation by G-protein-coupled receptors requires metalloproteinase cleavage of proHB-EGF. *Nature* **402**:884, 1999.

183. Schuchardt A, D'Agati V, Larsson-Blomberg L, Costantini F, Pachnis V: RET-deficient mice: An animal model for Hirschsprung's disease and renal agenesis. *J Intern Med* **238**:327, 1995.

184. Lo L, Anderson DJ: Postmigratory neural crest cells expressing c-RET display restricted developmental and proliferative capacities. *Neuron* **15**:527, 1995.

185. Hearn CJ, Murphy M, Newgreen D: GDNF and ET-3 differentially modulate the numbers of avian enteric neural crest cells and enteric neurons *in vitro*. *Dev Biol* **197**:93, 1998.

186. Saxen L, Sariola H: Early organogenesis of the kidney. *Pediatr Nephrol* **1**:385, 1987.

187. Pavan W, Tilghman SM: Piebald lethal (sl) acts early to disrupt the development of neural crest-derived melanocytes. *Proc Natl Acad Sci U S A* **91**:7159, 1994.

188. Shin M, Levorse JM, Ingram RS, Tilghman SM: The temporal requirement for endothelin receptor-B signaling during neural crest development. *Nature* **402**:496, 1999.

189. Sakurai T, Yanagisawa M, Takuwa Y, Miyazaki H, Kimura S, Goto K, Masaki T: Cloning of a cDNA encoding a non-isopeptide-selective subtype of the endothelin receptor. *Nature* **348**:732, 1990.

190. Pavan W, Mac S, Cheng M, Tilghman SM: Quantitative trait loci that modify the severity of spotting in piebald mice. *Genome Res* **5**:29, 1995.

191. Kapur RP, Livingston R, Doggett B, Sweetser DA, Siebert JR, Palmiter RD: Abnormal microenvironmental signals underlie intestinal aganglionosis in Dominant megacolon mutant mice. *Dev Biol* **174**:360, 1996.

192. Kapur R, Sweester, D, Dogget B, Siebert J, Palmiter R: Intercellular signals downstream of endothelin receptor-B mediate colonization of the large intestine by enteric neuroblasts. *Development* **121**:3787, 1995.

193. Bourne H: Signal transduction. Team blue sees red. *Nature* **376:**727, 1995.

194. van Biesen T, Hawes BE, Luttrell DK, Krueger KM, Touhara K, Porfiri E, Sakaue M, Luttrell LM, Lefkowitz RJ: Receptor-tyrosine-kinase and G beta gamma-mediated MAP kinase activation by a common signaling pathway. *Nature* **376**:781, 1995.

195. Auricchio A, Griseri P, Carpentieri ML, Betsos N, Staiano A, Tozzi A, Priolo M, et al: Double Heterozygosity for a *RET* Substitution Interfering with Splicing and an *EDNRB* Missense Mutation in Hirschsprung Disease. *Am J Hum Genet* **64**:1216, 1999.

196. Tennyson V, Gershon MD, Wade PR, Crotty DA, Wolgemuth DJ: Fetal development of the enteric nervous system of transgenic mice that overexpress the Hoxa-4 gene. *Dev Dyn* **211**:269, 1998.

197. Hatano M, Iitsuka Y, Yamamoto H, Dezawa M, Yusa S, Kohno Y, Tokuhisa T: Ncx, a Hox11 related gene, is expressed in a variety of tissues derived from neural crest cells. *Anat Embryol* **195**:419, 1997.

198. Pritchard C, Bolin L, Slattery R, Murray R, McMahon M: Post-natal lethality and neurological and gastrointestinal defects in mice with targeted disruption of the A-Raf protein kinase gene. *Curr Biol* **6**:614, 1996.

199. Qiu M, Bulfone A, Martinez S, Meneses JJ, Shimamura K, Pedersen RA, Rubenstein JL: Null mutation of Dlx-2 results in abnormal morphogenesis of proximal first and second branchial arch derivatives and abnormal differentiation in the forebrain. *Genes Dev* **9**:2523, 1995.

200. Sakai T, Ohtani N, McGee TL, Robbind PD, Dryja TP: Oncogenic germ-line mutations in Sp1 and ATF sites in the human retinoblastoma gene. *Nature* **353**:83, 1991.

201. Otterson G, Chen W, Coxon AB, Khleif SN, Kaye FJ: Incomplete penetrance of familial retinoblastoma linked to germ-line mutations that result in partial loss of RB function. *Proc Natl Acad Sci U S A* **94**:12036, 1997.

202. Cass D: Aganglionosis: associated anomalies. *J Paediatr Child Health* **26**:351, 1990.

203. Rarey KE, Davis LE: Inner ear anomalies in Waardenburg's syndrome associated with Hirschsprung's disease. *Int J Pediatr Otorhinolaryngol* **8**:181, 1984.

204. Bonnet JP, Till M, Edery P, Attie T, Lyonnet S: Waardenburg-Hirschsprung disease in two sisters: A possible clue to the genetics of this association? *Eur J Pediatr Surg* **6**:245, 1996.

205. Bidaud C, Salomon R, Van Camp G, Pelet A, Attie T, Eng C, Bonduelle M, et al: Endothelin-3 gene mutations in isolated and syndromic Hirschsprung disease. *Eur J Hum Genet* **5**:247, 1997.

206. Syrris P, Carter ND, Patton MA: Novel nonsense mutation of the endothelin-B receptor gene in a family with Waardenburg-Hirschsprung disease. *Am J Med Genet* **87**:69, 1999.

207. Dow E, Cross S, Wolgemuth DJ, Lyonnet S, Mulligan LM, Mascari M, Ladda R, et al: Second locus for Hirschsprung disease/Waardenburg syndrome in a large Mennonite kindred. *Am J Med Genet* **53**:75, 1994.

208. Jacobs JM, Wilson J: An unusual demyelinating neuropathy in a patient with Waardenburg's syndrome. *Acta Neuropathol (Berl)* **83**:670, 1992.

209. Inoue K, Tanabe Y, Lupski JR: Myelin deficiencies in both the central and the peripheral nervous systems associated with a *SOX10* mutation. *Ann Neurol* **46**:313, 1999.

210. Touraine RL, Attié-Bitach T, Manceau E, Korsch E, Sarda P, Pingault V, Encha-Razavi F, et al: Neurological phenotype in Waardenburg type 4 syndrome correlates with novel *SOX10* truncating mutations and expression in developing brain. *Am J Hum Genet* **66**:1496, 2000.

211. Bondurand N, Kuhlbrodt K, Pingault V, Enderich J, Sajus M, Tommerup N, Warburg M, et al: A molecular analysis of the Yemenite deaf-blind hypopigmentation syndrome: *SOX10* dysfunction causes different neurocristopathies. *Hum Mol Genet* **8**:1785, 1999.

212. Gross A, Kunze J, Maier RF, Stoltenburg-Didinger G, Grimmer I, Obladen M: Autosomal-recessive neural crest syndrome with albinism, black lock, cell migration disorder of the neurocytes of the gut, and deafness: ABCD syndrome. *Am J Med Genet* **56**:322, 1995.

213. Kaplan P, de Chaderevian JP: Piebaldism-Waardenburg syndrome: Histopathologic evidence for a neural crest syndrome. *Am J Med Genet* **31**:679, 1988.

214. Weese-Mayer DE, Silvestri JM, Marazita ML, Hoo JJ: Congenital central hypoventilation syndrome: inheritance and relation to sudden infant death syndrome. *Am J Med Genet* **47**:360, 1993.

215. Bolk S, Angrist M, Xie J, Yanagisawa M, Silvestri JM, Weese-Mayer, DE, Chakravarti A: Endothelin-3 frameshift mutation in congenital central hypoventilation syndrome [Letter]. *Nat Genet* **13**:395, 1996.

216. Sakai T, Wakizaka A, Matsuda H, Nirasawa Y, Itoh Y: Point mutation in exon 12 of the receptor tyrosine kinase proto-oncogene *RET* in Ondine-Hirschsprung syndrome. *Pediatrics* **101**:924, 1998.

217. Amiel J, Salomon R, Attié T, Pelet A, Trang H, Mokhtari M, Gaultier C, et al: Mutations of the *RET*-GDNF signaling pathway in Ondine's curse. *Am J Hum Genet* **62**:715, 1998.

218. Haddad, GG, Mazza NM, Defendini R, Blanc WA, Driscoll JM, Epstein MA, Epstein RA, et al: Congenital failure of automatic control of ventilation, gastrointestinal motility and heart rate. *Medicine (Baltimore)* **57**:517, 1978.

219. Verloes A, Elmer C, Lacombe D, Heinrichs C, Rebuffat E, Demarquez JL, Moncla A, et al: Ondine-Hirschsprung syndrome (Haddad syndrome). Further delineation in two cases and review of the literature. *Eur J Pediatr* **152**:75, 1993.

220. Croaker GD, Shi E, Simpson E, Cartmill T, Cass DT: Congenital central hypoventilation syndrome and Hirschsprung's disease. *Arch Dis Child* **78**:316, 1998.

221. Borst MJ, VanCamp JM, Peacock ML, Decker RA: Mutational analysis of multiple endocrine neoplasia type 2A associated with Hirschsprung's disease. *Surgery* **117**:386, 1995.

222. Caron P, Attie T, David D, Amiel J, Brousset F, Roger P, Munnich A, et al: C618R mutation in exon 10 of the *RET* proto-oncogene in a kindred with multiple endocrine neoplasia type 2A and Hirschsprung's disease. *J Clin Endocrinol Metab* **81**:2731, 1996.

223. Peretz H, Luboshitsky R, Baron E, Biton A, Gershoni R, Usher S, Grynberg, E et al: Cys 618 Arg mutation in the *RET* proto-oncogene associated with familial medullary thyroid carcinoma and maternally transmitted Hirschsprung's disease suggesting a role for imprinting. *Hum Mutat* **10**:155, 1997.

224. Decker RA, Peacock ML, Watson P: Hirschsprung disease in MEN 2A: Increased spectrum of *RET* exon 10 genotypes and strong genotype-phenotype correlation. *Hum Mol Genet* **7**:129, 1998.

225. Inoue K, Shimotake T, Tokiwa K, Iwai N: Mutational analysis of the *RET* proto-oncogene in a kindred with multiple endocrine neoplasia type 2A and Hirschsprung's disease. *J Pediatr Surg* **34**:1552, 1999.

226. Romeo G, Ceccherini I, Celli J, Priolo M, Betsos N, Bonardi G, Seri M, et al: Association of multiple endocrine neoplasia type 2 and Hirschsprung disease. *J Intern Med* **243**:515, 1998.

227. Sijmons RH, Hofstra RM, Wijburg FA, Links, TP, Zwierstra RP, Vermey A, Aronson DC, et al: Oncological implications of *RET* gene mutations in Hirschsprung's disease. *Gut* **43**:542, 1998.

228. Gaisie G, Oh KS, Young LW: Coexistent neuroblastoma and Hirschsprung's disease — Another manifestation of the neurocristopathy? *Pediatr Radiol* **8**:161, 1979.

229. Michna BA, McWilliams NB, Krummel TM, Hartenberg MA, Salzberg AM: Multifocal ganglioneuroblastoma coexistent with total colonic aganglionosis. *J Pediatr Surg* **23**:57, 1988.

230. Roshkow JE, Haller JO, Berdon WE, Sane SM: Hirschsprung's disease Ondine's curse, and neuroblastoma — Manifestations of neurocristopathy [Comments]. *Pediatr Radiol* **19**:45, 1988.

231. Merkler RG, Solish SB, Scherzer AL: Meningomyelocele and Hirschprung disease: Theoretical and clinical significance. *Pediatrics* **76**:299, 1985.

232. Clausen N, Andersson P, Tommerup N: Familial occurrence of neuroblastoma, von Recklinghausen's neurofibromatosis, Hirschsprung's aganglionosis and jaw-winking syndrome. *Acta Paediatr Scand* **78**:736, 1989.

233. Goldberg RB, Shprintzen RJ: Hirschsprung megacolon and cleft palate in two sibs. *J Craniofac Genet Dev Biol* **1**:185, 1981.

234. Fryer AE: Goldberg-Shprintzen syndrome: Report of a new family and review of the literature. *Clin Dysmorphol* **7**:97, 1998.

235. Hurst JA, Markiewicz M, Kumar D, Brett EM: Unknown syndrome: Hirschsprung's disease, microcephaly, and iris coloboma: A new syndrome of defective neuronal migration. *J Med Genet* **25**:494, 1988.

236. Halal F, Morel J: The syndrome of Hirschsprung disease, microcephaly, unusual face, and mental retardation. *Am J Med Genet* **37**:106, 1990.
237. Santos H, Mateus J, Leal MJ: Hirschsprung disease associated with polydactyly, unilateral renal agenesis, hypertelorism, and congenital deafness: A new autosomal recessive syndrome. *J Med Genet* **25**:204, 1988.
238. al-Gazali LI, Donnai D, Mueller RF: Hirschsprung's disease, hypoplastic nails, and minor dysmorphic features: A distinct autosomal recessive syndrome? *J Med Genet* **25**:758, 1988.
239. Huang T, Elias ER, Mulliken JB, Kirse DJ, Holmes LB: A new syndrome: Heart defects, laryngeal anomalies, preaxial polydactyly, and colonic aganglionosis in sibs. *Genet Med* **1**:104, 1999.
240. Reish O, Gorlin RJ, Hordinsky M, Rest EB, Burke B, Berry SA: Brain anomalies, retardation of mentality and growth, ectodermal dysplasia, skeletal malformations, Hirschsprung disease, ear deformity and deafness, eye hypoplasia, cleft palate, cryptorchidism, and kidney dysplasia/hypoplasia (BRESEK/BRESHECK): New X-linked syndrome? *Am J Med Genet* **68**:386, 1997.
241. Radetti G, Frick R, Pasquino B, Mengarda G, Savage MO: Hypothalamic-pituitary dysfunction and Hirschsprung's disease in the Bardet-Biedl syndrome. *Helv Paediatr Acta* **43**:249, 1988.
242. Lorda-Sanchez I, Ayuso C, Ibanez A: Situs inversus and Hirschsprung disease: Two uncommon manifestations in Bardet-Biedl syndrome [Citation]. *Am J Med Genet* **90**:80, 2000.
243. Davenport M, Taitz LS, Dickson JA: The Kaufman-McKusick syndrome: Another association. *J Pediatr Surg* **24**:1192, 1989.
244. Verloes A, Gillerot Y, Langhendries JP, Fryns JP, Koulischer L: Variability versus heterogeneity in syndromal hypothalamic hamartoblastoma and related disorders: Review and delineation of the cerebro-acro-visceral early lethality (CAVE) multiplex syndrome. *Am J Med Genet* **43**:669, 1992.
245. LeMerrer M, Briard ML, Girard S, Mulliez N, Moraine C, Imbert MC: Lethal acrodysgenital dwarfism: A severe lethal condition resembling Smith-Lemli-Opitz syndrome. *J Med Genet* **25**:88, 1988.
246. Patterson K, Toomey KE, Chandra RS: Hirschsprung disease in a 46,XY phenotypic infant girl with Smith-Lemli-Opitz syndrome. *J Pediatr* **103**:425, 1983.
247. Makitie O, Sulisalo T, de la Chapelle A, Kaitila I: Cartilage-hair hypoplasia. *J Med Genet* **32**:39, 1995.
248. Mandel H, Brik R, Ludatscher R, Braun J, Berant M: Congenital muscular dystrophy with neurological abnormalities: Association with Hirschsprung disease. *Am J Med Genet* **47**:37, 1993.
249. Kim JJ, Armstrong DD, Fishman MA: Multicore myopathy, microcephaly, aganglionosis, and short stature. *J Child Neurol* **9**:275, 1994.
250. Mallory SB, Haynie LS, Williams ML, Hall W: Ichthyosis, deafness, and Hirschsprung's disease. *Pediatr Dermatol* **6**:24, 1989.
251. Kaplan P: X-linked recessive inheritance of agenesis of the corpus callosum. *J Med Genet* **20**:122, 1983.
252. Okamoto N, Wada, Y, Goto M: Hydrocephalus and Hirschsprung's disease in a patient with a mutation of L1CAM. *J Med Genet* **34**:670, 1997.
253. Jespers A, Buntinx I, Melis K, Vaerenberg M, Janssens G: Two siblings with midline field defects and Hirschsprung disease: Variable expression of Toriello-Carey or new syndrome? *Am J Med Genet* **47**:299, 1993.
254. Sayed M, al-Alaiyan S: Agenesis of corpus callosum, hypertrophic pyloric stenosis and Hirschsprung disease: Coincidence or common etiology? *Neuropediatrics* **27**:204, 1996.
255. Azizi E, Berlowitz I, Vinograd I, Reif R, Mundel G: Congenital megacolon associated with familial dysautonomia. *Eur J Pediatr* **142**:68, 1984.
256. Emanuel B, Padorr M, Swenson O: Mongolism associated with Hirschsprung's disease. *J Pediatr* **66**:437, 1965.
257. Quinn FM, Surana R, Puri P: The influence of trisomy 21 on outcome in children with Hirschsprung's disease. *J Pediatr Surg* **29**:781, 1994.
258. Sakai T, Wakizaka A, Nirasawa Y, Ito Y: Point nucleotidic changes in both the *RET* proto-oncogene and the endothelin-B receptor gene in a Hirschsprung disease patient associated with Down syndrome. *Tohoku J Exp Med* **187**:43, 1999.
259. Lurie IW, Supovitz KR, Rosenblum-Vos LS, Wulfsberg EA: Phenotypic variability of del(2) (q22-q23): Report of a case with a review of the literature. *Genet Couns* **5**:11, 1994.
260. Mowat DR, Croaker GD, Cass DT, Kerr BA, Chaitow J, Ades LC, Chia NL, et al: Hirschsprung disease, microcephaly, mental retardation, and characteristic facial features: Delineation of a new syndrome and identification of a locus at chromosome 2q22-q23. *J Med Genet* **35**:617, 1998.
261. Webb GC, Keith CG, Campbell NT: Concurrent de novo interstitial deletion of band 2p22 and reciprocal translocation (3;7)(p21;q22). *J Med Genet* **25**:125, 1988.
262. Fewtrell MS, Tam PK, Thomson AH, Fitchett M, Currie J, Huson SM, Mulligan LM: Hirschsprung's disease associated with a deletion of chromosome 10 (q11.2q21.2): A further link with the neurocristopathies? *J Med Genet* **31**:325, 1994.
263. Carnevale A, Frias S, Alcantar R: Interstitial deletion of long arm of chromosome 13. *Ann Genet* **27**:49, 1984.
264. Kerstjens-Frederikse WS, Hofstra RM, van Essen AJ, Meijers JH, Buys CH: A Hirschsprung disease locus at 22q11? *J Med Genet* **36**:221, 1999.
265. Mahboubi S, Templeton JM Jr: Association of Hirschsprung's disease and imperforate anus in a patient with "cat-eye" syndrome. A report of one case and review of the literature. *Pediatr Radiol* **14**:441, 1984.
266. Beedgen B, Nutzenadel W, Querfeld U, Weiss-Wichert P: "Partial trisomy 22 and 11" due to a paternal 11;22 translocation associated with Hirschsprung disease. *Eur J Pediatr* **145**:229, 1986.
267. Bottani A, Dahoun-Hadorn S, D'Amato L, Antonarakis S: Hirschsprung disease and agenesis of the corpus callosum in a newborn with a de novo unbalanced translocation (7p22;14q11.2): Potential mapping of either or both phenotypes? Personal communication, 1995.
268. Michaelis RC, Skinner SA, Deason R, Skinner C, Moore CL, Phelan MC: Intersitial deletion of 20p: New candidate region for Hirschsprung disease and autism? *Am J Med Genet* **71**:298, 1997.
269. Edward E, Ecker J, Christakis N, Folkman J: Hirschsprung's disease: Associated Abnormalities and Demography. *J Pediatr Surg* **27**:76, 1992.
270. Ikeda K, Goto S: Additional anomalies in Hirschsprung's disease: An analysis based on the nationwide survey in Japan. *Z Kinderchir* **41**:279, 1986.
271. Russell MB, Russell CA, Niebuhr E: An epidemiological study of Hirschsprung's disease and additional anomalies. *Acta Paediatr* **83**:68, 1994.
272. Sarioglu A, Tanyel FC, Buyukpamukcu N, Hicsonmez A: Hirschsprung-associated congenital anomalies. *Eur J Pediatr Surg* **7**:331, 1997.
273. Johnson JF, Dean BL: Hirschsprung's disease coexisting with colonic atresia. *Pediatr Radiol* **11**:97, 1981.
274. Watanatittan S, Suwatanaviroj A, Limprutithum T, Rattanasuwan T: Association of Hirschsprung's disease and anorectal malformation. *J Pediatr Surg* **26**:192, 1991.
275. Sinnassamy P, Yazbeck S, Brochu P, O'Regan S: Renal anomalies and agenesis associated with total intestinal aganglionosis. *Int J Pediatr Nephrol* **7**:1, 1986.
276. Whalen TV Jr, Asch MJ: Report of two patients with hypertrophic pyloric stenosis and Hirschsprung's disease. Coincident or common etiology? *Am Surg* **51**:480, 1985.
277. Janik JP, Wayne ER, Janik JS, Price MR: Ileal atresia with total colonic aganglionosis. *J Pediatr Surg* **32**:1502, 1997.
278. Staiano A, Santoro L, De Marco R, Miele E, Fiorillo F, Auricchio A, Carpentieri ML, et al: Autonomic dysfunction in children with Hirschsprung's disease. *Dig Dis Sci* **44**:960, 1999.
279. Stone DL, Slavotinek A, Bouffard GG, Banerjee-Basu S, Baxevanis AD, Barr M, Biesecker LG: Mutation of a gene encoding a putative chaperonin causes McKusick-Kauffman syndrome. *Nat Genet* **25**:79, 2000.

# The Oculocerebrorenal Syndrome of Lowe (Lowe Syndrome)

*Robert L. Nussbaum* ■ *Sharon F. Suchy*

1. The oculocerebrorenal syndrome of Lowe (OCRL) is a multisystem disorder with major abnormalities in the eyes, the nervous system, and the kidneys. Prenatal development of cataracts is universal, and other ocular abnormalities, including glaucoma, microphthalmos, decreased visual acuity, and corneal keloid formation, are frequent. Neonatal or infantile hypotonia, intellectual impairment, and are-flexia are also cardinal features. Mental retardation, although very common, is not universal. Stereotypic behaviors, including tantrums and aggressiveness, are some of the more difficult management problems in the disease. Fanconi syndrome of the renal tubule (bicarbona-turia, renal tubular acidosis, aminoaciduria, phosphaturia, tubular proteinuria, and impaired urine-concentrating ability) is also a major feature, but the severity and age of onset of the tubular dysfunction are variable. Slowly progressive renal failure can also occur in the second to fourth decade of life. Musculoskeletal abnormalities such as joint hypermobility, dislocated hips, and fractures may develop as secondary consequences of hypotonia or renal tubular acidosis and hypophosphatemia, but nontender joint swelling and subcutaneous nodules are also frequently seen and may reflect a primary abnormality of excessive connective tissue growth.

2. OCRL is a rare X-linked disorder with an estimated prevalence of only a few cases per 100,000 males. The only significant manifestation in carriers is in the lens and is characterized by many smooth, off-white micropunctate cataracts clustered in a radial wedge pattern, and, occasionally, a dense posterior cortical cataract. The sensitivity of carrier detection by slit-lamp exam is >90 percent but, as with most X-linked conditions, penetrance is unlikely to ever be 100 percent in female carriers because the proportion of cells in the lens that have an inactivated Lowe syndrome allele can vary by chance between carriers. Germ line or somatic mosaicism has been documented.

3. The gene for OCRL, termed *OCRL1*, located at Xq25-q26, was identified by positional cloning in the Xq25-q26 region of the X chromosome, and encodes a phosphatidylinositol (4,5) bisphosphate 5-phosphatase (PtdIns(4,5)P$_2$) localized to the Golgi complex. How a deficiency of this enzyme results in the clinical phenotype remains obscure.

4. Clinical diagnosis of OCRL depends on the cardinal ophthalmologic, neurologic, and renal abnormalities, while X-linked inheritance is extremely helpful when present. Carrier detection by slit-lamp examination has high but not perfect sensitivity. Biochemical assay for deficiency of PtdIns(4,5)P$_2$ 5-phosphatase is the definitive laboratory test for diagnosing patients and for prenatal diagnosis, but its role in carrier detection is unproved.

5. Over two dozen mutations have been described in the *OCRL1* gene in Lowe syndrome patients. Most are unique to a family and are either nonsense mutations or deletions that cause frameshifts and premature termination, although missense mutations in domains conserved among all the known PtdIns(4,5)P$_2$ 5-phosphatases are also seen. Carrier detection can be done by direct detection of mutations when known and by linked markers when the mutation is unknown.

6. Treatment includes cataract extraction, refraction for aphakia, control of glaucoma, speech and physical therapy for developmental delay, anticonvulsants or behavior-modifying medications if needed, and replacement of urinary bicarbonate, water, and phosphate losses if indicated by the development of acidosis or bone disease.

## HISTORICAL FEATURES

OCRL was first described as a discrete entity by Lowe and colleagues in 1952[1] in an infant with organic aciduria, decreased renal ammonia production, hydrophthalmos, and mental retardation. The renal Fanconi syndrome associated with Lowe syndrome was recognized in 1954,[2] and a number of additional reports confirmed and expanded the clinical phenotype.[3,4]

X-linked recessive inheritance was convincingly demonstrated in 1965.[5] Ocular manifestations that could identify female carriers were identified a decade later.[6,7] The combination of X-linked inheritance and reliable heterozygote detection allowed gene mapping[8] and, ultimately, gene identification using positional cloning techniques.[9] Current work now focuses on determining the function of the product of the gene for OCRL and the pathogenesis of the phenotype. The bibliography in the chapter on Lowe syndrome in the seventh edition of *The Metabolic and Molecular Bases of Inherited Disease* contains a more complete listing of historical references.[10]

## CLINICAL FEATURES

The oculocerebrorenal syndrome is so-named because of the prominent involvement in this disorder of three organ systems: the eye, the central nervous system, and the kidney. However,

---

A list of standard abbreviations is located immediately preceding the index in each volume. Additional abbreviations used in this chapter include: PtdIns(4,5)P$_2$ = phosphatidylinositol (4,5) bisphosphate; INPP5B = human platelet inositol polyphos-phate 5-phosphatase; inpp5bp = enzyme encoded by INPP5B; OCRL = oculocerebrorenal syndrome of Lowe; *OCRL1* = gene for OCRL identified by positional cloning; ocrl1p = enzyme encoded by the *OCRL1* gene.

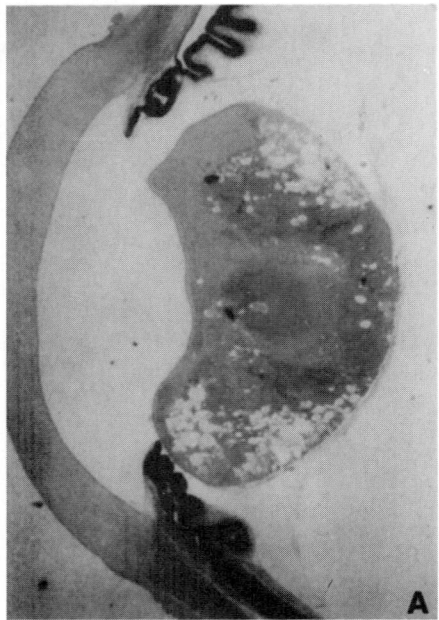
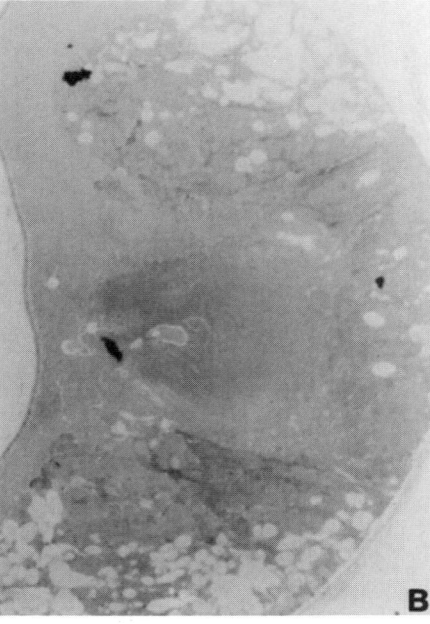

Fig. 252-1 *A.* Sagittal section through anterior portion of the eye including cornea, anterior chamber, lens, and ciliary bodies of a 20-week OCRL fetus (×24). *B.* Higher magnification of lens (×40). Note abnormal anterior concave shape with central fluid-filled space and necrotic cells in the fetal lens nucleus location. Remaining lens cells above and below the fetal nucleus are large, frequently swollen, and disorganized, without a regular parallel distribution. (Courtesy of M.M. Padilla, MD.)

connective tissue, bone, gonads, muscle, and skin may be involved with what are characteristic and, in some cases, unique clinical features.

## Ophthalmologic Abnormalities

The hallmark of this condition is the presence of congenital cataracts, which develop prenatally and are always present prior to birth. Abnormal lens formation in OCRL begins at 7 to 9 weeks' gestation and is due to disordered migration of the embryonic lens epithelium[11] as a primary defect rather than a secondary effect of systemic metabolic imbalance. Pathologic changes in the ocular lens have been described in 20- and 24-week fetuses. In the 20-week fetus, lens size was normal but there was abnormal concavity of the anterior portion of the lens and necrosis of the embryonic lens nucleus with disorganized architecture and swelling of the residual lens cells[12] (Fig. 252-1). In the other fetus studied, a cone-shaped opacity at the posterior pole caused loss of light transmission and additional aberrant developmental changes included disorganized nests of epithelial cells directly beneath the anterior lens capsule and swelling of the anterior lens fibers.[13] Histologically, the posterior lens capsule was incomplete, with protrusion of lens material and a cellular reaction surrounding the protruding material. It is not known if this histologic appearance results from abnormal formation of the lens capsule with secondary protrusion of material or if it is due to primary dysmigration. No glaucomatous changes were found, and the globes and anterior chambers were otherwise unremarkable in both fetuses.

Later in development there is continued protrusion of the posterior polar material through the posterior lens capsule, producing poor demarcation between the lens nucleus and cortex, marked thinning of the lens, and adherence of the vitreous to the posterior pole.[11,14,15] Calcification is frequent, with calcific excrescences of both anterior and posterior capsule, and hyperplasia of capsular epithelium. Microphthalmia and enophthalmos secondary to the lens abnormality are often also present.

Glaucoma, either with or without buphthalmos, is quite frequent, occurring in 50 to 60 percent of patients in some series. It is usually bilateral and is a characteristic feature of the disorder rather than a reflection of the surgical technique used for cataract extraction. (16-17). Glaucoma is typically detected in the first year of life, but may appear as late as the second or third decade.

Impaired visual acuity is almost universally present. Corrected visual acuity is rarely better than 20/100 despite optimal manage-

ment, and the impairment represents both the morphologic changes in the eye caused by congenital cataract and a primary retinal dysfunction caused by the underlying disorder. Nystagmus develops postnatally secondary to the poor visual acuity and is virtually always present in older OCRL patients.

Corneal scarring and keloids are additional features of OCRL that probably develop spontaneously without trauma[18] (Fig. 252-2). Keloids may develop in up to 25 percent of OCRL patients, usually after age 5, and are bilateral in about half of affected patients.[17] Keloids are often stable and do not interfere with central vision, but they may cause significant visual impairment.

## Nervous System Abnormalities

Both the central and the peripheral nervous system are involved in OCRL, causing the greatest disease burden of the illness. A prominent feature is cognitive impairment, but neonatal hypotonia with delay in motor milestones is the initial neurologic manifestation and a cardinal feature of the disorder. In addition, areflexia, seizures, neuropathologic and neuroimaging abnormalities, and behavioral disturbances may also be present.

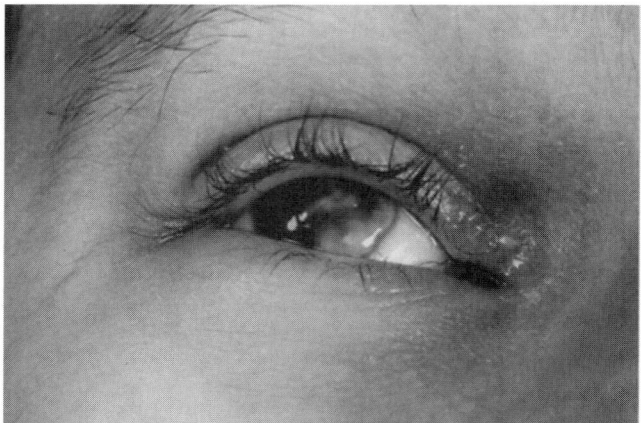

Fig. 252-2 Corneal keloid of the right eye in a 14-year-old boy without known eye-poking behavior or use of contact lenses. The keloid has its densest portion at the limbus and extends centrally to partially obscure central vision in this eye.

**Cognitive Outcome.** Mental retardation, though common, is not a cardinal feature because the diagnosis of OCRL is compatible with normal intelligence.[19] A more accurate description of the cognitive outcome is intellectual impairment; that is, functioning below what would be an individual's predicted intellectual level in the absence of OCRL. Approximately 10 percent of OCRL patients have intelligence within the normal range, typically borderline or low normal. The median IQ is in the moderately retarded range, and one-third of affected individuals appear to be profoundly retarded. These estimates for intelligence suffer from the use of testing techniques that inappropriately penalize OCRL patients for their visual impairment and for behavioral disturbances that may impair accurate testing.[19] Socioeconomic status, maternal intelligence, MRI findings, and even the specific mutation causing the disorder appear to have little predictive value for intellectual outcome.[20–22] Intelligence appears to be stable over the life span of the individual, and deterioration in cognitive performance, occasionally reported in OCRL,[23] most likely represents decline due to progressive renal disease or another intercurrent illness.

**Behavioral Abnormalities.** Behavioral disturbances may be the most troublesome feature for caregivers. Studies confirmed a high incidence of stereotypic behavioral disturbances including self-injury, episodic outbursts (Lowe tantrum), aggression, irritability, and repetitive nonpurposeful movements that interfered with function.[19,24,25] A specific behavioral phenotype for OCRL consisting of stubbornness, temper tantrums, rigidity of thought, and unacceptable stereotypic behavior emerged when age, gender, visual impairment, and cognitive function were controlled for.[25] This behavioral phenotype is reminiscent of the obsessive-compulsive disorder spectrum and warrants further study.

**Neuromuscular Abnormalities.** Neonatal or infantile hypotonia are cardinal manifestations of OCRL and may persist into childhood. A neuromuscular cause of hypotonia is suggested by the mildly elevated creatine kinase values and areflexia, but the improvement with age and the absence of reproducible and significant nerve or muscle pathology in most patients is more consistent with a central nervous system origin. Other than the deep tendon reflex, nerve conduction and motor amplitudes are normal. These data do not support the presence of a progressive peripheral neuropathy in OCRL.

**Central Nervous System Abnormalities.** *Seizures.* Seizures occur in up to 50 percent of patients with OCRL.[10] There is no characteristic seizure type, and infantile spasms with hypsarrhythmia, myoclonic seizures, partial complex seizures, and generalized convulsions have all been reported or observed in the series of OCRL patients studied at the NIH. "Febrile" seizures appear to occur at a higher frequency than in the general population (9 percent versus 1 percent), and approximately one-third of these patients will progress to a true seizure disorder. Most seizures occur before age 6, although some patients have developed seizures as late as age 19. Severe, early onset seizure disorders carry a poor prognosis for intellectual development and seizure control, as they do in the general population.

*Neuropathology and Neuroimaging.* Cranial MRI demonstrates mild ventriculomegaly in approximately one-third of patients, as well as areas of increased signal intensity on T2-weighted scans (which are particularly sensitive for water) in a periventricular and centrum semiovale distribution, without involvement of other myelinated areas (corpus callosum, cortical U-fibers, brainstem, or cerebellum).[24,26] These areas correspond to cysts of variable size and number[27,28] (Fig. 252-3). The signal is undetectable until cerebral myelination is well advanced, but it is uncertain whether cysts are present at birth and not detectable or whether they develop as myelination proceeds. Cysts appear to be stable in size

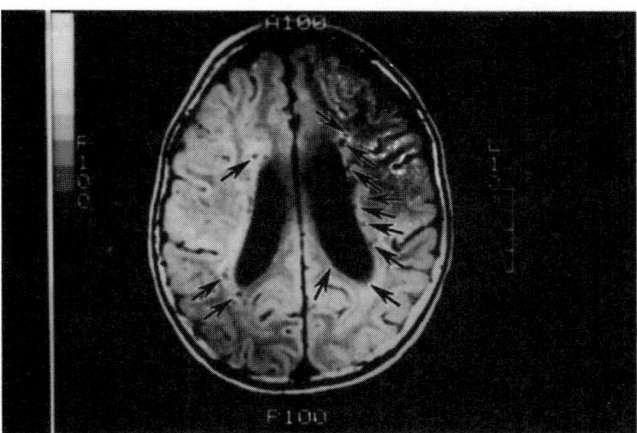

**Fig. 252-3** Multiple periventricular cysts and ventriculomegaly in an 18-year-old boy with OCRL, more prominent in the left hemisphere in this section.

and location over a several-year observation period, and their size, location, and number have no clinical significance.

Results of neuropathologic examination of the brain in OCRL were normal in some reports, while in others, a number of different abnormalities were found. These abnormalities include diffuse or focal myelin pallor without myelin breakdown; ventriculomegaly; mild cerebral abnormalities; isolated cases of subependymal cysts; mesencephalic proencephaly; postencephalitic changes; blunted and foreshortened frontal lobes; acute pontine necrosis; cerebellar hypoplasia; and aberrant neuronal migration.[10,23,27,29,30] Multiple tiny cysts without inflammatory changes were found in the cerebral white matter of one patient with typical evidence of such cysts on MRI (Wendy Shertz, MD, personal communication).

## Renal Manifestations

**Tubular Defect.** Abnormal kidney function is part of the clinical triad on which the diagnosis of OCRL is based.[31,32] Renal function and histology are apparently normal *in utero*, although the observation that amniotic fluid and maternal serum α-fetoprotein levels are elevated in some affected pregnancies with a male fetus suggests that there may be a defect in the fetal kidney with resulting leakage of serum protein.[33] The most striking renal abnormality is found postnatally, with the onset of proximal tubular acidosis, aminoaciduria, phosphaturia, and proteinuria.[31,34] The renal tubular dysfunction, in contrast to the cataracts, is not always present at birth and may require a few weeks to months to become apparent. Renal tubular dysfunction is quite variable in severity and clinical significance and may not require medical intervention, but is usually stable in older patients once established.

Acidosis is clearly of the proximal renal tubular type with bicarbonate wasting[4,5,31] and leads to the failure to thrive, recurrent infections, and metabolic collapse seen in early case reports when the disease was poorly recognized and untreated. Water resorption is also defective, as reflected in elevated 24-h volumes and low urine osmolality.[31] Clinically significant hypokalemia or hypocalcemia requiring replacement therapy occurs in a minority of patients and may be part of a preterminal exacerbation of tubular dysfunction.

The aminoaciduria is generalized, with greater elevations of basic amino acids and cysteine and relative sparing of branched-chain residues, but the profile is variable, with the degree of aminoaciduria (amino acid index) ranging from just above the upper limit of normal to 15 times the upper limit of normal.[4,31] In OCRL, as in other forms of the renal Fanconi syndrome, the pattern of aminoaciduria is not diagnostic of any particular etiology of the renal tubular dysfunction.[35]

Proteinuria is very frequently seen, but the amount of urinary protein loss and age of onset are both highly variable. Proteinuria is usually present in infancy but can occur first later in childhood. When present, protein losses can be substantial (1.38 to 10.77 g/m²/day; normal < 0.1 g/m²/day) and are composed of roughly equal proportions of tubular proteinuria (molecular mass < 40 kDa) and albuminuria, with little to no protein of higher molecular weight. Glycosuria is generally not a feature of the renal tubular dysfunction seen in OCRL.

Hyperphosphaturia is also frequent but variable, and may lead to osteomalacia, renal rickets, and pathologic fractures if untreated. It probably does not contribute significantly to the short stature seen in the syndrome.[31] In approximately half of patients, fractional excretions of phosphate are elevated despite low-normal serum phosphate levels, and there appears to be a progressive worsening of tubular phosphate wasting with age. Severe hypophosphatemia has been detected preterminally in several patients and may have contributed to their demise. Nephrolithiasis and nephrocalcinosis may occur in OCRL either because of hyperphosphaturia and hypercalciuria or as a complication of calcium and vitamin D therapy for rickets.[36] The frequency with which these complications occur is unknown.

**Progressive Renal Failure.** In addition to renal tubular dysfunction, gradual loss of creatine clearance reflecting progressive renal failure is a feature seen in OCRL patients in the second and third decades of life. The rate and extent of deterioration of renal function is, however, open to interpretation. In a series of 13 OCRL patients ranging in age from 10 to 31 years of age, there was a statistically significant linear correlation between the reciprocal of the serum creatinine concentration and age, similar to what is seen in many forms of chronic renal failure in children.[37,38] However, with the small sample size, it remains possible that the rate of loss of renal function was actually biphasic, with more rapid loss in children under age 15 and relative stability of function after that. Thus, although gradual loss of glomerular filtration has been seen in OCRL, the average age of onset of renal insufficiency and its severity have not been clearly defined in a large enough population of patients.

**Renal Pathology.** Results of histologic examination by light microscopy are usually normal in very young infants, but dilatation, atrophy, loss of brush border, and accumulation of proteinaceous material in the tubule lumen appear in the first few months of life.[4,5,34,39] These tubular abnormalities have been documented in a number of studies, including some in which serial biopsy specimens from the same patients were examined, and affect predominantly the proximal tubules; some involvement of Henle's loop, the distal tubules, and the conducting system is occasionally reported as well. Glomeruli are frequently normal in young children, even when proximal tubular lesions are present. After the first few years of life, however, glomerular lesions can be seen. These include thickening of basement membranes, focal fibrosis, and sclerosis. By electron microscopy, swelling of mitochondria in renal tubules was reported in a 22-month-old who showed no glomerular abnormalities.[4] When the same child was biopsied 7 years later, distinctive glomerular changes, including podocyte fusion and basement membrane thickening, were apparent.[34]

## Musculoskeletal Complications

Musculoskeletal complications of OCRL can occur either as complications of cardinal features of the illness — that is, hypotonia and renal disease — or as specific and possibly unique manifestations of the underlying disorder. Reported complications include joint hypermobility; recurrent fractures; genu valgum; joint contractures; scoliosis; kyphosis; platyspondylia; dislocated and/or subluxated hips; and cervical spine anomalies; as well as tenosynovitis and a nonspecific arthropathy.[40-44] Hypotonia contributes to joint hypermobility, decreased movement fosters the development of contractures, and inadequately treated rickets can lead to genu valgum deformities. Coxa valga deformity and hip contractures were found in a 16-year-old, profoundly retarded male who lost the ability to walk at age 13 years, but the hips were neither subluxated nor dislocated.[26] Joint laxity leading to varus deformity or hyperextension of the knee has also been seen. Osteopenia can be worsened by untreated renal phosphate wasting, but it is almost always present, with variable severity, despite adequate phosphate replacement, and it appears to be a specific manifestation of OCRL. Some of the patients studied in the NIH series had mildly increased cervical spine mobility without subluxation, and three had asymptomatic bone cysts,[24] but platyspondylisis, hip dislocation or subluxation, and cervical spine anomalies are quite uncommon in most series.[24] In contrast, scoliosis is widely reported in OCRL[10,17,24,41] and may be progressive postpubertally, suggesting that it is a specific feature of OCRL.

Tenosynovitis, joint swelling, and arthritis or arthropathy appear to be frequent and striking primary complications of OCRL and probably represent the same underlying disorder of excessive growth of fibroblasts. This manifestation was initially reported as palmar and plantar fibrosis[43] and later as thickened articular joint surfaces with nonspecific tenosynovitis, flexion contractures of the digits, and swelling of the interphalangeal and metacarpophalangeal joints;[44] the first detailed investigation described four additional patients with similar joint manifestations and varying degrees of nontender swelling of multiple joints. In some cases, the periarticular areas and joints of the fingers and wrist were involved, with erosion of the carpal bones. Results of laboratory studies were normal. A synovial biopsy found rubbery tissue with loss of the normal glistening surface, sparse synovial lining cells, no inflammatory cell infiltrate, fibrous connective tissue containing mature collagen and thin fibrils, and large amounts of finely fibrillar material and a granular basement membrane-like substance around the small vessels.[44] Similar diffuse swellings of the fingers, wrists, ankles, and feet without evidence of an inflammatory arthritis and similar joint changes are reported in 50 percent of OCRL patients over 20 years of age.[17] The spectrum of joint involvement is quite broad, presenting as nontender joint swelling involving both small and large joints, focal nodules (Fig. 252-4) on the finger, or bilateral plantar masses (Fig. 252-5). On occasion, these masses become painful and require resection.[24] It seems likely that these changes are the manifestation of abnormal, excessive growth of fibroblasts from periarticular tissue or tendons.

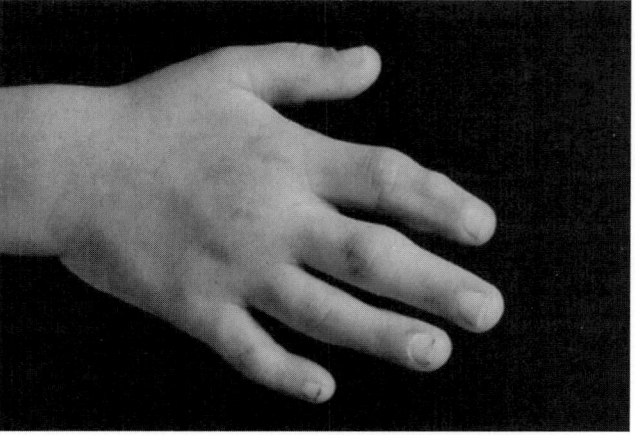

**Fig. 252-4 Hand of a 7-year-old boy showing nontender, diffuse swelling of the second and third proximal interphalangeal joints and a subcutaneous nodule on the second digit over the distal interphalangeal joint. There was no history of trauma to this area.**

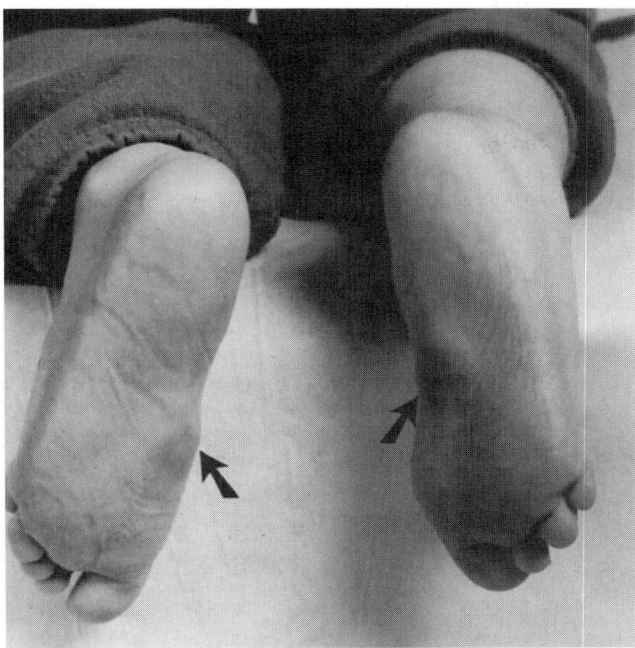

Fig. 252-5 Bilateral plantar masses (arrows) in a 12-year-old boy. The masses are firm and are attached to underlying connective tissue, but they are nontender and do not interfere with ambulation.

## Sexual Development

The onset and progression of puberty occur at a normal age in OCRL patients, producing Tanner V genitalia and axillary and facial hair. Testosterone levels are normal. Sexual interest among older males varies, but there is a notable lack of a strong sexual drive in comparison with other similarly intellectually compromised adults. Fertility may also be reduced owing to the peritubular fibrosis and azoospermia associated with OCRL.[23]

## Other Clinical Manifestations

Cryptorchidism is a common occurrence in OCRL, up to 40 percent in one report[16] and 15 percent in a more comprehensive survey.[17] Dental cysts during primary tooth eruption and enamel hypoplasia have been reported[45] and, in older individuals, sebaceous cysts on the buttocks and perineum appear to occur frequently.[17] Constipation of variable severity is frequent in OCRL and usually improves with age,[17] although it may persist and cause a protuberant abdomen or diarrhea with stooling around a fecal impaction.

## Growth

The mean length and weight are within the normal range at birth, typically above the 50th percentile, but fall from the normal curve with age. Mean height falls to the third percentile by 3 years of age, and continues to show a relative fall throughout adolescence. Mean final height is less than the third percentile, but OCRL patients continue to grow into early adulthood. Bone age lags slightly behind height age, and epiphyses fuse at adult height. Mean weight shows a similar profile, with a late plateau phase into the early twenties and a final weight less than the third percentile. Head circumference of OCRL patients is within the normal range, with a mean adult head circumference at the 50th percentile.[31]

## Cause of Death

OCRL patients have been reported to succumb to renal failure or infection in their second or third decade[16] but infection as a cause of death has become infrequent with more aggressive medical intervention. Other causes of death include status epilepticus, refractory renal tubular wasting of electrolytes, respiratory compromise from scoliosis, and sudden, unexplained death. The oldest OCRL patient in the United States expired at age 41. The expected life span with current medical practice has not been defined.

## GENETICS

From the first, patients with OCRL were overwhelmingly male and the inheritance X-linked, with multiple-affected males in pedigrees related to each other through asymptomatic, unaffected female carriers.[5,10] Two interesting female patients were described with classical OCRL in association with balanced X;autosome translocations involving, in both cases, the Xq26 region of the X chromosome with two different autosomes.[46,47] Because the normal X chromosome is generally inactive when there is a balanced X;autosome translocation, females carrying such translocations can develop full expression of an X-linked disorder if the translocation breakpoint disrupts the disease locus. Female patients with translocations proved instrumental in allowing the identification and characterization of the OCRL gene.

## THE GENE FOR OCRL

In 1992, positional cloning isolated *OCRL1*, the gene for OCRL.[9] The gene contains 24 exons with one small (24 bp) alternatively spliced exon.[48] The protein encoded by *OCRL1*, ocrl1p, has striking homology to a human enzyme involved in inositol phosphate metabolism, a 75-kDa inositol polyphosphate 5-phosphatase (inpp5bp) described in platelets and cloned from platelet and placenta cDNA libraries.[49] Inpp5bp cleaves the 5-phosphate specifically from inositol (1,4,5)-trisphosphate and inositol (1,3,4,5)-tetrakisphosphate although it also can dephosphorylate the 5′ position of the phospholipid substrates PtdIns(4,5)P$_2$ and PtdIns(3,4,5)P$_3$.[50] The two proteins show 53 percent identity and 71 percent similarity in primary amino acid sequence, but are distinct in their map location: *INPP5B*, the gene encoding inpp5bp, maps to chromosome 1p (51) whereas *OCRL1* is X-linked.

The strong similarity between ocrl1p and inpp5bp suggested that OCRL might also encode an inositol phosphate or phosphatidylinositol phosphate 5-phosphatase, which is, indeed, the case.[50,52] A specific deficiency of the *OCRL1*-encoded PtdIns(4,5)P$_2$ was demonstrated in fibroblasts from OCRL patients when assayed under the appropriate substrate and detergent concentrations that distinguish the activity of ocrl1p from inpp5bp.[52,53] This makes OCRL the first inherited defect of phosphatidylinositol metabolism in higher eukaryotes and allows biochemical diagnosis for Lowe syndrome.

### Molecular Characterization of Mutations in OCRL Patients

Twenty-two different mutations have been found in 28 unrelated OCRL patients to date[20–22,54] (Fig. 252-6). They cluster in 9 exons, particularly in exon 15. Most mutations are family specific, but four mutations have been seen in more than one unrelated OCRL patient. A frameshift mutation, a GT deletion in exon 21, and a missense mutation, CGA > CAA in exon 15, were found in three unrelated patients. Two other recurrent mutations are a nonsense mutation arg > stop in exon 22 observed in two patients and a splice junction mutation resulting in skipping of exon 22 in two patients. Approximately 75 percent of patients for whom there is western blot data have no antigenic cross-reacting material. Of the remaining 25 percent, the underlying mutations are missense mutations in domains conserved among many PtdIns polyphosphate 5-phosphatases and the amount of protein is usually (but not always) reduced on western analysis.[20–22,54] Thus, the syndrome appears to result from loss of function of the enzyme and not from any particular mutant allele. No obvious phenotype-genotype correlation can be made between severity or pleiotropy and the mutant allele present; in fact, patients with

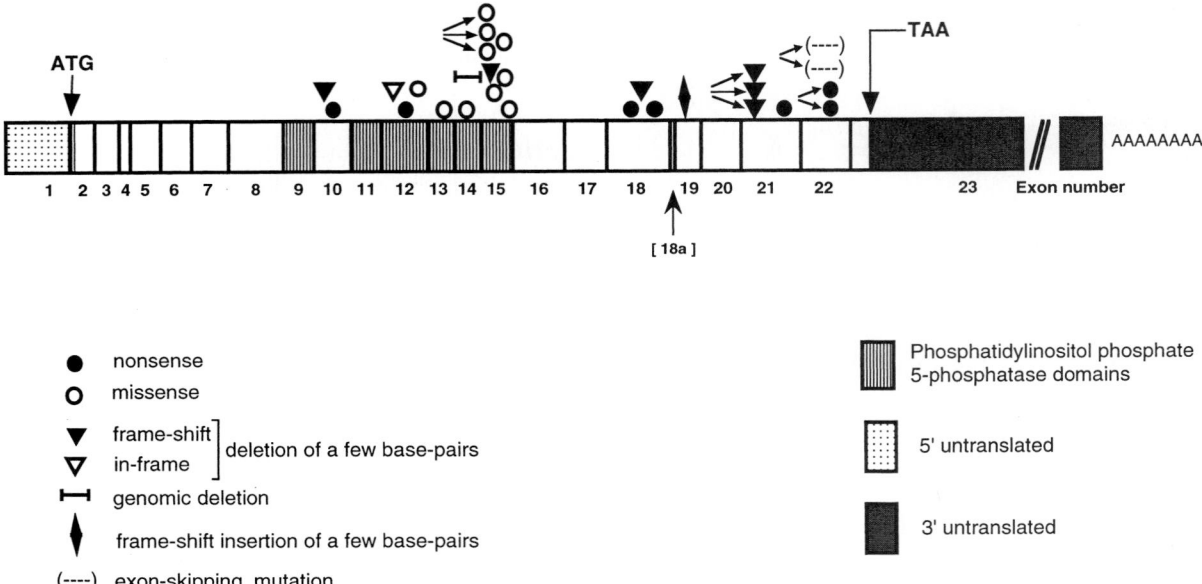

nonsense

missense

frame-shift
in-frame  } deletion of a few base-pairs

genomic deletion

frame-shift insertion of a few base-pairs

(----) exon-skipping mutation

Phosphatidylinositol phosphate 5-phosphatase domains

5' untranslated

3' untranslated

**Fig. 252-6 Spectrum of mutations in Lowe syndrome shown on a map of the mRNA of the *OCRL1* gene.**

different clinical courses have been found to have the same mutation.[20]

## Subcellular Localization and Possible Function of ocrl1p

Immunofluorescence micrography of normal fibroblasts using an affinity-purified polyclonal antibody to ocrl1p reveals a staining pattern characteristic of that for Golgi proteins.[55] This pattern is absent from fibroblasts of an OCRL patient without detectable *OCRL1* mRNA, indicating that ocrl1p is a Golgi-associated protein. This subcellular localization of the ocrl1p protein has been confirmed by subcellular fractionation experiments in fibroblasts that demonstrate that ocrl1p is predominantly in the microsomal fraction (Golgi, endosomes, and endoplasmic reticulum) (Suchy and Nussbaum, unpublished data). Simultaneous double-labeling experiments with antibodies to known Golgi proteins β-COP and γ-adaptin, with or without Golgi perturbation by brefeldin-A, provide further evidence that ocrl1p is located in the Golgi, particularly in the *trans*-Golgi network, and endosomal compartment, in a variety of cell types including fibroblasts and cultured proximal tubular cells (reference 55; Dressman, Suchy, and Nussbaum, unpublished data). This information provides important clues to understanding the cellular role of this 5-phosphatase.

The substrate for PtdInsP$_2$ 5-phosphatase, PtdInsP$_2$, is an effector of two proteins known to be involved in the regulation of Golgi vesicular transport, ADP ribosylation factor GTPase-activating protein (ARF-GAP) and phospholipase D.[57-59] In the Golgi apparatus, ARF-GAP is stimulated directly by PtdInsP$_2$ and indirectly via phospholipase D.[58] Furthermore, there is also substantial evidence from in vitro vesicle reconstruction experiments using defined, protein-free artificial lipid vesicles that the binding of coatmer proteins depends on the presence of acidic phosphatidylinositol polyphosphates in the vesicle membranes.[60,61] Thus, PtdInsP$_2$ in the Golgi appears to be involved in regulating Golgi vesicle formation or protein trafficking. It is possible that in Lowe syndrome, a deficiency of PtdInsP$_2$ 5-phosphatase may lead to elevated levels of PtdInsP$_2$ and result in abnormal Golgi transport.

PtdInsP$_2$ is also involved in cytoskeleton assembly, by interacting with actin-binding proteins such as profilin and gelsolin and regulating their interactions with actin.[62-64] Actin assembly in the region of the Golgi apparatus may be involved in protein transport by directing secretory vesicles to the plasma membrane.

An elevated level of PtdInsP$_2$ due to a deficiency of the ocrl1 protein may also affect polymerization of the actin cytoskeleton.

Currently it is not clear how the deficiency of ocrl1p produces the Lowe syndrome phenotype. But the localization of ocrl1p to the Golgi apparatus combined with evidence of an elevation of PtdInsP$_2$ in Lowe syndrome cells[65] and the role of PtdInsP$_2$ in vesicular trafficking leads to the speculation that ocrl1p plays a role in regulating protein trafficking or other aspects of vesicle formation. However, because OCRL1 is widely expressed in different tissues,[55] it is predicted that a generalized defect in protein targeting is highly detrimental to many tissues in the developing organism. It is unclear why Lowe syndrome has a phenotype limited to only a few tissues. It is possible that one or more PtdInsP$_2$ 5-phosphatase(s) may compensate for the defect in some tissues. It is also possible that the defect in Golgi functions may be one of dysregulation instead of complete loss of function and may affect cell-surface transport of only certain proteins. The resulting changes in cell membrane composition may disrupt the interactions between cells, or between cells and the substratum that are required for normal cell migration and differentiation in only some tissues, such as the epithelium of the lens or in tight junctions of the renal epithelium. Further studies are necessary to test these hypotheses.

## DIAGNOSIS

### Diagnostic Criteria

Clinical diagnosis relies on the cardinal clinical features of OCRL: congenital cataracts, neonatal or infantile hypotonia with later cognitive impairment and areflexia, and, eventually, renal tubular dysfunction. Confirming features include glaucoma (either congenital or developing postoperatively); buphthalmos; megalocornea; cryptorchidism; characteristic appearance; and abnormalities in serum and urine electrolytes and protein (see below). Cataracts are congenital in the strict sense, being present at birth with the characteristic thin lens and complete visual occlusion. Neonatal hypotonia is typically obvious. Demonstration of renal tubular dysfunction may be difficult initially and may require quantitative determination of amino acid or protein excretion as well as of impaired water-concentrating ability.

The differential diagnosis of neonatal hypotonia and cataracts includes congenital rubella, peroxisomal disorders such as

**Table 252-1** PtdIns (4, 5) P$_2$ 5-phosphatase Activity*
in Human Tissues

|  | OCRL | Control | | |
|---|---|---|---|---|
|  | Fibroblasts | Fibroblasts | Amniocytes | CVS cells |
| Mean | 0.49 | 6.41 | 6.78 | 6.45 |
| (+ SD†) | (+0.31) | (+0.81) | (+1.62) | (+0.73) |
| N‡ | 31 | 7 | 10 | 10 |

* = nmol/min/mg protein; † = standard deviation; ‡ = number of samples

Zellweger syndrome, congenital myotonic dystrophy, and Smith-Lemli-Opitz syndrome. Among these various disorders, however, the very dense congenital cataracts and the absence of the striking additional findings of the peroxisomal disorders or Smith-Lemli-Opitz, limit the diagnosis practically to rubella or OCRL. Serology, intracranial calcifications, and other clinical features may distinguish these two. Congenital myotonic dystrophy presents with severe neonatal hypotonia; lenticular opacities may also be present, but these cataracts are clinically subtle, metachromatic, and easily distinguished from the cataract in OCRL.

Definitive diagnosis of OCRL can now be done using an assay for the PtdInsP$_2$ 5-phosphatase activity of ocrl1p in cultured fibroblasts (Table 252-1). Fibroblasts from Lowe syndrome patients have < 10 percent of the activity seen in normal fibroblasts; there is no overlap between the distributions of normal and affected fibroblasts up to 5 standard deviations from the normal and affected mean values.

### Prenatal Diagnosis

Prenatal diagnosis by molecular methods using linked markers has been reported,[66] and even better tightly linked flanking markers are now available,[48] but the approach is limited to informative families. Prenatal diagnosis by fetal ultrasound detection of cataracts has also been done,[12] but the sensitivity of ultrasound detection of cataracts in fetuses at risk for OCRL may be low because directed prenatal ultrasound examination in two similar situations at experienced centers was unsuccessful in identifying the abnormal lens at 18 and 20 weeks, respectively (D. Steele and R. Miller, personal communication). Not all patients have abnormalities in their mRNA detectable by northern blot,[9] which limits this approach to a subset of families. Different mutations (deletion, missense, and nonsense) along the *OCRL1* gene have been observed in Lowe syndrome patients,[20–22] making direct molecular prenatal diagnosis tedious, and only practical for families in which the mutation is known.

Ocrl1p is expressed in amniocytes and chorionic villi, thus allowing direct prenatal diagnosis by biochemical testing.[68] The PtdInsP$_2$ 5-phosphatase activity in control amniocyte and chorionic villus cultures (15.5 to 20 and 9 to 11 gestational weeks, respectively) is similar to the activity in control fibroblasts from unrelated individuals (Table 252-1). There is no evidence of a correlation between enzyme activity in either amniocytes or chorionic villus cultures and gestational age ($r^2 = 0.087$, $p > 0.4$ and $r^2 = 0.249$, $p > 0.14$, respectively). Although the number of samples analyzed to date is very small, this result indicates that gestational age (during the weeks tested) does not have a substantial effect on PtdInsP$_2$ 5-phosphatase activity in these tissues.[68]

### Carrier Detection

Female carriers of OCRL are usually asymptomatic and have no significant renal or neurologic defects detectable on clinical or laboratory examination. Ophthalmologic evaluation, however, reveals one of two distinctive lenticular changes in most heterozygotes.[69,70] The most common finding on slit-lamp examination is numerous punctate, white-to-gray opacities, which are present in all layers of the lenticular cortex except the nucleus

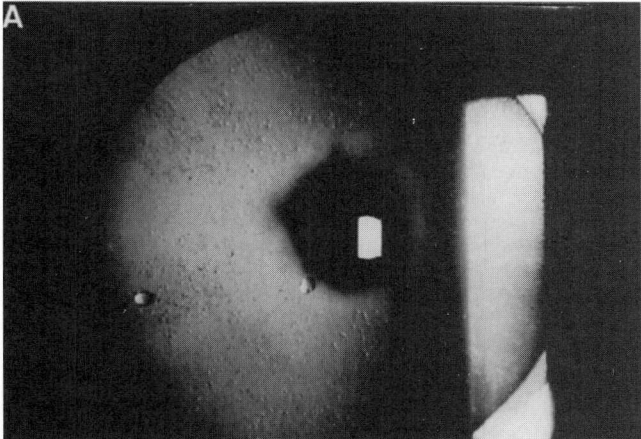

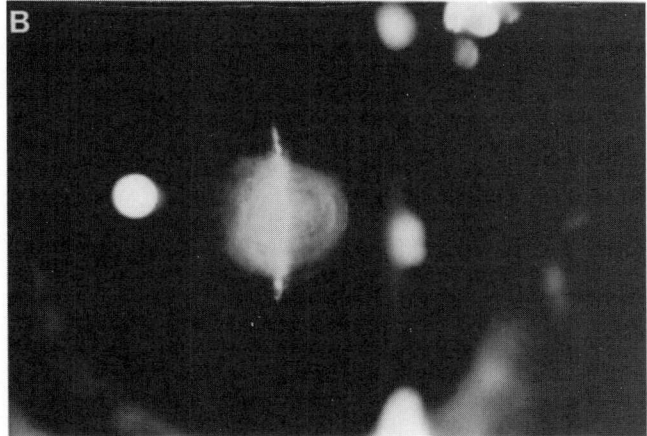

**Fig. 252-7 Slit-lamp examination of female carriers of Lowe syndrome. *A.* The typical pattern of hundreds of micropunctate, gray opacities in a radial distribution in the lens. *B.* A single dense posterior cataract as seen in some OCRL heterozygotes. (Courtesy of R. A. Lewis, MD.)**

and are distributed in a radial, spoke-like pattern (Fig. 252-7A). The distribution of opacities just outside the nucleus suggests that the opacities develop very early in life, while the more superficial opacities must arise in adulthood. There are usually more than 15 of these opacities, and there may be hundreds. A few female carriers show a single subcapsular dense cataract in the posterior pole (Fig. 252-7B). This form of cataract may be present congenitally and become clinically more apparent with age, eventually requiring surgery. The pattern of the lens changes in female carriers suggests that the defect is expressed in a cell-autonomous manner; that is, groups of cells in which the X chromosome carrying the normal OCRL allele is inactivated express the defect and cannot be "cross-corrected" by neighboring cells that have an active normal allele.

The sensitivity (penetrance) and specificity of lens opacities for carrier detection has been evaluated in families in whom female carriers were diagnosed using flanking linked markers.[71,72] In one study, slit-lamp examination could detect 31 of 33 (94 percent) of carriers, as determined by linked markers, and no false positives. Because of the uncertainty introduced by possible recombinations between the linked markers and *OCRL1* gene, a follow-up of this study was performed using direct detection of the specific mutation. Ophthalmologic evaluation of 31 at-risk females in three families with Lowe syndrome yielded only one false negative in a young girl age 5 years and no false positives among 31 females members examined.[70]

Controversy exists concerning the specificity and sensitivity of the lens changes in OCRL carrier females. Specificity has been questioned because of confusion between the OCRL carrier state and the changes that are seen with increasing age in normal individuals. Specificity can be markedly improved by taking into account not only the number of such opacities but also their characteristic distribution, particularly if one concentrates on females of child-bearing age who are most appropriate for carrier detection for genetic counseling. Sensitivity of carrier detection by slit lamp examination is demonstrably quite high, but unlikely to ever be 100 percent because of random X-inactivation. Sensitivity also appears to be reduced in children, but carrier testing in this age group is controversial because of concerns with protecting children's rights to make autonomous decisions about genetic testing.

## TREATMENT

### Vision

The visual defects in OCRL patients constitute a major obstacle to the ability of these patients to reach their developmental potential. A detailed discussion of ophthalmologic therapy and procedures is beyond the scope of this chapter, and early ophthalmologic consultation and therapy are mandated to aid in diagnosis and institution of therapy.[69] Cataracts should be removed when diagnosed, and the resulting aphakia treated with glasses. Glaucoma, a frequent component of the disease, may be difficult to control medically, and goniotomy or trabeculotomy to control intraocular pressure is often required. Corneal keloid formation is another serious complication that usually develops after age 5. Opinions differ as to whether corneal trauma or the use of contact lenses contributes to keloid development. For this reason, glasses are preferred over contact lenses, especially because younger patients are less likely to lose or damage glasses. The fact that the keloids involve the full thickness of the cornea makes lamellar keratoplasty ineffective. Even with early ophthalmologic intervention, including treatment of cataracts and glaucoma, some degree of impairment of visual acuity is usually present, and nystagmus is a common finding.

### Nervous System

The treatment of neurologic manifestations in OCRL is largely symptomatic. Hypotonia and developmental delay are treated with a combination of speech, physical, and occupational therapy beginning at an early age. Such interventions are designed to facilitate the progress of each child according to the child's ability, and the use of appropriate testing techniques and specialized environments appears to offer a better-than-expected outcome in some cases. Areflexia is a medical curiosity and does not warrant therapy. Seizures are treated according to current standards, depending on the seizure type and precipitating features. Phenobarbital, carbamazepine, phenytoin, and valproic acid, as well as the benzodiazepines, have all been used with success in patients with OCRL.[73]

Stereotypic behaviors that frequently interfere with normal function and the inability to change a pattern without precipitating a temper tantrum (rigidity, stubbornness) are frequently the most difficult treatment issues facing the clinician. Many psychopharmaceuticals (neuroleptics, stimulants, benzodiazepines, tricyclic antidepressants, and serotonin reuptake inhibitors) have been used without a clear pattern of success. Some improvement of stereotypic behavior and stubbornness following treatment with clomipramine or paroxetine has been seen. Drug therapy for this disorder must be tailored to the specific patient and is largely empirical.

### Renal Disease

Periodic monitoring for renal complications of OCRL should begin at the first suggestion of the diagnosis and continue every 3 months thereafter during the first 2 years of life in anticipation of development of significant tubular wasting of small molecules.

The renal tubular Fanconi syndrome is similar, although less severe, than that seen in cystinosis, and treatment guidelines have been modified from the cystinosis experience (see Chap. 200). All individuals have impaired water-concentrating ability and should have free access to fluids to replace urinary water losses. Alkalinizing therapy to counter renal bicarbonate losses should begin when serum bicarbonate drops below 20 mEq/liter, using either a tricitrate solution (Polycitra, Bicitra) or sodium bicarbonate starting at a dose of 2 to 3 mEq/kg/day given every 6 to 8 h, and adjusted once or twice a week until serum bicarbonate is above 20 mEq/liter. Typically, patients can be corrected to values of 23 to 24 mEq/liter, but more refractory patients may require higher doses with administration every 6 h. Hypokalemia is not usually encountered in OCRL, but administration of Polycitra, with 1 mEq of potassium and 1 mEq of sodium per milliequivalent of citric acid, may avoid this problem. Urinary phosphorus losses are variable and may be elevated without requiring phosphate supplementation.

The easiest and most reliable indicator for phosphorus supplementation is serum alkaline phosphatase, which increases as bone resorption occurs to maintain normal phosphorus levels. Clinical or radiographic evidence of rickets are late findings, and serum phosphate levels are maintained within the normal range until there is severe bone demineralization. Sodium or potassium phosphate administration should be initiated at between 1 and 4 g/day in divided doses, and serum alkaline phosphatase monitored at 2- to 4-month intervals to follow normalization. A vitamin D preparation may be a useful adjunct to increase intestinal phosphate absorption, although it should be used cautiously because of the potential to overstimulate intestinal calcium absorption, leading to increased urinary calcium excretion with the potential for nephrocalcinosis or nephrolithiasis. Calcium replacement is infrequently required in OCRL, and care should be taken to avoid precipitation of calcium phosphate in the renal collecting system.

Limitation of protein intake is recommended by some nephrologists to decrease the likelihood of renal insufficiency in the long term. Although this approach may be beneficial to adults with chronic renal failure, its efficacy in OCRL has not been demonstrated. Nitrogen losses from proteinuria and aminoaciduria in OCRL are significant, and severe protein restriction without consideration of these losses may lead to a protein intake that is inadequate for growth.

The efficacy of L-carnitine replacement in OCRL has not been systematically studied. Carnitine deficiency defined as plasma values greater than 2 standard deviations below the mean have been documented in OCRL, and a transient clinical benefit from carnitine supplementation has been reported in only one patient.[74] Normalization of plasma carnitine following oral supplementation is easily demonstrated, but there is no objective evidence of benefit. The major complications from L-carnitine supplementation are the expense of the medication, which is frequently available at health food stores, and the social stigma of a fishy odor due to tertiary amine release from carnitine breakdown.

Administration of recombinant human growth hormone (rhGH) to increase linear growth in OCRL should be limited to those individuals who have demonstrable growth hormone deficiency. Although there is no data for OCRL, the use of rhGH in cystinosis with renal tubular dysfunction and renal insufficiency has been reported to be associated with acceleration of renal disease,[75] although recent, larger multicenter studies have reported no adverse effect.[76]

### Musculoskeletal Abnormalities and Other Clinical Findings

The treatment of most of the musculoskeletal problems associated with OCRL is straightforward. Contractures are avoided by maintaining mobility, and astute management of the renal disease can prevent osteopenia and fractures. Scoliosis should be anticipated and treated using standard methods, including the use of rods. The proper management of joint swelling and fibroid tumors is less clear, but minimizing discomfort, maintaining mobility, and judicious use of surgery for relief of pain are reasonable guidelines. Undescended testes should be managed using standard criteria.

## ACKNOWLEDGMENTS

The authors acknowledge the officers and members of the Lowe Syndrome Association for their support, cooperation, and patience. We also thank W. Shertz, M. Norman, K. Armfield, D. Steele, R. Miller, E. Rawnlsey, M. M. Padilla, and R. A. Lewis for making patient information and photographs available.

## REFERENCES

1. Lowe CU, Terrey M, MacLachan EA: Organic aciduria, decreased renal ammonia production, hydrophthalmos, and mental retardation: A clinical entity. *Am J Dis Child* **83**:164, 1952.
2. Bickel H, Thursby-Pelham DC: Hyper-amino-aciduria in Lignac-Fanconi disease, in galactosaemia and in an obscure syndrome. *Arch Dis Child* **29**:224, 1954.
3. Falls HG: Ocular manifestations of the chronic renal tubular insufficiency syndromes. *Arch Ophthalmol* **62**:188, 1959.
4. Schoen EJ, Young G: "Lowe's syndrome": Abnormalities in renal tubular function in combination with other congenital defects. *Am J Med* **27**:781, 1959.
5. Richards W, Donnell GN, Wilson WA, Stowens D, Perry T: The oculocerebrorenal syndrome of Lowe. *Am J Dis Child* **109**:185, 1965.
6. Brown N, Gardner RJM: Lowe syndrome: Identification of the carrier state. *Birth Defects* **12(3)**:579, 1976.
7. Delleman JW, Bleeker-Wagemakers EM, van Veelen AWC: Opacities of the lens indicating carrier status in the oculo-cerebro-renal (Lowe) syndrome. *J Pediatr Ophthalmol* **14**:205, 1976.
8. Silver DN, Lewis RA, Nussbaum RL: Mapping the Lowe oculocerebrorenal syndrome to Xq24-q26 by use of restriction fragment length polymorphisms. *J Clin Invest* **79**:282, 1987.
9. Attree O, Olivos IM, Okabe I, Bailey LC, Nelson DL, Lewis RA, McInnes RR, Nussbaum RL: The Lowe oculocerebrorenal syndrome gene encodes a novel protein highly homologous to inositol polyphosphate-5-phosphatase. *Nature* **358**:239, 1992.
10. Charnas L, Nussbaum RL: Oculocerebrorenal syndrome of Lowe, in Scriver CR, Beaudet AL, Sly WS, Valle D (eds): *The Metabolic and Molecular Bases of Inherited Disease*, 7th ed. New York, McGraw-Hill, p 3705, 1995.
11. Ginsberg J, Bove KE, Fogelson MH: Pathological features of the eye in the oculocerebrorenal (Lowe) syndrome. *J Pediatr Ophthalmol Strabismus* **18**:16, 1981.
12. Gaary EA, Rawnsley E, Marin-Padilla JM, Morse CL, Crow HC: In utero detection of fetal cataracts. *Ultrasound Med* **12(4)**:234, 1993.
13. Endres W, Schaub J, Stefani FH, Wirtz A, Zahn V: Cataract in a fetus at risk for oculocerebrorenal syndrome. *Klin Wochenschr* **55**:141, 1977.
14. Curtin VT, Joyce EE, Ballin N: Ocular pathology in the oculo-cerebrorenal syndrome of Lowe. *Am J Opthalmol* **64**:533, 1967.
15. Tripathi RC, Cibis GW, Tripathi BJ: Pathogenesis of cataracts in patients with Lowe's syndrome. *Ophthalmology* **93**:1046, 1986.
16. Abbassi V, Lowe CU, Calcagno PL: Oculo-cerebro-renal syndrome. *Am J Dis Child* **115**:145, 1968.
17. McSpadden K: *Report of the Lowe's Syndrome Comprehensive Survey.* West Lafayette, IN, Lowe's Syndrome Association, 1991.
18. Cibis GW, Tripathi RC, Tripathi BJ, Harris DJ: Corneal keloid in Lowe's syndrome. *Arch Ophthalmol* **100**:1795, 1982.
19. Kenworthy L, Park T, Charnas LR: Cognitive and behavioral profile of the oculocerebrorenal syndrome of Lowe. *Am J Med Genet* **46**:297, 1993.
20. Leahey AM, Charnas LR, Nussbaum RL: Nonsense mutations in the OCRL-1 gene in patients with the oculocerebrorenal syndrome of Lowe. *Hum Mol Genet* **4**:461, 1993.
21. Lin T, Orrison BM, Leahey AM, Suchy SF, Bernard DJ, Lewis RA, Nussbaum RL: Spectrum of mutations in the OCRL1 gene in the oculocerebrorenal syndrome. *Am J Hum Genet* **60**:1384,1997.
22. Lin, T, Orrison BM, Suchy SF, Lewis RA, Nussbaum RL: Mutations are not uniformly distributed throughout the OCRL1 gene in Lowe syndrome patients. *Molec Genet Metab* **64**:58, 1998.
23. Matin MA, Sylvester PE: Clinicopathologic studies of oculocerebrorenal syndrome of Lowe, Terry and MacLachlan. *J Ment Defic Res* **24**:1, 1980.
24. Charnas LR, Gahl WA: The oculocerebrorenal syndrome of Lowe. *Adv Pediatr* **31**:75, 1991.
25. Kenworthy L, Charnas L: Evidence for a discrete behavioral phenotype in the oculocerebrorenal syndrome of Lowe. *Am J Med Genet* **59**:283, 1995.
26. Charnas L, Bernar J, Pezeshkpour GH, Dalakas M, Harper GS, Gahl WA: MRI findings and peripheral neuropathy in Lowe syndrome. *Neuropediatrics* **19**:7, 1988.
27. Demmer LA, Wippold FJ II, Dowton SB: Periventricular white matter cystic lesions in Lowe (oculocerebrorenal) syndrome. *Pediatr Radiol* **22**:76, 1992.
28. Carroll WJ, Woodruff WW, Cadman TE: MR findings in oculocerebrorenal syndrome. *Am J Neuroradiol* **14**:449, 1993
29. Banerjee AK, Allen IV, McKee P: Oculo-cerebro-renal syndrome: Failure to demonstrate specific neuropathological abnormalities in four cases. *Ir J Med Sci* **15**:42, 1982.
30. Ono J, Harada K, Mano T, Yamamoto T, Okada S: MR findings and neurologic manifestations in Lowe oculocerebrorenal syndrome. *Pediatr Neurol* **14**:162, 1996.
31. Charnas L, Bernardini I, Rader D, Hoeg J, Gahl WA: Clinical and laboratory findings in the oculocerebrorenal syndrome of Lowe, with special reference to growth and renal function. *N Engl J Med* **324**:1318, 1991.
32. Pueschel SM, Brem AS, Nittoli P: Central nervous system and renal investigations in patients with Lowe syndrome. *Child Nerv Syst* **8**:45, 1992.
33. Miller, RC, Wolf, EJ, Gould, M, Macri C, Charnas LR: Fetal oculocerebrorenal syndrome of Lowe associated with elevated maternal serum and amniotic fluid alpha-fetoprotein. *Obstet Gynecol* **84**:77, 1994.
34. Witzleben CL, Schoen EJ, Tu WH, McDonald LW: Progressive morphologic renal changes in the oculo-cerebro-renal syndrome of Lowe. *Am J Med* **44**:319, 1968.
35. Manz F, Bremer HJ, Brodehl J: Renal transport of amino acids in children with oculocerebrorenal syndrome. *Helv Paediatr Acta* **33**:37, 1978.
36. Sliman GA, Winters WD, Shaw DW, Avner ED: Hypercalciuria and nephrocalcinosis in the oculocerebrorenal syndrome. *J Urol* **153**:1244, 1995.
37. Arbus GS, Bacheyie GS: Method for predicting when children with progressive renal disease may reach high serum creatinine levels. *Pediatrics* **67**:871, 1981.
38. Reimold EW: Chronic progressive renal failure: Rate of progression monitored by change of serum creatinine concentration. *Am J Dis Child* **135**:1039, 1981.
39. Van Acker KJ, Roels H, Beelaerts W, Pasternack A, Valcke R: The histologic lesions of the kidney in the oculo-cerebro-renal syndrome of Lowe. *Nephron* **4**:193, 1967.
40. Athreya B, Schumacher HR, Getz HD, Norman ME, Borden S IV, Witzleben CL: Arthropathy of Lowe's (oculocerebrorenal) syndrome. *Arthritis Rheum* **26**:728, 1983.
41. Holtgrewe JL, Kalen V: Orthopedic manifestations of the Lowe (oculocerebrorenal) syndrome. *J Pediatr Orthop* **6**:165, 1986.
42. Rosenblatt D, Holmes LB: Development of arthritis in Lowe's syndrome. *J Pediatr* **84**:924, 1974.
43. Phelip X, Bocquet B, Gras JP, Bouvier M, Cabanel G, Lejeune E: Fibrose palmo-plantaire extensive au cours d'un syndrome de Lowe. *Rev Rhum Mal Osteoartic* **40**:597, 1973.
44. Elliman D, Woodley A: Tenosynovitis in Lowe syndrome. *J Pediatr* **103**:1011, 1983.
45. Roberts MW, Blakey GH, Jacoway JR, Chen SC, Morris CR: Enlarged dental follicles, a follicular cyst, and enamel hypoplasia in a patient with Lowe syndrome. *Oral Med Oral Pathol* **77**:264, 1994.
46. Hodgson SV, Heckmatt JZ, Hughes E, Crolla JA, Dubowitz V, Bobrow M: A balanced de novo X/autosome translocation in a girl with manifestation of Lowe syndrome. *Am J Med Genet* **23**:837, 1986.
47. Mueller OT, Hartsfield JK Jr, Gallardo LA, Essig Y-P, Miller KL, Papenhausen PR, Tedesco TA: Lowe oculocerebrorenal syndrome in a female with a balanced X;20 translocation: Mapping of the X chromosome breakpoint. *Am J Hum Genet* **49**:804, 1991.
48. Nussbaum RL, Orrison BM, Janne PA, Charnas L, Chinault AC: Physical mapping and genomic structure of the Lowe syndrome gene OCRL1. *Hum Genet* **99**:145, 1997.

49. Ross TS, Jefferson AB, Mitchell CA, Majerus PW: Cloning and expression of human 75-kDa inositol polyphosphate-5-phosphatase. *J Biol Chem* **266**:20283, 1991.
50. Zhang X, Jefferson AB, Auethavekiat V, Majerus PW: The protein deficient in Lowe syndrome is a phosphatidylinositol-4,5-bisphosphate 5-phosphatase. *Proc Natl Acad Sci U S A* **92**:4853, 1995.
51. Jänne P, Dutra AS, Dracapoli NC, Charnas L, Puck JM, Nussbaum RL. Localization of a type II inositol polyphosphate 5-phosphatase to human chromosome 1p34. *Cytogenet Cell Genet* **66**:164, 1994.
52. Suchy SF, Olivos-Glander IM, and Nussbaum RL: Lowe's syndrome, a deficiency of a phosphatidylinositol 4,5 bisphosphate 5-phosphatase in the Golgi apparatus. *Human Molec Genet* **4**:2245, 1995.
53. Jänne PA, Suchy SF, Bernard D, MacDonald M, Crawley J, Grinberg A, Wynshaw-Boris A, et al.: Functional overlap between murine Inpp5b and Ocrl1 may explain why deficiency of the murine ortholog for OCRL1 does not cause Lowe syndrome in mice. *J Clin Invest* **101**:2042, 1998.
54. Kawano T, Indo Y, Nakazato H, Shimadzu M, and Matsuda I: Oculocerebrorenal syndrome of Lowe: Three mutations in the OCRL1 gene derived from three patients with different phenotypes. *Am J Med Genet* **77**:348,1998.
55. Olivos-Glander IM, Jänne PA, and Nussbaum RL: The oculocerebrorenal syndrome gene product is a 105 kd protein localized to the golgi complex, *Am J Hum Genet* **57**:817, 1995.
56. Matzaris M, Jackson SP, Laxminarayan KM, Speed CJ, Mitchell CA: Identification and characterization of the phosphatidyl-(4,5)-biphosphate 5-phosphatase in human platelets. *J Biol Chem* **269**:3397, 1994.
57. Liscovitch M, Chalifa V, Pertile P, Chen C-S, Cantley LC: Novel function of phosphatidylinositol 4,5 bisphosphate as a cofactor for membrane phospholipase. *J Biol Chem* **269**:21403, 1994.
58. Randazzo PA and Kahn RA: GTP hydrolysis by ADP-ribosylation factor is dependent on both an ADP-ribosylation factor GTPase-activating protein and acid phospholipids. *J Biol Chem* **269**:10758, 1994.
59. Pertile P, Liscovitch M, Chalifa V, Cantley LC: Phosphatidylinositol 4,5 bisphosphate synthesis is required for activation of phospholipase D in U937 cells. *J Biol Chem* **270**:5130, 1995.
60. Takei K, Haucke V, Slepnev V, Farsad K, Salazar M, Chen H, De Camilli P: Generation of coated intermediates of clathrin-mediated endocytosis on protein-free liposomes. *Cell* **94**:131, 1998.
61. Matsuoka K, Orci L, Amherdt M, Bednarek SY, Hamamoto S, Schekman R, Yeung T: COPII-coated vesicle formation reconstituted with purified coat proteins and chemically defined liposomes. *Cell* **93**:263, 1998.
62. Janmey PA: Phosphoinositides and calcium as regulators of cellular actin assembly and disassembly. *Annu Rev Physiol* **56**:169, 1994.
63. Stossel TP: From signal to pseudopod. How cells control cytoplasmic actin assembly. *J Biol Chem* **264**:18261, 1989.
64. Yu F-X: Identification of a polyphosphoinositide-binding sequence in an actin monomer-binding domain of gelsolin. *J Biol Chem* **267**:14616, 1992.
65. Zhang X, Hartz PA, Philip E, Racusen LC, Majerus PW: Cell lines from kidney proximal tubules of a patient with Lowe syndrome lack OCRL inositol polyphosphate 5-phosphatase and accumulate phosphatidylinositol 4,5-bisphosphate. *J Biol Chem* **273**:1574, 1998.
66. Gazit E, Brand N, Harel Y, Lotan D, Barkai G: Prenatal diagnosis of Lowe's syndrome: A case report with evidence of de novo mutation. *Prenat Diagn* **10**:257, 1990.
67. Hayashi Y, Hanioka K, Kanomata N, Imai Y, Itoh H: Clinicopathologic and molecular-pathologic approaches to Lowe's syndrome. *Pediatr Pathol Lab Med* **15**:389, 1995.
68. Suchy SF, Lin T, Horwitz JA, O'Brien WE, Nussbaum RL: First report of prenatal biochemical diagnosis of Lowe syndrome. *Prenat Diagn* **18**:1117, 1998.
69. Cibis GW, Tripathi RC, Tripathi BJ: Lowe's oculocerebrorenal syndrome, in Gold DH, Weingeist TA (eds): *The Eye in Systemic Disease*. Philadelphia, Lippincott, 1990, p 504.
70. Lin T, Lewis RA, Nussbaum RL: Molecular confirmation of carriers for Lowe syndrome. *Ophthalmology* **106**:119, 1999.
71. Reilly DS, Lewis RA, Ledbetter DH, Nussbaum RL: Tightly linked flanking markers for the Lowe oculocerebrorenal syndrome with application to carrier assessment. *Am J Hum Genet* **42**:748, 1988.
72. Wadelius C, Fagerholm P, Pettersson U, Anneren G: Lowe oculocerebrorenal syndrome: DNA-based linkage of the gene to Xq24-26, using tightly linked flanking markers and the correlation to lens examination in carrier diagnosis. *Am J Hum Genet* **44**:241, 1989.
73. Charnas L: Seizures in the oculocerebrorenal syndrome of Lowe. *Neurology* **39(Suppl 1)**:362, 1989.
74. Bernardini I, Rizzo WB, Dalakas M, Bernar J, Gahl WA: Plasma and muscle free carnitine deficiency due to renal Fanconi syndrome. *J Clin Invest* **75**:1124, 1985.
75. Andersson HC, Markello T, Schneider JA, Gahl WA: Effect of growth hormone treatment on serum creatinine concentration in patients with cystinosis and chronic renal disease. *J Pediatr* **120**:716, 1992.
76. The European Study Group on Growth Hormone Treatment in Short Children with Nephropathic Cystinosis. Treatment with recombinant human growth hormone in short children with nephropathic cystinosis: no evidence for increased deterioration rate of renal function. *Pediatr Res* **43**:484, 1998.

# Campomelic Dysplasia/Autosomal Sex Reversal/*SOX9*

*Alan J. Schafer*

1. Campomelic dysplasia (CD) is a rare, dominant, and usually neonatal lethal chondrodysplasia clinically and radiologically defined by a number of skeletal and extra-skeletal phenotypes, the most conspicuous of which is angulation of the long bones. Bent or bowed limbs occur in other skeletal malformation syndromes and are not pathognomonic for CD. Major diagnostic radiologic features include bowed or angulated femora and tibiae, hypoplastic scapulae, vertically narrow iliac wings, and nonmineralized thoracic pedicles. No single feature is diagnostic, but each of these appears with high frequency, and no other syndrome has this combination of features. Additional common radiologic features are facial hypoplasia, abnormal cervical vertebrae, slender ribs, 11 pairs of ribs, small chest, dislocated hips, a variety of pelvic abnormalities, and short first metacarpal. Common clinical features include micrognathia, respiratory distress, flat nasal bridge, pretibial dimples, macrocephaly, and talipes equinovarus.

2. More than two-thirds of 46,XY campomelic dysplasia patients are sex reversed, developing as phenotypic females due to a failure to form testes. The degree of sex reversal can vary, with the most common outcome being normal phenotypic female with dysgenic ovaries.

3. Dominant mutations in the transcription factor *SOX9* are responsible for both the skeletal and the sex development phenotypes. Mutation analysis and functional assays suggest that the phenotypes result from haploinsufficiency due to loss-of-function mutations of a single *SOX9* allele. *SOX9* mutations apparently do not cause sex reversal in the absence of CD skeletal defects.

4. *SOX9* appears to be a critical component of the developmental pathways of both cartilage formation and testis formation, functioning independently in the development of these two dissimilar tissues. *SOX9* mutations cause a loss of protein function that leads to a failure to propagate the appropriate developmental signals in both chondrogenic tissue and the indifferent gonad.

5. Expression of *SOX9* is the earliest marker of cartilage differentiation and is required for cartilage formation. The SOX9 protein is expressed during embryonic chondrogenesis and directly regulates type II collagen gene expression in chondrocytes. *SOX9* may also be directly involved in regulation of type XI collagen, which is coexpressed with type II collagen, both collagens being essential for normal cartilage development and skeletal morphogenesis. In chimeric mice, cells with homozygous deletions of *Sox9* are excluded from all cartilages and do not express chondrocyte-specific markers, showing the essential role of *Sox9* in chondrogenesis and cartilage formation.

6. During mouse gonadal development, *Sox9* is expressed in both XX and XY embryos in the undifferentiated genital ridge. In XY embryos, *Sox9* is up-regulated coincident with the onset of expression of *Sry*, the Y chromosome testis determination factor, and continues to be expressed at high levels in developing testes, with expression limited to the Sertoli cells. At the corresponding time in XX embryos, *Sox9* expression is down-regulated. This is the earliest difference in gene expression known between males and females other than that of *Sry* itself. *SOX9* appears to act as a partner of *SF1* in activating the Sertoli cell-specific expression of anti-Müllerian hormone (AMH), a hormone that promotes regression of the Müllerian ducts, the primordia of female-specific sex organs. The timing and sexually dimorphic expression of *Sox9* in differentiating gonads, and its involvement in transactivation of a testis-specific gene, suggests a critical role for *SOX9* in testis determination.

## HISTORICAL

### Definition of the Syndrome

In 1970, Spranger, Langer, and Maroteaux called attention to what they perceived to be an increasing frequency of a syndrome of multiple osseous defects, primarily affecting the craniofacial skeleton, the tubular bones of the lower extremities, and the axial skeleton.[1] Most cases resulted in neonatal death. In addition to describing eight cases that they had recently observed, they cited an additional five previously reported cases that showed similar features.[2–6] Subsequently, additional earlier cases came to light.[7–10] Detailed descriptions of some of these cases and examination of new patients allowed quick elucidation of the clinical and radiologic phenotypes defining the newly recognized syndrome.[11] The names "le syndrome campomélique" (campomelic syndrome) and "camptomelic dwarfism" were simultaneously and independently proposed to describe the newly recognized condition.[11,12] Both names derive from the Greek, noting the curved or bent (campo/campto) limbs (melia) commonly found in CD. The multiple designations led to confusion that different conditions may exist, and complicated literature review. Indeed, the same condition has also been described as "syndrome of multiple osseous defects,"[1] "multiple osseous defects with pretibial dimple,"[13] "congenital bowing of the long bones,"[4,14] and "long-limbed campomelic syndrome."[15] In 1977, at the Paris meeting for International Nomenclature of

Constitutional Disease of the Bone, the term "campomelic dysplasia" (CD) was selected to specify the syndrome.[16]

Worldwide, hundreds of additional cases have been described, allowing refinement of the CD diagnostic criteria by description of additional associated phenotypes. An important early observation was the association of 46,XY sex reversal as a common feature of CD.[9,10,13,17] 46,XY sex reversal is a full or partial failure of testes development in individuals with a Y chromosome, where dysgenic ovaries develop due to a failure in induction of the testis development pathway. In these individuals, the absence of endocrine events mediated by the testes leads to development of female internal and external genitalia. Male to female 46,XY sex reversal is a common feature of CD.[18,19]

## Incidence

Although it was initially suggested that the frequency of CD was increasing, possibly due to an exogenous cause,[1] the increase in number of observed cases of CD appears to have a basis in increased recognition due to heightened awareness of the diagnostic criterion. The finding of a genetic basis for the disease, that CD is caused by (usually *de novo*) mutations in the *SOX9* gene,[20,21] makes it unlikely that the disease occurrence is increasing. Population studies have found campomelic dysplasia to occur with an incidence of 0.5 to 1 per 100,000 births,[22,23] although 4 cases were found in 18,350 live births in Norway, suggesting that the syndrome may be underdiagnosed or may vary between different populations.[24]

## SYNDROME MANIFESTATIONS AND POSTNATAL DIAGNOSIS

At birth, infants with campomelic dysplasia present with a variety of skeletal and extraskeletal abnormalities. Nearly all clinically exhibit bowing or angulation of the long bones, often accompanied by pretibial skin dimples. Radiologic examination often reveals bowed or angulated femora or tibiae, hypoplastic scapulae, vertically narrow iliac wings, and nonmineralized thoracic pedicles as well as a variety of additional skeletal and extraskeletal malformations (Fig. 253-1). No single feature is pathognomonic and descriptions of "acampomelic" CD patients demonstrate that bending of the limbs is not a mandatory feature of the disease.[19,25–32] Compilation of information from detailed reports of clinical, radiographic, and autopsy findings has allowed identification of anomalies that occur at a high frequency in CD patients (Table 253-1).

Taking account of common features of CD, diagnostic criteria for CD have been established, most recently described by Mansour et al.[19] (Table 253-2). Importantly, the criteria allow differential diagnosis from other limb-shortening syndromes involving bowing of the limbs such as osteogenesis imperfecta congenita, hypophosphatasia, thanatophoric dwarfism, and achondroplasia,[33,34] and differentiation of classic, long-limb CD from similar but distinct short-limb campomelic dwarfism syndromes.[15]

Histologic examination of affected bones in CD patients reveals aberrant endochondral ossification consistent with defective maturation of cartilage cells.[4,15,25,35–46] The bending of the long bones occurs in the diaphyses, which exhibit parallel masses of periosteal bone arising from the concave side of the bend and extending into the medullary cavity at right angles to the axis of the bone.[15,41] The periosteum is thickened at the concave side of the bend.[41,42] The direct cause of the bent bones and limb shortening (micromelia) in CD is not known. One mechanism of shortening could be retardation in endochondral growth. The zone of provisional calcification and the metaphyseal bone usually have a normal appearance, but some reports describe the proliferating and hypertrophic zones of the growth plate appearing reduced in height.[35,37,39,42,44] However, consistent irregularities are not seen[15,40] (W. Wilcox, unpublished observations). In one case, fractures observed in the epiphyseal ends of the femur and tibia in the growth plate region were interpreted as indicative of disturbed

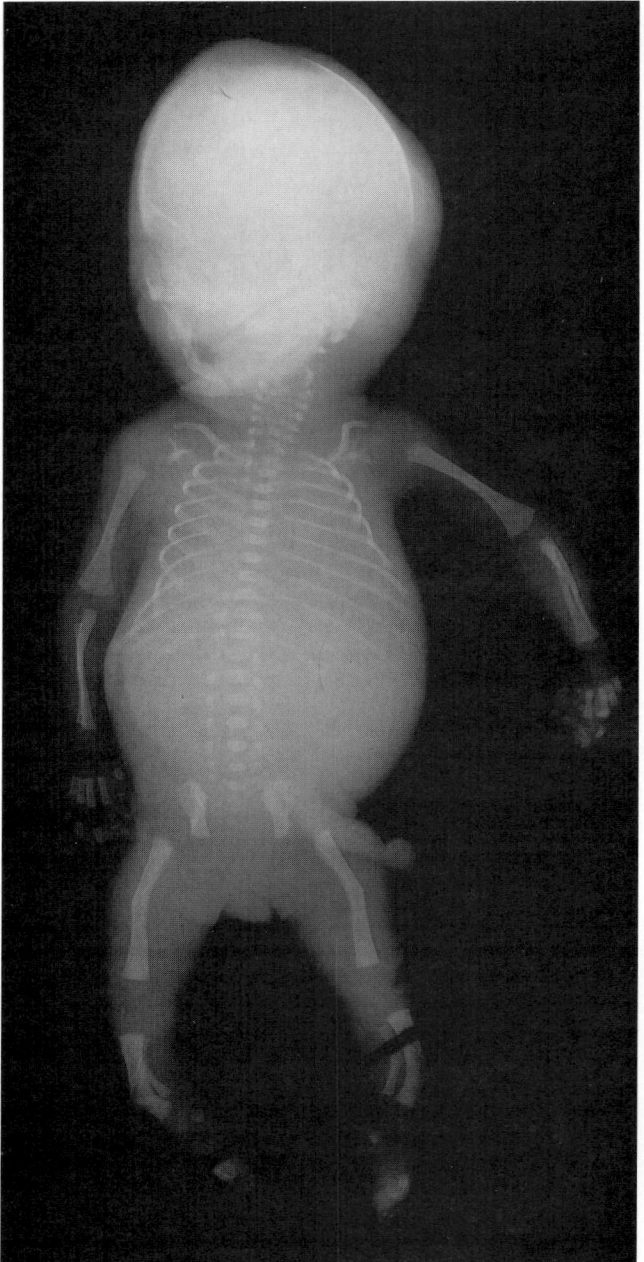

**Fig. 253-1** Radiologic features of a fetus with campomelic dysplasia, showing hypoplastic scapulae, nonmineralization of the thoracic pedicles, 11 pairs of ribs, bowed femora, bowed tibiae, and vertical, narrow iliac wings. (*From Mansour et al.[19] Used by permission.*)

collagen synthesis.[25] Few histologic studies have been reported for bones of the axial skeleton; one particularly striking observation is the lack of chondrocytes in the endochondral layer of the otic capsule in the two patients examined.[38,45]

Secondary sexual characteristics in 46,XY CD individuals can be normal male, ambiguous internal and external genitalia of varying male and female sexual differentiation, or normal female.[10,17–19,25,37,42,46–61] The differences in sexual differentiation reflect the variable lack of development of the testes, which normally produce hormones to direct male internal and external differentiation. In 46,XY individuals that develop normal testes, normal male development ensues; in cases of complete failure to form a testis, a dysgenic ovary develops accompanied by female

**Table 253-1** Clinical, Radiologic, and Extraskeletal Findings in Patients with Campomelic Dysplasia

| | Present | Absent | Total | % |
|---|---|---|---|---|
| **Clinical Feature** | | | | |
| Micrognathia | 54 | 2 | 56 | **96%** |
| Respiratory distress | 27 | 1 | 28 | **96%** |
| Bowed tibia | 31 | 3 | 34 | **91%** |
| Flat nasal bridge | 19 | 2 | 21 | **90%** |
| Pretibial skin dimples | 22 | 3 | 25 | **88%** |
| Congenital dislocation of hips | 23 | 5 | 28 | **82%** |
| Macrocephaly | 47 | 11 | 58 | **81%** |
| Talipes equinovarus | 53 | 19 | 72 | **74%** |
| Bowed femora | 18 | 8 | 26 | **69%** |
| Low-set ears | 40 | 21 | 61 | **66%** |
| Cleft palate | 37 | 21 | 58 | **64%** |
| **Radiologic Feature** | | | | |
| Facial hypoplasia | 33 | 5 | 38 | **87%** |
| ***Thorax*** | | | | |
| Hypoplastic scapulae | 52 | 3 | 55 | **95%** |
| Absent mineralization of sternum | 11 | 2 | 13 | **85%** |
| Slender ribs | 42 | 12 | 54 | **78%** |
| 11 ribs | 25 | 15 | 40 | **63%** |
| Small chest | 27 | 21 | 48 | **56%** |
| ***Spine*** | | | | |
| Non-mineralized thoracic pedicles | 17 | 5 | 22 | **77%** |
| Abnormal cervical vertebrae | 27 | 10 | 37 | **73%** |
| Flattened vertebral bodies | 13 | 6 | 19 | **68%** |
| Kyphosis or scoliosis | 26 | 27 | 53 | **49%** |
| Hypoplastic vertebral bodies | 8 | 33 | 41 | **20%** |
| ***Pelvis*** | | | | |
| Poorly developed pubic bones | 50 | 1 | 51 | **98%** |
| Vertically narrow iliac bones | 52 | 2 | 54 | **96%** |
| Abnormal ischial bones | 49 | 2 | 51 | **96%** |
| Dislocated hips | 47 | 10 | 57 | **82%** |
| ***Lower limbs*** | | | | |
| Delayed ossification of proximal femoral epiphyses | 51 | 2 | 53 | **96%** |
| Bowed femora | 61 | 3 | 64 | **95%** |
| Bowed tibiae | 55 | 5 | 60 | **92%** |
| Hypoplastic fibulae | 47 | 8 | 55 | **85%** |
| Delayed ossification of distal femoral epiphyses | 42 | 11 | 53 | **79%** |
| Absent talus | 34 | 12 | 46 | **74%** |
| ***Upper limbs*** | | | | |
| Short 1st metacarpal | 12 | 0 | 12 | **100%** |
| Dislocated radial head | 10 | 10 | 20 | **50%** |
| Bowed radii or ulnae | 10 | 39 | 49 | **20%** |
| Bowed humeri | 9 | 45 | 54 | **17%** |
| **Autopsy** | | | | |
| Small thorax | 18 | 19 | 37 | **49%** |
| Tracheomalacia | 14 | 25 | 39 | **36%** |
| Renal abnormality | 14 | 27 | 41 | **34%** |
| Congenital heart disease | 11 | 29 | 40 | **28%** |
| Absence of olfactory tract or bulb | 5 | 18 | 23 | **22%** |
| Hydrocephalus | 6 | 33 | 39 | **15%** |

Data compiled from Austin et al.[39] and Mansour et al.[19]

**Table 253-2** Diagnostic Criteria for Campomelic Dysplasia

**Radiologic**

3 or more of:
  Hypoplastic scapulae
  Bowed femora (marked or mild)
  Bowed tibiae (marked or mild)
  Vertically narrow iliac wings
  Non-mineralized thoracic pedicles

**Clinical**

7 or more of:
  Macrocephaly
  Micrognathia
  Cleft palate
  Flat nasal bridge
  Low-set ears
  Talipes equinovarus
  Congenital dislocation of hips
  Bowed femora
  Bowed tibiae
  Pretibial skin dimples
  Respiratory distress
or:
  Sex reversal and bowed lower limbs

From Mansour et al.[19] Used by permission.

commonly reported phenotype of sex-reversed CD patients is of dysgenic gonads positioned as ovaries, composed of ovarian-like stroma with a few primordial follicles, and accompanied by normal female external genitalia.[17–19,25,37,46,49,50,53,55,56] In some cases, dysgenic gonads show histologic suggestions of testicular development,[13,47,52,59,60] and a case of a true hermaphrodite (an individual with both ovarian and testicular tissue) has been described.[61] Another sex-reversed CD patient developed a gonadoblastoma,[59] a common occurrence in dysgenic gonads associated with other 46,XY sex reversal syndromes. Gonadal abnormalities in 46,XX female CD patients have not been reported. A mild case of CD was reported in a woman who gave birth to a severely affected child, suggesting that CD does not affect gonadal development in 46,XX individuals.[62] Radiographic examination is essential for accurate diagnosis of CD, and karyotypic analysis of phenotypic females or patients with ambiguous genitalia for 46,XY sex reversal can be important in correctly identifying the syndrome. More than two-thirds of 46,XY CD patients develop as phenotypic females or with ambiguous genitalia (Table 253-3).

Campomelic dysplasia commonly involves multiple systems. In addition to the gonadal defects in most 46,XY patients, nonskeletal aberrations involving the renal, cardiac, and the central nervous systems are common (Table 253-1). Additional extraskeletal features that occur in one or a few cases of CD have been noted. These include brain malformations;[63] nerve, muscle, and vasculature anomalies;[42,46] anorectal atresia;[64] cystic hygroma;[65] deafness;[66] and Potter type I polycystic disease and cardiosplenic syndrome.[67]

## *IN UTERO* DIAGNOSIS

The development of ultrasonic imaging and its application to fetal monitoring has led to *in utero* detection of skeletal anomalies and with increasing frequency to the prenatal diagnosis of CD. The initial cases detected by ultrasound resulted from careful monitoring of fetal development in mothers at risk due to previous delivery of CD-affected infants,[68–70] but prenatal diagnosis in mothers without a known risk has also been accomplished by ultrasound.[19,58,71–73] Although a definitive diagnosis may not be

internal and external genitalia. In some cases, testis formation is incomplete, and an intersex phenotype (ambiguous genitalia) can result, manifesting in a variety of phenotypes including hypospadias,[19,46,51] bifid scrotum,[19,51] hypoplastic penis,[46,51] enlarged clitoris,[18,19,48] and missing internal sex organs.[18] The most

Table 253-3 46,XY Sex Reversal and Campomelic Dysplasia

**A. Phenotypic sex and karyotype of 133 patients with campomelic dysplasia**

| | Karyotype | | | |
|---|---|---|---|---|
| Phenotypic sex | 46,XX | 46,XY | Unknown | Total |
| Female | 31 | 29 | 33 | 93 |
| Male | 0 | 14 | 16 | 30 |
| Ambiguous genitalia | 0 | 5 | 5 | 10 |
| Total | 31 | 48 | 54 | 133 |

Data compiled from Houston et al.[18] and Mansour et al.[19]

**B. Proportion of sex-reversed 46,XY campomelic dysplasia patients**

| | |
|---|---|
| 46,XY with female or ambiguous genitalia | 34 |
| Total 46,XY CD patients | 48 |
| % sex-reversed 46,XY CD patients | 71 |

Data compiled from Houston[18] and Mansour.[19]

possible, *in utero* detection of CD-associated abnormalities is important in management of pregnancy.[55,74,75] However, abnormalities may not be evident or may be unclear by ultrasound, and the condition in a fetus can be missed[70,76] or misdiagnosed.[66] When detected, the CD congenital abnormalities are usually noted in the late second or early third trimester,[77] although diagnosis has been made as early as 18 weeks' gestation.[57,70] The frequency of prenatal diagnosis is not known, but in one recent report, 6 of 36 cases reviewed were detected by routine antenatal ultrasound scan.[19] In all six cases, the decision was made to terminate pregnancy. The features most commonly evident are shortening and bowing of the lower limbs, but additional abnormalities may be observed, including polyhydramnios, which is seen at a high frequency with fetal anomalies including CD.[4,35,68,72,76,78] Ultrasound can be used to reliably establish fetal sex at 20 weeks;[79] coupled with amniocentesis or chorionic villi sampling which provide a source of fetal chromosomes, female phenotype fetuses suspected of having CD can be tested for 46,XY sex reversal as further evidence for diagnosis.

Although mutations in the *SOX9* gene are known to be the cause of CD,[20,21] prenatal DNA diagnosis is not feasible, as most known mutations are unique and spread throughout the gene, requiring sophisticated and laborious DNA mutation-scanning techniques to be applied for detection of the mutation. Although under appropriate test conditions a high proportion of *SOX9* mutations in CD patients can be detected,[80] some are missed due to technical aspects of the screen, or because the mutations lie outside of the region tested. Chromosomal translocations outside of the *SOX9* RNA coding region are known to cause CD and lie scattered over a region of several hundred kilobase pairs.[29,32,81–84] Some of these can be detected by karyotyping, but small deletions or rearrangements will not be detected by chromosome analysis, and the region in which CD-associated translocations are known to occur is too large to practically test by molecular mutation scanning techniques.

## PROGNOSIS

Neonatal death of CD-affected individuals is usual, and survival past 1 year of age is uncommon.[1,11,14,18,19,85,86] Deficiency in tracheobronchial cartilages including reduced number, fused, soft, easily collapsible, or even absent cartilages in smaller bronchi is prevalent.[18,33,35,86–88] As a result, most patients die of severe respiratory distress or tracheomalacia, although cardiac, renal, and central nervous system anomalies, including hydrocephalus, can contribute to their demise. No difference in longevity between sex-

reversed and non-sex-reversed individuals is seen.[19] However, there is some indication that patients with chromosomal translocations associated with the disease are less severely affected and may have a greater chance of survival,[19–21] although it is clearly not always the case.[32,81] Some patients do survive and can live to adulthood.[1,11,18,19,57,85,86] Surviving individuals suffer from the effects of skeletal maldevelopment, exhibiting scoliosis, kyphosis, or both.[44,89] The spinal abnormalities often progress to affect cardiopulmonary function at an early age, further compromising impaired respiratory function. Surgical intervention for skeletal problems can be performed but has serious attendant risks.[44,89]

## ETIOLOGY

Congenital angulation of the tibia and other long bones has been known clinically for many years.[90,91] Early explanations focused on a mechanical origin, that *in utero* "packing" applied physical pressure to the limbs, which caused angulation or bowing to arise during fetal growth.[3,7,92,93] A second mechanical explanation was that the primary defect was talipes equinus, which was apparently produced and maintained by calf muscle shortening, and the long bone bending was a secondary effect due to bone stress resulting from progressive contraction.[2] Recognition of the generalized conditions of bone malformations[5] led to explanations for the multiple effects being sought. Spranger[1] suggested an unspecified exogenous cause based on a suspected increase in frequency of the disease. A variety of potential teratogens were implicated by other investigators, including exposure to oral contraceptives,[10,13,60,94] folic acid agonists,[95] drugs of an unknown nature,[96] organic solvents,[96] and intrauterine infection.[97] Discernment of the malformations as an intrinsic abnormality in ossification probably arising from an abnormal cartilaginous axial skeleton[4,5] and the absence of a consistent exogenous exposure promoted the consideration of a genetic basis for the congenital malformations in CD.[12]

### Genetics

For many years, the genetics of CD was uncertain at least in part as a result of the few cases described. The rare incidence and severity of the disease along with descriptions of familial cases implicated a disease of monogenic origin. Reports of consanguinity and multiple occurrences within families suggested autosomal recessive inheritance[25,49,50,52,65,69,70,98–102] and one report hypothesized X linkage.[48] Dominant transmission was suggested by numerous investigators.[12,18,19,36,62] Supporting evidence for this mode of inheritance was found in a case in which three affected offspring were born to two different fathers,[36] in a case in which an apparently affected mother delivered an affected offspring,[36,62] and in segregation analysis of CD cases.[18,19] Identification of heterozygous mutations in patients firmly established CD as an autosomal dominant disease.[20,21]

### Molecular Genetics

Evidence as to the genomic location of the CD locus came with the discovery in patients of chromosomal translocations and rearrangements sharing a common cytogenetic breakpoint. Although a familial balanced chromosome translocation t(5;8) had been reported in a sex-reversed campomelic dysplasia patient, the description of two *de novo* chromosome rearrangements of the long arm of chromosome 17 implicated this chromosome in CD and in the associated sex reversal.[81,82] Subsequently, using *de novo* reciprocal translocations, Tommerup et al.[83] localized the campomelic dysplasia locus 1 (*CMPD1*) and the sex reversal, autosomal 1 locus (*SRA1*) to human chromosome 17q24.3-q25.1 with the genes growth hormone (*GH1*) and thymidine kinase (*TK1*) as flanking markers. Investigation of a translocation patient followed by screening of karyotypically normal patients[20] and a candidate gene approach[21] independently led to the discovery of heterozygous mutations in *SOX9*, a gene located adjacent to the chromosome 17 breakpoints found in CD patients. The presence of *SOX9* mutations in sex-reversed CD patients identified *SOX9* as both *CMPD1* and *SRA1*, and demonstrated that the pleiotropic effects are the result of mutations in a single gene. The identification of *SOX9* mutations in the majority of CD patients investigated suggests that most if not all cases of CD are likely to be caused by mutations in *SOX9*.[80,103]

## *SOX9* Mutations

To date, 25 different *SOX9* mutations have been described in 30 CD patients.[20,21,61,80,103–107] Twenty-nine patients have heterozygous mutations; a single compound heterozygote has been described, although in this individual it is believed that one allele represents a neutral polymorphism[21] (Table 253-4). Other than this single exception, the mutations are predicted to result in loss of function of the protein translated from the mutated allele, and include missense, nonsense, and splice-junction mutations. *SOX9* belongs to the *SOX* family of transcription factors,[108] the archetype of which is the Y chromosome-located mammalian testis-determining factor *SRY*. The protein encoded by *SRY* contains an 80-amino-acid DNA-binding domain ("HMG box")[109] that binds to specific DNA sequences in vitro. A large number of genes have been identified that encode proteins containing regions with greater than 60 percent amino acid similarity to the *SRY* HMG box region, and these comprise the *SOX* (*SRY* HMG box) gene family.[108,110–113] The *SOX9* cDNA contains an open reading frame (ORF) that is predicted to code for a protein of 509 amino acids, containing an HMG box that is 71 percent similar to the *SRY* HMG box that exhibits specific binding in vitro to DNA target sequences similar to those of SRY or other SOX proteins.[114,115] The functional relevance of the *SOX9* DNA binding domain is evident in its sensitivity to phenotype-causing mutations: one-third of the known *SOX9* mutations have been found in this domain (Table 253-4), although it comprises only 16 percent of the ORF. In addition, 7 of the 10 reported HMG box mutations are missense mutations, and comprise the only known *SOX9* missense mutations. All seven of the *SOX9* HMG box missense mutations have been investigated for in vitro binding affinity. One shows near wild-type binding, three have reduced binding (one displaying altered sequence specificity), and three exhibit negligible or abolished binding[103,107] (Table 253-4). A feature of HMG box DNA binding is bending of the bound DNA, a function thought to be important for transactivation of target genes. *SOX9* induces bending of a 48-target sequence.[116] Although some *SRY* HMG box mutations have been shown to alter target DNA bending,[117] the three missense *SOX9* mutations tested induce normal bending in *SOX9* target sequences, including the one with altered specificity and the one that shows near wild-type binding.[107] In vitro assays have identified a domain in the C-terminal end of the protein that functions as a transcriptional activator.[107,114,118] Many *SOX9* mutations remove or truncate the transactivation domain (Table 253-4), and transactivation function is lost,[103,107,118] suggesting that the loss of *SOX9* function and, in specific cases, augmentation of loss by dominant negative activity of the mutated protein,[116] leads to failure of activation of downstream genes.

In cases in which parental DNA has been available for testing, most mutations are found to arise *de novo* in the CD patients.[20,21,80,103] Several examples of transmission from apparently unaffected parents have been described.[21,61,107] In one case, paternal germ-line mosaicism was demonstrated,[61] but whether other instances represent mosaicism or nonexpressivity of the mutation is not known. In one case, a mildly affected mother with a mutant *SOX9* allele gave birth to a severely affected daughter[62] (I. Barroso, A. Schafer, unpublished observations).

## Haploinsufficiency of *SOX9*

Haploinsufficiency diseases result from the loss of functional activity of one of the two alleles of a gene.[119] Several lines of evidence support the idea that the CD skeletal and sex-reversal phenotypes result from haploinsufficiency of *SOX9* rather than from dominant-negative effects of the mutant allele. Mutations are found in single alleles of *SOX9*, and are predicted to inactivate protein function (Table 253-4). These mutations could be hypothesized to produce proteins with a gain of function that causes CD (and sex reversal, when present), but this seems unlikely. First, comprehensive mutation analysis in sex-reversed CD chromosome 17 translocation patients has not revealed any mutations in the *SOX9* ORF (Table 253-5). Presumably, no mutated SOX9 protein is present in these patients to act in a gain-of-function manner. In these individuals, the disease is likely to result from loss of appropriate spatial or temporal expression of *SOX9* from the translocation-associated allele, support for which comes from transgenic mouse studies showing reduced human *SOX9* expression associated with deletion of genomic sequences 5′ and distal to *SOX9*.[120] Second, in genes for which mutations change the protein structure and cause a dominant gain of function, the mutations usually result in a common type of mutated protein.[121] In CD, the *SOX9* mutations are distributed throughout the ORF and do not obviously result in any common type of altered protein. Mutations are found that affect DNA binding and others that truncate or extend the predicted protein via frameshifts, translational stops, or inappropriate splicing of the transcript. Additional genetic evidence comes from the description of apparent[122] or clinically diagnosed[123] CD individuals hemizygous for *SOX9* as a result of chromosome 17 deletions encompassing the *SOX9* locus. These individuals are likely to be affected due to haploinsufficiency resulting from the loss of one copy of *SOX9*, although in the absence of mutation screening of the remaining *SOX9* locus, it is formally possible that the remaining allele has mutations that additionally compromise function.

## Mutation / Phenotype Correlations

Variability in the CD phenotype is seen to some degree in the extent and severity of skeletal malformations and, more profoundly, in the wide range of sexual phenotypes of 46,XY patients. A wide variation of phenotype such as this is often seen in haploinsufficiency syndromes.[119] Examination of the type and location of *SOX9* mutations with regard to the variation in phenotypes has not revealed any genotype-phenotype correlations. A notable variation in the skeletal phenotype of CD is the absence of characteristic angulation of the long bones (acampomelia) in a small number of CD patients. Although it has been suggested that other genes may play a role in this phenotypic variation,[124] an acampomelic patient with a *SOX9* mutation has been identified.[107] This mutation is located in the *SOX9* DNA-binding domain and appears unremarkable, although additional mutations in acampomelic patients are necessary to draw any conclusions about genotype-phenotype relationships for this phenotype. Identification of the same *SOX9* mutation in different patients exhibiting markedly different sex phenotypes shows that the sex phenotype variability is not a result of the *SOX9* mutation type (Table 253-4). Two unrelated 46,XY individuals were found to have the same mutation; one exhibited a (sex-reversed) female phenotype, while the other developed as a normal male.[80] A different *SOX9* mutation was found in three unrelated individuals. These individuals were a 46,XY (sex-reversed) female, a 46,XY male, and a 46,XX female.[21,103,105] Finally, a familial mutation in three sibs at yet another position in *SOX9* resulted in a 46,XY hermaphrodite, a 46,XY (sex-reversed) female, and a 46,XX female.[61] The variable expressivity of the sex-reversal phenotype of 46,XY CD individuals remains to be explained. The differences may be due to threshold dosage effects, or may result primarily from factors other than the *SOX9* mutation, such as differences in genetic background.

*SOX9* mutations have not been described in individuals without clinical characteristics of CD. Most instances of 46,XY female sex reversal occur in the absence of extragonadal-related anomalies, and a minority have been explained by mutation of other genes involved in sex determination. To assess whether *SOX9* mutations

**Table 253-4 SOX9 Mutations in Campomelic Dysplasia Patients**

| Codon* | Nucleotide† | Base Change | Effect on Protein | Karyotype/Sex Phenotype | 46,XY Sex-Reversed? | Located in Functional Domain? | Reference | In Vitro DNA Binding | Target DNA Bending? |
|---|---|---|---|---|---|---|---|---|---|
| 86 | 258 | G > A | Trp > Stop | 46,XX; female | No | DNA-binding domain | 103 | abolished[103] | nt |
| 108 | 323 | C > T | Pro > Leu | 46,XY; female | Yes | DNA-binding domain | 103 | abolished[103] | normal bending[106] |
| 112 | 334 | T > C | Phe > Leu | 46,XY; male | No | DNA-binding domain | 80 | abolished/negligible[107] | normal bending[106] |
| 112 | 334 | T > C | Phe > Leu | 46,XY; male | No | DNA-binding domain | 106 | abolished/negligible[107] | normal bending[106] |
| 117 | 349 | C > T | Gln > Stop | 46,XY; female | Yes | DNA-binding domain | 103 | nt | nt |
| 119 | 356 | C > T | Ala > Val | 46,XX; female | No | DNA-binding domain | 80 | wt | normal bending[106] |
| 143 | 427 | T > C | Trp > Arg | 46,XY; female | Yes | DNA-binding domain | 103 | abolished[103] | nt |
| 143 | 430 | A > C | Intron 1 AG > CG; 3' splice acceptor | 46,XY; female | Yes | DNA-binding domain | 80 | nt | nt |
| 148 | 442 | G > T | Glu > Stop | 46,XY; female | Yes | DNA-binding domain | 21 | nt | nt |
| 152 | 456 | G > C | Arg > Pro | 46,XX; female | No | DNA-binding domain | 103 | reduced[103] | nt |
| 165 | 493 | C > T | His > Tyr | 46,XY; male | No | DNA-binding domain | 107 | reduced/minimal[106] | normal bending[106] |
| 170 | 509 | C > G | Pro > Arg | 46,XY, inv(9), male | No | DNA-binding domain | 103 | reduced;[103] reduced, altered specificity[106] | normal bending[106] |
| 195 | 583 | C > T | Gln > Stop | 46,XX; female | No | | 20 | nt | nt |
| 229 | 685 | G > A | Intron 2 GT > AT; 5' splice acceptor | 46,XY; female | Yes | | 21 | nt | nt |
| 246 | 736 | C Insertion | Frameshift causes stop at codon 251 | 46,XY; hermaphrodite | Yes | | 61 | nt | nt |
| 246 | 736 | C Insertion | Frameshift causes stop at codon 251 | 46,XY; female | Yes | | 61 | nt | nt |
| 246 | 736 | C Insertion | Frameshift causes stop at codon 251 | 46,XX; female | No | | 61 | nt | nt |
| 261–263 | 783–788 | G Insertion | Frameshift causes stop at codon 294 | 46,XY; female | Yes | | 20 | nt | nt |
| 277 | 829 | 10 basepair deletion | Frameshift causes stop at codon 294 | 46,XX; female | No | | 20 | nt | nt |
| 286–287 | 858 | 4 basepair Insertion | Frameshift causes stop at codon 294 | 46,XY; female | Yes | | 103 | nt | nt |
| 329 | 985 | G Insertion* | Frameshift adds 248 amino acids | 46,XY; female | Yes | | 21 | nt | nt |
| 353–357 | 1059 | 9 basepair in-frame deletions‡ | Pro-Ala-Pro deletions‡ | 46,XY; female | Yes | | 21 | nt | nt |
| 357 | 1069 | 43 basepair deletion | Frameshift adds 208 amino acids | 46,XY; female | Yes | | 103 | nt | nt |
| 368 | 1103 | A Insertion | Frameshift adds 208 amino acids | 46,XY; male | No | | 80 | nt | nt |
| 368 | 1103 | A Insertion | Frameshift adds 208 amino acids | 46,XY; female | Yes | | 80 | nt | nt |
| 375 | 1123 | C > T | Gln > Stop | 46,XY; female | Yes | | 103 | nt | nt |
| 400 | 1198 | G > T | Glu > Stop | 46,XY; male | No | | 103 | nt | nt |
| 440 | 1320 | C > G | Tyr > Stop | 46,XY; female | Yes | Transactivation domain | 21 | nt | nt |
| 440 | 1320 | C > G | Tyr > Stop | 46,XX; female | No | Transactivation domain | 103 | nt | nt |
| 440 | 1320 | C > G | Tyr > Stop | 46,XY; male | No | Transactivation domain | 105 | nt | nt |
| 507 | 1519 | 4 basepair Insertion | Frameshift adds 51 amino acids | 46,XY; female | Yes | Transactivation domain | 80 | nt | nt |

* Nucleotide 1 is the first nucleotide of the open reading frame.
† Amino acid 1 is the first codon (ATG) of the open reading frame.
‡ Found in a compound heterozygous patient. This is thought to be a neutral mutation.[21]
* Found in a compound heterozygote; this is thought to be the causative allele.[21]
Multiple occurrences of the same mutation found in different individuals is indicated by gray shading.

**Table 253-5** Chromosome 17 Translocations in CD Patients

| Karyotype | Sex Phenotype | 46,XY Sex Reversal? | SOX9 Screened for Mutations? | Patient Designation | Reference | Distance 5′ from *SOX9* | Notes |
|---|---|---|---|---|---|---|---|
| 46,XX inv(17)(q12;q25) | female | no | nr | none | 81 | unknown | |
| 46,XY t(2;17)(q35;q23-24) | female | yes | yes | patient E | 82, 20 | 88 kb | |
| 46,XY t(7;17)(q32;q24.2 or q25.1) | female | yes | yes | Case 1 | 21, 83, 130 | 50 kb | |
| 46,XY t(13;17)(q22;q25.1) | female | yes | yes | C 799, Case 2 | 9, 21, 83, 130 | 130–690 kb | |
| 46,XY t(1;17)(q42.13;q24.3 or q25.1) | female | no | yes | Case 3 | 21, 83, 130 | 130–400 kb | |
| 46,XY inv(17)(q11.2;q24.3-25.1) | female | yes | yes | patient V, cu002 | 19, 80, 120 | 75–350 kb | |
| 46,XX t(4;17)(q21.3;q23.3) | female | no | yes* | patient Z | 19 | unknown | |
| 46,XY t(12:17)(q21.32;q24.3 or q25.1) | female | yes | nr | none | 29 | unknown | acampomelic |
| 46,XY t(6;17)(q14;q24) | female | yes | yes | C.R. | 130 | >130 kb | |
| 46,XX t(5;17)(q13.3;q24.2) | nr | nr | yes | none | 84 | 295–350 kb | |
| 46,XY t(17;22)(q25.1;p11.2) | nr | nr | yes | none | 84 | >600 kb | |
| 46,XX t(5;17)(q15;q25.1) | female | no | nr | none | 32 | unknown | acampomelic |
| 46,XY t(9;17)(p13;q23.3 or 24.1) | male | no | yes* | cu004 | 120 | 110–140 kb | |

* Inês Barroso and Alan Schafer, unpublished results.
nr=not reported

cause 46,XY sex reversal in the absence of skeletal malformation, Kwok et al.[125] performed a *SOX9* mutation screen on a cohort of thirty 46,XY individuals with variable aberrations of sexual development, including gonadal dysgenesis (Swyer syndrome), partial gonadal dysgenesis (with and without testicular regression), and incomplete masculinization associated with low testosterone levels. Meyer et al.[103] screened eighteen 46,XY female Swyer syndrome patients. None of the tested individuals were known to have skeletal abnormalities. No *SOX9* mutations were found, providing evidence that *SOX9* mutations do not usually result in XY sex reversal without skeletal malformations.

## Relationship of the Translocation Breakpoints to *SOX9*

Multiple instances of chromosome 17 translocations identified the genomic region involved in the etiology of CD, yet the mechanism by which the translocations cause the disease is not fully resolved. Heterozygous mutations in the *SOX9* gene (located in this chromosomal region) cause CD, but *SOX9* mutations have not been found in translocation patients (Table 253-5). The *SOX9* mutations in nontranslocation CD patients appear to inactivate a single allele of *SOX9*, so the simplest explanation is that the translocations interfere with the adjacent *SOX9* allele to abrogate or abolish normal function. One possibility is that the breakpoints interrupt the *SOX9* transcription unit, but the breakpoints all map 5′ to the known *SOX9* transcription start site, and rather than being clustered are scattered over a wide region, making this explanation unlikely. Molecular mapping has localized translocation breakpoints at distances ranging from 50 kb 5′ to *SOX9* to greater than 600 kb 5′ to *SOX9*, with other breakpoints located at various points within this interval (Table 253-5). A single 5′ end of the *SOX9* transcript has been defined and cDNA analysis defines a complete transcript of 3.95 kilobases, while northern blot analysis of testis RNA identifies a slightly longer *SOX9* transcript of approximately 4.3 kb.[20,21] The larger than predicted transcript size may result from polyadenylation of the *SOX9* transcript or may reflect inaccurate sizing of the transcript. It is also possible that additional 5′ transcribed sequences remain unidentified and that 5′ exons are interrupted by the chromosome breaks. Examination of *SOX9* RNA from fetal chondrogenic and gonadal tissues is necessary to determine whether these tissues use upstream promoters that produce a transcript containing sequences potentially interrupted by the translocations. Given that the translocations are unlikely to directly interrupt the *SOX9* transcript, it is possible that another gene is interrupted by the breakpoints and causes CD. The spatial distribution of the breakpoints and the implication of *SOX9* as the

CD gene argue strongly against this, although it remains a formal possibility. There have been no reports of transcripts interrupted by any of the breakpoints. However, one report describes isolation of a partial testis-specific cDNA adjacent to one breakpoint from an acampomelic CD patient.[124] The 3.5-kb sequence known of the 3.7-kb transcript detected by northern analysis contains no long ORF and does not produce a peptide in in vitro translation experiments, suggesting that its normal function, if any, is mediated directly via the RNA. It was suggested that this transcript may contribute to the variable campomelic phenotype, specifically with regard to the acampomelia, but the finding of a *SOX9* mutation in an acampomelic CD patient without a chromosomal translocation argues against this possibility.[107] A second report has described the use of exon trapping to discover three putative exons between two translocation breakpoints, suggesting that additional genes may lie in the translocation breakpoint regions.[84]

An alternative to the translocations directly interrupting a transcript is that they may exert translocation-induced negative effects on transcription at the adjacent *SOX9* allele. This could result from a juxtapositioning of silencer or heterochromatin elements, or by interruption or deletion of upstream *SOX9* control sequences, leading to loss of expression, or inappropriate temporal or spatial expression. Instances of haploinsufficiency diseases involving transcription factors associated with distal chromosomal rearrangements leading to position effects acting at distances comparable to those observed in CD translocation patients have been reported for several genes.[126–129] Establishing reduced transcription of *SOX9* from a translocation haplotype requires the use of an allele-specific assay. Wirth et al.[130] used such an analysis to measure expression of *SOX9* from both alleles of a translocation patient in an established lymphoblastoid cell line. In this experiment, comparable amounts of transcript were detected from both *SOX9* alleles. Although this demonstrates that expression is possible from the translocation-associated allele, the results should not be extended to indicate that the translocations do not interfere with appropriate expression in developing tissue as the cells tested were from an adult tissue not related to chondrogenesis or testis development and the levels detected were relatively low. Functional studies support the hypothesis that CD patient translocations remove distal control elements necessary for appropriate *SOX9* expression. In transgenic mice containing human YACs encompassing *SOX9* and containing variable amounts of 5′ upstream sequence, similar to those observed in CD patients (deletion of sequences 350 kb 5′ to *SOX9*), one sees a substantial reduction in human *SOX9* expression, especially in chondrogenic tissues.[120] The longest construct, with 600 kb of 5′ *SOX9* sequence, exhibited human *SOX9* expression in most developing skeletal tissues comparable to that of the endogenous mouse *Sox9* genes. However, no corresponding expression was seen in developing gonadal tissue, indicating that the gonadal and skeletal tissue control elements are distinct, or that species-specific elements are involved in the activation of *SOX9* in the sex-determination pathway. Investigation of nearly 7 kb of the proximal 5′ sequences of the mouse *Sox9* gene suggests that sequences located within a few hundred bases of the transcription initiation site are in part responsible for the sex and tissue-specific expression of the gene, but that additional distal elements contribute to in vivo regulation of *Sox9*.[131] These observations are consistent with translocations further upstream disrupting control elements and resulting in CD.

## *SOX9* FUNCTION

### Pleiotropy

The finding that mutation of *SOX9* can cause both abnormal skeletal formation and abnormal testis formation raises the question as to how mutations in a single gene affect the development of such dissimilar tissues as cartilage and gonads. Molecular data and biochemistry suggest that *SOX9* functions as a transactivator of other genes, and CD phenotypes indicate a role as initiators or key components of the skeletal and gonadal developmental programs. At the stage in which the mutations appear to exert their phenotypes, the two affected tissues are well diverged from their shared mesoderm precursor. The spatial separation of the two tissues at this point also suggests that direct cell-cell interactions are not involved. The simplest explanation is that *SOX9* functions independently in the two developing tissues, and that mutations in *SOX9* cause a loss of protein function, which leads to a failure to propagate the appropriate developmental signals within both chondrogenic tissue and the indifferent gonad. Although *SOX9* is expressed in multiple human fetal tissues, in nearly all adult human tissue tested,[21] and in nongonadal, nonskeletal sites in developing mouse embryos,[114,120,132,133] a broader role for *SOX9* in these tissues is not evident. In vitro and in vivo experiments are consistent with a fundamental role primarily in chondrogenesis and testis determination.

### *SOX9* and Chondrogenesis

**Expression in Developing Bone.** Most bones of the mammalian embryo are initially laid down as a scaffold of hyaline cartilage by the process of chondrogenesis. This involves mesenchymal condensation to assume the approximate shape of the bone, differentiation of chondroblasts within this structure, and synthesis of the extracellular matrix. These cartilage models are subsequently transformed into bone by deposition of calcium salts during ossification. Expression of *SOX9* at sites of chondrogenesis at particular developmental stages can be construed as evidence of involvement of *SOX9* in this process. This pattern is seen in both developing human and mouse skeletons. In humans, Wagner et al.[21] showed by *in situ* hybridization of *SOX9* RNA that developing long bone of 7-week human embryos shows strong expression in the perichondrium and chondrocytes of resting, proliferative, and upper hypertrophic zones with reduced expression toward the mineralized zone in the area of the diaphyseal calcification. Significant expression was also seen in hypertrophic rib chondrocytes.

Extensive investigation of *Sox9* expression in the developing mouse shows a clear correlation with cartilage formation, with *Sox9* being expressed at sites of chondrogenesis.[114,132–134] *In situ* hybridization experiments on mouse embryos show that *Sox9* is strongly expressed at sites where skeletal components are being laid down as cartilage. Expression is predominantly in mesenchymal condensations just preceding and during cartilage deposition with expression of *Sox9* ceasing in these regions following the

formation of cartilage. Similar patterns are seen in developing chick embryos.[135] These expression patterns provide support for a role of *SOX9* in chondrogenesis. Mouse *Sox9* expression has been closely correlated with the onset of expression of the pro-αI(II) collagen (type II collagen) gene *Col2a1*, the predominant collagen found in cartilage. In precartilaginous condensing mesenchyme and maturing cartilage, *Sox9* and *Col2a1* are expressed in parallel, showing a correlation in expression levels.[114,133,134] This relationship is also seen in primary chondrocytes and fibroblasts in culture, with the additional observation of parallel down-regulation of *Sox9* and *Col2a1* in spontaneously de-differentiating chondrocytes.[116] In addition, application of compressive forces to dissociated mouse embryonic limb bud mesenchymal cells induces chondrogenesis with a concomitant up-regulation of *Sox9*.[136] In contrast, the expression and accumulation of IL-1$\beta$, a transcriptional repressor of type II collagen, is down-regulated.

**Targets of *SOX9*.** In vitro and in vivo experiments clearly demonstrate that Sox9/SOX9 directly regulates the type II collagen gene. Sox9/SOX9 binds to an enhancer element in the first intron of the *Col2a1/COL2A1* gene that is essential for chondrocyte-specific expression, activating expression through these elements.[114,116,137,138] Point mutations in these regulatory sequences abolish both Sox9/SOX9 binding and transactivation.[116,137,138] The effect specifically requires *Sox9*, as other *Sox* genes tested do not individually transactivate *Col2a1*.[116] However, transcripts for a new form of *Sox5*, called L-*Sox5*, and *Sox6* are coexpressed with *Sox9* in all chondrogenic sites of mouse embryos.[139] L-*Sox5* forms homodimers and heterodimers with *Sox6*. Transfection experiments show that L-*Sox5*, *Sox6*, and *Sox9* bind to the *Col2a1* enhancer and cooperatively activate expression of *Col2a1* in nonchondrogenic cells, suggesting that multiple classes of *Sox* transcription factors may function coordinately with each other in controlling expression of *Col2a1* and possibly other genes of the chondrocytic program.[139]

Type XI collagen (Col11a2) is coexpressed with type II collagen in all cartilage, and both types are essential for normal cartilage differentiation and skeletal morphogenesis. Two chondrocyte-specific enhancer elements located in the 5′ portion of the type XI collagen gene influence chondrocyte-specific expression in transgenic mice. These Col11a2-enhancer elements, like the Col2a1 enhancer, bind and are activated by SOX9.[140] The interactions of SOX9 with both type II and type XI collagen control elements implicate participation of *SOX9* in the coordinate regulation of expression of these genes in the chondrocyte differentiation pathway.

Studies of chimeric knockout mice containing inactivated copies of *Sox9* have been most conclusive in showing the key role of *Sox9* in cartilage formation.[134] At odds with the abnormal cartilage phenotype in CD patients with heterozygous mutations, in mouse, cells that are heterozygous null for *Sox9* appear to differentiate into chondrocytes that are functionally equivalent to wild-type cells. However, cells that are homozygous null for *Sox9* are excluded from all cartilages and do not express chondrocyte-specific markers. Histologic examination by *in situ* expression analysis at various stages of mouse development suggests that mesenchymal cell migration appears to be unaffected, but prechondrocytic mesenchymal cells that lack *Sox9* are unable to differentiate into chondrocytes.[134]

**Activators of *SOX9*.** Additional experiments have examined the relationship of *Sox9* expression to upstream signaling molecules and transcription factors in developing tissues. The morphoregulator Bmp-4 (bone morphogenic protein 4) induces ectopic chondrogenesis in embryonic mouse mandibular explants when applied to the posterior portion of the mandible head, but no induction occurs when applied to the anterior portion. *Sox9* is induced at all sites of Bmp-4-induced chondrogenesis, while the repressor *Msx-2* is induced more strongly at anterior than posterior positions.[141] These results suggest that *Sox9* and *Msx-2* are mediators of Bmp-4-induced chondrogenesis and that their combined actions are dependent on temporal and positional information. Further development of the mandible involves the differentiation of multiple cell lineages into different tissues, including bone, cartilage, and teeth. A role for *Sox9* in tooth development is suggested by expression in the epithelial components and, to a lesser degree, in the condensed mesenchyme of the developing teeth.[142] *Hoxa-2* directs proper skeletal formation in the second branchial arch by preventing chondrogenesis and intramembranous ossification. In normal mouse embryos, *Hoxa-2* is expressed throughout the second arch mesenchyme, but is excluded from the chondrogenic condensations. In the absence of *Hoxa-2*, chondrogenesis is activated ectopically within the rostral *Hoxa-2* expression domain to form a mutant set of cartilages. In *Hoxa-2* −/− embryos the Sox9 expression domain is shifted into the normal *Hoxa-2* domain, indicating that *Hoxa-2* acts at early stages of the chondrogenic pathway, upstream of *Sox9* induction.[143] The chondrogenic pathway is initiated in diverse developmental milieu; undoubtedly the upstream signals that induce chondrogenesis will be varied and involve many different or additional factors to the ones described above. Likely, but unproven, candidates include additional bone morphogenic proteins (BMPs), which appear to control the pattern formation of skeletal structures,[144] and Sonic hedgehog (*Shh*), a gene that plays an important role in sclerotome formation.[145] Regardless of the upstream inducing signals, all available evidence supports a role of *SOX9* as a critical juncture in initiation of the chondrocyte-differentiation pathway.

## *SOX9* and Gonadal Development

The sexual phenotype of a mammal is determined by the sex chromosome content established at fertilization. In the presence of the Y chromosome, the indifferent gonads are induced to form as testes; in its absence, ovarian development occurs. The developmental decision to form testes is pivotal: the differentiation of male internal ducts and external genitalia are secondary, resulting from endocrine functions of the testes. In the absence of testes, female internal and external genitalia develop, regardless of the presence or absence of ovaries. Sex determination can thus be equated with determination of testis formation. The Y chromosome inducer of testis formation, *SRY*, is a transcription factor that initiates the developmental cascade that induces the indifferent gonad to form testes rather than ovaries. *SOX9* is a member of a large family of transcription factors of which *SRY* is the prototype. The *SOX* gene family is defined by high sequence similarity of the common DNA-binding domain between the genes; outside of this region, the genes are divergent in sequence content and structure, reflecting quite varied roles in many developmental processes.[146] The partial molecular similarity of *SOX9* to *SRY* taken alone is not strong evidence of a role in sex determination in light of the diversity of *SOX* gene function and given the apparent absence of a function in sex determination of those genes for which function has been ascribed (other than *SRY*). However, multiple lines of evidence indicate a pivotal role of *SOX9* in testis formation.

*SOX9* **Mutations, Dosage, and Sex Phenotype.** The discovery of *de novo* mutations in sex-reversed CD patients links *SOX9* to the skeletal malformations seen in campomelic dysplasia as well as to the sex-reversal phenotype. The degree of sexual differentiation exhibited in CD patients varies (Table 253-3), reflecting the variable lack of development of the testes that normally produce hormones to direct male internal and external differentiation. No correlation is seen between the type or location of *SOX9* mutation, and the presence or absence, or variable expressivity of the sex-reversal phenotype. In vivo expression studies and in vitro demonstration of *SOX9* activation of testes-specific genes (below) provide compelling evidence for a direct role of *SOX9* in testis development. As the sex-reversal phenotype results from haploinsufficiency of *SOX9*, it is possible that the variable gonadal development results from variation in expression of the non-

mutated allele in developing gonad (and is likely influenced by other loci), or in residual activity of the mutated protein. Interestingly, Huang et al.[147] identified an SRY-negative (non-CD) 46,XX sex-reversed (female to male) individual with a duplication of *SOX9*. This study suggests that an extra dose of *SOX9* may be sufficient to initiate testis differentiation in the absence of *SRY*, although a previously reported 46,XX individual trisomic for 17q, including the region containing *SOX9*, did not exhibit sex reversal, developing instead as a phenotypic female.[148] Another locus involved in sex determination, *DSS* (dosage-sensitive sex reversal),[149] also exhibits dosage sensitivity. *DSS* is X-linked and 46,XY males contain a single copy of the gene. However, the presence of two *DSS* copies (encoding the *DAX1* [DSS-AHC critical region on the X chromosome] gene) in 46,XY individuals causes male to female sex reversal involving varying degrees of masculinization.[150,151] The sensitivity of testis formation to the levels of *DSS* and *SOX9* could reflect an ancestral dose-dependent sex determination mechanism, such as those seen in *Caenorhabditis* and *Drosophila*, that only becomes apparent in humans under abnormal circumstances.

*SOX9* **Gonadal Expression.** In vivo assessment of *SOX9/Sox9* in developing gonads of humans and mice reveals patterns consistent with a role in mammalian testis formation. In human tissue, some expression is observed in developing male gonad in the area of the rete testis and seminiferous tubules of an 18-week human male fetus.[21] Expression of *SOX9* in 46,XY fetuses is preceded by *SRY* and extends beyond the period of morphologic testicular differentiation, suggesting that *SRY* directly or indirectly induces *SOX9* expression in the developing gonad.[152] More extensive investigation has been performed in developing mice,[133,153,154] where *Sox9* is expressed in the undifferentiated genital ridge (which, upon further differentiation, forms the ovaries or testes) in both XX and XY mice. Expression is up-regulated in the XY gonad shortly after or coincident with *Sry* expression. As testes differentiate, expression is restricted to the developing Sertoli cells, and represents the earliest Sertoli cell marker known. The gonadal phenotype in sex-reversed CD patients is consistent with Sertoli cell failure and, as Sertoli cell differentiation in mouse is closely associated with testis development, *Sox9* may be essential for Sertoli cell development. In contrast, *Sox9* expression is down-regulated in the developing XX gonad.

In chickens, there is no evidence for an *Sry* gene, and the female rather than male sex contains the dimorphic pair of sex chromosomes. Male-specific expression of chicken *cSOX9* mRNA during the sex determination period is also observed in chicken genital ridges.[153,154] No *cSOX9* expression is seen at any stage by *in situ* hybridization in the developing ovary. In contrast to the chromosomal sex determination mechanism evident in mammals and birds, many reptiles exhibit temperature-dependent sex determination (TSD) where the egg incubation temperature triggers sex determination. Expression of *SOX9* during gonadogenesis in the American alligator (*Alligator mississippiensis*) shows that during TSD, alligator *SOX9* is expressed in the embryonic testis but not in the ovary.[155] In the TSD reptile the red-eared slider turtle, *Trachemys scripta*, *Sox9* is expressed in the undifferentiated gonads of embryos incubated at both the male- and the female-permissive temperatures.[156] At the stage of testis differentiation, only embryos at the male-permissive temperature expressed *Sox9* at a high level. In addition, there were two transcripts of *Sox9* at all stages, but the relative proportion of the two transcripts differed at the two temperatures. The conservation of sexually dimorphic expression in multiple vertebrate classes that have significant differences in their sex determination mechanisms points to a fundamental role for *Sox9* in testis determination in vertebrates.

*SOX9* **Gonadal Targets.** Genetic analysis of XY sex-reversed patients has led to the identification of a number of genes involved in sex determination.[157,158] The genes *WT1* (Wilms tumor 1), *SF1* (steroidogenic factor 1), and *Lhx9* (LIM homeobox protein 9) have been demonstrated to be involved in the formation of the gonads prior to their differentiation as testes or ovaries, while subsequent sex-specific gonadal differentiation appears to be mediated by the *SRY* and *SOX9* genes in the testis, and the *DAX1* gene appears to mediate ovarian development. Following *SRY* induction of testis development, anti-Müllerian hormone (*AMH*) expression occurs in Sertoli cells of the maturing testis in a tightly regulated fashion to promote regression of the Müllerian ducts, the primordia of female-specific sex organs. A DNA-binding element for the *SF1*, a member of the orphan nuclear receptor family, located in the AMH proximal promoter is essential for AMH gene activation.[159] The presence of conserved *cis* DNA-binding elements in the AMH promoter as well as the requirement for a specific promoter environment for *SF1* activation suggests that *SF1* is a member of a combinatorial protein-protein and protein-DNA complex. SOX9 binds to a canonical SOX-binding site within the human AMH proximal promoter, and *SOX9* and *SF1* interact directly via this DNA-binding domain, acting cooperatively in gene activation.[160] Thus, *SOX9* appears to act as a partner of *SF1* in the Sertoli cell-specific expression of *AMH* during embryogenesis. This link may provide the basis for the variable sex-reversal phenotypes seen in CD patients, as altered *SOX9* activity due to reduced levels in these patients may not be sufficient or be partially sufficient to induce *AMH* expression.

In nonmammalian species, a role of *SOX9* in activation of *AMH* is questionable. Comparison of the expression of *AMH* and cSOX9 in the gonads of chick embryos using *in situ* hybridization shows that *AMH* is expressed in both sexes at stage 25, 1 day before the first cSOX9 transcripts appear in the male gonads.[161] Although these results oppose the hypothesis that cSOX9 could trigger the expression of testicular *AMH* in the chick, they do not exclude a later role in testis development. Additionally, in the American alligator, SOX9 up-regulation in male embryos coincides with the structural organization of the testis, which is not consistent with a role for this gene in the early stages of alligator sex determination.[155] However, the relationship between *SOX9* and *AMH* expression in this animal is currently unknown.

## REFERENCES

1. Spranger J, Langer LO, Maroteaux P: Increasing frequency of a syndrome of multiple osseous defects? *Lancet* 2:716, 1970.
2. Middleton DS: Studies on prenatal lesions of muscle as a cause of congenital deformity. *Edinburgh Med J* 41:401, 1934.
3. Bound JP, Finlay HVL, Rose FC: Congenital anterior angulation of the tibia. *Arch Dis Child* 27:179, 1952.
4. Bain AD, Barrett HS: Congenital bowing of the long bones: Report of a case. *Arch Dis Child* 34:516, 1959.
5. Williams ER: Two congenital deformities of the tibia: Congenital angulation and congenital pseudoarthrosis. *Br J Radiol* 16:371, 1943.
6. Schudel P: Morphology of congenital bowing of thighs and lower legs. *Helv Paediatr Acta* 23:659, 1968.
7. Angle CR: Congenital bowing and angulation of the long bones. *Pediatrics* 13:257, 1954.
8. Kučera J, Benešová D: Poruchy Poruchy Nitroděložního vývoje člověka zpusobené pokusem o potrat. *Cesk Pediatr* 17:483, 1962.
9. Engel W, Reinwein H, Bombel D, Ritter H, Wolf U: Multiple misbildungen bei einem mädchen mit dem karyotypus 46,XY, 17q+. *Humangenetik* 6:311, 1968.
10. Gardner LI, Assemany SR, Neu RL: 46,XY female: Anti-andrenergic effect of oral contraceptive? *Lancet* 2:667, 1970.
11. Maroteaux P, Spranger J, Opitz JM, Kučera J, Lowry RB, Schimke RN, Kagan SM: Le syndrome campomélique. *Presse Med* 79:1157, 1971.
12. Bianchine JW, Risemberg HM, Kanderian SS, Harrison HE: Camptomelic dwarfism. *Lancet* 1:1017, 1971.
13. Gardner LI, Assemany SR, Neu RL: Syndrome of multiple osseous defects with pretibial dimples. *Lancet* 2:98, 1971.
14. Bain AD, Barrett HS: Congenital bowing of the long bones. *Lancet* 1:1244, 1971.
15. Khajavi A, Lachman RS, Rimoin DL, Schimke RN, Dorst JP, Ebbin AJ, Handmaker S, Perreault G: Heterogeneity in the campomelic syndromes: Long and short bone varieties. *Birth Defects Orig Artic Ser* 12:93, 1976.
16. International nomenclature of constitutional diseases of bone. Revision—May 1977. *J Pediatr* 93:615, 1978.
17. Hoefnagel D, Wurster D, Carey D, Harris GJ, Pilliod J: Camptomelic dwarfism. *Lancet* 1:1068, 1972.
18. Houston CS, Opitz JM, Spranger JW, Macpherson RI, Reed MH, Gilbert EF, Herrmann J, Schinzel A: The campomelic syndrome: Review, report of 17 cases, and follow-up on the currently 17-year-old boy first reported by Maroteaux et al. in 1971. *Am J Med Genet* 15:3, 1983.
19. Mansour S, Hall CM, Pembrey ME, Young ID: A clinical and genetic study of campomelic dysplasia. *J Med Genet* 32:415, 1995.
20. Foster JW, Dominguez-Steglich MA, Guioli S, Kowk C, Weller PA, Stevanovic M, Weissenbach J, Mansour S, Young ID, Goodfellow PN, Brook JD, Schafer AJ: Campomelic dysplasia and autosomal sex reversal caused by mutations in an *SRY*-related gene. *Nature* 372:525, 1994.
21. Wagner T, Wirth J, Meyer J, Zabel B, Held M, Zimmer J, Pasantes J, Bricarelli FD, Keutel J, Hustert E, Wolf U, Tommerup N, Schempp W, Scherer G: Autosomal sex reversal and campomelic dysplasia are caused by mutations in and around the SRY-related gene *SOX9*. *Cell* 79:1111, 1994.
22. Camera G, Mastroiacovo P: Birth prevalence of skeletal dysplasias in the Italian Multicultural Monitoring System for Birth Defects, in Papadatos CJ, Bartsocas CS (eds): *Skeletal Dysplasias*. New York, Alan R. Liss, 1982, p 441.
23. Connor JM, Connor RA, Sweet EM, Gibson AA, Patrick WJ, McNay MB, Redford DH: Lethal neonatal chondrodysplasias in the West of Scotland 1970–1983 with a description of a thanatophoric, dysplasia-like, autosomal recessive disorder, Glasgow variant. *Am J Med Genet* 22:243, 1985.
24. Normann EK, Pedersen JC, Stiris G, van der Hagen CB: Campomelic dysplasia—An underdiagnosed condition? *Eur J Pediatr* 152:331, 1993.
25. Dagna Bricarelli F, Fraccaro M, Lindsten J, Muller U, Baggio P, Carbone LD, Hjerpe A, Lindgren F, Mayerova A, Ringertz H, Ritzen EM, Rovetta DC, Sicchero C, Wolf U: Sex-reversed XY females with campomelic dysplasia are H-Y negative. *Hum Genet* 57:15, 1981.
26. Macpherson RI, Skinner SA, Donnenfeld AE: Acampomelic campomelic dysplasia. *Pediatr Radiol* 20:90, 1989.
27. Decsi T, Botykai A: Campomelic dysplasia without campomelia. *Padiatr Padol* 27:29, 1992.
28. Friedrich U, Schaefer E, Meinecke P: Campomelic dysplasia without overt campomelia. *Clin Dysmorphol* 1:172, 1992.
29. Ninomiya S, Narahara K, Tsuji K, Yokoyama Y, Ito S, Seino Y: Acampomelic campomelic syndrome and sex reversal associated with de novo t(12;17) translocation. *Am J Med Genet* 56:31, 1995.
30. Glass RB, Rosenbaum KN: Acampomelic campomelic dysplasia: Further radiographic variations. *Am J Med Genet* 69:29, 1997.
31. Ahmad A, Miller C, Goldstein R, Kishnani P: Camptomelic dysplasia and acampomelic camptomelic dysplasia—A continuous spectrum. *Am J Hum Genet* 61:496, 1997.
32. Savarirayan R, Bankier A: Acampomelic campomelic dysplasia with de novo 5q;17q reciprocal translocation and severe phenotype. *J Med Genet* 35:597, 1998.
33. Storer J, Grossman H: The campomelic syndrome. Congenital bowing of limbs and other skeletal and extraskeletal anomalies. *Radiology* 111:673, 1974.
34. Segre A, Beluffi G, Peretti G: Camptomelic syndrome. A rare type of congenital dwarfism associated with skeletal and other abnormalities. *Ital J Orthop Traumatol* 4:237, 1978.
35. Lee FA, Isaacs H Jr, Strauss J: The "campomelic" syndrome. Short life-span dwarfism with respiratory distress, hypotonia, peculiar facies, and multiple skeletal and cartilaginous deformities. *Am J Dis Child* 124:485, 1972.
36. Thurmon TF, DeFraites EB, Anderson EE: Familial camptomelic dwarfism. *J Pediatr* 83:841, 1973.
37. Hövmoller ML, Osuna A, Eklof O, Fredga K, Hjerpe A, Linsten J, Ritzen M, Stanescu V, Svenningsen N: Camptomelic dwarfism. A genetically determined mesenchymal disorder combined with sex reversal. *Hereditas* 86:51, 1977.
38. Tokita N, Chandra-Sekhar HK, Daly JF, Becker MH, Aleksic S: The campomelic syndrome. Temporal bone, histopathologic features and otolaryngologic manifestations. *Arch Otolaryngol* 105:449, 1979.

39. Austin GE, Gold RH, Mirra JM, Perry S, Moedjono S: Long-limbed campomelic dwarfism. A radiologic and pathologic study. *Am J Dis Child* **134**:1035, 1980.

40. Roth SI, Jimenez JF, Husted S, Seibert JJ, Haynes DW: The histopathology of camptomelia (bent limbs), a dyschondrogenesis. *Clin Orthop* **167**:152, 1982.

41. Nogami H, Oohira A, Kuroyanagi M, Mizutani A: Congenital bowing of long bones: Clinical and experimental study. *Teratology* **33**:1, 1986.

42. Lazjuk GI, Shved IA, Cherstvoy ED, Feshchenko SP: Campomelic syndrome: Concepts of the bowing and shortening in the lower limbs. *Teratology* **35**:1, 1987.

43. Pazzaglia UE, Beluffi G: Radiology and histopathology of the bent limbs in campomelic dysplasia: Implications in the aetiology of the disease and review of theories. *Pediatr Radiol* **17**:50, 1987.

44. Coscia MF, Bassett GS, Bowen JR, Ogilvie JW, Winter RB, Simonton SC: Spinal abnormalities in camptomelic dysplasia. *J Pediatr Orthop* **9**:6, 1989.

45. Takahashi H, Sando I, Masutani H: Temporal bone histopathological findings in campomelic dysplasia. *J Laryngol Otol* **106**:361, 1992.

46. Rodriguez JI: Vascular anomalies in campomelic syndrome. *Am J Med Genet* **46**:185, 1993.

47. Hoefnagel D, Wuster-Hill DH, Dupree WB, Benirschke K, Fuld GL: Camptomelic dwarfism associated with XY-gonadal dysgenesis and chromosome anomalies. *Clin Genet* **13**:489, 1978.

48. Schimke RN: XY sex-reversed campomelia: Possibly an X-linked disorder? *Clin Genet* **16**:62, 1979.

49. Moedjono SJ, Crandall BF, Sparkes RS, Feldman GM, Austin GE, Perry S: The campomelic syndrome in a singleton and monozygotic twins. *Clin Genet* **18**:397, 1980.

50. Fraccaro M, Zuffardi O, Baggio P, Console V, Valagussa E: Campomelic dysplasia and sex reversal, in Spranger J, Tolksdorf M (eds): *Genetik in der Pädiatrie. II. Symposium, Mainz 1979.* Stuttgart, G. Thieme, 1980, p 62.

51. Pauli RM, Pagon RA: Abnormalities of sexual differentiation in campomelic dwarfs. *Clin Genet* **18**:223, 1980.

52. Puck SM, Haseltine FP, Francke U: Absence of H-Y antigen in an XY female with campomelic dysplasia. *Hum Genet* **57**:23, 1981.

53. Hall BD, Spranger JW: Campomelic dysplasia. Further elucidation of a distinct entity. *Am J Dis Child* **134**:285, 1980.

54. Shah KN, Patel ZM, Desai AP, Kulkarni MV, Ambani LM: Campomelic syndrome in phenotypic females with 46,XY chromosomes: Evidence of genetic heterogeneity. *Clin Pediatr (Phila)* **20**:214, 1981.

55. Slater CP, Ross J, Nelson MM, Coetzee EJ: The campomelic syndrome — Prenatal ultrasound investigations. A case report. *S Afr Med J* **67**:863, 1985.

56. Cooke CT, Mulcahy MT, Cullity GJ, Watson M, Srague P: Campomelic dysplasia with sex reversal: Morphological and cytogenetic studies of a case. *Pathology* **17**:526, 1985.

57. Gillerot Y, Vanheck CA, Foulon M, Podevain A, Koulischer L: Campomelic syndrome: Manifestations in a 20-week fetus and case history of a 5-year-old child. *Am J Med Genet* **34**:589, 1989.

58. Yang SP, Curry CJR, Roby JD, Smith JC, Yu CW, Lin CC: Prenatal diagnosis of camptomelic dysplasia with sex reversal. *Clin Res* **38**:A189, 1990.

59. Hong JR, Barber M, Scott CI, Guttenberg M, Wolfson PJ: Three-year-old phenotypic female with campomelic dysplasia and bilateral gonadoblastoma. *J Pediatr Surg* **30**:1735, 1995.

60. Kim MR, Qazi QH, Anderson VM, Valencia GB: A genetic male infant with female phenotype in camptomelic syndrome: A possible relationship to exposure to oral contraceptives during pregnancy. *Am J Obstet Gynecol* **172**:1042, 1995.

61. Cameron FJ, Hageman RM, Cooke-Yarborough C, Kwok C, Goodwin LL, Sillence DO, Sinclair AH: A novel germ line mutation in *SOX9* causes familial campomelic dysplasia and sex reversal. *Hum Mol Genet* **5**:1625, 1996.

62. Lynch SA, Gaunt ML, Minford AM: Campomelic dysplasia: Evidence of autosomal dominant inheritance. *J Med Genet* **30**:683, 1993.

63. Bentivoglio M, Di Trapani G, Mastroiacovo PP, Macchi G: Brain malformations in a case of camptomelic syndrome. *Acta Neurol (Napoli)* **31**:51, 1976.

64. Rebage Moises V, Arnal Alonso JM, Perez Gascon M, Baldellow Vazquez A, Anton Jimenez R, Used Aznar MM, Romo Montejo A, Marco Tello A: Campomelic dysplasia associated with anorectal atresia. *An Esp Pediatr* **31**:483, 1989.

65. Tricoire J, Sarramon MF, Rolland M, Lefort G: Familial cystic hygroma. Report of 8 cases in 3 families. *Genet Couns* **4**:265, 1993.

66. Randolph LM: Deafness in campomelic dysplasia of the long-limbed type — A previously unreported feature. *Am J Hum Genet* **49**:158, 1991.

67. Myong NH, Chi JG: Campomelic syndrome associated with Potter's syndrome and cardiosplenic syndrome. *Cong Anom* **33**:45, 1993.

68. Hobbins JC, Grannum PA, Berkowitz RL, Silverman R, Mahoney MJ: Ultrasound in the diagnosis of congenital anomalies. *Am J Obstet Gynecol* **134**:331, 1979.

69. Fryns JP, van den Berghe K, van Assche A, van den Berghe H: Prenatal diagnosis of campomelic dwarfism. *Clin Genet* **19**:199, 1981.

70. Winter R, Rosenkranz W, Hofmann H, Zierler H, Becker H, Borkenstein M: Prenatal diagnosis of campomelic dysplasia by ultrasonography. *Prenat Diagn* **5**:1, 1985.

71. Balcar I, Bieber FR: Sonographic and radiologic findings in campomelic dysplasia. *AJR Am J Roentgenol* **141**:481, 1983.

72. Redon JY, Le Grevellec JY, Marie F, Le Coq E, Le Guern H: Prenatal diagnosis of camptomelic dysplasia. *J Gynecol Obstet Biol Reprod (Paris)* **13**:437, 1984.

73. Cordone M, Lituania M, Zampatti C, Passamonti U, Magnano GM, Toma P: In utero ultrasonographic features of campomelic dysplasia. *Prenat Diagn* **9**:745, 1989.

74. Ohba S: Systemic air embolism associated with campomelic dysplasia. *Rinsho Hoshasen* **31**:725, 1986.

75. Tennstedt C, Bartho S, Bollmann R, Schwenke A, Nitz I, Rothe K: Osteochondrodysplasias. Prenatal diagnosis and pathological-anatomic findings. *Zentralbl Pathol* **139**:71, 1993.

76. Wong WS, Filly RA: Polyhydramnios associated with fetal limb abnormalities. *AJR Am J Roentgenol* **140**:1001, 1983.

77. Tretter AE, Saunders RC, Meyers CM, Dungan JS, Grumbach K, Sun CC, Campbell AB, Wulfsberg EA: Antenatal diagnosis of lethal skeletal dysplasias. *Am J Med Genet* **75**:518, 1998.

78. Hall BD, Spranger JW: Familial congenital bowing with short bones. *Radiology* **132**:611, 1979.

79. Elejalde BR, de Elejalde MM, Heitman T: Visualization of the fetal genitalia by ultrasonography: A review of the literature and analysis of its accuracy and ethical implications. *J Ultrasound Med* **4**:633, 1985.

80. Kwok C, Weller PA, Guioli S, Foster JW, Mansour S, Zuffardi O, Punnett HH, Dominguez-Steglich MA, Brook JD, Young ID, Goodfellow PN, Schafer AJ: Mutations in *SOX9*, the gene responsible for campomelic dysplasia and autosomal sex reversal. *Am J Hum Genet* **57**:1028, 1995.

81. Maraia R, Saal HM, Wangsa D: A chromosome 17q de novo paracentric inversion in a patient with campomelic dysplasia; case report and etiologic hypothesis. *Clin Genet* **39**:401, 1991.

82. Young ID, Zuccollo JM, Maltby EL, Broderick NJ: Campomelic dysplasia associated with a de novo 2q;17q reciprocal translocation. *J Med Genet* **29**:251, 1992.

83. Tommerup N, Schempp W, Meinecke P, Pedersen S, Bolund L, Brandt C, Goodpasture C, Guldberg P, Held KR, Reinwein H, Saugstad OD, Scherer G, Skjeldal O, Toder R, Westvik J, van der Hagen CB, Wolf U: Assignment of an autosomal sex reversal locus (SRA1) and campomelic dysplasia (CMPD1) to 17q24.3-q25.1. *Nat Genet* **4**:170, 1993.

84. Pfeifer D, Kist R, Meyer J, Zimmer J, Korniszewski L, Stankiewicz P, Back E, Scherer G: Campomelic dysplasia translocation patients have breakpoints scattered over more than 600 kb proximal to SOX9. *Am J Hum Genet* **61**:2009, 1997.

85. Beluffi G, Fraccaro M: Genetical and clinical aspects of campomelic dysplasia. *Prog Clin Biol Res* **104**:53, 1982.

86. Ray S, Bowen JR: Orthopaedic problems associated with survival in campomelic dysplasia. *Clin Orthop* **185**:77, 1984.

87. Grad R, Sammut PH, Britton JR, Goodrich P, Hoyme HE, Dambro NN: Bronchoscopic evaluation of airway obstruction in campomelic dysplasia. *Pediatr Pulmonol* **3**:364, 1987.

88. Shinwell ES, Hengerer AS, Kendig JW: A third case of bronchoscopic diagnosis of tracheobronchomalacia in campomelic dysplasia. *Pediatr Pulmonol* **4**:192, 1988.

89. Thomas S, Winter RB, Lonstein JE: The treatment of progressive kyphoscoliosis in camptomelic dysplasia. *Spine* **22**:1330, 1997.

90. Proudfoot L: Case of compound fracture of the tibia *in utero* and congenital talipes talus. *NY St J Med* **7**:199, 1846.

91. Kirmisson E: *Traité des Maladies Chirurgicales d'origine congénitale.* Paris, Masson, 1898.

92. Chapple CC, Davidson DT: A study of the relationship between fetal position and certain congenital deformities. *J Pediatr* **18**:483, 1941.

93. Caffey J: Prenatal bowing and thickening of tubular bones, with multiple cutaneous dimples in arms and legs: A congenital syndrome of mechanical origin. *Am J Dis Child* **75**:543, 1947.

94. Papp Z, Gardo S: Effect of exogenous hormones on the fetus. *Lancet* **1**:753, 1971.

95. Blessinger GM: Syndrome of multiple osseus deformaties. *Lancet* **ii**:982, 1970.

96. Kučera J: Syndrome of multiple osseous defects. *Lancet* **1**:260, 1972.

97. Krous HF, Turbeville DF, Altshuler GP: Campomelic syndrome— Possible role of intrauterine viral infection. *Teratology* **19**:9, 1979.

98. Stüve A, Wiedemann HR: Congenital bowing of the long bones in two sisters. *Lancet* **2**:495, 1971.

99. Cremin BJ, Orsmond G, Beighton P: Autosomal recessive inheritance in camptomelic dwarfism. *Lancet* **1**:488, 1973.

100. Shafai T: Camptomelic syndrome in siblings [Letter]. *J Pediatr* **89**:512, 1976.

101. Mellows HJ, Pryse-Davies J, Bennett MJ, Carter CO: The camptomelic syndrome in two female siblings. *Clin Genet* **18**:137, 1980.

102. Pavone L, Grasso S, Mazzone D, Sciacca F: Camptomelic dwarfism associated with camptodactyly in a new-born infant from consanguineous parents. *Acta Paediatr Belg* **33**:129, 1980.

103. Meyer J, Sudbeck P, Held M, Wagner T, Schmitz ML, Bricarelli FD, Eggermont E, Friedrich U, Haas OA, Kobelt A, Leroy JG, Van Maldergem L, Michel E, Mitulla B, Pfeiffer RA, Schinzel A, Schmidt H, Scherer G: Mutational analysis of the *SOX9* gene in campomelic dysplasia and autosomal sex reversal: Lack of genotype/phenotype correlations. *Hum Mol Genet* **6**:91, 1997.

104. Cameron FJ, Sinclair AH: Mutations in *SRY* and *SOX9*: Testis-determining genes. *Hum Mutat* **9**:388, 1997.

105. Hageman RM, Cameron FJ, Sinclair AH: Mutation analysis of the *SOX9* gene in a patient with campomelic dysplasia. *Hum Mutat* **Suppl 1**:S112, 1998.

106. Goji K, Nishijima E, Tsugawa C, Nishio H, Pokharel RK, Matsuo M: Novel missense mutation in the HMG box of SOX9 gene in a Japanese XY male resulted in campomelic dysplasia and severe defect in masculinization. *Hum Mutat* **Suppl 1**:S114, 1998.

107. McDowall S, Argentaro A, Ranganathan S, Weller P, Mertin S, Mansour S, Tolmie J, Harley V: Functional and structural studies of wild type *SOX9* and mutations causing campomelic dysplasia. *J Biol Chem* **274**:24023, 1999.

108. Gubbay J, Collignon J, Koopman P, Capel B, Economou A, Münsterberg A, Vivian N, Goodfellow P, Lovell-Badge R: A gene mapping to the sex-determining region of the mouse Y chromosome is a member of a novel family of embryonically expressed genes. *Nature* **346**:245, 1990.

109. Baxevanis AD, Landsman D: The HMG-1 box protein family: Classification and functional relationships. *Nucleic Acids Res* **23**:1604, 1995.

110. Denny P, Swift S, Brand N, Dabhade N, Barton P, Ashworth A: A conserved family of genes related to the testis determining gene, *SRY*. *Nucleic Acids Res* **20**:2887, 1992.

111. Laudet V, Stehelin D, Clevers H: Ancestry and diversity of the HMG box superfamily. *Nucleic Acids Res* **21**:2493, 1993.

112. Prior HM, Walter MA: *SOX* genes: Architects of development. *Mol Med* **2**:405, 1996.

113. Soullier S, Jay P, Poulat F, Vanacker JM, Berta P, Laudet V: Diversification pattern of the *HMG* and *SOX* family members during evolution. *J Mol Evol* **48**:517, 1999.

114. Ng LJ, Wheatley S, Muscat GE, Conway-Campbell J, Bowles J, Wright E, Bell DM, Tam PP, Cheah KS, Koopman P: SOX9 binds DNA, activates transcription, and coexpresses with type II collagen during chondrogenesis in the mouse. *Dev Biol* **183**:108, 1997.

115. Mertin S, McDowall SG, Harley VR: The DNA-binding specificity of SOX9 and other SOX proteins. *Nucleic Acids Res* **27**:1359, 1999.

116. Lefebvre V, Huang W, Harley VR, Goodfellow PN, de Crombrugghe B: *SOX9* is a potent activator of the chondrocyte-specific enhancer of the pro alpha1(II) collagen gene. *Mol Cell Biol* **17**:2336, 1997.

117. Pontiggia A, Rimini R, Harley VR, Goodfellow PN, Lovell-Badge R, Bianchi ME: Sex-reversing mutations affect the architecture of SRY-DNA complexes. *EMBO J* **13**:6115, 1994.

118. Sudbeck P, Schmitz ML, Baeuerle PA, Scherer G: Sex reversal by loss of the C-terminal transactivation domain of human SOX9. *Nat Genet* **13**:230, 1996.

119. Fisher E, Scambler P: Human haploinsufficiency—One for sorrow, two for joy. *Nat Genet* **7**:5, 1994.

120. Wunderle VM, Critcher R, Hastie N, Goodfellow PN, Schedl A: Deletion of long-range regulatory elements upstream of *SOX9* causes campomelic dysplasia. *Proc Natl Acad Sci U S A* **95**:10649, 1998.

121. Wilkie AO: The molecular basis of genetic dominance. *J Med Genet* **31**:89, 1994.

122. Bridge J, Sanger W, Mosher G, Buehler B, Nelson R, Welsh M, Newland J, Kafka M: Partial deletion of distal 17q. *Am J Med Genet* **21**:225, 1985.

123. Olney PN, Kean LS, Graham D, Elsas LJ, May KM: Campomelic syndrome and deletion of *SOX9*. *Am J Med Genet* **84**:20, 1999.

124. Ninomiya S, Isomura M, Narahara K, Seino Y, Nakamura Y: Isolation of a testis-specific cDNA on chromosome 17q from a region adjacent to the breakpoint of t(12;17) observed in a patient with acampomelic campomelic dysplasia and sex reversal. *Hum Mol Genet* **5**:69, 1996.

125. Kwok C, Goodfellow PN, Hawkins JR: Evidence to exclude *SOX9* as a candidate gene for XY sex reversal without skeletal malformation. *J Med Genet* **33**:800, 1996.

126. Vortkamp A, Gessler M, Grzeschik KH: *GLI3* zinc-finger gene interrupted by translocations in Greig syndrome families. *Nature* **352**:539, 1991.

127. Bedell MA, Brannan CI, Evans EP, Copeland N, Jenkins NA, Donovan PJ: DNA rearrangements located over 100 kb 5′ of the *Steel (Sl)*-coding region in *Steel-panda* and *Steel-contrasted* mice deregulate *Sl* expression and cause female sterility by disrupting ovarian follicle development. *Genes Dev* **9**:455, 1995.

128. Fantes J, Redeker B, Breen M, Boyle S, Brown J, Fletcher J, Jones S, Bickmore W, Fukushima Y, Mannens M, Danes S, van Heyningen V, Hanson I: Aniridia-associated cytogenetic rearrangements suggest that a position effect may cause the mutant phenotype. *Hum Mol Genet* **4**:415, 1995.

129. Engelkamp D, van Heyningen V: Transcription factors in disease. *Curr Opin Genet Dev* **6**:334, 1996.

130. Wirth J, Wagner T, Meyer J, Pfeiffer RA, Tietze HU, Schempp W, Scherer G: Translocation breakpoints in three patients with campomelic dysplasia and autosomal sex reversal map more than 130 kb from *SOX9*. *Hum Genet* **97**:186, 1996.

131. Kanai Y, Koopman P: Structural and functional characterization of the mouse *SOX9* promoter: Implications for campomelic dysplasia. *Hum Mol Genet* **8**:691, 1999.

132. Wright E, Hargrave MR, Christiansen J, Cooper L, Kun J, Evans T, Gangadharan U, Greenfield A, Koopman P: The Sry-related gene *Sox9* is expressed during chondrogenesis in mouse embryos. *Nat Genet* **9**:15, 1995.

133. Zhao Q, Eberspaecher H, Lefebvre V, De Crombrugghe B: Parallel expression of *Sox9* and *Col2a1* in cells undergoing chondrogenesis. *Dev Dyn* **209**:377, 1997.

134. Bi W, Deng JM, Zhang Z, Behringer RR, de Crombrugghe B: *Sox9* is required for cartilage formation. *Nat Genet* **22**:85, 1999.

135. Healy C, Uwanogho D, Sharpe PT: Expression of the chicken *Sox9* gene marks the onset of cartilage differentiation. *Ann N Y Acad Sci* **785**:261, 1996.

136. Takahashi I, Nuckolls GH, Takahashi K, Tanaka O, Semba I, Dashner R, Shum L, Slavkin HC: Compressive force promotes *Sox9*, type II collagen and aggrecan and inhibits IL-1beta expression resulting in chondrogenesis in mouse embryonic limb bud mesenchymal cells. *J Cell Sci* **111**:2067, 1998.

137. Bell DM, Leung KK, Wheatley SC, Ng LJ, Zhou S, Ling KW, Sham MH, Koopman P, Tam PP, Cheah KS: *SOX9* directly regulates the type-II collagen gene. *Nat Genet* **16**:174, 1997.

138. Zhou G, Lefebvre V, Zhang Z, Eberspaecher H, de Crombrugghe B: Three high mobility group-like sequences within a 48-base pair enhancer of the col2a1 gene are required for cartilage-specific expression in vivo. *J Biol Chem* **273**:14989, 1998.

139. Lefebvre V, Li P, de Crombrugghe B: A new long form of *Sox5* (*L-Sox5*), *Sox6* and *Sox9* are coexpressed in chondrogenesis and co-operatively activate the type II collagen gene. *EMBO J* **17**:5718, 1998.

140. Bridgewater LC, Lefebvre V, de Crombrugghe B: Chondrocyte-specific enhancer elements in the *Col11a2* gene resemble the *Col2a1* tissue-specific enhancer. *J Biol Chem* **273**:14998, 1998.

141. Nonaka K, Shum L, Takahashi K, Takahashi I, Nuckolls GH, Semba I, Slavkin HC: *Bmp4* induced chondrogenesis by upregulation of an activator *Sox9* and a repressor *Msx2*. *J Dent Res* **77**:376, 1998.

142. Mitsiadis TA, Mucchielli ML, Raffo S, Proust JP, Koopman P, Goridis C: Expression of the transcription factors *Otlx2*, *Barx1* and *Sox9* during mouse odontogenesis. *Eur J Oral Sci* **106(Suppl 1)**:112, 1998.

143. Kanzler B, Kuschert SJ, Liu YH, Mallo M: Hoxa-2 restricts the chondrogenic domain and inhibits bone formation during development of the branchial area. *Development* **125**:2587, 1998.

144. Hogan BL: Bone morphogenetic proteins: Multifunctional regulators of vertebrate development. *Genes Dev* **10**:1580, 1996.

145. Bumcrot DA, McMahon AP: Somite differentiation. Sonic signals somites. *Curr Biol* **5**:612, 1995.

146. Wegner M: From head to toes: The multiple facets of Sox proteins. *Nucleic Acids Res* **27**:1409, 1999.

147. Huang B, Wang S, Ning Y, Lamb AN, Bartley J: Autosomal XX sex reversal caused by duplication of *SOX9*. *Am J Med Genet* **87**:349, 1999.

148. Lenzini E, Leszl A, Artifoni L, Casellato R, Tenconi R, Baccichetti C: Partial duplication of 17 long arm. *Ann Genet* **31**:175, 1988.

149. Bardoni B, Zanaria E, Guioli S, Floridia G, Worley KC, Tonini G, Ferrante E, Chiumello G, McCabe ERB, Fraccaro M, Zuffardi O, Camerino G: A dosage-sensitive locus at chromosome Xp21 is involved in male to female sex reversal. *Nat Genet* **7**:497, 1994.

150. Zanaria E, Bardoni B, Dabovic B, Calvari V, Fraccaro M, Zuffardi O, Camerino G: Xp duplications and sex reversal. *Philos Trans R Soc Lond B Biol Sci* **350**:291, 1995.

151. Swain A, Narvaez V, Burgoyne P, Camerino G, Lovell-Badge R: Dax1 antagonizes Sry action in mammalian sex determination. *Nature* **391**:761, 1998.

152. Hanley NA, Hagan DM, Ostrer H, Guillen-Navarro E, Wilson DI, Bullen P, Lindsay S, Robson S, Clement-Jones M, Strachan T: Spatiotemporal expression patterns of the sex determining genes, *SRY, SOX9, & WT1*, during early human development. *Am J Hum Genet* **61**:SS878, 1997.

153. Kent J, Wheatley SC, Andrews JE, Sinclair AH, Koopman P: A male-specific role for *SOX9* in vertebrate sex determination. *Development* **122**:2813, 1996.

154. Morais da Silva S, Hacker A, Harley V, Goodfellow P, Swain A, Lovell-Badge R: *Sox9* expression during gonadal development implies a conserved role for the gene in testis differentiation in mammals and birds. *Nat Genet* **14**:62, 1996.

155. Western PS, Harry JL, Graves JA, Sinclair AH: Temperature-dependent sex determination: Upregulation of *SOX9* expression after commitment to male development. *Dev Dyn* **214**:171, 1999.

156. Spotila LD, Spotila JR, Hall SE: Sequence and expression analysis of WT1 and Sox9 in the red-eared slider turtle, *Trachemys scripta*. *J Exp Zool* **281**:417, 1998.

157. Schafer AJ: Sex determination and its pathology in man, in Hall JC, Dunlap JC (eds): *Advances in Genetics*. San Diego, Academic Press, 1995, p 275.

158. Lim HN, Hawkins JR: Genetic control of gonadal differentiation. *Baillieres Clin Endocrinol Metab* **12**:1, 1998.

159. Shen WH, Moore CC, Ikeda Y, Parker KL, Ingraham HA: Nuclear receptor steroidogenic factor 1 regulates the mullerian inhibiting substance gene: A link to the sex determination cascade. *Cell* **77**:651, 1994.

160. De Santa Barbara P, Bonneaud N, Boizet B, Desclozeaux M, Moniot B, Sudbeck P, Scherer G, Poulat F, Berta P: Direct interaction of SRY-related protein SOX9 and steroidogenic factor 1 regulates transcription of the human anti-Müllerian hormone gene. *Mol Cell Biol* **18**:6653, 1998.

161. Oreal E, Pieau C, Mattei MG, Josso N, Picard JY, Carre-Eusebe D, Magre S: Early expression of *AMH* in chicken embryonic gonads precedes testicular *SOX9* expression. *Dev Dyn* **212**:522, 1998.

# Hereditary Hearing Loss

*Christine Petit* ▪ *Jacqueline Levilliers*
*Sandrine Marlin* ▪ *Jean-Pierre Hardelin*

1. **There is a high prevalence of hearing loss at any age. The conductive forms of deafness are defined as being due to external and/or middle ear defects, and the sensorineural forms as being due to an abnormal response to sound from the inner ear to the cortex. The various forms of deafness are classified into two categories, syndromic and nonsyndromic (also termed isolated). In the introduction, we provide background information on the structure of the ear, its functioning, its development, and the auditory pathway. Finally, we discuss the causes of hearing loss. About 80 percent of the prelingual cases are of genetic origin in developed countries.**

2. **Syndromic forms of deafness are almost exclusively hereditary in developed countries; several hundreds of syndromes including hearing loss have been described. Table 254-1 summarizes the data concerning the 100 or so syndromic forms of deafness for which the causative gene has been isolated. They are distributed into three classes: (a) the forms with external and middle ear anomalies, with or without a sensorineural component to the deafness; (b) the forms with middle ear anomalies, with or without sensorineural deafness; and (c) the sensorineural forms. It is noteworthy that several genes underlying a syndromic deafness also underlie one, or sometimes two, genetic forms of isolated deafness.**

3. **The core of the review concerns the nonsyndromic forms of deafness. These are genetically highly heterogeneous and appear to be almost exclusively monogenic diseases. A hundred or so genes are supposed to underlie this deficit. Fifty-three loci have presently been reported. The 17 deafness forms for which the genes have been identified are presented. Each form is introduced by a brief history of how the gene was discovered, followed by the description of its clinical features and the established or putative role of the encoded protein, as well as the current hypotheses concerning the associated pathophysiological processes. Deaf mouse mutants involving the orthologous genes are discussed at the same time. In addition, four genes that have been implicated in deafness in the mouse, but not yet in humans, are discussed.**

4. **From the molecular data presently available, three main epidemiologic results emerge: (a) Mutations in the gene encoding a gap junction protein, connexin 26, account for about half of the cases of prelingual isolated deafness in Caucasian populations; (b) Defects of the gene responsible for Pendred syndrome (hearing loss and thyroid dysfunction), encoding a iodide-chloride transporter, may also account for an underestimated proportion of isolated deafness (DFNB4), which is characterized by the presence of particular inner ear anomalies; and (c) Mutations in the mitochondrial gene encoding the 12S ribosomal RNA underlie aminoglycoside-induced hearing loss, and may** also account for a high proportion of the cases of genetic deafness in the absence of any exposure to these antibiotics.

## GENERAL CONSIDERATIONS

Hearing loss is the most frequent of the sensory defects. It can appear at any age and with any degree of severity. The personal and social consequences of hearing impairment are greatly influenced by the severity of the hearing defect and by the age of onset. If the defect is severe and presents in early childhood, it has dramatic effects on speech acquisition and thereby may have an impact on cognitive and psychosocial development. Severe hearing defect appearing at a later age seriously compromises the quality of life as it results in the isolation of the affected individual.

Hearing impairments can be classified according to the degree of severity of the hearing loss for the better hearing ear: mild, moderate, severe, and profound hearing impairment corresponds to a loss of 20 to 39 decibels hearing level (dBHL), 40 to 69 dB, 70 to 89 dB, and equal or superior to 90 dB, respectively (see example illustrated in Fig. 254-1). They can also be classified according to the site of the defect. Conductive hearing loss refers to external and/or middle ear defects and sensorineural hearing loss refers to a transmission anomaly of the sound signal from the inner ear to the cortical auditory centers of the brain (see "The Structure of the Ear" and "The Auditory Pathway"). In fact, most cases of sensorineural hearing loss are due to inner ear defects. Finally, hearing impairment can be classified according to whether it is associated with other symptoms or anomalies (syndromic deafness, see example in Fig. 254-2) or not (nonsyndromic or isolated deafness).

Approximately 1 in 1000 individuals is affected by severe or profound deafness at birth or during early childhood, that is, the prelingual period. Syndromic deafness contributes to about 30 percent of the cases of prelingual deafness. These syndromic forms may be conductive, sensorineural, or mixed. In contrast, the nonsyndromic forms of prelingual deafness are almost exclusively sensorineural. An additional 1 in 1000 children becomes deaf before adulthood. These forms are usually less severe and progressive. Finally, 0.3 percent and 2.3 percent of the population manifests a hearing loss greater than 65 dB between the ages of 30 and 50 years and between 60 and 70 years, respectively. The late onset forms are often conductive, with otosclerosis, defined as a fixation of the stapes footplate to the oval window, accounting for a large proportion of them (see "The Structure of the Ear" below). As a whole, in developed countries, 6 to 8 percent of the population suffers from hearing loss.

This chapter presents the advances made in the past few years in our understanding of human hereditary deafness in terms of basic science and medical implications. Although the research concerning the nonsyndromic forms has only recently emerged, rapid progress has been made. The structure and functioning of the ear is briefly reviewed, as well as the prevalence of the various types of deafness. The genes currently known to be

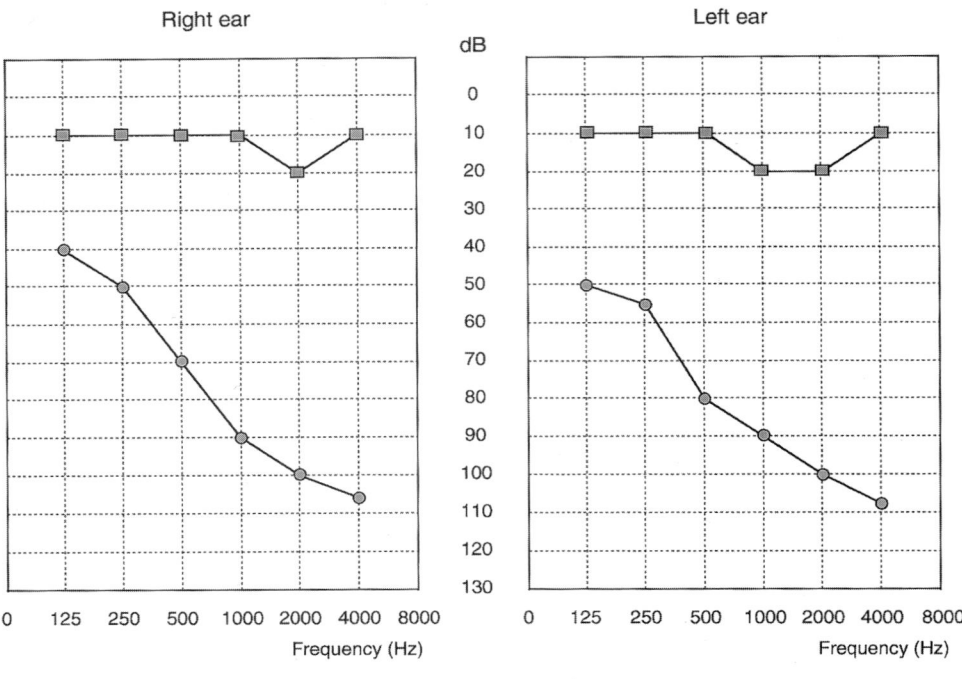

Right ear      Left ear

Fig. 254-1 Pure tone audiograms of the right and left ears. Air conduction hearing thresholds (in dBHL) have been determined for all indicated sound frequencies, in a normal hearing individual (squares) and in an individual affected by severe-profound hearing loss (circles).

responsible for human deafness are presented, with the main focus on those genes that cause nonsyndromic forms. The study of mouse deaf mutants not only constitutes a valuable approach to clone human deafness genes but also is expected to be particularly helpful to understand the underlying pathophysiological processes. Thus, mouse models for human nonsyndromic forms of deafness are discussed. Finally, although not yet characterized at the molecular level, zebrafish mutants with inner ear defects are also promising animal models for insight into the pathogenesis of human hereditary deafness.

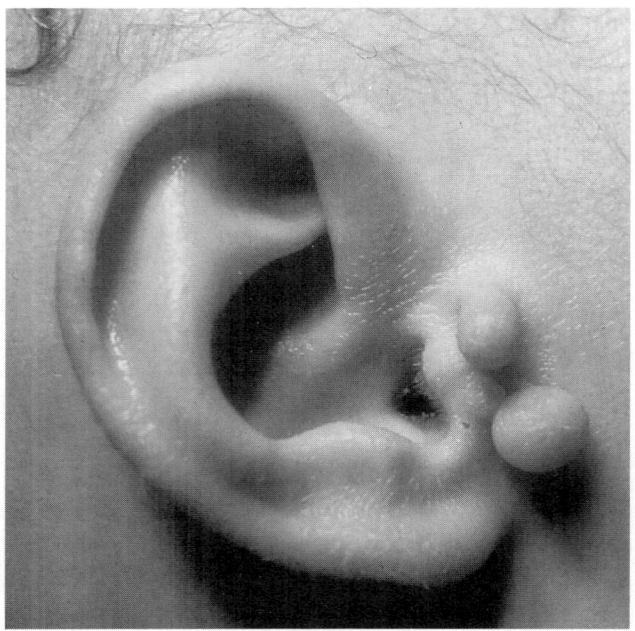

Fig. 254-2 Branchial anomalies in the branchio-oto-renal syndrome. Two preauricular tags corresponding to branchial residues can be seen in this child affected by the branchio-oto-renal syndrome.

## THE STRUCTURE OF THE EAR

The human ear is made up of three compartments, the external, middle, and inner ear (Fig. 254-3A). The external ear comprises the auricle and the external auditory canal, and is closed by the tympanic membrane. The middle ear consists of an air cavity containing a chain of three ossicles, namely the malleus, incus, and stapes. The proximal portion of this cavity forms the auditory (eustachian) tube, through which the tympanic cavity communicates with the pharynx. The inner ear is a complex membranous labyrinth present in a cavity of the temporal bone (bony labyrinth). This membranous labyrinth is filled with a liquid, the endolymph, and immersed in another liquid, the perilymph. The inner ear comprises six mechanosensory organs, namely the snail-shaped cochlea, which is the auditory sense organ, and the five vestibular end organs, which are responsible for balance. The human cochlea detects sound frequencies between 20 Hz and 20 kHz. The vestibule is composed of the saccule and the utricle, which respond to vertical and horizontal linear acceleration, respectively, and the three semicircular canals (located in approximately perpendicular planes), which respond to angular acceleration elicited by the rotation of the head. The cochlea and the vestibule both derive from the otic placode (see "Embryonic Development of the Ear," below) and share several histologic and physiological features. Finally, at the junction between the utricle and the saccule is located the endolymphatic canal (ending with the endolymphatic sac), an outgrowth of the membranous labyrinth that ensures the resorption of the endolymph and that drains into the venous sinus of the dura layer.

The six sensory patches of the inner ear, namely the organ of Corti in the cochlea, the maculae of the utricle and saccule, and the ampullar cristae of the semicircular canals, are composed of sensory cells (Fig. 254-3C) and various types of supporting cells. The inner ear sensory cells are termed hair cells in reference to the bundle of stiff actin-filled microvilli, improperly named stereocilia, present at their apical surface. Thirty to 300 stereocilia form the hair bundle, the mechanoreceptive structure of the hair cells. The stereocili always form into "staircase" or organ-pipe arrays, in which each stereociliar tip is connectd to the next taller stereocilium by a tip link (Fig. 254-4). In addition, many connecting strands are observed along the length of the stereocilia (lateral

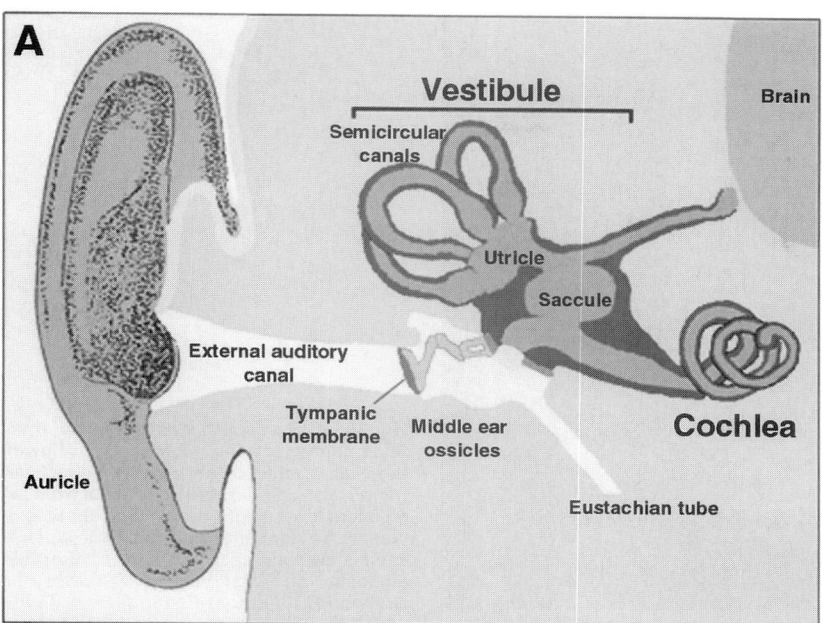

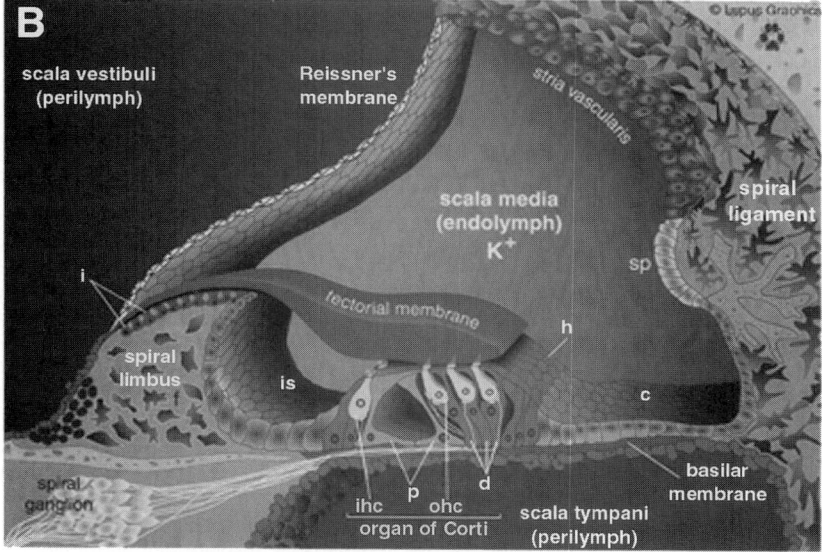

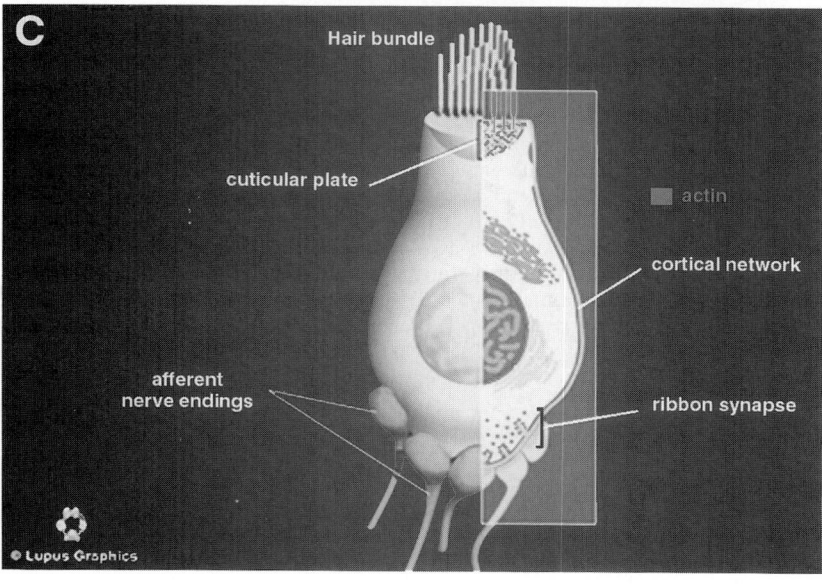

Fig. 254-3 *A*, Representation of the human inner ear. The mammalian ear is composed of three compartments: the outer ear made up of the auricle and external auditory canal; the middle ear made up of the ossicles within the tympanic cavity; and the inner ear which consists of six sensory organs, namely the five vestibular end organs (saccule, utricle, and three semicircular canals) and the cochlea. *B*, Cross-section through the cochlear duct. The membranous labyrinth of the cochlea (cochlear duct) divides the bony labyrinth into three canals: the scala vestibuli and the scala tympani, both filled with perilymph, and the scala media, filled with endolymph. The organ of Corti, which is the auditory transduction apparatus, protrudes in the scala media. This organ is made up of (a) an array of sensory cells, that is, the single row of inner hair cells (ihc) and three rows of outer hair cells (ohc), and (b) different types of supporting cells (p, d, h). An acellular gel, the tectorial membrane, covers it. The organ of Corti is flanked by the epithelial cells of the inner sulcus (is) on the medial side and by the Claudius' cells (c) on the lateral side. The stria vascularis, on the lateral wall of the cochlear duct, is responsible for the secretion of $K^+$ into the endolymph. Different types of fibrocytes surround the cochlear epithelium. Other abbreviations are: i = interdental cells; p = pillar cells; d = Deiter's cells; h = Hensen's cells; sp = spiral prominence. (*Modified from Kalatzis V, Petit C.*[35] *Used with permission.*). *C*, Representation of a sensory inner hair cell. Note the highly organized hair bundle, made of several rows of stereocilia, at the apical pole of the cell. The ribbon synapse has particular structural and functional features. Three specific structures of the actin cytoskeleton are shown, namely (a) the filaments of the stereocilia, (b) the cuticular plate, a dense meshwork of horizontal filaments running parallel to the apical cell surface, and (c) the cortical network, beneath the plasma membrane.

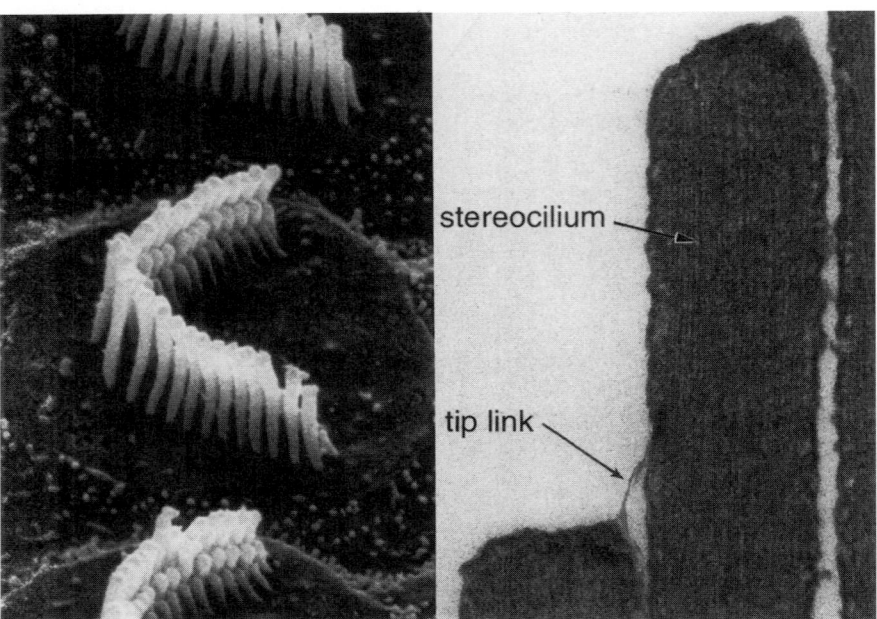

stereocilium

tip link

**Fig. 254-4 Stereocilia and their tip links.** Scanning electron microscopy showing the hair bundle of an outer hair cell (*left panel*), and detail of the stereocilia from two adjacent rows (*right panel*). The tip link, an elastic filament that connects the apex of each stereocilium to the side of the taller adjacent one, is visible. (*Courtesy of Romand R, Clermont-Ferrand, France.*)

links). The organ of Corti (Fig. 254-3*B*) lies on the basilar membrane. It possesses two types of sensory hair cells. The inner hair cells (IHC) organized in a single row are the genuine sensory cells accounting for most of the cochlear nerve influx sent to the auditory centers. The outer hair cells (OHC), which are organized in three rows, are contractile cells. The OHC amplify the auditory stimulus (see "The Functioning of the Ear"). The sensory cells of the mammalian vestibular end organs are of two types, type I and type II, so far mainly distinguished by their cytologic and innervation characteristics. The stereocilia of the hair cells are bathed by the endolymph. The apical parts of the lateral walls of the hair cells are sealed to that of surrounding supporting cells by tight junctions, forming the reticular lamina. As a result, the apical and the remaining surface of the hair cells are isolated from each other, and immersed in liquids of completely different ionic composition, the endolymph and the perilymph, respectively. The endolymph has an ionic composition unusual for an extracellular liquid, in the sense that it is potassium-rich (about 150 mM), almost devoid of sodium (1 mM), and poor in calcium (0.02 mM). The perilymph has a low K$^+$ concentration (3.5 mM), a high Na$^+$ concentration (140 mM), and a higher Ca$^{2+}$ concentration (1 mM) than the endolymph. This results in a large difference of potential of about +80 mV between the endolymph and the perilymph, named the endocochlear potential. Acellular membranes, namely the tectorial membrane in the cochlea, the otoconial membranes in the saccule and utricle, and the cupulae in the semicircular canals, cover the different sensory patches. In addition, the otoconial membranes are overlaid with dense crystal-shaped biominerals, the otoconia. A great variety of epithelial cells line the membranous labyrinth of the cochlea (see legend to Fig. 254-3). Some of these cells form a particular secretory structure, the stria vascularis, in the lateral wall of the cochlea. The stria vascularis consists of two cell barriers formed by the marginal cells and the basal cells. Each barrier consists of a continuous sheet of cells joined by tight junctional complexes. Between these barriers is the intrastrial space with the special capillary bed for which the tissue is named, and a discontinuous layer of intermediate cells. The tight junctions connecting the marginal cells, the basal cells, and the endothelial cells make the intrastrial space a separate fluid compartment. The basal cells are joined with gap junctions to intermediate cells and to fibrocytes of the adjacent connective tissue,[1] suggesting a level of cooperation among these three cell types. In contrast, strial marginal cells are not coupled to each other or to other cells by gap

junctions. The stria vascularis is responsible for secretion of K$^+$ into the cochlear endolymph and for production of the endo-cochlear potential (Fig. 254-5). In the vestibule, K$^+$ is secreted by the dark cells of the utricle and semicircular canals.

## THE FUNCTIONING OF THE EAR

The external ear collects sound, that is, air wave pressure, and transfers it to the tympanic membrane (Fig. 254-3*A*). The vibrations of the tympanic membrane are picked up by the three ossicles of the middle ear that transmit them to another membrane covering a hole in the bony labyrinth, the oval window. The vibrations of the membrane of the oval window induce liquid waves in the inner ear, which themselves result in the vibration of the basilar membrane. The basilar membrane vibration peaks at a location dependent on the sound frequency.[2] It is transferred to the organ of Corti and thereby to the hair cells. The relative motion between the hair cell body and the overlaying tectorial membrane leads to the deflection of the stereocilia bundle. Similarly, the vestibular stimuli result in the relative displacement of the sensory epithelia with regard to the overlaying acellular membranes, hence in the bending of the stereocilia bundle. According to the current view, the tension of the tip links increases; it follows an opening of the cationic mechanotransduction channels located near the stereociliar tips.[3,4] The transducer current is mainly carried by an influx of K$^+$ ions along the 150 mV or so electric gradient between the endolymph and the hair cell cytoplasm (the mean resting potential of the sensory hair cells being $-40$ mV for IHC and $-70$ mV for OHC). This current results in the depolarization of the hair cell (receptor potential); the depolarization induces a Ca$^{2+}$ influx that triggers the fusion of the synaptic vesicles with the plasma membrane. Upon neurotransmitter (probably gluta-mate) release, an afferent nerve fiber at the base of the hair cell transmits a pattern of action potentials encoding different characteristics of the stimulus to the brain, including intensity, time course, and frequency (low frequencies elicit a neuronal phase-locked response and fibers devoted to the high frequencies use the tonotopy to code sound frequency). Two other characteristics of the functioning of the mammalian inner ear deserve special comment: the spectral analysis of sound frequencies and the amplification of the auditory stimulus by the OHC. The spectral analysis of sound frequency relies not only on the biophysical characteristics of the basilar membrane, but also on

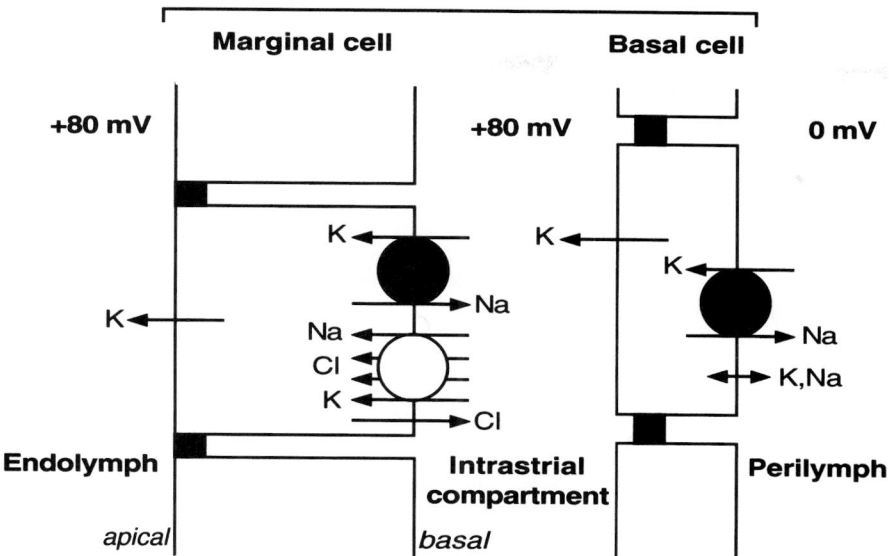

**Stria vascularis**

Fig. 254-5 Model of ion transport by the stria vascularis. The marginal cell epithelium secretes K⁺ into the endolymph, and the basal cell layer produces the voltage (endocochlear potential) between endolymph and perilymph. The ion transport processes ascribed to the marginal cells have a strong experimental basis. The transport processes proposed in the model of the basal cells have not yet been experimentally demonstrated and may be distributed among basal cells, intermediate cells of the stria vascularis, and fibrocytes of the spiral ligament, which are all connected by gap junctions. Arrows: ion channels; open circles: ion transporters; filled circles: primary-active ion "pump." (*From Wangemann P. Comparison of ion transport mechanisms between dark cells and strial marginal cells. Hearing Res 90:149, 1995. Used with permission.*)

the tuning response of each hair cell to a particular frequency. Hair cells respond to gradually varying frequencies and are linearly positioned along the longitudinal axis of the cochlea, thus forming a tonotopic map. High frequencies are analyzed at the base of the cochlea and low frequencies at the apex. These properties of the hair cells are underscored by their cytologic and biophysical characteristics (i.e., the length of their cell body and the length and flexibility of their stereocilia), which also vary along the cochlea. Experimental damage to OHC has established the role of these cells in the sensitivity and the selectivity of the cochlear response to sound stimulation.[5] These cells display a fast contraction of their lateral membrane in response to the depolarization caused by the sound wave. These cyclic length changes of the OHC amplify the acoustic stimulation by boosting the sound induced vibration of the basilar membrane.

## THE AUDITORY PATHWAY

The auditory pathway is complex; we present here a simplified view. The afferent fibers of the IHC, which send nerve impulses to the brain, come from about 95 percent of the neurons of the cochlear ganglion. Their axonal processes form the auditory nerve, which ends up in the ipsilateral cochlear nucleus of the brain stem, in an orderly fashion, thus perpetuating the cochlear tonotopic organization. Each part of the cochlear nucleus (ventral and dorsal) has complex relationships with different brain centers. Some neurons of the cochlear nucleus connect to both the ipsilateral and the contralateral olivary nuclear complexes in the brain stem; this is essential for the binaural localization of sounds in space. Others, as well as the axonal projections of the olivary nuclear neurons, ascend in the lateral lemniscus and synapse in the inferior colliculus; postsynaptic neurons send their axons to the medial geniculate nucleus of the thalamus. The axonal projections from the thalamus end in the auditory cortical areas on the dorsal aspect of the temporal lobe, where the tonotopic representation is preserved.

## EMBRYONIC DEVELOPMENT OF THE EAR

The inner ear develops from the otic placode, a thickening of the surface ectoderm, which is located in close apposition to rhombomeres 5 and 6, and appears at embryonic day 22 (E22) in humans (E8 in mouse). The chordomesoderm and the hindbrain exert inductive effects on the developing otic primordium that are needed for otic placode specification and invagination. During the fourth week, the otic placode invaginates to form the otic pit. By the end of the fourth week (E9.5 in the mouse), the pit becomes deeper and closes to form the otic vesicle (otocyst), which is covered by the surface ectoderm and completely surrounded by mesenchymal tissue of mesodermal origin. Reciprocal interactions between the epithelium of the otic vesicle and the periotic mesenchyme have been demonstrated to be essential for the differentiation of these tissues.[6] At the same period, cells delaminate from the ventromedial part of the vesicle to constitute the statoacoustic ganglion.[7] A group of neural crest cells migrate through the periotic mesenchyme; they will eventually form the intermediate cells of the stria vascularis in the cochlea and the dark cells in the vestibular end organs. During the fifth week, the otic vesicle elongates and the endolymphatic canal buds off the medial wall. The periotic mesenchyme starts to condense to form the otic capsule. The otic vesicle then enlarges and forms two pouches, the dorsal one, which gives rise to the three semicircular canals, and the ventral one to the cochlea. The area in between will divide to form the utricle and the saccule. By 7 weeks, the cochlear duct has formed $1\frac{1}{4}$ turns, and by 9 weeks, the full $2\frac{1}{2}$ turns have been achieved. In the mouse, there is only $1\frac{3}{4}$ cochlear turns, which are formed at E18. The nerve fibers enter the epithelium during the seventh week and the morphologic differentiation of the hair cells begins at the eleventh week. Differentiation proceeds from the base to the apex of the cochlea, and from inside to outside. The adult size of the cochlea is reached at the sixteenth week of embryonic development (postnatal day 14 in the mouse). The onset of hearing appears at the twentieth week, that is when the synapses of the IHC are mature, whereas the synapses of the OHC will mature later. The final differentiation of the human cochlea is reached at the end of the gestation period (thirty-second week) (but only at postnatal day 20 in the mouse).

The tympanic cavity and three ossicles (middle ear) are of endodermal and mesodermal origin, respectively. The tympanic cavity forms from the first pharyngeal pouch. Its distal portion reaches the region of the tympanic membrane, to which it provides the internal epithelium. The malleus and the incus derive from the mesenchyme of the first pharyngeal arch, the stapes from the mesenchyme of the second arch, both of neural crest origin.[8] The ossicles lie above the tympanic cavity in loose connective tissue until the eighth month. At that time, the connective tissue begins to disappear and the tympanic cavity gradually increases and finally houses the three ossicles. The oval window has been proposed to derive from the otic capsule, which breaks down into a fibrous tissue around the footplate of the stapes, as early as the ninth week of development.[9]

The external auditory canal and the auricle derive from the ectoderm of the first pharyngeal cleft and surrounding arches, respectively. The sides of the cleft develop by the fifth week (E11.5 in mouse) and form six mesenchymal hillocks. The fusion of these swellings into an auricle is complete at the eighth week. The tympanic membrane thus has a triple origin, from outside to inside, the ectoderm of the first pharyngeal cleft, the mesenchyme of the adjacent arches, and the ectoderm of the first pharyngeal pouch.

## THE CAUSES OF HEARING LOSS

With the exception of embryopathies due to rubella, toxoplasmosis, or cytomegalovirus infection, which can lead to polymalformations including hearing loss, the syndromic forms of deafness have a genetic origin. The nonsyndromic forms of deafness can be due to environmental, genetic, or a combination of both causes. The environmental causes vary with age.[10] Among the prenatal causes, infections, especially with cytomegalovirus, and exposure to ototoxic drugs (aminoglycoside and furosemide) during pregnancy are the most frequent in developed countries. During the perinatal period, several environmental factors can cause deafness, essentially anoxia and kernicterus related to high prematurity. Finally, postnatal environmental causes of deafness are mainly bacterial meningitis and administration of ototoxic drugs. Other rarer causes are fracture of the petrous temporal bone, noise or pressure trauma, infectious labyrinthitis, mumps, chronic otitis, and tumors. The hereditary nature of nonsyndromic forms of deafness was reported as early as the sixteenth century by Johannes Schenck.[11,12] In 1621, the papal physician Paolus Zacchias recommended that deaf people should not marry because of the risk of them having deaf children.[13] Early interest in the mode of inheritance of hearing loss arose from observations by Pierre Ménière in 1846.[14] In a lecture entitled "Upon marriage between relatives considered as the cause of congenital deafmutism," P. Ménière (professor at the Faculty and physician at the Institut Impérial des Sourds-muets) questioned the causes of deaf-mutism,[15] and acknowledged for the first time the autosomal recessive origin of deaf-mutism:

> **Given a deaf-mute, is it possible to determine the causes which led to this so serious disability?... From these documents emerges a general fact, namely that the number of deaf-mutes is largely variable in each country; sometimes it is estimated to be one affected individual in 3000, sometimes one in 2000 and some villages have as many as one in 200 individuals affected or even more...If in restricted, isolated villages, one marries his first cousin or an uncle marries his niece, as the scarcity of matrimonial elements may render it necessary,...it is within these populations that one observes...inborn deaf-mutism....**

It is now well-established that the vast majority of the nonsyndromic forms of congenital hereditary deafness are transmitted on the autosomal recessive mode. In developed countries, where most of the cases of prelingual, nonsyndromic deafness present as sporadic cases, we could recently estimate that more than two-thirds of these forms have a genetic origin[16] (see "Connexin 26 Defects: Clinical Features of DFNB1," below). This leads to a calculation that more than 80 percent of all congenital deafness cases are of genetic origin in these countries. The late onset forms of deafness were generally considered to result from a combination of genetic and environmental causes. However, an ever-increasing number of families with late onset deafness are being reported, indicating that the genetic contribution to late onset forms of deafness has undoubtedly been underestimated. Among these, otosclerosis deserves to be highlighted, as recent evidence has shown a significant genetic basis.[17]

To date, all the hereditary forms of deafness that have been analyzed, with few exceptions,[18–20] present as monogenic diseases. However, the phenotypic heterogeneity most frequently observed for a given mutation argues for the contribution of modifier genes.

## SYNDROMIC DEAFNESS

The 100 or so syndromes with hearing loss for which the causative gene has been identified are presented in Table 254-1. Data concerning the nature and the function of the encoded molecule, the mode of inheritance, as well as a short description of the organs most frequently affected and main clinical signs are included. The syndromic forms of deafness are classified in three categories: (a) conductive deafness due to middle ear and external ear defects, with or without a sensorineural component to the hearing loss; (b) conductive deafness due to middle ear defects, with or without a sensorineural component to the hearing loss, and (c) sensorineural deafness due to cochlear or retrocochlear defects.

Several syndromes (e.g., Waardenburg syndrome and Usher syndrome) are genetically heterogenous. Conversely, a single gene can underlie different syndromic deafness (see Table 254-1). In addition, several genes that underlie syndromic forms of deafness are also responsible for isolated forms of deafness. The following examples illustrate this: Pendred syndrome[21] and a recessive form of isolated deafness,[22] Stickler syndrome (type II)[23] and a dominant form of isolated deafness,[24] Usher syndrome1B[25] and two genetic forms of isolated deafness,[26–28] and Vohwinkel syndrome[29] and two genetic forms of isolated deafness[30,31] (see text and Table 254-2). In most instances, no direct correlation can be drawn between the type of the mutations and the association with a syndromic or a nonsyndromic form of hearing loss.

## NONSYNDROMIC (ISOLATED) DEAFNESS

The nonsyndromic forms of hereditary deafness are classified according to their mode of inheritance: DFN, DFNA, and DFNB refer to deafness forms inherited on the X chromosome-linked, autosomal dominant and autosomal recessive modes of transmission, respectively. The specific difficulties encountered by the chromosomal mapping of these forms explain why the identification of the causative genes began only a few years ago. These difficulties were mainly due to (a) the extreme genetic heterogeneity of these deficits, (b) the absence of clinically distinctive signs for the various gene defects, (c) the tendency of deaf people to marry together in developed countries.[32] These difficulties were circumvented mainly by studying deaf families living in geographic isolates. The first two genes responsible for autosomal dominant and autosomal recessive forms of nonsyndromic deafness were mapped in families from Costa Rica[33] and Tunisia,[34] respectively. Today, 53 loci have been identified: 21 for the DFNA forms, 26 for the DFNB forms, 4 for the DFN forms, and 2 linked to the mitochondrial genome. Only the forms with an identified gene are considered here. Together, several reviews[35–37] and the OMIM (www.ncbi.nlm.nih.gov) and "hereditary hearing loss homepage" (http://hgins.uia.ac.be/dnalab/hhh) websites provide regularly updated lists of identified loci for the isolated forms of deafness, the underlying genes and associated mutations. We focus on those of the auditory defects for which enough additional information has been obtained after the gene identification to provide some insight into the underlying pathogenesis. Much attention will also be paid to forms for which the discovery of the gene has clinical implications. The deafness forms for which the primary target of the inner ear defect is known are presented first. They are divided into three categories according to whether the primary target is the sensory hair cells, nonsensory cell types, or the acellular tectorial membrane. Table 254-2 summarizes the data presently obtained on these nonsyndromic deafness forms. The forms of deafness with an identified gene but without additional data are briefly presented thereafter.

Several mouse mutants present with an isolated inner ear defect. For all of these mutants, with the exception of one,

**Table 254-1 Syndromic Deafness**

Syndromic deafness with external and middle ear anomalies, with (+) or without (−) a sensorineural component to the Hearing Loss

| Syndrome | SN* | Gene | Protein | Function | Inheritance† | Chromosomal localization | Syndrome (gene) MIM number | Other affected organs & clinical signs | References |
|---|---|---|---|---|---|---|---|---|---|
| Branchio-oto-renal | + | EYA1 | EYA1 | transcriptional coactivator | AD | 8q13.3 | | preauricular pits & tags branchial fistulas | |
| | | | | | | | 113650 | with renal anomalies | 327 |
| | | | | | | | 602588 | without renal anomaly | 328 |
| Trichorhinophalangeal type I | + | TRPS1 | TRPS1 | putative transcription factor | AD | 8q24.12 | 190350 | short stature clinodactyly cone-shaped epiphyses craniofacial anomalies | 329 |
| Townes-Brocks | + | SALL1 | SALL1 | transcription factor | AD | 16q12.1 | 107480 | preaxial polydactyly imperforate/malpositioned anus preauricular pits & tags foot anomalies renal anomalies cardiac malformations | 330 |
| Mandibulofacial dysostosis (Treacher Collins-Franceschetti) | − | TCOF1 | Treacle | nucleolar transporter | AD | 5q32–33.1 | 154500 | microtia mandibular hypoplasia cleft palate eyelid coloboma | 331 |
| Fanconi pancytopenia | − | FAA | FAA | DNA repair | AR | 16q24.3 | 227650 | generalized pancytopenia pigmentary anomalies | 332 |
| | | FAC | FAC | DNA repair | AR | 9q22.3 | 227645 | urogenital & cardiac defects limb malformations high leukemia incidence | 333 |

*(Continued on next page)*

*The presence (+) or absence (−) of a sensorineural (SN) component to the hearing loss is indicated.
AD = autosomal dominant; AR = autosomal recessive.

6287

# Table 254-1 (Continued)

Syndromic deafness with middle ear anomalies, with (+) or without (−) a sensorineural component to the hearing loss

| Syndrome | SN* | Gene | Protein | Function | Inheritance† | Chromosomal localization | Syndrome (gene) MIM number | Other affected organs & clinical signs | References |
|---|---|---|---|---|---|---|---|---|---|
| Crouzon craniofacial dysostosis | − | FGFR2 | FGFR2 | fibroblast growth factor receptor | AD | 10q26 | 123500 | craniosynostosis, craniofacial malformations, hypertelorism, exophthalmos | 334, 335 |
| (+ acanthosis nigricans) | | FGFR3 | FGFR3 | | | 4p16.3 | | + hyperkeratosis, + hyperpigmentation | 336 |
| Acrocephalosyndactyly type V (Pfeiffer) | − | FGFR1 | FGFR1 | fibroblast growth factor receptor | AD | 8p11.1 | 101600 | craniosynostosis, craniofacial malformations | 337 |
| | | FGFR2 | FGFR2 | fibroblast growth factor receptor | | 10q26 | | broad thumb & toe, hypertelorism | 338, 339 |
| Acrocephalosyndactyly type I (Apert) | − | FGFR2 | FGFR2 | fibroblast growth factor receptor | AD | 10q26 | 101200 | craniosynostosis & spine malformations, short stature, hand & foot syndactyly, mental retardation, hypertelorism | 340 |
| Jackson-Weiss craniosynostosis | + | FGFR2 | FGFR2 | fibroblast growth factor receptor | AD | 10q26 | 123150 | craniosynostosis, craniofacial, hand & foot malformations, hypertelorism | 334 |
| Achondroplasia | + | FGFR3 | FGFR3 | fibroblast growth factor receptor | AD | 4p16.3 | 100800 | craniofacial & skeletal malformations, short-limb dwarfism | 341, 342 |
| Muenke craniosynostosis | +/− | FGFR3 | FGFR3 | fibroblast growth factor receptor | AD | 4p16.3 | 602849 | craniosynostosis, craniofacial & limb malformations | 343 |
| Acrocephalosyndactyly type III (Saethre-Chotzen) | + | TWIST | TWIST | transcription factor | AD | 7p21 | 101400 (601622) | craniofacial & limb malformations, syndactyly | 344–346 |
| | | FGFR2 | FGFR2 | fibroblast growth factor receptor | | 10q26 | (176943) | eyelid ptosis, strabism | 347 |
| | | FGFR3 | FGFR3 | fibroblast growth factor receptor | | 4p16.3 | (134934) | hypertelorism | 346 |
| Cleidocranial dysostosis | + | CBFA1 | CBFA1 | transcription factor | AD | 6p21 | 119600 | craniofacial & skeletal malformations (clavicles hypoplasia), dental anomalies | 348 |

| Disease | | Gene | Protein | Function | Inheritance | Location | OMIM | Clinical features | Ref. |
|---|---|---|---|---|---|---|---|---|---|
| Dyschondrosteosis (Leri-Weill) | — | SHOX | | transcription factor | XD | Xpter-22.32 | 127300 | forearm malformations, mesomelic dwarfism | 349, 350 |
| Campomelic dysplasia | ? | SOX9 | | transcription factor | AD | 17q24.3–25.1 | 114290 | craniofacial & skeletal malformations, mental retardation, sex reversal, respiratory deficiency, early death | 351, 352 |
| Osteogenesis imperfecta type I | +/− | COL1A1 | collagen I α1 chain | cartilage collagen | AD | 17q21–22 | 166200 (120150) | bone fragility, skeletal deformity, joint hyperextensibility | 353 |
| | V | COL1A2 | collagen 1 α2 chain | | | 7q22.1 | (120160) | eye blue sclerae, valvular insufficiency | 354 |
| type IV | +/− | COL1A1 | collagen I α1 chain | | AD | 17q21–22 | 166220 (120150) | bone fragility, skeletal deformity, joint hyperextensibility, dentinogenesis imperfecta | 355 |
| | | COL1A2 | collagen I α2 chain | | | 7q22.1 | (120160) | | 356 |
| Spondyloepiphyseal dysplasia congenita | + | COL2A1 | collagen II α1 chain | cartilage collagen | AD | 12q13.1–13.3 | 183900 | skeletal dysplasia, short stature, myopia | 357 |
| Kniest metatropic dysplasia | +/− | COL2A1 | collagen II α1 chain | cartilage collagen | AD | 12q13.1–13.3 | 156550 (120140) | skeletal dysplasia, dwarfism, stiff + enlarged joints, facial anomalies, cleft palate, myopia | 358 |
| Stickler arthroophthalmopathy type I | + | COL2A1 | collagen II α1 chain | cartilage collagen | AD | 12q13.1–13.3 | 108300 (120140) | facial & skeletal anomalies, cardiac malformations, cleft palate, severe myopia | 359 |
| type III | V + | COL11A1 | collagen XI α1 chain | fibrillar collagen | AD | 1p21 | (120280) | | 360 |
| Marshall | +/− | COL11A1 | collagen XI α1 chain | | AD | | 154780 (120280) | flat midface & hypertelorism | 361, 362 |
| type II | + | COL11A2 | collagen XI α2 chain | | AD | 6p21.3 | 184840 (120290) | without eye anomalies | 23 |
| neonatal form (Weissenbacher-Zweymuller) | +/− | | | | AR | | 277610 (120290) | fetal chondrodysplasia, with eye anomalies | 287 |
| Otospondylo-megaepiphyseal dysplasia (Nance-Insley/Sweeney) | +/− | | | | AR | | 215150 (120290) | with saddle nose | 23 |
| Ehlers-Danlos type VI | + | PLOD | protocollagen lysyl hydroxylase | collagen crosslinking | AR | 1p36.2–.3 | 225400 | spine deformation, joint laxity, heart & vascular defects, fragile skin, keratoconus, myopia | 363 |

(Continued on next page)

6289

Table 254-1 (Continued)

| Syndrome | SN* | Gene | Protein | Function | Inheritance† | Chromosomal localization | Syndrome (gene) MIM number | Other affected organs & clinical signs | References |
|---|---|---|---|---|---|---|---|---|---|
| Mucopolysaccharidosis type I (Hurler, Scheie) | + | IDUA | α-L-iduronidase | lysosomal enzyme | AR | 4p16.3 | 252800 | craniofacial & skeletal malformations corneal opacity hepatosplenomegaly mental retardation & early death (Hurler) | 364 |
| Mucopolysaccharidosis type II (Hunter) | +/− | IDS | iduronate 2-sulfatase | lysosomal enzyme | XR | Xq27.3 | 309900 | craniofacial & skeletal malformations cardiovascular defects hepatosplenomegaly mental retardation & early death (severe) | 365 |
| Mucopolysaccharidosis type III (Sanfilippo A) (Sanfilippo B) | + | HSS | sulfamidase | lysosomal enzyme | AR | 17q25.3 | 252900 | facial anomalies mental retardation | 366 |
| | | NAGLU | N-acetyl-α-glucosaminidase | lysosomal enzyme | AR | 17q21 | 252920 | facial anomalies mental retardation | 367, 368 |
| Mucopolysaccharidosis type IV (Morquio A) (Morquio B) | +/− | GALNS | galactosamine 6-sulfatase | lysosomal enzyme | AR | 16q24.3 | 253000 | facial & skeletal malformations corneal opacity dental anomalies | 369 |
| | | β-GAL | β-galactosidase | lysosomal enzyme | AR | 3p14–21 | 253010 | without dental anomalies | 370 |
| Mucopolysaccharidosis type VI (Maroteaux-Lamy) | + | ARSB | arylsulfatase B | lysosomal enzyme | AR | 5q11–13 | 253200 | facial & skeletal malformations hepatosplenomegaly corneal opacity heart defect | 371 |
| Mucopolysaccharidosis type VII (Sly) | + | GUSB | β-glucuronidase | lysosomal enzyme | AR | 7q21.11 | 253220 | facial & skeletal malformations hepatosplenomegaly | 372 |
| Symphalangism | − | NOG | noggin | transforming growth factor antagonist | AD | 17q22 | 185800 | multiple vertebral & limbs synostoses carpal & tarsal bone fusion | 373 |
| Facioaudio-symphalangism (Herrmann) | | | | | | | 186500 | + abnormal facies & long nose brachydactyly | 373 |
| Metaphyseal chondrodysplasia (Murk Jansen) | − | PTHR | parathyroid hormone receptor | hormone receptor | AD | 3p21.1–22 | 156400 | short limb dwarfism skeletal, facial & cranial dysplasia | 374 |

| Syndrome | Hearing defect* | Gene | Protein | Function | Inheritance† | Chromosomal localization | Syndrome (gene) MIM number | Other affected organs & clinical signs | References |
|---|---|---|---|---|---|---|---|---|---|
| Chondrodysplasia punctata 1 | ? | CDPX1 | arylsulfatase E | vitamin K metabolism? | XR | Xp22.3 | 302950 | distal phalanges & nasal hypoplasia atrophic & pigmentary skin lesions short stature | 375 |
| Chondrodysplasia punctata 2 (Conradi-Hünermann) | ? | EBP | hydroxysteroid -Δ8- isomerase (emopamil-binding protein) | sterol biosynthesis | XD | Xp11.22–.23 | 302960 | with short proximal limbs with cataract | 376, 377 |
| Keutel | +/– | MGP | γ-carboxyglutamic acid protein | extracellular matrix protein | AR | 12p12.3–13 | 245150 | midfacial hypoplasia ENT cartilage calcification brachytelephalangism pulmonary stenosis | 378 |
| Polyostotic fibrous dysplasia (McCune-Albright) | + | GNAS1 | guanine nucleotide-binding protein | adenylate cyclase stimulatory G-protein | AD | 20q13.1 | 174800 | skeletal asymmetry craniofacial anomalies café-au-lait spots endocrine hyperfunction blindness | 379 |
| Osteopetrosis with renal tubular acidosis | + | CA2 | CA2 | carbonic anhydrase | AR | 8q22 | 259730 | osteosclerosis cerebral calcification short stature hepatosplenomegaly optic nerve atrophy | 380, 381 |

*The presence (+) or absence (–) of a sensorineural (SN) component to the hearing loss is indicated.
†AD = autosomal dominant; AR = autosomal recessive; XD = dominant X chromosome-linked; XR = recessive X chromosome-linked.
Minor external ear anomalies such as low-set ears and/or minor malformed auricles may be occasionally associated with some of these syndromes.

## Sensorineural syndromic deafness

| Syndrome | Hearing defect* | Gene | Protein | Function | Inheritance† | Chromosomal localization | Syndrome (gene) MIM number | Other affected organs & clinical signs | References |
|---|---|---|---|---|---|---|---|---|---|
| G$_{M2}$ gangliosidosis (Tay-Sachs) | ? | HEXA | hexosaminidase A | lysosomal enzyme | AR | 15q23–24 | 272800 | psychomotor degeneration seizures nystagmus blindness recurrent infections early death | 382 |
| Globoid cell leukodystrophy (Krabbe) | ? | GALC | galacto-cerebrosidase | lysosomal enzyme | AR | 14q31 | 245200 | psychomotor degeneration optic atrophy retinal cherry-red spots early death | 383–385 |
| Aspartyl glucosaminuria | ? | AGU | Aspartyl glucosaminidase | lysosomal enzyme | AR | 4q32–33 | 208400 | mental retardation coarse facies frequent infections | 386, 387 |

(Continued on next page)

6291

**Table 254-1 (Continued)**

| Syndrome | Hearing defect* | Gene | Protein | Function | Inheritance† | Chromosomal localization | Syndrome (gene) MIM number | Other affected organs & clinical signs | References |
|---|---|---|---|---|---|---|---|---|---|
| α-Mannosidosis | ? | MANB | α-mannosidase | lysosomal enzyme | AR | 19cen–q12 | 248500 | mental retardation<br>ataxia<br>dysostosis<br>coarse facies<br>frequent infections<br>lens opacities | 388 |
| β-Mannosidosis | ? | MANB1 | β-mannosidase | lysosomal enzyme | AR | 4q22–25 | 248510 | mental retardation<br>coarse facies<br>frequent infections | 389 |
| Sialidosis | ? | NEU | neuraminidase | lysosomal enzyme | AR | 6p21.3 | 256550 | coarse facies<br>dysostosis<br>skeletal dysplasia<br>*late-onset (type I):* myoclonus,<br>macular cherry-red spots<br>*infantile-onset (type II):* seizures,<br>mental retardation,<br>hepatosplenomegaly | 390, 391 |
| Galactosialidosis (Goldberg) | ? | PPCA | cathepsin A | serine protease | AR | 20q13.1 | 256540 | mental retardation<br>coarse facies<br>dysostosis<br>myoclonus<br>macular cherry-red spots | 392 |
| α-Galactosidase deficiency (Fabry) | ?<br>V | GLA | α-galactosidase | lysosomal enzyme | XR | Xq22.1 | 301500 | angiokeratoma<br>cataract<br>pain attack<br>cardiac anomalies<br>nephropathy | 393 |
| Fucosidosis | ? | FUCA1 | α-L-fucosidase | lysosomal enzyme | AR | 1p34 | 230000 | coarse facies<br>dysostosis<br>angiokeratoma<br>mental & growth retardation<br>seizures<br>recurrent infections<br>visceromegaly | 394 |
| Niemann-Pick (type C) | IE, RC | NPC1 | NPC1 | lysosome transport membrane protein | AR | 18q11–12 | 257220 | ataxia<br>seizures<br>neurological degeneration<br>hepatosplenomegaly<br>early death | 395 |

| Disease | Defect | Gene | Gene product | Inheritance | Location | MIM No. | Phenotype | Ref. |
|---|---|---|---|---|---|---|---|---|
| Gaucher-like | IE | GBA | β-glucosidase (lysosomal enzyme) | AR | 1q21 | 231005 | heart valves calcification, corneal opacities, hydrocephalus | 396, 397 |
| Myopathy, encephalomyopathy, lactic acidosis, & strokelike episodes (MELAS) | IE, RC | MTTL1 | tRNA$^{leu(UUR)}$ | mito | mito | 540000 (590050) | encephalopathy, myopathy (ragged-red fibers), lactic acidosis, strokelike episodes, short stature | 398, 399 |
| | | ND4 (MTND4) | NADH dehydrogenase | mito | mito | (516003) | | 400 |
| Ballinger-Wallace | IE, V | del 10.4 kb ± 4.6 kb duplication | | mito | mito | 520000 | non-insulin-dependent diabetes, external ophthalmoplegia | 401 |
| Diabetes-deafness | | MTTL1 | tRNA$^{leu(UUR)}$ | mito | mito | (590050) | seizures | 402, 403 |
| Kearns-Sayre | IE, V | large deletions | | mito | mito | 530000 | ophthalmoplegia, retinitis pigmentosa, cardiac conduction defect, cerebellar dysfunction | 404 |
| | | MTTL2 | tRNA$^{leu(CUN)}$ | mito | mito | (590055) | | 405 |
| Cardiomyopathy-deafness | ? | MTTI | tRNA$^{ile}$ | mito | mito | 510000 (590045) | cardiomyopathy | 406 |
| | | MTTL1 | tRNA$^{leu(UUR)}$ | mito | mito | (590050) | myopathy (ragged-red fibers) + encephalomyopathy | 407 |
| | | MTTK | tRNA$^{lys}$ | mito | mito | (590060) | | 408 |
| Myoclonic epilepsy with ragged-red fibers (MERRF) | RC | MTTK | tRNA$^{lys}$ | mito | mito | 545000 (590060) | myoclonic epilepsy, myopathy (ragged-red fibers), encephalopathy, ataxia | 409 |
| | | MTTL1 | tRNA$^{leu(UUR)}$ | mito | mito | (590050) | pyruvic ± lactic acidosis | 410 |
| Cardiomyopathy-diabetes-deafness | ? | MTTL1 | tRNA$^{leu(UUR)}$ | mito | mito | (590050) | diabetes mellitus, cardiomyopathy, renal dysfunction | 411 |
| Ataxia-myoclonus-deafness | IE, RC | MTTS1 | tRNA$^{ser(UCN)}$ | mito | mito | (590080) | ataxia, myoclonus | 319 |
| Palmoplantar keratoderma-deafness | IE | MTTS1 | tRNA$^{ser(UCN)}$ | mito | mito | 148350 | palmoplantar keratoderma | 318 |
| Retinitis pigmentosa-deafness | ? | MTTS2 | tRNA$^{ser(AGY)}$ | mito | mito | 601850 (590085) | retinitis pigmentosa | 412 |
| Myoneurogastrointestinal encephalomyopathy (MNGIE) | RC | deletions | | mito | mito | 550900 | gastrointestinal dysfunction, leukoencephalopathy, neuropathy | 413, 414 |
| | | TP | thymidine phosphorylase (nucleoside synthesis) | AR | 22q13-ter | 603041 | myopathy (ragged-red fibers), ophthalmoplegia | 415 |
| Leber optic atrophy | ? | ND1 (MTND1) | NADH dehydrogenase | mito | mito | 535000 | optic neuropathy, dystonia, cardiac dysrhythmia | 416 |

*(Continued on next page)*

## Table 254-1 (Continued)

| Syndrome | Hearing defect* | Gene | Protein | Function | Inheritance† | Chromosomal localization | Syndrome (gene) MIM number | Other affected organs & clinical signs | References |
|---|---|---|---|---|---|---|---|---|---|
| Wolfram/diabetes insipidus & mellitus with optic atrophy (DIDMOAD)‡ | IE, RC | *deletions* | | | mito | mito | 598500 | diabetes mellitus + insipidus optic atrophy | 417 |
| | | *ND* | MTND | NADH dehydrogenase | | | (516003) | blood cytopenia urinary tract hypotonia | 418, 419 |
| | | *WFS* | wolframin | transmembrane protein | AR | 4p16.1 | 222300 | mental retardation psychiatric disorders | 420, 421 |
| Adrenoleukodystrophy | RC | *ALD* | ALDP | peroxisomal membrane transporter | XR | Xq28 | 300100 | adrenal insufficiency neurological degeneration peripheral neuropathy blindness hyperpigmentation | 422 |
| Cerebro-hepato-renal (Zellweger)‡ | RC | *PEX1* | peroxin 1 | peroxisomal membrane ATPase | AR | 7q21–22 | 214100 | mental retardation seizures hypotonia dysmorphism retinopathy hepatomegaly | 423–425 |
| | | *PEX2* | PAF1 (peroxin2) | peroxisomal membrane Zn-binding transporter | | 8q21.1 | | | 426 |
| | | *PEX5* | peroxin5 | PTS1 receptor | | 12p13.3 | | | 427 |
| | | *PEX10* | peroxin10 | peroxisomal membrane transporter | | ? | | | 428, 429 |
| | | *PEX12* | peroxin12 | peroxisomal membrane Zn-binding transporter | | ? | | | 430, 431 |
| | | *PEX13* | peroxin13 | peroxisomal SH3-domain membrane protein | | 2p15 | | | 432 |
| | | *PEX19* | peroxin19 | peroxisomal membrane protein | | 1q22 | | | 433 |
| | | *PXMP1* | PMP70 | peroxisomal membrane protein | | 1p21–22 | | | 434 |
| Neonatal adrenoleukodystrophy‡ | RC | *PEX1* | peroxin1 | peroxisomal membrane ATPase | AR | 7q21–22 | 202370 | mental retardation seizures dysmorphism retinopathy hepatomegaly | 423–425 |
| | | *PEX5* | peroxin5 | PTS1 receptor | | 12p13.3 | | | 427 |
| | | *PEX10* | peroxin10 | peroxisomal membrane transporter | | ? | | | 428, 429 |

| Disease | | Gene | Protein | Function | | Location | OMIM | Clinical features | Ref. |
|---|---|---|---|---|---|---|---|---|---|
| | | *PEX12* | peroxin12 | peroxisomal membrane Zn-binding transporter | | ? | | adrenal insufficiency | 430, 431 |
| | | *PEX13* | peroxin13 | peroxisomal SH3-domain membrane protein | | 2p15 | | | 432 |
| Phytanic acid oxidase deficiency (Refsum) | IE, RC | *PAHX/PHYH* | phytanoyl-CoA hydroxylase | lipid metabolism | AR | 10pter-11.2 | 266500 | neuropathy, ataxia, skeletal abnormalities, pigmentary retinopathy, cataract, ichthyosis, cardiac defect, anosmia | 435, 436 |
| Refsum infantile‡ | RC | *PEX1* | peroxin1 | peroxisomal membrane ATPase | AR | 7q21–22 | 266510 | mental retardation, ataxia, pigmentary retinopathy, dysmorphism, hepatomegaly | 423, 424 |
| | | *PEX12* | peroxin12 | peroxisomal membrane Zn-binding transporter | | ? | | | 430, 431 |
| Pseudoneonatal adrenoleukodystrophy | RC | *ACOX1* | acylCoA oxidase | peroxisomal enzyme | AR | 17q25 | 264470 | mental retardation, hypotonia, seizures, dysmorphism, hepatomegaly | 437 |
| Adrenal hypoplasia (Addison) | ? | *DAX1* | DAX1 | nuclear hormone receptor | XR | Xp21.2–21.3 | 300200 | hypogonadotrophic hypogonadism | 438, 439 |
| Cockayne A | RC | *CKN1 ERCC8* | CSA | DNA repair | AR | 5 | 216400 | skin & eye UV-sensitivity → tumors, retinal degeneration, dysmorphism, neuropathy, growth & mental retardation | 440 |
| Cockayne B | RC | *CSB ERCC6* | CSB | DNA-simulated ATPase | AD | 10q11 | 133540 | + dementia, + early death | 441 |
| Xeroderma pigmentosum A | RC | *XPA* | XPA | DNA repair | AR | 9q22.3–31 | 278700 | | 442, 443 |
| Cockayne/Xeroderma pigmentosum B+ | | *XPB ERCC3* | XPB | DNA repair helicase | AD | 2q23 | 133510 | | 444 |
| Cockayne/Xeroderma pigmentosum D | | *XPD ERCC2* | XPD | DNA repair helicase | AR | 19q13.2 | 278730 | | 445 |
| Cockayne/Xeroderma pigmentosum G | | *XPG ERCC5* | XPG | DNA endonuclease | AR | 13q33 | 278780 | | 446 |

*(Continued on next page)*

**Table 254-1 (Continued)**

| Syndrome | Hearing defect* | Gene | Protein | Function | Inheritance† | Chromosomal localization | Syndrome (gene) MIM number | Other affected organs & clinical signs | References |
|---|---|---|---|---|---|---|---|---|---|
| Juberg-Marsidi | IE | XH2/XNP | X-helicase-2 | nucleotide excision repair | XR | Xq13 | 309590 | mental & growth retardation microgenitalism ocular anomalies | 447 |
| Biotinidase deficiency | RC | BTD | biotinidase | biotin metabolism | AR | 3p25 | 253260 | developmental retardation ataxia seizures optic atrophy skin anomalies ketolactic acidosis | 448 |
| Multiple carboxylase deficiency (biotin responsive) | ? | HLCS | holocarboxylase synthetase | biotin metabolism | AR | 21q22.1 | 253270 | idem neonatal onset | 449 |
| Hypophosphatemia vitamin D-resistant rickets | IE | PHEX | PHEX (phosphate regulating with homologies to endopeptidases on X chromosome) | endopeptidase | XD | Xp22.1–22.2 | 307800 | vitamin D-resistant rickets progressive ankylosis | 450 |
| type I | V | | | | | | | | |
| type II | ? | CLCN5 | CLCN5 | chloride channel | XD | Xp11.22 | 307810 | | 451 |
| Primary hypomagnesemia | ? | PCLN1 | paracellin-1 | tight junction protein | AR | 3q | 248250 | nephrocalcinosis hypomagnesemia hypercalciuria seizures ocular anomalies | 452 |
| Renal tubular acidosis | IE | ATP6B1 | H⁺-ATPase B1-subunit | proton pump | AR | 2cen–q13 | 267300 | renal tubular acidosis nephrocalcinosis rickets/osteomalacia | 453 |
| Pendred | IE V | PDS | pendrin | chloride-iodide transporter | AR | 7q31 | 274600 | goiter +/– hypothyroidism petrous bone malformation | 246 |
| Generalized thyroid hormone resistance (Refetoff) | IE | THRB | THRB | thyroid hormone β subunit receptor | AD | 3p24.3 | 190160 | hypothyroidism +/– goiter stippled epiphysis | 454 |
| | | | | | AR | | 274300 | idem | 455 |
| Hyperuricemia-deafness (Rosenberg) | IE V | PRPS1 | phosphoribosyl phosphate synthetase I | purine biosynthesis | X semiD | Xq22–24 | 311850 | hyperuricemia ataxia psychomotor retardation cardiac anomalies | 456 |
| Cofin-Lowry | IE | RSK2 | RPS6KA3 | ribosome kinase | XD | Xp22.1–22.2 | 303600 | severe psychomotor retardation coarse facies & hands | 457 |

| Disease | | Gene | Protein | Function | Inh. | Location | OMIM | Clinical features | Ref. |
|---|---|---|---|---|---|---|---|---|---|
| Acetylaspartic aciduria (Canavan) | RC | ASPA | aspartoacylase | aspartate metabolism | AR | 17p13-ter | 271900 | progressive skeletal deformations / severe psychomotor retardation / hypotonia / megalencephaly / optic atrophy / early death | 458 |
| Mohr-Mageroy | IE | DDP | DDP (deafness dystonia peptide) | mitochondrial import protein | X | Xq22 | 304700 | blindness / dystonia / mental retardation | 253, 307 |
| Myotonic dystrophy (Steinert) | IE, RC | DMPK | DMPK | protein kinase | AD | 19q13.2–13.3 | 160900 | myotonia / muscular dystrophy / cardiac conduction defects / hypogonadism / cataract | 459 |
| Oculopharyngeal muscular dystrophy | IE | PABP2 | poly(A)-binding protein-2 | DNA binding protein | AD / AR | 14q11.2–13 | 164300 / 257950 | oculopharyngeal myopathy / dysphagia | 460 |
| Friedreich ataxia | RC V | FRDA | frataxin | mitochondrial ATP production | AR | 9q13 | 229300 | spinocerebellar degeneration / optic atrophy / cardiomyopathy | 461 |
| Charcot-Marie-Tooth (HMSN1) & deafness | IE | PMP22 | PMP22 | peripheral myelin protein | AD | 17p11.2 | 118300 | motor & sensory neuropathy / hypotonia | 462 |
| Hypertrophic neuropathy of Dejerine-Sottas (HMSN3) | ? | | | | | | 145900 | skeletal & limb extremity deformities | 463 |
| Hereditary neuropathy with liability to pressure palsies (HNPP) | | | | | | | 162500 | *idem* + pressure palsies | 464 |
| Charcot-Marie-Tooth (HMSN1) X-linked CMTX1 | ? | GJB1 (CX32) | connexin32 | gap junction protein | XD | Xq13.1 | 302800 | *idem* | 185 |
| Mutilating keratoderma & deafness (Vohwinkel) | IE | GJB2 (CX26) | connexin26 | gap junction protein | AD | 13q11 | 124500 | hyperkeratosis / constrictions of fingers & toes | 29 |
| Long QT syndrome (Jervell & Lange-Nielsen) | IE | KCNQ1/ KvLQT1 | KCNQ1 | K$^+$ channel | AR | 11p15.5 | 220400 | long QT interval / arrhythmia | 95 |
| | | KCNE1/ISK | KCNE1 | K$^+$ channel | | 21q22.1-22.2 | (176261) | sudden death | 216, 465 |
| Nephropathy & deafness (Alport) | IE | COL4A3 | collagen IV α3 chain | basement membrane collagen | AR | 2q36–37 | 203780 (120070) | glomerulonephritis / hematuria | 466, 467 |
| | V | COL4A4 | collagen IV α4 chain | idem | AR | 2q36–37 | 203780 (120131) | | 467 |

*(Continued on next page)*

**Table 254-1 (Continued)**

| Syndrome | Hearing defect* | Gene | Protein | Function | Inheritance† | Chromosomal localization | Syndrome (gene) MIM number | Other affected organs & clinical signs | References |
|---|---|---|---|---|---|---|---|---|---|
|  |  | COL4A5 | collagen IV α5 chain | idem | XD | Xq22 | 301050 (303630) | + anterior lenticonus + esophageal leiomyomatosis | 468, 469 |
| Neurofibromatosis type I (von Recklinghausen) | RC | NF1 | neurofibromin | tumor suppressor | AD | 17q11.2 | 162200 | neurofibromas various tumors café-au-lait spots Lisch nodules optic glioma scoliosis | 470–472 |
| Neurofibromatosis type II | RC V | NF2 V | merlin/ schwannomin | cytoskeleton-membrane interacting protein | AD | 22q12.2 | 101000 | schwannomas nervous system tumors cataract | 473, 474 |
| von Hippel-Lindau | ? | VHL | pVHL | tumor suppressor (multiprotein complex) | AD | 3p25–26 | 193300 | retinal angiomata cerebellar hemangioblastoma renal carcinoma pheochromocytoma pancreatic cysts | 475 |
| Waardenburg type I | IE V | PAX3 | PAX3 | transcription factor | AD | 2q35 | 193500 | dystopia canthorum broad & high nasal root white forelock congenital leukoderma heterochromia iridis | 476–478 |
| type II | IE | MITF | MITF | pigmentation transcription factor | AD | 3p12.3–14.1 | 193510 | without dystopia canthorum | 479 |
| type III (Klein-Waardenburg) | IE | PAX3 | PAX3 | transcription factor | AD | 2q35 | 148820 | with dystopia canthorum upper limb contractures mental retardation | 480 |
| Craniofacial-deafness-hand syndrome |  |  |  |  |  |  | 122880 | flat face ulnar deviation of hands | 481 |
| type IV (Hirschsprung-Shah-Waardenburg) | IE | EDN3 EDNRB SOX10 | endothelin-3 EDNRB SOX10 | vasoactive peptide endothelin receptor transcription factor | AR | 20q13.2–13.3 13q22 22q13 | 277580 (131242) (131244) (602229) | white forelock isochromia iridis neonatal intestinal obstruction | 482, 483 484 485 |
| Waardenburg type II & ocular albinism | IE V | MITF + TYR | MITF & tyrosinase | pigmentation transcription factor & melanin biosynthesis enzyme | AD | 3p12.3–14.1 & 11q14–21 | 103470 | heterochromia iridis visual acuity loss strabismus unpigmented hair & skin patches | 18 |

| Syndrome | Defect* | Gene | Protein | Inheritance† | Locus | OMIM | Associated features | Reference |
|---|---|---|---|---|---|---|---|---|
| Piebaldism | IE | KIT | KIT | growth factor receptor tyrosine kinase | AD | 4q12 | 172800 | unpigmented hair & skin patches, white forelock, heterochromia iridis | 486 |
| Kallmann | IE | KAL-1 | anosmin-1 | extracellular matrix protein | XR | Xp22.3 | 308700 | hypogonadotropic hypogonadism, anosmia, renal agenesis, mirror movements, high-arched palate | 487, 488 |
| Usher type I | IE, V | USH1B/MYO7A | myosin VIIA | unconventional myosin | AR | 11q13.5 | 276903 | retinitis pigmentosa (1st decade onset) | 25 |
|  |  | USH1C | harmonin | PDZ domains-containing protein | AR | 11p15.1 | 276904 | vestibular areflexia | 489 |
| type II | IE | USH2A | USH2A | extracellular matrix component | AR | 1q41 | 276901 | retinitis pigmentosa (late 2nd decade onset) | 490 |
| Norrie | IE | NDP | norrin | extracellular matrix component | XR | Xp11.4 | 310600 | mental retardation, microphthalmia, iris atrophy | 491–493 |
| Megaloblastic anemia thiamine-responsive (Rogers) | ? | THTR1/SLC19A2 | THTR1/SLC19A2 | transmembrane thiamine transporter | AR | 1q23.2–.3 | 249270 | diabetes mellitus, aminoaciduria, situs inversus | 494–496 |

*IE = inner ear defect; RC = retrocochlear defect; ? = unknown. V indicates vestibular dysfunction.
†AD = autosomal dominant; AR = autosomal recessive; XD = dominant X chromosome-linked; XR = recessive X chromosome-linked; mito = mitochondrial.
‡The ascription of the hearing loss to some of these genetic forms is uncertain.

**Table 254-2** Identified Gene Defects in Isolated Deafness

| Target | Gene | Protein | Human deafness | Mouse mutant | Type of molecule |
|---|---|---|---|---|---|
| Sensory hair cells | | | DFNB2 | | |
| | MYO7A | myosin VIIA | DFNA11 | shaker-1 | Motor protein |
| | | | Usher 1B* | | |
| | MYO15 | myosin XV | DFNB3 | shaker-2 | Motor protein |
| | Myo6 | myosin VI | | Snell's waltzer | Motor protein |
| | KCNQ4 | KCNQ4 | DFNA2 | | Potassium channel |
| | OTOF | otoferlin | DFNB9 | | Vesicle fusion protein? |
| | POU4F3 | POU4F3 | DFNA15 | $Brn3c^{-/-}$† | Transcription factor |
| | Atp2b2/Pmca2 | $Ca^{2+}$-ATPase type 2 | | deafwaddler | Calcium pump |
| Non sensory cells | | | DFNB1 | | |
| | CX26/GJB2 | connexin 26 | DFNA3 | | Gap junction protein |
| | | | Vohwinkel* | | |
| | CX30/GJB6 | connexin 30 | DFNA3' | | Gap junction protein |
| | CX31/GJB3 | connexin 31 | DFNA2' | | Gap junction protein |
| | | | DFNBi | | |
| | Slc12a2/Nkcc1 | $Na^+K^+2Cl^-$ cotransporter | | $sy^{ns}$ | Ion transporter |
| | | | | $Nkcc1^{-/-}$† | |
| | PDS | pendrin | DFNB4 | | Iodide-chloride transporter |
| | | | Pendred* | | |
| | POU3F4 | POU3F4 | DFN3 | $Brn4^{-/-}$† | Transcription factor |
| | COCH | cochlin | DFNA9 | | Extracellular matrix component |
| Tectorial membrane | COL11A2 | collagen XI (α2 chain) | DFNA13 | $Col11a2^{-/-}$† | Extracellular matrix component |
| | | | Stickler* | | |
| | TECTA | α-tectorin | DFNA8/12 | | Extracellular matrix component |
| | | | DFNB21 | | |
| | Otog | otogelin | | $Otog^{-/-}$† | Extracellular matrix component |
| Unknown | DIAPH1 | diaphanous-1 | DFNA1 | | Regulator of actin cytoskeleton |
| | DFNA5 | | DFNA5 | | ? |
| | 12S RNA | | MTRNR1 | | Mitochondrial ribosomal RNA |
| | tRNA$^{ser(UCN)}$ | | MINSD | | Mitochondrial transfer RNA |

*Syndromic deafness due to a defect in the same gene.
†Deaf mouse mutant obtained by targeted disruption of the gene.
See text for references.

*deafness (dn),*[38] the deafness is accompanied by vestibular dysfunction. The behavior of these mutants is characterized by circling behavior, head tossing, and an inability to swim. Such an association of vestibular symptoms associated with hearing loss is not surprising considering the high histologic and physiological similarities of the auditory and vestibular sensory organs. However, in humans, hereditary deafness is rarely associated with abnormal vestibular tests and patients exceptionally complain of balance problems. This discrepancy between the human and murine vestibular symptomatologies likely results from a more efficient cerebral compensation of peripheral vestibular defects in man. The rapid adaptive response of the human brain is evidenced by the rapid improvement (i.e., within a few days) of the acute vertigo provoked by a unilateral vestibular defect. The sensory substitution is based on the inputs of the visual and proprioceptive systems, which greatly contribute to balance in humans.

The mouse mutants with only an inner ear defect and which involve a gene orthologous to a human deafness gene are discussed jointly with the corresponding human forms of deafness. Mutants for which the human orthologous gene has not yet been implicated in deafness are presented separately, according to the target of the deficit (see Table 254-2).

## Forms of Deafness Caused by a Sensory Hair Cell Defect

**Myosin VIIA Defects: DFNB2, DFNA11, and USH1B Syndrome.** We mapped the second reported locus responsible for an autosomal recessive form of sensorineural deafness, DFNB2

(MIM 600060), to a 6 cM interval on chromosome 11q13.5 through the study of a highly consanguineous family living in the central part of Tunisia.[39] This region was homologous to the locus in the mouse genome to which the *shaker-1* phenotype (*sh-1*) had been assigned.[40] Seven *sh-1* alleles have been described.[41,42] Mutant animals exhibit head-tossing, circling behavior, and hyperactivity due to vestibular defects and a rapidly progressive hearing loss accompanied by neuroepithelial degeneration.[43] The locus for the Usher 1B syndrome (USH1B) in humans had also been mapped to this region of chromosome 11.[44] Usher syndrome is the most frequent cause of deafness associated with blindness. This syndrome is clinically and genetically heterogeneous. Three clinical subtypes (USH1, USH2, and USH3) have been distinguished.[45] The USH1 form, which is characterized by congenital sensorineural deafness, vestibular dysfunction, and retinitis pigmentosa beginning with a loss of night vision in late childhood or early adolescence, is the most severe. The USH1B locus had been evaluated to account for 75 percent of the Usher type I forms.[46] The colocalization of USH1B and DFNB2 suggested that a single gene could be responsible for both diseases. Thereafter, DFNA11 (MIM 601317), a progressive form of autosomal dominant sensorineural deafness was also mapped to the same chromosomal interval.[47]

Positional cloning of *sh-1* in the mouse led to the identification of a gene, *Myo7a*, predicted to encode an unconventional myosin, myosin VIIA. Because unconventional myosins were expected to play a role in the auditory mechanotransduction,[48,49] the myosin VIIA gene was considered to be a promising candidate for both

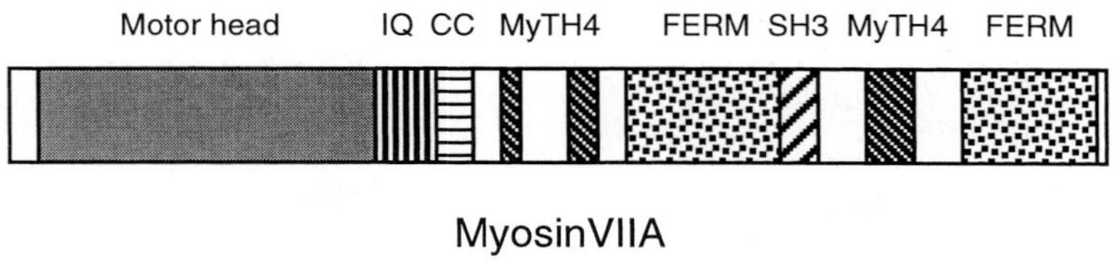

Motor head     IQ CC MyTH4     FERM SH3 MyTH4   FERM

## MyosinVIIA

**Fig. 254-6 Representation of myosin VIIA. This unconventional myosin consists of a motor head containing ATP- and actin-binding sequences, a neck region composed of five isoleucine-glutamine (IQ) motifs expected to bind to calmodulin, and a long tail of 1360 amino acids. The tail begins with a short coiled-coil (cc) domain, which is implicated in the formation of homodimers. The coiled-coil domain is followed by two large repeats, each containing a MyTH4** (myosin tail homology 4) and a FERM (4.1, ezrin, radixin, moesin) domains, which are separated by a poorly conserved SH3 (src homology-3) domain. The head of the protein moves along actin microfilaments. The functional specificity of each unconventional myosin is determined by its tail which greatly differs from one myosin to the other.

*sh-1* and the human USH1B and DFNB2 diseases. Mutations in exons encoding the motor head of myosin VIIA were detected concurrently in *sh-1* mutants[50] and in USH1B patients.[25] The mouse mutants, however, do not exhibit the retinal degeneration of the USH1B syndrome. Distinct *MYO7A* mutations were subsequently shown to be responsible for DFNB2 and DFNA11 (see "Pathogenesis," below).

Unconventional myosins form a large family that has been divided into 15 classes. These motor proteins move along the actin filaments using the energy generated by the hydrolysis of ATP. The N-terminal motor head possesses actin and ATP-binding sites, and is highly conserved between the various members of the family. The head is followed by a neck region expected to link to calmodulin and a tail that differs from one myosin to another. The tail sequence determines the functional specificity of each myosin because it contains various putative protein-protein interacting domains that bind to cargo molecules, regulatory factors, and components of the transduction pathways. Unconventional myosins have been implicated in the formation and the movements of cytoplasmic expansions, in the movements of vesicles, and in signal transduction.[51–53]

The human myosin VIIA (Fig. 254-6), 2215 amino acids in length (254 kDa), consists of a motor head domain of 729 amino acids, containing ATP- and actin-binding sequences, a neck region of 126 amino acids, composed of 5 IQ (isoleucine-glutamine) motifs expected to bind calmodulin, and a long tail of 1360 amino acids.[54] The tail begins with a short coiled-coil domain (78 amino acids), which is implicated in the formation of homodimers.[27] The coiled-coil domain is followed by two large repeats of about 460 amino acids, each containing a MyTH4 (myosin tail homology 4) and a FERM (4.1, ezrin, radixin, moesin)[55] domain, which are separated by a poorly conserved SH3 (src homology 3) domain.[56,57] The *MYO7A* gene consists of 48 coding exons (17 for the head, 3 for the neck, and 28 for the tail).[54]

***Clinical Features of DFNB2.*** Only three affected families have been reported. In each family, at least some patients complained of balance problems and/or had abnormal vestibular tests (calorimetric tests). The hearing loss was severe to profound and congenital, except in the originally described affected family in which the age of onset ranged from birth to 16 years. Furthermore, the mutation was not fully penetrant in this family.

***Clinical Features of DFNA11.*** In the single DFNA11 family reported to date, patients presented with a moderate bilateral hearing loss on all frequencies, which appeared in the first decade and then progressed. Vestibular anomalies were detected in some of the individuals.

***Pathogenesis.*** Most of the *Myo7a* mutations in *sh-1* mouse mutants affect the stability of the protein. Interestingly, in the various mutants, the severity of the phenotype and the histopathologic anomalies are well correlated with the level of protein preserved.[58] In humans, since the original report in 1995, dozens of

mutations have been found in USH1B-affected patients. Taking into account only the results obtained by mutation screenings covering all the coding exons, half of the mutations are missense or in-frame insertions/deletions.[59–63] In the original DFNB2 family,[39] a G > A substitution in the last nucleotide of exon 15 was observed.[27] Such a mutation is expected to result in the skipping of the mutated exon in a large proportion of the mature transcripts.[64] It is believed that the small amount of normal myosin VIIA that would be preserved in the patients is sufficient for the function in the retina but not in the inner ear. Two other mutations in *MYO7A* were concomitantly reported in two Chinese families affected with an autosomal recessive form of deafness.[26] One family was homozygous for a mutation leading to an amino acid substitution in the motor head. This mutation probably impairs the motor activity of the protein, but may preserve enough of it to permit normal function in the retina. Affected members of the second Chinese family were compound heterozygotes with a 1-bp insertion leading to a frameshift and truncation in the motor head on one allele and an acceptor splice site mutation on the other one. The absence of a retinal phenotype in this family is more difficult to explain, because the two mutations detected should lead to the complete absence of the normal protein.[26] This suggests an influence of the genetic background on the phenotypic expression. Finally, in the single DFNA11 family reported, a 9-bp in-frame deletion located in the dimerization domain of myosin VIIA tail was detected.[28] This mutation is likely to have a dominant negative effect.

Myosin VIIA is expressed in the photoreceptor cells and pigment epithelial cells of the retina, the hair cells of the inner ear, and a variety of epithelial cell types, which, in most cases, harbor apical microvilli.[65] In the mouse inner ear, myosin VIIA is expressed as early as E10,[65] and is thereafter exclusively detected in all the sensory hair cells.[66,67] Myosin VIIA is present all along the stereocilia, near the junction between hair cells and supporting cells[68] and in the synaptic region of the hair cells.[67] On the basis of the sublocalization of the protein, it has been proposed that myosin VIIA plays a role in (a) the anchoring of the lateral links, that is, fibrous material that connects each stereocilium to its neighbor in the hair bundle,[68] and (b) the trafficking of synaptic vesicles.[67] In the *shaker-1* mouse mutants, two types of hair cell anomalies have been detected by histologic analyses. In the most severely affected mutants, there is a disorganization of the hair bundle with clumps of stereocilia that project outside instead of forming the highly ordered U- or W-shaped structure. This suggests that myosin VIIA is involved in the normal arrangement of the stereocilia, a function that could be, at least in part, mediated by its role at the level of the lateral links. In addition, the kinocilium has an erratic position, thus indicating a role of myosin VIIA in the polarity of the hair bundle.[69] Moreover, it has been shown that inner and outer hair cells from *sh-1* mice, unlike those of the wild-type, do not uptake aminoglycosides.[70] This is indicative of a role of myosin VIIA in endocytosis. The identification of the molecules binding to the tail of myosin VIIA should help clarify the role of myosin VIIA in the formation and stabilization of the hair bundle and in the fluid phase endocytosis involved in aminoglycoside uptake. Other roles of

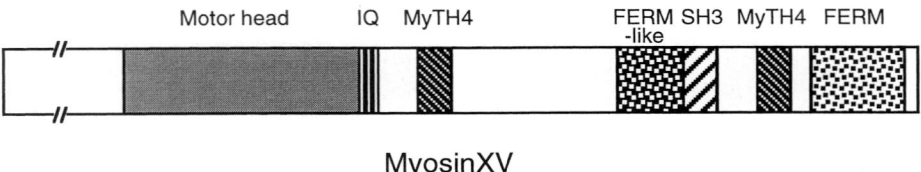

MyosinXV

Fig. 254-7 Representation of myosin XV. This unconventional myosin has a motor head containing ATP- and actin-binding sequences, a neck region containing two isoleucine-glutamine (IQ) motifs expected to bind to calmodulin, and a long tail of 1587 amino acids that comprises two MyTH4 (myosin tail homology 4) domains, one FERM (4.1, ezrin, radixin, moesin) domain and one FERM-like, and a SH3 (src homology-3) domain.

myosin VIIA have been documented. In the eye, myosin VIIA is implicated in the distribution of melanosomes by the pigment epithelium,[71] and participates in the transport of opsin through the kinocilium in the photoreceptors.[72] Finally, a class VII unconventional myosin in *Dictyostelium discoideum* amoeba has been shown to be involved in phagocytosis.[73] These results point to the existence of multiple cellular roles for myosin VIIA, which is not surprising, considering the various putative domains of protein-protein interaction that are present in the tail of this myosin.

The finding that mutations in *MYO7A* cause Usher1B, DFNB2, and DFNA11 was the first demonstration that a single gene can underlie both syndromic and nonsyndromic forms of deafness. This situation could extend to other genetic forms of Usher syndrome because the chromosomal intervals defined for several other DFNB and USH loci are overlapping, namely DFNB12 (MIM 601386)[74] and USH1D,[75] DFNB15 (MIM 601869)[76] and USH3,[77] DFNB18 (MIM 602902)[78] and USH1C.[79]

**Myosin XV Defect: DFNB3.** The identification of the locus responsible for the DFNB3 form (MIM 600316) represents a unique situation because it was characterized through the analysis of the population of a small village in Bali, in which 2.2 percent of the persons were deaf. Using allele frequency-dependent homozygosity mapping, the locus was assigned to an interval of about 5 cM on chromosome 17p11.2.[80] Based on conserved synteny, the deaf mouse mutant *shaker-2* (*sh-2*) was proposed to be affected in the orthologue of the DFNB3 gene.[81] Rescue of hearing and balance in *sh-2* mice was obtained by transgenesis of a bacterial artificial chromosome (BAC) covering the candidate region.[82] Sequencing of this BAC revealed a new unconventional myosin gene, *Myo15*, which, after the discovery that *MYO7A/Myo7a* (see above) and *Myo6* (see below) (Table 254-2) underlie deafness, was considered as a promising candidate gene. A missense mutation concerning a highly conserved amino acid residue of the motor head of this myosin was found in the *sh-2* mutant.[82] Recently, a deletion of *Myo 15* that removes the last 6 exons of the gene, was reported in *shaker-2^J*, another *shaker-2* mouse mutant.[497] Three different mutations in *MYO15* (MIM 602666), two missense and one nonsense, in the tail of the protein, were detected in three unrelated DFNB3 families, that is, the one originally described and two others from India.[83]

This new myosin was divergent enough from the other unconventional myosins to define a new class, which was designated myosin XV. This classification is further supported by recent results which show that some isoforms of myosin XV contain an additional sequence of 1223 amino acids upstream of the motor head. Myosin XV is composed of 3530 amino acids (395 kDa). The neck contains two IQ motifs. The tail is 1587 amino acid long and comprises two MyTH4 domains, one FERM-like and one FERM domain, and an SH3 domain between the FERM-like domain and the C-terminal MyTH4 domain (Fig. 254-7). The gene contains 65 coding exons[84].

***Clinical Features of DFNB3.*** Clinical features of DFNB3 have so far only been described in the individuals of the three DFNB3-affected families mentioned above. Deafness was sensorineural,

profound, congenital, bilateral, and affected all frequencies. No apparent vestibular defect has been reported.

***Pathogenesis.*** In the inner ear, the *Myo15/MYO15* expression seems to be restricted to the hair cells. The protein was mainly detected in the stereocilia and within the apical cell body, in the region of the cuticular plate,[84] that is, a dense meshwork of horizontal actin filaments that run parallel to the apical cell surface (Fig. 254-8 and see Fig. 254-3C). This site of expression is consistent with the histopathologic findings in the *sh-2* mouse mutants. Even though the global organization of the hair bundle seems to be normal in these mutants, the stereocilia are particularly short. Moreover, the actin filaments of the stereocilia, unlike those from wild-type mice, extend a long distance under the apical surface of the cell. These anomalies suggest that myosin XV is involved in the regulation of actin polymerization. In addition to its expression in the inner ear, *Myo15/MYO15* is expressed in a few other tissues, including the pituitary gland.[84]

**Myosin VI Defect: *Snell's Waltzer* Mouse Mutants.** Two *Snell's waltzer* mouse mutants have been described: one (*sv*) is a spontaneous mutant[85] and the other (*se^sv*) was induced by irradiation. Using a positional cloning strategy that took advantage of a chromosomal rearrangement present in the *se^sv* mutant, the gene encoding the unconventional myosin VI was recognized as underlying this phenotype.[86] An intragenic 130-bp deletion located at the beginning of the neck region of the protein was detected in the *sv* mutant. The cDNA sequence predicts a 1266-amino-acid protein (Fig. 254-9). The tail begins with a coiled-coil region, suggesting that this myosin forms a dimer, and ends by a globular structure. Myosin VI is characterized by a hydrophobic stretch of 53 amino acids located between the motor head and the single IQ motif. This sequence, called converter, is responsible for a property unique to myosin VI, namely its movement in a direction opposite to that of all other types of myosins. Myosin VI moves toward the minus end of the actin track (the positive end being defined as the end where actin subunits are added at high rate).[87] In mammalian hair cells, myosin VI is concentrated in the cuticular plate (see Fig. 254-3C). It is also present in the region surrounding the cuticular plate.[68] Although present in the stereocilia of frog hair cells, this myosin is absent from mammalian stereocilia. Histopathologic analysis revealed that the hair cells of the Snell's waltzer mutant do not survive in mice older than 6 weeks and neither do the supporting cells thereafter. In these mice, the hair bundle of stereocilia is disorganized and the adjacent stereocilia progressively fuse.[88] Several hypotheses have been proposed to account for this observation. An attractive one is that myosin VI is normally anchored to the apical membrane by its tail and thereby acts to pin this membrane down between the stereocilia; hence, the tendency of the stereocilia to fuse in the absence of myosin VI. Interestingly, the binding of some actin filaments of the cuticular plate to the apical surface has been demonstrated in the chicken.[89] The orthologous human gene, *MYOVI*, located in the centromeric region of chromosome 6, has been characterized.[90] However, no human deafness locus has yet been reported in this chromosomal region.

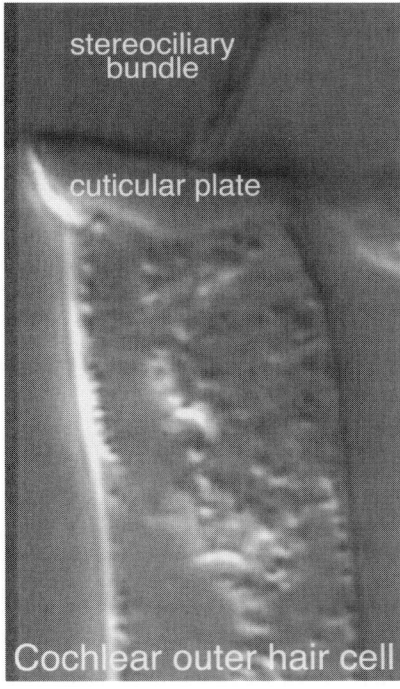

Fig. 254-8 Distribution of myosin XV in the outer hair cells of the cochlea (guinea pig). The structure of the apical region of the cell is presented on the left. The right panel shows the myosin XV immunoreactivity of the cuticular plate and stereocilia.

**KCNQ4 Potassium Channel Defect: DFNA2.** The DFNA2 locus was identified through the study of three families from Indonesia, the Netherlands, and the United States, which were affected by a progressive form of sensorineural deafness involving preferentially the high frequencies (MIM 600101). This locus was initially mapped to the short arm of chromosome 1[91] and the localization was subsequently refined to 1p34.[92] The discovery of a gene encoding a new member of the KCNQ voltage-dependent K+-channel family,[93] *KCNQ4*, which mapped to the DFNA2 chromosomal interval and was expressed in the inner ear, led us to consider this gene as a candidate for DFNA2. The finding of a missense mutation (G285S) that (a) affects the GYG consensus sequence required for the K+ selectivity of the channel pore,[94] and (b) abolishes, in cotransfected *Xenopus* oocytes, the potassium current through the normal KCNQ4 channel subunits, established that *KCNQ4* underlies DFNA2.[93]

KCNQ4 is the second member of the KCNQ voltage-dependent K+-channel family to be involved in deafness (see Table 254-1, the autosomal recessive Jervell and Lange-Nielsen syndrome involving *KCNQ1* (or *KvLQT1*) (MIM 220400)[95]). This family of K+ channels is characterized by six transmembrane

domains with an intramembrane P loop between domains 5 and 6, and by cytoplasmic N- and C-terminal regions. The P loop forms the K+ selective pore and the fourth transmembrane domain contains the voltage sensor. These channels are either homomultimeric or heteromultimeric. Heteromeric channels are composed of either different KCNQ subunits[96] or one KCNQ and one KNCE (also termed Isk or minK) subunits.[97,98]

The *KCNQ4* cDNA encodes a predicted 695-amino acid protein with a structure typical of voltage-dependent K+ channels (Fig. 254-10), and a predicted molecular mass of 77 kDa. The gene consists of 14 coding exons[93].

***Clinical Features of DFNA2.*** Of the three DFNA2 families initially analyzed,[91] two were shown to carry a mutation in

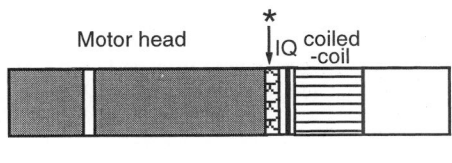

## MyosinVI

Fig. 254-9 Representation of myosin VI. This unconventional myosin has a motor head containing ATP- and actin-binding sequences, a neck region containing a single isoleucine-glutamine (IQ) motif expected to bind to calmodulin, and a short tail that begins with a coiled-coil region and ends by a globular structure. Myosin VI is characterized by a hydrophobic stretch of amino acids located between the motor head and the IQ motif (*). This sequence, called converter, is responsible for the movement of myosin VI toward the minus end of the actin track (that is in a direction opposite to that of all other known myosins).

## KCNQ4 potassium channel

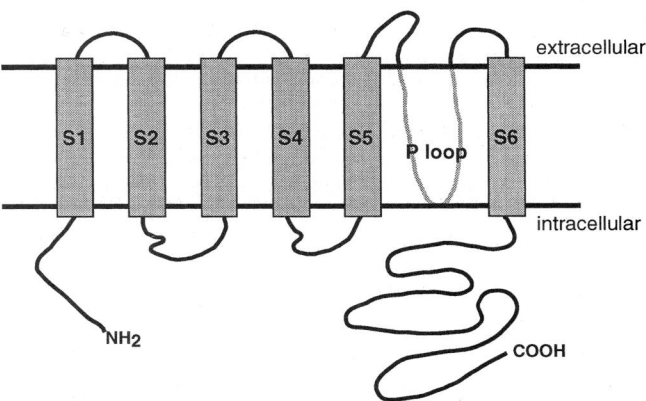

Fig. 254-10 Representation of the voltage-dependent K+ channel KCNQ4. This potassium channel subunit has a predicted structure typical of voltage-dependent K+ channels, with six transmembrane domains and an intramembrane P loop between domains 5 and 6. The P loop underlies the K+ selectivity of the pore and the 4th transmembrane domain (S4) contains the voltage sensor.

*KCNQ4.*[99] The deafness segregating in the third family turned out to be linked to an adjacent locus. A total of five families with an identified mutation in *KCNQ4* have been clinically analyzed.[91,93,100,101] In all of them, the hearing loss was sensorineural, initially predominating on high frequencies and then progressing to affect all frequencies. The progression has been estimated at about 1 dBHL per year for all frequencies.[100] The severity of the hearing loss was mild to profound, and the age of onset varied from birth to 30 years. Important intrafamilial variations of the phenotype were observed. Several patients complain of tinnitus, that is, a sensation of ringing sounds in the ears.

**Pathogenesis.** Five distinct mutations have been reported in DFNA2 patients. Two missense mutations result in the substitution of the same glycine residue (G285) of the P loop domain by a serine[93] or a cysteine.[99] Two other missense mutations were found in the P loop and sixth transmembrane domain, respectively. Finally, a small deletion before the first transmembrane domain is predicted to create a truncated protein.[99]

By voltage-clamp experiments in the *Xenopus* oocyte expression system, KCNQ4 was shown to form a channel selective for the potassium ion.[93] In the cochlea, KCNQ4 is expressed by the OHC, in a decreasing gradient from the base to the apex of the cochlea. In the vestibular end organs, KCNQ4 was only detected in type I hair cells. In OHC, KCNQ4 has a basal localization, whereas it is present in nearly the entire basolateral membrane of the type I hair cells, as well as in the facing postsynaptic membrane.[102] Several lines of evidence suggest that KCNQ4 underlies the $I_{K,n}$ and $I_{K,L}$ currents that have been described in the outer and type I hair cells, respectively. These currents are expected to be active already at the resting potentials of these cells and to influence their electrical properties.[103–106] Intriguingly, KCNQ4 was also detected in many nuclei of the auditory pathway including ventral cochlear nuclei, superior olivary complex, nuclei of the lateral lemniscus and inferior colliculus.[102] The expression of the protein also in the auditory pathway raises the possibility that the DFNA2 form of deafness involves not only a defect of the peripheral sensory organ, but also a central defect.

**Otoferlin Defect: DFNB9.** The DFNB9 locus was identified through the analysis of a consanguineous family from Northern Lebanon, which was affected by a profound prelingual hearing loss (MIM 601071). The causative gene had been assigned to a 2-cM interval on chromosome 2p23.1.[107] We cloned the responsible gene, *OTOF* (MIM 603681), by a candidate gene approach, using a subtracted murine cochlear cDNA library.[108] The reconstituted cDNA predicts a 1977-amino-acid (227-kDa) protein, otoferlin,[109,498] which exhibits homology with the spermatogenesis factor, fer-1, described in *Caenorhabditis elegans*[110] (and see "Pathogenesis"). A homozygous nonsense mutation (Y730X) was detected in the original DFNB9 family, as well as in three other families from Lebanon.[109] Two other *OTOF* mutations have since been reported in splice sites.[498,499]

Sequence analysis predicts a protein with a transmembrane domain close to the C-terminal end. It also indicates that the rest of the protein is cytoplasmic and composed of either three or six C2 domains (see "Pathogenesis") (Fig. 254-11).

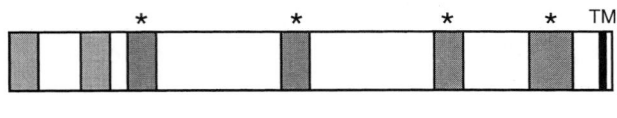

Otoferlin

**Fig. 254-11 Representation of otoferlin. The six predicted C2 domains of the protein are represented by gray boxes. Only the last four domains (indicated by asterisks) are expected to bind calcium. TM indicates the predicted transmembrane domain.**

Approximately 100 C2 domains have been described in various proteins, and for one of them, the C2A domain of rat synaptotagmin-1,[114] the three-dimensional structure has been established as well as its $Ca^{2+}$ binding sites.[115] Sequence comparison predicts that four of the six C2 domains of otoferlin bind $Ca^{2+}$. The isolation of several cDNA clones has revealed alternatively spliced forms.[498] Otoferlin belongs to the same protein family as dysferlin, a protein defective in Miyoshi myopathy and limb girdle muscular dystrophy type 2B,[111,112] and myoferlin.[113] The gene is approximately 90 kb long and is composed of 48 coding exons.[498]

**Clinical Features of DFNB9.** In all DFNB9 families examined, including a family from Eastern Turkey linked to this locus but with a yet-unidentified mutation,[116] deafness has been described as sensorineural, severe or profound, fully penetrant, affecting all frequencies and with an age of onset before 2 years.

**Pathogenesis.** The orthologous murine gene, *Otof*, is expressed at low levels in several tissues. Strong expression is restricted to the inner ear and the brain. In the mature cochlea, the *Otof* transcript is restricted to IHC. However, transient weak expression was detected in OHC during early postnatal life. In the vestibular organs, the gene is mainly expressed in type I hair cells.[109]

The C2-domain proteins are known to interact with phospholipids and proteins[117] and fall into two functional categories; they may be implicated either in the generation of the lipid second messengers involved in transduction pathways, or in membrane trafficking. This second category includes several proteins such as synaptotagmins, rabphilin 3A, munc 13, DOC2 proteins, and RIM, which are involved in the docking of the synaptic vesicles to the plasma membrane and/or their fusion.[118–124] Even though the function of *C. elegans* fer-1 is not yet entirely elucidated, this protein seems to be required for the final step of the fusion between vesicles and the plasma membrane.[110] Based on the expression of *Otof* in the sensory hair cells, the well-established interactions of C2 domains with phospholipids, and the impaired cellular process in *C. elegans fer-1* mutants, we hypothesized that otoferlin is involved in $Ca^{2+}$-triggered fusion of synaptic vesicles to the plasma membrane. The synapses of cochlear and vestibular hair cells, termed ribbon synapses (see Fig. 254-3C), have particular structural features (an electron-dense matrix surrounded by neurotransmitter vesicles), as well as specific functional[125] and biochemical[126] characteristics (e.g., they are devoid of synaptotagmins I and II). Therefore, otoferlin may have a crucial role in the synaptic vesicular trafficking of these particular synapses.

**POU4F3 Transcription Factor Defect: DFNA15.** In a family from Libya affected by an autosomal dominant form of deafness, the responsible locus, DFNA15 (MIM 602459), was mapped to 5q31.[127] The presence in the same chromosomal region of *POU4F3* that encodes the transcription factor POU4F3 (MIM 602460) known to be required for the survival of the sensory hair cells, prompted the authors to search for a mutation in this gene. A small deletion observed in affected individuals implicated *POU4F3* as the causative gene for DFNA15. The POU4F3 transcription factor is a 338-amino-acid protein belonging to the POU family; it is encoded by two exons.

**Clinical Features of DFNA15.** In the single DFNA15-affected family reported, hearing loss was detected between 18 and 30 years of age.[127] The auditory defect, which was sensorineural, moderate to severe, initially affected the mid and high frequencies, and progressively affected all frequencies. The mutation was fully penetrant.

**Pathogenesis.** The POU domain protein family is a subclass of homeodomain proteins that exhibit cell-specific expression and control early differentiation processes in certain cell lineages. The POU domain (Fig. 254-12) is a bipartite DNA-binding domain, composed of a POU-specific domain (POU$_S$, approximately 75

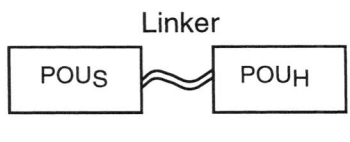

## POU Domain

**Fig. 254-12 Representation of the POU DNA-binding domain. The POU domain, which characterizes POU transcription factors, is a bipartite DNA-binding domain composed of a POU-specific domain (POU$_S$) and a POU-homeodomain (POU$_H$), joined by a hypervariable linker, between 15 and 56 amino acids in length. Cooperation of the POU$_S$ and POU$_H$ domains increases the binding affinity and specificity of these transcription factors for their target DNA.**

amino acids) and a POU-homeodomain (POU$_H$, 60 amino acids), both of which are highly conserved. These two segments are joined by a hypervariable linker sequence between 15 and 56 amino acids long. The POU$_S$ and POU$_H$ domains both contain helix-turn-helix motifs. Cooperation of the two domains increases the binding affinity and specificity for their target DNA. The POU-domain proteins are classified into seven classes (POU I to VII) based on the sequence of the POU$_H$ domain and linker region. Outside the POU-domain, the divergence between members of a given group is considerable. *POU4F3* belongs to class IV.

The *POU4F3* 8-bp deletion that was detected in the DFNA15 family predicts a truncated protein with a partial deletion of the POU$_H$ domain including its DNA-binding site.[127] The role of the murine orthologue of *POU4F3*, *Brn-3.1* (or *Brn-3c*), in the survival of cochlear and vestibular hair cells was established by the study of the expression profile of the gene and the study of mouse mutants with a targeted null mutation of the gene. *Brn-3.1* has a restricted expression pattern; it is expressed in a few neuronal cell populations and in the inner ear. In the inner ear, the transcript is found exclusively in postmitotic sensory hair cells.[128,129] In *Brn-3.1* null mice, no mature cochlear and vestibular hair cells can be detected.[128,130] However, some immature hair cells are present (without hair bundles); they eventually undergo apoptosis, followed by degeneration of auditory and vestibular ganglion neurons. This indicates that *POU4F3* is not involved either in the commitment of precursor cells to develop into hair cells or in their early differentiation. Rather, it seems to be required for the migration of the hair cells from the supporting cell layers to the luminal hair cell layer, and for their maturation and survival.[129] The target genes of POU4F3 are presently unknown.

**Ca$^{2+}$-ATPase Type 2 Pump Defect: *Deafwaddler* Mouse Mutant and Targeted Disruption of *Pmca2*.** The deafwaddler (*dfw*) mouse mutant is deaf and displays vestibular imbalance. Two deafwaddler alleles, *dfw* and *dfw$^2$* have been described.[131,132] The causative gene was mapped to a region of the murine chromosome 6 to which the *Atp2b2/Pmca2* gene encoding the Ca$^{2+}$-ATPase type 2 pump, had also been assigned. This Ca$^{2+}$-ATPase has 10 putative transmembrane domains (T) with the intracellular loop between T2 and T3 forming the transduction domain that couples ATP hydrolysis with Ca$^{2+}$ translocation, the large intracellular loop between T4 and T5 being involved in the ATP binding, and the intracellular C-terminus binding to several regulatory molecules[133,134] (Fig. 254-13). Considering the role of Ca$^{2+}$ in the sensory hair cells (see below), *Atp2b2* was considered an excellent candidate gene. In *dfw*, a missense mutation was found in the transduction domain. In *dfw$^{2J}$*, a 2-bp deletion was detected, creating a frameshift and predicted to result in a protein truncated at the level of T4. In the *dfw$^{2J}$* homozygotes, a paucity of stereocilia bundles was noted.[135]

In addition, a null mutant has been generated by targeted disruption of the *Pmca2* gene.[136] As in *dfw* natural mutants, homozygous null mutants exhibit hearing and balance deficits. The balance deficit of *Pmca2$^{-/-}$* mice could be correlated with an absence of otoconia in the vestibular system, thereby indicating a crucial role of the plasma membrane Ca$^{2+}$-ATPase in the formation of these calcitic biominerals. In the cochlea, regions in which the organ of Corti was almost normal coexisted with regions in which the cell architecture was markedly altered. Analysis of auditory-evoked brain stem responses also revealed that heterozygous *Pmca2$^{+/-}$* mice have a significant hearing loss.

The mechanism of the hearing and balance deficits in the *Atp2b2/Pmca2* mutant mice is still unclear. Based on the detection of this Ca$^{2+}$-ATPase type 2 pump in vestibular and cochlear sensory hair cells by *in situ* hybridization[137] and/or immunohistochemistry,[135] it has been suggested that these cells are the primary target cells of the genetic defect.[135] At the apical pole of the hair cells, the opening of the mechanotransduction channel results in a significant increase of the Ca$^{2+}$ concentration in the stereocilia despite the low Ca$^{2+}$ concentration in the endolymph.[138] The Ca$^{2+}$ concentration in the stereocilia is thought to control the adaptation process, namely the decrease of the

## Ca$^2$+ ATPase type 2 pump

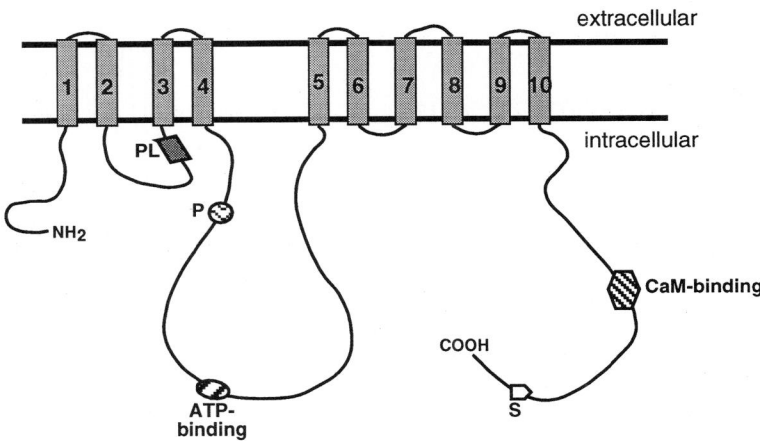

**Fig. 254-13 Representation of the Ca$^{2+}$-ATPase type2 pump. This Ca$^{2+}$-ATPase has 10 putative transmembrane domains (T1 to T10). Three main domains are believed to protrude into the cytoplasm: one between T2 and T3, the second (the largest) between T4 and T5, and the third from T10. Because of this membrane arrangement about 80 percent of the pump is found in the cytoplasm. The internal loop between T2 and T3 forms the transduction domain that couples ATP hydrolysis with Ca$^{2+}$ translocation. The ATP-binding site is located in the large loop between T4 and T5, and P indicates the site of phosphoenzyme formation. The protein is characterized by its long C-terminal cytoplasmic fragment, that contains most of the sites involved in the multifarious regulation of the pump; only the calmodulin (CaM)-binding domain and the site of phosphorylation by protein kinase A (S) are represented. In addition, a phospholipid-responsive site of regulation (PL) in the internal loop between T2 and T3 is indicated.**

transduction current which is observed in response to sustained stimulation. $Ca^{2+}$ is believed to modulate, via its binding to calmodulin, the activity of a myosin that gates the mechanotransduction channel. In the absence of an intracellular compartment that can sequester $Ca^{2+}$ (i.e., mitochondria, endoplasmic reticulum) within the stereocilia, the $Ca^{2+}$-ATPase located in the membrane of the stereocilia[139,140] is thought to play a crucial role in the extrusion of $Ca^{2+}$.[141] However, whereas the physiological significance of adaptation is clear for vestibular hair cells, where prolonged static displacements naturally occur during which sensitivity to transient stimuli must be maintained, the function of adaptation in the mammalian cochlea is less obvious.[142] At the basal pole of the hair cells, $Ca^{2+}$ mediates neurotransmitter vesicle exocytosis. The $Ca^{2+}$-ATPase pump, which is also located in the basolateral membrane of the hair cells, is thought to play a role in clearing the synaptic cell region of the $Ca^{2+}$ that has entered this subregion (via voltage-dependent $Ca^{2+}$ channels) upon membrane depolarization induced in response to mechanical stimulation. However, a possible contribution to the mutant phenotype of other inner ear structures that also express the *Pmca2* gene (e.g., the cochlear ganglion, the Reissner's membrane, and the inner sulcus of the cochlea[137]), should also be considered. Finally, some behavioral anomalies have been reported in *deafwaddler* mice, which may be accounted for by the presence of this $Ca^{2+}$ pump in the brain.[135]

No deafness locus has so far been identified in the human 3p25-26 chromosomal region homologous to the murine region containing *Atp2b2/Pmca2*.

### Forms of Deafness Caused by Nonsensory Cell Defects

**Connexin 26 Defects: DFNB1, DFNA3, and Vohwinkel Syndrome.** In 1994, we reported the first locus for an autosomal recessive form of deafness, DFNB1 (MIM 220290), on chromosome 13q12, through the study of two Tunisian families affected by profound prelingual sensorineural deafness.[34] Subsequently, we localized to the same chromosomal region a gene that is implicated in a family affected by a dominant form of deafness, DFNA3 (MIM 601544).[143] We thus suggested that defects in a single gene could underlie both DFNB1 and DFNA3. In 1997, the gene encoding connexin 26, *GJB2* or *CX26* (MIM 121011), was considered a candidate gene for these two deafness forms as it maps to 13q12 and had been shown to be expressed in the inner ear.[1] Two distinct nonsense mutations were discovered in three consanguineous deaf Pakistani families, thus establishing that *GJB2* is responsible for DFNB1.[30] In the same article, a heterozygous nucleotide change responsible for the amino acid substitution M34T was reported in a small family affected by a dominant form of hearing impairment. The causality of this mutation in hearing loss is still controversial. Indeed, on the one hand, the nucleotide change was found in several normal-hearing individuals, arguing in favor of an asymptomatic polymorphism.[31,144,145] On the other hand, when the mutated allele was tested in the *Xenopus* oocyte expression system,[146] electrical intercellular communication could not be detected.[147] In 1998, another missense mutation, W44C, was detected in the original DFNA3 family.[31]

*GJB2* has also been tentatively implicated in dominant forms of deafness with skin anomalies. A missense mutation, R75W, was found in members of a family affected by prelingual deafness and a diffuse fissured keratoderma, but the implication of this mutation in the phenotype was unclear as the mutation was also present in an unaffected member of the family.[148] Recently, another missense mutation, D66H, was discovered as segregating with a syndromic form of deafness, the Vohwinkel syndrome (MIM 124500), in three unrelated families.[29] This syndrome is characterized by mutilating keratoderma and moderate sensorineural deafness. Together, the present results demonstrate that *GJB2* underlies DFNB1, DFNA3, and Vohwinkel syndrome. The involvement of the gene in deafness associated with

diffuse fissured keratoderma, although very likely, still awaits confirmation.

***Clinical Features of DFNB1.*** The major feature concerning DFNB1 is the high prevalence of this form of deafness. First evidence arose soon[149] after the identification of the locus.[34] By studying small families affected by an autosomal recessive form of sensorineural deafness from New Zealand, a genetic linkage consistent with the involvement of the DFNB1 locus was observed in half of the families.[149] Thereafter, segregation analysis performed in patients from Spain and Italy, affected by sensorineural autosomal recessive deafness, established a linkage to the DFNB1 locus in 79 percent of them.[150] Upon the identification of *GJB2* as responsible for DFNB1, mutation screening confirmed the high prevalence of *GJB2* defects in the deaf populations. Soon after, a particular mutation named 30delG or 35delG was found to account for the majority of mutant alleles, in Mediterranean European populations (Italy, Spain, and France).[151,152] This mutation deletes a guanine (G) in a sequence of six G extending from nucleotide position 30 to 35 (Fig. 254-14), which results in a premature stop codon at codon position 13. The following picture is emerging. Among the autosomal recessive forms of isolated sensorineural deafness, a *CX26* defect is

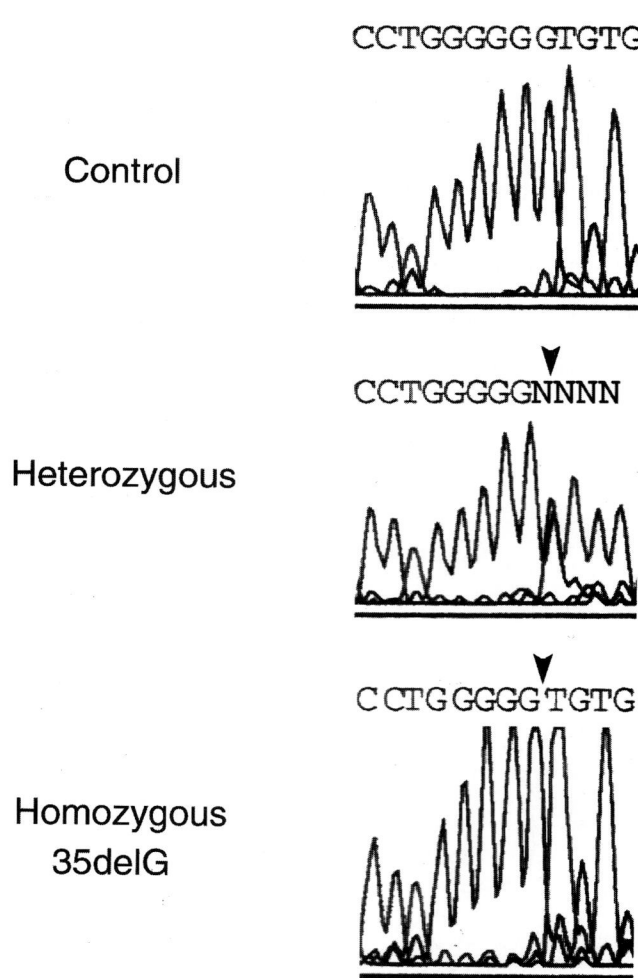

**Fig. 254-14 Electrophoregram profiles showing the 35delG mutation of *CX26* (*GJB2*) in an individual with recessively inherited hearing loss, and in his heterozygous parents. Mutations of the gene encoding connexin 26 account for about half of the cases of prelingual isolated deafness in Caucasian populations. The 35delG mutation is by far the most frequent of the *CX26* mutations in Mediterranean European countries.**

implicated in 56 percent of the cases in France,[16] 35 to 42 percent in Italy and Spain,[153,154] 40 to 58 percent in the United States,[144,155] 28 percent in the United Kingdom,[156] 41 percent in Israel,[157] and 12 to 33 percent in Japan.[158,159]

The 35delG mutation was established to account for up to 85 percent of the *CX26* mutations detected in deaf children in Mediterranean European countries,[16,153] 70 percent in the United States,[155] and 58 percent in Israel.[157] As a result of this finding, the frequency of this mutation has been estimated in various normal-hearing populations. This mutation was found in 4 percent of the general population from Italy, 2.3 percent from Spain,[153] 3.5 percent from Greece,[160] 2.3 percent from Belgium,[161] and between 0.58 percent and 2.5 percent in the Caucasian population from United States.[144,155,162] However, this mutation has not been observed in deaf children from Japan,[158,159] nor in African American or Asian populations. Due to the nature of this mutation, namely a deletion within a stretch of six G (that may favor the slippage of the polymerase) as well as the existence of several different haplotypes associated with the mutation, its high frequency was initially thought related to a mutational hot spot. The data obtained later concerning its geographic distribution argue in favor of an ancestral mutation that initially spread out around the Mediterranean Sea. Two other mutations are particularly frequent in specific populations. The 167delT mutation is frequently detected among deaf Ashkenazi Jews.[163] In Israel, this mutation represents 42 percent of the *CX26* mutations.[164] The 167delT mutation is associated with a specific haplotype, thus indicating a single origin of the mutation. Four percent of the normal-hearing Ashkenazi Jewish population were found to be carriers. Finally, the 235delG mutation, although less documented, seems to account for a large proportion of the *CX26* mutations in the Japanese population.[158,159] As a whole, the worldwide high frequency of the *CX26* mutations, compared to those of *CX30* and *CX31*, is puzzling. It raises the possibility that *CX26* mutations confer a selective advantage to carrier individuals. A great number of other mutations have been detected in *CX26*; these are presented on the CX26 homepage (http://hgins.uia.ac.be/dnalab/hhh/). For some of the missense mutations, whether they are responsible for hearing loss is still being debated. For several deaf patients, a *CX26* mutation was detected on one allele only, indicating either the existence of another *CX26* mutation in the unexplored region of the gene or the possible coimplication of another connexin gene (i.e., a digenic origin of the hearing loss related to the putative formation of heteromeric connexons or heterotypic channels).

Efforts to characterize the clinical features of DFNB1 have led to the following picture: *CX26* mutations have so far been exclusively associated with prelingual forms of sensorineural deafness.[16,157,159] Several investigators have observed that the degree of severity of deafness associated with *CX26* defects varies from mild to profound. Thus, the severity of the hearing loss in 35delG homozygous individuals may vary greatly, even between siblings.[16,155,165] Audiometric curves (see Fig. 254-1) are either flat or sloping with a preferential loss at high frequencies. High-resolution temporal bone computerized tomography did not reveal any anomaly, and the vestibular tests, when performed, were normal.[16] Finally, the hearing loss has been reported as nonprogressive in about two-thirds of the cases.[16,165] These findings have important implications for genetic counseling. In general, the request for a genetic counseling comes from hearing parents who have a single deaf child and who wish to be informed of the risk of having other affected children. Because of the high prevalence of *CX26* mutations, and the ease of the molecular diagnosis, in such families, the genetic origin of the hearing loss can be established in a high proportion of the cases, even in the absence of any suggestive family history. If *CX26* underlies the hearing loss, families can be informed about the possible variability of the severity of the deficit amongst siblings and about its probable absence of progression in affected individuals. The high prevalence of the *CX26* mutations in the autosomal recessive forms has made it possible to estimate the proportion of

the sporadic cases that are of genetic origin. In France, Italy, Spain, and the United States, about 35 to 40 percent of the congenital sporadic cases of deafness were found to present bi-allelic *CX26* mutations. Taking into account these bi-allelic mutations only, this results in a minimal estimation of about 65 percent to 80 percent of cases of sporadic deafness being of genetic origin.

***Clinical Features of DFNA3.*** Only two families unambiguously affected by DFNA3, have been described.[31,166] Their phenotypes were different. In the initially reported one, affected individuals were suffering from a sensorineural severe to profound hearing impairment, with a prelingual onset. In the other family, the hearing loss was detected between 10 and 20 years of age in most of the affected individuals. The degree of severity of the hearing loss was variable between affected individuals. The defect was restricted to high frequencies during the first decade, and progressed to mid-frequencies between 10 and 50 years of age.

***Pathogenesis.*** Most adjacent cells communicate via membrane channels tightly packed in aggregates at the level of gap junction plaques. In vertebrates, these channels are composed of two hemichannels, the connexons, which are hexamers of connexins. The connexons contributed by two neighboring cells, after docking, form a channel allowing the intercellular exchange of small diffusible molecules such as ions, metabolites, and second messengers (cyclic AMP, inositol 1,4,5-triphosphate, $Ca^{2+}$) up to a molecular mass of 1 kDa;[167] this communication between adjacent cells is essential for functional synchronization, for example, for the electrical activity of the myocardium and some neurons, for growth, and for differentiation. Fifteen members of the connexin family, with an expected molecular mass ranging from 26 to 60 kDa and a common predicted structure[168] are known. Connexins have four transmembrane domains; their N- and C-terminal regions are intracytoplasmic (Fig. 254-15).

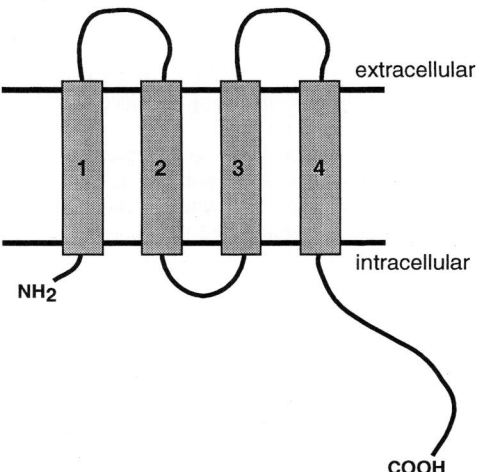

## Connexins 26, 30, 31

**Fig. 254-15** Representation of connexins 26, 30, and 31. Connexins associate into homo- or heterohexamers to form connexons. The connexons contributed by two neighboring cells form a channel allowing the intercellular exchange of ions, metabolites and second messengers up to a molecular mass of 1000 daltons. Connexins have four predicted transmembrane domains. The extracellular loops mediate interactions between connexons. Connexins 26, 30, and 31 belong to the GJ$\beta$ group of connexins, that is connexins having a short intracellular loop. The intracytoplasmic C-terminal region, which is an interacting domain, is different in size for each connexin. To date, little is known about the functional properties of the various connexins.

Each of the two extracellular loops contains three cysteine residues involved in intramolecular disulfide bonds. The extracellular loops mediate interconnexon interactions via noncovalent bonds. The intracellular loop is of a variable size. Whereas the current nomenclature of the connexins is based on their molecular weight deduced from their sequence, another one classifies the connexins into two groups, GJα and GJβ, characterized by long and short intracellular loops, respectively. The intracytoplasmic C-terminal region, which is an interacting domain, is different in size for each connexin.[169] Connexin 26 (or GJB2) has both a short intracellular loop and a short C-terminal region. The connexons are generally homomeric structures in which the six identical connexins are linked together through noncovalent bonds. However, some different connexins, such as Cx26 and Cx32, can assemble to form an heteromeric connexon.[170] Connexons of adjacent cells, which contribute to the formation of a given channel, can be composed of identical or different connexins, thus forming a homotypic or a heterotypic channel. The formation of heterotypic channels is limited by the compatibility between the connexins; for example, connexin 26 can form a channel with Cx32, Cx46, Cx50, but not with Cx31, Cx31.1, Cx37, Cx40, Cx43, and Cx45. The different connexins and their various combinations confer unique properties to the formed channels with regard to conductance, size and charge of the molecules exchanged,[171–175] and regulation of their gating (by transjunctional voltage, phosphorylation, cytosolic pH, $Ca^{2+}$, and cyclic nucleotides).[176–179] These properties have so far been mainly characterized in *Xenopus* oocyte assays and have been tentatively correlated with particular domains or residues of the protein.[169] Connexin 26 exhibits a greater permeability for positively versus negatively charged ions or molecules.[180] It has no consensus sequences for a phosphorylation by kinases.[181] The first extracellular loop[182] and proline-87 of the second transmembrane domain[183] have been implicated in the voltage control of its activity.

Connexins are differently expressed in tissues as well as during development.[184] Mutations in connexin genes underlie various inherited human disorders, including X-linked Charcot-Marie-Tooth (MIM 302800; *CX32* or *GJB1*),[185] two forms of zonular pulverulent cataract (CZP1, MIM 116200; *CX50* (*GJA8*)[186] and CZP3, MIM 601885; *CX46* (*GJA3*)[187]), erythrokeratodermia variabilis (MIM 133200;*CX31*) (see "Connexin 31 Defects," below)[188] and deafness (*CX26, CX30*, and *CX31*) (see "Connexin 31 Defects," below). The proposed role of *CX43* (*GJA1*) in heart malformations and defects of laterality (visceroatrial heterotaxy, MIM 208530)[189] is uncertain.[190]

The different connexin genes are remarkably similar and simple, with the first exon corresponding to the 5′-untranslated region and the second exon containing the complete open reading frame, as well as the 3′-untranslated region.

The *Cx26* cDNA was first isolated in the rat[191] and then in man.[192,193] The human *CX26* is composed of a first exon of 160 bp, the second exon (2136 bp) begins with 22 bp of 5′-untranslated region followed by an open reading frame of 624 bp and a 1490 bp 3′-untranslated region. The single intron is 3149 bp long. The gene encodes a predicted 208-amino-acid protein.

The rodent connexin 26 is expressed in several tissues including spleen, kidney, lung, pancreas, stomach, testis, leptomeninx, uterus, placental chorionic villi, and several endocrine (hypophysis, thyroid, parathyroid, pineal) and exocrine (mammary, salivary) glands. The transcript and/or the protein are particularly abundant in the liver and the inner ear.[1,191,194–200] No expression has been observed in the heart, skeletal muscle, prostate, and adrenal gland.[191,198]

*Cx26* has been shown to suppress the tumorigenicity in HeLa cells.[201] The tumor-suppressor activity of *Cx26* in human breast cancer has also been predicted[193] and was observed by transfection of the *Cx26* gene in human mammary carcinoma cells.[202] However, the role of the connexin in this process is far from being understood.[203]

Gap junctions in the inner ear were first reported in 1969, in the supporting cells of the saccular macula of the goldfish.[204] Gap junctions have been analyzed in the rat cochlea by light microscopy upon immunostaining of connexin 26 and by electron microscopy.[1] Because light microscopy detected connexin 26 labeling where electron microscopy showed gap junctions, it was concluded that connexin 26 enters in the composition of all gap junction plaques of the inner ear.[1]

Connexin 26 is expressed by all epithelial cells of the inner ear with the exception of the sensory hair cells, the epithelial cells of the spiral prominence, the cells of the Reissner's membrane, and the marginal cells of the stria vascularis. It is also expressed by the fibrocytes surrounding the epithelium of the membranous canal, that is, in the limbal and supra limbal regions as well as in the spiral ligament[1] (see Fig. 254-3*B*). Such networks of cells communicating by Cx26-positive gap junctions have been proposed to be the structural basis for a transcellular circulation of the perilymphatic $K^+$ and the $K^+$ released from the sensory hair cells, towards the endolymph.[1,205,206] Indeed, the endolymph most likely originates from the perilymph and not from the plasma.[207,208] The potassium of the perilymph is hypothesized to be taken up by the fibrocytes in closest proximity with the perilymph, thanks to their $Na^+$, $K^+$-ATPase. Thereafter, it is believed to be transferred to the basal cells of the stria vascularis, through the Cx26-positive fibrocyte network of the spiral ligament, along an electrochemical gradient. Likewise, the $K^+$ released from stimulated sensory hair cells has been hypothesized to be recycled across the Cx26 positive communicating epithelial cells of the neuroepithelium[209] and then to enter the fibrocyte network of the spiral ligament up to the stria vascularis.[1,205,206]

Within the stria vascularis, a $K^+$ gradient is generated, leading to a high secretion of $K^+$ in the endolymph by the marginal cells (see Fig. 254-5). The transport of $K^+$ in the marginal cells and its secretion in the endolymph are well documented. $Na^+$,$K^+$-ATPase (subunits $\alpha 1$ and $\beta 2$)[210,211] and the secretory isoform of $Na^+$-$K^+$-$2Cl^-$ cotransporter, both localized in the basolateral membrane of the marginal cells, take up the $K^+$ of the intrastrial compartment (i.e., between marginal and intermediate cells).[93,212,213] In the marginal cells, the secretion of $K^+$ in the endolymph is driven by the apical membrane potential (approximately $+10$ mV) via a voltage-dependent channel formed of two different subunits, KCNQ1 and KCNE1.[214] However, the precise cellular site of the generation of the endocochlear potential is still much debated. In the two-cell model (Fig. 254-5), the endocochlear potential is assumed to be generated by a $K^+$ conductance of the basal cells of the stria vascularis.[215] Interestingly, the genes encoding KCNQ1 and KCNE1 underlie deafness in man (Jervell and Lange-Nielsen syndrome),[95,216] and the $Na^+$-$K^+$-$2Cl^-$ cotransporter gene is responsible for deafness in mouse (*sy* and *sy*[ns] mutants and knockout mice)[217,218] (see "$Na^+$-$K^+$-$2Cl^-$ Cotransporterand Defects" and Table 254-2).

A role of CX26 in the transport of $K^+$ would account for the deafness because (a)$K^+$ carries most of the mechanotransduction current in hair cells and (b) the accumulation of the $K^+$ released from the hair cells is thought to be toxic for neighboring cells. However, it is worth noting that although connexins are surely involved in the transport of $K^+$ in the spiral ligament, the exact role of CX26 remains to be established. Furthermore, the role of the connexins of the neuroepithelium-supporting cells in the transport of the $K^+$ released from the sensory hair cells is presently entirely hypothetical. The *GJB2* knockout in the mouse is expected to contribute to clarify the pathogenesis of the defect. However, this knockout, which had already been achieved before the implication of CX26 in prelingual deafness was known,[219] is lethal early in embryonic life (E10). In the homozygous mutant mice, lethality is due to a deficient uptake of glucose through the placenta. Indeed, contrary to the human placenta, which contains one giant syncytiotrophoblast, the murine placenta consists of two layers of syncytiotrophoblast, interconnected by gap junctions that mediate the transport of nutrients such as glucose.[220] Therefore, only conditional or inducible knockouts in the inner ear could shed light on the role of connexin 26 in the development and functioning of the inner ear.

**Connexin 31 Defects: DFNA2′ and a DFNB Form.** Following the discovery of *GJB2* as the causative gene for DFNB1/DFNA3, an increasing attention was paid to other connexin genes as possible candidates for deafness. In this way, the implication of *GJB3*, encoding connexin 31, was found. The mouse[221] and rat[222] connexin 31 cDNAs were first isolated, and thereafter, the human orthologue was isolated.[223,224] The human gene encodes a 270-amino-acid (31-kDa)-predicted protein. In two small Chinese families affected by a dominant form of isolated deafness, two mutations in *GJB3* (*CX31*) were detected.[224] *GJB3* maps to the candidate gene interval of DFNA2 on 1p33-35 in which another deafness gene, *KCNQ4* (MIM 603537) (see "KCNQ4 Potassium Channel Defect: DFNA2," above) was identified; hence, the *CX31* (MIM 603324) associated form of deafness is referred to as DFNA2′. Recently, in two small Chinese families affected by an autosomal recessive form of deafness (named DFNBi in Table 254-2), deaf children were found to be compound heterozygotes for *GJB3* mutations establishing that *GJB3*, as does *GJB2*, underlies both dominant and recessive forms of deafness.[225] Interestingly, *CX31* has also been recognized as responsible for erythrokeratodermia variabilis (MIM 133200), but without association to deafness.[188] Thus, just like *CX26*, *CX31* underlies skin and inner ear defects, although no association of the two diseases in a syndromic form of deafness has yet been reported for *CX31*. The existence of these two independent diseases due to mutated *CX31* argues for distinct functions or regulations of this connexin in inner ear and skin.

*Clinical Features.* In the two DFNA2′-affected families described, the hearing loss starts after the second decade, is sensorineural, and affects only frequencies above 2000 Hz. In both families, the hearing loss appears not fully penetrant and it was noticed that females carrying a mutated allele had a normal audition, although tinnitus could be present.

Children affected by the autosomal recessive form[225] have sensorineural bilateral, either severe or moderate, hearing loss affecting all frequencies. No auditory defect was observed in their parents.

*Pathogenesis.* The two mutations reported in DFNA2′ affected families were one missense mutation at the boundary between the second extracellular loop and the fourth transmembrane domain (see Fig. 254-15), and a nonsense mutation three codons upstream. In the two families affected by the autosomal recessive form, the same mutations were observed, namely a 3-bp deletion leading to the loss of an isoleucine in the third transmembrane domain on one allele and a valine for isoleucine substitution at the same emplacement on the other allele. Based on the normal hearing of the parents in these families, the hypothesis of a dominant negative effect of the mutation present in the DFNA2′ form has been put forward.[225]

Besides *GJB3* expression in the inner ear[224] and the keratinocytes,[222,223] the transcript is also detected in several other tissues, including the placenta, eye,[222] kidney,[226] spinal cord and cerebral cortex.[224] In the inner ear, it is not known yet whether the protein is present in all gap junctions. Homozygous null mutant mice have been obtained by gene knockout, but it is still not known whether these mice have a hearing loss.[227]

**Connexin 30 Defect: DFNA3′.** In some families with a deafness linked to the chromosomal region 13q12, no mutation in *GJB2* had been detected. *GJB6*, the gene encoding connexin 30 (a 261-amino-acid protein), maps only 0.8 Mb centromeric to *GJB2*. Because connexin 30 is expressed in the rat cochlea,[228] and two

connexin genes had already been recognized as underlying deafness (*GJB2* and *GJB3*), *GJB6* was considered as a good candidate gene. By direct mutation screening performed on deaf individuals, a missense mutation was detected in one family affected by a dominant form of deafness (here named DFNA3′ because it maps near DFNA3).[229]

*Clinical Features.* In the single DFNA3′ family reported so far, the hearing loss was sensorineural and of a variable degree of severity.

*Pathogenesis.* The mutation identified in the DFNA3′ family substitutes a methionine for a threonine (T5M) in the N-terminal region (see Fig. 254-15) of connexin 30.[229] Electrophysiological studies performed on *Xenopus* oocytes expressing the mutated *GJB6* allele, showed an absence of electric coupling between oocytes. Moreover, the mutation exhibited a dominant negative effect in this system, when the mutated allele was coexpressed with the wild-type allele.[229] Sequence comparison indicates that among the various connexins, connexin 30 and connexin 26 have the closest relationship (77 percent amino acid identity).[230] They can form an heterotypic pairing together and with connexin 32. In rodents, both *Gjb2* and *Gjb6* are expressed in the brain, skin, uterus, and cochlea. However, *Gjb6* is not expressed in the liver and pancreas. In addition, whereas the brain expression of *Gjb2* decreases after birth, that of *Gjb6* becomes important in adults.[230] In the cochlea, the two connexins have the same cellular distribution.[228] Thus, the pathophysiological hypotheses concerning these two distinct auditory defects are similar.

**Na⁺-K⁺-2Cl⁻ Cotransporter Defects: *shaker-with-no-syndactylism* (*sy^{ns}*) Mouse Mutant and Targeted Disruption of *Slc12a2/Nkcc1*.** The involvement of the $Na^+$-$K^+$-$2Cl^-$ cotransporter (Fig. 254-16) in the $K^+$ homeostasis of the inner ear had previously been established, mainly using diuretics, such as furosemide, which act to block the transporter. These drugs decrease the $K^+$ concentration of the endolymph and the endocochlear potential.[231,232] The secretory isoform of the $Na^+$-$K^+$-$2Cl^-$ transporter, Nkcc1, has been detected in the basolateral membrane of the marginal cells of the stria vascularis,[213,233] (Fig. 254-5) as well as in the basal part of the spiral ligament and the spiral limbus. This transporter is involved in the initial steps of the $K^+$ secretion from the perilymph to the endolymph as well as in the final step of this process, namely the $K^+$ uptake from the intrastrial compartment by the marginal cells, which will secrete it into the endolymph. Two groups generated the targeted disruption of the corresponding gene,[218,234] and showed that homozygous mutant mice have profound hearing loss and balance troubles. A third group concomitantly reported the presence of a single base insertion creating a premature stop codon in the *shaker-with-no-syndactylism* mouse mutant, *sy^{ns}*, that had long been known to be affected by hearing loss and vestibular dysfunction.[217] Histopathologic analysis of both natural and induced mutants showed the collapse of the Reissner's membrane which results from the decrease in endolymph pressure due to the diminution of endolymphatic $K^+$ and associated water. A loss of hair and supporting cells, thin and collapsed semicircular canals were also observed. The human orthologous gene, *NKCC1*, is located on chromosome 5q31-33, in the DFNA1 region.[235] Because the *DFNA1* gene has already been identified (see "DIAPH1 Defect: DFNA1," below), this indicates the possible existence of an additional deafness gene in this region.

Interestingly, mutations in the $Na^+$-$K^+$-$2Cl^-$ cotransporter gene *NKCC2*, a putative paralogue of *NKCC1*, are responsible for the antenatal form of Bartter syndrome,[236] a disease characterized by hypokaliemic alkalosis with hypercalciuria (MIM 241200) but not associated with deafness. Three other forms or variants of Bartter syndrome are each caused by a defect in a cotransporter or

## Na⁺ K⁺ 2 Cl⁻ cotransporter

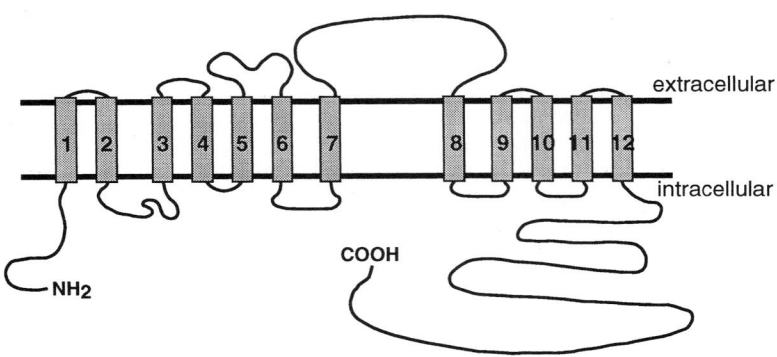

Fig. 254-16 Representation of the Na⁺-K⁺-2Cl⁻ cotransporter Nkcc1. This transporter has 12 predicted transmembrane domains. It is generally agreed that acute regulation of Na⁺-K⁺-2Cl⁻ cotransport occurs mainly through phosphorylation/ dephosphorylation mechanisms, but the precise regulatory domains of this cotransporter are still unknown.

an ionic channel. Therefore, another as yet unidentified Na⁺-K⁺-2Cl⁻ cotransporter gene might underlie the infantile form of Bartter syndrome with deafness (MIM 602522), which has been mapped on 1p31.[237]

**Iodide-Chloride Transporter (Pendrin) Defect: DFNB4 and Pendred Syndrome.** The DFNB4 (MIM 600791) locus was first described in an Israeli Druze deaf family on chromosome 7q21-34.[238] When the Pendred syndrome was subsequently assigned to the same chromosomal region,[239,240] this family was clinically reexamined and diagnosed as Pendred syndrome (MIM 274600). The autosomal recessive Pendred syndrome was initially defined as the association of a thyroid goitre developing before puberty with congenital deafness.[241] The thyroid goitre in Pendred syndrome is due to intrinsic defect in iodide organification,[240] which, in medical practice, is detected using the perchlorate discharge test.[242] However, the thyroid disease is extremely variable, even within a given family. The thyroid enlargement can be absent, and when present, is accompanied by either normal or decreased serum levels of T3 and T4. In addition, an increasing number of authentic Pendred cases are reported without abnormal perchlorate tests.[243] The hearing loss is sensorineural, profound, and prelingual. Some patients also have abnormal vestibular function (caloric tests). Computed tomography and magnetic resonance imaging easily detect morphologic anomalies of the inner ear. The enlargement of the vestibular aqueduct (which houses the endolymphatic canal) is the most common anomaly[244] (Fig. 254-17). An undercoiling of the cochlea, termed Mondini malformation, is also frequently observed.[244] Even though the exact prevalence of Pendred syndrome is still unknown, it seems to be the most common form of syndromic deafness,[242] and has been proposed to account for up to 20 percent of all deafness cases.[245]

The causative gene, *PDS*, has been identified by the detection, in three affected families, of one missense mutation on a highly conserved amino acid residue and two single base pair deletions predicting truncated proteins.[246] *PDS* comprises 21 exons. It encodes pendrin, a 780-amino-acid (86-kDa) protein that possesses 11 putative transmembrane domains[246] (Fig. 254-18).

As expected from the intrafamilial variation of the thyroid defect in Pendred syndrome, *PDS* also underlies an isolated deafness form, DFNB4,[22] a sensorineural hearing loss that is also associated with an enlarged vestibular aqueduct[247] (Fig. 254-17). Finally, a fluctuating form of hearing loss with enlarged vestibular aqueduct is also caused by mutations in *PDS*.[248]

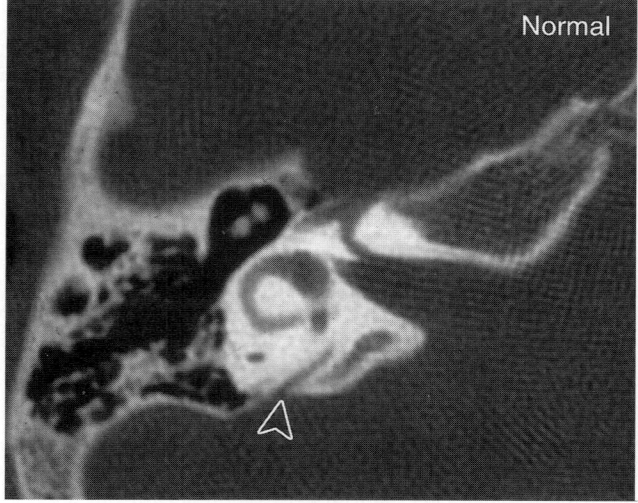
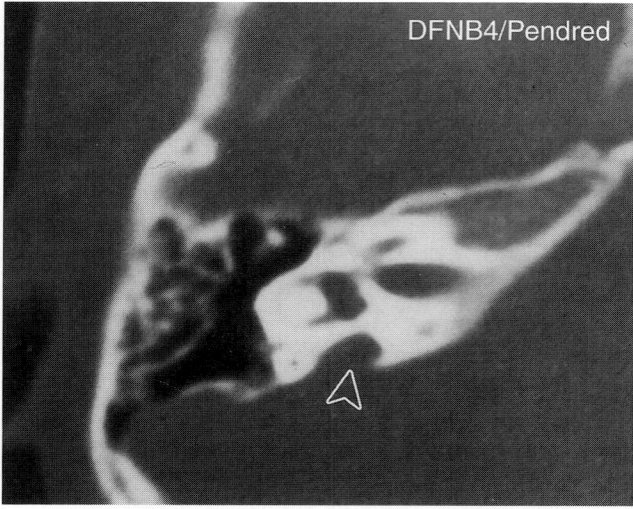

Fig. 254-17 Enlarged vestibular aqueduct in Pendred syndrome and DFNB4 isolated deafness, shown by computerized tomography of the temporal petrous bone.

# Pendrin iodide-chloride transporter

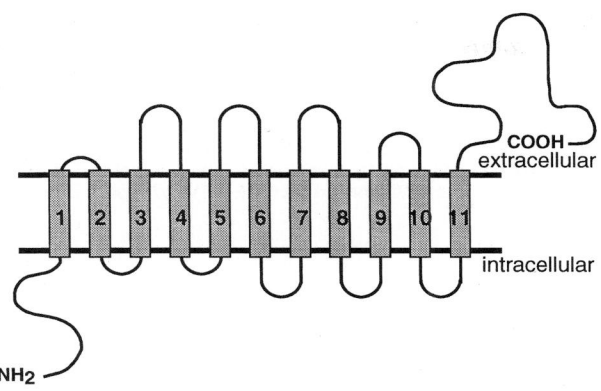

**Fig. 254-18 Representation of the iodide-chloride transporter pendrin. This 780-amino-acid protein has 11 putative transmembrane domains and a predicted C-terminal extracellular domain. Little is known about the structure-function relationship.**

***Clinical Features.*** DFNB4 presents as a congenital, sensorineural deafness. The hearing loss is sometimes progressive and it affects all frequencies but often predominates on high frequencies; it can fluctuate. Patients, occasionally complain of vertigo. Enlarged vestibular aqueduct (Fig. 254-17) seems to be very frequent, but its exact prevalence is still unknown.

***Pathogenesis.*** Several missense mutations as well as frameshift mutations have been described in DFNB4 affected patients with enlarged vestibular aqueduct.[247] Some of these mutations have also been reported in Pendred-affected patients, thus indicating the intervening role of modifier genes. The expression of pendrin in *Xenopus* oocytes and in insect cells has established that this protein is a chloride and iodide transporter.[249] Furthermore, in the *Xenopus* oocytes expression system, pendrin mediates chloride/formate exchange.[250]

In the mouse inner ear, *Pds* is strongly expressed, from E13 onward, in the endolymphatic duct and sac. *Pds* is also expressed in specific nonsensory areas of the utricle, saccule, and cochlea.[251] The expression of *Pds* in epithelial cells of the endolymphatic duct and sac, which are known to be involved in endolymph resorption, in conjunction with the aforementioned analyses showing that pendrin is a chloride-iodide transporter, strongly argues for a direct role of this protein in inner ear fluid ionic homeostasis. In particular, such a role would account for the fluctuation of the hearing loss that is observed in certain DFNB4-affected patients. In the context of this hypothesis, the enlarged vestibular aqueduct, which houses the endolymphatic duct, makes sense. However, the absence of endolymphatic hydrops (distension of the membranous labyrinth) in affected individuals is suggestive of a compensatory mechanism that would develop after the morphogenesis of the inner ear. The undercoiling of the cochlea has also been proposed to result from an increased endolymphatic pressure during the formation of the cochlea.[251] The recent finding that pendrin is functionally related to the renal chloride/formate exchanger[250] may provide some insight into the mechanism of the inner ear morphogenetic anomalies in DFNB4 and Pendred syndrome. In the proximal tubule of the kidney, chloride/formate exchange provides a mechanism for NaCl and volume reabsorption.[252] Therefore, a loss of chloride transport within the embryonic inner ear could lead to abnormal salt and water flux, with subsequent dilatation of the vestibular aqueduct and loss of the normal architecture of the cochlea.

**POU3F4 Transcription Factor Defect: DFN3.** The X chromosome-linked DFN3 locus (MIM 304400) was the second locus for an isolated form of deafness to be identified, because DFN1 (MIM 304700) actually corresponds to a syndromic form of deafness[253] (see "Mitochondrial Gene Defects," below, and Table 254-1). DFN3 was first mapped to Xq21 by linkage analysis,[254,255] and the interval was subsequently narrowed thanks to the molecular analysis of a variety of deletions of this chromosomal region associated with complex phenotypes that may or may not involve deafness.[256,257] The DFN3 gene was the first gene responsible for an isolated form of deafness to be identified.[258] This gene, *POU3F4* (MIM 300039), encodes a 361-amino-acid POU-domain transcription factor of class III, and consists of a single exon. In the DFN3-affected individuals, about half of the DNA anomalies are located within the gene and the other half upstream of the gene.[259–262]

***Clinical Features of DFN3.*** The DFN3 form of deafness was first described in 1971.[263] The hearing loss was reported to be mixed, that is, both conductive and sensorineural, with vestibular anomalies and perilymphatic gusher when surgical ablation of the stapes was attempted. Males generally have a progressive hearing loss that starts during youth with a conductive component predominating on the lower frequencies. The sensorineural component is rapidly progressive, resulting in severe to profound deafness.[264] Vestibular dysfunction can be detected by caloric tests.[263] High resolution computerized tomography (CT) reveals anomalies consisting mainly of stapes fixation and dilatation of the cochlea. The internal auditory meatus, which lets the auditory nerve pass towards the brain stem, is also dilated. Heterozygous females can also present with mixed hearing loss, but without CT scan-detectable anomalies.

***Pathogenesis.*** The orthologues of *POU3F4* that have been isolated in mouse (*Brn4*),[265] rat,[266,267] and *X. laevis*[268] have highly conserved sequences.

Among the mutations located within this gene, the two-thirds are missense mutations that, interestingly, are all clustered in the POU$_H$ and POU$_S$ domains (see Fig. 254-12). The DNA anomalies located outside the gene overlap on an 8-kb interval, about 900 kb upstream of the gene. This interval contains sequences that are highly conserved between species, and that are therefore likely to correspond to regulatory transcription elements.[269]

Although *Brn4/Pou3f4* is expressed in various mouse tissues,[267,270] both DFN3-affected individuals and *Brn4* null mouse mutants only present with an ear defect.[271–273] The expression of *Brn4/Pou3f4* in the developing ear is restricted to the mesenchyme of the inner ear.[274] The transcript appears at E10.5 when the mesenchyme starts to condense to give rise to the otic capsule, and the expression of the gene persists in the condensed mesenchyme. Interestingly, the Pou3f4 protein remains in the nucleus of the mesenchymal cells that will form the otic capsule, but shifts to the perinuclear space in the cells from regions that will cavitate in the temporal bone to form the scala vestibularis, the scala tympani, and the internal auditory meatus.[274] In adults, the gene is expressed in the three types of fibrocytes that compose the spiral ligament.[271]

To date, three mouse models of DFN3 have been described. Two are the result of a targeted gene disruption,[271,272] and one of an inversion in a radiation mutagenesis.[273] The three mutants present with hearing losses, which however differ in their degrees of severity. Curiously, these mutants, which are on different genetic backgrounds, differ both by their phenotypes and by their histopathologic anomalies in several respects. Two of them have severe balance dysfunction, with a vertical head bobbing which is likely due to the presence of a constriction of the superior semicircular canal,[272,273] whereas the third one has no vestibular dysfunction.[271] The first two mutants also have middle and inner ear morphogenetic anomalies. The stape is flattened, but is not fixed to the oval window as it is in the DFN3 individuals. A dilatation of the internal auditory meatus is also observed. Several of the inner ear anomalies, such as the reduction of the size of the scala tympani and scala vestibularis, dysplasia of the temporal bone, indicate a defect in the embryonic remodeling. In addition, the spiral ligament is reduced and thinner and an hydropsis was observed (the Reissner's membrane was distended). In contrast, in the third mutant, none of these middle and inner ear anomalies was observed,[271] and the defect only concerns the fibrocytes of the spiral ligament. Massive anomalies of the three types of fibrocytes are found with a reduction of the endocochlear potential (no collapse or distension of the Reissner's membrane is reported). Therefore, from one mutant to another, the deficit seems to predominate either at the mesenchymal stage or later, exclusively in the fibrocytes of the spiral ligament. These differences are still unexplained. To progress in the understanding of the role of *Brn4/POU3F4* in ear development, the target genes of this transcription factor, as well as the genes controlling its own expression in the ear, have to be identified.

**Cochlin Defect: DFNA9.** The DFNA9 locus was identified through the analysis of a U.S. family affected by a progressive form of sensorineural deafness (MIM 601369) and mapped on 14q12-13.[275] A very abundant cochlear cDNA, *COCH* (MIM 603196), which had been isolated from a subtracted human cochlear cDNA library, was subsequently assigned to this chromosomal region.[276,277] Three *COCH* missense mutations were found in DFNA9 individuals, therefore establishing *COCH* as the causative gene.[278] *COCH* contains 11 coding exons. The gene encodes a predicted 550-amino-acid protein, cochlin.

*Clinical Features.* The clinical descriptions have been reported for most of these families,[279–283] as well as the existence of very specific histologic findings in some of them. The following features characterize this form of deafness. The age of onset varies from adolescence to mature adulthood. The hearing loss initially predominates on the high frequencies with a variable degree of severity, and thereafter extends to all frequencies with a rapid progression of 3 to 5 dBHL per year. The mutations described so far are fully penetrant. Some of the patients suffer from vestibular dysfunction, namely recurrent episodes of vertigo, instability especially in the dark at the onset of hearing loss, and head movement-dependent oscillopsia, with vestibular areflexia or hyporeflexia. Patients also complain of aural fullness, tinnitus. Similar vestibular symptoms are observed in Ménière disease, a frequent disease due to "endolymphatic hydrops." Although the hearing loss associated with Ménière disease is fluctuating and affects low or all frequencies, the authors suggest that some defects classified as Ménière disease are due to *COCH* mutations.[278,282,283]

*Pathogenesis.* Cochlin possesses a signal peptide and no domain for anchoring to the cell membrane. The protein is composed of two consecutive von Willebrand factor (vWF) type A-like domains. A region containing several cysteine residues precedes each of these domains.[278] The overall sequence is indicative of an extracellular protein and the presence of the vWF type A domains[284,285] suggests a matrix component (Fig. 254-19). The protein sequence is highly conserved between species.[278]

After the initial discovery of the three missense mutations,[278] all located in the N-terminal cysteine-rich region, another missense mutation, in the same region, was reported in several Dutch[282,283] and Belgian[283] families, thus indicating a founder effect.

Histopathologic analyses of temporal bones of DFNA9-affected patients have revealed acidophilic deposits along the osseous spiral lamina (where the auditory nerve penetrates the membranous labyrinth), as well as in the spiral limbus and the spiral ligament (see Fig. 254-3B). Degeneration of the organ of Corti is detected in aged patients. A striking correlation is observed between the location of these deposits and the sites of

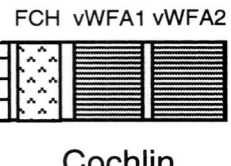

FCH vWFA1 vWFA2

### Cochlin

**Fig. 254-19 Representation of cochlin. Cochlin is a predicted extracellular matrix protein. The N-terminal signal peptide (horizontal bars) is followed by a region of *Limulus* factor C homology (FCH), and two von Willebrand factor (vWF)-like type A domains.**

expression of *COCH*, thus suggesting that cochlin might be a component of these deposits. Mutated forms of cochlin may show abnormal folding, impairing their stability or their interaction with other extracellular matrix components. The deposits that are present in the temporal bone are unlikely to explain the deafness, whereas those associated with the fibrocytes of the spiral limbus and spiral ligament (both involved in the transfer of $K^+$ from the perilymph towards the endolymph) or with the spiral lamina could account for the cochlear and vestibular defects.

### Forms of Deafness Caused by a Tectorial Membrane Anomaly

**COLXI (α2 Chain) Defect: DFNA13 and Stickler Syndrome.** The DFNA13 locus has been mapped to chromosome 6p21 through the study of a large family of American-European origin affected with progressive postlingual hearing loss.[286] *COL11A2*, the gene that encodes the α2 chain of collagen type XI, located at 6p21.3, underlies two forms of syndromic deafness, namely the autosomal dominant Stickler syndrome without ocular anomalies (Stickler type II, MIM 184840)[23] and the autosomal recessive Weissenbacher-Zweymuller syndrome (MIM 277610)[287] (see Table 254-1). Considering these data and the fact that collagen XI is a component of the cochlear tectorial membrane (see Fig. 254-3B), *COL11A2* was considered as an excellent candidate gene for DFNA13. Indeed, two distinct mutations were detected in this gene in two DFNA13 families.[24]

*Clinical Features.* Deafness was reported as sensorineural, mild to moderately severe, and with a preferential mid-frequency loss (U-shaped audiogram curve). No symptomatic vestibular dysfunction was observed. However, in the only family extensively analyzed, half of the patients showed abnormal vestibular tests (caloric tests) and a vestibular areflexia.

*Pathogenesis.* The murine orthologous gene has been disrupted by homologous recombination. *Col11a2$^{-/-}$* mice showed moderate to severe hearing impairment, whereas no hearing defect could be detected in *Col11a2$^{+/-}$* animals. The tectorial membrane is an acellular membrane composed of several collagens (type II, V, IX, and XI), noncollagenous proteins, and proteoglycans. It is involved in the deflexion of the hair bundle of the cochlear hair cells upon sound stimulation, and thus plays a crucial role in the mechanotransduction process. Electron microscopy of the tectorial membrane in *Col11a2* homozygous null mutants revealed a disorganization of its fibrillar structure.[24] No results on the vestibular function and the structure of the vestibular acellular membranes of these mice have yet been reported. Collagen XI is composed of three chains, α1, α2, and α3, which interact by the repeated tripeptide G-X-Y, where G is glycine and X and Y are often proline and hydroxyproline. The two DFNA13 mutations substitute either a cysteine or a glutamate for the glycine in one G-X-Y motif, and are thus expected to impair the trimerization of the protein.

**α-Tectorin Defects: DFNA8/12 and DFNB21.** Two groups have independently identified a locus on chromosome 11q22-24 as

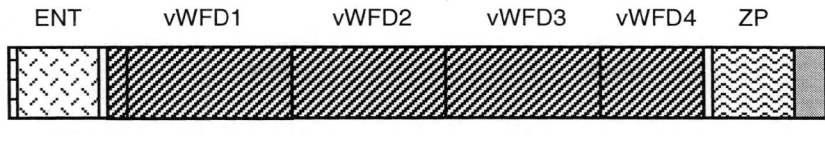

α-tectorin

**Fig. 254-20 Representation of α-tectorin.** α-Tectorin is a component of the acellular tectorial membrane of the cochlea. The N-terminal signal peptide (horizontal bars) is followed by a region homologous to the first globular domain of entactin (ENT), four von Willebrand factor (vWF)-like type D domains, a zona pellucida (ZP) domain, known as an interacting domain, and a hydrophobic C-terminal region (in gray).

underlying a dominant form of prelingual, nonprogressive sensorineural deafness; hence, its two denominations, DFNA8 (MIM601543)[288] and DFNA12 (MIM601842).[21]

*TECTA* (MIM 602574), a gene that encodes α-tectorin, a specific component of the cochlear tectorial membrane (see Fig. 254-3*B*), was located within the candidate chromosomal interval for DFNA8/12. α-Tectorin had been isolated upon the generation of antibodies directed against components of the tectorial membrane. *TECTA* was thus an excellent candidate for this nonsyndromic form of deafness. *TECTA* contains 23 exons encoding a predicted 2155-amino-acid modular protein. Missense mutations were detected in the two DFNA8/12-affected families originally described.[289] Later we mapped the locus responsible for a recessive form of deafness in a consanguineous Lebanese family, DFNB21 (MIM 603629), to the same chromosomal region, and discovered a homozygous splice site mutation in this family.[290]

***Clinical Features of DFNA8/12.*** Only three DFNA8/12-affected families with a *TECTA* identified mutation have been reported.[289,291] Their clinical features were different. The degree of severity of the hearing loss varied from mild to severe with large intrafamilial variations. In the first two families, the hearing loss was stable,[21,288] whereas in the third one, it was progressive.[291] The onset was either prelingual or during early childhood. The hearing defect either involved mid[289] or high[291] frequencies preferentially, or concerned all the frequencies.[288]

***Clinical Features of DFNB21.*** A single family has been reported, with severe to profound prelingual sensorineural hearing loss affecting all frequencies.[290]

***Pathogenesis.*** The *TECTA* cDNA sequence predicts a 2155-amino-acid (240-kDa)-secreted protein with 33 *N*-glycosylation sites. It also predicts that α-tectorin is synthesized as a precursor anchored to the plasma membrane via glycosylphosphatidylinositol; α-tectorin would be subsequently released from the membrane by proteolytic cleavage of the precursor. Several domains have been recognized in the protein (Fig. 254-20). The N-terminal region is homologous to the first globular domain of entactin. It is followed by three full and two partial repeats homologous to the D domain of the prepro-vonWillebrand factor. In the von Willebrand factor, the D domain is involved in the multimerization of the protein. Such a domain has also been found in numerous proteins that form filaments or gels.[292] Finally, the C-terminal region of α-tectorin contains a zona pellucida (ZP) domain, that has been recognized as an interacting domain, and hydrophobic residues at the very end. The human α-tectorin sequence shares 95 percent identity with the mouse one.

In the three DFNA8/12-affected families, different missense mutations have been reported, of which two are located in the ZP domain,[289] and the third one in the fourth vWF-like D domain.[291] The latter is the substitution of a serine for the first cysteine of the CGLC motif, which is presumably implicated in an oligomerization process. In the DFNB21-affected family, the donor splice site mutation is expected to create a protein truncated at the level of the second vWF type D domain.[290] Based on the normal auditory function of the heterozygous carriers in the DFNB21-affected family, half of the normal amount of α-tectorin seems to be sufficient to preserve the mechanical properties of the tectorial membrane.[293] Accordingly, the missense mutations found in DFNA8/12-affected patients should have a dominant negative effect. This provides genetic evidence supporting the idea that α-tectorin is involved in homo- or heteromeric structures, as suggested by Legan et al.[294]

Because α-tectorin is a major noncollagenous component of the tectorial membrane, its absence in the DFNB21 form of deafness is likely to impair the formation of this acellular membrane. The mouse α-tectorin is synthesized by a variety of supporting cells of the cochlear and vestibular neuroepithelia.[294,295] The generation of mouse mutants lacking a functional *Tecta* gene should lead to a better understanding of the contribution of α-tectorin to the formation and the biophysical properties of the tectorial membrane.

**Otogelin Defect: Targeted Disruption of *Otog*.** Two noncollagenous proteins have been identified by a biochemical approach in the cochlear tectorial membrane, namely α-tectorin[294] (see "α-Tectorin Defects: DFNA8/12 and DFNB21" above) and β-tectorin[296]. The gene encoding a third one, otogelin, has been isolated by generation of a subtracted cDNA library.[108] All three proteins are specific of the acellular membranes of the inner ear.

Otogelin is a predicted 2910-amino-acid-secreted protein related to mucins.[108] It contains a threonine-, serine-, and proline-rich central region (TSP region), flanked by an N- and a C-terminal cysteine-rich regions. The N-terminal region is made up of three complete and one incomplete vWF-like D domains. The C-terminal region is composed of a complete vWF D domain, followed by five VWF-like B domains, and ended by a fragment having similarity with domains present in the transforming growth factor-*β*2 and the protein defective in Norrie disease (Fig. 254-21). We have generated mice with a targeted disruption of the *Otog* gene.[297] Homozygous null mice present with a bilateral hearing loss and severe imbalance. Histopathologic analysis of the vestibular end organs showed that the utricular and saccular otoconial membranes and the cupulae of the ampullar cristae detached from their neuroepithelia a few days and a few weeks after birth, respectively. This indicated that otogelin is required to maintain the anchoring of the vestibular acellular membranes to the underlying epithelia. In contrast, anomalies of the tectorial membrane were only revealed by electron microscopy. In some mice, a delay in the age of onset of the hearing loss was observed, which indicates that otogelin is dispensable for the initial function of the tectorial membrane, and suggests that the resistance of the tectorial membrane to the mechanical stresses generated as a result of sound wave pressure is reduced in the absence of otogelin.

The human *OTOG* maps to 11p14.3. To this chromosomal region has been assigned the locus for the autosomal recessive deafness DFNB18. *OTOG* should thus be considered as a candidate gene for DFNB18.

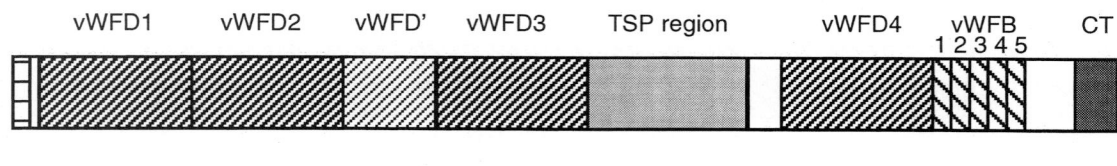

## Otogelin

**Fig. 254-21 Representation of otogelin. Otogelin is a component of the tectorial membrane. The N-terminal signal peptide (horizontal bars) is followed by four von Willebrand factor (vWF)-like type D domains, a threonine-, serine-, proline-rich (TSP) region, a fifth vWF D domain, five vWF-like type B domains, and a C-terminal (CT) region.**

### Deafness Forms of Unknown Cell Origin

**DIAPH1 Defect: DFNA1.** The first identification of a locus for an isolated form of deafness occurred in 1992.[33] In a large family from Costa Rica, a dominantly transmitted deafness, DFNA1 (MIM 124900), has been traced back through eight generations.[298] Genetic linkage analysis in 99 individuals mapped the responsible gene to chromosome 5q31 in a 5-cM interval.[33]

The candidate gene, *DIAPH1*, was identified on the reduction of the candidate interval followed by its complete sequencing.[299] *DIAPH1* was predicted to encode a protein sharing homology with the *Drosophila* diaphanous protein. A nucleotide substitution in a donor splice site was detected in the patients, which results in a 4-bp insertion in the transcript, leading to a premature stop codon.

*Clinical Features of DFNA1.* A single DFNA1 family has been reported so far. The hearing loss was sensorineural, progressive, and initially affected only low frequencies. By age 30, it was severe and concerned all frequencies; by age 40, the deafness was profound. Intriguingly, the early low frequency hearing loss in this family was associated with electrocochleographic findings suggestive of endolymphatic hydrops.[300]

*Pathogenesis.* *DIAPH1* encodes a predicted protein of 2152 amino acids (139 kDa), diaphanous-1, which belongs to a family of formin-related proteins. Diaphanous-1 contains a RhoGTPase-binding domain, a polyproline region, and the highly conserved formin-homology FH2 domain (Fig. 254-22). Expression of the human diaphanous-1 protein has been detected in all the tissues tested, including the cochlea.[299] The genes of the formin gene family are involved in cell polarization and cytokinesis.[301–303] The mouse diaphanous-1 has been shown to interact with the GTP-bound form of Rho and with profilin.[304] The formation of this complex ensures the targeting of profilin at specific plasma membrane emplacements where profilin promotes actin polymerization. The target cells of the *DIAPH1* defect in the inner ear are presently not known, but given the critical role of the actin cytoskeleton in auditory mechanotransduction, they could well be the hair cells themselves. Generation of a mouse model of DFNA1 should help clarify this point and contribute to elucidate in which developmental and/or differentiation process, the diaphanous protein is involved.

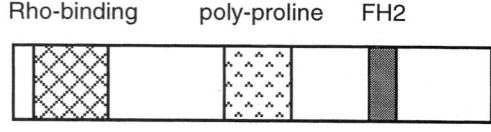

## Diaphanous-1

**Fig. 254-22 Representation of diaphanous-1. Diaphanous-1 belongs to a family of formin-related proteins. It contains a predicted RhoGTPase-binding domain, a polyproline region, and the highly conserved formin-homology FH2 domain.**

**DFNA5.** The DFNA5 locus has been assigned to chromosome 7p15 through the study of a large Dutch family affected by an autosomal dominant progressive form of deafness (MIM 600994).[305] The age of onset of the hearing loss was between 5 and 15 years, and only response to high frequencies was initially defective. By about 50 years, the hearing impairment became severe, and concerned also low frequencies. This family is the only DFNA5 family known so far. A candidate gene was isolated in the chromosomal interval defined for DFNA5.[306] The identification, in the affected individuals, of a complex deletion/insertion in intron 7, leading to the skipping of the downstream exon and thereby expected to encode a truncated protein, validated this gene as the causative gene.[306] The gene consists of 10 exons and encodes a 496-amino-acid protein.

The protein-deduced sequence did not give any information on its putative function. RT-PCR indicated that the gene is transcribed in the stria vascularis of the cochlea (see Fig. 254-3B).

**Mitochondrial Gene Defects.** The mitochondrial DNA (mtDNA) encodes 13 mRNAs translated into 13 proteins that interact with approximately 60 nuclear DNA-encoded proteins to form the 5 enzymatic complexes required for oxidative phosphorylation. It also encodes 2 ribosomal RNAs (rRNA) and 22 transfer RNAs (tRNA). mtDNA-linked diseases are transmitted to both sexes but only through maternal line (see Chaps. 104 and 105).

Several syndromic deafness forms are associated with mutations in mtDNA, among which Kearns-Sayre syndrome (chronic progressive external ophthalmoplegia; MIM 530000), myoclonic epilepsy with ragged-red fibers (MIM 545000), MELAS (myopathy, encephalopathy, lactic acidosis, and stroke-like episodes; MIM 540000) and some forms of diabetes mellitus associated with hearing loss (see Table 254-1). In contrast, a single syndromic deafness form involving a mitochondrial protein encoded by the nuclear genome has so far been reported. The gene[253] encodes DDP (deafness/dystonia peptide), a protein implicated in the import of carrier proteins from the intermembrane space into the inner membrane of the mitochondria,[307] and is responsible for the X-linked Mohr-Tranebjaerg syndrome (MIM 304700), an early childhood sensorineural hearing loss associated with progressive dystonia, spasticity, mental deterioration, and cortical blindness (DFN1) (see Table 254-1).

The first evidence for an isolated deafness form of mtDNA origin arose in 1992, through the study of a large Arab-Israeli family affected by hearing loss. In this family, at least two mutations were implicated, a mitochondrial one and an autosomal recessive one. A homoplasmic 1555A > G mutation was detected in the 12SrRNA gene.[308] The autosomal contributor gene(s) has(ve) not yet been mapped.[309] In this family, most of the individuals carrying the 1555A > G mutation were affected by severe to profound hearing loss during infancy; a few had onset during adulthood, and some were normal hearing.[310] This mutation was also observed in three families affected by a maternally inherited deafness induced by aminoglycoside antibiotics.[308,311] Since then, several studies have reported the presence of the 1555A > G mutation in deaf subjects, some of whom had not been exposed to aminoglycosides. Two independent studies on Spanish deaf individuals reported a high incidence (up to 25 percent) of the 1555A > G mutation among families affected by sensorineural hearing loss in whom most of the affected members had not been treated with aminoglycosides[312,313] (del Castillo, personal communication). The absence of such a high proportion of the 1555A > G mutation reported in other countries is puzzling, especially because haplotype analysis performed on Spanish individuals suggested that this mutation arose from numerous independent mutational events.[314] However, a recent study on the Japanese population put forward that 10 percent of profoundly deaf individuals without a history of aminoglycoside treatment carry the 1555A > G mutation.[500] Aminoglycosides are known to inhibit mRNA translation by the ribosomes in bacteria, through binding to a specific G of the 16SrRNA. The 1555A > G mutation concerns the nucleotide analogue in the mitochondrial 12SrRNA. More directly, this 12SrRNA mutated form has been shown to bind aminoglycosides with high affinity unlike the normal one.[315] Another mutation, 961delT, in the 12SrRNA gene was discovered in a family with a hearing loss induced by aminoglycosides.[316] However, no direct interaction between this nucleotide and aminoglycosides has yet been reported.

Three point mutations have been detected in *MTTS1*, which encodes the mitochondrial tRNA$^{\text{ser(UCN)}}$. First, a A7445G mutation was initially reported in a Scottish family affected with an isolated form of deafness;[317] the same mutation was thereafter detected in two pedigrees, in a syndromic form of deafness associated with palmoplantar keratoderma (MIM 148350)[318] (see Table 254-1). Second, an insertion of a C at nucleotide position 7472 (7472insC) has been shown to be responsible for a syndromic form of deafness including ataxia and myoclonus;[319] the same mutation was observed in a deaf family in which most of the patients presented with only hearing loss.[320] Finally, a T7511C mutation was found in patients suffering only from hearing loss, even though they present a cytochrome c oxidase deficiency in muscle.[321] The reason why a deficiency in the mitochondrial tRNA$^{\text{ser}}$ or 12SrRNA would result in hearing loss is not understood. The hair cell is presumed to be the target cell of the defect, according to the hair cell damage observed upon aminoglycoside exposure.[322–324] However, other inner ear cell types that are rich in mitochondria could as well be implicated. In the absence of mouse models for mitochondrial defects, this issue is difficult to clarify. Finally, some findings argue in favor of increasing mitochondrial DNA deletions and mutations in some patients affected by presbyacousis.[325,326]

As a result of the findings presented here, physicians who suspect a familial history of aminoglycoside-induced deafness can be helped in their diagnosis by the search for the 1555A > G and 961delT mutations in the 12S rRNA mitochondrial gene. In the future, this molecular test should become systematic prior to any prescription of aminoglycosides.

## CONCLUSION

Over the last 5 years, the molecular bases of nonsyndromic deafness in humans have started to be unraveled. Fifty or so loci have been identified and 17 genes underlying isolated deafness discovered. Amongst these genes, several have been recognized as responsible for both dominant and recessive forms of deafness and some also underlie a syndromic deafness. Taking into account the human genome sequencing program, it can be confidently predicted that, in a period of less than 10 years, the quasi-totality of the genes responsible for congenital or early onset forms of nonsyndromic deafness will have been identified. However, there are still large areas almost unexplored, such as the late onset forms of hereditary hearing loss and the genetic factors predisposing the ear to aging and/or to noise damage.

The results obtained so far already have significant medical implications. In particular, the detection of the highly prevalent connexin 26 mutation, that underlies about 50 percent of

prelingual forms of deafness in European and North American populations, has considerably improved genetic counseling. A screening for the mutations of the mitochondrial gene encoding the 12s ribosomal RNA, which underlie aminoglycoside-induced hearing loss, should lead to the eradication of a large proportion of this iatrogenic deafness. Future improvement relies on a more precise clinical description of the deafness forms that can be distinguished molecularly.

Over the last 40 or so years, understanding of the functioning of inner ear has benefited from some remarkable biophysical and cellular biologic studies. However, a description in molecular terms was missing. The small number of each type of cells present in this sensory organ has hindered a biochemical approach. Thus, the genetic approach was the method of choice to discover the molecules playing a crucial role in the function of this organ. Amongst the genes recognized as responsible for deafness, certain encode proteins which were already known to be involved in the auditory function (for example, the Na$^+$-K$^+$-2Cl$^-$ cotransporter), and in such cases, the value of the genetic approach is to reveal whether or not the protein is indispensable for the auditory function. Other deafness genes have brought to light a crucial role for certain molecules, even certain classes of molecules, for example, the role of several unconventional myosins in the morphologic differentiation and the functioning of the sensory cells. Finally, the structure and function of some identified molecules, such as that encoded by the *DFNA5* gene, remain unknown.

Beyond this initial step, remains a large and exciting amount of work aimed at integrating the information obtained for each of these molecules into our knowledge of the biologic processes taking place in the various inner ear cell types, and eventually into the physiology of the whole sensory organ. It is this kind of comprehension that can aid the research of targeted therapeutics, which is liable to take over from the prosthetics in use today. Despite the diversity of the mechanisms that underlie nonsyndromic deafness in humans, one can hope that, at least for some genetic forms, specific treatments will be discovered in near future.

## ACKNOWLEDGMENTS

The authors thank Sébastien Chardenoux for his help in the drawing of the protein schemes. The studies from the Unité de Génétique des Déficits Sensoriels are supported by grants from the European Community (QLG2-CT-1999-00988), Fondation pour la Recherche Médicale and Association Française contre les Myopathies.

## REFERENCES

1. Kikuchi T, Kimura RS, Paul DL, Adams JC: Gap junctions in the rat cochlea: Immunohistochemical and ultrastructural analysis. *Anat Embryol (Berl)* **191**:101, 1995.
2. von Békésy G: *Experiments in Hearing.* New York, McGraw-Hill, 1960.
3. Assad JA, Shepherd GM, Corey DP: Tip-link integrity and mechanical transduction in vertebrate hair cells. *Neuron* **7**:985, 1991.
4. Markin VS, Hudspeth AJ: Gating-spring models of mechanoelectrical transduction by hair cells of the internal ear. *Annu Rev Biophys Biomol Struct* **24**:59, 1995.
5. Ryan A, Dallos P: Effect of absence of cochlear outer hair cells on behavioural auditory threshold. *Nature* **253**:44, 1975.
6. Van de Water TR, Frenz DA, Giraldez F, Represa J, Lefebvre PP, Rogister B, Moonen G: Growth factors and development of the stato-acoustic system, in Romand R (ed): *Development of Auditory and Vestibular Systems,* vol 2. Amsterdam, Elsevier, 1992, p 1.
7. Van de Water TR: Tissue interactions and cell differentiation: neurone-sensory cell interaction during otic development. *Development* **103**:185, 1988.
8. Le Douarin NM, Ziller C, Couly GF: Patterning of neural crest derivatives in the avian embryo: in vivo and in vitro studies. *Dev Biol* **159**:24, 1993.

9. Mallo M: Embryological and genetic aspects of middle ear development. *Int J Dev Biol* **42**:11, 1998.
10. Vartiainen E, Kemppinen P, Karjalainen S: Prevalence and etiology of bilateral sensorineural hearing impairment in a Finnish childhood population. *Int J Pediatr Otorhinolaryngol* **41**:175, 1998.
11. Goldstein MA: *Problems of the Deaf.* St Louis, MO, The Laryngoscope Press, 1933.
12. Stephens SDG: Genetic hearing loss: A historical overview. *Adv Audiol* **3**:3, 1985.
13. Cranefield PF, Federn W: Paulus Zacchias on mental deficiency and on deafness. *Bull N Y Acad Med* **46**:3, 1970.
14. Ménière P: Recherches sur l'origine de la surdi-mutité. *Gaz Méd Paris* **3**:223, 1846.
15. Ménière P: Du mariage entre parents considéré comme cause de la surdi-mutité congénitale. *Gaz Méd Paris* **3**:303, 1856.
16. Denoyelle F, Marlin S, Weil D, Moatti L, Chauvin P, Garabédian -N, Petit C: Clinical features of the prevalent form of childhood deafness, *DFNB1*, due to a connexin26 gene defect: Implications for genetic counselling. *Lancet* **353**:1298, 1999.
17. Tomek MS, Brown MR, Mani SR, Ramesh A, Srisailapathy CR, Coucke P, Zbar RI, Bell AM, McGuirt WT, Fukushima K, Willems PJ, Van Camp G, Smith RJ: Localization of a gene for otosclerosis to chromosome 15q25-q26. *Hum Mol Genet* **7**:285, 1998.
18. Morell R, Spritz RA, Ho L, Pierpont J, Guo W, Friedman TB, Asher JH Jr: Apparent digenic inheritance of Waardenburg syndrome type 2 (WS2) and autosomal recessive ocular albinism (AROA). *Hum Mol Genet* **6**:659, 1997.
19. Balciuniene J, Dahl N, Borg E, Samuelsson E, Koisti MJ, Pettersson U, Jazin EE: Evidence for digenic inheritance of nonsyndromic hereditary hearing loss in a Swedish family. *Am J Hum Genet* **63**:786, 1998.
20. Adato A, Kalinski H, Weil D, Chaïb H, Korostishevsky M, Bonné-Tamir B: Possible interaction between USH1B and USH3 gene products as implied by apparent digenic deafness inheritance. *Am J Hum Genet* **65**:261, 1999.
21. Verhoeven K, Van Camp G, Govaerts PJ, Balemans W, Schatteman I, Verstreken M, Van Laer L, Smith RJH, Brown MR, Van de Heyning PH, Somers T, Offeciers FE, Willems PJ: A gene for autosomal dominant nonsyndromic hearing loss (DFNA12) maps to chromosome 11q22-24. *Am J Hum Genet* **60**:1168, 1997.
22. Li XC, Everett LA, Lalwani AK, Desmukh D, Friedman TB, Green ED, Wilcox ER: A mutation in *PDS* causes non-syndromic recessive deafness. *Nat Genet* **18**:215, 1998.
23. Vikkula M, Mariman ECM, Lui VCH, Zhidkova NI, Tiller GE, Goldring MB, van Beersum SEC, de Waal Malefijt MC, van den Hoogen FHJ, Ropers H-H, Mayne R, Cheah KSE, Olsen BR, Warman ML, Brunner HG: Autosomal dominant and recessive osteochondrodysplasia associated with the *COL11A2* locus. *Cell* **80**:431, 1995.
24. McGuirt WT, Prasad SD, Griffith AJ, Kunst HPM, Green GE, Shpargel KB, Runge C, Huybrechts C, Mueller RF, Lynch E, King M-C, Brunner HG, Cremers CWRJ, Takanosu M, Li S-W, Arita M, Mayne R, Prockop DJ, Van Camp G, Smith RJH: Mutations in *COL11A2* cause non-syndromic hearing loss (DFNA13). *Nat Genet* **23**:413, 1999.
25. Weil D, Blanchard S, Kaplan J, Guilford P, Gibson F, Walsh J, Mburu P, Varela A, Levilliers J, Weston MD, Kelley PM, Kimberling WJ, Wagenaar M, Levi-Acobas F, Larget-Piet D, Munnich A, Steel KP, Brown SDM, Petit C: Defective myosin VIIA gene responsible for Usher syndrome type 1B. *Nature* **374**:60, 1995.
26. Liu X-Z, Walsh J, Mburu P, Kendrick-Jones J, Cope MJTV, Steel KP, Brown SDM: Mutations in the myosin VIIA gene cause non-syndromic recessive deafness. *Nat Genet* **16**:188, 1997.
27. Weil D, Küssel P, Blanchard S, Lévy G, Levi-Acobas F, Drira M, Ayadi H, Petit C: The autosomal recessive isolated deafness, DFNB2, and the Usher 1B syndrome are allelic defects of the myosin-VIIA gene. *Nat Genet* **16**:191, 1997.
28. Liu X-Z, Walsh J, Tamagawa Y, Kitamura K, Nishizawa M, Steel KP, Brown SDM: Autosomal dominant non-syndromic deafness caused by a mutation in the myosin VIIA gene. *Nat Genet* **17**:268, 1997.
29. Maestrini E, Korge BP, Ocana-Sierra J, Calzolari E, Cambiaghi S, Scuder PM, Hovnanian A, Monaco AP, Munro CS: A missense mutation in connexin 26, D66H, causes mutilating keratoderma with sensorineural deafness (Vohwinkel's syndrome) in three unrelated families. *Hum Mol Genet* **8**:1237, 1999.
30. Kelsell DP, Dunlop J, Stevens HP, Lench NJ, Liang JN, Parry G, Mueller RF, Leigh IM: Connexin 26 mutations in hereditary non-syndromic sensorineural deafness. *Nature* **387**:80, 1997.
31. Denoyelle F, Lina-Granade G, Plauchu H, Bruzzone R, Chaïb H, Levi-Acobas F, Weil D, Petit C: Connexin26 gene linked to a dominant deafness. *Nature* **393**:319, 1998.
32. Petit C: Genes responsible for human hereditary deafness: Symphony of a thousand. *Nat Genet* **14**:385, 1996.
33. Leon PE, Raventos H, Lynch E, Morrow J, King M-C: The gene for an inherited form of deafness maps to chromosome 5q31. *Proc Natl Acad Sci U S A* **89**:5181, 1992.
34. Guilford P, Ben Arab S, Blanchard S, Levilliers J, Weissenbach J, Belkahia A, Petit C: A non-syndromic form of neurosensory, recessive deafness maps to the pericentromeric region of chromosome 13q. *Nat Genet* **6**:24, 1994.
35. Kalatzis V, Petit C: The fundamental and medical impacts of recent progress in research on hereditary hearing loss. *Hum Mol Genet* **7**:1589, 1998.
36. Lalwani AK, Castelein CM: Cracking the auditory genetic code: Nonsyndromic hereditary hearing impairment. *Am J Otol* **20**:115, 1999.
37. Steel KP, Bussoli TJ: Deafness genes expression of surprise. *Trends Genet* **15**:207, 1999.
38. Keats BJB, Nouri N, Huang J-M, Money M, Webster DB, Berlin CI: The deafness locus (*dn*) maps to mouse chromosome 19. *Mamm Genome* **6**:8, 1995.
39. Guilford P, Ayadi H, Blanchard S, Chaïb H, Le Paslier D, Weissenbach J, Drira M, Petit C: A human gene responsible for neurosensory, non-syndromic recessive deafness is a candidate homologue of the mouse *sh-1* gene. *Hum Mol Genet* **3**:989, 1994.
40. Brown KA, Sutcliffe MJ, Steel KP, Brown SDM: Close linkage of the olfactory marker protein gene to the mouse deafness mutation *shaker-1*. *Genomics* **13**:189, 1992.
41. Deol MS: The anatomy and development of the mutants pirouette, shaker-1 and waltzer in the mouse. *Proc R Soc London B Biol Sci* **145**:206, 1956.
42. Rinchik EM, Carpenter DA, Selby PB: A strategy for fine-structure functional analysis of a 6- to 11-centimorgan region of mouse chromosome 7 by high-efficiency mutagenesis. *Proc Natl Acad Sci U S A* **87**:896, 1990.
43. Kikuchi K, Hilding DA: The defective organ of Corti in shaker-1 mice. *Acta Otolaryngol* **60**:287, 1965.
44. Kimberling WJ, Möller CG, Davenport S, Priluck IA, Beighton PH, Greenberg J, Reardon W, Weston MD, Kenyon JB, Grunkemeyer JA, Pieke Dahl S, Overbeck LD, Blackwood DJ, Brower AM, Hoover DM, Rowland P, Smith RJH: Linkage of Usher syndrome type I gene (USH1B) to the long arm of chromosome 11. *Genomics* **14**:988, 1992.
45. El-Amraoui A, Petit C: Towards a molecular understanding of the pathophysiology of Usher syndrome. *J Audiol Med* **6**:170, 1997.
46. Boughman JA, Vernon M, Shaver KA: Usher syndrome: Definition and estimate of prevalence from two high-risk populations. *J Chronic Dis* **36**:595, 1983.
47. Tamagawa Y, Kitamura K, Ishida T, Ishikawa K, Tanaka H, Tsuji S, Nishizawa M: A gene for a dominant form of non-syndromic sensorineural deafness (*DFNA11*) maps within the region containing the *DFNB2* recessive deafness gene. *Hum Mol Genet* **5**:849, 1996.
48. Howard J, Hudspeth AJ: Mechanical relaxation of the hair bundle mediates adaptation in mechanoelectrical transduction by the bull-frog's saccular hair cell. *Proc Natl Acad Sci U S A* **84**:3064, 1987.
49. Gillespie PG, Wagner MC, Hudspeth AJ: Identification of a 120-kd hair-bundle myosin located near stereociliary tips. *Neuron* **11**:581, 1993.
50. Gibson F, Walsh J, Mburu P, Varela A, Brown KA, Antonio M, Beisel KW, Steel KP, Brown SDM: A type VII myosin encoded by the mouse deafness gene *Shaker-1*. *Nature* **374**:62, 1995.
51. Mermall V, Post PL, Mooseker MS: Unconventional myosins in cell movement, membrane traffic, and signal transduction. *Science* **279**:527, 1998.
52. Oliver TN, Berg JS, Cheney RE: Tails of unconventional myosins. *Cell Mol Life Sci* **56**:243, 1999.
53. Titus MA, Gilbert SP: The diversity of molecular motors: An overview. *Cell Mol Life Sci* **56**:181, 1999.
54. Weil D, Lévy G, Sahly I, Levi-Acobas F, Blanchard S, El-Amraoui A, Crozet F, Philippe H, Abitbol M, Petit C: Human myosin VIIA responsible for the Usher 1B syndrome: A predicted membrane-associated motor protein expressed in developing sensory epithelia. *Proc Natl Acad Sci U S A* **93**:3232, 1996.

55. Chishti AH, Kim AC, Marfatia SM, Lutchman M, Hanspal M, Jindal H, Liu SC, Low PS, Rouleau GA, Mohandas N, Chasis JA, Conboy JG, Gascard P, Takakuwa Y, Huang SC, Benz EJ Jr, Bretscher A, Fehon RG, Gusella JF, Ramesh V, Solomon F, Marchesi VT, Tsukita S, Hoover KB, et al: The FERM domain: A unique module involved in the linkage of cytoplasmic proteins to the membrane. *Trends Biochem Sci* **23**:281, 1998.

56. Chen Z-Y, Hasson T, Kelley PM, Schwender BJ, Schwartz MF, Ramakrishnan M, Kimberling WJ, Mooseker MS, Corey DP: Molecular cloning and domain structure of human myosin-VIIa, the gene product defective in Usher syndrome 1B. *Genomics* **36**:440, 1996.

57. Mburu P, Liu XZ, Walsh J, Saw D, Cope MJTV, Gibson F, Kendrick-Jones J, Steel KP, Brown SDM: Mutation analysis of the mouse myosin VIIA deafness gene. *Genes Function* **1**:191, 1997.

58. Hasson T, Walsh J, Cable J, Mooseker MS, Brown SD, Steel KP: Effects of shaker-1 mutations on myosin-VIIa protein and mRNA expression. *Cell Motil Cytoskeleton* **37**:127, 1997.

59. Adato A, Weil D, Kalinski H, Pel-Or Y, Ayadi H, Petit C, Korostishevsky M, Bonné-Tamir B: Mutation profile of all 49 exons of the human myosin VIIA gene, and haplotype analysis, in Usher 1B families from diverse origins. *Am J Hum Genet* **61**:813, 1997.

60. Lévy G, Levi-Acobas F, Blanchard S, Gerber S, Larget-Piet D, Chenal V, Liu X-Z, Newton V, Steel KP, Brown SDM, Munnich A, Kaplan J, Petit C, Weil D: Myosin VIIA gene: Heterogeneity of the mutations responsible for Usher syndrome type IB. *Hum Mol Genet* **6**:111, 1997.

61. Liu XZ, Newton VE, Steel KP, Brown SD: Identification of a new mutation of the myosin VII head region in Usher syndrome type 1. *Hum Mutat* **10**:168, 1997.

62. Cuevas JM, Espinos C, Millan JM, Sanchez F, Trujillo MJ, Ayuso C, Beneyto M, Najera C: Identification of three novel mutations in the MYO7A gene. *Hum Mutat* **14**:181, 1999.

63. Janecke AR, Meins M, Sadeghi M, Grundmann K, Apfelstedt-Sylla E, Zrenner E, Rosenberg T, Gal A: Twelve novel myosin VIIA mutations in 34 patients with Usher syndrome type I: Confirmation of genetic heterogeneity. *Hum Mutat* **13**:133, 1999.

64. Weil D, Bernard M, Combates N, Wirtz MK, Hollister DW, Steinmann B, Ramirez F: Identification of a mutation that causes exon skipping during collagen pre-mRNA splicing in an Ehlers-Danlos syndrome variant. *J Biol Chem* **263**:8561, 1988.

65. Sahly I, El-Amraoui A, Abitbol M, Petit C, Dufier J-L: Expression of myosin VIIA during mouse embryogenesis. *Anat Embryol (Berl)* **196**:159, 1997.

66. Hasson T, Heintzelman MB, Santos-Sacchi J, Corey DP, Mooseker MS: Expression in cochlea and retina of myosin VIIa, the gene product defective in Usher syndrome type 1B. *Proc Natl Acad Sci U S A* **92**:9815, 1995.

67. El-Amraoui A, Sahly I, Picaud S, Sahel J, Abitbol M, Petit C: Human Usher IB/mouse *shaker-1*; the retinal phenotype discrepancy explained by the presence/absence of myosin VIIA in the photoreceptor cells. *Hum Mol Genet* **5**:1171, 1996.

68. Hasson T, Gillespie PG, Garcia JA, MacDonald RB, Zhao Y, Yee AG, Mooseker MS, Corey DP: Unconventional myosins in inner-ear sensory epithelia. *J Cell Biol* **137**:1287, 1997.

69. Self T, Mahony M, Fleming J, Walsh J, Brown SD, Steel KP: Shaker-1 mutations reveal roles for myosin VIIA in both development and function of cochlear hair cells. *Development* **125**:557, 1998.

70. Richardson GP, Forge A, Kros CJ, Fleming J, Brown SD, Steel KP: Myosin VIIA is required for aminoglycoside accumulation in cochlear hair cells. *J Neurosci* **17**:9506, 1997.

71. Liu X, Ondek B, Williams DS: Mutant myosin VIIa causes defective melanosome distribution in the RPE of shaker-1 mice. *Nat Genet* **19**:117, 1998.

72. Liu X, Udovichenko IP, Brown SD, Steel KP, Williams DS: Myosin VIIa participates in opsin transport through the photoreceptor cilium. *J Neurosci* **19**:6267, 1999.

73. Titus MA: A class VII unconventional myosin is required for phagocytosis. *Curr Biol* **9**:1297, 1999.

74. Chaïb H, Place C, Salem N, Dodé C, Chardenoux S, Weissenbach J, El Zir E, Loiselet J, Petit C: Mapping of DFNB12, a gene for a non-syndromal autosomal recessive deafness, to chromosome 10q21-22. *Hum Mol Genet* **5**:1061, 1996.

75. Wayne S, Der Kaloustian VM, Schloss M, Polomeno R, Scott DA, Hejtmancik JF, Sheffield VC, Smith RJH: Localization of the Usher syndrome type 1D gene (Ush1D) to chromosome 10. *Hum Mol Genet* **5**:1689, 1996.

76. Chen AH, Wayne S, Bell A, Ramesh A, Srisailapathy CRS, Scott DA, Sheffield VC, Van Hauwe P, Zbar RIS, Ashley J, Lovett M, Van Camp

77. Sankila E-M, Pakarinen L, Kääriäinen H, Aittomäki K, Karjalainen S, Sistonen P, de la Chapelle A: Assignment of an Usher syndrome type III (USH3) gene to chromosome 3q. *Hum Mol Genet* **4**:93, 1995.

78. Jain PK, Lalwani AK, Li XC, Singleton TL, Smith TN, Chen A, Deshmukh D, Verma IC, Smith RJH, Wilcox ER: A gene for recessive nonsyndromic sensorineural deafness (*DFNB18*) maps to the chromosomal region 11p14-p15.1 containing the Usher syndrome type 1C gene. *Genomics* **50**:290, 1998.

79. Keats BJ, Nouri N, Pelias MZ, Deininger PL, Litt M: Tightly linked flanking microsatellite markers for the Usher syndrome type I locus on the short arm of chromosome 11. *Am J Hum Genet* **54**:681, 1994.

80. Friedman TB, Liang Y, Weber JL, Hinnant JT, Barber TD, Winata S, Arhya IN, Asher JH: A gene for congenital, recessive deafness DFNB3 maps to the pericentromeric region of chromosome 17. *Nat Genet* **9**:86, 1995.

81. Liang Y, Wang A, Probst FJ, Arhya IN, Barber TD, Chen KS, Deshmukh D, Dolan DF, Hinnant JT, Carter LE, Jain PK, Lalwani AK, Li XC, Lupski JR, Moeljopawiro S, Morell R, Negrini C, Wilcox ER, Winata S, Camper SA, Friedman TB: Genetic mapping refines DFNB3 to 17p11.2, suggests multiple alleles of DFNB3, and supports homology to the mouse model *shaker-2*. *Am J Hum Genet* **62**:904, 1998.

82. Probst FJ, Fridell RA, Raphael Y, Saunders TL, Wang A, Liang Y, Morell RJ, Touchman JW, Lyons RH, Noben-Trauth K, Friedman TB, Camper SA: Correction of deafness in *shaker-2* mice by an unconventional myosin in a BAC transgene. *Science* **280**:1444, 1998.

83. Wang A, Liang Y, Fridell RA, Probst FJ, Wilcox ER, Touchman JW, Morton CC, Morell RJ, Noben-Trauth K, Camper SA, Friedman TB: Association of unconventional myosin MYO15 mutations with human nonsyndromic deafness DFNB3. *Science* **280**:1447, 1998.

84. Liang Y, Wang A, Belyantseva IA, Anderson DW, Probst FJ, Barber TD, Miller W, Touchman JW, Jin L, Sullivan SL, Sellers JR, Camper SA, Lloyd RV, Kachar B, Friedman TB, Fridell RA: Characterization of the human and mouse unconventional myosin XV genes responsible for hereditary deafness DFNB3 and Shaker-2. *Genomics* **61**:243, 1999.

85. Deol MS, Green MC: Snell's waltzer, a new mutation affecting behaviour and the inner ear in the mouse. *Genet Res* **8**:339, 1966.

86. Avraham KB, Hasson T, Steel KP, Kingsley DM, Russell LB, Mooseker MS, Copeland NG, Jenkins NA: The mouse Snell's waltzer deafness gene encodes an unconventional myosin required for structural integrity of inner ear hair cells. *Nat Genet* **11**:369, 1995.

87. Wells AL, Lin AW, Chen L-Q, Safer D, Cain SM, Hasson T, Carragher BO, Milligan RA, Sweeney HL: Myosin VI is an actin-based motor that moves backwards. *Nature* **401**:505, 1999.

88. Self T, Sobe T, Copeland NG, Jenkins NA, Avraham KB, Steel KP: Role of myosin VI in the differentiation of cochlear hair cells. *Dev Biol* **214**:331, 1999.

89. Hirokawa N, Tilney LG: Interactions between actin filaments and between actin filaments and membranes in quick-frozen and deeply etched hair cells of the chick ear. *J Cell Biol* **95**: 261, 1982.

90. Avraham KB, Hasson T, Sobe T, Balsara B, Testa JR, Skvorak AB, Morton CC, Copeland NG, Jenkins NA: Characterization of unconventional MYO6, the human homologue of the gene responsible for deafness in Snell's waltzer mice. *Hum Mol Genet* **6**:1225, 1997.

91. Coucke P, Van Camp G, Djoyodiharjo B, Smith SD, Frants RR, Padberg GW, Darby JK, Huizing EH, Cremers CWRJ, Kimberling WJ, Oostra BA, Van de Heyning PH, Willems PJ: Linkage of autosomal dominant hearing loss to the short arm of chromosome 1 in two families. *N Engl J Med* **331**:425, 1994.

92. Van Camp G, Coucke PJ, Kunst H, Schatteman I, Van Velzen D, Marres H, van Ewijk M, Declau F, Van Hauwe P, Meyers J, Kenyon J, Smith SD, Smith RJ, Djelantik B, Cremers CW, Van de Heyning PH, Willems PJ: Linkage analysis of progressive hearing loss in five extended families maps the DFNA2 gene to a 1.25-Mb region on chromosome 1p. *Genomics* **41**:70, 1997.

93. Kubisch C, Schroeder BC, Friedrich T, Lütjohann B, El-Amraoui A, Marlin S, Petit C, Jentsch TJ: KCNQ4, a novel potassium channel expressed in sensory outer hair cells, is mutated in dominant deafness. *Cell* **96**:437, 1999.

94. Heginbotham L, Lu Z, Abramson T, MacKinnon R: Mutations in the K$^+$ channel signature sequence. *Biophys J* **66**:1061, 1994.

95. Neyroud N, Tesson F, Denjoy I, Leibovici M, Donger C, Barhanin J, Fauré S, Gary F, Coumel P, Petit C, Schwartz K, Guicheney P: A novel mutation in the potassium channel gene *KVLQT1* causes the Jervell and Lange-Nielsen cardioauditory syndrome. *Nat Genet* **15**:186, 1997.

96. Wang HS, Pan Z, Shi W, Brown BS, Wymore RS, Cohen IS, Dixon JE, McKinnon D: KCNQ2 and KCNQ3 potassium channel subunits: Molecular correlates of the M-channel. *Science* **282**:1890, 1998.

97. Barhanin J, Lesage F, Guillemare E, Fink M, Lazdunski M, Romey G: K(V)LQT1 and lsK (minK) proteins associate to form the I(Ks) cardiac potassium current. *Nature* **384**:78, 1996.

98. Sanguinetti MC, Curran ME, Zou A, Shen J, Spector PS, Atkinson DL, Keating MT: Coassembly of K(V)LQT1 and minK (IsK) proteins to form cardiac I(Ks) potassium channel. *Nature* **384**:80, 1996.

99. Coucke PJ, Van Hauwe P, Kelley PM, Kunst H, Schatteman I, Van Velzen D, Meyers J, Ensink RJ, Verstreken M, Declau F, Marres H, Kastury K, Bhasin S, McGuirt WT, Smith RJH, Cremers CWRJ, Van de Heyning P, Willems PJ, Smith SD, Van Camp G: Mutations in the *KCNQ4* gene are responsible for autosomal dominant deafness in four DFNA2 families. *Hum Mol Genet* **8**:1321, 1999.

100. Marres H, van Ewijk M, Huygen P, Kunst H, van Camp G, Coucke P, Willems P, Cremers C: Inherited nonsyndromic hearing loss. An audiovestibular study in a large family with autosomal dominant progressive hearing loss related to DFNA2. *Arch Otolaryngol Head Neck Surg* **123**:573, 1997.

101. Kunst H, Marres H, Huygen P, Ensink R, Van Camp G, Van Hauwe P, Coucke P, Willems P, Cremers C: Nonsyndromic autosomal dominant progressive sensorineural hearing loss: Audiologic analysis of a pedigree linked to DFNA2. *Laryngoscope* **108**:74, 1998.

102. Kharkovets T, Hardelin J-P, Safieddine S, Schweizer M, El-Amraoui A, Petit C, Jentsch TJ: KCNQ4, a K+-channel mutated in a form of dominant deafness, is expressed in the inner ear and in the central auditory pathway. *Proc Natl Acad Sci U S A* **97**:4333, 2000.

103. Rennie KJ, Ashmore JF: Ionic currents in isolated vestibular hair cells from the guinea-pig crista ampullaris. *Hear Res* **51**:279, 1991.

104. Housley GD, Ashmore JF: Ionic currents of outer hair cells isolated from the guinea-pig cochlea. *J Physiol* **448**:73, 1992.

105. Nakagawa T, Kakehata S, Yamamoto T, Akaike N, Komune S, Uemura T: Ionic properties of IK,n in outer hair cells of guinea pig cochlea. *Brain Res* **661**:293, 1994.

106. Marcotti W, Kros CJ: Developmental expression of the potassium current $I_{K,n}$ contributes to maturation of mouse outer hair cells. *J Physiol* **520**:653, 1999.

107. Chaïb H, Place C, Salem N, Chardenoux S, Vincent C, Weissenbach J, El Zir E, Loiselet J, Petit C: A gene responsible for a sensorineural nonsyndromic recessive deafness maps to chromosome 2p22-23. *Hum Mol Genet* **5**:155, 1996.

108. Cohen-Salmon M, El-Amraoui A, Leibovici M, Petit C: Otogelin: A glycoprotein specific to the acellular membranes of the inner ear. *Proc Natl Acad Sci U S A* **94**:14450, 1997.

109. Yasunaga S, Grati M, Cohen-Salmon M, El-Amraoui A, Mustapha M, Salem N, El-Zir E, Loiselet J, Petit C: A mutation in *OTOF*, encoding otoferlin, a FER-1 like protein, causes DFNB9, a nonsyndromic form of deafness. *Nat Genet* **21**:363, 1999.

110. Achanzar WE, Ward S: A nematode gene required for sperm vesicle fusion. *J Cell Sci* **110**:1073, 1997.

111. Bashir R, Britton S, Strachan T, Keers S, Vafiadaki E, Lako M, Richard I, Marchand S, Bourg N, Argov Z, Sadeh M, Mahjneh I, Marconi G, Passos-Bueno MR, de S Moreira E, Zatz M, Beckmann J, Bushby K: A gene related to *Caenorhabditis elegans* spermatogenesis factor *fer-1* is mutated in limb-girdle muscular dystrophy type 2B. *Nat Genet* **20**:37, 1998.

112. Liu J, Aoki M, Illa I, Wu C, Fardeau M, Angelini C, Serrano C, Urtizberea JA, Hentati F, Ben Hamida M, Bohlega S, Culper EJ, Amato AA, Bossie K, Oeltjen J, Bejaoui K, McKenna-Yasek D, Hosler BA, Schurr E, Arahata K, de Jong PJ, Brown RHJ: Dysferlin, a novel skeletal muscle gene, is mutated in Miyoshi myopathy and limb-girdle muscular dystrophy. *Nat Genet* **20**:31, 1998.

113. Belt Davis D, Delmonte AJ, Ly CT, McNally EM: Myoferlin, a candidate gene and potential modifier of muscular dystrophy. *Hum Mol Genet* **9**:217, 2000.

114. Matthew WD, Tsavaler L, Reichardt LF: Identification of a synaptic vesicle-specific membrane protein with a wide distribution in neuronal and neurosecretory tissue. *J Cell Biol* **91**:257, 1981.

115. Sutton RB, Davletov BA, Berghuis AM, Südhof TC, Sprang SR: Structure of the first C2 domain of synaptotagmin I: a novel Ca2+/ phospholipid-binding fold. *Cell* **80**:929, 1995.

116. Leal SM, Apaydin F, Barnwell C, Iber M, Kandogan T, Pfister M, Braendle U, Cura O, Schwalb M, Zenner H-P, Vitale E: A second Middle Eastern kindred with autosomal recessive non-syndromic hearing loss segregates DFNB9. *Eur J Hum Genet* **6**:341, 1998.

117. Rizo J, Südhof TC: C2-domains, structure and function of a universal Ca2+ -binding domain. *J Biol Chem* **273**:15879, 1998.

118. Perin MS, Fried VA, Mignery GA, Jahn R, Südhof TC: Phospholipid binding by a synaptic vesicle protein homologous to the regulatory region of protein kinase C. *Nature* **345**:260, 1990.

119. Clark JD, Lin LL, Kriz RW, Ramesha CS, Sultzman LA, Lin AY, Milona N, Knopf JL: A novel arachidonic acid-selective cytosolic PLA2 contains a Ca(2+)-dependent translocation domain with homology to PKC and GAP. *Cell* **65**:1043, 1991.

120. Shirataki H, Kaibuchi K, Sakoda T, Kishida S, Yamaguchi T, Wada K, Miyazaki M, Takai Y: Rabphilin-3A, a putative target protein for smg p25A/rab3A p25 small GTP-binding protein related to synaptotagmin. *Mol Cell Biol* **13**:2061, 1993.

121. Li C, Takei K, Geppert M, Daniell L, Stenius K, Chapman ER, Jahn R, De Camilli P, Südhof TC: Synaptic targeting of rabphilin-3A, a synaptic vesicle Ca2+/phospholipid-binding protein, depends on rab3A/3C. *Neuron* **13**:885, 1994.

122. Brose N, Hofmann K, Hata Y, Südhof TC: Mammalian homologues of Caenorhabditis elegans unc-13 gene define novel family of C2-domain proteins. *J Biol Chem* **270**:25273, 1995.

123. Verhage M, de Vries KJ, Roshol H, Burbach JP, Gispen WH, Südhof TC: DOC2 proteins in rat brain: complementary distribution and proposed function as vesicular adapter proteins in early stages of secretion. *Neuron* **18**:453, 1997.

124. Wang Y, Okamoto M, Schmitz F, Hofmann K, Südhof TC: Rim is a putative Rab3 effector in regulating synaptic-vesicle fusion. *Nature* **388**:593, 1997.

125. Parsons TD, Lenzi D, Almers W, Roberts WM: Calcium-triggered exocytosis and endocytosis in an isolated presynaptic cell: Capacitance measurements in saccular hair cells. *Neuron* **13**:875, 1994.

126. Safieddine S, Wenthold RJ: SNARE complex at the ribbon synapses of cochlear hair cells: analysis of synaptic vesicle- and synaptic membrane-associated proteins. *Eur J Neurosci* **11**:803, 1999.

127. Vahava O, Morell R, Lynch ED, Weiss S, Kagan ME, Ahituv N, Morrow J, Lee MK, Skvorak AB, Morton CC, Blumenfeld A, Frydman M, Friedman TB, King M-C, Avraham KA: Mutation in transcription factor *POU4F3* associated with inherited progressive hearing loss in humans. *Science* **279**:1950, 1998.

128. Xiang M, Gan L, Li D, Chen ZY, Zhou L, O'Malley BWJ, Klein W, Nathans J: Essential role of POU-domain factor Brn-3c in auditory and vestibular hair cell development. *Proc Natl Acad Sci U S A* **94**:9445, 1997.

129. Xiang M, Gao W-Q, Hasson T, Shin JJ: Requirement for Brn-3c in maturation and survival, but not in fate determination of inner hair cells. *Development* **125**:3935, 1998.

130. Erkman L, McEvilly RJ, Luo L, Ryan AK, Hooshmand F, O'Connell SM, Keithley EM, Rapaport DH, Ryan AF, Rosenfeld MG: Role of transcription factors Brn-3.1 and Brn-3.2 in auditory and visual system development. *Nature* **381**:603, 1996.

131. Street VA, Robinson LC, Erford SK, Tempel BL: Molecular genetic analysis of distal mouse chromosome 6 defines gene order and positions of the deafwaddler and opisthotonos mutations. *Genomics* **29**:123, 1995.

132. Noben-Trauth K, Zheng QY, Johnson KR, Nishina PM: *mdfw*: A deafness susceptibility locus that interacts with deaf waddler (*dfw*). *Genomics* **44**:266, 1997.

133. Carafoli E, Stauffer T: The plasma membrane calcium pump: Functional domains, regulation of the activity, and tissue specificity of isoform expression. *J Neurobiol* **25**:312, 1994.

134. Carafoli E: Biogenesis: Plasma membrane calcium ATPase: 15 years of work on the purified enzyme. *FASEB J* **8**:993, 1994.

135. Street VA, McKee-Johnson JW, Fonseca RC, Tempel BL, Noben-Trauth K: Mutations in a plasma membrane Ca2+-ATPase gene cause deafness in deafwaddler mice. *Nat Genet* **19**:390, 1998.

136. Kozel PJ, Friedman RA, Erway LC, Yamoah EN, Liu LH, Riddle T, Duffy JJ, Doetschman T, Miller ML, Cardell EL, Shull GE: Balance and hearing deficits in mice with a null mutation in the gene encoding plasma membrane Ca2+-ATPase isoform 2. *J Biol Chem* **273**:18693, 1998.

137. Furuta H, Luo L, Hepler K, Ryan AF: Evidence for differential regulation of calcium by outer versus inner hair cells: Plasma membrane Ca-ATPase gene expression. *Hear Res* **123**:10, 1998.

138. Lumpkin EA, Marquis RE, Hudspeth AJ: The selectivity of the hair cell's mechanoelectrical-transduction channel promotes $Ca^{2+}$ flux at low $Ca^{2+}$ concentrations. *Proc Natl Acad Sci U S A* **94**:10997, 1997.

139. Crouch JJ, Schulte BA: Expression of plasma membrane Ca-ATPase in the adult and developing gerbil cochlea. *Hear Res* **92**:112, 1995.

140. Apicella S, Chen S, Bing R, Penniston JT, Llinas R, Hillman DE: Plasmalemmal ATPase calcium pump localizes to inner and outer hair bundles. *Neuroscience* **79**:1145, 1997.

141. Yamoah EN, Lumpkin EA, Dumont RA, Smith PJ, Hudspeth AJ, Gillespie PG: Plasma membrane $Ca^{2+}$-ATPase extrudes $Ca^{2+}$ from hair cell stereocilia. *J Neurosci* **18**:610, 1998.

142. Kros CJ: Physiology of mammalian cochlear hair cells, in Dallos P, Popper AN, Fay RR (eds): *The Cochlea*. New York, Springer-Verlag, 1996, p 318.

143. Chaïb H, Lina-Granade G, Guilford P, Plauchu H, Levilliers J, Morgon A, Petit C: A gene responsible for a dominant form of neurosensory non-syndromic deafness maps to the *NSRD1* recessive deafness gene interval. *Hum Mol Genet* **3**:2219, 1994.

144. Kelley PM, Harris DJ, Comer BC, Askew JW, Fowler T, Smith SD, Kimberling WJ: Novel mutations in the connexin 26 gene (GJB2) that cause autosomal recessive (DFNB1) hearing loss. *Am J Hum Genet* **62**:792, 1998.

145. Scott DA, Kraft ML, Stone EM, Sheffield VC, Smith RJH: Connexin mutations and hearing loss. *Nature* **391**:32, 1998.

146. Dahl G, Miller T, Paul D, Voellmy R, Werner R: Expression of functional cell-cell channels from cloned rat liver gap junction complementary DNA. *Science* **236**:1290, 1987.

147. White TW, Deans MR, Kelsell DP, Paul DL: Connexin mutations in deafness. *Nature* **394**:630, 1998.

148. Richard G, White TW, Smith LE, Bailey RE, Compton JG, Paul DL, Bale SJ: Functional defects of Cx26 resulting from a heterozygous missense mutation in a family with dominant deaf-mutism and palmoplantar keratoderma. *Hum Genet* **103**:393, 1998.

149. Maw MA, Allen-Powell DR, Goodey RJ, Stewart IA, Nancarrow DJ, Hayward NK, McKinlay Gardner RJ: The contribution of the DFNB1 locus to neurosensory deafness in a Caucasian population. *Am J Hum Genet* **57**:629, 1995.

150. Gasparini P, Estivill X, Volpini V, Totaro A, Castellvi-Bel S, Goeva N, Mila M, Della Monica M, Ventruto V, De Benedetto M, Stanziale P, Zelante L, Mansfield ES, Sandkuijl L, Surrey S, Fortina P: Linkage of DFNB1 to non-syndromic neurosensory autosomal-recessive deafness in Mediterranean families. *Eur J Hum Genet* **5**:83, 1997.

151. Denoyelle F, Weil D, Maw MA, Wilcox SA, Lench NJ, Allen-Powell DR, Osborn AH, Dahl H-HM, Middleton A, Houseman MJ, Dodé C, Marlin S, Boulila-ElGaïed A, Grati M, Ayadi H, BenArab S, Bitoun P, Lina-Granade G, Godet J, Mustapha M, Loiselet J, El-Zir E, Aubois A, Joannard A, Levilliers J, Garabédian E-N, Mueller RF, McKinlay Gardner RJ, Petit C: Prelingual deafness: High prevalence of a 30delG mutation in the connexin 26 gene. *Hum Mol Genet* **6**:2173, 1997.

152. Zelante L, Gasparini P, Estivill X, Melchionda S, D'Agruma L, Govea N, Mila M, Della Monica M, Lutfi J, Shohat M, Mansfield E, Delgrosso K, Rappaport E, Surrey S, Fortina P: Connexin26 mutations associated with the most common form of non-syndromic neurosensory autosomal recessive deafness (DFNB1) in Mediterraneans. *Hum Mol Genet* **6**:1605, 1997.

153. Estivill X, Fortina P, Surrey S, Rabionet R, Melchionda S, D'Agruma L, Mansfield E, Rappaport E, Govea N, Milà M, Zelante L, Gasparini P: Connexin-26 mutations in sporadic and inherited sensorineural deafness. *Lancet* **351**:394, 1998.

154. Murgia A, Orzan E, Polli R, Martella M, Vinanzi C, Leonardi E, Arslan E, Zacchello F: Cx26 deafness: Mutation analysis and clinical variability. *J Med Genet* **36**:829, 1999.

155. Green GE, Scott DA, McDonald JM, Woodworth GG, Sheffield VC, Smith RJ: Carrier rates in the midwestern United States for *GJB2* mutations causing inherited deafness. *JAMA* **281**:2211, 1999.

156. Lench N, Housemam M, Newton V, Van Camp G, Mueller R: Connexin-26 mutations in sporadic non-syndromal sensorineural deafness. *Lancet* **351**:415, 1998.

157. Sobe T, Vreugde S, Shahin H, Berlin M, Davis N, Kanaan M, Yaron Y, Orr-Urtreger A, Frydman M, Shohat M, Avraham KB: The prevalence and expression of inherited connexin 26 mutations associated with nonsyndromic hearing loss in the Israeli population. *Hum Genet* **106**:50, 2000.

158. Abe S, Usami S-i, Shinkawa H, Kelley PM, Kimberling WJ: Prevalent connexin 26 gene (GJB2) mutations in Japanese. *J Med Genet* **37**:41, 2000.

159. Kudo T, Ikeda K, Kure S, Matsubara Y, Oshima T, Watanabe K-I, Kawase T, Narisawa K, Takasaka T: Novel mutations in the connexin 26 gene (GJB2) responsible for childhood deafness in the Japanese population. *Am J Med Genet* **90**:141, 2000.

160. Antoniadi T, Rabionet R, Kroupis C, Aperis GA, Economides J, Petmezakis J, Economou-Petersen E, Estivill X, Petersen MB: High prevalence in the Greek population of the 35delG mutation in the connexin 26 gene causing prelingual deafness. *Clin Genet* **55**:381, 1999.

161. Storm K, Willocx S, Flothmann K, Van Camp G: Determination of the carrier frequency of the common GJB2 (connexin-26) 35delG mutation in the Belgian population using an easy and reliable screening method. *Hum Mutat* **14**:263-266, 1999.

162. Scott DA, Kraft ML, Carmi R, Ramesh A, Elbedour K, Yairi Y, Srisailapathy CR, Rosengren SS, Markham AF, Mueller RF, Lench NJ, Van Camp G, Smith RJ, Sheffield VC: Identification of mutations in the connexin 26 gene that cause autosomal recessive nonsyndromic hearing loss. *Hum Mutat* **11**:387, 1998.

163. Morell RJ, Kim HJ, Hood LJ, Goforth L, Friderici K, Fisher R, Van Camp G, Berlin CI, Oddoux C, Ostrer H, Keats B, Friedman TB: Mutations in the connexin 26 gene (GJB2) among Ashkenazi Jews with nonsyndromic recessive deafness. *N Engl J Med* **339**:1500, 1998.

164. Sobe T, Erlich P, Berry A, Korostichevsky M, Vreugde S, Avraham KB, Bonné-Tamir B, Shohat M: High frequency of the deafness-associated 167delT mutation in the connexin 26 (*GJB2*) gene in Israeli Ashkenazim. *Am J Med Genet* **86**:499, 1999.

165. Cohn ES, Kelley PM, Fowler TW, Gorga MP, Lefkowitz DM, Kuehn HJ, Schaefer GB, Gobar LS, Hahn FJ, Harris DJ, Kimberling WJ: Clinical studies of families with hearing loss attributable to mutations in the connexin 26 gene (GJB2/DFNB1). *Pediatrics* **103**:546, 1999.

166. Morlé L, Bozon M, Alloisio N, Latour P, Vandenberghe A, Plauchu H, Collet L, Edery P, Godet J, Lina-Granade G: A novel C202F mutation in the connexin26 gene (*GJB2*) associated with autosomal dominant isolated hearing loss. *J Med Genet* **37**:368, 2000.

167. Kumar NM, Giludla NB: The gap junction communication channel. *Cell* **84**:381, 1996.

168. Unger VM, Kumar NM, Gilula NB, Yeager M: Three-dimensional structure of a recombinant gap junction membrane channel. *Science* **283**:1176, 1999.

169. Bruzzone R, White TW, Paul DL: Connections with connexins: The molecular basis of direct intercellular signaling. *Eur J Biochem* **238**:1, 1996.

170. Lee MJ, Rhee SK: Heteromeric gap junction channels in rat hepatocytes in which the expression of connexin 26 is induced. *Mol Cells* **8**:295, 1998.

171. Brissette JL, Kumar NM, Gilula NB, Hall JE, Dotto GP: Switch in gap junction protein expression is associated with selective changes in junctional permeability during keratinocyte differentiation. *Proc Natl Acad Sci U S A* **91**:6453, 1994.

172. Steinberg TH, Civitelli R, Geist ST, Robertson AJ, Hick E, Veenstra RD, Wang HZ, Warlow PM, Westphale EM, Laing JG, et al.: Connexin 43 and connexin 45 form gap junctions with different molecular permeabilities in osteoblastic cells. *EMBO J* **13**:744, 1994.

173. Elfgang C, Eckert R, Lichtenberg-Frate H, Butterweck A, Traub O, Klein RA, Hulser DF, Willecke K: Specific permeability and selective formation of gap junction channels in connexin-transfected HeLa cells. *J Cell Biol* **129**:805, 1995.

174. Veenstra RD, Wang HZ, Beblo DA, Chilton MG, Harris AL, Beyer EC, Brink PR: Selectivity of connexin-specific gap junctions does not correlate with channel conductance. *Circ Res* **77**:1156, 1995.

175. Bevans CG, Kordel M, Rhee SK, Harris AL: Isoform composition of connexin channels determines selectivity among second messengers and uncharged molecules. *J Biol Chem* **273**:2808, 1998.

176. Dhein S: Gap junction channels in the cardiovascular system: Pharmacological and physiological modulation. *Trends Pharmacol Sci* **19**:229, 1998.

177. Warn-Cramer BJ, Cottrell GT, Burt JM, Lau AF: Regulation of connexin-43 gap junctional intercellular communication by mitogen-activated protein kinase. *J Biol Chem* **273**:9188, 1998.

178. Bevans CG, Harris AL: Direct high affinity modulation of connexin channel activity by cyclic nucleotides. *J Biol Chem* **274**:3720, 1999.

179. Bevans CG, Harris AL: Regulation of connexin channels by pH. Direct action of the protonated form of taurine and other aminosulfonates. *J Biol Chem* **274**:3711, 1999.

180. Cao F, Eckert R, Elfgang C, Nitsche JM, Snyder SA, DF Hu, Willecke K, Nicholson BJ: A quantitative analysis of connexin-specific permeability differences of gap junctions expressed in HeLa transfectants and *Xenopus* oocytes. *J Cell Sci* **111**:31, 1998.

181. Saez JC, Nairn AC, Czernik AJ, Spray DC, Hertzberg EL, Greengard P, Bennett MV: Phosphorylation of connexin 32, a hepatocyte gap-junction protein, by cAMP-dependent protein kinase, protein kinase C and Ca2+/calmodulin-dependent protein kinase II. *Eur J Biochem* **192**:263, 1990.

182. Rubin JB, Verselis VK, Bennett MV, Bargiello TA: Molecular analysis of voltage dependence of heterotypic gap junctions formed by connexins 26 and 32. *Biophys J* **62**:183, 1992.

183. Suchyna TM, Xu LX, Gao F, Fourtner CR, Nicholson BJ: Identification of a proline residue as a transduction element involved in voltage gating of gap junctions. *Nature* **365**:847, 1993.

184. Simon A, Goodenough D: Diverse functions of vertebrate gap junctions. *Trends Cell Biol* **8**:477, 1998.

185. Bergoffen J, Scherer SS, Wang S, Oronzi Scott M, Bone LJ, Paul DL, Chen K, Lensch MW, Chance PF, Fischbeck KH: Connexin mutations in X-linked Charcot-Marie-Tooth disease. *Science* **262**:2039, 1993.

186. Shiels A, Mackay D, Ionides A, Berry V, Moore A, Bhattacharya S: A missense mutation in the human connexin50 gene (*GJA8*) underlies dominant "zonular pulverulent" cataract, on chromosome 1q. *Am J Hum Genet* **62**:526, 1998.

187. Mackay D, Ionides A, Kibar Z, Rouleau G, Berry V, Moore A, Shiels A, Bhattacharya S: Connexin 46 mutations in autosomal dominant congenital cataract. *Am J Hum Genet* **64**:1357, 1999.

188. Richard G, Smith LE, Bailey RA, Itin P, Hohl D, Epstein EH, DiGiovanna JJ, Compton JG, Bale SJ: Mutations in the human connexin gene GJB3 cause erythrokeratodermia variabilis. *Nat Genet* **20**:366, 1998.

189. Britz-Cunningham SH, Shah MM, Zuppan CW, Fletcher WH: Mutations of the connexin 43 gap-junction gene in patients with heart malformations and defects of laterality. *N Engl J Med* **332**:1323, 1995.

190. Penman Splitt M, Tsai MY, Burn J, Goodship JA: Absence of mutations in the regulatory domain of the gap junction protein connexin 43 in patients with visceroatrial heterotaxy. *Heart* **77**:369, 1997.

191. Zhang JT, Nicholson BJ: Sequence and tissue distribution of a second protein of hepatic gap junctions, Cx26, as deduced from its cDNA. *J Cell Biol* **109**:3391, 1989.

192. Lee SW, Tomasetto C, Sager R: Positive selection of candidate tumor-suppressor genes by subtractive hybridization. *Proc Natl Acad Sci U S A* **88**:2825, 1991.

193. Lee SW, Tomasetto C, Paul D, Keyomarsi K, Sager R: Transcriptional downregulation of gap-junction proteins blocks junctional communication in human mammary tumor cell lines. *J Cell Biol* **118**:1213, 1992.

194. Dermietzel R, Traub O, Hwang TK, Beyer E, Bennett MV, Spray DC, Willecke K: Differential expression of three gap junction proteins in developing and mature brain tissues. *Proc Natl Acad Sci U S A* **86**:10148, 1989.

195. Traub O, Look J, Dermietzel R, Brummer F, Hulser D, Willecke K: Comparative characterization of the 21-kD and 26-kD gap junction proteins in murine liver and cultured hepatocytes. *J Cell Biol* **108**:1039, 1989.

196. Risek B, Gilula NB: Spatiotemporal expression of three gap junction gene products involved in fetomaternal communication during rat pregnancy. *Development* **113**:165, 1991.

197. Kuraoka A, Iida H, Hatae T, Shibata Y, Itoh M, Kurita T: Localization of gap junction proteins, connexins 32 and 26, in rat and guinea pig liver as revealed by quick-freeze, deep-etch immunoelectron microscopy. *J Histochem Cytochem* **41**:971, 1993.

198. Meda P, Pepper MS, Traub O, Willecke K, Gros D, Beyer E, Nicholson B, Paul D, Orci L: Differential expression of gap junction connexins in endocrine and exocrine glands. *Endocrinology* **133**:2371, 1993.

199. Winterhager E, Grummer R, Jahn E, Willecke K, Traub O: Spatial and temporal expression of connexin 26 and connexin 43 in rat endometrium during trophoblast invasion. *Dev Biol* **157**:399, 1993.

200. Salomon D, Masgrau E, Vischer S, Ullrich S, Dupont E, Sappino P, Saurat JH, Meda P: Topography of mammalian connexins in human skin. *J Invest Dermatol* **103**:240, 1994.

201. Mesnil M, Krutovskikh V, Piccoli C, Elfgang C, Traub O, Willecke K, Yamasaki H: Negative growth control of HeLa cells by connexin genes: connexin species specificity. *Cancer Res* **55**:629, 1995.

202. Hirschi KK, Xu CE, Tsukamoto T, Sager R: Gap junction genes Cx26 and Cx43 individually suppress the cancer phenotype of human mammary carcinoma cells and restore differentiation potential. *Cell Growth Differ* **7**:861, 1996.

203. Duflot-Dancer A, Mesnil M, Yamasaki H: Dominant-negative abrogation of connexin-mediated cell growth control by mutant connexin genes. *Oncogene* **15**:2151, 1997.

204. Hama K: A study on the fine structure of the saccular macula of the gold fish. *Zeitschr Zellforsch Mikroskop Anat* **94**:155, 1969.

205. Spicer SS, Schulte BA: Differentiation of inner ear fibrocytes according to their ion transport related activity. *Hear Res* **56**:53, 1991.

206. Spicer SS, Schulte BA: The fine structure of spiral ligament cells relates to ion return to the stria and varies with place-frequency. *Hear Res* **100**:80, 1996.

207. Sterkers O: Origin and electrochemical composition of endolymph in the cochlea, in Dresscher D (ed): *Audiology Biochemistry.* Springfield, IL, CC Thomas, 1985, p 473.

208. Salt AN, Thalmann R, Marcus DC, Bohne BA: Direct measurement of longitudinal endolymph flow rate in the guinea pig cochlea. *Hear Res* **23**:141, 1986.

209. Oesterle EC, Dallos P: Intercellular recordings from supporting cells in the guinea-pig cochlea: DC potentials. *J Neurophysiol* **64**:617, 1990.

210. Kuijpers W, Bonting SL: Studies on (Na+-K+)-activated ATPase. XXIV. Localization and properties of ATPase in the inner ear of the guinea pig. *Biochim Biophys Acta* **173**:477, 1969.

211. Fina M, Ryan A: Expression of mRNAs encoding alpha and beta subunit isoforms of Na,K-ATPase in the vestibular labyrinth and endolymphatic sac of the rat. *Mol Cell Neurosci* **5**:604, 1994.

212. Goto S, Oshima T, Ikeda K, Ueda N, Takasaka T: Expression and localization of the Na-K-2Cl cotransporter in the rat cochlea. *Brain Res* **765**:324, 1997.

213. Mizuta K, Adachi M, Iwasa KH: Ultrastructural localization of the Na-K-Cl cotransporter in the lateral wall of the rabbit cochlear duct. *Hear Res* **106**:154, 1997.

214. Vetter DE, Mann JR, Wangemann P, Liu J, McLaughlin KJ, Lesage F, Marcus DC, Lazdunski M, Heinemann SF, Barhanin J: Inner ear defects induced by null mutation of the *isk* gene. *Neuron* **17**:1251, 1996.

215. Wangemann P, Schacht J: Homeostatic mechanisms in the cochlea, in Dallos P, Popper AN, Fay RR (eds): *The Cochlea.* New York, Springer-Verlag, 1996, p 130.

216. Schulze-Bahr E, Wang Q, Wedekind H, Haverkamp W, Chen Q, Sun Y: *KCNE1* mutations cause Jervell and Lange-Nielsen syndrome. *Nat Genet* **17**:267, 1997.

217. Dixon J, Gazzard J, Chaudhry SS, Sampson N, Schulte BA, Steel KP: Mutation of the Na-K-Cl co-transporter gene *Slc12a2* results in deafness in mice. *Hum Mol Genet* **8**:1579, 1999.

218. Delpire E, Lu J, England R, Dull C, Thorne T: Deafness and imbalance associated with inactivation of the secretory Na-K-2Cl co-transporter. *Nat Genet* **22**:192, 1999.

219. Gabriel HD, Jung D, Butzler C, Temme A, Traub O, Winterhager E, Willecke K: Transplacental uptake of glucose is decreased in embryonic lethal connexin 26-deficient mice. *J Cell Biol* **140**:1453, 1998.

220. Takata K: Structural basis of glucose transport in the placental barrier: Possible role of GLUT1 and the gap junction. *Endocrine J* **41**:S3, 1994.

221. Hennemann H, Schwarz HJ, Willecke K: Characterization of gap junction genes expressed in F9 embryonic carcinoma cells: Molecular cloning of mouse connexin 31 and -45 cDNAs. *Eur J Cell Biol* **57**:51, 1992.

222. Hoh JH, John SA, Revel JP: Molecular cloning and characterization of a new member of the gap junction gene family, connexin-31. *J Biol Chem* **266**:6524, 1991.

223. Wenzel K, Manthey D, Willecke K, Grzeschik KH, Traub O: Human gap junction protein connexin31:molecular cloning and expression analysis. *Biochem Biophys Res Commun* **248**:910, 1998.

224. Xia J-h, Liu C-y, Tang B-s, Pan Q, Huang L, Dai H-p, Zhang B-r, Xie W, Hu D-x, Zheng D, Shi X-l, Wang D-a, Xia K, Yu K-p, Liao X-d, Feng Y, Yang Y-p, Xiao J-y, Xie D-h, Huang J-Z: Mutations in the gene encoding gap junction protein β-3 associated with autosomal dominant hearing impairment. *Nat Genet* **20**:370, 1998.

225. Liu X-Z, Xia XJ, Xu LR, Pandya A, Liang CH, Blanton SH, Brown SDM, Steel KP, Nance WE: Mutations in connexin 31 underlie recessive as well as dominant non-syndromic hearing loss. *Hum Mol Genet* **9**:63, 2000.

226. Tucker MA, Barajas L: Rat connexins 30.3 and 31 are expressed in the kidney. *Exp Cell Res* **213**:224, 1994.

227. Plum A, Hallas G, Winterhager E, Rosentreter B, Traub O, Willecke K: Decreased embryonic survival of connexin 31-deficient mice, in *International Gap Junction Conference 89,* Gwatt, Switzerland, 1999.

228. Lautermann J, ten Cate WJ, Altenhoff P, Grummer R, Traub O, Frank H, Jahnke K, Winterhager E: Expression of the gap-junction connexins 26 and 30 in the rat cochlea. *Cell Tissue Res* **294**:415, 1998.

229. Grifa A, Wagner CA, D'Ambrosio L, Melchionda S, Bernardi F, Lopez-Bigas N, Rabionet R, Arbones M, Monica MD, Estivill X, Zelante L, Lang F, Gasparini P: Mutations in *GJB6* cause nonsyndromic autosomal dominant deafness at DFNA3 locus. *Nat Genet* **23**:16, 1999.

230. Dahl E, Manthey D, Chen Y, Schwarz HJ, Chang YS, Lalley PA, Nicholson BJ, Willecke K: Molecular cloning and functional expression of mouse connexin-30, a gap junction gene highly expressed in adult brain and skin [Published erratum appears in *J Biol Chem* 271(42):26444, 1996]. *J Biol Chem* **271**:17903, 1996.

231. Ferrary E, Bernard C, Oudar O, Loiseau A, Sterkers O, Amiel C: *N*-ethylmaleimide-inhibited electrogenic K+ secretion in the ampulla of the frog semicircular canal. *J Physiol* **461**:451, 1993.

232. Wangemann P, Liu J, Marcus DC: Ion transport mechanisms responsible for K+ secretion and the transepithelial voltage across marginal cells of stria vascularis *in vitro*. *Hear Res* **84**:19, 1995.

233. Crouch JJ, Sakaguchi N, Lytle C, Schulte BA: Immunohistochemical localization of the Na-K-Cl co-transporter (NKCC1) in the gerbil inner ear. *J Histochem Cytochem* **45**:773, 1997.

234. Flagella M, Clarke LL, Miller ML, Erway LC, Giannella RA, Andringa A, Gawenis LR, Kramer J, Duffy JJ, Doetschman T, Lorenz JN, Yamoah EN, Cardell EL, Shull GE: Mice lacking the basolateral Na-K-2Cl cotransporter have impaired epithelial chloride secretion and are profoundly deaf. *J Biol Chem* **274**:26946, 1999.

235. Payne JA, Xu JC, Haas M, Lytle CY, Ward D, Forbush B 3rd: Primary structure, functional expression, and chromosomal localization of the bumetanide-sensitive Na-K-Cl cotransporter in human colon. *J Biol Chem* **270**:17977, 1995.

236. Simon DB, Karet FE, Hamdan JM, DiPietro A, Sanjad SA, Lifton RP: Bartter's syndrome, hypokalaemic alkalosis with hypercalciuria, is caused by mutations in the Na-K-2Cl cotransporter NKCC2. *Nat Genet* **13**:183, 1996.

237. Brennan TM, Landau D, Shalev H, Lamb F, Schutte BC, Walder RY, Mark AL, Carmi R, Sheffield VC: Linkage of infantile Bartter syndrome with sensorineural deafness to chromosome 1p. *Am J Hum Genet* **62**:355, 1998.

238. Baldwin CT, Weiss S, Farrer LA, De Stefano AL, Adair R, Franklyn B, Kidd KK, Korostishevsky M, Bonne-Tamir B: Linkage of congenital, recessive deafness (DFNB4) to chromosome 7q31 and evidence for genetic heterogeneity in the Middle Eastern Druze population. *Hum Mol Genet* **4**:1637, 1995.

239. Coyle B, Coffey R, Armour JAL, Gausden E, Hochberg Z, Grossman A, Britton K, Pembrey M, Reardon W, Trembath R: Pendred syndrome (goitre and sensorineural hearing loss) maps to chromosome 7 in the region containing the nonsyndromic deafness gene *DFNB4*. *Nat Genet* **12**:421, 1996.

240. Sheffield VC, Kraiem Z, Beck JC, Nishimura D, Stone EM, Salameh M, Sadeh O, Glaser B: Pendred syndrome maps to chromosome 7q21-34 and is caused by an intrinsic defect in thyroid iodine organification. *Nat Genet* **12**:424, 1996.

241. Pendred V: Deaf mutism and goitre. *Lancet* **i**:352, 1896.

242. Fraser GR: Association of congenital deafness with goiter (Pendred's syndrome). A study of 207 families. *Ann Hum Genet* **28**:201, 1965.

243. Reardon W, Coffey R, Chowdhury T, Grossman A, Jan H, Britton K, Kendall-Taylor P, Trembath R: Prevalence, age of onset, and natural history of thyroid disease in Pendred syndrome. *J Med Genet* **36**:595, 1999.

244. Phelps PD, Coffey RA, Trembath RC, Luxon LM, Grossman AB, Britton KE, Kendall-Taylor P, Graham JM, Cadge BC, Stephens SG, Pembrey ME, Reardon W: Radiological malformations of the ear in Pendred syndrome. *Clin Radiol* **53**:268, 1998.

245. Cremers WR, Bolder C, Admiraal RJ, Everett LA, Joosten FB, van Hauwe P, Green ED, Otten BJ: Progressive sensorineural hearing loss and a widened vestibular aqueduct in Pendred syndrome. *Arch Otolaryngol Head Neck Surg* **124**:501, 1998.

246. Everett LA, Glaser B, Beck JC, Idol JR, Buchs A, Heyman M, Adawi F, Hazani E, Nassir E, Baxevanis A, Sheffield VC, Green ED: Pendred syndrome is caused by mutations in a putative sulphate transporter gene (*PDS*). *Nat Genet* **17**:411, 1997.

247. Usami S, Abe S, Weston MD, Shinkawa H, Van Camp G, Kimberling WJ: Non-syndromic hearing loss associated with enlarged vestibular aqueduct is caused by *PDS* mutations. *Hum Genet* **104**:188, 1999.

248. Abe S, Usami S, Hoover DM, Cohn E, Shinkawa H, Kimberling WJ: Fluctuating sensorineural hearing loss associated with enlarged vestibular aqueduct maps to 7q31, the region containing the Pendred gene. *Am J Med Genet* **82**:322, 1999.

249. Scott DA, Wang R, Kreman TM, Sheffield VC, Karniski LP: The Pendred syndrome gene encodes a chloride-iodide transport protein. *Nat Genet* **21**:440, 1999.

250. Scott DA, Karniski LP: Human pendrin expressed in *Xenopus laevis* oocytes mediates chloride/formate exchange. *Am J Physiol* **278**:C207, 2000.

251. Everett LA, Morsli H, Wu DK, Green ED: Expression pattern of the mouse ortholog of the Pendred's syndrome gene (Pds) suggests a key role for pendrin in the inner ear. *Proc Natl Acad Sci U S A* **96**:9727, 1999.

252. Wang TG, Giebisch G, Aronson PS: Efects of formate and oxalate on volume absorption in rat proximal tubule. *Am J Physiol* **263**:F37, 1992.

253. Jin H, May M, Tranebjaerg L, Kendall E, Fontan G, Jackson J, Subramony SH, Arena F, Lubs H, Smith S, Stevenson R, Schwartz C, Vetrie D: A novel X-linked gene, *DDP*, shows mutations in families with deafness (DFN-1), dystonia, mental deficiency and blindness. *Nat Genet* **14**:177, 1996.

254. Brunner HG, van Bennekom CA, Lambermon EMM, Oei TL, Cremers CWRJ, Wieringa B, Ropers H-H: The gene for X-linked progressive mixed deafness with perilymphatic gusher during stapes surgery (DFN3) is linked to PGK. *Hum Genet* **80**:337, 1988.

255. Wallis C, Ballo R, Wallis G, Beighton P, Goldblatt J: X-linked mixed deafness with stapes fixation in a Mauritian kindred: Linkage to Xq probe pDP34. *Genomics* **3**:299, 1988.

256. Nussbaum RL, Lesko JG, Lewis RA, Ledbetter SA, Ledbetter DH: Isolation of anonymous DNA sequences from within a submicroscopic X chromosomal deletion in a patient with choroideremia, deafness, and mental retardation. *Proc Natl Acad Sci U S A* **84**:6521, 1987.

257. Bach I, Brunner HG, Beighton P, Ruvalcaba RHA, Reardon W, Pembrey ME, van der Velde-Visser SD, Bruns GAP, Cremers CWRJ, Cremers FPM, Ropers H-H: Microdeletions in patients with gusher-associated, X-linked mixed deafness (DFN3). *Am J Hum Genet* **50**:38, 1992.

258. de Kok YJM, van der Maarel SM, Bitner-Glindzicz M, Huber I, Monaco AP, Malcolm S, Pembrey ME, Ropers H-H, Cremers FPM: Association between X-linked mixed deafness and mutations in the POU domain gene *POU3F4*. *Science* **267**:685, 1995.

259. Bitner-Glindzicz M, Turnpenny P, Höglund P, Kääriäinen H, Sankila E-M, van der Maarel SM, de Kok YJM, Ropers H-H, Cremers FPM, Pembrey M, Malcolm S: Further mutations in *Brain 4* (POU3F4) clarify the phenotype in the X-linked deafness, DFN3. *Hum Mol Genet* **4**:1467, 1995.

260. de Kok YJ, Cremers CW, Ropers HH, Cremers FP: The molecular basis of X-linked deafness type 3 (DFN3) in two sporadic cases: Identification of a somatic mosaicism for a POU3F4 missense mutation. *Hum Mutat* **10**:207, 1997.

261. Friedman RA, Bykhovskaya Y, Tu G, Talbot JM, Wilson DF, Parnes LS, Fischel-Ghodsian N: Molecular analysis of the POU3F4 gene in patients with clinical and radiographic evidence of X-linked mixed deafness with perilymphatic gusher. *Ann Otol Rhinol Laryngol* **106**:320, 1997.

262. Hagiwara H, Tamagawa Y, Kitamura K, Kodera K: A new mutation in the POU3F4 gene in a Japanese family with X-linked mixed deafness (DFN3). *Laryngoscope* **108**:1544, 1998.

263. Nance WE, Setleff R, McLeod A, Sweeney A, Cooper C, McConnell F: X-linked mixed deafness with congenital fixation of the stapedial footplate and perilymphatic gusher. *Birth Defects* **07**:64, 1971.

264. Glasscock ME: The stapes gusher. *Arch Otolaryngol* **98**:82, 1973.

265. Hara Y, Rovescalli AC, Kim Y, Nirenberg M: Structure and evolution of four POU domain genes expressed in mouse brain. *Proc Natl Acad Sci U S A* **89**:3280, 1992.

266. Le Moine C, Young WSd: RHS2, a POU domain-containing gene, and its expression in developing and adult rat. *Proc Natl Acad Sci U S A* **89**:3285, 1992.

267. Mathis JM, Simmons DM, He X, Swanson LW, Rosenfeld MG: Brain 4: A novel mammalian POU domain transcription factor exhibiting restricted brain-specific expression. *EMBO J* **11**:2551, 1992.

268. Witta SE, Agarwal VR, Sato SM: XIPOU 2, a noggin-inducible gene, has direct neuralizing activity. *Development* **121**:721, 1995.

269. de Kok YJM, Vossenaar ER, Cremers CWRJ, Dahl N, Laporte J, Hu LJ, Lacombe D, Fischel-Ghodsian N, Friedman RA, Parnes LS, Thorpe P, Bitner-Glindzicz M, Pander H-J, Heilbronner H, Graveline J, den Dunnen JT, Brunner HG, Ropers H-H, Cremers FPM: Identification of a hot spot for microdeletions in patients with X-linked deafness type 3 (DFN3) 900 kb proximal to the DFN3 gene *POU3F4*. *Hum Mol Genet* **5**:1229, 1996.

270. Dominov JA, Miller JB: POU homeodomain genes and myogenesis. *Dev Genet* **19**:108, 1996.

271. Minowa O, Ikeda K, Sugitani Y, Oshima T, Nakai S, Katori Y, Suzuki M, Furukawa M, Kawase T, Zheng Y, Ogura M, Asada Y, Watanabe K, Yamanaka H, Gotoh S, Nishi-Takeshima M, Sugimoto T, Kikuchi T, Takasaka T, Noda T: Altered cochlear fibrocytes in a mouse model of DFN3 nonsyndromic deafness. *Science* **285**:1408, 1999.

272. Phippard D, Lu L, Lee D, Saunders JC, Crenshaw EB: Targeted mutagenesis of the POU-domain gene *Brn4/Pou3f4* causes developmental defects in the inner ear. *J Neurosci* **19**:5980, 1999.

273. Phippard D, Boyd Y, Reed V, Fisher G, Masson WK, Evans EP, Saunders JC, Crenshaw EB: The *sex-linked fidget* mutation abolishes *Brn4/Pou3f4* gene expression in the embryonic inner ear. *Hum Mol Genet* **9**:79, 2000.

274. Phippard D, Heydemann A, Lechner M, Lu L, Lee D, Kyin T, Crenshaw EB: Changes in the subcellular localization of the *Brn4* gene product precede mesenchymal remodeling of the otic capsule. *Hear Res* **120**:77, 1998.

275. Manolis EN, Yandavi N, Nadol JBJ, Eavcy RD, McKenna M, Rosenbaum S, Khetarpal U, Halpin C, Merchant SN, Duyck GM, MacRae C, Seidman CE, Seidman JG: A gene for non-syndromic autosomal dominant progressive postlingual sensorineural hearing loss maps to chromosome 14q12-13. *Hum Mol Genet* **5**:1047, 1996.

276. Robertson NG, Khetarpal U, Gutierrez-Espeleta GA, Bieber FR, Morton CC: Isolation of novel and known genes from a human fetal cochlear cDNA library using subtractive hybridization and differential screening. *Genomics* **23**:42, 1994.

277. Robertson NG, Skvorak AB, Yin Y, Weremowicz S, Johnson KR, Kovatch KA, Battey JF, Bieber FR, Morton CC: Mapping and characterization of a novel cochlear gene in human and in mouse: A positional candidate gene for a deafness disorder, DFNA9. *Genomics* **46**:345, 1997.

278. Robertson NG, Lu L, Heller S, Merchant SN, Eavey RD, McKenna M, Nadol JB, Myamoto RT, Linthicum FHJ, Lubianca Neto JF, Hudspeth AJ, Seidman CE, Morton CC, Seidman JG: Mutations in a novel cochlear gene cause DFNA9, a human nonsyndromic deafness with vestibular dysfunction. *Nat Genet* **20**:299, 1998.

279. Khetarpal U, Schuknecht HF, Gacek RR, Holmes LB: Autosomal dominant sensorineural hearing loss. Pedigrees, audiologic findings, and temporal bone findings in two kindreds. *Arch Otolaryngol Head Neck Surg* **117**:1032, 1991.

280. Khetarpal U: Autosomal dominant sensorineural hearing loss. Further temporal bone findings. *Arch Otolaryngol Head Neck Surg* **119**:106, 1993.

281. Halpin C, Khetarpal U, McKenna M: Autosomal dominant progressive hearing loss in a large North American family. *Am J Audiol* **5**:105, 1996.

282. de Kok YJM, Bom SJH, Brunt TM, Kemperman MH, van Beusekom E, van der Velde-Visser SD, Robertson NG, Morton CC, Huygen PLM, Verhagen WIM, Brunner HG, Cremers CWRJ, Cremers FPM: A Pro51Ser mutation in the *COCH* gene is associated with late onset autosomal dominant progressive sensorineural hearing loss with vestibular defects. *Hum Mol Genet* **8**:361, 1999.

283. Fransen E, Verstreken M, Verhagen WIM, Wuyts FL, Huygen PLM, D'Haese P, Robertson NG, Morton CC, McGuirt WT, Smith RJH, Declau F, van de Heyning PH, Van Camp G: High prevalence of symptoms of Ménière's disease in three families with a mutation in the *COCH* gene. *Hum Mol Genet* **8**:1425, 1999.

284. Colombatti A, Bonaldo P: The superfamily of proteins with von Willebrand factor type A-like domains: One theme common to components of extracellular matrix, hemostasis, cellular adhesion, and defense mechanisms. *Blood* **77**:2305, 1991.

285. Colombatti A, Bonaldo P, Doliana R: Type A modules: interacting domains found in several non-fibrillar collagens and in other extracellular matrix proteins. *Matrix* **13**:297, 1993.

286. Brown MR, Tomek MS, Van Laer L, Smith S, Kenyon JB, Van Camp G, Smith RJ: A novel locus for autosomal dominant nonsyndromic hearing loss, DFNA13, maps to chromosome 6p. *Am J Hum Genet* **61**:924, 1997.

287. Pihlajamaa T, Prockop DJ, Faber J, Winterpacht A, Zabel B, Giedion A, Wiesbauer P, Spranger J, Ala-Kokko L: Heterozygous glycine substitution in the COL11A2 gene in the original patient with the Weissenbacher-Zweymuller syndrome demonstrates its identity with heterozygous OSMED (nonocular Stickler syndrome). *Am J Med Genet* **80**:115, 1998.

288. Kirschhofer K, Kenyon JB, Hoover DM, Franz P, Weipoltshammer K, Wachtler F, Kimberling WJ: Autosomal-dominant congenital severe sensorineural hearing loss. Localisation of a disease gene to chromosome 11q by linkage in an Austrian family. *European Workgroup on Genetics of Hearing Impairment*, Milan, Italy, , October 11-13 1996.

289. Verhoeven K, Van Laer L, Kirschhofer K, Legan PK, Hughes DC, Schatteman I, Verstreken M, Van Hauwe P, Coucke P, Chen A, Smith RJH, Somers T, Offeciers FE, Van de Heyning P, Richardson GP, Wachtler F, Kimberling WJ, Willems PJ, Govaerts PJ, Van Camp G: Mutations in the human α-tectorin gene cause autosomal dominant non-syndromic hearing impairment. *Nat Genet* **19**:60, 1998.

290. Mustapha M, Weil D, Chardenoux S, Elias S, El-Zir E, Beckmann JS, Loiselet J, Petit C: An α-tectorin gene defect causes a newly identified autosomal recessive form of sensorineural pre-lingual non-syndromic deafness, DFNB21. *Hum Mol Genet* **8**:409, 1999.

291. Alloisio N, Morlé L, Bozon M, Godet J, Verhoeven K, Van Camp G, Plauchu H, Muller P, Collet L, Lina-Granade G: Mutation in the zonadhesin-like domain of α-tectorin associated with autosomal dominant non-syndromic hearing loss. *Eur J Hum Genet* **7**:255, 1999.

292. Greve JM, Wassarman PM: Mouse egg extracellular coat is a matrix of interconnected filaments possessing a structural repeat. *J Mol Biol* **181**:253, 1985.

293. Steel KP: Tectorial membrane, in Altschuler RA, Hoffman DW, Bobbin RP (eds): *Neurobiology of Hearing: The Cochlea.* New York, Raven Press, 1986, p 139.

294. Legan PK, Rau A, Keen JN, Richardson GP: The mouse tectorins. Modular matrix proteins of the inner ear homologous to components of the sperm-egg adhesion system. *J Biol Chem* **272**:8791, 1997.

295. Rau A, Legan PK, Richardson GP: Tectorin mRNA expression is spatially and temporally restricted during mouse inner ear development. *J Compar Neurol* **405**:271, 1999.

296. Killick R, Legan PK, Malenczak C, Richardson GP: Molecular cloning of chick β-tectorin, an extracellular matrix molecule of the inner ear. *J Cell Biol* **129**:535, 1995.

297. Simmler M-C, Cohen-Salmon M, El-Amraoui A, Guillaud L, Benichou J-C, Petit C, Panthier J-J: Targeted disruption of *Otogelin* results in deafness and severe imbalance. *Nat Genet* **24**:139, 2000.

298. Leon PE, Bonilla JA, Sanchez JR, Vanegas R, Villalobos M, Torres L, Leon F, Howell AL, Rodriguez JA: Low frequency hereditary deafness in man with childhood onset. *Am J Hum Genet* **33**:209, 1981.

299. Lynch ED, Lee MK, Morrow J, Welsh PL, Leon PE, King M-C: Nonsyndromic deafness DFNA1 associated with mutation of a human homolog of the *Drosophila* gene *diaphanous*. *Science* **278**:1315, 1997.

300. Lalwani AK, Jackler RK, Sweetow RW, Lynch ED, Raventos H, Morrow J, King M-C, Leon PE: Further characterization of the DFNA1 audiovestibular phenotype. *Arch Otolaryngol Head Neck Surg* **124**:669, 1998.

301. Castrillon DH, Wasserman SA: Diaphanous is required for cytokinesis in *Drosophila* and shares domains of similarity with the products of the limb deformity gene. *Development* **120**:3367, 1994.

302. Kohno H, Tanaka K, Mino A, Umikawa M, Imamura H, Fujiwara T, Fujita Y, Hotta K, Qadota H, Watanabe T, Ohya Y, Takai Y: Bni1p implicated in cytoskeletal control is a putative target of Rho1p small GTP binding protein in Saccharomyces cerevisiae. *EMBO J* **15**:6060, 1996.

303. Evangelista M, Blundell K, Longtine MS, Chow CJ, Adames N, Pringle JR, Peter M, Boone C: Bni1p, a yeast formin linking Cdc42p and the actin cytoskeleton during polarized morphogenesis. *Science* **276**:118, 1997.

304. Watanabe N, Madaule P, Reid T, Ishizaki T, Watanabe G, Kakizuka A, Saito Y, Nakao K, Jockusch BM, Narumiya S: p140mDia, a mammalian homolog of *Drosophila diaphanous*, is a target protein for Rho small GTPase and is a ligand for profilin. *EMBO J* **16**:3044, 1997.

305. van Camp G, Coucke P, Balemans W, van Velzen D, van de Bilt C, van Laer L, Smith RJ, Fukushima K, Padberg GW, Frants RR, Van de Heyning P, Smith SD, Huizing EH, Willems PJ: Localization of a gene for non-syndromic hearing loss (DFNA5) to chromosome 7p15. *Hum Mol Genet* **4**:2159, 1995.

306. Van Laer L, Huizing EH, Verstreken M, van Zuijlen D, Wauters JG, Bossuyt PJ, Van de Heyning P, McGuirt WT, Smith RJ, Willems PJ, Legan PK, Richardson GP, Van Camp G: Nonsyndromic hearing impairment is associated with a mutation in *DFNA5*. *Nat Genet* **20**:194, 1998.

307. Koehler CM, Leuenberger D, Merchant S, Renold A, Junne T, Schatz G: Human deafness dystonia syndrome is a mitochondrial disease. *Proc Natl Acad Sci U S A* **96**:2141, 1999.

308. Prezant TR, Agapian JV, Bohlman MC, Bu X, Öztas S, Arnos KS, Cortopassi GA, Jaber L, Rotter JI, Shohat M, Fischel-Ghodsian N: Mitochondrial ribosomal RNA mutation associated with both antibiotic-induced and non-syndromic deafness. *Nat Genet* **4**:289, 1993.

309. Bykhovskaya Y, Shohat M, Ehrenman K, Johnson D, Hamon M, Cantor RM, Aouizerat B, Bu X, Rotter JI, Jaber L, Fischel-Ghodsian N: Evidence for complex nuclear inheritance in a pedigree with nonsyndromic deafness due to a homoplasmic mitochondrial mutation. *Am J Med Genet* **77**:421, 1998.

310. Braverman I, Jaber L, Levi H, Adelman C, Arons KS, Fischel-Ghodsian N, Shohat M, Elidan J: Audiovestibular findings in patients with deafness caused by a mitochondrial susceptibility mutation and precipitated by an inherited nuclear mutation or aminoglycosides. *Arch Otolaryngol Head Neck Surg* **122**:1001, 1996.

311. Fischel-Ghodsian N, Prezant TR, Bu X, Oztas S: Mitochondrial ribosomal RNA gene mutation in a patient with sporadic aminoglycoside ototoxicity. *Am J Otolaryngol* **14**:399, 1993.

312. el-Schahawi M, Lopez de Munain A, Sarrazin AM, Shanske AL, Basirico M, Shanske S, DiMauro S: Two large Spanish pedigrees with nonsyndromic sensorineural deafness and the mtDNA mutation at nt 1555 in the 12s rRNA gene: Evidence of heteroplasmy. *Neurology* **48**:453, 1997.

313. Estivill X, Govea N, Barcelo E, Badenas C, Romero E, Moral L, Scozzri R, D'Urbano L, Zeviani M, Torroni A: Familial progressive sensorineural deafness is mainly due to the mtDNA A1555G mutation and is enhanced by treatment of aminoglycosides. *Am J Hum Genet* **62**:27, 1998.

314. Torroni A, Cruciani F, Rengo C, Sellitto D, LÂpez-Bigas N, Rabionet R, Govea N, LÂpez de Munain A, Sarduy M, Romero L, Villamar M, del Castillo I, Moreno F, Estivill X, Scozzari R: The A1555G mutation in the 12S rRNA gene of human mtDNA: Recurrent origins and founder events in families affected by sensorineural deafness. *Am J Hum Genet* **65**:1349, 1999.

315. Hamasaki K, Rando RR: Specific binding of aminoglycosides to a human rRNA construct based on a DNA polymorphism which causes aminoglycoside-induced deafness. *Biochemistry* **36**:12323, 1997.

316. Casano RA, Johnson DF, Bykhovskaya Y, Torricelli F, Bigozzi M, Fischel-Ghodsian N: Inherited susceptibility to aminoglycoside ototoxicity: Genetic heterogeneity and clinical implications. *Am J Otolaryngol* **20**:151, 1999.

317. Reid FM, Vernham GA, Jacobs HT: A novel mitochondrial point mutation in a maternal pedigree with sensorineural deafness. *Hum Mutat* **3**:243, 1994.

318. Sevior KB, Hatamochi A, Stewart IA, Bykhovskaya Y, Allen-Powell DR, Fischel-Ghodsian N, Maw MA: Mitochondrial A7445G mutation in two pedigrees with palmoplantar keratoderma and deafness. *Am J Med Genet* **75**:179, 1998.

319. Tiranti V, Chariot P, Carella F, Toscano A, Soliveri P, Girlanda P, Carrara F, Fratta GM, Reid FM, Mariotti C, Zeviani M: Maternally inherited hearing loss, ataxia and myoclonus associated with a novel point mutation in mitochondrial tRNA^Ser(UCN) gene. *Hum Mol Genet* **4**:1421, 1995.

320. Verhoeven K, Ensink RJH, Tiranti V, Huygen PLM, Johnson DF, Schatteman I, Van Laer L, Verstreken M, Van de Heyning P, Fischel-Ghodsian N, Zeviani M, Cremers CWRJ, Willems PJ, Van Camp G: Hearing impairment and neurological dysfunction associated with a mutation in the mitochondrial tRNA^Ser(UCN) gene. *Eur J Hum Genet* **7**:45, 1999.

321. Sue CM, Tanji K, Hadjigeorgiou G, Andreu AL, Nishino I, Krishna S, Bruno C, Hirano M, Shanske S, Bonilla E, Fischel-Ghodsian N, DiMauro S, Friedman R: Maternally inherited hearing loss in a large kindred with a novel T7511C mutation in the mitochondrial DNA tRNA(Ser(UCN)) gene. *Neurology* **52**:1905, 1999.

322. Caussé R: Action toxique vestibulaire et cochléaire de la streptomycine du point de vue expérimental. *Ann Otolaryngol (Paris)* **66**:518, 1949.

323. Hawkins JE Jr: Cochlear signs of streptomycin intoxication. *J Pharmacol Exp Ther* **100**:38, 1950.

324. Theopold HM: Comparative surface studies of ototoxic effects of various aminoglycoside antibiotics on the organ of Corti in the guinea pig. A scanning electron microscopic study. *Acta Otolaryngol (Stockh)* **84**:57, 1977.

325. Seidman MD, Bai U, Khan MJ, Murphy MJ, Quirk WS, Castora FL, Hinojosa R: Association of mitochondrial DNA deletions and cochlear pathology: A molecular biologic tool. *Laryngoscope* **106**:777, 1996.

326. Fischel-Ghodsian N, Bykhovskaya Y, Taylor K, Kahen T, Cantor R, Ehrenman K, Smith R, Keithley E: Temporal bone analysis of patients with presbycusis reveals high frequency of mitochondrial mutations. *Hear Res* **110**:147, 1997.

327. Abdelhak S, Kalatzis V, Heilig R, Compain S, Samson D, Vincent C, Weil D, Cruaud C, Sahly I, Leibovici M, Bitner-Glindzicz M, Francis M, Lacombe D, Vigneron J, Charachon R, Boven K, Bedbeder P, Van Regemorter N, Weissenbach J, Petit C: A human homologue of the *Drosophila eyes absent* gene underlies Branchio-Oto-Renal (BOR) syndrome and identifies a novel gene family. *Nat Genet* **15**:157, 1997.

328. Vincent C, Kalatzis V, Abdelhak S, Chaïb H, Compain S, Helias J, Vanecloo F-M, Petit C: BOR and BO syndromes are allelic defects of *EYA1*. *Eur J Hum Genet* **5**:242, 1997.

329. Momeni P, Glöckner G, Schmidt O, von Holtum D, Albrecht A, Gillessen-Kaesbach G, Hennekam R, Meinecke P, Zabel B, Rosenthal A, Horsthemke B, Lüdecke H-J: Mutations in a new gene, encoding a zinc-finger protein, cause tricho-rhino-phalangeal syndrome type I. *Nat Genet* **24**:71, 2000.

330. Kohlhase J, Wischermann A, Reichenbach H, Froster U, Engel W: Mutations in the *SALL1* putative transcription factor gene cause Townes-Brocks syndrome. *Nat Genet* **18**:81, 1998.

331. Treacher Collins Syndrome Collaborative Group: Positional cloning of a gene involved in the pathogenesis of Treacher Collins syndrome. *Nat Genet* **12**:130, 1996.

332. Fanconi Anaemia Breast Cancer Consortium: Positional cloning of the Fanconi anaemia group A gene. *Nat Genet* **14**:324, 1996.

333. Strathdee CA, Gavish H, Shannon WR, Buchwald M: Cloning of cDNAs for Fanconi's anaemia by functional complementation [Published erratum appears in *Nature* 358(6385):434, 1992]. *Nature* **356**:763, 1992.

334. Jabs EW, Li X, Scott AF, Meyers G, Chen W, Eccles M, Mao JI, Charnas LR, Jackson CE, Jaye M: Jackson-Weiss and Crouzon syndromes are allelic with mutations in fibroblast growth factor receptor 2 [Published erratum appears in *Nat Genet* 9(4):451, 1995]. *Nat Genet* **8**:275, 1994.

335. Reardon W, Winter RM, Rutland P, Pulleyn LJ, Jones BM, Malcolm S: Mutations in the fibroblast growth factor receptor 2 gene cause Crouzon syndrome. *Nat Genet* **8**:98, 1994.

336. Meyers GA, Orlow SJ, Munro IR, Przylepa KA, Jabs EW: Fibroblast growth factor receptor 3 (FGFR3) transmembrane mutation in Crouzon syndrome with acanthosis nigricans. *Nat Genet* **11**:462, 1995.

337. Muenke M, Schell U, Hehr A, Robin NH, Losken HW, Schinzel A, Pulleyn LJ, Rutland P, Reardon W, Malcolm S, Winter RM: A common mutation in the fibroblast growth factor receptor 1 gene in Pfeiffer syndrome. *Nat Genet* **8**:269, 1994.

338. Rutland P, Pulleyn LJ, Reardon W, Baraitser M, Hayward R, Jones B, Malcolm S, Winter RM, Oldridge M, Slaney SF, Poole MD, Wilkie AOM: Identical mutations in the FGFR2 gene cause both Pfeiffer and Crouzon syndrome phenotypes. *Nat Genet* **9**:173, 1995.

339. Schell U, Hehr A, Feldman GJ, Robin NH, Zackai EH, de Die-Smulders C, Viskochil DH, Stewart JM, Wolff G, Ohashi H, Price RA, Cohen MM Jr, Muenke M: Mutations in FGFR1 and FGFR2 cause familial and sporadic Pfeiffer syndrome. *Hum Mol Genet* **4**:323, 1995.

340. Wilkie AO, Slaney SF, Oldridge M, Poole MD, Ashworth GJ, Hockley AD, Hayward RD, David DJ, Pulleyn LJ, Rutland P, Malcolm S, Winter RM, Reardon W: Apert syndrome results from localized mutations of FGFR2 and is allelic with Crouzon syndrome. *Nat Genet* **9**:165, 1995.

341. Rousseau F, Bonaventure J, Legeai-Mallet L, Pelet A, Rozet JM, Maroteaux P, Le Merrer M, Munnich A: Mutations in the gene encoding fibroblast growth factor receptor-3 in achondroplasia. *Nature* **371**:252, 1994.

342. Shiang R, Thompson LM, Zhu YZ, Church DM, Fielder TJ, Bocian M, Winokur ST, Wasmuth JJ: Mutations in the transmembrane domain of FGFR3 cause the most common genetic form of dwarfism, achondroplasia. *Cell* **78**:335, 1994.

343. Muenke M, Gripp KW, McDonald-McGinn DM, Gaudenz K, Whitaker LA, Bartlett SP, Markowitz RI, Robin NH, Nwokoro N, Mulvihill JJ, Losken HW, Mulliken JB, Guttmacher AE, Wilroy RS, Clarke LA, Hollway G, Ades LC, Haan EA, Mulley JC, Cohen MM Jr, Bellus GA, Francomano CA, Moloney DM, Wall SA, Wilkie AO, Zackai EH: A unique point mutation in the fibroblast growth factor receptor 3 gene (*FGFR3*) defines a new craniosynostosis syndrome. *Am J Hum Genet* **60**:555, 1997.

344. El Ghouzzi V, Le Merrer M, Perrin-Schmitt F, Lajeunie E, Benit P, Renier D, Bourgeois P, Bolcato-Bellemin AL, Munnich A, Bonaventure J: Mutations of the TWIST gene in the Saethre-Chotzen syndrome. *Nat Genet* **15**:42, 1997.

345. Howard TD, Paznekas WA, Green ED, Chiang LC, Ma N, Ortiz de Luna RI, Garcia Delgado C, Gonzalez-Ramos M, Kline AD, Jabs EW: Mutations in TWIST, a basic helix-loop-helix transcription factor, in Saethre-Chotzen syndrome. *Nat Genet* **15**:36, 1997.

346. Rose CS, Patel P, Reardon W, Malcolm S, Winter RM: The *TWIST* gene, although not disrupted in Saethre-Chotzen patients with apparently balanced translocations of 7p21, is mutated in familial and sporadic cases. *Hum Mol Genet* **6**:1369, 1997.

347. Paznekas WA, Cunningham ML, Howard TD, Korf BR, Lipson MH, Grix AW, Feingold M, Goldberg R, Borochowitz Z, Aleck K, Mulliken J, Yin M, Jabs EW: Genetic heterogeneity of Saethre-Chotzen syndrome, due to *TWIST* and *FGFR* mutations. *Am J Hum Genet* **62**:1370, 1998.

348. Mundlos S, Otto F, Mundlos C, Mulliken JB, Aylsworth AS, Albright S, Lindhout D, Cole WG, Henn W, Knoll JH, Owen MJ, Mertelsmann R, Zabel BU, Olsen BR: Mutations involving the transcription factor CBFA1 cause cleidocranial dysplasia. *Cell* **89**:773, 1997.

349. Belin V, Cusin V, Viot G, Girlich D, Toutain A, Moncla A, Vekemans M, Le Merrer M, Munnich A, Cormier-Daire V: *SHOX* mutations in dyschondrosteosis (Leri-Weill syndrome). *Nat Genet* **19**:67, 1998.

350. Shears DJ, Vassal HJ, Goodman FR, Palmer RW, Reardon W, Superti-Furga A, Scambler PJ, Winter RM: Mutation and deletion of the pseudoautosomal gene SHOX cause Leri-Weill dyschondrosteosis. *Nat Genet* **19**:70, 1998.

351. Foster JW, Dominguez-Steglich MA, Guioli S, Kowk G, Weller PA, Stevanovic M, Weissenbach J, Mansour S, Young ID, Goodfellow PN, Brook JD, Schafer JD: Campomelic dysplasia and autosomal sex reversal caused by mutations in an SRY-related gene. *Nature* **372**:525, 1994.

352. Wagner T, Wirth J, Meyer J, Zabel B, Held M, Zimmer J, Pasantes J, Dagna Bricarelli F, Keutel J, Hustert E, Wolf U, Tommerup N, Schempp W, Scherer G: Autosomal sex reversal and campomelic dysplasia are caused by mutations in and around the SRY-related gene SOX9. *Cell* **79**:1111, 1994.

353. Willing MC, Cohn DH, Byers PH: Frameshift mutation near the 3' end of the COL1A1 gene of type I collagen predicts an elongated Pro alpha 1(I) chain and results in osteogenesis imperfecta type I [Published erratum appears in *J Clin Invest* 85(4):1338, 1990]. *J Clin Invest* **85**:282, 1990.

354. Zhuang J, Tromp G, Kuivaniemi H, Nakayasu K, Prockop DJ: Deletion of 19 base pairs in intron 13 of the gene for the pro alpha 2(I) chain of type-I procollagen (COL1A2) causes exon skipping in a proband with type-I osteogenesis imperfecta. *Hum Genet* **91**:210, 1993.

355. Marini JC, Grange DK, Gottesman GS, Lewis MB, Koeplin DA: Osteogenesis imperfecta type IV. Detection of a point mutation in one alpha 1(I) collagen allele (COL1A1) by RNA/RNA hybrid analysis. *J Biol Chem* **264**:11893, 1989.

356. Wenstrup RJ, Cohn DH, Cohen T, Byers PH: Arginine for glycine substitution in the triple-helical domain of the products of one alpha 2(I) collagen allele (COL1A2) produces the osteogenesis imperfecta type IV phenotype. *J Biol Chem* **263**:7734, 1988.

357. Lee B, Vissing H, Ramirez F, Rogers D, Rimoin D: Identification of the molecular defect in a family with spondyloepiphyseal dysplasia. *Science* **244**:978, 1989.

358. Winterpacht A, Hilbert M, Schwarze U, Mundlos S, Spranger J, Zabel BU: Kniest and Stickler dysplasia phenotypes caused by collagen type II gene (COL2A1) defect. *Nat Genet* **3**:323, 1993.

359. Ahmad NN, Ala-Kokko L, Knowlton RG, Jimenez SA, Weaver EJ, Maguire JI, Tasman W, Prockop DJ: Stop codon in the procollagen II gene (COL2A1) in a family with the Stickler syndrome (arthro-ophthalmopathy). *Proc Natl Acad Sci U S A* **88**:6624, 1991.

360. Richards AJ, Yates JR, Williams R, Payne SJ, Pope FM, Scott JD, Snead MP: A family with Stickler syndrome type 2 has a mutation in the COL11A1 gene resulting in the substitution of glycine 97 by valine in alpha 1 (XI) collagen. *Hum Mol Genet* **5**:1339, 1996.

361. Griffith AJ, Sprunger LK, Sirko-Osadsa DA, Tiller GE, Meisler MH, Warman ML: Marshall syndrome associated with a splicing defect at the COL11A1 locus. *Am J Hum Genet* **62**:816, 1998.

362. Shanske A, Bogdanow A, Shprintzen RJ, Marion RW: Marshall syndrome and a defect at the COL11A1 locus [Letter]. *Am J Hum Genet* **63**:1558, 1998.

363. Hyland J, Ala-Kokko L, Royce P, Steinmann B, Kivirikko KI, Myllyla R: A homozygous stop codon in the lysyl hydroxylase gene in two siblings with Ehlers-Danlos syndrome type VI. *Nat Genet* **2**:228, 1992.

364. Scott HS, Litjens T, Nelson PV, Thompson PR, Brooks DA, Hopwood JJ, Morris CP: Identification of mutations in the alpha-l-iduronidase gene (IDUA) that cause Hurler and Scheie syndromes. *Am J Hum Genet* **53**:973, 1993.

365. Wilson PJ, Morris CP, Anson DS, Occhiodoro T, Bielicki J, Clements PR, Hopwood JJ: Hunter syndrome: Isolation of an iduronate-2-sulfatase cDNA clone and analysis of patient DNA. *Proc Natl Acad Sci U S A* **87**:8531, 1990.

366. Scott HS, Blanch L, Guo XH, Freeman C, Orsborn A, Baker E, Sutherland GR, Morris CP, Hopwood JJ: Cloning of the sulphamidase gene and identification of mutations in Sanfilippo A syndrome. *Nat Genet* **11**:465, 1995.

367. Weber B, Blanch L, Clements PR, Scott HS, Hopwood JJ: Cloning and expression of the gene involved in Sanfilippo B syndrome (mucopolysaccharidosis III B). *Hum Mol Genet* **5**:771, 1996.

368. Zhao HG, Li HH, Bach G, Schmidtchen A, Neufeld EF: The molecular basis of Sanfilippo syndrome type B. *Proc Natl Acad Sci U S A* **93**:6101, 1996.

369. Fukuda S, Tomatsu S, Masue M, Sukegawa K, Iwata H, Ogawa T, Nakashima Y, Hori T, Yamagishi A, Hanyu Y, Morooka K, Kiman T, Hashimoto T, Orii T: Mucopolysaccharidosis type IVA. N-acetylga-lactosamine-6-sulfate sulfatase exonic point mutations in classical Morquio and mild cases. *J Clin Invest* **90**:1049, 1992.

370. Oshima A, Yoshida K, Shimmoto M, Fukuhara Y, Sakuraba H, Suzuki Y: Human β-galactosidase gene mutations in Morquio B disease. *Am J Hum Genet* **49**:1091, 1991.

371. Wicker G, Prill V, Brooks D, Gibson G, Hopwood J, von Figura K, Peters C: Mucopolysaccharidosis VI (Maroteaux-Lamy syndrome). An intermediate clinical phenotype caused by substitution of valine for glycine at position 137 of arylsulfatase B. *J Biol Chem* **266**:21386, 1991.

372. Tomatsu S, Fukuda S, Sukegawa K, Ikedo Y, Yamada S, Yamada Y, Sasaki T, Okamoto H, Kuwahara T, Yamaguchi S, Kiman T, Shintaku H, Isshiki G, Orii T: Mucopolysaccharidosis type VII: Characterization of mutations and molecular heterogeneity. *Am J Hum Genet* **48**:89, 1991.

373. Gong Y, Krakow D, Marcelino J, Wilkin D, Chitayat D, Babul-Hirji R, Hudgins L, Cremers CW, Cremers FP, Brunner HG, Reinker K, Rimoin DL, Cohn DH, Goodman FR, Reardon W, Patton M, Francomano CA, Warman ML: Heterozygous mutations in the gene encoding noggin affect human joint morphogenesis. *Nat Genet* **21**:302, 1999.

374. Schipani E, Kruse K, Juppner H: A constitutively active mutant PTH-PTHrP receptor in Jansen-type metaphyseal chondrodysplasia. *Science* **268**:98, 1995.

375. Franco B, Meroni G, Parenti G, Levilliers J, Bernard L, Gebbia M, Cox L, Maroteaux P, Sheffield L, Rappold GA, Andria G, Petit C, Ballabio A: A cluster of sulfatase genes on Xp22.3: Mutations in chondrodysplasia punctata (CDPX) and implications for warfarin embryopathy. *Cell* **81**:15, 1995.

376. Braverman N, Lin P, Moebius FF, Obie C, Moser A, Glossmann H, Wilcox WR, Rimoin DL, Smith M, Kratz L, Kelley RI, Valle D: Mutations in the gene encoding 3β-hydroxysteroid-$\Delta^8,\Delta^7$-isomerase cause X-linked dominant Conradi-Hünermann syndrome. *Nat Genet* **22**:291, 1999.

377. Derry JM, Gormally E, Means GD, Zhao W, Meindl A, Kelley RI, Boyd Y, Herman GE: Mutations in a $\Delta^8$-$\Delta^7$ sterol isomerase in the tattered mouse and X-linked dominant chondrodysplasia punctata. *Nat Genet* **22**:286, 1999.

378. Munroe PB, Olgunturk RO, Fryns JP, Van Maldergem L, Ziereisen F, Yuksel B, Gardiner RM, Chung E: Mutations in the gene encoding the human matrix Gla protein cause Keutel syndrome. *Nat Genet* **21**:142, 1999.

379. Weinstein LS, Gejman PV, Friedman E, Kadowaki T, Collins RM, Gershon ES, Spiegel AM: Mutations of the Gs α-subunit gene in Albright hereditary osteodystrophy detected by denaturing gradient gel electrophoresis. *Proc Natl Acad Sci U S A* **87**:8287, 1990.

380. Venta PJ, Welty RJ, Johnson TM, Sly WS, Tashian RE: Carbonic anhydrase II deficiency syndrome in a Belgian family is caused by a point mutation at an invariant histidine residue (107 His → Tyr): complete structure of the normal human CA II gene. *Am J Hum Genet* **49**:1082, 1991.

381. Roth DE, Venta PJ, Tashian RE, Sly WS: Molecular basis of human carbonic anhydrase II deficiency. *Proc Natl Acad Sci U S A* **89**:1804, 1992.

382. Myerowitz R, Hogikyan ND: Different mutations in Ashkenazi Jewish and non-Jewish French Canadians with Tay-Sachs disease. *Science* **232**:1646, 1986.

383. Sakai N, Inui K, Fujii N, Fukushima H, Nishimoto J, Yanagihara I, Isegawa Y, Iwamatsu A, Okada S: Krabbe disease: Isolation and characterization of a full-length cDNA for human galactocerebrosidase. *Biochem Biophys Res Commun* **198**:485, 1994.

384. Rafi MA, Luzi P, Chen YQ, Wenger DA: A large deletion together with a point mutation in the GALC gene is a common mutant allele in patients with infantile Krabbe disease. *Hum Mol Genet* **4**:1285, 1995.

385. Tatsumi N, Inui K, Sakai N, Fukushima H, Nishimoto J, Yanagihara I, Nishigaki T, Tsukamoto H, Fu L, Taniike M, Okada S: Molecular defects in Krabbe disease. *Hum Mol Genet* **4**:1865, 1995.

386. Fisher KJ, Aronson NN Jr: Characterization of the mutation responsible for aspartylglucosaminuria in three Finnish patients. Amino acid substitution Cys163 → Ser abolishes the activity of lysosomal glycosylasparaginase and its conversion into subunits. *J Biol Chem* **266**:12105, 1991.

387. Ikonen E, Baumann M, Gron K, Syvanen AC, Enomaa N, Halila R, Aula P, Peltonen L: Aspartylglucosaminuria: cDNA encoding human aspartylglucosaminidase and the missense mutation causing the disease. *EMBO J* **10**:51, 1991.

388. Nilssen O, Berg T, Riise HM, Ramachandran U, Evjen G, Hansen GM, Malm D, Tranebjaerg L, Tollersrud OK: α-Mannosidosis: Functional cloning of the lysosomal α-mannosidase cDNA and identification of a mutation in two affected siblings. *Hum Mol Genet* **6**:717, 1997.

389. Alkhayat AH, Kraemer SA, Leipprandt JR, Macek M, Kleijer WJ, Friderici KH: Human β-mannosidase cDNA characterization and first identification of a mutation associated with human β-mannosidosis. *Hum Mol Genet* **7**:75, 1998.

390. Bonten E, van der Spoel A, Fornerod M, Grosveld G, d'Azzo A: Characterization of human lysosomal neuraminidase defines the molecular basis of the metabolic storage disorder sialidosis. *Genes Dev* **10**:3156, 1996.

391. Pshezhetsky AV, Richard C, Michaud L, Igdoura S, Wang S, Elsliger MA, Qu J, Leclerc D, Gravel R, Dallaire L, Potier M: Cloning, expression and chromosomal mapping of human lysosomal sialidase and characterization of mutations in sialidosis. *Nat Genet* **15**:316, 1997.

392. Zhou XY, Galjart NJ, Willemsen R, Gillemans N, Galjaard H, d'Azzo A: A mutation in a mild form of galactosialidosis impairs dimerization of the protective protein and renders it unstable. *EMBO J* **10**:4041, 1991.

393. Bernstein HS, Bishop DF, Astrin KH, Kornreich R, Eng CM, Sakuraba H, Desnick RJ: Fabry disease: six gene rearrangements and an exonic point mutation in the alpha-galactosidase gene. *J Clin Invest* **83**:1390, 1989.

394. Kretz KA, Darby JK, Willems PJ, O'Brien JS: Characterization of EcoRI mutation in fucosidosis patients: A stop codon in the open reading frame. *J Mol Neurosci* **1**:177, 1989.

395. Carstea ED, Morris JA, Coleman KG, Loftus SK, Zhang D, Cummings C, Gu J, Rosenfeld MA, Pavan WJ, Krizman DB, Nagle J, Polymeropoulos MH, Sturley SL, Ioannou YA, Higgins ME, Comly M, Cooney A, Brown A, Kaneski CR, Blanchette-Mackie EJ, Dwyer NK, Neufeld EB, Chang TY, Liscum L, Tagle DA, et al: Niemann-Pick C1 disease gene: Homology to mediators of cholesterol homeostasis. *Science* **277**: 231, 1997.

396. Abrahamov A, Elstein D, Gross-Tsur V, Farber B, Glaser Y, Hadas-Halpern I, Ronen S, Tafakjdi M, Horowitz M, Zimran A: Gaucher's disease variant characterised by progressive calcification of heart valves and unique genotype [see comments]. *Lancet* **346**:1000, 1995.

397. Chabas A, Cormand B, Grinberg D, Burguera JM, Balcells S, Merino JL, Mate I, Sobrino JA, Gonzalez-Duarte R, Vilageliu L: Unusual expression of Gaucher's disease: Cardiovascular calcifications in three sibs homozygous for the D409H mutation. *J Med Genet* **32**:740, 1995.

398. Goto Y, Nonaka I, Horai S: A mutation in the tRNA(Leu)(UUR) gene associated with the MELAS subgroup of mitochondrial encephalomyopathies. *Nature* **348**:651, 1990.

399. Kobayashi Y, Momoi MY, Tominaga K, Momoi T, Nihei K, Yanagisawa M, Kagawa Y, Ohta S: A point mutation in the mitochondrial tRNA(Leu)(UUR) gene in MELAS (mitochondrial myopathy, encephalopathy, lactic acidosis and stroke-like episodes). *Biochem Biophys Res Commun* **173**:816, 1990.

400. Lertrit P, Noer AS, Jean-Francois MJ, Kapsa R, Dennett X, Thyagarajan D, Lethlean K, Byrne E, Marzuki S: A new disease-related mutation for mitochondrial encephalopathy lactic acidosis and strokelike episodes (MELAS) syndrome affects the ND4 subunit of the respiratory complex I. *Am J Hum Genet* **51**:457, 1992.

401. Ballinger SW, Shoffner JM, Hedaya EV, Trounce I, Polak MA, Koontz DA, Wallace DC: Maternally transmitted diabetes and deafness associated with a 10.4-kb mitochondrial DNA deletion. *Nat Genet* **1**:11, 1992.

402. Reardon W, Ross RJ, Sweeney MG, Luxon LM, Pembrey ME, Harding AE, Trembath RC: Diabetes mellitus associated with a pathogenic point mutation in mitochondrial DNA. *Lancet* **340**:1376, 1992.

403. van den Ouweland JM, Lemkes HH, Ruitenbeek W, Sandkuijl LA, de Vijlder MF, Struyvenberg PA, van de Kamp JJ, Maassen JA: Mutation in mitochondrial tRNA(Leu)(UUR) gene in a large pedigree with maternally transmitted type II diabetes mellitus and deafness. *Nat Genet* **1**:368, 1992.

404. Zeviani M, Moraes CT, DiMauro S, Nakase H, Bonilla E, Schon EA, Rowland LP: Deletions of mitochondrial DNA in Kearns-Sayre syndrome [see comments]. *Neurology* **38**:1339, 1988.

405. Fu K, Hartlen R, Johns T, Genge A, Karpati G, Shoubridge EA: A novel heteroplasmic tRNA^leu(CUN) mtDNA point mutation in a sporadic patient with mitochondrial encephalomyopathy segregates rapidly in skeletal muscle and suggests an approach to therapy. *Hum Mol Genet* **5**:1835, 1996.

406. Taniike M, Fukushima H, Yanagihara I, Tsukamoto H, Tanaka J, Fujimura H, Nagai T, Sano T, Yamaoka K, Inui K, Okada S: Mitochondrial tRNA(Ile) mutation in fatal cardiomyopathy. *Biochem Biophys Res Commun* **186**:47, 1992.

407. Zeviani M, Gellera C, Antozzi C, Rimoldi M, Morandi L, Villani F, Tiranti V, DiDonato S: Maternally inherited myopathy and cardiomyopathy: Association with mutation in mitochondrial DNA tRNA (Leu)(UUR). *Lancet* **338**:143, 1991.

408. Santorelli FM, Mak SC, El-Schahawi M, Casali C, Shanske S, Baram TZ, Madrid RE, DiMauro S: Maternally inherited cardiomyopathy and hearing loss associated with a novel mutation in the mitochondrial tRNA(Lys) gene (G8363A). *Am J Hum Genet* **58**:933, 1996.

409. Shoffner JM, Lott MT, Lezza AM, Seibel P, Ballinger SW, Wallace DC: Myoclonic epilepsy and ragged-red fiber disease (MERRF) is associated with a mitochondrial DNA tRNA(Lys) mutation. *Cell* **61**:931, 1990.

410. Moraes CT, Ciacci F, Bonilla E, Jansen C, Hirano M, Rao N, Lovelace RE, Rowland LP, Schon EA, DiMauro S: Two novel pathogenic mitochondrial DNA mutations affecting organelle number and protein synthesis. Is the tRNA^Leu(UUR) gene an etiologic hot spot? *J Clin Invest* **92**:2906, 1993.

411. Manouvrier S, Rotig A, Hannebique G, Gheerbrandt JD, Royer-Legrain G, Munnich A, Parent M, Grunfeld JP, Largilliere C, Lombes A, Bonnefont J-P: Point mutation of the mitochondrial tRNA(Leu) gene (A3243G) in maternally inherited hypertrophic cardiomyopathy, diabetes mellitus, renal failure, and sensorineural deafness. *J Med Genet* **32**:654, 1995.

412. Mansergh FC, Millington-Ward S, Kennan A, Kiang AS, Humphries M, Farrar GJ, Humphries P, Kenna PF: Retinitis pigmentosa and progressive sensorineural hearing loss caused by a C12258A mutation in the mitochondrial MTTS2 gene. *Am J Hum Genet* **64**:971, 1999.

413. Carrozzo R, Hirano M, Fromenty B, Casali C, Santorelli FM, Bonilla E, DiMauro S, Schon EA, Miranda AF: Multiple mtDNA deletions features in autosomal dominant and recessive diseases suggest distinct pathogeneses. *Neurology* **50**:99, 1998.

414. Papadimitriou A, Comi GP, Hadjigeorgiou GM, Bordoni A, Sciacco M, Napoli L, Prelle A, Moggio M, Fagiolari G, Bresolin N, Salani S, Anastasopoulos I, Giassakis G, Divari R, Scarlato G: Partial depletion and multiple deletions of muscle mtDNA in familial MNGIE syndrome. *Neurology* **51**:1086, 1998.

415. Nishino I, Spinazzola A, Hirano M: Thymidine phosphorylase gene mutations in MNGIE, a human mitochondrial disorder. *Science* **283**:689, 1999.

416. Howell N, Bindoff LA, McCullough DA, Kubacka I, Poulton J, Mackey D, Taylor L, Turnbull DM: Leber hereditary optic neuropathy: identification of the same mitochondrial ND1 mutation in six pedigrees. *Am J Hum Genet* **49**:939, 1991.

417. Rotig A, Cormier V, Chatelain P, Francois R, Saudubray JM, Rustin P, Munnich A: Deletion of mitochondrial DNA in a case of early-onset diabetes mellitus, optic atrophy, and deafness (Wolfram syndrome, MIM 222300). *J Clin Invest* **91**:1095, 1993.

418. Pilz D, Quarrell OW, Jones EW: Mitochondrial mutation commonly associated with Leber's hereditary optic neuropathy observed in a patient with Wolfram syndrome (DIDMOAD). *J Med Genet* **31**:328, 1994.

419. Hofmann S, Jaksch M, Bezold R, Mertens S, Aholt S, Paprotta A, Gerbitz KD: Population genetics and disease susceptibility: Characterization of central European haplogroups by mtDNA gene mutations, correlation with D loop variants and association with disease. *Hum Mol Genet* **6**:1835, 1997.

420. Inoue H, Tanizawa Y, Wasson J, Behn P, Kalidas K, Bernal-Mizrachi E, Mueckler M, Marshall H, Donis-Keller H, Crock P, Rogers D, Mikuni M, Kumashiro H, Higashi K, Sobue G, Oka Y, Permutt MA: A gene encoding a transmembrane protein is mutated in patients with diabetes mellitus and optic atrophy (Wolfram syndrome). *Nat Genet* **20**:143, 1998.

421. Strom TM, Hortnagel K, Hofmann S, Gekeler F, Scharfe C, Rabl W, Gerbitz KD, Meitinger T: Diabetes insipidus, diabetes mellitus, optic atrophy and deafness (DIDMOAD) caused by mutations in a novel gene (wolframin) coding for a predicted transmembrane protein. *Hum Mol Genet* **7**:2021, 1998.

422. Mosser J, Douar AM, Sarde CO, Kioschis P, Feil R, Moser H, Poustka AM, Mandel JL, Aubourg P: Putative X-linked adrenoleukodystrophy gene shares unexpected homology with ABC transporters. *Nature* **361**:726, 1993.

423. Portsteffen H, Beyer A, Becker E, Epplen C, Pawlak A, Kunau WH, Dodt G: Human *PEX1* is mutated in complementation group 1 of the peroxisome biogenesis disorders. *Nat Genet* **17**:449, 1997.

424. Reuber BE, Germain-Lee E, Collins CS, Morrell JC, Ameritunga R, Moser HW, Valle D, Gould SJ: Mutations in *PEX1* are the most common cause of peroxisome biogenesis disorders. *Nat Genet* **17**:445, 1997.

425. Tamura S, Okumoto K, Toyama R, Shimozawa N, Tsukamoto T, Suzuki Y, Osumi T, Kondo N, Fujiki Y: Human *PEX1* cloned by functional complementation on a CHO cell mutant is responsible for peroxisome-deficient Zellweger syndrome of complementation group I. *Proc Natl Acad Sci U S A* **95**:4350, 1998.

426. Shimozawa N, Tsukamoto T, Suzuki Y, Orii T, Shirayoshi Y, Mori T, Fujiki Y: A human gene responsible for Zellweger syndrome that affects peroxisome assembly. *Science* **255**:1132, 1992.

427. Dodt G, Braverman N, Wong C, Moser A, Moser HW, Watkins P, Valle D, Gould SJ: Mutations in the PTS1 receptor gene, PXR1, define complementation group 2 of the peroxisome biogenesis disorders. *Nat Genet* **9**:115, 1995.

428. Okumoto K, Itoh R, Shimozawa N, Suzuki Y, Tamura S, Kondo N, Fujiki Y: Mutations in PEX10 is the cause of Zellweger peroxisome deficiency syndrome of complementation group B. *Hum Mol Genet* **7**:1399, 1998.

429. Warren DS, Morrell JC, Moser HW, Valle D, Gould SJ: Identification of PEX10, the gene defective in complementation group 7 of the peroxisome-biogenesis disorders. *Am J Hum Genet* **63**:347, 1998.

430. Chang CC, Lee WH, Moser H, Valle D, Gould SJ: Isolation of the human PEX12 gene, mutated in group 3 of the peroxisome biogenesis disorders. *Nat Genet* **15**:385, 1997.

431. Okumoto K, Fujiki Y: PEX12 encodes an integral membrane protein of peroxisomes. *Nat Genet* **17**:265, 1997.

432. Shimozawa N, Suzuki Y, Zhang Z, Imamura A, Toyama R, Mukai S, Fujiki Y, Tsukamoto T, Osumi T, Orii T, Wanders RJ, Kondo N: Nonsense and temperature-sensitive mutations in *PEX13* are the cause of complementation group H of peroxisome biogenesis disorders. *Hum Mol Genet* **8**:1077, 1999.

433. Matsuzono Y, Kinoshita N, Tamura S, Shimozawa N, Hamasaki M, Ghaedi K, Wanders RJ, Suzuki Y, Kondo N, Fujiki Y: Human *PEX19*: cDNA cloning by functional complementation, mutation analysis in a patient with Zellweger syndrome, and potential role in peroxisomal membrane assembly. *Proc Natl Acad Sci U S A* **96**:2116, 1999.

434. Gartner J, Moser H, Valle D: Mutations in the 70KD peroxisomal membrane protein gene in Zellweger syndrome. *Nat Genet* **1**:16, 1992.

435. Jansen GA, Ofman R, Ferdinandusse S, Ijlst L, Muijsers AO, Skjeldal OH, Stokke O, Jakobs C, Besley GT, Wraith JE, Wanders RJ: Refsum disease is caused by mutations in the phytanoyl-CoA hydroxylase gene. *Nat Genet* **17**:190, 1997.

436. Mihalik SJ, Morrell JC, Kim D, Sacksteder KA, Watkins PA, Gould SJ: Identification of *PAHX*, a Refsum disease gene. *Nat Genet* **17**:185, 1997.

437. Fournier B, Saudubray JM, Benichou B, Lyonnet S, Munnich A, Clevers H, Poll-The BT: Large deletion of the peroxisomal acyl-CoA oxidase gene in pseudoneonatal adrenoleukodystrophy. *J Clin Invest* **94**:526, 1994.

438. Muscatelli F, Strom TM, Walker AP, Zanaria E, Recan D, Meindl A, Bardoni B, Guioli S, Zehetner G, Rabl W, Schwarz HP, Kaplan J-C, Camerino G, Meitinger T, Monaco AP: Mutations in the DAX-1 gene give rise to both X-linked adrenal hypoplasia congenita and hypogonadotropic hypogonadism. *Nature* **372**:672, 1994.

439. Zanaria E, Muscatelli F, Bardoni B, Strom TM, Guioli S, Guo W, Lalli E, Moser C, Walker AP, McCabe ER, Meitinger T, Monaco AP, Sassone-Corsi P, Camerino G: An unusual member of the nuclear hormone receptor superfamily responsible for X-linked adrenal hypoplasia congenita. *Nature* **372**:635, 1994.

440. Henning KA, Li L, Iyer N, McDaniel LD, Reagan MS, Legerski R, Schultz RA, Stefanini M, Lehmann AR, Mayne LV, et al: The Cockayne syndrome group A gene encodes a WD repeat protein that interacts with CSB protein and a subunit of RNA polymerase II TFIIH. *Cell* **82**:555, 1995.

441. Troelstra C, van Gool A, de Wit J, Vermeulen W, Bootsma D, Hoeijmakers JH: ERCC6, a member of a subfamily of putative helicases, is involved in Cockayne's syndrome and preferential repair of active genes. *Cell* **71**:939, 1992.

442. Tanaka K, Miura N, Satokata I, Miyamoto I, Yoshida MC, Satoh Y, Kondo S, Yasui A, Okayama H, Okada Y: Analysis of a human DNA excision repair gene involved in group A xeroderma pigmentosum and containing a zinc-finger domain. *Nature* **348**:73, 1990.

443. Satokata I, Tanaka K, Miura N, Miyamoto I, Satoh Y, Kondo S, Okada Y: Characterization of a splicing mutation in group A xeroderma pigmentosum. *Proc Natl Acad Sci U S A* **87**:9908, 1990.

444. Weeda G, van Ham RC, Vermeulen W, Bootsma D, van der Eb AJ, Hoeijmakers JH: A presumed DNA helicase encoded by ERCC-3 is involved in the human repair disorders xeroderma pigmentosum and Cockayne's syndrome. *Cell* **62**:777, 1990.

445. Frederick GD, Amirkhan RH, Schultz RA, Friedberg EC: Structural and mutational analysis of the xeroderma pigmentosum group D (XPD) gene. *Hum Mol Genet* **3**:1783, 1994.

446. Nouspikel T, Clarkson SG: Mutations that disable the DNA repair gene XPG in a xeroderma pigmentosum group G patient. *Hum Mol Genet* **3**:963, 1994.

447. Villard L, Gecz J, Mattei JF, Fontes M, Saugier-Veber P, Munnich A, Lyonnet S: XNP mutation in a large family with Juberg-Marsidi syndrome. *Nat Genet* **12**:359, 1996.

448. Pomponio RJ, Reynolds TR, Cole H, Buck GA, Wolf B: Mutational hotspot in the human biotinidase gene causes profound biotinidase deficiency. *Nat Genet* **11**:96, 1995.

449. Suzuki Y, Aoki Y, Ishida Y, Chiba Y, Iwamatsu A, Kishino T, Niikawa N, Matsubara Y, Narisawa K: Isolation and characterization of mutations in the human holocarboxylase synthetase cDNA. *Nat Genet* **8**:122, 1994.

450. Anonymous: A gene (PEX) with homologies to endopeptidases is mutated in patients with X-linked hypophosphatemic rickets. The HYP Consortium. *Nat Genet* **11**:130, 1995.

451. Lloyd SE, Pearce SH, Fisher SE, Steinmeyer K, Schwappach B, Scheinman SJ, Harding B, Bolino A, Devoto M, Goodyer P, Rigden SP, Wrong O, Jentsch TJ, Craig IW, Thakker RV: A common molecular basis for three inherited kidney stone diseases. *Nature* **379**:445, 1996.

452. Simon DB, Lu Y, Choate KA, Velazquez H, Al-Sabban E, Praga M, Casari G, Bettinelli A, Colussi G, Rodriguez-Soriano J, McCredie D, Milford D, Sanjad S, Lifton RP: Paracellin-1, a renal tight junction protein required for paracellular Mg$^{2+}$ resorption. *Science* **285**:103, 1999.

453. Karet FE, Finberg KE, Nelson RD, Nayir A, Mocan H, Sanjad SA, Rodriguez-Soriano J, Santos F, Cremers CW, Di Pietro A, Hoffbrand BI, Winiarski J, Bakkaloglu A, Ozen S, Dusunsel R, Goodyer P, Hulton SA, Wu DK, Skvorak AB, Morton CC, Cunningham MJ, Jha V, Lifton RP: Mutations in the gene encoding B1 subunit of H$^+$-ATPase cause renal tubular acidosis with sensorineural deafness. *Nat Genet* **21**:84, 1999.

454. Sakurai A, Takeda K, Ain K, Ceccarelli P, Nakai A, Seino S, Bell GI, Refetoff S, DeGroot LJ: Generalized resistance to thyroid hormone associated with a mutation in the ligand-binding domain of the human thyroid hormone receptor beta. *Proc Natl Acad Sci U S A* **86**:8977, 1989.

455. Takeda K, Balzano S, Sakurai A, DeGroot LJ, Refetoff S: Screening of nineteen unrelated families with generalized resistance to thyroid hormone for known point mutations in the thyroid hormone receptor beta gene and the detection of a new mutation. *J Clin Invest* **87**:496, 1991.

456. Roessler BJ, Nosal JM, Smith PR, Heidler SA, Palella TD, Switzer RL, Becker MA: Human X-linked phosphoribosylpyrophosphate synthetase superactivity is associated with distinct point mutations in the PRPS1 gene. *J Biol Chem* **268**:26476, 1993.

457. Trivier E, De Cesare D, Jacquot S, Pannetier S, Zackai E, Young I, Mandel JL, Sassone-Corsi P, Hanauer A: Mutations in the kinase Rsk-2 associated with Coffin-Lowry syndrome. *Nature* **384**:567, 1996.

458. Kaul R, Gao GP, Balamurugan K, Matalon R: Cloning of the human aspartoacylase cDNA and a common missense mutation in Canavan disease. *Nat Genet* 5:118, 1993.

459. Brook JD, McCurrach ME, Harley HG, Buckler AJ, Church D, Aburatani H, Hunter K, Stanton VP, Thirion JP, Hudson T, Sohn R, Zemelman B, Snell RG, Rundle SA, Crow S, Davies J, Shelbourne P, Buxton J, Jones C, Juvonen V, Johnson K, Harper PS, Shaw DJ, Housman DE: Molecular basis of myotonic dystrophy: Expansion of a trinucleotide (CTG) repeat at the 3′ end of a transcript encoding a protein kinase family member [Published erratum appears in *Cell* 69(2):385, 1992]. *Cell* 68:799, 1992.

460. Brais B, Bouchard JP, Xie YG, Rochefort DL, Chretien N, Tome FM, Lafreniere RG, Rommens JM, Uyama E, Nohira O, Blumen S, Korczyn AD, Heutink P, Mathieu J, Duranceau A, Codere F, Fardeau M, Rouleau GA: Short GCG expansions in the PABP2 gene cause oculopharyngeal muscular dystrophy [Published erratum appears in *Nat Genet* 19(4):404, 1998]. *Nat Genet* 18:164, 1998.

461. Campuzano V, Montermini L, Molto MD, Pianese L, Cossee M, Cavalcanti F, Monros E, Rodius F, Duclos F, Monticelli A, Zara F, Canizares J, Koutnikova H, Bidichandani SI, Gellera C, Brice A, Trouillas P, De Michele G, Filla A, De Frutos R, Palau F, Patel PI, Di Donato S, Mandel J-L, Cocozza S, Koenig M, Pandolfo M: Friedreich's ataxia: Autosomal recessive disease caused by an intronic GAA triplet repeat expansion. *Science* 271:1423, 1996.

462. Kovach MJ, Lin JP, Boyadjiev S, Campbell K, Mazzeo L, Herman K, Rimer LA, Frank W, Llewellyn B, Wang Jabs E, Gelber D, Kimonis VE: A unique point mutation in the *PMP22* gene is associated with Charcot-Marie-Tooth disease and deafness. *Am J Hum Genet* 64:1580, 1999.

463. Roa BB, Dyck PJ, Marks HG, Chance PF, Lupski JR: Dejerine-Sottas syndrome associated with point mutation in the peripheral myelin protein 22 (PMP22) gene. *Nat Genet* 5:269, 1993.

464. Nicholson GA, Valentijn LJ, Cherryson AK, Kennerson ML, Bragg TL, DeKroon RM, Ross DA, Pollard JD, McLeod JG, Bolhuis PA, Baas F: A frameshift mutation in the PMP22 gene in hereditary neuropathy with liability to pressure palsies [Published erratum appears in *Nat Genet* 7(1):113, 1994]. *Nat Genet* 6:263, 1994.

465. Tyson J, Tranebjaerg L, Bellman S, Wren C, Taylor JF, Bathen J, Aslaksen B, Sorland SJ, Lund O, Malcolm S, Pembrey M, Bhattacharya S, Bitner-Glindzicz M: IsK and KvLQT1: Mutation in either of the two subunits of the slow component of the delayed rectifier potassium channel can cause Jervell and Lange-Nielsen syndrome. *Hum Mol Genet* 6:2179, 1997.

466. Lemmink HH, Mochizuki T, van den Heuvel LP, Schroder CH, Barrientos A, Monnens LA, van Oost BA, Brunner HG, Reeders ST, Smeets HJ: Mutations in the type IV collagen alpha 3 (COL4A3) gene in autosomal recessive Alport syndrome. *Hum Mol Genet* 3:1269, 1994.

467. Mochizuki T, Lemmink HH, Mariyama M, Antignac C, Gubler MC, Pirson Y, Verellen-Dumoulin C, Chan B, Schroder CH, Smeets HJ, Reeders ST: Identification of mutations in the alpha 3(IV) and alpha 4(IV) collagen genes in autosomal recessive Alport syndrome. *Nat Genet* 8:77, 1994.

468. Barker DF, Hostikka SL, Zhou J, Chow LT, Oliphant AR, Gerken SC, Gregory MC, Skolnick MH, Atkin CL, Tryggvason K: Identification of mutations in the COL4A5 collagen gene in Alport syndrome. *Science* 248:1224, 1990.

469. Zhou J, Hostikka SL, Chow LT, Tryggvason K: Characterization of the 3′ half of the human type IV collagen alpha 5 gene that is affected in the Alport syndrome. *Genomics* 9:1, 1991.

470. Cawthon RM, Weiss R, Xu GF, Viskochil D, Culver M, Stevens J, Robertson M, Dunn D, Gesteland R, O'Connell P, White R: A major segment of the neurofibromatosis type 1 gene: cDNA sequence, genomic structure, and point mutations [Published erratum appears in *Cell* 62(3):608, 1990]. *Cell* 62:193, 1990.

471. Viskochil D, Buchberg AM, Xu G, Cawthon RM, Stevens J, Wolff RK, Culver M, Carey JC, Copeland NG, Jenkins NA, White R, O'Connell P: Deletions and a translocation interrupt a cloned gene at the neurofibromatosis type 1 locus. *Cell* 62:187, 1990.

472. Wallace MR, Marchuk DA, Andersen LB, Letcher R, Odeh HM, Saulino AM, Fountain JW, Brereton A, Nicholson J, Mitchell AL, Brownstein BH, Collins FS: Type 1 neurofibromatosis gene: Identification of a large transcript disrupted in three NF1 patients [Published erratum appears in *Science* 250(4988):1749, 1990]. *Science* 249:181, 1990.

473. Rouleau GA, Merel P, Lutchman M, Sanson M, Zucman J, Marineau C, Hoang-Xuan K, Demczuk S, Desmaze C, Plougastel B, Pulst SM, Lenoir G, Bijlsma E, Fashold R, Dumanski J, de Jong P, Parry D, Eldrige R, Aurias A, Delattre O, Thomas G: Alteration in a new gene encoding a putative membrane-organizing protein causes neurofibromatosis type 2. *Nature* 363:515, 1993.

474. Trofatter JA, MacCollin MM, Rutter JL, Murrell JR, Duyao MP, Parry DM, Eldridge R, Kley N, Menon AG, Pulaski K, Haase VH, Ambrose CM, Munroe D, Bove C, Haines JL, Martuza RL, MacDonald ME, Seizinger BR, Short MP, Buckler AJ, Gusella JF: A novel moesin-, ezrin-, radixin-like gene is a candidate for the neurofibromatosis 2 tumor suppressor. *Cell* 72:791, 1993.

475. Latif F, Tory K, Gnarra J, Yao M, Duh FM, Orcutt ML, Stackhouse T, Kuzmin I, Modi W, Geil L, Schmidt L, Zhou F, Li H, Wei MH, Chen F, Glenn G, Choyke P, Walther MM, Weng Y, Duan D-SR, Dean M, Glavac D, Richards FM, Crossey PA, Ferguson-Smith MA, Le Paslier D, Chumakov I, Cohen D, Chinault AC, Maher ER, Linehan WM, Zbar B, Lerman MI: Identification of the von Hippel-Lindau disease tumor suppressor gene. *Science* 260:1317, 1993.

476. Baldwin CT, Hoth CF, Amos JA, da-Silva EO, Milunsky A: An exonic mutation in the HuP2 paired domain gene causes Waardenburg's syndrome [see comments]. *Nature* 355:637, 1992.

477. Morell R, Friedman TB, Moeljopawiro S, Hartono, Soewito, Asher JH Jr: A frameshift mutation in the HuP2 paired domain of the probable human homolog of murine Pax-3 is responsible for Waardenburg syndrome type 1 in an Indonesian family. *Hum Mol Genet* 1:243, 1992.

478. Tassabehji M, Read AP, Newton VE, Harris R, Balling R, Gruss P, Strachan T: Waardenburg's syndrome patients have mutations in the human homologue of the *Pax-3* paired box gene. *Nature* 355:635, 1992.

479. Tassabehji M, Newton VE, Read AP: Waardenburg syndrome type 2 caused by mutations in the human microphtalmia (*MITF*) gene. *Nat Genet* 8:251, 1994.

480. Hoth CF, Milunsky A, Lipsky N, Sheffer R, Clarren SK, Baldwin CT: Mutations in the paired domain of the human PAX3 gene cause Klein-Waardenburg syndrome (WS-III) as well as Waardenburg syndrome type I (WS-I). *Am J Hum Genet* 52:455, 1993.

481. Asher JH Jr, Sommer A, Morell R, Friedman TB: Missense mutation in the paired domain of PAX3 causes craniofacial-deafness-hand syndrome. *Hum Mutat* 7:30, 1996.

482. Edery P, Attié T, Amiel J, Pelet A, Eng C, Hofstra RMW, Martelli H, Bidaud C, Munnich A, Lyonnet S: Mutation of the endothelin-3 gene in the Waardenburg-Hirschsprung disease (Shah-Waardenburg syndrome). *Nat Genet* 12:442, 1996.

483. Hofstra RMW, Osinga J, Tan-Sindhunata G, Wu Y, Kamsteeg E-J, Stulp RP, van Ravenswaaij-Arts C, Majoor-Krakauer D, Angrist M, Chakraverti A, Meijers C, Buys CHCM: A homozygous mutation in the endothelin-3 gene associated with a combined Waardenburg type 2 and Hirschsprung phenotype (Shah-Waardenburg syndrome). *Nat Genet* 12:445, 1996.

484. Attie T, Till M, Pelet A, Amiel J, Edery P, Boutrand L, Munnich A, Lyonnet S: Mutation of the endothelin-receptor B gene in Waardenburg-Hirschsprung disease. *Hum Mol Genet* 4:2407, 1995.

485. Pingault V, Bondurand N, Kuhlbrodt K, Goerich DE, Prehu MO, Puliti A, Herbarth B, Hermans-Borgmeyer I, Legius E, Matthijs G, Amiel J, Lyonnet S, Ceccherini I, Romeo G, Smith JC, Read AP, Wegner M, Goossens M: SOX10 mutations in patients with Waardenburg-Hirschsprung disease. *Nat Genet* 18:171, 1998.

486. Giebel LB, Spritz RA: Mutation of the KIT (mast/stem cell growth factor receptor) protooncogene in human piebaldism. *Proc Natl Acad Sci U S A* 88:8696, 1991.

487. Hardelin JP, Levilliers J, Blanchard S, Carel JC, Leutenegger M, Pinard-Bertelletto JP, Bouloux P, Petit C: Heterogeneity in the mutations responsible for X chromosome-linked Kallmann syndrome. *Hum Mol Genet* 2:373, 1993.

488. Hardelin J-P, Julliard AK, Moniot B, Soussi-Yanicostas N, Verney C, Schwanzel-Fukuda M, Ayer-Le Lièvre C, Petit C: Anosmin-1 is a regionally restricted component of basement membranes and interstitial matrices during organogenesis: Implications for the developmental anomalies of X chromosome-linked Kallmann syndrome. *Dev Dyn* 215:26, 1999.

489. Verpy E, Leibovici M, Zwaenepoel I, Liu X-Z, Gal A, Salem N, Mansour A, Blanchard S, Kobayashi I, Keats BJB, Slim R, Petit C: A defect in harmonin, a PDZ domain-containing protein expressed in the inner ear sensory hair cell, underlies Usher syndrome type 1C. *Nature Genet* 26:51, 2000.

490. Eudy JD, Weston MD, Yao S, Hoover DM, Rehm HL, Ma-Edmonds M, Yan D, Ahmad I, Cheng JJ, Ayuso C, Cremers C, Davenport S, Moller C, Talmadge CB, Beisel KW, Tamayo M, Morton CC, Swaroop A, Kimberling WJ, Sumegi J: Mutation of a gene encoding a protein with extracellular matrix motifs in Usher syndrome type IIa. *Science* **280**:1753, 1998.

491. Berger W, Meindl A, van de Pol TJ, Cremers FPM, Ropers HH, Doerner C, Monaco A, Bergen AA, Lebo R, Warburg M, Zergollern L, Lorenz B, Gal A, Bleeker-Wagemakers EM, Meitinger T: Isolation of a candidate gene for Norrie disease by positional cloning [Published erratum appears in *Nat Genet* 2(1):84, 1992]. *Nat Genet* **1**:199, 1992.

492. Chen ZY, Hendriks RW, Jobling MA, Powell JF, Breakefield XO, Sims KB, Craig IW: Isolation and characterization of a candidate gene for Norrie disease. *Nat Genet* **1**:204, 1992.

493. Meindl A, Berger W, Meitinger T, van de Pol D, Achatz H, Dorner C, Haasemann M, Hellebrand H, Gal A, Cremers F, Ropers H-H: Norrie disease is caused by mutations in an extracellular protein resembling C-terminal globular domain of mucins. *Nat Genet* **2**:139, 1992.

494. Diaz GA, Banikazemi M, Oishi K, Desnick RJ, Gelb BD: Mutations in a new gene encoding a thiamine transporter cause thiamine-responsive megaloblastic anaemia syndrome. *Nat Genet* **22**:309, 1999.

495. Fleming JC, Tartaglini E, Steinkamp MP, Schorderet DF, Cohen N, Neufeld EJ: The gene mutated in thiamine-responsive anaemia with diabetes and deafness (TRMA) encodes a functional thiamine transporter. *Nat Genet* **22**:305, 1999.

496. Labay V, Raz T, Baron D, Mandel H, Williams H, Barrett T, Szargel R, McDonald L, Shalata A, Nosaka K, Gregory S, Cohen N: Mutations in *SLC19A2* cause thiamine-responsive megaloblastic anaemia associated with diabetes mellitus and deafness. *Nat Genet* **22**:300, 1999.

497. Anderson DW, Probst FJ, Belyantseva IA, Fridell RA, Bayer L, Martin DM, Wu D, Kachar B, Friedman TB, Raphael Y, Camper SA: The motor and tail regions of myosin XV are critical for normal structure and function of auditory and vestibular hair cells. *Hum Mol Genet* **9**:1729, 2000.

498. Yasunaga S, Grati M, Chardenoux S, Smith TN, Friedman TB, Lalwani AK, Wilcox ER, Petit C: *OTOF* encodes multiple long and short isoforms: genetic evidence that the long ones underlie the recessive deafness DFNB9. *Am J Hum Genet* **67**:591, 2000.

499. Adato A, Raskin L, Petit C, Bonné-Tamir B: Deafness heterogeneity in a Druze isolate from the Middle East: novel *OTOF* and *PDS* mutations, low prevalence of *GJB2* 35delG mutation and indication for a new DFNB locus. *Eur J Hum Genet* **8**:437, 2000.

500. Usami S-i, Abe S, Akita J, Namba A, Shinkawa H, Ishii M, Iwasaki S, Hoshino T, Ito J, Dio K, Kubo T, Nakagawa T, Komiyama S, Tono T, Komune S: Prevalence of mitochondrial gene mutations among hearing impaired patients. *J Med Genet* **37**:38, 2000.

# Rett Syndrome

*Huda Y. Zoghbi* ■ *Uta Francke*

1. Rett syndrome (RTT) is an X-linked dominant neurodevelopmental disorder that afflicts females after 6 to 18 months of apparently normal development. Around this time, they enter a short period of developmental stagnation followed by rapid regression in language and motor development. A hallmark of RTT is the loss of purposeful hand use followed by repetitive, stereotyped hand movements. Additional features include autistic behavior, gait ataxia and apraxia, seizures, episodic apnea and/or hyperpnea, bruxism, and acquired microcephaly. After this period of rapid deterioration, the disease becomes relatively stable, but patients reaching the second or third decade may show additional neurologic abnormalities, such as seizures, dystonia, parkinsonism, spasticity, and kyphoscoliosis. X-linked inheritance explains the existence of a few males with severe neonatal encephalopathy born into families affected by RTT.

2. No laboratory findings have proven consistent enough to be diagnostically useful. The EEG is typically normal for the first 2 years of life, after which patients lose occipital dominant rhythm and background activity. CT and MRI show cortical atrophy and sometimes narrowing of the brain stem; PET reveals reduced cerebral blood flow in the prefrontal and temporoparietal association regions. Brains of RTT patients weigh less than age-matched controls; there is mild cortical and cerebellar atrophy but no evidence of neuronal loss. Select neuronal populations show reduced dendritic arborization, smaller neuronal size, and increased neuronal density.

3. Current effective management of RTT patients focuses on supportive and symptomatic therapy, for example, anticonvulsants for seizures, chloral hydrate for agitation, carbidopa/levodopa for rigidity, and melatonin for sleep disturbances. Nutritional management is important to ensure adequate caloric and fiber intake.

4. RTT is caused by any of various mutations in the *MECP2* gene, which encodes the methyl CpG-binding protein 2. This ubiquitous protein assists in transcriptional silencing by binding to symmetrically methylated single CpGs in double-stranded DNA. The transcriptional repression domain binds to the corepressor Sin3A and recruits histone deacetylases and other proteins to the silencing complex. When lysine residues of the core histones H3 and H4 become deacetylated, the chromatin structure changes and renders the DNA inaccessible to the transcriptional machinery. The heritability of the repressed state depends on maintenance of CpG methylation through replication by the maintenance methylase that acts on hemimethylated DNA.

5. The severity of the RTT phenotype is determined primarily by the female's pattern of X inactivation (XCI), but the type of mutation could also have an influence. Individuals who meet the diagnostic criteria for RTT have more or less random XCI. Rare cases with skewed XCI might be severely affected and lack a period of normal early development if the mutant X is predominantly active. Patients with the normal X predominantly active have milder presentation. Extreme skewing can cause nonspecific learning deficits in women for whom a diagnosis of RTT would not have been considered; so far, such women have been identified only because of relation to individuals with classic RTT. Indications for mutation testing extend beyond individuals with the clinical diagnosis of RTT to include females with partial phenotypes who do not meet diagnostic criteria for RTT and males with unexplained encephalopathy in the neonatal period or death during infancy.

## HISTORY AND CLINICAL FEATURES

### Defining the Syndrome

In 1966, the Viennese physician Andreas Rett described 22 girls with "cerebral atrophy and hyperammonemia," a progressive neurologic disorder characterized by autistic behavior, dementia, gait apraxia, loss of facial expression, and stereotypic hand movements.[1] Rett noted that the syndrome appeared only in girls some time after the first year of life. Fourteen years later, and unaware of Rett's findings, Bengt Hagberg of Sweden described "infantile autistic dementia and loss of hand use" in 16 Swedish girls.[2] Hagberg and colleagues described the disorder in greater detail in 1983 based on a study of 35 French, Portuguese, and Swedish female patients. By then having realized that their disorder was the same clinical entity as that discovered by Andreas Rett, they named it Rett syndrome (RTT; MIM 312750).[3] It was this report that brought this fascinating disorder to the attention of neurologists and geneticists around the world.

The prevalence of Rett syndrome is estimated to be from 1:15,000[4] to 1:10,000.[5] Affected girls usually have a normal birth and neonatal course followed by apparently normal psychomotor development during the first 6 to 18 months of life. Shortly thereafter, they enter a short period of developmental stagnation followed by rapid regression in language and motor development. Loss of purposeful hand use followed by repetitive stereotyped hand movements—anything from hand-wringing to clapping or waving—is one of the earliest and most common findings (Fig. 255-1). Additional features include autistic behavior, gait ataxia and apraxia, seizures, episodic apnea and/or hyperpnea, bruxism, and acquired microcephaly. After this period of rapid deterioration the disease becomes relatively stable, but patients reaching the second or third decade may show additional neurologic abnormalities such as dystonia, parkinsonism, spasticity, and kyphoscoliosis.[3,6–8]

A list of standard abbreviations is located immediately preceding the index in each volume. Additional abbreviations used in this chapter include: AS = Angelman syndrome; DSS = dosage-sensitive sex reversal; DZ = dizygotic; MBD = methyl-binding domain; *MECP2* = the gene that encodes methyl CpG-binding protein 2; MeCP2 = the protein; *Mecp2* = the mouse homolog of *MECP2*; MZ = monozygotic; NLS = nuclear localization signal; NREM = nonrapid eye movement; PTT = premature termination of translation; RTT = Rett syndrome; TRD = transcriptional repression domain; XCI = X chromosome inactivation.

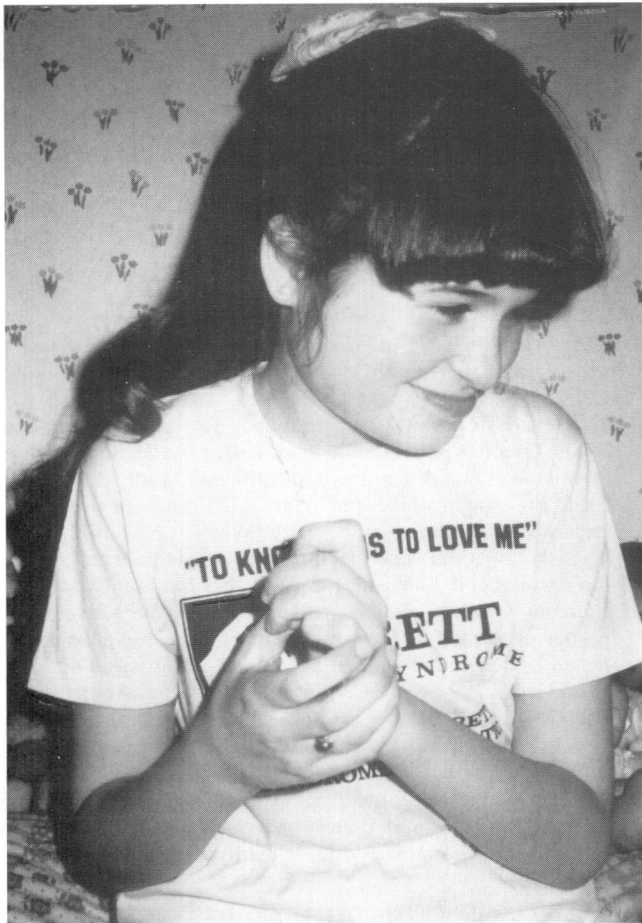

**Fig. 255-1** A 16-year-old Rett syndrome patient with the characteristic stereotyped hand-washing movements.

## Clinical Criteria and Differential Diagnosis

Diagnostic clinical criteria were set forth in 1988[9] and are summarized in Table 255-1. The limitation of clinical diagnosis is evidenced partly by the fact that diagnosis is considered tentative until 2 to 5 years of age, when most of the patients have gone through several stages of disease (Table 255-2).[10] A deteriorating infant with loss of motor skills and apparent dementia may be misdiagnosed as having neuronal ceroid lipofuscinosis, while an 18-month-old girl with loss of communication skills may be misdiagnosed as having autism. A disorder that is frequently in the

**Table 255-1** Diagnostic Criteria for Classic Rett Syndrome

- Apparently normal prenatal and perinatal period*
- Apparently normal development through the first 6 months*
- Normal head circumference at birth
- Deceleration of head growth between ages 5 and 48 months
- Loss of acquired hand skills and purposeful hand use between ages 5 and 30 months, with subsequent development of stereotyped hand movements
- Severe impairment of expressive and receptive language together with severe psychomotor retardation
- Development of gait apraxia and truncal ataxia between ages 12 and 48 months

*These clinical criteria may not be applicable to severely affected females; other criteria will not apply to those who are mildly affected by mutations in *MECP2*. Molecular diagnosis has broadened the relevant phenotypes since these criteria were set forth.

**Table 255-2** Clinical Stages in Classic Rett Syndrome

| | |
|---|---|
| I. Stagnation stage (6 to 18 months) | Developmental arrest<br>Deterioration of eye contact and possible loss of communication<br>Decreased play interest<br>Deceleration of head growth |
| II. Rapid destructive stage (1 to 4 years) | Developmental deterioration<br>Loss of purposeful hand use<br>Stereotyped hand movements<br>Autistic features<br>Gait ataxia and apraxia<br>Irregular breathing — hyperventilation<br>Seizures |
| III. Pseudostationary stage (Preschool to early school years) | Mental retardation<br>Autistic features decrease<br>Gait ataxia and apraxia prominent<br>Gross motor dysfunction<br>Seizures |
| IV. Late motor deterioration stage (5 to 25 years) | Decreasing mobility<br>Spasticity<br>Improved emotional contact<br>Scoliosis<br>Cachexia and growth retardation<br>Staring, unfathomable gaze |

differential diagnosis of Rett syndrome is Angelman syndrome (AS), in which patients also show mental deficiency, seizures, ataxia, and microcephaly. Careful history to establish developmental regression together with the stereotyped hand movements help distinguish RTT from AS clinically. In the older patient who is severely wasted, and who has spasticity and severe mental retardation, it is sometimes even more difficult to establish the diagnosis; these girls are often diagnosed as having cerebral palsy. Only detailed review of the developmental and early childhood history enables the correct diagnosis of RTT.

The issue of early "apparently normal" development is controversial. Very subtle developmental deficiencies may be easily missed; some patients have hypotonia from the first months of life, and others might have slight delay after the rolling-over stage at about 5 months.[11] Parents describe screaming fits and inconsolable crying by 18 months of age in the majority of patients.[12] Although the basis of this behavioral abnormality remains a mystery, there is no doubt of its high prevalence in RTT. In sum, it is best to say that early development appears grossly normal until this issue can be settled when more patients are diagnosed early in life using molecular approaches (see "Etiology and Genetics" below).

Seizures are reported to occur in 50 to 90 percent of RTT patients; generalized tonic-clonic seizures are the most common and partial complex seizures the second most common.[13] Additional clinical manifestations of seizure activities include focal clonic activity, head or eye deviation, and/or apnea.[14] Seizures occur more frequently in clinical stage III and often decrease when patients are in clinical stage IV. It is noteworthy that many reported seizures are not associated with epileptiform activity on the electroencephalogram (EEG), and that clinical events accompanying EEG epileptiform activities are not always recognized as seizures by the parents.[14] To obtain definitive information about the occurrence of seizures and the need for antiepileptic drugs, video/EEG monitoring is recommended.

Girls with Rett syndrome are not dysmorphic but they are quite small; 85 to 90 percent of them suffer from growth failure and wasting that worsen with age.[15,16] These patients have poor food intake primarily because of oropharyngeal and gastroesophageal incoordination.[17,18] Dysmotility of the bowel and functional megacolon are common in Rett syndrome, along with constipation and, in extreme cases, fecal impaction, volvulus, and intussusception.[15] Ample fluid intake and a high-fiber diet with occasional use of stool softeners can help prevent acute intestinal crises.

Rett syndrome patients typically survive into adulthood, but their life expectancy is short (three to four decades) and the incidence of sudden, unexplained death in RTT is significantly higher than controls of similar age.[19] This sudden death may partly be due to the higher incidence of longer corrected QT intervals, T wave abnormalities, and reduced heart rate variability in Rett patients.[20,21]

## Atypical Variants and Male Rett Patients

Atypical variants of Rett syndrome have been described. Some of these patients have a more severe phenotype characterized by absence of early normal development, congenital hypotonia, and massive infantile spasms. Patients with a milder phenotype ("forme fruste") demonstrate less severe regression in childhood, have mild mental retardation, some hand use, and usually do not have seizures.[22] Another variant includes those patients that have most of the usual features but a much milder course with preserved speech.[23] These patients have apparently normal development during the first 3 years of life, regress over several years, and have seizures. They always lose some hand skills, but they walk independently, and several are able to sing simple songs and say some words. All these patients have some degree of gait and hand apraxia, stereotyped hand movements, autistic features, and mild-moderate mental retardation. Given the X-linked genetic basis of Rett syndrome (see "Etiology and Genetics" below), it is not surprising that these variants occur; the clinical manifestations depend, at least in part, on the patterns of X chromosome inactivation in these girls. Indeed, one would expect that some patients have such a mild phenotype that they may not be diagnosed as having Rett syndrome (see "Mutations and Sequence Variants" below).

Some males have been reported to have clinical features similar to those seen in classic Rett syndrome. None of these males, however, meet all the diagnostic criteria for the disorder;[24,25] because all of them are sporadic cases, it is difficult to determine whether they have Rett syndrome or another disease with some overlapping manifestations. A male patient with a 47,XXY karyotype and a clinical phenotype of Rett and Klinefelter syndromes has been described.[26]

Of more interest are two males presenting with severe neonatal encephalopathy that were born into families with recurrent RTT. Both of these patients presented with congenital hypotonia, central apnea requiring mechanical ventilation, seizures, and severe gastroesophageal reflux.[27] Both patients acquired some milestones in early infancy (some head control, smiling, and recognizing parents). One of them had documented acquired microcephaly and suffered from severe intestinal dysfunction leading to obstruction. Both died before their second birthday from respiratory arrest. The clinical findings in these two patients raised the question whether males with RTT might present with a phenotype quite different form the classic syndrome owing to the X-linked dominant nature of the disease.[27] Recent genetic studies have now confirmed this hypothesis (see "Etiology and Genetics").[28]

## Laboratory Findings

Laboratory studies have not been useful in establishing the diagnosis because no consistent laboratory abnormalities have been found. Although Rett initially described hyperammonemia in some of his patients, later studies by both him and Hagberg revealed no hyperammonemia in the vast majority of cases.[3] Laboratory tests of serum amino acids, uric acid, lipids, copper, ceruloplasmin, urine organic acids, lactic and pyruvic acids, very long chain fatty acids, lysosomal enzymes, cerebrospinal fluid (CSF) glucose, protein, and cells all tend to be normal in Rett patients.[3,7,29] Although alterations in CSF biogenic amine metabolites and beta endorphins have been reported in Rett syndrome, none of these are consistently abnormal.[29]

# NEUROPHYSIOLOGY, NEUROIMAGING, AND NEUROPATHOLOGY

## Electroencephalography

The EEG is typically normal for the first 2 years of life without evidence of epileptiform activity. In early stage I, there is slowing of the occipital dominant rhythm and background activity with the occurrence of spike or sharp wave discharges during sleep. When the patients regress (stage II), the EEG is characterized by loss of occipital dominant rhythm, further slowing of background activity, loss of nonrapid eye movement (NREM) sleep characteristics, and frequent focal and generalized spike and sharp wave discharges. In stages III and IV, the EEG becomes markedly slow (theta and delta activity) with multifocal spike and wave discharges. In some older patients, the occipital dominant rhythm and NREM sleep characteristics reappear.[14] Video/EEG monitoring reveals that episodes of apnea and hyperventilation, laughing, screaming, and vacant staring spells often occur. Focal electrographic seizures are usually associated with focal clonic activity, head or eye deviation, and sometimes apnea. Generalized electrographic seizures are frequently accompanied by absence episodes or flexor spasms.

Although these EEG changes are common to many patients with RTT, they are not unique to this disorder, and thus are not diagnostic.

## Neuroimaging Studies

Routine computed tomography (CT) and magnetic resonance imaging (MRI) show cortical atrophy predominantly in the frontal area. MRI studies reveal no abnormalities in the white matter, basal ganglia, thalamus, or hippocampus. Narrowing of the brain stem occurs in some patients.[30] Photon emission CT demonstrates lower cerebral blood flow in the prefrontal and temporoparietal association regions with sparing of the sensorimotor regions.[31] The flow distribution in Rett patients is similar to that observed in infants of a few months of age, suggesting that this disorder is due to a neurodevelopmental abnormality rather than a neurodegenerative process.

## Neuropathology Studies

The brains of Rett syndrome patients consistently weigh less than age-matched controls, by 12 to 34 percent. Mild cortical and cerebellar atrophy without evidence of neuronal loss argues against a neurodegenerative process.[32,33] In the first extensive report on the neuropathology of Rett, Jellinger and Seitelberger[34] documented the decreased brain size and found that neurons of the pars compacta of the substantia nigra contained less melanin than age-matched control brains. In another study, neurons were smaller but more densely packed in the hippocampus and entorhinal cortex.[35] This is consistent with the reduced dendritic arborization observed in selected neuronal populations: using Golgi techniques, Armstrong noted a paucity of dendrites and simplified dendritic branching patterns in the premotor frontal cortex, motor cortex, inferior temporal cortex, and hippocampus.[33] Belichenko and colleagues reported subnormal numbers of dendrites in similar cortical regions using confocal microscopy.[36] These investigators also found "naked dendrites" that lacked spines in the pyramidal neurons. The paucity of dendritic spines was most prominent in the frontal cortex and was found to be a common feature in RTT.[37] Additional pathology studies revealed that the cardiac conduction system is immature in seven of seven RTT hearts. This immature pattern may explain the higher frequency of sudden death in RTT patients.[38]

Examination of glutamate and gamma-aminobutyric acid (GABA) receptor density using autoradiography in the basal ganglia of RTT patients revealed reduction in alpha-amino-3-hydroxy-5-methylisoxazole-4-propionic acid (AMPA) and N-methyl-D-aspartate (NMDA) receptor density in the putamen, and reduced kainate receptor density in the caudate. These changes were found in patients over 8 years of age. Younger RTT patients, in contrast, had increased ionic glutamate receptor and GABA receptors in the caudate.[39] Although the relationship of these findings to pathogenesis is unknown, the authors propose that age-specificalterations in amino acid neurotransmitter receptors in the basal ganglia may be relevant to the age-related clinical stages.

## MANAGEMENT OF RTT PATIENTS

At this time there is no treatment known to improve the neurologic outcome of RTT patients. Two double-blind randomized trials have been carried out: one using L-carnitine,[40] and the other using the oral opiate antagonist Naltrexone[41] (because elevated opioids had been observed in CSF).[42,43] Naltrexone promoted some decrease in the disorganized breathing during wakefulness, but its propulsion of some patients into a higher stage of disease rendered this drug inappropriate for RTT.[41] L-Carnitine did not lead to significant functional improvements, although parents and care-givers reported improvement in the "well-being" of the subjects. Additional studies using objective outcome measures will be necessary to establish the potential benefit of L-carnitine.

Current effective management of RTT patients focuses on supportive and symptomatic therapy, for example, anticonvulsants for seizures, chloral hydrate for agitation, carbidopa/levodopa for rigidity, and melatonin for sleep disturbances.[15] Nutritional management is important to insure adequate caloric and fiber intake. Antireflux agents, smaller and thickened feedings, and positioning help decrease the gastroesophageal reflex.

## ETIOLOGY AND GENETICS

The cause of RTT has been debated for more than a decade.[3,44–46] If it were genetic, the prevalence, estimated at 1 in 15, 000 females, with 99.5 percent of all cases being sporadic, would imply a high mutation rate.[4] Because RTT is limited to females and XXY males by clinical criteria, many different hypotheses about the disease-causing mechanism have been considered.

### Models Proposed

Uniparental disomy (UPD) of the X chromosome was formally excluded by several studies of RTT families.[45,47,48] Bi-allelic overexpression of an X-linked gene normally subject to inactivation could occur if a mutation in the gene causes it to be expressed from the inactive X chromosome.[49] Overexpression of X-linked genes due to small gene duplications can be disease-causing, as in the case of Pelizaeus-Merzbacher disease (caused by proteolipid protein gene duplication[50]) and dosage-sensitive sex reversal (DSS, due to an Xp21.1 duplication of the DSS region[51]). Autosomal gene mutations with sex-limited expression has been a frequently cited theoretical model, but aside from hormonally influenced disorders such as breast cancer and familial baldness, there is neither precedent nor an obvious mechanism to explain exclusive manifestation in females. Triplet-repeat expansion was considered as a mechanism when genealogic studies in Sweden traced ancestors of RTT patients to a small number of countries, suggesting the possibility of an inherited predisposition.[52] Hofferbert and colleagues, however, excluded this possibility using repeat expansion detection methodology.[53] Microdeletions mediated by recombination between highly homologous blocks of flanking sequences account for *de novo* recurrences of the Prader Willi/Angelman, Williams-Beuren, Smith-Magenis, and velocardiofacial syndromes;[54] a systematic search revealed no deletions greater than 100 kb in six unrelated RT patients,[55] but smaller deletions could not be excluded.

The favored hypothesis is X-linked dominant inheritance, with variability of expression in females explained by nonrandom X chromosome inactivation (XCI) patterns, and lethality (or different clinical manifestations) in males. Various lines of evidence support this hypothesis. First, twin data support a genetic etiology. Ten of 11 female monozygotic (MZ) pairs are concordantly affected, while 5 of 5 female dizygotic (DZ) pairs are discordant. In eight pairs of non-like-sex DZ twins, the male twins are normal (IRSA Registry). Migeon et al. found variable XCI patterns in affected MZ twins and extremely skewed XCI (with the paternal X active) in an unaffected member of the only discordant MZ twin pair known to date.[45] These results are consistent with a hypothesis of X-linked dominant inheritance; both MZ twins should be affected, but skewing of XCI in one twin, as may be more common in MZ than in DZ twins, would lead to differences in clinical presentation. This could vary from different degrees of severity to apparent discordance. If *de novo* mutations in the putative X-linked RTT gene were to occur exclusively in the male germline, only affected females would be expected.[56] Higher mutation rates for X-linked diseases in the male germ line have been established, especially in cases of small structural rearrangements, for example, DMD and hemophilia A.

Familial recurrence of RTT has been reported in a dozen instances. In Sweden, a girl with classic RTT gave birth to a similarly affected daughter, the first evidence of direct vertical transmission.[57] Six families with two affected full sisters are thought to represent germ line mosaicism in one parent. In two sets of half-sisters with a common mother, maternal mosaicism is assumed. Skewed XCI in one of the mothers suggests that she may be carrying the mutation in her somatic cells as well.[58] Skewed XCI (95 percent:5 percent) was also reported for the mother of three affected girls in a Brazilian family,[59] suggesting that she is a nonpenetrant carrier of the mutation. There are two families with an affected aunt and niece.[60,61] In one family, the putative transmitting (minimally affected) woman had a favorably skewed XCI pattern with mostly the paternal X active. X chromosome haplotype analysis revealed a grandmaternal origin of the mutation, probably by way of germ line mosaicism, because XCI pattern in her somatic tissue was random.[60]

An X-linked dominant hypothesis also allows us to answer the intriguing question raised by the males with severe encephalopathy born into RTT families (see above), such as those described by Schanen.[62] Other males with unexplained encephalopathy or neonatal death have been born into other sibships of RTT girls,[27] including the Brazilian family.[59,63] Although these latter cases are less well-documented, X-linked inheritance would produce males with RTT gene mutations who are much more severely affected than females. Hemizygosity produces a different phenotype than heterozygosity with random XCI. The recent finding of mutations in the families discussed above confirmed all these predictions (see "Identifying MECP2 as the Rett Gene" below).

### Mapping of the RTT Gene on the X Chromosome

Given the paucity of familial cases, the standard linkage mapping and positional cloning approach was not applicable and an exclusion mapping strategy was pursued. Genotyping of X-chromosomal markers in the families with affected maternal half-sisters identified the shared regions of the maternal X-chromosome and excluded the pericentromeric region from Xp21.3 to Xq22.3.[64–66] Typing new markers in the previously nonexcluded region extended the region of discordance to Xp22.13.[60] The discovery of a new family with affected aunt and niece provided several more informative meioses.[60,62] Marker typing left a small region in the Xp22.31 area and the distal long arm from Xq25-qter as possible sites for the RTT locus. Recently, data from a Brazilian family with three affected sisters[59] were added, leading to a single concordant region extending from the marker DXS998 in the Xq27.3 to the Xq pseudoautosomal region.[59,60,62,63]

### Identifying *MECP2* as the RTT Gene

The *MECP2* gene, which encodes a methyl CpG binding protein, had been mapped to Xq28 between L1CAM and RCP/GCP several years ago;[67,68] an abnormal methylation pattern serendipitously discovered in one RTT patient led investigators to search for mutations in this gene. The discovery of missense

**Table 255-3** *MECP2* Mutations and Normal Variants

| | Exon | Domain | Nucleotide change* | Amino acid change | Restriction enzyme (+)/(−) | CpG hotspot | Recurrent |
|---|---|---|---|---|---|---|---|
| Missense | | | | | | | |
| | 2 | MBD | 316C > T | R106W | NlaIII(+) | + | +(2x) |
| | 3 | MBD | 397C > T | R133C | None | + | − |
| | 3 | MBD | 464T > C | F155S | Tfil (+), Hinfl (+) | − | − |
| | 3 | MBD | 473C > T | T158M | NlaIII (+) | + | − |
| | 3 | TRD | 916C > T | R306C | HhaI (−), HinP (−) | + | − |
| PTT† | | | | | | | |
| | 3 | MBD | 411delG | Stop138 | None | − | − |
| | 3 | — | 502C > T | R168X | HphI (+) | + | +(7x) |
| | 3 | — | 620insT | Stop235 | BsgI (−) | − | − |
| | 3 | TRD | 763C > T | R255X | None | + | +(2x) |
| | 3 | TRD | 803delG | Stop288 | NlaIV (−) | − | − |
| Amino acid variant | 3 | — | 1189G > A | E397K | StyI (+), MnlI (−) | +(AS) | +(2x) |

*Numbered from the ATG initiator codon
†PTT: mutations leading to premature termination of translation
From Amir et al.[69] and Wan et al.[28] Used with permission.

and truncating mutations in *MECP2* identified it as the cause of RTT.[69]

The *MECP2* protein (MeCP2) serves as a molecular link between methylated DNA and compacted chromatin, assisting in transcriptional silencing and in epigenetic regulation. The methyl CpG-binding domain (MBD) of MeCP2 binds to symmetrically methylated single CpGs in double-stranded DNA. The transcriptional repression domain (TRD) binds to the corepressor Sin3A and recruits histone deacetylases and other proteins to the silencing complex.[70–72] When lysine residues of the core histones H3 and H4 become deacetylated, the chromatin structure changes and renders the DNA inaccessible to the transcriptional machinery. The heritability of the repressed state depends on maintenance of CpG methylation through replication by the maintenance methylase that acts on hemimethylated DNA.[73]

DNA methylation becomes essential at the stage of gastrulation when the specific tissue and developmental patterns of gene expression are established. DNA methyl transferase (*Dnmt*) deficient embryos die in midgestation,[74] and chimeras between normal and *Mecp2*-deficient ES cells have developmental defects and survive only if the proportion of mutant ES cells is low.[75] It is hypothesized that CpG methylation and associated histone modification are used to suppress the tissue-specific genes whose activity is not required in the particular cell type; alternatively, they may act as a global repressor system.

## Gene Structure and Transcripts

The *MECP2* protein is ubiquitously expressed, very abundant, located in the nucleus, and associated with 5-methylcytosine (5-mC)-rich heterochromatin.[75,76] Its 486 amino acids are encoded in 3 exons. The entire sequence, including the intron sequences, are available through the human genome sequencing project (GenBank AF030876). The third exon contains a large (>8.5 kb) untranslated region 3′ to the translational stop codon. It includes several polyadenylation sites that enable the generation of multiple transcripts of different lengths. Comparison with the mouse *Mecp2* sequence reveals at least eight regions of high sequence similarity in the 3′ UTR, the function of which is yet unknown. It has been suggested that these conserved sequences may be important for transcript stability and posttranscriptional regulation.[77] Some tissue preference for alternative transcript termination exists, with the largest 10.1-kb transcript being the one preferentially formed in fetal brain and the 1.8- and 5-kb transcripts being highest in fetal liver, although transcripts of all

sizes, including a 7.5-kb band, are visible in all tissues on northern blots.[67,77]

## Mutations and Sequence Variants

Mutation detection was performed on genomic DNA with a set of PCR primers that amplify overlapping segments of the coding region, including all splice junctions and part of the introns. Missense mutations in the functional domains as well as mutations leading to premature termination of translation (PTT) were identified[28,69] (Table 255-3). The most common mutation to date is a 502C → T transition that changes codon 168 from CGA (arginine) to a TGA stop in exon 3. Routine DNA sequencing found this mutation in six unrelated sporadic cases and in the Brazilian family with three affected sisters and a normal mother with a skewed XCI pattern.[28] This recurrent mutation, which occurs at a CpG dinucleotide, was not detected by the conformation sensitive gel electrophoresis (CSGE) heteroduplex screening method used in the initial study.[69] The presence of the R168X mutation can be assessed by *Hph*I restriction digest (Fig. 255-2A). Another recurrent nonsense mutation at a CpG hotspot, 763C → T leading to R255X, predicts a mutant protein that is truncated in the TRD.[28,69]

Frameshifts due to single nucleotide deletions or insertions were identified in three cases. The 411delG deletion at codon 137 creates a TGA stop codon at the next amino acid. This is the only truncation mutation within the MBD. The affected individual had incomplete diagnostic features of RTT and localized skin lesions resembling those seen in incontinentia pigmenti.[28] Deletion of one of four consecutive guanines (803delG) causes a frameshift and a stop codon at position 288 within the TRD following 19 missense amino acids. This mutation was identified in all affected members of a two-generation family: the aunt and niece diagnosed with classic RTT; the transmitting female with mild neurologic symptoms (poor motor coordination, apraxia, fine tremor), an IQ of 71 and favorably skewed X inactivation; and her son, who died from a neonatal encephalopathy.[62] The mutation is detected by digestion with *Nla*IV (Fig. 255-2B); its absence in generation I indicates germ line mosaicism. Presence of a truncating *MECP2* mutation in this family confirms that hemizygous males may be born alive. Furthermore, favorably skewed X inactivation mosaicism can lead to mild involvement in heterozygous females (e.g., individual II-4), while the same mutation causes classic RTT when associated with random X inactivation (individuals II-2 and III-1). The single nucleotide insertion 620insT leads to a stop codon after 27 missense amino acids at position 235.[69] This mutation was

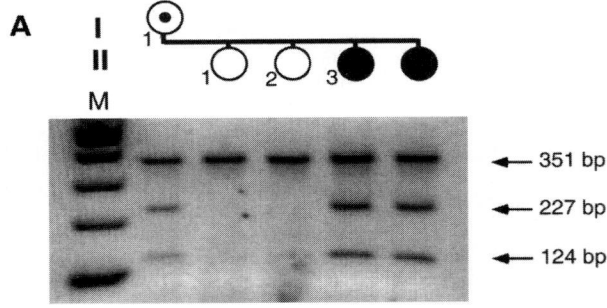

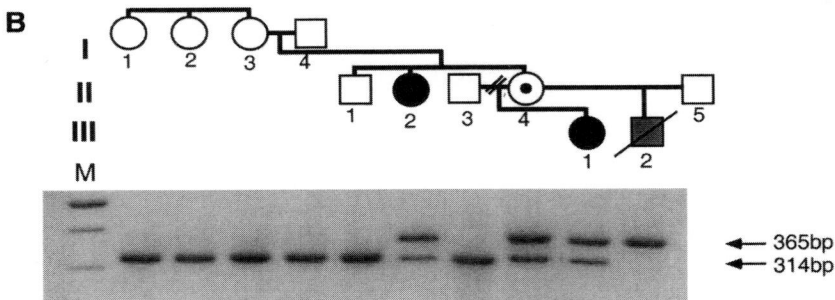

Fig. 255-2 Familial mutations in *MECP2* detected by restriction digests. *A*, The R168X mutation is identified by mutation-induced cleavage at a *Hph*I site. The clinically unaffected mother and two daughters with RTT are heterozygotes. *B*, The 803delG frameshift mutation is identified by loss of an *Nla*IV site. Two females with RTT, the obligate carrier, and the affected male are positive for the diagnostic 365-bp fragment. There is no evidence for somatic mosaicism in I-3, who transmitted the mutation to her two daughters. (*From Wan et al.*[28] *Used with permission.*)

found in a sporadic RTT patient whose father was not available for study.

Mutations causing amino acid substitutions involve highly conserved residues in one of the functional domains (Fig. 255-3). In the part of the MBD encoded by exon 2, a 316C → T transition leading to an R106W substitution was identified in a sporadic case as well as in affected half-sisters, but not in their common mother.[28,69] Unique *de novo* missense mutations found in sporadic cases include 397C → T (R133C), 464T → C (F155S), and 473C → T (T158M) in the part of the MBD encoded by exon 3,[69] and 916C → T (R306C) in the TRD.[28] All five of these

substituted amino acid residues are conserved in *MECP2* genes from *Xenopus laevis* to mammals.

Sequence variants of no clinical significance were also identified in the course of mutation searches. Two synonymous nucleotide substitutions were described in single families, 582C → T and 1233C → T (positions 656 and 1307, respectively, in the Amir paper; this revised nucleotide numbering system is according to the first nucleotide at the start methionine instead of the first nucleotide of GenBank 99686).[69] An 1189G → A transition leading to a lysine for glutamic acid substitution (E397K) in the C-terminal region was identified in the

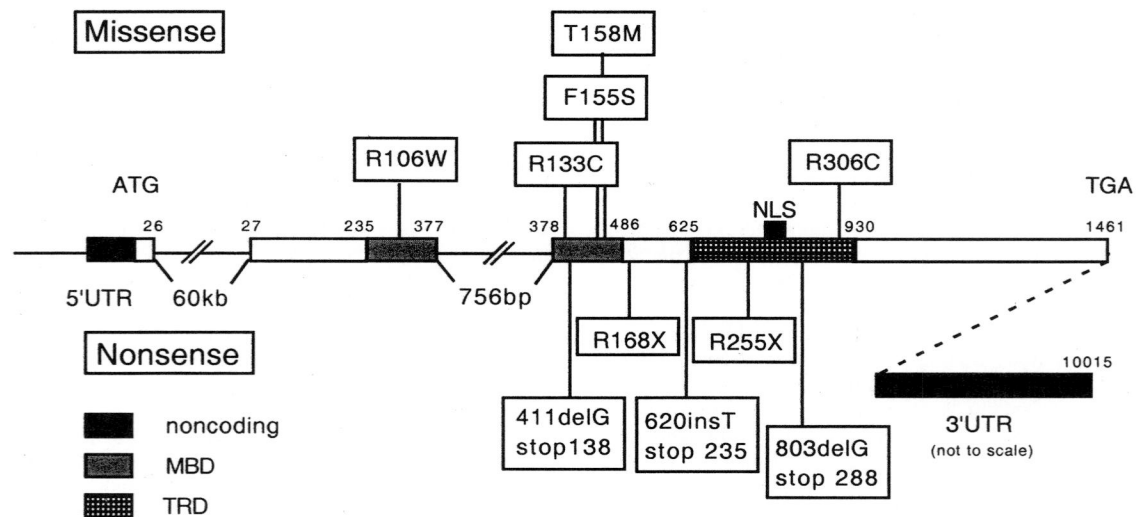

Fig. 255-3 *MECP2* mutations in Rett syndrome. The structure of the human *MECP2* gene is derived from the genomic sequence (GenBank AF030876). The functional domains were defined by Nan et al.[76,84] MBD = methyl-CpG binding domain; TRD = transcription repression domain; NLS = nuclear localization signal. (*Modified from Wan et al.*[28] *Used with permission.*)

heterozygous state in an RTT individual and in her unaffected sister, as well as in the hemizygous state in the normal father.[28] The substituted glutamic acid residue is outside of the functional domains and is not evolutionarily conserved. This amino acid variant was also present in a Caucasian family from the control population.[28] The 1189A (E397K) allele arises from a C → T transition at a CpG dinucleotide on the antisense strand. This coding SNP may be useful for association studies.

## Origin of *MECP2* Mutations

In the first 18 unrelated families studied, only 10 different mutations were identified because of the high frequency of independent *de novo* recurrences. Seven of the eight single nucleotide substitutions are C → T transitions at CpG sites caused by 5-methylation of cytosine by a methyltransferase and spontaneous deamination of 5-methylcytosine to thymine (Table 255-3). Because of this mechanism, CpG dinucleotides, although underrepresented in vertebrate genomes, are frequent sites of germline and somatic mutations.[78] C → T or G → A transitions (when the 5-methylcytosine deamination occurs on the antisense strand) constitute about 55 percent of single nucleotide substitutions in human genetic diseases overall,[79] but for some genes the frequencies are much higher. For example, almost all cases of achondroplasia are due to a G → A transition at a single CpG site in the *FGFR3* gene.[80,81] Because CpG hypermutability implies that the site is methylated in the germ line and thus prone to deamination, and male germ cells have high levels of CpG methylation while DNA in oocytes is markedly undermethylated, this type of mutation seems likely to occur preferentially during spermatogenesis. Indeed, an elevenfold male predominance was found for germ line CpG transition mutations in the factor IX gene causing hemophilia B.[82] Because the *MECP2* gene is not expressed in male germ cells, it is probably highly methylated because of its location on the condensed, hypermethylated X chromosome.

We thus predict that the majority of *MECP2* mutations leading to RTT stem from *de novo* 5mC → T deamination events in male germ cells. Once parental origin is established by haplotyping, we expect to find a preferential paternal origin for this type of mutation. A hypothesis of exclusively paternal origin of RTT mutations was previously proposed to explain the sex-limited occurrence,[56] but we have identified maternal mosaicism for *MECP2* mutations in two families. Of the 63 CpG dinucleotides in the *MECP2* coding sequence, 35 CpGs are potential mutational hotspots,[28] which are presented in a Table only in the online version of the reference (www.journals.uchicago.edu/AJHG/journal/issues/v65n6/991319/991319.html). Two of the five potential R → X mutations were already identified in RTT patients as recurrent nonsense mutations (Table 255-3). There are 9 possible amino acid substitutions in the MBD and 6 in the TRD; 4 of these 15 potential disease-causing mutations were identified among the first 18 families studied.[28] G → A transitions that are caused by C → T transitions at CpG sites on the antisense strand of the human *MECP2* gene could give rise to 9 different types of amino acid substitutions at 51 different codons. Many of these substitute similar amino acids such as val for ile or asp for asn. One of these predicted substitutions, E397K, was identified as a rare variant in the normal population.

The second most common type of *MECP2* mutation observed thus far involves a single nucleotide insertion or deletion. Often found at runs of the same nucleotide, these mutations are replication errors and their chance of occurrence goes up with increasing numbers of cell divisions. Paternal origin, associated with increased paternal age, is likely to correlate with this type of mutation.

## Consequences of *MECP2* Mutations

All frameshifts or stop codons leading to protein truncation involve the third and final exon. The mechanism of nonsense mediated-mRNA decay thus should not destroy the mRNA containing these mutations, and synthesis of truncated proteins is expected.[83] This prediction needs to be verified experimentally. The currently available antibodies[76] are not suitable for detecting truncated *MECP2* proteins in immunoblot analysis of total cellular proteins because of cross-reactivity with numerous other proteins.

Of all known *MECP2* mutations, L138X is the closest to a complete loss of function. The putative truncated product missing half of the MBD would be unable to bind methyl-CpG, because a truncated protein containing amino acids 1 to 156 did not bind a CpG-methylated oligonucleotide in a southwestern DNA binding assay.[84]

The other predicted truncated proteins have retained intact MBDs and may be able to bind 5-methyl CpG, but, lacking the TRD, they could not bind to Sin3A. Full-length MeCP2 is capable of binding to single methyl-CpG sites where it may protect up to 12 nucleotides.[84] Inactive promoters usually contain a higher density of CpGs than MeCP2 molecules can bind.[76] Therefore, smaller MBD-containing mutant protein molecules bound to multiple CpGs in CpG islands might accomplish partial silencing by steric hindrance of transcription factor binding or by recruiting a silencing complex by a TRD-independent mechanism. Because the nuclear localization signal (NLS) resides within the TRD,[85] truncated proteins lacking the NLS may remain largely in the cytoplasm. Indeed, the product of a transfected mutant construct containing the N-terminal 173 amino acids of the rat *MECP2* gene was located predominantly in the cytoplasm.[86] Because there are no consistent differences in the clinical presentations of the RTT individuals, truncating mutations may be functional null mutations.

The consequences of the missense mutations are less obvious, but their functional significance is suggested by the fact that they all replace highly conserved amino acids within one of the functional domains. Replacement of arginine by cysteine or substitutions of hydrophobic with polar amino acids may cause abnormal folding and instability of the polypeptide. The mutations in the MBD may reduce or abolish methyl-CpG binding, and those in the TRD may affect interactions with the proteins of the Sin3A/histone deacetylase silencing complex.

During organogenesis, *MECP2* is expressed throughout the embryo, and in postnatal life its expression remains ubiquitous, with highest levels in the hippocampus.[77] Although the RTT phenotype seems to primarily affect the brain, mutations in this gene would be expected to impair several organ systems. It is possible that functional redundancy of methyl-CpG-binding proteins protects other tissues. The function of a mutant MeCP2 might also be compensated for by related proteins that share a similar MBD but have no sequence similarity outside of this domain and no identifiable TRD (such as MBD2, MBD3, and MBD4[87]). MBD4 functions as a thymine glycosylase that corrects mismatches generated by C → T transitions, and MBD2 and MBD3 are components of the MeCP1 silencing complex.[88]

DNA methylation-dependent silencing is known to maintain X inactivation and gametic imprinting patterns. RTT patient cells are being studied for abnormalities in these epigenetic processes. Possible dysregulation of imprinted genes in RTT will need to be evaluated at the transcriptional or translational level, accompanied by histone acetylation studies at imprinted loci.[89] Because methyl-CpGs required for uniparental gene expression may also be located in introns of the expressed alleles, both over- and underexpression of imprinted genes may be anticipated as a consequence of *MECP2* mutations. Global assessments of gene expression levels using high-density microarrays representing all human genes will identify over- and underexpressed candidate genes for more detailed studies. Knowledge of the genes that are regulated by the MeCP2-containing protein complex is essential for understanding the pathogenetic steps that lead to neuronal dysfunction and for designing rational treatment strategies.

## Indications for *MECP2* Mutation Testing

The phenotypic spectrum associated with *MECP2* mutations far exceeds the criteria of RTT: it ranges from lethality to normality. A truncating *MECP2* mutation was identified in a hemizygous male with congenital encephalopathy who had multiple respiratory arrests and survived for 1 year.[27,62] That same mutation caused classic RTT in his sister and aunt, but only mild neurologic symptoms and learning problems in his mother, who had a favorably skewed X inactivation pattern. Another nonsense *MECP2* mutation was found in a completely normal woman who passed it on to three daughters who had RTT, and possibly to one son who died in the neonatal period.[59] These observations indicate that regardless of the type of mutation, the X chromosome inactivation pattern is the major determinant of the phenotype in females. It is likely that individuals who meet the diagnostic criteria for RTT[9] have more or less random XCI. Rare cases with skewed XCI might be severely affected and lack a period of normal early development if the mutant X is predominantly active. In cases in which the normal X is predominantly active, forme fruste[90] presentations would result. Extreme skewing can be present in women with nonspecific learning deficits for whom a diagnosis of RTT would not be considered. So far, such women have been identified only in the context of families with classically affected RTT individuals. Alternatively, incomplete clinical manifestations in females with milder variants of RTT could also be caused by missense mutations that have a more subtle effect on *MECP2* function. Indications for mutation testing extend beyond individuals with the clinical diagnosis of RTT to include women with partial phenotypes who do not meet diagnostic criteria for RTT, female infants with neurodevelopmental problems with or without a period of normal development, and males with unexplained encephalopathy in the neonatal period or death during infancy. The yield of *MECP2* mutations in these groups, predicted to be much lower than in classic RTT individuals, will need to be established by future studies.

## ADDENDUM

Since the submission of this chapter, more studies have been reported that significantly expand the number of known mutations and raise the percentage of Rett patients with documented *MECP2* mutations to as much as 80%. Interested readers are referred to the additional papers,[91–96] realizing that even more will be published by the time this chapter reaches press.

## REFERENCES

1. Rett A: *Über ein zerebral-atrophisches Syndrome bei Hyperammone-mie.* Vienna, Bruder Hollinek, 1966c.
2. Hagberg B: *Infantile autistic dementia and loss of hand use: A report of 16 Swedish girl patients.* Manchester England, Presented at the European Federation of Child Neurology Societies, 1980.
3. Hagberg B, Aicardi J, Dias K, Ramos O: A progressive syndrome of autism, dementia, ataxia, and loss of purposeful hand use in girls: Rett's syndrome: Report of 35 cases. *Ann Neurol* **14**:471, 1983.
4. Hagberg B: Rett's syndrome: Prevalence and impact on progressive severe mental retardation in girls. *Acta Paediatr Scand* **74**:405, 1985.
5. Hagberg B, Hagberg G: Rett syndrome: Epidemiology and geographical variability. *Eur Child Adolesc Psychiatry* **6**:5, 1997.
6. Al-Mateen M, Philippart M, Shields WD: Rett syndrome. A commonly overlooked progressive encephalopathy in girls. *Am J Dis Child* **140**:761, 1986.
7. Naidu S: Rett syndrome: A disorder affecting early brain growth [Published erratum appears in Ann Neurol 42(5):816, 1997]. *Ann Neurol* **42**:3, 1997.
8. FitzGerald PM, Jankovic J, Glaze DG, Schultz R, Percy AK: Extrapyramidal involvement in Rett's syndrome. *Neurology* **40**:293, 1990.
9. Trevathan E, et al: Diagnostic criteria for Rett syndrome. The Rett Syndrome Diagnostic Criteria Work Group. *Ann Neurol* **23**:425, 1988.
10. Hagberg B, Witt-Engerström I: Rett syndrome: A suggested staging system for describing impairment profile with increasing age towards adolescence. *Am J Med Genet* **24**:47, 1986a.
11. Nomura Y, Honda K, Segawa M: Pathophysiology of Rett syndrome. *Brain Dev* **9**:506, 1987.
12. Coleman M, Brubaker J, Hunter K, Smith G: Rett syndrome: A survey of North American patients. *J Ment Defic Res* **32**:117, 1988.
13. Witt-Engerström I: Age-related occurrence of signs and symptoms in the Rett syndrome. *Brain Dev* **14(Suppl)**:S11, 1992.
14. Glaze DG, Schultz RJ, Frost JD: Rett syndrome: characterization of seizures versus non-seizures. *Electroencephalogr Clin Neurophysiol* **106**:79, 1998.
15. Budden SS: Rett syndrome: Habilitation and management reviewed. *Eur Child Adolesc Psychiatry* **6**:103, 1997.
16. Motil KJ, Schultz RJ, Wong WW, Glaze DG: Increased energy expenditure associated with repetitive involuntary movement does not contribute to growth failure in girls with Rett syndrome. *J Pediatr* **132**:228, 1998.
17. Morton RE, Bonas R, Minford J, Kerr A, Ellis RE: Feeding ability in Rett syndrome. *Dev Med Child Neurol* **39**:331, 1997.
18. Motil KJ, Schultz RJ, Browning K, Trautwein L, Glaze DG: Oropharyngeal dysfunction and gastroesophageal dysmotility are present in girls and women with Rett syndrome. *J Pediatr Gastroenterol Nutr* **29**:31, 1999.
19. Kerr AM, Julu PO: Recent insights into hyperventilation from the study of Rett syndrome. *Arch Dis Child* **80**:384, 1999.
20. Sekul EA, Moak JP, Schultz RJ, Glaze DG, Dunn JK, Percy AK: Electrocardiographic findings in Rett syndrome: An explanation for sudden death? *J Pediatr* **125**:80, 1994.
21. Guideri F, Acampa M, Hayek G, Zappella M, Di Perri T: Reduced heart rate variability in patients affected with Rett syndrome. A possible explanation for sudden death. *Neuropediatrics* **30**:146, 1999.
22. Hagberg BA: Rett syndrome: Clinical peculiarities, diagnostic approach, and possible cause. *Pediatr Neurol* **5**:75, 1989.
23. Zappella M, Gillberg C, Ehlers S: The preserved speech variant: A subgroup of the Rett complex: A clinical report of 30 cases. *J Autism Dev Disord* **28**:519, 1998.
24. Philippart M: The Rett syndrome in males. *Brain Dev* **12**:33, 1990.
25. Christen HJ, Hanefeld F: Male Rett variant. *Neuropediatrics* **26**:81, 1995.
26. Salomao Schwartzman J, Zatz M, dos Reis Vasquez L, Ribeiro Gomes R, Koiffmann CP, Fridman C, Guimaraes Otto P: Rett syndrome in a boy with a 47,XXY karyotype. *Am J Hum Genet* **64**:1781, 1999.
27. Schanen NC, Kurczynski TW, Brunelle D, Woodcock MM, Dure LSt, Percy AK: Neonatal encephalopathy in two boys in families with recurrent Rett syndrome. *J Child Neurol* **13**:229, 1998b.
28. Wan M, Lee SS, Zhang X, Houwink-Manville I, Song HR, Amir RE, Budden S, et al: Rett Syndrome and beyond: Recurrent spontaneous and familial MECP2 mutations at CpG hotspots. *Am J Hum Genet* **65**:1520, 1999.
29. Percy AK: Neurobiology and neurochemistry of Rett syndrome. *Eur Child Adolesc Psychiatry* **6**:80, 1997.
30. Nihei K, Naitoh H: Cranial computed tomographic and magnetic resonance imaging studies on the Rett syndrome. *Brain Dev* **12**:101, 1990.
31. Nielsen JB, Friberg L, Lou H, Lassen NA, Sam IL: Immature pattern of brain activity in Rett syndrome. *Arch Neurol* **47**:982, 1990.
32. Oldfors A, Sourander P, Armstrong DL, Percy AK, Witt-Engerström I, Hagberg BA: Rett syndrome: Cerebellar pathology. *Pediatr Neurol* **6**:310, 1990.
33. Armstrong D, Dunn JK, Antalffy B, Trivedi R: Selective dendritic alterations in the cortex of Rett syndrome. *J Neuropathol Exp Neurol* **54**:195, 1995.
34. Jellinger K, Seitelberger F: Neuropathology of Rett syndrome. *Am J Med Genet Suppl* **1**:259, 1986.
35. Bauman ML, Kemper TL, Arin DM: Microscopic observations of the brain in Rett syndrome. *Neuropediatrics* **26**:105, 1995.
36. Belichenko PV, Oldfors A, Hagberg B, Dahlstrom A: Rett syndrome: 3-D confocal microscopy of cortical pyramidal dendrites and afferents. *Neuroreport* **5**:1509, 1994.
37. Belichenko PV, Dahlstrom A: Studies on the 3-dimensional architecture of dendritic spines and varicosities in human cortex by confocal laser scanning microscopy and Lucifer yellow microinjections. *J Neurosci Methods* **57**:55, 1995.
38. Kerr AM, Armstrong DD, Prescott RJ, Doyle D, Kearney DL: Rett syndrome: Analysis of deaths in the British survey. *Eur Child Adolesc Psychiatry* **6**:71, 1997.
39. Blue ME, Naidu S, Johnston MV: Altered development of glutamate and GABA receptors in the basal ganglia of girls with Rett syndrome. *Exp Neurol* **156**:345, 1999.

40. Ellaway C, Williams K, Leonard H, Higgins G, Wilcken B, Christodoulou J: Rett syndrome: randomized controlled trial of L-carnitine. *J Child Neurol* **14**:162, 1999.
41. Percy AK, Glaze DG, Schultz RJ, Zoghbi HY, Williamson D, Frost JD Jr, Jankovic JJ, et al: Rett syndrome: Controlled study of an oral opiate antagonist, naltrexone. *Ann Neurol* **35**:464, 1994.
42. Budden SS, Myer EC, Butler IJ: Cerebrospinal fluid studies in the Rett syndrome: Biogenic amines and beta-endorphins. *Brain Dev* **12**:81, 1990.
43. Nielsen JB, Bach FW, Buchholt J, Lou H: Cerebrospinal fluid beta-endorphin in Rett syndrome. *Dev Med Child Neurol* **33**:406, 1991.
44. Martinho PS, Otto PG, Kok F, Diament A, Marques-Dias MJ, Gonzalez CH: In search of a genetic basis for the Rett syndrome. *Hum Genet* **86**:131, 1990.
45. Migeon BR, Dunn MA, Thomas G, Schmeckpeper BJ, Naidu S: Studies of X inactivation and isodisomy in twins provide further evidence that the X chromosome is not involved in Rett syndrome. *Am J Hum Genet* **56**:647, 1995.
46. Zoghbi H: Genetic aspects of Rett syndrome. *J Child Neurol* **3**:S76, 1988.
47. Rivkin MJ, Ye Z, Mannheim GB, Darras BT: A search for X-chromosome uniparental disomy and DNA rearrangements in the Rett syndrome. *Brain Dev* **14**:273, 1992.
48. Webb T, Watkiss E, Woods CG: Neither uniparental disomy nor skewed X-inactivation explains Rett syndrome. *Clin Genet* **44**:236, 1993.
49. Brown CJ, Carrel L, Willard HF: Expression of genes from the human active and inactive X chromosomes. *Am J Hum Genet* **60**:1333, 1997.
50. Ellis D, Malcolm S: Proteolipid protein gene dosage effect in Pelizaeus-Merzbacher disease. *Nat Genet* **6**:333, 1994.
51. Swain A, Narvaez V, Burgoyne P, Camerino G, Lovell-Badge R: Dax1 antagonizes Sry action in mammalian sex determination. *Nature* **391**:761, 1998.
52. Akesson H-O, Hagberg B, Wahlstrom J, Witt-Engerström I: Rett syndrome: Search for gene sources. *Am J Med Genet* **42**:104, 1992.
53. Hofferbert S, Schanen NC, Budden SS, Francke U: Is Rett syndrome caused by a triplet repeat expansion? *Neuropediatrics* **28**:179, 1997a.
54. Lupski JR: Genomic disorders: structural features of the genome can lead to DNA rearrangements and human disease traits. *Trends Genet* **14**:417, 1998.
55. Fan F, Amir RD, Zhang S, Dahle EJ, Zoghbi H, Francke U: Search for X-chromosomal microdeletions in Rett syndrome. *Am J Hum Genet* **65**:1648, 1999.
56. Thomas GH: High male:female ratio of germ-line mutations: An alternative explanation for postulated gestational lethality in males in X-linked dominant disorders. *Am J Hum Genet* **58**:1364, 1996.
57. Engerström IW, Forslund M: Mother and daughter with Rett syndrome. *Dev Med Child Neurol* **34**:1022, 1992.
58. Zoghbi HY, Percy AK, Schultz RJ, Fill C: Patterns of X chromosome inactivation in the Rett syndrome. *Brain Dev* **12**:131, 1990.
59. Sirianni N, Naidu S, Pereira J, Pillotto RF, Hoffman EP: Rett syndrome: Confirmation of X-linked dominant inheritance, and localization of the gene to Xq28. *Am J Hum Genet* **63**:1552, 1998.
60. Schanen NC, Dahle EJ, Capozzoli F, Holm VA, Zoghbi HY, Francke U: A new Rett syndrome family consistent with X-linked inheritance expands the X chromosome exclusion map. *Am J Hum Genet* **61**:634, 1997.
61. Anvret M, Wahlstrom J, Skogsberg P, Hagberg B: Segregation analysis of the X-chromosome in a family with Rett syndrome in two generations. *Am J Med Genet* **37**:31, 1990.
62. Schanen C, Francke U: A severely affected male born into a Rett syndrome kindred supports X-linked inheritance and allows extension of the exclusion map. *Am J Hum Genet* **63**:267, 1998a.
63. Webb T, Clarke A, Hanefeld F, Pereira JL, Rosenbloom L, Woods CG: Linkage analysis in Rett syndrome families suggests that there may be a critical region at Xq28. *J Med Genet* **35**:997, 1998.
64. Archidiacono N, Lerone M, Rocchi M, Anvret M, Ozcelik T, Francke U, Romeo G: Rett syndrome: Exclusion mapping following the hypothesis of germinal mosaicism for new X-linked mutations. *Hum Genet* **86**:604, 1991.
65. Ellison KA, Fill CP, Terwilliger J, DeGennaro LJ, Martin-Gallardo A, Anvret M, Percy AK, et al: Examination of X chromosome markers in Rett syndrome: Exclusion mapping with a novel variation on multilocus linkage analysis. *Am J Hum Genet* **50**:278, 1992.
66. Curtis AR, Headland S, Lindsay S, Thomas NS, Boye E, Kamakari S, Roustan P, et al: X chromosome linkage studies in familial Rett syndrome. *Hum Genet* **90**:551, 1993.
67. D'Esposito M, Quaderi NA, Ciccodicola A, Bruni P, Esposito T, D'Urso M, Brown SD: Isolation, physical mapping, and northern analysis of the X-linked human gene encoding methyl CpG-binding protein, MECP2. *Mamm Genome* **7**:533, 1996.
68. Vilain A, Apiou F, Vogt N, Dutrillaux B, Malfoy B: Assignment of the gene for methyl-CpG-binding protein 2 (MECP2) to human chromosome band Xq28 by *in situ* hybridization. *Cytogenet Cell Genet* **74**:293, 1996.
69. Amir RE, Van den Veyver IB, Wan M, Tran CQ, Francke U, Zoghbi HY: Rett syndrome is caused by mutations in X-linked MECP2, encoding methyl-CpG-binding protein 2. *Nat Genet* **23**:185, 1999.
70. Jones PL, Veenstra GJ, Wade PA, Vermaak D, Kass SU, Landsberger N, Strouboulis J, et al: Methylated DNA and MeCP2 recruit histone deacetylase to repress transcription. *Nat Genet* **19**:187, 1998.
71. Nan X, Ng HH, Johnson CA, Laherty CD, Turner BM, Eisenman RN, Bird A: Transcriptional repression by the methyl-CpG-binding protein MeCP2 involves a histone deacetylase complex. *Nature* **393**:386, 1998a.
72. Ng HH, Bird A: DNA methylation and chromatin modification. *Curr Opin Genet Dev* **9**:158, 1999.
73. Bestor TH, Verdine GL: DNA methyltransferases. *Curr Opin Cell Biol* **6**:380, 1994.
74. Li E, Bestor TH, Jaenisch R: Targeted mutation of the DNA methyltransferase gene results in embryonic lethality. *Cell* **69**:915, 1992.
75. Tate P, Skarnes W, Bird A: The methyl-CpG binding protein MeCP2 is essential for embryonic development in the mouse. *Nat Genet* **12**:205, 1996.
76. Nan X, Campoy FJ, Bird A: MeCP2 is a transcriptional repressor with abundant binding sites in genomic chromatin. *Cell* **88**:471, 1997.
77. Coy JF, Sedlacek Z, Bachner D, Delius H, Poustka A: A complex pattern of evolutionary conservation and alternative polyadenylation within the long 3'-untranslated region of the methyl-CpG-binding protein 2 gene (MeCP2) suggests a regulatory role in gene expression. *Hum Mol Genet* **8**:1253, 1999.
78. Rideout WMd, Coetzee GA, Olumi AF, Jones PA: 5-Methylcytosine as an endogenous mutagen in the human LDL receptor and p53 genes. *Science* **249**:1288, 1990.
79. Krawczak M, Cooper DN: Single base-pair substitutions in pathology and evolution: Two sides to the same coin. *Hum Mutat* **8**:23, 1996.
80. Bellus GA, Hefferon TW, Ortiz de Luna RI, Hecht JT, Horton WA, Machado M, Kaitila I, et al: Achondroplasia is defined by recurrent G380R mutations of FGFR3. *Am J Hum Genet* **56**:368, 1995.
81. Wilkin DJ, Szabo JK, Cameron R, Henderson S, Bellus GA, Mack ML, Kaitila I, et al: Mutations in fibroblast growth-factor receptor 3 in sporadic cases of achondroplasia occur exclusively on the paternally derived chromosome. *Am J Hum Genet* **63**:711, 1998.
82. Ketterling RP, Vielhaber E, Bottema CD, Schaid DJ, Cohen MP, Sexauer CL, Sommer SS: Germ-line origins of mutation in families with hemophilia B: The sex ratio varies with the type of mutation. *Am J Hum Genet* **52**:152, 1993.
83. Carter MS, Li S, Wilkinson MF: A splicing-dependent regulatory mechanism that detects translation signals. *EMBO J* **15**:5965, 1996.
84. Nan X, Meehan RR, Bird A: Dissection of the methyl-CpG binding domain from the chromosomal protein MeCP2. *Nucleic Acids Res* **21**:4886, 1993.
85. Lewis JD, Meehan RR, Henzel WJ, Maurer-Fogy I, Jeppesen P, Klein F, Bird A: Purification, sequence, and cellular localization of a novel chromosomal protein that binds to methylated DNA. *Cell* **69**:905, 1992.
86. Kudo S: Methyl-CpG-binding protein MeCP2 represses Sp1-activated transcription of the human leukosialin gene when the promoter is methylated. *Mol Cell Biol* **18**:5492, 1998.
87. Hendrich B, Abbott C, McQueen H, Chambers D, Cross S, Bird A: Genomic structure and chromosomal mapping of the murine and human mbd1, mbd2, mbd3, and mbd4 genes. *Mamm Genome* **10**:906, 1999.
88. Bird AP, Wolffe AP: Methylation-induced repression — Belts, braces, and chromatin. *Cell* **99**:451, 1999.
89. Coffee B, Zhang F, Warren ST, Reines D: Acetylated histones are associated with FMR1 in normal but not fragile X-syndrome cells [Published erratum appears in *Nat Genet* 22(2):209, 1999]. *Nat Genet* **22**:98, 1999.
90. Hagberg B: Clinical delineation of Rett syndrome variants. *Neuropediatrics* **26**:62, 1995.

91. Amir RE, Van den Veyver IB, Schultz R, Malicki DM, Tran CQ, Dahle JE, Philippi A, Timar L, Percy AK, Motil KJ, Lichtarge O, O'Brian Smith E, Glaze DG, Zoghbi HY: Influence of Mutation Type and X Chromosome Inactivation on Rett Syndrome Phenotypes. *Ann Neurol* **47**:670, 2000.

92. Bienvenu T, Carrie A, de Roux N, Vinet MC, Jonveaux P, Couvert P, Villard L, Arzimanoglou A, Beldjord C, Fontes M, Tardieu M, Chelly J: MECP2 mutations account for most cases of typical forms of Rett syndrome. *Hum Mol Genet* **9**:1377, 2000

93. Cheadle JP, Gill H, Glemong N, Maynard J, Kerr A, Leonard H, Krawczak M, Cooper DN, Lynch S, Thomas N, Hughes H, Hulten M, Ravine D, Sampson JR, Clarke A: Long-read sequence analysos of the MECP2 gene in Rett syndrome patients: correlation of disease severity with mutation type and location. *Hum Mol Genet* **9**:1119, 2000.

94. Huppke P, Laccone F, Kramer N, Engel W, Hanefeld F: Rett syndrome: analysis of MECP2 and clinical characterization of 31 patients. *Hum Mol Genet* **9**:1369, 2000.

95. Kim SJ, Cook EH Jr: Novel de novo nonsense mutation of MECP2 in a patient with Rett syndrome. *Hum Mutat* **15**:382, 2000

96. Xiang F, Buervenich S, Nicolao P, Bailey M, Zhang Z, Anvret M: Mutation screening in Rett syndrome patients. *J Med Genet* **37**:250, 2000.

## STANDARD ABBREVIATIONS

| Abbreviation | Name | Abbreviation | Name |
|---|---|---|---|
| ACTH | corticotropin (adrenocorticotropin, adrenocorticotropic hormone) | ER | endoplasmic reticulum |
| ADA | adenosine deaminase | ES cells | embryonic stem cells |
| AdoMet | s-adenosylmethionine | FAD and | flavin-adenine dinucleotide and its |
| Ag | antigen | $FADH_2$ | fully reduced form |
| AIDS | acquired immunodeficiency syndrome | FISH | fluorescence *in situ* hybridization |
| ALT | alanine aminotransferase | FITC | fluorescein isothiocyanate |
| AMP, ADP, and ATP* | adenosine 5′-mono-, di-, and triphosphates | FMN | riboflavin 5′-phosphate |
| | | G, $G_i$, $G_s$ | guanine nucleotide binding protein, inhibitory form, stimulatory form |
| AP1, AP2 | activator protein 1, 2; transcription factors | G-6-PD | glucose 6-phosphate dehydrogenase |
| apo A-I | apolipoprotein A-I | GABA | $\gamma$-aminobutyric acid |
| apo A-II | apolipoprotein A-II | GC | gas chromatography |
| apo A-III | apolipoprotein A-III | GC/MS | gas chromatography/mass spectroscopy |
| apo B | apolipoprotein B | GERL | Golgi endoplasmic reticulum-like |
| apo C-I | apolipoprotein C-I | GFR | glomerular filtration rate |
| apo C-II | apolipoprotein C-II | GMP, GDP, and GTP* | guanosine 5′-mono-, di-, and triphosphates |
| apo C-III | apolipoprotein C-III | | |
| apo D | apolipoprotein D | GSH and GSSG | glutathione and its oxidized form |
| apo E | apolipoprotein E | Hb, HbCO, $HbO_2$ | hemoglobin, carbon monoxide hemoglobin, oxyhemoglobin |
| APRT | adenine phosphoribosyltransferase | | |
| ASO | allele-specific oligonucleotide | HDL | high density lipoprotein |
| AST | aspartate aminotransferase | HEPES | 4-(2-hydroxyethyl)-1-piperazine ethanesulfonic acid |
| ATPase | adenosine triphosphate | | |
| $\alpha_1$AT | $\alpha_1$-antitrypsin | Hep G2 | hepatocellular carcinoma human cell line |
| B cell | B lymphocyte | HIV | human immunodeficiency virus |
| BAC | bacterial artificial chromosome | HLA | human leukocyte antigens |
| cAMP, cGMP, etc. | cyclic AMP (adenosine 3′: 5′-monophosphate), etc. | HMG-CoA | 3-hydroxy-3-methylglutaryl-coenzyme A |
| | | HPLC | high performance (or pressure) liquid chromatography |
| CAT | chloramphenicol acetyltransferase | | |
| CD | cluster of differentiation or cluster determinant (e.g., CD34) | HPRT | hypoxanthine-guanine phosphoribosyltransferase |
| cDNA | complementary DNA | IDDM | insulin-dependent diabetes mellitus |
| CHO cells | Chinese hamster ovary cells | IFN | interferon |
| CoA (or CoASH) | coenzyme A | Ig | immunoglobulin |
| CoASAc | acetyl coenzyme A | IgA | gamma A immunoglobulin |
| cM | centimorgan | IgG | gamma G immunoglobulin |
| Cm-cellulose | O-(carboxymethyl)cellulose | IgM | gamma M immunoglobulin |
| CMP, CDP, and CTP* | cytidine 5′-mono-, di-, and triphosphates | IL | interleukin, including IL-1, IL-2, etc. |
| | | IM or i.m. | intramuscular |
| CNS | central nervous system | IMP, IDP, and ITP* | inosine 5′-mono-, di, and triphosphates |
| COS cells | CV-I origin, SV40; cells widely used for transfection studies | | |
| | | LDH | lactate dehydrogenase |
| CPK | creatine phosphokinase | LDL | low density lipoproteins |
| CRM, CRM+, CRM− | cross-reacting material, CRM positive, CRM negative | LINE | long interspersed repeat element |
| | | lod | logarithm of the odds |
| CT | computerized tomography | MCH | erythrocyte mean corpuscular hemoglobin |
| CVS | chorionic villus sampling | MCHC | erythrocyte mean corpuscular hemoglobin concentration |
| DEAE-cellulose | O-(diethylaminoethyl)cellulose | | |
| DNA | deoxyribonucleic acid | MCV | erythrocyte mean corpuscular volume |
| DNase | deoxyribonuclease | MHC | histocompatibility complex |
| DOPA | 3,4-dihydroxyphenylalanine | MPS | mucopolysaccharide or mucopolysaccharidosis |
| DPN, DPN+, DPNH+ | diphosphopyridine nucleotide and its oxidized and reduced forms | | |
| | | MRI | magnetic resonance imaging |
| DPT | diphtheria, pertussis, tetanus vaccine | mRNA | messenger RNA |
| dTMP, dTDP, and dTTP* | thymidine 5′-mono-, di-, and triphosphates | MS | mass spectrometry |
| | | mtDNA, mtRNA | mitochondrial DNA, RNA |
| DTT | dithiothreitol | | |
| EBV | Epstein-Barr virus | *Myc* | oncogene homologous to avian myelocytomatosis virus including c-*myc*, N-*myc*, and L-*myc* |
| EDTA | ethylenediaminetetraacetate | | |
| EEG | electroencephalogram | | |
| EGF | epidermal growth factor | NAD, NAD+, and NADH† | nicotinamide adenine dinucleotide and its oxidized and reduced forms |
| EGTA | [ethylenebis(oxyethylenenitrilo)] tetraacetic acid | NADP, NADP+, and NADPH† | nicotinamide adenine dinucleotide phosphate and its oxidized and reduced forms |
| EKG | electrocardiogram | | |
| ELISA | enzyme-linked immunosorbent assay | | |
| EM | electron microscopy or microscopic | NIDDM | non-insulin-dependent diabetes mellitus |

*(Continues)*

| Abbreviation | Name | Abbreviation | Name |
|---|---|---|---|
| NK cells | natural killer cells | SE | standard error |
| NMN | nicotinamide mononucleotide | SEM | standard error of mean |
| NMR | nuclear magnetic resonance | SER | smooth endoplasmic reticulum |
| p | probability | SH1, SH2, SH3 | Src homology domains 1, 2, 3 |
| $p_i$ | inorganic phosphate | | |
| PAC | P1-derived artificial chromosome | SNP | single nucleotide polymorphism |
| PAS | periodic acid Schiff | *src* | oncogene homologous to Rous sarcoma virus |
| PCR | polymerase chain reaction | SSCP | single strand conformational polymorphism |
| PEG | polyethylene glycol | STR | short tandem repeat |
| PFGE | pulsed-field gel electrophoresis | SV40 | Simian virus 40 |
| PKA | protein kinase A | $T_3$ | triiodothyronine |
| PKC | protein kinase C | $T_4$ | thyroxine |
| PKU | phenylketonuria | T cell | T lymphocyte |
| $PP_i$ | inorganic pyrophosphate | TMP, TDP, and TTP* | ribosylthymine 5′-mono-, di-, and triphosphates |
| PP-ribose-P | phosphoribosylpyrophosphate | | |
| *ras* | oncogenes homologous to sarcoma retroviruses including HRAS, KRAS, and NRAS, H-*ras*, K-*ras*, and N-*ras* | TNF | tumor necrosis factor (e.g. TNF-1) |
| | | TPN, TPN$^+$, TPNH$^†$ | triphosphopyridine nucleotide and its oxidized and reduced forms |
| RER | rough endoplasmic reticulum | Tris | tris(hydroxymethyl)aminomethane |
| RFLP | restriction fragment length polymorphism | tRNA | transfer RNA |
| RIA | radioimmunoassay | UDP-Gal | uridine diphosphogalactose |
| rRNA | ribosomal RNA | UDP-Glc | uridine diphosphoglucose |
| RNase | ribonuclease | UMP, UDP, and UTP* | uridine 5′-mono-, di-, and triphosphates |
| RT-PCR | reverse transcription-polymerase chain reaction | | |
| | | UV | ultraviolet light |
| SD | standard deviation | VLDL | very low density lipoprotein |
| SDS | sodium dodecyl sulfate | VNTR | variable number tandem repeat |
| SDS-PAGE | sodium dodecyl sulfate polyacrylamide gel electrophoresis | YAC | yeast artificial chromosome |

*The d prefix may be used to represent the corresponding deoxyribonucleoside phosphates, e.g., dADP.
†Note that DPN = NAD and TPN = NADP.

## AMINO ACID SYMBOLS

| Name | Symbols | | Name | Symbols | |
|---|---|---|---|---|---|
| alanine | Ala | A | leucine | Leu | L |
| arginine | Arg | R | lysine | Lys | K |
| asparagine | Asn | N | methionine | Met | M |
| aspartic acid | Asp | D | phenylalanine | Phe | F |
| cysteine | Cys | C | proline | Pro | P |
| glutamic acid | Glu | E | serine | Ser | S |
| glutamine | Gln | Q | threonine | Thr | T |
| glycine | Gly | G | tryptophan | Trp | W |
| histidine | His | H | tyrosine | Tyr | Y |
| isoleucine | Ile | I | valine | Val | V |

## CARBOHYDRATE SYMBOLS

| Name | Symbols | Name | Symbols |
|---|---|---|---|
| fructose | Fru | N-acetylgalactosamine | GalNAc |
| fucose | Fuc | N-acetylglucosamine | GlcNAc |
| galactose | Gal | N-acetylneuraminic acid | NeuAc |
| glucosamine | GlcN | ribose | Rib |
| glucose | Glc | sialic acid | Sia |
| glucuronic acid | GlcA | xylose | Xyl |
| mannose | Man | | |

# INDEX

Page numbers followed by an "f" indicate figures; numbers followed by a "t" indicate tables.

molecular biology, 4795
molecular genetics, 4796
pathophysiology, 4793f, 4795–4796
C4 protein, 4787, 4790–4791
C4a protein, 4787
C4b-binding protein deficiency, 4792t, 4802
  clinical expression, 4802
  molecular biology, 4802
  pathophysiology, 4802
C4b protein, 4787
C4b2a protein, 4787
C4bp protein, 4791
C4c protein, 4787
C4d protein, 4787
C5 deficiency, 79t, 4792–4793, 4792t, 4798
  animal models, 4798
  clinical expression, 4798
  molecular biology, 4798
  molecular genetics, 4798
  pathophysiology, 4798
C5 protein, 4787–4788, 4790
  activation, 4789
C6 deficiency, 66t, 4792–4793, 4792t, 4798–
    4799
  animal models, 4799
  clinical expression, 4798
  molecular biology, 4798
  molecular genetics, 4798–4799
  pathophysiology, 4798
C6 protein, 4788, 4790–4791
  activation, 4789
C7 deficiency, 66t, 4792–4793, 4792t, 4799
  C7 subtotal deficiency, 4799
  clinical expression, 4799
  molecular biology, 4799
  molecular genetics, 4799
  pathophysiology, 4799
C7 protein, 4788, 4790–4791
  activation, 4789
C8 binding protein, 4789
C8 deficiency, 4792–4793, 4792t, 4799
  clinical expression, 4799, 4799f
  molecular biology, 4799
  molecular genetics, 4799
  pathophysiology, 4799
  type I, 53t
  type II, 53t
C8 protein, 4788, 4790–4791
  activation, 4789
C9 deficiency, 66t, 4792, 4792t, 4794, 4800
  clinical expression, 4800
  molecular biology, 4800
  molecular genetics, 4800
  pathophysiology, 4800
C9 protein, 4788, 4790
  activation, 4789
*CACNA1A* gene, 5229–5230, 5231t, 5234.
    *See also* Spinocerebellar ataxia, type 6
*CACNA1A1* gene, 5743, 5747
*CAD* gene, 2665
Cadherins, 657, 6043
Cadmium, cause of Fanconi syndrome, 5025–
    5026
*Caenorhabditis elegans:*
  apoptosis, 632–633, 634f
  CHX10 protein, 6007
  genome analysis, 278
Café-au-lait spots, in neurofibromatosis 1, 878,
    878t, 879f, 890
Caffeine-halothane contracture test, 230–232,
    231f
  caffeine specific concentration, 231
CAG repeat expansion:
  AR gene in spinobulbar muscular atrophy,
    4147–4154

dentatorubropallidolusian atrophy, 5820
Huntington disease, 5677–5694
somatic stability in spinobulbar muscular
    atrophy, 4151
spinocerebellar ataxias, 5741–5754
CAH. *See* Congenital adrenal hyperplasia
Cajal body, 5836
CAK. *See* Cdk-activating kinase
Calbindin, 4226
Calciferol(s), 4223–4236
  history, 4223
  metabolism, 4224–4225
  normal actions, 4225–4226
  physiology, 4224–4226
  plasma and body pools, 4225t
  transcalciferin as binder, 4225
  turnover and requirements, 4225
Calciferol deficiency, 4227, 4228t, 4235
  clinical presentation, 4228
  generalized resistance to 1α,25-
    dihydroxyvitamin D, 4230–4235
  nomenclature, 4227
  pathophysiology, 4228–4229
  radiographic features, 4228
  response to vitamin D therapy, 4228
Calciferol excess, 4235–4236
Calcific periarthritis, 5317
Calcification, cerebral, in carbonic anhydrase II
    deficiency syndrome, 5331–5340
Calciosome, 460
Calcitonin, 4224
Calcium:
  calciferols, 4223–4236
  control of peptide release from β-cells, 1409–
    1410, 1410f
  effect on red cell membrane structure, 4679
  in ER-to-Golgi proteins transport, 459
  homeostasis, 5041
  intestinal transport, 4226
  metabolism, control by PTH and vitamin D,
    4206, 4206f
  in muscle contraction, 228
  regulation of proximal renal tubular transport,
    4989
Calcium channel:
  L-type, 5920
  regulation of nitric oxide synthase, 4283,
    4283f
  structure, 5225, 5226f
  voltage-gated, 5224
Calcium channel defect. *See also*
    Spinocerebellar ataxia, type 6
  in episodic ataxia, 5228–5230
  in hypokalemic periodic paralysis, 5227–
    5228, 5228t
  mouse models, 5229, 5816
Calcium deficiency, 4235
Calcium deprivation, 5041
Calcium-induced calcium release, 228
Calcium oxalate. *See also* Primary hyperoxaluria
  crystallization, 3324
  renal deposition in primary hyperoxaluria,
    3354
  solubilization, 3354
Calcium sensing receptor, mutation database,
    115t
Calcium supplementation, for
    pseudohypoparathyroidism, 4217
Caldesmon, red cell membrane, 4678
Calf hypertrophy, 5775
Callipyge locus, sheep, 3987
Calmodulin, 228, 5911
  effect on red cell membrane structure, 4679
  in phosphorylase kinase, 1525
Calnexin, 455

Caloric restriction, effect on life span, 219–
    220
Calpain-3 defect. *See also* Limb-girdle muscular
    dystrophy
  in limb-girdle muscular dystrophy 2A, 5504t,
    5505
Calreticulin, 4757
CAM(F)AK, 697
cAMP. *See* Cyclic AMP
cAMP-dependent protein kinase, 1524f, 1526,
    1677–1678. *See also* Protein kinase A
5α-Campestanol, 2979
Campesterol, 2965. *See also* Phytosterolemia;
    Plant sterols
Campomelic dysplasia (CD), 6267–6276, 6287t.
    *See also* SOX9 gene
  clinical manifestations, 6268–6269, 6268f,
    6269t
  definition of the syndrome, 6267–6268
  diagnosis, 6268–6269, 6268f, 6269t
  etiology, 6270
  genetics, 6270
  historical aspects, 6267–6268
  incidence, 6268
  molecular genetics, 6270
  mutation/phenotype correlations, 6271
  prenatal diagnosis, 6269–6270
  prognosis, 6270
Campomelic dysplasia (CD) with autosomal sex
    reversal, 98t, 1217
Camptodactyly-arthropathy-coxa vara-
    pericarditis syndrome, 56t
Camurati-Engelmann disease, 101t
Canale-Smith syndrome. *See* Autoimmune
    lymphoproliferative syndrome
Canavan disease. *See* Aspartoacylase deficiency
Canavanine resistance, 1929–1930
Cancer. *See also specific types and sites of
    cancer*
  age at onset, 147
  age-specific rates, 216
  aneuploidy in cancer cells, 611
  α1-antitrypsin deficiency and, 5575
  apoptosis, 631–639
  Bloom syndrome and, 737, 738t, 748
  CBP protein and, 6176
  chromosomal alterations, 529t, 575–590, 576t
  chromosomal instability, 611
  compared to other genetic diseases, 521, 522f
  cystic fibrosis and, 5134
  DNA alterations:
    amplifications, 523
    chromosome number changes, 522
    chromosome translocation, 523
    exogenous sequences, 523
    subtle alterations, 522
  in Fanconi anemia, 757, 758t
  Fanconi syndrome in, 5026
  Gaucher disease and, 3639
  gene amplification, 597–606
  gene therapy for, 185–186
  genetic testing. *See* Cancer gene tests
  genome imprinting, 525–533
    imprinted genes on 11p15, 530–531, 530f,
      530t
    loss of imprinting, 530–531, 530f, 530t
  in hepatorenal tyrosinemia, 1785–1786
  in hereditary nonpolyposis colorectal cancer,
    770t, 778, 778f
  HLA associations, 329
  Internet resources, 1070t
  invasive disease, 523
  in Li-Fraumeni syndrome, 849–859
  logic of disease, 147
  metastatic disease, 523

Fibrinoligase. *See* Factor XIII
Fibrinolysis inhibitors, abnormal, 4512–4513
Fibrinolytic system:
    cellular receptors, 4509
    disorders, 4505–4513
    genes, 4506–4507
    historical aspects, 4505
    lipoprotein(a) in, 2754f, 2760–2761
    plasminogen activation, 4505–4506, 4506f
    proteins, 4506–4507
    therapeutic modulation, 4513
Fibrinopeptides, removal from fibrinogen, 4347, 4348f
Fibroblast(s):
    in D-bifunctional protein deficiency, 3236
    cholesterol efflux in Tangier disease, 2947
    skin, transport of imino acids and glycine in iminoglycinuria, 4977
Fibroblast growth factor (FGF), 652
    in breast cancer, 1019
    cranial suture biology, 6138–6139, 6139f
    in multiple endocrine neoplasia type 1, 951
    signaling, proteoglycans and, 5197
Fibroblast growth factor receptor (FGFR), 5385–5386, 5386f, 6118. *See also* *FGFR* genes
    cranial suture biology, 6138–6139, 6139f
    function, 6131
    structure, 6131, 6131f–6132f
Fibroblast growth factor receptor (FGFR) defects. *See* Achondroplasia
Fibrodysplasia ossificans progressiva, 65t, 102t
Fibromatosis, gingival, 58t
Fibronectin, 4349
    crosslinking, 4354
Fibronectin defect, 5271
Fibrosing colonopathy, in cystic fibrosis, 5130, 5169
Fibrosis, in chronic iron toxicity, 3143
Fibrosis of extraocular muscles, 84t, 87t, 95t
*FIC1* gene, 3090
FIGLU. *See* Formiminoglutamic acid
Filaggrin, 5631
Filamen, 5881
Filament-producing collagen, 5246
Filamin 1 defect, in bilateral periventricular heteropia, 5814
Filensin, 6043
Filopodia, 6161
Fine-needle aspiration biopsy, in retinoblastoma, 824
Finishing process, 277
Finnish lethal neonatal metabolic syndrome, 60t
First-degree relatives, 31
FISH. *See* Fluorescence *in situ* hybridization
Fish eye disease, 95t, 2817, 2821, 2823t, 2824, 2952
    LCAT gene defects, 2822t–2823t, 2827
Fish-odor syndrome, 55t
Fish tapeworm, 1478
Fitness, 304
*FKHL7* gene, 6002, 6011
    in Axenfeld-Rieger syndrome, 6008–6009, 6070
    gene expression, 6009
    in glaucoma, 6008–6009, 6070
    identification, 6008
    in iridogonial dysgenesis, 6008–6009
    mutations, 6009, 6009f
FKHL7 protein:
    conservation, 6008, 6009f
    regulation of downstream target genes, 6009
    structure, 6008, 6009f
Flap endonuclease, 1268
Flavins, as nitric oxide synthase cofactors, 4278

FLDB. *See* Familial ligand-defective apolipoprotein B
Fletcher factor. *See* Prekallikrein
Fletcher factor deficiency, 66t
*FLI1* gene, 585–588
*FLN1* gene, 5814
Floating-Harbor syndrome, 6170
Floppy baby syndrome. *See* Multiple endocrine neoplasia type 2
Fludrocortisone, for adrenal hypoplasia congenita, 4265–4266
Fluid-phase endocytosis, 475
Fluorescence *in situ* hybridization (FISH), 17, 21, 264, 264f, 1293, 1294f
    detection of gene amplification, 606
Fluoride number, 236
Fluorometric analysis, of bilirubin, 3074
5-Fluorouracil:
    inhibition of UMP synthase, 2671
    pharmacogenetics, 2692
    toxicity, 2082–2083, 2085
        in dihydropyrimidine dehydrogenase deficiency, 2691–2692
        sensitivity to, 54t
Fluoxetine, for obesity, 4005
Fluphenazine, for Lesch-Nyhan disease, 2557–2558
Flush junction, 360
FMD. *See* Fukuyama muscular dystrophy
FMF. *See* Familial Mediterranean fever
*FMR1* gene. *See also* Fragile X syndrome
    allelic forms, 1259–1260, 1259f, 1259t
    expansions in families, 1261–1262, 1262t–1263t
    full mutation, 1260
    gene conservation, 1260–1261
    gene expression, 1260, 1260f
    identification, 1258
    "mosaics," 1260
    mutations other than repeat expansions, 1261
    premutation, 1259–1260, 1263
    repeat mutations, 1262–1263, 1264f
        ethnic variation, 1265
        haplotype-association studies, 1260f, 1266–1267, 1266f
        mechanisms of expansion, 1267–1268
        population dynamics, 1262t, 1265
        timing of expansion, 1263–1264
    structure, 1260, 1260f
*Fmr1* knockout mouse, 1279
FMRP protein:
    biochemistry, 1276–1279
    functional studies, 1278–1279, 1278f–1279f
    neurobiology, 1279
    nucleocytoplasmic localization, 1278
    protein domains and related genes, 1276–1277, 1277f
    ribosome association, 1277–1278
    RNA binding, 1277, 1277f
FMRP protein deficiency, 1257–1280. *See also* Fragile X syndrome
Foam cell. *See* Niemann-Pick cell
Foamy cells, 3614, 3614f, 3624
Focal adhesion kinase, 985
Folate:
    chemistry and physiology, 3898–3901, 3899f
    cobalamins and, 3914
    CSF, 1734t, 1735f, 1737
    in cystathionine β-synthase deficiency, 2037
    genome imprinting and, 427
    metabolic pathways and enzymes, 3900–3901, 3900f
    in methionine adenosyltransferase I/III deficiency, 2015
    transport, 3899

Folate-binding proteins. *See* Folate receptor
Folate deficiency, 2016, 2059
    sarcosinemia in, 2062
    in sickle cell anemia, 4590
Folate disorders:
    differential diagnosis, 3909, 3910t
    nutritional, 3901–3902, 3902f
Folate malabsorption, hereditary, 3902–3903, 3902f
Folate polyglutamates, 3898–3900
Folate receptor (FR), 3899
Folate receptor-α (FR-α), 3899
Folate receptor-β (FR-β), 3899
Folate supplementation:
    for cystathionine β-synthase deficiency, 2037
    in Lesch-Nyhan disease, 2557
    to prevent neural tube defects, 6113
Folate transport defects, 3902f, 3903
Folate trap hypothesis, 3914
Folinic acid:
    for methylenetetrahydrofolate reductase deficiency, 3906
    for tetrahydrobiopterin disorders, 1743
Follicle-stimulating hormone (FSH):
    in spinobulbar muscular atrophy, 4150
    in steroid 5α-reductase 2 deficiency, 4125
Follicular lymphoma, *BCL2* gene in, 560
Folylpolyglutamate synthase, 3899
Food cobalamin malabsorption, 3914, 3916. *See also* Cobalamin transport defects
Food intake, 3979
Forbes disease. *See* Glycogen storage disease, type III
Forebrain:
    holoprosencephaly, 6203–6223
    midline patterning, 6206
    ventral patterning, 6209–6210
Forkhead transcription factor, 1441, 1444
Formaldehyde, active, formation, 2058, 2058f
Formimino-tetrahydrofolate cyclodeaminase, 3900f, 3901
Formiminoglutamic acid (FIGLU), 2675
    urine, 3902, 3904
Formiminotransferase, 1808f, 1810
Formiminotransferase/cyclodeaminase deficiency, 2675, 2680
5-Formyl-tetrahydrofolate, 2057, 3899
10-Formyl-tetrahydrofolate, 3900
10-Formyl-tetrahydrofolate dehydrogenase, 3900f, 3901
10-Formyl-tetrahydrofolate synthase, 3900, 3900f
Forsius-Erickson ocular albinism. *See* Åland Island eye disease
*fos* gene family, 657, 659, 4032
    in breast cancer, 1019
    in hepatocellular carcinoma, 1160
Founder effect, 302, 308, 1694
Four-disulfide core domain, 5731
Fovea, 5957
Foveal hypoplasia, isolated, 83t
FPD/AML. *See* Familial platelet deficiency/ acute myelogenous anemia
FR. *See* Folate receptor
Fragile site, molecular basis, 1268
Fragile X syndrome, 110t, 367, 527, 1257–1280. See also *FMR1* gene
    antibody studies, 1276
    biochemistry of FMRP protein, 1259f, 1276–1279, 1277f–1279f
    clinical aspects, 1196
        behavior, 1269, 1272
        cognition deficits, 1270–1272
        full-mutation females, 1271–1272
        males with fragile X syndrome, 1268–1271

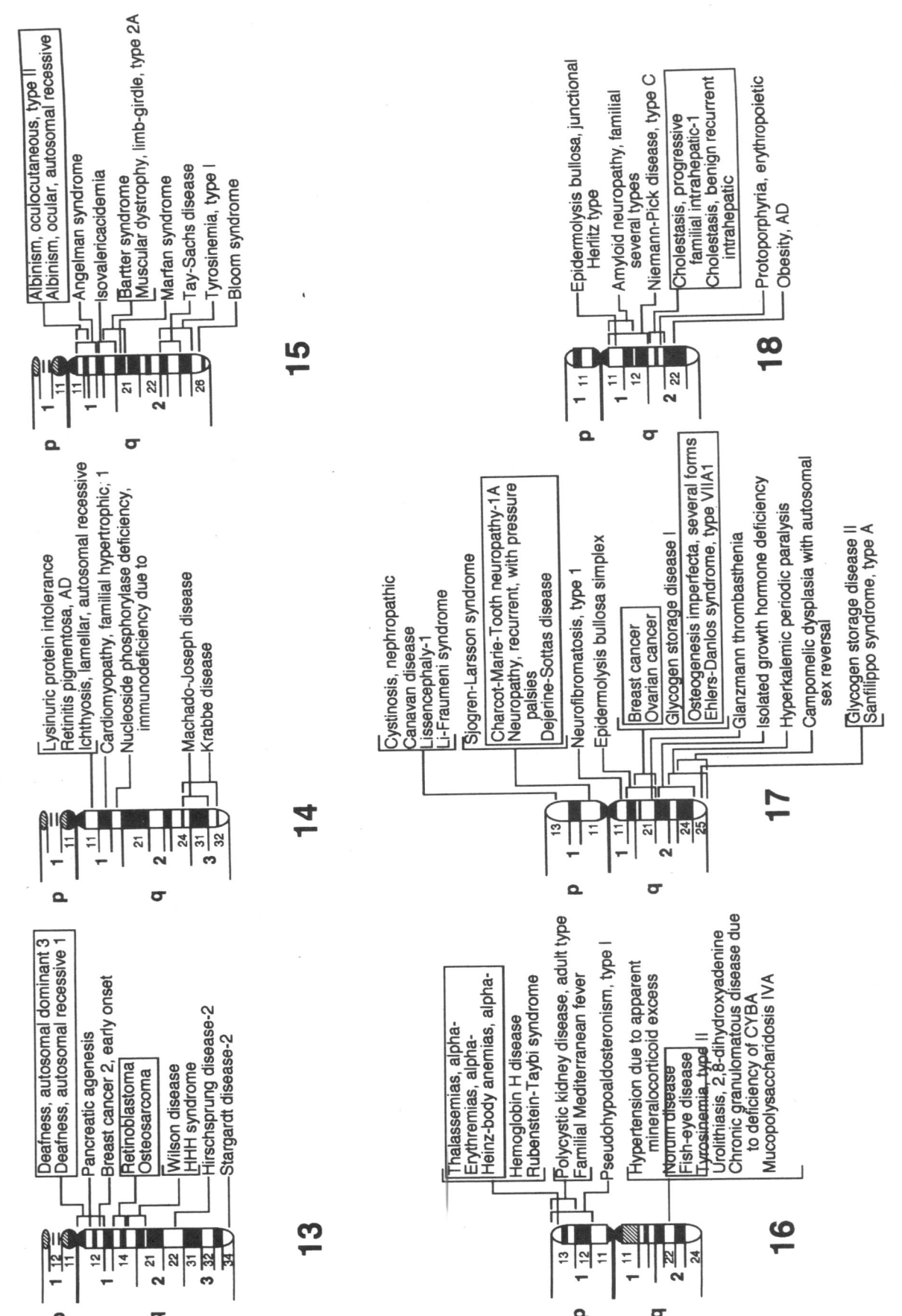